KAPLAN'S CARDIAC ANESTHESIA: THE ECHO ERA

Sixth Edition

Editor

Joel A. Kaplan, MD, CPE, FACC
Professor of Anesthesiology
University of California, San Diego
San Diego, California

Dean Emeritus, School of Medicine
Former Chancellor, Health Sciences Center
University of Louisville
Louisville, Kentucky

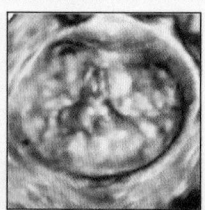

Associate Editors

David L. Reich, MD
Horace W. Goldsmith, Professor and Chair
Department of Anesthesiology
Mount Sinai School of Medicine
New York, New York

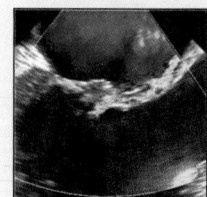

Joseph S. Savino, MD
Professor of Anesthesiology and Critical Care
Vice Chairman, Strategic Planning and Clinical Operations
University of Pennsylvania School of Medicine
Philadelphia, Pennsylvania

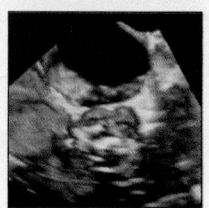

SAUNDERS
ELSEVIER

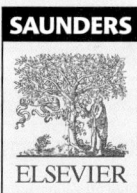

ELSEVIER
SAUNDERS

3251 Riverport Lane
St. Louis, Missouri 63043

KAPLAN'S CARDIAC ANESTHESIA: THE ECHO ERA, SIXTH EDITION   ISBN: 978-1-4377-1617-7

NOTICES

Knowledge and best practice in this field are constantly changing. As new research and experience broaden our understanding, changes in research methods, professional practices, or medical treatment may become necessary.

Practitioners and researchers must always rely on their own experience and knowledge in evaluating and using any information, methods, compounds, or experiments described herein. In using such information or methods they should be mindful of their own safety and the safety of others, including parties for whom they have a professional responsibility.

With respect to any drug or pharmaceutical products identified, readers are advised to check the most current information provided (i) on procedures featured or (ii) by the manufacturer of each product to be administered, to verify the recommended dose or formula, the method and duration of administration, and contraindications. It is the responsibility of practitioners, relying on their own experience and knowledge of their patients, to make diagnoses, to determine dosages and the best treatment for each individual patient, and to take all appropriate safety precautions.

To the fullest extent of the law, neither the Publisher nor the authors, contributors, or editors assume any liability for any injury and/or damage to persons or property as a matter of products liability, negligence or otherwise, or from any use or operation of any methods, products, instructions, or ideas contained in the material herein.

S8409

Previous editions copyrighted 2006, 1999, 1993, 1987, 1979

International Standard Book Number: 978-1-4377-1617-7

WO 470 KAP

Executive Publisher: Natasha Andjelkovic
Developmental Editor: Anne Snyder
Publishing Services Manager: Anne Altepeter
Project Manager: Cindy Thoms
Design Direction: Steven Stave

Printed in China

Last digit is the print number: 9   8   7   6   5   4   3   2   1

DEDICATION

To the pioneers of cardiac surgery and anesthesia who have led us to this exciting era of techniques and technologies that continue to improve our patient care.

Joel A. Kaplan, MD, CPE, FACC

CONTRIBUTORS

AHMAD ADI, MD
Department of Cardiothoracic Anesthesiology
Cleveland Clinic
Cleveland, Ohio

SHAMSUDDIN AKHTAR, MBBS
Associate Professor
Department of Anesthesiology
Yale University School of Medicine
New Haven, Connecticut

KORAY ARICA, MD
Clinical Assistant Professor
Department of Anesthesiology
SUNY Downstate Medical Center
Brooklyn, New York

JOHN G. AUGOUSTIDES, MD, FASE, FAHA
Associate Professor
Cardiovascular and Thoracic Section
Anesthesiology and Critical Care
University of Pennsylvania School of Medicine
Philadelphia, Pennsylvania

JAMES M. BAILEY, MD, PHD
Clinical Associate Professor
Department of Anesthesiology
Emory University School of Medicine
Atlanta, Georgia

DANIEL BAINBRIDGE, MD, FRCPC
Associate Professor
Anesthesia and Perioperative Medicine
Schulich School of Medicine
University of Western Ontario
London, Ontario, Canada

DALIA A. BANKS, MD
Associate Clinical Professor of Anesthesiology
Chief, Division of Cardiothoracic Anesthesia
Director of Cardiac Fellowship
Department of Anesthesiology
University of California, San Diego
La Jolla, California

PAUL G. BARASH, MD
Professor
Department of Anesthesiology
Yale University School of Medicine
New Haven, Connecticut

VICTOR C. BAUM, MD
Professor of Anesthesiology and Pediatrics
Executive Vice-Chair
Department of Anesthesiology
Director, Cardiac Anesthesia
University of Virginia
Charlottesville, Virginia

ELLIOTT BENNETT-GUERRERO, MD
Director of Perioperative Clinical Research
Duke Clinical Research Institute
Professor of Anesthesiology
Duke University Medical Center
Durham, North Carolina

DAN E. BERKOWITZ, MD
Professor, Department of Anesthesiology and Critical Care
  Medicine
Professor, Department of Biomedical Engineering
Johns Hopkins Medicine
Baltimore, Maryland

SIMON C. BODY, MBCHB, MPH
Associate Professor of Anesthesia
Harvard Medical School
Brigham and Women's Hospital
Boston, Massachusetts

T. ANDREW BOWDLE, MD, PHD
Professor of Anesthesiology and Pharmaceutics
Chief of the Division of Cardiothoracic Anesthesiology
Department of Anesthesiology
University of Washington
Seattle, Washington

MICHAEL K. CAHALAN, MD
Professor and Chair of Anesthesiology
University of Utah School of Medicine
Salt Lake City, Utah

ALFONSO CASTA, MD
Associate Professor
Anesthesia
Harvard University Medical School
Senior Associate in Cardiac Anesthesia
Children's Hospital Boston
Boston, Massachusetts

CHARLES E. CHAMBERS, MD
Professor of Medicine and Radiology
Milton S. Hershey Medical Center
Pennsylvania State University School of Medicine
Hershey, Pennsylvania

MARK A. CHANEY, MD
Professor
Director of Cardiac Anesthesia
Department of Anesthesia and Critical Care
University of Chicago Medical Center
Chicago, Illinois

ALYSSA B. CHAPITAL, MD, PHD
Assistant Professor of Surgery
Department of Critical Care Medicine
Division Head of Acute Care Surgery
Mayo Clinic
Phoenix, Arizona

ALAN CHENG, MD
Assistant Professor of Medicine
Doctor, Arrhythmia Device Service
Johns Hopkins University School of Medicine
Baltimore, Maryland

DAVY C.H. CHENG, MD, MSC, FRCPC, FCAHS
Distinguished University Professor and Chair
Department of Anesthesia and Perioperative Medicine
University of Western Ontario
Chief of Anesthesia and Perioperative Medicine
London Health Sciences Center and St. Joseph's Health Care
London, Ontario, Canada

ALBERT T. CHEUNG, MD
Professor
Anesthesiology and Critical Care
University of Pennsylvania
Philadelphia, Pennsylvania

JOANNA CHIKWE, MD
Assistant Professor
Department of Cardiothoracic Surgery
Mount Sinai Medical Center
New York, New York

DAVID J. COOK, MD
Professor
Department of Anesthesiology
Chair, Cardiovascular Anesthesiology
Mayo Clinic
College of Medicine
Rochester, Minnesota

DUNCAN G. DE SOUZA, MD, FRCPC
Assistant Professor
Anesthesiology
University of Virginia
Charlottesville, Virginia

KAREN B. DOMINO, MD, MPH
Professor
Vice Chair for Clinical Research
Department of Anesthesiology and Pain Medicine
University of Washington
Seattle, Washington

MARCEL E. DURIEUX, MD, PHD
Professor
Departments of Anesthesiology and Neurological Surgery
University of Virginia
Charlottesville, Virginia

HARVEY L. EDMONDS, JR., PHD
Emeritus Research Professor
Anesthesiology and Perioperative Medicine
University of Louisville School of Medicine
Louisville, Kentucky

MARK EDWARDS, MBCHB, FANZCA
Anaesthetist
Department of Cardiothoracic and ORL Anaesthesia
Auckland City Hospital
Auckland, New Zealand

LIZA J. ENRIQUEZ, MD
Departments of Anesthesiology
Montefiore Medical Center
Bronx, New York

GREGORY W. FISCHER, MD
Associate Professor of Anesthesiology
Director of Adult Cardiothoracic Anesthesia
Mount Sinai School of Medicine
New York, New York

LEE A. FLEISHER, MD, FACC, FAHA
Roberts D. Dripps Professor and Chair of Anesthesiology
Professor of Medicine
University of Pennsylvania School of Medicine
Philadelphia, Pennsylvania

VALENTIN FUSTER, MD, PHD, MACC
Director, Mount Sinai Heart
Mount Sinai Hospital
Professor of Medicine
Mount Sinai School of Medicine
New York, New York

MARIO J. GARCIA, MD, FACC, FACP
Chief, Division of Cardiology
Montefiore Medical Center
Professor of Medicine
Albert Einstein College of Medicine
Bronx, New York

JUAN GAZTANAGA, MD
Director, Cardiac MRI/CT Program
Winthrop University Hospital
Mineola, New York

DEAN T. GIACOBBE, MD
Anesthesiologist
University Medical Center at Princeton
Princeton, New Jersey

LEANNE GROBAN, MS, MD
Associate Professor
Department of Anesthesiology
Wake Forest University School of Medicine
Winston Salem, North Carolina

HILARY P. GROCOTT, MD, FRCPC, FASE
Professor of Anesthesia and Surgery
University of Manitoba
St. Boniface Hospital
Winnipeg, Manitoba, Canada

KELLY GROGAN, MD
Associate Professor
Department of Anesthesia and Perioperative Medicine
Medical University of South Carolina
Charleston, South Carolina

ROBERT C. GROOM, MS, CCP
Associate Vice President of Cardiac Services
Director of Cardiovascular Perfusion
Maine Medical Center
Portland, Maine

DAVID W. GROSSHANS, DO
Assistant Professor
Department of Anesthesiology
Wake Forest University School of Medicine
Winston Salem, North Carolina

MASAO HAYASHI, MD
Fellow, Cardiothoracic Anesthesiology
Mount Sinai School of Medicine
New York, New York

EUGENE A. HESSEL II, MD, FACS
Professor
Department of Anesthesiology
University of Kentucky College of Medicine
Lexington, Kentucky

BENJAMIN HIBBERT, MD, FRCPC
Vascular Biology Lab Research Fellow
Department of Biochemistry and Division of Cardiology
University of Ottawa Heart Institute
Ottawa, Ontario, Canada

THOMAS L. HIGGINS, MD, MBA, FACP, FCCM
Professor of Medicine, Surgery, and Anesthesiology
Tufts University School of Medicine
Boston, Massachusetts
Interim Chairman, Department of Medicine
Departments of Medicine and Surgery
Baystate Medical Center
Medical Director, Inpatient Informatics
Baystate Health
Springfield, Massachusetts

CHARLES W. HOGUE, JR., MD
Professor of Anesthesiology and Critical Care Medicine
Chief, Division of Adult Anesthesia
Johns Hopkins University School of Medicine
Johns Hopkins Hospital
Baltimore, Maryland

JIRI HORAK, MD
Assistant Professor
Anesthesia and Critical Care
University of Pennsylvania
Philadelphia, Pennsylvania

JAY HORROW, MD, MS, FAHA
Professor of Anesthesiology, Physiology, and Pharmacology
Drexel University College of Medicine
Professor of Epidemiology and Biostatistics
Drexel University School of Public Health
Philadelphia, Pennsylvania

PHILIPPE R. HOUSMANS, MD, PHD
Professor, Department of Anesthesiology
Mayo Clinic
Rochester, Minnesota

STUART W. JAMIESON, MB, FRCS
Endowed Chair and Distinguished Professor of Surgery
Chief, Division of Cardiovascular and Thoracic Surgery
Chair, Department of Cardiothoracic Surgery
University of California, San Diego
La Jolla, California

MANDISA-MAIA JONES-HAYWOOD, MD
Assistant Professor
Anesthesiology
Wake Forest University School of Medicine
Winston Salem, North Carolina

RONALD A. KAHN, MD
Professor
Department of Anesthesiology
Mount Sinai Medical Center
New York, New York

JOEL A. KAPLAN, MD, CPE, FACC
Professor of Anesthesiology
University of California, San Diego
San Diego, California
Dean Emeritus, School of Medicine
Former Chancellor, Health Sciences Center
University of Louisville
Louisville, Kentucky

JACK F. KERR, AIA
Senior Healthcare Architect
Array Healthcare Facilities Solutions
King of Prussia, Pennsylvania

KIM M. KERR, MD, FCCP
Clinical Professor of Medicine
Division of Pulmonary and Critical Care Medicine
University of California, San Diego
La Jolla, California

OKSANA KLIMKINA, MD
Department of Anesthesiology
University of Kentucky Medical Center
Lexington, Kentucky

COLLEEN KOCH, MD, MS, MBA
Professor of Anesthesiology
Lerner College of Medicine of Case Western Reserve University
Vice Chair of Research and Education
Department of Cardiothoracic Anesthesia
Cleveland Clinic
Cleveland, Ohio

STEVEN N. KONSTADT, MD, MBA, FACC
Chairman
Department of Anesthesiology
Maimonides Medical Center
Brooklyn, New York
Professor
Anesthesiology
Mount Sinai Medical Center
New York, New York

MARK KOZAK, MD
Associate Professor of Medicine
Milton S. Hershey Medical Center
Pennsylvania State University School of Medicine
Hershey, Pennsylvania

ADAM B. LERNER, MD
Assistant Professor of Anesthesia
Harvard Medical School
Director, Cardiac Anesthesia
Beth Israel Deaconess Medical Center
Boston, Massachusetts

JERROLD H. LEVY, MD, FAHA
Professor and Deputy Chair for Research
Emory University School of Medicine
Director of Cardiothoracic Anesthesiology
Cardiothoracic Anesthesiology and Critical Care
Emory Healthcare
Atlanta, Georgia

MARTIN J. LONDON, MD
Professor of Clinical Anesthesia
University of California at San Francisco
San Francisco, California

BARRY A. LOVE, MD
Assistant Professor of Pediatrics and Medicine
Director of Congenital Cardiac Catheterization Laboratory
Mount Sinai Medical Center
New York, New York

FEROZE MAHMOOD, MD
Director of Vascular Anesthesia and Perioperative Echocardiography
Department of Anesthesia and Critical Care
Beth Israel Deaconess Medical Center
Boston, Massachusetts

GERARD R. MANECKE, JR., MD
Clinical Professor of Anesthesiology
Chair, Department of Anesthesiology
University of California, San Diego
La Jolla, California

CHRISTINA T. MORA MANGANO, MD, FAHA
Professor, Department of Anesthesia
Stanford University
Chief, Division of Cardiovascular Anesthesia
Stanford University Medical Center
Palo Alto, California

VERONICA MATEI, MD
Fellow
Department of Anesthesiology
Yale University School of Medicine
New Haven, Connecticut

WILLIAM J. MAUERMANN, MD
Assistant Professor of Anesthesiology
Mayo Clinic
Rochester, Minnesota

TIMOTHY M. MAUS, MD
Assistant Clinical Professor of Anesthesiology
Director of Perioperative Transesophageal Echocardiography
University of California, San Diego
La Jolla, California

NANHI MITTER, MD
Assistant Professor
Adult Cardiothoracic Anesthesiology Fellowship Program, Director
Anesthesiology and Critical Care Medicine
Johns Hopkins Hospital
Baltimore, Maryland

ALEXANDER J.C. MITTNACHT, MD
Director, Pediatric Cardiac Anesthesia
Associate Professor
Department of Anesthesiology
Mount Sinai Medical Center
New York, New York

EMILE R. MOHLER, MD, MS
Associate Professor of Medicine
University of Pennsylvania
Director of Vascular Medicine
University of Philadelphia Health System
Philadelphia, Pennsylvania

JOHN M. MURKIN, MD, FRCPC
Professor of Anesthesiology (Senate)
Director of Cardiac Anesthesiology Research
Schulich School of Medicine
University of Western Ontario
London, Ontario, Canada

ANDREW W. MURRAY, MB, CHB
Assistant Professor
Department of Anesthesiology
University of Pittsburgh School of Medicine
Cardiac Anesthesiologist
University of Pittsburgh Medical Center–Presbyterian
Director of Cardio-Thoracic Anesthesiology
Veteran's Administration Medical Center–Oakland
Pittsburgh, Pennsylvania

MICHAEL J. MURRAY, MD, PHD
Professor of Anesthesiology
Mayo Clinic College of Medicine
Consultant
Department of Anesthesiology
Mayo Hospital
Scottsdale, Arizona

HOWARD J. NATHAN, MD, FRCPC
Professor and Vice Chairman (Research)
Department of Anesthesiology
University of Ottawa
Ottawa, Ontario, Canada

GREGORY A. NUTTALL, MD
Professor of Anesthesiology
Mayo Clinic
Rochester, Minnesota

DANIEL NYHAN, MD
Professor
Division Chief, Cardiothoracic Anesthesia
Anesthesia and Critical Care Medicine
Johns Hopkins University
Baltimore, Maryland

EDWARD R.M. O'BRIEN, MD
Professor of Medicine, Cardiology
Research Chair, Canadian Institutes of Health Research/Medtronic
University of Ottawa Heart Institute
Ottawa, Ontario, Canada

WILLIAM C. OLIVER, JR., MD
Professor
Department of Anesthesiology
College of Medicine
Mayo Clinic
Rochester, Minnesota

PAUL S. PAGEL, MD, PHD
Professor of Anesthesiology
Director of Cardiac Anesthesia
Medical College of Wisconsin
Clement J. Zablocki Veterans Affairs Medical Center
Milwaukee, Wisconsin

ENRIQUE J. PANTIN, MD
Assistant Professor
Department of Anesthesiology
University of Medicine and Dentistry of New Jersey
Robert Wood Johnson Medical School
New Brunswick, New Jersey

JOSEPH J. QUINLAN, MD
Professor
Department of Anesthesiology
University of Pittsburgh
Chief Anesthesiologist
University of Pittsburgh Medical Center–Presbyterian
Pittsburgh, Pennsylvania

JAMES G. RAMSAY, MD
Professor of Anesthesiology
Director, Anesthesiology Critical Care
Emory University School of Medicine
Atlanta, Georgia

KENT H. REHFELDT, MD
Consultant
Assistant Professor of Anesthesiology
Department of Anesthesiology
Mayo Clinic
Rochester, Minnesota

DAVID L. REICH, MD
Horace W. Goldsmith Professor and Chair
Department of Anesthesiology
Mount Sinai School of Medicine
New York, New York

ROGER L. ROYSTER, MD, FACC
Professor and Executive Vice Chairman
Department of Anesthesiology
Wake Forest University School of Medicine
Winston-Salem, North Carolina

MARC A. ROZNER, PHD, MD
Professor of Anesthesiology and Perioperative Medicine
Professor of Cardiology
University of Texas MD Anderson Cancer Center
Adjunct Assistant Professor of Integrative Biology and Pharmacology
University of Texas Houston Health Science Center
Houston, Texas

JOSEPH S. SAVINO, MD
Professor of Anesthesiology and Critical Care
Vice Chairman, Strategic Planning and Clinical Operations
University of Pennsylvania School of Medicine
Philadelphia, Pennsylvania

ALAN JAY SCHWARTZ, MD, MSED
Professor
Clinical Anesthesiology and Critical Care
University of Pennsylvania School of Medicine
Director of Education and Program Director
Pediatric Anesthesiology Fellowship
Department of Anesthesiology and Critical Care Medicine
Children's Hospital of Philadelphia
Philadelphia, Pennsylvania

ASHISH SHAH, MD
Assistant Professor of Surgery
Johns Hopkins University School of Medicine
Surgical Director, Lung Transplantation
Johns Hopkins Cardiac Surgery
Baltimore, Maryland

JACK S. SHANEWISE, MD, FASE
Professor and Director
Division of Cardiothoracic Anesthesiology
Columbia University College of Physicians and Surgeons
New York, New York

SONAL SHARMA, MD
Research Associate
Department of Anesthesiology
University of Virginia
Charlottesville, Virginia

STANTON K. SHERNAN, MD, FAHA, FASE
Associate Professor of Anesthesia
Director of Cardiac Anesthesia
Department of Anesthesiology, Perioperative, and Pain Medicine
Brigham and Women's Hospital
Harvard Medical School
Boston, Massachusetts

LINDA SHORE-LESSERSON, MD
Professor of Anesthesiology
Chief, Cardiothoracic Anesthesiology
Montefiore Medical Center
Bronx, New York

NIKOLAOS J. SKUBAS, MD, FASE
Associate Professor of Anesthesiology
Director, Cardiac Anesthesia
Weill Cornell Medical College
New York, New York

THOMAS F. SLAUGHTER, MD, MHA, CPH
Professor and Head, Section on Cardiothoracic Anesthesiology
Wake Forest University School of Medicine
Winston-Salem, North Carolina

BRUCE D. SPIESS, MD, FAHA
Professor of Anesthesiology and Emergency Medicine
Director of VCURES
VCU–Medical College of Virginia
Richmond, Virginia

MARK STAFFORD-SMITH, MD, CM, FRCPC
Professor of Anesthesiology
Director of Fellowship Education
Director of Cardiothoracic Anesthesia and Critical Care
   Medicine Fellowship
Division of Cardiothoracic Anesthesia and Critical Care Medicine
Department of Anesthesiology
Duke University Medical Center
Durham, North Carolina

ALFRED H. STAMMERS, MSA, CCP, PBMT
Director of Perfusion Services
Division of Cardiothoracic Surgery
Geisinger Health Systems
Danville, Pennsylvania

MARC E. STONE, MD
Associate Professor of Anesthesiology
Program Director, Fellowship in Cardiothoracic Anesthesiology
Mount Sinai School of Medicine
New York, New York

KENICHI TANAKA, MD, MSC
Associate Professor
Anesthesiology
Emory University School of Medicine
Atlanta, Georgia

MENACHEM WEINER, MD
Assistant Professor
Anesthesiology
Mount Sinai School of Medicine
New York, New York

STUART J. WEISS, MD, PHD
Associate Professor of Anesthesiology and Critical Care
University of Pennsylvania School of Medicine
Philadelphia, Pennsylvania

JEAN-PIERRE YARED, MD
Director, Critical Care Medicine in the Heart and Vascular Institute
Cleveland Clinic Foundation
Cleveland, Ohio

The Next Frontier in Cardiac Surgery and Interventions

Nothing endures but change.
Heraclitus

Medicine is in constant flux. Humans constantly are pushing the realm of scientific discovery into meaningful medical applications that ultimately alleviate suffering. The art and science of anesthesia care, as the practice of medicine, continues to progress significantly, especially in cardiac anesthesia. Our responsibilities have expanded beyond creating insensitivity to pain to the practice of sophisticated medical techniques based on fundamental scientific principles. As a specialty, we are much more involved in disease assessment and physiologic manipulation. The distinctions among anesthesiologist, diagnostician, and even interventionalist have blurred. The cardiac anesthesiologists' pivotal role constantly is growing in the successful outcome of a patient population that is becoming ever more complex.

These advances in our specialty come from our ever-expanding knowledge of cardiopulmonary physiology, biochemistry, pharmacology, and neuroscience. However, much of our deeper understanding has come from advancements in technology. This edition of *Kaplan's Cardiac Anesthesia* comes at a time that witnesses the practice of our subspecialty at a major crossroads. Cardiac surgery is undergoing a revolution in the way both simple and complex heart disease will be treated. Simultaneously, anesthesiology and cardiology are undergoing major advancements in imaging. Regional anesthesia now moves beyond the art of landmark assessment to the science of *looking* and *guiding*. In cardiology, it is fascinating to see that as new imaging or quantification technologies are brought online, new physiologic variables of the heart are discovered, rediscovered, or simply appreciated better. Moreover, newer imaging methodologies will serve as the eyes for catheter-guided hands in what can only be called a revolution in the development of new cardiac implantables and repair techniques that avoid sternotomy and cardiopulmonary bypass. Enter the "Echo Era."

We have moved away from an era of palpation of the post-mitral repair thrill to sophisticated techniques to quantify a myriad of cardiac physiologic parameters. We are also moving away from an era of opening the chest to operate on the still heart. Newer image-guided procedures ultimately will lead to less invasive incisions, less infection, and less end-organ insult from cardiopulmonary bypass. Cardiopulmonary bypass will still predominate over the next few years, but this decade will witness an explosion of newer catheter-based techniques that avoid reanimating the nonbeating heart. Imaging will be the cornerstone of these new minimally invasive procedures. Advances in materials science and microelectronics ultimately will put three-dimensional eyes onto the tips of catheters, and these procedures will be performed by physicians who now operate inside the beating heart. Valve surgery is changing in a major way with adult senile calcific stenosis. Progressive change is accelerating transcatheter aortic valve intervention (TAVI). More than 20,000 cases have been performed. These procedures already avoid sternotomy and cardiopulmonary bypass to the point at which some patients are treated without endotracheal intubation and general anesthesia. Time will tell whether this procedure can be done safely. Nonetheless, the course is set and clear; cardiopulmonary bypass has brought us into the 21st century and imaging will advance us in the decades to come. Cardiac anesthesiologists now face a career-changing decision: will they embrace being key members of the new interventional team, or will they be content to be sideline observers of these new procedures?

The pivotal role of echocardiography as both monitoring and diagnostic tool evidenced itself in the 1990s with mitral valve repair. The technology revolution is only going to accelerate. New advancements will include technologies that look at structures with more detail in space and time. Ultimately, newer parallel-processing algorithms in beamforming and automated machine analysis of cardiac images will allow assessment of 3D regurgitant volume, myocardial contraction, and full four-chamber and valvular quantification. Because computers have become more powerful, imaging will be embraced only as it progresses in simplicity.

This new echo era will advance both diagnostics and therapeutic guidance. I have been most privileged that my path from medical student to cardiac anesthesiologist has been mentored by Drs. Kaplan, Reich, and Savino. This edition's framework, penned by a world-renowned group of experts, not only is current and complete but also will equip its readers well for the dynamic ride to come.

Ivan S. Salgo, MD, MS
Chief of Cardiovascular Investigations, Ultrasound
Philips Healthcare
Andover, Massachusetts

PREFACE

The sixth edition of *Kaplan's Cardiac Anesthesia* has been written to further improve the anesthetic management of the patient with cardiac disease undergoing both cardiac and noncardiac surgery. Since publication of the first edition in 1979, at the beginning of the modern era of cardiac surgery, continued advances in the field have made cardiac anesthesia the leading subspecialty of anesthesiology. To maintain its place as the standard reference textbook in the field, this edition has been completely revised, expanded, and updated throughout to reflect the ongoing changes in cardiovascular care, especially the rapid growth and use of ultrasound and other imaging technologies. Significant contributions to the text have been made by leading cardiologists and cardiac surgeons to fully cover the broader aspects of the total care of the cardiac patient.

This edition is subtitled *The Echo Era* to emphasize today's expanded role of transesophageal echocardiography (TEE) and other ultrasound techniques in the perioperative period. The developments leading to the clinical use of TEE are described, and many of the authors discuss the expanding applications in monitoring and diagnosis by the modern cardiac anesthesiologist. Specific clinical situations are described using the decision-making process highlighted by Weiss and Savino: (1) framing the question asked of the anesthesiologist/echocardiographer; (2) collecting echocardiographic and nonechocardiographic information; (3) making the clinical decision based on integration of knowledge, framing, and information; and (4) implementing the recommendations after a full discussion with the surgeon and other clinicians (e.g., cardiologists).

These case discussions dealing with clinical decision making are augmented by the full-color presentation of the text, multiple color echo and Doppler images, cine clips, and supplementary material on the Expert Consult premium website accompanying the print version of the text. The website also will be used to update the book as new material appears between editions. Some of the new information will be provided by integrating key clinical areas first described in the *Journal of Cardiothoracic and Vascular Anesthesia*. The reader will be able to move seamlessly from the text to the new electronic information technology available with the book.

The content of the sixth edition ranges from the basic sciences through translational medicine to the clinical care of the sickest and most complex cardiac patients. The final section of this edition is entitled "Education in Cardiac Anesthesia" and emphasizes reducing errors to further improve the quality of our patient care. Training and certification in cardiovascular anesthesia are discussed, as well as the educational process and certification available for TEE. Because of the success of the new teaching aides used in the last edition, the Key Points of each chapter appear at the start of the chapters, and Teaching Boxes appear with many of the important "take-home messages." The emphasis throughout the book is on using the latest scientific developments to guide proper therapeutic interventions in the perioperative period.

Kaplan's Cardiac Anesthesia: The Echo Era was written by acknowledged experts in each specific area or related specialties. It is the most authoritative and up-to-date collection of material in the field. Each chapter aims to provide the scientific foundation in the area as well as the clinical basis for practice, and outcome information is included when it is available. All of the chapters have been coordinated in an effort to maximize the clinical utility. Whenever possible, material has been integrated from the fields of anesthesiology, cardiology, cardiac surgery, physiology, and pharmacology to present a complete clinical picture. Thus, this edition should continue to serve as the definitive text for cardiac anesthesia residents, fellows, attendings, practitioners, cardiologists, cardiac surgeons, intensivists, and others interested in the management of the patient with cardiac disease for either cardiac or noncardiac surgery.

Cardiac anesthesia is a complex and comprehensive field of medicine, incorporating many aspects of the specialties of anesthesiology, cardiology, and cardiac surgery. Monitoring modalities always have been an integral part of the practice and have provided us with data to improve our therapeutic interventions. Over the past 30 years, these monitors have become progressively more sophisticated. Many of these monitoring techniques have been adapted from cardiologists and then applied to the cardiac surgical setting. This has been true of electrocardiographic monitoring, with the introduction of the V_5 lead for the intraoperative detection of myocardial ischemia modified from its use during exercise tolerance testing. The pulmonary artery catheter (PAC) was developed for use in the coronary care unit by Dr. Swan, but as he told me, the perioperative use of the PAC in high-risk patients with heart failure and cardiogenic shock was a better role for it, and this use would outlast its role for cardiologists; it turned out to be very true!

Now, we have arrived at the echo era in which TEE—adapted from transthoracic echocardiography use in cardiology—is used widely in cardiac anesthesia for monitoring, diagnosis, and helping to guide the surgery in procedures such as mitral valve repairs. This technique certainly has led to changes in the operative procedures, as well as improvements in our care and choices of pharmacologic treatments, as pointed out in this edition. However, the practice of cardiac anesthesia is and always has been more than the interpretation of any one monitor. Those who believe and emphasize that obtaining certification in TEE makes an anesthesiologist into a cardiac anesthesiologist are sadly mistaken. The practice of cardiac anesthesia includes the use and interpretation of TEE, as it does with other monitors, but it also includes much, much more, and explains the overall size and depth of this book, incorporating all of the areas involved in the complete care of a cardiac surgical patient. It was this overall care in the perioperative period that led J. Willis Hurst, MD, one of the world's leading cardiologists, to state, in his foreword to the first edition of *Kaplan's Cardiac Anesthesia,* that "This cardiologist views the modern cardiac anesthesiologist with awe."

The editors gratefully acknowledge the contributions made by the authors of each of the chapters. They are the dedicated experts who have made the field of cardiac anesthesia what it is today and are the teachers of our young colleagues practicing anesthesiology around the world. This book would not have been possible without their hard work and expertise.

Joel A. Kaplan, MD, CPE, FACC

CONTENTS

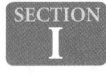

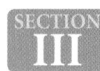
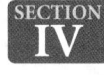

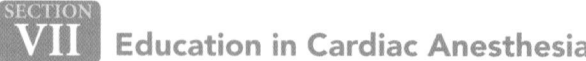

SECTION VII   Education in Cardiac Anesthesia

SECTION I

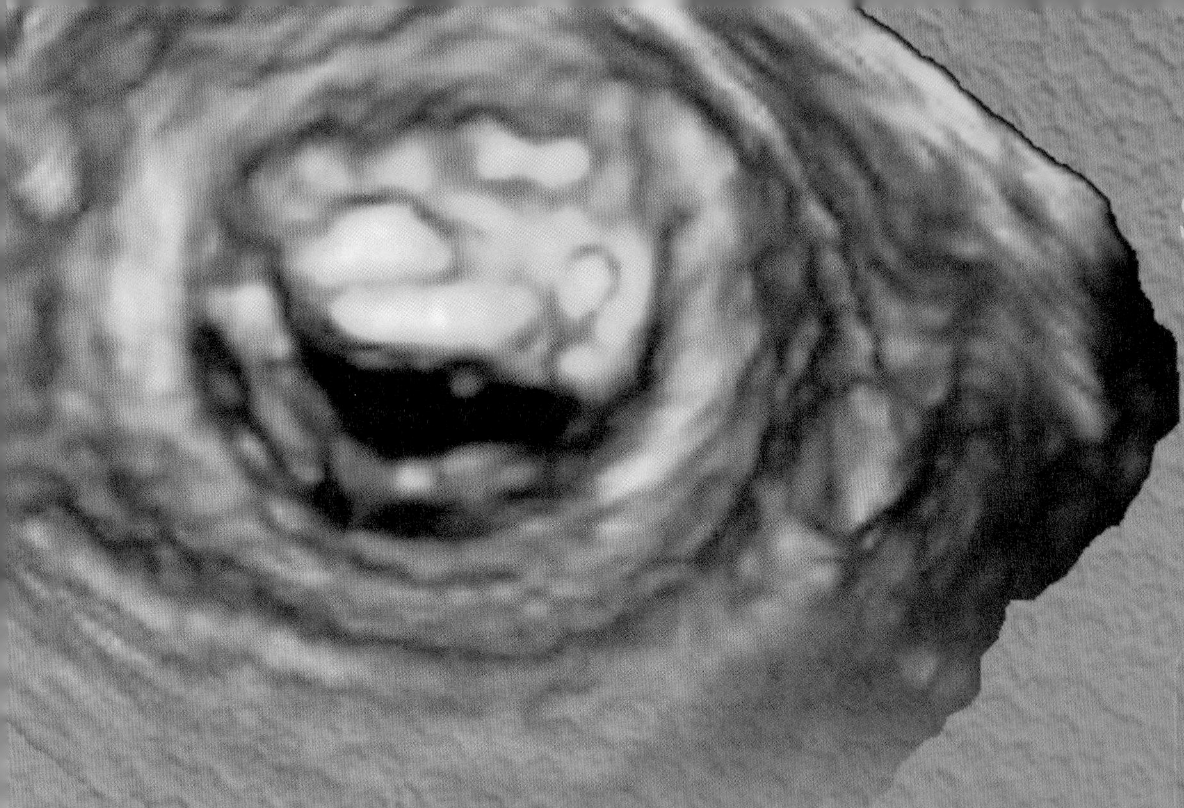

Preoperative Assessment and Management

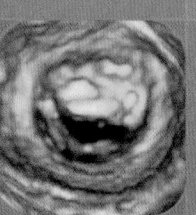

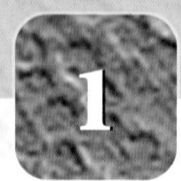

1

Assessment of Cardiac Risk and the Cardiology Consultation

JIRI HORAK, MD | EMILE R. MOHLER, MD, MS | LEE A. FLEISHER, MD, FACC, FAHA

KEY POINTS

1. Perioperative cardiac morbidity is multifactorial, and understanding these factors helps define individual risk factors.
2. Assessment of myocardial injury is based on the integration of information from myocardial imaging (e.g., echocardiography), electrocardiography (ECG), and serum biomarkers, with significant variability in the diagnosis based on the criteria selected.
3. Multivariate modeling has been used to develop risk indices that focus on preoperative variables, intraoperative variables, or both.
4. Key predictors of perioperative risk are dependent on the type of cardiac operation and the outcome of interest.
5. The factors used to construct a risk index are critical in determining whether it is applicable to a given population.
6. Although coronary angiography measures anatomy, stress myocardial imaging provides a better assessment of cardiac function.
7. New risk models have become available for valvular heart surgery or combined coronary and valvular cardiac procedures.

In the early 1980s, coronary artery bypass graft surgery (CABG) was characterized by operative mortality rates in the range of 1% to 2%. Over the ensuing years, however, urgent and emergent operations and "redo" procedures became common, and greater morbidity and mortality rates were observed. Percutaneous coronary interventions (PCIs) absorbed low-risk patients from the surgery pool, with the net result being that the operative mortality rate increased to the range of 5% to 6%. The trend toward PCI has continued, with recent trials demonstrating the safety of stenting even left main coronary artery disease (CAD).[1] This demographic shift has led hospital administrators to ask for justification of the observed increase in CABG mortality. This often has prompted a time-consuming and expensive chart review to identify the differences in the patient populations that led to the greater morbidity. Even with this information, it was difficult to *objectively* determine the impact of these new and compelling factors on mortality. The impetus for the development of a risk-adjusted outcome assessment/appropriate risk adjustment scoring system was the need to compare adult cardiac surgery results in different institutions and to benchmark the observed complication rates.[2] With the passage of healthcare reform, there is increased interest in publicly reporting perioperative outcomes, which requires optimal risk adjustment.

The first risk-scoring scheme for cardiac surgery was introduced by Paiement et al[3] at the Montreal Heart Institute in 1983. Since then,

multiple preoperative cardiac surgery risk indices have been developed. The patient characteristics that affected the probability of specific adverse outcomes were identified and weighed, and the resultant risk indices have been used to adjust for case-mix differences among surgeons and centers where performance profiles have been compiled. In addition to comparisons among centers, the preoperative cardiac risk indices have been used to counsel patients and their families in resource planning, in high-risk group identification for special care or research, to determine cost-effectiveness, to determine effectiveness of intervention, to improve provider practice, and to assess costs related to severity of disease.[4,5]

Anesthesiologists are interested in risk indices as a means of identifying patients who are at high risk for intraoperative cardiac injury and, together with the surgeon, to estimate perioperative risk for cardiac surgery to provide objective information to patients and their families during the preoperative discussion. This chapter approaches the preoperative evaluation from this perspective.

Sources of Perioperative Myocardial Injury in Cardiac Surgery

Myocardial injury, manifested as transient cardiac contractile dysfunction ("stunning") or acute myocardial infarction (AMI), or both, is the most frequent complication after cardiac surgery and is the single-most important cause of hospital complications and death. Furthermore, patients who have a perioperative myocardial infarction (MI) have poor long-term prognosis; only 51% of such patients remain free from adverse cardiac events after 2 years, compared with 96% of patients without MI.[6]

It is important to understand the pathogenesis of this morbidity and mortality to understand the determinants of perioperative risk. This is particularly important with respect to cardiac outcomes because the definition of *cardiac morbidity* represents a continuum rather than a discrete event. This understanding can help target the biologically significant risk factors, as well as interventions that may decrease irreversible myocardial necrosis.

Myocardial necrosis is the result of progressive pathologic ischemic changes that start to occur in the myocardium within minutes after the interruption of its blood flow, as seen in cardiac surgery (Box 1-1). The duration of the interruption of blood flow, either partial or complete, determines the extent of myocardial necrosis. This is consistent with the finding that both the duration of the period of aortic cross-clamping (AXC) and the duration of cardiopulmonary bypass (CPB) consistently have been shown to be the main determinants of postoperative outcomes in virtually all studies. This was further supported in a study with an average follow-up of 10 years after complex

BOX 1-1. DETERMINATIONS OF PERIOPERATIVE MYOCARDIAL INJURY

- Disruption of blood flow
- Reperfusion of ischemic myocardium
- Adverse systemic effects of cardiopulmonary bypass

cardiac surgery in which Khuri[7] observed a direct relation between the lowest mean myocardial pH recorded both during and after the period of AXC and long-term patient survival. Patients who experienced acidosis (pH < 6.5) had decreased survival compared with those who did not. Because myocardial acidosis reflects both myocardial ischemia and poor myocardial protection during CPB, this study demonstrated the relation of the adequacy of intraoperative myocardial protection to long-term outcome (see Chapters 3, 6, 18, and 28).

Reperfusion of an Ischemic Myocardium

Surgical interventions requiring interruption of blood flow to the heart must, out of necessity, be followed by restoration of perfusion. Numerous experimental studies have provided compelling evidence that reperfusion, although essential for tissue or organ survival, or both, is not without risk because of the extension of cell damage as a result of reperfusion itself. Myocardial ischemia of limited duration (< 20 minutes), followed by reperfusion, are accompanied by functional recovery without evidence of structural injury or biochemical evidence of tissue injury.[8,9]

Paradoxically, reperfusion of cardiac tissue, which has been subjected to an extended period of ischemia, results in a phenomenon known as *myocardial reperfusion injury*.[10–12] Thus, a paradox exists in that tissue viability can be maintained only if reperfusion is instituted within a reasonable time period, but only at the risk for extending the injury beyond that caused by the ischemic insult itself. This is supported by the observation that ventricular fibrillation was prominent when the regionally ischemic canine heart was subjected to reperfusion.[13] Jennings et al[14] reported adverse structural and electrophysiologic changes associated with reperfusion of the ischemic canine heart, and Hearse[15] introduced the concept of an oxygen paradox in noting cardiac muscle enzyme release and alterations in ultrastructure when isolated hearts were reoxygenated after a period of hypoxic perfusion.

Myocardial reperfusion injury is defined as the death of myocytes, alive at the time of reperfusion, as a direct result of one or more events initiated by reperfusion. Myocardial cell damage results from the restoration of blood flow to the previously ischemic heart, thereby extending the region of irreversible injury beyond that caused by the ischemic insult alone. The cellular damage that results from reperfusion can be reversible or irreversible, depending on the length of the ischemic insult. If reperfusion is initiated within 20 minutes after the onset of ischemia, the resulting myocardial injury is reversible and is characterized functionally by depressed myocardial contractility, which eventually recovers completely. Myocardial tissue necrosis is not detectable in the previously ischemic region, although functional impairment of contractility may persist for a variable period, a phenomenon known as *myocardial stunning*. Initiating reperfusion after a duration of ischemia of longer than 20 minutes, however, results in irreversible myocardial injury or cellular necrosis. The extent of tissue necrosis that develops during reperfusion is directly related to the duration of the ischemic event. Tissue necrosis originates in the subendocardial regions of the ischemic myocardium and extends to the subepicardial regions of the area at risk, often referred to as the *wavefront phenomenon*. The cell death that occurs during reperfusion can be characterized microscopically by explosive swelling, which includes disruption of the tissue lattice, contraction bands, mitochondrial swelling, and calcium phosphate deposits within mitochondria.[13]

The magnitude of reperfusion injury is directly related to the magnitude of the ischemic injury that precedes it. In its most severe form, it manifests in a "no-reflow" phenomenon. In cardiac surgery, prevention of myocardial injury after the release of the AXC, including the prevention of no reflow, is directly dependent on the adequacy of myocardial protection during the period of aortic clamping. The combination of ischemic and reperfusion injury is probably the most frequent and serious type of injury that leads to poor outcomes in cardiac surgery today (see Chapters 2, 3, 6, 12 to 14, 18, and 28).

Basic science investigations (in mouse, human, and porcine hearts) have implicated acidosis as a primary trigger of apoptosis. Acidosis, reoxygenation, and reperfusion, but not hypoxia (or ischemia) alone, are strong stimuli for programmed cell death, as well as the demonstration that cardiac apoptosis can lead to heart failure.[16,17] This suggests that apoptotic changes might be triggered in the course of a cardiac operation, thus effecting an injurious cascade of adverse clinical events that manifest late in the postoperative course.

Based on the previous discussion, it is clear that a significant portion of perioperative cardiac morbidity is related primarily to intraoperative factors. However, preoperative risk factors may influence ischemia/reperfusion injury.

Adverse Systemic Effects of Cardiopulmonary Bypass

In addition to the effects of disruption and restoration of myocardial blood flow, cardiac morbidity may result from many of the components used to perform cardiovascular operations, which lead to systemic insults that result from CPB circuit-induced contact activation. Inflammation in cardiac surgical patients is produced by complex humoral and cellular interactions, including activation, generation, or expression of thrombin, complement, cytokines, neutrophils, adhesion molecules, mast cells, and multiple inflammatory mediators.[18] Because of the redundancy of the inflammatory cascades, profound amplification occurs to produce multiorgan system dysfunction that can manifest as coagulopathy, respiratory failure, myocardial dysfunction, renal insufficiency, and neurocognitive defects. Coagulation and inflammation also are linked closely through networks of both humoral and cellular components, including proteases of the clotting and fibrinolytic cascades, as well as tissue factor. Vascular endothelial cells mediate inflammation and the cross-talk between coagulation and inflammation. Surgery alone activates specific hemostatic responses, activation of immune mechanisms, and inflammatory responses mediated by the release of various cytokines and chemokines (see Chapters 8 and 28 to 31). This complex inflammatory reaction can lead to death from nonischemic causes and suggests that preoperative risk factors may not predict morbidity. The ability to risk-adjust populations is critical to study interventions that may influence these responses to CPB.

Assessment of Perioperative Myocardial Injury in Cardiac Surgery

Unfortunately, the current clinical armamentarium is devoid of a means by which perioperative cardiac injury can be reliably monitored in real time, leading to the use of indicators of AMI after the event occurs. Generally, there is a lack of consensus regarding how to measure myocardial injury in cardiac surgery because of the continuum of cardiac injury. Electrocardiographic (ECG) changes, biomarker elevations, and measures of cardiac function have all been used, but all assessment modalities are affected by the direct myocardial trauma of surgery. The American College of Cardiology/European Society of Cardiology (ACC/ESC) published a definition of AMI in 2000, which includes a characteristic rise and fall in blood concentrations of cardiac troponins or creatine kinase (CK)-MB, or both, in the context of a coronary intervention, whereas other modalities are less sensitive and specific (Figure 1-1).[19] Subsequently, the Joint ESC/ACCF/American Heart Association/World Heart Federation Task Force's Universal Definition of Myocardial Infarction published a new "Universal Definition of Myocardial Infarction" in 2007.[20] Any of the following criteria meet the diagnosis for MI: Detection of rise/fall of cardiac biomarkers (preferably troponin) with at least one value above the 99th percentile of the upper reference limit (URL), together with evidence of myocardial ischemia with at least one of the following: symptoms of ischemia, ECG changes indicative of new ischemia (new ST-T changes or new left bundle branch block), development of pathologic Q waves in the ECG, or imaging evidence of new loss of viable myocardium or new regional wall motion abnormality (RWMA).

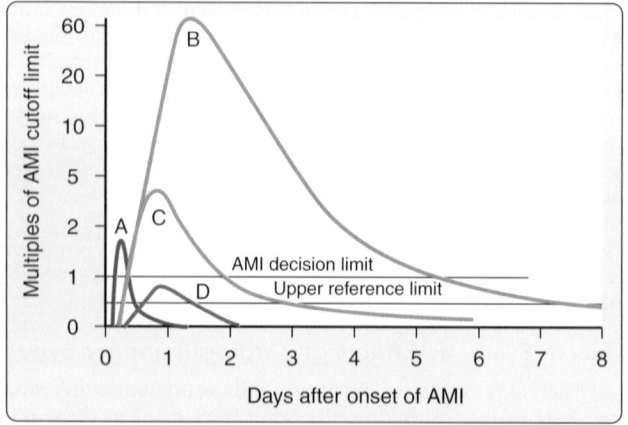

Figure 1-1   **Timing of release of various biomarkers after acute ischemic myocardial infarction.** Peak A, early release of myoglobin or creatine kinase (CK)-MB isoforms after acute myocardial infarction (AMI); peak B, cardiac troponin after AMI; peak C, CK-MB after AMI; peak D, cardiac troponin after unstable angina. Data are plotted on a relative scale, where 1.0 is set at the AMI cutoff concentration. *(From Apple FS, Gibler WB: National Academy of Clinical Biochemistry Standards of Laboratory Practice: Recommendations for the use of cardiac markers in coronary artery disease. Clin Chem 45:1104, 1999.)*

Traditionally, AMI was determined electrocardiographically (see Chapters 15 and 18). Biochemical measures have not been widely accepted because exact thresholds for myocardial injury have not been clearly defined. Cardiac biomarkers are increased after surgery and can be used for postoperative risk stratification, in addition to being used to diagnose acute morbidity (Box 1-2).

Assessment of Cardiac Function

Cardiac contractile dysfunction is the most prominent feature of myocardial injury, despite the fact that there are virtually no perfect measures of postoperative cardiac function.

The need for inotropic support, thermodilution cardiac output (CO) measurements, and transesophageal echocardiography (TEE) may represent practical intraoperative options for cardiac contractility evaluation. The need for inotropic support and CO measurements are not reliable measures because they depend on loading conditions and practitioner variability. Failure to wean from CPB, in the absence of systemic factors such as hyperkalemia and acidosis, is the best evidence of intraoperative myocardial injury or cardiac dysfunction; but it also may be multifactorial and, therefore, a less robust outcome measure.

RWMAs follow the onset of ischemia in 10 to 15 seconds. Echocardiography can, therefore, be a sensitive and rapid monitor for cardiac ischemia/injury.[21] If the RWMA is irreversible, this indicates irreversible myocardial necrosis (see Chapters 11 through 14). The importance of

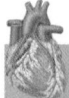

BOX 1-2. ASSESSMENT OF PERIOPERATIVE MYOCARDIAL INJURY

- Assessment of cardiac function
  - Echocardiography
- Nuclear imaging
- Electrocardiography
  - Q waves
  - ST-T wave changes
- Serum biomarkers
  - Myoglobin
  - CK
  - CK-MB
  - Troponin
  - Lactate dehydrogenase

TEE assessment of cardiac function is further enhanced by its value as a predictor of long-term survival.[22] In patients undergoing CABG, a postoperative decrease in left ventricular ejection fraction (LVEF) compared with preoperative baseline predicts decreased long-term survival.[23]

The use of TEE is complicated because myocardial stunning (post-ischemic transient ventricular dysfunction) is a common cause of new postoperative RWMAs, which are transient. However, the appearance of a new ventricular RWMA in the postoperative period, whether caused by irreversible AMI or by reversible myocardial stunning, is an indication of some form of inadequate myocardial protection during the intraoperative period and, therefore, of interest for the assessment of new interventions. Echocardiographic and Doppler systems also have the limitation of being sensitive to alterations in loading conditions, similar to the need for inotropic support and CO determinations.[24] The interpretation of TEE images is also operator dependent.[25] In addition, there are nonischemic causes of RWMAs, such as conduction abnormalities, ventricular pacing, and myocarditis, which confound the use of this outcome measure for the assessment of ischemic morbidity.

Electrocardiography Monitoring

The presence of new persistent Q waves of at least 0.03-second duration, broadening of preexisting Q waves, or new QS deflections on the postoperative ECG have been considered evidence of perioperative AMI.[26] However, new Q waves also may be caused by unmasking of an old MI and therefore not indicative of a new AMI. Crescenzi et al[27] demonstrated that the association of a new Q wave and high levels of biomarkers was strongly associated with postoperative cardiac events, whereas the isolated appearance of a new Q wave had no impact on the postoperative cardiac outcome. In addition, new Q waves may actually disappear over time.[28] Signs of non–Q-wave MI, such as ST-T wave changes, are even less reliable signs of AMI after cardiac surgery in the absence of biochemical evidence. ST-segment changes are even less specific for perioperative MI because they can be caused by changes in body position, hypothermia, transient conduction abnormalities, and electrolyte imbalances (see Chapter 15).

Serum Biochemical Markers to Detect Myocardial Injury

Serum biomarkers have become the primary means of assessing the presence and extent of AMI after cardiac surgery. Serum biomarkers that are indicative of myocardial damage include the following (with post-insult peak time given in parentheses): myoglobin (4 hours), total CK (16 hours), CK-MB isoenzyme (24 hours), troponins I and T (24 hours), and lactate dehydrogenase (LDH) (76 hours). The CK-MB isoenzyme has been used most widely, but studies have suggested that troponin I is the most sensitive and specific in depicting myocardial ischemia and infarction.[29–34]

With respect to CK-MB, the definition of an optimal cutoff has been defined best by the correlation of multiples of the upper limit of normal (ULN) for the laboratory and medium- and long-term outcomes. For example, Klatte et al[35] reported on the implications of CK-MB in 2918 high-risk CABG patients enrolled in a clinical trial of an anti-ischemic agent. The unadjusted 6-month mortality rates were 3.4%, 5.8%, 7.8%, and 20.2% for patients with a postoperative peak CK-MB ratio (peak CK-MB value/ULN for laboratory test) of less than 5, ≥5 to <10, ≥10 to < 20, and ≥20 ULN, respectively.[35] The relation remained statistically significant after adjustment for ejection fraction (EF), congestive heart failure (CHF), cerebrovascular disease, peripheral vascular disease, cardiac arrhythmias, and the method of cardioplegia delivery. In the Arterial Revascularization Therapies Study (ARTS), 496 patients with multivessel CAD undergoing CABG were evaluated by CK-MB testing and followed after surgery at 30 days and 1 year.[36] Patients with increased cardiac enzyme levels after CABG were at increased risk for both death and repeat AMI within the first 30 days. CK-MB increase also was independently related to late adverse outcome.

Studies suggest that postcardiac surgery monitoring of troponins can be used to assess myocardial injury and risk stratification. Increased cardiac-specific troponin I or T in patients after CABG has been associated with a cardiac cause of death and with major postoperative complications within 2 years after CABG.[37,38] The ACC/ESC definition includes biomarkers but does not include specific criteria for diagnosing post-CABG AMI using cardiac biomarkers.[19]

There are a few new biomarkers of perioperative cardiac injury or ischemia under development. Brain natriuretic peptide (BNP) could be detected in the early stages of ischemia and decreases shortly after ischemic insult, allowing better detection of reinjury.[39] BNP concentrations after CABG in the patients who had cardiac events within 2 years were significantly greater than those in the patients free of cardiac events.[40] Soluble CD40 ligand (sCD40L) is another early biomarker of myocardial ischemia,[41] and CPB causes an increase in the concentration of plasma sCD40L. A corresponding decrease in platelet CD40L suggests that this prothrombotic and proinflammatory protein was derived primarily from platelets and may contribute to the thrombotic and inflammatory complications associated with CPB.[42] Future research will be required to determine how these biomarkers will be used to assess outcome after cardiac surgery.

Variability in Diagnosis of Perioperative Myocardial Infarction

The variability in diagnosing perioperative AMI has been studied by Jain and colleagues,[43] who evaluated data from 566 patients at 20 clinical sites, collected as part of a clinical trial. The occurrence of AMI by Q-wave, CK-MB, or autopsy criteria was determined. Of the 25% of patients who met the Q-wave, CK-MB, or autopsy criteria for AMI, 19% had increased CK-MB concentrations, as well as ECG changes. Q-wave and CK-MB or autopsy criteria for AMI were met by 4% of patients. Multicenter data collection showed a substantial variation in the incidence of AMI and an overall incidence rate of up to 25%. The definition of perioperative AMI was highly variable depending on the definitions used.

Clinicians are still in search for a "gold standard" approach to diagnose perioperative AMI. Perioperative myocardial necrosis/injury ranges from mild to severe and can have ischemic and nonischemic origin in patients undergoing cardiac surgery. Perioperative ECG changes, including Q-waves, and new RWMAs on ECGs are less reliable than in the nonperioperative arena. Currently, troponin I or T is the best indicator of myocardial damage after cardiac surgery. The level of enzymes correlates with the extension of the injury, but there is no universal cutoff point defining perioperative MI.

■ Cardiac Risk Assessment and Cardiac Risk Stratification Models

In defining important risk factors and developing risk indices, each of the studies has used different primary outcomes. Postoperative mortality remains the most definitive outcome that is reflective of patient injury in the perioperative period. It is important to note that death can be cardiac and noncardiac, and if cardiac, may be ischemic or nonischemic in origin. Postoperative mortality rate is reported as either in-hospital or 30-day rate. The latter represents a more standardized definition, although more difficult to capture because of the cost-cutting push to discharge patients early after surgery. The value of developing risk-adjusted postoperative mortality models is the assessment of the comparative efficacy of various techniques in preventing myocardial damage, but it does not provide information that is useful in preventing the injury in real time.[44] The postoperative mortality rate also has been used as a comparative measure of quality of cardiac surgical care.[45,46]

Postoperative morbidity includes AMI and reversible events such as CHF and need for inotropic support. The problems of using AMI as an outcome of interest were described earlier. Because resource utilization has become such an important financial consideration for hospitals, length of intensive care unit (ICU) stay increasingly has been used in the development of risk indices (see Chapter 33).

Predictors of Postoperative Morbidity and Mortality

Clinical and angiographic predictors of operative mortality were initially defined from the Coronary Artery Surgery Study (CASS).[47,48] A total of 6630 patients underwent isolated CABG between 1975 and 1978. Women had a significantly greater mortality rate than men; mortality increased with advancing age in men, but this was not a significant factor in women. Increasing severity of angina, manifestations of heart failure, and number and extent of coronary artery stenoses all correlated with greater mortality, whereas EF was not a predictor. Urgency of surgery was a strong predictor of outcome, with those patients requiring emergency surgery in the presence of a 90% left main coronary artery stenosis sustaining a 40% mortality rate.

A risk-scoring scheme for cardiac surgery (CABG and valve) was introduced by Paiement et al[3] at the Montreal Heart Institute in 1983. Eight risk factors were identified: (1) poor left ventricular (LV) function, (2) CHF, (3) unstable angina or recent (within 6 weeks) MI, (4) age greater than 65 years, (5) severe obesity (body mass index > 30 kg/m²), (6) reoperation, (7) emergency surgery, and (8) other significant or uncontrolled systemic disturbances. Three classifications were identified: patients with none of these factors (normal), those presenting with one risk factor (increased risk), and those with more than one factor (high risk). In a study of 500 consecutive cardiac surgical patients, it was found that operative mortality increased with increasing risk (confirming their scoring system).

One of the most commonly used scoring systems for CABG was developed by Parsonnet and colleagues (Table 1-1).[49] Fourteen risk

TABLE 1-1	Components of the Additive Model	
Risk Factor	**Assigned Weight**
Female sex	1
Morbid obesity (≥ 1.5 × ideal weight)	3
Diabetes (unspecified type)	3
Hypertension (systolic BP > 140 mm Hg)	3
Ejection fraction (%):	
Good > 50)	0
Fair (30–49)	2
Poor (< 30)	4
Age (yr):	
70–74	7
75–79	12
≥ 80	20
Reoperation	
First	5
Second	10
Preoperative IABP	2
Left ventricular aneurysm	5
Emergency surgery after PTCA or catheterization complications	10
Dialysis dependency (PD or Hemo)	10
Catastrophic states (e.g., acute structural defect, cardiogenic shock, acute renal failure)*	10–50†
Other rare circumstances (e.g., paraplegia, pacemaker dependency, congenital HD in adult, severe asthma)*	2–10†
Valve surgery	
Mitral	5
PA pressure ≥ 60 mm Hg	8
Aortic	5
Pressure gradient > 120 mm Hg	7
CABG at the time of valve surgery	2

* On the actual worksheet, these risk factors require justification.
† Values were predictive of increased risk for operative mortality in univariate analysis.
BP, blood pressure; CABG, coronary artery bypass graft; HD, heart disease; Hemo, hemodialysis; IABP, intra-aortic balloon pump; PA, pulmonary artery; PD, peritoneal dialysis; PTCA, percutaneous transluminal coronary angioplasty.
From Parsonnet V, Dean D, Bernstein A: A method of uniform stratification of risk for evaluating the results of surgery in acquired adult heart disease. *Circulation* 79:13, 1989, by permission.

factors were identified for in-hospital or 30-day mortality after uni-variate regression analysis of 3500 consecutive operations. An additive model was constructed and prospectively evaluated in 1332 cardiac procedures. Five categories of risk were identified with increasing mortality rates, complication rates, and length of stay at the Newark Beth Israel Medical Center. The Parsonnet Index frequently is used as a benchmark for comparison among institutions. However, the Parsonnet model was created earlier than the other models and may not be representative of the current practice of CABG. During the period after publication of the Parsonnet model, numerous technical advances now in routine use have diminished CABG mortality rates.

Bernstein and Parsonnet[50] simplified the risk-adjusted scoring system in 2000 to provide a handy tool in preoperative discussions with patients and their families, and for preoperative risk stratification calculation. The authors developed a logistic regression model in which 47 potential risk factors were considered, and a method requiring only simple addition and graphic interpretation was designed for relatively easily approximating the estimated risk. The final estimates provided by the simplified model correlated well with the observed mortality (Figure 1-2).

O'Connor et al[51] used data collected from 3055 patients undergoing isolated CABG at five clinical centers between 1987 and 1989 to develop a multivariate numerical score. A regression model was developed in a training set and subsequently validated in a test set. Independent predictors of in-hospital mortality included patient age, body surface area, comorbidity score, prior CABG, EF, LV end-diastolic pressure, and priority of surgery. The validated multivariate prediction rule was robust in predicting the in-hospital mortality for an individual patient, and the authors proposed that it could be used to contrast observed and expected mortality rates for an institution or a particular clinician.

Higgins et al[52] developed a Clinical Severity Score for CABG at The Cleveland Clinic. A multivariate logistic regression model to predict perioperative risk was developed in 5051 patients undergoing CABG between 1986 and 1988, and subsequently validated in a cohort of 4069 patients. Independent predictors of in-hospital and 30-day mortality were emergency procedure, preoperative serum creatinine level of greater than 168 µmol/L, severe LV dysfunction, preoperative hematocrit of less than 34%, increasing age, chronic pulmonary disease, prior vascular surgery, reoperation, and mitral valve insufficiency. Predictors of morbidity (AMI and use of the intra-aortic balloon pump [IABP],

---

CARDIAC SURGERY:
PREOPERATIVE RISK-ESTIMATION WORKSHEET
(not intended for retrospective risk stratification)

Newark Beth Isreal Medical Center
Division of Surgical Research

Patient's Name: _____
Patient Number: _____
Date: _____

INSTRUCTIONS:

Step 1.   Fill in the blanks for existing risk factors, using the scores provided. (Note: Scores shown are in arbitrary units, and are not, by themselves, estimates of percent risk.)

Step 2.   Add the scores to obtain a total score. (Include common risk factors on this side of the page and less common risk factors on the other side.)

Step 3.   See reverse side to interpret the total score.

RISK FACTOR	SCORING (APPROXIMATE SYSTEM 97)		VALUE
Female gender		6	6
Age	70–75 76–79 80+	2.5 7 11	7
Congestive failure		2.5	
COPD, severe		6	
Diabetes		3	
Ejection fraction	30–42% <30%	6.5 8	
Hypertension	Over 140/90, or history of hypertension, or currently taking anti-hypertension medication	3	3
Left-main disease	Left-main stenosis is 50%	2.5	
Morbid obesity	Over 1.5 times ideal weight	1	1
Preoperative IABP	IABP present at time of surgery	4	
Reoperation	First reoperation Second or subsequent reoperation	10 20	
One valve, aortic	Procedure proposed	0	
One valve, mitral	Procedure proposed	4.5	
Valve + ACB	Combination valve procedure and ACB proposed	6	
Special conditions	*(see reverse side)*		

(See reverse side for risk estimation.)

TOTAL SCORE: 17

RISK VALUES FOR SPECIAL CONDITIONS

Cardiac

Cardiogenic shock (urinary output <10 cc/hr)	12
Endocarditis, active	5.5
Endocarditis, treated	0
LV aneurysm resected	1.5
One valve, incuspid: procedure proposed	5
Pacemaker dependency	0
Transmural acute MI within 48 hr	4
Ventricular septal defect, acute	12
Ventricular tachycardia, ventricular fibrillation, aborted sudden death	1

Pulmonary

Asthma	1
Endotracheal tube, preoperative	4
Idiopathic thrombocytopenic purpura	12
Pulmonary hypertension (mean pressure >30)	11

Hepato-renal

Cirrhosis	12.5
Dialysis dependency	13.5
Renal failure, acute or chronic	3.5

Vascular

Abdominal aortic aneurysm, asymptomatic	0.5
Cartoid disease (bilateral or 100% unilateral occlusion)	2
Peripheral vascular disease, severe	3.5

Miscellaneous

Blood products refused	11
Severe neurologic disorder (healed CVA, paraplegia, muscular dystrophy, hemiparesis)	5
PTCA or cathaterization failure	5.5
Substance abuse	4.5

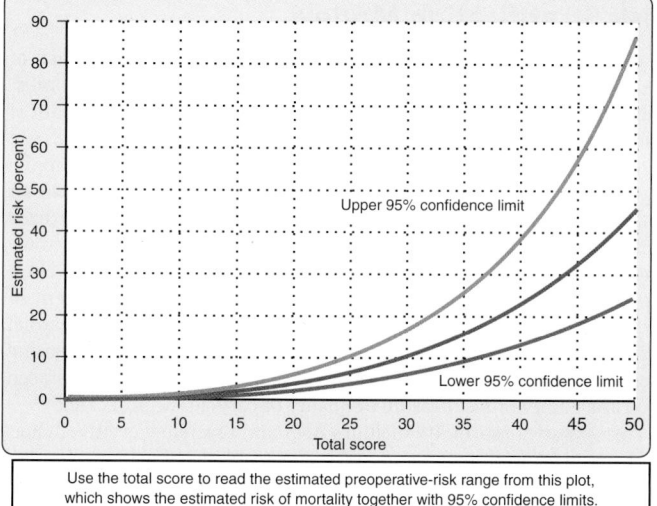

Use the total score to read the estimated preoperative-risk range from this plot, which shows the estimated risk of mortality together with 95% confidence limits.

Figure 1-2   Preoperative Risk-Estimation Worksheet. *(From Bernstein AD, Parsonnet V: Bedside estimation of risk as an aid for decision-making in cardiac surgery. Ann Thorac Surg 69:823, 2000, by permission from the Society of Thoracic Surgeons.)*

mechanical ventilation for ≥3 days, neurologic deficit, oliguric or anuric renal failure, or serious infection) included diabetes mellitus, body weight of 65 kg or less, aortic stenosis, and cerebrovascular disease. Each independent predictor was assigned a weight or score, with increasing mortality and morbidity associated with an increasing total score.

The New York State model of Hannan et al[53] collected data over the years of 1989 through 1992 with 57,187 patients in a study with 14 variables. It was validated in 30 institutions. The mortality definition was "in-hospital." The crude mortality rate was 3.1%; the receiver operating characteristic (ROC) curve was 0.7, with the Hosmer-Lemeshow (H-L) statistic less than 0.005. Observed mortality was 3.7%, and the expected mortality rate was 2.8%. They included only isolated CABG operations.

The Society of Thoracic Surgeons (STS) national database represents the most robust source of data for calculating risk-adjusted scoring systems. Established in 1989, the database has grown to include 892 participating hospitals in 2008. This provider-supported database allows participants to benchmark their risk-adjusted results against regional and national standards. This National Adult Cardiac Surgery Database (STS NCD) has become one of the largest in the world. New patient data are brought into the STS database on an annual and now semiannual basis. These new data have been analyzed, modeled, and tested using a variety of statistical algorithms. Since 1990, when more complete data collection was achieved, risk stratification models were developed for both CABG and valve replacement surgery. Models developed in 1995 and 1996 were shown to have good predictive value (Table 1-2; Figure 1-3).[54,55] In 1999, the STS analyzed the database for valve replacement with and without CABG to determine trends in risk stratification. Between 1986 and 1995, 86,580 patients were analyzed. The model evaluated the influence of 51 preoperative variables on operative mortality by univariate and multivariate analyses for the overall population and for each subset. After the significant risk factors were determined by univariate analysis, a standard logistic regression analysis was performed using the training-set population to develop a formal model. The test-set population then was used to determine the validity of the model. The preoperative risk factors associated with greatest operative mortality rates were salvage status, renal failure (dialysis dependent and nondialysis dependent), emergent status, multiple reoperations, and New York Heart Association class IV. The multivariate logistic regression analysis identified 30 independent preoperative risk factors among the 6 valvular models, isolated or in combination with CABG. The addition of CABG increased the mortality rate significantly for all age groups and for all subset models.[56]

There are currently three general STS risk models: CABG, valve (aortic or mitral), and valve plus CABG. These apply to seven specific, precisely defined procedures: the CABG model refers to an isolated CABG; the valve model includes isolated aortic or mitral valve replacement and mitral valve repair; and the valve and CABG model includes aortic valve replacement and CABG, mitral valve replacement and CABG, and mitral valve repair and CABG. Besides operative mortality, these models were developed for eight additional end points: reoperation, permanent stroke, renal failure, deep sternal wound infection, prolonged (> 24 hours) ventilation, major morbidity, and operative death, and finally short (< 6 days) and long (> 14 days) postoperative length of stay.[57–59] These models are updated periodically, every few years, and calibrated annually to provide an immediate and accurate tool for regional and national benchmarking, and have been proposed for public reporting. The calibration of the risk factors is based on the observed/expected (O/E) ratio, and calibration factors are updated quarterly. The expected mortality (E) is calibrated to obtain the national E/O ratio.

Tu et al[60] collected data from 13,098 patients undergoing cardiac surgery between 1991 and 1993 at all nine adult cardiac surgery institutions in Ontario, Canada. Six variables (age, sex, LV function, type of surgery, urgency of surgery, and repeat operation) predicted in-hospital mortality, ICU stay, and postoperative stay in days after cardiac surgery. Subsequently, the Working Group Panel on the Collaborative CABG Database Project categorized 44 clinical variables into 7 core,

TABLE 1-2	Risk Model Results
Variable	*Odds Ratio*
Age (in 10-year increments)	1.640
Female sex	1.157
Non-white	1.249
Ejection fraction	0.988
Diabetes	1.188
Renal failure	1.533
Serum creatinine (if renal failure is present)	1.080
Dialysis dependence (if renal failure is present)	1.381
Pulmonary hypertension	1.185
Cerebrovascular accident timing	1.198
Chronic obstructive pulmonary disease	1.296
Peripheral vascular disease	1.487
Cerebrovascular disease	1.244
Acute evolving, extending myocardial infarction	1.282
Myocardial infarction timing	1.117
Cardiogenic shock	2.211
Use of diuretics	1.122
Hemodynamic instability	1.747
Triple-vessel disease	1.155
Left main disease > 50%	1.119
Preoperative intra-aortic balloon pump	1.480
Status	
Urgent or emergent	1.189
Emergent salvage	3.654
First reoperation	2.738
Multiple reoperations	4.282
Arrhythmias	1.099
Body surface area	0.488
Obesity	1.242
New York Heart Association Class IV	1.098
Use of steroids	1.214
Congestive heart failure	1.191
Percutaneous transluminal coronary angioplasty within 6 hours of surgery	1.332
Angiographic accident with hemodynamic instability	1.203
Use of digitalis	1.168
Use of intravenous nitrates	1.088

From Shroyer AL, Plomondon ME, Grover FL, et al: The 1996 coronary artery bypass risk model: The Society of Thoracic Surgeons Adult Cardiac National Database. *Ann Thorac Surg* 67:1205, 1999, by permission of Society of Thoracic Surgeons.

13 level 1, and 24 level 2 variables, to reflect their relative importance in determining short-term mortality after CABG. Using data from 5517 patients undergoing isolated CABG at 9 institutions in Ontario in 1993, a series of models were developed. The incorporation of additional variables beyond the original six added little to the prediction of in-hospital mortality.

Spivack et al[61] collected data during 1991 and 1992 and included 513 patients with 15 variables, validated only in their institution. They used only an isolated CABG population, and the outcomes measured were mortality and morbidity. The morbidity definition was ventilator time and ICU days. Both prolonged mechanical ventilation and death were rare events (8.3% and 2.0%, respectively). The combination of reduced LVEF and the presence of selected preexisting comorbid conditions (clinical CHF, angina, current smoking, diabetes) served as modest risk factors for prolonged mechanical ventilation; their absence strongly predicted an uncomplicated postoperative respiratory course.

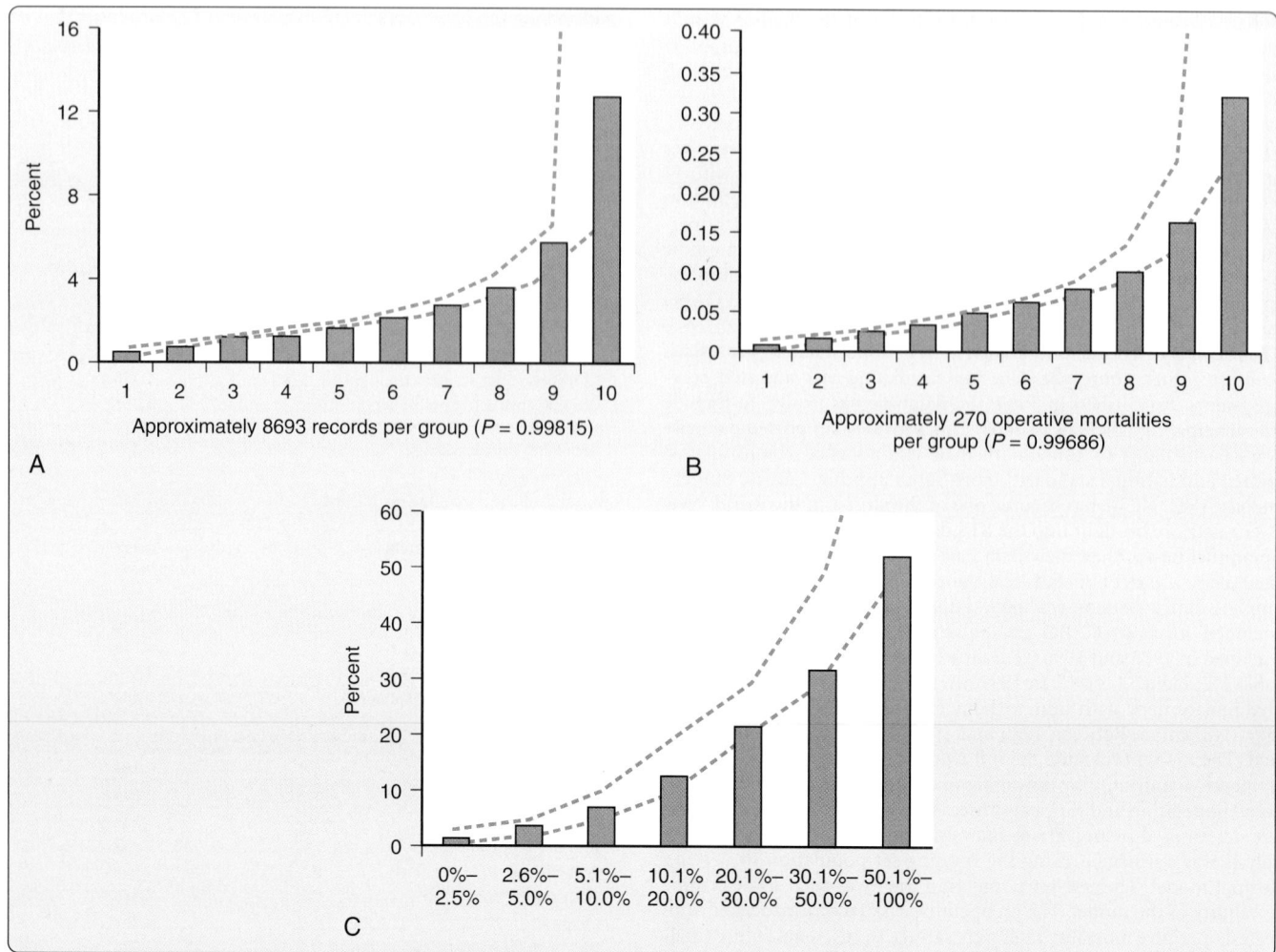

Figure 1-3   *A*, **Ordered risk deciles with equal number of records per group.** After the predicted risk for each patient in the test set was determined, the patient records were arranged sequentially in order of predicted risk. The population was divided into 10 groups of equal size. The predicted mortality rate was compared with the actual mortality for each of the 10 groups. *Dashed lines* represent range of predicted mortality for a group of patients; *bars* represent actual mortality for a group of patients. *B,* **Ordered risk deciles with equal number of deaths per group.** After the predicted risk for each patient in the test set was determined, the patient records were arranged sequentially in order of predicted risk. The population was divided into 10 groups with equal numbers of deaths in each group. The predicted mortality was compared with the actual mortality for each of the 10 groups. *Dashed lines* represent range of predicted mortality for a group of patients; *bars* represent actual mortality for a group of patients. *C,* **Ordered risk categories in clinically relevant groupings.** After the predicted risk for each patient in the test set was determined, the patient records were arranged sequentially in order of predicted risk. The population was divided into seven clinically relevant risk categories. The predicted mortality was compared with the actual mortality for each of the seven groups. *Dashed lines* represent range of predicted mortality for a group of patients; *bars* represent actual mortality for a group of patients. *(A–C, From Shroyer AL, Plomondon ME, Grover FL, et al: The 1996 coronary artery bypass risk model: The Society of Thoracic Surgeons Adult Cardiac National Database. Ann Thorac Surg 67:1205, 1999, by permission of the Society of Thoracic Surgeons.)*

The European System for Cardiac Operative Risk Evaluation (EuroSCORE) for cardiac operative risk evaluation was constructed from an analysis of 19,030 patients undergoing a diverse group of cardiac surgical procedures from 128 centers across Europe (Tables 1-3 and 1-4).[62,63] The following risk factors were associated with increased mortality: age, female sex, serum creatinine, extracardiac arteriopathy, chronic airway disease, severe neurologic dysfunction, previous cardiac surgery, recent MI, LVEF, chronic CHF, pulmonary hypertension, active endocarditis, unstable angina, procedure urgency, critical preoperative condition, ventricular septal rupture, noncoronary surgery, and thoracic aortic surgery.

EuroSCORE provided a unique opportunity to assess the true risk of cardiac surgery in the absence of any identifiable risk factors. For the purposes of this analysis, baseline mortality figures were calculated in patients in whom no preoperative risk factors could be identified (including risk factors that were not found to have a significant impact in this study, such as diabetes and hypertension). When all such patients were excluded, it was gratifying to note the extremely low current mortality for cardiac surgery in Europe: 0% for atrial septal defect repair, 0.4% for CABG, and barely more than 1% for single valve repair or replacement.

During the 2000s, this additive EuroSCORE has been used widely and validated across different centers in Europe and across the world, making it a primary tool for risk stratification in cardiac surgery.[64-75] Although its accuracy has been well established for CABG and isolated valve procedures, its predictive ability in combined CABG and valve procedures has been less well studied. Karthik et al[66] showed that, in patients undergoing combined procedures, the additive EuroSCORE significantly underpredicted the risk compared with the observed mortality. In this subset, they determined that the logistic EuroSCORE is a better and more accurate method of risk assessment.

TABLE 1-3	Risk Factors, Definitions, and Weights (Score)	
Risk Factors	*Definition*	*Score*
Patient-Related Factors		
Age	Per 5 years or part thereof over 60 years	1
Sex	Female	1
Chronic pulmonary disease	Long-term use of bronchodilators or steroids for lung disease	1
Extracardiac arteriopathy	Any one or more of the following: claudication, carotid occlusion or > 50% stenosis, previous or planned intervention on the abdominal aorta, limb arteries, or carotids	2
Neurologic dysfunction	Disease severely affecting ambulation or day-to-day functioning	2
Previous cardiac surgery	Requiring opening of the pericardium	3
Serum creatinine	> 200 µmol/L before surgery	2
Active endocarditis	Patient still under antibiotic treatment for endocarditis at the time of surgery	3
Critical preoperative state	Any one or more of the following: ventricular tachycardia or fibrillation or aborted sudden death, preoperative cardiac massage, preoperative ventilation before arrival in the anesthetic room, preoperative inotropic support, intra-aortic balloon counterpulsation or preoperative acute renal failure (anuria or oliguria < 10 mL/hr)	3
Cardiac-Related Factors		
Unstable angina	Rest angina requiring IV nitrates until arrival in the anesthetic room	2
Left ventricular dysfunction	Moderate or LVEF 30–50%	1
	Poor or LVEF > 30%	3
	Recent myocardial infarct (< 90 days)	2
Pulmonary hypertension	Systolic pulmonary artery pressure > 60 mm Hg	2
Surgery-Related Factors		
Emergency	Carried out on referral before the beginning of the next working day	2
Other than isolated CABG	Major cardiac procedure other than or in addition to CABG	2
Surgery on thoracic aorta	For disorder of ascending aorta, arch or descending aorta	3
Postinfarct septal rupture		4

CABG, coronary artery bypass graft surgery; LVEF, left ventricular ejection fraction.
From Nashef SA, Roques F, Michel P, et al: European system for cardiac operative risk evaluation (EuroSCORE). *Eur J Cardiothorac Surg* 16:9, 1999.

TABLE 1-5	Cardiac Anesthesia Risk Evaluation Score

1 = Patient with stable cardiac disease and no other medical problem. A noncomplex surgery is undertaken.

2 = Patient with stable cardiac disease and one or more controlled medical problems.[*] A noncomplex surgery is undertaken.

3 = Patient with any uncontrolled medical problem[†] or patient in whom a complex surgery is undertaken.[‡]

4 = Patient with any uncontrolled medical problem *and* in whom a complex surgery is undertaken.

5 = Patient with chronic or advanced cardiac disease for whom cardiac surgery is undertaken as a last hope to save or improve life.

E = Emergency: surgery as soon as diagnosis is made and operating room is available.

[*]Examples: controlled hypertension, diabetes mellitus, peripheral vascular disease, chronic obstructive pulmonary disease, controlled systemic diseases, others as judged by clinicians.
[†]Examples: unstable angina treated with intravenous heparin or nitroglycerin, preoperative intra-aortic balloon pump, heart failure with pulmonary or peripheral edema, uncontrolled hypertension, renal insufficiency (creatinine level > 140 µmol/L, debilitating systemic diseases, others as judged by clinicians).
[‡]Examples: reoperation, combined valve and coronary artery surgery, multiple valve surgery, left ventricular aneurysmectomy, repair of ventricular septal defect after myocardial infarction, coronary artery bypass of diffuse or heavily calcified vessels, others as judged by clinicians.
From Dupuis JY, Wang F, Nathan H, et al: The cardiac anesthesia risk evaluation score: A clinically useful predictor of mortality and morbidity after cardiac surgery. *Anesthesiology* 94:194, 2001, by permission.

Dupuis et al[76] attempted to simplify the approach to risk of cardiac surgical procedures in a manner similar to the original American Society of Anesthesiologists (ASA) physical status classification. They developed a score that uses a simple continuous categorization, using five classes plus an emergency status (Table 1-5). The Cardiac Anesthesia Risk Evaluation (CARE) score model collected data from 1996 to 1999 and included 3548 patients to predict both in-hospital mortality and a diverse group of major morbidities. It combined clinical judgment and the recognition of three risk factors previously identified by multifactorial risk indices: comorbid conditions categorized as controlled or uncontrolled, the surgical complexity, and the urgency of the procedure. The CARE score demonstrated similar or superior predictive characteristics compared with the more complex indices.

Nowicki et al[77] used data on 8943 cardiac valve surgery patients aged 30 years and older from eight northern New England medical centers from 1991 through 2001 to develop a model to predict in-hospital mortality. In the multivariate analysis, 11 variables in the aortic model (older age, lower body surface area, prior cardiac operation, increased creatinine, prior stroke, NYHA class IV, CHF, atrial fibrillation, acuity, year of surgery, and concomitant CABG) and 10 variables in the mitral model (female sex, older age, diabetes, CAD, prior cerebrovascular accident, increased creatinine, NYHA class IV, CHF, acuity, and valve replacement) remained independent predictors of the outcome. They developed a look-up table for mortality rate based on a simple scoring system.

TABLE 1-4	Application of EuroSCORE Scoring System			
			95% Confidence Limits for Mortality	
EuroSCORE	*Patients (n)*	*Died (n)*	*Observed*	*Expected*
0–2 (low risk)	4529	36 (0.8%)	0.56–1.10	1.27–1.29
3–5 (medium risk)	5977	182 (3.0%)	2.62–3.51	2.90–2.94
6 plus (high risk)	4293	480 (11.2%)	10.25–12.16	10.93–11.54
Total	14,799	698 (4.7%)	4.37–5.06	4.72–4.95

EuroSCORE, European System for Cardiac Operative Risk Evaluation.
From Nashef SA, Roques F, Michel P, et al: European system for cardiac operative risk evaluation (EuroSCORE). *Eur J Cardiothorac Surg* 16:9, 1999, by permission.

Hannan and colleagues[78] also evaluated predictors of mortality after valve surgery but used data from 14,190 patients from New York State. A total of 18 independent risk factors were identified in the 6 models of differing combinations of valve and CABG. Shock and dialysis-dependent renal failure were among the most significant risk factors in all models. The risk factors and odds ratios are shown in Tables 1-6, 1-7, and 1-8. They also studied which risk factors are associated with early readmission (within 30 days) after CABG. Of 16,325 total patients, 2111 (12.9%) were readmitted within 30 days for reasons related to CABG. Eleven risk factors were found to be independently associated with greater readmission rates: older age, female sex, African American race, greater body surface area, previous AMI within 1 week, and six comorbidities. After controlling for these preoperative patient-level risk factors, two provider characteristics (annual surgeon CABG volume < 100 and hospital risk-adjusted mortality rate in the highest decile) and two postoperative factors (discharge to nursing home or rehabilitation/acute care facility and length of stay during index CABG admission of ≥5 days) also were related to greater readmission rates. The development of several excellent risk models for cardiac valve surgery provides a powerful new tool to improve patient care, select procedures, counsel patients, and compare outcomes (see Chapter 19).[79]

Consistency Among Risk Indices

Many different variables have been found to be associated with the increased risk during cardiac surgery, but only a few variables consistently have been found to be major risk factors across multiple and very diverse study settings. Age, female sex, LV function, body habitus, reoperation, type of surgery, and urgency of surgery were some variables consistently present in most of the models (Box 1-3).

Although a variety of investigators have found different comorbid diseases to be significant risk factors, no diseases have been shown to be consistent risk factors, with the possible exception of renal dysfunction and diabetes. These two comorbidities have been shown to be important risk factors in a majority of the studies (Box 1-4).

Applicability of Risk Indices to a Given Population

It is critical to understand how these indices were created to understand how best to apply a given risk index to a specific patient or population. Specifically, the application of these risk models must be done with caution and after careful study for any specific population. One issue is that the profile of patients undergoing cardiac surgery is constantly changing, and patients who previously would not have been considered for surgery (and thus not included in the development data set) are now undergoing surgery. Therefore, the models require continuous updating and revision. In addition, cardiac surgery itself is changing with the increasing use of off-pump and less invasive procedures, which may change the nature of the influence of preexisting conditions.

One critical factor in the choice of model to use for a given practice is to understand the clinical goals used in the original development process. In addition, despite extensive research and widespread use of

TABLE 1-6	Significant Independent Risk Factors for In-Hospital Mortality for Isolated Aortic Valve Replacement and for Aortic Valvuloplasty or Valve Replacement Plus Coronary Artery Bypass Graft Surgery			
	Isolated Aortic Valve Replacement (C = 0.809)		Aortic Valvuloplasty or Valve Replacement Plus CABG (C = 0.727)	
Risk Factor	OR	95% CI for OR	OR	95% CI for OR
Age ≥ 55 years	1.06	1.04–1.08	1.04	1.02–1.06
Hemodynamic instability	3.97	1.85–8.51	NS	
Shock	8.68	2.76–27.33	9.09	3.82–21.62
CHF in same admission	2.26	1.54–3.30	NS	
Extensively calcified ascending aorta	1.96	1.22–3.15	1.56	1.16–2.08
Diabetes	2.52	1.67–3.81	NS	
Dialysis-dependent renal failure	5.51	2.58–11.73	3.17	1.70–5.90
Pulmonary artery systolic pressure ≥ 50 mm Hg	2.35	1.61–3.41	2.28	1.75–2.96
Body surface area	NS		0.28	0.16–0.50
Previous cardiac operation	NS		2.13	1.54–2.96
Renal failure, no dialysis	NS		2.36	1.32–4.21
Aortoiliac disease	NS		1.88	1.26–2.82

CABG, coronary artery bypass graft; CHF, congestive heart failure; CI, confidence interval; NS, not significant; OR, odds ratio.
From Hannan EL, Racz MJ, Jones RH, et al: Predictors of mortality for patients undergoing cardiac valve replacements in New York State. *Ann Thorac Surg* 70:1212, 2000, by permission of the Society of Thoracic Surgeons.

TABLE 1-7	Significant Independent Risk Factors for In-Hospital Mortality for Isolated Mitral Valve Replacement and for Mitral Valve Replacement Plus Coronary Artery Bypass Graft Surgery			
	Isolated Mitral Valve Replacement (C = 0.823)		Mitral Valve Replacement Plus CABG (C = 0.718)	
Risk Factor	OR	95% CI for OR	OR	95% CI for OR
Age ≥ 55 years	1.08	1.06–1.11	1.07	1.05–1.09
Carotid disease	2.98	1.65–5.39	1.81	1.21–2.70
Shock	9.17	4.17–20.16	5.29	3.03–9.22
CHF in same admission	3.03	2.01–4.56	NS	
Dialysis-dependent renal failure	5.07	1.98–12.97	NS	
Endocarditis	4.28	2.49–7.36	NS	
Ejection fraction < 30%	NS		1.76	1.23–2.51
Hemodynamic instability	NS		3.40	2.16–5.36
Extensively calcified ascending aorta	NA		1.94	1.27–2.96

CABG, coronary artery bypass graft; CHF, congestive heart failure; CI, confidence interval; NA, not available; NS, not significant; OR, odds ratio.
From Hannan EL, Racz MJ, Jones RH, et al: Predictors of mortality for patients undergoing cardiac valve replacements in New York State. *Ann Thorac Surg* 70:1212, 2000, by permission of the Society of Thoracic Surgeons.

TABLE 1-8	Significant Independent Risk Factors for In-Hospital Mortality for Multiple Valvuloplasty or Valve Replacement and for Multiple Valvuloplasty or Valve Replacement Plus Coronary Artery Bypass Graft Surgery				
	Multiple Valvuloplasty or Valve Replacement (C = 0.764)			Multiple Valvuloplasty or Valve Replacement Plus CABG (C = 0.750)	
Risk Factor	OR	95% CI for OR		OR	95% CI for OR
Age ≥ 55 years	1.05	1.03–1.07		1.05	1.10–1.08
Aortoiliac disease	3.55	1.17–10.72		4.63	2.12–10.10
CHF in same admission	2.18	1.44–3.29		NS	
Malignant ventricular arrhythmia	2.62	1.19–5.78		NS	
Extensively calcified ascending aorta	2.13	1.13–4.00		NS	
Diabetes	1.87	1.13–3.10		2.49	1.46–4.24
Renal failure without dialysis	3.55	1.88–6.72		NS	
Dialysis-dependent renal failure	9.37	4.10–21.40		NS	
Female sex	NS	1.95		1.20–3.18	
Hemodynamic instability	NS	3.65		1.50–8.86	
Shock	NS	50.19		6.08–414.44	
Hepatic failure	NS	8.21		1.84–36.66	
Endocarditis	NS	4.70		1.59–13.87	

CABG, coronary artery bypass graft; CHF, congestive heart failure; CI, confidence interval; NA, not available; NS, not significant; OR, odds ratio.
From Hannan EL, Racz MJ, Jones RH, et al: Predictors of mortality for patients undergoing cardiac valve replacements in New York State. *Ann Thorac Surg* 70:1212, 2000, by permission of the Society of Thoracic Surgeons.

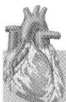

BOX 1-3. COMMON VARIABLES ASSOCIATED WITH INCREASED RISK FOR CARDIAC SURGERY

- Age
- Female sex
- Left ventricular function
- Body habitus
- Reoperation
- Type of surgery
- Urgency of surgery

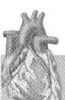

BOX 1-4. MEDICAL CONDITIONS ASSOCIATED WITH INCREASED RISK

- Renal dysfunction
- Diabetes (inconsistent)
- Recent acute coronary syndromes

risk models in cardiac surgery, there are methodologic problems. The extent of the details in the reports varies greatly. Different conclusions can be reached depending on the risk model used. Processes critical to the development of risk models are shown in Figure 1-4.

The underlying assumption in the development of any risk index is that specific factors (disease history, physical findings, laboratory data, nature of surgery) cannot be modified with respect to their influence on outcome; that is, the perioperative period is essentially a black box. If a specific factor is left untreated, it could lead to major morbidity or mortality. For example, the urgency of the planned surgical procedure and baseline comorbidities cannot be changed. However, the models themselves depend on the appropriate selection of baseline variables or risk factors to study, and their prevalence in the population of interest is critical for them to affect outcome. For example, referral patterns to a given institution may result in an absence of certain patient populations and, therefore, the risk factor would not appear in the model. Also, the use of multivariate logistic regression may eliminate biologically important risk factors, which are not present in sufficient numbers to achieve statistical significance.

In developing a risk index, it is also important to validate the model and to benchmark it against other known means of assessing risks. It is important to determine whether the index predicts morbidity, mortality, or both. Typically, a model's performance is first evaluated on

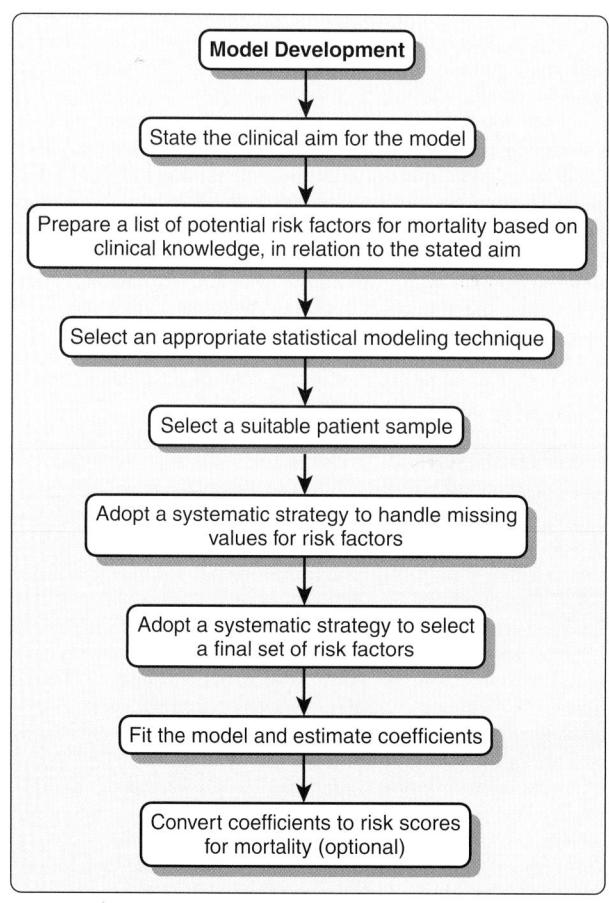

Figure 1-4 Risk model development. *(From Omar RZ, Ambler G, Royston P, et al: Cardiac surgery risk modeling for mortality: A review of current practice and suggestions for improvement. Ann Thorac Surg 77:2232, 2004, by permission of the Society of Thoracic Surgeons.)*

the developmental data, evaluating its goodness of fit. Alternatively, the original data can be split and the model can be built on half of the data and validated on the other half. This reduces the total number of patients and outcomes available to create the model. This method is best suited to situations in which data on tens of thousands of patients are available. This internal validation does not provide the practitioner with information on the generalizability of the model. External validation on a large, completely independent test dataset is the best approach to satisfying this requirement.

In addition to validation, calibration refers to a model's ability to predict mortality accurately. Numerous tests can be applied, the most common being the H-L test. If the *P* value from an H-L test is greater than 0.05, the current practice of the developers is to claim that the model predicts mortality accurately.

Discrimination is the ability of a model to distinguish patients who die from those who survive. The area under the ROC is the common method of assessing this facet of the model. In brief, the test is determined by evaluating all possible pairs of patients, determining whether the predicted probability of death should ideally be greater for the patient who died than for the one who survived. The ROC area is the percentage of pairs for which this is true. The current practice in cardiac surgery is to conclude that a model discriminates well if the ROC area is greater than 0.7. If predictions are used to identify surgical centers or surgeons with unexpectedly high or low rates, achieving a high ROC area alone is not adequate, but good calibration is also critical. A poorly calibrated model may cause large numbers of institutions or surgeons to reveal excessively high or low rates of mortality, when, in fact, the fault lies with the model, not the clinical performance. If predictions are used to stratify patients by disease severity to compare treatments or to decide on patient management, both calibration and discrimination aspects are important.

A key problem in the development of cardiac surgery risk stratification models is the evolving practice of surgery. This includes new procedures, or variations on older procedures, which may affect perioperative risk and not be accounted for in the data used to develop the model. Despite these limitations, calibrated and validated risk model remains the most objective tool currently available. Clinicians need to understand the specific model, its strengths and weaknesses, to appropriately apply the model in academic research, patient counseling, benchmarking, and management of resources.

Specific Risk Conditions

Renal Dysfunction

Renal dysfunction has been shown to be an important risk factor for surgical mortality in patients undergoing cardiac surgery.[80-82] However, the spectrum of what constitutes renal dysfunction is broad, with some models defining it as increased creatinine levels and others defining it as dialysis dependency.

The Northern New England Cardiovascular Study Group reported a 12.2% in-hospital mortality rate after CABG in patients on chronic dialysis versus a 3.0% mortality rate in patients not on dialysis.[83] However, the incidence of dialysis dependency in the cardiac surgical population is sufficiently low (e.g., 0.5% in New York State) so that it may not enter into many of the models developed.

Acute kidney injury (AKI) after cardiac surgery carries significant morbidity and mortality. Patients who experienced development of severe renal dysfunction (defined as glomerular filtration rate [GFR] < 30 mL/min) after CABG had an almost 10% mortality rate compared with 1% mortality in those with normal renal function.[84] Poor outcome associated with perioperative AKI has led to development of predictive models of AKI to identify patients at risk. One of the recent models predicts need for renal replacement therapy (RRT) after cardiac surgery. Wijeysundera et al[85] retrospectively studied a cohort of 20,131 cardiac surgery patients at 2 hospitals in Ontario, Canada. Multivariate predictors of RRT were preoperative estimated GFR, diabetes mellitus requiring medication, LVEF, previous cardiac surgery, procedure, urgency of surgery, and preoperative IABP. An estimated GFR less than or equal to 30 mL/min was assigned 2 points; other components were assigned 1 point each: estimated GFR of 31 to 60 mL/min, diabetes mellitus, EF less than or equal to 40%, previous cardiac surgery, pro-

cedure other than CABG, IABP, and nonelective case. Among the 53% of patients with low risk scores (≤1), the risk for RRT was 0.4%; by comparison, this risk was 10% among the 6% of patients with high-risk scores (≥4). Another group developed a robust prediction rule to assist clinicians in identifying patients with normal, or near-normal, preoperative renal function who are at high risk for development of severe renal insufficiency.[86] In a multivariate model, the preoperative patient characteristics most strongly associated with postoperative severe renal insufficiency included age, sex, white blood cell count > 12,000, prior CABG, CHF, peripheral vascular disease, diabetes, hypertension, and preoperative IABP.

A major issue with respect to the development of indices to predict perioperative renal failure is that the pathophysiology of perioperative AKI includes inflammatory, nephrotoxic, and hemodynamic insults. This multifactorial nature of AKI might be one of the reasons that a limited single-strategy approach has not been successful.[87] Contrast agents used for angiography before cardiac surgery represent one of the modifiable nephrotoxic factors perioperatively. Delaying cardiac surgery beyond 24 hours after the exposure and minimizing the contrast agent load can decrease the incidence of AKI in elective cardiac surgery cases.[88]

Uniformity of AKI definition (Risk of renal dysfunction, Injury to the kidney, Failure of kidney function, Loss of kidney function, and End-stage kidney disease; RIFLE) improved risk stratification models and utilization of early biomarkers of AKI hopefully will provide tools to design clinical trials addressing this important issue.[89,90]

Diabetes

The association between diabetes and mortality with cardiac surgery has been inconsistent, with some studies supporting the association, whereas other studies do not.[91-98] Several recent trials have evaluated outcome between CABG and PCI in patients with diabetes. In the CARDia (Coronary Artery Revascularization in Diabetes) trial,[99] a total of 510 patients with diabetes with multivessel or complex single-vessel CAD from 24 centers were randomized to PCI plus stenting (and routine abciximab) or CABG. At 1 year of follow-up, the composite rate of death, MI, and stroke was 10.5% in the CABG group and 13.0% in the PCI group (hazard ratio [HR]: 1.25; 95% CI: 0.75 to 2.09; *P* = 0.39), all-cause mortality rates were 3.2% and 3.2%, and the rates of death, MI, stroke, or repeat revascularization were 11.3% and 19.3% (HR: 1.77; 95% CI: 1.11 to 2.82; *P* = 0.02), respectively. The Bypass Angioplasty Revascularization Investigation 2 Diabetes (BARI 2D) trial randomized 2368 patients with both type 2 diabetes and heart disease to undergo either prompt revascularization with intensive medical therapy or intensive medical therapy alone, and to undergo either insulin-sensitization or insulin-provision therapy.[100] In patients with more extensive CAD, similar to those enrolled in the CABG stratum, prompt CABG, in the absence of contraindications, intensive medical therapy, and an insulin sensitization strategy appears to be a preferred therapeutic strategy to reduce the incidence of MI.[101]

Acute Coronary Syndrome

Patients with a recent episode of non–ST-segment elevation acute coronary syndrome before CABG have greater rates of operative morbidity and mortality than do patients with stable coronary syndromes.[102] However, a recent report of the American College of Cardiology Foundation, in collaboration with numerous other societies, has published appropriateness for coronary revascularization.[103] There are numerous Class A recommendations for revascularization and, therefore, many patients may come to the operating room directly after coronary angiography and potentially after attempted stent placement with antiplatelet agents. There is evidence to suggest that delaying CABG for 3 to 7 days in patients after ST-elevation myocardial infarction (STEMI) or non–ST-elevation myocardial infarction (NSTEMI) is beneficial in selected stable patients with contraindications to PCI. In addition, patients with a hemodynamically significant right ventricular MI should be allowed to recover the injured ventricle.[104]

Cardiovascular Testing

Patients who present for cardiac surgery have extensive cardiovascular imaging before surgery to guide the procedure. Coronary angiography provides a static view of the coronary circulation, whereas exercise and pharmacologic testing provide a more dynamic view. Because both tests may be available, it is useful to review some basics of cardiovascular imaging (Box 1-5) (see Chapters 2, 3, 6, 11 to 14, and 18).

In patients with a normal baseline ECG without a prior history of CAD, the exercise ECG response is abnormal in up to 25% and increases up to 50% in those with a prior history of MI or an abnormal resting ECG. In the general population, the usefulness of an exercise ECG test is somewhat limited. The mean sensitivity and specificity are 68% and 77%, respectively, for detection of single-vessel disease, 81% and 66% for detection of multivessel disease, and 86% and 53% for detection of three-vessel or left main CAD.[105–108]

The level at which ischemia is evident on exercise ECG can be used to estimate an "ischemic threshold" for a patient to guide perioperative medical management, particularly in the prebypass period.[109,110] This may support further intensification of perioperative medical therapy in high-risk patients, which may have an impact on perioperative cardiovascular events (see Chapters 2, 3, 6, 10, 12 to 15, and 18).

All patients referred for cardiac surgery should have had a transthoracic echocardiogram. In addition to the primary reason for surgery (e.g., CABG), other incidental findings (e.g., valve disease) should be considered in the preoperative assessment of the patient. There are clinical scenarios in which a TEE should be obtained before surgery. These include endocarditis and anticipated mitral valve repair or replacement. A TEE commonly is obtained for assessment of ascending aortic dissection and congenital anomalies. However, other imaging modalities such as magnetic resonance (MR) and computed tomography (CT) imaging are increasingly being used for more detailed assessment of specific congenital problems such as right-sided defects and right ventricular function. MR and CT imaging are particularly useful for assessment of the pulmonary venous system.

The absolute indications for preoperative carotid duplex ultrasound imaging are not clear but should be considered in patients with an audible bruit, or other conditions such as severe peripheral arterial disease, or a previous stroke or transient ischemic attack. The presence of an underlying critical carotid or vertebral artery lesion would herald more caution regarding mean arterial pressure during and after CPB.

Nonexercise (Pharmacologic) Stress Testing

Pharmacologic stress testing has been advocated for patients in whom exercise tolerance is limited, both by comorbid diseases and by symptomatic peripheral vascular disease. Often, these patients may not stress themselves sufficiently during daily life to provoke symptoms of myocardial ischemia or CHF. Pharmacologic stress testing techniques either increase myocardial oxygen demand (dobutamine)[111] or produce coronary vasodilatation leading to coronary flow redistribution (dipyridamole/adenosine).[112] Echocardiographic or nuclear scintigraphic imaging (SPECT) are used in conjunction with the pharmacologic therapy to perform myocardial perfusion imaging for risk stratification and myocardial viability assessment (Box 1-6) (see Chapters 2, 3, 6, 11 to 15, and 18).

BOX 1-6. INDICATIONS FOR MYOCARDIAL PERFUSION IMAGING

- Risk stratification
- Myocardial viability assessment
- Preoperative evaluation
- Evaluation after PCI or CABG
- Monitoring medical therapy in CAD

Dipyridamole-Thallium Scintigraphy

Dipyridamole works by blocking adenosine reuptake and increasing adenosine concentration in the coronary vessels. Adenosine is a direct coronary vasodilator. After infusion of the vasodilator, flow is preferentially distributed to areas distal to normal coronary arteries, with minimal flow to areas distal to a coronary stenosis.[113,114] A radioisotope, such as thallium or 99-technetium sestamibi, then is injected. Normal myocardium will show up on initial imaging, whereas areas of either myocardial necrosis or ischemia distal to a significant coronary stenosis will demonstrate a defect. After a delay of several hours, or after infusion of a second dose of 99-technetium sestamibi, the myocardium is again imaged. Those initial defects that remain as defects are consistent with old scar, whereas those defects that demonstrate normal activity on subsequent imaging are consistent with areas at risk for myocardial ischemia. Several strategies have been suggested to increase the predictive value of the test. The redistribution defect can be quantitated, with larger areas of defect being associated with increased risk.[114] In addition, both increased lung uptake and LV cavity dilation have been shown to be markers of ventricular dysfunction with ischemia (Box 1-7).

Dobutamine Stress Echocardiography

Dobutamine stress echocardiography (DSE) involves the identification of new or worsening RWMAs using two-dimensional echocardiography during infusion of intravenous dobutamine. It has been shown to have the same accuracy as dipyridamole thallium scintigraphy for the detection of CAD.[115,116] There are several advantages to DSE compared with dipyridamole thallium scintigraphy: the DSE study also can assess LV function and valvular abnormalities, the cost of the procedure is significantly lower, there is no radiation exposure, the duration of the study is significantly shorter, and results are immediately available.

Conclusions

Preoperative cardiac risk assessment and stratification in patients undergoing cardiac surgery are distinct from those in patients undergoing noncardiac surgery. In the noncardiac surgery patients, the main goal is to identify a high-risk group of patients who would benefit from either noninvasive or invasive cardiac evaluation and appropriate perioperative medical management or interventional therapy. In patients undergoing cardiac surgery, extensive cardiac evaluation is part of the routine preoperative workup for the procedure, and the patient is having corrective therapy for the underlying disease.

The main goal of cardiac risk assessment in this group of patients, from the anesthesiologist's perspective, is to provide risk-adjusted

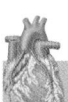

BOX 1-5. PREOPERATIVE CARDIOVASCULAR TESTING

- Coronary angiography
- Exercise electrocardiography
- Nonexercise (pharmacologic) stress testing
- Dipyridamole thallium scintigraphy
- Dobutamine stress echocardiography

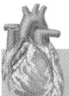

BOX 1-7. SCINTIGRAPHIC FINDINGS OF HIGH RISK WITH CORONARY ARTERY DISEASE

- Increased lung uptake
- LV dilatation
- Increased end-diastolic and end-systolic volumes
- Stress-induced ischemia
- Multiple perfusion defects

mortality rates for the preoperative patient and family counseling and identification of the high-risk group for a perioperative cardiac event. Various complex or simplified risk-adjusted morbidity and mortality models can serve as a tool for the preoperative discussion with the patient, but even a well-calibrated model with good discrimination has to be used with caution when applied to individual counseling. First, it is difficult for any model to predict morbidity/mortality, which occurs at a low incidence. Second, it has to be clear that the scoring system provides only the probability of death or major complication, but the individual patient experiences only one of the outcomes.

Clinicians are unable to reliably monitor cardiac injury intraoperatively or in real time. There is also a lack of consensus regarding the definition and quantification of AMI in the perioperative and early postoperative periods. In contrast, postoperative mortality is easy to define. Therefore, deviation of expected mortality from observed mortality has been used as a "gold standard." However, it is important to recognize that late outcome and survival may also be reflective of intraoperative events. Preoperative cardiac risk assessment of patients undergoing cardiac surgery would ideally lead to identification of a group of patients at risk for increased morbidity and mortality because of perioperative myocardial injury. Based on individual risk factors, perioperative care would then be modified to improve the patient's outcome. To achieve this goal, a clear definition and quantification of myocardial injury in cardiac surgery patients are required. Clinicians need to be able to monitor intraoperative ischemia and intervene to prevent loss of myocardium. Anesthesiologists also need to follow both short- and long-term outcomes of cardiac surgical patients, as well as the impact of different preoperative and intraoperative strategies, on short- and long-term outcomes. Evidence-based medicine has led to an unprecedented growth in the scientific approach to decision making in the belief that it will translate into benefits for patients to decrease their risk and improve outcomes.[117]

REFERENCES

1. Kang SH, Park KH, Choi DJ, et al: Coronary artery bypass grafting versus drug-eluting stent implantation for left main coronary artery disease (from a two-center registry), Am J Cardiol 105:343, 2010.
2. Kouchoukos NT, Ebert PA, Grover FL, et al: Report of the Ad Hoc Committee on Risk Factors for Coronary Artery Bypass Surgery, Ann Thorac Surg 45:348, 1988.
3. Paiement B, Pelletier C, Dyrda I, et al: A simple classification of the risk in cardiac surgery, Can Anaesth Soc J 30:61, 1983.
4. Pinna-Pintor P, Bobbio M, Sandrelli L, et al: Risk stratification for open heart operations: Comparison of centers regardless of the influence of the surgical team, Ann Thorac Surg 64:410, 1997.
5. Smith PK, Smith LR, Muhlbaier LH: Risk stratification for adverse economic outcomes in cardiac surgery, Ann Thorac Surg 64:S61, 1997 discussion S80.
6. Guiteras Val P, Pelletier LC, Hernandez MG, et al: Diagnostic criteria and prognosis of perioperative myocardial infarction following coronary bypass, J Thorac Cardiovasc Surg 86:878, 1983.
7. Khuri SF: Evidence, sources, and assessment of injury during and following cardiac surgery, Ann Thorac Surg 72:S2205, 2001.
8. Heyndrickx GR, Millard RW, McRitchie RJ, et al: Regional myocardial functional and electrophysiological alterations after brief coronary artery occlusion in conscious dogs, J Clin Invest 56:978, 1975.
9. Bolli R: Mechanism of myocardial "stunning," Circulation 82:723, 1990.
10. Hearse DJ, Bolli R: Reperfusion-induced injury: Manifestations, mechanisms, and clinical relevance, Cardiovasc Res 26:101, 1992.
11. Opie LH: Reperfusion injury and its pharmacologic modification, Circulation 80:1049, 1989.
12. Braunwald E, Kloner RA: Myocardial reperfusion: A double-edged sword? J Clin Invest 76:1713, 1985.
13. Park JL, Lucchesi BR: Mechanisms of myocardial reperfusion injury, Ann Thorac Surg 68:1905, 1999.
14. Jennings RB, Sommers HM, Smyth GA, et al: Myocardial necrosis induced by temporary occlusion of a coronary artery in the dog, Arch Pathol 70:68, 1960.
15. Hearse DJ: Ischemia, reperfusion, and the determinants of tissue injury, Cardiovasc Drugs Ther 4 (Suppl 4):767, 1990.
16. Webster KA, Discher DJ, Kaiser S, et al: Hypoxia-activated apoptosis of cardiac myocytes requires reoxygenation or a pH shift and is independent of p53, J Clin Invest 104:239, 1999.
17. Thatte HS, Rhee JH, Zagarins SE, et al: Acidosis-induced apoptosis in human and porcine heart, Ann Thorac Surg 77:1376, 2004.
18. Levy JH, Tanaka KA: Inflammatory response to cardiopulmonary bypass, Ann Thorac Surg 75:S715, 2003.
19. Alpert JS, Thygesen K, Antman E, et al: Myocardial infarction redefined—a consensus document of The Joint European Society of Cardiology/American College of Cardiology Committee for the redefinition of myocardial infarction, J Am Coll Cardiol 36:959, 2000.
20. Thygesen K, Alpert JS, White HD, et al: Universal definition of myocardial infarction, Circulation 116:2634, 2007.
21. Comunale ME, Body SC, Ley C, et al: The concordance of intraoperative left ventricular wall-motion abnormalities and electrocardiographic S-T segment changes: Association with outcome after coronary revascularization. Multicenter Study of Perioperative Ischemia (McSPI) Research Group, Anesthesiology 88:945, 1998.
22. Royster RL, Butterworth JF, Prough DS, et al: Preoperative and intraoperative predictors of inotropic support and long-term outcome in patients having coronary artery bypass grafting, Anesth Analg 72:729, 1991.
23. Jacobson A, Lapsley D, Tow DE, et al: Prognostic significance of change in resting left ventricular ejection fraction early after successful coronary artery bypass surgery: A long-term follow-up study, J Am Coll Cardiol 184A, 1995.
24. Fleisher LA, Tuman KJ: What can we learn from provoking ischemia? Anesth Analg 84:1177, 1997.
25. Griffin M, Edwards B, Judd J, et al: Field-by-field evaluation of intraoperative transoesophageal echocardiography interpretative skills, Physiol Meas 21:165, 2000.
26. Brewer DL, Bilbro RH, Bartel AG: Myocardial infarction as a complication of coronary bypass surgery, Circulation 47:58, 1973.
27. Crescenzi G, Bove T, Pappalardo F, et al: Clinical significance of a new Q wave after cardiac surgery, Eur J Cardiothorac Surg 25:1001, 2004.
28. Sztajzel J, Urban P: Early and late Q wave regression in the setting of acute myocardial infarction, Heart 83:708, 2000.
29. Alyanakian MA, Dehoux M, Chatel D, et al: Cardiac troponin I in diagnosis of perioperative myocardial infarction after cardiac surgery, J Cardiothorac Vasc Anesth 12:288, 1998.
30. Carrier M, Pellerin M, Perrault LP, et al: Troponin levels in patients with myocardial infarction after coronary artery bypass grafting, Ann Thorac Surg 69:435, 2000.
31. Etievent JP, Chocron S, Toubin G, et al: Use of cardiac troponin I as a marker of perioperative myocardial ischemia, Ann Thorac Surg 59:1192, 1995.
32. Greenson N, Macoviak J, Krishnaswamy P, et al: Usefulness of cardiac troponin I in patients undergoing open heart surgery, Am Heart J 141:447, 2001.
33. Mair J, Larue C, Mair P, et al: Use of cardiac troponin I to diagnose perioperative myocardial infarction in coronary artery bypass grafting, Clin Chem 40:2066, 1994.
34. Vermes E, Mesguich M, Houel R, et al: Cardiac troponin I release after open heart surgery: A marker of myocardial protection? Ann Thorac Surg 70:2087, 2000.
35. Klatte K, Chaitman BR, Theroux P, et al: Increased mortality after coronary artery bypass graft surgery is associated with increased levels of postoperative creatine kinase-myocardial band isoenzyme release: Results from the GUARDIAN trial, J Am Coll Cardiol 38:1070, 2001.
36. Costa MA, Carere RG, Lichtenstein SV, et al: Incidence, predictors, and significance of abnormal cardiac enzyme rise in patients treated with bypass surgery in the Arterial Revascularization Therapies Study (ARTS), Circulation 104:2689, 2001.
37. Fellahi JL, Gue X, Richomme X, et al: Short- and long-term prognostic value of postoperative cardiac troponin I concentration in patients undergoing coronary artery bypass grafting, Anesthesiology 99:270, 2003.
38. Lehrke S, Steen H, Sievers HH, et al: Cardiac troponin T for prediction of short- and long-term morbidity and mortality after elective open heart surgery, Clin Chem 50:1560, 2004.
39. Baxter GF: Natriuretic peptides and myocardial ischaemia, Basic Res Cardiol 99:90, 2004.
40. Watanabe M, Egi K, Hasegawa S, et al: Significance of serum atrial and brain natriuretic peptide release after coronary artery bypass grafting, Surg Today 33:671, 2003.
41. Vishnevetsky D, Kiyanista VA, Gandhi PJ: CD40 ligand: A novel target in the fight against cardiovascular disease, Ann Pharmacother 38:1500, 2004.
42. Nannizzi-Alaimo L, Rubenstein MH, Alves VL, et al: Cardiopulmonary bypass induces release of soluble CD40 ligand, Circulation 105:2849, 2002.
43. Jain U, Laflamme CJ, Aggarwal A, et al: Electrocardiographic and hemodynamic changes and their association with myocardial infarction during coronary artery bypass surgery. A multicenter study. Multicenter Study of Perioperative Ischemia (McSPI) Research Group, Anesthesiology 86:576, 1997.
44. Fleisher LA: Risk indices: What is their value to the clinician and patient? Anesthesiology 94:191, 2001.
45. Hannan EL, Kilburn H Jr, Racz M, et al: Improving the outcomes of coronary artery bypass surgery in New York State, JAMA 271:761, 1994.
46. Mukamel DB, Mushlin AI: Quality of care information makes a difference: An analysis of market share and price changes after publication of the New York State Cardiac Surgery Mortality Reports, Med Care 36:945, 1998.
47. Coronary Artery Surgery Study (CASS): A randomized trial of coronary artery bypass surgery. Survival data, Circulation 68:939, 1983.
48. Alderman EL, Fisher LD, Litwin P, et al: Results of coronary artery surgery in patients with poor left ventricular function (CASS), Circulation 68:785, 1983.
49. Parsonnet V, Dean D, Bernstein A: A method of uniform stratification of risk for evaluating the results of surgery in acquired adult heart disease, Circulation 79:I–13, 1989.
50. Bernstein AD, Parsonnet V: Bedside estimation of risk as an aid for decision-making in cardiac surgery, Ann Thorac Surg 69:823, 2000.
51. O'Connor G, Plume S, Olmstead E, et al: Multivariate prediction of in-hospital mortality associated with coronary artery by-pass graft surgery, Circulation 85:2110, 1992.
52. Higgins T, Estafanous F, Loop F, et al: Stratification of morbidity and mortality outcome by preoperative risk factors in coronary artery bypass patients, JAMA 267:2344, 1992.
53. Hannan EL, Kilburn H Jr, O'Donnell JF, et al: Adult open heart surgery in New York State. An analysis of risk factors and hospital mortality rates, JAMA 264:2768, 1990.
54. Shroyer AL, Grover FL, Edwards FH: 1995 Coronary artery bypass risk model: The Society of Thoracic Surgeons Adult Cardiac National Database, Ann Thorac Surg 65:879, 1998.
55. Shroyer AL, Plomondon ME, Grover FL, et al: The 1996 coronary artery bypass risk model: The Society of Thoracic Surgeons Adult Cardiac National Database, Ann Thorac Surg 67:1205, 1999.
56. Jamieson WR, Edwards FH, Schwartz M, et al: Risk stratification for cardiac valve replacement. National Cardiac Surgery Database. Database Committee of the Society of Thoracic Surgeons, Ann Thorac Surg 67:943, 1999.
57. Shahian DM, O'Brien SM, Filardo G, et al: The Society of Thoracic Surgeons 2008 cardiac surgery risk models: Part 1—coronary artery bypass grafting surgery, Ann Thorac Surg 88:S2, 2009.
58. O'Brien SM, Shahian DM, Filardo G, et al: The Society of Thoracic Surgeons 2008 cardiac surgery risk models: Part 2—isolated valve surgery, Ann Thorac Surg 88:S23, 2009.
59. Shahian DM, O'Brien SM, Filardo G, et al: The Society of Thoracic Surgeons 2008 cardiac surgery risk models: Part 3—valve plus coronary artery bypass grafting surgery, Ann Thorac Surg 88:S43, 2009.
60. Tu JV, Jaglal SB, Naylor CD: Multicenter validation of a risk index for mortality, intensive care unit stay, and overall hospital length of stay after cardiac surgery. Steering Committee of the Provincial Adult Cardiac Care Network of Ontario, Circulation 91:677, 1995.
61. Spivack SD, Shinozaki T, Albertini JJ, et al: Preoperative prediction of postoperative respiratory outcome. Coronary artery bypass grafting, Chest 109:1222, 1996.
62. Nashef SA, Roques F, Michel P, et al: European system for cardiac operative risk evaluation (EuroSCORE), Eur J Cardiothorac Surg 16:9, 1999.
63. Roques F, Nashef SA, Michel P, et al: Risk factors and outcome in European cardiac surgery: Analysis of the EuroSCORE multinational database of 19030 patients, Eur J Cardiothorac Surg 15:816, 1999, discussion 822.
64. Al-Ruzzeh S, Nakamura K, Athanasiou T, et al: Does off-pump coronary artery bypass (OPCAB) surgery improve the outcome in high-risk patients? A comparative study of 1398 high-risk patients, Eur J Cardiothorac Surg 23:50, 2003.
65. Ghosh P, Djordjevic M, Schistek R, et al: Does gender affect outcome of cardiac surgery in octogenarians? Asian Cardiovasc Thorac Ann 11:28, 2003.

66. Karthik S, Srinivasan AK, Grayson AD, et al: Limitations of additive EuroSCORE for measuring risk stratified mortality in combined coronary and valve surgery, *Eur J Cardiothorac Surg* 26:318, 2004.
67. Kasimir MT, Bialy J, Moidl R, et al: EuroSCORE predicts mid-term outcome after combined valve and coronary bypass surgery, *J Heart Valve Dis* 13:439, 2004.
68. Kurki TS, Jarvinen O, Kataja MJ, et al: Performance of three preoperative risk indices CABDEAL, EuroSCORE and Cleveland models in a prospective coronary bypass database, *Eur J Cardiothorac Surg* 21:406, 2002.
69. Nakamura Y, Nakano K, Nakatani H, et al: Hospital and mid-term outcomes in elderly patients undergoing off-pump coronary artery bypass grafting—comparison with younger patients, *Circ J* 68:1184, 2004.
70. Nilsson J, Algotsson L, Hoglund P, et al: Early mortality in coronary bypass surgery: The EuroSCORE versus The Society of Thoracic Surgeons risk algorithm, *Ann Thorac Surg* 77:1235, 2004, discussion 1239.
71. Riha M, Danzmayr M, Nagele G, et al: Off pump coronary artery bypass grafting in EuroSCORE high and low risk patients, *Eur J Cardiothorac Surg* 21:193, 2002.
72. Swart MJ, Joubert G: The EuroSCORE does well for a single surgeon outside Europe, *Eur J Cardiothorac Surg* 25:145, 2004, author reply 146.
73. Toumpoulis IK, Anagnostopoulos CE, DeRose JJ, et al: European system for cardiac operative risk evaluation predicts long-term survival in patients with coronary artery bypass grafting, *Eur J Cardiothorac Surg* 25:51, 2004.
74. Toumpoulis IK, Anagnostopoulos CE, Swistel DG, et al: Does EuroSCORE predict length of stay and specific postoperative complications after cardiac surgery? *Eur J Cardiothorac Surg* 27:128, 2005.
75. Ugolini C, Nobilio L: Risk adjustment for coronary artery bypass graft surgery: An administrative approach versus EuroSCORE, *Int J Qual Health Care* 16:157, 2004.
76. Dupuis JY, Wang F, Nathan H, et al: The cardiac anesthesia risk evaluation score: A clinically useful predictor of mortality and morbidity after cardiac surgery, *Anesthesiology* 94:194, 2001.
77. Nowicki ER, Birkmeyer NJ, Weintraub RW, et al: Multivariable prediction of in-hospital mortality associated with aortic and mitral valve surgery in Northern New England, *Ann Thorac Surg* 77:1966, 2004.
78. Hannan EL, Racz MJ, Jones RH, et al: Predictors of mortality for patients undergoing cardiac valve replacements in New York State, *Ann Thorac Surg* 70:1212, 2000.
79. Gardner S, Grunwald G, Rumsfeld J, et al: Comparison of short-term mortality risk factors for valve replacement vs. coronary artery bypass graft surgery, *Ann Thorac Surg* 77:549, 2004.
80. Brandrup-Wognsen G, Haglid M, Karlsson T, et al: Preoperative risk indicators of death at an early and late stage after coronary artery bypass grafting, *Thorac Cardiovasc Surg* 43:77, 1995.
81. Conlon PJ, Little MA, Pieper K, et al: Severity of renal vascular disease predicts mortality in patients undergoing coronary angiography, *Kidney Int* 60:1490, 2001.
82. Hayashida N, Chihara S, Tayama E, et al: Coronary artery bypass grafting in patients with mild renal insufficiency, *Jpn Circ J* 65:28, 2001.
83. Liu JY, Birkmeyer NJ, Sanders JH, et al: Risks of morbidity and mortality in dialysis patients undergoing coronary artery bypass surgery. Northern New England Cardiovascular Disease Study Group, *Circulation* 102:2973, 2000.
84. Cooper WA, O'Brien SM, Thourani VH, et al: Impact of renal dysfunction on outcomes of coronary artery bypass surgery: Results from the Society of Thoracic Surgeons National Adult Cardiac Database, *Circulation* 113:1063, 2006.
85. Wijeysundera DN, Karkouti K, Dupuis JY, et al: Derivation and validation of a simplified predictive index for renal replacement therapy after cardiac surgery, *JAMA* 297:1801, 2007.
86. Brown JR, Cochran RP, Leavitt BJ, et al: Multivariable prediction of renal insufficiency developing after cardiac surgery, *Circulation* 116:I139, 2007.
87. Rosner MH, Portilla D, Okusa MD: Cardiac surgery as a cause of acute kidney injury: Pathogenesis and potential therapies, *J Intensive Care Med* 23:3, 2008.
88. Ranucci M, Ballotta A, Kunkl A, et al: Influence of the timing of cardiac catheterization and the amount of contrast media on acute renal failure after cardiac surgery, *Am J Cardiol* 101:1112, 2008.
89. Bellomo R, Ronco C, Kellum JA, et al: Acute renal failure: Definition, outcome measures, animal models, fluid therapy and information technology needs: The Second International Consensus Conference of the Acute Dialysis Quality Initiative (ADQI) Group, *Crit Care* 8:R204, 2004.
90. Bennett M, Dent CL, Ma Q, et al: Urine NGAL predicts severity of acute kidney injury after cardiac surgery: A prospective study, *Clin J Am Soc Nephrol* 3:665, 2008.
91. Yamamoto T, Hosoda Y, Takazawa K, et al: Is diabetes mellitus a major risk factor in coronary artery bypass grafting? The influence of internal thoracic artery grafting on late survival in diabetic patients, *Jpn J Thorac Cardiovasc Surg* 48:344, 2000.
92. Clement R, Rousou JA, Engelman RM, et al: Perioperative morbidity in diabetics requiring coronary artery bypass surgery, *Ann Thorac Surg* 46:321, 1988.
93. Devineni R, McKenzie FN: Surgery for coronary artery disease in patients with diabetes mellitus, *Can J Surg* 28:367, 1985.
94. Engelman RM, Bhat JG, Glassman E, et al: The influence of diabetes and hypertension on the results of coronary revascularization, *Am J Med Sci* 271:4, 1976.
95. Herlitz J, Wognsen GB, Emanuelsson H, et al: Mortality and morbidity in diabetic and nondiabetic patients during a 2-year period after coronary artery bypass grafting, *Diabetes Care* 19:698, 1996.
96. Magee MJ, Dewey TM, Acuff T, et al: Influence of diabetes on mortality and morbidity: Off-pump coronary artery bypass grafting versus coronary artery bypass grafting with cardiopulmonary bypass, *Ann Thorac Surg* 72:776, 2001 discussion 780.
97. Salomon NW, Page US, Okies JE, et al: Diabetes mellitus and coronary artery bypass. Short-term risk and long-term prognosis, *J Thorac Cardiovasc Surg* 85:264, 1983.
98. Thourani VH, Weintraub WS, Stein B, et al: Influence of diabetes mellitus on early and late outcome after coronary artery bypass grafting, *Ann Thorac Surg* 67:1045, 1999.
99. Kapur A, Hall RJ, Malik IS, et al: Randomized comparison of percutaneous coronary intervention with coronary artery bypass grafting in diabetic patients: 1-year results of the CARDia (Coronary Artery Revascularization in Diabetes) trial, *J Am Coll Cardiol* 55:432, 2010.
100. Frye RL, August P, Brooks MM, et al: A randomized trial of therapies for type 2 diabetes and coronary artery disease, *N Engl J Med* 360:2503, 2009.
101. Chaitman BR, Hardison RM, Adler D, et al: The Bypass Angioplasty Revascularization Investigation 2 Diabetes randomized trial of different treatment strategies in type 2 diabetes mellitus with stable ischemic heart disease: Impact of treatment strategy on cardiac mortality and myocardial infarction, *Circulation* 120:2529, 2009.
102. Marso SP, Bhatt DL, Roe MT, et al: Enhanced efficacy of eptifibatide administration in patients with acute coronary syndrome requiring in-hospital coronary artery bypass grafting. PURSUIT Investigators, *Circulation* 102:295, 2000.
103. Patel MR, Dehmer GJ, Hirshfeld JW, et al: ACCF/SCAI/STS/AATS/AHA/ASNC 2009 Appropriateness Criteria for Coronary Revascularization: A Report of the American College of Cardiology Foundation Appropriateness Criteria Task Force, Society for Cardiovascular Angiography and Interventions, Society of Thoracic Surgeons, American Association for Thoracic Surgery, American Heart Association, and the American Society of Nuclear Cardiology: Endorsed by the American Society of Echocardiography, the Heart Failure Society of America, and the Society of Cardiovascular Computed Tomography, *Circulation* 119:1330, 2009.
104. Eagle KA, Guyton RA, Davidoff R, et al: ACC/AHA 2004 guideline update for coronary artery bypass graft surgery: A report of the American College of Cardiology/American Heart Association Task Force on Practice Guidelines (Committee to Update the 1999 Guidelines for Coronary Artery Bypass Graft Surgery), *Circulation* 110:e340, 2004.
105. Connolly HM, Oh JK, Schaff HV, et al: Severe aortic stenosis with low transvalvular gradient and severe left ventricular dysfunction: Result of aortic valve replacement in 52 patients, *Circulation* 101:1940, 2000.
106. Horacek BM, Wagner GS: Electrocardiographic ST-segment changes during acute myocardial ischemia, *Cardiol Electrophysiol Rev* 6:196, 2002.
107. Schneider RM, Seaworth JF, Dohrmann ML, et al: Anatomic and prognostic implications of an early treadmill exercise test, *Am J Cardiol* 50:682, 1982.
108. Weiner DA, McCabe CH, Ryan TJ: Prognostic assessment of patients with coronary artery disease by exercise testing, *Am Heart J* 105:749, 1983.
109. Myers J, Prakash M, Froelicher V, et al: Exercise capacity and mortality among men referred for exercise testing, *N Engl J Med* 346:793, 2002.
110. Balady GJ: Survival of the fittest: More evidence, *N Engl J Med* 346:852, 2002.
111. Carstensen S: Dobutamine-atropine stress echocardiography, *Heart Drug* 5:101, 2005.
112. Grossman GB, Alazraki N: Myocardial perfusion imaging in coronary artery disease, *Cardiology* 10:1, 2004.
113. Klocke FJ, Baird MG, Bateman TM, et al: ACC/AHA/ASNC guidelines for the clinical use of cardiac radionucleotide imaging: Executive summary, *Circulation* 108:1404, 2003.
114. Beller GA: Clinical value of myocardial perfusion imaging in coronary artery disease, *J Nucl Cardiol* 10:529, 2003.
115. Armstrong WF, Pellikka PA, Ryan T, et al: Stress echocardiography: Recommendations for performance and interpretation, *J Am Soc Echocardiogr* 11:97, 1998.
116. Marwick TH: Quantitative techniques for stress echocardiography, *Eur J Echocardiogr* 3:171, 2002.
117. Cheng DC, Martin JE: Raising the bar: A primer on evidence-based decision-making, *Semin Cardiothoracic Vasc Anesth* 9:1, 2005.

Cardiovascular Imaging

JUAN GAZTANAGA, MD | VALENTIN FUSTER, MD, PHD, MACC | MARIO J. GARCIA, MD, FACC, FACP

KEY POINTS

1. Echocardiography and invasive angiography remain the most widely used modalities for evaluation of left ventricular function, valvular and ischemic heart disease.
2. Computed tomography coronary angiography and cardiac magnetic resonance (CMR) are increasingly utilized when there are conflicting results or when further information is required in the patient evaluated before surgery.
3. CMR is able to evaluate ventricular and valvular function, atherosclerosis, and plaque composition.
4. CMR is the gold standard for quantitative assessment of ventricular volumes, ejection fraction (EF), and mass.
5. CMR is the most accurate method for assessment of RVEF and volumes.
6. Myocardial perfusion imaging can be performed using both SPECT and PET.
7. CT angiography is most commonly used for the diagnosis of aortic aneurysms and dissections.
8. Cardiac CT can clearly depict mechanical valvular prosthesis when echocardiography cannot clearly show abnormalities.

Preoperative cardiac diagnostic evaluation for cardiac surgery traditionally has been performed by echocardiography and invasive catheterization. Similarly, preoperative risk-assessment before noncardiac surgery has been supported by resting and stress echocardiography and single-photon emission computed tomography (SPECT). Since the early 1990s, there has been an explosion in new imaging technology that has seen the introduction of cardiac computed tomography (CCT), cardiac magnetic resonance (CMR), and positron emission tomography (PET) in the clinical setting. In the field of preoperative evaluation, these new imaging modalities have complemented more than supplemented traditional imaging. Echocardiography remains the most widely used noninvasive cardiac imaging test and so far the only one currently available in the intraoperative setting. The role of echocardiography is discussed at length in many chapters of this book. This chapter focuses on the use of advanced imaging modalities for perioperative evaluation of patients undergoing cardiac surgery, as well as those with suspected or known coronary artery disease (CAD) planning to undergo noncardiac surgery.

BASIC PRINCIPLES AND INSTRUMENTATION

Myocardial Nuclear Scintigraphy

SPECT uses the principles of radioactive decay to evaluate the myocardium and its blood supply. It is able to detect the presence of flow-limiting coronary artery stenosis, as well as myocardial infarction.

The stability of the nucleus for emitting radiation depends on the ratio of neutrons to protons and on the nuclide's atomic number (Z). The sources used for this are known as radionuclides, which are nuclides with neutron-proton ratios that are not on the stable nuclei curve and are unstable and, therefore, radioactive. There are several types of radioactive decay. The least penetrating radiation is called an *alpha particle* (α), which corresponds to the heaviest radiation. An alpha particle is composed of the nuclei of a helium atom (2 protons + 2 neutrons) with positive charge. A second type of radioactive decay is known as beta (β) particle emission, which is moderate penetrating radiation. Beta particles are lighter than alpha particles and are actually electrons emitted from the nucleus. Positron (β^+) particles, which are positive electrons, have similar penetration to beta particles but are made of antimatter and emitted from positron tracers. Lastly, the highest energy emission particles are known as gamma (γ) rays and are the same as particles emitted from an X-ray tube.

The radionuclides that are used in SPECT are technetium-99m (Tc^{99m}) and thallium-201 (Tl^{201}). Tc^{99m} is a large radionuclide that emits a single photon or γ-ray per radioactive decay, with a half-life of 6 hours. The energy of the emitted photon is 140,000 electron volts, or keV. Thallium-201 is less commonly used and decays by electron capture. It has a much longer half-life than Tc^{99m} of 73 hours, and the energy emitted is between 69 and 83 keV. To obtain images, the gamma rays that are released by decay from the body must be captured and modified by a detector or gamma camera. The standard camera is composed of a collimator, scintillating crystals, and photomultiplier tubes. When a radionuclide emits gamma rays, it does so in all directions. A collimator made of lead with small, elongated holes is used as a filter to accept only those gamma rays traveling from the target organ toward the camera. Once the selected gamma rays have reached the scintillating crystals, they are converted to visible light and then into electrical signals by the photomultiplier tubes. These electrical signals are then processed by a computer to form images. Myocardial regions that are infarcted or ischemic after stress will have relatively decreased tracer uptake and, therefore, decreased signal or counts in the processed images.

PET is similar to SPECT in that it uses radioisotopes and the properties of radioactive decay to produce and acquire images. The most common radioisotopes used for cardiac evaluation are rubidium-82, N-ammonia-13, and fluorine-18 (F^{18}). F^{18} is a much smaller radionuclide than Tc^{99m}. It emits a positron (β^+) antiparticle. This ionized antiparticle travels until it interacts with an electron. The electron and the positron are antiparticles of each other, meaning they have the same mass but are opposite in charge. When this occurs, both particles disintegrate and are converted into energy in the form of two photons traveling in opposite directions. Both photons have the same energy, 511 keV. This phenomenon is known as pair annihilation, which is used to create the images in PET. PET cameras also differ from SPECT cameras in that they capture only incoming photons that travel in opposite directions and arrive at a circular detector around the body at precisely the same time. PET detectors have much higher sensitivity than SPECT cameras because they do not require a collimator. Like in SPECT, PET cameras also use scintillating crystals and photomultiplier tubes. Recently, PET systems have been combined with computed tomography (CT) and magnetic resonance imaging (MRI) systems to simultaneously display PET metabolic images with their corresponding anatomic information.

Cardiac Computed Tomography

CCT has grown significantly in clinical use since the early 2000s with the advent of multidetector CT scanners with submillimeter resolution allowing evaluation of the coronary anatomy. The X-ray tube produces beams that traverse the patient and are received by a detector array on the opposite side of the scanner. The X-ray tube and detector array are coupled to each other and rotate around the patient at a velocity of 250 to 500 msec/rotation. Initially, in 1999, the first multidetector CT scan used for coronary imaging had four rows of detectors and had a scanning coverage of 2 cm per slice rotation. Breath-holds on the order of 10 to 20 seconds were required to cover the entire heart. Artifacts produced by the patient's respiration and heart rate variability rendered many studies nondiagnostic for the assessment of coronary stenosis. Technology has advanced at a rapid pace to the point that 64-slice systems are standard, and 320-slice systems with 16 cm of coverage are able to capture the entire heart in one heartbeat and rotation.

CCT utilizes ionizing radiation for the production of images. Concern over excessive medical radiation exposure has been raised in recent years. Although several techniques, such as prospective electrocardiogram (ECG)-gated acquisition, may be implemented[1–3] to reduce radiation dose, a risk-benefit assessment must be done for the selection of patients who have appropriate indications for CCT. The patient's heart rate must be lowered to less than 65 beats/min to achieve adequate results imaging the coronaries with CCT. This usually requires the administration of oral or intravenous β-blockers. After the scan has been completed, images are reconstructed at different intervals of the cardiac cycles and analyzed in a computer workstation.

Cardiovascular Magnetic Resonance Imaging

Cardiovascular magnetic resonance is a robust and versatile imaging modality. It is able to evaluate multiple elements of cardiac status: function, morphology, flow, tissue characterization, perfusion, angiography, and/or metabolism. CMR is able to do this using its unique ability to distinguish morphology by taking advantage of the different molecular properties of tissues. This is achieved without the use of any radiation, by using the influence of magnetic fields on the abundance of hydrogen atoms in the human body. This is one of the main advantages of CMR over other imaging modalities. Multicontrast CMR uses the intrinsic properties of organs and takes advantage of the three imaging contrasts: T1, T2, and proton density without the need for gadolinium contrast. T1-weighted imaging is utilized for the imaging of lipid content and fat deposition appears bright or hyperintense. T2-weighted imaging is used for the evaluation of edema[4] and fibrous tissue,[5] which also appears hyperintense. Dynamic contrast-enhanced CMR uses the paramagnetic contrast agent gadolinium, which enhances the magnetization (T1) of protons of nearby water and creates a stronger signal. In addition, gadolinium contrast permeates through the intercellular space in necrotic or fibrotic myocardium, which is the basis for myocardial scar detection seen on late gadolinium enhancement.

CMR is able to evaluate both ventricular and valvular function. It also can evaluate atherosclerosis[6] in large vessels and is capable of imaging morphology and distinguishing between different elements of atherosclerotic plaque composition including fibrous tissue, lipid core, calcification, and hemorrhage.[7] In addition to vascular plaque assessment, CMR may be used for the evaluation of ischemia after the administration of gadolinium contrast agents. First-pass perfusion is evaluated at rest and after the administration of a pharmacologic stressor such as adenosine or dobutamine for the evaluation of myocardial infarction and ischemia.

Vascular Ultrasound

Vascular ultrasound has been in existence clinically since the 1950s. It is versatile and relatively inexpensive when compared with other imaging modalities. It is one of the few imaging techniques that may be performed at the patient's bedside. In addition, there is no use of ionizing radiation, as opposed to CT or nuclear cardiology. For these reasons, vascular ultrasound can never be replaced in the clinical setting.

Vascular ultrasound is composed of several techniques or modes, which include grayscale imaging (also known as B-mode), pulsed- and continuous-wave Doppler imaging, and color Doppler imaging. Each of these provides different information. Duplex ultrasound uses both B-mode and pulsed-wave Doppler to acquire vessel anatomy, as well as hemodynamic data. This includes peak and mean velocities of blood flow in addition to pressure gradients caused by stenosis. Duplex is also used for the evaluation of aneurysms and dissections. Color-flow Doppler allows for the visualization and direction of blood flow through vessels. Typically, the color scale is from red (flow toward transducer) to blue (flow away from transducer; see Chapter 12). Many times it aids in the localization and identification of vessels when duplex is inadequate. Vascular ultrasound is used for the evaluation of the aorta; carotid, renal, celiac, and mesenteric arteries; the lower extremity arterial system; and the peripheral venous system. More recently, it also has come into clinical use for the evaluation of atherosclerosis by measuring carotid intima-media thickness.

EVALUATION OF CARDIAC FUNCTION

Left Ventricular Systolic Function

Perhaps the most important factor that contributes to surgical outcome is cardiac function, specifically left ventricular (LV) systolic function. Systolic dysfunction is directly related to patient outcome after surgery. Preoperative knowledge of LV systolic dysfunction is crucial for the anesthesiologist to prepare and anticipate perioperative and postoperative complications. Patients with systolic dysfunction who undergo coronary artery bypass graft (CABG) surgery require more inotropic support after cardiopulmonary bypass (CPB).[8,9] In addition, systolic dysfunction is a good prognosticator for postsurgical mortality.[10–12] In patients who are known to have CAD and are scheduled to have CABG surgery, the cause of systolic dysfunction is, most often than not, ischemic heart disease. In patients who are scheduled to have elective noncardiac surgery and are found to have newly diagnosed systolic dysfunction, it is important to do further testing to find the cause and exclude critical coronary stenosis and ischemia.

Transthoracic echocardiography (TTE) is the most widely used modality for this evaluation because it is inexpensive, portable, and readily available. However, limited acoustic windows may limit the accuracy of echocardiographic assessment of global and regional LV function in a significant number of patients.[13]

Nuclear scintigraphic methods, including both SPECT and PET myocardial perfusion imaging, can be used to evaluate global and segmental LV systolic function. This is achieved by implementing ECG gating during data acquisition. Most often, eight frames or phases are acquired per cardiac cycle. The left ventricular ejection fraction (LVEF) is measured using absolute end-diastolic (EDV) and end-systolic volumes (ESV), where LVEF = LVEDV − LVESV/LVEDV.

Gated images can be acquired at both rest and after stress; however, rest images typically have less radiation dose and the images may be noisy. In most institutions, gated imaging is done using poststress images because of the higher radioisotope dose and, thus, less noise. This does have its limitation for accurate LV systolic analysis in the circumstance of stress-induced ischemia, in which myocardial stunning can transiently reduce the LVEF. Another limitation of ECG-gated SPECT or PET is arrhythmias, specifically frequent premature ventricular contractions (PVCs) or atrial fibrillation.[14] In patients who have extensive myocardial infarction, assessment of LV function also may be inaccurate because there is absence of isotope in the scar regions; thus, the endocardial border cannot be defined. Gated-blood pool scans (multiple gated acquisition; MUGA) image the cardiac "blood pool" with high resolution during the cardiac cycle. Ventricular function, as well as various temporal parameters, can be measured using this technique.[15] There is good correlation between echocardiography and MUGA for the evaluation of LVEF. However, MUGA has demonstrated better intraobserver and interobserver reproducibility than echocardiography.[16]

CCT, with its excellent spatial and temporal resolution, allows for an accurate assessment of LV function when compared with echocardiography, invasive ventriculography, and cardiac MRI.[17-19] CCT also uses real three-dimensional volumes to calculate the LV systolic function. Functional analysis can be evaluated only when retrospective scanning is used because the entire cardiac cycle (both systole and diastole) is necessary. The raw dataset must be reconstructed in intervals or cardiac phases of 10%, from 0% (early systole) to 90% (late diastole). Advanced computer workstations allow for cine images to be reconstructed and displayed in multiple planes (Figure 2-1). Segmental wall motion analysis may be performed using the 17-segment model recommended by the American Heart Association/American College of Cardiology (AHA/ACC)[20] (Figure 2-2).

The main limitation to using CCT for LV systolic function assessment is the required radiation exposure. Because retrospective ECG gating is required to image the entire cardiac cycle, radiation exposure is relatively high. In comparison, CCT studies performed with prospective ECG gating expose the patient to radiation during only 10% to 15% of the cardiac cycle. Thus, in most clinical scenarios, LV functional information usually is not acquired to reduce radiation exposure.

CMR is considered the gold standard for the quantitative assessment of biventricular volumes, EF, and mass, whereas also offering excellent reproducibility.[21] CMR also has excellent spatial and temporal resolution allowing for cine imaging. Typically, a stack of 10 to 14 contiguous two-dimensional slices are acquired and used for LV functional analysis.[22] The acquisition of each of these images generally requires a breath-hold of at least 10 to 20 seconds. In a computer workstation, the endocardial and epicardial contours of the LV can be traced in each short-axis slice at the phases of maximal and minimal ventricular dimensions. The software then calculates the volume of ventricular cavity per slice as the product of the area enclosed within the endocardial contour multiplied by the slice thickness. The data are then combined to calculate EDV and ESV and EF. In addition, cine images may be acquired in the four-, three-, and two-chamber views for LV segmental wall analysis (Figure 2-3).

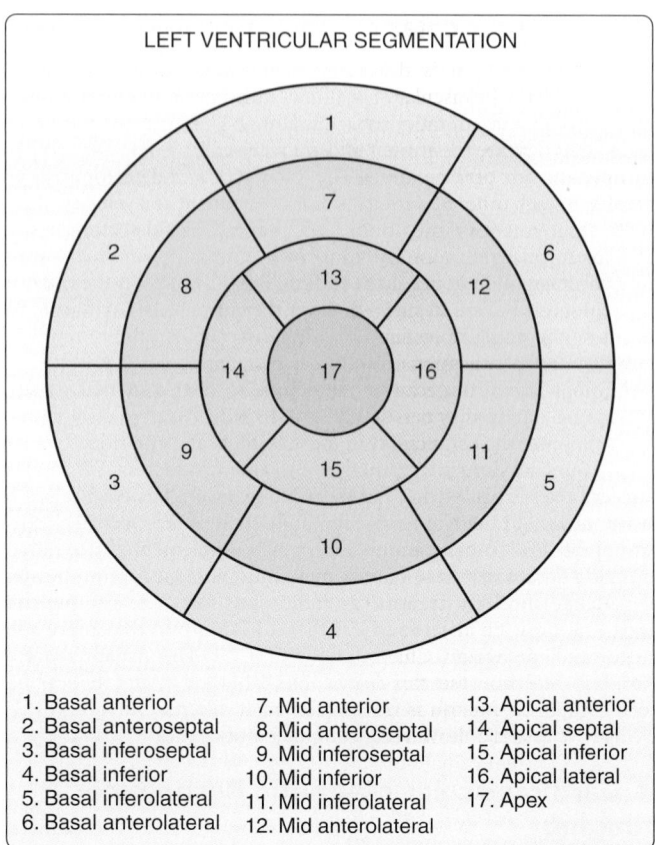

LEFT VENTRICULAR SEGMENTATION

1. Basal anterior
2. Basal anteroseptal
3. Basal inferoseptal
4. Basal inferior
5. Basal inferolateral
6. Basal anterolateral
7. Mid anterior
8. Mid anteroseptal
9. Mid inferoseptal
10. Mid inferior
11. Mid inferolateral
12. Mid anterolateral
13. Apical anterior
14. Apical septal
15. Apical inferior
16. Apical lateral
17. Apex

Figure 2-2   American Heart Association/American College of Cardiology (AHA/ACC)–recommended 17-segment model for left ventricular segmental wall motion analysis. *(From Cerqueira MD, Weissman NJ, Dilsizian V, et al: Standardized myocardial segmentation and nomenclature for tomographic imaging of the heart: A statement for healthcare professionals from the Cardiac Imaging Committee of the Council on Clinical Cardiology of the American Heart Association. Circulation 105:539–542, 2002.)*

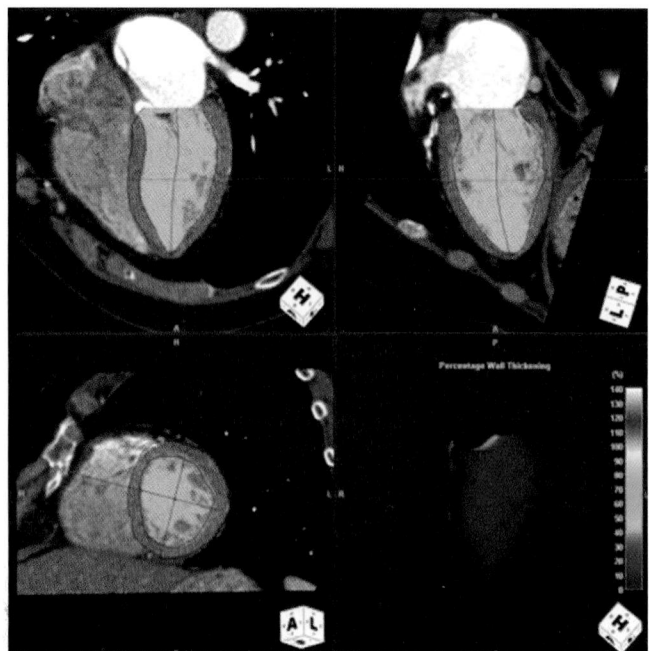

Figure 2-1   Computed tomography angiography: left ventricular (LV) functional analysis in three orthogonal planes using specialized workstation. It allows for the evaluation of LV end-diastolic and end-systolic volumes, mass, and ejection fraction.

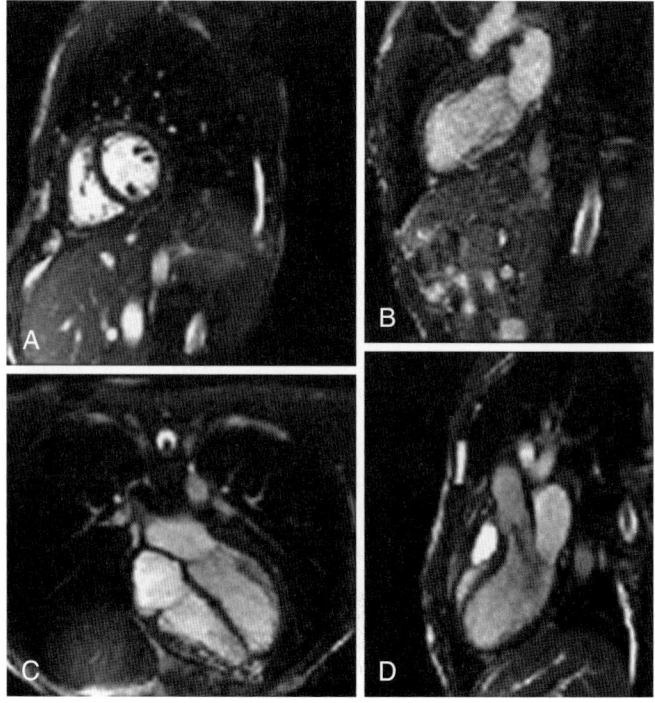

Figure 2-3   Cardiac magnetic resonance demonstrating *(A)* short-axis, *(B)* two-chamber, *(C)* four-chamber, and *(D)* three-chamber views.

Left Ventricular Diastolic Function

Diastolic dysfunction is the most common abnormality found in patients with cardiovascular disease.[23,24] Patients with diastolic dysfunction may be asymptomatic[25] or may have exercise-induced dyspnea or overt heart failure.[26] Until recently, the profound impact of diastolic dysfunction on perioperative management and postoperative outcome has been underestimated. In fact, the prevalence of diastolic dysfunction in patients undergoing surgery is significant. A recent study demonstrated that in more than 61% of patients with normal LV systolic function undergoing surgery, diastolic filling abnormalities were present.[27] This is critical information for the anesthesiologist because patients with diastolic dysfunction who undergo CABG require more time on CPB, as well as more inotropic support up to 12 hours after surgery.[28] This may be because of deterioration of diastolic dysfunction after CABG, which may persist for several hours.[29–31] Taking all this into account, diastolic dysfunction increases the risk for perioperative morbidity and mortality.[32]

In 85% of patients with diastolic dysfunction, hypertension is the primary cause. Diastolic function requires a complex balance among several hemodynamic parameters that interact with each other to maintain LV filling with low atrial pressure, including LV relaxation, LV stiffness, aortic elasticity, atrioventricular and intraventricular electrical conduction, left atrial contractility, pericardial constraint, and neurohormonal activation. Changes in preload, afterload, stroke volume, and heart rate can upset this delicate balance.[33–35]

LV diastolic function is most easily and commonly assessed with echocardiography; however, different aspects of diastolic function also can be evaluated by SPECT and CMR. At least 16 phases of the cardiac cycle need to be acquired to evaluate diastolic dysfunction using SPECT. This is because diastolic functional analysis, as opposed to systolic function, is dependent on heart rate changes during acquisition and processing. The two main parameters that can be measured by SPECT are LV peak filling rate and time to peak filling rate. It is measured in EDV/sec, and is normally more than 2.5. The normal time to peak filling rate is less than 180 milliseconds. Heart rate, cardiovascular medications, and adrenergic state may alter these parameters.[36]

Velocity-encoded (phase-contrast) cine-CMR is capable of measuring intraventricular blood flow accurately and is able to quantify mitral valve (MV) and pulmonary vein flow, which are hemodynamic parameters of diastolic function. It has been shown that in patients with amyloidosis, echocardiography and velocity-encoded cine imaging correlate significantly in estimating pulmonary vein systole/diastole ratios, LV filling E/A ratio, and E deceleration times, which are all diastolic functional indices.[37] In addition to measuring blood flow and velocity through the MV and pulmonary vein, CMR-tagging is able to measure myocardial velocities of the walls and MV similar to strain rate and tissue Doppler in echocardiography. CMR-delayed enhancement imaging also is used for the diagnosis of diastolic dysfunction. The presence and severity of fibrosis seen on delayed-enhancement imaging correlate significantly with severity of diastolic dysfunction.[38]

Right Ventricular Function

In preoperative evaluation, knowledge of right ventricular (RV) dysfunction is critical for intraoperative management of the patient. RV dysfunction is an independent risk factor for clinical outcomes in patients with cardiovascular disease.[39–41] Patients with RV dysfunction in the presence of LV ischemic cardiomyopathy who undergo CABG surgery have increased risk for postoperative and long-term morbidity and mortality.[42] Patients with RV dysfunction often require postoperative inotropic and mechanical support, resulting in longer surgical intensive care unit and hospital stays.[42] In patients who undergo mitral and mitral/aortic valve surgery, RV dysfunction is a strong predictor of perioperative mortality.[43] In addition, RV dysfunction is associated with postoperative

circulatory failure.[44] If RV dysfunction is detected before or after surgery, further evaluation is necessary. In the case of preoperative RV dysfunction, pulmonary hypertension (PH) is a common cause that negatively impacts perioperative and postoperative outcome. PH significantly increases morbidity and mortality in patients undergoing both cardiac[45,46] and noncardiac surgery.[47,48] Patients with acute onset of RV dysfunction without an explained cause must be evaluated for pulmonary emboli. Recent studies have demonstrated that the incidence rate of pulmonary emboli after CABG surgery can be as high as 3.9%.[49–51]

The RV is designed to sustain circulation to the pulmonary system while preserving a low central venous pressure. Patients with RV dysfunction can maintain relatively normal functional capacity unless pulmonary vascular resistance is increased, at which point RV function is critical for pulmonary circulation. RV failure is characterized by venous congestion (i.e., hepatomegaly, ascites, edema), as well as decreasing LV preload and cardiac output. There is also an interdependence between the RV and LV imposed by the pericardium that can negatively affect LV filling. There are several mechanisms for RV dysfunction including primary causes like RV infarction and RV dysplasia, as well as secondary causes because of LF dysfunction. The severity of RV dysfunction may be difficult to evaluate by TTE at times because of suboptimal acoustic windows. Furthermore, the ability to derive accurate and reproducible estimations of RVEF by echocardiography is limited by the complex changes in RV geometry that occur as the right ventricle dilates.

CMR is the most accurate method for the assessment of RVEF and volumes.[52,53] The RV is evaluated in a similar manner to the LV by CMR, where short-axis cine slices from ventricular base to apex are obtained and measured in a computer workstation. CMR is the gold standard for the diagnosis of RV dysplasia, providing assessment of global and regional function, as well as detecting the presence of myocardial fat infiltration and scarring.[54,55]

Global and segmental RV function also may be evaluated using first-pass radionuclide angiography (FPRNA). RVEF obtained by FPRNA has been shown to have good correlation with CMR.[56]

CCT also is very accurate for RV functional assessment when compared with CMR.[57,58] The protocol used to acquire RV data is different from that used for coronary artery evaluation. A biphasic contrast injection is used to opacify the RV. In addition, retrospective ECG gating must be utilized to acquire the entire cardiac cycle for functional evaluation. CCT is, therefore, not frequently used primarily for RV functional assessment because the radiation dose is generally higher than for FPRNA and CMR.

RV dysfunction is a common cause of post- and perioperative hypotension and is associated with poor outcomes, regardless of its cause. New onset of RV dysfunction may be caused by RV infarction, pulmonary embolism, or acute respiratory failure (cor pulmonale). Echocardiography is more suitable than other imaging modalities in these cases because it is a portable imaging technique. Moreover, echocardiography allows estimation of RV systolic pressure, which is usually elevated in pulmonary embolism and respiratory failure, and low or normal in RV infarction.

EVALUATION OF MYOCARDIAL PERFUSION

Exercise versus Pharmacologic Testing

Preoperative assessment for ischemic burden in patients with CAD or those at risk for CAD who are to have elective noncardiac surgery is important. Figure 2-4 indicates the ACC/AHA algorithm for preoperative cardiac evaluation and care before noncardiac surgery. Nuclear myocardial perfusion imaging is the most common test used in the United States for preoperative evaluation. Patients can be stressed using exercise or pharmacologic agents. The preferred modality is exercise, which is most often done on a treadmill and less commonly on a stationary bike.[59] For an exercise stress test to be

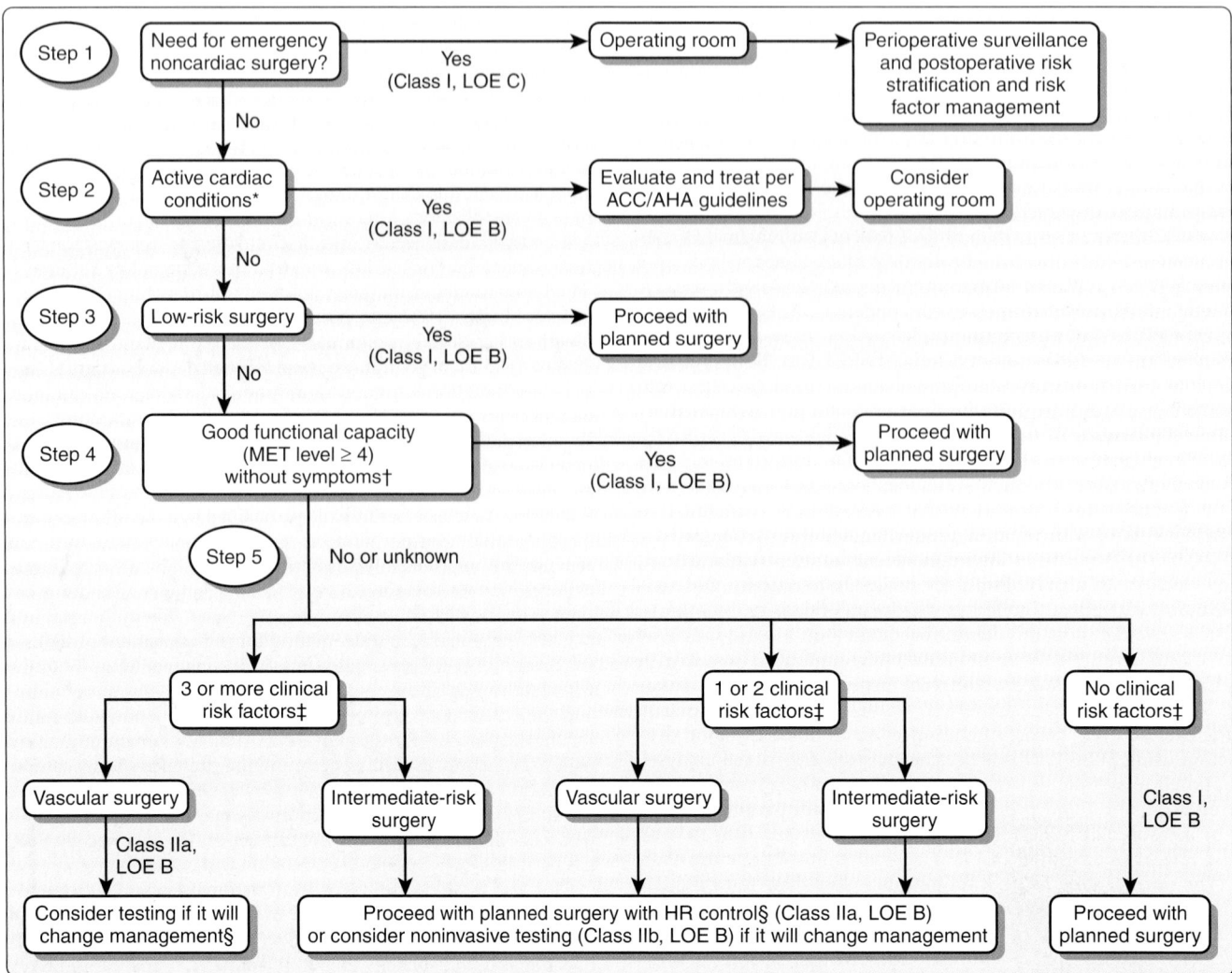

Figure 2-4 American Heart Association/American College of Cardiology (AHA/ACC) algorithm for preoperative evaluation for patients planning to go for noncardiac surgery. HR, heart rate; LOE, level of evidence. (*From Fleisher LA, Beckman JA, Brown KA, et al: ACC/AHA 2007 Guidelines on perioperative cardiovascular evaluation and care for noncardiac surgery: Executive summary: A report of the American College of Cardiology/American Heart Association Task Force on Practice Guidelines [Writing Committee to Revise the 2002 Guidelines on Perioperative Cardiovascular Evaluation for Noncardiac Surgery] developed in collaboration with the American Society of Echocardiography, American Society of Nuclear Cardiology, Heart Rhythm Society, Society of Cardiovascular Anesthesiologists, Society for Cardiovascular Angiography and Interventions, Society for Vascular Medicine and Biology, and Society for Vascular Surgery. J Am Coll Cardiol 50:1707–1732, 2007.*)

adequate, a patient must exercise for at least 6 minutes and reach at least 85% of their maximum predicted heart rate (MPHR) adjusted for their age (MPHR= 220 − age). Uniform treadmill protocols are used to compare with peers and serial testing. The most common protocols used are Bruce and modified Bruce. In addition, exercise stress tests are symptom limited. Exercise as a stressor has robust prognostic data for the risk for future cardiac events. There are several types of scores that predict a patient's risk for cardiovascular disease. The most commonly used score is known as the Duke treadmill score, which uses exercise time in minutes, maximum ST-segment deviation on the ECG, and anginal symptoms during exercise. Heart rate recovery to baseline after exercise is also a strong predictor for cardiovascular disease. In general, exercise stress testing is safe as long as testing guidelines are followed carefully. The risk for a major complication is 1 in 10,000.

For myocardial perfusion imaging, a radioisotope must be injected during exercise. When using Tc^{99m}, it must be injected once the patient has reached peak heart rate and the patient must exercise for at least 1 minute afterward to allow sufficient time for the radioisotope to circulate through the myocardium.

Pharmacologic stress testing is a negative prognosticator in itself because patients who, for one reason or another, are not able to do sufficient physical activity to attempt an exercise stress test have greater incidences of cardiovascular disease and other comorbidities. Pharmacologic stress testing is also preferred in patients with a left bundle branch block, Wolf-Parkinson-White (WPW) pattern, and ventricular pacing on ECG. There are two types of pharmacologic agents available on the market today: vasodilators that include dipyridamole, adenosine, and regadenoson; and the chronotropic agent, dobutamine. They each have their advantages and disadvantages. Dipyridamole was the original stressor used for myocardial perfusion imaging. It is an indirect coronary vasodilator that prevents the breakdown and increases intravascular concentration of adenosine. It is contraindicated in those patients with asthma and those with chronic obstructive pulmonary disease (COPD) who have active wheezing. Adenosine is used more widely now because it produces fewer side effects compared with dipyridamole. It induces coronary vasodilation directly by binding to the A2A receptor. Adenosine has similar contraindications to dipyridamole. Known side effects include bronchospasm, as well as high-degree AV block; however, because the half-life is seconds, it is usually enough just to discontinue the adenosine infusion and symptoms resolve without further treatment. If the patient is able to walk slowly on the treadmill, adenosine is given while the patient walks at a constant slow pace to alleviate the severity of potential side effects. In addition, image quality is improved with low-level exercise because there is less tracer uptake in the gastrointestinal system. Regadenoson is a relatively new agent to the market. It is a selective adenosine analog. It is given as a single intravenous (IV) bolus and has less incidence of significant AV block. However, it also may cause bronchospasm in patients with asthma or active COPD.[60]

Dobutamine is a chronotropic agent that is more often used during stress echocardiography. Dobutamine may be used as a stressor during myocardial perfusion imaging if the patient is not able to exercise or if the patient cannot use a vasodilator secondary to asthma or COPD exacerbation. It also should not be used in patients with left bundle branch block or WPW. Dobutamine causes the heart rate and blood pressure to increase. After the radioisotope is injected, when the patient reaches at least 85% of MPHR, dobutamine infusion must be continued for an additional 2 minutes. In case of ischemia or severe side effects, short-acting β-blockers (esmolol) should be given to counteract the effects.

Single-Photon Emission Computed Tomography versus Positron Emission Tomography Myocardial Perfusion Imaging

Myocardial perfusion imaging can be performed using both SPECT and PET. They are based on LV myocardial uptake of the radioisotope at rest and after stress. Myocardial uptake will be reduced after stress

in corresponding myocardial regions where significant coronary artery stenosis is present. The images are displayed in three different orientations for proper LV wall-segment analysis. The three LV orientations are short-axis, horizontal long-axis, and vertical long-axis, with the stress images to the corresponding rest images directly above. Resting images are acquired to differentiate between normal myocardium and infarcted myocardium (Figure 2-5). PET scanners have inherently less attenuation and higher resolution, making them more desirable than SPECT.[61] PET myocardial perfusion tests usually use pharmacologic stressors because of the very short half-life of PET radioisotopes. The sensitivity and specificity of SPECT for the detection of obstructive CAD is 91% and 72%, respectively. The use of PET improves the specificity of diagnosing obstructive CAD to 90%.[61] Patients with normal SPECT and Rb PET have less than 1% and 0.4% probability of annual cardiac events, respectively. The use of myocardial perfusion tests is recommended in those patients with an intermediate risk based on CAD risk factors.

Once the patient has completed the examination, a decision must be made about what to do with the results. If the stress test is normal, then the risk for cardiovascular events is low and the patient is considered ready for surgery. If the stress test demonstrates ischemia, but the patient requires nonelective surgery, data support better outcomes with medical management. Several trials have examined the benefit of revascularization compared with medical management in patients with CAD who require noncardiac surgery. The Coronary Artery Revascularization Prophylaxis (CARP) trial evaluated more than 500 patients with significant but stable CAD who were undergoing major elective vascular disease. Percutaneous intervention was performed in 59% and CABG in 41% of the revascularization group. At 30 days after surgery,

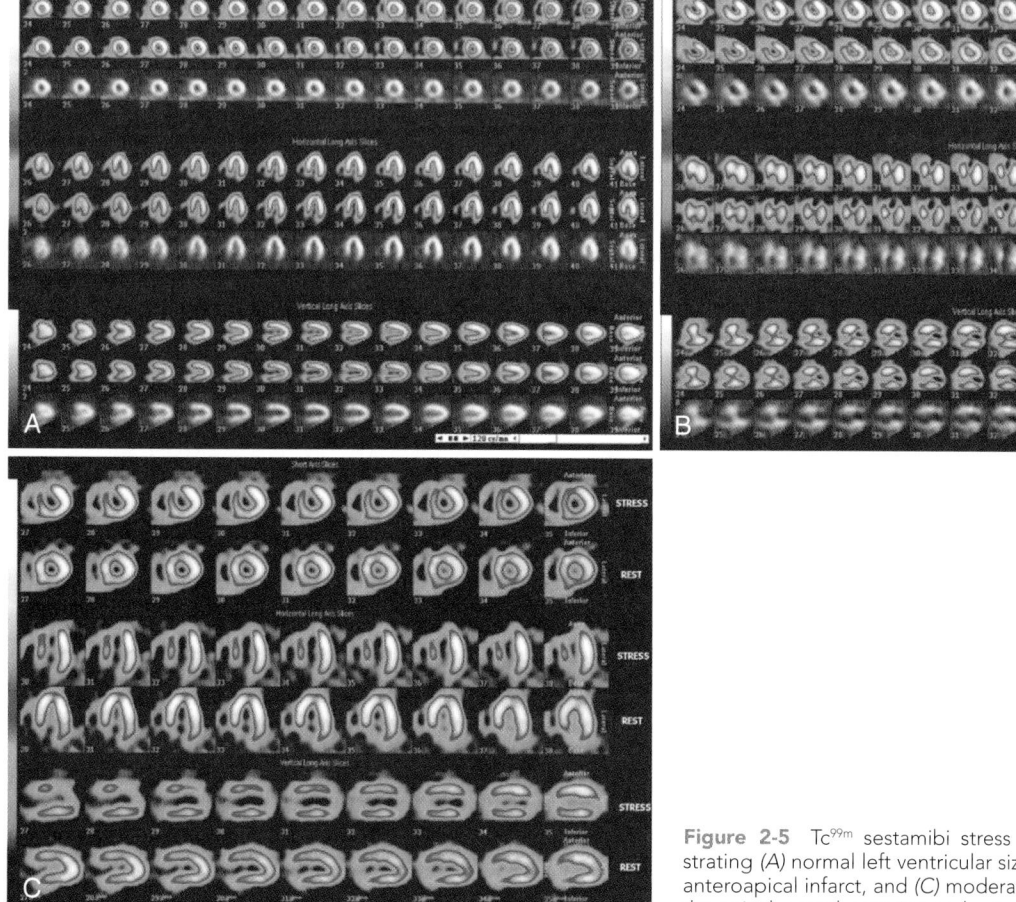

Figure 2-5 Tc^{99m} sestamibi stress myocardial perfusion demonstrating (A) normal left ventricular size and perfusion, (B) apical and anteroapical infarct, and (C) moderate-to severe ischemia involving the apical, septal, anterior, and anteroseptal walls.

there were no differences in postoperative myocardial infarction, death, or length of hospital stay between the revascularization group and the medical management group. At 2.7 years, there was still no difference in mortality between both groups.[62] The DECREASE-V study showed similar results. In this study, 430 high-risk patients were enrolled to undergo revascularization versus medical management before high-risk vascular surgery. Among the high-risk patients, 23% had extensive myocardial ischemia on stress testing. Again at 30 days and at 1 year, there were no differences in postoperative myocardial infarction or mortality between the revascularization and medical management groups.[63]

With respect to the use of perioperative β-blockers, they should be continued in those patients who are already taking them. In those patients who are at high risk because of known CAD or have ischemia on preoperative testing, β-blockers may be started and titrated to blood pressure and heart rate, while avoiding bradycardia and hypotension.[64,65]

Magnetic Resonance Perfusion Imaging

CMR perfusion imaging is evaluated by the first pass of IV gadolinium contrast through the myocardium. ECG-gated images are acquired generally using three LV short-axis slices (base, mid, and apical) and, possibly, a four-chamber image depending on the heart rate. As the contrast is being injected, it is being tracked through the right side of the heart and, subsequently, the LV cavity and the LV myocardium. The assessment of perfusion requires imaging during several consecutive heartbeats during which the contrast bolus completes its first pass through the myocardium. This is done during a breath-hold. First-pass perfusion images are acquired at rest, then repeated during adenosine infusion. The same slice positions (between 3 or 4) are used for both rest and stress for comparison (Figure 2-6). Perfusion defects appear as areas of delayed and/or decreased myocardial enhancement and are interpreted visually.

The accuracy of stress MRI perfusion has been validated in several trials. In one trial, which evaluated 147 consecutive women with chest pain or other symptoms suggestive of CAD, MRI perfusion was compared with invasive angiography. The CMR perfusion stress test had a sensitivity, specificity, and accuracy of 84%, 88%, and 87%, respectively.[66] Another study comparing stress perfusion MRI to invasive angiography examined 102 subjects. CMR demonstrated a sensitivity of 88% and specificity of 82% for the diagnosis of significant flow-limiting stenosis.[67] A negative MRI perfusion stress test also confers significant prognostic information. Patients with a normal stress MRI have a 3-year event-free survival rate of 99.2%.[68]

EVALUATION OF MYOCARDIAL METABOLISM

Stunned and Hibernating Myocardium

Myocardial stunning occurs during acute ischemic injury in which the cardiac myocytes that are on the border of the myocardial infarction are underperfused and sustain temporary loss of function. In theory,

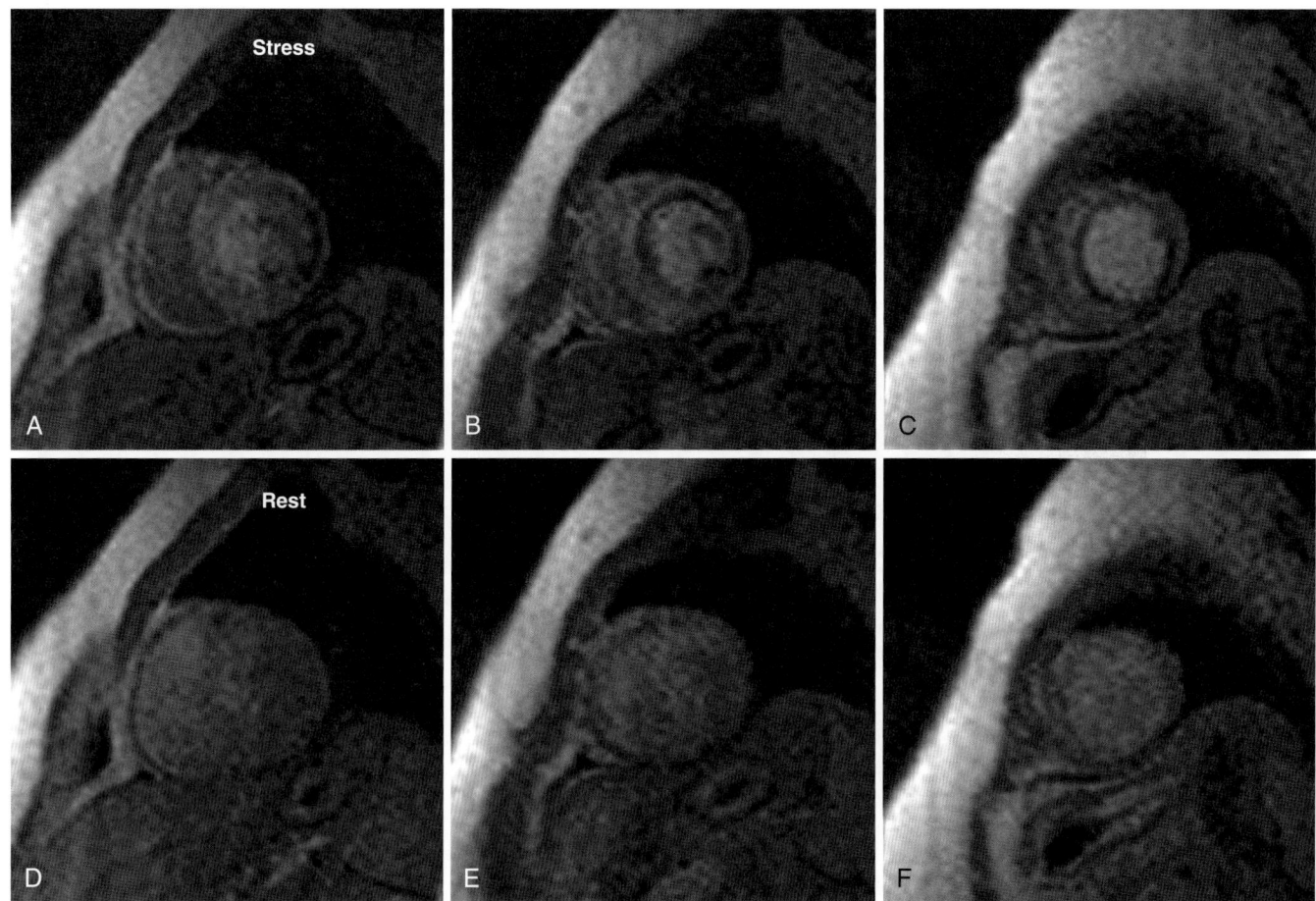

Figure 2-6   Adenosine cardiac magnetic resonance perfusion stress test of a 45-year-old woman with chest pain who had a normal nuclear perfusion stress test and was found to have triple-vessel disease on catheterization. Figure demonstrates short-axis views of the *(A)* left ventricular (LV) base, *(B)* LV midcavity, and *(C)* LV apex at stress with corresponding segments below *(D–F)* at rest. Stress images show diffuse circumferential subendocardial decreased myocardial enhancement in the LV midcavity and apex and partial subendocardial decreased myocardial enhancement in the LV base, which are not present at rest. This corresponds to balanced ischemia caused by three-vessel disease.

function to these myocytes returns once the acute phase of injury resolves; however, this depends on duration of ischemic injury and time to recovery of blood flow to the artery. On rest perfusion imaging, this area would be normal.[69] If blood flow is not returned to normal levels or if repetitive stunning occurs, the myocardium enters a chronic state of hibernation. About 24% to 82% of hibernating myocardial segments can recover function after target-vessel revascularization; in different series, anywhere between 38% and 88% of patients with hibernating myocardium experience improvement in LVEF.[69,70] Several studies indicate meaningful improvement of LV systolic function occurs; at least 20% to 30% of the myocardium should be hibernating or ischemic.

Thallium-201 is used frequently for viability assessment with SPECT imaging, taking advantage of this isotope's long half-life (73 hours). Thallium uptake is dependent on several physiologic factors, including blood flow and sarcolemmal intercellular integrity. Thallium is taken up in a short time in normal myocardium, but may take up to 24 hours in hibernating myocardium that still has metabolic activity. Patients are injected with thallium radioisotope and imaged the same day for baseline images. They are brought back after 24 hours without any further injection and reimaged. Baseline images are compared with the 24-hour images. Defects that are present at baseline and fill in at 24 hours represent viability (Figure 2-7). Technetium radioisotopes also can be used for the evaluation of viable myocardium using different protocols.

PET imaging is more sensitive than SPECT and is considered by many experts as the gold standard for assessment of viability. PET has the ability to identify the presence of preserved metabolic activity in areas of decreased perfusion using 18-fluorodeoxyglucose (FDG). PET imaging uses both FDG and either rubidium or ammonia radioisotopes for quantification of energy utilization by the myocardium, as well as for evaluating patterns of blood flow. Areas with reduced blood flow and reduced FDG uptake are considered scar and infarcted.

Areas with reduced blood flow (> 50%) and normal FDG uptake are considered viable.[69] A recent meta-analysis analyzing more than 750 patients demonstrated a sensitivity of 92% and specificity of 63% for regional functional recovery with positive and negative predictive values of 74% and 87%.[71] When viable myocardium is detected by PET, it is important to revascularize as soon as possible because recovery of function decreases as revascularization is delayed.[72,73]

Myocardial Scar Imaging

Myocardial viability is unlikely to occur in the presence of extensive scarring because scar is necrotic tissue that cannot regain function. The importance of identifying scar in hypokinetic areas will determine whether revascularization will benefit the patient.

CMR has taken over as the gold standard for evaluation of myocardial scarring. Delayed-enhancement (DE) imaging is achieved by administering gadolinium contrast intravenously and imaging 5 to 10 minutes later. Gadolinium contrast accumulates extracellularly; however, in normal myocardium, there is not sufficient space for gadolinium deposition. In the setting of chronic scar, the volume of gadolinium distribution increases because of an enlarged interstitium in the presence of extensive fibrosis.[74] Hence, normal or viable myocardium appears as nulled or dark, whereas scar appears bright (Figure 2-8). The advantage of delayed enhancement imaging is that it allows for the assessment of transmural extent of the scar. The percentage of scar-to-wall thickness is the basis for prognosis of viability and segmental functional recovery. Generally, identical LV short-axis images used for function are acquired for DE imaging. This allows for side-by-side comparison of function and DE evaluation. DE imaging is analyzed visually, and the thickness of scarring is quantified as percentages (none, 1–25%, 26–50%, 51–75%, 75–100%). A wall segment is considered to be viable and has a high probability of functional recovery if the scar thickness is ≤ 50% of the wall.[75]

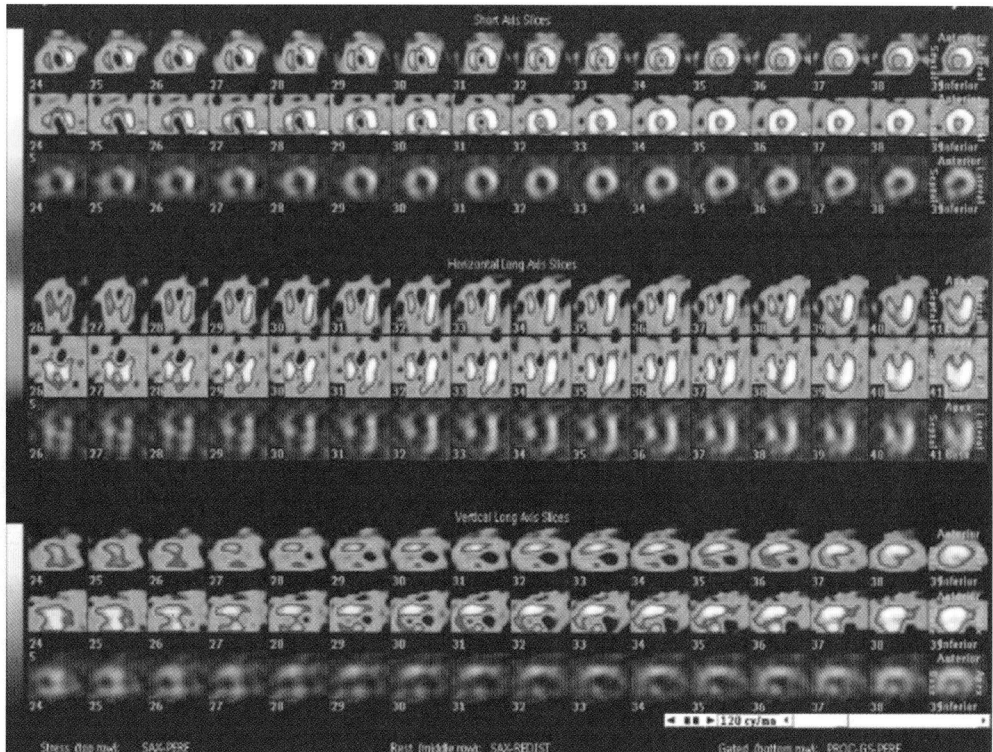

Figure 2-7 Thallium rest-redistribution scan demonstrating hibernating myocardium involving apical-basal anteroseptum, midbasal inferior, midbasal inferoseptum, and midbasal inferolateral wall segments. There is infarction of the apex, inferoapical, and apical-lateral wall segments.

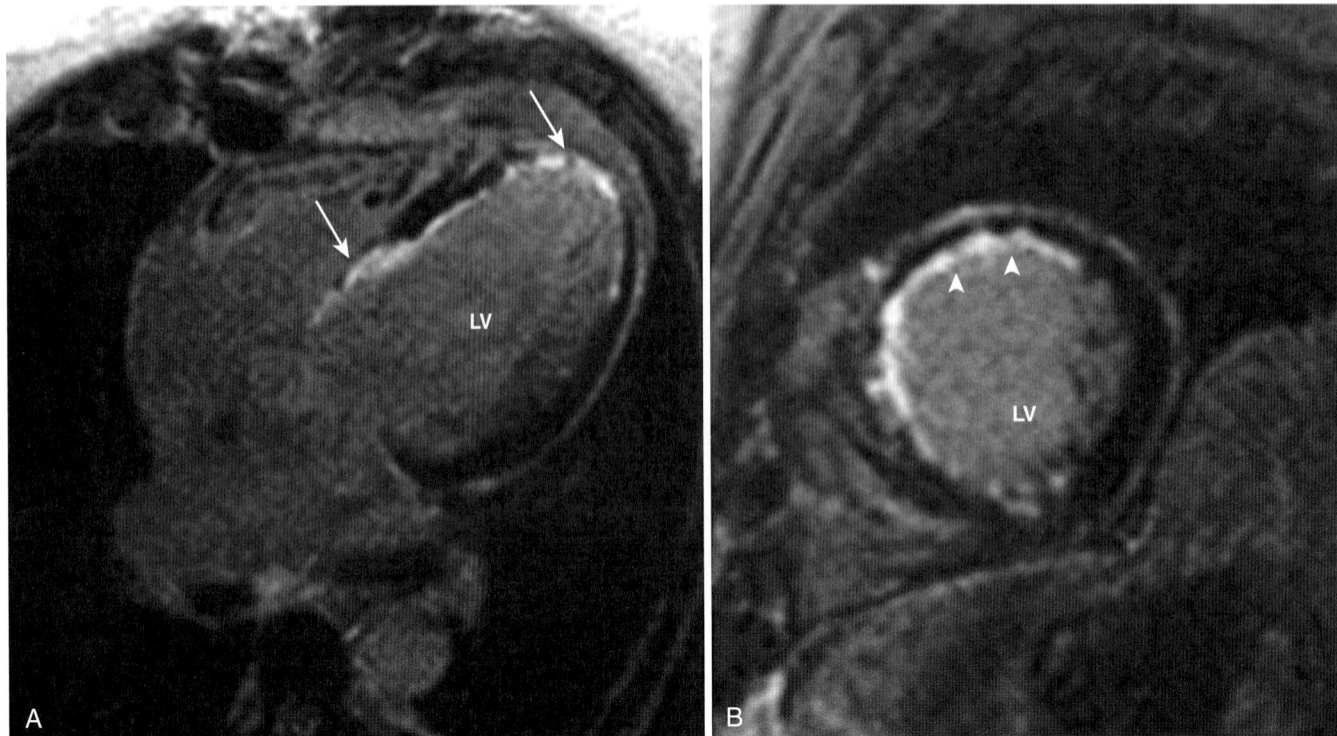

Figure 2-8 Cardiac magnetic resonance (CMR) demonstrating delayed enhancement imaging of (A) four-chamber view with transmural scars (arrows) appearing bright in the septum and apex; (B) short-axis view shows partial scar with viability (arrowheads) of the anterior wall. LV, left ventricle.

Autonomic Innervation

Myocardial infarction causes denervation of the scar and subsequent interruption of sympathetic nerves induces denervation of adjacent viable myocardium.[76,77] Sympathetic nerves are very sensitive to ischemia and usually become dysfunctional after repeated episodes of ischemia that do not result in irreversible myocyte injury.[78,79] Matsunari et al.[80] demonstrated that the area of denervation is larger than the area of scar and corresponds to the area at risk for ischemia. In addition, Bulow et al.[81] showed that denervation of myocytes occurs in the absence of previous infarction. Myocyte sympathetic innervation is measured by PET using the radioisotope ^{11}C-hydroxyephedrine (HED). This is compared with PET resting perfusion to determine the area of the scar. Areas of normal resting perfusion and reduced HED retention indicate viable myocardium. In addition, SPECT imaging of myocardial uptake of ^{123}I-mIBG, which is an analog of the sympathetic neurotransmitter norepinephrine, provides an assessment of β-receptor density. Reduced ^{123}I-mIBG uptake is associated with adverse outcomes in patients with heart failure and has been proposed as a marker of response to treatment.[82]

VALVULAR HEART DISEASE

Aortic Valve Disease

Transthoracic and transesophageal echocardiography (TEE) are the principal imaging modalities for valvular heart disease; however, on several occasions, additional imaging adds important information. Aortic stenosis (AS) is a common cause for valve replacement. There are several different mechanisms for AS. For patients younger than 75, congenital bicuspid aortic valve (BAV) is the most common cause. They have a high incidence of calcification and stenosis. In patients older than 75, senile degenerative calcification of the aortic valve is the leading cause, which is most frequently seen in men.[83] Patients with degenerative aortic valve disease typically have concurrent CAD

because they both have common risk factors including hypertension, active tobacco smoking, increased low-density lipoprotein (LDL), and lipoprotein (a) levels. In addition, patients with metabolic syndrome have increased incidence of aortic calcification.[84] Aortic calcification is directly related to the development of AS. CCT is an excellent tool for the evaluation of aortic valve calcification (Figure 2-9). This can be achieved by noncontrast CCT using the same protocol as calcium

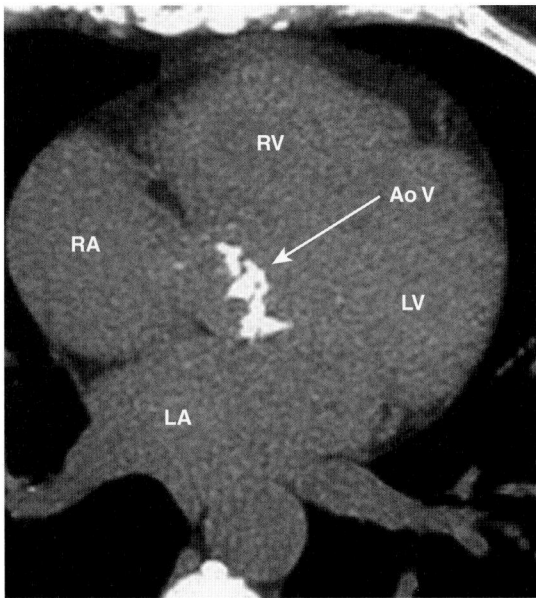

Figure 2-9 Noncontrast computed tomography (CT) demonstrating a severely calcified aortic valve (AoV). LA, left atrium; LV, left ventricle; RA, right atrium; RV, right ventricle.

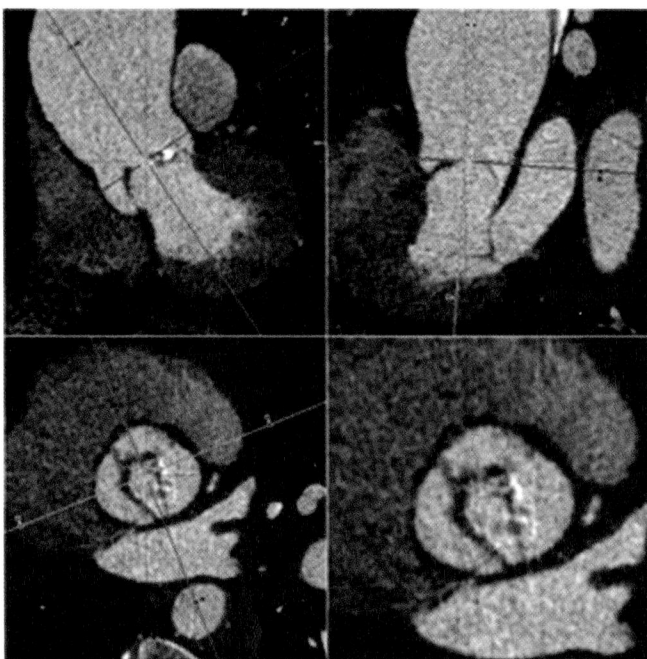

Figure 2-10 Computed tomographic (CT) angiography. Bicuspid aortic valve (BAV) and ascending aortic aneurysm in orthogonal views displaying the BAV in short-axis for the evaluation of the valve area by planimetry.

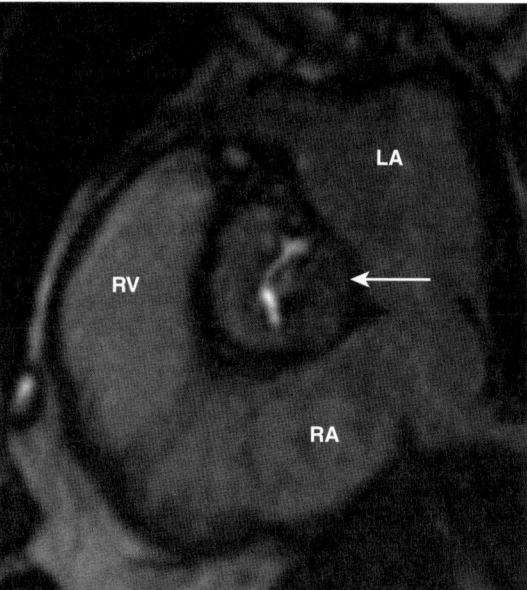

Figure 2-11 Cardiac magnetic resonance demonstrating a short-axis view of a stenotic bicuspid aortic valve. LA, left atrium; RA, right atrium; RV, right ventricle.

TABLE 2-1	Aortic and Mitral Valve Regurgitant Fractions and Corresponding Severity	
Regurgitant Fraction (%)	*Severity of Regurgitation*
≤ 15	Mild
16–25	Moderate
26–48	Moderate-to-severe
> 48	Severe

scoring of the coronary arteries. Coronary artery calcium is measured using the Agatston method. An aortic valve calcium score of ≥ 1100 has a 93% sensitivity and 82% specificity for severe AS.[85] Contrast-enhanced CCT allows for excellent visualization of the aortic valve and accurately differentiates between bicuspid and tricuspid aortic valves[86] (Figure 2-10). Aortic valve area (AVA) also can be evaluated by CCT using planimetry. AVAs measured by CCT have a strong correlation with valve areas and transvalvular gradients obtained by echocardiography.[87–91]

CCT also can be used for the evaluation of aortic regurgitation (AR). CCT can elucidate the potential mechanism for the AR, including inadequate leaflet coaptation during diastole, leaflet prolapse, cusp perforation, or interposition of an intimal flap in cases of type A aortic dissection.

Regurgitant orifice areas measured by CCT have an excellent correlation to AR severity parameters, including vena contracta width and regurgitant/left ventricular outflow tract (LVOT) height ratio obtained by TTE.[92,93]

CMR, like CCT, allows for excellent evaluation of valvular morphology, but it also has advantages over CCT including blood-flow analysis, as well as no radiation exposure. CMR allows for differentiation between BAV and TAV using cine imaging. AS severity can be quantified using phase-encoding imaging. Similarly to echocardiography, phase-encoding imaging allows for the measurement of velocities through the AV, which, in turn, can be used to derive mean and peak AV gradients by implementing the modified Bernoulli equation ($\Delta P = 4V^2$). The effective AVA also can be obtained by measuring the LVOT area and using the continuity equation: $\text{Area}_{valve} = \text{Area}_{LVOT} [\text{VTI}_{LVOT}/\text{VTI}_{valve}]$.[94] Another approach to calculation of the AVA is by direct planimetry of the AV using cine images[95] (Figure 2-11).

CMR also uses phase-encoded imaging for the evaluation of AR. Phase-encoded imaging is acquired just above the AV, and the velocity and the volume of blood per heartbeat are measured in the forward and reverse directions. This allows for measurement of the exact amount of blood that exits the AV, as well as the amount of blood that regurgitates back through the valve. From this the regurgitant amount and regurgitant fraction are obtained (Table 2-1).

Mitral Valve Disease

The most common cause of mitral stenosis (MS) worldwide continues to be rheumatic heart disease. In the United States, it rarely is seen except for in the immigrant population. Visualization of the valvular apparatus in rheumatic valvular disease demonstrates retraction, thickening, and calcification of the mitral leaflets, chordae, and, occasionally, papillary muscles. Accurate assessment of MV morphology is performed by examining cine imaging using ECG-gated, contrast-enhanced CCT.[96,97] Calcium scoring of the MV also is possible, but it has lower reproducibility than for the AV.[98] The degree of MV calcification correlates significantly with the severity of stenosis seen on TTE.[99] MV areas obtained by planimetry also correlate significantly with TTE data of MS.[100]

Mitral regurgitation is the most common cause for valve surgery. MV prolapse is a frequent cause of mitral regurgitation. It can be diagnosed by evaluating cine loops of the MV, and visualization of which scallops of the leaflets prolapsed can aid in the planning before surgery.

Severity of the mitral regurgitation can be assessed by planimetry of the regurgitant orifice, which in a recent study has been shown to correlate with TEE.[101] In addition, the presence of calcification of the MV annulus and leaflets will determine whether the valve can be repaired or needs to be replaced.

CMR also allows for excellent morphologic evaluation of rheumatic MVs. Planimetry of the MV using cine images is also feasible. MV insufficiency can be quantified using phase-encoded imaging and the LV stroke volume calculated by functional analysis. Mitral regurgitant volume is measured by subtracting the volume of forward flow through the AV acquired by phase contrast (PC) imaging from the LV stroke volume. Once the regurgitant volume is calculated, the regurgitant fraction is easily obtained by dividing the regurgitant volume by the total stroke volume.

Tricuspid Valve Disease

The tricuspid valve (TV) is the atrioventricular valve on the right side of the heart. In general, pathology of the TV is not of clinical significance, unless it is congenital or involves endocarditis. TV pathology is best imaged using TTE and TEE, but on occasion a patient may have poor TTE windows and the TEE also may be insufficient. Tricuspid stenosis (TS) occurs in less than 1% of the population in the United States. In patients with rheumatic heart disease, TS becomes clinically significant only 5% of the time. In cases of congenital TS, either CCT or CMR should be done to evaluate for additional congenital abnormalities.

Mild tricuspid regurgitation (TR) is present in approximately 70% of the normal population. Mild TR is clinically insignificant, and clinically significant TR occurs in only 0.9% of the population. Functional TR is most often a result of PH, mitral disease, or severe LV dysfunction. The degree of TR severity can be quantified by using CMR. Similar to mitral regurgitation evaluation, by using PC imaging of the pulmonary artery (PA) just above the PV, RV outflow volume is measured. This can be subtracted from the RV systolic volume acquired by cine imaging, to give TR regurgitant volume and fraction. CMR also is important for morphologic valve evaluation in patients with Ebstein's anomaly. In the instance in which CMR cannot be performed, CCT is also excellent for morphologic evaluation of the TV in Ebstein's anomaly.

Pulmonic Valve Disease

The pulmonic valve is generally not well visualized on either TTE or TEE. Pulmonic stenosis (PS) usually occurs as isolated valvular, subvalvular, or supravalvular stenosis. It also may be associated with more complex congenital disorders. Significant PS in congenital heart disease presents in infancy or early childhood. Acquired PS affects morbidity and mortality only when it becomes severe. Both CMR and CCT are appropriate for anatomic evaluation of the PV apparatus. CMR has the advantage of measuring velocities and gradients across the stenosis using PC imaging.

Trivial or mild pulmonary regurgitation is physiologic and normal. Severe PR is rare and is typically secondary to PH or repair of congenital PS. PR can be calculated using CMR by PC imaging of the PA just above the PV and measuring forward and reverse flow through the PV.

Prosthetic Valves

The visualization of mechanical prosthetic valves is difficult with TTE and TEE because of metal-related artifacts. CCT has the ability to clearly depict the mechanical prosthesis and detect any abnormality including valve thrombosis. This is done by using retrospective scanning and acquiring the entire cardiac cycle to play the cine movie and visualize the leaflets through systole and diastole. The mechanical valves that are used today consist of two disks that open symmetrically (Figure 2-12). The valve function of the two-disk prosthesis, as well as opening and closing angles, was evaluated by CCT and then compared with fluoroscopy and echocardiography. CCT correlated significantly with both imaging modalities for two-disk mechanical valves.[102] The role of CT in the assessment of bioprosthetic valves is similar because the metallic ring causes artifact on echo and often is difficult to assess.

In general, echocardiography is the gold standard for imaging valvular disease; however, when TTE or TEE is technically difficult or there are discrepancies between tests, advanced imaging is recommended. CMR offers more functional data than CCT; however, CCT may be used when further anatomic information about a valve is required. For evaluating prosthetic valves, CCT is usually superior to CMR because of metallic artifact from the valve, which is seen on CMR (see Chapters 12, 13, and 19).

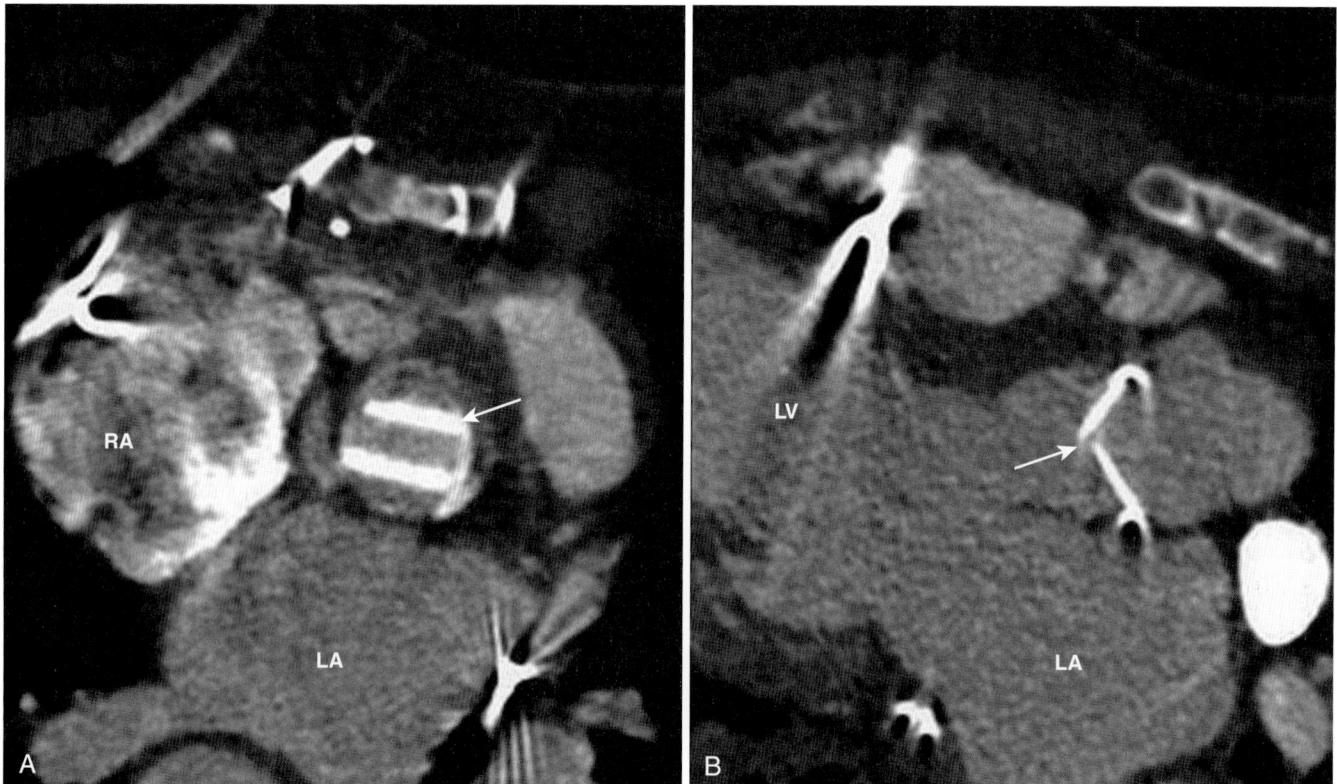

Figure 2-12   Computed tomography angiography of an aortic mechanical valve in (A) short-axis view and (B) three-chamber view. LA, left atrium; LV, left ventricle; RA, right atrium.

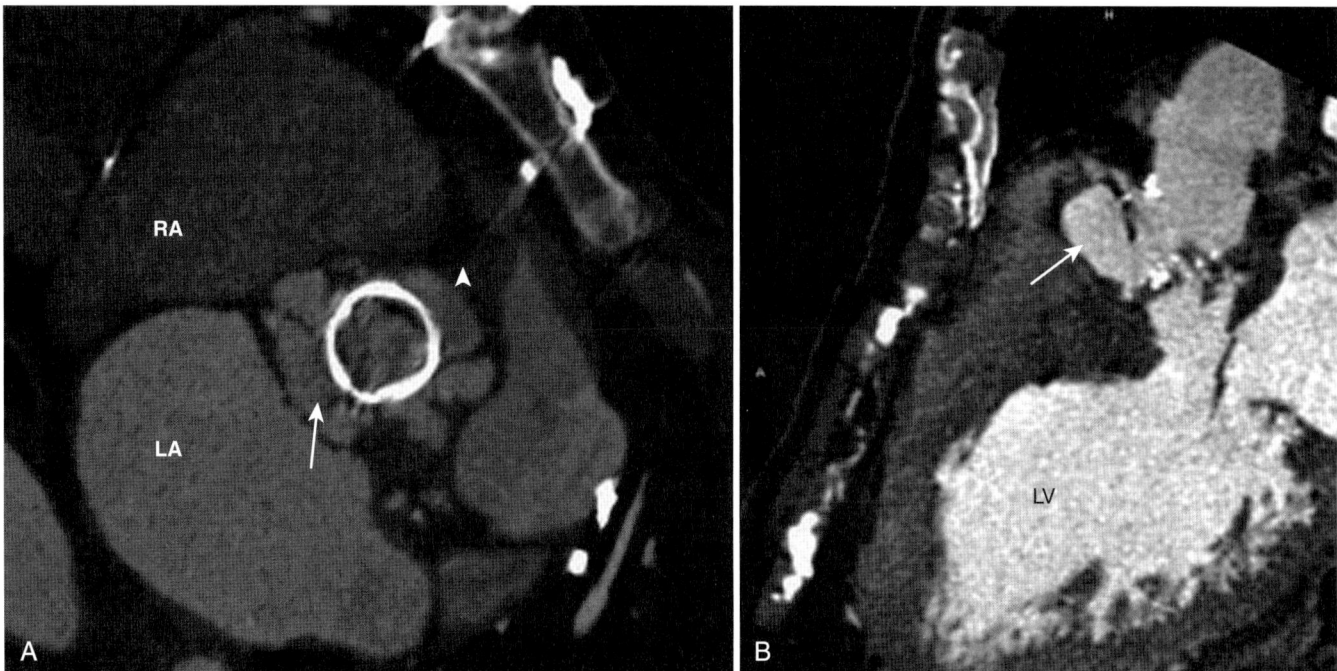

Figure 2-13 Computed tomography angiography of a bioprosthetic aortic valve *(arrowhead)* with a perivalvular abscess *(arrow)* in the *(A)* short-axis view and *(B)* three-chamber view. LA, left atrium; LV, left ventricle; RA, right atrium.

Infective Endocarditis

Bacterial endocarditis is a cause for valve replacement of native and prosthetic valves and is a life-threatening disease. Valvular endocarditis is associated with a mortality of up to 40%.[103] Diagnosis is usually made by visualization of vegetations by TEE, which is the gold standard for diagnosis. In severe cases of endocarditis, perivalvular abscesses are present and are an indication for valve replacement. CCT is excellent for the diagnosis of abscesses. They appear as perivalvular fluid-filled collections on CCT and are imaged by acquiring a delayed scan approximately 1 minute after contrast is given. Contrast is retained within the abscess after the contrast washes out of the circulation[104] (Figure 2-13). A recent study comparing multidetector computed tomography (MDCT) with intraoperative TEE for the detection of suspected infective endocarditis and abscesses demonstrated excellent correlation. CCT correctly identified 96% of patients with valvular vegetations and 100% of patients with abscesses. In addition, CCT performed better than TEE in the characterization of abscesses.[105]

Preoperative Coronary Evaluation before Valve Surgery

Coronary computed tomography angiography (CCTA) has been used in many centers for the evaluation of CAD in patients with low-to-intermediate CAD risk before valve surgery to avoid invasive testing. CCTA has been well-studied in the diagnosis of CAD in patients without known ischemic heart disease, demonstrating a sensitivity of 94% and a negative predictive value of 99%[106] (Figure 2-14). Several studies have examined the use of CCTA for preoperative evaluation before valve surgery. One such study used 64-slice MDCT in 50 patients, who had a mean age of 54 years, undergoing valve replacement for AR. CCTA demonstrated a sensitivity of 100%, specificity of 95%, and a negative predictive value of 100%, respectively, when compared with invasive catheterization. In addition, it was determined that 70% of the patients could have avoided invasive catheterization.[107] Two further studies used preoperative 16- and 64-slice CCTA in patients with AS. The mean ages of the patients were 68 and 70 years, respectively. Both the sensitivity and negative predictive value for each study were

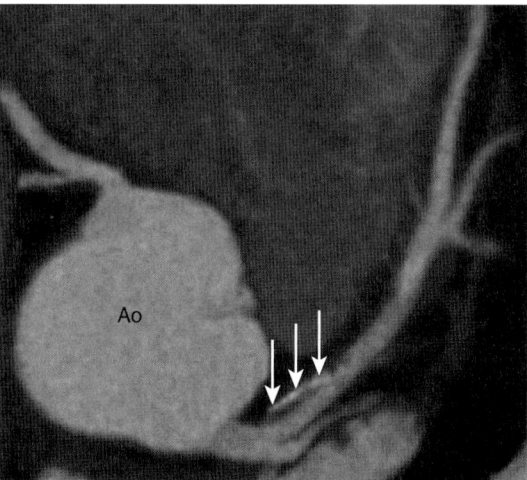

Figure 2-14 Computed tomography angiography demonstrating a long, nonobstructive, mixed eccentric plaque *(arrows)* in the proximal LAD artery. Ao, aorta; LAD, left anterior descending.

100% for the detection of significant stenosis.[108,109] These studies show that preoperative coronary evaluation with CCTA is safe and accurate. It is important that only patients with no known CAD or those with low-to-intermediate risk are referred for CCTA. In general, patients with degenerative AS are older and have greater risk for CAD.[110] Patients who undergo valve surgery for mitral regurgitation because of MV prolapse are usually younger and are excellent candidates for CCTA (Table 2-2).

VASCULAR DISEASE

Carotid Artery Stenosis

Stroke is a severely debilitating disease, and extracranial atherosclerotic disease, specifically carotid artery stenosis, is the major cause. Atherosclerotic plaques most often form in the proximal internal

TABLE 2-2	Appropriate Indications for the Use of Computed Tomography Angiography[141]

1. Evaluation of chest pain syndrome in patients with an intermediate pretest probability of CAD
2. Evaluation of coronary anomalies
3. Evaluation of acute chest pain in patients with an intermediate pretest probability of CAD
4. Evaluation of chest pain syndrome in patients with an equivocal or uninterpretable stress test
5. Evaluation of cause of new-onset heart failure
6. Evaluation of complex congenital heart disease
7. Evaluation of cardiac masses
8. Evaluation of pericardial disease
9. Evaluation of pulmonary vein anatomy before atrial fibrillation ablation
10. Evaluation of cardiac structures, coronary arteries, and bypass grafts before coronary artery bypass graft redo
11. Evaluation of possible aortic dissection
12. Evaluation for pulmonary embolus

CAD, coronary artery disease.

carotid artery; however, the common carotid artery is also the culprit at times. In patients who have had a carotid endarterectomy, the distal common carotid artery is a frequent location for plaque formation. Generally, stroke occurs as the first symptom of the disease, and often a carotid bruit is the only sign that can be seen on physical examination. The two main predictors for stroke are previous symptoms (transient ischemic attack and recent stroke) and severity of stenotic lesions.[111] For this reason, diagnosis is critical for the prevention of stroke. Several imaging modalities can be used for diagnosis. CTA has excellent spatial and contrast resolution for plaque detection, as well as morphology. It is able to detect plaque at the bifurcation of the internal and external carotid arteries, and is used to define vascular anatomy proximal and distal to a stenotic plaque.

CT, however, is not used as the initial screening test. Vascular ultrasound is easily accessible and can be brought to the patient's bedside. It is inexpensive, risk-free, and excellent for the evaluation of carotid anatomy and flow dynamics. B-mode ultrasound is used for the anatomic definition of the arteries, whereas severity of plaques are evaluated by Doppler, which measures the velocity and pressure gradients across a lesion. There are limitations of Doppler imaging, which can give false measurements. Anything that decreases the velocity of the blood from the heart to the carotid arteries can interfere with accurate estimation of carotid stenosis. Most commonly, severe LV dysfunction, valvular heart disease, and aortic disease are the culprits. Highly calcified plaques also may cause artifact on ultrasound that may interfere with accurate assessment.

Magnetic resonance angiography (MRA) is another tool for carotid artery assessment. It is more expensive than the previous two modalities, but it is relatively safe and provides anatomy, as well as plaque morphology. "Black-blood" imaging is a magnetic resonance sequence in which blood is black and vessel walls are enhanced to highlight and define plaque morphology (Figure 2-15). Angiography can be performed without gadolinium contrast by using "time-of-flight" sequence, which provides high-intensity signals for flowing blood. In addition, PC imaging also can give blood flow velocity pressure information across stenotic lesions. In general, CT and MRI are

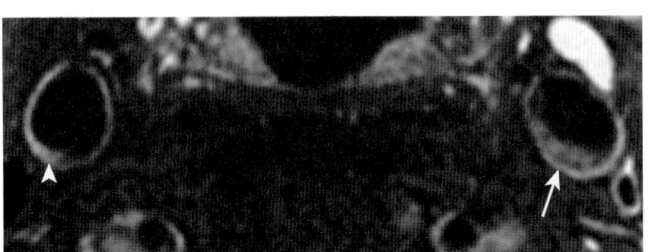

Figure 2-15 Cardiac magnetic resonance demonstrating "black-blood" imaging of a left common carotid artery with significant atherosclerosis (*arrow*) and right common carotid artery with mild atherosclerosis (*arrowhead*).

used only in the cases in which vascular ultrasound is limited or when a patient requires carotid endarterectomy for carotid artery stenosis.

Aortic Aneurysm and Dissection

The aorta is composed of three different layers: the intima, which is a thin delicate inner layer; the media, which is a thick middle layer; and the adventitia, which is a thin outer layer. Aortic aneurysm is a dilatation of a segment or various segments of the aorta. Aneurysm refers to a dilatation of more than 1.5 times the normal size. Ascending aortic aneurysms usually occur because of cystic medial degeneration. These aneurysms frequently involve the aortic root and cause AR. There are also several connective tissue diseases that predispose a patient to aortic aneurysms, including Marfan and Ehler–Danlos syndromes; in addition, patients with Turner syndrome or congenital BAV are also at greater risk (see Chapter 21).[112]

Descending aortic aneurysms are mostly caused by atherosclerosis. They are associated with the same risk factors as CAD. In addition, patients with a history of tobacco smoking are recommended to have prophylactic screening for abdominal aortic aneurysms. Abdominal aneurysms are more common than thoracic aortic aneurysms. Aortic aneurysms are generally diagnosed as accidental findings on examinations performed for other reasons.

Aortic dissection is one of the true emergencies and needs to be diagnosed and treated surgically when it involves the ascending or aortic arch. In aortic dissections there is a tear in the intima that forms a communication with the aortic true lumen. The media is exposed to blood flow and a false lumen typically forms, and the dissection extends antegradely or retrogradely.[113,114]

On occasion, the blood in the false lumen coagulates and thromboses if there is not a reentry site or other communication at the distal portion of the dissection. Aortic dissections most commonly originate in one of two locations that experience greatest stress: in the ascending aorta just above the sinuses of Valsalva and in the descending aorta just distal to the subclavian artery. Aortic dissections take place most often in the ascending aorta, where they occur 65% of the time. Twenty percent occur in the descending aorta, 10% in the aortic arch, and 5% in the abdominal arch.

Computed tomography angiography (CTA) is most commonly used for the diagnosis of aortic aneurysms and dissections. Similar protocols used for CCTAs also can be used for the evaluation of the aorta. It is important to have the scan gated to the patient's ECG because the ascending aorta has significant motion during the cardiac cycle. Nongated CTAs have inherent motion artifact that can be confused with a dissection. On some occasions, ascending aortic dissections can include the ostia of the coronary arteries, so visualization of the root and arteries is crucial. In addition, ECG-gated scans using prospective ECG-gating may be performed with low radiation exposure.

Once the images are on the specialized CT workstation, the aorta is evaluated and measured. The aorta is lined up in multiple orthogonal views to get a true short-axis at any point along the aorta to get correct measurements. The excellent spatial and contrast resolution is useful for the evaluation of dissection. Entry points of dissection, as well as intimal flap location, false lumen, and abdominal aortic circulation, are easily visualized.

CMR is also an excellent tool for the evaluation of aortic aneurysms and dissections. It has no radiation and is ideal for serial evaluation of the aorta. Black-blood imaging provides great morphologic information of the aortic wall. CMR is also ECG gated to compensate for the cardiac movement. Bright blood cine sequences provide alternative anatomic assessment. Delayed enhancement imaging also aids in the diagnosis of false lumen thrombosis. Three-dimensional images also can be acquired and transferred to a workstation for evaluation, and measurements, similar to CTA analysis.

Renal Artery Stenosis

Renal artery stenosis (RAS) is the most common cause of secondary hypertension. It can be caused by atherosclerosis, fibromuscular dysplasia, or systemic disease, which affects the renal arteries. Atherosclerosis is responsible for approximately 90% of all RAS cases.[115,116] Fibromuscular dysplasia is the most common cause in young and middle-aged women and is responsible for 10% of all cases. Atherosclerotic RAS is associated with similar CAD risk factors including diabetes, hypertension, and dyslipidemia. The clinical presentation can appear as renal involvement or extrarenal involvement. RAS can cause renovascular hypertension in addition to systemic hypertension and causes renal damage, renal atrophy, and the creatinine level to increase. Extrarenal effects range from angina, myocardial infarction, to hypertension-induced stroke and flash pulmonary edema.

The initial diagnostic tool used is vascular ultrasound because of its advantages mentioned previously. Using B-mode and Doppler ultrasound, renal artery anatomy and flow velocities can be accurately analyzed. Ultrasound is a good tool to monitor the renal artery after percutaneous or surgical intervention. Common limitations to ultrasound for the visualization of renal arteries are patient obesity and gas in the gastrointestinal system. This affects 15% to 20% of all studies. In addition, mild stenosis and accessory renal arteries may be completely missed.

CTA of the renal arteries has the same advantages as seen for coronary evaluation. Data can be reconstructed and visualized on workstations that allow two-dimensional analysis of the renal arteries in any desired plane. One of the main disadvantages is that patients with RAS often have abnormal renal function and iodine contrast is contraindicated.

MRA is an excellent tool for the diagnosis of RAS. Using multicontrast and contrast-enhanced magnetic resonance, the sensitivity and specificity for the diagnosis of RAS are 100% and 99%, respectively.[117–124] In addition, the renal artery assessment, anatomic, and perfusion evaluation of the kidneys are also performed.

Peripheral Arterial Disease

Peripheral arterial disease (PAD) refers to noncoronary atherosclerosis but is considered a CAD equivalent. Cerebrovascular and renovascular disease are generally considered separate entities, and PAD usually refers to lower extremity disease. Because atherosclerosis is a systemic disease, patients with coronary atherosclerosis should be assumed to have PAD as well and vice versa. However, a history of cigarette smoking confers two to three times more risk for PAD than CAD.[125] Eighty percent of all patients with PAD are active smokers or have smoked cigarettes in the past.[126,127] In the PARTNERS study, almost 7000 patients were evaluated for the prevalence of PAD. Ankle–brachial indices (ABIs) were used for PAD diagnosis. The study included subjects older than 70 years of age or subjects between the age of 50 and 69 with either history of tobacco smoking or diabetes. PAD was found in 29% of this population.[128] PAD most often is asymptomatic, with a relatively small percentage of patients experiencing intermittent claudication.[129–131]

Vascular ultrasound is generally the first modality used once PAD has been diagnosed or suspected clinically. It has very high sensitivity and specificity (90% and 95%) for the detection of a ≥ 50% stenosis from the iliac artery to the popliteal artery.

CTA and MRA may be the preferred modalities in the cases in which percutaneous or surgical intervention is planned. CTA because of its excellent spatial resolution has a sensitivity and specificity of greater than 92.9% and greater than 96.2%, respectively, for the detection of obstructions greater than 50%.[132,133]

MRA also is accurate for the detection of PAD (Figure 2-16). It has a sensitivity and specificity between 90% and 100% for the detection of greater than 50% stenosis when compared with conventional angiography.[134] When MRA is compared with CTA, MRA demonstrates greater interobserver agreement.[135,136]

Pulmonary Arterial Disease

Pulmonary arterial disease is important for preoperative evaluation and postoperative care. The two principal entities are PH and pulmonary embolus (PE). PH is a very complex disease and increases

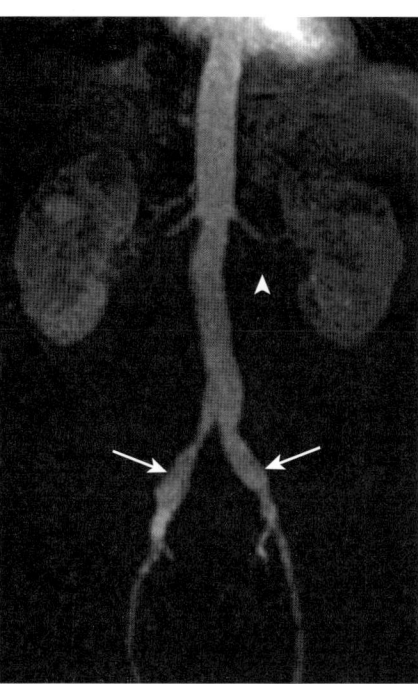

Figure 2-16 Magnetic resonance angiography demonstrating abdominal aorta *(arrowhead)* and common iliac arteries *(arrows)* with severe atherosclerosis.

the risk for perioperative morbidity and mortality. It is defined as a chronic elevation of mean pulmonary arterial pressure to greater than 25 mm Hg at rest or greater than 30 mm Hg with exercise. Patients who require CABG are increasingly sicker people who often have several comorbidities including significant PH. It commonly is diagnosed by echocardiography or by invasive right-heart catheterization. CTA also can evaluate signs of PH by analyzing RV function, RV and RA volumes, RV hypertrophy, enlarged proximal pulmonary vessels, and pruning of distal ones. ECG-gated CTA is required to assess RV function and volumes. CMR is the gold standard for RV functional analysis; however, 64-MDCT was recently compared with CMR for RV function and RV volumes and was found to have excellent correlation.[137] CMR, in addition to its analysis of the RV, PC imaging of the PA can be used to evaluate severity of PH. This is performed by measuring the velocity of blood in the PA, as well as the elasticity of the PA.

PE is usually caused by migration of a deep venous thrombosis (DVT) to the pulmonary arterial system. DVTs occur more frequently after surgery, and 80% of the time PEs are caused from lower extremity DVTs. In the United States, 2.5 million cases of DVT occur annually. Approximately 25% of all untreated DVTs will embolize and cause a PE. Vascular ultrasound is the imaging modality of choice for the diagnosis of DVT. The sensitivity and specificity for the detection of lower extremity DVTs are 90.6% and 94.6%, respectively.[138]

The test of choice for the diagnosis of PE is MDCT angiography (Figure 2-17). It has a sensitivity and specificity of 83% and 96%, respectively, for the detection of acute PE. Including a lower extremity CT venogram increased the sensitivity and specificity for PE diagnosis to 90% and 95%, respectively. However, this is accompanied by a much higher level of ionizing radiation exposure[139] (see Chapter 24).

CTA has largely replaced nuclear ventilation/perfusion imaging (also known as lung scintigraphy or V/Q scan) because the latter has limited use in patients with chronic lung disease and a high number of V/Q scans (> 72%) are found to have intermediate probability, with a 20% to 80% likelihood of PE. When CTA cannot be performed because of an increased creatinine level, a V/Q scan may be used alternatively.

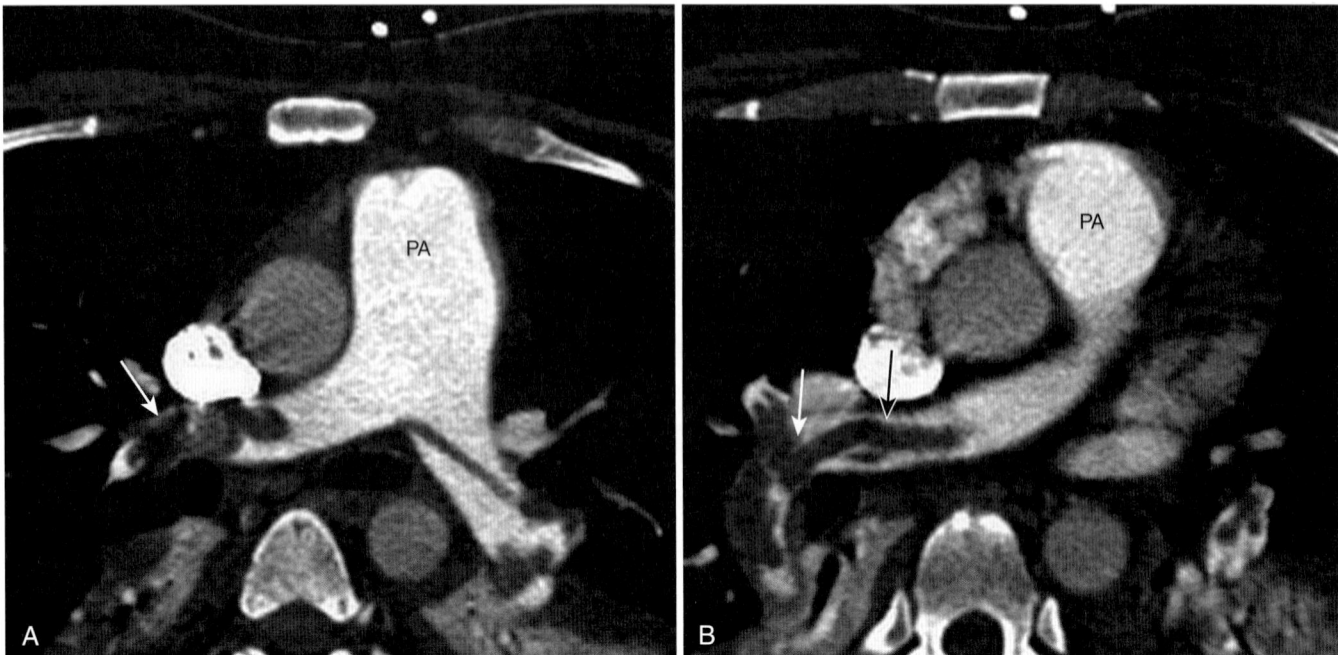

Figure 2-17   Computed tomography angiography showing large pulmonary emboli *(arrows)*. PA, pulmonary artery.

Peripheral Venous Insufficiency

Chronic venous insufficiency includes a large array of symptoms. It occurs more often with increased age and also has a greater incidence in women than men. Common clinical symptoms include limb pain, swelling, stasis skin changes, itching, restless legs, nocturnal leg cramps, and ulceration. In general, most cases of deep venous disease have either a nonthrombotic or post-thrombotic cause. Both types can involve reflux, obstruction, or a combination. Vascular inflammation, most notably by way of several cytokine mechanisms, causes tissue damage and, thus, chronic venous insufficiency.[140] Vascular ultrasound is commonly used for diagnosis of venous disease. In addition to previously mentioned DVT diagnosis, it also is accurate for the detection of venous post-thrombotic changes, patterns of obstructive flow, and reflux.

SUMMARY

Echocardiography and invasive angiography remain the most widely used modalities for evaluation of LV function, valvular and ischemic heart disease. CCTA and CMR are increasingly utilized when there are conflicting results or when further information is required in the patient evaluated before surgery.[142-144] It is important for the anesthesiologist to understand the advantages and limitations of all these imaging modalities and to use them to complement each other for the overall benefit of the patient; taking into account accuracy, cost, time, and potential radiation exposure, whose long-term effects are still not clearly understood.

REFERENCES

1. Shuman WP, Branch KR, May JM, et al: Prospective versus retrospective ECG gating for 64-detector CT of the coronary arteries: Comparison of image quality and patient radiation dose, *Radiology* 248:431–437, 2008.
2. Scheffel H, Alkadhi H, Leschka S, et al: Low-dose CT coronary angiography in the step-and-shoot mode: Diagnostic performance, *Heart* 94:1132–1137, 2008.
3. Hirai N, Horiguchi J, Fujioka C, et al: Prospective versus retrospective ECG-gated 64-detector coronary CT angiography: Assessment of image quality, stenosis, and radiation dose, *Radiology* 248:424–430, 2008.
4. Aletras AH, Tilak GS, Natanzon A, et al: Retrospective determination of the area at risk for reperfused acute myocardial infarction with T2-weighted cardiac magnetic resonance imaging: Histopathological and displacement encoding with stimulated echoes (DENSE) functional validations, *Circulation* 113:1865–1870, 2006.
5. Larose E, Yeghiazarians Y, Libby P, et al: Characterization of human atherosclerotic plaques by intravascular magnetic resonance imaging, *Circulation* 112:2324–2331, 2005.
6. Fayad ZA, Fuster V, Fallon JT, et al: Noninvasive in vivo human coronary artery lumen and wall imaging using black-blood magnetic resonance imaging, *Circulation* 102:506–510, 2000.
7. Fayad ZA, Fuster V: Characterization of atherosclerotic plaques by magnetic resonance imaging, *Ann N Y Acad Sci* 902:173–186, 2000.
8. Royster RL, Butterworth JFt, Prough DS, et al: Preoperative and intraoperative predictors of inotropic support and long-term outcome in patients having coronary artery bypass grafting, *Anesth Analg* 72:729–736, 1991.
9. Lewis KP: Early intervention of inotropic support in facilitating weaning from cardiopulmonary bypass: The New England Deaconess Hospital experience, *J Cardiothorac Vasc Anesth* 7:40–45, 1993.
10. Winkel E, Piccione W: Coronary artery bypass surgery in patients with left ventricular dysfunction: Candidate selection and perioperative care, *J Heart Lung Transplant* 16:S19–S24, 1997.
11. Higgins TL, Yared JP, Ryan T: Immediate postoperative care of cardiac surgical patients, *J Cardiothorac Vasc Anesth* 10:643–658, 1996.
12. Rao V, Ivanov J, Weisel RD, et al: Predictors of low cardiac output syndrome after coronary artery bypass, *J Thorac Cardiovasc Surg* 112:38–51, 1996.
13. Bellenger NG, Burgess MI, Ray SG, et al: Comparison of left ventricular ejection fraction and volumes in heart failure by echocardiography, radionuclide ventriculography and cardiovascular magnetic resonance; are they interchangeable? *Eur Heart J* 21:1387–1396, 2000.
14. Germano GB: Nuclear Cardiac Imaging: Principles and Applications, ed 3, New York, 2003, Oxford University Press.
15. Green MV, Ostrow HG, Douglas MA, et al: High temporal resolution ECG-gated scintigraphic angiocardiography, *J Nucl Med* 16:95–98, 1975.
16. van Royen N, Jaffe CC, Krumholz HM, et al: Comparison and reproducibility of visual echocardiographic and quantitative radionuclide left ventricular ejection fractions, *Am J Cardiol* 77:843–850, 1996.
17. Henneman MM, Schuijf JD, Jukema JW, et al: Assessment of global and regional left ventricular function and volumes with 64-slice MSCT: A comparison with 2D echocardiography, *J Nucl Cardiol* 13:480–487, 2006.
18. Hundt W, Siebert K, Wintersperger BJ, et al: Assessment of global left ventricular function: Comparison of cardiac multidetector-row computed tomography with angiocardiography, *J Comput Assist Tomogr* 29:373–381, 2005.
19. Wu YW, Tadamura E, Yamamuro M, et al: Estimation of global and regional cardiac function using 64-slice computed tomography: A comparison study with echocardiography, gated-SPECT and cardiovascular magnetic resonance, *Int J Cardiol* 128:69–76, 2008.
20. Cerqueira MD, Weissman NJ, Dilsizian V, et al: Standardized myocardial segmentation and nomenclature for tomographic imaging of the heart: A statement for healthcare professionals from the Cardiac Imaging Committee of the Council on Clinical Cardiology of the American Heart Association, *Circulation* 105:539–542, 2002.
21. Pujadas S, Reddy GP, Weber O, et al: MR imaging assessment of cardiac function, *J Magn Reson Imaging* 19:789–799, 2004.
22. Roussakis A, Baras P, Seimenis I, et al: Relationship of number of phases per cardiac cycle and accuracy of measurement of left ventricular volumes, ejection fraction, and mass, *J Cardiovasc Magn Reson* 6:837–844, 2004.

23. Fischer M, Baessler A, Hense HW, et al: Prevalence of left ventricular diastolic dysfunction in the community. Results from a Doppler echocardiographic-based survey of a population sample, *Eur Heart J* 24:320–328, 2003.

24. Kuznetsova T, Herbots L, Lopez B, et al: Prevalence of left ventricular diastolic dysfunction in a general population, *Circ Heart Fail* 2:105–112, 2009.

25. Yturralde RF, Gaasch WH: Diagnostic criteria for diastolic heart failure, *Prog Cardiovasc Dis* 47: 314–319, 2005.

26. Aurigemma GP, Gaasch WH: Clinical practice. Diastolic heart failure, *N Engl J Med* 351:1097–1105, 2004.

27. Phillip B, Pastor D, Bellows W, Leung JM: The prevalence of preoperative diastolic filling abnormalities in geriatric surgical patients, *Anesth Analg* 97:1214–1221, 2003.

28. Bernard F, Denault A, Babin D, et al: Diastolic dysfunction is predictive of difficult weaning from cardiopulmonary bypass, *Anesth Analg* 92:291–298, 2001.

29. McKenney PA, Apstein CS, Mendes LA, et al: Increased left ventricular diastolic chamber stiffness immediately after coronary artery bypass surgery, *J Am Coll Cardiol* 24:1189–1194, 1994.

30. Ekery DL, Davidoff R, Orlandi QG, et al: Imaging and diagnostic testing: Diastolic dysfunction after coronary artery bypass grafting: A frequent finding of clinical significance not influenced by intravenous calcium, *Am Heart J* 145:896–902, 2003.

31. Skarvan K, Filipovic M, Wang J, et al: Use of myocardial tissue Doppler imaging for intraoperative monitoring of left ventricular function, *Br J Anaesth* 91:473–480, 2003.

32. Apostolakis EE, Baikoussis NG, Parissis H, et al: Left ventricular diastolic dysfunction of the cardiac surgery patient; a point of view for the cardiac surgeon and cardio-anesthesiologist, *J Cardiothorac Surg* 4:67, 2009.

33. Gaasch WH, LeWinter MM: Left Ventricular Diastolic Dysfunction and Heart Failure, Philadelphia, 1994, Lea & Febiger.

34. Katz AM: Physiology of the Heart, New York, 1992, Raven Press.

35. Grossman W: Diastolic Relaxation of the Heart, Boston, 1988, Martinez Nijhoff.

36. Arrighi JA, Soufer R: Left ventricular diastolic function: Physiology, methods of assessment, and clinical significance, *J Nucl Cardiol* 2:525–543, 1995.

37. Rubinshtein R, Glockner JF, Feng D, et al: Comparison of magnetic resonance imaging versus Doppler echocardiography for the evaluation of left ventricular diastolic function in patients with cardiac amyloidosis, *Am J Cardiol* 103:718–723, 2009.

38. Moreo A, Ambrosio G, De Chiara B, et al: Influence of myocardial fibrosis on left ventricular diastolic function: Noninvasive assessment by cardiac magnetic resonance and echo, *Circ Cardiovasc Imaging* 2:437–443, 2009.

39. Polak JF, Holman BL, Wynne J, Colucci WS: Right ventricular ejection fraction: An indicator of increased mortality in patients with congestive heart failure associated with coronary artery disease, *J Am Coll Cardiol* 2:217–224, 1983.

40. de Groote P, Millaire A, Foucher-Hossein C, et al: Right ventricular ejection fraction is an independent predictor of survival in patients with moderate heart failure, *J Am Coll Cardiol* 32:948–954, 1998.

41. Mehta SR, Eikelboom JW, Natarajan MK, et al: Impact of right ventricular involvement on mortality and morbidity in patients with inferior myocardial infarction, *J Am Coll Cardiol* 37:37–43, 2001.

42. Maslow AD, Regan MM, Panzica P, et al: Precardiopulmonary bypass right ventricular function is associated with poor outcome after coronary artery bypass grafting in patients with severe left ventricular systolic dysfunction, *Anesth Analg* 95:1507–1518, 2002, table of contents.

43. Pinzani A, de Gevigney G, Pinzani V, et al: [Pre- and postoperative right cardiac insufficiency in patients with mitral or mitral-aortic valve diseases], *Arch Mal Coeur Vaiss* 86:27–34, 1993.

44. Haddad F, Denault AY, Couture P, et al: Right ventricular myocardial performance index predicts perioperative mortality or circulatory failure in high-risk valvular surgery, *J Am Soc Echocardiogr* 20:1065–1072, 2007.

45. Bernstein AD, Parsonnet V: Bedside estimation of risk as an aid for decision-making in cardiac surgery, *Ann Thorac Surg* 69:823–828, 2000.

46. Nashef SA, Roques F, Michel P, et al: European system for cardiac operative risk evaluation (EuroSCORE), *Eur J Cardiothorac Surg* 16:9–13, 1999.

47. Yeo TC, Dujardin KS, Tei C, et al: Value of a Doppler-derived index combining systolic and diastolic time intervals in predicting outcome in primary pulmonary hypertension, *Am J Cardiol* 81:1157–1161, 1998.

48. Ramakrishna G, Sprung J, Ravi BS, et al: Impact of pulmonary hypertension on the outcomes of noncardiac surgery: Predictors of perioperative morbidity and mortality, *J Am Coll Cardiol* 45:1691–1699, 2005.

49. Josa M, Siouffi SY, Silverman AB, et al: Pulmonary embolism after cardiac surgery, *J Am Coll Cardiol* 21:990–996, 1993.

50. Goldhaber SZ, Hirsch DR, MacDougall RC, et al: Prevention of venous thrombosis after coronary artery bypass surgery (a randomized trial comparing two mechanical prophylaxis strategies), *Am J Cardiol* 76:993–996, 1995.

51. Pouplard C, May MA, Iochmann S, et al: Antibodies to platelet factor 4-heparin after cardiopulmonary bypass in patients anticoagulated with unfractionated heparin or a low-molecular-weight heparin: Clinical implications for heparin-induced thrombocytopenia, *Circulation* 99:2530–2536, 1999.

52. Mogelvang J, Stubgaard M, Thomsen C, Henriksen O: Evaluation of right ventricular volumes measured by magnetic resonance imaging, *Eur Heart J* 9:529–533, 1988.

53. Grothues F, Moon JC, Bellenger NG, et al: Interstudy reproducibility of right ventricular volumes, function, and mass with cardiovascular magnetic resonance, *Am Heart J* 147:218–223, 2004.

54. Tandri H, Saranathan M, Rodriguez ER, et al: Noninvasive detection of myocardial fibrosis in arrhythmogenic right ventricular cardiomyopathy using delayed-enhancement magnetic resonance imaging, *J Am Coll Cardiol* 45:98–103, 2005.

55. Hunold P, Wieneke H, Bruder O, et al: Late enhancement: A new feature in MRI of arrhythmogenic right ventricular cardiomyopathy? *J Cardiovasc Magn Reson* 7:649–655, 2005.

56. Johnson LL, Lawson MA, Blackwell GG, et al: Optimizing the method to calculate right ventricular ejection fraction from first-pass data acquired with a multicrystal camera, *J Nucl Cardiol* 2:372–379, 1995.

57. Lembcke A, Dohmen PM, Dewey M, et al: Multislice computed tomography for preoperative evaluation of right ventricular volumes and function: Comparison with magnetic resonance imaging, *Ann Thorac Surg* 79:1344–1351, 2005.

58. Koch K, Oellig F, Oberholzer K, et al: Assessment of right ventricular function by 16-detector-row CT: Comparison with magnetic resonance imaging, *Eur Radiol* 15:312–318, 2005.

59. Gibbons RJ, Balady GJ, Bricker JT, et al: ACC/AHA 2002 guideline update for exercise testing: summary article: A report of the American College of Cardiology/American Heart Association Task Force on Practice Guidelines (Committee to Update the 1997 Exercise Testing Guidelines), *Circulation* 106:1883–1892, 2002.

60. Iskandrian AE, Bateman TM, Belardinelli L, et al: Adenosine versus regadenoson comparative evaluation in myocardial perfusion imaging: Results of the ADVANCE phase 3 multicenter international trial, *J Nucl Cardiol* 14:645–658, 2007.

61. Vesely MR, Dilsizian V: Nuclear cardiac stress testing in the era of molecular medicine, *J Nucl Med* 49:399–413, 2008.

62. McFalls EO, Ward HB, Moritz TE, et al: Coronary-artery revascularization before elective major vascular surgery, *N Engl J Med* 351:2795–2804, 2004.

63. Poldermans D, Schouten O, Vidakovic R, et al: A clinical randomized trial to evaluate the safety of a noninvasive approach in high-risk patients undergoing major vascular surgery: The DECREASE-V Pilot Study, *J Am Coll Cardiol* 49:1763–1769, 2007.

64. Poldermans D, Boersma E, Bax JJ, et al: The effect of bisoprolol on perioperative mortality and myocardial infarction in high-risk patients undergoing vascular surgery. Dutch Echocardiographic Cardiac Risk Evaluation Applying Stress Echocardiography Study Group, *N Engl J Med* 341:1789–1794, 1999.

65. Boersma E, Poldermans D, Bax JJ, et al: Predictors of cardiac events after major vascular surgery: Role of clinical characteristics, dobutamine echocardiography, and beta-blocker therapy, *JAMA* 285:1865–1873, 2001.

66. Klem I, Greulich S, Heitner JF, et al: Value of cardiovascular magnetic resonance stress perfusion testing for the detection of coronary artery disease in women, *JACC Cardiovasc Imaging* 1:436–445, 2008.

67. Plein S, Radjenovic A, Ridgway JP, et al: Coronary artery disease: Myocardial perfusion MR imaging with sensitivity encoding versus conventional angiography, *Radiology* 235:423–430, 2005.

68. Jahnke C, Nagel E, Gebker R, et al: Prognostic value of cardiac magnetic resonance stress tests: Adenosine stress perfusion and dobutamine stress wall motion imaging, *Circulation* 115:1769–1776, 2007.

69. Camici PG, Prasad SK, Rimoldi OE: Stunning, hibernation, and assessment of myocardial viability, *Circulation* 117:103–114, 2008.

70. Wijns W, Vatner SF, Camici PG: Hibernating myocardium, *N Engl J Med* 339:173–181, 1998.

71. Schinkel AF, Bax JJ, Poldermans D, et al: Hibernating myocardium: Diagnosis and patient outcomes, *Curr Probl Cardiol* 32:375–410, 2007.

72. Beanlands RS, Hendry PJ, Masters RG, et al: Delay in revascularization is associated with increased mortality rate in patients with severe left ventricular dysfunction and viable myocardium on fluorine 18-fluorodeoxyglucose positron emission tomography imaging, *Circulation* 98:II51–II56, 1998.

73. Tarakji KG, Brunken R, McCarthy PM, et al: Myocardial viability testing and the effect of early intervention in patients with advanced left ventricular systolic dysfunction, *Circulation* 113:230–237, 2006.

74. Mahrholdt H, Wagner A, Judd RM, Sechtem U: Assessment of myocardial viability by cardiovascular magnetic resonance imaging, *Eur Heart J* 23:602–619, 2002.

75. Bondarenko O, Beek AM, Nijveldt R, et al: Functional outcome after revascularization in patients with chronic ischemic heart disease: A quantitative late gadolinium enhancement CMR study evaluating transmural scar extent, wall thickness and periprocedural necrosis, *J Cardiovasc Magn Reson* 9:815–821, 2007.

76. Barber MJ, Mueller TM, Henry DP, et al: Transmural myocardial infarction in the dog produces sympathectomy in noninfarcted myocardium, *Circulation* 67:787–796, 1983.

77. Kramer CM, Nicol PD, Rogers WJ, et al: Reduced sympathetic innervation underlies adjacent noninfarcted region dysfunction during left ventricular remodeling, *J Am Coll Cardiol* 30:1079–1085, 1997.

78. Gutterman DD, Morgan DA, Miller FJ: Effect of brief myocardial ischemia on sympathetic coronary vasoconstriction, *Circ Res* 71:960–969, 1992.

79. Pettersen MD, Abe T, Morgan DA, Gutterman DD: Role of adenosine in postischemic dysfunction of coronary innervation, *Circ Res* 76:95–101, 1995.

80. Matsunari I, Schricke U, Bengel FM, et al: Extent of cardiac sympathetic neuronal damage is determined by the area of ischemia in patients with acute coronary syndromes, *Circulation* 101:2579–2585, 2000.

81. Bulow HP, Stahl F, Lauer B, et al: Alterations of myocardial presynaptic sympathetic innervation in patients with multi-vessel coronary artery disease but without history of myocardial infarction, *Nucl Med Commun* 24:233–239, 2003.

82. Merlet P, Pouillart F, Dubois-Rande JL, et al: Sympathetic nerve alterations assessed with 123I-MIBG in the failing human heart, *J Nucl Med* 40:224–231, 1999.

83. Stewart BF, Siscovick D, Lind BK, et al: Clinical factors associated with calcific aortic valve disease. Cardiovascular Health Study, *J Am Coll Cardiol* 29:630–634, 1997.

84. Katz R, Budoff MJ, Takasu J, et al: Relationship of metabolic syndrome with incident aortic valve calcium and aortic valve calcium progression: The Multi-Ethnic Study of Atherosclerosis (MESA), *Diabetes* 58:813–819, 2009.

85. Messika-Zeitoun D, Aubry MC, Detaint D, et al: Evaluation and clinical implications of aortic valve calcification measured by electron-beam computed tomography, *Circulation* 110:356–362, 2004.

86. Pouleur AC, le Polain, de Waroux JB, Pasquet A, et al: Aortic valve area assessment: Multidetector CT compared with cine MR imaging and transthoracic and transesophageal echocardiography, *Radiology* 244:745–754, 2007.

87. Feuchtner GM, Dichtl W, Friedrich GJ, et al: Multislice computed tomography for detection of patients with aortic valve stenosis and quantification of severity, *J Am Coll Cardiol* 47:1410–1417, 2006.

88. Alkadhi H, Wildermuth S, Plass A, et al: Aortic stenosis: Comparative evaluation of 16-detector row CT and echocardiography, *Radiology* 240:47–55, 2006.

89. Bouvier E, Logeart D, Sablayrolles JL, et al: Diagnosis of aortic valvular stenosis by multislice cardiac computed tomography, *Eur Heart J* 27:3033–3038, 2006.

90. Piers LH, Dikkers R, Tio RA, et al: A comparison of echocardiographic and electron beam computed tomographic assessment of aortic valve area in patients with valvular aortic stenosis, *Int J Cardiovasc Imaging* 23:781–788, 2007.

91. Feuchtner GM, Muller S, Bonatti J, et al: Sixty-four slice CT evaluation of aortic stenosis using planimetry of the aortic valve area, *AJR Am J Roentgenol* 189:197–203, 2007.

92. Alkadhi H, Desbiolles L, Husmann L, et al: Aortic regurgitation: Assessment with 64-section CT, *Radiology* 245:111–121, 2007.

93. Jassal DS, Shapiro MD, Neilan TG, et al: 64-slice multidetector computed tomography (MDCT) for detection of aortic regurgitation and quantification of severity, *Invest Radiol* 42:507–512 .

94. Caruthers SD, Lin SJ, Brown P, et al: Practical value of cardiac magnetic resonance imaging for clinical quantification of aortic valve stenosis: Comparison with echocardiography, *Circulation* 108:2236–2243, 2003.

95. Kupfahl C, Honold M, Meinhardt G, et al: Evaluation of aortic stenosis by cardiovascular magnetic resonance imaging: Comparison with established routine clinical techniques, *Heart* 90:893–901, 2004.

96. Alkadhi H, Bettex D, Wildermuth S, et al: Dynamic cine imaging of the mitral valve with 16-MDCT: A feasibility study, *AJR Am J Roentgenol* 185:636–646, 2005.

97. Willmann JK, Kobza R, Roos JE, et al: ECG-gated multi-detector row CT for assessment of mitral valve disease: Initial experience, *Eur Radiol* 12:2662–2669, 2002.

98. Budoff MJ, Takasu J, Katz R, et al: Reproducibility of CT measurements of aortic valve calcification, mitral annulus calcification, and aortic wall calcification in the multi-ethnic study of atherosclerosis, *Acad Radiol* 13:166–172, 2006.

99. Nkomo VT, Gardin JM, Skelton TN, et al: Burden of valvular heart diseases: A population-based study, *Lancet* 368:1005–1011, 2006.

100. Messika-Zeitoun D, Serfaty JM, Laissy JP, et al: Assessment of the mitral valve area in patients with mitral stenosis by multislice computed tomography, *J Am Coll Cardiol* 48:411–413, 2006.

101. Alkadhi H, Wildermuth S, Bettex DA, et al: Mitral regurgitation: Quantification with 16-detector row CT—initial experience, *Radiology* 238:454–463, 2006.

102. Konen E, Goitein O, Feinberg MS, et al: The role of ECG-gated MDCT in the evaluation of aortic and mitral mechanical valves: Initial experience, *AJR Am J Roentgenol* 191:26–31, 2008.

103. Bashore TM, Cabell C, Fowler V Jr: Update on infective endocarditis, *Curr Probl Cardiol* 31:274–352, 2006.
104. Gilkeson RC, Markowitz AH, Balgude A, Sachs PB: MDCT evaluation of aortic valvular disease, *AJR Am J Roentgenol* 186:350–360, 2006.
105. Feuchtner GM, Stolzmann P, Dichtl W, et al: Multislice computed tomography in infective endocarditis: Comparison with transesophageal echocardiography and intraoperative findings, *J Am Coll Cardiol* 53:436–444, 2009.
106. Budoff MJ, Dowe D, Jollis JG, et al: Diagnostic performance of 64-multidetector row coronary computed tomographic angiography for evaluation of coronary artery stenosis in individuals without known coronary artery disease: Results from the prospective multicenter ACCURACY (Assessment by Coronary Computed Tomographic Angiography of Individuals Undergoing Invasive Coronary Angiography) trial, *J Am Coll Cardiol* 52:1724–1732, 2008.
107. Scheffel H, Leschka S, Plass A, et al: Accuracy of 64-slice computed tomography for the preoperative detection of coronary artery disease in patients with chronic aortic regurgitation, *Am J Cardiol* 100:701–706, 2007.
108. Gilard M, Cornily JC, Pennec PY, et al: Accuracy of multislice computed tomography in the preoperative assessment of coronary disease in patients with aortic valve stenosis, *J Am Coll Cardiol* 47:2020–2024, 2006.
109. Meijboom WB, Mollet NR, Van Mieghem CA, et al: Pre-operative computed tomography coronary angiography to detect significant coronary artery disease in patients referred for cardiac valve surgery, *J Am Coll Cardiol* 48:1658–1665, 2006.
110. Bonow RO, Carabello BA, Chatterjee K, et al: 2008 Focused update incorporated into the ACC/AHA 2006 guidelines for the management of patients with valvular heart disease: A report of the American College of Cardiology/American Heart Association Task Force on Practice Guidelines (Writing Committee to Revise the 1998 Guidelines for the Management of Patients with Valvular Heart Disease): Endorsed by the Society of Cardiovascular Anesthesiologists, Society for Cardiovascular Angiography and Interventions, and Society of Thoracic Surgeons, *Circulation* 118:e523–e661, 2008.
111. Inzitari D, Eliasziw M, Gates P, et al: The causes and risk of stroke in patients with asymptomatic internal-carotid-artery stenosis. North American Symptomatic Carotid Endarterectomy Trial Collaborators, *N Engl J Med* 342:1693–1700, 2000.
112. Nistri S, Sorbo MD, Marin M, et al: Aortic root dilatation in young men with normally functioning bicuspid aortic valves, *Heart* 82:19–22, 1999.
113. Baumgartner D, Baumgartner C, Matyas G, et al: Diagnostic power of aortic elastic properties in young patients with Marfan syndrome, *J Thorac Cardiovasc Surg* 129:730–739, 2005.
114. Rousseau H, Verhoye J-P, Heautot J-F: *Thoracic Aortic Diseases*, Berlin, 2006, Springer.
115. McLaughlin K, Jardine AG, Moss JG: ABC of arterial and venous disease. Renal artery stenosis, *BMJ* 320:1124–1127, 2000.
116. Safian RD, Textor SC: Renal-artery stenosis, *N Engl J Med* 344:431–442, 2001.
117. Bakker J, Beek FJ, Beutler JJ, et al: Renal artery stenosis and accessory renal arteries: Accuracy of detection and visualization with gadolinium-enhanced breath-hold MR angiography, *Radiology* 207:497–504, 1998.
118. De Cobelli F, Vanzulli A, Sironi S, et al: Renal artery stenosis: Evaluation with breath-hold, three-dimensional, dynamic, gadolinium-enhanced versus three-dimensional, phase-contrast MR angiography, *Radiology* 205:689–695, 1997.
119. Fain SB, King BF, Breen JF, et al: High-spatial-resolution contrast-enhanced MR angiography of the renal arteries: A prospective comparison with digital subtraction angiography, *Radiology* 218:481–490, 2001.
120. Hany TF, Debatin JF, Leung DA, Pfammatter T: Evaluation of the aortoiliac and renal arteries: Comparison of breath-hold, contrast-enhanced, three-dimensional MR angiography with conventional catheter angiography, *Radiology* 204:357–362, 1997.
121. Rieumont MJ, Kaufman JA, Geller SC, et al: Evaluation of renal artery stenosis with dynamic gadolinium-enhanced MR angiography, *AJR Am J Roentgenol* 169:39–44, 1997.
122. Tello R, Thomson KR, Witte D, et al: Standard dose Gd-DTPA dynamic MR of renal arteries, *J Magn Reson Imaging* 8:421–426, 1998.
123. Thornton J, O'Callaghan J, Walshe J, et al: Comparison of digital subtraction angiography with gadolinium-enhanced magnetic resonance angiography in the diagnosis of renal artery stenosis, *Eur Radiol* 9:930–934, 1999.
124. Volk M, Strotzer M, Lenhart M, et al: Time-resolved contrast-enhanced MR angiography of renal artery stenosis: Diagnostic accuracy and interobserver variability, *AJR Am J Roentgenol* 174:1583–1588, 2000.
125. Price JF, Mowbray PI, Lee AJ, et al: Relationship between smoking and cardiovascular risk factors in the development of peripheral arterial disease and coronary artery disease: Edinburgh Artery Study, *Eur Heart J* 20:344–353, 1999.
126. Meijer WT, Hoes AW, Rutgers D, et al: Peripheral arterial disease in the elderly: The Rotterdam Study, *Arterioscler Thromb Vasc Biol* 18:185–192, 1998.
127. Smith GD, Shipley MJ, Rose G: Intermittent claudication, heart disease risk factors, and mortality. The Whitehall Study, *Circulation* 82:1925–1931, 1990.
128. Hirsch AT, Criqui MH, Treat-Jacobson D, et al: Peripheral arterial disease detection, awareness, and treatment in primary care, *JAMA* 286:1317–1324, 2001.
129. Criqui MH, Fronek A, Barrett-Connor E, et al: The prevalence of peripheral arterial disease in a defined population, *Circulation* 71:510–515, 1985.
130. Hiatt WR, Marshall JA, Baxter J, et al: Diagnostic methods for peripheral arterial disease in the San Luis Valley Diabetes Study, *J Clin Epidemiol* 43:597–606, 1990.
131. Fowkes FG, Housley E, Macintyre CC, et al: Reproducibility of reactive hyperaemia test in the measurement of peripheral arterial disease, *Br J Surg* 75:743–746, 1988.
132. Lawrence JA, Kim D, Kent KC, et al: Lower extremity spiral CT angiography versus catheter angiography, *Radiology* 194:903–908, 1995.
133. Rieker O, Duber C, Schmiedt W, et al: Prospective comparison of CT angiography of the legs with intraarterial digital subtraction angiography, *AJR Am J Roentgenol* 166:269–276, 1996.
134. Nelemans PJ, Leiner T, de Vet HC, van Engelshoven JM: Peripheral arterial disease: Meta-analysis of the diagnostic performance of MR angiography, *Radiology* 217:105–114, 2000.
135. Ouwendijk R, de Vries M, Pattynama PM, et al: Imaging peripheral arterial disease: A randomized controlled trial comparing contrast-enhanced MR angiography and multi-detector row CT angiography, *Radiology* 236:1094–1103, 2005.
136. Ouwendijk R, Kock MC, Visser K, et al: Interobserver agreement for the interpretation of contrast-enhanced 3D MR angiography and MDCT angiography in peripheral arterial disease, *AJR Am J Roentgenol* 185:1261–1267, 2005.
137. Plumhans C, Muhlenbruch G, Rapaee A, et al: Assessment of global right ventricular function on 64-MDCT compared with MRI, *AJR Am J Roentgenol* 190:1358–1361, 2008.
138. Wartski M, Collignon MA: Incomplete recovery of lung perfusion after 3 months in patients with acute pulmonary embolism treated with antithrombotic agents. THESEE Study Group. Tinzaparin ou Heparin Standard: Evaluation dans l'Embolie Pulmonaire Study, *J Nucl Med* 41:1043–1048, 2000.
139. Stein PD, Fowler SE, Goodman LR, et al: Multidetector computed tomography for acute pulmonary embolism, *N Engl J Med* 354:2317–2327, 2006.
140. Bergan JJ, Schmid-Schonbein GW, Smith PD, et al: Chronic venous disease, *N Engl J Med* 355:488–498, 2006.
141. Hendel RC, Patel MR, Kramer CM, et al: ACCF/ACR/SCCT/SCMR/ASNC/NASCI/SCAI/SIR 2006 appropriateness criteria for cardiac computed tomography and cardiac magnetic resonance imaging: A report of the American College of Cardiology Foundation Quality Strategic Directions Committee Appropriateness Criteria Working Group, American College of Radiology, Society of Cardiovascular Computed Tomography, Society for Cardiovascular Magnetic Resonance, American Society of Nuclear Cardiology, North American Society for Cardiac Imaging, Society for Cardiovascular Angiography and Interventions, and Society of Interventional Radiology, *J Am Coll Cardiol* 48:1475–1497, 2006.
142. Min J, Shaw L, Berman D: The present state of coronary computed tomography angiography, *J Am Coll Cardiol* 55:957–965, 2010.
143. Mark D, Kong D: Cardiac computed tomographic angiography: What is the prognosis? *J Am Coll Cardiol* 55:1029–1031, 2010.
144. Kato S, Kitagawa K, Ishida N, et al: Assessment of coronary artery disease using magnetic resonance coronary angiography, *J Am Coll Cardiol* 56:983–991, 2010.

3

Cardiac Catheterization Laboratory: Diagnostic and Therapeutic Procedures in the Adult Patient

MARK KOZAK, MD | CHARLES E. CHAMBERS, MD

KEY POINTS

1. The cardiac catheterization laboratory has evolved from a diagnostic facility to a therapeutic one. Despite improvements in equipment, the quality of the procedure depends on well-trained and experienced physicians with proper certification, adequate procedural volume, and personnel committed to the continuous quality improvement process.
2. Guidelines for diagnostic cardiac catheterization have established indications and contraindications, as well as criteria to identify high-risk patients. Careful evaluation of the patient before the procedure is necessary to minimize risks.
3. Interventional cardiology began in the late 1970s as balloon angioplasty, with a success rate of 80% and emergent coronary artery bypass graft surgery (CABG) rates of 3% to 5%. Although current success rates exceed 95%, with CABG rates less than 1%, the failed percutaneous coronary intervention (PCI) presents a challenge for the anesthesiologist because of hemodynamic problems, concomitant medications, and the underlying cardiac disease of the patient.
4. Thrombosis is a major cause of complications during PCI, and platelets are primary in this process. Thrombotic complications have declined with combination pharmacotherapy. This antithrombotic therapy can complicate surgical procedures.
5. In the stent era, acute closure from coronary dissection has diminished significantly. Restenosis rates have fallen precipitously since the introduction of the drug-eluting stents (DESs).
6. For patients with acute myocardial infarction, PCI is preferable if it is readily available.
7. In multivessel disease, the advantage of CABG over PCI is narrowing, and DESs may reverse this advantage.
8. Extensive thrombus, heavy calcification, degenerated saphenous vein grafts (SVGs), and chronic total occlusions (CTOs) present specific challenges in PCI. Various specialty devices have been developed to address these problems, with varying degrees of success.
9. The reach of the interventional cardiologist is extending beyond the coronary vessels, and now includes closure of congenital defects and percutaneous treatment of aortic and valvular disease. These long and complex procedures are more likely to require general anesthesia.

The cardiac catheterization laboratory began as a diagnostic unit. In the 1980s, percutaneous transluminal coronary angioplasty (PTCA) started the gradual shift to therapeutic procedures. Concomitantly, noninvasive modalities of echocardiography, computed tomography (CT), and magnetic resonance imaging (MRI) improved and, in some cases, obviated the need for diagnostic catheterization studies. Some experts predict the imminent demise of diagnostic cardiac catheterization studies.[1,2] Of course, the promise of PTCA led to various atherectomy and aspiration devices and stents, with or without drug elution. The evolution of the cardiac catheterization laboratory has continued, with many laboratories commonly performing procedures for the diagnosis and treatment of peripheral and cerebral vascular disease.[3] There also has been an expansion of the treatment of noncoronary forms of cardiac disease in the catheterization laboratory. Closure devices for patent foramen ovale (PFO)/atrial septal defect (ASD)/ventricular septal defect (VSD) are emerging as alternatives to cardiac surgery. Balloon valvuloplasty is well established, and percutaneous valve replacement/repair is in development. A variety of devices for circulatory support are now available for implantation by percutaneous methods. Finally, the era of "hybrid laboratories" has begun. Hybrid procedures include implantation of aortic stent grafts and performance of combined coronary artery bypass/stenting procedures (see Chapter 26). Such procedures require "routine" involvement of anesthesiologists in the catheterization laboratory.

Where and how did this entity called *cardiac catheterization* begin? In 1929, Dr. Werner Forssmann was a resident in the Auguste Viktoria Hospital at Eberswald near Berlin. At that time, cardiac arrests during anesthesia and surgery were not uncommon. Treatment included heroic measures such as intracardiac injection of epinephrine, which often resulted in fatal intrapericardial hemorrhage. In an effort to identify a safer route for delivery of medicine directly into the heart, Dr. Forssmann asked a colleague to place a catheter in his arm. The catheter was successfully passed to his axilla, at which time Dr. Forssmann, under radioscopic guidance and using a mirror, advanced the catheter into his own right atrium (RA). His mentor, Professor Ferdinand Sauerbruch, a leading surgeon in Berlin at the time, was quoted as saying, "I run a clinic, not a circus!" Dr. Forssmann subsequently practiced in a small town in the Rhine Valley, but eventually shared the Nobel Prize in 1956 for this procedure.[4]

Fortunately, the remainder of the world quickly acknowledged Forssmann's accomplishments[5] with right-heart catheterization; in 1930, Dewey measured cardiac output (CO) using the Fick method. In 1941, André Cournand published his work on right-sided heart catheterization in the *Proceedings of the Society of Experimental Biology and Medicine*. Dexter and his colleagues first reported cardiac catheterization in the pediatric population in 1947, and first documented correlation between the pulmonary capillary wedge pressure (PCWP) and the left atrial pressure (LAP). Zimmerman and Mason first performed arterial retrograde heart catheterization in 1950, and Seldinger developed his percutaneous approach in 1953. Ross[6] and Cope developed transseptal catheterization in 1959. The first coronary angiogram was performed inadvertently by Mason Sones in October 1958. While performing angiography of the aorta, the catheter moved during x-ray equipment placement, and Dr. Sones injected 50 mL of contrast into the right coronary artery (RCA). Expecting cardiac arrest from this amount of contrast and with no external defibrillator available in 1958, Dr. Sones jumped to his feet and grabbed a scalpel to perform a thoracotomy. Fortunately, asystole lasted only 5 seconds, the patient awoke perplexed by the commotion, and the birth of selective coronary angiography happened.[7]

Diagnostic catheterization led to interventional therapy in 1977 when Andreas Gruentzig performed his first PTCA. Refinements in both diagnostic and interventional equipment occurred over the next 15 to 20 years, but the focus remained on coronary artery disease (CAD). Over the past decade or so, cardiologists have expanded into the diagnosis and treatment of peripheral vascular disease and treatment of structural heart disease. In the near future, clinicians expect to see advances in all of these interventional areas, as well as the emergence of percutaneous valve replacement or repair. Endovascular treatment of aortic disease is expanding as the relative merits of this approach are clarified. Such treatment requires the services of a multidisciplinary team that includes an anesthesiologist. The percutaneous treatment of valvular heart disease will require a similar multidisciplinary approach. Hybrid bypass procedures are performed in some institutions with internal mammary artery grafting to the left anterior descending (LAD) artery via a limited incision and percutaneous treatment of other vessels.[8] Many newer catheterization laboratories are designed for these multidisciplinary procedures with the necessary access, ventilation, and lighting. Because anesthesiologists will work in these suites, it seems intuitive that they should participate in their design.

This brief historical background serves as an introduction to the discussion of diagnostic and therapeutic procedures in the adult catheterization laboratory.[9] The reader must realize the dynamic nature of this field. Although failed percutaneous coronary interventions (PCIs) once occurred in up to 5% of coronary interventions, most centers now report procedural failure rates of less than 1%. Simultaneously, the impact on the anesthesiologist has changed. The high complication rates of years past required holding an operating room (OR) open for all PCIs, and many almost expected to see the patient in the OR. Current low complication rates lead to complacency, together with amazement and perhaps confusion when a PCI patient comes emergently to the OR. In addition, the anesthesiologist may find the information in this chapter useful in planning the preoperative management of a patient undergoing a cardiac or noncardiac surgical procedure based on diagnostic information obtained in the catheterization laboratory. Finally, it is the goal of these authors to provide a current overview of this field so that the collaboration between the anesthesiologist and the interventional cardiologist will be mutually gratifying.

CATHETERIZATION LABORATORY FACILITIES: RADIATION SAFETY, IMAGE ACQUISITION, AND PHYSICIAN CREDENTIALING

Room Setup/Design/Equipment

The setup and design for the hybrid cardiac catheterization OR is covered separately in Chapter 26. This section reviews the importance of radiation safety and physician credentialing. For the individual laboratory, the monitoring suite is separated from the x-ray imaging equipment by lead-lined glass, as well as lead-lined walls. Voice communication from the

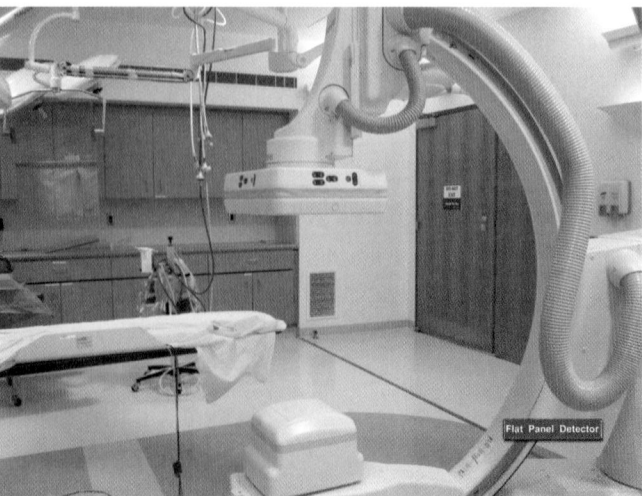

Figure 3-1 **A representative cardiac catheterization laboratory.** The x-ray tube is located below the table, and the flat-panel detector is located above the table, both mounted on a "C" arm. Shielding, image monitors, and emergency equipment can also be seen.

central area is maintained with each catheterization laboratory to coordinate tasks performed in the central area (e.g., monitoring and recording data, activated coagulation time [ACT] determination), thereby minimizing staff radiation exposure.[10] A picture of a representative catheterization laboratory is shown in Figure 3-1.

Radiation Safety

Radiation safety must be considered at all times in the catheterization laboratory, from room design to everyday practice.[11] Lead-lined walls, lead-glass partitions, and mobile lead shielding are useful in limiting the daily exposure of personnel.

A thermoluminescent film badge must be worn at all times by any personnel exposed to the X-ray equipment, with levels monitored regularly. In the past, anesthesiologists responding to emergencies in the catheterization laboratory were exposed to radiation briefly and infrequently (if at all). With the requirement for anesthesiologists in many of the newer multidisciplinary procedures, the inclusion of anesthesiologists in formal monitoring programs may be appropriate. Radiation levels should not exceed 5 rem per calendar year, and 1.25 rem per calendar quarter, or approximately 100 mrem per week.[12] Operator and staff radiation have been assessed for years. However, only recently has the issue of radiation toxicity to the patient gained attention. With long PCI and electrophysiology procedures, radiation injury to the patient has been identified, and the need for monitoring dose delivery to the patient is now appreciated.[13] Contemporary equipment estimates radiation doses to the patient, and recordings of theses doses are made. Lead aprons are mandatory for all personnel in the procedure suite. For those who need shielding for extended periods, lead apron and vest combinations may be more comfortable. Often cumbersome, these shields protect the gonads and about 80% of the active bone marrow.[11] Thyroid and eye shielding also should be considered, particularly for those working in close proximity to the x-ray source.[14]

It is not in the scope of this chapter to cover all aspects of radiation. For a more complete review of this topic, a consensus document was published by the American College of Cardiology/American Heart Association/Heart Rhythm Society/Society of Cardiovascular Angiography and Interventions.[15]

Several aspects of radiation safety require a brief review. The duration of the procedure will increase exposure. Cine imaging (i.e., making a permanent recording) requires about 10 times the radiation of fluoroscopy. Although newer equipment may narrow this ratio and permanently record fluoroscopic images, limiting cine imaging will decrease exposure.

Proximity to the x-ray tube, usually situated below the patient, is directly related to exposure. The bulk of the radiation exposure to medical personnel is the result of scattered x-rays coming from the patient. When working in an environment where x-rays are in use, clinicians should always remember the simple rule of radiation dose: The amount of radiation exposure is related to the square of the distance from the source. No body part should ever be placed in the imaging field when fluoroscopy/cine is being performed. Finally, the cardiologist can decrease x-ray scatter by placing the imaging equipment as close to the patient as possible, thereby decreasing personnel exposure.[16]

The anesthesiologist should recognize x-ray use in the catheterization laboratory and take appropriate precautions. For multidisciplinary procedures, this requires some attention to the location of equipment and the use of portable shields. It also is worth noting that most lead aprons have openings in the back, and protect best when the wearer is facing the source of the x-rays. Emergent situations, when the anesthesiologist is asked to resuscitate a critically ill patient during a procedure, may require the cardiologist to use fluoroscopic imaging while the anesthesiologist is within feet of, and often even straddling, the x-ray tube. With 96% of the x-ray beam scatter stopped with 0.5 mm of lead, aprons and thyroid shields clearly are neccessary to protect the anesthesiologist while at the head of the patient.[11] The use of x-rays can almost always be interrupted to protect personnel; patient care may require the interruptions to be brief. A collaborative effort between the cardiologist and the anesthesiologist is necessary, and communication is essential. The goal of the anesthesiologist should be to treat the patient while protecting himself or herself from excess radiation.[15]

Filmless Imaging/Flat-Panel Technology

Essentially all modern laboratories use filmless or digital recording. Radiation is required to generate an image and recordings are made at various frequencies (frames/sec). The best image quality for film is produced at x-ray frame rates of more than 30 frames/sec. Digital imaging decreases radiation exposure in the laboratory by allowing for image acquisition at lower frame rates, 15 frames/sec (half the radiation dose), while still maintaining excellent image quality. Cost savings have been achieved by the elimination of the purchasing, processing, and storage of film. Film imaging was an analog technique, and a single recording was made. Copies rarely were made because of cost and degradation of image quality. If films were loaned, lost, or misplaced, the study could not be reviewed. With the current digital technology, images are archived on a central server and can be viewed on remote workstations.[17] An infinite number of copies can be made at low cost and with no loss of image quality.

Data compression for storage is required to be 2:1 ("lossless") compression. Although "lossless" compression on a CD-ROM is the standard for the transfer of images between institutions, similar standards do not exist for long-term archival (no media standard) and data transfer options within a single institution (no compression standard).[18] Large amounts of memory and bandwidth are required for storage and transfer of the images in "lossless" compression. At remote viewing stations, such as those in the OR, it is essential that the viewer be aware of the type of image compression used to transfer data. If significant image compression is used, image quality will decrease. It is essential that improper decisions not be made because of inferior image quality.

The evolution of angiographic recording has extended beyond recording formats. Charged-couple device cameras and flat-panel detectors (FPDs) are ubiquitous in modern laboratories.[19] x-rays are generated from below the patient by the x-ray tube, pass through the patient, and are captured by the FPD. In this system, the x-rays are both acquired and digitally processed by the flat panel.[15] The flat panel is above the patient (analogous to the image intensifier), and the x-rays are generated below the patient, as before. This current generation of imaging in the catheterization laboratory delivers an improved image quality because the dynamic range of the image (number of shades of gray) is improved. It has the potential to decrease radiation exposure by providing immediate feedback to the x-ray generator. In laboratories

designed for peripheral vascular work, including many of the hybrid ones, the sizes of the FPD above the patient can be quite large and may limit access to the patient's face.

Facility Caseload

All catheterization facilities must maintain appropriate patient volume to assure competence. ACC/AHA guidelines recommend that a minimum of 300 adult diagnostic cases and 75 pediatric cases per facility per year be performed to provide adequate care.[12] A caseload of at least 200 PCIs per year, with an ideal volume of 400 cases annually, is recommended.[20-22]

Facilities performing PCIs without in-house surgical backup are becoming more prevalent.[23,24] Despite this, national guidelines still recommend that both elective and emergent PCIs be performed in centers with surgical capabilities.[22,25] Although emergent coronary artery bypass graft surgery (CABG) is infrequent in the stent era, when emergent CABG is required, the delays inherent in the transfer of patients to another hospital would compromise the outcomes of these compromised patients.[22] Primary PCI for acute myocardial infarction (AMI) is the accepted standard treatment for the following patients: (1) those in cardiogenic shock, (2) those who have contraindications to thrombolytic therapy, and (3) those who do not respond to thrombolytic therapy. It is preferred therapy for those who present late in the course of an infarction, and is probably the optimal treatment for all myocardial infarctions (MIs), provided that it can be performed in a timely manner.[26-28] When a patient presents with an AMI to a facility without cardiac surgical capabilities, management is controversial. Although national guidelines do not endorse the performance of PCI in this setting, they state that the operator should be qualified. In practice, this means that he or she performs elective and emergent PCIs at another facility and the total laboratory case volume should be at least 36 AMI procedures per year.[26]

Although minimal volumes are recommended, no regulatory control currently exists. In a study of volume-outcome relationships published for New York State, a clear inverse relation between laboratory case volume and procedural mortality and CABG rates was identified.[29] In a nationwide study of Medicare patients, low-volume centers had a 4.2% 30-day mortality rate, whereas the high-volume centers' mortality rate was 2.7%.[30] The ACC clinical competence statement for PCI summarizes these studies.[21] Centers of excellence, based on physician and facility volume, as well as overall services provided, may well be the model for cardiovascular care in the future.[31]

Physician Credentialing

The more experience an operator has with a particular procedure, the more likely this procedure will have a good outcome. The American College of Cardiology (ACC) Task Force has established guidelines for the volume of individual operators in addition to the facility volumes mentioned earlier.[12] The current recommendations for competence in diagnostic cardiac catheterization require a fellow to perform a minimum of 300 angiographic procedures, with at least 200 catheterizations as the primary operator, during his or her training.

Prior guidelines have recommended a cardiologist perform a minimum of 150 diagnostic cases per year to maintain clinical expertise after fellowship training.[12,32] Of note, when physicians have performed more than 1000 cases independently, the individual case volume may decline for a limited period with the operator still maintaining a high level of expertise. The ideal case volume should not exceed 500 to 600 procedures per year for physicians committed to cardiac catheterization. For the physician performing pediatric procedures, annual volumes should equal or exceed 50 cases.[12] Ultimately, each hospital's quality assurance/peer review program is responsible for setting its own standards and maintaining them through performance improvement reviews.[33,34]

In 1999, the American Board of Internal Medicine established board certification for interventional cardiology. To be eligible, a physician has to complete 3 years of a cardiology fellowship, complete a (minimum) of a 1-year fellowship in interventional cardiology, and obtain board certification in general cardiology. In addition to the diagnostic catheterization experience discussed earlier, a trainee must perform at least 250 coronary interventional procedures. Board certification requires renewal every 10 years, and initially was offered to practicing interventionalists with or without formal training in intervention. In 2004, the "grandfather" pathway ended, and a formal interventional fellowship is required for board certification in interventional cardiology. After board certification, the physician should perform at least 75 PCIs as a primary operator annually. Operators who perform fewer than 75 cases per year should operate only in facilities that perform more than 600 PCIs annually. In addition to caseload, the physician should attend at least 30 hours every 2 years in interventional cardiology continuing education.[22] With the establishment of board certification for PCI and the correlation of outcomes to PCI volumes, it is likely that high-volume, board-certified interventional cardiologists will displace low-volume PCI operators, and improved outcomes will result.[23,24]

The performance of peripheral interventions in the cardiac catheterization laboratory is increasing. Vascular surgeons, interventional radiologists, and interventional cardiologists all compete in this area. The claim of each subspecialty to this group of patients has merits and limitations. Renal artery interventions are the most common peripheral intervention performed by interventional cardiologists, but distal peripheral vascular interventions are performed in many laboratories. Stenting of the carotid arteries looks favorable when compared with carotid endarterectomy.[35] Guidelines are being developed with input from all subspecialties. These guidelines and oversight by individual hospitals will be necessary to ensure that the promise of clinical trials is translated into quality patient care.

With this in mind, internal peer review is essential for the catheterization laboratory. Although separate from credentialing, the peer review process is designed to identify quality issues for the purpose of improving patient care. This involves education, clinical practice standardization, feedback and benchmarking, professional interactions, incentives, decision-support systems, and administrative interventions.[12,34] An internal peer review process allows the physicians to establish and maintain in-hospital practice standards essential for quality patient care.

PATIENT SELECTION FOR CATHETERIZATION

Indications for Cardiac Catheterization in the Adult Patient

Table 3-1 lists generally agreed-on indications for cardiac catheterization. With respect to CAD, approximately 15% of the adult population studied will have normal coronary arteries.[12] This reflects limitations of the specificity of the clinical criteria and noninvasive tests used to select patients for catheterization. However, as the sensitivity and specificity of the noninvasive studies have improved, this percentage of normal studies has progressively declined.[36] Despite this, coronary angiography is, for the moment, still considered the gold standard for defining CAD. With advances in MRI and multislice CT scanning, the next decade may well see a further evolution of the catheterization laboratory to an interventional suite with fewer diagnostic responsibilities.[1]

Patient Evaluation before Cardiac Catheterization

Diagnostic cardiac catheterization in the 21st century universally is considered an outpatient procedure except for the patient at high risk. Therefore, the precatheterization evaluation is essential for quality patient care. Evaluation before cardiac catheterization includes diagnostic tests that are necessary to identify the high-risk patient. An electrocardiogram (ECG) must be performed on all patients shortly before catheterization. Necessary laboratory studies before catheterization

TABLE 3-1	Indications for Diagnostic Catheterization in the Adult Patient
Coronary Artery Disease	
Symptoms	
Unstable angina	
Postinfarction angina	
Angina refractory to medications	
Typical chest pain with negative diagnostic testing	
History of sudden death	
Diagnostic Testing	
Strongly positive exercise tolerance test	
Early positive, ischemia in ≥ 5 leads, hypotension, ischemia present for ≥ 6 minutes of recovery	
Positive exercise testing after myocardial infarction	
Strongly positive nuclear myocardial perfusion test	
Increased lung uptake or ventricular dilation after stress	
Large single or multiple areas of ischemic myocardium	
Strongly positive stress echocardiographic study	
Decrease in overall ejection fraction or ventricular dilation with stress	
Large single area or multiple or large areas of new wall motion abnormalities	
Valvular Disease	
Symptoms	
Aortic stenosis with syncope, chest pain, or congestive heart failure	
Aortic insufficiency with progressive heart failure	
Mitral insufficiency or stenosis with progressive congestive heart failure symptoms	
Acute orthopnea/pulmonary edema after infarction with suspected acute mitral insufficiency	
Diagnostic Testing	
Progressive resting left ventricular dysfunction with regurgitant lesion	
Decreasing left ventricular function and/or chamber dilation with exercise	
Adult Congenital Heart Disease	
Atrial Septal Defect	
Age > 50 with evidence of coronary artery disease	
Septum primum or sinus venosus defects	
Ventricular Septal Defect	
Catheterization for definition of coronary anatomy	
Coarctation of the aorta	
Detection of collaterals	
Coronary arteriography if increased age and/or risk factors are present	
Other	
Acute myocardial infarction therapy—consider primary percutaneous coronary intervention	
Mechanical complication after infarction	
Malignant cardiac arrhythmias	
Cardiac transplantation	
Pretransplant donor evaluation	
Post-transplant annual coronary artery graft rejection evaluation	
Unexplained congestive heart failure	
Research studies with institutional review board review and patient consent	

include a coagulation profile (prothrombin time [PT], partial thromboplastin time [PTT], and platelet count), hemoglobin, and hematocrit. Electrolytes are obtained together with a baseline blood urea nitrogen (BUN) and creatinine (Cr) to assess renal function. Recent guidelines express a preference for estimation of glomerular filtration rate (GFR) using accepted formulae. Many clinical laboratories now report this value routinely. Urinalysis and chest radiograph may provide useful information but are no longer routinely obtained by all operators. Prior catheterization reports should be available. If the patient had prior PCI or CABG surgery, this information also must be available.

The precatheterization history is important to delineate the specifics that may place the patient at increased risk. Proper identification of prior contrast exposure with or without contrast allergic reaction must be recorded. If a true contrast reaction (rash, breathing difficulties, angioedema, and so forth) occurred with prior contrast exposure, premedication with glucocorticoids is required. Diabetes, preexisting renal insufficiency, and heart failure are widely accepted risk factors for contrast-induced nephropathy (CIN). A Cr level greater than 1.5 mg/dL, particularly in a patient with diabetes, or a GFR less than 60 mL/min should prompt special precautions.[37] The study can be canceled or delayed. If the indication for catheterization is strong, prehydration, avoidance of certain medication (e.g., nonsteroidal anti-inflammatory drugs), and limiting the volume of contrast (i.e., assessing ventricular function by echocardiography and omitting ventriculography) will reduce the risk for worsening renal function.[12]

A review of the noninvasive cardiac evaluation before cardiac catheterization allows the cardiologist to formulate objectives for the procedure. In patients with hypotension on the exercise stress test, left main coronary lesions should be suspected. Knowing the location of either perfusion or wall-motion abnormalities in a particular coronary distribution, the cardiologist must specifically identify or exclude coronary lesions in these areas during the procedure. Finally, in patients with echocardiographic evidence of left ventricular (LV) thrombus, left ventriculography may not be performed.

Patient medications must be addressed. On the morning of the catheterization, antianginal and antihypertensive medications are routinely continued, whereas diuretic therapy is withheld. Diabetic patients are scheduled early, if possible. As breakfast is withheld, no short-acting insulin is given. Patients on oral anticoagulation should stop warfarin sodium (Coumadin) therapy 48 to 72 hours before catheterization (international normalized ratio ≤ 1.8) if femoral arterial access is used. Radial arterial access is considered an option without discontinuation of Coumadin.[38] This, however, may present its own challenges and laboratory protocols should be established to address this. In patients who are anticoagulated for mechanical prosthetic valves, the patient may be managed best with intravenous heparin before and after the procedure, when the warfarin effect is not therapeutic. Low-molecular-weight heparins (LMWHs) are used in this setting, but this is controversial. LMWHs vary in their duration of action, and their effect cannot be monitored by routine tests. This effect needs to be considered, particularly with regard to hemostasis at the vascular access site. Intravenous heparin is routinely discontinued 2 to 4 hours before catheterization, except in the patient with unstable angina (UA). Aspirin therapy for patients with angina or in patients with prior CABG is often continued, particularly in patients with UA.[39]

Contraindications, High-Risk Patients, and Postcatheterization Care

Despite advances in facilities, equipment, technique, and personnel, the precatheterization evaluation must identify those patients at increased risk for complications. In a modern facility with an experienced staff, the only absolute contraindication would be the refusal by a competent patient or an incompetent patient unable to provide informed consent. Relative contraindications are listed in Box 3-1; the primary operator is responsible for this assessment.[12]

Box 3-2 lists criteria for identifying the high-risk patient before catheterization. Procedural alterations based on this assessment may include avoidance of crossing an aortic valve or performing ventriculography.[40] Regardless of the risk, determination as to whether a patient is a candidate for catheterization must be based on the risk versus benefit for each individual.

With the increased emphasis on outpatient procedures in medicine today, outpatient diagnostic catheterization is the standard of care for stable patients. Unstable and postinfarction patients are already hospitalized, and catheterization usually is performed before discharge. Planned PCI usually requires admission. Even when outpatient catheterization is planned, assessment of the patient after catheterization is required. Some patients, particularly those with left main CAD, critical aortic stenosis, uncontrolled hypertension, significant LV dysfunction with congestive heart failure, or significant postprocedural complications such as a large groin hematoma will require hospital admission.[12]

In addition to the high-risk cardiac patient, patients with renal insufficiency may require overnight hydration before and after

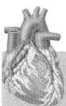

BOX 3-1 RELATIVE CONTRAINDICATIONS TO DIAGNOSTIC CARDIAC CATHETERIZATION

1. Uncontrolled ventricular irritability: the risk for ventricular tachycardia/fibrillation during catheterization is increased if ventricular irritability is uncontrolled
2. Uncorrected hypokalemia or digitalis toxicity
3. Uncorrected hypertension: predisposes to myocardial ischemia and/or heart failure during angiography
4. Intercurrent febrile illness
5. Decompensated heart failure; especially acute pulmonary edema
6. Anticoagulation state; international normalized ratio > 1.8, femoral approach
7. Severe allergy to radiographic contrast agent
8. Severe renal insufficiency and/or anuria; unless dialysis is planned to remove fluid and radiographic contrast load

Modified from Baim DS, Grossman W: *Cardiac Catheterization, Angiography, and Intervention*, 6th ed. Philadelphia: Lippincott Williams & Wilkins, 2000.

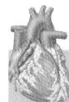

BOX 3-2 HIDENTIFICATION OF THE HIGH-RISK PATIENT FOR CATHETERIZATION

- Age
  - Infant: < 1 year old
  - Elderly: > 70 years old
- Functional class
  - Mortality ↑ 10-fold for class IV patients compared with I and II
- Severity of coronary obstruction
  - Mortality ↑ 10-fold for left main disease compared with one- or two-vessel disease
- Valvular heart disease
  - As an independent lesion
  - Greater risk when associated with coronary artery disease
- Left ventricular dysfunction
  - Mortality ↑ 10-fold in patients with low ejection fraction (< 30%)
- Severe noncardiac disease
- Renal insufficiency
- Insulin-requiring diabetes
- Advanced peripheral and cerebral vascular disease
- Severe pulmonary insufficiency

Modified from Baim DS, Grossman W: *Cardiac Catheterization, Angiography, and Intervention*, 6th ed. Philadelphia: Lippincott Williams & Wilkins, 2000; from Mahrer PR, Young C, Magnusson PT: Efficacy and safety of outpatient cardiac catheterization. *Cathet Cardiovasc Diagn* 13:304, 1987.

catheterization. Patients on chronic anticoagulation with warfarin (Coumadin) require measurement of the coagulation status and may require heparinization before and/or after the procedure. Day-of-procedure ambulation and discharge are planned for patients undergoing outpatient catheterization.[37] Radial catheterization is increasing in popularity and is associated with a reduction of vascular complications.[38,41] For a variety of reasons, the sheaths used for radial access are not suitable for long-term monitoring purposes and should be removed at the conclusion of the procedure. For patients undergoing catheterization via the percutaneous femoral approach, the use of smaller catheters (4 French) for the arterial puncture may hasten ambulation.[42] Alternatively, a variety of vascular closure devices are approved for use.[43] Vascular closure devices differ in the material that is used (and left in the patient). Some devices (i.e., Angio-Seal, St. Jude Medical) use an intraluminal anchor made of bioabsorbable material. However, it is recommended that the treated vessel not be used for repeat arterial access for up to 3 months, to permit absorption of the anchor and limit the risk for embolization. Protocols for early ambulation may permit the patient to be out of bed 2 to 4 hours after hemostasis, or even earlier if a closure device is used.[42]

CARDIAC CATHETERIZATION PROCEDURE

Whether the procedure is elective or emergent, diagnostic or interventional, coronary or peripheral, certain basic components are relatively constant in all circumstances. Variations are dependent on the specific situation and are discussed separately in this chapter.

Patient Preparation

All patients receive a thorough explanation of the procedure, often including pamphlets and videotapes. A full explanation of technique and potential risks minimizes patient anxiety, and is similar to the preoperative anesthesia visit. It is important for the cardiologist to meet the patient before the study. This relaxes the patient while allowing the physician to be better acquainted with the patient, aiding in the decision process. Although some laboratories do allow the patient to have a clear liquid breakfast up to 2 to 3 hours before the procedure, outpatients are routinely asked to have no oral intake for 8 hours before the procedure, except for oral medications.

Patients with previous allergic reactions to iodinated contrast agents require adequate prophylaxis.[44] Greenberger et al.[45] studied 857 patients with a prior history of an allergic reaction to contrast media. In this study, 50 mg of prednisone was administered 13, 7, and 1 hour before the procedure. Diphenhydramine (50 mg intramuscularly) also was administered 1 hour before the procedure. Although no severe anaphylactic reactions occurred, the overall incidence of urticarial reactions in known high-risk patients was 10%. The use of nonionic contrast agents may further decrease reactions in patients with known contrast allergies.[44] The administration of H_2 blockers (300 mg cimetidine) is less well-studied.[44] For patients undergoing emergent cardiac catheterization with known contrast allergies, 200 mg of hydrocortisone is administered intravenously immediately and repeated every 4 hours until the procedure is completed. Diphenhydramine (50 mg intravenously) is recommended 1 hour before the procedure.[44]

CIN is defined as an increase in serum Cr concentration of more than 0.5 mg/dL or 25% above baseline level within 48 hours.[37] Although infrequent, occurring in less than 5% of PCIs, when it does occur, its impact on patient morbidity and mortality is significant.[46] Total contrast doses less than 4 mL/kg are recommended in patients with normal renal function, and lower doses are recommended for those with preexisting renal dysfunction, particularly in diabetic patients (Cr > 1.5).[37] A study in more than 8000 PCI patients identified 8 risk factors for CIN: hypotension, intra-aortic balloon pump, congestive heart failure, chronic kidney disease, diabetes, age older than 75, anemia, and contrast volume.[47] It is, therefore, essential that the patient at high risk be identified and properly treated. In addition, renal function should be monitored for at least 48 hours in patients at high risk for CIN, particularly if surgery or other interventions are planned.

Several methods have been used to decrease renal toxicity from contrast agents. The two most important measures are minimizing contrast dose and adequate hydration with 0.9% saline at a rate of 1 mL/kg/hr for 12 hours before and after the procedure, if tolerated.[37] Low osmolar contrast agents are recommended.[48] Iso-osmolar contrast agents, treatment with *N*-acetylcysteine (Mucomyst) and sodium bicarbonate infusions, have yielded mixed results.[37,49,50] Fenoldopam, a dopamine agonist, has been studied and has shown no benefit.[51] Ultrafiltration dialysis has been beneficial in small studies.[37]

Patient Monitoring/Sedation

Standard limb leads with one chest lead are used for ECG monitoring during cardiac catheterization. One inferior and one anterior ECG lead are monitored during diagnostic catheterization. During an interventional procedure, two ECG leads are monitored in the same coronary artery distribution as the vessel undergoing PCI. Radiolucent ECG leads permit monitoring without interfering with angiographic data.

Cardiac catheterization laboratories routinely monitor arterial oxygen saturation by pulse oximetry (Spo_2) in all patients. Utilizing pulse oximetry, Dodson et al.[52] demonstrated that 38% of 26 patients undergoing catheterization had episodes of hypoxemia ($Spo_2 < 90\%$), with a mean duration of 53 seconds. Variable amounts of premedication were administered to the patients.

Sedation in the catheterization laboratory, either from preprocedural administration or intravenous administration during the procedure, may lead to hypoventilation and hypoxemia. The administration of midazolam, 1 to 5 mg intravenously, with fentanyl, 25 to 100 µg, is common practice. Institutional guidelines for conscious sedation typically govern these practices. Light-to-moderate sedation is beneficial to the patient, particularly for angiographic imaging and interventional procedures. Deep sedation, in addition to its widely recognized potential to cause respiratory problems, poses distinct problems in the catheterization laboratory. Deep sedation often requires supplemental oxygen, and this complicates the interpretation of oximetry data and may alter hemodynamics. Furthermore, deep sedation may exacerbate respiratory variation altering hemodynamic measurements.

Sparse data exist regarding the effect of sedation on hemodynamic variables and respiratory parameters in the cardiac catheterization laboratory. One study examined the cardiorespiratory effects of diazepam sedation and flumazenil reversal of sedation in patients in the cardiac catheterization laboratory.[53] A sleep-inducing dose of diazepam was administered intravenously in the catheterization laboratory; this produced only slight decreases in mean arterial pressure, PCWP, and LV end-diastolic pressure (LVEDP), with no significant changes in intermittently sampled arterial blood gases. Flumazenil awakened the patient without significant alterations in either hemodynamic or respiratory variables.

More complex interventions have resulted in longer procedures. Although hospitals require conscious sedation policies, individual variation in the type and degree of sedation is common. Although general anesthesia rarely is required for coronary procedures, it is necessary more frequently for percutaneous valve procedures, ASD closure, and aortic endografts. Advancements in intracardiac echocardiography have decreased the need for intubation and transesophageal echocardiography (TEE) in certain patients and procedures.[54] Pediatric procedures require general anesthesia more frequently than those in adults. As the frequency of noncoronary procedures increases, the presence of an anesthesiologist in the catheterization laboratory will be required more frequently.

Left-Sided Heart Catheterization

Catheterization Site and Anticoagulation

Left-sided heart catheterization traditionally has been performed by either the brachial or femoral artery approach. In the 1950s, the brachial approach was first introduced utilizing a cutdown with brachial arteriotomy. The brachial arteriotomy is often time-consuming, can seldom be performed more than three times in the same patient, and has greater complication rates. This led operators to adopt the femoral approach, which became nearly universal. The percutaneous radial artery approach has been used for more than 15 years. Only a small fraction of procedures are performed via the radial approach, but that fraction is increasing slowly.[41,55] The percutaneous radial approach is also more time-consuming than the femoral approach but is associated with fewer complications.[55] This approach may be preferred in patients with significant peripheral vascular disease, recent (<6 months) femoral/abdominal aortic surgeries, significant hypertension, taking oral anticoagulants with international normalized ratio greater than 1.8, or who are morbidly obese. With increasing utilization of the radial artery as a conduit for CABG, care must be taken if this vessel has been used for radial access during catheterization.[56]

It is beyond the scope of this chapter to provide a detailed description of the brachial arteriotomy, which rarely is utilized in the catheterization laboratory with the advancement of the radial approach. The percutaneous radial approach is similar to the insertion of a radial arterial cannula for the measurement of blood pressure. The Allen test, though not performed by all, is considered an important part of the precatheterization evaluation by most experts. Standard access kits with needles, wires, and sheaths are available to further simplify this approach. Once the sheath is in place, intravenous calcium channel-blocker therapy is given to prevent spasm. Although standard catheters may be used from the radial/brachial approach, specific catheters also are available.

The percutaneous femoral artery approach is performed using catheters that allow for operator ease and speed of performance. The landmarks for the percutaneous femoral approach are illustrated in Figure 3-2. The percutaneous approach uses the Seldinger technique or modifications thereof with a Cook needle, which does not have an internal obturator. Once the wire is successfully inserted into the vessel, standard sheaths (4 to 8 French) are placed in the femoral artery. Through these sheaths, separate coronary artery catheters are inserted to perform left and then right coronary cineangiography, and left ventriculography is performed using a pigtail catheter. These standard catheters and a sheath are illustrated in Figure 3-3.

In patients with synthetic grafts in the femoral area, arterial access is possible after the grafts are a few months old, and complication rates are similar to those seen with native vessels. An additional problem can be encountered with aortofemoral grafts. If the native iliac system or distal aorta is occluded, it can be a challenge to advance the catheters through the bypass conduit.

At the completion of the catheterization from the femoral approach, a closure device may be inserted in the catheterization laboratory. If so, femoral arteriography typically is performed via the sheath to assess the adequacy for the use of the device. If hemostasis will be obtained with manual compression, the patient is returned to the preprocedural/postprocedural area for sheath removal. If a right-heart catheterization is performed, arterial and venous sheaths should be removed separately to avoid the formation of an atrioventricular (AV) fistula.[57] Pressure is applied manually or by a compression device. The duration of bed rest depends on the size of the sheath.[58] Closure devices provide for more

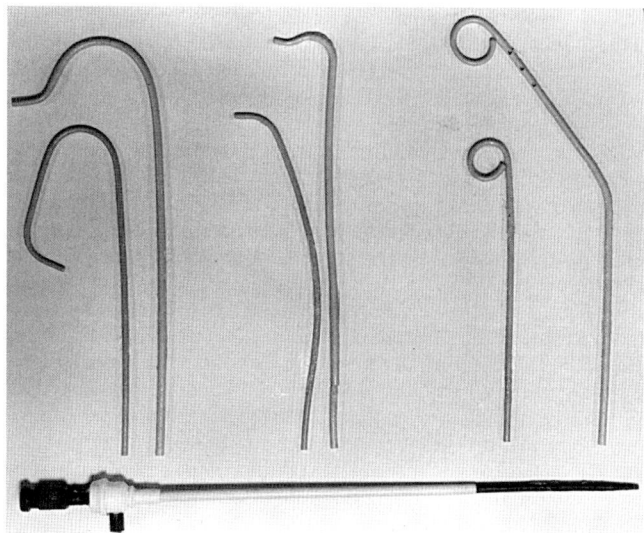

Figure 3-3 **Femoral arterial catheters and sheath.** *Left,* Standard left coronary artery catheters. *Middle,* Standard right coronary artery catheters. *Right,* Standard ventricular pigtail catheters. *Bottom,* Femoral artery sheath.

rapid hemostasis after the procedure, allowing for earlier ambulation and discharge. However, complication rates have not decreased with these devices.[12] Closure devices include collagen plugs placed within the artery that require avoidance of the site for repeat puncture for 3 months, external arterial/subcutaneous plugs that do not hinder repeat access, topical patches that elute coagulants to the puncture site, and suture devices that perform percutaneous arteriotomy closure.[43] For radial closure, wristbands are utilized to hold compression until hemostasis is achieved.[38]

Once hemostasis has been achieved, pulse and bleeding checks should be performed on a regular basis. Sandbag placement is seldom used. In most instances, for outpatient diagnostic studies, patients are ambulatory and ready to be discharged 2 to 4 hours after the procedure.[42,58]

Systemic heparinization with 5000 units was the standard of care in the early days of left-sided heart catheterization.[59] Heparin was used because of the theoretic risk for thrombus formation on catheters. Eventually, heparin doses were reduced to facilitate sheath removal. When various doses of heparin were compared, a doubling of the PTT was achieved with a dose of 3000 units, with no embolic events reported.[59] In contemporary practice, routine anticoagulation for diagnostic procedures from the femoral approach often is omitted because of the limited arterial access times, unproven need for anticoagulation, and risks for reversing anticoagulation and/or potential delay in sheath removal. If a sheath is to be left in place for more than 30 to 60 minutes (i.e., to confer about management or to transfer a patient), then anticoagulation is recommended. Heparinization is used routinely during brachial or radial catheterization to prevent thrombosis of the smaller arm arteries that may be obstructed by the sheath. Dosing is typically with a bolus of about 50 to 60 units/kg. Hemostasis is not compromised because the brachial arteriotomy is repaired with a suture, and radial compression devices can be left in place until hemostasis is achieved.

Contrast Agents

Adverse reactions have been the major disadvantage of the ionic contrast agents since their introduction for urinary tract visualization in 1923.[44] The two major classifications of contrast agents used today for cardiovascular imaging are based on their ability to either dissociate into ionic particles in solution (ionic media) or not dissociate (nonionic). The ionic agents were the first group developed, with sodium diatrizoate and iothalamate anions as the iodine carriers. Commercially available agents using meglumine and sodium salts of diatrizoic acid include Renografin, Hypaque, and Angiovist. In 1975,

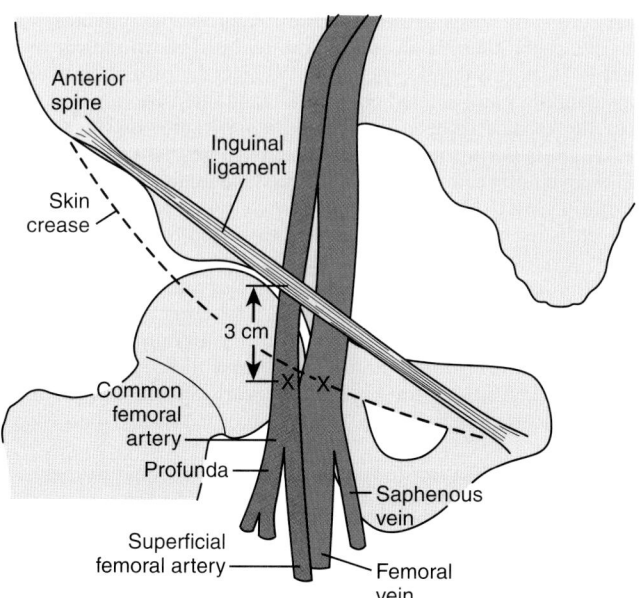

Figure 3-2 **Relevant anatomy for percutaneous catheterization of femoral artery and vein.** The right femoral artery and vein run underneath the inguinal ligament, which connects the anterior-superior iliac spine and pubic tubercle. The arterial puncture (indicated by X) should be made approximately 1.5 to 2 fingerbreadths (3 cm) below the inguinal ligament and directly over the femoral artery pulsation. The venous puncture should be made at the same level, but approximately 1 fingerbreadth medial. *(From Baim DS, Grossman W: Percutaneous approach. In Grossman W [ed]: Cardiac Catheterization and Angiography, 3rd ed. Philadelphia: Lea & Febiger, 1986, p 60.)*

Shehadi[60] reported on a prospective survey of 30 university hospitals in the United States, Canada, Europe, and Australia, involving 112,003 patients, using ionic contrast for cardiovascular diagnosis. The overall rate of adverse reactions was 5.65%, with 0.02% having severe reactions and eight patients dying.

The next generation of contrast agents began to impact clinical practice in the 1980s. These agents, listed in Table 3-2, are predominantly monomeric, nonionic agents with the exception of the two dimers: ioxaglate (ionic) and iodixanol (nonionic). These agents, particularly the nonionic dimer iodixanol, have lower osmolarity and potentially lower systemic toxicity.[48]

Several areas must be discussed when comparing ionic and nonionic contrast agents. First, the ECG effects (transient heart block, QT and QRS prolongation), depression of LV contractility, and systemic hypotension from peripheral vasodilation are more pronounced with the ionic agents, but only marginally statistically different from that of the nonionic compounds.[61] The hemodynamic effects of the nonionic dimer, iodixanol, were compared with the nonionic monomer, iohexol, in 48 patients. Although both agents caused an increase in LVEDP, this was significantly less in the iodixanol group.[62] In addition, the iodine content may vary among agents, resulting in variations in opacification. Also, for patients who have had previous anaphylactoid reactions to iodinated contrast, nonionic contrast decreases the incidence of an anaphylactoid reaction with repeat contrast exposure.[44,48] Finally, the nonionic agents and dimers are more expensive than the ionic agents. When first introduced, this difference was large and slowed the adoption of the newer agents. Current price differences are less dramatic, and nonionic agents are used in most laboratories.[48]

Both ionic and nonionic agents have anticoagulant and antiplatelet effects, these being pronounced with ionic agents. A comparison of the nonionic agents iohexol (monomer) and iodixanol with the ionic dimer, ioxaglate, demonstrated a clear distinction, with the in vivo antiplatelet effect of the ionic agent, ioxaglate, 65% greater than the nonionic agent.[63] Regardless of the agent used, these differences are unlikely to be important for diagnostic procedures. Although minute thrombi may form when blood and nonionic contrast remain in a syringe, clinical sequelae have not been noted.[64]

Patients with impaired renal function (Cr > 1.5 mg/dL; GFR < 60 mL/min), particularly if diabetic, most likely would be at risk for renal impairment after contrast administration.[37] The effects of contrast agents on the kidneys are more pronounced when larger volumes are delivered near the renal arteries. Thus, arteriography of the renal arteries or abdominal aorta would be the procedures in which the choice of contrast is most important. In fact, abdominal arteriography can be done with digital subtraction techniques and the intra-arterial injection of gaseous carbon dioxide, thus avoiding the use of any iodinated contrast.

Two large, multicenter trials have compared ionic and nonionic agents in patients undergoing cardiovascular diagnostic imaging.[65,66] One performed in 109,546 patients in Australia and another in 337,647 patients in Japan demonstrated severe adverse reactions in the ionic group of 0.9% and 0.25%, respectively, whereas severe adverse reactions occurred in the nonionic group at rates of 0.02% and 0.04%, respectively. For the patient undergoing intervention, a recent trial compared the iso-osmolar nonionic dimer, iodixanol, with the ionic dimer, ioxaglate, in 856 PCI patients at high risk and noted a 45% reduction in major adverse cardiac events (MACEs) in the iodixanol group.[67] The iso-osmolar contrast agent, iodixanol (Visipaque), has been compared with low-osmolar contrast agents in attempts to limit nephrotoxicity, with mixed results.

Minimizing the use of contrast is the surest way to limit nephrotoxicity. For patients at greatest risk, this might require that procedures be staged; for instance, performing a diagnostic study on one day and an interventional procedure at a later date. An additional concern is that iodinated contrast is administered frequently for other purposes, such as CT. If staging of procedures or repeat contrast administration is required, delaying these additional studies 72 hours and/or until renal dysfunctional has recovered is recommended.[37]

Right-Heart Catheterization

Indications

The Cournand catheter initially was used to measure right-sided heart pressures but required fluoroscopic guidance for placement. The Cournand catheter permitted the measurement of CO by the Fick method. Clinical applications of right-sided heart hemodynamic monitoring changed greatly in 1970 with the flow-directed, balloon-tipped, pulmonary artery catheter (PAC) developed by Swan and Ganz. This balloon flotation catheter allowed the clinician to measure pulmonary artery (PA) and wedge pressures without fluoroscopic guidance. It also incorporated a thermistor, making the repeated measurement of CO feasible. With this development, the PAC left the cardiac catheterization laboratory and entered both the OR and intensive care unit.[68]

In the cardiac catheterization laboratory, right-sided heart catheterization is performed for diagnostic purposes. The routine use of right-sided heart catheterization during standard left-sided heart catheterization was studied by Hill et al.[69] Two hundred patients referred for only left-sided heart catheterization for suspected CAD also underwent right-sided heart catheterization. This resulted in an additional 6 minutes of procedure time and 90 seconds of fluoroscopy. Abnormalities were detected in 35% of the patients. However, management was altered in only 1.5% of the patients. With this in mind, routine right-sided heart catheterization cannot be recommended. Table 3-3 outlines acceptable indications for right-sided heart catheterization during left-sided heart catheterization.

TABLE 3-2	Contrast Agents (Nonionic and/or Dimeric)		
Product	Type of Contrast Agent	Concentration (mg/mL)	Osmolality (mOsm/kg water)
Monomers			
Iohexol (Omnipaque)	Nonionic LOCM	350	844
Iopamidol (Isovue)	Nonionic LOCM	370	796
Ioxilan (Oxilan)	Nonionic LOCM	350	695
Iopromide (Ultravist)	Nonionic LOCM	370	774
Ioversol (Optiray)	Nonionic LOCM	350	792
Dimers			
Iodixanol (Visipaque)	Nonionic IOCM	320	290
Ioxaglate (Hexabrix)	Ionic LOCM	320	600

Omnipaque and Visipaque are registered trademarks of Nycomed Inc. Isovue is a registered trademark of Bracco Diagnostics. Ultravist is a registered trademark of Berlex Laboratories. Optiray is a registered trademark of Mallinckrodt Medical, Inc. Hexabrix is a registered trademark of Guerbet, S.A.
IOCM, iso-osmolar contrast media; LOCM, low-osmolality contrast media.

TABLE 3-3	Indications for Diagnostic Right-Heart Catheterization during Left-Heart Catheterization
Significant valvular pathology	
Suspected intracardiac shunting	
Acute infarct—differentiation of free wall versus septal rupture	
Evaluation of right- and/or left-heart failure	
Evaluation of pulmonary hypertension	
Severe pulmonary disease	
Evaluation of pericardial disease	
Constrictive pericarditis	
Restrictive cardiomyopathy	
Pericardial effusion	
Pretransplant assessment of pulmonary vascular resistance and response to vasodilators	

CO measurements during right-sided heart catheterization using the thermodilution technique allow for a further assessment of ventricular function.[70] This obviously is helpful in the setting of an AMI to delineate high-risk groups and to measure the effect of cardiac medications.[71,72] Measurement of CO can differentiate high-output failure states (hyperthyroidism, Paget disease, beriberi, anemia, AV malformations, or AV fistulas) from those secondary to a low CO. In patients with congenital heart disease, right-sided heart catheterization allows for measurement of oxygen saturation in various cardiac chambers and calculation of intracardiac shunting. In patients with ASDs, the right-sided heart catheter passes through the defect into the left atrium (LA), allowing for complete saturation and pressure measurements. The thermodilution technique cannot be used to measure CO in the setting of intracardiac shunting; in such cases, the Fick method must be used. With significant tricuspid regurgitation or very low COs, the Fick method provides a more accurate measurement of CO and is preferred. As the pharmacologic therapy for pulmonary hypertension has become more effective, right-heart catheterization is used to confirm the diagnosis of pulmonary *arterial* hypertension and differentiate it from pulmonary *venous* hypertension. A response to vasodilators predicts the response to some therapies, so vasodilators (including inhaled nitric oxide) are sometimes given during right-heart catheterization.[73]

Procedure

The brachial, femoral, and internal jugular venous approaches are used most commonly for right-sided heart catheterization in the catheterization laboratory. The brachial approach for right-sided heart catheterization may be done percutaneously or via venotomy. One pitfall in the brachial approach is identification of the proper vein for insertion. The basilic and brachial veins are preferable, whereas the cephalic vein on the radial aspect of the arm is tortuous in the axilla and should be avoided for catheter insertion. When the left brachial (or left internal jugular) approach is considered, the operator must be aware of the possibility of an anomalous left-sided superior vena cava (SVC). This empties into the coronary sinus, hindering catheter passage into the right ventricle (RV). Whenever the peripheral arm veins are entered, the catheter or sheath must be moist and inserted quickly to decrease venous spasm.

The femoral approach for PAC insertion is performed under fluoroscopic guidance using one of two approaches: The catheter can be advanced against the lateral wall of the atrium creating a loop in the RA, and the balloon is then inflated and advanced across the tricuspid and pulmonic valves to the PCWP position; or the catheter is passed from the RA into the RV; with clockwise rotation and balloon inflation, the catheter enters the pulmonary outflow tract and is advanced into the PA and PCWP positions.

Shunt Calculations

Although it is common to obtain oxygen saturation from the PA during right-sided heart catheterization, a complete oxygen saturation assessment is required in patients with suspected left-to-right shunts. In the adult population, ASDs and postinfarction VSDs are the most common left-to-right shunts requiring identification. In these patients, 0.5 to 1.0 mL blood is obtained in the following locations: high and low SVC; high and low inferior vena cava (IVC); high, mid, and low RA; RV apex and outflow tract; and main PA (rarely, right and left PA). These saturations are obtained on entry with the PAC, with repeat sampling during pullback if the data are ambiguous. These samples must be obtained in close temporal proximity to avoid systemic factors affecting oxygen saturation (e.g., hypoventilation). A step-up in saturation identifies the level at which the shunt is occurring. Right-to-left shunts are suspected when the arterial blood is not fully saturated, even with maximal oxygen supplementation; obviously, this must be differentiated from intrapulmonary shunting.

Pulmonic and systemic flows are calculated as modifications of the Fick equation for CO determination.[74] It is important that measurements be made during steady state. The Q_p/Q_s ratio is calculated for patients with left-to-right shunting by the following equation:

$$Q_p/Q_s = (SAo_2 - Mvo_2)/(Pvo_2 - PAo_2)$$

where Q_p is pulmonary flow, Q_s is systemic flow, Pvo_2 is pulmonary venous oxygen saturation, SAo_2 is systemic arterial oxygen saturation, PAo_2 is PA oxygen saturation, and Mvo_2 is mixed venous oxygen saturation.

In the presence of an RA step-up, an estimated resting Mvo_2 sample is obtained by the following weighted average:

$$[3 \times (SVC\ saturation) + 1 \times (IVC\ saturation)] / 4$$

Saturation values are measured in high and low regions of both the SVC and IVC and are normally the same. If anomalous pulmonary venous drainage is present, regional differences in saturation in either the SVC or IVC may occur. Calculation of the Q_p/Q_s ratio does not require the measurement of oxygen consumption and can be calculated with any stable level of oxygen supplementation. Calculation of the absolute values of pulmonary and systemic flow does require this measurement, and it can be complicated to measure if supplemental oxygen is required.

Correction of the defect is required when the Q_p/Q_s ratio is greater than 2 and is unnecessary when the Q_p/Q_s ratio is less than 1.5. Ratios of 1.5 to 2.0 require additional confirmatory evidence and clinical assessment before a decision to intervene can be made.

The following example demonstrates a sample calculation of left-to-right shunting in a patient with an ASD:

$$Oxygen\ saturations: IVC = 68\%;\ SVC = 60\%;\ mid\text{-}RA = 77\%;$$
$$mid\text{-}RV = 77\%;\ PAo_2 = 77\%;\ and\ SAo_2 = 92\%$$

$$Q_p/Q_s = (92 - 62)/(92 - 77) = 30/15 = 2/1 : Q_p/Q_s = 2/1$$

Significant bidirectional and/or right-to-left shunting are unusual in adult patients. These occur in the setting of congenital heart disease, typically after the development of pulmonary arterial disease. As more children with corrected or partially corrected congenital heart disease reach adulthood, the likelihood of encountering an adult with a complicated shunt will increase. These encounters may be complicated by the development of adult cardiology problems, mainly CAD. However, about 25% of the population has a PFO, and right-to-left shunting through the PFO with systemic oxygen desaturation can occur if the RA pressures become increased. This may occur after pulmonary emboli or after an RV infarction, among other causes.

Calculation of bidirectional shunting involves determination of the effective blood flow. Effective blood flow (Q_{eff}) represents the flow if no right-to-left or left-to-right shunting exists.[74] With Q_{eff}, right-to-left shunting is equal to $Q_s - Q_{eff}$, and left-to-right shunting is equal to $Q_p - Q_{eff}$, using the following formulas derived from the Fick equation for CO:

$$Q_S(L/min) = O_2\ consumption\ (mL/min)/SAo_2$$
$$(mL/L) - Mvo_2\ (mL/L)$$

$$Q_p(L/min) = O_2\ consumption\ (mL/min)/Pvo_2$$
$$(mL/L) - PAo_2\ (mL/L)$$

$$Q_{eff}(L/min) = O_2\ consumption\ (mL/min)/Pvo_2$$
$$(mL/L) - MVo_2\ (mL/L)$$

Right-sided heart pressure may be obtained either on entry or on pullback (Figure 3-4). Catheter placement using the femoral approach may be time-consuming, with expedited passage necessary to prevent catheter softening. Therefore, pressure measurements often are obtained during catheter pullback to assure temporal proximity. As with all invasive procedures, complications can occur with right-heart catheterization, requiring that risks and benefits be assessed before undertaking this and any procedure[75] (see Chapter 14).

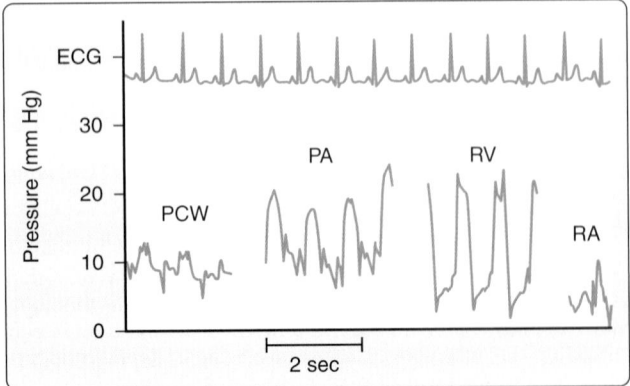

Figure 3-4   A pullback tracing obtained using a pulmonary artery catheter (PAC) from the pulmonary capillary wedge (PCW) position, to the pulmonary artery (PA), right ventricle (RV), and right atrium (RA). ECG, electrocardiogram.

Endomyocardial Biopsy

Endomyocardial biopsy is the most (only) reliable method to detect rejection in the transplanted heart. However, its role in the management of other cardiovascular diseases in the adult and pediatric patient remains controversial. In 2007, the ACC/AHA/European Society of Cardiology published recommendations on endomyocardial biopsy.[76] Either internal jugular (most common in the United States) or femoral (more common in Europe) veins are the preferred approaches with subclavian and even brachial approaches utilized. Complications are infrequent and are related to the access site in 2%, arrhythmia/conduction abnormalities in 1% to 2%, and perforation in 0.5%. Death, a rare event, is related to perforation. Histologic evaluation of the tissue is the purpose of the procedure and must be done by experienced pathologists to justify the risks.

Indications are controversial, but most groups agree that important information can be obtained in the setting of new-onset heart failure for both the less than 2-week group and the 2- to 3-month group unresponsive to therapy.[76] Other potential indications include unexplained restrictive cardiomyopathy, anthracycline cardiomyopathy, suspected cardiac tumor, unexplained arrhythmias, and heart failure associated with hypertrophic cardiomyopathy, but these are less clear. A complete review of potential scenarios is found in the 2007 scientific statement.[76]

▉ Diagnostic Catheterization Complications

Although adult diagnostic catheterization with selective coronary cineangiography had been performed since the late 1950s, complication rates were not followed until 1979 when the Society for Cardiac Angiography and Interventions established the first registry to prospectively monitor the performance of participating laboratories. In 1982, the first publication from this registry reported complication rates from a study population of more than 50,000 patients.[77] This was updated in 1989 with a report on 222,553 patients who underwent selective coronary arteriography between 1984 and 1987.[78] When compared with the earlier report, similar complication rates were noted. Complications are related to multiple factors, but severity of disease is important. Mortality rates are shown in Table 3-4. Complications are specific for both right- and left-heart catheterization (Table 3-5). The registry reported incidences of major complications as follows: death 0.1%, MI 0.06%, cerebrovascular accident 0.07%, arrhythmia 0.47%, contrast reaction 0.23%, and vascular complications 0.46%.[78] Infectious complications are infrequent; this may reflect underreporting. Guidelines for infection control are based more on extrapolation from ORs than randomized control data from the catheterization laboratory.[79] Although advances in technology continue, similar complication rates still are

TABLE 3-4	Cardiac Catheterization Mortality Data
Patient Characteristics*	**Mortality Rate (%)**
Overall mortality from cardiac catheterization	0.14
Age-related mortality	
< 1 yr	1.75
> 60 yr	0.25
Coronary artery disease	
One-vessel disease	0.03
Three-vessel disease	0.16
Left main disease	0.86
Congestive heart failure	
NYHA functional class I or II	0.02
NYHA functional class III	0.12
NYHA functional class IV	0.67
Valvular heart disease	
All valvular disease patients	0.28
Mitral valve disease	0.34
Aortic valve disease	0.19

*Other reported high-risk characteristics include unstable angina, acute myocardial infarction, renal insufficiency, ventricular arrhythmias, cyanotic congenital heart disease (including arterial desaturation and pulmonary hypertension). Detailed data from large-scale studies on these characteristics are unavailable.
From Pepine CJ, Allen HD, Bashore TM, et al: ACC/AHA guidelines for cardiac catheterization and cardiac catheterization laboratories. *J Am Coll Cardiol* 18:1149, 1991.

TABLE 3-5	Complications from Diagnostic Catheterization
Left Heart	
<u>Cardiac</u>	
Death	
Myocardial infarction	
Ventricular fibrillation	
Ventricular tachycardia	
Cardiac perforation	
<u>Noncardiac</u>	
Stroke	
Peripheral embolization	
Air	
Thrombus	
Cholesterol	
Vascular surgical repair	
Pseudoaneurysm	
AV fistula	
Embolectomy	
Repair of brachial arteriotomy	
Evacuation of hematomas	
Contrast related	
Renal insufficiency	
Anaphylaxis	
Right Heart	
<u>Cardiac</u>	
Conduction abnormality	
RBBB	
Complete heart block (RBBB superimposed on LBBB)	
Arrhythmias	
Valvular damage	
Perforation	
<u>Noncardiac</u>	
Pulmonary artery rupture	
Pulmonary infarction	
Balloon rupture	
Paradoxic (systemic) air embolus	

AV, arteriovenous; LBBB, left` bundle branch block; RBBB, right bundle branch block.

present today, most likely because of the higher-risk patient undergoing catheterization.[12] The current registries for identifying complications are primarily focused on percutaneous interventions. In addition to institutional and regional databases, such as those of the Cleveland Clinic and Northern New England, the ACC maintains the National Cardiovascular Data Registry (NDCR).

Vascular complications from the percutaneous femoral approach occur in less than 1% of diagnostic procedures, with the most common being pseudoaneurysms.[43] This risk is greater for the obese patient in whom compression is more difficult. Therapy for pseudoaneurysms includes either ultrasound-directed thrombin injection or surgical repair. In patients with aortic regurgitation (AR), an increased incidence of femoral arteriovenous fistulas is seen due to the widened pulse pressure.[57] Many small arteriovenous fistulas will close spontaneously. If large or if the fistula is associated with high output (rare) or edema of the affected leg, surgical correction is indicated. Thrombosis of the femoral artery occurs rarely, and underlying atherosclerotic disease usually is severe. Emergent restoration of flow is essential, with a surgical approach used at some hospitals and a percutaneous one at others.

Arrhythmic complications during left-sided heart catheterization are more frequent with ionic contrast than with nonionic contrast, and they occur during coronary injection. Surprisingly, the presence of the catheter in the LV rarely causes a sustained arrhythmia. Early contrast media containing potassium produced ventricular fibrillation during coronary arteriography. However, current contrast materials are potassium-free and contain added calcium, resulting in an incidence rate of significant ventricular arrhythmias of 0.47%.[78]

Anaphylactoid reactions occurred in approximately 5% to 8% of cases when nonionic contrast was used. The definition of reaction severity, as well as the differential diagnosis for severe reactions is listed in Table 3-6. If a severe anaphylactoid reaction to contrast media occurs with hypotension refractory to rapid fluid resuscitation, and/or significant bronchospasm, immediate therapy with intravenous epinephrine, 0.1 mL of 1:10,000 solution (10 µg) every minute, is recommended. Subcutaneous doses of 0.3 mL of 1:1000 solutions can be administered for moderate reactions, whereas diphenhydramine is effective for mild reactions.[44]

Cholesterol embolization can occur after catheter manipulation, and has been described after cardiac catheterization.[80] Although the femoral approach can be used in patients with unrepaired abdominal aortic aneurysms, an increased incidence of cholesterol emboli syndrome may occur in this population.[81] Cholesterol embolization produces small-vessel arterial occlusion by cholesterol crystals, resulting in a serious clinical presentation including livedo reticularis, acrocyanosis of the lower extremities, renal insufficiency, and accelerated hypertension. The clinical course is variable, does not respond to anticoagulation, and has the potential for an insidious development of progressive renal failure, accelerating hypertension, and a fatal outcome.

VALVULAR PATHOLOGY

In 2006, the ACC/AHA published updated practice guidelines for the management of patients with valvular heart disease.[82] These guidelines cover the invasive and noninvasive evaluation of valvular problems, as well as therapeutic approaches. Each type of valvular pathology has its own particular hemodynamic "fingerprint," the character of which depends on the severity of the pathology, as well as its duration (see Chapters 12, 13, and 19).

Stenotic Lesions

The transvalvular gradient, as well as the transvalvular flow, must be quantified to assess the severity of stenotic lesions. For a given amount of stenosis, hydraulic principles state that as flow increases, so also will the pressure decline across the orifice. Both the CO and the HR determine flow; it is during the systolic ejection period (SEP) that flow occurs through the semilunar valves and during the diastolic filling period (DFP) for the AV valves.

Gorlin and Gorlin[83] derived a formula from fluid physics to relate valve area with blood flow and blood velocity:

$$\text{Valve area} \propto \text{Blood flow/Blood velocity}$$

In general, as a valve orifice becomes increasingly stenotic, the velocity of flow must progressively increase if total flow across the valve is to be maintained. Flow velocity can be measured by the Doppler principle to estimate valve area; however, in the catheterization laboratory, this is not as practical as measuring blood *pressures* on either side of the valve.

As described by Gorlin and Gorlin,[83] the velocity of blood flow is related to the square root of the pressure drop across the valve:

$$P_1 - P_2 \propto (\text{Blood velocity})^2$$

Stated another way, for any given orifice size, *the transvalvular pressure gradient is a function of the square of the transvalvular flow rate.* For example, with mitral stenosis (MS), as the valve area progressively decreases, a modest increase in the rate of flow across the valve causes progressively larger increases in the pressure gradient across the valve (Figure 3-5).

The actual time of the cardiac cycle in which flow occurs must be known to complete the calculation. For semilunar valves (aortic and pulmonic), flow occurs during the SEP; for AV valves (mitral and tricuspid), flow occurs during the DFP. The SEP occurs during ventricular contraction when the aortic valve is open, and the DFP occurs while the mitral valve is open (Figure 3-6). The HR determines the duration of the SEP or DFP over an entire minute. Also present in the Gorlin formula is a coefficient that quantifies the conversion of potential energy (pressure energy) to kinetic energy (velocity). This term also contains an empirically derived factor, which accounts for the difference between calculated and measured valve areas at the time of surgery or postmortem.

The final Gorlin formula then becomes:

$$\text{Valve area} = CO \div [(\text{DFP or SEP})(HR)] / 44.3 \bullet C \bullet (P_1 - P_2)^{1/2}$$

where CO is cardiac output (mL/min), DFP or SEP is diastolic filling period or systolic ejection period in seconds per beat, HR is heart rate in beats per minute, C is orifice constant (aortic, C = 1.0; mitral, C = 0.85; tricuspid, C = 0.7), and $P_1 - P_2$ is the mean pressure difference across the orifice using computer-assisted analysis or area blanketing. The 44.3 term is derived from the energy calculation.

TABLE 3-6	Contrast-Induced Anaphylactoid Reactions	
	Severity Classification	
Minor	*Moderate*	*Severe*
Urticaria (limited)	Urticaria (diffuse)	Cardiovascular shock
Pruritus	Angioedema	Respiratory arrest
Erythema	Laryngeal edema	Cardiac arrest
	Bronchospasm	
Differential Diagnosis (Severe Reactions)		
Cardiac	*Noncardiac*	
Vasovagal reaction	Hypovolemia	
Cardiogenic shock	Dehydration	
Right ventricular infarction	Blood loss—gastrointestinal, vascular, external	
Cardiac tamponade	Drug related	
Cardiac rupture	Narcotic, benzodiazepine, protamine	
Bezold–Jarich reflex	Sepsis	

Adapted from Goss J, Chambers C, Heupler F, et al: Systemic anaphylactoid reactions to iodinated contrast media during cardiac catheterization procedures. *Cathet Cardiovasc Diagn* 34:99, 1995.

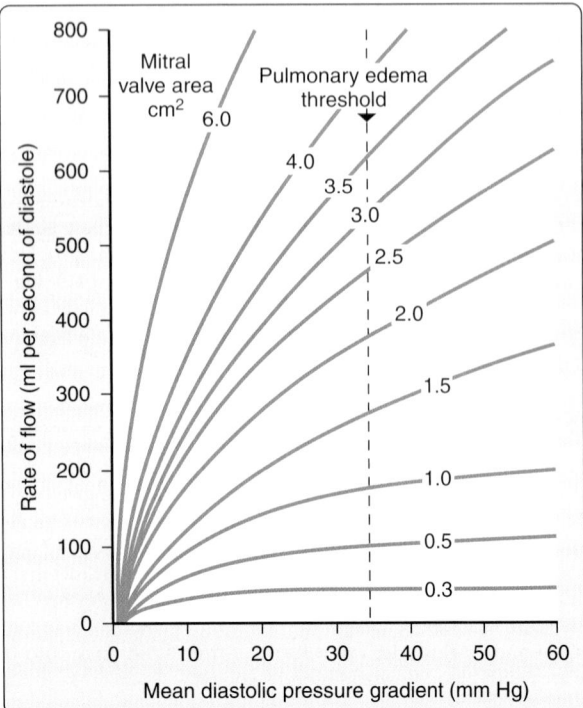

Figure 3-5 **Rate of flow in diastole versus mean pressure gradient for several degrees of mitral stenosis.** The pressure gradient is directly proportional to the square of the flow rate, such that as the degree of stenosis progresses, modest increases in flow (as with light exercise) will require large increases in the pressure gradient. As an example, a cardiac output (CO) of 5.2 L/min, heart rate (HR) of 60 beats/min, and diastolic filling time of 0.5 second result in a 200-mL/sec flow during diastole. For mild mitral stenosis (valve area = 2.0 cm²), the required pressure gradient remains small (< 10 mm Hg). In the case of severe stenosis (valve area < 1.0 cm²), the resultant gradient is high enough to place the patient past the threshold for pulmonary edema. *(From Wallace AG: Pathophysiology of cardiovascular disease. In Smith LH Jr, Thier SO [eds]: Pathophysiology: The Biological Principles of Disease. The International Textbook of Medicine, Vol. 1. Philadelphia: WB Saunders Company, 1981, p 1192.)*

Aortic Stenosis

The normal adult aortic valve area is 2.6 to 3.5 cm², which corresponds to a normal aortic valve index of 2.0 cm²/m². As the valve area decreases to a range of 1.5 to 2.0 cm² (or a valve index of 1.0 cm²/m², the major hemodynamic finding is an increase in the LV systolic pressure to maintain a normal aortic systolic pressure. An elevation in LVEDP also may be observed, which is merely a reflection of the decrease in compliance of the hypertrophied ventricle (see Chapter 19).

As the stenosis becomes moderate and the valve area decreases to 1.0 to 1.5 cm², symptoms can occur. At this point, the LV exhibits a more rounded appearance at its peak systolic pressure, and a progressive increase in the LVEDP occurs. As the LV hypertrophies, its filling becomes more dependent on the contraction of the LA; this is reflected as an augmented A wave on the ventricular tracing. At this point, the increased LA pressure makes atrial fibrillation (AF) more likely, and the decreasing compliance of the LV makes it poorly tolerated. Widening of the systolic pressure gradient from the LV to the aorta, a decrease in the rate of rise of the upstroke of the aortic pressure tracing, and a delay in the time-to-peak aortic pressure also are seen (Figure 3-7).

In the case of severe AS with a valve area of less than 1.0 cm² and a valve area index of less than 0.5 cm²/m², a decrease in systolic function of the LV can occur. Increases in PAP, PCWP, and right atrial pressure

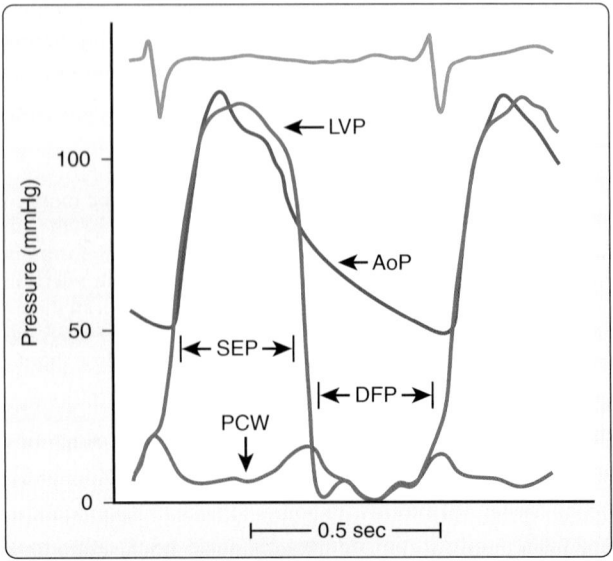

Figure 3-6 **Simultaneous left ventricular (LVP), aortic (AoP), and left atrial pressure (PCW) waveforms.** The systolic ejection period (SEP) is defined as the period during which the aortic valve is open (from when LVP crosses over AoP at the beginning of systole to when AoP crosses over LVP near the end of systole) and forward blood flow is present in the aorta (see also Figure 3-2). Diastolic filling period (DFP) is defined as that period during which the mitral valve is open (from the crossover of LVP by PCW to the crossover of PCW by LVP) and blood is flowing through the mitral valve. *(Modified from Grossman W, Baim DS [eds]: Cardiac Catheterization, Angiography, and Intervention, 4th ed. Philadelphia: Lea & Febiger, 1991, p 153.)*

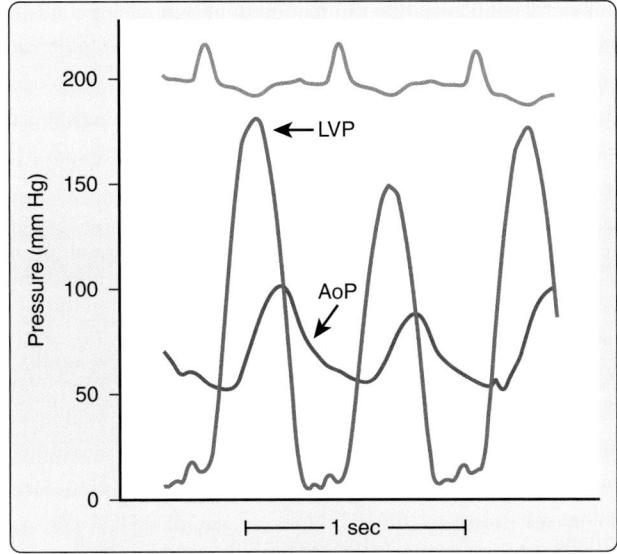

Figure 3-7 **Left ventricular (LVP) and aortic (AoP) pressure waveforms in patient with aortic stenosis.** Of note is the large pressure gradient from left ventricle to aorta at peak systolic pressure, the delay to the onset of aortic upstroke, and the decrease in the rate of rise of the aortic pressure. End-diastolic pressure is still normal at this stage of the disease.

(RAP) also are observed. These latter changes often are accompanied by symptoms of congestive heart failure. The diagnosis and potential therapy for the patient with low-flow/low-gradient aortic stenosis is always challenging. Among patients with low-gradient AS, dobutamine infusions may help to identify those who will benefit from aortic valve replacement.[84]

Mitral Stenosis

In normal adults, the mitral valve orifice is 4 to 6 cm². Mild MS is considered to be present when the mitral valve orifice is reduced to less than 2.0 cm². In this condition, the typical hemodynamic finding is that of an elevation in either LAP or PCWP. The increase in LAP will tend to maintain normal flow across the valve. As the mitral valve orifice becomes reduced to less than 1.0 cm², considered to be critical MS, a much larger LA-to-LV gradient is required to maintain reasonable flow across the valve (Figure 3-8). An increase in LAP during diastole leads to early opening of the mitral valve, as well as slightly delayed closure of the same valve (Figure 3-9). It is easy to understand why a slow HR in the presence of MS is preferred, because a maximal DFP is necessary to maintain reasonable flow and maintain CO across the mitral valve. Another hemodynamic hallmark in patients with MS is the reduced increase in LV pressure during early diastole. Normally, a fairly rapid increase is seen during the rapid filling phase of diastole, but the slope of this pressure increase is delayed in the presence of severe MS. In the presence of severe MS, increases in right-sided heart pressures are common. In severe long-standing MS, the PAP can reach or exceed systemic arterial pressure. Dilation of the LA commonly leads to chronic AF in these patients.

Doppler echocardiography has reduced the importance of catheterization in the evaluation of valvular disease (see Chapter 12). In stenoses of borderline severity, data from the catheterization laboratory are still important for clinical decision making. Performance of exercise or administration of inotropic agents increases the CO. In addition to confirmation of inotropic reserve, this increase in output increases the flow across the valves and increases the gradient exponentially. When both the gradient across the valve and the CO are low, augmentation of flow can help to distinguish severe stenosis with reversible ventricular failure from mild stenosis with irreversible ventricular failure.

■ Regurgitant Lesions

The severity of regurgitant lesions is quantified angiographically (see later). However, several hallmark changes occur in the presence of regurgitant lesions of either the semilunar or AV valves. As an example of semilunar valve regurgitation, the aortic valve is discussed, and the mitral valve is used as an example of AV valve regurgitation or incompetence (see Chapters 12, 13, and 19).

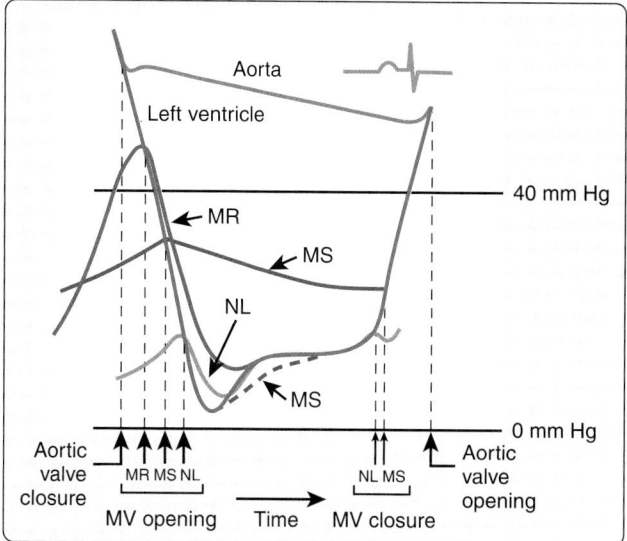

Figure 3-9 Idealized diagram summarizing mitral valve disorders, concentrating on the diastolic filling period. In mitral stenosis (MS), the increase in left atrial pressure (— -) versus normal atrial pressure (— -) causes early mitral valve (MV) opening and a slight delay in MV closure. Left ventricular rapid filling is delayed, which delays the increase of ventricular pressure (— — -) from that seen during normal diastole (—). In mitral regurgitation (MR), the left atrial pressure (..) has a large V wave, because the atrium fills with blood from the pulmonary veins and with blood regurgitating through the MV. Thus, the MV opens early. NL, normal. *(From Braunwald E: Valvular heart disease. In Braunwald E [ed]:* Heart Disease: A Textbook of Cardiovascular Medicine, *3rd edition. Philadelphia, WB Saunders Company, 1988, p 1024.)*

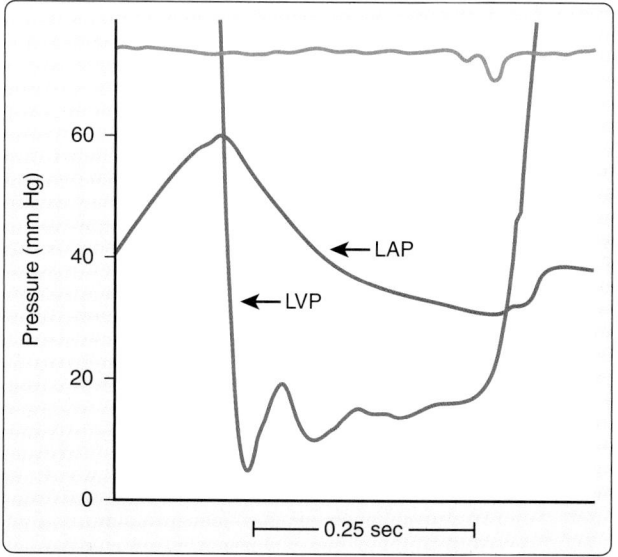

Figure 3-8 Mitral stenosis, with pressures measured at catheterization. Note the gradient during diastole between the left atrial (LAP) and the left ventricular (LVP) pressures, and the increase in the LAP.

Aortic Regurgitation

Acute AR or insufficiency (AI) is uncommon, unless there is aortic dissection, sudden failure of a valve prosthesis, or if there is native valve destruction in the setting of bacterial endocarditis. In the presence of acute AR, there are sudden increases in systolic and end-diastolic volumes (EDVs) and pressures. Thus, the normal ventricle suddenly is faced with an increased load and generates greater pressure. During relaxation, because the ventricle is filling with blood from the aorta, there is a delay in the isovolumic pressure decline, accompanied by rapid increases in ventricular diastolic pressures, both because of continued valve regurgitation. The wide pulse pressure, a characteristic of chronic AR, may not be seen in the acute setting. In addition, the dicrotic notch, which usually occurs with aortic valve closure, is absent in severe AR. A condition called *pulsus bisferiens* is a common finding in the presence of AR, and this condition is due to the "tidal-wave effect" as regurgitant blood entering the ventricle during early diastole causes a reflected pressure wave that is seen in the aorta. In the PCWP tracing, an accentuated V wave commonly is seen in the presence of AR, presumably a reflection of the decrease in compliance of the ventricles.

Chronic AR can be caused by aortic root dilation, bicuspid valves, rheumatic fever, failing prostheses, endocarditis, and other conditions. With chronic AR, the LV dilates and becomes more compliant, reflected as a lower LVEDP, than in the acute phase. End-diastolic pressure may even be in the normal range until terminal failure is present. The systolic arterial pressure increases, and the diastolic pressure decreases. The former is due to the greater ventricular pressures generated, and the latter is due to continued runoff from the arterial system into the ventricle (Figure 3-10). AI imposes both a pressure load and a volume load on the left ventricle. Accordingly, the mass of the left ventricle can increase markedly if the condition is chronic.

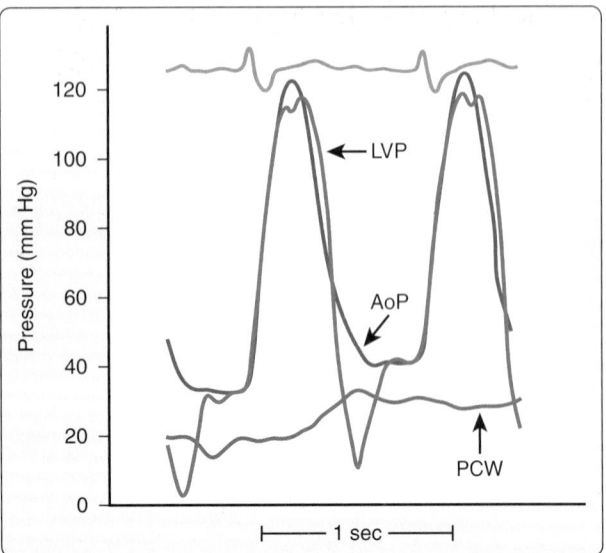

Figure 3-10 Aortic regurgitation. Simultaneous aortic (AoP), left ventricular (LVP), and pulmonary wedge (PCW) pressures demonstrate a wide aortic pulse pressure with absence of dicrotic notch, a rapid increase in LVP during early diastole caused by regurgitation, and increased PCW, reflective of increased left ventricular end-diastolic pressure. *(Modified from Grossman W, Baim DS: Profiles in valvular heart disease. In Grossman W [ed]: Cardiac Catheterization, Angiography, and Intervention, 4th ed. Philadelphia: Lea & Febiger, 1991, p 575.)*

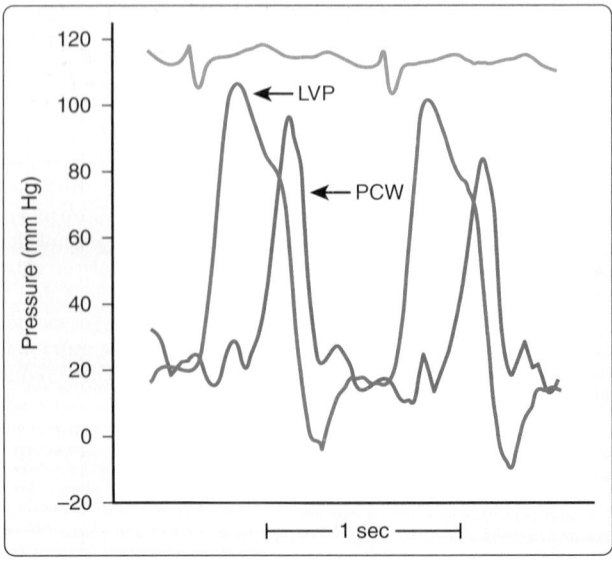

Figure 3-11 Acute mitral regurgitation caused by chordae tendineae rupture. Simultaneous left ventricular (LVP) and pulmonary wedge (PCW) pressures demonstrate large V wave caused by severe regurgitation into a normal-sized left atrium. Note that the V wave is delayed temporally from that shown in Figure 13-2. This delay is due to the time required for the pressure wave to travel through the compliant pulmonary venous and capillary beds to the pulmonary artery catheter. *(Modified from Grossman W, Baim DS [eds]: Profiles in valvular heart disease. In Grossman W [ed]: **Cardiac** Catheterization, Angiography, and Intervention, 4th ed. Philadelphia: Lea & Febiger, 1991, p 564.)*

Mitral Regurgitation

Mitral regurgitation either can be acute or chronic in nature. Acute mitral regurgitation usually is secondary to a condition such as acute ischemia leading to dysfunction of the papillary muscles of the mitral valve, or frank rupture of the structures after a significant MI. Rupture of the chordae tendineae can occur in the setting of endocarditis or spontaneously and cause acute mitral regurgitation (Figure 3-11). In this instance, it is not uncommon to see an enormously large V wave in the PCWP or LAP tracing, as ventricular blood freely flows back into a small, normal, and, thus, noncompliant LA. This also is accompanied by acute increases in the PAP and RAP, which can lead to significant clinical signs and symptoms.

In the setting of chronic mitral regurgitation, the LA can become quite large, nonfunctional, and compliant. Thus, a significant regurgitant fraction can exist in the presence of a minimal V wave on the pressure tracing.

Prosthetic Valves

The assessment of the function of a bioprosthetic valve is similar to the assessment of a native valve. However, the assessment of a mechanical prosthesis differs in several regards. First, patients with mechanical prostheses require chronic anticoagulation, and this typically needs to be interrupted for the catheterization procedure. Second, mechanical valves should not be crossed with catheters or wires, as doing so could cause sudden and severe valvular regurgitation. Finally, the leaflets of a mechanical prosthesis are (slightly) radioopaque, and leaflet motion can be assessed by fluoroscopy. The normal angles of opening and closing are specific to each valve model, size, and location, and such values are available from the manufacturer. Restricted mobility implies that pannus or thrombus has covered the leaflet(s). Videos 1 and 2 show such use of fluoroscopy. Similarly, if a mechanical prosthesis is unstable, it usually can be detected by fluoroscopy (see Video 3). Echocardiography also is used to evaluate prosthetic valves. However, transthoracic studies do not reliably view prosthetic mitral leaflets, and fluoroscopy can be repeated serially with little risk or inconvenience to the patient.

ANGIOGRAPHY

Ventriculography

Ejection Fraction Determination

Ventriculography routinely is performed in the single-plane 30-degree right anterior oblique (RAO) or biplane 60-degree left anterior oblique (LAO) and 30-degree RAO projections using 20 to 45 mL contrast with injection rates of 10 to 15 mL/sec (Box 3-3). Complete opacification of the ventricle without inducing ventricular extrasystoles is necessary for accurate assessment during ventriculography. These premature contractions not only alter the interpretation of mitral regurgitation, but result in a false increase in the global ejection fraction (EF).

The EF is a global assessment of ventricular function and is calculated as follows:

$$EF = [EDV - ESV]/EDV = SV/EDV$$

where EF is ejection fraction, EDV is end-diastolic volume, ESV is end-systolic volume, and SV is stroke volume.

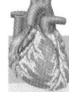

BOX 3-3 ANGIOGRAPHY

- Coronary anatomy
  - Left anterior descending coronary artery with diagonal and septal branches
  - Circumflex artery with marginal branches
  - Right coronary artery with conus, sinoatrial nodal, AV nodal, and right ventricular branches
  - Dominant circulation (posterior descending): 10% circumflex; 90% right coronary artery
- Coronary collaterals
- Coronary anomaly
- Ventriculography/aortography
- EF calculation
- Valvular regurgitation

The primary clinical method for calculation of ventricular volumes necessary for determining the EF utilizes the area length method described by Dodge et al. in 1960.[85] Before calculation, visual identification is the outer margin of the ventricular silhouette in both the RAO and LAO projections for both end-systole and end-diastole is necessary. The ventricle is approximated as an ellipsoid to facilitate volume calculations (Figure 3-12). Using biplane ventriculography to define major (L) and minor (M, N) axes, the following standard geometric formula for the area of an ellipsoid is used[86]:

$$A_{rao} = \pi[L_{rao}/2][M/2]$$

$$A_{lao} = \pi[L_{lao}/2][N/2]$$

Using planimetry, the area (A) is obtained in both LAO and RAO projections with volume (V) calculated as follows:

$$V = [8/3\pi][A_{rao}(A_{lao}/L_{min})]$$

with L_{min} being the shorter of L_{rao} and L_{lao}.

Single-plane calculation in the 30-degree RAO assumes M = N and L is the true long axis. Using the ellipsoid volume calculation V = π/6

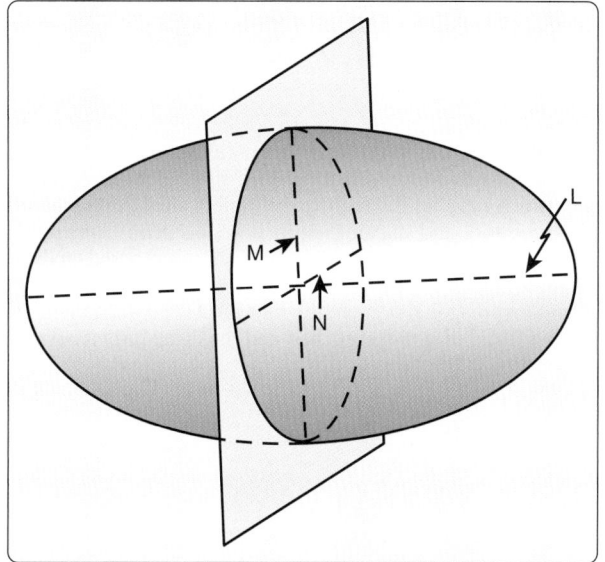

Figure 3-12 Ellipsoid used as reference figure for the left ventricle. The long axis (L) and the short axes (M and N) are shown. *(From Fifer MA, Grossman W: Measurement of ventricular volumes, ejection fraction, mass, and wall stress. In Grossman W [ed]: Cardiac Catheterization and Angiography, 3rd ed. Philadelphia: Lea & Febiger, 1986, p 284.)*

LMN, with M the planimetered area A and M = 4A/πL, the following formula is obtained:

$$V = [8A^2/3\pi L]$$

Calculation of EF does not require correction for magnification, but measurement of dimensions or calculation of volumes does. Such correction can be made using a calibrated grid imaged after cineangiography, or a part of the catheter that is in the ventricle can be used for calibration. Catheters with precise calibration markings are available. Contemporary software permits calibration that is based on the height of the table and detector. Mathematical equations for ventricular volume overestimate true volume; therefore, regression equations are used to correct for this.[86] This method or a variation has been incorporated into software on most modern systems.

There are problems with the use of EF as a measure of ventricular function. EFs calculated by various techniques (e.g., echocardiography, ventriculography, gated blood pool scanning) may not be identical because of the mathematical modeling involved. When single-plane ventriculography is used to calculate the EF, dysfunction of a nonvisualized segment (e.g., the lateral wall in an RAO ventriculogram) and global function may be overestimated. Most importantly, the EF is a load-dependent measure of ventricular function. Changes in preload, afterload, and contractility can significantly alter the EF determination. Thus, the EF can vary over time without any change in the myocardium, if the loading conditions or the inotropic conditions change. Identification of a load-independent measure of LV function has been the quest of many cardiologists over the years. The best approximation requires pressure-volume analysis at varying loading conditions to generate a series of curves. Although not used in routine clinical practice, pressure-volume curve analysis provides assessment of the systolic and diastolic properties of the ventricle and has been a valuable research tool (see Chapters 5 and 14). In addition to EF calculations, ventriculography allows for estimation of wall stress and LV mass.

Abnormalities in Regional Wall Motion

Segmental wall motion abnormalities are defined in both the RAO and LAO projections. A 0 to 5 grading scale may be used with hypokinesis (decreased motion), akinesis (no motion), and dyskinesis (paradoxic or aneurysmal motion). This scale is as follows: 0 = normal; 1 = mild hypokinesis; 2 = moderate hypokinesis; 3 = severe hypokinesis; 4 = akinesis; 5 = dyskinesis (aneurysmal). Each wall segment is identified as outlined in Figure 3-13 for both the LAO and RAO projections. These segments correspond roughly to vascular territories.

In addition to the information listed earlier, other things occasionally can be learned from the ventriculogram. Filling defects, particularly in akinetic or dyskinetic segments, can be seen and are suggestive of intracavitary thrombus. VSDs can be detected and localized. Obliteration of the LV cavity or outflow tract during systole suggests intracavitary obstruction.

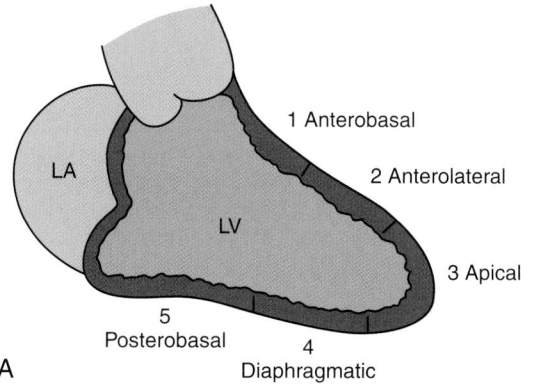

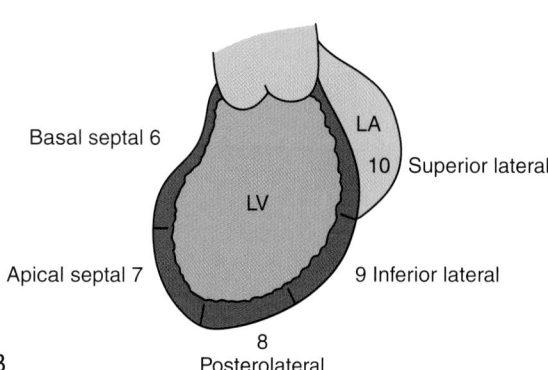

Figure 3-13 *A,* Terminology for left ventricular segments 1 through 5 analyzed from right anterior oblique ventriculogram. *B,* Terminology for left ventricular segments 6 through 10 analyzed from left anterior oblique ventriculogram. LA, left atrium; LV, left ventricle. *(A, B, from Principal Investigators of CASS and Their Associates: National Heart, Lung, and Blood Institute Coronary Artery Surgery Study. Circulation 63[suppl II]:1, 1981.)*

Assessment of Mitral Regurgitation

The qualitative assessment of the degree of mitral regurgitation can be made with LV angiography. It is dependent on proper catheter placement outside of the mitral apparatus in the setting of no ventricular ectopy. The assessment is, by convention, done on a scale of 1+ to 4+, with 1+ being mild and 4+ being severe mitral regurgitation. As defined by ventriculography, 1+ regurgitation is that in which the contrast clears from the LA with each beat, never causing complete opacification of the LA. Moderate or 2+ mitral regurgitation is present when the opacification does not clear with one beat, leading to complete opacification of the LA after several beats. In 3+ mitral regurgitation (moderately severe), the LA becomes completely opacified, becoming equal in opacification to the LV after several beats. In 4+ or severe regurgitation, the LA densely opacifies with one beat and the contrast refluxes into the pulmonary veins.

By combining data from left ventriculography and right-heart catheterization, a more quantitative assessment of mitral regurgitation can be made by calculating the regurgitant fraction. This can be effectively calculated by measuring the following: end-diastolic LV volume (EDV), end-systolic LV volume (ESV), and the difference between these two, or the total LV stroke volume (TSV). The TSV (stroke volume calculated from angiography) may be quite high, but it must be remembered that in the setting of significant mitral regurgitation, a significant portion of this volume will be ejected backward into the LA. The forward stroke volume (FSV) must be calculated from a measurement of forward CO by the Fick or thermodilution method. The regurgitant stroke volume (RSV) then can be calculated by subtracting the FSV from the TSV (TSV − FSV). The regurgitant fraction (RF) is then calculated as the RSV divided by the TSV:

$$RF = (RSV) / (TSV)$$

A regurgitant fraction less than 20% is considered mild, 20% to 40% is considered moderate, 40% to 60% is considered moderately severe, and greater than 60% is considered severe mitral regurgitation.

Aortography

The primary indication for aortography performed in the cardiac catheterization laboratory is to delineate the extent of AR. Secondary indications include defining supravalvular lesions and determining the origins of saphenous vein grafts (SVGs). Studies to differentiate proximal and distal dissections may be performed in the catheterization laboratory. However, TEE, MRI, and CT scanning with contrast are more commonly utilized today to make this diagnosis.[87]

Similar to mitral regurgitation, AR is graded 1+ to 4+ based on the degree of contrast dye present in the LV chamber during aortography. As with mitral regurgitation, assessment of AR is dependent on proper catheter placement free of the valve leaflets but not too high in the ascending aorta. Mild (1+) is transient filling of the LV cavity by contrast dye clearing after each systolic beat; moderate (2+) is a small amount of contrast dye regurgitated into the LV, but present throughout the subsequent systolic beat; moderately severe AR (3+) is a significant amount of contrast dye present in the LV throughout systole, but not the intensity of that in the aorta; severe AR (4+) is contrast dye in the LV consistent with the intensity of that in the aorta with rapid ventricular opacification and delayed clearance after aortic injection.

Coronary Arteriography

Description of Coronary Anatomy

The left main coronary artery is variable in length (Figure 3-14). The left main bifurcates into the circumflex (CX) and LAD arteries. Occasionally, the CX and LAD arteries may arise from separate ostia or the left main may trifurcate, creating a middle branch, the ramus intermedius, which supplies the high lateral wall of the left ventricle. Both septal perforators and diagonal branch vessels arise from the LAD, which is described as proximal, mid, and distal vessel based on the location of these branch vessels. The proximal LAD artery is before the first septal and first diagonal branch; the mid LAD is between the first and second septal and diagonal branches; and the distal LAD is beyond the

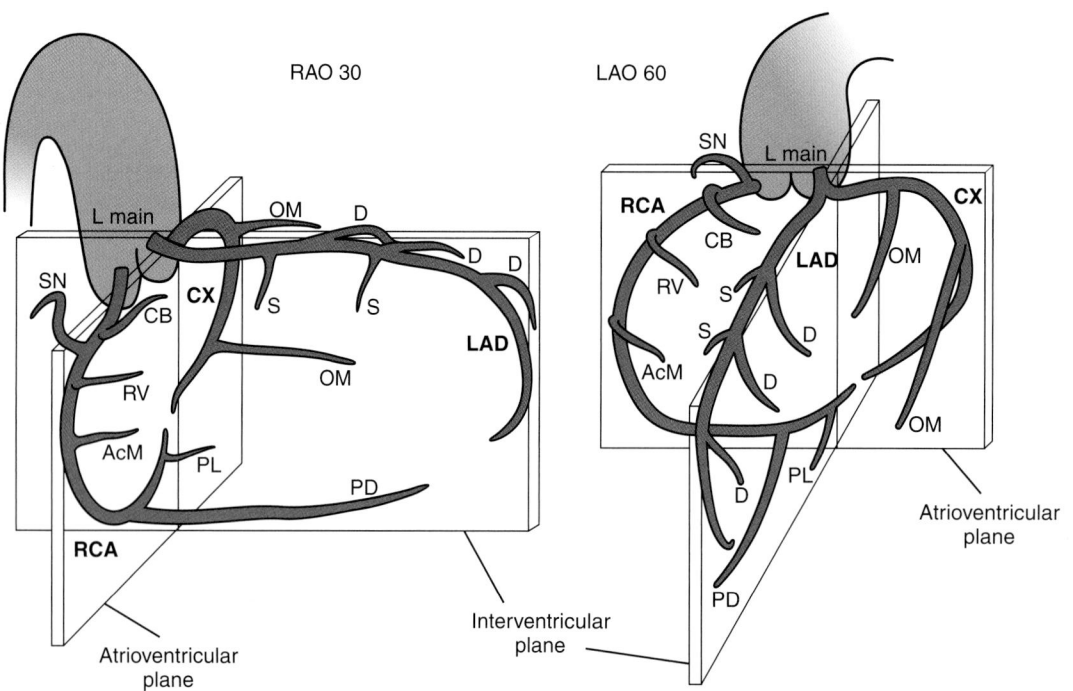

Figure 3-14 **Representation of coronary anatomy relative to the interventricular and arterioventricular valve planes.** Coronary branches are as indicated: AcM, acute marginal; CB, conus branch; CX, circumflex; D, diagonal; L main, left main; LAD, left anterior descending; OM, obtuse marginal; PD, posterior descending; PL, posterolateral left ventricular; RCA, right coronary; RV, right ventricular branch; S, septal; SN, sinus node branch. LAO, left anterior oblique; RAO, right anterior oblique. *(From Baim DS, Grossman W: Coronary angiography. In Grossman W, Baim DS [eds]: Cardiac Catheterization, Angiography, and Intervention, 4th ed. Philadelphia: Lea & Febiger, 1991, p 200.)*

major septal and large diagonal vessels. The distal LAD provides the apical blood supply in two thirds of patients, with the distal RCA supplying the apex in the remaining third (see Chapters 6 and 18).

The CX artery is located in the AV groove and is angiographically identified by its location next to the coronary sinus. The latter is seen as a large structure that opacifies during delayed venous filling after left coronary injections. Marginal branches arise from the CX artery and are the vessels in this coronary artery system usually bypassed. The CX artery in the AV groove is often not surgically approachable.

The dominance of a coronary system is defined by the origin of the posterior descending artery (PD), through which septal perforators supply the inferior one third of the ventricular septum. The origin of the AV nodal artery often is near the origin of the PD artery. In 85% to 90% of patients, the PD originates from the RCA. In the remaining 10% to 15% of patients, the CX artery creates the PD. Codominance, or a contribution from both the CX and RCA, can occur and is defined when septal perforators from both vessels arise and supply the posterior-inferior aspect of the left ventricle. Surgical bypass of this region may be difficult when this anatomy exists.

Coronary Anomalies

The coronary anomalies most frequently encountered during coronary angiography are listed in Table 3-7. Anomalous coronary origins are seldom of clinical or surgical significance, but are potentially time-consuming during coronary angiography. Rarely, anomalous coronary arteries arising from the opposite cusp and traversing between the PA and aorta may produce vessel compression and ischemia. The Bland–Garland–White syndrome occurs when the LAD arises from the PA. Although most patients present early in life, young adults with this syndrome also may present with sudden cardiac death or ischemic cardiomyopathy.[88] Coronary-cameral fistulas are not rare. Most are small and of no clinical significance.[89]

A variety of classification systems have been proposed for coronary anomalies. Some classification systems try distinguishing significant anomalies from minor ones, whereas other classification systems consider all anomalies anatomically, independent of clinical or hemodynamic repercussions.[90] The reported incidence of coronary anomalies varies. Unfortunately, the life-threatening anomalies, particularly an anomalous origin of the left coronary artery from the right sinus, often are diagnosed at autopsy.[90]

Assessing the Degree of Stenosis

By convention, the severity of a coronary stenosis is quantified as percentage diameter reduction. Multiple views of each vessel are recorded, and the worst narrowing is recorded and used to make clinical decisions. Diameter reductions can be used to estimate area reductions; for instance, 50% and 70% diameter reductions would result in 75% and 91% cross-sectional area reductions, respectively, if the narrowing were circumferential. Using the reduction in diameter as a measure of

lesion severity is difficult when diffuse CAD creates difficulty in defining "normal" coronary diameter. This is particularly true in patients with insulin-dependent diabetes, as well as in individuals with severe lipid disorders. In addition, the use of percentage diameter reduction does not account for the length of the stenosis.

Qualitative estimates of percentage of diameter reduction are highly variable among different observers, and not reflective of coronary flow. Using a Doppler velocity probe, White et al.[91] demonstrated that lesion severity was underestimated in the overwhelming majority of cases. When visual interpretation is required for clinical decisions, as opposed to research purposes, there may be a systematic bias toward overestimation of lesion severity. Quantitative coronary angiography was developed to overcome the pitfalls of qualitative visual interpretation of lumen reduction. Although cumbersome in its early iterations, most contemporary imaging systems include a usable quantification program.[92] Even with quantification, the limitations of angiography remain.[93] Accurate interpretation of coronary angiography and quantitation are possible only when high-quality images are obtained. Contrast injections must be forceful to fully opacify the artery, whereas pressure tracings are closely observed to prevent coronary artery dissection. When smaller catheters are used, injection may require smaller syringes or power injection for adequate coronary opacification. Branch vessels must clearly be separated utilizing cranial and caudal angulations. Periodic assessment of image quality is required to assure properly functioning imaging equipment.[15]

Intravascular ultrasound (IVUS) is a newer imaging modality that uses a miniature transducer in the lumen of the artery to generate a two-dimensional, cross-sectional image of the vessel. Although electronic (phased-array) transducers exist, the most commonly used intracoronary systems use mechanical rotation to provide 360-degree imaging. This rotation introduces the potential for artifacts that must be recognized as such. Refinements to these systems permit a transducer diameter of about 1 mm with an imaging frequency of 40 megahertz (MHz) for coronary arteries. However, the transducer is placed into the coronary (or peripheral) artery over a 0.014-inch guidewire. Thus, it entails more risk than angiography, and anticoagulation is mandatory. The transducer is placed distally in the vessel, and a mechanical system is used to withdraw the transducer at a controlled rate, typically 0.5 mm/sec, while a recording is made. Software permits reconstruction of serial cross-sectional images into longitudinal views, and volumetric analysis is possible. Both the lumen and the vessel wall can be imaged. The apposition of stent struts can be confirmed, and small dissections can be seen. Wall constituents, such as calcium and pooled lipids can be identified. Modifications permit analysis of "virtual histology." IVUS has been a critical research tool. For instance, early stent implantation was associated with a high risk for subacute thrombosis that seemed refractory to anticoagulants. IVUS identified incomplete expansion of many stents using the existing deployment techniques and incomplete apposition of the struts to the vessel wall. Deployment techniques were modified to include higher pressures and larger balloon diameters, and subacute thrombosis receded. The volumetric measurements with IVUS are sufficiently reproducible to measure the effects of medication on the progression of atherosclerotic plaque. IVUS is used clinically in selected situations. In a study comparing IVUS findings with quantitative angiography, the plaque burden at maximal obstruction frequently were underestimated by quantitative angiography.[93] Thus, IVUS can be used when angiography is equivocal. It also is useful in certain segments of the coronary tree, like the left main and bifurcations, where angiography may be limited. IVUS reports contain information on the diameter reductions and area reductions, which translate to angiographic values. However, an important value in the IVUS report is the minimal luminal area (MLA). Generally, an MLA less than 4.0 mm² in a proximal coronary vessel correlates with an ischemic response during perfusion imaging. An MLA less than 6.0 mm² in the left main correlates with ischemia. Finally, IVUS can be used to ensure optimal stent sizing and deployment. Similar equipment exists for peripheral vessels, although the role of IVUS in the periphery remains to be determined.

TABLE 3-7	Coronary Anomalies

Anomalous Coronary Origin

Left main coronary artery from right sinus of Valsalva separately or with right coronary artery

Circumflex artery as a separate origin off right cusp or with common origin with right coronary artery

Right coronary artery as a separate vessel from left cusp as separate ostia or as common ostia with circumflex as branch

Coronary Artery from Pulmonary Artery

Left coronary artery (Bland–Garland–White syndrome)

Right coronary artery

Fistula Formation from Normal Coronary Origin

Coronary branch vessels drain directly into right ventricle, pulmonary artery, coronary sinus, superior vena cava, pulmonary vein

Anatomic information usually is used to guide management decisions. However, recent work suggests that revascularization may offer no advantage over medical therapy when it is guided by anatomic data.[94] This has prompted a renewed interest in the physiologic assessment of coronary stenoses.[95] One method uses a Doppler probe that is incorporated into a standard, 0.014-inch angioplasty wire (Volcano Therapeutics, San Diego, CA). The Doppler probe is placed distal to the coronary stenosis, and baseline velocity is recorded. An intracoronary (or intravenous) agent is administered to produce maximal coronary dilation, and the velocity is recorded again. A normal response is about a fourfold increase in velocity, but for clinical use, a value of twofold is used. The stability of velocity recordings varies, and accurate readings require careful placement of the probe into the middle of the vessel. These concerns have limited the use of the Doppler wire in clinical practice. An alternative is the Pressure Wire (St. Jude Medical, St. Paul, MN), in which a micromanometer is incorporated into a standard angioplasty wire. Again, the micromanometer is placed distal to the stenosis, and maximal coronary dilation is induced with the administration of an intracoronary or intravenous vasodilator. The ratio of the distal pressure to the aortic pressure (measured at the tip of the guiding catheter) is calculated at peak vasodilation and is termed the *fractional flow reserve* (FFR). Correlation with nuclear stress testing has been good for both techniques. For instance, a ratio of distal pressure to proximal pressure after adenosine vasodilation (FFR < 0.75) predicts an abnormal nuclear perfusion scan result. This can aid in the assessment of an angiographically "borderline" stenosis. Clinical outcomes have been good for those with a greater ratio (FFR).[96,97] Moreover, when PCI is guided by pressure-wire measurements, as opposed to angiography, fewer stents are implanted and clinical outcomes are superior.[98,99]

Coronary Collaterals

Common angiographically defined coronary collaterals are described in Table 3-8. Although present at birth, these vessels become functional and enlarge only if an area of myocardium becomes hypoperfused by the primary coronary supply.[100] Angiographic identification

TABLE 3-8	Collateral Vessels

Left Anterior Descending Coronary Artery (LAD)

Right-to-Left

Conus to proximal LAD

Right ventricular branch to mid-LAD

Posterior descending septal branches at midvessel and apex

Left-to-Left

Septal to septal within LAD

Circumflex-OM to mid-distal LAD

Circumflex Artery (Cx)

Right-to-Left

Posterior descending artery to septal perforator

Posterior lateral branch to OM

Left-to-Left

Cx to Cx in AV groove (left atrial circumflex)

OM to OM

LAD to OM via septal perforators

Right Coronary (RCA)

Right-to-Right

Kugels—proximal RCA to AV nodal artery

RV branch to RV branch

RV branch to posterior descending

Conus to posterior lateral

Left-to-Right

Proximal mid and distal septal perforators from distal LAD OM to posterior lateral

OM to AV nodal

AV groove Cx to posterior lateral

AV, atrioventricular; OM, obtuse marginal; RV, right ventricular.

of collateral circulation requires both the knowledge of potential collateral source and prolonged imaging to allow for coronary collateral opacification.

The increased flow from the collateral vessels may be sufficient to prevent ongoing ischemia. A stenosis in a main coronary or branch vessel must reduce the luminal diameter by 80% to 90% to recruit collaterals for an ischemic area. Clinical studies suggest that collateral flow can double within 24 hours during an episode of acute ischemia.[101] However, well-developed collaterals require time to develop and only these respond to nitroglycerin (NTG). The RCA is a better collateralized vessel than the left coronary. Areas that are supplied by good collaterals are less likely to be dyskinetic or akinetic.

CATHETERIZATION REPORT

The promise of the electronic medical record is the timely availability of patients' medical information at sites that need it. Most catheterization laboratories have integrated the catheterization reports into the record system of the hospital, facilitating its retrieval in preoperative anesthesia clinics. However, it must be remembered that the information obtained in the cardiac catheterization laboratory is representative of the patient's pathophysiologic process at only one point in time. Therefore, these data are static and not dynamic. In addition, alterations in fluid and medication management before catheterization can influence the results obtained. The hemodynamic information usually is obtained after the patient has fasted for 8 hours. Particularly in patients with dilated, poorly contractile hearts, the diminished filling pressures seen in the fasted state may reduce the CO. In other circumstances, fluid status will be altered in the opposite direction. Patients with known renal insufficiency are hydrated overnight before contrast administration. In these instances, the right- and left-sided heart hemodynamics may not reflect the patient's usual status. In addition, medications may be withheld before catheterization, particularly diuretics. Acute β-blocker withdrawal can produce a rebound tachycardia, altering hemodynamics and potentially inducing ischemia.[102] These should be noted in interpreting the catheterization data.

Sedation may falsely alter blood gas and hemodynamic measurements if hypoxia occurs. Patients with chronic lung disease or Down syndrome may be particularly sensitive to sedatives, and respiratory depression may result in hypercapnia and hypoxia. Careful notations in the catheterization report must be made of medications administered, as well as the patient's symptoms. Ischemic events during catheterization may dramatically affect hemodynamic data. In addition, therapy for ischemia (e.g., NTG) may affect both angiographic and hemodynamic results.

Technical factors may influence coronary arteriography and ventriculography. The table in the catheterization laboratory may not hold very heavy patients. Patient size may limit X-ray tissue penetration and visualization and may prevent proper angulations. Stenosis at vessel bifurcations may not be identified in the hypertensive patient with tortuous vessels. Catheter-induced coronary spasm, most commonly seen proximally in the RCA, must be recognized, treated with NTG, and not reported as a fixed stenosis.[103] Myocardial bridging results in a dynamic stenosis seen most commonly in the mid-LAD during systole. This is seldom of clinical significance and should not be confused with a fixed stenosis present throughout the cardiac cycle. With ventriculography, frequent ventricular ectopy or catheter placement in the mitral apparatus may result in nonpathologic (artificial) mitral regurgitation. This must be recognized to avoid inappropriate therapy.

Finally, catheterization reports often are unique to institutions and often are purely computer generated, including valve area calculations. Familiarity with the catheterization report at each institution and discussions with cardiologists are essential to allow for a thorough understanding of the information and its location in the report, and the potential limitations inherent in any reporting process.

INTERVENTIONAL CARDIOLOGY: PERCUTANEOUS CORONARY INTERVENTION

This section is designed to present the current practice of interventional cardiology (Box 3-4). Although begun by Andreas Gruentzig in September 1977 as PTCA, catheter-based interventions have expanded dramatically beyond the balloon to include a variety of PCIs.[104] Worldwide, this field has expanded to include approximately 900,000 PCI procedures annually.[22]

The interventional cardiology section is divided into two subsections. The first subsection consists of a general discussion of issues that relate to all catheter-based interventions. This includes a general discussion of indications, operator experience, equipment and procedures, restenosis, and complications. Anticoagulation and controversial issues in interventional cardiology also are reviewed. The second subsection is devoted to a discussion of the various catheter-based systems for PCI. Beginning with the first, PTCA, most devices are presented, including current technology and devices in development. With this review, the cardiac anesthesiologist may better understand the current practice and future direction of interventional cardiology.

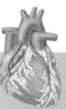

General Topics for All Interventional Devices

Indications

Throughout the history of PCI, both technology and operator expertise have improved continually. With the proper credentialing, experience, and current technology, the interventionalist now has the capabilities to go places in the coronary tree "where no man (or woman) has gone before." This is reflected in the expanded role for PCI. Although first restricted to patients with single-vessel disease and normal ventricular function who had a discrete, noncalcified lesion in the proximal vessel, PCI now is performed as preferred therapy in many groups of patients, including select patients with unprotected (no bypass grafts) left main stenosis.[22,105]

Box 3-5 provides a summary of current clinical indications for PCI. Primary PCI is the standard of care for patients with STEMI with or without cardiogenic shock.[28,106] Although initially reserved only for those patients considered suitable candidates for CABG, PCI routinely is performed in patients who are not candidates for CABG in both emergent and nonemergent settings.[22] In considering both the indications and the appropriateness of PCI, the physician must review the patient's historic presentation, including functional class, treadmill results with or without perfusion data, and wall motion assessment. Demonstrating ischemia noninvasively, either before procedure or with an intraprocedural physiologic assessment, avoids inappropriate procedures prompted by the "ocular-dilatory reflex" (lesion seen = lesion dilated).[97,107,108]

Absolute contraindications are few. Unprotected left-main stenosis in a patient who is a surgical candidate, diffusely diseased native vessels, or a single remaining conduit for myocardial circulation is approached by PCI only after a significant discussion with patient and surgeon.[22] Several series of unprotected left-main PCIs have been published, and this topic is in evolution.[105,109] Although the procedural risk may be low,

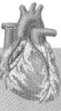

BOX 3-5 CLINICAL INDICATIONS FOR PERCUTANEOUS TRANSLUMINAL CORONARY INTERVENTIONAL PROCEDURES

Cardiac Symptoms
- Unstable angina pectoris/non–ST-segment myocardial infarction
- Angina refractory to antianginal medications
- Postmyocardial infarction angina
- Sudden cardiac death

Diagnostic Testing
- Early positive exercise tolerance testing
- Positive exercise tolerance test despite maximal antianginal therapy
- Large areas of ischemic myocardium on perfusion or wall motion studies
- Positive preoperative dipyridamole or adenosine perfusion study
- Electrophysiologic studies suggestive of arrhythmia related to ischemia

Acute Myocardial Infarction
- Cardiogenic shock
- Unsuccessful thrombolytic therapy in unstable patient with large areas of myocardium at risk
- Contraindication to thrombolytic therapy
- Cerebral vascular event
- Intracranial neoplasm
- Uncontrollable hypertension
- Major surgery < 14 days previously
- Potential for uncontrolled hemorrhage
- Probably preferred for all ST-elevation acute myocardial infarction (STEMI)

most left-main PCIs still are performed in patients who are not operative candidates; this is discussed in more detail later in the chapter. By definition, they are high-risk patients, and they continue to have a high rate of late events.[110] Multivessel PCI frequently is performed and remains a reasonable alternative to CABG in selected patients.[111] However, CABG remains the preferred therapy for many patients, particularly patients with diabetes. Finally, though currently performed, the role of PCI at facilities without onsite surgical capability is controversial.[22,24]

In addition to indications and contraindications, there is the concept of "appropriateness." The SCAI, Society of Thoracic Surgeons, American Academy of Thoracic Surgeons, the ACC, and the AHA published a consensus document on coronary revascularization in 2009.[112] This document attempted to identify the "appropriate" therapy for a given patient scenario, based on presentation, anatomy, medication, and noninvasive and invasive testing. For each scenario, revascularization was considered appropriate, inappropriate, or uncertain. Though far from all-inclusive, and not replacing the physician's judgment for the individual patient, this document provides an overview of potential appropriateness of medical therapy, PCI, and CABG.

Equipment and Procedure

Significant advances have been and will continue to be made with all aspects of PCI. Although the femoral artery is still the most commonly utilized access site, the radial artery is utilized more frequently for coronary interventions. Despite numerous advances, all PCIs still involve sequential placement of the following: guiding catheter in the ostium of the vessel, guiding wire across the lesion and into the distal vessel, and device(s) of choice at the lesion site. Routine central venous access is not required, as it increases access site complications. Its use is reserved for situations in which peripheral venous access is limited, temporary pacing may be required, or hemodynamic monitoring may be helpful.

Guiding catheters are available in multiple shapes and sizes for coronary and graft access, device support, and radial artery entry.[22,104] Guiding wires offer flexible tips for placement into tortuous vessels, as well as stiffer shafts to allow for the support of the newer devices during passage within the vessel. Separate guidewire placement within branch vessels may be required for coronary lesions at vessel bifurcations (Figure 3-15).

BOX 3-4 INTERVENTIONAL CARDIOLOGY TIMELINE

1977 Percutaneous transluminal coronary angioplasty
1991 Directional atherectomy
1993 Rotational atherectomy
1994 Stents with extensive antithrombotic regimen
1995 Abciximab approved
1996 Simplified antiplatelet regimen after stenting
2001 Distal protection
2003 Drug-eluting stents

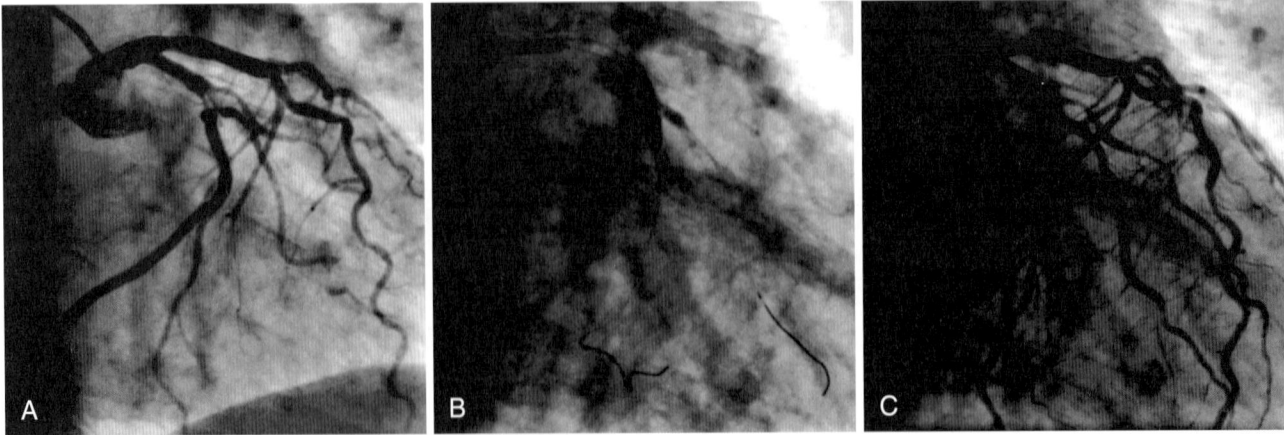

Figure 3-15 **Complex percutaneous coronary intervention.** *A*, Stenosis at bifurcation in circumflex. *B*, Kissing balloon inflation after "culotte" stent implantation in main circumflex and marginal branch. *C*, Final result is good in both branches.

In selecting the appropriate device for the lesion, quantitative angiography and/or IVUS may be used to determine the size of the vessel and composition of the lesion.[113,114]

While a device is in a coronary artery, blood flow is impeded to varying degrees. In vessels supplying large amounts of myocardium (e.g., proximal LAD), prolonged obstruction of flow is poorly tolerated. However, when smaller areas of myocardium are jeopardized or the distal vessel is well-collateralized, longer occlusion times are possible. Distal protection devices, which involve balloon occlusion, may result in loss of flow down the vessel for up to 5 minutes. However, with current technology, occlusion times seldom exceed 1 minute.

The performance of PCI immediately after a diagnostic procedure is known as "ad hoc intervention." Obviously preferred in emergent situations, this strategy is increasing in popularity for elective cases as well.[22] Ad hoc PCI requires careful preparation. The patient and family must understand not only the risks and benefits of the diagnostic procedure, but the risks and benefits of various revascularization strategies.[115] This requires that informed consent be obtained for all potential procedures before sedation is given. The cardiologist must carefully assess each clinical situation and must have a collegial relationship with his or her surgical colleagues, if expedited consultation is required to avoid operator bias, and with anesthesiology colleagues, for the rare occasions when emergency surgery is required. Finally, a flexible schedule must allow for the additional time required for the PCI within the catheterization laboratory.[115]

Anti-ischemic medications may permit longer periods of vessel occlusion before signs and symptoms of ischemia become limiting.[116] This additional time could permit the completion of a complex case or allow the use of distal protection devices. Most centers use either intracoronary or intravenous NTG at some point during the procedure to treat or prevent coronary spasm. Intracoronary calcium channel blockers frequently are used to treat vasospasm and the "no-reflow" phenomenon.[117] The latter term describes an absence of flow in a coronary vessel when there is no epicardial obstruction. No-reflow is associated with a variety of adverse outcomes; it is seen when acutely occluded vessels are opened during an MI or when PCI is performed in old saphenous vein bypass grafts. The cause is believed to be microvascular obstruction from embolic debris or microvascular spasm, or both. Intracoronary calcium antagonists may help to restore normal flow, and nicardipine is preferred for its relative lack of hemodynamic and conduction effects.[118] NTG therapy rarely is necessary after PCI unless signs of heart failure or ongoing ischemia are noted.

After the PCI procedure, the patient is transferred to the appropriate unit for the level of care required. The ST-elevation acute myocardial infarction (STEMI) patient is admitted to the cardiac care unit, the inpatient with an acute coronary syndrome (ACS) often returns to the previous level of care, and the outpatient returns to the equivalent of the pre/post holding area. As the field of interventional cardiology has changed since the 1970s, so has the care of the patient after PCI.[119] Multiple factors enter into the location and duration of post-PCI care. Hospitals must work with physicians and patients to create the appropriate pathways to provide quality patient care.

Restenosis

Once PTCA/PCI became an established therapeutic option for treating patients with CAD, it was soon realized that there were two major limitations: acute closure and restenosis. Stents and antiplatelet therapy significantly decreased the incidence of acute closure. Before stents were available, restenosis occurred in 30% to 40% of PTCA procedures. With stent use, this figure decreased to about 20%. Thus, restenosis remained the Achilles heel of intracoronary intervention until the current drug-eluting stent (DES) era.

Restenosis usually occurs within the first 6 months after an intervention and has three major mechanisms: vessel recoil, negative remodeling, and neointimal hyperplasia.[120] Vessel recoil is caused by the elastic tissue in the vessel and occurs early after balloon dilation. It is no longer a significant contributor to restenosis because metal stents are nearly 100% effective in preventing any recoil.[121] Negative remodeling refers to late narrowing of the external elastic lamina and adjacent tissue. This accounted for up to 75% of lumen loss in the past.[120] This process also is prevented by metal stents and no longer contributes to restenosis. Neointimal hyperplasia is the major component of in-stent restenosis. Neointimal hyperplasia is exuberant in the diabetic patient, and this serves to explain the increased incidence of restenosis in this population.[122] DESs limit neointimal hyperplasia and have dramatically reduced the frequency of in-stent restenosis.[123,124]

Establishing the true rate of restenosis requires a uniform definition. Clinical restenosis is defined as recurrence of angina or a positive stress test that results in a repeat procedure. Angiographic restenosis is defined at repeat catheterization and has greater rates than clinical restenosis. To be classified as a restenotic lesion at follow-up catheterization, at least a 50% reduction in luminal diameter must be present visually with a decrease of 0.72 mm quantitatively from the postpercutaneous transluminal coronary intervention result.[125] IVUS can measure cross-sectional area and also may be used in assessing restenosis.[120] Because restenosis occurs within 6 to 12 months after intervention, symptoms occurring thereafter more commonly represent progression of atherosclerotic disease.[125]

Several clinical factors have been linked to restenosis. These include cigarette smoking, diabetes mellitus, male sex, absence of prior infarction, and UA. Of these, only diabetes consistently has shown a statistically significant association with restenosis.[125] Lesion characteristics proved to predict restenosis are lesion location, baseline stenosis diameter and length, postpercutaneous transluminal coronary intervention stenosis severity, and adjacent artery diameter.[125] In the stent era, baseline stenosis is no longer a predictor, whereas a large reference vessel diameter is associated with a lower risk for restenosis.[126]

Medical therapy to decrease restenosis has been unrewarding.[127] Aspirin decreases the risk for acute occlusion but does not significantly decrease the risk for restenosis.[128] Radiation therapy can be delivered from a source within the vessel lumen (vascular brachytherapy) and is discussed in more detail later. Brachytherapy has been useful to treat in-stent restenosis, but results for prophylactic treatment have been disappointing.[129,130]

The major gains in combating restenosis have been in the area of stenting.[131] Intracoronary stents maximize the increase in lumen area during the PCI procedure and decrease late lumen loss by preventing recoil and negative remodeling. However, neointimal hyperplasia is enhanced due to a "foreign body-like reaction" to the stents. Different stent designs, as well as varying strut thickness, lead to different restenosis rates.[132,133] Systemic administrations of antiproliferative drugs decrease restenosis but cause significant systemic side effects. DESs, with a polymer utilized to attach the antiproliferative drug to the stent, have shown the best results to date for decreasing restenosis.[123,124,134]

In the days of balloon angioplasty, the risk for acute vessel closure was in the 5% to 10% range, but these events occurred almost exclusively in the catheterization laboratory or within the first 24 hours. Acute closure was related to dissection, thrombosis, or both. Emergent bypass surgery was frequently necessary to salvage myocardium. Bare metal stents (BMSs) reduced the incidence of acute closure dramatically but introduced a less-common phenomenon, subacute thrombosis.[135] Any thrombosis that occurs outside of the catheterization laboratory is likely to cause MI, and death is common if it occurs outside of the hospital. Subacute thrombosis is defined as thrombosis occurring more than 24 hours but less than 30 days after stent implantation. Adequate stent deployment and thienopyridine therapy reduced the frequency of subacute stent thrombosis (SST) to about 1%. By 1 month, neointima covered the stent struts, and the risk for thrombosis became very low, permitting discontinuation of thienopyridine treatment.[136]

Important lessons were learned when stent placement was accompanied by brachytherapy. Late stent thrombosis (> 30 days) was recognized as an important problem, and it was related to damaged neointima with delayed coverage of the stent struts. Prolonged use of thienopyridines seemed to reduce the likelihood of late thrombosis.[137]

In anticipation of a similar situation, namely, delayed stent coverage by neointima, the clinical trials of DESs incorporated prolonged thienopyridine therapy. In these clinical trials of predominantly low-risk patients treated with a 3- to 6-month course of thienopyridines, the risk for stent thrombosis was noted to be identical to that seen with BMSs, at least out to 1 year.[138] However, case reports and registry reports began to describe a new phenomenon with DESs, "very late stent thrombosis," defined as stent thrombosis occurring more than 1 year after implantation. Pathologic reports described incomplete tissue coverage of DESs at late time points.[139] In response to this information, the U.S. Food and Drug Administration (FDA) convened a panel to evaluate the problem in December 2006. Several specialty organizations responded by recommending that the course of clopidogrel be extended to 1 year after implantation of a DES, if no contraindications existed.[140,141] Many controversies are related to this topic, such as the relationship of off-label use to "very late stent thrombosis" and whether newer DESs carry the same risk. These are beyond the scope of this chapter, but it is sufficient to say that discontinuation of antiplatelet therapy should be approached with caution.

Anticoagulation

Thrombosis is a major component in ACSs, as well as acute complications during PCI; its management has evolved since its inception and will continue to evolve in the future[142,143] (Box 3-6). Proper anticoagulation regimens are essential to limit bleeding complications, as well as thrombotic complications, both of which negatively impact prognosis.[144] This is most important with interventional procedures, in which the guiding catheter, wire, and device in the coronary artery serve as nidi for thrombus. In addition, catheter-based interventions disrupt the vessel wall, exposing thrombogenic substances to blood. Table 3-9 summarizes the current anticoagulation agents utilized in the setting of PCI (see Chapter 31).

The primary pathway for clot formation during PCI has proved to be platelet mediated. This has prompted a focus on aggressive antiplatelet therapy. Aspirin was developed in the late 19th century and subsequently found to block platelet activation by irreversible acetylation of cyclooxygenase. It remains the foundation of antiplatelet therapy for PCI patients. When administered at least 24 and preferably up to 72 hours before the intervention in doses of 81 to 1500 mg, aspirin decreases thrombotic complications.[142] Aspirin resistance and combination therapy with nonsteroidal anti-inflammatory drugs are controversial.[145] Cilostazol, a phosphodiesterase inhibitor with antiplatelet effects, has been used in peripheral vascular disease; data on the use of cilostazol after coronary intervention remain inconclusive.[146]

The thienopyridines, ticlopidine (Ticlid), clopidogrel (Plavix), and prasugrel (Effient), block platelet activation by irreversibly binding to

BOX 3-6   ANTICOAGULATION

- Antithrombin agents used
  - Heparin (IV during PCI)
  - Enoxaparin (SQ before, IV during PCI)
  - Bivalirudin (IV during PCI)
  - Argatroban (IV during PCI)
  - Warfarin (PO after PCI—rarely)
- Antiplatelet agents used
  - Aspirin (PO before and after PCI)
  - Ticlopidine (PO before and after PCI)
  - Clopidogrel (PO before and after PCI—preferred)
  - Prasugrel (PO before and after PCI—new)
  - Ticagrelor (PO before and after PCI—awaiting approval)
  - Abciximab (IV during PCI bolus + 12-hour infusion)
  - Eptifibatide (IV during PCI bolus + 18-hour infusion)
  - Tirofiban (IV before, during, and after PCI)

TABLE 3-9	Anticoagulation in Interventional Cardiology			
Medication	*Dose*	*Mechanism of Action*	*Duration of Treatment*	*Binding*
Antiplatelet Agents				
Aspirin	75–325 mg	Acetylates cyclooxygenase	Indefinite	Irreversible
Thienopyridines (clopidogrel)	300–600 mg load 75 mg/day	Binds platelet ADP	1–12 mo	Irreversible
GPIIB/IIIA Inhibitors				Receptor
Anticoagulants				
Heparin	Agent-specific receptor ACT specific	Platelet IIB/IIIA receptor Indirect inhibition of thrombin	12–18 hr after PTCI During PCI	60–90 min after infusion
Low-molecular-weight heparin	Agent specific	Inhibition of factor Xa	During PCI	8–12 hr
Direct thrombin inhibitors	Agent specific	Direct inhibition of thrombin	During PCI	Slowly reversible

ACT, activated coagulation time; ADP, adenosine diphosphate; GP, glycoprotein; PCI, percutaneous coronary intervention; PTCI, percutaneous transluminal coronary intervention.

the ADP ($P2Y_{12}$) receptors. Ticlopidine was the initial thienopyridine used for PCI patients. However, side effects, including dyspepsia, neutropenia, and a small but clinically significant incidence of thrombotic thrombocytopenic purpura (TTP), led to its replacement by clopidogrel, which has a lower incidence of TTP.[147,148] Clopidogrel has been shown to be beneficial in patients with ACSs for up to 9 months of therapy, both with and without PCI.[149] A 1-month course of clopidogrel is standard therapy after implantation of a BMS for stable disease. An extended course of therapy is used when BMSs are implanted for ACSs.[150] At least 1 year of clopidogrel therapy is recommended when a DES is implanted for any indication.[140] Because clopidogrel (and ticlopidine and prasugrel) is a prodrug, its onset of action is slow unless a loading dose is used. A loading dose of 300 mg of clopidogrel ideally is given at least 4 hours before the procedure. Recent work has shown it is possible to achieve more rapid platelet inhibition when a 600-mg bolus is administered.[151] The relative efficacy and safety of clopidogrel have been established in men and women; however, the variability in individual responsiveness has raised concerns.[152,153]

Prasugrel (Effient) recently was approved for use in the United States. Like clopidogrel and ticlopidine, it is a prodrug that is converted into an irreversible antagonist of the ADP ($P2Y_{12}$) receptor. However, its onset of action is faster and less variable. When compared with clopidogrel in patients with ACSs, prasugrel reduced ischemic complications (nonfatal MI, need for urgent revascularization, and stent thrombosis), but caused more bleeding complications. An unfavorable risk/benefit ratio was identified for three groups: age $\geq$ 75 years, body weight less than 60 kg, or history of stroke or transient ischemic attack (TIA). Bleeding related to CABG was significantly greater with prasugrel, and surgery should be delayed to permit recovery of platelet function, if possible.[154]

Several additional issues should be discussed regarding antiplatelet therapy. Clopidogrel therapy for ACSs decreases cardiac events, but concerns have been raised about bleeding should CABG be necessary. The consistency and magnitude of this observation have not been sufficient to limit its use in these situations.[155] Management of patients undergoing invasive, noncardiac procedures on dual antiplatelet therapy is complicated and requires consideration of all options. The risks for drug discontinuation (stent thrombosis, MI, death) must be weighed against the risks of continuation of medicines (bleeding) and the risks of cancellation or deferral of the procedure.[156] All antiplatelet and anticoagulant medications increase the risk for bleeding, and dual-antiplatelet therapy increases the risk more than single therapy. The ACC, the American College of Gastroenterology, and the AHA published a Clinical Expert Consensus Document in 2008. This document recommended therapy with a proton pump inhibitor (PPI) for virtually all patients receiving dual-antiplatelet therapy.[157] More recently, observational data suggested that the combination of clopidogrel and a PPI was associated with a greater rate of ischemic events, and ex-vivo studies showed that the combination was associated with less inhibition of platelet function than was clopidogrel alone. This led to an FDA warning about the combination (11/17/2009). Other data suggest that the clinical risk of adding a PPI to clopidogrel may be negligible,[154] but the issue remains contentious.[158] Finally, combining antiplatelet and antithrombin therapy increases bleeding risks. This requires careful consideration of the indications for each therapy as the risks and benefits of combination therapy are weighed.[154,159]

Unfractionated heparin (UFH) has been used since the inception of PTCA. Traditional anticoagulant therapy for PCI was an initial heparin dose of 10,000 units. Currently, weight-adjusted heparin administration is routine. The ACT is used to guide additional heparin therapy with the ACT in the range of 300 to 350 seconds for patients not receiving glycoprotein IIb/IIIa inhibitors (GPIs) and 200 to 250 seconds for patients receiving these inhibitors of platelet aggregation[160] (see Chapter 17). Protamine is not used routinely, and the femoral sheaths are removed once the ACT is 150 seconds or less. Limitations of UFH include a variable antithrombotic effect requiring frequent ACT monitoring, inability to inhibit clot-bound thrombin, and concerns regarding heparin-induced thrombocytopenia syndrome. This has led to the search for a replacement for UFH.[161]

As an alternative to heparin, direct thrombin inhibitors have been investigated in the setting of PCI. The synthetic compound, bivalirudin (Angiomax; The Medicines Company), is the best studied of these agents. The advantage of the direct thrombin inhibitors is the direct dose response and the shorter half-life, allowing for earlier sheath removal and less frequent bleeding complications. The Bivalirudin Angioplasty Trial randomized 2161 patients and supported the hypothesis that bivalirudin reduces ischemic complications marginally, but reduces bleeding dramatically during PCI, compared with UFH.[162] REPLACE-2 trial (Randomized Evaluation in PCI Linking Angiomax to Reduced Clinical Events) randomized 6010 patients undergoing PCI (primarily stenting) to bivalirudin or UFH with glycoprotein (GP) IIb/IIIa inhibition.[163] MACEs were similar between the two groups, but major bleeding was significantly less in the bivalirudin group. ACUITY (Acute Catheterization and Urgent Intervention Triage strategY) trial studied 13,819 patients with ACSs undergoing PCI, comparing bivalirudin alone with either UFH or enoxaparin and a GPIIa/IIIb inhibitor. One-year results showed no difference in composite ischemia or mortality among the three groups.[164] The HORIZONS-AMI trial randomized 3602 STEMI patient undergoing PCI to bivalirudin or UFH with GPIIb/IIIa inhibitor. The bivalirudin had fewer clinical events, a lower mortality (cardiac and total), and less major bleeding at 1 year.[165]

Argatroban is another direct thrombin inhibitor and also is approved for use during PCI, although fewer data are available. Although easier to use than heparin, the direct thrombin inhibitors are more expensive than UFH, but similar in cost to the combination of UFH and a GP IIb/IIIa inhibitor. There currently is no known agent to reverse the effects of these new compounds (see Chapter 31). In patients with normal renal function, coagulation can be expected to return to normal in about 2 hours.

LMWHs are obtained by depolymerization of standard UFH. LMWHs were developed to overcome the limitations of UFH.[166] Enoxaparin (Lovenox) has been studied extensively in patients with ACSs. Overall, enoxaparin use leads to a slight reduction in the occurrence of MI when compared with UFH and has a similar side-effect profile.[167] In PCI, the NICE (National Investigators Collaborating on Enoxaparin) trials were registries of patients treated with enoxaparin instead of UFH during PCI.[168] In addition, the SYNERGY (Superior Yield of the New strategy of Enoxaparin, Revascularization, and GlYcoprotein IIb/IIIa Inhibitors) trial was a randomized comparison of enoxaparin and UFH in patients with an ACS in whom early catheterization was planned; about half of both groups underwent PCI.[169] Based on these and other smaller trials, enoxaparin and UFH seem to be associated with similar rates of cardiac events and bleeding complications when used during PCI. Thus, most interventionalists are comfortable with the use of enoxaparin for ACSs and the management of patients receiving enoxaparin in the periprocedural period. However, UFH offers several advantages in the patient who arrives in the laboratory without prior antithrombin therapy: a shorter half-life, facilitating sheath removal; the ability to easily monitor its effect with the ACT; and the ability to reverse its effect with protamine.

The OASIS 5 trial studied 20,078 patients with ACS randomized to enoxaparin or fondaparinux. Fondaparinux is a synthetic pentasaccharide thought to bind to the high-affinity binding site of the anticoagulant factor, antithrombin III, increasing the anticoagulant activity of antithrombin III 1000-fold. In patients receiving fondaparinux plus either GPIIb/IIIa agents or thienopyridines, bleeding was reduced and net clinical outcomes were improved compared with enoxaparin.[170]

Arterial thrombi are rich in platelets. Prevention of these thrombi is complicated by the fact that platelets aggregate in response to many stimuli. Aspirin inhibits only one of these pathways. The final common aggregation pathway is the IIb/IIIa GP on the platelet surface. Fibrinogen can bind to two IIb/IIIa receptors on separate platelets to permit aggregation. Several compounds target this receptor. The monoclonal antibody, abciximab (ReoPro) was the first GPIIb/IIIa inhibitor approved. Abciximab is used as a bolus followed by a 12-hour infusion. Bleeding times increase to more than 30 minutes with ex vivo platelet aggregation nearly abolished. The platelet binding of this compound essentially is irreversible, requiring more than 48 hours for normal platelet function to return. During the clinical trials of this agent, patients requiring emergency CABG experienced no significant increase in adverse events with platelet transfusions used to restore normal platelet function. In the EPIC (European Prospective Investigation into Cancer and Nutrition) study of high-risk PCI patients, abciximab reduced early ischemic complications by 35% and late events by 26%, with an increase in vascular complications.[171] In the EPILOG (Evaluation in PTCA to improve long-term outcome with Abciximab GP IIb/IIIa blockade) study, a similar benefit in lower risk interventional patients was seen.[172] In addition, fewer vascular complications occurred when adjunctive heparin was used in lower doses and vascular access site management improved. Abciximab is more expensive than the other IIb/IIIa inhibitors, and its repeated use may lead to thrombocytopenia.[173]

The other GPIIb/IIIa inhibitor compounds, eptifibatide (Integrilin) and tirofiban (Aggrastat), are not antibodies but rather synthetic agents that bind reversibly to the IIb/IIIa receptor. Both have half-lives of approximately 1.5 hours in patients with normal renal function with normal hemostasis returning in under 6 hours after cessation of the medication.[174] Standard doses lead to very high plasma concentrations of these medicines; thus, platelet transfusion is less effective in correcting the hemostatic defect than with abciximab. Studies have identified the superiority of eptifibatide plus UFH to UFH alone in stable patients undergoing PCI, the superiority of abciximab plus UFH to UFH alone, as well as the superiority of abciximab to tirofiban in more unstable patients undergoing PCI.[175,176] GPIs have not been proved beneficial in SVG interventions.[177] Currently, the choice of GPIIb/IIIa inhibitor for the patient undergoing PCI is controversial. They are all expensive, but abciximab is the most expensive. A variety of factors, including patient acuity, presence or absence of diabetes, renal function, pretreatment with clopidogrel, use of bivalirudin, and cost enter into the decision of which, if any, GPIIb/IIIa inhibitor should be used. For ACS patients, including those with STEMI, adequate pretreatment with clopidogrel may provide a benefit in low-risk patients that is comparable with that from GPIs at a fraction of the cost.[178,179] Several oral IIb/IIIa inhibitors were used in clinical trials, but results were disappointing for reasons that remain unclear.[180]

Thrombolytic therapy has been used for the treatment of STEMI since the 1980s. Although some of the early studies used intracoronary administration of thrombolytics, the need for a catheterization laboratory precluded widespread adoption, and intravenous administration of thrombolytics became standard treatment for STEMI. Several agents have been used for intravenous treatment of STEMI, including streptokinase, anistreplase, alteplase, reteplase, and tenecteplase.[181] Alteplase, reteplase, and tenecteplase are recombinant variations of tissue plasminogen activator, and are all specific for fibrin (as opposed to fibrinogen). They differ primarily in their half-lives, a difference that affects the dosing regimens. Since the early 1990s, emergent or primary PCI has evolved as an alternative and often preferable treatment to intravenous thrombolytics. With both therapies, time to treatment correlates with myocardial salvage and clinical outcome.[182] In the setting of planned primary PCI, adjunctive thrombolytic agents, classified as facilitated PCI, have not proved beneficial and may be detrimental.[28,183] In patients with unsuccessful thrombolytic therapy, rescue PCI is beneficial, but not without risk, whereas repeat thrombolysis is ineffective.[28,184]

Outcomes: Success and Complications

An important component of an interventional cardiology program is quality assessment. This is not just a score card of complications; it is a process in which risk-adjusted outcomes are compared with national standards, and the comparisons are used to identify avenues for improvement.[33,34] The tracking of outcome data has been a feature of interventional cardiology since its beginning and contributed to the rapid developments in the field. The history of interventional cardiology has been marked by an increase in success rates with a simultaneous decrease in adverse events. This reflects both significant

technologic advancement and increased operator skill, both of which were facilitated by the systematic collection of outcomes data. PCI once was considered successful when the luminal narrowing was reduced to less than 50% residual stenosis.[185] In current practice with stent placement, seldom is a residual stenosis greater than 20% accepted, and excellent stent expansion without edge dissection is required before termination of the procedure.[127] The initial National Heart, Lung, and Blood Institute (NHLBI) PTCA registry from 1979 to 1983 reported a success rate of 61% and a major coronary event rate of 13.6%. The 1985 to 1986 NHLBI registry reported a success rate of 78%, with the incidence of AMI rate as 4.3% and emergency CABG rate as 3.4%.[186] In the stent era, success rates are more than 90% and emergent surgery rates less than 1% in laboratories performing more than 400 PCIs.[186] In a multicenter study of more than 8000 angioplasty patients from the 1980s, an overall cardiac mortality rate of 0.16% in elective cases was reported.[187] The Society for Cardiac Angiography and Interventions' registry data were published for the years 1991 to 1996. This showed a success rate of 95%, an emergent CABG rate of 1.5%, and a mortality rate of 0.5%.[188]

The ACC developed the National Cardiovascular Data Registry (NCDR) in the 1990s. Currently, at least 700 of the more than 2100 laboratories in the United States participate. Participation in ACC/NCDR is voluntary currently and requires a facility to dedicate an employee to data entry. Outcomes for both diagnostic and interventional procedures are tabulated, adjusted for baseline risk, and provided to the participating facility. Results from an ACC/NCDR publication are listed in Table 3-10.

Recent plateaus in the rates of success and complications reflect not only the maturity of the field and changes in demographics but the scope of practice of PCI. As older patients with more comorbidities undergo PCI, further statistical improvements will be harder to achieve, but risk-adjusted outcomes must be studied. From et al[189] looked at a 19-year experience with PCI in nonagenarians (≥ 90 years). In these 138 patients, there was a high technical success rate and relatively low morbidity and mortality rate when the patients were properly selected. Patients with vessels that have been totally occluded for more than 3 months have been studied. In an era of increased technical advances, these patients have seen improved procedural success, long-term vessel patency, and survival outcomes.[190] Patients more than 3 days after MI with vessel occlusion have been similarly studied. This study, the Occluded Artery Trial (OAT), entered 2201 of these patients, followed them for more than 3 years, and demonstrated no benefit across various risk categories when PCI was performed.[191] Continued attention to outcomes data will help to identify the limits of PCI.

The incidence of procedure-related MI is controversial and depends on the definition of MI (new Q waves, total creatine kinase [CK] increase, CK-isoform elevation, troponin elevation).[192] Increased CK levels occur in approximately 15% of catheter-based interventional procedures, with significant increases (threefold baseline) present in 8%.[192] These figures are even greater for interventions in SVGs and

TABLE 3-10	Morbidity and Mortality for the Percutaneous Coronary Intervention Patient	
Complication	Outcome
Dissection	5%
Abrupt closure	1.9%
Successful reopening	41%
Angiographic success	94.5%
Postpercutaneous coronary intervention myocardial infarction	0.4%
Coronary artery bypass graft	1.9%
Death	1.4%
Clinical success	92.2%
No adverse events	96.5%

From Anderson HV, Shaw R, Brindis RG, et al: A contemporary overview of percutaneous coronary interventions, the American College of Cardiology-National Cardiovascular Registry Data (ACC-NCDR). *J Am Coll Cardiol* 39:1096, 2002.

with some devices. For years, routine enzymatic assessment of interventional procedural infarctions has been at the discretion of the operator. Some studies suggest that long-term outcome is adversely related to even small periprocedural increases of CK ("infarctlets").[192] These increases are reduced by GPIs.[158] Stone et al[193] published data from 7143 PCI patients. In this study, CK-MB increases of more than eight times the upper limit of normal were predictive of death in the subsequent 2-year follow-up. However, smaller enzyme increases, including a threefold increase of enzymes seen in 17.9% of patients, proved to have no impact on survival.[193]

In 1988 and then revised in 1993, the ACC/AHA task force developed a lesion morphology classification in an attempt to correlate the complexity of lesions with outcomes. This anatomic characterization of lesion complexity is outlined in Table 3-11. However, as operators gained experience and equipment improved, complication rates have decreased across all subsets. A 1998 study of more than 1000 consecutive lesions identified success rates for A, B1, and B2 lesions as approximately equal (95–96%), with only C lesions having success rates of less than 90% (88%).[194] The Mayo Clinic devised a risk score for PCI and recently compared this with the ACC/AHA criteria in 5064 PCIs. They found that the ACC/AHA criteria better predicted success, whereas complications were better predicted with the Mayo classification.[195]

Bleeding after PCI has been studied extensively.[196] Various anticoagulation regimens have been studied; in particular, the use of bivalirudin compared with heparin and a GPIIb/IIIa agent in both elective and emergent primary PCI. Significantly less bleeding occurred in patients receiving bivalirudin.[197] In addition, radial artery access has been compared with femoral access. Though complications can occur with the radial approach, bleeding is significantly reduced when radial atesy access is utilized rather than the femoral approach.[41] This is particularly important because mortality is increased when significant bleeding complications occur or blood transfusions are required, or both.[144,196]

Iatrogenic pericardial effusion and tamponade are infrequent complications of PCI but may be life-threatening if a large perforation occurs or a small perforation goes unrecognized.[198] Because this is most commonly an acute event, relatively small amounts of blood can cause hemodynamic compromise. The incidence during PCI varies and commonly is reported as occurring in ≤ 1% of cases. However, it is dependent on guidewire, and interventional devices with hydrophilic wires and atherectomy catheters are more likely to be involved. Tamponade can occur in non-PCI procedures, such as AF ablation, pacemaker placement, valvuloplasty, percutaneous closure devices, and percutaneous valve replacement. Prompt recognition of tamponade is required after PCI or other cardiac procedures, and can be facilitated with emergent echocardiography. Pericardiocentesis is life-saving and should be performed without delay.[198]

Intimal dissection was a significant issue in the present era, occurring in up to 10% of all PTCAs. Propagation of the intimal dissection is the leading cause of vessel occlusion during an intervention. Normally initiated by arterial disruption by the PCI device, it also may be caused by the guiding catheter or wire (Figure 3-16). Stenting significantly reduces these events by approximating the intimal dissection flap and reestablishing flow down the true lumen.

Bifurcation lesions have become a significant area of interest in the stent era. With side-branch occlusion from displacement of plaque from the primary vessel lesion occurring in 1% to 20% of patients, bifurcation lesions often require attention to both the primary and secondary (branch) vessel. Various techniques have been used to protect the side branch, ranging from primary vessel stenting with balloon dilation of the branch vessel through the stent struts to different types of branch-vessel stenting. The "crush" technique involves stenting both the primary and branch vessels, with excellent initial success rates, but side-branch restenosis may be a problem[199] (see Figure 3-23). New T-shaped stents are under development.[200] Different debulking devices, including rotational atherectomy and the cutting balloon, have been utilized in attempts to reduce the plaque volume and prevent shifting.

TABLE 3-11	Lesion-Specific Characteristics of Type A, B, and C Lesions*	
Type A Lesions (Least Complex)		
Discrete (<10 mm length)	Little or no calcification	
Concentric	Less than totally occlusive	
Readily accessible	Nonostial in location	
Nonangulated segment, < 45 degrees	No major branch involvement	
Smooth contour	Absence of thrombus	
Type B Lesions (Intermediate)		
Tubular (10–20 mm in length)	Moderate to heavy calcification	
Eccentric		
Moderate tortuosity of proximal segment	Total occlusions < 3 mo old	
	Ostial in location	
Moderately angulated, > 45 segment degrees, < 90 degrees	Bifurcation lesions requiring double guidewires	
Irregular contour	Some thrombus present	
Type C Lesions (Most Complex)		
Diffuse (> 2 cm in length)	Total occlusions > 3 mo old	
Excessive tortuosity of proximal segment	Inability to protect major side branches	
Extremely angulated segments > 90 degrees	Degenerated vein grafts with friable lesions	

*American Heart Association/American College of Cardiology classification of lesion type. From Ryan TJ, Bauman WB, Kennedy JW, et al: Guidelines for percutaneous transluminal angioplasty. *J Am Coll Cardiol* 22:2033, 1993.

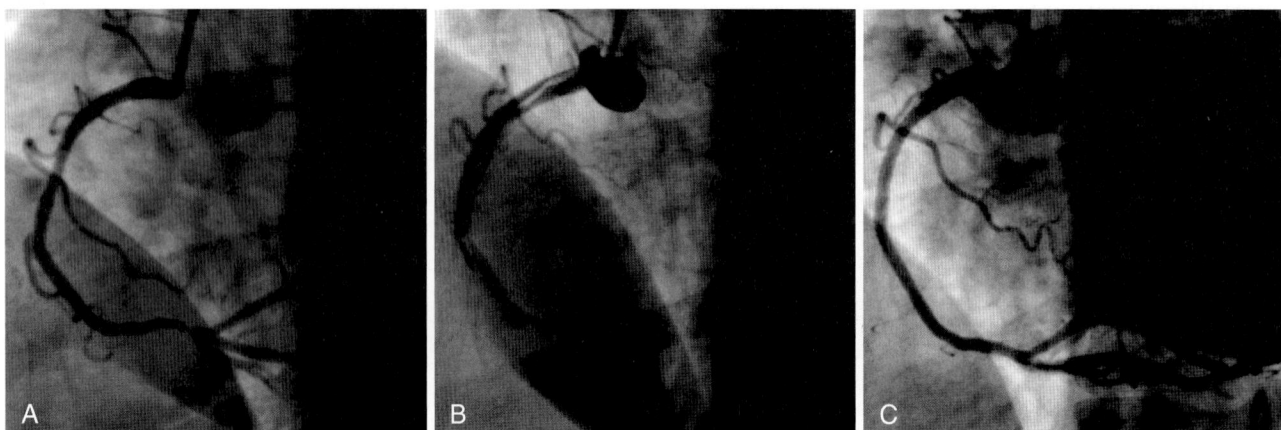

Figure 3-16 *A,* Initial image shows a severe stenosis in the distal right coronary artery (RCA). *B,* The guiding catheter caused a dissection in the proximal RCA with impairment of flow. Note retrograde propagation into aortic sinus. *C,* Normal flow is restored after placement of multiple stents. The persistent dissection in the aortic sinus healed uneventfully.

The recognition of high-risk lesion and patient characteristics allows the cardiologist to better predict which patient is at increased risk for catheter-based interventional therapy.[110] In current interventional practice, when the high-risk patient is identified, the cardiologist should share this information with the surgeon and anesthesiologist so that patient care is not compromised in the event of an emergency.

Operating Room Backup

When PTCA was introduced, all patients were considered candidates for CABG. The physicians' learning curve in the early 1980s was considered 25 to 50 cases; increased complications were seen during these initial cases.[20,21,104] All PCI procedures had immediate OR availability, with the anesthesiologist often in the catheterization laboratory. In the 1990s, OR backup was necessary less often. First, perfusion catheter technology developed to allow for longer inflation times with less ischemia.[201] The role for perfusion balloons and OR backup has diminished with the use of stents. With the current low incidence of emergent CABG at 0.3 to 0.6% of PCI procedures, few institutions maintain a cardiac room on standby for routine coronary interventions.

Infrequently, high-risk interventional cases still may require a cardiac room on immediate standby. This may occur in an emergent situation in which a STEMI patient requires assist support during primary PCI,[202] or more electively when a patient is identified as high risk but is not a candidate for a hybrid laboratory or no such facility is available.[8] Preoperative anesthetic evaluation, which allows for preoperative assessment of the overall medical condition, past anesthetic history, current drug therapy, allergic history, and a physical examination concentrating on airway management considerations, is reserved for these high-risk cases.

Because a less-stringent policy for OR backup is required, PCI without cardiac surgery onsite is becoming more frequent.[24] Initially begun in an effort to provide emergent primary PCI for STEMI patients in remote areas, PCI without onsite cardiac surgery now is being performed in more elective, low-risk patients. Transfer agreements with established oversite hospitals with onsite cardiac surgery are required with both minimal requirements established for operators and institutions, as well as a comprehensive quality assurance program in place.[24] Despite these modifications, this is not standard practice and remains controversial.[22,24,26]

Regardless of the location of the interventional procedure, when an emergency CABG is required, it is essential to provide enough "lead" time to adequately prepare an OR. These patients often are very ill, with ongoing myocardial injury and circulatory collapse. Time is critical to limit the damage and prevent death. Therefore, the sooner the anesthesiologist, staff, and OR are aware of an arriving "potential disaster," the better for all involved. In addition, because this happens infrequently, cooperation among the interventionalist, surgeon, and anesthesiologist is essential for optimal patient care in this critically ill population.

General Management for Failed Percutaneous Coronary Intervention

Several possible scenarios may result from a failed PCI (Box 3-7). First, the interventional procedure may not successfully open the vessel, but no coronary injury has occurred; the patient often remains in the hospital until CABG can be scheduled. The second type of patient has a patent vessel with an unstable lesion. This most often occurs when a dissection cannot be contained by stents but the vessel remains open. The third patient type has an occluded coronary vessel after a failed PCI with stenting either not an option or unsuccessful. In this instance, myocardial ischemia/infarction ensues dependent on the degree of collateralization.[203] This patient most commonly requires emergent surgical intervention.

In preparation for the OR, a perfusion catheter, pacemaker, and/or PAC may be inserted, dependent on patient stability, OR availability, and patient assessment by the cardiologist, CT surgeon, and anesthesiologist. Although intended to better stabilize the patient, these procedures are at the expense of ischemic time. An intra-aortic balloon pump or one of the newer support devices may be placed. Although these devices can reduce the myocardial oxygen requirements, myocardial

BOX 3-7 FAILED INTERVENTION

- Perform usual preoperative evaluation for emergent procedure
- Inventory of vascular access sites: pulmonary artery catheter, intra-arterial balloon pump
- Defer removal of sheaths
- Review medicines administered
  - Boluses may linger even if infusion stopped (e.g., abciximab)
  - Check medicines before catheterization laboratory (e.g., enoxaparin, clopidogrel)
- Confirm availability of blood products

necrosis still will occur in the absence of coronary or collateral blood flow. Once in the OR, decisions on the placement of catheters for monitoring should take several details into consideration. If perfusion has been reestablished, and the degree of coronary insufficiency is mild (no ECG changes, absence of angina), time can be taken to place an arterial catheter and a PAC. *Remember, however, that these patients usually have received significant anticoagulation with heparin and often GPIIb/IIIa platelet receptor inhibitors; attempts at catheter placement should not be undertaken when direct pressure cannot be applied to a vessel.* The most experienced individual should perform these procedures.

The worst scenario is the patient who arrives in the OR either in profound circulatory shock or full cardiopulmonary arrest. In these patients, cardiopulmonary bypass (CPB) should be established as quickly as possible. No attempt should be made to establish access for monitoring that would delay the start of surgery. The only real requirement to start a case such as this is to have good intravenous access, a five-lead ECG, airway control, a functioning blood pressure cuff, and arterial access from the PCI procedure.

In many cases of emergency surgery, the cardiologist has placed femoral artery sheaths for access during the PCI. *These should not be removed,* again because of heparin (or bivalirudin) and, possibly, GPIIb/IIIa inhibitor therapy during the PCI. A femoral artery sheath will provide extremely accurate pressures, which closely reflect central aortic pressure. Also, a PAC may have been placed in the catheterization laboratory, and this can be adapted for use in the OR.

Several surgical series have looked for associations with mortality in patients who present for emergency CABG after failed PCI. The presence of complete occlusion, urgent PCI, and multivessel disease have all been associated with an increased mortality.[204] In addition, long delays lead to increases in morbidity and mortality. The paradigm shift in cardiovascular medicine toward PCI will be negatively impacted if significant numbers of serious complications occur because of prolonged delays in arranging emergent cardiac surgical care for the infrequent patient after failed PCI.[205,206] As the frequency of PCI at institutions with no onsite cardiac surgery increases, cooperation among specialties and facilities will be required to assure that timely transfer can be arranged after a failed PCI. Important time will be lost unless formal arrangements are in place ahead of time.[24]

Support Devices for High-Risk Angioplasty

Numerous support devices for high-risk angioplasty have been used, including intra-aortic balloon pumps and partial CPB via femoral cannulae. National registries of elective angioplasty during partial CPB have reported that 95% of attempted vessels were successfully dilated with bypass support, but 39% of the patients incurred vascular complications.[207] In addition, 43% of the patients required transfusions. Tierstein et al[208] compared cardiopulmonary support for high-risk angioplasty versus standby support. Three hundred sixty-three patients were placed on cardiopulmonary support during angioplasty and 92 underwent standby support. The mortality rate in both groups was 6%.

Several mechanical support devices may be used in the high-risk intervention patient or in the patient with cardiogenic shock. The TandemHeart (CardiacAssist, Inc., Pittsburgh, PA) received CE mark approval in Europe and FDA 510(k) clearance in 2003. This device uses a cannula that is inserted percutaneously into the LA via a femoral vein and puncture of the interatrial septum. An extracorporeal pump then returns oxygenated blood to the arterial system, thereby unloading the left ventricle. The Impella Recover LP 2.5 System (Abiomed, Danvers, MA) is a 12.5-French catheter that is placed in the left ventricle. This device is inserted percutaneously and uses a transaxial flow pump to transfer up to 2.5 L/min of blood from the left ventricle to the ascending aorta.[209,210]

Some centers use extracorporeal membrane oxygenation systems to provide circulatory support for cardiogenic shock or during high-risk PCI (see Chapters 27–29). To date, mechanical support devices have been shown to improve hemodynamic parameters when compared with the IABP, but provide no clinical benefit.[211] Improved equipment and technique have made PCI safer. Although this should reduce the need for mechanical support, it also permits sicker patients to be candidates for PCI (Figure 3-17). Accordingly, the future role of mechanical support in the interventional suite remains to be determined.

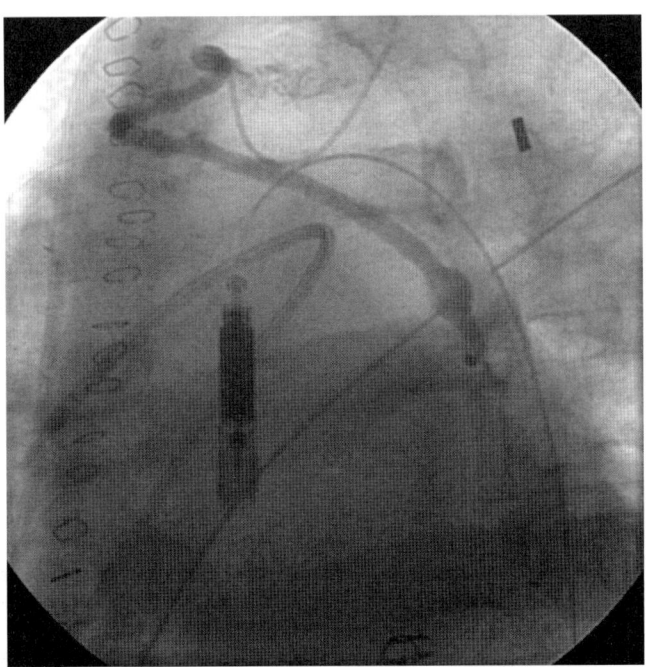

Figure 3-17 High-risk percutaneous coronary intervention with patient supported by the Impella system. A 62-year-old man, after coronary artery bypass graft, presented with acute myocardial infarction and severe hemodynamic instability refractory to maximal pressor therapy, as well as an intra-aortic balloon pump. Impella device in place during saphenous vein graft intervention of the left anterior descending artery is shown.

Controversies in Interventional Cardiology

Therapy for acute myocardial infarction: primary percutaneous coronary intervention versus thrombolysis

Thrombolytic therapy was introduced for AMI patients in the 1970s (Box 3-8). Multiple multicenter trials have compared the following benefits: (1) thrombolytic therapy versus no thrombolytic therapy, (2) one thrombolytic agent compared with another, (3) different adjunctive medications given with thrombolytic therapy (platelet GPIs, LMWHs, direct thrombin inhibitors), and (4) thrombolytic therapy versus primary PCI (bringing the patient directly to the catheterization laboratory).[28] Table 3-12 lists the currently available drugs used for thrombolytic therapy in AMI patients.

Before discussing thrombolytic therapy versus primary PCI for AMI, several issues must be considered. With contraindications to thrombolysis in approximately 60% of all AMI patients, PCI often is the only alternative to establish arterial patency in this group.[212] PCI has proved beneficial in patients with cardiogenic shock.[106,213] For patients who have not shown evidence of coronary reperfusion within 45 to 60 minutes after thrombolysis, cardiac catheterization and rescue PCI may be performed, particularly when large areas of myocardium are at risk (Figure 3-18). This is preferable to repeat thrombolytics.[184] Rescue PCI may improve outcome, particularly if done early.[214,215] However, several studies have suggested mixed results with rescue PCI after failed thrombolysis in the nonshock patient.[214,216] In 2009, the 1-year follow-up results for the REACT (Rescue Angioplasty Versus Conservative Treatment or Repeat Thrombolysis) trial were published. Compared with either conservative strategies or repeat thrombolytics, PCI showed a significant improvement in 1-year event-free survival.[216] Identification of reperfusion using noninvasive tests is difficult.[217] Resolution of ST-segment elevation may be the most accurate and rapid of the noninvasive markers of reperfusion, and it predicts mortality and reinfarction.[218] In patients with recurrent pain or clinical instability, cardiac catheterization after thrombolysis often is required.[28]

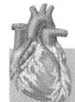

BOX 3-8 CORONARY INTERVENTION IN ACUTE MYOCARDIAL INFARCTION (PRIMARY PERCUTANEOUS CORONARY INTERVENTION)

- Thrombolytics preferred
  - Symptoms < 3 hours
  - No contraindications
  - Would take > 90 minutes until PCI (actual balloon inflation)
- Primary PCI preferred
  - Contraindications to thrombolytics (e.g., after surgery)
  - Cardiogenic shock
  - PCI (balloon inflation) < 90 minutes
  - Late presentations (probably)
  - Elderly (possibly)

TABLE 3-12	Current Thrombolytic Therapy			
Characteristics	*Streptokinase*	*Alteplase*	*Reteplase*	*Tenecteplase*
Abbreviation	SK	t-PA	r-PA	TNKase
Dose (> 90 kg)	1.5 million U	100 mg	20 units	50 mg
$t_{1/2}$	23 min	< 5 min	13–16 min	20–24 min
Infusion time	60 min	1.5 hr (double bolus)	30 min (double bolus)	Single bolus
Fibrin specificity	+	++	++	+++
Antigenicity	Yes	No	No	No
Concomitant heparin	No	Yes	Yes	Yes

Source: Lexi-Comp Online, www.lexi.com

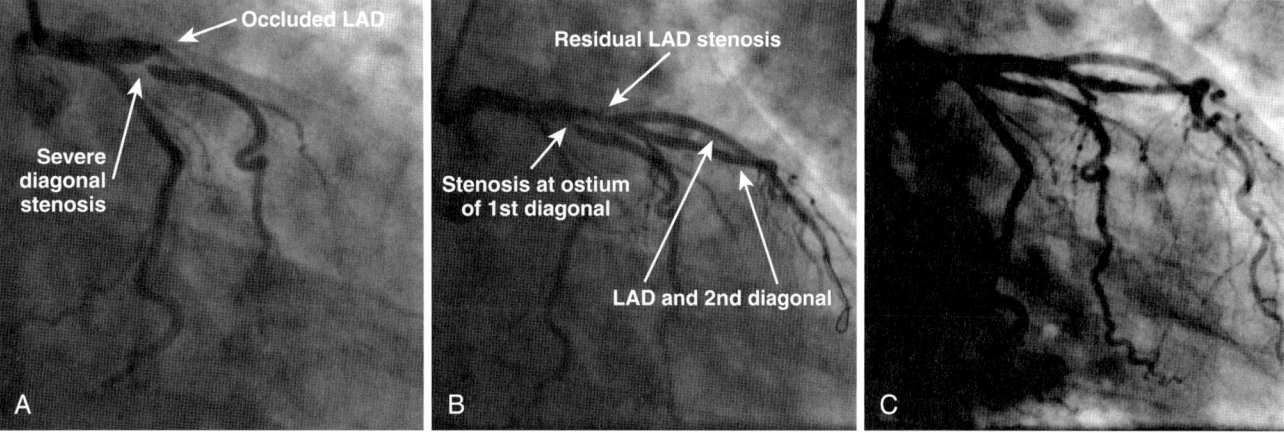

Figure 3-18 **Primary percutaneous coronary intervention for an acute anterior ST-elevation acute myocardial infarction (STEMI).** *A*, Complete occlusion of the left anterior descending artery (LAD) and high-grade stenosis of the first diagonal. *B*, After thrombectomy, antegrade flow is restored in the LAD and a second diagonal, but severe stenosis persists in the LAD. *C*, After stenting of the LAD and first diagonal.

Time to reperfusion is important, as long-term mortality is lowest and ventricular function improves the most when reperfusion occurs within 2 to 3 hours of symptom onset.[219] Postinfarction prognosis also is related to infarct artery patency. Thus, strategies to promote early reperfusion are imperative and may include prehospital protocols.[220] Transfer strategies for patients arriving in hospitals without interventional capabilities have been studied, and successful outcomes were seen when transfer times were less than 90 minutes.[28,221]

The 2004 guidelines by the ACC/AHA on management of patients with STEMI emphasized early reperfusion and discussed the choice between thrombolytic therapy and primary PCI.[222] If a patient presented within 3 hours of symptom onset, the guidelines expressed no preference for either strategy with the following caveats: Primary PCI was preferred if (1) door-to-balloon time was less than 90 minutes and was performed by skilled personnel (operator annual volume more than 75 cases and laboratory volume more than 200 cases with 36 primary PCIs); (2) thrombolytic therapy was contraindicated; or (3) the patient was in cardiogenic shock. Thrombolytic therapy was to be considered if symptom onset was less than 3 hours and door-to-balloon time was more than 90 minutes. Individual assessment was recommended for patients older than 75 years, because they had a higher mortality from the MI and a greater risk for complications, particularly intracranial bleeding, with thrombolytic therapy.

The 2007 ACC/AHA update to the guidelines for the management of STEMI recommended primary PCI at capable facilities for all patients with STEMI.[222] This recommendation was based on older comparisons with thrombolytic therapy and on data that process refinement was crucial to the provision of timely reperfusion.[28,223] This update did not materially change the recommendations for timely reperfusion. However, for patients receiving fibrinolytic therapy (at a non-PCI hospital), it was recommended that those deemed at high risk should receive appropriate antithrombotic therapy and be moved immediately to a PCI-capable facility for diagnostic catheterization and possible PCI.[224] It was anticipated that some patients would require emergent surgery, and their coagulation would be impaired at multiple levels. If not at high risk, the patient could be moved to a PCI-capable facility after receiving antithrombotic therapy or could be observed in the initial facility.

In the postoperative period, most patients will have contraindications to thrombolytic therapy. Thus, primary PCI is usually their best option. However, primary PCI requires the use of a short course of heparin and a long course of aspirin. If these medicines cannot be given, primary PCI may not be possible. Ideally, primary PCI would include a GPIIb/IIIa inhibitor and stent placement, and the latter would include a course of clopidogrel. *If primary PCI is chosen, only the infarct-related artery should be treated in the acute setting.*[26,28,222] This prevents the

small potential for complications arising from other "elective lesions," compromising an already critically ill patient.

Facilitated PCI involves the administration of thrombolytic therapy, usually a reduced dose, with the intention of proceeding to PCI.[183,225] Early studies of this approach failed to show a benefit compared with primary PCI alone.[220] Although later studies were more encouraging,[226–228] the recent guidelines recognized some uncertainty in the designations "rescue" and "facilitated." As such, the focus was on systems to promote timely reperfusion as noted earlier.[28]

The recent guidelines give a class IIa recommendation to insulin-based glucose control in the setting of an STEMI, with the goal of maintaining glucose levels less than 180 mg/dL without causing hypoglycemia.[28] As the diabetic population increases, this recommendation is likely to increase the number of patients receiving intravenous insulin therapy in the catheterization laboratory. Frequent monitoring of blood glucose levels will be necessary, both in the catheterization laboratory and in any venues that receive such patients.

Although hypothermia has been used in the OR for many years, there has been recent expansion of its use in other settings. Of particular interest to this chapter is the use of hypothermia in patients resuscitated from sudden cardiac arrest. Many of these patients will continue to the catheterization laboratory. A recent review covered the potential benefits and pitfalls of the expanded use of hypothermia.[229] Although the benefits appear substantial, the logistics of an extended period of hypothermia are significant.

All patients require risk stratification after MI regardless of the method of reperfusion and even, or perhaps especially, if they have not received reperfusion therapy. This includes an assessment of LV function and residual burden of CAD. The incidence and extent of CAD in patients after thrombolysis were compiled from several large studies. In these patients, the following significant coronary lesions were present: left main in 5%, multivessel disease in 30%, single-vessel open in 35%, single-vessel closed in 15%, and minimal lesion in 15%. Obviously, the state of the other coronary arteries is assessed at the time of primary PCI. For patients treated with thrombolytic therapy or no reperfusion therapy, angiography or stress testing are alternative methods to assess the residual ischemic burden. The electrical stability of the heart must be addressed. In patients with a low EF after an MI, prophylactic implantation of a defibrillator results in a 30% reduction in total mortality over 20 months.[230] Finally, modification of risk factors for CAD must be undertaken.

The development of systems of care for STEMI involves community-wide coordination of prehospital care and available hospital services.[28] In this environment, primary PCI has supplanted fibrinolytic therapy. This has led to more frequent performance of PCI in catheterization laboratories without OR backup.[24,231] Many patients undergo thrombolytic therapy or present late and do not receive reperfusion therapy. If such patients are hemodynamically or electrically unstable, or if they have recurrent symptoms, a consensus would favor catheterization and revascularization. If such patients are stable, their management is controversial, although many cardiologists in the United States would recommend catheterization and revascularization.

Therapy for Acute Coronary Syndromes (Non–ST-Elevation Myocardial Infarction and Unstable Angina): Primary Percutaneous Coronary Intervention versus Medical Therapy

The ACSs of non–ST-elevation myocardial infarction (NSTEMI) and UA have similar presentations, and often can be distinguished only in retrospect.[149] STEMI has received much attention of late with a variety of efforts promoted to foster early reperfusion.[28] However, presentation with ACS is more frequent, and high-risk subgroups have a prognosis that is similar to that in STEMI.[231] Accordingly, guidelines for the management of ACS have embraced an aggressive approach, including the early administration of antiplatelet agents.[149] As many of these patients proceed to cardiac catheterization, the potential need for emergent cardiac surgery presents similar problems as with STEMI patients.

Percutaneous Coronary Intervention versus Coronary Artery Bypass Graft

The choice of therapy for multivessel CAD must be made by comparing PCI with CABG and medical therapy. In the 1970s, CABG was compared with medical therapy in several randomized trials. A survival benefit for CABG was seen in only a few subgroups, such as those with left main disease and those with three-vessel disease and impaired LV function. Both CABG and medical therapy have improved since that time, but few recent comparisons have been made. Comparisons of PCI to medical therapy in patients with stable CAD generally have shown improved symptoms without a reduction of hard end points.[94,232]

In the mid-1980s, when PCI consisted only of balloon PTCA, the first comparisons of catheter intervention to CABG were begun. By the early to mid-1990s, nine randomized clinical trials had been published comparing PTCA with CABG in patients with significant CAD. Only the Bypass Angioplasty Revascularization Investigation (BARI) trial was statistically appropriate for assessing mortality.[233] These are summarized in Figure 3-19. The conclusions of these studies included similarities between the two approaches with respect to relief of angina and 5-year mortality. Costs were initially lower in the PCI group, but by 5 years had converged because of repeat PCI procedures precipitated by restenosis, occurring in 20% to 40% of the PCI group.[234]

The only clear difference between PCI and CABG for patients with multivessel disease was identified in the diabetic patient subset of the BARI trial.[233] A difference in mortality was seen in a subgroup analysis of the BARI trial in which both insulin-dependent and non–insulin-dependent diabetic patients with multivessel disease had a lower 5-year mortality rate with CABG (19.4%) than with PCI (34.5%).[235]

Regretfully, these trials were outdated by the time of their publication. For the patient undergoing PCI, stents had become the norm, with a significant decrease in emergent CABG because of reduced acute closure, as well as a decrease in repeat procedures because of less restenosis.[125] For the patient undergoing CABG, off-pump bypass became more common during this time period with its potential to decrease complications.[236] In addition, the importance of arterial grafting with its favorable impact on long-term graft patency was recognized.[237]

To address the changes in PCI and CABG therapy, four more randomized trials were undertaken, and these are included in Figure 3-19. The results of these newer studies were similar to the results of the earlier ones. In the Arterial Revascularization Therapy Study (ARTS) trial, diabetic patients had poorer outcomes with PCI. Repeat procedures, though higher in the PCI group at 20%, were significantly lower than with the earlier trials. CABG patients also had improved outcomes; for instance, cognitive impairment occurred in fewer patients in the recent studies.[234] A meta-analysis of all 13 randomized trials identified a 1.9% absolute survival advantage at 5 years in the CABG patients, but no significant difference at 1, 3, or 8 years.[238] As with the first generation of PCI versus CABG trials, the second-generation trials were outdated before publication because of the advent of the DESs.

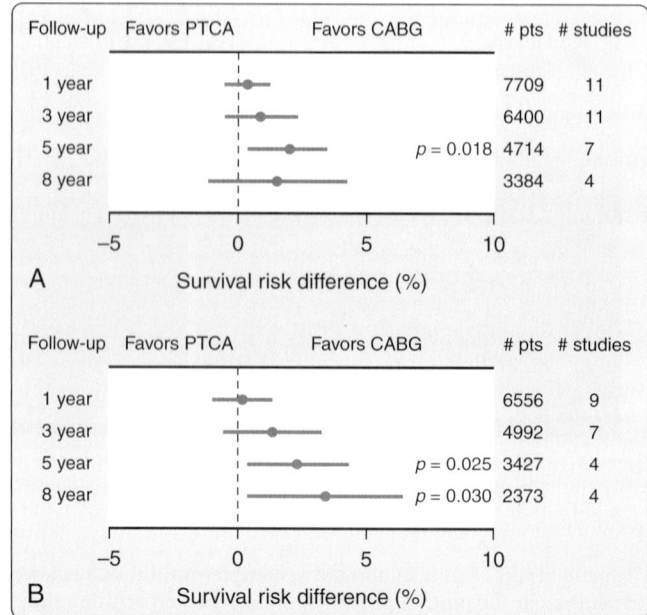

Figure 3-19 Randomized trials of coronary artery bypass graft surgery (CABG) versus coronary angioplasty (PTCA) in patients with multivessel coronary disease showing risk difference for all-cause mortality for Years 1, 3, 5, and 8 after initial revascularization. *A,* All trials. *B,* Multivessel trials. (Redrawn from Hoffman SN, TenBrook JA, Wolf MP, et al: A meta-analysis of randomized controlled trials comparing coronary artery bypass graft with percutaneous transluminal coronary angioplasty: One- to eight-year outcomes. J Am Coll Cardiol 41:1293, 2003. Copyright 2003, with permission from The American College of Cardiology Foundation.)

The SYNTAX trial randomized 1800 patients with three-vessel CAD and/or left main stenosis to either CABG or treatment with paclitaxel-eluting stents with the intention of obtaining complete revascularization. Patients were eligible regardless of clinical presentation, if complete revascularization was believed feasible by both techniques. By 1 year, 17.8% of the PCI patients versus 12.4% of the CABG patients had experienced a MACE (*P* = 0.002). Although this difference was driven primarily by a greater need for repeat revascularization in the PCI group, the rate of death was nonsignificantly greater in the PCI group at 4.4% versus 3.5% in the CABG group. The rate of stroke was significantly greater in the CABG group at 2.2% versus 0.6% (*P* = 0.003). Of the patients who gave consent, 1275 were not eligible for randomization because complete revascularization was not believed feasible by both techniques; of these, 1077 underwent CABG.[239]

Other contentious issues exist in the management of CAD. Concerns for potential deleterious effects on CABG outcomes in patients with prior PCI have not proved to be warranted.[240] The roles of staged PCI procedures in patients with multivessel disease, ad hoc PCI, and combination procedures (LIMA [left internal mammary artery] to LAD and PCI of other vessels) have generated debate within the interventional and surgical communities. The performance of PCI for left main disease is performed frequently in other countries but remains controversial in the United States.[241] In the 2009 update to the ACC/AHA guidelines, PCI has been moved from a class III (contraindicated) recommendation to class IIb ("may be considered").[28]

In conclusion, the physician must weigh the data and explain the advantages and disadvantages of both techniques to the individual patient. CABG offers a more complete revascularization with survival advantages in selected groups and a decreased need for repeat procedures.[239,242] The disadvantages of CABG are the greater early risk, longer hospitalization and recovery, initial expense, increased difficulty of second procedures, morbidity associated with leg incisions, increased risk for stroke, and the limited durability of venous grafts. The cost of

DESs may negate the initial cost advantage of PCI if multiple stents are used. From the perspective of a hospital administrator in the United States, current reimbursement policies favor CABG over the placement of multiple DESs.[243]

SPECIFIC INTERVENTIONAL DEVICES

Interventional Diagnostic Devices

Three intravascular diagnostic tools for the interventionalist currently are available. Angioscopy, the least applied of the three, offers the most accurate assessment of intravascular thrombus.[244] Cineangiography and IVUS often are inadequate for visualization of thrombus. Although useful as an investigative technique, angioscopy has not entered into routine interventional practice.

IVUS permits visualization of the vessel wall in vivo.[93] A miniature transducer mounted on the tip of a 3-French catheter is advanced over the standard guidewire into the coronary artery. The IVUS transducer is about 1 mm in diameter, with frequencies of 30 to 40 MHz. These high frequencies allow for excellent resolution of the vessel wall. By comparison, contrast angiography images only the lumen, with the status of the vessel wall inferred from the image of the lumen.[245] IVUS is useful in evaluating equivocal left-main lesions, ostial stenoses, and vessels overlapping angiographically (Figure 3-20).[246] IVUS is superior to angiography in the early detection of the diffuse, immune-mediated, arteriopathy of cardiac transplant allografts.[247]

IVUS has been used extensively in research because it allows an excellent assessment of the post-PCI result and a precise quantitative assessment of restenosis.[114,248] As an adjunct to PCI, clinicians have utilized IVUS for years to assess the adequacy of stent deployment, the extent of vessel calcification, and the presence of edge dissections.[249] The quantitative capability of IVUS has been indispensable to researchers in preventive cardiology. It has allowed these researchers to document the benefits of aggressive lipid reduction using smaller numbers of patients and less time than would be possible with other techniques, as in the Pravastatin or Atorvastatin Evaluation and Infection Therapy (PROVE-IT) and Reversal of Atherosclerosis with Aggressive Lipid Lowering (REVERSAL) trials.[250,251]

Various physiologic measurements can be made in the catheterization laboratory during clinical diagnostic or interventional procedures.[95] The Doppler flow wire (Volcano, San Diego, CA) was the first tool available for the interventionalist to determine the physiologic significance of an anatomic stenosis in the catheterization laboratory. Utilizing a 12-MHz piezoelectric ultrasound transducer on a 0.014-inch wire, it allows the measurement of coronary flow and coronary flow reserve.[252] By comparing this information with normal values, physiologic significance can be determined; these data compare favorably with stress-nuclear perfusion imaging. The interventionalist can then decide, during the diagnostic procedure, whether to proceed with PCI.[253]

In the mid-1990s, the pressure wire was introduced by Radi (now part of St. Jude Medical). This wire has a pressure transducer near its tip and permits measurement of a gradient across a stenosis. This gradient is measured during vasodilation after the administration of intracoronary adenosine. Fractional flow reserve (FFR), has also been used to assess successful stent placement and can identify inadequate stent results predictive of restenosis.[97] Finally, a strategy of deferring PCI in patients with an FFR more than 0.75 has been tested and found to be associated with good clinical outcomes.[98]

Cardiovascular optical coherence tomography (OCT) is another catheter-based invasive diagnostic imaging system. OCT uses light rather than ultrasound. First utilized clinically to visualize the retina, this low-coherence reflectometry was named OCT and expanded in the early 1990s to numerous biomedical and clinical applications. In the catheterization laboratory, it provides high-resolution images of the coronary arteries and deployed stents. For imaging without signal attenuation, blood must be removed from the coronary artery. This is achieved by proximal balloon inflation with proper sizing of a nontraumatic balloon within the coronary artery with occlusion times limited to 30 seconds or less. OCT provides the invasive cardiologist with accurate measurements of luminal architecture including stent apposition, neointimal thickening, and course of stent dissolution with the new-generation bioabsorbable stents.[254]

Percutaneous Transluminal Coronary Angioplasty

When Andreas Gruentzig performed his first PTCA in 1977, the equipment was so large and bulky that he could dilate only proximal lesions and, even then, this equipment would not cross severe narrowings.[104] Since that time, balloon, guidewire, and guide-catheter technology have advanced to allow the interventional cardiologist to place balloon catheters nearly anywhere in the arterial tree. Despite the development of new devices, POBA (plain old balloon angioplasty) is still an important component of the interventional procedure as it "paves the way" for stent implantation.

The mechanism by which balloon inflation leads to vessel patency must be understood to better understand balloon angioplasty. Although four mechanisms have been described to explain the efficacy of this procedure (i.e., plaque splitting, stretching of the arterial wall, plaque compression, and plaque desquamation), the primary mechanism is *discrete* intimal dissection, which results in plaque compression into the media. Desquamation and distal embolization of superficial

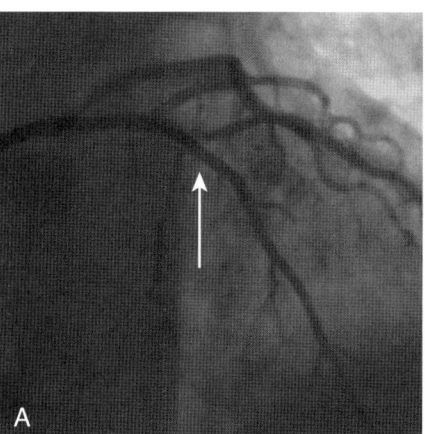
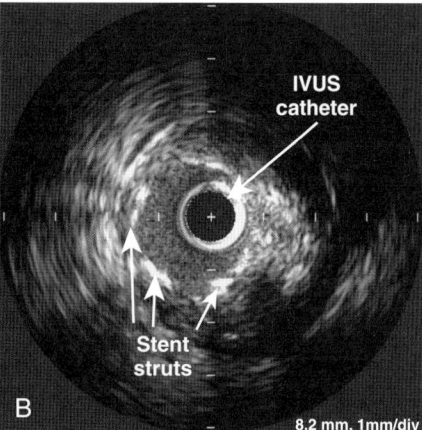
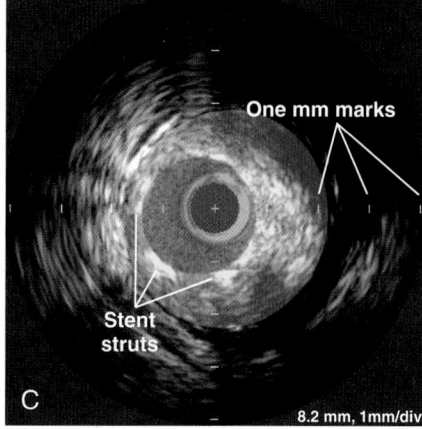

Figure 3-20 **Intravascular ultrasound (IVUS).** *A,* Angiography shows mild stenosis in stented segment of left anterior descending artery (LAD) in patient with recurrent symptoms. *B,* By IVUS, the 3.0-mm stent is underexpanded with a diameter of only 2.2 mm. *C,* Red area is lumen, about 3.8 mm². Blue area is that bounded by the external elastic lamina, about 12.5 mm². The difference is atherosclerotic plaque.

plaque components have been observed; however, experimental studies demonstrate this to be a minor contributor to the procedure's efficacy.[122] Propagation of the intimal dissection is the primary cause of vessel occlusion during angioplasty (see Figure 3-16).

Although the mechanism of balloon angioplasty has not changed, equipment and operator expertise have improved to the point that procedural success rates now exceed 90%.[188] These advances allow for the treatment of sicker patients and more complex coronary lesions, whereas success rates continue to improve and complication rates decrease.[186]

Atherectomy Devices: Directional and Rotational

Atherectomy devices are designed to remove some amount of plaque or other material from an atherosclerotic vessel. Of these devices, directional coronary atherectomy (DCA) became the first nonballoon technology to gain FDA approval in 1991. DCA removes tissue from the coronary artery, thus "debulking" the area of stenosis. Although tissue removal is an attractive concept, application of DCA was limited. Trials comparing DCA with PTCA did not show improved angiographic restenosis rates, and greater rates of acute complications were seen with DCA.[255–257]

The FDA approved rotational coronary atherectomy in 1993. The Rotablator® catheter (Boston Scientific Corp, Natick, MA) is designed to differentially remove nonelastic tissue, utilizing a diamond-studded burr rotating at 140,000 to 160,000 rpm. Designed to alter lesion compliance, particularly in heavily calcified vessels, rotational atherectomy often is used before balloon dilation to permit full expansion of the vessel.[258] The ablated material is emulsified into 5-μm particles, which pass through the distal capillary bed. Heavily calcified lesions commonly are chosen for rotational atherectomy (Figure 3-21). In addition, restenotic (in-stent), bifurcation, ostial, or nondilatable lesions are candidates for the Rotablator.[259] Contraindications to the Rotablator include tortuous anatomy, poor ventricular function, thrombus, poor runoff, and lesions within SVGs.[260]

The main limitation of rotational atherectomy is the "no-reflow" phenomenon.[117] Thought secondary to particle load, this effect is associated with myocardial ischemia and occasionally infarction. Hemodynamic problems can occur, particularly in patients with depressed LV function. The frequency of "no reflow" has been reduced by shorter, slower ablation passes and variation in medications within the flush solution.[260] In heavily calcified vessels, rotational atherectomy may be the only device that can change the compliance of an artery and permit complete expansion of balloons and stents. However, rotational atherectomy is more cumbersome and time consuming than balloon dilation. It is rarely used alone, and stent placement usually is necessary to achieve an adequate result. Therefore, though available in most interventional laboratories, rotational atherectomy is a niche item primarily relegated to vessels with significant calcification.

Cutting Balloon

Vessel wall damage during interventional procedures generally is considered the initiating factor for neointimal proliferation, which ultimately can lead to restenosis. All interventional technologies damage the vessel wall to varying degrees. In an attempt to decrease intimal injury, the cutting balloon (Boston Scientific Corp) introduced the concept of microsurgical dilation. Whereas standard balloon PCI

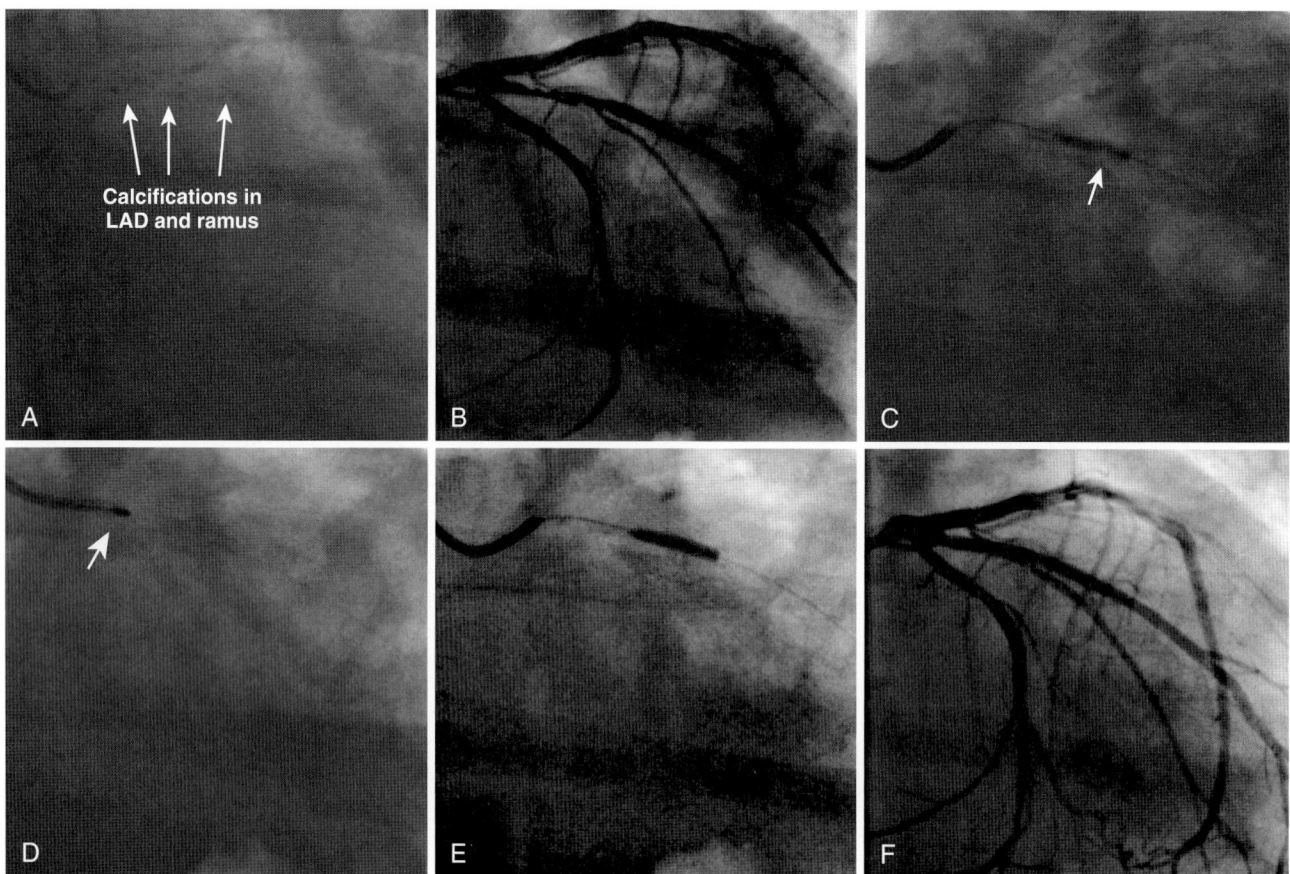

Figure 3-21 Rotational coronary atherectomy. *A,* Fluoroscopy shows calcification of the ramus intermedius. *B,* Angiography shows a severe stenosis. *C,* Percutaneous transluminal coronary angioplasty balloon cannot be expanded. *D,* 1.5-mm rotational atherectomy burr advanced at 140,000 rpm. *E,* Balloon expands fully after rotationally atherectomy. *F,* Final result after stent placement.

dilates haphazardly and can severely injure the arterial wall, the cutting balloon permits vessel expansion with lower pressure and less wall injury, thereby reducing the stimulus for restenosis.

This device is a noncompliant balloon with three or four blades, depending on balloon size. These blades are 10 to 15 mm in length and 0.25 mm in size and are attached to the balloon by a proprietary bond-to-bond manufacturing process. Once inflated, the balloon introduces these blades into the coronary intima, producing a series of tiny longitudinal incisions before balloon dilation. These microscopic cuts permit less traumatic vessel expansion. The safety and efficacy of this technique have been validated; however, there was no benefit compared with POBA when tested in a large group of patients. The cutting balloon is currently utilized for decreasing plaque shift in bifurcating lesions, for changing artery compliance, and in treating in-stent restenosis.[261]

Intracoronary Laser

Excimer laser coronary angioplasty (Spectranetics, Colorado Springs, CO) uses xenon chloride (XeCl) and operates in the ultraviolet range (308 nm) to photochemically ablate tissue. Currently, excimer laser coronary angioplasty is indicated for use in lesions that are long (>2 mm in length), ostial, in saphenous vein bypass grafts, and unresponsive to PTCA. With the development of the eccentric directional laser, treatment of eccentric or bifurcation lesions can be approached with increased success. Also, in-stent restenosis can be effectively treated with the excimer laser.[259] The Prima FX laser wire (Spectranetics, Colorado Springs, CO) is a 0.018-inch wire with the ability to deliver excimer laser energy to areas of chronic, total occlusion. With conventional equipment, failure to cross such lesions with a guidewire is frequent. The Prima FX has CE mark approval in Europe but is investigational in the United States. The optimal wavelength for the treatment of coronary atheroma has yet to be determined. In current practice, laser interventions rarely are used in the coronary arteries.

Intracoronary Stent

The term *stent* was used first in reference to a dental mold developed by an English dentist, Charles Thomas Stent, in the mid-19th century.[262] The word evolved to describe various supportive devices used in medicine.[248] To date, the introduction of intracoronary stents has had a larger impact on the practice of interventional cardiology than any other development.[263]

The use of intracoronary stents exploded during the mid-1990s[264] (Box 3-9). Receiving FDA approval in April 1993, the Gianturco-Roubin (Cook Flex stent), a coiled balloon-expandable stent, was approved for the treatment of acute closure after PCI. Use of the Gianturco-Roubin stent was limited by difficulties with its delivery and high rates of restenosis. The first stent to receive widespread clinical application was

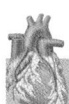

BOX 3-9 STENTS

- Antiplatelet therapy after stent placement
  - Indefinite aspirin therapy plus:
  BMS: clopidogrel 4 weeks (12 months for ACSs)
  DES: clopidogrel 12 months
- With BMSs, thienopyridines reduce subacute thrombosis from 3% to < 1%
- DES never tested without clopidogrel
- Concern with DES is delay in endothelial coverage of stent, similar to brachytherapy
- With clopidogrel, subacute and late thrombosis rates of DES and BMS are identical
- Very late thrombosis rates are greater with DES
- Stents and elective surgery:
  - Delay until clopidogrel completed: recommended
  - Perform during clopidogrel therapy: accept bleeding risk
  - Discontinue clopidogrel early: not recommended

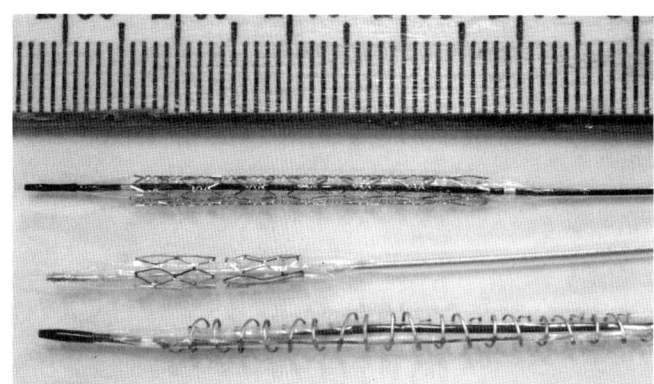

Figure 3-22 Evolution of stents: Three balloon-expandable bare metal stents are shown mounted on their delivery balloons with the above ruled marking in millimeters. *Bottom,* This is the first stent type introduced, the Gianturco-Roubin Flex-stent (Cook Cardiology, Bloomington, IN). The thick but pliable struts and low metal-to-artery ratio limited its effectiveness. *Middle,* The Palmaz-Schatz stent (Cordis/J&J, Warren, NJ) was the next stent type to be U.S. Food and Drug Administration approved for use other than acute closure. This consisted of two 8-mm relatively stiff slotted tube stents connected by a central strut. Although its introduction revolutionized PCI, its stiff structure and sheath covering limited delivery. *Top,* Newer stent designs produced smaller struts with increased flexibility for improved deliverability while maintaining the support structure required for long-term patency.

the Palmaz-Schatz (Johnson & Johnson, New Brunswick, NJ) tubular slotted stent approved for the treatment of de novo coronary stenosis in 1994.[265] Throughout the 1990s, multiple stents were introduced with improved support, flexibility, and thinner struts, resulting in improved delivery and decreased restenosis rates (Figure 3-22).[132,133]

As discussed earlier, the major limitations of catheter-based interventions had been acute vessel closure and restenosis. Stents offered an option for stabilizing intimal dissections while limiting late lumen loss, major components of acute closure, and restenosis, respectively. Clinical trials have demonstrated the ability of stents not only to salvage a failed PTCA, thus avoiding emergent CABG (see Figure 3-16), but also to reduce restenosis.[132,266] Multiple studies demonstrated the benefit of stenting compared with PTCA alone in a variety of circumstances, including long lesions, vein grafts, chronic occlusions, and the thrombotic occlusions of AMI. Only in small vessels did stenting not demonstrate a restenosis benefit when compared with balloon angioplasty.[267] Clinical restenosis rates declined from 30% to 40% with PTCA to less than 20% with BMSs.[265]

Stent technology improved in incremental fashion. Modifications in coil geometry, alterations in the articulation sites, and the use of mesh-like stents offered minor advantages.[131] Different metals, such as tantalum and nitinol, were used and various coatings were applied, such as heparin, polymers, or even human cells.[132] In addition, the delivery systems that are used to implant stents have decreased in size.[133] Stent procedures, once requiring 9-French guiding catheters, can now be done through 5- to 6-French catheters. This even permits coronary stenting to be done through the radial artery.[268]

When first introduced, stents were used sparingly primarily because of the aggressive anticoagulation regimens recommended. These regimens included intravenous heparin and dextran, together with oral aspirin, dipyridamole, and warfarin. This required long hospitalizations and led to bleeding problems at vascular access sites. These complicated combinations of medicines were used in the clinical trials that led to the approval of the stents, and were chosen based on the fear of thrombosis and limited animal data. Despite the use of these drugs, stent thrombosis still occurred in 3% to 5% of patients. The use of intracoronary ultrasound improved stent deployment by demonstrating incomplete expansion with conventional deployment techniques.

This led to high-pressure balloon inflations, complete stent expansion, and simplified pharmacologic therapy.[114,136]

Initially, aspirin and ticlopidine (Ticlid) were used instead of warfarin, but clopidogrel (Plavix) replaced ticlopidine because it has a better side-effect profile. The combination of a thienopyridine and aspirin has markedly reduced thrombotic events and vascular complications.[150] The timing and dosing of clopidogrel therapy are still evolving with doses of 300 to 600 mg given at least 2 to 4 hours before PCI.[151] Given that PCI is often performed immediately after a diagnostic study, some cardiologists begin clopidogrel therapy before diagnostic studies. PCI can be performed immediately after the diagnostic study, with a reduction in adverse events that is comparable with that seen with GPIs but at a fraction of the cost.[178] However, if the diagnostic study indicates a need for CABG, bleeding complications will be increased if clopidogrel has been given during the 5 days before CABG.[155]

With the realization that restenosis involves poorly regulated cellular proliferation, researchers focused on medicines that had antiproliferative effects. Many of these medicines are toxic when given systemically, a tolerable situation in oncology, but not for a relatively benign condition like restenosis. For such medicines, local delivery was attractive, and the stent provided a vehicle.

Rapamycin, a macrolide antibiotic, is a natural fermentation product produced by *Streptomyces hygroscopicus*, which was originally isolated in a soil sample from Rapa Nui (Easter Island).[269] Rapamycin was soon discovered to have potent immunosuppressant activities, making it unacceptable as an antibiotic but attractive for prevention of transplant rejection. Rapamycin works through inhibition of a protein kinase called the *mammalian target of rapamycin* (mTOR), a mechanism that is distinct from other classes of immunosuppressants. Because mTOR is central to cellular proliferation, as well as immune responses, this agent was an inspired choice for a stent coating. The terms *rapamycin* and *sirolimus* often are used interchangeably. A metal stent does not hold drugs well and permits little control over their release. These limitations required that polymers be developed to attach a drug to the stent and to allow the drug to slowly diffuse into the wall of the blood vessel, whereas eliciting no inflammatory response.[270] The development of DESs would not have been possible without these (proprietary) polymers. This led to the true revolution in PCI, which occurred with the approval in April 2003 of the first DES,[127] the Cypher (Johnson & Johnson/Cordis). This is their Velocity stent and polymer, which elutes sirolimus over 14 days; the drug is completely gone by 30 days after implantation.[269]

A European trial randomized 238 patients to receive either a sirolimus-eluting stent (SES) or a BMS. Remarkably, there was no restenosis in the group that received an SES.[271] A larger American trial randomized 1058 patients to an SES or a BMS. At 9 months, restenosis rates were 8.9% in the SES group and 36.3% in the BMS group, with no difference in adverse events. Clinically driven repeat procedures were required in 3.9% and 16.6%,[271] respectively. This benefit was sustained, if not slightly improved, at 12 months.[272] Although initially approved only for use in de novo lesions in native vessels of stable patients, subsequent publications have shown similar benefits in every clinical scenario that has been studied.[273–277] Initial concerns regarding SST have proved unjustified, with the rate of SST approximately 1%, equal to that seen in BMS patients.[140,141,269]

The next DES to receive FDA approval in March 2004 was the Taxus stent (Boston Scientific Corp). The Taxus stent uses a polymer coating to deliver paclitaxel, a drug that also has many uses in oncology. This is a lipophilic molecule, derived from the Pacific yew tree *Taxus brevifolia*. It interferes with microtubular function, affecting mitosis and extracellular secretion, thereby interrupting the restenotic process at multiple levels.[278] The Taxus IV study randomized 1314 patients to the Taxus stent or a BMS. Angiographic restenosis was reduced from 26.6% in the BMS group to 7.9% in the Taxus group, with no significant difference in adverse events. Clinically driven repeat procedures were required in 12.0% and 4.7%, respectively.[124]

Two more DESs are approved in the United States, the zotarolimus-eluting stent (Endeavor; Medtronic, Minneapolis, MN) and the everolimus-eluting stent (Xience; Abbott, Abbott Pask, IL; Promus; Boston Scientific Corp). The newer stents use different drugs, polymers, and stent platforms. Comparisons of different DESs have shown differences in some angiographic end points, but similar clinical outcomes. Polymer-free and bioabsorbable stents are under investigation.

Currently, stents are placed at the time of most PCI procedures, if the size and anatomy of the vessel permit (Figure 3-23). Multiple studies have been performed comparing BMS with DES in various clinical scenarios.[279,280] There are several reasons not to use a DES in every procedure. First, DESs are available in fewer sizes and the polymer makes them more rigid. Second, a longer course of thienopyridine is required, and this may not be desirable if a surgical procedure is urgently needed, as it requires an uncomfortable choice between bleeding and increased risk for cardiac events.[281] Stent thromboses, MIs, and deaths have been reported when antiplatelet therapy is interrupted.[282,283] Finally, the cost of a DES is about three times that of a BMS, and this increment is not fully reflected in reimbursement. It was hoped that the arrival of additional DESs on the market would lead prices to decline. However, price declines have been modest to date. With the significant reduction in restenosis, DESs were anticipated to give PCI an advantage over CABG

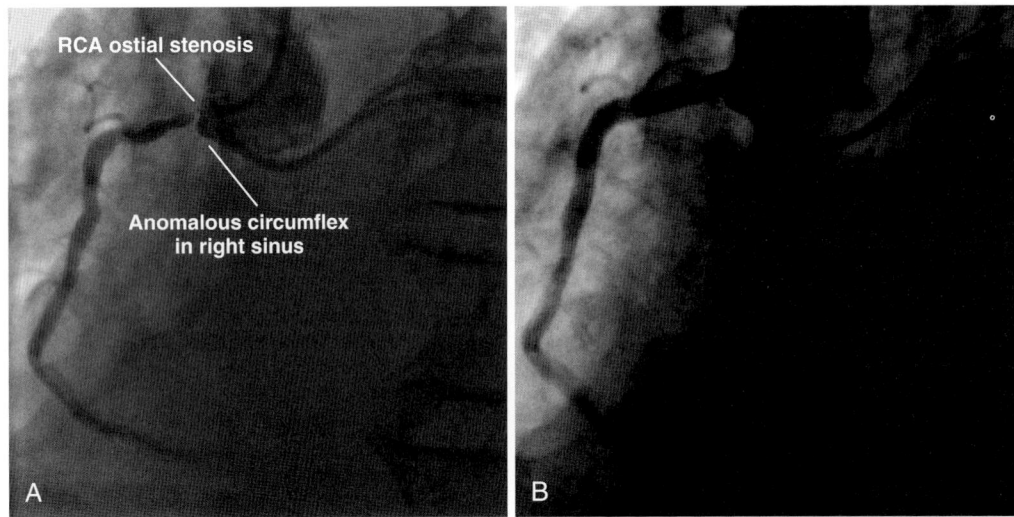

Figure 3-23 **Stenting at the ostium of the right coronary.** *A,* Anomalous circumflex originates near the right coronary artery (RCA). True ostial stenosis requires stent struts to protrude into lumen. *B,* After stenting there is little residual narrowing. Anomalous circumflex is unchanged.

in multivessel disease.[124] The potential consequences of this provoked some anxiety among cardiac surgeons and hospital administrators.[284]

Intravascular Brachytherapy

Brachytherapy is the use of a radioisotope placed at the site where its effects are desired. It was first introduced and developed for the treatment of malignant disease. In an attempt to decrease the neointimal proliferative process associated with restenosis, brachytherapy has been applied to the coronary artery. Two types of radiation are utilized in the coronary arteries: gamma and beta. Gamma radiation, such as that from Ir-192, has no mass, only energy; therefore, there is limited tissue attenuation.[285] Beta-emitters, such as P-32 and Y-90, lose an orbiting electron or positron; the mass of this particle permits significant tissue attenuation.[285]

Radiation safety for the patient, staff, and operator is essential for intravascular brachytherapy. For the staff and the operator, radiation exposure is related to both the energy of the isotope and the type of emission. Staff exposure is much greater with gamma-emitters than with the beta-emitters because of its insignificant tissue attenuation.[286] From the patient's perspective, brachytherapy is prescribed to provide a specific dose to the target vessel. Total body exposure is greater with gamma radiation, again because attenuation is minimal. Because gamma radiation requires significant extra shielding and requires the staff to leave the room during delivery of therapy, beta radiation is used more commonly. In addition, the long-term effects remain a concern.[285] Finally, significant expertise is required for intracoronary brachytherapy. In addition to the interventionalist, a radiation oncologist, medical physicist, and radiation safety officer must participate in these procedures.[286]

Brachytherapy, using either a gamma- or beta-emitter, was effective for the treatment of in-stent restenosis in BMSs.[287,288] After brachytherapy, clopidogrel must be continued for at least 6 to 12 months to prevent late stent thrombosis that occurs because of delayed endothelialization of the stent. The future for brachytherapy in the era of DESs is unknown.[127] DESs have significantly decreased in-stent restenosis. If restenosis does occur with a DES, whether brachytherapy should be undertaken or repeat DES insertion performed is unclear.[130] Because of the benefit of DESs in reducing restenosis and the complexity of brachytherapy, its use in the interventional suite currently is limited to a few centers in the country.

Thrombosuction/Thrombolysis

The transluminal extraction catheter (TEC) was released for use in 1993 as the first device designed to mechanically remove thrombus or other loose debris and was designed primarily for degenerated SVGs. The TEC device was a hollow tube with a propeller-like blade on its tip that applied proximal suction so it cut and aspirated as it was advanced into the lesion. Although an important tool when first introduced, newer thrombectomy devices have replaced this tool in the interventional suite.[289]

The AngioJet rheolytic thrombectomy system (Possis Medical, Minneapolis, MN) creates a Venturi effect utilizing six high-velocity saline jets distally at a pressure of 2500 psi and a flow rate of 50 mL/min to generate a low-pressure zone (< 600 mm Hg) and cause a powerful vacuum effect. The catheter is a multilumen 4-French system and may be passed through a 6-French guiding catheter. One lumen delivers the saline, a second lumen is for guidewire passage, and a third permits thrombus evacuation utilizing a roller pump.[289]

The system creates a recirculation pattern at the catheter tip. This emulsifies and removes thrombus without embolization. Rheolytic thrombectomy was first approved for SVGs, utilizing a larger 6-French catheter. It can remove thrombus from native arteries and SVGs; however, some trials suggest that it may be less effective than alternative therapies for SVGs.[290,291] Although initial studies in small patient populations were encouraging for AMI patients,[292] a larger trial of 480 patients presenting within 12 hours of the onset of MI demonstrated greater mortality in the rheolytic

thrombectomy group.[293] The Rescue Catheter (Boston Scientific/Scimed. Inc., Maple Grove, MN) is a thrombectomy system with vacuum withdrawal that similarly showed possible deleterious effects with routine use in primary PCI.[294] Despite these findings, this therapy remains an option in lesions with a significant thrombus burden.[295]

Ultrasound thrombolysis is under development for the treatment of degenerated SVGs. However, the ATLAS (Acolysis during Treatment of Lesions Affecting Saphenous vein bypass grafts) trial in patients with ACSs and undergoing interventions in SVGs showed a greater incidence of ischemic complications with ultrasound thrombolysis.[296]

Simple aspiration devices have been developed to facilitate thrombus removal, particularly in the setting of AMI.[297] The prototype was the Export catheter (Medtronic). This is simply a tube with two lumens. One lumen tracks over a guidewire that has been advanced through the thrombotic area. The second lumen is connected to a syringe. Negative pressure is generated with the syringe. The TAPAS trial (Thrombus Aspiration during Percutaneous coronary intervention in acute myocardial infarction Study) randomized 1071 patients undergoing primary PCI for AMI to either PCI alone or thrombus aspiration with the Export catheter, followed by PCI. Mortality at 1 year was 3.6% in the group that had thrombus aspiration and 6.7% in the control group ($P = 0.02$).[298] This would seem to make manual aspiration the preferred adjunctive therapy in primary PCI (Figure 3-24).

Distal Protection Devices

PCI in degenerative vein grafts is complicated by a significant incidence of MI that is thought to result from embolization of debris. GPIIb/IIIa inhibition has not decreased MI in this situation.[177] Although other factors, such as spasm in the distal arterial bed, may contribute to the complications during PCI in SVGs, most efforts to address this problem have focused on devices that are designed to capture potential embolic debris released as the probable cause of the "no-reflow" phenomenon during PCI.[117] These distal protection devices come in two types: vessel occlusive and vessel nonocclusive.

Vessel-occlusive devices use a soft, compliant balloon that is incorporated into a wire. The wire is passed distal to the stenosis and inflated during the PCI. A column of blood is trapped, which includes the debris liberated during PCI. The blood and debris are aspirated before deflation of the distal balloon and restoration of flow. The GuardWire is an FDA-approved device of this type (Medtronic). In the SAFER (Saphenous vein graft Angioplasty Free of Emboli Randomized) trial, 801 patients undergoing PCI in SVGs were randomized to distal protection with the GuardWire or no distal protection. The composite end point of death, MI, and repeat target vessel revascularization were 9.6% in the GuardWire group and 16.5% in the standard care group. MI was reduced by 42% in the distal protection group.[290]

A learning curve exists with this device to maximize prevention of emboli and minimize ischemic time. Patients with large areas of myocardium supplied by the SVG undergoing PCI may not be candidates because of the inability to tolerate ischemia. Also, distal lesions in an SVG may not allow for placement of the large balloon. The Enhanced Myocardial Efficacy and Removal by Aspiration of Liberated Debris (EMERALD) trial tested the GuardWire in the setting of primary PCI

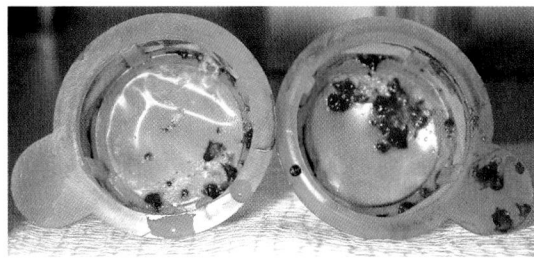

Figure 3-24 The Export catheter was used to aspirate this thrombotic material in the setting of an acute myocardial infarction.

of native vessels during AMI. The thrombotic AMI lesion seemed likely to benefit from aspiration of debris. However, this study showed no benefit from the device, a result attributed to the presence of side branches that are not present in SVGs.[299]

Nonocclusive devices include various forms of filters, as well as the thrombolysis or thrombectomy devices discussed earlier.[300,301] The Filter Wire (Boston Scientific) was the first filter approved. This is a 0.014-inch guidewire that incorporates a nonoccluding, polyurethane, porous membrane filter (80-μm pores). The system includes a retrieval catheter that fits over the device after PCI is completed (Figure 3-25). Two clinical trials, the first compared with PCI alone and the second randomizing the Filter Wire EX to the GuardWire, have been completed to date.[301,302] The Filter Wire was superior to PCI alone and noninferior to the GuardWire system.

Therapy for Chronic Total Occlusions

Despite steady progress in most areas of interventional cardiology, therapy for chronic total occlusions (CTOs) appeared to lag behind until several recent advances.[303] CTOs are defined as vessels that have been occluded for more than 3 months. They often are associated with significant collateral flow from other vessels and often are treated conservatively (medical therapy). Guidewires with stiff tips, improved techniques, and operator experience have led to success rates greater

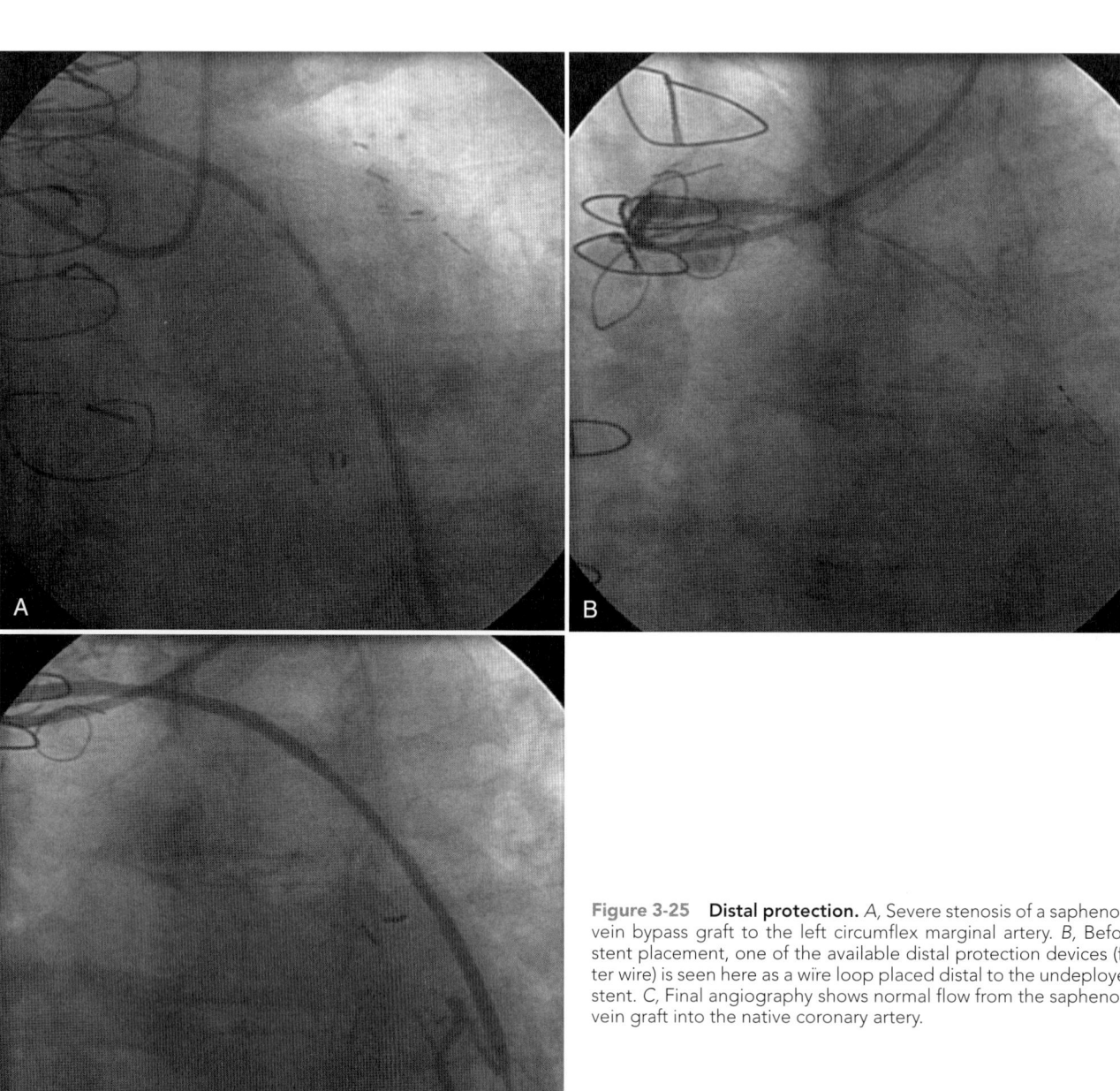

Figure 3-25 **Distal protection.** *A,* Severe stenosis of a saphenous vein bypass graft to the left circumflex marginal artery. *B,* Before stent placement, one of the available distal protection devices (filter wire) is seen here as a wire loop placed distal to the undeployed stent. *C,* Final angiography shows normal flow from the saphenous vein graft into the native coronary artery.

than 80% in high-volume centers.[304] Patients with CTO who were successfully revascularized had better long-term outcomes than those who could not be revascularized.[305,306]

Other devices for CTO are in various stages of development. The Frontrunner (LuMend, Inc., Redwood City, CA) is a bioptome-like cutting device designed to selectively remove fibrous tissue from within the lumen.[307] This is approved for peripheral interventions but not coronary interventions. The Prima FX laser wire (Spectranetics, Colorado Springs, CO) has the ability to deliver excimer laser energy from the tip of the wire. The Prima FX has CE mark approval in Europe but is investigational in the United States. With these continued advances in technology, changing techniques including retrograde wire approaches and more experienced operators forming "CTO" clubs, CTO interventions will continue to expand with improved procedural outcomes.[303]

OTHER CATHETER-BASED PERCUTANEOUS THERAPIES

Percutaneous Valvular Therapy

Mitral Balloon Valvuloplasty

Percutaneous mitral valvuloplasty (PMV) was first performed in 1982 as an alternative to surgery for patients with rheumatic MS. The procedure usually is performed via an antegrade approach and requires expertise in transseptal puncture. During the early years of PMV, the simultaneous inflation of two balloons in the mitral apparatus was required to obtain an adequate result. The development of the Inoue balloon (Toray, Inc., Houston, TX) in the 1990s simplified this procedure. This single balloon, with a central waist for placement at the valve, does not require wire placement across the aortic valve.[308] The key to mitral valvuloplasty is patient selection. Absolute contraindications to mitral valvuloplasty include a known LA thrombus or recent embolic event within the preceding 2 months, and severe cardiothoracic deformity or bleeding abnormality preventing transseptal catheterization. Relative contraindications include significant mitral regurgitation, pregnancy, concomitant significant aortic valve disease, or significant CAD.[309]

All patients must undergo TEE to exclude LA thrombus, as well as transthoracic echocardiography, to classify the patient by anatomic groups. The most widely used classification, the Wilkins score, addresses leaflet mobility, valve thickening, subvalvular thickening, and valvular calcification. These scoring systems, as well as operator experience, predict outcomes. In experienced hands, the procedure is successful in 85% to 99% of cases. Risks for PMV include a procedural mortality of 0% to 3%, hemopericardium in 0.5% to 12%, and embolism in 0.5% to 5%. Severe mitral regurgitation occurs in 2% to 10% of procedures and often requires emergent surgery.[310] Although peripheral embolization occurs in up to 4% of patients, long-term sequelae are rare.

The procedure requires a large puncture in the interatrial septum, and this does not close completely in all patients. However, a clinically significant ASD with Q_p/Q_s of 1.5 or greater occurs in 10% or fewer cases; surgical repair is seldom necessary. Advances in patient selection, operator experience, and equipment have significantly reduced procedural complications.[310] Restenosis rates are dependent on the degree of commissural calcium.[308] TEE or intracardiac echocardiography is helpful during balloon mitral valvuloplasty.[54] These imaging modalities offer guidance with the transseptal catheter placement, verification of balloon positioning across the valve, and assessment of procedural success.[310] Long-term results have been good.[311]

Aortic Balloon Valvuloplasty

Percutaneous aortic balloon valvuloplasty was introduced in the 1980s. This procedure usually is performed via a femoral artery, using an 11-French sheath and 18- to 23-mm balloons. Some advocate the double-balloon technique for aortic valvuloplasty to decrease restenosis with a balloon placed through each femoral artery and inflated simultaneously.

Symptomatic improvement does occur with at least a 50% reduction in gradient in more than 80% of cases.[312] Complications include femoral artery repair in up to 10% of patients, a 1% incidence rate of stroke, and a less than 1% incidence rate of cardiac fatality.[312] Contraindications to aortic balloon valvuloplasty are significant peripheral vascular disease and moderate-to-severe AI. AI usually increases at least one grade during valvuloplasty. The development of severe AR acutely leads to pulmonary congestion and possibly death, as the hypertrophied ventricle is unable to dilate.

Initial success rates are acceptable, but restenosis occurs as early as 6 months after the procedure and nearly all patients will have restenosis by 2 years. Therefore, the use of aortic valvuloplasty has waned. Current indications include the following: inoperable patient willing to accept the restenosis rate for temporary reduction in symptoms; noncardiac surgery patient hoping to decrease the surgical risk; and patient with poor LV function, in an attempt to improve ventricular function for further consideration of aortic valve replacement. The latter is the most common current indication for aortic valvuloplasty, which has seen a recent resurgence as preparation for percutaneous aortic valve implantation.[313]

Percutaneous Valve Replacement and Repair

Surgical valve replacement is performed for regurgitant and stenotic valves. Although surgical morbidity and mortality continue to improve, the risks remain prohibitive for some patients. Catheter-based alternatives to surgical valve replacement have been explored since the 1960s but were not successful until 2000, when percutaneous pulmonic valve replacement was performed.[314] The Melody transcatheter pulmonary valve (Medtronic) was approved in Canada and Europe in 2006. It recently received humanitarian device exemption approval from the FDA and is available for treatment of failed pulmonary valve conduits.[315] The procedures are performed under general anesthesia with fluoroscopic and echocardiographic guidance. A bovine jugular valve is sutured onto a platinum-iridium stent and delivered on a balloon. The stent compresses the native valve against the wall of the annulus. Large 22-French delivery systems are used. The results in high-risk patients have been promising, and the device is now being tested in a lower-risk group, that is, as a true alternative to surgery. The success of percutaneous pulmonic valve replacement prompted interest in the aortic and mitral valves.[316,317]

The first percutaneous aortic valve replacement in humans was performed in France in 2002. This valve was created by shaping bovine pericardium into leaflets and mounting them within a short, balloon-expandable stent.[318] Retrograde, antegrade, and transapical approaches have been used. The size of the delivery system is large, requiring surgical entry and repair of the vascular access sites. Many patients with aortic valve disease, particularly those at high risk for traditional surgical valve replacement, have severe vascular disease that would not permit delivery passage of the large systems required for percutaneous valve replacement. For such patients, the transapical approach using a small thoracotomy incision may be most suitable. This approach requires that general anesthesia be administered to a patient with critical aortic stenosis and may pose particular challenges for the anesthesiologist.[319]

The Edwards SAPIEN percutaneous valve (Edwards Lifesciences, Irvine, CA) has received regulatory approval in Europe, and clinical trials are in progress in the United States. A second system, the CoreValve Revalving system (Medtronic), has received regulatory approval in Europe, and clinical trials are planned in the United States. This system consists of a long, self-expanding nitinol stent with an attached valve constructed from porcine pericardium. Early results were encouraging with both systems, as improvements in symptoms and ventricular function were seen after percutaneous aortic valve replacement.[319] To date, results have been obtained in patients who were deemed at high risk for surgical valve replacement.[316] The high rate of observed complications was tolerable when compared with the projected outcome with surgery. There is some controversy as to the determination of risk status.[320] Further improvements will be necessary before percutaneous techniques can replace surgical valve replacement in lower-risk groups.

The percutaneous approach for mitral regurgitation includes both attempts to replace as well as to repair the mitral valve.[82,317] Preliminary work to date has included two approaches. The first approach involves placement of a device composed of a distal and proximal anchor placed within the coronary sinus. This device can then be shortened to decrease the size of the mitral annulus and decrease mitral regurgitation, similar to a surgically placed annuloplasty ring.[321] The second approach involves percutaneous suturing of the mitral leaflets with the MitraClip (Evalve, Menlo Park, CA). The result is similar to the surgical Alfieri operation. Flow from the LA continues through both orifices, whereas prolapse of the leaflets and regurgitation are minimized. Accordingly, the device is suitable for functional mitral regurgitation and mitral regurgitation from degenerative disease, but less so with restriction from ischemia or other causes. A report on 107 patients described procedural success in 74%, with a 9% rate of major adverse events (none lethal) in a high-risk cohort.[322] Trials comparing the device with surgical repair are in progress. The device has received regulatory approval in Europe. Finally, both temporary and permanent mitral valve implantations have been attempted but are early in the experimental process.[317]

Although still experimental, percutaneous valve replacement and repair are exciting and offer a new dimension in catheter-based therapy. Experience to date is limited compared with the years of work and thousands of patients with surgical intervention. Although initial outcomes are encouraging,[316,322] enthusiasm should still be tempered.[323] However, as this field expands, the role of the cardiac anesthesiologist in the catheterization laboratory for these complex procedures likely will expand (see Chapters 19 and 26).

OTHER CATHETER-BASED INTRACARDIAC PROCEDURES

■ Alcohol Septal Ablation

Hypertrophic cardiomyopathy is a genetic disorder that can present with sudden cardiac death or symptoms of heart failure. A minority of patients will have asymmetric septal hypertrophy that leads to dynamic outflow tract obstruction and produces severe symptoms. When these patients are refractory to medical therapy, a surgical procedure for septal tissue removal, and often mitral valve repair or replacement, may be required. Since the mid-1990s, percutaneous methods have been studied to induce a controlled infarction and selectively ablate this overgrown septal tissue[324] (see Chapter 22).

Through a standard guiding catheter, a guidewire is placed in the large proximal septal perforator. A balloon catheter is placed over the wire, into the septal perforator, and inflated to occlude flow. The wire is removed and ethanol, 1 to 3 mL, is injected through the balloon into the septal perforator and left in place for 5 minutes. Temporary pacing is required in all patients, and a permanent pacemaker is required occasionally. When performed by experienced operators, morbidity and mortality are limited, the gradient is reduced, and symptoms are improved.[325,326] Controversy persists regarding the role of alcohol septal ablation compared with surgical septal myectomy, with the specific procedure selection best based on the individual patient.[327,328]

■ Left Atrial Appendage Occlusion

AF is responsible for up to 20% of strokes. These strokes are caused by embolization of an atrial clot, most of which arise in the LA appendage. Warfarin therapy is effective for stroke prevention but is associated with morbidity and mortality, and many patients have contraindications to warfarin. The PLAATO system (Appriva Medical, Inc., Sunnyvale, CA) is a self-expanding nitinol cage, 5 to 32 mm in diameter, covered with an occlusive polytetrafluoroethylene membrane. Placed via the transseptal approach under TEE guidance, this device is designed to occlude the atrial appendage, as well as become incorporated into the appendage, preventing both clot formation and embolization. An observational study of 64 patients with permanent or paroxysmal AF who were at high risk for stroke reported one major complication from the implantation procedure.[329] After up to 5 years of follow-up, the annualized stroke/TIA rate was 3.8%. The anticipated stroke/TIA rate ($CHADS_2$ method) was 6.6%/year.

The WATCHMAN left atrial appendage system (Atritech Inc., Plymouth, MN) is a similar, covered, nitinol device implanted percutaneously to seal the appendage. The PROTECT AF trial (WATCHMAN Left Atrial Appendage System for Embolic PROTECTion in Patients with Atrial Fibrillation) randomized 707 patients with permanent, persistent, or paroxysmal AF at high risk for a stroke to appendage occlusion with the WATCHMAN device or warfarin therapy in a 2:1 ratio. The annual stroke rate was 2.3% in the device group and 3.2% in the warfarin group. Pericardial drainage was required in 5% of patients undergoing implantation, although no deaths occurred. Periprocedural stroke and device embolization occurred in 1.1% and 0.6% of patients, respectively.[330] The WATCHMAN has received regulatory approval in Europe but is awaiting regulatory action in the United States. In the treatment of AF, individual patient decisions will need to be made by weighing the proven long-term benefits and risks of rate control with warfarin against those of invasive therapies like catheter ablation and left atrial appendage occlusion.

■ Percutaneous Closure of Patent Foramen Ovale and Atrial Septal Defect

The Amplatzer device (AGA Medical Corp., Golden Valley, MN) is FDA approved and is preferred to surgical closure for isolated secundum defects. A newer device, the Helex septal occluder (Gore Medical, Flagstaff, AZ), is an alternative for some smaller defects.[331] Echocardiographic guidance is required, either transesophageal or intracardiac.[54] Accordingly, general anesthesia is used frequently to permit prolonged transesophageal imaging. In appropriately selected patients, success rates are near 100%, and complications are rare (see Videos 4–6).

Two devices, the Amplatzer PFO Occluder (AGA Medical, Plymouth, MN) and the CardioSEAL (NMT Medical, Inc., Boston, MA), had been available under the Humanitarian Device Exemption in the United States for use in the patient with a PFO who had a recurrent stroke while receiving warfarin. The devices were withdrawn from the market in 2006 for a variety of reasons, primarily the fact that their use had expanded outside of the approved indication without data to support such expanded use. Clinical trials are in progress to determine whether the devices are more effective than anticoagulation in preventing recurrent stroke after the first event (Figure 3-26). Improvement in migraine after PFO closure has been reported.[332] Surgical closure has been relegated to the few patients whose anatomy precludes percutaneous closure[333] (see Chapters 20 and 22).

Percutaneous Transmyocardial Laser Revascularization

Surgical transmyocardial laser revascularization was introduced in the late 1990s. This procedure produces a series of channels from the epicardium to the endocardium, either as a primary procedure or in conjunction with CABG, in patients with refractory angina and proved ischemia who cannot be revascularized by standard techniques. Transmyocardial laser revascularization can improve angina in these patients, although the mechanism is not clear.[334,335] In an attempt to avoid the risks of a thoracotomy, percutaneous transmyocardial laser revascularization was developed to create these channels from the endocardial surface. A randomized clinical trial in 141 patients with class III or IV angina was performed to determine whether this technique was more effective in decreasing ischemia than a sham procedure. Unfortunately, this study failed to show a benefit of percutaneous transmyocardial laser revascularization, and its future is uncertain.[336]

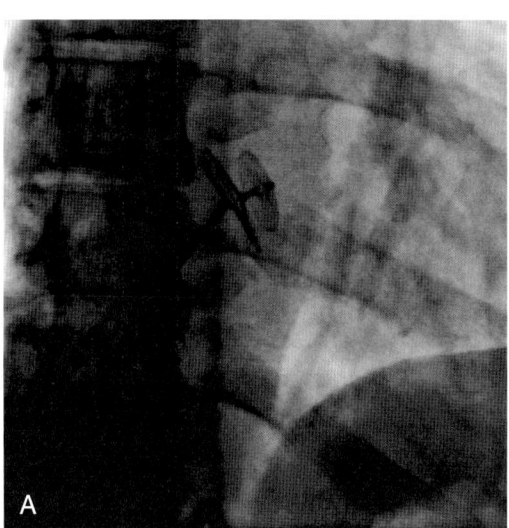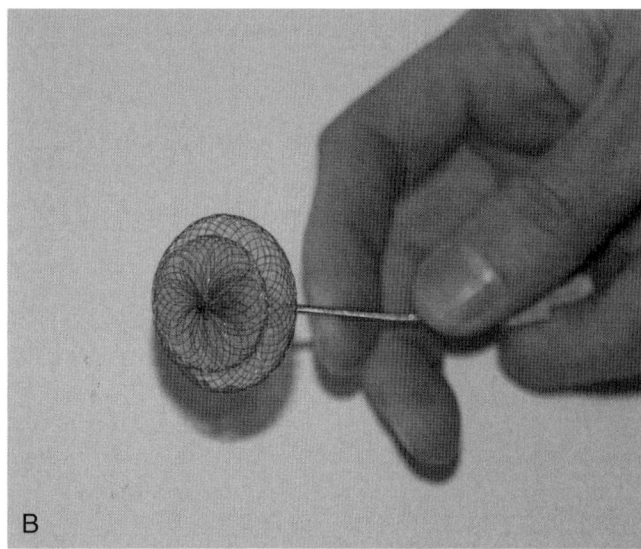

Figure 3-26 *A,* Deployment of a patent foramen ovale (PFO) closure device. *B,* PFO closure device.

THE CATHETERIZATION LABORATORY AND THE ANESTHESIOLOGIST

The objective of this chapter has been to provide a broad overview of the catheterization laboratory for the anesthesiologist. As success rates for coronary interventions have increased and complication rates have decreased, there have been fewer opportunities for the invasive/interventional cardiologist and the anesthesiologist to interact in the

catheterization suite. However, in the 21st century, the role of the anesthesiologist in the catheterization laboratory and the location of the invasive cardiac procedures are destined to change. Whether it is the anesthesiologist traveling to the catheterization laboratory for percutaneous valve insertion or the cardiologist "visiting" the hybrid OR suite for combined stent/surgical procedures, the invasive cardiologist and the anesthesiologist will likely be reunited in this ever-changing field of invasive cardiac care.

REFERENCES

1. Achenbach S, Ludwig J: Is CT the better angiogram? Coronary interventions and CT imaging, *J Am Coll Cardiol* 3:29, 2010.
2. Kim WY, Danias PG, Stuber M, et al: Coronary magnetic resonance angiography for the detection of coronary stenoses, *N Engl J Med* 345:1863, 2001.
3. Bittl JA, Hirsch AT: Concomitant peripheral arterial disease and coronary artery disease: Therapeutic opportunities, *Circulation* 109:3136, 2004.
4. Verel D, editor: *Cardiac Catheterization and Angiocardiography,* ed 3, London, 1978, Churchill Livingstone.
5. Forssmann-Falch R: Werner Forssman: A pioneer of cardiology, *Am J Cardiol* 79:651, 1997.
6. Ross J: Transseptal left heart catheterization, *J Am Coll Cardiol* 51:2107, 2008.
7. Bruschke A, Sheldon W, Shirey E, et al: A half century of selective coronary anatomy, *J Am Coll Cardiol* 54:2139, 2009.
8. Byrne J, Leacche M, Vaughan D, et al: Hybrid cardiovascular procedures, *J Am Coll Cardiol* 1:459, 2008.
9. Braunwald E: Cardiology: The past, the present, and the future, *J Am Coll Cardiol* 42:2031, 2003.
10. Balter S, Moses J: Managing patient dose in interventional cardiology, *Catheter Cardiovasc Interv* 70:244–249, 2007.
11. Johnson LW, Moore RJ, Balter S: Review of radiation safety in the cardiac catheterization laboratory, *Cathet Cardiovasc Diagn* 25:186, 1992.
12. Bashore TM, Bates ER, Berger PB, et al: ACC/SCA&I expert consensus document on cardiac catheterization laboratory standards, *J Am Coll Cardiol* 37:2170, 2001.
13. Mettler FA, Voelz GL: Major radiation exposure—what to expect and how to respond, *N Engl J Med* 346:1554, 2002.
14. Stecker MS, Balter S, Towbin RB, et al: Guidelines for patient radiation management, *J Vasc Interv Radiol* 20:S263–S273, 2009.
15. Hirshfeld JW, Balter S, Brinker JA, et al: ACCF/AHA/NASPE-HRS/SCAI clinical competence statement on physician knowledge to optimize patient safety and image quality in fluoroscopically guided invasive cardiovascular procedures, *J Am Coll Cardiol* 44:2259, 2004.
16. Klein LW, Miller DL, Balter S, et al: Occupational health hazards in the interventional laboratory: Time for a safer environment, *Catheter Cardiovasc Interv* 73:432, 2009.
17. ACC/ACR/NEMA Ad Hoc Group: American College of Cardiology, American College of Radiology and industry develop standard for digital transfer of angiographic images, *J Am Coll Cardiol* 25:800, 1995.
18. American College of Cardiology Cardiac Catheterization Committee: Cardiac angiography without cine film: Erecting a "Tower of Babel" in the cardiac catheterization laboratory, *J Am Coll Cardiol* 24:834, 1994.
19. Holmes DR, Laskey WK, Wondrow MA, et al: Flat-panel detectors in the cardiac catheterization laboratory: Revolution or evolution—What are the issues? *Catheter Cardiovasc Interv* 63:324, 2004.
20. Ryan TJ, Klocke FJ, Reynolds WA: Clinical competence in percutaneous transluminal coronary angioplasty: A statement for physicians from the ACP/ACC/AHA Task Force on Clinical Privileges in Cardiology, *Circulation* 81:2041, 1990.
21. King S, Aversano T, Ballard W, et al: ACCF/AHA/SCAI 2007 Update of the Clinical Competence Statement on Cardiac Interventional Procedures, *J Am Coll Cardiol* 50:82, 2007.
22. Smith SC Jr, Feldman TE, Hirshfeld JW Jr, et al: ACC/AHA/SCAI 2005 guideline update for percutaneous coronary intervention: A report of the American College of Cardiology/American Heart Association Task Force on Practice Guidelines (ACC/AHA/SCAI Writing Committee to Update the 2001 Guidelines for Percutaneous Coronary Intervention), *J Am Coll Cardiol* 47:e1–e121, 2006.
23. Wennberg DE, Lucas FL, Siewers AE, et al: Outcomes of percutaneous coronary interventions performed at centers without and with onsite coronary artery bypass graft surgery, *JAMA* 292:1961, 2004.
24. Kutcher M, Klein L, et al: Percutaneous coronary interventions in facilities without cardiac surgery on site: A report from the National Cardiovascular Data Registry (NCDR), *J Am Coll Cardiol* 54:15, 2009.
25. Lotfi M, Mackie K, Dzavik V, et al: Impact of delays to cardiac surgery after failed angioplasty and stenting, *J Am Coll Cardiol* 43:337, 2004.
26. King SB, Smith SC, Hirshfeld JW, et al: 2007 Writing Group to Review the Evidence and Update the ACC/AHA/SCAI 2005 Guideline Update for Percutaneous Coronary Intervention. 2007 Focused Update of the ACC/AHA/SCAI 2005 Guideline Update for Percutaneous Coronary Intervention. A report of the American College of Cardiology/American Heart Association Task Force on Practice Guidelines, *J Am Coll Cardiol* 51:172, 2008.
27. Krumholz H, Anderson J, Fesmire F, et al: ACC/AHA clinical performance measures for adult with ST-elevation and non-ST-elevation myocardial infarction, *Circulation* 113:732, 2006.
28. Kushner F, Hand M, Smith S, et al: 2009 focused updates: ACC/AHA guidelines for the management of patients with ST-elevation myocardial infarction (updating the 2004 guideline and 2007 focused update) and ACC/AHA/SCAI guidelines on percutaneous coronary intervention (updating the 2005 guideline and 2007 focused update), *J Am Coll Cardiol* 54:2205, 2009.
29. Vakili BA, Kaplan R, Brown DL: Volume-outcome relation for physicians and hospitals performing angioplasty for acute myocardial infarction in New York State, *Circulation* 104:2171, 2001.
30. Jollis JG, Peterson ED, DeLong ER, et al: The relation between the volume of coronary angioplasty procedures at hospitals treating Medicare beneficiaries and short-term mortality, *N Engl J Med* 334:1625, 1994.
31. Epstein AJ, Rathore SS, Volpp KGM, et al: Hospital percutaneous coronary intervention volume and patient mortality, 1998 to 2000. Does the evidence support current procedure volume minimums? *J Am Coll Cardiol* 43:1755, 2004.
32. Beller G, Bonow R, Fuster V: ACCP 2008 Recommendations for Training in Adult Cardiovascular Medicine Core Cardiology Training (COCATS 3), *J Am Coll Cardiol* 51:335, 2008.
33. Klein LW, Kolm P, Krone RJ, et al: A longitudinal assessment of coronary interventional program quality. A report from the ACC-NCDR, *JACC Cardiovasc Interv* 2:136, 2009.
34. Heupler FA Jr, Chambers CE, Dear WE, et al: Guidelines for internal peer review in the cardiac catheterization laboratory, *Cathet Cardiovasc Diagn* 40:21, 1997.
35. Yadav JS, Wholey MH, Kuntz RE, et al: Protected carotid-artery stenting versus endarterectomy in high-risk patients, *N Engl J Med* 351:1493, 2004.
36. ACC/AHA guidelines for exercise testing: A report of the American College of Cardiology/American Heart Association task force on practice guidelines (committee on exercise testing), *J Am Coll Cardiol* 30:260, 1997.
37. Schweiger MJ, Chambers CE, Davidson CJ, et al: Prevention of contrast induced nephropathy: Recommendations for the high risk patient undergoing cardiovascular procedures, *Catheter Cardiovasc Interv* 69:135, 2007.
38. Brueck M, Bandorski D, Kramer W, et al: A randomized comparison of transradial versus transfemoral approach for coronary angiography and angioplasty, *JACC Cardiovasc Interv* 2:1047, 2009.
39. Brouwer MA, Freek VW: Oral anticoagulation for acute coronary syndromes, *Circulation* 105:1270, 2002.
40. Heyder O, Schmidt H, Hackenbroch M, et al: Silent and apparent cerebral embolism after retrograde catheterization of the aortic valve in valvular stenosis: A prospective, randomized study, *Lancet* 361:1241, 2003.

41. Jolly S, Amlani S, Hamon M, et al: Radial versus femoral access for coronary angiography or intervention and the impact on major bleeding and ischemic events: A systematic review and meta-analysis of randomized trials, *Am Heart J* 157:132, 2009.
42. Steffenino G, Dellavalle A, Ribichini F, et al: Ambulation three hours after elective cardiac catheterization through the femoral artery, *Heart* 75:477, 1996.
43. Dauerman H, Applegate R, Cohen D: Vascular closure devices, *J Am Coll Cardiol* 50:1617, 2007.
44. Goss JE, Chambers CE, Heupler FA, et al: Systemic anaphylactoid reactions to iodinated contrast media during cardiac catheterization procedures: Guidelines for prevention, diagnosis, and treatment, *Cathet Cardiovasc Diagn* 34:99, 1995.
45. Greenberger PA, Patterson R, Tapio CM: Prophylaxis against repeated radiocontrast media reactions in 857 cases, *Ann Intern Med* 145:2197, 1985.
46. Rihal CS, Textor SC, Grill DE, et al: Incidence and prognostic importance of acute renal failure after percutaneous coronary intervention, *Circulation* 105:2259, 2002.
47. Mehran R, Aymong ED, Nikolsky E, et al: A simple risk score for prediction of contrast-induced nephropathy after percutaneous coronary intervention, *J Am Coll Cardiol* 44:1393, 2004.
48. American College of Cardiology Cardiovascular Imaging Committee: Use of nonionic or low osmolar contrast agents in cardiovascular procedures, *J Am Coll Cardiol* 21:269, 1993.
49. Heinrich M, Haberle L, Muller V, et al: Nephrotoxicity of iso-osmolar iodizanol compared with nonionic low-osmolar contrast media: Meta-analysis of randomized controlled trials, *Radiology* 250:68, 2009.
50. Brown J, Block C, Malenka D, et al: Sodium bicarbonate plus N-acetylcysteine prophylaxis, *J Am Coll Cardiol* 2:1117, 2009.
51. Briguori C, Colombo A, Airoldi F, et al: N-acetylcysteine versus fenoldopam mesylate to prevent contrast agent-associated nephrotoxicity, *J Am Coll Cardiol* 44:762, 2004.
52. Dodson SR, Hensley FA Jr, Martin DE, et al: Continuous oxygen saturation monitoring during cardiac catheterization in adults, *Chest* 94:28, 1988.
53. Geller E, Halpern P, Chernilas J, et al: Cardiorespiratory effects of antagonism of diazepam sedation with flumazenil in patients with cardiac disease, *Anesth Analg* 72:207, 1991.
54. Kim S, Hijazi Z, Lang R, et al: The use of intra-cardiac echocardiography and other intracardiac imaging tools to guide non-coronary cardiac interventions, *J Am Coll Cardiol* 53:2117, 2009.
55. Rao S, Ou F, Wang T, et al: Trends in the prevalence and outcomes of radial and femoral approaches to percutaneous coronary intervention, *J Am Coll Cardiol* 1:379, 2008.
56. Wakeyama T, Ogawa H, Iida H, et al: Intima-media thickening of the radial artery after transradial intervention, *J Am Coll Cardiol* 41:1109, 2003.
57. Kron J, Sutherland D, Rosch J, et al: Arteriovenous fistula: A rare complication of arterial puncture for cardiac catheterization, *Am J Cardiol* 55:1445, 1985.
58. Kern MJ, Cohen M, Talley JD, et al: Early ambulation after 5-French diagnostic cardiac catheterization: Results of a multicenter trial, *J Am Coll Cardiol* 15:1475, 1990.
59. Vacek JL, Bellinger RL, Phelix J: Heparin bolus therapy during cardiac catheterization, *Am J Cardiol* 62:1314, 1988.
60. Shehadi WH: Adverse reactions to intravascularly administered contrast media: A comprehensive study based on prospective survey, *Am J Radiol* 124:145, 1975.
61. Salem DN, Konstam MA, Isner JM, et al: Comparison of the electrocardiographic and hemodynamic responses to ionic and nonionic radiocontrast media during left ventriculography: A randomized double-blind study, *Am Heart J* 111:533, 1986.
62. Bergstra A, VanDijk RB, Brekke O, et al: Hemodynamic effects of iodixanol and iohexol during ventriculography in patients with compromised left ventricular function, *Catheter Cardiovasc Interv* 50:314, 2000.
63. Markou CP, Chronos NAF, Hanson SR: Antithrombotic effects of ionic and nonionic contrast media in nonhuman primates, *J Thromb Haemost* 85:488, 2001.
64. Grabowski EF: A hematologist's view of contrast media, clotting in angiography syringes, and thrombosis during coronary angiography, *Am J Cardiol* 66:23F, 1990.
65. Katayama H: *Report of the Japanese committee on the safety of contrast media*, Presented at the Radiological Society of North America Meeting, November, 1988.
66. Palmer FJ: The RACR survey of intravenous contrast media reactions: A preliminary report, *Australas Radiol* 32:8, 1988.
67. Davidson CJ, Laskey WK, Hermiller JB, et al: Randomized trial of contrast media utilization in high-risk PTCA. The COURT Trial, *Circulation* 101:2172, 2000.
68. Robin ED: The cult of the Swan-Ganz catheter, *Ann Intern Med* 103:445, 1985.
69. Hill JA, Miranda AA, Keim SG, et al: Value of right-sided cardiac catheterization in patients undergoing left-sided cardiac catheterization for evaluation of coronary artery disease, *Am J Cardiol* 65:590, 1990.
70. Ganz W, Donoso R, Marcus HS, et al: A new technique for measurement of cardiac output by thermodilution in man, *Am J Cardiol* 27:392, 1971.
71. Forrester JS, Diamond G, Chatterjee K, et al: Medical therapy of acute myocardial infarction by application of hemodynamic subsets (first of two parts), *N Engl J Med* 295:1356, 1976.
72. Forrester JS, Diamond G, Chatterjee K, et al: Medical therapy of acute myocardial infarction by application of hemodynamic subsets (second of two parts), *N Engl J Med* 295:1404, 1976.
73. Chin K, Rubin L: Pulmonary arterial hypertension, *J Am Coll Cardiol* 51:1527, 2008.
74. Grossman W: Shunt detection and measurement. In Grossman W, Baim DS, editors: *Cardiac Catheterization, Angiography, and Intervention*, ed 4, Philadelphia, 1991, Lea & Febiger, pp 166.
75. Polanczyk CA, Rohde LE, Goldman L, et al: Right-heart catheterization and cardiac complications in patients undergoing noncardiac surgery. An observational study, *JAMA* 286:309, 2001.
76. Cooper LT, Baughman KL, Feldman AM, et al: The role of endomyocardial biopsy in the management of cardiovascular disease: A scientific statement from the American Heart Association, the American College of Cardiology, and the European Society of Cardiology. Endorsed by the Heart Failure Society of America and the Heart Failure Association of the European Society of Cardiology, *J Am Coll Cardiol* 50:1914, 2007.
77. Kennedy JW: The Registry Committee of the Society for Cardiac Angiography: Complications associated with cardiac catheterization and angiography, *Cathet Cardiovasc Diagn* 8:5, 1982.
78. Johnson W, Lozner EC, Johnson S, et al: Coronary angiography 1984: A report of the Registry of the Society for Cardiac Angiography and Interventions. I. Results and complications, *Cathet Cardiovasc Diagn* 17:5, 1989.
79. Chambers CE, Eisenhauer MD, McNicol LB, et al: Infection control guidelines for the cardiac catheterization laboratory, *Catheter Cardiovasc Interv* 67:78, 2006.
80. Colt HG, Begg RJ, Saporito J, et al: Cholesterol emboli after cardiac catheterization, *Medicine* 67:389, 1988.
81. Hendel RC, Cuenoud HF, Giansiracusa DF, et al: Multiple cholesterol emboli syndrome: Bowel infarction after retrograde angiography, *Arch Intern Med* 149:2371, 1989.
82. Bonow R, Carabello B, Chatterjee K, et al: ACC/ACHA 2006 Practice Guidelines for the Management of Patients with Valvular Heart Disease: Executive summary, *J Am Coll Cardiol* 48:596, 2006.
83. Gorlin R, Gorlin G: Hydraulic formula for calculation of area of stenotic mitral valve, other cardiac values, and central circulatory shunts, *Am Heart J* 41:1, 1951.
84. Levy F, Laurent M, Monin JL, et al: Aortic valve replacement for low-flow/low-gradient aortic stenosis, *J Am Coll Cardiol* 51:1464, 2008.
85. Dodge HT, Sandler H, Ballew DW, et al: The use of biplane angiocardiography for the measurement of left ventricular volume in man, *Am Heart J* 60:762, 1960.
86. Fifer MA, Grossman W: Measurement of ventricular volumes, ejection fraction, mass, wall stress, and regional wall motion. In Grossman W, Baim DS, editors: *Cardiac Catheterization, Angiography, and Intervention*, Philadelphia, 1991, Lea & Febiger, pp 300.
87. Peterson GE, Brickner E, Reimold SC: Transesophageal echocardiography. Clinical indications and applications, *Circulation* 107:2398, 2003.
88. Moodie DS, Fyfe D, Gill CC, et al: Anomalous origin of the left coronary artery from the pulmonary artery (Bland-White-Garland syndrome) in adult patients: Long-term follow-up after surgery, *Am Heart J* 106:381, 1983.
89. Chaitman BR, Lesperance J, Saltiel J, et al: Clinical, angiographic, and hemodynamic findings in patients with anomalous origin of the coronary arteries, *Circulation* 53:122, 1976.
90. Angelini P: Congenital heart disease for the adult cardiologist-coronary artery anomalies, *Circulation* 115:1296, 2007.
91. White CW, Wright CB, Doty DB, et al: Does visual interpretation of the coronary arteriogram predict the physiologic importance of a coronary stenosis? *N Engl J Med* 310:819, 1984.
92. Mancini GBJ: Quantitative coronary arteriographic methods in the interventional catheterization laboratory: An update and perspective, *J Am Coll Cardiol* 17:23B, 1991.
93. Brown G: A direct comparison if intravascular ultrasound and quantitative coronary arteriography, *Circulation* 115:1824, 2007.
94. Boden WE, O'Rourke RA, Teo KK, et al: Optimal medical therapy with or without PCI for stable coronary disease, *N Engl J Med* 356:1503, 2007.
95. Kern M, Samady H: Current concepts of integrated coronary physiology in the catheterization laboratory, *J Am Coll Cardiol* 55:173, 2010.
96. Tonino PAL, De Bruyne B, Pijls NHJ, et al: Fractional flow reserve versus angiography for guiding percutaneous coronary intervention, *N Engl J Med* 360:213, 2009.
97. Tobis J, Azarbal B, Slavin L: Assessment of intermediate severity coronary lesions in the catheterization laboratory, *J Am Coll Cardiol* 49:839, 2007.
98. Pijls NHJ, van Schaardenburgh P, Manoharan G, et al: Percutaneous coronary intervention of functionally nonsignificant stenosis: 5-year follow-up of the DEFER study, *J Am Coll Cardiol* 49:2105, 2007.
99. Tonino P, Bruyne B, Pijls NHJ, et al: Fractional flow reserve versus angiography for guiding percutaneous coronary intervention, *N Engl J Med* 360:213, 2009.
100. Pellinen TJ, Virtanen KS, Toivonen L, et al: Coronary collateral circulation, *Clin Cardiol* 14:111, 1991.
101. Gregg DE, Patterson RE: Functional importance of the coronary collaterals, *N Engl J Med* 303:1404, 1980.
102. Nattel S, Rangno RE, Van Loon G: Mechanism of propranolol withdrawal phenomena, *Circulation* 59:1158, 1979.
103. Deckelbaum LI, Isner JM, Konstam MA, et al: Catheter-induced versus spontaneous spasm. Do these coronary bedfellows deserve to be estranged? *Am J Med* 79:1, 1985.
104. King SB: Percutaneous transluminal coronary angioplasty, *J Am Coll Cardiol* 34:615, 1999.
105. Kandzari D, Colombo A, Park SJ, et al: Revascularization for unprotected left main disease, *J Am Coll Cardiol* 54:1574, 2009.
106. Singh M, White J, Hasdai D, et al: Long-term outcome and its predictors among patients with ST-segment elevation myocardial infarction complicated by shock, *J Am Coll Cardiol* 50:1750, 2007.
107. Katritsis D, Meier B: Percutaneous coronary intervention for stable coronary artery disease, *J Am Coll Cardiol* 52:889, 2008.
108. Pijls NHJ, van Schaardenburgh P, Manoharan G, et al: Percutaneous coronary intervention of functionally nonsignificant stenosis, *J Am Coll Cardiol* 49:2105, 2007.
109. Buszman PE, Buszman PP, Kiesz RS, et al: Early and long-term results of unprotected left main coronary artery stenting, *J Am Coll Cardiol* 54:1498, 2009.
110. Chowdhary S, Ivanov J, Mackie K, et al: The Toronto score for in-hospital mortality after percutaneous coronary intervention, *Am Heart J* 157:156, 2009.
111. Daemen J, Kuck K, Macaya C, et al: Multivessel coronary revascularization in patients with and without diabetes mellitus, *J Am Coll Cardiol* 52:1957, 2008.
112. ACCF/SCAI/STS/AATS/AHA/ASNC: 2009 Appropriateness Criteria for Coronary Revascularization. Technical panel member, *J Am Coll Cardiol* 56:6, 2009.
113. Hodgson J, Reddy KG, Suneja R: Intracoronary ultrasound imaging: Correlation of plaque morphology with angiography, clinical syndrome and procedural results in patients undergoing coronary angioplasty, *J Am Coll Cardiol* 21:35, 1993.
114. Mintz G, Weissman N: Intravascular ultrasounds in the drug-eluting stent era, *J Am Coll Cardiol* 48:421, 2006.
115. Krone RJ, Shaw RE, Klein LW, et al: Ad hoc percutaneous coronary interventions in patients with stale coronary artery disease—a study of prevalence, safety, and variation in use from the American College of Cardiology National Cardiovascular Data Registry (AAA-NCDR), *Catheter Cardiovasc Interv* 68:696, 2006.
116. Fleischmann K, Beckman JA, Buller CE, et al: 2009 ACCF/AHA focused update on perioperative beta blockade, *J Am Coll Cardiol* 54:2102, 2009.
117. Niccoli G, Burzotta F, Galliuto L, et al: Myocardial no-reflow in humans, *J Am Coll Cardiol* 54:281, 2009.
118. Fugit MD, Rubal BJ, Donovan DJ: Effects of intracoronary nicardipine, diltiazem, and verapamil on coronary blood flow, *J Invasive Cardiol* 12:80, 2000.
119. Chambers CE, Dehmer G, Cox D, et al: Defining the level of care following percutaneous coronary intervention. An expert consensus document from the Society of Cardiovascular Angiography and Interventions, *Catheter Cardiovasc Interv* 73:847, 2009.
120. Mintz GS, Popma JJ, Pichard AD: Arterial remodeling after coronary angioplasty. A serial intravascular ultrasound study, *Circulation* 94:35, 1996.
121. Peters RJG, Kok WEM, DiMario C: Prediction of restenosis after coronary balloon angioplasty, *Circulation* 95:2254, 1997.
122. Kornowski R, Mintz GS, Kent KM, et al: Increased restenosis in diabetes mellitus after coronary interventions is due to exaggerated intimal hyperplasia, *Circulation* 95:1366, 1997.
123. Moses JW, Leon MB, Popma JJ, et al: Sirolimus-eluting stents versus standard stents in patients with stenosis in a native coronary artery, *N Engl J Med* 349:1315, 2003.
124. Stone GW, Ellis SG, Cox DA, et al: A polymer-based, paclitaxel-eluting stent in patients with coronary artery disease, *N Engl J Med* 350:221, 2004.
125. Mercado N, Boersma E, Wijns W, et al: Clinical and quantitative coronary angiographic predictors of coronary restenosis. A comparative analysis from the balloon-to-stent era, *J Am Coll Cardiol* 38:645, 2001.
126. Ruygrok PN, Webster MW, deValk V, et al: Clinical and angiographic factors associated with asymptomatic restenosis after percutaneous coronary intervention, *Circulation* 104:2289, 2001.
127. King SB: Restenosis. The mouse that roared, *Circulation* 108:248, 2003.
128. Schwartz L, Bourassa MG, Lesperance J, et al: Aspirin and dipyridamole in the prevention of restenosis after percutaneous transluminal coronary angioplasty, *N Engl J Med* 318:1714, 1988.
129. Williams DO: Intracoronary brachytherapy, *Circulation* 105:2699, 2002.
130. Holmes D, Teirstein P, Satler L, et al: 3-year follow-up of the SISR (Sirolimus-Eluting Stents Versus Vascular Brachytherapy for IN-Stent Restenosis) Trial, *JACC Cardiovasc Interv* 1:439, 2008.
131. Holmes DR, Hirshfield J, Faxon D, et al: ACC expert consensus document on coronary artery stents. Document of the American College of Cardiology, *J Am Coll Cardiol* 32:1471, 1998.

132. Escaned J, Goicolea J, Alfonso F, et al: Propensity and mechanisms of restenosis in different coronary stent designs. Complementary value of the analysis of the luminal gain-loss relationship, *J Am Coll Cardiol* 34:1490, 1999.
133. Pache J, Kastrati A, Mehilli J, et al: Intracoronary stenting and angiographic results: Strut thickness effect on restenosis outcome (ISAR-STEREO) trial, *J Am Coll Cardiol* 41:1283, 2003.
134. Sousa JE, Serruys PW, Costa MA: New frontiers in cardiology. Drug-eluting stents: Part I, *Circulation* 107:2274, 2003.
135. Kukreja N, Onuma Y, Garcia-Garcia HM, et al: The risk of stent thrombosis in patients with acute coronary syndromes treated with bare-metal and drug-eluting stents, *JACC Cardiovasc Interv* 2:533, 2009.
136. Leon MB, Baim DS, Popma JJ, et al: A clinical trial comparing three antithrombotic-drug regimens after coronary-artery stenting, *N Engl J Med* 338:1665–1671, 1999.
137. Waksman R, Ajani AE, Pinnow E, et al: Twelve versus six months of clopidogrel to reduce major cardiac events in patients undergoing gamma-radiation therapy for in-stent restenosis: Washington Radiation for In-Stent restenosis Trial (WRIST) 12 versus WRIST PLUS, *Circulation* 106:776, 2002.
138. Chen J, Hou D, Pendyala L, et al: Drug-eluting stent thrombosis, *JACC Cardiovasc Interv* 2:583, 2009.
139. Cook S, Wenaweser P, Togni M, et al: Incomplete stent apposition and very late stent thrombosis after drug-eluting stent implantation, *Circulation* 115:2426, 2007.
140. Hodgson JM, Stone GW, Lincoff AM, et al: Late stent thrombosis: Considerations and practical advice for the use of drug-eluting stents: A report from the Society for Cardiovascular Angiography and Interventions Drug-eluting Stent Task Force, *Catheter Cardiovasc Interv* 327:327–333, 2007.
141. Holmes D, Kereiakes D, Laskey WK, et al: Thrombosis and drug-eluting stents, *J Am Coll Cardiol* 50:109, 2007.
142. Boston DR, Malouf A, Barry WH: Management of intracoronary thrombosis complicating coronary angioplasty, *Circulation* 76:125, 1987.
143. Marin F, Gonzalez-Conejero R, Capranzano P, et al: Pharmacogenetics in cardiovascular antithrombotic therapy, *J Am Coll Cardiol* 54:1041, 2009.
144. Nikolsky E, Mehran R, Sadeghi HM, et al: Prognostic impact of blood transfusion after primary angioplasty for acute myocardial infarction, *JACC Cardiovasc Interv* 2:622, 2009.
145. Freedman J: The aspirin resistance controversy clinical entity or platelet heterogeneity? *Circulation* 113:2865–2867, 2006.
146. Schleintz M, Olkin I, Heidenreich PA: Cilostazol, clopidogrel or ticlopidine to prevent sub-acute stent thrombosis: A meta-analysis of randomized trials, *Am Heart J* 148:990, 2004.
147. Ochoa AB, Wolfe M, Lewis P, et al: Ticlopidine-induced neutropenia mimicking sepsis early after intracoronary stent placement, *Clin Cardiol* 21:304, 1998.
148. Bennett CL, Connors JM, Carwile JM, et al: Thrombotic thrombocytopenic purpura associated with clopidogrel, *N Engl J Med* 342:1773, 2000.
149. Anderson J, et al: ACC/AHA 2007 guidelines for the management of patients with unstable angina/non-ST-elevation myocardial infarction-executive summary, *J Am Coll Cardiol* 50:649, 2007.
150. Mishkel GJ, Aguirre FV, Ligon RW, et al: Clopidogrel as adjunctive antiplatelet therapy during coronary stenting, *J Am Coll Cardiol* 34:1884, 1999.
151. Kastrati A, von Beckerath N, Joost A, et al: Loading with 600mg clopidogrel in patients with coronary artery disease with and without chronic clopidogrel therapy, *Circulation* 110:1916, 2004.
152. Berger J, Bhatt D, Cannon CP, et al: The relative efficacy and safety of clopidogrel in women and men, *J Am Coll Cardiol* 54:1935, 2009.
153. Angiolillo D, Fernandez-Ortiz A, Bernardo E, et al: Variability in individual responsiveness to clopidogrel, *J Am Coll Cardiol* 49:1505, 2007.
154. Wiviott SD, Braunwald E, McCabe CH, et al: Prasugrel versus clopidogrel in patients with acute coronary syndromes, *N Engl J Med* 357:1–15, 2009.
155. Ebrahimi R, Dyke C, Mehran R, et al: Outcomes following pre-operative clopidogrel administration in patients with acute coronary syndromes undergoing coronary artery bypass surgery, *J Am Coll Cardiol* 53:1965, 2009.
156. Becker R, Scheiman J, Dauerman H, et al: Management of platelet-directed pharmacotherapy in patients with atherosclerotic coronary artery disease undergoing elective endoscopic gastrointestinal procedures, *J Am Coll Cardiol* 54:2261, 2009.
157. Bhatt DL, Scheiman J, Abraham NS, et al: ACCF/ACG/AHA 2008 expert consensus document on reducing the gastrointestinal risks of antiplatelet therapy and NSAID use: A report of the American College of Cardiology Foundation Task Force on clinical expert consensus documents, *J Am Coll Cardiol* 52:1502, 2008.
158. Gilard M, Arnaud B, Cornily JC, et al: Influence of omeprazole on antiplatelet action of clopidogrel associated with aspirin, *J Am Coll Cardiol* 51:256, 2008.
159. Holmes D, Kereiakes D, Kleiman NS, et al: Combining antiplatelet and anticoagulant therapies, *J Am Coll Cardiol* 54:95, 2009.
160. Varga ZA, Papp L: Hemochron versus HemoTec activated coagulation time target values during percutaneous transluminal coronary angioplasty, *J Am Coll Cardiol* 25:803, 1995.
161. Antman EM: The search for replacements for unfractionated heparin, *Circulation* 103:2310, 2001.
162. Bittl JA, Chaitman BR, Feit F, et al: Bivalirudin versus heparin during coronary angioplasty for unstable or postinfarction angina: Final report reanalysis of the bivalirudin angioplasty study, *Am Heart J* 142:952, 2001.
163. Lincoff AM, Kleiman NS, Kereiakes DJ, et al: Long-term efficacy of bivalirudin and provisional glycoprotein IIb/IIIa blockade vs heparin and planned glycoprotein IIb/IIIa blockade during percutaneous coronary revascularization. REPLACE randomized trial, *JAMA* 292:696, 2004.
164. White H, Ohman M, Lincoff AM, et al: Safety and efficacy of bivalirudin with and without glycoprotein llb/llla inhibitors in patients with acute coronary syndromes undergoing percutaneous coronary intervention, *J Am Coll Cardiol* 52:807, 2008.
165. Mehran R, Lansky A, Witzenbichler B, et al: Bivalirudin in patients undergoing primary angioplasty for acute myocardial infarction (HORIZON-AMI): 1-year results of a randomized controlled trial, *Lancet* 374:1149, 2009.
166. Beguin S, Mardiguian J, Lindhout T, et al: The mode of action of low molecular weight heparin preparation (PK10169) and two of its major components on thrombin generation in plasma, *Thromb Haemost* 61:30, 1989.
167. Petersen JL, Mahaffey KW, Hasselblad V, et al: Efficacy and bleeding complications among patients randomized to enoxaparin or unfractionated heparin for antithrombin therapy in nonST-segment elevation acute coronary syndromes: A systematic overview, *JAMA* 292:89, 2004.
168. Young JJ, Kereiakes DJ, Grines CL, et al: Low-molecular-weight heparin therapy in percutaneous coronary intervention: The NICE 1 and NICE 4 trials, *J Invasive Cardiol* 12(Suppl E):E14, 2000.
169. Ferguson JJ, Califf RM, Antman EM, et al: Enoxaparin vs unfractionated heparin in high-risk patients with nonST-segment elevation acute coronary syndromes managed with an intended early invasive strategy: Primary results of the SYNERGY randomized trial, *JAMA* 292:45, 2004.
170. Jolly S, Faxon D, Fox K, et al: Efficacy and safety of fondaparinux versus enoxaparin in patients with acute coronary syndromes treated with glycoprotein llb/llla inhibitors or thienopyridines, *J Am Coll Cardiol* 54:468, 2009.
171. The EPIC Investigators: Use of a monoclonal antibody directed against the platelet glycoprotein II_B/III_A receptor in high-risk coronary angioplasty, *N Engl J Med* 330:956, 1996.
172. The EPILOG Investigators: Platelet glycoprotein IIb/IIIa receptor blockade and low-dose heparin during percutaneous coronary revascularization, *N Engl J Med* 336:1689, 1997.
173. Mark DB, Talley JD, Topol EJ, et al: Economic assessment of platelet glycoprotein IIb/IIIa inhibition for prevention of ischemic complications of high-risk coronary angioplasty, *Circulation* 94:629, 1996.
174. Kereiakes DJ, Kleiman NS, Ambrose J, et al: Randomized, double-blind, placebo-controlled dose-ranging study of tirofiban (MK) platelet IIb/IIIa blockade in high risk patients undergoing angioplasty, *J Am Coll Cardiol* 27:536, 1996.
175. The ESPRIT Investigators: Novel dosing regimen of eptifibatide in planned coronary stent implantation (ESPRIT): A randomized, placebo-controlled trial, *Lancet* 356:2037, 2000.
176. The EPISTENT Investigators: Randomized placebo-controlled and balloon-angioplasty-controlled trial to assess safety of coronary stenting with use of platelet glycoprotein-IIb/IIIa blockade, *Lancet* 352:87, 1998.
177. Kereiakes DJ: Platelet glycoprotein IIb/IIIa inhibition and atheroembolism during bypass graft angioplasty. A cup half full, *Circulation* 106:2994, 2002.
178. Kastrati A, Mehilli J, Schuhlen H, et al: Intracoronary Stenting Antithrombotic Regimen-Rapid Early Action for Coronary Treatment Study Investigators. A clinical trial of abciximab in elective percutaneous coronary intervention after pretreatment with clopidogrel, *N Engl J Med* 350:232, 2004.
179. Dangas G, Mehran R, Guagliumi G, et al: Role of clopidogrel loading dose in patients with ST-segment elevation myocardial infarction undergoing primary angioplasty, *J Am Coll Cardiol* 54:1438, 2009.
180. Second SYMPHONY Investigators: Randomized trial of aspirin, sibrafiban, or both for secondary prevention after acute coronary syndromes, *Circulation* 103:1727–1733, 2001.
181. Armstrong PW, Collen D: Fibrinolysis for acute myocardial infarction. Current status and new horizons for pharmacological reperfusion, Part I, *Circulation* 103:2862, 2001.
182. Nallamothu B, Bradley E, Krumholz HM, et al: Time to treatment in primary percutaneous coronary intervention, *N Engl J Med* 357:1631, 2007.
183. Elli S, Tendera M, de Belder MA, et al: Facilitated PCI in patients with ST-elevation myocardial infarction, *N Engl J Med* 358:2205, 2008.
184. Wijeysundera H, Vijayaraphavan R, Nallamothu, et al: Rescue angioplasty or repeat fibrinolysis after failed fibrinolytic therapy for ST-segment myocardial infarction, *J Am Coll Cardiol* 49:420, 2007.
185. Roubin GS, Douglas JS, King SB, et al: Influence of balloon size on initial success, acute complications, and restenosis after percutaneous transluminal coronary angioplasty, *Circulation* 78:557, 1988.
186. Williams DO, Holubkov R, Yeh W, et al: Percutaneous coronary intervention in the current era compared with 1985. The National Heart, Lung, and Blood Institute Registries, *Circulation* 102:2945, 2000.
187. Ellis SG, Roubin GS, King SB III, et al: In-hospital cardiac mortality after acute closure after coronary angioplasty: Analysis of risk factors from 8,207 procedures, *J Am Coll Cardiol* 11:211, 1988.
188. Krone RJ, Laskey W, Babb J, et al: Four-year trends in coronary interventions, a report from the registry of the society for coronary angiography and interventions (abstract), *Cathet Cardiovasc Diagn* 41:98, 1997.
189. From A, Rihal C, Lennon R, et al: Temporal trends and improved outcomes of percutaneous coronary revascularization in nonagenarians, *JACC Cardiovasc Interv* 1:692, 2008.
190. Prasad A, Rihal C, Lennon R, et al: Trends in outcomes after percutaneous coronary intervention for chronic total occlusions, *J Am Coll Cardiol* 49:1611, 2007.
191. Kruk M, Kadziela J, Reynolds H, et al: Predictors of outcomes and the lack of effect of percutaneous coronary intervention across the risk strata in patients with persistent total occlusion after myocardial infarction, *JACC Cardiovasc Interv* 1:511, 2008.
192. Califf RM, Abdelmeguid AE, Kuntz RE, et al: Myonecrosis after revascularization procedures, *J Am Coll Cardiol* 31:241, 1998.
193. Stone GW, Mehran R, Dangas G, et al: Differential impact on survival of electrocardiographic Q-wave versus enzymatic myocardial infarction after percutaneous intervention. A device-specific analysis of 7147 patients, *Circulation* 104:642, 2001.
194. Zaacks SM, Allen JE, Calvin JE, et al: Value of the American College of Cardiology/American Heart Association stenosis morphology classification for coronary interventions in the late 1990s, *Am J Cardiol* 82:43, 1998.
195. Singh M, Rihal CS, Lennon RJ, et al: Comparison of Mayo Clinic risk score and American College of Cardiology/American Heart Association lesion classification in the prediction of adverse cardiovascular outcome following percutaneous coronary interventions, *J Am Coll Cardiol* 44:357, 2004.
196. Ndrepepa G, Berger P, Behilli J, et al: Periprocedural bleeding and 1-year outcome after percutaneous coronary interventions, *J Am Coll Cardiol* 51:689, 2008.
197. Manoukian S, Feit F, Mehran SV, et al: Impact of major bleeding on 30-day mortality and clinical outcomes in patients with acute coronary syndromes, *J Am Coll Cardiol* 49:1361, 2007.
198. Holmes D, Mishimura R, Fountain R, et al: Iatrogenic pericardial effusion and tamponade in the percutaneous intra-cardiac intervention era, *JACC Cardiovasc Interv* 2:705, 2009.
199. Ormiston JA, Currie E, Webster MW, et al: Drug-eluting stents for coronary bifurcations: Insights into the crush technique, *Catheter Cardiovasc Interv* 63:332, 2004.
200. Yamashita T, Nishida T, Adamian MG, et al: Bifurcation lesions: Two stents versus one stent—immediate and follow-up results, *J Am Coll Cardiol* 35:1145, 2000.
201. Stack RS, Quigley PJ, Collins G, et al: Perfusion balloon catheter, *Am J Cardiol* 61:77G, 1988.
202. Seyfarth M, Sibbing D, Bauer R, et al: A randomized clinical trial to evaluate the safety and efficacy of a percutaneous left ventricular assist device versus intra-aortic balloon pumping for treatment of cardiogenic shock caused by myocardial infarction, *J Am Coll Cardiol* 52:1583, 2008.
203. Blanke H, Cohen M, Karsch KR, et al: Prevalence and significance of residual flow to the infarct zone during the acute phase of myocardial infarction, *J Am Coll Cardiol* 5:827, 1985.
204. Greene MA, Gray LA, Slater AD, et al: Emergency aortocoronary bypass after failed angioplasty, *Ann Thorac Surg* 51:194, 1991.
205. Lotfi M, Mackie K, Dzavik V, Seidelin PH: Impact of delays to cardiac surgery after failed angioplasty and stenting, *J Am Coll Cardiol* 43:337, 2004.
206. Baratke MS, Bannon PG, Hughes CF, et al: Emergency surgery after unsuccessful coronary angioplasty: A review of 15 years of experience, *Ann Thorac Surg* 75:1400, 2003.
207. Vogel RA, Shawl FA: Report of the National Registry of Elective Supported Angioplasty: Comparison of the 1988 and 1989 results, *Circulation* 82(Suppl II):II, 1989.
208. Tierstein PS, Bogel RA, Dorros G, et al: Prophylactic vs standby cardiopulmonary support for high-risk PTCA, *Circulation* 82(Suppl III):680, 1990.
209. Satler LF: A minimally invasive, mechanical cardiovascular support system. Cath lab digest talks with Lowell F. Satler, M.D, about his experience with the Impella Recover LP 2.5 System, *Cath Lab Digest* 12:1, 2004.
210. Aziz T, Singh G, Popjes, et al: Initial experience with CentriMag extra-corporal membrane oxygenation for support of critically ill patients with refractory cardiogenic shock, *J Heart Lung Transplant* 29:66, 2010.
211. Cheng JM, den Uil CA, Hoeks SE, et al: Percutaneous left ventricular assist devices vs. intra-aortic balloon pump counterpulsation for treatment of cardiogenic shock: A meta-analysis of controlled trials, *Eur Heart J* 30(17):2102–2108, 2009.
212. International Society and Federation of Cardiology and World Health Organization Task Force on Myocardial Reperfusion: Reperfusion in acute myocardial infarction, *Circulation* 90:2091, 1994.
213. Sanborn TA, Sleeper LA, Webb JG, et al: Correlates of one-year survival in patients with cardiogenic shock complicating acute myocardial infarction. Angiographic findings from the SHOCK Trial, *J Am Coll Cardiol* 42:1373, 2003.

214. Sutton AG, Campbell PG, Graham R, et al: A randomized trial of rescue angioplasty versus a conservative approach for failed fibrinolysis in ST-segment elevation myocardial infarction: The Middlesbrough Early Revascularization to Limit INfarction (MERLIN) trial, *J Am Coll Cardiol* 44:287, 2004.
215. The TIMI Study Group: Comparison of invasive and conservative strategies after treatment with intravenous tissue plasminogen activator in acute myocardial infarction. Results of the thrombolysis in myocardial infarction (TIMI) Phase II Trial, *N Engl J Med* 320:618, 1989.
216. Carver A, Refelt S, Gershlick, et al: Longer-term follow-up of patients recruited to the REACT (Rescue Angioplasty Versus Conservative Treatment or Repeat Thrombolysis) Trial, *J Am Coll Cardiol* 54:11, 2009.
217. Califf RM, O'Neil W, Stack RS, et al: Failure of simple clinical measurements to predict perfusion status after intravenous thrombolysis, *Ann Intern Med* 108:658, 1988.
218. McLaughlin MG, Stone GW, Aymong E, et al: Prognostic utility of comparative methods for assessment of ST-segment resolution after primary angioplasty for acute myocardial infarction. The controlled abiximab and device investigation to lower late angioplasty complications (CADILLAC) trial, *J Am Coll Cardiol* 44:1215, 2004.
219. Gingliano RP, Braunwald E: Selecting the best reperfusion strategy in ST-elevation myocardial infarction. It's all a matter of time, *Circulation* 108:2828, 2003.
220. Danchin N, Blanchard D, Steg PG, et al: Impact of prehospital thrombolysis for acute myocardial infarction on 1-year outcome. Results from the French nationwide USIC 2000 registry, *Circulation* 110:1909, 2004.
221. Francone M, Bucciarelli-Ducci C, et al: Impact of primary coronary angioplasty delay on myocardial salvage, infarct size, and micro-vascular damage in patients with ST-segment elevation myocardial infarction, *J Am Coll Cardiol* 54:2145, 2009.
222. Antman EM, Hand M, Armstrong PW, et al: 2007 Focused update of the ACC/AHA 2004 guidelines for the management of patients with ST-elevation myocardial infarction, *Circulation* 117:296–329, 2008.
223. Ross AM, Coyne KS, Reiner JS, et al: A randomized trial comparing primary angioplasty with a strategy of short-acting thrombolysis and immediate planned rescue angioplasty in acute myocardial infarction: The PACT Trial, *J Am Coll Cardiol* 34:1954, 1999.
224. Nallamothu BK, Wang Y, Magid DJ, et al: Relation between hospital specialization with primary percutaneous coronary intervention and clinical outcomes in ST-segment elevation myocardial infarction: National Registry of Myocardial Infarction-4 analysis, *Circulation* 113:222–229, 2006.
225. Gersh BJ, Stone GW, White HD, et al: Pharmacological facilitation of primary percutaneous intervention for acute myocardial infarction, *JAMA* 293:979, 2005.
226. Di Mario C, Dudek D, Piscione F, et al: Immediate angioplasty versus standard therapy with rescue angioplasty after thrombolysis in the Combined Abciximab REteplase Stent Study in Acute Myocardial Infarction (CARESS-in-AMI): An open, prospective, randomized, multicentre trial, *Lancet* 371:559–568, 2008.
227. Cantor WJ, Fitchett D, Borgundvaag B, et al: Routine early angioplasty after fibrinolysis for acute myocardial infarction, *N Engl J Med* 360:2705–2718, 2009.
228. Ellis S, Tendera M, de Belder MA, et al: 1-Year survival in a randomized trial of facilitated reperfusion, *JACC Cardiovasc Interv* 2:909, 2009.
229. Polderman KH: Induced hypothermia and fever control for prevention and treatment of neurological injuries, *Lancet* 371:1955, 2008.
230. Moss AJ, Zareba W, Hall WJ, et al: Prophylactic implantation of a defibrillator in patients with myocardial infarction and reduced ejection fraction, *N Engl J Med* 346:877, 2002.
231. Eagle KA, Lim MJ, Dabbous OH, et al: A validated prediction model for all forms of acute coronary syndrome: Estimating the risk of 6-month post-discharge death in an international registry, *JAMA* 291:2727, 2004.
232. Hueb W, Lopes NH, Gersh BJ, et al: Five-Year Follow-Up of the Medicine, Angioplasty, or Surgery Study (MASS II): A randomized controlled clinical trial of 3 therapeutic strategies for multi-vessel coronary artery disease, *Circulation* 115:1082, 2007.
233. Bypass Angioplasty Revascularization Investigation (BARI) Investigators: Comparison of coronary bypass surgery with angioplasty in patients with multivessel disease, *N Engl J Med* 335:217, 1995.
234. Casey C, Faxon DP: Multi-vessel coronary disease and percutaneous coronary intervention, *Heart* 90:341, 2004.
235. Holmes DR: Randomized clinical trials: Do they really make a difference? BARI and diabetes mellitus, *Cathet Cardiovasc Diagn* 37:351, 1996.
236. Khan NE, DeSouza A, Mister R, et al: A randomized comparison of off-pump and on-pump multivessel coronary-artery bypass surgery, *N Engl J Med* 350:21, 2004.
237. Zacharias A, Habib RH, Schwann TA, et al: Improved survival with radial artery versus vein conduits in coronary bypass surgery with left internal thoracic artery to left anterior descending artery grafting, *Circulation* 109:1489, 2004.
238. Hoffman SN, TenBrook JA, Wolf MP, et al: A meta-analysis of randomized controlled trials comparing coronary artery bypass graft surgery with percutaneous transluminal coronary angioplasty: One- to eight-year outcomes, *J Am Coll Cardiol* 41:1293, 2003.
239. Surreys PW, Morice MC, Kappetein AP, et al: Percutaneous coronary intervention versus coronary artery bypass grafting for severe coronary artery disease, *N Engl J Med* 360:961, 2009.
240. Yap C, Yan B, Akowuah E, et al: Dose prior percutaneous coronary intervention adversely affect early and mid-term survival after coronary artery surgery? *JACC Cardiovasc Interv* 2:758, 2009.
241. Seung K, Park D, Kim YH, et al: Stents versus coronary-artery bypass grafting for left main coronary artery disease, *N Engl J Med* 358:1781, 2008.
242. Leavitt BJ, O'Connor GT, Olmstead EM, et al: Use of the internal mammary artery graft and in-hospital mortality and other adverse outcomes associated with coronary artery bypass surgery, *Circulation* 103:507, 2001.
243. Holmes DR, Firth BG, Wood DL: Paradigm shifts in cardiovascular medicine, *J Am Coll Cardiol* 43:507, 2004.
244. Heijer P, Foley DP, Escaned J, et al: Angioscopic versus angiographic detection of intimal dissection and intracoronary thrombus, *J Am Coll Cardiol* 24:649, 1994.
245. vonBirgelen C, Hartmann M, Mintz GS, et al: Relationship between cardiovascular risk as predicted by established risk scores versus plaque progression as measured by serial intravascular ultrasound in left main coronary arteries, *Circulation* 110:1579, 2004.
246. Abizaid A, Mintz GS, Abizaid A., et al: One-year follow-up after intravascular ultrasound assessment of moderate left main coronary artery disease in patients with ambiguous angiograms, *J Am Coll Cardiol* 34:707, 1999.
247. St Goar FG, Pinto FJ, Alderman EL, et al: Intracoronary ultrasound in cardiac transplant recipients, *Circulation* 85:979, 1992.
248. Sousa JE, Costa MA, Sousa AGMR., et al: Two-year angiographic and intravascular ultrasound follow-up after implantation of sirolimus-eluting stents in human coronary arteries, *Circulation* 107:381, 2003.
249. Mudra H, diMario C, deJaegere P, et al: Randomized comparison of coronary stent implantation under ultrasound or angiographic guidance to reduce stent restenosis (OPTICUS Study), *Circulation* 104:1343, 2001.
250. Cannon CP, Braunwald E, McCabe CH, et al: Comparison of intensive and moderate lipid lowering with statins after acute coronary syndromes, *N Engl J Med* 350:15, 2004.
251. Nissen SE, Tuzcu EM, Schoenhagen P, et al: Effect of intensive compared with moderate lipid-lowering therapy on progression of coronary atherosclerosis. A randomized controlled trial, *JAMA* 291:1071, 2004.
252. Spaan J, Piek J, Hoffman J, Siebes M: Physiological basis of clinically used coronary hemodynamic indices, *Circulation* 113:446–455, 2006.
253. Miller DD, Donohue TJ, Younis LT, et al: Correlation of pharmacological (99m)Tc-sestamibi myocardial perfusion imaging with post-stenotic coronary flow reserve in patients with angiographically intermediate coronary artery stenosis, *Circulation* 89:2150, 1996.
254. Bezerra H, Costa M, Cuaglunmi G, et al: Intracoronary optical coherence tomography: A comprehensive review, *JACC Cardiovasc Interv* 2:1035, 2009.
255. Topol EJ, Leya F, Pinkerton CA, et al: A comparison of directional atherectomy with coronary angioplasty in patients with coronary artery disease, *N Engl J Med* 329:221, 1993.
256. Holmes DR, Topol EJ, Califf RM, et al: A multicenter, randomized trial of coronary angioplasty versus directional atherectomy for patients with saphenous vein bypass graft lesions. CAVEAT-II Investigators, *Circulation* 91:1966, 1995.
257. Tsuchikane E, Sumitsuji S, Awata N, et al: Final results of the Stent versus Directional Coronary Atherectomy Randomized Trial (START), *J Am Coll Cardiol* 34:1050, 1999.
258. Bowers TR, Stewart RE, O'Neill WW, et al: Effect of Rotablator atherectomy and adjunctive balloon angioplasty on coronary blood flow, *Circulation* 95:1157, 1997.
259. Mehran R, Dangas G, Mintz GS, et al: Treatment of in-stent restenosis with eximer laser coronary angioplasty versus rotational atherectomy. Comparative mechanisms and results, *Circulation* 101:2484, 2000.
260. Reisman M: Technique and strategy of rotational atherectomy, *Cathet Cardiovasc Diagn* (Suppl 3):2, 1996.
261. Albiero R, Silber S, DiMario C, et al: Cutting balloon versus conventional balloon angioplasty for the treatment of in-stent restenosis. Results of the Restenosis Cutting Balloon Evaluation Trial (RESCUT), *J Am Coll Cardiol* 43:943, 2004.
262. Ring M: How a dentist's name became a synonym for a life saving device: The story of Dr. Charles Stent, *J Hist Dent* 49:1, 2001.
263. Ellis S: Refining the art and science of coronary stenting, *N Engl J Med* 360:292, 2009.
264. Pepine CJ, Holmes DR: Coronary artery stents, *J Am Coll Cardiol* 28:782, 1996.
265. Kiemeneij F, Serruys PW, Macaya C, et al: Continued benefit of coronary stenting versus balloon angioplasty: Five-year clinical follow-up of Benestent-I trial, *J Am Coll Cardiol* 37:1598, 2001.
266. George B, Voorhees W, Roubin G: Multicenter investigation of coronary stenting to treat acute or threatened closure after percutaneous transluminal coronary angioplasty: Clinical and angiographic outcomes, *J Am Coll Cardiol* 22:135, 1993.
267. Doucet S, Schalij MJ, Vrolix MCM, et al: Stent placement to prevent restenosis after angioplasty in small coronary arteries, *Circulation* 104:2029, 2001.
268. Bertrand O, Larose E, Rodes-Cabau J, et al: Incidence, predictors, and clinical impact of bleeding after transradial coronary stenting and maximal antiplatelet therapy, *Am Heart J* 157:164, 2009.
269. Serruys P, Daemen J: Are drug-eluting stents associated with a higher rate of late thrombosis than bare metal stents? *Circulation* 115:1433, 2007.
270. Schwartz RS, Chronos NA, Virmani R, et al: Preclinical restenosis models and drug-eluting stents, *J Am Coll Cardiol* 44:1373, 2004.
271. Morice MC, Serruys PW, Sousa JE, et al: A randomized comparison of a sirolimus-eluting stent with a standard stent for coronary revascularization, *N Engl J Med* 346:1773, 2002.
272. Holmes DR, Leon MB, Moses JW, et al: Analysis of 1-year clinical outcomes in the SIRUS trial. A randomized trial of a sirolimus-eluting stent versus a standard stent in patients at high risk for coronary restenosis, *Circulation* 109:634, 2004.
273. Lemos PA, Saia F, Hofma SH, et al: Short- and long-term clinical benefit of sirolimus-eluting stents compared with conventional bare stents for patients with acute myocardial infarction, *J Am Coll Cardiol* 43:704, 2004.
274. Schampaert E, Cohen EA, Schluter M, et al: The Canadian study of the sirolimus-eluting stent in the treatment of patients with long de nova lesions in small native coronary arteries (C-SIRIUS), *J Am Coll Cardiol* 43:1110, 2004.
275. Colombo A, Moses JW, Morice MC, et al: Randomized study to evaluate sirolimus-eluting stents implanted at coronary bifurcation lesions, *Circulation* 109:1244, 2004.
276. Iakovou I, Ge L, Michev I, et al: Clinical and angiographic outcome after sirolimus-eluting stent implantation in aorto-ostial lesions, *J Am Coll Cardiol* 44:967, 2004.
277. Hoye A, Tanabe K, Lemos PA, et al: Significant reduction in restenosis after the use of sirolimus-eluting stents in the treatment of chronic total occlusions, *J Am Coll Cardiol* 43:1954, 2004.
278. Grube E, Silber S, Hauptmann KE, et al: TAXUS I. Six- and twelve-month results from a randomized, double-blind trial on a slow-release paclitaxel-eluting stent for de nova coronary lesions, *Circulation* 107:38, 2003.
279. Lee M, Kobashigawa K, Tobis J: Comparison of percutaneous coronary intervention with bare-metal and drug-eluting stents for cardiac allograft vasculopathy, *JACC Cardiovasc Interv* 1:709, 2008.
280. Brodie B, Wilson H, Stuckey T, et al: Outcomes with drug-eluting versus bare-metal stents in saphenous vein graft intervention, *JACC Cardiovasc Interv* 2:1105, 2009.
281. Rabbitts J, Nuttall G, Brown MJ, et al: Cardiac risk of non-cardiac surgery after percutaneous coronary intervention with drug-eluting stents, *Anesthesiology* 109:596, 2008.
282. Wilson SH, Fasseas P, Orford JL, et al: Clinical outcome of patients undergoing noncardiac surgery in the two months following coronary stenting, *J Am Coll Cardiol* 42:234, 2003.
283. McFadden EF, Stabile E, Regar E, et al: Late thrombosis in drug-eluting coronary stents after discontinuation of antiplatelet therapy, *Lancet* 364:1519, 2004.
284. Lemos PA, Serruys PW, Sousa JE: Drug-eluting stents. Cost versus clinical benefit, *Circulation* 107:3003, 2003.
285. Nag S: *High-dose-rate brachytherapy: A textbook*, Armonk, NY, 1994, Futura Publishing.
286. Teirstein P: β-Radiation to reduce restenosis, too little, too soon? *Circulation* 95:1095, 1997.
287. Waksman R, White RL, Chan RC, et al: Intracoronary β-radiation therapy after angioplasty inhibits recurrence in patients with in-stent restenosis, *Circulation* 2165:2000.
288. Waksman R, Bhargava B, White L, et al: Intracoronary β-radiation therapy inhibits recurrence of in-stent restenosis, *Circulation* 101:1895, 2000.
289. Safian RD, May MA, Lichtenberg A: Detailed clinical and angiographic analysis of transluminal extraction coronary atherectomy for complex lesions in native coronary arteries, *J Am Coll Cardiol* 25:848, 1995.
290. Cohen DJ, Murphy SA, Baim DS, et al: Cost-effectiveness of distal embolic protection for patients undergoing percutaneous intervention of saphenous vein bypass grafts. Results from the SAFER trial, *J Am Coll Cardiol* 44:1801, 2004.
291. deFeyter PJ: Percutaneous treatment of saphenous vein bypass graft obstructions. A continuing obstinate problem, *Circulation* 107:2284, 2003.
292. Antoniucci D, Valenti R, Migliorini A, et al: Comparison of rheolytic thrombectomy before direct infarct artery stenting versus direct stenting alone in patients undergoing percutaneous coronary intervention for acute myocardial infarction, *Am J Cardiol* 93:1033, 2004.
293. Ali A, Cox D, Dib N, et al: Rheolytic thrombectomy with percutaneous coronary intervention for infarct size reduction in acute myocardial infarction: 30-day results from a multicenter randomized study, *J Am Coll Cardiol* 48:244, 2006.

294. Kaltoft A, Bottcher M, Nielsen S, et al: Routine thrombectomy in percutaneous coronary intervention for acute ST-segment-elevation myocardial infarction: A randomized, controlled trial, *Circulation* 114:40, 2006.

295. Gaitonde RS, Sharm N, Von Lohe E, et al: Combined distal embolization protection and rheolytic thrombectomy during percutaneous revascularization of totally occluded grafts, *Catheter Cardiovasc Interv* 60:212, 2003.

296. Singh M, Rosenschein U, Ho KKL, et al: Treatment of saphenous vein bypass grafts with ultrasound thrombolysis. A randomized study (ATLAS), *Circulation* 107:2331, 2003.

297. Sardella G, Mancome M, Bucciarelli-Ducci C, et al: thrombus aspiration during primary percutaneous coronary intervention improves myocardial reperfusion and reduces infarct size, *J Am Coll Cardiol* 53:309, 2009.

298. Vlaar PJ, Svilaas T, van der Horst IC, et al: Cardiac death and reinfarction after 1 year in the Thrombus Aspiration during Percutaneous coronary intervention in acute myocardial infarction Study (TAPAS): A 1-year follow-up study, *Lancet* 371:1915, 2008.

299. Stone GW, Webb J, Cox DA, et al: Primary angioplasty in acute myocardial infarction with distal protection of the microcirculation: Principal results from the prospective, randomized EMERALD trial, *J Am Coll Cardiol* 43(Suppl 2):A285, 2004.

300. Li SSL, Lam CW, So YC, et al: The use of distal occlusion balloon protection device in acute coronary syndrome, *Int J Cardiol* 92:281, 2003.

301. Limbruno U, Micheli A, DeCarlo M, et al: Mechanical prevention of distal embolization during primary angioplasty. Safety, feasibility, and impact on myocardial reperfusion, *Circulation* 108:171, 2003.

302. Stone GW, Rogers C, Hermiller J, et al: Randomized comparison of distal protection with a filter-based catheter and a balloon occlusion and aspiration system during percutaneous intervention of diseased saphenous vein aorto-coronary bypass grafts, *Circulation* 108:548, 2003.

303. Grantham J, Marso S, Spertus J, et al: Chronic total occlusion angioplasty in the United States, *JACC Cardiovasc Interv* 2:479, 2009.

304. Rathore S, Matsuo H, Terashima M, et al: Procedural and in-hospital outcomes after percutaneous coronary intervention for chronic total occlusions of coronary arteries 2002-2008, *JACC Cardiovac Interv* 2:489, 2009.

305. Suero JA, Marso SP, Jones PG, et al: Procedural outcomes and long-term survival among patients undergoing percutaneous coronary intervention of a chronic total occlusion in native coronary arteries: A 20-year experience, *J Am Coll Cardiol* 38:409, 2001.

306. Olivari Z, Rubartelli P, Piscione F, et al: Immediate results and one-year clinical outcome after percutaneous coronary interventions in chronic total occlusions. Data from a multicenter, prospective, observational study (TOAST-GISE), *J Am Coll Cardiol* 41:1672, 2003.

307. Whitlow PL, Selmon M, O'Neill W, et al: Treatment of uncrossable chronic total occlusions with the Frontrunner: Multicenter experience, *J Am Coll Cardiol* 39(Suppl 1):29, 2002.

308. Cannan CR, Nishimura RA, Reeder GS, et al: Echocardiographic assessment of commissural calcium: A simple predictor of outcome after percutaneous mitral balloon valvotomy, *J Am Coll Cardiol* 29:175, 1997.

309. Iung B, Cormier B, Ducimetiere P, et al: Immediate results of percutaneous mitral commissurotomy: A predictive model on a series of 1514 patients, *Circulation* 94:2124, 1996.

310. Vahanian A, Palacios IF: Percutaneous approaches to valvular disease, *Circulation* 109:1572, 2004.

311. Hernandez R, Banuelos C, Alfonso F, et al: Long-term clinical and echocardiographic follow-up after percutaneous mitral valvuloplasty with the Inoue balloon, *Circulation* 99:1580, 1999.

312. Kuntz RE, Tosteson ANA, Berman AD, et al: Predictors of event-free survival after balloon aortic valvuloplasty, *N Engl J Med* 325:17, 1991.

313. Masson J, Kovac J, Schuler G, et al: Transcatheter aortic valve implantation, *J Am Coll Cardiol Cardiovasc Interv* 2:811, 2009.

314. Bonhoeffer P, Boudjemline Y, Qureshi SA, et al: Percutaneous insertion of the pulmonary valve, *J Am Coll Cardiol* 39:1664, 2002.

315. Momenah T, Oakley R, Najashi KA, et al: Extended application of percutaneous pulmonary valve implantation, *J Am Coll Cardiol* 53:1859, 2009.

316. Zajarias A, Cribier A: Outcomes and safety of percutaneous aortic valve replacement, *J Am Coll Cardiol* 53:1829, 2009.

317. Piazza N, Asgar A, Ibrahim R, et al: Transcatheter mitral and pulmonary valve therapy, *J Am Coll Cardiol* 53:1837, 2009.

318. Cribier A, Eltchaninoff H, Bash A, et al: Percutaneous transcatheter implantation of an aortic valve prosthesis for calcific aortic stenosis. First human case description, *Circulation* 106:3006, 2002.

319. Himbert D, Descoutures F, Al-Attar N, et al: Results of transfemoral or transapical aortic valve implantation following a uniform assessment in high-risk patients with aortic stenosis, *J Am Coll Cardiol* 54:303, 2009.

320. Osswald BR, Gegouskov V, Badowski-Zyla D: Overestimation of aortic valve replacement risk by EuroSCORE: Implications for percutaneous valve replacement, *Eur Heart J* 30:74, 2009.

321. Maniu CV, Patel JB, Reuter DG, et al: Acute and chronic reduction of functional mitral regurgitation in experimental heart failure by percutaneous mitral annuloplasty, *J Am Coll Cardiol* 44:1652, 2004.

322. Feldman T, Kar S, Rinaldi M, et al: Percutaneous mitral repair with the MitraClip system: Safety and midterm durability in the initial EVEREST (Endovascular Valve Edge-to-Edge REpair Study) cohort, *J Am Coll Cardiol* 54:686, 2009.

323. Fish RD: Percutaneous heart valve replacement, *Circulation* 110:1876, 2004.

324. Hess OM, Sigwart U: New treatment strategies for hypertrophic obstructive cardiomyopathy. Alcohol ablation of the septum: The new gold standard? *J Am Coll Cardiol* 44:2054, 2004.

325. Chang SM, Lakkis NM, Franklin J, et al: Predictors of outcome after alcohol septal ablation therapy in patients with hypertrophic obstructive cardiomyopathy, *Circulation* 109:824, 2004.

326. Kwon D, Kapadia S, Tuzcu EM, et al: Long-terms outcomes in high-risk symptomatic patients with hypertrophic cardiomyopathy undergoing alcohol septal ablation, *JACC Cardiovasc Interv* 1:430, 2008.

327. Valeti U, Nishimura R, Holmes DR, et al: Comparison of surgical septal myectomy and alcohol septal ablation with cardiac magnetic resonance imaging in patient with hypertrophic obstructive cardiomyopathy, *J Am Coll Cardiol* 49:348, 2007.

328. Maron B: Is septal ablation preferable to surgical myomectomy for obstructive hypertrophic cardiomyopathy? *Circulation* 116:196, 2007.

329. Block PC, Burstein S, Casale PN, et al: Percutaneous left atrial appendage occlusion for patients in atrial fibrillation suboptimal for warfarin therapy: 5-year results of the PLAATO (Percutaneous Left Atrial Appendage Transcatheter Occlusion) Study, *JACC Cardiovasc Interv* 2:594, 2009.

330. Holmes DR, Reddy VY, Turi ZG, et al: Percutaneous closure of the left atrial appendage versus warfarin therapy for prevention of stroke in patients with atrial fibrillation: A randomized non-inferiority trial, *Lancet* 374:534, 2009.

331. Jones T, Latson L, Zahn E, et al: Results of the U.S. Multicenter Pivotal Study of the HELEX Septal Occluder for Percutaneous Closure of Secundum Atrial Septal Defects, *J Am Coll Cardiol* 49:2215, 2007.

332. Vigna C, Marchese N: Improvement of migraine after patent foramen ovale percutaneous closure in patients with subclinical brain lesion, *JACC Cardiovasc Interv* 2:107, 2009.

333. Martin F, Sanchez PL, Doherty E, et al: Percutaneous transcatheter closure of patent foramen ovale in patients with paradoxical embolism, *Circulation* 106:1121, 2002.

334. Aaberge L, Rootwelt K, Blomhoff S, et al: Continued symptomatic improvement three to five years after transmyocardial revascularization with CO_2, *J Am Coll Cardiol* 39:1588, 2002.

335. Saririan M, Eisenberg MJ: Myocardial laser revascularization for the treatment of end-stage coronary artery disease, *J Am Coll Cardiol* 41:173, 2003.

336. Stone GW, Teirstein PS, Rubenstein R, et al: A prospective, multicenter, randomized trial of percutaneous transmyocardial laser revascularization in patients with nonrecanalizable chronic total occlusions, *J Am Coll Cardiol* 39:1581, 2002.

4

Cardiac Electrophysiology: Diagnosis and Treatment

ALAN CHENG, MD | ASHISH SHAH, MD | CHARLES W. HOGUE, JR., MD

KEY POINTS

1. Cardiac arrhythmias are common and mechanistically occur as a result of an ectopic focus or the result of reentry.
2. Surgical and catheter-based ablative therapies aim to abolish origins of arrhythmias by interposition of scar tissue along the reentrant pathway or by isolating an area of ectopy.
3. Supraventricular arrhythmias can be hemodynamically unstable, especially when occurring in the setting of structural heart disease. In some cases, persistent tachycardia can lead to tachycardia-induced cardiomyopathy.
4. Accessory pathways are now typically interrupted using percutaneous catheter-based techniques with high success rates and minimal complications.
5. Atrioventricular (AV) nodal reentrant tachycardia is due to altered electrophysiologic properties of the anterior fast pathway and posterior slow pathway fibers, providing input to the AV node; interruption of involved pathway is curative.
6. Atrial flutter typically involves a reentrant circuit that circles the tricuspid valve, crossing the myocardial isthmus between the inferior vena cava and the tricuspid valve; catheter ablation of this region can prevent the arrhythmia.
7. Paroxysmal atrial fibrillation often is due to ectopy arising from the pulmonary veins; pulmonary vein isolation with catheter ablative energy is indicated in patients who have not responded positively to antiarrhythmic therapy and are either symptomatic or have evidence of structural heart disease that is thought secondary to atrial fibrillation.
8. Catheter ablation of persistent or longstanding atrial fibrillation is less effective (as compared with paroxysmal atrial fibrillation). Although pulmonary vein isolation is still recommended, adjuvant ablation strategies also are used, including abatement of complex fractionated atrial electrograms and targeting areas of ganglionated plexuses.
9. Surgical treatment for atrial fibrillation ("Maze procedure") has been used with good success and has been modified to avoid the sinus node in an effort to minimize occurrences of chronotropic incompetence.
10. In adults, most episodes of sudden cardiac death are the result of ventricular tachyarrhythmias secondary to ischemic and nonischemic cardiomyopathy. Other conditions associated with an increased risk for sudden death include infiltrative cardiac diseases (e.g., cardiac sarcoidosis, amyloidosis) and other genetically based abnormalities such as hypertrophic cardiomyopathy, long QT syndrome, Brugada syndrome, catecholaminergic polymorphic ventricular tachycardia (VT), and arrhythmogenic right ventricular dysplasia.
11. Substantial evidence supports cardioverter-defibrillator implantation for primary and secondary prevention of sudden cardiac death.

Cardiac rhythm disturbances are common and an important source of morbidity and mortality.[1,2] Supraventricular tachycardias (SVTs) have an estimated incidence from 35 per 100,000 person-years for paroxysmal SVT to 5 to 587 per 100,000 person-years for atrial flutter for individuals age 50 years versus those older than 80 years, respectively.[3,4] But it is atrial fibrillation that has proved to be the most common sustained cardiac arrhythmia in the general population, affecting more than 2.3 million Americans.[5] The prevalence of atrial fibrillation is strongly related to age, occurring in fewer than 1% of individuals younger than 55 years but in nearly 10% of those older than 80 years.[5] The occurrence of atrial fibrillation increases health resource utilization, heightens the risk for stroke, and is associated with long-term mortality.[6]

There has been a major shift in the treatment of cardiac arrhythmias since the 1980s; this is due, in part, to advances made in catheter- and surgical-based ablations, as well as widely held views that pharmacologic treatments have limited efficacy and, in some instances, may actually increase risk for mortality. These latter observations are mostly due to the negative inotropic and proarrhythmic effects of these drugs.[7,8] Data from prospective randomized trials showing improved survival for patients with implantable cardioverter-defibrillators (ICDs) compared with those given antiarrhythmic drugs have further contributed to a shift to nonpharmacologic treatments.[9]

Given improvements made in the management of cardiac arrhythmias, a greater breadth of therapeutic options are currently available, including surgical ablation and catheter-based ablation techniques using various types of energy sources. The underlying principle, however, remains the same: identification of the electrophysiologic mechanism of the arrhythmia followed by ablation of the involved myocardium with surgical incisions, cryothermy, or radiofrequency (RF) current. As these techniques become more complex and time-intensive, a growing need for anesthesia support has emerged. The fundamentals for the anesthetic care of patients undergoing these procedures require familiarization with the anatomy of the normal cardiac conduction system, the electrophysiologic basis for common cardiac rhythm disorders, and the approaches to their ablative treatment. This chapter discusses these basic principles, together with special anesthetic considerations when unique to a particular form of treatment.

BASIC ELECTROPHYSIOLOGIC PRINCIPLES

Anatomy and Physiology of the Cardiac Pacemaker and Conduction Systems

Sinus Node

The sinoatrial node (SAN; Figure 4-1) is a spindle-shaped structure composed of highly specialized cells located in the right atrial sulcus terminalis, lateral to the junction of the superior vena cava (SVC) and the right atrium[10,11] (see Box 4-1 for a summary of the anatomy of the cardiac pacemaker and conduction system). Three cell types have been identified in the SAN (nodal, transitional, and atrial muscle cells), but no single cell appears to be solely responsible for initiating the pacemaker impulse. Rather, multiple cells in the SAN discharge synchronously through complex interactions.[12–14] Rather than a discrete and isolated structure, studies suggest that the SAN consists of three distinct regions, each responsive to a separate group of neural and circulatory stimuli.[15] The interrelationship of these three regions appears to determine the ultimate rate of output of the SAN. Although the SAN is the

BOX 4-1. ANATOMY OF THE CARDIAC PACEMAKER AND CONDUCTION SYSTEM

- Sinus node
- Internodal conduction
- Atrioventricular junction
- Intraventricular conduction system
  - Left bundle branch
    - Anterior fascicle
    - Posterior fascicle
  - Right bundle branch
  - Purkinje fibers

site of primary impulse formation, subsidiary atrial pacemakers located throughout the right and left atria also can initiate cardiac impulses.[16–18] In a series of studies both in dogs and humans, it was confirmed that there is an extensive system of atrial pacemakers widely distributed in the right and left atria, as well as in the atrial septum.[15,19–21] Because the atrial pacemaker system occupies a much larger area than the SAN, it can be severed during arrhythmia surgery, resulting in impaired rate responsiveness.[10] However, it is extremely difficult to completely abolish SAN activity through catheter-based ablation techniques.

The arterial supply to the SAN (SAN artery) is provided from either the right coronary artery (RCA; in 60% of the population) or the left circumflex coronary artery (see Figure 4-1). The SAN is richly innervated with postganglionic adrenergic and cholinergic nerve terminals. Vagal stimulation, by releasing acetylcholine, slows SA nodal automaticity and prolongs intranodal conduction time, whereas adrenergic stimulation increases the discharge rate of the SAN.[10]

Internodal Conduction

For many years, there has been much controversy concerning the existence of specialized conduction pathways connecting the SAN to the atrioventricular (AV) node. Most electrophysiologists now agree that preferential conduction is unequivocally present, and that spread of activation from the SAN to the AV node follows distinct routes by necessity because of the peculiar geometry of the right atrium.[10] The orifices of the superior and inferior cavae, the fossa ovalis, and the ostium of the coronary sinus divide the right atrium into muscle bands, thus limiting the number of routes available for internodal conduction (see Figure 4-1). These routes, however, do not represent discrete bundles of histologically specialized internodal tracts comparable with the ventricular bundle branches.[22] It has been suggested that a parallel arrangement of myocardial cells in bundles, such as the crista terminalis and the limbus of the fossa ovalis, may account for preferential internodal conduction. Although electrical impulses travel more rapidly through these thick atrial muscle bundles, surgical transection will not block internodal conduction because alternate pathways of conduction through atrial muscle are available.[23]

Atrioventricular Junction and Intraventricular Conduction System

The AV junction (Figure 4-2) corresponds anatomically to a group of discrete specialized cells, morphologically distinct from working myocardium and divided into a transitional cell zone, compact portion, and penetrating AV bundle (bundle of His).[24] Based on animal experiments, the transitional zone appears to connect atrial myocardium with the compact AV node.[25] The compact portion of the AV node is located superficially, anterior to the ostium of the coronary sinus above the insertion of the septal leaflet of the tricuspid valve. The longitudinal segment of the compact AV node penetrates the central fibrous body and becomes the bundle of His. As the nodal-bundle axis descends into the ventricular musculature, it gradually becomes completely isolated by collagen and is no longer in contact with atrial fibers.

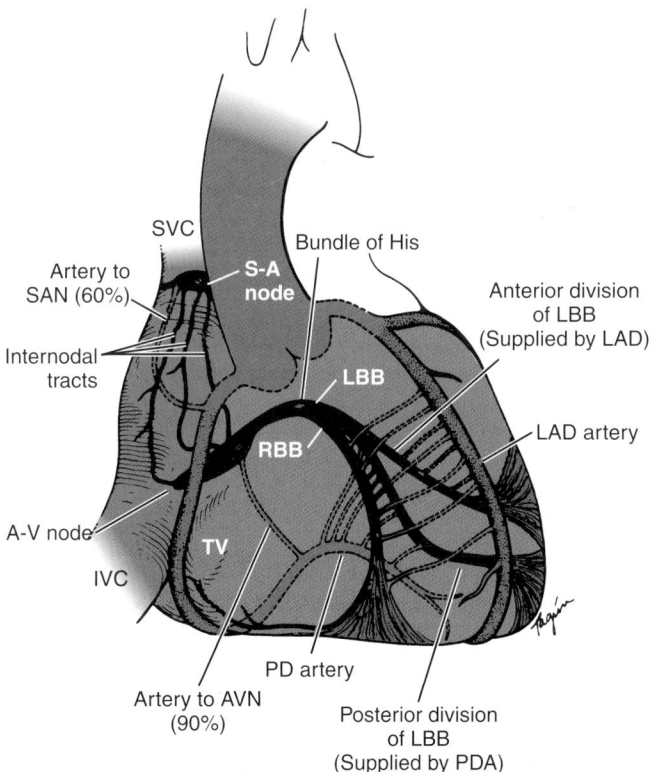

Figure 4-1   Drawing of the anatomy of the cardiac conduction system including arterial blood supply. In 60% of patients the sinoatrial (S-A) nodal artery is a branch of the right coronary artery, whereas in the remainder it arises from the circumflex artery. The atrioventricular node (AVN) is supplied by a branch from the right coronary artery or posterior descending artery. A-V, atrioventricular; IVC, inferior vena cava; LAD, left anterior descending coronary artery; LBB, left bundle branch; PD, posterior descending; PDA, posterior descending artery; RBB, right bundle branch; SAN, sinoatrial node; SVC, superior vena cava; TV, tricuspid valve. *(From Harthorne JW, Pohost GM: Electrical therapy of cardiac arrhythmias. In Levine HJ [ed]: Clinical Cardiovascular Physiology. New York: Grune & Stratton, 1976, p 854.)*

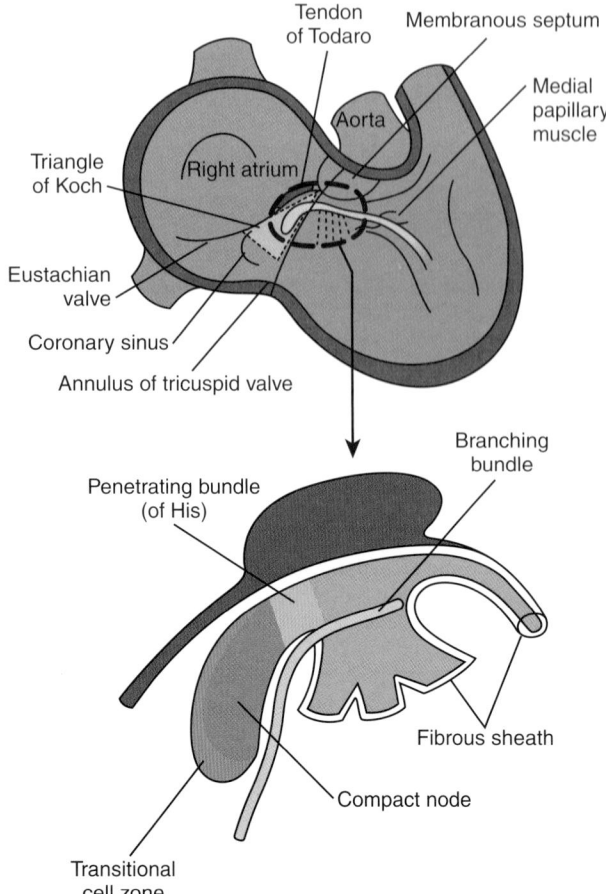

Figure 4-2 Anatomic relation of the atrioventricular junction in relation to other cardiac structures. *(From Harrison DC [ed]: Cardiac Arrhythmias: A Decade of Progress. Boston: GK Hall Medical Publishers, 1981.)*

The AV junction is contained within the triangle of Koch, an anatomically discrete region bounded by the tendon of Todaro, the tricuspid valve annulus, and the ostium of the coronary sinus (Figure 4-3). This triangle is avoided in all cardiac operative procedures to prevent surgical damage to AV conduction. Individual variability in the specific

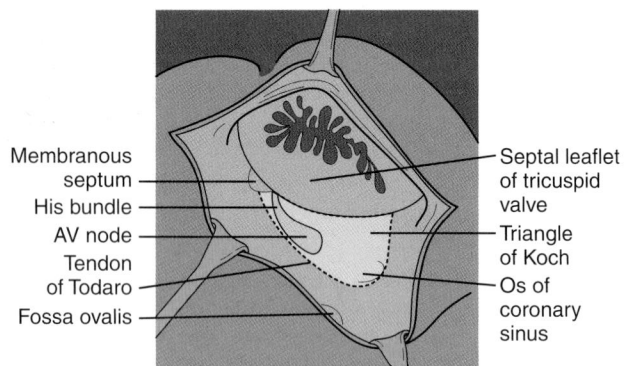

Figure 4-3 View of right atrial septum via a right atriotomy incision (superior is to the left). The triangle of Koch is an important anatomic area that includes the atrioventricular (AV) node and proximal portion of the bundle of His. This anatomic region is contained in the area between the tendon of Todaro, the tricuspid valve annulus, and a line connecting the two at the level of the os of the coronary sinus. *(From Cox JL, Holman WL, Cain ME: Cryosurgical treatment of atrioventricular node reentry tachycardia. Circulation 76:1331, 1987.)*

anatomy of the AV nodal area is dependent on the degree of central fibrous body development.[10]

The branching of the nodal-bundle axis begins at the superior margin of the muscular interventricular septum. At this level, the bundle of His emits a broad band of fasciculi, forming the left bundle branch that extends downward as a continuous sheet into the left side of the septum beneath the noncoronary aortic cusp (see Figure 4-1). The left bundle divides into smaller anterior and broader posterior fascicles, although this is not a consistent anatomic delineation. The right bundle branch usually originates as the final continuation of the bundle of His, traveling subendocardially on the right side of the interventricular septum toward the apex of the right ventricle. The distal branches of the conduction system connect with an interweaving network of Purkinje fibers, expanding broadly on the endocardial surface of both ventricles. Blood supply to the AV node is mostly from the RCA (in 85% of the population) or from the left circumflex artery. The bundle of His is supplied by branches from the anterior and posterior descending coronary arteries. Innervation to the SA and AV nodes is complex because of substantial overlapping of vagal and sympathetic nerve branches. Stimulation of the right cervical vagus nerve causes sinus bradycardia, whereas stimulation of the left vagus produces prolongation of AV nodal conduction. Stimulation of the right stellate ganglion speeds SA nodal discharge rate, whereas stimulation of the left ganglion produces a shift in the pacemaker from the SAN to an ectopic site.[26]

Basic Arrhythmia Mechanisms

The mechanisms of cardiac arrhythmias are broadly classified as: (1) focal mechanisms that include automatic or triggered arrhythmias, or (2) reentrant arrhythmias (Box 4-2). Cells that display automaticity lack a true resting membrane potential and, instead, undergo slow depolarization during diastole (Figures 4-4 and 4-5). Diastolic depolarization results in the transmembrane potential becoming more positive between successive action potentials until the threshold potential is reached, leading to cellular excitation. Cells possessing normal automaticity can be found in the SAN, subsidiary atrial foci, AV node, and His-Purkinje system.[10,13,27-29] The property of slow diastolic depolarization is termed *spontaneous diastolic,* or phase 4 depolarization. Factors that may modify spontaneous diastolic depolarization are shown in Figure 4-5 and include alterations in the maximum diastolic potential, threshold potential, and rate or slope of diastolic depolarization. The net effect of these factors is to influence the rate (increased or decreased) at which the threshold potential is achieved, resulting in either an increase or a decrease in automaticity. The ionic mechanism of diastolic depolarization involves the "funny" current, which, in turn, may involve a decrease in net outward K^+ movement and/or an increase in net inward Na^+ movement.[26,30-33] Pacemaker cells with the fastest rate of phase 4 depolarization become dominant in initiating the cardiac impulse, with other automatic foci subject to overdrive suppression.

BOX 4-2. ARRHYTHMIA MECHANISMS

- Focal mechanisms
  - Automatic
  - Triggered
- Reentrant arrhythmias
- Normal automaticity
  - Sinoatrial node
  - Subsidiary atrial foci
  - Atrioventricular node
  - His-Purkinje system
- Triggered mechanisms occur from repetitive delayed or early afterdepolarizations
- Reentry
  - Unidirectional block is necessary
  - Slowed conduction in the alternate pathway exceeds the refractory period of cells at the site of unidirectional block

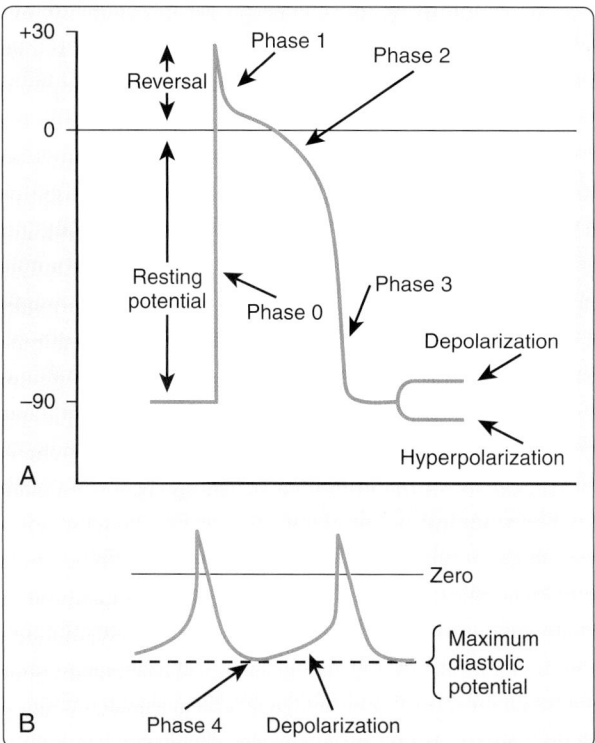

Figure 4-4 Graph depicting the cardiac cellular action potential from fast-response fiber (*A*) and slow-response fiber (*B*). The slow-response fiber similar to that found in the sinoatrial node lacks the rapid upstroke of phase 0. (*From Ferguson TB Jr: Anatomic and electrophysiologic principles in the surgical treatment of cardiac arrhythmias. Cardiac Surg 4:19, 1990.*)

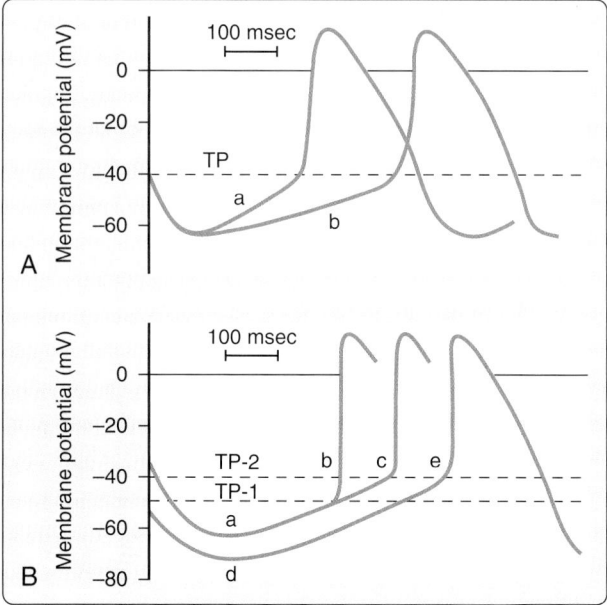

Figure 4-5 **Transmembrane potential from sinus node.** *A*, A decrease in the slope of phase 4 or diastolic depolarization (from *a* to *b*) will increase the time to reach threshold potential (TP), thus slowing the heart rate. *B*, Heart rate slowing occurs by changing from TP-1 to TP-2, such that a longer interval is needed to reach TP (*b* to *c*). Increasing maximum diastolic potential (*a* to *d*) will also slow heart rate by increasing the time to reach TP (*b* to *c*). (*From Atlee JL III: Perioperative Cardiac Arrhythmias: Mechanisms, Recognition, Management, 2nd edition. Chicago: Year Book Medical Publishers, 1990, p 36.*)

When cells that normally display automaticity (e.g., SAN, AV node, Purkinje fibers) change the rate of pacemaker firing, altered normal automaticity is said to occur. Although the ionic mechanisms resulting in altered normal automaticity are unchanged, other factors such as those seen in Figure 4-5 can contribute to an increase in automaticity. In contrast, automaticity resulting from abnormal ionic mechanisms, even if occurring in cells that are usually considered automatic (e.g., Purkinje fibers), is referred to as "abnormal automaticity." Abnormal automaticity also may occur in cells in which automaticity is not normally observed (e.g., ventricular myocardium).

Arrhythmias arising from a "triggered" mechanism are initiated from cells that experience repetitive afterdepolarizations. Afterdepolarizations are oscillations in the transmembrane potential that occur either before (early afterdepolarizations) or after (delayed afterdepolarizations) membrane repolarization. Different ionic mechanisms are responsible for each form of afterdepolarization, and if the oscillations in membrane potential reach the threshold potential, a triggered cardiac impulse can be generated.[13] Triggered activity is often considered an abnormal form of automaticity. However, because triggered activity requires a prior cardiac impulse (in contrast with automaticity), this abnormal electrophysiologic event cannot purely be considered a form of automaticity.

Reentry is a condition in which a cardiac impulse persists to reexcite myocardium that is no longer refractory.[10] Unidirectional block of impulse conduction is a necessary condition for reentry. This unidirectional block may be in the form of differences in membrane refractoriness (dispersion of refractoriness) such that some areas of myocardium are unexcitable, whereas other areas allow impulse propagation. On repolarization, previously refractory membranes will be available for depolarization if the initial impulse has found an alternate route of propagation and returns to the prior site of conduction block. For reentry to occur, slowed conduction in the alternate pathway must exceed the refractory period of cells at the site of unidirectional block. Partial depolarization of fast-response fibers (depressed fast response) results in reduced Na^+ channel availability with consequent reduced rate of phase 0 of the action potential. This reduced rate of action potential upstroke of phase 0 can result in slowed conduction and contribute to the above conditions conducive to reentry. Arrhythmias produced by reentrant or triggered mechanisms, but not those secondary to increased automaticity, can be induced with programmed stimulation in the setting of a diagnostic electrophysiology study (EPS). Pacemaker-induced overdrive suppression is a characteristic of arrhythmias produced by automaticity (see Chapter 25).

Diagnostic Evaluation

The history of symptoms often can provide clues in determining the cause of a patient's palpitations. Abrupt onset and abrupt termination of regular palpitations, for example, are consistent with a paroxysmal SVT most often caused by atrioventricular nodal reentrant tachycardia (AVNRT), atrioventricular reentrant tachycardia (AVRT) associated with an accessory AV bypass tract, or atrial tachycardia. Although a history of syncope does not definitively point toward a ventricular or supraventricular cause, its presence is helpful in determining how urgently this condition should be evaluated. Whether palpitations are regular or irregular is useful in differentiating atrial fibrillation as a cause of the symptoms. Precipitating events, number and duration of episodes, presence of dyspnea, fatigue, or other constitutional symptoms should be sought from the history (Box 4-3).

A 12-lead electrocardiogram (ECG) should be obtained during tachycardia whenever possible and compared with baseline sinus rhythm ECGs. It also is helpful to run a rhythm strip during periods of intervention such as carotid sinus massage or adenosine administration. Patients with a history of pre-excitation presenting with an arrhythmia should be evaluated immediately because atrial fibrillation in the presence of an accessory pathway can lead to sudden death. For all patients undergoing evaluation of an arrhythmia, an echocardiogram is essential to evaluate for cardiac structural abnormalities and ventricular function. The latter is particularly germane for patients with persistent

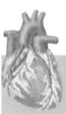

BOX 4-3. DIAGNOSTIC EVALUATION OF ARRHYTHMIAS

- History of palpitations, syncope, and constitutional symptoms; physical examination
- 12-Lead electrocardiogram at baseline and during tachycardia, if available
- Two-dimensional echocardiogram
- 24-Hour Holter monitoring of patient-triggered events
- Invasive electrophysiologic testing

tachycardia because this can lead to tachycardia-associated cardiomyopathy.[34] Twenty-four-hour Holter monitoring of patient-triggered events also may be useful in some patients with frequent but transient symptoms. Other evaluations such as exercise or pharmacologic stress testing also have been used to elicit episodes of tachycardia or determine how robust pre-excitation is present with increasing heart rates.

The ultimate diagnosis of the underlying mechanisms of the arrhythmia may require invasive electrophysiologic testing. These studies involve percutaneous introduction of catheters capable of electrical stimulation and recording of electrograms from various intracardiac sites. Initial recording sites often include the high right atrium, bundle of His, coronary sinus, and the right ventricle[10,35] (Figures 4-6 and

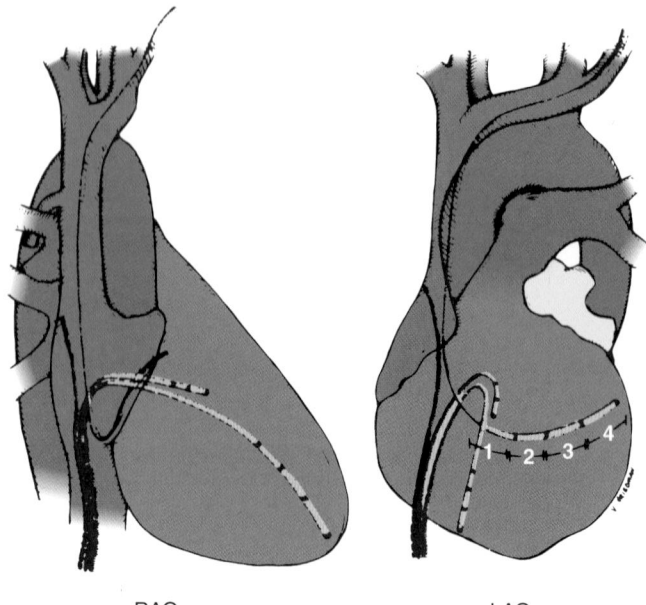

RAO   LAO

Figure 4-7 Electrophysiologic study in patient with Wolff–Parkinson–White syndrome is schematically depicted. Catheter with multiple recording/pacing electrodes is positioned in the high right atrium, coronary sinus, bundle of His region, and right ventricular apex. Right anterior oblique (RAO) projections differentiate anterior from posterior sites. Left anterior oblique (LAO) projections differentiate septal from lateral sites. Numbered zones in the LAO projection regionalize electrode positions in the coronary sinus (*4,* posterolateral; *3,* posterior; *2,* posterior; *1,* posteroseptal). *(From Cain ME, Cox JL: Surgical treatment of supraventricular tachyarrhythmias. In Platia EV [ed]: Management of Cardiac Arrhythmias: The Nonpharmacologic Approach. Philadelphia: JB Lippincott, 1987, p 307.)*

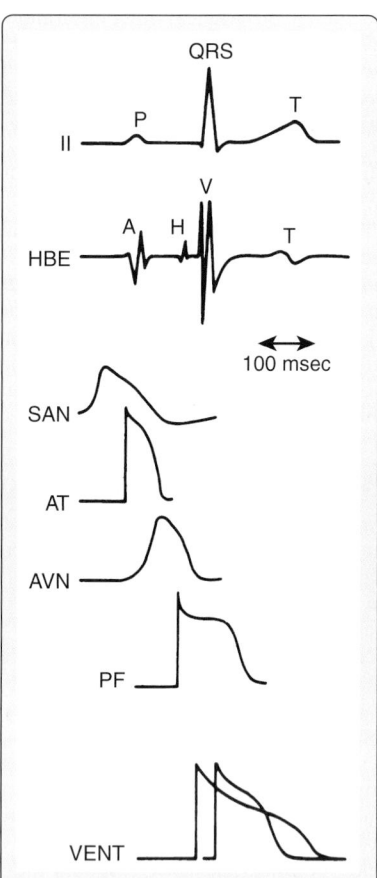

Figure 4-6 Electrograms from leads placed in various cardiac locations in reference to the surface electrocardiogram (ECG). Note rapid upstroke of action potential (phase 0) in fast-response fibers compared with slower upstroke of slow-response fibers. Sequences of action potentials from various cardiac tissues are presented in relation to surface ECG and bundle of His electrogram. AT, atrium; AVN, atrioventricular node; HBE, His-bundle region; PF, Purkinje fiber; SAN, sinoatrial node; VENT, ventricle. *(From Atlee JL III: Perioperative Cardiac Arrhythmias: Mechanisms, Recognition, Management, 2nd ed. Chicago: Year Book Medical Publishers, 1990, p 27.)*

4-7). The sequence of cardiac activation can be discerned from these recordings together with the surface ECG. This is illustrated in Figure 4-8 from a patient undergoing evaluation for an accessory AV conduction pathway. The sequence of the activation is observed by noting the timing of depolarization recorded by the respective electrodes positioned fluoroscopically at various anatomic sites. An example of a recording obtained during diagnostic evaluation of a patient with a ventricular arrhythmia is shown in Figure 4-9.

The catheters are most often introduced via the femoral vessels under local anesthesia. Systemic heparinization is required, particularly when catheters are introduced into the left atrium or left ventricle. The most common complications from electrophysiologic testing are those associated with vascular catheterization.[10,36] Other complications include hypotension (in 1% of patients), hemorrhage, deep venous thrombosis (in 0.4% of patients), embolic phenomena (0.4%), infection (0.2%), and cardiac perforation (0.1%).[10,37] Proper application of adhesive cardioversion electrodes before the procedure facilitates rapid cardioversion/defibrillation in the event of persistent or hemodynamically unstable tachyarrhythmia resulting from stimulation protocols.

The principles of intraoperative electrophysiologic mapping are similar to those used in the cardiac catheterization suite. These procedures have evolved from early single-point epicardial mapping systems with a handheld electrode to sophisticated multichannel computerized systems. The latter are capable of acquiring and storing multiple epicardial, intramural, and endocardial electrograms from a single depolarization. Multichannel, computerized mapping allows for rapid identification of arrhythmia pathways (e.g., accessory pathways) before initiation of cardiopulmonary bypass (CPB), reducing the need for excessive cardiac manipulations necessary with a handheld electrode, thus promoting stable conduction.

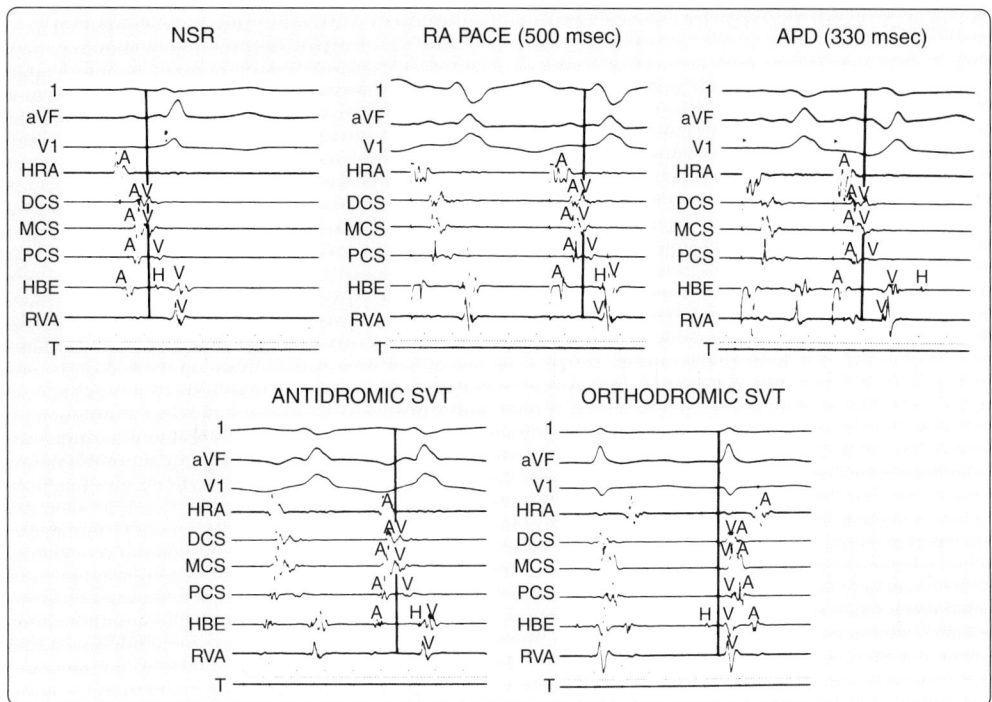

Figure 4-8 Surface electrocardiogram (ECG; leads I, aVF, and V₁) and electrograms at various intracardiac sites during sinus rhythm, pacing from the right atrium (RA), after an atrial premature depolarization (APD), and during antidromic and orthodromic supraventricular tachycardia (SVT). The left free wall accessory pathway is identified by noting the earliest onset of ventricular depolarization at the distal coronary sinus catheter (DCS) in relation to the delta wave on the surface ECG *(solid vertical line)*. This is followed closely by activation in the mid (MCS) and proximal coronary sinus (PCS) sites. Other catheter locations are the high right atrium (HRA), His-bundle region (HBE), and right ventricular apex (RVA). Conduction is followed during supraventricular tachycardia by noting the pattern of cardiac activation from the right atrium *(solid vertical line)* to the ventricles. NSR, normal sinus rhythm. *(From Cain ME, Cox JL: Surgical treatment of supraventricular tachyarrhythmias. In Platia EV [ed]: Management of Cardiac Arrhythmias. Philadelphia: JB Lippincott, 1987, p 308.)*

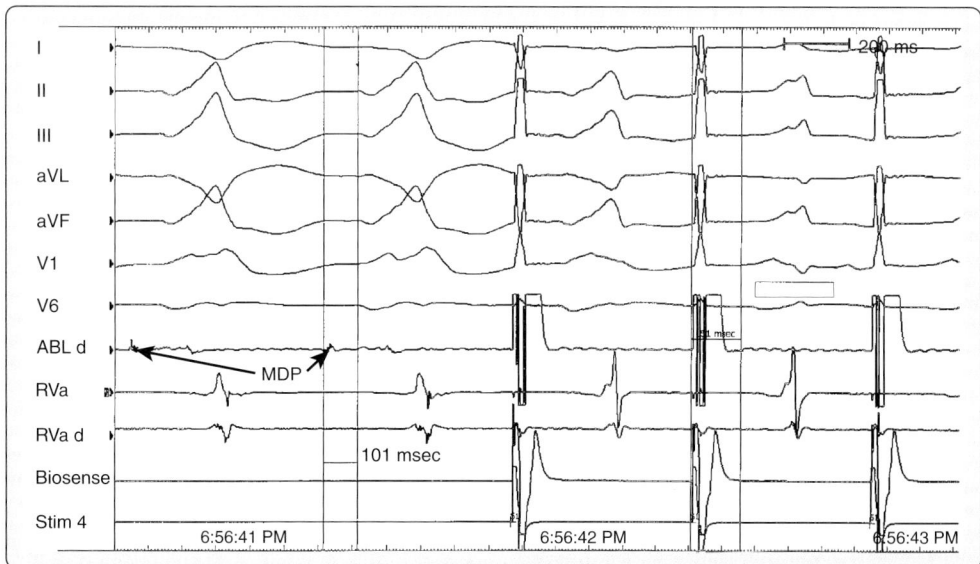

Figure 4-9 **Endocardial mapping of ventricular tachycardia.** Surface electrocardiograms and selected endocardial electrograms are shown during sustained ventricular tachycardia in a patient with a severe ischemic tachycardia. The mapping catheter distal electrode (ABL d) has been positioned at an endocardial site that records a mid-diastolic potential (MDP) that precedes the QRS by 101 milliseconds. Pacing at a cycle length slightly faster than the tachycardia cycle length results in ventricular capture with a QRS morphology that is slightly different from the native tachycardia. The interpretation of this maneuver is that the endocardial pacing site is not at a favorable location for catheter ablation. Pacing at an optimal site for catheter ablation produces an identical QRS morphology to the native tachycardia.

Principles of Electrophysiologic Treatment

The paradigm for ablative treatment of cardiac arrhythmias evolved from the surgical treatment of Wolff–Parkinson–White (WPW) syndrome and then ventricular tachycardia (VT) developed by Sealy, Boineau, and colleagues.[38-40] The fundamental paradigm for this approach is precise localization of the electrophysiologic substrate for the arrhythmia and then ablating the pathway. In the case of WPW syndrome, the accessory pathway is identified with intraoperative electrophysiologic mapping that initially used handheld electrodes.[10,41] Development of multichannel computer-based mapping systems allowed for the identification of both the mechanisms for many arrhythmias, including VT, and their termination by interruption of the underlying substrate. Experience and insights into arrhythmia mechanisms led to the development of catheter-based methods now routinely used for a variety of supraventricular and ventricular arrhythmias. General indications for ablative treatments include drug-resistant arrhythmias, drug intolerance, severe symptoms, and desire to avoid lifelong drug treatments (Box 4-4).

Manipulation of catheter electrodes in the heart for precise mapping and treatment of arrhythmias can be laborious and time consuming. Newer catheters, as well as robotically and magnetically driven navigational systems, have been developed to facilitate this process and improve both catheter positioning and stability. With these navigational systems, the catheter tip is localized with three-dimensional fluoroscopy and/or advanced three-dimensional mapping applications and precisely moved to the myocardial area of interest using either a robotic arm or a magnetic field[42] (Figure 4-10).

Given the two predominant mechanisms of arrhythmias, surgical and catheter-based treatments often focus on either identifying the site of earliest electrical activity (in the case of focal automatic or triggered arrhythmias) or identifying the critical "isthmus" responsible for perpetuating reentrant arrhythmias. Ablation of atrial fibrillation, however, deviates from this traditional paradigm and focuses on isolating the critical anatomic substrate (often the pulmonary veins) responsible for both its initiation and its perpetuation. But as a general rule, the aim of electrophysiologic treatments is to interpose scar tissue within the conduction pathway of the arrhythmia. This is accomplished with a properly placed surgical incision or by inducing myocardial injury by application of an energy source from a precisely placed catheter. Various energy sources have been used including laser energy, microwave energy, RF, and cryoablation. The most common energy source is RF energy that destroys myocardium by resistive heating. Success is determined by the volume and depth of tissue injured by RF and is a function of how much power is delivered during energy application. This, in turn, is affected by both the catheter tip size and the amount of convective cooling that occurs during energy delivery. Measurement of tissue impedance during application of bipolar RF energy ensures that transmural injury occurs. Because transmural scarring may not occur depending on the thickness of the tissue, measurement of conduction across the lesion is recommended. Failure to conduct an applied electrical stimulus indicates pathway interruption.

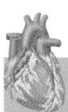

BOX 4-4. ELECTROPHYSIOLOGIC ABLATIVE TREATMENT INDICATIONS

- Drug-resistant arrhythmias
- Drug intolerance
- Severe symptoms
- Avoiding lifelong treatments

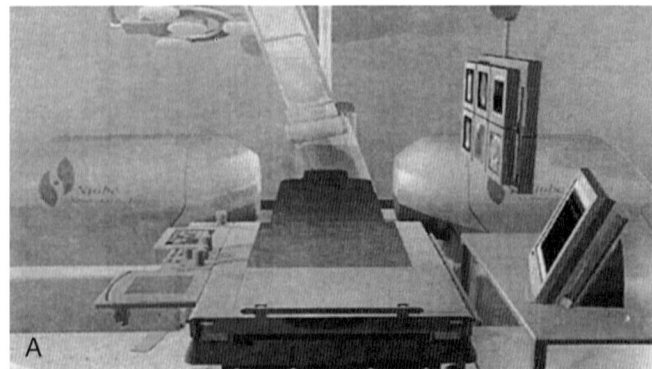
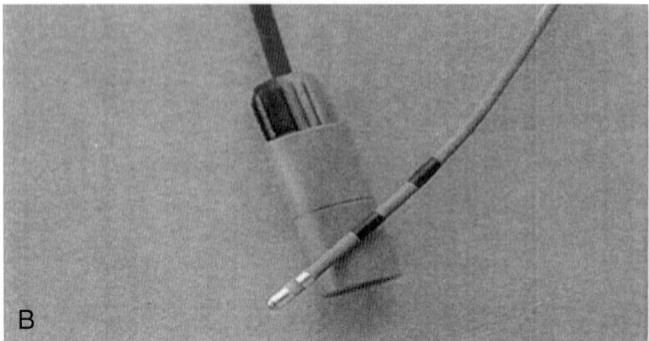

Figure 4-10 Stereotaxis magnetic catheter navigation system. *A,* The Stereotaxis system consists of two permanent magnetic arrays positioned on either side of a standard fluoroscopy table and digital fluoroscopy together with a computer control system. The magnetic arrays project a composite magnetic field of 0.08 T in the region of a patient's heart to control the position of a magnetic catheter. *B,* A 7-French magnetic catheter that is used with the Stereotaxis system is shown. The catheter has two distal electrodes for endocardial pacing, recording, and radiofrequency ablation. An internal permanent magnet allows the catheter to interact with the prevailing magnetic field for motion control.

SPECIFIC ARRHYTHMIAS

Supraventricular Tachyarrhythmias

Supraventricular arrhythmias are defined as cardiac rhythms with a heart rate greater than 100 beats/min originating above the division of the common bundle of His. These arrhythmias are often seen as a narrow-complex tachycardia and, in some cases, can be hemodynamically unstable in the presence of structural heart disease. Further, persistent tachycardias for weeks to months may lead to tachycardia-associated cardiomyopathy and to disabling symptoms.[34] The differential diagnosis of SVTs includes atrioventricular reciprocating tachycardia (AVRT), AVNRT, atrial tachycardia, inappropriate sinus tachycardia or sinus node reentry, atrial flutter, and atrial fibrillation. Antiarrhythmic medications traditionally have been used with mixed success. Hence surgical and catheter-based procedures have been developed for the management of these arrhythmias.

Atrioventricular Reciprocating Tachycardia

Accessory pathways are abnormal strands of myocardium connecting the atria and ventricles across the AV groove, providing alternate routes for conduction that bypass the AV node and bundle of His (Box 4-5). Various classifications are used to describe accessory pathways and are based on their location (e.g., tricuspid, mitral), whether they are manifest or concealed on a surface ECG, and the conduction properties

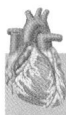

exhibited by the pathway (e.g., antegrade, retrograde, decremental, nondecremental).[42] Decremental conduction along any myocardial tissue refers to the concept that conduction through that tissue is slower as the frequency of impulses reaching it increases. Accessory pathways are more often nondecremental, meaning that regardless of how quickly impulses reach the pathway, the conduction velocity across the pathway remains the same. Concealed pathways refer to the situation in which the accessory pathway only exhibits retrograde conduction; thus, there is no conduction from the atrium to the ventricles through the pathway, thereby showing no evidence of ventricular pre-excitation. This is in contrast with manifest pathways displaying antegrade conduction from the atrium to the ventricles. Because electrical signals can enter the ventricles both from the AV node and the accessory pathway, ventricular pre-excitation will be "manifest" on the surface ECG as delta waves. Manifest pathways typically conduct in both antegrade and retrograde directions. The presence of a manifest pathway allows for the ventricle to be depolarized or "pre-excited" before that occurring via the normal route of conduction through the AV node (Figures 4-11 and 4-12). During pre-excitation, an activation wavefront propagates simultaneously to the ventricles across the bundle of His and the accessory pathway. Because anterograde conduction is delayed at the AV node but not the accessory pathway, the impulse passing through the accessory pathway initiates ventricular depolarization before the

impulse traveling via the normal AV conduction system. The ventricle is thus pre-excited, resulting in a delta wave preceding the QRS complex (see Figure 4-11). These ECG findings (short PR interval and delta wave) were noted by Wolff, Parkinson, and White in the 1930s in association with SVT.[44] WPW syndrome describes the condition of pre-excitation when accompanied by tachyarrhythmias caused by reentry via the accessory pathway. Not all individuals with the classic WPW ECG findings experience tachyarrhythmias. In fact, it is estimated that about 30% of individuals with WPW ECG findings exhibit tachyarrhythmias. Individuals with WPW ECG findings but without tachyarrhythmias are said to have the WPW signature. AVRT occurs in the absence of the WPW syndrome when the pathway is concealed, and not all tachyarrhythmias in patients with WPW result from the AVRT mechanism.

By noting polarity of the delta wave (QRS axis) and precordial R-wave progression, the resting 12-lead ECG can provide clues about the location of the accessory pathway in either the left lateral, left posterior, posterior septal, right free wall, or anterior septal regions[45] (Table 4-1). Precise localization, though, is dependent on EPS. Additional information provided by such investigation includes documentation of the mechanism for the arrhythmia (AV vs. other mechanism) and the conduction properties of the accessory pathways. The atrial and ventricular insertion sites of the accessory pathway are identified by observing ventricular activation patterns during sinus rhythm and during atrial pacing (see Figure 4-11). In the presence of an accessory pathway, the interval between the deflection denoting activation of the bundle of His and the earliest ventricular activation (delta wave) is less than the H-V interval. The area with the shortest delta-to-V interval localizes the accessory pathway's ventricular insertion. More than one accessory pathway may be present, which is suggested by observing different delta-wave morphology with increasing atrial pacing rates or with introduced atrial premature beats (see Figure 4-12). Observing atrial activation patterns during ventricular pacing, after a ventricular premature beat or during induced orthodromic SVT, can identify the location of the atrial insertion sites.

AVRT can occur in one of two fashions: orthodromic reciprocating tachycardia (ORT) and antidromic reciprocating tachycardia (ART)[46-48] (Figure 4-13). ORT is by far the most common type and involves antegrade conduction via the normal AV nodal conduction system and retrograde conduction via the accessory pathway. ART, in contrast, involves antegrade conduction down the accessory pathway and retrograde conduction via the AV node. As suggested by these mechanisms,

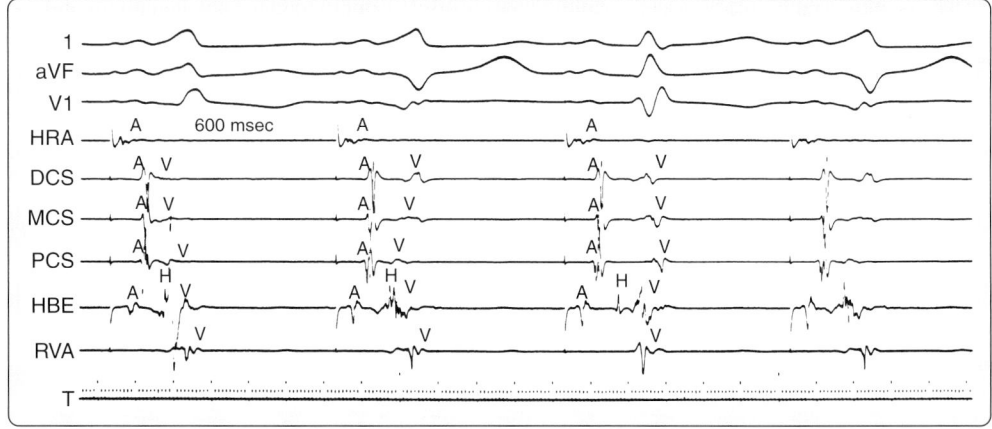

Figure 4-11 The presence of two accessory pathways is shown during pacing. The site of earliest ventricular activation is noted with the distal coronary sinus (DCS) electrode, indicating left free-wall accessory pathway. The second paced beat shows the site of earliest ventricular activation from the proximal coronary sinus (PCS) electrode, indicating posterior septal accessory pathway. After the third paced beat, neither site is activated due to anterograde conduction block. In this instance, conduction follows the normal AV-His bundle and bundle-branch pathways. Surface electrocardiogram leads and intracardiac electrograms are organized as in Figure 4-8. HBE, His-bundle region; HRA, high right atrium; MCA, mid-coronary sinus; RVA, right ventricular apex. *(From Cain ME, Cox JL: Surgical treatment of supraventricular tachyarrhythmias. In Platia EV [ed]: Management of Cardiac Arrhythmias. Philadelphia: JB Lippincott, 1987, p 312.)*

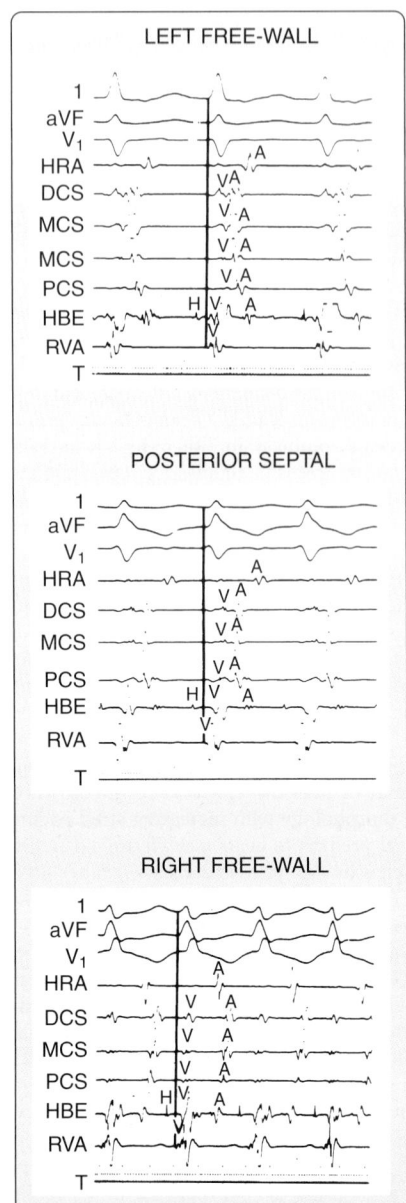

Figure 4-12 Atrial activation recordings from three different patients during orthodromic tachycardia via accessory pathways at distinct locations. Using the *solid vertical line* as a reference for the QRS complex from the surface electrocardiogram (ECG), the first example demonstrates the earliest atrial activation at the distal coronary sinus (DCS) site, indicating a left free-wall accessory pathway. The posterior septal accessory pathway is indicated by earliest activation of the electrode located in the proximal coronary sinus (PCS). In the last example, atrial activation at the high right atrium (HRA) and bundle of His area (HBE) occurs before all the coronary sinus recording sites, indicative of a right free-wall accessory pathway. Surface ECG leads and intracardiac electrograms are organized as in Figure 4-8. MCA, mid-coronary sinus; RVA, right ventricular apex. *(From Cain ME, Cox JL: Surgical treatment of supraventricular tachyarrhythmias. In Platia EV [ed]: Management of Cardiac Arrhythmias. Philadelphia: JB Lippincott, 1987, p 313.)*

ORT appears as a narrow-complex tachycardia, whereas ART appears as a wide-complex tachycardia that at times can be difficult to distinguish from VT. Importantly, atrial fibrillation occurring in patients with a pathway capable of conducting in an antegrade fashion run the risk for rapid conduction to the ventricles and development of ventricular fibrillation and sudden death. The potential for sudden death caused

TABLE 4-1	Electrocardiogram Patterns Common with Different Anatomic Locations of Accessory Pathways		
Region	*Negative Delta Wave*	*QRS Frontal Axis*	*R > S*
Left lateral free wall	I and/or aVL	Normal	V_1 to V_3
Left posterior free wall	III and aVF	−75 to +75	V_1
Posterior septal	III and aVF	0 to −90	V_2 to V_4
Right free wall	aVR	Normal	V_3 to V_5
Anterior septal	V_1 and V_2	Normal	V_3 to V_5

R > S refers to progression of the R wave in the precordial electrocardiogram leads.
Adapted from Lindsay BD, Crossen KL, Cain ME: Concordance of distinguishing electrocardiographic features during sinus rhythm with the location of accessory pathways in the Wolff-Parkinson-White syndrome. *Am J Cardiol* 59:1093, 1987.

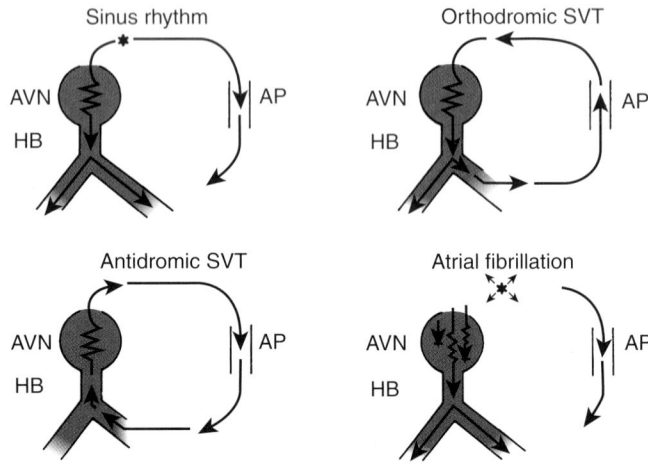

Figure 4-13 Schematic representation of conduction through an accessory pathway (AP) and the normal conduction system (AVN HB) during sinus rhythm, orthodromic supraventricular tachycardia (SVT), antidromic SVT, and atrial fibrillation. *(From Lindsay BD, Branyas NA, Cain ME: The preexcitation syndrome. In El-Sherif N, Samet P [eds]: Cardiac Pacing and Electrophysiology, 3rd ed. Orlando, FL: Grune & Stratton, 1990.)*

by atrial fibrillation in patients with WPW provides an argument for aggressive ablative treatment when the procedure can be performed in centers with low periprocedural morbidity.

Catheter-Based Therapy for Accessory Pathways

Percutaneous catheter ablation of accessory pathways has largely supplanted the surgical approach to treatment. RF ablation is typically performed during EPS once the accessory pathway has been localized. Transseptal or retrograde aortic catheter approaches are used to ablate left-sided accessory pathways, and right-heart catheterization via a venous approach is used to ablate right-sided pathways. Success rates of 95% have been reported using these methods.[43,49–51] Recurrence rates after successful catheter ablation of an accessory pathway are generally less than 5% and are a function of pathway location, as well as stability of the catheter during energy delivery. Overall, reported complications are low and include those related to vascular access such as hematoma and AV fistula. Other complications are related to catheter manipulations of the left- and right-sided circulation such as valvular or cardiac damage from the catheter, systemic and cerebral embolization caused by catheter manipulation in the aorta, coronary sinus damage, coronary thrombosis and dissection, cardiac perforation, and cardiac tamponade. Complete AV block, cardiac perforation, and coronary spasm caused by RF also may occur. A 1995 survey involving

5427 patients reported serious complications from catheter ablation of accessory pathways in 1.8% of patients and procedure-related mortality in 0.08%.[43,49] Complete AV block is more common with ablation of accessory pathways close to the bundle of His. Procedural success with catheter ablation methods is reported to be 87% to 99%.[43,50,51] In a randomized study comparing ablation with drug treatment, quality of life, symptom scores, and exercise performance were improved with successful RF ablation.[52]

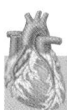

Atrioventricular Nodal Reentrant Tachycardia

AVNRT is due to altered electrophysiologic properties of the anterior fast pathway and posterior slow pathway fibers providing input to the AV node.[10,43,51] In the past, the only treatment for recurrent SVT caused by AVNRT was total ablation of the His bundle and permanent pacemaker insertion. Surgical techniques developed in the 1980s provided an alternate treatment that was associated with high procedural success, acceptable morbidity, and preservation of AV conduction.[53-56] Fundamentals developed with this surgical approach and increased understanding of the physiologic basis of AVNRT led to the development of percutaneous catheter-based treatments. Interruption of either the slow or fast pathway with RF ablation can eliminate AVNRT, with greater success rates reported for ablation of the slow pathway (slow-pathway ablation [68% to 100%] vs. fast-pathway ablation [46% to 94%]).[43,57-60] Complication rates are lower with slow-pathway RF ablation and include AV block requiring pacemaker insertion (1%)[43] (Box 4-6).

BOX 4-6. ATRIOVENTRICULAR NODAL REENTRANT TACHYCARDIA

- Altered electrophysiologic properties of the anterior fast and posterior slow pathways provide input to the atrioventricular node
- Successful fast-pathway ablation occurs when the PR interval is prolonged or fast-pathway conduction eliminated
- Successful slow-pathway ablation occurs when induced atrioventricular nodal reentrant tachycardia is eliminated
- Surgical techniques involve selective cryoablation

Catheter-Based Therapy for Atrioventricular Nodal Reentrant Tachycardia

Historically, fast-pathway ablation is performed by positioning the catheter adjacent to the AV node–His bundle anterosuperior to the tricuspid valve annulus. The catheter is withdrawn until the atrial electrogram is larger than the ventricular electrogram and the His recording small or absent. The ECG is closely monitored as RF energy is applied for PR prolongation/heart block. The energy is delivered until there is PR prolongation or the retrograde fast-pathway conduction is eliminated. Noninducibility of AVNRT then is confirmed. Given the increased incidence of complete heart block with fast-pathway ablation, most electrophysiologists have adopted ablation of the slow pathway as a safer alternative. Slow-pathway ablation is performed by identifying the pathway along the posteromedial tricuspid annulus near the coronary sinus. One approach using fluoroscopy is to divide the level of the coronary sinus os and His bundle recordings into six anatomic regions[61] (Figure 4-14). Lesions then are placed beginning with the most posterior region moving anteriorly. Rather than the anatomic approach, the slow pathway can be mapped and then ablated by performing ventricular pacing. The end point of slow-pathway ablation is elimination of induced AVNRT.[43,57-60] The development of junctional ectopy during RF ablation of the slow pathway is associated with successful slow-pathway ablation.[10]

Focal Atrial Tachycardia

Focal atrial tachycardia accounts for less than 15% of patients undergoing evaluation for SVT.[62] The arrhythmia is due to atrial activation from a discrete atrial area, resulting in heart rates between 100 and 250 beats/min.[63] Although the 12-lead ECG might provide clues to the origin of the tachycardia based on P-wave axis, localization of the site of atrial tachycardia is made by electrophysiologic investigations and tends to "cluster" in certain anatomic zones.[43] Right-sided tachycardias typically originate along the crista terminalis from the SAN to the AV node and left-sided ones from the pulmonary veins, atrial septum, or mitral valve annulus.[63,64] The mechanisms for atrial tachycardia include abnormal automaticity, triggered activity, or microreentry. Characteristics of the arrhythmia might provide clues to the underlying mechanisms. Abrupt onset and offset suggest a reentrant mechanism, whereas a gradual onset ("warm-up") and offset ("cooldown") pattern suggests automaticity (Box 4-7).

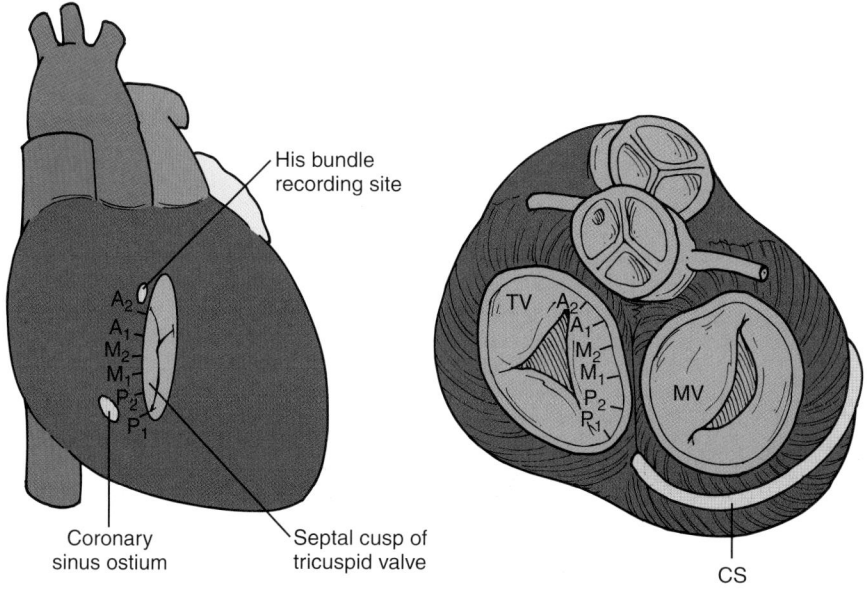

His bundle recording site

Coronary sinus ostium

Septal cusp of tricuspid valve

TV   MV   CS

Figure 4-14 Schematic representation of sites for atrioventricular (AV) nodal modification in relation to other anatomic structures. The posterior location is usually first targeted for ablation of the slow-pathway with subsequent ablative lesions placed more anteriorly depending on the response. CS, coronary sinus; MV, mitral valve; TV, tricuspid valve. *(From Akhtar M, Jazayeri MR, Sra JS, et al: Atrioventricular nodal reentry: Clinical, electrophysiologic, and therapeutic considerations. Circulation 88:282, 1993.)*

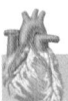

BOX 4-7. FOCAL ATRIAL TACHYCARDIA

- Mechanisms include abnormal automaticity, triggered activity, or microreentry
- Catheter-based treatment is with radiofrequency ablation
- Surgical-based treatment is with incision and cryoablation

Catheter-Based Therapy for Focal Atrial Tachycardia

Because of the discrete localized area involved in generating atrial tachycardia, the approach to catheter ablation is the same regardless of the mechanisms for the arrhythmia. The site of tachycardia onset is identified with electrophysiologic mapping and then isolated from the remaining atrium by application of RF current. Success of this approach is reported to be 86%, and recurrence rates, 8%.[43,64-68] Complications reported in these series occur in 1% to 2% of cases and include rare myocardial perforation, phrenic nerve injury, and sinus node dysfunction.[69]

Inappropriate Sinus Tachycardia

Sinus tachycardia is deemed inappropriate when it occurs in the absence of physiologic stressors (e.g., increased body temperature, hypovolemia, anemia, hyperthyroidism, anxiety, postural changes, drugs), indicating failure of normal mechanisms controlling sinus rate. Proposed mechanisms are enhanced sinus node automaticity or abnormal autonomic regulation, or both. Clinically, this entity is seen most often in female health-care providers. The diagnosis is made based on nonparoxysmal, persistent resting sinus tachycardia and excessive increases in response to normal physiologic stressors and nocturnal normalization of the rate based on Holter monitoring.[51] The P-wave morphology and endocardial activation are consistent with a sinus origin and secondary causes have been excluded. Catheter-based or surgical treatments are considered for a minority of patients not responding to β-blockers and when symptoms are truly disabling. The aim of this treatment is RF ablative modification of the sinus node to promote dominance of slower depolarizing sinus nodal tissues. An esophageal electrode is placed and connected to the operating room ECG monitor to guide treatment. The end point of application of RF energy is change in the P-wave morphology. Reported complications include need for permanent pacemaker, SVC syndrome, phrenic nerve injury, and pericarditis.[43,70] Acute and long-term reported success rates are 76% and 66%, respectively.[43,70]

Sinus Node Reentrant Tachycardia

Reentrant pathways involving the sinus node may lead to paroxysmal tachycardia, in contrast with the nonparoxysmal inappropriate sinus tachycardia.[71] The P-wave morphology is similar to that occurring during sinus rhythm. Similar to other reentrant tachycardias, the arrhythmia is usually triggered by a premature atrial beat. Endocardial activation sequence during EPS is in the high right atrium and is similar to sinus rhythm. The arrhythmia can be initiated with a premature pace beat and is terminated by vagal maneuvers or adenosine.[43] Clinically, the arrhythmia also is responsive to β-blockers, nonhydropyridine calcium channel antagonists, and amiodarone. RF ablation of the identified reentrant pathway can be used for frequently occurring tachycardia episodes not responsive to other treatments.[72]

Atrial Flutter

Atrial flutter usually presents with acute onset of symptoms (e.g., palpitations, shortness of breath, fatigue) accompanied by tachycardia and typical "flutter" waves on the ECG (Box 4-8). Fixed 2:1 conduction is usually present with flutter rate of 300 beats/min and ventricular rate of 150 beats/min. When AV conduction is fixed, the heart rate is regular, but varying AV conduction results in an irregular rhythm. Rapid AV conduction can occur with exercise, in patients with accessory

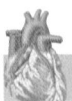

BOX 4-8. ATRIAL FLUTTER

- Reentry occurs because of a large anatomic circuit
- Macroreentrant pathway is amenable to catheter ablation

pathways, and, paradoxically, after administration of class 1C antiarrhythmic drugs.[43] This results from the antiarrhythmic drugs slowing the atrial flutter rate, thus allowing the AV node to support more rapid conduction to the ventricles. This maneuver requires coadministration of drugs with AV conduction-slowing properties (e.g., β-blockers).

Atrial flutter is due to reentry that is referred to as "macroreentry" because the anatomic circuit is large. "Typical" atrial flutter occupies a circuit that circles the tricuspid valve, crossing the myocardial isthmus between the inferior vena cava (IVC) and the tricuspid valve[43,62] (Figure 4-15). Counterclockwise rotation through the cava-tricuspid region is usually observed, although other patterns such as clockwise rotation, double waves, and "lower-loop" reentry (i.e., reentry around the IVC) might be observed.[43,73,74] Polarity of the flutter waves on the 12-lead ECG provides insight into the pattern of atrial flutter. Counterclockwise rotation is associated with negative flutter waves in the inferior leads and positive flutter waves in V_1, whereas the opposite is observed with clockwise rotation.[43]

The anatomic location of this macroreentrant pathway is amenable to catheter ablation and cure of atrial flutter by creating a linear conduction block across the tricuspid-IVC isthmus. Testing for bidirectional conduction block through the cavo-tricuspid region after application of RF energy enhances success.[75,76]

Atrial flutter and atrial fibrillation may coexist, complicating success with catheter ablation methods. Procedural success with pure atrial flutter is reported in 80% to 100% of cases, with recurrence occurring in 16% of patients.[77-81] In a prospective, randomized trial, catheter ablation resulted in sinus rhythm in 80% of patients, compared with 36% of patients treated with antiarrhythmic drugs (mean follow-up, 21 months).[81] Fewer hospitalizations and higher scores on quality-of-life surveys are reported after catheter ablation compared with drug treatment. In the absence of atrial fibrillation, subsequent RF ablation procedures may result in successful elimination of atrial flutter. Even when not present during initial treatment, atrial fibrillation may develop after successful catheter ablation for atrial flutter in 8% to 12% of patients.[43,79]

Atrial scar tissue from prior cardiac surgery (e.g., congenital heart surgery, mitral valve surgery, Maze procedure) may provide an area for reentry leading to atrial flutter.[64,82-85] Reentrant circuits involving the cavo-tricuspid area may coexist, leading to complicated, multiple reentry pathways.[43,85] Characterization of the reentry circuit with electrophysiologic mapping studies may allow for successful RF ablation in these circumstances.

Anesthetic Considerations for Supraventricular Arrhythmia Surgery/ Ablation Procedures

The approach to the care of patients undergoing percutaneous therapies for supraventricular arrhythmias involves similar basic principles (Box 4-9). Patients with WPW are usually young and free of other cardiac disease, although the syndrome can be accompanied by Ebstein's anomaly in up to 10% of cases.[41,86] Anesthesiologists must be familiar with preoperative EPS results and the characteristics of associated supraventricular arrhythmias (rate, associated hemodynamic disturbances, syncope, etc.), including treatments. Tachyarrhythmias might recur at any time during surgical and percutaneous treatments. Transcutaneous cardioversion/defibrillation adhesive pads are placed before anesthesia induction and connected to a defibrillator/cardioverter. The development of periprocedural tachyarrhythmias is unrelated to any single anesthetic or adjuvant drug.

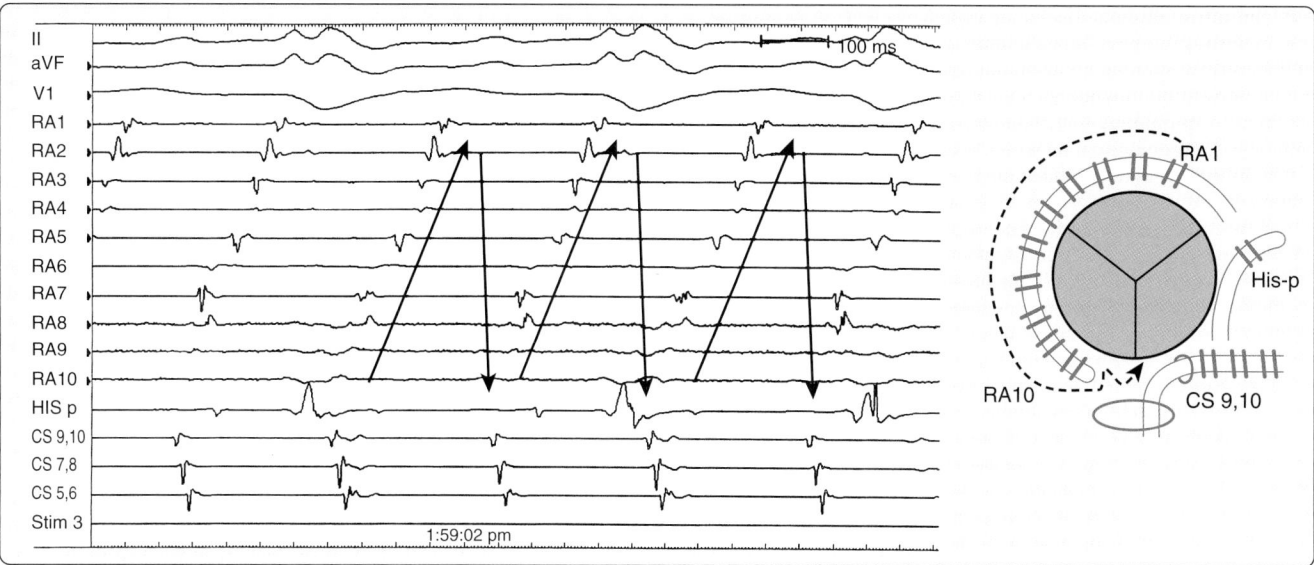

Figure 4-15 Endocardial mapping of typical atrial flutter. Endocardial signals recorded from diagnostic catheters are shown in a patient with typical atrial flutter. The anatomic basis for this circuit is an electrical wavefront circulating in a counterclockwise direction around the tricuspid valve annulus. A 20-pole catheter has been positioned around the tricuspid valve to record the passage of the activation wavefront by adjacent electrode pairs RA1 to RA10. The wavefront then proceeds across the isthmus connecting the inferior vena cava and the tricuspid valve before passing the ostium of the coronary sinus (CS), recorded by CS electrodes 9 and 10 and the His bundle recording catheter (His-p). The progress of the activation wavefront is indicated by the schematic *arrows* and by the diagram on the right.

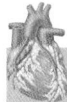

BOX 4-9. ANESTHETIC CONSIDERATIONS FOR SUPRAVENTRICULAR ARRHYTHMIA SURGERY AND ABLATION PROCEDURES

- Familiarity with electrophysiologic study results and associated treatments
- Transcutaneous cardioversion/defibrillation pads placed before induction
- Hemodynamically tolerated tachyarrhythmias treated by slowing conduction across accessory pathway as opposed to atrioventricular node
- Hemodynamically significant tachyarrhythmias treated with cardioversion
- Avoiding sympathetic stimulation

Treatment of hemodynamically tolerated tachyarrhythmias is aimed at slowing conduction across the accessory pathway as opposed to the AV node. Therapy directed at slowing conduction across the AV node (e.g., β-adrenergic–blocking drugs, verapamil, digoxin) may enhance conduction across accessory pathways and should be used only if proved safe by prior EPS. Drugs that are recommended include amiodarone and procainamide. A consideration is that antiarrhythmic drugs may interfere with electrophysiologic mapping. Hemodynamically significant tachyarrhythmias developing before mapping are usually treated with cardioversion.

Accessory pathway ablation is typically performed under conscious sedation, with general anesthesia reserved for selected patients such as those unable to tolerate the supine position. There is considerable experience with anesthetizing patients with WPW for surgical ablation when this treatment approach was prevalent. The effects of anesthetics on accessory pathway conduction have been investigated mostly to evaluate whether these agents might interfere with electrophysiologic mapping. Droperidol has been demonstrated to depress accessory pathway conduction, but the clinical significance of small antiemetic doses is likely minimal.[87,88] Opioids and barbiturates have no proven electrophysiologic effect on accessory pathways and have

been shown to be safe in patients with WPW syndrome.[89–92] Normal AV conduction is depressed by halothane, isoflurane, and enflurane, and preliminary evidence suggests that these volatile anesthetics also may depress accessory pathway conduction.[92,93] Although muscle relaxants with anticholinergic effects (e.g., pancuronium) have been used safely in patients with WPW, drugs lacking autonomic side effects are most often chosen.[94]

The major goal of the management of patients undergoing supraventricular ablative procedures is to avoid sympathetic stimulation and the development of tachyarrhythmias. Clinical studies have evaluated the efficacy of various anesthetic techniques in maintaining intraoperative hemodynamic stability and in preventing arrhythmias in patients with WPW syndrome.[10,95,96] An opioid-based anesthetic technique with supplemental volatile anesthetics is typically used.

Atrial Fibrillation

Atrial fibrillation, the most common sustained cardiac arrhythmia in the general population, can lead to palpitations, shortness of breath, chest discomfort, or anxiety because of the irregular-irregular heart rate pattern[5] (Box 4-10). The treatment aims for atrial fibrillation include anticoagulation to decrease the risk for stroke, and heart rate control to limit symptoms and reduce the risk for tachycardia-associated cardiomyopathy. Restoration of sinus rhythm with cardioversion, antiarrhythmic drugs, or both are considered in some instances, but data suggest this strategy is no more effective than a

BOX 4-10. ATRIAL FIBRILLATION FEATURES

- Associated with multiple reentrant circuits
- May originate from automatic foci in pulmonary vein or vena cava
- Treatment with catheter ablation
  - Atrioventricular node ablation with pacemaker placement
  - Curative ablation to restore sinus rhythm
- Surgical therapy with the Maze procedure

strategy of anticoagulation/heart rate control for improving mortality in *certain* populations.[97] Because antiarrhythmic drugs are associated with life-threatening proarrhythmic side effects, speculation exists that any benefits of restoring sinus rhythm might be outweighed by mortality caused by drug-induced ventricular arrhythmias.[7,8] Regardless, the increasing prevalence of atrial fibrillation and the limitations of pharmacologic treatments have led to much interest in nonpharmacologic treatments.

A growing understanding of the mechanisms of atrial fibrillation has led to the introduction of surgical and catheter-based procedures to restore sinus rhythm. Experimental and clinical investigations demonstrate that atrial fibrillation is associated with multiple reentrant circuits in the atrium ("multiple wavelets") that rapidly and unpredictably change their anatomic location.[98–101] Intraoperative electrophysiologic mapping of a patient in sinus rhythm (Figure 4-16), and then after atrial fibrillation was induced by introducing atrial ectopic beats (Figure 4-17), demonstrates the random and fleeting nature of the reentrant circuits.[10,101] The rapidly changing nature of the reentrant circuits precludes a map-directed surgical or ablative strategy for atrial fibrillation. Nonetheless, the realization that certain cardiac structures (e.g., pulmonary veins, valve annulus, vena cava) were necessary substrates for the fibrillatory reentrant circuits led to the development of an anatomically based surgical procedure for atrial fibrillation (the Cox–Maze procedure), whereby macroreentrant circuits are interrupted by a series of atrial incisions and cryoablation lesions.[10,101,102]

Investigators have demonstrated that atrial fibrillation in some instances originates from automatic foci in the pulmonary veins or vena cava and that isolating these sites may restore sinus rhythm[103] (Figure 4-18). Other data have demonstrated focal sources of atrial fibrillation in patients with mitral valve disease.[104,106] These findings are supported by laboratory investigations showing that atrial fibrillation can be maintained by a single atrial source of fibrillatory waves moving away from the originating circuit.[106,107] These and other findings, together with advances in computer-based electrophysiologic mapping systems, open up the possibility of map-guided strategies to eliminate the substrate for atrial fibrillation in some patients.[108–118] The latter strategy would have the benefit of perhaps greater success rates and lower complications than what occur with current procedures.

Catheter-Based Therapy for Atrial Fibrillation

Catheter ablation approaches for atrial fibrillation include AV node ablation with permanent pacemaker placement to control ventricular rate and catheter ablation procedures that aim to restore sinus rhythm. AV node ablation is used for medically refractory tachycardia caused by atrial fibrillation or to eliminate intolerable symptoms caused by an irregular heart rate. The procedure requires pacemaker implantation, does not aim to restore sinus rhythm, and does not eliminate the need for anticoagulation. In this latter class of procedures, many different strategies are employed, but all tend to involve electrical isolation of the pulmonary veins. It is thought that myocardial sleeves involving the os of the pulmonary veins can initiate atrial fibrillation because of their inherently different electrophysiologic properties. By electrically isolating them, the goal is to prevent atrial fibrillation from developing. Pulmonary vein isolation can be achieved in one of two ways. In the first, complete electrical isolation is achieved by sequential, segmental application of RF ablation at each pulmonary vein ostium.[103,119] An alternate strategy is to regionally isolate the posterior left atrium by encircling not only the pulmonary vein ostia but the surrounding posterior left atrial wall by a circular pattern of adjacent RF ablation lesions.[105] A randomized comparison of these two strategies has demonstrated a significantly greater success rate with the regional isolation strategy; 88% of patients were free of atrial fibrillation at 6 months compared with 67% free of atrial fibrillation at 6 months with the segmental isolation strategy.[112] The regional isolation procedure also reduces the risk for creating pulmonary venous stenosis that can be associated with the segmental isolation procedure.

Research into methods emulating the surgical Maze procedure continues to evolve but remains investigative (see later). Linear ablation techniques involve RF energy application along critical sites for the maintenance of atrial fibrillation.[113–116,118,120] Success has been limited with

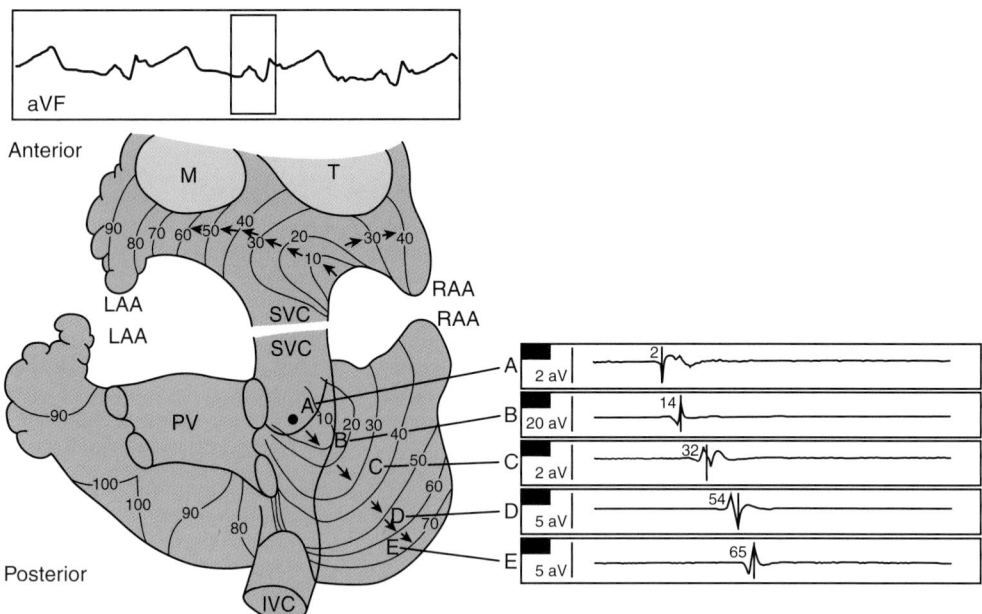

Figure 4-16   **Atrial activation sequence map of a single beat during sinus rhythm in a human.** Isochronous lines are in 10-millisecond increments across the anterior and posterior atrium. The top left panel is the lead aVF from the surface electrocardiogram (ECG), and the window denotes the P wave chosen to obtain atrial mapping data. The labels on each electrogram A to E correspond to the letters on the map denoting the five electrode positions shown. The time of activation from the electrodes is used to generate the isochronous representation of atrial depolarization. IVC, inferior vena cava; LAA, left atrial appendage; M, mitral valve; PV, pulmonary veins; RAA, right atrial appendage; SVC, superior vena cava; T, tricuspid valve. *(From Cox JL, Canavan TE, Schuessler RB, et al: The surgical treatment of atrial fibrillation. II. Intraoperative electrophysiologic mapping and description of the electrophysiologic basis of atrial flutter and atrial fibrillation. J Thorac Cardiovasc Surg 101:406, 1991.)*

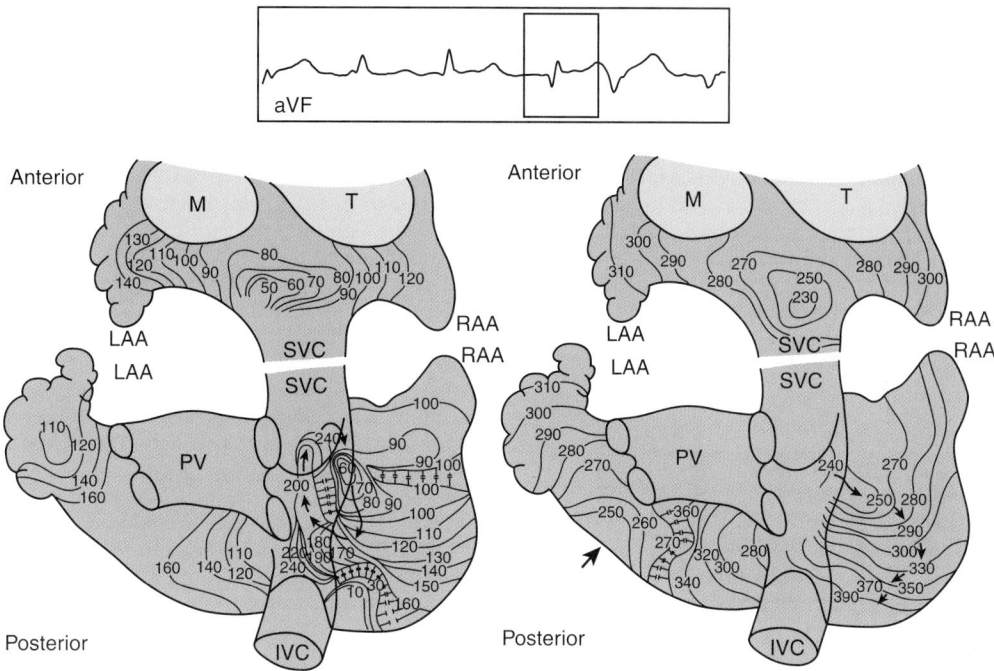

Figure 4-17 Atrial activation mapping from a human during atrial fibrillation indicating a single reentrant circuit. Recordings and isochronous mapping are the same as in Figure 4-20. The map on the left shows the first 240 milliseconds, with 230 to 400 milliseconds in the right map. The beat spreads along the anterior and posterior atria *(left)*. Posteriorly, the beat encounters several areas of conduction block, but as it spreads, it encounters myocardium now repolarized and capable of sustaining conduction. The clockwise, rotating reentrant circuit circulates around natural obstacles such as the orifices of the vena cava. IVC, inferior vena cava; LAA, left atrial appendage; M, mitral valve; PV, pulmonary veins; RAA, right atrial appendage; SVC, superior vena cava; T, tricuspid valve. *(From Cox JL, Canavan TE, Schuessler RB, et al: The surgical treatment of atrial fibrillation. II. Intraoperative electrophysiologic mapping and description of the electrophysiologic basis of atrial flutter and atrial fibrillation. J Thorac Cardiovasc Surg 101:406, 1991.)*

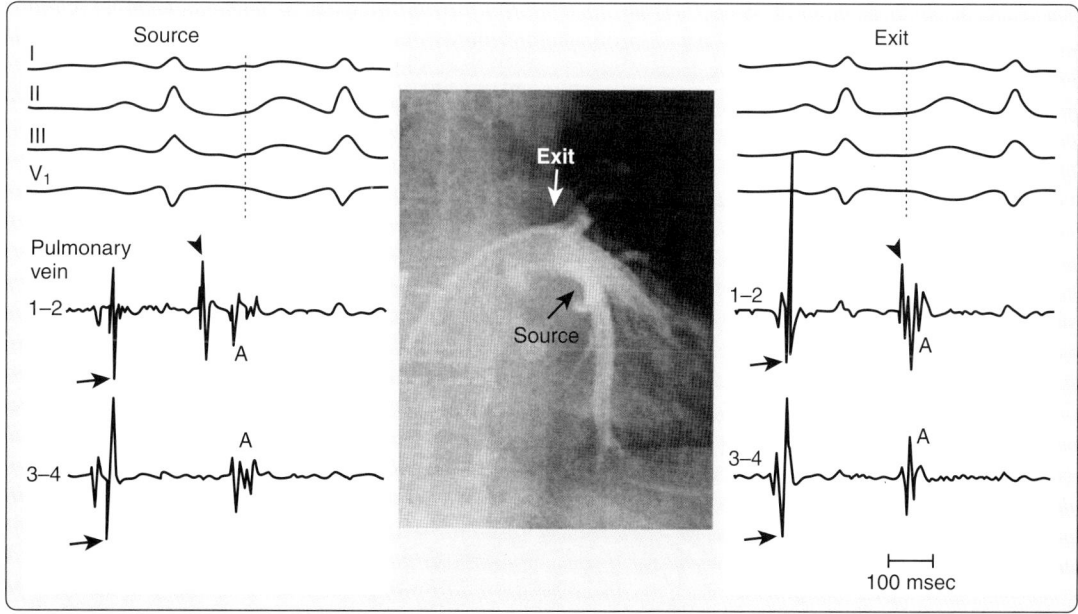

Figure 4-18 Electrophysiologic recordings and venous angiogram of the left inferior pulmonary vein from a patient with paroxysmal atrial fibrillation. Positioning of the distal catheter toward the source of ectopic beats results in progressively delayed activation in relation to the P wave during sinus rhythm *(left, arrows)*. Ectopic activity is recorded earlier *(arrowhead)*. The catheter electrode positioned at the exit of the pulmonary vein *(right)* shows the spike to be less delayed in sinus rhythm *(arrows)* and later after an ectopic beat *(arrowhead)*. *Center*, Pulmonary vein angiogram demonstrating the position of the catheter. *Vertical lines* indicate the onset of an atrial ectopic beat. A, Near-field electrical activity. Radiofrequency ablation of the ectopic source resulted in cure of atrial fibrillation. *(From Haissaguerre M, Pierre J, Shah DC, et al: Spontaneous initiation of atrial fibrillation by ectopic beats originating in the pulmonary veins. N Engl J Med 339:659, 1998.)*

this approach (28% to 57%), and the procedures are associated with long procedure duration and associated radiation exposure. Further, complication rates remain high (4% to 50%).

Surgical Therapy for Atrial Fibrillation

The growing understanding of the underlying mechanisms for atrial fibrillation led to the development of a surgical procedure developed by Cox et al termed the *Maze procedure*.[101,102,121–125] This moniker stems from the basic design of the operation to surgically create a "Maze" of functional myocardium, allowing propagation of atrial depolarization throughout the atrium to the AV node while interposed scar tissue interrupts possible routes of reentry (Figure 4-19). The principal goals of the Maze procedure are (a) to interrupt the electrophysiologic sub-

strate for atrial fibrillation (reentrant circuits) restoring sinus rhythm; (b) to maintain sinus nodal–to–AV nodal conduction, thus preserving AV synchrony; and (c) to preserve atrial mechanical function ("atrial kick") to improve hemodynamic function.

The Maze procedure has evolved from the original procedure (Maze I) introduced in the early 1990s. The Maze I procedure consisted of multiple atrial incisions around the SAN including an incision anterior to the atrial-SVC junction[102–104,124] (Figure 4-20). The latter incision is through the sinus tachycardia region of the SAN, resulting in the unintended consequence of blunted heart rate response to exercise and obtunded atrial mechanical function.[125–127] Subsequently, the procedure was modified (Maze II procedure) to include an incision on the anterior right atrium while allowing the sinus impulse to travel anteriorly across the left atrium but preventing it from reentering the right atrial–SVC junction (Figure 4-21). Although successfully addressing the limitations with the original procedure, the Maze II procedure was technically challenging, particularly the approach to the left atrium that necessitated division and then reapproximation of the SVC. This was addressed by moving the left atrial incision to a more posterior location (Figure 4-22). These and other modifications led to the introduction of the Maze III procedure, which reduced the frequency of chronotropic incompetence, improved atrial transport function, and shortened the procedure.[124]

Surgery for atrial fibrillation continues to advance in two fundamental forms: ablative procedures concomitant to another cardiac operation or as a stand-alone procedure specifically for terminating atrial fibrillation. Newer energy sources and devices have allowed much simpler execution. The availability of such devices has resulted in the modern Maze procedure becoming a hybrid operation using catheter/device-delivered RF energy and properly placed incisions. These advances shorten surgical time, allowing the Maze procedure to be performed with other surgeries such as mitral valve surgery. Shortened surgical times and lower complexity further allow for expansion of eligibility criteria and foster the development of less-invasive surgical approaches such as minimally invasive and beating-heart surgeries.

The combination of conduction blocks imparted surgically for treating atrial fibrillation is called the *lesion set*, which consists of three basic components: pulmonary vein isolation alone, pulmonary vein isolation with connecting lesions to the mitral valve, and lesions involving the right atrium. The Cox–Maze III represents the gold standard of lesion sets in atrial fibrillation surgery. As shown in Figure 4-22, the pulmonary veins are isolated with connection lesions to the mitral annulus and left atrial appendage (LAA). This constitutes the "left-sided" lesion set. On the right side, the SVC and IVC line is combined with

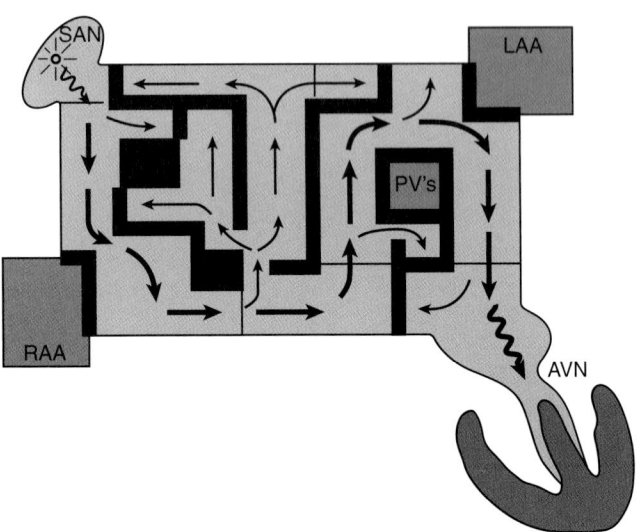

Figure 4-19 Schematic representation of the Maze I procedure for atrial fibrillation designed to allow for conduction of an impulse from the sinus nodal complex to the atria and atrioventricular node (AVN), whereas interposing scar tissue interrupts the multiple reentrant circuits of atrial fibrillation. Atrial appendages are excised and the pulmonary veins are isolated. LAA, left atrial appendage; PVs, pulmonary veins; RAA, right atrial appendage; SAN, sinoatrial node. *(From Cox JL, Schuessler RB, D'Agostino HJ Jr, et al: The surgical treatment of atrial fibrillation. III. Development of a definitive surgical procedure.* J Thorac Cardiovasc Surg *101:569, 1991.)*

Figure 4-20 Depiction of surgical incisions and resultant conduction pathways of the Maze I procedure. *Left,* The atria are shown splayed open such that the anterior surface is superior and the posterior surface inferior. *Right,* The atria are divided in a sagittal plane showing the right atrial septum. Incisions are placed at sites most commonly associated with reentrant circuits of atrial fibrillation to eliminate the arrhythmia. At the same time, bridges of myocardium are left intact to allow the spread of conduction across the atria and to the atrioventricular (AV) node, preserving atrial transport function and facilitating sinus rhythm. The pulmonary veins are isolated to eliminate potential conduction of premature beats. *(From Cox JL: Evolving applications of the Maze procedure for atrial fibrillation [invited editorial].* Ann Thorac Surg *55:578–580, 1993.)*

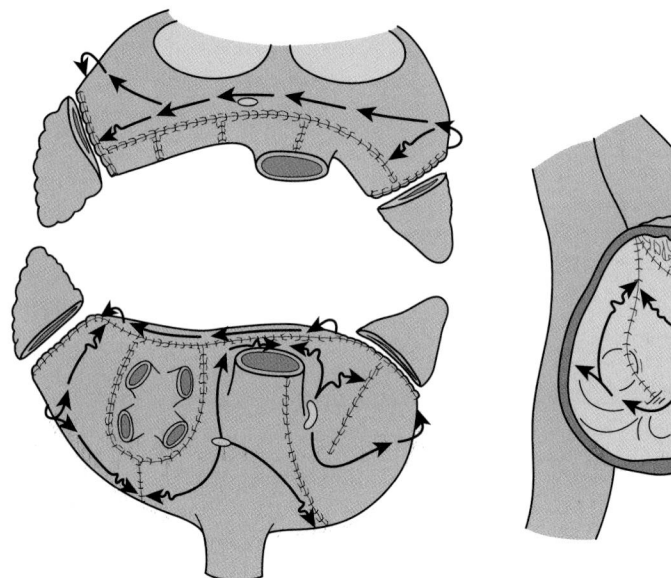

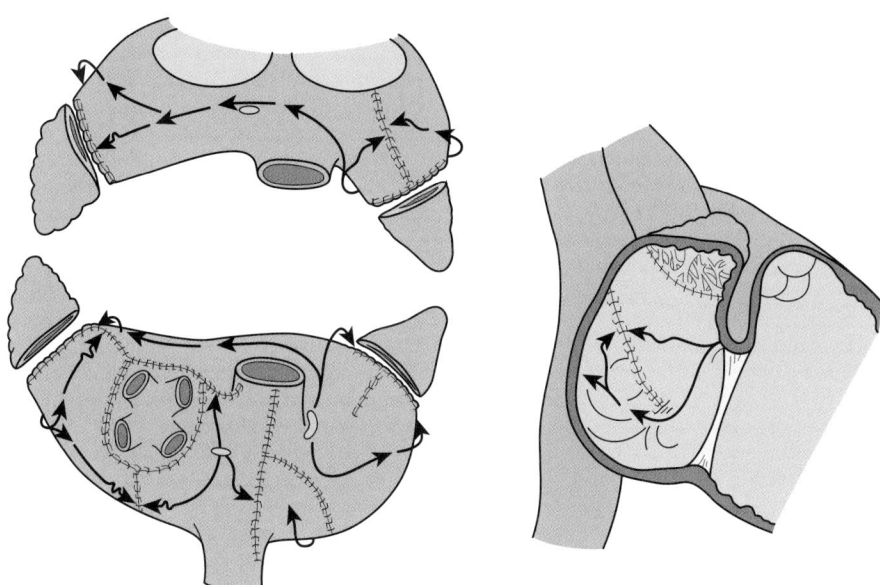

Figure 4-21 **Representation of surgical incisions and conduction pathways of the Maze II procedure (similar views as in Figure 4-24).** The procedure is modified to eliminate incisions through the sinus tachycardia region of the sinus nodal complex performed in the Maze I procedure to address chronotropic incompetence. A transverse incision across the dome of the left atrium is moved posteriorly. *(From Cox JL: Evolving applications of the Maze procedure for atrial fibrillation [invited editorial]. Ann Thorac Surg 55:578–580, 1993. Reprinted with permission from the Society of Thoracic Surgeons. Copyright 1993, Society of Thoracic Surgeons.)*

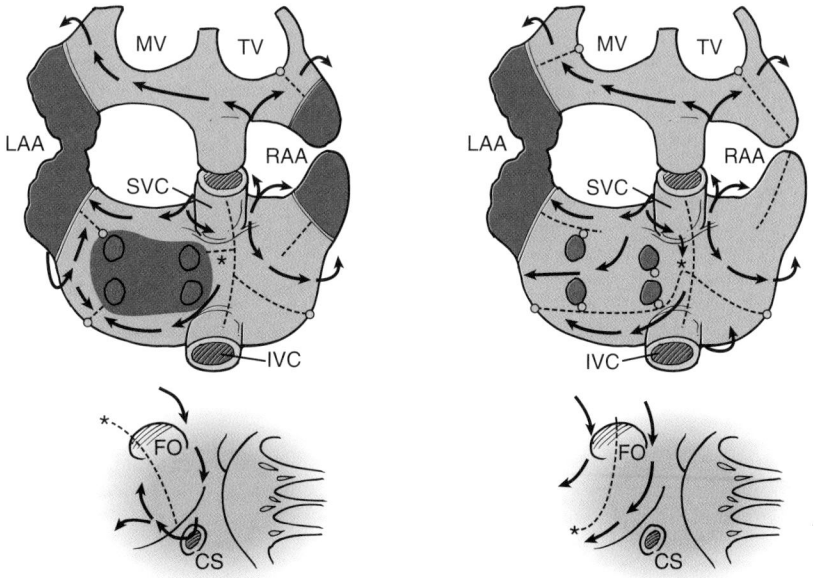

Figure 4-22 The Maze III procedure is shown using the same views. Modification of the posterior incisions to the vena cava and placement of the septal incision posterior to the orifice of the superior vena cava (SVC) are noted. CS, coronary sinus; FO, foramen ovale; IVC, inferior vena cava; LAA, left atrial appendage; MV, mitral valve; RAA, right atrial appendage; SAN, sinoatrial node; TV, tricuspid valve. *(From Cox JL: Evolving applications of the Maze procedure for atrial fibrillation [invited editorial]. Ann Thorac Surg 55:578–580, 1993. Copyright 1993, Society of Thoracic Surgeons.)*

connecting lesions to the tricuspid annulus and right atrial appendage. The coronary sinus is ablated in one spot using cryothermy and both atrial appendages are removed. The complexity of this procedure combined with alternative energy sources has motivated surgeons to use other combinations of lesion sets. These other combinations are collectively called "modified Maze" procedures.

Based on Haissaguerre's[103] seminal article in 1998, electrical isolation of the pulmonary veins has been used extensively. With modern devices, pulmonary vein isolation is straightforward and may be performed epicardially and without CPB. In patients with paroxysmal atrial fibrillation, most centers report that up to 80% of patients remain free of atrial fibrillation 6 months after surgery. For persistent

atrial fibrillation, sinus rhythm is reported to be successfully restored in 30% to 40% of patients. The addition of connecting lesions increases the efficacy of the modified Maze. This is particularly true in patients with persistent or permanent atrial fibrillation.

The right-sided lesion set appears to be important for patients with permanent atrial fibrillation. These lesions also decrease the risk for atrial flutter. Typical atrial flutter arises from the tricuspid isthmus: an area between the coronary sinus, tricuspid annulus, and Eustachian valve. Some surgeons omit the right-sided lesion and, if the patient develops atrial flutter after surgery, will complete the ablation using a catheter-based strategy because it is a straightforward procedure in the electrophysiology laboratory.

The LAA is a primary source of intracardiac thrombus in patients with atrial fibrillation, and its exclusion or elimination presumably decreases the thrombotic risk to the patient. There are several strategies to manage the LAA. The appendage may be ligated or stapled externally. Because LAA morphology varies, the results can be suboptimal. Left atrial tissue also is very friable, and bleeding from this area can be problematic. The appendage may be completely resected and the base of the appendage oversewn with suture. The LAA also may be excluded from within the atrium. This is easily accomplished with a running suture at the opening of the appendage, but obviously requires an atriotomy.

There continues to be great investigative interest in the development of different energy sources for surgical atrial fibrillation ablation therapies. Currently, the fundamental requirement for treatment is generation of a transmural lesion that leads to conduction block while minimizing collateral tissue damage. Though the issue of transmurality is somewhat controversial at this time, it remains a basic goal.

To simplify the Cox-Maze III operation, Cox et al[157] proposed cryothermy. Tissue is exposed to −60°C temperature using a handheld probe, which leads to a consistent transmural scar despite being applied only to the heart surface. A variety of flexible and colder probes is available that allows the creation of all lesion sets.

Another energy form for surgical arrhythmia ablation is RF energy in which alternating electrical current is used to generate thermal injury and, thus, localized atrial scar. Unipolar RF, however, can be associated with collateral atrial injury and tissue charring. This has led to the development of bipolar probes that minimize this risk. Although bipolar RF energy may be used epicardially for pulmonary vein isolation, any other ablative lesions require opening the heart. The latter can be accomplished via a small incision using a purse-string technique. Because of the generated heat, contiguous structures like the esophagus have been injured with pulmonary vein isolation (PVI) or posterior atrial lesion generation.[128] Thus, when RF energy is used, it is advised to retract the transesophageal echocardiography probe to hopefully decrease the risk for this complication. Nonetheless, esophageal injury from RF energy may occur regardless of whether TEE is used during surgery. Monitoring esophageal temperature using a probe fluoroscopically placed behind the left atrium may provide guidance to the operator.

Another energy source for arrhythmia ablative procedures is ultrasound. This form of energy involves focusing high-intensity ultrasound signals resulting in myocardial injury and scar. Ultrasound energy may be delivered at varying depths with minimal collateral tissue injury and protection of the coronary arteries. Delivery systems under development involve epicardial application and are potentially amenable to a minimally invasive approach.

Conventional and partial median sternotomy allow excellent exposure for all lesion sets. The atrium may be opened via a left atriotomy or trans-septal approach. As a concomitant procedure with mitral valve surgery, the MAZE is performed first, then the mitral valve procedure. This allows for access to the mitral annulus before placement of a prosthesis. Similarly, when an atrial fibrillation procedure is combined with coronary artery bypass grafting, the lesions are created before cardioplegic arrest. However, the left-sided pulmonary veins may be difficult to ablate with the beating heart and may be approached after cardioplegic arrest but before bypass graft construction. The left atrium may be reduced in size by resecting atrial tissue between the inferior pulmonary vein and mitral annulus.

Atrial fibrillation procedures may be performed using minimally invasive techniques. A right anterior thoracotomy and femoral cannulation allow access to the left atrium and mitral valve. Alternatively, a bilateral thoracoscopic and off-pump approach has been used.

Overall, the choice of atrial fibrillation operation (lesion set and surgical approach) depends on several factors, including the duration and classification of atrial fibrillation, size of the left atrium, and need for concomitant procedure. For example, a patient with paroxysmal atrial fibrillation undergoing coronary artery bypass grafting is well served by simple epicardial pulmonary vein isolation using a bipolar RF ablation device. Alternatively, a patient with heart failure and persistent atrial fibrillation who requires mitral valve intervention is better treated with pulmonary vein isolation and connecting lesions. Finally, a patient with symptomatic permanent atrial fibrillation and stroke who has not responded successfully to medical and catheter-based therapy is best treated with a full Cox–Maze III.

Operative results from multiple centers show that greater than 90% of patients remain free of atrial fibrillation after the classic Maze procedure.[127] Episodes of atrial flutter during the immediate perioperative period do not alter the long-term success of restoration of sinus rhythm.[127] Procedure-specific complications have included an attenuated heart rate response to exercise resulting in the need for permanent pacemaker implantation.[127] The frequency of these complications is less with newer versions of the procedure. Fluid retention is a common problem after the Maze procedure, which is attributed to reduced secretion of atrial natriuretic peptide and increase of antidiuretic hormone, as well as aldosterone.[129,130] Furosemide, spironolactone, or both perioperatively can limit the consequences of this complication.[131]

An intended goal of the Maze procedure is preservation of atrial transport function. Follow-up of patients early in the experience at Washington University School of Medicine demonstrated that this was achieved in 98% of patients for the right atrium but only in 86% of patients for the left atrium.[132] More detailed analyses further demonstrated that even when left atrial contraction was present, quantitative mechanical function was lower compared with control patients.[133,134] The latter consequence was believed to be related to the incisions used to isolate the pulmonary veins that resulted in isolating nearly 30% of the left atrium myocardium from excitation.[135] A new approach to the Maze procedure was developed whereby incisions radiate from the SAN (Figure 4-23) along the path of coronary arteries supplying the atrium (rather than across as in the Maze III procedure), to better preserve left atrial transport function.[136,137] This modification is termed the *radial procedure* and is further designed to preserve the right atrial appendage, which is an important source of atrial natriuretic peptide.[138] Compared with the standard Maze III procedure, the radial approach results in a more synchronous activation sequence of the left atrium, preserving atrial transport function, although it is equally effective in eliminating the reentrant circuits of atrial fibrillation.

Anesthetic Considerations

Anesthesiology teams increasingly are asked to care for patients undergoing catheter-based atrial fibrillation ablative procedures. Monitored anesthesia care may be possible in some situations, but general anesthesia is typically chosen because of the duration of the procedure and the demand for no patient movement during critical lesion placement. The care of the patient undergoing either catheter-based therapy or

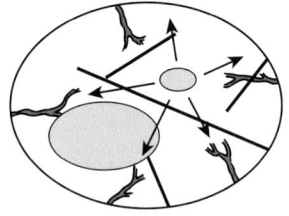 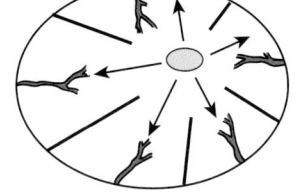

Maze procedure   Radial approach

Figure 4-23 Contrasting concepts for the Maze procedure *(left)* and radial approach *(right)*. *Small circle* in the middle indicates the sinus node, *outer circle* the atria, and *shaded area* the atrial myocardium isolated by the incisions. The atrial arterial supply is depicted. *Arrows* indicate propagation of the depolarizing wavefront. The radial approach preserves atrial arterial blood supply and a more physiologic activation sequence. With the Maze procedure, some arteries are divided and the atrial activation sequence disrupted. *(From Nitta T, Lee R, Schuessler RB, et al: Radial approach: A new concept in surgical treatment of atrial fibrillation. I. Concept, anatomic and physiologic bases and development of a procedure. Ann Thorac Surg 67:27, 1999. Copyright 1999, Society of Thoracic Surgeons.)*

surgical atrial fibrillation surgery is similar. Preparation of the patient includes review of preoperative cardiac testing, assessment of the characteristics of the patient's arrhythmia, and review of surgical plan and whether concomitant procedures will accompany the Maze procedure (e.g., coronary artery bypass grafting, valve replacement, repair of congenital lesions).

Anesthetics chosen are based on the patient's general physical condition, including comorbid conditions and ventricular dysfunction. Anesthetic requirements for catheter-based procedures are minimal and consist of small doses of an opioid, an induction agent, intermediate-duration skeletal muscle relaxants, and a volatile agent. For the most part, the anesthetic chosen for the surgical patient is aimed at early tracheal extubation and consists of a lower dose, opioid-based technique supplemented with volatile anesthetics and skeletal muscle relaxants.

LAA thrombus must be excluded with TEE before proceeding with catheter-based ablation and surgical manipulations. Monitoring of patients undergoing catheter-ablation atrial fibrillation procedures includes direct arterial pressure monitoring and esophageal temperature monitoring. With the latter, acute increases in temperature of even 0.1°C are communicated to the electrophysiologist. Immediately terminating RF energy and cooling the catheter tip via intraprobe saline at room temperature limit spread of myocardial heating. Heparin is administered during the procedure, necessitating monitoring of the ACT. Constant vigilance for pericardial tamponade is mandated. Immediate transthoracic echocardiography should be performed when abrupt hypotension develops. Percutaneous pericardial drainage, which typically restores blood pressure, is emergently performed. Continued collection of pericardial blood after protamine reversal of heparin anticoagulation may necessitate transfer of the patient to the operating room for sternotomy and repair of the atrial defect.

Patient monitoring modalities for the surgical procedures are similar to those used for other cardiac surgical procedures including TEE to evaluate for ventricular and valvular function, monitor for new wall motion abnormalities, and assist in evacuation of air from the cardiac chambers at the conclusion of surgery. Ventricular dysfunction (right more often than left ventricle), at least transiently, as well as echocardiographic and ECG ischemic changes (inferiorly more often), is common.[10] The proposed cause includes coronary artery air embolization or inadequate myocardial protection, or both. Because the Maze procedure entails placement of multiple atrial incisions, initial atrial compliance and performance of the atria appear altered. TEE evaluation of atrial activity is performed after separation from the extracorporeal circulation and decannulation.[10]

VENTRICULAR ARRHYTHMIAS

As with supraventricular arrhythmias, the treatment of ventricular fibrillation and VT is aimed at addressing underlying mechanisms (e.g., myocardial ischemia, drug induced, electrolyte, or metabolic abnormalities). In most patients with life-threatening ventricular arrhythmias and structural heart disease, ICD placement is the standard of care with or without concomitant antiarrhythmic drug therapy.[139] In patients with significant structural heart disease, catheter ablation is considered as an adjuvant therapy for medically refractory monomorphic VT. Rarely, VT occurs in the setting of a structurally normal heart. This syndrome of a primary electrical disorder is typically due to a focal, triggered mechanism that occurs mostly in younger patients and originates from the right ventricular outflow tract or apical septum[140–142] (Box 4-11). ICDs are typically not indicated in these individuals.

Catheter Ablation Therapy for Ventricular Tachycardia

The mechanism for VT can be identified in the electrophysiology laboratory using programmed stimulation.[143,144] Single or multiple extrastimuli are introduced during the vulnerable period of cardiac repolarization (near T wave) until sustained VT develops that is similar

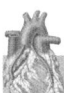

BOX 4-11. VENTRICULAR ARRHYTHMIAS

- A majority of episodes of ventricular tachycardia or fibrillation result from coronary artery disease and dilated or hypertrophic cardiomyopathy.
- Implantable cardioverter-defibrillator placement is the standard of care with or without medical treatment in life-threatening ventricular arrhythmias and structural heart disease.
- Catheter ablation is adjuvant therapy for medically refractory monomorphic ventricular tachycardia.
- Surgical therapy includes endocardial resection with cryoablation.
- Anesthetic considerations focus on preoperative catheterization, echocardiogram, and electrophysiologic testing.
- Monitoring of surgical patients is dictated by the underlying cardiac disease.

in morphology to that of the spontaneous arrhythmia. The diagnostic hallmark of VT caused by a reentrant circuit is the ability to entrain the tachycardia by pacing slightly faster than the tachycardia cycle length.[145] Traditional catheter mapping techniques for guiding catheter ablation of VT serve to position the ablation catheter within a protected isthmus of the reentrant circuit. The pathologic characteristics of this site are thought to be viable myocardium surrounded by scar tissue that is electrically isolated from the bulk of the ventricular myocardium except at the entrance and exit sites. Important shortcomings of these techniques are that most VTs are not hemodynamically stable enough for mapping, and that multiple morphologies of inducible VT are commonly present in a single patient. As a result, newer strategies that rely on three-dimensional computerized mapping techniques attempt to identify important areas of myocardial scar, of which the perimeter may participate in reentrant circuits. By strategic placement of areas of conduction block guided by these maps, significant cure rates have been obtained without the necessity of mapping individual reentrant circuits.[146] In rare instances, the VT circuits might involve the conduction system as in bundle-branch reentry or fascicular VT that is easily ablated with RF energy.[147]

There are no data from prospective randomized trials of VT ablation, but results from case series report success rates ranging from 37% to 86%.[129,147–153] The latter represent mostly patients with drug-resistant VT or multiple VT morphologies and the treatment performed as a "last-ditch effort" to control the arrhythmia. Reported success rates are greater after RF ablation for primary VT. Major complications from catheter ablation procedures for VT in the setting of structural heart disease include stroke, myocardial infarction, heart failure exacerbation, vascular injury, and death. The incidence of these complications appears to be low despite the lengthy procedure times that are commonly required.[146]

Anesthetic Considerations

Anesthetic management of patients undergoing catheter-based procedures to ameliorate ventricular arrhythmias is primarily based on the patient's underlying cardiac disease and other comorbidities. Candidates often have underlying coronary artery disease, severely impaired left ventricular function, and other secondary organ dysfunction (e.g., hepatic and renal dysfunction) and are receiving multiple medications that may potentially interact with anesthetics (e.g., vasodilation from angiotensin-converting enzyme inhibitors). Consequently, a thorough review of the patient's underlying conditions and treatments is mandated. Special attention is given to cardiac catheterization results and preoperative echocardiogram findings. Information regarding characteristics of the patient's arrhythmia such as ventricular rate, hemodynamic tolerance, and method of arrhythmia termination should be sought.

Prior or current treatment with amiodarone is a particular concern. The long elimination half-life (about 60 days) of amiodarone requires that potential side effects such as hypothyroidism be considered perioperatively.[154] The α- and β-adrenergic properties of amiodarone might lead to hypotension during anesthesia, but most anesthesiologists in contemporary practice are familiar with the management of these complications. Much attention has been given to bradycardia associated with amiodarone during anesthesia that might be resistant to atropine.[155–159] Methods for temporary cardiac pacing should be readily available to care for patients receiving long-term amiodarone. Retrospective reports further suggest a greater need for inotropic support for patients receiving preoperative amiodarone therapy because a low systemic vascular resistance has been observed in these patients.[156,157] Pulmonary complications speculated to be related to pulmonary toxicity from amiodarone have also been reported.[106,159] In a series of 67 patients receiving preoperative amiodarone, 50% experienced development of acute respiratory distress syndrome that could not be attributed to other factors including intraoperative Fio_2 (see Chapter 10).[159]

Monitoring includes direct arterial pressure monitoring, and central venous access is necessary for administration of vasoactive drugs, if needed. Means for rapid cardioversion/defibrillation should be readily available when inserting any central venous catheter. Self-adhesive electrode pads are most often used and connected to a cardioverter/defibrillator before anesthesia induction. Premature ventricular beats induced during these procedures can easily precipitate the patient's underlying ventricular arrhythmia that might be difficult to convert to sinus rhythm.[157,160] Selection of anesthetics for arrhythmia ablation is dictated mostly by the patient's underlying physical state. General anesthesia with endotracheal intubation is typically chosen because of the duration of the procedures. Because anesthetics can influence cardiac conduction and arrhythmogenesis, there is a concern about the potential of anesthetics to alter the electrophysiologic mapping procedures.[161,162] The effects of the various volatile anesthetics on ventricular arrhythmias vary among the experimental models and, importantly, because of the mechanism of the arrhythmia. Data showing proarrhythmic, antiarrhythmic, and no effects of volatile anesthetics on experimental arrhythmias have been reported.[13,161–168] Nonetheless, the small doses administered during ablative procedures may have minimal effects on electrophysiologic mapping. Opioids have been shown to have no effects on inducibility of VT.[165,168,169]

IMPLANTABLE CARDIOVERTER-DEFIBRILLATOR

Considerable progress has occurred with the ICD, including decreased device size, improved battery life, and improved treatment algorithms, all contributing to enhanced reliability (Box 4-12). Current ICDs are capable of providing tiered therapy consisting of antitachycardia

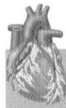

BOX 4-12. IMPLANTABLE CARDIOVERTER-DEFIBRILLATOR

- Implantable cardioverter-defibrillators (ICDs) are capable of pacing, as well as providing tiered therapy for tachyarrhythmias (e.g., shocks, antitachycardia pacing).
- Insertion of modern devices is almost exclusively via percutaneous techniques.
- ICDs are indicated for the primary or secondary prevention of sudden cardiac death.
- ICDs have been shown to reduce the incidence of total mortality versus standard treatment alone.
- ICDs are indicated for individuals surviving sudden death without a reversible cause, individuals with ischemic cardiomyopathy with an ejection fraction ≤ 30%, and individuals with ischemic or nonischemic cardiomyopathy with an ejection fraction ≤ 35% and New York Heart Association Class II or III heart failure symptoms.

pacing and shocks to terminate potentially life-threatening ventricular arrhythmias. All ICDs also have the ability to pace the heart to treat bradycardia either as a single-chamber, dual-chamber, or biventricular system. Advances in lead technology, as well as the implementation of a biphasic waveform, have considerably reduced defibrillation energy requirements.[170,171] These improvements have led to simplification of lead implantation for the use of transvenous insertion methods rather than epicardial patch electrodes used in prior generations. As a result, insertion of modern devices is nearly exclusively via percutaneous techniques rather than more invasive median sternotomy, except in cases in which the body habitus would preclude this approach (e.g., pediatric population).

The ICD consists of a pulse generator and transvenous leads that continuously monitor the heart rate. When the heart rate exceeds a programmable limit, therapy is initiated that might include a brief burst of rapid pacing (i.e., antitachycardia pacing) followed by a biphasic shock if the arrhythmia persists. Electrogram storage capabilities allow for review of appropriateness of delivered treatments, as well as changes in ventricular arrhythmia characteristics. The style of ICD, either one, two, or three leads, is chosen based on a patient's requirement for antibradycardia pacing (single- or dual-lead devices) or cardiac resynchronization therapy, also known as biventricular pacing, when medically refractory heart failure and interventricular conduction delay are present (see Chapter 25).

Technologic aspects of ICDs have been reviewed and are discussed in more detail in Chapter 25.[170] Defibrillation voltage is much greater than can be delivered with existing batteries, necessitating the use of storage capacitors and transformers. Once the ICD has detected an arrhythmic event, the device begins to charge its capacitor. During charging and immediately after the capacitor has been fully charged, continued presence of the arrhythmia is confirmed and, if present, the device delivers therapy. If during the charge or immediately after charging is complete the arrhythmia spontaneously terminates, the energy is then dumped to avoid unnecessary energy delivery. If energy is delivered, the device enters into a redetection algorithm to assess whether the arrhythmia was successfully terminated. If the arrhythmia persists, then the device recharges its capacitor and repeats the process. If the arrhythmia has terminated, then the episode is declared complete. Although much of the ICD's ability to determine whether an arrhythmia needs therapy is based on the rate, all ICDs have the ability to apply various algorithms to discriminate whether the arrhythmia is ventricular or supraventricular. These include criteria for abruptness of onset, intracardiac signal morphology, and rate stability (stable with VT but irregular with atrial fibrillation).[170] Presence of an atrial lead can sometimes enhance the discrimination of atrial fibrillation with rapid ventricular response from VT.[170]

Guidelines for implantation of ICDs have been issued by the American College of Cardiology, the American Heart Association, and the Heart Rhythm Society[172] (Table 4-2). In general, ICDs are indicated for the primary or secondary prevention of sudden cardiac death. These recommendations are based on data from large, multicenter investigations that have compared ICD therapy with standard care including antiarrhythmic drugs. For patients with prior cardiac arrest caused by VT or ventricular fibrillation (secondary prevention), the data show that ICDs reduce the risk for subsequent mortality by 20% to 30% compared mostly with amiodarone or β-adrenergic receptor blockers.[172–175] Similarly, relative mortality is reduced by 49% to 54% with ICD treatment for patients with nonsustained VT or inducible ventricular arrhythmias with programmed stimulation compared with standard care or serial drug testing in patients with ischemic left ventricular dysfunction.[176,177]

The most convincing data regarding primary prevention of sudden death with ICD treatment for patients with ischemic and nonischemic cardiomyopathy come from the MADIT II (Multicenter Automatic Defibrillator Implantation Trial II)[176] and SCD-HeFT (Sudden Cardiac Death in Heart Failure Trial)[178] trials. In contrast with other studies, these two randomized trials did not require a history of inducible or spontaneous ventricular arrhythmias. Rather, enrollment criteria were based on the ejection fraction alone (≤ 30%) in the presence of ischemic cardiomy-

TABLE 4-2	American College of Cardiology/American Heart Association/Heart Rhythm Society Guidelines for Insertion of ICD[216]

Class I
- Survivors of cardiac arrest caused by VF or sustained VT after reversible causes have been excluded
- Patients with structural heart disease and spontaneous sustained VT regardless of whether hemodynamically stable or unstable
- Patients with syncope of undetermined origin with clinically relevant sustained VT or VF induced at electrophysiology study
- Patients with LVEF ≤ 35% because of prior MI who are at least 40 days after MI and NYHA functional Class II or III
- Patients with nonischemic dilated cardiomyopathy who have LVEF ≤ 35% and NYHA functional Class II or III
- Patients with LV dysfunction because of prior MI who are at least 40 days after MI with LVEF ≤ 30% and who are NYHA Class I
- Patients with nonsustained VT because of prior MI with LVEF ≤ 40% with inducible VF or sustained VT at electrophysiology study

Class IIa
- Patients with unexplained syncope, LV dysfunction, and nonischemic cardiomyopathy
- Patients with sustained VT and normal LV function
- Patients with hypertrophic cardiomyopathy and at least one risk factor for sudden cardiac death
- Patients with arrhythmogenic RV dysplasia with at least one risk factor for sudden cardiac death
- Patients with long QT syndrome with syncope and/or sustained VT while on β-blockers
- Nonhospitalized patients awaiting heart transplant
- Patients with Brugada syndrome who have syncope or with documented VT not resulting in cardiac arrest
- Patients with catecholaminergic polymorphic VT who have syncope and/or documented sustained VT while receiving β-blockers
- Patients with cardiac sarcoidosis, giant cell myocarditis, or Chagas disease

Class IIb
- Patients with nonischemic heart disease who have LVEF ≤ 35% and who are NYHA Class I
- Patients with long QT syndrome and risk factors for sudden cardiac death
- Patients with syncope and structural heart disease when evaluation has failed to define a cause
- Patients with familial cardiomyopathy associated with sudden cardiac death
- Patients with LV noncompaction

Class III
- ICD implantation is not indicated for patients whose reasonable life expectancy at an acceptable functional status is < 1 year even if they meet other criteria

Class I indications: evidence or general agreement that the treatment is useful and effective

Class IIa indications: weight of the data of evidence favors benefit of the therapy

Class IIb: conditions usefulness/efficacy of the treatment is less well established

Class III: intervention is not indicated

ICD, implantable cardioverter-defibrillator; LV, left ventricular; LVEF, left ventricular ejection fraction; MI, myocardial infarction; NYHA, New York Heart Association; RV, right ventricular; VF, ventricular fibrillation; VT, ventricular tachycardia.

opathy (MADIT II) or the ejection fraction (≤ 35%) with New York Heart Association Class II/III heart failure symptoms in the presence of any type of end-stage cardiomyopathy (SCD-HeFT).[178] Patients were continued on conventional treatments including β-blockers, angiotensin-converting enzyme inhibitors, and 3-hydroxy-3-methylglutaryl-coenzyme

A (hMG-CoA) reductase inhibitors ("statins"). After more than 4 years of follow-up, ICD treatment was associated with a significant reduction in all-cause mortality compared with those randomized to only conventional treatment. Other conditions such as inherited long QT syndrome, hypertrophic cardiomyopathy, Brugada syndrome, arrhythmogenic right ventricular dysplasia, and infiltrative disorders including cardiac sarcoidosis may warrant ICD insertion for prevention of sudden cardiac death, although data from large randomized studies are lacking because of the relative rarity of the conditions. In the future, genetic screening might provide valuable information about the risk for sudden death for patients with these less common entities.[179,180]

Anesthetic Considerations

Insertion of ICDs is mostly performed in the catheterization suite. The procedure typically includes defibrillation testing to ensure an acceptable margin of safety for the device. VT or ventricular fibrillation is induced by the introduction of premature beats timed to the vulnerable repolarization period. External adhesive pads are placed before the procedure and connected to an external cardioverter/defibrillator to provide "back-up" shocks should the device be ineffective. Monitored anesthesia care is typically chosen, but a brief general anesthetic given for defibrillation testing can be considered. General anesthesia may be chosen for patients with severe concomitant diseases (e.g., chronic lung disease, sleep apnea) when control of the airway is desired. Simultaneous insertion of biventricular pacing systems with an ICD is performed for an increasing population of patients with impaired left ventricular dysfunction with or without ventricular conduction delay.

In addition to standard patient monitoring, continuous arterial blood pressure monitoring might be considered even during monitored anesthesia care to rapidly assess for return of blood pressure after defibrillation testing. Defibrillation testing was demonstrated to be associated with ischemic electroencephalographic (EEG) changes 7.5 ± 1.8 seconds (mean ± SD) after arrest.[181] These changes were transient and not associated with persistent ischemic EEG changes or exacerbation of an existing neurologic deficit, nor was significant deterioration in neuropsychometric performance detected. Repeated defibrillation testing is usually well tolerated without deterioration of cardiac function even in patients with left ventricular ejection fractions less than 35%. Nonetheless, means of pacing must be available should bradycardia develop after cardioversion/defibrillation. Often, however, restoration of circulatory function after defibrillation testing is accompanied by tachycardia and hypertension, necessitating treatment with a short-acting β-blocker or vasoactive drugs, or both.

Complications associated with ICD insertion include those related to insertion and those associated specifically with the device. Percutaneous insertion is typically via the subclavian vein, predisposing to pneumothorax. Cardiac injury including perforation is a remote possibility. Cerebrovascular accident and myocardial infarction have been reported, but mostly with older device insertion methods.[10] Device-related complications include those associated with multiple shocks that may lead to myocardial injury or refractory hypotension.[182,183] Device infections are particularly difficult to manage, often requiring device and lead explantation.

REFERENCES

1. National Center for Health Statistics: Report of final mortality statistics, 1995, *Monthly Vital Stat Rep* 45(Suppl 2):1997.
2. Gillum RE: Sudden coronary death in the United States: 1980-1985, *Circulation* 79:756, 1989.
3. Orejarena LA, Vidailles H Jr, DeStefano F, et al: Paroxysmal supraventricular tachycardia in the general population, *J Am Coll Cardiol* 31:150, 1998.
4. Granada J, Uribe W, Chyou PH, et al: Incidence and predictors of atrial flutter in the general population, *J Am Coll Cardiol* 36:2242, 2000.
5. Sra J, Dhala A, Blanck Z, et al: Atrial fibrillation: Epidemiology, mechanisms, and management, *Curr Probl Cardiol* 25:405, 2000.
6. Benjamin EJ, Wolf PA, D'Agostino RB, et al: Impact of atrial fibrillation on the risk of death: The Framingham Heart Study, *Circulation* 98:946, 1998.
7. The Cardiac Arrhythmia Suppression Trial (CAST) Investigators: Preliminary report: Effect of encainide and flecainide on mortality in a randomized trial of arrhythmia suppression after myocardial infarction, *N Engl J Med* 321:406, 1989.
8. Ben-David J, Zipes DP: Torsades de pointes and proarrhythmia, *Lancet* 341:1578, 1993.
9. Zipes DP: Implantable cardioverter-defibrillator: A Volkswagen or Rolls Royce? *Circulation* 103:1372, 2001.
10. Andritsos M, Faddis M, Hogue Jr, CW: Cardiac electrophysiology: Diagnosis and treatment. In *Kaplan's Cardiac Anesthesia*, 2006, WB Saunders, 355–382.
11. Anderson KR, Ho SY, Anderson RH: The location and vascular supply of the sinus node in the human heart, *Br Heart J* 41:28, 1979.
12. Cranefield PF: Action potentials, afterpotentials and arrhythmias, *Circ Res* 41:415, 1977.
13. Atlee JL, Bosnjak ZJ: Mechanism for cardiac arrhythmias during anesthesia, *Anesthesiology* 72:347, 1990.
14. Fozzard HA, Gunn RB: Membrane transport. In Fozzard HA, Haber E, Jennings RB, et al, editors: *The Heart and Cardiovascular System*, New York, 1986, Raven Press, pp 1–30.
15. Boineau JP, Schuessler RB, Mooney CR, et al: Multicentric origin of the atrial depolarization wave: The pacemaker complex, *Circulation* 58:1036, 1978.
16. Goldberg JM: Intra-SA-nodal pacemaker shifts induced by autonomic nerve stimulation in the dog, *Am J Physiol* 229:1116, 1975.
17. Randall WC, Talano J, Kaye MP, et al: Cardiac pacemakers in absence of the SA node: Responses to exercises and autonomic blockade, *Am J Physiol* 234:H465, 1978.
18. Sealy WC, Bache RJ, Seaber AV, Bhattacharga SK: The atrial pacemaking site after surgical exclusion of the sinoatrial node, *J Thorac Cardiovasc Surg* 65:841, 1973.

19. Sealy WC, Seaber AV: Surgical isolation of the atrial septum from the atria: Identification of an atrial septal pacemaker, *J Thorac Cardiovasc Surg* 80:742, 1980.
20. Boineau JP, Schuessler RB, Hackel DB, et al: Widespread distribution and rate differentiation of the atrial pacemaker complex, *Am J Physiol* 239:H406, 1980.
21. Boineau JP, Miller CB, Schuessler RB, et al: Activation sequence and potential distribution maps demonstrating multicentre atrial impulse origin in dogs, *Circ Res* 54:332, 1984.
22. Hoffman BF: Fine structure of internodal pathways, *Am J Cardiol* 44:385, 1979.
23. Cox JL: The surgical treatment of cardiac arrhythmias. In Sabiston DC Jr, editors: *Textbook of Surgery*, Philadelphia, 1991, WB Saunders, p 2058.
24. Anderson RH, Davies MJ, Becker AE: Atrioventricular ring specialized tissue in the normal heart, *Eur J Cardiol* 2:219, 1974.
25. Anderson RH, Becker AE: Anatomy of conducting tissues revisited, *Br Heart J* 40:2, 1979.
26. Zipes DP: Genesis of cardiac arrhythmias: Electrophysiologic considerations. In Braunwald E, editor: *Heart Disease*, ed 3, Philadelphia, 1990, WB Saunders, pp 581–620.
27. Kreitner D: Electrophysiological study of the two main pacemaker mechanisms in the rabbit sinus node, *Cardiovasc Res* 19:304, 1985.
28. Rozanski GJ, Lipsius SL: Electrophysiology of functional subsidiary pacemakers in canine right atrium, *Am J Physiol* 249:H504, 1985.
29. Watanabe Y, Dreifus LS: Sites of impulse formation within the atrioventricular junction of the rabbit, *Circ Res* 22:717, 1968.
30. DiFrancesco D: A new interpretation of the pacemaker current in calf Purkinje fibers, *J Physiol (Lond)* 314:359, 1981.
31. Noble D, Tsien RW: The kinetics and rectifier properties of the slow potassium current in cardiac Purkinje fibers, *J Physiol (Lond)* 195:185, 1968.
32. Vassalle M: Cardiac pacemaker potentials at different extracellular and intracellular K^+ concentrations, *Am J Physiol* 208:770, 1965.
33. Vassalle M: Analysis of cardiac pacemaker potential using "voltage clamp" technique, *Am J Physiol* 210:1335, 1966.
34. Wu EB, Chia HM, Gill JS: Reversible cardiomyopathy after radiofrequency ablation of lateral free-wall pathway-mediated incessant supraventricular tachycardia, *PACE Pacing Clin Electrophysiol* 23:1308, 2000.
35. Cain ME, Lindsay BD: The preoperative electrophysiologic study, *Cardiac Surg* 4:53, 1990.
36. DiMarco JP, Garan H, Ruskin JN: Complications in patients undergoing cardiac electrophysiologic procedures, *Ann Intern Med* 97:490, 1982.
37. Horowitz LN, Kay HR, Kutalek SP, et al: Risks and complications of clinical cardiac electrophysiologic studies: A prospective analysis of 1,000 consecutive patients, *J Am Coll Cardiol* 9:1261, 1987.
38. Cobb FR, Blumenschein SD, Sealy WC, et al: Successful surgical interruption of the bundle of Kent in a patient with Wolff-Parkinson-White syndrome, *Circulation* 38:1018, 1968.
39. Sealy WC, Boineau JP, Wallace AG: The identification and division of the bundle of Kent for premature ventricular excitation and supraventricular tachycardia, *Surgery* 68:1009, 1970.
40. Boineau JP, Moore EN, Sealy WC, Kasell JH: Epicardial mapping in Wolff-Parkinson-White syndrome, *Arch Intern Med* 135:422, 1975.
41. Cox JL, Gallagher JJ, Cain ME: Experience with 118 consecutive patients undergoing surgery for the Wolff-Parkinson-White syndrome, *J Thorac Cardiovasc Surg* 90:490, 1985.
42. Faddis MN, Chen J, Osborn J, et al: Magnetic guidance system for cardiac electrophysiology: A prospective trial of safety and efficacy in humans, *J Am Coll Cardiol* 42:1952, 2003.
43. Blomström-Lundqvist C, Scheinman MM, Aliot EM, et al: ACC/AHA/ESC guidelines for the management of patients with supraventricular arrhythmias, *J Am Coll Cardiol* 108:1871, 2003.
44. Wolff L, Parkinson J, White PD: Bundle-branch block with short P-R interval in healthy young people prone to paroxysmal tachycardia, *Am Heart J* 5:685, 1930.
45. Lindsay BD, Crossen KJ, Cain ME: Concordance of distinguishing electrocardiographic features during sinus rhythm with the location of accessory pathways in the Wolff-Parkinson-White syndrome, *Am J Cardiol* 59:1093, 1987.
46. Gallagher JJ, Pritchett ELC, Sealy WC, et al: The preexcitation syndromes, *Prog Cardiovasc Dis* 20:285, 1978.
47. Bardy GH, Packer DL, German LD, et al: Pre-excited reciprocating tachycardia in patients with Wolff-Parkinson-White syndrome: Incidence and mechanisms, *Circulation* 70:377, 1984.
48. Kuck K, Brugada P, Wellens HJ: Observations on the antidromic type of circus movement tachycardia in the Wolff-Parkinson-White syndrome, *J Am Coll Cardiol* 2:1003, 1983.
49. Scheinman MM, Huang S: The 1998 NASPE prospective catheter ablation registry, *PACE Pacing Clin Electrophysiol* 23:1020, 2000.
50. Calkins H, Yong P, Miller JM, et al: For the Atakr Multicenter Investigator Group: Catheter ablation of accessory pathways, atrioventricular nodal re-entrant tachycardia, and the atrioventricular junction: Final results of a prospective, multicenter clinical trial, *Circulation* 99:262, 1999.
51. Yee R, Connolly S, Noorani H: Clinical review of radiofrequency catheter ablation for cardiac arrhythmias, *Can J Cardiol* 19:1273, 2003.
52. Lau CP, Tai YT, Lee PW: The effects of radiofrequency ablation versus medical therapy on the quality-of-life and exercise capacity in patients with accessory pathway-mediate supraventricular tachycardia: A treatment comparison study, *PACE Pacing Clin Electrophysiol* 18:424, 1995.
53. Holman W, Ikeshita M, Lease J, et al: Elective prolongation of atrioventricular conduction by multiple discrete cryolesions: A new technique for the treatment of paroxysmal supraventricular tachycardia, *J Thorac Cardiovasc Surg* 84:554, 1982.
54. Holman WL, Ikeshita M, Lease JG, et al: Alteration of antegrade atrioventricular conduction by cryoablation of periatrioventricular nodal tissue, *J Thorac Cardiovasc Surg* 88:67, 1984.
55. Holman WL, Ikeshita M, Lease JG, et al: Cryosurgical modification of retrograde atrioventricular conduction: Implications for the surgical treatment of atrioventricular node reentry tachycardia, *J Thorac Cardiovasc Surg* 91:826, 1986.
56. Cox JL, Holman WL, Cain ME: Cryosurgical treatment of atrioventricular node reentry tachycardia, *Circulation* 76:1329, 1987.
57. Stein KM, Lerman BB: Evidence for functionally distinct dual atrial inputs to the human AV node, *Am J Physiol* 267:H2333, 1994.
58. Langberg JJ, Leon A, Borganelli M, et al: A randomized, prospective comparison of anterior and posterior approaches to radiofrequency catheter ablation of atrioventricular nodal reentry tachycardia, *Circulation* 87:1551, 1993.
59. Jazayeri MR, Akhtar M: Electrophysiological behavior of atrioventricular node after selective fast or slow pathway ablation in patients with atrioventricular nodal reentrant tachycardia, *PACE Pacing Clin Electrophysiol* 16:623, 1993.
60. Chen SA, Chiang CE, Tsang WP, et al: Selective radiofrequency catheter ablation of fast and slow pathways in 100 patients with atrioventricular nodal reentrant tachycardia, *Am Heart J* 125:1, 1993.
61. Akhtar M, Jazayeri MR, Sra JS, et al: Atrioventricular nodal reentry: Clinical, electrophysiologic and therapeutic considerations, *Circulation* 88:282, 1993.
62. Steinbeck G, Hoffmann E: 'True' atrial tachycardia, *Eur Heart J* 19:E–10, 1998.
63. Saoudi N, Cosio F, Waldo A, et al: A classification of atrial flutter and regular atrial tachycardia according to electrophysiological mechanism and anatomical bases: A statement from a joint expert group from The Working Groups of Arrhythmias of the European Society of Cardiology and the North American Society of Pacing and Electrophysiology, *Eur Heart J* 22:1162, 2001.
64. Hoffmann E, Reithmann C, Nimmermann P, et al: Clinical experience with electroanatomic mapping of ectopic atrial tachycardia, *PACE Pacing Clin Electrophysiol* 25:49, 2002.
65. Lai LP, Lin JL, Chen TF, et al: Clinical, electrophysiological characteristics, and radiofrequency catheter ablation of atrial tachycardia near the apex of Koch's triangle, *PACE Pacing Clin Electrophysiol* 21:367, 1998.
66. Chen SA, Tai CT, Chiang CE, et al: Focal atrial tachycardia: Reanalysis of the clinical and electrophysiologic characteristics and prediction of successful radiofrequency ablation, *J Cardiovasc Electrophysiol* 9:355, 1998.
67. Schmitt C, Zrenner B, Schneider M, et al: Clinical experience with a novel multielectrode basket catheter in right atrial tachycardia, *Circulation* 99:2414, 1999.
68. Natale A, Breeding L, Tomassoni G, et al: Ablation of right and left ectopic atrial tachycardia using a three-dimensional nonfluoroscopic mapping system, *Am J Cardiol* 82:989, 1998.
69. Anguera I, Brugada J, Roba M, et al: Outcomes after radiofrequency catheter ablation of atrial tachycardia, *Am J Cardiol* 87:886, 2001.
70. Man KC, Knight B, Tse HF, et al: Radiofrequency catheter ablation of inappropriate sinus tachycardia guided by activation mapping, *J Am Coll Cardiol* 35:451, 2000.
71. Cossu SF, Steinberg JS: Supraventricular tachyarrhythmias involving the sinus node: Clinical and electrophysiologic characteristics, *Prog Cardiovasc Dis* 41:51, 1998.
72. Goya M, Iesaka Y, Takahashi A, et al: Radiofrequency catheter ablation for sinoatrial node reentrant tachycardia: Electrophysiologic features of ablation sites, *Jpn Circ J* 63:177, 1999.
73. Cheng J, Scheinman MM: Acceleration of typical atrial flutter due to double-wave reentry induced by programmed electrical stimulation, *Circulation* 97:1589, 1998.
74. Cheng J, Cabeen WR Jr, Scheinman MM: Right atrial flutter due to lower loop reentry: Mechanism and anatomic substrates, *Circulation* 99:1700, 1999.
75. Willems S, Weiss C, Ventura R, et al: Catheter ablation of atrial flutter guided by electroanatomic mapping (CARTO): A randomized comparison to the conventional approach, *J Cardiovasc Electrophysiol* 11:1223, 2000.
76. Kottkamp H, Hugl B, Krauss B, et al: Electromagnetic versus fluoroscopic mapping of the inferior isthmus for ablation of typical atrial flutter: A prospective randomized study, *Circulation* 102:2082, 2000.
77. Ward DE, Xie B, Rowland E: Ablation of atrial flutter using the anatomical method: Results and long-term follow-up, *J Interv Cardiol* 8:697, 1995.
78. Tai CT, Chen SA, Chiang CE, et al: Long-term outcome of radiofrequency catheter ablation for typical atrial flutter: Risk prediction of recurrent arrhythmia, *J Cardiovasc Electrophysiol* 9:115, 1998.
79. Lee SH, Tai CT, Yu WC, et al: Effects of radiofrequency catheter ablation on quality of life in patients with atrial flutter, *Am J Cardiol* 84:278, 1999.
80. Anselmen F, Saoudi N, Poty H, et al: Radiofrequency catheter ablation of common atrial flutter: Significance of palpitations and quality-of-life evaluation in a patient with proven isthmus block, *Circulation* 99:534, 1999.
81. Natale A, Newby KH, Pisano E, et al: Prospective randomized comparison of antiarrhythmic therapy versus first-line radiofrequency ablation in patients with atrial flutter, *J Am Coll Cardiol* 35:1898, 2000.
82. Nakagawa H, Shah N, Matsudaira K, et al: Characterization of re-entrant circuit in macro-re-entrant right atrial tachycardia after surgical repair of congenital heart disease: Isolated channels between scars allow "focal" ablation, *Circulation* 103:699, 2001.
83. Shah D, Jais P, Takahashi A, et al: Dual-loop intra-atrial re-entry in humans, *Circulation* 101:631, 2000.
84. Duru F, Hindricks G, Kottkamp H: Atypical left atrial flutter after intraoperative radiofrequency ablation of chronic atrial fibrillation: Successful ablation using three-dimensional electroanatomic mapping, *J Cardiovasc Electrophysil* 12:602, 2001.
85. Akar JG, Kok LC, Haines DE, et al: Coexistence of type I atrial flutter and intra-atrial reentrant tachycardia in patients with surgically corrected congenital heart disease, *J Am Coll Cardiol* 38:377, 2001.
86. Lev M, Gibson S, Miller DA: Ebstein's disease with Wolff-Parkinson-White syndrome, *Am Heart J* 49:724, 1955.
87. Henzi I, Sonderegger J, Tramer MR: Efficacy, dose-response, and adverse effects of droperidol for prevention of postoperative nausea and vomiting, *Can J Anesth* 47:537–551, 2000.
88. Bertolo L, Novakovic BS, Penna M: Antiarrhythmic effects of droperidol, *Anesthesiology* 29:529, 1972.
89. Gomez-Arnau J, Mones JM, Auello F: Fentanyl and droperidol effects on the refractoriness of the accessory pathway in the Wolff-Parkinson-White syndrome, *Anesthesiology* 58:307, 1983.
90. Sadowski AR, Moyers JR: Anesthetic management of the Wolff-Parkinson-White syndrome, *Anesthesiology* 51:553, 1979.
91. Suppan P: Althesin in the Wolff-Parkinson-White syndrome, *Br J Anaesth* 51:69, 1979.
92. Sharpe MD, Dobkowski WB, Murkin JM: The electrophysiologic effects of volatile anesthetics on the normal AV conduction system and accessory pathways in WPW, *Anesthesiology* 80:63–70, 1994.
93. Dobkowski WB, Murkin JM, Sharpe MD, et al: The effect of enflurane (IMAC) on the normal AV conduction system and accessory pathways, *Anesth Analg* 72:550, 1991.
94. Geha GD, Rozelle BC, Raessler KL, et al: Pancuronium bromide enhances atrioventricular conduction in halothane-anesthetized dogs, *Anesthesiology* 46:342, 1977.
95. Kumazawa T: Wolff-Parkinson-White syndrome and anesthesia, *Jpn J Anesthesiol* 19:68, 1970.
96. Van der Starr PJA: Wolff-Parkinson-White syndrome during anesthesia, *Anesthesiology* 48:369, 1978.
97. Wyse DG, Waldo AL, DiMarco JP, et al: Atrial Fibrillation Follow-up Investigation of Rhythm Management (AFFIRM) Investigators. A comparison of rate control and rhythm control in patients with atrial fibrillation, *N Engl J Med* 347:1825, 2002.
98. Moe GK: On the multiple wavelet hypothesis of atrial fibrillation, *Arch Int Pharmacodyn* 140:183, 1962.
99. Boineau JP, Schuessler RB, Mooney CR, et al: Natural and evoked atrial flutter due to circus movement in dogs: Role of abnormal atrial pathways, slow conduction, nonuniform refractory period distribution and premature beats, *Am J Cardiol* 45:1167, 1980.
100. Allessie MA, Bonke FIM, Schopman FG: Circus movement in rabbit atrial muscle as a mechanism of tachycardia. II. The role of nonuniform recovery of excitability in the occurrence of unidirectional block as studied with multiple microelectrodes, *Circ Res* 39:168, 1976.
101. Cox JL, Boineau JP, Schuessler RB, et al: Successful surgical treatment of atrial fibrillation. Review and clinical update, *JAMA* 266:1976, 1991.
102. Cox JL, Boineau JP, Schuessler RB, et al: Operations for atrial fibrillation, *Clin Cardiol* 14:827, 1991.
103. Haissaguerre M, Jais P, Shah DC, et al: Spontaneous initiation of atrial fibrillation by ectopic beats originating in the pulmonary veins, *N Engl J Med* 339:659, 1998.
104. Yamauchi S, Tanaka S, Asano T, et al: Efficacy of combining mapping with surgery for atrial fibrillation, *Rinsho Kyobu Geka* 14:344–345, 1994.
105. Harada A, Sasaki K, Fukushima T, et al: Atrial activation during chronic atrial fibrillation in patients with isolated mitral valve disease, *Ann Thorac Surg* 61:104, 1996.
106. Schuessler RB, Grayson TM, Bromberg BI, et al: Cholinergically mediated tachyarrhythmias induced by a single extrastimulus in the isolated canine right atrium, *Circ Res* 71:1254, 1992.
107. Yamauchi S, Boineau JP, Schuessler RB, Cox JL: Varying types of circus movement reentry with both normal and dissociated contralateral conduction causing different right and left atrial rhythms in canine atrial flutter, *Jpn Circ J* 62:201, 1998.

108. Nitta T, Ishii Y, Miyagi Y, et al: Concurrent multiple left atrial focal activations with fibrillatory conduction and right atrial focal or reentrant activation as the mechanisms in atrial fibrillation, *J Thorac Cardiovasc Surg* 127:770, 2004.
109. Schuessler RB: Do we need a map to get through the Maze? *J Thorac Cardiovasc Surg* 127:627, 2004.
110. Haissaguerre M, Shah DC, Jais P, et al: Electrophysiological breakthroughs from the left atrium to the pulmonary veins, *Circulation* 102:2463, 2000.
111. Pappone C, Rosario S, Oreto G, et al: Circumferential radiofrequency ablation of pulmonary vein ostia: A new anatomic approach for curing atrial fibrillation, *Circulation* 102:2619, 2000.
112. Oral H, Scharf C, Chugh A, et al: Catheter ablation for paroxysmal atrial fibrillation: Segmental pulmonary vein ostial ablation versus left atrial ablation, *Circulation* 108:2355, 2003.
113. Haissaguerre M, Jais P, Shah DC, et al: Right and left atrial radiofrequency catheter therapy of paroxysmal atrial fibrillation, *J Cardiovasc Electrophysiol* 7:1132, 1996.
114. Jais P, Shah DC, Haissaguerre M, et al: Efficacy and safety of septal and left-atrial linear ablation for atrial fibrillation, *Am J Cardiol* 84:R139, 1999.
115. Natale A, Leonelli F, Bheiry S, et al: Catheter ablation approach on the right side only for paroxysmal atrial fibrillation therapy: Long-term results, *PACE Pacing Clin Electrophysiol* 23:224, 2000.
116. Shah DC, Haissaguerre M, Jais P, et al: Electrophysiological endpoint for catheter ablation of atrial fibrillation initiated from multiple pulmonary venous foci, *Circulation* 101:1409, 2000.
117. Hsieh MH, Chen SA, Tai CT, et al: Double multi-electrode mapping catheters facilitate radiofrequency catheter ablation of focal atrial fibrillation originating from pulmonary veins, *J Cardiovasc Electrophysiol* 10:136, 1999.
118. Chen SA, Hsieh MH, Tai CT, et al: Initiation of atrial fibrillation by ectopic beats originating from the pulmonary veins: Electrophysiological characteristics, pharmacological response, and effect of radiofrequency ablation, *Circulation* 100:1879, 1999.
119. Haissaguerre M, Jais P, Shah DC, et al: Electrophysiological end point for catheter ablation of atrial fibrillation initiated from multiple pulmonary venous foci, *Circulation* 101:1409–1417, 2000.
120. Hsieh MH, Chem SA, Tai CT, et al: Double multielectrode mapping catheters facilitate radiofrequency catheter ablation of focal atrial fibrillation originating from pulmonary veins, *J Cardiovasc Electrophysiol* 10:136–144, 1999.
121. Cox JL, Canavan TE, Schuessler RB, et al: The surgical treatment of atrial fibrillation. II. Intraoperative electrophysiologic mapping and description of the electrophysiologic basis of atrial flutter and atrial fibrillation, *J Thorac Cardiovasc Surg* 101:406, 1991.
122. Cox JL, Schuessler RB, D'Agostino HJ, et al: The surgical treatment of atrial fibrillation. III. Development of a definitive surgical procedure, *J Thorac Cardiovasc Surg* 101:569, 1991.
123. Cox JL: The surgical treatment of atrial fibrillation. IV. Surgical technique, *J Thorac Cardiovasc Surg* 101:584, 1991.
124. Cox JL, Boineau JP, Schuessler RB, et al: Modification of the Maze procedure for atrial flutter and atrial fibrillation. I. Rationale and surgical results, *J Thorac Cardiovasc Surg* 110:473, 1995.
125. Cox JL, Jaquiss RDB, Schuessler RB, et al: Modification of the Maze procedure for atrial flutter and atrial fibrillation. II. Surgical technique of the Maze III procedure, *J Thorac Cardiovasc Surg* 110:485, 1995.
126. Pasic M, Musci M, Siniawski HK, et al: Transient sinus node dysfunction after the Cox-Maze III procedure in patients with organic heart disease and chronic fixed atrial fibrillation, *J Am Coll Cardiol* 32:1040, 1998.
127. Gillinov AM, Blackstone EH, McCarthy PM: Atrial fibrillation: Current surgical options and their assessment, *Ann Thorac Surg* 74:2210, 2002.
128. Doll N, Borger MA, Fabricius A, et al: Esophageal perforation during left atrial radiofrequency ablation: Is the risk too high? *J Thorac Cardiovasc Surg* 125:836, 2003.
129. Kim YH, Sosa-Suarez G, Trouton TG, et al: Treatment of ventricular tachycardia by transcatheter radiofrequency ablation in patients with ischemic heart disease, *Circulation* 89:1094, 1994.
130. Albâge A, van der Linden J, Bengtsson L, et al: Elevations in antidiuretic hormone and aldosterone as possible causes of fluid retention in the Maze procedure, *Ann Thorac Surg* 72:58, 2001.
131. Ad N, Suyderhoud JP, Kim YD, et al: Benefits of prophylactic continuous infusion of furosemide after the Maze procedure for atrial fibrillation, *J Thorac Cardiovasc Surg* 123:232, 2002.
132. Cox JL, Schuessler RB, Lappas DG, Boineau JP: An 8 1/2-year clinical experience with surgery for atrial fibrillation, *Ann Surg* 224:267, 1996.
133. Isobe F, Kawashima Y: The outcome and indications of the Cox Maze III procedure for chronic atrial fibrillation with mitral valve disease, *J Thorac Cardiovasc Surg* 116:220, 1998.
134. Feinberg MS, Waggoner AD, Kater KM, et al: Restoration of atrial function after the Maze procedure for patients with atrial fibrillation: Assessment by Doppler echocardiography, *Circulation* 90(Suppl II):II–285, 1994.
135. Tsui SS, Grace AA, Ludman PF, et al: Maze 3 for atrial fibrillation: Two cuts too few? *PACE Pacing Clin Electrophysiol* 17:2163, 1994.
136. Nitta T, Lee R, Schuessler RB, et al: Radial approach: A new concept in surgical treatment for atrial fibrillation. I. Concept, anatomic and physiologic bases and development of the procedure, *Ann Thorac Surg* 67:27, 1999.
137. Nitta T, Lee R, Watanabe H, et al: Radial procedure: A new concept in surgical treatment for atrial fibrillation. II. Electrophysiologic effects and atrial contribution to ventricular filling, *Ann Thorac Surg* 67:36, 1999.
138. Omari BO, Nelson RJ, Robertson JM: Effect of right atrial appendectomy on the release of atrial natriuretic hormone, *J Thorac Cardiovasc Surg* 102:272, 1991.
139. The Antiarrhythmics Versus Implantable Defibrillator (AVID) Investigators: A comparison of antiarrhythmic-drug therapy with implantable defibrillators in patients resuscitated from near-fatal ventricular arrhythmias, *N Engl J Med* 337:1576, 1997.
140. Calkins H, Kalbfleisch SJ, el-Atassi R, et al: Relation between efficacy of radiofrequency catheter ablation and site of origin of idiopathic ventricular tachycardia, *Am J Cardiol* 71:827, 1993.
141. Coggins DL, Lee RJ, Sweeney J, et al: Radiofrequency catheter ablation as a cure for idiopathic tachycardia of both left and right ventricular origin, *J Am Coll Cardiol* 23:1333, 1994.
142. Thakur RK, Klein GJ, Sivaram CA, et al: Anatomic substrate for idiopathic left ventricular tachycardia, *Circulation* 93:497, 1996.
143. Prystowsky EN, Miles WM, Evans JJ, et al: Induction of ventricular tachycardia during programmed electrical stimulation: Analysis of pacing methods, *Circulation* 73(Suppl II):II–132, 1986.
144. Bigger JT, Reiffel JA, Livelli FD Jr, et al: Sensitivity, specificity, and reproducibility of programmed ventricular stimulation, *Circulation* 73(Suppl II):II, 1986.
145. Stevenson WG, Sager PT, Friedman PL: Entrainment techniques for mapping atrial and ventricular tachycardias, *J Cardiovasc Eletrophysiol* 6:201, 1995.
146. Marchlinski FE, Callans DJ, Gottlieb CD, et al: Linear ablation lesions for control of unmappable ventricular tachycardia in patients with ischemic and nonischemic cardiomyopathy, *Circulation* 101:1288, 2000.
147. Mehdirad AA, Keim S, Rist K, Tchou P: Long-term clinical outcome of right bundle branch radiofrequency catheter ablation for treatment of bundle branch reentrant ventricular tachycardia, *Pacing Clin Electrophysiol* 18:2135, 1995.
148. Rothman SA, Hsia HH, Cossu SF, et al: Radiofrequency catheter ablation of postinfarction ventricular tachycardia: Long-term success and the significance of inducible nonclinical arrhythmias, *Circulation* 96:3499, 1997.
149. Callans DJ, Zado E, Sarter BY, et al: Efficacy of radiofrequency catheter ablation for ventricular tachycardia in healed myocardial infarction, *Am J Cardiol* 82:42, 1998.
150. Stevenson WG, Friedman PL, Kocovic D, et al: Radiofrequency catheter ablation of ventricular tachycardia after myocardial infarction, *Circulation* 98:308, 1998.
151. Stevenson WG, Khan H, Sage P, et al: Identification of reentry circuit sites during catheter mapping and radiofrequency ablation of ventricular tachycardia late after myocardial infarction, *Circulation* 88:1647, 1993.
152. Gonska BD, Cao K, Schaumann A, et al: Catheter ablation of ventricular tachycardia in 136 patients with coronary artery disease: Result and long-term follow-up, *J Am Coll Cardiol* 24:1506, 1994.
153. Jadonath RL, Snow JS, Goldner BG, Cohen TJ: Radiofrequency catheter ablation as primary therapy for symptomatic ventricular tachycardia, *J Invasive Cardiol* 6:289, 1994.
154. Haffajee C, Love J, Canada A, et al: Clinical pharmacokinetics and efficacy of amiodarone for refractory tachyarrhythmias, *Circulation* 67:1347–1355, 1981.
155. Gallagher JD, Lieberman RW, Meranze J, et al: Amiodarone-induced complications during coronary artery surgery, *Anesthesiology* 55:186, 1981.
156. Liberman BA, Teasdale SJ: Anesthesia and amiodarone, *Can Anaesth Soc J* 32:629, 1985.
157. Feinberg BI, LaMantia KR: Ventricular tachyarrhythmias during placement of pulmonary artery catheters in patients with recurrent ventricular tachycardia, *Mt Sinai J Med* 53:545, 1986.
158. Schmid JP, Rosengant TK, McIntosh CL, et al: Amiodarone-induced complications after cardiac operation for obstructive hypertrophic cardiomyopathy, *Ann Thorac Surg* 48:359, 1989.
159. Greenspon AJ, Kidwell GA, Hurley W, Mannion J: Amiodarone-related postoperative adult respiratory distress syndrome, *Circulation* 84(Suppl III):III–1407, 1991.
160. Eliot GC, Zimmerman GA, Clemmen TP: Complications of pulmonary artery catheterization in the case of critically ill patients, *Chest* 76:647, 1979.
161. Kroll DA, Knight PR: Antifibrillatory effects of volatile anesthetics in acute occlusion/reperfusion arrhythmias, *Anesthesiology* 61:657, 1984.
162. Turner LA, Bosnjak ZJ, Kampine JP: Electrophysiological effects of halothane on Purkinje fibers from normal and infarcted canine hearts, *Anesthesiology* 67:619, 1987.
163. Hunt GB, Ross DL: Comparison of effects of three anesthetic agents on induction of ventricular tachycardia in a canine model of myocardial infarction, *Circulation* 78:221, 1988.
164. Deutsch N, Huntler CB, Tait AR, et al: Suppression of ventricular arrhythmias by volatile anesthetics in a canine model of chronic myocardial infarction, *Anesthesiology* 72:1012, 1990.
165. MacLeod BA, Augerean P, Walker MJA: Effects of halothane anesthesia compared with fentanyl anesthesia and no anesthesia during coronary ligation in rats, *Anesthesiology* 58:44, 1983.
166. Denniss AR, Richards DA, Taylor AT, Uther JB: Halothane anesthesia reduces inducibility of ventricular tachyarrhythmias in chronic canine myocardial infarction, *Basic Res Cardiol* 84:5, 1989.
167. Atlee JL: Halothane: Cause or cure for arrhythmias, *Anesthesiology* 67:617, 1987.
168. Saini V, Carr DB, Hagestod EL, et al: Antifibrillatory action of the narcotic agonist fentanyl, *Am Heart J* 115:598, 1988.
169. DeSilva RA, Verrier RL, Lown B: Protective effect of the vagotonic action of morphine sulphate or ventricular vulnerability, *Cardiovasc Res* 12:167, 1978.
170. Atlee JL, Bernstein AD: Cardiac rhythm management devices. Part I, *Anesthesiology* 95:1265, 2001.
171. Saksena S, An H, Mehra R, et al: Prospective comparison of biphasic and monophasic shocks for implantable cardioverter-defibrillators using endocardial leads, *Am J Cardiol* 70:304, 1992.
172. Epstein AE: An update on implantable cardioverter-defibrillator guidelines, *Curr Opin Cardiol* 19:23–25, 2004.
173. The Antiarrhythmics Versus Implantable Defibrillator (AVID) Investigators: A comparison of antiarrhythmic drug therapy with implantable defibrillators in patients resuscitated for near-fatal ventricular arrhythmias, *N Engl J Med* 337:1576, 1997.
174. Connolly SJ, Gent M, Roberts RS, et al: Canadian Implantable Defibrillator Study (CIDS): A randomized trial of the implantable cardioverter-defibrillator against amiodarone, *Circulation* 101:129, 2000.
175. Kuck KH, Capitol R, Seibel J, et al: Randomized comparisons of anti-arrhythmic drug therapy with implantable defibrillators in patients resuscitated from cardiac arrest: The Cardiac Arrest Study Hamburg (CASH), *Circulation* 102:748, 2000.
176. Moss AJ, Hall WJ, Cannon DS, et al: Improved survival with an implanted defibrillator in patients with coronary disease at high risk for ventricular arrhythmia: Multicenter Automatic Defibrillator Implantation Trial Investigators, *N Engl J Med* 335:1933, 1996.
177. Buxton AE, Lee KL, Fisher JD, et al: A randomized study of the prevention of sudden death in patients with coronary artery disease: Multicenter Unsustained Tachycardia Trial Investigators, *N Engl J Med* 341:1882, 1999.
178. Bardy GH, Lee KL, Mark DB, et al: Amiodarone or an implantable cardioverter-defibrillator for congestive heart failure, *N Engl J Med* 352:225–237, 2005.
179. Zareba W, Moss AJ, Schwartz PJ, et al: Influence of genotype on the clinical course of the long-QT syndrome: International Long-QT Syndrome Registry Research Group, *N Engl J Med* 339:960, 1998.
180. Watkins H, McKenna WJ, Thierfelder L, et al: Mutations in the genes for cardiac troponin T and alpha-tropomyosin in hypertrophic cardiomyopathy, *N Engl J Med* 332:1058, 1995.
181. Adams DC, Heyer EJ, Emerson RG, et al: Implantable cardioverter-defibrillator. Evaluation of clinical neurologic outcome and electroencephalographic changes during implantation, *J Thorac Cardiovasc Surg* 109:565, 1995.
182. Meyer J, Mollhoff T, Seifert T, et al: Cardiac output is not affected during testing of the AICD, *J Cardiovasc Electrophysiol* 7:211, 1996.
183. Hurst TM, Hinrichs M, Breidenbach C, et al: Detection of myocardial injury during transvenous implantation of automatic cardioverter-defibrillators, *J Am Coll Cardiol* 34:402, 1999.

Cardiovascular Physiology, Pharmacology, Molecular Biology, and Genetics

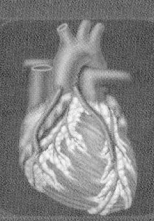

5

Cardiac Physiology

PAUL S. PAGEL, MD, PHD

The heart is an electrically self-actuated, phasic, variable speed, hydraulic pump composed of two dual-component, elastic muscular chambers, each consisting of an atrium and a ventricle, connected in series that simultaneously provide an equal quantity of blood to the pulmonary and systemic circulations. All four chambers of the heart are responsive to stimulation rate, muscle stretch immediately before contraction (preload), and the forces resisting further muscle shortening after this event has begun (afterload). The heart efficiently provides its own energy supply through an extensive network of coronary arterial blood vessels. The heart rapidly adapts to changing physiologic conditions by altering its inherent mechanical properties (Frank–Starling relation) and by responding to neurohormonal and reflex-mediated signaling determined primarily by the balance of sympathetic and parasympathetic nervous system activity. The overall performance of the heart is determined not only by the contractile characteristics of its atria and ventricles (systolic function), but by the ability of its chambers to effectively collect blood at normal filling pressures before the subsequent ejection (diastolic function). This innate duality implies that heart failure (HF) may occur as a consequence of abnormalities in either systolic or diastolic function. At an average heart rate (HR) of 75 beats/min, the heart will contract and relax more than 3 billion times during a typical human life expectancy, thereby supplying the rest of the body with the oxygen and nutrients necessary to meet its metabolic requirements. This chapter discusses the fundamentals of cardiac physiology with a primary emphasis on the determinants of mechanical function that readily allow the heart to achieve this truly remarkable performance. A thorough understanding of cardiac physiology is essential for the practice of cardiac anesthesia.

FUNCTIONAL IMPLICATIONS OF GROSS ANATOMY

Structure

The anatomic design of the heart determines many of its major mechanical capabilities and limitations. The annuli of the cardiac valves, the aortic and pulmonary arterial roots, the central fibrous body, and the left and right fibrous trigones form the skeletal base of the heart. This flexible but very strong cartilaginous structure is located at the superior (termed *basal* in opposition to the left ventricular [LV] apex) aspect of the heart; provides support for the translucent, macroscopically avascular valves; resists the forces of developed pressure and blood flow within the chambers; and provides a site of insertion for superficial subepicardial muscle.[1] Most of the atrial and ventricular muscle is not directly connected to this central fibrous skeleton, but instead arises from and inserts within adjacent surrounding myocardium consistent with the well-known embryologic derivation of the heart from an expanded arterial blood vessel.[2] An interstitial collagen fiber network (composed of thick type I collagen cross-linked with thin type III collagen) also provides important structural support to the myocardium. The protein elastin is closely associated with this collagen matrix, thereby imparting additional flexibility and elasticity to the heart without compromising its strength. In contrast with William Harvey's original assertion,[3] atrial and ventricular myocardium cannot be separated into distinct bands or layers* using an "unwinding" dissection technique[4,5] and, instead, is a continuum of interconnecting cardiac muscle fibers. The left and right atria (LA and RA, respectively) are composed of two relatively thin, orthogonally oriented layers of myocardium. The right ventricular (RV) and, to an even greater extent, the LV walls are thicker (approximately 5 and 10 mm, respectively) than those of the atria and consist of three muscle layers: interdigitating deep sinospiral, the superficial sinospiral, and the superficial bulbospiral. Well-ordered, differential alterations in fiber angle extending from the endocardium to the epicardium are especially apparent in ventricular myocardium and are spatially conserved despite the substantial alterations in wall thickness that occur with contraction and relaxation during the cardiac cycle (Figure 5-1).[6] Subendocardial and subepicardial muscle fibers of the LV follow perpendicular, oblique, and helical routes from the base to the apex, but orientation of these interdigitating sheets of cardiac muscle also reverses direction at approximately the midpoint of the LV. Thus, LV fiber architecture resembles a flattened "figure of eight" (Figure 5-2). Contraction of obliquely arranged subepicardial and subendocardial fibers causes LV chamber shortening along its longitudinal axis and is accompanied by a characteristic "twisting" action that increases the magnitude of force generated by the LV during systole above that produced by basal-apical muscle fiber shortening alone. Indeed, a transition of this primarily helical geometry into a more

Endocardium

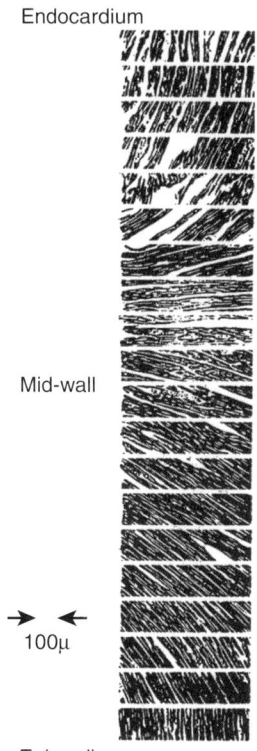

Mid-wall

100μ

Epicardium

Figure 5-1 Sequence of photomicrographs depicting myocardial fiber angles at successive sections from the endocardial *(top)* to the epicardial surface *(bottom)* through the thickness of the left ventricular anterior wall. Note the transition in myocardial fiber orientation relative to wall thickness from the subendocardium (perpendicular) to the midmyocardium (parallel). A mirror image transition in fiber orientation is observed from the midmyocardium to the subepicardium. *Katz AM:* Physiology of the Heart, *3rd ed. Lippincott Williams and Wilkins, 2001.*

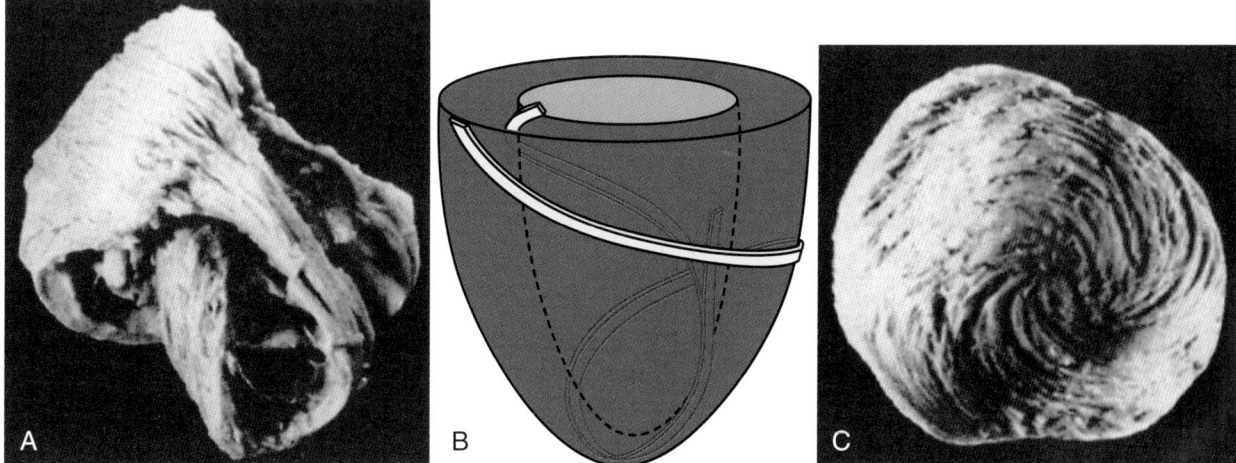

Figure 5-2 Photograph *(A)* and schematic illustration *(B)* depicting the spiral orientation of fiber continuity in the left ventricle (LV). The photograph in *A* demonstrates a dissection of the human LV anterior and lateral walls showing spiral cardiac muscle bundles sweeping from the base to the apex. This helical orientation is schematically represented in *B*. Another photograph *(C)* shows a dissection of endocardial fiber orientation at the left ventricular apex and also demonstrates this spiral fiber structure. *Katz AM:* Physiology of the Heart, *3rd ed. Lippincott Williams and Wilkins, 2001.*

*The term *layer* is used as a metaphor throughout this section.

spherical configuration has been proposed to directly contribute to the reduction in ejection fraction (EF) observed during evolving HF.[7] Elastic recoil of this systolic "wringing" motion during LV relaxation is also an important determinant of diastolic suction, a critical factor that preserves LV filling during profound hypovolemia and strenuous exercise.[8,9] In contrast with the subepicardial and subendocardial layers, most fibers within the midmyocardium are circumferentially oriented around the diameter of the LV cavity, and their contraction reduces chamber diameter.

The LV free walls are thickest near the base and gradually thin toward the apex because of a progressive decline in relative number of midmyocardial fibers. Subendocardial layers of both the left and right ventricles and combine with LV midmyocardium extending from the LV free wall to create the interventricular septum.[1] Thus, structural elements derived primarily from the LV form the septum and, as a result, the septum normally thickens toward the LV chamber during contraction. Nevertheless, systolic movement of the interventricular septum toward the RV chamber may be observed in pathologic conditions, such as acute RV distention or chronic pressure-overload RV hypertrophy. Similar to the LV free wall, a gradual decrease in the number of midmyocardial fibers produces a characteristic basal-to-apical reduction in interventricular septum thickness. The LV apical free wall is composed of subendocardial and subepicardial fibers, but the apical interventricular septum contains only LV and RV subendocardium. These regional differences in LV wall thickness and laminar myocardial fiber orientation have been shown to contribute to load-dependent alterations in LV mechanics.[10] Irregular ridges of subendocardium, termed *trabeculae carneae,* are commonly observed along the apical LV chamber border and within the RV, but the precise physiologic implications of these structural features remain unclear. Endocardial endothelium lines the subendocardium on the LV chamber surface and may play a minor role in the regulation of myocardial function.[11]

The LV apex and interventricular septum remain relatively fixed in three-dimensional (3D) space within the mediastinum during contraction. In contrast, the lateral and posterior walls move toward the anterior and the right during contraction, thereby displacing the LV longitudinal axis from a plane oriented toward the mitral valve (which favors LV filling during diastole) to a position more parallel to the LV outflow tract (which facilitates ejection during systole). The anterior-right movement of lateral and posterior LV walls during contraction also produces the point of maximum impulse, which is normally palpated on the anterior chest wall in the left fifth or sixth intercostal space in the midclavicular line. Subendocardial and subepicardial fiber shortening, papillary muscle contraction, and mechanical recoil resulting from ejection of blood into the aortic root also cause the LV base to descend toward the apex during systole. Thus, synchronous contraction of LV myocardium shortens the LV long axis, decreases the LV chamber diameter, and rotates the apex in an anterior-right direction toward the chest wall. LV ejection is also associated with an apex-to-base gradient in wall tension, thereby creating the intraventricular pressure gradient required to efficiently transfer stroke volume (SV) from the left ventricle into the proximal aorta.

The right ventricle is located in a more right-sided, anterior position than the left ventricle within the mediastinum. Unlike the thicker-walled, ellipsoidal-shaped left ventricle that propels oxygenated blood from the pulmonary venous circulation into the high-pressure systemic arterial vascular tree, the thinner-walled, crescent-shaped right ventricle pumps deoxygenated venous blood into a substantially lower pressure, more compliant pulmonary arterial bed. The right ventricle is composed of embryologically distinct inflow and outflow tracts and, as a result, contracts in a peristaltic manner, whereas the activation sequence of the left ventricle is temporally uniform. The right ventricle moves toward the interventricular septum with a "bellows-like" action. The interventricular septum and left ventricle provide a "splint" against which the RV free wall shortens during contraction. LV contraction also makes an important contribution to RV systolic function (systolic ventricular interdependence).[12] These factors give the less muscular right ventricle the mechanical advantage necessary to propel an SV equivalent to that of the left ventricle. However, the right ventricle is substantially more vulnerable than the left ventricle to acutely decompensate with modest increases in afterload because the more muscular left ventricle is able to generate pressure-volume work (stroke work [SW]) that is five- to seven-fold greater in magnitude than that produced by the right ventricle. Conversely, the right ventricle is more compliant and accommodates volume overload more easily than the left ventricle. The atrioventricular (AV) groove separating the RA and the RV and the adjacent tricuspid valve annular plane shorten toward the RV apex during contraction. This motion may be used as an index of RV contractile function by echocardiographic quantification of RV free-wall tricuspid annular plane systolic excursion.[13]

Valves

Two pairs of valves assure unidirectional blood flow through the right and left sides of the heart. The pulmonic and aortic valves are trileaflet structures located at RV and LV outlets, respectively, and operate passively with changes in hydraulic pressure gradients. The pulmonic valve leaflets are identified by their simple anatomic positions (right, left, and anterior), whereas the name of each aortic valve leaflet is derived from the presence or absence of an adjacent coronary artery ostium (right coronary cusp located adjacent to the right coronary artery [RCA] ostium, left coronary cusp located adjacent to the left main coronary artery ostium, and noncoronary cusp without a coronary ostium). The pulmonic and aortic valves open as a consequence of RV and LV ejection, respectively. The effective orifice area of each of these valves during maximal systolic blood flow is only modestly less than total cross-sectional area of the respective valve annulus. The proximal aortic root contains dilated segments, known as the sinuses of Valsalva, located immediately behind each leaflet. The sinuses of Valsalva prevent the aortic valve leaflets from closely approaching or adhering to the aortic wall by facilitating the formation of eddy currents of blood flow during ejection, thereby preventing the right and left coronary leaflets from occluding their respective coronary ostia. The eddy currents within the sinuses of Valsalva also assist with aortic valve closure at the end of ejection by assuring that the leaflets remain fully mobile during early diastole.[14] In addition, the normal velocity of blood flow through the aortic valve (approximately 1.0 m/sec) creates vortices of flow between the aortic valve leaflets and the sinuses of Valsalva that serve to further prevent leaflet-aortic wall contact.[15] In contrast with the aortic root, the proximal pulmonary artery does not contain sinuses.

The thin, flexible, and very strong mitral valve separates the LA from the LV. The mitral valve is a saddle-shaped structure containing two leaflets, identified as anterior and posterior on the basis of their anatomic location. The valve leaflets coapt in the middle of the annulus in a simple central curve in which the anterior mitral leaflet forms the convex border. The anterior mitral leaflet is oval and occupies a greater central diameter across the annulus, whereas the posterior mitral leaflet is crescent shaped and extends farther around the annular circumference. As a result, the cross-sectional area of each leaflet is similar. The leaflets are physically joined at anterior-lateral and posterior-medial commissures that are located superior to corresponding papillary muscles. The leaflets thicken slightly along the line of coaptation. The pressure gradient between the LA and LV chambers near the end of LV relaxation combined with LV mechanical recoil cause opening of the mitral valve, whereas retrograde blood flow toward the valve during LV contraction forces the previously open valve leaflets in a superior direction and produces coaptation. Thin fibrous threads, termed *chordae tendineae,* attach to the papillary muscles and prevent inversion of the valve leaflets during contraction. Primary and secondary chordae tendineae insert into the valve edges and the clear and rough zones of the valve bodies (located approximately one third of the distance between the valve edge and the annulus), respectively, of the leaflets. Tertiary chordae tendineae extend from the posteromedial papillary muscle and insert into the posterior mitral leaflet or the adjacent myocardium near the annulus. Each papillary muscle is an outpouching of subendocardial myocardium that provides chordae tendineae to both mitral valve leaflets and contracts synchronously with the main LV. Papillary muscle contraction tightens the chordae tendineae, thereby inhibiting excessive leaflet motion beyond the normal coaptation zone and preventing regurgitation of blood into the LA.[16] The mitral annular circumference also decreases modestly during LV contraction through a sphincter-like action of the surrounding subepicardial myocardium that reduces the total orifice area and assists in valve closure.[17] The importance of the functional integrity of the mitral valve apparatus to overall cardiac performance cannot be overemphasized. The apparatus not only assures unidirectional blood flow from the LA to the LV by preventing regurgitant flow into the LA and proximal pulmonary venous circulation, but also contributes to LV systolic function through papillary muscle contributions to LV apical posteromedial and anterolateral contraction. For example, loss of native chordae tendinea-papillary muscle attachments associated with mitral valve replacement is invariably associated with a modest decrease in global LV contractile function. Similarly, papillary muscle ischemia or infarction frequently causes mitral regurgitation and also may contribute to the development of LV systolic dysfunction.

The anterior (also known as anterosuperior), posterior (inferior or mural), and septal (medial) leaflets and their corresponding chordae tendineae and papillary muscles comprise the tricuspid valve that regulates blood flow from the RA to the RV. The anterior and septal leaflets are usually larger than the posterior leaflet. The presence of a septal papillary muscle distinguishes the morphologic RV from the LV in patients with certain forms of congenital heart disease (e.g., transposition of the great vessels). A lateral band of myocardium, known as the moderator band, connects the apical anterior and septal papillary muscles, and demarcates the RV inflow and outflow tracts. Relatively fine trabeculations characterize the LV subendocardial surface, but the RV contains a large quantity of coarse trabeculae carneae throughout the chamber. The reasons for this difference in trabeculation are unknown. Unlike the mitral valve, the tricuspid valve does not have a clearly defined collagenous annulus. Instead, the RA myocardium is separated from the RV by the AV groove that lies immediately above, may fold into the origin of the tricuspid leaflets, and contains the proximal portion of the RCA.

Blood Supply

Blood flow to the heart is supplied by the left anterior descending, left circumflex, and right coronary arteries (LAD, LCCA, and RCA, respectively). Most of the blood flow to the LV occurs in diastole when aortic blood pressure exceeds the LV chamber pressure, thereby establishing a positive-pressure gradient in each coronary artery. All three major coronary arteries contribute to the blood supply of the LV. As a result, acute myocardial ischemia resulting from a critical coronary artery stenosis or abrupt occlusion causes a predictable pattern of LV injury based on the known distribution of blood supply. In brief, the LAD and its branches (including septal perforators and diagonals) supply the medial half of the LV anterior wall, the apex, and the anterior two thirds of the interventricular septum. The LCCA and its obtuse marginal branches supply the anterior and posterior aspects of the lateral wall, whereas the RCA and its distal branches supply the medial portions of the posterior wall and the posterior one third of the interventricular septum. The coronary artery that supplies blood to the posterior descending coronary artery (PDA) defines the right or left "dominance" of the coronary circulation. Right dominance (PDA supplied by the RCA) is observed in approximately 80% of patients, whereas left dominance (PDA supplied by the LCCA) occurs in the remainder. Anastomoses between the distal regions of the coronary arteries or collateral blood vessels between the major coronary arteries also may exist that provide an alternative route of blood flow to myocardium distal to a severe coronary artery stenosis or complete occlusion. Either the RCA (approximately two thirds of patients) or the LCCA provides the sole blood supply to the posteromedial papillary muscle, which renders this crucial structure particularly vulnerable to acute ischemia or infarction. However, one third of patients may have a dual blood supply (RCA and LCCA) to the posterior papillary

muscle.[18] Both the LAD and the LCCA usually provide coronary blood flow to the anterolateral papillary muscle, and as a result, ischemic dysfunction of this papillary muscle is relatively uncommon.

In contrast with the LV, coronary blood flow to the RA, LA, and RV occurs throughout the cardiac cycle because both systolic and diastolic aortic blood pressures are greater than the pressure within these chambers. The RCA and its branches supply the majority of the RV, but the RV anterior wall also may receive blood from branches of the LAD. As a result, RV dysfunction may occur because of RCA or LAD ischemia. Coronary arterial blood supply to the LA is derived from branches of the LCCA.[19,20] Thus, augmented LA contractile function usually occurs in the presence of acute myocardial ischemia or infarction resulting from LAD occlusion,[21] but such a compensatory response may not be observed during compromise of LCCA blood flow concomitant with LA ischemia.[22] Branches of the RCA and the LCCA provide coronary blood flow to the RA.[19] For example, a nodal artery from the RCA (55% of patients) or the LCCA (45%) supplies blood to the sinoatrial (SA) node. Similarly, the RCA or, less commonly, the LCCA branches supply blood flow to the AV node concomitant with the right or left dominance of the coronary circulation. As a result, a critical stenosis or acute occlusion in either of these two perfusion territories may adversely affect the proximal conduction system of the heart and produce hemodynamically significant bradyarrhythmias.

Conduction

The mechanism by which the heart is electrically activated plays a crucial role in its mechanical performance.[23] The SA node is the primary cardiac pacemaker in the absence of marked decreases in firing rate, conduction delays or blockade, or accelerated firing of secondary pacemakers (e.g., AV node, bundle of His). The anterior, middle (Wenckebach), and posterior (Thorel) internodal pathways transmit the initial SA node depolarization rapidly through the RA myocardium to the AV node (Table 5-1). A branch (Bachmann's bundle) of the anterior internodal pathway also transmits the SA node depolarization from the RA to the LA across the atrial septum. The internodal pathways may be demonstrated in the electrophysiology laboratory, but microscopic examination of tissue histology usually fails to differentiate anatomically discernible bundles of morphologically distinct cardiac cells capable of more rapid impulse conduction than the atrial myocardium itself. The cartilaginous skeleton of the heart isolates the atria from the ventricles by acting as an electrical insulator. Thus, atrial depolarization is not indiscriminately transmitted throughout the heart, but instead is directed solely to the ventricles through the AV node and its distal conduction pathway, the bundle of His. This electrical isolation between the atrial and ventricular chambers and the temporal transmission delay occurring within the slowly conducting AV node establishes the normal sequential pattern of atrial followed by ventricular contraction. Abnormal accessory pathways (e.g., bundle of Kent) between the atria and ventricles may bypass the AV node and contribute to the development of reentrant supraventricular tachyarrhythmias (e.g., Wolff–Parkinson–White syndrome). The bundle of His pierces the connective tissue insulator of the cartilaginous cardiac skeleton and transmits the AV depolarization signal through the

TABLE 5-1	Cardiac Electrical Activation Sequence	
Structure	Conduction Velocity (m/sec)	Pacemaker Rate (beats/min)
Sinoatrial node	< 0.01	60–100
Atrial myocardium	1.0–1.2	None
Atrioventricular node	0.02–0.05	40–55
Bundle of His	1.2–2.0	25–40
Bundle branches	2.0–4.0	25–40
Purkinje network	2.0–4.0	25–40
Ventricular myocardium	0.3–1.0	None

Katz AM: *Physiology of the Heart*, 3rd ed. Lippincott Williams and Wilkins, 2001.

right and left bundle branches to the RV and LV myocardium, respectively, via an extensive Purkinje network located within the inner third of the ventricular walls. The bundle of His, the bundle branches, and the Purkinje network are composed of His-Purkinje fibers that assure rapid, coordinated distribution of depolarization throughout the RV and LV myocardium. This ingenious electrical design allows synchronous ventricular contraction and efficient, coordinated ejection. In contrast, artificial cardiac pacing that bypasses the normal conduction system (e.g., epicardial RV pacing) produces dyssynchronous LV activation, causes a contraction pattern that may result in suboptimal LV systolic function, and is a frequent cause of a new regional wall motion abnormality after cardiopulmonary bypass in cardiac surgical patients. This form of contractile dyssynchrony is also associated with chronic RV apical pacing (e.g., used for the treatment of sick-sinus syndrome or an AV conduction disorder) and is known to cause detrimental effects on LV chamber geometry and function.[24] Furthermore, recognition of the crucial relation between a normal electrical activation sequence and LV contractile synchrony forms the basis for the successful use of cardiac resynchronization therapy in some patients with congestive HF.[25]

CARDIAC MYOCYTE ANATOMY AND FUNCTION

▓ Ultrastructure

The ultrastructure of the cardiac myocyte is a remarkably elegant example of the architectural principle "form follows function." The external membrane of the cardiac muscle cell is known as the sarcolemma. This bilayer lipid membrane contains ion channels (e.g., Na^+, K^+, Ca^{2+}, Cl^-), active and passive ion transporters (e.g., Na^+-K^+ ATPase, Ca^{2+}-ATPase, Na^+-Ca^{2+} or -H^+ exchangers), receptors (e.g., β_1-adrenergic, muscarinic cholinergic, adenosine, opioid), and transport enzymes (e.g., glucose transporter) that modulate intracellular ion concentrations, regulate homeostasis of electrophysiology, mediate signal transduction, and provide substrates for metabolism. Deep sarcolemmal invaginations, termed *transverse* ("T") *tubules,* penetrate the myoplasm and facilitate rapid, synchronous transmission of cellular depolarization (Figure 5-3). The myocyte contains very large numbers of mitochondria responsible for the generation of high-energy phosphates (e.g., adenosine triphosphate [ATP], creatine phosphate) required for contraction and relaxation. The sarcomere is the contractile unit of cardiac myocyte and contains myofilaments arranged in parallel cross-striated bundles of thin (containing actin, tropomyosin, and the troponin complex) and

thick (primarily composed of myosin and its supporting proteins) fibers. Sarcomeres are connected in series, and as a result, the long and short axes of each myocyte simultaneously shorten and thicken, respectively, during contraction. Light and electron microscopic observations form the basis for the description of sarcomere structure. Thick and thin fibers functionally interact in an area known as the "A" band that becomes wider (indicating more pronounced overlap) as the sarcomere shortens. The sarcomere region containing thin filaments alone is termed the "I" band; the width of this band is reduced during myocyte contraction. A "Z" (derived from the German *zuckung*, meaning "twitch") line bisects each "I" band. The "Z" line denotes the border at which two adjacent sarcomeres are joined. Thus, an "A" band and two half "I" bands (between the "Z" lines) describe the length of each sarcomere. The "A" band also contains a central "M" band composed of thick filaments oriented in a cross-sectional hexagonal arrangement by myosin binding protein C.

Each cardiac myocyte contains a highly intertwined sarcoplasmic reticulum (SR) network that surrounds the contractile protein bundles. The SR serves as the primary calcium (Ca^{2+}) reservoir of the cardiac myocyte, and its extensive distribution assures almost homogenous dispersal and subsequent reaccumulation of activator Ca^{2+} throughout the myofilaments during contraction and relaxation, respectively. The SR contains specialized structures, known as subsarcolemmal cisternae, located adjacent to the sarcolemma and T tubules. These subsarcolemmal cisternae contain a dense concentration of ryanodine receptors that function as the SR's primary Ca^{2+} release channel and facilitate Ca^{2+}-induced Ca^{2+} release immediately on sarcolemmal depolarization. The contractile apparatus and the mitochondria that supply its energy comprise more than 80% of the myocyte's total volume, whereas the cytosol and nucleus occupy less than 15%. This observation emphasizes that contraction, and not de novo protein synthesis, is the predominant function of the cardiac myocyte. Intercalated disks not only mechanically join adjacent myocytes via the fascia adherens (which links actin molecules at each Z line) and desmosomes, but also create electrical transparency between myocytes through gap junctions that allow diffusion of ions and small molecules.

▓ Proteins of the Contractile Apparatus

The contractile apparatus is composed of six major components: myosin, actin, tropomyosin, and the three-protein troponin complex. Myosin (molecular weight = 500 kDa; length = 0.17 μm) contains a pair of intertwined α-helical proteins (tails), each with a globular head that binds the actin molecule, and two adjoining pairs of light chains. Enzymatic digestion of myosin reveals the presence of "light"

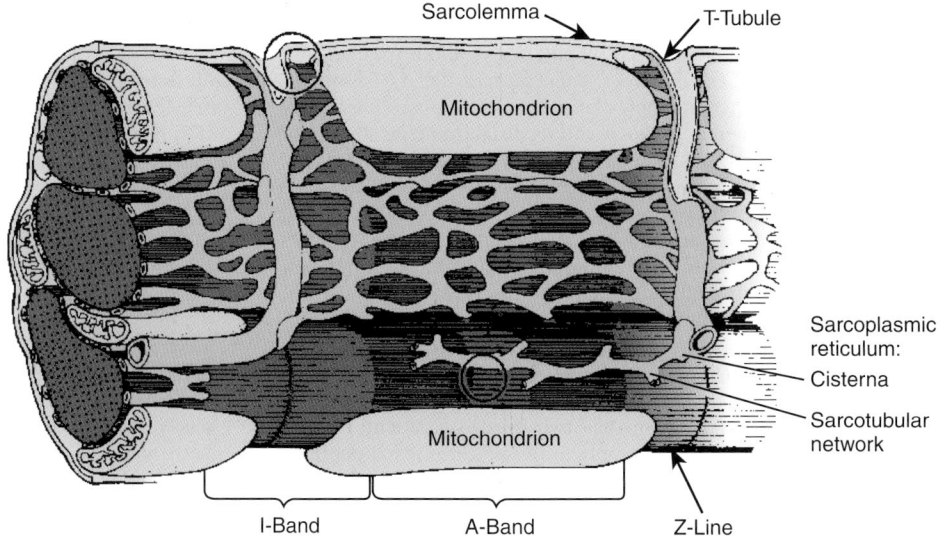

Figure 5-3   Arnold Katz's schematic illustration depicting the ultrastructure of the cardiac myocyte. *Katz AM: Physiology of the Heart, 3rd ed. Lippincott Williams and Wilkins, 2001.*

(composed of the tail sections) and "heavy" (containing the globular heads and the light chains) meromyosin. The primary structural support of the myosin molecule is the elongated tail section ("light" meromyosin). The globular heads of the myosin dimer contain two "hinges" that are located at the distal light chain tail–double helix junction. These hinges are responsible for myofilament shortening during contraction. The binding of the myosin head to the actin molecule stimulates a cascade of events initiated by activation of a myosin ATPase that mediates both hinge rotation and actin release during contraction and relaxation, respectively. The activity of this actin-activated myosin ATPase is a major determinant of the maximum velocity of sarcomere shortening. Of note, several different myosin ATPase isoforms have been identified in adult and neonatal atrial and ventricular myocardium that are distinguished by their relative ATPase activity. Myosin molecules are oriented in series along the length of the thick filament and are joined "tail to tail" in the filament's center at the M line. Such an orientation produces equivalent shortening of each half of the sarcomere as the actin molecules are pulled toward the center.

The four light chains in the myosin complex are considered "regulatory" or "essential." Regulatory myosin light chains affect the interaction between myosin and actin by modulating the phosphorylation state of Ca^{2+}-dependent protein kinases. In contrast, essential light chains serve vital, but currently undefined, roles in myosin activity because their removal denatures the myosin molecule. Notably, LV hypertrophy is characterized by myosin light chain isoform alterations from ventricular to atrial forms that may play an important role in the contractile dysfunction associated with this disorder.[26] These interesting data suggest that genetic modulation of light-chain isoform expression may form the basis for pathologic changes in function in some cardiac disease states. Thick filaments are not only composed of myosin and its binding protein, but also contain titin, a long elastic molecule that attaches myosin to the Z lines. Titin is an important contributor to myocardial elasticity and, similar to a bidirectional spring, acts as a "length sensor" by establishing greater passive restoring forces as sarcomere length approaches its maximum or minimum.[27] Titin compression and stretching are observed during decreases and increases in load that serve to limit additional shortening and lengthening of the sarcomere, respectively. Thus, titin is another important elastic element (in addition to actin and myosin) that mediates the stress-strain biomechanical properties of cardiac muscle.[28]

Actin is the major component of the thin filament and is composed of a 42-kDa oval-shaped, globular protein (known as the "G" form; diameter = 5.5 nm). Actin exists in a polymerized filamentous configuration ("F" form) wound in double-stranded helical chains of G-actin monomers that resemble two intertwined strands of pearls. Each complete helical revolution of F-actin contains 14 G-actin monomers and is 77 nm in length. F-actin does not directly hydrolyze high-energy nucleotides (e.g., ATP), but the molecule does bind adenosine diphosphate (ADP) and divalent cations such as Ca^{2+} and Mg^{2+}. Actin functions as the "activator" (hence its name) of myosin ATPase through its reversible binding with myosin. This actin-myosin complex is capable of hydrolyzing ATP, thereby supplying the energy required to cause the conformational changes in the myosin heads that mediate the cycle of contraction and relaxation within the sarcomere. Tropomyosin (weight = 68 and 72 kDa; length = 40 nm) is a major inhibitor of the interaction between actin and myosin, and consists of a rigid double-stranded α-helix protein linked by a single disulfide bond. Human tropomyosin contains both α and β isoforms (34 and 36 kDa, respectively), and may exist as either a homodimer or heterodimer.[29] The Ca^{2+}-dependent interaction of tropomyosin with the troponin complex is the primary mechanism by which excitation-contraction coupling occurs; that is, the association between sarcolemmal membrane depolarization and the resultant binding of actin and myosin that is responsible for contraction of the cardiac myocyte. Tropomyosin also stiffens the thin filament through its position within the longitudinal cleft between the interwoven F-actin helices. Several cytoskeletal proteins (e.g., α- and β-actinin, nebulette) anchor the thin filaments to the Z lines of the sarcomere.[30]

The troponin complex consists of three proteins that are critical regulators of the contractile apparatus. Each troponin protein serves a distinct role.[31] Troponin complexes are interspersed at 40-nm intervals along the thin filament. A highly conserved, single isoform of troponin C (named for the molecule's Ca^{2+} binding ability) exists in cardiac muscle. The structure of this protein consists of a central nine-turn α helix separating two globular regions that contain four discrete divalent cation-binding amino acid sequences, two of which (termed "sites I and II") are Ca^{2+} specific. As a result, the troponin C molecule is able to directly respond to the acute changes in intracellular Ca^{2+} concentration that accompany contraction and relaxation. Troponin I ("I" for "inhibitor"; 23 kDa) exists in a single isoform in cardiac muscle. Troponin I alone weakly interferes with actin-myosin interaction, but becomes the major inhibitor of actin-myosin binding when combined with tropomyosin. This inhibition is responsive to receptor-operated signal transduction, as the troponin I molecule contains a serine residue that is susceptible to protein kinase A (PKA)–mediated phosphorylation through the intracellular second messenger cyclic adenosine monophosphate. Such phosphorylation of this serine residue reduces the ability of troponin C to bind Ca^{2+}, an action that facilitates relaxation during administration of positive inotropic drugs including β-adrenoceptor agonists (e.g., dobutamine) and phosphodiesterase fraction III (PDE III) inhibitors (e.g., milrinone). Troponin T (the "T" identifies the protein's ability to bind other troponin molecules and tropomyosin) is the largest of the troponin proteins and has four major human isoforms. Troponin T serves as an anchor for the other troponin molecules and also may influence the relative Ca^{2+} sensitivity of the troponin C.[32]

Ca^{2+}-Myofilament Interaction

Ca^{2+}-troponin C binding produces a sequence of conformational changes in the troponin-tropomyosin complex that expose the specific myosin-binding site on actin (Figure 5-4). Small amounts of Ca^{2+} are bound to troponin C when intracellular Ca^{2+} concentration is low during diastole (10^{-7} M). Under these conditions, the troponin complex confines each tropomyosin molecule to the outer region of the groove between F-actin filaments, thereby effectively preventing the interaction of myosin and actin by blocking the formation of cross-bridges between these proteins. This resting inhibitory state is rapidly transformed by the 100-fold increase in intracellular Ca^{2+} concentration (to 10^{-5} M) occurring as a consequence of sarcolemmal depolarization that opens L- and T-type Ca^{2+} channels, allows Ca^{2+} influx from the extracellular space, and stimulates ryanodine receptor–mediated, Ca^{2+}-induced Ca^{2+} release from the SR. Ca^{2+}-troponin C binding occurs under these conditions, and this action not only elongates the troponin C protein but enhances its interactions with troponin T and I. Such

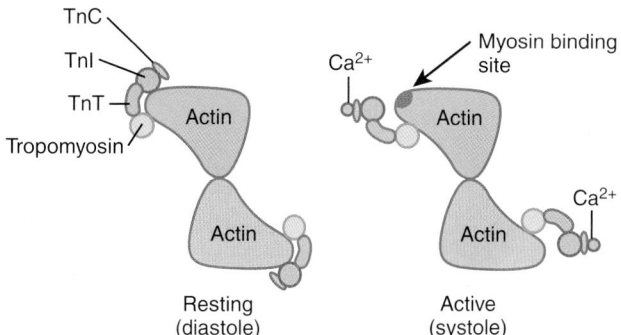

Figure 5-4 Cross-sectional schematic illustration demonstrates the structural relationship between the troponin-tropomyosin complex and the actin filament under resting conditions (diastole; *left*) and after Ca^{2+} binding (systole; *right*). Ca^{2+} binding produces a conformational shift in the troponin-tropomyosin complex toward the groove between the actin molecules, thereby exposing the myosin binding site on actin. TnC, troponin C; TnI, troponin I; TnT, troponin T. *Katz AM: Physiology of the Heart, 3rd ed. Lippincott Williams and Wilkins, 2001.*

Ca^{2+}-mediated allosteric alterations in the structure of the troponin complex weaken the interaction between troponin I and actin, promote repositioning of the tropomyosin molecule relative to the F-actin filaments, and minimize the previously described inhibition of actin-myosin binding by tropomyosin that is observed during low intracellular Ca^{2+} concentrations.[33] Thus, Ca^{2+}-troponin C binding stimulates a sequence of alterations in the chemical conformation of the regulatory proteins that reveal the binding site for myosin on the actin molecule and allow cross-bridge formation and contraction to occur. Subsequent dissociation of Ca^{2+} from troponin C fully reverses this antagonism of inhibition, prevents further myosin-actin interaction, and facilitates relaxation by rapidly restoring of the original conformation of the troponin-tropomyosin complex on F-actin.

An energy-dependent ion pump (Ca^{2+}-ATPase) located in the SR membrane (abbreviated as "SERCA" for SR Ca^{2+}-ATPase) removes most Ca^{2+} ions from the myofilaments and the myoplasm after the sarcolemmal membrane is repolarized. This activator Ca^{2+} is stored in the SR at a concentration of approximately 10^{-3} M and is transiently bound to calsequestrin and calrectulin until the next sarcolemmal depolarization occurs and ryanodine receptor–activated SR channels open again. Another Ca^{2+}-ATPase and a Na$^+$/Ca^{2+} exchanger passively driven by ion concentration gradients, each located in the sarcolemmal membrane, also play roles in the removal of substantially smaller amounts of Ca^{2+} from the myoplasm after repolarization. Phospholamban is a small protein (6 kDa) located in the SR membrane that modulates the activity of SERCA by partially inhibiting the dominant form (type 2a) of this main Ca^{2+} pump under baseline conditions. However, PKA-induced phosphorylation of phospholamban antagonizes this baseline inhibition and enhances SERCA-mediated Ca^{2+} uptake into the SR.[34] Thus, drugs such as dobutamine and milrinone that act by modifying PKA-mediated signal transduction enhance the rate and extent of relaxation by facilitating Ca^{2+} reuptake (positive lusitropic effect), while simultaneously increasing the amount of Ca^{2+} available for the next contractile activation (positive inotropic effect).

Biochemistry of Myosin-Actin Interaction

A four-component kinetic model is most often used to describe the biochemistry of cardiac muscle contraction (Figure 5-5).[35] High-affinity binding of ATP to the catalytic domain of myosin initiates a coordinated sequence of events that results in sarcomere shortening. The myosin ATPase enzyme hydrolyzes the ATP molecule into ADP and inorganic phosphate. These products remain bound to myosin, thereby forming an "active" complex that retains the reaction's chemical energy as potential energy. In the absence of actin, ADP and phosphate eventually dissociate from myosin and the muscle remains relaxed. The activity of myosin ATPase is substantially enhanced when the myosin-ADP-phosphate complex is bound to actin, and under these conditions, the energy released by ATP hydrolysis is translated into mechanical work. Myosin binding to actin releases the phosphate anion from the myosin head, thereby producing a tension-inducing molecular conformation within the cross-bridge.[36] Release of ADP and potential energy from this "activated" orientation combine to rotate the cross-bridge ("power stroke") at the hinge point separating the helical tail from the globular head of the myosin molecule. Each cross-bridge rotation generates approximately 3.5 × 10^{-12} newtons of force, and myosin moves 11 nm along the actin molecule.[37] The myosin-active complex does not immediately dissociate after rotation of the myosin head rotation and ADP release, but instead remains in a low-energy bound ("rigor") state. Subsequent dissociation of the myosin and actin molecules occurs only when a new ATP molecule binds to myosin. This four-step process is then repeated, assuming an adequate ATP supply and lack of inhibition of the myosin-binding site on actin by the troponin-tropomyosin complex.

Several factors may affect cross-bridge biochemistry and the sarcomere shortening that it produces. There is a direct relation between the maximal velocity of unloaded muscle shortening (V$_{max}$) and myosin ATPase activity. The 100-fold increase in intracellular Ca^{2+} concentration associated with sarcolemmal depolarization enhances myosin ATPase activity by a factor of 5 before it interacts with actin, thereby increasing V$_{max}$. The extent of sarcomere shortening during contraction is also dependent on sarcomere length before sarcolemmal depolarization. This length-dependent activation is known as the Frank–Starling effect in the intact heart, and may be related to an increase in myofilament Ca^{2+} sensitivity, more optimal spacing between actin and myosin, or titin-induced elastic recoil. Abrupt increases in load during shortening (termed the *Anrep effect*) or after an extended pause between a series of contractions (known as the *Woodworth phenomenon*) cause transient increases in contractile force through such a length-dependent activation mechanism. An increase in stimulation frequency also augments

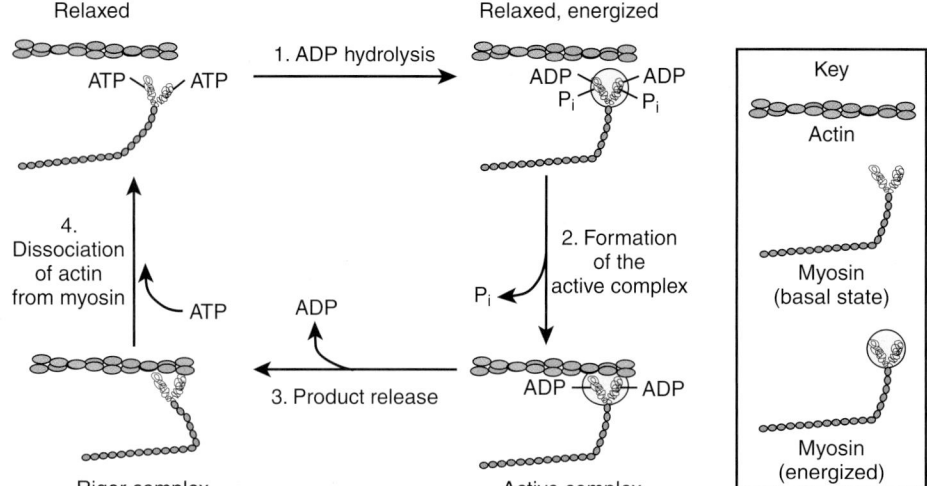

Figure 5-5 Schematic illustration demonstrates the four-step reaction mechanism for actin-myosin adenosine triphosphatase (ATPase). The reaction begins with ATP bound to the myosin heads (top left). The hydrolysis of this myosin-bound ATP energizes the myosin heads, which retain the products of the reaction (adenosine diphosphate [ADP] and inositol phosphate [P$_i$]) as potential energy. At this stage, the muscle remains relaxed because myosin is not attached to actin (top right). Dissociation of phosphate occurs when the activated myosin heads bind to the actin filament (bottom right). The dissociation of ADP from the myosin heads releases the chemical energy of the ATP hydrolysis and shifts the position of the myosin crossbridge, thereby performing mechanical work (bottom left). Binding of new ATP molecules to the myosin head dissociates this "rigor complex" and completes the cycle. *Katz AM: Physiology of the Heart, 3rd ed. Lippincott Williams and Wilkins, 2001.*

shortening through enhanced myofilament Ca^{2+} sensitivity and more pronounced release of Ca^{2+} from the SR.

LAPLACE'S LAW

It is clear based on the previous discussion that the sarcomere generates tension and shortens during contraction, and thereafter it releases this developed tension and lengthens during relaxation. However, the intact heart produces pressure on and causes ejection of a volume of blood. Thus, the alterations in muscle tension and length observed in the sarcomere require transformation into the phasic changes in pressure and volume that occur in the intact heart.[38] Laplace's law facilitates this conversion of the contractile behavior of individual sarcomeres or isolated, linear cardiac muscle preparations in vitro into three-dimensional (3-D) chamber function in vivo, thereby permitting a systematic examination of the intact heart's ability to function as a hydraulic pump. The relation between myocyte length and chamber volume (V) may be modeled as a pressurized, spherical shell (Figure 5-6),[39] where volume is proportional to the cube of the radius (r) such that $V = 4\pi r^3/3$. This model may be pedagogically useful and will be used for the following discussion, but the LV and the atria are more precisely described using prolate ellipsoidal geometry, which defines three axes corresponding to the anterior-posterior, septal-lateral, and long-axis diameters $(D_{AP}, D_{SL},$ and D_{LA}, respectively), such that $V = \pi D_{AP} D_{SL} D_{LA}/6$. This technique of measuring LV or atrial volume more closely approximates anatomic reality and has been validated extensively in experimental animals[40,41] and humans.[42,43] However, such a method does not apply when attempting to describe RV volume because of the unique bellows-shaped structure of this chamber.[44]

The relation between wall stress (defined as tension exerted over a cross-sectional area) and pressure within a cardiac chamber is complex. Laplace's law relates wall stress to pressure and chamber geometry, which may be determined based on three major suppositions[38]: First, the chamber is assumed to be spherical with a uniform wall thickness (h) and an internal radius (r); second, the stress (σ) throughout the thickness of the chamber wall is assumed to be constant; and finally, the chamber remains in static equilibrium (i.e., is not actively contracting). Tension development within each sarcomere causes a corresponding increase in wall stress that is translated into the generation of hydraulic pressure within the chamber. Within this context, internal pressure (P) is defined as an orthogonal distending force exerted against the chamber walls, whereas wall stress is a shear force exerted around the

circumference of the chamber.[38] Bisecting the chamber into two equal halves exposes the internal forces within it (see Figure 5-6). The product of internal pressure and wall cross-sectional area (πr^2) represents the total force tending to repel the chamber hemispheres. In contrast, the total force within the chamber walls resists this distracting force and is equal to the σ times the cross-sectional wall area. The two forces must balance for the chamber to remain in equilibrium such that $P\pi r^2 = \sigma[\pi(r + h)^2 - \pi r^2]$. This equation may be algebraically simplified to the form $Pr = \sigma h(2 + h/r)$ by removal of the redundant terms. The chamber wall is normally thin relative to its internal radius. As a result, the h/r term may be neglected and the remaining expression may be rearranged to become the more familiar $\sigma = Pr/2h$. This simple derivation of Laplace's law indicates that wall stress varies directly with internal pressure and radius, and inversely with wall thickness. Despite the observation that the ratio of wall thickness to radius is not entirely negligible at LV end-diastole ($h/r = 0.4$),[45] Laplace's law for a thin-walled sphere provides a useful description of the factors that contribute to changes in LV or atrial wall stress. For example, LV dilation associated with chronic aortic insufficiency increases global LV wall stress that reflects greater tension on each sarcomere within the chamber wall.[46] Similarly, the persistent increase of LV pressure observed in the presence of severe aortic stenosis also produces greater stress on the LV wall. Such increases in wall stress resulting from chronic volume or pressure overload are directly translated into greater myocardial oxygen demand because the myofilaments require more energy to develop this degree of enhanced tension. In contrast, an increase in wall thickness causes a reduction in global wall stress and tension developed by individual sarcomeres. Thus, Laplace's law predicts that hypertrophy is a critically important compensatory response to chronically altered chamber load that serves to reduce the tension generated by each muscle fiber. Prolate ellipsoidal models of chamber geometry and those incorporating orthogonal radial, circumferential, and meridional components of wall stress require more complex derivations of Laplace's law[47] that may be corrected with dimensional measurements obtained using echocardiography.[48] Formal derivations of these models are beyond the scope of the current chapter but are available elsewhere.[49,50]

In contrast with the assumption used in the derivation of Laplace's law for a simple sphere, wall stress is not uniformly distributed across LV thickness in the intact heart,[51] but instead is greatest in the subendocardium and progressively declines to a minimum at the epicardial surface. These regional differences in wall stress become especially important in LV pressure overload hypertrophy (e.g., aortic stenosis, severe hypertension),[52] as the subendocardium is exposed to more pronounced increases in intraventricular pressure concomitant with greater myocardial oxygen demand that make it more susceptible to ischemia. The combination of increased subendocardial wall stress and oxygen demand is particularly deleterious in the presence of a flow-limiting coronary artery stenosis and may contribute to the relatively common occurrence of subendocardial myocardial infarction in the absence of complete coronary occlusion in patients with severe LV hypertrophy.

CARDIAC CYCLE

The cardiac cycle describes a highly coordinated, temporally related series of electrical, mechanical, and valvular events (Figure 5-7).[53] A single cardiac cycle occurs in 0.8 second at a HR of 75 beats/min. Synchronous depolarization of RV and LV myocardium (as indicated by the electrocardiogram QRS complex) initiates contraction of and produces a rapid increase in pressure within these chambers (systole). Closure of the tricuspid and mitral valves occurs when RV and LV pressures exceed the corresponding atrial pressures and cause the first heart sound (S_1). LV systole is divided into isovolumic contraction, rapid ejection, and slower ejection phases. LV isovolumic contraction describes the time interval between mitral valve closure and aortic valve opening during which LV volume remains constant. Nevertheless, global LV geometry is transformed from an ellipsoidal shape at end-diastole to a more spherical configuration during isovolumic contraction because the

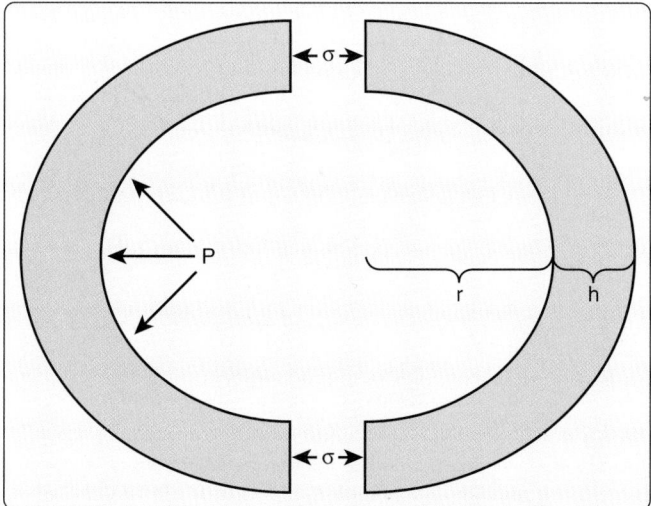

Figure 5-6 Schematic diagram depicts the opposing forces within a theoretical left ventricular (LV) sphere that determine Laplace's law. LV pressure *(P)* tends to push the sphere apart, whereas wall stress (σ) holds the sphere together. h, LV thickness; r, LV radius.

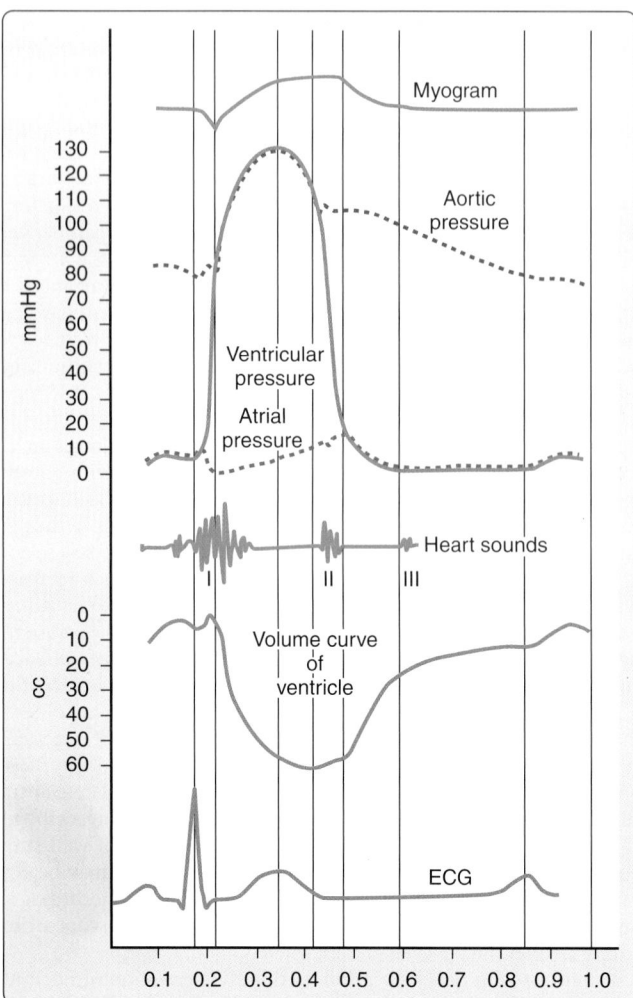

Figure 5-7   Carl Wiggers' original figure depicts the electrical, mechanical, and audible events of the cardiac cycle including the electrocardiogram (ECG); aortic, left ventricular, and left atrial pressure waveforms; left ventricular volume waveform; and heart tones associated with mitral and aortic valve closure. *Wiggers CJ: The Henry Jackson Memorial Lecture. Dynamics of ventricular contraction under abnormal conditions,* Circulation *5:321–348, 1952.*

length of the longitudinal axis (base-apex) shortens and LV wall thickness increases.[54] The maximum rate of increase of LV pressure (dP/dt_{max}) occurs during LV isovolumic contraction and may be used to estimate myocardial contractility in vivo.[55] True isovolumic contraction most likely does not occur in the RV because of the sequential nature of contraction of the inflow and outflow tracts.[55] The pressures in the aortic and pulmonic roots decline to their minimum value immediately before the corresponding valves open. Rapid ejection occurs when LV and RV pressures exceed aortic and pulmonary arterial pressures, respectively. Approximately two thirds of the end-diastolic volume of each ventricle is ejected during this rapid-ejection phase. Dilation of the elastic aorta and proximal great vessels, and to a lesser extent, the pulmonary artery and its proximal branches, occurs concomitant with this rapid increase in volume as the kinetic energy of LV and RV contraction is transferred to the aorta and pulmonary artery, respectively, as potential energy. The compliance of the proximal systemic and pulmonary arterial vessels determines the amount of potential energy that may be stored and subsequently released to their respective distal vascular beds during diastole. Further ejection of additional blood from the LV and RV declines precipitously as the pressures within the aorta and pulmonary artery reach their maximum values. Ejection ceases entirely when the LV and RV begin to repolarize and the arterial forces resisting

further ejection are greater than the ventricular forces continuing to drive blood flow forward. As the period of slower ejection comes to an end, aortic and pulmonary artery pressures briefly exceed LV and RV pressures. These pressure gradients cause the aortic and pulmonic valves to close, an action that produces the second heart sound (S_2), signifying the end of systole and the beginning of diastole. The aortic valve closes slightly before the pulmonic valve during inspiration because RV ejection is modestly prolonged by augmented venous return, thereby causing normal physiologic splitting of S_2. The normal end-diastolic and end-systolic volumes (V_{ed} and V_{es}) are approximately 120 and 40 mL, respectively. Thus, SV (the difference between V_{ed} and V_{es}) is 80 mL and EF (the ratio of SV to V_{ed}) is 67%.[56]

LV diastole is divided into isovolumic relaxation, early ventricular filling, diastasis, and atrial systole. LV isovolumic relaxation defines the period between aortic valve closure and mitral valve opening during which LV volume remains constant. LV pressure rapidly declines as the myofilaments relax. When LV pressure declines to less than LA pressure, the mitral valve opens, and blood volume stored in the LA enters the LV driven by the initial pressure gradient between the chambers. Notably, LV pressure continues to decline after mitral valve opening as sarcomere relaxation is completed and myocardial elastic components recoil (Figure 5-8).[57–59] These factors contribute to the creation of a time-dependent pressure gradient between the LA and LV that extends to the apex.[58] The rate and extent of LV pressure decline and the LA pressure when the mitral valve opens determine the initial magnitude of the pressure gradient between these chambers.[60] Early LV filling occurs rapidly, as indicated by the observation that the peak blood flow velocity across the mitral valve during this phase of diastole may exceed the flow rate across the aortic valve during LV contraction.[61] Vortex formation from the primary mitral blood flow jet also facilitates selective filling of the LV outflow tract.[62,63] Delays in LV relaxation may occur as a consequence of age or disease processes (e.g., ischemia, hypertrophy) and are a common cause of attenuated early LV filling because the initial LA-LV pressure gradient is reduced under these circumstances.[64] After the mitral valve opens, the pressure gradient between the LA and the LV is temporally dependent on the relative pressure in each chamber. Notably, most of the increase in LV volume observed during early ventricular filling occurs while LV pressure continues to decrease. In fact, LV pressure has been shown to decrease to a subatmospheric level if blood flow across

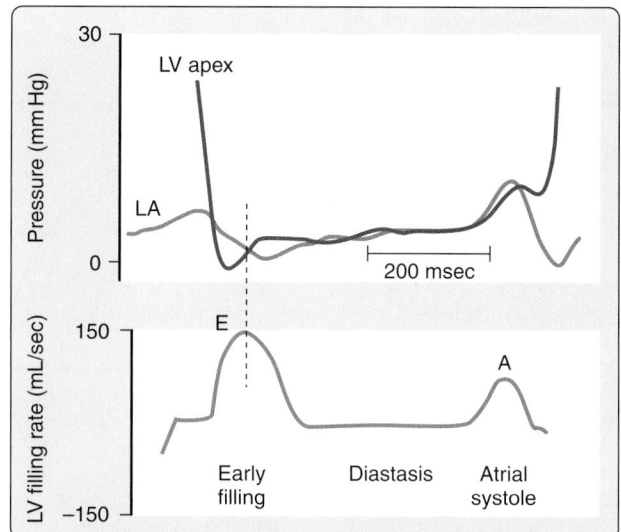

Figure 5-8   Diagram depicts the relation between left ventricular (LV) and left atrial (LA) pressure (top) and the corresponding LV filling rate (bottom) during early filling *(E)*, diastasis, and atrial systole *(A)*. Note that LV pressure initially decreases to less than LA pressure, thereby creating a pressure gradient between the chambers that causes early LV filling. *Little WC, Oh JK: Echocardiographic evaluation of diastolic function can be used to guide clinical care,* Circulation *120:802–809, 2009.*

the mitral valve is completely obstructed.[8,65] These data imply that the LV ventricle will continue to fill through this "diastolic suction" mechanism even if LA pressure is zero.[66,67] The early filling phase of diastole normally provides 70% to 75% of the total SV ejected during the subsequent LV contraction and ends when LA and LV pressures equilibrate or the gradient between these chambers transiently reverses. The mitral valve remains open and pulmonary venous blood flow directly traverses the LA into the LV after the LA and LV pressures have equalized. Thus, the LA acts as a simple conduit during this diastasis phase of diastole, and LV filling markedly slows as a result. The small amount of blood flow from pulmonary veins occurring during diastasis usually adds less than 5% to the total LV SV.[68] Progressive increases in HR shorten and may completely eliminate diastasis, but such a response to tachycardia has little, if any, effect on overall LV filling. Atrial systole is the final phase of diastole. LA contraction increases the pressure in this chamber, thereby again creating a positive pressure gradient for blood flow from the LA and the LV. The peristaltic pattern of LA contraction and the unique anatomy of the pulmonary venous-LA junction largely prevent retrograde blood flow into the pulmonary veins during atrial systole at normal LA pressures.[69] Atrial systole usually accounts for between 15% and 25% of total left ventricular stroke volume (LVSV), but this LA "kick" becomes especially important to the maintenance of LV filling in pathologic states characterized by delayed LV relaxation or reduced LV compliance.[70] Similarly, improperly timed LA contraction or the onset of atrial tachyarrhythmias (e.g., atrial fibrillation) may cause profound hemodynamic compromise in patients with myocardial ischemia or pressure-overload hypertrophy who are particularly dependent on atrial systole for LV filling. Descriptions of RV diastole are similar to those used to characterize LV diastole, with the exception that true isovolumic relaxation most likely does not occur in the RV.

The LA pressure waveform is composed of three major deflections during normal sinus rhythm. The LA contracts immediately after the P wave of atrial depolarization is recorded on the electrocardiogram, producing the "a" wave of atrial systole. This wave may be enhanced by an increase in LA preload or contractile state. The rate of deceleration of the a wave has been shown to be an index of LA relaxation.[71] LV contraction with the onset of systole causes a pressure wave to be transmitted to the LA in retrograde fashion by closure of the mitral valve, resulting in a small increase in LA pressure. This "c" wave may become more pronounced in the presence of mitral valve prolapse. During late LV isovolumic contraction, LV ejection, and the majority of LV isovolumic relaxation, pulmonary venous blood progressively fills the LA and gradually increases LA pressure, resulting in the LA "v" wave. This v wave may be augmented in the presence of mitral regurgitation or reductions in LA compliance.[72] RA pressure waveform deflections are similar to those observed in the LA. This RA a-c-v waveform morphology is transmitted to the jugular veins and may be clinically observed in the neck during routine physical examination in the supine position. In contrast with the biphasic nature of LA and RA pressure waveforms, the volume waveforms of these chambers are essentially monophasic. For example, minimum LA volume occurs immediately after the completion of LA contraction and corresponds closely to the mitral valve closure, whereas maximal LA volume is observed immediately before the mitral valve opens.

PRESSURE-VOLUME DIAGRAMS

A time-dependent, two-dimensional (2D) plot of continuous LV pressure and volume throughout a single cardiac cycle creates a phase space diagram that provides a useful framework for the analysis of LV systolic and diastolic function in the ejecting heart (Figure 5-9). Otto Frank initially described the theoretic foundations of this technique at the end of the 19th century,[73,74] but Hiroyuki Suga and Kiichi Sagawa[†] were the first

---

[†]The reader should consult the definitive textbook by these investigators and their collaborators for a detailed description of pressure-volume analysis of cardiac function: Sagawa K, Maughan L, Suga H, Sunagawa K: *Cardiac Contraction and the Pressure-Volume Relationship.* New York: Oxford University Press, 1988.

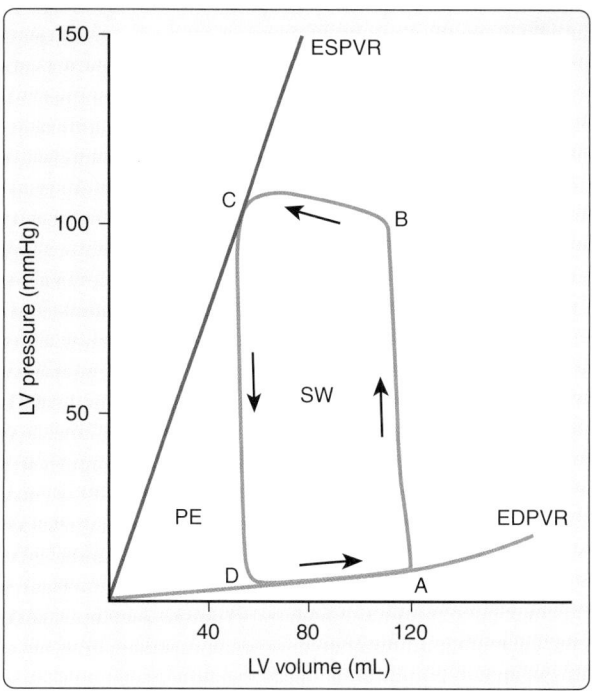

Figure 5-9 Steady-state left ventricular (LV) pressure-volume diagram. The cardiac cycle proceeds in a time-dependent counterclockwise direction *(arrows)*. Points A, B, C, and D correspond to LV end-diastole (closure of the mitral valve), opening of the aortic valve, LV end-systole (closure of the aortic valve), and opening of the mitral valve, respectively. Segments AB, BC, CD, and DA represent isovolumic contraction, ejection, isovolumic relaxation, and filling, respectively. The LV is constrained to operate within the boundaries of the end-systolic and end-diastolic pressure-volume relations (ESPVR and EDPVR, respectively). The area inscribed by the LV pressure-volume diagram is stroke work (SW; kinetic energy) performed during the cardiac cycle. The area to the left of the LV pressure-volume diagram between ESPVR and EDPVR is the remaining potential energy (PE) of the system. The sum of SW and PE is pressure-volume area.

to widely apply pressure-volume analysis after technologic advances enabled the continuous measurement of high-fidelity LV pressure (e.g., using a miniature micromanometer implanted in the chamber) and LV volume (e.g., sonomicrometry, conductance catheter).[75–77] Alterations in LV pressure with respect to volume occur in a counterclockwise fashion over time. The cardiac cycle begins at end-diastole (point A, Figure 5-9). An abrupt increase in LV pressure at constant LV volume occurs during isovolumic contraction. Opening of the aortic valve occurs when LV pressure exceeds aorta pressure (point B, Figure 5-9) and ejection begins. LV volume decreases rapidly as blood is ejected from the LV into the aorta and proximal great vessels. When LV pressure declines below aortic pressure at the end of ejection, the aortic valve closes (point C, Figure 5-9). This event is immediately followed by a rapid decline in LV pressure in the absence of changes in LV volume (isovolumic relaxation). The mitral valve opens when LV pressure decreases to less than LA pressure (point D, Figure 5-9), thereby initiating LV filling. The LV pressure-volume diagram is completed as the LV refills its volume for the next contraction concomitant with relatively small increases in pressure during early filling, diastasis, and LA systole.

The steady-state LV pressure-volume diagram provides advantages over temporal plots of individual LV pressure and volume waveforms when recognizing major cardiac events without electrocardiographic correlation (e.g., aortic or mitral valve opening or closing) or identifying acute alterations in LV loading conditions. For example, end-diastolic and end-systolic volumes may immediately be recognized as the lower right (point A) and upper left (point C) corners of Figure 5-9, respectively, allowing rapid calculation of SV and EF. Movement of the right

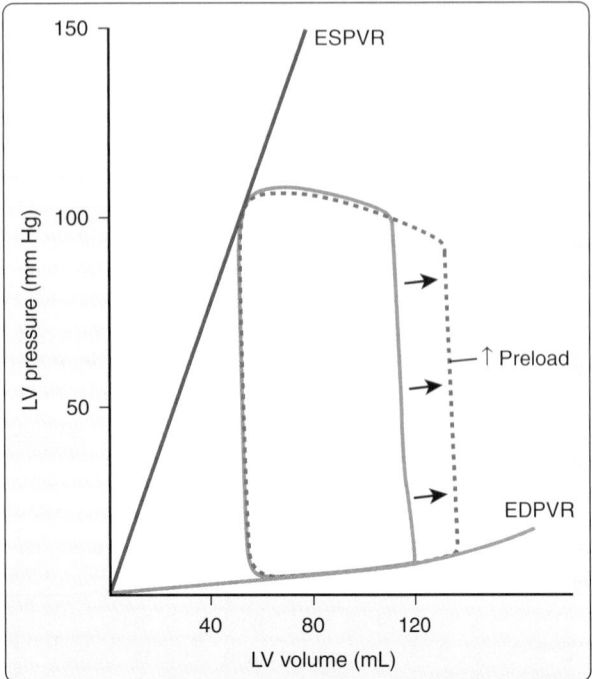 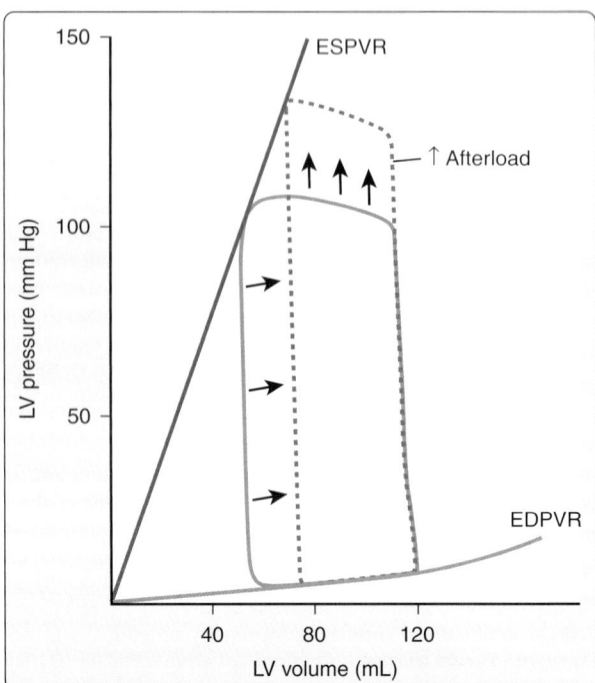

Figure 5-10 Schematic illustrations demonstrate alterations in the steady-state left ventricular (LV) pressure-volume diagram produced by a pure theoretical increase in LV preload (*left*) and afterload (*right*). Additional preload causes direct increases in stroke volume and LV end-diastolic pressure, whereas an acute increase in afterload produces greater LV pressure but also reduces stroke volume. EDPVR, end-diastolic pressure-volume relation; ESPVR, end-systolic pressure-volume relation.

side of the pressure-volume diagram to the right is characteristic of an increase in preload concomitant with larger SV, whereas an increase in afterload causes the pressure-volume diagram to become taller (greater LV pressure) and narrower (decreased SV; Figure 5-10). The area of the diagram precisely defines the LV pressure-volume (stroke) work (kinetic energy) for a single cardiac cycle. As illustrative as a single LV pressure-volume diagram may be for obtaining basic physiologic information, it is the dynamic changes of a series of these LV pressure-volume diagrams occurring during an acute alteration in LV load over several consecutive cardiac cycles that truly provide unique insight into LV systolic and diastolic function. Such a series of differentially loaded LV pressure-volume diagrams may be generated by transient changes in preload or afterload using mechanical (e.g., vena caval or aortic constriction, respectively) or pharmacologic (e.g., sodium nitroprusside or phenylephrine infusions, respectively) techniques. This nested set of diagrams allows calculation of relatively HR- and load-insensitive estimates of myocardial contractility in vivo such as the end-systolic pressure-volume relation (ESPVR; the slope of the relation is termed *end-systolic elastance* [E_{es}])[77] and the SW–end-diastolic volume relation (a linear Frank–Starling analog also known as "preload recruitable stroke work")[78]. This family of pressure-volume diagrams also describes the end-diastolic pressure-volume relation (EDPVR) that characterizes LV compliance and is a primary determinant of LV filling.[38] Thus, the ESPVR and EDPVR define the operative constraints of the LV (see Figures 5-9 and 5-10). The ESPVR and the EDPVR are determined by the intrinsic properties of the LV during systole and diastole, respectively, but the relative positions of the end-diastolic and end-systolic points that lie along these lines for any given cardiac cycle are established primarily by venous return and arterial vascular tone (i.e., preload and afterload).[79] This essential unifying concept emphasizes that analysis of overall cardiovascular performance in vivo must not consider the LV or the systemic circulation with which it interacts as an independent entity.[80] The area to the left of the steady-state LV pressure-volume diagram that lies between the ESPVR and the EDPVR is the remaining potential energy of the system (see Figure 5-9) and is an important factor in determining the LV mechanical energetics and efficiency.[81] RV systolic and diastolic function also may be quantified using the principles of this pressure-volume theory.[82]

The pressure-volume plane also provides a valuable illustration of the pathophysiology of LV systolic or diastolic dysfunction as underlying causes for congestive HF.[83] For example, a decrease in the ESPVR slope indicates that a reduction in myocardial contractility has occurred consistent with pure LV systolic dysfunction. Such an event is accompanied by a compensatory LV dilation (movement of the pressure-volume diagram to the right) along a normal EDPVR (Figure 5-11). This increase in preload may preserve SV and cardiac output (CO) but occurs at the cost of greater LV filling and pulmonary venous pressures.[79] In contrast, an increase in the EDPVR denotes a reduction in LV compliance such that LV diastolic pressure is greater at each LV volume. Under these circumstances, myocardial contractility may remain relatively normal (the ESPVR does not change), but LV filling pressures are increased, thereby producing pulmonary venous congestion and clinical symptoms (see Figure 5-11). Simultaneous depression of the ESPVR and elevation of the EDPVR indicate the presence of both LV systolic and diastolic dysfunction. SV and CO may be severely reduced because available compensatory changes in preload or afterload, depicted by movement of the steady-state LV pressure-volume diagram within the ESPVR and the EDPVR boundaries, are quite limited under such conditions.

The pressure-volume plane may be extrapolated to a single region or dimension of the LV, and analogous LV pressure-dimension relationships may then be analyzed.[84–86] For example, ultrasonic transducers placed within the LV wall may be used in the laboratory to measure changes in segment length[87] or LV diameter[88] during the cardiac cycle. Such transducers also may be placed on the LV epicardial and endocardial surfaces to measure continuous changes in wall thickness.[86] The time for ultrasound to be transmitted between a pair of these transducers is directly proportional to the length between them (Doppler principle). Thus, segment length or chamber diameter normally increases during diastole and shortens during systole analogous to changes in continuous LV volume, whereas myocardial wall thickness decreases in diastole and increases during systole. Acute changes in LV loading conditions may then be used to generate a series of diagrams for measurement of LV end-systolic and end-diastolic pressure-segment length, pressure-wall thickness, or

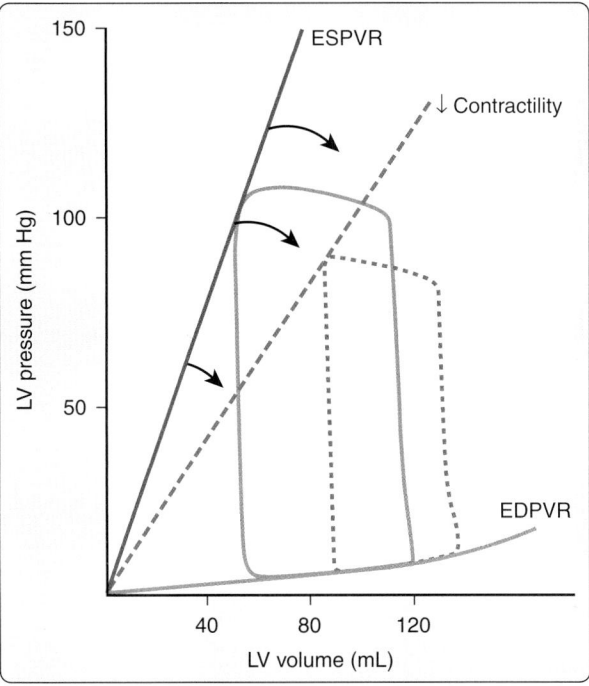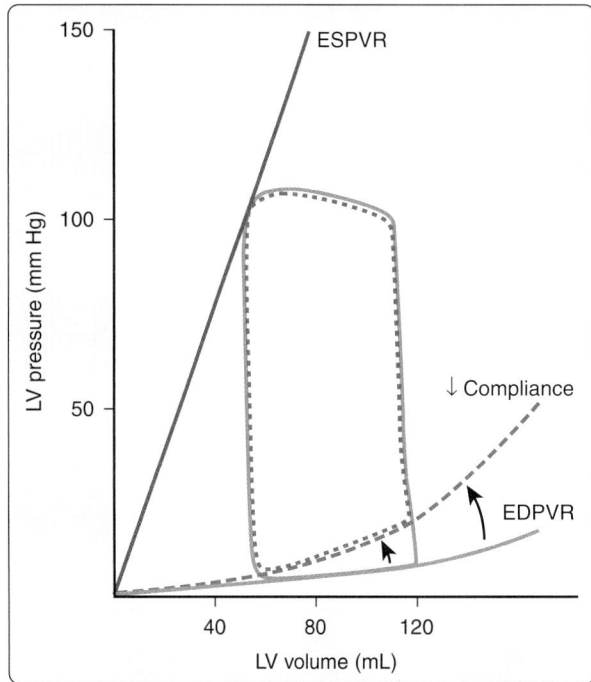

Figure 5-11 Schematic illustrations demonstrate alterations in the steady-state left ventricular (LV) pressure-volume diagram produced by a reduction in myocardial contractility as indicated by a decrease in the slope of the end-systolic pressure-volume relation (ESPVR; right) and a decrease in LV compliance as indicated by an increase in the position of the end-diastolic pressure-volume relation (EDPVR; right). These diagrams emphasize that heart failure may result from LV systolic or diastolic dysfunction independently.

pressure-dimension relationships. The use of regional compared with global LV pressure-volume analysis is particularly advantageous when studying the mechanical consequences of myocardial ischemia.[89] For example, acute occlusion of a major coronary artery produces a time-dependent collapse of the steady-state LV pressure-length diagram in

the central ischemic zone consistent with a rapidly progressing decline and eventual complete absence of effective regional SW (Figure 5-12). In contrast, the LV pressure-segment length diagram tilts to the right in a moderately ischemic area such as a border zone surrounding a central ischemic region. This diagram may be divided into three regions

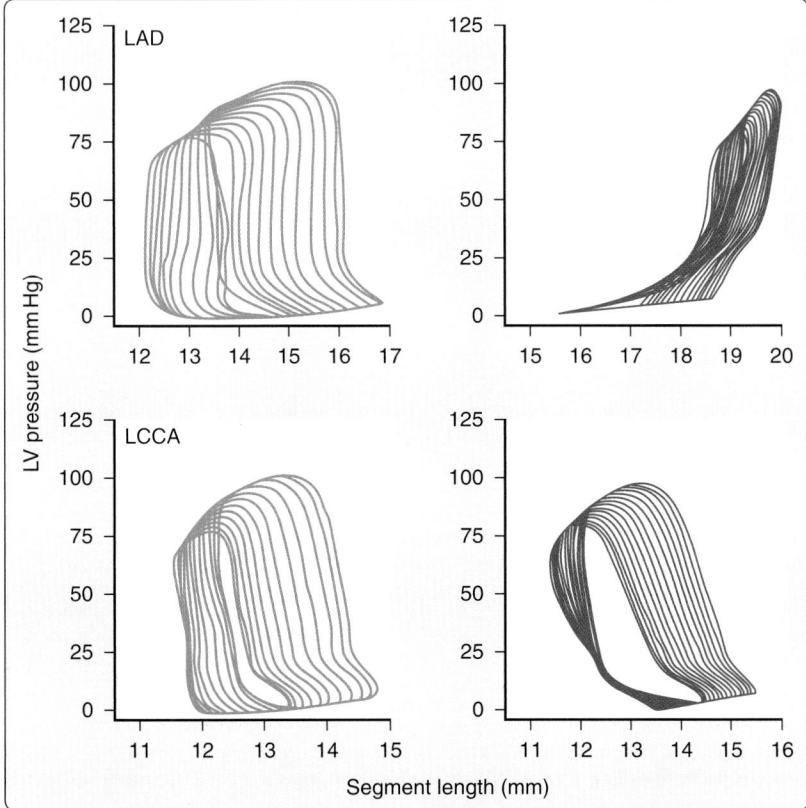

Figure 5-12 Differentially loaded left ventricular (LV) pressure-segment length diagrams resulting from abrupt occlusion of the inferior vena cava in the left anterior descending (LAD) and left circumflex coronary artery (LCCA) perfusion territories before *(left panels)* and during *(right panels)* a 2-minute occlusion of the LAD in a conscious, chronically instrumented dog. Aneurysmal systolic lengthening, postsystolic shortening, loss of effective stroke work, and diastolic creep (segment expansion) occur in the LAD LV pressure-segment length diagram in response to ischemia in this region. Corresponding isovolumic shortening and early diastolic lengthening in the LCCA LV pressure-segment length diagram also occur as the contraction and relaxation of nonischemic zone myocardium and partially compensate for the adjacent dyskinetic region. *Pagel et al. Anesthesiology 83:1021–1035, 1995.*

that correspond to systolic lengthening (because of paroxysmal systolic aneurysmal bulging of the ischemic zone), postsystolic shortening (shortening in the ischemic zone that occurs after ejection as a result of tethering to adjacent normal myocardium), and a variable area between the two that contributes to functional regional LV SW (Figure 5-13). These parameters may be used to quantify the relative intensity of regional myocardial ischemia.[90]

Pressure-volume analysis also may be applied to the study of atrial function. In contrast with the nearly rectangular shape of the LV pressure-volume diagram, the steady-state LA (or RA) pressure-volume diagram is composed of two intersecting loops arranged in a horizontal "figure-of-eight" pattern that incorporates active ("A" loop) and passive ("V" loop) components of LA function (Figure 5-14).[91] The unusual shape of the LA pressure-volume diagram results primarily from the biphasic morphology of the LA pressure waveform. Beginning at the end of LV diastasis (corresponding to LA end-diastole), the active component of the diagram traces a counterclockwise outline during atrial systole as the LA ejects its contents into the LV through the open mitral valve. LA end-systole (corresponding to LV end-diastole) marks the end of atrial contraction and is defined by minimum LA volume. Thus, identification of LA end-diastole and end-systole on the LA pressure-volume diagram facilitates calculation of LASV and emptying fraction (analogous to LVEF). After the mitral valve closes, LA filling occurs during LV systole and isovolumic relaxation. LA pressure and volume gradually increase as the chamber is filled with pulmonary venous blood during this reservoir phase, thereby forming the bottom portion of the A loop and the upper portion of the V loop. The area of the A loop represents active LA SW[92] (analogous to

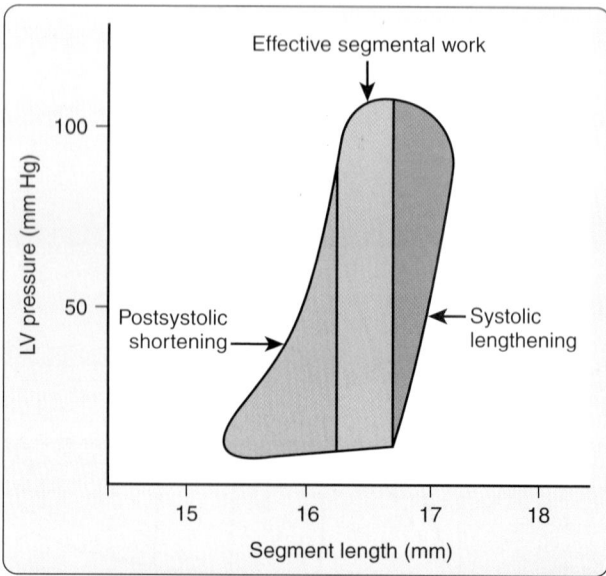

Figure 5-13 Steady-state left ventricular (LV) pressure-segment length diagram measured within the border zone of the central ischemia region during acute occlusion of the left anterior descending coronary artery in a dog. Areas of systolic lengthening (right) and postsystolic shortening (left) produced by partial ischemia and tethering to the central ischemia zone do not contribute to segmental work, but a small area of the diagram (center) demonstrates effective segment shortening that contributes to global LV stroke work.

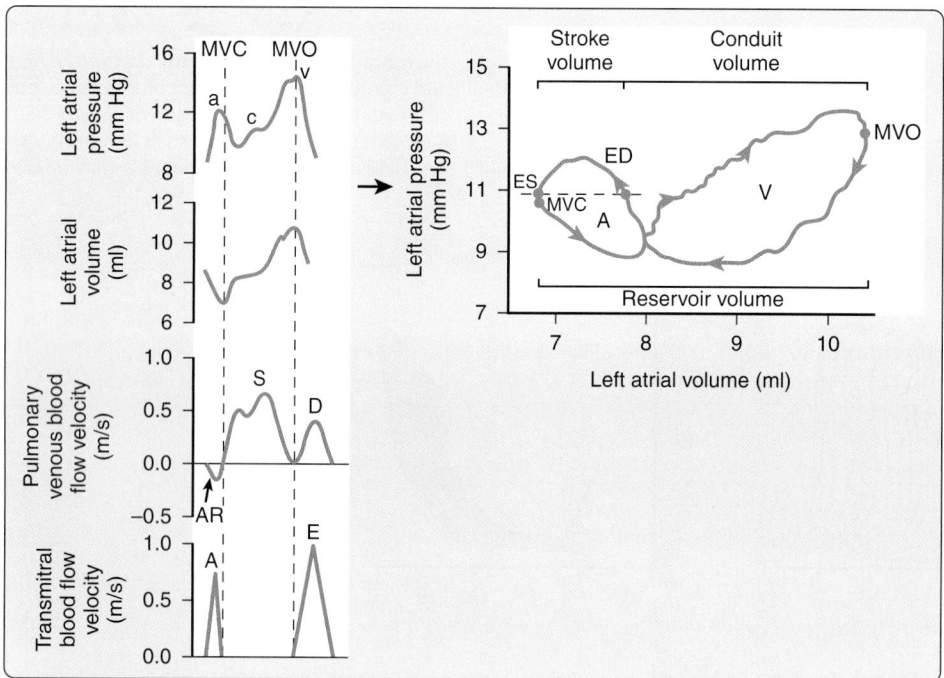

Figure 5-14 Left atrial (LA) pressure and volume waveforms (left) and the corresponding steady-state LA pressure-volume diagram (right) inscribed in phase space by these waveforms during a single cardiac cycle. The corresponding schematic pulmonary venous and transmitral blood flow velocity waveforms are also depicted (left). The "a" wave of LA pressure corresponds to atrial systole, the "c" wave represents the small increase in LA pressure that occurs during early left ventricular (LV) isovolumic contraction, and the "v" wave identifies the increase in LA pressure associated with LA filling. In contrast with this biphasic LA pressure waveform, the morphology of the LA volume waveform is monophasic. The resulting LA pressure-volume diagram is shaped in a horizontal figure-of-eight pattern. *Arrows* indicate the time-dependent direction of movement around the diagram. The "A" portion of the diagram (left loop of the figure of eight) incorporates active LA contraction and temporally proceeds in a counterclockwise fashion. The "V" portion of the diagram (right loop) represents passive LA reservoir function and proceeds in a clockwise manner over time. Mitral valve closure and opening (MVC and MVO, respectively) also are depicted on the individual waveforms and the LA pressure-volume diagram. Left atrial end-diastole (ED) is defined as the time point immediately before LA contraction at which LA pressure corresponds to LA end-systolic (ES) pressure *(horizontal dashed line)*. LV isovolumic contraction, ejection, and the majority of isovolumic relaxation occur between MVC and MVO illustrated on the LA pressure-volume diagram. The pulmonary venous blood flow velocity waveform consists of an atrial reversal ("AR") wave, a biphasic "S" wave that occurs during LV systole, and a "D" wave that is observed with opening of the mitral valve. The corresponding atrial systole (A) and early LV filling (E) waves of transmitral blood flow velocity are also illustrated. The AR and D waves of pulmonary venous blood flow velocity occur in conjunction with the A and E waves of transmitral blood flow velocity, respectively. *Pagel PS, Kehl F, Gare M, et al: Mechanical function of the left atrium: New insights based on analysis of pressure-volume relations and Doppler echocardiography,* Anesthesiology 98:975–994, 2003.

LV SW defined as the area inscribed by the LV pressure-volume diagram). The passive component (V loop) of the LA pressure-volume diagram proceeds in a clockwise direction as a consequence of external forces acting on the LA during this period of the cardiac cycle. Total LA reservoir volume is easily determined from the steady-state LA pressure-volume diagram as the difference between maximum and minimum LA volumes.[71] The V loop area represents the total passive elastic energy stored by the LA during the reservoir phase and, thus, is an index of reservoir function.[93] The slope of the line between minimum LA pressure of the A loop and maximum LA pressure in the V loop has been used as an index of static LA compliance. Regional myocardial ischemia[22] or severe LV dysfunction[94] increase the slope of this line, indicating that a decrease in compliance is present. LA emptying after mitral valve opening causes a rapid decline in LA volume that forms the bottom portion of the V loop. Additional pulmonary venous return also enters the LA during LV diastasis, but this blood flow does not alter LA volume because the mitral valve is open. Thus, the LA conduit phase is defined between mitral valve opening and LA end diastole, and LA conduit volume is calculated as the difference between maximum and end-diastolic volumes (see Figure 5-14). The interrelation among LA loading conditions, LA and LV contractile state, the rate and extent of LA relaxation, LA elastic properties, and pulmonary venous blood flow combine to determine the relative areas of the A and V loops and the point of intersection between them.[91] Analogous to the observations in the LV, acute alterations in LA loading conditions may be used to assess LA myocardial contractility and dynamic compliance using LA end-systolic and end-reservoir pressure-volume relations.[41,95,96]

DETERMINANTS OF PUMP PERFORMANCE

The ability of each cardiac chamber to function as a hydraulic pump depends on how effectively it is able to collect (diastolic function) and eject (systolic function) blood. For the sake of this discussion, the focus is on the LV, but the principles that determine LV pump performance are equally applicable to the RA, LA, and RV as well. From a clinical perspective, LV systolic function is most often quantified using CO (the product of HR and SV) and EF. These variables are dependent not only on the intrinsic contractile properties of the LV myocardium itself, but the quantity of blood the chamber contains immediately before contraction commences (preload) and the external resistance to emptying with which it is confronted (afterload). This complex interaction among preload, afterload, and myocardial contractility establishes the SV and EF generated during each cardiac cycle (Figure 5-15). When combined with HR and rhythm, preload, afterload, and myocardial contractility determine the volume of blood that the LV is capable of pumping per minute (CO) assuming adequate venous return. Malfunction of the mitral and aortic valves (e.g., regurgitation) or the presence of an anatomically abnormal route of intracardiac blood flow (e.g., ventricular septal defect with left-to-right shunt) reduces effective forward flow, thereby limiting the use of SV, CO,

and EF as indices of LV systolic performance. Thus, the structural integrity of the LV is also a key determinant of its systolic function. Pulmonary venous blood flow, LA function, mitral valve integrity, pericardial restraint, and the active (relaxation) and passive elastic (compliance) mechanical properties of the LV during diastole determine its ability to properly fill. LV diastolic function is considered to be normal when these factors combine to provide the LV preload that is adequate to establish sufficient CO required for cellular metabolism while maintaining normal pulmonary venous and mean LA pressures (approximately 10 mm Hg for each).[97] In contrast, LA or mitral valve dysfunction, delayed LV relaxation, reduced LV compliance, or increased pericardial pressure may substantially restrict the ability of the LV to properly fill unless pulmonary venous and LA pressures are increased. Thus, LV diastolic dysfunction is invariably associated with increases in pulmonary venous and LA pressures, and may lead to the development of signs and symptoms of congestive HF independent of changes in LV systolic function.

Heart Rate

An alteration in the stimulation frequency of isolated cardiac muscle produces a parallel change in LV contractile state. The Bowditch, "staircase," or "treppe" (German for "stair") phenomenon or "force-frequency" relation has been demonstrated in the isolated[98] and intact LV.[99] Enhanced Ca^{2+} cycling efficiency and myofilament Ca^{2+} sensitivity are responsible for this stimulation-rate dependence of contractile state. Maximal contractile force occurs at 150 to 180 stimulations per minute during isometric contraction of isolated cardiac muscle. From a clinical perspective, this "treppe"-induced increase in LV contractility is especially important during exercise by matching CO to venous return at HRs approaching 175 beats/min in highly trained endurance athletes. However, contractility deteriorates above this HR because the intracellular mechanisms responsible for Ca^{2+} removal from the contractile apparatus are overwhelmed and LV diastolic filling time is markedly attenuated.[100] These factors directly contribute to the development of hypotension during tachyarrhythmias or very rapid pacing. An increase in HR within the normal physiologic range has little effect on overall pump performance despite the modestly associated increase in LV contractile state,[101] but tachycardia and its resultant "treppe"-induced enhanced contractility are essential compensatory mechanisms that serve to maintain CO during disease states characterized by severely restricted LV filling (e.g., pericardial tamponade, constrictive pericarditis).[102] Myocardial hypertrophy decreases the stimulation rate at which the peak "treppe" effect occurs, whereas this phenomenon may be completely abolished in failing myocardium. Another example of the force-frequency relation occurs when a prolonged delay is observed between beats (e.g., associated with an AV conduction abnormality) or after an LV extrasystole. Under these conditions, the force of the subsequent LV contraction is enhanced. This phenomenon is termed the *interval-strength* effect. A time-dependent increase in the amount of Ca^{2+} available for contractile activation and an increase in preload resulting from greater diastolic filling are most likely responsible for the interval-strength effect.[103,104]

Preload

A definition of preload as sarcomere length immediately before the onset of myocyte contraction is certainly useful, but such a definition may be of limited practical utility in an ejecting heart because of the dynamic, 3D changes in geometry that occur in each chamber during the cardiac cycle. As a result, preload is most often defined as the volume of blood contained within each chamber at its end-diastole.[‡] This blood volume effectively establishes the length of each LV sarcomere immediately before isovolumic contraction and is directly related to LV end-diastolic wall stress.[105] Nevertheless,

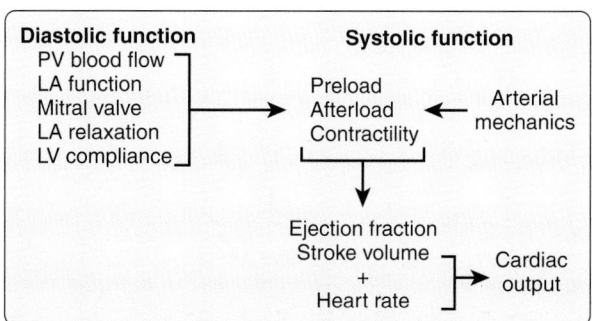

Figure 5-15 **The major factors that determine left ventricular (LV) diastolic (left) and systolic (right) function.** Note that pulmonary venous (PV) blood flow, left atrial (LA) function, mitral valve integrity, LA relaxation, and LV compliance combine to determine LV preload.

---

‡The author refers primarily to the LV for the purposes of this discussion of preload.

precise real-time measurement of continuous LV volume through-out the cardiac cycle (including LV volume at end-diastole) remains technically challenging.[106] Continuous LV volume may be approximated using ultrasonic sonomicrometers implanted in a 3D orthogonal array in the LV subendocardium,[107] and mathematical models may then be applied to generate remarkably accurate estimates of LV volume in the laboratory. The conductance catheter is another extensively validated method of measuring continuous LV volume in experimental animals[108] and patients in the cardiac catheterization laboratory.[109,110] This technique involves placement of a multiple-electrode catheter within the LV cavity to establish a series of cylindrical electric current fields and measure time-varying voltage potentials from which intraventricular conductance is determined and LV volume is estimated.[111] As discussed later, continuous LV volume waveforms derived using either sonomicrometry or conductance catheter techniques are beneficial for formal pressure-volume analysis of LV systolic and diastolic function in vivo, but the use of such invasive methods to determine LV end-diastolic volume is obviously impractical in patients undergoing cardiac surgery. Similarly, LV volume may be accurately measured using noninvasive methods such as radionuclide angiography or dynamic magnetic resonance imaging (MRI), but these techniques also cannot be used in the operating room. Instead, cardiac anesthesiologists most often rely on dimensional approximations of LV end-diastolic volume using 2D transesophageal echocardiography (TEE). The transgastric LV midpapillary short-axis imaging plane is particularly useful for estimating LV end-diastolic area or diameter. For example, an acute decrease in LV preload may be easily recognized by a corresponding reduction in the end-diastolic area and diameter of the chamber concomitant with physical contact ("kiss") between the anterior-lateral and posterior-medial papillary muscles. Real-time 3D TEE also may be used to quantify LV end-diastolic volume, but this technology has only recently become commercially available.

LV preload may be estimated using a variety of other methods, each of which has inherent limitations (Figure 5-16). LV end-diastolic pressure may be measured invasively in the cardiac catheterization laboratory or during surgery by advancing a fluid-filled or pressure transducer-tipped catheter from the aorta across the aortic valve or through the LA across the mitral valve into the LV chamber. LV end-diastolic pressure is related to end-diastolic volume based on the nonlinear EDPVR and, as a result, may not accurately quantify end-diastolic volume.[112] Other estimates of LV end-diastolic volume commonly used by cardiac anesthesiologists are dependent on measurements obtained further "upstream" from the LV. Mean LA, pulmonary capillary occlusion (wedge), pulmonary arterial diastolic, RV end-diastolic, and RA (central venous) pressures may be used to approximate LV preload. These estimates of LV end-diastolic volume are affected by functional integrity of the structures that separate each

measurement location from the LV itself. For example, a correlation between RA and LV end-diastolic pressures assumes that the fluid column between the RA and LV has not been adversely influenced by pulmonary disease, airway pressure during respiration, RV or pulmonary vascular pathology, LA dysfunction, mitral valve abnormalities, or LV compliance. The complex relation between these structures may be fully intact in healthy subjects, but this may not be the case in patients with significant pulmonary or cardiac disease who, in particular, may require accurate assessment of LV preload to assure optimal cardiac performance. The correlation among LV end-diastolic volume, pulmonary artery occlusion pressure, and RA pressure is notoriously poor in patients with compromised LV systolic function,[113] and measurement of such pressures "upstream" from the LV may be of limited clinical use in the assessment of LV preload under these circumstances. The author uses the terms *preload* and *end-diastolic volume* as synonyms in the remainder of this chapter unless otherwise noted.

Afterload

Afterload is defined as the additional load to which cardiac muscle is subjected immediately after the onset of contraction. This definition of afterload is intuitively clear and easily quantified in an isolated cardiac muscle preparation, but is more difficult to envision and measure in the intact cardiovascular system even under tightly controlled experimental conditions (Table 5-2). Impedance to LV or RV ejection by the mechanical properties of the systemic or pulmonary arterial vasculature provides the foundation for a definition of afterload in vivo. Several approaches have been used to quantify afterload. Aortic input impedance [$Z_{in}(\omega)$; the complex ratio of aortic pressure (the forces acting on the blood) to blood flow (the resultant motion)] is derived from power spectral or Fourier series analysis of simultaneous, high-fidelity measurements of aortic pressure and blood flow, and provides a comprehensive description of LV afterload that incorporates arterial viscoelasticity, frequency dependence, and wave reflection.[114,115] $Z_{in}(\omega)$ is characterized by modulus and phase angle spectra expressed in the frequency domain (Figure 5-17).[116] $Z_{in}(\omega)$ is most often interpreted using an electrical three-element Windkessel model[117] of the arterial circulation that describes characteristic aortic impedance (Z_c), total arterial compliance (C), and total arterial resistance (R; Figure 5-18).[118] Z_c represents aortic resistance to LV ejection; C is determined primarily by the compliance of the aorta and proximal great vessels; and represents the energy storage component of the arterial circulation, and R equals the combined resistances of the remaining arterial vasculature. The three-element Windkessel model has been shown to closely approximate $Z_{in}(\omega)$ under a variety of physiologic conditions.[117-119] RV afterload also has been described using pulmonary input impedance spectra interpreted using a similar Windkessel model.

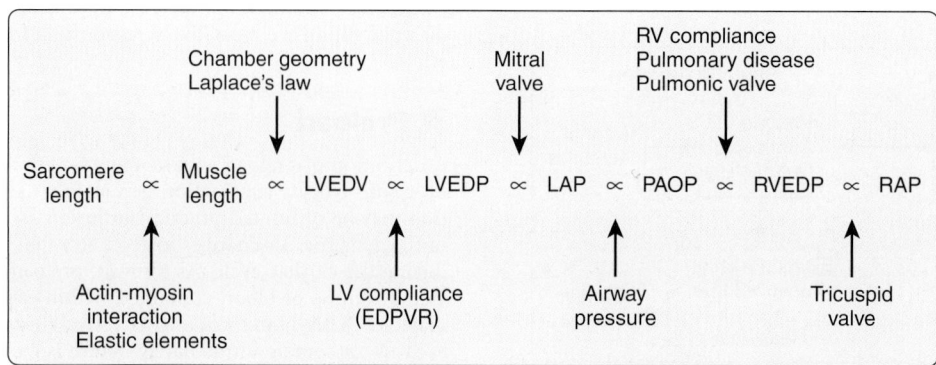

Figure 5-16   Schematic diagram depicts factors that influence experimental and clinical estimates of sarcomere length as a pure index of the preload of the contracting left ventricular (LV) myocyte. EDPVR, end-diastolic pressure-volume relation; LAP, left atrial pressure; LVEDV, left ventricular end-diastolic volume; LVEDP, left ventricular end-diastolic pressure; PAOP, pulmonary artery occlusion pressure; RAP, right atrial pressure; RV, right ventricle; RVEDP, right ventricular end-diastolic pressure.

TABLE 5-2	Indices of Left Ventricular Afterload

Aortic input impedance (magnitude and phase spectra)
Windkessel parameters
    Characteristic aortic impedance (Z_c)
    Total arterial compliance (C)
    Total arterial resistance (R)
End-systolic pressure
End-systolic wall stress
Effective arterial elastance (E_a)
Systemic vascular resistance

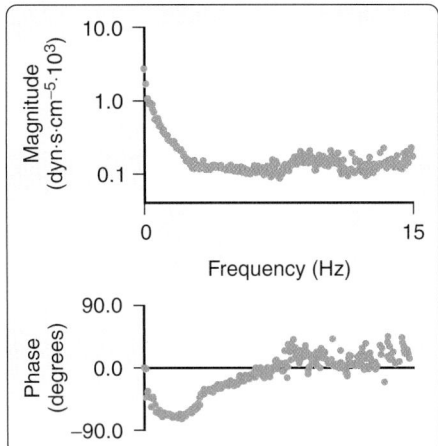

Figure 5-17 A typical aortic input impedance [$Z_{in}(\omega)$] spectrum obtained from a conscious, chronically instrumented dog. $Z_{in}(\omega)$ has frequency-dependent magnitude (top) and phase (bottom) components. The $Z_{in}(\omega)$ magnitude at 0 Hz is equal to total arterial resistance. The average of the $Z_{in}(\omega)$ magnitude spectrum between 2 and 15 Hz determines characteristic aortic impedance (Z_c). Nichols WW, O'Rourke MF: McDonald's Blood Flow in Arteries: Theoretic, Experimental and Clinical Principles, Philadelphia, 1990, Lea & Febiger.

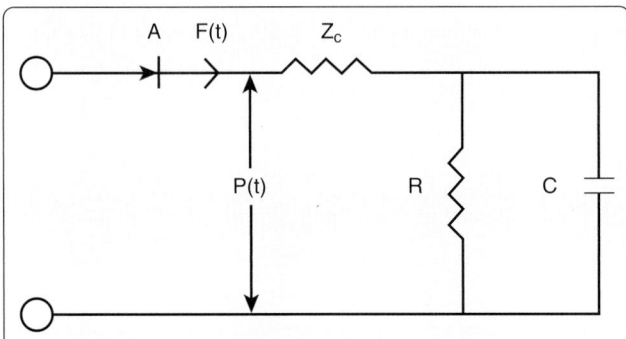

Figure 5-18 Electrical analog of the three-element Windkessel model of aortic input impedance [$Z_{in}(\omega)$]. The diode "A" represents the aortic valve. Time-dependent blood flow [F(t)] entering the arterial system from the LV first encounters the resistance of the proximal aorta and great vessels [characteristic aortic impedance (Z_c)]. Total arterial resistance (R) and total arterial compliance (C; the energy storage component of the arterial vasculature) determine further arterial blood flow, which is associated with a time-dependent change in arterial pressure [P(t)] from the aortic root to the capillary bed. Nichols WW, O'Rourke MF: McDonald's Blood Flow in Arteries: Theoretic, Experimental and Clinical Principles, Philadelphia, 1990, Lea & Febiger.

The mechanical forces to which the LV is subjected during ejection also may be used to define LV afterload as LV end-systolic wall stress. Increases in LV pressure and wall thickness occur during isovolumic contraction and are accompanied by a large reduction in LV volume (radius) after the aortic valve opens. These factors combine

to cause a dramatic increase in LV systolic wall stress as predicted by Laplace's law. LV systolic wall stress reaches a maximum during early LV ejection and declines thereafter.[47] Such changes in continuous LV systolic wall stress have several important physiologic consequences. For example, peak LV systolic wall stress is a major stimulus of LV concentric hypertrophy in disease states characterized by chronic pressure overload (e.g., poorly controlled essential hypertension, aortic stenosis).[47,120] The integral of LV systolic wall stress with respect to time is an important determinant of myocardial oxygen demand.[121] The relation between LV end-systolic wall stress and the HR-corrected maximal velocity of circumferential fiber shortening (V_{cfs}) during contraction has been used as a relatively HR- and load-independent index of contractile state in humans because each parameter may be derived noninvasively using echocardiography.[122] LV end-systolic wall stress identifies the magnitude of force that prevents further fiber shortening at the end of ejection, thereby determining the degree of LV emptying that may occur at a fixed inotropic state. Thus, LV end-systolic wall stress defines the maximal isometric value of instantaneous myocardial force at end ejection for each chamber size, thickness, and pressure, and incorporates both internal cardiac forces and those external to the heart (the arterial system) that oppose it.[123–125] As suggested in the previous discussion of Laplace's law, the use of LV end-systolic wall stress as a quantitative index of LV afterload may be complicated by LV geometry assumptions, the nonlinear force distribution between the subendocardium and subepicardium, and the nonuniformity of wall thickness throughout the LV.[51] Such difficulties may become especially important when abnormal regional wall motion is present (e.g., critical coronary artery stenosis or occlusion, LV remodeling after infarction).

Optimal transfer of energy from the LV to the arterial circulation during ejection requires coupling of these mechanical systems and provides another interpretation of LV afterload.[126,127] LV-arterial coupling most often has been described using a series elastic chamber model of the cardiovascular system in which LV elastance (E_{es}) and effective arterial elastance (E_a) are determined in the pressure-volume plane using the slopes of the LV ESPVR and aortic end-systolic pressure-SV relation, respectively (Figure 5-19).[128] The ratio of E_{es} to E_a formally defines coupling between the LV and the arterial circulation,[129,130] identifies the SV that may be transferred between these elastic components, and provides a useful foundation from which to study energetics and myocardial efficiency.[81] As such, E_a is strictly a composite coupling variable that is affected by total arterial resistance and total arterial compliance, but this parameter also has been suggested as a measure of LV afterload that is somewhat analogous to LV end-systolic wall stress.[126] The product of E_a and HR also approximates systemic vascular resistance (SVR). Nevertheless, E_a alone most likely should not be used to quantify LV afterload because this variable does not strictly incorporate alterations in characteristic aortic impedance, an important high-frequency component of arterial mechanical behavior, nor does it consider arterial wave reflection properties.

The magnitude of $Z_{in}(\omega)$ is primarily dependent on total arterial resistance[131] and, thus, may be reasonably approximated by SVR, the most commonly used estimate of LV afterload in clinical anesthesiology. SVR is a simple ratio of pressure to flow (analogous to Ohm's law) that is calculated using the familiar formula (MAP − RAP)80/CO, where MAP and RAP are mean arterial and right atrial pressures, respectively, CO is cardiac output, and 80 is a constant that converts mm Hg/min/L to dynes · sec · cm⁻⁵. However, SVR is an inadequate quantitative description of LV afterload because this parameter ignores the mechanical characteristics of the blood (e.g., viscosity, density) and arterial walls (e.g., compliance); does not consider the frequency-dependent, phasic nature of arterial blood pressure and blood flow; and fails to incorporate arterial wave reflection. The phasic contributions to arterial load become especially important in the presence of advanced age, peripheral vascular disease, and tachycardia.[132,133] As a result, SVR cannot be reliably used to quantify changes in LV afterload produced by vasoactive

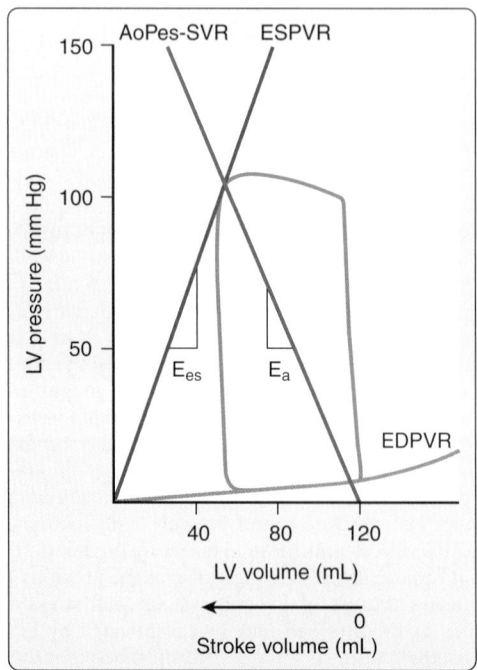

Figure 5-19 Schematic diagram illustrates the left ventricular (LV) end-systolic pressure-volume (ESPVR) and aortic end-systolic pressure-stroke volume relations (AoPes-SVR) used to determine LV-arterial coupling as the ratio of end-systolic elastance (E$_{es}$; the slope of ESPVR) and effective arterial elastance (E$_a$; the slope of A$_o$P$_{es}$-SVR). EDPVR, end-diastolic pressure-volume relation.

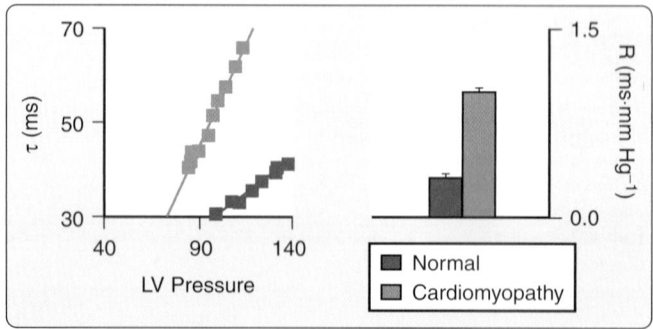

Figure 5-20 Linear relation between the time constant of isovolumic relaxation (τ) and left ventricular (LV) end-systolic pressure during inferior vena caval occlusion *(left)* in a conscious dog before *(purple squares)* and after *(green squares)* the development of rapid LV pacing-induced cardiomyopathy. The histogram illustrates the slope *(R)* of the τ-LV end-systolic pressure relation before *(purple)* and after *(green)* chronic rapid pacing and indicates that the LV isovolumic relaxation is more sensitive to alterations in LV pressure in this model of heart failure. *Pagel et al.* Anesthesiology *87:952–962, 1997.*

afterload, respectively. A model of LA afterload based on analogous descriptions of LV-arterial coupling also has been developed using combined LA and LV pressure-volume analysis and has been used to characterize LA compensatory responses to alterations in LA afterload.[94,96]

drugs or cardiovascular disease and, instead, should be used as a nonparametric estimate of LV afterload.[134]

It is clear based on the previous discussion that four major components mediate LV afterload in the intact cardiovascular system: (1) the physical properties (e.g., diameter, elasticity) of arterial blood vessels; (2) LV end-systolic wall stress (determined by LV pressure development and the geometric changes in the LV chamber required to produce it); (3) total arterial resistance (determined primarily by arteriolar smooth muscle tone); and (4) the volume and physical properties (e.g., rheology, viscosity, density) of blood. An acute increase in LV afterload is most often well tolerated in the presence of normal LV systolic function, but the performance of the failing LV is more sensitive to an increase in afterload (Figure 5-20),[135,136] and such an event may precipitate further LV dysfunction. Reflex activation of the sympathetic nervous system occurs in response to LV systolic dysfunction, but this compensatory mechanism also inadvertently increases LV afterload and may further decrease CO, especially when combined with pathologic abnormalities that reduce arterial compliance (e.g., atherosclerosis). LV hypertrophy is an important adaptive response to chronic increases in LV afterload that serves to reduce LV end-systolic wall stress by increasing wall thickness and thereby may preserve LV systolic function, but the greater mass of LV myocardium associated with hypertrophy also substantially increases the risk for myocardial ischemia and contributes to the development of LV diastolic dysfunction (Figures 5-21 and 5-22). Thus, the primary therapeutic objective in the management of acutely or chronically increased LV afterload is directed at reduction of the inciting stress.

Descriptions of RV afterload are similar to those described for the LV with two important differences: The pulmonary arterial vasculature is more compliant than its systemic arterial counterpart, and the RV is more sensitive to acute changes in afterload than the LV. The ability of the AV valves to open freely and the compliance of the LV and RV are the primary determinants of LA and RA

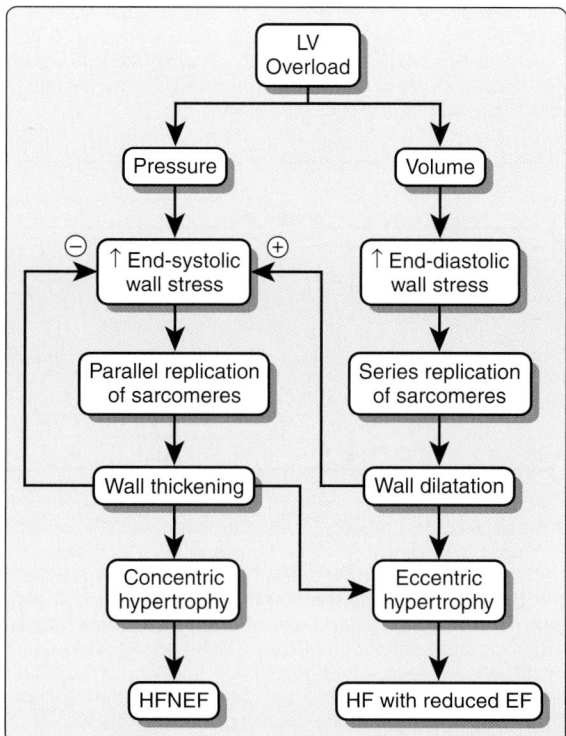

Figure 5-21 Left ventricular (LV) pressure and volume overload produce compensatory responses based on the nature of the inciting stress. Wall thickening reduces (−), whereas chamber dilation (+) increases, end-systolic wall stress as predicted by Laplace's law. LV pressure-overload hypertrophy has been linked to heart failure with normal ejection fraction (HFNEF), but LV volume overload most often causes heart failure (HF) with reduced ejection fraction (EF).

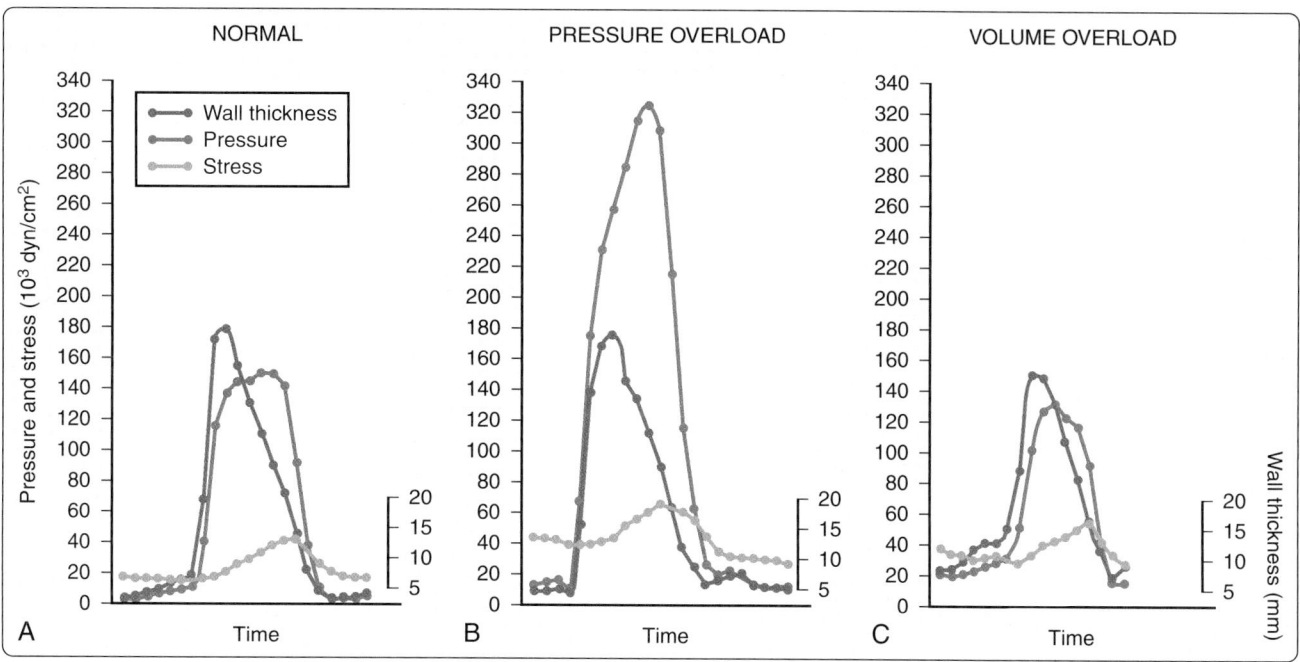

Figure 5-22 Left ventricular (LV) pressure *(red circles)*, wall thickness *(purple circles)*, and wall stress *(green circles)* during the cardiac cycle. Compared with the normal LV *(A)*, LV pressure-overload hypertrophy *(B)* occurs concomitant with dramatic increases in LV pressure, but compensatory increases in wall thickness maintain wall stress in the reference range and configuration. In contrast, end-diastolic stress is markedly increased in LV volume-overload hypertrophy *(C)*. Grossman W, Jones D, McLaurin LP: Wall stress and patterns of hypertrophy in the human left ventricle, J Clin Invest 56:56–64, 1975.

Myocardial Contractility

Rigid control of loading conditions and measurement of the velocity, force, and extent of muscle shortening facilitate accurate determination of myocardial contractility in isolated cardiac muscle preparations, but quantifying inotropic state in the intact heart has proved to be challenging. The ability to precisely assess LV or RV contractility remains an important objective that may allow the cardiac anesthesiologist to reliably evaluate the effects of pharmacologic interventions or pathologic processes on LV or RV systolic performance. To date, a "gold standard" of myocardial contractility in vivo has yet to be developed, and all contractile indices proposed, including those derived from pressure-volume analysis, have significant limitations because contractile state and loading conditions are fundamentally interrelated at the level of the sarcomere.[137,138] Many indices of myocardial contractility have been suggested that may be classified into four broad categories (Table 5-3): pressure-volume relations, isovolumic contraction, ejection phase, and power analysis.

End-Systolic Pressure-Volume Relations

The relation between LV pressure and volume may be described in terms of time-varying elastance (the ratio of pressure to volume).[75,76] LV elastance increases during systole as LV pressure increases and LV volume declines. Maximum LV elastance (E_{max}) occurs at or very near end-systole for each cardiac cycle and usually corresponds to the left upper corner of the steady-state LV pressure-volume diagram. Analogously, minimum LV elastance is observed at end-diastole. Thus, $E(t) = P(t)/[V(t) - V_0]$, where $E(t)$ is the time-varying elastance, $P(t)$ and $V(t)$ are the time-dependent changes in LV pressure and volume, respectively, during the cardiac cycle, and V_0 is LV volume at 0 mm Hg LV pressure (unstressed volume). The relation between each F_{max} of a differentially loaded series of LV pressure-volume diagrams is linear within the normal physiologic range at a constant inotropic state and establishes the ESPVR. The slope (E_{es}; designating "end-systolic elastance") of the ESPVR is a quantitative index of LV contractile state that incorporates afterload because the analysis is conducted at end-systole (Figure 5-23). As a result, the time-varying elastance equation may be rewritten at

TABLE 5-3	Indices of Left Ventricular Contractility

Pressure-Volume Analysis
End-systolic pressure-volume relation (E_{es})
Stroke work—end-diastolic volume relation (M_{sw})

Isovolumic Contraction
dP/dt_{max}
$dP/dt_{max}/50$
$dP/dt_{max}/P$
dP/dt_{max}/end-diastolic volume relation (dE/dt_{max})

Ejection Phase
Stroke volume
Cardiac output
Ejection fraction
Fractional area change
Fractional shortening
Wall thickening
Velocity of shortening

Ventricular Power
PWR_{max}
PWR_{max}/EDV^2

dE/dt_{max}, slope of the dP/dt_{max}–end-diastolic volume relation; dP/dt_{max}, maximum rate of increase of left ventricular pressure; EDV, end-diastolic volume; E_{es}, end-systolic elastance; M_{sw}, slope of the stroke work–end-diastolic volume relation; P, peak left ventricular pressure; PWR_{max}, maximum left ventricular power (product of aortic pressure and blood flow).

end-systole as $P_{es} = E_{es}(V_{es} - V_0)$, where P_{es} and V_{es} are LV end-systolic pressure and volume, respectively. Thus, an increase in the magnitude of E_{es} produced by a positive inotropic drug (e.g., epinephrine) quantifies the increase in LV contractility that has occurred. Regional LV contractility may also be determined using pressure-dimension relations based on determinations of continuous segment length, LV midpapillary short-axis diameter, or wall thickness,[84,86,139] and usually reflects global LV systolic function in the absence of wall motion abnormalities.[107] LV ESPVR or dimension relations have been derived noninvasively using radionuclide angiography[140] or 2D echocardiography[141]

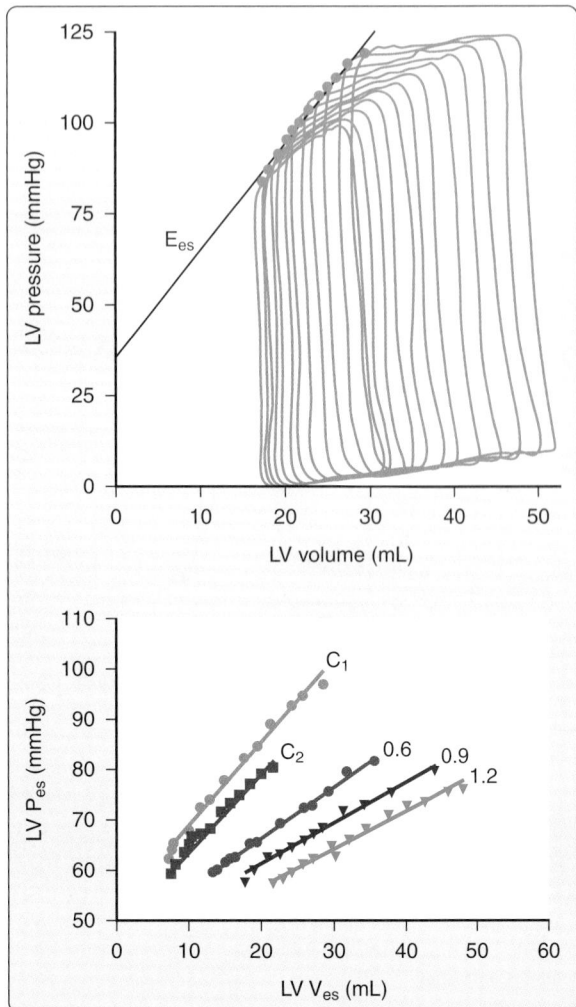

Figure 5-23 Illustration depicts method used to derive the left ventricular (LV) end-systolic pressure-volume relation (ESPVR) from a series of differentially loaded LV pressure-volume diagrams generated by abrupt occlusion of the inferior vena cava in a canine heart in vivo. The maximal elastance (E_{max}; pressure/volume ratio) for each pressure-volume diagram is identified as its left upper corner, and a linear regression analysis is used to define the slope (E_{es}; end-systolic elastance) and volume intercept of the ESPVR (*top*). *Bottom*, Effects of isoflurane (0.6, 0.9, and 1.2 minimum alveolar concentration) on the ESPVR. C_1, control 1 (before isoflurane); C_2, control 2 (after isoflurane). *Hettrick DA, Pagel PS, Warltier DC: Desflurane, sevoflurane, and isoflurane impair canine left ventricular-arterial coupling and mechanical efficiency, Anesthesiology 85:403–413, 1996.*

with automated border detection[142] to measure continuous LV volume or area. In addition, single-beat estimates of E_{es} (determined as the simple ratio of P_{es} to V_{es} or derived using a modified time-varying elastance method) were proposed that may provide quantitative information about contractile state assuming that the value V_0 remains small.[143,144] The principle of time-varying elastance also has been successfully applied to the study of RV[82] and atrial contractility[41] (Figure 5-24) in the intact heart.

The simplicity and elegance of time-varying elastance model of LV contractility may be particularly attractive from an engineering perspective, but a number of potential pitfalls were subsequently identified after its initial description that may limit the use of E_{es} as a clinical index of inotropic state. The position of unstressed volume (V_0) does not consistently remain constant during alterations in contractility.[77,145] For example, administration of dobutamine not only increases E_{es}, but also shifts the ESPVR to the left (decrease in V_0),[145] whereas acute coronary artery occlusion-induced regional LV dysfunction has the opposite effect.[146]

Thus, both E_{es} and V_0 may reflect alterations in LV contractility, and an index of inotropic state based on the combined effects of these variables was proposed as a result.[147] Several consecutive LV pressure diagrams must be obtained over a range of LV loading conditions to accurately define E_{es} and V_0, but this necessary intervention may inadvertently produce baroreceptor reflex–mediated increases in HR and contractility during generation of the ESPVR by activating the sympathetic nervous system.[148] E_{max} or aortic valve closure may not occur precisely at end-systole in the presence of markedly increased or reduced LV afterload and may be delayed or occur earlier, respectively.[149] Thus, E_{max} may deviate from its normal position in the left upper corner of the LV pressure-volume diagram, thereby introducing errors into the derivation of ESPVR. The units of E_{es} are millimeters of mercury per milliliter (mm Hg/mL), and as a result, E_{es} is inherently dependent on chamber size despite efforts to standardize its measurement.[150,151] This volume dependence of E_{es} may complicate direct comparison of contractile state between patients with different LV sizes. Other potential limitations of the use of E_{es} as an index of contractile state include lack of measurement precision,[152] nonlinearity,[153] load sensitivity,[154] dependence on underlying autonomic nervous system balance[155] or ejection-mediated alterations on LV pressure generation,[156] and interaction with LV diastolic function.[157] Despite these concerns, the ESPVR is a superb conceptual tool with which to examine contractile state and its interactions with loading conditions in vivo.

Stroke Work–End-Diastolic Volume Relations

Early studies by Frank[73] and Starling[158] initially defined a fundamental relation between LV pump performance (e.g., CO) and preload determined using indirect indices of LV filling (e.g., central venous pressure). Sarnoff and Berglund[159] extended these seminal investigations in his landmark description of LV or RV function curves that relate estimates of SW to filling pressures. In this familiar framework, movement of an LV function curve upward or to the left indicated that an increase in contractile state had occurred because the LV was now able to effectively generate more SW at an equivalent preload. Unfortunately, these LV function curves were inherently nonlinear and difficult to quantify because the technology available to Sarnoff at the time precluded his ability to precisely measure LV SW and end-diastolic volume. Glower et al[78] used a high-fidelity LV micromanometer and 3D orthogonal endocardial sonomicrometers to measure continuous LV pressure and volume, respectively, in a pressure-volume reexamination of Sarnoff's original hypothesis. These investigators demonstrated that the relationship between each LV SW–end-diastolic volume (V_{ed}) pair obtained from a series of differentially loaded LV pressure-volume diagrams was indeed linear such that $SW = M_{sw}(V_{ed} - V_{sw})$, where M_{sw} and V_{sw} were the slope and volume intercept of the relation (Figure 5-25). Thus, M_{sw} was shown to quantify alterations in LV inotropic state in a relatively load-independent manner because preload is already incorporated and, unlike the ESPVR, its determination does not occur solely at end-systole. Similar linear relations between regional work and dimensional measurements (e.g., segment length, wall thickness) also may be used to quantify changes in regional contractile state. Notably, LV SW-V_{ed} relations may be calculated with the same series of pressure-volume diagrams used to determine the ESPVR.

The SW-V_{ed} relation offers several advantages over the ESPVR for the determination of LV or RV contractility. The SW-V_{ed} relation is highly linear and reproducible over a wide variety of loading conditions, arterial blood pressures, and contractile states because LV pressure and volume data from the entire cardiac cycle are incorporated into its calculation.[78,152] Conversely, the ESPVR displays more pronounced curvilinear behavior and may be more susceptible to instrument noise because it is determined at a single instantaneous time point (end-systole).[154] The ESPVR may also demonstrate some degree of afterload sensitivity,[160] but the SW-V_{ed} relation is essentially afterload-independent over a wide physiologic range.[78] Unlike E_{es}, the unit of M_{sw} is millimeters of mercury (mm Hg); therefore, quantification of LV contractile state may be performed independent of chamber size. Thus, M_{sw} allows direct comparisons of contractility to be made between patients with

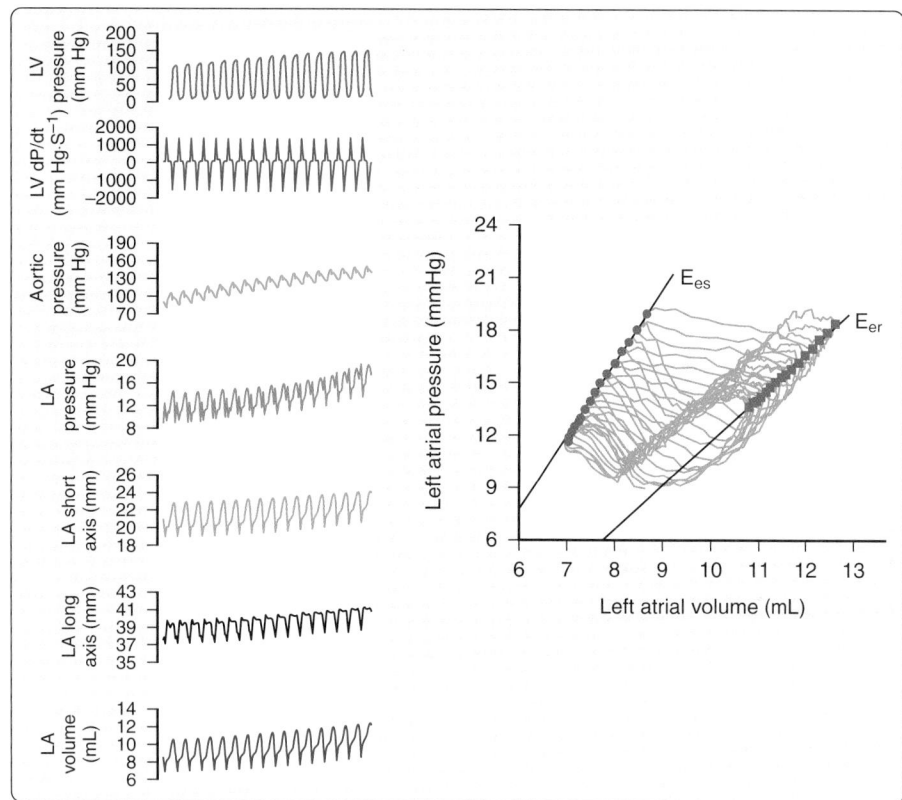

Figure 5-24 Continuous left ventricular (LV) pressure, LV dP/dt, aortic pressure, left atrial (LA) pressure, LA short- and long-axis dimensions, and LA volume waveforms *(left)* and corresponding LA pressure-volume diagrams *(right)* resulting from intravenous administration of phenylephrine (200 μg) in a canine heart in vivo. The LA maximal elastance *(solid circles)* and end-reservoir pressure and volume *(solid squares)* for each pressure-volume diagram were used to obtain the slopes (E_{es} and E_{er}) and extrapolated volume intercepts of the LA end-systolic and end-reservoir pressure-volume relations to quantify LA contractile state and chamber stiffness, respectively. *Pagel PS, Kehl F, Gare M, et al: Mechanical function of the left atrium: New insights based on analysis of pressure-volume relations and Doppler echocardiography, Anesthesiology 98:975–994, 2003.*

varying LV size. Nevertheless, the SW-V_{ed} relation has two disadvantages compared with the ESPVR. First, integration of data from the entire cardiac cycle implies that the SW-V_{ed} relation does not strictly separate LV systolic events from those that occur during diastole. Thus, a reduction in LV compliance without a simultaneous change in the ESPVR (as may be observed in the presence of LV pressure-overload hypertrophy) may introduce errors into the calculation of LV contractile state using the SW-V_{ed} relation.[138] Second, partial collapse of the LV pressure-volume diagram during regional myocardial ischemia[90] makes calculation of LV contractility more difficult using the SW-V_{ed} relation compared with the ESPVR.[161] Despite these relatively minor potential shortcomings, the SW-V_{ed} relation provides a useful index of LV or RV contractile function in the intact heart that has been successfully applied in a variety of laboratory settings and in patients with heart disease.

Isovolumic Indices of Contractility

The maximum rate of increase of LV pressure (dP/dt_{max}) is the most commonly derived index of global LV contractile state during isovolumic contraction. Precise determination of LV dP/dt_{max} requires high-fidelity, invasive measurement of continuous LV pressure and usually is performed in the cardiac catheterization laboratory. LV dP/dt_{max} also may be noninvasively estimated using TEE in patients undergoing cardiac surgery by analysis of the continuous-wave Doppler mitral regurgitation waveform.[162] LV dP/dt_{max} is very sensitive to acute alterations in contractile state[163] but is probably most useful when quantifying directional changes in contractility rather than establishing an absolute baseline value.[164] LV dP/dt_{max} is essentially afterload-independent because the peak rate of increase of LV pressure occurs before the aortic valve opens unless severe myocardial depression or pronounced arterial

vasodilation is present.[165] However, LV preload profoundly affects dP/dt_{max}, and an increase in LV dP/dt_{max} produced by either greater preload or enhanced contractile state may be virtually indistinguishable. LV mass, chamber size, and mitral or aortic valve disease also affect LV dP/dt_{max}. In addition, LV dP/dt_{max} may not detect changes in contractile state produced by regional myocardial ischemia because LV dP/dt_{max} is an index of global LV systolic function. The failure of LV dP/dt_{max} to detect such an alteration in regional dysfunction resulting from compromised coronary perfusion may occur because of a compensatory increase in contractility in the remaining normal myocardium through activation of the Frank–Starling mechanism or an increase in sympathetic nervous system activity. The rate of increase of LV pressure at a fixed developed pressure [e.g., dP/dt measured at 50 mm Hg (dP/dt_{50})] and the ratio of dP/dt to peak developed LV pressure (dP/dt/P) also have been proposed as isovolumic indices of contractility. These measures of LV contractile state may be somewhat less preload dependent than LV dP/dt_{max}, but neither provides any truly unique additional information compared with LV dP/dt_{max}.

The preload dependence of LV dP/dt_{max} may be used to derive another index of myocardial contractility based on the pressure-volume framework. Similar to the SW-V_{ed} relation, the relation between each pair of LV dP/dt_{max} and V_{ed} values obtained from a differentially loaded series of LV pressure-volume diagrams was shown to be linear such that LV $dP/dt_{max} = dE/dt_{max}(V_{ed} - V_0)$, where dE/dt_{max} is the slope and V_0 is the volume intercept of the relation.[166] Like E_{es} and M_{sw}, alterations in dE/dt_{max} produced by inotropic drugs or cardiac disease may be used to quantify changes in LV contractile state. For example, the LV dP/dt_{max}-V_{ed} relation was shown to precisely determine alterations in contractility in the normal and regionally ischemic LV.[166,167] Furthermore, LV dE/dt_{max} and E_{es} are mathematically related,[166] and interventions that shift

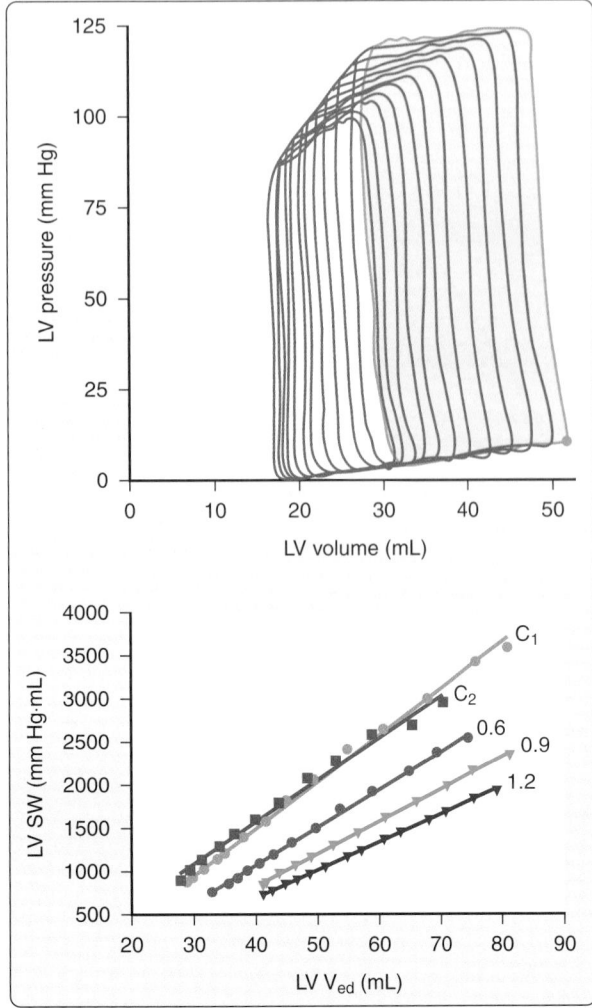

Figure 5-25 Illustration demonstrates the method used to derive the left ventricular (LV) stroke work (SW)-end-diastolic volume (V_{ed}) relation from a series of differentially loaded LV pressure-volume diagrams generated by abrupt occlusion of the inferior vena cava in a canine heart in vivo. The area of each LV pressure-volume diagram (*shaded area* corresponding to SW) is plotted against the corresponding V_{ed} (*top*), and a linear regression analysis is used to define the SW-V_{ed} relation (*bottom*). *Bottom*, Effects of isoflurane (0.6, 0.9, and 1.2 minimum alveolar concentration) on the SW-V_{ed} relation. C_1, control 1 (before isoflurane); C_2, control 2 (after isoflurane). *Hettrick DA, Pagel PS, Warltier DC: Desflurane, sevoflurane, and isoflurane impair canine left ventricular-arterial coupling and mechanical efficiency,* Anesthesiology 85:403–413, 1996.

the ESPVR without altering E_{es} also shift the volume intercept of the LV dP/dt_{max}-V_{ed} relation without changing dE/dt_{max} as well.[138] Similar to the ESPVR, the LV dP/dt_{max}-V_{ed} relation becomes more curvilinear at greater LV volumes or contractile states, a finding that is predicted based on isolated cardiac muscle mechanics.[168] Direct comparison among the ESPVR, the SW-V_{ed} relations, and the LV-dP/dt_{max} relation also indicated that dE/dt_{max} may be more variable than either E_{es} or M_{sw} during acute changes in contractile state.[152] RV dP/dt_{max}-V_{ed} relations also have been described.[44]

Ejection Phase Indices of Contractility

Examination of the degree (e.g., EF, SV) or the rate (e.g., velocity of shortening) of LV ejection forms the basis of all currently used ejection phase indices of LV contractile state, including newer echocardiography parameters derived from tissue Doppler imaging, myocardial stress-strain relations, speckling tracking technology, and endocardial color kinesis. From a clinical perspective, the most common ejection phase index of LV contractility is EF, where $EF = V_{ed}$-V_{es}/V_{ed}. LVEF may be calculated using a variety of noninvasive techniques (e.g., radionuclide angiography, functional MRI, echocardiography). Cardiac anesthesiologists most often measure LVEF using 2D TEE. Midesophageal four- or two-chamber images are obtained at LV end-systole and end-diastole and are subsequently analyzed by applying Simpson's rule of disks (Figure 5-26). This method of measuring LVEF is simple, but it is rather time-consuming and may be impractical during rapidly changing hemodynamic conditions. As a result, two closely related parameters, fractional shortening (FS) and fractional area of change, are often calculated as surrogate measures of LVEF in the midpapillary short-axis plane using images obtained at end-systole and end-diastole. FS is calculated from endocardial measurements of anterior-posterior (or septal-lateral) wall diameter as $FS = D_{ed} - D_{es}/D_{ed}$, where D_{ed} and D_{es} are endocardial end-diastolic and end-systolic diameters, respectively (Figure 5-27). Fractional area change (FAC) may be determined using the same midpapillary short-axis images by manually tracing the endocardial borders (the papillary muscles are most often excluded) at end-systole and end-diastole (see Figure 5-27). Computer software automatically integrates the end-systolic and end-diastolic areas (A_{es} and A_{ed}, respectively) within each endocardial tracing, and FAC is calculated as $A_{ed} - A_{es}/A_{ed}$. These and all other ejection phase indices are inherently dependent on both LV contractile state and loading conditions.[80] Because preload is incorporated into the denominators of EF, FAC, and FS (V_{ed}, A_{ed}, and D_{ed}, respectively), these indices are relatively unaffected by moderate preload alterations in the presence of normal mitral and aortic valve function.[169] Myocardial stress-strain relations or speckle tracking techniques also may include similar modifications (e.g., Lagrangian or natural strain) designed to minimize such intrinsic preload dependency. Nevertheless, EF, FAC, FS, and related variables derived from newer technologies decrease linearly with increases in

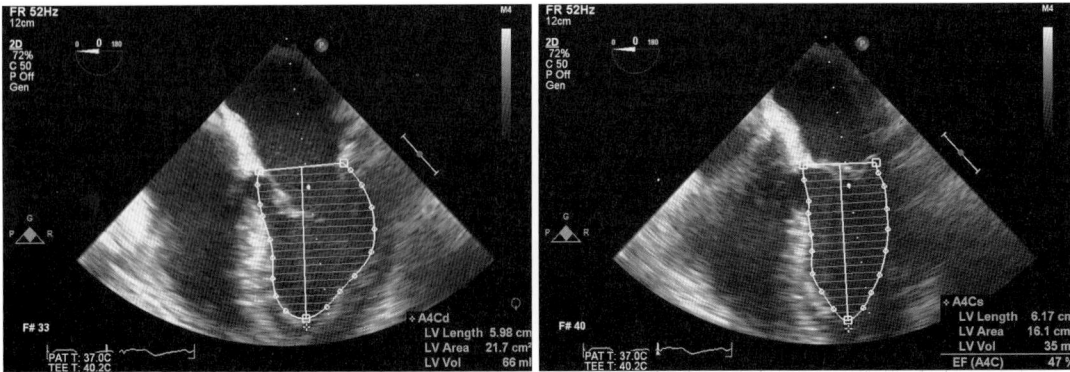

Figure 5-26 Calculation of ejection fraction from midesophageal four-chamber images obtained at left ventricular (LV) end-diastole (*left*) and end-systole (*right*) using Simpson's rule. After the LV endocardial border is identified in each image, the software generates a series of thin cylindrical disks and determines the volume based on their sum. LV ejection fraction is then calculated using the standard formula. In this example, the LV ejection fraction is 47%.

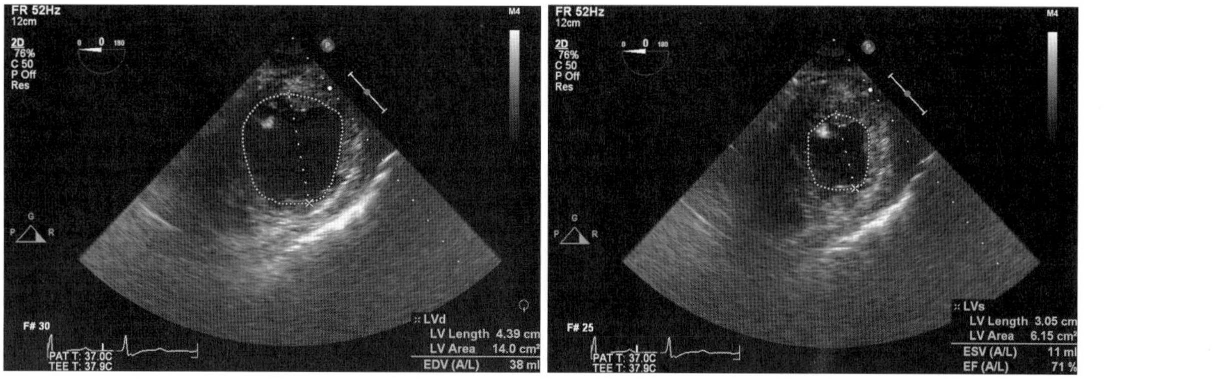

Figure 5-27 Calculation of fractional area change and fractional shortening from left ventricular (LV) midpapillary short-axis images obtained at end-diastole (*left*) and end-systole (*right*). The LV endocardial border is manually traced (excluding the papillary muscles). The software integrates the area inscribed and determines the diameter of the LV chamber. In this example, fractional area change is 56% and fractional shortening is 31%.

afterload and also vary inversely with HR, and as a result, are relatively insensitive indices of LV contractile state. Similar to the observations with LV dP/dt_{max}, EF and FAC are global measures of pump performance that may not adequately reflect regional contractile dysfunction produced by myocardial ischemia or infarction. Ejection phase indices also may provide inaccurate information about contractility in the presence of mitral or aortic valvular disease, LV chamber enlargement, or LV hypertrophy.[120,170,171] Similar difficulties with load and HR dependency are encountered when ejection phase indices are used in an attempt to quantify RV or atrial contractile state.

The rate of myocardial fiber shortening also provides information about the LV contractile state during ejection. Maximal or mean velocity of circumferential fiber shortening may be determined using a variety of invasive and noninvasive techniques. The midpapillary short-axis view on TEE is especially useful for cardiac anesthesiologists measuring these variables in the operating room. Maximal velocity of circumferential fiber shortening (V_{cfs}) is calculated as the ratio of FS to ejection time and may be more sensitive to changes in contractile state than EF because the velocity, rather than the magnitude, of shortening is evaluated. Nevertheless, V_{cfs} also varies directly with HR and inversely with changes in afterload similar to other ejection phase indices.[165] Methods for correcting the inherent HR and afterload dependency of V_{cfs} have been proposed that are based on the force-velocity behavior of isolated cardiac muscle. For example, a linear relation was demonstrated between LV end-systolic wall stress and HR-corrected V_{cfs}, and the slope of this relation provided a relatively HR- and afterload-independent index of LV contractile state in healthy patients[123] and those with hypertension or valve disease.[120,122] A similar relation between EF and effective arterial elastance also was described.[172] Unfortunately, these and other analogous techniques[173] have not achieved widespread clinical application because extensive analysis is required after data have been acquired.

Contractile Indices Based on Ventricular Power

The product of LV or RV pressure and aortic or pulmonary blood flow defines LV or RV power, respectively. Maximal LV power (PWR_{max}) and the rate of increase of LV power during ejection are sensitive to alterations in contractile state,[174,175] but these indices are also profoundly affected by LV preload. In contrast, the ratio of LV PWR_{max} to the square of end-diastolic volume (PWR_{max}/V_{ed}^2) largely eliminates this preload dependence and allows the rapid calculation of LV contractile state from data obtained during a single cardiac cycle.[176] Alterations in LV contractile state determined using this preload-adjusted maximal power technique correlate with those calculated with the ESPVR (E_{es}) and the LV dP/dt_{max}-V_{ed} relation (dE/dt_{max}), and also may be measured using noninvasive arterial blood pressure (e.g., tonometry, oscillometry) concomitant with 2D and Doppler echocardiography to define its pressure, flow, and dimension variables without the need for

formal pressure-volume analysis.[177,178] A regional power quotient using end-diastolic segment length (SL_{ed}) also correlated with the regional SW-SL_{ed} (M_{sw}) and accurately quantified depression of LV contractility produced by volatile anesthetics.[179]

COUPLING, ENERGETICS, AND EFFICIENCY

The pressure-volume framework is useful for the description of the sequential transfer of kinetic energy (SW) between two elastic chambers. This mechanical "coupling" defines the blood volume that may be actively ejected from one chamber into the next. Coupling between the LV and arterial circulation is most often described, but similar relationships between the LA and the LV[96] or analogous structures on the right side of the heart[180] also have been characterized. As described previously in the discussion of afterload, LV-arterial coupling is defined by the ratio of the slopes of the ESPVR (E_{es}) and the aortic end-systolic pressure-SV relation (E_a; see Figure 5-19) that denote their respective elastances.[127] Ideal coupling between the normal LV and the arterial circulation indicates optimal transfer of SW between the chambers and occurs when their elastances are equal ($E_{es}/E_a = 1$) under resting conditions[129] and during exercise.[181,182] LV contractile dysfunction (indicated by a decrease in E_{es}) or greater resistance to LV ejection (an increase in E_a) reduce the E_{es}/E_a ratio to less than 1, indicating that the efficiency of kinetic energy transfer between these chambers is no longer optimal.[183] An E_{es}/E_a ratio less than 1 often occurs in the presence of a large acute myocardial infarction because global LV contractile state is depressed and compensatory activation of the sympathetic nervous system produces arterial vasoconstriction.[184] In fact, the severity of abnormal LV-arterial coupling correlates with serum B-type natriuretic peptide concentration (a biochemical marker of LV systolic dysfunction), and an E_{es}/E_a ratio less than 0.68 predicts long-term mortality in patients after myocardial infarction.[185] Tachycardia also increases E_a and worsens LV-arterial coupling in the failing heart.[186] In contrast, positive inotropic drugs and vasodilators improve LV-arterial coupling in HF by increasing E_{es} and reducing E_a, respectively.[187] LV-arterial coupling is relatively preserved in the presence of a low end-tidal concentration of desflurane, sevoflurane, or isoflurane (0.6 minimum alveolar concentration; Figure 5-28), but kinetic energy transfer from the LV to the proximal arterial vasculature degenerates when greater concentrations are used because the magnitude of anesthetic-induced vasodilation (decrease in E_a) is unable to compensate for more profound LV contractile depression (decrease in E_{es}).[128] Interestingly, the ratio of E_{es} to E_a may be mathematically related to EF such that $E_{es}/E_a = EF/(1 - EF)$, and as a result, optimal LV-arterial coupling occurs when EF equals 50%.[188] This simple relation between the coupling ratio and EF predicts that EF will be reduced when E_{es}/E_a is less than 1 because SW is less efficiently transferred from the LV to the arterial vasculature.

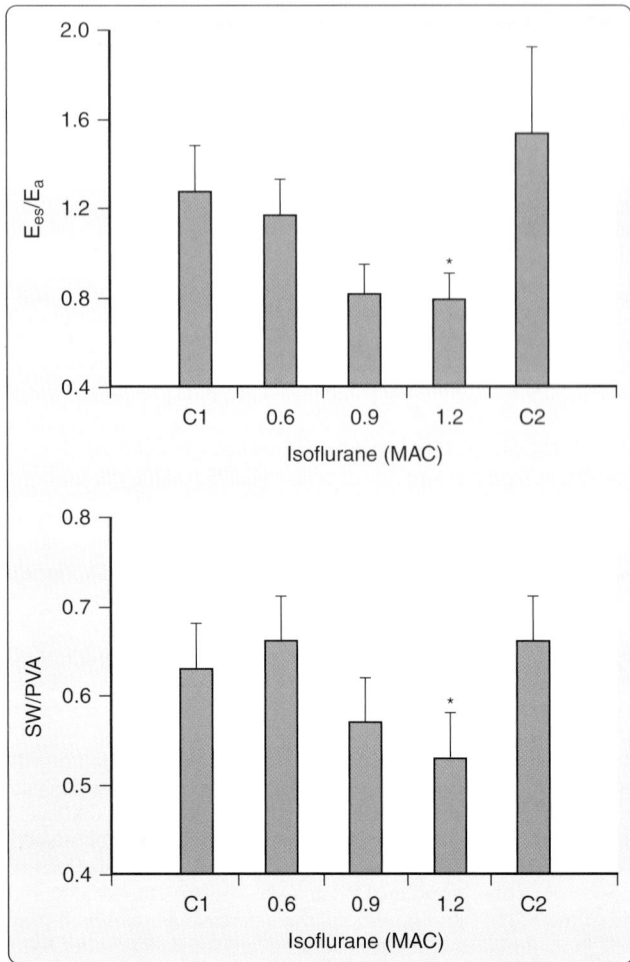

Figure 5-28 Histograms illustrating the effects of isoflurane (0.6, 0.9, and 1.2 minimum alveolar concentration [MAC]) on left ventricular (LV)-arterial coupling (LV end-systolic elastance/effective arterial elastance [E_{es}/E_a]; *top*) and energy transfer efficiency (stroke work/pressure volume area [SW/PVA]; *bottom*). Isoflurane reduces LV-arterial coupling and energy transfer efficiency in a dose-related manner. C_1, control 1 (before isoflurane); C_2, control 2 (after isoflurane). *Hettrick DA, Pagel PS, Warltier DC: Desflurane, sevoflurane, and isoflurane impair canine left ventricular-arterial coupling and mechanical efficiency, Anesthesiology 85:403–413, 1996.*

LV energetics also has been modeled in pressure-volume phase space. Total mechanical energy is defined as the sum of the SW generated during a single cardiac cycle and the potential energy that remains in the chamber wall at end-systole as a result of compression of myocardial elastic elements.[81] The triangular area bounded above by the ESPVR, below by the EDPVR, and to the right by the isovolumic relaxation portion of the steady-state LV pressure-volume diagram defines the remaining potential energy (see Figure 5-9). This potential energy has the same units as SW (mm Hg • mL = 1.33 • 10^{-4} joules) and is converted into heat during diastole.[189] The sum of the kinetic and potential energy components is termed *pressure-volume area* (PVA)[190] and linearly related to measured myocardial oxygen consumption (MVO_2) such that $MVO_2 = \alpha(PVA) + \delta$, where α is the slope of the relation and δ denotes basal metabolism in the absence of contraction (MVO_2 when PVA equals zero).[191-193] Thus, the area beneath the MVO_2-PVA line includes the sum of kinetic and potential energies associated with contraction and relaxation (excitation-contraction coupling) combined with the energy required for the maintenance of vital cellular function. Alterations in LV contractile state produced by positive or negative inotropic drugs cause the MVO_2-PVA relation to shift up or down, respectively, in a parallel manner without a change in the slope of the relation.[192,194] This intriguing observation allows the relation between MVO_2 and PVA to be rewritten as $MVO_2 = \alpha(PVA) + \beta (E_{es}) + \delta$, where β is the sensitivity of the MVO_2-PVA relation to E_{es} and indicates that the total energy consumed for excitation-contraction coupling increases or decreases during enhanced or reduced LV contractile state, respectively.[192] Notably, the relative contribution of kinetic and potential energy (PVA) to MVO_2 remains constant because the slope (α) of the relation does not change, suggesting that the actual biochemistry of conversion of high-energy phosphates (e.g., ATP) into mechanical activity at the myofilament level is not affected by alterations in inotropic state.[192] Perhaps not surprisingly, alterations in LV compliance (as indicated by the EDPVR) do not substantially affect MVO_2 even though PVA may be modestly affected because kinetic and potential energy generated during systole are the predominant factors that determine MVO_2.[189]

LV efficiency also may be accurately described using pressure-volume analysis.[129,195] The SW/PVA ratio indicates the mechanical energy that is converted into external work and is an index of energy transfer efficiency.[130,196] The SW/PVA ratio responds predictably to alterations in LV contractile state and afterload. For example, an increase in E_{es} produced by a positive inotropic drug or exercise enhances the amount of mechanical energy that is converted into work, and hence the SW/PVA ratio becomes larger.[182] In contrast, an increase in LV afterload decreases SW and energy transfer efficiency.[196] These observations make it readily apparent that LV-arterial coupling is the primary determinant of the SW/PVA ratio,[197] such that SW/PVA = 1/[1 + 0.5(E_a/E_{es})].[198] Administration of a volatile anesthetic causes a dose-related decrease in SW/PVA because LV E_{es} is depressed to a greater extent than E_a (see 5-28).[128] Because E_{es}/E_a is related to EF,[188] the ratio of SW to PVA may be rewritten as 2/[(1/EF) − 1]. This simple equation demonstrates that a decrease in EF is associated with less efficient conversion of total mechanical energy into external work regardless of the underlying cause. The ratio of PVA to measured MVO_2 provides a useful index of the conversion of metabolic to mechanical energy,[199] whereas the product of SW/PVA and PVA/MVO_2 (SW/MVO_2) indicates the efficiency with which the LV transfers its metabolic energy into physical work. The ratio of SW to MVO_2 increases in the presence of positive inotropic drugs[200] and during exercise[182] but is substantially reduced[201] and predicts mortality[202] in patients with HF.

EVALUATION OF DIASTOLIC FUNCTION

The ability of each chamber to efficiently fill under normal pressure conditions is essential to assure the best possible overall cardiac performance. LV diastolic function has been studied most extensively, but the relaxation, filling, and distensibility characteristics of the more compliant RV and the atrial chambers also have been described. This section focuses almost exclusively on LV diastolic function, but many of the techniques used to quantify LV diastolic function also may be applied to the study of RV "diastology." As previously discussed, LV diastole encompasses a complicated sequence of temporally related, heterogeneous events (see Figure 5-15; Table 5-4), and as such, no single index of LV diastolic function devised to date is capable of comprehensively describing this period of the cardiac cycle in its entirety or selectively identifying patients at greatest risk for development of clinical signs and symptoms of HF resulting from filling abnormalities.[203] In addition, most indices of LV diastolic function are dependent on HR, loading conditions, and myocardial contractility, and as a result, alterations in these variables require interpretation within the constraints of these limitations. Despite such inherent difficulties, the crucial nature of LV diastolic function is emphasized by the striking observation that as many as 50% of patients with HF do not have a substantial reduction in LVEF.[204,205] This "heart failure with normal ejection fraction" (HFNEF; previously termed "diastolic heart failure") occurs most frequently in hypertensive elderly women concomitant with obesity, renal insufficiency, anemia, general deconditioning, or atrial fibrillation.[206] Many of these risk factors contribute to the progressive development

TABLE 5-4	Determinants of Left Ventricular Diastolic Function

Heart rate and rhythm
LV systolic function
Wall thickness
Chamber geometry
Duration, rate, and extent of myocyte relaxation
LV untwisting and elastic recoil
Magnitude of diastolic suction
LA-LV pressure gradient
Passive elastic properties of LV myocardium
Viscoelastic effects (rapid LV filling and atrial systole)
LA structure and function
Mitral valve structure and function
Pulmonary venous blood flow
Pericardial restraint
RV loading conditions and function
Ventricular interdependence
Coronary blood flow and vascular engorgement
Compression by mediastinal masses

LA, left atrium; LV, left ventricle; RV, right ventricle.

TABLE 5-6	Common Causes of Left Ventricular Diastolic Dysfunction

Age > 60 yr
Acute myocardial ischemia (supply or demand)
Myocardial stunning, hibernation, or infarction
Ventricular remodeling after infarction
Pressure-overload hypertrophy (e.g., aortic stenosis, hypertension)
Volume-overload hypertrophy (e.g., aortic or mitral regurgitation)
Hypertrophic obstructive cardiomyopathy
Dilated cardiomyopathy
Restrictive cardiomyopathy (e.g., amyloidosis, hemochromatosis)
Pericardial diseases (e.g., tamponade, constrictive pericarditis)

of LV hypertrophy and fibrosis that adversely affect LV filling characteristics and increase the risk for overt HF.[206] The pathophysiology of HFNEF appears to be multifactorial (Table 5-5), and involves not only delayed LV relaxation and reduced compliance,[207,208] but also abnormal ventricular-arterial stiffening.[209,210] Regardless of the underlying cause (Table 5-6), diastolic dysfunction is a ubiquitous feature in HFNEF and also is observed in all patients with HF resulting from LV contractile dysfunction.[211] Notably, the severity of LV diastolic dysfunction with or without LV systolic compromise and its response to medical therapy are important determinants of exercise tolerance[212] and mortality[213] in patients with chronic HF. From the perspective of the cardiac anesthe-

siologist, LV diastolic dysfunction has significant implications in determining the LV response to acute alterations in loading conditions that commonly occur during the perioperative setting. Cardiopulmonary bypass temporally exacerbates preexisting LV diastolic dysfunction in cardiac surgical patients.[214] Further, volatile and intravenous anesthetics are known to alter LV relaxation and filling properties in the normal and failing heart.[215] Thus, assessing the presence and severity of LV diastolic dysfunction remains an important objective in the management of patients undergoing cardiac surgery.

Invasive Evaluation of Diastolic Function

Isovolumic Relaxation

Based on the previous discussions of intracellular Ca^{2+} homeostasis and myosin-actin interaction, it is readily apparent that relaxation of the cardiac myocyte is an active, energy-dependent process requiring removal of activator Ca^{2+} from the myoplasm, resulting in rapid dissociation of contractile proteins and recoil of elastic elements compressed during contraction. Delays in relaxation may be envisioned as a form of "active" elasticity because failure of actin-myosin cross-bridges to dissociate occurs when energy supply is inadequate or intracellular Ca^{2+} homeostasis is dysfunctional.[216,217] Such a delay in relaxation is of paramount importance because early LV filling may be substantially attenuated and, thus, overall LV filling may become increasingly dependent on LA systole. In fact, the subsequent loss of LA contraction occurring with the onset of atrial fibrillation often precipitates acute signs and symptoms of congestive HF in patients with diseases in which delayed LV relaxation is an especially prominent feature (e.g., severe pressure-overload hypertrophy, hypertrophic obstructive cardiomyopathy [HCM]). Delayed global LV relaxation produced as a consequence of hypoxemia[218] or regional myocardial ischemia in a relatively large perfusion territory also may translate into reduced LV compliance (upward shift of the EDPVR).[219,220] In addition, LV relaxation delays have been shown to compromise early diastolic subendocardial coronary blood flow because failure to complete actin-myosin dissociation and facilitate elastic recoil prolong the compression of intramyocardial coronary arterioles.[221] Thus, evaluation of LV isovolumic relaxation provides essential information about early diastolic mechanical behavior that directly influences subsequent events during filling.

An invasively implanted, high-fidelity pressure transducer is required to precisely determine the rate and extent of LV pressure decline during isovolumic relaxation. Analogous to the use of LV dP/dt_{max} as an index of inotropic state during isovolumic contraction, the peak rate of LV pressure decrease (dP/dt_{min}) has been used to quantify isovolumic relaxation during this early phase of diastole. LV dP/dt_{min} is generally regarded as an unreliable index of relaxation because the parameter is highly dependent on the magnitude of LV end-systolic pressure[222] and examines only a single time point near the onset of relaxation. Instead, LV relaxation is most often described based on the observation that LV pressure decline follows an exponential time course between aortic valve closure and mitral valve opening, and thus

TABLE 5-5	Left Ventricular Structure and Function in Chronic Heart Failure	
Characteristics	*LV Systolic Heart Failure*	*LV Diastolic Heart Failure*
Remodeling		
End-diastolic volume	Increased	Normal
End-systolic volume	Increased	Normal
LV mass	Increased	Increased
Geometry	Eccentric	Concentric
Cardiac myocyte	Increased length	Increased diameter
Extracellular matrix	Decreased collagen	Increased collagen
LV Systolic Properties		
Stroke volume	Decreased (or normal)	Normal (or decreased)
Stroke work	Decreased	Normal
M_{sw}	Decreased	Normal
E_{es}	Decreased	Normal (or increased)
Ejection fraction	Decreased	Normal
dP/dt_{max}	Decreased	Normal
Preload reserve	Exhausted	Limited
LV Diastolic Properties		
End-diastolic pressure	Increased	Increased
τ	Increased	Increased
β	Normal (or increased)	Increased

β, myocardial stiffness constant; τ, time constant of LV isovolumic relaxation; dP/dt_{max}, maximum rate of increase of LV pressure; E_{es}, slope of the LV end-systolic pressure-volume relation; LV, left ventricle; M_{sw}, slope of the LV stroke work-end-diastolic volume relation.
Aurigemma GP. et al. *Circulation* 113:296–304, 2006.

may be described using a time constant (τ) derived from the equation $P(t) = P_0 e^{-t/\tau}$, where $P(t)$ is time-dependent LV pressure, P_0 is LV pressure at end-systole, e is the natural exponent, and t is time (msec) after LV end-systole. This simple model mathematically constrains LV pressure to decline to 0 mm Hg, but LV pressure may decrease to subatmospheric pressures during marked hypovolemia or intense exercise,[65] or remain greater than 0 mm Hg when forces outside the LV are acting on it (e.g., pericardial tamponade, constrictive pericarditis).[223] As a result, a more physiologically relevant model of isovolumic relaxation allows the calculation of τ assuming a nonzero asymptote of LV pressure decay such that $P(t) = P_0 e^{-t/\tau} + P_a$, where P_a is the true asymptote to which pressure declines.[224] Regardless of the method used to derive the time constant, increases in τ quantify delays in LV relaxation that occur during disease processes such as myocardial ischemia,[225] pressure-overload hypertrophy,[226] or HCM,[227] or as a consequence of negative inotropic drugs including volatile anesthetics.[228] Conversely, reductions in τ indicate that more rapid LV relaxation may be observed during tachycardia, sympathetic nervous system activation, or administration of positive inotropic drugs. Interpretation of alterations in τ produced by drugs or disease requires qualification because LV loading conditions affect the time constant.[38] For example, LV preload and τ are directly related[224,229] unless arterial pressure remains relatively constant.[230] Similarly, τ is linearly related to afterload because afterload affects the duration, rate, and extent of LV ejection.[38] The afterload dependence of LV relaxation is enhanced in the failing heart (see Figure 5-20).[136,231] This observation has important clinical ramifications because afterload reduction may not only enhance LV systolic function, but may facilitate LV relaxation and improve early LV filling dynamics in patients with HF.[135] These findings emphasize that interpretation of changes in the time constant of LV isovolumic relaxation requires consideration of the loading conditions under which τ is measured.[232] Invasive quantification of LA relaxation also has been described using methods similar to those characterized in the LV.[71]

Filling

Invasive measurement of continuous LV volume is useful for the calculation of indices of LV filling. Accurate LV volume waveforms also may be obtained noninvasively using echocardiography with automated border detection, radionuclide angiography, and dynamic MRI. The first derivative of the LV volume signal with respect to time (dV/dt) produces a biphasic waveform characterized by peaks corresponding to early LV filling and LA systole (E and A waves, respectively). This dV/dt waveform is closely related to the transmitral blood flow and annular velocity signals obtained using conventional pulse-wave and tissue Doppler echocardiography, respectively. In fact, it is easily demonstrated using the continuity equation that products of the time-velocity integrals of transmitral blood flow velocity E and A signals (TVI_E and TVI_A) and the mitral valve area are identical to the areas inscribed by the E and A waves obtained from differentiation of the LV volume waveform, respectively. A wide variety of filling parameters may be determined using the dV/dt waveform, including E and A wave peak filling rates, E/A ratio, the areas (obtained by integration) of the E and A waves (corresponding to early LV filling and LA systole blood volumes, respectively), the ratio of early LV filling to total LV end-diastolic volumes (percentage of early LV filling), and measurements of time intervals of these events. Notably, progressive development of congestive HF produces similar changes in the morphology of the dV/dt compared with the transmitral blood flow velocity waveforms as indicated by the transition of "delayed relaxation" through "pseudonormal" to "restrictive" filling patterns (Figure 5-29).[233] An analogous set of parameters also may be derived from continuous measurement of LV dimension (e.g., segment length, wall thickness),[234] but the relative accuracy with which such variables describe global LV filling characteristics are dependent on implicit geometric assumptions, the LV region that is examined, and the absence of regional wall motion abnormalities.[203]

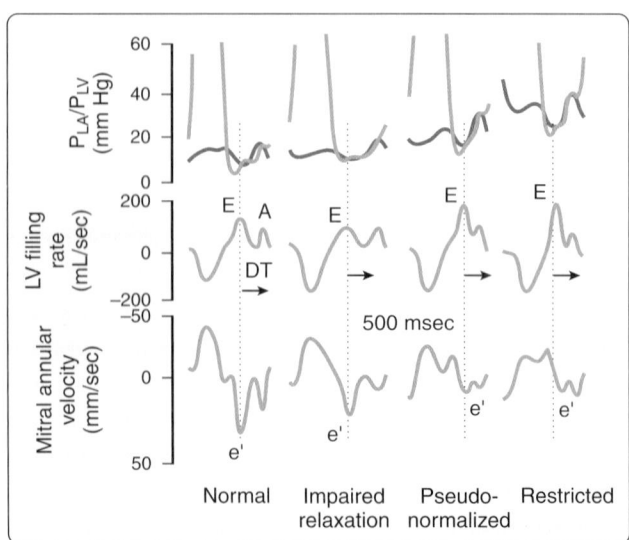

Figure 5-29 Illustration depicts the simultaneous relationships between left atrial (LA) and left ventricular (LV) pressures (P_{LA} and P_{LV}, respectively; top), LV filling rate during early filling (E) and atrial systole (A; middle), and early mitral annular velocity (e'; bottom) under normal conditions and during evolving diastolic dysfunction (impaired relaxation, pseudonormal, and restrictive). Note the initial lengthening of E-wave deceleration time (DT) during impaired relaxation and the subsequent shortening of DT as diastolic function worsens. *Little WC, Oh JK: Echocardiographic evaluation of diastolic function can be used to guide clinical care, Circulation 120:802–809, 2009.*

Passive Mechanical Behavior

Derived from a series of differentially loaded LV pressure-volume diagrams, the EDPVR describes the overall passive elastic compliance of the LV. This relation between end-diastolic pressure (P_{ed}) and volume (V_{ed}) is nonlinear and may be described using an exponential relationship such that $P_{ed} = Ae^{KV_{ed}} + B$, where K is the modulus of chamber stiffness (end-diastolic elastance) and A and B are curve-fitting constants (Figure 5-30). Thus, an increase in K produced by a disease process such as pressure-overload hypertrophy indicates that the LV chamber has become less compliant; that is, it demonstrates a greater LV pressure for a given filling volume. The modulus of chamber stiffness also may

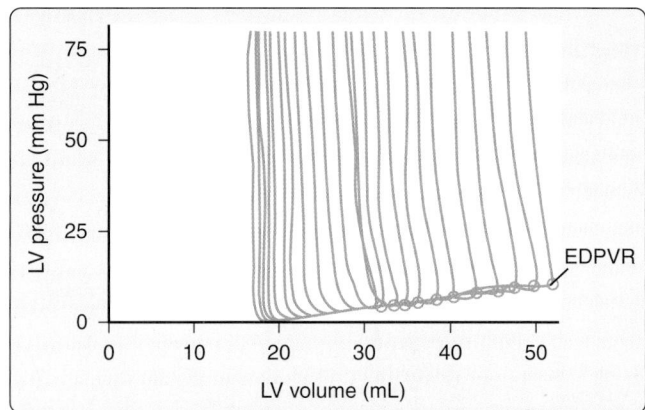

Figure 5-30 Illustration demonstrates the method used to derive the left ventricular (LV) end-diastolic pressure-volume relation (EDPVR) from a series of differentially loaded LV pressure-volume diagrams generated by abrupt occlusion of the inferior vena cava in a canine heart in vivo. The end-diastolic pressure and volume data from of each diagram (right bottom corner) are related by a monoexponential relationship such that $P_{ed} = Ae^{KV_{ed}} + B$, where P_{ed} and V_{ed} are end-diastolic pressure and volume, respectively, K is the modulus of stiffness, and A and B are curve-fitting constants.

be derived from a single LV pressure-volume diagram by using pairs of diastolic pressure and volume data points obtained after relaxation is complete (during diastasis and LA systole) to avoid viscoelastic effects[235] and also may be estimated noninvasively using the deceleration time of the transmitral blood flow velocity E wave.[236] The EDPVR provides a simple model of LV compliance that is intuitively useful, but its interpretation is subject to important limitations. LV geometry, mass, and wall thickness influence the modulus of chamber stiffness, and comparison of changes in K between patients requires appropriate normalization of these variables as a result.[232] Because the relationship between end-diastolic pressure and end-diastolic volume is exponential, comparisons of the modulus of chamber stiffness between patients or interventions should be made using a similar range of pressure and volume. Notably, measurements of the modulus of chamber stiffness do not strictly consider parallel shifts in the EDPVR.[38] For example, an acute increase in pericardial pressure causes a parallel upward shift of the EDPVR, thereby indicating that LV pressure is greater at each LV volume.[83] Thus, the relative position of the EDPVR, and not the magnitude of the modulus of chamber stiffness per se, is probably more important in defining overall LV passive mechanical characteristics because shifts in the relation up or to the left indicate that a greater LV pressure is required to distend the LV to a given volume.[237] Similar descriptions of LA compliance also have been reported using differentially loaded end-reservoir pressure-volume diagrams.[96]

The distinct material properties of the myocardium itself independent of size, geometry, and external forces may also be determined by the derivation of stress-strain relations from the EDPVR. Myocardium exhibits the physical characteristics of an elastic material (Hooke's law) by developing a resisting force (stress; σ) as muscle length (strain; ε) increases during LV filling. Thus, the forces resisting further increases in length increase as the muscle is stretched. Strain is defined as the percentage change in muscle length (L) from unstressed muscle length (L_0) determined at LV pressure of 0 mm Hg. Lagrangian [$\varepsilon = (L - L_0)/L_0$] or natural ($\varepsilon = L/L_0$) strain is most often used to normalize muscle lengths. The stress-strain relation is exponential such that $\sigma = \alpha(e_{\beta\varepsilon} - 1)$, where α is the coefficient of gain and β is the modulus of myocardial stiffness.[235] A shift of the nonlinear stress-strain relationship up and to the left is consistent with an increase in β that is known to occur in diseases such as HCM, amyloidosis, and hemochromatosis. Myocardium is not only an elastic material, but also demonstrates viscous properties. Viscoelasticity is observed when the forces resisting further alterations in length are dependent on both the magnitude of the change in length and rate with which this change occurs. Viscoelastic effects are most evident in the intact heart during early LV filling when the rate of change of LV volume is greatest, but also may be observed during LA systole. Stress-strain relations incorporating viscoelastic properties may be described using the equation $\sigma = \alpha(e_{\beta\varepsilon} - 1) + \eta(d\varepsilon/dt)$, where η is the viscoelastic constant and $d\varepsilon/dt$ is the rate of change of strain.[238] An increase in viscous effects may modestly attenuate but certainly is not a major determinant of early LV filling in the normal heart.[239] The clinical use of myocardial stress-strain relations (with or without viscous corrections) for the invasive evaluation of passive mechanical behavior in vivo has been quite limited because analysis is complicated and time-consuming.

Noninvasive Evaluation of Diastolic Function

Isovolumic Relaxation

Isovolumic relaxation time (IVRT) is defined as the duration between aortic valve closure and mitral valve opening and is the most commonly used noninvasive surrogate of invasively derived indices of LV relaxation (e.g., dP/dt$_{min}$, τ). IVRT may be measured with M-mode echocardiography or continuous wave Doppler echocardiography as the interval between the cessation of aortic blood flow and the onset of transmitral blood flow in the modified midesophageal five-chamber or deep transgastric TEE imaging planes. The rate of LV relaxation and the difference between LV end-systolic pressure and LA pressure at mitral valve opening are the major determinants of IVRT in the absence of mitral or aortic valve disease.[240] As a result, IVRT is dependent on not only the relaxation behavior of LV myocardium, but also LV loading conditions. For example, an increase in LV afterload prolongs IVRT by increasing LV pressure at aortic valve closure, whereas an increase in LA pressure shortens IVRT. In an attempt to partially circumvent this load dependence of IVRT, Doppler echocardiographic analysis of mitral or aortic regurgitant jet velocity has been used in combination with the modified Bernoulli equation ($\Delta P = 4v^2$, where ΔP is the pressure gradient and v is regurgitant blood flow velocity in m/sec) to noninvasively estimate the time constant of LV relaxation.[241] However, this technique has not been widely applied in clinical echocardiography because, as previously discussed, τ is also load dependent.

Transmitral Blood Flow Velocity

Pulse-wave Doppler echocardiographic evaluation of the pattern of transmitral blood flow velocity is the foundation on which noninvasive analysis of LV diastolic function is based.[242] RV filling properties also may be assessed using pulse-wave Doppler analysis of transtricuspid blood flow velocity. Cardiac anesthesiologists most often use the midesophageal four-chamber view to record the transmitral blood flow velocity profile by placing a small (1 to 3 mm³) pulse-wave Doppler echocardiography sample volume between the tips of the mitral leaflets during diastole to obtain a sharp, high-quality spectral envelope. Similar to the invasively derived dV/dt waveform described earlier, the normal pattern of transmitral blood flow velocity contains two peaks associated with early LV filling and LA systole (E and A waves, respectively; Figure 5-31).[243] The ratio of peak E to peak A wave velocities (E/A ratio) is used to characterize the relative contributions of early and late filling to final LV end-diastolic volume. Time-velocity integrals of the E

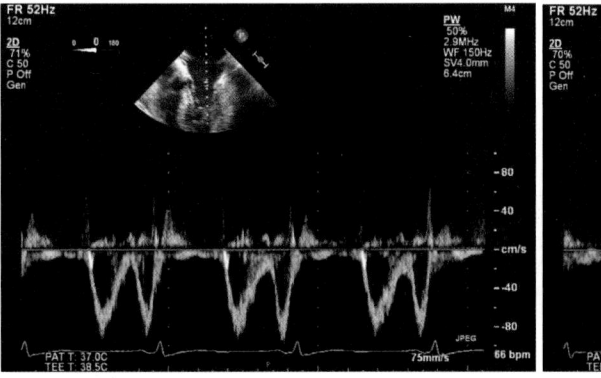
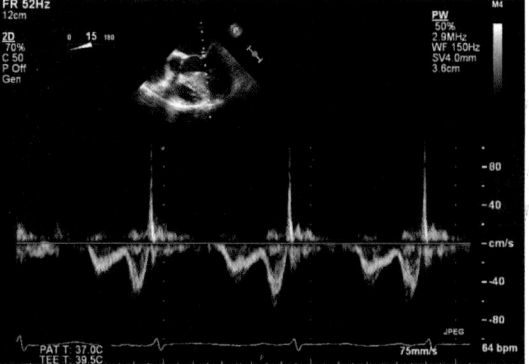

Figure 5-31 Transmitral blood flow velocity waveforms obtained using pulse-wave Doppler echocardiography under normal conditions (*left*) and during delayed relaxation (*right*).

TABLE 5-7	Stages of Left Ventricular Diastolic Dysfunction				
	Normal Age 21–49	*Normal Age >50*	*Delayed Relaxation*	*Pseudonormal Filling*	*Restrictive Filling*
E/A	> 1	≥ 1	< 1	1–2	> 2
DT (msec)	< 220	< 220	> 220	150–200	< 150
IVRT (msec)	< 100	< 100	> 100	60–100	< 60
S/D	< 1	≥ 1	≥ 1	< 1	< 1
Ar (cm/sec)	< 35	< 35	< 35	≥ 35*	≥ 25*
V_p (cm/sec)	> 55	> 45	< 45	< 45	< 45
e' (cm/sec)	> 10	> 8	< 8	< 8	< 8

*Unless left atrial failure is present.
Ar, pulmonary venous atrial reversal blood flow velocity; DT, early left ventricular filling deceleration time; e', peak early diastolic annular myocardial velocity; E/A, transmitral early left ventricular filling-to-atrial systole blood flow velocity ratio; IVRT, isovolumic relaxation time; S/D, pulmonary venous systolic-to-diastolic blood flow velocity ratio; V_p, color M-mode transmitral blood flow propagation velocity.
Garcia MJ, Thomas JD, Klein AL: New Doppler echocardiographic applications for the study of diastolic function, *J Am Coll Cardiol* 32:865–875, 1998.

and A waves (TVI_E and TVI_A, respectively) may be combined with measurements of mitral valve area to quantify the magnitude of blood flow (volume) by application of the continuity equation. The time required for deceleration of the E wave (deceleration time) also is commonly measured as an indicator of the influence of LV relaxation on the pressure gradient between the LA and LV that determines the magnitude and extent of early LV filling. The normal values of these variables are age dependent and demonstrate a gradual slowing of LV relaxation as age increases (Table 5-7). Thus, E-wave velocity and E/A ratio decrease with advancing age, whereas IVRT, deceleration time, and A-wave velocity increase.[244] These changes predispose elderly patients to the development of HF and occur because of progressive stiffening of the myocardial cartilaginous structure, loss of myocyte elasticity, increased LV muscle mass, and increased arterial pressure.[245,246]

The alterations in transmitral blood flow velocity related to age are indicative of "delayed relaxation," the least severe of three major abnormal LV filling patterns that characterize the continuum of LV diastolic dysfunction (see Figure 5-29). Clinical symptoms, exercise tolerance, New York Heart Association (NYHA) functional class, and mortality are closely correlated with the relative severity of LV diastolic dysfunction demonstrated using this simple method.[247] A reduction in early LV filling and a greater contribution of LA systole to overall LV filling are the pathognomonic findings in this "delayed relaxation" pattern. Thus, the E/A ratio is less than 1, and deceleration time is prolonged because a delay in LV relaxation reduces the initial LV-LA pressure gradient and extends the duration of early LV filling, respectively.[233] The enhanced contribution of LA systole occurs primarily through a Frank–Starling mechanism, increases A-wave size, and compensates for the reduction in early LV filling, thereby preserving relatively normal LV end-diastolic volume. In addition to advanced age, the "delayed relaxation" pattern frequently is observed in patients with essential hypertension, pressure-overload LV hypertrophy, and ischemic heart disease.

A "pseudonormal" pattern of transmitral blood flow velocity appears after the "delayed relaxation" profile as the underlying disease worsens. The E/A ratio increases to a value greater than 1 and, in fact, this "pseudonormal" pattern may be virtually indistinguishable from a normal LV filling pattern when other indices of diastolic dysfunction (e.g., pulmonary venous blood flow velocity pattern, tissue Doppler imaging, color M-mode echocardiography) are not examined or maneuvers to acutely alter loading conditions (e.g., Valsalva, nitroglycerin infusion) are not performed.[248] Increased LA pressure restores the normal LA-LV pressure gradient on mitral valve opening and thereby increases E-wave velocity to a normal value despite the continued presence of an LV relaxation abnormality. The "pseudonormal" pattern of LV filling may be recognized by the presence of a shorter E-wave deceleration time (< 200 msec; consistent with a reduction in early diastolic LV compliance[236]) or by the reappearance of the "delayed relaxation" pattern during a decrease in preload.[249] In contrast, the "delayed relaxation" profile does not appear when preload is reduced in patients with normal LV diastolic function. The "restrictive pattern" denotes the presence of severe, end-stage LV

diastolic dysfunction. LA pressure is profoundly increased, and the LA-LV pressure gradient is augmented far beyond what is necessary to compensate for the LV relaxation delay as a result. This LA hypertension also contributes to progressive LA contractile dysfunction and eventual failure. Thus, the peak E-wave velocity becomes markedly greater than its A-wave counterpart, and the E/A exceeds a value of 2. E-wave deceleration time also becomes very rapid (< 150 msec) as LV compliance is further reduced (see Table 5-7).

The "restrictive" filling pattern frequently is observed in patients with NYHA Class IV HF resulting from a variety of underlying causes,[250,251] and is also a characteristic finding in those with severe constrictive pericarditis,[252] restrictive cardiomyopathy,[253] or rejection of a transplanted heart[254] independent of changes in LV systolic function. Failure of such a "restrictive" filling pattern to revert to a less severe "pseudonormal" or "delayed relaxation" profile in response to a diuretic or a vasodilator is associated with a particularly grim prognosis.[242] Thus, two opposing parabolic curves describing changes in E/A ratio and deceleration time may be used to illustrate changes in LV diastolic function related to age or progressive deterioration from "delayed relaxation" to "restrictive" physiology (Figure 5-32).

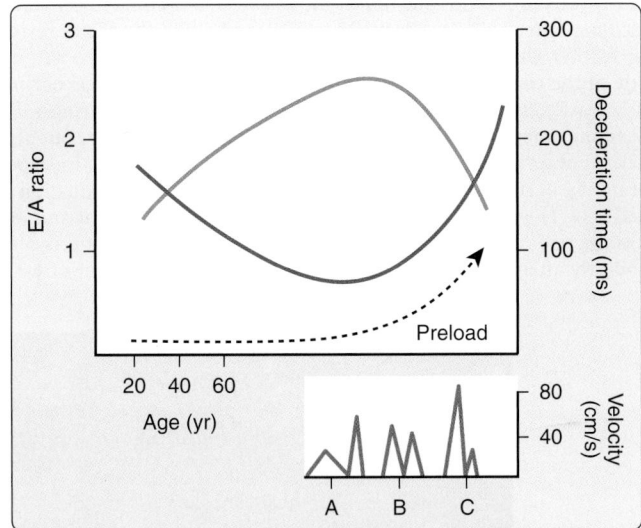

Figure 5-32 Schematic diagram illustrates changes in the ratio of transmitral blood flow velocity during early left ventricular filling and atrial systole (E/A ratio; left axis; *purple curve*) and deceleration time (right axis; *green curve*) associated with age and the development of left ventricular diastolic dysfunction. *Dashed line* represents left ventricular preload, which increases as diastolic dysfunction worsens. The accompanying diagram depicted in the lower right demonstrates impaired relaxation (A), pseudonormal (B), and restrictive (C) left ventricular filling patterns of diastolic dysfunction measured using pulse-wave Doppler echocardiography.

In addition to load dependence, several other factors, including HR, abnormal AV conduction, atrial arrhythmias, and mitral valve disease, may adversely affect evaluation of transmitral blood flow velocity patterns. For example, sinus tachycardia and first-degree AV block produce partial or complete fusion of E and A waves, thereby complicating assessment of individual peak velocities, time-velocity integrals, or deceleration time. Atrial flutter produces variably loaded LA contractions depending on the extent of the accompanying AV block, whereas atrial fibrillation eliminates the active LA contribution to LV filling altogether. Severe mitral stenosis clearly limits LV filling and the transmitral blood flow velocity measurements obtained in the presence of this pathology are obviously unreliable for LV diastolic function analysis. Mitral regurgitation increases LA pressure independent of changes in LV diastolic function, and this action makes isolated recognition of LV diastolic dysfunction difficult, if not impossible. Thus, normal sinus rhythm and the absence of hemodynamically significant mitral valve disease are most often required when the morphology of transmitral blood flow velocity is used for the analysis of LV diastolic function.

Pulmonary Venous Blood Flow Velocity

Analysis of the pulmonary venous blood flow velocity pattern is used to noninvasively determine LV diastolic dysfunction,[255] quantify the degree of mitral regurgitation,[256] or estimate pulmonary capillary occlusion and mean LA pressures.[257] Analogously, the pattern of hepatic venous blood flow velocity provides important information about the relative severity of RV diastolic dysfunction or tricuspid regurgitation. Cardiac anesthesiologists most often interrogate pulmonary venous blood flow velocity by placing a small pulse-wave Doppler sample volume between 0.5 and 1.0 cm into the right or left superior pulmonary vein in a modified midesophageal bicaval or four-chamber TEE imaging plane, respectively, to obtain a crisp velocity profile.[258] Color-flow Doppler mapping is especially useful to identify the best position to place the pulse-wave Doppler sample volume. TEE is the preferred method for pulmonary venous blood flow velocity analysis because the anatomic proximity of the right and left upper pulmonary veins to the esophagus provides optimal imaging windows with minimal ultrasound scatter by intervening tissue compared with a transthoracic approach.[259] As observed when using transmitral blood flow velocity patterns to evaluate LV diastolic function, it is important to recognize that the pulmonary venous blood flow velocity profile is highly dependent on not only LV relaxation, filling, and compliance, but also HR, LA and LV loading conditions, and LA function.[260] Thus, conclusions about LV diastolic function derived using this methodology require interpretation with these potential limitations in mind. In general, the pulmonary venous blood flow velocity profile is used primarily as an adjunctive tool in combination with the transmitral LV filling pattern and not as an independent prognostic indicator of disease progression.[261]

The normal pulmonary venous blood flow velocity pattern is composed of a single small negative deflection that indicates retrograde flow from the LA chamber into the pulmonary veins, termed the atrial reversal ("Ar") wave, and two large positive deflections that demonstrate forward flow from the pulmonary veins into the LA.[262] LA preload, LA contractile state, and LV pressure during late diastole affect the magnitude and duration of the Ar wave.[263] The first positive deflection is known as the "S" (systolic) wave and occurs during LV systole and isovolumic relaxation when the mitral valve is closed. This S wave displays a biphasic morphology ("S_1" and "S_2"; these notations are not equivalent to the first and second heart sounds) originating from a series of LA, LV, and RV events.[264] LA relaxation after contraction and the consequent reduction in LA pressure facilitates forward blood flow from the pulmonary veins into the LA during early LV isovolumic contraction.[263] Mitral annular descent toward the apex during LV systole (approximately 1.3 cm in healthy individuals) also causes a piston-like effect that acts to draw additional blood from the pulmonary veins into the LA.[265] These actions combine to produce S_1. Mitral annular descent may be markedly attenuated in patients with reduced LV systolic function, emphasizing that LV contractility directly influences the degree of LA filling.[266] Transmission of the RV systolic pressure pulse through the pulmonary circulation contributes to additional LA filling later during LV contraction to produce S_2. S_1 and S_2 are most often combined into a single S wave when using pulmonary venous blood flow velocity patterns to assess LV diastolic function. The second positive deflection ("D" wave) of the pulmonary venous blood flow velocity pattern occurs immediately after the opening of the mitral valve because the rapid decline in LA pressure that accompanies early LV filling allows subsequent blood flow from the pulmonary veins into the LA to occur (Figure 5-33). The peak velocity and time-velocity integral of the D wave are dependent on LV compliance and the extent of early LV filling.[267] As a result, factors that attenuate early LV filling (e.g., delayed LV relaxation, reduced LV compliance, mitral stenosis) cause decreases in D-wave velocity.[268]

Similar to the pattern of transmitral blood flow velocity, the pulmonary venous blood flow velocity profile is also age dependent. The S/D ratio, the peak Ar velocity, and the Ar duration increase with age,[243] consistent with the enhanced importance of LA systole to LV filling during the gradual development of delayed LV relaxation. However, the compensatory increase in LA pressure that serves to restore E-wave velocity and E/A ratio in "pseudonormal" physiology attenuates systolic pulmonary venous blood flow and begins to produce pulmonary venous congestion. As a result, the S wave becomes progressively blunted and the S/D ratio declines to less than 1, whereas the magnitude and duration of the Ar wave continue to increase, thereby allowing an easily recognizable distinction between otherwise morphologically similar "normal" and "pseudonormal" transmitral blood flow velocity patterns.[255] As "restrictive" LV diastolic dysfunction develops, these changes are more pronounced concomitant with further increases in LV diastolic and LA pressures. The S/D ratio declines as systolic LA filling is further attenuated and the D-wave deceleration time becomes more rapid as the LV becomes less compliant (see Figure 5-33). The Ar blood flow velocity exceeds 35 cm/sec, and the duration of the Ar wave becomes greater than that of the corresponding transmitral A wave unless overt LA failure occurs.[269] An Ar-A duration greater than 30 msec is strongly predictive of increased LV end-diastolic pressure.[270] As observed with transmitral blood flow velocity profiles, atrial arrhythmias, AV conduction abnormalities, and mitral valve disease limit the use of pulmonary venous blood flow patterns for the evaluation of LV diastolic function.

Tissue Doppler Imaging

Interrogation of septal or lateral mitral annular motion using low-velocity (10 to 15 cm/sec) pulse-wave Doppler echocardiography provides additional information about the relative severity of LV diastolic dysfunction (see Figure 5-29).[271] Mitral annular motion is an index of the

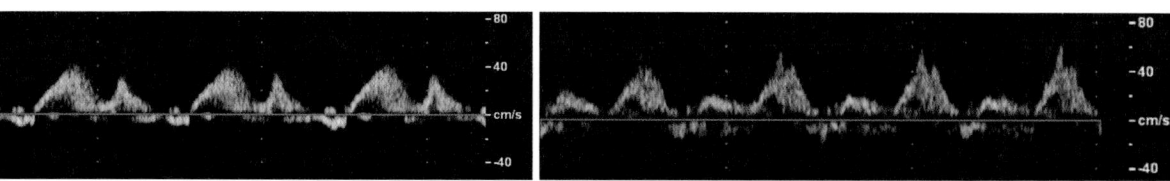

Figure 5-33 Pulmonary venous blood flow velocity waveforms obtained using pulse-wave Doppler echocardiography under normal conditions (*left*) and in the presence of increased left atrial pressure (*right*).

relative LV long-axis lengthening rate during filling. Averaging of septal and lateral tissue Doppler imaging is recommended to account for the effects of regional differences in function.[272] Cardiac anesthesiologists most often use the midesophageal four-chamber TEE view to acquire tissue Doppler waveforms during LV filling. Similar to the transmitral blood flow velocity profile, the tissue Doppler waveform demonstrates peak velocities associated with early LV filling and LA systole (e' and a', respectively), and the e'/a' ratio demonstrates the relative contributions of these events to final LV end-diastolic volume. The ratio of transmitral E to tissue Doppler e' waves (E/e') has been shown to be a reliable estimate of LV filling pressure.[273] For example, a septal E/e' ratio less than 8 strongly suggests that LV filling pressure is normal, but an E/e' ratio greater than 15 usually indicates that LV end-diastolic pressure is markedly increased.[274] The E/e' ratio is especially useful for establishing the diagnosis of HFNEF.[275,276] The determinants of tissue Doppler e' and a' velocities are similar to those described for transmitral E and A velocities, respectively. The rate and extent of LV isovolumic relaxation, LV systolic function, and LV preload are the major hemodynamic factors that determine tissue Doppler e' velocity in humans. Notably, tissue Doppler e' velocity appears to be less affected by preload than transmitral E velocity, especially when LV relaxation is delayed.[277] As a result, the e'/a' ratio is less likely to display overt "delayed relaxation" and subsequent "pseudonormal" profiles than its transmitral E/A counterpart as LV diastolic dysfunction progresses and LA pressure increases. This relative Doppler e' preload independence during abnormal LV relaxation also increases the time interval between the onset of the transmitral E and tissue Doppler e' velocities ($T_{E-e'}$), which has been shown to be a noninvasive estimate of the time constant (τ) of LV isovolumic relaxation in humans.[278] Unlike transmitral E-wave velocity, tissue Doppler e' velocity is also particularly useful in distinguishing between constrictive pericarditis (e' is normal) and restrictive cardiomyopathy (e' is decreased).[279] LA contractile function and LV diastolic pressure are the primary factors that influence the magnitude of tissue Doppler a' velocity. As observed with transmitral and pulmonary venous blood flow velocities, tissue Doppler velocities are age dependent such that e' velocity and e'/a' ratio decrease, whereas a' velocity and E/e' increase with age. In addition to age, the use of tissue Doppler imaging to quantify LV diastolic dysfunction also may be limited by mitral annular calcification, the presence of a prosthetic mitral valve or ring, or mitral valve disease, as well as technical difficulties obtaining a reproducible, clean envelope of low-velocity annular motion during diastole.[243]

Color M-Mode Propagation Velocity

The flow propagation velocity (V_p) of the blood column extending from the mitral valve to the apex during early LV filling is reliably obtained using color M-mode echocardiography and is another frequently measured index of LV diastolic function.[280] V_p is relatively preload insensitive,[281] is particularly useful for evaluating LV relaxation abnormalities,[282] and correlates with invasively derived indices of LV relaxation (e.g., τ).[280] The midesophageal four-chamber imaging plane allows the cardiac anesthesiologist to acquire a color Doppler M-mode envelope by placing the M-mode scan line into the center of LV inflow aligned from base to apex. After adjusting the Nyquist limit to assure that the highest velocity is blue, V_p is determined as the slope of the first aliasing velocity (Figure 5-34).[243] A V_p value greater than 50 cm/sec is normal and quantifies the rapid movement of blood from the mitral valve to the apex, mediated by the pressure gradient between these intraventricular regions (termed *apical suction*) during early LV filling.[280,283] The extent of relaxation and the elastic recoil of the LV are the primary determinants of V_p. Thus, clinical conditions (e.g., myocardial ischemia, HCM) in which these factors are attenuated reduce V_p by decreasing the apical suction during early LV filling.[284,285] However, the use of V_p as a quantitative index of LV diastolic dysfunction may be limited by other factors, including alterations in chamber geometry, contractile dyssynchrony, and blood flow vortex formation, that become increasingly important in determining the magnitude of apical suction as HF progresses.[286] The ratio of transmitral E-wave velocity to

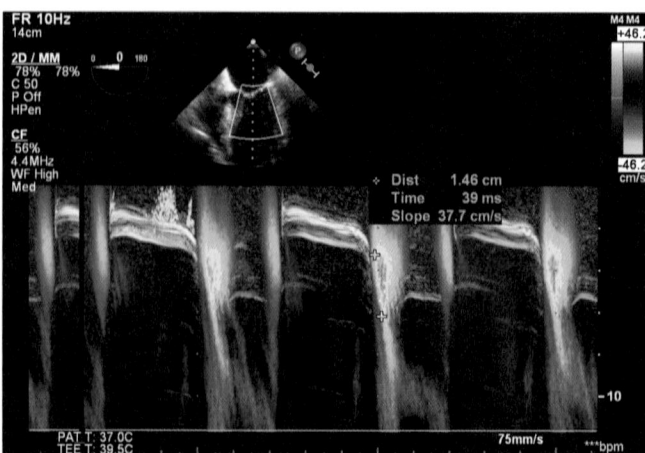

Figure 5-34 Determination of color M-mode mitral valve blood flow propagation velocity (V_p). A color Doppler M-mode envelope is obtained by placing the M-mode scan line into the center of LV inflow aligned from base to apex, and V_p is determined as the slope of the first aliasing velocity. A value of V_p less than 45 cm/sec suggests that early left ventricular (LV) filling is attenuated consistent with LV diastolic dysfunction.

V_p (E/V_p) is related to LV filling pressure and has been used as a noninvasive surrogate of pulmonary capillary occlusion pressure.[283] For example, an E/V_p ratio greater than 2.5 indicates that "wedge" pressure is greater than 15 mm Hg and is common in the presence of "restrictive" physiology.[278]

PERICARDIAL FORCES

The pericardium is a sac that encloses the heart, proximal great vessels, and distal vena cavae and pulmonary veins. The smooth surface of the visceral pericardium combined with the lubrication provided by between 15 and 35 mL pericardial fluid (composed of plasma ultrafiltrate, myocardial interstitial fluid, and a small quantity of lymph) and surfactant phospholipids reduce friction and facilitate normal cardiac movement during systole and diastole. The pericardium also acts as a mechanical barrier that separates the heart from other mediastinal structures and limits abnormal displacement of the heart through its inferior (diaphragmatic) and superior (great vessels) attachments. The fibrous layer of the parietal pericardium determines the J-shaped pericardial pressure-volume relation (Figure 5-35), which indicates that the pericardium is substantially less compliant than the LV myocardium. As a result of this lack of elasticity, the pericardium has limited volume reserve and thus is capable of accommodating only a small increase in volume before a large increase in pressure occurs.[287] Pericardial pressure is usually subatmospheric (range, −5 to 0 mm Hg), varies with changes in intrathoracic pressure, and produces little, if any, mechanical effect in a normal heart under euvolemic conditions.[288] However, the pericardium exerts a critical restraining force on the filling of all four cardiac chambers,[289] and this effect is exaggerated during pericardial compression (e.g., tamponade, constrictive pericarditis) or acute increases in chamber dimension (e.g., volume loading). Pericardial restraint is most apparent in the thinner-walled atria and RV and is the primary determinant of the diastolic pressure and volume of these chambers. Thus, the pericardium resists further increases in atrial and RV chamber size during volume loading, and pressure within these chambers increases more rapidly than predicted on the basis of myocardial elastic properties alone. The pericardium also plays an important role in LV filling,[290] as an acute increase in pericardial pressure causes a parallel upward shift of the LV EDPVR.[291] The elevation of the EDPVR combined with more pronounced diastolic ventricular interdependence (interaction) is responsible for the severely restricted LV filling observed during pericardial tamponade. Conversely, atrial

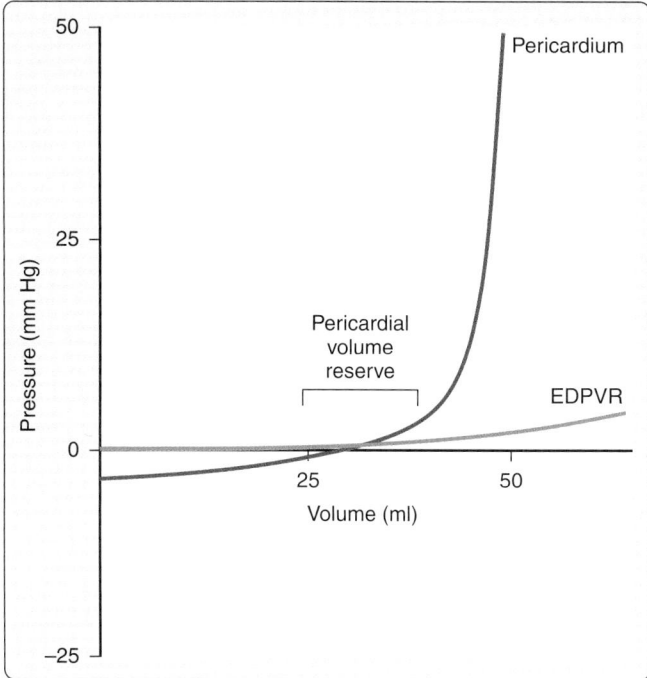

Figure 5-35 Pressure-volume relation of the pericardium (*purple line*) compared with the left ventricular end-diastolic pressure-volume relation (EDPVR; *green line*). Note that large increases in pericardial pressure occur after reserve volume is exceeded.

volume, RV and LV end-diastolic volumes, SV, and CO increase after pericardiectomy because pericardial restraining forces are no longer present and the myocardium solely determines the compliance of each chamber. In contrast with the effects of an acute increase in pericardial or cardiac chamber volume, a chronic pericardial effusion or chamber enlargement progressively stretches the pericardium, thereby increasing its compliance and attenuating or abolishing its restraining effects. This compensatory response to a gradual, chronic increase in pericardial load explains why hemodynamic instability does not occur in the presence of a very large (> 1000 mL) pericardial effusion or profound biventricular dilatation that would otherwise precipitate severe hemodynamic instability.

The pericardium plays an essential role in ventricular interdependence (the influence of the pressure and volume of one ventricle on the mechanical behavior of the other). The pericardium restrains both the RV and the LV equally despite the inherent differences in compliance between the chambers. Hence, an increase in RV size (e.g., ischemia, volume overload) causes pericardial pressure to increase, thereby reducing LV compliance and restricting LV filling.[292] Similarly, acute LV distention (e.g., application of an aortic cross clamp) encroaches on the RV, shifts its EDPVR up and to the left, and limits RV filling.[293] These observations emphasize that the relative position and direction of movement of the interventricular septum are not the only factors that determine ventricular interdependence. Evidence for diastolic ventricular interaction is readily apparent using pulse-wave Doppler echocardiography to determine changes in RV and LV filling during spontaneous ventilation.[294] Inspiration decreases intrathoracic pressure, enhances systemic venous return, and causes modest RV distention. These actions mildly reduce LV filling by decreasing compliance of the chamber, resulting in small declines in CO and mean arterial pressure. Conversely, RV filling is attenuated and LV filling is augmented during expiration through a similar ventricular interaction mechanism. Compression of the ventricular chambers during pericardial tamponade[295] or constrictive pericarditis[296] markedly exaggerates these respiratory changes in RV and LV filling and causes pulsus paradoxus. Nevertheless, maintenance of spontaneous ventilation

is critical under these circumstances because negative intrathoracic pressure preserves venous return to some degree. In contrast, positive-pressure ventilation of the lungs may rapidly cause cardiovascular collapse during acute pericardial tamponade by profoundly limiting venous return.

DETERMINANTS OF ATRIAL FUNCTION

The maximum velocity of shortening of LA myocardium is equivalent to or greater than LV myocardium under similar loading conditions.[297,298] LA emptying fraction is primarily dependent on LA preload and contractile state in vivo unless the LA dilates and its myofilaments are extended beyond optimal operating length.[299] Under these circumstances, emptying fraction falls precipitously and LA contraction no longer makes a meaningful contribution to final LV end-diastolic volume. Alterations in the activity of the autonomic nervous system produce similar changes in LA compared with LV contractile state.[300] For example, increases in LA emptying fraction and the LA contribution to LV filling occur as a result of sympathetic nervous system activation,[301] whereas parasympathetic stimulation causes a direct negative inotropic effect. Volatile anesthetics also cause a similar degree of myocardial depression in LA compared with LV myocardium in vivo.[96,302] LV compliance and pressure during late diastole determine the afterload to which the LA is subjected during its contraction. Thus, LV diastolic dysfunction increases LA afterload and the amount of energy the LA must expend to perform similar pressure-volume work. Analogous to the changes in myofilament composition occurring in response to chronic increases in LV afterload, upregulation of the β-myosin isoform in atrial myocardium serves as an important compensatory response to increased LA afterload that preserves LA emptying fraction.[303] However, the LA, like the RV, has less muscle mass and operates at lower pressures than the LV. Thus, the LA is substantially more susceptible to afterload mismatch than the LV, and as a result, increases in LA afterload and energy utilization produced by impaired LV filling often lead to LA contractile failure.[268] For example, an initial increase in LA emptying fraction may be observed early in the course of developing LV failure, but LA contractile dysfunction eventually occurs as LV compliance declines and end-diastolic pressure increases.[304] Conversely, drug therapy for chronic hypertension reduces LA and LV afterload, and improves the active contribution of the LA to LV filling.[305] Notably, remodeling and reduced compliance of the LA also occur in response to LV diastolic dysfunction. These effects further restrict pulmonary venous blood flow into the LA during the reservoir and conduit phases, and may lead to the development of pulmonary edema.

Several factors determine LA reservoir and conduit function. LA relaxation after contraction normally facilitates forward flow from the pulmonary veins during early LV isovolumic contraction,[263] whereas relaxation abnormalities produced by LA ischemia, hypertrophy, or dilation attenuate the ability of the chamber to function effectively as a reservoir. Descent of the LV base toward the apex during LV systole is also an important determinant of LA reservoir function.[265] This action is markedly attenuated in the presence of severe LV contractile dysfunction. As a result, LA reservoir function decreases because pulmonary venous return during the S_1 phase is markedly reduced or entirely absent.[266] Transmission of RVSV through the pulmonary circulation contributes blood to the LA during the late reservoir phase (S_2)[306] and, thus, RV systolic dysfunction also adversely affects LA reservoir function. In addition to these factors, LA compliance plays a crucial role in the ability of the chamber to act as a reservoir and a conduit. LA diseases in which compliance is reduced are clearly associated with impaired LA filling.[72,30] Pressure-volume analysis has demonstrated that the LA appendage is more compliant than the main body of the chamber[308,309] and plays a crucial role in LA filling. Temporary LA appendage exclusion[310] or permanent removal[309] reduces the compliance of the remaining LA, thereby attenuating reservoir function and blunting subsequent early LV filling. These effects are particularly important in the presence of LA dilation or hypertension. The pericardium also limits LA passive filling as pericardiectomy was shown to increase LA compliance, enhance early LV filling rate, and augment conduit and, to a lesser extent, reservoir function.[95]

Exercise and age produce characteristic changes in LA function. LA contractility and reservoir function are enhanced during exercise.[311] The increase in reservoir capacity contributes to the formation of a larger LA-LV pressure gradient during early LV filling, thereby increasing LV SV and CO. An increase in conduit function also has been observed in endurance athletes compared with normal subjects.[312] In contrast with these findings, LA dilation and declines in passive emptying occur in healthy elderly subjects[313] concomitant with a compensatory increase in LA ejection force[314] and augmentation of LA contribution to LV end-diastolic volume.[315] LA dilation also increases storage fraction (ratio of LA reservoir to LV SV),[316] but this dilation may contribute to further increases in LA wall stress and eventual LA contractile dysfunction in the elderly.[317]

REFERENCES

1. Greenbaum RA, Ho SY, Gibson DG, et al: Left ventricular fibre architecture in man, *Br Heart J* 45:248–263, 1981.
2. Keith A: Harveian Lecture on the functional anatomy of the heart, *Br J Med* 1:361–363, 1918.
3. Harvey W: An anatomical disquisition on the motion of the heart and blood in animals (1628). In Willis FA, Keys TE, editors: *Cardiac Classics*, London, 1941, Henry Kimpton, pp 19–79.
4. Mall FP: On the muscular architecture of the ventricles of the human heart, *Am J Anat* 11:211–278, 1911.
5. Robb JS, Robb RD: The normal heart: Anatomy and physiology of the structural units, *Am Heart J* 23:455–467, 1942.
6. Streeter DD Jr, Spotnitz HM, Patel DP, et al: Fiber orientation in the canine left ventricle during diastole and systole, *Circ Res* 24:339–347, 1969.
7. Buckberg GD, Coghlan HC, Torrent-Guasp F: The structure and function of the helical heart and its buttress wrapping. VI. Geometric concepts of heart failure and use for structural correction, *Semin Thorac Cardiovasc Surg* 13:386–401, 2001.
8. Yellin EL, Hori M, Yoran C, et al: Left ventricular relaxation in the filling and nonfilling intact canine heart, *Am J Physiol* 250:H620–H629, 1986.
9. Cheng C-P, Noda T, Nozawa T, et al: Effect of heart failure on the mechanism of exercise-induced augmentation of mitral valve flow, *Circ Res* 72:795–806, 1993.
10. Takayama Y, Costa KD, Covell JW: Contribution of laminar myofiber architecture to load-dependent changes in mechanics of LV myocardium, *Am J Physiol Heart Circ Physiol* 282:H1510–H1520, 2002.
11. De Hert SG, Gillebert TC, Andries LC, et al: Role of the endocardial endothelium in the regulation of myocardial function: Physiologic and pathophysiologic implications, *Anesthesiology* 79:1354–1366, 1993.
12. Feneley MP, Gavaghan TP, Baron DW, et al: Contribution of left ventricular contraction to the generation of right ventricular systolic pressure in the human heart, *Circulation* 71:473–480, 1985.
13. Hammarstrom E, Wranne B, Pinto FJ, et al: Tricuspid annular motion, *J Am Soc Echocardiogr* 4:131–139, 1991.
14. Stein PD, Munter WA: New functional concept of valvular mechanics in normal and diseased aortic valves, *Circulation* 44:101–108, 1971.
15. Gharib M, Rambod E, Kheradvar A, et al: Optimal vortex formation as an index of cardiac health, *Proc Natl Acad Sci U S A* 103:6305–6308, 2006.
16. Lam JHC: Morphology of the human mitral valve. I. Chordae tendinae: A new classification, *Circulation* 41:449, 1970.
17. Perloff JK, Roberts WC: The mitral apparatus. Functional anatomy of mitral regurgitation, *Circulation* 46:227–239, 1972.
18. Voci P, Bilotta F, Caretta Q, et al: Papillary muscle perfusion pattern. A hypothesis for ischemic papillary muscle dysfunction, *Circulation* 91:1714–1718, 1995.
19. James TN, Burch GE: The atrial coronary arteries in man, *Circulation* 17:90–98, 1958.
20. Porter WT: The influence of the heart beat on the flow of blood through the walls of the heart, *Am J Physiol* 1:145–163, 1898.
21. Rahimtoola SH, Ehsani A, Sinno MZ, et al: Left atrial transport function in myocardial infarction. Importance of its booster pump function, *Am J Med* 59:686–694, 1975.
22. Stefanadis C, Dernellis J, Tsiamis E, et al: Effects of pacing-induced and balloon coronary occlusion ischemia on left atrial function in patients with coronary artery disease, *J Am Coll Cardiol* 33:687–696, 1999.
23. James TN: Cardiac innervation: Anatomic and pharmacologic relations, *Bull N Y Acad Med* 43:1041–1086, 1967.
24. Tops LF, Schalij MJ, Bax JJ: The effects of right ventricular apical pacing on ventricular function and dyssynchrony implications for therapy, *J Am Coll Cardiol* 54:764–776, 2009.
25. Epstein AE, DiMarco JP, Ellenbogen KA, et al: ACC/AHA/HRS 2008 guidelines for device-based therapy of cardiac rhythm abnormalities: a report of the American College of Cardiology/American Heart Association Task Force on Practice Guidelines (Writing Committee to Revise the ACC/AHA/NASPE 2002 Guideline Update for Implantation of Cardiac Pacemakers and Antiarrhythmia Devices): Developed in collaboration with the American Association for Thoracic Surgery and Society of Thoracic Surgeons, *Circulation* 117:e350–e408, 2008.
26. Schaub MC, Hefti MA, Zuellig RA, et al: Modulation of contractility in human cardiac hypertrophy by myosin essential light chain isoforms, *Cardiovasc Res* 37:381–404, 1998.
27. Cazorla O, Vassort G, Garnier D, et al: Length modulation of active force in rat cardiac myocytes: Is titin the sensor? *J Mol Cell Cardiol* 31:1215–1227, 1999.
28. Helmes M, Trombitas K, Granzier H: Titin develops restoring force in rat cardiac myocytes, *Circ Res* 79:619–626, 1996.
29. Schiaffino S, Reggiani C: Molecular diversity of myofibrillar proteins: Gene regulation and molecular significance, *Physiol Rev* 76:371–423, 1996.
30. Moncman CL, Wang K: Nebulette: A 107 kD nebulin-like protein in cardiac muscle, *Cell Motil Cytoskel* 32:205–225, 1995.
31. Solaro RJ, Rarick HM: Troponin and tropomyosin. Proteins that switch on and tune in the activity of cardiac myofilaments, *Circ Res* 83:471–480, 1998.
32. Tobacman LS: Thin filament-mediated regulation of cardiac contraction, *Annu Rev Physiol* 58:447–481, 1996.
33. Solaro RJ, Van Eyk J: Altered interactions among thin filaments proteins modulate cardiac function, *J Mol Cell Cardiol* 28:217–230, 1999.
34. Luo W, Grupp IL, Harrer J, et al: Targeted ablation of the phospholamban gene is associated with markedly enhanced myocardial contractility and loss of β-agonist stimulation, *Circ Res* 75:401–409, 1994.
35. Rayment I, Holden HM, Whittaker M: Structure of the actin-myosin complex and its implications for muscle contraction, *Science* 261:58–65, 1993.
36. Dominguez R, Freyzon Y, Trybus KM, et al: Crystal structure of a vertebrate smooth muscle myosin motor domain and its complex with the essential light chain: Visualization of the prepower stroke state, *Cell* 94:559–571, 1998.
37. Finer JT, Simmons RM, Spudich JA: Single myosin molecule mechanics: Piconewton forces and nanometer steps, *Nature* 368:113–119, 1994.
38. Gilbert JC, Glantz SA: Determinants of left ventricular filling and of the diastolic pressure-volume relation, *Circ Res* 64:827–852, 1989.
39. Stillwell GK: The law of Laplace: Some clinical applications, *Mayo Clin Proc* 48:863–869, 1973.
40. Cheng CP, Igarashi Y, Little WC: Mechanism of augmented rate of left ventricular filling during exercise, *Circ Res* 70:9–19, 1992.
41. Hoit BD, Shao Y, Gabel M, et al: In vivo assessment of left atrial contractile performance in normal and pathological conditions using a time-varying elastance model, *Circulation* 89:1829–1838, 1994.
42. Hermann HJ: Left ventricular volumes by angiocardiography: Comparison of methods and simplification of techniques, *Cardiovasc Res* 2:404–414, 1968.
43. Stefanadis C, Dernellis J, Stratos C, et al: Assessment of left atrial pressure-area relation in humans by means of retrograde left atrial catheterization and echocardiographic automatic boundary detection: Effect of dobutamine, *J Am Coll Cardiol* 31:426–436, 1998.
44. Karunanithi MK, Michniewicz J, Copeland SE, et al: Right ventricular preload recruitable stroke work, end-systolic pressure-volume, and dP/dt_{max}-end-diastolic volume relations compared as indexes of right ventricular contractile performance in conscious dogs, *Circ Res* 70:1169–1179, 1992.
45. Sandler H, Dodge HT: Left ventricular tension and stress in man, *Circ Res* 13:91–104, 1963.
46. Florenzano F, Glantz SA: Left-ventricular mechanical adaptation to chronic aortic regurgitation in intact dogs, *Am J Physiol* 252:H969–H984, 1987.
47. Grossman W, Jones D, McLaurin LP: Wall stress and patterns of hypertrophy in the human left ventricle, *J Clin Invest* 56:56–64, 1975.
48. Borow KM, Lang RM, Neumann A, et al: Physiologic mechanisms governing hemodynamic responses to positive inotropic therapy in patients with dilated cardiomyopathy, *Circulation* 77:625–637, 1988.
49. Regen DM: Calculation of left ventricular wall stress, *Circ Res* 67:245–252, 1990.
50. Regen DM, Anversa P, Capasso JM: Segmental calculation of left ventricular wall stresses, *Am J Physiol* 264:H1411–H1421, 1993.
51. Mirsky I: Review of various theories for the evaluation of left ventricular wall stresses. In Mirsky I, Ghista DN, Sandler H, editors: *Cardiac mechanics: Physiological, clinical, and mathematical considerations*, New York, 1974, Wiley, pp 381–409.
52. Grossman W: Cardiac hypertrophy: Useful adaptation or pathologic process? *Am J Med* 69:576–584, 1980.
53. Wiggers CJ: The Henry Jackson Memorial Lecture. Dynamics of ventricular contraction under abnormal conditions, *Circulation* 5:321–348, 1952.
54. Sandler H, Alderman E: Determination of left ventricular size and shape, *Circ Res* 34:1–8, 1974.
55. Haddad F, Couture P, Tousignant C, et al: The right ventricle in cardiac surgery, a perioperative perspective: I. Anatomy, physiology, and assessment, *Anesth Analg* 108:407–421, 2009.
56. Fifer MA, Grossman W: Measurement of ventricular volumes, ejection fraction, mass, wall stress, and regional wall motion. In Grossman W, editor: *Cardiac catheterization, angiography, and intervention*, ed 4 Philadelphia, 1991, Lea and Febiger, pp 300–318.
57. Sabbah HN, Stein PD: Negative diastolic pressure in the intact canine right ventricle. Evidence of diastolic suction, *Circ Res* 49:108–113, 1981.
58. Courtois M, Kovacs SJ Jr, Ludbrook PA: Transmitral pressure-flow velocity relation. Importance of regional pressure gradients in the left ventricle during diastole, *Circulation* 78:661–671, 1988.
59. Cheng C-P, Freeman GL, Santamore WP, et al: Effect of loading conditions, contractile state, and heart rate on early diastolic left ventricular filling in conscious dogs, *Circ Res* 66:814–823, 1990.
60. Ishida Y, Meisner JS, Tsujioka K, et al: Left ventricular filling dynamics: Influence of left ventricular relaxation and left atrial pressure, *Circulation* 74:187–196, 1986.
61. Little WC, Oh JK: Echocardiographic evaluation of diastolic function can be used to guide clinical care, *Circulation* 120:802–809, 2009.
62. Kilner PJ, Yang GZ, Wilkes AJ, et al: Asymmetric redirection of flow through the heart, *Nature* 404:759–761, 2000.
63. Kheradvar A, Gharib M: On mitral valve dynamics and its connection to early diastolic flow, *Ann Biomed Eng* 37:1–13, 2009.
64. Brutsaert DL, Rademakers FE, Sys SU, et al: Analysis of relaxation in the evaluation of ventricular function of the heart, *Prog Cardiovasc Dis* 28:143–163, 1985.
65. Yellin EL, Nikolic S, Frater RWM: Left ventricular filling dynamics and diastolic function, *Prog Cardiovasc Dis* 32:247–271, 1990.
66. Suga H, Goto Y, Igarashi Y, et al: Ventricular suction under zero source pressure for filling, *Am J Physiol* 251:H47–H55, 1986.
67. Suga H, Yasumura Y, Nozawa T, et al: Pressure-volume relation around zero transmural pressure in excised cross-circulated dog left ventricle, *Circ Res* 63:361–372, 1988.
68. Keren G, Meisner JS, Sherez J, et al: Interrelationship of mid-diastolic mitral valve motion, pulmonary venous flow, and transmitral flow, *Circulation* 74:36–44, 1986.
69. Little RC: Volume pressure relationships of the pulmonary-left heart vascular segment. Evidence for a "valve-like" closure of the pulmonary veins, *Circ Res* 8:594–599, 1960.
70. Ruskin J, McHale PA, Harley A, et al: Pressure-flow studies in man: Effect of atrial systole on left ventricular function, *J Clin Invest* 49:472–478, 1970.
71. Barbier P, Solomon SB, Schiller NB, et al: Left atrial relaxation and left ventricular systolic function determine left atrial reservoir function, *Circulation* 100:427–436, 1999.
72. Mehta S, Charbonneau F, Fitchett DH, et al: The clinical consequences of a stiff left atrium, *Am Heart J* 122:1184–1191, 1991.
73. Frank O: Zur dynamik des herzmuskels, *Z Biol* 32:370–437, 1895.
74. Frank O: Die grundform des arteriellen pulses, *Z Biol* 39:483–526, 1898.
75. Suga H, Sagawa K: Instantaneous pressure-volume relationships and their ratio in the excised, supported canine left ventricle, *Circ Res* 35:117–126, 1974.
76. Suga H, Sagawa K, Shoukas AA: Load-independence of the instantaneous pressure-volume ratio of the canine left ventricle and effects of epinephrine and heart rate on the ratio, *Circ Res* 32:314–322, 1973.
77. Sagawa K: The end-systolic pressure-volume relation of the ventricle: Definition, modifications and clinical use, *Circulation* 63:1223–1227, 1981.
78. Glower DD, Spratt JA, Snow ND, et al: Linearity of the Frank-Starling relationship in the intact heart: The concept of preload recruitable stroke work, *Circulation* 71:994–1009, 1985.

79. Katz AM: Influence of altered inotropy and lusitropy on ventricular pressure-volume loops, *J Am Coll Cardiol* 11:438–445, 1988.
80. Kass DA, Maughan WL, Guo ZM, et al: Comparative influence of load versus inotropic states on indexes of ventricular contractility: Experimental and theoretical analysis based on pressure-volume relationships, *Circulation* 76:1422–1436, 1987.
81. Suga H: Ventricular energetics, *Physiol Rev* 70:247–277, 1990.
82. Brown KA, Ditchey RV: Human right ventricular end-systolic pressure-volume relation defined by maximal elastance, *Circulation* 78:81–91, 1988.
83. Grossman W: Diastolic dysfunction and congestive heart failure, *Circulation* 81(Suppl 2):III1–III7, 1990.
84. Aversano T, Maughan WL, Hunter WC, et al: End-systolic measures of regional ventricular performance, *Circulation* 73:938–950, 1986.
85. Kaseda S, Tomoike H, Ogata I, et al: End-systolic pressure-volume, pressure-length, and stress-strain relations in canine hearts, *Am J Physiol* 249:H648–H654, 1985.
86. Lee JD, Tajimi T, Widmann TF, et al: Application of end-systolic pressure-volume and pressure-wall thickness relations in conscious dogs, *J Am Coll Cardiol* 9:136–146, 1987.
87. Pagel PS, Kampine JP, Schmeling WT, et al: Comparison of end-systolic pressure-length relations and preload recruitable stroke work as indices of myocardial contractility in the conscious and anesthetized, chronically instrumented dog, *Anesthesiology* 73:278–290, 1990.
88. Mahler F, Covell JW, Ross J Jr: Systolic pressure-diameter relations in the normal conscious dog, *Cardiovasc Res* 9:447–455, 1975.
89. Foex P, Francis CM, Cutfield GR, et al: The pressure-length loop, *Br J Anaesth* 60(8 Suppl 1):65S–71S, 1988.
90. Safwat A, Leone BJ, Norris RM, et al: Pressure-length loop area: Its components analyzed during graded myocardial ischemia, *J Am Coll Cardiol* 17:790–796, 1991.
91. Pagel PS, Kehl F, Gare M, et al: Mechanical function of the left atrium: New insights based on analysis of pressure-volume relations and Doppler echocardiography, *Anesthesiology* 98:975–994, 2003.
92. Matsuda Y, Toma Y, Ogawa H, et al: Importance of left atrial function in patients with myocardial infarction, *Circulation* 67:566–571, 1983.
93. Matsuzaki M, Tamitani M, Toma Y, et al: Mechanism of augmented left atrial pump function in myocardial infarction and essential hypertension evaluated by left atrial pressure dimension relation, *Am J Cardiol* 67:1121–1126, 1991.
94. Dernellis JM, Stefanadis CI, Zacharoulis AA, et al: Left atrial mechanical adaptation to long-standing hemodynamic loads based on pressure-volume relations, *Am J Cardiol* 81:1138–1143, 1998.
95. Hoit BD, Shao Y, Gabel M, et al: Influence of pericardium on left atrial compliance and pulmonary venous flow, *Am J Physiol* 264:H1781–H1787, 1993.
96. Gare M, Schwabe DA, Hettrick DA, et al: Desflurane, sevoflurane, and isoflurane affect left atrial active and passive mechanical properties and impair left atrial-left ventricular coupling in vivo. Analysis using pressure-volume relations, *Anesthesiology* 95:689–698, 2001.
97. Little WC, Downes TR: Clinical evaluation of left ventricular diastolic performance, *Prog Cardiovasc Dis* 32:273–290, 1990.
98. Maughan WL, Sunagawa K, Burkhoff D, et al: Effect of heart rate on the canine end-systolic pressure-volume relationship, *Circulation* 72:654–659, 1985.
99. Freeman GL, Little WC, O'Rourke RA: Influence of heart rate on left ventricular performance in conscious dogs, *Circ Res* 61:455–464, 1987.
100. Mitchell JH, Wallace AG, Skinner NS: Intrinsic effects of heart rate on left ventricular performance, *Am J Physiol* 205:41–48, 1963.
101. Vatner SF: Sympathetic mechanisms regulating myocardial contractility in conscious animals. In Fozzard HA, Haber E, Jennings RB, et al, edited: *The Heart and Cardiovascular System: Scientific Foundations*, ed 2, New York, 1991, Raven Press, pp 1709–1728.
102. Spodick DH: The normal and diseased pericardium: Current concepts of pericardial physiology, diagnosis, and treatment, *J Am Coll Cardiol* 1:240–251, 1983.
103. Wier W, Yue DT: Intracellular [Ca++] transients underlying the short-term force-interval relationship in ferret ventricular myocardium, *J Physiol (Lond)* 376:507–530, 1986.
104. Yue DT, Burkhoff D, Franz MR, et al: Postextrasystolic potentiation of the isolated canine left ventricle: Relationship to mechanical restitution, *Circ Res* 56:340–350, 1985.
105. Spotnitz HM, Sonnenblick EH, Spiro D: Relation of ultrastructure to function in the intact heart: Sarcomere structure relative to pressure volume curves of intact left ventricles of dog and cat, *Circ Res* 18:49–66, 1966.
106. Burkhoff D: The conductance method of left ventricular volume estimation. Methodologic limitations put into perspective, *Circulation* 81:703–706, 1990.
107. Little WC, Freeman GL, O'Rourke RA: Simultaneous determination of left ventricular end-systolic pressure-volume and pressure-dimension relationships in closed-chest dogs, *Circulation* 71:1301–1308, 1985.
108. Applegate RJ, Cheng C-P, Little WC: Simultaneous conductance catheter and dimension assessment of left ventricle volume in the intact animal, *Circulation* 81:638–648, 1990.
109. Baan J, Van der Velde ET, De Bruin HG, et al: Continuous measurement of left ventricular volume in animals and humans by conductance catheter, *Circulation* 70:812–823, 1984.
110. Kass DA: Clinical evaluation of left heart function by conductance catheter techique, *Eur Heart J* 13(Suppl E):57–64, 1993.
111. Baan J, Jong TT, Kerkhof PLM, et al: Continuous stroke volume and cardiac output from intra-ventricular dimensions obtained with impedance catheter, *Cardiovasc Res* 15:328–334, 1981.
112. Alderman EL, Glantz SA: Acute hemodynamic interventions shift the diastolic pressure-volume curve in man, *Circulation* 54:662–671, 1976.
113. Hansen RM, Viquerat CE, Matthay MA, et al: Poor correlation between pulmonary arterial wedge pressure and left ventricular end-diastolic volume after coronary artery bypass graft surgery, *Anesthesiology* 64:764–770, 1986.
114. Milnor WR: Arterial impedance as ventricular afterload, *Circ Res* 36:565–570, 1975.
115. Nichols WW, O'Rourke MF: *McDonald's Blood Flow in Arteries: Theoretic, Experimental and Clinical Principles*, Philadelphia, 1990, Lea & Febiger.
116. Noble MIM: Left ventricular load, arterial impedance and their interrelationship, *Cardiovasc Res* 13:183–198, 1979.
117. Burkhoff D, Alexander J, Schipke J: Assessment of Windkessel as a model of aortic input impedance, *Am J Physiol* 255:H742–H753, 1988.
118. Wesseling KH, Jansen JRC, Settels JJ, et al: Computation of aortic flow from pressure in humans using a nonlinear, three element model, *J Appl Physiol* 74:2566–2573, 1993.
119. Hettrick DA, Pagel PS, Warltier DC: Differential effects of isoflurane and halothane on aortic input impedance quantified using a three element Windkessel model, *Anesthesiology* 83:361–373, 1995.
120. Borow KM, Colan SD, Neumann A: Altered left ventricular mechanics in patients with valvular aortic stenosis and coarctation of the aorta: Effects on systolic performance and late outcome, *Circulation* 72:515–522, 1985.
121. Weber KT, Janicki JS: Myocardial oxygen consumption: The role of wall force and shortening, *Am J Physiol* 233:H421–H430, 1977.
122. Colan SD, Borow KM, Neumann A: The left ventricular end-systolic wall stress-velocity of fiber shortening relation: A load independent index of myocardial contractility, *J Am Coll Cardiol* 4:715–724, 1984.

123. Borow KM, Green LH, Grossman W, et al: Left ventricular end-systolic stress-shortening and stress-length relations in humans: Normal values and sensitivity to inotropic states, *Am J Cardiol* 50:1301–1308, 1982.
124. Carabello BA, Spann JF: The uses and limitations of end-systolic indexes of left ventricular function, *Circulation* 69:1058–1064, 1984.
125. Ross J Jr: Applications and limitations of end-systolic measures of ventricular performance, *Fed Proc* 43:2418–2422, 1984.
126. Sunagawa K, Maughan WL, Burkhoff D, et al: Left ventricular interaction with arterial load studied in isolated canine ventricle, *Am J Physiol* 245:H773–H780, 1983.
127. Sunagawa K, Maughan WL, Sagawa K: Optimal arterial resistance for the maximal stroke work studied in isolated canine left ventricle, *Circ Res* 56:586–595, 1985.
128. Hettrick DA, Pagel PS, Warltier DC: Desflurane, sevoflurane, and isoflurane impair canine left ventricular-arterial coupling and mechanical efficiency, *Anesthesiology* 85:403–413, 1996.
129. Little WC, Cheng CP: Left ventricular-arterial coupling in conscious dogs, *Am J Physiol* 261:H70–H76, 1991.
130. Starling MR: Left ventricular-arterial coupling relations in the normal human heart, *Am Heart J* 125:1659–1666, 1993.
131. Kenner T: Some comments on ventricular afterload, *Basic Res Cardiol* 82:209–215, 1987.
132. Nichols WW, Nicolini FA, Pepine CJ: Determinants of isolated systolic hypertension in the elderly, *J Hypertens* 10:S73–S77, 1992.
133. Chen CH, Nakayama M, Nevo E, et al: Coupled systolic-ventricular and vascular stiffening with age: Implications for pressure regulation and cardiac reserve in the elderly, *J Am Coll Cardiol* 32:1221–1227, 1998.
134. Lang RM, Borow KM, Neumann A, et al: Systemic vascular resistance: An unreliable index of left ventricular afterload, *Circulation* 74:1114–1123, 1986.
135. Little WC: Enhanced load dependence of relaxation in heart failure. Clinical implications, *Circulation* 85:2326–2328, 1992.
136. Ishizaka S, Asanoi H, Wada O, et al: Loading sequence plays an important role in enhanced load sensitivity of left ventricular relaxation in conscious dogs with tachycardia-induced cardiomyopathy, *Circulation* 92:3560–3567, 1995.
137. de Tombe PP, Little WC: Inotropic effects of ejection are myocardial properties, *Am J Physiol* 266:H1202–H1213, 1994.
138. Kass DA, Maughan WL: From 'E$_{max}$' to pressure-volume relations: A broader view, *Circulation* 77:1203–1212, 1988.
139. Kaseda S, Tomoike H, Ogata I, et al: End-systolic pressure-length relations during changes in regional contractile state, *Am J Physiol* 247:H768–H774, 1984.
140. Iskandrian AS, Hakki AH, Bemis CE, et al: Left ventricular end-systolic pressure-volume relation. A combined radionuclide and hemodynamic study, *Am J Cardiol* 51:1057–1061, 1983.
141. Magorien DJ, Shaffer P, Bush CA, et al: Assessment of left ventricular pressure-volume relations using gated radionuclide angiography, echocardiography, and micromanometer pressure recordings. A new method for serial measurements of systolic and diastolic function in man, *Circulation* 67:844–853, 1983.
142. Gorcsan IIIJ., Romand JA, Mandarino WA, et al: Assessment of left ventricular performance by on-line pressure-area relations using echocardiographic automated border detection, *J Am Coll Cardiol* 23:242–252, 1994.
143. Pirwitz MJ, Lange RA, Willard JE, et al: Use of left ventricular peak systolic pressure/end-systolic volume ratio to predict symptomatic improvement with valve replacement in patients with aortic regurgitation and enlarged end-systolic volume, *J Am Coll Cardiol* 24:1672–1677, 1994.
144. Senzaki H, Chen CH, Kass DA: Single-beat estimation of end-systolic pressure-volume relation in humans. A new method with the potential for noninvasive application, *Circulation* 94:2497–2506, 1996.
145. Kass DA, Beyar R, Lankford E, et al: Influence of contractile state on curvilinearity of in situ end-systolic pressure-volume relations, *Circulation* 79:167–178, 1989.
146. Little WC, O'Rourke RA: Effect of regional ischemia on the left ventricular end-systolic pressure-volume relation in chronically instrumented dogs, *J Am Coll Cardiol* 5:297–302, 1985.
147. Crottogini AJ, Willshaw P, Barra JG, et al: Inconsistency of the slope and the volume intercept of the end-systolic pressure-volume relationship as individual indexes of inotropic state in conscious dogs: Presentation of an index combining both variables, *Circulation* 76:1115–1126, 1987.
148. Crottogini AJ, Willshaw P, Barra JG, et al: Left ventricular end-systolic elastance is incorrectly estimated by the use of stepwise afterload variations in conscious, unsedated, autonomically intact dogs, *Circulation* 90:1431–1440, 1994.
149. Brickner ME, Starling MR: Dissociation of end systole from end ejection in patients with long-term mitral regurgitation, *Circulation* 81:1277–1286, 1990.
150. Belcher P, Boerboom LE, Olinger GN: Standardization of end-systolic pressure-volume relation in the dog, *Am J Physiol* 249:H547–H553, 1985.
151. Burkhoff D, Mirsky I, Suga H: Assessment of systolic and diastolic ventricular properties via pressure-volume analysis: A guide for clinical, translational, and basic researchers, *Am J Physiol Heart Circ Physiol* 289:H501–H512, 2005.
152. Little WC, Cheng CP, Mumma M, et al: Comparison of measures of left ventricular contractile performance derived from pressure-volume loops in conscious dogs, *Circulation* 80:1378–1387, 1989.
153. Burkhoff D, Sugiura S, Yue DT, et al: Contractility-dependent curvilinearity of end-systolic pressure-volume relations, *Am J Physiol* 252:H1218–H1227, 1987.
154. Van der Velde ET, Burkhoff D, Steendijk P, et al: Nonlinearity and load sensitivity of end-systolic pressure-volume relation of canine left ventricle in vivo, *Circulation* 83:315–327, 1991.
155. Spratt JA, Tyson GS, Glower DD, et al: The end-systolic pressure-volume relationship in conscious dog, *Circulation* 75:1295–1309, 1987.
156. Burkhoff D, De Tombe PP, Hunter WC: Impact of ejection on magnitude and time course of ventricular pressure-generating capacity, *Am J Physiol Heart Circ Physiol* 265:H899–H909, 1993.
157. Zile MR, Izzi G, Gaasch WH: Left ventricular diastolic dysfunction limits use of maximum systolic elastance as an index of contractile function, *Circulation* 83:674–680, 1991.
158. Patterson SW, Piper H, Starling E: Regulation of the heart beat, *J Physiol (Lond)* 48:465–513, 1914.
159. Sarnoff SJ, Berglund E: Ventricular function. I. Starling's law of the heart studied by means of simultaneous right and left ventricular function curves in the dog, *Circulation* 9:706–718, 1954.
160. Freeman GL, Little WC, O'Rourke RA: The effect of vasoactive agents on the left ventricular end-systolic pressure-volume relation in closed chest dogs, *Circulation* 74:1107–1113, 1986.
161. Glower DD, Spratt JA, Kabas JS, et al: Quantification of regional myocardial dysfunction after acute ischemic injury, *Am J Physiol* 255:H85–H93, 1988.
162. Chen C, Rodriguez L, Guerrero JL, et al: Noninvasive estimation of the instantaneous first derivative of left ventricular pressure using continuous-wave Doppler echocardiography, *Circulation* 83:2101–2110, 1991.
163. Mason DT: Usefulness and limitations of the rate of rise of intraventricular pressure (dP/dt) in the evaluation of myocardial contractility in man, *Am J Cardiol* 23:516–527, 1969.
164. Peterson KL, Skloven D, Ludbrook P, et al: Comparison of isovolumic and ejection phase indices of myocardial performance in man, *Circulation* 49:1088–1101, 1974.
165. Quinones MA, Gaasch WH, Alexander JK: Influence of acute changes in preload, afterload, contractile state, and heart rate on ejection and isovolumic indices of myocardial contractility in man, *Circulation* 53:293–302, 1976.

166. Little WC: The left ventricular dP/dt$_{max}$-end-diastolic volume relation in closed-chest dogs, *Circ Res* 56:808–815, 1985.
167. Little WC, Park RC, Freeman GL: Effects of regional ischemia and ventricular pacing on LV dP/dt$_{max}$-end-diastolic volume relation, *Am J Physiol* 252:H933–H940, 1987.
168. Noda N, Cheng CP, De Tombe PP, et al: Curvilinearity of LV end-systolic pressure-volume and dP/dt$_{max}$-end-diastolic volume relations, *Am J Physiol* 265:H910–H917, 1993.
169. Nixon JV, Murray RG, Leonard PD, et al: Effect of large variations in preload on left ventricular performance characteristic in normal subjects, *Circulation* 65:698–703, 1982.
170. Douglas PS, Reichek N, Hackney K, et al: Contribution of afterload, hypertrophy and geometry to left ventricular ejection fraction in aortic valve stenosis, pure aortic regurgitation and idiopathic dilated cardiomopathy, *Am J Cardiol* 59:1398–1404, 1987.
171. Wisenbaugh T: Does normal pump function belie muscle dysfunction in patients with chronic severe mitral regurgitation? *Circulation* 77:515–525, 1988.
172. Devlin WH, Petrusha J, Briesmiester K, et al: Impact of vascular adaptation to chronic aortic regurgitation on left ventricular performance, *Circulation* 99:1027–1033, 1999.
173. Banerjee A, Brook MM, Klautz RJ, et al: Nonlinearity of the left ventricular end-systolic wall stress-velocity of fiber shortening relation in young pigs: A potential pitfall in its use as a single-beat index of contractility, *J Am Coll Cardiol* 23:514–524, 1994.
174. Snell RE, Luchsinger PC: Determination of the external work and power of the intact left ventricle in intact man, *Am Heart J* 69:529–537, 1965.
175. Stein PD, Sabbah HN: Rate of change of ventricular power: An indicator of ventricular performance during ejection, *Am Heart J* 91:219–227, 1976.
176. Kass DA, Beyar R: Evaluation of contractile state by maximal ventricular power divided by the square of end-diastolic volume, *Circulation* 84:1698–1708, 1991.
177. Sharir T, Feldman MD, Haber H, et al: Ventricular systolic assessment in patients with dilated cardiomyopathy by preload-adjusted maximal power. Validation and noninvasive application, *Circulation* 89:2045–2053, 1994.
178. Nakayama M, Chen CH, Nevo E, et al: Optimal preload adjustment of maximal ventricular power index varies with cardiac chamber size, *Am Heart J* 136:281–288, 1998.
179. Pagel PS, Nijhawan N, Warltier DC: Quantitation of volatile anesthetic-induced depression of myocardial contractility using a single beat index derived from maximal ventricular power, *J Cardiothorac Vasc Anesth* 7:688–695, 1993.
180. Fourie PR, Coetzee AR, Bollinger CT: Pulmonary artery compliance: Its role in right ventricular-arterial coupling, *Cardiovasc Res* 26:839–844, 1992.
181. Little WC, Cheng CP: Effect of exercise on left ventricular-arterial coupling assessed in the pressure-volume plane, *Am J Physiol* 264:H1629–H1633, 1993.
182. Nozawa T, Cheng CP, Noda T, et al: Effect of exercise on left ventricular mechanical efficiency in conscious dogs, *Circulation* 90:3047–3054, 1994.
183. Borlaug BA, Kass DA: Ventricular-vascular interaction in heart failure, *Heart Fail Clin* 4:23–26, 2008.
184. Ahmet I, Krawczyk M, Heller P, et al: Beneficial effects of chronic pharmacological manipulation of beta-adrenoceptor subtype signaling in rodent dilated ischemic cardiomyopathy, *Circulation* 110:1083–1090, 2004.
185. Antonini-Camterin F, Enache R, Popescu BA, et al: Prognostic value of ventricular-arterial coupling and B-type natriuetic peptide in patients after myocardial infarction: A five-year follow-up study, *J Am Soc Echocardiogr* 22:1239–1245, 2009.
186. Ohte N, Cheng CP, Little WC: Tachycardia exacerbates abnormal left ventricular-arterial coupling in heart failure, *Heart Vessels* 18:136–141, 2003.
187. Binkley PF, Van Fossen DB, Nunziata E, et al: Influence of positive inotropic therapy on pulsatile hydraulic load and ventricular-vascular coupling in congestive heart failure, *J Am Coll Cardiol* 15:1127–1135, 1990.
188. Little WC, Pu M: Left ventricular-arterial coupling, *J Am Soc Echocardiogr* 22:1246–1248, 2009.
189. Suga H, Goto Y, Yamada O, et al: Independence of myocardial oxygen consumption from pressure-volume trajectory during diastole in canine left ventricle, *Circ Res* 55:734–739, 1984.
190. Suga H: Total mechanical energy of a ventricle model and cardiac oxygen consumption, *Am J Physiol* 236:H498–H505, 1979.
191. Suga H, Hayashi T, Suehiro S, et al: Equal oxygen consumption rates of isovolumic and ejecting contractions with equal systolic pressure volume areas in canine left ventricle, *Circ Res* 49:1082–1091, 1981.
192. Suga H, Hisano R, Goto Y, et al: Effect of positive inotropic agents on the relation between oxygen consumption and systolic pressure volume area in canine left ventricle, *Circ Res* 53:306–318, 1983.
193. Vanoverschelde JLJ, Wijns W, Essamri B, et al: Hemodynamic and mechanical determinants of myocardial O_2 consumption in normal human heart: Effects of dobutamine, *Am J Physiol* 265:H1884–H1892, 1993.
194. Burkhoff D, Yue D, Oikawa Y, et al: Influence of ventricular contractility on non-work-related myocardial oxygen consumption, *Heart Vessel* 3:66–72, 1987.
195. Suga H, Igarashi Y, Yamada O, et al: Mechanical efficiency of the left ventricle as a function of preload, afterload, and contractility, *Heart Vessel* 1:3–8, 1985.
196. Nozawa T, Yasumura Y, Futaki S, et al: Efficiency of energy transfer from pressure-volume area to external mechanical work increases with contractile state and decreases with afterload in the left ventricle of the anesthetized closed-chest dog, *Circulation* 77:1116–1124, 1988.
197. Nozawa T, Yasumura Y, Futaki S, et al: The linear relation between oxygen consumption and pressure-volume area can be reconciled with the Fenn effect in dog left ventricle, *Circ Res* 65: 1380–1389, 1989.
198. Burkhoff D, Sagawa K: Ventricular efficiency predicted by an analytical model, *Am J Physiol* 250:R1021–R1027, 1986.
199. Nozawa T, Wada O, Ishizaka S, et al: Dobutamine improves afterload-induced deterioration of mechanical efficiency toward maximal, *Am J Physiol* 263:H1201–H1207, 1992.
200. Pagel PS, Hettrick DA, Warltier DC: Comparison of the effects of levosimendan, pimobendan, and milrinone in canine left ventricular-arterial coupling and mechanical efficiency, *Basic Res Cardiol* 91:296–307, 1996.
201. Eichhorn EJ, Heesch CM, Barnett JH, et al: Effect of metoprolol on myocardial function and energetics in patients with nonischemic dilated cardiomyopathy: A randomized, double-blind, placebo-controlled study, *J Am Coll Cardiol* 24:1310–1320, 1994.
202. Kim IS, Izawa H, Sobue T, et al: Prognostic value of mechanical efficiency in ambulatory patients with idiopathic dilated cardiomyopathy in sinus rhythm, *J Am Coll Cardiol* 39:1264–1268, 2002.
203. Yew WYW: Evaluation of left ventricular diastolic function, *Circulation* 79:1393–1397, 1989.
204. Kitzman DW, Little WC, Brubaker PH, et al: Pathophysiological characterization of isolated diastolic heart failure in comparison to systolic heart failure, *JAMA* 288:2144–2150, 2002.
205. Gaasch WH, Zile MR: Left ventricular diastolic dysfunction and diastolic heart failure, *Annu Rev Med* 55:373–394, 2004.
206. Maeder MT, Kaye DM: Heart failure with normal left ventricular ejection fraction, *J Am Coll Cardiol* 53:905–918, 2009.
207. Zile MR, Baicu CF, Gaasch WH: Diastolic heart failure—abnormalities in active relaxation and passive stiffness of the left ventricle, *N Engl J Med* 350:1953–1959, 2004.
208. Westermann D, Kasner M, Steendijk P, et al: Role of left ventricular stiffness in heart failure with normal ejection fraction, *Circulation* 117:2051–2060, 2008.
209. Kawaguchi M, Hay I, Fetics B, et al: Combined ventricular systolic and arterial stiffening in patients with heart failure and preserved ejection fraction: Implications for systolic and diastolic reserve limitations, *Circulation* 107:714–720, 2003.
210. Bench T, Burkhoff D, O'Connell JB, et al: Heart failure with normal ejection fraction: Consideration of mechanisms other than diastolic dysfunction, *Curr Heart Fail Rep* 6:57–64, 2009.
211. Futuka H, Little WC: Contribution of systolic and diastolic abnormalities to heart failure with a normal or reduced ejection fraction, *Prog Cardiovasc Dis* 49:229–240, 2007.
212. Grewal J, McCully RB, Kane GC, et al: Left ventricular function and exercise capacity, *JAMA* 301:286–294, 2009.
213. Traversi E, Pozzoli M, Cioffi G, et al: Mitral flow velocity changes after 6 months of optimized therapy provides important hemodynamic and prognostic information in patients with heart failure, *Am Heart J* 132:809–819, 1996.
214. De Hert SG, Rodrigus IE, Haenen LR, et al: Recovery of systolic and diastolic left ventricular function early after cardiopulmonary bypass, *Anesthesiology* 85:1063–1075, 1996.
215. Pagel PS, Farber NE, Pratt PF Jr, et al: Cardiovascular pharmacology. In Miller RD, editor: *Miller's Anesthesia*, ed 7 Philadelphia, 2009, Elsevier Churchill Livingstone, pp 595–632.
216. Grossman W: Why is left ventricular diastolic pressure increased during angina pectoris? *J Am Coll Cardiol* 5:607–608, 1985.
217. Morgan JP, Erny RE, Allen PD, et al: Abnormal intracellular calcium handling, a major cause of systolic and diastolic dysfunction in ventricular myocardium from patients with heart failure, *Circulation* 81(Suppl III):21–32, 1990.
218. Apstein CS, Grossman W: Opposite initial effects of supply and demand ischemia on left ventricular diastolic compliance: The ischemia-diastolic paradox, *J Mol Cell Cardiol* 19:119–128, 1987.
219. Aroesty JM, McKay RG, Heller GV, et al: Simultaneous assessment of left ventricular systolic and diastolic dysfunction during pacing-induced ischemia, *Circulation* 71:889–900, 1985.
220. Carroll JD, Hess OM, Hirzel HO, et al: Left ventricular systolic and diastolic function in coronary artery disease: Effects of revascularization on exercise-induced ischemia, *Circulation* 72:119–129, 1985.
221. Doyle RL, Foex P, Ryder WA, et al: Effects of halothane on left ventricular relaxation and early diastolic coronary blood flow in the dog, *Anesthesiology* 70:660–666, 1989.
222. Weisfeldt ML, Scully HE, Frederiksen J, et al: Hemodynamic determinants of maximum negative dP/dt and periods of diastole, *Am J Physiol* 227:613–621, 1974.
223. Frais MA, Bergman DW, Kingma I, et al: The dependence of the time constant of left ventricular isovolumic relaxation (tau) on pericardial pressure, *Circulation* 81:1071–1080, 1990.
224. Raff GL, Glantz SA: Volume loading slows left ventricular isovolumic relaxation rate: Evidence of load-dependent relaxation in the intact dog heart, *Circ Res* 48:813–824, 1981.
225. Serizawa T, Vogel WM, Apstein CS, et al: Comparison of acute alterations in left ventricular relaxation and diastolic chamber stiffness induced by hypoxia and ischemia. Role of myocardial oxygen supply-demand imbalance, *J Clin Invest* 68:91–102, 1981.
226. Eichhorn P, Grimm J, Koch R, et al: Left ventricular relaxation in patients with left ventricular hypertrophy secondary to aortic valve disease, *Circulation* 65:1395–1404, 1982.
227. Paulus WJ, Lorell BH, Craig WE, et al: Comparison of the effects of nitroprusside and nifedipine on diastolic properties in patients with hypertrophic cardiomyopathy: Altered left ventricular loading or improved muscle relaxation? *J Am Coll Cardiol* 2:879–886, 1983.
228. Pagel PS, Kampine JP, Schmeling WT, et al: Alteration of left ventricular diastolic function by desflurane, isoflurane, and halothane in the chronically instrumented dog with autonomic nervous system blockade, *Anesthesiology* 74:1103–1114, 1991.
229. Gaasch WH, Carroll JD, Blaustein AS, et al: Myocardial relaxation: effects of preload on the time course of isovolumetric relaxation, *Circulation* 73:1037–1041, 1986.
230. Varma SK, Owen RM, Smucker ML, et al: Is τ a preload-independent measure of isovolumetric relaxation? *Circulation* 80:1757–1765, 1989.
231. Eichhorn EJ, Willard JE, Alvarez L, et al: Are contraction and relaxation coupled in patients with and without congestive heart failure? *Circulation* 85:2132–2139, 1992.
232. Smith VE, Zile MR: Relaxation and diastolic properties of the heart. In Fozzard HA, Haber E, Jennings RB, et al: *The Heart and Cardiovascular System: Scientific Foundations*, ed 2 New York, 1991, Raven, pp 1353–1367.
233. Ohno M, Cheng C-P, Little WC: Mechanism of altered patterns of left ventricular filling during the development of congestive heart failure, *Circulation* 89:2241–2250, 1994.
234. Lew WYW, LeWinter MM: Regional circumferential lengthening patterns in the canine left ventricle, *Am J Physiol* 245:H741–H748, 1983.
235. Mirsky I: Assessment of diastolic function: Suggested methods and future considerations, *Circulation* 69:836–841, 1984.
236. Little WC, Ohno M, Kitzman DW, et al: Determination of left ventricular chamber stiffness from the time of deceleration of early left ventricular filling, *Circulation* 92:1933–1939, 1995.
237. Glantz SA: Computing indices of diastolic stiffness has been counterproductive, *Fed Proc* 39:162–168, 1980.
238. Rankin JS, Arentzen CE, McHale PA, et al: Viscoelastic properties of the diastolic left ventricle in the conscious dog, *Circ Res* 41:37–45, 1977.
239. Nikolic SD, Tamura K, Tamura T, et al: Diastolic viscous properties of the intact canine left ventricle, *Circ Res* 67:352–359, 1990.
240. Myreng Y, Smiseth OA: Assessment of left ventricular relaxation by Doppler echocardiography. Comparison of isovolumic relaxation time and transmitral flow velocities with time constant of isovolumic relaxation, *Circulation* 81:260–266, 1990.
241. Nishimura RA, Schwartz RS, Tajik AJ, et al: Noninvasive measurement of rate of left ventricular relaxation by Doppler echocardiography. Validation with simultaneous cardiac catheterization, *Circulation* 88:146–155, 1993.
242. Nishimura RA, Tajik AJ: Evaluation of diastolic filling of left ventricle in health and disease: Doppler echocardiography is the clinician's Rosetta stone, *J Am Coll Cardiol* 30:8–18, 1997.
243. Nagueh SF, Appleton CP, Gillebert TC, et al: Recommendations for the evaluation of left ventricular diastolic function by echocardiography, *J Am Soc Echocardiogr* 22:107–133, 2009.
244. Klein AL, Burstow DJ, Tajik AJ, et al: Effects of age on left ventricular dimensions and filling dynamics in 117 normal persons, *Mayo Clin Proc* 69:212–224, 1994.
245. Genovesi-Ebert A, Marabotti C, Palombo C, et al: Left ventricular filling: Relationship with arterial blood pressure, left ventricular mass, age, heart rate, and body build, *J Hypertens* 9:345–353, 1991.
246. Rittoo D, Monaghan M, Sadiq T, et al: Echocardiographic and Doppler evaluation of left ventricular hypertrophy and diastolic function in black and white hypertensive patients, *J Hum Hypertens* 4: 113–115, 1990.
247. Cohen GI, Petrolungo JF, Thomas JD, et al: A practical guide to assessment of ventricular diastolic function using Doppler echocardiography, *J Am Coll Cardiol* 27:1753–1760, 1996.
248. Hurrell DG, Nishimura RA, Ilstrup DM, et al: Utility of preload alteration in assessment of left ventricular filling pressure by Doppler echocardiography: A simultaneous catheterization and Doppler echocardiographic study, *J Am Coll Cardiol* 30:459–467, 1997.
249. Farias CA, Rodriguez L, Garcia MJ, et al: Assessment of diastolic function by tissue Doppler echocardiography: Comparison with standard transmitral and pulmonary venous flow, *J Am Soc Echocardiogr* 12:609–617, 1999.
250. Pinamonte B, Zecchin M, Di Lenarda A, et al: Persistence of restrictive left ventricular filling pattern in dilated cardiomyopathy: An ominous prognostic sign, *J Am Coll Cardiol* 29:604–612, 1997.

251. Moller JE, Sondergaard E, Poulsen SH, et al: Pseudonormal and restrictive filling patterns predict left ventricular dilation and cardiac death after a first myocardial infarction: A serial color M-mode Doppler echocardiographic study, *J Am Coll Cardiol* 36:1841–1846, 2000.
252. Oh JK, Hatle LK, Seward JB, et al: Diagnostic role of Doppler echocardiography in constrictive pericarditis, *J Am Coll Cardiol* 23:154–162, 1994.
253. Klein AL, Hatle LK, Taliercio CP, et al: Prognostic significance of Doppler measures of diastolic function in cardiac amyloidosis. A Doppler echocardiographic study, *Circulation* 83:808–816, 1991.
254. Valantine HA, Appleton CP, Hatle LK, et al: A hemodynamic and Doppler echocardiographic study of ventricular function in long-term cardiac allograft recipients. Etiology and prognosis of restrictive-constrictive physiology, *Circulation* 79:66–75, 1989.
255. Rakowski H, Appleton C, Chan KL, et al: Canadian consensus recommendations for the measurement and reporting of diastolic dysfunction by echocardiography: From the Investigators of Consensus on Diastolic Dysfunction by Echocardiography, *J Am Soc Echocardiogr* 9:736–760, 1996.
256. Klein AL, Obarski TP, Stewart WJ, et al: Transesophageal Doppler echocardiography of pulmonary venous flow: A new marker of mitral regurgitation severity, *J Am Coll Cardiol* 18:518–526, 1991.
257. Kuecherer HF, Muhiudeen IA, Kusumoto FM, et al: Estimation of mean left atrial pressure from transesophageal pulsed Doppler echocardiography of pulmonary venous flow, *Circulation* 82: 1127–1139, 1990.
258. Hofman T, Keck A, Van Ingen G, et al: Simultaneous measurement of pulmonary venous flow by intravascular catheter Doppler velocimetry and transesophageal Doppler echocardiography: Relation to left atrial pressure and left atrial and left ventricular function, *J Am Coll Cardiol* 26:239–249, 1995.
259. Castello R, Pearson AC, Lenzen P, et al: Evaluation of pulmonary venous flow by transesophageal echocardiography in subjects with a normal heart: Comparison with transthoracic echocardiography, *J Am Coll Cardiol* 18:65–71, 1991.
260. Appleton CP: Hemodynamic determinants of Doppler pulmonary venous flow velocity components: New insights from studies in lightly sedated normal dogs, *J Am Coll Cardiol* 30:1562–1574, 1997.
261. Dini FL, Dell'Anna R, Micheli A, et al: Impact of blunted pulmonary venous flow on the outcome of patients with left ventricular systolic dysfunction secondary to either ischemic or idiopathic dilated cardiomyopathy, *Am J Cardiol* 85:1455–1460, 2000.
262. Morkin E, Collins JA, Goldman HS, et al: Pattern of blood flow in the pulmonary veins of the dog, *J Appl Physiol* 20:1118–1128, 1965.
263. Keren G, Bier A, Sherez J, et al: Atrial contraction is an important determinant of pulmonary venous flow, *J Am Coll Cardiol* 7:693–695, 1986.
264. Smiseth OA, Thompson CR, Lohavanichbutr K, et al: The pulmonary venous systolic flow pulse. Its origin and relationship to left atrial pressure, *J Am Coll Cardiol* 34:802–809, 1999.
265. Fujii K, Ozaki M, Yamagishi T, et al: Effect of left ventricular contractile performance on passive left atrial filling: Clinical study using radionuclide angiography, *Clin Cardiol* 17:258–262, 1994.
266. Keren G, Sonnenblick EH, LeJemtel TH: Mitral annulus motion. Relation to pulmonary venous and transmitral flows in normal subjects and in patients with dilated cardiomyopathy, *Circulation* 78: 621–629, 1988.
267. Appleton CP, Gonzalez MS, Basnight MA: Relationship of left atrial pressure and pulmonary venous flow velocities: Importance of baseline mitral and pulmonary venous flow velocity patterns in lightly sedated dogs, *J Am Soc Echocardiogr* 7:264–275, 1994.
268. Prioli A, Marino P, Lanzoni L, et al: Increasing degrees of left ventricular filling impairment modulate left atrial function in humans, *Am J Cardiol* 82:756–761, 1998.
269. Appleton CP, Galloway JM, Gonzalez MS, et al: Estimation of left ventricular filling pressures using two-dimensional and Doppler echocardiography in adult patients with cardiac disease. Additional value of analyzing left atrial size, left atrial ejection fraction and the difference in duration of pulmonary venous and mitral flow velocity at atrial contraction, *J Am Coll Cardiol* 22:1972–1982, 1993.
270. Klein AL, Tajik AJ: Doppler assessment of pulmonary venous flow in healthy subjects and in patients with heart disease, *J Am Soc Echocardiogr* 4:379–392, 1991.
271. Garcia MJ, Thomas JD, Klein AL: New Doppler echocardiographic applications for the study of diastolic function, *J Am Coll Cardiol* 32:865–875, 1998.
272. Nagueh SF, Rao L, Soto J, et al: Haemodynamic insights into the effects of ischaemia and cycle length on tissue Doppler-derived mitral annulus diastolic velocities, *Clin Sci (Lond)* 106:147–154, 2004.
273. Nagueh SF, Middleton KJ, Kopelen HA, et al: Doppler tissue imaging: A noninvasive technique for evaluation of left ventricular relaxation and estimation of filling pressures, *J Am Coll Cardiol* 30: 1527–1533, 1997.
274. Ommen SR, Nishimura RA, Appleton CP, et al: Clinical utility of Doppler echocardiography and tissue Doppler imaging in the estimation of left ventricular filling pressures: A comparative simultaneous Doppler-catheterization study, *Circulation* 102:1788–1794, 2000.
275. Paulus WJ, Tschope C, Sanderson JE, et al: How to diagnose diastolic heart failure: A consensus statement on the diagnosis of heart failure with normal left ventricular ejection fraction by the Heart Failure and Echocardiography Associations of the European Society of Cardiology, *Eur Heart J* 28:2539–2550, 2007.
276. Kasner M, Westermann D, Steendijk P, et al: Utility of Doppler echocardiography and tissue Doppler imaging in the estimation of diastolic function in heart failure with normal ejection fraction: A comparative Doppler-conductance catheterization study, *Circulation* 116:637–647, 2007.
277. Nagueh SF, Sun H, Kopelen HA, et al: Hemodynamic determinants of mitral annulus diastolic velocities by tissue Doppler, *J Am Coll Cardiol* 37:278–285, 2001.
278. Rivas-Gotz C, Khoury DS, Manolios M, et al: Time interval between onset of mitral inflow and onset of early diastolic velocity by tissue Doppler: A novel index of left ventricular relaxation: Experimental studies and clinical application, *J Am Coll Cardiol* 42:1463–1470, 2003.
279. Garcia MJ, Rodriguez L, Ares M, et al: Differentiation of constrictive pericarditis from restrictive cardiomyopathy: Assessment of left ventricular diastolic velocities in longitudinal axes by Doppler tissue imaging, *J Am Coll Cardiol* 27:108–114, 1996.
280. Takatsuji H, Mikami T, Urasawa K, et al: A new approach for evaluation of left ventricular diastolic function: Spatial and temporal analysis of left ventricular filling flow propagation by color M-mode Doppler echocardiography, *J Am Coll Cardiol* 27:365–371, 1996.
281. Garcia MJ, Smedira NG, Greenberg NL, et al: Color M-mode Doppler flow propagation velocity is a preload insensitive index of left ventricular relaxation: Animal and human validation, *J Am Coll Cardiol* 35:201–208, 2000.
282. Brun P, Tribouilloy C, Duval AM, et al: Left ventricular flow propagation during early filling is related to wall relaxation: A color M-mode Doppler analysis, *J Am Coll Cardiol* 20:420–432, 1992.
283. Garcia MJ, Ares MA, Asher C, et al: An index of early left ventricular filling that combined with pulsed Doppler peak E velocity may estimate capillary wedge pressure, *J Am Coll Cardiol* 29:448–454, 1997.
284. Steine K, Stugaard M, Smiseth OA: Mechanisms of retarded apical filling in acute ischemic left ventricular failure, *Circulation* 99:2048–2054, 1999.
285. Nishihara K, Mikami T, Takatsuji H, et al: Usefulness of early diastolic flow propagation velocity measured by color M-mode Doppler technique for the assessment of left ventricular diastolic function in patients with hypertrophic cardiomyopathy, *J Am Soc Echocardiogr* 13:801–808, 2000.
286. Yotti R, Bermejo J, Antoranz JC, et al: A noninvasive method for assessing impaired diastolic suction in patients with dilated cardiomyopathy, *Circulation* 112:2921–2929, 2005.
287. Watkins MW, LeWinter MM: Physiologic role of the normal pericardium, *Annu Rev Med* 44:171–180, 1993.
288. Spodick DH: Macrophysiology, microphysiology, and anatomy of the pericardium: A synopsis, *Am Heart J* 124:1046–1051, 1992.
289. Maruyama Y, Ashikawa K, Isoyama S, et al: Mechanical interactions between four heart chambers with and without the pericardium in canine hearts, *Circ Res* 50:86–100, 1982.
290. Refsum H, Junemann M, Lipton MJ, et al: Ventricular diastolic pressure-volume relations and the pericardium. Effects of changes in blood volume and pericardial effusion in dogs, *Circulation* 64:997–1004, 1981.
291. Junemann M, Smiseth OA, Refsum H, et al: Quantification of effect of pericardium on LV diastolic PV relation in dogs, *Am J Physiol* 252:H963–H968, 1987.
292. Santamore WP, Dell'Italia LJ: Ventricular interdependence: Significant left ventricular contributions to right ventricular systolic function, *Prog Cardiovasc Dis* 40:289–308, 1998.
293. Weber KT, Janicki JS, Shroff S, et al: Contractile mechanics and interaction of the right and left ventricles, *Am J Cardiol* 47:686–695, 1981.
294. Gonzalez MS, Basnight MA, Appleton CP: Experimental cardiac tamponade: A hemodynamic and Doppler echocardiographic reexamination of the relation of right and left heart ejection dynamics to the phase of respiration, *J Am Coll Cardiol* 18:243–252, 1991.
295. Santamore WP, Heckman JL, Bove AA: Right and left ventricular pressure-volume response to elevated pericardial pressure, *Am Rev Respir Dis* 134:101–107, 1986.
296. Santamore WP, Bartlett R, Van Buren SJ, et al: Ventricular coupling in constrictive pericarditis, *Circulation* 74:597–602, 1986.
297. Goldman S, Olajos M, Morkin E: Comparison of left atrial and left ventricular performance in conscious dogs, *Cardiovasc Res* 18:604–612, 1984.
298. Wikman-Coffelt J, Refsum H, Hollosi G, et al: Comparative force-velocity relation and analyses of myosin of dog atria and ventricles, *Am J Physiol* 243:H391–H397, 1982.
299. Payne RM, Stone HL, Engelken EJ: Atrial function during volume loading, *J Appl Physiol* 31:326–331, 1971.
300. Williams JF Jr, Sonnenblick EH, Braunwald E: Determinants of atrial contractile force in the intact heart, *Am J Physiol* 209:1061–1068, 1965.
301. Dernellis J, Tsiamis E, Stefanadis C, et al: Effects of postural changes on left atrial function in patients with hypertrophic cardiomyopathy, *Am Heart J* 136:982–987, 1998.
302. Kehl F, LaDisa JF Jr, Hettrick DA, et al: Influence of isoflurane on left atrial function in dogs with pacing-induced cardiomyopathy: Evaluation with pressure-volume relations, *J Cardiothorac Vasc Anesth* 17:709–714, 2003.
303. Buttrick PM, Malhotra A, Brodman R, et al: Myosin isoenzyme distribution in overloaded human atrial tissue, *Circulation* 74:477–483, 1986.
304. Ito T, Suwa M, Kobashi A, et al: Reversible left atrial dysfunction possibly due to afterload mismatch in patients with left ventricular dysfunction, *J Am Soc Echocardiogr* 11:274–279, 1998.
305. Dernellis JM, Vyssoulis GP, Zacharoulis AA, et al: Effects of antihypertensive therapy on left atrial function, *J Hum Hypertens* 10:789–794, 1996.
306. Guntheroth WG, Gould R, Butler J, et al: Pulsatile flow in pulmonary artery, capillary, and vein in the dog, *Cardiovasc Res* 8:330–337, 1974.
307. Plehn JF, Southworth J, Cornwell GG III: Brief report: Atrial systolic failure in primary amyloidosis, *N Engl J Med* 327:1570–1573, 1992.
308. Hoit BD, Walsh RA: Regional atrial distensibility, *Am J Physiol* 262:H1356–H1360, 1992.
309. Hoit BD, Shao Y, Tsai LM, et al: Altered left atrial compliance after atrial appendectomy. Influence on left atrial and ventricular filling, *Circ Res* 72:167–175, 1993.
310. Tabata T, Oki T, Yamada H, et al: Role of left atrial appendage in left atrial reservoir function as evaluated by left atrial appendage clamping during cardiac surgery, *Am J Cardiol* 81:327–332, 1998.
311. Nishikawa Y, Roberts JP, Tan P, et al: Effect of dynamic exercise on left atrial function in conscious dogs, *J Physiol* 481:457–468, 1994.
312. Toutouzas K, Trikas A, Pitsavos C, et al: Echocardiographic features of left atrium in elite male athletes, *Am J Cardiol* 78:1314–1317, 1996.
313. Triposkiadis F, Tentolouris K, Androulakis A, et al: Left atrial mechanical function in the healthy elderly: New insights from a combined assessment of changes in atrial volume and transmitral flow velocity, *J Am Soc Echocardiogr* 8:801–809, 1995.
314. Manning WJ, Silverman DI, Katz SE, et al: Atrial ejection force: A noninvasive assessment of atrial systolic function, *J Am Coll Cardiol* 22:221–225, 1993.
315. Spencer KT, Mor-Avi V, Gorcsan J III, et al: Effects of aging on left atrial reservoir, conduit, and booster pump function: A multi-institution acoustic quantification study, *Heart* 85:272–277, 2001.
316. Nishigaki K, Arakawa M, Miwa H, et al: A study of left atrial transport function. Effect of age or left ventricular ejection fraction on left atrial storage function, *Angiology* 45:953–962, 1994.
317. Zuccala G, Cocchi A, Lattanzio F, et al: Effect of age on left atrial function in patients with coronary artery disease, *Cardiology* 85:8–13, 1994.

6

Coronary Physiology and Atherosclerosis

EDWARD R.M. O'BRIEN, MD | BENJAMIN HIBBERT, MD, FRCPC | HOWARD J. NATHAN, MD, FRCPC

KEY POINTS

1. To safely care for patients with coronary artery disease (CAD) in the perioperative period, the clinician must understand how the coronary circulation functions in health and disease.
2. Coronary endothelium modulates myocardial blood flow by producing factors that relax or contract the underlying vascular smooth muscle.
3. Vascular endothelial cells help maintain the fluidity of blood by elaborating anticoagulant, fibrinolytic, and antiplatelet substances.
4. One of the earliest changes in CAD, preceding the appearance of stenoses, is the loss of the vasoregulatory and antithrombotic functions of the endothelium.
5. The mean systemic arterial pressure and not the diastolic pressure may be the most useful and reliable measure of coronary perfusion pressure in the clinical setting.
6. Although sympathetic activation increases myocardial oxygen demand, activation of α-adrenergic receptors causes coronary vasoconstriction.
7. It is unlikely that one substance alone (e.g., adenosine) provides the link between myocardial metabolism and myocardial blood flow under a variety of conditions.
8. As coronary perfusion pressure decreases, the inner layers of myocardium nearest the left ventricular cavity are the first to become ischemic and display impaired relaxation and contraction.
9. The progression of an atherosclerotic lesion is similar to the process of wound healing.
10. Lipid-lowering therapy can help restore endothelial function and prevent coronary events.

When caring for patients with coronary artery disease (CAD), the anesthesiologist must prevent or minimize myocardial ischemia by maintaining optimal conditions for perfusion of the heart. This goal can be achieved only with an understanding of the many factors that determine myocardial blood flow in both health and disease. This chapter begins with an overview of the structure and function of coronary arteries. Rapid progress has been made in the past several decades in the understanding of the physiology of blood vessels, particularly the role of the endothelium in maintaining flow. Following this overview is an analysis of the major determinants of coronary blood flow.

Physiologic or pharmacologic interventions alter myocardial flow by their effects on these factors. The Coronary Pressure-Flow Relations section explains the important concepts of autoregulation and coronary reserve. Studies of the coronary circulation are sometimes misinterpreted because of an inadequate understanding of the complex interrelations among the heart, the coronary circulation, and the peripheral circulation. The discussion of pathophysiology begins with a description of the process of atherosclerosis and the current understanding of how this disease evolves and causes clinical events. Next, the anatomy and hemodynamic effects of a coronary stenosis are explained. Coronary collateral function and development are reviewed here. These concepts are the basis of predicting how significantly the stenoses seen on angiography impair myocardial perfusion. The topic of the final section is the pathophysiology of myocardial ischemia. The concepts learned in the preceding sections are applied in an analysis of clinical ischemic syndromes. The final section highlights future directions in the treatment of CAD.

ANATOMY AND PHYSIOLOGY OF BLOOD VESSELS

The coronary vasculature has been traditionally divided into three functional groups: large conductance vessels visible on coronary angiography, which offer little resistance to blood flow; small resistance vessels ranging in size from about 10 to 250 μm in diameter; and veins. Although it has been taught that arterioles (precapillary vessels < 50 μm) account for most of the coronary resistance, recent studies indicate that, under resting conditions, 45% to 50% of total coronary vascular resistance resides in vessels larger than 100 μm in diameter[1-3] (Figure 6-1). This may be due, in part, to the relatively great length of the small arteries. During intense pharmacologic dilation, the proportion of total coronary vascular resistance because of larger arteries and veins is even greater.[2] The regulation of tone in coronary arteries larger than 100 μm in diameter plays an important role in delivering adequate myocardial perfusion.[4] One of the early changes in CAD is a diminished ability of the endothelium of epicardial coronary arteries to dilate in response to increased flow (see Endothelium-Derived Relaxing Factors later in this chapter). Advances in technology have enabled measurement, in the beating heart, of diameters of coronary vessels as small as 15 μm. It is becoming evident that, in response to a given intervention, different size classes of coronary vessels can change diameter with different intensity or even in opposite directions.[5,6] This heterogeneity of response according to vessel size would be an important consideration in predicting the effects of vasoactive agents on myocardial perfusion. For example, a drug that dilated large vessels and collaterals but not arterioles would be beneficial to patients with CAD (see Coronary Steal later in this chapter).

■ Normal Artery Wall

The arterial lumen is lined by a monolayer of endothelial cells that overlies smooth muscle cells (Figure 6-2). The inner layer of smooth muscle cells, known as the *intima*, is circumscribed by the internal elastic lamina. Between the internal elastic lamina and external elastic lamina is another layer of smooth muscle cells, the media. Outside the external elastic lamina is an adventitia that is sparsely populated by cells and microvessels of the vasa vasorum.

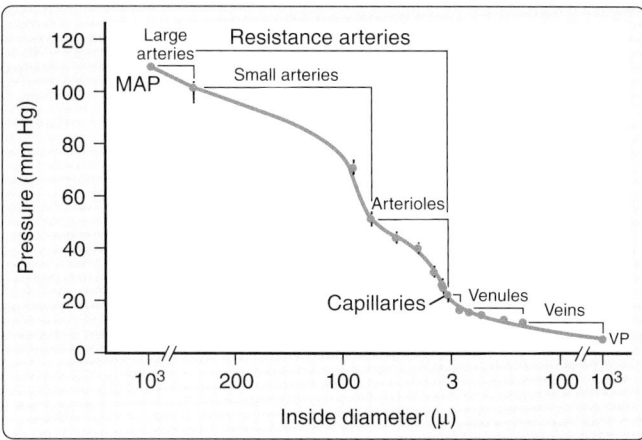

Figure 6-1 Pressure decline through the hamster cheek pouch circulation illustrates the resistance and nomenclature of various portions of the vascular bed. The important contribution of small arteries to vascular resistance is clearly shown here. Similar observations have been made in the coronary circulation. Error bars indicate standard error. MAP, mean arterial pressure; VP, venous pressure. *(From Davis MJ, Ferrer PN, Gore RW: Vascular anatomy and hydrostatic pressure profile in the hamster cheek pouch. Am J Physiol 250:H291, 1986.)*

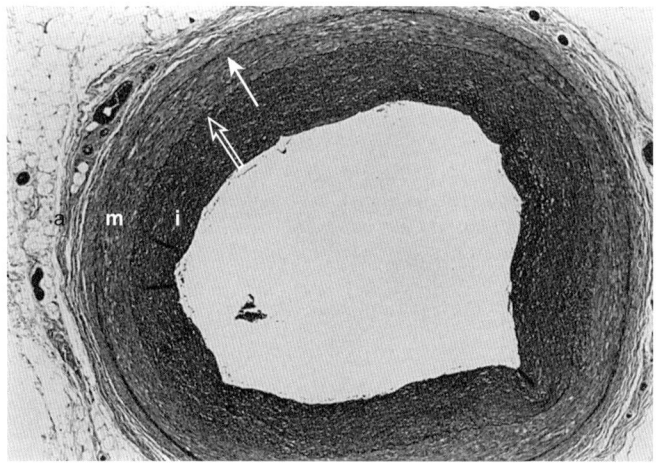

Figure 6-2 **Normal human coronary artery of a 32-year-old woman.** The intima *(i)* and media *(m)* are composed of smooth muscle cells. The adventitia *(a)* consists of a loose collection of adipocytes, fibroblasts, vasa vasorum, and nerves. The media is separated from the intima by the internal elastic lamina *(open arrow)* and the adventitia by the external elastic lamina *(closed arrow)*. (Movat's pentachrome-stained slide, original magnification, ×6.6.)

Intima

Traditionally, the intima has been considered the most important layer of the artery wall.[7] The intima can vary from a single endothelial layer to a more complex structure of an endothelium overlying a patchwork of extracellular matrix and vascular smooth muscle cells. As part of the normal development of many large arteries, smooth muscle cells populate this space and form a neointima. This diffuse form of intimal thickening consists of layers of smooth muscle cells and connective tissue, the thickness of which may vary considerably. For convenience, the intima/media ratio is often measured, and the reference range is 0.1 to 1.0. How this benign intima forms is not well understood. Presumably, the intima represents a physiologic adaptation to changes in arterial flow and wall tension. The intima is made up of two distinct layers.[8]

As seen by electron microscopy, the inner layer subjacent to the luminal endothelium contains an abundance of proteoglycan ground substance. Smooth muscle cells found in this layer are usually distributed as isolated cells in a sea of matrix, rather than in contiguous layers. A few macrophages also may be found in this layer underneath the endothelial monolayer. The outer, musculoelastic layer of the intima is adjacent to the internal elastic lamina and contains smooth muscle cells and elastic fibers.

Media

In normal adult arteries, several smooth muscle cell subpopulations with distinct lineages exist within the media.[9] These diverse cell populations likely fulfill different functions to maintain homeostasis in the artery wall. For example, in response to pressure elevations, increases in smooth muscle cell mass and extracellular matrix may be required. Alternatively, for arteries to be able to stretch both longitudinally and circumferentially, smooth muscle cells with variable orientations of cytoskeletal fibers must be present. These distinct cell types may be important not only in health but in disease. In certain experimental models of neointimal formation, proliferation and inward migration of subpopulations of medial smooth muscle cells occur.[10] The biologic determinants of medial smooth muscle cell diversity are unknown.[11]

Adventitia

The adventitia, the outermost layer of the artery wall, normally consists of a sparse collection of fibroblasts, microvessels (vasa vasorum), nerves, and few inflammatory cells. The majority of the vasa vasorum that nourish the inner layers of the artery wall originate in the adventitia. Traditionally, the adventitia has been ignored and is not thought to play a role in vascular lesion formation. However, more recent studies have elucidated the role of the adventitia as not only a source of inflammatory cells in the development of atherosclerosis, but a hub for paracrine signaling that can maintain vascular homeostasis in a variety of vascular diseases.[12]

Transmembrane and Transcellular Communication

Blood vessels respond to a multitude of neural, humoral, and mechanical stimuli in fulfilling their role in homeostasis. When norepinephrine, released from adrenergic nerve terminals in the adventitia, binds to receptors on the vascular smooth muscle cell membrane, a series of events takes place, culminating in a change in vessel diameter. Much progress has been made in understanding this transmembrane signaling since the discovery of cyclic adenosine monophosphate (cAMP) in the late 1950s. Hormones circulating in the blood must interact with receptors on endothelial cells before the message reaches the vascular smooth muscle cell. The mechanism of communication between cells has been one of the central themes of biologic research in the past decades. Future understanding of cardiovascular disease will likely be based on identification of abnormalities of the molecules involved in transmembrane and transcellular communication. A brief introduction to these topics is provided here.

Figure 6-3 illustrates examples of pathways of transmembrane signaling. Up to five components can be involved: receptor, G protein, effector producing a second messenger, phosphorylation of regulator protein, and the consequent change in cell behavior. G proteins (guanine nucleotide-binding regulatory proteins) are made up of three subunits (α, β, γ) and float in the cell membrane. On contact with a ligand-receptor complex, guanosine diphosphate (GDP) on the α subunit is replaced by guanosine triphosphate (GTP). The activated α subunit then dissociates from the beta-gamma complex and can interact with several membrane targets (see Figure 6-3B). For example, β-receptor activation results in the activation of G_s (s = stimulate), which will stimulate the synthesis of cAMP by adenylyl cyclase. Muscarinic receptor activation

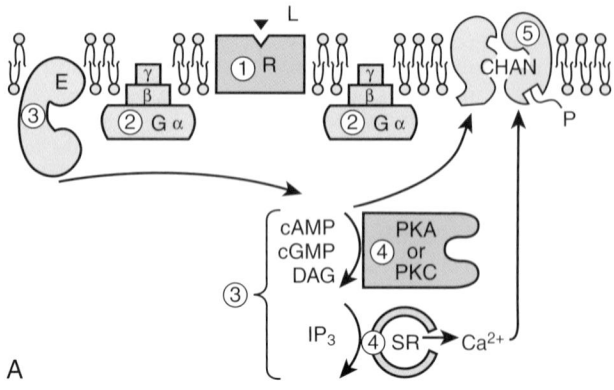

A

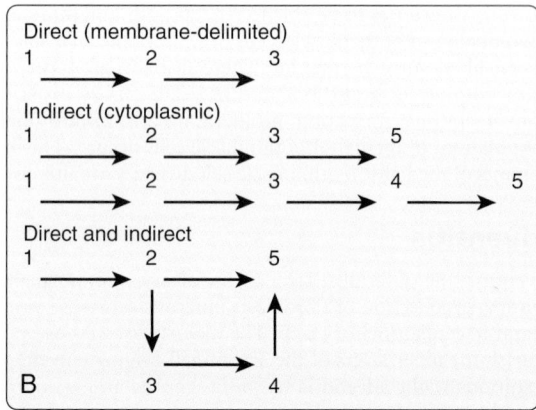

B

Figure 6-3 **Steps in the process whereby hormone-receptor binding results in a change in cell behavior.** In this example, the final result is the opening of an ion channel. *A*, A hormone or ligand (L) binds to a receptor (R) embedded in the cell membrane. The receptor-ligand complex interacts with G protein (G) floating in the membrane, resulting in activation of the α subunit (Gα). The activated α subunit can then follow different pathways *(B)*. Effector enzymes in the membrane (E), such as adenylyl cyclase, cyclic guanosine monophosphate (cGMP), phospholipase C, or phospholipase A$_2$, change the cytoplasmic concentration of their "messengers": cyclic adenosine monophosphate (cAMP), cGMP, diacylglycerol (DAG), and inositol 1,4,5-triphosphate (IP$_3$). These soluble molecules activate protein kinase A or C (PKA or PKC), or release Ca^{++} from sarcoplasmic reticulum (SR). Subsequently, cell behavior is changed by phosphorylation of an ionic channel on the cell membrane (CHAN) or by release of Ca^{++} from SR. *B*, Several pathways coupling receptor activation to final effect are illustrated. It is likely that multiple pathways are activated concomitantly, both facilitatory and inhibitory. In this way, the final response can be determined by the sum of the effects of several stimuli. *(A, B, From Brown AM, Birnbaumer L: Ionic channels and their regulation by G-protein subunits. Annu Rev Physiol 52:197, 1990.)*

activates a G$_i$ (i = inhibit) protein that inhibits adenylyl cyclase. A single G protein can interact with more than one effector. In this way, the G protein can be a branch point for the regulation of multiple effectors in response to a single signal. These proteins already have been implicated in human disease; cholera toxin covalently modifies G$_s$ so that it becomes persistently active in stimulating adenylyl cyclase in intestinal epithelial cells, likely causing the severe diarrhea of cholera.

Several second-messenger systems have been characterized. G$_s$ can directly enhance conductance through calcium channels, with the increased intracellular calcium acting as second messenger. The cyclic nucleotides, cAMP and guanosine monophosphate (GMP), act as second messengers. Their intracellular action is terminated when they are cleaved by phosphodiesterase enzymes, which, in turn, are regulated by stimuli and second messengers. The breakdown products of membrane phosphoinositide constitute another, more recently recognized set of second messengers.[13] In response to agonists such as vasopressin, G

protein is activated, leading to activation of the membrane-associated enzyme phospholipase C. This enzyme cleaves phosphatidylinositol 4,5-biphosphate on the inner leaflet of the plasma membrane, producing inositol 1,4,5-triphosphate (IP$_3$) and diacylglycerol (DAG). Both are second messengers. IP$_3$ diffuses through the cytoplasm and mobilizes calcium from intracellular stores. DAG remains within the plasma membrane and activates protein kinase C, which modulates cellular activity by phosphorylating intracellular proteins. In many cell types, activation of the same receptors that control phosphoinositide breakdown also results in the liberation of arachidonate and/or eicosanoids (prostaglandins, leukotrienes, and thromboxanes). The resultant change in cell behavior can be the opening of an ion channel, contraction or relaxation of smooth muscle, secretory activity, or initiation of cell division (see Chapter 7).

■ Endothelium

Although the vascular endothelium was once thought of as an inert lining for blood vessels, it is more accurately characterized as a very active, distributed organ with many biologic functions. It has synthetic (Table 6-1) and metabolic (Table 6-2) capabilities, and contains receptors for a variety of vasoactive substances (Table 6-3). Functions of the endothelium that may play an important role in the pathophysiology of ischemic heart disease are discussed.

Endothelium-Derived Relaxing Factors

The first vasoactive endothelial substance to be discovered was prostacyclin (PGI$_2$), a product of the cyclooxygenase pathway of arachidonic acid metabolism (Figure 6-4; Box 6-1).[14] The production of PGI$_2$ is activated by shear stress, pulsatility of flow, hypoxia, and a variety of vasoactive mediators. On production it leaves the endothelial cell and acts in the local environment to cause relaxation of the underlying smooth muscle or to inhibit platelet aggregation. Both actions are mediated by the stimulation of adenylyl cyclase in the target cell to produce cAMP.

In 1980, Furchgott and Zawadzki[15] observed that the presence of an intact endothelium was necessary for acetylcholine-induced vasodilation. Since that time it has been shown that many physiologic stimuli cause vasodilation by stimulating the release of a labile, diffusible,

TABLE 6-1	Substances Produced by Vascular Endothelium	
Antithrombotic Substances	*Procoagulants*
Prostacyclin	von Willebrand factor
Antithrombin III	Collagen
Plasminogen activator	Fibronectin
Protein C	Thromboplastin
α_2-Macroglobulin	Thrombospondin
Glycosaminoglycans (heparin)	Plasminogen inhibitors
	Platelet-activating factor
	Thromboxane A$_2$

From Bassenge E, Busse R: Endothelial modulation of coronary tone. *Prog Cardiovasc Dis* 30:349, 1988.

TABLE 6-2	Vasoactive Substances Processed by Vascular Endothelium	
Uptake and Metabolism	*Enzymatic Conversion or Degradation*
Norepinephrine	Angiotensin I to angiotensin II (ACE)
Serotonin	Angiotensin II to angiotensin III (angiotensinase)
Prostaglandins (E$_1$, E$_2$, E$_{2\alpha}$)	Bradykinin degradation (ACE)
Leukotrienes	Substance P degradation
Adenosine	

ACE, angiotensin-converting enzyme.

From Bassenge E, Busse R: Endothelial modulation of coronary tone. *Prog Cardiovasc Dis* 30:349, 1988.

TABLE 6-3	Stimulators of Endothelium-Mediated Vasodilation	
Transmitters	Adenosine diphosphate (ADP)
Acetylcholine	Adenosine
Norepinephrine	Serotonin
Peptides	Thrombin
Angiotensin	Trypsin
Bradykinin	**Local Hormones**
Vasopressin	Histamine
Oxytocin	Platelet-activating factor
Substance P	**Physicochemical Stimuli**
Vasoactive intestinal peptide	Shear stress (flow)
Calcitonin gene–related peptide	Mechanical stress (pulsatility)
Platelet or Blood Components	Hypoxia
Adenosine triphosphate (ATP)	

Modified from Bassenge E, Busse R: Endothelial modulation of coronary tone. *Prog Cardiovasc Dis* 30:349, 1988.

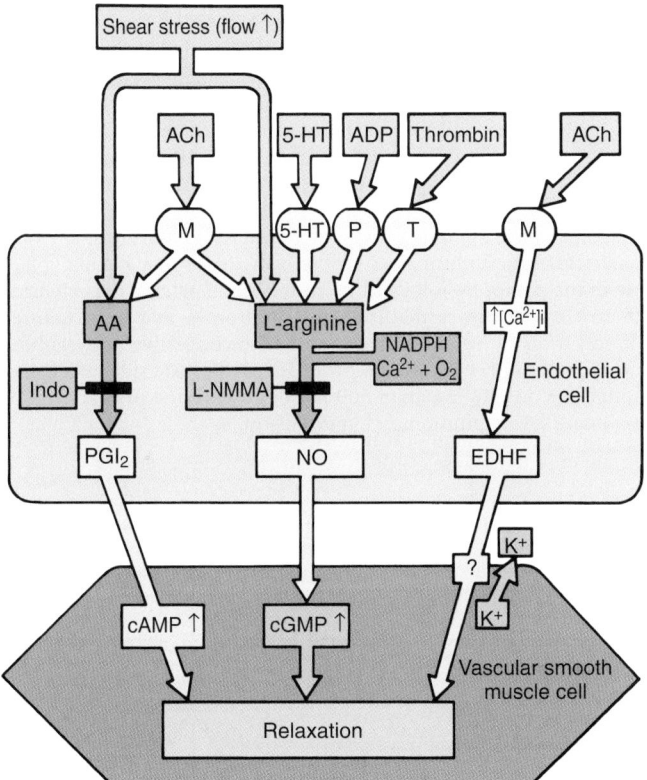

Figure 6-4 The production of endothelium-derived vasodilator substances. Prostacyclin (PGI_2) is produced via the cyclooxygenase pathway of arachidonic acid (AA) metabolism, which can be blocked by indomethacin (Indo) and aspirin. PGI_2 stimulates smooth muscle adenylyl cyclase and increases cyclic adenosine monophosphate (cAMP) production, which cause relaxation. Endothelium-derived relaxing factor (EDRF), now known to be nitric oxide (NO), is produced by the action of NO synthase on l-arginine in the presence of reduced nicotinamide adenine dinucleotide phosphate (NADPH), oxygen (O_2), and calcium and calmodulin. This process can be blocked by arginine analogs like N^G-monomethyl-l-arginine (l-NMMA). NO combines with guanylate cyclase in the smooth muscle cell to stimulate production of cyclic guanosine monophosphate (cGMP), which results in relaxation. Less well characterized is an endothelium-derived factor, which hyperpolarizes the smooth muscle membrane (EDHF) and probably acts via activation of potassium (K^+) channels. 5-HT, serotonin; ACh, acetylcholine; ADP, adenosine diphosphate; M, muscarinic receptor; P, purinergic receptor; T, thrombin receptor. *(From Rubanyi GM: Endothelium, platelets, and coronary vasospasm. Coron Artery Dis 1:645, 1990.)*

BOX 6-1. ENDOTHELIUM-DERIVED RELAXING AND CONTRACTING FACTORS

Healthy endothelial cells have an important role in modulating coronary tone by producing the following factors:

Vascular Muscle Relaxing Factors
- Prostacyclin
- Nitric oxide
- Hyperpolarizing factor

Vascular Muscle Contracting Factors
- Prostaglandin H_2
- Thromboxane A_2
- Endothelin

nonprostanoid molecule termed *endothelium-derived relaxing factor* (EDRF; see Figure 6-4), now known to be nitric oxide (NO). NO is the basis of a widespread paracrine signal transduction mechanism whereby one cell type can modulate the behavior of adjacent cells of different type.[16,17] NO is a very small lipophilic molecule that can readily diffuse across biologic membranes and into the cytosol of nearby cells. The half-life of the molecule is less than 5 seconds, so that only the local environment can be affected. NO is synthesized from the amino acid l-arginine by nitric oxide synthase (NOS). In vascular endothelium, the enzyme (endothelial NOS or NOS3) is always present (constitutive) and resides in the cytoplasm. Its function depends on the presence of Ca^{++} and calmodulin, as well as tetrahydrobiopterin. Serine phosphorylation is important for prolonged activity. The enzyme is activated in response to receptor occupancy or physical stimulation (see Table 6-3). When NO diffuses into the cytosol of the target cell, it binds with the heme group of soluble guanylate cyclase, resulting in a 50- to 200-fold increase in production of cyclic GMP, its second messenger. If the target cells are vascular smooth muscle cells, vasodilation occurs; if the target cells are platelets, adhesion and aggregation are inhibited. In vascular smooth muscle, cyclic GMP leads to activation of protein kinase G, which phosphorylates various intracellular target proteins, including the myosin light-chain regulatory subunit and proteins that control intracellular calcium.[18]

It is likely that NO is the final common effector molecule of nitrovasodilators (including sodium nitroprusside and organic nitrates such as nitroglycerin). The cardiovascular system is in a constant state of active vasodilation that is dependent on the generation of NO. The molecule is more important in controlling vascular tone in veins and arteries compared with arterioles. When the microcirculation dilates in response to metabolic myocardial demand (e.g., exercise), increased flow through epicardial coronary arteries increases shear stress at the endothelium. This leads to release of NO, which causes vascular smooth muscle relaxation and dilation of the conductance vessels, thereby facilitating the increase in flow. The importance of the loss of this mechanism in atherosclerosis is underlined by the fact that, in this situation, more than 50% of the resistance to flow in the coronary circulation resides in vessels larger than 100 μm in diameter (see Figure 6-1). Abnormalities in the ability of the endothelium to produce NO likely plays a role in diseases such as diabetes, atherosclerosis, and hypertension.[19,20] The venous circulation of humans appears to have a lower basal release of NO and an increased sensitivity to nitrovasodilators when compared with the arterial side of the circulation.[21]

Many agents, such as acetylcholine and norepinephrine, can cause contraction when applied directly to the vascular smooth muscle membrane instead of relaxation, which occurs when it is applied to the intact endothelium (Figure 6-5). The net effect of neural or humoral stimuli depends on a combination of direct effects mediated by binding to vascular smooth muscle receptors and indirect effects because of the ligand binding to endothelial receptors causing NO release from the endothelium. In the presence of healthy endothelium, vasodilation usually predominates. When the endothelium is absent (injured vessel) or diseased (atherosclerosis), vasoconstriction may be the net effect.

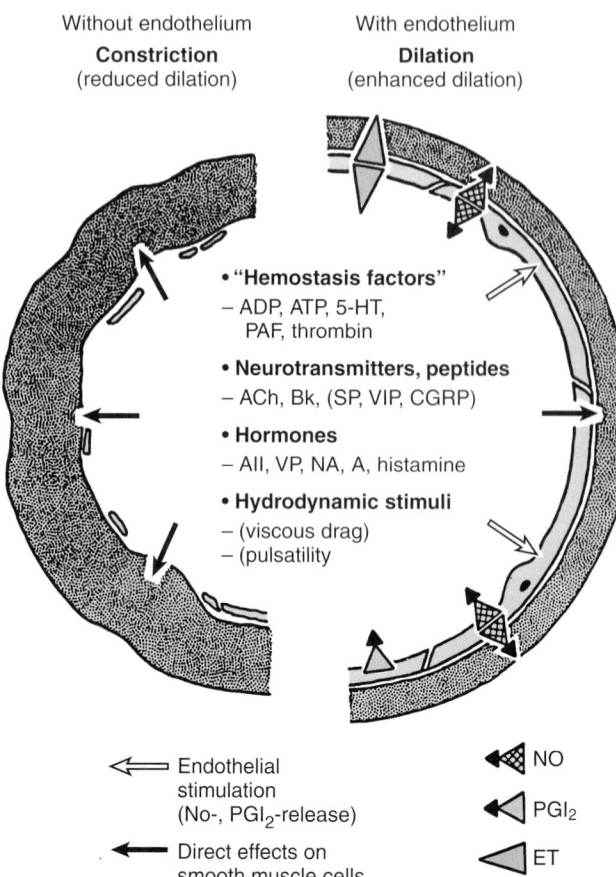

Without endothelium
Constriction
(reduced dilation)

With endothelium
Dilation
(enhanced dilation)

- **"Hemostasis factors"**
  – ADP, ATP, 5-HT,
    PAF, thrombin
- **Neurotransmitters, peptides**
  – ACh, Bk, (SP, VIP, CGRP)
- **Hormones**
  – AII, VP, NA, A, histamine
- **Hydrodynamic stimuli**
  – (viscous drag)
  – (pulsatility

⟸ Endothelial
    stimulation
    (No-, PGI₂-release)

◄ NO

← Direct effects on
   smooth muscle cells

◄ PGI₂

◄ ET

Figure 6-5   Role of endothelium in the control of coronary tone. Intact endothelium has an important modulatory role in the effect of numerous factors on vascular smooth muscle. In the absence of a functional endothelium (mechanical trauma, atherosclerosis), many factors act directly on smooth muscle to cause constriction (left). Under normal conditions (right), the release of nitric oxide (NO; endothelium-derived relaxing factor [EDRF]) and prostacyclin (PGI₂) stimulated by these same factors can attenuate constriction or cause dilation. PGI₂ release is predominantly into the lumen, whereas EDRF release is similar on both the luminal and abluminal sides. Substances in parentheses elicit only vasodilation. 5-HT, serotonin; A, adenosine; ACh, acetylcholine; ADP, adenosine monophosphate; AII, angiotensin II; ATP, adenosine triphosphate; Bk, bradykinin; CGRP, calcitonin gene–related peptide; ET, endothelin; NA, norepinephrine; PAF, platelet-activating factor; SP, substance P; VIP, vasoactive intestinal polypeptide; VP, vasopressin. *(From Bassenge E, Heusch G: Endothelial and neurohumoral control of coronary blood flow in health and disease. Rev Physiol Biochem Pharmacol 116:77, 1990.)*

NO has important roles in neurohumoral regulation of vascular tone, in preventing intravascular platelet aggregation, and in the structural adaptation of blood vessels to the demands of blood flow and pressure. Knowledge of its role in inflammation and atherosclerosis is rapidly expanding.

In addition to PGI₂ and NO, another less-well-understood pathway for receptor-mediated or mechanically induced endothelium-derived vasodilation exists that is associated with smooth muscle hyperpolarization. Both epoxyeicosatrienoic acid (a metabolite of cytochrome P450) and H_2O_2 have been suggested as possible endothelium-derived hyperpolarizing factors (EDHFs).[22,23] Smooth muscle relaxation is a result of hyperpolarization of the myocyte, which leads to decreased intracellular calcium concentration. EDHF-mediated vasodilation can be blocked by inhibition of calcium-dependent potassium channels. EDHF may have an important vasodilator role in the human coronary microcirculation.[24]

Endothelium-Derived Contracting Factors

Contracting factors produced by the endothelium include prostaglandin H_2, thromboxane A_2 (TxA_2; via cyclooxygenase), and the peptide endothelin (ET). ET is a potent vasoconstrictor peptide (100-fold more potent than norepinephrine)[25] with remarkable similarities to the toxin of the burrowing asp. Both have potent coronary constrictor activity to which the strong cardiac toxicity and lethality of the toxin are attributed.[26] Three closely related 21 amino acid peptides have been identified: endothelin-1 (ET-1), ET-2, and ET-3. The primary product of vascular endothelium is ET-1, which is synthesized from prepro-ET-1 within vascular endothelial cells by the action of ET-converting enzyme. It is not stored but rapidly synthesized in response to stimuli such as ischemia, hypoxia, and shear stress, and released predominantly abluminally (toward the underlying smooth muscle).[27] In vascular smooth muscle cells, ET-1 binds to specific membrane receptors (ET_A) and, via phospholipase C, induces an increase in intracellular calcium resulting in long-lasting contractions.[28] It is also linked via a G_i protein to voltage-operated calcium channels. This peptide has greater vasoconstricting potency than any other cardiovascular hormone, and in pharmacologic doses can abolish coronary flow, leading to ventricular fibrillation and death.[29] Another receptor subtype, ET_B, is expressed by both smooth muscle and endothelium and binds ET-1 and ET-3 equally well (Figure 6-6). When isolated vessels are perfused with ET-1, there is an initial NO-mediated vasodilation because of binding with ET_B receptors on the endothelial cells, followed by contraction because of binding of ET-1 to ET_A receptors on the vascular smooth muscle membrane. Studies utilizing bosentan, a combined ET_A- and ET_B-receptor antagonist, have demonstrated that ET exerts a basal coronary vasoconstrictor tone in humans.[30] There is evidence that ET may play a role in the pathophysiology of pulmonary and arterial hypertension, atherosclerosis, myocardial ischemic syndromes, and heart failure.[31] Clinical trials of bosentan in patients with congestive heart failure[32] and hypertension have shown promise, but hepatic side effects have limited the dose to less than 500 mg daily, with the primary indication being severe pulmonary hypertension.[33]

Vascular effects of endothelin and its receptors

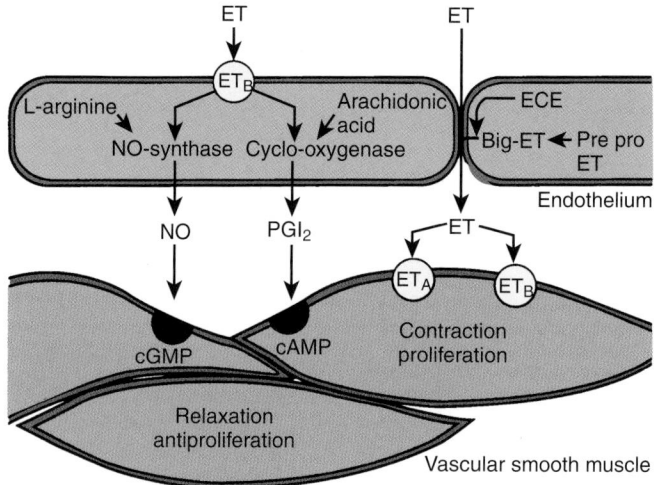

Figure 6-6 Endothelin (ET) released abluminally interacts with ET_A and ET_B receptors on vascular smooth muscle to cause contraction. Activators of ET_B receptors on endothelial cells cause vasodilation. cAMP, cyclic adenosine monophosphate; cGMP, cyclic guanosine monophosphate; ECE, endothelin-converting enzyme; NO, nitric oxide; PGI₂, prostacyclin. *(From Luscher TF: Do we need endothelin antagonists? Cardiovasc Res 29:2089, 1997; reproduced by permission of Elsevier Science-NL, Sara Burgerhartstraat 25, 1055 KV Amsterdam, the Netherlands.)*

Endothelial Inhibition of Platelets

A primary function of endothelium is to maintain the fluidity of blood. This is achieved by the synthesis and release of anticoagulant (e.g., thrombomodulin, protein C), fibrinolytic (e.g., tissue-type plasminogen activator), and platelet inhibitory (e.g., PGI$_2$, NO) substances (Box 6-2).[34] Mediators released from aggregating platelets stimulate the release of NO and PGI$_2$ from intact endothelium, which act together to increase blood flow and decrease platelet adhesion and aggregation (Figure 6-7), thereby flushing away microthrombi and maintaining the patency of the vessel.

With vital roles in modulating the tone of vascular smooth muscle, inhibiting platelets, and processing circulating chemicals, it seems clear that endothelial cell dysfunction would cause or contribute to ischemic syndromes. There is evidence of endothelial dysfunction in atherosclerosis, hyperlipidemia, diabetes, and hypertension.[35] Procedures such as coronary artery surgery and angioplasty disrupt the endothelium. The role of endothelium in the pathophysiology of myocardial ischemia is discussed later (see Dynamic Stenosis section).

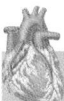

BOX 6-2. ENDOTHELIAL INHIBITION OF PLATELETS

Healthy endothelial cells have a role in maintaining the fluidity of blood by producing:
- Anticoagulant factors: protein C and thrombomodulin
- Fibrinolytic factor: tissue-type plasminogen activator
- Platelet inhibitory substances: prostacyclin and nitric oxide

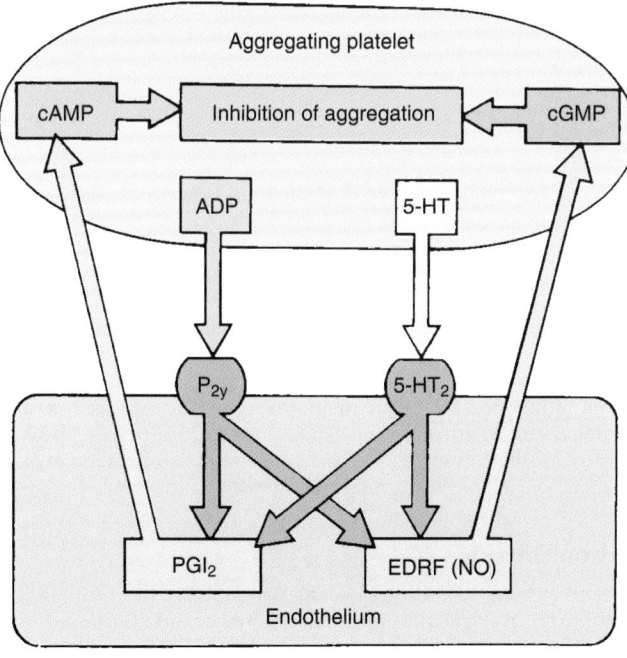

Figure 6-7 Inhibition of platelet adhesion and aggregation by intact endothelium. Aggregating platelets release adenosine diphosphate (ADP) and serotonin (5-HT), which stimulate the synthesis and release of prostacyclin (PGI$_2$) and endothelium-derived relaxing factor (EDRF; nitric oxide [NO]), which diffuse back to the platelets and inhibit further adhesion and aggregation, and can cause disaggregation. PGI$_2$ and EDRF act synergistically by increasing platelet cyclic adenosine monophosphate (cAMP) and cyclic guanosine monophosphate (cGMP), respectively. By inhibiting platelets and also increasing blood flow by causing vasodilation, PGI$_2$ and EDRF can flush away microthrombi and prevent thrombosis of intact vessels. P$_{2y}$, purinergic receptor. (*From Rubanyi GM: Endothelium, platelets, and coronary vasospasm. Coron Artery Dis 1:645, 1990.*)

DETERMINANTS OF CORONARY BLOOD FLOW

Under normal conditions, there are four major determinants of coronary blood flow: perfusion pressure, myocardial extravascular compression, myocardial metabolism, and neurohumoral control. Changes in myocardial perfusion caused by different interventions can be explained by analyzing the effects of those interventions on these four factors.

Perfusion Pressure and Myocardial Compression

Coronary blood flow is proportional to the pressure gradient across the coronary circulation (Box 6-3). This gradient is calculated by subtracting downstream coronary pressure from the pressure in the root of the aorta. The determination of downstream pressure is complicated because the intramural coronary vessels are compressed with each heartbeat.

During systole, the heart throttles its own blood supply. The force of systolic myocardial compression is greatest in the subendocardial layers, where it approximates intraventricular pressure. Resistance caused by extravascular compression increases with blood pressure, heart rate, contractility, and preload. Because it is difficult to measure intramyocardial pressure, the relative importance of these factors is controversial.[36,37] Flow is impeded both by direct compression and by shear caused by twisting of vessels as the heart contracts. Myocardial extravascular compression is less in the right ventricle, where pressures are lower and coronary perfusion persists during systole (Figure 6-8). In pathologic conditions associated with pulmonary hypertension, right coronary flow assumes a phasic pattern similar to left coronary flow. Under normal conditions, extravascular compression contributes only a small component (10% to 25%) to total coronary vascular resistance. When the coronary vessels are dilated by pharmacologic agents such as dipyridamole or during ischemia, the effects of extravascular compression on myocardial perfusion become more important (see Transmural Blood Flow section later in this chapter).

With each contraction, the intramural vessels are squeezed and blood is expelled forward into the coronary sinus and retrograde into the epicardial arteries. The large coronary arteries on the epicardial surface act as capacitors, charging with blood during systole and expelling blood into the coronary circulation during diastole.[38] Coronary capacitance likely explains the findings of Bellamy,[39] who reported that flow in the proximal left anterior descending coronary artery of the dog ceased when arterial pressure decreased to less than 45 mm Hg. It was suggested that flow throughout the coronary circulation stopped at pressures far in excess of the pressure at the coronary sinus. This pressure at which flow stopped was termed *critical closing pressure* or *zero-flow pressure* (P$_{zf}$). This had important implications in the calculation of coronary resistance because the effective downstream pressure would be P$_{zf}$ and not the much lower coronary venous pressure. This is analogous to a stream with a waterfall, where flow rate over the waterfall depends on the drop from the source to the waterfall edge and is unaffected by the distance to the bottom of the falls. It was later suggested that flow through the intramural coronary vessels continues after coronary inflow near the ostia (measured by Bellamy) has ceased.[40,41] There is evidence that antegrade movement of red blood

BOX 6-3. DETERMINANTS OF CORONARY BLOOD FLOW

The primary determinants of coronary blood flow are:
- Perfusion pressure
- Myocardial extravascular compression
- Myocardial metabolism
- Neurohumoral control

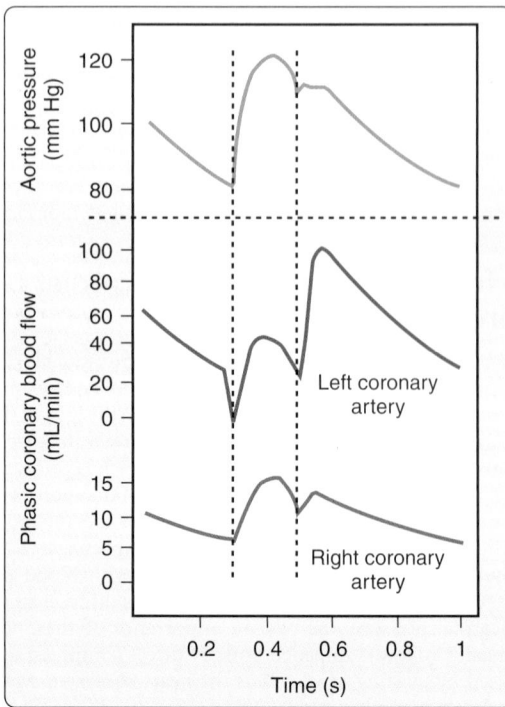

Figure 6-8 **Blood flow in the left and right coronary arteries.** The right ventricle is perfused throughout the cardiac cycle. Flow to the left ventricle is largely confined to diastole. *(From Berne RM, Levy MN: Special circulations. In Berne RM, Levy MN [eds]: Physiology. St. Louis: CV Mosby, 1988, pp 540–560.)*

cells in 20-μm arterioles continues until coronary pressure is only a few millimeters of mercury greater than coronary sinus pressure.[42] The concept of a critical closing pressure greatly in excess of coronary sinus pressure is probably not valid in the coronary circulation.

Although the true downstream pressure of the coronary circulation is likely close to the coronary sinus pressure, other choices may be more appropriate in clinical circumstances. In patients with CAD, the subendocardial layers of the left ventricle are at greatest risk for ischemia and necrosis (see Transmural Blood Flow section later in this chapter). Because this layer is perfused mostly when the aortic valve is closed, the most appropriate measure of the driving pressure for flow here is the average pressure in the aortic root during diastole. This can be approximated by aortic diastolic or mean pressure. Pressures monitored in peripheral arteries by routine methods in clinical settings can differ from central aortic readings. This is due to distortion of the pressure waveform as it is propagated through the arterial tree and inaccuracies associated with the hydraulic and electronic components of the monitoring system. Under these conditions, the mean arterial pressure may be the most reliable measure of coronary driving pressure. The true downstream pressure of the left ventricular subendocardium is the left ventricular diastolic pressure, which can be estimated by pulmonary artery occlusion pressure. When the right ventricle is at risk for ischemia (e.g., severe pulmonary hypertension), right ventricular diastolic pressure or central venous pressure may be more appropriate choices for downstream pressure.

Myocardial Metabolism

Myocardial blood flow, like flow in the brain and skeletal muscle, is primarily under metabolic control. Even when the heart is cut off from external control mechanisms (neural and humoral factors), its ability to match blood flow to its metabolic requirements is almost unaffected.[35] Because coronary venous oxygen tension is normally 15 to 20 mm Hg, there is only a small amount of oxygen available through increased extraction. A major increase in cardiac oxygen consumption

(M_{vo_2}) can occur only if oxygen delivery is increased by augmentation of coronary blood flow. Normally, flow and metabolism are closely matched so that over a wide range of oxygen consumption, coronary sinus oxygen saturation changes little.[43]

Despite intensive research over the last several decades, the mediator or mediators linking myocardial metabolism so effectively to myocardial blood flow are still unknown. Hypotheses of metabolic control propose that vascular tone is linked either to a substrate that is depleted, such as oxygen or adenosine triphosphate (ATP), or to the accumulation of a metabolite such as CO_2 or hydrogen ion (Box 6-4). Adenosine has been proposed in both categories. Feigl[43] has proposed six criteria for a chemical transmitter between the cardiac myocyte and the coronary vascular smooth muscle cell:

1. The transmitter is released under appropriate conditions and can be recovered from the tissue under those conditions.
2. Transmitter substance infused into the target tissue should faithfully mimic physiologic activation.
3. The biochemical apparatus for production of the proposed transmitter is present in the tissue in an appropriate location.
4. A mechanism for inactivation and/or uptake of the transmitter is present at an appropriate location in the tissue.
5. The action of various inhibitors and blocking agents on synthesis, release, target-organ receptor function, or transmitter inactivation should have effects consistent with the hypothesis. Blocking agents should give the same effect whether the transmitter is released physiologically or artificially applied.
6. Quantitative studies should indicate that the amount and time course of transmitter release under physiologic conditions are appropriate to give the indicated effect.

Many potential mediators of metabolic regulation have been proposed.[44] Although NO has a role in many coronary vasoregulatory pathways, it does not fulfill the role of metabolic regulator because blockade of NOS does not alter the increase in myocardial blood flow associated with an increase in myocardial oxygen demand.[45] The arguments for oxygen, carbon dioxide, and adenosine are briefly examined.

Oxygen

The coronary smooth muscle would have to be more sensitive to lack of oxygen than the working cardiocytes for oxygen to regulate coronary flow through a direct vascular action. Coronary microvessels in vitro do not relax until P_{O_2} is less than 5 mm Hg, a level well below the average P_{O_2} of 20 mm Hg in cardiac muscle cytosol.[46,47] With myocardial oxygen consumption (M_{vo_2}) held constant, increases in arterial oxygen content cause coronary flow to decrease, whereas decreases in arterial oxygen content cause flow to increase. These changes could explain only 40% of the increase in flow observed with tachycardia.[48] It is undecided whether the constancy of myocardial oxygen tension is the cause or the consequence of the excellent match between myocardial metabolism and myocardial blood flow.[49]

Carbon Dioxide

The end product of substrate oxidation is CO_2, the formation of which is directly related to the level of cardiac work. Carbon dioxide

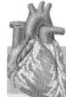

BOX 6-4. MYOCARDIAL METABOLISM

Several molecules have been proposed as the link between myocardial metabolism and myocardial blood flow, including:
• Oxygen
• Carbon dioxide
• Adenosine
  Current evidence suggests that a combination of local factors act together, each with differing importance during rest, exercise, and ischemia, to match myocardial oxygen delivery to demand.

is highly diffusible and can easily reach coronary smooth muscle cells. Unfortunately, it is difficult to separate the effects on coronary tone of increasing CO_2 from concomitant increases in other metabolites. Broten et al[48] pump-perfused the left main coronary artery of dogs and used an oxygenator in the perfusion circuit to alter coronary arterial Pco_2 and Po_2 at a constant level of myocardial metabolism. Increases in arterial and coronary sinus Pco_2 caused increases in coronary blood flow in the absence of changes in Mvo_2. Interestingly, there was a synergistic action of Pco_2 and Po_2: The increase in flow with elevation of Pco_2 was much greater at low Po_2 and vice versa. The effect of increasing CO_2, however, could not completely account for flow changes associated with an increase in Mvo_2.

Adenosine

Adenosine is a powerful coronary vasodilator via its activation of receptors on vascular endothelium and smooth muscle. In 1963, both Berne[50] and Gerlach[51] independently demonstrated the production of adenosine in ischemic heart muscle. They hypothesized that the release of adenosine may serve as a feedback signal inducing coronary vasodilation and augmenting coronary blood flow in proportion to myocardial metabolic needs. Initially, it was suggested that adenosine formation was coupled to myocardial oxygen tension.[50] A substrate theory has been proposed whereby adenosine production is linked to the cardiac energy state by the regulation of cytosolic AMP concentration to explain metabolic regulation by adenosine under both normoxic and ischemic conditions.[52] According to this theory, increases in cardiac work lead to a decline in ATP potential, which results in a quantitatively appropriate change in cytosolic AMP concentration, leading to increased adenosine release. In this way, the rate of adenosine production is determined by the myocardial oxygen supply/demand ratio. It is likely that adenosine causes coronary arteriolar dilation through stimulation of A_1 receptors directly coupled to ATP-sensitive K^+ (K^+_{ATP}) channels and A_2 receptor–mediated elevation of cAMP/protein kinase A, which lead to vasodilation, in part, by opening of K^+_{ATP} channels.[53,54]

Evidence against the adenosine hypothesis is accumulating. Adenosine deaminase is an enzyme that, when introduced in sufficient quantity into the myocardium, can significantly reduce the interstitial concentration of adenosine. Aminophylline and theophylline interfere with the coronary dilating effects of adenosine by acting on the receptor on vascular smooth muscle. Experiments using these agents to inhibit adenosine effect have shown that resting coronary blood flow, exercise-induced coronary dilation, autoregulation, and reactive hyperemia are largely unrelated to adenosine.[55–58] Measuring coronary microvessel diameters in beating hearts in situ, Kanatsuka et al[5] found that when Mvo_2 was doubled by pacing, vessels between 40 and 380 μm dilated, whereas when a similar increase in flow was induced by the infusion of adenosine or dipyridamole at constant Mvo_2, only vessels smaller than 150 μm dilated. Although adenosine does not seem to have an important role in metabolic regulation in the normal heart, adenosine blockade has been shown to cause a decrease in blood flow to hypoperfused myocardium sufficient to decrease systolic segment shortening.[59] Adenosine may have other important roles in ischemia, in which there is evidence of a cardioprotective action.[60,61]

Current evidence suggests that a combination of local factors act together, perhaps with differing importance in different situations, to match myocardial oxygen delivery to demand. The extreme difficulty of designing an experiment that can distinguish the effects of individual factors on coronary blood flow suggests that the exact mechanism of metabolic coronary regulation will not soon be elucidated.

◾ Neural and Humoral Control

Neural Control

The role of neural control in the regulation of myocardial blood flow is difficult to study because sympathetic or parasympathetic activation can cause profound changes in heart rate, blood pressure, and contractility. The resulting changes in coronary tone, mediated by metabolic regulation, can mask the concomitant direct effects of autonomic nerves on coronary smooth muscle. Studies of isolated vessels have given results that contradict in vivo studies, in part, because of damage to the endothelium during preparation. Despite these difficulties, there is much interest in exploring the role of autonomic control because it is implicated in the pathogenesis of myocardial ischemia.

Coronary Innervation

The heart is supplied with branches of the sympathetic and parasympathetic divisions of the autonomic nervous system. Thicker vagal fibers end in the adventitia of coronary vessels, whereas fine nonmedullated sympathetic fibers end on vascular smooth muscle cells.[62] Large and small coronary arteries, as well as veins, are richly innervated. The sympathetic nerves to the heart and coronary vessels arise from the superior, middle, and inferior cervical sympathetic ganglia, as well as the first four thoracic ganglia. The stellate ganglion (formed when the inferior cervical and first thoracic ganglia merge) is a major source of cardiac sympathetic innervation. The vagi supply the heart with efferent cholinergic nerves.

Parasympathetic Control

Vagal stimulation causes bradycardia, decreased contractility, and lower blood pressure. The resultant decline in Mvo_2 causes a metabolically mediated coronary vasoconstriction. When myocardial metabolism is held constant, however, cholinergic coronary dilation is consistently observed in response to exogenous acetylcholine, electrical vagal stimulation, and reflex activation through baroreceptors, chemoreceptors, and ventricular receptors.[35,43,63] These effects can be abolished by atropine.

In patients with angiographically normal coronary arteries, the response to intracoronary acetylcholine injection is predominantly dilation, whereas in atherosclerotic segments of epicardial arteries, constriction is observed.[64–66] Acetylcholine injected intraluminally binds to muscarinic receptors on the endothelium and stimulates the release of NO, which causes smooth muscle dilation. Acetylcholine is not normally found circulating in the blood but is released from vagal fibers and reaches the coronary smooth muscle from the adventitial side. Surprisingly, activation of muscarinic receptors on vascular smooth muscle cells causes constriction. Parasympathetic stimulation normally causes coronary vasodilation. This response depends on the ability of the coronary endothelium to elaborate NO and perhaps also EDHF (see earlier).[67,68] Parasympathetic control has not been shown to be important in the initiation of myocardial ischemia.

β-Adrenergic Coronary Dilation

β-Receptor activation causes dilation of both large and small coronary vessels even in the absence of changes in blood flow.[35,43] Studies in animals indicate that both $β_1$ and $β_2$ receptors are present throughout the coronary circulation, but $β_1$ receptors predominate in the conductance vessels, whereas $β_2$ receptors predominate in the resistance vessels. Mature canine coronary collaterals respond similarly to the conductance vessels.[69,70] β-Adrenergic coronary dilation may improve the speed and accuracy of coronary blood flow regulation during exercise.[71]

α-Adrenergic Coronary Constriction

Activation of the sympathetic nerves to the heart results in increases in heart rate, contractility, and blood pressure, which lead to a marked, metabolically mediated increase in coronary blood flow (Box 6-5). This suggested to early investigators that the effect of sympathetic coronary innervation is vasodilation. More recent investigation has demonstrated that the direct effect of sympathetic stimulation is coronary vasoconstriction, which is in competition with the metabolically mediated dilation of exercise or excitement. Whether adrenergic coronary constriction is powerful enough to further diminish blood flow in

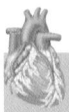

BOX 6-5. α-ADRENERGIC CORONARY CONSTRICTION

Sympathetic activation causes increased heart rate, contractility, and blood pressure, leading to a marked metabolically mediated increase in coronary blood flow. Surprisingly, the direct effect of sympathetic stimulation on the coronary vessels is vasoconstriction, sufficient to restrict the increase in blood flow and increase oxygen extraction.

ischemic myocardium or whether it can have some beneficial effect in the distribution of myocardial blood flow is controversial.

Classification

α-Adrenergic receptors can be classified anatomically as presynaptic or postsynaptic and also according to their pharmacologic properties as α_1 and α_2 (Table 6-4). The receptors can be further divided into subtypes according to their signal transduction mechanism (G-protein subtype) and second messenger (adenylyl cyclase, phospholipase C, etc.).[72]

Presynaptic α Receptors

α receptors on cardiac sympathetic nerve terminals mediate feedback inhibition of neuronal norepinephrine release. Both α_1 and α_2 receptors appear to be involved because exercise-induced increases in heart rate and contractility can be potentiated by either idazoxan (α_2-blockade) or prazosin (α_1-blockade).[73]

Cardiac Muscle Cells

Activation of myocardial α_1 receptors results in a positive inotropic effect that, in contrast with β-receptor activation, is associated with prolongation of contraction. Although normally of minor functional importance, this effect may serve as an inotropic reserve mechanism when β-receptor–mediated inotropy is impaired (e.g., hypothyroidism, cardiac failure, chronic propranolol treatment).[74] The importance of this mechanism in humans is uncertain. An increase in inotropy caused by stimulation of myocardial α receptors would result in increased Mvo_2 and a metabolically mediated coronary dilation.

Coronary Endothelium

Binding of norepinephrine to α_2 receptors on vascular endothelium stimulates the release of NO, which acts to relax vascular smooth muscle. The endothelium can also act to limit the effect of norepinephrine by metabolizing it. In these ways, the endothelium modulates the direct constrictive effects of α-adrenergic activation. Abnormal endothelial function in atherosclerosis may predispose to excessive α-adrenergic constriction and is implicated in the pathogenesis of myocardial ischemia (see Dynamic Stenosis later in this chapter).

TABLE 6-4	Classification of α-Adrenergic Receptor Subtypes in the Heart		
Selective Agonists	**Selective Antagonists**	**Effects of Activation**	
α_1			
Phenylephrine	Prazosin	*Presynaptic:* feedback inhibition of norepinephrine release	
Methoxamine		*Postsynaptic:* coronary vasoconstriction, increase in myocardial arrhythmias	
Inotropism			
α_2			
Clonidine	Yohimbine	*Presynaptic:* feedback inhibition of norepinephrine release	
Azepexole	Rauwolscine	*Postsynaptic:* coronary vasoconstriction, arrhythmias (?)	
BHT 920	Idazoxan		
UK 14, 304			

Norepinephrine is a nonselective agonist. Phentolamine and phenoxybenzamine are nonselective antagonists. Phenylephrine also causes β-receptor activation.
Modified from Heusch G: Alpha-adrenergic mechanisms in myocardial ischemia. *Circulation* 81:1, 1990.

Coronary Resistance

The magnitude of α-adrenergic vasoconstriction that occurs in the coronary bed is small compared with that which occurs in the skin and skeletal muscle. In the presence of β-blockade, intense sympathetic stimulation results in only a 20% to 30% increase in coronary resistance.[75] Mohrman and Feigl[76] examined the effect of sympathetic activation on coronary flow in the absence of β-blockade. The net effect of α-receptor vasoconstriction was to restrict the metabolically related flow increase by 30%, thereby increasing oxygen extraction and decreasing coronary sinus oxygen content.

Epicardial coronary diameter changes little during sympathetic stimulation.[77] α_1-Adrenergic and α_2-adrenergic receptors are found throughout the coronary circulation; however, α_1 receptors appear to be more important in the large epicardial vessels, whereas α_2 predominate in small coronary vessels less than 100 μm in diameter.[78] Studies of mature coronary collateral vessels in dogs have generally failed to provide evidence of α-receptor–mediated vasoconstriction.[79] After heart transplant, patients demonstrated a lesser increase in myocardial blood flow after a cold pressor test in denervated regions of the heart.[80] The authors argue that this was not due to increased myocardial metabolism secondary to myocardial β-receptor activation. They suggest that sympathetic innervation has an important role in coronary vessel dilation during stress.

Exercise

α-Adrenergic coronary constrictor tone during exercise is exerted predominantly by circulating catecholamines.[81] Numerous studies indicate that myocardial blood flow during exercise is limited by α vasoconstriction.[35] In a study of exercising dogs, Huang and Feigl[82] found that despite an increase in total coronary flow in an α-blocked region of myocardium, flow to the inner, subendocardial layer was diminished. These results suggest a beneficial effect of α-adrenergic coronary constriction on the distribution of blood flow within the myocardium.

Myocardial Ischemia

Buffington and Feigl[83] demonstrated the persistence of α-adrenergic coronary vasoconstriction distal to a moderate coronary stenosis during norepinephrine infusion. Investigations in dogs have demonstrated that, as coronary reserve is depleted by increasing stenosis severity, the response to sympathetic stimulation shifts from a metabolically induced coronary dilation to coronary constriction.[84,85] These observations suggest that sympathetic coronary vasoconstriction limits coronary blood flow even during myocardial ischemia, when autoregulatory reserve is exhausted (see Coronary Reserve later in this chapter). There is no consensus as to the importance of α_1 vs α_2 receptors in ischemic myocardium.[35] Using constant flow coronary perfusion in anesthetized dogs, Nathan and Feigl[86] compared the transmural distribution of myocardial blood flow in α-blocked and intact regions of myocardium during hypoperfusion. Surprisingly, α-blockade diverted blood flow from the subendocardium to the subepicardium. This suggests that α vasoconstriction had limited flow more in the subepicardium, thereby producing an antisteal effect, and improved perfusion of the more vulnerable inner layers of the left ventricle. Chilian and Ackell[87] found similar results in exercising dogs with an artificial coronary stenosis. In contrast, work from Heusch and colleagues[88,89] demonstrated improved subendocardial perfusion distal to a severe coronary stenosis with α_2-receptor blockade. This controversy is unresolved.[90] α-Receptor blockers have not been shown to have a role in the treatment of myocardial ischemia in patients with CAD.

Studies in Humans

Studies indicate that there is little α-adrenoceptor–mediated tone in resting humans.[91] Clinical studies have failed to provide convincing evidence that α-adrenergic coronary constriction plays an important role in Prinzmetal's variant angina (angina with ST-segment elevation at rest).[92] During sympathetic activation, however, there is evidence that α vasoconstriction can precipitate myocardial ischemia by further narrowing diseased coronary arteries. This has been shown during isometric exercise, dynamic exercise, and with the cold pressor test[93–98] (see Dynamic Stenosis later in this chapter).

Humoral Control

A complete understanding of the effects of circulating substances on the coronary vessels would require determining their effects on large versus small coronary vessels, while separating direct effects on coronary vessels from changes in tone mediated by changes in myocardial metabolism. This is further complicated by the critical role of an intact vascular endothelium in modulating these responses (see Endothelium earlier in this chapter). Some of the better studied agents are discussed briefly later.

The peptide hormones include vasopressin (arginine vasopressin [AVP] or antidiuretic hormone [ADH]), atrial natriuretic peptide (ANP), vasoactive intestinal peptide, neuropeptide Y, and calcitonin gene–related peptide.[44] Of these, AVP and ANP have been the most studied. It has been demonstrated in dogs that AVP, in concentrations 3 to 30 times those found in stressed patients, can cause vasoconstriction sufficient to produce myocardial ischemia.[99] In large coronary arteries, the dilator response (via NO) likely exceeded the constrictor response.[35] This was due to constriction of the small-resistance vessels. In physiologic concentrations, AVP acts primarily as an ADH with little effect on the coronary circulation. ANP can cause endothelium-dependent coronary dilation but is not known to have significant vascular effects in physiologic concentrations.[100]

Angiotensin-converting enzyme (ACE) is present on vascular endothelium and converts angiotensin I to angiotensin II (AII), which causes coronary vasoconstriction. AII also facilitates release of norepinephrine from presynaptic adrenergic nerve terminals. ACE inactivates bradykinin, which can attenuate vasoconstriction via NO stimulation. Thus, ACE inhibition can reduce coronary tone by suppressing AII formation and degrading bradykinin, and perhaps also by decreasing norepinephrine release. Despite these theoretical considerations, ACE inhibition has not been shown to be of benefit in human myocardial ischemia other than through control of afterload.[101]

PGI_2 and TxA_2 are synthesized from arachidonic acid in a reaction catalyzed by cyclooxygenase. PGI_2 is synthesized in the vascular endothelium and, in addition to inhibiting platelet aggregation, induces vasodilation (see Endothelium-Derived Relaxing Factors section earlier in this chapter). TxA_2 is mainly synthesized in platelets and causes platelet aggregation and vasoconstriction in the presence of damaged vascular endothelium. In response to TxA_2, the intact endothelium releases NO, causing both vasodilation and platelet disaggregation, mechanisms to maintain patency of normal vessels (see Endothelial Inhibition of Platelets section earlier in this chapter). Unlike platelets, the vascular endothelium can synthesize proteins de novo, and thus cyclooxygenase acetylation by aspirin administration has a lesser effect in reducing vascular PGI_2 than platelet TxA_2. Other than in platelet-vessel interactions and inflammation, prostaglandins are not known to have an important role in the regulation of coronary blood flow.[35] Serotonin (5-HT) is another platelet product that can cause endothelium-dependent dilation of coronary arterial vessels smaller than 100 μm, but causes constriction of larger epicardial coronary arteries.[102]

Histamine receptors are present in the coronary vessels. H_1 receptors are located on vascular smooth muscle cells of large and small coronary arteries, and mediate vasoconstriction. H_2 receptors are located on smooth muscle cells of arterioles and mediate vasodilation. H_1 receptors also are located on vascular endothelium and can mediate vasodilation via stimulation of NO release. In patients with vasospastic angina and endothelial dysfunction, administration of exogenous histamine can cause vasospasm.[103]

CORONARY PRESSURE-FLOW RELATIONS

▓ Autoregulation

Autoregulation is the tendency for organ blood flow to remain constant despite changes in arterial perfusion pressure.[104] Autoregulation can maintain flow to myocardium served by stenotic coronary arteries despite low perfusion pressure distal to the obstruction. This is a local

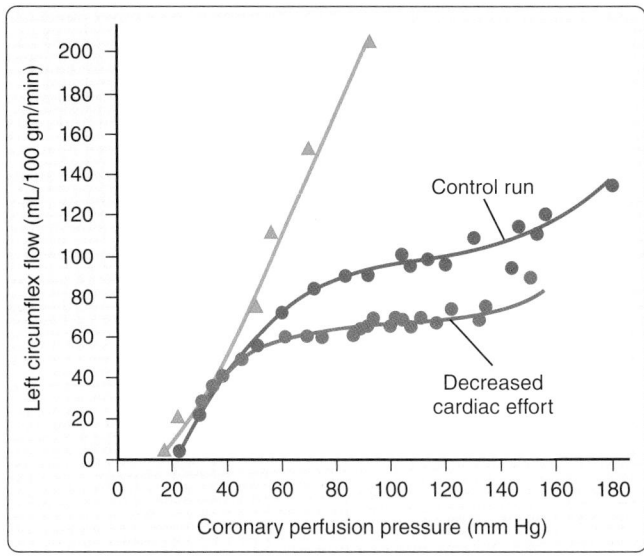

Figure 6-9 Autoregulation at two levels of myocardial oxygen consumption. Pressure in the cannulated left circumflex artery was varied independently of aortic pressure. When pressures were suddenly increased or decreased from 40 mm Hg, flow instantaneously increased with pressure (*steep line, green triangles*). With time, flow decreases to the steady-state level determined by oxygen consumption (*purple* and *red circles*). The vertical distance from the steady-state (autoregulating) line to the instantaneous pressure-flow line is the autoregulatory flow reserve. (*From Mosher P, Ross J Jr, McFate PA, Shaw RF: Control of coronary blood flow by an autoregulatory mechanism. Circ Res 14:250, 1964.*)

mechanism of control and can be observed in isolated, denervated hearts. If Mvo_2 is fixed, coronary blood flow will remain relatively constant between mean arterial pressures of 60 to 140 mm Hg. Figure 6-9 illustrates that, at a given cardiac workload, the level of flow (determined by metabolic regulation) is maintained constant over a broad range of pressure by autoregulation.

Coronary perfusion pressure must be varied while holding Mvo_2 constant to study autoregulation. This is difficult in the heart because changing aortic pressure changes both the perfusion pressure for the coronary arteries and the afterload of the left ventricle. Thus, changes in aortic pressure inevitably change Mvo_2. This problem is overcome by cannulating the coronary arteries and perfusing them with a pump. However, even when heart rate and aortic pressure are held constant, Mvo_2 changes with changing coronary pressure. This is because myocardial contractility and metabolism increase when coronary pressure is increased to more than the normal autoperfused level. This phenomenon is known as the Gregg effect and may be explained by the "garden hose" hypothesis of Lochner, whereby engorgement of the coronary vasculature elongates the myocardial sarcomere length during diastole and contractile strength is increased because of the Frank–Starling mechanism (for a detailed review, see Feigl[43] and Gregg[105]).

In addition to the Gregg effect, two other issues complicate studies of autoregulation: collateral flow and myocardial oxygen extraction. If pressure is lowered in the left coronary artery and not in the right, there will be a pressure gradient for flow from the right to left coronary artery via collateral vessels. Flow measured proximally in the left coronary artery will then underestimate flow reaching the myocardium. Normal coronary sinus oxygen tension (CSo_2) is less than 20 mm Hg. Dole[106] observed that autoregulation was effective when CSo_2 was less than 25 mm Hg, but was completely lost when CSo_2 exceeded 32 mm Hg. Autoregulation can be intensified by vasoconstriction (increased oxygen extraction) and attenuated by vasodilation (decreased oxygen extraction).[107] The degradation of autoregulation with α-receptor blockade suggests a benefit of adrenergic coronary vasoconstriction.[108]

Early reports indicated that autoregulation is less effective in the right ventricle than the left. More recently, it has been suggested that increases in right coronary pressures may produce large changes in Mvo_2, perhaps because of an exaggerated Gregg effect. When changes in myocardial metabolism are taken into account, autoregulation in the right and left ventricle is similar.[109,110]

Quantitation of the degree of autoregulation must involve a comparison of the observed change in vascular resistance to the change in resistance that would have occurred in the absence of flow autoregulation. Some degree of autoregulation exists when the relative change in flow ($\Delta F/F$) is less than the relative change in pressure ($\Delta P/P$). From these definitions, Dole[107] has derived an autoregulation index that can be used to quantify the effects of different agents on coronary autoregulation.[111]

Three theories have been proposed to explain coronary autoregulation: the tissue pressure theory, the myogenic theory, and the metabolic theory.[112] The tissue pressure hypothesis proposes that changes in perfusion pressure result in directionally similar changes in capillary filtration and, therefore, tissue pressure. In this way, extravascular resistance would oppose changes in flow with changes in perfusion pressure. Experimental evidence has shown, however, that there is no relation between the degree of autoregulation and the magnitude of change in tissue pressure. Arterial smooth muscle contracts in response to augmented intraluminal pressure; this is known as the *myogenic response*. Recently, this response has been demonstrated in coronary arterioles in the presence and absence of functioning endothelium.[113] The argument for myogenic regulation of coronary flow is that myocardial metabolic changes are not rapid enough to explain large decreases in resistance after coronary occlusions for one or two heartbeats. However, myocardial metabolic events have been shown to occur during the course of a single cardiac contraction.[114] The metabolic theory of autoregulation proposes that coronary arteriolar tone is determined by the balance of myocardial oxygen supply and demand. An increase in flow above the requirements of metabolism would wash out metabolites or cause accumulation of substrates, and this would be the signal for an appropriate change in coronary tone. Although metabolic regulation and autoregulation are separate phenomena, they may, therefore, have a common underlying mechanism. Metabolic regulation is discussed earlier (see Myocardial Metabolism). For an instructive, three-dimensional, graphic analysis of the interrelations among coronary artery pressure, myocardial metabolism, and coronary blood flow, see Feigl et al.[115]

Coronary Reserve

Myocardial ischemia causes intense coronary vasodilation. After a 10- to 30-second coronary occlusion, restoration of perfusion pressure is accompanied by a marked increase in coronary flow. This large increase in flow, which can be five or six times resting flow in the dog, is termed *reactive hyperemia*. Figure 6-10 illustrates that the repayment volume is greater than the debt volume. There is, however, no overpayment of the oxygen debt because oxygen extraction declines

during the hyperemia.[116] The presence of high coronary flows when coronary venous oxygen content is high suggests that mediators other than oxygen are responsible for this metabolically induced vasodilation.[43] The difference between resting coronary blood flow and peak flow during reactive hyperemia represents the autoregulatory coronary flow reserve: the further capacity of the arteriolar bed to dilate in response to ischemia. In Figure 6-9, the flow reserve is the vertical distance from the autoregulating pressure-flow curve (purple or red circles) to the nonautoregulating curve (triangles). The reserve is greater at higher perfusing pressure and lower Mvo_2. Unlike cannula-perfused preparations in which these data are obtained, in the clinical setting, increases in pressure increase both perfusing pressure and Mvo_2. Reactive hyperemia responses have been used in animals and humans to estimate coronary reserve in conditions such as obstructive coronary disease, aortic stenosis, and left ventricular hypertrophy[117-119]. The myocardial fractional flow reserve (FFR) is calculated by dividing the pressure in a coronary vessel distal to a stenosis during maximal pharmacologic dilation by the aortic root pressure. This ratio (FFR) easily can be measured in the angiography suite and has been recommended as a useful index of the functional severity of coronary stenoses of intermediate morphologic severity on angiography, as well as a measure of residual obstruction after interventions.[120] Indeed, the relevance of a reduction in the FFR is highlighted in a recent randomized, controlled study that demonstrated improved clinical outcomes in FFR-guided percutaneous coronary interventions as opposed to angiography alone.[121]

It has been generally accepted that the coronary resistance vessels are maximally dilated when coronary perfusion pressure is reduced sufficiently to cause myocardial ischemia. In fact, agents such as adenosine, carbochromene, and dipyridamole can cause further increases in coronary flow in the presence of intense ischemia, when autoregulatory reserve is believed to be exhausted. This pharmacologic vasodilator reserve is greater than the autoregulatory vasodilator reserve. If flow to ischemic myocardium can be increased by pharmacologic dilation of resistance vessels, the use of these agents should reverse ischemic dysfunction and metabolism. Arteriolar dilators have, in general, not been found to be beneficial during myocardial ischemia. Coronary blood flow in the different layers of the ventricle must be reviewed to understand why (Box 6-6).

Transmural Blood Flow

It is well-known that, when coronary perfusion pressure is inadequate, the inner one third to one fourth of the left ventricular wall is the first region to become ischemic or necrotic.[122] This increased vulnerability of the subendocardium may be caused by an increased demand for perfusion or a decreased supply, compared with the outer layers. There has been extensive study of the transmural distribution of oxygen consumption, use of oxidizable substrates, activity of glycolytic and mitochondrial enzymes, tissue contents of endogenous substrates, high-energy phosphates, lactate, isoforms of contractile proteins, and fiber stress and fiber shortening. In general, these studies indicate that

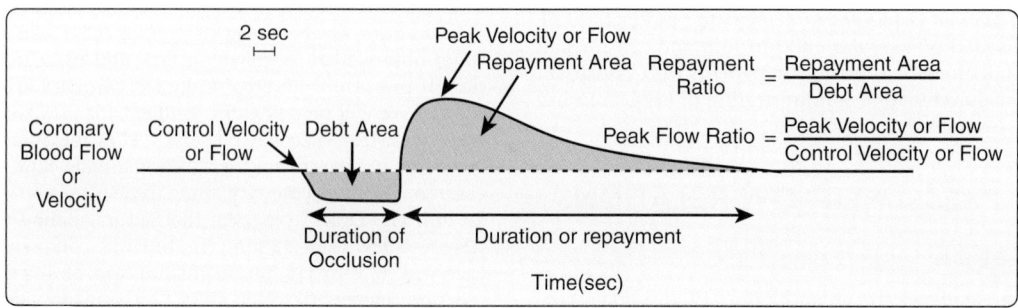

Figure 6-10 Schematic diagram of the reactive hyperemic response to a 10-second coronary occlusion. (*From Marcus ML: Metabolic regulation of coronary blood flow. In Marcus ML [ed]: The coronary circulation in health and disease. New York: McGraw-Hill, 1983, pp 65–92. Reproduced by permission of McGraw-Hill Companies.*)

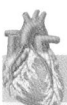

BOX 6-6. TRANSMURAL BLOOD FLOW

- When coronary perfusion pressure is inadequate, the inner third of the left ventricular wall is the first region to become ischemic or necrotic.
- During systole, intramyocardial pressure is greatest in the inner layers of the ventricle, and this restricts perfusion to that region.
- In concentric hypertrophy, this effect is exaggerated, and the subendocardium is at increased risk for ischemia.

if such differences exist between the layers of the left ventricle, they are unlikely to exceed 10% to 20%.[43,123] It is likely that preferential underperfusion of the subendocardium is the primary determinant of its increased vulnerability.

Regional blood flow in the myocardium is usually determined using radioactive microspheres. These plastic beads, labeled with a radioisotope, are injected into the bloodstream. The assumption is that they will mix uniformly with blood and be distributed in proportion to blood flow, as if they were red blood cells.[124] Because they are rigid and larger than red cells (9- or 15-μm diameters are usually chosen), they are trapped in the microcirculation. At the end of an experiment, the heart can be divided into small blocks and the amount of radioactivity in each piece measured in a gamma counter. The blood flow to each block of tissue will be proportional to the number of microspheres in each piece, which can be determined from its radioactivity. By using different radioisotopes as labels, several sets of microspheres can be injected during an experiment, giving "snapshots" of what flow was at the time of each injection. It is difficult to reduce the variability of the technique below 10%.[43,125] Subendocardial blood flow is found using this technique to be about 10% greater than subepicardial blood flow under normal circumstances. This gives a normal subendocardial/subepicardial or inner/outer (I/O) blood flow ratio of 1.10. This ratio is maintained at normal perfusing pressures even at heart rates greater than 200 beats/min.

If coronary pressure is gradually reduced, autoregulation is exhausted and flow decreases in the inner layers of the left ventricle before it begins to decrease in the outer layers (Figure 6-11). This indicates that there is less flow reserve in the subendocardium than in the subepicardium. The limits of autoregulation will depend on the level of cardiac work (see Autoregulation section earlier in this chapter) and on the experimental conditions. In conscious dogs, the mean coronary pressure at which evidence of subendocardial ischemia appeared was 38 mm Hg at a heart rate of 100 beats/min, and increased to 61 mm Hg at 200 beats/min. Subepicardial flow during tachycardia did not decline even at pressures as low as 33 mm Hg.[126] Because subepicardial flow is rarely inadequate, a subendocardial/subepicardial blood flow ratio close to 1.0 indicates adequate subendocardial flow and an appropriate matching of myocardial oxygen supply to oxygen demand. For this reason, the I/O ratio is often used as a measure of the adequacy of myocardial blood flow.

Three mechanisms have been proposed to explain the decreased coronary reserve in the subendocardium: differential systolic intramyocardial pressure, differential diastolic intramyocardial pressure, and interactions between systole and diastole. Because the force of systolic myocardial compression is greatest in the inner layers of the ventricle and is low at the subepicardium, it was believed that the outer layers of the heart were perfused throughout the cardiac cycle, whereas the subendocardium was perfused only during diastole. The subendocardium would have to obtain its entire flow during only a portion of the cycle and, therefore, would have to have a lower resistance. Recent studies, suggesting that there may be little systolic flow even to the outer layers, argue against this explanation.[127] The second mechanism is based on the high coronary pressures observed when coronary flow has ceased during a long diastole, P_{zf} (see Perfusion Pressure and Myocardial Compression earlier in this chapter).[39] The shape of the pressure-flow relation during a long diastole suggests that P_{zf} is higher in the subendocardium. This would mean that perfusion pressure for the subendocardium is lower in diastole compared with the outer layers of myocardium. Available evidence suggests that P_{zf} is not high in any layer and is unlikely to be more than 2 to 3 mm Hg greater in the subendocardium than in the subepicardium.[127] Hoffman[109,127] proposed an interaction between systole and diastole as the explanation for the increased vulnerability of the subendocardium to ischemia. During systole, intramyocardial pressure is high enough throughout most of the ventricular wall to squeeze blood out of the intramural vessels and into the extramural coronary veins and arteries. Because the compressive force is greatest in the subendocardium, vessels here are the narrowest at end systole. At the beginning of diastole, blood will be directed first to vessels with the lowest resistance, the larger vessels in the subepicardium, and last to the most narrowed vessels in the subendocardium. In this way, should the duration of diastole or the diastolic perfusion pressure be reduced, the subendocardial muscle would receive the least flow. Spaan[36] presents an interesting analysis of the interaction between arterial pressure and force of contraction as an intramyocardial pump. Although this theory is compatible with existing evidence, support for it will remain indirect until it becomes possible to measure phasic pressures and flows in separate layers of myocardium.

When the left ventricle hypertrophies in response to a pressure load (aortic stenosis, hypertension), myofibrillar growth outstrips the capillary network, resulting in decreased capillary density and increased diffusion distances. The net effect is to reduce coronary autoregulatory reserve.[128] The transmural gradient of reserve is exaggerated as well, so the subendocardium is at increased risk for ischemia in the hypertrophied heart compared with normal.[129]

In addition to the transmural gradient of coronary reserve from outer to inner layer of the left ventricle, there is also marked variation of reserve between small regions of myocardium within a layer.[130] This heterogeneity of flow reserve may explain why pharmacologic reserve exceeds autoregulatory reserve (see Coronary Reserve section earlier in this chapter). During hypoperfusion, regional myocardial blood flow is decreased, but in all layers some small pieces of muscle will have no flow reserve left, whereas adjacent pieces can have substantial reserve. Fewer pieces will retain reserve in the subendocardium than in the subepicardium. The increase in flow in response to an infusion of adenosine is due to increased flow in the small regions with reserve, with no change in the adjacent fully dilated regions.[131-133] These findings suggest

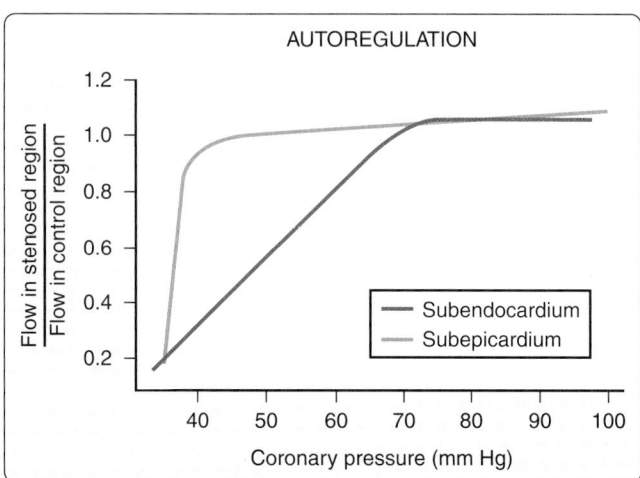

Figure 6-11 **Pressure-flow relations of the subepicardial and subendocardial thirds of the left ventricle in anesthetized dogs.** In the subendocardium, autoregulation is exhausted and flow becomes pressure dependent when pressure distal to a stenosis declines to less than 70 mm Hg. In the subepicardium, autoregulation persists until perfusion pressure declines to less than 40 mm Hg. Autoregulatory coronary reserve is less in the subendocardium. *(Redrawn from Guyton RA, McClenathan JH, Newman GE, Michaelis LL: Significance of subendocardial ST segment elevation caused by coronary stenosis in the dog. Am J Cardiol 40:373, 1977.)*

that ischemia causes maximal coronary vasodilation, and that increases in flow with adenosine or dipyridamole are due to dilation of vessels in nonischemic regions. Contrasting evidence is provided by Duncker and Bache,[54] who used a balloon occluder to simulate a coronary stenosis in exercising dogs. The occluder was adjusted to maintain distal coronary pressure constant at 43 mm Hg. During exercise, an intracoronary infusion of adenosine increased blood flow to all myocardial layers and improved regional systolic segment shortening. Although this is evidence of vasodilator reserve in ischemic myocardium, the constant distal pressure preparation does not faithfully mimic a coronary stenosis because it makes transmural steal impossible (see Coronary Steal later in this chapter). In general, pharmacologic dilation of resistance vessels has the potential to worsen ischemia by producing coronary steal. Dilation of larger penetrating vessels (50 to 500 μm in diameter) with nitrovasodilators could preferentially decrease resistance to blood flow to the subendocardium, and this may, in addition to favorable effects on the systemic circulation, explain the usefulness of nitrates in the treatment of angina.[54]

ATHEROSCLEROSIS

The atherosclerotic lesion consists of an excessive accumulation of smooth muscle cells in the intima, with quantitative and qualitative changes in the noncellular connective tissue components of the artery wall, and intracellular and extracellular deposition of lipoproteins and mineral components (e.g., calcium; Box 6-7). By definition, atherosclerosis is a combination of atherosis and sclerosis. The latter term, *sclerosis,* refers to the hard, collagenous material that accumulates in lesions and is usually more voluminous than the pultaceous "gruel" of the atheroma (Figure 6-12).

Stary and colleagues[134] note that the earliest detectable change in the evolution of coronary atherosclerosis in young people was the accumulation of intracellular lipid in the subendothelial region, creating lipid-filled macrophages or "foam cells." Grossly, a collection of foam cells may give the artery wall the appearance of a "fatty streak." In general, fatty streaks are covered by a layer of intact endothelium and are not characterized by excessive smooth muscle cell accumulation. At later stages of atherogenesis, extracellular lipoproteins accumulate in the musculoelastic layer of the intima, eventually forming an avascular core of lipid-rich debris that is separated from the central arterial lumen by a fibrous cap of collagenous material. Foam cells are not usually seen deep within the atheromatous core, but are frequently found at the periphery of the lipid core.

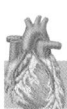 Atherogenesis

Certain human arteries are more prone to develop atherosclerosis than others. For example, the coronary, renal, and internal carotid arteries, as well as some areas of the aorta, are known to be common sites for lesion formation.[134] In the Pathobiological Determinants of Atherosclerosis in Youth (PDAY) study, the aorta and right coronary arteries of 1378 young people aged 15 to 34 who died as a result of

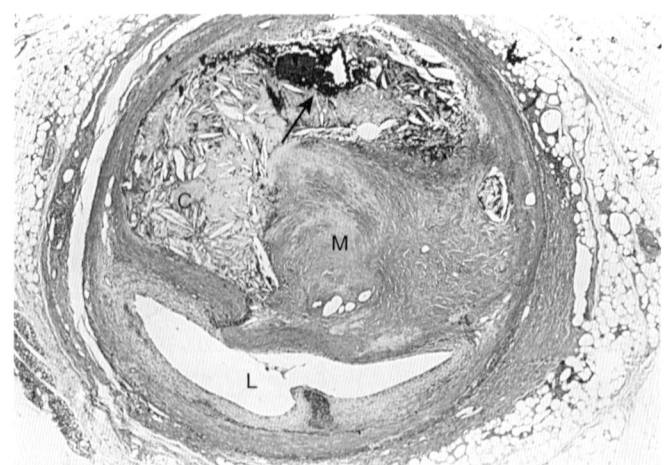

Figure 6-12 **Atherosclerotic human coronary artery of an 80-year-old man.** There is severe narrowing of the central arterial lumen (*L*). The intima consists of a complex collection of cells, extracellular matrix (*M*), and a necrotic core with cholesterol (*C*) deposits. Rupture of plaque microvessels has resulted in intraplaque hemorrhage (*arrow*) at the base of the necrotic core. (Movat's pentachrome-stained slide, original magnification ×40.)

trauma were studied.[135] Two-dimensional maps of lipid-laden fatty streaks, as well as fibrous plaques, were made for each vessel. Although atherosclerosis is usually clinically silent until middle age or later, these investigators found that the disease process begins in adolescence or childhood. Moreover, fatty streaks and fibrous plaques do not occur randomly in the circulation but follow a well-defined distribution pattern. For example, in the right coronary artery, fatty streaks were found with the highest probability in the proximal 2 cm of this vessel, which closely parallels the distribution of raised fibrous lesions. However, in the abdominal aorta, where aortic lesions are commonly found, the high prevalence of fatty streaks did not always correlate with the prevalence of raised fibrous lesions. Therefore, at least in the aorta, the role of childhood fatty streaks in the development of adult fibrous lesions is uncertain.

The atherogenic stimuli that promote the progression of early lesions to clinically relevant stenoses are not known. Currently, the development of CAD is associated with various risk factors. Dyslipidemias, hypertension, diabetes mellitus, cigarette smoking, and a family history of premature CAD are known to correlate with premature vascular disease. The association between lipid disorders and atherogenesis is best understood and is discussed later in this chapter. Unfortunately, little is known about how the remaining risk factors may contribute to lesion development.

Historically, there are two classical theories of atherogenesis. According to von Rokitansky's[136] thrombogenic (or encrustation) theory, fibrin is the initiating factor in lesion development. Later, Duguid[137] expanded on this theory by suggesting that atherosclerosis is the result of altered fibrinolysis, whereas more recent studies have documented the overexpression of prothrombotic factors, such as plasminogen activator inhibitor-1, in atherosclerotic plaques.[138] Alternatively, in 1856, Virchow's imbibition (or insudation) theory proposed that atherosclerotic lesions were the result of altered vessel wall permeability.[139] Variations of this theory have been suggested by others, and all support the concept that the accumulation of various plasma components, including lipoproteins, may be important during lesion formation. For example, Ross and Glomset[140] blended the concepts of these original hypotheses into the "response-to-injury" hypothesis in which both lipid infiltration and thrombus formation play important roles in atherogenesis. Similarly, Schwartz and colleagues[141] compared arterial narrowing in atherosclerotic arteries with the process of wound healing. This perspective has advantages, as it allows a multifactorial process such as atherosclerosis to be broken down into components of a more

---

BOX 6-7. ATHEROSCLEROSIS

- The atherosclerotic process begins in childhood and adolescence.
- The progression of an atherosclerotic lesion has many similarities to the process of wound healing.
- Inflammation, lipid infiltration, and smooth muscle proliferation have important roles in atherogenesis.
- Impairment of endothelial function is an early consequence of atherosclerosis.
- Statin therapy has been shown to improve endothelial function, impede development of atherosclerosis, and in some cases may reverse established disease.

completely understood process such as the biology of a skin wound. For example, wound healing of any form begins with the formation of a clot (fibrin- and fibronectin-containing gel) that fills the wound and provides a provisional matrix for inflammatory cells, fibroblasts, and newly formed microvessels.[142,143] This is followed by the proliferation and migration of fibroblasts into the wound.[144] By day 7 after injury, microvessels grow into the base of the wound and form granulation tissue. As the wound matures and undergoes contracture, these blood vessels regress and fibroblasts disappear. After resorption of microvessels, tissue hypoxia develops and likely plays a role in the completion of the final scarring process.[145] As discussed later, there is now ample evidence to suggest that many similar events take place during arterial wound healing; however, because atherosclerosis is a chronic process, it is likely that vascular lesion formation involves indolent levels of inflammation with ongoing cycles of injury and repair over many years.[142,146,147]

Arterial Wall Inflammation

A number of studies have demonstrated the presence of monocytes/macrophages and T lymphocytes in the arteries of not only advanced lesions but early atherosclerotic lesions of young adults.[148,149] Moreover, in experimental atherosclerosis, leukocyte infiltration into the vascular wall is known to precede smooth muscle cell hyperplasia.[150] Once inside the artery wall, mononuclear cells may play several important roles in lesion development. For example, monocytes may transform into macrophages and become involved in the local oxidation of low-density lipoproteins (LDLs) and accumulation of oxidized LDLs. Alternatively, macrophages in the artery wall may act as a rich source of factors that, for example, promote cell proliferation, migration, or the breakdown of local tissue barriers. The latter process of local tissue degradation may be important for the initiation of acute coronary artery syndromes because loss of arterial wall integrity may lead to plaque fissuring or rupture.[151]

Normally, the endothelium exhibits a low affinity for circulating leukocytes. Therefore, the transmigration of leukocytes into the artery wall must occur as a facilitated process. The release of proinflammatory cytokines such as interleukin-1 may promote the expression of leukocyte adhesive molecules.[152] For simplicity, the interaction between leukocytes and the endothelium can be considered to involve three steps.[153] First, leukocytes in the bloodstream must loosely associate and roll along the endothelium—a process that is mediated by selectins expressed on endothelial cells.[152] Second, firm adhesion of these leukocytes to endothelial cells occurs via the interaction between integrins, such as $\alpha_4\beta_1$ (also known as very late antigen-4 [VLA-4]), expressed on leukocytes, and counter-receptors, such as vascular cell adhesion molecule-1 (VCAM-1), on endothelial cells.[154] Finally, the transmigration of leukocytes into the subendothelial space is mediated by various migration-inducing factors, such as monocyte chemoattractant protein-1 (MCP-1).[155]

Dysfunction, discontinuity, or injury of the endothelial cell monolayer has been postulated to play a significant role in facilitating the transmigration of leukocytes into the intima and the development of intimal hyperplasia. However, the premise that regrowth of a healthy endothelium will limit neointimal accumulation is inconsistent with the results of several independent lines of investigation. For example, in experimental models, smooth muscle cell proliferation is not increased in arterial regions devoid of an endothelium.[156] Moreover, restoration of the endothelium, as might be achieved by seeding endothelial cells back into a denuded artery, does not decrease neointimal accumulation after vascular interventions.[157] Therefore, the presence of an endothelium in the central lumen of an artery and resistance to intimal growth do not appear to be inextricably linked. Finally, it is important to note that the endothelium is not restricted to the central lumen, as the artery wall is also invested with a rich supply of microvessels (i.e., vasa vasorum).[158–161] The vasa vasorum are likely another portal of entry for inflammatory cells into the artery wall, particularly because the expression of certain adhesion molecules is more abundant in the endothelium lining these microvessels than that of the central arterial lumen.[162]

Role of Lipoproteins in Lesion Formation

The clinical and experimental evidence linking dyslipidemias with atherogenesis is well established and need not be reviewed here. However, the exact mechanisms by which lipid moieties contribute to the pathogenesis of atherosclerosis remain elusive. Although the simple concept of cholesterol accumulating in artery walls until flow is obstructed may be correct in certain animal models, this theory is not correct for human arteries.

Much of the pioneering work in understanding cholesterol metabolism is based on seminal observations by Brown and Goldstein.[163] The work of these two investigators focused on LDL, the so-called bad form of cholesterol, and the absence (or deficient forms) of the LDL receptor that are seen in familial hypercholesterolemia (FH). Patients with FH have high levels of LDL cholesterol and suffer from accelerated forms of atherosclerosis as cholesterol moieties enter the cell via an alternate route. In the absence of a functional LDL receptor, LDL cholesterol is oxidized and taken up by scavenger receptors of monocytes and macrophages resident within the artery wall. Steinberg[164] and others have integrated these data into a theory of atherogenesis that highlights the central role of LDL oxidation and the formation of lipid-laden monocytes in fatty streaks.

One of the major consequences of cholesterol accumulation in the artery wall is thought to be the impairment of endothelial function. The endothelium is more than a physical barrier between the bloodstream and the artery wall. Under normal conditions, the endothelium is capable of modulating vascular tone (e.g., via nitrous oxide), thrombogenicity, fibrinolysis, platelet function, and inflammation. In the presence of traditional risk factors, particularly dyslipidemias, these protective endothelial functions are reduced or lost. Notably, the loss of these endothelial-derived functions may occur in the presence or absence of an underlying atherosclerotic plaque and may simply imply that atherogenesis has begun. Aggressive attempts to normalize atherosclerotic risk factors (e.g., diet and lipid-lowering therapies) may markedly attenuate endothelial dysfunction—even in the presence of extensive atherosclerosis. A number of clinical studies now demonstrate dramatic improvements in endothelial function, as well as cardiovascular morbidity and mortality, with the use of inhibitors of 3-hydroxy-3-methylglutaryl coenzyme A (HGM-CoA) reductase, or "statins."[165–167] Future studies may help clarify the exact mechanisms by which dyslipidemias (and other risk factors) alter endothelial function.

Smooth Muscle Cell Proliferation, Migration, and Arterial Remodeling

The dominant cell type in atherosclerotic lesions is the smooth muscle cell, and as lesions progress, the number of smooth muscle cells in the artery wall tends to increase. Therefore, smooth muscle replication must occur at some time during atherogenesis. Perhaps the first line of evidence that cell replication occurs in human arteries is from the observation that atherosclerotic plaques contain monoclonal cell populations. Elegant studies by Benditt and Benditt[168] demonstrated that groups (or clones) of cells that arise from a single progenitor cell are present in tissue from atherosclerotic coronary arteries of women who were deficient in glucose-6-phosphate dehydrogenase (G-6-PD). Because G-6-PD is an X-chromosome–linked enzyme that has two isoforms, cells would express only one isoform, with the other isoform being suppressed on the inactivated X chromosome. Therefore, groups of cells in an atherosclerotic plaque that contain only one isoform of G-6-PD are likely the result of proliferation of a single progenitor cell. More recently, Murry and colleagues[169] studied the monoclonality of atherosclerotic plaques using X-chromosome inactivation patterns. Using the polymerase chain reaction, they examined the monoclonality of plaques according to the methylation pattern of the human androgen receptor gene, a highly polymorphic locus on the X chromosome for which 90% of women are heterozygous. These investigators note that diseased and normal arteries contain monoclonal populations (or patches) of cells. Therefore, they speculate that the monoclonality of plaques might be caused by expansion of a preexisting monoclonal patch of cells, rather than mutation or selection of individual cells in the artery wall.

Little is known about when and why cells proliferate in the artery wall. However, it is known that early in life there is a rapid expansion in neointimal smooth muscle cell mass. Sims and Gavin[170,171] describe the accumulation of intimal smooth muscle cells in the left anterior descending coronary artery of neonates. Using electron microscopy, these investigators demonstrate interruptions in the internal elastic lamina in coronary arteries where a neointima had formed.[171] These interruptions in the internal elastic lamina are not present in all human arteries. Indeed, the internal mammary artery, which typically is devoid of atherosclerosis, has an intact internal elastic lamina. Therefore, it has been suggested that medial smooth muscle cells migrate inward through breaks in the internal elastic lamina to expand and form a neointima. The frequency and degree of smooth muscle cell replication in adult coronary arteries have been examined by various investigators. The majority of these studies have demonstrated very low replication rates in tissue from both normal and diseased arteries.[172–175] Whether these low cell replication rates are sufficient to gradually result in advanced lesions, or whether sporadic bursts of replication occur in response to injury, is unknown. Finally, it is recognized that programmed cell death, or apoptosis, occurs in the artery wall.[176] Therefore, the accumulation of cells in the artery wall is a function of not only cell proliferation, but also apoptosis.

The role of smooth muscle cell migration in adult CAD is poorly understood. It has been suggested, however, that like fibroblasts that migrate into the base of a wound, arterial wall smooth muscle cells migrate inward to expand plaque mass. Smooth muscle cell migration into the intima has been studied in various animal models of neointimal formation (e.g., rat carotid artery model).[11] The majority of these models demonstrate the inward migration of medial smooth muscle cells after normal arteries are subjected to balloon injury. A number of growth factors (e.g., platelet-derived growth factor) have been shown to play an important role in facilitating smooth muscle cell migration in these models.[177–179] Unfortunately, the clinical relevance of these experimental observations remains to be clarified, as the milieu for cell migration in complex human lesions appears to be very different from that of normal animal arteries that are subjected to injury. More information is required regarding the factors that regulate smooth muscle cell migration, as well as why smooth muscle cells differ in their propensity to migrate after injury.

Finally, it is important to point out that the buildup of atherosclerotic plaque does not always translate into the formation of arterial obstructions.[142] For example, Glagov[180] notes that human vessels can accumulate massive amounts of atherosclerotic plaque without encroaching on the central arterial lumen. Instead, abluminal expansion of the artery wall may occur until 40% of the area encompassed by the internal elastic lamina is occupied by plaque. Thereafter no further enlargement may occur, and luminal narrowing may ensue. Although this form of compensatory enlargement is referred to as "remodeling," the term is confusing because it holds different meaning in different contexts (Figures 6-13 and 6-14).[180–182] For example, remodeling has also been used to describe the arterial response to changes in blood flow (e.g., during pregnancy or in the neonatal period) or pressure (e.g., hypertension).[183] In addition, remodeling has been invoked as a key component of the response to arterial injury—however, with quite a different meaning.[184] In animal models of arterial injury, as well as studies of human coronary arteries that have undergone angioplasty (or percutaneous transluminal coronary angioplasty [PTCA]), "shrinkage" or constrictive remodeling of the artery wall is a major determinant of lumenal narrowing, whereas neointimal formation plays a minor role in this process.[185–192]

How arterial wall constriction is accomplished or why some, but not all, arteries undergo compensatory dilatation to preserve lumen area is incompletely understood.[193–195] Blood flow and shear stress are known to play a critical role in remodeling. The response of arteries to chronic alterations in blood flow are endothelium dependent.[196,197] For example, Langille and O'Donnell[196] demonstrated in rabbit carotid arteries that decreased blood flow results in narrowing of the vessel diameter that is unchanged with papaverine and likely caused by structural changes in the artery wall. However, when the endothelium is removed from these vessels, the response to reduced blood flow is abolished. In atherosclerotic arteries that contain a rich network of endothelial cell-lined microvessels or vasa vasorum, the role of the endothelium in regulating remodeling may be important.[198–200]

Assessment of Atherosclerosis by Intravascular Ultrasonography

A detailed description of both diagnostic and therapeutic procedures performed in the cardiac catheterization laboratory is provided in Chapter 3. However, given that an integral understanding of the anatomy of the coronary artery and the atherosclerotic lesion is necessary for the appropriate interpretation and use of these technologies, a brief review of new developments in invasive assessment of atherosclerosis by intravascular ultrasonography (IVUS) is included here.

Standard coronary angiography gives operators a two-dimensional representation of the lumen. By examining arteries in multiple views, the operator estimates coronary stenoses by comparison of the lumen diameter at the point of maximal narrowing to adjacent disease-free segments. However, as discussed earlier, development of the atherosclerotic plaque results not only in luminal encroachment but arterial remodeling,[201] meaning significant disease may be overlooked on traditional angiography. Thus, technologies, such as IVUS, are becoming more prevalent in the assessment of CAD.

IVUS of coronary arteries was first popularized in the 1990s,[202] with subsequent refinement of catheter delivery systems and commercialization making it now commonplace in the modern catheterization laboratory. Compatible with most guiding catheters, IVUS probes are delivered to the coronary arteries via standard angiography techniques, and both manual and mechanical pullback of the IVUS probe allows operators to assess real-time cross-sectional images. Complementary software can then allow users to generate either longitudinal or three-dimensional reconstructions of the interrogated vessel.

IVUS images demonstrate remarkable fidelity to cross-sectional histologic specimens and permit accurate visualization and measurement of the intima, media, and, in some instances, the adventitia (Figure 6-15). Arterial remodeling with significant intimal hyperplasia but relatively intact lumen diameter can thus identify occult disease not otherwise appreciated on standard angiography. One landmark article has noted that even if only minor luminal irregularities exist, atherosclerotic disease can be demonstrated throughout most other vessels in the coronary circulation, suggesting luminograms may be simply the tip of the atherosclerotic iceberg.[203] Indeed, IVUS is now commonly used to more accurately quantify lesions in cases of intermediate severity lesions,[204] or in regions that are otherwise difficult to assess on standard angiography, such as left main disease. As well, IVUS allows operators to assess arteries after percutaneous intervention for not only adequate stent deployment but also for complications, such as arterial dissection, which can be missed on standard angiography.[205] However, IVUS is not limited to simply documenting and quantifying atherosclerotic burden. Plaque composition also can be assessed qualitatively and classified based on acoustic impedance, allowing differentiation among fibromuscular "soft" lesions, dense "fibrous" lesions, and "calcified" hyperechoic lesions.[206] Although not yet reliably predictable, ongoing studies are aimed at identifying which plaques are "vulnerable" or susceptible to rupture, thus causing acute vessel closure and myocardial infarction.[207,208]

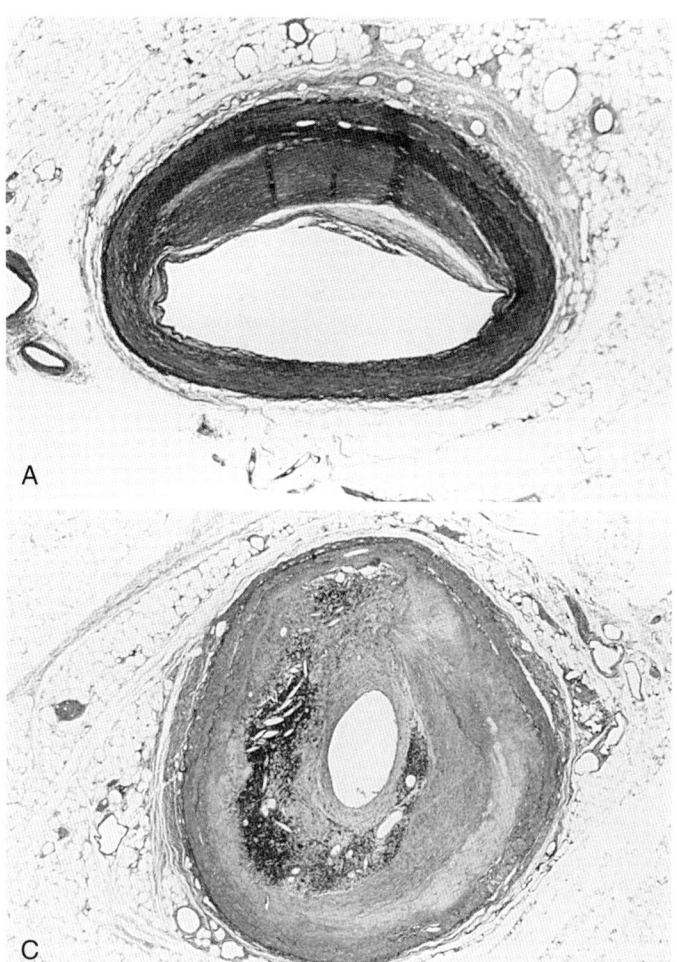

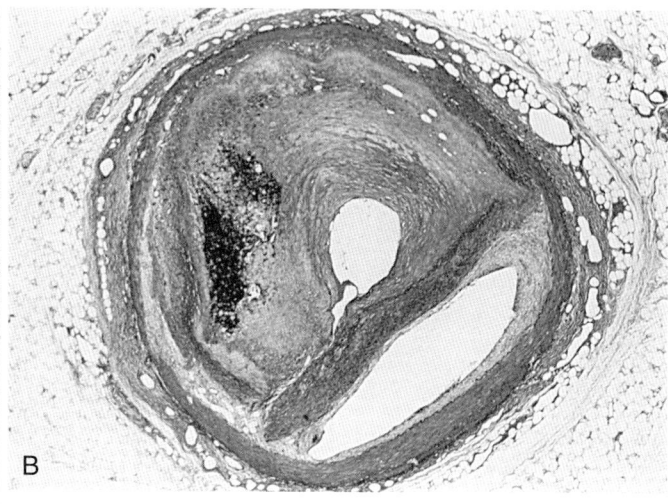

Figure 6-13 **Arterial remodeling.** Serial sections, proximal (A), mid (B), and distal (C), of an atherosclerotic human left circumflex coronary artery (Movat's pentachrome-stained slide, original magnification ×40). There is narrowing of the central arterial lumen in the mid and distal sections; however, the total arterial area of these sections is also larger than that of the proximal section. The ability of arteries to undergo compensatory enlargement is referred to as *arterial remodeling.*

PATHOPHYSIOLOGY OF CORONARY BLOOD FLOW

Coronary Artery Stenoses and Plaque Rupture

Coronary atherosclerosis is a chronic disease that develops over decades, remaining clinically silent for prolonged periods (Box 6-8). Clinical manifestations of CAD occur when the atherosclerotic plaque mass encroaches on the vessel lumen and obstructs coronary blood flow, causing angina. Alternatively, cracks or fissures may develop in the atherosclerotic lesions and result in acute thromboses that cause unstable angina or myocardial infarction.

On angiography, patients with stable angina typically have lesions with smooth borders. Only a minority of coronary lesions are concentric, most having a complex geometry varying in shape over their length. Eccentric stenoses, with a remaining pliable, musculoelastic arc of normal wall, can vary in diameter and resistance in response to changes in vasomotor tone or intraluminal pressure. Most human coronary stenoses are compliant.[209] The intima of the normal portion of the vessel wall is often thickened, making endothelial dysfunction probable (see Dynamic Stenosis section later in this chapter). In contrast, patients with unstable angina usually have lesions characterized by overhanging edges, scalloped or irregular borders, or multiple irregularities. These complicated stenoses likely represent ruptured plaque or partially occlusive thrombus, or both.[210] On angiography, these lesions may appear segmental, confined to a short segment of an otherwise normal proximal coronary artery. At autopsy, however, the most common pathologic finding is *diffuse* vessel involvement with superimposed segmental obstruction of greater severity.[211] In a diffusely narrowed vessel, even modest progression of luminal narrowing can be significant. In such a patient, rating the significance of the obstruction by the percentage of diameter reduction relative to adjacent vessel segments will underestimate its physiologic importance.[212,213] Therefore, understanding the characteristics of atherosclerotic plaques is of central importance to the management of acute coronary artery syndromes.

The intuitive notion that the severity of coronary artery stenoses should correlate with the risk for complications from CAD has been disproved by several key investigations. Ambrose and colleagues[214] reviewed the coronary angiograms of 38 patients who had had a Q-wave myocardial infarct in the interval between serial studies. On the preinfarct angiograms, the mean percentage stenosis at the coronary segment that was later responsible for infarction was only 34%. Similarly, Little and colleagues[215] reviewed the coronary angiograms of 42 patients who also had this procedure performed at an interval before and after myocardial infarction. Total occlusion of a previously patent artery was observed in 29 patients; yet, for 19 of these occluded arteries, the degree of stenosis was less than 50% on the initial angiogram. Therefore, although the revascularization of arteries with critical stenoses in target lesions is appropriately indicated to reduce symptoms and myocardial ischemia, the risk for further cardiac events remains because atherosclerosis is a diffuse process and mild or modest angiographic stenoses are more likely to result in subsequent myocardial infarction than are severe stenoses.

With this background comes the question of predicting which arterial segments with minimal angiographic disease will later develop new critical stenoses. Clues to the answer for this question are emerging

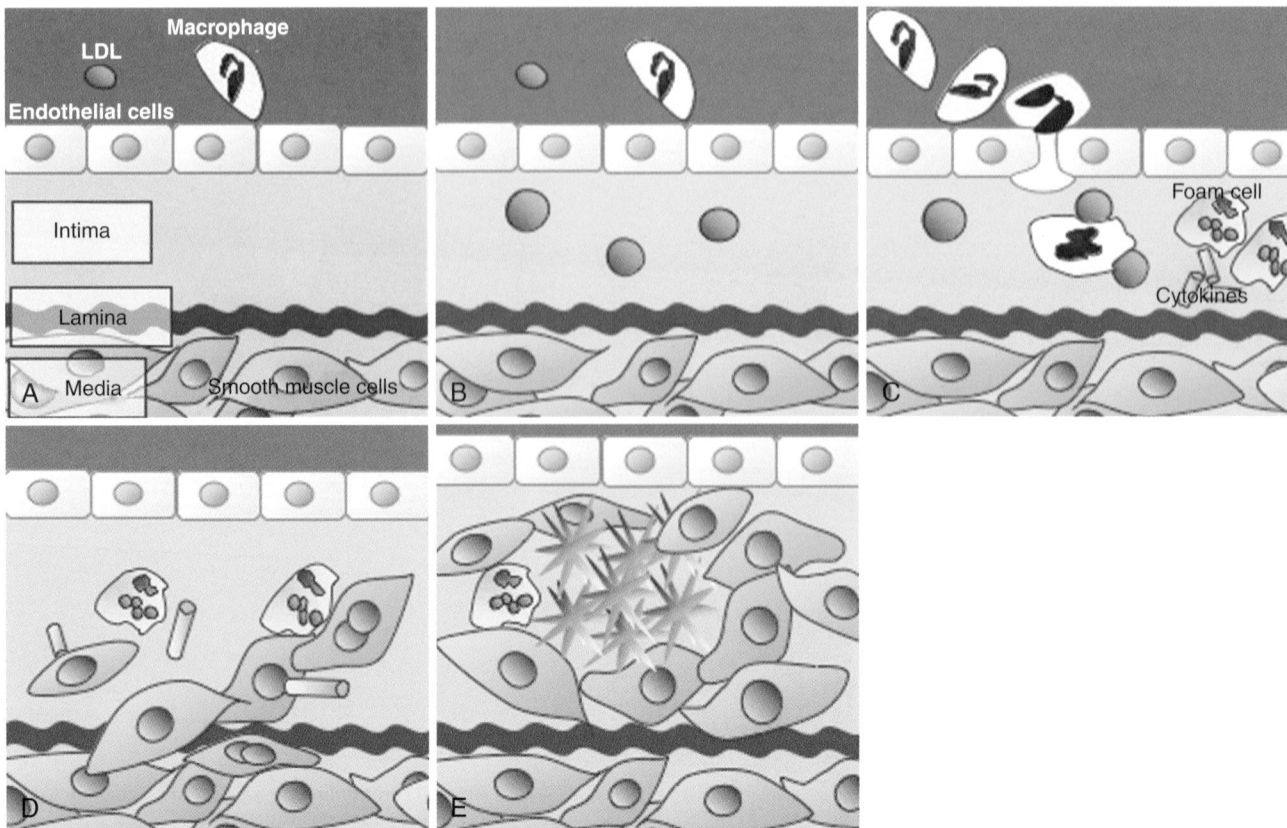

Figure 6-14 Model of atherogenesis in human coronary arteries. *A,* Normal coronary artery. *B,* Infiltration of the intima by particles containing low-density lipoproteins (LDLs) stimulates expression of adhesion molecules on the luminal surface of the endothelium. *C,* Monocyte/macrophage translocation into the intima. Once translocation is complete, uptake of LDL via scavenger receptors on macrophages creates foam cells that secrete proinflammatory cytokines, such as interleukin-1. *D,* Further inflammation promotes division and migration of medial and/or adventitial smooth muscle cells with ongoing accumulation of foam cells and extracellular matrix, resulting in intimal thickening. *E,* Local cell signaling via paracrine factors can lead to regional apoptosis and development of a necrotic core with accumulation of cholesterol deposits.

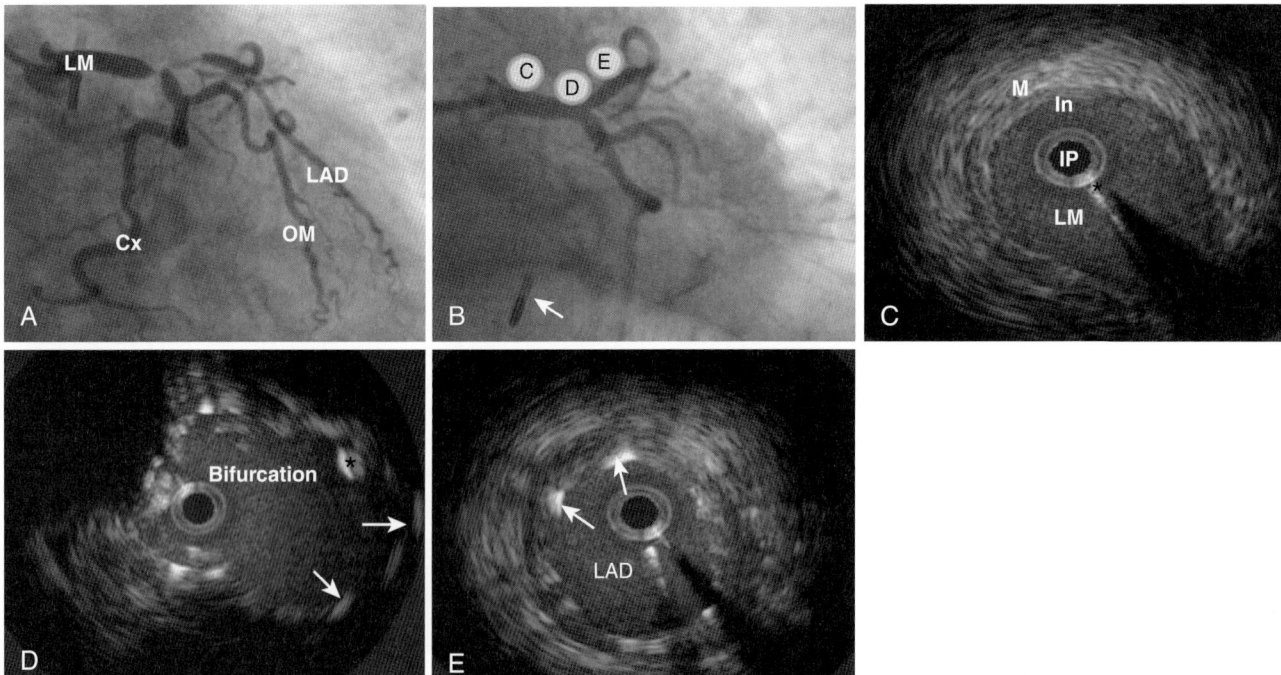

Figure 6-15 Intravascular ultrasonography (IVUS) for assessment of human coronary arteries. *A,* A right anterior oblique projection of the left coronary circulation. The left main artery (LM), left anterior descending artery (LAD), circumflex artery (Cx), and obtuse marginal artery (OM) are seen. A severe distal LM stenosis is seen bifurcating into the LAD and Cx. *B,* Postpercutaneous intervention angiogram demonstrates no residual stenosis. Drug-eluting stents were placed in the left main, LAD, and Cx. The tip of an aortic balloon pump can be seen *(arrow).* Letters indicate location of IVUS images for correlating panels. *C–E,* IVUS images of LM, LM bifurcation, and LAD, respectively. In, intima; IP, IVUS probe; M, media. *Asterisk* indicates guidewire; *arrows* indicate stent struts.

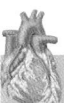

BOX 6-8. PATHOPHYSIOLOGY OF CORONARY BLOOD FLOW

- In the majority of patients experiencing a myocardial infarction, the coronary occlusion occurs at the site of < 50% stenosis.
- Plaque rupture leads to incremental growth of coronary stenoses and can cause coronary events.
- Plaque rupture occurs at the shoulder of the plaque where inflammatory cells are found.

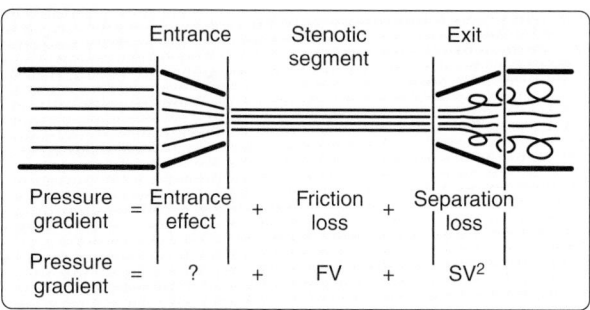

Figure 6-16 **Sources of energy loss across a stenosis.** Equations that (accurately) predict the pressure gradient across a stenosis usually ignore entrance effects. Frictional losses are proportional to blood velocity but are usually not important except in very long stenoses. Separation losses, caused by turbulence as blood exits the stenosis, increase with the square of blood velocity and account for more than 75% of energy loss. F, friction coefficient (Poiseuille); S, separation coefficient; V, blood velocity. *(From Marcus ML: The physiologic effects of a coronary stenosis. In Marcus ML [ed]: The coronary circulation in health and disease, New York: McGraw-Hill, 1983, pp 242–269. Reproduced by permission of McGraw-Hill Companies.)*

from careful pathologic studies of lesions by Davies and Thomas.[216] Superficial intimal injury (plaque erosions) and intimal tears of variable depth (plaque fissures) with overlying microscopic mural thrombosis are commonly found in atherosclerotic plaques. In the absence of obstructive luminal thrombosis, these intimal injuries do not cause clinical events. However, disruption of the fibrous cap, or plaque rupture, is a more serious event that typically results in the formation of clinically significant arterial thromboses. From autopsy studies, it is known that rupture-prone plaques tend to have a thin, friable fibrous cap.[217] The site of plaque rupture is thought to be the shoulder of the plaque, where substantial numbers of mononuclear inflammatory cells are commonly found.[218] The mechanisms responsible for the local accumulation of these cells at this location in the plaque are unknown; presumably, monocyte chemotactic factors, the expression of leukocyte cell adhesion molecules, and specific cytokines are involved.[162,219] Moreover, macrophages in plaques have been shown to express factors such as stromelysin, which promote the breakdown of the extracellular matrix, and thereby weaken the structural integrity of the plaque.[151] Currently, no effective strategies have been designed to limit the possibility of plaque rupture; however, as discussed later, aggressive lipid-lowering therapy may be a helpful preventative measure.

Hemodynamics

If accurate angiographic assessment of the geometry of a coronary stenosis is made, hydrodynamic principles can be used to estimate the physiologic significance of the obstruction.[220] Energy is lost when blood flows through a stenosis because of entrance effects, frictional losses in the stenotic segment, and separation losses caused by turbulence as blood exits the stenosis (Figure 6-16). The equation relating stenosis geometry to hemodynamic severity is:

$$\Delta P = fQ + sQ^2$$

where ΔP is the pressure decline across the stenosis, Q is the volume flow of blood, f is a factor accounting for frictional effects, and s accounts for separation effects. Based on the Poiseuille law for laminar flow:

$$f = \frac{8\pi\eta L A_n}{A_s^2}$$

where π is the blood viscosity, L is stenosis length, A_n is the cross-sectional area of the normal vessel, and A_s is the cross-sectional area of the stenosis. The separation or turbulence factor is:

$$s = \frac{\rho k}{2}\left(\frac{A_n}{A_s} - 1\right)^2$$

where ρ is blood density, and k is an experimentally determined coefficient. Thus, frictional losses are directly proportional to the first power of stenosis length but are inversely proportional to the square of the area (or fourth power of diameter). Separation losses are particularly prominent because they increase with the square of flow. Even at resting flows, more than 75% of energy loss is due to this turbulence when blood exits the stenosis. Except for very long stenoses, the frictional term can be neglected.[209] Thus, the amount of energy loss or pressure decline across the obstruction increases exponentially as flow rate increases. For this reason, exercise, anemia, and arteriolar vasodi-

lator drugs (e.g., dipyridamole) are poorly tolerated in the presence of a severe stenosis. Figure 6-17 illustrates that, although resting flow is unaffected until coronary diameter is reduced by more than 80%, maximal flow begins to decline when diameter is reduced by 50%.

Resting flow in Figure 6-17 remains constant as lumen diameter decreases because the coronary arterioles progressively dilate, thereby reducing the resistance of the distal coronary bed sufficiently to compensate for the resistance of the stenosis. As the severity of the stenosis increases further, the arteriolar bed can no longer compensate and flow begins to fall. This is an example of autoregulation: As stenosis severity increases, distal perfusion pressure decreases, arterioles dilate to maintain flow until autoregulation is exhausted (in the subendocardium first) and flow becomes pressure dependent. As illustrated in Figure 6-9, the distal pressure (or stenosis diameter) at which flow becomes pressure dependent is lower at low levels of myocardial metabolism (Mvo_2). The interpretation of normal resting flow can be difficult in the presence of CAD. A coronary artery supplying blood through collaterals to a large mass of myocardium will require high resting flow rates and even a mild stenosis may be flow limiting.

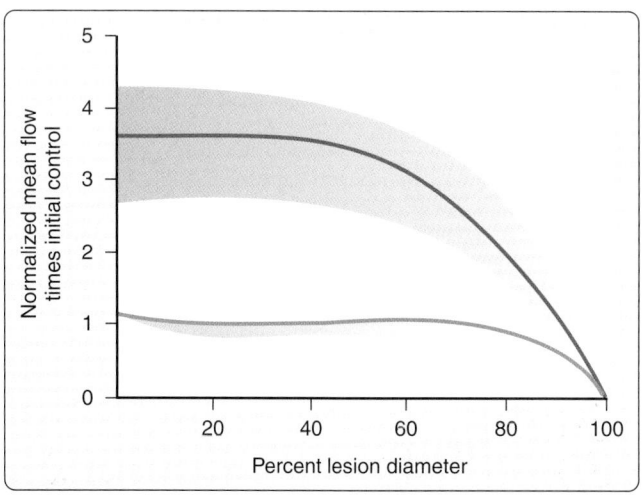

Figure 6-17 **Effect of increasing stenosis severity at resting and maximal coronary flows.** At rest, lumen diameter must be reduced by more than 80% before flow decreases *(green line)*. Because pressure drop across a stenosis increases exponentially with blood velocity, maximal coronary flow is restricted by a 50% diameter reduction *(purple line)*. *(From Gould KL, Lipscomb K: Effect of coronary stenoses on coronary flow reserve and resistance. Am J Cardiol 34:48, 1974.)*

The term *critical stenosis* is frequently used. This is usually defined as a coronary constriction sufficient to prevent an increase in flow over resting values in response to increased myocardial oxygen demands.[221] This is a greater degree of obstruction than an angiographically significant stenosis, which is usually defined as a reduction in cross-sectional area of 75%, which is equivalent to a 50% decrease in the diameter of a concentric stenosis.[212] A critical stenosis is demonstrated experimentally by blunting or abolishing reactive hyperemia (see Autoregulation section earlier in this chapter). This is evidence that autoregulation has been exhausted in at least the inner layer of myocardium (see Transmural Blood Flow section earlier in this chapter). Notably, the critical nature of the stenosis is relative to the resting Mvo₂. If oxygen demand decreases, some coronary autoregulatory reserve will be recovered and the stenosis will no longer be critical. The failure to recognize this fact has led to misinterpretation of studies designed to demonstrate coronary steal (see later).

Coronary Collaterals

Coronary collaterals are anastomotic connections, without an intervening capillary bed, between different coronary arteries or between branches of the same artery. In the normal human heart, these vessels are small and have little or no functional role. In patients with CAD, well-developed coronary collateral vessels may play a critical role in preventing death and myocardial infarction. Individual differences in the capability of developing a sufficient collateral circulation is a determinant of the vulnerability of the myocardium to coronary occlusive disease.[222] There is great interspecies variation in the ability of the collateral circulation to support myocardial perfusion after acute coronary occlusion; pigs and rats have little collateral circulation and infarct almost all the area at risk, whereas dogs and cats with better collateralization will infarct less than 75% of the area at risk.[223] In the guinea pig, collaterals are so well developed that coronary occlusion does not even decrease myocardial blood flow. There are also differences in the location of collateral vessels; in dogs, collaterals develop in a narrow subepicardial zone, at the border of the potentially ischemic region, whereas in pigs, a dense subendocardial plexus develops in response to coronary occlusion. In the presence of coronary disease, humans exhibit a small number of large epicardial collateral vessels and numerous small subendocardial vessels.

In response to coronary occlusion, native coronary collateral vessels do not passively stretch but undergo an active growth process that within 8 weeks, in the dog, can restore perfusion sufficient to support normal myocardial function, even during exercise. Human collaterals have a tortuous corkscrew-like pattern visible on angiography. This may be because of an embryonal pattern of vascular development in which longitudinal growth of smooth muscle cells occurs at the same time as radial growth. In the nongrowing adult heart, this increase in length results in tortuosity.[224] There is much interest in discovering the factors that control collateral vessel growth in the hope of providing therapy for patients who cannot be revascularized otherwise. Arteriogenesis refers to the transformation of preexisting collateral arterioles into functional arteries with a thick muscular coat and the acquisition of viscoelastic and vasomotor properties.[225] Fujita and Tambara[226] provide an overview of the process: A high-grade coronary stenosis decreases distal intraarterial pressure, resulting in an increased pressure gradient across the preexisting collateral network. Increased collateral blood flow results in increased shear stress at the endothelium, which upregulates cell adhesion molecules. This leads to adherence of monocytes, which transform into macrophage, and the production and release of growth factors such as granulocyte macrophage colony-stimulating factor (GM-CSF), MCP-1, and basic fibroblast growth factor (bFGF). Angiogenesis is not directly related to collateral vessel development but refers to the proliferation, migration, and tube formation of capillaries in the central area of ischemic regions.[227] The development of a treatment to promote collateral growth in patients with intractable CAD is currently a subject of intense investigation.

Evidence in dogs suggests that mature coronary collaterals respond differently to neurohumoral stimulation than normal coronary arteries. Collaterals do not constrict in response to α-receptor activation, but do dilate in response to β₁- or β₂-agonists. They constrict in response to prostaglandin F₂α (PGF₂α) and AII, but less so than normal vessels. Remarkably, collateral vessels constrict in response to vasopressin to a much greater extent than normal vessels. In vivo studies in dogs indicate that levels of vasopressin present during stress (hemorrhage, cardiopulmonary bypass) can diminish flow to collateral-dependent myocardium. This is likely due to constriction of collateral vessels, as well as enhanced vasoconstriction of the resistance vessels in the collateral-dependent myocardium.[79] It is possible that the endothelial cells of both types of vessel are dysfunctional.[228] Relaxation in response to nitroglycerin was enhanced. This is a further mechanism for the beneficial effects of nitroglycerin in CAD. The deleterious effects of coronary arteriolar dilators such as adenosine and dipyridamole are discussed later (see Coronary Steal).

It has been estimated that, in humans, perfusion via collaterals can equal perfusion via a vessel with a 90% diameter obstruction.[229] Although coronary collateral flow can be sufficient to preserve structure and resting myocardial function, muscle dependent on collateral flow usually becomes ischemic when oxygen demand increases above resting levels.[230] It is possible that evidence from patients with angina underestimates collateral function of the population of all patients with CAD. Perhaps individuals with coronary obstructions but excellent collateralization remain asymptomatic and are not studied.

Pathogenesis of Myocardial Ischemia

Ischemia is the condition of oxygen deprivation accompanied by inadequate removal of metabolites consequent to reduced perfusion.[231] Clinically, myocardial ischemia is a decline in the blood flow supply/demand ratio resulting in impaired function. There is no universally accepted "gold standard" for the presence of myocardial ischemia. In practice, symptoms, anatomic findings, and evidence of myocardial dysfunction must be combined before concluding that myocardial ischemia is present.[232] Conclusive evidence of anaerobic metabolism in the setting of reduced coronary blood flow (relative to demand) would be convincing. Such evidence is extremely difficult to obtain, even in experimental preparations.

Determinants of Myocardial Oxygen Supply/Demand Ratio

An increase in myocardial oxygen requirement beyond the capacity of the coronary circulation to deliver oxygen results in myocardial ischemia (Box 6-9). This is the most common mechanism leading to ischemic episodes in chronic stable angina and during exercise testing. Intraoperatively, the anesthesiologist must measure and control the determinants of Mvo₂ and protect the patient from "demand" ischemia. The major determinants of Mvo₂ are heart rate, myocardial contractility, and wall stress (chamber pressure × radius/wall thickness). Shortening, activation, and basal metabolic requirements are minor determinants of Mvo₂ (Figure 6-18).

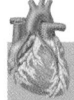

BOX 6-9. DETERMINANTS OF MYOCARDIAL OXYGEN SUPPLY/DEMAND RATIO

The major determinants of myocardial oxygen consumption are:
- Heart rate
- Myocardial contractility
- Wall stress (chamber pressure × radius/wall thickness)

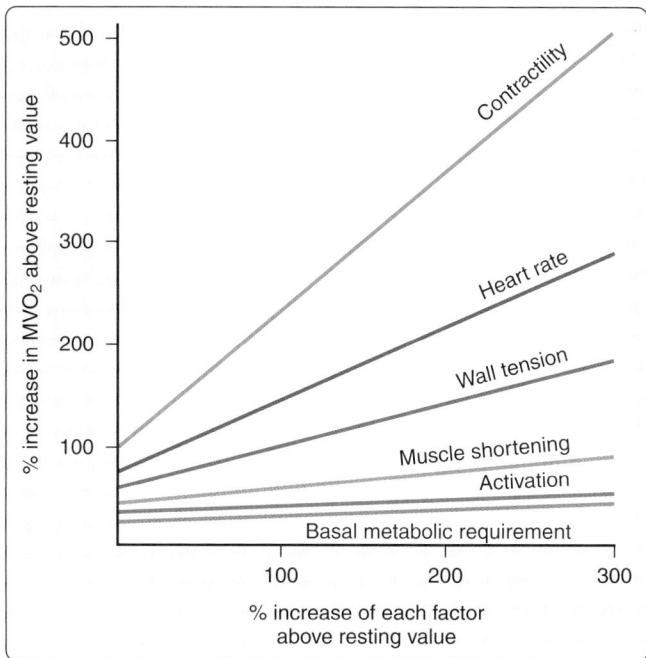

Figure 6-18 **Relative importance of variables that determine myocardial oxygen consumption (Mvo$_2$).** Each line roughly approximates the effect of manipulating one variable without changing the others. Most interventions cause changes in several of the variables at the same time. The importance of contractility, which is difficult to monitor in practice, is apparent. *(From Marcus ML: Metabolic regulation of coronary blood flow. In Marcus ML [ed]: The coronary circulation in health and disease. New York: McGraw-Hill, 1983, pp 65–92. Reproduced by permission of McGraw-Hill Companies.)*

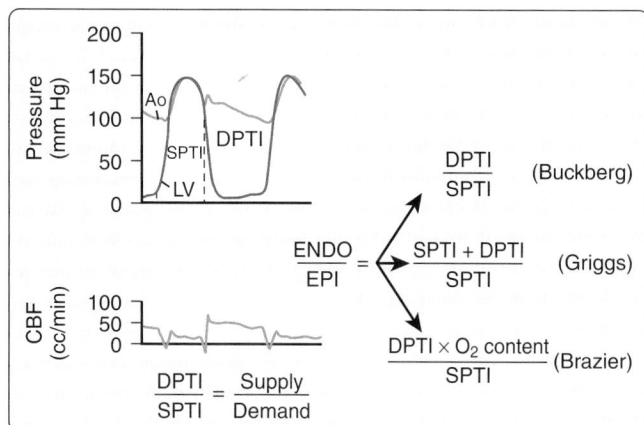

Figure 6-19 Three indices, proposed to predict the adequacy of subendocardial perfusion in normal dogs, illustrate the variables determining myocardial oxygen supply and demand. The systolic pressure-time index (SPTI) relates to oxygen demand. The diastolic pressure-time index (DPTI) relates to the supply of coronary blood flow (CBF) to the inner layers of the left ventricle. Arterial oxygen content (O$_2$ content) is important when there are large changes in hematocrit. Ao, aortic pressure; ENDO, subendocardial layer of left ventricle; EPI, subepicardial layer of left ventricle; LV, left ventricular pressure. *(From Hoffman JIE, Buckberg GD: Transmural variations in myocardial perfusion. In Yu PN, Goodwin JF [eds]: Progress in cardiology. Philadelphia: Lea & Febiger, 1976, p 37.)*

An increase in heart rate can reduce subendocardial perfusion by shortening diastole. Coronary perfusion pressure may decline because of reduced systemic pressure or increased left ventricular end-diastolic pressure. With the onset of ischemia, perfusion may be further compromised by delayed ventricular relaxation (decreased subendocardial perfusion time) and decreased diastolic compliance (increased left ventricular end-diastolic pressure). Anemia and hypoxia also can compromise delivery of oxygen to the myocardium. Several indices of myocardial oxygen supply/demand ratio have been proposed to guide therapy. The rate-pressure product (heart rate × systolic blood pressure) gives a good estimate of Mvo$_2$ but does not correlate well with ischemia. A patient with a systolic pressure of 160 and heart rate of 70 has a much lower likelihood of ischemia than a patient with a pressure of 70 and rate of 160, although both have a rate-pressure product of 11,200. The ratio of the diastolic pressure–time index (DPTI) to the systolic pressure–time index (SPTI) was devised to estimate subendocardial perfusion and takes into account determinants of oxygen delivery (Figure 6-19).[233–235] When blood oxygen content was included, the index became a good predictor of endocardial flow in animals with normal coronary arteries. More recently, the ratio of mean arterial pressure/heart rate has been proposed as a correlate of myocardial ischemia.[236] In dogs with moderate-to-severe coronary stenoses, systolic shortening was best with high pressures and low heart rate, and worst with low pressure and high heart rate. None of these indices has proved to be reliable in the clinical setting. Their major value is to bring attention to the important variables determining the supply/demand ratio. These variables should be measured (or estimated) and controlled individually.

Dynamic Stenosis

Patients with CAD can have variable exercise tolerance during the day and between days. Ambulatory monitoring of the electrocardiogram has demonstrated that ST-segment changes indicative of myocardial

ischemia, in the absence of changes in oxygen demand, are common.[237] These findings are explained by variations over time in the severity of the obstruction to blood flow imposed by coronary stenoses.

Although the term *hardening of the arteries* suggests rigid, narrowed vessels, in fact, most stenoses are eccentric and have a remaining arc of compliant tissue (Figure 6-20). A modest amount (10%) of shortening of the muscle in the compliant region of the vessel can cause dramatic changes in lumen caliber.[209] This was part of Prinzmetal's original proposal to explain coronary spasm. Maseri et al[238] suggest that the term *spasm* should be reserved for "situations where coronary constriction is

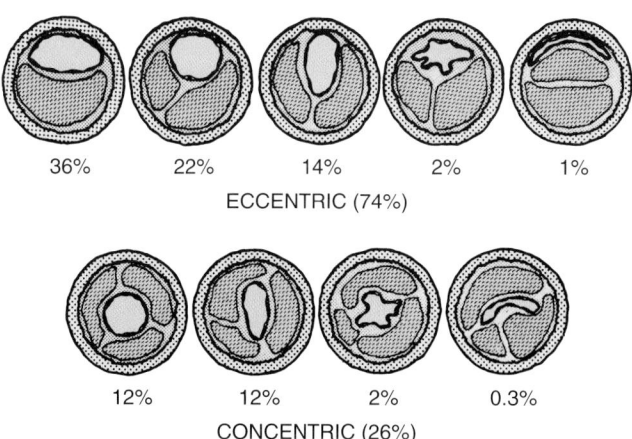

Figure 6-20 **Drawings and incidence of the various types of structure of stenoses observed in human coronary artery specimens.** In almost three quarters of vessels with greater than 50% narrowing, the residual arterial lumen was eccentric and partially circumscribed by an arc of normal arterial wall. In such lesions, a decline in intraluminal pressure or an increase in vasomotor tone can cause lumen diameter to decrease further and sufficiently to precipitate myocardial ischemia. *(From Brown BG, Bolson EL, Dodge HT: Dynamic mechanisms in human coronary stenosis. Circulation 70:917, 1984; redrawn from Freudenberg H, Lichtlen PR: The normal wall segment in coronary stenoses-a postmortem study. Z Kardiol 70:863, 1981.)*

both focal, sufficiently profound to cause transient coronary occlusion, and is responsible for reversible attacks of angina at rest" (i.e., variant angina). Although this syndrome is rare, lesser degrees of obstruction in response to vasoconstrictor stimuli are common among patients with CAD.

Sympathetic tone can be increased by the cold pressor test (immersing the arm in ice water) or isometric handgrip testing. In response to this maneuver, coronary resistance decreased in normal subjects but increased in patients with coronary disease, some of whom experienced angina.[239] This increase in resistance appears to be mediated by α receptors because it can be prevented by phentolamine. Studies using quantitative coronary angiography have documented reductions in caliber in diseased vessels in contrast with dilation of vessels in healthy subjects.[98,240] Zeiher et al[240] showed that the same vessel segments that constricted with the cold pressor test also constricted in response to an infusion of acetylcholine. Because the normal, dilatory response to acetylcholine is dependent on intact endothelium, these findings suggest that the abnormal response of stenotic coronary arteries is due to endothelial dysfunction.

Animal models of coronary vasospasm demonstrate that enhanced vascular smooth muscle reactivity also may underlie vasospasm.[241] Rho, a GTP-binding protein, sensitizes vascular smooth muscle cells to calcium by inhibiting myosin phosphatase activity through an effector protein called Rho-kinase. Upregulation of this pathway may be a mechanism of coronary vasospasm. Interestingly, Rho-kinase inhibitors have been shown to block agonist-induced vasoconstriction of internal thoracic artery segments from patients undergoing coronary artery surgery.[242]

It also has been noted that, in patients with coronary disease, some of the angiographically normal-appearing segments also respond abnormally.[243] It appears likely that, during the development of coronary atherosclerosis, endothelial dysfunction precedes the appearance of visible stenoses. In patients with angiographically smooth coronary arteries, Vita et al[244] found that an abnormal response to acetylcholine was correlated with serum cholesterol, male sex, age, and family history of coronary disease. The normal dilation of epicardial coronary arteries in response to increased blood flow (shear stress) has been shown to be absent in atherosclerotic vessels.[245] As well, it has been demonstrated that patients with coronary disease respond to 5-HT with coronary vasoconstriction instead of the normal vasodilatory response.[246,247] The concentrations of 5-HT used were within the range found in coronary sinus blood of patients with coronary disease. Very high concentrations of 5-HT may be found on the endothelium at the site of aggregating platelets.[246] All these findings point to the central role of endothelial dysfunction in the abnormal coronary vasomotion of patients with atherosclerosis[248] (see Endothelium section earlier in this chapter).

Coronary Steal

Steal occurs when the perfusion pressure for a vasodilated vascular bed (in which flow is pressure dependent) is lowered by vasodilation in a parallel vascular bed, both beds usually being distal to a stenosis. Two kinds of coronary steal are illustrated: collateral and transmural (Figure 6-21).

Collateral steal in which one vascular bed (R_3), distal to an occluded vessel, is dependent on collateral flow from a vascular bed (R_2) supplied by a stenotic artery is shown (see Fig 6-21A). Because collateral resistance is high, the R_3 arterioles are dilated to maintain flow in the resting condition (autoregulation). Dilation of the R_2 arterioles will increase flow across the stenosis, R_1, and decrease pressure, P_2. If R_3 resistance cannot further decrease sufficiently, flow there will decline, producing or worsening ischemia in the collateral-dependent bed. The values of all the resistances, including collaterals, and the baseline myocardial metabolic state will determine how powerful the vasodilator stimulus must be to produce ischemia in the collateral bed. Failure to recognize this has confounded studies of vasodilator drugs. If collateral vessels are very well developed or Mvo_2 is low, sufficient autoregulatory reserve may remain in the collateral-dependent bed to maintain adequate myocardial blood flow even with the administration of a moderately powerful vasodilator.

Transmural steal is also illustrated (see Figure 6-21B). Normally, vasodilator reserve is less in the subendocardium (see Transmural Blood Flow section earlier in this chapter). In the presence of a stenosis, flow may become pressure dependent in the subendocardium, whereas autoregulation is maintained in the subepicardium. This is illustrated in Figure 6-11, where at a perfusion pressure of 50 mm Hg, flow has declined in the subendocardium, whereas the subepicardium retains autoregulatory reserve. Dilation of the subepicardial arterioles, R_2, will then increase flow across the stenosis (R_1) causing P_2 to fall and resulting in decreased flow to the subendocardium as subepicardial flow increases.

The term *steal* is most appropriate when the vasodilation is caused by a pharmacologic agent (adenosine, dipyridamole) producing "luxury" flow (beyond metabolic requirements) in the vascular bed with coronary reserve (R_2). The same redistribution of blood flow also occurs during exercise in response to metabolically mediated vasodilation. The study of coronary steal demonstrates well the complex interrelations among the determinants of myocardial blood flow.

FUTURE DIRECTIONS

There is a major need not only to identify but to treat the vulnerable nonstenotic plaque that is prone to rupture. Although angiography is ideal for imaging the lumen of arteries, it provides little information

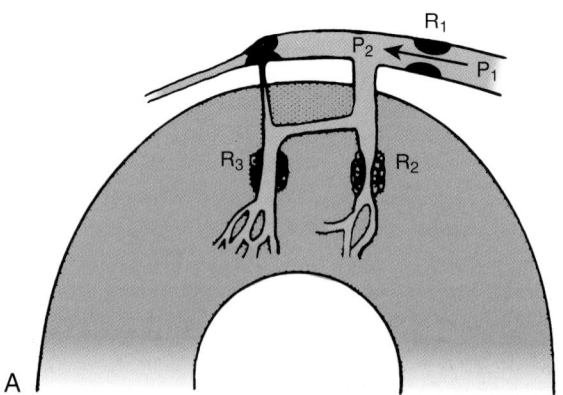
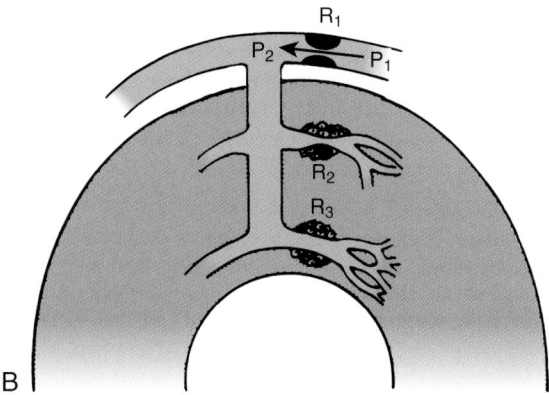

Figure 6-21 Conditions for coronary steal between different areas of the heart (collateral steal *[A]*) and between the subendocardial and the subepicardial layers of the left ventricle (transmural steal *[B]*). P$_1$, aortic pressure; P$_2$, pressure distal to the stenosis; R$_1$, stenosis resistance; R$_2$ and R$_3$, resistance of autoregulating cand pressure-dependent vascular beds, respectively. *(From Epstein SE, Cannon RO, Talbot TL: Hemodynamic principles in the control of coronary blood flow. Am J Cardiol 56:4E, 1985.)*

about the atherosclerotic process within the vessel wall. Unfortunately, newer imaging techniques, such as IVUS and electron beam computer tomography, have yet to evolve as practical predictive modalities that can be used to manage patients at risk for acute coronary syndromes secondary to plaque rupture.

Interestingly, clues to the biology of plaque rupture are indirectly emerging from clinical trials with statins, in that these trials show modest reductions in the angiographic degree of vessel stenoses but consistently demonstrate a significant decrease in acute ischemic events well before the effects of LDL cholesterol lowering should appear. For example, the MIRACL (Myocardial Ischemia Reduction with Acute Cholesterol Lowering) trial demonstrated that treating only 38 patients with acute coronary syndromes with high-dose atorvastatin could prevent one recurrent infarction, refractory angina, or death as early as 30 days after the index event. [249] Similarly, the ARMYDA (Atorvastatin for Reduction of Myocardial Damage during Angioplasty),[250] ARMYDA-ACS (Atorvastatin for Reduction of Myocardial Damage During Angioplasty–Acute Coronary Syndromes),[251] and ARMYDA RECAPTURE (Atorvastatin for Reduction of Myocardial Damage During Angioplasty)[252] studies have demonstrated that acute treatment with atorvastatin in patients undergoing percutaneous coronary interventions results in reductions in periprocedural myocardial infarctions when started just days before the procedure. Certainly, given the impressive clinical benefits, there is much interest in exploring the pleiotropic effects of statins that extend beyond lipid lowering and understanding how plaque stabilization is occurring.[253,254]

Most recently, there has become a renewed focus on the adventitia of the coronary artery and its role in initiation of inflammation in the vessel wall and subsequent development of atherosclerosis.[12,255] Although much effort has been devoted to studying the intima and media in development of vascular lesions, the adventitia is just now garnering the focus it may deserve. The adventitia is unique in that it houses the vaso vasorum, which provides nutrients and vasoactive factors and acts as a portal of entry for inflammatory cells into the media and intima of epicardial coronary arteries. As well, the adventitia is unique in that it alone supplies all neural input to the vessel wall—an input that has been implicated in plaque progression and destabilization.[256] Supporting this notion of an "outside-in" hypothesis to the development of atherosclerosis is that changes in the adventitial vaso vasorum often precede intimal changes.[257] In addition to atherosclerosis, the adventitia also has been implicated as a source of cells in neointimal development after vascular injury such as balloon angioplasty.[258] Given the dynamic nature of the adventitia in disease and the unique role it serves in vessel homeostasis, understanding of adventitial biology is lacking.

There also is a growing need to better understand the role of vascular progenitor cells in both arterial repair[259] and lesion formation after vascular injury.[260] Studies suggest that endothelial and smooth muscle cells appear to be derived from multiple sources such as circulating stem and progenitor cells, as well as tissue-resident progenitor cell populations.[259–261] A number of observational clinical studies have inversely correlated endothelial progenitor cell (EPC) number and cardiovascular risk, fueling the hypothesis that impaired progenitor cell–mediated repair of arteries is a risk factor for atherosclerosis and clinical events.[262,263] Moreover, reports of the involvement of vascular progenitor cells in the pathogenesis of other vascular lesions are also emerging. For example, observations from organ transplantations highlight the involvement of a blood-borne population of human vascular cells in development of transplant arteriosclerosis.[264] Circulating EPC levels also have been found to be lower or have impaired adhesion capacity in patients who develop in-stent restenosis compared with patients with patent stents or an absence of CAD. [265,266] Hence, taken together, the emerging data suggest that vascular progenitor cells may play a critical role, not only in maintaining the artery wall but in ensuring that appropriate repair mechanisms occur in the face of injury. Therapeutic strategies that target EPC mobilization, homing, and differentiation may prove beneficial. Already, early clinical trials have suggested potential benefit of progenitor cell transplantation after myocardial infarction in improving left ventricular ejection fraction,[267] and a combined clinical end point of death, recurrent myocardial infarction, or revascularization.[268] Although these early clinical studies are promising, significant progress in our understanding the role vascular progenitors play in the pathogenesis of a wide variety of vascular lesions remains hampered by the absence of a clear definition of what constitutes a true vascular stem cell.[269]

REFERENCES

1. Zweifach BW, Lipowsky HH: Pressure-flow relations in blood and lymph microcirculation. In Berne R, Sperelakis N, editors: *Handbook of Physiology, Section 2: The Cardiovascular System*, vol III, *Microcirculation*, Baltimore, 1984, William & Wilkins, pp 251–307.
2. Marcus ML, Chilian WM, Kanatsuka, et al: Understanding the coronary circulation through studies at the microvascular level, *Circulation* 82(1):1, 1990.
3. Mulvany MJ, Aalkjaer C: Structure and function of small arteries, *Physiol Rev* 70:921, 1990.
4. Merkus D, Chilian WM, Stepp DW: Functional characteristics of the coronary microcirculation, *Herz* 24:7, 1999.
5. Kanatsuka H, Lamping KG, Eastham CL, et al: Comparison of the effects of increased myocardial oxygen consumption and adenosine on the coronary microvascular resistance, *Circ Res* 65:1296, 1989.
6. Chilian WM, Layne SM, Eastham CL, et al: Heterogeneous microvascular coronary alpha-adrenergic vasoconstriction, *Circ Res* 64:376, 1989.
7. Schwartz SM, deBlois D, O'Brien ER: The intima: Soil for atherosclerosis and restenosis, *Circ Res* 77:445, 1995.
8. Stary HC, Blankenhorn DH, Chandler AB, et al: A definition of the intima of human arteries and of its atherosclerosis-prone regions, *Circulation* 85:391, 1992.
9. Frid MG, Moiseeva EP, Stenmark KR: Multiple phenotypically distinct smooth muscle cell populations exist in the adult and developing bovine pulmonary arterial media in vivo, *Circ Res* 75:669, 1994.
10. Clowes AW, Clowes MM, Reidy MA: Kinetics of cellular proliferation after arterial injury. I. Smooth muscle growth in the absence of endothelium, *Lab Invest* 49:327, 1983.
11. Clowes AW, Schwartz SM: Significance of quiescent smooth muscle migration in the injured rat carotid artery, *Circ Res* 56:139, 1985.
12. Maiellaro K, Taylor WR: The role of the adventitia in vascular inflammation, *Cardiovasc Res* 75:4, 2007.
13. Rana RS, Hokin LE: Role of phosphoinositides in transmembrane signaling, *Physiol Rev* 70:115, 1990.
14. Moncada S, Higgs EA, Vane JR: Human arterial and venous tissues generate prostacyclin (prostaglandin X), a potent inhibitor of platelet aggregation, *Lancet* I:18, 1977.
15. Furchgott RF, Zawadzki JV: The obligatory role of endothelial cells in the relaxation of arterial smooth muscle by acetylcholine, *Nature* 288:373, 1980.
16. Ignarro LJ: Nitric oxide. A novel signal transduction mechanism for transcellular communication, *Hypertension* 16:477, 1990.
17. Ignarro LJ: Biological actions and properties of endothelium-derived nitric oxide formed and released from artery and vein, *Circ Res* 65:1, 1989.
18. Lincoln TM, Dey N, Sellak H: Invited review: cGMP-dependent protein kinase signaling mechanisms in smooth muscle: From the regulation of tone to gene expression, *J Appl Physiol* 91:3, 2001.
19. Moncada S, Palmer RMJ, Higgs EA: Nitric oxide: Physiology, pathophysiology, and pharmacology, *Pharmacol Rev* 43:109, 1991.
20. Harrison DG, Cai H: Endothelial control of vasomotion and nitric oxide production, *Cardiol Clin* 21:3, 2003.
21. Vallance P, Collier J, Moncada S: Nitric oxide synthesised from L-arginine mediates endothelium-dependent dilatation in human veins, *Cardiovasc Res* 23:1053, 1989.
22. Miura H, Bosnjak JJ, Ning G, et al: Role for hydrogen peroxide in flow-induced dilation of human coronary arterioles, *Circ Res* 92:2, 2003.
23. Busse R, Edwards G, Feletou M, et al: EDHF: Bringing the concepts together, *Trends Pharmacol Sci* 23:8, 2002.
24. Miura H, Wachtel RE, Liu Y, et al: Flow-induced dilation of human coronary arterioles: Important role of Ca(2+)-activated K(+) channels, *Circulation* 103:15, 2001.
25. Miyauchi T, Tomobe Y, Shiba R, et al: Involvement of endothelin in the regulation of human vascular tonus. Potent vasoconstrictor effect and existence in endothelial cells, *Circulation* 81:6, 1990.
26. Lee SY, Lee CY, Chen YM, et al: Coronary vasospasm as the primary cause of death due to the venom of the burrowing asp Atractaspis engaddensis, *Toxicon* 24:285, 1986.
27. Goodwin AT, Yacoub MH: Role of endogenous endothelin on coronary flow in health and disease, *Coron Artery Dis* 12:6, 2001.
28. Hirata Y, Yoshimi H, Takata S: Cellular mechanism of action by a novel vasoconstrictor endothelin in cultured rat vascular smooth muscle cells, *Biochem Biophys Res Commun* 154:868, 1988.
29. Clozel J-P, Clozel M: Effects of endothelin on the coronary vascular bed in open-chest dogs, *Circ Res* 65:1193, 1989.
30. Wenzel RR, Fleisch M, Shaw S, et al: Hemodynamic and coronary effects of the endothelin antagonist bosentan in patients with coronary artery disease, *Circulation* 98:21, 1998.
31. Goodwin AT, Yacoub MH: Role of endogenous endothelin on coronary flow in health and disease, *Coron Artery Dis* 12:6, 2001.
32. Mylona P, Cleland JG: Update of REACH-1 and MERIT-HF clinical trials in heart failure. Cardionet Editorial Team, *Eur J Heart Fail* 1:2, 1999.
33. Humbert M, Sitbon O, Simonneau G: Treatment of pulmonary arterial hypertension, *N Engl J Med* 351:14, 2004.
34. Hoak JC: The endothelium, platelets, and coronary vasospasm, *Adv Intern Med* 34:353, 1989.
35. Bassenge E, Heusch G: Endothelial and neuro-humoral control of coronary blood flow in health and disease, *Rev Physiol Biochem Pharmacol* 116:77, 1990.
36. Spaan JA: Mechanical determinants of myocardial perfusion, *Basic Res Cardiol* 90:2, 1995.
37. Westerhof N: Physiological hypotheses—intramyocardial pressure. A new concept, suggestions for measurement, *Basic Res Cardiol* 85:105, 1990.
38. Mates RE, Klocke FJ, Canty JM Jr: Coronary capacitance, *Prog Cardiovasc Dis* 31(1):1, 1988.
39. Bellamy RF: Diastolic coronary artery pressure-flow relations in the dog, *Circ Res* 43:92, 1978.
40. Eng C, Jentzer JH, Kirk ES: The effects of coronary capacitance on the interpretation of diastolic pressure-flow relationships, *Circ Res* 50:334, 1982.

41. Messina LM, Hanley FL, Uhlig PN, et al: Effects of pressure gradients between branches of the left coronary artery on the pressure axis intercept and the shape of steady state circumflex pressure-flow relations in dogs, *Circ Res* 56:11, 1985.
42. Kanatsuka H, Ashikawa K, Suzuki T, et al: Diameter change and pressure-red blood cell velocity relations in coronary microvessels during long diastoles in the canine left ventricle, *Circ Res* 66:503, 1990.
43. Feigl EO: Coronary physiology, *Physiol Rev* 63:1, 1983.
44. Hoffman JI, Piedimonte G, Maxwell AJ, et al: Aspects of coronary vasomotor regulation, *Adv Exp Med Biol* 381:135, 1995.
45. Tune JD, Richmond KN, Gorman MW, et al: Control of coronary blood flow during exercise, *Exp Biol Med (Maywood)* 227:4, 2002.
46. Gellai M, Norton JM, Detar R: Evidence for direct control of coronary vascular tone by oxygen, *Circ Res* 32:279, 1973.
47. Weiss HR, Neubauer JA, Lipp JA: Quantitative determination of regional oxygen consumption in the dog heart, *Circ Res* 42:394, 1978.
48. Broten TP, Romson JL, Fullerton DA, et al: Synergistic action of myocardial oxygen and carbon dioxide in controlling coronary blood flow, *Circ Res* 68:531, 1991.
49. Spaan JA, Dankelman J: Theoretical analysis of coronary blood flow and tissue oxygen pressure-control, *Adv Exp Med Biol* 346:189, 1993.
50. Berne RM: Cardiac nucleotides in hypoxia: Possible role in regulation of coronary blood flow, *Am J Physiol* 204:317, 1963.
51. Gerlach E, Deuticke B, Dreisbach RH: Der Nucleotid-Abbau im Herzmuskel bei Sauerstoffmangel und seine mogliche Bedeutung fur die Coronardurchblutung, *Naturwissenschaften* 6:228, 1963.
52. Olsson RA, Bunger R: Metabolic control of coronary blood flow, *Prog Cardiovasc Dis* 29:369, 1987.
53. Standen NB, Quayle JM: K+ channel modulation in arterial smooth muscle, *Acta Physiol Scand* 164:4, 1998.
54. Duncker DJ, Bache RJ: Regulation of coronary vasomotor tone under normal conditions and during acute myocardial hypoperfusion, *Pharmacol Ther* 86:1, 2000.
55. Kroll K, Feigl EO: Adenosine is unimportant in controlling coronary blood flow in unstressed dog hearts, *Am J Physiol* 249:H1176, 1985.
56. Bache RJ, Dai X, Schwarts JS, et al: Role of adenosine in coronary vasodilation during exercise, *Circ Res* 62:846, 1988.
57. Dole WP, Yamada N, Bishop VS, et al: Role of adenosine in coronary blood flow regulation after reductions in perfusion pressure, *Circ Res* 56:517, 1985.
58. Saito D, Steinhard CR, Nixon DG, et al: Intracoronary adenosine deaminase reduces canine myocardial reactive hyperemia, *Circ Res* 49:1262, 1981.
59. Laxson DD, Homans DC, Bache RJ: Inhibition of adenosine-mediated coronary vasodilation exacerbates myocardial ischemia during exercise, *Am J Physiol* 5(Pt 2):265, 1993.
60. Baxter GF: Role of adenosine in delayed preconditioning of myocardium, *Cardiovasc Res* 55:3, 2002.
61. Zaugg M, Lucchinetti E, Uecker M, et al: Anaesthetics and cardiac preconditioning. Part I. Signalling and cytoprotective mechanisms, *Br J Anaesth* 91:4, 2003.
62. Woollard HH: The innervation of the heart, *J Anat Physiol* 60:345, 1926.
63. Van Winkle DM, Feigl EO: Acetylcholine causes coronary vasodilation in dogs and baboons, *Circ Res* 65:6, 1989.
64. Horio Y, Yasue H, Okumura KT, et al: Effects of intracoronary injection of acetylcholine on coronary arterial hemodynamics and diameter, *Am J Cardiol* 62:13, 1988.
65. Hodgson JM, Marshall JJ: Direct vasoconstriction and endothelium-dependent vasodilation. Mechanisms of acetylcholine effects on coronary flow and arterial diameter in patients with nonstenotic coronary arteries, *Circulation* 79:5, 1989.
66. Ludmer PL, Selwyn AP, Shook TL, et al: Paradoxical vasoconstriction induced by acetylcholine in atherosclerotic coronary arteries, *N Engl J Med* 315:1046, 1986.
67. Feigl EO: EDRF—a protective factor? *Nature* 331:490, 1988.
68. Feigl EO: Neural control of coronary blood flow, *J Vasc Res* 35:2, 1998.
69. Feldman RD, Christy JP, Paul ST, et al: β-adrenergic receptors on canine coronary collateral vessels: Characterization and function, *Am J Physiol* 257:H1634, 1989.
70. Mosher P, Ross J Jr, McFate PA, et al: Control of coronary blood flow by an autoregulatory mechanism, *Circ Res* 14:250, 1964.
71. Gorman MW, Tune JD, Richmond KN, et al: Feedforward sympathetic coronary vasodilation in exercising dogs, *J Appl Physiol* 89:5, 2000.
72. Holtz J: Alpha-adrenoceptor subtypes in the coronary circulation, *Basic Res Cardiol* 85(Suppl 1):81, 1990.
73. Guth BD, Thaulow E, Heusch G, et al: Myocardial effects of selective alpha-adrenoceptor blockade during exercise in dogs, *Circ Res* 66:1703, 1990.
74. Heusch G: Alpha-adrenergic mechanisms in myocardial ischemia, *Circulation* 81:1, 1990.
75. Kelley KO, Feigl EO: Segmental alpha-receptor-mediated vasoconstriction in the canine coronary circulation, *Circ Res* 43:908, 1978.
76. Mohrman DE, Feigl EO: Competition between sympathetic vasoconstriction and metabolic vasodilation in the canine coronary circulation, *Circ Res* 42:79, 1978.
77. Heusch G, Deussen A: Nifedipine prevents sympathetic vasoconstriction distal to severe coronary stenoses, *J Cardiovasc Pharmacol* 6:378, 1984.
78. Chilian WM: Adrenergic vasomotion in the coronary microcirculation, *Basic Res Cardiol* 85(Suppl 1):111, 1990.
79. Harrison DG, Sellke FW, Quillen JE: Neurohumoral regulation of coronary collateral vasomotor tone, *Basic Res Cardiol* 85(Suppl 1):121, 1990.
80. DiCarli MF, Tobes MC, Mangner T, et al: Effects of cardiac sympathetic innervation on coronary blood flow, *N Engl J Med* 336:1208, 1997.
81. Chilian WM, Harrison DG, Haws CW, et al: Adrenergic coronary tone during submaximal exercise in the dog is produced by circulating catecholamines. Evidence for adrenergic denervation supersensitivity in the myocardium but not in coronary vessels, *Circ Res* 58:68, 1986.
82. Huang AH, Feigl EO: Adrenergic coronary vasoconstriction helps maintain uniform transmural blood flow distribution during exercise, *Circ Res* 62:286, 1988.
83. Buffington CW, Feigl EO: Adrenergic coronary vasoconstriction in the presence of coronary stenosis in the dog, *Circ Res* 48:416, 1981.
84. Heusch G, Deussen A: The effects of cardiac sympathetic nerve stimulation on the perfusion of stenotic coronary arteries in the dog, *Circ Res* 53:8, 1983.
85. Bassenge E, Walter P, Doutheil U: Wirkungsmumkehr der adrenergischen coronargefassreakton in abhangigkeit vom coronargefasstonus, *Pflugers Arch* 297:146, 1967.
86. Nathan HJ, Feigl EO: Adrenergic coronary vasoconstriction lessens transmural steal during coronary hypoperfusion, *Am J Physiol* 250:H645, 1986.
87. Chilian WM, Ackell PH: Transmural differences in sympathetic coronary constriction during exercise in the presence of coronary stenosis, *Circ Res* 62:216, 1988.
88. Seitelberger R, Guth BD, Heusch G, et al: Intracoronary alpha 2-adrenergic receptor blockade attenuates ischemia in conscious dogs during exercise, *Circ Res* 62:436, 1988.
89. Baumgart D, Heusch G: Neuronal control of coronary blood flow, *Basic Res Cardiol* 90:2, 1995.
90. Feigl EO: Adrenergic control of transmural coronary blood flow, *Basic Res Cardiol* 85(Suppl 1):167, 1990.
91. Hodgson JMB, Cohen MD, Szentpetery S, et al: Effects of regional alpha- and beta-blockade on resting and hyperemic coronary blood flow in conscious, unstressed humans, *Circulation* 79:797, 1989.
92. Chierchia S, Davies G, Berkenboom G, et al: Alpha-adrenergic receptors and coronary spasm: An elusive link, *Circulation* 69:8, 1984.
93. Brown BG, Lee AB, Bolson EL, et al: Reflex constriction of significant coronary stenosis as a mechanism contributing to ischemic left ventricular dysfunction during isometric exercise, *Circulation* 70:18, 1984.
94. Berkenboom G, Unger P: Alpha-adrenergic coronary constriction in effort angina, *Basic Res Cardiol* 85(Suppl 1):359, 1990.
95. Berkenboom GM, Abramowicz M, Vandermoten P, et al: Role of alpha-adrenergic coronary tone in exercise induced angina pectoris, *Am J Cardiol* 57:195, 1986.
96. Gage JE, Hess OM, Murakami T, et al: Vasoconstriction of stenotic coronary arteries during dynamic exercise in patients with classic angina pectoris: Reversibility by nitroglycerin, *Circulation* 73:865, 1986.
97. Chilian WM, Layne SM: Coronary microvascular responses to reductions in perfusion pressure. Evidence for persistent arteriolar vasomotor tone during coronary hypoperfusion, *Circ Res* 66:1227, 1990.
98. Nabel EG, Ganz P, Gordon JB, et al: Dilation of normal and constriction of atherosclerotic coronary arteries caused by the cold pressor test, *Circulation* 77:43, 1988.
99. Maturi MF, Martin SE, Markle D, et al: Production of myocardial ischemia in dogs by constriction of nondiseased small vessels, *Circulation* 83:2111, 1991.
100. Chu A, Morris K, Kuehl W, et al: Effects of atrial natriuretic peptide on the coronary arterial vasculature in humans, *Circulation* 80:1627, 1989.
101. Linder C, Heusch G: ACE-inhibitors for the treatment of myocardial ischemia? *Cardiovasc Drugs Ther* 4:1375, 1990.
102. Lamping KG, Kanatsuka H, Eastham CL, et al: Nonuniform vasomotor responses of the coronary microcirculation to serotonin and vasopressin, *Circ Res* 65:2, 1989.
103. Ginsburg R, Bristow MR, Kantrowitz N, et al: Histamine provocation of clinical coronary artery spasm: Implications concerning pathogenesis of variant angina pectoris, *Am Heart J* 102:5, 1981.
104. Johnson PC: Autoregulation of blood flow, *Circ Res* 59:483, 1986.
105. Gregg DE: Effect of coronary perfusion pressure or coronary flow on oxygen usage of the myocardium, *Circ Res* 13:497, 1963.
106. Dole WP, Nuno DW: Myocardial oxygen tension determines the degree and pressure range of coronary autoregulation, *Circ Res* 59:202, 1986.
107. Dole WP: Autoregulation of the coronary circulation, *Prog Cardiovasc Dis* 29:293, 1987.
108. Jones CE, Liang IYS, Gwirtz PA: Effects of alpha-adrenergic blockade on coronary autoregulation in dogs, *Am J Physiol* 253:H365, 1987.
109. Hoffman JIE, Spaan JA: Pressure-flow relations in coronary circulation, *Physiol Rev* 70(2):331, 1990.
110. Feigl EO: Coronary autoregulation, *J Hypertens* 7(Suppl):S55, 1989.
111. Hickey RF, Sybert PE, Verrier ED, et al: Effects of halothane, enflurane, and isoflurane on coronary blood flow, autoregulation, and coronary vascular reserve in the canine heart, *Anesthesiology* 68:21, 1988.
112. Sestier FJ, Mildenberger RR, Klassen GA: Role of autoregulation in spatial and temporal perfusion heterogeneity of canine myocardium, *Am J Physiol* 235(1):H64, 1978.
113. Kuo L, Chilian WM, Davis MJ: Coronary arteriolar myogenic response is independent of endothelium, *Circ Res* 66:860, 1990.
114. Fossel ET, Morgan HE, Ingwall JS: Measurement of changes in high-energy phosphates in the cardiac cycle by using 31P nuclear magnetic resonance, *Proc Natl Acad Sci U S A* 77:3654, 1980.
115. Feigl EO, Neat GW, Huang AH: Interrelations between coronary artery pressure, myocardial metabolism and coronary blood flow, *J Mol Cell Cardiol* 22:375, 1990.
116. Ruiter JH, Spaan JAE, Laird JD: Transient oxygen uptake during myocardial reactive hyperemia in the dog, *Am J Physiol* 235:H87, 1978.
117. Marcus ML: Metabolic regulation of coronary blood flow. *In* Marcus ML (eds): *The Coronary Circulation in Health and Disease.* New York, McGraw-Hill, 1983, pp 65–92.
118. Bourdarias JP: Coronary reserve: Concept and physiological variations, *Eur Heart J* 16:2, 1995.
119. Nitenberg A, Antony I: Coronary vascular reserve in humans: A critical review of methods of evaluation and of interpretation of the results, *Eur Heart J* 16:7, 1995.
120. Aude YW, Garza L: How to prevent unnecessary coronary interventions: Identifying lesions responsible for ischemia in the cath lab, *Curr Opin Cardiol* 18:5, 2003.
121. Tonino PA, De BB, Pijls NH, et al: Fractional flow reserve versus angiography for guiding percutaneous coronary intervention, *N Engl J Med* 360:3, 2009.
122. Hoffman JIE: Transmural myocardial perfusion, *Prog Cardiovasc Dis* 29:429, 1987.
123. van der Vusse T, Arts, Glatz JF, et al: Transmural differences in energy metabolism of the left ventricular myocardium: Fact or fiction, *J Mol Cell Cardiol* 22:1, 1990.
124. Bassingthwaighte JB, Malone MA, Moffett TC, et al: Validity of microsphere depositions for regional myocardial flows, *Am J Physiol* 253:H184, 1987.
125. Buckberg GD, Luck JC, Payne DB, et al: Some sources of error in measuring regional blood flow with radioactive microspheres, *J Appl Physiol* 31:4, 1971.
126. Canty JM Jr, Giglia J, Kandath D: Effect of tachycardia on regional function and transmural myocardial perfusion during graded coronary pressure reduction in conscious dogs, *Circulation* 82:1815, 1990.
127. Hoffman JIE: Transmural myocardial perfusion, *Prog Cardiovasc Dis* 29:429–464, 1990.
128. Harrison DG, Florentine MS, Brooks LA, et al: The effect of hypertension and left ventricular hypertrophy on the lower range of coronary autoregulation, *Circulation* 77:1108, 1988.
129. Tomanek RJ: Response of the coronary vasculature to myocardial hypertrophy, *J Am Coll Cardiol* 15:528, 1990.
130. Hoffman JI: Heterogeneity of myocardial blood flow, *Basic Res Cardiol* 90:2, 1995.
131. Coggins DL, Flynn AE, Austin RE, et al: Nonuniform loss of regional flow reserve during myocardial ischemia in dogs, *Circ Res* 67:253, 1990.
132. Pantely GA, Bristow JD, Swenson LJ, et al: Incomplete coronary vasodilation during myocardial ischemia in swine, *Am J Physiol* 249:638, 1985.
133. Aversano T, Becker LC: Persistence of coronary vasodilator reserve despite functionally significant flow reduction, *Am J Physiol* 248:H403, 1985.
134. Stary HC: Evolution and progression of atherosclerotic lesions in coronary arteries of children and young adults, *Arteriosclerosis* 9(Suppl 1):I–19, 1989.
135. PDAY Research Group: Relationship of atherosclerosis in young men to serum lipoprotein cholesterol concentrations and smoking: A preliminary report from the Pathobiological Determinants of Atherosclerosis in Youth, *JAMA* 264:3018, 1990.
136. von Rokitansky C: *A manual of pathological anatomy.* London, The Sydenham Society, 1852.
137. Duguid JB: Thrombosis as a factor in atherogenesis, *J Pathol Bacteriol* 58:207, 1946.
138. Schneiderman J, Sawdey MS, Keeton MR, et al: Increased type 1 plasminogen activator inhibitor gene expression in atherosclerotic human arteries, *Proc Natl Acad Sci U S A* 89:6998, 1992.
139. Virchow R: *Gesammelte abhandlungen zur wissenschaftlichen medicin, phlogose und thrombose im gefassystem.* Berlin, Meidinger Sohn and Co, 1856, pp 458–463.
140. Ross R, Glomset JA: The pathogenesis of atherosclerosis, *N Engl J Med* 295:369, 1976.
141. Schwartz SM, Murry CE, O'Brien ER: Vessel wall response to injury, *Sci Med* 3:2, 1996.
142. Dvorak HF, Harvey VS, Estrella P, et al: Fibrin containing gels induce angiogenesis. Implications for tumor stroma generation and wound healing, *Lab Invest* 57:673, 1987.

143. Hunt TK, Knighton DR, Thakral KK, et al: Studies on inflammation and wound healing: Angiogenesis and collagen synthesis stimulated in vivo by resident and activated wound macrophage, *Surgery* 96(1):48, 1984.
144. Gabbiani G: The biology of the myofibroblast, *Kidney Int* 41:530, 1996.
145. Dvorak HF: Tumors: Wounds that do not heal. Similarities between tumor stroma generation and wound healing, *N Engl J Med* 315:26, 1986.
146. Ross R: The pathogenesis of atherosclerosis: A perspective for the 1990s, *Nature* 362:801, 1993.
147. Munro JM, Cotran RS: The pathogenesis of atherosclerosis: Atherogenesis and inflammation, *Lab Invest* 58:3, 1988.
148. Jonasson L, Holm J, Skalli O, et al: Regional accumulations of T cells, macrophages, and smooth muscle cells in the human atherosclerotic plaque, *Arteriosclerosis* 6:2, 1986.
149. Katsuda S, Boyd HC, Fligner C, et al: Human atherosclerosis: Immunocytochemical analysis of the cell composition of lesions of young adults, *Am J Pathol* 140:907, 1992.
150. Prescott MF, McBride CK, Court M: Development of intimal lesions after leukocyte migration into the vascular wall, *Am J Pathol* 135:5, 1989.
151. Henney AM, Wakeley PR, Davies MJ, et al: Localization of stromelysin gene expression in atherosclerotic plaques by in situ hybridization, *Proc Natl Acad Sci U S A* 88(18):8154, 1991.
152. Bevilacqua MP, Slengelin S, Gimbrone MAJ, et al: Endothelial leukocyte adhesion molecule 1: An inducible receptor for neutrophils related to complement regulatory proteins and lectins, *Science* 243:1160, 1989.
153. Springer TA: Traffic signals for lymphocyte recirculation and leukocyte emigration: The multistep paradigm, *Cell* 76:301, 1994.
154. Osborn L, Hession C, Tizard R, et al: Direct expression cloning of vascular cell adhesion molecules 1, a cytokine-induced endothelial protein that binds to lymphocytes, *Cell* 59:1203, 1989.
155. Nelken NA, Coughlin SR, Gordon D, et al: Monocyte chemoattractant protein-1 in human atheromatous plaques, *J Clin Invest* 88:1121, 1991.
156. Reidy MA, Silver M: Endothelial regeneration. Lack of intimal proliferation after defined injury to rat aorta, *Am J Pathol* 118:2, 1985.
157. Conte MS, Choudhry RP, Shirakowa M, et al: Endothelial cell seeding fails to attenuate intimal thickening in balloon-injured rabbit arteries, *J Vasc Surg* 21:413, 1995.
158. Winternitz MC, Thomas RM, LeCompte PM: *The biology of arteriosclerosis.* Springfield, IL, Charles C. Thomas, 1938.
159. Barger AC, Beeuwkes R, Lainey LL, et al: Hypothesis: Vasa vasorum and neovascularization of human coronary arteries, *N Engl J Med* 310:175, 1984.
160. O'Brien ER, Garvin MR, Dev R, et al: Angiogenesis in human coronary atherosclerotic plaques, *Am J Pathol* 145(4):883, 1994.
161. Pels K, Labinaz M, O'Brien ER: Arterial wall neovascularization: Potential role in atherosclerosis and restenosis, *Japan Circ J* 35:241, 1997.
162. O'Brien KD, McDonald TO, Chait A, et al: Neovascular expression of E-selection intercellular adhesion molecule-1, and vascular cell adhesion molecule-1 in human atherosclerosis and their relation to intimal leukocyte content, *Circulation* 93:672, 1996.
163. Brown MS, Goldstein JL: A receptor-mediated pathway for cholesterol homeostasis, *Science* 232:34, 1986.
164. Steinberg D: Antioxidant vitamins and coronary heart disease, *N Engl J Med* 328(20):1444, 1993.
165. The Scandinavian Simvastatin Survival Study Group: Randomised trial of cholesterol lowering in 4444 patients with coronary heart disease: The Scandinavian Simvastatin Survival Study (4S), *Lancet* 344:8934, 1994.
166. Treasure CB, Klein JL, Weintraub WS: Beneficial effects of cholesterol-lowering therapy on the coronary endothelium in patients with coronary artery disease, *N Engl J Med* 332:481, 1995.
167. Anderson TJ, Meredith IT, Yeung AC, et al: The effect of cholesterol-lowering and antioxidant therapy on endothelium-dependent coronary vasomotion, *N Engl J Med* 332:488, 1995.
168. Benditt EP, Benditt JM: Evidence for a monoclonal origin of human atherosclerotic plaques, *Proc Natl Acad Sci U S A* 70:1753, 1973.
169. Murry CE, Gipaya CT, Bartosek T, et al: Monoclonality of smooth muscle cells in human atherosclerosis, *Am J Pathol* 151:3, 1997.
170. Sims FH, Gavin JB, Vanderwee MA: The intima of human coronary arteries, *Am Heart J* 118:32, 1989.
171. Sims FH, Gavin JB: The early development of intimal thickening of human coronary arteries, *Coron Artery Dis* 1:205, 1990.
172. Gordon D, Reidy MA, Benditt EP, et al: Cell proliferation in human coronary arteries, *Proc Natl Acad Sci U S A* 87:4600, 1990.
173. O'Brien ER, Alpers CE, Stewart DK, et al: Proliferation in primary and restenotic coronary atherectomy tissue: Implications for anti-proliferative therapy, *Circ Res* 73(2):223, 1993.
174. Villaschi S, Spagnoli LG: Autoradiographic and ultrastructural studies on the human fibroatheromatous plaque, *Atherosclerosis* 48:95, 1983.
175. Spagnoli LG, Villaschi S, Neri L, et al: Autoradiographic studies of the smooth muscle cells in human arteries, *Artery Wall* 7:107, 1981.
176. Bennett MR, Evan GI, Schwartz SM: Apoptosis of human vascular smooth muscle cells derived from normal vessels and coronary atherosclerotic plaques, *J Clin Invest* 95:2266, 1995.
177. Lindner V, Olson NE, Clowes AW, et al: Heparin inhibits smooth muscle cell proliferation in injured rat arteries by displacing basic fibroblast growth factor, *J Clin Invest* 90:2044, 1992.
178. Jackson CL, Raines EW, Ross R, et al: Role of endogenous platelet-derived growth factor in arterial smooth muscle cell migration after balloon catheter injury, *Arterioscler Thromb* 13(8):1218, 1993.
179. Reidy MA, Irvin C, Lindner V: Migration of arterial wall cells. Expression of plasminogen activators and inhibitors in injured rat arteries, *Circ Res* 78:3, 1996.
180. Glagov S, Weisenberg E, Zarins CK, et al: Compensatory enlargement of human atherosclerotic coronary arteries, *N Engl J Med* 316:1371, 1987.
181. Folkow B: Physiological aspects of primary hypertension, *Physiol Rev* 62:347, 1982.
182. Jamal A, Bendeck M, Langille BL: Structural changes and recovery of function after arterial injury, *Arterioscler Thromb* 12:307, 1992.
183. Folkow B: "Structural factor" in primary and secondary hypertension, *Hypertension* 16:89, 1990.
184. Isner JM: Vascular remodeling: Honey, I think I shrunk the artery, *Circulation* 89(6):2937, 1994.
185. Lafont A, Guzman LA, Whitlow PL, et al: Restenosis after experimental angioplasty. Intimal, medial, and adventitial changes associated with constrictive remodeling, *Circ Res* 76:996, 1995.
186. Kakuta T, Currier JW, Haudenschild CC, et al: Differences in compensatory vessel enlargement, not intimal formation, account for restenosis following angioplasty in the hypercholesterolemic rabbit model, *Circulation* 89:2809, 1994.
187. Post MJ, Borst C, Kuntz RE: The relative importance of arterial remodeling compared with intimal hyperplasia in lumen renarrowing after balloon angioplasty. A study in the normal rabbit and the hypercholesterolemic Yucatan micropig, *Circulation* 89:2816, 1994.
188. Pasterkamp G, Borst C, Post MJ, et al: Atherosclerotic arterial remodeling in the superficial femoral artery. Individual variation in local compensatory enlargement response, *Circulation* 93:1818, 1996.
189. Kimura T, Kaburagi S, Tamura T, et al: Remodeling of human coronary arteries undergoing coronary angioplasty or atherectomy, *Circulation* 96:475, 1999.
190. Luo H, Nishioka T, Eigler NL, et al: Coronary artery restenosis after balloon angioplasty in humans is associated with circumferential coronary artery constriction, *Arterioscler Thromb Vasc Biol* 16:1393, 1999.
191. Mintz GS, Popma JJ, Pichard AD, et al: Arterial remodeling after coronary angioplasty. A serial intravascular ultrasound study, *Circulation* 94:35, 1996.
192. Pasterkamp G, de Kleijn D, Borst C: Arterial remodeling in atherosclerosis, restenosis and after alteration of blood flow: Potential mechanisms and clinical implications, *Cardiovasc Res* 45:843, 2000.
193. Schwartz SM, Murry CE, O'Brien ER: Vessel wall response to injury, *Sci Med* 3:2, 1996.
194. Shi Y, Pieniek M, Fard A, et al: Adventitial remodeling after coronary artery injury, *Circulation* 93:340, 1996.
195. Bryant SR, Bjercke RJ, Erichsen DA, et al: Vascular remodeling in response to altered blood flow is mediated by fibroblast growth factor-2, *Circ Res* 84:323, 1999.
196. Langille BL, O'Donnell F: Reductions in arterial diameter produced by chronic diseases in blood flow are endothelium-dependent, *Science* 231:405, 1986.
197. Jamal A, Bendeck M, Langille BL: Structural changes and recovery of function after arterial injury, *Arterioscler Thromb* 12:307, 1992.
198. Koester W: Endarteriitis and arteriitis, *Berl Klin Wochenschr* 13:454, 1876.
199. Geiringer E: Intimal vascularization and atherosclerosis, *J Pathol Bacteriol* 63:201, 1951.
200. Heistad DH, Armstrong ML: Blood flow through vasa vasorum of coronary arteries in atherosclerotic monkeys, *Arteriosclerosis* 6:326, 1986.
201. Glagov S, Weisenberg E, Zarins CK, et al: Compensatory enlargement of human atherosclerotic coronary arteries, *N Engl J Med* 316(22):1371, 1987.
202. Nissen SE, Gurley JC, Grines CL, et al: Intravascular ultrasound assessment of lumen size and wall morphology in normal subjects and patients with coronary artery disease, *Circulation* 84:3, 1991.
203. Topol EJ, Nissen SE: Our preoccupation with coronary luminology. The dissociation between clinical and angiographic findings in ischemic heart disease, *Circulation* 92:8, 1995.
204. Tobis J, Azarbal B, Slavin L: Assessment of intermediate severity coronary lesions in the catheterization laboratory, *J Am Coll Cardiol* 49:8, 2007.
205. Escolar E, Weigold G, Fuisz A, et al: New imaging techniques for diagnosing coronary artery disease, *CMAJ* 174:4, 2006.
206. Nissen SE: Application of intravascular ultrasound to characterize coronary artery disease and assess the progression or regression of atherosclerosis, *Am J Cardiol* 4A:89, 2002.
207. Virmani R, Burke AP, Kolodgie FD, et al: Pathology of the thin-cap fibroatheroma: A type of vulnerable plaque, *J Interv Cardiol* 16:3, 2003.
208. Ambrose JA: In search of the "vulnerable plaque": Can it be localized and will focal regional therapy ever be an option for cardiac prevention? *J Am Coll Cardiol* 51:16, 2008.
209. Brown BG, Bolson EL, Dodge HT: Dynamic mechanisms in human coronary stenosis, *Circulation* 70:917, 1984.
210. Levin DC, Gardiner GA: Coronary arteriography. *In* Braunwald E (ed): *Heart disease*, 3rd ed. Philadelphia, WB Saunders, 1988, pp 268–310.
211. Arnett EN, Isner JM, Redwood DR, et al: Coronary artery narrowing in coronary heart disease: Comparison of cineangiographic and necropsy findings, *Ann Intern Med* 91:350, 1979.
212. Wilson RF: Assessing the severity of coronary artery stenoses, *N Engl J Med* 334:1735, 1996.
213. Marcus ML: The physiologic effects of a coronary stenosis. *In* Marcus ML (ed): *The coronary circulation in health and disease.* New York, McGraw Hill,1983, pp 242–269.
214. Ambrose JA, Tannenbaum MA, Alexopoulos D, et al: Angiographic progression of coronary artery disease and the development of myocardial infarction, *J Am Coll Cardiol* 12(1):56, 1988.
215. Little WC, Constantinescu M, Applegate RJ, et al: Can coronary angiography predict the site of a subsequent myocardial infarction in patients with mild to moderate coronary artery disease? *Circulation* 78:1157, 1988.
216. Davies MJ, Thomas AC: Plaque fissuring—the cause of acute myocardial infarction, sudden ischemic death, and crescendo angina, *Br Heart J* 53(4):363, 1985.
217. Richardson PD, Davies MJ, Born GV: Influence of plaque configuration and stress distribution on fissuring of coronary atherosclerotic plaques, *Lancet* 2(8669):941, 1989.
218. Van der Wal AC, Becker AE, van der Loos CM, et al: Site of intimal rupture or erosion of thrombosed coronary atherosclerotic plaques is characterized by an inflammatory process irrespective of the dominant plaque morphology, *Circulation* 89:36, 1994.
219. Libby P, Hansson GK: Involvement of the immune system in human atherogenesis: Current knowledge and unanswered questions, *Lab Invest* 64:5, 1991.
220. Demer L, Gould KL, Kirkeeide R: Assessing stenosis severity; coronary flow reserve, collateral function, quantitative coronary arteriography, positron imaging, and digital subtraction angiography. A review and analysis, *Prog Cardiovasc Dis* 30(5):307, 1988.
221. Gould KL, Lipscomb K, Hamilton GW: Physiologic basis for assessing critical coronary stenosis, *Am J Cardiol* 33:87, 1974.
222. Koerselman J, van der Graaf Y, De Jaegere PP, Grobbee DE: Coronary collaterals: An important and underexposed aspect of coronary artery disease, *Circulation* 107:19, 2003.
223. Schaper W, Gorge G, Winkler B, et al: The collateral circulation of the heart, *Prog Cardiovasc Dis* 1:57, 1988.
224. Schaper W: Biological and molecular biological aspects of angiogenesis in coronary collateral development. *In* Nakamwa M, Vanhoutte PM (eds): *Coronary circulation in physiological and pathophysiological states.* Tokyo, Springer-Verlag, 1991, pp 21–27.
225. Conway EM, Collen D, Carmeliet P: Molecular mechanisms of blood vessel growth, *Cardiovasc Res* 49:3, 2001.
226. Fujita M, Tambara K: Recent insights into human coronary collateral development, *Heart* 90:3, 2004.
227. Carmeliet P: Mechanisms of angiogenesis and arteriogenesis, *Nat Med* 6:4, 2000.
228. Sellke FW, Quillen JE, Brooks LA, et al: Endothelial modulation of the coronary vasculature in vessels perfused via mature collaterals, *Circulation* 81:1938, 1990.
229. Verani MS: The functional significance of coronary collateral vessels: Anecdote confronts science, *Cathet Cardiovasc Diagn* 9:333, 1983.
230. Marcus ML: The coronary collateral circulation. *In* Marcus ML (ed): *The coronary circulation in health and disease.* New York, McGraw Hill, 1983, pp 221–241.
231. Braunwald E, Sobel BE: Coronary blood flow and myocardial ischemia. *In* Braunwald E (ed): *Heart disease*, 3rd ed. Philadelphia, WB Saunders, 1988, pp 1191–1221.
232. Hlatky MA, Mark DB, Califf RM, et al: Angina, myocardial ischemia and coronary disease: Gold standards, operational definitions and correlations, *J Clin Epidemiol* 42(5):381, 1989.
233. Buckberg GD, Fixler DE, Archie JP, et al: Experimental subendocardial ischemia in dogs with normal coronary arteries, *Circ Res* 30:67, 1972.
234. Griggs DM, Nakamura Y: Effects of coronary constriction on myocardial distribution of Iodoantipyrine I 131, *Am J Physiol* 215:1082, 1968.
235. Brazier J, Cooper N, Buckberg GD: The adequacy of subendocardial oxygen delivery: The interaction of determinants of flow, arterial oxygen content and myocardial oxygen need, *Circulation* 49:968, 1974.
236. Buffington CW: Hemodynamic determinants of ischemic myocardial dysfunction in the presence of coronary stenosis in dogs, *Anesthesiology* 63:651, 1985.
237. Stone PH: Mechanisms of silent myocardial ischemia: Implications for selection of optimal therapy, *Adv Cardiol* 37:328, 1990.
238. Maseri A, Newman C, Davies G: Coronary vasomotor tone: A heterogeneous entity, *Eur Heart J* 10(Suppl F):2, 1989.

239. Malacoff RF, Mudge GH, Holman BL, et al: Effect of cold pressor test on regional myocardial blood flow in patients with coronary artery disease, *Am Heart J* 106:78, 1983.
240. Zeiher AM, Drexler H, Wollschlaeger H, et al: Coronary vasomotion in response to sympathetic stimulation in humans: Importance of the functional integrity of the endothelium, *J Am Coll Cardiol* 14:1181, 1989.
241. Konidala S, Gutterman DD: Coronary vasospasm and the regulation of coronary blood flow, *Prog Cardiovasc Dis* 46:4, 2004.
242. Batchelor TJ, Sadaba JR, Ishola A, et al: Rho-kinase inhibitors prevent agonist-induced vasospasm in human internal mammary artery, *Br J Pharmacol* 132:1, 2001.
243. Werns SW, Walton JA, Hsia HH, et al: Evidence of endothelial dysfunction in angiographically normal coronary arteries of patients with coronary artery disease, *Circulation* 79:2, 1989.
244. Vita JA, Treasure CB, Nabel EG, et al: Coronary vasomotor response to acetylcholine relates to risk factors for coronary artery disease, *Circulation* 81:491, 1990.
245. Nabel EG, Selwyn AP, Ganz P: Large coronary arteries in humans are responsive to changing blood flow: An endothelium-dependent mechanism that fails in patients with atherosclerosis, *J Am Coll Cardiol* 16:349, 1990.
246. Golino P, Piscione F, Willerson JT, et al: Divergent effects of serotonin on coronary artery dimensions and blood flow in patients with coronary atherosclerosis and control patients, *N Engl J Med* 324:641, 1991.
247. McFadden EP, Clarke JG, Davies GJ, et al: Effect of intracoronary serotonin on coronary vessels in patients with stable angina and patients with variant angina, *N Engl J Med* 324:648, 1991.
248. Golino P, Maseri A: Serotonin receptors in human coronary arteries, *Circulation* 90:3, 1994.
249. Schwartz GG, Olsson AG, Ezekowitz MD, et al: Effects of atorvastatin on early recurrent ischemic events in acute coronary syndromes: The MIRACL study: A randomized controlled trial, *JAMA* 285:13, 2001.
250. Pasceri V, Patti G, Nusca A, et al: Randomized trial of atorvastatin for reduction of myocardial damage during coronary intervention: Results from the ARMYDA (Atorvastatin for Reduction of MYocardial Damage during Angioplasty) study, *Circulation* 110:6, 2004.
251. Patti G, Pasceri V, Colonna G, et al: Atorvastatin pretreatment improves outcomes in patients with acute coronary syndromes undergoing early percutaneous coronary intervention: Results of the ARMYDA-ACS randomized trial, *J Am Coll Cardiol* 49:12, 2007.
252. Di SG, Patti G, Pasceri V, et al: Efficacy of atorvastatin reload in patients on chronic statin therapy undergoing percutaneous coronary intervention: Results of the ARMYDA-RECAPTURE (Atorvastatin for Reduction of Myocardial Damage During Angioplasty) Randomized Trial, *J Am Coll Cardiol* 54:6, 2009.
253. Schonbeck U, Libby P: Inflammation, immunity, and HMG-CoA reductase inhibitors: Statins as antiinflammatory agents? *Circulation* 109(Suppl 1):21, 2004.
254. Halcox JPJ, Deanfield JE: Beyond the laboratory: Clinical implications for statin pleiotropy, *Circulation* 109(Suppl 1):21, 2004.
255. Pagano PJ, Gutterman DD: The adventitia: The outs and ins of vascular disease, *Cardiovasc Res* 75:4, 2007.
256. Bot I, de Jager SC, Bot M, et al: The neuropeptide substance P mediates adventitial mast cell activation and induces intraplaque hemorrhage in advanced atherosclerosis, *Circ Res* 106:1, 2010.
257. Herrmann J, Lerman LO, Rodriguez-Porcel M, et al: Coronary vasa vasorum neovascularization precedes epicardial endothelial dysfunction in experimental hypercholesterolemia, *Cardiovasc Res* 51:4, 2001.
258. Shi Y, O'Brien J, Fard A, et al: Adventitial myofibroblasts contribute to neointimal formation in injured porcine coronary arteries, *Circulation* 94(7):1655, 1996.
259. Zampetaki A, Kirton JP, Xu Q: Vascular repair by endothelial progenitor cells, *Cardiovasc Res* 78:3, 2008.
260. Hibbert B, Olsen S, O'Brien ER: Involvement of progenitor cells in vascular repair, *Trends Cardiovasc Med* 13:8, 2003.
261. Ma X, Hibbert B, White D, et al: Contribution of recipient-derived cells in allograft neointima formation and the response to stent implantation, *PLoS ONE* 3:3, 2008.
262. Hill JM, Zalos G, Halcox JP, et al: Circulating endothelial progenitor cells, vascular function, and cardiovascular risk, *N Engl J Med* 348:7, 2003.
263. Werner N, Kosiol S, Schiegl T, et al: Circulating endothelial progenitor cells and cardiovascular outcomes, *N Engl J Med* 353:10, 2005.
264. Quaini F, Urbanek K, Beltrami AP, et al: Chimerism of the transplanted heart, *N Engl J Med* 346:1, 2002.
265. George J, Herz I, Goldstein E, et al: Number and adhesive properties of circulating endothelial progenitor cells in patients with in-stent restenosis, *Arterioscler Thromb Vasc Biol* 23:12, 2003.
266. Hibbert B, Chen Y-X, O'Brien ER: The opposing roles of c-kit immunopositive vascular progenitor cells and endothelial progenitor cells in human coronary in-stent restenosis, *Am J Physiol (Heart Circ Physiol)* 287:H518, 2004.
267. Assmus B, Honold J, Schachinger V, et al: Transcoronary transplantation of progenitor cells after myocardial infarction, *N Engl J Med* 355:12, 2006.
268. Schachinger V, Erbs S, Elsasser A, et al: Intracoronary bone marrow-derived progenitor cells in acute myocardial infarction, *N Engl J Med* 355:12, 2006.
269. Hirschi KK, Ingram DA, Yoder MC: Assessing identity, phenotype, and fate of endothelial progenitor cells, *Arterioscler Thromb Vasc Biol* 28:9, 2008.

7

Molecular and Genetic Cardiovascular Medicine

SONAL SHARMA, MD | MARCEL E. DURIEUX, MD, PHD

KEY POINTS

1. The rapid development of molecular biologic and genetic techniques has greatly expanded the understanding of cardiac functioning, and they are beginning to be applied to the clinic.
2. Cardiac ion channels form the machinery behind the cardiac rhythm; cardiac membrane receptors regulate cardiac function.
3. Na^+, K^+, and Ca^{++} channels are the main types involved in the cardiac action potential. Many subtypes exist, and their molecular structure is known in some detail, allowing a molecular explanation for phenomena such as voltage sensing, ion selectivity, and inactivation.
4. Muscarinic and adrenergic receptors, both of the G-protein–coupled receptor class, are the main regulators of cardiac function.
5. Adenosine plays important roles in myocardial preconditioning through an action on ATP-regulated K^+ channels and is an effective antiarrhythmic drug by its action on G-protein–coupled adenosine receptors.
6. Volatile anesthetics significantly affect Ca^{++} channels and muscarinic receptors.
7. Powerful genetic analysis techniques allow cardiovascular diagnosis through molecular approaches, but treatment through gene therapy has not yet become standard practice.

The past decades have witnessed what may be termed a revolution in the biomedical sciences, as molecular and genetic methodologies have suddenly jumped onto the clinical scene. Molecular biology originated in the 1950s, its birth most commonly identified with the description of the structure of deoxyribonucleic acid (DNA) by Watson and Crick.[1] For many years after, it was practiced almost exclusively in the research laboratory. Much of this research involved the laborious process of cloning: the identification of DNA molecules encoding specific proteins. Although at the time most people in the field realized that these advances would one day be of immense importance to clinical medicine, the exact place they would take was unclear.

Not generally appreciated was the rapidity with which molecular biology would advance. Now, more than a half century since the discovery of the structure of DNA, the human genome has been sequenced completely. Techniques for manipulating nucleic acids have been simplified enormously, and for many routine procedures, kits are available. The development of the polymerase chain reaction (PCR), a technique of remarkable simplicity and flexibility, has dramatically increased the speed with which many molecular biology procedures can be performed; in addition, it has allowed the invention of many new ones. Recent years have seen the development of techniques directed at screening large amounts of genetic material for changes associated with disease states. As a result of these and other developments, molecular biology has become a practical tool to study the expression and functioning of proteins in health and disease.

Cardiovascular medicine has been a major beneficiary of these advances. Not only have the electrophysiologic and pump function of the heart been placed on a firm molecular footing, but for a number of disease states, the pathophysiology has been determined, allowing progress in therapeutic development. Importantly, there is no indication that the pace of progress in molecular biology has slowed. If anything, the opposite is the case, and more dramatic advances may be expected in the years to come. Thus, techniques such as gene therapy may become available as therapeutic options in cardiac disease.

In this chapter, the most important aspects of molecular and genetic cardiovascular medicine are surveyed, with specific emphasis on medical issues relevant to the anesthesiologist. The myocyte membrane signaling proteins are of prime importance in this respect, and the two major classes—membrane channels and membrane receptors—are discussed. Simply stated, the channels form the machinery behind the cardiac rhythm, whereas the receptors are involved in regulation of cardiac function. This is, of course, an overgeneralization because close interactions among the various systems exist. In fact, these interactions have stimulated some of the more exciting areas of investigation in molecular cardiovascular medicine. In each of these sections, a brief overview of the general properties of the class of proteins is provided, and then several examples specific to the cardiovascular system are discussed. Each section ends with a discussion of some clinical correlates flowing from the material discussed.

The actions of anesthetics on these systems are also described. This is an area of active investigation. Much detail remains to be filled in, but it is clear now that anesthetics, at clinically relevant concentrations, interact with a number of cardiac signaling systems. Although it is too early to explain completely the cardiac effects of the various anesthetics through these mechanisms, there is no doubt that such interactions can be of significant clinical relevance. Considering the rapid pace of research in this area, rather than attempting to be all-inclusive, two examples in which a significant body of information is available, and in which clinical relevance appears likely, are emphasized. These examples are the cardiac Ca^{++} channels and the muscarinic acetylcholine receptors.

The final section looks at the role of genetics in cardiovascular medicine, again with emphasis on developments of relevance to anesthesiology. The authors discuss techniques for genetic diagnostic screening, and their applications in the clinical setting. In addition, the potential of genetic therapy is also described briefly, an area that at this time has not yet made it into clinical practice.

In addition to providing an overview of the current state of knowledge, this chapter demonstrates a few of the many methodologies that have been used to obtain these results, to enable the reader to access the current literature with more ease. In quoting the literature, the authors have, therefore, chosen to provide references to many of the original articles describing techniques and findings, complemented by references to recent review articles to provide a current viewpoint.

THE MACHINERY BEHIND THE CARDIAC RHYTHM: ION CHANNELS

The cardiac action potential results from the flow of ions through *ion channels,* which are the membrane-bound proteins that form the structural machinery behind cardiac electrical excitability. In response to changes in electrical potential across the cell membrane, ion channels open and allow the passive flux of ions into or out of the cell along their electrochemical gradients. This flow of charged ions results in a current, which will alter the cell membrane potential toward the potential at which the electrochemical gradient for the ion is zero and is called the *equilibrium potential* (E) for the ion. Depolarization of the cell could, in principle, result from an inward cation current or an outward anion current; for repolarization, the reverse is true. In excitable cells, action potentials are mainly caused by the flow of cation currents. Membrane depolarization results principally from the flow of Na^+ down its electrochemical gradient (E_{Na} is around +50mV), whereas repolarization results from the outward flux of K^+ down its electrochemical gradient (E_K is around −90 mV). Opening and closing of ion channels selective for a single ion result in an individual ionic current. The integrated activity of many different ionic currents, each activated over precisely regulated potential ranges and at different times in the cardiac cycle, results in the cardiac action potential. Ion channels are usually highly (but not uniquely) *selective* for a single ion (e.g., K^+ channels, Na^+ channels). Channels may *rectify,* that is, pass current in one direction across the membrane more easily than the other. Electrical and chemical stimuli, which lead to opening and closing of the channel, cause a conformational change in the channel molecule *(gating).* The rate of change of channel conformation *(gating kinetics)* may be rapid, in which case the channel will open *(activate)* almost immediately (e.g., Na^+ channels), or relatively slowly, which will result in a delay in channel activation (e.g., delayed rectifier K^+ channels). After activation, ion channels may stay open until closed by another stimulus (e.g., repolarization of the membrane) or may close *(inactivate)* in the face of a continued stimulus. Inactivated channels will usually not reopen on repeat stimulation until they have recovered from inactivation (Box 7-1).

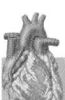 Patch Clamping

Much of the understanding of the molecular mechanisms behind the action potential has derived from the development and implementation of three techniques: *patch clamping,* a technique that allows recording of ion flow through individual channel molecules, *voltage clamping* of isolated cardiac cells, and *cloning and heterologous expression* of ion channel genes. Comparison of ionic currents recorded in isolated myocytes with currents recorded from cells expressing ion channel genes has resulted in the identification of many of the ion channel molecules that underlie the cardiac action potential.

The development of the voltage clamp technique in the early 1950s and its application to multicellular preparations of cardiac muscle allowed identification of the major ionic currents that underlie the cardiac action potential. The whole-cell currents recorded by the technique were smooth waveforms derived from summation of the activity of thousands of ion channels, and many different patterns of events at the single-channel level, arising from more than one molecular specie,

can summate to produce identical whole-cell current waveforms. Patch clamping allows resolution of events at the single-channel level. In this technique, small patches of cell membrane ($< 1 \mu m^2$) are isolated electrically and physically in the tip of a glass micropipette.[2] Single-channel events can then be resolved because there are only a few ion channel molecules present in the patch. Current flowing across the patch typically jumps between well-defined values corresponding to sudden opening or closing of the ion-conducting pore (Figure 7-1A). The whole-cell current will be the sum of the currents through all of the individual channels in the cell membrane; summation of the current flowing through a single channel during repeated stimuli will reproduce the macroscopic whole-cell current (see Figures 7-1A and B). As channel opening and closing in response to a stimulus are a stochastic phenomena, the regulation of ion flow, whether resulting from a change in membrane potential or from interaction with regulator molecules, is usually achieved by increasing the *probability* that the channel will be open. Thus, in Figure 7-1, which shows records from human cardiac muscle Na^+ channels, the channels open *(activate)* a few milliseconds after depolarization because the probability that the channel will be open increases. Similarly, as the channels spontaneously close *(inactivate)*, the open probability decreases.

An ion current with distinct electrical and pharmacologic properties indicates the presence of a population of identical ion channel molecules. Application of molecular techniques has allowed the identification of many ion channel molecules, and thus a better understanding of the currents that underlie the cardiac action potential. An as-yet unrealized dream would be tailoring of pharmacologic agents that interact with specific channel types to shape the action potential.

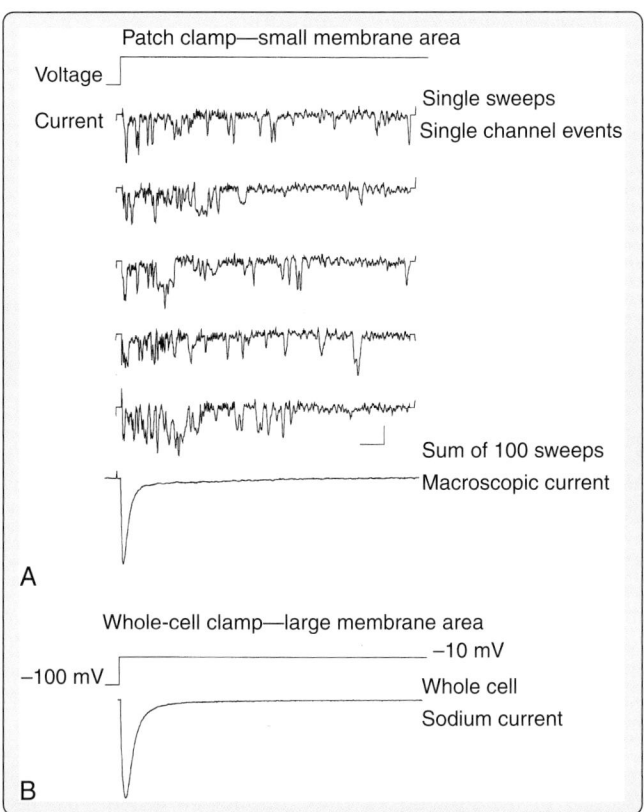

Figure 7-1   **Voltage clamp recordings from muscle Na^+ channels.** *A,* Patch-clamp recordings. Individual Na^+ channel openings are recorded as short-lived downward deflections. Note that openings are concentrated in the first part of the trace. The top five traces represent a single depolarizing clamp pulse. The sum of 100 such pulses (bottom trace) recreates the whole-cell current *(B).*

BOX 7-1. PROPERTIES OF ION CHANNELS

- Ion selectivity
- Rectification (passing current more easily in one direction than the other)
- Gating (mechanism for opening and closing the channel):
  - Activation (opening)
  - Inactivation (closing)

Electrical Events Underlying the Cardiac Action Potential

Figure 7-2 shows a diagram of a cardiac action potential with a summary of the ionic currents flowing during each phase. As far as has been determined, the probable molecular identity of the ion channels that underlie these currents is also given. This section examines the biophysical properties of these currents; subsequent sections focus on possible molecular mechanisms underlying the biophysical phenomena.

The Resting Membrane Potential and the Role of I_{K1}

The resting cardiac membrane potential is maintained close to the equilibrium potential for potassium (E_K) by a background, inwardly rectifying, highly selective K^+ current (I_{K1}). Under physiologic conditions, the E_K is around −90 mV, and displacement of the membrane potential from this value should result in an inward or outward current through I_{K1}, thus returning the membrane potential toward E_K. However, although I_{K1} passes significant *inward* current at potentials negative to E_K, at positive potentials, the channels display inward rectification (i.e., they pass inward current more easily than outward current), which limits outward current flow and reduces the tendency for I_{K1} to hyperpolarize the membrane. This has obvious significance for an excitable cell; inward rectification[3] allows the initiation of action potentials and limits cellular K^+ loss during the action potential. I_{K1} is large in ventricular cells, smaller in atrial cells, and almost absent in nodal tissue.[4] This explains why ventricular cells rest near E_K and have a high threshold for excitation, atrial cells have a more positive resting potential, and nodal cells have no defined resting potential.

Phase 0: Rapid Upstroke of the Cardiac Action Potential

The rapid upstroke of the cardiac action potential (phase 0) is caused by the flow of a large inward Na^+ current (I_{na}) (Box 7-2).[5] I_{Na} is activated by depolarization of the sarcolemma to a threshold potential of

BOX 7-2. CARDIAC ACTION POTENTIAL

- Phase 0 (rapid upstroke): primarily Na^+ channel opening
- Phase 1 (early rapid repolarization): inactivation of Na^+ current, opening of K^+ channels
- Phase 2 (plateau phase): balance between K^+ and Ca^{++} currents
- Phase 3 (final rapid repolarizations): activation of Ca^{++} channels
- Phase 4 (diastolic depolarization): balance between Na^+ and K^+ currents

−65 to −70 mV. I_{Na} activation, and hence the action potential, is an all-or-nothing response. Subthreshold depolarizations have only local effects on the membrane. After the threshold for activation of fast Na^+ channels is exceeded, Na^+ channels open (i.e., I_{Na} activates) and Na^+ ions enter the cell down their electrochemical gradient. This results in displacement of the membrane potential toward the equilibrium potential for Na^+ ions, around +50 mV. I_{Na} activation is transient, lasting at most 1 to 2 msec because, simultaneous with activation, a second, slightly slower conformational change in the channel molecule occurs (inactivation), which closes the ion pore in the face of continued membrane depolarization (see Figures 7-1*A* and *B*). The channel cannot open again until it has recovered from inactivation (i.e., regained its resting conformation), a process that requires repolarization to the resting potential for a defined period. Thus, the channels cycle through three states: *resting* (and available for activation), *open*, and *inactivated*. Although the channel is inactivated, it is absolutely refractory to repeated stimulation. Stimuli that occur during recovery from inactivation will result in opening of fewer Na^+ channels (because not all have recovered), and the resulting action potential will have a reduced maximal rate of depolarization and reduced conduction velocity. Na^+ channels do not need to open to become inactivated. If the resting membrane potential depolarizes for a time, inactivation will occur in some channels and subsequent stimulation will result in an action potential of reduced amplitude and conduction velocity.

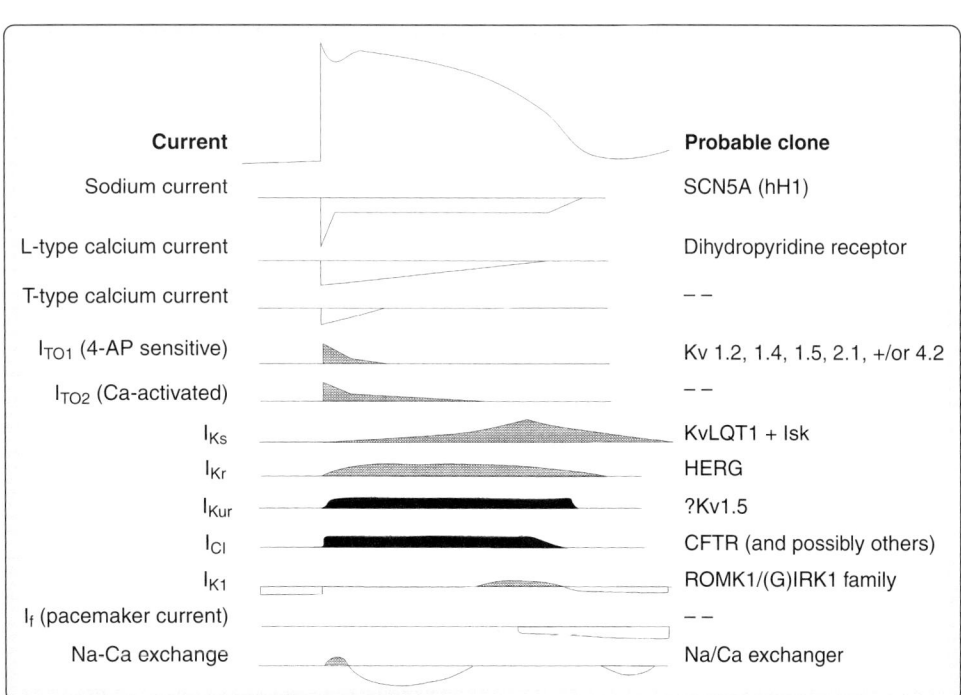

Figure 7-2 Ionic currents underlying the cardiac action potential. Currents are listed on the left, and the ion channel genes encoding the currents are listed on the right. 4-AP, 4-aminopyridine; CFTR, cystic fibrosis transmembrane regulator. (*From Roden DM, Lazzarra R, Rosen R, et al, for the SADS Foundation Task Force on LQTS: Multiple mechanisms in the long QT syndrome: Current knowledge, gaps and future directions. Circulation 94:1996, 1996.*)

Phase 1: Early Rapid Repolarization

The early rapid repolarization phase of the action potential, which follows immediately after phase 0, results both from rapid inactivation of the majority of the Na^+ current and from activation of a transient outward current (I_{TO}), carried mainly by K^+ ions. On depolarization of the membrane, I_{TO} opens rapidly, over about 20 msec, before spontaneously inactivating. I_{TO} comprises two separate currents: the rapidly inactivating I_{TO1}, which is activated by depolarization and blocked by 4-aminopyridine, and the slowly inactivating I_{TO2}, which is activated by elevated intracellular Ca^{++} (possibly explaining the observation that action potential duration tends to decrease with rapid heart rates and hypercalcemia)[6,7] (Figure 7-3).

In addition to its effect on phase 1, I_{TO}, in combination with the delayed rectifier potassium currents (I_{Kr} and I_{Ks}) and I_{K1}, also contributes to membrane repolarization. Arrhythmogenic prolongation of the action potential in myocardial cells recovered from patients with myocardial hypertrophy,[8] congestive cardiomyopathy,[6] and from the border zone of myocardial infarction in animals[9] appears to result from depression of I_{TO}.

Phases 2 and 3: Plateau Phase and Final Rapid Repolarization

The action potential plateau and final rapid repolarization are mediated by a balance between the slow inward current and outward, predominantly K^+ current. During the plateau phase, membrane conductance to all ions falls and very little current flows. Potassium conductance is low because of inward rectification of I_{K1} (i.e., inward current passes more easily than outward current), so little outward current flows despite the large outward electrochemical gradient for K^+ ions and the delayed onset of the outwardly rectifying K^+ currents (I_{Ks}, I_{Kr}, and I_{Kur}). The resulting small outward current is balanced by inward current, predominantly through L-type Ca^{++} channels (I_{Ca-L}), but also via a slowly inactivating population of Na^+ channels, and a small inward flux of chloride (Cl^-) ions, possibly carried by the cardiac variant of the ATP-dependent channel (abnormalities of which underlie cystic fibrosis).[10,11] Phase 3, regenerative rapid repolarization,

results from time-dependent inactivation of L-type Ca^{++} current and increasing outward current through delayed rectifier K^+ channels. The net membrane current becomes outward and the cell repolarizes.

Slow Inward Ca++ Current

The slow inward current (I_{Ca-L}) is activated by depolarization of the cell to potentials less negative than −40 to −50 mV. In ventricular and atrial myocytes and in Purkinje fibers, I_{Ca-L} is activated by the regenerative depolarization caused by I_{Na} during phase 0 of the action potential. I_{Ca-L} does not contribute significantly to phase 0 because, in comparison with I_{Na}, it activates much more slowly (over about 10 msec) and is smaller in amplitude. I_{Ca-L} also inactivates slowly and, therefore, contributes the major inward current during the plateau of the action potential. I_{Ca-L} flows through L-type (long-lasting) Ca^{++} channels, which are sensitive to block by dihydropyridines (e.g., nifedipine), and activation of contraction is related to the magnitude of the resulting calcium influx.[12] Gating of I_{Ca-L} is generally similar to I_{Na} in that channel opening and closing are dependent on membrane potential and time. Ca^{++} channels are also, importantly, dynamically regulated by the autonomic nervous system.[13] β agonists activate I_{Ca-L} (and hence increase myocardial contractility) indirectly by activating adenylyl cyclase via a guanosine triphosphate (GTP)–binding protein, G_s (Figure 7-4). The resulting increase in intracellular cyclic adenosine monophosphate (cAMP) activates protein kinase A (PKA), which phosphorylates the Ca^{++} channel. Phosphorylated channels open in response to membrane depolarization; nonphosphorylated channels do not, so the effect of β-adrenergic stimulation is to increase the number of functional channels. The electrophysiologic effect of this is illustrated in Figure 7-5, which shows enhancement of the slow inward current by increase of adenosine monophosphate (AMP) level in single-channel Ca^{++} channels and intact cells. β-Adrenergic effects on I_{Ca-L} are antagonized by acetylcholine, which, in myocardial cells, activates M_2 muscarinic receptors and inhibits adenylyl cyclase through activation of the GTP-binding protein G_i.

In the relatively depolarized pacemaker cells, which lack I_{K1}, I_{Na} is inactivated and the slow inward current is solely responsible for the upstroke of the action potential. I_{Ca-L} also can generate slowly propagated action potentials in diseased or damaged myocardial cells in which I_{Na} has been inactivated by depolarization. These *slow responses*, which may occur in the border zone of myocardial infarcts, are important because they may cause the slow conduction that can lead to reentrant arrhythmias.

Delayed Rectifier K+ Currents

Delayed rectifier K^+ channels are present in all cardiac myocytes. They open slowly (over 200 to 300 msec) after depolarization of the membrane to the plateau level (−10 mV and greater), producing a K^+-selective outward current, I_K. I_K does not inactivate on prolonged depolarization (unlike I_{Na} and I_{Ca-L}), and the channels close on repolarization of the membrane. Unlike I_{K1}, I_K displays outward rectification; that is, it passes outward current more easily than inward current. This is the expected behavior for a K^+-selective channel because both the concentration and electrical gradients for potassium are outward. Thus, for any depolarizing displacement of membrane potential from E_K, the driving force will be larger in an outward direction. Similar to I_{Ca-L}, I_K is under autonomic control (see Figure 7-4). β-Adrenergic stimulation enhances I_K by a mechanism similar to that of the enhancement of I_{Ca-L}, thus ensuring repolarization of the cell in the face of increased inward Ca^{++} current.[14]

Three components of I_K, carried by different channel molecules, can be distinguished. A rapidly activating component, I_{Kr}, is blocked by the compound E4031 (a Class III antiarrhythmic agent), which leaves a slower activating component, I_{Ks}, unaffected.[15] This is illustrated in Figure 7-6, which also emphasizes the importance of I_K in the regulation of repolarization, and hence of action potential duration. A third component, the ultra-rapidly activated delayed rectifier, I_{Kur}, can be distinguished in atrial (but not ventricular) myocytes.[16] This additional

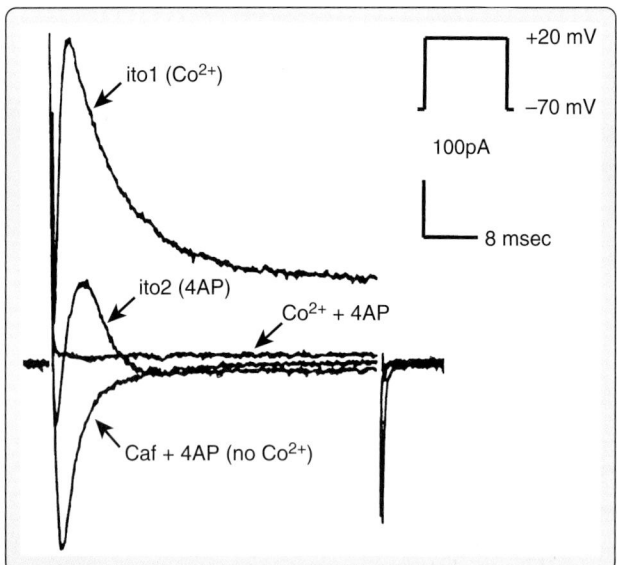

Figure 7-3 Voltage clamp recordings from an atrial myocyte showing pharmacologic separation of I_{TO1} (ito1) and I_{TO2} (ito2). In the presence of cobalt ions, only I_{TO1} is seen. When cobalt is omitted and 4-aminopyridine (4-AP) is added, I_{TO2} is revealed. Caffeine (Caf) eliminates I_{TO2}, leaving the underlying inward calcium current. In the presence of both 4-AP and cobalt ions, all outward currents are inhibited. (From Wang Z, Fermini B, Nattel S: Delayed rectifier outward current and repolarization in human atrial myocytes. Circ Res 73:276, 1993.)

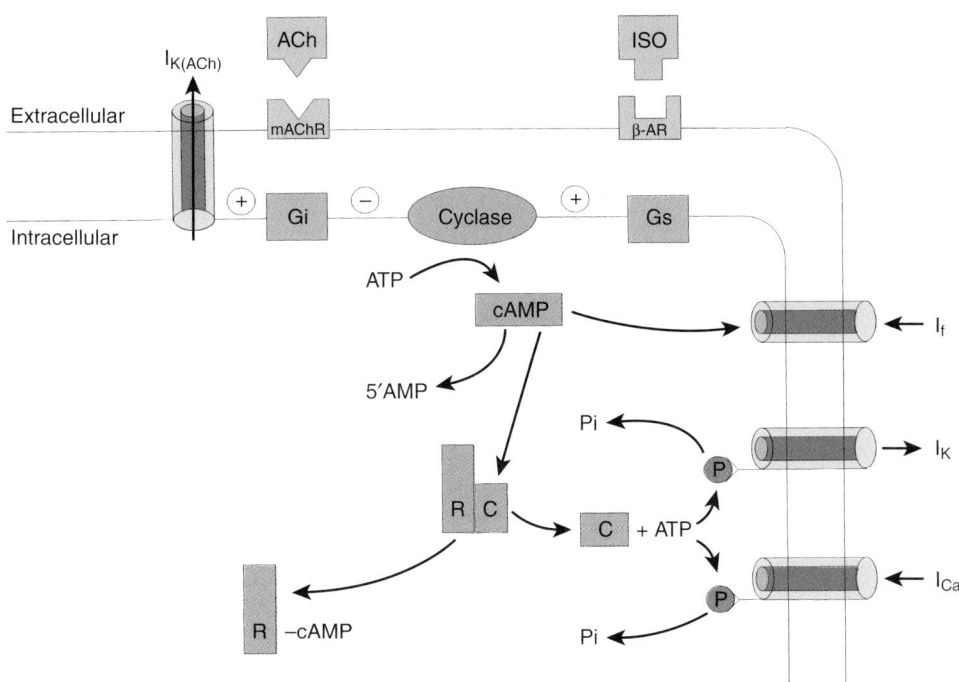

Figure 7-4 **Autonomic regulation of ion currents.** ACh, acetylcholine; 5′AMP, adenosine 5′ monophosphate; β-AR, β-adrenergic receptor; ATP, adenosine triphosphate; cAMP, cyclic adenosine monophosphate; Cyclase, adenylyl cyclase; Gi and Gs, guanosine triphosphate–binding proteins; ISO, isoproterenol; mAChR, M2 muscarinic receptor; Pi, pyrophosphate; R and C, regulatory and catalytic subunits, respectively, of protein kinase A.

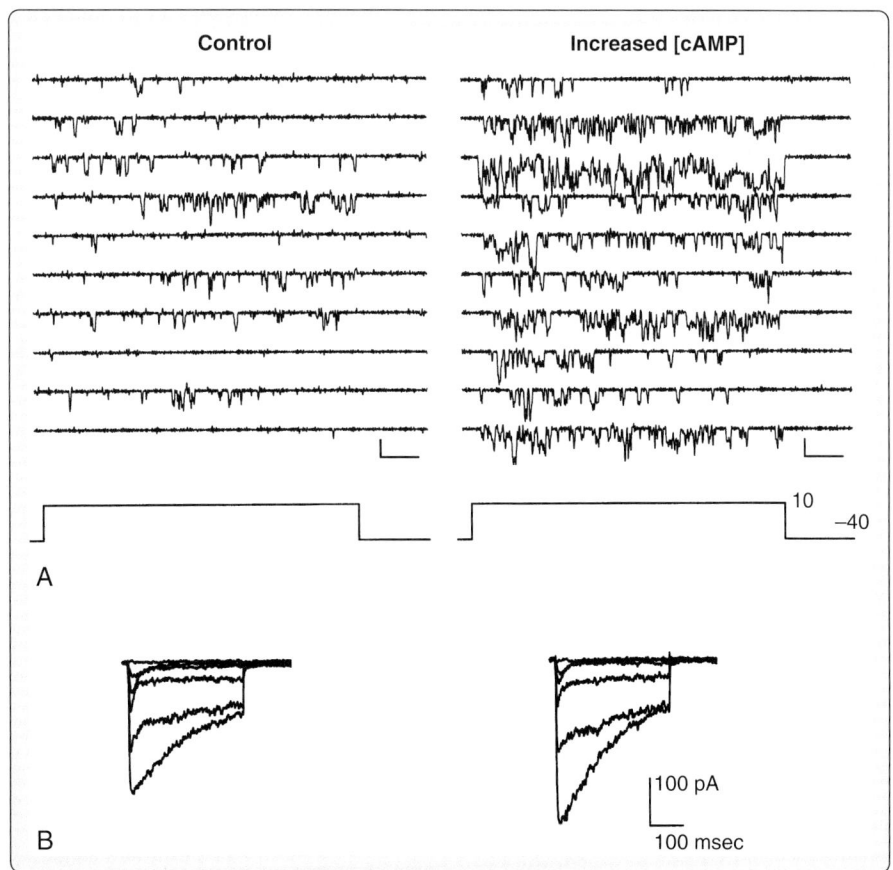

Figure 7-5 **Effects of elevated cyclic adenosine monophosphate (cAMP) on cardiac calcium channels.** *A*, Single-channel recordings; *B*, whole-cell currents. Left panels are control recordings; right panels show the effect of elevation of intracellular cAMP (in this case, induced by exposure to parathyroid hormone). Note the increased probability of channel opening and resulting increase in whole-cell current in the presence of increased cAMP. (A, B, *Modified from Rampe D, Lacerda AE, Dage RC, Brown AM: Parathyroid hormone: An endogenous modulator of cardiac calcium channels. Am J Physiol 261[6 Pt 2]:H1945, 1991.*)

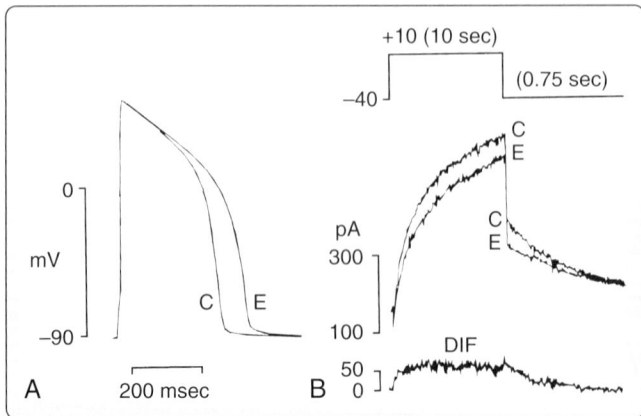

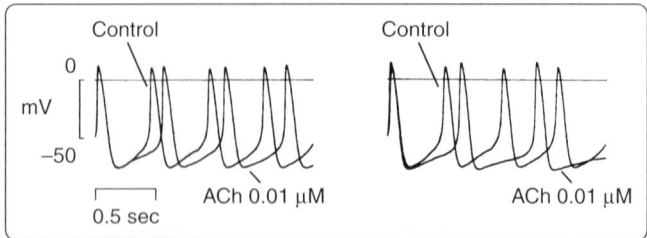

Figure 7-7 Effect of acetylcholine on spontaneous pacemaker activity in isolated sinoatrial (SA) node cells. Pacemaker activity in control solution is compared with activity in increasing doses of acetylcholine (ACh). Note the slowing of diastolic depolarization and resultant slowing of heart rate. *(From DiFrancesco D: Current I and the neuronal modulation of heart rate. In Zipes DP, Jaliffe J [eds]: Cardiac electrophysiology from cell to bedside. Philadelphia: WB Saunders Company, 1990, p 28.)*

Figure 7-6 *A,* Effect on action potential duration of blockade of I_{Kr} by E4031 in isolated guinea pig ventricular myocytes. After application of E4031, outward repolarizing currents are inhibited and action potential duration is increased. *B,* Voltage clamp records showing separation of I_{Kr} and I_{Ks} by E4031. The control delayed rectifier K^+ current (C) is partially inhibited by E4031 (E), and the difference between the two currents (DIF) represents I_{Ks}. *(A, B, From Sanguinetti MC, Jurkiewicz NK: Two components of cardiac delayed rectifier K+ current. Differential sensitivity to block by class III antiarrhythmic agents. J Gen Physiol 96:195, 1990. Reproduced from The Journal of General Physiology by copyright permission of The Rockefeller University Press.)*

repolarizing current explains, in part, the enhancement of repolarization in atrial myocardium when compared with ventricle and Purkinje fibers.

Repolarization in Different Cardiac Tissue Types

Phase 3 repolarization in atrium and pacemaker tissues, but not in ventricular myocardium, is also enhanced by the presence of a large outward repolarizing K^+ current ($I_{K[ACh]}$).[17,18] This potential independent current is activated indirectly by stimulation of muscarinic (M2-type) receptors by acetylcholine or purinergic (A-type) receptors by adenosine.[19] This channel is potential independent and is activated via binding of an activated, membrane-bound GTP-binding protein (G_i), as discussed later.[20]

There is variability in action potential duration between cells in normal ventricle.[21] A gradient in action potential duration exists across the myocardium (from epicardium to endocardium), and specialized mid-myocardial cells (M cells) have been identified, which exhibit prolongation of action potential duration at slow stimulation rates, possibly as a result of a decrease in I_{Ks}.

Phase 4: Diastolic Depolarization and I_f

Phase 4 diastolic depolarization, or normal automaticity, is a normal feature of cardiac cells in the sinus and atrioventricular (AV) nodes, but subsidiary pacemaker activity is also observed in the His-Purkinje system and in some specialized atrial and ventricular myocardial cells (see Chapter 4). Pacemaker discharge from the sinus node normally predominates because the rate of diastolic depolarization in the sinoatrial (SA) node is faster than in other pacemaker tissues. Pacemaker activity results from a slow net gain of positive charge, which depolarizes the cell from its maximal diastolic potential to threshold.

Pacemaker cells in the sinus node are relatively depolarized, with a maximal diastolic potential of -60 to -70 mV and a threshold potential of -40 mV. Rapid regenerative depolarization (phase 0) is dependent on opening of T-type and then L-type Ca^{++} channels. Repolarization is dependent on activation of delayed rectifier K^+ channels, and the maximum diastolic potential is around -80 mV. Pacemaker channels are activated by hyperpolarization to this potential and produce a slow inward Na^+ current, I_f. This flows against slowly inactivating delayed rectifier K^+ currents and results in diastolic depolarization.[22] Because the current is nonselective among cations, its reversal potential lies

between E_K and E_{Na}, at around -10 mV, and activation of I_f will tend to depolarize the cell toward this value. Similar to I_{Ca-L}, I_f is under autonomic control (see Figure 7-4) through GTP-dependent binding proteins G_s and G_i, which regulate cAMP production by adenylyl cyclase.[23,24] β-Adrenergic stimulation shifts the voltage dependence of activation of I_f to more depolarized potentials, so for any hyperpolarizing stimulus, more I_f will be activated and diastolic depolarization will be enhanced. Acetylcholine has the opposite effect (Figure 7-7).

Molecular Biology of Ion Channels

The preceding sections have focused on the electrical events that underlie cardiac electrical excitability, and on the identification of cardiac ionic currents on the basis of their biophysical properties. Here the molecular structures behind these electrical phenomena are reviewed. The first step in understanding the molecular physiology of cardiac electrical excitability is to identify the ion channel proteins responsible for the ionic currents. Figure 7-2 gives the current classification of the ion channel responsible for each of the cardiac ionic currents. There are firm molecular candidates for voltage-gated Na^+ and L-type Ca^{++} channels. Similarly, channel molecules with properties similar to delayed rectifier K^+ channels, the 4-aminopyridine–sensitive component of I_{TO}, the inward rectifier I_{K1}, the ligand-gated K^+ channel $I_{K(ACh)}$, and the pacemaker current I_f have been cloned. Figure 7-8 shows diagrams of the predicted membrane topology of some of these channels. Voltage-gated Na^+, Ca^{++}, and K^+ channels exist as conglomerates of molecules, consisting of a large α subunit and several accessory subunits (labeled β, δ, and γ in Figure 7-8). The α subunit alone is usually sufficient to induce channel activity in biologic membranes, but its activity is modulated by the presence of the accessory subunits. The diagrams in Figure 7-8 were deduced from hydrophobicity analysis of the primary structure of the major channel polypeptides. Regions of the polypeptides predicted to span the membrane are those that contain a high concentration of hydrophobic amino acids, whereas peptides linking these transmembrane sections are hydrophilic. Similarities among the various channels strongly suggest a common evolutionary ancestry. Na^+ and Ca^{++} channel α subunits (see Figures 7-8A and B) are strikingly similar, each consisting of four homologous transmembrane domains (labeled I to IV), linked by cytoplasmic peptides. Each homologous domain contains six linked membrane-spanning segments (labeled S1 to S6). These large polypeptides, containing more than 2000 amino acids, form a tetrameric structure and generate Na^+ or Ca^{++} channel activity in biologic membranes. Voltage-gated K^+ channel α subunits, in contrast, are much smaller (see Figure 7-8C) and consist of a single transmembrane domain with six membrane-spanning segments, an arrangement similar to one of the individual domains of Na^+ and Ca^{++} channels. Four molecules are noncovalently linked in the membrane to produce a tetrameric structure, similar to a Na^+ or Ca^{++} channel, to produce K^+ channel activity. The structure of the inwardly rectifying K^+ channel molecules, I_{K1} and $I_{K(ACh)}$, is dissimilar to other K^+ channels

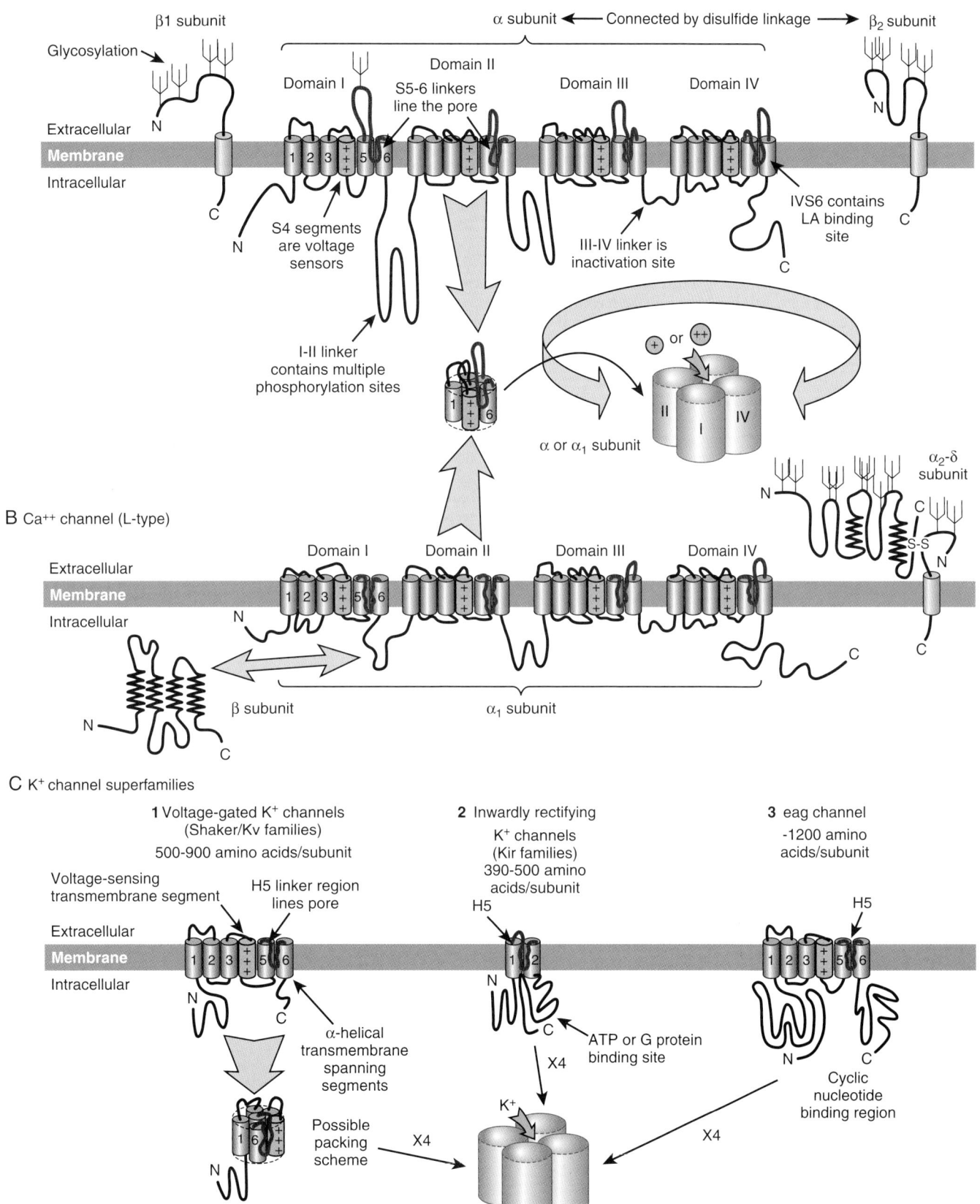

Figure 7-8 **Diagrams of ion channel molecular structure.** *A,* Na+ channel. *B,* Ca++ channel. *C,* K+ channels. ATP, adenosine triphosphate.

(see Figure 7-8C). The molecules are much less complex, having only two membrane-spanning segments, although these segments share considerable homology with the S5 and S6 segments of the classic voltage-gated K+ channel.

Voltage-gated ion channel activity requires that the channel molecule should sense and respond to changes in membrane potential, form an ion-selective membrane pore, and (in some cases) inactivate despite continuing depolarization. The molecular mechanisms for these phenomena are examined in separate sections later.

Molecular Mechanisms

The Voltage Sensor

Channel proteins respond to changes in electrical potential across the cell membrane by conformational changes *(gating)*, which result from electrostatic interactions between charged portions of the molecule and the membrane electric field (Box 7-3). Gating of the channel is associated with a measurable flow of electrical charge through the membrane lipid bilayer (called *gating current*), as a zone of the molecule rich in electrical charge moves within the membrane.[25] This charge movement is linked to opening of the channel pore. The voltage sensor of voltage-dependent ion channels resides in the mobile S4 membrane-spanning segments, α-helical structures unusually rich in positively charged amino acids.[26] At rest, each of the positive charges in the S4 segment is balanced by fixed negative charges in other segments of the molecule. The resting membrane potential (negative inside) forces the (mobile) positive charges inward and the fixed negative charges outward. This dynamic equilibrium holds the channel pore closed. On depolarization, the force pulling the positive charge inward is relieved; positive charges (the S4 segments) are repelled outward and assume new partners with the fixed negative membrane charges. This charge movement comprises the *gating current*. If the depolarizing stimulus is short, repolarization of the membrane is followed by a gating current of equal and opposite magnitude as the S4 segment relaxes to its original position. If the depolarizing stimulus is prolonged, however, the movement of the S4 segments induces a conformational change in the channel molecule, which prohibits easy return to baseline. This conformational change in the channel molecule is manifested as activation (or channel opening), and this is closely coupled to channel closing (or inactivation; see later) in channels that inactivate. Thus, small changes in the membrane electric field cause conformational changes in the channel molecule, which result in opening (and closing) of the channel pore. An S4 segment rich in positive charge is a remarkably consistent feature of voltage-gated ion channels from a variety of different species and with a variety of ion selectivities. The dependence of channel activation on membrane potential is proportional to the density of positive charge in the S4 segment.

Ion Channel Pore and Selectivity Filter

The presence of four homologous domains in voltage-gated Na+ and Ca++ channels suggests that basic ion channel architecture consists of a transmembrane pore surrounded by the four homologous domains arranged symmetrically (see Figure 7-8). The membrane-spanning segments each form an α helix so that the walls of the pore will be derived from α-helical segments from each of the four domains. A pore formed from four such α helices would have limiting dimensions of 3 by 5 Angstrom units, similar to the size inferred for the Na+ channel pore by measurement of the permeability of cations of different sizes.[27,28]

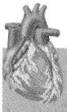

BOX 7-3. MOLECULAR MECHANISMS OF ION CHANNELS

- Voltage sensor
- Gating mechanism (activation and inactivation)
- Ion pore
- Selectivity filter

The selectivity filter is formed by the S5 and S6 membrane-spanning segments of each domain together with their peptide linker.[29] As emphasized in Figure 7-8, unlike the hydrophilic extracellular linkers between other membrane-spanning segments, the S5/S6 linker is sufficiently hydrophobic to place it (at least partially) within the membrane lipid bilayer. The channel pore is lined both by the S5/S6 linker and the S5 and S6 membrane-spanning segments. Point mutations in the S5/S6 linker have dramatic effects on channel ion selectivity and reduce channel conductance to its primary ion. Extensive site-directed mutagenesis experiments of the S5/S6 linkers from a variety of channels suggest that they form a funnel that allows the passage of a specific ion into the pore. In Na+ channels, selectivity is imposed by two rings of negatively charged amino acids at the outer mouth of the funnel, which collect Na+ ions for transmission into the cell.[27]

Channel Inactivation

Inactivation gating is the process by which ion channels close in the face of continuing depolarization. Inactivation is characteristic of voltage-gated Na+ and Ca++ channels, as well as the K+ channels underlying I_{TO}. Inactivation begins after activation gating, as a second, slower conformational change in the molecule that halts the ion flux through the channel. Inactivation gating is thus closely coupled to activation gating, and ionic current flows only while both the activation and inactivation gates are open simultaneously. In Na+ channels, the inactivation gate is formed by the intracellular peptide linker between homologous domains III and IV (Figure 7-9A).[30] This peptide is postulated to act as a hinged lid, which moves upward to plug the ion pore (and thus halt current flow) shortly after membrane depolarization.[26] For the channel to recover from inactivation (i.e., to be ready to open in response to a new depolarizing stimulus), the III/IV linker peptide must resume its resting position, a process that requires hyperpolarization of the membrane to the resting potential for a finite period. Site-directed mutagenesis of the III/IV linker peptide has revealed a trio of hydrophobic amino acid residues (isoleucine, I; phenylalanine, F; and methionine, M), near to

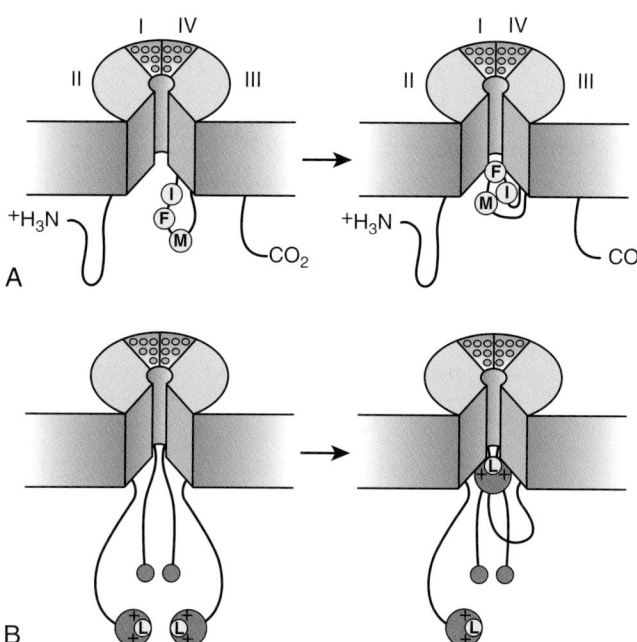

Figure 7-9   **Mechanism of inactivation of Na+ and K+ channels.** *A,* Hinged-lid mechanism of Na+-channel inactivation. *B,* Ball-and-chain mechanism of K+-channel inactivation. F, phenylalanine; I, isoleucine; M, methionine. *(A, B, From Catterall WA: Structure and function of voltage-gated ion channels. Annu Rev Biochem 64:493, 1995, by permission of the Annual Review of Biochemistry, Volume 64, ©1995, by Annual Reviews, Inc.)*

the domain III end of the peptide, which are crucial for normal channel inactivation. Replacement of just one of these residues (the phenylalanine) almost completely removes inactivation. These residues are postulated to latch on to a receptor in the channel pore to close the channel. The molecular basis of inactivation in K⁺ channels is rather different from Na⁺ channels. Because the four domains of K⁺ channels are formed by noncovalently linked molecules, there are no interdomain linkers to plug the channel pore. In K⁺ channels, a picture of an N-terminal ball-and-chain mechanism has emerged (see Figure 7-9B).[31] The terminal 20 or so amino acids are very hydrophobic and are postulated to swing up and attach to the open pore. The next few amino acids contain a number of positively charged residues that draw the whole N-terminal end up to the membrane. These two domains act as a ball. The remaining amino acids, up to the beginning of the transmembrane S1 segment, act as a chain. If the chain is made longer, inactivation is slower, and vice versa.

Clinical Correlates

Ion Channels and Antiarrhythmic Drugs

Drug therapy of cardiac arrhythmias would ideally be targeted at an individual ionic current, tailoring the cardiac action potential in such a way that abnormal excitability was reduced but normal rhythmicity was unaffected. This remains an as-yet unrealized goal. The prototype antiarrhythmic agents (e.g., disopyramide and quinidine) have diverse effects on cardiac excitability and, similar to agents introduced more recently, frequently exhibit significant proarrhythmic activity with potentially fatal consequences. In the Cardiac Arrhythmia Suppression Trial (CAST), mortality among asymptomatic postmyocardial infarction patients was approximately doubled by treatment with the potent Na⁺-channel–blocking agents encainide and flecainide—an effect likely attributable to slowing of conduction velocity with a consequent increase in fatal reentrant arrhythmias.[32] The results of the CAST prompted efforts to approach antiarrhythmic drug therapy by prolonging action potential duration (e.g., dofetilide)—a strategy with some support from animal studies, but one that also may cause proarrhythmia through induction of polymorphic ventricular tachycardia (the acquired long QT syndrome [LQTS]).[33] Drugs that prolong action potential duration all block I_{Kr}, and it is not clear that this therapeutic goal will result in arrhythmia control without induction of clinically significant proarrhythmia. The only drugs currently available that definitely prolong life by reducing fatal arrhythmias are β-blockers (e.g., ISIS-1, 1997), and these agents have no channel-blocking effects.

Ion Channels in Disease

Elucidation of the molecular mechanisms of the cardiac action potential is beginning to have direct impact on patient management. This is most obvious in patients with inherited genetic abnormalities of ion channels leading to cardiac sudden death, and two groups of diseases serve to illustrate this point: the LQTS and Brugada syndrome. An understanding of the molecular mechanism of cardiac electrical excitability is also starting to lead to the emergence of gene therapies and stem cell therapies that may in the future allow manipulation of cardiac rhythm and function.

Long QT Syndromes

This rare group of ion-channel abnormalities causes abnormal prolongation of the cardiac action potential, resulting in early afterdepolarizations (i.e., oscillations in the action potential during the plateau phase) and death from polymorphic ventricular tachycardia (torsades de pointes type). To date, six LQTS subtypes have been identified on the basis of the affected gene. They are numbered sequentially according to the date of discovery (Table 7-1), and all the loci so far identified encode ion channels except for LQT4. LQTS occurs because of disruption of cardiac repolarization, and in principle this can occur either from enhancement of inward depolarizing current or reduction of outward current. LQT3 is a gain-of-function mutation of the cardiac

TABLE 7-1	Spectrum of Long QT Syndrome			
Type	Gene	Current	Chromosome	Comment
LQT1	KCNQ1 (KvLQT1)	I_{Ks}	11	Induced by stress and exercise
LQT2	KCNH2 (hERG)	I_{Kr}	7	Noise, emotional stress
LQT3	SCN5A	I_{Na}	3	Sleep, β-blockers less effective
LQT4	ANKB	—	4	Ankyrin B, transporter accessory protein
LQT5	KCNE1 (minK)	I_{Ks}	21	Associated congenital deafness
LQT6	KCNE2 (MiRP1)	I_{Kr}	21	Drugs, exercise

Na⁺ channel that results in failure of channel inactivation, most commonly from a deletion of three amino acids from the inactivation gate. LQT1 and LQT2 result from mutations of the delayed rectifier K channels that underlie I_{Ks} and I_{Kr}, and LQT5 and LQT6 result in reductions of I_{Kr} and I_{Ks} through mutations in channel accessory subunits. Loss of repolarizing current results in prolongation of the QT interval, and this leads to the syndrome. LQT4 is unique in that it results from a mutation in ankyrin B, an adapter protein that binds to the Na⁺ pump and Na⁺/Ca⁺⁺ exchanger. The resulting effects on cellular Ca⁺⁺ homeostasis cause ventricular arrhythmias.[34] Identification of the molecular substrate for LQTS will allow detection of the disease in asymptomatic carriers and may in the future allow targeted gene therapy; these issues are discussed in more detail later in the Genetic Cardiovascular Medicine section.

Brugada Syndrome

The Brugada syndrome also is a group of ion-channel abnormalities that affect cardiac repolarization and result in cardiac sudden death. It is characterized by incomplete right bundle-branch block and persistent ST-segment elevation in the anterior precordial leads of the electrocardiogram (ECG).[35] Cases for which the genotype is available appear to result from channel mutations that reduce depolarizing Na⁺ current. This results in loss of the action potential dome, an effect that is most marked in the right ventricular epicardium where the transient outward current I_{TO1} is strongly expressed (hence the ST-segment elevation in the anterior chest ECG leads). Early repolarization of the epicardial action potential results in a transmural repolarization gradient, and this can lead to reentry and sudden cardiac death.[36] In more than two thirds of patients with Brugada syndrome, the genetic locus is unknown, and much work remains to be done to elucidate the mechanism of this condition.

CONTROLLING CARDIAC FUNCTIONING: RECEPTORS

Receptors are membrane proteins that transduce signals from the outside to the inside of the cell. When a *ligand*—a hormone carried in blood, a neurotransmitter released from a nerve ending, or a local messenger released from neighboring cells—binds to the receptor, it induces a conformational change in the receptor molecule. This changes the configuration of the intracellular segment of the receptor and results in activation of intracellular systems, with a variety of potential effects, ranging from enhanced phosphorylation and changes in intracellular (second) messenger concentrations to activation of ion channels.

Receptors

Receptors are grouped in several broad classes, the *protein tyrosine kinase receptors* and the *G-protein–coupled receptors* (GPCRs) being the most important ones. The protein tyrosine kinase receptors are large molecular

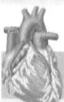

BOX 7-4. G-PROTEIN–COUPLED RECEPTORS

- β-Adrenergic receptors
- α-Adrenergic receptors
- Muscarinic acetylcholine receptors
- Adenosine A_1 receptors
- ATP receptors
- Histamine H_2 receptors
- Vasoactive intestinal peptide receptors
- Angiotensin II receptors

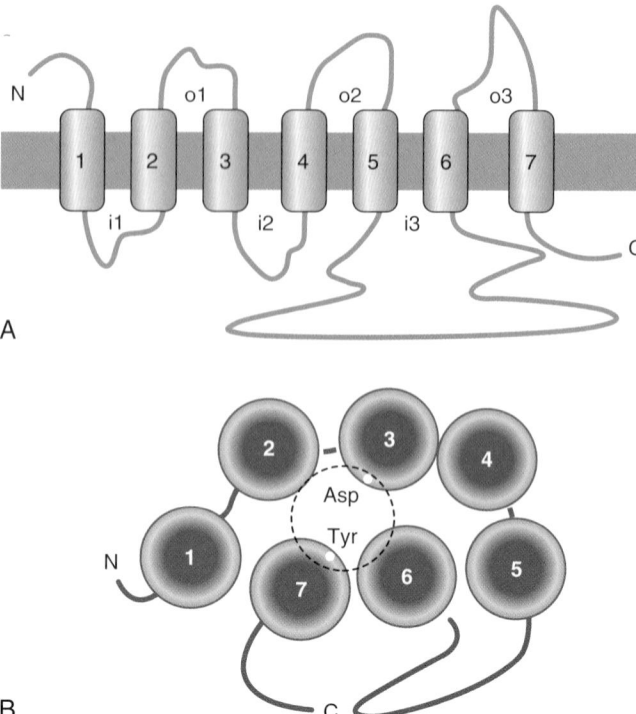

Figure 7-10 **Model of G-protein–coupled receptor.** *A,* Linear model. Seven hydrophobic stretches of approximately 20 amino acids are present, presumably forming α helices that pass through the cell membrane, thus forming seven transmembrane domains. (t1–t7). Extracellularly, the amino terminus (N) and three outside loops (o1 through o3) are found; intracellularly there are similarly three loops (i1 through i3) and the carboxy-terminus (C). *B,* Top-down view. Although in *(A),* the molecule is pictured as a linear complex, the transmembrane domains are thought to be in close proximity, forming an ellipse with a central ligand-binding cavity *(dashed circle).* Asp and Tyr refer to two amino acids important for ligand interaction. G-protein binding takes place at the i3 loop and the carboxy terminus.

complexes that incorporate phosphorylating enzyme activity in the intracellular segment. Ligand binding induces activation of this enzyme activity. Because phosphorylation is one of the major mechanisms of cellular regulation (see, for example, the phosphorylation of the Ca^{++} channel described earlier), such receptors can have a variety of cellular effects (Box 7-4). GPCRs are much smaller than protein tyrosine kinase receptors. Ligand binding results in activation of an associated protein *(G protein)* that subsequently influences cellular processes. The receptors discussed in this section all belong to the GPCR superfamily, and the properties of this class are discussed in some detail.

The number of GPCRs is large. For more than 100 receptors, the function has been defined. In addition, the olfactory epithelium expresses hundreds of GPCRs, which are thought to mediate the sense of smell, and another large group, with unknown function, is expressed on sperm cells. Taken together, the superfamily has more than 1000 members.

All of these have similar molecular characteristics. They are generally several hundred to 1000 amino acids in length and contain 7 stretches of 20 to 25 hydrophobic amino acids. These hydrophobic domains are thought to form α helices and traverse the membrane, thus anchoring the receptor to the cell (Figure 7-10). For this reason, the family is often referred to as the "seven transmembrane" family. Although crystallographic data are not yet available for the clinically relevant GPCRs, it is thought that the seven-transmembrane domains arrange in a funnel-like structure, the inside of which forms the ligand-binding domain. The intracellular domains, particularly the third intracellular loop and the C terminus, bind to the G protein.

The heart and blood vessels express a variety of GPCRs, the most important of which are discussed later. The β-adrenergic and muscarinic acetylcholine receptors are those most important for regulation of cardiac functioning, but a number of others play relevant modulatory roles. These include the α-adrenergic, adenosine A_1, ATP, histamine H_2, vasoactive intestinal peptide (VIP), and angiotensin II receptors.

G Proteins

As do the receptors, G proteins (GTP-binding proteins) also come in two families: the small (cytoplasmic) G proteins and the heterotrimeric (membrane) G proteins. Common to both groups is their mechanism of function. In their resting state, they bind a molecule of guanosine diphosphate (GDP). When activated by a GPCR (in the case of heterotrimeric G proteins) or by an intracellular messenger (in the case of cytoplasmic G proteins), this GDP is exchanged for a GTP molecule. The activated G protein can now perform functions within the cell, as discussed later, until it is inactivated when an intrinsic enzyme activity hydrolyzes the GTP to a GDP. The critical point about this hydrolytic activity is that it is (molecularly speaking) very slow, on the order of seconds. As a result, brief activation of a receptor (on the order of milliseconds) can lead to more prolonged activation of the intracellular signaling machinery.

GPCRs bind to *heterotrimeric* G proteins, so called because they consist of three subunits: α, β, and γ. Of these, the β and γ subunits are so tightly associated that, for practical purposes, they can be viewed as a single unit, often termed the βγ unit. The α subunit contains both the GDP-GTP binding domain and the hydrolytic activity, and it was classically thought to be the "business end" of the molecule, with the βγ unit

roaming freely and inactively, serving as an anchor and a sink of free α units. This turns out not to be the case; the βγ subunit has activating functions as well, as is discussed later in relation to the muscarinic K^+ channel.

Several classes of heterotrimeric G proteins exist, indicated by subscripts (Box 7-5). The classic types are G_s and G_i, which stimulate and inhibit, respectively, the enzyme adenylate cyclase, thereby leading to changes in cytoplasmic cAMP concentrations. G_q proteins (and G_o in brain) activate phospholipase C (PLC) and thereby induce the generation of inositol-1,4,5-triphosphate (IP_3) and diacylglycerol (DAG) from phosphatidylinositol bisphosphate (PIP_2). IP_3 acts on its own receptor/channel complex on intracellular Ca^{++} storage sites and induces release of Ca^{++} from these sites, thereby increasing intracellular Ca^{++} concentrations. DAG activates protein kinase C (PKC), leading to phosphorylation of a variety of targets (including the receptors that initiated the cascade). In recent years,

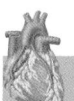

BOX 7-5. G-PROTEIN CLASSES

- G_s: activates adenylate cyclase
- G_i: inhibits adenylate cyclase
- G_q: activates phospholipase C
- G_o: subtype of G_i, found mostly in brain, Ca^{++} also activates phospholipase C
- G_k: subtype of G_i, linked to K^+ channels

cloning efforts have shown each of these classes of G proteins to consist of a number of members, but their functional differences are as yet incompletely defined.

Adrenergic Receptors and Signaling Pathways

Adrenergic Receptors

Main control over cardiac contractility is provided by the β-adrenergic signaling pathways, which can be activated by circulating catecholamines (derived from the adrenal glands) or those released locally from adrenergic nerve endings on the myocardium.

The two main subtypes of β-adrenergic receptors are the β_1 and β_2 subclasses. A β_3 subtype exists as well, but its role in the cardiovascular system is unclear[37]; its most important role is in fat cells. Both β_1 and β_2 receptors are present in the heart, and both contribute to the increased contractility induced by catecholamine stimulation (this is different from the situation in vascular muscle, where β-adrenergic stimulation induces relaxation). Under normal conditions, the relative ratio of β_1 to β_2 receptors in heart is approximately 70:30, but as discussed later, this ratio can be changed dramatically by cardiac disease.

Structurally, as well as functionally, the various β-adrenergic receptors are closely related. Both couple to G_s proteins and, as described earlier, thereby activate adenylate cyclase, leading to increased intracellular levels of cAMP. Some differences in their intracellular signaling are likely, however. For example, it has been suggested that β_2 receptors couple more effectively than β_1 receptors and induce greater changes in cAMP levels.[38] In addition to their effect on cAMP signaling, β receptors may couple to myocardial Ca channels.[39] However, these additional actions are species specific, and care should be taken in extrapolating animal data to humans.

The inotropic and electrophysiologic effects of β-adrenergic signaling are an indirect result of increases in intracellular cAMP levels. cAMP activates a specific protein kinase (PKA) that, in turn, is able to phosphorylate several important cardiac ion channels (including L-type Ca^{++} channels, Na^+ channels, voltage-dependent K^+ channels, and Cl^- channels). Phosphorylation alters channel functioning, and it is these changes in membrane electrophysiologic events that modify myocardial behavior.

The α-adrenergic receptors, like their β-receptor counterparts, can be divided into two groups: the α_1 and α_2 receptors. Both of these groups consist of several closely related subtypes, with different tissue distributions and functions that are as yet not very well differentiated. In general, α_1 receptors couple to G_q proteins, thereby activating PLC, which results in increases in intracellular Ca^{++} concentrations. α_2 receptors couple to G_i, which inhibits adenylate cyclase, thereby reducing intracellular cAMP concentrations.

The primary role of α receptors is in the vasculature, where α_1 receptors on vascular smooth muscle are the main mediators of neuronally mediated vasoconstriction. α_2 receptors on the neurons themselves function in a negative feedback loop to control α-adrenergic vasoconstriction.

In the heart, the primary subtype present is α_1. Activation of these receptors leads to a modest increase in cardiac contractility.[40]

Regulation of β-Receptor Functioning

Whereas β-receptor stimulation allows the dramatic increases in cardiac output of which the human heart is capable, it is clearly intended to be a temporary measure. Prolonged adrenergic stimulation has highly detrimental effects on the myocardium; the pronounced increases in cAMP levels are followed by increases in intracellular Ca^{++} concentration, reductions in RNA and protein synthesis, and finally, cell death. Thus, β-receptor modulation is best viewed as part of the "fight-or-flight" response: beneficial in the short term, but detrimental if depended on for too long. Cardiac failure, in particular, has been shown to be associated with prolonged increases in adrenergic stimulation—even to the extent that norepinephrine "spillover" from cardiac nerve endings can be detected in the blood of patients in heart failure.[41]

For this reason, the regulation of β-receptor functioning has received significant attention, and it is now known that a number of mechanisms exist that are capable of modifying adrenergic responsiveness of the myocyte. Unfortunately, it appears that the reduction of adrenergic responsiveness necessary to prevent cell death in the face of adrenergic overstimulation may be in large part responsible for the decreased myocardial performance that is the hallmark of cardiac failure.

One mechanism for decreasing β-receptor functioning is the *downregulation* (i.e., decrease in density) of receptors. In cardiac failure, receptor levels are reduced up to 50%. β_1 receptors downregulate more than β_2 receptors do, resulting in a change in the β_1:β_2 ratio. As mentioned earlier, the normal ratio is approximately 4:1; in the failing heart, it is approximately 3:2.[42] Various molecular mechanisms exist for this downregulation. In the long term, receptors are degraded and permanently removed from the cell surface. In the short term, receptors can be temporarily removed from the cell membrane and "stored" in intracellular vesicles, where they are not accessible by an agonist. These receptors are, however, fully functional and can be recycled to the membrane when adrenergic overstimulation has ceased.[43]

An additional method by which β-adrenergic receptor functioning can be modified is through phosphorylation of the agonist-occupied receptor by a specific β-adrenergic receptor kinase (β-ARK, which can itself be activated by $\beta\gamma$ subunits).[44] Phosphorylation by this kinase allows binding to the receptor of a protein, β-arrestin, that inhibits receptor functioning.[45] In addition, the β receptor can be phosphorylated by PKA, which itself can be activated by several other receptors. The detrimental actions of adrenergic overstimulation can also be modified by activation of muscarinic receptors, as discussed in the next section.

Despite the existence of these various regulatory mechanisms and the known detrimental effects of adrenergic overstimulation, paradoxic increases in β-receptor functioning occur in clinical disease states. For example, under ischemic conditions, β receptors are upregulated, so that after periods of ischemia as brief as 15 minutes, significant increases in expressed and functional receptor levels are found. Interestingly, reperfusion rapidly decreases the number of receptors back to their normal levels.

Muscarinic Receptors and Signaling Pathways

Muscarinic Acetylcholine Receptors

The second major receptor type involved in cardiac regulation is the muscarinic receptor. Although five subtypes of muscarinic receptors exist, only one of these (M2) is present in cardiac tissue. Most of these muscarinic receptors are present on the atria. Indeed, it was thought until recently that there was no vagal innervation of the ventricles, but this view turns out to be incorrect. The ventricles are innervated by the vagus, and muscarinic receptors are, in fact, present in the ventricles, albeit at lower concentrations than in the atria; the amount of muscarinic receptor protein in atrium is approximately twofold greater than in ventricle (200 to 250 vs. 70 to 100 fmol/mg protein).[46] Thus, although the primary function of cardiac muscarinic signaling is heart rate control through actions at the atrial level, vagal stimulation is, in fact, able to directly influence ventricular functioning.

M2-muscarinic receptors couple to G_i proteins, thereby inhibiting adenylate cyclase and decreasing intracellular levels of cAMP. In fact, the M2 receptors have been used as an elegant model to determine the site of G-protein binding to the receptor. Exchanging approximately 20 amino acids of the third intracellular loop (i3) (see Figure 7-10) between M2 and M3 receptors resulted in altered coupling; M2 receptors mutated in this manner were now able to release Ca^{++} from intracellular IP_3-sensitive stores by coupling to G_q.[47]

In the impulse-generating system of the heart, a more important signaling mechanism than changes in cAMP is opening of an inwardly rectifying K^+ channel (K_{ACh}) in the plasma membrane. The coupling between M2 receptor and K_{ACh} is performed by G_K, a member of the

G_i class of G proteins. Interestingly, it is not the α subunit of G_K that activates K_{ACh}, but rather the $\beta\gamma$ subunit.[48] As discussed later, cardiac adenosine receptors couple to this channel as well.

Whereas the adenylate cyclase system is ubiquitous, differential expression of K_{ACh} determines the actions of muscarinic signaling on the heart. K_{ACh} is largely absent from ventricular tissue. Therefore, in the ventricle, muscarinic signaling will primarily involve decreases in cAMP levels, and because these are low under resting conditions, little effect will be seen unless the heart has been stimulated previously by adrenergic agents. In other words, in the absence of adrenergic stimulation, acetylcholine will have little effect on the ventricle; in conditions of high adrenergic tone, however, muscarinic stimulation can modify the adrenergic effects, as discussed in the next section.

Regulation of Muscarinic Acetylcholine Receptors

Whereas the role of atrial muscarinic receptors in impulse generation and the conduction system is straightforward, the role of ventricular muscarinic receptors is not as clear. It appears that under nonstressed conditions, muscarinic signaling has little influence on cardiac contractility. In contrast, the system might act as a brake on overstimulation by adrenergic receptors (see earlier discussion). The effects of muscarinic signaling, which virtually all oppose those induced by adrenergic signaling (because muscarinic receptors couple to G_i and adrenergic receptors couple to G_s), may counteract adrenergic effects and thereby preserve cardiac functioning during prolonged stress responses.

Unfortunately, these compensatory mechanisms may not be available in the old heart. Increased age is accompanied by changes in cardiac muscarinic receptor expression that might make it more difficult for the heart to respond to adrenergic stress. In senescent rats, muscarinic receptor density was decreased by approximately 50%.[49] Adrenergic receptor levels also were decreased, but to a lesser extent. As a result, the adrenergic/muscarinic receptor ratio is increased, from 0.29 in young adults to 0.42 in senescent animals. Although the physiologic implications of these changes are not well known, the data at least suggest that the muscarinic systems in the aged heart might not be as well prepared to react to prolonged adrenergic stimulation, such as observed in hypertension and cardiac failure.

With the exception of age, muscarinic receptors are little affected in settings that profoundly modify β-receptor expression. There are, for example, no consistent data supporting changes in muscarinic receptor expression in hypertension, cardiac failure, or ischemic heart disease.[50,51] Therefore, imbalances between adrenergic and muscarinic stimulation might occur in each of these situations.

■ Regulation of G-Protein Functioning

In view of the profound changes in GPCR expression that occur in various disease states, the expression and function of G proteins in cardiovascular disease have been studied with interest. G_s proteins appear unchanged in cardiac failure, both in expression level and in function. With G_i proteins, the situation is more interesting, because $G_{i\alpha}$ is considered to have a secondary role in addition to its inhibition of adenylate cyclase. Under normal conditions, G_i is present in greater amounts than G_s. Activation of receptors coupled to G_i would, therefore, lead to the release of a large number of free $\beta\gamma$ subunits. These could combine with any free $G_{s\alpha}$, thereby making it unavailable for activation of adenylate cyclase.[52] In addition, these $\beta\gamma$ units can enhance the phosphorylation of β receptors by β-ARK.[53] In failing human cardiac tissue, the amount of G_i (as assessed by ADP-ribosylation by pertussis toxin) is increased.[54] Although this would be expected to make muscarinic signaling more efficacious (thereby helping counteract the adrenergic overstimulation), it has been difficult to correlate these changes with alterations in adenylate cyclase functioning. It is similarly unclear whether the reported increases in G_i levels are a result of increased mRNA expression or increased stability of the G protein itself.

The catalytic subunit of adenylate cyclase appears little influenced by cardiac disease. Pressure overload is the only situation in which a consistent decrease in its activity has been observed.[55]

■ Other Receptors

As stated earlier, the heart and vasculature express a large variety of GPCRs apart from the adrenergic and muscarinic receptors. A few examples are mentioned here. Angiotensin receptors mediate hormonal vasoconstriction in the vascular tree and are also present in the heart, although their function there is not fully defined. Receptors for several purinergic compounds are expressed in the heart as well and are the subject of intense investigation, as discussed in the next section. In addition, histamine H_2 and VIP receptors are present, the former mediating the inotropic action of histamine.

Although less is understood about the role and regulation of these receptors than about their adrenergic and cholinergic counterparts, it is clear that some are affected by cardiovascular disease. For example, VIP receptors are downregulated by 70% in idiopathic dilated cardiomyopathy (DCM), whereas histamine receptors are unaffected.[56] In general, receptors coupled to G_i show little alteration in expression and function during disease states, whereas G_s-coupled receptors are affected more profoundly.

■ Clinical Correlates

Understanding of the role of adenosine in cardiac regulation has expanded significantly over the past years. Its established use as an antiarrhythmic compound and its probable role in cardiac preconditioning are two examples of clinical advances resulting from this increase in understanding. Adenosine acts through a GPCR, activating several intracellular signaling systems. This section discusses the molecular aspects of adenosine signaling, as well as their clinical implications. More detailed recent reviews on the topic are available.[57,58]

■ Adenosine Signaling

Although adenosine can be generated by several pathways, in the heart, it is usually found as a dephosphorylation product of AMP.[59] Because AMP accumulation is a sign of a low cellular energy charge, an increased adenosine concentration is a marker of unbalanced energy demand and supply; thus, ischemia, hypoxemia, and increased catecholamine concentrations are all associated with increased adenosine release.[60] Adenosine is rapidly degraded by various pathways, both intracellularly and extracellularly. As a result, its half-life is extremely short, on the order of 1 second.[61] Therefore, it is not only a marker of a cardiac "energy crisis," but its concentrations will fluctuate virtually instantly with the energy balance of the heart; it provides a real-time indication of the cellular energy situation.

Adenosine signals through GPCR of the purinergic receptor family. Two subclasses of purinoceptors exist: P_1 (high affinity for adenosine and AMP) and P_2 (high affinity for ATP and ADP). The P_1 receptor class can be divided into two main receptor subtypes: A_1 and A_2. A_1 receptors are present mostly in the heart and, when activated, inhibit adenylate cyclase; A_2 receptors are present in the vasculature and, when activated, stimulate adenylate cyclase. The A_2 receptors mediate the vasodilatory actions of adenosine. The A_1 receptors mediate its complex cardiac effects, and they are the topic of the remainder of this section.

The A_1 adenosine receptor couples to (at least) two intracellular signaling systems. Both of these actions are mediated by G proteins of the G_i class. The first intracellular system is one already encountered: the K_{ACh} channel. Presumably, through the same G_K protein, adenosine activates this channel in the same way as does M2 muscarinic stimulation, and the cardiac electrophysiologic effects of acetylcholine and adenosine are therefore quite similar. The specific effect of adenosine depends on the cardiac tissue studied because K_{ACh} expression varies with location. As has been discussed, whereas the channel is present in large amounts in the atrial conduction system and atrial myocardium, it is virtually absent in the ventricle. Therefore, in the unstimulated heart, adenosine shortens the atrial action potential, decreases atrial refractoriness and decreases atrial contractile force, but it is almost without effect on the ventricle.[62]

The second intracellular signaling system activated is a G_i protein that inhibits adenylate cyclase. As cAMP levels are quite low under resting conditions, this mechanism plays little role until cAMP concentrations are increased by adrenergic stimulation of the heart. Therefore, cAMP-mediated cardiac actions of adenosine are observed only under conditions of adrenergic drive. Because the adenylate cyclase system is present throughout the heart, its effects are widespread; L-type Ca^{++} channel functioning is diminished (by inhibiting cAMP-induced phosphorylation of the channel) in atrium as well as ventricle, resulting in decreased inotropy and shortening of the action potential.[63]

Antiarrhythmic Actions of Adenosine

From these molecular actions of adenosine, its clinical effects easily can be deduced. The antiarrhythmic actions are largely a result of its activation of K_{ACh}. Recalling the tissue distribution of K_{ACh}, it could be anticipated that adenosine will be much more effective in the treatment of supraventricular arrhythmias than ventricular arrhythmias, and such is indeed the case. Because of its negative chronotropic effects on the atrial conduction system, the compound is most effective in treating supraventricular tachycardias that contain a reentrant pathway involving the AV node. The efficacy of adenosine in terminating such tachycardias has been reported as greater than 90%.[64] In contrast, it is consistently ineffective in tachycardias not involving the AV node.[65]

Most ventricular tachycardias are insensitive to adenosine. The only exception is again easily deduced from the compound's molecular mechanism of action; a rare form of exercise- or catecholamine-induced ventricular tachycardia responds promptly to adenosine.[66] Presumably, in this setting, adenosine-mediated inhibition of adenylate cyclase counteracts the stimulatory effects of catecholamines.

Occasionally, adenosine may be useful because of its ability to differentiate between true ventricular tachycardia and supraventricular tachycardia with aberrant conduction. In view of concerns that the often already precarious cardiovascular status of patients in ventricular tachycardia could be temporarily worsened by vasodilatation, many clinicians have been hesitant to use adenosine for this purpose. In contrast, it has been found very useful as a diagnostic agent for supraventricular tachycardias. Care should be taken, however, in the patient with Wolff–Parkinson–White syndrome, who may respond with increases in ventricular rate and hemodynamic deterioration.

The side effects of adenosine would be significant if the half-life of the compound was not as short as it is. Many of the adverse effects result from activation of A_2 receptors in the vascular system: flushing, headache, and light-headedness. Chest pain, anxiety, nausea, vomiting, and occasional bronchospasm are seen as well. However, these effects are usually short-lived, and if the patient has been adequately warned about their occurrence, they are rarely of significance. Profound but brief electrophysiologic responses are observed on the ECG, ranging from premature atrial and ventricular beats to short periods of asystole. Again, these are rarely of significance.

Adenosine and Myocardial Preconditioning

Myocardial preconditioning is the phenomenon in which brief exposure of the myocardium to ischemic conditions will allow it to withstand a subsequent, more prolonged, exposure. The phenomenon has received much attention because its application in the clinical setting might allow the heart to better withstand, for instance, the insults of cardiac surgery. Thus, the mechanisms of this effect were investigated in the hope that they might be activated directly, without the need for ischemia. A variety of mechanisms might account for preconditioning, as has been reviewed recently.[58,67]

A G-protein–linked K^+ channel located on the mitochondrial membrane, the mitochondrial K_{ATP} channel (mitoK_{ATP}), is a key mediator in myocardial preconditioning. Opening of this channel using compounds that selectively open mitoK_{ATP} without affecting other cellular K_{ATP} channels[68] has been shown to have a protective effect, whereas inhibition of the channel (with the channel blocker glibenclamide) increases

ischemic damage to the myocardium. For example, abolishment by glibenclamide of preconditioning could be shown in a study measuring ST-segment changes and cardiac pain in patients undergoing balloon angioplasty.[69] Similar findings have been observed in various animal studies. K_{ATP}, like K_{ACh}, belongs to the class of G-protein–coupled inward rectifier-type channels; its structure is indicated in Figure 7-10. In contrast with K_{ACh}, however, it appears to be modulated primarily by changes in intracellular ATP derivatives. For example, intracellular increases in ATP levels have a direct inhibitory effect on the channel. In addition, K_{ATP} can be modulated by PKC, which phosphorylates the channel. PKC can be activated directly by ischemic conditions or by activation of α-adrenergic and adenosine receptors. In addition, adenosine also may be able to influence behavior of K_{ATP} in the same manner that it regulates K_{ACh}: through a G_i protein.[70] The mechanisms by which mitoK_{ATP} opening is protective are still a focus of investigation. Potential beneficial effects involve inhibition of mitochondrial Ca^{++} uptake, regulation of mitochondrial volume, and modulation of the generation of reactive oxygen species. Of interest from the anesthesiologist's point of view are observations that volatile anesthetics induce preconditioning by similar mechanisms. For example, sevoflurane preconditions human myocardium against hypoxia through activation of K_{ATP} channels and activation of A_1-adenosine receptors.[71] Similarly, lidocaine was shown to induce protection against inflammatory stimulation of endothelial and vascular smooth muscle cells by affecting mitoK_{ATP}.[72]

ANESTHETIC ACTIONS

Although the functioning and the physiologic role of the receptors and channels described are of obvious importance to the anesthesiologist, from a practical perspective, the interactions between anesthetic drugs and these signaling molecules are at least as relevant. As mentioned at the end of the previous section, effects of anesthetics on such proteins may be beneficial to the cardiovascular system. However, detrimental interactions may exist as well.

Volatile anesthetics are administered in extremely high concentrations as compared with most other pharmacologic agents. Most commonly used drugs are administered in doses that result in micromolar blood concentrations. This reflects the fact that these compounds are sufficiently potent so that a half-maximal effect on the site of action requires only low micromolar concentrations. Anesthetics, in contrast, require low millimolar concentrations in blood to be effective, almost a thousand times as much. Although they commonly are referred to as "potent agents," they are certainly not very potent as compared with other pharmacologic compounds. As a result, it is not surprising that they have a wide range of actions in addition to their primary effect site (which, of course, is still not completely defined). In addition, volatile anesthetics are lipophilic compounds, and if, under laboratory conditions, concentrations are increased even further, they can be found to interact with almost any preparation exhibiting a certain degree of lipophilicity. As a result, data exist demonstrating interactions between volatile anesthetics and virtually every component of the cardiovascular system. The issue, then, is not with which channels and receptors the anesthetics interact, but which of all these interactions are clinically important, and this has been difficult to determine. A first test that should be applied, of course, is that of reasonable concentrations; if effects are not observed at 1 to 2 minimal alveolar concentration (MAC) equivalents, it is unlikely that an interaction has clinical relevance. As many experiments are performed at temperatures below 37°C, temperature correction of anesthetic solubility is an important issue. It is also important that actions are shown in several models. Effects observed in an isolated system may not necessarily be reproduced in an organ or whole-animal model; in that case, the relevance of the finding is in doubt. This issue has been reviewed in some detail.[73]

Injected anesthetics are less troublesome in this regard. Most of these act at defined sites (the γ-aminobutyric acid [$GABA_A$] receptor/channel complex for most of them; ketamine's primary action on the N-methyl-D-aspartate [NMDA] receptor/channel is an exception), they are more potent, and they are therefore active at significantly lower concentrations. However, this does not necessarily mean that they are without other interactions, as their various side-effect profiles show.

This section focuses on some of the interactions between anesthetics and the molecular systems described in previous sections; those interactions for which there is most support in the literature, and which, in addition, help explain some of the specific side effects of anesthetic drugs. Thus, rather than providing a detailed overview of all interactions reported, several well-described examples with probable clinical relevance are presented. Unfortunately, many of these interactions have not yet been described in the molecular and submolecular detail desired. Although it may be known that an anesthetic inhibits functioning of a receptor or channel type, it is usually not defined where in the molecule this interaction takes place. Most times it cannot even be ascertained that the interaction occurs with the protein itself, rather than with the lipid membrane environment surrounding the protein. More detailed site-directed mutagenesis and the study of chimeric molecules are likely to shed light on these issues.

Interactions with Channels: Ca^{++} Channels

Of the variety of ion channels present in the heart, those most likely to be significantly affected by anesthetics in the clinical setting are the voltage-gated Ca^{++} channels. Although interactions with other cardiac channel types may also be relevant (particularly with K^+ channels, such as the K_{ATP} channel, described earlier), they have not yet received as much research attention, and it is not yet possible to draw firm conclusions about the clinical relevance of these interactions. Hence, in this section, the focus is on Ca^{++} channels only.

Anesthetic actions on cardiac Ca^{++} channels have been studied in a variety of models. The original observations that halothane blocked Ca^{++} flux into heart cells date back approximately 30 years,[74] and much specific information has been gained since. In particular, voltage-clamp and patch-clamp studies have contributed significantly to the understanding of the interactions between anesthetics and Ca^{++} channels, and have elegantly described the effects of anesthetics on electrophysiologic behavior. However, it is not straightforward to assign the observed electrophysiologic effects to a molecular substrate. This issue is only beginning to be addressed with the use of recombinant technology.

Almost all volatile anesthetics inhibit L-type Ca^{++} channels.[75,76] Inhibition is modest, approximately 25% to 30% at 1 MAC anesthetic, but certainly sufficient to account for the physiologic changes induced by the anesthetics. Volatile anesthetics decrease peak current and, in addition, tend to increase the rate of inactivation.[77] Hence maximal Ca^{++} current is depressed, and duration of Ca^{++} current is shortened. Together, these actions significantly limit the Ca^{++} influx into the cardiac myocyte. However, some specific actions may depend on the particular compound studied. In the presence of β-adrenergic stimulation, halothane, but not sevoflurane, is associated with a long-lasting enhancement of Ca^{++} channel function that may contribute to its proarrhythmic effects.[78] Xenon is without effect on cardiac Ca^{++} channels, explaining, in large part, its lack of effect on myocardial contractility. Other types of Ca^{++} channels have different sensitivities. Neuronal (N-type) channels have been shown to be quite resistant to volatile anesthetics. T-type channels in general tend to be much more sensitive than L-type channels; at clinical concentrations of most volatile anesthetics, T currents are inhibited 50% or more.

The effects of volatile anesthetics on cardiac Ca^{++} channels can be modulated greatly by concurrent interactions of the compounds on other cardiac signaling systems. As discussed later, volatile anesthetics inhibit function of several types of muscarinic acetylcholine receptor systems. Because Ca channel function can be inhibited by muscarinic signaling, as discussed earlier, clinicians would anticipate additional interactions when this system is exposed to volatile anesthetics, and such is the case. Halothane and isoflurane further inhibited currents through Ca^{++} channels when either volatile anesthetic was applied after inhibition produced by prior muscarinic stimulation. However, when muscarinic receptors were stimulated after administration of volatile anesthetic, its effect was reduced. Thus, whereas volatile anesthetics directly inhibit L-type channels, they also interfere with channel modulation by GPCR.[79]

Not only volatile but also injected anesthetics have been reported to inhibit cardiac L-type Ca^{++} channels in some models. However, the concentrations used generally exceed those used in clinical practice. Thiopental and methohexital block L-type Ca^{++} currents.[76,80] Similarly, propofol has been reported to inhibit these channels, but at concentrations well beyond the clinical range.

Interactions with Receptors: Muscarinic Receptors

As with cardiac channels, anesthetic interactions with a variety of GPCRs may be of potential relevance to cardiovascular side effects of anesthetic compounds. However, most of these potential interactions have not been described in significant detail. The two main control systems of myocardial functioning, the muscarinic and adrenergic systems, have been studied to some extent, and a generalizing conclusion can be that muscarinic receptors are and adrenergic receptors are not sensitive to many anesthetics. Hence the focus is on muscarinic receptors in this section.

Determination of anesthetic effects on GPCR is in some ways more complex than determination of the effects on channels. Although the receptors are smaller and consist of a single subunit only, they are only one part of very complex signaling pathways. Therefore, it is not sufficient to determine the effects on the receptor itself; actions on intracellular signaling should be investigated as well.

There is no doubt that at least some volatile anesthetics interfere with muscarinic signaling. Unfortunately, most of these investigations have not studied the heart, or even looked specifically at the M2 receptor, the only subtype expressed in cardiac tissue.

Aronstam et al[81] published a series of articles reporting the effect of various anesthetics on muscarinic receptor binding. A summary of their findings has appeared in print as well. Several studies investigated the effect of halothane on agonist and antagonist binding.[82,83] The conclusions drawn from this work were: (1) the anesthetic enhanced antagonist binding by slowing the rate of ligand dissociation, and (2) the anesthetic inhibited agonist binding (by 48%, using 10% halothane).

The site of action of these effects was studied in more detail by investigating the interactions of anesthetics with G-protein functioning.[84] As discussed earlier, G proteins are activated by GDP-GTP exchange. An intrinsic, but remarkably slow, enzyme activity hydrolyzes GTP back to GDP, thereby inactivating the G protein after several seconds. While active, the G protein is no longer able to couple to the receptor, and uncoupled receptors exhibit a decreased affinity for their agonist. This decrease in activity can be induced in the experimental setting by including a nonhydrolyzable analog of GTP [such as Gpp(NH)p] in the reaction mixture, resulting in irreversibly activated G proteins. This effect is known as the GTP shift in receptor affinity. Halothane shifts the Gpp(NH)p concentration–response relation to the right. In other words, a greater concentration of the GTP analog was necessary to induce a similar decrease in agonist binding. In the absence and presence of 5% halothane, the half-maximal inhibitory concentration (IC_{50}) values for the inhibitory effect on agonist binding of Gpp(NH)p were 0.7 and 83 μM, respectively—a 100-fold difference. These findings were interpreted as an ability of halothane to stabilize high-affinity G-protein–receptor complexes.

Therefore, it appears that halothane affects receptor binding, as well as receptor–G-protein interaction. In a subsequent study, the effect of the anesthetic on G-protein functioning—its ability to hydrolyze bound GTP—was investigated. Halothane was found not to inhibit binding of radiolabeled GTP analog to G proteins.[82] However, the anesthetic completely blocked the stimulation of G-protein GTPase activity induced by acetylcholine, with a half-maximal effect at the clinically relevant halothane concentration of 0.3 mM. The site of this effect was not determined. Largely similar findings were obtained with other anesthetics. Halothane also has been shown to interfere with G-protein–mediated

Ca++ sensitization in airway smooth muscle by inhibiting G proteins.[85] More recently, however, the interaction between halothane and purified, recombinant G_i was investigated. In contrast with the findings described earlier, no effect of the anesthetic on G_i protein function was found.[86] Hence the earlier results might have been contaminated by interactions with other G-protein subtypes that are less relevant to muscarinic M2-receptor signaling. The conclusion to be drawn from these studies is that anesthetics may interfere with several components of the muscarinic signaling pathway. However, the following should be kept in mind: (1) most times a mixture of muscarinic receptor subtypes was studied; (2) the anesthetics were administered in relatively high, and clinically unequal, concentrations; and (3) anesthetic effects on functional properties of the receptor–G-protein unit were not specifically addressed. Magyar and Szabo,[87] using the patch-clamp technique, have investigated the effects of halothane (0.9 mM) and isoflurane (0.8 mM) on acetylcholine (10 μM)-induced activation of the muscarinic K+ channel in frog atrial myocytes. They found that if anesthetic and agonist were administered at the same time, a reduction in the peak K+ current was observed, which was greater with halothane than with isoflurane. However, pretreatment with the anesthetic was found to have a significant, time-dependent, additional effect: 25-minute exposure to halothane restored the peak and significantly increased the steady-state current, whereas exposure to isoflurane decreased both. As equilibration of the anesthetic with the direct signaling pathway should be complete within milliseconds to seconds, the prolonged time course of these effects appears to indicate that additional intracellular pathways (such as PKC-mediated phosphorylation) are involved. Exposure of the membrane patches to the nonhydrolyzable GTP analog GTPγS, thereby irreversibly activating G_K, prolonged the current. When single-channel measurements were performed, halothane was found to enhance the frequency of channel opening without significantly affecting the single-channel conductance. Isoflurane was without effect. Therefore, halothane affects the signaling pathway downstream of the muscarinic receptor in this model. Whether this action is on the G protein or on the channel itself cannot be conclusively determined from these studies. When the time considerations are taken into account, it appears likely that the initial action of halothane on the system is inhibiting, whereas that of isoflurane is less so. After prolonged exposure, halothane is found to enhance signaling, whereas isoflurane inhibits it. These results are probably due to various effects of the anesthetics on intracellular systems that modify the signaling properties of the muscarinic pathway. In addition, halothane, but not isoflurane, has a direct activating effect downstream of the muscarinic receptor. The latter is consistent with findings of halothane effect on Ca++ channels mentioned earlier.

Genetic Cardiovascular Medicine

Over the past few decades, considerable progress has been made in the identification and understanding of the genetic basis of cardiovascular disease. More than 40 cardiovascular disorders are now known to be caused directly by gene defects. These disorders, spanning all aspects of cardiovascular disease and affecting all parts of the heart structure, can be divided into two groups (Box 7-6). *Monogenic disorders* are (usually rare) Mendelian disorders for which single gene changes are implicated in the disease process and which usually exhibit characteristic inheritance patterns. Examples include familial hypercholesterolemia, hypertrophic cardiomyopathies (HCM), DCMs, and the LQTSs.[88] More commonly, however, multiple genes influence the disease process by enhancing disease susceptibility or by augmenting the impact of environmental risk factors. The genetic component in those *multigenic disorders* comprises a collection of gene variants such as single nucleotide mutations, referred to as *single nucleotide polymorphisms* (SNPs). Each individual SNP may have a modest effect on the quantity or function of a translated protein product. However, when individual SNPs aggregate and interact with environmental risk factors, they may have a major impact on disease biology. Common diseases postulated to follow this paradigm include coronary artery disease (CAD), hypertension, and atherosclerosis.[89]

BOX 7-6. IMPORTANT CARDIOVASCULAR DISORDERS WITH A GENETIC BASIS

- Monogenic disorders
  - Familial hypercholesterolemia
  - Hypertrophic cardiomyopathy
  - Dilated cardiomyopathy
  - Long QT syndrome
- Multigenic disorders
  - Coronary artery disease
  - Hypertension
  - Atherosclerosis

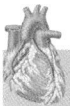

BOX 7-7. MAJOR GENETIC DIAGNOSTIC TECHNIQUES

- Monogenic disorders
  - Southern blotting
  - Polymerase chain reaction
  - Microarray
  - Chip
- Multigenic disorders
  - Linkage analysis
  - Whole-genome association
  - Gene expression profiling (functional genomics)

This section discusses the current status of genetic diagnosis of monogenic and complex cardiovascular disorders, as well as the main techniques used to perform such diagnostic testing (Box 7-7).

Monogenic Cardiovascular Disorders

Great progress has been made in the identification and characterization of the disease genes specific to Mendelian cardiovascular diseases,[88,90] but several factors complicate these investigative efforts. *Locus heterogeneity* (many genes causing the same disease) is one of those.[91] The channelopathies, encompassing the LQTS and related genetic arrhythmogenic disorders, are accounted for by more than 10 genes. Whereas HCM genes *MYH7, MYBPC3,* and *TNNT2* (encoding the β-myosin heavy chain, cardiac myosin-binding protein C, and cardiac troponin T genes, respectively) account for 70% to 80% of HCM as diagnosed by molecular genetic approaches,[92] an additional 19 genes have been implicated to cause the HCM phenotype.[93] In addition, more than 20 genes have been implicated in DCM.[91] A second, related factor complicating genetic diagnosis is that not all disease loci have been identified, which diminishes the sensitivity of molecular testing. Whereas it has been estimated that a mutation causing LQTS can be identified in up to three quarters of index patients, this is not true for other cardiovascular single-gene disorders. For example, only 30% to 60% of the genetic causes of HCM[94] and only 20% to 30% of genetic causes for DCM have been identified.[90,91] Further complicating diagnostic strategies is *allelic heterogeneity* (many mutations within a single gene). As an example, MYH7 consists of 40 exons encoding the β-myosin heavy chain protein, and 194 mutations in this structure have been reported to be associated with HCM. For diagnostic purposes, this necessitates sequencing the entire coding sequence and intron/exon boundaries of each gene, making sequencing a time- and effort-intensive undertaking.

Methodologies for Identifying Mutations: Sequencing and Microarrays

Techniques for identifying gene sequences have evolved from the classic Southern blotting procedure into highly automated systems that can rapidly screen hundreds of thousands of gene sequences. Southern

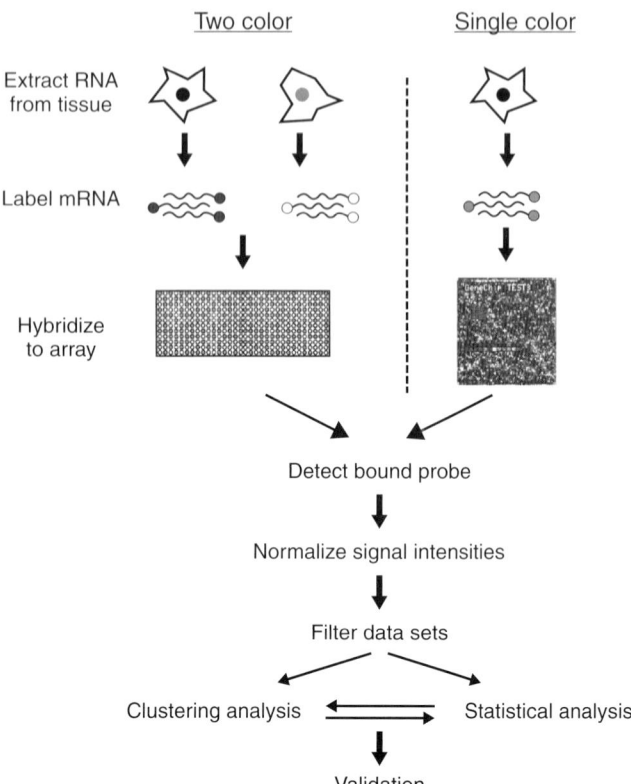

Figure 7-11 Schematic representation of a microarray experiment. RNA is extracted from the tissue(s) of interest, labeled, and then hybridized (competitively, two color arrays; noncompetitively, one color arrays) to the DNA microarray where it binds complementary sequences. Bound sequences are identified by their position on the array. Signal intensities are normalized allowing interarray comparisons. Normalized datasets are filtered and subjected to computational analysis. Finally, differentially regulated transcripts should be prospectively validated and/or confirmed using independent methods. (*From Cook SA, Rosenzweig A: DNA microarrays: Implications for cardiovascular medicine. Circ Res 91: 559–564, 2002.*)

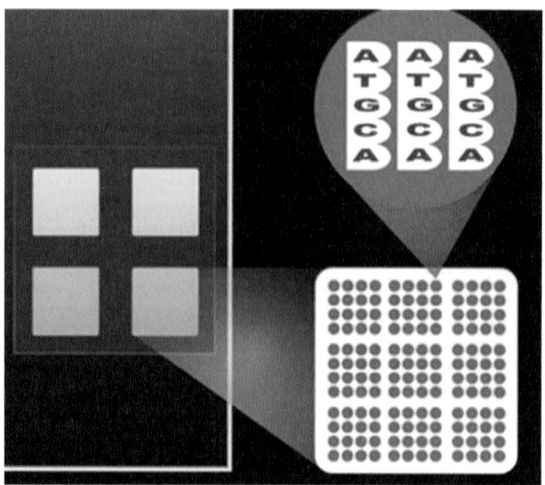

Figure 7-12   Chip method of sequencing combines chromatin immunoprecipitation (ChIP) with massively parallel DNA sequencing, allowing improved speed and efficiency. (*From* Central European Journal of Medicine, *1895–2058 (print) 1644–3640 (online), 2009, vol 4, No.1, pp 1–10.*)

TABLE 7-2	Clinical Applicability of Genetic Testing in Monogenic Cardiac Diseases				
	Success Rate	Identification of Silent Carriers/ Diagnosis	Reproductive Risk Assessment	Prognosis	Therapy
HCM	60–65%	+	+	±	−
DCM	Na	+	+	−	−
ARVC	< 10%	+	+	−	−
MFS	80–90%	+	+	−	−
LQTS	60–65%	+	+	+	+
BrS	20%	+	+	−	−
CPVT	50%	+	+	+	−
NS	40%	+	+	−	−

Only conditions in which consistent epidemiologic data are available have been listed.
ARVC, arrhythmogenic right ventricular cardiomyopathy; BrS, Brugada syndrome; CPVT, catecholaminergic polymorphic ventricular tachycardia; DCM, dilated cardiomyopathy; HCM, hypertrophic cardiomyopathy; LQTS, long QT syndrome; MFS, Marfan syndrome; NA, not applicable; NS, Noonan syndrome.
(From Camm AJ, Lüscher TF, Serruys PW: *The ESC Textbook of Cardiovasular Medicine*, 2nd ed. New York, Oxford University Press Inc., 2009.)

blotting, invented in the mid-1970s, is based on the transfer to nitrocellulose of DNA molecules separated on gels and their subsequent identification with DNA probes. It allows detection of small mutations, as well as large deletions, duplications, and gene rearrangements. The principle was expanded and automated in the development of DNA microarrays (Figure 7-11), which consist of series of thousands of microscopic spots of DNA oligonucleotides, each containing tiny amounts of a specific DNA sequence. The arrays are printed on a platform, usually a glass slide. A DNA probe, encoding a specific sequence, is then used to bind to and identify homologous nucleic acids, as detected by fluorophore-labeled targets whose signal is proportional to the relative abundance of nucleic acid sequences in the target. This makes it possible to examine the relative abundance of thousands of genes at any given time. Newer chip-based sequencing methods, designed to improve speed and efficiency, enable simultaneous sampling of 25,000 genes (Figure 7-12).

Clinical Applications

The ability of these techniques to identify diseases before they become clinically manifest allows preventive treatment as summarized in Table 7-2. For example, implantable cardioverters-defibrillators (ICDs) can prevent sudden cardiac death, improve quality of life, and prolong the time to cardiac transplantation (or avoid it altogether) in patients with genetic cardiomyopathies and arrhythmias[95–97] (Figure 7-13). Medical therapy may ameliorate the progression of genetic DCM. Prospective identification of those patients yet asymptomatic, but at greater risk for development of the disease, enables close surveillance and early

intervention. Knowledge of the LQTS genotype may be used to tailor the treatment plan (Figure 7-14). For instance, LQT3 patients benefit less from β-blockers, so a lower threshold for ICD implantation is advised in LQT3 patients.[98] In addition, the triggers for malignant arrhythmias have been found to differ based on gene involved, and, for example, patients with LQT1 can be asked to avoid vigorous activities such as exercise and competitive sports.[99]

Multigenic Cardiovascular Disorders

Identifying the gene variants associated with the development and progression of multigenic diseases allows them to be used to assess treatment response or serve as targets for novel treatment strategies. The obvious challenge is to identify the genes and gene variants that collectively contribute to the disease. Several genomic technologies allow researchers to study the genetic components of multigenic disorders like CAD.

Methodologies for Multigenic Genetic Screening: Linkage Analysis, Whole-Genome Association, and Gene Expression Profiling

Linkage analysis is a nonbiased and powerful approach for identifying causative genes underlying complex diseases.[100] The analysis is conducted after a priori identification of potential candidate genes or their chromosomal locations. It then looks for DNA markers that

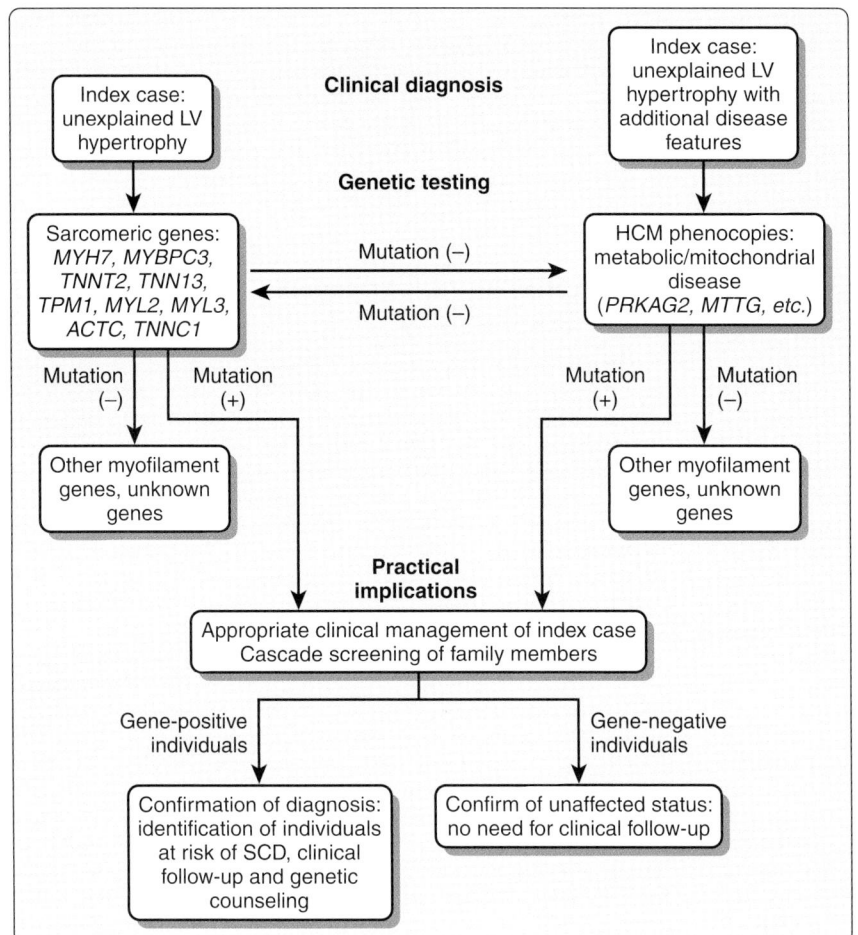

Figure 7-13 **Proposed sequence of genetic testing for patients with hypertrophic cardiomyopathy.** *HCM, hypertrophic cardiomyopathy; LV, left ventricular; SCD, sudden cardiac death. (From Keren A, Syrris P, McKenna WJ: Hypertrophic cardiomyopathy: The genetic determinants of clinical disease expression.* Nat Clin Pract Cardiovasc Med 5:158–168, 2008.)

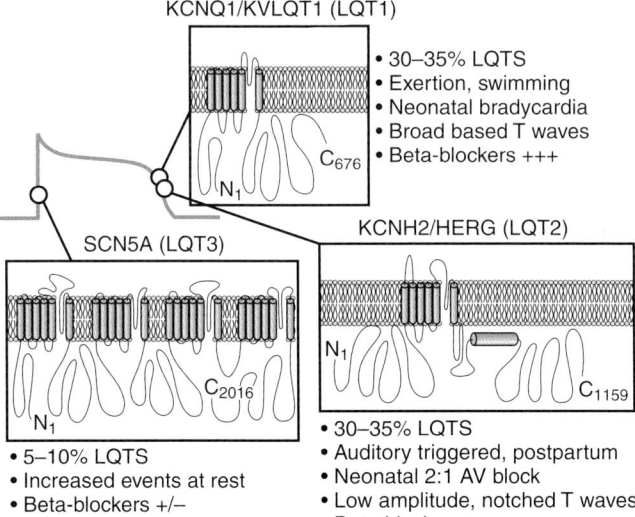

Figure 7-14 **Genotype-phenotype relations seen in LQT1, LQT2, and LQT3.** The linear topologies for the three principal cardiac channels that account for two thirds of long QT syndromes (LQTSs) are superimposed on the cardiac action potential of a ventricular myocyte. The inset next to each channel summarizes some of the signature phenotypes associated with the three most common LQTS-causing genotypes. AV, atrioventricular. *(From Ackerman, Michael J: Genetic testing for risk stratification in hypertrophic cardiomyopathy and long QT syndrome: Fact or fiction?* Curr Opin Cardiol 20:175–181, 2005.)

cosegregate with the disease phenotype between affected family members at a rate that is statistically greater than random chance. The chromosomal region containing the DNA markers can then be examined in further detail to look for potential candidate genes. Several successful studies have been performed using CAD as a model.[101-103]

Genetic association studies are performed to determine whether a genetic variant is associated with a disease or trait; if association is present, a particular allele, genotype, or haplotype of a polymorphism or polymorphism(s) will be seen more often than expected by chance in an individual carrying the trait. Thus, a person carrying one or two copies of a high-risk variant is at increased risk for development of the associated disease or having the associated trait. Using modern genomic technologies, researchers can now assay hundreds and thousands of SNPs simultaneously in a single individual using "SNP chips," the principle of which is the same as previously described for gene arrays. Two recent studies performed whole-genome association to identify SNPs associated with the development and progression of myocardial infarctions.[104,105]

Gene expression profiling (functional genomics) is another approach to identify genes and pathways that contribute to the development and progression of complex cardiovascular diseases such as coronary atherosclerosis. This approach analyzes disease in relevant tissues to look for changes in the abundance of transcribed genes or messenger RNA (mRNA) that correlate with a disease state, clinical outcome, or therapeutic response.[106,107]

Clinical Application

As in single-gene disorders, genetic information is used in multigenic disorders to establish disease susceptibility by defining a person's individual risk beyond currently available clinical and laboratory assessment tools. Several commercially available tests fall in this category, including tests for susceptibility to atrial fibrillation[108] and myocardial infarction.[104,105] Higher risk individuals, once identified, can then receive more intensive preventive medical treatments to delay or prevent disease development. However, there are several issues to consider before using genetic testing in this set of patients.[109] The first concern is the interpretation of results. Unlike single-gene disorders, the results of a positive or negative test provide no concrete diagnostic or prognostic information. A positive test simply means that a patient has an increased risk for development of the disorder—it is not a near certainty. Similarly, a negative test does not guarantee that the patient will not ultimately develop the disease. A second issue is the clinical interventions that should be administered given the test results. For example, if genotyping indicates that the individual is at risk for a future myocardial infarction, should intensive medical therapies be prescribed? Approaches such as blood pressure reduction, augmented antiplatelet therapy, and aggressive cholesterol lowering have all been shown to substantially reduce risk for CAD and are considered safe, but universal administration of these therapies is financially unfeasible and would lead to unavoidable side effects. Theoretically, with the use of more precise genomic information, it may be possible to identify disease-susceptible individuals for whom intensive prevention is cost effective, but this remains to be proven. Will the benefits of interventions applied in response to a positive genomic test outweigh the risks for unnecessary treatment and financial costs and result in durable and cost-effective improvements in health? On the other hand, given that there is no guarantee of a disease-free future, will a negative test lead to a false sense of security and encourage the maintenance or resumption of prior deleterious behaviors? Further evaluation of the utility of these tests through carefully designed disease outcome trials is needed. Finally, potentially problematic legal and ethical issues surround the clinical genetic testing for complex diseases. Although the results of the test provide no concrete diagnostic or prognostic information, they may have potentially significant effects on health insurance premiums or employment.

Another application of genetic testing in multigenic disorders lies in the development of new diagnostic and prognostic tools. This can be exemplified by its use in cardiac transplantation, in which it can identify subtle changes in peripheral blood mononuclear cells, allowing the detection of organ rejection much earlier than traditional histopathology.[110] In this example, genetic testing can be thought of as an extension of currently available biochemical and histopathologic approaches that aids in clinical decision making or determining prognosis by virtue of providing more detailed molecular phenotype information. Unfortunately, there are currently no genetic tests that meet these criteria with respect to more common disorders such as CAD.

Finally, an additional way to translate new genetic information into clinical practice is through the identification of targets for drug development or more precise indications for currently used medications. This is a straightforward idea, but a number of hurdles need to be overcome. The primary problem is to provide convincing evidence that a gene contributes to disease development and progression. In the case of linkage studies, it is sometimes difficult to determine the dominant candidate genes. Often, these studies identify chromosomal regions associated with disease that are 10 cM (roughly 10 million nucleotides) in length. A region of this size may contain 100 to 300 potential genes, making it challenging to identify the causal gene(s). For whole-genome association studies, an associated SNP is not necessarily functionally relevant and may simply be tightly linked with the real (but unidentified) causal gene. In some cases, the SNP may not even lie within a known or putative gene. For candidate genes identified by functional genomic studies, the difficulty is in determining whether gene expression levels are altered because the genes are contributing to disease biology or whether the genes are altered as a consequence of the disease process. There are success stories, however. The information on genes obtained from genome-wide association studies has been used

successfully to study the variations in response to some critical drugs such as warfarin. Warfarin has a narrow therapeutic window and shows large variations in dose requirements between patients. Patients with CYP29*2 and CYP29*3 allele variants seem to require lower doses of warfarin to achieve an optimal state of anticoagulation.[111] In 2005, the U.S. Food and Drug Administration (FDA) changed the label of warfarin to point out the potential relevance of genetic information to prescribing decisions.[112]

Perioperative Genomics in Cardiac Surgery

Despite advances in surgical, anesthetic, and cardioprotective strategies, the incidence of perioperative adverse events in cardiac surgery continues to be significant and is associated with reduced short- and long-term survival.[113] Because all surgical patients are exposed to perturbations that potentially activate inflammation, coagulation, and other stress-related pathways, but only a subset experience adverse perioperative events (even after controlling for coexistent disease), a genetic component is likely to be involved[114-116] (Figure 7-15). Perioperative genomics is a new field that uses functional genomic approaches to discover underlying biologic mechanisms that explain why similar patients have dramatically different outcomes after surgery.[117]

Genetic variants have been found for adverse events such as myocardial ischemia,[118] postoperative arrhythmias,[119] vein graft restenosis,[118] renal compromise,[120] neurocognitive dysfunction,[121] stroke,[122] and death,[118] as well as more systemic outcomes such as bleeding,[123] thrombosis,[124] inflammatory responses, and severe sepsis[125-128] (Figure 7-16). The Duke Perioperative Genomics investigative team initiated a prospective study (the Perioperative Genomics And Safety Study, US [PEGASUS]) in 2001. In recent years, broader multi-institutional perioperative genomics groups have been formed in the United States (PeriGReN) and internationally (iPEGASUS). The goal of the PEGASUS group is to use genetic variability to determine which individuals are at risk for adverse events after surgery. As an example of the power of perioperative genetic/genomic approaches, the PEGASUS group recently examined the perioperative myocardial injury/infarction (PMI) end point by genotyping 48 polymorphisms from 23 candidate genes in a prospective cohort of 434 patients undergoing elective cardiac surgery with cardiopulmonary bypass.[129] After adjusting for multiple comparisons and clinical risk factors, three polymorphisms were found as independent predictors of PMI. These represent SNPs in genes encoding IL-6 and 2 adhesion molecules, intercellular adhesion molecule 1 (ICAM-1) and E-selectin. In contrast, one mutation (SELE98G>T) decreased the risk for PMI in the study. The investigators concluded that functional genetic variants in cytokine and leukocyte-endothelial interaction pathways are independently associated with severity of myonecrosis after cardiac surgery.

Do these genetic/genomic studies result in practical information capable of facilitating therapeutic interventions designed to improve outcome? A study of the effects of a 5-lipoxygenase-activating protein (FLAP) inhibitor on biomarkers associated with increased risk for myocardial infarction demonstrated that, by defining at-risk patients using two genes in the leukotriene pathway, it can be predicted who will respond to targeted drug therapy.[130] Use of the FLAP inhibitor DG-031 in patients with these variants leads to significant and dose-dependent suppression of biomarkers associated with increased risk for myocardial infarction events. Although this study did not take place during surgery, similar principles would be expected to be operational in the perioperative period. These findings may soon translate into prospective risk assessment incorporating genomic profiling of markers important in inflammatory, thrombotic, vascular, and neurologic responses to perioperative stress, with implications ranging from individualized additional preoperative testing and physiologic optimization, to perioperative decision making, options for monitoring approaches, and critical care resource utilization.

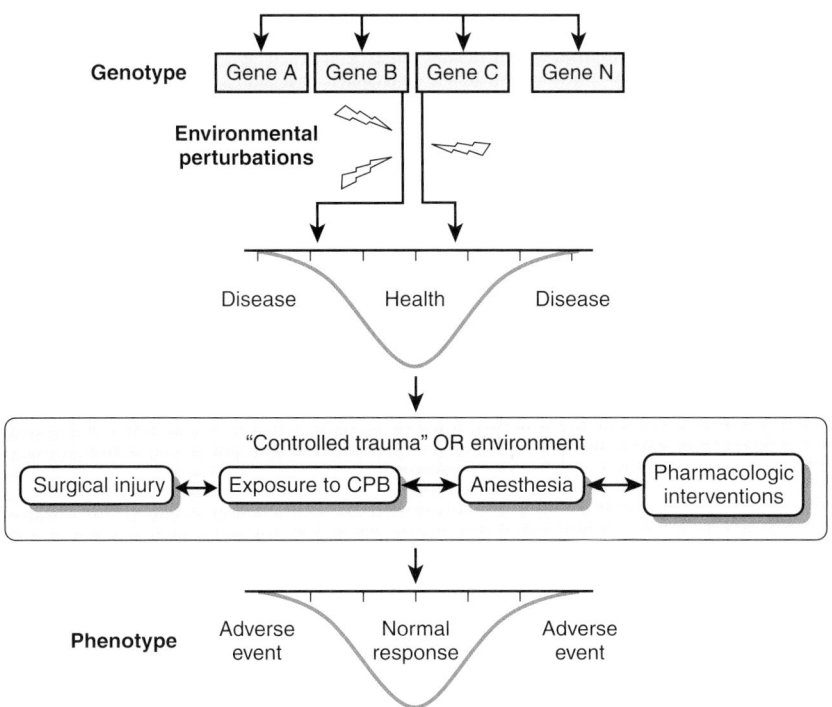

Figure 7-15 Diagram illustrating how genetic factors in combination with perioperative insults may play a role in adverse postoperative outcomes. CPB, cardiopulmonary bypass; OR, operating room.

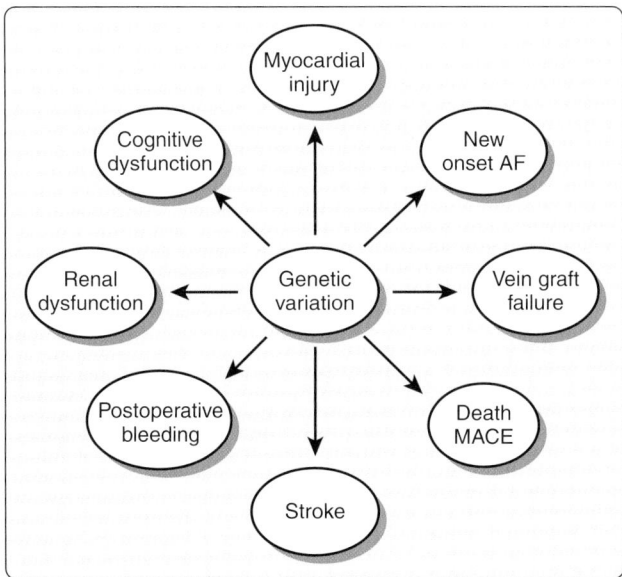

Figure 7-16 Genetic variation linked to various postoperative outcomes. AF, atrial fibrillation; MACE, major adverse cardiac event. (Reproduced with permission from http://anesthesia.mc.duke.edu/modules/anes_genes/index.php?id=5.)

Gene Therapy

Whereas molecular diagnosis is here, molecular therapy appears just tantalizingly out of reach—and has seemed that way for much of the past decade. The concepts are clear. The application, however, has been fraught with much more difficulty than at first appreciated.

Gene therapy attempts to modify expression of genetic material. Although a myriad of approaches have been suggested, those with the most promise are replacement of lacking or defective genes and selective inhibition of gene expression by antisense treatment. Another approach, further removed from clinical practice at this time, is the targeting of drug delivery to specific tissues using molecular techniques.

Replacement of genes is by now a routine technique in laboratory cell cultures, and can be performed with reasonable ease in animal models such as transgenic animals. Application in the clinical setting has been difficult, however. Obviously, it is most times not necessary to replace a gene in every cell of the body. In cystic fibrosis, for example, a disease in which gene therapy is probably closest to succeeding, the main target tissue will be the pulmonary system. The main issue then becomes the delivery of the functional gene to the target tissue in such a manner that it will be consistently expressed at adequate levels. A variety of experimental techniques exists. Cells can be removed from the patient's body, changed in culture, and then be returned to the patient. Alternatively, the gene can be incorporated in an otherwise innocuous virus that then is used to infect the patient's tissues. Both approaches show promise, but the technical difficulties indicate that this is still a considerable time away from routine clinical application. Nonetheless, several clinical trials are in progress.[131,132]

Inhibition of gene expression by antisense treatment is similarly full of promise.[133–135] The technique is based on the fact that mRNA can no longer be translated efficiently into protein when bound to a complementary strand of nucleic acid, a so-called antisense strand. Thus, by introducing specific antisense DNA into cells, expression of a selected gene product can be inhibited. The problem here, again, is efficient targeting of the tissue of interest. Remarkably, cells are able to take up antisense material from the extracellular environment without degrading it, but the material still has to be brought in contact with the tissue of interest. A second technical problem involves the stability of the antisense DNA. Because most diseases for which this technique seems suitable require constant inhibition of gene expression over long periods, the antisense construct has to be highly stable, and this degree of stability has not been consistently achieved yet.

Thus, molecular therapy seems feasible but is not quite ready for the clinic yet. Several times clinicians have believed that a breakthrough would be achieved rapidly; each time they have been disappointed. It would, therefore, be dangerous to predict that these techniques will find practical clinical application in the next few years. Nonetheless, the concepts appear sound, and have been proved in animal models. It appears to be only a matter of time before patients will be treated with these methods.

Somatic Gene Therapy for Cardiac Arrhythmias

Somatic gene therapy means addition of genes as either DNA or RNA to cells other than eggs or sperm, with the goal of treating or preventing a disease. Potential delivery strategies include replication-deficient viruses, and physicochemical techniques such as liposomes and direct injection. Viral transfection of an inhibitory G protein into the AV node of pigs has been used to control the ventricular response to atrial fibrillation.[136] The rationale for this strategy was that overexpression of an inhibitory G protein would, in effect, create a localized β receptor blockade. The success of this strategy may point to human trials in the future.

Stem Cell Therapy

Stem cells are immature tissue precursor cells that are undifferentiated and can differentiate into specialized cells including cardiomyocytes and cardiac rhythm-generating tissue. Stem cells may be isolated from the fetus, but limited supply and ethical considerations have mandated a search for a more easily accessible source. Skeletal myoblasts, endothelial progenitor cells, and adult mesenchymal stem cells have all been used. There are early reports of the use of stem cells for cellular cardiomyoplasty in patients with end-stage heart failure after myocardial infarction, but there remain concerns about incorporation of the cells into the myocardium and the possibility of arrhythmogenesis.[137] Prospective randomized trials are awaited. Human mesenchymal stem cells transfected with HCN2, a pacemaker channel, have been incorporated into canine myocardium. These cells have been shown to form gap junctions with the myocardium and to generate rhythmic activity after AV nodal blockade.[138] These experiments offer the distant prospect of a biologic cardiac pacemaker.

Acknowledgments

The authors thank J. Paul Mounsey, MD, PhD, for his contributions to earlier editions of this chapter, and Logan Reeves, MD, for his assistance in preparing this edition.

REFERENCES

1. Watson JD, Crick FH: Molecular structure of nucleic acids; a structure for deoxyribose nucleic acid, *Nature* 171:737–738, 1953.
2. Hamill OP, Marty A, Neher E, et al: Improved patch-clamp techniques for high-resolution current recording from cells and cell-free membrane patches, *Pflugers Arch* 391:85–100, 1981.
3. Sakmann B, Trube G: Voltage-dependent inactivation of inward-rectifying single-channel currents in the guinea-pig heart cell membrane, *J Physiol* 347:659–683, 1984.
4. Hume JR, Uehara A: Ionic basis of the different action potential configurations of single guinea-pig atrial and ventricular myocytes, *J Physiol* 368:525–544, 1985.
5. Moorman JR: Sodium channels. In Yaksh T, et al, editors: *Anesthesia: Biologic foundations*, Philadelphia, 1997, Lippincott-Raven Publishers, pp 145.
6. Coraboeuf E, Carmeliet E: Existence of two transient outward currents in sheep cardiac Purkinje fibers, *Pflugers Arch* 392:352–359, 1982.
7. Hiraoka M, Kawano S: Calcium-sensitive and insensitive transient outward current in rabbit ventricular myocytes, *J Physiol* 410:187–212, 1989.
8. Li Q, Keung EC: Effects of myocardial hypertrophy on transient outward current, *Am J Physiol* 266:H1738–H1745, 1994.
9. Lue WM, Boyden PA: Abnormal electrical properties of myocytes from chronically infarcted canine heart. Alterations in Vmax and the transient outward current, *Circulation* 85:1175–1188, 1992.
10. Attwell D, Cohen I, Eisner D, et al: The steady state TTX-sensitive ("window") sodium current in cardiac Purkinje fibres, *Pflugers Arch* 379:137–142, 1979.
11. Grant AO, Starmer CF: Mechanisms of closure of cardiac sodium channels in rabbit ventricular myocytes: Single-channel analysis, *Circ Res* 60:897–913, 1987.
12. Tsien RW, Bean BP, Hess P, et al: Mechanisms of calcium channel modulation by beta-adrenergic agents and dihydropyridine calcium agonists, *J Mol Cell Cardiol* 18:691–710, 1986.
13. Reuter H: Calcium channel modulation by neurotransmitters, enzymes and drugs, *Nature* 301: 569–574, 1983.
14. Bennett P, McKinney L, Begenisich T, Kass RS: Adrenergic modulation of the delayed rectifier potassium channel in calf cardiac Purkinje fibers, *Biophys J* 49:839–848, 1986.
15. Sanguinetti MC, Jurkiewicz NK: Two components of cardiac delayed rectifier K^+ current. differential sensitivity to block by class III antiarrhythmic agents, *J Gen Physiol* 96:195–215, 1990.
16. Wang Z, Fermini B, Nattel S: Sustained depolarization-induced outward current in human atrial myocytes. Evidence for a novel delayed rectifier K^+ current similar to Kv1.5 cloned channel currents, *Circ Res* 73:1061–1076, 1993.
17. Trautwein W, Taniguchi J, Noma A: The effect of intracellular cyclic nucleotides and calcium on the action potential and acetylcholine response of isolated cardiac cells, *Pflugers Arch* 392:307–314, 1982.
18. Giles W, Noble SJ: Changes in membrane currents in bullfrog atrium produced by acetylcholine, *J Physiol* 261:103–123, 1976.
19. Ragazzi E, Wu SN, Shryock J, Belardinelli L: Electrophysiological and receptor binding studies to assess activation of the cardiac adenosine receptor by adenine nucleotides, *Circ Res* 68:1035–1044, 1991.
20. Pfaffinger PJ, Martin JM, Hunter DD, et al: GTP-binding proteins couple cardiac muscarinic receptors to a K channel, *Nature* 317:536–538, 1985.
21. Liu DW, Gintant GA, Antzelevitch C: Ionic bases for electrophysiological distinctions among epicardial, midmyocardial, and endocardial myocytes from the free wall of the canine left ventricle, *Circ Res* 72:671–687, 1993.
22. DiFrancesco D: The onset and autonomic regulation of cardiac pacemaker activity: Relevance of the f current, *Cardiovasc Res* 29:449–456, 1995.
23. DiFrancesco D, Tortora P: Direct activation of cardiac pacemaker channels by intracellular cyclic AMP, *Nature* 351:145–147, 1991.
24. Yatani A, Okabe K, Codina J, et al: Heart rate regulation by G proteins acting on the cardiac pacemaker channel, *Science* 249:1163–1166, 1990.
25. Armstrong CM, Bezanilla F: Currents related to movement of the gating particles of the sodium channels, *Nature* 242:459–461, 1973.
26. Catterall WA: Molecular properties of voltage gated ion channels in the heart. In Fozzard HA, Haber E, Jennings R, editors: *The heart and cardiovascular system—scientific foundations*, New York, 1992, Raven Press, pp 945–962.
27. Lipkind GM, Fozzard HA: A structural model of the tetrodotoxin and saxitoxin binding site of the Na^+ channel, *Biophys J* 66:1–13, 1994.
28. Hille B: The permeability of the sodium channel to organic cations in myelinated nerve, *J Gen Physiol* 58:599–619, 1971.
29. Tomaselli GF, Backx PH, Marban E: Molecular basis of permeation in voltage-gated ion channels, *Circ Res* 72:491–496, 1993.
30. Armstrong CM, Bezanilla F, Rojas E: Destruction of sodium conductance inactivation in squid axons perfused with pronase, *J Gen Physiol* 62:375–391, 1973.
31. Korn SJ, Trapani JG: Potassium channels, *IEEE Trans Nanobioscience* 4:21–33, 2005.
32. Echt DS, Liebson PR, Mitchell LB, et al: Mortality and morbidity in patients receiving encainide, flecainide, or placebo. The Cardiac Arrhythmia Suppression Trial, *N Engl J Med* 324:781–788, 1991.
33. Riera AR, Uchida AH, Ferreira C, et al: Relationship among amiodarone, new class III antiarrhythmics, miscellaneous agents and acquired long QT syndrome, *J Cardiol* 15:209–219, 2008.
34. Mohler PJ, Schott JJ, Gramolini AO, et al: Ankyrin-B mutation causes type 4 long-QT cardiac arrhythmia and sudden cardiac death, *Nature* 421:634–639, 2003.
35. Brugada P, Brugada J: Right bundle branch block, persistent ST segment elevation and sudden cardiac death: A distinct clinical and electrocardiographic syndrome. A multicenter report, *J Am Coll Cardiol* 20:1391–1396, 1992.
36. Benito B, Brugada R, Brugada J, Brugada P: Brugada syndrome, *Prog Cardiovasc Dis* 51:1–22, 2008.
37. Rozec B, Gauthier C: Beta3-adrenoceptors in the cardiovascular system: Putative roles in human pathologies, *Pharmacol Ther* 111:652–673, 2006.
38. Bristow MR, Hershberger RE, Port JD, et al: Beta 1- and beta 2-adrenergic receptor-mediated adenylate cyclase stimulation in nonfailing and failing human ventricular myocardium, *Mol Pharmacol* 35: 295–303, 1989.
39. Lipsky R, Potts EM, Tarzami ST, et al: Beta-adrenergic receptor activation induces internalization of cardiac Cav1.2 channel complexes through a beta-arrestin 1-mediated pathway, *J Biol Chem* 283:17221–17226, 2008.
40. Bristow MR, Minobe W, Rasmussen R, et al: Alpha-1 adrenergic receptors in the nonfailing and failing human heart, *J Pharmacol Exp Ther* 247:1039–1045, 1988.
41. Hasking GJ, Esler MD, Jennings GL, et al: Norepinephrine spillover to plasma in patients with congestive heart failure: Evidence of increased overall and cardiorenal sympathetic nervous activity, *Circulation* 73:615–621, 1986.
42. Harding SE, Brown LA, Wynne DG, et al: Mechanisms of beta adrenoceptor desensitisation in the failing human heart, *Cardiovasc Res* 28:1451–1460, 1994.
43. Maisel AS, Ziegler MG, Carter S, et al: In vivo regulation of beta-adrenergic receptors on mononuclear leukocytes and heart. Assessment of receptor compartmentation after agonist infusion and acute aortic constriction in guinea pigs, *J Clin Invest* 82:2038–2044, 1988.
44. Chen CY, Dion SB, Kim CM, Benovic JL: Beta-adrenergic receptor kinase. Agonist-dependent receptor binding promotes kinase activation, *J Biol Chem* 268:7825–7831, 1993.
45. Lohse MJ, Benovic JL, Codina J, et al: Beta-arrestin: A protein that regulates beta-adrenergic receptor function, *Science* 248:1547–1550, 1990.
46. Deighton NM, Motomura S, Borquez D, et al: Muscarinic cholinoceptors in the human heart: Demonstration, subclassification, and distribution, *Naunyn Schmiedebergs Arch Pharmacol* 341: 14–21, 1990.
47. Lechleiter J, Hellmiss R, Duerson K, et al: Distinct sequence elements control the specificity of G protein activation by muscarinic acetylcholine receptor subtypes, *EMBO J* 9:4381–4390, 1990.
48. Logothetis DE, Kurachi Y, Galper J, et al: The beta gamma subunits of GTP-binding proteins activate the muscarinic K^+ channel in heart, *Nature* 325:321–326, 1987.
49. Swynghedauw B, Besse S, Assayag P, et al: Molecular and cellular biology of the senescent hypertrophied and failing heart, *Am J Cardiol* 76:2D–7D, 1995.
50. Schmitz W, Boknik P, Linck B, Muller FU: Adrenergic and muscarinic receptor regulation and therapeutic implications in heart failure, *Mol Cell Biochem* 157:251–258, 1996.
51. Bohm M, Gierschik P, Jakobs KH, et al: Increase of Gi alpha in human hearts with dilated but not ischemic cardiomyopathy, *Circulation* 82:1249–1265, 1990.
52. Fleming JW, Wisler PL, Watanabe AM: Signal transduction by G proteins in cardiac tissues, *Circulation* 85:420–433, 1992.
53. Pitcher JA, Inglese J, Higgins JB, et al: Role of beta gamma subunits of G proteins in targeting the beta-adrenergic receptor kinase to membrane-bound receptors, *Science* 257:1264–1267, 1992.
54. Feldman AM, Jackson DG, Bristow MR, et al: Immunodetectable levels of the inhibitory guanine nucleotide-binding regulatory proteins in failing human heart: Discordance with measurements of adenylate cyclase activity and levels of pertussis toxin substrate, *J Mol Cell Cardiol* 23:439–452, 1991.
55. Bristow MR, Minobe W, Rasmussen R, et al: Beta-adrenergic neuroeffector abnormalities in the failing human heart are produced by local rather than systemic mechanisms, *J Clin Invest* 89:803–815, 1992.
56. Hershberger RE, Anderson FL, Bristow MR: Vasoactive intestinal peptide receptor in failing human ventricular myocardium exhibits increased affinity and decreased density, *Circ Res* 65:283–294, 1989.
57. Mustafa SJ, Morrison RR, Teng B, Pelleg A: Adenosine receptors and the heart: Role in regulation of coronary blood flow and cardiac electrophysiology, *Handb Exp Pharmacol* 193:161–188, 2009.
58. Murphy E, Steenbergen C: Mechanisms underlying acute protection from cardiac ischemia-reperfusion injury, *Physiol Rev* 88:581–609, 2008.
59. Schutz W, Schrader J, Gerlach E: Different sites of adenosine formation in the heart, *Am J Physiol* 240:H963–H970, 1981.
60. Schrader J: Metabolism of adenosine and sites of production in the heart. In Berne RM, Rall TW, Rubio R, editors: *Regulatory functions of adenosine*, Martinus Nijhoff, 1983, The Hague, p 133.
61. Moser GH, Schrader J, Deussen A: Turnover of adenosine in plasma of human and dog blood, *Am J Physiol* 256:C799–C806, 1989.
62. Visentin S, Wu SN, Belardinelli L: Adenosine-induced changes in atrial action potential: Contribution of Ca and K currents, *Am J Physiol* 258:H1070–H1078, 1990.

63. Dobson JG Jr: Mechanism of adenosine inhibition of catecholamine-induced responses in heart, *Circ Res* 52:151–160, 1983.
64. Innes JA: Review article: Adenosine use in the emergency department, *Emerg Med Australas* 20:209–215, 2008.
65. diMarco JP, Sellers TD, Lerman BB, et al: Diagnostic and therapeutic use of adenosine in patients with supraventricular tachyarrhythmias, *J Am Coll Cardiol* 6:417–425, 1985.
66. Shen WK, Hamill SC: Cardiac arrhythmias. In *Mayo clinic practice of cardiology*, ed 3, St. Louis, 1996, CV Mosby.
67. Huffmyer J, Raphael J: Physiology and pharmacology of myocardial preconditioning and postconditioning, *Semin Cardiothorac Vasc Anesth* 13:5–18, 2009.
68. Sato T, Sasaki N, Seharaseyon J, et al: Selective pharmacological agents implicate mitochondrial but not sarcolemmal K(ATP) channels in ischemic cardioprotection, *Circulation* 101:2418–2423, 2000.
69. Tomai F, Crea F, Gaspardone A, et al: Ischemic preconditioning during coronary angioplasty is prevented by glibenclamide, a selective ATP-sensitive K^+ channel blocker, *Circulation* 90:700–705, 1994.
70. Kirsch GE, Codina J, Birnbaumer L, Brown AM: Coupling of ATP-sensitive K^+ channels to A1 receptors by G proteins in rat ventricular myocytes, *Am J Physiol* 259:H820–H826, 1990.
71. Yvon A, Hanouz JL, Haelewyn B, et al: Mechanisms of sevoflurane-induced myocardial preconditioning in isolated human right atria in vitro, *Anesthesiology* 99:27–33, 2003.
72. de Klaver MJ, Buckingham MG, Rich GF: Lidocaine attenuates cytokine-induced cell injury in endothelial and vascular smooth muscle cells, *Anesth Analg* 97:465, 2003.
73. Huneke R, Fassl J, Rossaint R, Luckhoff A: Effects of volatile anesthetics on cardiac ion channels, *Acta Anaesthesiol Scand* 48:547–561, 2004.
74. Porsius AJ, van Zwieten PA: Influence of halothane on calcium movements in isolated heart muscle and in isolated plasma membranes, *Arch Int Pharmacodyn Ther* 218:29–39, 1975.
75. Bosnjak ZJ, Supan FD, Rusch NJ: The effects of halothane, enflurane, and isoflurane on calcium current in isolated canine ventricular cells, *Anesthesiology* 74:340–345, 1991.
76. Yamakage M, Hirshman CA, Croxton TL: Inhibitory effects of thiopental, ketamine, and propofol on voltage-dependent Ca^{2+} channels in porcine tracheal smooth muscle cells, *Anesthesiology* 83:1274–1282, 1995.
77. Pancrazio JJ: Halothane and isoflurane preferentially depress a slowly inactivating component of Ca^{2+} channel current in guinea-pig myocytes, *J Physiol* 494:91–103, 1996.
78. Fassl J, Halaszovich CR, Huneke R, et al: Effects of inhalational anesthetics on L-type Ca^{2+} currents in human atrial cardiomyocytes during beta-adrenergic stimulation, *Anesthesiology* 99:90–96, 2003.
79. Kamatchi GL, Durieux ME, Lynch C 3rd: Differential sensitivity of expressed L-type calcium channels and muscarinic M(1) receptors to volatile anesthetics in Xenopus oocytes, *J Pharmacol Exp Ther* 297:981–990, 2001.
80. Ikemoto Y, Yatani A, Arimura H, Yoshitake J: Reduction of the slow inward current of isolated rat ventricular cells by thiamylal and halothane, *Acta Anaesthesiol Scand* 29:583–586, 1985.
81. Aronstam RS, Dennison RL Jr: Anesthetic effects on muscarinic signal transduction, *Int Anesthesiol Clin* 27:265–272, 1989.
82. Aronstam RS, Anthony BL, Dennison RL Jr: Halothane effects on muscarinic acetylcholine receptor complexes in rat brain, *Biochem Pharmacol* 35:667–672, 1986.
83. Dennison RL Jr, Anthony BL, Narayanan TK, Aronstam RS: Effects of halothane on high affinity agonist binding and guanine nucleotide sensitivity of muscarinic acetylcholine receptors from brainstem of rat, *Neuropharmacology* 26:1201–1205, 1987.
84. Krnjevic K, Puil E: Halothane suppresses slow inward currents in hippocampal slices, *Can J Physiol Pharmacol* 66:1570–1575, 1988.
85. Kai T, Jones KA, Warner DO: Halothane attenuates calcium sensitization in airway smooth muscle by inhibiting G-proteins, *Anesthesiology* 89:1543–1552, 1998.
86. Streiff J, Jones K, Perkins WJ, et al: Effect of halothane on the guanosine 5′ triphosphate binding activity of G-protein alpha subunits, *Anesthesiology* 99:105–111, 2003.
87. Magyar J, Szabo G: Effects of volatile anesthetics on the G protein-regulated muscarinic potassium channel, *Mol Pharmacol* 50:1520–1528, 1996.
88. Robin NH, Tabereaux PB, Benza R, Korf BR: Genetic testing in cardiovascular disease, *J Am Coll Cardiol* 50:727–737, 2007.
89. Nabel EG: Cardiovascular disease, *N Engl J Med* 349:60–72, 2003.
90. Cowan J, Morales A, Dagua J, Hershberger RE: Genetic testing and genetic counseling in cardiovascular genetic medicine: Overview and preliminary recommendations, *Congest Heart Fail* 14:97–105, 2008.
91. Burkett EL, Hershberger RE: Clinical and genetic issues in familial dilated cardiomyopathy, *J Am Coll Cardiol* 45:969–981, 2005.
92. Ho CY, Seidman CE: A contemporary approach to hypertrophic cardiomyopathy, *Circulation* 113:e858–e862, 2006.
93. Bos JM, Poley RN, Ny M, et al: Genotype-phenotype relationships involving hypertrophic cardiomyopathy-associated mutations in titin, muscle LIM protein, and telethonin, *Mol Genet Metab* 88:78–85, 2006.
94. Van Driest SL, Ommen SR, Tajik AJ, et al: Yield of genetic testing in hypertrophic cardiomyopathy, *Mayo Clin Proc* 80:739–744, 2005.
95. Nishimura RA, Holmes DR Jr: Clinical practice. Hypertrophic obstructive cardiomyopathy, *N Engl J Med* 350:1320–1327, 2004.
96. Semsarian C: CSANZ Cardiovascular Genetics Working Group: Guidelines for the diagnosis and management of hypertrophic cardiomyopathy, *Heart Lung Circ* 16:16–18, 2007.
97. Maron BJ, McKenna WJ, Danielson GK, et al: American College of Cardiology/European Society of Cardiology clinical expert consensus document on hypertrophic cardiomyopathy. A report of the American College of Cardiology Foundation task force on clinical expert consensus documents and the European Society of Cardiology Committee for practice guidelines, *J Am Coll Cardiol* 42:1687–1713, 2003.
98. Priori SG, Napolitano C, Schwartz PJ, et al: Association of long QT syndrome loci and cardiac events among patients treated with beta-blockers, *JAMA* 292:1341–1344, 2004.
99. Schwartz PJ, Priori SG, Spazzolini C, et al: Genotype-phenotype correlation in the long-QT syndrome: Gene-specific triggers for life-threatening arrhythmias, *Circulation* 103:89–95, 2001.
100. Ott J, Bhat A: Linkage analysis in heterogeneous and complex traits, *Eur Child Adolesc Psychiatry* 3:43–46, 1999.
101. Wang L, Fan C, Topol SE, et al: Mutation of MEF2A in an inherited disorder with features of coronary artery disease, *Science* 302:1578–1581, 2003.
102. Broeckel U, Hengstenberg C, Mayer B, et al: A comprehensive linkage analysis for myocardial infarction and its related risk factors, *Nat Genet* 30:210–214, 2002.
103. Hauser ER, Crossman DC, Granger CB, et al: A genomewide scan for early-onset coronary artery disease in 438 families: The GENECARD study, *Am J Hum Genet* 75:436–447, 2004.
104. Helgadottir A, Thorleifsson G, Manolescu A, et al: A common variant on chromosome 9p21 affects the risk of myocardial infarction, *Science* 316:1491–1493, 2007.
105. McPherson R, Pertsemlidis A, Kavaslar N, et al: A common allele on chromosome 9 associated with coronary heart disease, *Science* 316:1488–1491, 2007.
106. Bell J: Predicting disease using genomics, *Nature* 429:453–456, 2004.
107. Tuomisto TT, Binder BR, Yla-Herttuala S: Genetics, genomics and proteomics in atherosclerosis research, *Ann Med* 37:323–332, 2005.
108. Gudbjartsson DF, Arnar DO, Helgadottir A, et al: Variants conferring risk of atrial fibrillation on chromosome 4q25, *Nature* 448:353–357, 2007.
109. Rockhill B, Kawachi I, Colditz GA: Individual risk prediction and population-wide disease prevention, *Epidemiol Rev* 22:176–180, 2000.
110. Horwitz PA, Tsai EJ, Putt ME, et al: Detection of cardiac allograft rejection and response to immunosuppressive therapy with peripheral blood gene expression, *Circulation* 110:3815–3821, 2004.
111. Cooper GM, Johnson JA, Langaee TY, et al: A genome-wide scan for common genetic variants with a large influence on warfarin maintenance dose, *Blood* 112:1022–1027, 2008.
112. FDA releases final guidance for pharmacogenomic data, *Pharmacogenomics* 6:209, 2005.
113. Newby LK, Alpert JS, Ohman EM, et al: Changing the diagnosis of acute myocardial infarction: Implications for practice and clinical investigations, *Am Heart J* 144:957–980, 2002.
114. Fox AA, Shernan SK, Body SC: Predictive genomics of adverse events after cardiac surgery, *Semin Cardiothorac Vasc Anesth* 8:297–315, 2004.
115. Stuber F, Hoeft A: The influence of genomics on outcome after cardiovascular surgery, *Curr Opin Anaesthesiol* 15:3–8, 2002.
116. Ziegeler S, Tsusaki BE, Collard CD: Influence of genotype on perioperative risk and outcome, *Anesthesiology* 99:212–219, 2003.
117. Donahue BS, Balser JR: Perioperative genomics. Venturing into uncharted seas, *Anesthesiology* 99:7–8, 2003.
118. Zotz RB, Klein M, Dauben HP, et al: Prospective analysis after coronary-artery bypass grafting: Platelet GP IIIa polymorphism (HPA-1b/PIA2) is a risk factor for bypass occlusion, myocardial infarction, and death, *Thromb Haemost* 83:404–407, 2000.
119. Gaudino M, Andreotti F, Zamparelli R, et al: The -174G/C interleukin-6 polymorphism influences postoperative interleukin-6 levels and postoperative atrial fibrillation. Is atrial fibrillation an inflammatory complication? *Circulation* 108:195–199, 2003.
120. Stafford-Smith M, Podgoreanu M, Swaminathan M, et al: Association of genetic polymorphisms with risk of renal injury after coronary bypass graft surgery, *Am J Kidney Dis* 45:519–530, 2005.
121. Mathew JP, Rinder CS, Howe JG, et al: Platelet PlA2 polymorphism enhances risk of neurocognitive decline after cardiopulmonary bypass. Multicenter study of perioperative ischemia (McSPI) research group, *Ann Thorac Surg* 71:663–666, 2001.
122. Grocott HP, White WD, Morris RW, et al: Genetic polymorphisms and the risk of stroke after cardiac surgery, *Stroke* 36:1854–1858, 2005.
123. Welsby IJ, Podgoreanu MV, Phillips-Bute B, et al: Genetic factors contribute to bleeding after cardiac surgery, *J Thromb Haemost* 3:1206–1212, 2005.
124. Donahue BS, Gailani D, Higgins MS, et al: Factor V leiden protects against blood loss and transfusion after cardiac surgery, *Circulation* 107:1003–1008, 2003.
125. Burzotta F, Iacoviello L, Di Castelnuovo A, et al: Relation of the -174 G/C polymorphism of interleukin-6 to interleukin-6 plasma levels and to length of hospitalization after surgical coronary revascularization, *Am J Cardiol* 88:1125–1128, 2001.
126. Grocott HP, Newman MF, El-Moalem H, et al: Apolipoprotein E genotype differentially influences the proinflammatory and anti-inflammatory response to cardiopulmonary bypass, *J Thorac Cardiovasc Surg* 122:622–623, 2001.
127. Roth-Isigkeit A, Hasselbach L, Ocklitz E, et al: Inter-individual differences in cytokine release in patients undergoing cardiac surgery with cardiopulmonary bypass, *Clin Exp Immunol* 125:80–88, 2001.
128. Galley HF, Lowe PR, Carmichael RL, Webster NR: Genotype and interleukin-10 responses after cardiopulmonary bypass, *Br J Anaesth* 91:424–426, 2003.
129. Podgoreanu MV, White WD, Morris RW, et al: Inflammatory gene polymorphisms and risk of postoperative myocardial infarction after cardiac surgery, *Circulation* 114:I275–I281, 2006.
130. Hakonarson H, Thorvaldsson S, Helgadottir A, et al: Effects of a 5-lipoxygenase-activating protein inhibitor on biomarkers associated with risk of myocardial infarction: A randomized trial, *JAMA* 293:2245–2256, 2005.
131. Alexander BL, Ali RR, Alton EW, et al: Progress and prospects: Gene therapy clinical trials (part 1), *Gene Ther* 14:1439–1447, 2007.
132. Aiuti A, Bachoud-Levi AC, Blesch A, et al: Progress and prospects: Gene therapy clinical trials (part 2), *Gene Ther* 14:1555–1563, 2007.
133. Aboul-Fadl T: Antisense oligonucleotides: The state of the art, *Curr Med Chem* 12:2193–2214, 2005.
134. Nath RK, Xiong W, Humphries AD, Beri R: Treatment with antisense oligonucleotide reduces the expression of type I collagen in a human-skin organ-wound model: Implications for antifibrotic gene therapy, *Ann Plast Surg* 59:699–706, 2007.
135. Takeshima Y, Yagi M, Wada H, et al: Intravenous infusion of an antisense oligonucleotide results in exon skipping in muscle dystrophin mRNA of Duchenne muscular dystrophy, *Pediatr Res* 59:690–694, 2006.
136. Donahue JK, Heldman AW, Fraser H, et al: Focal modification of electrical conduction in the heart by viral gene transfer, *Nat Med* 6:1395–1398, 2000.
137. Lee MS, Makkar RR: Stem-cell transplantation in myocardial infarction: A status report, *Ann Intern Med* 140:729–737, 2004.
138. Potapova I, Plotnikov A, Lu Z, et al: Human mesenchymal stem cells as a gene delivery system to create cardiac pacemakers, *Circ Res* 94:952–959, 2004.

8

Systemic Inflammation

ELLIOTT BENNETT-GUERRERO, MD

KEY POINTS

1. Mortality and morbidity are relatively common after major surgery.
2. Postoperative morbidity often involves multiple organ systems, which implies a systemic process.
3. A large body of evidence suggests that excessive systemic inflammation is a cause of postoperative organ dysfunction.
4. No interventions have been proved in large, randomized clinical trials to protect patients from systemic inflammation–mediated morbidity.

Numerous advances in perioperative care have allowed increasingly high-risk patients to safely undergo cardiac surgery. Although mortality rates of 1% are quoted for "low-risk" cardiac surgery, results from large series of patients older than 65 years suggest that mortality rates are actually more substantial.[1] For example, Birkmeyer et al[1] reviewed a large number ($n = 474,108$) of "all-comers" undergoing coronary artery bypass surgery (CABG) or aortic valve surgery in the Medicare Claims Database. Notably, 30-day all-cause mortality was in the range of 4.0% to 5.4% after CABG and 6.5% to 9.1% after aortic valve replacement. The patient population studied, although elderly (age > 65), would not be considered to be particularly high risk by today's standards. These data do not point to the cause of death. Nevertheless, they indicate that outcome after routine cardiac surgery is poor for many patients. Outcome after these procedures is even worse if the extent of postoperative complications is considered. Postoperative morbidity is common,[2] and complications include atrial fibrillation, poor ventricular function requiring inotropic agents, and noncardiac-related causes such as infection, gastrointestinal dysfunction, acute lung injury, stroke, and renal dysfunction. For example, in Rady et al's[3] large series of patients ≥ 75 years of age undergoing cardiac surgery ($n = 1,157$), the mortality rate was 8%. The rate of serious complications, however, exceeded 50%.

Many postoperative complications appear to be caused by an exaggerated systemic proinflammatory response to surgical trauma.[4–6] The most severe form of this inflammatory response leads to multiple organ dysfunction syndrome and death.[5,6] Milder forms of a proinflammatory response cause less severe organ dysfunction, which does not lead to admission to an intensive care unit (ICU), but nevertheless causes suffering, increased hospital length of stay, and increased cost. The cause and clinical relevance of systemic inflammation after cardiac surgery are poorly understood. Systemic inflammation is a multifactorial process and has profound secondary effects on both injured and normal tissues. Proinflammatory mediators can have beneficial as well as deleterious effects on multiple organ systems. According to most theories, tissue injury, endotoxemia, and contact of blood with the foreign surface of the cardiopulmonary bypass (CPB) circuit are some of the major factors postulated to initiate a systemic inflammatory response. Nevertheless, controversy surrounds the cause and pathogenesis of inflammation in the perioperative period.

TERMINOLOGY

The terminology of *inflammation* is confusing and has hampered effective communication among scientists and clinicians. Despite attempts to standardize the terminology, variation in usage still exists in the scientific literature, as well as the clinical setting.[7] Much of the confusion relates to the term *inflammation,* defined as "a fundamental pathologic process consisting of a dynamic complex of cytologic and chemical reactions that occur in the affected blood vessels and adjacent tissues in response to an injury or abnormal stimulation caused by a physical, chemical, or biologic agent, including (1) the local reactions and resulting morphologic changes, (2) the destruction or removal of the injurious material, (3) the responses that lead to repair and healing."[8] This definition acknowledges the potential role of noninfectious causative factors; that is, infection is not a prerequisite for the development of *inflammation.* The American College of Chest Physicians/Society of Critical Care Medicine Consensus Conference has developed definitions for terms related to inflammation (Table 8-1). Figure 8-1 demonstrates the possible interrelations among many of these terms.

In particular, the *systemic inflammatory response syndrome* (SIRS) refers to an inflammatory process that can arise from or in the absence of infection. A viewpoint consistent with the recommended terminology is that systemic inflammation is a spectrum from mild systemic inflammation without organ dysfunction to a more severe form characterized by multisystem organ failure and death. There are three reasons why many clinicians do not routinely think of systemic inflammation as a clinical entity: (1) There are no universally accepted tests, for example, physical diagnosis or laboratory assays, which can reliably and accurately measure the degree of systemic inflammation; (2) even if such a test existed and it is known that a patient has "severe" SIRS, the clinician still would not be able to predict (a) whether organs will fail, (b) which organ(s) will fail, and (c) when organ(s) will fail; and (3) even if SIRS could be diagnosed accurately, currently, there are no therapies in widespread clinical use for the prevention or treatment of systemic inflammation.

In the surgical population, the use of the phrase and definition for SIRS has generated some controversy.[9] This controversy relates to the fact that almost all patients after major surgery fulfill the criteria for SIRS. Most patients, however, clearly do not develop clinically significant organ dysfunction from their systemic inflammation. Critics may argue that the use of the term *SIRS* in cardiac surgery patients, therefore, is meaningless because it does not differentiate patients who will have a benign versus a complicated postoperative course. For these reasons, SIRS is used more commonly by investigators than by practicing physicians. Use of the phrase *SIRS,* nevertheless, has the benefit of increasing awareness regarding the many noninfectious causes of inflammation.

The distinction of systemic versus local inflammation is important. Local inflammation has several beneficial purposes. Invasion of the injured or infected tissue by inflammatory cells, that is, neutrophils and macrophages, results in high concentrations of cells involved in host defense. Local mediator-induced edema and clotting of lymphatics by fibrinogen result in the effective "walling off" of the injured area. In contrast, systemic inflammation is not limited to the initial area of infection or injury. The systemic elaboration of inflammatory mediators may be beneficial by heightening the host's general defenses.

TABLE 8-1	**Definitions Related to Inflammation**

Infection = microbial phenomenon characterized by an inflammatory response to the presence of microorganisms or the invasion of normally sterile host tissue by those organisms.

Bacteremia = the presence of viable bacteria in the blood.

Systemic inflammatory response syndrome (SIRS) = the systemic inflammatory response to a variety of severe clinical insults. The response is manifested by two or more of the following conditions: (1) temperature > 38°C or < 36°C; (2) heart rate > 90 beats per minute; (3) respiratory rate > 20 breaths per minute or $PaCO_2$ < 32 mm Hg; and (4) white blood cell count > 12,000/mm³, < 4000/mm³, or > 10% immature (band) forms.

Sepsis = the systemic response to infection, manifested by two or more of the following conditions as a result of infection: (1) temperature > 38°C or < 36°C; (2) heart rate > 90 beats per minute; (3) respiratory rate > 20 breaths per minute or $PaCO_2$ < 32 mm Hg; and white blood cell count > 12,000/mm³, < 4000/mm³, or > 10% immune (band) forms.

Severe sepsis = sepsis associated with organ dysfunction, hypoperfusion, or hypotension. Hypoperfusion and perfusion abnormalities may include, but are not limited to, lactic acidosis, oliguria, or an acute alteration in mental status.

Septic shock = sepsis-induced with hypotension despite adequate fluid resuscitation together with the presence of perfusion abnormalities that may include, but are not limited to, lactic acidosis, oliguria, or an acute alteration in mental status. Patients who are receiving inotropic or vasopressor agents may not be hypotensive at the time that perfusion abnormalities are measured.

Sepsis-induced hypotension = a systolic blood pressure < 90 mm Hg or a reduction of ≥ 40 mm Hg from baseline in the absence of other causes for hypotension.

Multiple organ dysfunction syndrome (MODS) = presence of altered organ function in an acutely ill patient such that homeostasis cannot be maintained without intervention.

From Bone RC, Balk RA, Cerra FB, et al: Definitions for sepsis and organ failure and guidelines for the use of innovative therapies in sepsis: ACCP/SCCM consensus conference. *Chest* 101:1644–1655, 1992.

It, however, may lead to the "autodestruction" of the host through secondary damage to tissues/organs not originally affected by the primary injury or infection.

The *acute-phase response* to tissue injury and infection is characterized by leukocytosis, fever, increased vascular permeability, a negative nitrogen balance, changes in plasma steroid and metal concentrations, and increased synthesis of hepatic acute-phase proteins. Examples of these proteins include haptoglobin, fibrinogen, C-reactive protein (CRP), complement factors (C3, factor B), serum amyloid A, α_1-acid glycoprotein, and α_1-antichymotrypsin.[10] The terms *acute-phase response* and *systemic inflammation* often are used interchangeably.

A common misconception relates to the terms *bacteremia* and *endotoxemia*. Whereas *bacteremia* refers to the presence of viable bacteria in the blood, *endotoxemia* refers to the presence of endotoxin in the blood. Endotoxin, also known as lipopolysaccharide (LPS), is a component of the cell membranes of gram-negative bacteria, and hence its presence does not require the existence of viable organisms. In fact, it has been clearly established that cardiac surgical patients have a high incidence of intraoperative endotoxemia despite simultaneously exhibiting a low incidence of culture-proven bacteremia. This observation is consistent with the observation that "sterile" instruments and solutions, including intravenous fluids and the CPB circuit, may be contaminated with endotoxin.[11]

SYSTEMIC INFLAMMATION AND CARDIAC SURGERY

The systemic inflammatory response after cardiac surgery is multifactorial. As described earlier, the term *SIRS* is not particularly helpful in clarifying the pathophysiology of inflammation in cardiac surgery.[9] A schematic of the inflammatory process is depicted in Figure 8-2. There does not appear to be much disagreement with the statement that all of these processes may happen and may be responsible for causing complications in cardiac surgical patients. Tissue injury, endotoxemia, and contact of blood with the foreign surface of the CPB circuit are thought to initiate a systemic inflammatory response after cardiac surgery. What is least understood and of most controversy is the issue of which of these many processes is the most clinically relevant. It appears as if major surgery is an important cause of systemic inflammation,

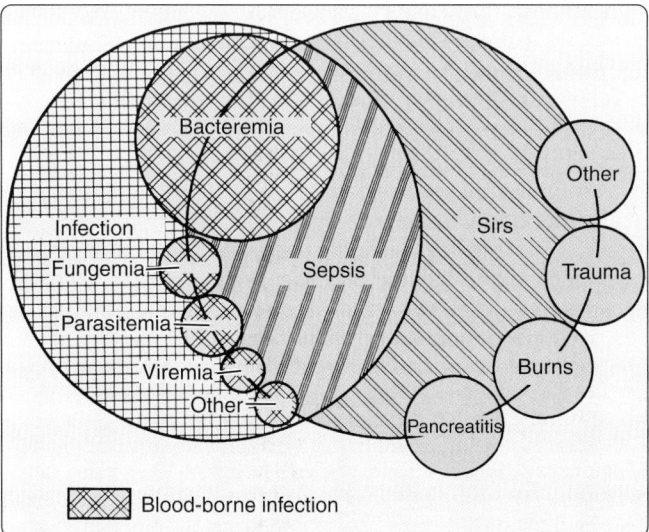

Figure 8-1 The interrelations among systemic inflammatory response syndrome (SIRS), sepsis, and infection. *(From Bone RC, Balk RA, Cerra FB, et al: Definitions for sepsis and organ failure and guidelines for the use of innovative therapies in sepsis: ACCP/SCCM Consensus Conference. Chest 101:1644–1655, 1992.)*

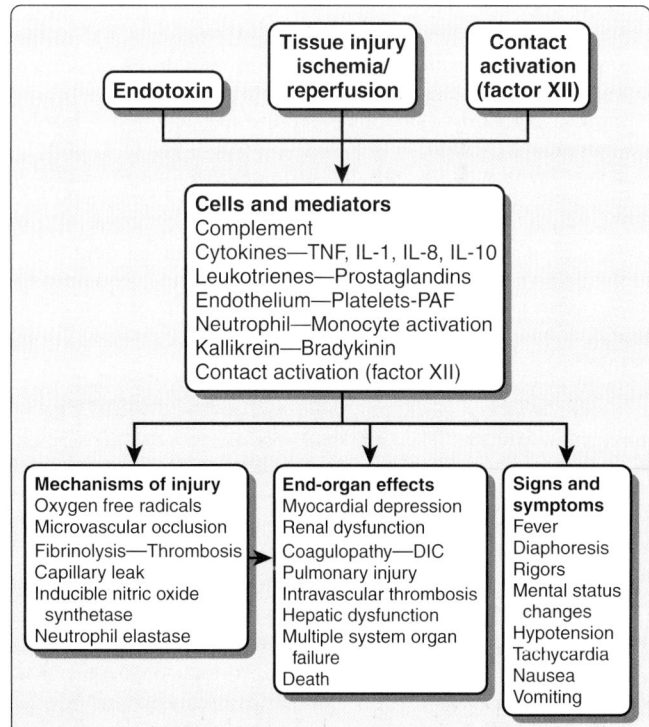

Figure 8-2 Overview of inflammation. DIC, disseminated intravascular coagulation; IL, interleukin; PAF, platelet-activating factor; TNF, tumor necrosis factor.

and that CPB further exacerbates the elaboration of proinflammatory mediators. Various causes and mediators of inflammation are reviewed in the subsequent sections.

Mechanisms of Inflammation-Mediated Injury

It is not entirely clear how inflammation ultimately damages cells and organ systems. Activation of neutrophils and other leukocytes is central to most theories regarding inflammation-induced injury.[6,12–15] Neutrophil activation leads to the release of oxygen radicals, intracellular proteases, and fatty acid (i.e., arachidonic acid) metabolites. These products, as well as those from activated macrophages and platelets, can cause or exacerbate tissue injury.

In localized areas of infection, oxygen free radicals liberated by activated neutrophils aid in the destruction of pathogens.[16] Complement, in particular, C5a, results in activation of leukocytes and oxygen free radical formation.[17] These activated neutrophils liberate toxic amounts of oxygen free radicals such as hydrogen peroxide, hydroxyl radicals, and superoxide anion. Oxygen free radicals are thought to cause cellular injury, ultimately through damage to the lipid membrane.[18–20] Increased levels of lipid peroxidation products, that is, products of oxidation of membrane lipids such as malondialdehyde, are thought to reflect the severity of free radical cellular damage.[21] Consistent with this model of injury, Royston et al[22] demonstrated increased levels of peroxidation products in cardiac surgical patients. In another study, oxygen free radicals were found to be increased in 21 patients undergoing cardiac surgery; however, the clinical relevance of these changes was not studied.[21]

A related mechanism of injury results from the degranulation of neutrophils. Activated neutrophils release granules that contain myeloperoxidase, as well as other toxic digestive enzymes such as neutrophil elastase, lactoferrin, β-glucuronidase, and N-acetyl-β-glucosaminidase.[23–26] Release of these intracellular enzymes not only causes tissue damage but also reduces the number of cells that can participate in bacterial destruction. In one study, cardiac surgical patients who developed splanchnic hypoperfusion, a possible cause of inflammation, demonstrated increased neutrophil degranulation and increased plasma neutrophil elastase concentrations.[26]

Another mechanism of inflammation-mediated injury involves microvascular occlusion. Activation of neutrophils leads to adhesion of leukocytes to endothelium and formation of clumps of inflammatory cells, that is, microaggregates.[14,27] Activated leukocytes have less deformable cell membranes, which affects their ability to pass through capillaries.[28] Microaggregates can cause organ dysfunction through microvascular occlusion and reductions in blood flow and oxygen at the local level.[22,28,29] After the disappearance of these microaggregates and restoration of microvascular flow, reperfusion injury may occur.

Finally, activated leukocytes release leukotrienes such as leukotriene B_4. Leukotrienes are arachidonic acid metabolites generated by the lipoxygenase pathway. They markedly increase vascular permeability and are potent arteriolar vasoconstrictors. These leukotriene-mediated effects account for some of the clinical signs of systemic inflammation, in particular, generalized edema, as well as "third-space losses." Prostaglandins, generated from arachidonic acid via the cyclooxygenase pathway, also act as mediators of the inflammatory process.

Physiologic Mediators of Inflammation

Cytokines

Cytokines are believed to play a pivotal role in the pathophysiology of acute inflammation associated with cardiac surgery.[30,31] Cytokines are proteins released from activated macrophages, monocytes, fibroblasts, and endothelial cells, which have far-reaching regulatory effects on cells.[32] They are small proteins that exert their effects by binding to specific cell-surface receptors. Many of these proteins are called *interleukins* because they aid in the communication between white blood cells (leukocytes).

Cytokines are an important component of the acute-phase response to injury or infection. The acute-phase response is the host's physiologic response to tissue injury or infection and is intended to fight infection, as well as contain areas of diseased or injured tissue. Cytokines mediate this attraction of immune system cells to local areas of injury or infection. They also help the host through activation of the immune system, thus providing for an improved defense against pathogens. For example, cytokines enhance the function of both B and T lymphocytes, therefore improving both humoral and cell-mediated immunity. Most cytokines are proinflammatory, whereas others appear to exert an anti-inflammatory effect, suggesting a complex feedback system designed to limit the amount of inflammation. Excessive levels of cytokines, however, may result in an exaggerated degree of systemic inflammation, which may lead to greater secondary injury. Numerous cytokines (tumor necrosis factor [TNF], interleukin-1 [IL-1] to -16), as well as other protein mediators (e.g., transforming growth factors, macrophage inflammatory proteins), have been described and may play an important role in the pathogenesis of postoperative systemic inflammation. The cytokines that have received the most attention related to cardiac surgery include TNF and IL-1, interleukin-1 receptor antagonist (IL-1ra), IL-6, IL-8, and IL-10.

Tumor Necrosis Factor

TNF is one of the earliest cytokines detected in the blood after the activation of macrophages and other proinflammatory cells. One factor complicating studies of TNF relates to the fact that there are two similar forms of TNF, TNF-α and TNF-β, as well as two distinct receptors, TNFR-I and TNFR-II. TNF appears to be pivotal in initiating the complex inflammatory cascade. Endotoxin is a potent stimulus for TNF production.

Endotoxemia unequivocally results in initiation of proinflammatory pathways, most likely through stimulation of TNF.[33–36] Michie et al[33] administered endotoxin intravenously to human volunteers and detected peak levels of TNF 90 to 180 minutes later. Peak concentrations of TNF correlated with increased temperature and heart rate (HR), as well as circulating levels of adrenocorticotropic hormone and epinephrine. In this and other studies, TNF levels soon appear after a proinflammatory stimulus and disappear quickly, which helps explain a common finding from clinical studies. TNF levels are often not increased when measured in patients with systemic inflammation, probably because test samples are obtained long after exposure to the primary inflammatory stimulus. This issue of sampling time may partially account for the fact that some cardiac surgical studies have detected increased TNF levels, whereas others have not.[37–53]

Interleukins

After the appearance of TNF, levels of IL-1 increase in cardiac surgical patients.[47,50,52,54] Measured levels are low and may peak within several hours after CPB.[54] Others have demonstrated maximum levels 1 day after cardiac surgery, which may explain the inability of some investigators to detect IL-1 during the intraoperative period.[50] IL-1 may decrease systemic vascular resistance after CPB through induction of nitric oxide synthesis in vascular endothelial cells.[55] Although IL-1 appears to be important in the initiation and propagation of the inflammatory cascade, it is not clear whether IL-1 levels cause deleterious effects or even serve as a marker for patients who will develop organ dysfunction after cardiac surgery. Some of the reported effects of IL-1 may be due instead to other cytokines, in particular, TNF, which are detected at the same time.

IL-8 is also believed to be an important component of the proinflammatory cascade. It is a potent chemoattractant of neutrophils to the site of injury or infection. IL-8 also is responsible for the activation, priming, and degranulation of neutrophils.[56,57] The relevance of increases in IL-8 levels to outcome after cardiac surgery has not been established.[42–44,46,47,51,53,58,59] Rothenburger et al[60,61] observed a significant association between prolonged mechanical ventilation and postoperative IL-8 levels but not IL-6 levels.

IL-6 levels have been shown to increase in the setting of cardiac surgery, although this is not a universal finding.[10,42,43,45–48,51–54,58,62–65] Peak levels of this cytokine appear after maximum values for TNF and IL-1. For example, Steinberg et al[54] measured plasma cytokine levels in 29 patients undergoing CPB. IL-6 levels peaked at 3 hours after separation from CPB and remained increased 24 hours after surgery. No association was found between IL-6 levels and hemodynamic parameters or postoperative pulmonary function.

Anti-inflammatory Cytokines

The regulation of inflammation is complex and involves a balance between proinflammatory and anti-inflammatory cytokines. IL-10 is a potent inhibitor of the synthesis of TNF, IL-1, IL-6, and IL-8, and increases in the perioperative period.[44,66–68] McBride et al[68] obtained blood samples perioperatively from 20 patients undergoing cardiac surgery. Before and during CPB, increases were observed in the proinflammatory cytokines TNF, IL-1, and IL-8. At the same time that proinflammatory cytokine levels began to decrease, increases in the anti-inflammatory cytokines IL-10 and IL-1ra were observed. The authors suggest that the balancing effects of these two types of cytokines may determine whether a patient suffers from the effects of excessive systemic inflammation (i.e., postoperative organ dysfunction) or the effects of inadequate immune system enhancement (i.e., postoperative infection and poor wound healing). Using this theory to improve outcome has not been translated yet into a clinical trial involving surgical patients. One concern related to potentially deleterious effects of inhibiting proinflammatory mediators has been borne out in sepsis trials in which mortality was increased in the group given an anti-inflammatory agent.[69] An understanding of the interaction between proinflammatory and anti-inflammatory mediators may result in the development of an effective and safe approach to reducing complications related to excessive systemic inflammation.

Complement System

The complement system describes at least 20 plasma proteins and is involved in the chemoattraction, activation, opsonization, and lysis of cells. Complement also is involved in blood clotting, fibrinolysis, and kinin formation. These proteins are found in the plasma, as well as in the interstitial spaces, mostly in the form of enzymatic precursors.

The complement cascade is illustrated in Figure 8-3. The complement cascade can be triggered by either the *classic pathway* or the *alternate pathway*. In the alternate pathway, C3 is activated by contact of complement factors B and D with complex polysaccharides, endotoxin, or exposure of blood to foreign substances such as the CPB circuit. *Contact activation* (Figure 8-4) describes contact of blood with a foreign surface with resulting adherence of platelets and activation of factor XII (Hageman factor). Activated factor XII has numerous effects, including initiation of the coagulation cascade through factor XI and conversion of prekallikrein to kallikrein. Kallikrein leads to generation of plasmin, which is known to activate the complement and the fibrinolytic systems. Kallikrein generation also activates the kinin-bradykinin system.

The classic pathway involves the activation of C1 by antibody-antigen complexes. In the case of cardiac surgery, there are two likely mechanisms for the activation of the classic pathway. Endotoxin can be detected in the serum of almost all patients undergoing cardiac surgery. Endotoxin forms an antigen-antibody complex with antiendotoxin antibodies normally found in serum, which can then activate C1. The administration of protamine after separation from CPB has been reported to result in heparin/protamine complexes, which also can activate the classic pathway[70,71] (see Chapters 28 through 31). Others, however, have not observed this effect.[72] Contact activation leads to activation of factor XII, which results in the generation of

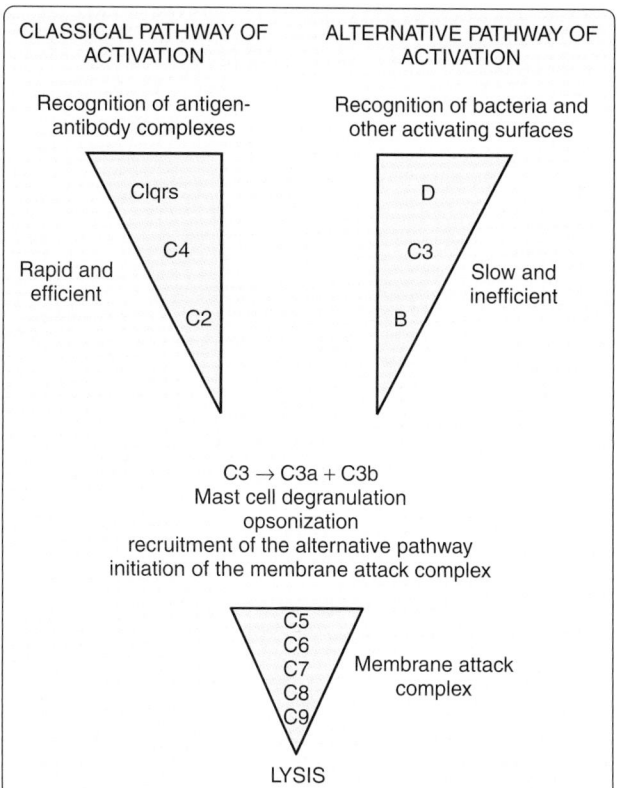

Figure 8-3 **Simplified components of the complement system.** *(From Haynes BF, Fauci AS: Introduction to clinical immunology. In Braunwald E, Isselbacher KJ, Petersdorf RG, et al [eds]: Harrison's principles of internal medicine, 11th ed. New York: McGraw-Hill, 1987, pp 328–337.)*

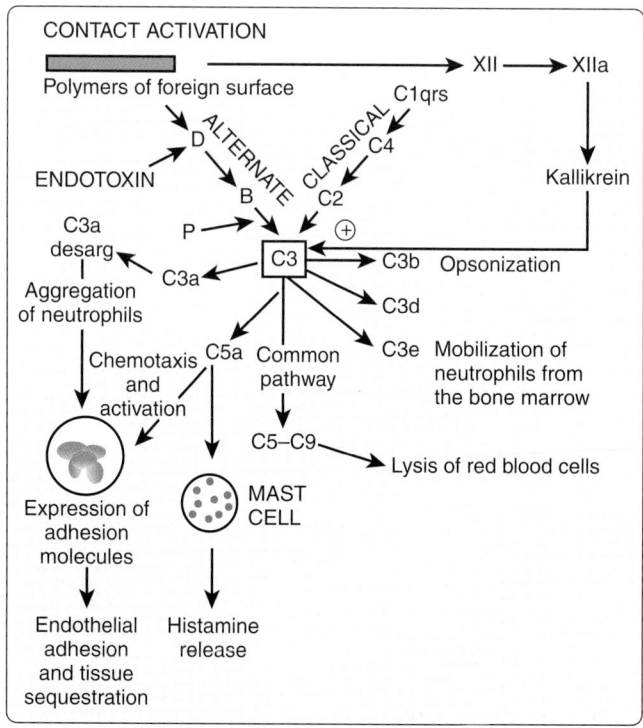

Figure 8-4 Contact activation of the complement cascade during cardiopulmonary bypass. Activation of complement occurs primarily through the alternate pathway. *(From Ohri SK: The effects of cardiopulmonary bypass on the immune system. Perfusion 8:121, 1993.)*

TABLE 8-2	Biologically Significant Effects of the Various Complement-Split Products	
Biologic Effect	**Complement-Split Products**
Mast cell degranulation, contraction of smooth muscle, increased vascular permeability	C3a, C5a
Chemotaxis of neutrophils	C5a, C5a des Arg
Neutrophil aggregation	C5a, C5a des Arg
Lysosomal enzyme release	C5a, C3b
Leukocytosis	C3e
Immune adherence/opsonization	C3b, C4b
Membrane lysis	C5b-9 (membrane attack complex)

From Knudsen F, Anderson LW: Immunological aspects of cardiopulmonary bypass. *J Cardiothorac Anesth* 4:245, 1990.

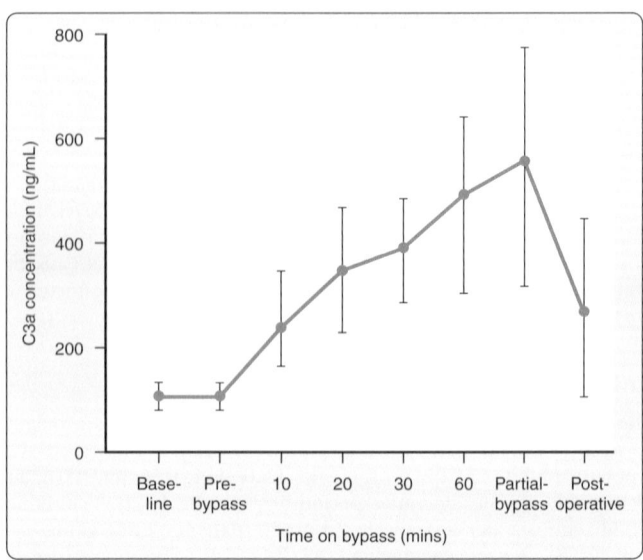

Figure 8-5 **Plasma levels of C3a in patients undergoing cardiopulmonary bypass.** Levels were unaffected by routine surgical procedures (prebypass) but displayed a time-dependent increase during cardiopulmonary bypass. Postoperative levels remained increased. Each point represents the mean (± standard deviation) of observations in 15 patients. *(From Chenowith DE, Cooper SW, Hugli TE, et al: Complement activation during cardiopulmonary bypass: Evidence for generation of C3a and C5a anaphylatoxins. N Engl J Med 304:497, 1981. Copyright 1981 Massachusetts Medical Society. All rights reserved.)*

plasmin. Plasmin is capable of activating complement factors C1 and C3. Table 8-2 is a summary of the physiologic effects of the complement system.

Activated C3, as well as other complement factors downstream in the cascade, have several actions. The effects of activated complement fragments on mast cells and their circulating counterparts, the basophil cells, may be relevant to the development of postoperative complications potentially attributable to complement activation. Fragments C3a and C5a (also called *anaphylatoxins*) lead to the release of numerous mediators including histamine, leukotriene B_4, platelet-activating factor, prostaglandins, thromboxanes, and TNF. These mediators, when released from mast cells, result in endothelial leak, interstitial edema, and increased tissue blood flow. Complement factors such as C5a and C3b complexed to microbes stimulate macrophages to secrete inflammatory mediators such as TNF. C3b activates neutrophils and macrophages, and enhances their ability to phagocytose bacteria. The lytic complex, composed of complement factors C5b, C6, C7, C8, and C9, is capable of directly lysing cells. Activated complement factors make invading cells "sticky," such that they bind to one another, that is, agglutinate. The complement-mediated process of capillary dilation, leakage of plasma proteins and fluid, and accumulation and activation of neutrophils make up part of the acute inflammatory response.

Although some elements of complement activation have been elucidated, clinicians are only now learning about the clinical relevance of this process to patients undergoing cardiac surgery. Several studies have reported increased complement levels during cardiac surgery.[38,58,73-78] Chenoweth et al[73] measured plasma C3a and C5a levels at different time points in 15 adults undergoing cardiac surgery with CPB. Although C3a levels were not affected by surgical stimulation, complement activation increased significantly during CPB (Figure 8-5). This and other studies did not test the association between increased complement levels and adverse postoperative outcome. Thus, they do not provide any evidence that complement activation causes clinically significant systemic inflammation. Kirklin et al.[75] measured plasma C3a levels in 116 patients undergoing cardiac surgery with CPB and 12 patients undergoing operations without CPB. In this study, an increase of complement activation during CPB was associated with postoperative morbidity. Patients undergoing procedures without CPB did not demonstrate increases in complement. This result suggests that a factor unique to CPB causes activation of complement. This study, however, did not pinpoint the clinical relevance of complement activation or of the CPB circuit, in part because even patients without postoperative morbidity had increased complement levels. Furthermore, confounding factors capable of causing SIRS, such as endotoxin, were not measured and accounted for in this study.

The results from several large, randomized clinical trials in which complement activation was selectively blocked have become available.[79-81] These studies indicate that attenuation of complement activation results in less myocardial injury; however, there did not appear to be an impact on complications such as pulmonary and renal dysfunction and severe vasodilation. These results suggest that complement activation may not play as large a role in the development of systemic inflammation-mediated morbidity as previously thought. These trials are discussed in more detail later in this chapter.

Endotoxin

Endotoxin, also called *LPS,* is a component of the cell membrane of gram-negative bacteria. It is a potent activator of complement and cytokines, and appears to be one of the initial triggers of systemic inflammation, as summarized in Figure 8-2.[12,82-84] Although the LPS constituent varies from one bacterial species to another, it generally may be described with reference to Figure 8-6 as consisting of three structural regions: (a) lipid A, (b) core, and (c) O-polysaccharide outer region. The lipid region of lipid A is embedded in the outer leaflet of the outer membrane. The oligosaccharide core region is positioned between lipid A and the O-polysaccharide outer region. Lipid A has the same basic structure in practically all gram-negative bacteria and is the toxic component of endotoxin. The LPS core region shows a high degree of similarity among various bacteria. It usually consists of a limited number of sugars. For example, the inner core region is constituted of heptose and 3-deoxy-d-*manno*-2-octulosonate (KDO) residues, whereas the outer core region comprises galactose, glucose, or *N*-acetyl-d-glucosamine residues displayed in various manners depending on the strain. The O-polysaccharide outer region (also called *O-specific antigen* or *O-specific side chain*) is highly variable and is composed of one or more oligosaccharide repeating units characteristic of the serotype.

ENDOTOXEMIA

Endotoxemia refers to the presence of endotoxin in the blood. Endotoxemia is common in cardiac surgical patients.[10,11,38,41,60,64,65,85-95] It is not surprising that some investigators have failed to detect endotoxemia during cardiac surgery given its transient and intermittent nature, although differences in endotoxin-assaying techniques used also may contribute to this discrepancy.[51,52,96,97] Andersen et al[11] measured circulating endotoxin levels in 10 patients undergoing cardiac surgery.

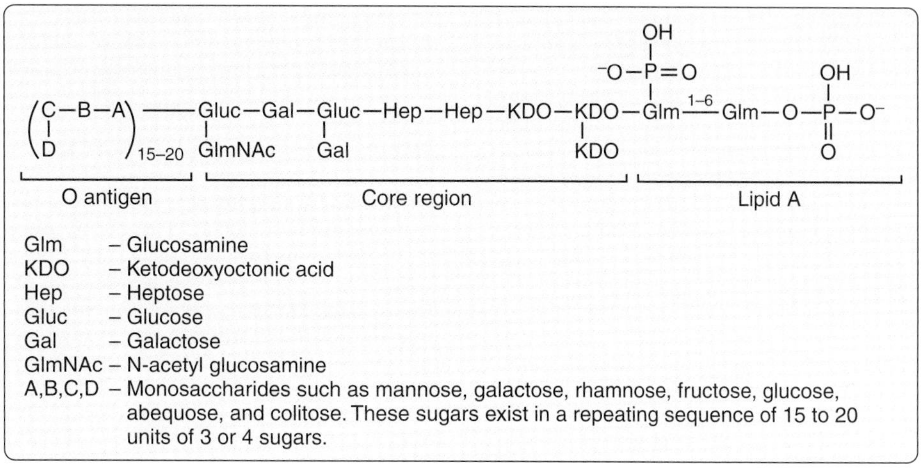

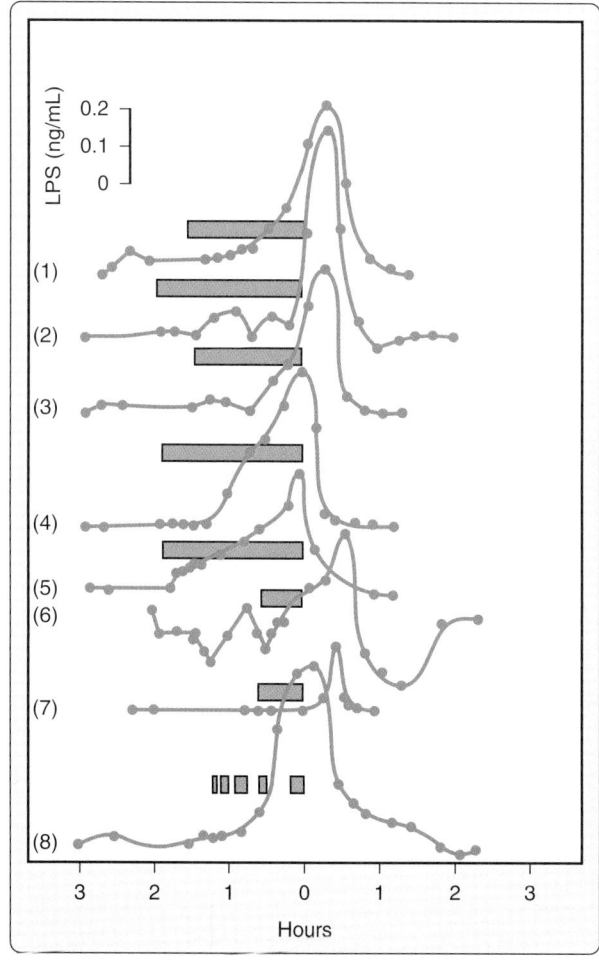

Figure 8-6 **Schematic structure of one unit of *Salmonella* cell wall lipopolysaccharide (LPS; endotoxin).** The structure of the cell wall LPS may vary slightly from one genus of gram-negative organism to another, but as far as is known, all contain three general regions, as shown. Although not shown here, all free hydroxyl groups of the glucosamines in lipid A are esterified with fatty acids. The serologic differences between different strains within a genus lie in the kinds of sugars and their linkages that exist in the O-antigen region. *(From Volk WA, Benjamin DC, Kadner RJ, Parsons JT [eds]: Essentials of medical microbiology, 3rd ed. Philadelphia: JB Lippincott Company, 1986, p 399.)*

All preoperative blood samples were free of endotoxin; however, substantial levels of endotoxin were detected intraoperatively. Blood endotoxin levels from eight typical patients undergoing cardiac surgery are presented in Figure 8-7.[85] Although endotoxin can be found in sterile fluids administered to patients, it is believed that the majority of endotoxin arises through a patient's impaired gut barrier.[11] Rothenburger et al[60] studied the association of endotoxin levels with prolonged mechanical ventilation in 78 cardiac surgical patients. Endotoxin levels were three times greater in patients with a postoperative mechanical ventilation time longer than 24 hours (*n* = 13) compared with patients with ventilator time less than 24 hours.

Normally, intestinal flora contain a large amount of endotoxin from gram-negative microorganisms.[98] The average human colon contains approximately 25 billion nanograms of endotoxin, which is an enormous quantity when 300 ng endotoxin is toxic to humans.[33,34] The leakage of live bacterial cells into the bloodstream can result in infection as these viable bacteria multiply.[99] However, many of the bacteria in the intestine are dead, and thus endotoxin also can enter the bloodstream contained within cell membrane fragments of dead bacteria. In this case, infection per se does not develop. Instead, endotoxin may initiate a systemic inflammatory response through potent activation of macrophages and other proinflammatory cells.[100] A plasma endotoxin concentration of only 1 ng/mL has been reported to be lethal in humans.[101]

On entry to the bloodstream, endotoxin forms complexes with numerous intravascular compounds including high-density lipoprotein, LPS-binding protein, and endotoxin-specific immunoglobulins. Endotoxin has been linked to dysfunction in every organ system of the body and may be the key initiating factor in the development of systemic inflammation.[12,82–84,93]

Normal Host Defenses against Endotoxemia

Early Tolerance

If endotoxemia is deleterious to patients, it would be logical to assume that patients have defense mechanisms against this ubiquitous toxin. Tolerance to endotoxin was studied extensively by Greisman and Hornick in the early 1970s.[102] Two distinct types of tolerance to endotoxin exist and are classified as *early tolerance* and *late tolerance*.[102] Early tolerance to endotoxin represents a reduction in the proinflammatory effects of LPS when administered several hours after a prior infusion

Figure 8-7 Time course of plasma lipopolysaccharide (LPS) concentrations during cardiopulmonary bypass procedures for Patients 1 to 8. *Hatched boxes* indicate the period of aortic crossclamping. For clarity, records were offset and aligned at the time of removal of the aortic clamp. *(From Rocke DA, Gaffin SL, Wells MT, et al: Endotoxemia associated with cardiopulmonary bypass. J Thorac Cardiovasc Surg 93:832, 1987.)*

of LPS.[103] It appears to be due to an LPS-induced refractory state of macrophages in which they release less TNF in response to endotoxin. This early refractive state shows no LPS specificity and can be overcome with increased doses of endotoxin. The degree of this tolerance is directly proportional to the dose, and hence intensity of the initial LPS-induced inflammatory state. Early tolerance begins within hours of LPS exposure and decreases almost to baseline within 2 days. It cannot be transferred with plasma. Early tolerance may protect the host from lethal systemic inflammation after an overwhelming exposure of LPS.

Late Tolerance

Late tolerance to endotoxin is due to the synthesis of immunoglobulins, that is, antibodies, directed against the offending LPS.[102] Late tolerance begins approximately 72 hours after exposure to LPS, which correlates with the appearance of the early-appearing IgM class of antibodies. This form of tolerance persists for at least 2 weeks and correlates with the presence of serum immunoglobulins. In contrast with early tolerance, the late response is not proportional to the intensity of the initial LPS-induced inflammatory response but is related to the immunogenicity of the initial LPS. Furthermore, late tolerance does not generally protect against a subsequent challenge with a dissimilar type of LPS. In other words, late tolerance is most pronounced when the same, that is, homologous, LPS serotype is used for both the initial and the subsequent challenge. It is not definitively understood how antiendotoxin antibodies responsible for late tolerance confer protection from LPS-induced systemic inflammation. Proposed mechanisms include increased clearance of endotoxin into the reticuloendothelial system, as well as direct neutralization through binding.

Understanding of the host's normal humoral defense against endotoxin is further complicated because of the numerous serotypes of endotoxin.[98] Serotype-specific antibodies, that is, antibodies synthesized in response to a particular LPS, exhibit high-affinity binding to and protection from the specific serotype of endotoxin. These serotype, that is, O-specific, antiendotoxin antibodies, however, do not recognize the many possible variations of endotoxin O-polysaccharide side chains, and thus are ineffective at conferring protection against the numerous serotypes of endotoxin likely to be encountered in the clinical setting. Antibodies, however, directed against the well-conserved inner core structure of endotoxin should theoretically be cross-reactive against many clinically relevant serotypes of endotoxin. Cardiac surgical patients are exposed to a wide variety of endotoxin types. For example, at least 164 O-antigens exist for *Escherichia coli*, the gram-negative bacteria most commonly isolated in high-risk surgical and ICU patients.[104,105]

Criticisms of Endotoxin as a Causative Factor

There are several criticisms of the theory that endotoxemia is an important cause of postoperative morbidity. A common criticism relates to the low incidence of culture-proven bacteremia in surgical and ICU patients.[106–109] Endotoxemia, however, is clearly prevalent in these patients and usually exists in the setting of negative blood cultures.[10,11,24,38,41,64,65,85–95] In fact, studies attempting to detect endotoxemia probably underestimate its incidence given its intermittent nature.

The failure of two anti-lipid A monoclonal antibodies (HA-1A, Centocor, Malvern, PA; and E5, Xoma, Berkeley, CA) to improve outcome on an "intention-to-treat" basis in ICU patients with established sepsis also has been used to suggest that endotoxemia is not clinically relevant.[110,111] These monoclonal antibodies may not bind to endotoxin with high affinity, which may explain, in part, their lack of demonstrable efficacy.[112] In addition, they were tested in patients with established sepsis and organ failure, which is an entirely different setting from elective surgical patients, who are more likely to benefit from prophy-

laxis with endotoxin-neutralizing drugs. Arguing against the clinical relevance of endotoxin is the negative result from a trial of prophylactic administration of a lipid A antagonist (E5564) in cardiac surgery.[113]

SPLANCHNIC PERFUSION

Splanchnic hypoperfusion appears to be an important cause of systemic inflammation.[114–117] The gut is one of the most susceptible organs to hypoperfusion during conditions of trauma or stress.[117–119] In the 1960s, Price et al[118] removed 15% of the blood volume from healthy volunteers, causing a 40% reduction in splanchnic blood volume. In this study, cardiac output (CO), blood pressure (BP), and HR did not change from baseline. A study was conducted by Hamilton-Davies et al, in which 25% of the blood volume was removed from six healthy volunteers.[120] Gastric mucosal perfusion, as measured by saline tonometry, was the first variable to decline (in five of the six subjects). Stroke volume (SV) also decreased; however, routinely measured cardiovascular variables such as HR, BP, and CO did not change significantly enough from baseline values to cause suspicion of a hypovolemic state. Based on these types of studies, the Advanced Trauma Life Support (ATLS) course teaches that a 15% blood loss (Class I hemorrhage) rarely results in changes in HR, BP, or urine output.[121] Significant decreases in systolic BP are a late sign of shock, which typically occurs after Class III hemorrhage (30–40% blood loss).

These studies suggest that during periods of hypovolemia, the gut vasoconstricts, thus shunting blood toward "more vital organs" such as the heart and brain.[117–119] In addition to hypovolemia, endogenously released vasoconstrictors during CPB, such as angiotensin II, thromboxane A$_2$, and vasopressin, also may result in decreased splanchnic perfusion.[122–125] Vasoconstrictors, such as phenylephrine, are routinely administered by anesthesiologists and perfusionists to increase BP and are likely to further reduce gut perfusion. Oudemans-van Straaten et al[89] measured intestinal permeability and endotoxin levels in 23 patients during cardiac surgery. Intestinal leak was measured by the amount of orally administered cellobiose present in the patients' urine. Intestinal permeability increased during surgery and correlated with circulating endotoxin levels. Administration of ephedrine, low central venous pressures, and less fluid balance during surgery also were associated with intestinal permeability, confirming the theory that gut perfusion is reduced by vasoconstrictors, as well as hypovolemia. There is also evidence that systemic endotoxemia may worsen intestinal permeability, thus exacerbating splanchnic hypoperfusion and initiating a vicious circle.[126]

Several studies have observed a high incidence of splanchnic hypoperfusion during cardiac surgery, with some showing an association between abnormal gut perfusion during cardiac surgery and postoperative complications.[10,87,88,127–130] Fiddian-Green and Baker[127] used saline tonometry to measure gastric mucosal perfusion in 85 cardiac surgical patients. Half (49%) of these patients developed evidence of abnormal perfusion, and all serious postoperative complications (eight patients, including five deaths) developed in this group. Gastric tonometry was shown in this and in two other studies to be a more sensitive predictor of adverse postoperative outcome compared with more routinely used global measures such as CO, BP, HR, and urine output.[128,130] A study using air tonometry demonstrated an increased gastric mucosal Pco$_2$ in 52% of cardiac surgical patients. Thirty-five percent of these patients with abnormal perfusion developed postoperative complications, in contrast with 5% in the group without evidence of hypoperfusion.[130]

Studies that have failed to demonstrate an association between splanchnic hypoperfusion and adverse postoperative outcome are limited, in part, by small sample size, insensitive measures of postoperative morbidity, and deviation from validated methodology of tonometry.[87,88] Tonometric measurements of gastric mucosal perfusion during hypothermic CPB have not been validated in terms of their ability to predict postoperative morbidity.

POSTOPERATIVE COMPLICATIONS ATTRIBUTABLE TO INFLAMMATION

Types of Complications

Many postoperative complications appear to be caused by an exaggerated systemic proinflammatory response to surgical trauma. A common misunderstanding relates to the types of postoperative complications that may be attributable to systemic inflammation and, in particular, splanchnic hypoperfusion. Many of the complications that are thought to be linked to splanchnic hypoperfusion do not involve the gastrointestinal system. Because splanchnic hypoperfusion may cause injury through a systemic inflammatory response, it would be expected that every organ system of the body potentially would be involved.[131] For example, endotoxin has been reported to have adverse effects on the pulmonary, renal, cardiac, and vascular systems.[41,46,83,84,132–135] It affects the coagulation system and may be both antihemostatic, potentially explaining bleeding, and prothrombotic.[83,132,136] Prothrombotic effects may account for some cases of postoperative stroke, deep venous thrombosis, and pulmonary emboli. There is also circumstantial evidence that systemic inflammation may worsen neurologic injury.[137] Activation of inflammatory cascades has been shown to worsen neurologic injury in numerous animal models.

Infections are common after cardiac surgery and increase hospital length of stay and cost.[107,138,139] Infecting bacteria may arise from translocation across the patient's gastrointestinal tract.[107,114,116] Surgical wounds (sternum and lower extremity) and the respiratory tract are common sources of postoperative infection.[140] Infections of prosthetic heart valves are less common but represent a devastating complication.[141] Infections are probably not caused by the direct effects of inflammation, but instead through secondary effects on host immunity.[142]

Widespread activation of the complement system results in depletion of complement factors, which are crucial to the effective opsonization of bacterial pathogens.[143,144] Systemic activation and degranulation of neutrophils render these cells less capable of destroying bacteria via phagocytosis. CPB leads to reductions in immunoglobulin levels through denaturation of these and other proteins.[144–148] Antibody production by B lymphocytes (plasma cells) is depressed after cardiac surgery.[149] Cell-mediated immunity, revealed by decreased T-lymphocyte function, appears to be impaired after cardiac surgery.[150] Thus, reduced antibody levels, as well as reduced B- and T-cell function in the post-CPB period, may lead to increased infection rates after cardiac surgery.

Incidence of Complications

The "low" mortality rate after cardiac surgery also has been cited as evidence that splanchnic hypoperfusion, endotoxemia, and systemic inflammation only result in "rare" complications. As discussed earlier, it is clear that mortality[1] and morbidity[3,151] are still significant problems after cardiac surgery. In addition, many studies only report frank organ failures or catastrophes and do not take into account less severe forms of organ dysfunction, which do not lead to admission to an ICU but nevertheless cause suffering and increase hospital length of stay.

For example, a series by Huddy et al[152] of 4473 cases involving CPB demonstrated a very low incidence rate (0.78%) of "gastrointestinal complications." In a series of 3129 patients, Christenson et al[153] reported an incidence rate of 2.3% for major gastrointestinal complications after coronary artery bypass graft surgery. The low incidence of major gastrointestinal complications (i.e., perforation, necrotic bowel, major gastrointestinal bleed) is often used to call into question the clinical relevance of splanchnic hypoperfusion. There is growing evidence, however, that less severe forms of splanchnic dysfunction (e.g., ileus, nausea, anorexia, and abdominal distention) are clinically relevant and increase hospital length of stay.

Some series of postoperative complications have broadened their scope. In a series of 572 patients, Corwin et al[154] reported the incidence of renal failure requiring dialysis (1%), as well as the incidence of renal dysfunction not requiring dialysis (6.3%). This study demonstrates that organ dysfunction is common after surgery, despite a low incidence of organ failure.

Similarly, the incidence rate of acute respiratory distress syndrome after cardiac surgery has been reported to be very low (< 2%) in several series.[155,156] The incidence, however, of less severe pulmonary dysfunction appears to be much greater, with as many as 7% of patients requiring supplemental oxygen 11 days after surgery.[157] Furthermore, a high incidence of postoperative pulmonary dysfunction, as measured by diagnostic tests, gives further support to the hypothesis that many patients have abnormal pulmonary physiology potentially attributable to systemic inflammation.[158–160]

Potential Therapies for the Prevention of Inflammation-Related Complications

Numerous strategies and pharmacologic agents have been postulated to reduce the severity and incidence of systemic inflammation. Often, interventions have demonstrated reductions in intermediate end points, for example, laboratory indices of complement activation and cytokinemia. Many of these studies, however, have been too small to detect improvements in clinically meaningful postoperative outcomes. Several of these interventions have failed in phase II and III trials. There are studies that show an improvement in outcome using an intervention that is postulated to reduce inflammation but do not actually document that there is less systemic inflammation in the treated group. Therefore, it cannot be determined whether the better outcome was attributable to reduced inflammation versus some other potential mechanism. Currently, there are no therapies in widespread clinical use for the prevention or treatment of organ dysfunction resulting from systemic inflammation; however, several approaches are discussed.

Steroid Administration

Several attempts have been made to prevent increases in proinflammatory cytokines and complement activation with steroids during cardiac surgery.[37,86,161–169] In a randomized, double-blind study of 25 cardiac surgical patients, dexamethasone administration (1 mg/kg on induction of anesthesia) prevented increases in TNF, as well as reduced postoperative hyperthermia and hypotension.[162] There was a trend toward improved outcome in the treatment group; however, the small sample size prevented any conclusions from being drawn regarding clinically relevant outcomes.

Inaba et al[163] randomized 17 patients undergoing cardiac surgery to placebo or methylprednisolone, 30 mg/kg given immediately before the initiation of CPB. In this study, glucocorticoid administration minimized intraoperative increases in both plasma endotoxin and IL-6 levels; however, no improvement in postoperative outcome was reported.

Cavarocchi et al[161] randomized 91 patients undergoing CPB to a bubble oxygenator without methylprednisolone (Group 1), bubble oxygenator with 30 mg/kg methylprednisolone (Group 2), or membrane oxygenator (Group 3). C3a levels increased in all three groups during CPB but were greater in Group 1 than in the other two groups. This study suggests that complement activation may be reduced by specific medical interventions. Andersen et al[86] randomized 16 patients to receive, at induction of anesthesia, either methylprednisolone (30 mg/kg) or placebo. This study demonstrated a reduction of complement activation in the protocol group.

Randomized clinical trials by Chaney et al[170,171] evaluated the effects of methylprednisolone (30 mg/kg) or placebo in cardiac surgical patients. Patients randomized to the steroid groups exhibited statistically significantly prolonged extubation times and received more vasoconstrictors. The investigators also observed significantly more hyperglycemia in the postoperative period in the methylprednisolone-treated patients. In another study, cardiac surgical patients randomized to steroid administration did not show benefit compared with placebo; however, a third study arm randomized to ultrafiltration without steroids did show a reduction in time to extubation.[172] A 2008 meta-analysis of 44 randomized trials involving 3,205 patients demonstrated a reduction of new-onset atrial fibrillation, postoperative bleeding, and ICU length of stay.[173] There were less pronounced reductions in hospital length of stay and mortality, and no safety concerns were identified. Therefore, although there are conflicting data on this issue, there is some evidence that there may be some benefit to steroid administration.

Role of Cardiopulmonary Bypass Technique

Although heparin-coated circuits have many theoretic advantages, there is little evidence that their use during cardiac surgery results in fewer clinically significant adverse complications. Steinberg et al[54] found no difference in cytokine levels or markers of complement activation between patients randomized to a heparin-coated circuit or to a traditional circuit. Borowiec et al,[25] however, observed lower levels of myeloperoxidase and lactoferrin (markers of inflammation) in patients undergoing CPB with a heparin-coated circuit. Other investigators have reported reduced plasma levels of cytokines and/or neutrophil proteases in patients subjected to CPB using heparin-coated circuits; however, no improvement in outcome was observed in these small studies[23,53,174,175] (see Chapters 28 and 29). A meta-analysis involving 3,434 patients from 41 randomized trials demonstrated reductions in blood transfusion and durations of mechanical ventilation, ICU and hospital length of stays, which provides some support for this intervention.[176]

Centrifugal vortex blood pumping has been shown to result in reduced complement and neutrophil activation, as well as reduced hemolysis during cardiac surgery compared with standard roller blood pumping.[177,178] Centrifugal vortex blood pumping, however, did not significantly prevent increases in cytokines in 17 pediatric patients randomized to this bypass technique.[58]

A randomized study of 15 patients suggested that pulsatile flow CPB may result in less endotoxemia than CPB involving nonpulsatile flow.[94] Levine et al[125] randomized 20 patients to pulsatile versus nonpulsatile flow and observed a less marked increase in vasopressin levels (an endogenous vasoconstrictor) in patients perfused with pulsatile flow. Taylor et al[122] demonstrated increased levels of the endogenously produced vasoconstrictor angiotensin II in patients ($N = 24$) randomized to nonpulsatile flow CPB as compared with pulsatile flow. Watkins et al[124] observed fewer marked alterations in thromboxane B_2 and prostacyclin levels in patients ($N = 16$) randomized to pulsatile CPB. These studies evaluating pulsatile flow suggest that splanchnic perfusion may be better preserved with pulsatile flow because of less endogenously mediated vasoconstriction. Quigley et al,[52] however, reported a lack of endotoxemia and pathologic cytokinemia in an uncontrolled study of patients who underwent nonpulsatile CPB. They claimed that the use of "adequate flow and perfusion pressures" during CPB accounted for their findings.

The role of membrane oxygenators as a means of reducing systemic inflammation-related complications also is controversial. Less complement activation has been observed with the use of membrane oxygenators; however, other studies have found no difference.[62,74,161,179-183] The use of membrane oxygenators was associated with better pulmonary function as compared with the use of a bubble oxygenator; however, it is unclear whether the difference observed reflected reduced systemic inflammation in the protocol group.[181] Butler et al[62] randomized 20 patients undergoing cardiac surgery to either a membrane or bubble oxygenator. IL-6 levels peaked 4 hours after surgery, yet there were no significant differences between groups in IL-1 or IL-6 levels, or in intrapulmonary shunting. This study failed to show a difference in postoperative outcome, possibly because of short CPB durations (< 1 hour), as well as the small sample size, which makes detecting a clinically significant difference in postoperative complications unlikely. Host defenses may be better maintained with the use of membrane oxygenators.[182]

There also is controversy whether hypothermia during CPB worsens systemic inflammation.[40,51,76,184-186] Hypothermia has been shown to reduce markers of complement activation.[76] Another study demonstrated reduced markers of inflammation, such as TNF and IL-6,

as well as reduced neutrophil activation in the hypothermia group.[185] In contrast, another study randomized 30 cardiac surgical patients to either normothermic or hypothermic CPB.[40] They found no association between CPB temperature and plasma TNF levels at any time point in the perioperative period, suggesting a limited role for temperature as an independent cause of proinflammatory cytokine release. In one of the largest randomized trials to date, 300 elective CABG patients were randomized to either normothermic (35.5°C to 36.5°C) or hypothermic (28°C to 30°C) CPB.[187] No differences were seen in either short-term or longer term outcome, suggesting no benefit to intraoperative hypothermia. There is evidence, however, that perioperative hyperthermia may be detrimental to the brain.[188] These investigators also observed an association between greater levels of the proinflammatory cytokine IL-6 and postoperative hyperthermia, suggesting a potential role of inflammation in the increases in temperature commonly observed after major surgery.

Finally, current data suggest that the use of CPB for cardiac surgery may not in and of itself be more deleterious than cardiac surgery without the use of CPB. Results from initial randomized clinical trials did not suggest that outcomes were substantially different in patients undergoing on- versus off-pump CABG surgery.[189-193] Given the importance of this question, 2203 cardiac surgical patients were enrolled at 18 Veterans Affairs medical centers from 2002-2008 and randomized to on- or off-pump CABG. No benefit was found with regard to outcomes such as duration of mechanical ventilation, lengths of stay in the ICU or hospital, renal failure, or a composite end point of complications.[194] Systemic inflammation was not specifically studied in this important trial, but these data suggest that systemic inflammation attributable to CPB may have a more modest role in determining clinical outcome than previously thought. Another plausible conclusion, however, is that hemodynamic instability and use of potent vasoactive agents associated with the off-pump technique may be an equivalent insult to the use of CPB.

Complement Inhibition

The results from several large, randomized clinical trials in which complement activation is selectively blocked have become available.[79-81] For example, in the largest randomized, double-blind clinical trial conducted to date, 3099 adults undergoing CABG surgery at 205 hospitals in North America and Western Europe were enrolled.[80] Patients were randomized to placebo or to a 24-hour infusion of pexelizumab, which is a recombinant, humanized, single-chain antibody fragment that binds to human C5 complement and prevents its activation. The administration of pexelizumab resulted in rapid and complete inhibition of complement activation. The primary outcome variable (death or myocardial infarction within 30 days) did not achieve statistical significance ($p = 0.07$). The subset of patients undergoing CABG plus valve did demonstrate a statistically significant difference ($p = 0.03$) in this outcome. This finding is somewhat contradictory to the previous phase IIb trial ($n = 914$) that enrolled patients undergoing CABG and/or valve surgery and did not show a significant difference with regard to the end point of death or myocardial infarction.[79] This previous trial did achieve significance in the subset undergoing isolated CABG, which was the apparent justification for studying isolated CABG surgeries in the larger phase III trial. These studies indicate that attenuation of complement activation results in less myocardial injury; however, there did not appear to be an impact on complications such as pulmonary and renal dysfunction and severe vasodilation. These results suggest that complement activation may not play as large a role in the development of systemic inflammation-mediated morbidity as previously thought.

Ultrafiltration

Removal of excess fluid with ultrafiltration has been proposed as a method for removing proinflammatory mediators during cardiac surgery, particularly in the pediatric population.[46,195] It is unclear in studies performed thus far whether beneficial effects of ultrafiltration are due to one or some combination of the following factors: prevention of initiation of inflammation, removal of inflammatory mediators, or removal of excessive fluid alone. In one study, Journois et al[196] randomized 20 pediatric cardiac surgical patients to either a control group or to high-volume, zero-fluid balance ultrafiltration. Measured TNF, IL-1, IL-10, myeloperoxidase, and C3a levels were lower in the protocol group compared with the control group. The authors suggested that hemofiltration may have some beneficial effects that are not due to water removal alone. Patients in the ultrafiltration group had less postoperative fever, reduced perioperative blood loss, reduced time to extubation, and reduced postoperative alveolar-arterial oxygen gradient, which suggests, yet does not prove, a causal relation between proinflammatory cytokinemia and several clinically meaningful end points. The small sample size of this study precludes any conclusions from being made regarding other outcomes such as the incidence of multiple organ dysfunction syndrome or hospital length of stay.

In an interesting study, 192 cardiac surgical patients were randomized to placebo (no steroids or ultrafiltration), steroid administration without ultrafiltration, or hemofiltration without steroids.[172] The study arm randomized to ultrafiltration without steroids showed a reduction in time to extubation; however, steroid administration was not effective compared with placebo. These data are promising, but the small number of subjects per arm and limited number of positive outcomes reported make it unclear whether ultrafiltration should be used more routinely.

Leukocyte Depletion

Removal of leukocytes during CPB with an inline leukocyte filter has been proposed as a method for reducing the concentration of activated leukocytes. This, in turn, may prevent inflammatory-mediated postoperative complications. This technology has been nicely reviewed by Warren et al,[197] who, in their review of 63 studies, concluded that there may be some modest benefits, but that the low quality of evidence from the predominantly small trials precluded any definitive conclusions on this matter. For example, patients randomized to leukocyte depletion ($n = 20$) had better oxygenation after CPB; however, there were no differences in other outcomes measured.[198] A prospective randomized study of patients ($N = 50$) receiving inline leukocyte filtration demonstrated decreased leukocytes; however, postoperative arterial blood gases, pulmonary vascular resistance, ventilator time, and hospital length of stay were no different between groups.[199] Another study demonstrated no difference in postoperative complications or in the plasma levels of neutrophil proteases in patients undergoing leukocyte depletion with an inline filter.[200]

Davies et al[201] used another method of leukocyte depletion in which they removed platelets and leukocytes by plasmapheresis from patients before cardiac surgery. These patients, compared with the control group, demonstrated reduced postoperative thoracic drainage, reduced allogeneic blood product administration, and improved pulmonary function. This technique is not in widespread clinical use because of a lack of studies confirming its findings, as well as the time and cost involved in performing plasmapheresis (see Chapters 28 through 31).

The techniques described earlier differ from the issue of administration of leukocyte-reduced packed red blood cells. This method of minimizing a patient's exposure to leukocytes involves the filtering of the collected blood either at the time of donation (fresh filtered) or before its release by the blood bank (stored filtered).[202] Van de Watering and colleagues[203] reported results from a large ($n = 914$) randomized clinical trial in which patients undergoing cardiac surgery were randomized to receive allogeneic red cells without buffy coat, fresh-filtered allogeneic red cells, or stored filtered units. Patients randomized to either filtration group experienced a significant reduction in postoperative mortality ($P = 0.015$); however, this effect was most robust in patients administered more than three transfusions. It should be noted that differences between groups in the incidence of infection did not achieve statistical significance ($P = 0.13$). No differences between groups were found in ICU or hospital length of stay in those patients in the overall study population or in the subset administered more than three units. These data are from a randomized trial and, therefore, should be more

heavily weighted. Data from some retrospective cohort studies have shown no benefit to leukocyte reduction.[204,205]

Aprotinin and Other Serine Protease Inhibitors

Aprotinin, a 58-amino-acid serine protease inhibitor isolated from bovine lung, has been shown in numerous studies to decrease bleeding associated with cardiac surgery. It antagonizes numerous proteolytic enzymes including plasmin and kallikrein, and may have some anti-inflammatory effects,[14,206] although a recent meta-analysis found no beneficial effect of aprotinin on systemic markers of inflammation.[207] Aprotinin's blood-sparing effects were apparently discovered serendipitously while it was being evaluated as an anti-inflammatory agent in cardiac surgical patients. Despite more than 45 randomized clinical trials conducted to date, there are little data to support the hypothesis that aprotinin administration reduces postoperative complications attributable to excessive systemic inflammation. In these trials, numerous surrogate markers of postoperative morbidity, such as the duration of postoperative tracheal intubation, ICU stay, and hospital length of stay, were not reported to be improved in aprotinin-treated patients. A large trial was recently completed in 2,331 cardiac surgical patients at 19 Canadian centers.[208] Patients were randomized to aprotinin, aminocaproic acid, or tranexamic acid. No benefit of aprotinin was observed with regard to complications such as respiratory failure, renal failure, or multisystem organ failure, and the study was terminated early because of an increase in mortality in aprotinin-treated patients. The findings from this trial, as well as several previous observational studies, led to market withdrawal of aprotinin.

It is worth noting that several novel drugs are under development that are postulated to reduce inflammation and blood loss, while being free of potential adverse effects associated with aprotinin. These include the synthetic serine protease inhibitors CU-2010 and CU-2020[209] and DX-88/ecallantide, a plasma kallikrein inhibitor.[210]

Tumor Necrosis Factor Antagonists

Soluble TNF receptor proteins antagonize the toxic effects of LPS-induced lethality in mice.[211] These agents are ineffective in the treatment of sepsis/septic shock but have not been tested in the setting of cardiac surgery.[212] Anti-TNF monoclonal antibodies have been studied in septic ICU patients as well; however, they have not yet been tested prophylactically in cardiac surgical patients.[69] A study involving prophylactic administration would allow for the antibody to be present before the TNF and thus determine whether TNF has overall harmful or beneficial effects. If TNF and other cytokines are essential to the healing process, complete inhibition of their effects may result in worse rather than improved postoperative outcome. Well-designed, large clinical trials could resolve these controversial issues.

E5564

E5564 is a synthetically derived lipid A analog that is a potent Toll-like receptor 4–directed endotoxin antagonist.[213] It does not have lipid A agonist properties, and even in high doses does not cause signs or symptoms of endotoxemia or systemic inflammation in humans and animals. Healthy volunteers were administered E5564 before a standard challenge dose of reference endotoxin (4 ng/kg). Single E5564 doses of 50 to 250 µg blocked or attenuated all of the effects of LPS in a dose-dependent manner. All E5564 dose groups had statistically significant reductions in increased temperature, HR, CRP levels, white blood cell count, and cytokine levels (TNF-α and IL-6), compared with placebo ($P < 0.01$).[213] This drug has shown promising results in critically ill patients with sepsis; however, results from a phase II trial in cardiac surgical patients were disappointing.[113] In this trial, 152 cardiac surgical patients at 9 U.S. centers were randomized to receive placebo or ascending doses of E5564. Blocking lipid A with eritoran did not result in any overt beneficial effects on markers of systemic inflammation (IL-6, IL-8, or CRP) or measures of organ injury. These results call into question the potential clinical relevance of lipid A in this setting.

Pentoxifylline

Pentoxifylline is a nonspecific phosphodiesterase inhibitor similar in chemical structure to theophylline, a common anti-inflammatory used to treat asthma. Pentoxifylline has multiple rheologic and anti-inflammatory properties, but the exact mechanism of its pharmacologic effects is poorly understood. Clinically, pentoxifylline is approved by the U.S. Food and Drug Administration to treat intermittent claudication, presumably by increasing red cell deformability, which may improve oxygen delivery to ischemic tissues. Animal studies have shown that treatment with pentoxifylline significantly attenuates endothelial damage and the formation of oxygen radicals after ischemia/reperfusion, prevents fever after the administration of LPS, and prevents leakage of bacteria from the gut during hemorrhagic shock. Clinical research studies using pentoxifylline have been performed in the setting of lung transplantation, cardiac surgery, and anemia requiring red blood cell transfusion.

In an initial study, Hoffman et al[214] randomized 40 patients with an Acute Physiology and Chronic Health Enquiry (APACHE) II score ≥ 19 after cardiac surgery to placebo or pentoxifylline (1.5 mg/kg/hr for 48 hours). In this study, patients administered pentoxifylline had significantly fewer days on mechanical ventilation, less need for hemofiltration, and a shorter ICU length of stay. In a historic control study, Thabut et al[215] administered pentoxifylline to 23 consecutive patients undergoing lung transplantation. Compared with historic controls, patients administered pentoxifylline experienced less allograft dysfunction and a significant reduction in 60-day mortality was noted. These findings need to be confirmed in a prospective, randomized clinical trial.

Boldt et al[216,217] randomized 30 elderly (> 80 years) patients undergoing cardiac surgery to placebo or pentoxifylline (300 mg bolus administered immediately after induction of general anesthesia followed by a continuous infusion of 1.5 mg/kg/hr for 48 hours). In this study, pentoxifylline administration minimized intraoperative and postoperative increases in plasma CRP, polymorphonuclear elastase, IL-6, and IL-8 levels. Duration of mechanical ventilation was significantly lower in patients randomized to pentoxifylline. This study was not powered to detect differences in rare but serious complications. Other small studies also suggested possible benefit[218,219]; however, these results have not been confirmed in a large, multicenter trial.

Ethyl pyruvate

This is a novel anti-inflammatory agent.[220,221] It has been shown to protect the intestinal mucosa from mesenteric ischemia and reperfusion in rats and improve survival in murine models of acute endotoxemia and bacterial peritonitis. Results from a phase II trial in cardiac surgical patients were disappointing.[222] In this trial, 102 high-risk cardiac surgical patients were randomized to receive placebo or ethyl pyruvate at 13 U.S. centers. Administration of ethyl pyruvate did not result in any overt beneficial effects on markers of systemic inflammation (TNF-α, IL-6, or CRP) or measures of organ injury.

Statins

Statins are routinely used to reduce cholesterol levels in patients at risk for cardiovascular disease; however, their anti-inflammatory effects have received significant attention.[223] It has been speculated that prophylactic statin administration before surgery may have beneficial effects. A recently published trial randomized 497 vascular surgical patients to placebo or fluvastatin daily from randomization to 30 days after surgery.[224] Patients randomized to the statin exhibited lower levels of the inflammatory markers IL-6 and CRP, and also reduced myocardial ischemia ($P = 0.01$). All-cause mortality was lower in statin-treated patients (2.4% vs. 4.9%); however, this difference did not achieve statistical significance ($P = 0.14$). There are no similar large trials in cardiac surgery, but a meta-analysis was recently completed of 8 trials involving a total of 638 such patients.[225] This analysis showed that statin use decreased levels of IL-6, IL-8, CRP, and TNF-α; however, no improvement in clinical outcomes was reported. At this point, the use of statins in cardiac surgery must be investigational until additional data are obtained to support this indication.

N-acetylcysteine

This is used to prevent radiocontrast-induced nephropathy and as an antidote for acetaminophen overdose. Its anti-inflammatory and antioxidant properties have been studied in the ICU setting and in cardiac surgical patients, with mixed results. A meta-analysis of N-acetylcysteine to ameliorate postoperative morbidity was recently published and included 1,338 patients from 13 trials.[226] This analysis suggested that N-acetylcysteine may have a beneficial effect with regard to postoperative atrial fibrillation but did not appear to be beneficial with regard to other postoperative complications.

Other Potential Antiendotoxin or Anti-Inflammatory Agents

Other potential approaches to preventing endotoxin-related complications involve the use of either synthetic or naturally occurring antiendotoxin compounds. *Bactericidal/permeability-increasing protein (BPI)* is a neutrophil granule protein and has been shown to have endotoxin-neutralizing and bactericidal activity in animal models. A human recombinant version, rBPI$_{21}$, neutralized endotoxin-mediated toxicity in humans. A recombinant version of an antiendotoxin factor, *endotoxin-neutralizing protein,* is another agent that has been shown to protect animals from endotoxin-mediated toxicity.[227] Reconstituted high-density lipoprotein (rHDL) neutralized some of endotoxin's toxic effects during an experimental model of human endotoxemia.[228] Polymyxin B neutralizes the toxic effects of endotoxin, although toxicity has prevented prophylactic intravenous use.[229] *Dextran-polymyxin B* is a variation of polymyxin B that has been reported to have antiendotoxin properties, as well as minimal toxicity in animal models. *Soluble TNF receptor proteins* antagonize the toxic effects of LPS-induced lethality in mice. This agent was not effective in the treatment of sepsis/septic shock but has not been tested in the setting of cardiac surgery.[211]

Role of Anesthetic Agents and Vasoactive Agents

Anesthetic agents, defined here as drugs that induce hypnosis, amnesia, muscle relaxation, or regional anesthesia, have not been shown to result in clinically meaningful reductions in systemic inflammation after cardiac surgery. Numerous studies have evaluated the effect of these agents on the immune system with varied results; however, no studies have reported a difference in outcome with one technique versus another. Ketamine is a promising agent that has been studied largely as an adjunct to reduce postoperative pain in noncardiac surgery. In an initial study in cardiac surgery, administration of a low dose (0.25 mg/kg) of ketamine before CPB prevented an increase in IL-6 for 7 days after surgery.[230] In addition, ketamine administration inhibited TNF production and leukocyte adherence in animal models and suppressed oxygen radical production in vitro. These results were confirmed in another small study of patients undergoing CPB.[231] However, there are no outcome data from large outcome trials, so it is unknown whether this intervention reduces clinically relevant complications.

All general anesthetics can reduce splanchnic perfusion indirectly through a depression of myocardial function and a reduction in CO, and hence oxygen delivery to the splanchnic mucosa.[232,233] Isoflurane theoretically may be better than halothane, enflurane, or propofol because of its vasodilating properties, which may preserve splanchnic blood flow and blood volume.[232-235] A prospective randomized study of cardiac surgical patients demonstrated better splanchnic perfusion in patients maintained with isoflurane in contrast with propofol or enflurane.[236]

Although not definitively supported yet, there is evidence that splanchnic hypoperfusion and endotoxin-induced inflammation can be prevented in the operating room by strategies familiar to clinicians. Strategies involve the use of fluid loading to maximize SV,[129] as well as the use of adequate levels of vasodilating volatile anesthetics. Inodilating agents, such as milrinone, amrinone, dopamine, and dobutamine, may be more protective of splanchnic perfusion than inoconstricting agents such as epinephrine, norepinephrine, and dopamine. Patients randomized to enoximone administration during cardiac surgery demonstrated lower endotoxin levels, suggesting a beneficial effect on the barrier function of the gut.[91] Endotoxemia is probably a more sensitive marker of loss of barrier function than gastric mucosal hypoperfusion because these patients still demonstrated decreases in calculated gastric mucosal pH (pHi). When tested in vitro, amrinone was a potent inhibitor of endotoxin-induced TNF production at clinically relevant drug concentrations, suggesting an additional advantage to the use of this phosphodiesterase inhibitor.[237] Dopamine is often touted as preserving splanchnic blood flow; however, responses to this agent are unpredictable, with vascular resistance increasing in some patients at low doses (3–5 μg/kg/min).

Selective Digestive Decontamination

Selective digestive decontamination represents a possible approach to limiting the incidence and severity of systemic inflammation. The technique attempts to reduce the total amount of endotoxin exposure by reducing the reservoir of endotoxin normally contained within the gut. Martinez-Pellús et al[65] conducted a prospective, open, randomized, controlled trial in 80 cardiac surgical patients. Patients were randomized to either a control group or up to 3 days of preoperative selective digestive decontamination accomplished with the administration of oral nonabsorbable antibiotics (polymyxin E, tobramycin, amphotericin B). Patients in the protocol group demonstrated much lower gut bacterial counts, as well as lower blood levels of endotoxin and the proinflammatory cytokine IL-6 in the operating room and the postoperative unit. The study was not designed with sufficient power to determine whether this technique affects outcomes such as mortality and morbidity. Nevertheless, it is interesting to note that there was a trend toward improved outcome (mortality, hospital length of stay) in the protocol group. In contrast, Bouter et al[238] found no beneficial effects of selective digestive decontamination on clinical outcome or blood levels of TNF-α, IL-6, or IL-10 in 78 cardiac surgical patients.

Summary

A very large body of circumstantial evidence strongly suggests that systemic inflammation is an important cause of mortality and morbidity after cardiac surgery. Although several strategies appear promising, there are little data from large randomized trials to support the widespread use of a particular intervention at the current time.

REFERENCES

1. Birkmeyer JD, Stukel TA, Siewers AE, et al: Surgeon volume and operative mortality in the United States, *N Engl J Med* 349(22):2117–2127, 2003.
2. Hammermeister KE, Burchfiel C, Johnson R, Grover FL: Identification of patients at greatest risk for developing major complications at cardiac surgery, *Circulation* 82(Suppl 5):IV380–IV389, 1990.
3. Rady MY, Ryan T, Starr NJ: Perioperative determinants of morbidity and mortality in elderly patients undergoing cardiac surgery, *Crit Care Med* 26(2):225–235, 1998.
4. Goris RJ, te Boekhorst TP, Nuytinck JK, Gimbrere JS: Multiple-organ failure. Generalized autodestructive inflammation? *Arch Surg* 120(10):1109–1115, 1985.
5. Bone RC, Balk RA, Cerra FB, et al: Definitions for sepsis and organ failure and guidelines for the use of innovative therapies in sepsis. The ACCP/SCCM Consensus Conference Committee. American College of Chest Physicians/Society of Critical Care Medicine, *Chest* 101(6):1644–1655, 1992.
6. Schlag G, Redl H, Hallstrom S: The cell in shock: The origin of multiple organ failure, *Resuscitation* 21(2–3):137–180, 1991.
7. American College of Chest Physicians/Society of Critical Care Medicine Consensus Conference: Definitions for sepsis and organ failure and guidelines for the use of innovative therapies in sepsis, *Crit Care Med* 20(6):864–874, 1992.
8. *Stedman's Medical Dictionary*, ed 26, Baltimore, 1995, Williams & Wilkins.
9. Vincent JL: Dear SIRS, I'm sorry to say that I don't like you, *Crit Care Med* 25(2):372–374, 1997.
10. Berendes E, Mollhoff T, Van Aken H, et al: Effects of dopexamine on creatinine clearance, systemic inflammation, and splanchnic oxygenation in patients undergoing coronary artery bypass grafting, *Anesth Analg* 84(5):950–957, 1997.
11. Andersen LW, Baek L, Degn H, et al: Presence of circulating endotoxins during cardiac operations, *J Thorac Cardiovasc Surg* 93(1):115–119, 1987.
12. Doran JE: Biological effects of endotoxin, *Curr Stud Hematol Blood Transfus* 59:66–99, 1992.
13. Herskowitz A, Mangano DT: Inflammatory cascade. A final common pathway for perioperative injury? *Anesthesiology* 85(5):957–960, 1996.
14. Royston D: Preventing the inflammatory response to open-heart surgery: The role of aprotinin and other protease inhibitors, *Int J Cardiol* 53(Suppl):S11–S37, 1996.
15. Miller BE, Levy JH: The inflammatory response to cardiopulmonary bypass, *J Cardiothorac Vasc Anesth* 11(3):355–366, 1997.
16. Weiss SJ: Tissue destruction by neutrophils, *N Engl J Med* 320(6):365–376, 1989.
17. Webster RO, Hong SR, Johnston RB Jr, Henson PM: Biologial effects of the human complement fragments C5a and C5ades Arg on neutrophil function, *Immunopharmacology* 2(3):201–219, 1980.
18. Freeman BA, Crapo JD: Biology of disease: free radicals and tissue injury, *Lab Invest* 47(5):412–426, 1982.
19. Meerson FZ, Kagan VE, Kozlov Yu P, et al: The role of lipid peroxidation in pathogenesis of ischemic damage and the antioxidant protection of the heart, *Basic Res Cardiol* 77(5):465–485, 1982.
20. Halliwell B, Guiteridge M: *Oxygen radical and tissue damage*, Bologna, Italy, 1982, Cooperativa Libraria Iniversitavia Editrice.
21. Prasad K, Kalra J, Bharadwaj B, Chaudhary AK: Increased oxygen free radical activity in patients on cardiopulmonary bypass undergoing aortocoronary bypass surgery, *Am Heart J* 123(1):37–45, 1992.
22. Royston D, Fleming JS, Desai JB, et al: Increased production of peroxidation products associated with cardiac operations. Evidence for free radical generation, *J Thorac Cardiovasc Surg* 91(5):759–766, 1986.
23. Fosse E, Moen O, Johnson E, et al: Reduced complement and granulocyte activation with heparin-coated cardiopulmonary bypass, *Ann Thorac Surg* 58(2):472–477, 1994.
24. Kharazmi A, Andersen LW, Baek L, et al: Endotoxemia and enhanced generation of oxygen radicals by neutrophils from patients undergoing cardiopulmonary bypass, *J Thorac Cardiovasc Surg* 98(3):381–385, 1989.
25. Borowiec J, Thelin S, Bagge L, et al: Heparin-coated circuits reduce activation of granulocytes during cardiopulmonary bypass. A clinical study, *J Thorac Cardiovasc Surg* 104(3):642–647, 1992.
26. Mythen MG, Purdy G, Mackie IJ, et al: Postoperative multiple organ dysfunction syndrome associated with gut mucosal hypoperfusion, increased neutrophil degranulation and C1- esterase inhibitor depletion, *Br J Anaesth* 71(6):858–863, 1993.
27. Bjork J, Hugli TE, Smedegard G: Microvascular effects of anaphylatoxins C3a and C5a, *J Immunol* 134(2):1115–1119, 1985.
28. Liu B, Belboul A, al-Khaja N, et al: Effect of high-dose aprotinin on blood cell filterabiltiy in association with cardiopulmonary bypass, *Coron Artery Dis* 3:129, 1992.
29. Blauth C, Arnold J, Kohner EM, Taylor KM: Retinal microembolism during cardiopulmonary bypass demonstrated by fluorescein angiography, *Lancet* 2(8511):837–839, 1986.
30. Sheeran P, Hall GM: Cytokines in anaesthesia, *Br J Anaesth* 78(2):201–219, 1997.
31. Tonnesen E, Christensen VB, Toft P: The role of cytokines in cardiac surgery, *Int J Cardiol* 53(Suppl):S1–S10, 1996.
32. Baumann H, Gauldie J: The acute phase response, *Immunol Today* 15(2):74–80, 1994.
33. Michie HR, Manogue KR, Spriggs DR, et al: Detection of circulating tumor necrosis factor after endotoxin administration, *N Engl J Med* 318(23):1481–1486, 1988.
34. Michie HR, Spriggs DR, Manogue KR, et al: Tumor necrosis factor and endotoxin induce similar metabolic responses in human beings, *Surgery* 104(2):280–286, 1988.
35. Tracey KJ, Lowry SF, Fahey TJ 3rd, et al: Cachectin/tumor necrosis factor induces lethal shock and stress hormone responses in the dog, *Surg Gynecol Obstet* 164(5):415–422, 1987.
36. Hesse DG, Tracey KJ, Fong Y, et al: Cytokine appearance in human endotoxemia and primate bacteremia, *Surg Gynecol Obstet* 166(2):147–153, 1988.
37. Jansen NJ, van Oeveren W, van Vliet M, et al: The role of different types of corticosteroids on the inflammatory mediators in cardiopulmonary bypass, *Eur J Cardiothorac Surg* 5(4):211–217, 1991.
38. Jansen NJ, van Oeveren W, Gu YJ, et al: Endotoxin release and tumor necrosis factor formation during cardiopulmonary bypass, *Ann Thorac Surg* 54(4):744–747, 1992 discussion 747–748.
39. Abe K, Nishimura M, Sakakibara T: Interleukin-6 and tumour necrosis factor during cardiopulmonary bypass, *Can J Anaesth* 41(9):876–877, 1994.
40. Tonz M, Mihaljevic T, von Segesser LK, et al: Normothermia versus hypothermia during cardiopulmonary bypass: A randomized, controlled trial, *Ann Thorac Surg* 59(1):137–143, 1995.
41. te Velthuis H, Jansen PG, Oudemans-van Straaten HM, et al: Myocardial performance in elderly patients after cardiopulmonary bypass is suppressed by tumor necrosis factor, *J Thorac Cardiovasc Surg* 110(6):1663–1669, 1995.
42. Hennein HA, Ebba H, Rodriguez JL, et al: Relationship of the proinflammatory cytokines to myocardial ischemia and dysfunction after uncomplicated coronary revascularization, *J Thorac Cardiovasc Surg* 108(4):626–635, 1994.
43. Wan S, Marchant A, DeSmet JM, et al: Human cytokine responses to cardiac transplantation and coronary artery bypass grafting, *J Thorac Cardiovasc Surg* 111(2):469–477, 1996.
44. Seghaye M, Duchateau J, Bruniaux J, et al: Interleukin-10 release related to cardiopulmonary bypass in infants undergoing cardiac operations, *J Thorac Cardiovasc Surg* 111(3):545–553, 1996.
45. Deng MC, Dasch B, Erren M, et al: Impact of left ventricular dysfunction on cytokines, hemodynamics, and outcome in bypass grafting, *Ann Thorac Surg* 62(1):184–190, 1996.
46. Millar AB, Armstrong L, van der Linden J, et al: Cytokine production and hemofiltration in children undergoing cardiopulmonary bypass, *Ann Thorac Surg* 56(6):1499–1502, 1993.
47. Furunaga A: Measurement of cytokines at cardiopulmonary-bypass, *Nippon Kyobu Geka Gakkai Zasshi* 42(12):2200–2206, 1994.
48. Kawamura T, Wakusawa R, Okada K, Inada S: Elevation of cytokines during open heart surgery with cardiopulmonary bypass: Participation of interleukin 8 and 6 in reperfusion injury, *Can J Anaesth* 40(11):1016–1021, 1993.
49. Markewitz A, Faist E, Lang S, et al: Regulation of acute phase response after cardiopulmonary bypass by immunomodulation, *Ann Thorac Surg* 55(2):389–394, 1993.
50. Haeffner-Cavaillon N, Roussellier N, Ponzio O, et al: Induction of interleukin-1 production in patients undergoing cardiopulmonary bypass, *J Thorac Cardiovasc Surg* 98(6):1100–1106, 1989.
51. Frering B, Philip I, Dehoux M, et al: Circulating cytokines in patients undergoing normothermic cardiopulmonary bypass, *J Thorac Cardiovasc Surg* 108(4):636–641, 1994.
52. Quigley RL, Caplan MS, Perkins JA, et al: Cardiopulmonary bypass with adequate flow and perfusion pressures prevents endotoxaemia and pathologic cytokine production, *Perfusion* 10(1):27–31, 1995.
53. Steinberg BM, Grossi EA, Schwartz DS, et al: Heparin bonding of bypass circuits reduces cytokine release during cardiopulmonary bypass, *Ann Thorac Surg* 60(3):525–529, 1995.
54. Steinberg JB, Kapelanski DP, Olson JD, Weiler JM: Cytokine and complement levels in patients undergoing cardiopulmonary bypass, *J Thorac Cardiovasc Surg* 106(6):1008–1016, 1993.
55. Kilbourn RG, Belloni P: Endothelial cell production of nitrogen oxides in response to interferon gamma in combination with tumor necrosis factor, interleukin-1, or endotoxin, *J Natl Cancer Inst* 82(9):772–776, 1990.
56. Finn A, Naik S, Klein N, et al: Interleukin-8 release and neutrophil degranulation after pediatric cardiopulmonary bypass, *J Thorac Cardiovasc Surg* 105(2):234–241, 1993.
57. Huber AR, Kunkel SL, Todd RF 3rd, Weiss SJ: Regulation of transendothelial neutrophil migration by endogenous interleukin-8, *Science* 254(5028):99–102, 1991.
58. Ashraf SS, Tian Y, Cowan D, et al: Proinflammatory cytokine release during pediatric cardiopulmonary bypass: Influence of centrifugal and roller pumps, *J Cardiothorac Vasc Anesth* 11(6):718–722, 1997.
59. Kawahito K, Kawakami M, Fujiwara T, et al: Proinflammatory cytokine levels in patients undergoing cardiopulmonary bypass. Does lung reperfusion influence the release of cytokines? *ASAIO J* 41(3):M775–M778, 1995.
60. Rothenburger M, Soeparwata R, Deng MC, et al: Prediction of clinical outcome after cardiac surgery: The role of cytokines, endotoxin, and anti-endotoxin core antibodies, *Shock* 16(Suppl 1):44–50, 2001.
61. Rothenburger M, Tjan TD, Schneider M, et al: The impact of the pro- and anti-inflammatory immune response on ventilation time after cardiac surgery, *Cytometry* 53B(1):70–74, 2003.

62. Butler J, Chong GL, Baigrie RJ, et al: Cytokine responses to cardiopulmonary bypass with membrane and bubble oxygenation, *Ann Thorac Surg* 53(5):833–838, 1992.
63. Almdahl SM, Waage A, Ivert T, Vaage J: Release of bioactive interleukin-6 but not of tumor necrosis factor-alpha after elective cardiopulmonary bypass, *Perfusion* 8:233, 1993.
64. Cremer J, Martin M, Redl H, et al: Systemic inflammatory response syndrome after cardiac operations, *Ann Thorac Surg* 61(6):1714–1720, 1996.
65. Martinez-Pellús AE, Merino P, Bru M, et al: Can selective digestive decontamination avoid the endotoxemia and cytokine activation promoted by cardiopulmonary bypass? *Crit Care Med* 21(11):1684–1691, 1993.
66. de Waal Malefyt R, Abrams J, Bennett B, et al: Interleukin 10(IL-10) inhibits cytokine synthesis by human monocytes: An autoregulatory role of IL-10 produced by monocytes, *J Exp Med* 174(5):1209–1220, 1991.
67. Bogdan C, Vodovotz Y, Nathan C: Macrophage deactivation by interleukin 10, *J Exp Med* 174(6): 1549–1555, 1991.
68. McBride WT, Armstrong MA, Crockard AD, et al: Cytokine balance and immunosuppressive changes at cardiac surgery: Contrasting response between patients and isolated CPB circuits, *Br J Anaesth* 75(6):724–733, 1995.
69. Fisher CJ Jr, Agosti JM, Opal SM, et al: Treatment of septic shock with the tumor necrosis factor receptor:Fc fusion protein. The Soluble TNF Receptor Sepsis Study Group, *N Engl J Med* 334(26):1697–1702, 1996.
70. Best N, Sinosich MJ, Teisner B, et al: Complement activation during cardiopulmonary bypass by heparin-protamine interaction, *Br J Anaesth* 56(4):339–343, 1984.
71. Kirklin JK, Chenoweth DE, Naftel DC, et al: Effects of protamine administration after cardiopulmonary bypass on complement, blood elements, and the hemodynamic state, *Ann Thorac Surg* 41(2):193–199, 1986.
72. Chiu RC, Samson R: Complement (C3, C4) consumption in cardiopulmonary bypass, cardioplegia, and protamine administration, *Ann Thorac Surg* 37(3):229–232, 1984.
73. Chenoweth DE, Cooper SW, Hugli TE, et al: Complement activation during cardiopulmonary bypass: Evidence for generation of C3a and C5a anaphylatoxins, *N Engl J Med* 304(9):497–503, 1981.
74. Hammerschmidt DE, Stroncek DF, Bowers TK, et al: Complement activation and neutropenia occurring during cardiopulmonary bypass, *J Thorac Cardiovasc Surg* 81(3):370–377, 1981.
75. Kirklin JK, Westaby S, Blackstone EH, et al: Complement and the damaging effects of cardiopulmonary bypass, *J Thorac Cardiovasc Surg* 86(6):845–857, 1983.
76. Moore FD Jr, Warner KG, Assousa S, et al: The effects of complement activation during cardiopulmonary bypass. Attenuation by hypothermia, heparin, and hemodilution, *Ann Surg* 208(1):95–103, 1988.
77. Riegel W, Spillner G, Schlosser V, Horl WH: Plasma levels of main granulocyte components during cardiopulmonary bypass, *J Thorac Cardiovasc Surg* 95(6):1014–1019, 1988.
78. Bonser RS, Dave JR, Davies ET, et al: Reduction of complement activation during bypass by prime manipulation, *Ann Thorac Surg* 49(2):279–283, 1990.
79. Shernan SK, Fitch JC, Nussmeier NA, et al: Impact of pexelizumab, an anti-C5 complement antibody, on total mortality and adverse cardiovascular outcomes in cardiac surgical patients undergoing cardiopulmonary bypass, *Ann Thorac Surg* 77(3):942–949, 2004 discussion 949–950.
80. Verrier ED, Shernan SK, Taylor KM, et al: Terminal complement blockade with pexelizumab during coronary artery bypass graft surgery requiring cardiopulmonary bypass: A randomized trial, *JAMA* 291(19):2319–2327, 2004.
81. Fitch JC, Rollins S, Matis L, et al: Pharmacology and biological efficacy of a recombinant, humanized, single-chain antibody C5 complement inhibitor in patients undergoing coronary artery bypass graft surgery with cardiopulmonary bypass, *Circulation* 100(25):2499–2506, 1999.
82. Morrison DC, Cochrane CG: Direct evidence for Hageman factor (factor XII) activation by bacterial lipopolysaccharides (endotoxins), *J Exp Med* 140(3):797–811, 1974.
83. Morrison DC, Ryan JL: Endotoxins and disease mechanisms, *Annu Rev Med* 38:417–432, 1987.
84. Natanson C, Eichenholz PW, Danner RL, et al: Endotoxin and tumor necrosis factor challenges in dogs simulate the cardiovascular profile of human septic shock, *J Exp Med* 169(3):823–832, 1989.
85. Rocke DA, Gaffin SL, Wells MT, et al: Endotoxemia associated with cardiopulmonary bypass, *J Thorac Cardiovasc Surg* 93(6):832–837, 1987.
86. Andersen LW, Baek L, Thomsen BS, Rasmussen JP: Effect of methylprednisolone on endotoxemia and complement activation during cardiac surgery, *J Cardiothorac Anesth* 3(5):544–549, 1989.
87. Andersen LW, Landow L, Baek L, et al: Association between gastric intramucosal pH and splanchnic endotoxin, antibody to endotoxin, and tumor necrosis factor-alpha concentrations in patients undergoing cardiopulmonary bypass, *Crit Care Med* 21(2):210–217, 1993.
88. Riddington DW, Venkatesh B, Boivin CM, et al: Intestinal permeability, gastric intramucosal pH, and systemic endotoxemia in patients undergoing cardiopulmonary bypass, *JAMA* 275(13):1007–1012, 1996.
89. Oudemans-van Straaten HM, Jansen PG, Hoek FJ, et al: Intestinal permeability, circulating endotoxin, and postoperative systemic responses in cardiac surgery patients, *J Cardiothorac Vasc Anesth* 10(2):187–194, 1996.
90. Oudemans-van Straaten HM, Jansen PG, Velthuis H, et al: Endotoxaemia and postoperative hypermetabolism in coronary artery bypass surgery: The role of ketanserin, *Br J Anaesth* 77(4):473–479, 1996.
91. Loick HM, Mollhoff T, Berendes E, et al: Influence of enoximone on systemic and splanchnic oxygen utilization and endotoxin release following cardiopulmonary bypass, *Intensive Care Med* 23(3):267–275, 1997.
92. te Velthuis H, Jansen PG, Oudemans-van Straaten HM, et al: Circulating endothelin in cardiac operations: Influence of blood pressure and endotoxin, *Ann Thorac Surg* 61(3):904–908, 1996.
93. Bowles CT, Ohri SK, Klangsuk N, et al: Endotoxaemia detected during cardiopulmonary bypass with a modified Limulus amoebocyte lysate assay, *Perfusion* 10(4):219–228, 1995.
94. Watarida S, Mori A, Onoe M, et al: A clinical study on the effects of pulsatile cardiopulmonary bypass on the blood endotoxin levels, *J Thorac Cardiovasc Surg* 108(4):620–625, 1994.
95. Nilsson L, Kulander L, Nystrom SO, Eriksson O: Endotoxins in cardiopulmonary bypass, *J Thorac Cardiovasc Surg* 100(5):777–780, 1990.
96. Myles P, Buckland M, Cannon G, et al: The association among gastric mucosal pH, endotoxemia, and low systemic vascular resistance after cardiopulmonary bypass, *J Cardiothorac Vasc Anesth* 10(2):195–200, 1996.
97. Imai T, Shiga T, Saruki N, et al: Change in plasma endotoxin titres and endotoxin neutralizing activity in the perioperative period, *Can J Anaesth* 43(8):812–819, 1996.
98. Lebek G, Cottier H: Notes on the bacterial content of the gut, *Curr Stud Hematol Blood Transfus* 59:1–18, 1992.
99. Fink MP: Effect of critical illness on microbial translocation and gastrointestinal mucosa permeability, *Semin Respir Infect* 9(4):256–260, 1994.
100. Daniel M: Response of man to endotoxin, *Immunobiology* 187:403, 1993.
101. Rubin J, Robbs JV, Gaffin SL, Wells MT: Plasma lipopolysaccharide increase after aortic aneurysm resection, *S Afr Med J* 74(4):193, 1988.
102. Greisman SE, Hornick RB: Mechanism of endotoxin tolerance with special reference to man, *J Infect Dis* 128(S):265, 1973.
103. Astiz ME, Rackow EC, Still JG, et al: Pretreatment of normal humans with monophosphoryl lipid A induces tolerance to endotoxin: A prospective, double-blind, randomized, controlled trial, *Crit Care Med* 23(1):9–17, 1995.
104. Luderitz O, Staub AM, Westphal O: Immunochemistry of O and R antigens of *Salmonella* and related *Enterobacteriaceae*, *Bacteriol Rev* 30(1):192–255, 1966.
105. Volk WBDKR.: In *Medical microbiology*, Philadelphia, 1986, Lippincott, pp 396–398.
106. DeCamp MM, Demling RH: Posttraumatic multisystem organ failure, *JAMA* 260(4):530–534, 1988.
107. Ford EG, Baisden CE, Matteson ML, Picone AL: Sepsis after coronary bypass grafting: Evidence for loss of the gut mucosal barrier, *Ann Thorac Surg* 52(3):514–517, 1991.
108. Moore FA, Moore EE, Poggetti R, et al: Gut bacterial translocation via the portal vein: A clinical perspective with major torso trauma, *J Trauma* 31(5):629–636, 1991 discussion 636–628.
109. Rush BF Jr, Sori AJ, Murphy TF, et al: Endotoxemia and bacteremia during hemorrhagic shock. The link between trauma and sepsis? *Ann Surg* 207(5):549–554, 1988.
110. Ziegler EJ, Fisher CJ Jr, Sprung CL, et al: Treatment of gram-negative bacteremia and septic shock with HA-1A human monoclonal antibody against endotoxin. A randomized, double-blind, placebo-controlled trial. The HA-1A Sepsis Study Group, *N Engl J Med* 324(7):429–436, 1991.
111. Greenman RL, Schein RM, Martin MA, et al: A controlled clinical trial of E5 murine monoclonal IgM antibody to endotoxin in the treatment of gram-negative sepsis. The XOMA Sepsis Study Group, *JAMA* 266(8):1097–1102, 1991.
112. Warren HS, Amato SF, Fitting C, et al: Assessment of ability of murine and human anti-lipid A monoclonal antibodies to bind and neutralize lipopolysaccharide, *J Exp Med* 177(1):89–97, 1993.
113. Bennett-Guerrero E, Grocott HP, Levy JH, et al: A phase II, double-blind, placebo-controlled, ascending-dose study of Eritoran (E5564), a lipid A antagonist, in patients undergoing cardiac surgery with cardiopulmonary bypass, *Anesth Analg* 104(2):378–383, 2007.
114. Deitch EA, Berg R: Bacterial translocation from the gut: a mechanism of infection, *J Burn Care Rehabil* 8(6):475–482, 1987.
115. Deitch EA: Bacterial translocation of the gut flora, *J Trauma* 30(Suppl 12):S184–S189, 1990.
116. Deitch EA: The role of intestinal barrier failure and bacterial translocation in the development of systemic infection and multiple organ failure, *Arch Surg* 125(3):403–404, 1990.
117. Mythen MG, Webb AR: The role of gut mucosal hypoperfusion in the pathogenesis of post-operative organ dysfunction, *Intensive Care Med* 20(3):203–209, 1994.
118. Price HL, Deutsch S, Marshall BE, et al: Hemodynamic and metabolic effects of hemorrhage in man, with particular reference to the splanchnic circulation, *Circ Res* 18(5):469–474, 1966.
119. Lundgren O: Physiology of intestinal circulation. In Martson AF-GR, editor: *Splanchnic ischemia and multiple organ failure*, St. Louis, 1989, Mosby, pp 29–40.
120. Hamilton-Davies C, Mythen MG, Salmon JB, et al: Comparison of commonly used clinical indicators of hypovolaemia with gastrointestinal tonometry, *Intensive Care Med* 23(3):276–281, 1997.
121. American College of Surgeons: *Advanced Trauma Life Support*, Chicago, 1993, American College of Surgeons.
122. Taylor KM, Bain WH, Russell M, et al: Peripheral vascular resistance and angiotensin II levels during pulsatile and no-pulsatile cardiopulmonary bypass, *Thorax* 34(5):594–598, 1979.
123. Richardson PD, Withrington PG: The effects of intraportal injections of noradrenaline, adrenaline, vasopressin and angiotensin on the hepatic portal vascular bed of the dog: Marked tachyphylaxis to angiotensin, *Br J Pharmacol* 59(2):293–301, 1977.
124. Watkins WD, Peterson MB, Kong DL, et al: Thromboxane and prostacyclin changes during cardiopulmonary bypass with and without pulsatile flow, *J Thorac Cardiovasc Surg* 84(2):250–256, 1982.
125. Levine FH, Philbin DM, Kono K, et al: Plasma vasopressin levels and urinary sodium excretion during cardiopulmonary bypass with and without pulsatile flow, *Ann Thorac Surg* 32(1):63–67, 1981.
126. Fink MP, Antonsson JB, Wang HL, Rothschild HR: Increased intestinal permeability in endotoxic pigs. Mesenteric hypoperfusion as an etiologic factor, *Arch Surg* 126(2):211–218, 1991.
127. Fiddian-Green RG, Baker S: Predictive value of the stomach wall pH for complications after cardiac operations: Comparison with other monitoring, *Crit Care Med* 15(2):153–156, 1987.
128. Mythen MG, Webb AR: Intra-operative gut mucosal hypoperfusion is associated with increased post-operative complications and cost, *Intensive Care Med* 20(2):99–104, 1994.
129. Mythen MG, Webb AR: Perioperative plasma volume expansion reduces the incidence of gut mucosal hypoperfusion during cardiac surgery, *Arch Surg* 130(4):423–429, 1995.
130. Bennett-Guerrero E, Panah MH, Bodian CA, et al: Automated detection of gastric luminal partial pressure of carbon dioxide during cardiovascular surgery using the Tonocap, *Anesthesiology* 92(1): 38–45, 2000.
131. Martich GD, Boujoukos AJ, Suffredini AF: Response of man to endotoxin, *Immunobiology* 187(3–5): 403–416, 1993.
132. Braude AI, Douglas H, Davis CE: Treatment and prevention of intravascular coagulation with antiserum to endotoxin, *J Infect Dis* 128(Suppl):157–164, 1973.
133. Suffredini AF, Fromm RE, Parker MM, et al: The cardiovascular response of normal humans to the administration of endotoxin, *N Engl J Med* 321(5):280–287, 1989.
134. Cunnion RE, Parrillo JE: Myocardial dysfunction in sepsis, *Crit Care Clin* 5(1):99–118, 1989.
135. Hollenberg SM, Cunnion RE, Parrillo JE: The effect of tumor necrosis factor on vascular smooth muscle. In vitro studies using rat aortic rings, *Chest* 100(4):1133–1137, 1991.
136. Clauss M, Ryan J, Stern D: Modulation of endothelial cell hemostatic properties by TNF: Insights into the role of endothelium in the host response to inflammatory stimuli. In Beutler B, editor: *Tumor necrosis factors: The molecules and their emerging role in medicine*, New York, 1992, Raven, pp 49–63.
137. Arvin B, Neville LF, Barone FC, Feuerstein GZ: The role of inflammation and cytokines in brain injury, *Neurosci Biobehav Rev* 20(3):445–452, 1996.
138. Loop FD, Lytle BW, Cosgrove DM, et al: J. Maxwell Chamberlain memorial paper. Sternal wound complications after isolated coronary artery bypass grafting: Early and late mortality, morbidity, and cost of care, *Ann Thorac Surg* 49(2):179–186, 1990 discussion 186–177.
139. Weintraub WS, Jones EL, Craver J, et al: Determinants of prolonged length of hospital stay after coronary bypass surgery, *Circulation* 80(2):276–284, 1989.
140. Sarr MG, Gott VL, Townsend TR: Mediastinal infection after cardiac surgery, *Ann Thorac Surg* 38(4):415–423, 1984.
141. Miholic J, Hudec M, Domanig E, et al: Risk factors for severe bacterial infections after valve replacement and aortocoronary bypass operations: Analysis of 246 cases by logistic regression, *Ann Thorac Surg* 40(3):224–228, 1985.
142. Kress HG, Scheidewig C, Engelhardt W, et al: Prediction and prevention, by immunological means, of septic complications after elective cardiac surgery, *Prog Clin Biol Res* 308:1031–1035, 1989.
143. Collett B, Alhaq A, Abdullah NB, et al: Pathways to complement activation during cardiopulmonary bypass, *Br Med J (Clin Res Ed)* 289(6454):1251–1254, 1984.
144. Parker DJ, Cantrell JW, Karp RB, et al: Changes in serum complement and immunoglobulins following cardiopulmonary bypass, *Surgery* 71(6):824–827, 1972.
145. van Oeveren W, Kazatchkine MD, Descamps-Latscha B, et al: Deleterious effects of cardiopulmonary bypass. A prospective study of bubble versus membrane oxygenation, *J Thorac Cardiovasc Surg* 89(6):888–899, 1985.
146. Hairston P, Manos JP, Graber CD, Lee WH Jr: Depression of immunologic surveillance by pump-oxygenation perfusion, *J Surg Res* 9(10):587–593, 1969.

147. Lee WH Jr, Krumhaar D, Fonkalsrud EW, et al: Denaturation of plasma proteins as a cause of morbidity and death after intracardiac operations, *Surgery* 50:29–39, 1961.

148. van Velzen-Blad H, Dijkstra YJ, Schurink GA, et al: Cardiopulmonary bypass and host defense functions in human beings: I. Serum levels and role of immunoglobulins and complement in phagocytosis, *Ann Thorac Surg* 39(3):207–211, 1985.

149. Eskola J, Salo M, Viljanen MK, Ruuskanen O: Impaired B lymphocyte function during open-heart surgery. Effects of anaesthesia and surgery, *Br J Anaesth* 56(4):333–338, 1984.

150. Markewitz A, Faist E, Lang S, et al: Successful restoration of cell-mediated immune response after cardiopulmonary bypass by immunomodulation, *J Thorac Cardiovasc Surg* 105(1):15–24, 1993.

151. Welsby IJ, Bennett-Guerrero E, Atwell D, et al: The association of complication type with mortality and prolonged stay after cardiac surgery with cardiopulmonary bypass, *Anesth Analg* 94(5):1072–1078, 2002 table of contents.

152. Huddy SP, Joyce WP, Pepper JR: Gastrointestinal complications in 4473 patients who underwent cardiopulmonary bypass surgery, *Br J Surg* 78(3):293–296, 1991.

153. Christenson JT, Schmuziger M, Maurice J, et al: Gastrointestinal complications after coronary artery bypass grafting, *J Thorac Cardiovasc Surg* 108(5):899–906, 1994.

154. Corwin HL, Sprague SM, DeLaria GA, Norusis MJ: Acute renal failure associated with cardiac operations. A case-control study, *J Thorac Cardiovasc Surg* 98(6):1107–1112, 1989.

155. Fowler AA, Hamman RF, Good JT, et al: Adult respiratory distress syndrome: Risk with common predispositions, *Ann Intern Med* 98(5 Pt 1):593–597, 1983.

156. Messent M, Sullivan K, Keogh BF, et al: Adult respiratory distress syndrome following cardiopulmonary bypass: Incidence and prediction, *Anaesthesia* 47(3):267–268, 1992.

157. Bennett-Guerrero E: Unpublished data

158. Geha AS, Sessler AD, Kirklin JW: Alveolar-arterial oxygen gradients after open intracardiac surgery, *J Thorac Cardiovasc Surg* 51(5):609–615, 1966.

159. el-Fiky MM, Taggart DP, Carter R, et al: Respiratory dysfunction following cardiopulmonary bypass: Verification of a non-invasive technique to measure shunt fraction, *Respir Med* 87(3):193–198, 1993.

160. Turnbull KW, Miyagishima RT, Gerein AN: Pulmonary complications and cardiopulmonary bypass: A clinical study in adults, *Can Anaesth Soc J* 21(2):181–194, 1974.

161. Cavarocchi NC, Pluth JR, Schaff HV, et al: Complement activation during cardiopulmonary bypass. Comparison of bubble and membrane oxygenators, *J Thorac Cardiovasc Surg* 91(2):252–258, 1986.

162. Jansen NJ, van Oeveren W, van den Broek L, et al: Inhibition by dexamethasone of the reperfusion phenomena in cardiopulmonary bypass, *J Thorac Cardiovasc Surg* 102(4):515–525, 1991.

163. Inaba H, Kochi A, Yorozu S: Suppression by methylprednisolone of augmented plasma endotoxin-like activity and interleukin-6 during cardiopulmonary bypass, *Br J Anaesth* 72(3):348–350, 1994.

164. Niazi Z, Flodin P, Joyce L, et al: Effects of glucocorticosteroids in patients undergoing coronary artery bypass surgery, *Chest* 76(3):262–268, 1979.

165. Miranda DR, Stoutenbeek C, Karliczek G, Rating W: Effects of dexamethason on the early postoperative course after coronary artery bypass surgery, *Thorac Cardiovasc Surg* 30(1):21–27, 1982.

166. Jorens PG, De Jongh R, De Backer W, et al: Interleukin-8 production in patients undergoing cardiopulmonary bypass. The influence of pretreatment with methylprednisolone, *Am Rev Respir Dis* 148(4 Pt 1):890–895, 1993.

167. Tabardel Y, Duchateau J, Schmartz D, et al: Corticosteroids increase blood interleukin-10 levels during cardiopulmonary bypass in men, *Surgery* 119(1):76–80, 1996.

168. Tennenberg SD, Bailey WW, Cotta LA, et al: The effects of methylprednisolone on complement-mediated neutrophil activation during cardiopulmonary bypass, *Surgery* 100(2):134–142, 1986.

169. Toledo-Pereyra LH, Lin CY, Kundler H, Replogle RL: Steroids in heart surgery: A clinical double-blind and randomized study, *Am Surg* 46(3):155–160, 1980.

170. Chaney MA, Durazo-Arvizu RA, Nikolov MP, et al: Methylprednisolone does not benefit patients undergoing coronary artery bypass grafting and early tracheal extubation, *J Thorac Cardiovasc Surg* 121(3):561–569, 2001.

171. Chaney MA: Corticosteroids and cardiopulmonary bypass: A review of clinical investigations, *Chest* 121(3):921–931, 2002.

172. Oliver WC Jr, Nuttall GA, Orszulak TA, et al: Hemofiltration but not steroids results in earlier tracheal extubation following cardiopulmonary bypass: A prospective, randomized double-blind trial, *Anesthesiology* 101(2):327–339, 2004.

173. Whitlock RP, Chan S, Devereaux PJ, et al: Clinical benefit of steroid use in patients undergoing cardiopulmonary bypass: A meta-analysis of randomized trials, *Eur Heart J* 29(21):2592–2600, 2008.

174. Weerwind PW, Maessen JG, van Tits LJ, et al: Influence of Duraflo II heparin-treated extracorporeal circuits on the systemic inflammatory response in patients having coronary bypass, *J Thorac Cardiovasc Surg* 110(6):1633–1641, 1995.

175. Ovrum E, Mollnes TE, Fosse E, et al: Complement and granulocyte activation in two different types of heparinized extracorporeal circuits, *J Thorac Cardiovasc Surg* 110(6):1623–1632, 1995.

176. Mangoush O, Purkayastha S, Haj-Yahia S, et al: Heparin-bonded circuits versus nonheparin-bonded circuits: An evaluation of their effect on clinical outcomes, *Eur J Cardiothorac Surg* 31(6):1058–1069, 2007.

177. Jakob H, Hafner G, Iversen S, et al: Reoperation and the centrifugal pump? *Eur J Cardiothorac Surg* 6(Suppl 1):S59–S63, 1992.

178. Driessen JJ, Dhaese H, Fransen G, et al: Pulsatile compared with nonpulsatile perfusion using a centrifugal pump for cardiopulmonary bypass during coronary artery bypass grafting. Effects on systemic haemodynamics, oxygenation, and inflammatory response parameters, *Perfusion* 10(1):3–12, 1995.

179. Tamiya T, Yamasaki M, Maeo Y, et al: Complement activation in cardiopulmonary bypass, with special reference to anaphylatoxin production in membrane and bubble oxygenators, *Ann Thorac Surg* 46(1):47–57, 1988.

180. Jones HM, Matthews N, Vaughan RS, Stark JM: Cardiopulmonary bypass and complement activation. Involvement of classical and alternative pathways, *Anaesthesia* 37(6):629–633, 1982.

181. Byrick RJ, Noble WH: Postperfusion lung syndrome. Comparison of Travenol bubble and membrane oxygenators, *J Thorac Cardiovasc Surg* 76(5):685–693, 1978.

182. van Oeveren W, Dankert J, Wildevuur CR: Bubble oxygenation and cardiotomy suction impair the host defense during cardiopulmonary bypass: A study in dogs, *Ann Thorac Surg* 44(5):523–528, 1987.

183. Videm V, Fosse E, Mollnes TE, et al: Complement activation with bubble and membrane oxygenators in aortocoronary bypass grafting, *Ann Thorac Surg* 50(3):387–391, 1990.

184. Croughwell ND, Newman MF, Lowry E, et al: Effect of temperature during cardiopulmonary bypass on gastric mucosal perfusion, *Br J Anaesth* 78(1):34–38, 1997.

185. Menasche P, Peynet J, Lariviere J, et al: Does normothermia during cardiopulmonary bypass increase neutrophil-endothelium interactions? *Circulation* 90(5 Pt 2):II275–279, 1994.

186. Ohata T, Sawa Y, Kadoba K, et al: Normothermia has beneficial effects in cardiopulmonary bypass attenuating inflammatory reactions, *ASAIO J* 41(3):M288–M291, 1995.

187. Grigore AM, Mathew J, Grocott HP, et al: Prospective randomized trial of normothermic versus hypothermic cardiopulmonary bypass on cognitive function after coronary artery bypass graft surgery, *Anesthesiology* 95(5):1110–1119, 2001.

188. Grocott HP, Mackensen GB, Grigore AM, et al: Postoperative hyperthermia is associated with cognitive dysfunction after coronary artery bypass graft surgery, *Stroke* 33(2):537–541, 2002.

189. van Dijk D, Nierich AP, Jansen EW, et al: Early outcome after off-pump versus on-pump coronary bypass surgery: Results from a randomized study, *Circulation* 104(15):1761–1766, 2001.

190. Puskas JD, Williams WH, Mahoney EM, et al: Off-pump vs conventional coronary artery bypass grafting: Early and 1-year graft patency, cost, and quality-of-life outcomes: A randomized trial, *JAMA* 291(15):1841–1849, 2004.

191. Nathoe HM, van Dijk D, Jansen EW, et al: A comparison of on-pump and off-pump coronary bypass surgery in low-risk patients, *N Engl J Med* 348(5):394–402, 2003.

192. Khan NE, De Souza A, Mister R, et al: A randomized comparison of off-pump and on-pump multivessel coronary-artery bypass surgery, *N Engl J Med* 350(1):21–28, 2004.

193. Racz MJ, Hannan EL, Isom OW, et al: A comparison of short- and long-term outcomes after off-pump and on-pump coronary artery bypass graft surgery with sternotomy, *J Am Coll Cardiol* 43(4):557–564, 2004.

194. Shroyer AL, Grover FL, Hattler B, et al: On-pump versus off-pump coronary-artery bypass surgery, *N Engl J Med* 361(19):1827–1837, 2009.

195. Andreasson S, Gothberg S, Berggren H, et al: Hemofiltration modifies complement activation after extracorporeal circulation in infants, *Ann Thorac Surg* 56(6):1515–1517, 1993.

196. Journois D, Israel-Biet D, Pouard P, et al: High-volume, zero-balanced hemofiltration to reduce delayed inflammatory response to cardiopulmonary bypass in children, *Anesthesiology* 85(5):965–976, 1996.

197. Warren O, Alexiou C, Massey R, et al: The effects of various leukocyte filtration strategies in cardiac surgery, *Eur J Cardiothorac Surg* 31(4):665–676, 2007.

198. Gu YJ, de Vries AJ, Boonstra PW, van Oeveren W: Leukocyte depletion results in improved lung function and reduced inflammatory response after cardiac surgery, *J Thorac Cardiovasc Surg* 112(2):494–500, 1996.

199. Lust RM, Bode AP, Yang L, et al: In-line leukocyte filtration during bypass. Clinical results from a randomized prospective trial, *ASAIO J* 42(5):M819–M822, 1996.

200. Mihaljevic T, Tonz M, von Segesser LK, et al: The influence of leukocyte filtration during cardiopulmonary bypass on postoperative lung function. A clinical study, *J Thorac Cardiovasc Surg* 109(6):1138–1145, 1995.

201. Davies GG, Wells DG, Mabee TM, et al: Platelet-leukocyte plasmapheresis attenuates the deleterious effects of cardiopulmonary bypass, *Ann Thorac Surg* 53(2):274–277, 1992.

202. Vamvakas EC: Meta-analysis of randomized controlled trials investigating the risk of postoperative infection in association with white blood cell-containing allogeneic blood transfusion: The effects of the type of transfused red blood cell product and surgical setting, *Transfus Med Rev* 16(4):304–314, 2002.

203. van de Watering LM, Hermans J, Houbiers JG, et al: Beneficial effects of leukocyte depletion of transfused blood on postoperative complications in patients undergoing cardiac surgery: A randomized clinical trial, *Circulation* 97(6):562–568, 1998.

204. Llewelyn CA, Taylor RS, Todd AA, et al: The effect of universal leukoreduction on postoperative infections and length of hospital stay in elective orthopedic and cardiac surgery, *Transfusion* 44(4):489–500, 2004.

205. Dzik WH, Anderson JK, O'Neill EM, et al: A prospective, randomized clinical trial of universal WBC reduction, *Transfusion* 42(9):1114–1122, 2002.

206. Soeparwata R, Hartman AR, Frerichmann U, et al: Aprotinin diminishes inflammatory processes, *Int J Cardiol* 53(Suppl):S55–S63, 1996.

207. Brown JR, Toler AW, Kramer RS, Landis RC: Anti-inflammatory effect of aprotinin: A meta-analysis, *J Extra Corpor Technol* 41(2):79–86, 2009.

208. Fergusson DA, Hebert PC, Mazer CD, et al: A comparison of aprotinin and lysine analogues in high-risk cardiac surgery, *N Engl J Med* 358(22):2319–2331, 2008.

209. Szabo G, Veres G, Radovits T, et al: Effects of novel synthetic serine protease inhibitors on postoperative blood loss, coagulation parameters, and vascular relaxation after cardiac surgery, *J Thorac Cardiovasc Surg* 139(1):181–188, 2010 discussion 188.

210. Lehmann A: Ecallantide (DX-88), a plasma kallikrein inhibitor for the treatment of hereditary angioedema and the prevention of blood loss in on-pump cardiothoracic surgery, *Expert Opin Biol Ther* 8(8):1187–1199, 2008.

211. Lesslauer W, Tabuchi H, Gentz R, et al: Recombinant soluble tumor necrosis factor receptor proteins protect mice from lipopolysaccharide-induced lethality, *Eur J Immunol* 21(11):2883–2886, 1991.

212. Abraham E, Glauser MP, Butler T, et al: p55 Tumor necrosis factor receptor fusion protein in the treatment of patients with severe sepsis and septic shock. A randomized controlled multicenter trial. Ro 45-2081 Study Group, *JAMA* 277(19):1531–1538, 1997.

213. Lynn M, Rossignol DP, Wheeler JL, et al: Blocking of responses to endotoxin by E5564 in healthy volunteers with experimental endotoxemia, *J Infect Dis* 187(4):631–639, 2003.

214. Hoffmann H, Markewitz A, Kreuzer E, et al: Pentoxifylline decreases the incidence of multiple organ failure in patients after major cardio-thoracic surgery, *Shock* 9(4):235–240, 1998.

215. Thabut G, Brugiere O, Leseche G, et al: Preventive effect of inhaled nitric oxide and pentoxifylline on ischemia/reperfusion injury after lung transplantation, *Transplantation* 71(9):1295–1300, 2001.

216. Boldt J, Brosch C, Lehmann A, et al: Prophylactic use of pentoxifylline on inflammation in elderly cardiac surgery patients, *Ann Thorac Surg* 71(5):1524–1529, 2001.

217. Boldt J, Brosch C, Piper SN, et al: Influence of prophylactic use of pentoxifylline on postoperative organ function in elderly cardiac surgery patients, *Crit Care Med* 29(5):952–958, 2001.

218. Heinze H, Rosemann C, Weber C, et al: A single prophylactic dose of pentoxifylline reduces high dependency unit time in cardiac surgery: A prospective randomized and controlled study, *Eur J Cardiothorac Surg* 32(1):83–89, 2007.

219. Cagli K, Ulas MM, Ozisik K, et al: The intraoperative effect of pentoxifylline on the inflammatory process and leukocytes in cardiac surgery patients undergoing cardiopulmonary bypass, *Perfusion* 20(1):45–51, 2005.

220. Fink MP: Ringer's ethyl pyruvate solution: A novel resuscitation fluid for the treatment of hemorrhagic shock and sepsis, *J Trauma* 54(Suppl 5):S141–S143, 2003.

221. Fink MP: Ethyl pyruvate: A novel anti-inflammatory agent, *Crit Care Med* 31(Suppl 1):S51–S56, 2003.

222. Bennett-Guerrero E, Swaminathan M, Grigore AM, et al: A phase II multicenter double-blind placebo-controlled study of ethyl pyruvate in high-risk patients undergoing cardiac surgery with cardiopulmonary bypass, *J Cardiothorac Vasc Anesth* 23(3):324–329, 2009.

223. Devaraj S, Rogers J, Jialal I: Statins and biomarkers of inflammation, *Curr Atheroscler Rep* 9(1):33–41, 2007.

224. Schouten O, Boersma E, Hoeks SE, et al: Fluvastatin and perioperative events in patients undergoing vascular surgery, *N Engl J Med* 361(10):980–989, 2009.

225. Morgan C, Zappitelli M, Gill P: Statin prophylaxis and inflammatory mediators following cardiopulmonary bypass: A systematic review, *Crit Care* 13(5):R165, 2009.

226. Baker WL, Anglade MW, Baker EL, et al: Use of N-acetylcysteine to reduce post-cardiothoracic surgery complications: A meta-analysis, *Eur J Cardiothorac Surg* 35(3):521–527, 2009.

227. Nelson D, Kuppermann N, Fleisher GR, et al: Recombinant endotoxin neutralizing protein improves survival from Escherichia coli sepsis in rats, *Crit Care Med* 23(1):92–98, 1995.

228. Pajkrt D, Doran JE, Koster F, et al: Antiinflammatory effects of reconstituted high-density lipoprotein during human endotoxemia, *J Exp Med* 184(5):1601–1608, 1996.

229. Palmer JD, Rifkind D: Neutralization of the hemodynamic effects of endotoxin by polymyxin B, *Surg Gynecol Obstet* 138(5):755–759, 1974.

230. Roytblat L, Talmor D, Rachinsky M, et al: Ketamine attenuates the interleukin-6 response after cardiopulmonary bypass, *Anesth Analg* 87(2):266–271, 1998.

231. Bartoc C, Frumento RJ, Jalbout M, et al: A randomized, double-blind, placebo-controlled study assessing the anti-inflammatory effects of ketamine in cardiac surgical patients, *J Cardiothorac Vasc Anesth* 20(2):217–222, 2006.

232. Debaene B, Goldfarb G, Braillon A, et al: Effects of ketamine, halothane, enflurane, and isoflurane on systemic and splanchnic hemodynamics in normovolemic and hypovolemic cirrhotic rats, *Anesthesiology* 73(1):118–124, 1990.

233. Stoelting RK: *Pharmacology and physiology in anesthetic practice*, Philadelphia, 1991, JB Lippincott.

234. Gelman S, Fowler KC, Smith LR: Regional blood flow during isoflurane and halothane anesthesia, *Anesth Analg* 63(6):557–565, 1984.

235. Conzen PF, Peter K: Volatile anesthetics and organ blood flow. In Torri G, Damin G, editors: *Update on modern inhalation anesthetics*, New York, 1989, Worldwide Medical Communications, pp 29–35.

236. Mythen MGW, Webb AR: There is no correlation between gastric mucosal perfusion (tonometer pHi) and arterial hemoglobin concentration during major surgery, *Med Intensiva* 17:S44, 1993.

237. Giroir BP, Beutler B: Effect of amrinone on tumor necrosis factor production in endotoxic shock, *Circ Shock* 36(3):200–207, 1992.

238. Bouter H, Schippers EF, Luelmo SA, et al: No effect of preoperative selective gut decontamination on endotoxemia and cytokine activation during cardiopulmonary bypass: A randomized, placebo-controlled study, *Crit Care Med* 30(1):38–43, 2002.

9

Pharmacology of Anesthetic Drugs

NANHI MITTER, MD | KELLY GROGAN, MD | DANIEL NYHAN, MD | DAN E. BERKOWITZ, MD

KEY POINTS

1. In patients, the observed acute effect of any specific anesthetic agent on the cardiovascular system represents the net effect on the myocardium, coronary blood flow, electrophysiologic behavior, the vasculature, and neurohormonal reflex function. Anesthetic agents may differ from one another, quantitatively and/or qualitatively, even within the same category, with respect to any of these variables. Moreover, the acute response to an anesthetic agent may be modulated by a patient's underlying pathology, pharmacologic treatment, or both.

2. Volatile agents cause dose-dependent decreases in systemic blood pressure that for halothane and enflurane are mainly due to depression of contractile function and for isoflurane, desflurane, and sevoflurane are mainly due to decreases in systemic vascular responses. Volatile anesthetic agents cause dose-dependent depression of contractile function mediated at a cellular level by attenuating calcium currents and decreasing calcium sensitivity. Decreases in systemic vascular responses reflect variable effects on both endothelium-dependent and -independent mechanisms.

3. The net effect of volatile agents on coronary blood flow is determined by several variables, including anesthetic effects on systemic hemodynamics, myocardial metabolism, and direct effects on the coronary vasculature. When confounding variables are controlled, studies of volatile agents, including isoflurane, indicate that they exert only mild direct vasodilatory effects on the coronary vasculature.

4. In addition to causing acute coronary syndromes, myocardial ischemia can manifest itself as myocardial stunning, preconditioning, or hibernating myocardium. Volatile anesthetic agents have been demonstrated to attenuate myocardial ischemia development by mechanisms that are independent of myocardial oxygen supply and demand, and to facilitate functional recovery in stunned myocardium. Volatile agents also can simulate ischemic preconditioning, a phenomenon described as anesthetic preconditioning, and the underlying mechanisms are similar to but not necessarily identical to those underlying ischemic preconditioning.

5. The intravenous induction agents/hypnotics belong to different drug classes (barbiturates, benzodiazepines, N-methyl-d-aspartate receptor antagonists, and α_2-adrenergic receptor agonists). Although they all induce hypnosis, their sites of action and molecular targets differ based on their class. Furthermore, their cardiovascular effects are, to some degree, dependent on the class to which they belong.

6. In general, studies in isolated cardiac myocytes, cardiac muscle tissue, and vascular tissue demonstrate that induction agents inhibit cardiac contractility and relax vascular tone by inhibiting mechanisms that increase intracellular Ca^{++}. This effect may be offset by mechanisms that increase myofilament Ca^{++} sensitivity in both the cardiac myocyte and vascular smooth muscle. Although these effects may contribute to or modulate cardiovascular changes, the cumulative effects of the induction agents on contractility and vascular resistance and capacitance are mediated predominantly by their sympatholytic effects. It is for this reason that these agents should be used judiciously and with extreme caution in patients with shock, heart failure, or other pathophysiologic circumstances in which the sympathetic nervous system is paramount in maintaining myocardial contractility and arterial and venous tone.

7. Opioids exhibit diverse chemical structures, but all retain an essential T-shaped component necessary stereochemically for the activation of the different opioid receptors (the μ, κ, and δ receptors). The latter are not confined to the nervous system and also have been identified in the myocardium and in blood vessels where endogenous opioid proteins can be synthesized.

8. Acute exogenous opioid administration modulates multiple determinants of central and peripheral cardiovascular regulation. However, the predominant clinical effect is mediated by attenuation of central sympathetic outflow.

9. Activation of the δ-opioid receptor can elicit preconditioning, and this is mediated via a variety of signaling pathways that involve G-protein–coupled protein kinases, caspases, and nitric oxide, to name a few. The role of these mechanisms in both physiologic and pathophysiologic conditions is currently an area of active investigation. In contrast with ischemia in homeotherms, hibernation is, by definition, well tolerated in certain species. This latter phenomenon may be partially dependent on mechanisms that are activated by opioids or opioid-like molecules.

An enormous body of literature has been accumulated describing the protean effects of the different anesthetic agents on the heart and the pulmonary and systemic regional vascular beds. The effects on the heart, especially, have spawned innumerable publications. More recently, this has been because of the great interest in anesthesia-induced preconditioning (APC). However, even before the initial description of APC, the literature detailing the influence of anesthetic agents on the myocardium was prodigious and not always consistent.[1–3] This likely reflected not only the challenges inherent in quantitating the direct effects of volatile agents on the myocyte/myocardium, but the presence of several potential confounding variables including effects on coronary blood flow (CBF), the systemic vasculature, and the baroreceptor reflex arc. This chapter divides the discussion of the effects of volatile agents, fixed agents, and narcotics on the cardiovascular system (CVS) into those that involve acute and delayed effects. Under acute effects, the influence of anesthetic agents is described on: (1) myocardial function, (2) electrophysiology, (3) coronary vasoregulation, (4) systemic and pulmonary vasoregulation, and (5) the baroreceptor reflex. Within delayed effects, the focus is on APC.

VOLATILE AGENTS

Acute Effects

Myocardial Function

The influence of volatile anesthetics on contractile function has been investigated extensively in several animal species and in humans using various in vitro and in vivo models.[4–11] In general, it is now widely agreed that volatile agents cause dose-dependent depression of contractile function (Box 9-1). Moreover, different volatile agents are not identical in this regard and the preponderance of information indicates that halothane and enflurane exert equal but more potent myocardial depression than do isoflurane, desflurane, or sevoflurane. This reflects, in part, reflex sympathetic activation with the latter agents. It is also widely accepted that in the setting of preexisting myocardial depression, volatile agents have a greater effect than in normal myocardium.[12,13] Early studies indicating that volatile agents may not have a deleterious effect on function in the setting of acute myocardial infarction (AMI) likely reflected the fact that the limited infarction did not compromise overall myocardial function.[14,15] At the cellular level, volatile anesthetics

exert their negative inotropic effects, mainly by modulating sarcolemmal (SL) L-type Ca++ channels, the sarcoplasmic reticulum (SR), and the contractile proteins. L-type Ca++ currents are decreased and, secondarily, SR Ca++ release is depressed (Figures 9-1 and 9-2).[16] Moreover, the contractile response to lower Ca++ levels is further attenuated in the presence of volatile agents in that the response is decreased by volatile agents at any given Ca++ level; that is, volatile agents also decrease Ca++ sensitivity (Figure 9-3).[16] However, the mechanisms whereby anesthetic agents modify ion channels are not completely understood. Ion channels usually are studied in ex vivo circumstances in which, by definition, multiple modulating influences of the specific channel under study may be altered. Moreover, these studies frequently are undertaken in nonhuman tissue. Well-recognized species differences make extrapolation to humans difficult.[17] Nitrous oxide causes direct mild myocardial depression but also causes sympathetic activation.[18]

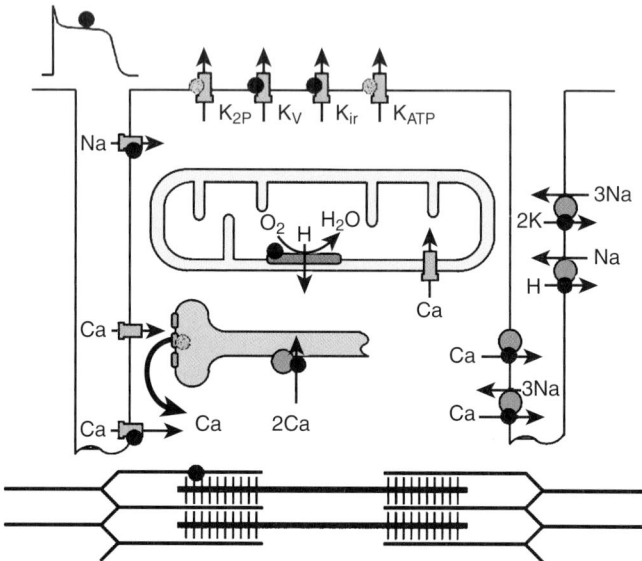

Figure 9-1 Sites of action of volatile anesthetics in a ventricular myocyte. *Dark spots* indicate inhibitory actions; *light spots* indicate stimulatory actions. (*From Hanley PJ, ter Keurs HEDJ, Cannell MB: Excitation-contraction in the heart and the negative inotropic action of volatile anesthetics,* Anesthesiology *101:999, 2004.*)

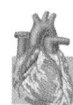

BOX 9-1. VOLATILE ANESTHETIC AGENTS

- All volatile anesthetic agents cause dose-dependent decreases in systemic blood pressure, which for halothane and enflurane are predominantly due to attenuation of myocardial contractile function, and which for isoflurane, desflurane, and sevoflurane are predominantly due to decreases in systemic vascular resistance. Moreover, volatile agents obtund all components of the baroreceptor reflex arc.
- The effects of volatile agents on myocardial diastolic function are not yet well characterized and await the application of "bedside" emerging technologies that have the sensitivity to quantitate indices of diastolic function.
- Volatile anesthetics lower the arrhythmogenic threshold to catecholamines. However, the underlying molecular mechanisms are not well understood.
- When confounding variables are controlled (e.g., systemic blood pressure), isoflurane does not cause "coronary steal" by a direct effect on coronary vasculature.
- The effects of volatile agents on systemic regional vascular beds and on the pulmonary vasculature are complex and depend on variables that include, but are not confined to, the specific anesthetic under study, the specific vascular bed, the vessel size, and whether endothelial-dependent or -independent mechanisms are being investigated.

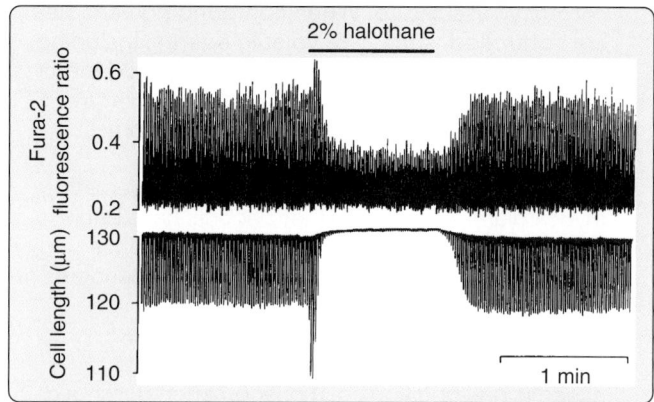

Figure 9-2 Fura-2 fluorescence (*top trace*), an index of Ca++, and cell length (*bottom trace*), an index of contraction, were measured simultaneously in an electrically stimulated rat ventricular myocyte. Application of halothane initially induced a transient increase in the Ca++ transient and twitch force before both the Ca++ signals and contraction decreased. (*From Harrison SM, Robinson M, Davies LA, et al: Mechanisms underlying the inotropic action of halothane on intact rat ventricular myocytes,* Br J Anaesth *82:609, 1999.*)

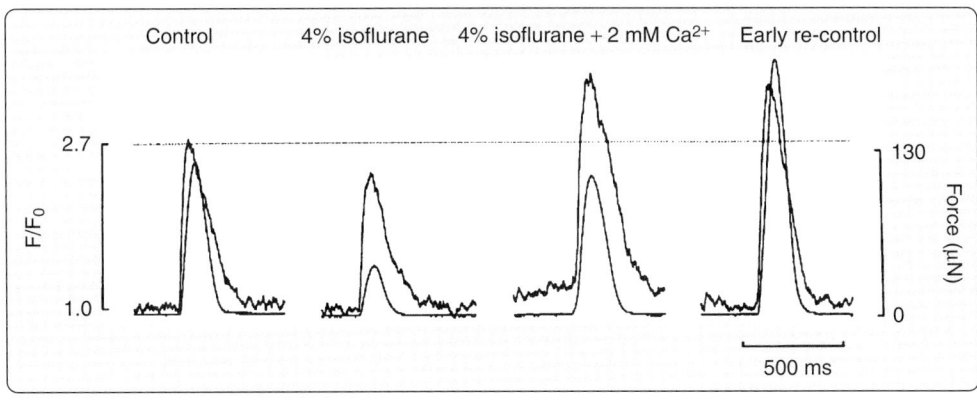

Figure 9-3 Simultaneous measurement of force and fluo-3 fluorescence, an index of Ca^{++}, in a rat cardiac trabecula. Application of isoflurane decreased force and Ca^{++}. Restoration of the Ca^{++} transient amplitude by increase of external Ca^{++} did not recover force, indicating that, in addition to decreasing Ca^{++} availability, the anesthetic decreased Ca^{++} responsiveness of the contractile proteins. *(From Hanley PJ, Loiselle DS: Mechanisms of force inhibition of halothane and isoflurane in intact rat cardiac muscle, J Physiol 506:231, 1998.)*

It is well recognized that even in the setting of normal systolic function, diastolic dysfunction occurs with increasing frequency in the elderly and is an important cause of congestive heart failure (CHF).[19-25] Diastolic dysfunction and its more severe clinical counterpart, diastolic heart failure, have protean causative factors and can be mechanistically complex[23] (Table 9-1). However, the mechanisms underlying these conditions can be categorized into those involving alterations in myocardial relaxation (e.g., SR Ca^{++} handling, phospholamban), those related to intrinsic properties of myocardial tissue (e.g., myocyte cytoskeletal elements), and those that are extramyocardial (e.g., loading conditions). Indices of diastolic function were not readily and reliably measured noninvasively in the past; hence the relatively more recent recognition and description of diastolic dysfunction and diastolic heart failure compared with perturbations in systolic function. This likely also explains the relative paucity of literature detailing the modulating effects of volatile agents on diastolic function. There is reasonable agreement in the literature that volatile agents prolong isovolumic relaxation and do so in a dose-dependent manner.[21,22,26-30] The effects of volatile agents on chamber stiffness are more controversial; for example, halothane has been reported to both decrease compliance and have no effect on myocardial stiffness.[21,22,26,28-31] The effect of nitrous oxide on diastolic function has not been investigated in a manner that critically rules out confounding variables. At a molecular level, alterations in relaxation likely reflect modulation of Ca^{++} currents, including SR Ca^{++} reuptake mechanisms. Paradoxically, in the setting of reperfusion injury and Ca^{++} overload, the volatile agent sevoflurane improves indices of diastolic relaxation and attenuates myoplasmic Ca^{++} overload.[32]

Cardiac Electrophysiology

Volatile anesthetic agents reduce the arrhythmogenic threshold for epinephrine. Moreover, not all volatile agents are similar, with the order of sensitization being: halothane > enflurane > sevoflurane > isoflurane = desflurane.

The molecular mechanisms underlying this effect of volatile anesthetics are poorly understood. Anesthetic agent–induced modulation of ion channels is important mechanistically in excitation-contraction coupling (vide supra), in preconditioning (vide infra), and in modulating automaticity and arrhythmia generation[17] (Table 9-2). Although the effects of any particular volatile agent on a specific cardiac ion channel may have been characterized, this does not allow a ready extrapolation into clinical situations. This partly reflects those issues already discussed (species differences, ex vivo studies) but also the recognition that it is impossible to predict the arrhythmogenic effect that might ensue after modulation with a particular volatile agent. This should be one of the lessons garnered from the experience with the antiarrhythmic drugs such as encainide and flecainide.[33] Moreover, even in the clinical setting, not all volatile agents have the same effect.[34]

Coronary Vasoregulation

Volatile anesthetic agents modulate several determinants of both myocardial oxygen supply and demand. Moreover, it is now established that

TABLE 9-1	Diastolic Heart Failure: Mechanisms and Causes
Abnormalities of myocardial relaxation	
Ischemia	
Hypertrophy	
Hypertension	
Valvular heart disease	
Abnormalities of myocardial compliance	
Aging	
Fibrosis	
Hypertrophy	
Diabetes mellitus	
Metabolic syndrome	
Infiltrative disorders—amyloidosis	
Cardiomyopathies	
Constrictive pericarditis	

TABLE 9-2	Summary of the Actions of Volatile Anesthetics on Various Ion Currents in the Heart and the Most Important Side Effects of the Drugs		
Target	*Effect*	*Anesthetic Gas*	*Cardiac Side Effects*
L-type Ca^{++} current	Inhibition	Halothane, isoflurane, sevoflurane	Reduced contractility,* shortened AP and refractory time
β-Adrenergic regulation of L-type Ca^{++} current	Complex interference	Halothane	Enhanced proarrhythmicity in comparison with sevoflurane?
Voltage-dependent transient outward K^+ current	Inhibition	Halothane, isoflurane, xenon	Shortened AP duration, AP duration mismatch within the heart
Voltage-dependent sustained outward K^+ current	Inhibition	Halothane, isoflurane, sevoflurane	Delayed repolarization, mismatch of AP duration*
ATP-dependent K^+ current	Enhancement	Isoflurane, sevoflurane	Myocardial preconditioning
Fast Na^+ current	Inhibition	Halothane, isoflurane, sevoflurane	Slowed conduction,* induction of tachyarrhythmias?

*Effects of paramount importance. AP, Action potential.
From Huneke R, Fassl J, Rossaint R, et al: Effects of volatile anesthetics on cardiac ion channels, *Acta Anaesthesiol Scand* 48:547, 2004.

volatile agents also directly modulate the myocytes' response to ischemia. Thus, studies investigating the effects of volatile agents on coronary vasoregulation should be interpreted in this context.

Animal studies indicate that halothane has little direct effect on the coronary vasculature.[35–37] Likewise, clinical studies investigating the effect of halothane indicate that it has either minimal or mild coronary vasodilator effects.[38–41] The effect of isoflurane on coronary vessels was controversial and dominated much of the literature in this area in the 1980s and early 1990s. The current assessments of the effects of isoflurane have been succinctly detailed by Tanaka et al.[42] Several reports have indicated that it caused direct coronary arteriolar vasodilatation in vessels of 100 μm or less, and that isoflurane could cause "coronary steal" in patients with "steal-prone" coronary anatomy; that is, in patients with significant coronary stenosis in a vessel subserving a region of ischemic myocardium, when, presumably, vessels were maximally dilated because of local metabolic autoregulation, and in whom isoflurane-induced vasodilatation in adjacent vessels resulted in diversion of coronary flow away from the ischemic region.[43,44] Several animal and human studies in which potential confounding variables were controlled indicated clearly that isoflurane did not cause coronary steal.[45–51] Studies of sevoflurane and desflurane showed similar results and are consistent with a mild direct coronary vasodilator effect of these agents.[52,53]

Ultimately, CBF (in the setting of normal systemic hemodynamics) is controlled by coronary vascular smooth muscle tone, which can be modulated directly (endothelium-independent) or indirectly via the endothelium (endothelium-dependent). Teleologically, it can be predicted that in vital organs, control of blood flow is predominantly local, acting through either endothelium-dependent or -independent mechanisms. Thus, volatile agents have the capacity to modulate mechanisms underlying vascular tone: (1) Halothane and isoflurane have been shown to attenuate endothelial-dependent tone (by receptor-dependent and receptor-dependent plus -independent mechanisms, respectively) in coronary microvessels[54]; (2) several volatile agents cause coronary vasodilation via K^+_{ATP}-channel–dependent mechanisms[54–57]; and (3) sevoflurane induced K^+- and Ca^{++}-channel–mediated increases in coronary collateral blood flow.[58] The effects in vivo are likely to be modest because local control mechanisms are likely to predominate.

Systemic Regional and Pulmonary Vascular Effects

Vascular tone can be modulated by volatile agents. However, the specific result can be influenced not only by the agent under study but by the vascular bed being investigated, the vessel size/type within that vascular bed, the level of preexisting vascular tone, age, and indirect effects of the agents, such as anesthesia-induced hypotension and reflex autonomic nervous system (ANS) activation.

All volatile anesthetic agents decrease systemic blood pressure (BP) in a dose-dependent manner. With halothane and enflurane, the decrease in systemic BP primarily is due to decreases in stroke volume (SV) and cardiac output (CO), whereas isoflurane, sevoflurane, and desflurane decrease overall systemic vascular resistance (SVR) while maintaining CO. However, these overall effects belie the multiple effects in the various regional vascular beds. Within the systemic noncoronary vasculature, aortic and mesenteric vessels have been the best studied.

Reversible inhibition of endothelium-dependent relaxation in aortic and femoral vessels was first demonstrated for halothane and also has been demonstrated for enflurane, isoflurane, and sevoflurane in both capacitance and resistance vessels.[54,59–63] However, these observations mask the differential effects of volatile agents on underlying endothelium-dependent mechanisms. Halothane and enflurane decrease agonist (bradykinin) and ATP-induced Ca^{++} increases in bovine endothelial cells, whereas isoflurane does not.[64] In contrast, isoflurane does attenuate histamine-induced Ca^{++} influx into human endothelial cells.[65] Alterations in endothelium-dependent mechanisms by volatile agents are not confined to attenuation of agonist-dependent and -independent activation of endothelial nitric oxide synthase (eNOS) and nitric

oxide (NO) release but also may extend to other mechanisms. For example, the effects of sevoflurane on endothelial cell function may be partially because of sevoflurane-induced changes in endothelin-1 (ET-1) production and in the redox milieu of the endothelial cells (i.e., increased superoxide anion production).[66]

The effect of volatile agents on vascular smooth muscle mechanisms is equally complex and varies among agents. In endothelial cell–denuded aortic rings, halothane decreases both SL Ca^{++} influx via voltage-dependent calcium channels and SR Ca^{++} release, but sevoflurane does not.[67] Sevoflurane also inhibits angiotensin II–induced vascular smooth muscle contraction in aortic rings.[68] In mesenteric vessels, sevoflurane accentuates endothelium-dependent mechanisms and attenuates endothelium-independent mechanisms in the presence of norepinephrine.[69] Studies of the influence of volatile agents on vascular smooth muscle Ca^{++} currents indicate that both halothane and enflurane stimulate SR release and reuptake from the caffeine-sensitive pool. In contrast, halothane, enflurane, and isoflurane all increase calcium-induced calcium release (CICR) mechanisms, but sevoflurane decreases CICR mechanisms.[70] Finally, volatile agents also have been demonstrated to modulate Ca^{++} sensitivity. In mesenteric vessels, halothane relaxation is largely mediated by Ca^{++} and myosin light-chain desensitizing mechanisms.[71]

The pulmonary circulation has unique features that must be taken into account when interpreting studies of this vascular bed. In addition to those issues that also apply to systemic vascular beds (vessel size, etc.), the pulmonary vasculature is a low-resistance bed (requiring preconstriction to access vasoactive effects), is not rectilinear (thus, changes in flow per se can change certain parameters used to calculate resistance), is contained within the chest (and thus subject to extravascular pressures, which are not atmospheric and change during the respiratory cycle), and exhibits the unique vascular phenomenon of hypoxia-induced vasoconstriction. It is clear that volatile agents modulate not only the baseline pulmonary vasculature but also multiple vasoactive mechanisms that control pulmonary vascular tone. Moreover, the effect of volatile agents is agent specific. For example, halothane causes flow-independent pulmonary vasoconstriction.[72] In contrast, the hypoxic pulmonary vasoconstrictor response does not appear to be altered by at least two currently used volatile agents: sevoflurane and desflurane.[73] The pulmonary vascular endothelial response appears to be impaired by the volatile agents halothane and isoflurane.[74,75] Finally, pulmonary vascular smooth muscle regulatory mechanisms also can be modified by volatile agents. Halothane, enflurane, and isoflurane all attenuate pulmonary vasodilatation induced by K^+_{ATP} channel activation.[76,77] Although the effects of the different volatile agents on K^+_{ATP}-channel activation are similar, β-adrenergic receptor–induced pulmonary vasodilatation is differently modulated. Halothane and isoflurane potentiate the vasodilatory response, but enflurane has no effect.[78]

Baroreceptor Reflex

All volatile agents attenuate the baroreceptor reflex. Baroreceptor reflex inhibition by halothane and enflurane is more potent than that observed with isoflurane, desflurane, or sevoflurane, each of which has a similar effect.[79,80] Each component of the baroreceptor reflex arc (afferent nerve activity, central processing, efferent nerve activity) is inhibited by volatile agents. Inhibition of afferent nerve traffic results, in part, from baroreceptor sensitization,[81,82] whereas attenuation of efferent activity is due, in part, to ganglionic inhibition as manifest by differential preganglionic and postganglionic nerve activity.[81–83]

Delayed Effects

Reversible Myocardial Ischemia

Prolonged ischemia results in irreversible myocardial damage and necrosis (Box 9-2). Shorter durations of myocardial ischemia can, depending on the duration and sequence of ischemic insults, lead to either preconditioning or myocardial stunning (Figure 9-4).[84] Stunning, first described in 1975, occurs after brief ischemia and is characterized

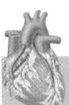

BOX 9-2. VOLATILE AGENTS AND MYOCARDIAL ISCHEMIA

- Volatile anesthetic agents have been demonstrated to attenuate the effects of myocardial ischemia (acute coronary syndromes).
- Nonacute manifestations of myocardial ischemia include hibernating myocardium, stunning, and preconditioning.
- Halothane and isoflurane facilitate the recovery of stunned myocardium.
- Preconditioning, a profoundly important adaptive protective mechanism in biologic tissues, can be provoked by protean nonlethal stresses, including but not confined to ischemia.
- Volatile anesthetic agents can mimic preconditioning (anesthetic preconditioning), an observation that could have important clinical implications, as well as provide insight into the cellular mechanisms of action of volatile agents.

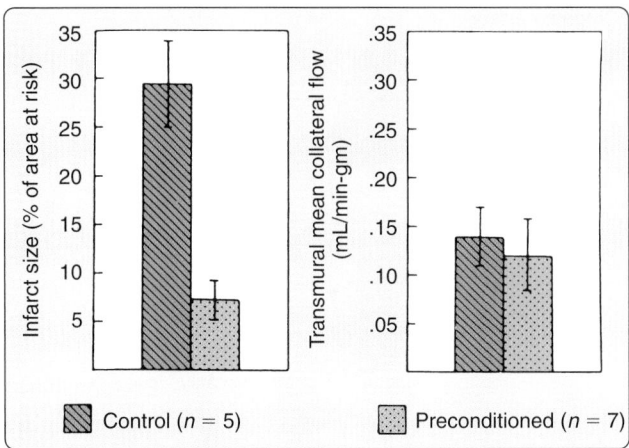

Figure 9-5 **Infarct size and collateral blood flow in the 40-minute study.** *Left,* Infarct size, as a percentage of the anatomic area at risk, in the control *(striped bar)* and preconditioned *(stippled bar)* hearts. Infarct size in control animals averaged 29.4% of the area at risk. Infarct size in preconditioned hearts averaged only 7.3% of the area at risk (preconditioned vs. control, P < 0.001). Transmural mean collateral blood flow *(right)* was not significantly different in the two groups. Thus, the protective effect of preconditioning was independent of the two major baseline predictors of infarct size, area at risk and collateral blood flow. Bars represent group mean ± standard error of the mean. *(From Warltier DC, al-Wathiqui MH, Kampine JP, et al: Recovery of contractile function of stunned myocardium in chronically instrumented dogs is enhanced by halothane or isoflurane,* Anesthesiology *69:552, 1988.)*

by myocardial dysfunction in the setting of normal restored blood flow and by an absence of myocardial necrosis.[85] Ischemic preconditioning (IPC) was first described by Murry et al[86] in 1986 and is characterized by an attenuation in infarct size after sustained ischemia, if this period of sustained ischemia is preceded by a period of brief ischemia (Figure 9-5). Moreover, this effect is independent of collateral flow. Thus, short periods of ischemia followed by reperfusion can lead to either stunning or preconditioning with a reduction in infarct size (Figure 9-6).[84]

As discussed previously, work in the 1970s indicated that volatile anesthetic agents attenuated ST-segment elevations in the setting of short-duration ischemia and limited infarct size and lactate production after prolonged ischemia.[87,88] Moreover, these effects seemed to be independent of the main determinants of myocardial oxygen supply and demand, and suggested that the volatile agents may be exerting a beneficial effect at the level of the myocyte. On resolution of the iso-flurane "coronary steal" controversy, the first description of the salutary effects of volatile agents on the consequences of brief ischemia was made in 1988. Warltier and coworkers[89] described the beneficial effects of halothane and isoflurane in facilitating the recovery of contractile function in stunned myocardium (Figure 9-7). However, it was almost

a decade later before the effects of volatile agents on preconditioning were outlined[2,3] and the term *APC* was used[1] (Figure 9-8).

The phenomenon of and the mechanisms underlying IPC are the focus of extensive investigation. IPC has the following characteristics: (1) results in two periods (termed *windows*) of protection—the first (termed *early* or *classic*) occurs at 1 to 3 hours, and the second (termed *late* or *delayed*) occurs 24 to 96 hours after the preconditioning stimulus; (2) occurs also in noncardiac tissue, such as brain

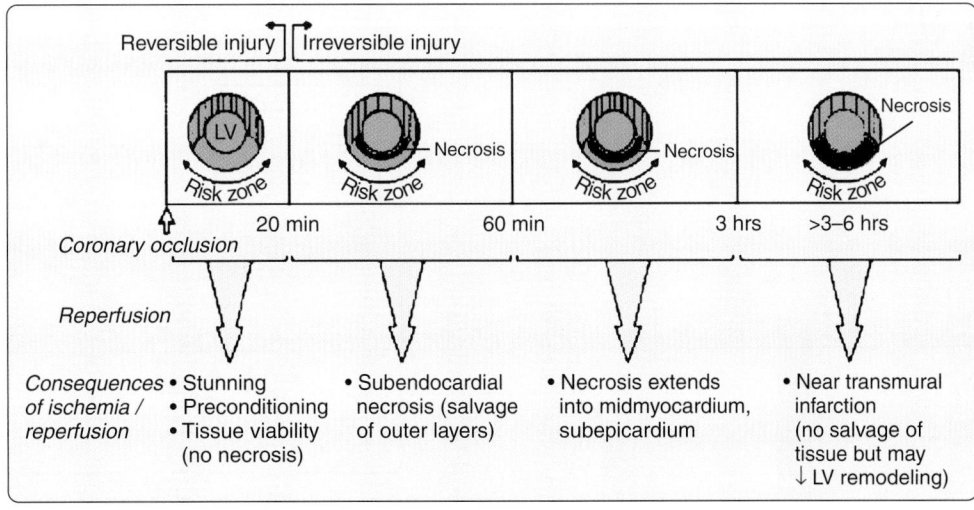

Figure 9-4   Effects of ischemia and reperfusion on the heart based on studies in anesthetized canine model of proximal coronary artery occlusion. Brief periods of ischemia of less than 20 minutes followed by reperfusion are not associated with development of necrosis (reversible injury). Brief ischemia/reperfusion results in the phenomenon of stunning and preconditioning. If duration of coronary occlusion is extended beyond 20 minutes, a wavefront of necrosis marches from subendocardium to subepicardium over time. Reperfusion before 3 hours of ischemia salvages ischemic but viable tissue. (This salvaged tissue may demonstrate stunning.) Reperfusion beyond 3 to 6 hours in this model does not reduce myocardial infarct size. Late reperfusion may still have a beneficial effect on reducing or preventing myocardial infarct expansion and left ventricular (LV) remodeling. *(From Kloner RA, Jennings RB: Consequences of brief ischemia: stunning, preconditioning, and their clinical implications, Part I,* Circulation *104:2981, 2001.)*

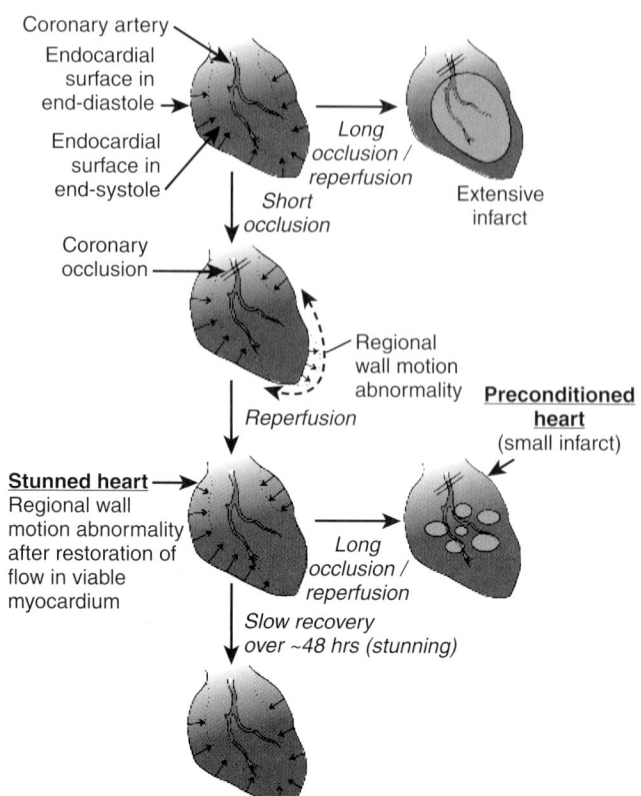

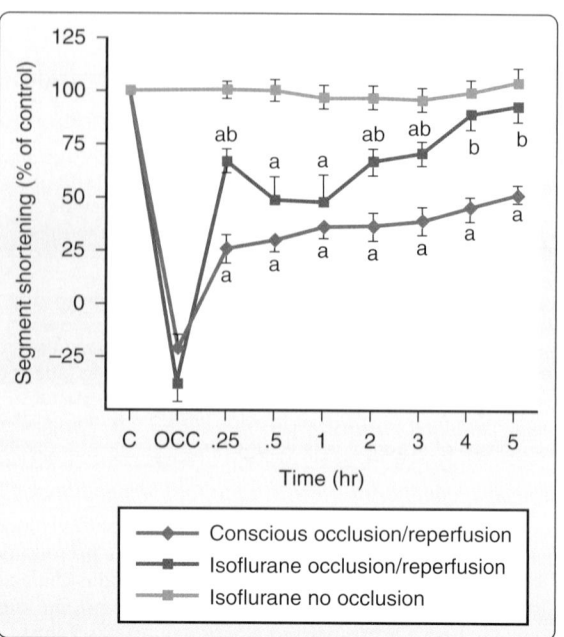

Figure 9-6 **Schematic of stunning and preconditioning.** Short coronary artery occlusions result in stunning, in which there is prolonged regional wall motion abnormality, despite presence of reperfusion and viable myocardial cells. Brief episodes of ischemia/reperfusion also precondition the heart. When the heart is then exposed to a longer duration of ischemia and reperfusion, myocardial infarct size is reduced. *(From Kloner RA, Jennings RB: Consequences of brief ischemia: stunning, preconditioning, and their clinical implications, Part I, Circulation 104:2981, 2001.)*

Figure 9-7 Segment shortening data (expressed as a percentage of control mean ± standard error of the mean during coronary artery occlusion (OCC) and at various times after reperfusion in conscious dogs (Group 1, *diamonds*) and in those dogs anesthetized with isoflurane (Group 7, *dark squares*). Comparisons are made at various time points with those animals anesthetized with isoflurane but not undergoing coronary artery occlusion and reperfusion (Group 6, *light squares*). [a]Significant ($P < 0.05$) difference, Group 6 (anesthetized without occlusion) versus 1 (conscious occlusion) or 7 (occlusion during anesthesia). [b]Significant ($P < 9.95$) difference, Group 1 (conscious occlusion) versus 7 (occlusion during anesthesia). Note that the control state (C) indicates either the awake, unsedated state (Group 1) or after a stable hemodynamic state after 2 hours of isoflurane anesthesia (Groups 6 and 7). *(From Warltier DC, al-Wathiqui MH, Kampine JP, et al: Recovery of contractile function of stunned myocardium in chronically instrumented dogs is enhanced by halothane or isoflurane, Anesthesiology 69:552, 1988.)*

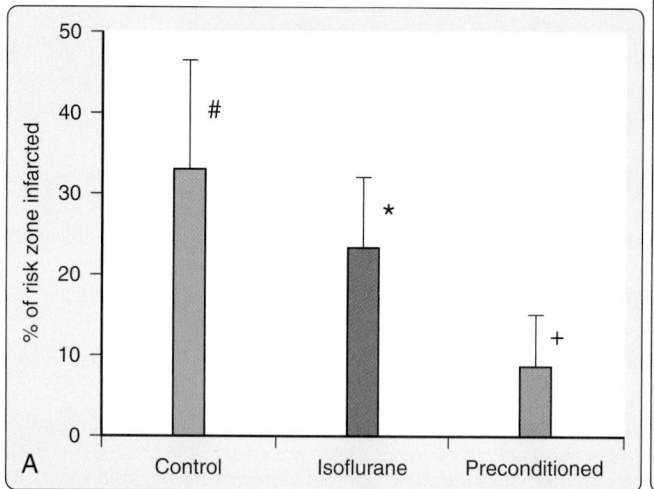

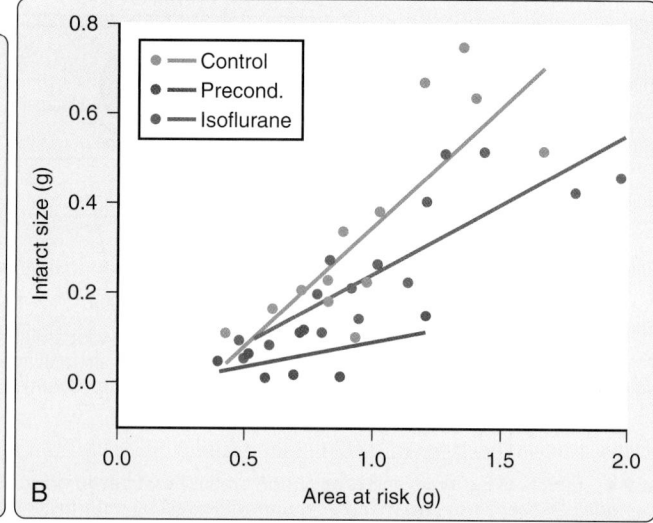

Figure 9-8 *A,* Infarct size (mean ± standard deviation) expressed as a percentage of area at risk in rabbit hearts that were not pretreated (control: $N = 13$), exposed to 5 minutes of preconditioning (ischemic preconditioned: $N = 8$), or exposed to 15 minutes of 1.1% isoflurane (isoflurane: $N = 15$) before 30 minutes of anterolateral coronary occlusion. #,*,+Statistical analysis showed that the relation between infarct size and area at risk was different in each group ($P < 0.05$). *B,* Relation between infarct size and myocardium at risk for the three groups. All three regression lines were statistically different because of differences in line elevation. *(From Cason BA, Gamperi AK, Slocum RE, et al: Anesthetic-induced preconditioning: previous administration of isoflurane decreases myocardial infarct size in rabbits, Anesthesiology 87:1182, 1997.)*

and kidney; (3) is ubiquitous across species; (4) is most pronounced in larger species with lower metabolism and slower heart rates (HRs); (5) seems to be important clinically because angina within the 24-hour period preceding an AMI is associated with an improved outcome (Figure 9-9)[90]; and (6) is mediated by multiple endogenous signaling pathways[91] (Figure 9-10).[92] As might be predicted from the time

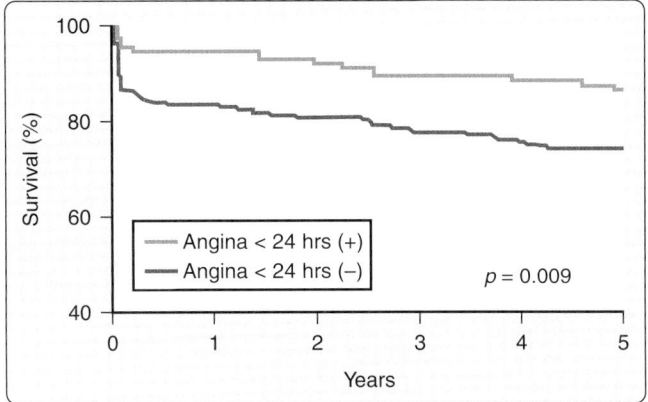

Figure 9-9   Five-year survival curves for patients with [angina < 24 hours (+)] versus those without [angina < 24 hours (−)] prodromal angina in the 24 hours before infarction. *(From Ishihara M, Sato K, Tateishi H, et al: Implications of prodromal angina pectoris in anterior wall acute myocardial infarction: acute angiographic findings and long-term prognosis,* J Am Coll Cardiol *30:970, 1997.)*

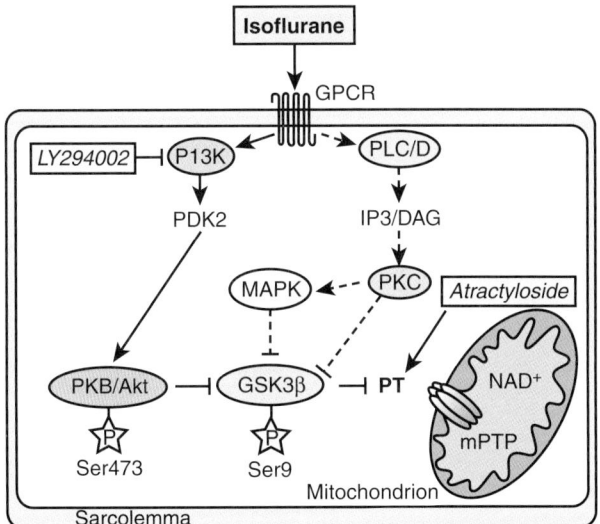

Figure 9-10   **Investigated signaling pathways** *(full lines)*. During early reperfusion, multiple signaling cascades inhibit the master switch kinase glycogen synthase kinase-3β (GSK-3β), which converges the prosurvival pathways and prevents permeability transition (PT) in mitochondria. Beside other kinases, protein kinase B (PKB)/Akt represents a key enzyme in the reperfusion injury salvage kinase cascade requiring phosphorylation at Ser473 for full activation. Phosphorylated PKB/Akt subsequently inactivates its downstream target GSK-3β by phosphorylation at Ser9. LY294002 specifically inhibits phosphatidylinositol 3-kinase (PI3K). Atractyloside induces opening of the mitochondrial permeability transition pore (mPTP). *Arrows* indicate positive activity; *lines with blunted ends* indicate inhibition. DAG, diacylglycerol; GPCR, G-protein–coupled receptor; IP3, inositol triphosphate; MAPK, mitogen-activated protein kinases; NAD+, nicotinamide adenine dinucleotide; PDK2, phosphatidylinositol-dependent kinase 2, also called Ser473 kinase; PKC, protein kinase C; PLC/D, phospholipase C/D. *(From Feng J, Lucchinetti E, Ahuja P, et al: Isoflurane postconditioning prevents opening of the mitochondrial permeability transition pore through inhibition of glycogen synthase kinase 3β,* Anesthesiology *103:987–995, 2005.)*

frame of delayed IPC, it is mediated, at least in part, by transcriptional and posttranslational mechanisms[91] (Figure 9-11). Finally, and of the utmost importance, preconditioning can be triggered by events other than ischemia (cellular stress of various forms, pharmacologic agonists, anesthetic agents; see Figure 9-11).[91] Moreover, the benefits of IPC are not necessarily confined to and may not include limitation of infarct size, and depend on the specific trigger for IPC, the species under study, and classic versus delayed IPC. For example, rapid pacing affords protection against arrhythmias but not against infarct evolution. In contrast, cytokine-induced IPC limits infarct size but has no effect on arrhythmias.[91] Different triggers of IPC modulating different end points suggest that, although there are fundamental mechanisms common to various triggers of IPC, there also exist mechanistic differences across triggers. Thus, APC may not be identical to IPC mechanistically.

Anesthetic Agents: Pre- and Post-Conditioning

This is an area of intense investigation as reflected by two issues of *Anesthesiology* being devoted predominantly to the subject.[93,94] After the initial description of APC,[1–3] subsequent investigations have indicated that volatile agents can elicit delayed (late), as well as classic (early), preconditioning.[95,96] Moreover, APC is dose dependent,[97–99] exhibits synergy with ischemia in affording protection,[100,101] and perhaps not surprisingly, in view of differential uptake and distribution of volatile agents, has been demonstrated to require different time intervals between exposure and the maintenance of a subsequent benefit that is agent dependent[42] (see Chapters 6 and 7).

The contributions of both SL and mitochondrial K+$_{ATP}$ channels in IPC have been extensively investigated, and it is now widely agreed that mitochondrial K+$_{ATP}$ channels play a critical role in this process. Volatile agents that exhibit APC activate mitochondrial K+$_{ATP}$ channels, and this effect is blocked by specific mitochondrial K+$_{ATP}$ channel antagonists. However, the precise relative contributions of SL versus mitochondrial K+$_{ATP}$ channel activation to APC remain to be elucidated (Figure 9-12).[42] The original descriptions of APC indicated that volatile agents can trigger preconditioning without concurrent ischemia during the "triggering" period[1–3] (see Figure 9-8). However, studies of mitochondrial activation (via mitochondrial K+$_{ATP}$ channels) indicate that volatile agents on their own do not activate mitochondria but do potentiate the effects of direct mitochondrial K+$_{ATP}$ channel openers[99] (Figure 9-13). These apparent inconsistencies are likely explained by the presence of multiple parallel and redundant pathways activated during APC (and IPC)[96] (see Figure 9-12). For example, it is now well established that the adenosine A-1 and δ$_1$ opioid G-coupled receptors can trigger IPC. Moreover, pharmacologic blockade of these receptors attenuates the positive effects of volatile agents.[98,102] Protein kinase C (PKC) and the nuclear signaling pathway, mitogen-activated protein kinase (MAPK), are important signaling pathways in preconditioning, and volatile agents have been shown to modulate at least PKC translocation.[103] Oxidant stress is a central feature of reperfusion and, depending on the specific moiety, the enzymatic source and, most importantly, the oxidant stress load may trigger preconditioning on the one hand or mediate reperfusion injury on the other. Both indirect and direct evidence indicate that volatile agents can increase oxidant stress to levels that trigger preconditioning.[104–106]

Activation of eNOS also has been shown to play a role, as has depolarization of the mitochondrial internal membrane.[107] This may prevent the opening of the mitochondrial permeability transition pore (MPTP) and inhibit Na+-H+ exchange, attenuating Ca+2 overload and cell edema.[107] Inhibition of mitochondrial permeability by APC has been suggested to decrease myocyte death, and PKC also has been thought to play a role in IPC-induced delay of MPTP opening.[108,109] For the first time, a recent study demonstrates that isoflurane has been shown to activate PKC-dependent signaling pathways resulting in the delay of MPTP opening,[110] suggesting a possible mechanism for isoflurane in APC. With respect to postconditioning, Ge et al[111] demonstrated that NO may, in fact, act as both a trigger and a mediator for

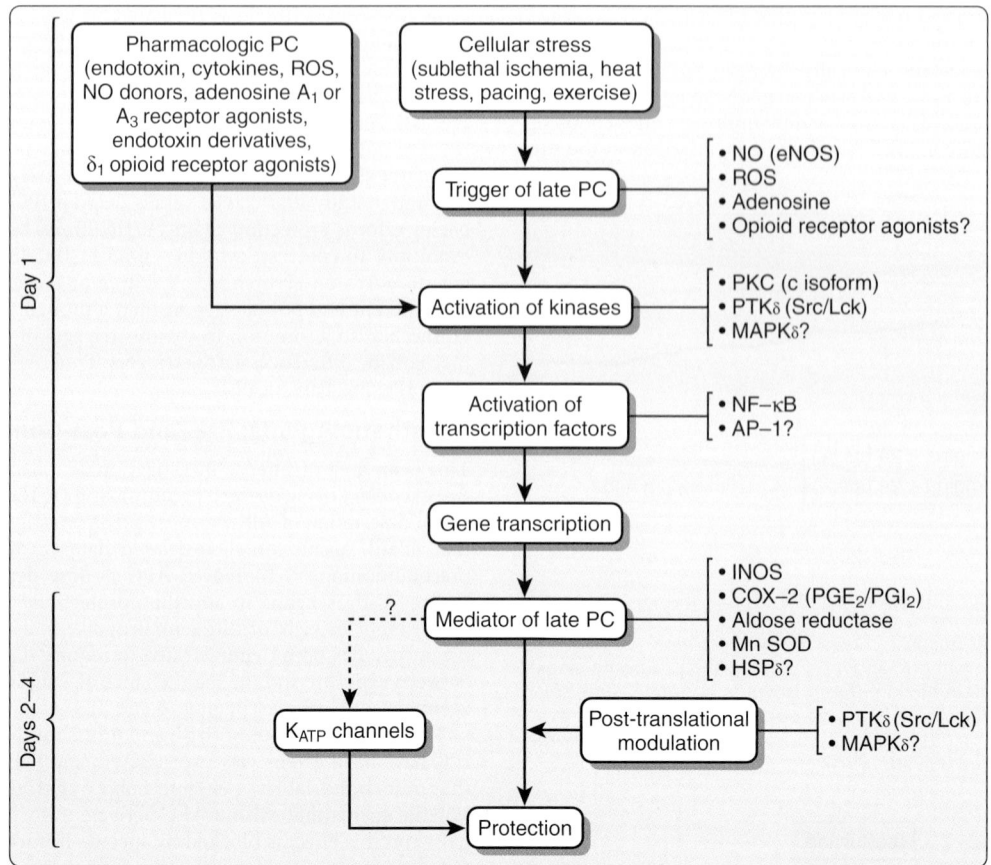

Figure 9-11   **Schematic representation of the cellular mechanisms underlying late preconditioning (PC).** A nonlethal cellular stress (such as reversible ischemia, heat stress, ventricular pacing, or exercise) causes release of chemical signals (nitric oxide [NO], reactive oxygen species [ROS], adenosine, and possibly opioid receptor agonists) that serve as triggers for the development of late PC. These substances activate a complex signal transduction cascade that includes protein kinase C (PKC) (specifically, the ε isoform), PTKs (specifically, Src and/or Lck), and probably other as yet unknown kinases. A similar activation of PKC and downstream kinases can be elicited pharmacologically by a wide variety of agents, including naturally occurring, and often noxious, substances (such as endotoxin, interleukin-1, tumor necrosis factor-α [TNF-α], TNF-β, leukemia inhibitor factor, or ROS), as well as clinically applicable drugs (NO donors, adenosine A1- or A3-receptor agonists, endotoxin derivatives, or δ₁-opioid receptor agonists). The recruitment of PKC and distal kinases leads to activation of nuclear factor (NF)-κB and almost certainly other transcription factors, resulting in increased transcription of multiple cardioprotective genes and synthesis of multiple cardioprotective proteins that serve as comediators of protection 2 to 4 days after the PC stimulus. The mediators of late PC identified thus far include inducible nitric oxide synthase (iNOS), cyclooxygenase-2 (COX-2), aldose reductase, and manganese superoxide dismutase (MnSOD). Among the products of COX-2, prostaglandin E_2 (PGE_2) and/or PGI_2 appear to be the most likely effectors of COX-2–dependent protection. Increased synthesis of heat shock proteins (HSPs) is unlikely to be a mechanism of late PC, although the role of post-translational modification of preexisting HSPs remains to be determined. In addition, the occurrence of cardioprotection on days 2 to 4 requires the activity of PTKs and possibly p38 mitogen-activated protein kinases (MAPKs), potentially because iNOS and other mediators need to undergo post-translational modulation to confer protection against ischemia. Opening of K^+_{ATP} channels is also essential for the protection against infarction (but not against stunning) to become manifest. The exact interrelationships among iNOS, COX-2, aldose reductase, MnSOD, and K^+_{ATP} channels are unknown, although recent evidence suggests that COX-2 may be downstream of iNOS (i.e., COX-2 is activated by NO). AP-1, activator protein 1; PTK, protein tyrosine kinases. *(From Bolli R: The late phase of preconditioning,* Circ Res 87:972, 2000.)

isoflurane-induced cardiac protection in mouse hearts. This implies that an eNOS-dependent mechanism prevents the opening of the MPT pore, although other pathways including glycogen synthase kinase-3β also have been implicated (Figure 9-14).[92,111]

It is clear that mitochondrial activation attenuates ischemia-induced oxidant stress, favorably modulates mitochondrial energetics, decreases cytochrome *c* egress into the cytoplasm, and attenuates mitochondrial and cytoplasmic Ca^{++} overload. Mitochondrial cytochrome *c* release is one of the important mechanisms underlying caspase activation, and thus the apoptotic process[112] (Figure 9-15). Whether by Ca^{++}-mediated or by apoptotic mechanisms, or both, volatile agents clearly attenuate cell death in models of APC[101] (Figure 9-16). Although the mechanisms underlying mitochondrial activation have been aggressively studied, they remain incompletely understood. Finally, these salutary effects of volatile agents seem to have a clinical correlate[101] (Figure 9-17).

The use of volatile anesthetics also can alter outcomes after cardiac surgery. A meta-analysis by Landoni et al[113] demonstrated a significant reduction in postoperative myocardial infarction after cardiac surgery, as well as significant advantages with respect to postoperative cardiac troponin release, inotrope requirements, time to extubation, intensive care unit stay, hospital stay, and survival. Furthermore, another meta-analysis by Bignami et al[114] demonstrated that the use of volatile anesthetics may, in fact, have a beneficial role with respect to mortality after cardiac surgery. The duration of the volatile anesthetic exposure seemed to have some impact—the longer the exposure, the greater the effect. De Hert et al[115] demonstrated the cardioprotective effects of volatile anesthetics if used throughout the surgical procedure rather than only before and after cardiopulmonary bypass (CPB).

Further studies are necessary to delineate the role of the anesthetic regimen on outcomes after cardiac surgery and elucidate the

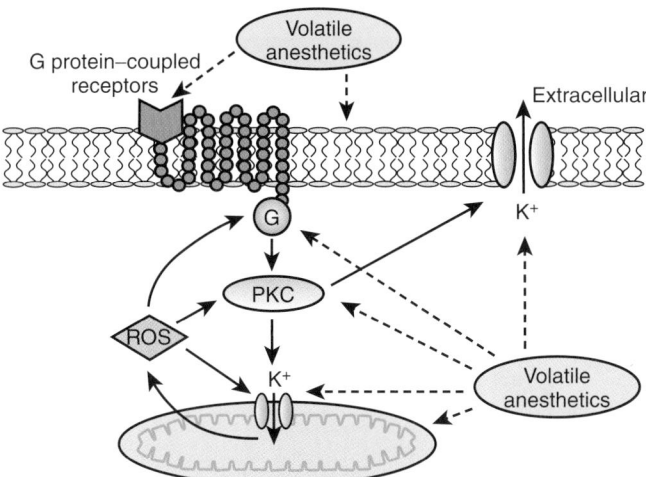

Figure 9-12 Multiple endogenous signaling pathways mediate volatile anesthetic-induced myocardial activation of an end-effector that promotes resistance against ischemic injury. Mitochondrial K^+_{ATP} channels have been implicated as the end-effector in this protective scheme, but sarcolemmal K^+_{ATP} channels may also be involved in this mechanism of protection. A trigger initiates a cascade of signal transduction events, resulting in the protection. Volatile anesthetics signal through adenosine and opioid receptors, modulate G proteins, stimulate protein kinase C (PKC) and other intracellular kinases, or have direct effects on mitochondria to generate reactive oxygen species (ROS) that ultimately enhance K^+_{ATP} channel activity. Volatile anesthetics may also directly facilitate K^+_{ATP} channel opening. *Dotted arrows* delineate the intracellular targets that may be regulated by volatile anesthetics; *solid arrows* represent potential signaling cascades. *(From Tanaka K, Ludwig LM, Kersten JR, et al: Mechanisms of cardioprotection by volatile anesthetics, Anesthesiology 100:707, 2004.)*

mechanisms behind this protection. Whether it involves mechanisms that are associated with APC continues to remain unclear.

INTRAVENOUS INDUCTION AGENTS

The drugs discussed in this section are all induction agents and hypnotics. These drugs belong to different classes (barbiturates, benzodiazepines, *N*-methyl-d-aspartate [NMDA] receptor antagonists, and α₂-adrenergic receptor agonists). Their effects on the CVS are, therefore, dependent on the class to which they belong. As with the inhalation anesthetic agents, the basic research that has emerged to explain the mechanisms that underlie the integrated cardiovascular effects observed in the intact organism is discussed. These effects have been studied at a cellular, tissue, organ, and whole-animal level. Although a detailed discussion of the molecular mechanisms underlying each agent is far beyond the scope of this chapter, a focused appraisal of well-established effects of specific drugs is given. At one level, sophisticated pharmacologic studies dissecting the signal transduction pathways may provide insights into mechanisms, but they cannot fully predict the response of the intact organisms. Because propofol is the most common induction agent, literature for this agent is used as the paradigm for discussing mechanisms by which cardiovascular regulation is altered by intravenous agents. A discussion summarizing the cardiovascular effects of each induction agent follows later in the chapter.

Unlike the inhalation anesthetic agents that augment IPC, there is no good evidence that the intravenous hypnotic agents demonstrate these protective effects. There is, however, emerging evidence that propofol, the mainstay of induction agents, may enhance antioxidant activity in the heart and thus may prevent lipid peroxidation after ischemia/reperfusion, offering a potential protective effect on the heart.[116]

Acute Cardiac Effects

Myocardial Contractility

To understand the effect of intravenous anesthetics on integrated cardiovascular responses is to understand the effect on the different factors that regulate the force of contraction of the heart. If the heart in isolation is considered (not coupled to the vasculature and not regulated by the autonomic system), the best methodologies for examining the effects of anesthetic agents involve using isolated myocytes and muscle tissue preparations in which the effect of the anesthetic drugs on contractile force/tension or myocyte/sarcomere shortening can be determined. With regard to propofol, the studies remain controversial whether there is a direct effect on myocardial contractile function at clinically relevant concentrations. However, the weight of evidence suggests that the drug has a modest negative inotropic effect, which may be mediated by inhibition of L-type Ca^{++} channels or modulation of Ca^{++} release from the SR. Thus, the effect of propofol may be mediated at multiple sites in the cardiac myocytes.

The effect of the agents may be species dependent, thus further confounding the literature regarding mechanism. For instance, van Klarenbosch et al[117] demonstrated that in contrast with rat, propofol directly depresses myocardial contractility in isolated muscle preparations from guinea pig, probably by decreasing trans-SL Ca^{++} influx. However, there was little influence of propofol on Ca^{++} handling by the SR or on the contractile proteins in rat. In one of the few human studies using isolated atrial muscle tissue (Figure 9-18), no inhibition of myocardial contractility was found in the clinical concentration ranges of propofol, midazolam, and etomidate. In contrast, thiopental showed strong negative inotropic properties, whereas ketamine showed slight negative inotropic properties (Figure 9-19). Thus, negative inotropic effects may explain, in part, the cardiovascular depression on induction of anesthesia with thiopental but not with propofol, midazolam, and etomidate. Improvement of hemodynamics after induction of anesthesia with ketamine cannot, therefore, be explained by intrinsic cardiac stimulation but is a function of sympathoexcitation.[118]

The effect of drugs such as propofol also may be affected by the underlying myocardial pathology.[119,120] For instance, Sprung et al[120] determined the direct effects of propofol on the contractility of human nonfailing atrial and failing atrial and ventricular muscles obtained from the failing human hearts of transplant patients or from nonfailing hearts of patients undergoing coronary artery bypass graft surgery (CABG). They concluded that propofol exerts a direct negative inotropic effect in nonfailing and failing human myocardium, but only at concentrations larger than typical clinical concentrations. Negative inotropic effects are reversible with β-adrenergic stimulation, suggesting that propofol does not alter the contractile reserve but may shift the dose responsiveness to adrenergic stimulation. The negative inotropic effect of propofol is at least partially mediated by decreased Ca^{++} uptake into the SR; however, the net effect of propofol on contractility is insignificant at clinical concentrations because of a simultaneous increase in the sensitivity of the myofilaments to activator Ca^{++}.[120]

Molecular Mechanisms: Adrenergic Signaling, Ca^{++} Influx, and Ca^{++} Sensitivity

There are a number of suggested molecular mechanisms by which a drug such as propofol may alter cardiac contractility. Propofol may inhibit cardiac L-type calcium current by interacting with the dihydropyridine-binding site[121] (Figure 9-20A), with resultant alteration in developed tension (see Figure 9-20B). Furthermore, as mentioned earlier, propofol may alter adrenergic signaling in cardiac myocytes. Experiments in membranes and cardiac preparations isolated from rat heart demonstrate that relatively high concentrations of propofol (25 to 200 μmol/L) are required to antagonize β-adrenoceptor binding and tissue responsiveness.[122] Kurokawa et al[123] observed that clinically relevant concentrations of propofol attenuated β-adrenergic signal transduction in cardiac myocytes via inhibition of cyclic adenosine

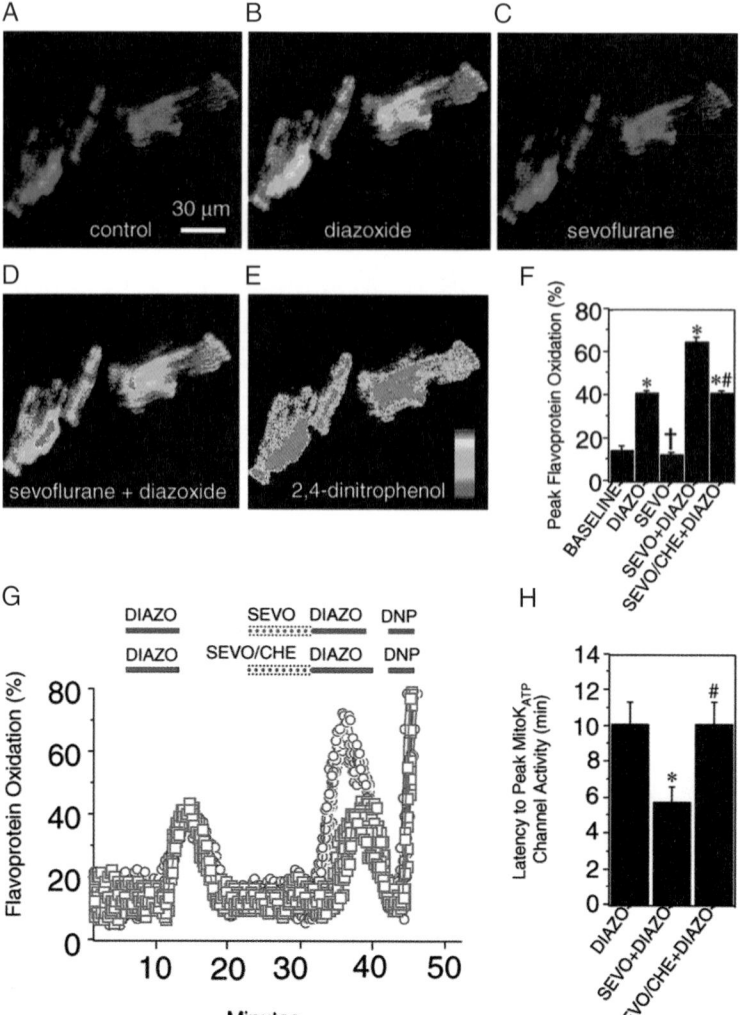

Figure 9-13 Effect of sevoflurane (SEVO; 2.8% [vol/vol]) on diazoxide (DIAZO)-induced flavoprotein oxidation in myocytes excited at 480 nm. Similar results were obtained for isoflurane. An artificial color scale was used to visualize the relative intensity of emitted fluorescence at 530 nm (dark blue indicates reduced flavoproteins; red indicates fully oxidized flavoproteins). *A,* At baseline. *B,* At 100 μm DIAZO (same cells). *C,* At 2 minimal alveolar concentration (MAC) SEVO. *D,* At 100 μm DIAZO preceded by 2 MAC SEVO. Red color indicates intense local oxidation by mitochondrial clusters. *E,* At 100 μm 2,4-dinitrophenol (DNP). *F,* Mean percentages of peak flavoprotein fluorescence depending on the drugs exposed to myocytes. *$P < 0.0001$ versus baseline or SEVO + DIAZO versus DIAZO alone. #P value not significantly different from DIAZO; †P value not significantly different from baseline. SEVO/CHE indicates concomitant treatment of myocytes with SEVO and chelerythrine (CHE) at 2 μm before exposure to DIAZO. *G,* Time-lapse analysis of alterations in fluorescence intensity in individual myocytes expressed as percentage of DNP-induced fluorescence. *Blue squares* and *red circles* indicate values from eight different experiments. *H,* Latency to peak activation of mitoK$^+_{ATP}$ channels in response to the various treatment regimens. *$P < 0.001$ versus DIAZO; #P value not significant versus DIAZO. Data are mean ± standard deviation. *(From Zaugg M, Lucchinetti E, Spahn DR, et al: Volatile anesthetics mimic mitochondrial cardiac preconditioning by priming the activation of mitochondrial KATP channels via multiple signaling pathways, Anesthesiology 97:4, 2002.)*

monophosphate (cAMP) production (Figure 9-21). The inhibitory site of action of propofol appears to be upstream of adenylyl cyclase and involves activation of PKCα.

Although propofol may decrease contractile response to adrenergic stimulation, there is emerging evidence that it may enhance myofilament sensitivity to Ca^{++}. Propofol caused a leftward shift in the extracellular Ca^{++}-shortening relationship, suggesting that propofol increases the sensitivity of myofibrillar actomyosin ATPase to Ca^{++} (i.e., increases myofilament Ca^{++} sensitivity; Figure 9-22). This is mediated, at least in part, by increasing pH via PKCc-dependent activation of Na$^+$-H$^+$ exchange[124] or by a PKC-dependent pathway involving the phosphorylation of MLC2.[124]

Figure 9-14 Concentration-dependent decreases in myocardial infarct size by isoflurane postconditioning (IsoPC) in wild-type mice subjected to 30 minutes of coronary occlusion followed by 2 hours of reperfusion. *A,* Area at risk expressed as a percentage of left ventricle area. *B,* Myocardial infarct size expressed as a percentage of area at risk. IsoPC was produced by 0.5, 1.0, or 1.5 minimum alveolar concentration of isoflurane (ISO$_{0.5}$, ISO$_{1.0}$, or ISO$_{1.5}$) administered during the last 5 minutes of ischemia and first 3 minutes of reperfusion. *$P < 0.05$ versus control (*n* = 8–10 mice/group). *(From Ge Z, Pravdic D, Bienengraeber M, et al: Isoflurane postconditioning protects against reperfusion injury by preventing mitochondrial permeability transition by an endothelial nitric oxide synthase-dependent mechanism. Anesthesiology 112:73–85, 2010.)*

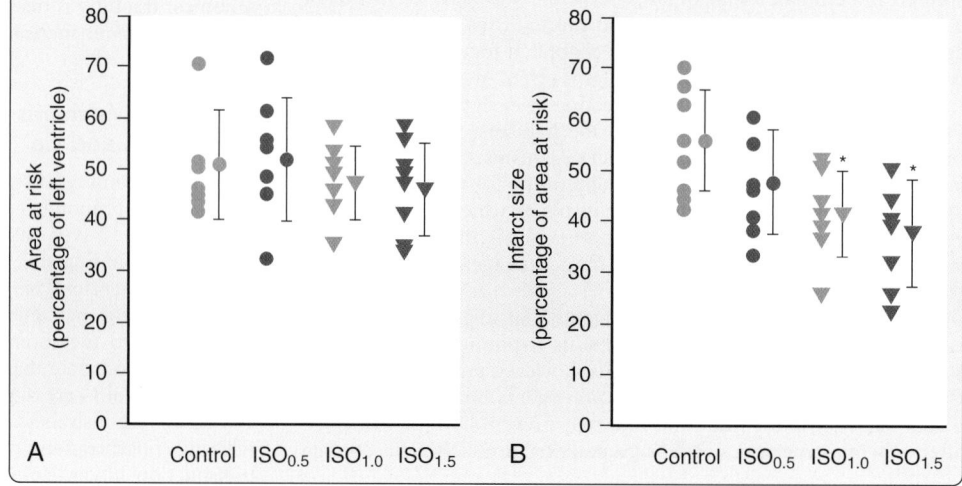

MITOCHONDRION: CENTER STAGE

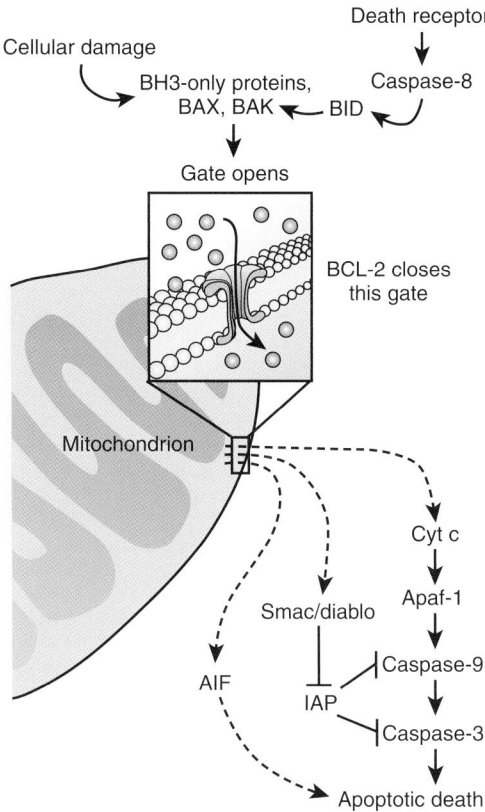

Figure 9-15 **Center stage in apoptosis.** In this view, numerous cell-death stimuli work through the mitochondria. They cause proapoptotic members of the BCL-2 family, such as BAX and BAK, to either open new pores or modify existing channels in the mitochondrial membrane, releasing cytochrome *c* (Cyt c) and other proteins that lead to caspase activation and cell death. BCL-2 itself, which is antiapoptotic, somehow blocks the pore or channel opening. *AIF*, apoptosis-inducing factor; *IAP*, inhibitors of apoptosis. *(Reprinted from Finkel E: The mitochondrion: is it central to apoptosis?* Science *292(5517):624–626, 2001. Illustration: C. Slayden, Copyright 2001 AAAS.)*

Integrated Cardiovascular Responses

The use of combined conductance-manometric catheters, which allows the simultaneous measurement of pressure and volume in the ventricle, has enabled the precise determination of the effects of anesthetic agents on integrated cardiovascular responses. These parameters include load-independent measures of contractility (slope of the end-systolic pressure-volume relation [ESPVR], E_{es}), as well as indices of ventricular-vascular coupling (ratio of arterial elastance to ventricular elastance [E_a/E_{es}]; see Chapters 5 and 14). In a study, the effects of propofol and pentobarbital on integrated cardiovascular function were assessed in pigs both at baseline and after an acute increase in ventricular afterload.[125] At baseline, E_{es} was lower during pentobarbital versus propofol anesthesia, suggesting a greater negative inotropic effect of barbiturates versus propofol (Figure 9-23). On the other hand, the responses to ventricular afterload induced by aortic banding were maintained in the pentobarbital-anesthetized animals, whereas the responses were markedly attenuated in the propofol-anesthetized pigs, suggesting an attenuation of the baroreflex responses with propofol. Furthermore, a decrease in arterial pressure with propofol is consistent with this drug acting as a vasodilator.

One of the questions with regard to intravenous induction agents is: What represents a clinically relevant dose? As would be predicted, with regard to the myocardial depressant effects, the coronary concentrations of propofol have been shown to be the major contributor to the

cardiac depression caused by propofol, but were a less significant contributor to the hypotension caused by this drug.[126]

The effects of propofol on cardiac contractility are manifest not only on ventricular but also atrial function.[127] Propofol depresses contractile function of left atrial myocardium and reduces the active left atrial contribution to left ventricular filling in vivo. Compensatory decreases in chamber stiffness, however, contribute to relative maintenance of left atrial reservoir function during the administration of propofol.

Oxidative Stress

Oxidative stress remains an important pathophysiologic mechanism for cellular injury in critically ill patients and represents an imbalance between the production of these radicals and the enzymatic defense system that removes them (Box 9-3). This has potential therapeutic implications because these agents are used routinely for sedation in the intensive care unit, in which disease processes associated with increased oxidative stress are treated.

Animal data also suggest that propofol decreases postischemic myocardial mechanical dysfunction, infarct size, and histologic evidence of injury[128–132] (Figure 9-24). On further analysis, it becomes clear that propofol has a chemical structure similar to that of phenol-based free radical scavengers, such as vitamin E, and may therefore act as a free radical scavenger.[133,134] Studies by Tsuchiya et al[135,136] demonstrated in vitro the potential for both propofol and midazolam to act as free radical scavengers at near-therapeutic doses. Propofol also impairs the activity of neutrophils by inhibiting the oxidative burst and supports a potential role for propofol in modulating injury at the critical phase of reperfusion by reducing free radicals, Ca^{++} influx, and neutrophil activity.[137] Furthermore, microsomes prepared from animals anesthetized with propofol demonstrate a significantly increased resistance to lipid peroxidation.[138] The evidence does not support propofol as an APC-inducing agent because protection was observed when the heart was treated with propofol solely during reperfusion rather than before or during the ischemic insult,[131] although the addition of glibenclamide, a K^+_{ATP} channel blocker, does not abolish the protection afforded by propofol.[132] There is little evidence for other intravenous induction agents having protective effects on the heart. In fact, ketamine may block IPC[139–141] by deactivating SL K^+_{ATP} channels.[142]

Vasculature

As with the heart, the cumulative physiologic effects in the vasculature represent a summation of the effects of the agents on the central ANS, as well as the direct effects of these agents on the vascular smooth muscle, and the modulating effects on the underlying endothelium. An exhaustive review of the effects of each agent on isolated and integrated vascular function is beyond the scope of the chapter; however, a global overview of the effect of some of the most commonly used agents on vasoregulation is presented.

Although there clearly are effects of anesthetic agents on vascular smooth muscle and endothelial function, controversy and diversity regarding mechanisms arise because of the species of animals studied, the vessel bed examined, and the drug dosage used. In addition, the effects may be significantly different in vessels from animals that develop disease phenotypes, such as hypertension and diabetes. Furthermore, although effects of these anesthetic agents on a variety of signal transduction pathways are invariably seen with high concentrations of agents, the clinical relevance of these effects remains unclear.

Systemic Vasoregulation

It is now well established that propofol decreases SVR in humans. This was demonstrated in a patient with an artificial heart in whom the CO remained fixed.[143] As discussed later, the effect is predominantly mediated by alterations in sympathetic tone; however, in isolated arteries, propofol decreases vascular tone and agonist-induced contraction. The mechanism by which propofol mediates these effects has been attributed, in part, to inhibition of Ca^{++} influx through voltage- or

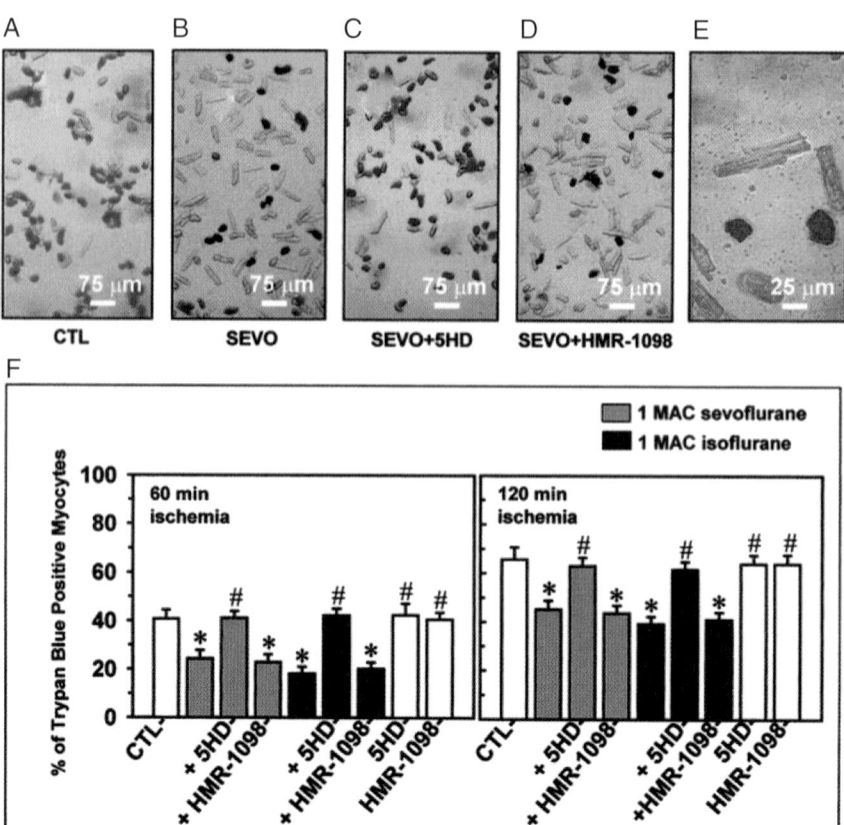

Figure 9-16 Effects of the specific mitochondrial K⁺$_{ATP}$ (mitoK⁺$_{ATP}$) channel blocker 5-hydroxy-decanoate (5HD) and the specific sarcolemmal K⁺$_{ATP}$ (sarcK⁺$_{ATP}$) channel blocker HMR-1098 on sevoflurane (SEVO)- and isoflurane (ISO)-mediated protection at 1 minimal alveolar concentration (MAC) against 60 or 120 minutes of ischemia in myocytes as assessed by trypan blue staining. *A,* Control myocytes after 60 minutes of ischemia. Myocytes staining dark blue indicate irreversible cell damage. *B,* Myocytes exposed to SEVO before ischemia. Most myocytes retain their rod-shaped morphology. *C,* Myocytes exposed to 5HD and SEVO before ischemia. The protective effect of SEVO is abolished. *D,* Myocytes exposed to HMR-1098 and SEVO before ischemia. The protection by SEVO is unaffected. *E,* Representative trypan blue–positive and –negative myocytes after exposure to ischemia seen at higher magnification. *F,* Trypan blue–positive myocytes are indicated as percentage of total viable myocytes before ischemia. CTL indicates control group and represents myocytes exposed to 60 or 120 minutes of ischemia alone. Data are mean ± standard deviation. *$P < 0.0001$ versus respective CTL; #P value not significant versus respective CTL. *(From Zaugg M, Lucchinetti E, Spahn DR, et al: Volatile anesthetics mimic cardiac preconditioning by priming the activation of mitochondrial KATP channels via multiple signaling pathways, 97:4, 2002.)*

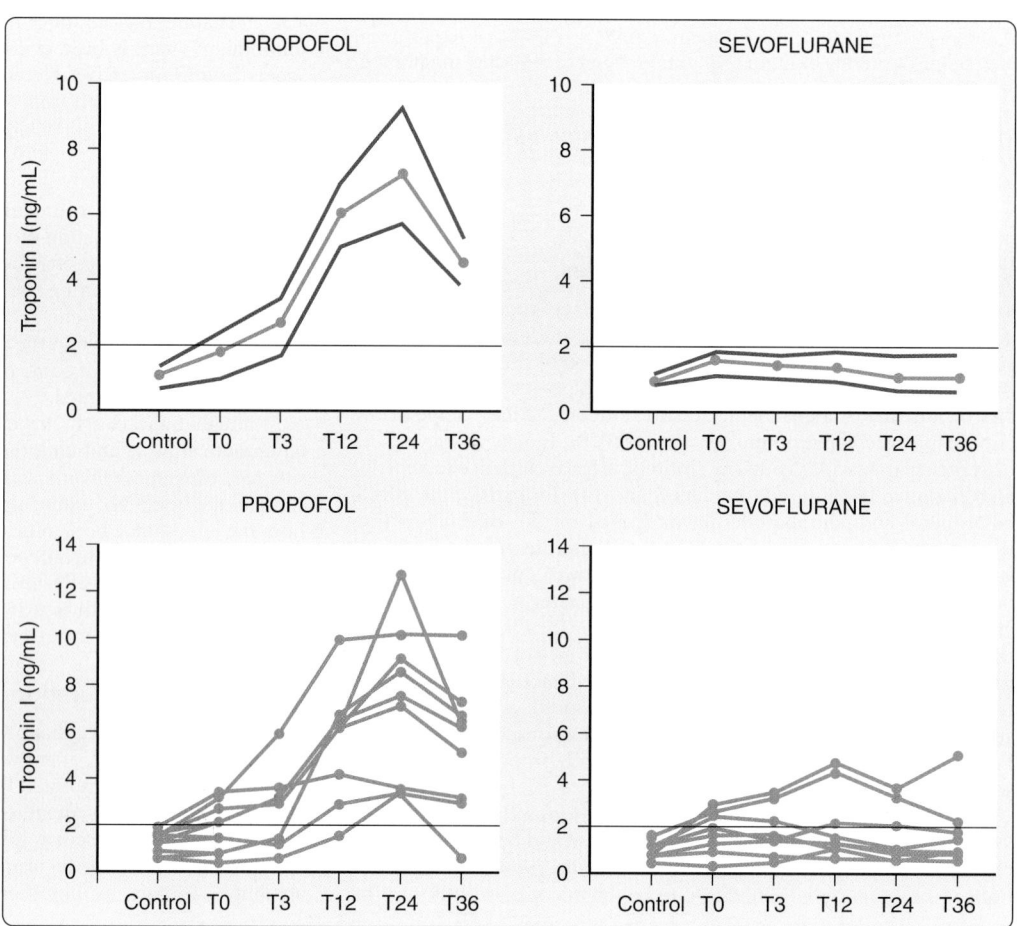

Figure 9-17 Cardiac troponin I concentrations in the propofol and sevoflurane groups before surgery (control), at arrival in the intensive care unit (T0), and after 3 (T3), 12 (T12), 24 (T24), and 36 (T36) hours. *Top panels,* Median values *(green)* with 95% confidence intervals *(purple). Bottom panels,* Evolution of the individual values. Concentrations were significantly greater with propofol. In the propofol group, all patients had troponin concentrations greater than the cutoff value of 2 ng/mL *(gray line). (From de Hert S, ten Broecke PW, Mertens E, et al: Sevoflurane but not propofol preserves myocardial function in coronary surgery patients,* Anesthesiology 97:42, 2002.)

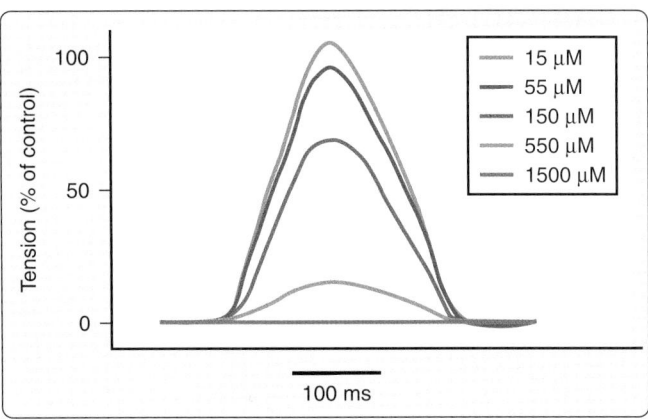

Figure 9-18 Typical experiment showing the force traces of an isometric twitch of human atrial tissue during exposure to increasing concentrations of propofol (15 to 1500 µmol/L). *(From Gelissen HP, Epema AH, Henning RH, et al: Inotropic effects of propofol, thiopental, midazolam, etomidate, and ketamine on isolated human atrial muscle, Anesthesiology 84:397, 1996.)*

receptor-gated Ca^{++} channels, as well as inhibition of Ca^{++} release from intracellular Ca^{++} stores regulated by the ryanodine receptor.[144-147] Much of the experimental data obtained in isolated studies have focused on conduit arteries (rat aorta); however, some properties of the resistance arteries differ from the rat bioassay. Modulation of vasoconstriction by vascular smooth muscle may be mediated by (1) an alteration in endothelium-independent vasodilation[145] or (2) an alteration in the sensitivity of the myofilaments to Ca^{++}, primarily mediated by the rho activation, and thereby the activation of Rho kinase. In an elegant

study examining the effects of propofol on resistance arteries, Imura et al[148] examined the effect of propofol on simultaneous measurements of force and in mesenteric resistance arteries. The authors concluded that propofol attenuates norepinephrine-induced contraction through an inhibition of Ca^{++} release, as well as Ca^{++} influx through L-type Ca^{++} channels, thus partially explaining the effects of propofol on vascular adrenergic signaling (Figure 9-25). Propofol also may modulate vascular tone by interfering with other signaling pathways involved in vasoregulation, such as ET-1.[148,149] In addition, propofol also may attenuate the myogenic tone/response in pressure-flow autoregulation.[150]

Pulmonary Vasoregulation

The effects of induction agents on pulmonary vasoregulation may have important implications for the management of patients whose primary pathologies involve the pulmonary circulation when they present for cardiothoracic surgery (primary pulmonary hypertension for lung transplantation and chronic thromboembolic disease for pulmonary endarterectomy). In addition, the effects may be of importance in patients with right ventricular failure.[151] Furthermore, the effect of these agents in modulating hypoxic pulmonary vasoconstriction may have an effect on intraoperative A-a (alveolar-arterial) gradients, particularly during one-lung ventilation. Murray and colleagues[152,153] have systematically studied the effects of anesthetic agents on pulmonary vasoregulation. Specifically, they have demonstrated that propofol attenuates endothelium-dependent vasodilatation[152] via a mechanism that involves NO and endothelium-dependent hyperpolarizing factor.[153] With regard to the vascular smooth muscle, the effect appears somewhat different in the pulmonary circulation. Rather than attenuate vasoconstriction and thereby decrease tone, propofol appears to increase the sensitivity of the contractile myofilaments to Ca^{++},[154] and thereby potentiates the effect of catecholamines on pulmonary artery smooth muscle cells[155] (Figure 9-26).

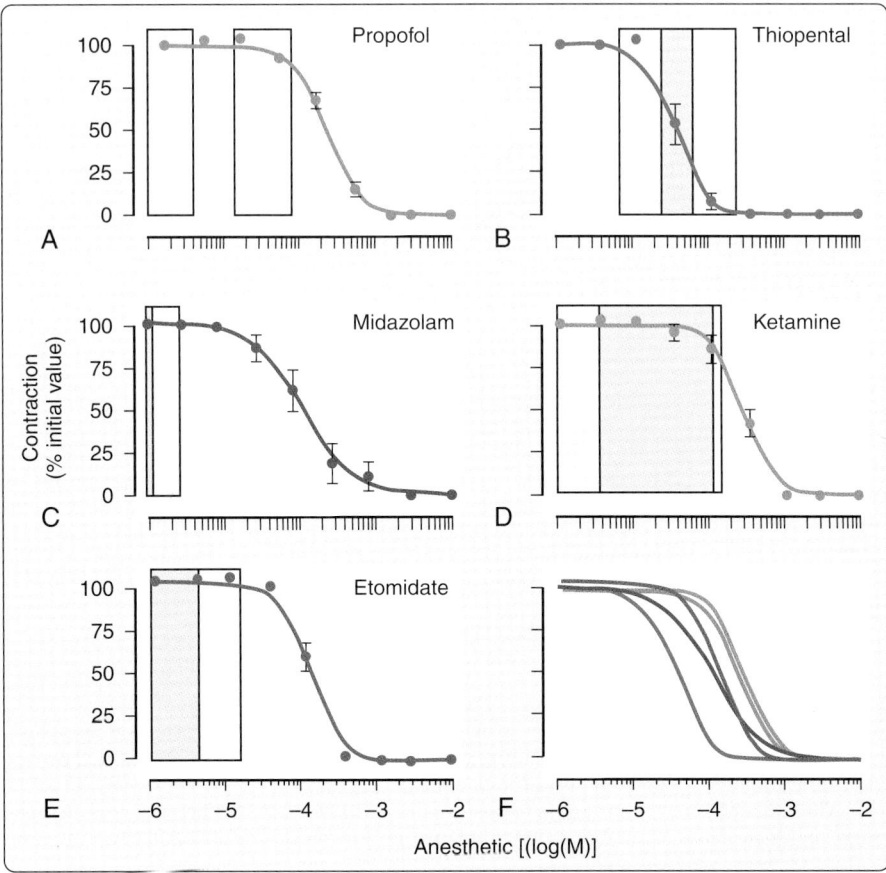

Figure 9-19 Comparative effects of increasing concentrations of anesthetic on isometric contractions of human atrial tissue induced by field stimulation. Data are mean ± standard error of the mean. Curves were plotted using logistic regression. *Squares* indicate the clinical concentration range during anesthesia. Tan hatching *(left)* represents the total concentration and white hatching *(right)* shows the free fraction. *A,* Propofol (n = 16). *B,* Thiopental (n = 7). *C,* Midazolam (n = 7). *D,* Ketamine (n = 9). *E,* Etomidate (n = 9). *F,* Combined plot showing the concentration–response curve of the five anesthetics. *(From Gelissen HP, Epema AH, Henning RH, et al: Inotropic effects of propofol, thiopental, midazolam, etomidate, and ketamine on isolated human atrial muscle, Anesthesiology 84:397, 1996.)*

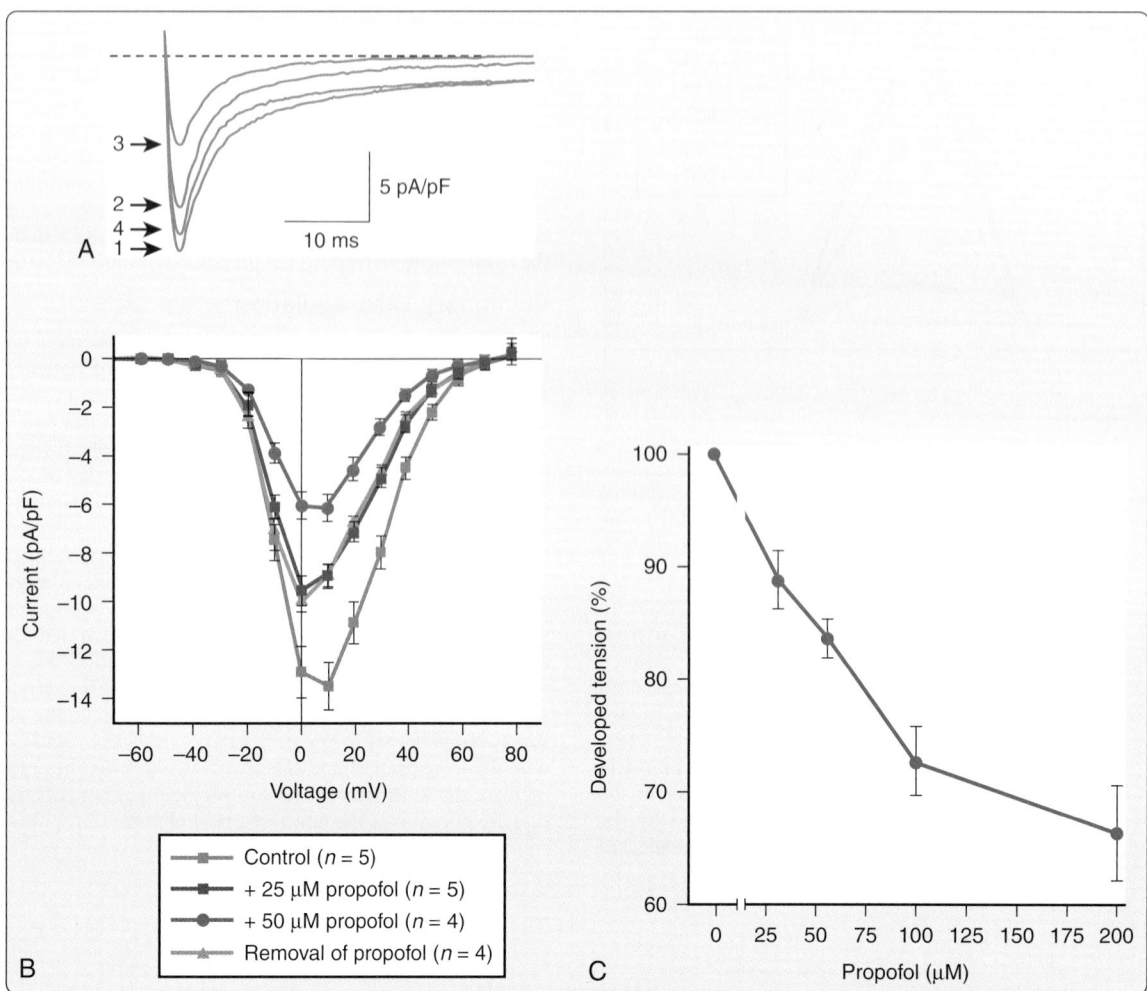

Figure 9-20 *A,* Representative current traces of I$_{Ca,L}$ in response to depolarizing pulses to 0 μmol/L from a holding potential of −70 μV. These traces were obtained before exposure to propofol *(light squares),* during treatment with 25 *(dark squares)* and 50 μmol/L *(circles)* propofol, and after recovery *(triangles). B,* Current-voltage (I-V) relation of peak I$_{Ca,L}$ as monitored before and during exposure to propofol. Cultured rat ventricular myocytes were clamped at −70 μV. I$_{Ca,L}$ was elicited by 200-millisecond pulses from the holding potential of −70 μV to potentials between −60 and +80 μV in 10-μV increments. Propofol dose-dependently decreases calcium current. *C,* Effects of propofol on developed tension in papillary muscle isolated from the rat heart. Preparations (*n* = 4) were bathed in an oxygenated Krebs–Henseleit solution at 37°C and paced electrically at 1 Hz. The anesthetic was added to the bathing solution cumulatively. *Vertical bars* represent standard error of the mean. Values on the ordinate are presented as a percentage of the developed tension recorded immediately before adding propofol (0.64 ± 0.15 g). Propofol dose-dependently decreases twitch tension. *(From Zhou W, Fontenot HJ, Liu S, et al: Modulation of cardiac calcium channels by propofol,* Anesthesiology *86:670, 1997.)*

Endothelial Function

Propofol modulates the function of the endothelium, thus altering the underlying tone of the vessels. The data as to the direction and mechanism underlying this effect are widely divergent and are dependent on the vascular bed, species, and experimental conditions. Early studies suggested that propofol-mediated vasodilatation was a function of stimulation of NO and vasodilator prostanoids from the endothelium.[140] Other studies have demonstrated an inhibitory effect of propofol and ketamine, but not of midazolam, on endothelium-dependent relaxation.[156] Moreover, the suppressive effect of ketamine on endothelium-dependent relaxation appears to be mediated by suppression of NO formation, whereas that of propofol may be mediated, at least partly, by suppression of NO function. In a rabbit mesenteric resistance artery preparation, Yamashita et al[157] demonstrated that propofol inhibits prostacyclin-mediated endothelium-dependent vasodilatation by inhibition of vascular hyperpolarization (Figure 9-27). This inhibition of hyperpolarization, and thereby inhibition of relaxation, appears to be mediated by the blockade of ATP-sensitive K⁺ channels. The clinical implications of these findings are unclear;

however, it may be predicted, based on the data, that the effects of propofol on the vasculature may be significantly different in patients in whom endothelial dysfunction, such as hypertension and atherosclerosis, is a significant factor.

With respect to vasorelaxation, Gursoy et al[158] described the dose-dependent vasorelaxation produced by intravenous anesthetic agents on human radial artery grafts. Thiopental and ketamine were found to be more potent than etomidate and propofol with respect to relaxant properties. These observations may have implications for the perioperative management of coronary artery graft vasospasm.[158]

Sympathetic and Parasympathetic Nervous System

In human in vivo studies, it appears that the cumulative effects of propofol on peripheral arterial venous capacitance are mediated primarily, but not solely, by its effects on the sympathetic nervous system (SNS). In a well-designed study in which the effect of local infusion of propofol into the brachial artery was compared with systemic intravenous administration with induction of anesthesia, it was demonstrated that direct brachial infusion had little effect on resistance and

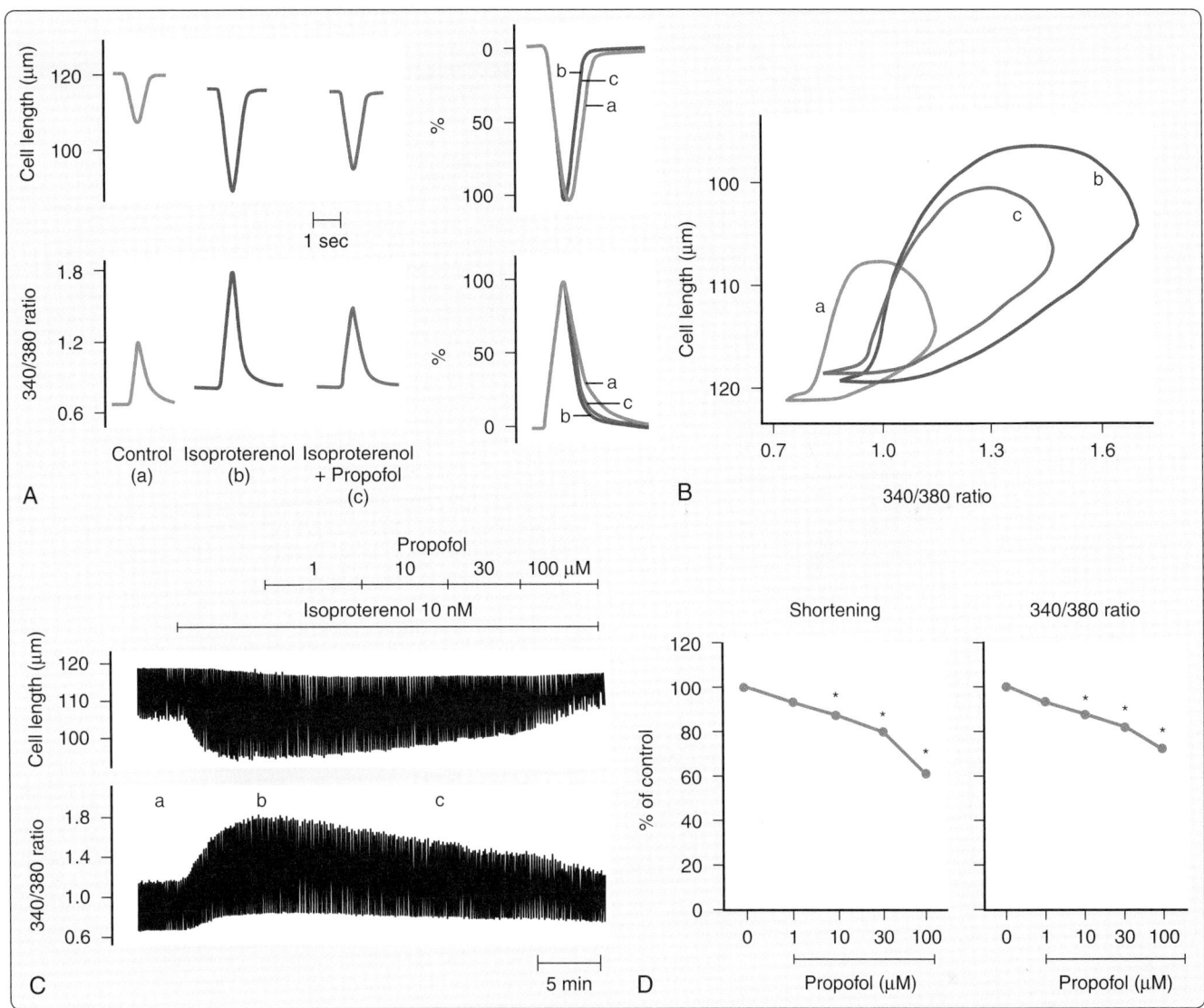

Figure 9-21 *A and B,* Original traces depicting the dose-dependent effects of propofol on shortening and intracellular Ca^{++} concentration ([Ca^{++}]$_i$) after exposure to isoproterenol (10 nm) in a rat isolated ventricular myocyte. *C and D,* Summarized data for the effects of propofol on isoproterenol-stimulated increases in shortening and [Ca^{++}]$_i$. Results are expressed as percentage of control. Propofol inhibits β-adrenergic–mediated contractility in a dose-dependent system. *, significant changes shown. *(From Kurokawa H, Murray PA, Damron DS: Propofol attenuates beta-adrenoreceptor-mediated signal transduction via a protein kinase c-dependent pathway in cardiomyocytes,* Anesthesiology *96(3):688–698, 2002.)*

capacitance, whereas the effect of intravenous administration was similar to the effect observed with sympathectomy induced by stellate ganglion block (Figure 9-28). Thus, the peripheral vascular effects of propofol appear to be primarily mediated by reduced sympathetic vasoconstrictor nerve activity.[159] In another elegant study, Sellgren et al[160] measured the effect of propofol on the SNS using percutaneous recordings of muscle sympathetic nerve activity. The authors demonstrated a profound decrease in SNS activity with a reciprocal increase in blood flow (measured by laser Doppler) with propofol-induced anesthesia. Furthermore, sympathetic baroreflex sensitivities were also depressed by propofol, highlighting the profound effect of this agent on central sympathetic modulation of integrated cardiovascular function. The precise locations of the central modulation by propofol have been investigated by Yang et al,[161,162] who demonstrated that propofol principally inhibits the vasomotor mechanism in the dorsomedial and ventrolateral medulla to effect its hypotensive actions. The implications of these effects are significant in that this sympathoinhibition is amplified in patients in whom SNS activity is high. Thus, caution is indicated

in the administration of these agents to patients with shock, CHF, or other pathophysiologic circumstances in which the SNS is paramount in maintaining arterial and venous tone.

Remodeling and Cell Proliferation

Emerging literature suggests that the effects of intravenous anesthetic agents may not be solely mediated by direct modulation of vascular tone through alteration of the contractile state of the vascular smooth muscle. New studies suggest that intravenous anesthetic agents may alter vascular smooth muscle proliferation, as well as modulate pathways that are important in angiogenesis. For example, Shiga et al[163] demonstrated the effect of ketamine (but not propofol) on inhibiting vascular smooth muscle proliferation through a PKC-dependent pathway. On the other hand, midazolam, but not ketamine, was demonstrated to release vascular endothelial growth factor, a growth factor important in angiogenesis and cellular proliferation from vascular smooth muscle cells.[164] The clinical importance of these findings remains unstudied and unclear. However, they serve

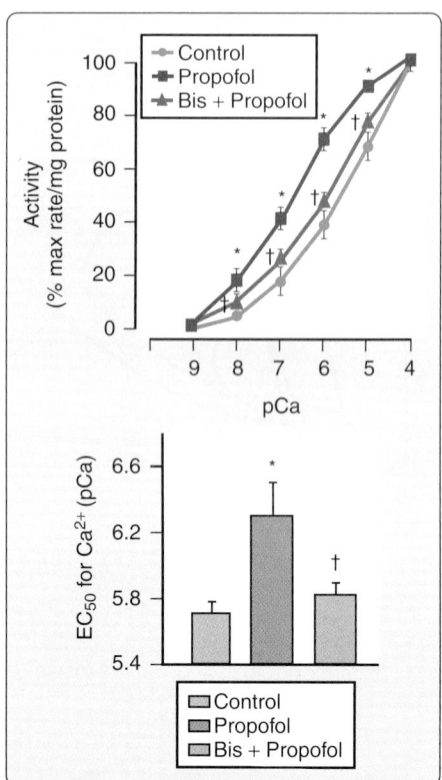

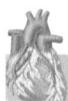

Figure 9-22 *Top,* Summarized data depicting the effects of Bis/aprotinin kinase C inhibition on the propofol-induced (30 μm) leftward shift in actomyosin ATPase activity in isolated myofibrils. *Bottom,* Summarized data depicting the increase (*$P < 0.05$ vs. control) in the median effective concentration (EC_{50}) value for Ca^{++} induced by propofol and inhibition of this effect ($^{†}P < 0.05$ vs. propofol) after pretreatment with Bis. Propofol increased myofilament Ca^{++} sensitivity by a protein kinase C–dependent receptor. *(From Kanaya N, Gable B, Murray PA, et al: Propofol increases phosphorylation of troponin I and myosin light chain 2 via protein kinase C activation in cardiomyocytes,* Anesthesiology 98:1363, 2003.)

to emphasize that the administration of these agents (and others) by the anesthesiologist may have effects that last well after the drug has disappeared from the core.

INDIVIDUAL AGENTS

Thiopental

General Characteristics

Thiopental has survived the test of time as an intravenous anesthetic drug (Box 9-4). Since Lundy introduced it in 1934, thiopental has become the most widely used induction agent because of the rapid hypnotic effect (one arm-to-brain circulation time), highly predictable

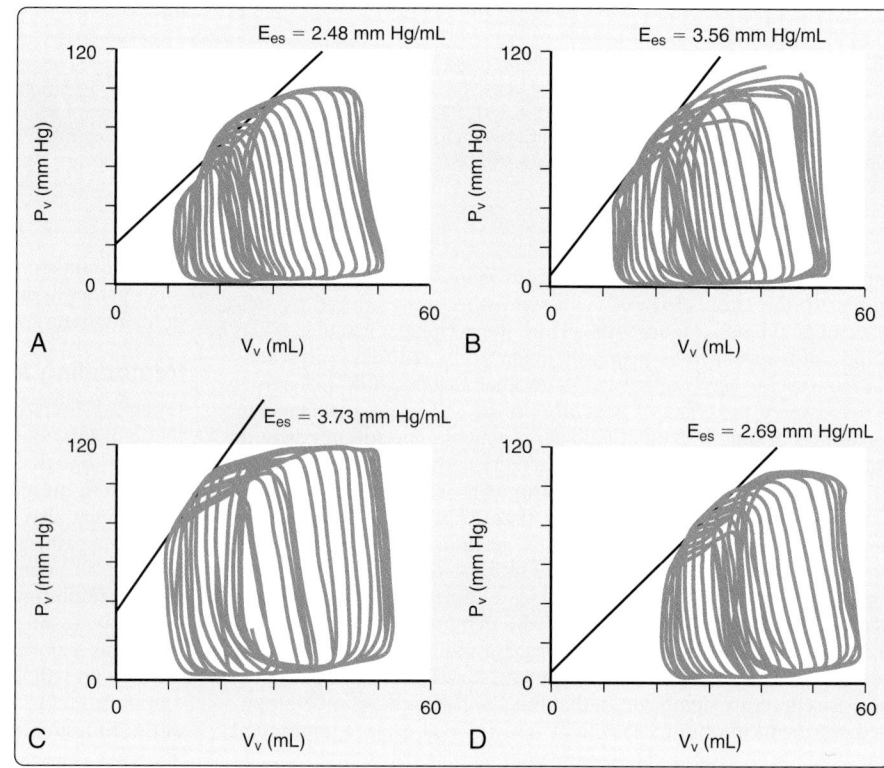

Figure 9-23 Typical pressure-volume loop recordings under pentobarbital anesthesia, at baseline (*A*) and during aortic banding (*C*); under propofol anesthesia, at baseline (*B*); and during aortic banding (*D*). *(From Kolh P, Lambermont B, Ghuysen A, et al: Comparison of the effects of propofol and pentobarbital on left ventricular adaptation to an increased afterload,* J Cardiovasc Pharmacol 44:294, 2004.)

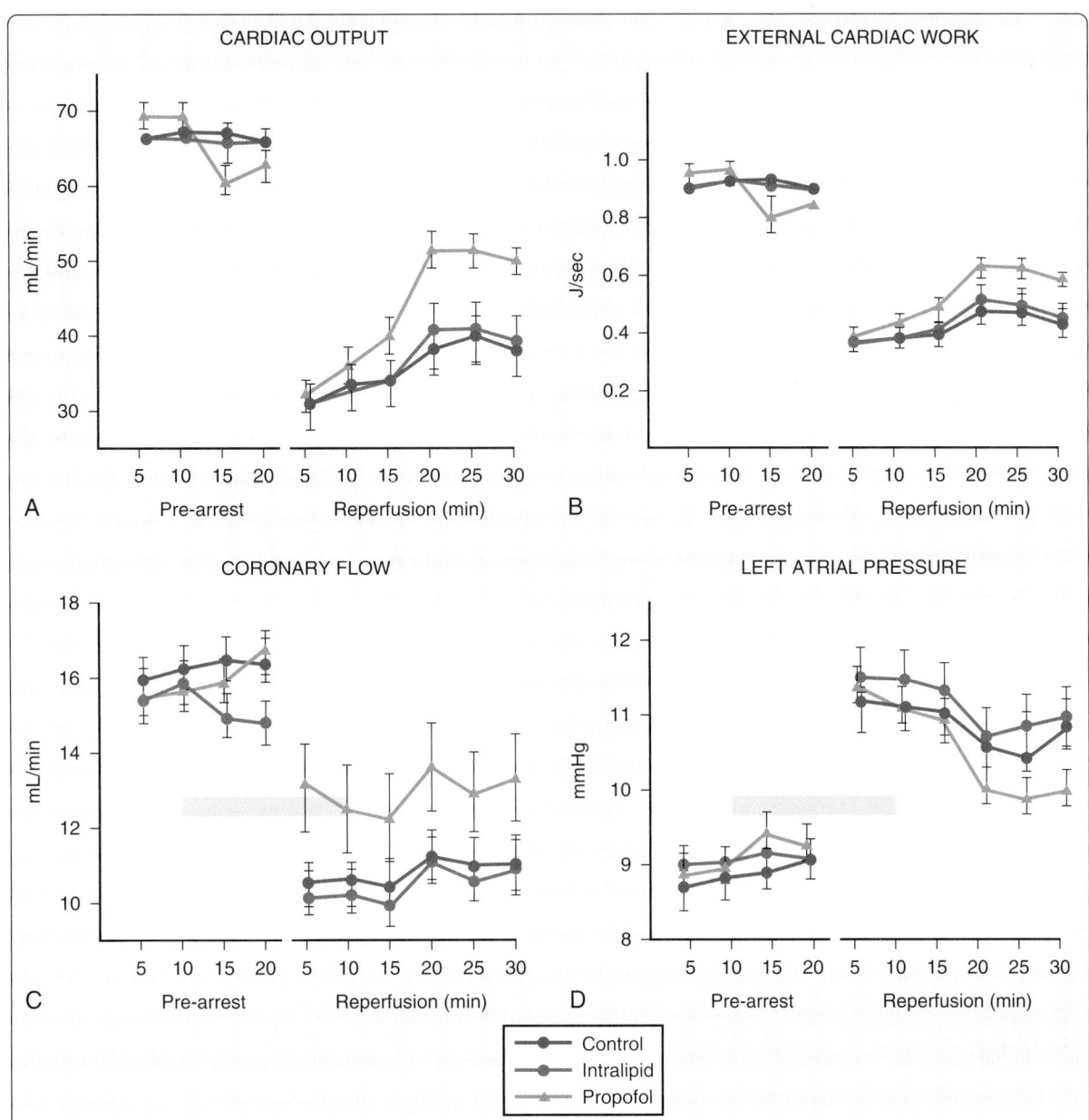

Figure 9-24 Cardiac function of the isolated working rat heart subjected to cold cardioplegic arrest and subsequent reperfusion. Propofol (4 g/mL dissolved in intralipid emulsion) or intralipid alone was added 10 minutes after initiation of the working heart mode and washed out after 10 minutes into working heart reperfusion. Data are plotted as mean ± standard error of the mean (as error bars) for the separate heart preparations: control, intralipid, and propofol (n = 12, 12, and 14, respectively). *Shaded area* represents the period when test agents were present. The break in the plots represents 60-minute cold cardioplegic arrest and 10 minutes of initial Langendorff reperfusion. An increase in cardiac output *(A)* and a decrease in left atrial pressure *(D)* in propofol-perfused hearts are apparent in the protective effect of the drug. *(From Ko SH, Yu CW, Lee SK, et al: Propofol attenuates ischemia-reperfusion injury in the isolated rat heart,* Anesth Analg 85:719, 1997.)

effect, lack of vascular irritation, and general overall safety.[165] The induction dose of thiopental is less for older than for younger healthy patients.[166] Pharmacokinetic analyses[167–169] confirm the findings from the early classic studies of Brodie and Mark[170] relating the awakening from thiopental to rapid redistribution. Thiopental has a distribution half-life ($t_{1/2}\alpha$) of 2.5 to 8.5 minutes, and the total body clearance varies, according to sampling times and techniques, from 0.15 to 0.26 L/kg/hr.[159–161,163,164] The elimination half-life ($t_{1/2}\beta$) varies from 5 to 12 hours.[168,169,171,172] Barbiturates[173] and drugs such as propofol[174] have increased volumes of distribution (V_d) when used during CPB. Young (< 13 years old) patients seem to have a greater total clearance and quicker plasma thiopental clearance than do adults, which theoretically might result in earlier awakening, especially after multiple doses.[175]

Because of the affinity of fat for this drug, its relatively large V_d, and its low hepatic clearance, thiopental can accumulate in tissues, especially if given in large doses over a prolonged period.

Cardiovascular Effects

The hemodynamic changes produced by thiopental have been studied in healthy patients[166,176–182] and in patients with cardiac disease (Table 9-3).[183–188] The principal effect is a decrease in contractility,[180,181,189] which results from reduced availability of calcium to the myofibrils.[190] There is also an increase in HR.[166,177,179–181,186–189] The cardiac index (CI) is unchanged[177,185–188] or reduced,[176,178,181] and the mean aortic pressure (MAP) is maintained[177,187,188,191] or slightly reduced.[178,179,185–187] In the dose range studied, no relation between plasma thiopental and

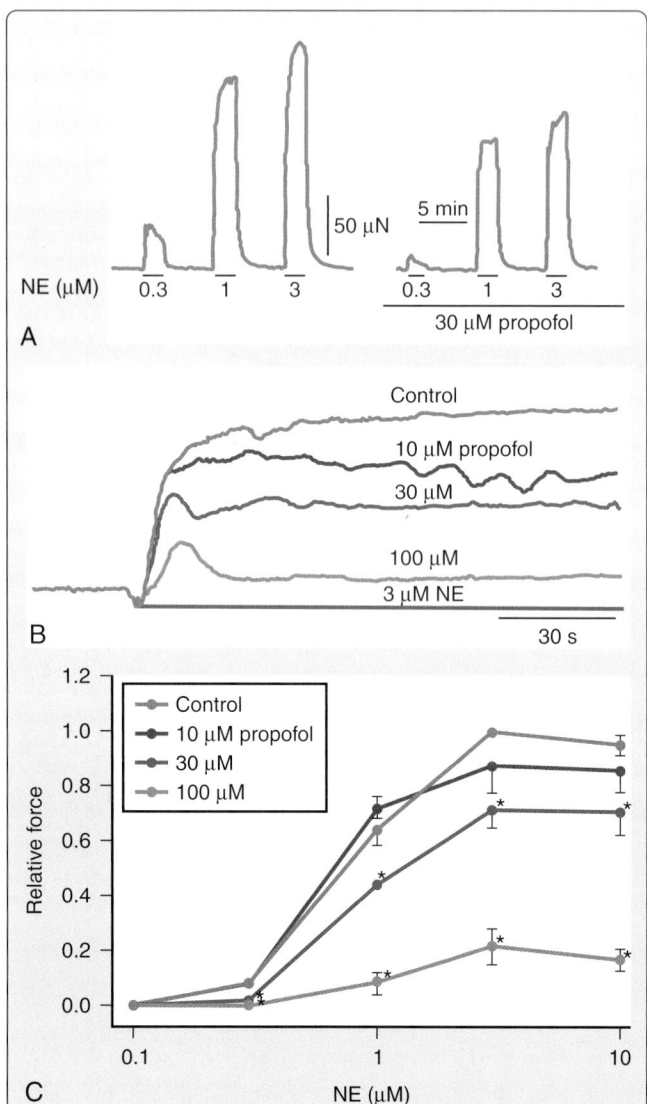

Figure 9-25 Effect of propofol on norepinephrine (NE)-induced increases in intracellular Ca++ concentration ([Ca++]) and force in smooth muscle of the rabbit mesenteric resistance artery. *(From Imura N, Shiraishi Y, Katsuya H, et al: Effect of propofol on norepinephrine-induced increases in [Ca++] and force in smooth muscle of the rabbit mesenteric resistance artery, Anesthesiology 88:1566, 1998.)*

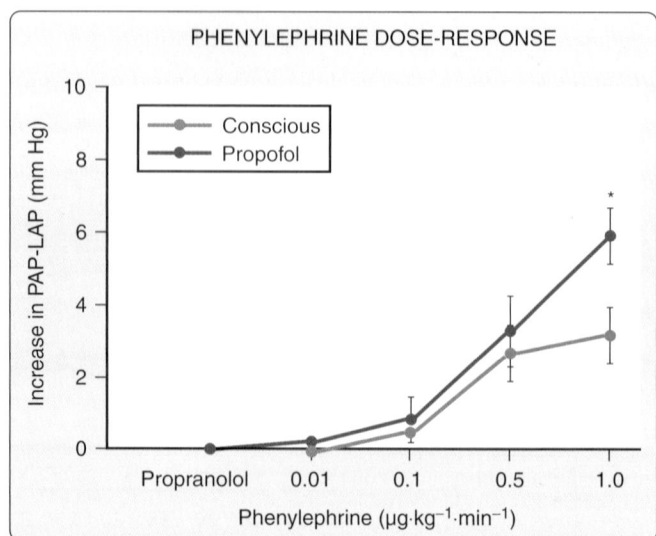

Figure 9-26 Pulmonary vascular effects of propofol at baseline, during elevated vasomotor tone, and in response to sympathetic and adrenoreceptor activation. PAP, pulmonary artery pressure; LAP, left atrial pressure. *(From Kondo U, Kim SO, Nakayama M, et al: Pulmonary vascular effects of propofol at baseline, during elevated vasomotor tone, and in response to sympathetic alpha- and beta-adrenoreceptor activation, Anesthesiology 94:815, 2001.)*

Despite the well-known potential for cardiovascular depression when thiopental is given rapidly in large doses, this drug has minimal hemodynamic effects in healthy patients and in those who have heart disease when it is given slowly or by infusion. Significant reductions in cardiovascular parameters occur in patients who have impaired ventricular function. When thiopental is given to patients with hypovolemia, there is a significant reduction in CO (69%), as well as a large decrease in BP, which indicate that patients without adequate compensatory mechanisms may have serious hemodynamic depression with a thiopental induction.[195] Clearly, thiopental produces greater changes in BP and HR than does midazolam when used for induction of American Society of Anesthesiologists (ASA) Class III and IV patients.

Uses in Cardiac Anesthesia

Thiopental can be used safely for the induction of anesthesia in normal patients and in those who have compensated cardiac disease. Because of the negative inotropic effects, increase in venous capacitance, and dose-related decrease in CO, caution should be used when thiopental is given to patients who have left or right ventricular failure, cardiac tamponade, or hypovolemia. The development of tachycardia is a potential problem in patients with ischemic heart disease.

A possible additional use for thiopental infusion is cerebral protection during CPB in patients undergoing selected cardiac operations.[196] However, the cerebral protective effect of thiopental during CPB has been challenged by Zaidan et al,[197] who demonstrated no differences in outcome between thiopental and control patients undergoing hypothermic CPB for CABG. Although the administration of a barbiturate during CPB may result in myocardial depression, necessitating additional inotropic support, Ito et al's[198] study suggested beneficial effects of a thiopental infusion during CPB in maintaining peripheral perfusion, which allowed more uniform warming, decreased base deficit, and decreased requirements for postoperative pressor support.

■ Midazolam

General Characteristics

Midazolam (Versed; Figure 9-29), a water-soluble benzodiazepine, was synthesized in the United States in 1975, in contrast with most new anesthetic drugs, which are synthesized and first tested in European countries. It is unique among benzodiazepines because of its rapid

hemodynamic effect has been found.[166] Early hemodynamic investigations demonstrated that thiopental (100 to 400 mg) significantly decreased CO (24%) and systemic BP (10%), presumably by reducing venous return, because of an increase in venous capacitance.[178,192]

Mechanisms for the decrease in CO include (1) direct negative inotropic action; (2) decreased ventricular filling, resulting from increased venous capacitance; and (3) transiently decreased sympathetic outflow from the central nervous system (CNS). The increase in HR (10% to 36%) that accompanies thiopental administration probably results from the baroreceptor-mediated sympathetic reflex stimulation of the heart. Thiopental produces dose-related negative inotropic effects that appear to result from a decrease in calcium influx into the cells with a resultant diminished amount of calcium at sarcolemma sites.[193,194] Patients who had compensated heart disease and received 4 mg/kg thiopental had a greater (18%) BP decline than did other patients without heart disease. The increase in HR (11% to 36%) encountered in patients with CAD, anesthetized with thiopental (1 to 4 mg/kg), is potentially deleterious because of the obligatory increase in myocardial oxygen consumption (Mvo_2).

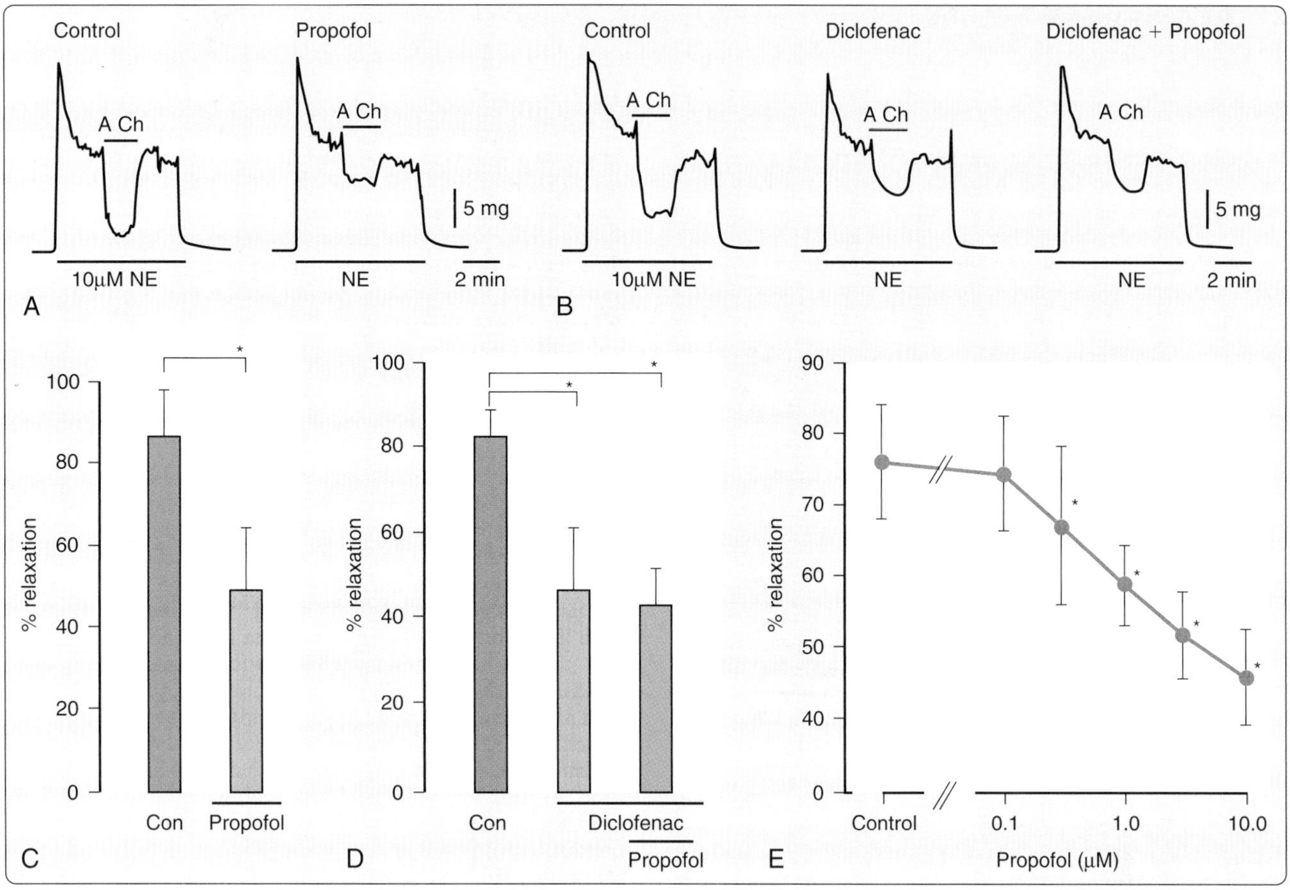

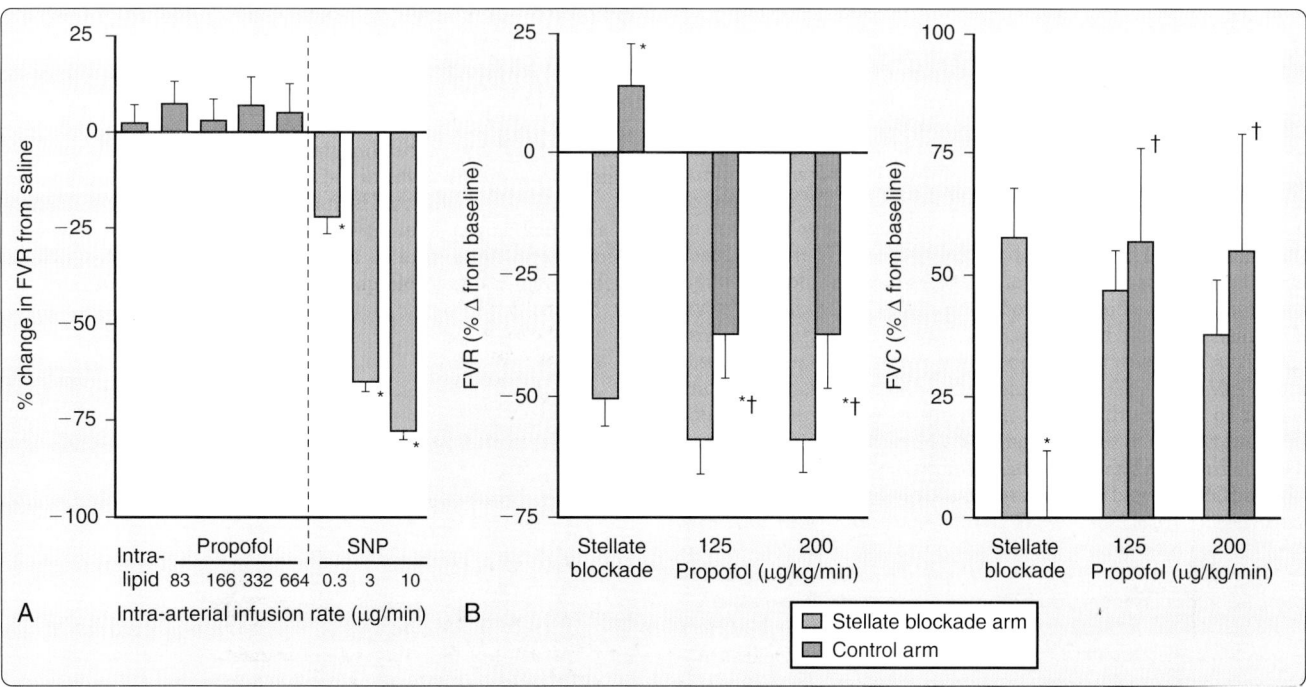

Figure 9-27 Inhibitory effects of propofol on acetylcholine (ACh)-induced, endothelium-dependent relaxation and prostacyclin synthesis in rabbit mesenteric resistance arteries. Con, control; NE, norepinephrine; *, Significant difference from control ($P < 0.05$). *(From Yamashita A, Kajikuri J, Ohashi M, et al: Inhibitory effects of propofol on acetylcholine-induced, endothelium-dependent relaxation and prostacyclin synthesis in rabbit mesenteric resistance arteries, Anesthesiology 91:1080, 1999.)*

Figure 9-28 A, Change in forearm vascular resistance (FVR) during brachial artery infusions of intralipid, propofol, and sodium nitroprusside (SNP). Intra-arterial infusions of propofol did not change FVR, whereas intra-arterial infusions of SNP significantly reduced FVR. Data are expressed as the percentage change from saline and are shown as mean ± standard error of the mean (SEM). *$P < 0.05$ indicates significant change from saline. B, Percentage changes from awake baseline in FVR and forearm venous compliance (FVC) in the left arm after stellate blockade and in the control unblocked arm before and during propofol anesthesia. Stellate blockade decreased FVR and increased FVC on the side of the blockade. During propofol anesthesia, there was no further arterial or venous dilation in the sympathectomized arm, but significant dilation occurred in the unblocked control arm. Data are mean ± SEM. *$P < 0.05$ indicates significant difference between arms; †$P < 0.05$ indicates significant change from prepropofol baseline. *(From Robinson BJ, Ebert TJ, O'Brien TJ, et al: Mechanisms whereby propofol mediates peripheral vasodilation in humans. Sympathoinhibition or direct vascular relaxation? Anesthesiology 86:64, 1997.)*

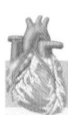

BOX 9-4. INTRAVENOUS ANESTHETICS

- Thiopental decreases cardiac output by:
  A direct negative inotropic action
  Decreased ventricular filling, resulting from increased venous capacitance
  Transiently decreasing sympathetic outflow from the central nervous system
  Because of these effects, caution should be used when thiopental is given to patients who have left or right ventricular failure, cardiac tamponade, or hypovolemia.
- Midazolam
  There are only small hemodynamic changes after the intravenous administration of midazolam.
- Etomidate
  Etomidate is described as the drug that changes hemodynamic variables the least. Studies in noncardiac patients and those who have heart disease document the remarkable hemodynamic stability after administration of etomidate.
  Patients who have hypovolemia, cardiac tamponade, or low cardiac output probably represent the population for whom etomidate is better than other induction drugs, with the possible exception of ketamine.
- Ketamine
  A unique feature of ketamine is stimulation of the cardiovascular system with the most prominent hemodynamic changes including significant increases in heart rate, CI, systemic vascular resistance, pulmonary artery pressure, and systemic artery pressure. These circulatory changes cause an increase in myocardial oxygen consumption (Mvo_2) with an appropriate increase in coronary blood flow.
  Studies have demonstrated the safety and efficacy of induction with ketamine in hemodynamically unstable patients, and it is the induction drug of choice for patients with cardiac tamponade physiology.
- Dexmedetomidine
  Dexmedetomidine is a highly selective, specific, and potent adrenoreceptor agonist.
  α_2-Adrenergic agonists can safely reduce anesthetic requirements and improve hemodynamic stability. These agents may enhance sedation and analgesia without producing respiratory depression or prolonging recovery period.

onset, short duration of action, and relatively rapid plasma clearance.[199] Although controversial, the dose for induction of general anesthesia is between 0.05 and 0.2 mg/kg, and depends on the premedication and speed of injection.[200-203]

The pharmacokinetic variables of midazolam reveal that it is cleared significantly more rapidly than are diazepam and lorazepam. The rapid redistribution of midazolam, as well as high liver clearance, accounts for its relatively short hypnotic and hemodynamic effects. The $t_{1/2}\beta$ is about 2 hours, which is at least 10-fold less than for diazepam.[204-208]

Cardiovascular Effects

The hemodynamic effects of midazolam have been investigated in healthy subjects,[179,209,210] in ASA Class III patients,[211] and in patients who have ischemic[212-219] and valvular[211] heart disease (VHD). Table 9-3 summarizes the hemodynamic changes after induction of anesthesia with midazolam. In general, there are only small hemodynamic changes after the intravenous administration of midazolam (0.2 mg/kg) in premedicated patients who have coronary artery disease (CAD).[215,217] Changes of potential importance include a decrease in MAP of 20% (from 102 to 81 mm Hg) and an increase in HR of 15% (from 55 to 64 beats/min).[215] The CI is maintained.[215,217] Filling pressures are either unchanged or decreased in patients who have normal ventricular function,[215,217] but are significantly decreased in patients who have an increased pulmonary capillary wedge pressure (PCWP; ≥ 18 mm Hg).[216] There seems to be little effect of differences in doses on hemodynamics: 0.2,[217] 0.25,[214] and 0.3 mg/kg[219] all produce similar effects. Sedation with midazolam (0.05 mg/kg) in patients undergoing cardiac catheterization is devoid of any hemodynamic effect.[212] Marty et al showed that induction with 0.2 mg/kg produced a 24% reduction in CBF and a 26% reduction in Mvo_2 in patients with CAD.[213] As in patients with ischemic heart disease, the induction of anesthesia in patients with VHD is associated with minimal changes in CI, HR, and MAP after midazolam.[212] When intubation follows anesthesia induction with midazolam, significant increases in HR and BP occur, because midazolam is not an analgesic.[179,217-219] Adjuvant analgesic drugs are required to block the response to noxious stimuli.

There is a suggestion that midazolam affects the capacitance vessels more than diazepam does, at least during CPB, when decreases in venous reservoir volume of the pump are greater with midazolam than with diazepam. In addition, diazepam decreases SVR more than midazolam during CPB.[220]

TABLE 9-3	Induction Agents and Hemodynamic Changes				
Parameter	Thiopental	Midazolam	Etomidate	Propofol	Ketamine
Heart rate	0% to +36%	−14% to +21%	0% to +22%	−6% to +12%	0% to +59%
MAP	−18% to +8%	−12% to −26%	0% to −20%	0% to −47%	0% to +40%
Systemic vascular resistance	0% to +19%	0% to −20%	0% to −17%	−9% to −25%	0% to +33%
Pulmonary artery pressure	Unchanged	Unchanged	0% to −17%	−4% to +8%	+44% to +47%
Pulmonary vascular resistance	Unchanged	Unchanged	0% to +27%	—	0% to +33%
LAP/PAOP	Unchanged	0% to −25%	—	—	—
Left ventricular end-diastolic pressure/PAOP	—	—	0% to −11%	+13%	Unchanged
Right atrial pressure	0% to +33%	Unchanged	Unchanged	−8% to −21%	+15% to +33%
Cardiac index	0% to −24%	0% to −25%	0% to +14%	−6% to −26%	0% to +42%
Stroke volume	−12% to −35%	0% to −18%	0% to −15%	−8% to −18%	0% to −21%
Left ventricular stroke work index	0% to −26%	−28% to −42%	0% to −27%	−15% to −40%	0% to +27%
Right ventricular stroke work index	NR	−41% to −57%	—	—	—
dP/dt	−14%	0% to −12%	0% to −18%	—	Unchanged
1/PEP²	−18% to −28%	—	—	—	—
Systolic time interval	—	—	Unchanged	—	NR

LAP, left atrial pressure; MAP, mean arterial pressure; NR, not reported; PAOP, pulmonary artery occlusion pressure; PEP, pre-ejection period.

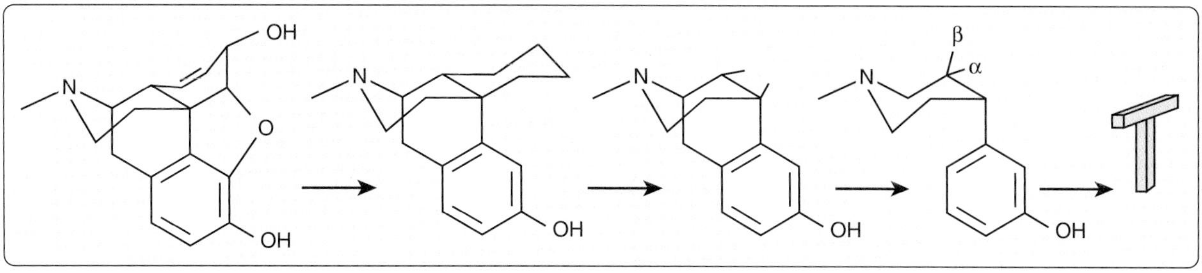

Figure 9-29 Synthetic opioids are produced by successive removal of ring structures from the five-ring phenanthrene structure of morphine. However, a common core, envisaged as a T shape, is shared by all opioids. A piperidine ring (which is believed to confer opioid-like properties to a compound) forms the crossbar, and a hydroxylated phenyl group forms the vertical axis. (*From Ferrante FM: Opioids. In Ferrante FM, VadeBoncouer TR, editors:* Postoperative pain management, *New York: Churchill Livingstone, 1992, p 149, by permission.*)

Midazolam (0.15 mg/kg) and ketamine (1.5 mg/kg) have proved to be a safe and useful combination for a rapid-sequence induction for emergency surgery.[182] This combination was superior to thiopental alone because it caused less cardiovascular depression, more amnesia, and less postoperative somnolence. If midazolam is given to patients who have received fentanyl, significant hypotension may occur, as seen with diazepam and fentanyl.[221] However, midazolam routinely is combined with fentanyl for induction and maintenance of general anesthesia during cardiac surgery without adverse hemodynamic sequelae.[222,223]

Uses

Midazolam is distinctly different from the other benzodiazepines because of its rapid onset, short duration, water solubility, and failure to produce significant thrombophlebitis; it is, therefore, one of the mainstays of anesthesia in the cardiac operating room.

▮ Etomidate

General Characteristics

Etomidate is a carboxylated imidazole derivative synthesized by Godefroi et al[224] in 1965. In animal experiments, it was found that etomidate has a safety margin four times greater than the safety margin for thiopental.[225] The recommended induction dose of 0.3 mg/kg has pronounced hypnotic effects. Etomidate is moderately lipid soluble[226] and has a rapid onset (10 to 12 seconds) and a brief duration of action.[227–229] It is hydrolyzed primarily in the liver and in the blood as well.[230]

The administration of etomidate in a buffered solution was accompanied by a significant incidence of a burning sensation (about 40%) and myoclonic movements (about 40% to 50%).[229] The myoclonic movements were not associated with an epileptiform pattern on the electroencephalogram.[226]

Reports have shown that etomidate infusion and single injections directly suppress adrenocortical function, which, in turn, interferes with the normal stress response.[231–233] Blockade of 11-β-hydroxylation mediated by the imidazole radical of etomidate results in decreased biosynthesis of cortisol and aldosterone.[234] The clinical significance of etomidate-induced adrenal suppression remains undetermined.

Cardiovascular Effects

In comparative studies with other anesthetic drugs, etomidate is usually described as the drug that changes hemodynamic variables the least.[235–241] Studies in noncardiac patients[237,240,242] and those who have heart disease[187,235,238,239,243,244] document the remarkable hemodynamic stability after administration of etomidate (see Table 9-3). In healthy subjects or patients who have compensated ischemic heart disease, HR, pulmonary artery pressure (PAP), PCWP, left ventricular end-diastolic pressure, right atrial pressure (RAP), CI, SVR, pulmonary vascular resistance (PVR), dP/dt, and systolic time intervals

(STIs) are not significantly changed after doses of 0.15 to 0.30 mg/kg.[187,235,236,242,244] In comparison with other anesthetics, etomidate produces the least change in the balance of myocardial oxygen demand and supply. Systemic BP remains unchanged in most series[235,236,238–241] but may be decreased 10% to 19%[239,243,245] in patients who have VHD. Ammon et al[235] found modest dose-related decreases in MAP and left ventricular stroke work index (LVSWI). Doses of 0.3, 0.45, and 0.6 mg/kg caused greater decreases in mean BP and LVSWI but had no effect on HR, PAP, PCWP, CVP, CI, SV, or SVR. Therefore, although there was a small dose-related effect on hemodynamics, the remarkable fact is that there is hemodynamic stability despite the twofold increase in dose. Dose-related changes have been demonstrated in the dog and were attributed to three possible causes: (1) decreased CNS sympathetic stimulation, (2) autoregulation secondary to decreased regional O_2 consumption, and (3) decreased SV secondary to reduced venous return.[246]

A dose-dependent direct negative inotropic effect of etomidate was demonstrated in dogs, although at equianesthetic doses, it was half as pronounced as that of thiopental.[193] To determine the effects of anesthetic agents on myocardial contractility is difficult in vivo because of concomitant changes in HR, preload, and afterload. In contrast, the effects may be evaluated in vitro, although this does not accurately represent what is occurring in the myocardium as a whole. Riou et al[247] studied the effect of etomidate on intrinsic myocardial contractility, using left ventricular papillary muscle and an electromagnetic lever system. Etomidate induced a slightly positive inotropic effect, as manifested by increased maximum shortening velocity. It appears, however, that propylene glycol, the solvent in which etomidate is available, may result in SR dysfunction with a slight negative inotropic effect in some clinical conditions.

Etomidate (0.3 mg/kg intravenously), used to induce general anesthesia in patients with AMI undergoing percutaneous coronary angioplasty, did not alter HR, MAP, and rate-pressure product, demonstrating the remarkable hemodynamic stability of this agent.[248] However, the presence of VHD may influence the hemodynamic responses to etomidate. Whereas most patients can maintain their BP, patients with both aortic and mitral VHD had significant decreases of 17% to 19% in systolic and diastolic BP,[239,243] as well as decreases of 11% and 17% in PAP and PCWP, respectively.[243] CI in patients who had VHD and received 0.3 mg/kg either remained unchanged[186,239] or decreased 13%.[243] There was no difference in response to etomidate between patients who had aortic valve disease and those who had mitral valve disease.[243]

Wauquier et al[249] anticipated the widespread clinical use of etomidate in their investigation, in which they compared the effects of etomidate and thiopental in hypovolemic dogs. In a hemorrhagic shock model, dogs were bled to an MAP of 40 to 45 mm Hg and then given either etomidate (1 mg/kg) or thiopental (10 mg/kg). There was significantly more hemodynamic depression in the thiopental group and increased survival in the etomidate group. Whether this is true in humans is not known, but certainly clinical evidence suggests that etomidate is useful in patients with hypovolemia.

Uses

There are certain situations in which the advantages of etomidate outweigh the disadvantages. Emergency uses include situations in which rapid induction is essential. Patients who have hypovolemia, cardiac tamponade, or low CO probably represent the population for whom etomidate is better than other drugs, with the possible exception of ketamine. The fact that the hypnotic effect is brief means that additional analgesic and/or hypnotic drugs must be administered. Etomidate offers no real advantage over most other induction drugs for patients undergoing elective surgical procedures.

▓ Ketamine

General Characteristics

Ketamine is a phencyclidine derivative whose anesthetic actions differ so markedly from barbiturates and other CNS depressants that Corssen and Domino[250] labeled its effect *dissociative anesthesia*. The properties of ketamine and its use in anesthesia have been completely reviewed.[191] Although ketamine produces rapid hypnosis and profound analgesia, respiratory and cardiovascular functions are not depressed as much as with most other induction agents. Disturbing psychotomimetic activity (described as vivid dreams, hallucinations, or emergence phenomena) remains a problem. Interestingly, preliminary data suggest the possibility of a protective effect against postoperative cognitive dysfunction in patients undergoing cardiac surgery, and a recent study conducted by Hudetz et al suggests that ketamine attenuates the postoperative delirium noted in cardiac surgical patients after surgery.[251]

Cardiovascular Effects

The hemodynamic effects of ketamine have been examined in noncardiac patients,[239,252-257] critically ill patients,[258] geriatric patients,[259] and patients who have a variety of heart diseases.[254,260-270] Table 9-3 contains the range of hemodynamic responses to ketamine. One unique feature of ketamine is stimulation of the CVS. The most prominent hemodynamic changes are significant increases in HR, CI, SVR, PAP, and systemic artery pressure. These circulatory changes cause an increase in Mvo$_2$ with an apparently appropriate increase in CBF.[260,269] Although global increases in Mvo$_2$ occur, there is some evidence that the increased work may be borne primarily by the right ventricle, because of significantly greater increases in PVR than SVR[271]; however, both ventricles certainly demonstrate increased work. The hemodynamic changes observed with ketamine are not dose related in the relatively small dose ranges examined; there is no significant difference between changes after administration of 0.5 and 1.5 mg/kg intravenously.[272] It is interesting that a second dose of ketamine produces hemodynamic effects opposite to those of the first.[268] Thus, the cardiovascular stimulation seen after ketamine induction of anesthesia (2 mg/kg) in a patient who has VHD is not observed with the second administration, which is accompanied instead by decreases in the BP, PCWP, and CI.

Ketamine produces similar hemodynamic changes in healthy patients and in patients who have ischemic heart disease.[256] In patients who have increased PAP (as with mitral valvular disease), ketamine appears to cause a more pronounced increase in PVR than in SVR. The presence of marked tachycardia after administration of ketamine and pancuronium also can complicate the induction of anesthesia in patients who have CAD or VHD with atrial fibrillation.[273] In a recent study of patients undergoing elective coronary artery bypass grafting, the use of S-(+)-ketamine did not lead to increased cardiac troponin T levels after surgery when used in combination with propofol.[274]

The mechanism responsible for ketamine's stimulation of the circulatory system remains enigmatic. The direct effects of ketamine on the myocardium remain controversial. Riou et al[275] demonstrated that ketamine has a dual opposing action on the myocardium: (1) a positive inotropic effect, probably secondary to increased Ca^{++} influx; and (2) an impairment of SR function. This impairment is significant only at supratherapeutic ketamine concentrations or in cardiomyopathic

myocardium,[276] and overcomes this positive inotropic effect only under these circumstances. Myocardial depression has been demonstrated in isolated rabbit hearts,[277] intact dogs, and isolated dog heart preparations.[278,279] Although the precise site of cardiovascular stimulation is still unknown, Ivankovich and colleagues[280] showed that small doses of ketamine injected directly into the CNS result in immediate hemodynamic stimulation. Ketamine also causes the sympathoneuronal release of norepinephrine, which can be measured in venous blood.[260,272,281] Blockade of this effect is possible with barbiturates, benzodiazepines,[272,280-282] and droperidol.[261] Animal work supports the hypothesis that the primary hemodynamic effect of ketamine is central and not peripheral.[283-290] The role of ketamine's cocaine-like neuronal inhibition of norepinephrine reuptake has yet to be defined in its overall influence on the CVS.[291,292] It also is unknown whether ketamine exerts the same effect centrally, preventing reuptake of norepinephrine in the brain.

One of the most common and successful approaches to blocking ketamine-induced hypertension and tachycardia is the prior administration of benzodiazepines. Diazepam, flunitrazepam, and midazolam all successfully attenuate the hemodynamic effects of ketamine.[182,262,265,282,293-295] For example, in a study involving 16 patients with VHD, ketamine (2 mg/kg) did not produce significant hemodynamic changes when preceded by diazepam (0.4 mg/kg).[262] Indeed, HR, MAP, and rate-pressure product were unchanged; however, there was a slight but significant decrease in CI.[262] Hatano and associates[294] reported their experience with 200 cardiac surgical patients in whom the administration of diazepam (0.3 to 0.5 mg/kg) and then a ketamine infusion (0.7 mg/kg/hr) provided a stable hemodynamic course during induction, intubation, and incision. In fact, the combination of diazepam and ketamine rivals the high-dose fentanyl technique with regard to hemodynamic stability. No patient had hallucinations, although 2% had dreams and 1% had recall of events in the operating room.[294] Levanen et al[296] suggested that premedication with 2.5 μg/kg intramuscular dexmedetomidine before ketamine-based anesthesia is as effective as midazolam in blocking the hemodynamic effects of ketamine and was more effective in reducing adverse CNS effects. Because of the propensity of dexmedetomidine to produce bradycardia, concomitant use of an anticholinergic agent was suggested.

Studies have demonstrated the safety and efficacy of induction with ketamine (2 mg/kg) in hemodynamically unstable patients who required emergency operations.[258,297,298] Most of these patients were hypovolemic because of trauma or massive hemorrhage. Ketamine induction was accompanied in the majority of patients by the maintenance of BP and, presumably, of CO as well.[258,297] In patients who have an accumulation of pericardial fluid, with or without constrictive pericarditis, induction with ketamine (2 mg/kg) maintains CI and increases BP, SVR, and RAP.[299,300] The HR in this group of patients was unchanged by ketamine, probably because cardiac tamponade already produced a compensatory tachycardia.

Uses

In adults, ketamine is probably the safest and most efficacious drug for patients who have decreased blood volume or cardiac tamponade. Undesired tachycardia, hypertension, and emergence delirium may be attenuated with benzodiazepines.

▓ Propofol

Propofol is the most recent intravenous anesthetic to be introduced into clinical practice. It is an alkylphenol with hypnotic properties. The pharmacokinetics of propofol have been evaluated by numerous investigators and have been described by both two-compartment[301,302] and three-compartment[303,304] models.

Cardiovascular Effects

The hemodynamic effects of propofol have been investigated in healthy ASA Class I and II patients,[305] elderly patients,[306,307] patients with CAD and good left ventricular function,[308,309] and patients with impaired left ventricular function (see Table 9-3). Numerous studies also have compared the cardiovascular effects of propofol with the most commonly used induction drugs, including the thiobarbiturates and etomidate.[310–314] Comparison of the findings between investigators is, however, difficult because of the variations in the anesthetic techniques used, doses of drugs administered, and techniques used for measuring data. It is clear that with propofol, systolic arterial pressure declines 15% to 40% after intravenous induction with 2 mg/kg and maintenance infusion with 100 μg/kg/min. Similar changes are seen in both diastolic arterial pressure and MAP.

The effect of propofol on HR is variable. The majority of studies have demonstrated significant reductions in SVR (9% to 30%), CI, SV, and LVSWI after propofol. Although controversial, the evidence points to a dose-dependent decrease in myocardial contractility. Bendel et al,[315] in a double-blind, randomized, controlled trial, compared the effects of propofol and etomidate in patients undergoing elective aortic valve surgery for aortic stenosis. They concluded that propofol was twice as likely to result in hypotension during the induction of patients with severe aortic stenosis compared with etomidate.[315] Finally, it has been suggested that propofol increases triglyceride levels.[316–318] Oztekin et al[319] conducted a study evaluating the effect of propofol and midazolam on lipid levels early in the postoperative period in patients undergoing CABG surgery. Serum triglyceride levels and very-low-density lipoproteins were significantly increased in patients receiving intraoperative propofol infusions 4 hours after surgery. It remains to be seen what effect this increase has on clinical outcomes and postoperative course.[319]

Uses

In a study of the cerebral physiologic effects of propofol during CPB, Newman et al[320] demonstrated that when given during nonpulsatile CPB, propofol produced statistically significant reductions in cerebral blood flow and cerebral metabolic rate in a coupled manner without adverse effects on cerebral arteriovenous oxygen content difference or jugular bulb venous saturation. The coupled reductions in cerebral blood flow and cerebral metabolic rate suggest the potential for propofol to reduce cerebral exposure to emboli during CPB.

The effect of propofol on hypoxic pulmonary vasoconstriction was minimal in thoracic surgical patients undergoing one-lung ventilation. In comparison with isoflurane, maintenance of anesthesia with propofol resulted in lower CI and right ventricular ejection fraction, but avoided the threefold increase in shunt fraction observed with isoflurane on commencement of one-lung ventilation.[321]

Dexmedetomidine

Dexmedetomidine, the pharmacologically active d-isomer of medetomidine, is a highly selective, specific, and potent adrenoreceptor agonist. Medetomidine has a considerably greater α_2/α_1 selectivity ratio than does the classic prototype α_2-adrenergic agonist clonidine in receptor-binding experiments. In comparison with clonidine, it is more efficacious as an α_2-adrenoreceptor agonist. It has been shown to effectively reduce volatile anesthetic requirements in experimental animals, as measured by minimal alveolar concentration (MAC), and can even be a complete anesthetic in sufficiently high doses. The exact mechanism of action and reduction of anesthetic requirement are unknown but are thought to involve an action at both presynaptic and postsynaptic α_2-adrenoreceptors in the CNS.

Cardiovascular Effects

The cardiovascular effects of dexmedetomidine are dose related. Furst and Weinger[322] demonstrated that an increase in systemic BP was associated with the pretreatment of rats with high-dose dexmedetomidine, and that dexmedetomidine had little effect on arterial blood gases in spontaneously ventilating rats, consistent with minimal respiratory depression. Canine studies with medetomidine in doses of 30 μg/kg intravenously or 80 μg/kg intramuscularly showed decreases in HR

and CO with increased SVR after drug administration. The intravenous administration of 5 to 10 μg/kg medetomidine to anesthetized, autonomically blocked dogs suggested that the decline in CO was not mediated by decreased contractility but rather by the effects of increased vascular resistance and decreased HR. At high doses, the increase in SVR is most likely due to the activation of peripheral postsynaptic α_2-adrenoreceptors in vascular smooth muscle.

In human studies, ASA Class I women who received low-dose premedication with 0.5 μg/kg dexmedetomidine demonstrated modest decreases in BP and HR. Intramuscular dexmedetomidine in a dose of 2.5 μg/kg administered 45 minutes before induction of a ketamine/N_2O/oxygen anesthetic resulted in effective attenuation of the cardiostimulatory effects of ketamine but also resulted in increased intraoperative and postoperative bradycardia.[296] The use of perioperative intravenous infusions of low-dose dexmedetomidine in vascular patients at risk for CAD produced lower preoperative HR and systolic BP, and less postoperative tachycardia, but also resulted in a greater intraoperative requirement for pharmacologic intervention to support BP and HR. The precise cause of this effect is unknown, but it is possibly due to the attenuation of sympathetic outflow from the CNS.

Some controversy exists whether the hemodynamic effects of dexmedetomidine are influenced by the background anesthetic. In conscious animals, the hypotensive effect of the drug dominates; however, with the addition of potent inhalation anesthetics, MAP remains unchanged or increased, which implies a different mechanism of interaction of inhalation agent with this class of anesthetics. Dexmedetomidine has little effect on respiration, with minimal increase in arterial carbon dioxide tension ($Paco_2$) after administration to spontaneously ventilating dogs; thus, it has a potential advantage over other respiratory depressant anesthetics. Antinociceptive effects of medetomidine are mediated by suppression of responses of the pain-relay neurons in the dorsal horn of the spinal cord.

Uses

Clinical studies have suggested that α_2-adrenergic agonists can safely reduce anesthetic requirements and improve hemodynamic stability. These agents may enhance sedation and analgesia without producing respiratory depression or prolonging the recovery period. Barletta et al[323] compared postoperative opioid requirements in patients undergoing cardiac surgery who received intraoperative propofol versus dexmedetomidine. Although dexmedetomidine resulted in lower opioid use compared with propofol, it did not translate to a shorter duration of mechanical ventilation but did result in significantly greater sedation-related costs.[323] Levanen et al[296] suggested that dexmedetomidine may be an effective alternative to benzodiazepines in attenuating the postanesthetic delirium effects of ketamine. Because α_2-adrenergic agonists potentially inhibit opiate-induced rigidity, it is clear that they may be of use as adjuvants with high-dose opioid anesthetics for cardiac surgery. In contrast with other anesthetic adjuvants, such as the benzodiazepines, the α_2-adrenoreceptor agonist dexmedetomidine does not further compromise cardiovascular or respiratory status in the presence of high-dose opioids. The use of dexmedetomidine as a sedative adjunct in the management of patients after surgery in the intensive care unit is becoming increasingly popular.[324] In general, the concept whereby the type and amount of agent used intraoperatively can influence the postoperative course, specifically the neuropsychologic events, is emerging as an important paradigm.[325] The management of patients after surgery is covered extensively in Chapters 33, 35, 36, and 37. In summary, pharmacologic evidence suggests dexmedetomidine may be useful as an adjuvant in cardiac anesthesia.

OPIOIDS IN CARDIAC ANESTHESIA

Terminology and Classification

Various terms are commonly used to describe morphine-like drugs that are potent analgesics. The word *narcotic* is derived from the Greek word for "stupor" and refers to any drug that produces sleep. In legal terminology, it refers to any substance that produces addiction and physical dependence. Its use to describe morphine or morphine-like drugs is misleading and should be discouraged. Opiates refer to alkaloids and related synthetic and semisynthetic drugs that interact stereospecifically with one or more of the opioid receptors to produce a pharmacologic effect. The more encompassing term, *opioid*, also includes the endogenous opioids and is used in this chapter. Opioids may be agonists, partial agonists, or antagonists.

A wide diversity in chemical structure exists among the naturally occurring, semisynthetic, and synthetic opioids. Opium contains several important alkaloid constituents, which may vary markedly in their pharmacologic actions. The five major alkaloid constituents of opium can be separated into two groups based on differences in their chemical structure. The phenanthrene derivatives include morphine and codeine, as well as the convulsogenic compound thebaine, which is used as a chemical precursor in the development of many clinically useful semisynthetic opioid compounds like oxycodone. The benzylisoquinoline derivatives of opium include the phosphodiesterase inhibitor, smooth muscle relaxant papaverine, and the antitussive compound noscapine.

Modification of the morphine molecule, although simultaneously preserving the basic five-ring structure, will result in semisynthetic compounds that also exhibit analgesic effects (e.g., hydromorphone, heroin). Progressive removal of these rings results in synthetic opioids. As long as the common core or T shape is retained stereochemically and is shared by these synthetic derivatives, opioid properties will be retained. The piperidine ring forms the crossbar and the hydroxyl phenyl group forms the vertical axis of the T shape (see Figure 9-29).

Opioid Receptors

The postulation of opioid receptor existence was stated in the pioneering work of Beckett and Casy,[326] which, in 1965, allowed Portoghese[327] to theorize the existence of separate opioid receptors by correlating analgesic activity to the chemical structure of many opioid compounds (Box 9-5). The idea of multiple opioid receptors is an accepted concept, and a number of subtypes for each class of opioid receptors have been identified. Through biochemical and pharmacologic methods, the μ, δ, and κ receptors have been characterized.[328–330] Pharmacologically, it is well-known that δ-opioid receptors consist of two subtypes: δ_1 and δ_2.[331–334] Table 9-4 lists the opioid receptors and their associated agonists and antagonists.

The μ-, κ-, and δ-opioid receptors have all been cloned, and experimental data indicate that they belong to the family of G-protein–coupled receptors.[335–338] Three steps have been identified in the opioid-induced transmembrane signaling process: (1) recognition by the receptor of the extracellular opioid agonist, (2) signal transduction mediated by G pro-

TABLE 9-4	List of Opioid-Receptor Agonist and Antagonist Drugs for the μ-, κ-, and δ-Opioid Receptors	
Opioid Receptor	**Agonist**	**Antagonist**
μ	Morphine	Naloxone
	Fentanyl	Naltrexone
	Levorphanol	β-Funaltrexamine*
	Methadone	Nalbuphine†
κ	U-50,488H	Nor-BNI
	EKC	MR-2266
	U-62,066E (spiradoline)	Naloxone
	U-69,593	
δ	(−)TAN-67	Naltrindole
	SIOM‡	BNTX
	SNC 80§	Naltriben

*β-FNA is an irreversible opioid receptor antagonist.
†Nalbuphine is an opioid receptor antagonist with partial agonist properties.
‡7-Spiroindinooxymorphone.
§(+)-4-[((αR)-α(2S,5R)-4-Allyl-2,5-dimethyl-1-piperazinyl)-3-methoxy-benzyl]-N, N-diethylbenzamide chloride.
BNTX, 7-benzylidene naltrexone; Nor-BNI, nor-binaltorphimine.

tein, and (3) altered production of an intracellular second messenger (Figure 9-30). The opioid receptors preferentially couple to a pertussis toxin–sensitive G protein (G_i/G_o) to influence one or more of three second-messenger pathways: cytoplasmic-free Ca^{++} $[Ca^{++}]_i$, the phosphatidylinositol-$[Ca^{++}]_i$ system, and the cyclic nucleotide cAMP. The actions of opioids are primarily inhibitory. Opioids close N-type, voltage-operated Ca^{++} channels and open Ca^{++}-dependent inwardly rectifying K^+ channels. This results in hyperpolarization and a reduction in

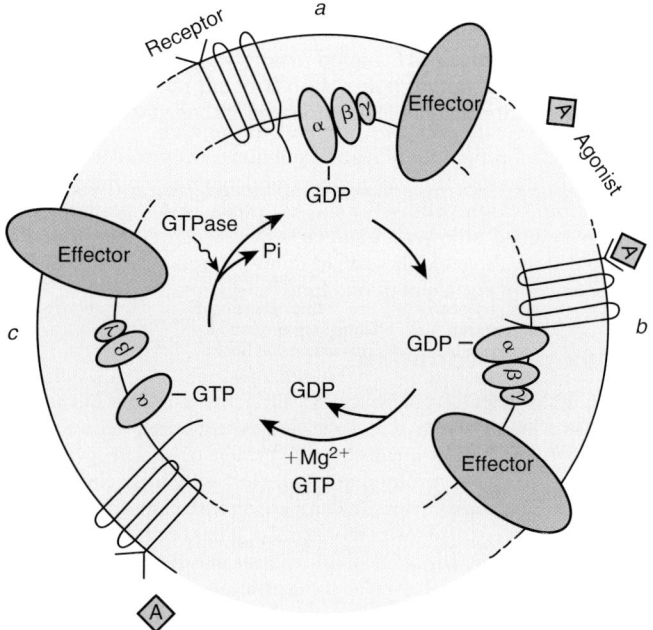

Figure 9-30 Simple scheme for G-protein signal transduction. From the unliganded state (*a*), receptor binds agonist A (e.g., epinephrine/acetylcholine), which produces a change (*b*) in receptor–G protein interaction, allowing GTP in the presence of Mg++, to replace GDP on the α subunit. The activated α-GTP subunit and the βγ subunits dissociate and one or both interact with effectors (e.g., adenylyl cyclase, K+ channel). Alternatively, free βγ may bind other α subunits. The intrinsic GTPase activity of the α subunit hydrolyzes GTP to GDP, releasing inorganic phosphate (P_i), and α-GDP recombines with βγ (*c*), ending the activation cycle. Nonhydrolyzable analogs of GTP, such as Gpp(NH)p or GTP-γS, produce persistent activation of α subunits and persistent dissociations of α from βγ because activation cannot be reversed by hydrolysis of these nucleotide analogs to GDP.

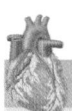

BOX 9-5. OPIOIDS

- The μ-, κ-, and δ-opioid receptors and endogenous opioid precursors have been identified in both cardiac and vascular tissue.
- The functional roles of opioid precursors/opioid receptors in the cardiovascular system in physiologic and pathophysiologic conditions (e.g., congestive heart failure, arrhythmia development) are areas of ongoing investigation.
- The predominant cardiovascular effect of exogenously administered opioids is to attenuate central sympathetic outflow.
- Endogenous opioids and opioid receptors, especially the δ1 receptor, are likely important contributors in effecting both early and delayed preconditioning in the heart.
- Plasma drug concentrations are profoundly altered by cardiopulmonary bypass as a result of hemodilution, altered plasma protein binding, hypothermia, exclusion of the lungs from the circulation, and altered hemodynamics that likely modulate hepatic and renal blood flow. The specific effects are drug dependent.

neuronal excitability.[339] κ receptors may only act on Ca[++] channels.[340] Evidence has been reported that P/Q-type Ca[++] channels may be inhibited by μ-, but not δ-, receptor opioids.[341] These effects may be mediated via a direct coupling between G protein and the ion channels or indirectly via changes in intracellular Ca[++]. Both Ca[++] fluxes and the consequences of these fluxes, such as calmodulin activation, are altered by opioids. Ca[++] ions are essential in nociception, and Ca[++]-channel blockers potentiate opioid analgesia[342,343] and reduce fentanyl requirements during cardiac surgery.[344] Opioid-induced inhibition of adenylyl cyclase, and the resultant decrease in the concentration of cAMP, may be responsible for modulation of neurotransmitter release (e.g., substance P).

Opioids also have excitatory effects that involve both disinhibition of interneurons and direct excitation of neurons themselves. Nanomolar concentrations, acting via G proteins, stimulate adenylyl cyclase activity in certain neurons.[345] Another important stimulatory effect is a transient increase in cytoplasmic-free Ca[++] secondary to Ca[++] influx via L-type Ca[++] channel opening, as well as mobilization of Ca[++] from inositol triphosphate–sensitive intracellular stores.[346] Mu-agonists also may stimulate Ca[++] entry into neurons via G-protein–coupled activation of phospholipase C to increase inositol-1,4,5-triphosphate formation, secondary to Ca[++] influx via L-type Ca[++] channel opening.[346–348]

Opioid receptors involved in regulating the CVS have been localized centrally to the cardiovascular and respiratory centers of the hypothalamus and brainstem, and peripherally to cardiac myocytes, blood vessels, nerve terminals, and the adrenal medulla. It generally is accepted that opioid receptors are differentially distributed between atria and ventricles. The highest specific receptor density for binding of κ-agonists is in the right atrium and least in the left ventricle.[349,350] As with the κ-opioid receptor, the distribution of the δ-opioid receptor favors atrial tissue and the right side of the heart more than the left.[351] The data confirming the presence of the μ-opioid receptor subtype in the heart are less conclusive, and most conclude that this receptor subtype is not present in cardiac tissue.[349,350,352,353] Whether these differences in receptor location are important cannot be determined, as it has not been shown whether these receptors are differentially located in cardiac muscle or cardiac nerves, or are expressed on immunomodulatory cells within the heart. Based on these studies, the ability of opioid agonists to produce cardioprotection is most likely the effect of δ- and κ-receptor stimulation, and the current studies appear to support a role for the δ-opioid receptor as the primary receptor responsible for IPC.

Endogenous Opioids in the Heart

Myocardial cells are capable of the synthesis, storage, and release of peptides, such as opioid receptor peptides.[354] Opioid-receptor peptides may be either secreted from nerves that innervate the heart or produced in myocardial tissue. Regardless of the manner of production, these peptides are devoid of activity until they undergo enzymatic proteolysis of the precursor by convertases into one (or more) active peptide products. These large stores of endogenous opioid peptide (EOP) precursors, which reside in the myocardial tissue, include proenkephalin, proendorphin, and prodynorphin.

The EOP system consists of the peptides endorphin, dynorphin, and enkephalin, and their associated μ-, δ-, and κ-opioid receptors (Table 9-5). These opioid peptides and receptors are widely distributed in the body, and all have complex actions. In the heart, κ- and δ-receptor agonists have been shown to inhibit ventricular contractility without altering atrial function.[351] A study of the actions of peptides on both electrical and mechanical properties of the isolated rat heart has shown that δ- and κ-opioid receptor agonists can directly depress cardiac function.[355] The rate of vagal firing has been shown to be regulated by opioid peptides.[356] Vagal bradycardia is inhibited by the administration of the intrinsic cardiac opioid heptapeptide MERF (met-enkephalin-arg-phe), presumably by the activation of δ-opioid receptors on prejunctional cardiac vagal nerves or parasympathetic ganglia, reducing acetylcholine release.[357] Therefore, EOPs can mediate direct and indirect actions in

TABLE 9-5	Endogenous Opioid Peptide Precursors and Some of Their Active Opioid Peptide Products Involved in Cardiovascular Regulation and Function	
Precursor	*Opioid Peptide*	*Receptor**
Proenkephalin[†]	[Met]Enkephalin	δ > μ >>> κ
	[Leu]Enkephalin	
POMC[‡]	β-Endorphin	μ ≈ δ >> δ
Prodynorphin[§]	Dynorphin A	κ >>> μ > δ
	Dynorphin A$_{(1–8)}$	κ >> μ > δ
	Dynorphin B	κ >>> μ > δ
Pronociception	Nociception	ORL$_1$

*The efficacy of the opioid peptide to its receptor is only qualitatively described in this table for the μ-, κ-, and δ-opioid receptor subtypes found in the central nervous system.[534]
[†]An additional opioid peptide product from this precursor that exhibits relevant cardiovascular actions in MERF (Zhang et al, 1996).
[‡]An additional POMC peptide cleavage product is adrenocorticotropic hormone, which is converted to α-melanocyte–stimulating hormone-related peptides in cardiac tissue (Millington et al, 1999).
[§]Additional active peptides include leumorphin, α-neoendorphin, and β-neoendorphin.[534]
ORL$_1$, opiod receptor-like-1; POMC, proopiomelanocortin.

various regions of the heart. Thus, in addition to complex differences in the general tissue distribution of opioid receptors, cardiac opioid peptide function is complicated by the fact that receptor expression is modulated by both physiologic states and disease.

A number of investigators have demonstrated that certain opioid peptides are released during stressful situations into the peripheral circulation.[358–361] These peptides can result in the modulation of the ANS.[362] In the heart, opioid peptides (leu- and met-enkephalins) have been shown to increase with age,[363–365] as well as disease.[366–369] EOPs are involved in the modulation of hypertension and other cardiovascular conditions such as CHF and appear to be involved in arrhythmogenesis.[370] Myocardial ischemia/reperfusion has been shown to induce synthesis and release of opioid peptides.[369,371–376] In fact, several studies in humans have demonstrated that levels of circulating β-endorphins are greater in patients with acute myocardial ischemia or those undergoing angioplasty.[371,374,375,377] Although κ-receptor agonists have no effect on cardiovascular indices in healthy humans,[378] activation of δ and κ receptors during CHF decreases myocardial mechanical performance and alters regional blood flow distribution.[372] The mechanism for the negative inotropic effects is thought to be an increase of intracellular free Ca[++] by increasing the mobilization of calcium from intracellular stores subsequent to increased production of inositol-1,4,5-triphosphate. The increase in Ca[++] may manifest in cardiac arrhythmias, whereas depletion of Ca[++] from intracellular stores is responsible for a reduction in contractility.[372,379]

In patients with acute heart failure, the concentrations of EOPs are increased,[380] whereas the concentrations are decreased in patients with chronic heart failure. This has been interpreted as exhaustion of the opioid system.[381] Many studies suggest that EOPs mediate depression of myocardial function in CHF states.[359,380,382,383] Clinically, increased levels of EOPS (β-endorphin, met-enkephalin, and dynorphin) have been found in CHF patients, and these may correlate with severity. Naloxone administration to these CHF patients increased BP and HR, suggesting a homeostatic regulatory role for EOPs in CHF. However, not all clinical studies suggest that inhibition of opioid peptides is of benefit to patients with acute and chronic heart failure.[381] Oldroyd et al[384] found that plasma levels of β-endorphins were normal in patients with acute and chronic heart failure, and did not correlate with the severity of heart failure observed in their study.[384] They also found that naloxone administration did not alter cardiopulmonary exercise in these patients, and suggest that EOP inhibition is not likely to have any therapeutic potential.

Cardiac Effects of Opioids

At clinically relevant doses, the cardiovascular actions of narcotic analgesics are limited. The role that endogenously or exogenously administered opioids play in the regulation of the CVS is difficult to interpret because the physiologic effects they impart depend on pharmacologic variables such as dose, site, and route of administration, as well as receptor specificity and species. The actions opioids exhibit are mediated both by opioid receptors located centrally in specific areas of the brain and nuclei that regulate the control of cardiovascular function and peripherally by tissue-associated opioid receptors. The opioids, in general, exhibit a variety of complex pharmacologic actions on the CVS[359] (Figure 9-31).

Most of the hemodynamic effects of opioids in humans can be related to their influence on the sympathetic outflow from the CNS. Current evidence shows that sympathetic overactivity favors the genesis of life-threatening ventricular tachyarrhythmias, and its control has protective effects during acute myocardial ischemia.[385] Moreover, an imbalance of the ANS, characterized by increased sympathetic activity and reduced vagal activity, results in myocardial electrical instability and promotes the occurrence of ischemic events. The pharmacologic modulation of the sympathetic activity by centrally or peripherally acting drugs elicits cardioprotective effects. Opioid-receptor agonists such as fentanyl are known to exhibit significant central sympathoinhibitory effects.[386]

Fentanyl and sufentanil enhance the calcium current that occurs during the plateau phase (phase 2) of the cardiac action potential and depress the outward potassium current responsible for terminal repolarization,[387] resulting in a significant prolongation of the duration of the action potential. Blair et al[388] suggested that the cardiac electrophysiologic effects of fentanyl and sufentanil represented a direct membrane effect resembling that produced by Class III antiarrhythmic drugs. In patients, large doses of opioids prolong the QT interval of the electrocardiogram.[387] This may explain the reported antiarrhythmic properties of opioids, particularly in the presence of myocardial ischemia.[284] Fentanyl, 60 μg/kg, and sufentanil, 10 μg/kg, significantly increased the ventricular fibrillation threshold in dogs after coronary artery occlusion.[389]

All opioids, with the exception of meperidine, produce bradycardia, although morphine given to unpremedicated healthy subjects may cause tachycardia. The mechanism of opioid-induced bradycardia is central vagal stimulation. Premedication with atropine can minimize but not totally eliminate opioid-induced bradycardia, especially in patients taking β-adrenoceptor antagonists. Although severe bradycardia should be avoided, moderate slowing of the HR may be beneficial in patients with CAD by decreasing myocardial oxygen consumption.

Isolated heart or heart-muscle studies have demonstrated dose-related inotropic effects for morphine, meperidine, fentanyl, and

alfentanil.[390-393] However, these effects occurred at concentrations one hundred to several thousand times those found clinically. In canine hearts, the direct intracoronary injection of fentanyl in concentrations up to 240 ng/mL produced no changes in myocardial mechanical functions.[394]

Morphine produced dose-related decreases in the contractility of atria obtained from nonfailing and failing human hearts, but the concentration–response curve was significantly shifted to the right in preparations from failing hearts[395] (Figure 9-32). The negative inotropic effects induced by morphine in both failing and nonfailing preparations were not antagonized by naloxone, indicating that opioid receptors do not play a part in this cardiac effect of morphine. One explanation could be an interaction with β-adrenoceptors, unrelated to the binding of opioids to opioid receptors. Opioids inhibit β-adrenoceptor–sensitive adenylyl cyclase.[396]

Hypotension can occur after even small doses of morphine and is primarily related to decreases in SVR. The most important mechanism responsible for these changes is probably histamine release. The amount of histamine release is reduced by slow administration (< 10 mg/min). Pretreatment with a histamine H_1 or H_2 antagonist does not block these reactions, but they are significantly attenuated by combined H_1 and H_2 antagonist pretreatment.[397] Neither morphine nor fentanyl, in clinically relevant concentrations, blocks α-adrenergic receptors in isolated vascular tissue studies.[398,399] Opioids also may have a direct action on vascular smooth muscle, independent of histamine release. In the isolated hind limbs of dogs anesthetized with halothane, high doses of alfentanil (500 μg/kg), fentanyl (50 μg/kg), and sufentanil (6 μg/kg) caused significant decreases in SVR of 48%, 48%, and 44%, respectively. Neither pretreatment with naloxone nor denervation changed the responses, and it was concluded that the three opioids produced vasodilation by a direct action on vascular smooth muscle.[400] Although fentanyl-induced relaxation in the rat aorta may be mediated

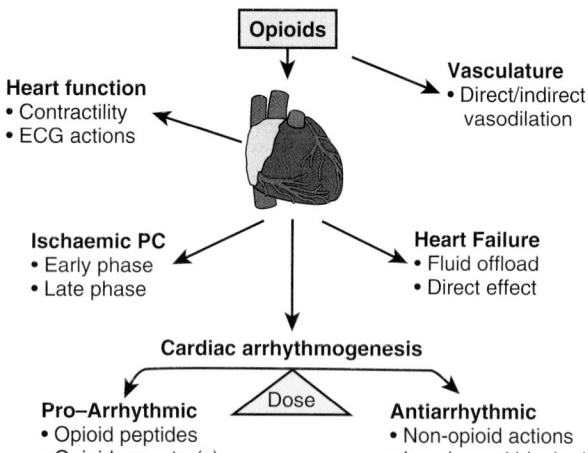

Figure 9-31 **Some of the actions of opioids on the heart and cardiovascular system.** Opioid actions may either involve direct opioid receptor–mediated actions, such as the involvement of the δ-opioid receptor in ischemic preconditioning (PC), or indirect, dose-dependent, nonopioid-receptor–mediated actions such as ion channel blockade associated with the antiarrhythmic actions of opioids. ECG, electrocardiogram.

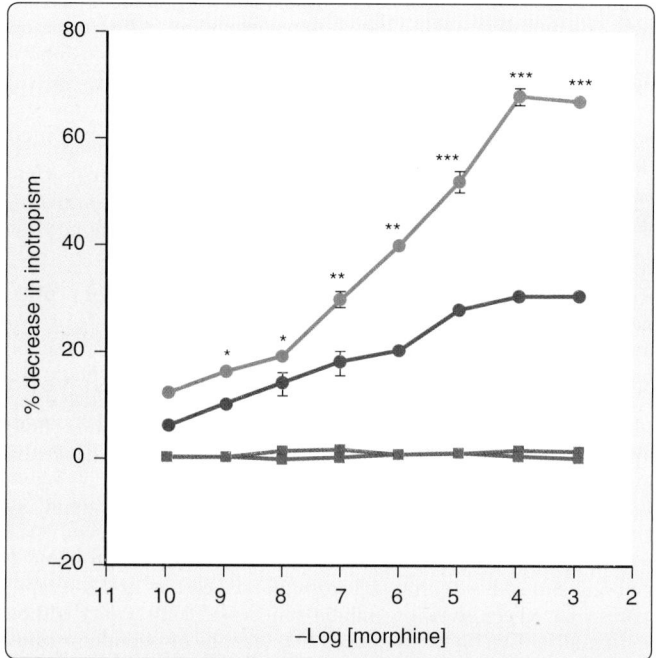

Figure 9-32 Concentration–response curves for morphine (*circles*) in isolated electrically stimulated human right atrial strips from nonfailing (*filled symbols*) and failing (*open symbols*) hearts (*squares* indicate control). Average auricular inotropism (mean [standard error of the mean (SEM)]) for nonfailing hearts was 0.90 (0.05) g, and 0.89 (0.02) g for failing hearts. *P < 0.05; **P < 0.01; ***P < 0.001 versus failing heart. Each point represents the mean (SEM) of eight experiments for each experimental group.

by α-adrenergic receptors, this effect occurs only at concentrations several hundred times greater than those encountered clinically.[401]

The effects of κ-agonists on BP have been examined[402] and been shown to be dose, species, and route dependent.[402,403] U-50,488H, for example, displays a markedly different cardiovascular profile when injected intravenously as compared with injected directly into the CNS. In anesthetized dogs, κ-agonists produce dose-related decreases in BP, HR, peak systolic pressure, and cardiac contractility when administered intravenously. The cardiovascular responses to both opioid agonists were abolished by previous administration of naloxone.[404] In addition to causing a reduction in BP, κ-opioid agonist dose-dependently reduced the HR in anesthetized rats.[402] This is suggestive of an effect on either the reflex mechanisms that regulate the HR during hypotension or direct action on the electrical or mechanical properties responsible for normal cardiac contractility. κ-Agonists cause slight depressant action on the HR and BP at low doses that is not inhibited by naloxone, suggesting a lack of involvement of opioid receptors and a possible direct effect on cardiac muscle.[403] In anesthetized rats, the cardiovascular responses to κ-opioid agonists in the presence of opioid antagonists were not changed.[403,405,406] It was concluded from these studies and others[407] that because opioid receptor antagonists did not block these responses, they were not mediated by opioid receptors.

Opioid-receptor agonists and antagonists have been shown to block ion channels that constitute the genesis of the action potential in neurons. Voltage-gated Na^+ channels are responsible for the initiation of membrane depolarization and the conduction of action potentials in electrically excitable cells, resulting in contraction of the heart or transmission of electrical impulses in nerves. K^+ channels are responsible for repolarization of the cell membrane and cessation of action potentials in excitable cells. Morphine and naloxone have been shown to block the propagation of action potentials in many nerve and cardiac muscle preparations by directly inhibiting voltage-dependent Na^+ and K^+ currents. In addition to the opioid-receptor–independent–mediated actions of U-50,488H and related κ-agonists on BP and HR (i.e., actions not blocked by opioid-receptor antagonist), these drugs produce changes in the electrocardiogram indicative of a drug interaction with cardiac ion channels.[402,408] Table 9-6 summarizes the action of several κ-opioid agonists and their actions on BP, HR, and the PR, QRS, RSh, and Q-T intervals on rat electrocardiograms. The electrocardiographic changes, including PR interval prolongation, QRS widening, and increased amplitude of the RSh, are indicative of cardiac Na^+ channel blockade. The widening of the Q-T interval, an index of cardiac repolarization, is suggestive of K^+-channel blockade.

The results of studies with opioid drugs, such as sufentanil[387] and morphine,[409] corroborate the suggestion of interaction of κ-opioids with cardiac K^+ channels. However, the opioid receptor–independent

nature of the ion-channel blockade may not be isolated to Na^+ and K^+ channels and also may include L-type Ca^+ channels found in cardiac muscle. The use of Ca^{++} fluorescent techniques for measurement of cardiac myocyte contractility suggested that the negative inotropic actions for κ-opioid agonists also may be because of inhibition of L-type Ca^{++} currents.[410,411] While investigating the possible cardiotoxic effects produced by opioids in human poisoning, Wu et al[412] found that opioids, like meperidine and dextropropoxyphene, exert negative inotropic actions in cardiac muscle by blockade of Ca^{++} currents in myocytes in the presence of naloxone.

Ischemic Preconditioning

Myocardial IPC is a phenomenon that occurs in cardiac muscle in which brief periods of ischemia (usually < 5 minutes) render the muscle tolerant to tissue damage that occurs during a subsequent period of ischemia, after an interlude of perfusion[86] (Figure 9-33). Such a phenomenon has been shown to occur in many species and is known to be mediated by a well-defined intracellular cascade.[413] The intercellular mediator or IPC-induction trigger appears to be diverse and has been shown to involve opioids and other substances. Thus, the nature of IPC may not be consistent between the species examined, despite a common end result.

In vivo studies show that IPC can reduce the size of an infarct resulting from prolonged ischemia.[414] There also is a reduction in damage to myocardial intracellular structure, a decrease in the dysfunction of the cardiac contractile machinery, and a direct reduction in arrhythmias associated with IPC.[414,415] The ability of IPC to limit myocardial damage occurs chronologically in two distinct phases. The first (or early) phase provides a window of protection to the heart muscle that occurs soon after IPC and declines with time during the first 3 hours of reperfusion. The second, late (or delayed) phase of IPC provides a second window of protection to heart muscle that emerges after 24 hours of reperfusion and may last up to 72 hours[416–418] (see Chapters 3, 6, and 18).

Importance of Opioid Receptors in Early Preconditioning

The involvement of opioids in IPC resulted from the recognition of their value at increasing survival time and tissue preservation before surgical transplantation, and their possible role in enhancing tolerance to hypoxia.[419,420] The first evidence to demonstrate a role for opioids in early IPC was published by Schultz et al[421] in the intact blood-perfused rat heart. These investigators demonstrated that the nonselective opioid receptor antagonist naloxone completely antagonized the ability of IPC to reduce infarct size whether administered before the IPC stimulus or after the IPC stimulus just before the index ischemia. These results suggested that endogenous opioids serve as both a trigger and end-effector of IPC in rat hearts (Figure 9-34). Chien and Van Winkle[422] found similar results in the rabbit heart with the use of the active enantiomer, (−)naloxone. Furthermore, Schulz et al[423] determined the role of endogenous opioids in mediating IPC and myocardial hibernation in pig hearts, and observed that naloxone blocked IPC but not the effects of short-term hibernation. These data clearly suggest that an opioid receptor is mediating the effect of endogenous opioids to elicit IPC in the rat, rabbit, and pig.

Takashi et al[424] performed a study in isolated adult rabbit cardiomyocytes to determine which EOPs are responsible for the cardioprotective effect observed during and after IPC. They found that metenkephalin, leuenkephalin, and met enkephalin-ang-phe (MEAP) produced a reduction in the incidence of cell death, suggesting that the enkephalins are the most likely candidates that serve as triggers and distal effectors of IPC in the rabbit heart. Huang et al[425,426] studied the role of δ-opioid-receptor activation in reducing myocardial infarct size in human and rat hearts. Their studies indicated that endogenous adrenergic-receptor activation and downstream signaling were important mediators in attenuating infarct size.[425,426]

TABLE 9-6	D_{25} Drug Doses of Arylacetamide κ-Opioid Agonists in Intact Rats: Effects on Heart Rate, Blood Pressure, and Electrocardiogram Measures					
		ECG Measures (msec)				
Drug	Heart Rate	Blood Pressure	PR	QRS	RSh	Q-T
U-50,488H	1.5	> 32	20	> 32	16	32
U-62,066E	4.0	8.0	15	25	2.0	10
PD117,302	5.5	0.50	3.0	7.5	1.0	6.0

The nonopioid actions of structurally related arylacetamide κ-opioid receptor agonists were examined in pentobarbital-anesthetized rats. Heart rate, blood pressure, and electrocardiogram (ECG) measures were determined as D_{25}, the dose (μmol/kg/min IV) producing a 25% change in the given response. This measure allowed for a determination of the differential actions of the arylacetamides on ECG measures, an index of drug action on cardiac ion channels ($n = 6$). The drug dose produced a 25% change from control in intact animals for six determinations per measure. All drugs consistently reduced the heart rate but had varying D_{25} doses for blood pressure reduction. PD117,302 [(±)-N-methyl-N-[2-(1-pyrrolidinyl)cyclohexyl]benzo[b]thiophene-4-acetamide monohydrochloride] produced evidence of sodium channel blockade (changes in the PR, QRS, and RSh measures) and potassium-channel blockade (changes in the Q-T interval) at lower D_{25} values than either of the other two drugs.

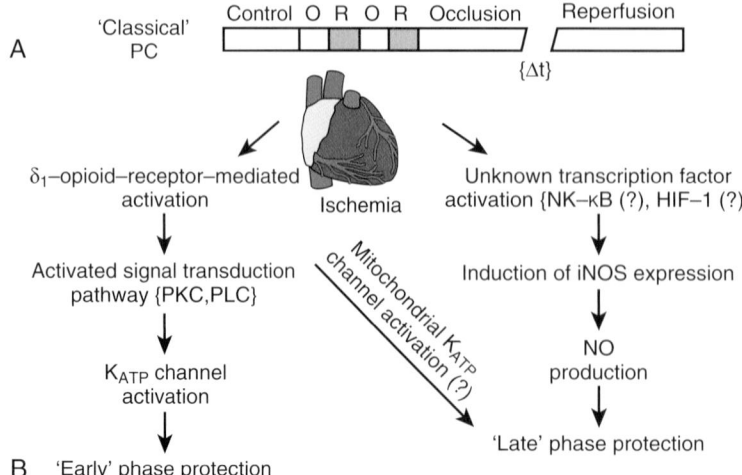

Figure 9-33 *A,* A "typical" protocol bar that may be used in experiments that investigate the effects of agents on ischemic preconditioning (PC) in the heart. Similar protocols have been used to study opioid receptor–mediated cardioprotective mechanisms in the rat and other mammalian species. Studies may investigate the effects of ischemic PC on ischemia and/or reperfusion arrhythmias of various durations in length (Δt). Ischemic PC usually involves a sequence of coronary artery occlusion (O), followed by reperfusion (R) cycles. Two cycles are depicted before coronary artery occlusion followed by reperfusion. *Note that this type of protocol may be easily amenable to modification; the protocol shown is a simplified protocol bar. B,* Schematic diagram that describes the molecular pathways involved in the protective effects of ischemic PC in the heart. Brief periods of ischemia provide both an "early" and "late" phase of protection to the heart from subsequent episodes of prolonged or permanent ischemia. The activation of G-protein–coupled δ_1-opioid receptors has been shown to be involved in both protective phases. The activation of the δ_1-opioid receptor activates intracellular signal transduction pathways (including protein kinase C [PKC], phospholipase C [PLC], and related kinase pathways). Activation of these pathways results in the phosphorylation of certain proteins such as the K_{ATP} channel present both on the myocyte cell surface, as well as the myocyte mitochondrial cell surface. The opening of these ion channels mediates the "early" phase of cardioprotection that lasts 2 to 3 hours after the ischemic episode. The "late" phase of cardioprotection that results from the brief episodes of ischemia may be mediated by the activation of oxygen-sensitive transcription factors (such as nuclear factor [NF]-κB and HIF-1). These factors subsequently induce the expression of inducible nitric oxide synthase (iNOS) and the production of NO, the putative mediator of the protective effect on the heart observed 24 to 48 hours after the ischemic episode. Recently, it has been shown that δ_1-opioid–receptor stimulation also may produce a "late" cardioprotective effect that may result from activation of mitochondrial K^+_{ATP} channels. *(From Murry CE, Jennings RB, Reimer KA: Preconditioning with ischemia: A delay of lethal cell injury in ischemic myocardium, Circulation 74:1124, 1986.)*

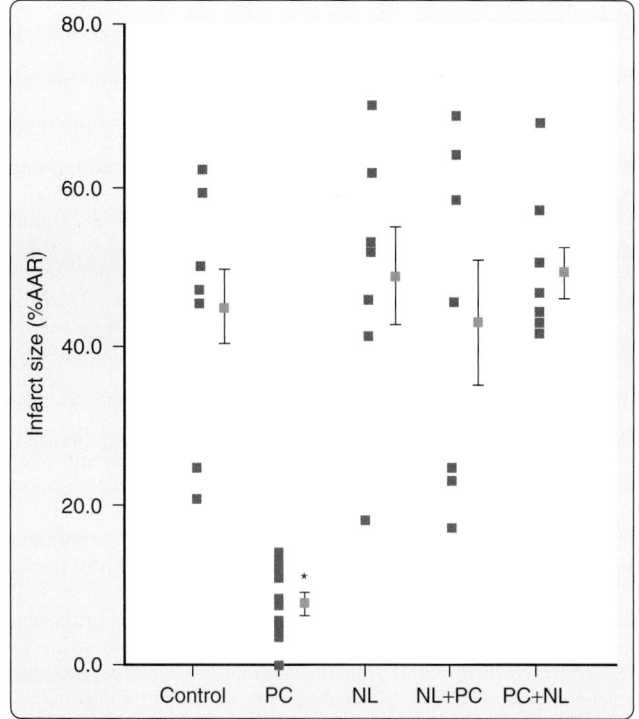

Figure 9-34 Infarct size (IS) expressed as a percentage of the area at risk (AAR) in intact rat hearts subjected to vehicle (control), ischemic preconditioning (PC), naloxone (NL) in the absence of PC, NL treatment before PC (NL + PC), and NL treatment after PC (PC + NL) before the index ischemic period. *Filled squares* are the mean ± standard error of the mean of each group. *$P < 0.05$ versus the control group. *(From Schultz JJ, Rose E, Yao Z, et al: Evidence for involvement of opioid receptors in ischemic preconditioning in rat heart, Am J Physiol 268:157, 1995.)*

Cardioprotective Effects of Exogenous Opioid Agonists

In 1996, Schultz and colleagues[427] were the first to demonstrate that an opioid could attenuate ischemia/reperfusion damage in the heart. Morphine, at the dose of 300 µg/kg, was given before left anterior descending coronary artery occlusion for 30 minutes in rats in vivo. Infarct area/area at risk was diminished from 54% to 12% by this treatment. The infarct-reducing effect of morphine has been shown in hearts in situ, isolated hearts, and cardiomyocytes.[424,428,429] Morphine also improved postischemic contractility.[430] It is now well accepted that morphine provides protection against ischemia/reperfusion injury. Furthermore, Gross et al[431] reported a significant reduction in infarct development in rats after administration of morphine or a selective δ-receptor ligand at reperfusion. The authors reported that the effects are mediated via a glycogen synthase kinase β and the phosphatidylinositol-3 kinase pathway.[431] There is also some evidence to suggest that remifentanil, when added to a standard anesthetic regimen, may reduce myocardial damage after coronary artery bypass surgery (Figure 9-35).[432]

Fentanyl has been studied in a limited fashion and has had mixed results as far as its ability to protect the myocardium.[430,433,434] This may be because of differences in species studied, fentanyl concentrations, or both. Pentazocine and buprenorphine improved postischemic contractility in rabbits in vitro.[430] Overall, the effects of opioids other than morphine have not been sufficiently investigated to allow conclusions to be drawn.

Schultz et al[435] also demonstrated that the effect of IPC to reduce infarct size was mediated by the δ_1-receptor but not the δ_2, µ, or κ receptor, because the effects of IPC were blunted by the selective δ_1-receptor antagonist BNTX (7-benzylidenenaltrexone) but not the δ_2-antagonist naltriben. They also showed that cardioprotection was not induced by the administration of the selective µ-agonist DAMGO (D-Ala[2], N-Me-Phe, (4) glycerol[5-enkephaline]) and that IPC was not attenuated by the µ-antagonist B-FNA (beta-funaltrexamine).[435] In that same study, they excluded the involvement of the κ receptor because a κ-selective antagonist could not reverse the effects of IPC to reduce

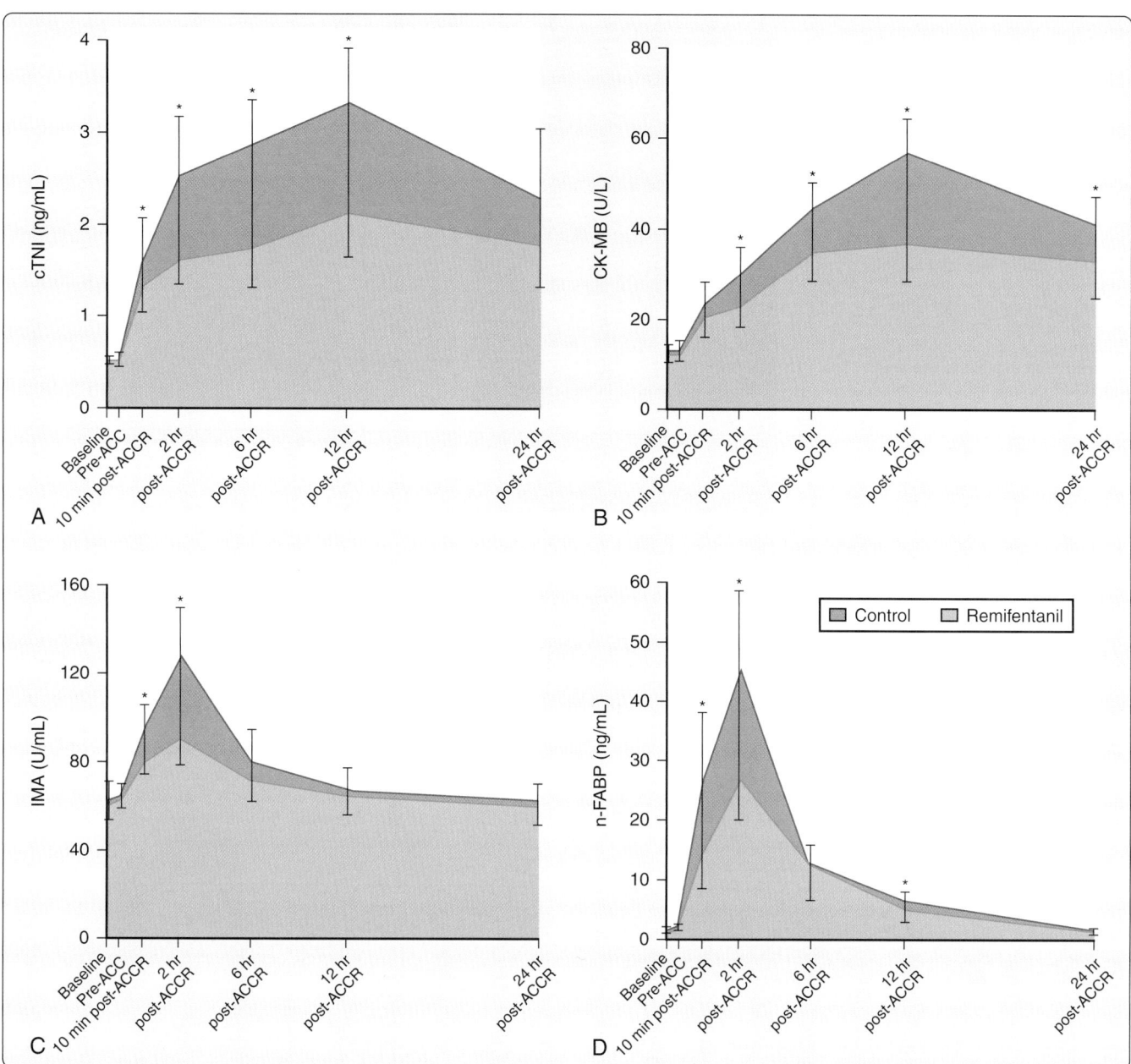

Figure 9-35 Blood levels of biochemical markers over time. Values are plotted as median (error bars = interquartile range). ACCR, aortic cross-clamp release; post-ACC, period after aortic cross-clamp was applied; pre-ACC, period before aortic cross-clamp was applied. *$P < 0.05$. CK-MD, creatinine kinase; cTNI, cardiac troponin 1; IMA, ischemia-modified albumin; n-FABP, heart-type fatty-acid bonding protein. *(From Wong GT, Huang Z, Ji S, et al: Remifentanil reduces the release of biochemical markers of myocardial damage after coronary artery bypass surgery: A randomized trial.* J Cardiothorac Vasc Anesth 2010; 24:790–796.)

infarct size. These data suggest that the δ_1-opioid receptor appears to be the primary opioid receptor involved in IPC in the intact rat heart.

Although the exogenous activation of the δ-opioid receptor subtype by highly specific agonists before ischemia has been shown to reduce infarct size in a number of species, including rats,[435] rabbits,[436] and swine,[437] the role of the κ-opioid receptors in preconditioning has been a subject of much controversy. Cao et al[438,439] demonstrated that the cardioprotective effects caused by κ-opioid receptor stimulation were abolished with a calcium-activated potassium-channel (K_{Ca}) blocker. This is consistent with previous reports that the κ-receptor protective effects are mediated via a K_{Ca}-channel pathway as seen in IPC.[438,439] It has also been reported that preischemic administration of selective κ-agonists will reduce infarct size and ischemia-induced arrhythmias in the isolated rat heart. Conversely, specific activation of the κ-opioid receptor before ischemia also has been shown to increase infarct size[419] and arrhythmias[440] and induce an "antipreconditioning"-like state in rats.

It has been proposed that the κ-opioid receptor agonists exert a biphasic effect on the myocardium, producing proarrhythmic and antiarrhythmic effects in the rat.[385] Therefore, it is unclear whether selective or nonselective activation of the κ-opioid-receptor subtype is beneficial during preconditioning, and although such conflicting information exists for the rat, the role of opioid receptor subtypes in IPC and pharmacologic preconditioning in other species is even more limited. Further studies are needed to address the role of the κ receptor in arrhythmias.

Signaling Pathways Involved in Opioid-Induced Cardioprotection

Opioid-induced cardioprotection and IPC appear to share a common pathway, in that the δ-opioid receptor and the mitochondrial K^+_{ATP} channel appear to be involved in the beneficial effects observed. Additional studies show that the cardioprotective effect of IPC and δ_1-opioid-receptor activation were both mediated via a G_i-protein–coupled

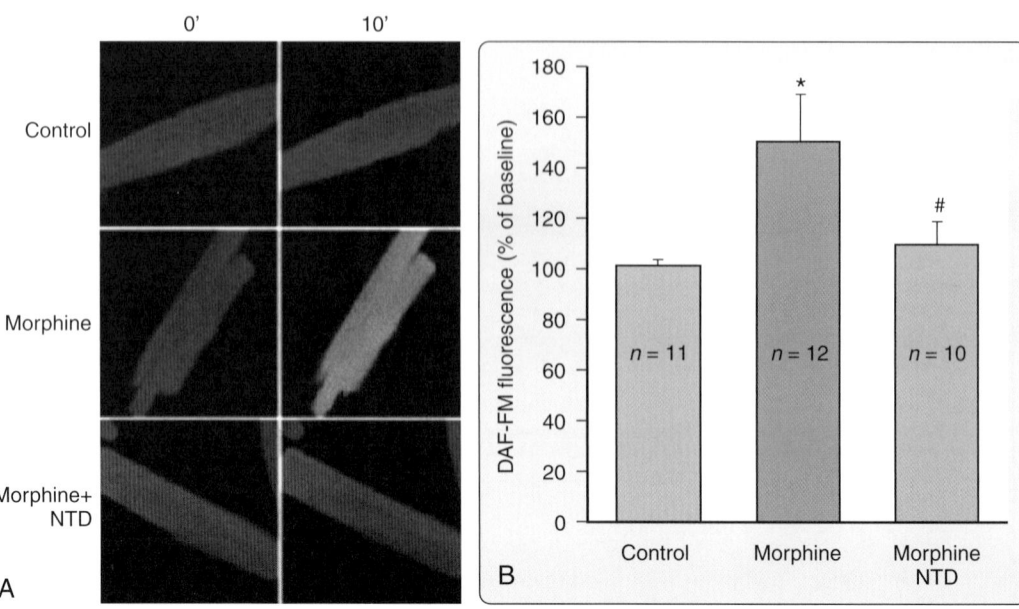

Figure 9-36 *A*, Confocal fluorescence images of 4-amino-5-methylamino-2′,7′-difluorofluorescein (DAF-FM) at the baseline and 10 minutes after exposure to morphine in rat cardiomyocytes. Morphine (1 µm) increased nitric oxide production in cardiomyocytes, which was blocked by naltrindole (NTD, 5 µm). *B*, Summarized data for DAF-FM fluorescence intensity 10 minutes after exposure to morphine expressed as a percentage of the baseline. *$P < 0.05$ versus control; #$P < 0.05$ versus morphine. *(From Jang Y, Xi J, Wang H, et al: Postconditioning prevents reperfusion injury by activating delta-opioid receptors, Anesthesiology 108:243–250, 2008.)*

receptor and may involve NO.[435,441,442] G-protein receptors have an established role in the attenuation of ischemic-reperfusion injury mainly by the activation of κ and δ receptors.[443,444] The mechanisms underlying this effect involve apoptotic pathways and restriction of internucleosomal DNA fragmentation.[445] To further address potential signaling pathways involved in opioid-induced protection, it was observed that morphine produced a cardioprotective effect in isolated rabbit hearts that was blocked by pretreatment with a nonselective PKC inhibitor. Jang et al[441] demonstrated the activation of δ-opioid receptors and their role in postconditioning. This effect occurs via modulation of the MPTP and signaling via a NO and PKG-mediated pathway (Figure 9-36). In summary, the beneficial effects were eliminated by a G_i-protein inhibitor, a PKC inhibitor,[429,433,446,447] and a selective mitochondrial K^+_{ATP} channel blocker.[428,433,446,448-451] Furthermore, studies also have demonstrated the role of iNOS as an upstream mediator of COX-2. In iNOS gene knockout mice, this morphine-mediated cardioprotection is attenuated and some reports suggest iNOS and COX-2 are required only during the mediation phase and not the trigger phase.[452,453] Figure 9-37 is a schematic summary of the major pathways thought to be involved in acute opioid-induced cardioprotection.

Role of Opioids in Delayed Preconditioning

It appears that opioid receptors are involved in delayed cardioprotection via activation of the δ- and κ-opioid receptors. Fryer et al[449] demonstrated that TAN-67, a $δ_1$-opioid agonist, also could induce cardioprotection during the "second window" of IPC. They found no protective effect to reduce infarct size 12 hours after administration of the selective $δ_1$-opioid agonist; however, it produced a marked cardioprotective effect at 24 to 48 hours after drug administration, which disappeared at 72 hours (Figure 9-38). The cardioprotective effects were blocked by pretreatment with a selective $δ_1$-antagonist, a nonselective K^+_{ATP}-channel antagonist, and a mitochondrial-selective K^+_{ATP}-channel blocker. These results suggest that $δ_1$-opioid receptor activation 24 to 48 hours before an ischemic insult results in a delayed cardioprotective effect that appears to be mediated by the mitochondrial K^+_{ATP} channel. Wu and colleagues[454] demonstrated that κ-opioid-receptor–induced cardioprotection occurred via two phases: the first window occurred about 1 hour after receptor activation, and the second developed 16 to 20 hours after administration in isolated ventricular myocytes.

Opioids and Cardioprotection in Humans

Although the animal and cell work reviewed imply a cardioprotective effect of opioid receptor activation, it is important to demonstrate that

a similar system exists in humans if these basic studies can be extrapolated to the clinical world. Tomai et al[455] have demonstrated that naloxone could abolish the reduction in ST-segment elevation normally observed during a second balloon inflation during coronary angioplasty. In addition, they demonstrated that in naloxone-treated patients, the severity of cardiac pain and time to onset at the end of the second balloon inflation were similar to that of the first inflation, whereas in the placebo-treated patients, the severity of cardiac pain during the second inflation was reduced and the time to onset of pain was lengthened versus the first inflation. This suggests a preconditioning-like effect in humans undergoing coronary angioplasty that could be attenuated by the opioid antagonist naloxone. Similarly, Xenopoulos and coworkers[456] have shown that intracoronary morphine (15 µg/kg) mimics IPC, as assessed by changes in ST-segment shifts in humans undergoing percutaneous transluminal coronary angioplasty. Finally, Bell et al[448] also demonstrated that δ-opioid-receptor stimulation mimics IPC in human atrial trabeculae via K^+_{ATP} channel activation. These

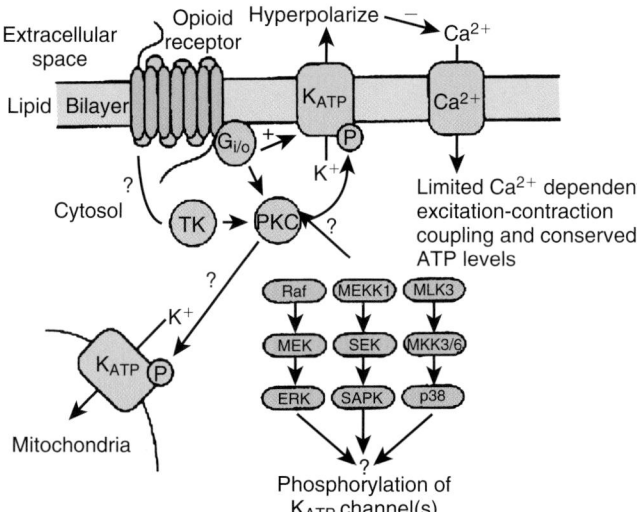

Figure 9-37 Schematic diagram of some of the major pathways thought to be involved in acute opioid-induced cardioprotection. PKC, protein kinase C. *(From Schultz J, Gross GJ: Opioids and cardiac protection, Pharmacology and Therapeutics 89:123–137, 2001.)*

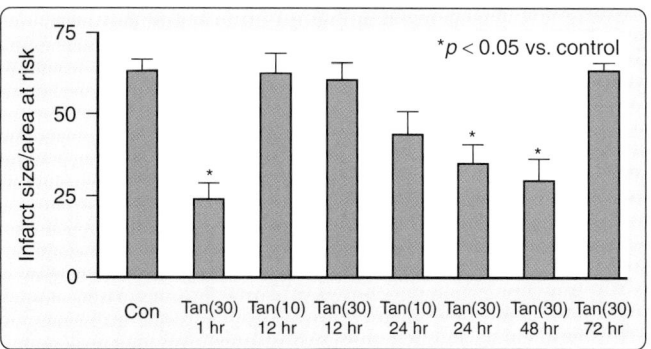

Figure 9-38 Infarct size expressed as a percentage of the area at risk in rats administered 10 or 30 mg/kg TAN-67, either 1, 12, 24, 48, or 72 hours before 30 minutes of ischemia and 2 hours of reperfusion. A 1-hour pretreatment with TAN-67 produced a significant reduction in infarct size/area at risk. Pretreatment with both doses of TAN-67 12 hours before ischemia/reperfusion or low-dose TAN-67 24 hours before ischemia/reperfusion had no significant effect on infarct size/area at risk. However, pretreatment with the large dose of TAN-67 24 to 48 hours before ischemia/reperfusion significantly reduced infarct size/area at risk. This cardioprotective effect was lost after 72 hours of pretreatment. All values are the mean ± standard error of the mean. *P < 0.05. (From Fryer RM, Hsu AK, Ells JT, et al: Opioid-induced second window of cardioprotection. Potential role of mitochondrial KATP channels, Circ Res 84:846, 1999.)

results are encouraging and may suggest a possible clinical use for opioids in the therapy of acute or chronic myocardial ischemia.[448]

Cardioplegia and hypothermia provide considerable myocardial protection against the induced ischemia of cardiac surgery. However, in certain high-risk subgroups and, to some extent, in all patients, current methods of cardioprotection are still suboptimal, and there continues to be poor myocardial tolerance to ischemia. This myocardial ischemia often is evidenced by perioperative ventricular dysfunction, myocardial stunning, and poor functional recovery after an ischemic episode, which may lead to poor surgical outcome (see Chapters 28 and 32). Postsurgical myocardial ischemic changes include hypothermia, intracellular acidosis, hypoxia, depletion of energy stores, and cellular volume shifts, all of which adversely affect myocardial contractility. Hibernating animals demonstrate similar cellular and molecular cardiac changes during hibernation that closely parallel those seen in hypothermic cardioplegic arrest. However, these changes are well tolerated in the myocardium of the hibernating mammals for months at a time, whereas the duration of induced ischemia tolerated surgically is limited. This process is induced by a hibernation-induction-trigger molecule, which has been shown to have an opioid basis.[457] It has been shown that opioid peptides can induce mammalian hibernation and may provide protection against the adverse effects of hypothermic myocardial ischemia, providing potential therapeutic applications during CPB and protection of organs for heart transplantation.

In animal studies, Bolling et al[458,459] showed the δ-opioid-receptor agonist DADLE protected hearts that were subjected to 18 hours of cold storage at 4°C or 2 hours of global ischemia, respectively, in the presence of a standard cardioplegic solution. Another study[460] provided evidence that pentazocine, a δ-opioid agonist, enhanced the myocardial protection of standard cardioplegia at temperatures ranging from 0°C to 34°C. Subsequently, Kevelaitis et al[450] showed that stimulation of δ-opioid receptors improved recovery of cold-stored rat hearts to a state similar to IPC. These investigators showed that this opioid-induced cardioprotection is mediated through K^+_{ATP}-channel activation.[450]

Although the initial success of cardiopulmonary resuscitation (CPR) is, on average, 39% (13% to 59%), a majority of victims die within 72 hours, primarily because of heart failure, recurrent ventricular fibrillation, or both. CPR, therefore, yields a functional survival rate of only

1.4% to 5%.[461–463] Myocardial function is substantially impaired after successful resuscitation from cardiac arrest. This has led to the investigation of the use of opioid-receptor agonists to improve functional outcome. Tang and colleagues[464] demonstrated that pharmacologic activation of δ-opioid receptors significantly reduced Mvo_2 during the global myocardial ischemia of cardiac arrest. A follow-up study in rats demonstrated that the nonselective δ-opioid-receptor agonist pentazocine strikingly reduced the severity of postresuscitation myocardial dysfunction and increased the duration of postresuscitation survival.[464]

Opioid analgesics are used widely for the treatment of pain. Although these agents are predominantly μ-opioid-receptor agonists, cross talk with δ-opioid receptors has been demonstrated. However, the U.S. Food and Drug Administration has not approved these drugs for use in patients with unstable angina or who are predisposed to myocardial infarction. This is likely due to the limited research in humans concerning the importance of opioid receptors in the myocardium and the high potential for dependence, abuse, and respiratory depression. Future avenues of research should focus on the identification of orally active compounds with high δ-opioid-receptor affinity to be used as cardioprotective agents because these drugs are currently lacking.

Opioids in Cardiac Anesthesia

A technique of anesthesia for cardiac surgery involving high doses of morphine was developed in the late 1960s and early 1970s. This was based on Lowenstein et al's[465] observation that patients requiring mechanical ventilation after surgery for end-stage VHD tolerated large doses of morphine for sedation without discernible circulatory effects. When they attempted to administer equivalent doses of morphine as the anesthetic for patients undergoing cardiac surgery, they discovered serious disadvantages including inadequate anesthesia, even at doses of 8 to 11 mg/kg, episodes of hypotension related to histamine release, and increased intraoperative and postoperative blood and fluid requirements. Attempts to overcome these problems by combining lower doses of morphine with a variety of supplements (such as N_2O, halothane, or diazepam) proved unsatisfactory, resulting in significant myocardial depression, with decreases in CO and hypotension.[466] However, recently, Murphy et al[467] demonstrated that morphine, compared with fentanyl, resulted in better myocardial function after CABG surgery. Specifically, with regard to the protective effects mediated by IPC, it appears that morphine may have some benefit over fentanyl.[467] The use of morphine, however, has to be weighed against the multitude of other deleterious effects during the management of cardiac surgical patients.

Because of the above problems associated with the use of morphine, several other opioids were investigated in an attempt to find a suitable alternative. The use of fentanyl in cardiac anesthesia was first reported by Stanley and Webster in 1978.[468] Since then there have been extensive investigations of fentanyl, as well as sufentanil and alfentanil, in cardiac surgery. The fentanyl group of opioids has proved to be the most reliable and effective for producing anesthesia for patients with valvular disorders and CABG (see Chapters 18 and 19).

A major advantage of fentanyl and its analogs for patients undergoing cardiac surgery is their lack of cardiovascular depression. This is of particular importance during the induction of anesthesia, when episodes of hypotension can be critical. Cardiovascular stability may be less evident during surgery; in particular, the period of sternotomy, pericardiectomy, and aortic root dissection may be associated with significant hypertension and tachycardia. During and after sternotomy, arterial hypertension increases in SVR and decreases in CO frequently occur.[469,470] The variability in the hemodynamic responses to surgical stimulation, even with similar doses of fentanyl, is probably a reflection of differences in the patient populations studied by different authors. One factor is the influence of β-blocking agents. In patients anesthetized with fentanyl undergoing CABG, 86% of those not taking β-blockers became hypertensive during sternal spread versus only 33% of those who were taking β-blockers.[471]

There may be differences among the opioids with regard to hemodynamic stability during surgery. One study concluded that both fentanyl and sufentanil provide similar hemodynamic stability during induction, whereas alfentanil causes hemodynamic instability and myocardial ischemia.[472] Alfentanil also may be less effective in suppressing reflex sympathetic and hemodynamic responses to stimuli than fentanyl or sufentanil.[473] In patients undergoing valvular surgery, all three opioids provided satisfactory anesthesia.[474] However, controversy still surrounds the best choice of anesthetic, at least for CABG. Two studies involving more than 2000 patients anesthetized with inhalation agents, fentanyl or sufentanil, came to the conclusion that the choice of anesthetic did not significantly influence the outcome after CABG, although the type of anesthetic continues to remain a topic of controversy with respect to postoperative outcomes.[113-115,475,476]

The degree of myocardial impairment also will influence the response. Critically ill patients or patients with significant myocardial dysfunction appear to require lower doses of opioid for anesthesia. This may reflect altered pharmacokinetics in those patients. A decrease in liver blood flow consequent to decreased CO and CHF reduces plasma clearance. Thus, patients with poor left ventricular function may develop greater plasma and brain concentrations for a given loading dose or infusion rate than patients with good left ventricular function. In addition, patients with depressed myocardial function may lack the ability to respond to surgical stress by increasing CO in the face of progressive increases in SVR.[477]

An infusion of alfentanil (125-μg/kg bolus followed by 0.5 mg/kg/hr) has been compared with fentanyl, 100 μg/kg, or sufentanil, 20 μg/kg, by bolus injection, as the sole anesthetic for patients undergoing valvular surgery.[474] No differences in hemodynamic effects were found in the study, and it was concluded that all three opioids can provide satisfactory anesthesia for valve replacement surgery (see Chapter 19).

Sufentanil appears to offer more stable anesthesia with less hemodynamic disturbance than fentanyl,[478] and it has been used successfully for cardiac transplantation.[479,480] In patients undergoing mitral or aortic valve surgery, sufentanil (total dose, 9.0 ± 0.4 μg/kg) resulted in less need for supplements and vasodilators than fentanyl, 113 ± 11 μg/kg, but sufentanil produced more hypotension during induction.[481] Howie et al[482] compared a fentanyl/isoflurane/propofol regimen with remifentanil/isoflurane/propofol for fast-track anesthesia. Significantly more patients in the fentanyl regimen experienced hypertension during skin incision and maximum sternal spread compared with patients in the remifentanil regimen. There was no difference between groups in time to extubation, discharge from the intensive care unit, electrocardiographic changes, catecholamine levels, or cardiac enzymes. The remifentanil-based anesthetic (bolus followed by continuous infusion) resulted in less need for anesthetic interventions compared with the fentanyl regimen.[482]

Samuelson et al[483] compared hemodynamic and stress responses in patients with CAD anesthetized with either sufentanil-oxygen or enflurane-nitrous oxide and oxygen. Both techniques were satisfactory and resulted in stable hemodynamics, but considerable "fine tuning" was required when enflurane was administered. The postoperative hemodynamic effects were compared in patients who received sufentanil, 25 μg/kg, or fentanyl, 100 μg/kg, for anesthesia for CABG.[484] Patients who received sufentanil had a more stable course, with higher CO, lower SVR, and a lower incidence of hypertension. The two groups had similar values for time to awakening, response to verbal commands, and extubation.

Collard et al[485] compared the intraoperative hemodynamic profiles and recovery characteristics of propofol-alfentanil versus a fentanyl-midazolam anesthetic in elective coronary artery surgery. Cardiovascular parameters and time to extubation were recorded. Throughout surgery, hemodynamic profiles were comparable between groups except after intubation, when the MAP was significantly lower in the propofol-alfentanil group. This group also required less inotropic support, and extubation was performed earlier in this group.

EFFECTS OF CARDIOPULMONARY BYPASS ON PHARMACOKINETICS AND PHARMACODYNAMICS

The pharmacokinetics of drugs in cardiac anesthesia is well covered by Wood.[486] This section focuses on the effects of CPB on pharmacokinetics as the most relevant area for the cardiac anesthesiologist.

The institution of CPB has profound effects on the plasma concentration, distribution, and elimination of administered drugs. The major factors responsible for this are hemodilution and altered plasma protein binding, hypotension, hypothermia, pulsatile versus nonpulsatile flow, isolation of the lungs from the circulation, and uptake of anesthetic drugs by the bypass circuit. These changes result in altered blood concentrations, which also are dependent on particular pharmacokinetics of the drug in question (Table 9-7).

Hemodilution

At the onset of CPB, the circuit priming fluid is mixed with the patient's blood. In adults, the priming volume is 1.5 to 2 L, and the prime may be crystalloid or crystalloid combined with blood or colloid. The overall result is a reduction in the patient's packed cell volume (PCV) to approximately 25% with an increase in plasma volume of 40% to 50%. This will decrease the total blood concentration of any free drug present in the blood. At the time of initiation of CPB, there is an immediate reduction in the levels of circulating proteins such as albumin and α_1-acid glycoprotein. This affects the protein binding of drugs because of alteration in the ratio of bound-to-free drug in the circulation.

In the blood, drugs exist as free (unbound) drug in equilibrium with bound (i.e., bound to plasma proteins) drug. It is the free drug that interacts with the receptor to produce the drug effect (Figure 9-39). Drugs primarily are bound to plasma protein albumin and α_1-acid glycoprotein. Changes in protein binding are of clinical significance only for drugs that are highly protein bound. The degree of drug-protein binding depends on the total drug concentration, the affinity of the protein for the drug, and the presence of other substances that may compete

TABLE 9-7	Effects of Cardiopulmonary Bypass on Drug Disposition	
Pharmacokinetic Process	*Pathophysiology*	*Pharmacokinetic Sequelae*
Absorption	Hypotension and alterations in regional blood flow/perfusion	Reduced oral or intramuscular absorption
Distribution	Lung sequestration	Decreased volume of distribution
	Decreased pulmonary blood flow	Decreased pulmonary drug distribution and increase in systemic drug levels
	Hypotension, altered regional blood flow	Decreased volume of distribution
	Decreased protein binding	Increased volume of distribution
	Hemodilution	
	Dilution of binding proteins	
	Postoperative ↑ AAG	Decreased volume of distribution
	Postoperative ↑ protein binding	Interpretation of postoperative drug levels difficult
Elimination	Decreased hepatic blood flow	Decreased drug clearance
	Hypothermia	Decreased intrinsic clearance (↓ hepatic metabolism)
	Decreased renal blood flow and hypothermia	Decreased renal function

AAG, α_1 acid glycoprotein.

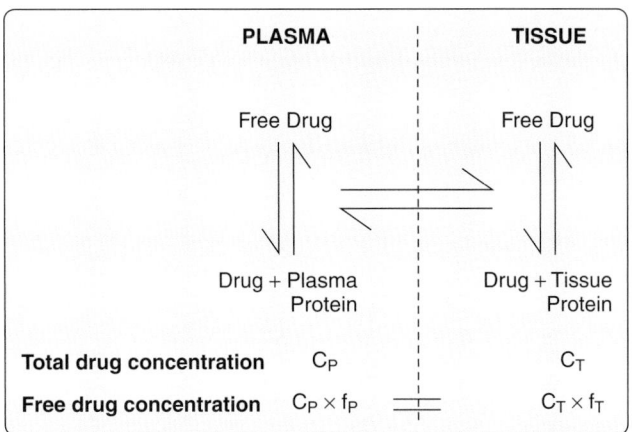

	PLASMA	TISSUE
	Free Drug	Free Drug
	Drug + Plasma Protein	Drug + Tissue Protein
Total drug concentration	C_P	C_T
Free drug concentration	$C_P \times f_P$	$C_T \times f_T$

Figure 9-39 **Relation between free drug concentration in plasma and tissue.** The free concentration in plasma equals the total concentration (C_p) × the free fraction in plasma (f_p). The free concentration in tissue equals the total concentration in tissue (C_T) × the free fraction in tissue (f_t).

with the drug or alter the drug's binding site. If the drug in question has high plasma protein binding, then hemodilution results in a potentially relatively larger increase in free fraction than for a drug with low plasma protein binding.

The effect of heparin administration on plasma protein binding is of importance. Heparin results in lipoprotein lipase and hepatic lipase release, which, in turn, hydrolyzes plasma triglycerides into nonesterified fatty acids. These can bind competitively to plasma proteins and result in displacement of bound drug, increasing its concentration.[486]

The consequences of acute hemodilution by the pump prime on drug disposition can be summarized as follows:

1. Because plasma drug concentration is reduced without any change in the amount of drug in the body, the apparent V_d increases acutely but by a relatively small amount.
2. After acute hemodilution, drug redistribution from tissues may occur to bring free drug concentrations in plasma and tissues back into equilibrium. The magnitude of this flux of drug depends on the relative amounts in tissues and plasma and on the degree of protein binding change.
3. Focus on total drug concentration of the free fraction and free concentration change may give misleading information on the expected change in the drug effect.
4. For drugs whose plasma/red cell partitioning is not equal, blood and plasma clearance will no longer bear the same relation to each other after hemodilution and must be distinguished.
5. Heparin has an effect on measurement of drug protein binding.

There may be marked changes in acid-base balance during CPB, resulting in changes in ionized and unionized drug concentrations, again affecting drug binding. CPB may be conducted using pH-stat or alpha-stat blood gas management. The change in pH with either management scheme may affect organ blood flow.[487,488] pH management may affect the degree of ionization and protein binding of certain drugs, leading to either increased or decreased free (active) drug concentrations.

Blood Flow

Hepatic, renal, cerebral, and skeletal perfusion have been shown to be reduced during CPB, and the use of vasodilators and vasoconstrictor agents to regulate arterial pressure may further change regional blood flow. These alterations in regional blood flow distribution have implications for drug distribution and metabolism. The combination of hypotension, hypothermia, and nonpulsatile blood flow has significant impact on distribution of the circulation, with a marked reduction in peripheral flow and relative preservation of the central circulation.[489,490]

CPB may be conducted with or without pulsatile perfusion. Nonpulsatile perfusion is associated with altered tissue perfusion.[491] Nonpulsatile flow and decreased peripheral perfusion from CPB and hypothermia, as well as the administration of vasoconstrictors, may result in cellular hypoxia and probable intracellular acidosis. This may affect the tissue distribution of drugs whose tissue binding is sensitive to pH. On reperfusion, rewarming, and the re-establishment of normal cardiac (pulsatile) function, redistribution of drugs from poorly perfused tissue is likely to add to the systemic plasma concentration because basic drugs will have been "trapped" in acidic tissue. The degree to which pulsatile perfusion alters drug pharmacokinetics is not well studied.

Hypothermia

Hypothermia commonly is used and has been shown to reduce hepatic and possibly renal enzyme function.[492] Hypothermia depresses metabolism by inhibiting enzyme function and reduces tissue perfusion by increasing blood viscosity and activation of autonomic and endocrine reflexes to produce vasoconstriction. Hepatic enzymatic activity is decreased during hypothermia, and in addition there is marked intrahepatic redistribution of blood flow with the development of significant intrahepatic shunting. Hypothermia thus reduces metabolic drug clearance and has been shown to reduce the metabolism of propranolol and verapamil.

Altered renal drug excretion occurs as a result of decreased renal perfusion, glomerular filtration rate, and tubular secretion. In dogs, glomerular filtration rate is decreased by 65% at 25°C.[493]

Sequestration

When normothermia is re-established, reperfusion of tissue might lead to washout of drug sequestered during the hypothermic CPB period. This may be one explanation for the increase in opioid plasma levels during the rewarming period.[494–496]

Many drugs bind to components of the CPB circuit, and their distribution may be affected by changes in circuit design, for example, the use of membrane versus bubble oxygenators. In vitro, various oxygenators bind lipophilic agents such as volatile anesthetic agents, propofol, opioids, and barbiturates.[488,497–501] This phenomenon has never been demonstrated to be important in vivo, likely because any drug removed by the circuit is replaced from the much larger tissue reservoir.

During CPB, the lungs are isolated from the circulation with the pulmonary artery blood flow being interrupted. Basic drugs (lidocaine, propranolol, fentanyl) that are taken up by the lungs are, therefore, sequestered during CPB, and the lungs may serve as a reservoir for drug release when systemic reperfusion is established.[494] After the onset of CPB, plasma fentanyl concentrations decrease acutely and then plateau. However, when mechanical ventilation of the lungs is instituted before separation from CPB, plasma fentanyl concentrations increase. During CPB, pulmonary artery fentanyl concentrations exceed radial artery levels; but when mechanical ventilation resumes, the pulmonary artery/radial ratio is reversed, suggesting that fentanyl is being washed out from the lungs.

Specific Agents

Opioids

All opioids show a decrease in total drug concentration on commencing CPB (Table 9-8). The degree of decrease is greater with fentanyl because a significant proportion of the drug adheres to the surface of the CPB circuit.[488,499,502] Inadequate anesthesia has been described when fentanyl was used as the major "anesthetic" agent.[503] There is high first-pass uptake of fentanyl by the lungs,[490,504] and reperfusion of the lungs at the end of CPB has been shown to result in increases in fentanyl concentrations (Figures 9-40 and 9-41).

TABLE 9-8	Effect of Cardiopulmonary Bypass on the Disposition of Opioids				
	Concentration				
Opioid	Start of CPB	During CPB	Clearance	Half-life	Volume of Distribution
Fentanyl	Decreased	Relatively stable or increased toward end of CPB		Increased	
Alfentanil	Decrease in total alfentanil concentration; no change in free concentration	Gradual increase in total concentration toward end of CPB	Unchanged	Increased	Increased
Sufentanil	Decreased	Gradual increase			

CPB, cardiopulmonary bypass.
Data from Buylaert WA, Herregods LL, Mortier EP, Bogaert MG: Cardiopulmonary bypass and the pharmacokinetics of drugs, *Clin Pharmacokinet* 17:10, 1989.

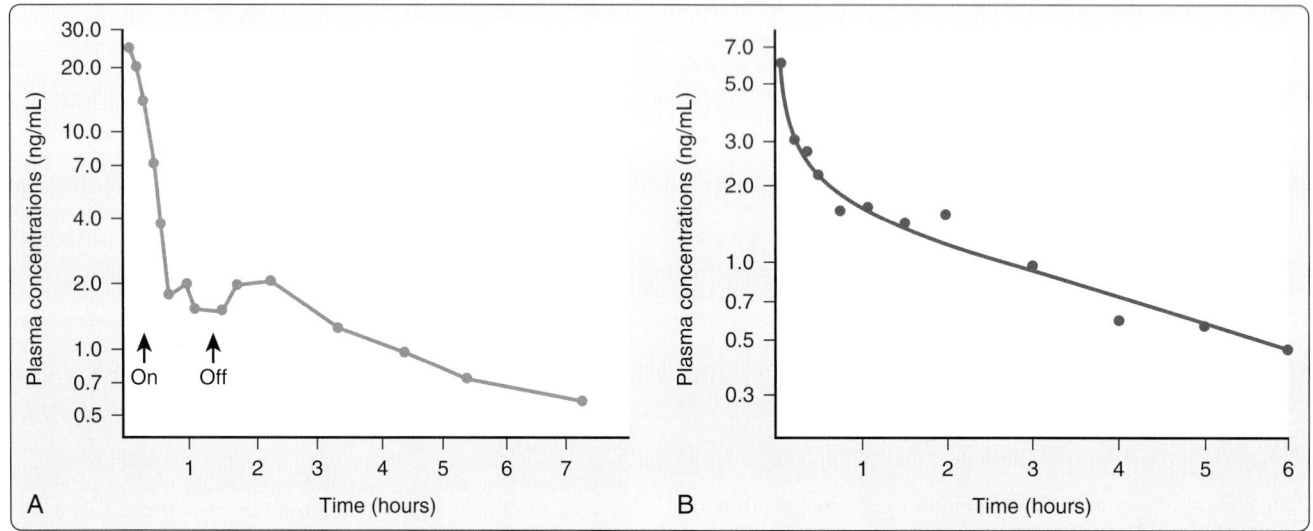

Figure 9-40 Effect of cardiopulmonary bypass (CPB) on the disposition of a single bolus injection of fentanyl. The time course of plasma fentanyl concentrations after injection of a 500-μg intravenous bolus at time zero. *A,* Data from a cardiac surgery patient. Times of CPB are indicated by *arrows. B,* Data from a vascular surgery control patient. *(Reproduced from Koska AJ, Romagnole A, Karmer WG: Effect of cardiopulmonary bypass on fentanyl distribution and elimination,* Clin Pharmacol Ther *29:100, 1981.)*

The decrease in total drug concentration is seen least with opioids that have a high V_d, when the addition of the prime volume is less important, and in those drugs that can equilibrate rapidly to minimize dilutional effect. In this respect, sufentanil, which has the most stable total drug concentrations, may offer advantages. Studies of free alfentanil concentrations have shown that these remain relatively stable throughout CPB and, therefore, the pharmacologically active concentration remains unchanged. It is the bound concentration that changes, reflecting changes in both albumin and α_1-acid glycoprotein concentrations to which alfentanil is predominantly bound.[505–507] Elimination of fentanyl and alfentanil has been shown to be prolonged by CPB, whereas that of morphine was unchanged. There are inadequate data available on the elimination of sufentanil after CPB. From the pharmacokinetic information currently available, alfentanil may be the most suitable opioid for CPB because free concentrations have been shown to be stable during CPB and the prolongation of its half-life is much less than that of fentanyl.

Benzodiazepines

The benzodiazepines show a decrease in total concentration on commencing CPB. However, because these drugs are more than 90% protein bound, changes in free concentrations are greatly influenced by changes in protein concentrations or in factors such as acid-base balance that influence protein binding. This is particularly pertinent in the context of CPB, but no studies have commented on free versus total concentrations of benzodiazepines. Diazepam has a very long elimination half-life, even in non-CPB patients, and has been shown to be cumulative after CPB.[508] Midazolam has a shorter elimination half-life.

This increases with age and also is significantly longer for CPB patients than for patients undergoing other types of major surgery (Figure 9-42). The elimination half-life is prolonged in a subset (6%) of patients.[509,510] However, the half-life of midazolam is shorter than that of the other benzodiazepines; and, in small doses, elimination was rapid in most patients. For this reason, it is the suitable benzodiazepine for use by repeated boluses of infusion. The elimination half-life of lorazepam was unchanged by CPB but was longer than that of midazolam.

Intravenous Anesthetic Agents

Thiopental and methohexital show a decrease in total drug concentration on commencing CPB, but the active free concentrations are remarkably stable[506,511] (Figure 9-43). Clearance of thiopental is halved during CPB, but elimination after CPB is not known. Elimination of methohexital remains unchanged. Conflicting results have been obtained for propofol[512,513] (Figure 9-44). The total concentration of propofol may decrease on commencing CPB with an increase in the free fraction, or the total concentration may remain unchanged. A prolonged elimination half-life has been demonstrated in one study,[512] but the redistribution half-life was short, concentrations decreased rapidly after stopping the drug, and patients made a rapid recovery. In general, the free active concentrations of these drugs remain unchanged, but their actions may be prolonged.

Volatile Anesthetic Agents

The effect of CPB on MAC remains uncertain. Some authors have shown that CPB reduces the MAC of enflurane by as much as 30% in

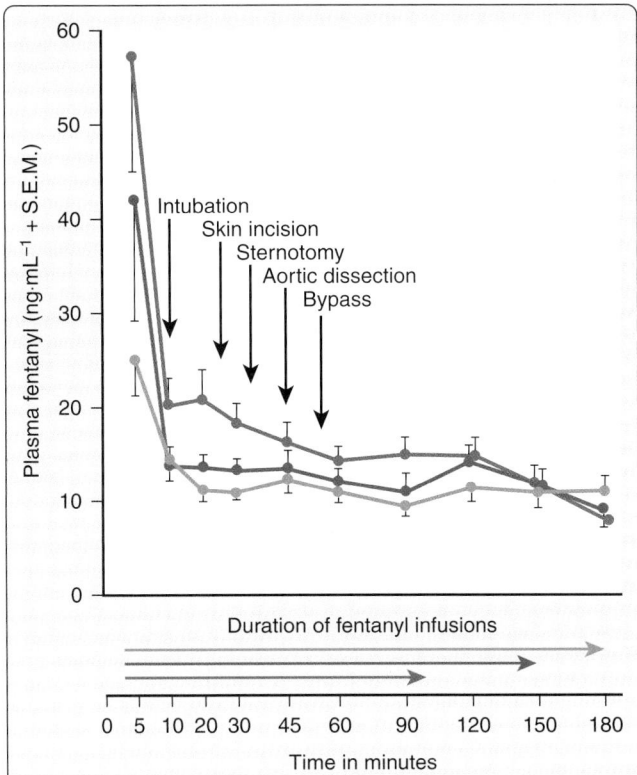

Figure 9-41 Effect of cardiopulmonary bypass (CPB) on plasma fentanyl concentrations when fentanyl is administered at various constant rate infusions for aortocoronary surgery. Plasma fentanyl concentrations and duration of fentanyl infusion for three groups of patients: those given 30 μg/kg followed by 0.3 μg/kg/min (*green line*); those given 40 μg/kg followed by 0.4 μg/kg/min (*purple line*); and those given 50 μg/kg followed by 0.5 μg/kg/min (*red line*). S.E.M., standard error of the mean. (*Reproduced from Sprigge JS, Wynands JE, Whalley DG, et al: Fentanyl infusion anesthesia for aortocoronary bypass surgery: Plasma levels and hemodynamic response,* Anesth Analg *61:972, 1982.*)

animal studies, whereas others have failed to demonstrate any reduction.[514-516] Several groups have shown variation in MAC with temperature and with reduced volatile concentrations required at lower temperatures.[515,517-519]

The effect of CPB with cooling on the uptake of volatile anesthetics administered to the oxygenator is dependent on three factors: (1) the blood-gas solubility of the agent and the opposing effects of cooling in increasing blood-gas solubility of blood versus hemodilution, which decreases blood-gas solubility of volatile anesthetic agents[520]; (2) the increased solubility in tissue of volatile anesthetics secondary to hypothermia; and (3) uptake by the oxygenator.[521] CPB produces changes in the blood-gas partition coefficient dependent on the prime used and the temperature. Factors that alter the solubility of volatile anesthetic agents in blood and other tissues include lipid concentration, osmolarity, and PCV. The changes in blood composition after the addition of a crystalloid prime tend to decrease blood solubility, favoring a more rapid attainment of steady state and a lower blood concentration of volatile agent for a given inspired concentration. However, hemodilution with a plasma prime increases solubility because volatile agents are more soluble in albumin than red cells.[522] Blood solubility also is inversely proportional to temperature. This relation is linear, but different for individual agents, with a range of 4% to 4.9% per degree Celsius decrease in body temperature.[523] Thus, hemodilution with a crystalloid prime and hypothermia have opposite effects on the blood-gas partition coefficient. The predicted net change in solubility for isoflurane when PCV is reduced from 40% to 20% and temperature is reduced from 37°C to 28°C is +2%.[524]

Volatile agents have been shown to bind to a variety of plastics,[525] and this may account for some of the decrease in concentrations on commencing bypass. A volatile agent started during hypothermic CPB takes longer to equilibrate, and agents already in use need to re-equilibrate, potentially changing the depth of anesthesia, until equilibration is complete. Because these agents are metabolized to a small degree and washout is fast, the duration of action is not prolonged after CPB.[526,527]

Neuromuscular Blockers

It has been demonstrated that hypothermic CPB influences the concentration and the response relations of neuromuscular blockers during hypothermia.[528] In general, the requirements for neuromuscular

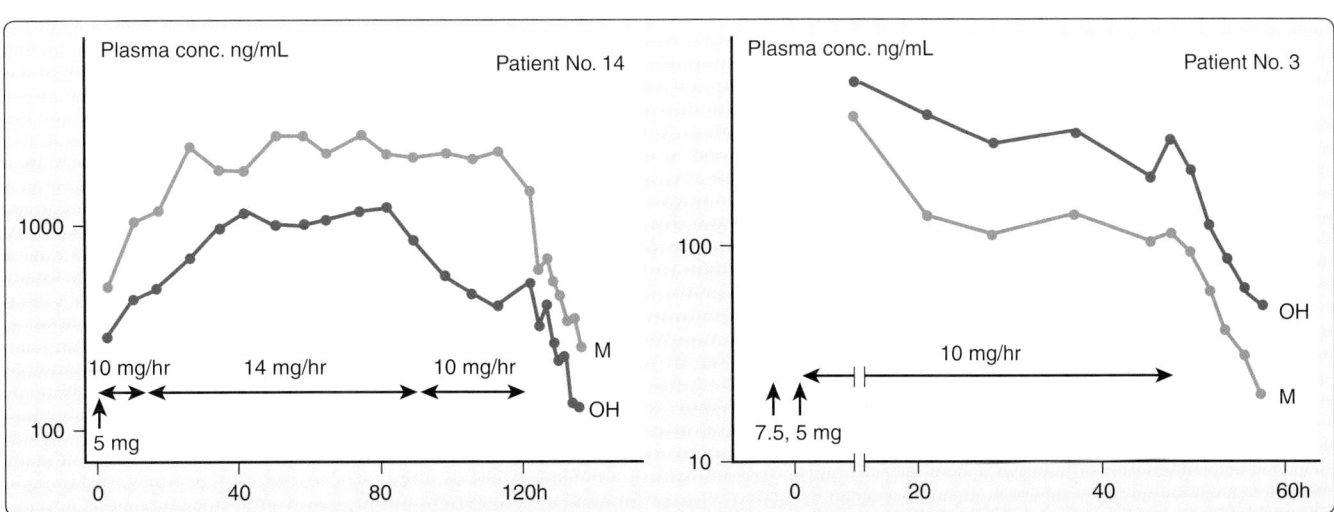

Figure 9-42 Variability of concentrations of midazolam and its metabolite in the intensive care unit. Note the difference in the two scales for concentration for the left and right panels. *Left,* Concentrations of midazolam (M) are slightly higher than those of its metabolite (OH). *Right,* Midazolam concentrations are lower than those of the metabolite. (*Reproduced from Vree TB, Shimoda M, Driessen JJ, et al: Decreased plasma albumin concentration results in increased volume of distribution and increased elimination of midazolam in intensive care patients,* Clin Pharmacol Ther *46:537, 1989.*)

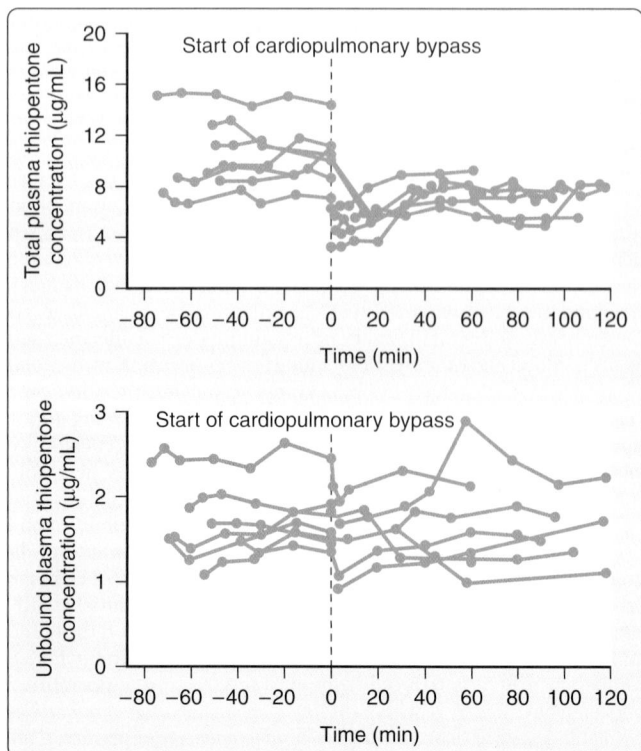

Figure 9-43 **Effect of cardiopulmonary bypass on plasma thiopental concentrations during continuous infusion.** *Top*, Total plasma thiopental concentrations. *Bottom*, Unbound (free) plasma thiopental concentrations. The point of reference (zero time) is taken as the start of bypass. (*Reproduced from Morgan DJ, Crankshaw DP, Prideaux PR, et al: Thiopentone levels during cardiopulmonary bypass: Changes in plasma protein binding during continuous infusion, Anaesthesia 41:4, 1986.*)

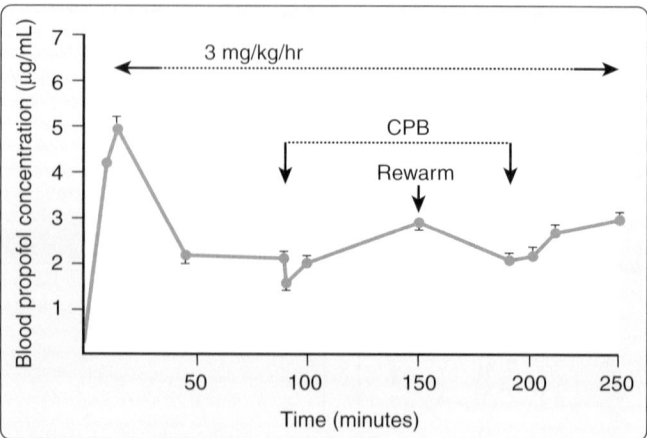

Figure 9-44 **Blood propofol concentrations during coronary artery surgery and cardiopulmonary bypass (CPB).** A two-stage propofol infusion (10 mg/kg/hr for 30 minutes followed by 3 mg/kg/hr thereafter) was administered. Time scale shows the mean time taken to specific events, such as the onset of cardiopulmonary bypass (CPB), induced hypothermia (25°C to 27°C), and the end of bypass. Bars represent mean concentrations ± standard error of the mean. (*Reproduced from Russell GN, Wright EL, Fox MA, et al: Propofol-fentanyl anaesthesia for coronary artery surgery and cardiopulmonary bypass,* Anaesthesia 44:205, 1989)

blockade are found to be significantly reduced as a result of a number of both pharmacokinetic and pharmacodynamic effects. Specifically, cooling influences nerve conduction in the mobilization of acetylcholine from the nerve vesicles,[529] as well as modifying cholinergic receptors. Furthermore, the effect of cooling is manifest on cholinesterase enzyme activity, which is temperature dependent. The most important effect of cooling, however, is a decrease in the mobilization of acetylcholine that has been demonstrated both in vitro and in animal models.[530,531] Thus, during hypothermia, fewer muscle relaxants are needed to obtain the same amount of muscle relaxation. In addition, cooling alters the mechanical properties of the muscle, as well as having potentially significant effects on electrolytes, which modulate the contractile response.

CPB causes hemodilution, which may result in an initial decrease in the free drug concentration. However, there also is an associated

decrease in the albumin concentration during CPB, so that although the total drug concentration may be decreased as a result of hemodilution, if the drug is partially bound to albumin, the free drug concentration may actually be increased. This phenomenon may occur with neuromuscular blockers such as rocuronium.[532]

Hypothermia inhibits the hepatic clearance of steroidal neuromuscular blocking agents, although it seems to promote renal clearance. This may explain why the time course of action of steroidal neuromuscular blocking agents such as rocuronium and vecuronium, which are dependent on liver clearance, are relatively more prolonged under hypothermic conditions than those that are dependent on renal clearance, such as pancuronium and pipecuronium.[533]

Acknowledgments

The authors thank Cheryl Dewyre and Mary Ann Anderson for their enthusiasm and knowledgeable administrative skills in the preparation of this chapter. The authors also thank all of the authors of the previous chapters: Kyung W. Park, MD, J. Michael Haering, MD, Sebastian Reiz, MD, Edward Lowenstein, MD, James G. Bovill, MD, PhD, Fred Boer, MD, PhD, J. G. Reves, MD, Steven Hill, MD, Matthew R. Belmont, MD, Ralph P. F. Scott, MD, and Margaret Wood, MD, some of whose work has been reproduced in this chapter.

REFERENCES

1. Cason BA, Gamperi AK, Slocum RE, et al: Anesthetic-induced preconditioning: Previous administration of isoflurane decreases myocardial infarct size in rabbits, *Anesthesiology* 87(5):1182–1190, 1997.
2. Kersten JR, Lowe D, Hettrick DA, et al: Glyburide, a KATP channel antagonist, attenuates the cardioprotective effects of isoflurane in stunned myocardium, *Anesth Analg* 83(1):27–33, 1996.
3. Kersten JR, Schmeling TJ, Pagel PS, et al: Isoflurane mimics ischemic preconditioning via activation of K(ATP) channels: Reduction of myocardial infarct size with an acute memory phase, *Anesthesiology* 87(2):361–370, 1997.
4. Bernard J, Wouters PF, Doursout M, et al: Effects of sevoflurane and isoflurane on cardiac and coronary dynamics in chronically instrumented dogs, *Anesthesiology* 72(4):659–662, 1990.
5. DeTraglia MC, Komai H, Rusy BF: Differential effects of inhalation anesthetics on myocardial potentiated-state contractions in vitro, *Anesthesiology* 68(4):534–540, 1988.
6. Harkin CP, Pagel PS, Kersten JR, et al: Direct negative inotropic and lusitropic effects of sevoflurane, *Anesthesiology* 81(1):156–167, 1994.
7. Housmans PR, Murat I: Comparative effects of halothane, enflurane, and isoflurane at equipotent anesthetic concentrations on isolated ventricular myocardium of the ferret. I. Contractility, *Anesthesiology* 69(4):451–463, 1988.
8. Kikura M, Ikeda K: Comparison of effects of sevoflurane/nitrous oxide and enflurane/nitrous oxide on myocardial contractility in humans. Load-independent and noninvasive assessment with transesophageal echocardiography, *Anesthesiology* 79(2):235–243, 1993.
9. Lynch C 3rd: Differential depression of myocardial contractility by halothane and isoflurane in vitro, *Anesthesiology* 64(5):620–631, 1986.

10. Pagel PS, Kampine JP, Schmeling TJ, et al: Influence of volatile anesthetics on myocardial contractility in vivo: Desflurane versus isoflurane, *Anesthesiology* 74(5):900–907, 1991.
11. Pagel PS, Kampine JP, Schmeling WT, et al: Evaluation of myocardial contractility in the chronically instrumented dog with intact autonomic nervous system function: Effects of desflurane and isoflurane, *Acta Anaesthesiol Scand* 37(2):203–210, 1993.
12. Kemmotsu O, Hashimoto Y, Shimosato S: Inotropic effects of isoflurane on mechanics of contraction in isolated cat papillary muscles from normal and failing hearts, *Anesthesiology* 39(5):470–477, 1973.
13. Kemmotsu O, Hashimoto Y, Shimosato S: The effects of fluroxene and isoflurane on contractile performance of isolated papillary muscles from failing hearts, *Anesthesiology* 40(3):252–260, 1974.
14. Lowenstein E, Foëx P, Francis CM, et al: Regional ischemic ventricular dysfunction in myocardium supplied by a narrowed coronary artery with increasing halothane concentration in the dog, *Anesthesiology* 55(4):349–359, 1981.
15. Prys-Roberts C, et al: Interaction of anesthesia, beta-receptor blockade, and blood loss in dogs with induced myocardial infarction, *Anesthesiology* 45(3):326–329, 1976.
16. Hanley PJ, ter Keurs HE, Cannell MB: Excitation-contraction coupling in the heart and the negative inotropic action of volatile anesthetics, *Anesthesiology* 101(4):999–1014, 2004.
17. Huneke R, Fassl J, Rossaint R, et al: Effects of volatile anesthetics on cardiac ion channels, *Acta Anaesthesiol Scand* 48(5):547–561, 2004.
18. Pagel PS, Kampine JP, Schmeling TJ, et al: Effects of nitrous oxide on myocardial contractility as evaluated by the preload recruitable stroke work relationship in chronically instrumented dogs, *Anesthesiology* 73(6):1148–1157, 1990.

19. Brogan WC 3rd, Hillis LD, Flores ED, et al: The natural history of isolated left ventricular diastolic dysfunction, *Am J Med* 92(6):627–630, 1992.
20. Judge KW, Pawitan Y, Caldwell J, et al: Congestive heart failure symptoms in patients with preserved left ventricular systolic function: Analysis of the CASS registry, *J Am Coll Cardiol* 18(2):377–382, 1991.
21. Pagel PS, Hettrick DA, Warltier DC: Amrinone enhances myocardial contractility and improves left ventricular diastolic function in conscious and anesthetized chronically instrumented dogs, *Anesthesiology* 79(4):753–765, 1993.
22. Pagel PS, Kampine JP, Schmeling TJ, et al: Reversal of volatile anesthetic-induced depression of myocardial contractility by extracellular calcium also enhances left ventricular diastolic function, *Anesthesiology* 78(1):141–154, 1993.
23. Zile MR, Brutsaert DL: New concepts in diastolic dysfunction and diastolic heart failure: Part II: Causal mechanisms and treatment, *Circulation* 105(12):1503–1508, 2002.
24. Aurigemma GP, Gottdiener JS, Shemanski L, et al: Predictive value of systolic and diastolic function for incident congestive heart failure in the elderly: The cardiovascular health study, *J Am Coll Cardiol* 37(4):1042–1048, 2001.
25. Dauterman KW, Massie BM, Gheorghiade M: Heart failure associated with preserved systolic function: A common and costly clinical entity, *Am Heart J* 135(6 Pt 2 Suppl):S310–S319, 1998.
26. Graham M, Thiessen D, Mutch W: Isoflurane and halothane impair both systolic and diastolic function in the newborn pig, *Can J Anesth* 43(5):495–502, 1996.
27. Humphrey LS, Stinson DC, Humphrey MJ, et al: Volatile anesthetic effects on left ventricular relaxation in swine, *Anesthesiology* 73(4):731–738, 1990.
28. Ihara T, Shannon RP, Komamura K, et al: Effects of anaesthesia and recent surgery on diastolic function, *Cardiovasc Res* 28(3):325–336, 1994.
29. Pagel PS, Kampine JP, Schmeling WT, et al: Alteration of left ventricular diastolic function by desflurane, isoflurane, and halothane in the chronically instrumented dog with autonomic nervous system blockade, *Anesthesiology* 74(6):1103–1114, 1991.
30. Yamada T, Takeda J, Koyama K, et al: Effects of sevoflurane, isoflurane, enflurane, and halothane on left ventricular diastolic performance in dogs, *J Cardiothorac Vasc Anesth* 8(6):618–624, 1994.
31. Sohma A, Foex P, Ryder WA: Regional distensibility, chamber stiffness, and elastic stiffness constant in halothane and propofol anesthesia, *J Cardiothorac Vasc Anesth* 7(2):188–194, 1993.
32. Varadarajan SG, An J, Novalija E, et al: Sevoflurane before or after ischemia improves contractile and metabolic function while reducing myoplasmic Ca2+ loading in intact hearts, *Anesthesiology* 96(1):125–133, 2002.
33. Echt DS, Liebson PR, Mitchell LB: Mortality and morbidity in patients receiving encainide, flecainide, or placebo. The Cardiac Arrhythmia Suppression Trial, *N Engl J Med* 324(12):781–788, 1991.
34. Guler N, Kati I, Demirel CB, et al: The effects of volatile anesthetics on the Q-Tc interval, *J Cardiothorac Vasc Anesth* 15(2):188–191, 2001.
35. Hickey RF, Sybert PE, Verrier ED, et al: Effects of halothane, enflurane, and isoflurane on coronary blood flow autoregulation and coronary vascular reserve in the canine heart, *Anesthesiology* 68(1):21–30, 1988.
36. Tarnow J, Eberlein HJ, Oser G, et al: Haemodynamik, myokardkontraktilitaat, ventrikelvolumnia, and sauerstoffversorgung des herzens unter verschiedenen inhalations-anaesthetika, *Anaesthetist* 26:220, 1977.
37. Verrier ED, Edelist G, Macke C, et al: Greater coronary vascular reserve in dogs anesthetized with halothane, *Anesthesiology* 53(6):445–459, 1980.
38. Moffitt EA, Sethna DH, Gary RJ, et al: Nitrous oxide added to halothane reduces coronary flow and myocardial oxygen consumption in patients with coronary disease, *Can Anaesth Soc J* 30(1):5–9, 1983.
39. Reiz S, Balfors E, Gustavsson B, et al: Effects of halothane on coronary haemodynamics and myocardial metabolism in patients with ischaemic heart disease and heart failure, *Acta Anaesthesiol Scand* 26(2):133–138, 1982.
40. Sonntag H, Merin RG, Donath U, et al: Myocardial metabolism and oxygenation in man awake and during halothane anesthesia, *Anesthesiology* 51(3):204–210, 1979.
41. Wilkinson PL, Hamilton WK, Moyers JR, et al: Halothane and morphine-nitrous oxide anesthesia in patients undergoing coronary artery bypass operation. Patterns of intraoperative ischemia, *J Thorac Cardiovasc Surg* 82(3):372–382, 1981.
42. Tanaka K, Ludwig LM, Kersten JR, et al: Mechanisms of cardioprotection by volatile anesthetics, *Anesthesiology* 100(3):707–721, 2004.
43. Buffington CW, Romson JL, Levine A, et al: Isoflurane induces coronary steal in a canine model of chronic coronary occlusion, *Anesthesiology* 66(3):280–292, 1987.
44. Priebe HJ, Foex P: Isoflurane causes regional myocardial dysfunction in dogs with critical coronary artery stenoses, *Anesthesiology* 66(3):293–300, 1987.
45. Diana P, Tullock WC, Gorcsan J, et al: Myocardial ischemia: A comparison between isoflurane and enflurane in coronary artery bypass patients, *Surv Anesthesiol* 38(2):80, 1994.
46. Hartman JC, Kampine JP, Schmeling WT, et al: Actions of isoflurane on myocardial perfusion in chronically instrumented dogs with poor, moderate, or well-developed coronary collaterals, *J Cardiothorac Anesth* 4(6):715–725, 1990.
47. Hartman JC, Kampine JP, Schmeling WT, et al: Steal-prone coronary circulation in chronically instrumented dogs: Isoflurane versus adenosine, *Anesthesiology* 74(4):744–756, 1991.
48. Hartman JC, Kampine JP, Schmeling WT, et al: Alterations in collateral blood flow produced by isoflurane in a chronically instrumented canine model of multivessel coronary artery disease, *Anesthesiology* 74(1):120–133, 1991.
49. Leung JM, Goehner P, O'Kelly BF, et al: Isoflurane anesthesia and myocardial ischemia: Comparative risk versus sufentanil anesthesia in patients undergoing coronary artery bypass graft surgery, *Anesthesiology* 74(5):838–847, 1991.
50. Moore PG, Kien ND, Reitan JA, et al: No evidence for blood flow redistribution with isoflurane or halothane during acute coronary artery occlusion in fentanyl-anesthetized dogs, *Anesthesiology* 75(5):854–865, 1991.
51. Pulley DD, Kirvassilis GV, Kelermenos N, et al: Regional and global myocardial circulatory and metabolic effects of isoflurane and halothane in patients with steal-prone coronary anatomy, *Anesthesiology* 75(5):756–766, 1991.
52. Glower DD, Spratt JA, Kabas JS, et al: Quantification of regional myocardial dysfunction after acute ischemic injury, *Am J Physiol* 255(1 Pt 2):H85–H93, 1988.
53. Glower DD, Spratt JA, Snow ND, et al: Linearity of the Frank-Starling relationship in the intact heart: The concept of preload recruitable stroke work, *Circulation* 71(5):994–1009, 1985.
54. Park KW, Dai HB, Lowenstein E, et al: Isoflurane and halothane attenuate endothelium-dependent vasodilation in rat coronary microvessels, *Anesth Analg* 84(2):278–284, 1997.
55. Hartman JC, Pagel PS, Kampine JP, et al: Influence of desflurane on regional distribution of coronary blood flow in a chronically instrumented canine model of multivessel coronary artery obstruction, *Anesth Analg* 72(3):289–299, 1991.
56. Kersten JR, Brayer AP, Pagel PS, et al: Perfusion of ischemic myocardium during anesthesia with sevoflurane, *Anesthesiology* 81(4):995–1004, 1994.
57. Kitahata H, Kawahito S, Nozaki J, et al: Effects of sevoflurane on regional myocardial blood flow distribution: Quantification with myocardial contrast echocardiography, *Anesthesiology* 90(5):1436–1445, 1999.
58. Kehl F, Krolikowski JG, Tessmer JP, et al: Increases in coronary collateral blood flow produced by sevoflurane are mediated by calcium-activated potassium (BKCa) channels in vivo, *Anesthesiology* 97(3):725–731, 2002.
59. Akata T, Nakamura K, Kodama K, et al: Effects of volatile anesthetics on acetylcholine-induced relaxation in the rabbit mesenteric resistance artery, *Anesthesiology* 82(1):188–204, 1995.
60. Muldoon SM, Hart JL, Bowen KA, et al: Attenuation of endothelium-mediated vasodilation by halothane, *Anesthesiology* 68(1):31–37, 1988.
61. Toda H, Nakamura K, Hatano Y, et al: Halothane and isoflurane inhibit endothelium-dependent relaxation elicited by acetylcholine, *Anesth Analg* 75(2):198–203, 1992.
62. Uggeri MJ, Proctor GJ, Johns RA: Halothane, enflurane, and isoflurane attenuate both receptor- and non-receptor-mediated EDRF production in rat thoracic aorta, *Anesthesiology* 76(6):1012–1017, 1992.
63. Yoshida K, Okabe E: Selective impairment of endothelium-dependent relaxation by sevoflurane: Oxygen free radicals participation, *Anesthesiology* 76(3):440–447, 1992.
64. Pajewski TN, Miao N, Lynch C, et al: Volatile anesthetics affect calcium mobilization in bovine endothelial cells, *Anesthesiology* 85(5):1147–1156, 1996.
65. Tas PW, Stobetael C, Roewer N: The volatile anesthetic isoflurane inhibits the histamine-induced Ca2+ influx in primary human endothelial cells, *Anesth Analg* 97(2):430–435, table of contents, 2003.
66. Arriero MM, Alameda LM, Lopez-Farre A, et al: Sevoflurane reduces endothelium-dependent vasorelaxation: Role of superoxide anion and endothelin, *Can J Anaesth* 49(5):471–476, 2002.
67. Vinh VH, Enoki T, Hirata S, et al: Comparative contractile effects of halothane and sevoflurane in rat aorta, *Anesthesiology* 92(1):219, 2000.
68. Yu J, Tokinaga Y, Ogawa K, et al: Sevoflurane inhibits angiotensin II-induced, protein kinase C-mediated but not Ca2+-elicited contraction of rat aortic smooth muscle, *Anesthesiology* 100(4):879–884, 2004.
69. Izumi K, Akata T, Takahashi S: The action of sevoflurane on vascular smooth muscle of isolated mesenteric resistance arteries (part 1): Role of endothelium, *Anesthesiology* 92(5):1426–1440, 2000.
70. Akata T, Nakashima M, Izumi K: Comparison of volatile anesthetic actions on intracellular calcium stores of vascular smooth muscle: Investigation in isolated systemic resistance arteries, *Anesthesiology* 94(5):840–850, 2001.
71. Tsuneyoshi I, Zhang D, Boyle WA III: Ca2+- and myosin phosphorylation-independent relaxation by halothane in K+-depolarized rat mesenteric arteries, *Anesthesiology* 99(3):656–666, 2003.
72. Chen BB, Nyhan D, Fehr DM, et al: Halothane anesthesia causes active flow-independent pulmonary vasoconstriction, *Am J Physiol* 259(1 Pt 2):H74–H83, 1990.
73. Lesitsky MA, Davis S, Murray PA: Preservation of hypoxic pulmonary vasoconstriction during sevoflurane and desflurane anesthesia compared to the conscious state in chronically instrumented dogs, *Anesthesiology* 89(6):1501–1508, 1998.
74. Gambone LM, Fujiwara Y, Murray PA: Endothelium-dependent pulmonary vasodilation is selectively attenuated during isoflurane anesthesia, *Am J Physiol Heart Circ Physiol* 272(1):H290–H298, 1997.
75. Oshima Y, Ishibe Y, Okazaki N, et al: Isoflurane inhibits endothelium-mediated nitric oxide relaxing pathways in the isolated perfused rabbit lung, *Can J Anaesth* 44(10):1108–1114, 1997.
76. Fujiwara Y, Murray PA: Effects of isoflurane anesthesia on pulmonary vascular response to K+ ATP channel activation and circulatory hypotension in chronically instrumented dogs, *Anesthesiology* 90(3):799–811, 1999.
77. Seki S, Sato K, Nakayama M, et al: Halothane and enflurane attenuate pulmonary vasodilation mediated by adenosine triphosphate-sensitive potassium channels compared to the conscious state, *Anesthesiology* 86(4):923–935, 1997.
78. Sato K, Seki S, Murray PA: Effects of halothane and enflurane anesthesia on sympathetic [beta]-adrenoreceptor-mediated pulmonary vasodilation in chronically instrumented dogs, *Anesthesiology* 97(2):478–487, 2002.
79. Ebert TJ, Harkin CP, Muzi M: Cardiovascular responses to sevoflurane: A review, *Anesth Analg* 81(Suppl 6):S11–S22, 1995.
80. Muzi M, Ebert TJ: A comparison of baroreflex sensitivity during isoflurane and desflurane anesthesia in humans, *Anesthesiology* 82(4):919–925, 1995.
81. Seagard JL, Elegbe EO, Hopp FA, et al: Effects of isoflurane on the baroreceptor reflex, *Anesthesiology* 59(6):511–520, 1983.
82. Seagard JL, Hopp FA, Donegan JH, et al: Halothane and the carotid sinus reflex: Evidence for multiple sites of action, *Anesthesiology* 57(3):191–202, 1982.
83. Boban N, McCallum JB, Schedewie HK, et al: Direct comparative effects of isoflurane and desflurane on sympathetic ganglionic transmission, *Anesth Analg* 80(1):127–134, 1995.
84. Kloner RA, Jennings RB: Consequences of brief ischemia: Stunning, preconditioning, and their clinical implications: Part 2, *Circulation* 104(25):3158–3167, 2001.
85. Heyndrickx GR, Millard RW, McRitchie RJ, et al: Regional myocardial functional and electrophysiological alterations after brief coronary artery occlusion in conscious dogs, *J Clin Invest* 56(4):978–985, 1975.
86. Murry CE, Jennings RB, Reimer KA: Preconditioning with ischemia: A delay of lethal cell injury in ischemic myocardium, *Circulation* 74(5):1124–1136, 1986.
87. Bland JH, Lowenstein E: Halothane-induced decrease in experimental myocardial ischemia in the non-failing canine heart, *Anesthesiology* 45(3):287–293, 1976.
88. Davis RF, DeBoer LW, Rude RE, et al: The effect of halothane anesthesia on myocardial necrosis, hemodynamic performance, and regional myocardial blood flow in dogs following coronary artery occlusion, *Anesthesiology* 59(5):402–411, 1983.
89. Warltier DC, al-Wathiqui MH, Kampine JP, et al: Recovery of contractile function of stunned myocardium in chronically instrumented dogs is enhanced by halothane or isoflurane, *Anesthesiology* 69(4):552–565, 1988.
90. Ishihara M, Sato K, Tateishi H, et al: Implications of prodromal angina pectoris in anterior wall acute myocardial infarction: Acute angiographic findings and long-term prognosis, *J Am Coll Cardiol* 30(4):970–975, 1997.
91. Bolli R: The late phase of preconditioning, *Circ Res* 87(11):972–983, 2000.
92. Feng J, Lucchinetti E, Ahuja P, et al: Isoflurane postconditioning prevents opening of the mitochondrial permeability transition pore through inhibition of glycogen synthase kinase 3β, *Anesthesiology* 103:987–995, 2005.
93. Warltier DC, Kersten JR, Pagel PS, et al: Editorial view: Anesthetic preconditioning: Serendipity and science, *Anesthesiology* 97(1):1–3, 2002.
94. Todd MM: Special issue on preconditioning: Work presented at the October 2003 journal symposium, *Anesthesiology* 100(3):469, 2004.
95. de Klaver MJM, Buckingham M-G, Rich GF: Isoflurane pretreatment has immediate and delayed protective effects against cytokine-induced injury in endothelial and vascular smooth muscle cells, *Anesthesiology* 99(4):896–903, 2003.
96. Tanaka K, Ludwig LM, Krolikowski JG, et al: Isoflurane produces delayed preconditioning against myocardial ischemia and reperfusion injury: Role of cyclooxygenase-2, *Anesthesiology* 100(3):525–531, 2004.
97. Kehl F, Krolikowski JG, Mraovic B, et al: Is Isoflurane-induced preconditioning dose related? *Anesthesiology* 96(3):675–680, 2002.
98. Ludwig LM, Patel HH, Gross GJ, et al: Morphine enhances pharmacological preconditioning by isoflurane: Role of mitochondrial KATP channels and opioid receptors, *Anesthesiology* 98(3):705–711, 2003.

99. Zaugg M, Lucchinetti E, Spahn DR, et al: Volatile anesthetics mimic cardiac preconditioning by priming the activation of mitochondrial KATP channels via multiple signaling pathways, *Anesthesiology* 97(1):4–14, 2002.
100. Mullenheim J, Ebel D, Bauer M, et al: Sevoflurane confers additional cardioprotection after ischemic late preconditioning in rabbits, *Anesthesiology* 99(3):624–631, 2003.
101. Toller WG, Kersten JR, Pagel PS, et al: Sevoflurane reduces myocardial infarct size and decreases the time threshold for ischemic preconditioning in dogs, *Anesthesiology* 91(5):1437–1446, 1999.
102. Kersten JR, Orth KG, Pagel PS, et al: Role of adenosine in isoflurane-induced cardioprotection, *Anesthesiology* 86(5):1128–1139, 1997.
103. Hemmings HC Jr, Adamo AI: Activation of endogenous protein kinase C by halothane in synaptosomes, *Anesthesiology* 84(3):652–662, 1996.
104. Mullenheim J, Ebel D, Frassdorf J, et al: Isoflurane preconditions myocardium against infarction via release of free radicals, *Anesthesiology* 96(4):934–940, 2002.
105. Novalija E, Varadarajan SG, Camara AK, et al: Anesthetic preconditioning: Triggering role of reactive oxygen and nitrogen species in isolated hearts, *Am J Physiol Heart Circ Physiol* 283(1):H44–H52, 2002.
106. Tanaka K, Weihrauch D, Kehl F, et al: Mechanism of preconditioning by isoflurane in rabbits: A direct role for reactive oxygen species, *Anesthesiology* 97(6):1485–1490, 2002.
107. Landoni G, Fochi O, Torri G: Cardiac protection by volatile anaesthetics: A review, *Curr Vasc Pharmacol* 6:108–111, 2008.
108. Bouwman RA, Musters RJ, van Beek-Harmsen BJ, et al: Sevoflurane-induced cardioprotection depends on PKC-alpha activation via production of reactive oxygen species, *Br J Anaesth* 99:639–645, 2007.
109. Juhaszova M, Zorov DB, Kim SH, et al: Glycogen synthase kinase-3beta mediates convergence of protection signaling to inhibit the mitochondrial permeability transition pore, *J Clin Invest* 113:1535–1549, 2004.
110. Pravdic D, Sedlic F, Mio Y, et al: Anesthetic-induced preconditioning delays opening of mitochondrial permeability transition pore via protein kinase C-epsilon-mediated pathway, *Anesthesiology* 111:267–274, 2009.
111. Ge Z, Pravdic D, Bienengraeber M, et al: Isoflurane postconditioning protects against reperfusion injury by preventing mitochondrial permeability transition by an endothelial nitric oxide synthase-dependent mechanism, *Anestheisology* 112:73–85, 2010.
112. Finkel E: The mitochondrion: Is it central to apoptosis? *Science* 292(5517):624–626, 2001.
113. Landoni G, Biondi-Zoccai G, Zangrillo A, et al: Desflurane and sevoflurane in cardiac surgery: A meta-analysis of randomized clinical trials, *J Cardiothorac Vasc Anesth* 21:502–511, 2007.
114. Bignami E, Biondi-Zoccai G, Landoni G, et al: Volatile anesthetics reduce mortality in cardiac surgery, *J Cardiothorac Vasc Anesth* 23:594–599, 2009.
115. De Hert SG, Van der Linden P, Cromheecke S, et al: Cardioprotective properties of sevoflurane in patients undergoing coronary surgery with cardiopulmonary bypass are related to the modalities of its administration, *Anesthesiology* 101:299–310, 2004.
116. Kato R, Foex P: Myocardial protection by anesthetic agents against ischemia-reperfusion injury: An update for anesthesiologists, *Can J Anaesth* 49(8):777–791, 2002.
117. van Klarenbosch J, Stienen GJ, de Ruijter W, et al: The differential effect of propofol on contractility of isolated myocardial trabeculae of rat and guinea-pig, *Br J Pharmacol* 132(3):742–748, 2001.
118. Gelissen HP, Epema AH, Henning RH, et al: Inotropic effects of propofol, thiopental, midazolam, etomidate, and ketamine on isolated human atrial muscle, *Anesthesiology* 84(2):397–403, 1996.
119. Hebbar L, Dorman BH, Clair MJ, et al: Negative and selective effects of propofol on isolated swine myocyte contractile function in pacing-induced congestive heart failure, *Anesthesiology* 86(3):649–659, 1997.
120. Sprung J, Ogletree-Hughes ML, McConnell BK, et al: The effects of propofol on the contractility of failing and nonfailing human heart muscles, *Anesth Analg* 93(3):550–559, 2001.
121. Zhou W, Fontenot HJ, Liu S, et al: Modulation of cardiac calcium channels by propofol, *Anesthesiology* 86(3):670–675, 1997.
122. Zhou W, Fontenot HJ, Wang SN, et al: Propofol-induced alterations in myocardial beta-adrenoceptor binding and responsiveness, *Anesth Analg* 89(3):604–608, 1999.
123. Kurokawa H, Murray PA, Damron DS: Propofol attenuates beta-adrenoreceptor-mediated signal transduction via a protein kinase C-dependent pathway in cardiomyocytes, *Anesthesiology* 96(3):688–698, 2002.
124. Kanaya N, Gable B, Murray PA, et al: Propofol increases phosphorylation of troponin I and myosin light chain 2 via protein kinase C activation in cardiomyocytes, *Anesthesiology* 98(6):1363–1371, 2003.
125. Kolh P, Lambermont B, Ghuysen A, et al: Comparison of the effects of propofol and pentobarbital on left ventricular adaptation to an increased afterload, *J Cardiovasc Pharmacol* 44(3):294–301, 2004.
126. Zheng D, Upton RN, Martinez AM: The contribution of the coronary concentrations of propofol to its cardiovascular effects in anesthetized sheep, *Anesth Analg* 96(6):1589–1597, table of contents, 2003.
127. Kehl F, Kress TT, Mraovic B, et al: Propofol alters left atrial function evaluated with pressure-volume relations in vivo, *Anesth Analg* 94(6):1421–1426, table of contents, 2002.
128. Javadov SA, Lim KH, Kerr PM, et al: Protection of hearts from reperfusion injury by propofol is associated with inhibition of the mitochondrial permeability transition, *Cardiovasc Res* 45(2):360–369, 2000.
129. Ko SH, Yu CW, Lee SK, et al: Propofol attenuates ischemia-reperfusion injury in the isolated rat heart, *Anesth Analg* 85(4):719–724, 1997.
130. Kokita N, Hara A: Propofol attenuates hydrogen peroxide-induced mechanical and metabolic derangements in the isolated rat heart, *Anesthesiology* 84(1):117–127, 1996.
131. Kokita N, Hara A, Arakawa J, et al: Propofol improves functional and metabolic recovery in ischemic reperfused isolated rat hearts, *Anesth Analg* 86(2):252–258, 1998.
132. Mathur S, Farhangkhgoee P, Karmazyn M: Cardioprotective effects of propofol and sevoflurane in ischemic and reperfused rat hearts: Role of K(ATP) channels and interaction with the sodium-hydrogen exchange inhibitor HOE 642 (cariporide), *Anesthesiology* 91(5):1349–1360, 1999.
133. Kahraman S, Demiryurek AT: Propofol is a peroxynitrite scavenger, *Anesth Analg* 84(5):1127–1129, 1997.
134. Murphy PG, Myers DS, Davies MJ, et al: The antioxidant potential of propofol (2,6-diisopropylphenol), *Br J Anaesth* 68(6):613–618, 1992.
135. Tsuchiya M, Asada A, Kasahara E, et al: Antioxidant protection of propofol and its recycling in erythrocyte membranes, *Am J Respir Crit Care Med* 165(1):54–60, 2002.
136. Tsuchiya M, Asada A, Maeda K, et al: Propofol versus midazolam regarding their antioxidant activities, *Am J Respir Crit Care Med* 163(1):26–31, 2001.
137. Murphy PG, Ogilvy AJ, Whiteley SM: The effect of propofol on the neutrophil respiratory burst, *Eur J Anaesthesiol* 13(5):471–473, 1996.
138. Murphy PG, Bennett JR, Myers DS, et al: The effect of propofol anaesthesia on free radical-induced lipid peroxidation in rat liver microsomes, *Eur J Anaesthesiol* 10(4):261–266, 1993.
139. Molojavyi A, Preckel B, Comfere T, et al: Effects of ketamine and its isomers on ischemic preconditioning in the isolated rat heart, *Anesthesiology* 94(4):623–629, discussion 5A6A, 2001.
140. Mullenheim J, Frässdorf J, Preckel B, et al: Ketamine, but not S (+)-ketamine, blocks ischemic preconditioning in rabbit hearts in vivo, *Anesthesiology* 94(4):630–636, 2001.
141. Mullenheim J, Rulands R, Wietschorke T, et al: Late preconditioning is blocked by racemic ketamine, but not by S(+)-ketamine, *Anesth Analg* 93(2):265–270, 2001.
142. Ko SH, Lee SK, Han YJ, et al: Blockade of myocardial ATP-sensitive potassium channels by ketamine, *Anesthesiology* 87(1):68–74, 1997.
143. Rouby JJ, Andreev A, Leger P, et al: Peripheral vascular effects of thiopental and propofol in humans with artificial hearts, *Anesthesiology* 75(1):32–42, 1991.
144. Biddle NL, Gelb AW, Hamilton JT: Propofol differentially attenuates the responses to exogenous and endogenous norepinephrine in the isolated rat femoral artery in vitro, *Anesth Analg* 80(4):793–799, 1995.
145. Chang KSK, Davis RF: Propofol produces endothelium-independent vasodilation and may act as a Ca2+ channel blocker, *Anesth Analg* 76(1):24–32, 1993.
146. Gelb AW, Zhang C, Hamilton JT: Propofol induces dilation and inhibits constriction in guinea pig basilar arteries, *Anesth Analg* 83(3):472–476, 1996.
147. Park WK, Lynch C 3rd, Johns RA: Effects of propofol and thiopental in isolated rat aorta and pulmonary artery, *Anesthesiology* 77(5):956–963, 1992.
148. Imura N, Shiraishi Y, Katsuya H, et al: Effect of propofol on norepinephrine-induced increases in [Ca2+] (i) and force in smooth muscle of the rabbit mesenteric resistance artery, *Anesthesiology* 88(6):1566–1578, 1998.
149. Tanabe K, Kozawa O, Kaida T, et al: Inhibitory effects of propofol on intracellular signaling by endothelin-1 in aortic smooth muscle cells, *Anesthesiology* 88(2):452–460, 1998.
150. MacPherson RD, Rasiah RL, McLeod LJ: Propofol attenuates the myogenic response of vascular smooth muscle, *Anesth Analg* 76(4):822–829, 1993.
151. Berkowitz DE, Gaine S: Overview of the perioperative management of the patient with primary pulmonary hypertension, *Probl Anesth* 13:224, 2001.
152. Horibe M, Ogawa K, Sohn JT, Murray PA: Propofol attenuates acetylcholine-induced pulmonary vasorelaxation: Role of nitric oxide and endothelium-derived hyperpolarizing factors, *Anesthesiology* 93(2):447–455, 2000.
153. Kondo U, Kim SO, Murray PA: Propofol selectively attenuates endothelium-dependent pulmonary vasodilation in chronically instrumented dogs, *Anesthesiology* 93(2):437–446, 2000.
154. Tanaka S, Kanaya N, Homma Y, et al: Propofol increases pulmonary artery smooth muscle myofilament calcium sensitivity: Role of protein kinase C, *Anesthesiology* 97(6):1557–1566, 2002.
155. Kondo U, Kim SO, Nakayama M, et al: Pulmonary vascular effects of propofol at baseline, during elevated vasomotor tone, and in response to sympathetic [alpha]- and [beta]-adrenoreceptor activation, *Anesthesiology* 94(5):815–823, 2001.
156. Miyawaki I, Nakamura K, Terasako K, et al: Modification of endothelium-dependent relaxation by propofol, ketamine, and midazolam, *Anesth Analg* 81(3):474–479, 1995.
157. Yamashita A, Kajikuri J, Ohashi M, et al: Inhibitory effects of propofol on acetylcholine-induced, endothelium-dependent relaxation and prostacyclin synthesis in rabbit mesenteric resistance arteries, *Anesthesiology* 91(4):1080–1089, 1999.
158. Gursoy S, Berkan O, Bagcivan I, et al: Effects of intravenous anesthetics on the human radial artery used as a coronary artery bypass graft, *J Cardiothorac Vasc Anesth* 21:41–44, 2007.
159. Robinson BJ, Ebert TJ, O'Brien TJ, et al: Mechanisms whereby propofol mediates peripheral vasodilation in humans. Sympathoinhibition or direct vascular relaxation? *Anesthesiology* 86(1):64–72, 1997.
160. Sellgren J, Ejnell H, Elam M, et al: Sympathetic muscle nerve activity, peripheral blood flows, and baroreceptor reflexes in humans during propofol anesthesia and surgery, *Anesthesiology* 80(3):534–544, 1994.
161. Yang CY, Luk HN, Chen SY, et al: Propofol inhibits medullary pressor mechanisms in cats, *Can J Anaesth* 44(7):775–781, 1997.
162. Yang CY, Wu WC, Chai CY, et al: Propofol inhibits neuronal firing activities in the caudal ventrolateral medulla, *Chang Gung Med J* 26(8):570–577, 2003.
163. Shiga Y, Minami K, Segawa K, et al: The inhibition of aortic smooth muscle cell proliferation by the intravenous anesthetic ketamine, *Anesth Analg* 99(5):1408–1412, table of contents, 2004.
164. Tanabe K, Dohi S, Matsuno H, et al: Midazolam stimulates vascular endothelial growth factor release in aortic smooth muscle cells: Role of the mitogen-activated protein kinase superfamily, *Anesthesiology* 98(5):1147–1154, 2003.
165. Olesen AS, Huttel MS, Hole P: Venous sequelae following the injection of etomidate or thiopentone I.V, *Br J Anaesth* 56(2):171–173, 1984.
166. Christensen J, Andreasen F, Jansen J: Pharmacokinetics and pharmacodynamics of thiopentone: A comparison between young and elderly patients, *Anaesthesia* 37:398, 1982.
167. Christensen JH, Andreasen F, Jansen JA: Pharmacokinetics of thiopentone in a group of young women and a group of young men, *Br J Anaesth* 52(9):913–918, 1980.
168. Ghoneim MM, Van Hamme MJ: Pharmacokinetics of thiopentone: Effects of enflurane and nitrous oxide anaesthesia and surgery, *Br J Anaesth* 50(12):1237–1242, 1978.
169. Morgan DJ, Blackman GL, Paull JD, et al: Pharmacokinetics and plasma binding of thiopental. I: Studies in surgical patients, *Anesthesiology* 54(6):468–473, 1981.
170. Brodie BB, Mark LC: The fate of thiopental in man and a method for its estimation in biological material, *J Pharmacol Exp Ther* 98(1):85–96, 1950.
171. Christensen JH, Andreasen F, Jansen JA: Influence of age and sex on the pharmacokinetics of thiopentone, *Br J Anaesth* 53(11):1189–1195, 1981.
172. Heikkila H, Jalone J, Arola M, et al: Midazolam as adjunct to high-dose fentanyl anaesthesia for coronary artery bypass grafting operation, *Acta Anaesthesiol Scand* 28:683, 1984.
173. Lehot J, Boulieu R, Foussadier A, et al: Comparison of the pharmacokinetics of methohexital during cardiac surgery with cardiopulmonary bypass and vascular surgery, *J Cardiothorac Vasc Anesth* 7(1):30–34, 1993.
174. Bailey JM, Mora CT, Shafer SL: Pharmacokinetics of propofol in adult patients undergoing coronary revascularization. The Multicenter Study of Perioperative Ischemia Research Group, *Anesthesiology* 84(6):1288–1297, 1996.
175. Sorbo S, Hudson RJ, Loomis JC: The pharmacokinetics of thiopental in pediatric surgical patients, *Anesthesiology* 61(6):666–670, 1984.
176. Christensen JH, Andreasen F, Kristoffersen MB: Comparison of the anaesthetic and haemodynamic effects of chlormethiazole and thiopentone, *Br J Anaesth* 55(5):391–397, 1983.
177. Filner BE, Karliner JS: Alterations of normal left ventricular performance by general anesthesia, *Anesthesiology* 45(6):610–621, 1976.
178. Flickinger H, Fraimow W, Cathcart R, et al: Effect of thiopental induction on cardiac output in man, *Anesth Analg* 40:693–700, 1961.
179. Nauta J, Stanley TH, de Lange S, et al: Anaesthetic induction with alfentanil: Comparison with thiopental, midazolam, and etomidate, *Can Anaesth Soc J* 30(1):53–60, 1983.
180. Seltzer JL, Gerson JI, Allen FB: Comparison of the cardiovascular effects of bolus v. incremental administration of thiopentone, *Br J Anaesth* 52(5):527–530, 1980.
181. Sonntag H, Hellberg K, Schenk H, et al: Effects of thiopental (Trapanal) on coronary blood flow and myocardial metabolism in man, *Acta Anaesthesiol Scand* 19(1):69–78, 1975.
182. White PF: Comparative evaluation of intravenous agents for rapid sequence induction—thiopental, ketamine, and midazolam, *Anesthesiology* 57(4):279–284, 1982.
183. Fischler M, Dubois C, Brodaty D, et al: Circulatory responses to thiopentone and tracheal intubation in patients with coronary artery disease. Effects of pretreatment with labetalol, *Br J Anaesth* 57(5):493–496, 1985.
184. Lyons SM, Clarke RS: A comparison of different drugs for anaesthesia in cardiac surgical patients, *Br J Anaesth* 44(6):575–583, 1972.

185. Milocco BA, Löf, William-Olsson G, et al: Haemodynamic stability during anaesthesia induction and sternotomy in patients with ischaemic heart disease, *Acta Anaesthesiol Scand* 29(5):465–473, 1985.
186. Reiz S, Balfors E, Friedman A, et al: Effects of thiopentone on cardiac performance, coronary hemodynamics and myocardial oxygen consumption in chronic ischemic heart disease, *Acta Anaesthesiol Scand* 25(2):103–110, 1981.
187. Tarabadkar S, Kopriva CJ, Sreenivasan N, et al: Hemodynamic impact of induction in patients with decreased cardiac reserve, *Anesthesiology* 53(3):S43, 1980.
188. Tarnow J, Hess W, Klein W: Etomidate, alfathesin and thiopentone as induction agents for coronary artery surgery, *Can J Anesth* 27(4):338–344, 1980.
189. Toner W, Howard P, McGowan W, et al: Another look at acute tolerance to thiopentone, *Br J Anaesth* 52(10):1005–1009, 1980.
190. Frankl WS, Poole-Wilson PA: Effects of thiopental on tension development, action potential, and exchange of calcium and potassium in rabbit ventricular myocardium, *J Cardiovasc Pharmacol* 3(3):554–565, 1981.
191. White PF, Way WL, Trevor AJ: Ketamine—its pharmacology and therapeutic uses, *Anesthesiology* 56(2):119–136, 1982.
192. Eckstein JW, Hamilton WK, Mc CJ: The effect of thiopental on peripheral venous tone, *Anesthesiology* 22:525–528, 1961.
193. Kissin I, Motomura S, Aultman D, et al: Inotropic and anesthetic potencies of etomidate and thiopental in dogs, *Anesth Analg* 62(11):961–965, 1983.
194. Komai H, Rusy BF: Differences in the myocardial depressant action of thiopental and halothane, *Anesth Analg* 63(3):313–318, 1984.
195. Pedersen T, Engbaek J, Klausen N, et al: Effects of low-dose ketamine and thiopentone on cardiac performance and myocardial oxygen balance in high-risk patients, *Acta Anaesthesiol Scand* 26(3):235–239, 1982.
196. Nussmeier NA, Arlund C, Slogoff S: Neuropsychiatric complications after cardiopulmonary bypass: Cerebral protection by a barbiturate, *Anesthesiology* 64(2):165–170, 1986.
197. Zaidan J, Klochany A, Martin W, et al: Effect of thiopental on neurologic outcome following coronary artery bypass grafting, *Anesthesiology* 74(3):406–411, 1991.
198. Ito S, Tanaka A, Arakawa M, et al: [Influence of thiopental administration on peripheral circulation during cardiac surgery with extracorporeal circulation], *Masui* 41(1):59–66, 1992.
199. Reves J, Fragen R, Vinik H, et al: Midazolam: Pharmacology and uses, *Anesthesiology* 62(3):310–324, 1985.
200. Dundee JW, Kawar P: Consistency of action of midazolam, *Anesth Analg* 61(6):544–545, 1982.
201. Gross JB, Caldwell CB, Edwards MW: Induction dose-response curves for midazolam and ketamine in premedicated ASA class III and IV patients, *Anesth Analg* 64(8):795–800, 1985.
202. Reves JG, Kissin I, Smith LR: The effective dose of midazolam, *Anesthesiology* 55(1):82, 1981.
203. Reves J, Samuelson P, Vinik H: Consistency of midazolam, *Anesth Analg* 61:545, 1982.
204. Allonen H, Ziegler G, Klotz U: Midazolam kinetics, *Clin Pharmacol Ther* 30(5):653–661, 1981.
205. Brown CR, Sarnquist FH, Canup CA, et al: Clinical, electroencephalographic, and pharmacokinetic studies of a water-soluble benzodiazepine, midazolam maleate, *Anesthesiology* 50(5):467–470, 1979.
206. Greenblatt D, Loeniskar A, Ochs H, et al: Automated gas chromatography for studies of midazolam pharmacokinetics, *Anesthesiology* 55(2):176–179, 1981.
207. Heizmann P, Eckert M, Ziegler WH: Pharmacokinetics and bioavailability of midazolam in man, *Br J Clin Pharmacol* 16(Suppl 1):43S–49S, 1983.
208. Puglisi CV, Meyer JC, D'Arconte L, et al: Determination of water soluble imidazo-1,4-benzodiazepines in blood by electron-capture gas—liquid chromatography and in urine by differential pulse polaragraphy, *J Chromatogr* 145(1):81–96, 1978.
209. Forster A, Gardaz JP, Suter PM, et al: I.V. midazolam as an induction agent for anaesthesia: A study in volunteers, *Br J Anaesth* 52(9):907–911, 1980.
210. Lebowitz P, Cote M, Daniels A, et al: Comparative cardiovascular effects of midazolam and thiopental in healthy patients, *Anesth Analg* 61(9):771–775, 1982.
211. Lebowitz P, Cote M, Daniels A, et al: Cardiovascular effects of midazolam and thiopentone for induction of anaesthesia in ill surgical patients, *Can Anaesth Soc J* 30(1):19–23, 1983.
212. Fragen R, Meyers S, Barresi V, et al: Hemodynamic effects of midazolam in cardiac patients, *Anesthesiology* 51(3):S104, 1979.
213. Marty J, Nitenberg A, Blancet F, et al: Effects of midazolam on the coronary circulation in patients with coronary artery disease, *Anesthesiology* 64(2):206–210, 1986.
214. Massaut J, d'Hollander A, Barvais L, et al: Haemodynamic effects of midazolam in the anaesthetized patient with coronary artery disease, *Acta Anaesthesiol Scand* 27(4):299–302, 1983.
215. Reves J, Samuelson P, Lewis S: Midazolam maleate induction in patients with ischaemic heart disease: Haemodynamic observations, *Can J Anesth* 26(5):402–409, 1979.
216. Reves J, Samuelson P, Linnan M: Effects of midazolam maleate in patients with elevated pulmonary artery occluded pressure. In Aldrete J, Stanley T, editors: *Trends in intravenous anesthesia*, Miami, USA: Symposia Specialists Inc., 1980, p 253.
217. Samuelson P, Reves J, Kouchoukos N, et al: Hemodynamic responses to anesthetic induction with midazolam or diazepam in patients with ischemic heart disease, *Anesth Analg* 60(11):802–809, 1981.
218. Schulte-Sasse UWE, Hess W, Tarnow J: Haemodynamic responses to induction of anaesthesia using midazolam in cardiac surgical patients, *Br J Anaesth* 54(10):1053–1058, 1982.
219. Kwar P, Carson I, Clarke R, et al: Haemodynamic changes during induction of anaesthesia with midazolam and diazepam (Valium) in patients undergoing coronary artery bypass surgery, *Anaesthesia* 40(8):767–771, 1985.
220. Samuelson PN, Reves JG, Smith LR, et al: Midazolam versus diazepam: Different effects on systemic vascular resistance. A randomized study utilizing cardiopulmonary bypass constant flow, *Arzneimittelforschung* 31(12a):2268–2269, 1981.
221. Tomichek R, Rosow C, Schneider R, et al: Cardiovascular effects of diazepam-fentanyl anesthesia in patients with coronary artery disease, *Anesth Analg* 61:217, 1982.
222. Newman M, Reves J: Pro: midazolam is the sedative of choice to supplement narcotic anesthesia, *J Cardiothorac Vasc Anesth* 7:615, 1993.
223. Theil D, Stanley T, White W, et al: Midazolam and fentanyl continuous infusion anesthesia for cardiac surgery: A comparison of computer-assisted versus manual infusion systems, *J Cardiothorac Vasc Anesth* 7(3):300–306, 1993.
224. Godefroi EF, Janssen PA, Vandereycken CA, et al: DL-1-(1-Arylalkyl)imidazole-5-carboxylate esters. A novel type of hypnotic agents, *J Med Chem* 8(2):220–223, 1965.
225. Kissin I, McGee T, Smith LR: The indices of potency for intravenous anaesthetics, *Can Anaesth Soc J* 28(6):585–590, 1981.
226. Ghoneim MM, Yamada T: Etomidate: A clinical and electroencephalographic comparison with thiopental, *Anesth Analg* 56(4):479–485, 1977.
227. Fragen RJ, Caldwell N: Comparison of a new formulation of etomidate with thiopental—side effects and awakening times, *Anesthesiology* 50(3):242–244, 1979.
228. Horrigan RW, Moyers JR, Johnson BH, et al: Etomidate vs. thiopental with and without fentanyl: A comparative study of awakening in man, *Anesthesiology* 52(4):362–364, 1980.
229. Schuermans V, Dom J, Dony J, et al: Multinational evaluation of etomidate for anesthesia induction. Conclusions and consequences, *Anaesthesist* 27(2):52–59, 1978.
230. Ghoneim MM, Van Hamme MJ: Hydrolysis of etomidate, *Anesthesiology* 50(3):227–229, 1979.
231. Fragen R, Shanks C, Molteni A, et al: Effects of etomidate on hormonal responses to surgical stress, *Anesthesiology* 61(6):652–656, 1984.
232. Wagner RL, White PF: Etomidate inhibits adrenocortical function in surgical patients, *Anesthesiology* 61(6):647–651, 1984.
233. Wanscher M, Tønnesen E, Hüttel M, et al: Etomidate infusion and adrenocortical function. A study in elective surgery, *Acta Anaesthesiol Scand* 29(5):483–485, 1985.
234. Schrag S, Pawlik M, Mohn U, et al: The role of ascorbic acid and xylitol in etomidate-induced adrenocortical suppression in humans, *Eur J Anaesthesiol* 13(4):346–351, 1996.
235. Ammon J, Fogdall R, Garman J: *Hemodynamic effects of etomidate and thiopental in patients undergoing cardiac surgery*, Palo Alto, CA, Stanford University. Unpublished manuscript.
236. Doenicke A, Gabanyi D, Lemcke H, et al: Circulatory behaviour and myocardial function after the administration of three short-acting IV hypnotics: Etomidate, propanidid, and methohexital, *Anaesthetist* 23:108, 1974.
237. Firestone S, Kleinman CS, Jaffe CC, et al: Human research and noninvasive measurement of ventricular performance: An echocardiographic evaluation of etomidate and thiopental, *Anesthesiology* 51(3):S23, 1979.
238. Hempelmann G, Piepenbrock S, Hempelmann W: Influence of althesin and etomidate on blood gases (continuous PO2 monitoring) and hemodynamics in man, *Acta Anaesthesiol Belg* 25:402, 1974.
239. Kettler D, Sonntag H, Wolfram-Donath U, et al: Haemodynamics, myocardial function, oxygen requirement, and oxygen supply of the human heart after administration of etomidate. In DA, editors: *Anaesthesiology and resuscitation*, Berlin: Springer-Verlag, 1977.
240. Lamalle D: Cardiovascular effects of various anesthetics in man. Four short-acting intravenous anesthetics: Althesin, etomidate, methohexital and propanidid, *Acta Anaesthesiol Scand* 27:2008, 1976.
241. Patschke D, Pruckner J, Eberlein J, et al: Effects of althesin, etomidate and fentanyl on haemodynamics and myocardial oxygen consumption in man, *Can Anaesth Soc J* 24(1):57–69, 1977.
242. Gooding JM, Corssen G: Effect of etomidate on the cardiovascular system, *Anesth Analg* 56(5):717–719, 1977.
243. Colvin M, Savege T, Newland P, et al: Cardiorespiratory changes following induction of anaesthesia with etomidate in patients with cardiac disease, *Br J Anaesth* 51(6):551–556, 1979.
244. Gooding JM, Weng JT, Smith RA, et al: Cardiovascular and pulmonary responses following etomidate induction of anesthesia in patients with demonstrated cardiac disease, *Anesth Analg* 58(1):40–41, 1979.
245. Criado A, Maseda J, Navarro E, et al: Induction of anaesthesia with etomidate: Haemodynamic study of 36 patients, *Br J Anaesth* 52(8):803–806, 1980.
246. Prakash O, Dhasmana KM, Verdouw PD, et al: Cardiovascular effects of etomidate with emphasis on regional myocardial blood flow and performance, *Br J Anaesth* 53(6):591–600, 1981.
247. Riou B, Lecarpentier Y, Chemla D, et al: In vitro effects of etomidate on intrinsic myocardial contractility in the rat, *Anesthesiology* 72(2):330–340, 1990.
248. Kates R, Stack R, Hill R, et al: General anesthesia for patients undergoing percutaneous transluminal coronary angioplasty during acute myocardial infarction, *Anesth Analg* 65(7):815–818, 1986.
249. Wauquier A, HC, Van den Brock W, et al: *Resuscitative drugs effects in hypovolemic-hypotensive animals. Part I. Comparative cardiovascular effects of an infusion of saline, etomidate, thiopental or pentobarbital in hypovolemic dogs*, Unpublished observations.
250. Corssen G, Domino EF: Dissociative anesthesia: Further pharmacologic studies and first clinical experience with the phencyclidine derivative Cl-581, *Anesth Analg* (45):29, 1966.
251. Hudetz JA, Patterson KM, Iqbal Z, et al: Ketamine attenuated delirium after cardiac surgery with cardiopulmonary bypass, *J Cardiothorac Vasc Anesth* 23:651–657, 2009.
252. Nishimura K, Kitamura Y, Hamai R, et al: Pharmacological studies of ketamine hydrochloride in the cardiovascular system, *Osaka City Med J* 19(1):17–26, 1973.
253. Stanley TH: Blood-pressure and pulse-rate responses to ketamine during general anesthesia, *Anesthesiology* 39(6):648–649, 1973.
254. Stanley V, Hunt J, Willis KW, et al: Cardiovascular and respiratory function with CI-581, *Anesth Analg* 47(6):760–768, 1968.
255. Tweed WA, Minuck M, Mymin D: Circulatory responses to ketamine anesthesia, *Anesthesiology* 37(6):613–619, 1972.
256. Tweed WA, Mymin D: Myocardial force-velocity relations during ketamine anesthesia at constant heart rate, *Anesthesiology* 41(1):49–52, 1974.
257. Virtue RW, Alanis JM, Mori M, et al: An anesthetic agent: 2-orthochlorophenyl, 2- methylamino cyclohexanone HCl (CI-581), *Anesthesiology* 28(5):823–833, 1967.
258. Lippman M, Appel P, Mok M, et al: Sequential cardiorespiratory patterns of anesthetic induction with ketamine in critically ill patients, *Crit Care Med* 11(9):730–734, 1983.
259. Stefansson T, Wickstrom I, Haljamae H: Hemodynamic and metabolic effects of ketamine anesthesia in the geriatric patient, *Acta Anaesthesiol Scand* 26(4):371–377, 1982.
260. Balfors E, Haggmark S, Nyhman H, et al: Droperidol inhibits the effects of intravenous ketamine on central hemodynamics and myocardial oxygen consumption in patients with generalized atherosclerotic disease, *Anesth Analg* 62(2):193–197, 1983.
261. Corssen G, Moustapha I, Varner E: The role of dissociative anaesthesia with ketamine in cardiac surgery: A preliminary report based on 253 patients. In *Asia-Australian Congress of Anaesthesiologists*, Singapore, 1974.
262. Dhadphale PR, Jackson APF, Alseri S: Comparison of anesthesia with diazepam and ketamine vs. morphine in patients undergoing heart-valve replacement, *Anesthesiology* 51(3):200–203, 1979.
263. Greeley W, Bushman G, Davis D: *Comparative effects of two induction techniques in arterial oxygen saturation during pediatric cardiovascular surgery*, Society of Cardiovascular Anesthesiologists, Richmond, VA.
264. Hobika G, Evers J, Mostert J, et al: Comparison of hemodynamic effects of glucagon and ketamine in patients with chronic renal failure, *Anesthesiology* 37(6):654–658, 1972.
265. Jackson A, Dhadphale P, Callaghan M, et al: Haemodynamic studies during induction of anaesthesia for open-heart surgery using diazepam and ketamine, *Br J Anaesth* 50:375, 1978.
266. Lyons S, Clarke R, Dundee J: Some cardiovascular and respiratory effects of four non-barbiturate anesthetic induction agents, *Eur J Clin Pharmacol* 6:61, 1974.
267. Morray J, Lynn A, Stamm S, et al: Hemodynamic effects of ketamine in children with congenital heart disease, *Anesth Analg* 63(10):895–899, 1984.
268. Savage T, Colvin M, Weaver E, et al: A comparison of some cardiorespiratory effects of althesin and ketamine when used for induction of anaesthesia in patients with cardiac disease, *Br J Anaesth* 48(11):1071–1081, 1976.
269. Sonntag H, Knoll HHD: Coronary blood flow and myocardial oxygen consumption in patients during induction of anesthesia with droperidol/fentanyl or ketamine, *Z Kreislaufforsch* 61:1092, 1972.
270. Spotoft H, Korshin J, Sorensen M, et al: The cardiovascular effects of ketamine used for induction of anaesthesia in patients with valvular heart disease, *Can J Anesth* 26(6):463–467, 1979.
271. Gooding J, Dimick A, Tavakoli M, et al: A physiologic analysis of cardiopulmonary responses to ketamine anesthesia in noncardiac patients, *Anesth Analg* 56(6):813–816, 1977.
272. Zsigmond E: Guest discussion, *Anesth Analg* 53:931, 1974.
273. McIntyre JW, Dobson D, Aitken G: Ketamine with pancuronium for induction of anaesthesia, *Can Anaesth Soc J* 21(5):475–481, 1974.
274. Neuhauser C, Preiss V, Feurer MK, et al: Comparison of S-(+)-ketamine with sufentanil-based anaesthesia for elective coronary artery bypass graft surgery: Effect on troponin T levels, *Br J Anesth* 100:765–771, 2008.

275. Riou B, Lecarpentier Y, Viars P: Inotropic effect of ketamine on rat cardiac papillary muscle, *Anesthesiology* 71(1):116–125, 1989.
276. Riou B, Viars P, Lecarpentier Y: Effects of ketamine on the cardiac papillary muscle of normal hamsters and those with cardiomyopathy, *Anesthesiology* 73(5):910–918, 1990.
277. Dowdy EG, Kaya K: Studies of the mechanism of cardiovascular responses to CI-581, *Anesthesiology* 29(5):931–942, 1968.
278. Urthaler F, Walker AA, James TN: Comparison of the inotropic action of morphine and ketamine studied in canine cardiac muscle, *J Thorac Cardiovasc Surg* 72(1):142–149, 1976.
279. Valicenti J, Newman W, Bagwell E, et al: Myocardial contractility during induction and steady-state ketamine anesthesia, *Anesth Analg* 52(2):190–194, 1973.
280. Ivankovich A, Miletich D, Reimann C, et al: Cardiovascular effects of centrally administered ketamine in goats, *Anesth Analg* 53(6):924–933, 1974.
281. Zsigmond E, Kothary S, Matsuki A, et al: Diazepam for prevention of he rise of plasma catecholamines caused by ketamine, *Clin Pharmacol Ther* 15:223, 1974.
282. Kumar SM, Kothary SP, Zsigmond EK: Plasma free norepinephrine and epinephrine concentrations following diazepam-ketamine induction in patients undergoing cardiac surgery, *Acta Anaesthesiol Scand* 22(6):593–600, 1978.
283. Clanachan AS, McGrath JC, MacKenzie JE: Cardiovascular effects of ketamine in the pithed rat, rabbit and cat, *Br J Anaesth* 48(10):935–939, 1976.
284. Saini V, Carr DB, Hagestad EL, et al: Antifibrillatory action of the narcotic agonist fentanyl, *Am Heart J* 115(3):598–605, 1988.
285. Slogoff S, Allen GW: The role of baroreceptors in the cardiovascular response to ketamine, *Anesth Analg* 53(5):704–707, 1974.
286. Traber DL, Wilson RD: Involvement of the sympathetic nervous system in the pressor response to ketamine, *Anesth Analg* 48(2):248–252, 1969.
287. Traber DL, Wilson RD, Priano LL: Differentiation of the cardiovascular effects of CI-581, *Anesth Analg* 47(6):769–778, 1968.
288. Traber DL, Wilson RD, Priano LL: Blockade of the hypertensive response to ketamine, *Anesth Analg* 49(3):420–426, 1970.
289. Traber DL, Wilson RD, Priano LL: The effect of beta-adrenergic blockade on the cardiopulmonary response to ketamine, *Anesth Analg* 49(4):604–613, 1970.
290. Traber DL, Wilson RD, Priano LL: A detailed study of the cardiopulmonary response to ketamine and its blockade by atropine, *South Med J* 63(9):1077–1081, 1970.
291. Hill G, Wong K, Shaw C, et al: Interactions of ketamine with vasoactive amines at normothermia and hypothermia in the isolated rabbit heart, *Anesthesiology* 48:315, 1978.
292. Miletich D, Ivankovich A, Albrecht R, et al: The effect of ketamine on catecholamine metabolism in the isolated perfused rat heart, *Anesthesiology* 39(3):271–277, 1973.
293. Freuchen I, Ostergaard J, Kuhl J, et al: Reduction of psychotomimetic side effects of Ketalar (ketamine) by Rohypnol (flunitrazepam), *Acta Anaesthsiol Scand* 20:97, 1976.
294. Hatano S, Keane D, Boggs R, et al: Diazepam-ketamine anaesthesia for open heart surgery: a "micro-mini" drip administration technique, *Can Anaesth Soc J* 23:648, 1976.
295. Pedersen T, Engbaek J, Ording H, et al: Effect of vecuronium and pancuronium on cardiac performance and transmural myocardial perfusion during ketamine anaesthesia, *Acta Anaesthesiol Scand* 28:443, 1984.
296. Levanen J, Makela ML, Scheinin H: Dexmedetomidine premedication attenuates ketamine-induced cardiostimulatory effects and postanesthetic delirium, *Anesthesiology* 82(5):1117–1125, 1995.
297. Corssen G, Reves J, Carter J: Neurolept anesthesia, dissociative anesthesia, and hemorrhage, *Int Anesthesiol Clin* 12:145, 1974.
298. Nettles DC, Herrin TJ, Mullen JG: Ketamine induction in poor-risk patients, *Anesth Analg* 52(1):59–64, 1973.
299. Kingston H, Bretherton K, Halloway A, et al: A comparison between ketamine and diazepam as induction agents for pericardiectomy, *Anaesth Intensive Care* 6:66, 1978.
300. Patel K, Gelman S, McElvein R: Ketamine in patients with pericarditis: Hemodynamic effects. In *VI European Congress of Anaesthesiology,* 427, 1982.
301. Adam H, Briggs L, Bahar M, et al: Pharmacokinetic evaluation of ICI 35 868 in man. Single induction doses with different rates of injection, *Br J Anaesth* 55(2):97–103, 1983.
302. Simons P, Cockshott I, Douglas E, et al: Blood concentrations, metabolism and elimination after a subanesthetic dose of 4C-propofol (Diprivan) to volunteers, *Postgrad Med J* 61:64, 1985.
303. Kay NH, Sear JW, Uppington J, et al: Disposition of propofol in patients undergoing surgery: A comparison in men and women, *Br J Anaesth* 58(10):1075–1079, 1986.
304. Kirkpatrick T, Cockshott I, Douglas E, et al: Pharmacokinetics of propofol (diprivan) in elderly patients, *Br J Anaesth* 60(2):146–150, 1988.
305. Coates DP, Monk CR, Prys-Roberts C, et al: Hemodynamic effects of infusions of the emulsion formulation of propofol during nitrous oxide anesthesia in humans, *Anesth Analg* 66(1):64–70, 1987.
306. Claeys MA, Gepts E, Camu F: Haemodynamic changes during anaesthesia induced and maintained with propofol, *Br J Anaesth* 60(1):3–9, 1988.
307. Monk CR, Coates DP, Prys-Roberts C, et al: Haemodynamic effects of a prolonged infusion of propofol as a supplement to nitrous oxide anaesthesia: Studies in association with peripheral arterial surgery, *Br J Anaesth* 59(8):954–960, 1987.
308. Stephan H, Sonntag H, Schenk H, et al: Effects of propofol on cardiovascular dynamics, myocardial blood flow and myocardial metabolism in patients with coronary artery disease, *Br J Anaesth* 58(9):969–975, 1986.
309. Vermeyen K, Erpels F, Janssen L, et al: Propofol-fentanyl anaesthesia for coronary bypass surgery in patients with good left ventricular function, *Br J Anaesth* 59(9):1115–1120, 1987.
310. Brussel T, Theissen J, Vigfusson G, et al: Hemodynamic and cardiodynamic effects of propofol and etomidate: Negative inotropic properties of propofol, *Anesth Analg* 69(1):35–40, 1989.
311. De Hert SG, Vermeyen KM, Adriaensen HF: Influence of thiopental, etomidate, and propofol on regional myocardial function in the normal and acute ischemic heart segment in dogs, *Anesth Analg* 70(6):600–607, 1990.
312. Mulier J, Wouters P, van Aken H, et al: Cardiodynamic effects of propofol in comparison with thiopental: Assessment with a transesophageal echocardiographic approach, *Anesth Analg* 72(1): 28–35, 1991.
313. Patrick MR, Blair IJ, Feneck RO, et al: A comparison of the haemodynamic effects of propofol ('Diprivan') and thiopentone in patients with coronary artery disease, *Postgrad Med J* 61(Suppl 3):23–27, 1985.
314. Profeta J, Guffin A, Mikula S, et al: The hemodynamic effects of propofol and thiamylal sodium for induction in coronary artery surgery, *Anesth Analg* 66:S142, 1987.
315. Bendel S, Ruokonen E, Polonen P, et al: Propofol causes more hypotension than etomidate in patients with severe aortic stenosis: A double-blind, randomized study comparing propofol and etomidate, *Acta Anaesthesiol Scand* 51:284–289, 2007.
316. Carrasco G, Molina R, Costa J, et al: Propofol vs midazolam in short-, medium-, and long-term sedation of critically ill patients: A cost-benefit analysis, *Chest* 103:557–564, 1993.
317. Mateu J, Barrachina F: Hypertriglyceridaemia associated with propofol sedation in critically ill patients, *Intensive Care Med* 22:834–835, 1996.
318. Theilen H, Adams S, Albrecht MD, et al: Propofol in a medium- and long-chain triglyceride emulsion: Pharmacological characteristics and potential beneficial effects, *Anesth Analg* 4:923–929, 2002.
319. Oztekin I, Gökdo an S, Ozenkin DS, et al: Effects of propofol and midazolam on lipids, glucose, and plasma osmolality during and in the early postoperative period following coronary artery bypass graft surgery: A randomized trial, *Yakugaku Zasshi* 127:173–182, 2007.
320. Newman MF, Murkin JM, Roach G, et al: Cerebral physiologic effects of burst suppression doses of propofol during nonpulsatile cardiopulmonary bypass. CNS Subgroup of McSPI, *Anesth Analg* 81(3):452–457, 1995.
321. Kellow N, Scott A, White S, et al: Comparison of the effects of propofol and isoflurane anaesthesia on right ventricular function and shunt fraction during thoracic surgery, *Br J Anaesth* 75(5):578–582, 1995.
322. Furst SR, Weinger MB: Dexmedetomidine, a selective [alpha]2-agonist, does not potentiate the cardiorespiratory depression of alfentanil in the rat, *Anesthesiology* 72(5):882–888, 1990.
323. Barletta JF, Miedema SL, Wiseman D, et al: Impact of dexmedetomidine on analgesic requirements in patients after cardiac surgery in a fast-track recovery room setting, *Pharmacotherapy* 29:1427–1432, 2009.
324. Gerlach AT, Murphy C, Dasta JF: An updated focused review of dexmedetomidine in adults, *Ann Pharmacother* 43:2064–2074, 2009.
325. Seiber FE, Zakriya K, Gottschalk A, et al: Sedation depth during spinal anesthesia and the development of postoperative delirium in elderly patients undergoing hip fracture repair, *Mayo Clin Proc* 85:18–26, 2010.
326. Beckett AH, Casy AF: Synthetic analgesics: Stereochemical considerations, *J Pharm Pharmacol* 6(12):986–1001, 1954.
327. Portoghese PS: A new concept on the mode of interaction of narcotic analgesics with receptors, *J Med Chem* 8(5):609–616, 1965.
328. Dhawan BN, Cesselin F, Raghubir R, et al: International Union of Pharmacology. XII. Classification of opioid receptors, *Pharmacol Rev* 48(4):567–592, 1996.
329. Martin WR: Pharmacology of opioids, *Pharmacol Rev* 35(4):283–323, 1983.
330. Paterson SJ, Robson LE, Kosterlitz HW: Classification of opioid receptors, *Br Med Bull* 39(1):31–36, 1983.
331. Jiang Q, Takemori AE, Sultana M, et al: Differential antagonism of opioid delta antinociception by [D-Ala2,Leu5,Cys6]enkephalin and naltrindole 5′-isothiocyanate: Evidence for delta receptor subtypes, *J Pharmacol Exp Ther* 257(3):1069–1075, 1991.
332. Mattia A, Vanderah T, Mosberg HI, et al: Lack of antinociceptive cross-tolerance between [D-Pen2, D-Pen5]enkephalin and [D-Ala2]deltorphin II in mice: Evidence for delta receptor subtypes, *J Pharmacol Exp Ther* 258(2):583–587, 1991.
333. Sofuoglu M, Portoghese PS, Takemori AE: Differential antagonism of delta opioid agonists by naltrindole and its benzofuran analog (NTB) in mice: Evidence for delta opioid receptor subtypes, *J Pharmacol Exp Ther* 257(2):676–680, 1991.
334. McDonald J, Lambert DG: Opioid receptors, *Contin Educ Anaesth Crit Care Pain* 5(1):22–25, 2005.
335. Chen Y, Mestek A, Liu J, et al: Molecular cloning and functional expression of a mu-opioid receptor from rat brain, *Mol Pharmacol* 44(1):8–12, 1993.
336. Evans CJ, Keith DE Jr, Morrison H, et al: Cloning of a delta opioid receptor by functional expression, *Science* 258(5090):1952–1955, 1992.
337. Kieffer BL, Befort K, Gaveriaux-Ruff C, et al: The delta-opioid receptor: Isolation of a cDNA by expression cloning and pharmacological characterization, *Proc Natl Acad Sci U S A* 89(24):12048–12052, 1992.
338. Minami M, Toya T, Katao Y, et al: Cloning and expression of a cDNA for the rat kappa-opioid receptor, *FEBS Lett* 329(3):291–295, 1993.
339. McFadzean I: The ionic mechanisms underlying opioid actions, *Neuropeptides* 11(4):173–180, 1988.
340. North R: Opioid receptor types and membranes on ion channels, *Trends Neurosci* 9:114–117, 1986.
341. Rhim H, Miller RJ: Opioid receptors modulate diverse types of calcium channels in the nucleus tractus solitarius of the rat, *J Neurosci* 14(12):7608–7615, 1994.
342. Carta F, Bianchi M, Argenton S, et al: Effect of nifedipine on morphine-induced analgesia, *Anesth Analg* 70(5):493–498, 1990.
343. Santillan R, Maestre JM, Hurle MA, et al: Enhancement of opiate analgesia by nimodipine in cancer patients chronically treated with morphine: A preliminary report, *Pain* 58(1):129–132, 1994.
344. Boldt J, von Bormann B, Kling D, et al: Low-dose fentanyl analgesia modified by calcium channel blockers in cardiac surgery, *Eur J Anaesthesiol* 4(6):387–394, 1987.
345. Crain SM, Shen KF: Opioids can evoke direct receptor-mediated excitatory effects on sensory neurons, *Trends Pharmacol Sci* 11:77, 1990.
346. Smart D, Smith G, Lambert DG: Mu-opioids activate phospholipase C in SH-SY5Y human neuroblastoma cells via calcium-channel opening, *Biochem J* 305(Pt 2):577–581, 1995.
347. Smart D, Smith G, Lambert DG: Mu-opioid receptor stimulation of inositol (1,4,5)triphosphate formation via a pertussis toxin-sensitive G protein, *J Neurochem* 62:1009, 1994.
348. Wandless AL, Smart D, Lambert DG: Fentanyl increases intracellular Ca2+ concentrations in SH-SY5Y cells, *Br J Anaesth* 76(3):461–463, 1996.
349. Krumins SA, Faden AI, Feuerstein G: Opiate binding in rat hearts: Modulation of binding after hemorrhagic shock, *Biochem Biophys Res Commun* 127(1):120–128, 1985.
350. Tai KK, Jin WQ, Chan TK, et al: Characterization of [3H]U69593 binding sites in the rat heart by receptor binding assays, *J Mol Cell Cardiol* 23(11):1297–1302, 1991.
351. Barron BA: Opioid peptides and the heart, *Cardiovasc Res* 43(1):13–16, 1999.
352. Ela C, Barg J, Vogel Z, et al: Distinct components of morphine effects on cardiac myocytes are mediated by the kappa and delta opioid receptors, *J Mol Cell Cardiol* 29(2):711–720, 1997.
353. Ventura C, Bastagli L, Bernardi P, et al: Opioid receptors in rat cardiac sarcolemma: Effect of phenylephrine and isoproterenol, *Biochim Biophys Acta* 987(1):69–74, 1989.
354. Barron BA, Jones CE, Caffrey JL: Pericardial repair depresses canine cardiac catecholamines and met-enkephalin, *Regul Pept* 59(3):313–320, 1995.
355. Vargish T, Beamer KC: Delta and mu receptor agonists correlate with greater depression of cardiac function than morphine sulfate in perfused rat hearts, *Circ Shock* 27:245, 1989.
356. Pokrovsky VM, Osadchiy OE: Regulatory peptides as modulators of vagal influence on cardiac rhythm, *Can J Physiol Pharmacol* 73:1235, 1995.
357. Caffrey JL: Enkephalin inhibits vagal control of heart rate, contractile force and coronary blood flow in the canine heart in vivo, *J Auton Nerv Syst* 76(2–3):75–82, 1999.
358. Akil H, Watson S, Young E, et al: Endogenous opioids: Biology and function, *Annu Rev Neurosci* 7:223, 1984.
359. Holaday J: Cardiovascular effects of endogenous opiate systems, *Annu Rev Pharmacol Toxicol* 23:541, 1983.
360. Howlett T, Tomlin S, Ngahfoong L: Release of beta-endorphin and met-enkephalin during exercise in normal women response to training, *Br Med J* 288:1950, 1984.
361. Lewis JW, Tordoff MG, Sherman JE, et al: Adrenal medullary enkephalin-like peptides may mediate opioid stress analgesia, *Science* 217(4559):557–559, 1982.
362. Xiao RP, Pepe S, Spurgeon HA, et al: Opioid peptide receptor stimulation reverses beta-adrenergic effects in rat heart cells, *Am J Physiol* 272(2 Pt 2):H797–H805, 1997.
363. Boluyt MO, Younes A, Cappey JL, et al: Age-associated increase in rat cardiac opioid production, *Am J Physiol* 265(1 Pt 2):H212–H218, 1993.
364. Caffrey JL, Boluyt MO, Younes A, et al: Aging, cardiac proenkephalin mRNA and enkephalin peptides in the Fisher 244 rat, *J Mol Cell Cardiol* 26:701, 1994.
365. McLaughlin PJ, Wu Y: Opioid gene expression in the developing and adult rat heart, *Dev Dyn* 211(2):153–163, 1998.

366. Dumont M, Lemaire S: Increased content of immunoreactive Leu-enkepahlin and alteration of delta opioid receptor in hearts of spontaneously hypertensive rats, *Neurosci Lett* 24:114, 1988.
367. Forman LJ, Hock C, Harwell M, et al: The results of exposure to immobilization, hemorrhagic shock, and cardiac hypertrophy on beta-endorphin in rat cardiac tissue, *Proc Soc Exp Biol Med* 206:124, 1994.
368. Ouellette M, Brakier-Gingras L: Increase in the relative abundance of preproenkephalin messenger RNA in the ventricles of cardiomyopathic hamsters, *Biochem Biophys Res Comm* 155:449, 1988.
369. Paradis P, Dumont M, Belicahrd P, et al: Increased preproenkephalin A gene expression in the rat heart after induction of a myocardial infarction, *Biochem Cell Biol* 70:593, 1992.
370. Lee AY: Endogenous opioid peptides and cardiac arrhythmias, *Int J Cardiol* 27(2):145–151, 1990.
371. Falcone C, Guasti L, Ochan M, et al: Beta-endorphins during coronary angioplasty in patients with silent or symptomatic myocardial ischemia, *J Am Coll Cardiol* 22(6):1614–1620, 1993.
372. Imai N, Kashiki M, Woolf PD, et al: Comparison of cardiovascular effects of mu- and delta-opioid receptor antagonists in dogs with congestive heart failure, *Am J Physiol* 267(3 Pt 2):H912–H917, 1994.
373. Maslov LN, Lishmanov YB: Change in opioid peptide level in the heart and blood plasma during acute myocardial ischaemia complicated by ventricular fibrillation, *Clin Exp Pharmacol Physiol* 22(11):812–816, 1995.
374. Miller PJ, Light KC, Bragdon EE, et al: Beta-endorphin response to exercise and mental stress in patients with ischemic heart disease, *J Psychosom Res* 37(5):455–465, 1993.
375. Oldroyd KG, Harvey K, Gray CE, et al: Beta endorphin release in patients after spontaneous and provoked acute myocardial ischaemia, *Br Heart J* 67(3):230–235, 1992.
376. Wu JP, Chen YT, Lee AYS: Opioids in myocardial ischaemia: Potentiating effects of dynorphin on ischaemic arrhythmia, bradycardia and cardiogenic shock following coronary artery occlusion in the rat, *Eur Heart J* 14(9):1273–1277, 1993.
377. Slepushkin VD, Pavlenko VS, Zoloyez GK, et al: The role of enkephalins in the pathogenesis of acute myocardial infarction, *Exp Pathol* 35(2):129–131, 1988.
378. Rimoy GH, Wright DM, Bhaskar NK, et al: The cardiovascular and central nervous system effects in the human of U-62066E. A selective opioid receptor agonist, *Eur J Clin Pharmacol* 46(3):203–207, 1994.
379. Ventura C, Spurgeon H, Lakatta EG, et al: Kappa and delta opioid receptor stimulation affects cardiac myocyte function and Ca++ release from an intracellular pool in myocytes and neurons, *Circ Res* 70:66, 1992.
380. Fontana F, Bernardi P, Pich EM, et al: Relationship between plasma atrial natriuretic factor and opioid peptide levels in healthy subjects and in patients with acute congestive heart failure, *Eur Heart J* 14:219, 1993.
381. Lowe H: [Role of endogenous opioids in heart failure], *Z Kardiol* 80(Suppl 8):47–51, 1991.
382. Barron BA, Gu H, Gaugl JF, et al: Screening for opioids in dog heart, *J Mol Cell Cardiol* 24(1):67–77, 1992.
383. Llobel F, Laorden ML: Effects of mu-, delta- and kappa-opioid antagonists in atrial preparations from nonfailing and failing human hearts, *Gen Pharmacol* 28(3):371–374, 1997.
384. Oldroyd KG, Gray GE, Carter R, et al: Activation and inhibition of the endogenous opioid system in human heart failure, *Br Heart J* 73(1):41–48, 1995.
385. Airaksinen KE: Autonomic mechanisms and sudden death after abrupt coronary occlusion, *Ann Med* 31(4):240–245, 1999.
386. Flacke JW, Flacke WE, Bloor BC, et al: Effects of fentanyl, naloxone, and clonidine on hemodynamics and plasma catecholamine levels in dogs, *Anesth Analg* 62(3):305–313, 1983.
387. Pruett JK, Adams BJ, RJ: Cellular and subcellular actions of opioids in the heart. In EF, editors: *Opioids in anesthesia*, Boston, Butterworth-Heinemann, 1991, p 61.
388. Blair JR, Pruett JK, Introna RP, et al: Cardiac electrophysiologic effects of fentanyl and sufentanil in canine cardiac Purkinje fibers, *Anesthesiology* 71(4):565–570, 1989.
389. Hess L, Vrana M, Vranova Z, et al: The antifibrillatory effect of fentanyl, sufentanil and carfentanil in the acute phase of local myocardial ischaemia in the dog, *Acta Cardiol* 44(4):303–311, 1989.
390. Goldberg AH, Padget CH: Comparative effects of morphine and fentanyl on isolated heart muscle, *Anesth Analg* 48(6):978–982, 1969.
391. Strauer BE: Contractile responses to morphine, piritramide, meperidine, and fentanyl: A comparative study of effects on the isolated ventricular myocardium, *Anesthesiology* 37(3):304–310, 1972.
392. Sullivan DL, Wong KC: The effects of morphine on the isolated heart during normothermia and hypothermia, *Anesthesiology* 38(6):550–556, 1973.
393. Zhang CC, Su JY, Calkins D: Effects of alfentanil on isolated cardiac tissues of the rabbit, *Anesth Analg* 71(3):268–274, 1990.
394. Kohno K, Takaki M, Ishioka K, et al: Effects of intracoronary fentanyl on left ventricular mechanoenergetics in the excised cross-circulated canine heart, *Anesthesiology* 86(6):1350–1358, discussion 7A–8A, 1997.
395. Llobel F, Laorden ML: Effects of morphine on atrial preparations obtained from non-failing and failing human hearts, *Br J Anaesth* 76(1):106–110, 1996.
396. Van Vliet BJ, Ruuls SR, Drukarch B, et al: Beta-adrenoceptor-sensitive adenylate cyclase inhibited by activation of μ-opioid receptors in rat striated neurons, *Eur J Pharmacol* 195:295, 1991.
397. Philbin DM, Moss J, Akins CW, et al: The use of H1 and H2 histamine antagonists with morphine anesthesia: A double-blind study, *Anesthesiology* 55(3):292–296, 1981.
398. Muldoon SM, Otto J, Freas W, et al: The effects of morphine, nalbuphine, and butorphanol on adrenergic function in canine saphenous veins, *Anesth Analg* 62(1):21–28, 1983.
399. Rorie DK, Muldoon SM, Tyce GM: Effects of fentanyl on adrenergic function in canine coronary arteries, *Anesth Analg* 60(1):21–27, 1981.
400. White DA, Reitan JA, Kien ND, et al: Decrease in vascular resistance in the isolated canine hindlimb after graded doses of alfentanil, fentanyl, and sufentanil, *Anesth Analg* 71(1):29–34, 1990.
401. Karasawa F, Iwanov V, Moulds RFW: Effects of fentanyl on the rat aorta are mediated by alpha-adrenoceptors rather than by the endothelium, *Br J Anaesth* 71(6):877–880, 1993.
402. Pugsley MK, Penz WP, Walker MJ, et al: Cardiovascular actions of U-50,488H and related kappa agonists, *Cardiovasc Drug Rev* 11:151, 1993.
403. Pugsley MK, Penz WP, Walker MJ, et al: Cardiovascular actions of the kappa receptor agonist, U-50,488H, in the absence and presence of opioid receptor blockade, *Br J Pharmacol* 105:521, 1992.
404. Hall ED, Wolf DL, McCall RB: Cardiovascular depressant effects of the kappa opioid receptor agonist U-50,488H and spiradoline mesylate, *Circ Shock* 26:409, 1988.
405. Kaschube M, Brasch H: Negative chronotropic but no antiarrhythmic effect of (+) and (−) naloxone in rats and guinea pigs, *Cardiovasc Res* 25:230, 1991.
406. Brasch H: Influence of the optical isomers (+)- and (−)-naloxone on beating frequency, contractile force and action potentials of guinea-pig isolated cardiac preparations, *Br J Pharmacol* 88(4):733–740, 1986.
407. Pugsley MK, Saint D, Penz WP, et al: Electrophysiological and antiarrhythmic actions of the kappa agonist PD129290, and its R,R(+) enantiomer, PD 129289, *Br J Pharmacol* 110:1579, 1993.
408. Pugsley MK, Hayes ES, Saint DA, et al: Do related kappa agonists produce similar effects on cardiac ion channels? *Proc West Pharmacol Soc* 38:25, 1995.
409. Helgesen KG, Refsum H: Arrhythmogenic, antiarrhythmic and inotropic properties of opioids. Effects of piritramide, pethidine, and morphine compared on heart muscle isolated from rats, *Pharmacology* 35:121, 1987.
410. Kasper E, Ventura C, Ziman BD, et al: Effect of U-50,488H on the contractile response of cardiomyopathic hamster ventricular myocytes, *Life Sci* 50:2029, 1992.
411. Lakatta EG, Xiao R, Ventura C, et al: Negative feedback of opioid peptide receptor stimulation of beta-adrenergic effects in heart cells, *J Mol Cell Cardiol* 24:S25, 1992.
412. Wu C, Fry C, Henry J: The mode of action of several opioids on cardiac muscle, *Exp Physiol* 82:261, 1997.
413. Dana A, Yellon DM: Angina: Who needs it? Cardioprotection in the preconditioning era, *Cardiovasc Drug Ther* 12:515, 1998.
414. Gross GJ, Fryer RM: Sarcolemmal versus mitochondrial ATP-sensitive K+ channels and myocardial preconditioning, *Circ Res* 84:973, 1999.
415. Light PE: Cardiac KATP channels and ischemic preconditioning: Current perspectives, *Can J Cardiol* 15(10):1123–1130, 1999.
416. Bolli R, Dawn B, Tang XL, et al: The nitric oxide hypothesis of late preconditioning, *Basic Res Cardiol* 93(5):325–338, 1998.
417. Bolli R, Marban E: Molecular and cellular mechanisms of myocardial stunning, *Physiol Rev* 79(2):609–634, 1999.
418. Guo Y, Wu W, Qiu Y, et al: Demonstration of an early and a late phase of ischemic preconditioning in mice, *Am J Physiol* 275(4 Pt 2):H1375–H1387, 1998.
419. Chien CC, Brown G, Pan YX, et al: Blockade of U50,488H analgesia by antisense oligodeoxynucleotides to a kappa-opioid receptor, *Eur J Pharmacol* 253(3):R7–R8, 1994.
420. Mayfield KP, D'Alecy LG: Role of endogenous opioid peptides in the acute adaptation to hypoxia, *Brain Res* 582(2):226–231, 1992.
421. Schultz JE, Rose E, Yao Z, et al: Evidence for involvement of opioid receptors in ischemic preconditioning in rat hearts, *Am J Physiol* 268(5 Pt 2):H2157–H2161, 1995.
422. Chien GL, Van Winkle DM: Naloxone blockade of myocardial ischemic preconditioning is stereoselective, *J Mol Cell Cardiol* 28(9):1895–1900, 1996.
423. Schulz R, Gres P, Heusch G: Role of endogenous opioids in ischemic preconditioning but not in short-term hibernation in pigs, *Am J Physiol Heart Circ Physiol* 280(5):H2175–H2181, 2001.
424. Takashi Y, Wolff RA, Chien GL, et al: Met5-enkephalin protects isolated adult rabbit cardiomyocytes via delta-opioid receptors, *Am J Physiol* 277(6 Pt 2):H2442–H2450, 1999.
425. Huang MH, Nguyen V, Wu Y, et al: Reducing ischaemia/reperfusion injury through δ-opoiod-regulated intrinsic cardiac adrenergic cells: Adrenopeptidergic co-signalling, *Cardiovasc Res* 84:452–460, 2009.
426. Huang MH, Wang H, Roeske WR, et al: Mediating δ-opiod-initiated heart protection via the β2-adrenergic receptor: Role of the intrinsic cardiac adrenergic cell, *Am J Physiol Heart Circ Physiol* 293:H376–H384, 2007.
427. Schultz JE, Hsu AK, Gross GJ: Morphine mimics the cardioprotective effect of ischemic preconditioning via a glibenclamide-sensitive mechanism in the rat heart, *Circ Res* 78(6):1100–1104, 1996.
428. Liang BT, Gross GJ: Direct preconditioning of cardiac myocytes via opioid receptors and KATP channels, *Circ Res* 84(12):1396–1400, 1999.
429. Miki T, Cohen MV, Downey JM: Opioid receptor contributes to ischemic preconditioning through protein kinase C activation in rabbits, *Mol Cell Biochem* 186(1–2):3–12, 1998.
430. Benedict PE, Benedict MB, Su TP, et al: Opiate drugs and delta-receptor-mediated myocardial protection, *Circulation* 100(Suppl 19):II357–II360, 1999.
431. Gross E, Hsu A, Gross GJ: Opioid-induced cardioprotection occurs via glycogen synthase kinase β inhibition during reperfusion in intact rat hearts, *Circ Res* 94:960–966, 2004.
432. Wong GT, Huang Z, Ji S, et al: Remifentanil reduces the release of biochemical markers of myocardial damage after coronary artery bypass surgery: A randomized trial, *J Cardiothorac Vasc Anesth* (in press).
433. Kato R, Foex P: Fentanyl reduces infarction but not stunning via delta-opioid receptors and protein kinase C in rats, *Br J Anaesth* 84(5):608–614, 2000.
434. Kato R, Ross S, Foex P: Fentanyl protects the heart against ischaemic injury via opioid receptors, adenosine A1 receptors and KATP channel linked mechanisms in rats, *Br J Anaesth* 84(2):204–214, 2000.
435. Schultz JE, Hsu AK, Gross GJ: Ischemic preconditioning in the intact rat heart is mediated by delta1- but not mu- or kappa-opioid receptors, *Circulation* 97(13):1282–1289, 1998.
436. Bolling SF, Badhwar V, Schwartz CF, et al: Opioids confer myocardial tolerance to ischemia: Interaction of delta opioid agonists and antagonists, *J Thorac Cardiovasc Surg* 122(3):476–481, 2001.
437. Sigg DC, Coles JA, Oeltgen PR, et al: Role of delta-opioid receptor agonists on infarct size reduction in swine, *Am J Physiol Heart Circ Physiol* 282(6):H1953–H1960, 2002.
438. Cao CM, Chen M, Wong TM: The K_{Ca} channel as a trigger for the cardioprotection induced by kappa-opioid receptor stimulation—its relationship with protein kinase, *Br J Pharmacol* 145:984–991, 2005.
439. Cao CM, Xia Q, Gao Q, et al: Calcium-activated potassium channel triggers cardioprotection of ischemic preconditioning, *J Pharmacol Exp Ther* 312:644–650, 2005.
440. Wong TM, Lee AY, Tai KK: Effects of drugs interacting with opioid receptors during normal perfusion or ischemia and reperfusion in the isolated rat heart—an attempt to identify cardiac opioid receptor subtype(s) involved in arrhythmogenesis, *J Mol Cell Cardiol* 22(10):1167–1175, 1990.
441. Jang Y, Xi J, Wang H, et al: Postconditioning prevents reperfusion injury by activating δ-opioid receptors, *Anesthesiology* 108:243–250, 2008.
442. Kim SF, Huri D, Snyder S: Inducible nitric oxide synthase binds, S-nitrosylates, and activates cyclooxygenase-2, *Science* 310:1966–1969, 2005.
443. Cheng L, Ma S, Wei LX, et al: Mechanism of cardioprotective and antiarrhythmic effect of U50488H in ischemia/reperfusion rat heart, *Heart Vessels* 22:335–344, 2007.
444. Okubo S, Tanabe Y, Takeda K, et al: Ischemic preconditioning and morphine attenuate myocardial apoptosis and infarction after ischemia-reperfusion in rabbits: Role of the δ-opioid receptor, *Am J Physiol Heart Circ Physiol* 287:1786–1791, 2004.
445. Rong F, Peng Z, Ming-Xiang Y, et al: Myocardial apoptosis and infarction after ischemia/reperfusion are attenuated by κ-opioid receptor agonist, *Arch Med Res* 40:227–234, 2009.
446. Huh J, Gross GJ, Nagase H, et al: Protection of cardiac myocytes via delta(1)-opioid receptors, protein kinase C, and mitochondrial K(ATP) channels, *Am J Physiol Heart Circ Physiol* 280(1):H377–H383, 2001.
447. Wang GY, Wu S, Pei JM, et al: Kappa- but not delta-opioid receptors mediate effects of ischemic preconditioning on both infarct and arrhythmia in rats, *Am J Physiol Heart Circ Physiol* 280(1):H384–H391, 2001.
448. Bell SP, Sack MN, Patel A, et al: Delta opioid receptor stimulation mimics ischemic preconditioning in human heart muscle, *J Am Coll Cardiol* 36(7):2296–2302, 2000.
449. Fryer RM, Hsu AK, Eells JT, et al: Opioid-induced second window of cardioprotection: Potential role of mitochondrial KATP channels, *Circ Res* 84(7):846–851, 1999.
450. Kevelaitis E, Peynet J, Mouas C, et al: Opening of potassium channels: The common cardioprotective link between preconditioning and natural hibernation? *Circulation* 99(23):3079–3085, 1999.
451. McPherson BC, Yao Z: Signal transduction of opioid-induced cardioprotection in ischemia-reperfusion, *Anesthesiology* 94(6):1082–1088, 2001.
452. Patel HH, Hsu AK, Gross GJ: COX-2 and iNOS in opioid-induced delayed cardioprotection in the intact rat, *Life Sci* 75(2):129–140, 2004.
453. Peart JN, Gross E, Gross GJ: Opioid induced preconditioning: Recent advances and future perspective, *Vasc Pharmacol* 42:211–218, 2005.
454. Wu S, Li HY, Wong TM: Cardioprotection of preconditioning by metabolic inhibition in the rat ventricular myocyte. Involvement of kappa-opioid receptor, *Circ Res* 84(12):1388–1395, 1999.

455. Tomai F, Crea F, Gaspardone A, et al: Effects of naloxone on myocardial ischemic preconditioning in humans, *J Am Coll Cardiol* 33(7):1863–1869, 1999.
456. Xenopoulos NP, Leeser M, Bolli R: Morphine mimics ischemic preconditioning in human myocardium during PTCA, *J Am Coll Cardiol* 31(Suppl):65A, 1998.
457. Horton ND, Kaftani DJ, Bruce DS, et al: Isolation and partial characterization of an opioid-like 88 kDa hibernation-related protein, *Comp Biochem Physiol B Biochem Mol Biol* 119(4):787–805, 1998.
458. Bolling SF, Su TP, Childs KF, et al: The use of hibernation induction triggers for cardiac transplant preservation, *Transplantation* 63(2):326–329, 1997.
459. Bolling SF, Tramontini NL, Kilgore KS, et al: Use of "natural" hibernation induction triggers for myocardial protection, *Ann Thorac Surg* 64(3):623–627, 1997.
460. Schwartz CF, Georges AJ, Gallagher MA, et al: Delta opioid receptors and low temperature myocardial protection, *Ann Thorac Surg* 68(6):2089–2092, 1999.
461. Becker LB, Ostrander MP, Barrett J, et al: Outcome of CPR in a large metropolitan area—where are the survivors? *Ann Emerg Med* 20(4):355–361, 1991.
462. Brown CG, Martin DR, Pepe PE, et al: A comparison of standard-dose and high-dose epinephrine in cardiac arrest outside the hospital. The Multicenter High-Dose Epinephrine Study Group, *N Engl J Med* 327(15):1051–1055, 1992.
463. Lombardi G, Gallagher J, Gennis P: Outcome of out-of-hospital cardiac arrest in New York City. The Pre-Hospital Arrest Survival Evaluation (PHASE) Study, *Jama* 271(9):678–683, 1994.
464. Fang X, Tang W, Sun S, et al: Mechanism by which activation of delta-opiod receptor reduces the severity of post resuscitation myocardial dysfunction. *Crit Care Med* 34(10):2607–2612, 2010.
465. Lowenstein E, Hallowell P, Levine FH, et al: Cardiovascular response to large doses of intravenous morphine in man, *N Engl J Med* 281(25):1389–1393, 1969.
466. Lowenstein E: Morphine "anesthesia"—a perspective, *Anesthesiology* 35(6):563–565, 1971.
467. Murphy GS, Szokol J, Marymont JH, et al: Opioids and cardioprotection: The impact of morphine and fentanyl on recovery of ventricular function after cardiopulmonary bypass, *J Cardiothorac Vasc Anesth* 20(4):493–502, 2006.
468. Stanley TH, Webster LR: Anesthetic requirements and cardiovascular effects of fentanyl-oxygen and fentanyl-diazepam-oxygen anesthesia in man, *Anesth Analg* 57(4):411–416, 1978.
469. Sebel PS, et al: Cardiovascular effects of high-dose fentanyl anaesthesia, *Acta Anaesthesiol Scand* 26(4):308–315, 1982.
470. Waller JL, Bovill JG, Boekhorst RA, et al: Hemodynamic changes during fentanyl—oxygen anesthesia for aortocoronary bypass operation, *Anesthesiology* 55(3):212–217, 1981.
471. de Lange S, Boscoe MJ, Stanley TH, et al: Comparison of sufentanil—O2 and fentanyl—O2 for coronary artery surgery, *Anesthesiology* 56(2):112–118, 1982.
472. Miller DR, Wellwood M, Teasdale SJ, et al: Effects of anesthetic induction on myocardial function and metabolism: A comparison of fentanyl, sufentanil and alfentanil, *Can J Anaesth* 35(3 Pt 1):219–233, 1988.
473. Swenzen GO, Chakrabarti MK, Sapsed-Byrne S, et al: Selective depression by alfentanil of group III and IV somatosympathetic reflexes in the dog, *Br J Anaesth* 61(4):441–445, 1988.
474. Bovill JG, Warren PJ, Schuller JL, et al: Comparison of fentanyl, sufentanil, and alfentanil anesthesia in patients undergoing valvular heart surgery, *Anesth Analg* 63(12):1081–1086, 1984.
475. Slogoff S, Keats AS: Randomized trial of primary anesthetic agents on outcome of coronary artery bypass operations, *Anesthesiology* 70(2):179–188, 1989.
476. Tuman KJ, McCarthy RJ, Speiss BD, et al: Does choice of anesthetic agent significantly affect outcome after coronary artery surgery? *Anesthesiology* 70(2):189–198, 1989.
477. Wynands JE, Townsend GE, Wong P, et al: Blood pressure response and plasma fentanyl concentrations during high- and very high-dose fentanyl anesthesia for coronary artery surgery, *Anesth Analg* 62(7):661–665, 1983.
478. Butterworth JFt, Bean VE, Royster RL: Sufentanil is preferable to etomidate during rapid-sequence anesthesia induction for aortocoronary bypass surgery, *J Cardiothorac Anesth* 3(4):396–400, 1989.
479. Berberich JJ, Fabian JA: A retrospective analysis of fentanyl and sufentanil for cardiac transplantation, *J Cardiothorac Anesth* 1(3):200–204, 1987.
480. Gutzke GE, Shah KB, Glisson SN, et al: Cardiac transplantation: A prospective comparison of ketamine and sufentanil for anesthetic induction, *J Cardiothorac Anesth* 3(4):389–395, 1989.
481. Stanley TH, de Lange S: Comparison of sufentanil-oxygen and fentanyl-oxygen anesthesia for mitral and aortic valvular surgery, *J Cardiothorac Anesth* 2(1):6–11, 1988.
482. Howie MB, Cheng D, Newman MF, et al: A randomized double-blinded multicenter comparison of remifentanil versus fentanyl when combined with isoflurane/propofol for early extubation in coronary artery bypass graft surgery, *Anesth Analg* 92(5):1084–1093, 2001.
483. Samuelson PN, Reves JG, Kirklin JK, et al: Comparison of sufentanil and enflurane-nitrous oxide anesthesia for myocardial revascularization, *Anesth Analg* 65(3):217–226, 1986.
484. Howie MB, Smith DF, Reilley TE, et al: Postoperative course after sufentanil or fentanyl anesthesia for coronary artery surgery, *J Cardiothorac Vasc Anesth* 5(5):485–489, 1991.
485. Collard E, Delire V, Mayne A, et al: Propofol-alfentanil versus fentanyl-midazolam in coronary artery surgery, *J Cardiothorac Vasc Anesth* 10(7):869–876, 1996.
486. Wood M: Pharmacokinetics and principles of drug infusions in cardiac patients. In Kaplan, Reich, Konstadt, eds. *Cardiac anesthesia*, Philadelphia: WB Saunders Company, 1999, p 670.
487. Schell RM, Kern FH, Greeley WJ, et al: Cerebral blood flow and metabolism during cardiopulmonary bypass, *Anesth Analg* 76(4):849–865, 1993.
488. Skacel M, Knott C, Reynolds F, et al: Extracorporeal circuit sequestration of fentanyl and alfentanil, *Br J Anaesth* 58(9):947–949, 1986.
489. Boer F, Engbers FH, Bovill JG, et al: First-pass pulmonary retention of sufentanil at three different background blood concentrations of the opioid, *Br J Anaesth* 74(1):50–55, 1995.
490. Roerig DL, Kotrly KJ, Vucins EJ, et al: First pass uptake of fentanyl, meperidine, and morphine in the human lung, *Anesthesiology* 67(4):466–472, 1987.
491. Hornick P, Taylor K: Pulsatile and nonpulsatile perfusion: The continuing controversy, *J Cardiothorac Vasc Anesth* 11(3):310–315, 1997.
492. McAllister RG Jr, Tan TG: Effect of hypothermia on drug metabolism. In vitro studies with propranolol and verapamil, *Pharmacology* 20(2):95–100, 1980.
493. Boylan JW, Hong SK: Regulation of renal function in hypothermia, *Am J Physiol* 211(6):1371–1378, 1966.
494. Bentley JB, Conahan TJ 3rd, Cork RC: Fentanyl sequestration in lungs during cardiopulmonary bypass, *Clin Pharmacol Ther* 34(5):703–706, 1983.
495. Caspi J, Klausner JM, Safadi T, et al: Delayed respiratory depression following fentanyl anesthesia for cardiac surgery, *Crit Care Med* 16(3):238–240, 1988.
496. Okutanil R, Philbin DM, Rosow CE, et al: Effect of hypothermic hemodilutional cardiopulmonary bypass on plasma sufentanil and catecholamine concentrations in humans, *Anesth Analg* 67(7):667–670, 1988.
497. Booth BP, Henderson M, Milne B, et al: Sequestration of glyceryl trinitrate (nitroglycerin) by cardiopulmonary bypass oxygenators, *Anesth Analg* 72(4):493–497, 1991.
498. Hickey S, Gaylor JD, Kenny GN: In vitro uptake and elimination of isoflurane by different membrane oxygenators, *J Cardiothorac Vasc Anesth* 10(3):352–355, 1996.
499. Hynynen M: Binding of fentanyl and alfentanil to the extracorporeal circuit, *Acta Anaesthesiol Scand* 31(8):706–710, 1987.
500. Hynynen M, Hammaren E, Rosenberg PH: Propofol sequestration within the extracorporeal circuit, *Can J Anaesth* 41(7):583–588, 1994.
501. Rosen DA, Rosen KR: Elimination of drugs and toxins during cardiopulmonary bypass, *J Cardiothorac Vasc Anesth* 11(3):337–340, 1997.
502. Rosen DA, Rosen KR, Davidson B, et al: Absorption of fentanyl by the memprane oxygenator, *Anesthesiology* 63(3):A281, 1985.
503. Hug CC Jr, Moldenhauer CC: Pharmacokinetics and dynamics of fentanyl infusions in cardiac surgical patients, *Anesthesiology* 57(3):A45, 1982.
504. Taeger K, Weninger E, Franke N, et al: Uptake of fentanyl by human lung, *Anesthesiology* 61(3):A246, 1984.
505. Hug CC Jr, Burm AG, de Lange S: Alfentanil pharmacokinetics in cardiac surgical patients, *Anesth Analg* 78(2):231–239, 1994.
506. Hynynen M, Hynninen M, Soini H, et al: Plasma concentration and protein binding of alfentanil during high-dose infusion for cardiac surgery, *Br J Anaesth* 72(5):571–576, 1994.
507. Kumar K, Crankshaw DP, Morgan DJ, et al: The effect of cardiopulmonary bypass on plasma protein binding of alfentanil, *Eur J Clin Pharmacol* 35(1):47–52, 1988.
508. Lowry KG, Dundee JW, McClean E, et al: Pharmacokinetics of diazepam and midazolam when used for sedation following cardiopulmonary bypass, *Br J Anaesth* 57(9):883–885, 1985.
509. Dundee JW, Collier PS, Carlisle RJ, et al: Prolonged midazolam elimination half-life, *Br J Clin Pharmacol* 21(4):425–429, 1986.
510. Harper KW, Collier PS, Dundee JW, et al: Age and nature of operation influence the pharmacokinetics of midazolam, *Br J Anaesth* 57(9):866–871, 1985.
511. Bjorksten AR, Crankshaw DP, Morgan DJ, et al: The effects of cardiopulmonary bypass on plasma concentrations and protein binding of methohexital and thiopental, *J Cardiothorac Anesth* 2(3):281–289, 1988.
512. Massey NJ, Sherry KM, Oldroyd S, et al: Pharmacokinetics of an infusion of propofol during cardiac surgery, *Br J Anaesth* 65(4):475–479, 1990.
513. Russell GN, Wright EL, Fox MA, et al: Propofol-fentanyl anaesthesia for coronary artery surgery and cardiopulmonary bypass, *Anaesthesia* 44(3):205–208, 1989.
514. Antognini JF, Kien ND: Cardiopulmonary bypass does not alter canine enflurane requirements, *Anesthesiology* 76(6):953–957, 1992.
515. Doak GJ, Gefeng L, Hall RI, et al: Does hypothermia or hyperventilation affect enflurane MAC reduction following partial cardiopulmonary bypass in dogs? *Can J Anaesth* 40(2):176–182, 1993.
516. Hall RI, Sullivan JA: Does cardiopulmonary bypass alter enflurane requirements for anesthesia? *Anesthesiology* 73(2):249–255, 1990.
517. Hall RI, Hawwa R: The enflurane-sparing effect of hypothermia, *Can J Anaesth* 36(S114), 1989.
518. Steffey EP, Eger EI 2nd: Hyperthermia and halothane MAC in the dog, *Anesthesiology* 41 (4):392–396, 1974.
519. Vitez TS, White PF, Eger EI 2nd: Effects of hypothermia on halothane MAC and isoflurane MAC in the rat, *Anesthesiology* 41(1):80–81, 1974.
520. Nussmeier NLambert M, Moskowitz G, et al: Washin and washout of three volatile anesthetics concurrently administered during cardiopulmonary bypass, *Anesthesiology* 14(A84), 1988.
521. Stern R, Weiss C, Steinbach J, et al: Isoflurane uptake and elimination are delayed by absorption of anesthetic by the Scimed membrane oxygenator, *Anesth Analg* 69(5):657–662, 1989.
522. Lerman J, Gregory GA, Eger EI 2nd: Hematocrit and the solubility of volatile anesthetics in blood, *Anesth Analg* 63(10):911–914, 1984.
523. Eger RR, Eger EI 2nd: Effect of temperature and age on the solubility of enflurane, halothane, isoflurane, and methoxyflurane in human blood, *Anesth Analg* 64(6):640–642, 1985.
524. Feingold A: Crystalloid hemodilution, hypothermia, and halothane blood solubility during cardiopulmonary bypass, *Anesth Analg* 56(5):622–626, 1977.
525. Targ AG, Yasuda N, Eger EI: Anesthetic plastic solubility, *Anesthesiology* 14(A297), 1988.
526. Nussmeier N, Lambert DG, Moskowitz G, et al: Washin and washout of isoflurane administered via bubble oxygenators during hypothermic cardiopulmonary bypass, *Anesthesiology* 71(4):519–525, 1989.
527. Price SL, Brown DL, Carpenter RL, et al: Isoflurane elimination via a bubble oxygenator during extracorporeal circulation, *J Cardiothorac Anesth* 2(1):41–44, 1988.
528. Smeulers NJ, Wierda MKH, van den Broek L, et al: Effects of hypothermic cardiopulmonary bypass on the pharmacodynamics and pharmacokinetics of rocuronium, *J Cardiothorac Vasc Anesth* 9(6):700–705, 1995.
529. Miller R: Factors affect the action of neuromuscular blacking drugs. In Agoston SBW, editor: *Muscle relaxants*, Amsterdam, 1990, Elsevier, pp 181–197.
530. Boyd IA, Martin AR: Spontaneous subthreshold activity at mammalian neural muscular junctions, *J Physiol* 132(1):61–73, 1956.
531. Hubbard JI, Jones SF, Landau EM: The effect of temperature change upon transmitter release, facilitation and post-tetanic potentiation, *J Physiol* 216(3):591–609, 1971.
532. Wierda J.M.K.H., Proost JH, Muir AW, et al: Design of drugs for rapid onset, *Anaesth Pharmacol Rev* 1:57, 1993.
533. Buzello W, Schluermann D, Schindler M, et al: Hypothermic cardiopulmonary bypass and neuromuscular blockade by pancuronium and vecuronium, *Anesthesiology* 62(2):201–204, 1985.
534. Fowler CV, Fraser GL: Mu-, delta-, kappa-opioid receptors and their subtypes. A critical review with emphasis on radiologand binding experiments, *Neurochem Int* 24:401, 1994.

10

Cardiovascular Pharmacology

ROGER L. ROYSTER, MD, FACC | LEANNE GROBAN, MS, MD | DAVID W. GROSSHANS, DO |
MANDISA-MAIA JONES-HAYWOOD, MD | THOMAS F. SLAUGHTER, MD, MHA, CPH

KEY POINTS

Anti-Ischemic Drug Therapy

1. Ischemia during the perioperative period demands immediate attention by the anesthesiologist. The impact of ischemia may be both acute (impending infarction, hemodynamic compromise) and chronic (a marker of previously unknown cardiac disease, a prognostic indicator of poor outcome).
2. Nitroglycerin is indicated in nearly all conditions of perioperative myocardial ischemia. Mechanisms of action include coronary vasodilation and favorable alterations in preload and afterload. Nitroglycerin is contraindicated when hypotension is present.
3. Perioperative β-blockade may reduce the incidence of perioperative myocardial ischemia via a number of mechanisms. Favorable hemodynamic changes associated with β-blockade include a blunting of the stress response and reduced heart rate, blood pressure, and contractility. All of these conditions improve myocardial oxygen supply/demand ratios.
4. Calcium channel blockers reduce myocardial oxygen demand by depression of contractility, heart rate, and/or decreased arterial blood pressure. Calcium channel blockers often are administered in the perioperative period for longer term antianginal symptomatic control.

Drug Therapy for Systemic Hypertension

1. Current guidelines suggest seeking a target blood pressure of less than 140/85 mm Hg to minimize long-term risk for adverse cardiovascular morbidity and mortality.
2. For patients with diabetes, renal impairment, or established cardiovascular diseases, a lower target of less than 130/80 mm Hg is recommended.
3. Mild-to-moderate hypertension does not represent an independent risk factor for perioperative complications; however, a diagnosis of hypertension necessitates preoperative assessment for target organ damage.
4. Patients with poorly controlled preoperative hypertension experience more labile blood pressures in the perioperative setting with greater potential for hypertensive or hypotensive episodes, or both.

Pharmacotherapy for Acute and Chronic Heart Failure

1. The signs, symptoms, and treatment of chronic heart failure are as related to the neurohormonal response as they are to the underlying ventricular dysfunction.
2. Current treatments for chronic heart failure are aimed at prolonging survival, not just relief of symptoms.
3. The low-cardiac-output syndrome seen after cardiac surgery has a pathophysiology, treatment, and prognosis that differ from those of chronic heart failure, with which it is sometimes compared.

Pharmacotherapy for Cardiac Arrhythmias

1. Physicians must be cautious in administering antiarrhythmic drugs because of the proarrhythmic effects that can increase mortality in certain subgroups of patients.
2. Amiodarone has become a popular intravenous antiarrhythmic drug for use in the operating room and critical care areas because it has a broad range of effects for ventricular and supraventricular arrhythmias.
3. β-Adrenergic receptor antagonists are very effective but underused antiarrhythmics in the perioperative period because many arrhythmias are adrenergically mediated because of the stress of surgery and critical illness.
4. Managing electrolyte abnormalities and treating underlying disease processes such as hypervolemia and myocardial ischemia are critical treatment steps before the administration of any antiarrhythmic agent.

ANTI-ISCHEMIC DRUG THERAPY

Anti-ischemic drug therapy during anesthesia is indicated whenever evidence of myocardial ischemia exists. The treatment of ischemia during anesthesia is complicated by the ongoing stress of surgery, blood loss, concurrent organ ischemia, and the patient's inability to interact with the anesthesiologist. Nonetheless, the fundamental principles of treatment remain the same as in the unanesthetized state. All events of myocardial ischemia involve an alteration in the oxygen supply/demand balance (Table 10-1). The American College of Cardiology/American Heart Association (ACC/AHA) Guidelines on the Management and Treatment of Patients with Unstable Angina and Non-ST-Segment Elevation Myocardial Infarction provide an excellent framework for the treatment of patients with ongoing myocardial ischemia.[1] These guidelines detail the initial evaluation, management, hospital care, and coronary revascularization strategies in the nonanesthetized patient

TABLE 10-1	Myocardial Ischemia: Factors Governing O₂ Supply and Demand	
O₂ Supply		*O₂ Demand*
Heart rate*		Heart rate*
O₂ content		Contractility
Hgb, SAT%, Pao₂		Wall tension
Coronary blood flow		Afterload
CPP = DP − LVEDP*		Preload (LVEDP)*
CVR		

*Affects both supply and demand.

CPP, coronary perfusion pressure; CVR, coronary vascular resistance; DP, diastolic blood pressure; Hgb, hemoglobin; LVEDP, left ventricular end-diastolic pressure; SAT%, percent oxygen saturation.

Modified from Royster RL: Intraoperative administration of inotropes in cardiac surgery patients. *J Cardiothorac Anesth* 6(suppl 5):17, 1990.

with an acute coronary syndrome. In the anesthetized patient with evidence of myocardial ischemia, initiation of anti-ischemic drug therapy is indicated. This section reviews the common agents used for this purpose (see Chapter 18).

Nitroglycerin

Nitroglycerin (NTG) is clinically indicated as initial therapy in nearly all types of myocardial ischemia.[2] Chronic exertional angina, de novo angina, unstable angina, Prinzmetal's angina (vasospasm), and silent ischemia respond to NTG administration.[2–6] NTG therapy decreases the incidence of anginal attacks and improves exercise tolerance before angina symptoms.[7] During therapy with intravenous (IV) NTG, if blood pressure (BP) declines and ischemia is not relieved, the addition of phenylephrine will allow coronary perfusion pressure (CPP) to be maintained while allowing greater doses of NTG to be used for ischemia relief.[8] If reflex increases in heart rate (HR) and contractility occur, combination therapy with β-adrenergic blockers may be indicated to blunt this undesired increase in HR. Combination therapy with nitrates and calcium channel blockers may be an effective anti-ischemic regimen in selected patients; however, excessive hypotension and reflex tachycardia may be a problem, especially when a dihydropyridine calcium antagonist is used.[9]

Mechanism of Action

NTG enhances myocardial oxygen delivery and reduces myocardial oxygen demand. NTG is a smooth muscle relaxant that causes vasculature dilation. Nitrate-mediated vasodilation occurs with or without

intact vascular endothelium.[10] Nitrites, organic nitrites, nitroso compounds, and other nitrogen oxide–containing substances (e.g., nitroprusside) enter the smooth muscle cell and are converted to reactive nitric oxide (NO) or S-nitrosothiols, which stimulate guanylate cyclase metabolism to produce cyclic guanosine monophosphate (cGMP)[11–13] (Figure 10-1). A cGMP-dependent protein kinase is stimulated with resultant protein phosphorylation in the smooth muscle. This leads to a dephosphorylation of the myosin light chain and smooth muscle relaxation.[14,15] Vasodilation is also associated with a reduction of intracellular calcium.[16] Sulfhydryl (SH) groups are required for formation of NO and the stimulation of guanylate cyclase. When excessive numbers of SH groups are metabolized by prolonged exposure to NTG, vascular tolerance occurs.[17] The addition of N-acetylcysteine, an SH donor, reverses NTG tolerance.[18] The mechanism by which NTG compounds are uniquely better venodilators, especially at lower serum concentrations, is unknown but may be related to increased uptake of NTG by veins compared with arteries.[19]

Physiologic Effects

Two important physiologic effects of NTG are systemic and regional venous dilation (Figure 10-2). Venodilation can markedly reduce venous pressure, venous return to the heart, and cardiac filling pressures. Prominent venodilation occurs at lower doses and does not increase further as the NTG dose increases.[20] Venodilation results primarily in pooling of blood in the splanchnic capacitance system.[21] Mesenteric blood volume increases as ventricular size, ventricular pressures, and intrapericardial pressure decrease.[21]

NTG increases the distensibility and conductance of large arteries without changing systemic vascular resistance (SVR) at low doses.[22] Improved compliance of the large arteries does not necessarily imply afterload reduction. At greater doses, NTG dilates smaller arterioles and resistance vessels, reducing afterload and BP[23] (see Figure 10-2). Reductions in cardiac dimension and pressure reduce myocardial oxygen consumption (MVO₂) and improve myocardial ischemia[24] (Figure 10-3). NTG may preferentially reduce cardiac preload, while maintaining systemic perfusion pressure, an important hemodynamic effect in myocardial ischemia. However, in hypovolemic states, greater doses of NTG may markedly reduce systemic BP to dangerous levels. A reflex increase in HR may occur at arterial vasodilating doses.

NTG causes vasodilation of pulmonary arteries and veins and predictably decreases right atrial (RAP), pulmonary artery (PAP), and pulmonary capillary wedge pressures (PCWP).[23] Pulmonary artery hypertension may be reduced in various disease states and in

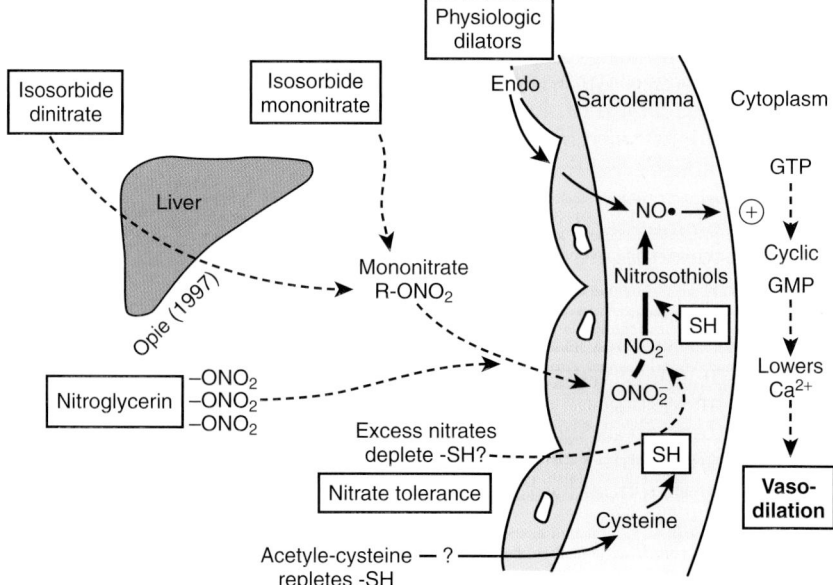

Figure 10-1 Mechanisms of the effects of nitrates in the generation of nitric oxide (NO•) and the stimulation of guanylate cyclase (+) and cyclic guanosine monophosphate (cGMP), which mediates vasodilation. Sulfhydryl (SH) groups are required for the formation of NO• and the stimulation of guanylate cyclase. Isosorbide dinitrate is metabolized by the liver, whereas this route of metabolism is bypassed by the mononitrates. GTP, guanosine triphosphate. *(Redrawn from Opie LH: Drugs for the heart, 4th ed. Philadelphia: WB Saunders, 1995, p 33.)*

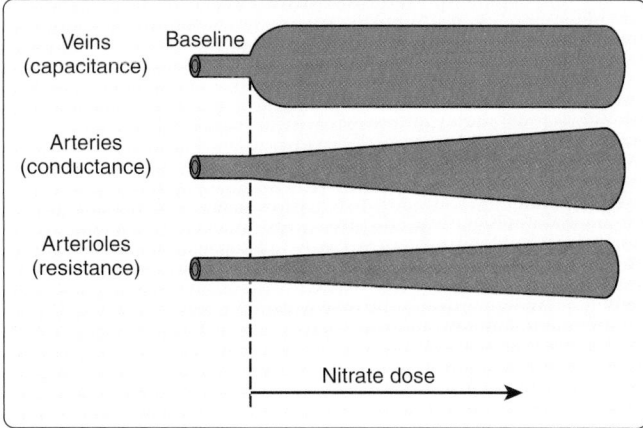

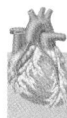

Figure 10-2 Actions of organic nitrates on the major vascular beds and relation of vasodilation to the size of the administered dose. The venous capacitance system dilates maximally with very low doses of organic nitrates. Increasing the amount of drug does not cause appreciable additional venodilation. Arterial dilation and enhanced arterial conductance begin at low doses of nitrates, with further vasodilation as the dosage is increased. With high plasma concentrations of nitrates, the arteriolar resistance vessels dilate, resulting in decreases in systemic and regional vascular resistances. *(Modified from Abrams J: Hemodynamic effects of nitroglycerin and long-acting nitrates. Am Heart J 110(part 2):216, 1985; and Abrams J: Nitrates. In Chatterjee K, Cheitlin MD, Karliner J, et al [eds]: Cardiology: An illustrated text/reference, vol 1. Philadelphia: JB Lippincott, 1991, pp 275–290.)*

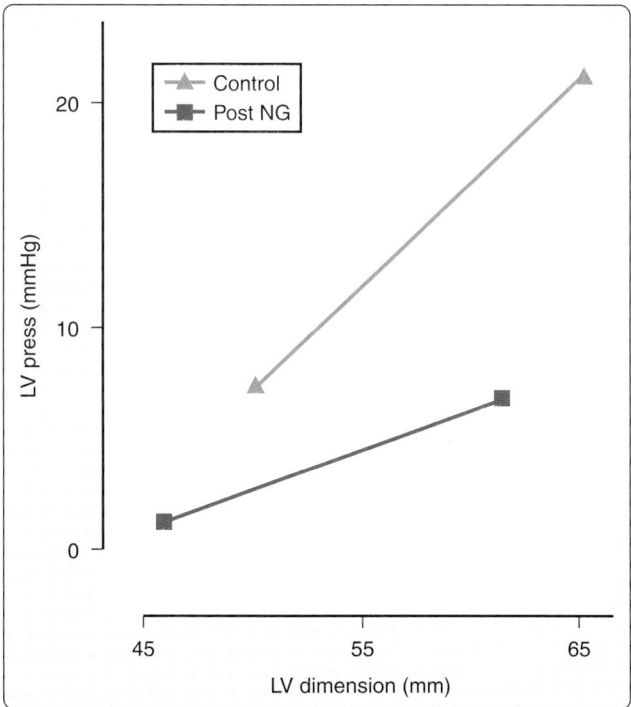

Figure 10-3 Effect of sublingual nitroglycerin (NG) on the left ventricular (LV) diastolic pressure-dimension relation in a patient with chronic aortic regurgitation. Dimensions (from an echocardiogram) and pressure data points were obtained in early diastole (minimal pressure) and at end-diastole (peak of QRS). After the administration of nitroglycerin, the pressure-dimension curve is shifted to the left. *Triangles* represent control; *squares* represent post-NG. *(From Smith ER, Smiseth OA, Kingma I, et al: Mechanism of action of nitrates. Role of changes in venous capacitance and in the left ventricular diastolic pressure-volume relation. Am J Med 76:14, 1984. copyright 1984 with permission from Excerpta Medical Inc.)*

BOX 10-1. EFFECTS OF NITROGLYCERIN AND ORGANIC NITRATES ON THE CORONARY CIRCULATION

Epicardial coronary artery dilation: small arteries dilate proportionately more than larger arteries
Increased coronary collateral vessel diameter and enhanced collateral flow
Improved subendocardial blood flow
Dilation of coronary atherosclerotic stenoses
Initial short-lived increase in coronary blood flow, later reduction in coronary blood flow as MVO$_2$ decreases
Reversal and prevention of coronary vasospasm and vasoconstriction

(Modified from Abrams J: Hemodynamic effects of nitroglycerin and long-acting nitrates. Am Heart J 110[pt 2]:216, 1985.)

congenital heart disease with NTG.[25,26] Renal arteries, cerebral arteries, and cutaneous vessels also dilate with NTG.[27] Blood flow to the kidney and brain may decrease if adequate renal and cerebral perfusion pressures are not maintained.

NTG has several important effects on the coronary circulation (Box 10-1). NTG is a potent epicardial coronary artery vasodilator in both normal and diseased vessels. Stenotic lesions dilate with NTG, reducing the resistance to coronary blood flow (CBF) and improving myocardial ischemia.[28,29] Smaller coronary arteries may dilate relatively more than larger coronary vessels; however, the degree of dilation may depend on the baseline tone of the vessel.[30] NTG effectively reverses or prevents coronary artery vasospasm.[31]

Total CBF may initially increase but eventually decreases with NTG despite coronary vasodilation[32] (Figure 10-4). Autoregulatory mechanisms probably result in decreases in total flow as a result of reductions in wall tension and myocardial oxygen consumption.[23] However, regional myocardial blood flow may improve by vasodilation of intercoronary collateral vessels or reduction of subendocardial compressive forces[33] (Figure 10-5). Coronary arteriographic studies in humans demonstrate that coronary collateral vessels increase in size after NTG administration.[34] This effect may be especially important when epicardial vessels have subtotal or total occlusive disease.[35] Improvement in collateral flow also may be protective in situations in which coronary artery steal may occur with other potent coronary vasodilator agents. The improvement in blood flow to the subendocardium, the most vulnerable area to the development of ischemia, is secondary to both improvement in collateral flow and reductions in left ventricular end-diastolic pressure (LVEDP), which reduce subendocardial resistance to blood flow.[36] With the maintenance of an adequate CPP (e.g., with administration of phenylephrine), NTG can maximize subendocardial blood flow[8] (see Figures 10-4 and 10-5). The ratio of endocardial to epicardial blood in transmural segments is enhanced with NTG.[36] Inhibition of platelet aggregation also occurs with NTG; however, the clinical significance of this action is unknown.[37]

Pharmacology

Organic nitrates are biotransformed by reduction hydrolysis catalyzed by the hepatic enzyme glutathione-organic nitrate reductase.[15] The rate of hepatic denitrification is characteristic of each nitrate and is further dependent on hepatic blood flow or presence of hepatic disease.[15] Common organic nitrates for clinical use are shown in Table 10-2.

Sublingual Nitroglycerin

Sublingual NTG (0.15- to 0.6-mg tablets) achieves blood levels adequate to cause hemodynamic changes within several minutes; physiologic effects last 30 to 45 minutes.[38] Sublingual bioavailability is approximately 80% and bypasses the high first-pass biodegradation in the liver (90%) by nitrate reductase to glycerol dinitrate

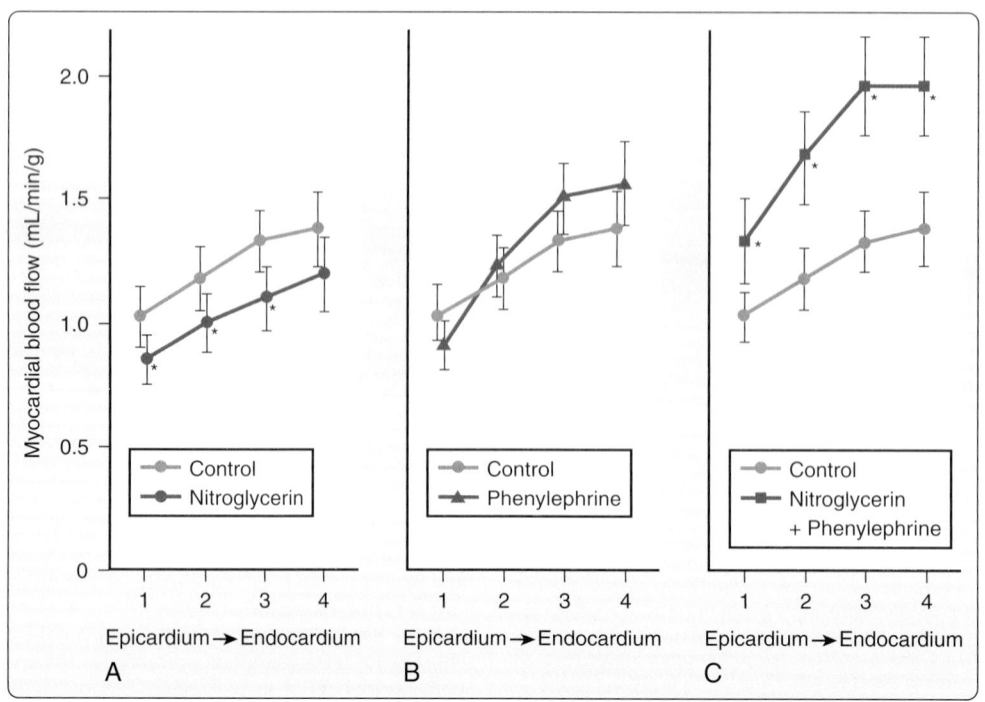

Figure 10-4 Mean blood flow (mL/min/g) ± standard error to four transmural layers of anterior nonischemic myocardium during occlusion of the circumflex coronary artery in animals. Data are reported during control conditions, during infusion of nitroglycerin (0.015 mg/kg/min) *(A)*, during administration of phenylephrine to increase mean arterial pressure to 153 ± 6 mm Hg *(B)*, and during simultaneous administration of nitroglycerin and phenylephrine *(C)*. Nitroglycerin decreases blood flow, and phenylephrine generally increases blood flow in normal myocardium. The combination markedly augments flow. *P < 0.05 in comparison with control measurements. *Light circles* represent control; *dark circles* represent nitroglycerin; *triangles* represent phenylephrine; *squares* represent nitroglycerin + phenylephrine. *(From Bache RJ: Effect of nitroglycerin and arterial hypertension on myocardial blood flow following acute coronary artery occlusion in the dog. Circulation 57:557, 1978. copyright 1978 American Heart Association.)*

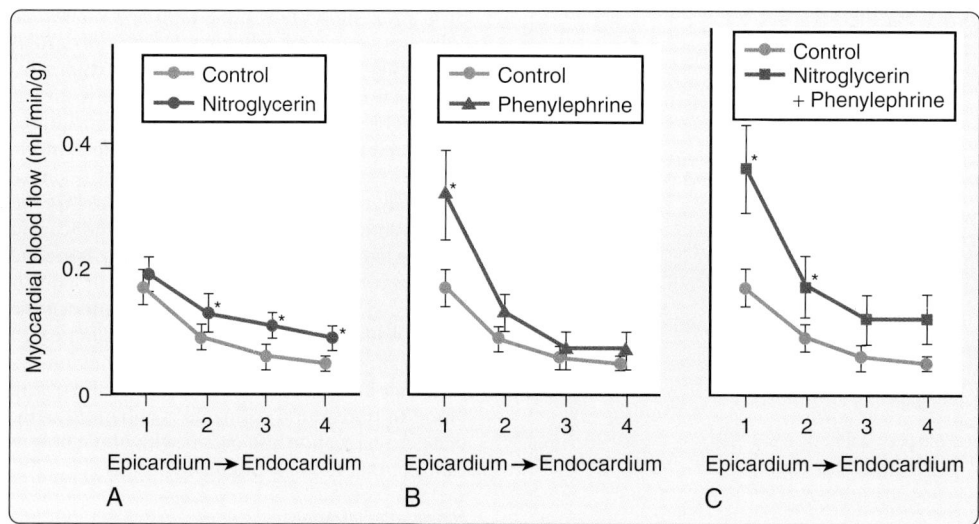

Figure 10-5 Mean blood flow (mL/min/g) ± standard error to four transmural layers of the central ischemic zone during occlusion of the circumflex coronary artery in animals. Data are reported during control conditions, during infusion of nitroglycerin (0.015 mg/kg/min) *(A)*, during administration of phenylephrine to increase mean arterial pressure to 153 ± 6 mm Hg *(B)*, and during simultaneous administration of nitroglycerin and phenylephrine *(C)*. Coronary blood flow to all layers of ischemic myocardium is enhanced with the combination. *P < 0.05 in comparison with control measurements. *Light circles* represent control; *dark circles* represent nitroglycerin; *triangles* represent phenylephrine; *squares* represent nitroglycerin + phenylephrine. *(From Bache RJ: Effect of nitroglycerin and arterial hypertension on myocardial blood flow following acute coronary artery occlusion in the dog. Circulation 57:557, 1978. copyright 1978 American Heart Association.)*

and nitrite, which are excreted renally. Plasma half-life of sublingual NTG is 4 to 7 minutes. NTG spray has pharmacokinetics and pharmacodynamics equivalent to those of a 0.4-mg sublingual tablet; however, it has a longer shelf half-life compared with the tablets, which decompose in air and warm temperatures.[39] A tablet that adheres to the buccal area between the upper lip and teeth has rapid onset and has the advantage of longer half-life than sublingual tablets.[40] Although NTG is readily absorbed through the gastric mucosa, the high rate of liver metabolism makes oral administration highly unpredictable.

TABLE 10-2	Nitroglycerin and Nitrates in Angina		
Compound	*Route*	*Dose/Dosage*	*Duration of Effect*
Nitroglycerin	Sublingual tablets	0.3–0.6 mg up to 1.5 mg	1–7 min
	Spray	0.4 mg as needed	Similar to sublingual tablets
	Transdermal	0.2–0.8 mg/h every 12 hr	8–12 hr during intermittent therapy
	Intravenous	5–200 μg/min	Tolerance in 7–8 hr
Isosorbide dinitrate	Oral	5–80 mg, 2 or 3 times daily	Up to 8 hr
	Oral, slow release	40 mg 1 or 2 times daily	Up to 8 hr
Isosorbide mononitrate	Oral	20 mg twice daily	12–24 hr
	Oral, slow release	60–240 mg once daily	
Pentaerythritol tetranitrate	Sublingual	10 mg as needed	Not known
Erythritol tetranitrate	Sublingual	5–10 mg as needed	Not known
	Oral	10–30 mg 3 times daily	Not known

Adapted from Gibbons RJ, Chatterjee K, Daley J, Douglas JS: ACC/AHA/ACP-ASIM guidelines for the management of patients with chronic stable angina: A report of the American College of Cardiology/American Heart Association Task Force on Practice Guidelines (Committee on Management of Patients with Chronic Stable Angina). *J Am Coll Cardiol* 33:2092–2197, 1999; Table 28.

Nitroglycerin Ointment and Patches

NTG ointment (2%) is readily absorbed through the skin, with this method of administration providing longer-lasting effects.[41] Adequate NTG blood levels are reached within 20 to 30 minutes, and duration of action is 4 to 6 hours.[41] Ointment is administered in inches (15 mg/inch), but the surface area of application and not the amount administered determines the blood level achieved. NTG ointment is messy, requires application four times a day, and is most appropriate for nursing administration in special care units.[42]

NTG patches contain either liquid NTG or NTG bonded to a polymer gel and slowly released to the skin through a semipermeable membrane.[43] The pharmacokinetics approach that of a consistent IV infusion.[43] Blood levels are reached within 20 to 30 minutes, and a steady state is reached within 2 hours. Blood levels may be maintained up to 24 hours and are largely determined by patch size. Patches or disks contain an NTG concentration per square centimeter, and dosages of 0.2 to 0.8 mg/hr usually are required for relief of myocardial ischemia. Although convenient for patients, tolerance may be a problem with these sustained-release preparations.[41] Intermittent therapy is recommended to avoid tolerance.[44]

Intravenous Nitroglycerin

NTG has been available since the early 1980s as an injectable drug with stable shelf half-life in a 400-μg/mL solution of D_5W (5% dextrose in water). Blood levels are achieved instantaneously, and arterial dilating doses with resulting hypotension may quickly occur. If the volume status of the patient is unknown, initial dosages of 5 to 10 μg/min are recommended. The dosage necessary for relieving myocardial ischemia may vary from patient to patient, but relief is usually achieved with 75 to 150 μg/min. In a clinical study of 20 patients with rest angina, a mean dosage of 72 μg/min reduced or abolished ischemic episodes in 85% of patients.[45] However, doses as high as 300 to 400 μg/min may be necessary for ischemic relief in some patients. Arterial dilation becomes clinically apparent at doses around 50 μg/min. Drug offset after discontinuation of an infusion is rapid (2 to 5 minutes). The dosage of NTG available is less when administered in plastic bags and polyvinylchloride tubing because of NTG absorption by the bag and tubing, although this is not a significant clinical problem because the drug is titrated to effect.[46]

Adverse Effects

The metabolism of NTG by liver nitrate reductase produces a nitrite that oxidizes the ferrous iron of hemoglobin to the ferric form of methemoglobin. The ferric iron does not bind or release oxygen.[47] Methemoglobin is formed normally and is reduced by enzyme systems within the red blood cell.[48] Normally, methemoglobin levels do not exceed 1%, but may increase when direct oxidants are present in the serum (nitrates, sulfonamides, aniline dye derivates). Methemoglobinemia with levels up to 20% is not a clinical problem.

Documented increases in methemoglobin blood levels occur with IV NTG, averaging 1.5% in one study of 50 patients receiving NTG for longer than 48 hours.[49] NTG dosages of 5 mg/kg/day orally should be avoided to prevent significant methemoglobinemia.[50] However, rare instances of smaller doses causing clinically significant problems have been reported.[51] Nitrates are effective in producing methemoglobin to bind cyanide in sodium nitroprusside toxicity.

Several mechanisms of nitrate tolerance have been proposed, including a depletion of SH groups, neurohumoral activation, volume expansion, and/or downregulation of nitrate receptors.[52-57] Tolerance may occur with all forms of nitrate administration that maintain continuous blood levels of the drug.[17,58-61] Discontinuation of the drug after prolonged exposure may result in a rebound phenomenon, possibly resulting in coronary vasospasm and myocardial ischemia or infarction.[62] Tolerance to NTG apparently does not occur in all patients.[63] If tolerance develops after prolonged exposure, physiologic responsiveness may be achieved with greater dosages of NTG, an important observation during NTG administration in cardiac surgery.[64] Intermittent dosing with a nitrate-free interval each day or night can maintain NTG responsiveness.[44,65]

NTG interferes with platelet aggregation.[66] The ability of the platelet to adhere to damaged intima is reduced.[67] Primary and secondary wave aggregation of platelets is also attenuated.[68] Previously formed platelet plugs are disaggregated.[69] A clinical study of 10 patients with coronary artery disease (CAD) demonstrated that a mean dosage of NTG (1.19 μg/kg/min) inhibited platelet aggregation by 50%, with a return to baseline platelet aggregation 15 minutes after the infusion was discontinued[70] (Figure 10-6). NO production increases cGMP, which modulates intracellular platelet calcium and reduces platelet secretion of proaggregatory factors.[71] The clinical significance of these actions remains unclear. As with other potent vasodilators, NTG may increase intrapulmonary shunting of blood and reduce arterial oxygen tension.

NTG may induce resistance to the anticoagulant effects of heparin.[72] During simultaneous infusions of NTG and heparin, an increase in the NTG infusion caused the activated partial thromboplastin time to decrease.[73] Becker et al[74] reported NTG-induced heparin resistance at NTG infusion rates greater than 350 μg/min. The authors suggested a qualitative problem with antithrombin III (AT III) because AT III levels did not decrease. Others have suggested that NTG interferes with AT III binding to heparin by *N*-desulfation of the heparin molecule at the AT III binding sites.[75] *N*-desulfation of heparin reduces its anticoagulant activity.[76]

NTG is contraindicated in patients who have used sildenafil, vardenafil, or tadalafil, or in patients who are hypotensive. These drugs for erectile dysfunction inhibit the phosphodiesterase (PDE5) that degrades cGMP, and the cGMP mediates vascular smooth muscle relaxation by NO. NTG-mediated vasodilation is markedly enhanced and prolonged, resulting in cases of profound hypotension, myocardial infarction (MI), and death.[77] Small doses of NTG have been used, but

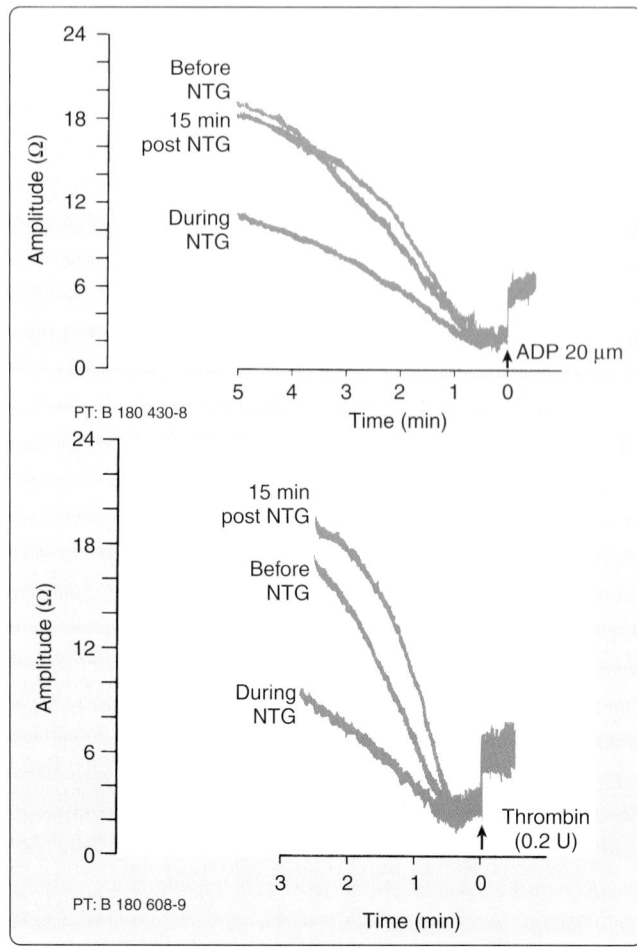

Figure 10-6 Typical examples of aggregation responses to *(top)* adenosine diphosphate (ADP) and to *(bottom)* thrombin before, during, and after infusion of nitroglycerin (NTG) in patients with coronary artery disease. The amplitude of the curve is calibrated in ohms using a dual-channel impedance aggregometer. Nitroglycerin inhibits platelet aggregation to both reagents, and the effect is rapidly reversible after discontinuation of the drug. *(Modified from Diodati J, Theroux P, Latour JG, et al: Effects of nitroglycerin at therapeutic doses on platelet aggregation in unstable angina pectoris and acute myocardial infarction. Am J Cardiol 66:683, 1990.)*

the amount of time that must elapse after a patient's last dose of one of these medications before regular doses of nitrates may be safely administered is unclear.[78–80]

Summary

NTG remains a first-line agent for the treatment of myocardial ischemia. Special care must be taken in patients with signs of hypovolemia or hypotension because the vasodilating effects of the drug may worsen the clinical condition. Recent ACC/AHA Guidelines address the prophylactic intraoperative use of NTG and suggest that its usefulness in preventing myocardial ischemia and cardiac morbidity in high-risk patients undergoing noncardiac surgery is unclear.[81]

β-Adrenergic Blockers

β-Adrenergic blockers have multiple favorable effects in treating the ischemic heart during anesthesia (Box 10-2). β-Adrenergic blockers reduce oxygen consumption by decreasing HR, BP, and myocardial contractility. HR reduction increases diastolic CBF. Increased collateral blood flow and redistribution of blood to ischemic areas may occur with β-blockers. More free fatty acids may be available for substrate

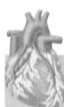

BOX 10-2. EFFECTS OF β-ADRENERGIC BLOCKERS ON MYOCARDIAL ISCHEMIA

- Reductions in myocardial oxygen consumption
- Improvements in coronary blood flow
- Prolonged diastolic perfusion period
- Improved collateral flow
- Increased flow to ischemic areas
- Overall improvement in supply/demand ratio
- Stabilization of cellular membranes
- Improved oxygen dissociation from hemoglobin
- Inhibition of platelet aggregation
- Reduced mortality after myocardial infarction

consumption by the myocardium. Microcirculatory oxygen delivery improves, and oxygen dissociates more easily from hemoglobin after β-adrenergic blockade. Platelet aggregation is inhibited. β-Blockers should be started early in patients with ischemia in the absence of contraindications.[1] Many patients at high risk for perioperative cardiac morbidity should be started on β-blockers before surgery and continued for up to 30 days after surgery.[82–84] The choice of which β-blocker for any individual patient is based on clinician familiarity and desired pharmacologic profile. There is no evidence that one specific agent is superior to another; however, β-blockers without intrinsic sympathomimetic activity (ISA) are preferable when treating acute myocardial ischemia.

β-Blockers administered during MI reduce myocardial infarct size.[85] In addition, a reduction in morbidity has been shown to occur with acute IV metoprolol during MI.[85] Similar findings with reductions in mortality extending up to 3 years after MI have been shown in numerous trials with β-adrenergic blockers[86,87] (Figure 10-7). The mechanisms for mortality reduction are unclear. In the absence of contraindications, β-blockers should be a routine part of care in patients with all forms of CAD, including unstable angina and recent MI.

Data confirm the important role of β-blockade in treating patients after acute MI and in reducing mortality in high-risk populations. Immediate β-blockade after thrombolytic therapy in patients with acute MI significantly decreased recurrent early myocardial ischemia and reinfarction.[88] Early β-blockade is indicated in the treatment of MI[89,90] (Box 10-3). In fact, β-blocker therapy after MI may be greatly underused in patients older than 65 years.[91] Atenolol has been found to reduce ischemia and adverse outcome in patients with mildly symptomatic ischemia.[92] Multiple studies have shown that perioperative administration of β-adrenergic blockers reduces both mortality and morbidity when given to patients at high risk for CAD who must undergo noncardiac surgery[82–84,93,94] (Figures 10-8 to 10-10). These data suggest that intermediate- and high-risk patients presenting for noncardiac surgery should receive perioperative β-adrenergic blockade to reduce postoperative cardiac mortality and morbidity. However, in the Perioperative Ischemic Evaluation Study (POISE) trial, the use of higher dose metoprolol started in patients on the day of noncardiac surgery was associated with increased risk for severe stroke and greater total mortality.[95] These findings have led to increased scrutiny of perioperative β-blockade usage. Recent ACC/AHA recommendations on the perioperative use of β-adrenergic blockade for noncardiac surgery are given in Box 10-4.[81]

β Receptor

The β receptor was conceptualized by Ahlquist,[96] who divided various physiologic effects of catecholamine stimulation into α and β responses. The β receptor has been identified biochemically as a polypeptide chain of approximately 50,000 to 60,000 kDa.[97] The receptor's structure is common to most receptor proteins that have been identified: seven transmembrane crossings with two extramembranous terminal ends[98] (Figure 10-11). All receptors that transduce a signal

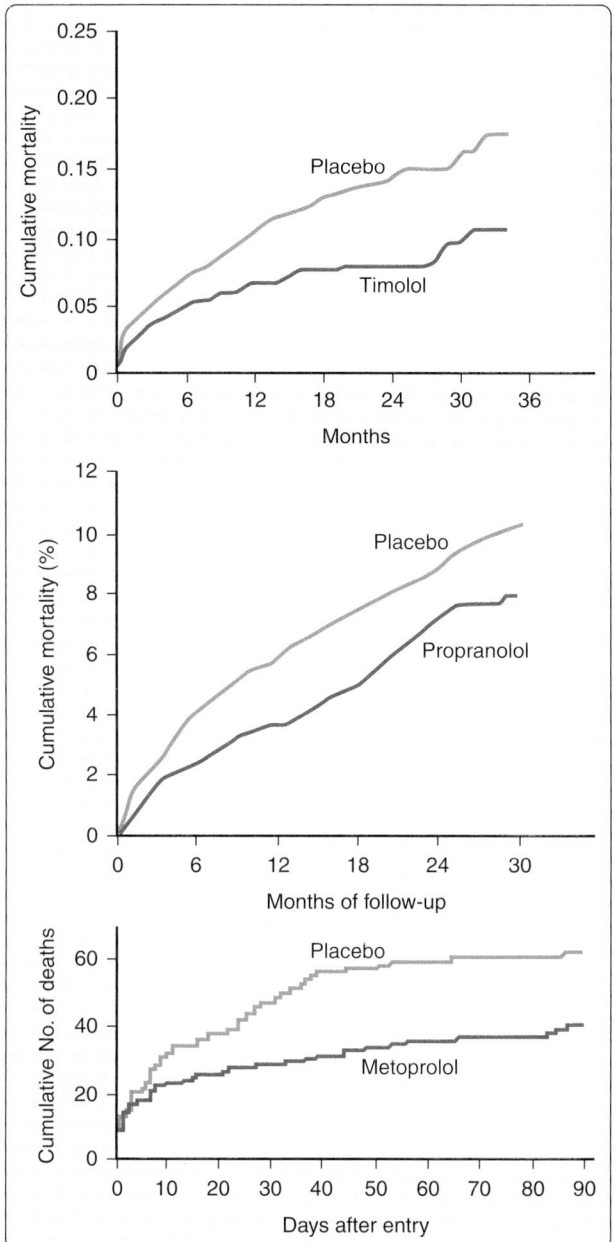

Figure 10-7 Cumulative mortality curves for timolol (top), propranolol (center), and metoprolol (bottom) after myocardial infarction mortality reduction trials. (Modified from Turi ZG, Braunwald E: The use of β-blockers after myocardial infarction. JAMA 249:2512, 1983. copyright 1983 American Medical Association.)

through G proteins share this basic structure.[99] There are three extracellular and intracellular loops connecting the intramembranous portion of the receptor.[98] Agonist-antagonist binding occurs at the intramembranous portion, whereas the intracellular loops modulate interaction with the G-protein complex.[100,101] The terminal intracellular end contains amino acid residues that undergo phosphorylation, which relates to desensitization and downregulation of the receptor.[102]

Receptor stimulation activates a G protein, which stimulates adenylyl cyclase. The G-protein complex is composed of both stimulatory (G_s) and inhibitory (G_i) intermediary proteins.[99] Adenylyl cyclase converts adenosine triphosphate (ATP) to cyclic adenosine monophosphate (cAMP), which phosphorylates a protein kinase and produces the appropriate cellular response. A typical cascade of this sequence

leading to increases in myocardial contractility from β-receptor stimulation is illustrated in Figure 10-12.

β-Receptor numbers in any tissue may decrease with chronic stimulation (downregulation) or increase with chronic blockade (upregulation). The process of desensitization of the adrenergic response in chronic stimulation (i.e., congestive heart failure [CHF]) may involve downregulation of the receptors but may involve either the G-protein complex or adenylyl cyclase. Desensitization may occur quickly, whereas downregulation with actual internalization of the receptor within the cell may take days to weeks.[103] Myocardial ischemia increases β-receptor density, although it remains controversial whether this upregulation results in greater adrenergic response.[104] Several studies have demonstrated that high-affinity β receptors in nonischemic tissue were shifted to a low-affinity state during ischemia.[105,106] Also, the levels of G_s and its activity are reduced during myocardial ischemia.[107] However, stimulation of these receptors with isoproterenol during ischemia does result in increases in cAMP production.[104,108]

There are two types of β receptors with a multitude of responses[109] (Table 10-3). Both $β_1$- and $β_2$-receptor stimulation primarily involve cardiac function (Figure 10-13). Responses of isolated human atrial tissue demonstrated greater inotropic response to $β_1$- than to $β_2$-receptor stimulation.[110] Endogenous norepinephrine produces inotropic responses in human atrial appendages and ventricular papillary muscle by $β_1$-receptor stimulation, whereas epinephrine produces its maximal inotropic effects on the atria by $β_2$-receptor stimulation and up to 50% of its maximal inotropic response in the ventricle by $β_2$-receptor stimulation.[111,112] Sinus node, atrioventricular (AV) node, the left and right bundle branches, and the Purkinje system contain higher densities of $β_2$ receptors.[113] Clearly, both receptor subtypes have cardiac inotropic, chronotropic, and dromotropic properties.

$β_2$-Adrenoceptors comprise 93% of the total population of β receptors in arterioles and 100% of receptors in epicardium, vena cava, aorta, and pulmonary artery.[112] $β_2$ receptors are found on the intimal surface of human internal mammary artery, but not on the saphenous vein,[114] the two vessels most commonly used for coronary artery bypass graft surgery (CABG). $β_2$-Stimulation results in vascular smooth muscle relaxation and vasodilation.

$β_1$-Receptor stimulation increases plasma renin production and aqueous humor production. $β_2$-Receptor stimulation relaxes smooth muscle and produces bronchodilation and uterine relaxation. $β_2$-Stimulation also increases insulin secretion, glycogenolysis, and lipolysis and shifts extracellular potassium to intracellular sites.

$β_3$-Adrenoceptors are found on visceral adipocytes, the gallbladder, and colon. Stimulation of $β_3$ receptors is thought to mediate lipolytic and thermic responses in brown and white adipose tissue.[115]

Physiologic Effects

Anti-ischemic Effects

β-Blockade on the ischemic heart may result in a favorable shift in the O_2 demand/supply ratio (see Table 10-1). The reductions in the force of contraction and HR reduce myocardial oxygen consumption and result in autoregulatory decreases in myocardial blood flow. Several studies have shown that blood flow to ischemic regions with propranolol is maintained; however, this is probably secondary to maintenance of α-vasoconstrictor tone of epicardial vessels and of a pressure gradient to the vasodilated endocardial areas of ischemia.[116,117] Reductions in blood flow in some patients with vasospastic angina may worsen with the administration of propranolol.[118] Intracoronary infusion of propranolol does not worsen stenotic lesions and actually increases the luminal size of the stenosis at rest and during exercise.[119]

Antihypertensive Effects

The exact mechanisms involved in BP reduction are not clear. Both $β_1$- and $β_2$-receptor blockers inhibit myocardial contractility and reduce HR; both effects should reduce BP. No acute decrease in BP occurs during acute administration of propranolol.[120] However, chronic BP reduction has been attributed to a chronic reduction in cardiac output (CO).[121] Reductions in high levels of plasma renin have

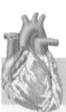

BOX 10-3. ACC/AHA GUIDELINES FOR EARLY USE OF β-ADRENOCEPTOR BLOCKING AGENTS AFTER STEMI

Early Therapy

*Class I***

1. Oral β-blocker therapy should be initiated in the first 24 hours for patients who do not have any of the following: 1) signs of heart failure, 2) evidence of low output state, 3) increased risk* for cardiogenic shock, or 4) other relative contraindications to β-blockade (PR interval > 0.24 sec), second- or third-degree heart block, active asthma, or reactive airway disease. (Level of Evidence: B)
2. Patients with contraindications within the first 24 hours of STEMI should be reevaluated for candidacy for β-blocker therapy as secondary prevention. (Level of Evidence: C)
3. Patients with moderate-to-severe LV failure should receive β-blocker therapy as secondary prevention with a gradual titration scheme. (Level of Evidence: B)

Class IIa:

1. It is reasonable to administer an IV β-blocker at the time of presentation to STEMI patients who are hypertensive and who do not have any of the following: 1) signs of heart failure, 2) evidence of a low output state, 3) increased risk* for cardiogenic shock, or 4) other relative contraindications to β-blockade (PR interval greater than 0.24 seconds, second- or third-degree heart block, active asthma, or reactive airway disease). (Level of Evidence: B)

Class III

1. IV β-blockers should not be administered to STEMI patients who have any of the following: 1) signs of heart failure, 2) evidence of a low output state, 3) increased risk* for cardiogenic shock, or 4) other relative contraindications to β-blockade (PR interval > 0.24 seconds, second- or third-degree heart block, active asthma, or reactive airway disease). (Level of Evidence: A)

*Risk factors for cardiogenic shock (the greater the number of risk factors present, the higher the risk of developing cardiogenic shock) are age older than 70 years, systolic blood pressure less than 120 mm Hg, sinus tachycardia greater than 110 bpm or heart rate less than 60 bpm, and increased time since onset of symptoms of STEMI.
STEMI, ST-segment elevation myocardial infarction.
Reproduced from Antman EM, Hand M, Armstrong PW, et al: 2007 focused update of the ACC/AHA 2004 guidelines for the management of patients with ST-elevation myocardial infarction: A report of the American College of Cardiology/American Heart Association Task Force on Practice Guidelines (Writing Group to Review New Evidence and Update the ACC/AHA 2004 Guidelines for the Management of Patients with ST-Elevation Myocardial Infarction). *Circulation* 117:296, 2008, by permission.[90]

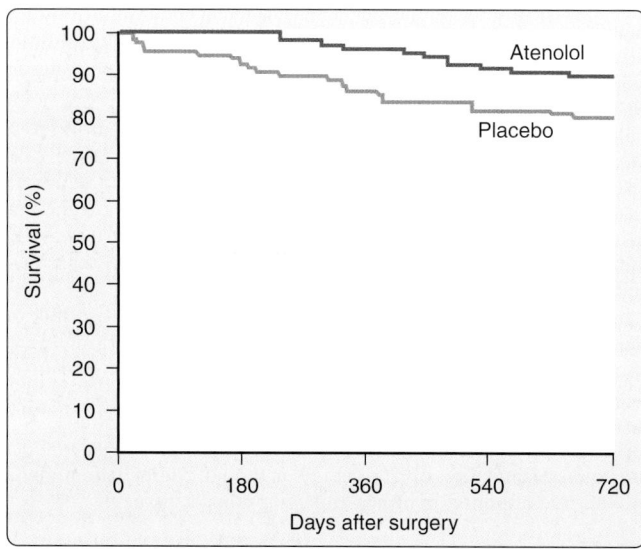
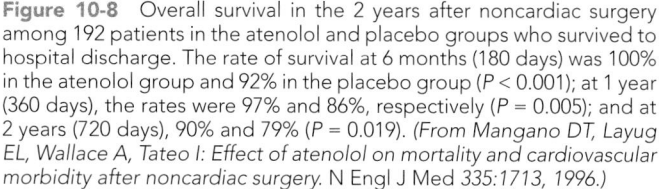

Figure 10-8 Overall survival in the 2 years after noncardiac surgery among 192 patients in the atenolol and placebo groups who survived to hospital discharge. The rate of survival at 6 months (180 days) was 100% in the atenolol group and 92% in the placebo group (P < 0.001); at 1 year (360 days), the rates were 97% and 86%, respectively (P = 0.005); and at 2 years (720 days), 90% and 79% (P = 0.019). *(From Mangano DT, Layug EL, Wallace A, Tateo I: Effect of atenolol on mortality and cardiovascular morbidity after noncardiac surgery. N Engl J Med 335:1713, 1996.)*

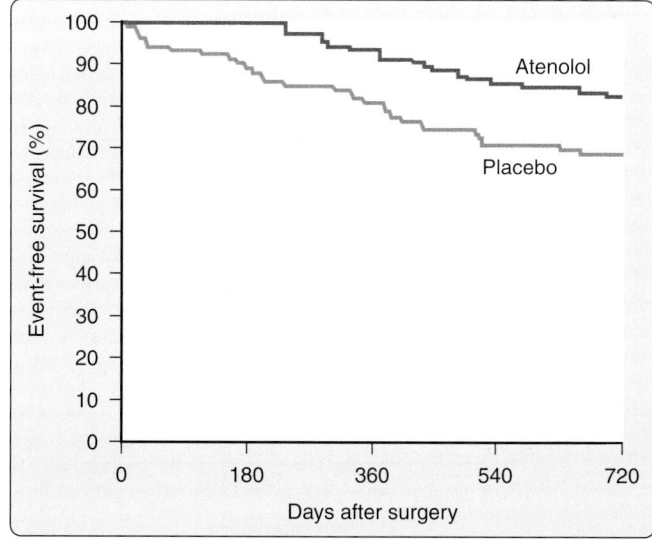

Figure 10-9 Event-free survival in the 2 years after noncardiac surgery among 192 patients in the atenolol and placebo groups who survived to hospital discharge. The outcome measure combined the following events: myocardial infarction, unstable angina, the need for coronary artery bypass surgery, and congestive heart failure. The rate of event-free survival at 6 months (180 days) was 100% in the atenolol group and 88% in the placebo group (P < 0.001); at 1 year (360 days), the rates were 92% and 78%, respectively (P = 0.003); and at 2 years (720 days), 83% and 68% (P = 0.008). *(From Mangano DT, Layug EL, Wallace A, Tateo I: Effect of atenolol on mortality and cardiovascular morbidity after noncardiac surgery. N Engl J Med 335:1713, 1996.)*

been suggested as effective therapy in controlling essential hypertension.[122] However, the relation between renin levels and hypertension is not established, and the decrease in BP in patients has no relation to the change in renin levels.[123,124] Stimulation of prejunctional β receptors results in norepinephrine release from postganglionic sympathetic fibers and increases in vascular tone to most major organ systems.[125] Prejunctional β-blockade reduces norepinephrine release, sympathetic nerve traffic, and vascular tone.[125]

Electrophysiologic Effects

Several β-blockers have potent local anesthetic activity at greater serum levels because of sodium-channel–blocking activity and result in depression of phase 0 of the cardiac action potential.[126] However,

this membrane-stabilizing or quinidine-like effect is of questionable clinical relevance because it is observed at concentrations far exceeding therapeutic levels.[127] Generalized slowing of cardiac depolarization results from reducing the rate of diastolic depolarization (phase 4). Action potential duration (APD) and the QT interval may shorten with β-adrenergic blockers.[126] The ventricular fibrillation (VF) threshold is increased with β-blockers.[128] These antiarrhythmic actions of β-blockers are enhanced in settings of catecholamine excess as in pheochromocytoma, acute MI, the perioperative period, and hyperthyroidism.

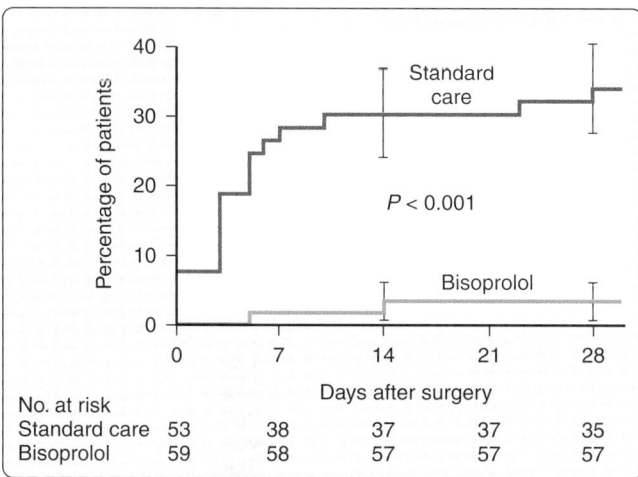

Figure 10-10 Kaplan–Meier estimates of the cumulative percentages of patients who died of cardiac causes or had a nonfatal myocardial infarction during the perioperative period and were at high risk for myocardial mortality with and without preoperative treatment of the β-adrenergic blocker bisoprolol. I bars indicate standard errors. The difference between groups was significant (P < 0.001 by the log-rank test). (From Poldermans D, Boersma E, Bax JJ, et al: The effect of bisoprolol on perioperative mortality and myocardial infarction in high-risk patients undergoing vascular surgery. N Engl J Med 341:1789, 1999. copyright ©1999 Massachusetts Medical Society. All rights reserved.)

Metabolic Effects

Although β₂-blockers are reported to reduce insulin release, the clinical significance of this reduction is questionable.[129] Catecholamines, however, promote glycogenolysis and mobilization of glucose in response to hypoglycemia. In the diabetic patient, nonselective β-blockade may impede this process, thereby worsening recovery from a hypoglycemic episode. Also, the usual hypoglycemic symptoms of tachycardia and anxiety may be suppressed when taking β-blockers, thus delaying detection. In fact, bradycardia and hypertension have been documented as side effects of hypoglycemia in the diabetic patient receiving propranolol because of unopposed β-receptor stimulation with catecholamine release.[130]

Stimulation of β₂-receptors increases the movement of potassium into skeletal muscle cells, reduces aldosterone secretion, and increases renal potassium loss, effects resulting in reduction of serum potassium. β₂-Receptor blockers aid in the maintenance of serum potassium levels by blocking the adrenergic-stimulated movement of potassium intracellularly.[131] β₂-Receptor blockers may cause mild increases in serum potassium concentration, which may be significant in patients with renal insufficiency.[132]

Inhibition of catecholamine-stimulated lipolysis may occur with β-blockers, which reduces the availability of free fatty acids to activate contracting muscle, such as the heart.[133] β-Adrenergic blockers produce increases in serum triglycerides, decreases in high-density lipoprotein cholesterol, and little change in low-density lipoprotein cholesterol. A proposed mechanism is an increase in the relative ratio of α- to β-activity receptors.[134] Increases in β-receptor activity result in increases in lipoprotein lipase and triglyceride levels.[135] These effects on blood lipids are concerns for patients receiving chronic therapy. However, animal studies have shown that β-blockers actually have a retarding effect on the development of atherosclerosis.[136] β-Blockers with ISA produce the smallest changes in the lipid profile.[137]

Intrinsic Sympathomimetic Activity

Several β-blockers (acebutolol, carteolol, penbutolol, pindolol) have agonist and antagonist properties, and are characterized as having ISA.[138] These agents are actually agonists that elicit a submaximal response and block the effects of endogenous catecholamines in a competitive fashion.[138] CO and HR are reduced less with ISA

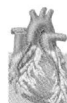

BOX 10-4. RECOMMENDATIONS FOR PERIOPERATIVE β-BLOCKER THERAPY

Class I
1. β-Blockers should be continued in patients undergoing surgery who are receiving β-blockers for treatment of conditions with American College of Cardiology (ACC)/American Heart Association Class I guideline indications for the drugs. (Level of Evidence: C)

Class IIa
1. β-Blockers titrated to heart rate and blood pressure are probably recommended for patients undergoing vascular surgery who are at high cardiac risk because of coronary artery disease or the finding of cardiac ischemia on preoperative testing. (Level of Evidence: B)
2. β-Blockers titrated to heart rate and blood pressure are reasonable for patients in whom preoperative assessment for vascular surgery identifies high cardiac risk, as defined by the presence of more than one clinical risk factor.* (Level of Evidence: C)
3. β-Blockers titrated to heart rate and blood pressure are reasonable for patients in whom preoperative assessment identifies coronary artery disease or high cardiac risk, as defined by the presence of more than one clinical risk factor,* who are undergoing intermediate-risk surgery. (Level of Evidence: B)

Class IIb
1. The usefulness of β-blockers is uncertain for patients who are undergoing either intermediate-risk procedures or vascular surgery in whom preoperative assessment identifies a single clinical risk factor in the absence of coronary artery disease.* (Level of Evidence: C)
2. The usefulness of β-blockers is uncertain in patients undergoing vascular surgery with no clinical risk factors* who are not currently taking β-blockers. (Level of Evidence: B)

Class III
1. β-Blockers should not be given to patients undergoing surgery who have absolute contraindications to β-blockade. (Level of Evidence: C)
2. Routine administration of high-dose β-blockers in the absence of dose titration is not useful and may be harmful to patients not currently taking β-blockers who are undergoing noncardiac surgery. (Level of Evidence: B)

*Clinical risk factors include history of ischemic heart disease, history of compensated or prior heart failure, history of cerebrovascular disease, diabetes mellitus, and renal insufficiency (defined in the Revised Cardiac Risk Index as a preoperative serum creatinine concentration greater than 2 mg/dL).
Adapted from Fleisher LA, Beckman JA, Brown KA, et al: 2009 ACCF/AHA focused update on perioperative beta blockade incorporated into the ACC/AHA 2007 guidelines on perioperative cardiovascular evaluation and care for noncardiac surgery: A report of the American College of Cardiology Foundation/American Heart Association Task Force on Practice Guidelines. Circulation 120:e169, 2009, by permission.

drugs.[139] Peripheral blood flow also is reduced less, making ISA agents attractive in patients with peripheral vascular disease.[140] ISA drugs also cause less bronchoconstriction and are advantageous in chronic obstructive pulmonary disease. Theoretically, differences in changes in β-receptor density should differ with ISA. The effects of ISA drugs reduce β-receptor density (similar to pure agonists), whereas non-ISA agents increase β-receptor density.[141] Although controversial, ISA drugs appear to have a role in mortality reduction after MI, similar to non-ISA β-blockers.[142]

General Pharmacology

Lipid-soluble β-blockers (propranolol, labetalol, metoprolol) are well absorbed after oral administration and attain high concentrations in the brain.[143] Lipid-soluble agents have a high incidence of central nervous system (CNS) side effects, such as depression, sleep disturbances,

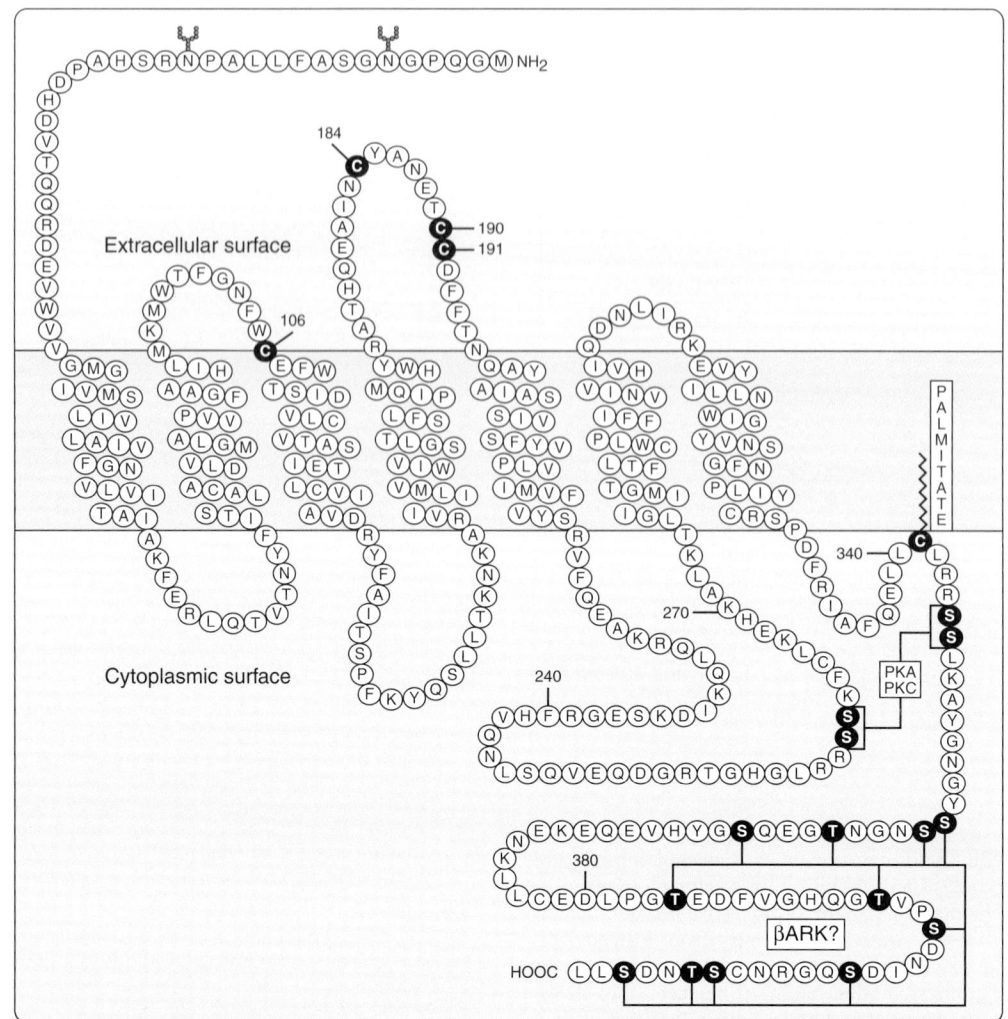

Figure 10-11   **Human β₂-adrenergic receptor (*darkened area* represents the cell membrane).** Depicted are two sites of extracellular *N*-linked glycosylation (Asn5, 16), four cysteine residues that may participate in disulfide bonds (Cys106, 184, 190, 191), an intracellular cysteine residue (Cys341) that may serve as a site of attachment for a palmitate membrane anchor, as well as multiple threonine and serine residues located in C-III and the cytoplasmic carboxyl terminus, which are potential sites of phosphorylation by protein kinase A (PKA), protein kinase C (PKC), or β-adrenergic receptor kinase (βARK). (*Reproduced from Raymond JR, Hnatowich M, Lefkowitz RJ, Caron MG: Adrenergic receptors. Models for regulation of signal transduction processes. Hypertension 15:119, 1990. copyright 1990 American Heart Association.*)

and impotence. First-pass hepatic metabolism after oral ingestion can be very high but varies from patient to patient and affects daily dosing schedules.[144] Cirrhosis, CHF, and cigarette smoking may reduce hepatic metabolism.[145] Lipophilic agents are highly protein bound. The hepatic metabolism of lipophilic agents is independent of protein binding, which is different from most drugs in which hepatic metabolism occurs only with the unbound drug.[146]

Lipid-insoluble or water-soluble agents (atenolol, nadolol, acebutolol, sotalol) are less well absorbed orally but are not hepatically metabolized. These drugs are almost entirely eliminated by renal excretion and must be used with caution in renal insufficiency. The incidence of CNS side effects is low because of lipid insolubility.

Pindolol and timolol have intermediate lipid solubility properties and are metabolized partially by the liver (50%) and excreted through the kidneys (50%). Acebutolol, which is water soluble, has an active metabolite, diacetolol, which is water soluble and excreted renally.[147] The plasma elimination of acebutolol is more rapid than that of diacetolol. For further information on the available oral and IV β-adrenergic blockers for treatment of myocardial ischemia, see Table 10-4. Additional β-blockers with other indications, such as carvedilol (for CHF) and sotalol (for arrhythmias), are covered later in this chapter.

Pharmacology of Intravenous β-Adrenergic Blockers

Propranolol

Propranolol has an equal affinity for β₁ and β₂ receptors, lacks ISA, and has no β-adrenergic receptor activity. It is the most lipid-soluble β-blocker and generally has the most CNS adverse effects. First-pass liver metabolism (90%) is very high, requiring much greater oral doses than IV doses for pharmacodynamic effect.[148] Although propranolol has an active metabolite (4-hydroxypropranolol), the metabolite's half-life is much shorter and does not add to the clinical effect.[149] Serum half-life of the drug after IV dosing is 3 to 4 hours.[150]

Because of the high hepatic extraction of propranolol, factors that affect hepatic blood flow markedly affect propranolol plasma levels. Because propranolol reduces hepatic blood flow, it can reduce its own metabolism, as well as the metabolism of other drugs.[151] This must be taken into consideration during anesthetic procedures in patients with liver disease, reduced CO states, and right ventricular (RV) heart failure (HF).

Propranolol serum levels of 100 ng/mL produce a maximum β-blocking effect in relation to reducing exercise-induced tachycardia.[144] Propranolol still produces a 50% reduction of exercise-induced

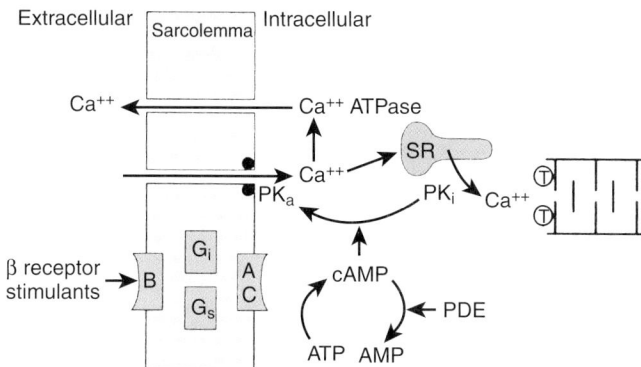

Figure 10-12 **The β-receptor, G protein, adenylyl cyclase system.** With β-receptor stimulation, dynamic changes occur in the G_i and G_s regulatory proteins. Ultimately, G_s stimulates adenylyl cyclase (AC) to convert adenosine triphosphate (ATP) to cyclic adenosine monophosphate (cAMP), which is metabolized by phosphodiesterase enzyme (PDE). An inactive protein kinase (PK_i) is activated (PK_a) by cAMP, which opens an energy-dependent receptor-operated calcium channel allowing calcium entry into the cell. Calcium cycling occurs with calcium actively pumped out of the cell by Ca^{2+} adenosine triphosphatase (ATPase). This calcium cycling causes a release of calcium from the sarcoplasmic reticulum (SR), allowing calcium to bind to troponin C (T) with subsequent activation of the actin-myosin complex. AMP, adenosine monophosphate. *(Modified from Royster RL: Intraoperative administration of inotropes in cardiac surgery patients. J Cardiothorac Anesth 4:17, 1990.)*

TABLE 10-3	Physiologic Effects of β₁- and β₂-Receptor Stimulation		
Physiologic Effect		*$β_1$ Response*	*$β_2$ Response*
Cardiac			
Increased heart rate		++	++
Increased contractility			
Atrium		+	++
Ventricle		++	++
Increased automaticity and conduction velocity			
Nodal tissue		++	++
His-Purkinje		++	++
Arterial relaxation			
Coronary			++
Skeletal muscle			++
Pulmonary			+
Abdominal			+
Renal		+	+
Venous relaxation			++
Smooth muscle relaxation			
Tracheal and bronchial			+
Gastrointestinal			+
Bladder			+
Uterus			+
Splenic capsule			+
Ciliary muscle			+
Metabolic			
Renin release		++	
Lipolysis		++	+
Insulin secretion			+
Glycogenolysis, gluconeogenesis			++
Cellular K^+ uptake			+
Antidiuretic hormone secretion (pituitary)		+	

Modified from Lefkowitz RJ, Hoffman BB, Taylor P: Neurohumoral transmission: The autonomic and somatic motor nervous systems. In Gilman AG, Rall TW, Niew AS, Taylor P (eds): *Goodman and Gilman's the pharmacological basis of therapeutics.* New York: Pergamon Press, 1990, pp 84–121, by permission of McGraw-Hill Companies.

tachycardia at serum levels of 12 ng/mL.[152] Reductions in HR with propranolol occur at lower serum levels than depression of myocardial contractility.[153] Accordingly, as drug levels decrease after discontinuation of therapy, reductions in the chronotropic response last much longer than reductions in inotropy.[153] This is an important concept in treating tachycardias in patients with significant ventricular dysfunction and CHF.

The usual IV dose of propranolol initially is 0.5 to 1.0 mg titrated to effect. A titrated dose resulting in maximum pharmacologic serum levels is 0.1 mg/kg. The use of continuous infusions of propranolol has been reported after noncardiac surgery in patients with cardiac disease.[154] A continuous infusion of 1 to 3 mg/hr can prevent tachycardia and hypertension but must be used with caution because of the potential of cumulative effects.

Metoprolol

Metoprolol was the first clinically used cardioselective β-blocker. Its affinity for $β_1$ receptors is 30 times greater than its affinity for $β_2$ receptors, as demonstrated by radioligand binding.[155] Metoprolol is lipid soluble, with 50% of the drug metabolized during first-pass hepatic metabolism and with only 3% excreted renally.[156] Protein binding is less than 10%. Metoprolol's serum half-life is 3 to 4 hours. Because of its lipophilic properties, metoprolol has been shown in animal studies to diffuse into ischemic tissue better than atenolol, a hydrophilic β-receptor blocker.[155]

As with any cardioselective β-blocker, greater serum levels may result in greater incidence of $β_2$-blocking effects. Metoprolol is administered intravenously in 1- to 2-mg doses, titrated to effect. The potency of metoprolol is approximately half that of propranolol. Maximum β-blocker effect is achieved with 0.2 mg/kg intravenously.

Esmolol

Esmolol's chemical structure is similar to that of metoprolol and propranolol, except it has a methylester group in the para position of the phenyl ring, making it susceptible to rapid hydrolysis by red blood cell esterases (9-minute half-life).[157] Esmolol is not metabolized by plasma cholinesterase. Hydrolysis results in an acid metabolite and methanol with clinically insignificant levels.[158] Ninety percent of the drug is eliminated in the form of the acid metabolite, normally within 24 hours.[158] A loading dose of 500 μg/kg given intravenously followed by a 50-to 300-μg/kg/min infusion will reach steady-state concentrations within 5 minutes. Without the loading dose, steady-state concentrations are reached in 30 minutes.[158]

Esmolol is cardioselective, blocking primarily $β_1$ receptors. It lacks ISA and membrane-stabilizing effects and is mildly lipid soluble. Esmolol produced significant reductions in BP, HR, and cardiac index after a loading dose of 500 μg/kg and an infusion of 300 μg/kg/min in patients with CAD, and the effects were completely reversed 30 minutes after discontinuation of the infusion.[159] Initial therapy during anesthesia may require significant reductions in both the loading and infusion doses.

Hypotension is a common side effect of IV esmolol. The incidence of hypotension was greater with esmolol (36%) than with propranolol (6%) at equal therapeutic end points.[160] The cardioselective drugs may cause more hypotension because of $β_1$-induced myocardial depression and the failure to block $β_2$ peripheral vasodilation. Esmolol appears safe in patients with bronchospastic disease. In another comparative study with propranolol, esmolol and placebo did not change airway resistance, whereas 50% of patients treated with propranolol experienced development of clinically significant bronchospasm.[161] Phlebitis may occur at the site of IV administration after prolonged infusion.[162]

Esmolol inhibits human plasma cholinesterase during in vitro studies, in which clinically insignificant prolongation of duration of succinylcholine action by esmolol was reported.[163] Digoxin levels may increase slightly with concomitant esmolol administration.[164] In addition, both esmolol and landiolol, a new short-acting $β_1$-receptor blocker, also suppress the bispectral index during general anesthesia.[165]

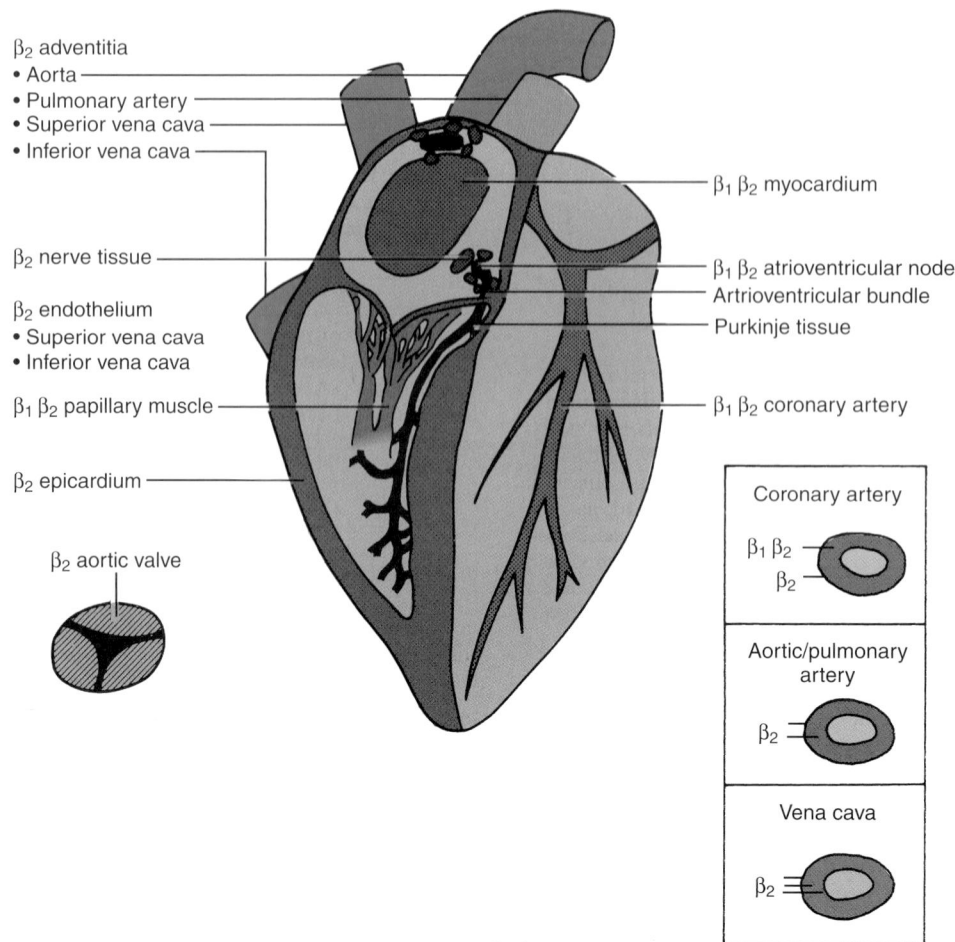

Figure 10-13 **Summary of locations of β₁- and β₂-adrenoceptors in rat, guinea pig, dog, and human hearts determined by autoradiography.** The β₁- and β₂-adrenoceptors are located on myocardium and specialized conducting tissue. A greater density of β₂-adrenoceptors is located on the atrioventricular node, bundle of His, and left and right bundle branches in comparison with surrounding myocardium in guinea pig. In addition, β₂-adrenoceptors are located on blood vessels, nerve tissue, epicardium, and the aortic valve. In large canine coronary arteries (0.5 to 2 mm in diameter), β₁-adrenoceptors account for 85% of the total population of β-adrenoceptors; in small arterioles (16 to 55 μm), β₂-adrenoceptors comprise 93% of the total population. *(Modified from Summers RJ, Molena-ar P, Stephenson JA: Autoradiographic localization of receptors in the cardiovascular system.* Trends Pharmacol Sci *8:272, 1987; and Jones CR: New views of human cardiac β-adrenoceptors.* J Mol Cell Cardiol *21:519, 1989.)*

TABLE 10-4	Properties of β-Blockers in Clinical Use		
Drug	*Selectivity*	*Partial Agonist Activity*	*Usual Dose for Angina*
Propranolol	None	No	20–80 mg twice daily
Metoprolol	β₁	No	50–200 mg twice daily
Atenolol	β₁	No	50–200 mg/day
Nadolol	None	No	40–80 mg/day
Timolol	None	No	10 mg twice daily
Acebutolol	β₁	Yes	200–600 mg twice daily
Betaxolol	β₁	No	10–20 mg/day
Bisoprolol	β₁	No	10 mg/day
Esmolol (intravenous)	β₁	No	50–300 μg • kg⁻¹ • min⁻¹
Labetalol*	None	Yes	200–600 mg twice daily
Pindolol	None	Yes	2.5–7.5 mg 3 times daily

*Labetalol is a combined α- and β-blocker.
Adapted from Gibbons RJ, Chatterjee K, Daley J, Douglas JS: ACC/AHA/ACP-ASIM guidelines for the management of patients with chronic stable angina: A report of the American College of Cardiology/American Heart Association Task Force on Practice Guidelines (Committee on Management of Patients with Chronic Stable Angina). *J Am Coll Cardiol* 33:2092–2197, 1999; Table 25.

Labetalol

Labetalol is an equal mixture of four stereoisomers with varying α- and β-blocking properties. Labetalol provides selective α₁-receptor blockade and nonselective β₁- and β₂-blockade. The potency of β-adrenergic blockade is 5- to 10-fold greater than α₁-adrenergic blockade.[15,165] Labetalol has partial β₂-agonist effects that promote vasodilation.[166] Labetalol is moderately lipid soluble and is completely absorbed after oral administration.[167] First-pass hepatic metabolism is significant with production of inactive metabolites.[167] Renal excretion of the unchanged drug is minimal. Elimination half-life is approximately 6 hours.[167]

In contrast with other β-blockers, clinically, labetalol should be considered a peripheral vasodilator that does not cause a reflex tachycardia. BP and systolic vascular resistance decrease after an IV dose.[168] Stroke volume (SV) and CO remain unchanged, with HR decreasing slightly.[169] The reduction in BP is dose related, and acutely hypertensive patients usually respond within 3 to 5 minutes after a bolus dose of 100 to 250 μg/kg.[170] However, the more critically ill or anesthetized patients should have their BP titrated beginning with 5- to 10-mg IV increments. Reduction in BP may last as long as 6 hours after IV dosing.

Significant Adverse Effects

CHF can be precipitated by β-adrenergic blockers, especially when other cardiac drugs with myocardial depressant properties are used, such as calcium blockers and disopyramide. β-Blockers blunt the usual reflex in sympathetic activity with these other depressant agents.[171] Similarly, these effects are additive on the conduction system, and heart block can occur. Propranolol reduces the clearance of many drugs that depend on hepatic metabolism by reducing hepatic blood flow (e.g., lidocaine).[172]

β_2-Blocker effects cause bronchospasm and peripheral vasoconstriction, which can exacerbate symptoms in patients with chronic pulmonary disease and peripheral vascular disease. Impotence is a problem in some patients. The lipophilic agents cause many CNS side effects such as depression, sleep disturbances, and fatigue. Hypoglycemia is a significant problem for patients with diabetes.

Sudden withdrawal of β-adrenergic blockers can precipitate a state of enhanced adrenergic activity, resulting in tachycardia, hypertension, arrhythmias, myocardial ischemia, and infarction.[173] Most studies indicated that this period of hypersensitivity occurs from 2 to 6 days after withdrawal of β -blockade. This corresponds to an increase in human lymphocyte β receptors during this period. Continuing β-receptor blockers before cardiac surgery results in a more stable anesthetic induction, intubation, and sternotomy sequence than performing anesthesia and surgery during a period of withdrawal hypersensitivity.[83,174] Furthermore, reinstitution of small doses of β-adrenergic blockade after cardiac surgery smooths the postoperative course and reduces the incidence of tachyarrhythmias.[175]

Summary

β-Adrenergic blockers are first-line agents in the treatment of myocardial ischemia. These agents effectively reduce myocardial work and oxygen demand. There is growing evidence that β-adrenergic–blocking agents may play a significant role in reducing perioperative cardiac morbidity and mortality in noncardiac surgery.[176]

Calcium Channel Blockers

Calcium channel blockers reduce myocardial oxygen demands by depression of contractility, HR, and/or decreased arterial BP.[177] Myocardial oxygen supply may be improved by dilation of coronary and collateral vessels. Calcium channel blockers are used primarily for symptom control in patients with stable angina pectoris. In an acute ischemic situation, calcium channel blockers (verapamil and diltiazem) may be used for rate control in situations when β-blockers cannot be used. The most important effects of calcium channel blockers, however, may be the treatment of variant angina. These drugs can attenuate ergonovine-induced coronary vasoconstriction in patients with variant angina, suggesting protection via coronary dilation.[178] Most episodes of silent myocardial ischemia, which may account for 70% of all transient ischemic episodes, are not related to increases in myocardial oxygen demands (HR and BP) but, rather, intermittent obstruction of coronary flow likely caused by coronary vasoconstriction or spasm.[179] All calcium channel blockers are effective at reversing coronary spasm, reducing ischemic episodes, and reducing NTG consumption in patients with variant or Prinzmetal's angina.[180] Combinations of NTG and calcium channel blockers, which also effectively relieve and possibly prevent coronary spasm, are currently rational therapy for variant angina. β-Blockers may aggravate anginal episodes in some patients with vasospastic angina and should be used with caution.[181] Preservation of CBF with calcium channel blockers is a significant difference from the predominant β-blocker anti-ischemic effects of reducing myocardial oxygen consumption.

Calcium channel blockers have proved effective in controlled trials of stable angina.[182-185] However, rapid-acting dihydropyridines such as nifedipine may cause a reflex tachycardia, especially during initial therapy, and exacerbate anginal symptoms. Such proischemic effects probably explain why the short-acting dihydropyridine nifedipine in high doses produced adverse effects in patients with unstable angina. The introduction of long-acting dihydropyridines such as extended-release nifedipine, amlodipine, felodipine, isradipine, nicardipine, and nisoldipine has led to fewer adverse events. These agents should be used in combination with β-blockers. Some patients may have symptomatic relief improved more with calcium channel blockers than with β-blocker therapy, although currently it is difficult to predict which patients respond better by other than empiric observation.

The causes of unstable angina may involve coronary vasospasm, accelerated atherosclerotic process, or enhanced platelet aggregation with fibrin clot formation. Calcium channel blockers have favorable effects in all three of the processes and are effective in the relief of symptoms of unstable angina.[186] There are no significant clinical differences in the response of patients with unstable angina to β-adrenergic blockers and calcium channel blockers.[187]

Calcium Channel

Calcium channels are functional pores in membranes through which calcium flows down an electrochemical gradient when the channels are open. Calcium channels exist in cardiac muscle, smooth muscle, and probably many other cellular membranes. These channels also are present in cellular organelle membranes such as the sarcoplasmic reticulum (SR) and mitochondria. Calcium functions as a primary generator of the cardiac action potential and an intracellular second messenger to regulate various intracellular events.[188]

Calcium enters cellular membranes through voltage-dependent channels or receptor-operated channels. The voltage-dependent channels depend on a transmembrane potential for activation (opening). Receptor-operated channels either are linked to a voltage-dependent channel after receptor stimulation or directly allow calcium passage through cell or organelle membranes independent of transmembrane potentials.

There are three types of voltage-dependent channels: the T (transient), L (long-lasting), and N (neuronal) channels.[189] The T and L channels are located in cardiac and smooth muscle tissue, whereas the N channels are located only in neural tissue. The T channel is activated at low voltages ($-50\,mV$) in cardiac tissue, plays a major role in cardiac depolarization (phase 0), and is not blocked by calcium antagonists.[190,191] The L channels are the classic "slow" channels, are activated at greater voltages ($-30\,mV$), and are responsible for phase 2 of the cardiac action potential. These channels are blocked by calcium antagonists.[190,191]

As mentioned previously, receptor-operated channels regulate calcium entry through voltage-regulated channels or through channels regulated by the receptor system per se. The β-adrenergic receptor operates an L-type voltage-dependent channel, which is activated by phosphorylation of a protein kinase by cAMP generated by the β-adrenergic receptor.[191] β_1-Receptor stimulation activates a G protein, which causes phospholipase C to hydrolyze phosphatidylinositol diphosphate to diacylglycerol (DAG) and inositol triphosphate (IP_3).[192] DAG activates protein kinase C that likely phosphorylates an L-type channel allowing calcium entry, whereas IP_3 is a second messenger that interacts with the SR and directly promotes calcium release from the SR through an intracellular calcium channel.[193] A receptor-operated channel also may increase calcium entry stimulated directly by a G protein. Both α_2-receptor and β-receptor stimulation may activate G-protein–regulated channels, which are not voltage dependent[194,195] (see Chapters 7 and 9).

Calcium channel blockers interact with the L-type calcium channel and are composed of drugs from four different classes: (1) the 1,4-dihydropyridine (DHP) derivatives (nifedipine, nimodipine, nicardipine, isradipine, amlodipine, and felodipine); (2) the phenylalkyl-amines, (verapamil); (3) the benzothiazepines (diltiazem); and (4) a diarylaminopropylamine ether (bepridil).[15] The L-type calcium channel has specific receptors, which bind to each of the different chemical classes of calcium channel blockers.[196] The binding to calcium blocker receptors by dihydropyridine derivatives (nifedipine) is voltage dependent.[197] Calcium channels transform from a closed resting form that can potentially open, to an activated open form, to an inactive conformation that cannot open, and finally back to the closed resting form. Nifedipine binds preferentially to the inactive receptor that has just recently undergone activation and cannot open. Nifedipine essentially acts as a plug to block the channel. Verapamil binds to the L-type channel preferentially when it is active or open.[198] The greater the period of activation of the channel, the more effective is the blockade (use dependent). Any repetitive activity, such as cardiac pacemaker activity, is sensitive to use-dependent agents.

Physiologic Effects

Hemodynamic Effects

Systemic hemodynamic effects of calcium channel blockers in vivo represent a complex interaction among myocardial depression, vasodilation, and reflex activation of the autonomic nervous system (Table 10-5).

Nifedipine, like all dihydropyridines, is a potent arterial dilator with few venodilating effects.[199] Reflex activation of the sympathetic nervous system (SNS) may increase HR. The intrinsic negative inotropic effect of nifedipine is offset by potent arterial dilation, which results in decline of BP and increase in CO in patients.[200] Dihydropyridines are excellent antihypertensive agents because of their arterial vasodilatory effects. Antianginal effects result from reduced myocardial oxygen requirements secondary to the afterload-reducing effect and to coronary vascular dilation, resulting in improved myocardial oxygen delivery.

Verapamil is a less potent arterial dilator than the dihydropyridines and results in less reflex sympathetic activation. In vivo, verapamil generally results in moderate vasodilation without significant change in HR, CO, or SV[201] (Table 10-6). IV administration of verapamil in the catheterization laboratory causes increases in RV pressure and LVEDP, decreases in SVR, improvement in ejection fraction (EF), and little change in PAPs.[202] Verapamil can significantly depress myocardial function in patients with preexisting ventricular dysfunction.[203]

Diltiazem is a less potent vasodilator and has fewer negative inotropic effects compared with verapamil. Studies in patients show reductions in SVR and BPs, with increases in CO, PAWP, and EF[204] (Figure 10-14). Diltiazem attenuates baroreflex increases in HR secondary to NTG and decreases in HR secondary to phenylephrine.[205] Regional blood flow to the brain and kidney increases, whereas skeletal muscle flow does not change.[206] In contrast with verapamil, diltiazem is not as likely to aggravate CHF, although it should be used carefully in these patients.[207]

Coronary Blood Flow

Coronary artery dilation occurs with the calcium channel blockers with increases in total CBF (Figure 10-15). Nifedipine is the most potent coronary vasodilator, especially in epicardial vessels, which are prone to

coronary vasospasm. Diltiazem is effective in blocking coronary artery vasoconstriction caused by a variety of agents, including α-agonists, serotonin, prostaglandin, and acetylcholine.[178,208,209]

Calcium channel blockers also may dilate the coronary artery at the stenotic site, thus reducing the pressure gradient across the coronary lesion.[178] Diltiazem preferentially dilates coronary arteries compared with other peripheral vessels.[210] Animal studies demonstrate that nifedipine, verapamil, and diltiazem increase coronary collateral flow distal to coronary ligation in animals and improve subendocardial flow relative to subepicardial flow[211-214] (Figure 10-16).

TABLE 10-6	Hemodynamic Effects of Intravenous Administration of Verapamil in 20 Patients with Coronary Artery Disease		
Characteristics	*Before Verapamil**	*After Verapamil**	*Significance (P)*
Heart rate (beats/min)	74 ± 12	75 ± 12	NS
Mean arterial pressure (mm Hg)	94 ± 17	82 ± 13	<0.0005
Right ventricular end-diastolic pressure (mm Hg)	4 ± 2	7 ± 2	<0.0005
Left ventricular end-diastolic pressure (mm Hg)	12 ± 4	14 ± 4	<0.25
Cardiac index (L/min/m²)	2.8 ± 0.6	3.1 ± 0.7	<0.0005
Stroke volume index (mL/m²)	57 ± 12	63 ± 13	<0.025
Systemic vascular resistance (dyne • sec • cm⁻⁵)	1413 ± 429	1069 ± 235	<0.0005
Ejection fraction (%)	55 ± 16	61 ± 18	<0.01

*Values are mean ± standard deviation.
NS, not significant.
Reproduced from Ferlinz J, Easthope JL, Aronow WS: Effects of verapamil on myocardial performance in coronary disease. *Circulation* 59:313, 1979, by permission. copyright 1979 American Heart Association.

TABLE 10-5	Calcium Channel Blocker Vasodilator Potency and Inotropic, Chronotropic, and Dromotropic Effects on the Heart			
Characteristics	*Amlodipine*	*Diltiazem*	*Nifedipine*	*Verapamil*
Heart rate	↑/0	↓	↑/0	↓
Sinoatrial node conduction	0	↓↓	0	↓
Atrioventricular node conduction	0	↓	0	↓
Myocardial contractility	↓0	↓	↓/0	↓↓
Neurohormonal activation	↑/0	↑	↑	↑
Vascular dilatation	↑↑	↑	↑↑	↑
Coronary flow	↑	↑	↑	↑

From Eisenberg MJ, Brox A, Bestawros AN: Calcium channel blockers: An update. *Am J Med* 116:35–43, 2004.

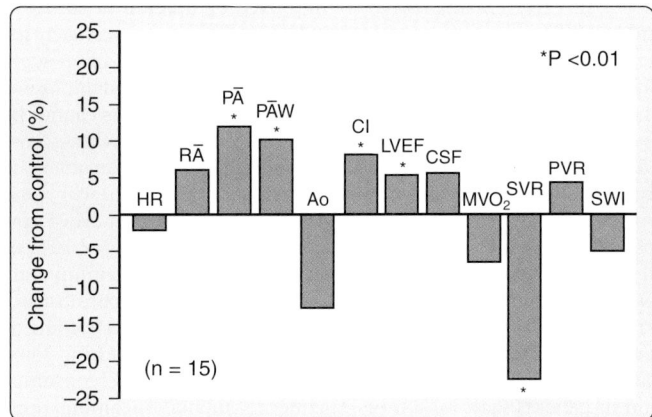

Figure 10-14 Effects of intravenous diltiazem on systemic and coronary hemodynamics and left ventricular ejection fraction in patients with coronary artery disease. Ao, mean aortic pressure; CI, cardiac index; CSF, coronary sinus flow; HR, heart rate; LVEF, left ventricular ejection fraction; MVO₂, myocardial oxygen consumption; P$\overline{A}$, mean pulmonary artery pressure; P$\overline{A}$W, mean pulmonary capillary wedge pressure; PVR, pulmonary vascular resistance; R$\overline{A}$, mean right atrial pressure; SVR, systemic vascular resistance; SWI, stroke work index. (*Modified from Josephson MA, Singh BN: Use of calcium antagonists for ventricular dysfunction. Am J Cardiol 55:81B, 1985; and Abrams J: Nitrates. In Chatterjee K, Cheitlin MD, Karliner J, et al [eds]: Cardiology: An illustrated text/reference, vol 1. Philadelphia: JB Lippincott, 1991, pp 2.75–2.90.*)

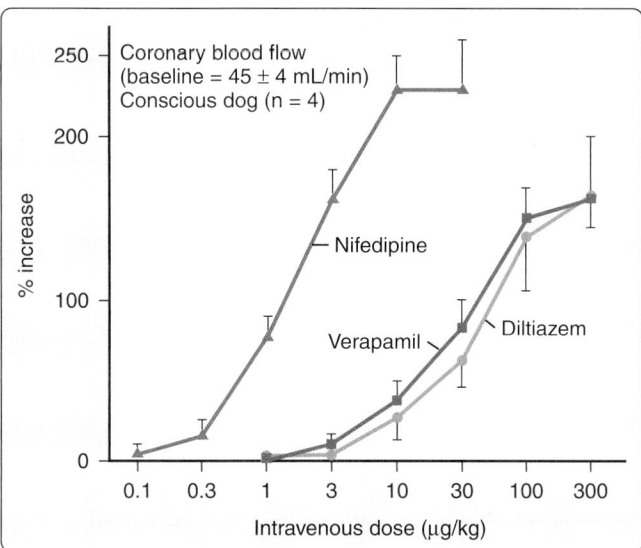

Figure 10-15 **Coronary blood flow responses to intravenous diltiazem, nifedipine, and verapamil in the conscious normal dog.** In contrast with nitroglycerin and β-blockers, calcium-channel blockers increase total coronary flow. Data are mean values ± standard error (n = 4). *(Reproduced by permission of Millard RW, Grupp G, Grupp IL, et al: Chronotropic, inotropic, and vasodilator actions of diltiazem, nifedipine, and verapamil. A comparative study of physiological responses and membrane receptor activity. Circ Res 52[Suppl I]:29, 1983. Copyright 1983 American Medical Association.)*

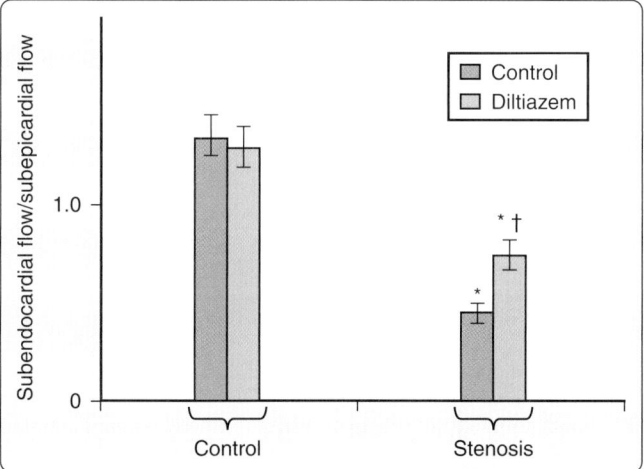

Figure 10-16 Ratio of subendocardial to subepicardial blood flow during resting control conditions and in the presence of proximal stenosis, which prevented arterial inflow from increasing above the preocclusion control after a 10-second coronary artery occlusion in animals. Diltiazem increased subendocardial to subepicardial blood flow ratio in the ischemic area. Values are mean ± standard error of the mean. *P < 0.05 compared with measurements during control conditions with unimpeded arterial inflow. †P < 0.05 compared with the control stenosis. *(From Bache RJ, Dymek DJ: Effect of diltiazem on myocardial blood flow. Circulation 65[Suppl I]:I, 1982. Copyright 1982 American Medical Association.)*

Electrophysiologic Effects

Calcium channel blockers exert their primary electrophysiologic effects on tissue of the conducting system that is dependent on calcium for generation of the action potential, primarily at the sinoatrial (SA) and AV nodes. They do not alter the effective refractory period (ERP) of atrial, ventricular, or His-Purkinje tissue. Diltiazem and verapamil exert these electrophysiologic effects in vivo and in vitro, whereas the electrophysiologic depression of dihydropyridines (nifedipine) is completely attenuated by reflex sympathetic activation. Nifedipine actually can enhance SA and AV node conduction, whereas verapamil and diltiazem slow conduction velocity and prolong refractoriness of nodal tissue.[215–217]

Atherosclerosis

Calcium is involved in the generation of atherosclerotic plaque and in damaged atherosclerotic tissue (calcification).[218] Verapamil and nifedipine have been found to have antiatherogenic effects.[218] Nifedipine has been shown to retard angiographic progression of CAD in humans.[219] Diltiazem also may reduce atherosclerotic progression after heart transplantation.[220] Diltiazem suppresses aortic atherosclerosis, but not that of coronary arteries, inhibits spontaneous calcinosis in hypertensive rats, and prevents vitamin D–induced calcinosis in arterial elastic tissue.[221–223] Diltiazem also suppresses necrosis of aortic smooth muscle cells by hyperlipidemia serum[224] and intimal thickening in rabbit carotid arteries.[225]

Platelet Aggregation

Calcium antagonists, nitrates, and β-adrenergic blockers all inhibit platelet aggregation. This could be a most important effect of all anti-ischemic drugs, especially in the treatment of chronic disease. Calcium is a mediator involved in the release of platelet aggregatory factors, such as ADP, and verapamil inhibits calcium-induced release of these factors.[226] Diltiazem inhibition of platelet aggregation correlates with changes in intracellular calcium levels.[227] In vivo, diltiazem inhibits platelet aggregation after 24 hours in healthy volunteers.[228] Similar antiaggregatory effects of diltiazem were seen in patients with unstable angina, but no inhibitory effect of platelet aggregation was found with verapamil. Diltiazem metabolites are even more effective in inhibiting platelet aggregation than diltiazem.[229]

Metabolic Effects

Nifedipine may be associated with decreases in serum glucose levels in patients with diabetes, but glucose levels in healthy volunteers generally increase slightly with nifedipine and in hypertensive patients with diltiazem.[230,231] Diltiazem reportedly has no effect on insulin, glucagon, growth hormone, or cortisol levels.[232,233] However, nifedipine apparently delays insulin release in patients with diabetes.[233]

Pharmacology

Table 10-7 illustrates pharmacokinetic parameters for the U.S. Food and Drug Administration–approved anti-ischemic calcium channel blockers.

Nifedipine

Nifedipine was the first dihydropyridine derivative to be used clinically. Other dihydropyridines available for clinical use include nicardipine, isradipine, amlodipine, felodipine, and nimodipine.[234] In contrast with the other calcium channel blockers, nimodipine is highly lipid soluble and penetrates the blood–brain barrier. It is indicated for vascular spasm after intracerebral bleeding.

Nifedipine's oral bioavailability is approximately 70%, with peak plasma levels occurring within 30 to 45 minutes. Protein binding is 95%, and elimination half-life is approximately 5 hours. Nifedipine is available for oral administration in capsular form. The compound degenerates in the presence of light and moisture, preventing commercially available IV preparations. Puncture of the capsule and sublingual administration provide an onset of effects in 2 to 3 minutes. Nifedipine GITS (GastroIntestinal Therapeutic System, Procardia XL), a long-acting, controlled-release delivery system, is available for single daily dosing and is now the preferred preparation. It has an onset of action of 20 minutes, with steady-state plasma levels being reached in 48 hours.

Nicardipine

Nicardipine is a dihydropyridine agent with a longer half-life than nifedipine and with vascular selectivity for coronary and cerebrovascular beds. Nicardipine may be the most potent overall relaxant of vascular smooth muscle among the dihydropyridines.[235] Peak plasma levels are

Drug	Usual Dose	Duration of Action	Side Effects
Dihydropyridines			
Nifedipine	Immediate release: 30–90 mg daily orally Slow release: 30–180 mg orally	Short	Hypotension, dizziness, flushing, nausea, constipation, edema
Amlodipine	5–10 mg once daily	Long	Headache, edema
Felodipine	5–10 mg once daily	Long	Headache, edema
Isradipine	2.5–10 mg twice daily	Medium	Headache, fatigue
Nicardipine	20–40 mg 3 times daily	Short	Headache, dizziness, flushing, edema
Nisoldipine	20–40 mg once daily	Short	Similar to nifedipine
Nitrendipine	20 mg once or twice daily	Medium	Similar to nifedipine
Miscellaneous			
Bepridil	200–400 mg once daily	Long	Arrhythmias, dizziness, nausea
Diltiazem	Immediate release: 30–80 mg 4 times daily Slow release: 120–320 mg once daily	Short Long	Hypotension, dizziness, flushing, bradycardia, edema
Verapamil	Immediate release: 80–160 mg 3 times daily Slow release: 120–480 mg once daily	Short Long	Hypotension, myocardial depression, heart failure, edema, bradycardia

TABLE 10-7 Properties of Calcium Antagonists in Clinical Use

From Gibbons RJ, Chatterjee K, Daley J, Douglas JS: ACC/AHA/ACP-ASIM guidelines for the management of patients with chronic stable angina: A report of the American College of Cardiology/American Heart Association Task Force on Practice Guidelines (Committee on Management of Patients with Chronic Stable Angina). J Am Coll Cardiol 33:2092–2197, 1999; Table 27.

reached 1 hour after oral administration, with bioavailability of 35%.[236] Plasma half-life is approximately 8 to 9 hours. Although the drug undergoes extensive hepatic metabolism with less than 1% of the drug excreted renally, greater renal elimination occurs in some patients.[237] Plasma levels may increase in patients with renal failure; reduction of the dose is recommended in these patients.[236]

Nicardipine is a potent cerebrovascular vasodilator and may prevent ischemia-related neuronal necrosis in animal studies.[238,239] Marked improvements in CBF occur with nicardipine.[240] Although coronary vasodilation is one explanation, positive inotropic effects with either PDE activity or calcium channel agonist (as well as antagonist) activity resulting in autoregulatory increases in blood flow may be an additional mechanism.[241]

Verapamil

The structure of verapamil is similar to that of papaverine. Verapamil exhibits significant first-pass hepatic metabolism, with a bioavailability of only 10% to 20%.[242] One hepatic metabolite, norverapamil, is active and has a potency approximately 20% of that of verapamil.[242] Peak plasma levels are reached within 30 minutes. Bioavailability markedly increases in hepatic insufficiency, mandating reduced doses.[242] IV verapamil achieves hemodynamic and dromotropic effects within minutes, peaking at 15 minutes and lasting up to 6 hours. Accumulation of the drug occurs with prolonged half-life during long-term oral administration.[243]

Verapamil's metabolism is dependent on hepatic blood flow and may decrease in the presence of H$_2$-receptor blockers. Increased metabolism may occur when hepatic enzyme-inducible agents like phenobarbital are given concomitantly. Seventy percent of verapamil's metabolites are recovered in the urine and 15% in feces.

Diltiazem

After oral dosing, the bioavailability of diltiazem is greater than verapamil's, varying between 25% and 50%.[244] Peak plasma concentration is achieved between 30 and 60 minutes, and elimination half-life is 2 to 6 hours.[244] Protein binding is approximately 80%. As with verapamil, hepatic clearance is flow dependent and major hepatic metabolism occurs, with metabolites having 40% of the clinical activity of diltiazem.[245,246] Hepatic disease may require decreased dosing, whereas renal failure does not affect dosing.[247]

Significant Adverse Effects

Most significant adverse hemodynamic effects can be predicted from the calcium channel blockers' primary effects of vasodilation, and negative inotropy, chronotropy, and dromotropy. Hypotension, HF, bradycardia and asystole, and AV nodal block have occurred with

calcium channel blockers.[248] These side effects are more likely to occur with combination therapy with β-blockers or digoxin, in the presence of hypokalemia.[248]

Verapamil increases digoxin levels, whereas diltiazem has variable effects and nifedipine no effect on digoxin levels.[249–251] Cimetidine and ranitidine increase calcium blockers' serum levels either by liver enzyme induction or reductions of hepatic blood flow.[252] The physiologic effects of calcium blockers may be additive to those of anesthetic agents in animal studies, but clinically significant effects are variable.[253,254] The cautious use of IV verapamil with a β-adrenergic receptor antagonist is necessary because of the increased risk for AV block or severe myocardial depression.

Paradoxic aggravation of myocardial ischemia may be seen with the short-acting dihydropyridines (nifedipine).[255] This may be secondary to decreased CPP with associated hypotension, selective vasodilation in the nonischemic region (coronary steal), or increased oxygen demand as a result of reflex sympathetic stimulation and tachycardia.

Case reports of a withdrawal syndrome similar to β-blocker withdrawal have been presented. Five of 143 patients had significant ST-segment changes after diltiazem or verapamil withdrawal.[256] MI and coronary spasm have been reported after diltiazem withdrawal.[257,258] One study comparing propranolol with verapamil withdrawal in patients with stable angina found that 2 of 20 patients had severe exacerbation of their angina with propranolol withdrawal, and no patients had hemodynamic or symptomatic evidence of a withdrawal phenomenon with verapamil.[259]

Summary

Calcium antagonists provide excellent symptom control in patients with unstable angina. In the absence of β-adrenergic blockade, the short-acting dihydropyridine nifedipine may increase the risk for MI or recurrent angina. When β-adrenergic blockers cannot be used, and HR slowing is indicated, verapamil and diltiazem may offer an alternative.

Drug Therapy for Systemic Hypertension

Systemic hypertension, long recognized as a leading cause of cardiovascular morbidity and mortality, accounts for enormous health-related expenditures. Nearly a fourth of the U.S. population has hypertensive vascular disease; however, 30% of these individuals are unaware of their condition, and another 30% to 50% are inadequately treated.[260,261] On a worldwide basis, nearly 1 billion individuals are hypertensive.[262] Based on data from the Framingham Heart Study, normotensive patients at age 55 can expect a 90% lifetime risk for subsequent development of hypertension.[263] Furthermore, hypertension management comprises the most common reason underlying adult visits to primary care physicians, and antihypertensive drugs are the most prescribed medication class.[264]

Despite the asymptomatic nature of hypertensive disease, with symptom onset delayed 20 to 30 years after development of systemic hypertension, substantial incontrovertible evidence demonstrates a direct association between systemic hypertension and increased morbidity and mortality. The World Health Organization estimates that hypertension underlies one in eight deaths worldwide, making elevated BP the third leading cause of mortality.[262] In fact, hypertension accounts for the single most treatable risk factor for MI, stroke, peripheral vascular disease, CHF, renal failure, and aortic dissection.[260] In prospective randomized trials, over the course of adult lifetimes, successful treatment of hypertension has been associated with 35% to 40% reductions in the incidence of stroke, 50% reductions in CHF, and 25% reductions in MIs.[260,262] Improved treatment of hypertension has been credited with the major reductions in stroke and cardiovascular mortality occurring since the 1970s in the United States.

Pathophysiologic mechanisms underlying predisposition to hypertension remain, for the most part, unclear. Undoubtedly, both genetic and environmental factors play contributory roles.[265] Concordance for hypertension is greater between monozygotic or dizygotic twins, and even siblings within a single family, than that observed between unrelated individuals, supporting a genetic component. However, by some estimates, genetic predeterminants account for only 30% to 40% of hypertensive disease.[265] As for environmental factors, a direct association between body mass index and hypertension has been reported, and dietary sodium intake is associated with long-term risk for development of hypertension.[266,267]

In most cases, no single reversible mechanism underlying systemic hypertensive disease can be identified—the so-called *primary or essential hypertension*. In a small subset, perhaps 5% of hypertensive patients, a distinct causative factor promoting systemic hypertension is identified. The most common causative factor underlying *secondary hypertension* is renal insufficiency. Other less common mechanisms include pheochromocytoma, renal artery stenosis, and hypertension resulting from adrenal cortical abnormalities such as primary aldosteronism or Cushing syndrome. Diagnostic clues suggestive of secondary hypertension include hypertensive disease refractory to medical therapy, unusually abrupt onset with severe associated symptoms, or occurrence of hypertension at a particularly young age.

Definitions for hypertension are somewhat arbitrary, although derived from clinical trials suggesting systemic pressures at which the benefits of treatment outweigh the risk for adverse effects related to antihypertensive therapy. BP varies with normal distribution across the population at large, and aging is associated with progressive increases in systolic pressure. After 50 years of age, reductions in diastolic pressure are commonly observed, resulting in widening of pulse pressure with age. Published evidence suggests that systolic and pulse pressures are better predictors for morbidity and mortality than diastolic pressure.[264] Most recently, the Seventh Report of the Joint National Committee on Prevention, Detection, Evaluation, and Treatment of High Blood Pressure (JNC-7 Report) defined systolic BPs (Table 10-8) exceeding 140 mm Hg and diastolic BPs exceeding 90 mm Hg as stage 1 hypertension. BPs less than 120/80 mm Hg were defined as normal, and those in between as consistent with "prehypertension."[260]

Although antihypertensive drug therapy is widely regarded as essential for BPs greater than 140/90 mm Hg, recent evidence suggests benefits to more aggressive BP reduction for certain patient subsets. The association between systemic BP and cardiovascular risk has been described as a "J-curve," with progressive cardiovascular risk reductions accompanying BP reductions until a critical threshold—after which the potential for myocardial ischemia and/or other organ injury increases.[268]

Risk for cardiovascular disease appears to increase at BPs greater than 115/75 mm Hg, with a doubling in risk associated with each 20/10-mm Hg increment in systemic pressure.[260] Thus, the most recent JNC-7 report recommends drug therapy for "prehypertensive" disease in patients with "compelling indications" such as chronic renal disease or diabetes. Antihypertensive therapy generally is targeted to achieve systemic BPs less than 140/90 mm Hg; however, for high-risk patients such as those with diabetes, renal, or cardiovascular disease, lower BP targets are suggested, typically more than 130/80 mm Hg.[260]

Medical Treatment for Hypertension

Currently, nearly 80 distinct medications are marketed for treatment of hypertension[264] (Table 10-9). Often, combined therapy with two or more classes of antihypertensive medications may be needed to achieve treatment goals[269] (Table 10-10). Although the specific drug selected for initial therapy now has been deemed less important than in the past, recognition that specific antihypertensive drug classes alleviate end-organ damage, beyond that simply associated with reductions in systemic BP, has led to targeted selection of antihypertensive drug combinations on the basis of coexisting risk factors such as recent MI, chronic renal insufficiency, or diabetes.

TABLE 10-8	Classification and Management of Blood Pressure for Adults Age 18 Years or Older					
					Management*	
					Initial Drug Therapy	
BP Classification	*Systolic BP* *(mm Hg)*		*Diastolic BP* *(mm Hg)*	*Lifestyle Modification*	*Without Compelling Indication*	*With Compelling Indication*
Normal	< 120	and	< 80	Encourage		
Prehypertension	120–139	or	80–89	Yes	No antihypertensive drug indicated	Drugs(s) for the compelling indications[†]
Stage 1 hypertension	140–159	or	90–99	Yes	Thiazide-type diuretics for most; may consider ACE inhibitor, ARB, β-blocker, CCB, or combination	Drug(s) for the compelling indications Other antihypertensive drugs (diuretics, ACE inhibitor, ARB, β-blocker, CCB) as needed
Stage 2 hypertension	≥ 160	or	≥ 100	Yes	Two-drug combination for most (usually thiazide-type diuretic and ACE inhibitor or ARB or β-blocker or CCB)[‡]	Drug(s) for the compelling indications Other antihypertensive drugs (diuretics, ACE inhibitor, ARB, β-blocker, CCB) as needed

*Treatment determined by highest blood pressure (BP) category.
[†]Treat patients with chronic kidney disease or diabetes to BP goal or <130/80 mm Hg.
[‡]Initial combination therapy should be used cautiously in those at risk for orthostatic hypotension.
ACE, angiotensin-converting enzyme; ARB, angiotensin-receptor blocker; CCB, calcium channel blocker.
Reproduced from Chobanian AV, Bakris, GL, Black HR, et al: Seventh report of the Joint National Committee on Prevention, Detection, Evaluation, and Treatment of High Blood Pressure: The JNC7 Report. *JAMA* 289:2560–2572, 2003, by permission.

TABLE 10-9	Oral Antihypertensive Drugs		
Class	Drug (Trade Name)	Usual Dosage Range (mg/day)	Usual Daily Frequency*
Thiazide diuretics	Chlorothiazide (Diuril)	125–500	1–2
	Chlorthalidone (generic)	12.5–25	1
	Hydrochlorothiazide (Microzide, HydroDIURIL†)	12.5–50	1
	Polythiazide (Renese)	2–4	1
	Indapamide (Lozol†)	1.25–2.5	1
	Metolazone (Mykrox)	0.5–1.0	1
	Metolazone (Zaroxolyn)	2.5–5	1
Loop diuretics	Bumetanide (Bumex†)	0.5–2	2
	Furosemide (Lasix†)	20–80	2
	Torsemide (Demadex†)	2.5–10	1
Potassium-sparing diuretics	Amiloride (Midamor†)	5–10	1–2
	Triamterene (Dyrenium)	50–100	1–2
Aldosterone receptor blockers	Eplerenone (Inspra)	50–100	1
	Spironolactone (Aldactone†)	25–50	1
β-Blockers	Atenolol (Tenormin†)	25–100	1
	Betaxolol (Kerlone†)	5–20	1
	Bisoprolol (Zebeta†)	2.5–10	1
	Metoprolol (Lopressor†)	50–100	1–2
	Metoprolol extended release (Toprol XL)	50–100	1
	Nadolol (Corgard†)	40–120	1
	Propranolol (Inderal†)	40–160	2
	Propranolol long-acting (Inderal LA†)	60–180	1
	Timolol (Blocadren†)	20–40	2
β-Blockers with intrinsic sympathomimetic activity	Acebutolol (Sectral†)	200–800	2
	Penbutolol (Levatol)	10–40	1
	Pindolol (generic)	10–40	2
Combined α-blockers and β-blockers	Carvedilol (Coreg)	12.5–50	2
	Labetalol (Normodyne, Trandate†)	200–800	2
ACEIs	Benazepril (Lotensin†)	10–40	1
	Captopril (Capoten†)	25–100	2
	Enalapril (Vasotec†)	5–40	1–2
	Fosinopril (Monopril)	10–40	1
	Lisinopril (Prinivil, Zestril†)	10–40	1
	Moexipril (Univasc)	7.5–30	1
	Perindopril (Aceon)	4–8	1
	Quinapril (Accupril)	10–80	1
	Ramipril (Altace)	2.5–20	1
	Trandolapril (Mavik)	1–4	1
Angiotensin II antagonists	Candesartan (Atacand)	8–32	1
	Eprosartan (Teveten)	400–800	1–2
	Irbesartan (Avapro)	150–300	1
	Losartan (Cozaar)	25–100	1–2
	Olmesartan (Benicar)	20–40	1
	Telmisartan (Micardis)	20–80	1
	Valsartan (Diovan)	80–320	1–2
CCBs-Nondihydropyridines	Diltiazem extended release (Cardizem CD, Dilacor XR, Tiazac†)	180–420	1
	Diltiazem extended release (Cardizem LA)	120–540	1
	Verapamil immediate release (Calan, Isoptin†)	80–320	2
	Verapamil long-acting (Calan SR, Isoptin SR†)	120–480	1–2
	Verapamil (Coer, Covera HS, Verelan PM)	120–360	1
CCBs-Dihydropyridines	Amlodipine (Norvasc)	2.5–10	1
	Felodipine (Plendil)	2.5–20	1
	Isradipine (Cynacirc CR)	2.5–10	2
	Nicardipine sustained release (Cardene SR)	60–120	2
	Nifedipine long-acting (Adalat CC, Procardia XL)	30–60	1
	Nisoldipine (Sular)	10–40	1
α₁-Blockers	Doxazosin (Cardura)	1–16	1
	Prazosin (Minipress†)	2–20	2–3
	Terazosin (Hytrin)	1–20	1–2

TABLE 10-9 Oral Antihypertensive Drugs—Cont'd

Class	Drug (Trade Name)	Usual Dosage Range (mg/day)	Usual Daily Frequency*
Central α₂-agonists and other centrally acting drugs	Clonidine (Catapres†)	0.1–0.8	2
	Clonidine patch (Catapres-TTS)	0.1–0.3	1 weekly
	Methyldopa (Aldomet†)	250–1000	2
	Reserpine (generic)	0.1–0.25	1
	Guanfacine (Tenex†)	0.5–2	1
Direct vasodilators	Hydralazine (Apresoline†)	25–100	2
	Minoxidil (Loniten†)	2.5–80	1–2

*In some patients treated once daily, the antihypertensive effect may diminish toward the end of the dosing interval (trough effect). Blood pressure (BP) should be measured just before dosing to determine whether satisfactory BP control is obtained. Accordingly, an increase in dosage or frequency may need to be considered. These dosages may vary from those listed in the *Physician's Desk Reference,* 51st ed.
†Available now or soon to become available in generic preparations.
CCB, calcium channel blocker.
Reproduced from Chobanian AV, Bakris GL, Black HR, et al: Seventh report of the Joint National Committee on Prevention, Detection, Evaluation, and Treatment of High Blood Pressure. *Hypertension* 42:1206–1252, 2003, by permission.

TABLE 10-10 Combination Drugs for Hypertension

Combination Type	Fixed-Dose Combination, mg*	Trade Name
ACEIs and CCBs	Amlodipine-benazepril hydrochloride (2.5/10, 5/10, 5/20, 10/20)	Lotrel
	Enalapril-felodipine (5/5)	Lexxel
	Trandolapril-verapamil (2/180, 1/240, 2/240, 4/240)	Tarka
ACEIs and diuretics	Benazepril-hydrochlorothiazide (5/6.25, 10/12.5, 20/12.5, 20/25)	Lotensin HCT
	Captopril-hydrochlorothiazide (25/15, 25/25, 50/15, 50/25)	Capozide
	Enalapril-hydrochlorothiazide (5/12.5, 10/25)	Vaseretic
	Fosinopril-hydrochlorothiazide (10/12.5, 20/12.5)	Monopril/HCT
	Lisinopril-hydrochlorothiazide (10/12.5, 20/12.5, 20/25)	Prinzide, Zestoretic
	Moexipril-hydrochlorothiazide (7.5/12.5, 15/25)	Uniretic
	Quinapril-hydrochlorothiazide (10/12.5, 20/12.5, 20/25)	Accuretic
ARBs and diuretics	Candesartan-hydrochlorothiazide (16/12.5, 32/12.5)	Atacand HCT
	Eprosartan-hydrochlorothiazide (600/12.5, 600/25)	Teveten-HCT
	Irbesartan-hydrochlorothiazide (150/12.5, 300/12.5)	Avalide
	Losartan-hydrochlorothiazide (50/12.5, 100/25)	Hyzaar
	Olmesartan medoxomil-hydrochlorothiazide (20/12.5, 40/12.5, 40/25)	Benicar HCT
	Telmisartan-hydrochlorothiazide (40/12.5, 80/12.5)	Micardis-HCT
	Valsartan-hydrochlorothiazide (80/12.5, 160/12.5, 160/25)	Diovan-HCT
BBs and diuretics	Atenolol-chlorthalidone (50/25, 100/25)	Tenoretic
	Bisoprolol-hydrochlorothiazide (2.5/6.25, 5/6.25, 10/6.25)	Ziac
	Metoprolol-hydrochlorothiazide (50/25, 100/25)	Lopressor HCT
	Nadolol-bendroflumethiazide (40/5, 80/5)	Corzide
	Propranolol LA-hydrochlorothiazide (40/25, 80/25)	Inderide LA
	Timolol-hydrochlorothiazide (10/25)	Timolide
Centrally acting drug and diuretic	Methyldopa-hydrochlorothiazide (250/15, 250/25, 500/30, 500/50)	Aldoril
	Reserpine-chlorthalidone (0.125/25, 0.25/50)	Demi-Regroton, Regroton
	Reserpine-chlorothiazide (0.125/250, 0.25/500)	Diupres
	Reserpine-hydrochlorothiazide (0.125/25, 0.125/50)	Hydropres
Diuretic and diuretic	Amiloride-hydrochlorothiazide (5/50)	Moduretic
	Spironolactone-hydrochlorothiazide (25/25, 50/50)	Aldactazide
	Triamterene-hydrochlorothiazide (37.5/25, 75/50)	Dyazide, Maxzide

ACEI, angiotensin-converting enzyme inhibitor; ARB, angiotensin-receptor blocker; BB, β-blocker; CCB, calcium channel blocker.
*Some drug combinations are available in multiple fixed doses. Each drug dose is reported in milligrams.
Reproduced from Chobanian AV, Bakris GL, Black HR, et al: Seventh report of the Joint National Committee on Prevention, Detection, Evaluation, and Treatment of High Blood Pressure. *Hypertension* 42:1206–1252, 2003, by permission.

Diuretics

Thiazide diuretic therapy comprises the cornerstone of most antihypertensive regimens.[270,271] Three classes of diuretics have proved efficacious in reducing systemic BP—the thiazide and related sulfonamide compounds, loop diuretics, and potassium-sparing agents. All classes of diuretics initially reduce BP by increasing urinary excretion of sodium, with resultant reductions in plasma volume and CO; however, over a period of 6 to 8 weeks, diuretic therapy leads to reductions in SVR—hypothesized to relate to activation of vascular endothelial potassium channels.

Thiazide diuretics remain the first-choice medical therapy for the majority of patients with hypertension.[272] Although the natriuretic effect achieved by blockade of sodium and chloride transport in the distal convoluted tubule is relatively weak, thiazide diuretics generally produce 10-mm Hg reductions in BP and have proved efficacious in numerous randomized trials to reduce morbidity and mortality related to hypertensive vascular disease.[264,269]

Loop diuretics, the most potent natriuretics of this class, block sodium, potassium, and chloride transport in the thick ascending loop of Henle. The loop diuretics typically are reserved for patients with renal insufficiency (serum creatinine > 2 mg/dL or creatinine clearance < 25 mL/min) or CHF, conditions for which thiazide diuretics are relatively ineffective. The short duration of action of loop diuretics (e.g., furosemide: 4 to 6 hours) and greater likelihood for adverse effects limit more widespread application.

Potassium-sparing and aldosterone-receptor–blocking diuretics are among the weakest natriuretics of this class. These drugs act by a variety of mechanisms to inhibit sodium reabsorption from the distal collecting duct while simultaneously reducing urinary potassium excretion. These drugs are most commonly administered in combination with a thiazide diuretic in an effort to reduce the incidence of hypokalemia or for their salutary effects in chronic HF.

Low doses of diuretic are well tolerated; however, common adverse effects related to this drug class include hypokalemia (secondary to renal potassium wasting), impaired glucose tolerance and insulin resistance, hyperuricemia, hypercalcemia, hyperlipidemia, and, rarely, hyponatremia. The potassium-sparing and aldosterone-receptor–blocking drugs are contraindicated in patients at risk for hyperkalemia, in particular, patients with renal insufficiency.

β-Blockers

β-Adrenergic receptor blockers, which reduce sympathetic stimulation of the heart and vasculature, comprise another common antihypertensive therapy, particularly in settings of CAD or CHF.[273–277] More specifically, β-blockers inhibit myocardial and peripheral β_1-adrenergic receptors to reduce CO. As well, β-blockers reduce renin release from renal juxtaglomerular cells and norepinephrine release by inhibition of prejunctional β_2-adrenergic receptors in the peripheral vasculature. β-Blockers traditionally are classified on the basis of cardioselectivity, lipid solubility, and intrinsic sympathetic activity, with first-generation agents such as propranolol nonselectively blocking both β_1- and β_2-adrenergic receptors. Second-generation agents (e.g., metoprolol or atenolol) exhibit a relatively cardioselective preference for β_1-adrenergic receptor blockade at low doses. Pindolol, a novel β-blocker with ISA, stimulates vasodilation by activation of β_2-adrenergic receptors. Combination agents, such as labetalol, provide mixed β- and α_1-adrenergic blocking properties resulting in inhibition of sympathetic activity, as well as direct vasodilatory effects.

As with the diuretics, β-blockers typically are well tolerated at low doses; however, the potential for nonselective blockade of β-adrenergic receptors may result in bronchospasm, Raynaud's phenomenon, depression, and HF or heart block. β-Blockers are relatively contraindicated in patients with asthma or reactive airways disease, heart block, or depression. Rapid withdrawal of β-blockers may be associated with rebound adrenergic stimulation and potential for exacerbating myocardial and/or peripheral vascular ischemia; therefore, β-blocker discontinuation must occur by gradual stepped reductions in dose.

Angiotensin-Converting Enzyme Inhibitors

Angiotensin-converting enzyme (ACE) inhibitors reduce peripheral vascular resistance by inhibiting conversion of angiotensin I (Ang I) to the highly vasoconstrictive angiotensin II (Ang II).[278] Recent evidence suggests that much of the long-term antihypertensive effect of ACE inhibitors derives from protective effects on bradykinin degradation. Bradykinin, a potent vasodilator under normal conditions, undergoes degradation by the action of ACE. Therefore, ACE inhibition results in increased plasma and tissue concentrations of bradykinin.

Persistent dry cough accounts for the most common adverse effect associated with ACE inhibitor administration. Attributed to increased concentrations of bradykinin, this side effect frequently leads to discontinuation of ACE inhibitor therapy. Much rarer, although substantially more serious, is the potential for angioedema, again attributable to increased bradykinin concentrations. Angioedema may occur at any time during therapy, occurs most frequently in African Americans, and

may prove fatal because of airway compromise. Increased potential for hyperkalemia occurs in patients with renal insufficiency and those receiving potassium supplements or potassium-sparing diuretics. ACE inhibitors have been reported to induce renal failure in patients with bilateral renal artery stenosis and may potentiate severe intractable hypotension in patients with particularly elevated renin activity (e.g., decompensated HF or intravascular volume depletion). Finally, ACE inhibitors pose a teratogenic risk and are therefore contraindicated in pregnancy.

Angiotensin II Antagonists

Ang II antagonists, or angiotensin-receptor blockers, are perhaps the best tolerated of all current antihypertensive therapies and rapidly are becoming a favored drug therapy for management of hypertensive vascular disease.[278] Ang II antagonists bind and competitively inhibit Ang II AT_1 receptors, thereby directly inhibiting the vasoconstrictive effects of Ang II.[279]

Similar concerns to those of ACE inhibitors exist with regard to administration of Ang II antagonists in the settings of bilateral renal artery stenosis or hypovolemia; however, Ang II antagonists typically are not associated with cough and are rarely implicated in angioedema. As with the ACE inhibitors, Ang II antagonists are contraindicated in pregnancy.

Calcium Channel Blockers

Calcium channel blockers, commonly classified as either dihydropyridines or nondihydropyridines, share a common mechanism of action in that they bind various sites on the α_1 subunit of the L-type voltage-dependent calcium channel to partially inhibit calcium entry into cells. Although all calcium channel blockers induce arterial vasodilation, the dihydropyridines more frequently induce a reflex tachycardia, whereas the nondihydropyridines (e.g., diltiazem and verapamil) may impair cardiac conduction or contractility, or both.[280]

Common side effects reported with calcium channel blockers, and relating to arterial vasodilation, include ankle edema, flushing, and headaches. Nondihydropyridines are most often contraindicated in patients with preexisting HF or cardiac conduction defects because of their potential for precipitating HF, heart block, or both. Controversy surrounding the safety of calcium channel blockers as antihypertensive therapy has been substantially negated by recent prospective randomized trials demonstrating the safety and efficacy of long-acting calcium channel blockers for treatment of hypertensive cardiovascular disease.[281–283] Administration of short-acting dihydropyridines (e.g., nifedipine) for rapid control of hypertension has been associated with an increased incidence of acute coronary events and is contraindicated in the acute treatment of severe hypertension.

α_1-Blockers

α_1-Adrenergic blockers competitively inhibit binding of norepinephrine to α_1-adrenergic receptors in the peripheral vasculature, thereby producing vasodilation and reducing BP. Prazosin and its congeners selectively block postsynaptic α_1-adrenergic receptors. Continued activity of the presynaptic α_1 receptors allows for downregulation of norepinephrine release, limits occurrence of tolerance, and reduces the incidence of compensatory tachycardia. In contrast, phenoxybenzamine, commonly used in the preoperative management of pheochromocytoma, blocks both presynaptic and postsynaptic α_1-adrenergic receptors.

Adverse effects associated with α_1-blockers include orthostatic hypotension, fluid retention, and reflex tachycardia.[284] Although rarely administered as monotherapy, α_1-blockers continue to prove useful in combination with other antihypertensives because of their lack of metabolic side effects and propensity to dilate urethral smooth muscle, alleviating symptoms of prostatism.[264]

Central α₂-Agonists and Other Centrally Acting Drugs

Centrally acting antihypertensive agents, such as clonidine and methyldopa, stimulate α₂-adrenergic and imidazoline receptors within the CNS to reduce sympathetic outflow and SVR. In the case of clonidine, activation of presynaptic α-adrenergic receptors inhibits norepinephrine release and subsequent catecholamine generation.[285] Reserpine differs from the α₂-agonists in that it inhibits reuptake of norepinephrine by storage vesicles in the postganglionic adrenergic neurons, depleting norepinephrine. As opposed to the α₂-agonists, reserpine's peripheral effects predominate over central activity.

More widespread use of centrally acting antihypertensives has been limited by CNS-mediated adverse effects including sedation, depression, and dry mouth. In addition, autoimmune hemolytic anemia has been reported with methyldopa. Despite these limitations, however, pregnancy-induced hypertension remains a common indication for this agent because long-term use has indicated no adverse effects toward the fetus. Abrupt discontinuation of clonidine frequently results in rebound hypertension, but this effect may be alleviated with transdermal clonidine patches or the longer-acting oral agent guanfacine. All centrally acting antihypertensives are contraindicated in the setting of depression.

Direct Vasodilators

Both hydralazine and minoxidil produce potent direct arterial vasodilation mediated by activation of ATP-sensitive potassium channels within the arterial vasculature. The relative lack of effect on venous capacitance vessels by direct vasodilators reduces the potential for orthostatic hypotension. The potency and relatively adverse side-effect profile for direct vasodilators limit applications to hypertensive disease resistant to standard pharmacologic approaches, most often in the setting of severe hypertension associated with chronic renal failure.

Both hydralazine and minoxidil cause peripheral edema formation and profound reflex sympathetic activation manifested as tachycardia, headaches, and flushing. Minoxidil, a more potent antihypertensive than hydralazine, frequently is associated with excessive growth of facial hair. Reflex sympathetic responses to direct vasodilators necessitate concomitant administration of diuretics and β-adrenergic blockers to alleviate the potential for fluid retention and myocardial ischemia.

Novel Approaches to Antihypertensive Therapy

Despite the array of antihypertensive medications currently available, heterogeneity of treatment effects and adverse effects of current drugs on quality-of-life measures suggest the need for alternative approaches to antihypertensive therapy.[286] Promising approaches include both aldosterone-receptor blockers and renin inhibitors. With the exception of potential for hyperkalemia, aldosterone-receptor inhibitors have proved well tolerated, and renin inhibitors administered in concert with Ang II inhibitors alleviated the compensatory increase in plasma renin activity. Third-generation β-blockers incorporating vasodilatory activity offer particular promise for treating hypertension in the setting of concomitant HF. Further modifications to endothelin-receptor antagonists and dual vasopeptidase inhibitors offer novel antihypertensive approaches for the future. Ultimately, gene therapy may prove the definitive solution to essential hypertension. It appears likely that environmental factors interacting with multiple genetic polymorphisms contribute to overall risk for hypertension. Gene therapy offers a viable approach to long-term management of hypertension but will prove dependent on further identification of target genes, improvements in gene transfer efficiency, and development of safer transfer vectors. Near term, advances in personalized medicine offer potential for DNA testing of genetic polymorphisms to identify antihypertensive drugs most likely to benefit specific patients.[287]

Management of Severe Hypertension

For purposes of characterizing treatment urgency, severe hypertension is characterized as either a hypertensive *emergency* with target-organ injury (e.g., myocardial ischemia, stroke, pulmonary edema) or hypertensive *urgency* with severe elevations in BP not yet associated with target-organ damage. Chronic increases in BP, even when of a severe nature, do not necessarily require urgent intervention and often may be managed with oral antihypertensive therapy on an outpatient basis. In contrast, a hypertensive emergency necessitates immediate therapeutic intervention, most often in an intensive care setting, with IV antihypertensive therapy and invasive arterial BP monitoring. In the most extreme cases of *malignant hypertension*, severe increases in BP may be associated with retinal hemorrhages, papilledema, and evidence of encephalopathy, which may include headache, vomiting, seizure, and/or coma. Progressive renal failure and cardiac decompensation are additional clinical features characteristic of the most severe hypertensive emergencies.

A common therapeutic approach to the hypertensive emergency includes a limited reduction in BP, of perhaps 10%, over the initial 1 to 2 hours of therapy, followed by further reductions to a target diastolic pressure (e.g., 110 mm Hg) during the initial 12 hours of therapy. Further reductions in BP to acceptable target levels should proceed over a period of days to minimize potential for inducing ischemic injury in the setting of altered autoregulatory flow to target organ vascular beds.[264,288]

The favored parenteral drug for rapid treatment of hypertensive emergencies remains sodium nitroprusside[264] (Table 10-11). An NO donor, sodium nitroprusside induces arterial and venous dilation, providing rapid and predictable reductions in systemic BP. Prolonged administration of large doses may be associated with cyanide or thiocyanate toxicity; however, rarely is this a concern in the setting of acute hypertensive emergencies. Although less potent and predictable than sodium nitroprusside, NTG, another NO donor, may be preferable in the setting of myocardial ischemia or after CABG. NTG preferentially dilates venous capacitance beds as opposed to arterioles; however, rapid onset of tolerance limits the efficacy of sustained infusions to maintain BP control. Nicardipine, a parenteral dihydropyridine calcium channel blocker, and fenoldopam, a selective dopamine₁-receptor antagonist, have been utilized increasingly in select patient populations after CABG and in the setting of renal insufficiency, respectively.

Several drugs remain available for intermittent parenteral administration in the setting of hypertensive emergencies or urgencies. Enalaprilat, an IV ACE inhibitor, has been administered in settings of severe hypertension complicated by HF. Hydralazine, labetalol, and esmolol provide additional therapeutic options for intermittent parenteral injection for hypertensive control. However, with the exception of sodium nitroprusside, the response to parenteral antihypertensive drugs remains unpredictable, posing the potential for delayed achievement of targeted BP goals or, conversely, severe hypotensive responses. In most cases of emergent or severe hypertension, a diuretic will be required to maintain the prolonged natriuresis needed to sustain an antihypertensive response. In the setting of renal insufficiency or failure, minoxidil and even acute dialysis may be necessary to attain BP control.

Compelling Indications for Specific Antihypertensive Drug Selection

Despite compelling evidence supporting the preferential administration of thiazide diuretics as agents of choice for treatment of hypertension, most patients will require addition of a second nondiuretic antihypertensive drug to achieve desired target BPs.[264] Selection of a complementary antihypertensive agent necessitates a thorough understanding of the mechanisms of action to optimize the additive effect of combined therapy. For example, β-blockers, ACE inhibitors, and Ang II antagonists inhibit renin release. Therefore, combinations of these

TABLE 10-11 Parenteral Drugs for Treatment of Hypertensive Emergencies

Drug	Dosage	Onset of Action	Duration of Action	Adverse Effects†	Special Indications
Vasodilators					
Sodium nitroprusside	0.25–10 μg/kg/min as intravenous infusion‡	Immediate	1–2 min	Nausea, vomiting, muscle twitching, sweating, thiocyanate and cyanide intoxication	Most hypertensive emergencies; caution with high intracranial pressure or azotemia
Nicardipine hydrochloride	5–15 mg/hr IV	5–10 min	15–30 min, may exceed 4 hr	Tachycardia, headache, flushing, local phlebitis	Most hypertensive emergencies except acute HF; caution with coronary ischemia
Fenoldopam mesylate	0.1–0.3 μg/kg/min intravenous infusion	<5 min	30 min	Tachycardia, headache, nausea, flushing	Most hypertensive emergencies; caution with glaucoma
Nitroglycerin	5–100 μg/min as intravenous infusion	2–5 min	5–10 min	Headache, vomiting, methemoglobinemia, tolerance with prolonged use	Coronary ischemia
Enalaprilat	1.25–5 mg every 6 hr IV	15–30 min	6–12 hr	Precipitous decline in pressure in high-renin states; variable response	Acute left ventricular failure; avoid in acute myocardial infarction
Hydralazine hydrochloride	10–20 mg IV	10–20 min IV	1–4 hr IV	Tachycardia, flushing, headache, vomiting, aggravation of angina	Eclampsia
	10–40 mg IM	20–30 min IM	4–6 hr IM		
Adrenergic Inhibitors					
Labetalol hydrochloride	20–80 mg IV bolus every 10 min 0.5–2.0 mg/min IV infusion	5–10 min	3–6 hr	Vomiting, scalp tingling, bronchoconstriction, dizziness, nausea, heart block, orthostatic hypotension	Most hypertensive emergencies except acute HF
Esmolol hydrochloride	250–500 μg/kg/min IV bolus, then 50–100 μg/kg/min by infusion; may repeat bolus after 5 min or increase infusion to 300 μg/min	1–2 min	10–30 min	Hypotension, nausea, asthma, first-degree heart block, HF	Aortic dissection, perioperative
Phentolamine	5–15 mg IV bolus	1–2 min	10–30 min	Tachycardia, flushing, headache	Catecholamine excess

These doses may vary from those in the *Physician's Desk Reference,* 51st ed.
†Hypotension may occur with all agents.
‡Requires special delivery system.
HF, heart failure; IM, intramuscularly; IV, intravenously.
Reproduced from Chobanian AV, Bakris GL, Black HR, et al: Seventh report of the Joint National Committee on Prevention, Detection, Evaluation, and Treatment of High Blood Pressure. Hypertension 42:1206–1252, 2003, by permission.

agents are unlikely to achieve a maximal additive antihypertensive response. Similarly, both the diuretics and dihydropyridine calcium channel blockers produce peripheral vasodilation such that combination with other antihypertensive drug classes may prove more efficacious. Increasingly, data derived from ongoing outcomes-based trials of antihypertensive therapy in patients with coexisting diseases suggest that specific antihypertensive drugs reduce morbidity beyond that expected for BP reduction alone[264] (Table 10-12).

For example, in patients with ischemic heart disease, and most especially a recent MI, β-blockers have been demonstrated to reduce mortality and morbidity related to subsequent cardiac events.[86,275,277,305] Although precise mechanisms remain unclear, reductions in overall sympathetic stimulation and antiarrhythmic effects presumably play contributory roles. In the setting of renal insufficiency, ACE inhibitors and Ang II antagonists delay progression of both diabetic and nondiabetic-associated renal disease.[305,308-310] Calcium channel blockers have proved efficacious in the setting of peripheral vascular diseases, such as Raynaud syndrome, and α_1-blockers favorably influence symptoms of prostatism. In the setting of hypertension and pregnancy, methyldopa and hydralazine remain preferred antihypertensives for management of chronic hypertension and preeclampsia, respectively.[260]

Perioperative Implications of Hypertension

There is little evidence to suggest that mild-to-moderate degrees of hypertension adversely affect morbidity and mortality in the perioperative setting. In fact, ACC/AHA guidelines state that mild-to-moderate hypertension does not represent an independent risk factor for perioperative cardiovascular complications.[314] However, given the strong association between hypertension and cardiovascular diseases, a preoperative diagnosis of hypertension necessitates preoperative assessment for evidence of target-organ damage (e.g., CAD, renal dysfunction, stroke, peripheral vascular disease).[315] In contrast with isolated hypertension, secondary cardiovascular diseases, in many cases, do pose increased risk for perioperative morbidity and mortality. In patients with a preoperative diagnosis of hypertension, an electrocardiogram (ECG) is performed (to assess for evidence of ischemia, prior MI, or left ventricular [LV] hypertrophy), and a urinalysis and plasma creatinine determination may be obtained to assess renal function. Specific antihypertensive therapies may necessitate additional evaluations such as assessment of plasma potassium and sodium in patients taking diuretics.

TABLE 10-12	Clinical Trial and Guideline Basis for Compelling Indications for Individual Drug Classes							
	Recommended Drugs							
*Compelling Indication**	*Diuretic*	*BB*	*ACEI*	*ARB*	*CCB*	*Aldo ANT*		*Clinical Trial Basis†*
Heart failure	•	•	•	•		•		ACC/AHA Heart Failure Guideline,[273] MERIT-HF,[274] COPERNICUS,[289] CIBIS,[276] SOLVD,[290] AIRE,[291] TRACE,[292] ValHEFT,[293] RALES,[294] CHARM[295]
Postmyocardial infarction		•	•			•		ACC/AHA Post-MI Guideline,[296] BHAT,[86] SAVE,[297] CAPRICORN,[275] EPHESUS (TS40)
High coronary disease risk	•	•	•		•			ALLHAT,[283] HOPE,[299] ANBP2,[300] LIFE,[301] CONVINCE,[302] EUROPA,[303] INVEST[304]
Diabetes	•	•	•	•	•			NKF-ADA Guideline,[305,306] UKPDS,[307] ALLHAT[283]
Chronic kidney disease			•	•				NKF Guideline,[305] Captopril Trial,[308] RENAAL,[309] IDNT,[310] REIN,[311] AASK[312]
Recurrent stroke prevention	•		•					PROGRESS[313]

*Compelling indications for antihypertensive drugs are based on benefits from outcome studies or existing clinical guidelines. The compelling indication is managed in parallel with the blood pressure.
†Conditions for which clinical trials demonstrate benefit of specific classes of antihypertensive drugs used as part of an antihypertensive regimen to achieve blood pressure goal to test outcomes.

ACEI, angiotensin-converting enzyme inhibitor; Aldo ANT, aldosterone antagonist; ARB, angiotensin receptor blocker; BB, β-blocker; CCB, calcium channel blocker.
Reproduced from Chobanian AV, Bakris GL, Black HR, et al: Seventh report of the Joint National Committee on Prevention, Detection, Evaluation, and Treatment of High Blood Pressure. *Hypertension* 42:1206, 2003, by permission.

In cases of mild-to-moderate hypertension, few controlled trials assessing the association between preoperative hypertension and perioperative morbidity and mortality are available. Most investigations have been observational in nature with no correction for potentially confounding risk factors. In many cases, the number of study participants has been inadequate to ensure statistical power to assess for relevant associations between outcomes and a preoperative diagnosis of hypertension. Howell et al[288] published a meta-analysis summarizing 30 studies including more than 12,995 patients for whom an association between hypertension and perioperative complications could be assessed. These authors calculated an odds ratio of 1.31, suggesting a slightly increased risk for perioperative cardiovascular complications in patients with preexisting hypertension; however, given limitations of the dataset, the authors further concluded that such a small odds ratio in the setting of a "low perioperative event rate" likely represents a clinically insignificant association between preexisting hypertension and cardiac risk. Other investigators have reported similar small associations between isolated systolic hypertension before surgery and subsequent perioperative morbidity.

As opposed to the apparently low perioperative risk posed by mild-to-moderate hypertension, cases of severe hypertension (diastolic BP > 110 mm Hg) frequently lead to questions whether elective surgery should be postponed to allow for titration of antihypertensive therapy to acceptable systemic BPs. Again, although there are little data to support conclusive recommendations regarding acceptable preoperative BPs or the length of antihypertensive therapy necessary to achieve a new "steady state," patients with poorly controlled BP experience more labile BP responses in the perioperative setting with greater potential for hypertensive or hypotensive episodes, or both.[315–317] Guidelines published by the ACC/AHA suggest that systemic BPs exceeding 180 mm Hg systolic and/or 110 mm Hg diastolic should be controlled before surgery.[314] In a review, Howell and colleagues[288] concluded that surgery need not be canceled in the setting of severe hypertension; however, a careful preoperative assessment for target organ damage (e.g., cardiovascular, renal, cerebrovascular disease) should be performed before surgery, and intraoperative arterial pressures should be maintained within 20% of preoperative BPs. At a minimum, in patients with severe hypertension, invasive monitoring of arterial pressure with strict control of perioperative BPs, continuing

into the postoperative setting, appears justified; given the predilection for CAD in these patients, perioperative therapy with β-blockers may be indicated.[93,94]

PHARMACOTHERAPY FOR ACUTE AND CHRONIC HEART FAILURE

Chronic HF is one major cardiovascular disorder that continues to increase in incidence and prevalence, both in the United States and worldwide. It affects nearly 550 million persons in the United States, and roughly 600,000 new cases are diagnosed each year.[318,319] Currently, 1% to 2% of those 40 to 59 years of age and 12% to 14% of individuals older than 80 have HF.[318] Because HF is primarily a disease of the elderly, its prevalence is projected to increase twofold to threefold over the next decade, as the median age of the U.S. population continues to increase.[320] The increasingly prolonged survival of patients with various cardiovascular disorders that culminate in ventricular dysfunction (e.g., patients with CAD are living longer rather than dying acutely with MI), and the greater diagnostic awareness further compound the HF epidemic. Despite improvements in the understanding of the neurohormonal mechanisms underlying its pathophysiology and remarkable advances made in pharmacologic therapy, HF continues to cost the United States an estimated $38 billion annually in medical expenditures,[321] and it contributes to approximately 292,000 deaths per year.[318] Given the public health impact of the disease and the rapid pace of therapeutic advances, it is essential that the perioperative physician remain aware of contemporary clinical practice for the benefit of those patients with chronic HF presenting to the operating room or intensive care unit.

Accordingly, the pharmacologic management of HF as it relates to guidelines published by the ACC/AHA is reviewed.[322] The focus is primarily on chronic HF associated with LV systolic dysfunction, although chronic HF with preserved systolic function (or diastolic heart failure [DHF]) and acute HF also are discussed. For each drug commonly used in clinical practice, the general format of presentation includes whether it alters the progression of myocardial damage (for agents administered chronically), its mechanism(s) of action, current clinical data on trials of its use for HF, and its current place in the treatment of HF. New, non-neurohormonal, pharmacologic options in HF management also are reviewed.

Heart Failure Classification

The ACC/AHA updated guidelines for evaluating and managing HF include a new, four-stage classification system emphasizing both the evolution and progression of the disease (Figure 10-17). It calls attention to patients with preclinical stages of HF to focus on halting disease progression. The staging system is meant to complement, not replace, the widely used New York Heart Association (NYHA) classification, a semi-quantitative index of functional classification that categorizes patients with HF by the severity of their symptoms (Box 10-5). NYHA classification remains useful clinically because it reflects symptoms, which, in turn, correlate with quality of life and survival.[323] The new classification

system for HF, recognizing its progressive course and identifying those who are at risk (e.g., the first two stages, A and B, clearly are not HF), reinforces the importance of determining the optimal strategy for neurohormonal antagonism in an attempt to improve the natural history of the syndrome. In this new staging approach, patients would only be expected to either not advance at all or to advance from one stage to the next, unless progression of the disease was halted by treatment. This is in contrast with the NYHA functional classification in which the severity of symptoms characteristically fluctuates depending on changes in diet and medications, even in the absence of measurable changes in LV structure and function.[318,322] The new HF staging approach may be comparable with that used in such disorders as cancer.

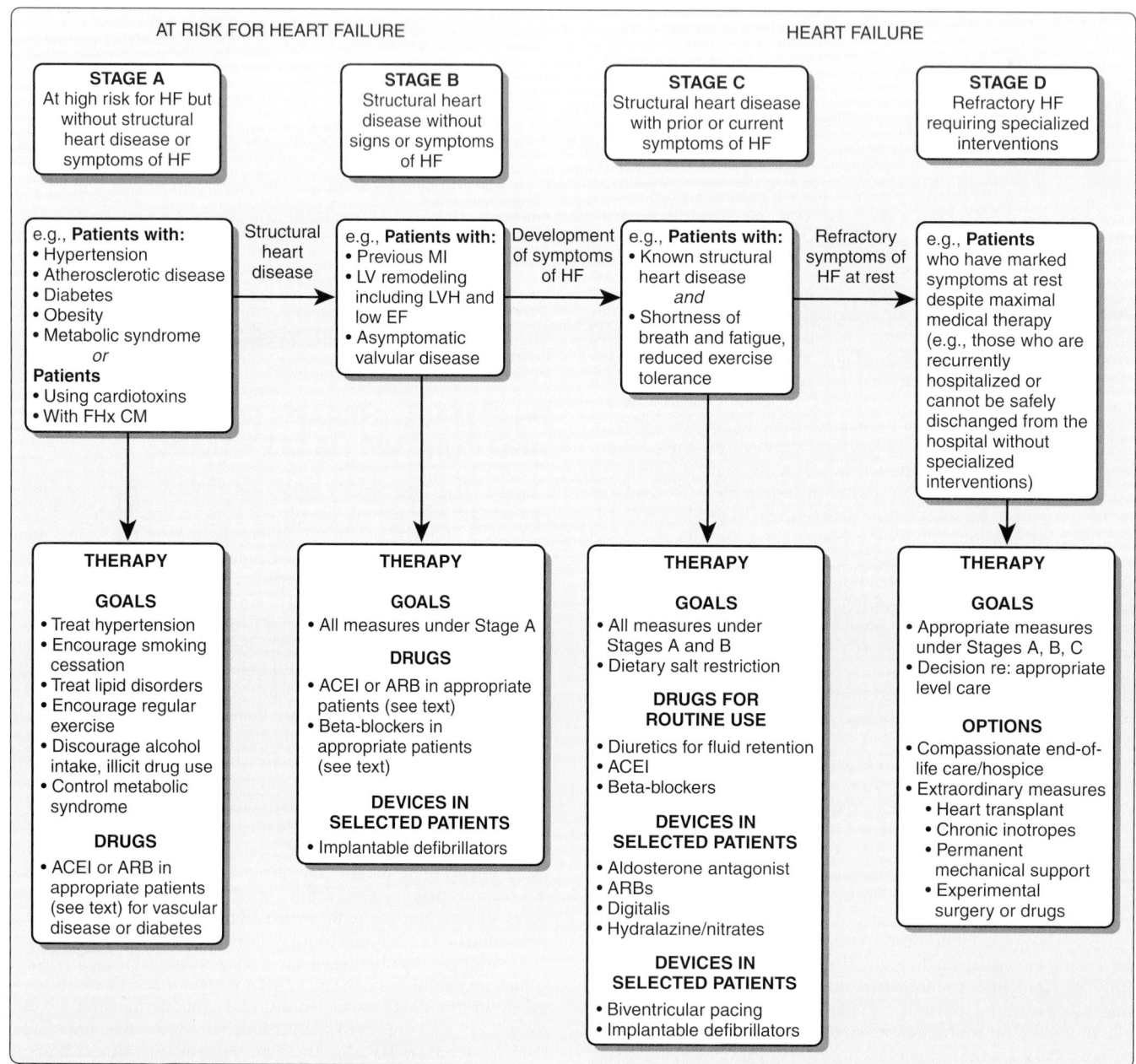

Figure 10-17 **American College of Cardiology/American Heart Association Four-Stage Classification and Management Recommendations.** Stages in the development of heart failure/recommended therapy. ACEI, angiotensin-converting enzyme inhibitors; ARB, angiotensin II receptor blocker; EF, ejection fraction; FHx CM, family history of cardiomyopathy; HF, heart failure; LVH, left ventricular hypertrophy; MI, myocardial infarction. *(Reprinted by permission of Hunt SA: 2009 focused update incorporated into the ACC/AHA 2005 Guidelines for the Diagnosis and Management of Heart Failure in Adults: A report of the American College of Cardiology Foundation/American Heart Association Task Force on Practice Guidelines: Developed in collaboration with the International Society for Heart and Lung Transplantation. Circulation 119:e391–e479, 2009; Figure 1.)*

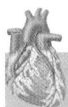

BOX 10-5. NEW YORK HEART ASSOCIATION FUNCTIONAL CLASS

Class I: No limitation of functional activity. Ordinary physical activity does not cause undue fatigue, palpitation, dyspnea, or anginal pain.

Class II: Slight limitation of physical activity. Comfortable at rest, but ordinary physical activity results in fatigue, palpitation, dyspnea, or anginal pain.

Class III: Marked limitation of physical activity. Comfortable at rest. Less than ordinary activity causes dyspnea, palpitation, fatigue, or anginal pain.

Class IV: Severe limitation in ability to carry on any physical activity without discomfort. Symptoms of heart failure or anginal pain are present even at rest. If any physical activity is undertaken, discomfort increases.

Although the pathophysiology of HF has been addressed elsewhere, it is important to mention key concepts as the basis of current pharmacologic therapy. To start, HF remains the final common pathway for CAD, hypertension, valvular heart disease, and cardiomyopathy, in which the natural history results in symptomatic or asymptomatic LV dysfunction (specifically, LV systolic dysfunction for the purposes of this discussion). The neurohormonal responses to impaired cardiac performance (salt and water retention, vasoconstriction, sympathetic stimulation) are initially adaptive but, if sustained, become maladaptive, resulting in pulmonary congestion and excessive afterload. This, in turn, leads to a vicious cycle of increases in cardiac energy expenditure and worsening of pump function and tissue perfusion (Table 10-13). Although the cardiorenal and cardiocirculatory branches of this neurohormonal hypothesis of HF were the original foundation for the use of diuretics, vasodilators, and inotropes, respectively, seminal information in the early 1990s emerged from large, randomized clinical trials that showed ACE inhibitors[324,325] and angiotensin receptor blockers,[293,326] but not most other vasodilators,[327] prolonged survival in patients with HF. In a similar fashion, the use of β-blockers, despite their negative inotropic effects, improved morbidity and mortality in randomized, controlled trials.[289,328,329]

The finding that low-dose aldosterone antagonists added to conventional therapy for HF reduce mortality in patients with severe HF suggests that there is more to the neurohormonal hypothesis of drug efficacy than cardiorenal and hemodynamic effects alone.[294,298] Taken together with evidence from basic investigations showing that Ang II is a growth factor and a vasoconstrictor,[330] the clinical data promoted a shift in focus from cardiorenal and cardiocirculatory processes toward cardiac remodeling as the central component in the progression of this neurohormone-mediated cardiac syndrome.[331] The renin-angiotensin-aldosterone system, excess sympathetic activity, endothelin, and various cytokines all have been implicated as stimuli of proliferative signaling that contribute to maladaptive cardiac growth. Accordingly, ventricular remodeling, or the structural alterations of the heart in the form of dilatation and hypertrophy (Boxes 10-6 and 10-7), in addition

BOX 10-6. PATHOBIOLOGY OF LEFT VENTRICULAR REMODELING

Alterations in Myocyte Biology
Excitation contraction coupling
Myosin heavy-chain (fetal) gene expression
β-Adrenergic desensitization
Hypertrophy
Myocytolysis
Cytoskeletal proteins

Myocardial Changes
Myocyte loss
  Necrosis
  Apoptosis
Alterations in extracellular matrix
  Matrix degradation
  Replacement fibrosis

Alterations in Left Ventricular (LV) Chamber Geometry
LV dilation
Increased LV sphericity
LV wall thinning
Mitral valve incompetence

From Mann DL: Mechanisms and models in heart failure: An approach. *Circulation* 100:999–1088, 1999.

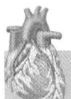

BOX 10-7. MECHANICAL DISADVANTAGE CREATED BY LEFT VENTRICULAR REMODELING

Increased wall stress (afterload)
Afterload mismatch
Episodic subendocardial hypoperfusion
Increased oxygen utilization
Sustained hemodynamic overloading
Worsening activation of compensatory mechanisms

From Mann DL: Mechanisms and models in heart failure: An approach. *Circulation* 100:999–1088, 1999.

to the counter-regulatory hemodynamic responses, lead to progressive ventricular dysfunction and represent the target of current therapeutic interventions (Figure 10-18).

Pathophysiologic Role of the Renin-Angiotensin System in Heart Failure

The renin-angiotensin system (RAS) is one of several neuroendocrine systems that are activated in patients with HF. The RAS is also an important mediator in the progression of HF. In the short term, the juxtaglomerular cells of the kidney release the proteolytic enzyme, renin, in response to a decrease in BP or renal perfusion (e.g., hemorrhage), generating Ang I from circulating angiotensinogen. ACE cleavage of Ang II from Ang I in the lung produces circulating Ang II. Acutely, Ang II acts as a potent arteriolar and venous vasoconstrictor to return BP and filling pressure to baseline, respectively. Ang II also stimulates the release of aldosterone from the adrenal cortex and antidiuretic hormone (ADH) from the posterior pituitary. Both contribute to increases in blood volume through their effects on the kidney to promote salt and water reabsorption, respectively. In the long term, increases in Ang II lead to sodium and fluid retention, and increases in SVR, which contribute to symptoms of HF, pulmonary congestion, and hemodynamic decompensation (Figure 10-19).

In addition to these cardiorenal and cardiocirculatory effects, most of the hormones and receptors of the RAS are expressed in the myocardium, where they contribute to maladaptive growth or remodeling,

TABLE 10-13	Neurohormonal Effects of Impaired Cardiac Performance and Their Effects on the Circulation	
Response	*Short-Term Effects*	*Long-Term Effects*
Salt and water retention	Augments preload	Pulmonary congestion, anasarca
Vasoconstriction	Maintains blood pressure for perfusion of vital organs (brain, heart)	Exacerbates pump dysfunction (excessive afterload), increases cardiac energy expenditure
Sympathetic stimulation	Increases heart rate and ejection	Increases energy expenditure

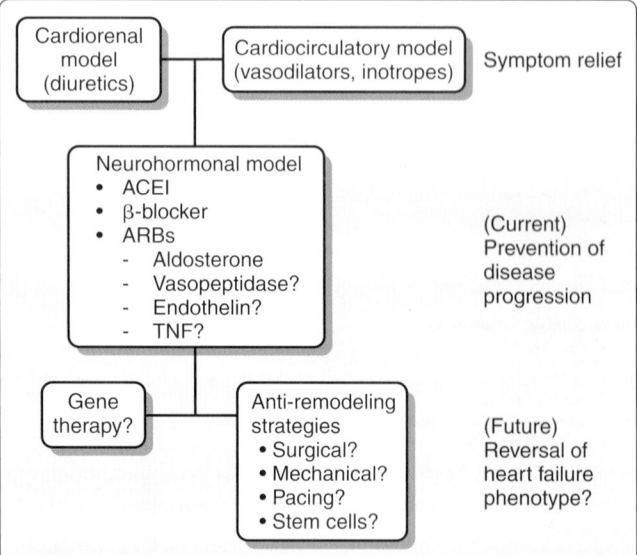

Figure 10-18 Current and future treatments of heart failure. Currently, heart failure therapies are focused on prevention of disease progression with drugs that antagonize neurohormonal systems. Future therapies may involve antagonists of other biologically active systems (e.g., endothelins, tumor necrosis factor [TNF]-α) and antiremodeling strategies that may reverse the heart failure phenotype. ACEI, angiotensin-converting enzyme inhibitor; ARB, angiotensin-receptor blocker; NEP, neutral endopeptidase blocker. *(Adapted from Mann DL: Mechanisms and model in heart failure: A combinatorial approach. Circulation 100:999, 1999.)*

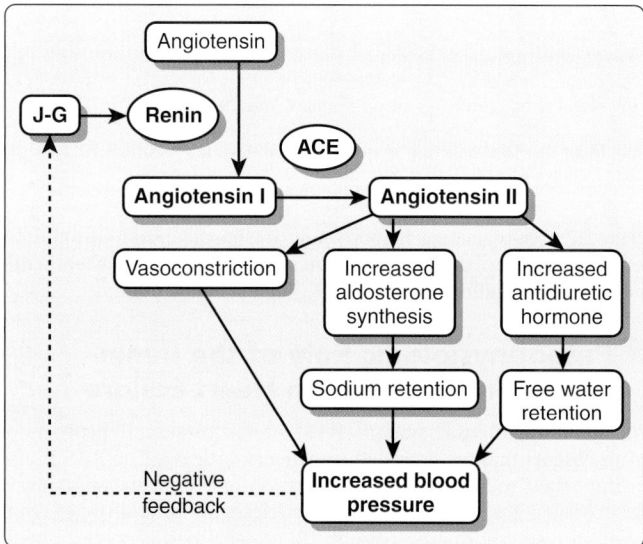

Figure 10-19 Basic pathway of the renin-angiotensin-aldosterone system. ACE, angiotensin-converting enzyme. *(From Jaski BE: Basis of heart failure: A problem solving approach. Boston: Kluwer Academic Publishers, 2000, by permission of Springer Science and Business Media.)*

key factors in the progression of HF. Increased expression of messenger RNA for angiotensinogen, ACE, and Ang II has been identified in the failing human heart.[332] Correspondingly, increased coronary sinus Ang II concentrations were measured in patients with dilated and ischemic cardiomyopathy, signifying a paracrine or autocrine action of the RAS. Moreover, progressive increases in coronary sinus Ang II production correlated with increases in NYHA functional classification of HF.[332] Taken together, these data provide evidence that intracardiac RAS is involved in the evolution of the disease process.

The effects of Ang II on its receptors, AT_1 and AT_2, are well appreciated. The AT_1 receptor is involved in several effects that lead to adverse cardiovascular outcomes. Activation of AT_1 receptors promotes aldosterone and vasopressin secretion with concomitant increases in salt and water reabsorption through the kidneys, vasoconstriction, catecholamine release, and cell growth and proliferation of cardiovascular tissue (Table 10-14). Stimulation of AT_2 receptors, in contrast, results in natriuresis, vasodilation, release of bradykinin and NO, and cell growth inhibition or apoptosis. The Ang II that is formed locally in the heart acts primarily through AT_1 receptors located on myocytes and fibroblasts, where it participates in the regulation of cardiac remodeling. Through complex cascades of intracellular signal transduction that activate protein transcription factors within the nucleus, initiating the creation of RNA transcripts, the long-term effects of intracardiac Ang II on the AT_1 receptor result in cardiomyocyte hypertrophy, fibroblast proliferation, and extracellular matrix deposition[333] (Figure 10-20). These processes contribute to progressive LV remodeling and LV dysfunction characteristic of HF.

Angiotensin-Converting Enzyme Inhibitors

Clinical Evidence
Evidence supporting the beneficial use of ACE inhibitors in HF patients comes from various randomized, placebo-controlled clinical trials (Table 10-15). Initially, this class of drugs was evaluated for

TABLE 10-14	Cellular and Physiologic Effects of AT_1 and AT_2 Stimulation That Lead to Tissue Remodeling	
AT_1 Receptor	**AT_2 Receptor**
Vasoconstriction	Vasodilation
Cell growth and proliferation	Cell growth inhibition/apoptosis
Positive inotropy	Negative chronotropy
Aldosterone secretion	Natriuresis
Catecholamine release	Bradykinin release

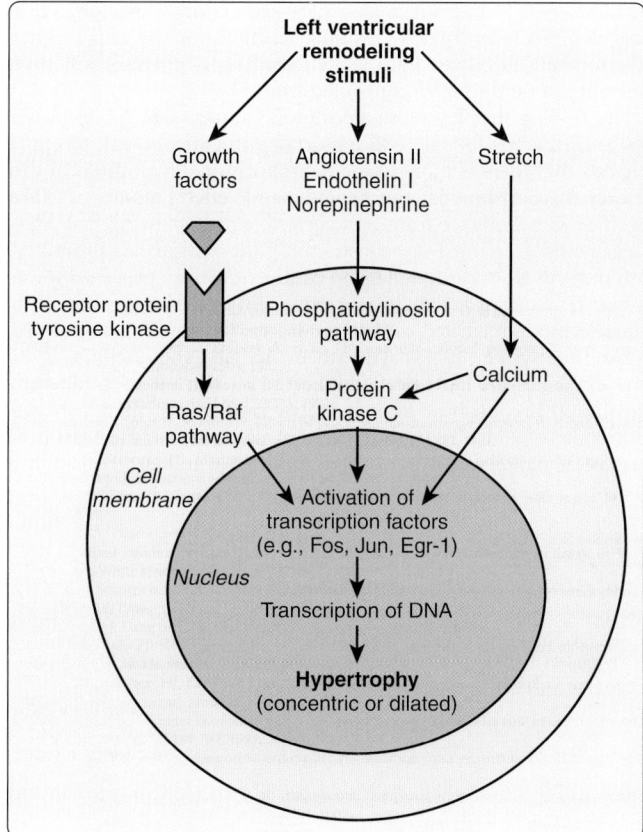

Figure 10-20 Left ventricular remodeling stimuli.

TABLE 10-15	Selected Clinical Trials of Angiotensin-Converting Enzyme Inhibitors in Heart Failure			
Patient Subset	Heart Failure Stage	Drug	Trial	
Heart Failure				
NYHA Class II and III	C	Enalapril	SOLVD (treat); V-HeFT II	
Class IV	D	Enalapril	CONSENSUS	
Asymptomatic LV Dysfunction				
EF < 35%	B	Enalapril	SOLVD (prevent)	
Post-MI (EF < 40%)	B	Captopril	SAVE	
Acute MI	B	Captopril Lisinopril	GISSI ISIS-4	
Asymptomatic High Risk				
History of DM, PVD, and coronary risk factors	A	Ramipril	HOPE	

DM, diabetes mellitus; EF, ejection fraction; HOPE, Heart Outcomes Prevention Evaluation; ISIS-4, Fourth International Study of Infarct Survival; LV, left ventricular; MI, myocardial infarction; NYHA, New York Heart Association; PVD, peripheral vascular disease; SAVE, Survival and Ventricular Enlargement; SOLVD, Studies Of Left Ventricular Dysfunction; V-HeFT II, second Vasodilator-Heart Failure Trial; CONSENSUS, Cooperative North Scandinavian Enalapril Survival Study; GISSI, Gruppo Italiano Studiso Pravvivenza Infartomi Ocardico.

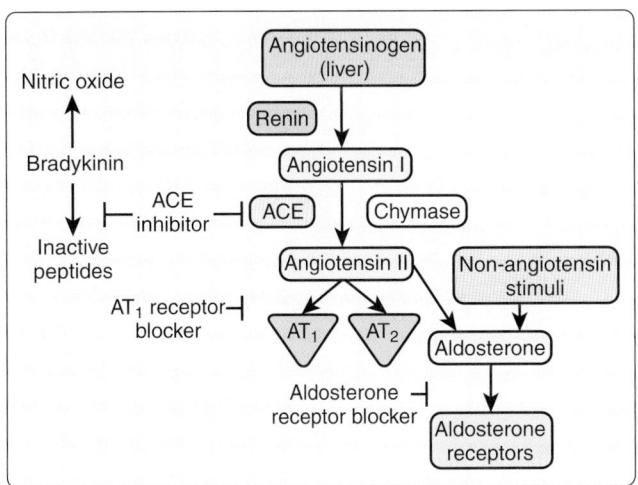

Figure 10-21 **Activation of the renin-angiotensin-aldosterone system.** ACE, angiotensin-converting enzyme. *(Redrawn from Mann DL: Heart therapy: A companion to Braunwald's Heart Disease. Philadelphia: Saunders, 2004.)*

treatment of symptomatic HF (Studies Of Left Ventricular Dysfunction [SOLVD], Vasodilator-Heart Failure Trial [V-HeFT], Cooperative North Scandinavian Enalapril Survival Study [CONSENSUS]). Patients with NYHA Class II to IV HF treated with ACE inhibitors had reductions in mortality rate ranging from 16% to 31%. Subsequently, ACE inhibitors also were found to improve outcome for asymptomatic patients with LV systolic dysfunction in the following categories: patients with EFs less than 35% because of cardiomyopathy,[333] patients within 2 weeks after MI with EFs less than 40%,[334] and patients presenting within the first 24 hours of MI regardless of EF.[335] Recent results from the Heart Outcomes Prevention Evaluation (HOPE) study have further expanded the indications for this class of agents to include asymptomatic, high-risk patients to prevent new-onset HF.[336] In patients with diabetes or peripheral vascular disease and an additional atherosclerotic risk factor, but without clinical HF or systolic dysfunction, ramipril (10 mg/day) reduced the HF risk by 23%. More recently, the Prevention of Events with Angiotensin Converting Enzyme (PEACE) trial evaluated the use of angiotensin converting enzyme-inhibitors (ACE-I) in addition to modern conventional therapy in patients with stable CAD with preserved LV function. The results of this trial did not demonstrate any decrease in mortality from cardiovascular causes or nonfatal MI compared with placebo.[337] As a result, the ACC/AHA committee has changed the level of recommendation for the use of ACE-I from Class I to Class IIa for patients with Stage A HF.[322] Together, these data endorse the use of ACE inhibitors as first-line therapy for a broad spectrum of patients including those with LV systolic dysfunction, with or without symptoms, and in high-risk patients with vascular disease, diabetes, or both, in addition to those with the traditional coronary risk factors. Indeed, the addition of ACE-I in patients with stable CAD, preserved LV systolic function, and at low risk for cardiovascular events also can be useful (Class IIa recommendation). Since the commencement of these trials, the rationale for the use of ACE inhibitors has expanded from a reduction in the progression of clinical HF through ACE inhibitor–mediated vasodilatory action, to acknowledgment that ACE inhibitors also directly affect the cellular mechanisms responsible for progressive myocardial pathology.

Mechanisms of Action
ACE inhibitors act by inhibiting one of several proteases responsible for cleaving the decapeptide, Ang I, to form the octapeptide, Ang II. Because ACE is also the enzyme that degrades bradykinin, ACE inhibitors lead to increased circulating and tissue levels of bradykinin (Figure 10-21). ACE inhibitors have several useful effects in chronic HF. They are potent vasodilators through decreasing Ang II and norepinephrine, and increasing bradykinin, NO, and prostacyclin.[338] By reducing the secretion of aldosterone and ADH, ACE inhibitors also reduce salt and

water reabsorption from the kidney. ACE inhibitors reduce release of norepinephrine from sympathetic nerves by acting on AT_1 receptors at the nerve terminal. Within tissue, ACE inhibitors inhibit Ang II production, and thus attenuate Ang II–mediated cardiomyocyte hypertrophy and fibroblast hyperplasia.[339,340] Clinical evidence supporting an ACE inhibitor–mediated role in cardiac remodeling comes from comparative studies of enalapril versus placebo (SOLVD trial) and enalapril versus hydralazine isosorbide dinitrate (VHeft II trial).[341,342] In a subset of the SOLVD study,[341] the placebo group exhibited LV dilation, whereas the enalapril group exhibited a decrease in chamber size for a given LV pressure. Correspondingly, in the VHeft II trial, survival was better with enalapril versus hydralazine-isosorbide dinitrate, despite improvements in exercise capacity in the latter group, suggesting that mechanisms other than vasodilation contribute to improved survival with ACE inhibitors.[341] Chymase also catalyzes the production of Ang II from Ang I within myocardial tissue. This serine protease has nearly 20-fold greater affinity for Ang I than ACE, and it is not influenced by ACE inhibitors.[343] Accordingly, Ang II receptor blockers (ARBs) may add to the inhibition by ACE inhibitors of angiotensin-promoted progression of HF (see Angiotensin II Receptor Blockers for Heart Failure).

ACE inhibitors attenuate insulin resistance, a common metabolic abnormality in patients with HF, independent of Ang II activity. Ang II receptor antagonists do not attenuate insulin resistance.[344] Both ACE inhibitors and ARBs have been shown to reduce proteinuria and slow the progression to renal failure in patients with hypertension (a common comorbidity in patients with HF).[309,345]

Drug Selection/Strategy for Clinical Practice
Treatment guidelines for the use of ACE inhibitors, including appropriate starting and target doses, and common side effects are shown in Table 10-16. Adherence to target doses of ACE inhibitors increases the likelihood of reproducing benefits demonstrated in large-scale HF trials (see Table 10-15). According to the AHA/ACC guidelines (see Table 10-13), it is reasonable to initiate ACE inhibitor therapy in high-risk patients (stage A)—those with diabetes, peripheral vascular disease, or both, though the committee now acknowledges that further objective studies are needed in this patient group. ACE-inhibitor therapy should be initiated in high-risk patients: Those with diabetes and/or peripheral vascular disease, asymptomatic patients with structural heart disease (stage A); those with previous MI and normal EFs (stage B); and all patients with EFs less than 40% (stages C and D) should receive ACE inhibitor therapy. The relative contraindications for the use of ACE inhibitors include (1) a history of intolerance or adverse reactions, for example, cough, angioedema, neutropenia, and rash; (2) persisting hyperkalemia > 5.5 mEq/L (that cannot be reduced by diet or diuretic

TABLE 10-16	Angiotensin-Converting Enzyme Inhibitors Proven Effective in Heart Failure and/or Left Ventricular Dysfunction					
Drug	Half-life (hr)	Dosing Interval	Start Dose (mg)	Target Dose (mg)	Relative Tissue Binding
Captopril	3	tid	6.25	50	+
Enalapril	11	bid	2.5–5	10	+
Lisinopril	12	qd	5	20	+
Ramipril	9–18	bid	2.5	5	++
Quinapril	2 (25)	bid	5	20	+++
Trandolapril	6	bid	1	1–2	NA*

*Not applicable

adjustment); (3) symptomatic hypotension; and (4) history of bilateral renal artery stenosis. Small doses of an agent with a short plasma half-life (e.g., captopril) are advocated when initiating therapy in patients with marginal BP (systolic BP < 90 mm Hg) or reduced renal function (baseline creatinine > 2.0 mg/dL). Once it is demonstrated that a patient tolerates inhibition of RAS, dosing should be adjusted to target doses of a longer-acting agent. In the Adjuvant Tamoxifen Longer Against Shorter (ATLAS) trial, lisinopril, 32.5 to 35 mg/day, had greater efficacy than 2.5 to 5.0 mg/day in patients with symptomatic HF and LV systolic dysfunction (EF < 35%).[346] Patients receiving "target doses" of ACE inhibitors are less frequently hospitalized than those receiving reduced doses.[347] The importance of differences in tissue binding among the various ACE inhibitors remains unclear.

Angiotensin II Receptor Blockers for Heart Failure

Pathophysiology/Mechanism of Action
Although ACE inhibitors reduce mortality, many patients will not tolerate their side effects. ACE inhibitors incompletely antagonize Ang II. These factors have prompted the development of specific ARBs in the pharmacologic treatment of HF[348] (see Figure 10-21). Non–ACE-generated Ang II within the myocardium contributes to LV remodeling and HF progression through AT_1-receptor effects (see Table 10-14). Selective AT_1 blockers prevent Ang II from acting on the cell, preventing vasoconstriction, sodium retention, release of norepinephrine, and delaying or preventing LV hypertrophy and fibrosis.[349] AT_2 receptors remain unaffected, and their actions, including NO release, remain intact.

Clinical Evidence
Outcome benefits from ARBs were first shown in the Evaluation of Losartan in the Elderly Study (ELITE) I trial, which showed, as a secondary end point, a significantly reduced risk for sudden death with losartan (4.8%) compared with captopril (8.7%),[350] despite no between-group differences in the primary end points, renal dysfunction, and hypotension. The follow-up ELITE II trial (Table 10-17), although having greater statistical power than ELITE I, failed to

confirm that losartan was superior to captopril in reducing mortality in older patients with HF.[351] Moreover, in subgroup analyses, the ELITE II trial patients on preexisting β-blockers tended to have less favorable outcomes with losartan, as opposed to captopril. The two more recent trials, Valsartan in Heart Failure (Val-HeFT) and Candesartan in Heart Failure Assessment in Reduction of Mortality (CHARM), were designed to evaluate whether ARBs plus conventional therapy (including β-blockers, ACE inhibitors, and diuretics) for symptomatic HF provide additional clinical benefit. Although the findings from the Val-HeFT support the use of this ARB in patients with chronic HF who are intolerant to ACE inhibitors, those patients already on ACE inhibitors and β-blockers (93% of their patient population) showed a trend toward an increased risk for death or hospitalization when valsartan was added to their treatment regimen[293] (Figure 10-22). This is in contrast with the CHARM-Added trial,[352] which showed safety with regard to use of candesartan in combination with ACE inhibitors and β-blockers (15% relative risk reduction in cardiovascular-related mortality or hospitalization), and in patients intolerant to ACE (alternative group), the relative risk reduction in mortality or hospitalization was 23%. In contrast, patients with EF greater than 40% not receiving ACE inhibition (preserved group) showed no difference in cardiovascular mortality and only a small reduction in HF hospitalizations.[353,354] In the CHARM-overall trial, both cardiovascular-related death and hospitalizations were significantly reduced with candesartan use (relative risk reduction for CV death was 16%).[326]

Clinical Practice
ARBs may be used as alternatives to ACE inhibitors for the treatment of patients with symptomatic HF if there are side effects to ACE inhibitors (e.g., persistent cough, angioedema, hyperkalemia, or worsening renal dysfunction) or persistent hypertension despite ACE inhibitors and β-blockers. Because ARBs do not affect bradykinin levels, cough and angioedema are rare side effects. Doses and dosing intervals for ARBs studied in large-scale trials are shown in Table 10-18. Similar to ACE inhibition, ARBs produce dose-dependent decreases in RAP, PCWP,

TABLE 10-17	Angiotensin-Receptor Blocker Trial in Heart Failure		
Trial	Agent	Population	Outcome
ELITE II	Losartan 50 mg qd	Age ≥ 60 NYHA Class II-IV EF ≤ 40%	• Losartan was not better than captopril • No difference in mortality • Losartan was better tolerated • Losartan + β-blocker had worse outcome
Val-HeFT	Valsartan 160 mg bid or placebo plus open-label ACE-I (93%)	NYHA Class II-IV EF < 40%	• No difference in all-cause mortality • 13% significant difference in combined morbidity/mortality • HF hospital decrease 27% • Most benefit observed in ACE-I intolerant patients (7% of study group) with 45% reduction in combined primary end points
CHARM	Candesartan 32 mg qd vs. placebo with or without open-label ACE-I	NYHA Class II-IV	
	Added	EF ≤ 40%	• 15% relative risk reduction in all-cause mortality
	Preserved	EF > 40%	• Mild reduction in HF-related hospitalizations
	Alternative	EF ≤ 40%	• 23% relative risk reduction in HF-related mortality or hospitalization
	Overall	ACE-I intolerant	• Significant difference in all-cause mortality

CHARM, Candesartan in Heart Failure Assessment in Reduction of Mortality; EF, ejection fraction; ELITE, Evaluation of Losartan in the Elderly Study; HF, heart failure; NYHA, New York Health Association; Val-HeFT, Valsartan in Heart Failure Trial.

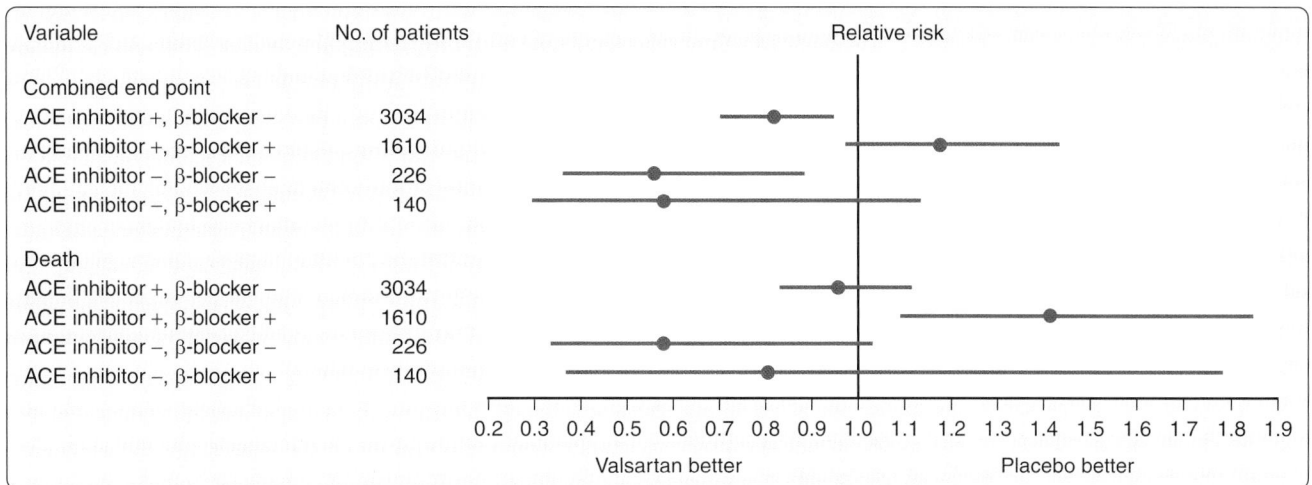

Figure 10-22 **Val-HeFT subgroups.** Relative risk for combined end point (cardiovascular-related mortality and hospitalization) and death. ACE, angiotensin-converting enzyme. *(From Cohn JN, Tognoni G; Valsartan Heart Failure Trial Investigators: A randomized trial of the angiotensin-receptor blocker valsartan in chronic heart failure. N Engl J Med 345:1667, 2001. copyright © 2001 Massachusetts Medical Society. All rights reserved.)*

and SVR. Unlike long-term ACE inhibition,[355] these hemodynamic effects and associated increases in cardiac index are sustained, and the plasma levels of Ang II remain suppressed with ARB therapy. Nevertheless, there is no convincing evidence that patients with HF benefit from addition of ARBs to standard therapy with ACE I and β-blockers.

TABLE 10-18	Angiotensin Receptor Blockers Evaluated in Large-Scale Trials			
Agent	*Half-life (hr)*	*Dosing Interval*	*Initial Dose*	*Target Dose*
Losartan	6–9	qd	25	50
Valsartan	9	bid	40	160
Irbesartan	11–15	qd	75	150
Candesartan	3.5–4	qd	4	32

Aldosterone Receptor Antagonists

Aldosterone, a mineralocorticoid, is another important component of the neurohormonal hypothesis of HF. Although it was previously assumed that treatment with an ACE inhibitor (or ARB) would block the production of aldosterone in patients with HF, increased levels of aldosterone have been measured despite inhibition of Ang II[356] (see Figure 10-21). Adverse effects of increased aldosterone levels on the cardiovascular system include sodium retention, potassium and magnesium loss, ventricular remodeling (e.g., collagen production, myocyte growth, and hypertrophy), myocardial norepinephrine release, and endothelial dysfunction[357] (Figure 10-23). Non–Ang II–mediated aldosterone production may, in part, be caused by the hypomagnesemia commonly seen in HF patients.[358] Low extracellular Mg^{2+}, common in chronic illness, as well as a result of loop diuretics,

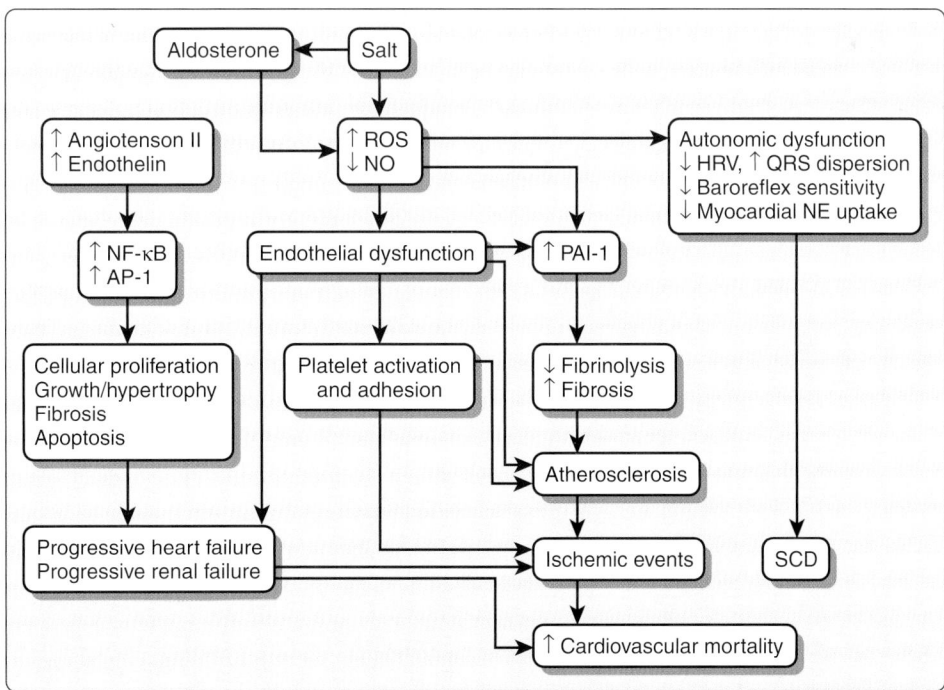

Figure 10-23 **Adverse effects of aldosterone and salt on the cardiovascular system.** HRV, heart rate variability; NE, norepinephrine; NF-κB, nuclear factor-κB; NO, nitric oxide; PAI-1, plasminogen activator inhibitor-1; ROS, reactive oxygen species; SCD, sudden cardiac death. *(From Pitt B, Rajagopalan A: The role of mineralocorticoid receptor blocking agents in patients with heart failure and cardiovascular disease. In McMurray JJ, Pfeffer MA [eds]: Heart failure updates. London: Martin Dunitz, 2003, p 129.)*

becomes a stimulus for adrenal aldosterone secretion.[359] Extra-adrenal production of aldosterone (e.g., in myocardial and vascular tissue) also may contribute to oxidative, proinflammatory, and prothrombotic signaling pathways (NF-κB, activator protein-I [AP-1], plasminogen activator inhibitor-1), and maladaptive processes such as LV dilatation, perivascular fibrosis, and atherosclerosis.[360–362] Aldosterone produced in the brain increases SNS activity, a central finding in HF.[363]

Given the multiple endocrine and auto/paracrine contributions of aldosterone to the neurohormonal hypothesis of HF, the possibility that aldosterone-receptor antagonism might halt disease progression became an increasingly attractive hypothesis. Besides the traditional mechanisms of mineralocorticoid receptor blockade, including natriuresis, diuresis, and kaliuresis,[358,364] beneficial nonrenal effects of aldosterone antagonism include decreased myocardial collagen formation,[365] increased myocardial norepinephrine uptake and decreased circulating norepinephrine levels,[365] normalization of baroreceptor function, increased HR variability,[366,367] and improved endothelial vasodilator dysfunction and basal NO bioactivity at the vascular level.[368]

Clinical Evidence

Two large-scale trials have demonstrated improved outcomes with aldosterone-receptor antagonism in chronic HF. The Randomized Aldactone Evaluation Study (RALES), conducted in more than 1600 symptomatic HF (e.g., stage C, NYHA Class III-IV) patients, showed the efficacy of spironolactone (26 mg/day) in combination with standard therapy: ACE inhibitor, loop diuretic with or without digoxin, and a β-blocker. Regardless of age, sex, and cause of HF, the treatment group experienced a 30% reduction in risk for all-cause mortality and in cardiovascular-related mortality compared with standard therapy[294] (Figure 10-24). Because β-blockers were used infrequently in this study (10% to 20%), the role of spironolactone in contemporary management of HF remains unclear. Indeed, studies have reported marked increases

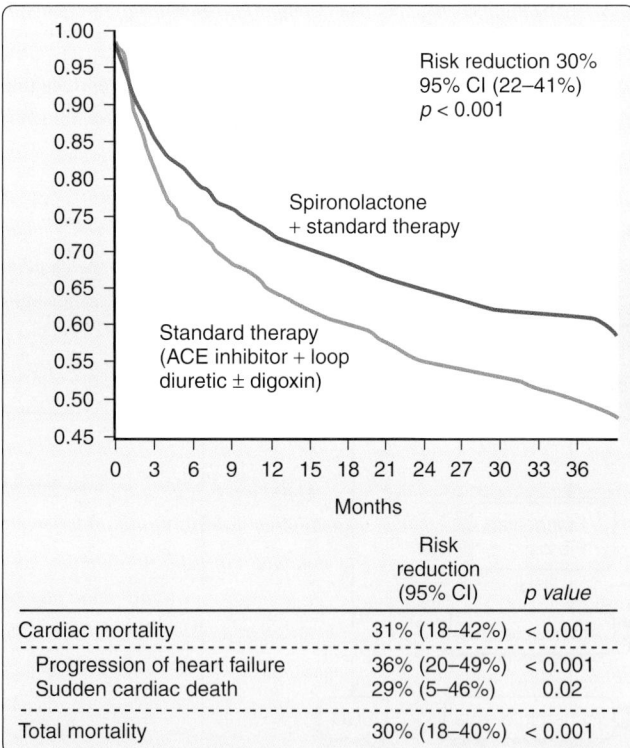

	Risk reduction (95% CI)	p value
Cardiac mortality	31% (18–42%)	< 0.001
Progression of heart failure	36% (20–49%)	< 0.001
Sudden cardiac death	29% (5–46%)	0.02
Total mortality	30% (18–40%)	< 0.001

Figure 10-24 Effect of spironolactone on morbidity and mortality in patients with severe heart failure. Randomized Aldactone Evaluation Study Investigators. ACE, angiotensin-converting enzyme; CI, confidence interval. *(From Pitt B, Rajagopalan A: The role of mineralocorticoid receptor blocking agents in patients with heart failure and cardiovascular disease. In McMurray JJ, Pfeffer MA [eds]: Heart failure updates. London: Martin Dunitz, 2003, p 118.)*

in hospital admission and death related to hyperkalemia subsequent to widespread use of spironolactone.[369] It has been speculated that the K⁺-sparing effect of spironolactone and its ability to reduce circulating norepinephrine[370] and increase NO availability[368] may have reduced the propensity for digitalis-related arrhythmias and the subsequent risk for sudden cardiac death reported in the digitalis trial.[371] Eplerenone is a new aldosterone antagonist that lacks some of spironolactone's common side effects.[372] The Eplerenone Post-acute Myocardial Infarction Heart Failure Efficacy and Survival Study (EPHSUS), conducted in more than 6600 patients with symptomatic HF within 3 to 14 days after MI, showed that eplerenone (25 to 50 mg/day) in combination with ACE inhibitor, loop diuretic, and β-blocker reduced all-cause mortality ($P = 0.008$), death from cardiovascular causes ($P = 0.0002$), and hospitalization for cardiovascular events.[298]

Although there are no large-scale trials examining the use of aldosterone receptor blockade in patients with mild-to-moderate systolic HF (NYHA Class II-III), pilot data suggest that aldosterone inhibition also may benefit these patients through improvements in endothelial function,[373] exercise tolerance, EF,[374] and attenuation of collagen formation. As noted previously, successful use of aldosterone antagonists mandates that close attention be paid to blood [K⁺].[373] Based on these data and the favorable effects of aldosterone antagonism in animal models of infarction,[360] it seems reasonable to expect that aldosterone-receptor blockers may find value even in patients with *asymptomatic* systolic LV dysfunction.

Clinical Practice

Current evidence supports aldosterone antagonists only for patients with severe symptomatic HF and patients with LV dysfunction after MI.[298] Aldosterone-receptor antagonists should be considered in addition to standard therapy (including ACE inhibitors) for patients with severe HF (NYHA stage IV) caused by LV systolic function. Spironolactone should be initiated at 12.5 to 25 mg/day. Patients should have a normal serum K⁺ (<5.0 mEq/L) and adequate renal function (creatinine ≤ 2.5 mg/dl in men, creatinine ≤ 2.0 mg/dl in women and creatinine clearance > 30). Regular measurement of electrolytes is mandatory to avoid hyperkalemia. In particular, dosages and/or dosing intervals should be reduced during episodes of potential dehydration (e.g., vomiting or diarrhea) and with concomitant use of pharmacologic agents that may predispose to impairments in renal function (e.g., steroidal anti-inflammatory agents). In the RALES trial, there was no significant increase in the incidence of severe hyperkalemia (K⁺ ≥ 6.0 mEq/L), and only one death related to hyperkalemia (in the placebo arm).[294] This is in marked contrast with a recent Canadian time-series analysis that showed an abrupt increase in hyperkalemia-associated morbidity and mortality in association with the publication of the RALES data.[369] Spironolactone can occupy androgen receptors, leaving unopposed estrogen receptors and, thus, predispose to estrogen-like effects such as painful gynecomastia and menstrual disorders. Because digoxin has estrogen-like properties, its use in combination with spironolactone also can predispose to gynecomastia.[375] This usually does not pose a problem in men because they do not have biologically significant amounts of estrogen. From the EPHESUS data, it appears that the newer aldosterone-receptor antagonist, eplerenone, has a lower incidence of hyperkalemia and no evidence of unopposed estrogen-receptor–like properties. Unfortunately, eplerenone is *many times more expensive* than spironolactone.

With regard to patients in stage B and C HF on baseline ACE inhibitor and β-blocker therapy, clinicians look forward to findings from large, randomized trials whether the addition of aldosterone antagonists to standard therapy will halt progression of the disease.

β-Adrenergic Receptor Antagonists

Sympathetic Nervous System Activation and Its Role in the Pathogenesis of Heart Failure

Activation of the SNS (e.g., after MI or with long-standing hypertension), much like increases in RAS activity, contributes to the pathophysiology of HF. In brief, SNS activation leads to pathologic

LV growth and remodeling. Myocytes thicken and elongate, with eccentric hypertrophy and increases in sphericity. Wall stress is increased by this architecture, promoting subendocardial ischemia, cell death, and contractile dysfunction. Persistent SNS activation leads to altered gene expression with a shift to a fetal-like phenotype (e.g., downregulation of cardiac α-actin and α-myosin heavy chain, and upregulation of fetal forms of β-myosin heavy chain). There is downregulation of calcium regulatory proteins, including SR calcium ATPase, and impairment of contractility and relaxation. The activated SNS also can be harmful to myocytes directly through programmed cell death. As myocytes are replaced by fibroblasts, the heart function deteriorates from this "remodeling."[376] The threshold for arrhythmias may also be lowered, contributing to a vicious, deteriorating cycle.

How β-Adrenergic Receptor Blockers Influence the Pathophysiology of Heart Failure

In chronic HF, the beneficial effects of long-term β-blockade include improved systolic function and myocardial energetics, and reversal of pathologic remodeling. A shift in substrate utilization from free fatty acids to glucose, a more efficient fuel in the face of myocardial ischemia, may partly explain the improved energetics and mechanics in the failing heart treated with β-blockade.[377] HR, a major determinant of myocardial oxygen consumption, is reduced by β_1-receptor blockade. β-Blockade also is associated with a change in the molecular phenotype of the heart. Systolic dysfunction of individual myocytes is associated with upregulation in gene expression of natriuretic peptides and fetal-like β-myosin heavy chain, and increased expression of SERCA2 and α-myosin heavy chain (the more efficient, faster, adult isoform).[376] β-Blockade reverses these changes in gene expression with concurrent improvements in LV function.[378] In a dog model of HF, β-blockade also reduces myocyte apoptosis.[379] Taken together, chronic β-blockade reduces the harmful effects of excessive SNS activation of the heart and can reverse LV remodeling.

β-Adrenergic blockade also may limit the disturbance of excitation-contraction (E-C) coupling and predisposition to ventricular arrhythmias associated with HF. In the normal heart, the "fight-or-flight" response activates the SNS. This, in turn, stimulates a β-adrenergic receptor signaling pathway in the myocyte that increases phosphorylation of three key components of E-C coupling: the voltage-gated Ca^{2+} channel (VGCC), the SR Ca^{2+} release channel (RYR2), and the Ca^{2+} uptake pathway (phosphorylation of phospholamban reduces inhibition of the Ca^{2+}-ATPase SERCA2a), ultimately resulting in increased contractility.[380] In the low-CO failing heart, the SNS is chronically activated. In this hyperadrenergically stimulated heart, excitation contraction coupling (ECC) becomes maladaptive because of "leaky" Ca^{2+} from the SR. This "leaky" Ca^{2+} is due to protein kinase A (PKA)–hyperphosphorylated RyR2 channels that cause a diastolic SR Ca^{2+} leak that conspires with reduced SERCA2a-mediated SR Ca^{2+} uptake (due, in part, to PKA-hypophosphorylated phospholamban that inhibits SERCA2a) to deplete SR Ca^{2+} and contribute to contractile dysfunction of cardiac muscle[381,382] (Figure 10-25). Depletion of SR Ca^{2+} stores explains, in part, the reduced contractility of failing cardiac muscle. The "leaky" Ca^{2+} also may explain the predisposition to ventricular arrhythmias thought to be initiated by delayed afterdepolarizations.[383] In brief, the cardiac RyR has a large cytoplasmic structure that serves as a scaffold for modulatory proteins that regulate the function of the channel. PKA phosphorylation of RyR2 dissociates the regulatory protein FKBP 12.6 and regulates the open probability of the channel. In failing hearts, RyR2 is PKA-hyperphosphorylated, resulting in defective channel function because of increased sensitivity of Ca^{2+}-induced activation. Interestingly, studies in animal models of HF show that chronic β-blockade may reverse the PKA hyperphosphorylated state and restore the structure and function of the RYR2 Ca^{2+} release channel.[384,385] Thus, another potential benefit of β-adrenergic receptor blockade in the failing heart may be normalization of E-C coupling, potentially reducing the propensity for arrhythmias.

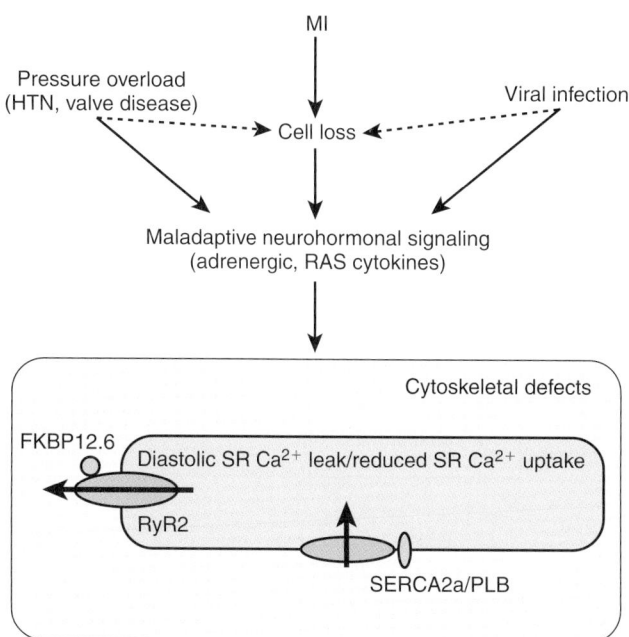

Figure 10-25 Remodeling of extracellular matrix (matrix metalloproteinases [MMPs] and tissue inhibitor of metalloproteinases [TIMPs]). MI, myocardial infarction; RAS, renin-angiotensin system; SR, sarcoplasmic reticulum. (*Redrawn from Marks AR: A guide for the perplexed: Towards an understanding of the molecular basis of heart failure. Circulation 107:1456, 2003.*)

An evolving concept in the pathophysiology of HF also relates to the negative inotropic action of catecholamines and, specifically, the role of β_3-adrenoreceptors. The failing heart is resistant to exogenous inotropic stimulation compared with hearts that are not failing. This has been attributed to a downregulation of β_1- and β_2-adrenoreceptors secondary to a hyperadrenergic state.[386,387] However, β_3-adrenoreceptors have been identified in the failing and nonfailing hearts of humans and other mammalian species.[388-390] Unlike the case for β_1- and β_2-adrenoreceptors, β_3-adrenoreceptors are upregulated in HF.[390-392] β_3-Activation decreases contractility. In contrast with the G_s-protein–coupled adenylyl cyclase activation and cAMP-dependent pathway of the β_1- and β_2-adrenoreceptors, the negative inotropy that results from stimulation of β_3-adrenoreceptors appears to be due to activation of an NO pathway and an increased intracellular cGMP.[393] However, an understanding of the role of β_3 receptors in the treatment and pathophysiology of HF will await the arrival of specific β_3-adrenoceptor antagonists.

Clinical Evidence

The use of β-blockers in patients with HF initially was accepted with skepticism related to the perceived risk for decompensation from transient negative inotropic effects. However, data from both human and animal studies have shown that β-blockers improve energetics and ventricular function, and reverse pathologic chamber remodeling. Although this beneficial biologic process takes 3 months or more to manifest (Figure 10-26), it translates into improved outcomes (reduced deaths and hospitalizations) in patients with HF. The available randomized trials show that metoprolol CR/XL, bisoprolol, and carvedilol (in conjunction with ACE inhibitors) reduce morbidity (hospitalizations) in symptomatic, stage C and D (not in cardiogenic shock) HF patients (NYHA Class II-IV)[328,329,394,395] (Table 10-19). Although β-blocker therapy is recommended for asymptomatic HF patients (stages A and B), evidence from randomized trials is still lacking.[322]

β-Blockers are classified as being first-, second-, or third-generation drugs based on specific pharmacologic properties. First-generation agents, such as propranolol and timolol, block both β_1- and β_2-adrenoreceptors, are considered nonselective, and have no ancillary

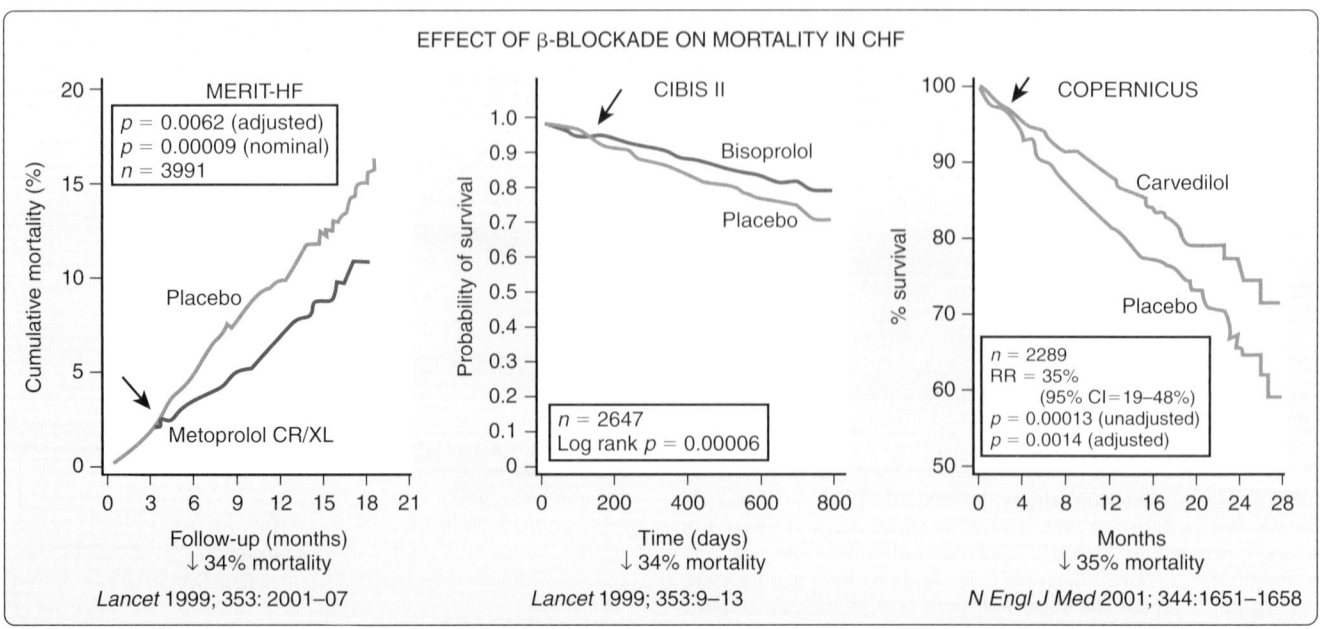

Figure 10-26 Kaplan–Meier analysis of the probability of survival among patients in the placebo and β-blocker groups in the Cardiac Insufficiency Bisoprolol Study II (CIBIS II), Metoprolol CR/XL Randomised Intervention Trial in Congestive Heart Failure (MERIT-HF), and Carvedilol Prospective Randomized Cumulative Survival (COPERNICUS) trials. *Arrows* denote 3-month lag phase of β-blocker benefit. CI, confidence interval; RR, relative risk. *(From Mann DL:* Heart failure: A companion to Braunwald's heart disease. *Philadelphia: Saunders, 2004.)*

TABLE 10-19	Large-Scale Placebo-Controlled Mortality Trials of β-Blockade in Heart Failure						
						Effect on All Causes	
Trial	*Agent*	*HF Severity*	*Patients* (n)	*Target Dose (mg)*		*Mortality*	*Hospitalization*
US Carvedilol	Carvedilol	NYHA II-III	1094	6.25–50 bid		↓ 65%	↓ 27%
CIBIS-II	Bisoprolol	EF ≤ 35; NYHA Class III-IV	2647	10 qd		↓ 34%	↓ 20%
MERIT-HF	Metoprolol CR/XL	EF ≤ 40; NYHA Class II-IV	3991	200 qd		↓ 34%	↓ 18%
BEST	Bucindolol	EF ≤ 35; NYHA Class III-IV	2708	50–100 bid		NS	↓ 8%
COPERNICUS	Carvedilol	EF ≤ 25; NYHA Class IV	2289	25 bid		↓ 35%	↓ 20%

BEST, Beta Blocker Evaluation of Survival Trial; CIBIS-II, Cardiac Insufficiency Bisoprolol Study II; COPERNICUS, Carvedilol Prospective Randomized Cumulative Survival; EF, ejection fraction; HF, heart failure; MERIT-HF, Metoprolol CR/XL Randomized Intervention Trial in Congestive Heart Failure; NS, not significant; NYHA, New York Heart Association; US, United States.

properties. Second-generation agents, such as metoprolol, bisoprolol, and atenolol, are specific for the β_1-adrenoreceptor subtype but lack additional mechanisms of cardiovascular activity. Third-generation agents, such as bucindolol, carvedilol, and labetalol, block both β_1- and β_2-adrenoreceptors, as well as possessing vasodilatory and other ancillary properties. Specifically, labetalol and carvedilol produce vasodilation by β_1-adrenoreceptor antagonism, whereas bucindolol produces mild vasodilation through a cGMP-mediated mechanism. Carvedilol increases insulin sensitivity,[396] possesses antioxidant effects,[397] and has β_3-adrenoreceptor selectivity.[398,399] Although it is not entirely clear whether these ancillary properties of the third-generation β-blockers translate into better outcomes as opposed to the second-generation agents, recent findings from the Carvedilol or Metoprolol European Trial (COMET) suggest that the beneficial effect from β-blockers is not a "drug-class" effect. The study compared carvedilol (25 mg twice a day) with metoprolol tartrate (50 mg twice a day) in symptomatic patients with EF ≤ 35% for 58 months and demonstrated that carvedilol reduced the risk for death significantly more than metoprolol tartrate (all-cause mortality risk reduction: 17%, $P = 0.0017$; cardiovascular death risk reduction: 20%, $P = 0.00004$).[400] Specifically, the superiority of carvedilol over metoprolol may reflect the importance of carvedilol's ancillary effects and/or pharmacodynamic (half-life) differences.[401] Findings from the BEST (Beta Blocker Evaluation of Survival Trial) confirm that not efit from carvedilol might not be a β_2-antagonistic effect, because there was no improvement with bucindolol compared with placebo.[395] Whether the selective β_1-specific agents bisoprolol and metoprolol CR/XL exert similar clinical benefits to carvedilol will require additional study. Nonetheless, based on the results of COMET, carvedilol is preferred to conventional metoprolol, not metoprolol CR/XL, for HF treatment. Interestingly, a recent metaregression analysis of β-blocker HF trials demonstrates that the magnitude of survival benefit seen with β-blockers is statistically significantly associated with the magnitude of HR reduction achieved but not the dosage of β-blocker administered. However, until HF trials randomly assign participants who receive β-blockers to different target HRs, an optimal HR (and thus target HR reduction) is unknown.[402]

Clinical Practice

Current evidence suggests that β-blockers should be given to all HF patients with reduced EF (EF < 0.40) who are stabilized on oral medications including ACE inhibitors and diuretics, unless there is a contraindication. This recommendation is endorsed by the ACC/AHA[322] and the European Society of Cardiology.[403] Specifically, long-term β-blockade is advocated in patients with HF in stages B to D in addition to ACE inhibition to limit disease progression and reduce mortality. Patients with ongoing decompensation (e.g., requiring IV inotropic or vasodilator therapy), overt fluid retention, or symptomatic hypotension should not receive β-blockers. There is no apparent decline in safety or efficacy when β-blockers are given to diabetics with HF. The long-term benefit of β-blocker therapy in patients with coexisting chronic obstructive pulmonary disease is uncertain, because these patients have been excluded from the major clinical trials.

The three agents with clinical trial evidence for improved morbidity and mortality in patients with HF are carvedilol, metoprolol CR/XL, and bisoprolol. Starting doses of β-blockers should be small to minimize worsening of HF symptoms, hypotension, and bradycardia. The dose should be doubled every 1 to 2 weeks, as tolerated, until target doses shown to be effective in large trials are achieved (Table 10-20). Although it is recommended that β-blocker therapy be continued indefinitely in patients with HF, if it is to be electively stopped, a slow down-titration is preferred. Acute withdrawal of β-blocker therapy in the face of high adrenergic tone may result in sudden cardiac death.[404] The adverse effects of β-blocker therapy include fatigue, dizziness, hypotension, and bradycardia. Because the absolute risk for adverse events is small compared with the overall risk reduction of cardiovascular death, few patients have been withdrawn from β-blocker therapy.[405] A practical guide to the use of β-blockers in patients with HF has been reported by McMurray et al[406]

Hydralazine-Isosorbide Dinitrate

Combination vasodilator therapy, hydralazine and isosorbide dinitrate, also has the potential to interfere with the mechanisms responsible for the progression of HF, particularly those that involve oxidative stress.[407] In addition to biochemical and molecular benefits, this isosorbide/hydralazine combination reduces preload and afterload, decreases mitral regurgitation, improves exercise capacity, increases left ventricular ejection fraction (LVEF), and prolongs survival in select HF populations.[408]

Clinical Evidence

Three major clinical studies have examined the effects of combination therapy with hydralazine and nitrates in the management of HF. In the first Vasodilator-Heart Failure Trial (V-HeFT I), combination vasodilator therapy with hydralazine and isosorbide dinitrate given to male patients with mild-to-severe HF improved survival compared with the ACE-I, prazosin, or placebo.[409] However, in V-HeFTII, enalapril had a major benefit on survival in NYHA Class II-III patients compared with the combination vasodilator therapy.[342] Because subanalyses performed on these studies showed that hydralazine-isosorbide dinitrate had a marked risk reduction in patients of black race,[410] the African-Americans Heart Failure (AheFT) was designed to prospectively examine the efficacy of this vasodilator combination. The AheFT randomized 1040 self-described African-Americans with HF and an abnormal LVEF (only 23% with ischemic heart disease) treated with diuretics, ACE inhibitors, and β-blockers to isosorbide dinitrate, 40 mg three time daily, plus hydralazine, 75 mg three times daily, or to placebo.[411] Because a significant reduction in mortality rate was observed in isosorbide dinitrate plus hydralazine–treated patients compared with placebo treatment (6% vs. 10%, respectively; HR, 0.52; $P = 0.02$), the study was terminated early and ACC/AHA recommendations were initiated.[411]

Clinical Practice

The combination of hydralazine and isosorbide dinitrate should be administered (Class I) to improve outcomes for patients self-described as African-American, with moderate-to-severe symptoms on optimal therapy with ACE inhibitors, β-blockers, and diuretics.[322] The benefit is presumed to be related to an increase in NO bioavailability. The addition of this combination vasodilator therapy is thought to be reasonable (Class IIa recommendation) in other stage C patients with HF with reduced LVEF who have persistent symptoms despite optimal medical therapy with ACE inhibitors and β-blockers. Whether hydralazine and isosorbide dinitrate have a significant benefit in those symptomatic patients with HF who are intolerant to ACE inhibitors, however, requires additional study (Class IIB recommendation).[322] The initial dosage of oral isosorbide dinitrate is 10 mg three times daily, with subsequent titration up to a maximum dosage of 40 mg three times daily. Nitrates should be given no more than three times daily, with daily nitrate washout intervals of 12 hours to prevent nitrate tolerance from developing. The initial dosage of oral hydralazine in patients with HF is 10 to 25 mg three times daily, with subsequent titration up to a maximum dose of 100 mg three times daily. Nonetheless, compliance with this regimen generally has been poor because of the large number of tablets required and the high incidence of adverse effects, including headache and dizziness.

Adjunctive Drugs

In addition to ACE inhibitors and β-blockers, diuretics and digoxin are often prescribed for patients with LV systolic dysfunction and symptomatic HF.

Diuretics

For most patients, volume status should be optimized before introduction of β-blockers and ACE inhibitors. Patients with pulmonary congestion often will require a loop diuretic in addition to standard therapy. Diuretics relieve dyspnea, decrease heart size and wall stress, and correct hyponatremia of volume overload. However, overly aggressive and especially unmonitored diuretic therapy can lead to metabolic abnormalities, intravascular depletion, hypotension, and neurohormonal activation. Loop diuretics inhibit tubular reabsorption of sodium along the ascending limb of the loop of Henle. Furosemide also reduces preload by increasing vascular capacity. Diuretics continue to have a role in the management of chronic HF, now generally added to ACE inhibitors, β-blockers, and aldosterone antagonists. However, no randomized, controlled trial has shown a survival benefit from diuretics in HF. Indeed, rates of hospitalization or death from worsening HF were significantly greater in HF patients receiving diuretics (other than aldosterone antagonists) than in those not receiving diuretics (relative risk, 1.31; 95% confidence interval, 1.09 to 1.57) in a large post hoc review of data from SOLVD.[412] Dosing recommendations and kinetic data for the commonly used loop diuretics are provided in Table 10-21. Common adverse effects of loop diuretics include electrolyte depletion (Na^+, K^+, Mg^{2+}, Ca^{2+}, Cl^-), prolonged action of nondepolarizing muscle relaxants, hyperglycemia, and insulin resistance. Less common adverse effects include skin rash, hyperuricemia, and ototoxicity.

Digoxin

Digoxin continues to be useful for patients with symptomatic HF and LV systolic dysfunction despite receiving ACE inhibitor, β-blocker, and diuretic therapy. Digoxin is the only positive inotropic drug approved for the management of chronic HF. Its indirect mechanism of positive inotropy begins with inhibition of the myocardial sarcolemmal Na^+/K^+-ATPase, resulting in increased intracellular Na^+. This, in turn, prompts the Na^+/Ca^{2+} exchanger to extrude Na^+ from the cell, increasing intracellular $[Ca^{2+}]$. The increased Ca^{2+} now available to the contractile proteins increases contractile function.[413] Besides its inotropic effects, digoxin has important vagotonic and sympatholytic effects.

TABLE 10-20	β-Blockers Proven Effective in Heart Failure		
Agent	*Receptor Selectivity*	*Start Dose (mg)*	*Target Dose (mg)*
Metoprolol CR/XL	β₁	12.5 qd	200 qd
Bisoprolol	β₁	1.25 qd	5–10 qd
Carvedilol	β₁ β₂≫β; α₂	3.125 qd	25–50 qd

TABLE 10-21 Loop Diuretics						
Drug	Equivalent Doses	Initial Dose	Maximal Dose	Onset (IV)	Diuresis Peak	Duration
Furosemide	40 mg	10–40 mg/day	240 mg twice a day	10–20 min	90 min	4–5 hr
Bumetanide	1 mg	0.5–1.0 mg/day	10 mg/day	Within 10 min	75–95 min	4–5 hr
Torsemide	20 mg	50 mg/day	200 mg twice a day	10 min	60 min	6–8 hr
Ethacrynic acid	25 mg	100 mg twice a day	100 mg twice a day	10–20 min	90 min	4–5 hr

The inhibition of Na^+/K^+-ATPase in the kidney also decreases sodium reabsorption in the renal tubules.[322] In atrial fibrillation (AF), digoxin slows the rate of conduction at the AV node. In patients with HF, it reduces sympathetic efferent nerve activity to the heart and peripheral circulation through direct effects on the carotid sinus baroreceptors.[414] Digoxin increases HR variability, an additional beneficial action on autonomic function in the patient with HF.[415] Although these properties are beneficial in controlling the ventricular rate in AF, digoxin has only a narrow therapeutic/toxicity ratio. Digoxin toxicity is dose dependent and modified by concurrent medications (nonpotassium-sparing diuretics) or conditions (renal insufficiency, myocardial ischemia). Ventricular arrhythmias consequent to digoxin toxicity may be caused by calcium-dependent afterpotentials. In patients with intoxication and life-threatening arrhythmias, purified antidigoxin FAB fragments from digoxin-specific antisera provide a specific antidote.[413]

The efficacy of digoxin for symptomatic HF was shown in randomized, controlled trials. The Digitalis Investigators Group (DIG) trial, enrolling more than 6500 patients with an average follow-up of 37 months, showed that digoxin reduced the incidence of HF exacerbations. Although the study showed no difference in survival in patients with EF less than 45% receiving either digoxin or placebo, the combined end point of death or hospitalization for HF was significantly reduced in patients who received digoxin (27% vs. 35%; relative risk, 0.72; 95% confidence interval, 0.66 to 0.79).[371] However, this study showed a greater incidence of suspected digoxin toxicity in the treatment group. Efficacy of digoxin in patients with mildly symptomatic HF was shown in pooled results from the Prospective Randomized Study of Ventricular Function (PROVED) and the Randomized Assessment of Digoxin and Inhibitors of Angiotensin-Converting Enzyme (RADIANCE) trials. Patients randomized to digoxin withdrawal had an increased likelihood of treatment failure compared with those who continued to receive digoxin, suggesting that patients with LV systolic dysfunction benefit from digoxin (or, at least, do *not* benefit from digoxin withdrawal), even when they have only mild symptoms.[416,417] Taken together with its narrow therapeutic window, digoxin is deemed reasonable to add to patients with HF with reduced EF who remain symptomatic despite optimal therapy (Class IIa recommendation). Ideally, serum digoxin concentration should remain between 0.7 and 1.1 ng/ml. In the elderly patient with renal insufficiency, severe conduction abnormalities, or acute coronary syndromes, even a low dose of 0.125 mg/day should be used with extra caution.

Other Pharmacologic Therapies for Chronic Heart Failure Management

Vasopressin Receptor Antagonists

Arginine vasopressin has been elucidated as one of the mediators involved in the progression of HF. Patients with HF have greater levels of arginine vasopressin than control subjects, and this has been shown to be a marker of increased cardiac-related mortality.[418] The effects of arginine vasopressin include vasoconstriction via the V1 receptor and antidiuresis via the V2 receptor in the kidney. The water retention that occurs in chronic HF because of the activation of the RAS currently is treated with diuretics. However, diuretics are associated with numerous adverse effects (electrolyte imbalance, renal insufficiency, and activation of the RAS). Vasopressin receptor antagonists, because of their ability to decrease water retention without activating the RAS, currently are being investigated for use in patients with HF.

Studies performed on patients with stage C HF comparing tolvaptan with placebo (e.g., EVEREST and ECLIPSE) have demonstrated its ability to decrease water retention, correct hyponatremia, improve patient-assessed clinical status, and decrease PCWP without causing renal injury. Vasopressin-receptor antagonists ultimately may come to replace the use of diuretics in patients with HF. However, further studies are necessary to determine whether this class of medication can produce an improvement in outcomes in patients with HF.

Anticytokines

In addition to the renin-angiotensin-aldosterone system and the SNS, an increasing number of other vasoactive mediators and growth factors have been implicated in the progression of HF. Production of inflammatory cytokines (including tumor necrosis factor-α and interleukin-6) is increased in patients with HF, and increased blood concentrations of these cytokines have been associated with poor short-term and long-term prognoses.[419] The value of anti–tumor necrosis factor-α therapy with etanercept, a tumor necrosis factor-α receptor fusion protein, has been studied in two trials: RENAISSANCE (Randomized Etanercept North American Strategy to Study Antagonism of Cytokines) and RECOVER (Research into Etanercept: Cytokine Antagonism in Ventricular Dysfunction), and in the combined analysis, RENEWAL (Randomized Etanercept Worldwide Evaluation). However, the trials were terminated prematurely after an interim data analysis showing lack of benefit. Etanercept had no effect on clinical status and had no effect on the death or HF hospitalization end points.[420] Accordingly, inhibition of anti-proinflammatory cytokines remains only a potential therapy for HF.

Endothelin-Receptor Antagonists

The endothelin system also may contribute to the progression of HF. Plasma levels of endothelin-1 (ET-1) are increased in patients with HF.[421] ET-1 produces vasoconstriction of the systemic, renal, pulmonary, and coronary vasculature, remodeling of the myocardium (including myocardial and vascular fibrosis), and neurohormonal activation, and has proarrhythmic and negative inotropic effects. Once the central role of endothelin in pathogenesis and beneficial effect of endothelin antagonists in treating experimental HF were defined, clinical studies with endothelin antagonists began.[422,423] To date, the clinical efficacy of endothelin receptor-antagonists (e.g., bosentan, enrasentan, and darusentan) have been investigated in four clinical trials: REACH-1, ENCOR, Endothelin Antagonist Bosentan for Lowering Cardiac Events in Heart Failure (ENABLE), and EARTH.[424–426] However, in none of these trials was there a significant difference between endothelin-receptor antagonists and placebo with regard to clinical status, all-cause mortality, or HF-related hospitalizations.

Vasopeptidase Inhibitors

In opposition to the endogenous vasoconstrictor systems (Ang II, the adrenergic system, ET-1, vasopressin, and aldosterone) are the endogenous vasodilator systems, including NO, endothelium-derived hyperpolarizing factor, prostaglandins, adrenomedullin, and natriuretic peptides. These vasodilating mediators not only reduce BP and improve sodium and water excretion, they reduce growth and fibrosis, inhibit coagulation, and reduce inflammation. However, in HF, there is an imbalance that favors vasoconstriction. Accordingly, the concept of neutral endopeptidase inhibition (the major enzymatic pathway for degradation of natriuretic peptides) for the treatment of chronic HF led to two large-scale, randomized, controlled trials, OCTAVE and Omapatrilat Versus Enalapril Randomized Trial of Utility in Reducing Events (OVERTURE), that compared the use of omapatrilat with ACE inhibition.[427,428] Although there was no statistically significant advantage with omapatrilat regarding total mortality, the secondary end point of cardiovascular death or HF hospitalizations was reduced in the omapatrilat group (hazard ratio, 0.91; 95% confidence interval, 0.82 to 0.98; $P = 0.012$). Concerns regarding the side-effect profile of omapatrilat (e.g., angioedema), however, will limit its use in the armamentarium of HF treatment.

Nonpharmacologic Therapy

In addition to the beneficial effects of the evidenced-based pharmacologic therapy for the management of HF, the use of cardiac resynchronization therapy has a Class Ia recommendation in patients with stage C HF.[322] In the Comparison of Medical Therapy, Pacing, and Defibrillation in Heart Failure (COMPANION) trial, cardiac resynchronization therapy with a pacemaker combined with an implantable defibrillator significantly decreased the likelihood of death or hospitalization for HF when compared with conventional pharmacologic therapy[429,430] (see Chapters 4, 13, and 25). Included in the guidelines for resynchronization therapy is the recommendation for implantable cardioverter-defibrillators for primary prevention to reduce mortality by a reduction in cardiac sudden death in patients with ischemic and nonischemic heart disease who are at least 40 days after MI, have an LVEF ≤ 35% with NYHA functional Class II-III symptoms while undergoing optimal medical therapy, and have reasonable expectation of survival (>1 year).[322]

Stem cell therapy is another potential treatment of HF (see Chapter 27). Stem cell therapy has shown promise in the treatment for ischemic heart disease both in the laboratory and in small clinical studies.[431,432] Autologous bone marrow and peripheral blood stem cells transplanted in patients with acute MI improved cardiac function.[433,434] Although fewer randomized trials of transplants of blood- or bone marrow–derived stem cells have been performed in the setting of chronic CAD and chronic HF,[435–438] the results show promise, including improvements in regional and global LV function, perfusion, and relief of angina pectoris.[439,440]

Pharmacologic Treatment of Diastolic Heart Failure

Abnormal diastolic ventricular function is a common cause of clinical HF. The incidence of HF with a normal or near-normal EF (HFNEF) (≥40%) includes up to 50% of the general HF population.[441] The risk for DHF increases with age, approaching 50% in patients older than 70 years.[442] DHF also is more common in female individuals and patients with hypertension or diabetes mellitus. The prognosis, in terms of morbidity and mortality, associated with the diagnosis of DHF is similar to that of systolic HF.[443–446] In the chronic state, abnormal increases in systolic BP and afterload may contribute to an impaired Frank–Starling response and the resultant symptoms of exercise intolerance. Because this syndrome carries substantial morbidity (exercise intolerance, hospital admissions) and mortality, and results in substantial annual health care expenditures, pharmacotherapy of DHF represents one of the current frontiers of clinical cardiovascular medicine.

In contrast with the large, randomized trials that have led to the treatment guidelines for systolic HF, the randomized, double-blind, placebo-controlled, multicenter trials performed in patients with DHF or HFNEF to date have not shown a survival benefit (Table 10-22). Consequently, the guidelines are based on clinical experience, small clinical studies, and an understanding of the pathophysiologic mechanisms. The general approach to treating DHF has three main components. First, treatment should reduce symptoms, primarily by reducing pulmonary venous pressure during rest and exercise

TABLE 10-22	Completed Clinical End-Point Trials of Heart Failure with Normal Ejection Fraction (HFNEF) or Heart Failure with Mildly Reduced Ejection Fraction	
Study Drug Primary End Point	*Inclusion Criteria*	*Results*
Calcium Channel Blockers		
N = 20 men, FU = 2 × 2 wk crossover, randomized, double blind (Setaro et al 1990)		
Verapamil PE not defined	EF > 45%, clinical heart failure > 3 mo, abnormal peak filling rate	Improvement in heart failure score ($P < .01$) and exercise duration (placebo-subtracted net effect +15%, $P < .01$). Increase in peak filling rate relative to baseline value (24%) not different from placebo because of suspected carryover effect
N = 15, FU = 2 × 3 mo crossover, randomized, double blind (Hung et al 2002)		
Verapamil PE not defined	EF > 50%, NYHA II/III, age ≥ 60 yr, Doppler echo criteria of abnormal relaxation or pseudonormalization	Improvement in heart failure score ($P < .05$), exercise duration (placebo-subtracted net effect +12%, $P < .05$) and Doppler echo criteria of diastolic function
β-Blockers		
N = 158, FU = 32 mo, randomized, open label (Aronow et al 1997)		
Propranolol PE not defined	EF ≥ 40%, NYHA II-III, age ≥ 62 yr, prior myocardial infarction, diuretics and ACEIs	Reduction of ACM (RRR 26%, $P = .007$) and ACM or NFMI (RRR 28%, $P = .002$). After 1 y greater increase in LVEF ($P < .0001$) and greater reduction in LV mass ($P = .0001$) with propranolol
SWEDIC (Bergström et al 2004), N = 97, FU = 6 mo, randomized, double blind		
Carvedilol Doppler diastolic function score	EF > 45%, heart failure signs ± symptoms, Doppler echo evidence of diastolic dysfunction	PE: no effect. SE: carvedilol increased E/A ratio ($P = .046$) but also increased left atrial size ($P < .05$) and BNP ($P < .05$). No difference in ACM, ACH, CVH, symptoms. Trend toward deterioration of NYHA class with carvedilol
SENIORS subset with EF > 35% (Flather et al 2005), N = 752, FU = 21 mo, randomized, double blind		
Nebivolol ACM or CVH	EF > 35%, age ≥ 70 yr, congestive heart failure hospitalization in prior 12 mo	PE reduction by 18% (95% CI, was 0.63–1.05). In the SENIORS echocardiographic substudy (Ghio et al 2006), nebivolol had no significant effect on LV volumes, EF, left atrial dimension, and function
N = 443, FU = 25 mo, prospective observational (Dobre et al 2007)		
β-Blockers ACM	EF ≥ 40%, heart failure hospitalization	PE reduction by 43% (95% CI, was 0.37–0.88) in multivariate analysis if β-blocker was given at hospital discharge

(Continued)

TABLE 10-22	Completed Clinical End-Point Trials of Heart Failure with Normal Ejection Fraction or Heart Failure with Mildly Reduced Ejection Fraction—Cont'd		
Study Drug Primary End Point	*Inclusion Criteria*		*Results*
Digitalis Glycosides			
DIG-PEF (Ahmed et al 2006), N = 988, FU = 37 mo, randomized double blind			
Digoxin HFH or HFM	EF > 45%, sinus rhythm, current or past clinical symptoms, signs or radiologic evidence of HF		PE: no effect. SE: no effect on ACM, HFM, CVM, CVM or HFH, CVH. Trend toward decreased HFH ($P = .094$) balanced by trend toward increase in hospitalizations for unstable angina ($P = .061$)
ACEIs			
N = 21, FU = 3 mo, randomized, open label (Aronow and Kronzon 1993)			
Enalapril PE not defined	EF > 50%, NYHA III, prior myocardial infarction, sinus rhythm, diuretics		Significant improvements for (placebo-subtracted net effects) NYHA class (−0.5 classes), cardiothoracic ratio (−0.02), exercise time (+19%), *E/A* ratio (+0.1), LV mass (−12%)
N = 416, FU = 2.6 yr, prospective observational (Grigorian Shamagian et al 2006)			
ACEIs PE not defined	EF ≥ 50%, hospitalized for heart failure		Significant prolongation of survival with the use of ACEIs (+1.57 yr, RRR 37%, $P = .012$ in multivariate analysis)
PEP-CHF (Cleland et al 2006), N = 846, FU = 26.2 mo, randomized, double blind			
Perindopril ACM or HFRH	EF ≥ 40%, age ≥ 70 yr, diuretics, three of nine clinical and two of four echo criteria, cardiovascular hospitalization in prior 6 mo		Generally, no effects on PE or SE for the entire duration of the study. One-year analysis: trend toward PE reduction (RRR 31%, $P = .055$), reduction of HFRH (RRR 37%, $P = .033$), CVM, or HFH (RRR 38%, $P = .018$), but no reduction in WHFE. After 1 yr improvement of NYHA class ($P = .03$) and 6-min walk distance (+14 m, $P = .011$)
Angiotensin II Receptor Antagonists			
CHARM-Preserved (Yusuf et al 2003), N = 3023, FU = 36.6 mo, randomized, double blind			
Candesartan CVM or HFH	EF > 40%, NYHA II-IV, prior cardiac hospitalization		PE: trend favoring candesartan (RRR, 11%, $P = .118$; in covariate-adjusted analysis RRR, 14%, $P = .051$). SE: no effect on CVM. HFH: RRR 15% ($P = .072$; covariate-adjusted RRR, 16%, $P = .047$). Pronounced effect in investigator reported end points: RRR 15% ($P = .028$) for the PE, RRR 18% ($P = .017$) for HFH
I-PRESERVE (Massie et al 2008), N = 4128, FU = 49.5 mo, randomized, double blind			
Irbesartan ACM or CVH	EF ≥ 45%, age ≥ 60 yr, NYHA II-IV, heart failure hospitalization in prior 6 mo or ongoing NYHA III/IV functional class		PE: no effect (RR for irbesartan, 0.95, with 95% CI, 0.86–1.05). SE: no effect on ACM (RR, 1.00; 95% CI, 0.88–1.14), CVH (RR, 0.95; 95% CI, 0.85–1.08), HFH (RR, 0.95; 95% CI, 0.81–1.10), heart failure-related quality of life ($P = .85$), change in NT-proBNP at 6 mo ($P = .14$)
Statins			
N = 137, FU = 21 mo, prospective observational (Fukuta et al 2005)			
Statins PE not defined	EF ≥ 50%, heart failure signs ± symptoms		Significant survival benefit with statin therapy (RRR 80%; $P = .005$ in multivariate analysis)
Others			
Hong Kong DHF Study (Yip et al 2008), N = 150, FU = 1 yr randomized, open label			
Diuretics alone plus irbesartan vs. ramipril QoL, tissue Doppler	EF > 45%, NYHA II-IV requiring diuretics, pulmonary venous congestion on chest x-ray		Diuretics significantly improved QoL with no significant additional effect of irbesartan or ramipril. Significant increase in early diastolic mitral annulus velocity and significant fall in NT-proBNP concentrations only with diuretics plus irbesartan or ramipril. No significant change in 6-min walk distance with either therapy

N indicates number of patients enrolled; FU, average follow-up time; PE, primary end point; SE, secondary end point. ACM/HFM/CVM, all-cause/heart failure/cardiovascular mortality; ACH/HFH/CVH, all-cause/heart failure/cardiovascular hospitalizations; HFRF, heart failure–related hospitalizations; WHFE, worsening heart failure events; NFMI, nonfatal myocardial infarction; RR, relative risk; RRR, relative risk reduction; NYHA, New York Heart Association functional class; *E/A*, ratio of peak early to peak late mitral valve blood flow velocity; QoL, quality of life; SWEDIC, Swedish Doppler-echocardiographic study; CI, confidence interval; SENIORS, Study of the Effects of Nebivolol Intervention on Outcomes and Rehospitalisation in Seniors with Heart Failure; DIG-PEF, Digitalis Investigation Group—Preserved Ejection Fraction; HF, heart failure; PEP-CHF, The perindopril in elderly people with chronic heart failure study; CHARM, Candesartan in Heart failure: Assessment of Reduction in Morality and morbidity; I-PRESERVE, The irbesartan in heart failure with preserved systolic function trial.

Reprinted from Kindermann M, Reil J-C, Pieske B, et al: Heart failure with normal left ventricular ejection fraction: What is the evidence? *Trends Cardiovasc Med* 18:280–292, 2008; Table 2A, by permission.

by carefully reducing LV volume, and maintaining AV synchrony or tachycardia control. Second, treatment should target the underlying diseases that cause DHF. Specifically, ventricular remodeling (e.g., myocardial hypertrophy and fibrosis) should be reversed by controlling hypertension, replacing stenotic aortic valves, treating ischemia, controlling glycemia in patients with diabetes, and body weight normalization in obese or overweight patients. Third, treatment should target the underlying mechanisms that are altered by the disease processes, mainly neurohormonal activation. Drug treatment of DHF with respect to these three goals is shown in Table 10-22.

Many of the drugs used to treat systolic HF also are used to treat DHF. However, the reason for their use and the doses used may be different for DHF. For instance, in DHF, β-blockers may be used to prevent tachycardia and thereby prolong diastolic filling and reduce left atrial pressure,[447] whereas in systolic HF, β-blockers are used to reverse heart remodeling (e.g., carvedilol). In fact, metoprolol-CR/XL may be a better β-blocker choice than carvedilol for DHF because too low a BP (as a consequence of carvedilol) may be detrimental for the DHF patient. However, because β-blocker therapy for the treatment of DHF has been challenged by recent exercise metabolic testing data indicating that impaired chronotropic response to exercise contributes to observed exercise intolerance,[448] it is less likely to be chosen as a stand-alone treatment for DHF. Similarly, diuretic and NTG doses for DHF are usually much smaller than for systolic HF because the DHF patient is very sensitive to large reductions in preload. Calcium channel blockers are not a part of the armamentarium in systolic HF treatment

TABLE 10-23	Upcoming Clinical End-Point Trials of Heart Failure with Normal Ejection Fraction		
Trial	**Inclusion Criteria**	**Primary End Point**	**N**
Efficacy and safety of Valsartan on exercise tolerance in patients with heart failure Valsartan (active, not recruiting)	DHF	Exercise tolerance	150
TOPCAT Spironolactone (currently recruiting)	EF ≥ 45%, age ≥ 50 yr, at least one heart failure symptom and sign, heart failure hospitalization in prior 12 mo, or elevated natriuretic peptides	CVM Aborted cardiac arrest HFRH	4500
Aldo-DHF Spironolactone (currently recruiting)	EF > 50%, age ≥ 50 yr, NYHA ≥ II, echocardiographic evidence of diastolic dysfunction, peak oxygen uptake ≤ 20 mL/kg per minute	Peak oxygen uptake change in E/E' ratio	420
PIE-II Spironolactone (active, not recruiting)	Age ≥ 60 yr, DHF	Exercise tolerance Quality of life	80
Novel treatment for DHF in women Spironolactone (currently recruiting)	Women, EF ≥ 50%, NYHA II/III, BNP ≥ 62 pg/mL, RR ≤ 155/95 mm Hg. Medication with ACEI or ARB for at least 4 wk	Not specified	?
Aldosterone antagonism in DHF Eplerenone (currently recruiting)	EF ≥ 50%, NYHA II/III, BNP ≥ 62 pg/mL, RR ≤ 155/95 mm Hg. Medication with ACEI or ARB for at least 4 wk	6-min walk distance	48
PREDICT Eplerenone (currently recruiting)	EF ≥ 45%, NYHA ≥ II, echocardiographic evidence of diastolic dysfunction, RR controlled	Not specified	80
ELANDD Nebivolol (currently recruiting)	EF > 45%, age ≥ 40 yr, NYHA II/III or pulmonary venous congestion on chest x-ray, echocardiographic evidence of diastolic dysfunction	6-min walk distance	150
J-DHF β-Blockers (currently recruiting)	EF > 40%, heart failure according to modified Framingham criteria	CVM or HFH	800

N indicates prospective number of enrolled patients; ACM/CVM, all-cause/cardiovascular mortality; HFH/CVH, heart failure/cardiovascular hospitalizations; HFRF, heart failure–related hospitalizations; E/E, ratio of early diastolic transmitral blood flow velocity and early diastolic mitral annular velocity; RR, blood pressure; ACEI, ACE inhibitor; ARB, angiotensin receptor blocker; TOPCAT, Trial of Aldosterone Antagonist Therapy with Adults with Preserved EF Congestive Heart Failure; Aldo-DHF, aldosterone receptor blockade in DHF; PIE-II, Pharmacological Intervention in the Elderly II; PREDICT, Parallel Design Study to Determine the Effectiveness of Inspra Reversing Diastolic Dysfunction, Improving Endothelial Function, and Suppressing Natriuretic Peptides and Collagen Turnover in Patients with DHF; ELANDD, Effects of the Long-Term Administration of Nebivolol on the Clinical Symptoms, Exercise Capacity and LV Function of Patients with Diastolic Dysfunction; J-DHF, Japanese DHF Trial.

Reprinted from Kindermann M, Reil J-C, Pieske B, et al: Heart failure with normal left ventricular ejection fraction: What is the evidence? *Trends Cardiovasc Med* 18:280–292, 2008, Table 2B, by permission.

but *may* be beneficial in DHF through effects on rate and BP control, specifically the long-acting dihydropyridine class of calcium channel blockers. With the exception of rate control in chronic AF, digoxin is not recommended for DHF.

Ongoing clinical trials focus on "mechanism-targeted" therapy for HF patients with preserved systolic function (Table 10-23). Two of the trials (CHARM and I-PRESERVE) examined the effects of treatment with angiotensin-receptor blockade, the PEP-CHF and Hong Kong Diastolic Heart Failure trials examined the effects of ACE-I, the SENIORS trial examined the role of β-blockers, and the MCC-135 trial examined the influence of modulation of calcium homeostasis at the SR and cellular membrane. In the ongoing Treatment of Preserved Cardiac Function Heart Failure with an Aldosterone Antagonist trial (TOPCAT) and Aldosterone in Diastolic Heart Failure (ALDO-DHF) trial, the role of spironolactone is under study, in regard to whether any antifibrotic intervention strategies are sufficient to improve the outcome in patients with DHF. Smaller studies are investigating the effects of physical activity, statins, ivabradine, PDE5 inhibitors, cross-link breaker,[449] pacing, or resynchronization therapeutic options in patients with DHF. Indeed, the beneficial effect of stem cells on diastolic function in patients after MI (B-naturetic peptide Observation Outcome Study [BOOST] trial)[450] will require further study to determine whether its usefulness holds in DHF patients without prior MI.

In 1999, a small trial showed that losartan, an angiotensin-receptor antagonist, improved exercise capacity in patients with DHF.[451] The CHARM-Preserved Trial data indicate that treatment with the angiotensin-receptor antagonist candesartan reduces hospitalization rates but does not alter mortality in patients with DHF.[354] Moreover, the assessment of the angiotensin-receptor blocker, irbesartan, in patients with DHF (I-Preserve trial) did not show a benefit, in part, because patients were already optimally treated with conventional therapies such as ACE-I, spironolactone, and β-adrenergic blockers.[452] In theory, the use of ACE inhibitors should be beneficial for patients with diastolic dysfunction by causing regression of hypertrophy, reduction of systemic BP, and prevention or modification of cardiac remod-

eling. Likewise, aldosterone antagonists have been proposed for use in patients with diastolic dysfunction because of their antifibrotic and antiremodeling effects.[294,298] Preliminary findings from ongoing studies suggest that aldosterone antagonists may improve exercise tolerance and quality of life in patients with DHF.[453] However, until validation from adequately powered, randomized, controlled trials is available, the treatment of chronic DHF remains empiric.

Except in the presence of acute DHF, positive inotropic and chronotropic agents should be avoided because they may worsen diastolic function by increasing contractile force and HR, or by increasing calcium concentrations in diastole. However, in the short-term management of acute diastolic dysfunction or HF (e.g., after cardiopulmonary bypass [CPB]), β-adrenergic agonists (e.g., epinephrine) and PDE inhibitors (e.g., milrinone) enhance calcium sequestration by the SR and thereby promote a more rapid and complete myocardial relaxation between beats.[454,455]

Management of Acute Exacerbations of Chronic Heart Failure

Patients with chronic HF, despite good medical management, may experience episodes of pulmonary edema or other signs of acute volume overload.[456] These patients may require hospitalization for intensive management if diuretics fail to relieve their symptoms. Other patients may experience exacerbations of HF associated with acute myocardial ischemia or infarction, worsening valvular dysfunction, infections (including myocarditis), or failure to maintain an established drug regimen. Fonarow et al[457] described a risk-stratification system for in-hospital mortality in acutely decompensated HF using data from a national registry. Low-, intermediate-, and high-risk patients with mortality rates ranging from 2.1% to 21.9% were identified using blood urea nitrogen, creatinine, and systolic BP on admission. These patients will require all the standard medications, as outlined in previous sections, and also may require infusions of vasodilators or positive inotropic drugs.

Vasodilators

IV vasodilators have long been used to treat the symptoms of low CO in patients with decompensated chronic HF. In general, vasodilators reduce ventricular filling pressures and SVR, while increasing SV and CO. NTG commonly is used for this purpose and has been studied in numerous clinical trials.[456] It is often initially effective at relatively small dosages (20 to 40 μg/min) but frequently requires progressively increasing doses to counteract tachyphylaxis. NTG is associated with dose-dependent arterial hypotension.[458]

Nesiritide

Brain natriuretic peptide (BNP) is a 32-amino acid peptide that is mainly secreted from the cardiac ventricles.[459] In healthy subjects, BNP concentrations in blood increase with age and are greater in female than male subjects. Physiologically, BNP functions as a natriuretic and a diuretic. It also serves as a counter-regulatory hormone to Ang II, norepinephrine, and endothelin by decreasing the synthesis of these agents and by direct vasodilation.

As the clinical severity of HF increases, the concentrations of BNP in blood also increase.[459] As a result, measurements of BNP in blood have been used to evaluate new onset of dyspnea (to distinguish between lung disease and HF). BNP concentrations in blood increase with decreasing LVEF; therefore, measurements of this mediator have been used to estimate prognosis. BNP concentrations decline in response to therapy with ACE inhibitors, Ang II antagonists, and aldosterone antagonists.

In addition, recombinant BNP has been released as a drug (nesiritide), indicated for patients with acute HF and dyspnea with minimal activity. Nesiritide produces arterial and venous dilatation through increasing cGMP. Nesiritide does not increase HR and has no effect on cardiac inotropy. It has a rapid onset of action and a short elimination half-life (15 minutes). In clinical studies, loading doses have ranged from 0.25 to 2 μg/kg, and maintenance doses have ranged from 0.005 to 0.03 μg/kg/min. Studies have shown that nesiritide reduces symptoms of acute decompensated HF similarly to NTG, without development of acute tolerance.[460] Patients receiving nesiritide experienced fewer adverse events than those receiving NTG.[461] However, the mortality rate at 6 months was greater in the patients receiving nesiritide than in the NTG group. Compared with dobutamine, nesiritide was associated with fewer instances of ventricular tachycardia (VT) or cardiac arrest.[462]

In the Acute Decompensated Heart Failure National Registry (ADHERE) registry of more than 65,000 episodes of acute decompensated HF, treatment with either nesiritide or a vasodilator was associated with a 0.59 odds ratio for mortality compared with either milrinone or dobutamine.[463] Recent data, however, suggest that nesiritide may *not* offer a compelling safety advantage but may be associated with an *increased* incidence of adverse side effects, including renal failure and mortality, when administered to patients with acutely decompensated chronic HF.[464,465] These data prompted the U.S. Food and Drug Administration to convene an expert panel that made several recommendations including that nesiritide be used only for hospitalized patients with acute decompensated HF, and that the agent not be used to enhance diuresis or "protect" the kidneys.[466] Indeed, findings from the Acute Study of Clinical Effectiveness of Nesiritide in Decompensated Heart Failure (ASCEND-HF) trial will establish whether nesiritide safely improves acute dyspnea, as well as morbidity and mortality, at 30 days in patients hospitalized for acute decompensated HF.[467]

Inotropes

Positive inotropic drugs, principally dobutamine or milrinone, have long been used to treat decompensated HF, despite the lack of data showing an outcome benefit to their use.[456] In the past, some patients with chronic HF would receive intermittent infusions of positive inotropic drugs as part of their maintenance therapy. Small studies consistently demonstrate improved hemodynamic values and reduced symptoms after administration of these agents to patients with HF. Studies comparing dobutamine with milrinone for advanced decompensated HF showed large differences in drug costs, favoring dobutamine, and only small hemodynamic differences, favoring milrinone.[468]

Nevertheless, placebo-controlled studies suggest that there may be no role whatsoever for discretionary administration of positive inotropes to patients with chronic HF.[469] In this study, 951 hospitalized patients with decompensated chronic HF who did not require IV inotropic support were assigned to receive a 48-hour infusion of either milrinone or saline. Meanwhile, all patients received ACE inhibitors and diuretics as deemed necessary. Total hospital days did not differ between groups; however, those receiving milrinone were significantly more likely to require intervention for hypotension or to have new atrial arrhythmias. A subanalysis of these results found that patients suffering from ischemic cardiomyopathy were particularly subject to adverse events from milrinone (a 42% incidence rate of death or rehospitalization vs. 36% for placebo).[470]

Currently, positive inotropic drug support can be recommended only when there is no alternative. Thus, dobutamine and milrinone continue to be used to treat low CO in decompensated HF, but only in selected patients.

Alternate Therapies

When drug treatment proves unsuccessful, patients with HF may require invasive therapy, including ventricular assist devices, biventricular pacing, CABG with or without surgical remodeling, or even cardiac orthotopic transplantation. These treatment options are beyond the scope of this chapter[471] (see Chapters 4, 13, 18, 19, 23, 25, 26 and 27).

■ Low-Output Syndrome

Acute HF is a frequent concern of the cardiac anesthesiologist, particularly at the time of separation from CPB. The new onset of ventricular dysfunction and a low CO state after aortic clamping and reperfusion are conditions with more pathophysiologic similarity to cardiogenic shock than to chronic HF and are typically treated with positive inotropic drugs, vasopressors (or vasodilators), if needed, and/or mechanical assistance.[472,473] The latter more commonly takes the form of intra-aortic balloon counterpulsation and less commonly includes one of the several available ventricular assist devices (see Chapters 27, 28, 32, and 34).

Causes

Most patients undergoing cardiac surgery with CPB experience a temporary decline in ventricular function, with a recovery to normal function in a period of roughly 24 hours. Thus, pathophysiologic explanations must acknowledge the (usual) temporary nature of the low-output syndrome after CPB. Most likely, this results from one of three processes, all related to inadequate oxygen delivery to the myocardium: acute ischemia, hibernation, or stunning. All three processes would be expected to improve with adequate revascularization and moderate doses of positive inotropic drugs, consistent with the typical progress of the cardiac surgery patient. All three processes would be expected to be more troublesome in patients with preexisting chronic HF, pulmonary hypertension, or arrhythmias.

Risk Factors for the Low-Output Syndrome after Cardiopulmonary Bypass

The need for inotropic drug support after CPB often can be anticipated based on data available in the preoperative medical history, physical examination, and imaging studies. In a series of consecutive patients undergoing elective CABG, it was observed that increasing age, decreasing LVEF, female sex, cardiac enlargement (on the chest radiograph), and prolonged duration of CPB were all associated with an increased likelihood that the patient would be receiving positive inotropic drugs on arrival in the intensive care unit.[474] Similarly, in a study of patients undergoing cardiac valve surgery, it was found that increasing age, reduced LVEF, and the presence of CAD all increased the likelihood that a patient would receive positive inotropic drug support.[475] The lack of a between-sex difference in the likelihood of inotropic drug support after cardiac valve surgery was consistent with there being no between-sex difference in pathophysiology of valve disease, unlike the between-sex difference in pathophysiology of CAD. This latter study also illustrated another important risk factor: practitioner bias. In this study from a single cardiac surgical unit, some anesthesiologists were more likely to administer positive inotropes than others, even after a statistical adjustment for other risk factors. Such differences are even more pronounced when one cardiac surgical unit is compared with another. In a survey of 40 cardiac surgical units participating in a University Health System Consortium benchmarking project of nonemergent coronary bypass surgery, use of positive inotropic drugs ranged almost linearly and continuously from 5% to 100% of patients.

Specific Drugs for Treating the Low-Output Syndrome

Although all positive inotropic drugs increase the strength of contraction in noninfarcted myocardium, mechanisms of action differ. These drugs can be divided into those that increase cAMP (directly or indirectly) for their mechanisms of action and those that do not. The agents that do not depend on cAMP form a diverse group, including cardiac glycosides, calcium salts, calcium sensitizers, and thyroid hormone. In contrast with chronic HF, cardiac glycosides are not used for this indication because of their limited efficacy and narrow margin of safety. Calcium salts continue to be administered for ionized hypocalcemia and hyperkalemia, common occurrences during and after cardiac surgery. Increased $[Ca^{2+}]$ in buffer solutions bathing cardiac muscle in vitro unquestionably increase inotropy. However, despite long-standing contrary opinions, available studies suggest that doses of $CaCl_2$ from 5 to 10 mg/kg do not increase cardiac index in patients recovering from cardiac surgery.[476,477]

Calcium sensitizers, specifically levosimendan, function by binding troponin C in a calcium-dependent fashion. Levosimendan does not increase intracellular Ca concentration and, therefore, does not impair diastolic cardiac function. Peripheral and coronary vasodilatation, because of its effects on ATP-K channels, provides afterload reduction and improved coronary perfusion. These combined effects result in an improvement of myocardial contractility without an increase in myocardial oxygen consumption. Another attractive feature of this relatively new inotropic agent is that its effects are not diminished by β-blockade.[478]

There are conflicting reports regarding the efficacy of levosimendan in patients with acute decompensated chronic HF. There have been four major clinical trials evaluating the ability of levosimendan to decrease mortality in these patients. Only two of these trials (the LIDO study and the RUSSLAN study) have shown a clear decrease in mortality in comparison with a placebo or dobutamine.[478,479] More recent trials, REVIVE II and SURVIVE,[480] have revealed concerning adverse effects of this drug, including hypotension, atrial arrhythmias, and tachycardia. These more recent trials have been questioned because of the concomitant administration of vasodilators and diuretics to its subjects without invasive monitoring to assess volume status, suggesting the possibility that hypovolemia was a contributing factor to their inability to show a clear benefit. Currently, levosimendan is an acceptable choice for patients with acute decompensated HF once hypovolemia, if present, has been corrected. Suggested dosing includes an infusion with or without a loading dose of 12 μg/kg for 10 minutes, followed by 0.005 to 2 μg/kg/min, for no more than 24 hours. Loading doses are not recommended for patients with low normal BP (e.g., systolic BP < 100). Without a loading dose, maximum effect of the drug will occur after 4 hours. Infusions should not continue for longer than 24 hours because of levosimendan's active metabolites, which can accumulate and produce refractory hypotension and tachycardia.

IV thyroid hormone (triiodothyronine [T_3], or liothyronine) has been studied extensively as a positive inotrope in cardiac surgery. There are multiple studies supporting the existence of euthyroid "sick" syndrome

with persistent reduced concentrations of T_3 in blood after cardiac surgery in both children and adults.[476] There are also data suggesting that after ischemia and reperfusion, T_3 increases inotropy faster than and as potently as isoproterenol.[481] Nevertheless, randomized, controlled clinical trials have failed to show efficacy of T_3 after CABG.[482,483]

cAMP-dependent agents are the mainstays of positive inotropic drug therapy after cardiac surgery. There are two main classes of agents: the PDE inhibitors and the β-adrenergic receptor agonists. There are many different PDEs in clinical use around the world, including enoximone, inamrinone, milrinone, olprinone, and piroximone. Comparisons among the agents have failed to demonstrate important hemodynamic differences.[484] Reported differences relate to pharmacokinetics and rare side effects, typically observed with chronic oral administrations during clinical trials. All members of the class produce rapid increases in contractile function and CO, and decreases in SVR. The effect on BP is variable, depending on the pretreatment state of hydration and hemodynamics; nevertheless, the typical response is a small decrease in BP. There is either no effect on HR or a small increase. Inamrinone and milrinone have been shown to be effective, first-line agents in patients with reduced preoperative LV function.[485,486] In one of the few studies in which outcome has been assessed after use of positive inotropic agents, it was confirmed that "prophylactic" use of milrinone in children undergoing correction of congenital heart disease improved outcomes in terms of length of stay and incidence of low-output syndrome.[487] Milrinone, the most commonly used member of the class, is most often dosed at a 50-μg/kg loading dose and 0.5-μg/kg/min maintenance infusion. It often is given in combination with a β-adrenergic receptor agonist.

Among the many β-adrenergic receptor agonists, the agents most often given to patients recovering from cardiac surgery are dopamine, dobutamine, and epinephrine. Dopamine has long been assumed to have dose-defined receptor specificity. At small doses (0.5 to 3 μg/kg/min), it is assumed to have an effect mostly on dopaminergic receptors. At intermediate doses, β-adrenergic effects are said to predominate; and at doses of 10 μg/kg/min or greater, β-adrenergic receptor effects predominate. Nevertheless, the relation between dose and blood concentration is poorly predictable, even in healthy volunteers, as shown by MacGregor et al.[488] This makes it unlikely that the dose–response relation is as consistent as has been described in textbooks. Moreover, dopamine is a relatively weak inotrope that has a predominant effect on HR rather than on SV.[489]

Dobutamine is a selective β-adrenergic receptor agonist. Most studies suggest that it causes less tachycardia and hypotension than isoproterenol.[490,491] It frequently has been compared with dopamine, where dobutamine's greater tendency for pulmonary and systemic vasodilation is evident.[489] Dobutamine has a predominant effect on HR, compared with SV; and as the dose is increased more than 10 μg/kg/min, there are further increases in HR without changes in SV.[492]

Epinephrine is a powerful adrenergic agonist and, like dopamine, demonstrates differing effects depending on the dose. At small doses (10 to 30 ng/kg/min), despite an almost pure β-adrenergic receptor stimulus, there is almost no increase in HR.[477,493] Clinicians have long assumed that epinephrine increases HR more than dobutamine administered at comparable doses. Nevertheless, in patients recovering from cardiac surgery, the opposite is true: Dobutamine increases HR more than epinephrine.[493]

Other β-adrenergic agonists are used in specific circumstances. For example, isoproterenol often is used after cardiac transplantation to exploit its powerful chronotropy and after correction of congenital heart defects to exploit its pulmonary vasodilatory effects.[494] Norepinephrine is exploited to counteract profound vasodilation.[495] Outside of North America, dopexamine, a weak dopaminergic and β-agonist with a pronounced tendency for tachycardia, is sometimes used.[496]

Left Atrial Drug Administration

Based on an appeal to "common sense," clinicians faced with severe cardiac depression in a severely ill patient undergoing cardiac surgery would sometimes administer potentially "vasoconstricting" agents (e.g., epinephrine or norepinephrine) into the left heart circulation (via a left atrial catheter) to avoid adverse effects on the pulmonary vascular resistance. Fullerton et al[497] have confirmed the usefulness of this approach in showing that left atrial administration of epinephrine produces a greater CO and a more reduced PAP than the same dose of epinephrine administered into the right atrium.

Assist Devices

A small fraction of patients undergoing cardiac surgery develop acute HF refractory to drug treatment. For these patients, available options include intra-aortic balloon counterpulsation, extracorporeal membrane oxygenation (or extracorporeal carbon dioxide elimination), and right- or left-heart assist devices either as "destination therapy" or as a bridge to transplantation.[471] (For a more detailed discussion of assist devices, see Chapters 27 and 32.)

▣ Current Clinical Practice

The pharmacotherapy of HF begins with primary prevention of LV dysfunction. Because hypertension and CAD are leading causes of LV dysfunction, adequate treatment of both hypertension and hypercholesterolemia has been endorsed after encouraging results in prevention trials.[260,455,498] Limitation of neurohormonal activation with ACE inhibitors, and possibly β-blockers, should be initiated in diabetic, hypertensive, and hypercholesterolemic patients (AHA/ACC, stage A HF) who are at increased risk for cardiovascular events, despite normal contractile function, to reduce the onset of new HF (HOPE trial). In patients with asymptomatic LV dysfunction (EF, 40%; stage B), treatment with ACE inhibitors and β-blockers can blunt the disease progression. In the symptomatic HF patient with reduced LVEF (stage C), diuretics are titrated to relieve symptoms of pulmonary congestion and peripheral edema, and achieve a euvolemic state (Class I, Level of Evidence C), whereas ACE inhibitors (or angiotensin-receptor antagonists) and β-blockers are recommended (Class I, Level of Evidence A) to blunt disease progression. In African-Americans with stage C HF with reduced LVEF and persistent HF symptoms, despite optimal treatment with ACE inhibitors and β-blockers, the addition of combination hydralazine and isosorbide dinitrate is recommended (Class I, Level of Evidence A). Although digoxin has no effect on patient survival, it may be considered in stage C if the patient remains symptomatic despite adequate doses of ACE inhibitors and diuretics. In general, the primary treatment objectives for stages A to C HF are (1) improve quality of life, (2) reduce morbidity, and (3) reduce mortality. At this time, the most important factor affecting long-term outcome in HF with reduced LVEF is blunting of neurohormonal stimulation because this mediates disease progression. Pharmacologic therapy in stage D, or patients with severe, decompensated HF, is based on hemodynamic status to alleviate symptoms with diuretics, vasodilators, and in palliative circumstances, IV inotropic infusions. ACE inhibitors and β-blockers also are incorporated in the treatment regimen to retard disease progression through reductions in ventricular enlargement, vascular hypertrophy, and ventricular arrhythmias[499] (Figure 10-27). Given the lack of evidence-based therapy to guide clinicians treating patients with DHF, the ACC/AHA guidelines have assigned all therapies (e.g., diuretics, agents controlling ventricular rate), aside from the treatment of hypertension, a "C" level of evidence (Tables 10-24 and 10-25).

PHARMACOTHERAPY FOR CARDIAC ARRHYTHMIAS

Perhaps the most widely used electrophysiologic and pharmacologic classification of antiarrhythmic drugs is that proposed by Vaughan Williams[500] (Table 10-26). There is, however, substantial overlap in pharmacologic and electrophysiologic effects of specific agents among the classes, and the linkage between observed electrophysiologic effects and the clinical antiarrhythmic effect is often tenuous. Likewise, especially in Class I, there may be considerable diversity within a single class. Moreover, other antiarrhythmic drugs are not included in this classification such as the classic antiarrhythmic for chronic AF, digitalis, or adenosine, a drug with potent antiarrhythmic effects mediated by a specific class of membrane receptors.[501,502]

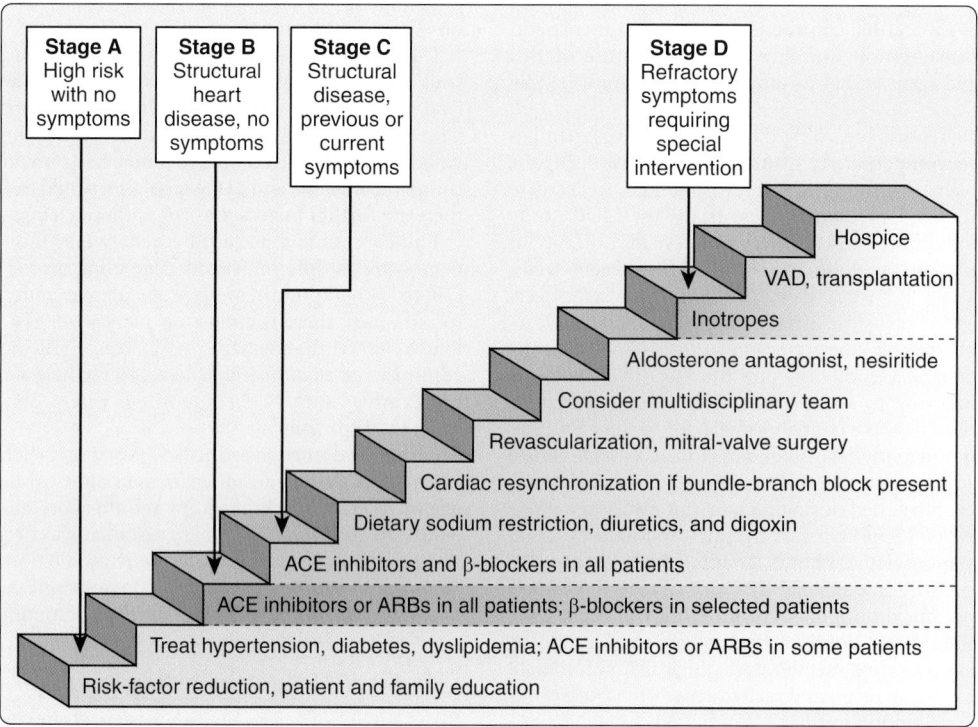

Figure 10-27 **Treatment options for the stages of heart failure.** ACE, angiotensin-converting enzyme; ARB, angiotensin II receptor blocker; VAD, ventricular assist device. (*Redrawn from Jessup M, Brozena S: Heart failure. N Engl J Med 348:2007, 2003, p 2013; Figure 3.*)

TABLE 10-24	Recommendations for Treatment of Patients with Heart Failure and Normal Ejection Fraction		
Recommendation		Class	Level of Evidence
Control systolic and diastolic hypertension according to published guidelines		I	A
Control ventricular rate in patients with atrial fibrillation		I	C
Use diuretics to control pulmonary congestion and peripheral edema		I	C
Coronary revascularization is reasonable in patients with coronary artery disease in whom symptoms or demonstrable myocardial ischemia is judged to be having an adverse effect on cardiac function		IIa	C
Restoration and maintenance of sinus rhythm in patients with atrial fibrillation might be useful to improve symptoms		IIb	C
The use of β-blockers, ACEIs, ARBs, or calcium channel antagonists in patients with controlled hypertension might be effective to minimize symptoms of heart failure		IIb	C
The use of digitalis to minimize symptoms of heart failure might be considered		IIb	C

From Hunt,[322] Table 8.

TABLE 10-25	Diastolic Heart Failure Treatments		
Goal	Management Strategy	Drugs/Recommended Doses	
Reduce the Congestive State	Salt restriction	<2 g sodium/day	
	Diuretics (avoid reductions in CO)	Furosemide, 10–120 mg Hydrochlorothiazide, 12.5–25 mg	
	ACE inhibitors	Enalapril, 2.5–40 mg Lisinopril, 10–40 mg	
	Angiotensin II-receptor blockers	Candesartan, 4–32 mg Losartan, 25–100 mg	
Target Underlying Cause			
Control hypertension	Antihypertensive agents (<130/80)	β-Blockers, ACE inhibitors, all receptor blockers according to published guidelines	
Restore sinus rhythm	Cardioversion of atrial fibrillation AV-sequential pacing		
Prevent tachycardia	β-Blockers, calcium channel blockers	Atenolol, 12.5–100 mg Metoprolol 25–100 mg Diltiazem, 120–540 mg	
Prevent/treat ischemia	Morphine, nitrates, oxygen, aspirin angioplasty or revascularization?		
Treat aortic stenosis	Aortic valve replacement		
Target Underlying Mechanisms			
Promote regression of hypertrophy and prevent myocardial fibrosis	(theoretical) Renin-angiotensin axis blockade	Enalapril, 2.5–40 mg Lisinopril, 10–40 mg Captopril, 25–150 mg Candesartan, 4–32 mg Losartan, 50–100 mg Spironolactone, 25–75 mg Eplerenone, 25–50 mg	

The Cardiac Arrhythmia Suppression Trial (CAST) questions the appropriateness of treating arrhythmias with antiarrhythmic agents in certain groups of patients.[503] The CAST study was designed to test the hypothesis that suppression of ventricular ectopy seen after MI reduces the subsequent incidence of sudden death. Patients were eligible for the study if they had ventricular ectopy without sustained VT after MI. The study required documented suppression of the ventricular ectopy with Class IC drugs encainide and flecainide. The primary study end points were death or cardiac arrest caused by arrhythmia. After 22 months of enrollment, of a planned 36 months, the Data and Safety Monitoring Board recommended discontinuation of the encainide and flecainide limbs of the study because of apparent excess mortality in those two treatment groups. Of the 1498 patients assigned to the encainide and flecainide groups, there were 89 deaths (63 in the active drug subgroups and 26 in the placebo subgroups; $P < 0.0001$). The mechanisms of the excess mortality were thought to be the precipitation of proarrhythmia secondary to facilitation of reentry, especially during ischemic episodes. After this study, the use of sodium-channel–blocking agents was not recommended, especially in low-risk patients after MI. Encainide is now no longer available; however, flecainide still is used for supraventricular tachyarrhythmias and documented life-threatening ventricular arrhythmias.

Although the Class I and especially subclass IC agents are most commonly known for their proarrhythmic effects, the other classes are not devoid of this side effect. Bretylium initially causes the release of norepinephrine, and an increased incidence of ventricular arrhythmias often is seen when therapy is initiated. In fact, in one study there was a significant arrhythmia frequency when different doses of bretylium were used.[504] Similarly, for the first week after initiation of sotalol, a nonspecific β-adrenergic blocker that is considered a Class III arrhythmic agent, there is an increased incidence of torsade de

pointes. The proarrhythmic effects appear to be increased in the presence of hypokalemia, bradycardia, CHF, and a history of sustained ventricular dysfunction (Box 10-8).[505]

Chronic antiarrhythmic therapy should be initiated only after careful evaluation of the risks and benefits of the intervention. The appropriate use of IV antiarrhythmic agents with sudden-onset arrhythmias is not clear. Obviously, life-threatening ventricular arrhythmias must be

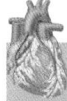

BOX 10-8. DRUGS THAT CAN PRODUCE TORSADES DE POINTES

- Amiodarone
- Disopyramide
- Dofetilide
- Ibutilide
- Procainamide
- Quinidine
- Sotalol

TABLE 10-26	Classification of Antiarrhythmic Drugs			
	Class			
Effect	I (Membrane Stabilizers)	II (β-Adrenergic Receptor Antagonists)	III (Drugs Prolonging Repolarization)	IV (Calcium Antagonists)
Pharmacologic	Fast channel (Na+) blockade	β-Adrenergic receptor blockade	Uncertain: possible interference with Na+ and Ca2+ exchange	Decreased slow-channel calcium conductance
Electrophysiologic	Decreased rate of V_{max}	Decreased V_{max}, increased APD, increased ERP, and increased ERP/APD ratio	Increased APD, increased ERP, increased ERP/ADP ratio	Decreased slow-channel depolarization; decreased ADP

APD, action potential duration; ERP, effective refractory period; V_{max}, maximal rate of depolarization.

treated. Patients at low risk for arrhythmic events may not benefit from therapy and, indeed, as learned from CAST, mortality may even increase with some of these agents. High-risk patients may be treated more safely in some cases by implantation of internal cardioverter-defibrillators.[506]

Class I Antiarrhythmic Drugs: Sodium Channel Blockers

Class I drugs have the common property of inhibiting the fast inward depolarizing current carried by sodium ion. Because of the diversity of other effects of the Class I drugs, a subgroup of the class has been proposed[507] (Table 10-27). Whether the depression of fast inward current of the sodium channel produces the primary antiarrhythmic effect of all Class I drugs is controversial. Other proposed mechanisms involve abolishing reentry by improving conduction in the reentry pathway; however, shortening the action potential duration (APD) in ventricular pathways and improving conduction of premature impulses by shortening the refractory period of the action potential also could decrease the likelihood for reentry.[508–510]

Class IA

Quinidine

In addition to the electrophysiologic effects summarized in Table 10-25, quinidine decreases the slope of phase 4 diastolic depolarization at low concentrations and increases threshold potential at high concentrations.[511] Quinidine depresses cardiac contractility, which in combination with an indirect α-adrenergic blockade can reduce arterial pressure. This hypotensive effect is the principal limitation to IV administration of quinidine.

Electrocardiographic effects of quinidine include an increase in sinus rate, which is perhaps a reflex response both to vasodilation and to cardiac depression. Conduction through the AV node may be enhanced, depressed, or may not change, depending on the interplay of the direct slowing effect and the anticholinergic effect of quinidine. Infranodal conduction is slowed and, at high concentrations, bundle-branch block, complete AV block, or asystole may result. The QT interval possibly is prolonged by sympathetic activation.[512]

Clinically, quinidine is used primarily in oral form to treat both atrial and ventricular arrhythmias. However, quinidine may substantially accelerate the ventricular response rate in AF or atrial flutter. Its use in these conditions should be preceded by β-blockade or digitalization. This acceleration of ventricular response rate is a function of the direct slowing of the atrial rate produced by quinidine and its indirect anticholinergic effects. The decreased frequency of atrial depolarization allows a greater percentage of impulses to be conducted through the AV node to depolarize the His bundle.

Quinidine may be administered orally or intramuscularly. The gastrointestinal absorption of quinidine is good, and plasma levels peak 1 to 2 hours after oral administration. Quinidine has an elimination half-life of 6 to 7 hours; therefore, a dose every 6 or 8 hours is appropriate, although shortening the dosage interval may maintain a stable plasma concentration more effectively than increasing the dosage. Typical maintenance doses are 300 to 600 mg, and therapeutic plasma concentrations range from 2 to 6 μg/mL.[513] Quinidine gluconate, 200 mg intramuscularly, is the preferred dose.

Quinidine is 70% to 80% protein bound in plasma, with much of that caused by hemoglobin. Administration of quinidine substantially increases the plasma concentrations of digoxin, probably by releasing the glycoside from protein-binding sites.[514] Elimination of quinidine is primarily by hepatic metabolism (hydroxylation), although about 20% is excreted unchanged by the kidney. Renal excretion is by both glomerular filtration and tubular secretion and depends on urinary pH; excretion is decreased up to 50% when urine is alkaline.[515]

The most serious toxic effect of quinidine is cardiac and is largely a function of its conduction effects. Monitoring both the QRS duration and QT interval is a useful guide to therapy; a 50% increment in either should prompt a reduction in dose. Various degrees of conduction block at both the atrial and ventricular levels may occur, including asystole. "Quinidine syncope" probably relates to a proarrhythmia produced by QT-interval prolongation and may not be dose related.[516] Symptoms of tinnitus, visual disturbance, and gastrointestinal irritation progressing to severe CNS symptoms (headache, diplopia, photophobia, confusion, or psychosis) are part of the spectrum of "cinchonism" produced by quinidine, by other cinchona alkaloids such as quinine, and by salicylates. Thrombocytopenia may occur with quinidine, and hypersensitivity to quinidine may appear as fever, anaphylaxis, or bronchospasm, which can be severe.

Procainamide

Electrophysiologic effects of procainamide include decreased V_{max} and amplitude during phase 0, decreased rate of phase 4 depolarization, and prolonged ERP and APD.[517] Clinically, procainamide prolongs conduction and increases the ERP in atrial and His-Purkinje portions of the conduction system, which may prolong PR interval and QRS complex durations; however, the QT interval is lengthened less than with quinidine. As with quinidine, AV nodal ERP may be decreased by indirect anticholinergic side effects.

Procainamide is used to treat ventricular arrhythmias and to suppress atrial premature beats to prevent the occurrence of AF and flutter. It has been useful for chronic suppression of premature ventricular contractions (PVCs), but may be supplanted in this use by Class IB drugs such as mexiletine. Both quinidine and procainamide are reported to reduce the frequency of short-coupling interval (< 400 msec) PVCs and thereby to reduce the frequency of VT or VF created by the R-on-T phenomenon.[518]

Administered intravenously, procainamide is an effective emergency treatment for ventricular arrhythmias, especially after lidocaine failure, but recently, amiodarone has become a more popular drug for IV suppression of ventricular arrhythmias. Dosage is 100 mg, or approximately 1.5 mg/kg given at 5-minute intervals until the therapeutic effect is obtained or a total dose of 1 g or 15 mg/kg is given (Tables 10-28 and 10-29). Arterial pressure and ECG should be monitored continuously during loading and administration stopped if significant hypotension occurs or if the QRS complex is prolonged by 50% or more. Maintenance infusion rates are 2 to 6 mg/min to maintain therapeutic plasma concentrations of 4 to 8 μg/ml.[517]

TABLE 10-27	Subgroup of Class I Antiarrhythmic Drugs		
	Subgroup		
Electrophysiologic Activity	**IA**	**IB**	**IC**
Phase 0	Decreased	Slight effect	Marked decrease
Depolarization	Prolonged	Slight effect	Slight effect
Conduction	Decreased	Slight effect	Markedly slowed
Effective refractory period (ERP)	Increased	Slight effect	Slight prolongation
Action potential duration (APD)	Increased	Decreased	Slight effect
ERP/APD ratio	Increased	Decreased	Slight effect
QRS duration	Increased	No effect during sinus rhythm	Marked increase
Prototype drugs	Quinidine, procainamide, disopyramide, diphenylhydantoin	Lidocaine, mexiletine, tocainide	Lorcainide, encainide, flecainide, aprindine

TABLE 10-28	Intravenous Supraventricular Antiarrhythmic Therapy
Class I	*Procainamide (IA)*—converts acute atrial fibrillation, suppresses PACs and precipitation of atrial fibrillation/flutter, converts accessory pathway SVT; 100 mg IV loading dose every 5 minutes until arrhythmia subsides or total dose of 15 mg/kg (rarely needed) with continuous infusion of 2 to 6 mg/min
Class II	*Esmolol*—converts or maintains slow ventricular response in acute atrial fibrillation; 0.5–1 mg/kg loading dose with each 50-μg/kg/min increase in infusion, with infusions of 50 to 300 μg/kg/min; hypotension and bradycardia are limiting factors
Class III	*Amiodarone*—converts acute atrial fibrillation to sinus rhythm; 5 mg/kg over 15 min IV *Ibutilide* (Convert)—converts acute atrial fibrillation and flutter Adults (>60 kg): 1 mg given over 10 minutes intravenously, may repeat once Adults (<60 kg) and Children: 0.01 mg/kg given over 10 minutes intravenously, may be repeated once
Class IV	*Verapamil*—slow ventricular response to acute atrial fibrillation, converts AV node reentry SVT; 75–150 μg/kg IV bolus *Diltiazem*—slow ventricular response in acute atrial fibrillation, converts AV node reentry SVT; 0.25 μg/kg bolus, then 100–300 μg/kg/hr infusion
Others	*Adenosine*—converts AV node reentry SVT and accessory pathway SVT; aids in diagnosis of atrial fibrillation and flutter Adults: 3–6 mg IV bolus, repeat with 6–12 mg bolus Children: 100 μg/kg IV bolus, repeat with 200 μg/kg bolus Increased dosage required with methylxanthines, decreased use required with dipyridamole. *Digoxin*—maintenance IV therapy for atrial fibrillation and flutter, slows ventricular response Adults: 0.25 mg IV bolus followed by 0.125 mg each 1–2 hours until rate controlled, not to exceed 10 μg/kg in 24 hours Children (age < 10 yr): 10–30 μg/kg load given in divided doses over 24 hr Maintenance: 25% of loading dose

IV, intravenous; PAC, premature atrial contraction; SVT, supraventricular tachyarrhythmia.

TABLE 10-29	Intravenous Ventricular Antiarrhythmic Therapy
Class I	*Procainamide (IA)*—100 mg IV loading dose every 5 min until arrhythmia subsides or total dose of 15 mg/kg (rarely needed) with continuous infusion of 2–6 mg/min *Lidocaine (IB)*—1.5 mg in divided doses given twice over 20 minutes with continuous infusion of 1–4 mg/min
Class II	*Propranolol*—0.5–1 mg given slowly up to a total β-blocking dose of 0.1 mg/kg; repeat bolus as needed *Metoprolol*—2.5 mg given slowly up to a total β-blocking dose of 0.2 mg/kg; repeat bolus as needed *Esmolol*—0.5–1.0 mg/kg loading dose with each 50 μg/kg/min increase in infusion, with infusions of 50–300 μg/kg/min; hypotension and bradycardia are limiting factors
Class III	*Bretylium*—5 mg/kg loading dose given slowly with a continuous infusion of 1–5 mg/min; hypotension may be a limiting factor with infusion *Amiodarone*—150 mg over 10 min intravenously, then 1 mg/min for 6 hours, then 0.5 mg/min for the next 18 hours; repeat bolus as needed
Others	*Magnesium*—2 g MgSO₄ over 5 min, then continuous infusion of 1 g/hr for 6–10 hours to restore intracellular magnesium levels

IV, intravenous.
From Royster RL: Diagnosis and management of cardiac disorders. ASA Refresher Course Lectures. Park Ridge, IL: American Society of Anesthesiologists, 1996, by permission.

Oral administration of procainamide has a 75% to 95% absorption rate, and plasma levels peak after 1 to 2 hours.[519] The elimination half-life of procainamide is 3 to 4 hours, and the oral dosage interval is similar; however, sustained-release preparations are available. Oral dose requirements are on the order of 50 mg/kg/24 hr or 400 to 600 mg every 3 to 4 hours.[520] Decreasing the dosage interval rather than increasing the dose may be a better method of producing a stable increase in plasma concentrations without creating peak levels that are toxic. Sustained-release forms of procainamide are available.

Procainamide has both hepatic and renal routes of elimination, with each route approximately equal in magnitude. Hepatic metabolism

is by acetylation and, therefore, will be either fast or slow in individual patients as a result of genetic variation.[521] The primary metabolite, *N*-acetylprocainamide, has antiarrhythmic effects, as well as toxic side effects, and is excreted almost entirely by the kidney.[522] The clinical importance is that patients with impaired hepatic or renal function, or with diminished perfusion of either organ, as in CHF, will have markedly impaired elimination of procainamide. Recommended dosages with renal impairment or CHF are a loading dose of 12 mg/kg given over 1 hour, with a maintenance dose of 1.4 mg/kg/hr.[523]

Toxic side effects of procainamide are dose related and primarily are related to plasma concentration, a function of both total dose and rate of administration during the loading technique. Serious cardiac toxicity generally requires plasma concentrations greater than 12 μg/ml. *N*-acetylprocainamide levels should be monitored as well. The likelihood of producing proarrhythmia as a result of QT_c prolongation is less with procainamide than with quinidine.[524] Procainamide also may produce gastrointestinal disturbances, CNS symptoms (headache and sleep disturbance), rash, and agranulocytosis. Among patients receiving procainamide chronically, antinuclear antibodies develop in 50% to 70%, and approximately half will suffer fever, myalgia, rash, pleuritis, or pericarditis similar to that seen with lupus erythematosus, although renal and CNS effects are rare.[525] They also are more common among patients who are slow acetylators. After discontinuation of the drug, lupus-like symptoms resolve slowly.

Intramyocardial distribution of procainamide, especially during ischemia or infarction, is an important component of its therapeutic effect. In a canine infarction model, procainamide increased ERP more in ischemic than in nonischemic myocardium.[526] The pharmacokinetics of procainamide has been shown to differ between ischemic and nonischemic regions of myocardium; tissue concentrations of procainamide decline more rapidly in the latter.[527]

Disopyramide

Although disopyramide is chemically different from quinidine and procainamide, electrophysiologic effects of the three drugs are similar. Conduction through the AV node may be facilitated slightly by disopyramide because of its indirect vagolytic effect.[528] Accessory pathway conduction may be slowed in patients with Wolff–Parkinson–White syndrome.[529] Disopyramide is a potent negative inotropic drug, and after IV use, SVR reflexively increases.[530]

Disopyramide is therapeutically effective against supraventricular and ventricular tachyarrhythmias. However, as with quinidine and procainamide, disopyramide should not be used for ventricular tachyarrhythmias caused by prolonged QT syndrome. The marked negative inotropic and anticholinergic effects limit the usefulness of the drug.

When given orally, 80% of disopyramide is absorbed, and steady-state therapeutic plasma concentrations of 2 to 4 μg/ml can be achieved with 100 to 200 mg orally every 6 hours.[531] The elimination half-life is approximately 7 hours, and elimination occurs equally by hepatic and renal mechanisms; hepatic or renal insufficiency may necessitate smaller doses.[532] Disopyramide is approximately 30% to 50% protein bound at plasma concentrations of 3 μg/ml.[533]

Toxicity of disopyramide is most frequently anticholinergic in origin, with symptoms of gastrointestinal upset, visual disturbance, and urinary tract obstruction, which may be marked in elderly men with prostatic hypertrophy. Unless there is LV failure, cardiovascular complications are infrequent; however, recurrent CHF is seen in up to 50% of patients with a history of CHF.[530] Conduction system toxicity resembles that with quinidine.

Class IB

Lidocaine

First introduced as an antiarrhythmic drug in the 1950s, lidocaine has become the clinical standard for the acute IV treatment of ventricular arrhythmias except those precipitated by an abnormally prolonged QT interval.[534–537] Lidocaine may, in fact, be one of the most useful drugs in clinical anesthesia because it has both local and general anesthetic properties, in addition to an antiarrhythmic effect.[538]

The direct electrophysiologic effects of lidocaine produce virtually all of its antiarrhythmic action. Lidocaine depresses the slope of phase 4 diastolic depolarization in Purkinje fibers and increases the VF threshold.[539] In Purkinje fibers, lidocaine increases transmembrane potassium conductance but does not affect resting membrane potential or threshold potential.[540] At less negative (partially depolarized) initial membrane potentials, lidocaine decreases fast-channel (Na) responses through an increase in background outward potassium flux, an effect directly related to extracellular potassium concentration.[541,542] Lidocaine may be ineffective in patients with hypokalemia.[543]

Conduction velocity is not affected by lidocaine in normal tissue, but it is significantly decreased in ischemic tissue.[544] The effects of lidocaine on APD vary by conduction system location. In atrial tissues, there is little or no effect. In contrast, in Purkinje fibers, APD is markedly decreased, and the magnitude of the decrease is directly proportional to normal APD.[509] Because lidocaine decreases APD, its antiarrhythmic effect has been attributed to improved conduction in ectopic foci, which would decrease the likelihood of reentry; however, it has been shown that lidocaine slows conduction in these areas and decreases reentrant ventricular ectopy after experimental infarction.[514,545]

The clinical pharmacokinetics of lidocaine is well described. Both distribution and elimination half-lives of lidocaine are short, approximately 60 seconds and 100 minutes, respectively.[546] Hepatic extraction of lidocaine is about 60% to 70%, and essentially all lidocaine is metabolized because the urine contains negligible amounts of unchanged lidocaine.[513] Hepatic metabolism produces monoethylglycine-xylidide and glycine-xylidide, both of which possess antiarrhythmic effects. Metabolic products are eliminated by the kidney, and accumulation of the monoethyl metabolite is related to the toxicity of IV lidocaine.[547-549] In patients with impaired hepatic function or blood flow (e.g., those with CHF), the dose requirement is approximately 50% of that in the healthy person (Figure 10-28; Tables 10-29 and 10-30).

Therapeutic plasma levels of lidocaine range from 1.5 to 5 μg/mL; signs of toxicity are frequent with concentrations greater than 9 μg/mL.[548] Various IV dosages can be used, but the important factor is to rapidly achieve steady-state therapeutic plasma concentrations. Thus, an initial bolus dose of 1 to 1.5 mg/kg should be followed immediately by a continuous infusion of 20 to 50 μg/kg/min to prevent the "therapeutic hiatus" produced by the rapid redistribution half-life of lidocaine. Likewise, infusion increments should be accompanied by additional bolus doses to immediately increase plasma level.

TABLE 10-30	Potential Effects of Pathophysiologic Changes in Congestive Heart Failure on Drug Disposition	
Pathology	**Pharmacokinetic Sequelae**
↓ Cardiac output and organ perfusion	↓ Hepatic and renal clearance
↑ Sympathetic activity	↓ Drug distribution
↑ Plasma norepinephrine Altered regional perfusion	↓ Intramuscular absorption
↓ Peripheral perfusion	
Changes in extracellular fluid volume and protein binding	↑↓ Volume of distribution
Visceral congestion	↓ Drug metabolism

The major toxic effect of lidocaine is associated with the CNS and is manifested by drowsiness and disorientation, which progress to agitation, muscle twitching, and hearing abnormalities and culminate in seizures. With regard to CNS toxicity, it is important to note that lidocaine can be an effective general anesthetic agent; cases of coma with electroencephalographic silence similar to brain death patterns have been produced by overdose of lidocaine and have resolved completely on discontinuation of the drug. Interestingly, the direct CNS effect of lidocaine and other local anesthetics is anticonvulsant.[550-552] Local anesthetic-induced seizures do not produce permanent damage to the CNS, as long as cardiovascular and respiratory complications of the seizure are prevented. Pharmacologically, benzodiazepines are superior to barbiturates (e.g., thiopental) for stopping local anesthetic-induced seizure activity. Drug therapy alone is insufficient; however, airway control, ventilation, and especially oxygenation are paramount to prevent CNS morbidity.

Mexiletine and Tocainide

Mexiletine and tocainide have electrophysiologic effects similar to those of lidocaine (decreases in APD and ERP, but little effect on conduction). Mexiletine has little effect on the QT interval. Hemodynamic effects are minor and consist primarily of small decreases of LV dP/dt and increases of LVEDP.[553] Small decreases of CO, SVR, and BP have been reported; however, even in patients with CAD, acute MI, or valvular heart disease, hemodynamic effects are clinically insignificant.[554-557]

The antiarrhythmic effects decrease the frequency of acute and chronic ventricular ectopy but not supraventricular arrhythmias. Mexiletine may decrease symptomatic ventricular arrhythmias in patients not responding to other therapy and may be more effective than lidocaine when used IV to suppress PVCs and VT in acute MI.[558-561] Mexiletine, administered orally, also may be effective prophylaxis for PVCs and VT, but it may less effectively suppress closely coupled PVCs.[562-564] Mexiletine may be used in children and in patients with a long QT syndrome.

Pharmacokinetics of orally administered mexiletine reveals a bioavailability of 85%, with 70% of the drug protein bound. The volume of distribution of mexiletine is 2.5 times that for other antiarrhythmics.[565] Elimination half-life is 10 hours and is suitable for two or three times per day dosage regimens.[566] Mexiletine is eliminated by hepatic metabolism, with less than 10% renally excreted unchanged in the urine. The hepatic metabolism is accelerated with microsomal enzyme induction and predictably decreased with hepatic disease, but overall metabolism is unaffected by renal failure.[567,568]

The usual dosage of mexiletine is 200 mg every 8 hours, which can be increased to 400 mg, but not to exceed 1200 mg/day. Effective plasma levels of mexiletine range from 0.5 to 2 μg/mL, but there is wide individual variation of the dosage required to achieve that concentration. Adverse effects of mexiletine include nausea, dysarthria, dizziness, paresthesia, tremor, vomiting, and sweating. Adverse reactions to mexiletine are dose related and may occur at serum concentrations at the high end of the therapeutic range, which requires careful titration of the drug in patients. The incidence rate of minor reactions is 30%, and the incidence rate of severe reactions (vomiting, confusion, and hypotension) is 19% when the plasma concentration is greater than 2 μg/mL.[569]

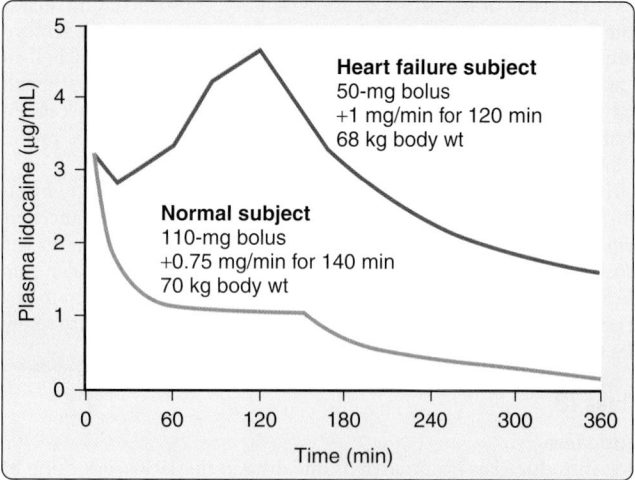

Figure 10-28 Difference between plasma level responses to infused lidocaine in a normal subject and a subject with heart failure. The accumulation of lidocaine in patients with depressed hepatic metabolism is dramatically illustrated. *(From Textbook of Cardiac Life Support, 1987. Copyright American Heart Association.)*

Diphenylhydantoin

Diphenylhydantoin (DPH) or phenytoin is unique among Class IA drugs in that it has a potent central sympatholytic effect that decreases cardiac sympathetic efferent nerve activity.[570,571] Its electrophysiologic effect in many ways bridges the IA and IB classification. In normal conduction system cells, DPH decreases V_{max} and the amplitude of phase 0, but this effect is weaker than with other Class IA drugs.[572] DPH does not decrease intraventricular conduction or prolong the QT interval, but shortens APD.[573] DPH effectively can abolish the delayed afterpotentials associated with digitalis intoxication.[574,575] In cells partially depolarized from cold, hypoxia, or cardiac glycoside administration, DPH increases maximal diastolic potential, V_{max} of phase 0, and the conduction velocity.[576] Thus, DPH exerts its antiarrhythmic effect by increasing the ERP/APD ratio and by decreasing automaticity, both of these effects being enhanced in partially depolarized cells.

The drug is useful to treat the atrial and ventricular arrhythmias produced by cardiac glycoside toxicity and in some patients with arrhythmias secondary to prolonged QT syndrome. It is less effective for other supraventricular arrhythmias and for suppressing chronic ventricular ectopy. The drug also is useful in children to prevent late postoperative arrhythmias after surgical correction of congenital heart disease such as junction ectopic tachycardia.[577]

IV loading of DPH is accomplished in much the same way as with procainamide. Doses of 50 to 100 mg (0.5 to 1.5 mg/kg) are given at 5-minute intervals until therapeutic effects are obtained, up to a total dose of 1 g (15 mg/kg); the usual therapeutic plasma concentration is 8 to 10 µg/mL.[578] The drug undergoes primary hepatic metabolism, with urinary excretion of unchanged DPH accounting for only 5% of the total dose.[579] Patients with impaired hepatic or renal function should be expected to have greater plasma concentrations of DPH for a given dose; therefore, the dose should be reduced to prevent toxicity.

With IV administration a depressor effect is seen with depressed contractile function and a moderate increase of LVEDP.[580,581] These effects may be, in part, because of the solvents used for the injectable preparation, propylene glycol and ethyl alcohol.[582] Infusion rates greater than 50 mg/min in adults have produced cardiovascular collapse, VF, and death.[583] Other side effects include visual disturbances (nystagmus and blurring), nausea, dysarthria, and cerebellar ataxia. Chronic DPH use produces gingival hyperplasia, macrocytic anemia, and dermatologic disorders.

Class IC

Flecainide

Flecainide depresses phase 0, delays repolarization in canine ventricular myocardium, and increases intracardiac monophasic APD in humans. The sodium channel depressant effects are slow onset and offset, and use dependent. It also can inhibit the slow calcium channel, so the drug has properties of multiple classes.[584] Minimal changes occur in ventricular or atrial refractoriness; however, the drug can markedly change accessory pathway refractoriness. The QT interval changes are also minimal.

This drug is indicated for life-threatening ventricular arrhythmias, supraventricular arrhythmias, and AF. It also is effective in patients with the Wolff–Parkinson–White syndrome. Chronic clinical studies have shown that PVCs and VT are effectively suppressed.[585] Flecainide is probably the most effective antiarrhythmic at eliminating premature depolarizations, but as CAST showed in certain patient populations, PVC suppression may not always be in the best interest of the patient. IV flecainide was effective in treating junctional ectopic tachycardia, converting all seven patients to sinus rhythm within 16 hours.[586]

Flecainide decreases LV dP/dt and CO experimentally.[587] Clinical studies have shown no effects of oral flecainide on BP, echocardiographic parameters, or exercise tolerance.[585,588,589] However, patients with depressed ventricular function may be more susceptible to the negative inotropic effects of flecainide.

Flecainide is well absorbed after oral administration, with a plasma half-life of 20 hours. The drug is 85% excreted renally either unchanged or as an inactive metabolite. Effective plasma concentrations range from 0.2 to 1.0 µg/mL. Dosages range from 100 to 200 mg twice a day. The dose should be reduced in renal failure or HF. Flecainide increases serum digoxin and propranolol levels, whereas propranolol, quinidine, and amiodarone can increase flecainide levels.

Adverse effects are usually minor at doses that have a significant therapeutic effect, but the QT interval has been prolonged with induction of polymorphic VT, and the CAST study showed definite increases in mortality after MI.[590] Confusion and irritability rarely occur.

Propafenone

Propafenone blocks the fast sodium current in a use-dependent manner. It also has a slow offset like flecainide. Propafenone also blocks β receptors and is a weak potassium channel blocker.[591] This drug generally slows conduction and prolongs refractoriness of most cardiac conduction system tissue. Propafenone is indicated for life-threatening ventricular arrhythmias, various supraventricular arrhythmias, and AF. In one study, a single 600-mg oral dose of propafenone converted 76% of patients in AF.[592] Propafenone was more effective than placebo in preventing atrial tachyarrhythmias after cardiac surgery with combined IV and oral therapy.[593]

Propafenone is well absorbed orally and is highly protein bound with an elimination half-life of 6 to 8 hours. Therapeutic serum levels are from 0.2 to 1.5 µg/mL. The metabolites of propafenone are active and demonstrate significant action potential and β-blocking effects. A small percentage of patients poorly metabolize the drug, and the metabolites of these patients exhibit greater β-blocking properties.

The drug has fewer proarrhythmic problems than flecainide likely because of the β-blocking effects, which tend to decrease arrhythmic traits of antiarrhythmic drugs. Worsening of bronchospastic lung disease has occurred, and in a small percentage of patients, dizziness, blurred vision, and taste issues, together with some gastrointestinal complaints, may develop.

Moricizine

Moricizine is a potent sodium channel blocker with mild potassium-blocking effects. It prolongs AV node, HV and QRS duration. It has little effect on atrial tissue. The drug is indicated for life-threatening ventricular arrhythmias and is as effective as some of the other Class I agents.

Moricizine is highly protein bound and its bioavailability is only 35%. Serum levels do not correlate with therapeutic activity. The elimination half-life is 1 to 3 hours, with the drug eliminated by both hepatic and renal routes. Dosage is 300 mg every 8 hours. Dosage may be changed to every 12 hours in patients with hepatic or renal disease or in patients with CHF.

Adverse effects include tremor, headache, vertigo, dizziness, and gastrointestinal side effects of nausea, vomiting, and diarrhea. Proarrhythmic episodes can occur in up to 15% of patients. In the CAST study, the moricizine limb was continued after the encainide and flecainide limbs were stopped, and analysis of the moricizine-treated patients showed an increase in mortality as well.[594]

Class II: β-Adrenergic Receptor Antagonists

β-Adrenergic receptor blockers are very effective antiarrhythmics in patients during the perioperative period or patients who are critically ill because many arrhythmias in these patients are adrenergically mediated.

Propranolol

Propranolol was the first major β-receptor-blocking drug to be used clinically. Propranolol is very potent but is nonselective for $β_{1/2}$-receptor subtypes. It possesses essentially no ISA. Because it interferes with the bronchodilating actions of epinephrine and the sympathetic stimulating effects of hypoglycemia, propranolol is less useful in patients with diabetes or bronchospasm. These difficulties with propranolol stimulated the search for β-receptor–blocking drugs with receptor subtype specificity, such as metoprolol, esmolol, and atenolol.

The electrophysiologic effects of β-receptor antagonism are decreased automaticity, increased APD, primarily in ventricular muscle, and a substantially increased ERP in the AV node. β-Blockade decreases the rate of spontaneous (phase 4) depolarization in the SA node; the magnitude of this effect depends on the background sympathetic tone. Although resting HR is decreased by β-blockade, the inhibition of the increase of HR in response to exercise or emotional stress is much more marked. Automaticity in the AV node and more distal portions of the conduction system is also depressed. β-Blockade affects the VF threshold variably, but it consistently reverses the fibrillation threshold-lowering effect of catecholamines.

In addition to β-blockade, propranolol decreases the background outward current of potassium and, at greater concentrations, also inhibits inward sodium current. Because of similarity to Class I activity, these effects have been termed *membrane-stabilizing activity* or quinidine-like effects. In very high concentrations (1000 to 3000 ng/mL), this effect increases depolarization threshold in Purkinje fibers.[126] Although effective β-blockade is achieved at propranolol concentrations of 100 to 300 ng/mL, concentrations of 1000 ng/mL may be required to control ventricular arrhythmias.[595] Propranolol decreases intramyocardial impulse conduction in acutely ischemic myocardium but does not do so in normal myocardium.[596]

Pharmacokinetics shows that absorption after oral administration is virtually 100%, but bioavailability is impaired by first-pass hepatic metabolism, which accounts for approximately two thirds of the administered dose. The degree of hepatic extraction is highly variable, which probably accounts for the great variability of the plasma concentration produced by a given oral dose of propranolol. The hepatic extraction of propranolol is a saturable process, and bioavailability improves with increased oral dose or with chronic therapy.[597] Propranolol is 90% to 95% protein bound in plasma, which further confounds the use of plasma concentration as a guide to therapy.[598] Propranolol is metabolized before excretion; one product, 4-hydroxypropranolol, has a β-blocking potency similar to that of propranolol, but a short half-life prevents this metabolic product from contributing significantly to the therapeutic effect of propranolol.[599] The elimination half-life of orally administered propranolol is 3 to 4 hours, but it is increased during chronic therapy as a result of saturation of hepatic metabolic processes.[600] CPB alters the kinetics of propranolol. Heparinization doubles the free fraction of propranolol, an effect that is reversed after protamine administration. This effect is thought to be due to an increase of free fatty acid concentration produced by heparin, which decreases the protein binding of propranolol.[601]

Major toxic side effects of propranolol relate to β-blockade per se. Cardiac toxicity includes CHF (uncommon without other causes of ventricular dysfunction) and depressed AV conduction. Both complete heart block and asystole have occurred in patients with preexisting AV nodal or intraventricular conduction abnormalities. In contrast, sudden discontinuation of β-blockade therapy may precipitate a withdrawal syndrome of excessive β-adrenergic activity, as a result of the altered sensitivity associated with chronic blockade; responses to normal levels of sympathetic activity are exaggerated as the β-blockade declines, likely because of an increased receptor density or upregulation of the β receptor.[602,603] Increased airway resistance results from β2-receptor blockade by propranolol, and this can precipitate severe pulmonary compromise in the asthmatic patient. The hypoglycemic action of insulin is accentuated by propranolol because the sympathomimetic effect of hypoglycemia is blocked. Adverse effects perhaps not related to β-receptor blockade include CNS disturbances such as insomnia, hallucinations, depression, and dizziness, and minor allergic manifestations such as rash, fever, and purpura.

An appropriate IV dose for acute control of arrhythmias is 0.5 to 1.0 mg titrated to therapeutic effect up to a total of 0.1 to 0.15 mg/kg. Stable therapeutic plasma concentrations of propranolol can be obtained with a continuous IV infusion. An effective level of β-blockade may be obtained with a continuous infusion approximating 3 mg/hr in adult postoperative patients previously receiving chronic treatment; however, with the availability of esmolol, the need for a propranolol infusion is no longer necessary.

Metoprolol

Metoprolol is a relatively selective β-receptor antagonist. The potency of metoprolol for β1-receptor blockade is equal to that of propranolol, but metoprolol exhibits only 1% to 2% of the effect of propranolol at β2 receptors.[604]

Like propranolol, metoprolol is rapidly and efficiently absorbed after oral administration; however, its first-pass extraction by the liver is lower, and 40% of the administered dose reaches the systemic circulation. Plasma half-life after oral administration is approximately 3 hours. Metoprolol is 90% metabolized, with hydroxylation and O-demethylation being the primary pathways. The metabolites lack β-receptor effects. As with acetylation of procainamide, the rate of hydroxylation of metoprolol is genetically determined. "Slow hydroxylators" show a markedly prolonged elimination of the parent drug and greater plasma concentrations.[605]

Toxicity of metoprolol is related primarily to its limited β2-antagonist activity. Metoprolol increases airway resistance and decreases the forced expiratory volume (FEV), in patients with asthma, although to a lesser extent than does propranolol at equipotent β1-antagonist doses. In contrast with propranolol, metoprolol does not inhibit the bronchodilation of isoproterenol. Metoprolol impairs β-receptor–mediated insulin release, and the signs of hypoglycemia will be masked as with propranolol. Other side effects of metoprolol are similar to those of propranolol.

Metoprolol is useful for treating supraventricular and ventricular arrhythmias that are adrenergically driven. The primary advantage of metoprolol is its relative lack of most of the bronchoconstrictive effects in patients with chronic obstructive pulmonary disease. Acute IV dosage is 1.0 mg titrated to therapeutic effect up to 0.1 to 0.2 mg/kg.

IV therapy may be more effective than oral therapy in preventing AF after cardiac surgery.[606] Another study compared oral carvedilol and oral metoprolol and found carvedilol more effective in preventing AF after on-pump CABG surgery.[607]

Esmolol

Esmolol is a cardioselective (β1) receptor antagonist with an extremely brief duration of action.[608] In anesthetized dogs, esmolol infused at 50 μg/kg/min produced a steady-state β-blockade that was completely reversed 20 minutes after stopping the infusion.[609] Esmolol has only minimal ISA and membrane-stabilizing activity and, in conscious dogs, has no effect on LVEDP, BP, HR, CO, or SVR; however, at 5 to 60 μg/kg/min, it does decrease LV dP/dt. The decreased contractility, however, fully resolves by 20 minutes after the infusion.

Electrophysiologic effects of esmolol are those of β-adrenergic receptor antagonism. In open-chest dogs, esmolol infused at 300 μg/kg/min increased SA node recovery time and AH conduction interval, but not HV interval. ERP was increased in the AV node, but this effect does not occur in vitro at β-blocking concentrations.

Esmolol is rapidly metabolized in blood by hydrolysis of its methyl ester linkage. Its half-life in whole blood is 12.5 to 27.1 minutes in dogs and humans, respectively. The acid metabolite possesses a slight degree (1500 times less than esmolol) of β-antagonism. Esmolol is not affected by plasma cholinesterase; the esterase responsible is located in erythrocytes and is not inhibited by cholinesterase inhibitors, but it is deactivated by sodium fluoride. Of importance to clinical anesthesia, no metabolic interactions between esmolol and other ester molecules are known. Specifically, esmolol dosages up to 500 μg/kg/min have not modified neuromuscular effects of succinylcholine.[157]

Clinically, in patients with asthma, esmolol (300 μg/kg/min) only slightly increases airway resistance. Also, in patients with chronic obstructive pulmonary disease who received esmolol, no adverse pulmonary effects occurred.[610] In a multicenter trial, in a comparison with propranolol for the treatment of paroxysmal supraventricular tachyarrhythmia (PSVT), esmolol was equally efficacious and had the advantage of a much faster termination of the β-blockade.[611] Esmolol has become a useful agent in controlling sinus tachycardia in the perioperative period, a time when a titratable and brief β-blockade is highly desirable.

Dosing begins at $25\,\mu g/kg/min$ and is titrated to effect up to $250\,\mu g/kg/min$. Doses greater than this may cause significant hypotension because of reduced CO in patients. Esmolol is especially effective in treating acute-onset AF or flutter perioperatively, and results in both acute control of the ventricular response and conversion of the arrhythmia back to sinus rhythm.

Landiolol, an ultrashort-acting β-blocker, similar to esmolol but with greater cardioselectivity and a shorter half-life (4 minutes), is currently undergoing investigation.[612] The drug is efficacious in converting 89% of patients who developed AF or flutter to sinus rhythm.[613] In addition, landiolol reduced the incidence of AF when given prophylactically after cardiac surgery.[614]

Class III: Agents That Block Potassium Channels and Prolong Repolarization

Amiodarone

Amiodarone is a benzofuran derivative initially introduced as an antianginal drug and was subsequently found to have antiarrhythmic effects. The drug has a wide spectrum of effectiveness including supraventricular,[615] ventricular,[616,617] and pre-excitation arrhythmias[615–618] (see Tables 10-28 and 10-29). It also may be effective against VT and VF refractory to other treatment.[619] Amiodarone has been approved by the AHA as the first-line antiarrhythmic in cardiopulmonary resuscitation.[620] Amiodarone may be effective prophylactically in preventing AF after surgery.[615] It also can decrease the number of shocks in patients who have internal cardioverter-defibrillators compared with other antiarrhythmic drugs.[621]

Amiodarone used in an isolated rabbit SA node preparation increased APD and decreased the slope of diastolic (phase 4) depolarization, which depressed SA node automaticity.[622] Amiodarone prolongs repolarization and refractoriness in the SA node, in atrial and ventricular myocardium, in the AV node, and in the His-Purkinje system.[623] Resting potential and myocardial automaticity are minimally affected, but both ERP and absolute refractory period are prolonged.[624] Amiodarone blocks inactive sodium channels in Purkinje fibers, which significantly depresses phase 0.[623] In anesthetized dogs, amiodarone decreases AV junctional and SA nodal automaticity and prolongs intranodal conduction.[625]

There are substantial differences in the electrophysiologic effects of acute and chronic amiodarone administration. Acutely, the drug slightly increases ERP of the His-Purkinje system and ventricular myocardium. The QTc is not prolonged by acute IV administration despite myocardial concentrations similar to those with chronic oral therapy.[626] However, chronic oral administration significantly increases QTc.[627] Although AV nodal ERP increases with acute IV amiodarone therapy, the increase is greater after chronic use. In other cardiac tissue, there is little or no change in ERP after IV administration; however, after chronic oral use, ERP is increased globally and both AH and HV conduction times are increased.[628]

The electrophysiologic effects of chronic amiodarone treatment mimic those of thyroid ablation.[629] Moreover, the repolarization effects of the drug are reversed by T_3 administration. This suggests that among the basic effects of amiodarone is the blockade of the cardiac effect of T_3; this mechanism has been proposed as an alternative to the active metabolite accumulation theory to account for the slow onset of the antiarrhythmic effect of amiodarone.[628]

Amiodarone increases the amount of electric current required to elicit VF (an increase in VF threshold). In most patients, refractory VT is suppressed by acute IV use of amiodarone. This effect has been attributed to a selectively increased activity in diseased tissue, as has been seen with lidocaine.[630] Amiodarone also has an adrenergic-receptor (α and β) antagonistic effect produced by a noncompetitive mechanism; the contribution of this effect to the antiarrhythmic action of the drug is not known.[631]

Hemodynamic effects of IV amiodarone (10 mg/kg) include decreased LV dP/dt, maximal negative dP/dt, mean aortic pressure, HR, and peak LV pressure after coronary artery occlusion in dogs. CO was increased despite the negative inotropic effect as a result of the more marked decrease of LV afterload.[632] Clinical effects are similar; a 5-mg/kg IV dose during cardiac catheterization decreased BP, LVEDP, and SVR and increased CO, but it did not affect HR. Chronic amiodarone therapy is not associated with clinically significant depression of ventricular function in patients without LV failure. Hemodynamic deterioration may occur in some patients with compensated CHF, perhaps because of the antiadrenergic effects of the drug.[633]

Pharmacokinetics of amiodarone is notable for the low bioavailability, very long elimination half-life, relatively low clearance, and large volume of distribution. Oral absorption of amiodarone is slow, with peak plasma levels occurring 3 to 7 hours after ingestion.[634] Bioavailability is variable and low, ranging from 22% to 50%. The hepatic extraction ratio, however, is only 0.13, so that the major limit to bioavailability may be incomplete absorption. Amiodarone has a large volume of distribution, variably estimated as 1.3 to 65.8 L/kg; plasma clearance rates range from 0.14 to 0.60 L/min.[635] Plasma half-life after chronic oral therapy is variably reported as from 14 to 107 days; therapeutic and steady-state plasma concentrations are slowly achieved with maintenance oral administration at 9.5 to 30 days, respectively.[636]

Because steady-state plasma levels are achieved slowly, loading techniques have been developed. Patient-specific pharmacokinetic data have been used to prescribe loading infusion rates from 0.5 to 3.9 mg/min and maintenance rates of 0.5 to 1.0 mg/min to produce plasma levels of 0.5 to $2.5\,\mu g/mL$ during maintenance infusion. This dosage reduced VT by 85%, paired PVCs by 74%, and isolated PVCs by 60%.[637] A comparison of onset of antiarrhythmic effect of oral loading (800 mg/day for 7 days, then 600 mg/day for 3 days) and IV (5 mg/kg for 30 minutes) plus oral (as for oral alone) administration demonstrated that the combined IV and oral loading technique had a more rapid therapeutic effect with a lower total amiodarone dose.[638] In acute situations with stable patients, a 150-mg IV bolus is followed by a 1.0-mg/min infusion for 6 hours and then 0.5 mg/min thereafter. In CPR, a 300-mg IV bolus is given and repeated with multiple boluses as needed if defibrillation is unsuccessful.

Adverse reactions to amiodarone are numerous. Photosensitivity of the skin occurs in 57% of patients without apparent relation to dose or plasma level.[639] Other skin manifestations include abnormal pigmentation (slate gray) and an erythematous, pruritic rash. Corneal microdeposits occur in most patients taking amiodarone chronically, although visual symptoms are uncommon.

Pulmonary side effects are more severe.[640–643] Clinical features include exertional dyspnea, cough, and weight loss. Hypoxia may occur; pulmonary function studies show decreased total lung capacity and diffusion rate. Chest radiographic findings are diffuse bilateral interstitial infiltrates, which histologically may be fibrosing alveolitis. Pulmonary effects may resolve with discontinuation of treatment or with dose reduction. The pathophysiologic mechanism of these pulmonary effects is not known but may relate to abnormal production of phospholipid. The overall incidence rate of pulmonary toxicity is up to 6%, with a mortality rate in those affected of 20% to 25%. There are case reports of an increased risk for acute respiratory distress syndrome when amiodarone is used before CPB, but this association has not been proved.

Thyroid abnormalities are associated with amiodarone; the frequencies of hyperthyroidism and hypothyroidism range from 1% to 5% and 1% to 2%, respectively.[631] Amiodarone contains two iodine atoms per molecule, or 75 mg organic iodide/200 mg drug, and 10% of that amount may become free iodine. The iodine alone does not account for the thyroid abnormalities because intake of an amount of inorganic iodine equivalent to that ingested with chronic amiodarone intake does not have the same effect. HR is not increased during hyperthyroidism associated with amiodarone, probably because of its antiadrenergic effects. Amiodarone therapy increases both thyroxine (T_4) and reverse T_3 but only slightly decreases T_3.[644,645]

Despite relatively widespread use of amiodarone, anesthetic complications infrequently have been reported. In two case reports, bradycardia and hypotension were prominent.[646,647] One of the reports described profound resistance to the vasoconstrictive effects of β-adrenergic agonists.[647] The slow decay of amiodarone in plasma and tissue makes such adverse reactions possible long after discontinuing its administration.

Because T_3 is reported to reverse electrophysiologic effects of amiodarone, T_3 possibly could be used to reverse hemodynamic abnormalities, such as those described in these two case reports, although this theory has not been tested. Epinephrine has been shown to be more effective than dobutamine or isoproterenol in reversing amiodarone-induced cardiac depression.[648]

A randomized, controlled study of amiodarone administered 6 days before and 6 days after cardiac surgery demonstrated significant reductions in atrial tachyarrhythmias and ventricular arrhythmias in different age patients and in different types of cardiac surgical procedures.[649] There were no differences in hospital mortality between groups. A study in CABG surgery patients showed amiodarone was more effective in converting AF than placebo.[650] All patients in this study received β-blockers. In children with postoperative junctional ectopic tachycardia, amiodarone was effective in either converting or slowing the HR in all 18 study patients.[651] Prophylactic amiodarone has also reduced the incidence of AF in lung resection[652] but did not reduce the incidence of AF in cardiac valvular surgery.[653]

Bretylium

Bretylium is a quaternary ammonium compound that produces a biphasic cardiac response after acute IV administration. Initially, norepinephrine is displaced from adrenergic nerve endings, and there are attendant increases in BP, SVR, and cardiac automaticity. After 20 to 30 minutes, this response wanes and the adrenergic-blocking effects of bretylium predominate.[654–656] These latter effects depend on uptake of bretylium by adrenergic neurons; however, inhibition of its adrenergic-blocking effects does not impair the antiarrhythmic effect.

The direct electrophysiologic effect of bretylium is prolongation of the ventricular ERP. In this regard, the electrophysiologic effect correlates with the myocardial rather than the plasma concentrations of bretylium.[657] Bretylium delays conduction of premature impulses from normal myocardium to the border of ischemic zones and decreases the disparity between the excitation thresholds of adjoining zones of ischemic and normal myocardium. Bretylium increases the electric current required to induce VF and may spontaneously convert VF to sinus rhythm.[658] The antiarrhythmic effect of bretylium is undiminished by cardiac denervation or chronic reserpine treatment, which indicates that the antiarrhythmic effects are dissociated from the antiadrenergic effects.[659,660] Bretylium also decreases the amount of electrical current required to produce defibrillation.[661]

Results of clinical trials of bretylium in acute cardiac arrest are inconsistent. In one study in which it was compared with lidocaine, bretylium did not have a better antiarrhythmic effect, improve resuscitation, or lower mortality.[662] In contrast, in another study, bretylium (10 mg/kg) was used as a first-line treatment for out-of-hospital VF and significantly improved the outcome from resuscitation; lidocaine administered after bretylium also decreased the incidence of recurrent VF.[663] In the acute setting, bretylium is effective prophylaxis against VF.[624,664–667]

Clinical indications for bretylium include refractory VT or VF. For VF, bretylium is administered as a 5- to 10-mg/kg IV bolus, which can be repeated to a total dose of 30 mg/kg if VF persists. The antifibrillatory effect may require some time to develop, so full resuscitative efforts should continue for at least 20 to 30 minutes after bretylium has been administered. Administration for recurrent VT is similar to that for VF. Continuous infusion of 2 mg/min may be used to maintain plasma levels. As with VF, the effect of bretylium in VT may take 20 to 30 minutes to manifest.

Adverse reactions to bretylium include nausea and vomiting in conscious patients. During chronic therapy, postural hypotension may develop, but it is reduced by tricyclic drugs, which block uptake of bretylium by adrenergic neurons.

Sotalol

Sotalol is classified as a Class III agent, but also has Class II β-adrenergic–blocking properties. Sotalol was first synthesized as a β-blocker and was initially used to treat angina and hypertension. The antiarrhythmic effect quickly was recognized and the antiarrhythmic actions then were evaluated. Sotalol prolongs refractoriness in both atrial and ventricular tissues because of blockade of the delayed rectifier potassium current. The β-blocking effects result in decreased HR and increased refractory periods at both the atrial and ventricular levels.[668] It is indicated for life-threatening ventricular arrhythmias and AF.

Sotalol exists as a mixture of the d- and l-isomers. These two isomers have different mechanisms of action. Sotalol can be administered orally or intravenously. Oral bioavailability is greater than 90%. The drug is poorly bound to plasma protein and undergoes renal excretion with an elimination half-life of 12 hours when renal function is normal. The usual starting oral dose is 80 to 160 mg every 12 hours. Peak plasma concentration is seen within 4 hours.[669]

Sotalol has been used to treat both supraventricular and ventricular tachyarrhythmias. Sotalol was found to be superior to Class I agents in preventing the recurrence of ventricular arrhythmias.[670] To investigate the contribution of the β-blocking property to the efficacy of sotalol, Class I agents with or without β-blocker were compared with sotalol.[671] Sotalol was more effective in preventing the recurrence of arrhythmias than Class I agents with or without β-blockers. However, the mortality rates were similar when sotalol was compared with the combined Class I and β-blocker regimen. Sotalol also is effective in the prevention of PSVTs.[672]

Sotalol administration is not without side effects. In fact, a large prospective study of d-sotalol (not the mixture of d- and l-isomers) in patients with reduced LV function was terminated early because of increased mortality in the treatment group.[673]

d-Sotalol lacks a significant β-adrenergic-receptor—blocking property, which may explain these findings. In addition, sotalol administration is associated with increased risk for torsades de pointes and QT-interval prolongation. Female patients and patients with renal failure are at increased risk for the proarrhythmic side effects.

Ibutilide

Ibutilide fumarate is a methanesulfonanilide antiarrhythmic agent that is approved for the conversion of atrial flutter and AF to sinus rhythm. Ibutilide prolongs the cardiac refractory period at both the atrial and ventricular levels by activating a slow inward sodium current.[674] In addition, ibutilide may cause the blockade of the rapid outward delayed rectifier potassium current, which also leads to prolongation of the cardiac refractory period.[675] In vitro and at high dose, ibutilide may shorten action potential, although this effect has not been observed clinically. Ibutilide may also predispose to the formation of afterdepolarizations, which may be involved in the development of torsades de pointes.

Ibutilide is administered intravenously, is 40% protein bound, and undergoes hepatic metabolism. There are eight metabolites, only one with slight antiarrhythmic activity. The pharmacokinetics of ibutilide is linear. There is rapid extravascular distribution and systemic clearance is high, with the elimination half-life ranging from 2 to 6 hours.[676] The usual dose is 1 mg administered over 10 minutes. This may be followed by a second dose of 0.5 to 1 mg.

In one study, ibutilide, 0.015 mg/kg, administered intravenously over 10 minutes, resulted in conversion to sinus rhythm of about 45% of patients with atrial flutter longer than 3 hours in duration or AF 3 hours to 90 days in duration.[677] The arrhythmia was terminated in 3% of patients receiving placebo. The mean time to termination of arrhythmia was 19 minutes from the start of the infusion. In this study, termination of arrhythmias was unaffected by an enlarged left atrium, decreased EF, presence of valvular heart disease, or the use of concomitant medications such as β-blocking agents and digoxin.

In another study, the safety and efficacy of repeated IV doses were evaluated.[678] The investigators found a similar conversion rate to the previously mentioned study. In addition, they found that efficacy was greater in atrial flutter than fibrillation (63% vs. 31%). In AF, conversion rates were greater in patients with shorter arrhythmia duration or a normal left atrial size. However, the duration of arrhythmias in all patients in this study was less than 45 days. Conversion rates of AF or flutter are enhanced with the concurrent use of magnesium.[679]

Cardiovascular side effects occur in about 25% of patients treated with ibutilide, compared with 7% for the placebo-treated group.[680] Torsades de pointes occurred in 4.3% of these patients. Most of the proarrhythmic activity was seen within 1 hour of termination of the infusion, reflecting the short half-life and lack of metabolites with significant antiarrhythmic properties. Bradycardia, low body weight, and a history of CHF were predictive of the occurrence of torsades de pointes. Electrolyte abnormalities and acquired prolonged QT interval should be corrected before ibutilide therapy.

Dofetilide

Dofetilide blocks the rapid component of the delayed rectifier potassium current of repolarization without slowing conduction. Similar to ibutilide, dofetilide has a profound effect on prolonging the QT interval. Atrial tissue is more affected by dofetilide's electrophysiologic effects than ventricular tissue. Thus, dofetilide is indicated for acute conversion and chronic suppression of AF.[681]

Dofetilide is only available orally and results in 90% bioavailability. About 50% of the drug is excreted in the urine with an elimination half-life of 8 to 12 hours. Several drugs have been shown to increase dofetilide serum concentrations including verapamil, cimetidine, and ketoconazole. These drugs should be avoided or used with caution in combination with dofetilide.

Dosing is from 0.125 to 0.5 mg twice a day and should be performed during electrocardiographic monitoring and measuring of the QT interval. QT prolongation with polymorphic VT may occur in up to 4% of patients. Any electrolyte abnormalities should be corrected before administering this drug. Patients with prolonged QT intervals or history of torsades de pointes should not receive chronic therapy. The concurrent use of magnesium enhanced the conversion of AF or atrial flutter with dofetilide and theoretically might reduce the incidence of QT prolongation.[682] No patients who received magnesium in this study developed torsades de pointes.

Class IV: Calcium Channel Antagonists

Although the principal direct electrophysiologic effects of the three main chemical groups of calcium antagonists (verapamil, a benzoacetonitrite; nifedipine, a dihydropyridine; and diltiazem, a benzothiazepine) are similar, verapamil and diltiazem are the primary antiarrhythmics.

As with other transmembrane ionic channels, the calcium channel is conceptualized as macromolecular protein that spans the ion-impermeable lipid bilayer of the membrane (Figure 10-29). Such channels exhibit selectivity both for a particular ionic species and for specific transmembrane electrical potential ranges to control the permeability of the pore.[198] The decreased membrane potential produced by depolarization increases the permeability of the Ca^{2+} channel for Ca^{2+}, which permits Ca^{2+} to pass down its concentration gradient into the cell. Conversely, the "gate" closes on repolarization. This mechanism has been termed the *voltage-dependent* or *voltage-gated* channel. In cardiac tissue, the Ca^{2+} channel is also controlled by membrane β-adrenergic receptors; activation of $β_1$ receptors recruits additional Ca^{2+} channels to the open or active state, and such channels are termed *receptor-operated* channels.[683]

Based on studies with the sodium channels in the giant axons of squid, three different activity states of the Ca^{2+} channel have been distinguished: resting, open, and inactive. The resting state of the Ca^{2+} channel is characterized by a closed activation (*d*) gate on the external surface of the membrane and an opened inactivation (*f*) gate on the internal surface[684] (Figure 10-30). Depolarization triggers the open state when the *d* gate relaxes to permit Ca^{2+} influx, and also triggers the slower closure of the *f* gate, which, when complete, blocks further Ca^{2+} influx; the resulting "inactive" state persists until complete repolarization resets both gates. For the Ca^{2+} channel, the time constant for the transition from the resting to the open state is 520 milliseconds, that from the open to the inactive state is 30 to 300 milliseconds, and that from the inactive to the resting state is also 30 to 300 milliseconds.[685]

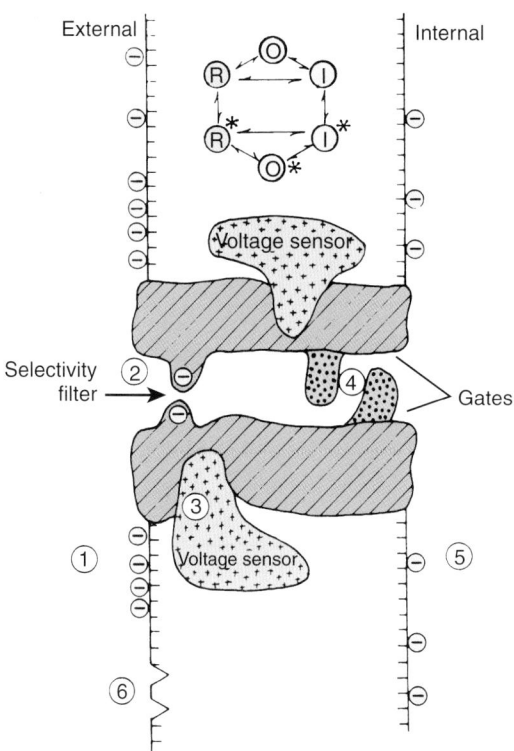

Figure 10-29 Schematic representation of a calcium channel depicted as a proteinaceous membrane pore. A selectivity filter *(2)* confers ion selectivity by specific molecular dimension and change density characteristics. Voltage sensor components *(3)* link membrane depolarization with channel opening and closing via the gating mechanism *(4)*. Negatively charged sites on the external surface serve as calcium binding sites *(1)*. (From Triggle DJ: Biochemical pharmacology of calcium blockers. In Flaim SF, Zelis R [eds]: Calcium blockers: Mechanisms of action and clinical applications. Baltimore: Urban and Schwarzenberg, 1982, pp 121–134.)

The "use dependence" noted with Ca^{2+} antagonists is the direct relation between the antagonist effect and the frequency of tissue activation. Thus, in cardiac tissue, the negative inotropic and Ca^{2+} channel-blocking properties of verapamil depend on both transmembrane potential and stimulation frequency; the inhibitory activity increases with increased frequency and with partial depolarization.[686] Such findings may indicate that verapamil interacts primarily with the inactive (depolarized) state of the Ca^{2+} channel. In contrast, the activation state of the membrane is less important for the inhibitory action of nifedipine.

The lipophilic nature of Ca^{2+} channel antagonists is important to their effect. In skinned cardiac cells, D600, a congener of verapamil, is ineffective, which would appear to indicate a primary effect of the drug at the plasma membrane.[687] Likewise, quaternary ammonium derivatives of D600 and nifedipine, which are highly ionized and therefore less lipophilic, are also less effective Ca^{2+} channel antagonists.[686] Such data indicate that perhaps the locus of activity of these Ca^{2+} channel antagonists is the internal surface of the channel or within the membrane itself.

In general, the drugs commonly classified as Ca^{2+} channel antagonists, typified by verapamil, diltiazem, nifedipine, and nicardipine, exhibit specificity for vascular smooth muscle and cardiac tissues; however, within the group, specificity for these tissues varies. Nifedipine and nicardipine (and other dihydropyridines) are more potent in smooth muscle than cardiac tissue, whereas verapamil and diltiazem are more potent in cardiac tissue.[688,689] Although Ca^{2+} channel antagonism is the dominant effect of these agents, at sufficiently high (>10⁶ M) concentrations, other effects become notable. For example, verapamil and D600 at concentrations greater than 10⁶ M inhibit sodium

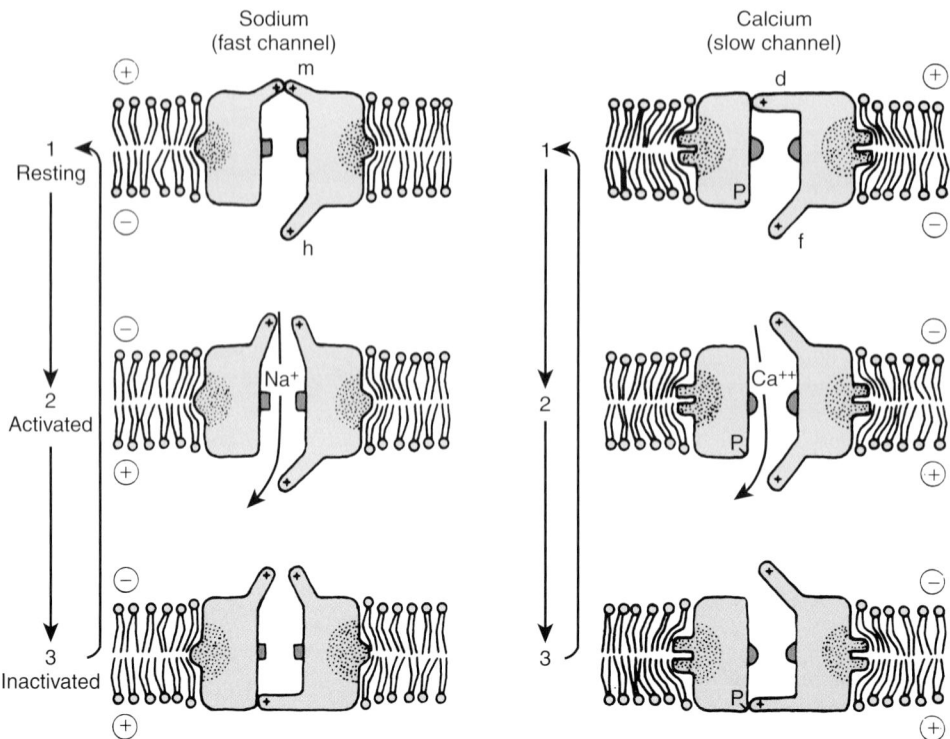

Figure 10-30 **Schematic depiction of the calcium channel in the sarcolemmal membrane.** The upstroke (phase 0) of the action potential, which allows rapid entry of sodium into the cell, produces the opening of the activation gates (m) in the sodium channel. The resulting change in trans-membrane potential closes the inactivation gate (h), which stops sodium influx but maintains a refractory state in the cell membrane until repolarization. Similar processes occur in the calcium-channel activation gate (d) and inactivation gate (f), except that at least some of the steps in slow channel activation require phosphorylation (P) by a cyclic adenosine monophosphate protein kinase. Changes in the conformation of the channel proteins provide the three functional states of the channel: (1) resting (closed and able to open); (2) activated (open); and (3) inactivated (closed and unable to open in response to depolarization). (From Katz AM, Messineo FC: Lipids and membrane function: Implications in arrhythmias. Hosp Pract 16:49, 1981.)

channel activity and receptor binding at muscarinic, adrenergic, and opiate receptors.[690] These latter effects do not exhibit stereoselectivity as does Ca^{2+}-channel–specific action.[691]

Verapamil and Diltiazem

Verapamil and diltiazem have been used extensively in the treatment of supraventricular arrhythmias, AF, and atrial flutter. They are especially effective at preventing or terminating PSVT by blocking impulse transmission through the AV node by prolonging AV nodal conduction and refractoriness.[692] They are also useful in the treatment of AF and atrial flutter by slowing AV nodal conduction and decreasing the ventricular response. The effect on ventricular response is similar to that of the cardiac glycosides, although the onset is more rapid and acutely effective for control of tachycardia in patients.[693,694]

In the perioperative period, verapamil is a useful antiarrhythmic agent. In one study of anesthetized patients, it successfully controlled a variety of supraventricular and ventricular arrhythmias.[694] However, verapamil should be used with caution intraoperatively because, in conjunction with inhalation anesthetics, significant cardiac depression may occur.[695,696]

A significant precaution in the use of verapamil and diltiazem to treat PSVT involves pre-excitation of the AV node in Wolff–Parkinson–White syndrome. If PSVT is orthodromic (anterograde conduction through the AV node and retrograde over the accessory pathway) with a narrow or normal QRS complex, verapamil has a high success rate by blocking anterograde AV nodal conduction. If the PSVT is antidromic (anterograde conduction through accessory pathway and retrograde over the AV node) with a widened QRS complex, successful blockade with verapamil is unlikely because it has little effect on refractoriness or conduction in accessory pathways. Atrial flutter and AF also may occur in Wolff–Parkinson–White syndrome. In this setting, agents that

shorten the ERP of the accessory pathway or increase the ERP in the AV node (e.g., digitalis, verapamil) often will increase ventricular response and may precipitate VF.[697] Type I and III drugs, such as procainamide or amiodarone, are more effective in slowing the ventricular response in AF with an accessory pathway (see Chapter 4).

Electrophysiologic effects of verapamil and diltiazem are seen predominantly in tissues in which phase 0 or 4 depolarization is largely calcium dependent, namely, SA and AV nodes. Discharge rate and recovery time in the SA, AV conduction time, and AV node ERP are prolonged. Clinically, the QRS complex and QT_c interval are not significantly affected, but AH (but not HV) conduction time is prolonged. Electrophysiologic effects of verapamil have been shown experimentally (in anesthetized dogs) to relate to plasma concentration; the AH interval was prolonged at lower concentrations than were necessary to slow the SA node or to produce AV block.[698]

As with several other antiarrhythmic drugs, the pharmacokinetics of intravenously and orally administered verapamil differ. The hepatic extraction of orally administered verapamil is extensive; as a result, its bioavailability, which is normally low, is increased significantly by liver disease.[242] After IV administration of verapamil, plasma clearance approximates splanchnic blood flow rate and, because of its lipophilic nature, the apparent volume of distribution is large. Elimination half-life of verapamil is approximately 5 hours, but it may be longer with chronic administration, perhaps because of saturation of hepatic metabolic pathways. Also, a principal metabolite, norverapamil, is biologically active, accumulates to concentrations equal to those of verapamil during chronic therapy, and has a longer half-life (8 to 13 hours).[699] Excretion of verapamil after metabolism is renal (65% to 70%), but 3% to 4% is excreted unchanged.[697] Metabolism involves n-dealkylation and O-demethylation with norverapamil (one eighth of the Ca^{2+}-channel–blocking potency of verapamil) as the major metabolite.[688] Verapamil and metabolites are highly protein bound (90%).

Verapamil dosage for acute IV treatment of PSVT is 0.07 to 0.15 mg/kg over 1 minute, with the same dose repeated after 30 minutes if the initial response is inadequate (10 mg maximum). Because the cardiovascular depressant effects of the inhalation anesthetics involve inhibition of calcium-related intracellular processes, the interaction of verapamil and these anesthetics is synergistic. In one large clinical series, verapamil given during steady-state halothane anesthesia transiently decreased BP and produced a 4% incidence of PR-interval prolongation.[700] In laboratory studies, verapamil interacts similarly with halothane, enflurane, and isoflurane to mildly depress ventricular function and to slow AV conduction (PR interval).[695] AV block can occur, however, and may be refractory. In addition, AV block can occur when verapamil is combined with β-blockers.

Diltiazem in doses of 0.25 to 0.30 mg/kg administered intravenously followed by a titratable IV infusion of 10 to 20 mg/hr has been shown to be rapid acting and efficacious in controlling ventricular response rate in new-onset AF and atrial flutter.[701,702] In addition, the prophylactic use of IV diltiazem has been shown to reduce the incidence of postoperative supraventricular arrhythmias after pneumonectomy and cardiac surgery.[703] Diltiazem also may have a role in treating ventricular arrhythmias. In an experimental model, diltiazem has been shown to be protective against VF with acute cocaine toxicity.[704]

Another adverse effect of verapamil is the potentiation of neuromuscular blockade. In two laboratory studies, verapamil depressed twitch height response to indirect stimulation.[705,706] Although the exact presynaptic versus postsynaptic site of the block was not determined, the qualitative similarity of the effect to that of pancuronium suggested an effect at the neuromuscular junction. At clinically relevant doses of verapamil, the effect is slight, but the clinical potential for synergistic interaction with residual muscle relaxants seems substantial. Cautious clinical attention to neuromuscular function is necessary to safely use verapamil in patients who are receiving or have recently received muscle relaxants.

Diltiazem proved equally as effective as amiodarone in managing postoperative AF occurring after lung resection surgery.[707] Another study in coronary artery surgery demonstrated diltiazem prophylaxis reduced the incidence of AF administered either intravenously or orally.[708]

Other Antiarrhythmic Agents

Digoxin

The primary therapeutic use of digitalis drugs is to slow the ventricular response during AF or atrial flutter, which occurs because of a complex combination of direct and indirect actions on the AV node. The primary direct pharmacologic effect of digitalis is inhibition of the membrane-bound Na-K–dependent ATPase. This enzyme provides the chemical energy necessary for the transport of sodium (out) and potassium (in) during repolarization. The glycosides bind to the enzyme in a specific saturable way that inhibits enzyme activity and impairs the active transport of sodium and potassium. The net result is a slight increase in intracellular sodium and a corresponding decrease in intracellular potassium concentration. The sodium exchanges for calcium, resulting in a relatively weak inotropic effect.

In Purkinje fibers, digoxin increases the slope of phase 4 depolarization and decreases resting potential or maximal diastolic potential so that the initiation of depolarization (phase 0) begins at a less negative potential; therefore, both the V_{max} and the conduction velocity of the action potential are lower. The phase 4 effect is inversely related to extracellular potassium concentration. At low concentrations of potassium, the increased rate of phase 4 depolarization is augmented and automaticity increases, which may partially explain the increased risk for digoxin-related toxicity during hypokalemia or pronounced potassium fluxes, such as during cardioversion or in the period immediately surrounding CPB. At concentrations approaching toxicity, digoxin produces delayed afterpotentials, which may be sufficient to reach threshold and trigger depolarization.[709-711] The direct action of therapeutic concentrations of digoxin in Purkinje fibers, therefore, decreases conduction velocity and increases ERP.

In specialized conduction fibers in the SA and AV nodes, similar electrophysiologic effects occur; in both of these regions, however, the dominant effects are indirect and mediated by the ANS. In atrial and ventricular muscle, direct effects resemble those in Purkinje fibers. The indirect effects of digitalis, notably a decreased APD, account for the decreased QT interval in the ECG; effects of this drug during phases 2 and 3 of the action potential account for the characteristic downward convexity of the ST segment.[712]

Digoxin increases vagal efferent activity, the origin of which may relate to increased sensitivity of arterial baroreceptors and an increased carotid sinus nerve activity, or to an effect on the central vagal nuclei.[713-715] In addition, SA node sensitivity to acetylcholine may be enhanced by digoxin. In high concentrations, digoxin may decrease SA and AV nodal sensitivities to catecholamines and sympathetic stimulation, although this may be because of increased sympathetic efferent activity produced by both the CNS (medulla) effects of digoxin and the inhibition of norepinephrine uptake at peripheral sympathetic nerve terminals.[714,715] The decreased sinus rate seen with digoxin is, therefore, due, in part, to both increased vagal efferent activity and decreased sympathetic tone.

The AV node is the portion of the conduction system most strongly influenced by both the direct and indirect effects of digoxin. Conduction through the AV node is slowed, and the ERP of the AV node is lengthened by digoxin. In toxic concentrations, digoxin can effectively block AV nodal transmission.

In atrial tissue, the direct and indirect (vagal) effects of digoxin are opposed. The direct effect is an increase in APD, but the indirect effect (mediated by acetylcholine release) is marked decreases in APD and ERP. At therapeutic concentrations, the indirect effect predominates, which makes the atria responsive to higher stimulation frequencies.[712] The frequency of atrial impulses arriving at the AV node generally is increased, which leads to frequent partial depolarization of the AV node *(concealed conduction)*. This effect, plus the increased AV nodal ERP (produced by direct effects, vagal effects, and sympatholytic effects), result in a net decrease in the frequency of impulses that successfully traverse the AV node to depolarize the His-Purkinje system.

The main preparation of cardiac glycosides available is digoxin. Digoxin reaches peak effects in 1.5 to 2 hours but has a significant effect within 5 to 30 minutes. For undigitalized patients, the initial dose is 0.5 to 0.75 mg digoxin, with subsequent doses of 0.125 to 0.25 mg. The usual total digitalizing dose ranges from 0.75 to 1.0 mg by the IV route. Digoxin is approximately 25% protein bound, and the therapeutic range of plasma concentrations is 0.5 to 2.0 ng/mL.

Adenosine

Adenosine is a virtually ubiquitous endogenous nucleoside that has potent electrophysiologic effects in addition to having a major physiologic role in regulation of vasomotor tone.[716] Adenosine is unique in that it is produced as an intermediate metabolite of adenosine monophosphate. It has an extremely short half-life in plasma (on the order of 1.5 to 2 seconds) because of metabolism by adenosine deaminase to inosine, or by adenosine kinase to adenosine monophosphate. Both enzymes are contained within the intracellular compartment (cytosolic), indicating a rapid transmembrane transport system for adenosine. Inhibition of this transport system by dipyridamole markedly enhances the cardiac effects of adenosine.

The important cardiac electrophysiologic effects of adenosine are mediated by the A_1 receptor and consist of negative chronotropic, dromotropic, and inotropic actions. Adenosine decreases SA node activity, AV node conductivity, and ventricular automaticity. In many ways, these effects mimic those of acetylcholine. The A_1 receptor is linked to the ionic channel for K^+ and Ca^{2+} and to adenylyl cyclase through guanine nucleotide–binding inhibitory protein (G_i). Activation of the A_1 receptor in the SA and AV nodes activates the outward acetylcholine-adenosine–regulated potassium current. In ventricular myocardium, adenosine antagonizes the stimulation of the inward Ca^{2+} current produced by catecholamines. The primary antiarrhythmic effect of adenosine is to interrupt reentrant AV nodal tachycardia, and this effect most likely relates to the potassium current effects.

For clinical use, adenosine must be administered by a rapid IV bolus in a dose of 100 to 200 μg/kg, although continuous IV infusions of 150 to 300 μg/kg/min have been used to produce controlled hypotension. For practical purposes, in adults, a dose of 3 to 6 mg is given by IV bolus followed by a second dose of 6 to 12 mg after 1 minute if the first dose was not effective. This therapy rapidly interrupts narrow-complex tachycardia caused by AV nodal reentry.[717] Comparison with verapamil has shown adenosine to be equally effective as an antiarrhythmic, but with the advantages of fewer adverse hemodynamic effects, a faster onset of action, and a more rapid elimination so that undesired effects are short-lived.[718] The median effective close range (MD$_{50}$) of adenosine for reentrant supraventricular arrhythmias in children is 100 to 150 μg/kg.[719]

Potassium

Because of the close relation between extracellular pH and potassium, the primary mechanism of pH-induced arrhythmias may be alteration of potassium concentration. Both hypokalemia and hyperkalemia are associated with cardiac arrhythmias; however, hypokalemia is more common perioperatively in cardiac surgical patients and is more commonly associated with arrhythmias.[720] Decreasing extracellular potassium concentration increases the peak negative diastolic potential, which would theoretically appear to decrease the likelihood of spontaneous depolarization. However, because the permeability of the myocardial cell membrane to potassium is directly related to extracellular potassium concentration, hypokalemia decreases cellular permeability to potassium. This prolongs the action potential by slowing repolarization, which, in turn, slows conduction and increases the dispersion of recovery of excitability, and thus predisposes to the development of arrhythmias. Electrocardiographic correlates of hypokalemia include appearance of a U wave and increased P-wave amplitude.[721] The arrhythmias most commonly associated with hypokalemia are premature atrial contractions, atrial tachycardia, and supraventricular tachycardia. Hypokalemia also accentuates the toxicity of cardiac glycosides.

Moderate hyperkalemia, in contrast, increases membrane permeability to potassium, which increases the speed of repolarization and decreases APD, thereby decreasing the tendency to arrhythmias. An increased potassium concentration also affects pacemaker activity. The increased potassium permeability caused by hyperkalemia decreases the rate of spontaneous diastolic depolarization, which slows HR and, in the extreme case, can produce asystole. The repolarization abnormalities of hyperkalemia lead to the characteristic ECG findings of T-wave peaking, prolonged PR interval, decreased QRS amplitude, and a widened QRS complex.[722] Both AV and intraventricular conduction abnormalities result from the slowed conduction and uneven repolarization.

Treatment of hyperkalemia is based on its magnitude and on the clinical presentation. For life-threatening, hyperkalemia-induced arrhythmias, the principle is rapid reduction of extracellular potassium concentration, a treatment that does not acutely decrease total body potassium content. Calcium chloride, 10 to 20 mg/kg, given by IV infusion, will directly antagonize the effects of potassium on the cardiac cell membranes. Sodium bicarbonate, 1 to 2 mEq/kg, or a dose calculated from acid-base measurements to produce moderate alkalinity (pH ≈7.45 to 7.50), will shift potassium intracellularly. A change in pH of 0.1 unit produces a 0.5- to 1.5-mEq/L change of potassium concentration in the opposite direction. An IV infusion of glucose and insulin has a similar effect; glucose at a dose of 0.5 to 2.0 g/kg with insulin in the ratio of 1 unit to 4 g glucose is appropriate. Sequential measurement of serum potassium is important with this treatment because marked hypokalemia can result. Loop diuretics and potassium-binding resins promote excretion of potassium, although the effects are less rapid than with the previously mentioned modalities (see Chapter 37).

With chronic potassium deficiency, the plasma level poorly reflects the total body deficit. Because only 2% of total body potassium is in plasma, and total body potassium stores may be 2000 to 3000 mEq, a 25% decline in serum potassium from 4 to 3 mEq/L indicates an equilibrium total body deficiency of 500 to 800 mEq, replacement of which should be undertaken slowly.

Acute hypokalemia frequently occurs after CPB as a result of hemodilution, urinary losses, and intracellular shifts,[723] the latter perhaps relating to abnormalities of the glucose-insulin system seen with nonpulsatile hypothermic CPB.[724] With frequent assessment of serum potassium concentrations and continuous ECG monitoring, potassium infusion at rates of up to 10 to 15 mEq/hr may be administered to treat serious hypokalemia.

Magnesium

Magnesium deficiency also is a relatively common electrolyte abnormality in critically ill patients, especially in chronic situations. Hypomagnesemia is associated with a variety of cardiovascular disturbances, including arrhythmias.[725,726] Sudden death from CAD, alcoholic cardiomyopathy, and CHF may involve magnesium deficiency.[725-727] Functionally, magnesium is required for the membrane-bound Na^+/K^+-ATPase, which is the principal enzyme that maintains normal intracellular potassium concentration. Not surprisingly, the ECG findings seen with magnesium deficiency mimic those seen with hypokalemia: prolonged PR and QT intervals, increased QRS duration, and ST-segment abnormalities. In addition, as with hypokalemia, magnesium deficiency predisposes to the development of the arrhythmias produced by cardiac glycosides.[728,729] Magnesium is effective as an adjuvant in therapy of patients with a prolonged QT syndrome and torsades de pointes.[730]

Arrhythmias induced by magnesium deficiency may be refractory to treatment with antiarrhythmic drugs and either electrical cardioversion or defibrillation. For this reason, adjunctive treatment of refractory arrhythmias with magnesium has been advocated even when magnesium deficiency has not been documented.[731] Magnesium deficiency is common in cardiac surgery patients because of the diuretic agents these patients are often receiving and because magnesium levels decrease with CPB because of hemodilution of the pump. Magnesium lacks a counter-regulatory hormone to increase magnesium levels during CPB in contrast with the hypocalcemia that is corrected by PTH. The results of magnesium administration trials involving CABG have been conflicting. Some studies have shown a benefit and others have not in regard to reducing the incidence of postoperative arrhythmias.

Magnesium has been studied alone and in combination with other drugs in the prophylaxis and treatment of perioperative arrhythmias. In younger patients with good LV function, magnesium reduced the incidence of AF after CABG surgery.[732] Magnesium supplementation after CPB in which the serum magnesium level returned to normal reduced the incidence of AF.[733] A protocol using magnesium as first-line therapy and amiodarone as backup therapy appears effective in management of arrhythmias after surgery, as well as in critically ill patients.[734,735] Combination therapy with magnesium and sotalol after coronary artery bypass reduced the incidence of AF.[736] A meta-analysis of 15 randomized, controlled trials showed magnesium to be effective at preventing AF in coronary artery surgery.[737] However, magnesium, when added to oral β-blocker prophylaxis, did not reduce the incidence of atrial arrhythmias.[738]

REFERENCES

1. Anderson JL, Adams CD, Antman EM, et al: ACC/AHA 2007 guidelines for the management of patients with unstable angina/non-ST-elevation myocardial infarction: A report of the American College of Cardiology/American Heart Association Task Force on Practice Guidelines (Writing Committee to Revise the 2002 Guidelines for the Management of Patient With Unstable Angina/Non-ST-Elevation Myocardial Infarction), *Circulation* 116:e148, 2007.
2. Rutherford JR: Medical management. In Fuster V, Topol E, Nabel E, editors: *Atherothrombosis and coronary artery disease,* Philadelphia, 2005, Lippincott, pp 1327–1337.
3. Horowitz JD: Role of nitrates in unstable angina pectoris, *Am J Cardiol* 70:64B, 1992.
4. Hill JA, Feldman RL, Pepine CJ, et al: Randomized double-blind comparison of nifedipine and isosorbide dinitrate in patients with coronary arterial spasm, *Am J Cardiol* 49:431, 1982.
5. Purcell H, Mulcahy D, Fox K: Nitrates in silent ischemia, *Cardiovasc Drugs Ther* 8:727, 1994.
6. Hoekenga D, Abrams J: Rational medical therapy for stable angina pectoris, *Am J Med* 76:309, 1984.
7. Abrams J: Usefulness of long-acting nitrates in cardiovascular disease, *Am J Med* 64:183, 1978.
8. Miller RR, Awan NA, DeMaria AN, et al: Importance of maintaining systemic blood pressure during nitroglycerin administration for reducing ischemic injury in patients with coronary disease. Effects on CBF, myocardial energetics and left ventricular function, *Am J Cardiol* 40:504, 1977.
9. Abrams J: Mechanisms of action of the organic nitrates in the treatment of myocardial ischemia, *Am J Cardiol* 70:30B, 1992.
10. Murad F: Cyclic guanosine monophosphate as a mediator of vasodilation, *J Clin Invest* 78:1, 1986.
11. Needleman P, Jakschik B, Johnson EM Jr: Sulfhydryl requirement for relaxation of vascular smooth muscle, *J Pharmacol Exp Ther* 187:324, 1973.

12. Galvas PE, DiSalvo J: Concentration and time-dependent relationships between isosorbide dinitrate-induced relaxation and formation of cyclic GMP in coronary arterial smooth muscle, *J Pharmacol Exp Ther* 224:373, 1983.
13. Anderson TJ, Meredith IT, Ganz P, et al: Nitric oxide and nitrovasodilators: Similarities, differences, and potential interactions, *J Am Coll Cardiol* 24:555, 1994.
14. Waldman SA, Murad F: Cyclic GMP synthesis and function, *Pharmacol Rev* 39:163, 1987.
15. Hardman JG, Limbird LE, editors: *Goodman and Gilman's the pharmacological basis of therapeutics*, New York, McGraw-Hill, 1996.
16. Opie LH, editor: *Drugs for the heart*, ed 6 Philadelphia, 2005, Elsevier, pp 33–49.
17. Armstrong PW, Moffat JA: Tolerance to organic nitrates: Clinical and experimental perspectives, *Am J Med* 74:73, 1983.
18. Packer M, Lee WH, Kassler PD, et al: Prevention and reversal of nitrate tolerance in patients with congestive heart failure, *N Engl J Med* 317:799, 1987.
19. Fung HL, Sutton SC, Kamiya A: Blood vessel uptake and metabolism of organic nitrates in the rat, *J Pharmacol Exp Ther* 228:334, 1984.
20. Imhof PR, Ott B, Frankhauser P, et al: Difference in nitroglycerin dose-response in the venous and arterial beds, *Eur J Clin Pharmacol* 18:455, 1980.
21. Smith ER, Smiseth OA, Kingma I, et al: Mechanism of action of nitrates. Role of changes in venous capacitance and in the left ventricular diastolic pressure-volume relation, *Am J Med* 76:14, 1984.
22. Simon AC, Levenson JA, Levy BY, et al: Effect of nitroglycerin on peripheral large arteries in hypertension, *Br J Clin Pharmacol* 14:241, 1982.
23. Abrams J: Hemodynamic effects of nitroglycerin and long-acting nitrates, *Am Heart J* 110:216, 1985.
24. McGregor M: Pathogenesis of angina pectoris and role of nitrates in relief of myocardial ischemia, *Am J Med* 74:21, 1983.
25. Pearl RG, Rosenthal MH, Schroeder JS, et al: Acute hemodynamic effects of nitroglycerin in pulmonary hypertension, *Ann Intern Med* 99:9, 1983.
26. Ilbawi MN, Idriss FS, DeLeon SY, et al: Hemodynamic effects of intravenous nitroglycerin in pediatric patients after heart surgery, *Circulation* 72:II–101, 1985.
27. Vatner SF, Pagani M, Rutherford JD, et al: Effects of nitroglycerin on cardiac function and regional blood flow distribution in conscious dogs, *Am J Physiol* 234:H244, 1978.
28. Brown G, Bolson E, Peterson RB, et al: The mechanisms of nitroglycerin action. Stenosis vasodilatation as a major component of drug response, *Circulation* 64:1089, 1981.
29. Conti CR, Feldman RL, Pepine CJ, et al: Effect of glyceryl trinitrate on coronary and systemic hemodynamics in man, *Am J Med* 74:28, 1983.
30. Feldman RL, Pepine CJ, Conti CR: Magnitude of dilatation of large and small coronary arteries by nitroglycerin, *Circulation* 64:324, 1981.
31. Ludmer PL, Selwyn AP, Shook TL, et al: Paradoxical vasoconstriction induced by acetylcholine in atherosclerotic coronary arteries, *N Engl J Med* 315:1046, 1986.
32. Panzenbeck MJ, Baez A, Kaley G: Nitroglycerin and nitroprusside increase CBF in dogs by a mechanism independent of prostaglandin release, *Am J Cardiol* 53:936, 1984.
33. Horwitz LD, Gorlin R, Taylor WJ, et al: Effects of nitroglycerin on regional myocardial blood flow in coronary artery disease, *J Clin Invest* 50:1578, 1971.
34. Cohen MV, Downey JM, Sonnenblick EH, et al: The effects of nitroglycerin on coronary collaterals and myocardial contractility, *J Clin Invest* 52:2836, 1973.
35. Feldman RL, Joyal M, Conti CR, et al: Effect of nitroglycerin on coronary collateral flow and pressure during acute coronary occlusion, *Am J Cardiol* 54:958, 1984.
36. Moir TW: Subendocardial distribution of CBF and the effect of antianginal drugs, *Circ Res* 30:621, 1972.
37. Munzel T, Mulsch A, Kleschyov A: Mechanisms underlying nitroglycerin-induced superoxide production in platelets, *Circulation* 106:170, 2002.
38. Armstrong PW, Armstrong JA, Marks GS: Blood levels after sublingual nitroglycerin, *Circulation* 59:585, 1979.
39. Parker JO, Vankoughnett KA, Farrell B: Nitroglycerin lingual spray: Clinical efficacy and dose-response relation, *Am J Cardiol* 57:1, 1986.
40. Reichek N, Priest C, Kienzle M, et al: Angina prophylaxis with buccal nitroglycerin: A rapid onset long-acting nitrate, *Adv Pharmacother* 1:2, 1982.
41. Reichek N, Goldstein RE, Redwood DR, et al: Sustained effects of nitroglycerin ointment in patients with angina pectoris, *Circulation* 50:348, 1974.
42. Armstrong PW, Mathew MT, Boroomand K, et al: Nitroglycerin ointment in acute myocardial infarction, *Am J Cardiol* 38:474, 1976.
43. Chien YW: Pharmaceutical considerations of transdermal nitroglycerin delivery: The various approaches, *Am Heart J* 108:207, 1984.
44. DeMots H, Glasser SP: Intermittent transdermal nitroglycerin therapy in the treatment of chronic stable angina, *J Am Coll Cardiol* 13:786, 1989.
45. DePace NL, Herling IM, Kotler MN, et al: Intravenous nitroglycerin for rest angina. Potential pathophysiologic mechanisms of action, *Arch Intern Med* 142:1806, 1982.
46. Young JB, Pratt CM, Farmer JA, et al: Specialized delivery systems for intravenous nitroglycerin. Are they necessary? *Am J Med* 76:27, 1984.
47. Darling RC, Roughton FJW: The effect of methemoglobin on the equilibrium between oxygen and hemoglobin, *Am J Physiol* 137:56, 1942.
48. Smith RP, Olson MV: Drug-induced methemoglobinemia, *Semin Hematol* 10:253, 1973.
49. Kaplan KJ, Taber M, Teagarden JR, et al: Association of methemoglobinemia and intravenous nitroglycerin administration, *Am J Cardiol* 55:181, 1985.
50. Harris JC, Rumack BH, Peterson RG, et al: Methemoglobinemia resulting from absorption of nitrates, *JAMA* 242:2869, 1979.
51. Zurick AM, Wagner RH, Starr NJ, et al: Intravenous nitroglycerin, methemoglobinemia, and respiratory distress in a postoperative cardiac surgical patient, *Anesthesiology* 61:464, 1984.
52. Axelsson KL, Anderson RGG: Tolerance towards nitroglycerin, induced in vivo, is correlated to a reduced cGMP response and an alteration in cGMP turnover, *Eur J Pharmacol* 88:71, 1983.
53. Thadani U: Role of nitrates in angina pectoris, *Am J Cardiol* 70:43B, 1992.
54. Parker JD, Farrell B, Fenton T, et al: Counter-regulatory responses to continuous and intermittent therapy with nitroglycerin, *Circulation* 84:2336, 1991.
55. Parker JD, Parker JO: Effect of therapy with an angiotensin-converting enzyme inhibitor of hemodynamic and counterregulatory responses during continuous therapy with nitroglycerin, *J Am Coll Cardiol* 21:1445, 1993.
56. Dupuis J, Lalonde G, Lemieux R, Rouleau JL: Tolerance to intravenous nitroglycerin in patients with congestive heart failure: Role of increased intravascular volume, neurohumoral activation and lack of prevention with N-acetylcysteine, *J Am Coll Cardiol* 16:923, 1990.
57. Watanabe H, Kakihana M, Ohtsuka S, et al: Platelet cyclic GMP. A potentially useful indicator to evaluate the effects of nitroglycerin and nitrate tolerance, *Circulation* 88:29, 1993.
58. Bassan MM: The daylong pattern of the antianginal effect of long-term three times daily administered isosorbide dinitrate, *J Am Coll Cardiol* 16:936, 1990.
59. Parker JO, Amies MH, Hawkinson RW, et al: Intermittent transdermal nitroglycerin therapy in angina pectoris. Clinically effective without tolerance or rebound, *Circulation* 91:1368, 1995.
60. Munzel T, Heitzer T, Kurz S, et al: Dissociation of coronary vascular tolerance and neurohormonal adjustments during long-term nitroglycerin therapy in patients with stable coronary artery disease, *J Am Coll Cardiol* 27:297, 1996.
61. Mangione NJ, Glasser SP: Phenomenon of nitrate tolerance, *Am Heart J* 128:137, 1994.
62. Lange RL, Reid MS, Tresch DD, et al: Nonatheromatous ischemic heart disease following withdrawal from chronic industrial nitroglycerin exposure, *Circulation* 46:666, 1972.
63. Elkayam V, Kulick D, McIntosh N, et al: Incidence of early tolerance to hemodynamic effects of continuous infusion of nitroglycerin in patients with coronary artery disease and heart failure, *Circulation* 76:577, 1987.
64. Thadani U, Fung HL, Darke AC, et al: Oral isosorbide dinitrate in angina pectoris: Comparison of duration of action and dose-response relationship during acute and sustained therapy, *Am J Cardiol* 49:411, 1982.
65. Parker JO: Eccentric dosing with isosorbide-5-mononitrate in angina pectoris, *Am J Cardiol* 72:871, 1993.
66. Stamler JS, Loscalzo J: The antiplatelet effects of organic nitrates and related nitroso compounds in vitro and in vivo and their relevance to cardiovascular disorders, *J Am Coll Cardiol* 18:1529, 1991.
67. Lam JYT, Chesebro JH, Fuster V: Platelets, vasoconstriction and nitroglycerin during arterial wall injury. A new antithrombotic role for an old drug, *Circulation* 78:712, 1988.
68. Mellion BT, Ignarro LJ, Myers CB, et al: Inhibition of platelet aggregation by S-nitrosothiols. Heme-dependent activation of soluble guanylate cyclase and stimulation of cyclic GMP accumulation, *Mol Pharmacol* 23:653, 1983.
69. Stamler JS, Vaughan DE, Loscalzo J: Synergistic disaggregation of platelets by tissue-type plasminogen activator, prostaglandin E_1, and nitroglycerin, *Circ Res* 65:796, 1989.
70. Diodati J, Theroux P, Latour JG, et al: Effects of nitroglycerin at therapeutic doses on platelet aggregation in unstable angina pectoris and acute myocardial infarction, *Am J Cardiol* 66:683, 1990.
71. Negrescu EV, Sazonova LN, Baldenkov GN, et al: Relationship between the inhibition of receptor-induced increase in cytosolic free calcium concentration and the vasodilator effects of nitrates in patients with congestive heart failure, *Int J Cardiol* 26:175, 1990.
72. Pizzulli L, Nitsch J, Luderitz B: Inhibition of the heparin effect by nitroglycerin, *Dtsch Med Wochenschr* 113:1837, 1988.
73. Habbab MA, Haft JI: Heparin resistance induced by intravenous nitroglycerin. A word of caution when both drugs are used concomitantly, *Arch Intern Med* 147:857, 1987.
74. Becker RC, Corrao JM, Bovill EG, et al: Intravenous nitroglycerin-induced heparin resistance: A qualitative antithrombin III abnormality, *Am Heart J* 119:1254, 1990.
75. Stanek EJ, Nair RN, Munger MA: Nitroglycerin-induced heparin resistance (letter), *Am Heart J* 121:1849, 1991.
76. Bjornsson TD, Schneider DE, Hecht AR: Effects of *N*-deacetylation and *N*-desulfation of heparin on its anticoagulant activity and in vivo disposition, *J Pharmacol Exp Ther* 245:804, 1988.
77. Cheitlin MD, Hutter AMJ, Brindis RG, et al: ACA/AHA expert consensus document of sildenafil in patients with cardiovascular disease: American College of Cardiology/American Heart Association, *J Am Coll Cardiol* 33:273, 1999.
78. Viagra® (package insert): New York, 2010, Pfizer Labs. Available at: http://www.pfizer.com/files/products/uspi_viagra.pdf Accessed February 23, 2010.
79. Cialis® (package insert): Indianapolis, IN, 2010, Eli Lilly and Company. Available at: http://pi.lilly.com/us/cialis-pi.pdf Accessed February 23, 2010.
80. Levitra® (package insert): Wayne, NJ, 2008, Bayer HealthCare Pharmaceuticals. Available at: http://www.univgraph.com/bayer/inserts/levitra.pdf Accessed February 23, 2010.
81. Fleisher LA, Beckman JA, Brown KA, et al: 2009 ACCF/AHA focused update on perioperative beta blockade incorporated into the ACC/AHA 2007 guidelines on perioperative cardiovascular evaluation and care for noncardiac surgery: A report of the American College of Cardiology Foundation/American Heart Association Task Force on Practice Guidelines, *Circulation* 120:e169, 2009.
82. Auerbach AD, Goldman L: Beta-blockers and reduction of cardiac events in noncardiac surgery, *JAMA* 287:1435–1444, 2002.
83. London MJ, Zaugg M, Schaub MC, Spahn DR: Perioperative beta-adrenergic receptor blockade, *Anesthesiology* 100:170, 2004.
84. Stevens RD, Burri H, Tramer MR: Pharmacologic myocardial protection in patients undergoing noncardiac surgery: A quantitative systematic review, *Anesth Analg* 97:623, 2003.
85. Peter T, Norris RM, Clarke ED, et al: Reduction of enzyme levels of propranolol after acute myocardial infarction, *Circulation* 57:1091, 1978.
86. β-Blocker Heart Attack Trial Research Group: A randomized trial of propranolol in patients with acute myocardial infarction: I. Mortality results, *JAMA* 247:1707, 1982.
87. Norwegian Multicenter Study Group: Timolol-induced reduction in mortality and reinfarction in patients surviving acute myocardial infarction, *N Engl J Med* 304:801, 1981.
88. Roberts R, Rogers WJ, Mueller HS, et al: Immediate versus deferred beta-blockade following thrombolytic therapy in patients with acute myocardial infarction. Results of the Thrombolysis in Myocardial Infraction (TIMI) II-B Study, *Circulation* 83:422, 1991.
89. Ryan TJ, Anderson JL, Antman EM, et al: ACC/AHA guidelines for the management of patients with acute myocardial infarction. A report of the American College of Cardiology/American Heart Association Task Force on Practice Guidelines, *J Am Coll Cardiol* 28:1328, 1996.
90. Antman EMHand M, Armstrong PW, et al: 2007 focused update of the ACC/AHA 2004 guidelines for the management of patients with ST-elevation myocardial infarction: A report of the American College of Cardiology/American Heart Association Task Force on Practice Guidelines (Writing Group to Review New Evidence and Update the ACC/AHA 2004 Guidelines for the Management of Patients With ST-Elevation Myocardial Infarction), *Circulation* 117:296, 2008.
91. Soumeral SB, McLaughlin TJ, Spiegelman D, et al: Adverse outcomes of underuse of β-blockers in elderly survivors of acute myocardial infarction, *JAMA* 277:115, 1997.
92. Pepine CJ, Cohn PF, Deedwania PC, et al: Effects of treatment on outcome in mildly symptomatic patients with ischemia during daily life. The Atenolol Silent Ischemia Study (ASIST), *Circulation* 90:762, 1994.
93. Poldermans D, Boersma E, Bax JJ, et al: The effect of bisoprolol on perioperative mortality and myocardial infarction in high risk patients undergoing vascular surgery, *N Engl J Med* 341:1789, 1999.
94. Mangano DT, Layug EL, Wallace A, Tateo I: Effect of atenolol on mortality and cardiovascular morbidity after noncardiac surgery, *N Engl J Med* 335:1713, 1996.
95. POISE Study Group: Effects of extended-release metoprolol succinate in patients undergoing non-cardiac surgery (POISE trial): A randomised controlled trial, *Lancet* 371:1838, 2008.
96. Ahlquist RP: A study of the adrenotropic receptors, *Am J Physiol* 153:586, 1948.
97. Benovic JL, Shorr RGL, Caron MG, et al: The mammalian β_2-adrenergic receptor: Purification and characterization, *Biochemistry* 23:4510, 1984.
98. Dixon RAF, Kobilka BK, Strader DJ, et al: Cloning of the gene and cDNA for mammalian β-adrenergic receptor and homology with rhodopsin, *Nature* 321:75, 1986.
99. Gilman AG: G proteins: Transducers of receptor-generated signals, *Annu Rev Biochem* 56:615, 1987.
100. Dohlman HG, Caron MG, Strader CD, et al: Identification and sequence of a binding site peptide of the β_2-adrenergic receptor, *Biochemistry* 27:1813, 1988.
101. O'Dowd BF, Hnatowich M, Regan JW, et al: Site-directed mutagenesis of the cytoplasmic domains of the human β_2-adrenergic receptor. Localization of regions involved in G protein-receptor coupling, *J Biol Chem* 263:15985–15992, 1988.
102. Bouvier M, Hausdorff WP, DeBlasi A, et al: Removal of phosphorylation sites from the β_2-adrenergic receptor delays onset of agonist-promoted desensitization, *Nature* 333:370, 1988.

103. Benovic JL, Bouvier M, Caron MG, et al: Regulation of adenylyl cyclase-coupled β-adrenergic receptors, *Annu Rev Cell Biol* 4:405, 1988.
104. Mukherjee A, Bush LR, McCoy KE, et al: Relationship between β-adrenergic receptor numbers and physiological responses during experimental canine myocardial ischemia, *Circ Res* 50:735, 1982.
105. Freissmuth M, Schütz W, Weindlmayer-Göttel M, et al: Effects of ischemia on the canine myocardial β-adrenoceptor-linked adenylate cyclase system, *J Cardiovasc Pharmacol* 10:568, 1987.
106. Vatner DE, Young MA, Knight DR, et al: β-Receptors and adenylate cyclase: Comparison of nonischemic and postmortem tissue, *Am J Physiol* 258:H140–H144, 1990.
107. Susanni EE, Manders WT, Knight DR, et al: One hour of myocardial ischemia decreases the activity of the stimulatory guanine nucleotide regulatory protein G_s, *Circ Res* 65:1145, 1989.
108. Maisel AS, Motulsky HJ, Insel PA: Externalization of beta-adrenergic receptors promoted by myocardial ischemia, *Science* 230:183, 1985.
109. Lands AM, Arnold A, McAuliff JP, et al: Differentiation of receptor systems activated by sympathomimetic amines, *Nature* 214:597, 1967.
110. Ablad B, Carlsson B, Carlsson E, et al: Cardiac effects of β-adrenergic antagonists, *Adv Cardiol* 12:290, 1974.
111. Lemoine H, Schönell H, Kaumann AJ: Contribution of $β_1$- and $β_2$-adrenoceptors of human atrium and ventricle to the effects of noradrenaline and adrenaline as assessed with (–)-atenolol, *Br J Pharmacol* 95:55, 1988.
112. Kaumann AJ, Lemoine H: $β_2$-Adrenoceptor-mediated positive inotropic effect of adrenaline in human ventricular myocardium. Quantitative discrepancies with binding and adenylate cyclase stimulation, *Naunyn Schmiedebergs Arch Pharmacol* 335:403, 1987.
113. Molena-ar P, Russell FD, Shimada T, et al: Function, characterization and autoradiographic localization and quantitation of beta-adrenoceptors in cardiac tissues, *Clin Exp Physiol Pharmacol* 16:529, 1989.
114. Molena-ar P, Malta E, Jones CR, et al: Autoradiographic localization and function of β-adrenoceptors on the human internal mammary artery and saphenous vein, *Br J Pharmacol* 95:225, 1988.
115. Lipworth BJ: Clinical pharmacology of $β_3$-adrenoreceptors, *Br J Clin Pharmacol* 42:291, 1996.
116. Lewis CM, Brink AJ: Beta-adrenergic blockade. Hemodynamics and myocardial energy metabolism in patients with ischemic heart disease, *Am J Cardiol* 21:846, 1968.
117. Becker LC, Fortuin NJ, Pitt B: Effect of ischemic and antianginal drugs on the distribution of radioactive microspheres in the canine left ventricle, *Circ Res* 28:263, 1971.
118. Kern MJ, Ganz P, Horowitz JD, et al: Potentiation of coronary vasoconstriction by beta-adrenergic blockade in patients with coronary artery disease, *Circulation* 67:1178, 1983.
119. Gaglione A, Hess OM, Corin WJ, et al: Is there coronary vasoconstriction after intracoronary beta-adrenergic blockade in patients with coronary artery disease? *J Am Coll Cardiol* 10:299, 1987.
120. Tarazi RC, Dustan HP: Beta-adrenergic blockade in hypertension. Practical and theoretical implications of long-term hemodynamic variations, *Am J Cardiol* 29:633, 1972.
121. Lund-Johansen P: Hemodynamic consequences of long-term beta-blocker therapy: A 5-year follow-up study of atenolol, *J Cardiovasc Pharmacol* 1:487, 1979.
122. Bühler FR, Laragh JH, Baer L, et al: Propranolol inhibition of renin secretion. A specific approach to diagnosis and treatment of renin-dependent hypertensive diseases, *N Engl J Med* 287:1209, 1972.
123. Hansson L: Beta-adrenergic blockade in essential hypertension. Effects of propranolol on hemodynamic parameters and plasma renin activity, *Acta Med Scand* 194:1, 1973.
124. Man in't Veld AJ, Schalekamp MA: Effects of 10 different beta-adrenoreceptor antagonists on hemodynamics, plasma renin activity, and plasma norepinephrine in hypertension: The key role of vascular resistance changes in relation to partial agonist activity, *J Cardiovasc Pharmacol* 5:S30–S45, 1983.
125. Yamaguchi N, de Champlain J, Nadeau RA: Regulation of norepinephrine release from cardiac sympathetic fibers in the dog by presynaptic α- and β-receptors, *Circ Res* 41:108, 1977.
126. Davis LD, Temte JV: Effects of propranolol on the transmembrane potentials of ventricular muscle and Purkinje fibers of the dog, *Circ Res* 22:661, 1968.
127. Henry JA, Cassidy SL: Membrane stabilizing activity: A major cause of fatal poisoning, *Lancet* 1:1414, 1986.
128. Venditti FJ Jr, Garan H, Ruskin JN: Electrophysiologic effects of beta-blockers in ventricular arrhythmias, *Am J Cardiol* 60:3D–9D, 1987.
129. Totterman K, Groop L, Groop PH, et al: Effect of beta-blocking drugs on beta-cell function and insulin sensitivity in hypertensive nondiabetic patients, *Eur J Clin Pharmacol* 26:13, 1984.
130. Ryan JR, LaCorte W, Jain A, et al: Hypertension in hypoglycemic diabetics treated with β-adrenergic antagonists, *Hypertension* 7:443, 1985.
131. Rosa RM, Silva P, Young JB, et al: Adrenergic modulation of extrarenal potassium disposal, *N Engl J Med* 302:431, 1980.
132. Traub YM, Rabinov M, Rosenfeld JB, et al: Elevation of serum potassium during beta-blockade: Absence of relationship to the renin-aldosterone system, *Clin Pharmacol Ther* 28:765, 1980.
133. Juhlin-Dannfelt A: Metabolic effects of β-adrenoceptor blockade on skeletal muscle at rest and during exercise, *Acta Med Scand* 665:113, 1982.
134. Day JL, Metcalfe J, Simpson CN: Adrenergic mechanisms in control of plasma lipid concentrations, *Br Med J* 284:1145, 1982.
135. Rohlfing JJ, Brunzell JD: The effects of diuretics and adrenergic-blocking agents on plasma lipids, *West J Med* 145:210, 1986.
136. Kaplan JR, Manuck SB, Adams MR, et al: The effects of beta-adrenergic blocking agents on atherosclerosis and its complications, *Eur Heart J* 8:928, 1987.
137. van Brummelen P: The relevance of intrinsic sympathomimetic activity for beta-blocker-induced changes in plasma lipids, *J Cardiovasc Pharmacol* 5:S51–S55, 1983.
138. Jaillon P: Relevance of intrinsic sympathomimetic activity for beta-blockers, *Am J Cardiol* 66:21C–23C, 1990.
139. Svendsen TL, Hartling OJ, Trap-Jensen J, et al: Adrenergic beta-receptor blockade: Hemodynamic importance of intrinsic sympathomimetic activity at rest, *Clin Pharmacol Ther* 29:711, 1981.
140. Ireland MA, Littler WA: The effects of oral acebutolol and propranolol on forearm blood flow in hypertensive patients, *Br J Clin Pharmacol* 12:363, 1981.
141. van den Meiracker AH, Man in't Veld AJ, Boomsma F, et al: Hemodynamic and β-adrenergic receptor adaptations during long-term β-adrenoceptor blockade. Studies with acebutolol, atenolol, pindolol, and propranolol in hypertensive patients, *Circulation* 80:903, 1989.
142. Multicentre International Study: Supplementary report. Reduction in mortality after myocardial infarction with long-term beta-adrenoceptor blockade, *Br Med J* 2:419, 1977.
143. Myers MG, Lewis PJ, Reid JL, et al: Brain concentration of propranolol in relation to hypotensive effect in the rabbit with observations on brain propranolol levels in man, *J Pharmacol Exp Ther* 192:327, 1975.
144. Nies AS, Shand DG: Clinical pharmacology of propranolol, *Circulation* 52:6, 1975.
145. Branch RA, Shand DG: Propranolol disposition in chronic liver disease: A physiological approach, *Clin Pharmacokinet* 1:264, 1976.
146. Wilkinson GR, Shand DG: Commentary: A physiological approach to hepatic drug clearance, *Clin Pharmacol Ther* 18:377, 1975.
147. Ryan JR: Clinical pharmacology of acebutolol, *Am Heart J* 109:1131, 1985.
148. Paterson JW, Conolly ME, Dollery CT, et al: The pharmacodynamics and metabolism of propranolol in man, *Pharmacol Clin* 2:127, 1970.
149. Walle T, Gaffney TE: Propranolol metabolism in man and dog: Mass spectrometric identification of six new metabolites, *J Pharmacol Exp Ther* 182:83, 1972.
150. Shand DG, Rangno RE: The disposition of propranolol. I. Elimination during oral absorption in man, *Pharmacology* 7:159, 1972.
151. Nies AS, Evans GH, Shand DG: The hemodynamic effects of beta-adrenergic blockade on the flow-dependent hepatic clearance of propranolol, *J Pharmacol Exp Ther* 184:716, 1973.
152. Chidsey C, Pine M, Favrot L, et al: The use of drug concentration measurements in studies of the therapeutic response to propranolol, *Postgrad Med J* 52:26, 1976.
153. Alderman EL, Davies RO, Crowley JJ, et al: Dose-response effectiveness of propranolol for the treatment of angina pectoris, *Circulation* 51:964, 1975.
154. Smulyan H, Weinberg SE, Howanitz PJ: Continuous propranolol infusion following abdominal surgery, *JAMA* 247:2539, 1982.
155. Abrahamsson T, Ek B, Nerme V: The $beta_1$- and $beta_2$-adrenoceptor affinity of atenolol and metoprolol. A receptor-binding study performed with different radioligands in tissues from the rat, the guinea pig and man, *Biochem Pharmacol* 37:203, 1988.
156. Åblad B, Borg KO, Carlsson E, et al: Animal and human pharmacological studies on metoprolol-α new selective adrenergic beta-1-receptor antagonist, *Acta Pharmacol Toxicol* 36:5, 1975.
157. Gorczynski RJ: Basic pharmacology of esmolol, *Am J Cardiol* 56:3F, 1985.
158. Sum CY, Yacobi A, Kartzinel R, et al: Kinetics of esmolol, an ultrashort-acting beta-blocker, and of its major metabolite, *Clin Pharmacol Ther* 34:427, 1983.
159. Thys D, Girard D, Kaplan JA, et al: Hemodynamic effects of esmolol during CABG, *Anesthesiology* 65:157, 1986.
160. Abrams J, Allen J, Allin D, et al: Efficacy and safety of esmolol versus propranolol in the treatment of supraventricular tachyarrhythmias: A multicenter double-blind clinical trial, *Am Heart J* 110:913, 1985.
161. Sheppard D, DeStefano S, Byrd RC, et al: Effects of esmolol on airway function in patients with asthma, *J Clin Pharmacol* 26:169, 1986.
162. The Esmolol Research Group: Intravenous esmolol for the treatment of supraventricular tachyarrhythmia: Results of a multicenter, baseline controlled safety and efficacy study of 160 patients, *Am Heart J* 112:498, 1986.
163. Murthy VS, Patel KD, Elangovan RG, et al: Cardiovascular and neuromuscular effects of esmolol during induction of anesthesia, *J Clin Pharmacol* 26:351, 1986.
164. Lowenthal DT, Porter RS, Saris SD, et al: Clinical pharmacology, pharmacodynamics and interactions with esmolol, *Am J Cardiol* 56:14F–18F, 1985.
165. Oda Y, Nishikawa K, Hase I, Asada A: The short-acting $β_1$-adrenoreceptor antagonists esmolol and candiolol suppress the bispectral index response to tracheal intubation during sevoflurane anesthesia, *Anesth Analg* 100:733, 2005.
166. Dage RC, Hsieh CP: Direct vasodilatation by labetalol in anaesthetized dogs, *Br J Pharmacol* 70:287, 1980.
167. Martin LE, Hopkins R, Bland R: Metabolism of labetalol by animal and man, *Br J Pharmacol* 3:695, 1976.
168. Kaplan NM: Treatment of hypertension: Drug therapy. In Kaplan NM, editor: *Clinical hypertension*, 8th ed, Philadelphia, 2002, Lippincott, pp 237–338.
169. Omvik P, Lund-Johansen P: Acute hemodynamic effects of labetalol in severe hypertension, *J Cardiovasc Pharmacol* 4:915, 1982.
170. Ronne-Rasmussen JO, Andersen GS, Bowel Jensen N, et al: Acute effect of intravenous labetalol in the treatment of systemic arterial hypertension, *Br J Clin Pharmacol* 3:805, 1976.
171. Packer M, Meller J, Medina N, et al: Hemodynamic consequences of combined beta-adrenergic and slow calcium channel blockade in man, *Circulation* 65:660, 1982.
172. Ochs HR, Carstens G, Greenblatt DJ: Reduction in lidocaine clearance during continuous infusion and by coadministration of propranolol, *N Engl J Med* 303:373, 1980.
173. Egstrup K: Transient myocardial ischemia after abrupt withdrawal of antianginal therapy in chronic stable angina, *Am J Cardiol* 61:1219, 1988.
174. Miklos D, Keertai M, Bax J, et al: Is there any reason to withhold beta-blockers from high-risk patients with coronary artery disease during surgery? *Anesthesiology* 100:4, 2004.
175. Silverman NA, Wright R, Levitsky S: Efficacy of low-dose propranolol in preventing postoperative supraventricular tachyarrhythmias: A prospective, randomized study, *Ann Surg* 196:194, 1982.
176. Giles J, Sear J, Foex P: Effect of chronic beta-blockade on perioperative outcome in patients undergoing noncardiac surgery, *Anaesthesia* 59:574, 2004.
177. Eisenberg MJ, Brox A, Bestawros AN: Calcium channel blockers: An update, *Am J Med* 116:35, 2004.
178. Brown BG, Bolson EL, Dodge HT: Dynamic mechanisms in human coronary stenosis, *Circulation* 70:917, 1984.
179. Singh BN, editor: Detection, quantification and clinical significance of silent myocardial ischemia in coronary artery disease, *Am J Cardiol*, 58(4): 1B–60B 1986.
180. Johnson SM, Mauritson DR, Willerson JT, et al: A controlled trial of verapamil in Prinzmetal's variant angina, *N Engl J Med* 304:862, 1981.
181. Robertson RH, Wood AJJ, Vaughan WK, et al: Exacerbation of vasotonic angina pectoris by propranolol, *Circulation* 65:281, 1982.
182. Strauss WE, McIntyre KM, Parisi AR, et al: Safety and efficacy of diltiazem hydrochloride for the treatment of stable angina pectoris: Report of a cooperative clinical trial, *Am J Cardiol* 49:560, 1982.
183. Pine MB, Citron PD, Bailly DJ, et al: Verapamil versus placebo in relieving stable angina pectoris, *Circulation* 65(Suppl I):17, 1982.
184. Pitt B, Byington R, Furberg C, et al: Effect of anesthesia on the progression of atherosclerosis and the occurrence of clinical events, *Circulation* 102:1503, 2000.
185. Subramanian VB, Bowles MJ, Khurmi NS, et al: Rationale for the choice of calcium antagonists in chronic stable angina. An objective double-blind placebo-controlled comparison of nifedipine and verapamil, *Am J Cardiol* 50:1173, 1982.
186. McCall D, Walsh RA, Frohlich ED, et al: Calcium entry blocking drugs: Mechanisms of action, experimental studies and clinical uses, *Curr Probl Cardiol* 10:1, 1985.
187. Theroux P, Taeymans Y, Morissette D, et al: A randomized study comparing propranolol and diltiazem in the treatment of unstable angina, *J Am Coll Cardiol* 5:717, 1985.
188. Zelis R, Moore R: Recent insights into the calcium channels, *Circulation* 80(Suppl IV):IV–114, 1989.
189. Nowycky MC, Fox AP, Tsien RW: Three types of neuronal calcium channel with different calcium agonist sensitivity, *Nature* 316:440, 1985.
190. Mitra R, Morad M: Two types of calcium channels in guinea pig ventricular myocytes, *Proc Natl Acad Sci U S A* 83:5340, 1986.
191. Hofmann F, Nastainczyk W, Rohrkasten A, et al: Regulation of the L-type calcium channel, *Trends Pharmacol Sci* 8:393, 1987.
192. Exton JH: Mechanisms of action of calcium-mobilizing agonists: Some variations on a young theme, *FASEB J* 2:2670, 1988.
193. Berridge MJ, Irvine RF: Inositol triphosphate, a novel second messenger in cellular signal transduction, *Nature* 312:315, 1984.
194. Van Meel JCA, de Jonge A, Kalkman HO, et al: Vascular smooth muscle contraction inhibited by postsynaptic $α_2$-adrenoceptor activation is induced by an influx of extracellular calcium, *Eur J Pharmacol* 69:205, 1981.

195. Armstrong DL: Calcium channel regulation by calcineurin, a Ca^{2+}-activated phosphatase in mammalian brain, *Trends Neurosci* 12:117, 1989.
196. Hosey MM, Lazdunski M: Calcium channels: Molecular pharmacology, structure and regulation, *J Membr Biol* 104:81, 1988.
197. Schmid A, Romey G, Barhanin J, et al: SR 33557, an indolizinsultone blocker of Ca^{2+} channels. Identification of receptor sites and analysis of its mode of action, *Mol Pharmacol* 35:766, 1989.
198. Triggle DJ, Swamy VC: Pharmacology of agents that affect calcium: Agonists and antagonists, *Chest* 78:174, 1980.
199. Robinson BF, Dobbs RJ, Kelsey CR: Effects of nifedipine on resistant vessels, arteries and veins in man, *Br J Clin Pharmacol* 10:433, 1980.
200. Serruys PW, Brower RW, Ten Katen JH, et al: Regional wall motion from radiopaque markers after intravenous and intracoronary injections of nifedipine, *Circulation* 63:584, 1981.
201. Singh BN, Roche AHG: Effects of intravenous verapamil on hemodynamics in patients with heart disease, *Am Heart J* 94:593, 1977.
202. Ferlinz J, Easthope JL, Aronow WS: Effects of verapamil on myocardial performance in coronary disease, *Circulation* 59:313, 1979.
203. Chew CYC, Hecht HS, Collett JT, et al: Influence of severity of ventricular dysfunction on hemodynamic responses to intravenously administered verapamil in ischemic heart disease, *Am J Cardiol* 47:917, 1981.
204. Josephson MA, Hopkins J, Singh BN: Hemodynamic and metabolic effects of diltiazem during coronary sinus pacing with particular reference to left ventricular ejection fraction, *Am J Cardiol* 55:286, 1985.
205. Giudicelli JF, Berdeaux A, Edouard A, et al: Attenuation by diltiazem of arterial baroreflex sensitivity in man, *Eur J Clin Pharmacol* 26:675, 1984.
206. Hof RP: Patterns of regional blood flow changes induced by five different calcium antagonists, *Prog Pharmacol* 5:71, 1983.
207. Walsh RA, Porter CB, Starling MR, et al: Beneficial hemodynamic effects of intravenous and oral diltiazem in severe congestive heart failure, *J Am Coll Cardiol* 3(4):1044, 1984.
208. Sato M, Ohashi M, Metz MZ, et al: Inhibitory effect of a calcium antagonist (diltiazem) on aortic and coronary contractions in rabbits, *J Mol Cell Cardiol* 14:741, 1982.
209. Taira N, Satoh K, Maruyama M, et al: Sustained coronary constriction and its antagonism by calcium-blocking agents in monkeys and baboons, *Circ Res* 52:I–40, 1983.
210. Nagao T, Sato M, Nakajima H, et al: Studies on a new 1,5-benzothiazepine derivative (CRD-401). II. Vasodilator actions, *Jpn J Pharmacol* 22:1, 1972.
211. Schmier J, VanAckern K, Bruckner U: Investigations on tachyphylaxis and collateral formation after nifedipine whilst taking into consideration the direction of flow and the mortality rate due to infarction. In Hashimoto K, Kimura E, Kobayashi T, editors: *The first nifedipine symposium*, Tokyo, 1975, Tokyo Press, pp 45–52.
212. Henry PD, Shuchleib R, Clark RE, et al: Effect of nifedipine on myocardial ischemia: Analysis of collateral flow, pulsatile heat and regional muscle shortening, *Am J Cardiol* 44:817, 1979.
213. da Luz PL, Monteiro de Barros LF, Leite JJ, et al: Effect of verapamil on regional coronary and myocardial perfusion during acute coronary occlusion, *Am J Cardiol* 45:269, 1980.
214. Bache RJ, Dymek DJ: Effect of diltiazem on myocardial blood flow, *Circulation* 65(Suppl I):I–19, 1982.
215. Rowland E, Evans T, Krikler D: Effect of nifedipine on atrioventricular conduction as compared with verapamil. Intracardiac electrophysiological study, *Br Heart J* 42:124, 1979.
216. Wellens HJJ, Tan SL, Bär FWH, et al: Effect of verapamil studied by programmed electrical stimulation of the heart in patients with paroxysmal re-entrant supraventricular tachycardia, *Br Heart J* 39:1058, 1977.
217. Sugimoto T, Ishikawa T, Kaseno K, et al: Electrophysiologic effects of diltiazem, a calcium antagonist, in patients with impaired sinus or atrio-ventricular node function, *Angiology* 31:700, 1980.
218. Henry PD: Atherosclerosis, calcium, and calcium antagonists, *Circulation* 72:456, 1985.
219. Lichtlen PR, Hugenholtz PG, Rafflenbeul W, et al: Retardation of angiographic progression of coronary artery disease by nifedipine. Results of the International Nifedipine Trial on Antiatherosclerotic Therapy (INTACT), *Lancet* 335:1109, 1990.
220. Schroeder JS, Gao SZ, Alderman EL, et al: A preliminary study of diltiazem in the prevention of coronary artery disease in heart transplant recipients, *N Engl J Med* 328:164, 1993.
221. Ginsburg R, Davis K, Bristow MR, et al: Calcium antagonists suppress atherogenesis in aorta but not in the intramural coronary arteries of cholesterol-fed rabbits, *Lab Invest* 49:154, 1983.
222. Frey M, Adelung C: Antihypertensive and anticalcinotic effects of calcium antagonists [abstract 167], *J Mol Cell Cardiol* 17, 1985.
223. Zorn J, Fleckenstein A: Anticalcinotic effects of calcium antagonists in cardiac, renal, intestinal and vascular tissues [abstract], *Pfluegers Arch* 403:R31, 1985.
224. Saito K, Birou H, Fukunaga H, et al: Diltiazem prevents the damage to cultured aortic smooth muscle cells induced by hyperlipidemic serum, *Experientia* 42:412, 1986.
225. Naito M, Asai K, Shibata K, et al: Anti-arteriosclerotic effect of diltiazem (III) [Japanese], *Yakuri To Chiryo* 13:1545, 1985.
226. Chierchia S, Crea F, Bernini W, et al: Antiplatelet effects of verapamil in man [abstract], *Am J Cardiol* 47:399, 1981.
227. Ware JA, Johnson PC, Smith M, et al: Inhibition of human platelet aggregation and cytoplasmic calcium response by calcium antagonists: Studies with aequorin and quin2, *Circ Res* 59:39, 1986.
228. Alusik S, Kubis M, Hrckova Y, et al: Antiagregacni ucinek diltiazemu, *Vnitr Lek* 31:877, 1985.
229. Kiyomoto A, Sasaki Y, Odawara A, et al: Inhibition of platelet aggregation by diltiazem. Comparison with verapamil and nifedipine and inhibitory potencies of diltiazem metabolites, *Circ Res* 52:I–115, 1983.
230. Charles S, Ketelslegers JM, Buysschaert M, et al: Hyperglycaemic effects of nifedipine, *Br Med J* 283:19, 1981.
231. Massie BM, MacCarthy EP, Ramanathan KB, et al: Diltiazem and propranolol in mild to moderate essential hypertension as monotherapy or with hydrochlorothiazide, *Ann Intern Med* 107:150, 1987.
232. Kindermann W, Schmitt W, Wolfing A: Physical performance capacity, metabolism and hormonal behavior as affected by diltiazem, *Z Kardiol* 75:99, 1986.
233. Ohneda A: Effect of diltiazem hydrochloride on glucose tolerance in diabetes mellitus, *Jpn J Clin Exp Med* 57:1, 1980.
234. Allen GS, Ahn HS, Preziosi TJ, et al: Cerebral arterial spasm-α-controlled trial of nimodipine in patients with subarachnoid hemorrhage, *N Engl J Med* 308:619, 1983.
235. Clarke B, Grant D, Patmore L: Comparative calcium entry blocking properties of nicardipine, nifedipine and Py-108068 on cardiac and vascular smooth muscle, *Br J Pharmacol* 79:333, 1983.
236. Clair F, Bellet M, Guerret M, et al: Hypotensive effect and pharmacokinetics of nicardipine in patients with severe renal failure, *Curr Ther Res* 38:74, 1985.
237. Dow RJ, Graham DJM: A review of the human metabolism and pharmacokinetics of nicardipine hydrochloride, *Br J Clin Pharmacol* 22:195S, 1986.
238. Gaab MR, Czech T, Korn A: Intracranial effects of nicardipine, *Br J Clin Pharmacol* 20:67S–74S, 1985.
239. Alps BJ, Haas WK: The potential beneficial effect of nicardipine in a rat model of transient forebrain ischemia, *Neurology* 37:809, 1987.
240. Pepine CJ, Lambert CR: Usefulness of nicardipine for angina pectoris, *Am J Cardiol* 59:13J–19J, 1987.
241. Thomas G, Gross R, Schramm M: Calcium channel modulation: Ability to inhibit or promote calcium influx resides in the same dihydropyridine molecule, *J Cardiovasc Pharmacol* 6:1170, 1984.
242. Somogyi A, Albrecht M, Kliems G, et al: Pharmacokinetics, bioavailability and ECG response of verapamil in patients with liver cirrhosis, *Br J Clin Pharmacol* 12:51, 1981.
243. McAllister RG Jr, Hamann SR, Blouin RA: Pharmacokinetics of calcium-entry blockers, *Am J Cardiol* 55:30B–40B, 1985.
244. Hermann P, Morselli PL: Pharmacokinetics of diltiazem and other calcium-entry blockers, *Acta Pharmacol Toxicol* 57:10, 1985.
245. Piepho RW: Comparative clinical pharmacokinetics of the calcium antagonists. In Hoffman BF, editor: *Calcium antagonists: The state of the art and role in cardiovascular disease. Symposia on the frontiers of pharmacology*, 2, Philadelphia, 1983, College of Physicians of Philadelphia, pp 159–174.
246. Rovei V, Gomeni R, Mitchard M, et al: Pharmacokinetics and metabolism of diltiazem in man, *Acta Cardiol (Brux)* 35:35, 1980.
247. Etoh A, Kohno K: Interactions by diltiazem (4). Relationship between first-pass metabolism of various drugs and absorption enhancement by diltiazem, *Yakugaku Zasshi* 103:581, 1983.
248. Hedner T: Calcium channel blockers: Spectrum of side effects and drug interactions, *Acta Pharmacol (Copenh)* 58:119, 1986.
249. Lang R, Klein HO, Weiss E, et al: Effect of verapamil on blood level and renal clearance of digoxin [abstract], *Circulation* 62(Suppl III):83, 1980.
250. Oyamar Y, Fuji S, Kana K, et al: Digoxin-diltiazem interaction, *Am J Cardiol* 53:1480, 1984.
251. Abernathy DR, Schwartz JB: Calcium antagonist drugs, *N Engl J Med* 341:1447, 1999.
252. Mazhar M, Popat KD, Sanders C: Effect of cimetidine on diltiazem blood levels [abstract], *Clin Res* 32:A741, 1984.
253. Kapur PA, Campos JH, Buchea OC: Plasma diltiazem levels, cardiovascular function, and coronary hemodynamics during enflurane anesthesia in the dog, *Anesth Analg* 65:918, 1986.
254. Henling CE, Slogoff S, Kodali SV, et al: Heart block after coronary artery bypass-effect of chronic administration of calcium-entry blockers and beta-blockers, *Anesth Analg* 63:515, 1984.
255. Egstrup K, Andersen PE Jr: Transient myocardial ischemia during nifedipine therapy in stable angina pectoris, and its relation to coronary collateral flow and comparison with metoprolol, *Am J Cardiol* 71:177, 1993.
256. Subramanian VB, Bowles MJ, Khurmi NS, et al: Calcium antagonist withdrawal syndrome: Objective demonstration with frequency-modulated ambulatory ST-segment monitoring, *Br Med J* 286:520, 1983.
257. Kozeny GA, Ragona BP, Bansal VK, et al: Myocardial infarction with normal results of coronary angiography following diltiazem withdrawal, *Am J Med* 80:1184, 1986.
258. Engelman RM, Hadji-Rousou I, Breyer RH, et al: Rebound vasospasm after coronary revascularization in association with calcium antagonist withdrawal, *Ann Thorac Surg* 37:469, 1984.
259. Frishman WH, Klein N, Strom J, et al: Comparative effects of abrupt withdrawal of propranolol and verapamil in angina pectoris, *Am J Cardiol* 50:1191, 1982.
260. Chobanian AV, Bakris GL, Black HR, et al: The Seventh Report of the Joint National Committee on Prevention, Detection, Evaluation, and Treatment of High Blood Pressure: The JNC 7 report, *JAMA* 289:2560, 2003.
261. Kaplan NM, Opie LH: Controversies in hypertension, *Lancet* 367:168, 2006.
262. Whitworth JA: 2003 World Health Organization (WHO)/International Society of Hypertension (ISH) statement on management of hypertension, *J Hypertens* 21:1983, 2003.
263. Vasan RS, Larson MG, Leip EP, et al: Assessment of frequency of progression to hypertension in nonhypertensive participants in the Framingham Heart Study: A cohort study, *Lancet* 358:1682, 2001.
264. Chobanian AV, Bakris GL, Black HR, et al: Seventh report of the Joint National Committee on Prevention, Detection, Evaluation, and Treatment of High Blood Pressure, *Hypertension* 42:1206, 2003.
265. Lifton RP, Gharavi AG, Geller DS: Molecular mechanisms of human hypertension, *Cell* 104:545, 2001.
266. Whelton PK, Appel LJ, Espeland MA, et al: Sodium reduction and weight loss in the treatment of hypertension in older persons: A randomized controlled trial of nonpharmacologic interventions in the elderly (TONE). TONE Collaborative Research Group, *JAMA* 279:839, 1998.
267. Sacks FM, Svetkey LP, Vollmer WM, et al: Effects on blood pressure of reduced dietary sodium and the Dietary Approaches to Stop Hypertension (DASH) diet. DASH-Sodium Collaborative Research Group, *N Engl J Med* 344:3, 2001.
268. Cruickshank JM: Coronary flow reserve and the J curve relation between diastolic blood pressure and myocardial infarction, *BMJ* 297:1227, 1988.
269. August P: Initial treatment of hypertension, *N Engl J Med* 348:610, 2003.
270. Appel LJ: The verdict from ALLHAT—thiazide diuretics are the preferred initial therapy for hypertension, *JAMA* 288:3039, 2002.
271. Psaty BM, Lumley T, Furberg CD, et al: Health outcomes associated with various antihypertensive therapies used as first-line agents: A network meta-analysis, *JAMA* 289:2534, 2003.
272. Staessen JA, Gasowski J, Wang JG, et al: Risks of untreated and treated isolated systolic hypertension in the elderly: Meta-analysis of outcome trials, *Lancet* 355:865, 2000.
273. Hunt SA, Baker DW, Chin MH, et al: ACC/AHA guidelines for the evaluation and management of chronic heart failure in the adult: executive summary. A report of the American College of Cardiology/American Heart Association Task Force on Practice Guidelines (Committee to revise the 1995 Guidelines for the Evaluation and Management of Heart Failure), *J Am Coll Cardiol* 38:2101, 2001.
274. Tepper D: Frontiers in congestive heart failure: Effect of metoprolol CR/XL in chronic heart failure: Metoprolol CR/XL Randomised Intervention Trial in Congestive Heart Failure (MERIT-HF), *Congest Heart Fail* 5:184, 1999.
275. Dargie HJ: Effect of carvedilol on outcome after myocardial infarction in patients with left ventricular dysfunction: The CAPRICORN randomised trial, *Lancet* 357:1385, 2001.
276. A randomized trial of beta-blockade in heart failure. The Cardiac Insufficiency Bisoprolol Study (CIBIS). CIBIS Investigators and Committees, *Circulation* 90:1765, 1994.
277. Ong HT: β blockers in hypertension and cardiovascular disease, *BMJ* 334:946, 2007.
278. Comfere T, Sprung J, Kumar MM, et al: Angiotensin inhibitors in a general surgical population, *Anesth Analg* 100:636, 2005.
279. Contreras F, de la Parte MA, Cabrera J, et al: Role of angiotensin II AT1 receptor blockers in the treatment of arterial hypertension, *Am J Ther* 10:401, 2003.
280. Israili ZH: The use of calcium antagonists in the therapy of hypertension in the elderly, *Am J Ther* 10:383, 2003.
281. Neal B, MacMahon S, Chapman N: Effects of ACE inhibitors, calcium antagonists, and other blood-pressure-lowering drugs: Results of prospectively designed overviews of randomised trials. Blood Pressure Lowering Treatment Trialists' Collaboration, *Lancet* 356:1955, 2000.
282. Brown MJ, Palmer CR, Castaigne A, et al: Morbidity and mortality in patients randomised to double-blind treatment with a long-acting calcium-channel blocker or diuretic in the International Nifedipine GITS study: Intervention as a Goal in Hypertension Treatment (INSIGHT), *Lancet* 356:366, 2000.
283. Major outcomes in high-risk hypertensive patients randomized to angiotensin-converting enzyme inhibitor or calcium channel blocker vs diuretic: The Antihypertensive and Lipid-Lowering Treatment to Prevent Heart Attack Trial (ALLHAT), *JAMA* 288:2981, 2002.

284. Major cardiovascular events in hypertensive patients randomized to doxazosin vs chlorthalidone: The antihypertensive and lipid-lowering treatment to prevent heart attack trial (ALLHAT). ALLHAT Collaborative Research Group, *JAMA* 283:1967, 2000.
285. van Zwieten PA: Centrally acting antihypertensive drugs. Present and future, *Clin Exp Hypertens* 21:859, 1999.
286. Materson BJ: Variability in response to antihypertensive drugs, *Am J Med* 120:S10, 2007.
287. Israili ZH, Hernandez-Hernandez R, Valasco M: In The future of antihypertensive treatment, 14, 121, 2007.
288. Howell SJ, Sear JW, Foex P: Hypertension, hypertensive heart disease and perioperative cardiac risk, *Br J Anaesth* 92:570, 2004.
289. Packer M, Coats AJ, Fowler MB, et al: Effect of carvedilol on survival in severe chronic heart failure, *N Engl J Med* 344:1651, 2001.
290. Effect of enalapril on survival in patients with reduced left ventricular ejection fractions and congestive heart failure. The SOLVD Investigators, *N Engl J Med* 325:293–302, 1991.
291. Effect of ramipril on mortality and morbidity of survivors of acute myocardial infarction with clinical evidence of heart failure. The Acute Infarction Ramipril Efficacy (AIRE) Study Investigators, *Lancet* 342:821–828, 1993.
292. Kober L, Torp-Pedersen C, Carlsen JE, et al: A clinical trial of the angiotensin-converting-enzyme inhibitor trandolapril in patients with left ventricular dysfunction after myocardial infarction. Trandolapril Cardiac Evaluation (TRACE) Study Group, *N Engl J Med* 333:1670–1676, 1995.
293. Cohn JN, Tognoni G: A randomized trial of the angiotensin-receptor blocker valsartan in chronic heart failure, *N Engl J Med* 345:1667, 2001.
294. Pitt B, Zannad F, Remme WJ, et al: The effect of spironolactone on morbidity and mortality in patients with severe heart failure. Randomized Aldactone Evaluation Study Investigators, *N Engl J Med* 341:709, 1999.
295. McMurray J, Ostergren J, Pfeffer M, et al: Clinical features and contemporary management of patients with low and preserved ejection fraction heart failure: Baseline characteristics of patients in the Candesartan in Heart failure-Assessment of Reduction in Mortality and morbidity (CHARM) programme, *Eur J Heart Fail* 5:261–270, 2003.
296. Braunwald E, Antman EM, Beasley JW, et al: ACC/AHA 2002 guideline update for the management of patients with unstable angina and non-ST-segment elevation myocardial infarction—summary article: A report of the American College of Cardiology/American Heart Association task force on practice guidelines (Committee on the Management of Patients With Unstable Angina), *J Am Coll Cardiol* 40:1366, 2002.
297. Hager WD, Davis BR, Riba A, et al: Absence of a deleterious effect of calcium channel blockers in patients with left ventricular dysfunction after myocardial infarction: The SAVE Study Experience. SAVE Investigators. Survival and Ventricular Enlargement, *Am Heart J* 135:406–413, 1998.
298. Pitt B, Remme W, Zannad F, et al: Eplerenone, a selective aldosterone blocker, in patients with left ventricular dysfunction after myocardial infarction, *N Engl J Med* 348:1309, 2003.
299. Yusuf S, Sleight P, Pogue J, et al: Effects of an angiotensin-converting-enzyme inhibitor, ramipril, on cardiovascular events in high-risk patients. The Heart Outcomes Prevention Evaluation Study Investigators, *N Engl J Med* 342:145–153, 2000.
300. Wing LM, Reid CM, Ryan P, et al: A comparison of outcomes with angiotensin-converting--enzyme inhibitors and diuretics for hypertension in the elderly, *N Engl J Med* 348:583, 2003.
301. Dahlof B, Devereux RB, Kjeldsen SE, et al: Cardiovascular morbidity and mortality in the Losartan Intervention For Endpoint reduction in hypertension study (LIFE): A randomised trial against atenolol, *Lancet* 359:995–1003, 2002.
302. Black HR, Elliott WJ, Grandits G, et al: Principal results of the Controlled Onset Verapamil Investigation of Cardiovascular End Points (CONVINCE) trial, *JAMA* 289:2073–2082, 2003.
303. Fox KM: Efficacy of perindopril in reduction of cardiovascular events among patients with stable coronary artery disease: Randomised, double-blind, placebo-controlled, multicentre trial (the EUROPA study), *Lancet* 362:782–788, 2003.
304. Pepine CJ, Handberg EM, Cooper-DeHoff RM, et al: A calcium antagonist vs a non-calcium antagonist hypertension treatment strategy for patients with coronary artery disease. The International Verapamil-Trandolapril Study (INVEST): A randomized controlled trial, *JAMA* 290:2805–2816, 2003.
305. K/DOQI clinical practice guidelines for chronic kidney disease: Evaluation, classification, and stratification, *Am J Kidney Dis* 39:S1–S266, 2002.
306. Arauz-Pacheco C, Parrott MA, Raskin P: Treatment of hypertension in adults with diabetes, *Diabetes Care* 26(Suppl 1):S80–S82, 2003.
307. Efficacy of atenolol and captopril in reducing risk of macrovascular and microvascular complications in type 2 diabetes: UKPDS 39. UK Prospective Diabetes Study Group, *BMJ* 317:713–720, 1998.
308. Lewis EJ, Hunsicker LG, Bain RP, Rohde RD: The effect of angiotensin-converting-enzyme inhibition on diabetic nephropathy. The Collaborative Study Group, *N Engl J Med* 329:1456, 1993.
309. Brenner BM, Cooper ME, de Zeeuw D, et al: Effects of losartan on renal and cardiovascular outcomes in patients with type 2 diabetes and nephropathy, *N Engl J Med* 345:861, 2001.
310. Lewis EJ, Hunsicker LG, Clarke WR, et al: Renoprotective effect of the angiotensin-receptor antagonist irbesartan in patients with nephropathy due to type 2 diabetes, *N Engl J Med* 345:851, 2001.
311. Randomised placebo-controlled trial of effect of ramipril on decline in glomerular filtration rate and risk of terminal renal failure in proteinuric, non-diabetic nephropathy. The GISEN Group (Gruppo Italiano di Studi Epidemiologici in Nefrologia), *Lancet* 349:1857–1863, 1997.
312. Wright JT Jr, Agodoa L, Contreras G, et al: Successful blood pressure control in the African American Study of Kidney Disease and Hypertension, *Arch Intern Med* 162:1636–1643, 2002.
313. PROGRESS Collaborative Group: Randomised trial of a perindopril-based blood-pressure-lowering regimen among 6,105 individuals with previous stroke or transient ischaemic attack, *Lancet* 358:1033–1041, 2001.
314. Eagle KA, Berger PB, Calkins H, et al: ACC/AHA guideline update for perioperative cardiovascular evaluation for noncardiac surgery—executive summary: A report of the American College of Cardiology/American Heart Association Task Force on Practice Guidelines (Committee to Update the 1996 Guidelines on Perioperative Cardiovascular Evaluation for Noncardiac Surgery), *Circulation* 105:1257, 2002.
315. Spahn DR, Priebe HJ: Editorial II: Preoperative hypertension: remain wary? "Yes"—cancel surgery? "No", *Br J Anaesth* 92:461, 2004.
316. Howell SJ, Hemming AE, Allman KG, et al: Predictors of postoperative myocardial ischaemia. The role of intercurrent arterial hypertension and other cardiovascular risk factors, *Anaesthesia* 52:107, 1997.
317. Williams B: Recent hypertension trials, *J Am Coll Cardiol* 45:813, 2005.
318. Lloyd-Jones D, Adams R: Heart disease and stroke statistics—2009 update: A report from the American Heart Association Statistics Committee and Stroke Statistics Subcommittee, *Circulation* 119:e21–e181, 2009.
319. Rosamond W, Flegal K, Furie K, et al: Heart disease and stroke statistics—2008 update: A report from the American Heart Association Statistics Committee and Stroke Statistics Subcommittee, *Circulation* 117:e25, 2008.
320. Wilhelmson L, Resengrew A, Eriksson H, et al: Heart failure in the general population on men: Morbidity, risk factors, and prognosis, *J Intern Med* 249:253, 2001.
321. O'Connell JB, Bristow MR: Economic impact of heart failure in the United States: Time for a different approach, *J Heart Lung Transplant* 13:S107–S112, 1994.
322. Hunt SA, Abraham WT, Chin MH, et al: 2009 focused update incorporated into the ACC/AHA 2005 Guidelines for the Diagnosis and Management of Heart Failure in Adults: A report of the American College of Cardiology Foundation/American Heart Association Task Force on Practice Guidelines: Developed in collaboration with the International Society for Heart and Lung Transplantation, *Circulation* 119:e391, 2009.
323. al-Kaade S, Hauptman PJ: Health-related quality of life measurement in heart failure: Challenges for the new millennium, *J Card Fail* 7:194, 2001.
324. Garg R, Yusuf S: Overview of randomized trials of angiotensin-converting enzyme inhibitors on mortality and morbidity in patients with heart failure, *JAMA* 273:1450, 1995.
325. Flather MD, Yusuf S, Kober L, et al: Long-term ACE inhibitor therapy in patients with heart failure or left ventricular dysfunction: A systematic overview of data from individual patients. ACE inhibitor Myocardial Infarction Collaborative Group, *Lancet* 355:1575, 2000.
326. Pfeffer MA, Swedberg K, Granger CB, et al: Effects of candesartan on mortality and morbidity in patients with chronic heart failure: The CHARM-Overall programme, *Lancet* 362:759, 2003.
327. Consensus recommendations for the management of chronic heart failure. On behalf of the membership of the advisory council to improve outcomes nationwide in heart failure, *Am J Cardiol* 83(Suppl 2A):1A–38A, 1999.
328. The Cardiac Insufficiency Bisoprolol Study II (CIBIS-II): A randomised trial, *Lancet* 353:9, 1999.
329. Effect of metoprolol CR/XL in chronic heart failure: Metoprolol CR/XL Randomised Intervention Trial in Congestive Heart Failure (MERIT-HF), *Lancet* 353:2001, 1999.
330. Katz AM: Angiotensin II: Hemodynamic regulator or growth factor? *J Mol Cell Cardiol* 22:739, 1990.
331. Cohn JN, Ferrari R, Sharpe N: Cardiac remodeling—concepts and clinical implications: A consensus paper from an international forum on cardiac remodeling, *J Am Coll Cardiol* 35:569, 2000.
332. Serneri GG, Boddi M, Cecioni I, et al: Cardiac angiotensin II formation in the clinical course of heart failure and its relationship with left ventricular function, *Circ Res* 88:961, 2001.
333. Dell'Italia LJ, Sabri A: Activation of the renin-angiotensin system in hypertrophy and heart failure. In Mann DL, editor: *Heart failure, a companion to Braunwald's Heart Disease*, Philadelphia, 2004, WB Saunders, pp 129–143.
334. Pfeffer MA, Braunwald E, Moye LA, et al: Effect of captopril on mortality and morbidity in patients with left ventricular dysfunction after myocardial infarction. Results of the survival and ventricular enlargement trial. The SAVE investigators, *N Engl J Med* 327:669, 1992.
335. ISIS-4: In A randomised factorial trial assessing early oral captorpil, oral mononitrate, and intravenous magnesium sulphate in 58,050 patients with suspected acute myocardial infarction. ISIS-4 (Fourth International Study of Infarct Survival) Collaborative Group, 345, 669, 1995.
336. Arnold JM, Yusuf S, Young J, et al: Prevention of heart failure in patients in the Heart Outcomes Prevention Evaluation (HOPE) Study, *Circulation* 107:1284, 2003.
337. Braunwald E, Domanski MJ, Fowler SE, et al: Angiotensin-converting-enzyme inhibition in stable coronary artery disease, *N Engl J Med* 351:2058, 2004.
338. Varin R, Mulder P, Tamion F, et al: Improvement of endothelial function by chronic angiotensin-converting enzyme inhibition in heart failure: Role of nitric oxide, prostanoids, oxidant stress, and bradykinin, *Circulation* 102:351, 2000.
339. Sadoshima J, Izumo S: Molecular characterization of angiotensin II-induced hypertrophy of cardiac myocytes and hyperplasia of cardiac fibroblasts. Critical role of the AT1 receptor subtype, *Circ Res* 73:413, 1993.
340. Kim S, Yoshiyama M, Izumi Y, et al: Effects of combination of ACE inhibitor and angiotensin-receptor blocker on cardiac remodeling, cardiac function, and survival in rat heart failure, *Circulation* 103:148, 2001.
341. Konstam MA, Kronenberg MW, Rousseau MF, et al: Effects of angiotensin-converting enzyme inhibitor, enalapril, on the long-term progression of left ventricular dilation in patients with asymptomatic systolic dysfunction, *Circulation* 88:2277, 1993.
342. Cohn JN, Johnson G, Ziesche S, et al: A comparison of enalapril with hydralazine-isosorbide dinitrate in the treatment of chronic congestive heart failure, *N Engl J Med* 325:303, 1991.
343. Dell'Italia LJ, Husain A: Dissecting the role of chymase in angiotensin II formation and heart and blood vessel diseases, *Curr Opin Cardiol* 17:374, 2002.
344. Fogari R, Zoppi A, Corradi L, et al: Comparative effects of lisinopril and losartan on insulin sensitivity in the treatment of nondiabetic hypertensive patients, *Br J Clin Pharmacol* 46:467, 1998.
345. Janssen JJ, Gans RO, van der Meulen J, et al: Comparison between the effects of amlodipine and lisinopril on proteinuria in nondiabetic renal failure: A double-blind, randomized prospective study, *Am J Hypertens* 11:1074, 1998.
346. Packer M, Poole-Wilson PA, Armstrong PW, et al: Comparative effects of low and high doses of the angiotensin-converting enzyme inhibitor, lisinopril, on morbidity and mortality in chronic heart failure. ATLAS Study Group, *Circulation* 100:2312, 1999.
347. Luzier AB, Forrest A, Feuerstein SG, et al: Containment of heart failure hospitalizations and cost by angiotensin-converting enzyme inhibitor dosage optimization, *Am J Cardiol* 86:519, 2000.
348. Mann DL, Deswal A, Bozkurt B, Torre-Amione G: New therapeutics for chronic heart failure, *Annu Rev Med* 53:59, 2002.
349. Burnier M, Brunner HR: Angiotensin II receptor antagonists, *Lancet* 355:637, 2000.
350. Pitt B, Segal R, Martinez FA, et al: Randomised trial of losartan versus captopril in patients over 65 with heart failure (Evaluation of Losartan in the Elderly Study, ELITE), *Lancet* 349:747, 1997.
351. Pitt B, Poole-Wilson PA, Segal R, et al: Effect of losartan compared with captopril on mortality in patients with symptomatic heart failure: Randomised trial—the Losartan Heart Failure Survival Study ELITE II, *Lancet* 355:1582, 2000.
352. McMurray JJ, Ostergren J, Swedberg K, et al: Effects of candesartan in patients with chronic heart failure and reduced left ventricular systolic function taking angiotensin-converting-enzyme inhibitors: The CHARM-Added trial, *Lancet* 362:767, 2003.
353. Granger CB, McMurray JJ, Yusuf S, et al: Effects of candesartan in patients with chronic heart failure and reduced left ventricular systolic function intolerant to angiotensin-converting-enzyme inhibitors: The CHARM-Alternative trial, *Lancet* 362:772, 2003.
354. Yusuf S, Pfeffer MA, Swedberg K, et al: Effects of candesartan in patients with chronic heart failure and preserved left ventricular ejection fraction: The CHARM-Preserved Trial, *Lancet* 362:777, 2003.
355. Roig E, Perez-Villa F, Morales M, et al: Clinical implications of increased plasma angiotensin II despite ACE inhibitor therapy in patients with congestive heart failure, *Eur Heart J* 21:53, 2000.
356. McKelvie RS, Yusuf S, Pericak D, et al: Comparison of candesartan, enalapril, and their combination in congestive heart failure: Randomized Evaluation of Strategies for Left Ventricular Dysfunction (RESOLVD) pilot study. The RESOLVD Pilot Study Investigators, *Circulation* 100:1056, 1999.
357. Pitt B, Rajagopalan A: The role of mineralocorticoid receptor blocking agents in patients with heart failure and cardiovascular disease. In McMurray JJ, Pfeffer MA, editors: *Heart failure updates*, London, 2003, Martin Dunitz, pp 115–140.
358. Weber KT: Aldosterone in congestive heart failure, *N Engl J Med* 345:1689, 2001.
359. Weber KT: Aldosteronism revisited: Perspectives on less well-recognized actions of aldosterone, *J Lab Clin Med* 142:71, 2003.
360. Delcayre C, Silvestre JS, Garnier A, et al: Cardiac aldosterone production and ventricular remodeling, *Kidney Int* 57:1346, 2000.
361. Weber KT: Fibrosis and hypertensive heart disease, *Curr Opin Cardiol* 15:264, 2000.
362. Rajagopalan S, Duquaine D, King S, et al: Mineralocorticoid receptor antagonism in experimental atherosclerosis, *Circulation* 105:2212, 2002.

363. Zhang ZH, Francis J, Weiss RM, Felder RB: The renin-angiotensin-aldosterone system excites hypothalamic paraventricular nucleus neurons in heart failure, *Am J Physiol* 283:H423–H433, 2002.
364. Stockand JD: New ideas about aldosterone signaling in epithelia, *Am J Physiol* 282:F559–F576, 2002.
365. Zannad F, Alla F, Dousset B, et al: Limitation of excessive extracellular matrix turnover may contribute to survival benefit of spironolactone therapy in patients with congestive heart failure: Insights from the randomized aldactone evaluation study (RALES). Rales Investigators, *Circulation* 102:2700, 2000.
366. Korkmaz ME, Muderrisoglu H, Ulucam M, Ozin B: Effects of spironolactone on heart rate variability and left ventricular systolic function in severe ischemic heart failure, *Am J Cardiol* 86:649, 2000.
367. Yee KM, Pringle SD, Struthers AD: Circadian variation in the effects of aldosterone blockade on heart rate variability and QT dispersion in congestive heart failure, *J Am Coll Cardiol* 37:1800, 2001.
368. Farquharson CA, Struthers AD: Spironolactone increases nitric oxide bioactivity, improves endothelial vasodilator dysfunction, and suppresses vascular angiotensin I/angiotensin II conversion in patients with chronic heart failure, *Circulation* 101:594, 2000.
369. Juurlink DN, Mamdani MM, Lee DS, et al: Rates of hyperkalemia after publication of the Randomized Aldactone Evaluation Study, *N Engl J Med* 351:543, 2004.
370. Barr CS, Lang CC, Hanson J, et al: Effects of adding spironolactone to an angiotensin-converting enzyme inhibitor in chronic congestive heart failure secondary to coronary artery disease, *Am J Cardiol* 76:1259, 1995.
371. The effect of digoxin on mortality and morbidity in patients with heart failure. The Digitalis Investigation Group, *N Engl J Med* 336:525, 1997.
372. Brown NJ: Eplerenone. Cardiovascular protection, *Circulation* 107:2512, 2003.
373. MacFadyen RJ, Barr CS, Struthers AD: Aldosterone blockade reduces vascular collagen turnover, improves heart rate variability and reduces early morning rise in heart rate in heart failure patients, *Cardiovasc Res* 35:30, 1997.
374. Cicoira M, Zanolla L, Rossi A, et al: Long-term, dose-dependent effects of spironolactone on left ventricular function and exercise tolerance in patients with chronic heart failure, *J Am Coll Cardiol* 40:304, 2002.
375. Weber KT: Efficacy of aldosterone receptor antagonism in heart failure: Potential mechanisms, *Curr Heart Fail Rep* 1:51, 2004.
376. Eichhorn EJ, Bristow MR: Antagonism of β-adrenergic receptors in heart failure. In Mann DL, editor: *Heart failure: A companion to Braunwald's Heart Disease*, Philadelphia, 2004, Saunders, pp 619–636.
377. Wallhaus TR, Taylor M, DeGrado TR, et al: Myocardial free fatty acid and glucose use after carvedilol treatment in patients with congestive heart failure, *Circulation* 103:2441, 2001.
378. Lowes BD, Gilbert EM, Abraham WT, et al: Myocardial gene expression in dilated cardiomyopathy treated with beta-blocking agents, *N Engl J Med* 346:1357, 2002.
379. Sabbah HN, Sharov VG, Gupta RC, et al: Chronic therapy with metoprolol attenuates cardiomyocyte apoptosis in dogs with heart failure, *J Am Coll Cardiol* 36:1698, 2000.
380. Marks AR: A guide for the perplexed: Towards an understanding of the molecular basis of heart failure, *Circulation* 107:1456, 2003.
381. Marx SO, Reiken S, Hisamatsu Y, et al: PKA phosphorylation dissociates FKBP12.6 from the calcium release channel (ryanodine receptor): Defective regulation in failing hearts, *Cell* 101:365, 2000.
382. Marks AR, Reiken S, Marx SO: Progression of heart failure: Is protein kinase a hyperphosphorylation of the ryanodine receptor a contributing factor? *Circulation* 105:272, 2002.
383. Schlotthauer K, Bers DM: Sarcoplasmic reticulum Ca(2+) release causes myocyte depolarization. Underlying mechanism and threshold for triggered action potentials, *Circ Res* 87:774, 2000.
384. Reiken S, Gaburjakova M, Gaburjakova J, et al: Beta-adrenergic receptor blockers restore cardiac calcium release channel (ryanodine receptor) structure and function in heart failure, *Circulation* 104:2843, 2001.
385. Doi M, Yano M, Kobayashi S: Propranolol prevents the development of heart failure by restoring FKBP12.6-mediated stabilization of ryanodine receptor, *Circulation* 105:1374, 2002.
386. Bristow MR, Ginsburg R, Minobe W, et al: Decreased catecholamine sensitivity and beta-adrenergic-receptor density in failing human hearts, *N Engl J Med* 307:205, 1982.
387. Ungerer M, Bohm M, Elce JS, et al: Altered expression of beta-adrenergic receptor kinase and beta1-adrenergic receptors in the failing human heart, *Circulation* 87:454, 1993.
388. Gauthier C, Tavernier G, Charpentier F, et al: Functional beta3-adrenoceptor in the human heart, *J Clin Invest* 98:556, 1996.
389. Gauthier C, Langin D, Balligand JL: Beta3-adrenoceptors in the cardiovascular system, *Trends Pharmacol Sci* 21:426, 2000.
390. Cheng HJ, Zhang ZS, Onishi K, et al: Upregulation of functional beta(3)-adrenergic receptor in the failing canine myocardium, *Circ Res* 89:599, 2001.
391. Morimoto A, Hasegawa H, Cheng HJ, et al: Endogenous beta3-adrenoreceptor activation contributes to left ventricular and cardiomyocyte dysfunction in heart failure, *Am J Physiol Heart Circ Physiol* 286:H2425–H2433, 2004.
392. Moniotte S, Kobzik L, Feron O, et al: Upregulation of beta(3)-adrenoceptors and altered contractile response to inotropic amines in human failing myocardium, *Circulation* 103:1649, 2001.
393. Gauthier C, Leblais V, Kobzik L, et al: The negative inotropic effect of beta3-adrenoceptor stimulation is mediated by activation of a nitric oxide synthase pathway in human ventricle, *J Clin Invest* 102:1377, 1998.
394. Packer M, Bristow MR, Cohn JN, et al: The effect of carvedilol on morbidity and mortality in patients with chronic heart failure. U.S. Carvedilol Heart Failure Study Group, *N Engl J Med* 334:1349, 1996.
395. Beta-Blocker Evaluation of Survival Trial Investigators: A trial of the beta-blocker bucindolol in patients with advanced chronic heart failure, *N Engl J Med* 344:1659, 2001.
396. Jacob S, Rett K, Wicklmayr M, et al: Differential effect of chronic treatment with two beta-blocking agents on insulin sensitivity: The carvedilol-metoprolol study, *J Hypertens* 14:489, 1996.
397. Dulin B, Abraham WT: Pharmacology of carvedilol, *Am J Cardiol* 93:3B–6B, 2004.
398. Hoffmann C, Leitz MR, Oberdorf-Ma-ass S, et al: Comparative pharmacology of human beta-adrenergic receptor subtypes—characterization of stably transfected receptors in CHO cells, *Naunyn Schmiedebergs Arch Pharmacol* 369:151, 2004.
399. Moniotte S, Balligand JL: Potential use of beta(3)-adrenoceptor antagonists in heart failure therapy, *Cardiovasc Drug Rev* 20:19, 2002.
400. Poole-Wilson PA, Swedberg K, Cleland JG, et al: Carvedilol or Metoprolol European Trial Investigators. Comparison of carvedilol and metoprolol on clinical outcomes in patients with chronic heart failure in the Carvedilol or Metoprolol European Trial (COMET): Randomised controlled trial, *Lancet* 362:7, 2003.
401. Di Lenarda A, Sabbadini G, Sinagra G: Do pharmacological differences among beta-blockers affect their clinical efficacy in heart failure? *Cardiovasc Drugs Ther* 18:91, 2004.
402. McAlister FA, Wiebe N, Ezekowitz JA, et al: Meta-analysis: beta-blocker dose, heart rate eduction, and death in patients with heart failure, *Ann Intern Med* 150:784, 2009.
403. Remme WJ, Swedberg K: Task Force for the Diagnosis and Treatment of Chronic Heart Failure, European Society of Cardiology. Guidelines for the diagnosis and treatment of chronic heart failure, *Eur Heart J* 22:1527, 2001.
404. Eichhorn EJ: Beta-blocker withdrawal: The song of Orpheus, *Am Heart J* 138:387, 1999.
405. Ko DT, Hebert PR, Coffey CS, et al: Adverse effects of beta-blocker therapy for patients with heart failure: A quantitative overview of randomized trials, *Arch Intern Med* 164:1389, 2004.
406. McMurray J, Cohen-Solal A, Dietz R, et al: Clinical Research Initiative in heart failure. Practical recommendations for the use of ACE inhibitors, beta-blockers and spironolactone in heart failure: Putting guidelines into practice, *Eur J Heart Fail* 3:495, 2001.
407. Keith M, Geranmayegan A, Sole MJ, et al: Increased oxidative stress in patients with congestive heart failure, *J Am Coll Cardiol* 31:1352, 1998.
408. Adorisio R, De Luca L, Rossi J, et al: Pharmacological treatment of chronic heart failure, *Heart Fail Rev* 11:109, 2006.
409. Cohn JN, Archibald DG, Ziesche S, et al: Effect of vasodilator therapy on mortality in chronic congestive heart failure. Results of a Veterans Administration Cooperative Study, *N Engl J Med* 314:1547, 1986.
410. Carson P, Ziesche S, Johnson G, et al: Racial differences in response to therapy for heart failure: Analysis of the vasodilator-heart failure trials. Vasodilator-Heart Failure Trial Study Group, *J Card Fail* 5:178, 1999.
411. Taylor AL, Ziesche S, Yancy C, et al: Combination of isosorbide dinitrate and hydralazine in blacks with heart failure, *N Engl J Med* 351:2049, 2004.
412. Domanski M, Norman J, Pitt B, et al: Diuretic use, progressive heart failure, and death in patients in the Studies Of Left Ventricular Dysfunction (SOLVD), *J Am Coll Cardiol* 42:705, 2003.
413. Gheorghiade M, Adams KF Jr, Colucci WS: Digoxin in the management of cardiovascular disorders, *Circulation* 109:2959, 2004.
414. Ferguson DW: Sympathetic mechanisms in heart failure: Pathophysiological and pharmacological implications, *Circulation* 87(Suppl VII):68, 1993.
415. Krum H, Bigger JT Jr, Goldsmith RL, et al: Effect of long-term digoxin therapy on autonomic function in patients with chronic heart failure, *J Am Coll Cardiol* 25:289, 1995.
416. Adams KF Jr, Gheorghiade M, Uretsky BF, et al: Patients with mild heart failure worsen during withdrawal from digoxin therapy, *J Am Coll Cardiol* 30:42, 1997.
417. Rahimtoola SH: Digitalis therapy for patients in clinical heart failure, *Circulation* 109:2942, 2004.
418. Oghlakian G, Klapholz M: Vasopressin and vasopressin receptor antagonists in heart failure, *Cardiol Rev* 17:10, 2009.
419. Rauchhaus M, Doehner W, Francis DP, et al: Plasma cytokine parameters and mortality in patients with chronic heart failure, *Circulation* 102:3060, 2000.
420. Mann DL, McMurray JJ, Packer M, et al: Targeted anticytokine therapy in patients with chronic heart failure: Results of the Randomized Etanercept Worldwide Evaluation (RENEWAL), *Circulation* 109:1594, 2004.
421. Ergul A, Grubbs AL, Zhang Y, et al: Selective upregulation of endothelin converting enzyme-1a in the human failing heart, *J Card Fail* 6:314, 2000.
422. Sakai S, Miyauchi T, Kobayashi M, et al: Inhibition of myocardial endothelin pathway improves long-term survival in heart failure, *Nature* 384:353, 1996.
423. Mishima T, Tanimura M, Suzuki G, et al: Effects of long-term therapy with bosentan on the progression of left ventricular dysfunction and remodeling in dogs with heart failure, *J Am Coll Cardiol* 35:222, 2000.
424. Teerlink JR: Recent heart failure trials of neurohormonal modulation (OVERTURE and ENABLE): Approaching the asymptote of efficacy? *J Card Fail* 8:124, 2002.
425. Kalra PR, Moon JC, Coats AJ: Do results of the ENABLE (Endothelin Antagonist Bosentan for Lowering Cardiac Events in Heart Failure) study spell the end for nonselective endothelin antagonism in heart failure? *Int J Cardiol* 85:195, 2002.
426. Neunteufl T, Berger R, Pacher R: Endothelin-receptor antagonists in cardiology clinical trials, *Expert Opin Investig Drugs* 11:431, 2002.
427. Packer M, Califf RM, Konstam MA, et al: Comparison of omapatrilat and enalapril in patients with chronic heart failure: The Omapatrilat Versus Enalapril Randomized Trial of Utility in Reducing Events (OVERTURE), *Circulation* 106:920, 2002.
428. Worthley MI, Corti R, Worthley SG: Vasopeptidase inhibitors: Will they have a role in clinical practice? *Br J Clin Pharmacol* 57:27, 2004.
429. Bristow MR, Saxon LA, Boehmer J, et al: Cardiac-resynchronization therapy with or without an implantable defibrillator in advanced chronic heart failure, *N Engl J Med* 350:2140, 2004.
430. Anand IS, Carson P, Galle E, et al: Cardiac resynchronization therapy reduces the risk of hospitalizations in patients with advanced heart failure: Results from the Comparison of Medical Therapy, Pacing and Defibrillation in Heart Failure (COMPANION) trial, *Circulation* 119:969, 2009.
431. Mathur A, Martin JF: Stem cells and repair of the heart, *Lancet* 364:183, 2004.
432. Segers VF, Lee RT: Stem-cell therapy for cardiac disease, *Nature* 451:937, 2008.
433. Wollert KM, Meyer GP, Lotz J, et al: Intracoronary autologous bone-marrow cell transfer after myocardial infarction: The BOOST randomised controlled clinical trial, *Lancet* 364:141, 2004.
434. Gersh BJ, Simari RD, Behfar A, et al: Cardiac cell repair therapy: A clinical perspective, *Mayo Clin Proc* 84:876, 2009.
435. Assmus B, Fischer-Rasokat U, Honold J, et al: Transcoronary transplantation of functionally competent BMCs is associated with a decrease in natriuretic peptide serum levels and improved survival of patients with chronic postinfarction heart failure: Results of the TOPCARE-CHD Registry, *Circ Res* 100:1234, 2007.
436. Erbs S, Linke A, Adams V, et al: Transplantation of blood-derived progenitor cells after recanalization of chronic coronary artery occlusion: First randomized and placebo-controlled study, *Circ Res* 97:756, 2005.
437. Tse HF, Thambar S, Kwong YL, et al: Prospective randomized trial of direct endomyocardial implantation of bone marrow cells for treatment of severe coronary artery diseases (PROTECT-CAD trial), *Eur Heart J* 28:2998, 2007.
438. Yao K, Huang R, Qian J, et al: Administration of intracoronary bone marrow mononuclear cells on chronic myocardial infarction improves diastolic function, *Heart* 94:1147, 2008.
439. Losordo DW, Schatz RA, White CJ, et al: Intramyocardial transplantation of autologous $CD34^+$ stem cells for intractable angina: A phase I/IIa double-blind, randomized controlled trial, *Circulation* 115:3165, 2007.
440. Seeger FH, Zeiher AM, Dimmeler S: Cell-enhancement strategies for the treatment of ischemic heart disease, *Nat Clin Pract Cardiovasc Med* 4(Suppl 1):S110, 2007.
441. Tschöpe C, Westermann D: Heart failure with normal ejection fraction. Pathophysiology, diagnosis, and treatment, *Herz* 34:89, 2009.
442. Zile MR, Brutsaert DL: New concepts in diastolic dysfunction and diastolic heart failure: Part I: diagnosis, prognosis, and measurements of diastolic function, *Circulation* 105:1387, 2002.
443. Bhatia RS, Tu JV, Lee DS, et al: Outcome of heart failure with preserved ejection fraction in a population-based study, *N Engl J Med* 355:260, 2006.
444. Owan TE, Hodge DO, Herges RM, et al: Trends in prevalence and outcome of heart failure with preserved ejection fraction, *N Engl J Med* 355:251, 2006.
445. Tribouilloy C, Rusinaru D, Mahjoub H, et al: Prognosis of heart failure with preserved ejection fraction: A 5 year prospective population-based study, *Eur Heart J* 29:339, 2008.
446. Fonarow GC, Stough WG, Abraham WT, et al: Characteristics, treatments, and outcomes of patients with preserved systolic function hospitalized for heart failure: A report from the OPTIMIZE-HF Registry, *J Am Coll Cardiol* 50:768, 2007.
447. Estep J: Diagnosis of heart failure with preserved ejection fraction, *JMDHVC* 4(3):8–12, 2008.
448. Brubaker PH, Joo KC, Stewart KP, et al: Chronotropic incompetence and its contribution to exercise intolerance in older heart failure patients, *J Cardiopulm Rehabil* 26:86, 2006.
449. Little WC, Zile MR, Kitzman DW, et al: The effect of alagebrium chloride (ALT-711), a novel glucose cross-link breaker, in the treatment of elderly patients with diastolic heart failure, *J Card Fail* 11:191, 2005.

450. Schaefer A, Meyer GP, Fuchs M, et al: Impact of intracoronary bone marrow cell transfer on diastolic function in patients after acute myocardial infarction: Results from the BOOST trial, *Eur Heart J* 27:929, 2006.
451. Warner JG Jr, Metzger DC, Kitzman DW, et al: Losartan improves exercise tolerance in patients with diastolic dysfunction and a hypertensive response to exercise, *J Am Cardiol* 33:1567, 1999.
452. Massie BM, Carson PE, McMurray JJ, et al: Irbesartan in patients with heart failure and preserved ejection fraction, *N Engl J Med* 359:2456, 2008.
453. Daniel KR, Wells G, Stewart K, et al: Effect of aldosterone antagonism on exercise tolerance, Doppler diastolic function, and quality of life in older women with diastolic heart failure, *Congest Heart Fail* 15:68, 2009.
454. Ga-asch WH, Zile MR: Left ventricular diastolic dysfunction and diastolic heart failure, *Annu Rev Med* 55:373, 2004.
455. Lobato E, Willert J, Looke T, et al: Effects of milrinone versus epinephrine on left ventricular relaxation after cardiopulmonary bypass following myocardial revascularization, *J Cardiothorac Vasc Anesth* 19:334–339, 2005.
456. DiDomenico RJ, Park HY, Southworth MR, et al: Guidelines for acute decompensated heart failure treatment, *Ann Pharmacother* 38:649, 2004.
457. Fonarow GC, Dams K, Abraham W, et al: Risk stratification for in-hospital mortality in acute decompensated heart failure, *JAMA* 293:572, 2005.
458. Loh E, Elkayam U, Cody R, et al: A randomized multicenter study comparing the efficacy and safety of intravenous milrinone and intravenous nitroglycerin in patients with advanced heart failure, *J Card Fail* 7:114, 2001.
459. de Denus S, Pharand C, Williamson DR: Brain natriuretic peptide in the management of heart failure: The versatile neurohormone, *Chest* 125:652, 2004.
460. Elkayam U, Akhter MW, Singh H, et al: Comparison of effects on left ventricular filling pressure of intravenous nesiritide and high-dose nitroglycerin in patients with decompensated heart failure, *Am J Cardiol* 93:237, 2004.
461. Publication Committee for the VMAC Investigators (Vasodilatation in the Management of Acute CHF): Intravenous nesiritide vs nitroglycerin for treatment of decompensated congestive heart failure: A randomized controlled trial, *JAMA* 287:1531, 2002.
462. Burger AJ, Horton DP, LeJemtel T, et al: Effect of nesiritide (B-type natriuretic peptide) and dobutamine on ventricular arrhythmias in the treatment of patients with acutely decompensated congestive heart failure: The PRECEDENT study, *Am Heart J* 144:1102, 2002.
463. Abraham WT, Adams KF, Fonarow GC, et al: In-hospital mortality in patients with acute decompensated heart failure requiring intravenous vasoactive medications: An analysis from the Acute Decompensated Heart Failure National Registry (ADHERE), *J Am Coll Cardiol* 46:57, 2005.
464. Sackner-Bernstein JD, Kowalski M, Fox M, et al: Short-term risk of death after treatment with nesiritide for decompensated heart failure: A pooled analysis of randomized controlled trials, *JAMA* 293:1900, 2005.
465. Sackner-Bernstein JD, Skopicki HA, Aaronson KD: Risk of worsening renal function with nesiritide in patients with acutely decompensated heart failure, *Circulation* 111:1487, 2005.
466. MedWatch-Natrecor®: *Dear Health Care Provider Letter*. Available at: http://www.fda.gov/downloads/Safety/MedWatch/SafetyInformation/SafetyAlertsforHumanMedicalProducts/UCM164672.pdf. Accessed January 20, 2010.
467. Hernandez AF, O'Connor CM, Starling RC, et al: Rationale and design of the Acute Study of Clinical Effectiveness of Nesiritide in Decompensated Heart Failure Trial (ASCEND-HF), *Am Heart J* 157:271, 2009.
468. Yamani MH, Haji SA, Starling RC, et al: Comparison of dobutamine-based and milrinone-based therapy for advanced decompensated congestive heart failure: Hemodynamic efficacy, clinical outcome, and economic impact, *Am Heart J* 142:998, 2001.
469. Cuffe MS, Califf RM, Adams KF Jr, et al: Short-term intravenous milrinone for acute exacerbation of chronic heart failure: A randomized controlled trial, *JAMA* 287:1541, 2002.
470. Felker GM, Benza RL, Chandler AB, et al: Heart failure etiology and response to milrinone in decompensated heart failure: Results from the OPTIME-CHF study, *J Am Coll Cardiol* 41:997, 2003.
471. Renlund DG: Building a bridge to heart transplantation, *N Engl J Med* 351:849, 2004.
472. Wernly JA: Ischemia, reperfusion, and the role of surgery in the treatment of cardiogenic shock secondary to acute myocardial infarction: An interpretative review, *J Surg Res* 117:6, 2004.
473. Hochman JS: Cardiogenic shock complicating acute myocardial infarction: Expanding the paradigm, *Circulation* 107:2998, 2003.
474. Royster R, Butterworth J, Prough D, et al: Preoperative and intraoperative predictors of inotropic support and long-term outcome in patients having coronary artery bypass grafting, *Anesth Analg* 72:729, 1991.
475. Butterworth J, Legrault C, Royster R, Hammon J: Factors that predict the use of positive inotropic drug support after cardiac valve surgery, *Anesth Analg* 86:461, 1998.
476. Butterworth JF, Prielipp RC: Endocrine, metabolic, and electrolyte responses. In Gravlee GP, Davis RF, Kurusz M, Utley JR, editors: *Cardiopulmonary bypass, principles and practice*, ed 2, Philadelphia, Lippincott Williams & Wilkins, 2000, pp 342–366.
477. Zaloga GP, Strickland RA, Butterworth J.F.I.V., et al: Calcium attenuates epinephrine's beta-adrenergic effects in postoperative heart surgery patients, *Circulation* 81:196, 1990.
478. Follath F, Cleland JG, Just H, et al: Efficacy and safety of intravenous levosimendan compared with dobutamine in severe low-output heart failure (the LIDO study): A randomised double-blind trial, *Lancet* 360:196, 2002.
479. Follath F: Newer treatments for decompensated heart failure: Focus on levosimendan, *Drug Des Devel Ther* 3:73, 2009.
480. Mebazaa A, Nieminen MS, Packer M, et al: Levosimendan vs dobutamine for patients with acute decompensated heart failure: The SURVIVE Randomized Trial, *JAMA* 297:1883, 2007.
481. Siirilia-Waris K, Suojaranta-Ylinen R, Harjola VP: Levosimendan in cardiac surgery, *J Cardiothorac Vasc Anesth* 19:345–349, 2005.
482. Ririe DG, Butterworth JF IV, Royster RL, et al: Triiodothyronine increases contractility independent of beta-adrenergic receptors or stimulation of cyclic-3 ,5 -adenosine monophosphate, *Anesthesiology* 82:1004, 1995.
483. Bennett-Guerrero E, Jimenez JL, White WD, et al: Cardiovascular effects of intravenous triiodothyronine in patients undergoing coronary artery bypass graft surgery. A randomized, double-blind, placebo-controlled trial. Duke T3 study group, *JAMA* 275:687, 1996.
484. Rathmell JP, Prielipp RC, Butterworth JF, et al: A multicenter, randomized, blind comparison of amrinone with milrinone after elective cardiac surgery, *Anesth Analg* 86:683, 1998.
485. Butterworth JF IV, Royster RL, Prielipp RC, et al: Amrinone in cardiac surgical patients with left ventricular dysfunction. A prospective, randomized placebo-controlled trial, *Chest* 104:1660, 1993.
486. Doolan LA, Jones EF, Kalman J, et al: A placebo-controlled trial verifying the efficacy of milrinone in weaning high-risk patients from cardiopulmonary bypass, *J Cardiothorac Vasc Anesth* 11:37, 1997.
487. Hoffman TM, Wernovsky G, Atz AM, et al: Efficacy and safety of milrinone in preventing low cardiac output syndrome in infants and children after corrective surgery for congenital heart disease, *Circulation* 107:996, 2003.
488. MacGregor DA, Smith TE, Prielipp RC, et al: Pharmacokinetics of dopamine in healthy male subjects, *Anesthesiology* 92:338, 2000.
489. DiSesa VJ, Gold JP, Shemin RJ, et al: Comparison of dopamine and dobutamine in patients requiring postoperative circulatory support, *Clin Cardiol* 9:253, 1986.
490. Tinker JH, Tarhan S, White RD, et al: Dobutamine for inotropic support during emergence from cardiopulmonary bypass, *Anesthesiology* 44:281, 1976.
491. Kersting F, Follath F, Moulds R, et al: A comparison of cardiovascular effects of dobutamine and isoprenaline after open heart surgery, *Br Heart J* 38:622, 1976.
492. Pellikka PA, Roger VL, McCully RB, et al: Normal stroke volume and cardiac output response during dobutamine stress echocardiography in subjects without left ventricular wall motion abnormalities, *Am J Cardiol* 76:881, 1995.
493. Butterworth JFIV, Prielipp RC, Royster RL, et al: Dobutamine increases heart rate more than epinephrine in patients recovering from aortocoronary bypass surgery, *J Cardiothorac Vasc Anesth* 6:535, 1992.
494. Jaccard C, Berner M, Rouge JC, et al: Hemodynamic effect of isoprenaline and dobutamine immediately after correction of tetralogy of Fallot. Relative importance of inotropic and chronotropic action in supporting cardiac output, *J Thorac Cardiovasc Surg* 87:862, 1984.
495. Leone M, Vallet B, Teboul JL, et al: Survey of the use of catecholamines by French physicians, *Intensive Care Med* 30:984, 2004.
496. MacGregor DA, Butterworth JFIV, Zaloga CP, et al: Hemodynamic and renal effects of dopexamine and dobutamine in patients with reduced cardiac output following coronary artery bypass grafting, *Chest* 106:835, 1994.
497. Fullerton DA, St Cyr JA, Albert JD, et al: Hemodynamic advantage of left atrial epinephrine administration after cardiac operations, *Ann Thorac Surg* 56:1263, 1993.
498. Shephard J, Cobbe SM, Ford I, et al: Prevention of coronary artery disease with pravastatin in men with hypercholesterolemia. West of Scotland Coronary Prevention Study Group, *N Engl J Med* 333:1301, 1995.
499. Liu P, Konstam M, Force T: Highlights of the 2004 Scientific Sessions of the Heart Failure Society of America, *J Am Coll Cardiol* 45:617, 2005.
500. Vaughan Williams EM: Classification of antiarrhythmic drugs, *J Cardiovasc Pharmacol* 20:51, 1992.
501. Singh S, Patrick J: Antiarrhythmic drugs, *Curr Treat Options Cardiovasc Med* 6:357, 2004.
502. Liang BT: Adenosine receptors and cardiovascular function, *Trends Cardiovasc Med* 2:100, 1992.
503. Echt DS, Liebson PR, Mitchell LB, et al: Mortality and morbidity in patients receiving encainide, flecainide, or placebo, *N Engl J Med* 324:781, 1991.
504. Duff HJ, Roden DM, Yacobi A, et al: Bretylium: Relations between plasma concentrations and pharmacological actions in high-frequency ventricular arrhythmias, *Am J Cardiol* 55:395, 1985.
505. Roden DM: Drug therapy: Drug-induced prolongation of this QT interval, *N Engl J Med* 350:1013, 2004.
506. Investigators AVID: A comparison of antiarrhythmic drug therapy with implantable defibrillators in patients resuscitated from near-fatal ventricular arrhythmias, *N Engl J Med* 337:1576, 1997.
507. Harrison DC, Winkle R, Sami M, et al: Encainide: A new and potent antiarrhythmic agent, *Am Heart J* 100:1046, 1980.
508. Scheinman M, Keung E: The year in clinical electrophysiology, *J Am Coll Cardiol* 45:790, 2005.
509. Wittig J, Harrison LA, Wallace AG: Electrophysiological effects of lidocaine on distal Purkinje fibers of canine heart, *Am Heart J* 86:69, 1973.
510. Vaughan Williams EM: A classification of antiarrhythmic actions reassessed after a decade of new drugs, *J Clin Pharmacol* 24:129, 1984.
511. Hoffman BF, Rosen MR, Wit AL: Electrophysiology and pharmacology of cardiac arrhythmias. VII. Cardiac effects of quinidine and procainamide, *Am Heart J* 90:117, 1975.
512. Darbar D, Fromm MF, Dellorto S, Roden DM: Sympathetic activation enhances QT prolongation by quinidine, *J Cardiovasc Electrophysiol* 12:9, 2001.
513. Kessler KM, Lowenthal DT, Warner H, et al: Quinidine elimination in patients with congestive heart failure or poor renal function, *N Engl J Med* 290:706, 1974.
514. Leahey EB Jr, Reiffel JA, Drusin RE, et al: Interaction between quinidine and digoxin, *JAMA* 240:533, 1978.
515. Gerhardt RE, Knouss RF, Thyrum PT, et al: Quinidine excretion in aciduria and alkaluria, *Ann Intern Med* 71:927, 1969.
516. Koster RW, Wellens HJJ: Quinidine-induced ventricular flutter and fibrillation without digitalis therapy, *Am J Cardiol* 38:519, 1976.
517. Rials SJ, Britchkow D, Marinchak RA, Kowey PR: Electropharmacologic effect of a standard dose of intravenous procainamide in patients with sustained ventricular tachycardia, *Clin Cardiol* 23:171, 2000.
518. Krone RJ, Miller JP, Kleiger RE, et al: The effectiveness of antiarrhythmic agents on early-cycle premature ventricular complexes, *Circulation* 63:664, 1981.
519. Graffner C, Johnsson G, Sjogren J: Pharmacokinetics of procainamide intravenously and orally as conventional slow release tablets, *Clin Pharmacol Ther* 17:414, 1975.
520. Collste P, Karlsson E: Arrhythmia prophylaxis with procainamide: Plasma concentrations in relation to dose, *Acta Med Scand* 194:405, 1973.
521. Reidenberg MM, Drayer DE, Levy M, et al: Polymorphic acetylation of procainamide in man, *Clin Pharmacol Ther* 17:722, 1975.
522. Woosley RL, Roden DM: Importance of metabolites in antiarrhythmic therapy, *Am J Cardiol* 52:3C–7C, 1983.
523. Dimarco J, Gersh B, Opie L: Antiarrhythmic drugs and strategies. In Opie L, Horsh G, editors: *Drugs for the heart*, ed 6, Philadelphia, Elsevier, 2005, pp 218–274.
524. Strasberg B, Sclarovsky S, Erdberg A, et al: Procainamide-induced polymorphous ventricular tachycardia, *Am J Cardiol* 47:1309, 1981.
525. Blomgren SE, Condemi JJ, Vaughn JH: Procainamide-induced lupus erythematosus: Clinical and laboratory observations, *Am J Med* 52:338, 1972.
526. Michelson EL, Spear JF, Moore EN: Effects of procainamide on strength-interval relations in normal and chronically infarcted canine myocardium, *Am J Cardiol* 47:1223, 1981.
527. Wenger TL, Browning DL, Masterton CE, et al: Procainamide delivery to ischemic canine myocardium following rapid intravenous administration, *Circ Res* 46:789, 1980.
528. Reid DS, Williams DO, Parashar SK: Disopyramide in the sick sinus syndrome—safe or not? *Br Heart J* 39:348, 1977.
529. Spurrell RA, Thorburn CW, Camm J, et al: Effects of disopyramide on electrophysiological properties of specialized conduction system in man and on accessory atrioventricular pathway in Wolff-Parkinson-White syndrome, *Br Heart J* 37:861, 1975.
530. Podrid PJ, Schoeneberger A, Lown B: Congestive heart failure caused by oral disopyramide, *N Engl J Med* 302:614, 1980.
531. Koch-Weser J: Drug therapy. Disopyramide, *N Engl J Med* 300:957, 1979.
532. Zipes DP, Troup PJ: New antiarrhythmic agents: Amiodarone, aprinidine, disopyramide, ethmozin, mexiletine, tocainide, verapamil, *Am J Cardiol* 41:1005, 1979.
533. Chien YW, Lambert HJ, Karim A: Comparative binding of disopyramide phosphate and quinidine sulfate to human plasma proteins, *J Pharm Sci* 63:1877, 1974.
534. Sadowski ZP: Multicenter randomized trial and systemic overview of lidocaine in acute myocardial infarction, *Am Heart J* 137:792, 1999.
535. Carden NL, Steinhaus JE: Lidocaine and cardiac resuscitation from ventricular fibrillation, *Circ Res* 4:680, 1956.
536. Dorian P, Cass D, Schwartz G, et al: Amiodarone compared with lidocaine for shock-resistant ventricular fibrillation, *N Engl J Med* 346:884, 2002.
537. Weiss WA: Intravenous use of lidocaine for ventricular arrhythmias, *Anesth Analg* 39:369, 1960.

538. DeClive-Lowe SG, Desmond J, North J: Intravenous lignocaine anaesthesia, *Anaesthesia* 13:138, 1958.
539. Gerstenblith G, Spear JF, Moore EN: Quantitative study of the effect of lidocaine on the threshold for ventricular fibrillation in the dog, *Am J Cardiol* 30:242, 1972.
540. Davis LD, Temte JV: Electrophysiological actions of lidocaine on canine ventricular muscle and Purkinje fibers, *Circ Res* 24:639, 1969.
541. Singh BN, Williams EM: Effect of altering potassium concentration on the action of lidocaine and diphenylhydantoin on rabbit atrial and ventricular muscle, *Circ Res* 29:286, 1971.
542. Obayashi K, Hayakawa H, Mandell WJ: Interrelationships between external potassium concentration and lidocaine: Effects on canine Purkinje fiber, *Am Heart J* 89:221, 1975.
543. Watanabe Y, Dreifus LS, Likoff W: Electrophysiological antagonism and synergism of potassium and antiarrhythmic agents, *Am J Cardiol* 12:702, 1963.
544. Kupersmith J, Antman EM, Hoffman BF: In vivo electrophysiological effects of lidocaine in canine acute myocardial infarction, *Circ Res* 36:84, 1975.
545. El-Sherif N, Scherlag BJ, Lazzara R, et al: Reentrant ventricular arrhythmias in the late myocardial infarction period. 4. Mechanism of action of lidocaine, *Circulation* 56:395, 1977.
546. Covino B: Pharmacology of local anesthetics, *Br J Anaesth* 58:701, 1986.
547. Blumer J, Strong JM, Atkinson AJ Jr: The convulsant potency of lidocaine and its o-dealkylated metabolites, *J Pharmacol Exp Ther* 186:31, 1973.
548. Collinsworth KA, Kalman SM, Harrison DC: The clinical pharmacology of lidocaine as an antiarrhythmic drug, *Circulation* 50:1217, 1974.
549. Smith ER, Duce BR: The acute antiarrhythmic and toxic effects in mice and dogs of 2-ethylamino-2,6-acetoxylidine (L-86), a metabolite of lidocaine, *J Pharmacol Exp Ther* 179:580, 1971.
550. Essman WB: Xylocaine-induced protection against electrically induced convulsions in mice, *Arch Int Pharmacodyn Ther* 157:166, 1965.
551. Bernheard CG, Bohm E: *Local anesthetics as anticonvulsants. A study on experimental and clinical epilepsy*, Stockholm, Almqvist & Wiksel, 1965.
552. Hood DD, Mecca RS: Failure to initiate electroconvulsive seizures in a patient pretreated with lidocaine, *Anesthesiology* 58:379, 1983.
553. Ikram H: Hemodynamic and electrophysiologic interactions between antiarrhythmic drugs and beta-blockers, with special reference to tocainide, *Am Heart J* 100:1076, 1980.
554. Kuhn P, Kroiss A, Klicpera M, et al: Antiarrhythmic and haemodynamic effects of mexiletine, *Postgrad Med J* 53(Suppl I):81, 1977.
555. Winkle RA, Anderson JL, Peters F, et al: The hemodynamic effects of intravenous tocainide in patients with heart disease, *Circulation* 57:787, 1978.
556. Nyquist O, Forssell G, Nordlander R, et al: Hemodynamic and antiarrhythmic effects of tocainide in patients with acute myocardial infarction, *Am Heart J* 100:1000, 1980.
557. Ryan WF, Karliner JS: Effects of tocainide on left ventricular performance at rest and during acute alterations in heart rate and systemic arterial pressure, *Br Heart J* 41:175, 1979.
558. Abinader EG, Cooper M: Mexiletine. Use and control of chronic drug-resistant ventricular arrhythmia, *JAMA* 242:337, 1979.
559. DiMarco JP, Garan H, Ruskin JN: Mexiletine for refractory-ventricular arrhythmias: Results using serial electrophysiologic testing, *Am J Cardiol* 47:131, 1981.
560. Podrid PJ, Lown B: Mexiletine for ventricular arrhythmias, *Am J Cardiol* 47:895, 1981.
561. Horowitz JD, Anavekar SN, Morris PM, et al: Comparative trial of mexiletine and lignocaine in the treatment of early ventricular tachyarrhythmias after acute myocardial infarction, *J Cardiovasc Pharmacol* 3:409, 1981.
562. Campbell RWF, Achuff SC, Pottage A, et al: Mexiletine in the prophylaxis of ventricular arrhythmias during acute myocardial infarction, *J Cardiovasc Pharmacol* 1:43, 1979.
563. Bell JA, Thomas JM, Isaacson JR, et al: A trial of prophylactic mexiletine in home coronary care, *Br Heart J* 48:285, 1982.
564. Chamberlain DA, Jewitt DE, Julian DG, et al: Oral mexiletine in high-risk patients after myocardial infarction, *Lancet* 2:1324, 1980.
565. Ryden L, Arnman K, Conradson TB, et al: Prophylaxis of ventricular tachyarrhythmias with intravenous and oral tocainide. In Harrison DC, editor: *Cardiac arrhythmias—a decade of progress*, Boston, 1981, GK Hall, pp 227–247.
566. Pottage A: Clinical profiles of newer class I antiarrhythmic agents-tocainide, mexiletine, encainide, flecainide, and lorcainide, *Am J Cardiol* 52:24C–31C, 1983.
567. Oltmanns D: Tocainid-pharmakokinetik bei chronischer lebererkrankung (abstract), *Z Kardiol* 71:172, 1982.
568. El Allaf D, Henrard L, Crochelet L, et al: Pharmacokinetics of mexiletine in renal insufficiency, *Br J Pharmacol* 14:431, 1982.
569. Campbell NP, Kelly JG, Adgey AA, et al: The clinical pharmacology of mexiletine, *Br J Clin Pharmacol* 6:103, 1978.
570. Gillis RA, McClellan JR, Sauer TS, et al: Depression of cardiac sympathetic nerve activity by diphenylhydantoin, *J Pharmacol Exp Ther* 179:599, 1971.
571. Evans DE, Gillis RA: Effect of diphenylhydantoin and lidocaine on cardiac arrhythmias induced by hypothalamic stimulation, *J Pharmacol Exp Ther* 191:506, 1974.
572. Singh BN: Explanation for the discrepancy in reported cardiac electrophysiological actions of diphenylhydantoin and lignocaine, *Br J Pharmacol* 41:385P, 1971.
573. Bigger JT Jr, Weinberg DI, Kovalik AT, et al: Effects of diphenylhydantoin on excitability and automaticity in the canine heart, *Circ Res* 26:1, 1970.
574. Rosen MR, Danilo P Jr, Alonso MB, et al: Effects of therapeutic concentrations of diphenylhydantoin on transmembrane potentials of normal and depressed Purkinje fibers, *J Pharmacol Exp Ther* 197:594, 1976.
575. Peon J, Ferrier GR, Moe GK: The relationship of excitability to conduction velocity in canine Purkinje tissue, *Circ Res* 43:125, 1978.
576. Bigger JT Jr, Bassett AL, Hollnian BF: Electrophysiological effects of diphenylhydantoin on canine Purkinje fibers, *Circ Res* 22:221, 1968.
577. Garson A Jr, Kugler JD, Gillette PC, et al: Control of late postoperative ventricular arrhythmias with phenytoin in young patients, *Am J Cardiol* 46:290, 1980.
578. Bigger JT Jr, Schmidt DH, Kutt H: Relationship between the plasma level of diphenylhydantoin sodium and its cardiac antiarrhythmic effects, *Circulation* 38:363, 1968.
579. Kutt H, Winters W, Kokenge R, et al: Diphenylhydantoin metabolism, blood levels, and toxicity, *Arch Neurol* 11:642, 1964.
580. Lieberson AD, Schumacher RR, Childress RH, et al: Effect of diphenylhydantoin on left ventricular function in patients with heart disease, *Circulation* 36:692, 1967.
581. Conn RD, Kennedy JW, Blackmon JR: The hemodynamic effects of diphenylhydantoin, *Am Heart J* 73:500, 1967.
582. Louis S, Kutt H, McDowell F: Cardiocirculatory changes caused by intravenous dilantin and its solvent, *Am Heart J* 74:523, 1967.
583. Unger AH, Sklaroff HJ: Fatalities following intravenous use of sodium diphenylhydantoin for cardiac arrhythmias, *JAMA* 200:335, 1967.
584. Olsson SB, Edvardsson N: Clinical electrophysiologic study of antiarrhythmic properties of flecainide: Acute intraventricular delayed conduction and prolonged repolarization in regular paced and premature beats using intracardiac monophasic action potentials with programmed stimulation, *Am Heart J* 102:864, 1981.
585. Duff HJ, Roden DM, Maffucci RJ, et al: Suppression of resistant ventricular arrhythmias by twice daily dosing with flecainide, *Am J Cardiol* 48:1133, 1981.
586. Bronzetti G, Formigari R, Giardini A, et al: Intravenous flecainide for the treatment of junctional ectopic tachycardia after surgery for congenital heart disease, *Ann Thorac Surg* 76:148, 2003.
587. Verdouw PD, Deckers JW, Conrad GJ: Antiarrhythmic and hemodynamic actions of flecainide acetate (R-818) in the ischemic porcine heart, *J Cardiovasc Pharmacol* 1:473, 1979.
588. Hodges M, Haugland JM, Granrud G, et al: Suppression of ventricular ectopic depolarization by flecainide acetate, a new antiarrhythmic agent, *Circulation* 65:879, 1982.
589. Anderson JL, Stewart JR, Perry BA, et al: Oral flecainide acetate for the treatment of ventricular arrhythmias, *N Engl J Med* 305:473, 1981.
590. Lui HK, Lee G, Dietrich P, et al: Flecainide-induced QT prolongation and ventricular tachycardia, *Am Heart J* 103:567, 1982.
591. Arias C, Gonzalez T, Moreno I, et al: Effects of propafenone and its main metabolite, 5-hydroxypropafenone, on HERG channels, *Cardiovasc Res* 57:660, 2003.
592. Boriani G, Martignani C, Biffi M, et al: Oral loading with propafenone for conversion of recent-onset atrial fibrillation: A review on in-hospital treatment, *Drugs* 62:415, 2002.
593. Mörike K, Kivistö KT, Schaeffeler E, et al: Propafenone for the prevention of atrial tachyarrhythmias after cardiac surgery: A randomized, double-blind placebo-controlled trial, *Clin Pharmacol Ther* 84:104, 2008.
594. Effect of the antiarrhythmic agent moricizine on survival after myocardial infarction. The Cardiac Arrhythmia Suppression Trial II Investigators, *N Engl J Med* 327:227, 1992.
595. Woosley RL, Shand D, Cornhauser B, et al: Relation of plasma concentration and dose of propranolol to its effect on resistant ventricular arrhythmias, *Clin Res* 25:262A, 1967.
596. Kupersmith J, Shiang H, Litwak RS, et al: Electrophysiological and antiarrhythmic effects of propranolol in canine acute myocardial ischemia, *Circ Res* 38:302, 1976.
597. Evans GH, Wilkinson GR, Shand DG: The disposition of propranolol. IV. A dominant role for tissue uptake in the dose-dependent extraction of propranolol by the perfused rat liver, *J Pharmacol Exp Ther* 186:447, 1973.
598. Evans GH, Nies AS, Shand DG: The disposition of propranolol. 3. Decreased half-life and volume of distribution as a result of plasma binding in man, monkey, dog, and rat, *J Pharmacol Exp Ther* 186:114, 1973.
599. Fitzgerald JD, O'Donnell SR: Pharmacology of 4-hydroxypropranolol, a metabolite of propranolol, *Br J Pharmacol* 43:222, 1971.
600. Shand DG: Drug therapy: Propranolol, *N Engl J Med* 293:280, 1975.
601. Wood M, Shand DG, Wood AJJ: Propranolol binding in plasma during cardiopulmonary bypass, *Anesthesiology* 51:512, 1979.
602. Miller RR, Olson HG, Amsterdam EA, et al: Propranolol-withdrawal rebound phenomenon. Exacerbation of coronary events after abrupt cessation of antianginal therapy, *N Engl J Med* 293:416, 1975.
603. Shiroff RA, Mathis J, Zelis R, et al: Propranolol rebound—a retrospective study, *Am J Cardiol* 41:778, 1978.
604. Ablad B, Carlsson E, Ek L: Pharmacological studies of two new cardioselective adrenergic beta-receptor antagonists, *Life Sci* 12:107, 1973.
605. Lennard MS, Silas JH, Freestone S, et al: Oxidation phenotype—a major determinant of metoprolol metabolism and response, *N Engl J Med* 307:1558, 1982.
606. Halonen J, Hakala T, Auvinen T, et al: Intravenous administration of metoprolol is more effective than oral administration in the prevention of atrial fibrillation after cardiac surgery, *Circulation* 114(1 Suppl):I1, 2006.
607. Haghjoo M, Saravi M, Hashemi MJ, et al: Optimal beta-blocker for prevention of atrial fibrillation after on-pump coronary artery bypass graft surgery: Carvedilol versus metoprolol, *Heart Rhythm* 4:1170, 2007.
608. Kaplan JA: Role of ultrashort-acting beta-blockers in the perioperative period, *J Cardiothorac Anesth* 2:683, 1988.
609. Gorczynski RJ, Shaffer JE, Lee RJ: Pharmacology of ASL, a novel beta-adrenergic receptor antagonist with an ultra short duration of action, *J Cardiovasc Pharmacol* 5:668, 1983.
610. Steck J, Sheppard D, Byrd RC, et al: Pulmonary effects of esmolol-an ultra short-acting beta-adrenergic blocking agent, *Clin Res* 33:472A, 1985.
611. Morganroth J, Horowitz LN, Anderson J, et al: Comparative efficacy and tolerance of esmolol to propranolol for control of supraventricular tachyarrhythmia, *Am J Cardiol* 56:33F–39F, 1985.
612. Harasawa R, Hayashi Y, Iwasaki M, et al: Bolus administration of landiolol, a short-acting, selective beta1-blocker, to treat tachycardia during anesthesia: A dose-dependent study, *J Cardiothorac Vasc Anesth* 20:793, 2006.
613. Wariishi S, Yamashita K, Nishimori H, et al: Postoperative administration of landiolol hydrochloride for patients with supraventricular arrhythmia: The efficacy of sustained intravenous infusion at a low dose, *Interact Cardiovasc Thorac Surg* 9:811, 2009.
614. Fujiwara H, Sakurai M, Namai A, et al: Effect of low-dose landiolol, an ultrashort-acting beta-blocker, on postoperative atrial fibrillation after CABG surgery, *Gen Thorac Cardiovasc Surg* 57:132, 2009.
615. Daoud EG, Strickberger SA, Man KC, et al: Preoperative amiodarone as prophylaxis against atrial fibrillation after heart surgery, *N Engl J Med* 337:1785, 1997.
616. Kaski JC, Girotti LA, Messuti H, et al: Long-term management of sustained, recurrent, symptomatic ventricular tachycardia with amiodarone, *Circulation* 64:273, 1981.
617. Nademanee K, Hendrickson JA, Cannom DS, et al: Control of refractory life-threatening ventricular tachyarrhythmias by amiodarone, *Am Heart J* 101:759, 1981.
618. Ward DE, Camm AJ, Spurrell RA: Clinical antiarrhythmic effects of amiodarone in patients with resistant paroxysmal tachycardias, *Br Heart J* 44:91, 1980.
619. Fogoros RN, Anderson KP, Winkle RA, et al: Amiodarone: Clinical efficacy and toxicity in 96 patients with recurrent, drug-refractory arrhythmias, *Circulation* 68:88, 1983.
620. American Heart Association: Guidelines for cardiopulmonary resuscitation emergency cardiovascular care, *Circulation* 102(Suppl I):I–1, 2000.
621. Dorian P, Mangat I: Role of amiodarone in the era of the implantable cardioverter defibrillator, *J Cardiovasc Electrophysiol* 14(Suppl 9):S78–S81, 2003.
622. Goupil N, Lenfant J: The effects of amiodarone on the sinus node activity of the rabbit heart, *Eur J Pharmacol* 39:23, 1976.
623. Rosen MR, Wit AL: Electropharmacology of antiarrhythmic drugs, *Am Heart J* 106:829, 1983.
624. Dhurandhar RW, Pickron J, Goldman AM: Bretylium tosylate in the management of recurrent ventricular fibrillation complicating acute myocardial infarction, *Heart Lung* 9:265, 1980.
625. Gloor HO, Urthaler F, James TN: Acute effects of amiodarone upon the canine sinus node and the atrioventricular junctional region, *J Clin Invest* 71:1457, 1983.
626. Singh BN: Amiodarone: Historical development and pharmacologic profile, *Am Heart J* 106:788, 1983.
627. Heger JJ, Prystowsky EN, Jackman WM, et al: Amiodarone: Clinical efficacy and electrophysiology during long-term therapy for recurrent ventricular tachycardia or fibrillation, *N Engl J Med* 305:539, 1981.
628. Zipes DP, Prystowsky EN, Heger JJ: Amiodarone: Electrophysiologic actions, pharmacokinetics, and clinical effects, *J Am Coll Cardiol* 3:1059, 1984.
629. Singh BN, Nademanee K: Amiodarone and thyroid function: Clinical implications during antiarrhythmic therapy, *Am Heart J* 106:857, 1983.

630. Hariman RJ, Gomes JAC, Kang PS, et al: Effects of intravenous amiodarone in patients with inducible repetitive ventricular responses and ventricular tachycardia, *Am Heart J* 107:1109, 1984.
631. Marcus FI, Fontaine GH, Frank R, et al: Clinical pharmacology and therapeutic applications of the antiarrhythmic agent amiodarone, *Am Heart J* 101:480, 1981.
632. DeBoer LWV, Nosta JJ, Kloner RA, et al: Studies of amiodarone during experimental myocardial infarction: Beneficial effects on hemodynamics and infarct size, *Circulation* 65:508, 1982.
633. Haffajee CI, Love JC, Alpert JS, et al: Efficacy and safety of long-term amiodarone in treatment of cardiac arrhythmias: Dosage experience, *Am Heart J* 106:935, 1983.
634. Canada AT, Lasko LG, Haffajee CI: Disposition of amiodarone in patients with tachyarrhythmias, *Curr Ther Res* 30:968, 1981.
635. Latini R, Tognoni G, Kates RE: Clinical pharmacokinetics of amiodarone, *Clin Pharmacokinet* 9:136, 1984.
636. Andreasen F, Agerbaek H, Bjerrega-ard P, et al: Pharmacokinetics of amiodarone after intravenous and oral administration, *Eur J Clin Pharmacol* 19:293, 1981.
637. Mostow ND, Rakita L, Vrobel TR, et al: Amiodarone: Intravenous loading for rapid suppression of complex ventricular arrhythmias, *J Am Coll Cardiol* 4:97, 1984.
638. Kerin NZ, Blevins RD, Frumin H, et al: Intravenous and oral loading versus oral loading alone with amiodarone for chronic refractory ventricular arrhythmias, *Am J Cardiol* 55:89, 1985.
639. Harris L, McKenna WJ, Rowland E, et al: Side effects and possible contraindications of amiodarone use, *Am Heart J* 106:916, 1983.
640. Rakita L, Sobol SM, Mostow N, et al: Amiodarone pulmonary toxicity, *Am Heart J* 106:906, 1983.
641. Marchlinski FE, Gansler TS, Waxman HL, et al: Amiodarone pulmonary toxicity, *Ann Intern Med* 97:839, 1982.
642. Kudenchuk PJ, Pierson DJ, Greene HL, et al: Prospective evaluation of amiodarone pulmonary toxicity, *Chest* 86:541, 1984.
643. Veltri EP, Reid PR: Amiodarone pulmonary toxicity: Early changes in pulmonary function tests during amiodarone rechallenge, *J Am Coll Cardiol* 6:802, 1985.
644. Burger A, Dinicher D, Nicod P, et al: Effect of amiodarone on serum triiodothyronine, reverse triiodothyronine, thyroxin and thyrotropin. A drug influencing peripheral metabolism of thyroid hormones, *J Clin Invest* 58:255, 1976.
645. Kerin NZ, Blevins RD, Benaderet D, et al: Relation of serum reverse T3 to amiodarone antiarrhythmic efficacy and toxicity, *Am J Cardiol* 57:128, 1986.
646. Buchser E, Chiolero R, Martin P, et al: Amiodarone-induced haemodynamic complications during anaesthesia, *Anaesthesia* 38:1008, 1983.
647. Gallagher JD, Lieberman RW, Meranze J, et al: Amiodarone-induced complications during coronary artery surgery, *Anesthesiology* 55:186, 1981.
648. Spotnitz WD, Nolan SP, Kaiser DL, et al: The reversal of amiodarone-induced perioperative reduction in cardiac systolic reserve in dogs, *J Am Coll Cardiol* 12:757, 1988.
649. Mitchell LB, Exner DV, Wyse DG, et al: Prophylactic oral amiodarone for the prevention of arrhythmias that begin early after revascularization, valve replacement, or repair: PAPABEAR: A randomized controlled trial, *JAMA* 294:3093, 2005.
650. Samuels LE, Holmes EC, Samuels FL: Selective use of amiodarone and early cardioversion for postoperative atrial fibrillation, *Ann Thorac Surg* 79:113, 2005.
651. Kovacikova L, Hakacova N, Dobos D, et al: Amiodarone as a first-line therapy for postoperative junctional ectopic tachycardia, *Ann Thorac Surg* 88:616, 2009.
652. Tisdale JE, Wroblewski HA, Wall DS, et al: A randomized trial evaluating amiodarone for prevention of atrial fibrillation after pulmonary resection, *Ann Thorac Surg* 88:886, 2009.
653. Beaulieu Y, Denault AY, Couture P, et al: Perioperative intravenous amiodarone does not reduce the burden of atrial fibrillation in patients undergoing cardiac valvular surgery, *Anesthesiology* 112:128, 2010.
654. Boura AL, Green AF: Actions of bretylium: Adrenergic neuron blocking and other effects, *Br Pharm Chemother* 14:536, 1959.
655. Chatterjee K, Mandel WJ, Vyden JK, et al: Cardiovascular effects of bretylium tosylate in acute myocardial infarction, *JAMA* 223:757, 1973.
656. Anderson JL, Patterson E, Wagner JG, et al: Clinical pharmacokinetics of intravenous and oral bretylium tosylate in survivors of ventricular tachycardia or fibrillation: Clinical application of a new assay for bretylium, *J Cardiovasc Pharmacol* 3:485, 1981.
657. Lucchesi BR: Rationale of therapy in the patient with acute myocardial infarction and life-threatening arrhythmias: A focus on bretylium, *Am J Cardiol* 54:14A–19A, 1984.
658. Kniffen FJ, Lomas TE, Counsell RE, et al: The antiarrhythmic and antifibrillatory actions of bretylium and its o-iodobenzyltrimethyl ammonium analog, UM-360, *J Pharmacol Exp Ther* 192:120, 1975.
659. Cervoni P, Ellis CH, Maxwell RA: Anti-arrhythmic action of bretylium in normal, reserpine-pretreated and chronically denervated dog hearts, *Arch Int Pharmacodyn Ther* 190:91, 1971.
660. Namm DH, Wang CM, El-Sayad S, et al: Effects of bretylium on rat cardiac muscle: The electrophysiological effects and its uptake and binding in normal and immunosympathectomized rat hearts, *J Pharmacol Exp Ther* 193:194, 1975.
661. Tacker WA Jr, Niebauer MJ, Babbs CF, et al: The effect of newer antiarrhythmic drugs on defibrillation threshold, *Crit Care Med* 8:177, 1980.
662. Haynes RE, Chinn TL, Copass MK, et al: Comparison of bretylium tosylate and lidocaine in management of out-of-hospital ventricular fibrillation: A randomized clinical trial, *Am J Cardiol* 48:353, 1981.
663. Nowak RM, Bodnar TJ, Dronen S, et al: Bretylium tosylate as initial treatment for cardiopulmonary arrest: Randomized comparison with placebo, *Ann Emerg Med* 10:404, 1981.
664. Terry G, Vellani CW, Higgins MR, et al: Bretylium tosylate in treatment of refractory ventricular arrhythmias complicating myocardial infarction, *Br Heart J* 32:21, 1970.
665. Bernstein JG, Koch-Weser J: Effectiveness of bretylium tosylate against refractory ventricular arrhythmias, *Circulation* 45:1024, 1972.
666. Holder DA, Sniderman AD, Fraser G, et al: Experience with bretylium tosylate by a hospital cardiac arrest team, *Circulation* 55:541, 1977.
667. MacAlpin RN, Zalis EG, Kivowitz CF: Prevention of recurrent ventricular tachycardia with oral bretylium tosylate, *Ann Intern Med* 72:909, 1970.
668. Woosley RL: Antiarrhythmic drugs. In Hurst JW, editor: *The heart*, ed 11, New York, 2004, McGraw-Hill, pp 949–974.
669. O'Callaghan PA, McGovern BA: Evolving role of sotalol in the management of ventricular tachyarrhythmias, *Am J Cardiol* 78:54, 1996.
670. Reiter MJ: The ESVEM trial: Impact on treatment of ventricular tachyarrhythmias. Electrophysiologic Study Versus Electrocardiographic Monitoring, *Pacing Clin Electrophysiol* 20:468, 1997.
671. Reiffel JA, Hahn E, Hartz V, Reiter MJ: Sotalol for ventricular tachyarrhythmias. ESVEM Investigators: Electrophysiologic Study Versus Electrocardiographic Monitoring, *Am J Cardiol* 79:1048, 1997.
672. Wanless RS, Anderson K, Joy M, Joseph SP: Multicenter comparative study of the efficacy and safety of sotalol in the prophylactic treatment of patients with paroxysmal supraventricular tachyarrhythmias, *Am Heart J* 133:441, 1997.
673. Waldo AL, Camm AJ, deRuyter H, et al: Effect of D-sotalol on mortality in patients with left ventricular dysfunction after recent and remote myocardial infarction. The SWORD Investigators, Survival with Oral D-Sotalol, *Lancet* 348:7, 1996.
674. Cropp JS, Antal EG, Talbert RL: Ibutilide: A new class III antiarrhythmic agent, *Pharmacotherapy* 17:1, 1997.
675. Yang T, Snyders DJ, Roden DM: Ibutilide, a methanesulfonailide antiarrhythmic, *Circulation* 91:1799, 1995.
676. Naccarelli GV, Lee KS, Gibson JK, VanderLugt JT: Electrophysiology and pharmacology of ibutilide, *Am J Cardiol* 78:12, 1996.
677. Ellenbogen KA, Stambler BS, Wood MA, et al: Efficacy of intravenous ibutilide for rapid termination of atrial fibrillation and atrial flutter: A dose-response study, *J Am Coll Cardiol* 28:130, 1996.
678. Stambler BS, Wood MA, Ellenbogen KA, et al: Efficacy and safety of repeated intravenous doses of ibutilide for rapid conversion of atrial flutter or fibrillation, *Circulation* 94:1613, 1996.
679. Tercius AJ, Kluger J, Coleman CI, et al: Intravenous magnesium sulfate enhances the ability of intravenous ibutilide to successfully convert atrial fibrillation or flutter, *Pacing Clin Electrophysiol* 30:1331, 2007.
680. Kowey PR, VanderLugt JT, Luderer JR: Safety and risk/benefit analysis of ibutilide for acute conversion of atrial fibrillation/flutter, *Am J Cardiol* 78:46, 1996.
681. Kalus JS, Mauro VF: Dofetilide: A class III-specific antiarrhythmic agent, *Ann Pharmacol Ther* 34:44, 2000.
682. Coleman CI, Sood N, Chawla D, et al: Intravenous magnesium sulfate enhances the ability of dofetilide to successfully cardiovert atrial fibrillation or flutter: Results of the Dofetilide and Intravenous Magnesium Evaluation, *Europace* 11:892, 2009.
683. Van Breemen C, Aaronson P, Loutzenhiser R: Sodium-calcium interactions in mammalian smooth muscle, *Pharmacol Rev* 30:167, 1978.
684. Katz AM, Messineo FC: Lipids and membrane function: Implications in arrhythmias, *Hosp Pract* 16:49, 1981.
685. Gettes LS: Possible role of ionic changes in the appearance of arrhythmias, *Pharmacol Ther [B]* 2:787, 1976.
686. Triggle DJ: Calcium antagonists: Basic chemical and pharmacological aspects. In Weiss GB, editor: *New perspectives on calcium antagonists*, Bethesda, MD, American Physiological Society, 1981, pp 1–18.
687. Fleckenstein A: Specific pharmacology of calcium in myocardium, cardiac pacemaker, and vascular smooth muscle, *Annu Rev Pharmacol Toxicol* 17:149, 1977.
688. Henry PD: Comparative pharmacology of calcium antagonists: Nifedipine, verapamil and diltiazem, *Am J Cardiol* 46:1047, 1980.
689. Kazda S, Garthoff B, Meyer H, et al: Pharmacology of a new calcium antagonist compound, isobutyl methyl 1,4-dihydro-2,6-dimethyl-4-(2-nitrofentyl)-3,5-pyridinedicarb oxylate (nisoldipine, k5552), *Arzneimittelforschung* 30:2144, 1980.
690. Triggle DJ: Biochemical pharmacology of calcium blockers. In Flaim SF, Xellis R, editors: *Calcium blockers: Mechanisms of action and clinical applications*, Baltimore, Urban and Swartzenberg, 1981.
691. Satoh K, Yanagisawa T, Taira N: Coronary vasodilator and cardiac effects of optical isomers of verapamil in the dog, *J Cardiovasc Pharmacol* 2:309, 1980.
692. Roy PR, Spurrell RA, Sowton GE: The effect of verapamil on the conduction system in man, *Postgrad Med J* 50:270, 1974.
693. Schlepper M, Weppner HG, Merle H: Haemodynamic effects of supraventricular tachycardias and their alterations by electrically and verapamil-induced termination, *Cardiovasc Res* 12:28, 1978.
694. Kopman EA: Intravenous verapamil to relieve pulmonary congestion in patients with mitral valve disease, *Anesthesiology* 58:374, 1983.
695. Kapur PA, Flacke WE, Olewine SK: Comparison of effects of isoflurane versus enflurane on cardiovascular and catecholamine responses to verapamil in dogs, *Anesth Analg* 61:193, 1982.
696. Kates RA, Kaplan JA, Guyton RA, et al: Hemodynamic interactions of verapamil and isoflurane in dogs, *Anesth Analg* 59:132, 1983.
697. Singh BN, Nademanee K, Feld G: Calcium blockers in the treatment of cardiac arrhythmias. In Flaim SF, Zelis R, editors: *Calcium blockers: Mechanisms of actions and clinical applications*, Baltimore, Urban and Swartzenberg, 1982, 258.
698. Mangiardi LM, Hariman RJ, McAllister RG Jr, et al: Electrophysiologic and hemodynamic effects of verapamil: Correlation with plasma drug concentrations, *Circulation* 57:366, 1978.
699. Kates RE, Keefe DLD, Schwartz J, et al: Verapamil disposition kinetics in chronic atrial fibrillation, *Clin Pharmacol Ther* 30:44, 1981.
700. Brichard G, Zimmermann PE: Verapamil in cardiac dysrrhythmias during anaesthesia, *Br J Anaesth* 42:1005, 1970.
701. Schreck DM, Rivera AR, Tricarico VJ: Emergency management of atrial fibrillation and flutter: Intravenous diltiazem versus intravenous digoxin, *Ann Emerg Med* 29:135, 1997.
702. Olshansky B: Management of atrial fibrillation after coronary artery bypass graft, *Am J Cardiol* 78:27, 1996.
703. Amar D, Roistacher N, Burt ME, et al: Effects of diltiazem versus digoxin on dysrhythmias and cardiac function after pneumonectomy, *Ann Thorac Surg* 63:1374, 1997.
704. Billman GE: Effect of calcium channel antagonists on cocaine-induced malignant arrhythmias: Protection against ventricular fibrillation, *J Pharmacol Exp Ther* 266:407, 1993.
705. Lawson NW, Kraynack BJ, Gintautas J: Neuromuscular and electrocardiographic responses to verapamil in dogs, *Anesth Analg* 62:50, 1983.
706. Kraynack BJ, Lawson NW, Gintautas J: Neuromuscular blocking action of verapamil in cats, *Can Anaesth Soc J* 30:242, 1983.
707. Bobbio A, Caporale D, Internullo E, et al: Postoperative outcome of patients undergoing lung resection presenting with new-onset atrial fibrillation managed by amiodarone or diltiazem, *Eur J Cardiothorac Surg* 31:70, 2007.
708. Dobrilovic N, Vadlamani L, Buchert B, et al: Diltiazem prophylaxis reduces incidence of atrial fibrillation after coronary artery bypass grafting, *J Cardiovasc Surg (Torino)* 46:457, 2005.
709. Davis LD: Effect of changes in cycle length on diastolic depolarization produced by ouabain in canine Purkinje fibers, *Circ Res* 32:206, 1973.
710. Ferrier GR, Saunders JH, Mendez C: A cellular mechanism for the generation of ventricular arrhythmias by acetylstrophanthidan, *Circ Res* 32:600, 1973.
711. Rosen MR, Gelband H, Merker C, et al: Mechanisms of digitalis toxicity: Effects of ouabain on phase 4 of canine Purkinje fiber transmembrane potentials, *Circ Res* 47:681, 1973.
712. Hoffman BF, Bigger JT Jr: Digitalis and allied cardiac glycosides. In Gilman AG, Goodman LS, Rall TW, et al (eds): The pharmacological basis of therapeutics, 7th ed. New York, Macmillan, 1985, pp 724–725.
713. Rosen MR, Wit AL, Hoffman BF: Electrophysiology and pharmacology of cardiac arrhythmias. IV. Cardiac antiarrhythmic and toxic effects of digitalis, *Am Heart J* 89:391, 1975.
714. Mudge GH Jr, Lloyd BL, Greenblatt DJ, et al: Inotropic and toxic effects of a polar cardiac glycoside derivative in a dog, *Circ Res* 43:847, 1978.
715. Gillis RA, Quest JA: The role of the central nervous system in the cardiovascular effects of digitalis, *Pharmacol Rev* 31:19, 1979.
716. Lerman BB, Belardinelli L: Cardiac electrophysiology of adenosine, basic and clinical concepts, *Circulation* 83:1499, 1991.
717. Camm AJ, Garratt CJ: Adenosine and supraventricular tachycardia, *N Engl J Med* 325:1621, 1991.
718. Hood MA, Smith WM: Adenosine versus verapamil in the treatment of supraventricular tachycardia: A randomized double-crossover trial, *Am Heart J* 123:1543, 1992.
719. Overholt ED, Rheuban KS, Gutgesell HP, et al: Usefulness of adenosine for arrhythmias in infants and children, *Am J Cardiol* 61:336, 1988.

720. Mohnle P, Schwann N, Vaughn W, et al: Perturbations in laboratory values after coronary artery bypass surgery with cardiopulmonary bypass, *J Cardiothorac Vasc Anesth* 19:19, 2005.
721. Eisenkraft J: Electrolyte disturbances and the electrocardiogram. In Thys D, Kapun JA, eds: *The ECG in anesthesia and critical care*, New York, 1987, Churchill-Livingstone, pp 167–180.
722. Chung EK: *Principles of cardiac arrhythmias*, ed 2, Baltimore, 1977, Williams & Wilkins, pp 25 32, 570, 651, 668, 672.
723. Pacifico AD, Digerness S, Kirklin JW: Acute alterations of body composition after open heart intracardiac operations, *Circulation* 41:331, 1970.
724. Mandelbaum I, Morgan CR: Effect of extracorporeal circulation upon insulin, *J Thorac Cardiovasc Surg* 55:526, 1968.
725. Burch GE, Giles TE: The importance of magnesium deficiency in cardiovascular disease, *Am Heart J* 94:649, 1977.
726. Aglio LS, Stanford GG, Maddi R, et al: Hypomagnesemia is common following cardiac surgery, *J Cardiothorac Vasc Anesth* 5:201, 1991.
727. Turlapaty PDMV, Altura BM: Magnesium deficiency produces spasm of coronary arteries. Relationship to etiology of sudden death and ischemic heart disease, *Science* 208:198, 1980.
728. Seller RH, Cangiano J, Kim KE, et al: Digitalis toxicity and hypomagnesemia, *Am Heart J* 79:57, 1970.
729. Specter MJ, Schweizer E, Goldman RH: Studies on magnesium's mechanism of action in digitalis-induced arrhythmias, *Circulation* 52:1001, 1975.
730. Gupta A, Lawrence AT, Krishnan K, et al: Current concepts in the mechanisms and management of drug-induced QT prolongation and torsade de pointes, *Am Heart J* 153:891, 2007.
731. Scheinman MM, Sullivan RW, Hyatt KH: Magnesium metabolism in patients undergoing cardiopulmonary bypass, *Circulation* 39:I235, 1969.
732. Kohno H, Koyanagi T, Kasegawa H, et al: Three-day magnesium administration prevents atrial fibrillation after coronary artery bypass grafting, *Ann Thorac Surg* 79:117, 2005.
733. Dabrowski W, Rzecki Z, Sztanke M, et al: The efficiency of magnesium supplementation in patients undergoing cardiopulmonary bypass: Changes in serum magnesium concentrations and atrial fibrillation episodes, *Magnes Res* 21:205, 2008.
734. Tiryakioglu O, Demirtas S, Ari H, et al: Magnesium sulphate and amiodarone prophylaxis for prevention of postoperative arrhythmia in coronary by-pass operations, *J Cardiothorac Surg* 4:8, 2009.
735. Sleeswijk ME, Tulleken JE, Van Noord T, et al: Efficacy of magnesium-amiodarone step-up scheme in critically ill patients with new-onset atrial fibrillation: A prospective observational study, *J Intensive Care Med* 23:61, 2008.
736. Aerra V, Kuduvalli M, Moloto AN, et al: Does prophylactic sotalol and magnesium decrease the incidence of atrial fibrillation following coronary artery bypass surgery: A propensity-matched analysis, *J Cardiothorac Surg* 1:6, 2006.
737. Shepherd J, Jones J, Frampton GK, et al: Intravenous magnesium sulphate and sotalol for prevention of atrial fibrillation after coronary artery bypass surgery: A systematic review and economic evaluation, *Health Technol Assess* 12:iii, 2008.
738. Cook RC, Humphries KH, Gin K, et al: Prophylactic intravenous magnesium sulphate in addition to oral {beta}-blockade does not prevent atrial arrhythmias after coronary artery or valvular heart surgery: A randomized, controlled trial, *Circulation* 120(Suppl 11):S163, 2009.

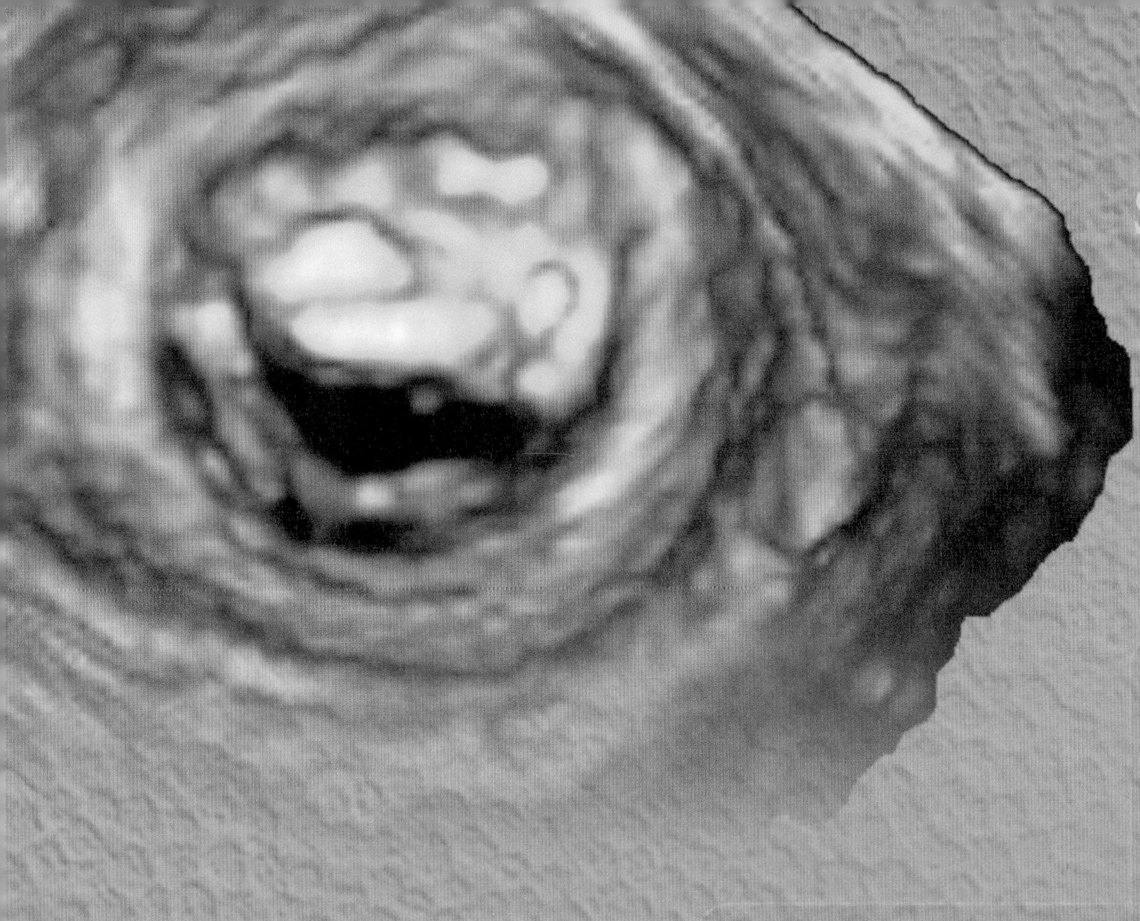

Monitoring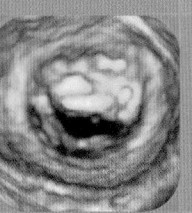

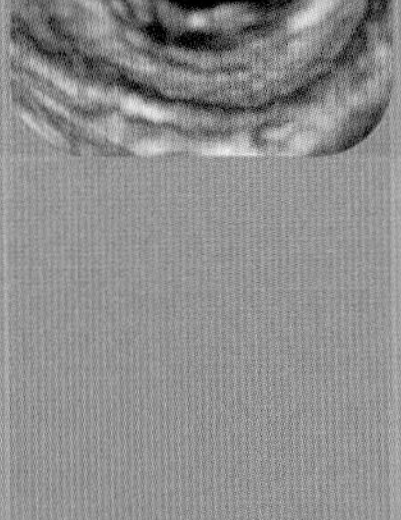

11

Evolution of Perioperative Echocardiography

EUGENE A. HESSEL II, MD, FACS | OKSANA KLIMKINA, MD | MICHAEL K. CAHALAN, MD

Many characteristics define a cardiac anesthesiologist, and these have evolved over time.[1] Some of these include intimate knowledge of cardiac diseases and the interaction of anesthesia with them, knowledge of the special techniques used by cardiac surgeons including, initially, pure moderate hypothermia and, subsequently, cardiopulmonary bypass (CPB), deep hypothermic circulatory arrest, cardioplegia, off-pump coronary artery bypass grafting, and minimally invasive and robotic surgery. But one of the cardinal characteristics of cardiac anesthesiologists has been their adoption and application of special monitoring techniques. Early on this involved electrocardiographic (ECG), electroencephalographic, arterial, central venous, and left atrial pressure monitoring, and use of arterial blood gases and tests of coagulation. In the 1970s, use of the pulmonary artery catheter (PAC) was introduced. Since about 1990, expertise with use of echocardiography has become one of the defining characteristics of the accomplished cardiac anesthesiologist. Today, few anesthesia or cardiac surgical groups would accept an anesthesiologist who wishes to provide anesthesia for cardiac cases if they have not been trained in perioperative echocardiography. Residents seeking fellowship training in cardiothoracic anesthesia view the quality of experience and teaching of echocardiography as critical criteria in selecting a fellowship. The authors believe that the introduction of echocardiography into cardiac surgery and anesthesia has contributed to the improved success and safety of cardiac surgery since the early 1990s.

Echocardiography, like the other special monitoring skills, has been transferred from the practice of cardiac anesthesia to the general practice of anesthesiology, including for noncardiac surgery in patients with cardiac disease, management of hemodynamic problems during noncardiac surgery, critical care, vascular access, and now into the practice of regional anesthesia and pain medicine. Subsequent chapters provide details on the basis and clinical application of various modalities of echocardiography. This chapter outlines how cardiac anesthesiologists arrived at the current state of practice.

As Feigenbaum[2] notes, the word *evolution* usually is reserved for changes of natural phenomena, but it is appropriate to use it in reference to the development of diagnostic ultrasound (e.g., echocardiography) because this represents an attempt to mimic a natural phenomenon. Some mammals (e.g., bats and aquatic mammals) use "diagnostic ultrasound" to visualize their environments, a phenomenon that was first recognized by Lazzaro Spallanzani (1729–1799). A number of previous articles and sections of other texts have reviewed the history of medical diagnostic ultrasound and echocardiography.[2–15] The authors have relied heavily on these prior works and frequently quote from them. What becomes immediately apparent in reviewing this history is that it has been an international effort with contributions from engineers, scientists, and clinicians from many different nations. The knowledge and experience of the authors of this chapter result in a particular emphasis on developments in North America, and they acknowledge that they may have unintentionally overlooked important contributions and events that have occurred elsewhere.

EARLY DEVELOPMENTS LEADING TO THE MEDICAL USE OF ULTRASOUND

The Roman architect Vitruvius coined the word *echo* (Table 11-1). The French friar Marin Mersenne (1588–1648) frequently is referred to as the "father of acoustics" because he first measured the velocity of sound, whereas the English physicist Robert Boyle (1627–1691) recognized that a medium was necessary for the propagation of sound.[13] The Italian Lazzaro Spallanzani (1729–1799) is sometimes referred to as the "father of ultrasound" because he deduced that bats must emit ultrasound waves (inaudible to humans) and listen to the echoes to navigate, based on his observations in the 1790s that bats navigate well when blindfolded but not when he plugged their ears. The Austrian mathematician and physicist Christian Johann Doppler (1803–1853) noted that the pitch of sound varied if the source of sound was moving and derived the mathematical relationship between change in pitch (frequency) and the relative motion (velocity) between the source and the observer. As an indication of the ingenuity of early scientific investigators, Buys Ballot at Utrecht in 1845 confirmed Doppler's theory and formula experimentally by having trumpeters play notes on railroad cars pulled at different speeds and employed musicians with perfect pitch to identify the frequencies they heard.[9] Doppler also predicted (which was later confirmed) that the frequency of light would decrease from a receding object (e.g., stars ["red shift"]) and increase (toward blue) if approaching. Interestingly, manufacturers of color-flow Doppler systems chose to use the opposite convention, using red to color-code flow moving toward the transducer and blue for flow moving away from the transducer ("Red returning, Blue away").

The creation and recording of ultrasound were made possible by the discovery of the piezoelectric effect by the French brothers Jacques and Pierre Curie. In 1880, they discovered that when certain quartz crystals were subjected to mechanical stress (compression), they developed an electrical charge. A year later, in 1881, they observed the converse: When crystals were placed in an alternating electrical field, they would rapidly change shape (vibrate).[9]

After the *Titanic* disaster in 1912, the British engineer Lewis F. Richardson suggested that an echo technique could be used to detect underwater objects. In 1917, the Frenchman Paul Langevin (1872–1946) conceived of the idea to use piezoelectric quartz crystal as both transmitter and receiver of ultrasound, which culminated in the development of SONAR (sound navigation and ranging) used to detect enemy submarines. In 1937, the Soviet scientist Sergei Sokolov and, in 1942, the American engineer Floyd Firestone described the use of reflected ultrasound to detect flaws in metals that, as explained later, ultimately led to the medical use of ultrasound in cardiac medicine.[11,13,14]

EARLY MEDICAL USE OF ULTRASOUND

The Austrian neurologist Karl T. Dussik (Figure 11-1), sometimes referred to as the "father of diagnostic ultrasound,"[11] is credited with being the first to apply ultrasound for medical diagnosis[16] (Table 11-2). In 1941, he reported on his use of transmission ultrasound to outline the ventricles of the brain.[17] He considered use of echo reflection but abandoned this approach when his idea was ridiculed.[11] In the 1940s, the German physicist W. D. Keidel used transmitted ultrasound through the chest (like X-rays) in an attempt to measure cardiac volumes.[11,18] Subsequently, both investigators appear to have abandoned their efforts.

TABLE 11-1	Early Developments Leading to Medical Use of Ultrasound	
Name	*Date**	*Development*
Marcus Vitruvius (Roman)	80–15 BC	Coined word *echo*
Marin Mersenne (French)	1588–1648	"Father of acoustics" Measured speed of sound
Robert Boyle (English)	1627–1691	Recognized a medium was necessary for propagation of sound
Lazzaro Spallanzani (Italian)	1727–1799	"Father of ultrasound" Demonstrated that bats navigated by echo reflection
Christian Doppler (Austrian)	1803–1853	In 1842, he described Doppler effect and mathematical relations between change in frequency (of sound and light) and relative motion
Jacque and Pierre Curie (French)	1880–1881	Discovered piezoelectric effect
Lewis F. Richardson (British)	1912	British engineer after the *Titanic* disaster suggested that an echo technique could be used to detect underwater objects
Paul Langevin (French)	WWI	Developed SONAR; used the piezoelectric effect to develop transmitters and receivers
Sergei Sokolov (Russian)	1929–1937	Used reflection of ultrasound to detect flaws in metal
Floyd Firestone (American)	1942	Flaw detection in metals

* Lifespan of first five; date of development for last five.

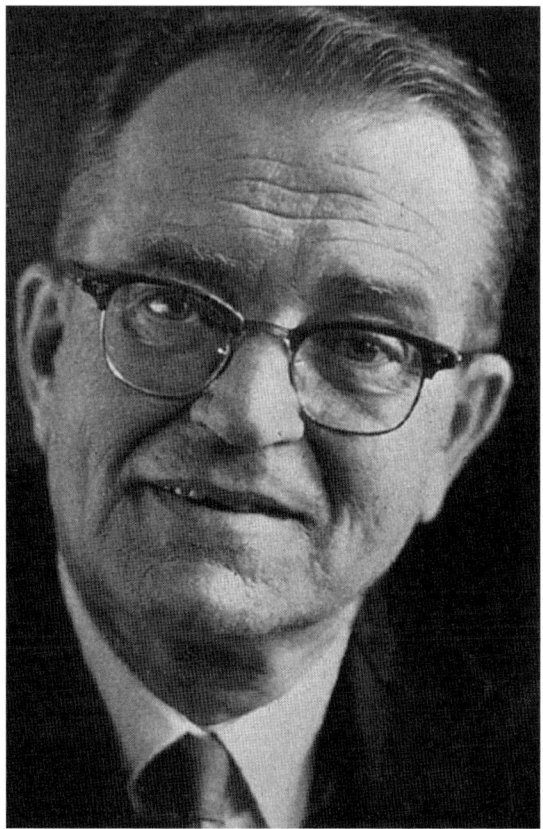

Figure 11-1 K. T. Dussik, the "father of diagnostic ultrasound," who first used transmission ultrasound to visualize the ventricles of the brain and suggested use of reflected ultrasound. *(From Roelandt JR: Seeing the invisible: A short history of cardiac ultrasound. Eur J Echocardiogr 1:8–11, 2000.)*

EARLY HISTORY OF CLINICAL ECHOCARDIOGRAPHY

Edler and Hertz and the Beginning of Clinical Echocardiography (Ultrasound Cardiography) and M-Mode Imaging

It was the collaboration between cardiologist Inge Edler (1911–2001) and physicist Carl Hellmuth Hertz (1920–1990) (Figure 11-2) at Lund University in Sweden in the early 1950s that is commonly accepted as the beginning of clinical echocardiography.[13]*

In a search of a better way to evaluate the mitral valve function before closed mitral commissurotomy, Edler considered the use of something like RADAR (see Table 11-2). He was referred to a young physicist at Lund University, C. Hellmuth Hertz. Hertz was the son of a Nobel Prize winner, and, remarkably, his uncle, Heinrich Hertz, had lent his name to the unit of frequency. Hertz thought that ultrasound (frequencies higher than that audible to the human ear) might be the solution to Edler's needs.[14] Hertz borrowed an ultrasonic reflectoscope used in nondestructive testing of metals at the ship-building yard in Malmo for a weekend, and Elder tested it on Hertz's chest and detected movement in the heart. The Siemens Corporation provided them with a reflectoscope in October 1953. They first studied isolated hearts in the laboratory with A-mode (static amplitude), but then devised a recording technique to display motion versus time (M-mode) by photographing the image off the oscilloscope (Figures 11-3 and 11-4). Their machine could produce ultrasound frequencies of 0.5, 1.0, 2.5, and 5.0 MHz, and Hertz opted to use 2.5 in humans as the optimal compromise between penetration and resolution. They first used this machine in a patient on October 29, 1953; they termed it "ultrasound cardiography" (UCG).[19] At first they attributed the reflectors to the posterior wall of the left ventricle and the anterior wall of the left atrium, but, subsequently, Edler demonstrated that the latter came from the anterior leaflet of the mitral valve. He determined this by passing an ice pick in the comparable direction through the chest at the time of an autopsy on a patient he had echoed shortly before death.[2] He subsequently used UCG to evaluate pericardial effusions and, in 1956, detected a left atrial myxoma (but this was not published until 1960).[12] However, his principal use of UCG was to evaluate mitral stenosis, and he described the value of the E-F slope in quantifying the severity of the stenosis. In the mid-1950s, Edler and Hertz actually experimented with *introducing a transducer into the esophagus* to overcome the attenuation in lung tissue, but they abandoned this effort because of difficulties in obtaining acoustic coupling between the transducer and the esophageal wall.[12] They published the first review article on UCG in *Acta Medica Scandinavia* in 1961.[20] Hertz left the field of cardiac ultrasound fairly early after he developed ink-jet technology, and Edler made few innovations after 1960.[2] In 1977, Edler and Hertz were awarded the Lasker Clinical Medicine Research Prize (often referred to as the American Nobel prize in Medicine).

Others Enter the Field

In the late 1950s, Schmidt and Braun, and Sven Effert in Germany separately began duplicating Elder and Hertz's work, and in 1959, Effert published the first report identifying an intra-atrial tumor by echocardiography. Between 1961 and 1965, workers in Shanghai and Wuhan, China began to report their use of echocardiography including fetal echocardiography.[13]

The American Experience

In 1957, engineers John Wild and John Reid at the University of Minnesota described ultrasonic echocardiographic imaging of excised hearts.[21] When Reid went to the University of Pennsylvania, he joined forces with cardiologist Claude Joyner, building an ultrasonoscope that they used to study mitral stenosis. Their report, which appeared in the

---

*The interested reader is referred to the tribute written by Singh and Goyal[14] and the historic review written by Edler himself and published posthumously.[12]

TABLE 11-2	Early History of Medical Use of Ultrasound and Clinical Echocardiography		
Investigator	*Year*	*Country*	*Contribution*
Karl Dussik	1941	Austria	Used ultrasound to outline ventricles of brain "Father of diagnostic ultrasound"[17]
W. D. Keidel	1950	Germany	Used transmission ultrasound to examine the heart[18]
Inge Edler and C. Hellmuth Hertz	1953	Sweden	Collaborated to use ultrasonoscope to examine the heart, commonly accepted as the beginning of clinical echocardiography[19]
Sven Effert, et al; W. Schmidt and H. Braun	Late 1950s	Germany	Separately duplicated Edler and Hertz's work
I. Edler et al.	1961	Sweden	First comprehensive review on cardiac ultrasound use in mitral and aortic stenosis, left atrial tumors, and pericardial effusions in *Acta Medica Scandinavia*[20]
C. C. Hsu; Y. Gao; X. F. Wang	1961–1964	China	Cardiac, fetal and contrast echo
J. Wild, H. D. Crawford, and J. Reid	1957	USA	First American article (*American Heart Journal*); described echocardiography of hearts[21]
J. Reid and Claude Joyner		USA	First American clinical effort (*Circulation*)[22]
H. Feigenbaum	1963	USA	Initiated clinical study of "cardiac ultrasound"
H. Feigenbaum	1965	USA	Published report on use of echo to diagnose pericardial effusion (*JAMA*)[23]
B. Segal	1966	USA	First to use term *echocardiography* in print (*JAMA*)[24]
S. Satomura et al.; T. Yoshida and Nimura	1950s	Japan	Used Doppler technology to examine heart
D. L. Franklin	1961	USA	Doppler shift to measure velocity of blood flow in vessels[38]
P. N. T. Wells; P. A. Peronneau, E. W. Baker	1969–1972	England, France, USA	Pulse Doppler
J. Holen; L. Hatle	1979	Norway	Applied modified Bernoulli equation to measure gradients across mitral[40] and aortic valve[41]
Nicholas Bom	1971	Netherlands	Linear two-dimensional (2D) scanner[31]
Griffith and Henry	1974	USA	Mechanical 2D scanner[33]
Eggleton and Feigenbaum	1974	USA	Commercially successful mechanical 2D scanner[34]
von Ramm and Thurstone	1976	USA	Phase-array 2D scanner[11,32]
Brandenstini	1979	Switzerland	M-mode multigated color-flow Doppler (CFD)
Namekawa, Kasaı, et al.	1982	Japan	Used autocorrelation to produce 2D CFD[42]
Bommer and Miller	1982	USA	Clinical application of CFD[43]
Omoto	1984	Japan	Used CFD to study valvular regurgitation[44]

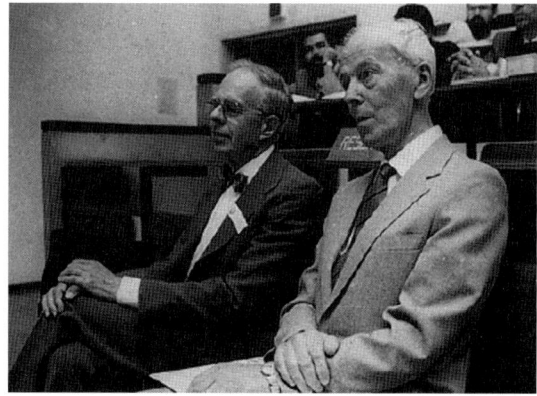

Figure 11-2 I. Edler (right) and C. H. Hertz (left) in 1979. They recorded the first M-mode echocardiogram of the heart in 1953 and are considered the "fathers of clinical echocardiography." (*From Roelandt JR: Seeing the invisible: A short history of cardiac ultrasound. Eur J Echocardiogr 1:8–11, 2000.*)

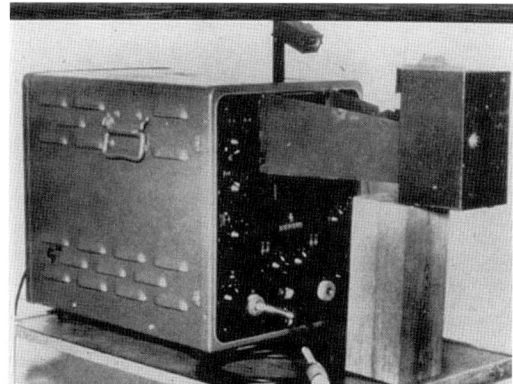

Figure 11-3 The ultrasonoscope initially used by Edler and Hertz for recording their early echocardiograms. (*From Feigenbaum H, Armstrong WF, Ryan T: Feigenbaum's echocardiography, 6th ed. Philadelphia: Lippincott Williams & Wilkins, 2005.*)

journal *Circulation* in 1963, was the first American publication on clinical echocardiography.[22] Harvey Feigenbaum in Indianapolis, author of one of the first (first published in 1972) and still published textbooks of echocardiography, first became interested in echocardiography in 1963 (Figure 11-5). He published his first article on use of ultrasound to diagnose pericardial effusions in 1965,[23] and as mentioned later, he collaborated with Reggie Eggleton to develop a mechanical two-dimensional (2D) scanner. Dr. Feigenbaum also may have been the first to train nonphysicians to do echocardiograms, leading to the development of cardiac sonographers.[13] Feigenbaum believes that Bernie Segal of Philadelphia was the first to use the term *echocardiography* in

print in an article published in 1966.[24,25] The senior author (E.A.H.) recalls cardiologists presenting their primitive, indistinct, and difficult to interpret M-mode images of the mitral valve at preoperative case conferences in the late 1960s and thinking that echocardiography did not have much future. How wrong he was!

Between the 1950s and the 1970s, M-mode was the only clinically useful format for echocardiography, and many advances and applications were described as the equipment and the skill of the echocardiographers improved, peaking in the late 1970s. But then its role rapidly declined with the development of 2D instrumentation.[9]

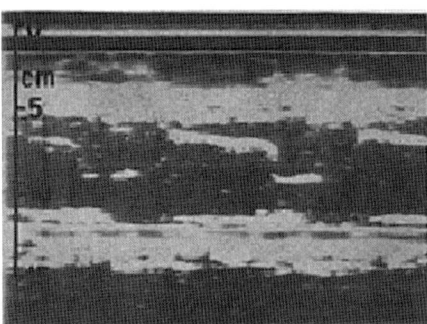

Figure 11-4 One of the earliest M-mode echocardiograms of the mitral valve recorded by Edler and Hertz in December 1953. *(From Roelandt JR: Seeing the invisible: A short history of cardiac ultrasound. Eur J Echocardiogr 1:8–11, 2000.)*

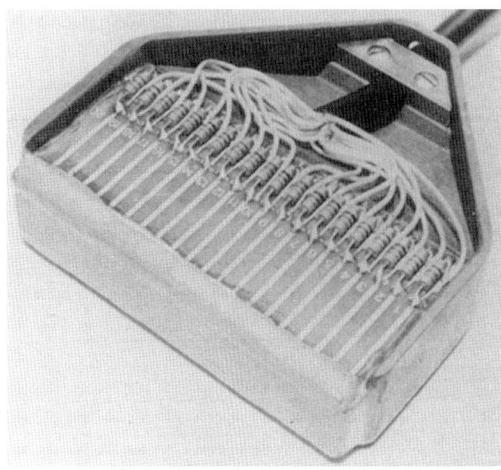

Figure 11-6 Twenty-element electronic linear two-dimensional transducer developed by N. Bom in Rotterdam circa 1972. *(From Feigenbaum H, Armstrong WF, Ryan T: Feigenbaum's echocardiography, 6th ed. Philadelphia: Lippincott Williams & Wilkins, 2005.)*

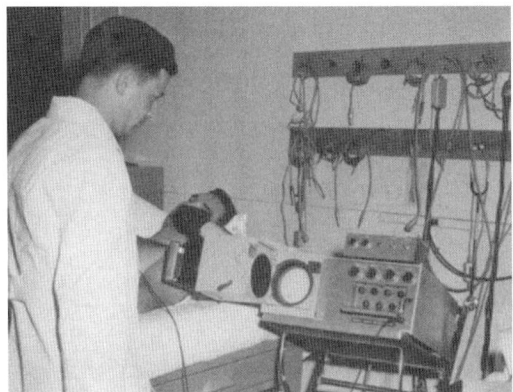

Figure 11-5 Feigenbaum using his early M-mode echocardiography, which used a Polaroid camera to record the echocardiogram. *(From Feigenbaum H, Armstrong WF, Ryan T: Feigenbaum's echocardiography, 6th ed. Philadelphia: Lippincott Williams & Wilkins, 2005.)*

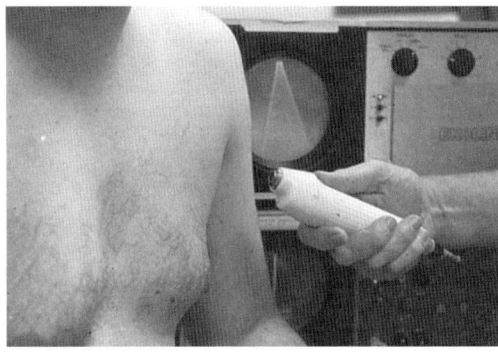

Figure 11-7 First practical handheld mechanical real-time sector scanner developed by Eggleton and Feigenbaum in the mid-1970s using a modified Sunbeam electric toothbrush. *(From Feigenbaum H: Evolution of echocardiography. Circulation 93:1321–1327, 1996.)*

Two-Dimensional Scanners

Work to develop real-time 2D scanners began in the 1960s, made possible by advances in sonar and radar technology and circuitry. Early pioneering work was done by the previously mentioned Americans Wild and Reid,[26] and Howry and Bliss[27] in the 1950s. In the later 1960s, Ebina[28] in Japan and Asberg[29] reported producing ultrasound-generated tomographic images of thoracic structures in humans. Their clinical application was limited because of transducer size.

In 1968, Somer[30] constructed the first electronic phased-array scanner based on the wavefront theory formulated in the 17th century by Huygens.[11] In 1971, this was followed by the description by Nicholas Bom[31] of Rotterdam of an electronic linear scanner (Figure 11-6) that generated a rectangular image and, in 1974, of an electronic phased-array scanner by F. L. Thurstone and O.T. von Ramm at Duke University.[11,32] At the same time, J. Griffith and W. Henry, at the National Institutes of Health, introduced a mechanical sector scanner.[11,33] This was said to be cumbersome to manipulate, and hence shortly thereafter Reggie Eggleton, working with Feigenbaum in Indianapolis, developed a handheld real-time mechanical 2D scanner[34] that was more "user friendly" and commercially successful[13] (Figure 11-7). In 1976 and 1977, Kisslo and colleagues[35,36] at Duke University reported on the clinical use of the von Ramm and Thurston phased-array scanner for 2D echocardiography (2DE).

Development of Vascular and Cardiac Doppler

In 1956, Satomura reported the application of the Doppler principle in the use of ultrasound to measure blood flow velocity.[11,37] However, in 1961, Franklin, at the University of Washington, was the first to measure Doppler shift of frequency, and hence velocity of flow of blood in vessels using a continuous-wave ultrasonic device.[38] Pulse-wave Doppler (in which flow at a defined depth could be analyzed) was nearly simultaneously introduced in 1969 and 1970 by P. N. T. Wells of England, P. A. Peronneau of France, and D. W. Baker in the United States.[11] In 1974, F. E. Barber, D. W. Baker, and colleagues at the University of Washington introduced the combination of pulse-wave Doppler with 2D scanning to produce the subsequently widely used "Duplex Scanner."[11,39] Subsequently, in Norway, but at different institutions, J. Holen[40] and L. Hatle[41] applied the Bernoulli principle to estimate the pressure decline across stenotic mitral and aortic valves, respectively.

Color-Flow (Doppler) Echocardiography

In 1978, the Swiss-born M. A. Brandestini, working at the University of Washington, described a method (based on pulse-wave Doppler) of color encoding flow velocity data and superimposing it on M-mode images.[13] His initial observations were extended by Namekawa et al[42] in Japan who described, in 1982, color Doppler flow imaging (CFI) utilizing autocorrelation to produce real-time images of flow in 2D sector scans. Bommer and Miller in the United States[43] and Omoto working with the Namekawa group[44] described clinical use of 2D color Doppler flow imaging.[9,11]

▦ Prelude to Perioperative Transesophageal Echocardiography

The first reported use of intraoperative echocardiography (IOE) was in 1972 when Johnson and his colleagues[45] at the University of Colorado reported on the use of intraoperative *epicardial* M-mode echocardiography to evaluate the results after open mitral commissurotomy. In 1976, Wexler and Pohost, of Massachusetts General Hospital, wrote a review article in the journal *Anesthesiology* on noninvasive techniques for hemodynamic monitoring, in which they described the basic principles and the potential application to anesthesia of the relatively new technique of "echocardiography."[46] At that time, this was limited to M-mode technology, but they anticipated that in the future 2D sector scanning would overcome some of the limitations of M-mode scanning. In that same year, at the annual meeting of the American Society of Anesthesiologists (ASA) in October in San Francisco, Rathod and colleagues,[47] at Cook County Hospital and Loyola University in Chicago, and Paul Barash and colleagues,[48] at Yale University, described use of *transthoracic M-mode* echocardiography to monitor the effects of anesthetics on cardiac function during anesthesia in 20 adults and 13 children, respectively. They concluded that this technique was a useful method to assess cardiac function, and Barash et al[48] predicted that it "has the potential to be a useful tool for clinical anesthesiology that may supplant the invasive monitors currently available."

In 1978, Strom and colleagues at Albert Einstein College of Medicine in Bronx, New York, published their experience with use of *intraoperative epicardial M-Mode scanning during* cardiac surgery,[49] which led to their investigations of transesophageal echocardiography (TEE; see later).

When superior handheld 2D transducers became available, they began to be used epicardially during cardiac surgery after gas sterilization or wrapping them in sterile sheaths. In the early 1980s, Spotnitz and colleagues,[51] at Columbia University College of Medicine in New York City (NYC), reported use of intraoperative epicardial 2D scanning after CPB to detect intracardiac air[50] and to assess left ventricular ejection fraction before and after cardiac surgery. In 1984, Goldman and colleagues, at Mount Sinai Medical Center in NYC, reported the use of intraoperative epicardial contrast 2DE to evaluate regurgitation after mitral valve surgery[52] and to assess myocardial perfusion during cardiac surgery.[53]

TRANSESOPHAGEAL ECHOCARDIOGRAPHY

TEE has had a profound effect on the practice of cardiac anesthesiology starting in the mid 1980s, and conversely, at least in North America, anesthesiologists played a key role in the introduction of this modality into the practice of cardiac anesthesia and cardiology[8] (Table 11-3).

▦ Intravascular Ultrasound

The development of TEE had its roots in the search for alternative ultrasound windows because of difficulties encountered in obtaining good ultrasound signals through the chest using the early insensitive transthoracic transducers.[7] In the early 1960s, this led to the investigation of intravascular probes. In 1960, Cieszynski[54] inserted a single-element transducer on a catheter into the jugular vein of dogs. In 1963, Omoto et al[55] reported obtaining static cross-sectional images in patients by slowly rotating a single-element transducer inserted into the right atrium,[7] and a year later, Kimoto et al[56] reported obtaining C-scans of the atrial septum in humans from an intravascular catheter.[9] In 1968, Carleton and Clark[57] reported similar studies. 1970, Reggie Eggleton[58] mounted four elements on a catheter and created the first cross-sectional images of intracardiac structures by computer reconstruction of images obtained by slow rotation and ECG triggering,[5] and in 1972, Nicholas Bom,[59] in Rotterdam, described a real-time intracardiac scanner using a 32-element circular electronically phased-array

TABLE 11-3	Notable Developments in Transesophageal Echocardiography	
Investigator (Reference)	*Year*	*Contribution*
Side and Gosling[60]	1971	Continuous-wave Doppler of the thoracic aorta mounted on a standard gastroscope
Duck[61]	1974	Pulse-wave Doppler of thoracic aortic blood flow with an esophageal probe
Daigle[62]	1975	Pulse-wave Doppler of thoracic aortic blood flow with an esophageal probe
Frazin[63]	1976	M-mode of heart via a cable-mounted transducer
Matsumoto, Oka, et al[64,65]	1979–1980	Transesophageal M-mode monitoring during cardiac surgery
Hisanaga[66]	1977–1980	Mechanical 2D scanner mounted on gastroscope
DiMagna[67]	1980	Electronic linear phased-array 2D scanner mounted on an endoscope mainly used to examine the gastrointestinal tract
Souquet[68]	1980–1982	Electronic phased-array 2D scanner mounted on gastroscope
Schulter, Hanrath, Sorquet[69]	1980–1982	Clinical evaluation of Sorquet's TEE probe
Goldman et al[93]	1976	TEE with color-flow Doppler
Takamoto et al[94]	1987	TEE with color-flow Doppler
deBruijn et al[95]	1987	TEE with color-flow Doppler
Omoto[98]; and others	~1989	Biplane probe
Roelandt[100]; and others	~1992	Multiplane probe

2D, two-dimensional; TEE, transesophageal echocardiography.

transducer placed at the tip of a 9 F-catheter. Thereafter, interest faded as sophisticated TEE probes became available, only to re-emerge in the late 1980s (see later).

▦ Transesophageal Ultrasound (Doppler and M-Mode)

Side and Gosling[60] were the first to use transesophageal (continuous-wave) Doppler (transducer mounted on a steerable gastroscope) to assess flow in the heart and aorta in 1971. This was followed by similar reports by Olson and Shelton in 1972. In 1974 and 1975, Duck et al[61] and Daigle et al[62] used transesophageal pulsed Doppler to measure flow in the thoracic aorta.[7] However, true TEE is said to have its embryonic beginnings in 1976 when Lee Frazin (a Chicago cardiologist) et al[63] reported recordings of M-mode echocardiograms of the aortic root and valve, mitral valve, and left atrium from the esophagus by attaching a nonfocused 3.5-mHz transducer attached to a 3-mm coaxial cable (Figure 11-8). They reported superior recordings compared with the

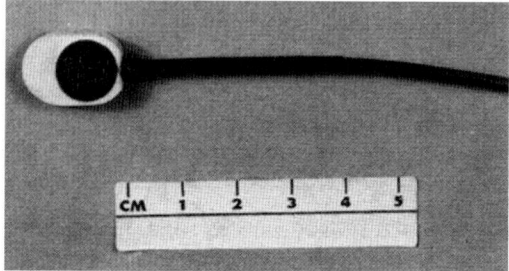

Figure 11-8 First clinically used transesophageal ultrasound probe used by Frazin and colleagues in the mid-1970s. Consisted of a nonfocused, 3.5-MHz M-mode transducer mounted on the end of a 3-mm coaxial cable. (*From Frazin L, Talano , Stephanides L, et al: Esophageal echocardiography. Circulation 54:102–108, 1976, Figure 1.*)

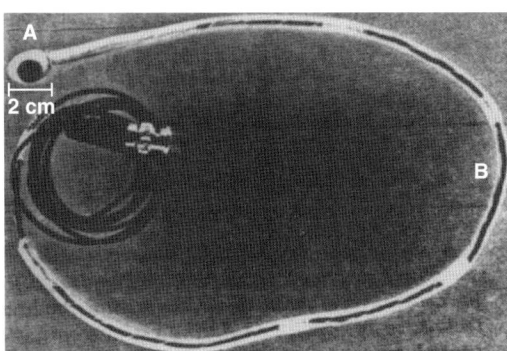

Figure 11-9 First "homemade" transesophageal M-mode probe used to monitor patients during cardiac surgery by Matsumoto and Oka in the Bronx, NY. The shaft consisted of a No. 4 sternal wire covered with a vinyl esophageal stethoscope catheter (A) KB-aerotech 3.5 MHz transducer; (B) Handmade cable. *(From Oka Y, Goldiner PL: Transesophageal echocardiography. Philadelphia: Lippincott, 1992, Figure 1. Originally from Matsumoto M, Oka Y, Lin YT, et al: Transesophageal echocardiography for assessing ventricular performance. N Y State J Med 79:19–21, 1979, Figure 1.)*

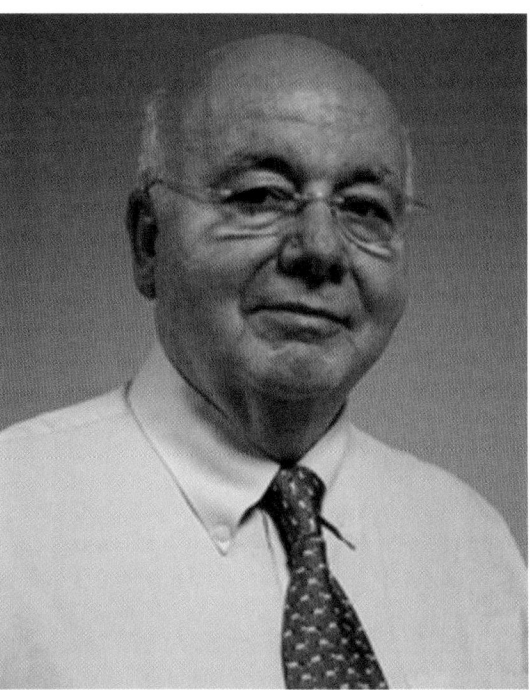

Figure 11-10 Jacques Souquet, PhD, a contemporary portrait. French ultrasound engineer working in both the United States and Europe, largely responsible for the design of the miniaturized phased-array two-dimensional transducer used in the early transesophageal echocardiography probes. *(From Image: A Conversation with...Jacques Souquet, PhD. Available at: http://www.rt-image.com/A_Conversation_with_Jacques_Souquet_PhD_The_diagnostic_capabilities_of_ShearWave/content=8504J05E48BE588440B6967644A0B0441.)*

transthoracic approach in 38 patients.[63] Following this lead, Matsumoto and Oka,[64] at Albert Einstein College of Medicine, fabricated a stiff transesophageal probe supporting an M-mode transducer (Figure 11-9). They first used this in 1979 to measure ventricular dimensions and volume during mitral valve surgery in a 65-year-old woman.[64] They subsequently reported intraoperative transesophageal M-mode monitoring in 21 patients undergoing cardiac surgery.[65] At that time, M-mode TEE was difficult to interpret except by the extremely sophisticated clinician and hence was not widely adopted. However, the development of a new generation of gastroscopes with steerable tips in the late 1960s, onto which echo transducers could be mounted, had a significant positive impact on the development of TEE by facilitating direct contact with the wall of the esophagus,[7] overcoming the problem encountered by Edler and Hertz a decade earlier.

Transesophageal Two-Dimensional Imaging

Although some primitive 2D TEE mechanical scanners and linear were described between 1977 and 1980 (e.g., Hisanaga et al[66] and DiMagno et al[67]), it was not until Jacques Souquet[68] (Figure 11-10), working in conjunction with the Varian Corporation, developed their phased-array transducer (Figure 11-11) mounted on the end of a gastroscope for their 2D sector scanner system (Figures 11-12 and 11-13) that TEE became a practical reality. These new TEE probes were evaluated clinically by cardiologists Michael Schluter and Peter Hanrath in Hamburg, Germany,[69] and their preliminary results were highlighted at an international conference held in Hamburg in 1981.[8] The early subsequent use of TEE took different directions in the United States and Europe. Cardiologists in Germany and the Netherlands rapidly began using TEE in awake patients to aid in the diagnosis of a variety of cardiac pathologies. In the United States, cardiologists seemed reluctant to adopt this new technology.[6] In the early 1980s, Peter Hanrath sent prototypes (first M-mode transducers and then with the 2D transducers mounted on gastroscopes) to cardiologists James Seward at Mayo Clinic and Nelson Schiller (Figure 11-14) at the University of California in San Francisco (UCSF), who passed them on to anesthesiologists. Schiller[70] spoke with William Hamilton, Chair of the Department of Anesthesiology at UCSF, who put him in contact with two young faculty members, Michael Cahalan and Michael Roizen. At that time (1981–1983), a cardiology fellow from Hanrath's group in Germany, Peter Kremer (Figure 11-15), came to UCSF and collaborated with Cahalan (Figure 11-16) and Roizen to investigate these new TEE instruments. At the 1982 annual meeting of the ASA, they started the American TEE "revolution" when they presented their results in monitoring cardiac and vascular surgery

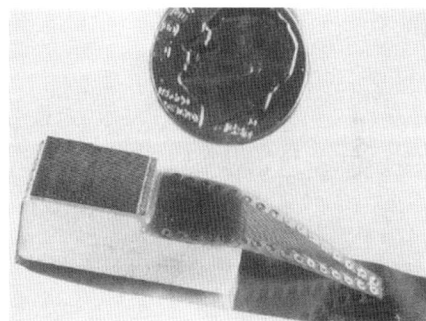

Figure 11-11 First 32-element 3.5-MHz phased-array transducer developed by Jacquet Souquet that was fitted on an Olympus gastroscope by Souquet. *(From Stumper O, Sutherland GR: Transesophageal echocardiography in congenital heart disease. London: Edward Arnold, 1994, Figure 1.2.)*

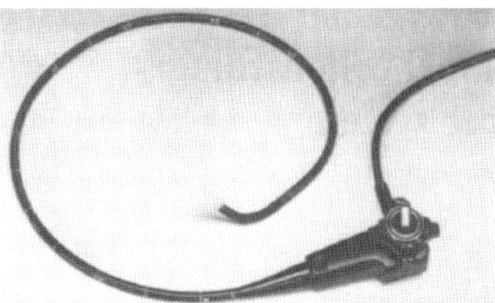

Figure 11-12 An early Souquet transesophageal echocardiography probe (Souquet phased-array transducer mounted on gastroscope) as used by Hanrath, Schluter, and Kremer in the early 1980s. *(From Schluter M, Langenstein BA, Polster J, et al: Transesophageal cross-sectional echocardiography with a phased array transducer system. Technique and initial clinical results. Br Heart J 48:67–72, 1982, Figure 1A.)*

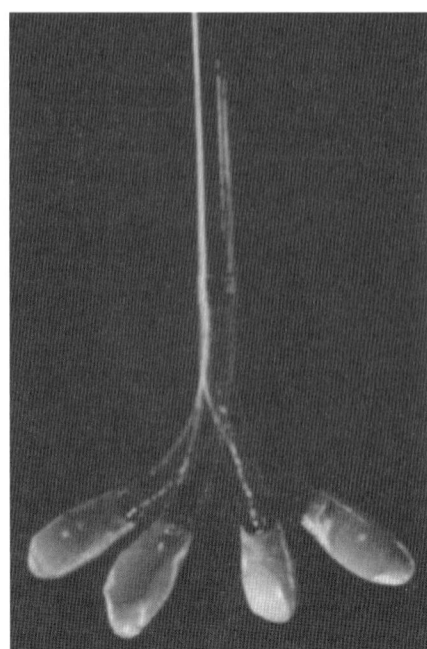

Figure 11-13 The ability to adjust the orientation of the transducer by the external controls on the gastroscope is a key innovative feature of the gastroscope mounted transesophageal echocardiography probe. *(From Schluter M, Langenstein BA, Polster J, et al: Transesophageal cross-sectional echocardiography with a phased array transducer system. Technique and initial clinical results. Br Heart J 48:67–72, 1982, Figure 1B.)*

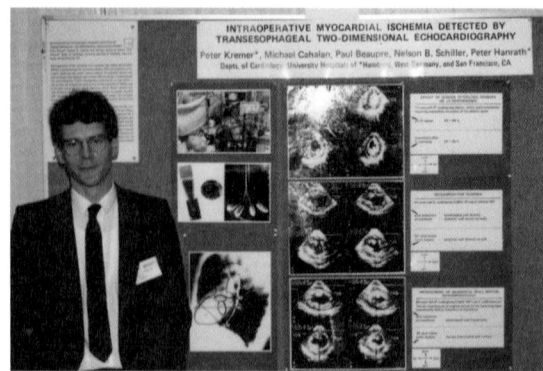

Figure 11-15 Peter Kremer, the cardiology fellow from Hanrath's group in Germany, who brought the probes to the University of California San Francisco (UCSF) and worked with them there for 2 years. Shown standing before a poster presentation of their work at a cardiology meeting circa 1982. *(Photograph courtesy M. K. Cahalan)*

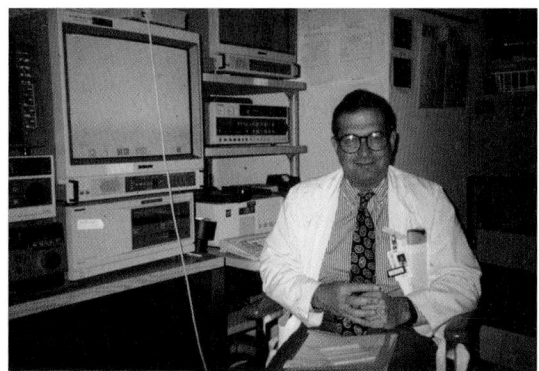

Figure 11-14 Nelson Schiller, MD, in 1983. He was the head of echo cardiology at the University of California San Francisco (UCSF) and was instrumental in promoting the work of Cahalan, Roizen, and Kremer and supporting their efforts to win acceptance of their publications. *(Photograph courtesy M. K. Cahalan.)*

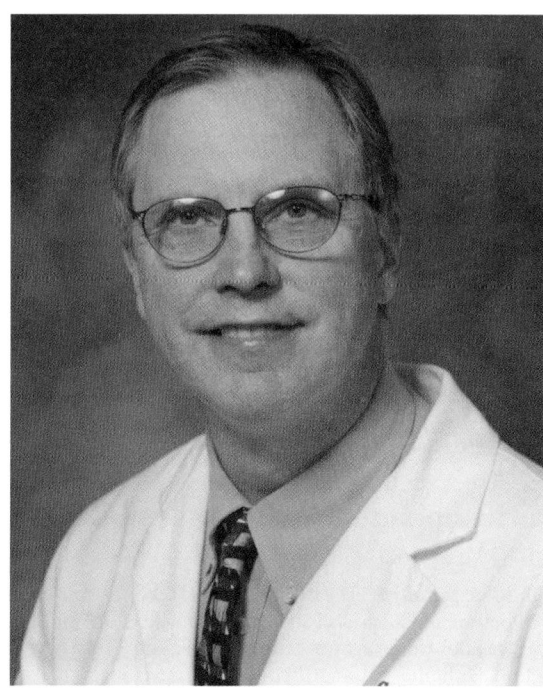

Figure 11-16 Michael K. Cahalan, Professor Anesthesiology, University of Utah. Pioneered use of transesophageal echocardiography (TEE) perioperatively (together with P. Kremer and M. Roizen) at the University of California in San Francisco in 1982 and helped introduce this modality to cardiologists, surgeons, and anesthesiologists in the United States. He facilitated the collaboration of anesthesiologists with echocardiologists (American Society of Echocardiography) and assisted with the development of postgraduate courses, guidelines, and certifying examinations in perioperative TEE. *(Photograph courtesy M. K. Cahalan.)*

patients with this new TEE probe, displaying the high-quality recordings and images obtained (Figures 11-17 and 11-18), and describing its usefulness in assessing filling and function of the left ventricle, and in detecting myocardial ischemia and intracardiac air.[71,72] Subsequently, they reported its superiority to PAC in assessing filling in the operating room[73] and usefulness in evaluating the hemodynamic changes during anaphylaxis[74] and during surgery for pheochromocytoma.[75] Topol and colleagues at Johns Hopkins University demonstrated its usefulness in determining the cause of hypotension immediately after CPB[76] and documented improvement in myocardial dysfunction immediately after coronary revascularization.[77] Cucchiara et al,[78] at the Mayo Clinic, described its usefulness in detecting air embolism during neurosurgery, whereas the UCSF group described its value in monitoring during vascular surgery[79,80] and its superiority over ECG in detecting myocardial ischemia.[81] In 1984, the Hamburg group and Cahalan published

an anatomic analysis of six standard TEE views,[82] which was expanded on a few years later by the Mayo Clinic group.[83] Meanwhile, the group at Mount Sinai Medical Center in NYC (Martin Goldman, Joel Kaplan, Daniel Thys, Zaharia Hillel, and Steven Konstadt) was quick to adopt and evaluate perioperative TEE, following the experience of Kaplan working with the early Diasonic TEE probes in the early 1980s.[84-88] In 1987, Cahalan et al[89] and Clements and deBruijn[90] at Duke University wrote review articles on the use of TEE in anesthesiology, whereas the group at Mayo Clinic reported on the reproducibility of measurements obtained during intraoperative TEE.[91] In that same year (1987), the second edition of this text edited by Kaplan on *Cardiac Anesthesia*

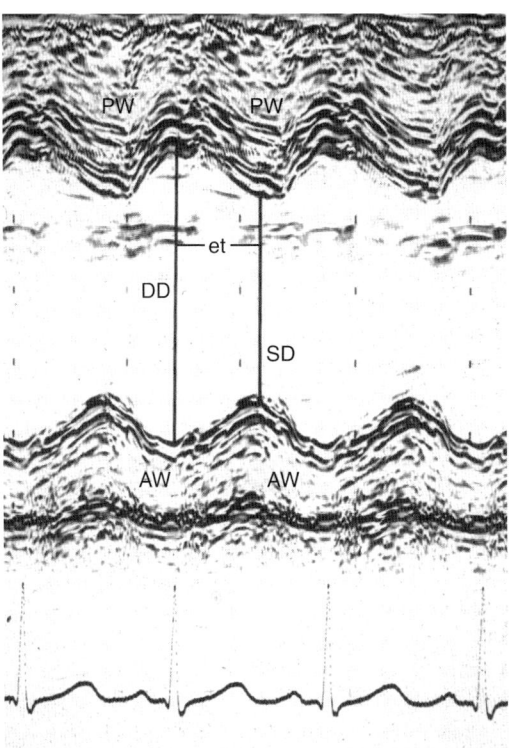

Figure 11-17 High-fidelity transesophageal M-mode echocardiogram from the first Hanrath-Souquet probe used in surgery at the University of California San Francisco (UCSF) circa 1981. AW, anterior wall; DD, diastolic distance; et, ejection time; PW, posterior wall; SD, systolic distance. (Courtesy M. K. Cahalan.)

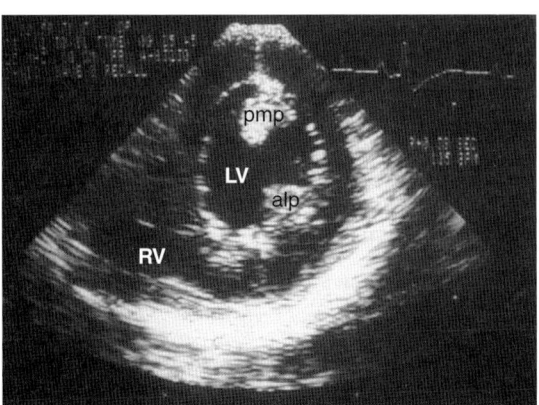

Figure 11-18 Two-dimensional (2D) image (transgastric midpapillary short-axis view) recording from the first 2D Hanrath-Souquet transesophageal echocardiographic probe used in surgery at the University of California San Francisco (UCSF) circa 1982. alp, anterior lateral papillary muscle; LV, left ventricle; pmp, posterior medial papillary muscle; RV, right ventricle. (Courtesy M. K. Cahalan.)

contained for the first time a 63-page thoroughly referenced chapter on Intraoperative Echocardiography.[92]

In 1986, Goldman and colleagues,[93] at Mount Sinai Medical Center in NYC, reported their experience with a new 2D TEE probe that also provided Doppler color-flow imaging (Aloka and Irex), as did a Japanese group.[94] That same year, the Hewlett-Packard Corporation also introduced a color-flow Doppler TEE probe; and in 1987, deBruijn and Clements, together with pioneering echocardiographer, Joseph Kisslo at Duke University, reviewed their early experience with this new technology.[95] In that same year, pulse-wave Doppler was added to 2D TEE probes,[96] although several years earlier the Hamburg group had described results of use of a TEE probe that combined pulse-wave Doppler with M-mode TEE.[97]

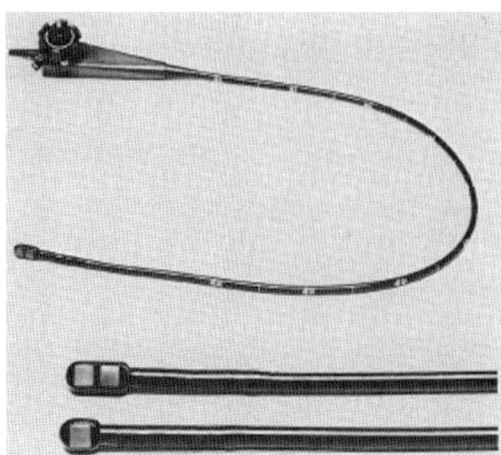

Figure 11-19 Photograph of single-plane (horizontal or transverse) and biplane (transverse and vertical) probes. The advent of biplane probes greatly increased the views available but were eventually superseded by multiplane probes. (From Matsuzaki M, Toma Y, Kusukawa R: Clinical applications of transesophageal echocardiography. Circulation 82:709–722, 1990, Figure 1.)

In 1989, biplane probes (Figure 11-19) first became available,[98] although prototypes had been described earlier,[99] and soon thereafter, multiplane single-transducer TEE probes[100] and smaller diameter probes suitable for pediatric use[101] appeared. In 1992, Pandian and colleagues, at Tufts-New England Medical Center, reviewed their early clinical experience with a 5-MHz phased-array multiplane TEE probe ("OmniPlane").[102]

A survey conducted of Society of Cardiovascular Anesthesiologists (SCA) members in early 1988 provides a "snap-shot" of the state of practice of IOE at that time[103]; 20% of the responders reported that IOE studies were being performed at their institutions. The majority of responders were practicing in large teaching hospitals. Anesthesiologists were involved 41% of the time and cardiologists in 33%, although in one third of the former group, cardiologists always assisted. TEE technique was used in 51%, epicardial in 37%, and transthoracic in 22% of cases. At the time of the survey, six manufactures made 2D TEE transducers—Hewlett-Packard, Aloka Toshiba, Diasonics, General Electric, Acusonics, and Hoffrel, but only the first three provide color-flow TEE. Most responders reported using either Diasonics (46%) or Hewlett-Packard (42%); 90% used the 2D mode, 75% M-mode, 60% pulsed-Doppler, 58% color-flow Doppler, and only 23% continuous-wave Doppler, whereas 97% believed that IOE had been or could have been helpful. The authors of the survey noted that few academic medical centers offered formal instruction and certification in IOE, and that a definite need for training had been identified.

Along this same line, in an editorial published in 1989, Kaplan[104] urged caution and restraint in the adoption of this new and complex technology that had the potential to cause numerous complications, and emphasized the need for anesthesiologists who aspire to be echocardiographers to obtain a high level of training.

In the late 1980s, the group at Duke University demonstrated the utility of routine *epicardial* echocardiography during surgery for congenital heart disease.[105-107] As soon as smaller probes that could be used in infants and children became available, these began to be used. In 1989, Kyo et al,[101] in Japan, were among the first to describe the use of TEE in pediatric cardiac surgery, a practice strongly supported by the work of the Seattle group about which they started publishing in 1993.[107-110] By the end of that decade, 98% of pediatric cardiac surgery centers used intraoperative TEE.[111]

Into the Mainstream

The 1990s witnessed the expansion of intraoperative TEE into the mainstream of clinical practice of cardiac surgery and anesthesia,[112] as well as into critical care and noncardiac surgery. From the beginning of perioperative TEE, its value to detect myocardial ischemia based on the appearance or regional wall motion abnormalities was recognized.[81] When only single-plane TEE transducers were available, the midpapillary transgastric short-axis view often was advocated for this purpose. With the appearance of biplane and multiplane probes in 1996, Cahalan's group[113] documented the limitations of the transgastric short-axis view and the need to use multiple views. In that same year, the group at UCSF also documented the value of TEE in assessing ischemia during CABG surgery[114]; whereas in 1997, the group at Cleveland Clinic documented the benefit of intraoperative TEE in high-risk CABG.[115] In 2000, Aronson and colleagues[116] reported on the use of intraoperative low-dose dobutamine echocardiography. Evidence of the increased importance of echocardiography to the practice of cardiac anesthesia is that with its first issue in 2001 (volume 15, number 1, February), *Journal of Cardiothoracic and Vascular Anesthesia* changed the logo on its cover from a PAC to echocardiographic images, and three TEE images graced the cover of Daniel Thys' *Textbook of Cardiothoracic Anesthesiology* published in 2001.[117]

OTHER DEVELOPMENTS

Contrast Echocardiography and Myocardial Contrast Echocardiography

Contrast enhancement of blood represents an important adjunct to echocardiography. It has been used to identify cardiac structures, enhance identification of the endocardial boarder, detect shunts and valvular regurgitation, and assess myocardial perfusion. Feinstein,[118] of Rush University in Chicago, and his international colleagues have reviewed the development of what they refer to as "contrast enhanced ultrasound" imaging and have identified important contributors over the years. Both the radiologist R. Gramiak, of University of Rochester,[13]* and the cardiologist C. R. Joyner, Jr., of the University of Pennsylvania,[9] have been credited as being the first to incidentally note dense echoes associated with the injection of normal saline or indocyanine green during M-mode echocardiography. Both of them subsequently described using saline contrast to help identify cardiac structures during M-mode echocardiography.[119] In 1975, Seward et al,[120] at the Mayo Clinic, described their initial experience with use of indocyanine green as an echocardiographic contrast agent in more than 300 cases, emphasizing its role in analyzing shunts. Bommer et al showed that when echocontrast agents were injected into coronary arteries during echocardiography, they produced myocardial opacification,[9] which led to the development of myocardial contrast echocardiography. The echo contrast of these agents was attributed to microbubbles. In these early media, the microbubbles were too large to pass through the capillaries including the lung, and hence direct injection into the left heart was necessary to image the structures in the left heart including the myocardium. In 1984, Feinstein et al described the use of ultrasonic energy ("sonication") to produce contrast agents consisting of relatively uniform, stable, and small gaseous microbubbles that could pass through capillary beds and allow imaging of the left heart chambers and myocardium via right-sided injection.[121] Over time, superior commercial contrast agents have been developed (e.g., Levovist, Albunex), and newer, more sophisticated agents are under development.[118]

In 1984, Goldman and colleagues[52] described the use of intraoperative contrast echocardiography to evaluate mitral regurgitation after mitral valve surgery by injecting saline into the left ventricle and monitoring for any regurgitation of contrast into the left atrium with epicardial 2D imaging. In that same year, this group also was the first to describe intraoperative myocardial contrast epicardial echocardiography (myocardial contrast produced by administration of cardioplegia into the aortic root) to predict the presence of coronary artery disease (CAD).[53] In the late 1980s and early 1990s, Aronson and colleagues at the University of Chicago, Kabas and Kisslo at Duke, and Spotnitz and Kaul at University of Virginia used intraoperative contrast echocardiography to assess coronary artery

surgery.[122–125] In 2000, Aronson[126] summarized the progress in measurement of myocardial perfusion by contrast echocardiography in the operating room, and in 2006, Dijkmans and his international colleagues[127] summarized the state of the development of myocardial contrast echocardiography. In 2007, the U.S. Food and Drug Administration called attention to concern about the safety of some of these agents, and in 2008, the American Society of Echocardiography (ASE) issued a consensus statement on "the clinical applications of ultrasonic contrast agents in echocardiography."[128]

Epicardial and Epiaortic Imaging

As noted earlier, Edler and Hertz first made epicardial ultrasound recordings of cadaver hearts in 1953, as did Wild and Reid in 1957.[21] Also, as mentioned earlier, in 1972, Johnson et al[45] reported on the use of intraoperative epicardial M-mode imaging to evaluate the results after mitral commissurotomy. In the early 1980s, the groups at Columbia University College of Medicine and the Mount Sinai Medical Center in NYC used intraoperative epicardial 2DE to detect intracardiac air,[50] assess left ventricular ejection fraction,[51] evaluate regurgitation after mitral valve surgery (after injection of contrast into the left ventricle),[52] and assess myocardial perfusion during cardiac surgery.[53] Because suitable small transesophageal probes were not available in the late 1980s and early 1990s, epicardial 2D scanning became the standard for echocardiographic surveillance during pediatric cardiac surgery in that era.[106]

With the introduction of TEE, epicardial imaging largely was discarded, but recently, both epicardial and epiaortic imaging have regained attention and are being utilized more frequently in situations in which TEE is not possible or adequate, and to assess the thoracic aorta, especially in the "blind spots" of the TEE.[129] The ASE/SCA have developed guidelines for epicardial[130] and epiaortic[131] applications.

Intracardiac Echocardiography

As reviewed earlier, intracardiac ultrasound was explored as an alternate method for examination of the heart during the era of limited transthoracic transducers. This approach largely was discarded with improved transthoracic instruments and, especially, the arrival of TEE. Recently, with improved miniaturization and technology of intravascular probes, and the increase in percutaneous intracardiac procedures (e.g., closure devices, percutaneous mitral valve surgery, electrophysiologic procedures), use of intracardiac ultrasound to monitor and aid in the safer performance of these procedures has become more popular.[132]

Intravascular Ultrasound

The circular-array catheter-mounted transducers ultimately were miniaturized (1 to 3 mm in diameter) and provided with sophisticated electronics so they could be placed into coronary arteries over a guidewire. Utilizing ultra-high frequencies (40 MHz), they permit a resolution of 150 µm to a depth of 2 to 3 cm. In the late 1980s, Nissen and colleagues,[133] at the University of Kentucky, were among the first to exploit these new intravascular ultrasound catheters to study CAD. Such technology is now used routinely to study CAD, and larger intravascular ultrasound probes are used to assist with placement of intracardiac devices, as well as to assess larger vessels.[13]

Echocardiography in Critical Care Medicine: In the Noncardiac Operating Room and Intensive Care Units

In Intensive Care Units and the Care of Critically Ill Patients

The value of transthoracic echocardiography (TTE) in the evaluation and management of critically ill patients was recognized as soon as 2D scanning became available. However, its common use was limited because of difficulty in obtaining adequate views by the transthoracic route in this patient population. As soon as TEE 2D probes arrived, their

---

*Goldberg, Gramiak, and Freimanis[4] have written a history of the contribution of American radiologists to the early development of diagnostic ultrasound.

usefulness and advantages over TTE in critical care situations became obvious. In 1986, groups at Erasmus University in the Netherlands and at the University of California in San Francisco collaborated in illustrating the role of 2D TEE in solving clinical problems.[134] In 1987, Erbel et al[136] in Mainz, Germany reported the superiority of TEE over TTE in detection of aortic dissection in 21 patients (100% vs. 29%),[135] which was followed by a report of a multicenter study comparing echocardiography (TTE and TEE) with CT scanning and angiography in 164 cases of aortic dissection (82 proved). Echocardiography was found to have a sensitivity and specificity, and positive and negative predictive values of 98% or greater, and was at least as good as the other diagnostic modalities. In 1988, Chan,[137] at the Ottawa Heart Institute, reported its usefulness in assessing the cause of hypotension after cardiac surgery in seven patients in whom TTE had failed to explain the problem (tamponade in three, ventricular septal rupture in one, and global LV failure in three). Reichert et al[138] of the Netherlands followed this with a report of use of TEE in 60 hypotensive patients after cardiac surgery and found it changed the clinical diagnosis in 60% of cases.

Between 1990 and 1994, the groups at St Louis University,[139] Mayo Clinic,[140] Cleveland Clinic,[141] UCSF,[142] National Taiwan University,[143] and Baylor College of Medicine[144] reported their initial results with use of TEE in more than 450 critically ill patients. In most of these series, TEE was performed because of unsatisfactory or suboptimal TTE, and the authors reported TEE to be invariably informative. Two groups directly compared use of TEE with TTE in intensive care units or the emergency department and found TEE to be vastly superior.[141,143] Many of these studies were done by cardiologists on patients with cardiologic issues. In 1998, the group at Mount Sinai Medical Center in NYC demonstrated the superiority of a goal-directed limited-scope TEE examination performed by surgical intensivists who had received limited goal-directed training in TEE, compared with conventional hemodynamic monitoring including use of the PAC.[145] Recent articles have reviewed the progress made in the use of TEE in the general intensive care unit.[146-148]

Intraoperative Transesophageal Echocardiography for Noncardiac Surgery

Although intraoperative TEE initially was adopted by cardiac anesthesiologists for use during cardiac surgery, early use during noncardiac surgery (vascular surgery, pheochromocytoma, and anaphylaxis) was reported by the group in UCSF.[72,74,75,79-81] The group at Duke emphasized the potential role of the anesthesiologist as a cardiac diagnostician.[149] Beginning in 1988, in a series of annual refresher course lectures given at the ASA annual meeting, Cahalan reviewed the benefits of intraoperative TEE for hemodynamic monitoring and advocated its adoption by all anesthesiologists caring for patients at risk for hemodynamic problems. The adoption of such practice had been limited by lack of educational opportunities (which is now being addressed; see later and Chapter 41) and maintenance of skills. A comprehensive review of the experience with use of TEE outside of the cardiac surgical operating room recently has been published by Mahmood et al,[148] whereas Goldstein[150] and Green et al[151] have debated whether the general anesthesiologist should be trained and certified in basic TEE.

RECENT DEVELOPMENTS

Since the early 2000s, many advances in digital technology and miniaturization, probe technology (including fully sampled matrix-array probes that have replaced the mechanically rotating multiplane probes), image-compression algorithms, high-density digital storage, and broadband communication networks have revolutionized storage and processing of TEE images (see Chapter 12). Secure digital servers have replaced videotape libraries of clinical studies, resulting in vastly faster and more convenient access to high-fidelity stored images even from remote locations.[152-155] Other areas that have seen considerable advancement include 3D and 4D, tissue Doppler, speckle tracking, regional wall motion detection, and handheld/hand-carried echocardiography (the "Echo-Stethoscope").

Three- and Four-Dimensional Echocardiography

Just as the limitations of 1DE (i.e., M-mode) led to the development of 2DE, the obvious limitations of the latter have led to the search and development of 3D imaging systems.

Transthoracic Three-Dimensional Echocardiography

History of 3D imaging in medicine starts in 1961 when Baum and Greenwood[156] used 3D ultrasonography for localization of orbital lesions. All early work in cardiac 3DE focused on methods of acquiring multiple 2D images by moving a standard 2D transducer in space and reconstructing the multiple 2D images into a 3D image. The first such publication came in 1974 from Stanford scientists Dekker, Piziali, and Dong[157] on a system for ultrasound imaging of the human heart in three dimensions. Dekker's group accomplished this by mounting the transducer onto a movable mechanical arm, which allowed alignment of multiple 2D images and creation of a 3D image (Figure 11-20).

In 1976, the spark-gap technique of 3D reconstruction of the heart was developed by Moritz and Shreve.[158] This technique involved measuring the transit times of spark-generated shock waves to obtain the spatial coordinates of the echocardiographic planes. The microprocessor controlled the operation of the system and performed all the computations required to determine the location and orientation of the ultrasound beam with respect to a known coordinate system. About this same time, Japanese engineers and clinicians with Matsumoto et al,[159] from Osaka University, described technology they used to process 3D images of left ventricle, atrium, and aorta: "We applied our newly developed computerized image processing system for 3-D echocardiographic display with binocular parallax shift and for constructing 2-D echocardiographic images in desired planes from sequential recordings of 2-D echocardiograms recorded with anteroposterior emission of ultrasound beams. This system mainly consisted of a flying spot scanner, a minicomputer and a display cathode ray tube....The frontal plane 2-D echocardiograms provided useful data."[159] In 1979, Raab et al[160] developed a magnetic locator that they attached to the transducer and to a central computer that located the transducer in space and subsequently followed its position.

Improvements on these methods led to the freehand imaging, allowing free movement of the transducer at a single or multiple acoustic

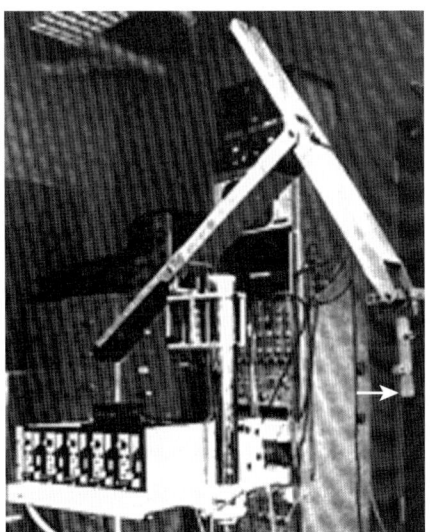

Figure 11-20 Dekker et al's mechanical arm described in 1974. The transducer *(arrow)* is held on the mechanical arm, and hence the location of the transducer is known. *(From Houck RC, Cooke JE, Gill EA: Live 3D echocardiography: A replacement for traditional 2D echocardiography? AJR Am J Roentgenol 187:1092–1106, 2006, Figure 2.)*

windows and resulting in a 3D wire-frame image. Images were acquired over short periods during held end-expiration with combination of angulated or rotated scans from parasternal or apical windows. Image quality depended on the patient's respiration. A magnetic field system was used to track the ultrasound scanhead. Images were digitized and registered with position data and image depth, as well as coordinated with independently acquired ECG. The borders of the left ventricle and associated anatomic structures were manually traced in the selected images.[160]

The 3D reconstruction of real-time transthoracic 2D images of the left ventricle, using an apical rotation method, was first described in 1982 by Ghosh and colleagues.[161] In their method, the transducer was placed on the patient's chest wall in the region of the apex to obtain the standard four-chamber view to record 2D left ventricular end-diastolic and end-systolic images. The transducer was then rotated in 30-degree increments from 0 to 180 degrees to obtain various planes passing through the apex. Using spatial coordinate data, 3D perspective images were plotted by the computer in any desired view. Three-dimensional reconstructed volumes closely correlated with those obtained by left ventricular angiography. In that same year, Geiser et al[162] described their technique of dynamic 3D echocardiographic reconstruction of the intact human left ventricle in patients.

The major limitation of these techniques was the inadequate delineation of the endocardium because of the nonperpendicular relation of the ultrasound beam to the left ventricular walls. Reconstruction from TTE images was restricted by the presence of chest wall artifacts, the limited number of acoustic windows, and inadequate image quality in some patients. Despite growing interest in 3DE, the clinical use of this technique was limited by time-consuming, complicated image acquisition and postprocessing, and hence was not available in real time.

Olaf von Ramm, professor of biomedical engineering at Duke University, with his colleague, Stephen Smith, pioneered the development of clinical 3D ultrasound scanners in the late 1980s. In 1987, they patented the first real-time high-speed 3D ultrasound system, capable of acquiring pyramidal volumetric data at frame rates (about 8 per second) sufficient to depict cardiac movement. Their transthoracic transducer, transmitting at frequency 2.5 to 3.5 MHz, included 256 elements configured in a "sparse array" pattern (not all the transducer head was used and connected to individual elements).[163] Later, this technique was developed commercially by Volumetrics Medical Imaging (Chapel Hill, NC) and existed for several years; however, it never made an impact on clinical practice because of poor image quality.

With real-time 3DE, an entire volume of the heart was obtained using one cardiac cycle, which was a major step up from the thin-slice sector of the 2D imaging. The limitations of the technique were poor image quality, motion artifact, low spatial resolution, low frame rates, limited dimensions of the 3D data set volume, and requirement of ECG and respiratory gating. Basically, images were computer-generated 2D slices derived from the 3D dataset. An off-line workstation had to be used to produce true 3D images.

Despite limitations, reconstructive techniques were used in numerous studies for determination of left ventricular volume, chamber size, mass, ejection fraction, and systolic function, particularly in patients with distorted ventricular shape or aneurysm. Comparison with angiography, thermodilution cardiac output measurements, radionuclide angiography, magnetic resonance imaging, conventional 2DTTE/TEE, and cine-ventriculography showed 3DE to be an accurate, if not superior, noninvasive technique.

In 1996, Hewlett-Packard Company began development of real-time 3DE. A rotational device was developed to be contained within the transducer. By 1998, Hewlett-Packard had a working prototype for transthoracic real-time 3DE and began showing it to customers by 1999. Moving beyond the "sparse array" transducer of van Ramm, in November 2002, Philips Medical Systems introduced the "Live 3D" imaging system, an advanced form of real-time 3D transthoracic imaging. The major advance of that system was improved image quality because of a fully sampled (matrix) or dense array configuration of

the transducer. The face of the transducer was completely sampled. This dense-array transducer, called a *matrix array*, consists of approximately 3000 elements compared with previous transducers with 256 elements. Increased computer processing power and hard drive capacity permitted the system to process, store, and analyze data. Even with this markedly improved ultrasound system, the size of the image volume is not enough to contain the whole left ventricle. Series of the four gated cycles had to be combined to create full-volume images, resulting in maximum frame rates of 25 Hz. 3D left atrial volume measurement could not be obtained from the patient with atrial fibrillation or those who could not hold their breath long enough to acquire a full-volume real-time 3D image. At the 2008 ASE meeting in Toronto, Siemens presented the Acuson SC2000 Volume Imaging Ultrasound System, which acquires full-volume 3D data pyramids—20 images/sec—in a single heartbeat. Acquiring a full pyramid in one heartbeat instead of four consecutive beats could be advantageous, because data would not require any restitching, reanimation, and regating.

Transesophageal Three-Dimensional Echocardiography

In the 1980s, when rapid development of TEE began, first attempts at 3D reconstruction from TEE were begun. The improved image resolution afforded by TEE was important for quality 3D image reconstruction. In 1986, Martin et al,[164] of the Department of Anesthesiology and Center for Bioengineering at the University of Washington, in Seattle, used a precision micromanipulator of a TEE-mounted transversely oriented 32-element 3.5-MHz ultrasonic array transducer to generate a 3D echocardiogram. This allowed them to obtain multiple multiplanar short-axis 2D images of the heart with known angular relations between them over a series of cardiac cycles. An off-line computer analysis of the images was used to form 3D reconstruction of the left ventricular cavity at end-diastole and end-systole from which stroke volume was determined.[164] In a canine study in 1989, Martin and Bashein[165] were able to demonstrate that the stroke volumes generated from their 3D reconstructed volumes were comparable with radionuclide and thermodilution measurements (Figure 11-21).

The next step in development of 3D TEE was when Wollschläger[166] et al reported on their system for TEE computer tomography. Their development was commercialized by TomTec Technology Company (Munich, Germany) and has found application in research and clinical practice. This technology was partially based on the rotational device used by Hewlett-Packard Corporation for their multiplane TEE probe that they introduced in 1992.

In 1992, Pandian et al,[167] at Tufts-New England Medical Center, were among the first to report clinical results with 3D TEE. They used a 5-MHz, 64-element, and phased-array TEE probe connected to a computer that directed transducer movement at 1-mm increments. A complete cardiac cycle was recorded at each tomographic level with ECG and respiration gating. These were then processed using dedicated 4D software and displayed as a dynamic 3D tissue image of the heart. In 1997, Chen et al,[168] at the Thorax Center in Rotterdam, Netherlands, published a study on the measurements of mitral valve orifice area with 3DE in patients with mitral stenosis. They had developed their own system for TEE acquisition, using TomTec software for off-line reconstruction. Transesophageal acquisition was performed in six patients with a custom-built transducer assembly; the transducer was rotated by a step motor that was commanded by computer algorithm that controlled the acquisition of cross sections within preset ranges of heart cycle length by ECG gating and respiratory phase.

From the mid-1990s to 2000, for most multiplane TEE probes, external acquisition and computer analysis from TomTec were used, but only Hewlett-Packard Corporation integrated the acquisition software into the ultrasound system itself. Hewlett-Packard had been working on the development of 3D TEE using the 2D reconstruction approach and had released such a system in 1995.

In 2007, Philips introduced its new "Live 3D TEE" probe with a matrix-array transducer (x7-2t, 2500 elements). This probe featured

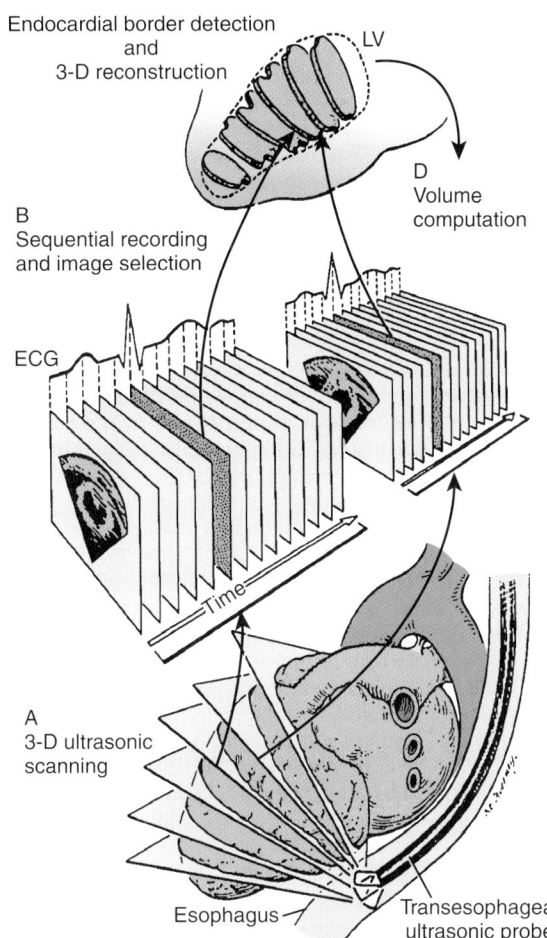

Figure 11-21 Martin and Bashein's method of measuring stroke volume in dogs with three-dimensional (3-D) transesophageal echocardiographic scanning. ECG, electrocardiogram; LV, left ventricle. *(From Martin RW, Bashein G: Measurement of stroke volume with three-dimensional transesophageal ultrasonic scanning: Comparison with thermodilution measurement.* Anesthesiology 70:470–476, 1989, Figure 1.)

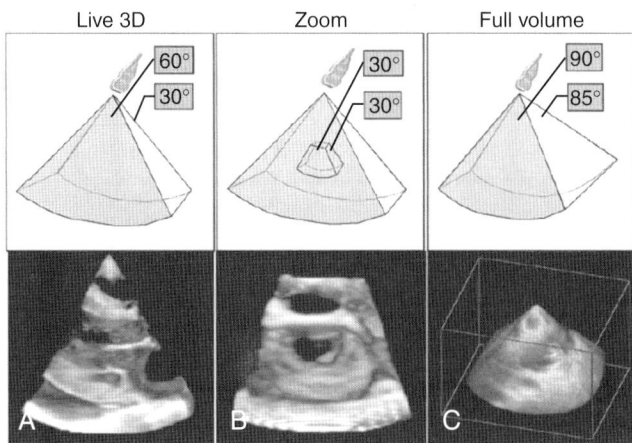

Figure 11-22 Three real-time three-dimensional (3D) imaging modes. *(From Hung J, et al: ASE Position Paper. 3D echocardiography: A review of current status and future directions.* J Am Soc Echocardiogr 20:213–233, 2007, Figure 3.)

the combination of two new novel technologies: xMATRIX (3D power) technology and "Pure Wave" crystal technology that resulted in improved image clarity. "Live 3DTEE" offers not only conventional imaging modes such as 2D multiplane imaging, M-mode, continuous- and pulse-wave Doppler, and color Doppler, but also real-time 3D imaging: Live 2D, 3D Zoom, Full Volume, and 3D Color Full Volume (Figure 11-22). *Live 3D* displays a fixed pyramidal data set determined by the depth of the initial 2D images and can be used to visualize any cardiac structures located in the near field. Movement of the probe results in real-time change of the 3D image. *3D Zoom* displays a truncated but magnified pyramidal data set of variable size. Placement of the probe over the region of interest with minimized sector width improved temporal resolution and optimized image quality. 3D zoom is used to view the left atrial appendage, interatrial septum, and mitral and tricuspid valves. *Full volume* provides a pyramidal data set that allows the inclusion of the larger cardiac volume at frame rate greater than 30 Hz. It combines a series of subvolumes acquired with ECG gating to create a final, larger, reconstructed full-volume image. This is the only one of these 3D modes that requires ECG-gated reconstruction. *3D color full volume* combines grayscale of full-volume data with color Doppler.

3DE has found particular application in measuring ventricular volumes (together with stroke volume, cardiac output, and ejection fraction), especially of the right ventricle (which is a particular problem

with 2DE because of its complex geometric shape), to evaluate mitral valve, aortic valve, and aortic root pathoanatomy, to evaluate complex congenital heart disease, and as a guide for percutaneous interventional procedures including placement of closure devices, transseptal puncture, ablation procedures, and placement of left atrial closure devices. In 2007, the ASE published a position article on the current status and future directions of 3DE[169] and, in 2008, published a practical guide for its use.[170]

Four-Dimensional Echocardiography

4DE or real-time 3DE, that is, 3DE plus time, is a recent addition to the volumetric cardiac imaging field, which is receiving significant clinical interest because it may replace the need for more expensive techniques (such as magnetic resonance imaging) and also suggests new areas of application for volumetric cardiac imaging (e.g., in interventions). The current approaches to 4D medical ultrasonic imaging can be separated into two categories: non–real-time and real-time imaging. Real-time imaging refers to the class of imaging that shows the rendering of the ultrasonic volume in a time frame that can be associated with other clinical monitoring technologies (such as the ECG). This property allows clinicians a more intuitive interface for capturing 4D images because movement of the probe is directly reflected in the imaging volume acquired.

Three-dimensional datasets often can be quite difficult to interpret and require considerable effort and time orienting the observer in relation to anatomic landmarks. When multiple measurements are necessary, as is the case with time-varying volumes, it often is helpful to have semiautomated or fully automated means of quantification, tools that are offered by 4D systems.

Real-time acquisition via 4D (3D plus time) ultrasound obviates the need for slice registration and reconstruction, leaving segmentation as the only barrier to an automated, rapid, and clinically applicable calculation of accurate left ventricular cavity volumes and ejection fraction. Tracking of mitral valve leaflets can determine whether they close fully or whether there is an opening for mitral regurgitation.

In the early 1990s, several studies investigated use of 4DE to study the dynamics of the heart over time utilizing myocardial motion phantoms that were constructed to simulate the motion of myocardial segments using various programmed waveforms and an ECG simulator that provided the necessary R-wave signal in synchrony with the phantom motion. This work was essential for evaluation of new acquisition techniques to provide an accurate method to quantify heart volumes from this type of data.

The next decade brought improvement in technology and new clinical studies. In 2005, Corsi et al[171] developed a volumetric analysis

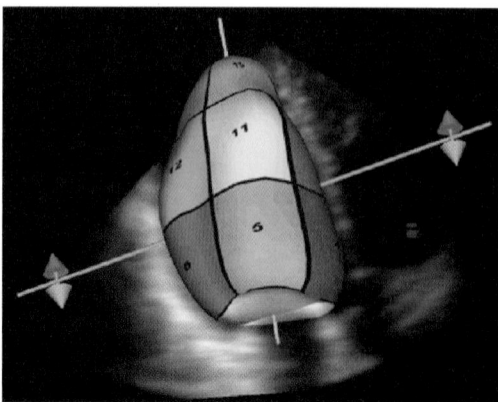

Figure 11-23 Four-dimensional echo visualization. Advanced automatic contour finding algorithms for an easy, fast, accurate, and highly reproducible functional analysis of the left ventricle. *(From www. emageon.com/downloads/Cardiology/HeartSuite_4D_Echo.pdf.)*

technique for quantification of global and regional LV function and studied patients with CAD, cardiomyopathy, and valvular disease. They concluded that volumetric analysis of real-time 3DE data was clinically feasible and allows fast, semiautomated, dynamic measurement of left ventricle volume and automated precise detection of regional wall motion abnormalities. More recent studies have used speckle tracking combined with 4DE to more accurately quantify regional LV strain for strain analysis.[172]

Because the left ventricle is a 3D structure with a complex pattern of wall motion, 4D imaging offers great potential for identification of dyssynchrony. It also could help to identify the optimum pacing site for resynchronization therapy. A recently published study described a novel approach for morphologic and functional quantification of the mitral valve based on a 4D model estimated from ultrasound data.[173] The 4D model's parameters are estimated for each patient using the latest discriminative learning and incremental searching techniques (Figure 11-23).

Tissue Doppler and Speckle Tracking

In 1989, Isaaz et al[174] described the application of Doppler echocardiography to evaluate myocardial motion, and tissue Doppler imaging was born.[175] By appropriate filtering, they examined the high-amplitude low-velocity signals reflected back from the myocardium instead of the blood with pulsed-wave Doppler. This information has been used to evaluate ventricular function (rate and pattern of filling, and emptying of the ventricle, strain, and strain rate) and to estimate filling pressures. In 1997, Nagueh et al[176] at Baylor University suggested that the ratio of early transmitral *blood* flow (E) to early movement of the basal *myocardium* as determined by tissue Doppler (Ea or E'), E/E', could give a clue to left atrial filling pressure. Color coding (mapping) of tissue Doppler velocities in various parts of the myocardium was introduced by the group at the Royal Infirmary of Edinburgh in 1994[177] and has been used to detect dyssynchrony.

Tissue Doppler recording has the same requirement of close alignment of the ultrasound beam with the movement being interrogated. This limitation has been overcome by the identification of small bright spots in the myocardium on the grayscale image because of backscattering from small structures within the myocardium (less than one wavelength) termed *Speckles*. This was first described by the innovative engineering group at Duke University in the late 1980s and early 1990s.[178] These speckles can be identified and tracked (i.e., *Speckle Tracking*) to generate similar information provided by tissue Doppler but without the alignment constraint. These techniques initially were introduced for TTE and are technically demanding but are being used for investigational purposes with clinical TEE, the clinical importance of which are being investigated.[154]

Regional Wall Motion and Endocardial Border Detection

The value of echocardiography in detecting regional wall motion abnormalities and especially for early detection of myocardial ischemia has been recognized for many years. This usually was accomplished by leisurely off-line analysis. With the development of perioperative applications (as well as echocardiographic monitoring of stress tests), more accurate online assessment was needed. One of the keys to accurate assessment of wall motion is accurate delineation of the endocardial border. Various techniques have been introduced to facilitate this. Initially, this included bloodstream and myocardial contrast (see earlier). In the early 1990s, Hewlett-Packard Corporation introduced a method of transesophageal real-time automatic (endocardial) border detection using backscatter imaging with lateral gain compensation, which they termed "acoustic quantification."[179] This subsequently was improved by adding color coding, termed "Color Kinesis" (CK) by the manufacturer.[180] Its use in perioperative TEE was assessed by the group at the University Hospital in Vienna.[181] More recently, tissue Doppler imaging enhanced by color coding,[182,183] and Speckle Tracking has been introduced to facilitate detection of abnormal regional myocardial function. Recently, dos Reis et al,[184] from University of Brasilia, briefly reviewed the history of attempts at semiautomatic border detection and proposed a new algorithm combining classic mathematical morphology for binary images, high-boost filtering, image segmentation, and motion estimation.

Handheld or Hand-Carried Echocardiography: The "Ultrasound-Stethoscope"

The concept and reality of a portable lightweight battery-operated echocardiograph machine was introduced by Roelandt et al in 1978,[185] who referred to this as the "Ultrasound-Stethoscope." Since then, industry has introduced more miniaturized but also more capable portable high-resolution devices that are now even the subject of television advertising. Their use is advocated to complement and expand the history and physical examination, especially in the age of decreased skills in the latter.[186] Mondillo et al[187] have classified these devices, based on their size, capabilities, and cost, into four categories. The top-level devices are now capable of providing 2D, M-mode, color-flow, pulse-wave, and continuous-wave and tissue Doppler. Mondillo et al[187] and Kobal et al[188] have reviewed the capability and limitations of the use of these devices. A key limiting factor is the capabilities of the person conducting and interpreting the examination,[189] and there are controversies about how much training and whether certification is required. Cost implications (vs. benefits) of acquiring the equipment and providing appropriate education are other issues. In 2002, the ASE, the American College of Cardiology, and the American Heart Association addressed the use of hand-carried echocardiography[190] and recommended that users should have a minimum of Level 1 training (75 supervised studies and 150 supervised interpretations), but strongly recommended that they have Level 2 training (150 supervised studies and 300 supervised interpretations), which are far beyond what other proponents of the use of this technology have suggested is necessary.[191]

ORGANIZATIONS, TRAINING, GUIDELINES, AND EXAMINATIONS

A unique feature of the development of the practice of perioperative echocardiography has been the close cooperation and collaboration between cardiologists and anesthesiologists. The former have welcomed and embraced the latter into their specialty, and the two groups have collaborated in training and educational activities, establishing standards for its use and certification, and the development of guidelines and examinations. The ASA and the SCA have cooperated and played key roles in the development of perioperative echocardiography. In 1974, Feigenbaum[192] addressed the educational problems in echocardiography, and these have largely been resolved in recent years. In 2001, Aronson and Thys[193] gave a historical review of the more recent developments in training and certification in perioperative echocardiography.

The first meeting dedicated to cardiac ultrasound was sponsored by the American College of Cardiology and held at Indiana University in Indianapolis on January 11 and 12, 1968. Among the approximately 50 who attended included Elder, Joyner, Reid, and Feigenbaum. The ASE was created in Indianapolis in 1975. *The Journal of the American Society of Echocardiography* began in 1988, and the first annual meeting of the ASE was held in Washington, DC, in 1990.[13]

The SCA has played a key role in the development of perioperative TEE. The SCA offered its first workshop on echocardiography in 1987, initiated the Annual Comprehensive Review on Perioperative Echocardiography in 1998, and in 1991 published a monograph on the *Intraoperative Use of Echocardiography*.[15,194] In 1994, the ASA and SCA embarked on jointly developing practice guidelines for perioperative TEE. The task force was led by Daniel Thys (Figure 11-24) and included representatives from both the American College of Cardiology (William Stewart) and the ASE (Alan Pearlman). These guidelines were published in 1996[195] and were updated in the fall of 2009.[15,200] This marked the beginning of collaborations with various organizations, especially the ASE, in producing a number of guidelines related to perioperative echocardiography (Table 11-4; see Chapter 41).

In 1993, the ASE launched an examination to test knowledge in echocardiography (ASeXAM). Although it contained questions on perioperative echocardiography, that was not its particular focus. Later that decade, the SCA developed an examination confined to perioperative TEE that was first administered on April 24, 1998. As

TABLE 11-4	Collaborative Practice Guidelines Related to Perioperative Echocardiography		
First Author	**Year Published**	**Topic**	**Collaborative Societies**
Thys[195]	1996	Perioperative TEE	ASA/SCA
Shanewise[196]	1999	Performing comprehensive intraoperative TEE examination	ASE/SCA
Cahalan[197]	2002	Training in perioperative TEE	SCAASE
Quiñones[198]	2003	Clinical competence statement	ASE/SCA/SPE/ ACC/AHA
Mathew[199]	2006	CQI in perioperative echocardiography	ASE/SCA
Reeves[130]	2007	Performing comprehensive epicardial echocardiography examination	ASE/SCA
Glas[131]	2008	Performance of comprehensive intraoperative epiaortic examination	ASE/SCA/STS

ACA, Society of Cardiovascular Anesthesiologists; ACC, American College of Cardiology; AHA, American Heart Association; ASA, American Society of Anesthesiologists; ASE, American Society of Echocardiography; STS, Society of Thoracic Surgery; TEE, transesophageal echocardiography.

a result of discussion with the ASeXAM, Inc., the National Board of Echocardiography was established on November 1, 1999, to develop and administer examinations in the field of clinical echocardiography.[15] Currently, three examinations are administered, one in adult echocardiography (ASCeXAM), another in advanced perioperative TEE (Advanced PTEeXAM), and, most recently, in basic perioperative TEE (Basic PTEeXAM). In 2002, Aronson and colleagues[201] reviewed the development and analyzed the results of the PTE examination. Physicians who successfully pass these examinations are recognized as "testamurs." As of 2009, 4091 have taken and 2966 have passed the advanced PTE examination.[15]

In 2003, the National Board of Echocardiography began issuing board certification in Advanced Perioperative TEE to candidates who are testamurs and have met the training and clinical experience requirements. As of 2009, 1111 physicians have become Diplomates in advanced perioperative TEE.[15] In 2010, the National Board of Echocardiography initiated a process for certification in Basic PTE.

In 2000, Morewood et al surveyed members of the SCA; 42% had completed fellowship training. The survey revealed that although 94% of those surveyed practiced in institutions that used intraoperative TEE, and 72% personally performed TEE, less than 30% had received formalized training, and only 19% had passed certifying examinations. Their use of TEE increased with the percentage of their practice devoted to cardiac anesthesia (56% utilization if 25% of practice was cardiac and 91% if more than 75% cardiac). They reported that TEE was performed most of the time or always in 90% of valve surgery, 41% of CABG, and only 1% of noncardiac surgery. Notably, less than 50% said their institutions had specific credentialing criteria.[202] It is interesting to compare these data with the results of the previously mentioned survey of the members of the SCA conducted 12 years earlier,[203] and it is unknown how contemporary practice differs from that reflected in Morewood's 2000 survey.

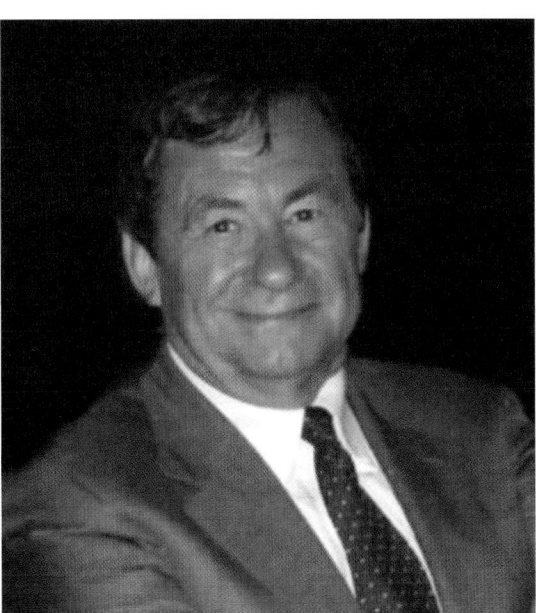

Figure 11-24 Daniel M. Thys, Professor (Emeritus) Anesthesiology Columbia University College of Physicians and Surgeons, New York City, President of the Society of Cardiovascular Anesthesiologists (SCA; 1999–2001), chaired the *ad hoc* Task Force of the ASA/SCA, which developed the Practice Guidelines for Perioperative TEE (1967, 2010). He was chair of the Council on Intraoperative Echocardiography of the American Society of Echocardiography (ASE; 1999–2001), and was on the editorial board of the *Journal of the American Society of Echocardiography*. He was founding member and president of the National Board of Echocardiography (NBE; 2005–2007). Gave the 2nd Annual Weyman Lecture on the history of cardiac anesthesiology emphasizing importance of echocardiography.[15] (*Courtesy D. M. Thys.*)

A CAUTIONARY NOTE

In 1970, Drs. Swan and Ganz introduced their balloon-tipped PAC,[204] which rapidly was adopted by cardiac anesthesiologists, critical care physicians, and all anesthesiologists because it provided hemodynamic information that they were sure was improving patient care. It was widely discussed at meetings of the SCA and the subject of an ASA practice guideline. Now, it has largely fallen into disrepute and its use has greatly diminished,[205] partly because of limitations of some of the data it provides (especially use of filling pressures to assess volume status), risks associated with its use (although with careful application these have found to be uncommon), but most importantly, because of lack of high-quality evidence that its use improves patient outcome. In fact, several recent randomized, controlled trials have failed to find evidence of benefit.[206,207] In an editorial entitled "The Pulmonary Artery Catheter, 1967-2007: Rest in Peace?" Rubenfeld and colleagues[208] conclude: "The 40-year story of the PA catheter is nearing its end. It is a cautionary tale of rapid adoption and slow evaluation of a monitoring device that when used correctly, provides exquisitely detailed physiological data that, regrettably, does not appear to benefit patients. Older clinicians will look back wistfully on the hours spent placing, troubleshooting, and debating the data from the PA catheter. Younger colleagues will just wonder what all the fuss was about." The authors of this chapter hope that the same will not be said about TEE 20 years from now. There is danger of being mesmerized by the new technology that has been developed and applied, without documenting its real clinical benefit and cost-effectiveness. Although clinicians are reasonably confident of the value and apparent clinical benefit that use of perioperative TEE has provided their patients, they recognize that much of the evidence supporting its use and showing its benefit is of a low level. Furthermore, having learned that filling pressures (e.g., central venous pressure [CVP] and pulmonary artery occlusion pressure [PAOP]) are poor predictors of volume status and fluid responsiveness, it is disheartening to encounter a study that also found no correlation between objective measures of right and left ventricular end-diastolic volume (per echocardiography and radionuclide cineangiography) and fluid responsiveness.[209] Thus, the reader is urged to look critically at the data. The clinical scientific community is urged to design and conduct valid studies to prove the benefit of these new technologies and modalities so that clinicians learn from history and do not repeat the errors of the past.

Acknowledgments

The senior author (E.A.H.) acknowledges and expresses his appreciation to the staff at Duke University, including Norbert de Bruijn, Fiona Clements, Gerald Reves, Mark Newman, Jonathan Mark, and the Cardiothoracic Fellows, and Joseph Kisslo, Thomas Ryan, and the ultrasonographers in the echocardiology laboratory, who helped him get started in echocardiography, and Mikel Smith, Director of Echocardiology at the University of Kentucky, who welcomed him and nurtured his growth in this field.

REFERENCES

1. Hessel EA II: Evolution of cardiac anesthesia and surgery. In Kaplan JA, Reich DL, Lake CL, Konstadt SN, editors: *Kaplan's cardiac anesthesia*, ed 5, Philadelphia, 2006, Saunders/Elsevier, pp 3–32.
2. Feigenbaum H: Evolution of echocardiography, *Circulation* 93:1321–1327, 1996.
3. Oka Y: Preface. In Yoka Y, Goldiner PL, editors: *Transesophageal echocardiography*, Philadelphia, 1992, JP Lippincott Company, pp xi–xvi.
4. Goldberg BB, Gramiak R, Freimanis AK: Early history of diagnostic ultrasound: The role of American radiologists, *AJR Am J Roentgenol* 160:189–194, 1993.
5. Wells PN: Milestones in cardiac ultrasound: Echoes from the past. History of cardiac ultrasound, *Int J Card Imaging* 9(Suppl 2):3–9, 1993.
6. Labovitz AJ: Pearson: Historical perspectives and technical considerations. In *Transesophageal echocardiography: Basic principles and clinical implications*, Philadelphia, 1993, Lea and Febiger, pp 1–11.
7. Roelandt J, Souquet J: The development of TEE: A historical review. In Stumper O, Sutherland GR, editors: *Transesophageal echocardiography in congenital heart disease*, London, 1994, Edward Arnold, pp 1–9.
8. Seward JB: Tranesophageal echocardiography. Past, present, future. In Freeman WK, Seward JB, Khandheria AJ, Tajak, editors: *Tranesophageal echocardiography*, Boston, 1994, Little Brown and Co, pp 1–8.
9. Weyman AE: *Principles and practice of echocardiography*, ed 2, Philadelphia, Lea & Febiger, 1994.
10. Newman PG, Rozycki GS: The history of ultrasound, *Surg Clin North Am* 78:179–195, 1998.
11. Roelandt JR: Seeing the invisible: A short history of cardiac ultrasound, *Eur J Echocardiogr* 1:8–11, 2000.
12. Edler I, Lindström K: The history of echocardiography, *Ultrasound Med Biol* 30:1565–1644, 2004.
13. Feigenbaum H: History of echocardiography. In Feigenbaum H, Armstrong WF, Ryan T, editors: *Feigenbaum's echocardiography*, ed 6 Philadelphia, 2005, Lippincott Williams & Wilkins, pp 1–10.
14. Singh S, Goyal A: The origin of echocardiography: A tribute to Inge Edler, *Tex Heart Inst J* 34:431–438, 2007.
15. Thys DM: Cardiac anesthesia: Thirty years later—the second annual Arthur, E. Weyman lecture, *Anesth Analg* 109:1782–1790, 2009.
16. Dussik KT: Uber die Moglichkeit Hochfrequente Mechanische Schwingungen als Diagnostisches Hilfsmitel zu Verwerten, *Z Neurol* 174:153, 1941.
17. Shampo MA, Kyle RA: Karl Theodore Dussik—pioneer in ultrasound, *Mayo Clin Proc* 70(12):1136, 1995.
18. Keidel WD: [New method of recording changes in volume of the human heart.], *Z Kreislaufforsch* 39(9–10):257–271, 1950.
19. Edler I, Hertz CH: The use of the ultrasonic reflectoscope for the continuous recordings of the movements of heart walls, *Kungl Fysiografiska Sallskapets I Lund Forhandlingar* 24:1–19, 1954.
20. Edler I, Gustafson A, Karlefors T, Christensson B: Ultrasoundcardiography, *Acta Med Scand Suppl* 370:5–124, 1961.
21. Wild JJ, Crawford HD, Reid JM: Visualization of the excised human heart by means of reflected ultrasound of echography; preliminary report, *Am Heart J* 54:903–906, 1957.
22. Joyner CR Jr, Reid JM, Bond JP: Reflected ultrasound in the assessment of mitral valve disease, *Circulation* 27(4 Pt 1):503–511, 1963.
23. Feigenbaum H, Waldhausen JA, Hyde LP: Ultrasound diagnosis of pericardial effusion, *JAMA* 191:711–734, 1965.
24. Segal BL, Likoff W, Kingsley B: Echocardiography. Clinical application in mitral stenosis, *JAMA* 195:161–166, 1966.
25. Feigenbaum H: The origin of echocardiography? (Letter), *Tex Heart Inst J* 35:87–88, 2008.
26. Wild JJ, Reid JM: Application of echo-ranging techniques to the determination of structure of biological tissues, *Science* 115(2983):226–230, 1952.
27. Howry DH, Bliss WR: Ultrasonic visualization of soft tissue structures of the body, *J Lab Clin Med* 40:579–592, 1952.
28. Ebina T, Oka S, Tanaka M, et al: The ultrasono-tomography for the heart and great vessels in living human subjects by means of the ultrasonic reflection technique, *Jpn Heart J* 8:331–353, 1967.
29. Asberg A: Ultrasonic cinematography of the living heart, *Ultrasonics* 5:113–117, 1967.
30. Somer JC: Electronic sector scanning for ultrasonic diagnosis, *Ultrasonics* 6:153–159, 1968.
31. Bom N, Lancée CT, Honkoop J, Hugenholtz PG: Ultrasonic viewer for cross-sectional analyses of moving cardiac structures, *Biomed Eng* 6:500–503, 5 1971.
32. vonRamm OT: Cardiac imaging using a phased array ultrasound system. I. System design, *Circulation* 53:258–262, 1976.
33. Griffith JM, Henry WL: A sector scanner for real time two-dimensional echocardiography, *Circulation* 49:1147–1152, 1974.
34. Eggleton RE, Fiegenbaum H, Johnson KW, et al: Visualization of cardiac dynamics with real time B-mode ultrasonic scanner (Abstract), *Circulation* 49–50(Suppl 3):26, 1974.
35. Kisslo J, von Ramm OT, Thurstone FL: Cardiac imaging using a phased array ultrasound system. II. Clinical technique and application, *Circulation* 53:262–267, 1976.
36. Kisslo JA, von Ramm OT, Thurstone FL: Dynamic cardiac imaging using a focused, phased-array ultrasound system, *Am J Med* 63:61–68, 1977.
37. Satomura S: A study on examining the heart with ultrasonics, *Jap Circ J* 20:227, 1956.
38. Franklin DL, Schlegel W, Rushmer RF: Blood flow measured by Doppler frequency shift of back-scattered ultrasound, *Science* 134:564–565, 1961.
39. Barber FE, Baker DW, Nation AW, et al: Ultrasonic duplex echo-Doppler scanner, *IEEE Trans Biomed Eng* 21:109–113, 1974.
40. Holen J, Aaslid R, Landmark K, Simonsen S: Determination of pressure gradient in mitral stenosis with a non-invasive ultrasound Doppler technique, *Acta Med Scand* 199:455–460, 1976.
41. Hatle L, Angelsen BA, Tromsdal A: Non-invasive assessment of aortic stenosis by Doppler ultrasound, *Br Heart J* 43:284–292, 1980.
42. Namekawa K, Kasai C, Tsukamoto M, Koyano A: Realtime bloodflow imaging system utilizing auto-correlation techniques, *Ultrasound Med Biol* (Suppl 2):203–208, 1983.
43. Bommer W, Miller L: Real-time two-dimensional color flow Doppler-enhanced imaging in the diagnosis of cardiovascular disease, *Am J Cardiol* 49:944, 1982.
44. Omoto R, Yokote Y, Takamoto S, et al: The development of real-time two-dimensional Doppler echocardiography and its clinical significance in acquired valvular diseases. With special reference to the evaluation of valvular regurgitation, *Jpn Heart J* 25:325–340, 1984.
45. Johnson ML, Holmes JH, Spangler RD, Paton BC: Usefulness of echocardiography in patients undergoing mitral valve surgery, *J Thorac Cardiovasc Surg* 64:922–934, 1972.
46. Wexler LF, Pohost GM: Hemodynamic monitoring: noninvasive techniques, *Anesthesiology* 45: 156–183, 1976.
47. Rathod R, Jacobs HK, Kramer NE, et al: Echocardiographic assessment of ventricular performance following induction with two anesthetics, *Anesthesiology* 49:86–90, 1978.
48. Barash PG, Glanz S, Katz JD, et al: Ventricular function in children during halothane anesthesia: An echocardiographic evaluation, *Anesthesiology* 49:79–85, 1978.
49. Strom J, Becker RM, Frishman W, et al: Effects of hypothermic hyperkalemic cardioplegic arrest on ventricular performance during cardiac surgery: Assessment by intraoperative echocardiography, *N Y State J Med* 78:2210–2213, 1978.
50. Rodigas PC, Meyer FJ, Haasler GB, et al: Intraoperative 2-dimensional echocardiography: Ejection of microbubbles from the left ventricle after cardiac surgery, *Am J Cardiol* 50:1130–1132, 1982.
51. Dubroff JM, Wong CY, et al: Left ventricular ejection fraction during cardiac surgery: A two-dimensional echocardiographic study, *Circulation* 68:95–103, 1983.
52. Goldman ME, Mindich BP, Teichholz LE, et al: Intraoperative contrast echocardiography to evaluate mitral valve operations, *J Am Coll Cardiol* 4:1035–1040, 1984.
53. Goldman ME, Mindich BP: Intraoperative cardioplegic contrast echocardiography for assessing myocardial perfusion during open heart surgery, *J Am Coll Cardiol* 4:1029–1034, 1984.
54. Cieszynski T: [Intracardiac method for the investigation of structure of the heart with the aid of ultrasonics.], *Arch Immunol Ther Exp (Warsz)* 8:551–557, 1960. Polish.
55. Omoto R: Ultrasonic tomography of the heart: An intracardiac scan method, *Ultrasonics* 5:80–83, 1967.
56. Kimoto S, et al: Ultrasonic tomography of the liver and detection of heart atrial septal defect with the aid of ultrasonic intravenous probes, *Ultrasonics* 2:82, 1964.
57. Carleton RA, Clark JG: Measurement of left ventricular diameter in the dog by cardiac catheterization. Validation and physiologic meaningfulness of an ultrasonic technique, *Circ Res* 22:545–558, 1968.
58. Eggleton RC, Townsend C, Herrick J, et al: Ultrasonic visualization of left ventricular dynamics, *Ultrasonics* 17:142–153, 1970.
59. Bom N, Lancée CT, Van Egmond FC: An ultrasonic intracardiac scanner, *Ultrasonics* 10:72–76, 1972.
60. Side CD, Gosling RG: Non-surgical assessment of cardiac function, *Nature* 232:335–336, 1971.
61. Duck FA, Hodson CJ, Tomlin PJ: An esophageal Doppler probe for aortic flow velocity monitoring, *Ultrasound Med Biol* 1:233–241, 1974.
62. Daigle RE, Miller CW, Histand MB, et al: Nontraumatic aortic blood flow sensing by use of an ultrasonic esophageal probe, *J Appl Physiol* 38:1153–1160, 1975.
63. Frazin L, Talano JV, Stephanides L, et al: Esophageal echocardiography, *Circulation* 54:102–108, 1976.

64. Matsumoto M, Oka Y, Lin YT, et al: Transesophageal echocardiography; for assessing ventricular performance, *N Y State J Med* 79:19–21, 1979.
65. Matsumoto M, Oka Y, Strom J, et al: Application of transesophageal echocardiography to continuous intraoperative monitoring of left ventricular performance, *Am J Cardiol* 46:95–105, 1980.
66. Hisanaga K, Hisanaga A, Hibi N, et al: High speed rotating scanner for transesophageal cross-sectional echocardiography, *Am J Cardiol* 46:837–842, 1980.
67. DiMagno EP, Buxton JL, Regan PT, et al: Ultrasonic endoscope, *Lancet* 1:629–631, 1980.
68. Souquet J, Hanrath P, Zitelli L, et al: Transesophageal phased array for imaging the heart, *IEEE Trans Biomed Eng* 29:707–712, 1982.
69. Schluter M, Langenstein BA, Polster J, et al: Transesophageal cross-sectional echocardiography with a phased array transducer system. Technique and initial clinical results, *Br Heart J* 48:67–72, 1982.
70. Schiller NB: *Intraoperative TEE: Its inception, development and future [Personal notes of the author (E.A.H.)]*, Chicago, Abbott Anesthesia Lecture 21st Annual Meeting of the Society of Cardiovascular Anesthesiologists, April 28. 1999,
71. Cahalan MK, Kremer P, Schiller NB, et al: Intraoperative monitoring with two-dimensional transesophageal echocardiography (Abstract), *Anesthesiology* 57:A–153, 1982.
72. Roizen MF, Kremer P, Cahalan M, et al: Monitoring with transesophageal echocardiography: Patients undergoing supraceliac aortic occlusion (Abstract), *Anesthesiology* 57:A–152, 1982.
73. Beaupre PN, Cahalan MK, Kremer PF, et al: Does pulmonary artery catheter occlusion pressure adequately reflect left ventricular filling during anesthesia and surgery? (Abstract), *Anesthesiology* 59:A3, 1983.
74. Beaupre PN, Roizen MF, Cahalan MK, et al: Hemodynamic and two-dimensional transesophageal echocardiographic analysis of an anaphylactic reaction in a human, *Anesthesiology* 60:482–484, 1984.
75. Roizen MF, Hunt TK, Beaupre PN, et al: The effect of alpha-adrenergic blockade on cardiac performance and tissue oxygen delivery during excision of pheochromocytoma, *Surgery* 94:941–945, 1983.
76. Topol EJ, Humphrey LA, Blanck TJJ, et al: Characterization of post-cardiopulmonary bypass hypotension with intraoperative transesophageal echocardiography, *Anesthesiology* 59:A2, 1983.
77. Topol EJ, Weiss JL, Guzman PA, et al: Immediate improvement of dysfunctional myocardial segments after coronary revascularization: Detection by intraoperative transesophageal echocardiography, *J Am Coll Cardiol* 4:1123–1134, 1984.
78. Cucchiara RF, Nugent M, Seward JB, Messick JM: Air embolism in upright neuro-surgical patients: Detection and localization by two-dimensional transesophageal echocardiography, *Anesthesiology* 60:353–355, 1984.
79. Roizen MF, Beaupre PN, Alpert RA, et al: Monitoring with two-dimensional transesophageal echocardiography. Comparison of myocardial function in patients undergoing supraceliac, suprarenal-infraceliac, or infrarenal aortic occlusion, *J Vasc Surg* 1:300–305, 1984.
80. Gewertz BL, Kremser PC, Zarins CK, et al: Transesophageal echocardiographic monitoring of myocardial ischemia during vascular surgery, *J Vasc Surg* 5:607–613, 1987.
81. Smith JS, Cahalan MF, Benfiel DJ, et al: Intraoperative detection of myocardial ischemia in high-risk patients: Electrocardiography versus two-dimensional transesophageal echocardiography, *Circ* 72:1015–1021, 1985.
82. Schlüter M, Hinrichs A, Thier W, et al: Transesophageal two-dimensional echocardiography: Comparison of ultrasonic and anatomic sections, *Am J Cardiol* 53:1173–1178, 1984.
83. Seward JB, Khandheria BK, Oh JK, et al: Transesophageal echocardiography: Technique, anatomic correlations, implementation, and clinical applications, *Mayo Clin Proc* 63:649–680, 1988.
84. Kaplan JA: Transesophageal echocardiography, *Mt Sinai J Med* 51:592–594, 1984.
85. Konstadt S, Goldman M, Thys D, et al: Intraoperative diagnosis of myocardial ischemia, *Mt Sinai J Med* 52:521–525, 1985.
86. Konstadt SN, Thys D, Mindich BP, et al: Validation of quantitative intraoperative transesophageal echocardiography, *Anesthesiology* 65:418–421, 1986.
87. Thys DM, Hillel Z, Goldman ME, et al: A comparison of hemodynamic indices derived by invasive monitoring and two-dimensional echocardiography, *Anesthesiology* 67:630–634, 1987.
88. Konstadt SN, Kaplan JA, Tannenbaum MA, et al: Case 5—1987. 45-year-old woman develops acute left ventricular ischemia and dysfunction after subxiphoid drainage of a pericardial tamponade, *J Cardiothorac Anesth* 1:469–478, 1987.
89. Cahalan MK, Litt L, Botvinick EH, Schiller NB: Advances in noninvasive cardiovascular imaging: Implication for the anesthesiologist, *Anesthesiology* 66:356–372, 1987.
90. Clements FM, deBruijn NP: Perioperative evaluation of regional wall motion by transesophageal two-dimensional echocardiography, *Anesth Analg* 66:249–261, 1987.
91. Abel MD, Nishimura RA, Callahan MJ, et al: Evaluation of intraoperative transesophageal two-dimensional echocardiography, *Anesthesiology* 66:64–68, 1987.
92. Thys DM, Hillel Z, Konstadt SN, Goldman ME: Intraoperative echocardiography. In Kaplan JA, editor: *Clinical anesthesia*, ed 2 Orlando, 1987, Grune & Stratton, pp 255–318.
93. Goldman ME, Thys D, Ritter S, et al: Transesophageal real time Doppler flow imaging: A new method for intraoperative cardiac evaluation, *Journal of the American College of Cardiology* 7: 1A 1986, .
94. Takamoto S, Omoto R: Visualization of thoracic dissecting aortic aneurysm by transesophageal Doppler color flow mapping, *Herz* 12:187–193, 1987.
95. deBruijn NP, Clements FM, Kisslo JA: Intraoperative color flow mapping: Initial experience, *Anesth Analg* 66:386–390, 1987.
96. Roewer N, Bednarz F, Schulte am Esch J: Continuous measurement of intracardiac and pulmonary blood flow velocities with transesophageal pulsed Doppler echocardiography: Technique and initial clinical experience, *J Cardiothorac Anesth* 1:418–428, 1987.
97. Schlüter M, Langenstein BA, Hanrath P, et al: Assessment of transesophageal pulsed Doppler echocardiography in the detection of mitral regurgitation, *Circulation* 66:784–799, 1982.
98. Omoto R, Kyo S, Matsumura M, et al: Bi-plane color transesophageal Doppler echocardiography (color TEE): Its advantages and limitations, *Int J Card Imaging* 4:57–58, 1989.
99. Curling PE, Newsom LR, Rogers A, et al: 2D transesophageal echocardiography: A bidirectional phased array probe with temperature monitoring, *Anesthesiology* 61:A159, 1984.
100. Roelandt JR, Thomson IR, Vletter WB, et al: Multiplane transesophageal echocardiography: Latest evolution in an imaging revolution, *J Am Soc Echocardiogr* 5:361–367, 1992.
101. Kyo S, Koike K, Takanawa E, et al: Impact of transesophageal Doppler echocardiography on pediatric cardiac surgery, *Int J Card Imaging* 4:41–42, 1989.
102. Pandian NG, Hsu TL, Schwartz SL, et al: Multiplane transesophageal echocardiography. Imaging planes, echocardiographic anatomy, and clinical experience with a prototype phased array OmniPlane probe, *Echocardiography* 9:649–666, 1992.
103. Hillel Z, Mikula S, Thys D: The current state of intraoperative echocardiography in North America: Results of a survey, *J Cardiothorac Anesth* 2:803–811, 1988.
104. Kaplan JA: Monitoring technology: Advances and restraints, *J Cardiothorac Anesth* 3:257–259, 1989.
105. Ungerleider RM, Kisslo JA, Greeley WJ, et al: Intraoperative prebypass and postbypass epicardial color flow imaging in the repair of atrioventricular septal defects, *J Thorac Cardiovasc Surg* 98:90–99, discussion 99–100, 1989.
106. Ungerleider RM, Greeley WJ, Sheikh KH, et al: Routine use of intraoperative epicardial echocardiography and Doppler color flow imaging to guide and evaluate repair of congenital heart lesions. A prospective study, *J Thorac Cardiovasc Surg* 100:297–309, 1990.
107. Ungerleider RM, Kisslo JA, Greeley WJ, et al: Intraoperative echocardiography during congenital heart operations: Experience from 1,000 cases, *Ann Thorac Surg* 60(6 Suppl):S539–S542, 1995.
108. Stevenson JG, Sorensen GK, Gartman DM, et al: Transesophageal echocardiography during repair of congenital cardiac defects: Identification of residual problems necessitating reoperation, *J Am Soc Echocardiogr* 6:356–365, 1993.
109. Stevenson JG, Sorensen GK: Proper probe size for pediatric transesophageal echocardiography, *Am J Cardiol* 72:491–492, 1993.
110. Stevenson JG: Role of intraoperative transesophageal echocardiography during repair of congenital cardiac defects, *Acta Paediatr Suppl* 410:23–33, 1995.
111. Stevenson JG: Utilization of intraoperative transesophageal echocardiography during repair of congenital cardiac defects: A survey of North American centers, *Clin Cardiol* 26:132–134, 2003.
112. Savage RM: Preface. In Savage RM, Aronson S, editors: *Comprehensive textbook of intraoperative transesophageal echocardiography*, Philadelphia, 2005, Lipppincott Williams & Wilkins, pp xiii.
113. Rouine-Rapp K, Ionescu P, Balea M: Detection of intraoperative segmental wall-motion abnormalities by transesophageal echocardiography: The incremental value of additional cross sections in the transverse and longitudinal planes, *Anesth Analg* 83:1141–1148, 1996.
114. Bergquist BD, Bellows WH, Leung JM: Transesophageal echocardiography in myocardial revascularization: II. Influence on intraoperative decision making, *Anesth Analg* 82:1139–1145, 1996.
115. Savage RM, Lytle BW, Aronson S, et al: Intraoperative echocardiography is indicated in high-risk coronary artery bypass grafting, *Ann Thorac Surg* 64:368–373, discussion 373–374, 1997.
116. Aronson S, Dupont F, Savage R, et al: Changes in regional myocardial function after coronary artery bypass graft surgery are predicted by intraoperative low-dose dobutamine echocardiography, *Anesthesiology* 93:685–692, 2000.
117. Thys DM, Hillel Z, Schwartz AJ: *Textbook of cardiothoracic anesthesiology*, New York, 2001, McGraw-Hill Companies.
118. Feinstein SB, Coll B, Staub D, et al: Contrast enhanced ultrasound imaging, *J Nucl Cardiol* 17:106–115, 2010.
119. Gramiak R, Shah PM: Echocardiography of the aortic root, *Invest Radiol* 3:356–366, 1968.
120. Seward JB, Tajik AJ, Spangler JG, Ritter DG: Echocardiographic contrast studies: Initial experience, *Mayo Clin Proc* 50:163–192, 1975.
121. Feinstein SB, Ten Cate FJ, Zwehl W, et al: Two-dimensional contrast echocardiography. I. In vitro development and quantitative analysis of echo contrast agents, *J Am Coll Cardiol* 3:14–20, 1984.
122. Aronson S, Savage R, Toledano A, et al: Identifying the cause of left ventricular systolic dysfunction after coronary artery bypass surgery: The role of myocardial contrast echocardiography, *J Cardiothorac Vasc Anesth* 12:512–518, 1998.
123. Kabas JS, Kisslo J, Flick CL, et al: Intraoperative perfusion contrast echocardiography. Initial experience during coronary artery bypass grafting, *J Thorac Cardiovasc Surg* 99:536–542, 1990.
124. Spotnitz WD, Kaul S: Intraoperative assessment of myocardial perfusion using contrast echocardiography, *Echocardiography* 7:209–228, 1990.
125. Aronson S, Lee BK, Wiencek JG, et al: Assessment of myocardial perfusion during CABG surgery with two-dimensional transesophageal contrast echocardiography, *Anesthesiology* 75:433–440, 1991.
126. Aronson S: Measurement of myocardial perfusion by contrast echocardiography: Application in the operating room, *Coron Artery Dis* 11:227–234, 2000.
127. Dijkmans PA, Senior R, Becher H, et al: Myocardial contrast echocardiography evolving as a clinically feasible technique for accurate, rapid, and safe assessment of myocardial perfusion: The evidence so far, *J Am Coll Cardiol* 48:2168–2177, 2006.
128. Mulvagh SL, Rakowski H, Vannan MA, et al: American Society of Echocardiography: American Society of Echocardiography Consensus 174. Statement on the Clinical Applications of Ultrasonic Contrast Agents in Echocardiography, *J Am Soc Echocardiogr* 21:1179–1201, 2008.
129. Whitley WS, Glas KE: An argument for routine ultrasound screening of the thoracic aorta in the cardiac surgery population, *Semin Cardiothorac Vasc Anesth* 12:290–297, 2008.
130. Reeves ST, Glas KE, Eltzschig H, et al: Council for Intraoperative Echocardiography of the American Society of Echocardiography; Society of Cardiovascular Anesthesiologists: Guidelines for performing a comprehensive epicardial echocardiography examination: Recommendations of the American Society of Echocardiography and the Society of Cardiovascular Anesthesiologists, *Anesth Analg* 105:22–28, 2007.
131. Glas KE, Swaminathan M, Reeves ST, et al: Council for Intraoperative Echocardiography of the American Society of Echocardiography; Society of Cardiovascular Anesthesiologists; Society of Thoracic Surgeons: Guidelines for the performance of a comprehensive intraoperative epiaortic ultrasonographic examination: Recommendations of the American Society of Echocardiography and the Society of Cardiovascular Anesthesiologists; endorsed by the Society of Thoracic Surgeons, *Anesth Analg* 106:1376–1384, 2008.
132. Foster GP, Picard MH: Intracardiac echocardiography: Current uses and future directions, *Echocardiography* 18:43–48, 2001.
133. Nissen SE, Grines CL, Gurley JC, et al: Application of a new phased-array ultrasound imaging catheter in the assessment of vascular dimensions. In vivo comparison to cineangiography, *Circulation* 81:660–666, 1990.
134. Gussenhoven EJ, Taams MA, Roelandt JR, et al: Transesophageal two-dimensional echocardiography: Its role in solving clinical problems, *J Am Coll Cardiol* 8:975–979, 1986.
135. Erbel R, Börner N, Steller D, et al: Detection of aortic dissection by transoesophageal echocardiography, *Br Heart J* 58:45–51, 1987.
136. Erbel R, Engberding R, Daniel W, et al: Echocardiography in diagnosis of aortic dissection, *Lancet* 1:457–461, 1989.
137. Chan K-L: Transesophageal echocardiography for assessing cause of hypotension after cardiac surgery, *Am J Cardiol* 62:1142–1143, 1988.
138. Reichert CL, Visser CA, Koolen JJ, et al: Transesophageal echocardiography in hypotensive patients after cardiac operations. Comparison with hemodynamic parameters, *J Thorac Cardiovasc Surg* 104:321–326, 1992.
139. Pearson AC, Castello R, Labovitz AJ: Safety and utility of transesophageal echocardiography in the critically ill patient, *Am Heart J* 119:1083–1089, 1990.
140. Oh JK, Seward JB, Khandheria BK, et al: Transesophageal echocardiography in critically ill patients, *Am J Cardiol* 66:1492–1495, 1990.
141. Foster E: The role of transesophageal echocardiography in critical care: UCSF experience, *J Am Soc Echocardiogr* 5:368–374, 1992.
142. Font VE, Obarski TP, Klein AL, et al: Transesophageal echocardiography in the critical care unit, *Cleve Clin J Med* 58:315–322, 1991.
143. Hwang JJ, Shyu KG, Chen JJ, et al: Usefulness of transesophageal echocardiography in the treatment of critically ill patients, *Chest* 104:861–866, 1993.
144. Khoury AF, Afridi I, Quiñones MA, Zoghbi WA: Transesophageal echocardiography in critically ill patients: Feasibility, safety, and impact on management, *Am Heart J* 127:1363–1371, 1994.
145. Benjamin E, Griffin K, Leibowitz AB, et al: Goal-directed transesophageal echocardiography performed by intensivists to assess left ventricular function: Comparison with pulmonary artery catheterization, *J Cardiothorac Vasc Anesth* 12:10–15, 1998.
146. Hüttemann E, Schelenz C, Kara F, et al: The use and safety of transoesophageal echocardiography in the general ICU—a minireview, *Acta Anaesthesiol Scand* 48:827–836, 2004.

147. Salem R, Vallee F, Rusca M, Mebazaa A: Hemodynamic monitoring by echocardiography in the ICU: The role of the new echo techniques, *Curr Opin Crit Care* 14:561–568, 2008.
148. Mahmood F, Christie A, Matyal R: Transesophageal echocardiography and noncardiac surgery, *Semin Cardiothorac Vasc Anesth* 12:265–289, 2008.
149. Hodgins L, Kisslo JA, Mark JB: Perioperative transesophageal echocardiography: The anesthesiologist as cardiac diagnostician, *Anesth Analg* 80:4–6, 1995.
150. Goldstein S: Pro: The general anesthesiologist should be trained and certified in transesophageal echocardiography, *J Cardiothorac Vasc Anesth* 24:183–188, 2010.
151. Green M: Con: General anesthesiologists should not be trained and certified in basic transesophageal echocardiography, *J Cardiothorac Vasc Anesth* 24:189–190, 2010.
152. Vezina DP, Johnson KB, Cahalan MK: Transesophageal echocardiography. In Miller RE, Eriksson LA, Fleisher, et al: *Miller's anesthesia*, ed 7 Philadelphia, Churchill Livingstone/Elsevier, 2010.
153. Yeates TM, Zimmerman JM, Cahalan MK: Perioperative echocardiography: Two-dimensional and three-dimensional applications, *Anesthesiol Clin* 26:419–435, 2008.
154. Marcucci C, Lauer R, Mahajan A: New echocardiographic techniques for evaluating left ventricular myocardial function, *Semin Cardiothorac Vasc Anesth* 12:228–247, 2008.
155. Weyman AE: Future directions in echocardiography, *Rev Cardiovasc Med* 10:4–13, 2009.
156. Baum G: Orbital lesion localization by three dimensional ultrasonography, *N Y State J Med* 61:4149–4157, 1961.
157. Dekker DL, Piziali RL, Dong E: A system for ultrasonically imaging the human heart in three dimensions, *Comput Biomed Res* 7:544–553, 1974.
158. Moritz WE: A microprocessor-based spatial locating system for use with diagnostic ultrasound, *IEEE Trans Biomed Eng* 64:966–974, 1976.
159. Matsumoto M, Matsuo H, Kitabatake A, et al: Three-dimensional echocardiograms and two-dimensional echocardiographic images at desired planes by a computerized system, *Ultrasound Med Biol* 3:163, 1977.
160. Raab FH, Blood EB, Steiner TO, et al: Magnetic position and orientation tracking system, *IEEE Trans Aerospace Elec Sys* AES-15:709–718, 1979.
161. Ghosh A, Maurer G: Three-dimensional reconstruction of echo-cardiographic images using the rotation method, *Ultrasound Med Biol* 8:655–661, 1982.
162. Geiser EA, Ariet M, Conetta DA, et al: Dynamic three-dimensional echocardiographic reconstruction of the intact human left ventricle: Technique and initial observations in patients, *Am Heart J* 103:1056–1065, 1982.
163. vonRamm OT, Smith SW: Real time volumetric ultrasound imaging system, *J Digit Imaging* 3:261–266, 1990.
164. Martin RW, Bashein G, Zimmer R, Sutherland J: An endoscopic micromanipulator for multiplanar transesophageal imaging, *Ultrasound Med Biol* 12:965–975, 1986.
165. Martin RW, Graham MM, Kao R, Bashein G: Measurement of left ventricular ejection fraction and volumes with three-dimensional reconstructed transesophageal ultrasound scans: Comparison to radionuclide and thermal dilution measurements, *J Cardiothorac Anesth* 3:260–268, 1989.
166. Wollschläger H, Zeiher AM, Klein HP, et al: [Transesophageal echo computer tomography (ECHO-CT): a new method of dynamic 3-D reconstruction of the heart], *Biomed Tech (Berl)* 34(Suppl):10–11, 1989.
167. Pandian NG, Schwartz SL, et al: Three-dimensional and four-dimensional transesophageal echocardiographic imaging of the heart and aorta in humans using a computed tomographic imaging probe, *Echocardiography* 9:677–687, 1992.
168. Chen Q, Nosir YF, Vletter WB, et al: Accurate assessment of mitral valve area in patients with mitral stenosis by three-dimensional echocardiography, *J Am Soc Echocardiogr* 10:133–140, 1997.
169. Hung J, Lang R, Flachskampf F, et al: ASE Position Paper: 3D echocardiography: A review of the current status and future directions, *J Am Soc Echocardiogr* 20:213–233, 2007.
170. Yang HS, Bansal RC, Mookadam F, et al: American Society of Echocardiography. Practical guide for three-dimensional transthoracic echocardiography using a fully sampled matrix array transducer, *J Am Soc Echocardiogr* 21:979–989, 2008.
171. Corsi C, Lang RM, Veronesi F, et al: Volumetric quantification of global and regional left ventricular function from real-time three-dimensional echocardiographic images, *Circulation* 112:1161–1170, 2005.
172. Nesser HJ, Mor-Avi V, Gorissen W, et al: Quantification of left ventricular volumes using three-dimensional echocardiographic speckle tracking: Comparison with MRI, *Eur Heart J* 30:1565–1573, 2009.
173. Voigt I, Ionasec RI, Georgescu B, Houle H, et al: Model-driven physiological assessment of the mitral valve from 4D TEE, *Progress in biomedical optics and imaging* 2009; 10(1), no 37:72610R.1–72610R.11.
174. Isaaz K, Thompson A, Ethevenot G, et al: Doppler echocardiographic measurement of low velocity motion of the left ventricular posterior wall, *Am J Cardiol* 64:66–75, 1989.
175. Marcucci C, Lauer R, Mahajan A: New echocardiographic techniques for evaluating left ventricular myocardial function, *Semin Cardiothorac Vasc Anesth* 12(4):228–247, 2008.
176. Nagueh SF, Middleton KJ, Kopelen HA, et al: Doppler tissue imaging: A noninvasive technique for evaluation of left ventricular relaxation and estimation of filling pressures, *J Am Coll Cardiol* 30:1527–1533, 1997.
177. Fleming AD, Xia X, McDicken WN, et al: Myocardial velocity gradients detected by Doppler imaging, *Br J Radiol* 67:679–688, 1994.
178. Bohs LN, Trahey GE: A novel method for angle independent ultrasonic imaging of blood flow and tissue motion, *IEEE Trans Biomed Eng* 38:280–286, 1991.
179. Pérez JE, Prater DM, et al: Automated, on-line quantification of left ventricular dimensions and function by echocardiography with backscatter imaging and lateral gain compensation, *Am J Cardiol* 70:1200–1205, 1992.
180. Lang RM, Vignon P, Weinert L, et al: Echocardiographic quantification of regional left ventricular wall motion with color kinesis, *Circulation* 93:1877–1885, 1996.
181. Hartmann T, Kolev N, Blaicher A, et al: Validity of acoustic quantification colour kinesis for detection of left ventricular regional wall motion abnormalities: A transoesophageal echocardiographic study, *Br J Anaesth* 79:482–487, 1997.
182. Gorcsan J 3rd, Gulati VK, Mandarino WA, Katz WE: Color-coded measures of myocardial velocity throughout the cardiac cycle by tissue Doppler imaging to quantify regional left ventricular function, *Am Heart J* 131:1203–1213, 1996.
183. Katz WE, Gulati VK, Mahler CM, Gorcsan J: Quantitative evaluation of the segmental left ventricular response to dobutamine stress by tissue Doppler echocardiography, *Am J Cardiol* 79:1036–1042, 1997.
184. dos Reis MdoC, da Rocha AF, Vasconcelos DF, et al: Semi-automatic detection of the left ventricular border, *Conf Proc IEEE Eng Med Biol Soc* 218–221, 2008.
185. Roelandt J, Ten Cate FJ, Hugenholtz P: The ultrasonic stethoscope: A miniature hand-held device for real time cardiac imaging, *Circulation* 58(II):II–79–II-81, 1978.
186. Roelandt JR: Ultrasound stethoscopy: A renaissance of the physical examination? *Heart* 89:971–973, 2003.
187. Mondillo S, Giannotti G, Innelli P, et al: Hand-held echocardiography: Its use and usefulness, *Int J Cardiol* 111:1–5, 2006.
188. Kobal SL, Atar S, Siegel RJ: Hand-carried ultrasound improves the bedside cardiovascular examination, *Chest* 126:693–701, 2004.
189. Alexander JH, Peterson ED, Chen AY, et al: Feasibility of point-of-care echocardiography by internal medicine house staff, *Am Heart J* 147:476–481, 2004.
190. Seward JB, Douglas PS, Erbel R, et al: Hand-carried cardiac ultrasound (HCU) device: Recommendations regarding new technology. A report from the Echocardiography Task Force on New Technology of the Nomenclature and Standards Committee of the American Society of Echocardiography, *J Am Soc Echocardiogr* 15:369–373, 2002.
191. Vignon P, Dugard A, Abraham J, et al: Focused training for goal-oriented hand-held echocardiography performed by noncardiologist residents in the intensive care unit, *Intensive Care Med* 33:1795–1799, 2007.
192. Feigenbaum H: Educational problems in echocardiography (Editorial), *Am J Cardiol* 34:741–742, 1974.
193. Aronson S, Thys DM: Training and certification in perioperative transesophageal echocardiography: A historical perspective, *Anesth Analg* 93:1422–1427, 2001.
194. deBruijn NP, Clements FM, editors: *Intraoperative use of echocardiography. A Society of Cardiovascular Anesthesiologists Monograph*, Philadelphia, JB Lippincott, 1991.
195. Thys DM, Abel M, Bollen BA, et al: Practice guidelines for perioperative transesophageal echocardiography. A report by the American Society of Anesthesiologists and the Society of Cardiovascular Anesthesiologists Task Force on Transesophageal Echocardiography, *Anesthesiology* 84:986–1006, 1996.
196. Shanewise JS, Cheung AT, Aronson S, et al: ASE/SCA guidelines for performing a comprehensive intraoperative multiplane transesophageal echocardiography examination: Recommendations of the American Society of Echocardiography Council for Intraoperative Echocardiography and the Society of Cardiovascular Anesthesiologists Task Force for Certification in Perioperative Transesophageal Echocardiography, *Anesth Analg* 89:870–884, 1999.
197. Cahalan MK, Stewart W, Pearlman A, et al: Society of Cardiovascular Anesthesiologists; American Society of Echocardiography Task Force. American Society of Echocardiography and Society of Cardiovascular Anesthesiologists task force guidelines for training in perioperative echocardiography, *J Am Soc Echocardiogr* 15:647 652, 2002.
198. Quiñones MA, Douglas PS, Foster E, et al: American Society of Echocardiography; Society of Cardiovascular Anesthesiologists; Society of Pediatric Echocardiography: ACC/AHA clinical competence statement on echocardiography: A report of the American College of Cardiology/American Heart Association/American College of Physicians-American Society of Internal Medicine Task Force on clinical competence, *J Am Soc Echocardiogr* 16:379–402, 2003.
199. Mathew JP, Glas K, Troianos CA, et al: Council for Intraoperative Echocardiography of the American Society of Echocardiography: ASE/SCA recommendations and guidelines for continuous quality improvement in perioperative echocardiography, *Anesth Analg* 103:1416–1425, 2006.
200. American Society of Anesthesiologists and Society of Cardiovascular Anesthesiologists Task Force on Transesophageal Echocardiography. Practice guidelines for perioperative transesophageal echocardiography. An updated report by the American Society of Anesthesiologists and the Society of Cardiovascular Anesthesiologists Task Force on Transesophageal Echocardiography, *Anesthesiology* 112(5):1084–1096, 2010.
201. Aronson S, Subhiyah R, et al: Development and analysis of a new certifying examination in perioperative transesophageal echocardiography, *Anesth Analg* 95:1476–1482, 2002.
202. Morewood GH, Gallgher ME, Conlay LA: Current practice patterns for perioperative transesophageal echocardiography in the United States (Abstract), *Anesth Analg* 92:SCA 94, 2001.
203. Hillel Z, Mikula S, Thys D: The current state of intraoperative echocardiography in North America: Results of a survey, *J Cardiothorac Anesth* 2(6):803–811, 1988.
204. Swan HJ, Ganz W, Forrester J, et al: Catheterization of the heart in man with use of a flow-directed balloon-tipped catheter, *N Engl J Med* 283:447–451, 1970.
205. Wiener RS, Welch HG: Trends in the use of the pulmonary artery catheter in the United States, 1993-2004, *JAMA* 298:423–429, 2007.
206. Shah MR, Hasselblad V, Stevenson LW, et al: Impact of the pulmonary artery catheter in critically ill patients: Meta-analysis of randomized clinical trials, *JAMA* 294:1664–1670, 2005.
207. Wheeler AP, Bernard GR, Thompson BT, et al: Pulmonary-artery versus central venous catheter to guide treatment of acute lung injury, *N Engl J Med* 354:2213–2224, 2006.
208. Rubenfeld GD, McNamara-Aslin E, Rubinson L: The pulmonary artery catheter, 1967-2007: Rest in peace? *JAMA* 298:458–461, 2007.
209. Kumar A, Anel R, Bunnell E, et al: Pulmonary artery occlusion pressure and central venous pressure fail to predict ventricular filling volume, cardiac performance, or the response to volume infusion in normal subjects, *Crit Care Med* 32:691–699, 2004.

12

Intraoperative Transesophageal Echocardiography

RONALD A. KAHN, MD | NIKOLAOS J. SKUBAS, MD, FASE | GREGORY W. FISCHER, MD | STANTON K. SHERNAN, MD, FAHA, FASE | STEVEN N. KONSTADT, MD, MBA, FACC

KEY POINTS

1. An ultrasound beam is a continuous or intermittent train of sound waves emitted by a transducer or wave generator that is composed of density or pressure. Ultrasound waves are characterized by their wavelength, frequency, and velocity.

2. Waves interact with the medium in which they travel and with one another, and the manner in which waves interact with a medium is determined by its density and homogeneity. When a wave is propagated through an inhomogeneous medium, it is partly absorbed, partly reflected, and partly scattered.

3. Doppler frequency shift analysis can be used to obtain blood flow velocity, direction, and acceleration of red blood cells, where the magnitude and direction of the frequency shift are related to the velocity and direction of the moving target.

4. Doppler shifts above the Nyquist limit will create artifacts described as "aliasing" or "wraparound," and blood flow velocities will appear in a direction opposite to the conventional one. The ultrasound frequency should be low, and the sampling frequency should be high to optimize Nyquist limits.

5. Normally, red blood cells scatter ultrasound waves weakly, resulting in a black appearance on ultrasonic examination. Contrast echocardiography uses gas microbubbles to present additional gas–liquid interfaces, which substantially increase the strength of the returning signal. This augmentation in signal strength may be used to better define endocardial borders, optimize Doppler envelope signals, and estimate myocardial perfusion.

6. *Axial resolution* is the minimum separation between two interfaces located in a direction parallel to the ultrasound beam so that they can be imaged as two different interfaces. *Lateral resolution* is the minimum separation of two interfaces aligned along a direction perpendicular to the beam. *Elevational resolution* refers to the ability to determine differences in the thickness of the imaging plane.

7. Absolute contraindications to transesophageal echocardiography in intubated patients include esophageal stricture, diverticula, tumor, recent suture lines, and known esophageal interruption. Relative contraindications include symptomatic hiatal hernia, esophagitis, coagulopathy, esophageal varices, and unexplained upper gastrointestinal bleeding.

8. Horizontal imaging planes are obtained by moving the transesophageal echocardiography probe up and down (upper esophageal: 20 to 25 cm; midesophageal: 30 to 40 cm; transgastric: 40 to 45 cm; deep transgastric: 45 to 50 cm). Multiplane probes may further facilitate interrogation of complex anatomic structures by allowing up to 180 degrees of axial rotation of the imaging plane without manual probe manipulation.

9. The dynamic assessment of ventricular function with echocardiography is based on derived indices of muscle contraction and relaxation. Echocardiography indices of left ventricular function that incorporate endocardial border outlines and Doppler techniques can be used to estimate cardiac output, stroke volume, ejection fraction, and parameters of ventricular relaxation and filling.

10. There are three primary stages of diastolic dysfunction: impaired relaxation, pseudonormalization, and restrictive cardiomyopathy. The evaluation of diastolic function may be performed using Doppler analysis of mitral valve inflow and pulmonary vein flow, color M-mode propagation velocities, and tissue Doppler analysis of the mitral valve annulus.

11. The summation of flow velocities in a given period is called the *velocity-time integral*. Flow across the orifice is equal to the product of the cross-sectional area of the orifice and the velocity-time integral.

Few areas in cardiac anesthesia have developed as rapidly as the field of intraoperative echocardiography. In the early 1980s, when transesophageal echocardiography (TEE) was first used in the operating room, its main application was the assessment of global and regional left ventricular (LV) function. Since that time, there have been numerous technical advances: biplane and multiplane probes; multifrequency probes; enhanced scanning resolution; color–flow Doppler (CFD), pulsed-wave (PW) Doppler, and continuous-wave (CW) Doppler; automatic edge detection; Doppler tissue imaging (DTI); three-dimensional (3D) reconstruction; and digital image processing. With these advances, the number of clinical applications of TEE has increased markedly. The common applications of TEE include: (1) assessment of valvular anatomy and function, (2) evaluation of the thoracic aorta, (3) detection of intracardiac defects, (4) detection of intracardiac masses, (5) evaluation of pericardial effusions, (6) detection of intracardiac air and clots, (7) assessment of biventricular systolic and diastolic function, and (8) evaluation of myocardial ischemia and regional wall motion abnormalities (RWMAs). In many of these evaluations, TEE is able to provide unique and critical information that previously was not available in the operating room (Box 12-1).

BASIC CONCEPTS

Properties of Ultrasound

In echocardiography, the heart and great vessels are insonated with ultrasound, which is sound above the human audible range. The ultrasound is sent into the thoracic cavity and is partially reflected by the cardiac structures. From these reflections, distance, velocity, and density of objects within the chest are derived.

An ultrasound beam is a continuous or intermittent train of sound waves emitted by a transducer or wave generator. It is composed of density or pressure waves and can exist in any medium with the exception of a vacuum (Figure 12-1). Ultrasound waves are characterized by their wavelength, frequency, and velocity.[1] *Wavelength* is the distance between the two nearest points of equal pressure or density in an ultrasound beam, and *velocity* is the speed at which the waves propagate through a medium. As the waves travel past any fixed point in an ultrasound beam, the pressure cycles regularly and continuously between a high and a low value. The number of cycles per second (Hertz) is called the *frequency* of the wave. Ultrasound is sound with frequencies above 20,000 Hz, which is the upper limit of the human audible range. The relationship among the frequency (f), wavelength (λ), and velocity (v) of a sound wave is defined by the following formula:

$$v = f \times \lambda$$

The velocity of sound varies with the properties of the medium through which it travels. In low-density gases, molecules must transverse long distances before encountering the adjacent molecules, so ultrasound velocity is relatively slow. In contrast, in solid, where molecules are constrained, ultrasound velocity is relatively high. For soft tissues, this velocity approximates 1540 m/sec but varies from 1475 to

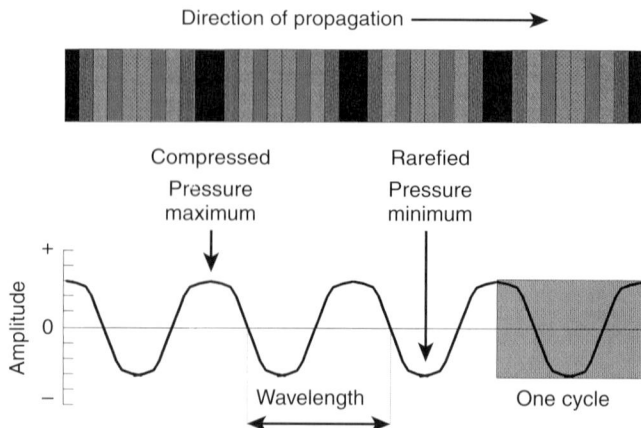

Direction of propagation ⟶

Figure 12-1   A sound wave is a series of compressions and rarefactions. The combination of one compression and one rarefaction represents one cycle. The distance between the onset (peak compression) of one cycle and the onset of the next is the wavelength. *(From Thys DM, Hillel Z: How it works: Basic concepts in echocardiography. In Bruijn NP, Clements F [eds]: Intraoperative use of echocardiography. Philadelphia: JB Lippincott, 1991.)*

1620 m/sec. In comparison, the velocity of ultrasound in air is 330 m/sec and 3360 m/sec in bone. Because the frequency of an ultrasound beam is determined by the properties of the emitting transducer, and the velocity through soft tissue is approximately constant, wavelengths are inversely proportional to the ultrasound frequency.

Ultrasound waves transport energy through a given medium; the rate of energy transport is expressed as "power," which is usually expressed in joules per second or watts.[1] Because medical ultrasound usually is concentrated in a small area, the strength of the beam usually is expressed as power per unit area or "intensity." In most circumstances, intensity usually is expressed with respect to a standard intensity. For example, the intensity of the original ultrasound signal may be compared with the reflected signal. Because ultrasound amplitudes may vary by a factor of 10^5 or greater, amplitudes usually are expressed using a logarithmic scale. The usual unit for intensity comparisons is the decibel, which is defined as:

$$\text{decibel (dB)} = 10 \bullet \log(I_1 / I_0)$$

where I_1 is the intensity of the wave to be compared and I_0 is the intensity of the reference waves.

Notably, positive values imply a wave of greater intensity than the reference wave, and negative values indicate a lower intensity. Increasing the wave's intensity by a factor of 10 adds 10 dB to the decibel measurement and doubling the intensity adds 3 dB.

Ultrasound Beam

Piezoelectric crystals convert between ultrasound and electrical signals. Most piezoelectric crystals that are used in clinical applications are the man-made ceramic ferroelectrics, the most common of which are barium titanate, lead metaniobate, and lead zirconate titanate. When presented with a high-frequency electrical signal, these crystals produced ultrasound energy; conversely, when they are presented with an ultrasonic vibration, they produce an electrical alternating current signal. Commonly, a short ultrasound signal is emitted from the piezoelectric crystal, which is directed toward the areas to be imaged. This pulse duration is typically 1 to 2 microseconds. After ultrasound wave formation, the crystal "listens" for the returning echoes for a given period and then pauses before repeating this cycle. This cycle length is known as the "pulse repetition frequency" (PRF). This cycle length must be long enough to provide enough time for a signal to travel to and return from a given object of interest. Typically, PRF varies from 1 to 10 kHz, which

BOX 12-1. COMMON APPLICATIONS OF TRANSESOPHAGEAL ECHOCARDIOGRAPHY

- Assessment of valvular anatomy and function
- Evaluation of the thoracic aorta
- Detection of intracardiac defects
- Evaluation of pericardial effusions
- Detection of intracardiac air, clots, or masses
- Assessment of biventricular systolic and diastolic function
- Evaluation of myocardial ischemia

results in 0.1 to 1 millisecond between pulses. When reflected ultrasound waves return to these piezoelectric crystals, they are converted into electrical signals, which may be appropriately processed and displayed. Electronic circuits measure the time delay between the emitted and received echo. Because the speed of ultrasound through tissue is a constant, this time delay may be converted into the precise distance between the transducer and tissue. The amplitude or strength of the returning ultrasound signal provides information about the characteristics of the insonated tissue.

The 3D shape of the ultrasound beam is dependent on both physical aspects of the ultrasound signal and the design of the transducer. An unfocused ultrasound beam may be thought of as an inverted funnel, where the initial straight columnar area is known as the "near field" (also known as Fresnel zone) followed by a conical divergent area known as the "far field" (also known as Fraunhofer zone). The length of the "near field" is directly proportional to the square of the transducer diameter and inversely proportional to the wavelength; specifically,

$$F_n = D^2/4\lambda$$

where F_n is the near-field length, D is the diameter of the transducer, and λ is the ultrasound wavelength. Increasing the frequency of the ultrasound increases the length of the near field. In this near field, most energy is confined to a beam width no greater than the transducer diameter. Long Fresnel zones are preferred with medical ultrasonography, which may be achieved with large-diameter transducers and high-frequency ultrasound. The angle of the "far-field" convergence (θ) is directly proportional to the wavelength and inversely proportional to the diameter of the transducer and is expressed by the equation:

$$\sin\theta = 1.22\lambda/D$$

Further shaping of the beam geometry may be adjusted using acoustic lenses or the shaping of the piezoelectric crystal. Ideally, imaging should be performed within the "near-field" or focused aspect of the ultrasound beam because the ultrasound beam is most parallel with the greatest intensity and the tissue interfaces are most perpendicular to these ultrasound beams.

Attenuation, Reflection, and Scatter

Waves interact with the medium in which they travel and with one another. Interaction among waves is called *interference*. The manner in which waves interact with a medium is determined by its density and homogeneity. When a wave is propagated through an inhomogeneous medium (and all living tissue is essentially inhomogeneous), it is partly reflected, partially absorbed, and partly scattered.

Ultrasound waves are reflected when the width of the reflecting object is larger than one fourth of the ultrasound wavelength. Because the velocity of sound in soft tissue is approximately constant, shorter wavelengths are obtained by increasing the frequency of the ultrasound beam (see Eq. 1). Large objects may be visualized using low frequencies (i.e., long wavelengths), whereas smaller objects require higher frequencies (i.e., short wavelength) for visualization. In addition, the object's ultrasonic impedance (Z) must be significantly different from the ultrasonic impedance in front of the object. The ultrasound impedance of a given medium is equal to the medium density multiplied by the ultrasound propagation velocity. Air has a low density and propagation velocity, so it has a low ultrasound impedance. Bone has a high density and propagation velocity, so it has a high ultrasound impedance. For normal incidence, the fraction of the reflected pulse compared with the incidence pulse is:

$$I_r = (Z_2 - Z_1)^2/(Z_2 + Z_1)^2$$

where I_r is intensity reflection coefficient, and Z_1 and Z_2 are acoustical impedance of the two media.

The greater the differences in ultrasound impedance between two objects at a given interface, the greater the ultrasound reflection. Because the ultrasound impedances of air or bone are significantly different from blood, ultrasound is strongly reflected from these interfaces, limiting the availability of ultrasound to deeper structures. Echo studies across lung or other gas-containing tissues or across bone are not feasible. Reflected echoes, also called "specular echoes," usually are much stronger than scattered echoes. A grossly inhomogeneous medium, such as a stone in a water bucket or a cardiac valve in a blood-filled heart chamber, produces strong specular reflections at the water–stone or blood–valve interface because of the significant differences in ultrasound impedances. Furthermore, if the interface between the two objects is not perpendicular, the reflected signal may be deflected at an angle and may not return to the transducer for imaging.

In contrast, if the objects are small compared with the wavelength, the ultrasound wave will be scattered. Media that are inhomogeneous at the microscopic level, such as muscle, produce more scatter than specular reflection because the differences in adjacent ultrasound impedances are low and the objects are small. These small objects will produce echoes that reflect throughout a large range of angles with only a small percentage of the original signal reaching the ultrasound transducer. Scattered ultrasound waves will combine in constructive and destructive fashions with other scattered waves, producing an interference pattern known as "speckle." Compared with specular echoes, the returning ultrasound signal amplitude will be lower and displayed as a darker signal. Although smaller objects can be visualized with higher frequencies, these higher frequencies result in greater signal attenuation, limiting the depth of ultrasound penetration.

Attenuation refers to the loss of ultrasound power as it transverses tissue. Tissue attenuation is dependent on ultrasound reflection, scattering, and absorption. The greater the ultrasound reflection and scattering, the less ultrasound energy is available for penetration and resolution of deeper structures; this effect is especially important during scanning with higher frequencies. In normal circumstances, however, absorption is the most significant factor in ultrasound attenuation.[2] Absorption occurs as a result of the oscillation of tissue caused by the transit of the ultrasound wave. These tissue oscillations result in friction, with the conversion of ultrasound energy into heat. More specifically, the transit of an ultrasound wave through a medium causes molecular displacement. This molecular displacement requires the conversion of kinetic energy into potential energy as the molecules are compressed. At the time of maximal compression, the kinetic energy is maximized and the potential energy minimized. The movement of molecules from their compressed location to their original location requires conversion of this potential energy back into kinetic energy. In most cases, this energy conversion (either kinetic into potential energy or vice versa) is not 100% efficient and results in energy loss as heat.[1]

The absorption is dependent both on the material through which the ultrasound is passing and the ultrasound frequency. The degree of attenuation through a given thickness of material, *x*, may be described by:

$$\text{Attenuation (dB)} = a \bullet \text{freq} \bullet x$$

where a is the attenuation coefficient in decibels (dB) per centimeter at 1 MHz, and freq represents the ultrasound frequency in megahertz (MHz).

Examples of attenuation coefficient values are given in Table 12-1. Whereas water, blood, and muscle have low ultrasound attenuation, air and bone have very high tissue ultrasound attenuation, limiting the ability of ultrasound to transverse these structures. Table 12-2 gives the distance in various tissues at which the intensity or amplitude of an ultrasound wave of 2 MHz is halved (the half-power distance).

IMAGING TECHNIQUES

M-Mode

The most basic form of ultrasound imaging is M-mode echocardiography. In this mode, the density and position of all tissues in the path of a narrow ultrasound beam (i.e., *along a single line*) are displayed as

TABLE 12-1	Attenuation Coefficients
Material	*Coefficient (dB/cm/MHz)*
Water	0.002
Fat	0.66
Soft tissue	0.9
Muscle	2
Air	12
Bone	20
Lung	40

TABLE 12-2	Half-Power Distances at 2 MHz
Material	*Half-Power Distance (cm)*
Water	380
Blood	15
Soft tissue (except muscle)	1–5
Muscle	0.6–1
Bone	0.2–0.7
Air	0.08
Lung	0.05

a scroll on a video screen. The scrolling produces an updated, continuously changing time plot of the studied tissue section several seconds in duration. Because this is a timed *motion display* (normal cardiac tissue is always in motion), it is called *M-mode*. Because only a limited part of the heart is being observed at any one time and because the image requires considerable interpretation, M-mode is not used currently as a primary imaging technique. This mode is, however, useful for the precise timing of events within the cardiac cycle and often is used in combination with CFD for the timing of abnormal flows (see later). Quantitative measurements of size, distance, and velocity also are easily performed in the M-mode without the need for sophisticated analysis stations. Because M-mode images are updated 1000 times per second,

they provide greater temporal resolution than two-dimensional (2D) echocardiography; thus, more subtle changes in motion or dimension can be appreciated.

B-Mode

The different reflectivities of various cardiac structures result in variations of the reflected ultrasound wave. The detected signals are translated from the amplitude of the reflected signal to luminance and displayed as a brightness-mode or B-mode image. By rapid, repetitive scanning along *many different radii* within an area in the shape of a fan (sector), echocardiography generates a 2D image of a section of the heart. This image, which resembles an anatomic section, can be interpreted more easily than an M-mode display. Information on structures and motion in the plane of a 2D scan is updated 20 to 40 times per second. This repetitive update produces a "live" (real–time) image of the heart. Scanning 2D echocardiography (2DE) devices usually image the heart using an electronically steered ultrasound beam (phased–array transducer).

Harmonic Imaging

Harmonic frequencies are ultrasound transmission of integer multiples of the original frequency. For example, if the fundamental frequency is 4 MHz, the second harmonic is 8 MHz, the third fundamental is 12 MHz, and so on. Harmonic imaging refers to a technique of B-mode imaging in which an ultrasound signal is transmitted at a given frequency but will "listen" at one of its harmonic frequencies.[3,4] As ultrasound is transmitted through a tissue, the tissue undergoes slight compressions and expansions that correspond to the ultrasound wave temporarily changing the local tissue density. Because the velocity of ultrasound transit is directly proportional to density, the peak amplitudes will travel slightly faster than the trough. This differential velocity transit of the peak with the trough wave results in distortion of the propagated sine wave, resulting in a more peaked wave. This peaked wave will contain frequencies of the fundamental frequency, as well as the harmonic frequencies (Figure 12-2). Although little distortion occurs in the near field, the amount of energy contained within these harmonics increases with ultrasound distance transversed as

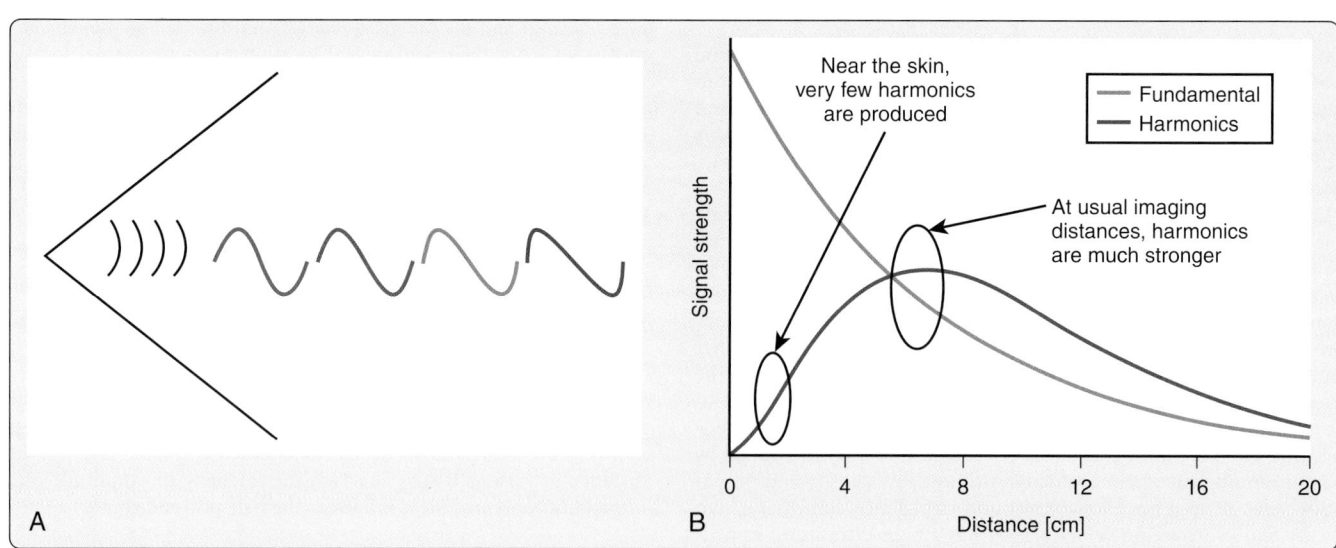

Figure 12-2 Harmonic imaging. *A,* Because the velocity of ultrasound transit is directly proportional to density, the peak amplitudes will travel slightly faster than the trough. With time, this differential velocity transit of the peak with the trough wave results in distortion of the propagated sin wave resulting in a more peaked wave. *B,* Relation between imaging distance and strength of fundamental and harmonics frequencies. As ultrasound pulse propagates, strength of fundamental frequency declines, whereas strength of harmonic frequency increases. At usual imaging distances for cardiac structures, strength of harmonic frequency is maximized. Note: Harmonic frequency strength is exaggerated in this schematic. Harmonic frequency signal strength is much lower than fundamental frequency signal strength. *(B, From Thomas JD, Rubin DN: Tissue harmonic imaging: Why does it work? J Am Soc Echocardiogr 11:803–808, 1998, by permission.)*

the ultrasound wave becomes more peaked. Eventually, the effects of attenuation will be more pronounced on these harmonic waves with subsequent decrease in harmonic amplitude. Because the effects of attenuation are greatest with high-frequency ultrasound, the second harmonic usually is used.

The use of tissue harmonic imaging is associated with improved B-mode imaging. Near-field scatter is common with fundamental imaging. Because the ultrasound wave has not yet been distorted, little harmonic energy is generated in the near field, minimizing near-field scatter when harmonic imaging is used. Because higher frequencies are used, greater resolution may be obtained. Finally, with tissue harmonic imaging, side-lobe artifacts are substantially reduced and lateral resolution is increased.

Doppler Techniques

Most modern echo scanners combine Doppler capabilities with their 2D imaging capabilities. After the desired view of the heart has been obtained by 2DE, the Doppler beam, represented by a cursor, is superimposed on the 2D image. The operator positions the cursor as parallel as possible to the assumed direction of blood flow and then empirically adjusts the direction of the beam to optimize the audio and visual representations of the reflected Doppler signal. Currently, Doppler technology can be utilized in at least four different ways to measure blood velocities: pulsed, high-repetition frequency, continuous wave, and color flow. Although each of these methods has specific applications, they are seldom available concurrently.

The Doppler Effect

Information on blood flow dynamics can be obtained by applying Doppler frequency shift analysis to echoes reflected by the moving red blood cells.[5,6] Blood flow velocity, direction, and acceleration can be instantaneously determined. This information is different from that obtained in 2D imaging, and hence complements it.

The Doppler principle as applied in echocardiography states that the frequency of ultrasound reflected by a moving target (red blood cells) will be different from the frequency of the reflected ultrasound. The magnitude and direction of the frequency shift are related to the velocity and direction of the moving target. The velocity of the target is calculated with the Doppler equation:

$$v = (cf_d) / (2f_0 \cos \theta)$$

where v = the target velocity (blood flow velocity); c = the speed of sound in tissue; f_d = the frequency shift; f_0 = the frequency of the emitted ultrasound; and θ = the angle between the ultrasound beam and the direction of the target velocity (blood flow). Rearranging the terms,

$$f_d = v(2f_0 \cos \theta)/c$$

As is evident in Equation 8, the greater the velocity of the object of interest, the greater the Doppler frequency shift. In addition, the magnitude of the frequency shift is directly proportional to the initial emitted frequency (Figure 12-3). Low emitted frequencies produce low Doppler frequency shifts, whereas higher emitted frequencies produce high Doppler frequency shifts. This phenomenon becomes important with aliasing, as is discussed later in this chapter. Furthermore, the only ambiguity in Equation 7 is that theoretically the direction of the ultrasonic signal could refer to either the transmitted or the received beam; however, by convention, Doppler displays are made with reference to the received beam; thus, if the blood flow and the reflected beam travel in the same direction, the angle of incidence is zero degrees and the cosine is +1. As a result, the frequency of the reflected signal will be higher than the frequency of the emitted signal.

Equipment currently used in clinical practice displays Doppler blood-flow velocities as waveforms. The waveforms consist of a spectral analysis of velocities on the ordinate and time on the abscissa.

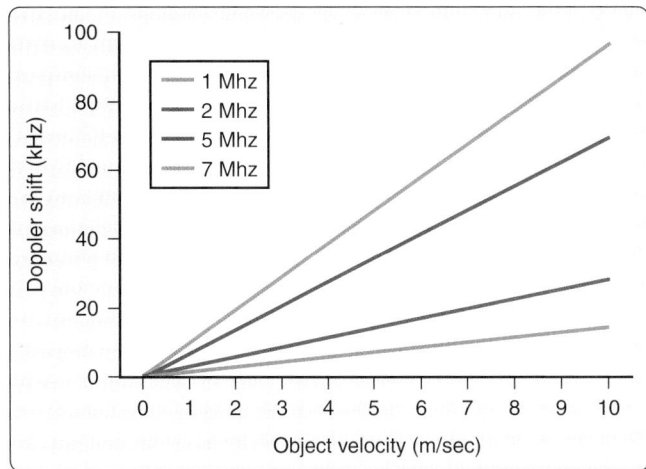

Figure 12-3 Graph of Doppler shift frequency versus velocity for various emitted ultrasound frequencies. A lower emitted ultrasound frequency will produce a lower Doppler frequency shift for a given velocity. This lower Doppler frequency shift will allow for a higher velocity measurement before aliasing occurs.

By convention, blood flow toward the transducer is represented above the baseline. If the blood flows away from the transducer, the angle of incidence will be 180 degrees, the cosine will equal −1, and the waveform will be displayed below the baseline. When the blood flow is perpendicular to the ultrasonic beam, the angle of incidence will be 90 or 270 degrees, the cosine of either angle will be zero, and no blood flow will be detected. Because the cosine of the angle of incidence is a variable in the Doppler equation, blood-flow velocity is measured most accurately when the ultrasound beam is parallel or antiparallel to the direction of blood flow. In clinical practice, a deviation from parallel of up to 20 degrees can be tolerated because this results in an error of only 6% or less.

Pulsed-Wave Doppler

In PW Doppler, blood-flow parameters can be determined at precise locations within the heart by emitting repetitive short bursts of ultrasound at a specific frequency (PRF) and analyzing the frequency shift of the reflected echoes at an identical sampling frequency (f_s). A time delay between the emission of the ultrasound signal burst and the sampling of the reflected signal determines the depth at which the velocities are sampled; the delay is proportional to the distance between the transducer and the location of the velocity measurements. To sample at a given depth (D), you must allow sufficient time for the signal to travel a distance of $2 \times D$ (from the transducer to the sample volume and back). The time delay, T_d, between the emission of the signal and the reception of the reflected signal, is related to D, and to the speed of sound in tissues (c), by the following formula:

$$D = cT_d/2$$

The operator varies the depth of sampling by varying the time delay between the emission of the ultrasonic signal and the sampling of the reflected wave. In practice, the sampling location or *sample volume* is represented by a small marker, which can be positioned at any point along the Doppler beam by moving it up or down the Doppler cursor. On some devices, it is also possible to vary the width and height of the sample volume.

The trade-off for the ability to measure flow *at precise locations* is that *ambiguous information* is obtained when flow velocity is very high. Information theory suggests that an unknown periodic signal must be sampled at least twice per cycle to determine even rudimentary information such as the fundamental frequency; therefore, the rate of PRF of PW Doppler must be at least twice the Doppler-shift frequency produced by flow.[7] If not, the frequency shift is said to be "undersampled." In other words, this frequency shift is sampled so infrequently that the frequency reported by the instrument is erroneously low.[1]

A simple reference to Western movies will clearly illustrate this point. When a stagecoach gets under way, its wheel spokes are observed as rotating in the correct direction. As soon as a certain speed is attained, rotation in the reverse direction is noted because the camera frame rate is too slow to correctly observe the motion of the wheel spokes. In PW Doppler, the ambiguity exists because the measured Doppler frequency shift (f_D) and the sampling frequency (f_s) are in the same frequency (kHz) range. Ambiguity will be avoided only if the f_D is less than half the sampling frequency:

$$f_D < f_s/2$$

The expression $f_s/2$ is also known as the Nyquist limit. Doppler shifts above the Nyquist limit will create artifacts described as "aliasing" or "wraparound," and blood-flow velocities will appear in a direction opposite to the conventional one (Figure 12-4). Blood flowing with high velocity toward the transducer will result in a display of velocities above and below the baseline. The maximum velocity that can be detected without aliasing is dictated by:

$$V_m = c^2/8Rf_0$$

where V_m = the maximal velocity that can be unambiguously measured; c = the speed of sound in tissue; R = the range or distance from the transducer at which the measurement is to be made; and f_0 = the frequency of emitted ultrasound.

Based on Equation 11, this "aliasing" artifact can be avoided by either minimizing R or f_0. Decreasing the depth of the sample volume in essence increases f_s. This higher sampling frequency allows for the more accurate determination of higher Doppler shifts frequencies (i.e., higher velocities). Furthermore, because f_0 is directly related to f_d (see Eq. 7), a lower emitted ultrasound frequency will produce a lower Doppler frequency shift for a given velocity (see Figure 12-3). This lower Doppler frequency shift will allow for a higher velocity measurement before aliasing occurs.

High-Pulse-Repetition Frequency Doppler

On some instruments, PW Doppler can be modified to a high-PRF mode. Whereas in conventional PW Doppler only a single burst of ultrasound is considered to be in the body at any given time, in high-PRF Doppler two to five sample volumes are simultaneously presented. Information coming back to the transducer may be coming back from depths of either two, three, or four times the initial sample volume depth. The returning signals can be a mix of signals that have been emitted previously and have traveled to distant gates and other signals that were just sent and returned from the first range gate.

The high-PRF mode allows increasing the sampling frequency because the scanner does not wait for the return of the information from distant gates; nonetheless, it receives information back within the specified time-gate period. Because higher sampling frequencies are used, higher velocities can be measured with this method than with PW Doppler; however, the exact gate from which the ultrasound signals are reflected is unknown (range ambiguity).

Continuous-Wave Doppler

The CW Doppler technique uses continuous, rather than discrete, pulses of ultrasound waves. Ultrasound waves are continuously being both transmitted and received by separate transducers. As a result, the region in which flow dynamics are measured cannot be precisely localized. Because of the large range of depths being simultaneously insonated, a large range of frequencies is returned to the transducer. This large frequency range corresponds to a large range of blood-flow velocities. This large velocity range is known as "spectral broadening." Spectral broadening during CW Doppler interrogation contrasts the homogenous envelope that is obtained with PW Doppler (Figure 12-5). Blood-flow velocity is, however, measured with great accuracy even at high flows because sampling frequency is very high. CW Doppler is particularly useful for the evaluation of patients with valvular lesions or congenital heart disease (CHD), in whom anticipated high-pressure/high-velocity signals are anticipated. It also is the preferred technique when attempting to derive hemodynamic information from Doppler signals (Box 12-2).

Color-Flow Doppler

Advances in electronics and computer technology have allowed the development of CFD ultrasound scanners capable of displaying real–time blood flow within the heart as colors while also showing 2D images in black and white. In addition to showing the location, direction, and velocity of cardiac blood flow, the images produced by these devices allow estimation of flow acceleration and differentiation of laminar and turbulent blood flow. CFD echocardiography is based on the principle of multigated PW Doppler in which blood-flow velocities are sampled at many locations along many lines covering the entire imaging sector.[8] At the same time, the sector also is scanned to generate a 2D image.

A location in the heart where the scanner has detected flow toward the transducer (the top of the image sector) is assigned the color red. Flow away from the direction of the top is assigned the color blue. This color assignment is arbitrary and determined by the equipment's manufacturer and the user's color mapping. In the most common color–flow coding scheme, the faster the velocity (up to a limit), the more intense the color. Flow velocities that change by more than a preset value within a brief time interval (flow variance) have an additional hue added to either the red or the blue. Both rapidly accelerating laminar flow (change in flow speed) and turbulent flow (change in flow direction) satisfy the criteria for rapid changes in velocity. In summary, the brightness of the red or blue colors at any location and time is usually proportional to the corresponding flow velocity, whereas the hue is proportional to the temporal rate of change of the velocity.

Three-Dimensional Reconstruction

Echocardiography has become a vital tool in the practice of contemporary cardiac anesthesiology. As with any technology, a considerable evolution has occurred since it was first introduced into the operating rooms in the early 1980s. Among the most important advances has

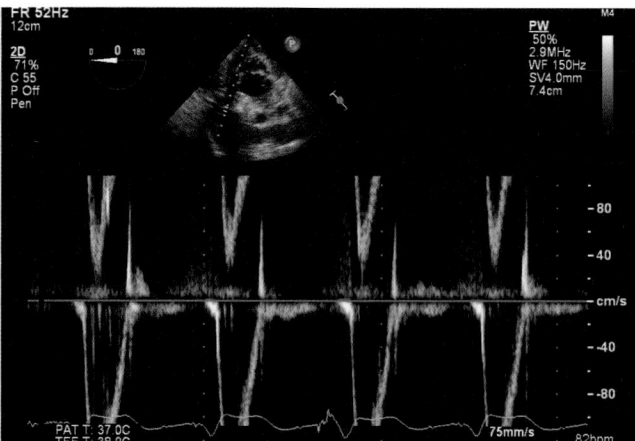

Figure 12-4 Example of aliasing. Pulse-wave Doppler spectrum through bioprosthetic aortic valve. Because the high-velocity blood through the bioprosthetic aortic valve results in a Doppler shift, which is greater than the Nyquist limit, the high-velocity flow away from the transducer is represented as flow toward the transducer. This effect is call *aliasing.*

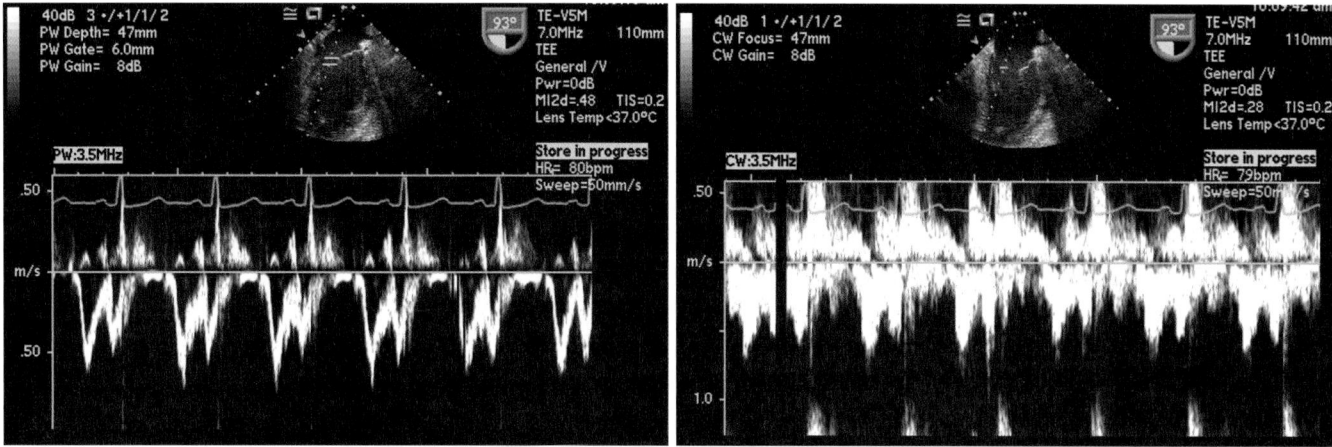

Figure 12-5 **Pulse-wave (PW) versus continuous-wave (CW) Doppler.** Both images are Doppler spectra through the mitral valve. *Left,* PW Doppler is used. Because a specific region of interest is defined by the Doppler gate, a clean envelope of transmitral flow is displayed. *Right,* CW Doppler is used. Because spatial specificity is lost, spectral broadening of velocities is displayed.

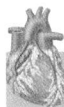

BOX 12-2. PULSED-WAVE VERSUS CONTINUOUS-WAVE DOPPLER ANALYSIS

- Pulsed-wave Doppler
  - Spatial specificity
  - Ambiguity in the measurement of high velocities
- Continuous-wave Doppler
  - Able to measure high velocities accurately
  - Spatial ambiguity

---

been the progression from one-dimensional (1D; e.g., M-mode) imaging to 2D imaging, as well as spectral Doppler and real-time color-flow mapping superimposed over a 2D image. The heart, however, remains a 3D organ. Although multiplane 2D images can be acquired easily with modern TEE probes by simply rotating the image plane electronically from 0 to 180 degrees, the final process occurs by the echocardiographer stitching the different 2D planes together and creating a "mental" 3D image. Transmitting this "mental" image to other members of the surgical team can sometimes be quite challenging. By directly displaying a 3D image onto the monitor, cardiac anatomy and function could be assessed more rapidly and communication between the echocardiographer and the cardiac surgeon facilitated before, during, and immediately after surgery.[9]

Historic Overview

Early concepts of 3D echocardiography (3DE) found their roots in the 1970s.[10] Because of the limitations of hardware and software capabilities in that era, the acquisition times required to create a 3D image prohibited widespread clinical acceptance, limiting its use for research purposes only. Technologic advances in the 1990s enabled 3D reconstruction from multiple 2D images obtained from different imaging planes. By capturing an image every 2 to 3 degrees as the probe rotated 180 degrees around a specific region of interest (ROI), high-powered computers were able to produce a 3D image, which could be refined further with postprocessing software. These multigated image planes must be acquired under electrocardiographic and respiratory gating to overcome motion artifact. The limitations of this technology are the time required to process and optimize the 3D image and the inability to obtain instantaneous, real-time imaging of the heart.

In 2007, a real-time 3D TEE probe with a matrix array of piezoelectric crystals within the transducer head was released on the market. This 3D imaging matrix array, as opposed to conventional 2D

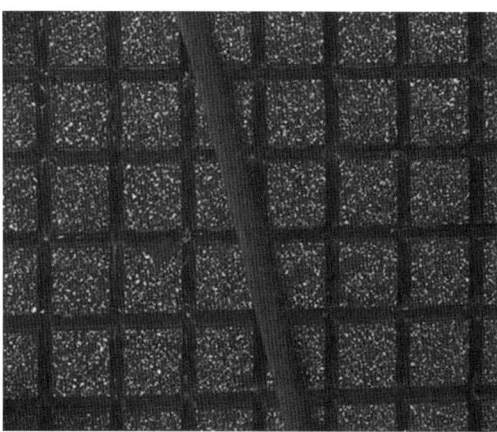

Figure 12-6 **Matrix array transducer consisting of 50 rows and 50 columns of piezoelectric elements.** A human hair demonstrates the size of each individual element.

imaging transducers, not only has columns in a single 1D plane but also rows of elements. That is, instead of having a single column of 128 elements, the matrix array comprises more than 50 rows and 50 columns of elements (Figure 12-6). Although this "matrix" technology was available for transthoracic (precordial) scanning, a breakthrough in engineering design was required before the technology could be transitioned into the limited space of the head of a TEE probe.

Limitations of Three-Dimensional Imaging

Notably, 3DE is subject to the same laws of acoustic physics as 2DE. Artifacts such as ringing, reverberations, shadowing, and attenuation occur in 3D, as well as 2D and M-mode. In addition, it is important to realize that the product of frame rate, sector/volume size, and imaging resolution equal a constant. That is, by increasing the requirements of one of these variables, a decrease in either one or both of the others will occur. An example would be, by increasing sector size, a loss in either frame rate or image resolution, or both, will occur. Modern ultrasound devices are equipped with incredible computing power, enabling them to display large 2D sectors while still maintaining excellent image resolution and high frame rates. Unfortunately, this does not apply for real-time instantaneous 3D imaging. The large amount of data that must be acquired and processed requires the echocardiographer to reduce sector size to maintain adequate resolution and frame rate. The rate-limiting factor in 3D imaging is no longer processing power but the speed of ultrasound in tissue.

Display of Three-Dimensional Images

The classic 20 views of 2D TEE are not required in 3DE because entire volumetric datasets are acquired that can be spatially orientated and cropped at the discretion of the echocardiographer. As previously stated, the limiting factor in 3DE is no longer processer performance, but the speed of sound traveling through tissue (1540 m/sec). Although the matrix configuration of the elements allows "live" and instantaneous scanning, the size of this sector is limited to guarantee adequate image resolution and frame rate. If larger sectors are to be scanned, the constraint of transmit time of ultrasound is sidestepped by stitching four to eight gated beats together, which enables wider volumes to be generated while maintaining frame rate and resolution. Several modes of 3DE are described in the following subsections.

Narrow Sector (Live 3D)—Real Time

In this mode, a 3D volume pyramid is obtained. The image shown in this mode is real time. The 3D image changes as the transducer is moved just as in live 2D imaging. Manipulations of the TEE probe (e.g., rotation, change in position) lead to instantaneous changes in the image seen on the monitor (Figure 12-7).

Wide Sector Focused (3D Zoom)—Real Time

If only a specific ROI requires imaging, the "zoom mode" can be used in a similar fashion as in 2DE. A typical example for this mode would be the mitral valve (MV) apparatus. The 3D zoom mode displays a small magnified pyramidal volume that may vary from 20 × 20 degrees up to 90 × 90 degrees, depending on the density setting. This small data set can be spatially orientated at the discretion of the echocardiographer. A key advantage to this mode is the fact that the real-time 3D images are devoid of rotational artifacts, as are commonly encountered with electrocardiogram (ECG)-gated 3D acquisitions (Figure 12-8).

Large Sector (Full Volume)—Gated

Because of insufficient time for sound to travel back and forth in large volumes while maintaining a frame rate greater than 20 Hz and reasonable resolution in live scanning modes, one maneuver to overcome this limitation entails stitching four to eight gates together to create a "full-volume" mode. These gated "slabs" or "subvolumes" represent a pyramidal 3D dataset as would be acquired in the live 3D mode. This technique can generate more than 90-degree scanning volumes at frame rates greater than 30 Hz. Increasing the gates from four to eight creates smaller 3D slabs; this can be used to maintain frame rates and/or resolution as the volumes (pyramids) become larger (Figure 12-9).

Unfortunately, as with any conventional gating technique, patients with arrhythmias are prone to motion artifacts when the individual datasets are combined; however, as long as the RR intervals fall within a reasonable range, a full-volume dataset still can be reconstructed (e.g., atrial fibrillation, electrocautery artifact). The acquired real-time 3D dataset subsequently can be cropped, analyzed, and quantified using integrated software in the 3D operating system (QLAB; Philips Healthcare, Andover, MA; Figure 12-10).

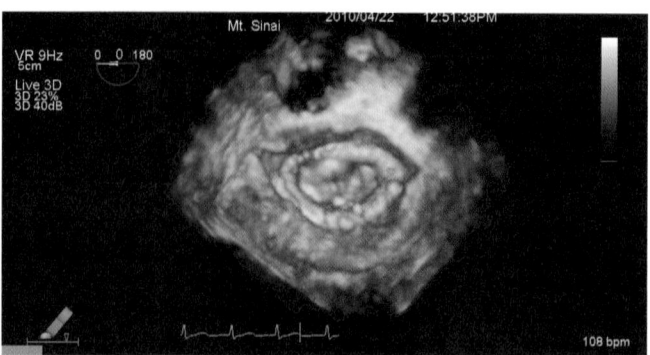

Figure 12-8 **Three-dimensional (3D) zoom mode acquisition of a mitral valve repair from the left atrial perspective.** Annuloplasty ring is easily visualized. In analogy to the live 3D mode, the 3D zoom mode acquires instantaneous images.

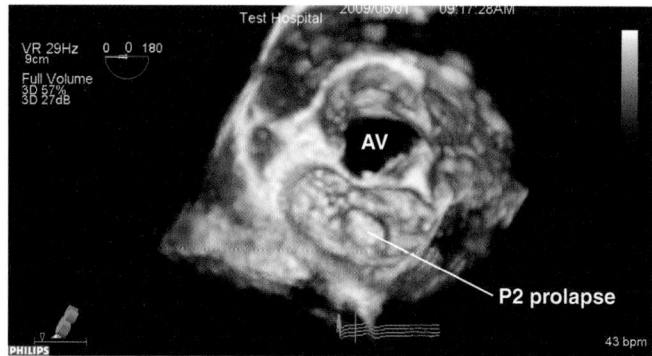

Figure 12-9 **Full-volume mode acquisition of the mitral valve from the left atrial perspective.** Although the sector size is similar to Figure 12-8, note the improvement in temporal resolution as a consequence of the four-beat acquisition (9 vs. 29 Hz). This mode does not permit instantaneous "live" imaging. AV, aortic valve.

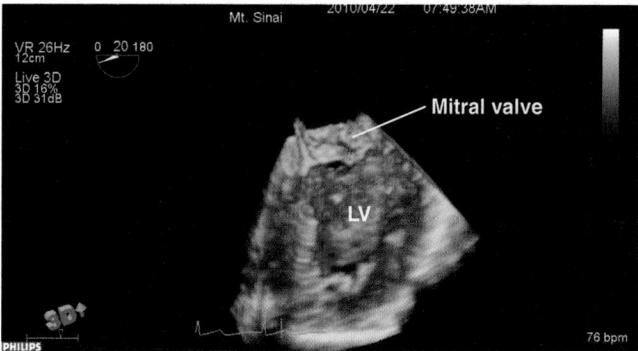

Figure 12-7 **Live three-dimensional image of mitral valve and left ventricle (LV).** Because of the matrix structure of the ultrasound transducer, this image represents a true live image. Change in transesophageal echocardiographic probe positioning by the echocardiographer will result in instantaneous changes in the volumetric data set.

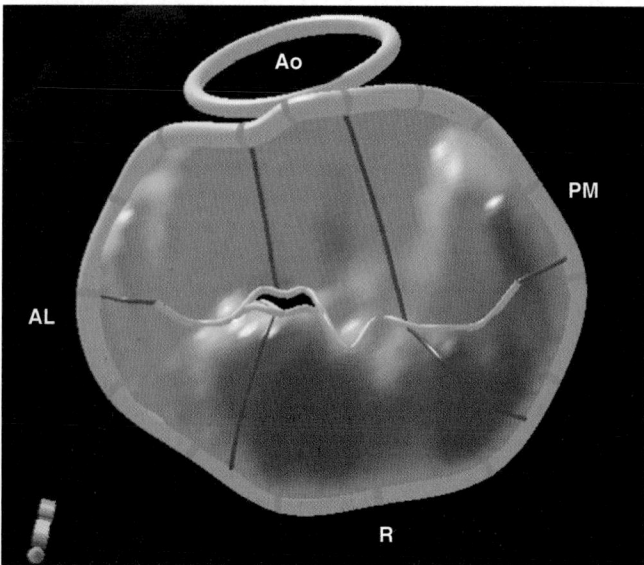

Figure 12-10 Mitral valve quantification (MVQ) of a mitral valve acquired with the full-volume mode. Red coloring of the leaflet indicates areas that exceed the annular plane (type II dysfunction). AL, anterolateral; Ao, aorta; PM, posteromedial.

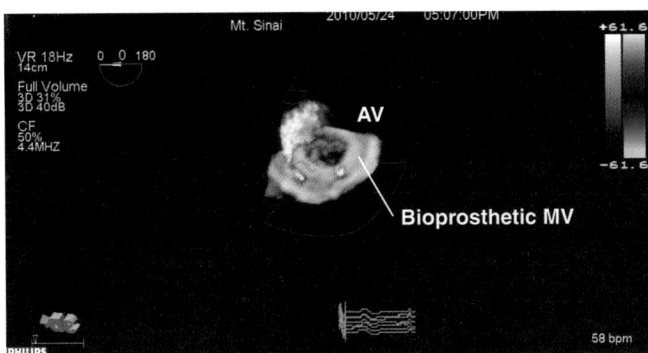

Figure 12-11 Color three-dimensional acquisition of a mitral valve (MV) bioprosthesis. The aortic valve (AV) is for orientation. Three paravalvular leaks can be identified.

BOX 12-3. DIAGNOSTIC APPLICATIONS FOR CONTRAST ECHOCARDIOGRAPHY

- Assessment of congenital heart disease
- Enhancement of endocardial borders for qualitative assessment of wall motion abnormalities
  - Measurement of left ventricular function
  - Quantification of valvular regurgitation
  - Enhancement of color-flow Doppler signals
- Assessment of myocardial perfusion
  - Measurements of perfusion area after coronary artery bypass graft surgery
  - Assessment of quality of coronary bypass grafts and cardioplegia distribution
  - Correct assessment of the results of surgery for ventricular septal defect

Three-dimensional Color Doppler—Gated

Because of the large amount of data that must be acquired with 3D color Doppler mode, a gating method must be utilized similar to that of the full-volume mode; however, because of the large amount of data required, 8 to 11 beats need to be combined to create an image. Jet direction, extent, and geometry easily can be recognized using this technique. Reports started emerging in the late 1990s showing that the strength of this methodology lies in its ability to quantitate severity of regurgitant lesions; 3D quantification of mitral regurgitation correlates better than 2D imaging, when using angiography as the gold standard.[11] In an experimental setting, 3D quantification was more accurate (2.6% underestimation) than 2D or M-mode methods, which had the tendency to underestimate regurgitant volumes (44.2% and 32.1%, respectively; Figure 12-11).[12]

Right Ventricle

The right ventricle is a complex, crescent-shaped structure that does not lend itself easily to geometric assumptions as its LV counterpart and has been the Achilles heel to 2D imaging. Because of the fact that numerous reports have linked right ventricular (RV) function to prognostic outcome in a variety of cardiopulmonary diseases, it would be of great interest to quantify its function echocardiographically.[13]

A preliminary report showed that 3DE marginally underestimated RV volumes when compared with cardiac magnetic resonance, and that correlation to cardiac magnetic resonance–measured volumes was as good as that obtained by cardiac computed tomography.[14] Further research in this field will undoubtedly lead to increased understanding of perioperative RV function.

Contrast Echocardiography

Normally, red blood cells scatter ultrasound waves weakly, resulting in their black appearance on ultrasonic examination. Contrast echocardiography is performed by injecting nontoxic solutions containing gaseous microbubbles. These microbubbles present additional gas-liquid interfaces, which substantially increase the strength of the returning signal. This augmentation in signal strength may be used to better define endocardial borders, optimize Doppler envelope signals, and estimate myocardial perfusion.

Gramiak and Shah[15] originally reported the use of contrast echocardiography in 1969. They described visualization of aortic valve (AV) incompetence during left-heart catheterization[15] (Box 12-3). Subsequently, contrast echocardiography has been used to image intracardiac shunts,[16] valvular incompetence,[17] and pericardial effusions.[18] In addition, LV injections of hand-agitated microbubble solutions have been used to identify semiquantitative LV endocardial edges,[19] cardiac output,[20] and valvular regurgitation.[21]

Contrast agents are microbubbles, consisting of a shell surrounding a gas. Initial contrast agents were agitated free air in either a saline or blood-saline solution. These microbubbles were large and unstable, so they were unable to cross the pulmonary circulation; they were effective only for right-heart contrast. Because of their thin shell, the gas quickly leaked into the blood with resultant dissolution of the microbubble. Agents with a longer persistence subsequently were developed.

More modern contrast agents have improved the shell surrounding the microbubble, as well as modification of the gas. The shell must inhibit the diffusion of gas into the blood and must enhance the pressure that a microbubble can tolerate before dissolving.[22] Gases with low shell diffusivity and blood saturation concentration result in a microbubble of increased survival because the gas would rapid equilibrate with blood, and the gas would tend to stay within the shell. Improvements in the shell both increase the tolerance of the microbubble to ultrasound energies and decrease the diffusion of the gas into the blood; both changes further increase the persistence of the microbubbles. At the same time, there must be an element of fragility; the microbubbles must be disrupted by ultrasound signals producing appropriate imaging effects. The use of high-molecular-weight and less-soluble gases further increases the persistence of the contrast agents. Currently, the perfluorocarbons are the most common gases used in contrast agents. The microbubbles need to be small enough to transverse the pulmonary circulation with a predominant size particle that approached the size of an erythrocyte. The number of larger particles needs to be minimized to reduce the risk for obstruction of pulmonary capillary flow. Because the reflected energy of contrast agents is high, attenuation of the ultrasound signal is common. This signal attenuation interferes with visualization of distal structures.

An ultrasound signal produces compression and rarefaction (expansion) of the medium through which it travels. When this compression and rarefaction impact a microbubble, the bubble is compressed and expanded, respectively.[23] These changes result in changes in the bubble volume, causing bubble vibrations with subsequent effects on the returning ultrasound signal. These bubble pulsations may result in changes in the bubble radius by a factor of 20 or more.[24]

The acoustic properties of these microbubbles depend on the amplitude of the ultrasound signal. The amplitude of an ultrasound signal usually is defined by its mechanical index, which is the peak negative pressure divided by the square root of the ultrasound frequency. Normally, when bubbles are insonated by ultrasound at their intrinsic resonant frequency, they vibrate; during the peak of the signal, they are compressed, and at the nadir of the signal, they expand. An ideal bubble would oscillate at the insonated ultrasound frequency.[25] At low ultrasound amplitudes (mechanical index < 0.1), the microbubbles oscillate at the frequency of the insonated signal with the degree of compression being equal to the degree of expansion. This is called *linear oscillation*. With fundamental imaging, no special contrast echo signals are produced.[26] With increasing signal amplitudes (mechanical index, 0.1 to 0.7), the degree of expansion exceeds the degree of compression, which results in nonlinear oscillations. These nonlinear oscillations result in the creation of ultrasound waves at harmonic frequencies of the delivered ultrasound waves. Although some bubble destruction will occur at all amplitudes, further increases in ultrasound amplitude (mechanical index, 0.8 to 1.9) result in more compression and expansion with subsequent extensive bubble destruction. This bubble destruction, called *scintillation,* results in a brief but high output signal appearing as swirling. Because of the extensive bubble destruction, intermittent imaging must be performed to allow contrast replenishment. The role of most contrast imaging modalities is to create and display these nonlinear components while suppressing the linear echoes from tissue and tissue motion.[27]

Further improvements in image acquisition can be achieved using harmonic imaging.[24] As explained previously, nonlinear oscillations result in the creation of harmonics. It was theorized that if the receiver was tuned to receive the first harmonic of the transmitted ultrasound signal, the signal-to-noise ratio can be improved by predominantly imaging signals from the microbubbles producing these harmonics. Because tissues also produce harmonics, tissue grayscale imaging also was enhanced. Further improvements may include subharmonic and ultraharmonic imaging, which may provide more specific contrast enhancement. Harmonic imaging with TEE improves endocardial visualization and allows partial assessment of myocardial perfusion.[28] Harmonic-power Doppler is more sensitive for detecting basilar perfusion in the far field compared with harmonic grayscale imaging.[29]

The first-generation agents were Albunex and Levovist. Currently, Optison (Mallinckrodt, St. Louis, MO) and Definity (DuPont Pharmaceuticals, Waltham, MA) are available in the United States for use; Levovist and Sonovue (Bracco Diagnostics, Princeton, NJ) are approved in Europe. Albunex is no longer available. Albunex utilized albumin encapsulation to stabilize a 4-μm air bubble that could opacify the left ventricle but did not result in good microvascular perfusion. Levovist uses an air microbubble within a fatty acid shell.

Optison is a refinement of Albunex, with the substitution of perfluoropropane within an albumin shell. Definity uses perfluoropropane within a liposome shell. SonoVue consists of hexafluoride with a phospholipid shell. New agents under development may use polymer shells whose flexibility and size can be controlled more precisely. These agents may be targeted to specific organs or vectors.

The safety of contrast echocardiography must be considered. The contrast agents themselves must have a high therapeutic index. Multiple large bubbles may obstruct pulmonary microcirculation. The disruption of microbubbles by high-amplitude ultrasound may rupture capillaries and injure surrounding tissue.[30] Rare allergic and life-threatening anaphylactic/anaphylactoid reactions occur at a rate of approximately 1 per 10,000.[27] Premature ventricular contractions have been described during high-intensity triggered imaging.[31] Other investigators were not able to demonstrate an increase in premature ventricular complex occurrence during or after imaging with triggered ultrasound at a mechanical index of 1.[32] Contraindications to the use of perflutren-containing agents include pulmonary hypertension, serious ventricular arrhythmias, severe pulmonary disease, cardiac shunting, or hypersensitivity to perflutren, blood, blood products, or albumin. If current recommendations are followed, contrast echocardiography rarely results in significant side effects.[22]

Uses

Diagnostic applications for contrast echocardiography include enhancement of endocardial borders from qualitative assessment of wall motion abnormalities, measurement of LV function, assessment of CHD, quantification of valvular regurgitation, enhancement of CFD signals, and assessment of myocardial perfusion. During cardiac surgery, the special and unique applications of myocardial contrast echocardiography include measurements of perfusion area after coronary artery bypass graft (CABG) surgery, assessment of quality of coronary bypass grafts and cardioplegia distribution, and correct assessment of the results of surgery for ventricular septal defect. Noncardiac intraoperative applications include assessment of

perfusion in the kidney and in skeletal muscle. Work is ongoing to investigate the potential for analyzing cerebral blood flow with contrast-echo techniques.

Enhancement of Right-Sided Structures
Hand-agitated saline solutions are still useful to enhance right-sided structures. These saline solutions can be prepared easily by hand agitation of saline between two 10-mL Luer lock syringes connected by a three-way stopcock; small amounts of blood or air may be added to improve right-sided opacification. This technique is used most commonly to opacify the right atrium (RA) and right ventricle, assisting in the diagnosis of intra-atrial and ventricular shunts, and to enhance pulmonary arterial Doppler signals. The most common indication is the detection of a patent foramen ovale (PFO). After obtaining a bicaval view, a Valsalva maneuver is induced and hand-agitated saline is injected into a large vein. After the RA is opacified, the Valsalva is released and the left atrium (LA) is examined for contrast.

Left Ventricular Opacification
The commercially available contrast agents allow for left ventricular opacification (LVO) as well. Relatively low mechanical index modes usually are used (<0.2), to allow for bubble detection without bubble destruction. The images are processed such that the linear scatters from tissue are completely eliminated, leaving only nonlinear scatters from the bubble contrast. The LVO allows enhancement of LV endocardial borders in patients in whom normal studies are challenging.[33,34] Such challenging studies include patients who are obese, with pulmonary disease, are critically ill, or on a ventilator.[27] The use of LVO substantially increases the accuracy of LV volume determination compared with electron beam computed tomography measurements, decreases interobserver variability associated with these measurements, and increases the number of myocardial segments that may be described accurately during stress echocardiography.[35,36] Underestimation of LV volume measurements, which is common with standard echocardiography, may be virtually eliminated with the use of LVO.[37] Finally, LVO provides greater visualization of structural abnormalities such as apical hypertrophy, noncompaction, ventricular thrombus, endomyocardial fibrosis, LV apical ballooning (Takotsubo), LV aneurysms or pseudoaneurysms, and myocardial rupture.[27]

Aortic Dissections
Echocardiographic contrast may be used to diagnose aortic dissections. Artifacts may be distinguished from true aortic dissection and artifact, by the homogenous distribution of contrast within the aortic lumen.[27] The intimal flap may be visualized, the entry and exit point may be identified, and the extension into major aortic branches may be more easily defined. The use of contrast further increases the successful differentiation between the true and false lumen.

Doppler Enhancement
The administration of contrast will enhance the echocardiographic Doppler spectrum, where the signal is weak or suboptimal.[38] The enhancement is particularly useful in the evaluation of aortic stenosis (AS) but also may be used with transmitral evaluation, pulmonary venous flow determination, or regurgitant tricuspid valvular flow (Figure 12-12). Whereas the threshold for detecting contrast is substantially less for Doppler compared with 2D imaging, contrast agents usually are used initially for the latter application.

Myocardial Perfusion
The second-generation agents allow for perfusion of the myocardial microcirculation. This perfusion allows for assessment of perfusion patterns, coronary artery stenosis, and myocardium at risk during acute coronary syndromes.[26] Currently, only Imagify has U.S. Food and Drug Administration approval for myocardial perfusion imaging.

Lindner et al[39] described a method for the quantification of myocardial blood flow using contrast echocardiography. If a contrast agent is administered at a steady rate, the blood concentration and myocardial

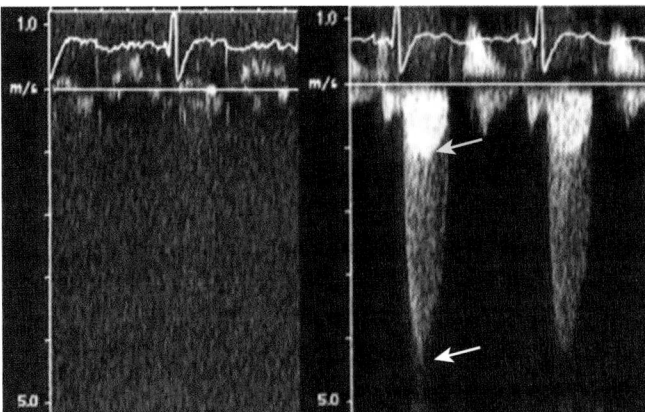

Figure 12-12 Doppler enhancement of aortic stenosis. Doppler spectrum through the left ventricular outflow tract in a patient with aortic stenosis is shown. The image on the left is without contrast, and the image on the right is after contrast enhancement. The contrast-enhanced image clearly demonstrates the high-velocity envelope consistent with aortic stenosis, which could not be visualized without contrast. *(Reproduced from Mulvagh SL, Rakowski H, Vannan MA, et al: American Society of Echocardiography Consensus Statement on the Clinical Applications of Ultrasonic Contrast Agents in Echocardiography. J Am Soc Echocardiogr 21:1179–1201, 2008, by permission.)*

concentration of the contrast agent will equilibrate. If a single high-amplitude (i.e., high mechanical index) ultrasound pulse is delivered to a myocardial ROI, the microbubbles will be destroyed; they will be replenished as the contrast-filled blood perfuses the myocardium. The rate of contrast replenishment in the myocardium is directly related to myocardial blood flow. Repeated ultrasound pulses are delivered at shorter frequencies until a maximum myocardial contrast-enhanced ultrasound signal is obtained. A time-myocardial contrast intensity curve is constructed. Myocardial-contrast echocardiographic-derived indications of myocardial perfusion rate have relatively good between-study and between-reading reproducibility.[40]

If contrast echocardiography is used in conjunction with traditional echocardiography, different flow patterns can be described as outlined in Table 12-3. A fixed myocardial deficit may be diagnosed with a perfusion deficit during rest and stress and with akinetic segments during both of these periods. An ischemic segment may be defined as a segment with normal perfusion and wall motion with rest, and a perfusion deficit during stress that is accompanied by a regional wall motion abnormality (RWMA). Myocardial stunning may be diagnosed if normal perfusion is observed during rest in the presence of a hypokinetic rest wall motion, and hibernation may be diagnosed with rest hypoperfusion and with hypokinetic rest wall motion. The addition of myocardial-contrast echocardiography (MCE) may increase the sensitivity, but not specificity, of dipyridamole-exercise echocardiography. Moir et al[41] combined MCE with dipyridamole-exercise echocardiography in 85 patients. They detected significant coronary artery stenosis in 43 patients involving 69 coronary areas. The addition of MCE improved sensitivity

for the detection of CAD (91% vs. 74%; $P = 0.02$) and accurate recognition of disease extent (87% vs. 65% of territories; $P = 0.003$).

Measurements of myocardial blood flow by MCE are comparable with other techniques. Senior et al[42] compared MCE and single-photon emission computerized tomography (SPECT) for the detection of coronary artery disease (CAD) in 55 patients with a medium probability of CAD. The sensitivity of MCE was significantly greater than that of SPECT for the detection of CAD (86% vs 43%; $P < 0.0001$); however, the specificities were not significantly different (88% and 93%; $P = 0.52$). In another investigation, quantitative real-time MCE with dipyridamole defined the presence and severity of CAD in a manner that compared favorably with quantitative SPECT.[43]

Microvascular perfusion is a prerequisite for ensuring viability early after acute myocardial infarction (AMI). For adequate assessment of myocardial perfusion, both myocardial blood volume and velocity need to be evaluated. Because of its high frame rate, low-power continuous MCE can assess both myocardial blood volume and velocity, allowing for assessment of microvascular perfusion.[44] To differentiate necrotic from viable myocardium after reperfusion therapy, Janardhanan et al[44] examined 50 patients with low-power continuous MCE 7 to 10 days after acute myocardial perfusion. Myocardial perfusion by contrast opacification was assessed over 15 cardiac cycles after the destruction of microbubbles, and wall thickening was assessed at baseline. Regional and global LV function were reassessed after 12 weeks. Of the segments without contrast enhancements, 93% showed no recovery of function; in the segments with contrast opacification, 84% exhibited functional recovery. The greater the extent and intensity of contrast opacification, the better the LV function at 3 months ($P < 0.001$; $r = -0.91$). Almost all patients (94%) with less than 20% perfusion in dysfunctional myocardium (assessing various cutoffs) failed to demonstrate an improvement in LV function.

Janardhanan et al[45] performed MCE in 70 patients with AMI after thrombolysis. Myocardial perfusion was examined in the akinetic areas in 20 patients with an occluded infarct-related artery that was subsequently revascularized. Contractile reserve was evaluated in these segments 12 weeks after revascularization with dobutamine–echocardiography. Of the 102 akinetic segments, 37 (36%) showed contractile reserve. Contractile reserve was present in 24 of the 29 segments (83%) with homogenous contrast opacification and absent in 60 of the 73 segments (82%) with reduced opacification. Quantitative measurements of myocardial blood flow were significantly greater ($P < 0.0001$) in the segments with contractile reserve than in those without contractile reserve. MCE may, thus, be used as a reliable bedside technique for the accurate evaluation of collateral blood flow in the presence of an occluded infarct-related artery after AMI. MCE performed early after percutaneous coronary interventions provides information on the extent of infarction, and hence the likelihood for recovery of contractile reserve. The presence of perfusion before this intervention predicts the maintenance of perfusion and recovery of systolic function.[46]

MCE may be a useful tool in the detection of myocardial viability before coronary revascularization. In Korosoglou et al's[47] study, contrast echocardiography was compared with low-dose dobutamine stress echocardiography and with combined technetium-99 sestamibi SPECT and fluorodeoxyglucose-18 positron emission tomography. Myocardial recovery was predicted by contrast echocardiography with a sensitivity of 86% and a specificity of 43%, by nuclear imaging with a sensitivity of 90% and specificity of 44%, whereas DSE was similarly sensitive (83%) but more specific (76%). A combination of quantitative MCE and dobutamine stress echocardiography provided the best diagnostic characteristics, with a sensitivity of 96%, a specificity of 63%, and an accuracy of 83%. Fukuda et al[48] performed myocardial contrast echocardiography on 28 patients with chronic stable CAD and LV dysfunction before and after coronary revascularization. Of the 101 revascularized dysfunctional segments, MCE was adequately visualized in 91 (90%) segments, and wall motion was recovered in 45 (49%) segments. Quantitative measurements of myocardial blood flow in the recovery segments were

TABLE 12-3	Diagnosis of Fixed Myocardial Deficits, Ischemia, Stunning, and Hibernation Based on Perfusion and Wall Motion Findings			
	Rest Perfusion	*Stress Perfusion*	*Rest Wall Motion*	*Stress Wall Motion*
Fixed deficit	Deficit	Deficit	Akinetic	Akinetic
Ischemia	Normal	Deficit	Normal	RWMA
Stunning	Normal		RWMA	
Hibernation	Hypoperfusion		Hypokinetic	

RWMA, regional wall motion abnormality.

significantly greater than that in nonrecovery segments. The investigators concluded that quantitative intravenous MCE can predict functional recovery after coronary revascularization.

ECHOCARDIOGRAPHIC SCANNERS

▣ Basic Principles

The conversion of reflected ultrasound echoes into 2D video images is a complicated process involving numerous electronic and digital manipulations. A 2D echo image is generated by scanning the heart every 17 msec, or 60 times each second. The image generated from a single 1/60th–second scan is called a *field*. A process called *interlacing* combines two scans or fields into a frame of 1/30th of a second. Because the eye cannot capture an image lasting 1/30th of a second, microprocessors further process the frame electronically in real time. The intrinsic persistence of the television screen enhances image quality, and the end result is a fairly smooth picture.

▣ Resolution

An ultrasound image may be described by its axial, lateral, and elevational resolution (Box 12-4). *Axial resolution* is the minimum separation between two interfaces located in a direction parallel to the beam so that they can be imaged as two different interfaces. The most precise image resolution is along this axial plane. The higher the frequency of the ultrasound signal, the greater the axial resolution, because ultrasound waves of shorter wavelengths may be utilized. Shorter bursts of ultrasound waves (i.e., short pulse length) provide greater axial resolution. Pulse length should be no more than two or three cycles. The range of frequencies contained within a given ultrasound transmission is referred to as the "frequency bandwidth." Generally, the shorter the pulse of the ultrasound produced, the greater the frequency bandwidth. Because of the relation between short pulse lengths and high bandwidths, high bandwidths are associated with better axial resolution. High transducer bandwidths also allow for better resolution of deeper structures.

Lateral resolution is the minimum separation of two interfaces aligned along a direction perpendicular to the ultrasound beam. The most important determinant of lateral resolution is the ultrasound beam width or ultrasound beam focusing; the narrower the beam, the better the lateral resolution. If a small object appears within the "near field," it can be resolved laterally accurately; however, if it appears within the "far field" the size of this small object will appear to increase with the increase in the width of the ultrasound beam. This increase in size associated with object resolution in the far field results in blurring of deeper structures. *Elevational resolution* refers to the ability to determine differences in the thickness of the imaging plane. The thickness of the ultrasound beam is a major determinant of elevational resolution.

▣ Preprocessing

Ultrasound echoes are received and converted to electronic signals by the transducer. On most modern echo scanners, the analog electronic signals undergo several modifications before being digitized and

eventually displayed as an image. Preprocessing describes the modifications performed on the analog and digital signal before storage.

Dynamic Range Manipulation

The intensity of echo signals spans a wide range from very weak to very strong. Very strong signals falling beyond the saturation level of the electronic circuitry and very weak signals below the sensitivity of the instrument are automatically eliminated. The dynamic range of the instrument is defined by the limits at which extremely strong or weak signals are eliminated; dynamic range is under operator control (Figure 12-13). In this manner, signals of low intensity that contain little useful information, and mostly noise, can be selectively rejected.

A wide dynamic range is necessary for high resolution, whereas a narrow range facilitates the discrimination between true image signals and noise. In clinical echocardiography, strong signals that arise from dense tissues (e.g., cardiac valves) and weaker signals arising from soft tissues (e.g., myocardium) are of interest. To give the weaker signals a greater representation in the dynamic range, an amplifier converts the linear signal intensity scale into a logarithmic scale. Although this increases the number of weaker signals detected, it also, unfortunately, tends to amplify noise.

Gain, Attenuation, and Damping

The gain and attenuation controls of a scanner increase and decrease the intensity of all signals in a proportional manner. As a result, they change the number of detected echo signals by bringing them above or below the rejection threshold of the dynamic range. To address the potential loss of image quality caused by the display of the larger number of insignificant echoes obtained at high settings, a "damping" adjustment exists. Damping does not modify the received signal directly, but it decreases the strength of the emitted ultrasound beam by limiting the duration of the pulses that form the beam. Because less power is sent toward the target, fewer noise signals are generated. Damping also enhances the image because it improves resolution by decreasing the number of cycles in each ultrasound pulse.

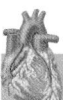

BOX 12-4. OPTIMIZATION OF RESOLUTION

- Axial
  - High ultrasound frequency
  - Short duration of ultrasound pulse
  - High-frequency bandwidth
- Lateral
  - Narrow beam width
- Elevational
  - Thickness of the ultrasound beam

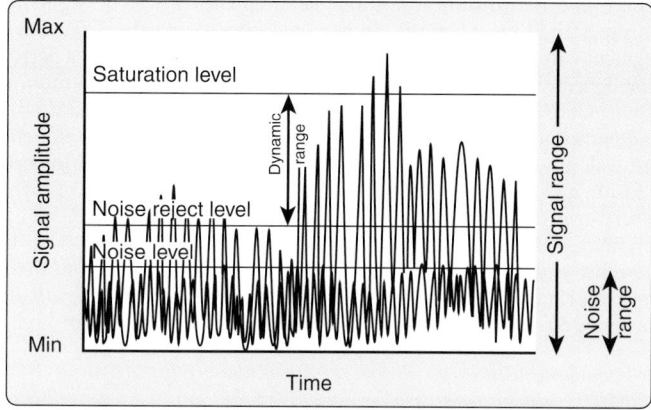

Figure 12-13 **Dynamic range of a representative echocardiographic display system.** All ultrasound signals begin at zero signal level and can increase in amplitude until they reach the signal "saturation" level. Many of the low-intensity signals fall within the range of the background noise and are, therefore, obscured. All systems have a built-in system reject, which eliminates both the system noise and the low-intensity echoes that lie just above the noise level. The dynamic range of the system is between the noise reject level and the saturation level. Signals within the dynamic range appear on the image display. *(From Thys DM, Hillel Z: How it works: Basic concepts in echocardiography. In Bruijn NP, Clements F [eds]: Intraoperative use of echocardiography. Philadelphia: JB Lippincott, 1991.)*

Lateral Gain Control

A recent innovation allows the application of gain control to selected sectors of the ultrasound image. This feature appears particularly useful for the enhancement of image strength of structures that are nearly parallel to the ultrasound beam (e.g., the septum and lateral wall on a short–axis (SAX) view at the level of the papillary muscles; Figure 12-14).

Time-Gain Compensation

Because any wave traveling through tissues is attenuated proportionally to the traveled distance, it is necessary to compensate for the fact that echoes returning from more distant objects will be weaker than those from equally dense objects closer to the transducer. A mechanism called *depth compensation* or *time-gain compensation* (TGC) is used to achieve this. The manner in which time-gain compensation is obtained is illustrated in Figure 12-15. Time-gain compensation can be manually or automatically controlled.

Leading-Edge Enhancement

Leading-edge enhancement, or differentiation, is another type of preprocessing used to sharpen the ultrasound image. The reflected echo signal undergoes half–wave rectification and is smoothed into a signal envelope (Figure 12-16A, B). An amplifier then differentiates the leading edge of the smoothed signal envelope from its first mathemati-

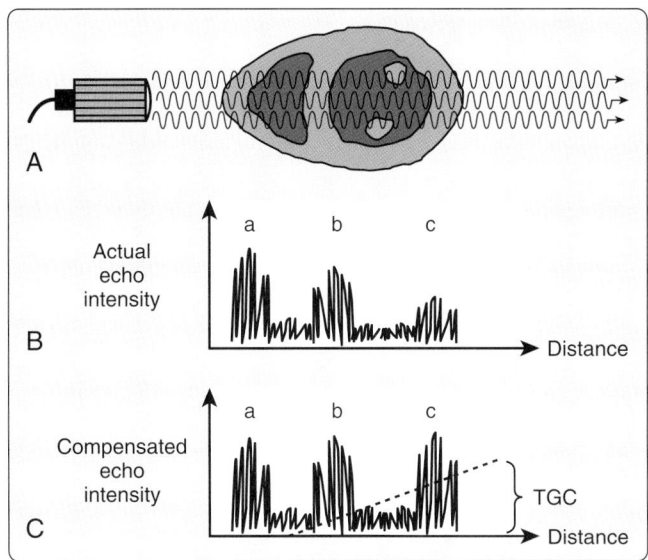

Figure 12-15   *A,* As an ultrasound beam is aimed across the heart, specular echoes are reflected at the right ventricular wall *(a),* the septum *(b),* and the left ventricular wall *(c). B,* The normal loss of echo strength is due to the decreasing intensity of the beam as it propagates through the heart. *C,* Time-gain compensation (TGC) allows the intensity of the far-field signals to be increased selectively. *(From Thys DM, Hillel Z: How it works: Basic concepts in echocardiography. In Bruijn NP, Clements F [eds]: Intraoperative use of echocardiography. Philadelphia: JB Lippincott, 1991.)*

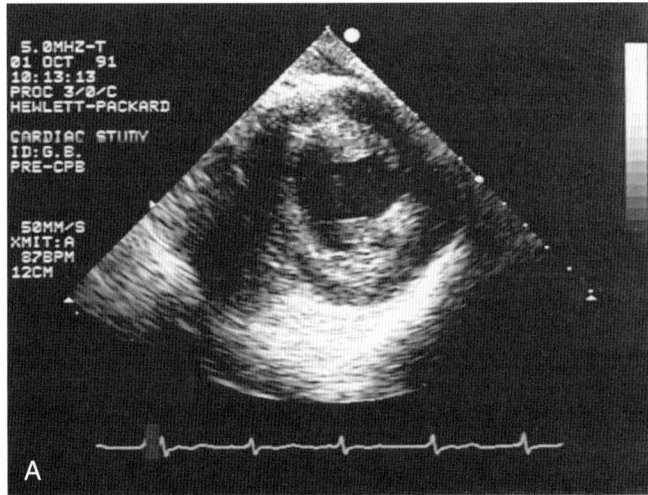

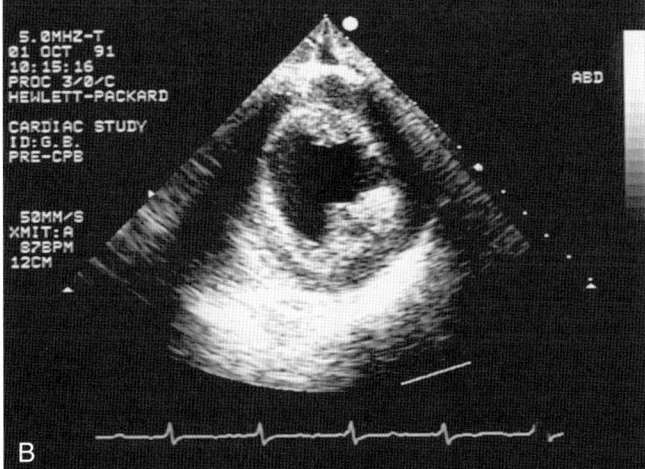

Figure 12-14   *A,* Standard two-dimensional short-axis view of the left ventricle at the level of the papillary muscles. Note that the image drops out in the septal and lateral walls (vertical portions of the wall). *B,* Identical view after application of lateral gain adjustments. The septal and lateral walls appear brighter and less dropout is seen.

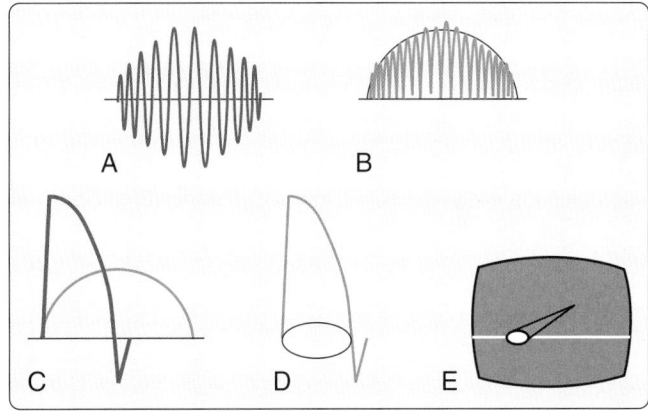

Figure 12-16   **Leading-edge enhancement techniques.** *A,* Radiofrequency (RF) type of echo display. *B,* This video represents the average height of the upper half of the RF signal. *C,* Differentiation is obtained by taking the first derivative of the video display. *D* and *E,* Intensity modulation represents the conversion of signal amplitude to intensity, changing the signal from a spike to a dot. *(From Thys DM, Hillel Z: How it works: Basic concepts in echocardiography. In Bruijn NP, Clements F [eds]: Intraoperative use of echocardiography. Philadelphia: JB Lippincott, 1991.)*

cal derivative (see Figure 12-16C), and a narrower and brighter image spot is formed (see Figure 12-16D). Because a 2D image is composed of multiple radially juxtaposed scan lines, excessive edge enhancement narrows bright spots in the direction of travel of the echo beam (i.e., axially but not laterally). For this reason, leading-edge enhancement primarily is performed on M-mode scans, whereas instruments with 2D mode capability use little or no edge enhancement in the 2D mode. Therefore, M-mode images often have better resolution than 2D images and are better suited for quantitative measurements.

Postprocessing

Digital Scan Conversion

After completing analog preprocessing, ultrasound devices digitize the image data with an analog-to-digital (A–D) converter (Figure 12-17). Further processing is done while data are stored in the digital memory (input processing) or as they are received from the memory (output processing). An early step in digital processing uses a scan converter to transform the information obtained as radial sector scan lines into a rectangular (Cartesian) format for television screen display.

The memory stores the information of two adjacent scan fields consisting of a total of 128 scan lines. Each scan line is assigned to one column of memory. There is also one row of memory for each of the 512 horizontal television image lines (raster lines). Therefore, a typical television display of an echo image consists of 128 columns by 512 rows for a total of 65,536 picture elements, or *pixels*. Although the monitor displays only 64 shades of gray for each pixel, the memory unit assigned to each pixel has the capacity to store 1024 degrees of brightness. Each pixel is assigned 10 binary bits of memory for a total of 2^{10} (1024) possible storage combinations.

Temporal Processing

As digital data are entered into memory, they can undergo temporal averaging in one of two modes. In the variable persistence mode, information from previous images is combined with current image data. A weighted average of the old and new data is then entered into memory as the new current data. A mechanism is built in to allow variable representation of old data into the new image. A different input–processing option calculates the arithmetic mean of the new data and up to nine frames of existing data.

Input processing mainly is used to improve the signal–to–noise ratio. In a 2D echo image, a lower signal-to-noise ratio means a less granular appearance (the result of microscopic scatter) and less echo dropout (the result of very weak signals that are difficult to detect on the screen). Time averaging is most useful for enhancing slowly varying images.

Histogram Equalization

The video image is generated from data retrieved from memory via the scan converter. During retrieval, data can be subjected to histogram equalization. This process redistributes the gray level assignment of each pixel according to the relative frequency of occurrence of the gray level in the entire image in an equalitarian manner. All levels of gray receive some representation even though the original image may have been formed from only a limited range of grays.

Grayscale Processing

Each unit of memory assigned to a pixel can store 1 to 24 values of echo intensity, whereas the pixel itself can display only 64 shades of gray; thus, each gray level represents multiple echo intensities. The gray level reassignment is done by transfer functions of variable shapes, slopes, and end points. An inverting transfer function allows the M-mode display to exist as a dark background with white lines or as a light background with dark lines. Grayscale processing greatly affects image quality.

Image Storage

All modern echo scanners allow the operator to store or "freeze" a single echo image on the display screen. This allows the scrutiny of any unusual transient anatomic or physiologic observations. Once frozen, an image also can be subjected to some simple quantitative measurements. With the continuous motion of the cardiac structures, it is often difficult, however, to capture the exact frame that is to be analyzed. For this reason, techniques to acquire several consecutive frames have been developed.

Cine Memory

When activated, this mode captures a sequence of several echo images in digital memory. Because of the digital storage technique, the quality of the stored images is high. They can be displayed again in several different ways. In one method, the frames are displayed one by one as the operator manually controls the transition from one frame to the next using a trackball. Any amount of time can be spent on a single frame. The images

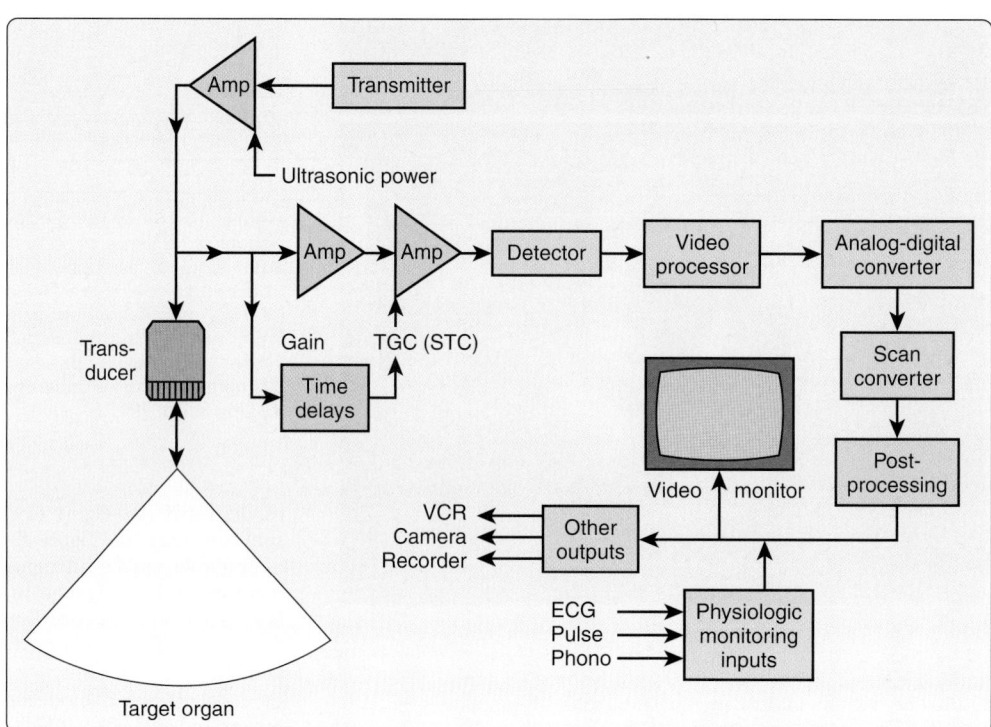

Figure 12-17 Schematic of a modern ultrasound scanner. *Arrows* indicate the directions for the flow of information or electronic power. Amp, electronic amplifier; ECG, electrocardiogram; TGC (STC), time-gain compensation; VCR, videocassette recorder. *(From Thys DM, Hillel Z: How it works: Basic concepts in echocardiography. In Bruijn NP, Clements F [eds]: Intraoperative use of echocardiography. Philadelphia: JB Lippincott, 1991.)*

also can be replayed continuously in repeated endless-loop fashion, at the same speed as the original recording speed or at a different speed.

Videotape

The video recorder is a commonly used long-term, mass-storage medium in echocardiography. Most echo scanners are equipped with 1/2-inch VHS, "super" VHS, or 3/4-inch videocassette recorders (VCRs). Their advantages include low cost and their ability to record multiple cardiac cycles, facilitating the creation of 3D images in the reviewer's mind.[49] Because VCRs store images in analog format, the quality of videotaped images currently is inferior to the real-time display, the digital cine memory replay, or digital storage. In the United States, videotape records images using NTSC (National Television Standards Committee) format. When videotape is used, resolution is limited by this NTSC format, which is not lost with digital storage.[49] Other disadvantages are the inability to randomly access parts of the current examination or previous examinations, difficulty sharing examinations with colleagues, as well as the degradation of videotape quality over time.[49]

Digital Storage

Digital image storage rapidly is becoming an alternative to videotape storage. Although the digital storage of echocardiographic images has increased the complexity of study storage, the American Society of Echocardiography (ASE) and others have suggested that digital storage has advantages over other modalities (Table 12-4).[50,51] These advantages include:

1. More efficient reading. With the use of VCR tapes, the echocardiographer needs to review the entire 10 to 30 minutes of the study, which includes both important and redundant information. Using digital storage, the echocardiographer can direct his or her attention to specific clips, data may accessed randomly, and the noncontributory segments of the study need not be viewed.
2. Because the studies are stored on a central server, the echocardiographer may read studies at any location that contains a workstation. When the storage system is properly configured, studies may be read on campus via institutional intranet connections or may even be read off site.
3. Because of study centralization indexing and archiving in digital storage systems, previous studies may be rapidly accessed for comparison with a current study. The need to rummage through racks of old videotapes and search for a specific study is eliminated. This centralization of studies decreases the inefficient use of clinical staff time retrieving and loading physical media such as VCR tapes or digital media. Because these older studies are more easily available, there is a decrease in unnecessary duplication of procedures and more optimal patient care.

4. Because the Digital Imaging and Communications in Medicine (DICOM) file header contains information about the acquisition of the study, spatial, temporal, and velocity calibration are included with each image, and quantification may be rapidly accomplished within the analysis program without special tools.
5. More convenient communication with the referring physician may be facilitated because the study images may be included easily with the report.
6. The standard resolution of VHS images is equivalent to 480 × 320 pixels, whereas the standard resolution of sVHS is equivalent to 560 × 480 pixels. Digital images provide a resolution of 640 × 480 pixels or higher, which are exactly as they are recorded by the ultrasound machine. There is no degradation in the transfer of images from the ultrasound machine to the digital storage systems, as will occur with videotape transfer.
7. Over time, videotape degrades. There is magnetic realignment of the VCR tape with resultant degradation of image quality. Digital echocardiographic storage provides a more stable image quality.
8. The physical storage of VCR tapes requires significant space, which is usually a premium in either a hospital or office environment.
9. The echocardiographic reports may be incorporated within the hospital's electronic medical record.
10. Because the highest quality images are available, more robust research may be performed. Communication with core laboratories is simplified.
11. A clinical quality-assurance program may be easily implemented, whereby echocardiograms can be re-reviewed randomly on a regular basis. If consultation is necessary, sharing studies with colleagues both within and outside of the institution can be easily accomplished over digital networks.
12. Because physicians may be directed to the important aspects of the echocardiographic examination, there are improved accuracy and reproducibility of echocardiographic examinations.
13. Because moving images can be easily incorporated into presentations, there is greater facilitation of medical education.
14. Because studies may be easily and reliably retrieved, medicolegal risk is reduced.

The increased efficiency of digital reading of echocardiographic studies has been demonstrated by Mathewson et al,[52] who timed study acquisition and analysis during approximately 750 pediatric echocardiograms. As a group, the digitally captured images contained more hemodynamic measurements and hence required more time for acquisition. The average times for study acquisition were 26.0 ± 8.9 minutes for videotape and 28.4 ± 11.5 minutes for the single-beat digital method. In contrast, interpretation of these studies was more rapid using digital methods, with an average interpretation time of 6.5 ± 3.7 minutes for the videotape compared with 4.6 ± 3.9 minutes for the digital method.

Image Terminology
Image Creation

A single static echocardiographic image is rendered by a number of dots or pixels on a screen. The image resolution is defined by the number of columns and rows of pixels displayed, which are typically 640 and 480, respectively, for medical ultrasound. Each pixel of the image is described by its red, green, and blue component, which are represented by three bytes of data; each of these bytes contains a number from 0 to 255, which represents the level of the pixels' primary colors. If there are 256 possible levels for each of these three primary colors, a total of 16.8 million colors (256^3) may be represented. A video clip consists of a series of sequentially displayed static images. Most echocardiographic video clips have approximately 30 frames per second. If no methods of compression are used, the storage requirements for digital storage of echocardiographic clips become huge. A single image would require 921,600 bytes of data (640 columns × 480 rows × 3 bytes per pixel). If a 30-frame/sec temporal resolution is used, an uncompressed 10-minute examination would require 16,588,800,000 bytes or 15.4 gigabytes (GB) of storage.

TABLE 12-4	Advantages of Digital Echocardiographic Storage[50,51]

1. More efficient reading
2. The ability to read studies in a variety of locations
3. Easy comparison with previous studies
4. Easier quantification
5. Ability to include images with reports to referring physicians
6. Higher image quality
7. No image degradation over time
8. Integration of the images and reports within the hospital's electronic medical record
9. More robust research
10. Easy implementation of a clinical performance improvement program
11. Improved accuracy and reproducibility overall
12. Greater facilitation of medical education
13. Decreases in medicolegal risk

Adapted from Thomas JD, Adams DB, Devries S, et al: Digital Echocardiography Committee of the American Society of Echocardiography. Guidelines and Recommendations for Digital Echocardiography: A report from the Digital Echocardiography Committee of the American Society of Echocardiography, *J Am Soc Echocardiogr* 18:287–297, 2005.
Thomas JD, Greenberg NL, Garcia MJ: Digital Echocardiography 2002: Now is the time, *J Am Soc Echocardiogr* 15:831–838, 2002.

Clinical Compression

Because of these space requirements, clinical examinations must be subject to compression. There are two major categories of compression: clinical and digital. During the performance of echocardiographic examinations, many cardiac cycles may be obtained during image acquisition. During standard analog storage of examinations using VCR technologies, the tape is allowed to run continuously, capturing the entire examination. With clinical compression, short clips are stored to represent each relevant echocardiographic view. Typically, either several seconds or several cardiac cycles are recorded, which may be played back in a loop when displayed for interpretation.

Does clinical compression affect the interpretation of echocardiographic examinations? Haluska et al[53] reported high concordance between video and digital echocardiographic interpretations of adult echocardiographic examinations. Most observed discordances were minor, with lesser values being reported with the digital method. For example, degrees of mitral regurgitation were reported to be milder by digital compared with video presentation. Most major discordances were cases of assessment of aortic and MV thickening and the degree of mitral regurgitation; the authors hypothesized that the major discordances were caused by undersampling and not image quality. The routine acquisition of longer video clips may not necessarily increase the accuracy of digital echocardiogram readings. Shah et al[54] evaluated 102 patients with regurgitant valvular disease, recording findings on videotape, as well as digitally, using one, two, and three cardiac cycles. They observed substantial agreement when the video and one-cycle digital presentations were compared. There were no increases in agreement when two or three cardiac cycles were presented digitally.

Digital Compression

There are two basic types of digital image compression: lossless and lossy. Lossless compression reduces the file size by replacing identical values in a given image data set with the single value and the number of repetitions. This type of digital compression allows for exact reconstruction of the data set and does not result in a loss of data. Because there is no data loss, there is no degradation of image quality. The creation of a lossless data set requires substantial processing power and may affect the speed of file manipulations. Lossless compression may allow for a threefold reduction in file size. In contrast, lossy compression reduces image size by permanently eliminating nonessential image information. Although the goal of lossy compression is image compression without the loss of image quality, excessive lossy compression may result in degradation of image quality. Lossy compression may provide a 20-fold reduction in image size.

In a comparison of quantitative measurements of sVHS- and digital MPEG-1–derived images, Garcia et al[55] demonstrated excellent agreement between linear, area, and Doppler measurements. The MPEG-1 measurements were reproducible and provided a higher quality compared with the sVHS images. Other studies have confirmed the diagnostic quality of images subjected to MPEG-1 compression.[56,57] Harris et al[58] compared the image quality of sVHS recording with MPEG-2 compressions, analyzing 80 matched examination interpretations among four echocardiographers. They reported an overall concordance rate of 94%. Most of the reported discrepancies (4% total) were minor. They concluded that MPEG-2 compression offers excellent concordance with sVHS image review. Similar high-quality compression may be seen with newer compression schemes such as MPEG-4.[59]

Digital Imaging and Communications in Medicine Standard

With the increased use of medical imaging, standardized formats for image storage were developed to allow for uniform acquisition, storage, and distribution of examinations. In 1983, the American College of Radiology and the National Electrical Manufacturers Association formed a joint committee to create a standard format for storing and transmitting these medical images, which was published in 1985. This original protocol was limited to single-frame grayscale images and required highly specific nonstandard hardware for information transfer and storage. Images were stored in a proprietary format, so image

viewing was difficult. Subsequently, this format has been further developed and renamed DICOM.[60] Its current version may be found on the National Electrical Manufacturers Association website (ftp://medical.nema.org/medical/dicom/2008/08_01pu.pdf); version 3.0 currently is being used.

Each DICOM file has both header and image data. The header data may contain a variety of patient demographic information, acquisition parameters, and image dimensions. Informational object definitions specify the source of the data, which supply the rules determining which data elements are required and which are optional, and they define the valid methods of data manipulation. In the case of echocardiography, 2D, color, and Doppler echocardiographic techniques are all supported. Calibration information for linear, temporal, and velocity data are available. Information may be exchanged using a variety of methods.

Image Acquisition, Transmission, Analysis, and Storage
Image Acquisition

Most modern ultrasonography machines have the ability to store electronic studies in a DICOM-compatible format for transmission to the PACS (Picture Archiving and Communication System), as well as modality worklist capability. This modality worklist capability enables a piece of imaging equipment to obtain details of patients and scheduled examinations electronically from the DICOM worklist server. Because of the need for image transmission, each ultrasound machine must be properly configured before its introduction into clinical service. The machine must be assigned an appropriate Application Entry (AE) Title and IP address, which will uniquely identify the machine to the network. The IP address of the gateway through which the machine is expected to communicate must be entered, as well as the IP addresses of both the PACS and DICOM worklist servers.

Before performing an examination, the patient must be properly identified. If a modality worklist capability is present on the ultrasound machine, the patient information already will have been prepopulated on the ultrasound machine. The minimum examination should consist of all 20 ASE/SCA (Society of Cardiovascular Anesthesiologists) recommended standard multiplane TEE views with the appropriate Doppler and color-Doppler spectra.[61] Most of these views are saved as clips, and the Doppler images are saved as static images. Calibration information for off-line analysis (such as length, time, and velocity) is automatically stored. Because ECG monitoring should be used, clips of a fixed number of cardiac cycles may be specified and automatically saved. Because electrocautery artifacts may interfere with cycle determination, an alternative fixed time (e.g., 1 to 2 seconds) may be specified. Although dependent on the number and duration of clips and images stored, the usual echocardiographic examination is between 50 and 100 MB. After conclusion of the study, all examination information may be sent via the LAN (local area network) to the PACS server.

Study Transmission

Normally, echocardiographic studies are initially stored on the internal hard drive of the ultrasound machine. These studies will normally be retained until deleted by the end-user. Because studies stored on these machines are not accessible via a global PACS, these studies must be transferred centrally. Although studies may be copied onto removable media, such as DVDs, CDs, USB devices, or magneto-optical devices, and manually transferred to a server ("sneaker-netted"), transmission via a LAN is most efficient.

LAN transmission speed will limit the speed of information exchange. Whereas older LANs may provide 10 megabits per second (Mbps) connectivity, a minimum of 100 Mbps is usually necessary between the ultrasound machines and the PACS server. A connection speed of 100 Mbps to 1 gigabit per second (Gbps) may be necessary to connect the PACS station to the review stations. In addition to transmission speed, network architecture (interconnectivity of gateways, bridges, switches, and servers) has an important role in the performance of a network. Most ultrasound devices will support a network switch with autonegotiate features, allowing for rapid transmission of information.

Some older devices may support only lower speeds of communications and/or less efficient duplex modes and may not function properly with a switch set for autonegotiate functionality. Several network connections may need to be left at a fixed setting to allow communication with these older devices.

Image Storage: PACS Server

After creation of a study entry by the DICOM worklist server, an acquisition number is assigned by the worklist server. As discussed earlier, this information is sent to the ultrasound machine but also may be sent to the PACS server. The important demographic information is stored, as well as the details of the expected echocardiographic examination. When the study has been completed, the study is sent from the ultrasound machine to the PACS server. Typically, the study will be stored on the PACS server for a short period (days) before it is sent to longer-term storage. In many cases, these data also will be mirrored to an off-site disaster recovery server and storage as well. The more recent studies (typically 6 months to a few years) usually are stored on redundant arrays of independent disks (RAID) for rapid retrieval of data, whereas the older studies (more than a few years) may be stored on cheaper, slower media such as DVDs, digital linear tape (DLT), or advanced intelligent tape (AIT). With the decreasing price of RAID storage, a greater number of studies may be stored on this fast-access medium.

Study Distribution and Analysis

Dedicated Workstations. The need for study analysis is heavily dependent on physician work flow. In the typical cardiac anesthesia practice, most studies will be performed, interpreted, and reported by the physician at the time of the examination. In contrast, most outpatient echocardiographic studies are done by a technician and sent to digital storage. They are then later recalled by the cardiologist for review, analysis, interpretation, and report generation. Nonetheless, most digital storage solutions will provide dedicated workstations for image review, analysis, and report-generation capability, and anesthesia providers have the option to utilize these resources. Typically, these workstations will have fast connections with the PACS server, allowing for rapid transmission of a particular study to a workstation for analysis. Multiple studies usually may be displayed for comparison. Image configurations may be adjusted by the user, and further off-line image adjustments (such as brightness and contrast) usually can be made. Clip playback speeds can be easily controlled, including the ability to start/stop and step through a study. Because calibration information has been incorporated into the study, off-line calculations may be performed. Images or clips can be selected for exportation as standard image or video files for incorporation into teaching material. Reporting software may be offered as an option for these image analysis workstations. Measurements and qualitative descriptions may be entered for generation of a study report, as well as population of a Structured Query Language (SQL) database, which may be used for performance improvement or research.

Off-site Distribution. Echocardiographic images may be distributed off site as well. It usually is most efficient to mirror the recently obtained studies on a separate server to handle all off-site distribution of studies (Web server). The distribution of studies is limited by two basic constraints: security and communication. Most off-site distribution of medical images utilizes an Internet browser application to both retrieve studies from the PACS and display these studies for the user. An open-access system through the public Internet may present challenges vis-à-vis the Health Insurance Portability and Accountability Act of 1996 (HIPAA) Privacy Rule. Security of this medical information must be assured. This security may be assured via either a login system allowing for auditing of access to patient information or via a virtual personal network (VPN), which is a method of providing remote access to an institutional LAN.

As discussed earlier, individual studies may be 50 to 100 MB in size. If high-speed network connectivity is available (such as 1 Gbps), a 50-MB study may be transmitted to a workstation in less than 1 second (Table 12-5). This high-speed connectivity is, however, not usually available

TABLE 12-5	Transmission Time Requirement for a 50-MB Study
Speed of Connectivity	*Study Download Time*
28.8 kbps modem	3.9 hours
112 kbps ISDN	1 hour
768 kbps DSL or cable modem	8.6 minutes
1.54 Mbps T1 line	4.4 minutes
10 Mbps Ethernet	40 seconds
100 Mbps Ethernet	4 seconds
1 Gbps Ethernet	0.4 second

Adapted from Thomas JD, Adams DB, Devries S, et al: Digital Echocardiography Committee of the American Society of Echocardiography. Guidelines and Recommendations for Digital Echocardiography. A Report from the Digital Echocardiography Committee of the American Society of Echocardiography. *J Am Soc Echocardiogr* 18:287–297, 2005.

to a user outside of the institutional LAN. If studies are to be accessed outside of an institution, the Internet must be used to download and view these studies; transmission speed may limit the speed of study display. An old-technology dial-up modem may require almost 4 hours to download a 50-MB study, whereas a 1.54-Mbps T1 line may require approximately 5 minutes. Because of these transmission speed issues, studies must be compressed before off-site study transmission. It is most common to use one of the lossy compression routines. Although there is generally some image degradation, image quality still may be reasonable for some diagnostic work. Because these compression routines are used and the actual DICOM image file is not sent, calibration information is lost; thus, off-line image measurements and calculation may be problematic.

EQUIPMENT

Because fat, bone, and air-containing lung interfere with sound-wave penetration, clear transthoracic echocardiogram views are particularly difficult to obtain in patients with obesity, emphysema, or abnormal chest wall anatomy. TEE transducers were developed to avoid these problems. Sound waves emitted from an esophageal transducer have to pass through only the esophageal wall and the pericardium to reach the heart, improving image quality and increasing the number of echocardiographic windows. Other advantages of TEE include the stability of the transducer position and the possibility of obtaining continuous recordings of cardiac activity for extended periods.

The first TEE examination was performed in 1975. The probe used allowed only M-mode imaging and had limited control of direction. Two-dimensional TEE was first performed with a mechanical system.[62] The system consisted of a vertical and a horizontal mechanical scanner connected to a 3.5-MHz ultrasonic transducer contained in a 12′20′6-mm oil bag. The transducers were rotated by a single-phase commutator motor via flexible shafts. Subsequently, phased-array transducers were mounted into gastroscope housings.[63,64] With their greater flexibility and control, these probes allowed 2D scanning of the heart through many planes, and the probes became the prototypes of the currently used models (see Chapter 11).

All TEE probes share several common features. All of the currently available probes use a multifrequency transducer that is mounted on the tip of a gastroscope housing. The majority of the echocardiographic examination is performed using ultrasound between 3.5 and 7 MHz. The tip can be directed by the adjustment of knobs placed at the proximal handle. In most adult probes, there are two knobs; one allows anterior and posterior movement, and the other permits side-to-side motion. Multiplane probes also include a control to rotate the echocardiographic array from 0 to 180 degrees. Thus, in combination with the ability to advance and withdraw the probe and to rotate it, many echocardiographic windows are possible. Another feature common to most probes is the inclusion of a temperature sensor to warn of possible heat injury from the transducer to the esophagus.

Currently, most adult echocardiographic probes are multiplane (variable orientation of the scanning plane), whereas pediatric probes are either multiplane or biplane (transverse and longitudinal orientation: parallel to the shaft). The adult probes usually have a shaft length of 100 cm and are between 9 and 12 mm in diameter. The tips of the probes vary slightly in shape and size but are generally 1 to 2 mm wider than the shaft. The size of these probes requires the patient to weigh at least 20 kg. Depending on the manufacturer, the adult probes contain between 32 and 64 elements per scanning orientation. In general, the image quality is directly related to the number of elements used. The pediatric probes are mounted on a narrower, shorter shaft with smaller transducers. These probes may be used in patients as small as 1 kg. Because of size limitations, these probes may not possess a lateral control knob. The question has been asked, Why not use the pediatric probe on all patients to decrease the risk for esophageal injury? The answer is that the smaller probes provide less diagnostic information. The number of elements is reduced, the aperture is smaller, there is less control of the tip, and the smaller transducer tip does not usually make good contact in the adult esophagus. These factors combine to significantly reduce image quality.

An important feature that is often available is the ability to alter the scanning frequency. A lower frequency, such as 3.5 MHz, has greater penetration and is more suited for the transgastric (TG) view. It also increases the Doppler velocity limits. Conversely, the higher frequencies yield better resolution for detailed imaging. One of the limitations of TEE is that structures very close to the probe are seen only in a very narrow sector. Newer probes also may allow a broader near-field view. Finally, newer probes possess the ability to scan simultaneously in more than one plane.

COMPLICATIONS

Complications resulting from intraoperative TEE can be separated into two groups: injury from direct trauma to the airway and esophagus and indirect effects of TEE (Box 12-5). In the first group, potential complications include esophageal bleeding, burning, tearing, dysphagia, and laryngeal discomfort. Many of these complications could result from pressure exerted by the tip of the probe on the esophagus and the airway. Although in most patients even maximal flexion of the probe will not result in pressure greater than 17 mm Hg, occasionally, even in the absence of esophageal disease, pressures greater than 60 mm Hg will result.[65] To look more closely at the effects on the esophagus, animal autopsy studies have been performed. In dogs as small as 5 kg on cardiopulmonary bypass (CPB) with full heparinization, no evidence of macroscopic or microscopic injury to the esophageal mucosa after 6 hours of maximally flexed probe positioning was noted.[66]

Further confirmation of the low incidence of esophageal injury from TEE is apparent in the few case reports of complications. In a study of 10,000 TEE examinations, there was one case of hypopharyngeal perforation (0.01%), two cases of cervical esophageal perforation (0.02%), and no cases of gastric perforation (0%).[67] Kallmeyer et al[68]

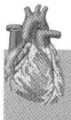

BOX 12-5. COMPLICATIONS FROM INTRAOPERATIVE TRANSESOPHAGEAL ECHOCARDIOGRAPHY

- Injury from direct trauma to the airway and esophagus
  - Esophageal bleeding, burning, tearing
  - Dysphagia
  - Laryngeal discomfort
  - Bacteremia
  - Vocal cord paralysis
- Indirect effects
  - Hemodynamic and pulmonary effects of airway manipulation
  - Distraction from patient

reported overall incidences of TEE-associated morbidity and mortality of 0.2% and 0%, respectively. The most common TEE-associated complication was severe odynophagia, which occurred in 0.1% of the study population, dental injury (0.03%), endotracheal tube malpositioning (0.03%), upper gastrointestinal hemorrhage (0.03%), and esophageal perforation (0.01%). Piercy et al[69] reported a gastrointestinal complication rate of approximately 0.1%, with a great frequency of injuries among patients older than 70 and women. If resistance is met while advancing the probe, the procedure should be aborted to avoid these potentially lethal complications.

Another possible complication of esophageal trauma is bacteremia. Studies have shown that the incidence rate of positive blood cultures in patients undergoing upper gastrointestinal endoscopy is 4% to 13%,[70,71] and that in patients undergoing TEE is 0% to 17%.[72-74] Even though bacteremia may occur, it does not always cause endocarditis. Antibiotic prophylaxis in accordance with the American Heart Association (AHA) guidelines is not routinely recommended but is optional in patients with prosthetic or abnormal valves, or who are otherwise at high risk for endocarditis.[75]

In one of the earliest studies using TEE, transient vocal cord paralysis was reported in two patients undergoing neurosurgery in the sitting position with the head maximally flexed and the presence of an armored endotracheal tube.[76] This complication was believed to be due to the pressure the TEE probe exerted against the larynx. Since this initial report, no further problems of this kind have been reported with the use of the newer equipment.

The second group of complications that result from TEE includes hemodynamic and pulmonary effects of airway manipulation and, particularly for new TEE operators, distraction from patient care. Fortunately, in the anesthetized patient, there are rarely hemodynamic consequences to esophageal placement of the probe, and no studies specifically address this question. More important for the anesthesiologist are the problems of distraction from patient care. Although these reports have not appeared in the literature, the authors have heard of several endotracheal tube disconnections that went unnoticed to the point of desaturation during TEE examination. In addition, there have been instances in which severe hemodynamic abnormalities have been missed because of fascination with the images or the controls of the echocardiograph machine. Clearly, new echo operators should enlist the assistance of an associate to watch the patient during the examination. This second anesthesiologist will become unnecessary after sufficient experience is gained. It also is important to be sure that all the respiratory and hemodynamic alarms are activated during the examination. One report that did appear in the literature was that, during TEE, an esophageal stethoscope was inadvertently pushed into the patient's stomach and was noticed to be missing only when the patient developed a small bowel obstruction.[77] There have been instances in which severe hemodynamic and ventilatory abnormalities have been missed because of fascination with the images or the controls of the echocardiograph machine.

▨ Safety Guidelines and Contraindications

To ensure the continued safety of TEE, the following recommendations have been made: The probe should be inspected before each insertion for cleanliness and structural integrity. If possible, the electrical isolation also should be checked. The probe should be inserted gently, and if resistance is met, the procedure aborted. Minimal transducer energy should be used and the image frozen when not in use. Finally, when not imaging, the probe should be left in the neutral, unlocked position to avoid prolonged pressure on the esophageal mucosa.

Absolute contraindications to TEE in intubated patients include esophageal stricture, diverticula, tumor, recent suture lines, and known esophageal interruption. Relative contraindications include symptomatic hiatal hernia, esophagitis, coagulopathy, esophageal varices, and unexplained upper gastrointestinal bleeding. Notably, despite these relative contraindications, TEE has been used in patients undergoing hepatic transplantation without reported sequelae.[78,79]

CREDENTIALING

This is an era in medicine in which the observance of guidelines for training, credentialing, certifying, and recertifying medical professionals has become increasingly common. Although there have been warnings[80] and objections[81] to anesthesiologists making diagnoses and aiding in surgical decision making, there is no inherent reason that an anesthesiologist cannot provide this valuable service to the patient. The key factors are proper training, extensive experience with TEE, and available backup by a recognized echocardiographer (see Chapter 41).

In 1990, a task force from the American College of Physicians, the American College of Cardiology (ACC), and the American Heart Association created initial general guidelines for echocardiography.[82] The ASE also provided recommendations for general training in echocardiography and has introduced a self-assessment test for measuring proficiency. These organizations recommended the establishment of three levels of performance with a minimum number of cases for each level: level 1, introduction and an understanding of the indications (120 2D and 60 Doppler cases); level 2, independent performance and interpretation (240 2D and 180 Doppler cases); and level 3, laboratory direction and training (590 2D and 530 Doppler cases).[81,83] However, these guidelines are limited because they are not based on objective data or achievement. Furthermore, because different individuals learn at different rates, meeting these guidelines does not ensure competence, nor does failure to meet these guidelines preclude competence.

Proficiency in echocardiography can be achieved more efficiently in a limited setting (i.e., the perioperative period) with fewer clinical applications (e.g., interpreting wall motion, global function, and mitral regurgitation severity) than in a setting that introduces every aspect of echocardiography. The American Society of Anesthesiologists (ASA) and the SCA have worked together to create a document on practice parameters for perioperative TEE.[84,85] The SCA then created a Task Force on Certification for Perioperative TEE to develop a process that acknowledged basic competence and offered the opportunity to demonstrate advanced competence as outlined by the SCA/ASA practice parameters. This process resulted in the development of the Examination of Special Competence in Perioperative Transesophageal Echocardiography (PTEeXAM). In 1998, the National Board of Echocardiography was formed. Currently, board certification in perioperative TEE may be granted by meeting the following requirements: (1) the holding of a valid license to practice medicine, (2) board certification in an approved medical specialty (e.g., anesthesiology), (3) training and/or experience in the perioperative care of surgical patients with cardiovascular disease, (4) the study of 300 echocardiographic examinations, and (5) the passing of the PTEeXAM (see the National Board of Echocardiography website for more information: http://www.echoboards.org/content/advanced-PTExam-certification).

TRAINING/QUALITY ASSURANCE

TEE training should begin with a dedicated training period. This is most easily accomplished during a cardiac anesthesia fellowship but can be done by postgraduate physicians as well. The subject can be approached through a combination of tutorials, scientific review courses, self–instruction with teaching tapes, interactive learning programs, and participation in echo reading sessions.[86,87] Frequently, a symbiotic relationship with the cardiology division can be established in which anesthesiologists can teach the fundamentals of airway management, operating room physiology, and the use of local anesthetics while learning the principles of echocardiography from the cardiologists.

Quality assurance is another area for which no specific guidelines currently exist for TEE. One model for quality assurance was proposed by Rafferty et al.[88] At the very least, each echocardiogram should be recorded in a standardized fashion and accompanied by a written report for inclusion in the patient's chart. Images also may be copied and included in the chart. Careful records of any complications should be maintained. To ensure that the proper images are being obtained and that the interpretations are correct, the studies should be periodically reviewed. This is another area in which the relation between cardiology and anesthesiology can be productive.

PRACTICE PARAMETERS

An updated report by the American Society of Anesthesiologists and the Society of Cardiovascular Anesthesiologists Task Force on Transesophageal Echocardiography was published in 2010.[85] This document updated the 1996 published guidelines for the perioperative use of TEE.[84] The major change that these guidelines recommend is that perioperative TEE should be utilized in all adult patients, without contraindications for TEE, presenting for cardiac or thoracic aortic procedures. A complete TEE examination should be performed in all patients with the following intent: (1) confirm and refine the preoperative diagnosis, (2) detect new or unsuspected pathology, (3) adjust the anesthetic and surgical plan accordingly, and (4) assess results of the surgical intervention.

For patients presenting to the catheterization laboratory, the use of TEE may be beneficial. Especially in the setting of catheter-based valve replacement and repair and transcatheter intracardiac procedures, both consultants and ASA members agree that TEE should be used. In the setting of noncardiac surgery, TEE may be beneficial in patients with known or suspected cardiovascular pathology, which potentially could lead to severe hemodynamic, pulmonary, or neurologic compromise. In life-threatening situations of circulatory instability, TEE remains indicated. A similar viewpoint is taken by the consultants and ASA members in regards to critically ill patients. TEE should be used to obtain diagnostic information that is expected to alter management in the ICU, especially when the quality of transthoracic images is poor or other diagnostic modalities are not obtainable in a timely manner.

Minhaj et al's[89] study found that in 30% of patients, the routine use of TEE during cardiac surgery revealed a previously undiagnosed cardiac pathology leading to change in surgical management in 25% of patients studied. Eltzschig et al[90] were able to confirm these findings in a much larger cohort, showing that the perioperative use of TEE may improve outcome. This group reported that 7% of 12,566 consecutive TEE examinations directly influenced surgical decision making. Combined procedures (CABG, valve) were most commonly influenced by perioperative TEE. In 0.05%, the surgical procedure was actually canceled as a direct result of the intraoperative TEE examination.

It is important to recognize that practice guidelines are systematically developed *recommendations* that assist the practitioner and patient in making decisions about health care. These recommendations may be adopted, modified, or rejected according to clinical needs and constraints. Practice guidelines are not intended as standards or absolute requirements, and their use cannot guarantee any specific outcome. Practice guidelines are subject to revisions from time to time as medical knowledge, technology, and technique evolve. Guidelines are supported by analysis of the current literature and by synthesis of expert opinion, open-forum commentary, and clinical feasibility data.

TECHNIQUE OF PROBE PASSAGE

Anesthesiologists may need to insert TEE probes in awake or anesthetized patients. Awake insertions are identical in technique to awake upper gastrointestinal endoscopy and should be performed when the patient has an empty stomach. It is also important to use a bite block. Probe insertion usually requires topical oral and pharyngeal anesthesia, as well as moderate sedation. The probe is well lubricated, and the function of the directional controls is tested before insertion. Most patients are able to assist the probe's passage through the pharynx with a swallowing action. The presence of a TEE probe, however, would complicate airway management during anesthetic induction. Thus, most anesthesiologists introduce TEE probes in anesthetized patients after tracheal intubation. It also is useful to evacuate the stomach via suction before probe insertion to improve image quality.

The passage of a TEE probe through the oral and pharyngeal cavities in anesthetized patients may be challenging at times. The usual technique is to place the well-lubricated probe in the posterior portion of the oropharynx with the transducer element pointing inferiorly and anteriorly. The remainder of the probe may be stabilized by looping the controls and the proximal portion of the probe over the operator's neck and shoulder. The operator's left hand then elevates the mandible by inserting the thumb behind the teeth, grasping the submandibular region with the fingers, and then gently lifting. The probe is then advanced against a slight but even resistance, until a loss of resistance is detected as the tip of the probe passes the inferior constrictor muscle of the pharynx. This usually occurs 10 cm past the lips in neonates to 20 cm past the lips in adults. Further manipulation of the probe is performed under echocardiographic guidance.

Difficult TEE probe insertion may be caused by the probe tip abutting the pyriform sinuses, vallecula, posterior tongue, or an esophageal diverticulum. Overinflation of the endotracheal tube cuff also could obstruct passage of the probe. Maneuvers that might aid the passage of the probe include changing the neck position, realigning the TEE probe, and applying additional jaw thrust by elevating the angles of the mandible. The probe also may be passed with the assistance of laryngoscopy. The probe should never be forced past an obstruction. This could result in airway trauma or esophageal perforation.

ANATOMY AND TEE VIEWS

Since the 1980s, perioperative TEE has become more recognized as a valuable hemodynamic monitor and diagnostic tool. In 1993, the ASE established the Council for Intraoperative Echocardiography (IOC) to address issues related to the rapidly increasing utility of TEE in the perioperative period and its important impact on anesthesia and surgical decision making. In 1997, the board members of the Council for Intraoperative Echocardiography decided to create the *ASE/SCA Guidelines for Performing a Comprehensive Intraoperative Multiplane Examination*,[61,91] which included the collective endorsement of a standard recommended set of anatomically directed cross-sectional views and the corresponding nomenclature. As implied in the original manuscript,[61,91] these guidelines were established with the following goals:

1. Facilitate training in intraoperative TEE by providing a framework in which to develop the necessary knowledge and skills.
2. Enhance and improve the technical quality and completeness of individual studies.
3. Facilitate the communication of intraoperative echocardiographic data between centers to provide a basis for multicenter investigations.
4. Standardize the description of intraoperative echocardiographic data to encourage industrial development of efficient and rapidly acquiring labeling, storage, and analysis systems.

The guidelines for the intraoperative TEE examination were not intended to be all-encompassing but rather to serve as a framework for a systematic and complete examination of cardiac and great vessel anatomy of the "normal patient and to serve as a baseline for later comparison."[61,91] This examination may require 20 minutes to complete by the beginner who must balance both comprehension and expedience in obtaining each 2D image and sequentially viewing one structure at a time. The experienced and competent echocardiographer, however, should be able to complete this examination in less than 10 minutes to provide timely and relevant diagnostic information. A more thorough intraoperative TEE examination, including the delineation of detailed intracardiac and extracardiac anatomy, description of congenital heart defects, and qualitative/quantitative Doppler analysis certainly is recommended and warranted in appropriate patients. Ideally, a complete intraoperative TEE examination not only provides information that is relevant to the particular diagnosis in question but also identifies unanticipated findings that may have a significant impact on

perioperative management (i.e., PFO, atrial thrombus, severe aortic atherosclerosis).

Multiplane Transesophageal Echocardiographic Probe Manipulation: Descriptive Terms and Technique

The process of obtaining a comprehensive intraoperative multiplane TEE examination begins with a fundamental understanding of the terminology and technique for probe manipulation (Figure 12-18). Efficient probe manipulation minimizes esophageal injury and facilitates the process of acquiring and sweeping through 2D image planes. Horizontal imaging planes are obtained by moving the TEE probe up and down (proximal and distal) in the esophagus at various depths relative to the incisors (*upper esophageal:* 20 to 25 cm; *midesophageal [ME]:* 30 to 40 cm; *TG:* 40 to 45 cm; *deep TG:* 45 to 50 cm; Table 12-6). Vertical planes are obtained by manually turning the probe to the patient's left or right. Further alignment of the imaging plane can be obtained by manually rotating one of the two control wheels on the probe handle that flexes the probe tip to the left or right direction or in the anterior or posterior plane. Multiplane probes may further facilitate interrogation of complex anatomic structures, such as the MV, by allowing up to 180 degrees of axial rotation of the imaging plane without manual probe manipulation.

The Comprehensive Intraoperative Transesophageal Echocardiographic Examination: Imaging Planes and Structural Analysis

Left and Right Ventricles

The left ventricle should be carefully examined for global and regional function using multiple transducer planes, depths, rotational, and angular orientations (Figure 12-19). Although a 17-segment model for assessing regional ventricular function has been developed,[92] the original comprehensive intraoperative TEE examination[61,91] proposed a regional assessment scheme that requires a systematic approach to evaluate each of the 16 individual LV segments: 6 basal, 6 mid, and 4 apical (Figure 12-20). Analysis of segmental function is based on a qualitative visual assessment that includes the following grading system of both LV wall thickness and motion (endocardial border excursion) during systole: 1 = normal (>30% thickening); 2 = mild hypokinesis (10% to 30% thickening); 3 = severe hypokinesis (<10% thickening); 4 = akinesis (no thickening); and 5 = dyskinesis (paradoxic motion). The *ME 4-chamber view* at 0 to 20 degrees (see Figure 12-19A) and *2-chamber* view at approximately 80 to 100 degrees (see Figure 12-19B) enable visualization of the septal and lateral, as well as the inferior and anterior, segments at the basal, mid, and apical level segments, respectively. The *ME long-axis (LAX) view* at 120 to 160 degrees (see Figure 12-19C) allows evaluation of the remaining anteroseptal and inferolateral LV segments. Because the left ventricle is usually oriented inferiorly to the true horizontal plane, slight retroflexion of the probe tip may be required to minimize LV foreshortening. The *transgastric mid-short-axis view (TG mid SAX)* at 0 to 20 degrees (see Figure 12-19D) is the most commonly utilized view for monitoring LV function because it allows a midpapillary assessment of the LV segments supplied by the corresponding coronary arteries (right, left circumflex, left anterior descending [LAD]). This view also enables qualitative and quantitative evaluation of pericardial effusions. Advancing or withdrawing the probe at the TG depth enables LV evaluation at the respective apical and basal levels (*TG basal SAX;* see Figure 12-19F). Further evaluation of the left ventricle can be obtained at the midpapillary TG depth by rotating the probe forward to the *TG 2-chamber* (80 to 100 degrees; see Figure 12-19E) and *TG LAX* (90 to 120 degrees; see Figure 12-19J). Global LV function requires assessment of dilatation (>6 cm at end-diastole), hypertrophy (>1.2 cm at end-diastole), and contractility. A more extensive quantitative evaluation of ventricular performance can be acquired by planimetry measurements of end-diastolic

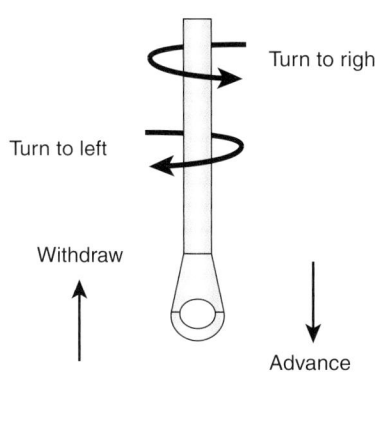

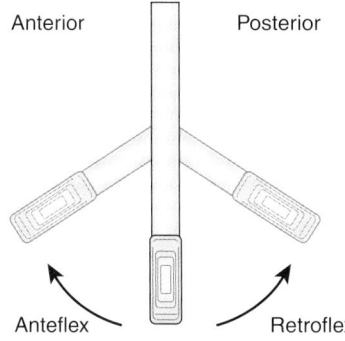

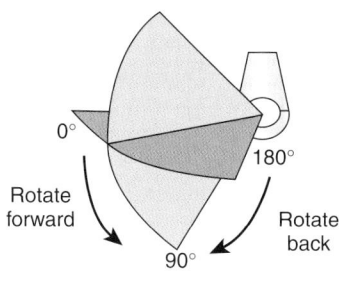

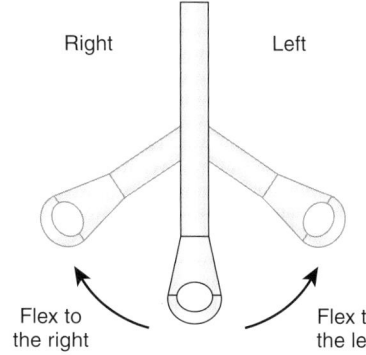

Figure 12-18 **Ways to adjust the probe.** *Top left,* Probe movement in the esophagus. *Top right,* Scanning angles obtained by crystal rotation. *Bottom left,* Movement of the tip forward and back. *Bottom right,* Movement of the tip from side to side.

TABLE 12-6	Comprehensive Intraoperative Multiplane Transesophageal Echocardiographic Examination
Probe Tip Depth (from lips) VIEW	*Upper Esophageal (20–25 cm)* AORTIC ARCH: LONG AXIS
Multiplane angle range	0 degrees
Anatomy imaged	Aortic arch; left brachiocephalic vein; left subclavian and carotid arteries; right brachiocephalic artery
Clinical utility	Ascending aorta and arch pathology: atherosclerosis, aneurysms and dissections; aortic CPB cannulation site evaluation
VIEW	AORTIC ARCH: SHORT AXIS
Multiplane angle range	90 degrees
Structures imaged	Aortic arch; left brachiocephalic vein; left subclavian and carotid arteries; right brachiocephalic artery Main pulmonary artery and pulmonic valve
Clinical utility	Ascending aorta and arch pathology: atherosclerosis, aneurysms and dissections; pulmonary embolus; pulmonary valve evaluation (insufficiency, stenosis, Ross procedure); pulmonary artery catheter placement
Probe Tip Depth VIEW	*Midesophageal (30–40 cm)* FOUR-CHAMBER
Multiplane angle range	0–20 degrees
Anatomy imaged	Left ventricle and atrium Right ventricle and atrium Mitral and tricuspid valves Interatrial and interventricle septa Left pulmonary veins: slight probe withdrawal and turning to left Right pulmonary veins: slight probe withdrawal and turning to right Coronary sinus: slight probe advancement and turn to right
Clinical utility	Ventricle function: global and regional Intracardiac chamber masses: thrombus, tumor, air; foreign bodies Mitral and tricuspid valve evaluation: pathology, pathophysiology Congenital or acquired interatrial and ventral septal defects Evaluation Hypertrophic obstructive cardiomyopathy evaluation Ventricular diastolic evaluation via transmitral and pulmonary vein Doppler flow profile analysis Pericardial evaluation: pericarditis; pericardial effusion Coronary sinus evaluation: coronary sinus catheter placement; dilation secondary to persistent left superior vena cava

(Continued)

TABLE 12-6	Comprehensive Intraoperative Multiplane Transesophageal Echocardiographic Examination—Cont'd
VIEW	**MITRAL COMMISSURAL**
Multiplane angle range	60–70 degrees
Anatomy imaged	Left ventricle and atrium
	Mitral valve
Clinical utility	Left ventricle function: global and regional
	Left ventricle and atrial masses: thrombus, tumor, air; foreign bodies
	Mitral valve evaluation: pathology, pathophysiology
	Ventricular diastolic evaluation via transmitral Doppler flow profile analysis
VIEW	**TWO-CHAMBER**
Multiplane angle range	80–100 degrees
Anatomy imaged	Left ventricle, atrium, and atrial appendage
	Mitral valve
	Left pulmonary veins: turning probe to left
	Coronary sinus (short axis or long axis by turning probe tip to left)
Clinical utility	Left ventricle function: global and regional
	Left ventricle and atrial masses: thrombus, tumor, air; foreign bodies
	Mitral valve evaluation: pathology, pathophysiology
	Ventricular diastolic evaluation via transmitral and pulmonary vein Doppler flow profile analysis
	Coronary sinus evaluation: coronary sinus catheter placement; dilation secondary to persistent left superior vena cava
VIEW	**LONG AXIS**
Multiplane angle range	120–160 degrees
Anatomy imaged	Left ventricle and atrium
	Left ventricular outflow tract
	Aortic valve
	Mitral valve
	Ascending aorta
Clinical utility	Left ventricle function: global and regional
	Left ventricle and atrial masses: thrombus, tumor, air; foreign bodies
	Mitral valve evaluation: pathology, pathophysiology;
	Ventricular diastolic evaluation via transmitral Doppler flow profile analysis
	Aortic valve evaluation: pathology, pathophysiology
	Ascending aorta pathology: atherosclerosis, aneurysms, dissections
	Hypertrophic obstructive cardiomyopathy evaluation
VIEW	**RIGHT VENTRICULAR INFLOW-OUTFLOW ("WRAPAROUND")**
Multiplane angle range	60–90 degrees
Anatomy imaged	Right ventricle and atrium
	Left atrium
	Tricuspid valve
	Aortic valve
	Right ventricular outflow tract
	Pulmonic valve and main pulmonary artery
Clinical utility	Right ventricle and atrial masses and left atrial: thrombus, embolus, tumor, foreign bodies
	Pulmonic valve and subpulmonic valve: pathology; pathophysiology
	Pulmonary artery catheter placement
	Tricuspid valve: pathology; pathophysiology
	Aortic valve: pathology; pathophysiology
VIEW	**AORTIC VALVE: SHORT AXIS**
Multiplane angle range	30–60 degrees
Anatomy imaged	Aortic valve
	Interatrial septum
	Coronary ostia and arteries
	Right ventricular outflow tract
	Pulmonary valve
Clinical utility	Aortic valve: pathology; pathophysiology
	Ascending aorta pathology: atherosclerosis, aneurysms and dissections
	Left and right atrial masses: thrombus, embolus, air, tumor, foreign bodies
	Congenital or acquired interatrial septal defects evaluation
VIEW	**AORTIC VALVE: LONG AXIS**
Multiplane angle range	120–160 degrees
Anatomy imaged	Aortic valve
	Proximal ascending aorta

TABLE 12-6	Comprehensive Intraoperative Multiplane Transesophageal Echocardiographic Examination—Cont'd
VIEW	**AORTIC VALVE: LONG AXIS**
	Left ventricular outflow tract
	Mitral valve
	Right pulmonary artery
Clinical utility	Aortic valve: pathology; pathophysiology
	Ascending aorta pathology: atherosclerosis, aneurysms and dissections
	Mitral valve evaluation: pathology, pathophysiology
VIEW	**BICAVAL**
Multiplane angle range	80–110 degrees
Anatomy imaged	Right and left atrium
	Superior vena cava (long axis)
	Inferior vena cava orifice: advance probe and turn to right to visualize inferior vena cava in the long axis, liver, hepatic and portal veins
	Interatrial septum
	Right pulmonary veins: turn probe to right
	Coronary sinus and thebesian valve
	Eustachian valve
Clinical utility	Right and left atrial masses: thrombus, embolus, air, tumor, foreign bodies
	Superior vena cava pathology: thrombus, sinus venosus atrial septal defect
	Inferior vena cava pathology (thrombus, tumor)
	Femoral venous line placement
	Coronary sinus catheter line placement
	Right pulmonary vein evaluation: anomalous return, Doppler evaluation for left ventricular diastolic function
	Congenital or acquired interatrial septal defects evaluation
	Pericardial effusion evaluation
VIEW	**ASCENDING AORTA: SHORT AXIS**
Multiplane angle range	0–60 degrees
Anatomy imaged	Ascending aorta
	Superior vena cava (short axis)
	Main pulmonary artery
	Right pulmonary artery
	Left pulmonary artery (turn probe tip to left)
	Pulmonic valve
Clinical utility	Ascending aorta pathology: atherosclerosis, aneurysms, and dissections
	Pulmonic valve: pathology; pathophysiology
	Pulmonary embolus/thrombus evaluation
	Superior vena cava pathology: thrombus, sinus venosus atrial septal defect
	Pulmonary artery catheter placement
VIEW	**ASCENDING AORTA LONG AXIS**
Multiplane angle range	100–150 degrees
Anatomy imaged	Ascending aorta
	Right pulmonary artery
Clinical utility	Ascending aorta pathology: atherosclerosis, aneurysms, and dissections
	Anterograde cardioplegia delivery evaluation
	Pulmonary embolus/thrombus
VIEW	**DESCENDING AORTA: SHORT AXIS**
Multiplane angle range	0 degrees
Anatomy imaged	Descending thoracic aorta
	Left pleural space
Clinical utility	Descending aorta pathology: atherosclerosis, aneurysms, and dissections
	Intra-aortic balloon placement evaluation
	Left pleural effusion
VIEW	**DESCENDING AORTA: LONG AXIS**
Multiplane angle range	90–110 degrees
Anatomy imaged	Descending thoracic aorta
	Left pleural space
Clinical utility	Descending aorta pathology: atherosclerosis, aneurysms, and dissections
	Intra-aortic balloon placement evaluation
	Left pleural effusion

(Continued)

TABLE 12-6	Comprehensive Intraoperative Multiplane Transesophageal Echocardiographic Examination—Cont'd
Probe Tip Depth	*Transgastric (40–45 cm)*
VIEW	BASAL SHORT AXIS
Multiplane angle range	0–20 degrees
Anatomy imaged	Left and right ventricle Mitral valve Tricuspid valve
Clinical utility	Mitral valve evaluation ("fish-mouth view"): pathology, pathophysiology Tricuspid valve evaluation: pathology, pathophysiology Basal left ventricular regional function Basal right ventricular regional function
VIEW	MID SHORT AXIS
Multiplane angle range	0–20 degrees
Anatomy imaged	Left and right ventricles Papillary muscles
Clinical utility	Mid-left and right ventricular regional and global function Intracardiac volume status
VIEW	TWO-CHAMBER
Multiplane angle range	80–100 degrees
Anatomy imaged	Left ventricle and atrium Mitral valve: chordae and papillary muscles Coronary sinus
Clinical utility	Left ventricular regional and global function (including apex) Left ventricular and atrial masses: thrombus, embolus, air, tumor, foreign bodies Mitral valve: pathology and pathophysiology
VIEW	LONG AXIS
Multiplane angle range	90–120 degrees
Anatomy imaged	Left ventricle and outflow tract Aortic valve Mitral valve
Clinical utility	Left ventricular regional and global function Mitral valve: pathology and pathophysiology Aortic valve: pathology and pathophysiology
VIEW	RIGHT VENTRICULAR INFLOW
Multiplane angle range	100–120 degrees
Anatomy imaged	Right ventricle and atrium Tricuspid valve: chordae and papillary muscles
Clinical utility	Right ventricular regional and global function Right ventricular and atrium masses: thrombus, embolus, tumor, foreign bodies Tricuspid valve: pathology and pathophysiology
Probe Tip Depth	*Deep Transgastric (45–50 cm)*
VIEW	LONG AXIS
Multiplane angle range	0–20 degrees (anteflexion)
Anatomy imaged	Left ventricle and outflow tract Interventricular septum Aortic valve and ascending aorta Left atrium Mitral valve Right ventricle Pulmonic valve
Clinical utility	Aortic valve and subaortic pathology and pathophysiology Mitral valve pathology and pathophysiology Left and right ventricle global function Left and right ventricle masses: thrombus, embolus, tumor Foreign bodies Congenital or acquired interventricular septal defect evaluation

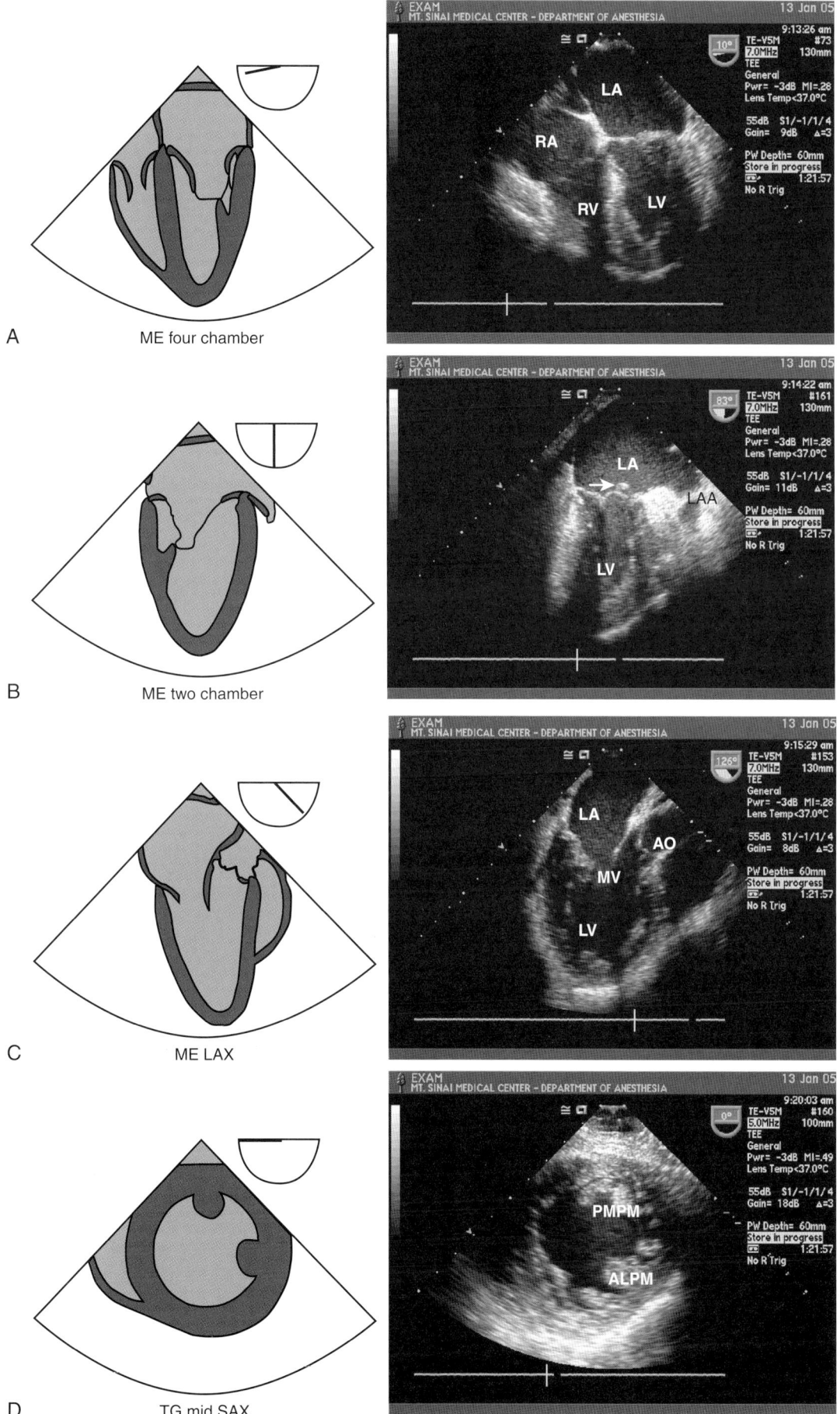

Figure 12-19 Schematic drawings of the comprehensive examination. *A,* Midesophageal (ME) four-chamber view. *B,* ME two-chamber view. *C,* ME long-axis (LAX) view. *D,* Transgastric (TG) mid short-axis (SAX) view.

(Continued)

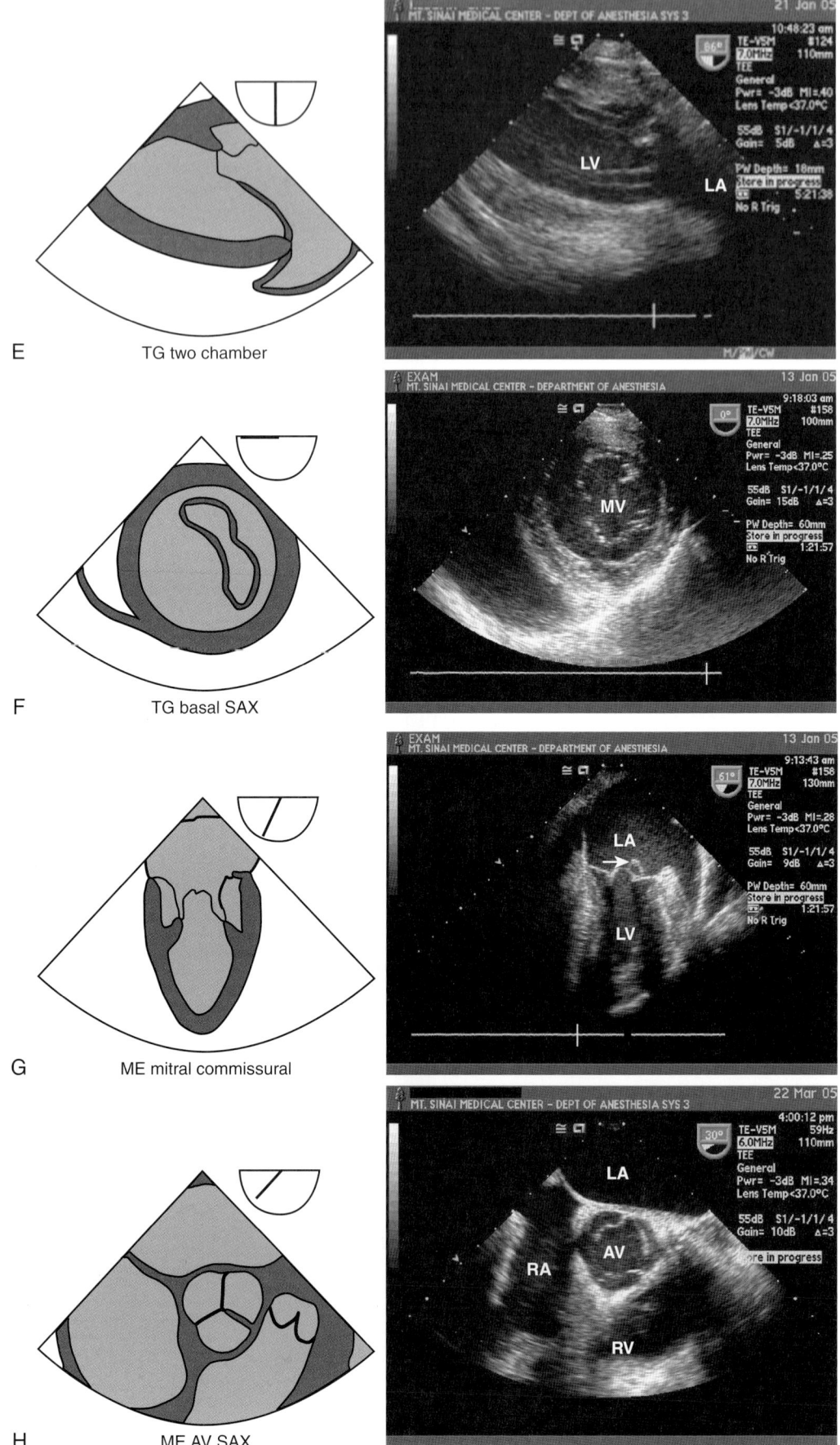

Figure 12-19—Cont'd   *E*, TG two-chamber view. *F*, TG basal SAX view. *G*, ME commissural. *H*, ME aortic valve (AV) SAX view.

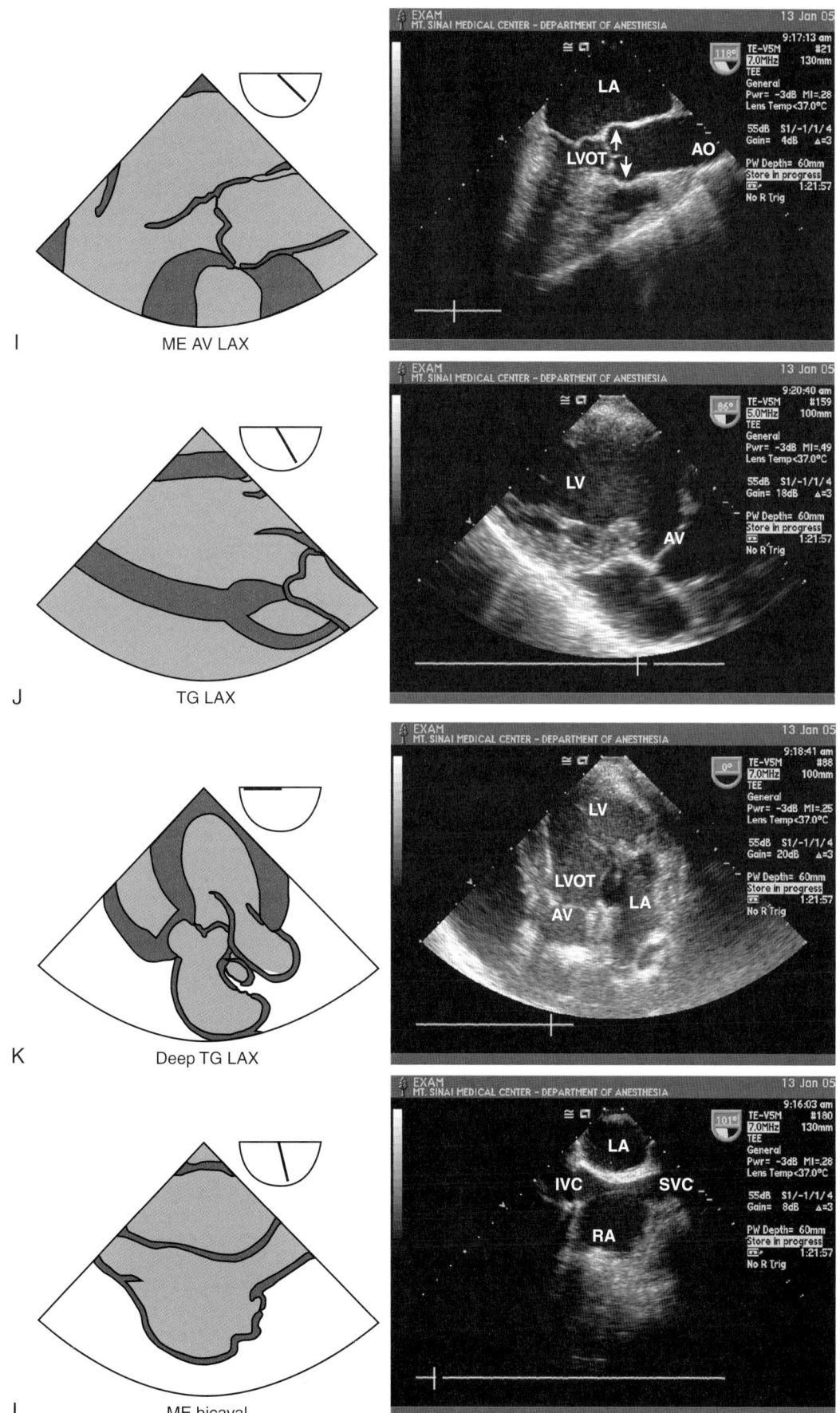

Figure 12-19—Cont'd *I*, ME AV LAX view. *J*, TG LAX view. *K*, Deep TG LAX view. *L*, ME bicaval.

(Continued)

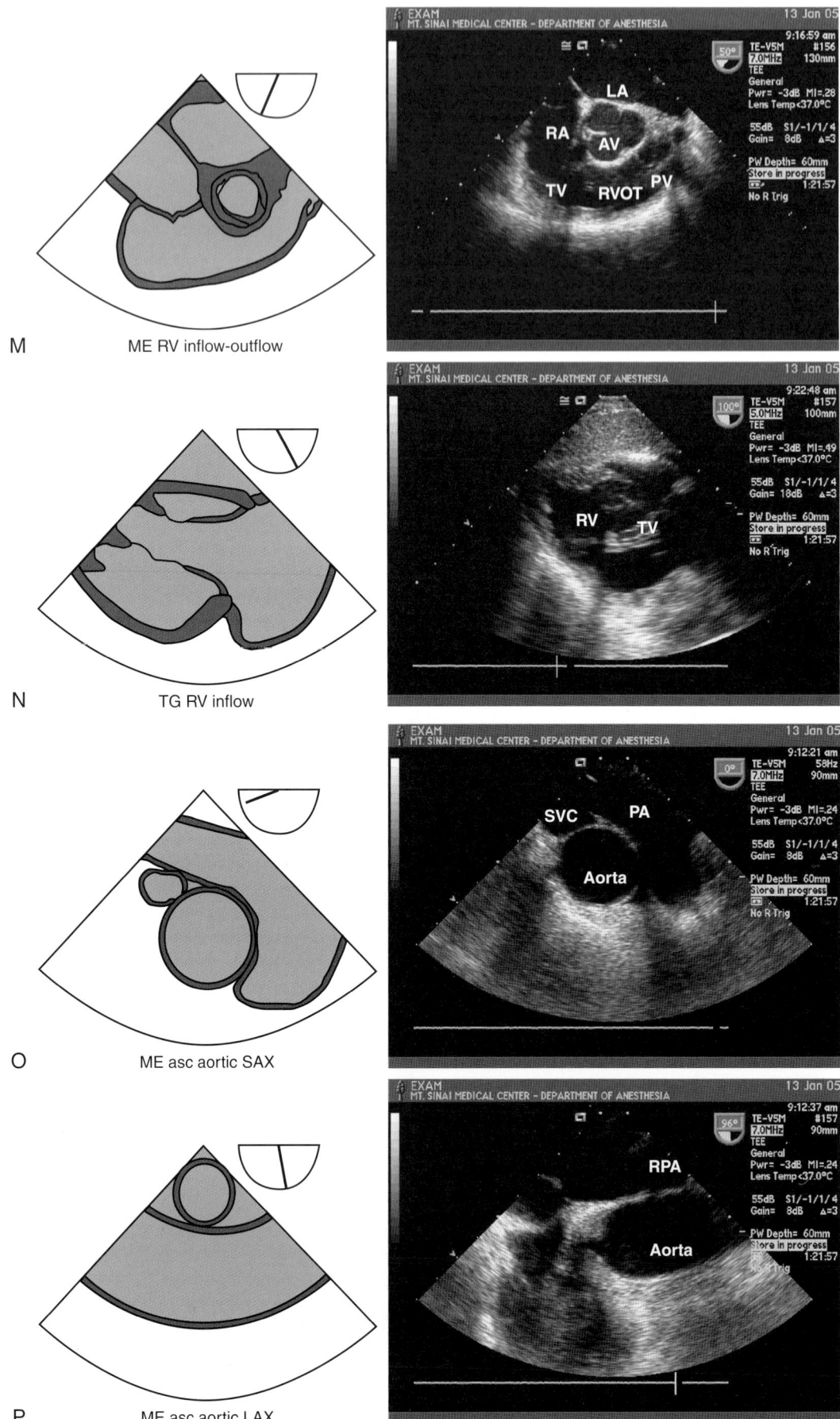

Figure 12-19—Cont'd *M*, ME RV inflow-outflow. *N*, TG RV inflow. *O*, ME ascending (Asc) aortic. *P*, ME Asc aortic LAX view.

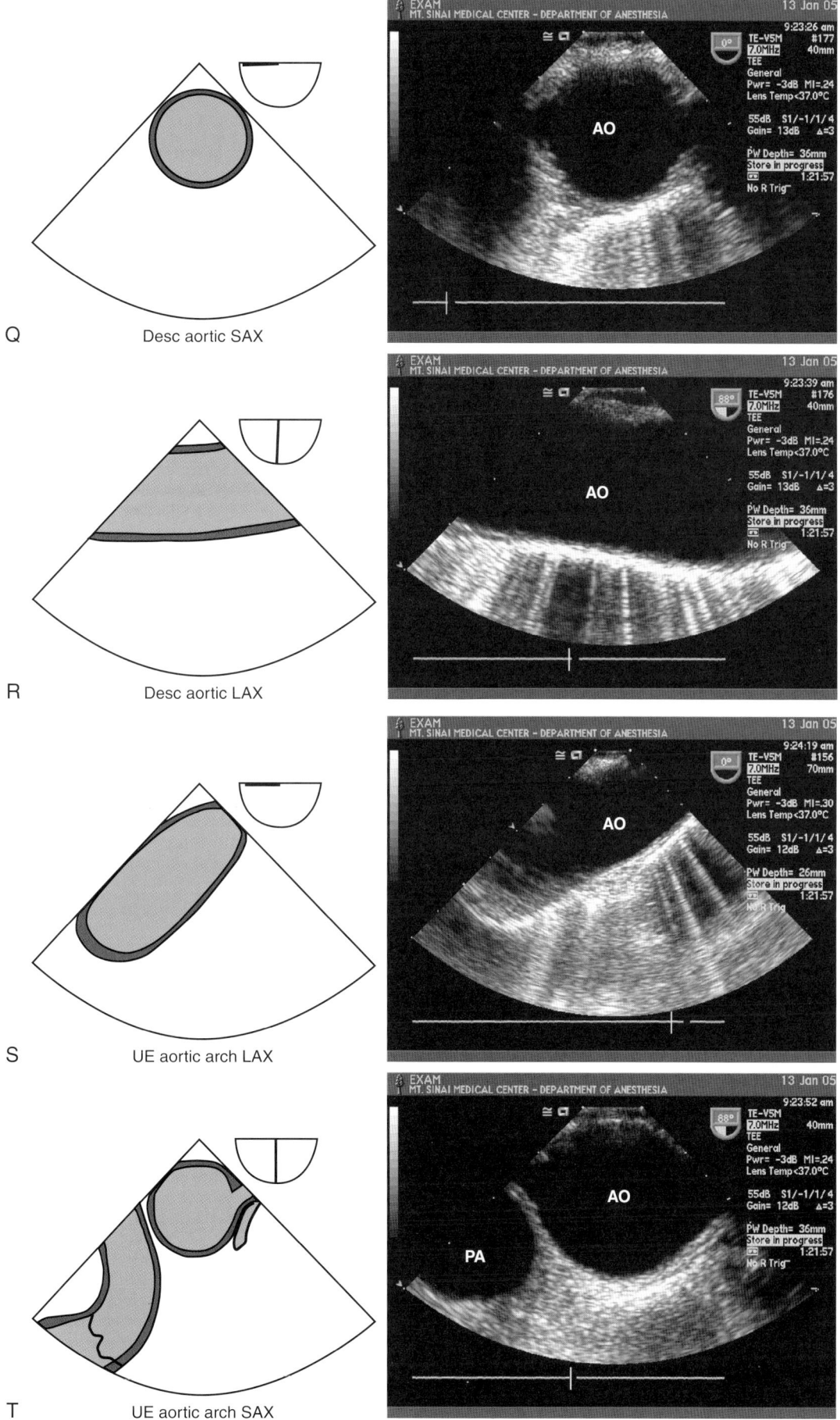

Figure 12-19—Cont'd *Q,* Descending (Desc) aortic SAX view. *R,* Desc aortic LAX view. *S,* Upper esophageal (UE) aortic arch LAX view. *T,* UE aortic arch SAX view. ALPM, anterior lateral papillary muscle; AO, aorta; IVC, inferior vena cava; LA, left atrium; LAA, left atrial appendage; LV, left ventricle; LVOT, left ventricular outflow tract; MV, mitral valve; PMPM, posterior medial papillary muscle; PV, pulmonic valve; RA, right atrium; RPA, right pulmonary artery; RV, right ventricle; RVOT, right ventricular outflow tract; SVC, superior vena cava; TV tricuspid valve.

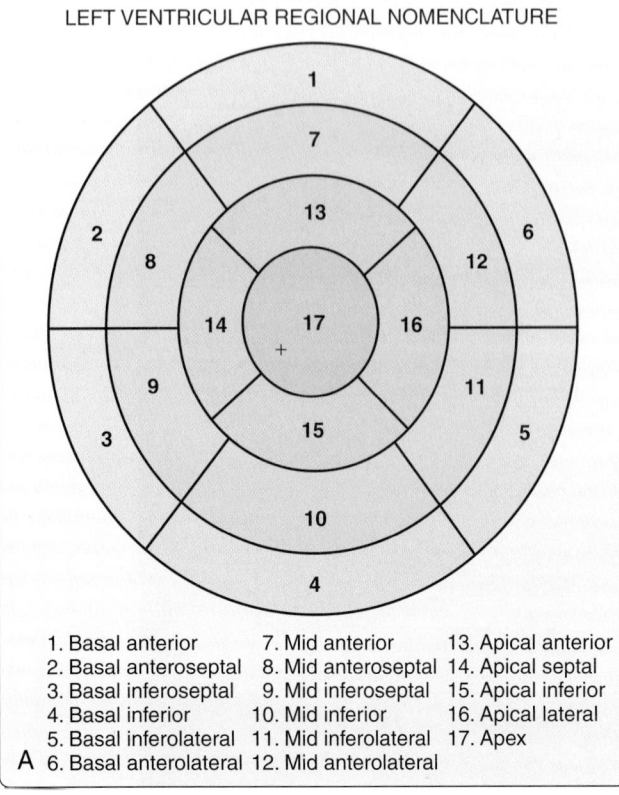

LEFT VENTRICULAR REGIONAL NOMENCLATURE

1. Basal anterior	7. Mid anterior	13. Apical anterior
2. Basal anteroseptal	8. Mid anteroseptal	14. Apical septal
3. Basal inferoseptal	9. Mid inferoseptal	15. Apical inferior
4. Basal inferior	10. Mid inferior	16. Apical lateral
5. Basal inferolateral	11. Mid inferolateral	17. Apex
6. Basal anterolateral	12. Mid anterolateral	

A

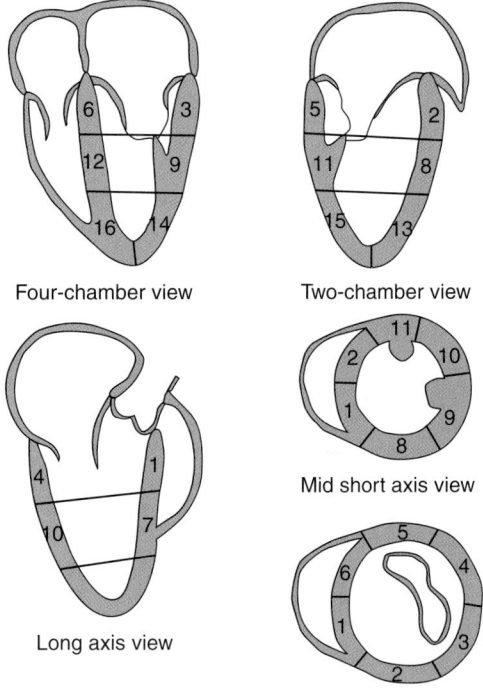

Four-chamber view   Two-chamber view

Long axis view

Mid short axis view

Basal short axis view

Basal segments	Mid segments	Apical segments
1 = Basal anteroseptal	7 = Mid anteroseptal	13 = Apical anterior
2 = Basal anterior	8 = Mid anterior	14 = Apical lateral
3 = Basal lateral	9 = Mid lateral	15 = Apical inferior
4 = Basal posterior	10 = Mid posterior	16 = Apical septal
5 = Basal inferior	11 = Mid inferior	
6 = Basal septal	12 = Mid septal	

B

Figure 12-20   Left ventricular segmental nomenclature. *A,* Seventeen segments; *B,* 16 segments.

and end-systolic areas from which ejection fractions (EFs), ventricular volumes, cardiac output, and mean circumferential shortening can be calculated.

RV regional and global function can be assessed from the *ME 4-chamber* view (see Figure 12-19A), which allows visualization of the septal and free walls. Although a formal segmental scheme has not been developed for the RV free wall, regional assessment of the septum can be performed. Turning the probe to the right and advancing slightly from the ME depth allows visualization of the tricuspid valve (TV), coronary sinus (CS), and RV apex. Rotating the probe between 60 and 90 degrees reveals the *ME RV inflow-outflow* view (see Figure 12-19M) in which the RA, TV, inferior RV free wall, right ventricular outflow tract (RVOT), pulmonic valve (PV), and main pulmonary artery (PA) can be viewed "wrapping around" the centrally oriented AV. This view often allows optimal Doppler beam alignment to evaluate the TV and also can be helpful for directing PA catheter floating and positioning. The *TG mid-SAX* view (see Figure 12-19D) displays the crescent-shaped, thinner-walled right ventricle to the left of the left ventricle (i.e., to the right side of the left ventricle). The *TG RV inflow* view (see Figure 12-19N) is developed by turning the probe to the right to center the right ventricle at this depth and rotating the multiplane angle forward to 100 to 120 degrees, thereby revealing the inferior RV free wall. Slight anteflexion, advancement, and rotation of the probe back toward 0 degrees often can reveal the RVOT and PV. Despite the asymmetric shape of the right ventricle, global function still can be assessed from the *ME 4-chamber, TG mid SAX, ME RV inflow-outflow,* and *TG RV inflow* views (see Figure 12-19A, D, M, N) using a quantitative evaluation scheme similar to that previously delineated for the left ventricle. Qualitative echocardiographic findings consistent with a diagnosis of global RV dysfunction include dilatation and hypertrophy, flattened or leftward shift of the atrial and ventricular septum, tricuspid regurgitation (TR), and a dilated CS.

Mitral Valve

The echocardiographic evaluation of the MV requires a thorough assessment of its leaflets (anterior and posterior), annulus, and the subvalvular apparatus (chordae tendineae, papillary muscles, and adjacent LV walls) to locate lesions and define the cause and severity of the pathophysiology. The mitral leaflets can be further divided into posterior leaflet scallops: lateral (P1), middle (P2), and medial (P3) that correspond with respective anterior leaflet sections: lateral third (A1), middle third (A2), and medial third (A3). The leaflets are united at the anterolateral and posteromedial commissures. The *ME 4-chamber view* (see Figure 12-19A) displays the larger appearing anterior leaflet (A3) to the left of the posterior leaflet (P1). Anteflexing the probe provides imaging of the anterolateral aspect of the MV, whereas gradual advancement of the probe and retroflexion shift the image plane to the posteromedial aspect of the MV. Maintaining the probe at the ME depth and rotating the multiplane angle forward to 60 to 70 degrees develops the *ME mitral commissural* view (see Figure 12-19G) in which A2 is flanked by P1 on the right and P3 on the left, giving A2 the appearance of a "trap-door" as it moves in and out of the imaging plane throughout the cardiac cycle. Further forward rotation of the probe to 80 to 100 degrees develops the *ME 2-chamber* view (see Figure 12-19B) revealing P3 to the left and A1 on the right. Final forward probe rotation to 120 to 160 degrees reveals the *ME LAX-view* (see Figure 12-19C), which images P2 on the left and A2 on the right. The *TG basal-SAX* view (see Figure 12-19F) enables visualization of both MV leaflets ("fish-mouth view") if the probe is anteflexed and withdrawn slightly from the mid-papillary level of the left ventricle. In this view, the posteromedial commissure is in the upper left, the anterolateral commissure to the lower right, the posterior leaflet is to the right, and anterior leaflet to the left of the displayed image. Rotation of the probe to 80 to 100 degrees develops the *TG 2-chamber* view (see Figure 12-19E) that is especially useful for evaluating the chordae tendineae and corresponding papillary muscles. Further functional evaluation of the MV requires a quantitative Doppler evaluation (PW Doppler, CW Doppler, and CFD) of transmitral and pulmonary venous flow for assessing MV regurgitation, stenotic lesions, and LV diastolic function.

Aortic Valve, Aortic Root, and Left Ventricular Outflow

The three cusps of the semilunar AV are best visualized simultaneously in the *ME AV-SAX* view (see Figure 12-19*H*), which is obtained by rotating the probe forward to 30 to 60 degrees. The noncoronary cusp is superior, lying adjacent to the atrial septum; the right cusp is inferiorly imaged; and the left cusp lies to the right, pointing in the direction of the left atrial appendage (LAA). This view permits planimetry of the AV orifice, evaluation of congenital anomalies of the AV (e.g., bicuspid AV), and qualitative assessment of aortic insufficiency (AI) when CFD is used. Withdrawing the probe slightly through the sinuses of Valsalva allows for imaging the right coronary artery inferiorly, as well as the left main coronary artery branching into the LAD and circumflex. The *ME AV-LAX* (see Figure 12-19*I*) view can be obtained at the same depth while rotating the probe to 120 to 160 degrees, allowing for visualization of the LVOT, AV annulus and leaflets (right and either noncoronary or left), sinuses of Valsalva, sinotubular junction, and proximal ascending aorta. This view is particularly useful for evaluating AI with CFD, systolic anterior motion of the MV, and proximal aortic pathology (dissections, aneurysms). Rotating the probe back to 90 to 120 degrees and advancing into the stomach to the TG level develops the *TG LAX*-view (see Figure 12-19*J*). In this view, the LVOT and AV are oriented to the right and inferiorly in the displayed image, thereby providing an optimal window for parallel Doppler beam alignment for the assessment of flows and pressure gradients (aortic stenosis [AS], hypertrophic obstructive cardiomyopathy). Rotating the probe back farther to 0 to 20 degrees, advancing deep into the stomach, and anteflexing the tip so that it lies adjacent to the LV apex allows for the development of the *deep TG LAX* view (see Figure 12-19*K*). This view provides optimal Doppler beam alignment for measuring trans-AV and LVOT flow velocities and also may provide an additional window for assessing flows through muscular ventricular septal defects and LV apical pathology (thrombus, aneurysms).

Tricuspid Valve

The echocardiographic evaluation of the TV requires a thorough assessment of its three leaflets (anterior, posterior, and septal), annulus, chordae tendineae, papillary muscles, and the corresponding RV walls. In the *ME 4-chamber* view (see Figure 12-19*A*), the septal TV leaflet is displayed on the right side and the posterior TV leaflet on the left side of the annulus. Rotating the multiplane angle to 60 to 90 degrees develops the *ME RV inflow-outflow* view (see Figure 12-19*M*), which displays the anterior TV leaflet on the left side of the image and the septal TV leaflet on the right side of the image adjacent to the AV. The *TG RV inflow* view (see Figure 12-19*N*) is obtained by advancing the probe into the stomach and rotating to 100 to 120 degrees. This view is ideal for visualizing the chordae tendineae and papillary muscles in the right ventricle. Rotating back to the *TG mid-SAX* at 0 to 20 degrees and slightly withdrawing the probe provides a cross-sectional view of the TV, displaying the anterior leaflet displayed in the far field, the posterior leaflet to the left in the near field, and the septal leaflet on the right side of the image. A more extensive quantitative analysis of TV pathophysiology requires the use of Doppler echocardiography (PW Doppler, CW Doppler, and CFD) by aligning the beam parallel to transtricuspid flow in either the *ME RV inflow-outflow* or *ME 4-chamber* views.

Pulmonic Valve and Pulmonary Artery

The PV is a trileaflet, semilunar valve. The *ME AV SAX* view (see Figure 12-19*H*) displays the transition between the RVOT and PV. Rotating the probe back toward 0 degrees and withdrawing slightly develops the *ME ascending aortic SAX* view (see Figure 12-19*O*), displaying the transition between the PV and main PA and its bifurcation. Although the right PA usually is easy to visualize by turning the probe to the right, the left PA often is obscured by the interposing, air-filled, left mainstem bronchus. This view can be used in the Doppler echocardiographic assessment of PV pathophysiology because of the parallel alignment of the beam relative to the flow and can be used to locate pulmonary emboli. The *ME RV inflow-outflow* (see Figure 12-19*M*) view also can be used to assess the PV and main PA, which lie on the right side of the

image adjacent to the AV, although the *upper esophageal aortic arch SAX* view (see Figure 12-19*T*), which displays the PV oriented to the left of the cross-sectional view of the aortic arch, usually provides a more parallel Doppler beam orientation for the evaluation of pulmonic regurgitation or stenosis. Withdrawing the probe slightly in the *deep TG LAX* view (see Figure 12-19*K*) in combination with slight anteflexion and turning to the right often can allow visualization of the RVOT and PV to the left in the far field and provide an alternative imaging plane for Doppler echocardiographic evaluation in patients with subpulmonic and pulmonary valve pathology.

Left Atrium, Left Atrial Appendage, Pulmonary Veins, and Atrial Septum

The left atrium (LA) is the closest cardiac structure to the TEE probe when positioned in the esophagus. Consequently, the LA usually is easily displayed in the superior aspect of the 2D image sector. The *ME 4-chamber view* (see Figure 12-19*A*) displays the LA almost in its entirety, with the LAA oriented to its superior and lateral aspect when the probe is slightly withdrawn. The muscular ridges of the pectinate muscles within the LAA should not be confused with thrombi. Slight further withdrawal of the probe and turning it to the left allow the left upper pulmonary vein to be imaged as it enters the LA from the anterior-to-posterior direction, separated from the lateral border of the LAA by the "warfarin ridge." In contrast with the left upper pulmonary vein, which is usually optimally aligned for parallel Doppler beam alignment, the left lower pulmonary vein enters the LA just below the left upper pulmonary vein in a lateral-to-medial direction and is more perpendicularly aligned. Pulmonary venous Doppler flow velocity profiles are useful for the qualitative and quantitative assessment of LV diastolic function. Turning the probe to the right at this depth reveals the right upper pulmonary vein entering the LA in an anterior-to-posterior direction. The right lower pulmonary vein sometimes can be visualized as it enters perpendicular to the long axis of the LA by slightly advancing the probe. The interatrial septum, consisting of thicker limbus regions flanking the thin fossa ovalis, also can be imaged in the *ME 4-chamber view* (see Figure 12-19*A*). Benign lipomatous hypertrophy of the interatrial septum must be distinguished from pathologic lesions such as atrial myxomas. The patency of the interatrial septum and presence of a PFO or congenital atrial septal defects should be assessed with Doppler echocardiography and intravenous injections of agitated saline. Advancing and rotating the probe to 80 to 100 degrees develops the *ME 2-chamber view* (see Figure 12-19*B*), which allows for further imaging of the LA from left to right. The LAA and left upper pulmonary vein can be seen by turning the probe slightly to the left. Rotating the probe to the right at this level and adjusting the multiplane angle to 80 to 110 degrees develop the *ME bicaval view* (see Figure 12-19*L*), which delineates the superior vena cava entering the RA to the right of the image and the inferior vena cava entering from the left. The interatrial septum can be seen in the middle of the image separating the LA and RA. The right upper pulmonary vein and right lower pulmonary vein usually can be seen if the probe is turned farther to the right just beyond the point at which the long axis of the superior vena cava can no longer be visualized. This transition of images also can be used in conjunction with Doppler echocardiography to identify sinus venosus atrial septal defects and anomalous pulmonary venous return.

Right Atrium and Coronary Sinus

The RA can be visualized most easily in the *ME four-chamber* view (see Figure 12-19*A*) by turning the probe to the patient's right side. In this view, the entire RA can be visualized for size, overall function, and presence of masses (thrombi, tumors). Rotating the multiplane angle to 80 to 110 degrees develops the *ME bicaval* view (see Figure 12-19*L*), which displays the RA and its internal structures (Eustachian valve, Chiari network, crista terminalis). The superior vena cava can be imaged entering the RA on the right, superior to the right atrial appendage, and the inferior vena cava enters the RA on the left of the display. Advancing and turning the probe to the right allow for a qualitative evaluation of the intrahepatic segment of the inferior vena cava and hepatic veins.

Pacemaker electrodes and central venous catheters for hemodynamic monitoring or CPB can be easily imaged in this view.

The CS lies posteriorly in the atrioventricular groove, emptying into the RA at the inferior extent of the atrial septum. The CS can be viewed in long axis entering the RA just superior to the tricuspid annulus by advancing and slightly retroflexing the probe from the *ME 4-chamber* view (see Figure 12-19A). The CS can be imaged cross sectionally in short axis in the *ME 2-chamber* (see Figure 12-19B) view in the upper left of the display. Turning the probe to the left in this view often allows visualization of the CS in long axis as it traverses the atrioventricular groove. The CS and thebesian valve also can be visualized in the *ME-bicaval* view (see Figure 12-19L) on the upper right of the image as it enters the RA at an obtuse angle, by turning the probe leftward simultaneously with retro and leftward flexion. Echocardiographic visualization of the CS can be useful for directing the placement of CS catheters used for CPB.

Thoracic Aorta

The proximal and mid-ascending thoracic aorta can be visualized in short axis in the *ME ascending aortic SAX* view (see Figure 12-19O). Advancing and withdrawing the probe should enable visualization of the thoracic aorta from the sinotubular junction to a point 4 to 6 cm superior to the AV and allow inspection for aneurysms and dissections. Rotating the multiplane angle to 100 to 150 degrees develops the *ME ascending aortic LAX* view (see Figure 12-19P), which optimally displays the parallel anterior and posterior walls for measuring proximal and mid-ascending aortic diameters. This view also can be obtained from the *ME AV LAX* view (see Figure 12-19I) by slightly withdrawing and turning the probe to the left.

TEE imaging of the aortic arch often is obscured by the interposing, air-filled trachea. The most optimal views of the aortic arch are obtained by withdrawing the probe from the *ME ascending aortic SAX* view at 0 degrees (see Figure 12-19O) and rotating to the left to obtain the *upper esophageal aortic arch LAX* view (see Figure 12-19S), which displays the proximal arch followed by the mid-arch, the great vessels (brachiocephalic, left carotid, and left subclavian artery), and distal arch before it joins the proximal descending thoracic aorta imaged in cross section. Alternatively, rotating the probe to 90 degrees develops the *upper esophageal aortic arch SAX* view (see Figure 12-19T). Turning the probe to the left in this view delineates the transition of the distal arch with the proximal descending thoracic aorta. Turning the probe to the right and slightly withdrawing allows for the mid-arch and great vessels to be imaged on the right side of the screen, followed by the distal ascending aorta when the probe is subsequently advanced and rotated forward to the 120-degree *ME ascending aortic long-LAX* view (see Figure 12-19P). Epiaortic aortic scanning may be particularly useful for assessing the extent of ascending aortic and arch pathology (i.e., aneurysms, dissection, atherosclerosis) to determine cross-clamping and cannulation sites for CPB.

A SAX image of the descending thoracic aorta is obtained by turning the probe leftward from the *ME 4-chamber* view (see Figure 12-19A) to produce the *descending aortic SAX* view (see Figure 12-19Q). Rotating the multiplane angle of the probe from 0 to 90 to 110 degrees produces a LAX image, the *descending aortic LAX* view (see Figure 12-19R). The descending thoracic aorta should be interrogated in its entirety, beginning at the distal aortic arch, by continually advancing the probe and turning slightly to the left until the celiac and superior mesenteric arteries are visualized branching tangentially from the anterior surface of the abdominal aorta when the probe is in the stomach. Thorough examination of the descending thoracic aorta may be necessary to evaluate the distal extent of an aneurysm or dissection. In addition, the *descending aortic SAX and LAX* views can be useful for confirming appropriate intra-aortic balloon positioning.

Epiaortic Ultrasonography

Neurologic injury after CPB remains a devastating complication of cardiac surgery. Possible causative factors include hypoperfusion, lack of pulsatile flow, and cerebral embolization of gaseous or particulate matter. The thoracic aorta is a potential source of such emboli because it often contains atherosclerotic plaques, and it may be instrumented multiple times during cardiac operations. TEE also can be used to detect aortic intraluminal thrombi and plaques. One major limitation is that the distal ascending and proximal transverse aorta are not well visualized by TEE.[93] Although the entire ascending aorta is not well visualized, TEE can serve as a screen to detect aortic atherosclerotic debris.[94] The presence of atherosclerotic disease in the visualized portions increases the likelihood of finding atherosclerotic changes in the nonvisualized portion of the aorta. Intraoperatively, this region can be scanned by placing a sterilely wrapped probe directly on the aorta to rule out pathology in the locations of planned instrumentation. Once the disease is defined, it often can be avoided during instrumentation, and hopefully, neurologic injury can be prevented. This epiaortic scanning is more sensitive than digital palpation in the detection of atherosclerotic disease, and its use has modified surgical management during the conduct of cardiac surgery.[95] Although epiaortic scanning may be justified for all patients presenting for cardiac surgery, its use should be seriously considered in those patients with increased risk for embolic stroke, including those patients with a history of cerebrovascular or peripheral vascular disease or those patients with evidence of aortic disease by any modality.[96] Phased-array probes generally are used for perioperative aortic scanning. Because of the fan-shaped sector displayed, the most anterior aspect of the aorta cannot be adequately visualized unless a standoff is used between the transducer and the aorta. It usually is most convenient to fill the pericardial cradle with saline and hold the probe approximately 1 cm anterior to the aorta while scanning.

A complete examination will include SAX views of the proximal, middle, and distal ascending aorta and LAX views of both the ascending aorta and arch. These views will allow for evaluation of the 12 areas of the aorta: anterior, posterior, left and right lateral walls of the proximal, middle, and distal ascending aorta. The proximal ascending aorta is defined as the region from the sinotubular junction to the proximal intersection of the right PA. The mid-ascending aorta includes that portion of the aorta that is adjacent to the right PA. The distal ascending aorta extends from the distal intersection of the right PA to the origin of the innominate artery. The severity of atherosclerosis may be graded according to the classification described by Katz et al[97] and is summarized in Table 12-7.

■ Three-Dimensional Views

Mitral Valve Apparatus

To ensure a high success rate of MV reconstruction, the cardiac anesthesiologist must have detailed understanding and insight into the mechanism responsible for regurgitant lesions and identify these echocardiographically. The MV apparatus can best be viewed by utilizing the 3D zoom mode. The data block should be spatially orientated to view the MV from the left atrial perspective, with the AV positioned at the top of the monitor (12 o'clock). This orientation, commonly referred to as the "surgeon's view," puts the MV in an anatomically correct position. This mode is especially useful in patients with atrial fibrillation, an arrhythmia frequently encountered in patients with MV disease, because it represents a live and instantaneous imaging mode

TABLE 12-7	Quantification of Aortic Atherosclerotic Disease	
Grade	Description
I	Normal to mild intimal thickening
II	Severe intimal thickening without protruding atheroma
III	Atheroma protruding < 5 mm into lumen
IV	Atheroma protruding ≥ 5 mm into lumen
V	Any thickness with mobile component or components

Adapted from Katz ES, Tunick PA, Rusinek H, et al: Protruding aortic atheromas predict stroke in elderly patients undergoing cardiopulmonary bypass: Experience with intraoperative transesophageal echocardiography. *J Am Coll Cardiol* 20:70–77, 1992.

not influenced by gating artifacts. Occasionally, in patients with Barlow disease, the valve is so grotesquely enlarged that temporal resolution suffers from the large sector required to image the entire valve. In these cases, a full-volume mode is best used, allowing the imager not only to visualize the entire valve but also maintain acceptable image and temporal resolution as well.

Although a comprehensive 2DE examination can identify the mechanism of regurgitation in most cases, 3DE can not only identify the mechanism but also provide information in regards to annular and leaflet geometry, which cannot be obtained by 2D imaging. Measurements that can be easily obtained include (1) the major anatomically oriented 3D axes of the annulus, anteroposterior (A-P) and anterolateral-posteromedial (AL-PM) diameters, as well as annular height; (2) 3D curvilinear leaflet lengths and areas of all segments (A1, A2, A3, P1, P2, P3); (3) total and functional anterior and posterior leaflet surface areas; and (4) the angle between the AV annulus and the MV annulus (aortomitral angle). A narrow angle should alert the imager to the possibility of systolic anterior motion during the postrepair period (Figure 12-21).

Aortic and Tricuspid Valves

Unlike the MV, acquiring high-quality images of the AV and TV represents a more difficult undertaking. The explanation lies, on the one hand, in the thinner leaflet tissue that generally comprises both the AV and TV and, on the other hand, on the orientation of the tissue as a reflector. Because these factors result in weaker acoustic signal strength, the 3D volume renderer is more apt to tag these as transparent and render the voxels as blood—that is, invisible. Caution must be taken by the echocardiographer not to misdiagnose these imaging artifacts as perforations.

Congenital and Interventional Procedures

CHD is complex and characterized by multiple variants. 3DE can enable improved understanding of CHD anatomy. The ability to spatially orient the data block to allow for views of atrial or ventricular septal defects and their relation to adjacent structures represents a milestone in improving understanding of these complex disease processes. The size and location of intracardiac shunts are crucial parameters when evaluating whether to pursue an interventional procedure. The understanding of congenital valvular pathology (e.g., cleft MV, Ebstein's anomaly) can be greatly enhanced by 3DE. Thus, real-time 3DE offers improved insight for diagnosing valve defects and predicting the success of a surgical valve repair (Figure 12-22).

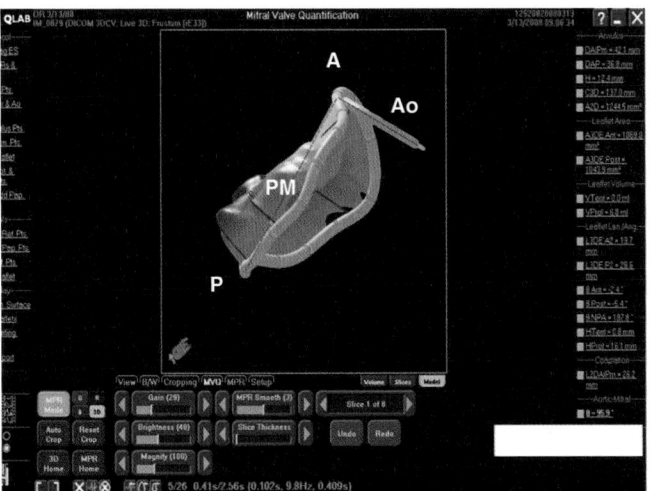

Figure 12-21 Mitral valve quantification (MVQ) showing the aortomitral angle of 95.9 degrees. Patient at increased risk for development of systolic anterior motion (SAM) after mitral valve repair surgery. A, anterior; Ao, aorta; P, posterior; PM, posteromedial.

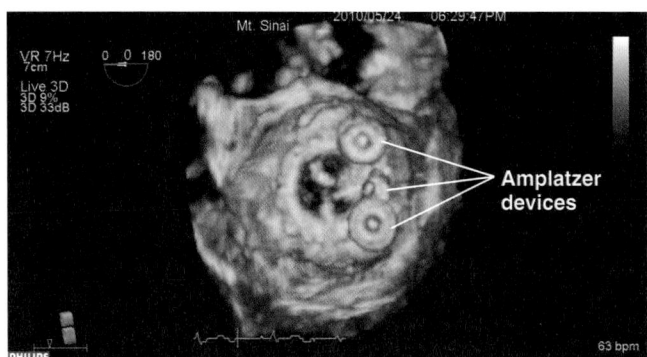

Figure 12-22 Patient with multiple paravalvular leaks. Percutaneous intervention successfully deploying three Amplatzer devices.

CLINICAL APPLICATIONS

Ventricular Function

Systolic Function

The echocardiographic assessment of global and regional LV function consists of 2D or Doppler evaluation of cardiac structures and their interaction with blood flow. The techniques used are mostly visual and subjective[98,99]; thus, they are not always accurate or error-free. Adequate visualization and accurate tracing of the endocardial–blood pool interface during the cardiac cycle,[100] precise measurement of an orifice diameter, and parallel orientation between the Doppler beam and direction of blood flow[101] are paramount in producing unidimensional (fractional shortening [FS]) or 2D estimates (fractional area change, stroke volume [SV], and EF),[102] as suggested by published guidelines.[100] The evaluation of regional LV function based on the degree of systolic myocardial thickening is highly subjective[99] and inaccurate if imaging is suboptimal (as happens in myocardial segments lying parallel to propagation of ultrasound, or when the epicardium is not seen). Furthermore, impairment of regional function does not cause reduction in LVEF unless several segments are involved.

Conventional TEE methods cannot discriminate the effects of load on contractility (i.e., impaired contractility and falsely high EF in severe mitral regurgitation, or intact contractility and falsely low EF in severe AS). Calculation of the rate of LV systolic pressure increase (LV + dP/dt) requires presence of a mitral regurgitation jet,[103] whereas contractility indices such as end-systolic elastance, preload-recruitable stroke work, or myocardial performance index are too complicated for clinical application.[104] In addition, all conventional echocardiographic methods examine only a single LV diameter or tomographic plane at a time. Taking into consideration the frequent LV foreshortening that occurs in the ME tomographic planes or the presence of segmental abnormalities (particularly in patients with CAD), it is easy to realize why true representation of global LV function is not always feasible with these methods.

Ejection-Phase Indices

Using echocardiography, contractility has been estimated most frequently with ejection-phase indices. A wide array of ejection-phase indices have been described, but all require that end–diastolic and end–systolic dimensions be measured. In M–mode echocardiography, these dimensions often will be simple, linear, internal dimensions of the LV cavity. The following ratio will yield percentage fractional shortening (FS), a basic ejection-phase index of contractility, with normal values between 25% and 45%:

$$FS = (LVIDD - LVISD)/LVIDD$$

where LVIDD = LV internal diastolic dimension, and LVISD = LV internal systolic dimension. The LV dimensions are measured at the level of the tips of the MV leaflets, and FS is considered representative of global LV systolic function in symmetrically contracting left ventricle.

With 2DE, multiple tomographic cuts can be obtained and utilized to calculate ventricular volumes using a variety of formula such as Simpson's rule.[105] Using the ventricular volumes, EF can be calculated using the standard formula:

$$EF = (LVEDV - LVESV)/LVEDV$$

where LVEDV = LV end-diastolic volume, and LVESV = LV end-systolic volume.

During intraoperative TEE, it is most convenient to monitor a single, TG SAX view at the level of the midpapillary muscles. Once the end-diastolic and end-systolic endocardial areas have been delineated with the help of tracing software, contractility may be estimated using the fractional area change (FAC), with normal values in the range of 60%:

$$FAC = (LVEDA - LVESA)/LVEDA$$

where LVEDA = LV end-diastolic area, and LVESA = LV end-systolic area.

Isovolumic Phase Indices

The standard isovolumic phase index, dP/dt, cannot be obtained using TEE. Some information on the isovolumic phase, however, can be gathered by measuring the length of the pre-ejection period. The pre-ejection period is the time between the onset of the Q wave on the ECG and the opening of the AV on M-mode echocardiography. The usefulness and limitations of pre-ejection period, as well as of the other systolic time intervals, have been extensively reviewed elsewhere.[106,107]

The maximal acceleration of blood flow in the aorta is another measurement related to the isovolumic phase of contraction.[108] Maximal blood flow acceleration occurs in the early part of LV ejection and can be measured by Doppler echocardiography. It is determined using transthoracic echocardiography by placing a Doppler transducer in the suprasternal notch and aiming the ultrasound beam at the AV. A variety of studies have demonstrated that maximum blood flow acceleration, sampled in this manner, provides information on LV contractility.[109-111] However, the currently available TEE imaging planes are not suitable for this type of measurement.

The circumferential fiber-shortening rate (Vcf) is an index of contractility that incorporates a time-related element and seems to be less preload dependent than EF:

$$Vcf = EDC - ESC / EDC \times LVET$$

where EDC and ESC are the end-diastolic and end-systolic circumferences of the left ventricle, respectively, measured at the TG SAX view; LVET is the LV ejection time obtained from a Doppler analysis of the left ventricular outflow tract (LVOT). Its value in normal individuals is 1.2 ± 0.1 circumferences/sec.

Strain, Strain Rate

The recent technologic advances in signal processing in Doppler (Doppler tissue imaging [DTI] and Doppler strain echocardiography) and ultrasound (2D speckle tracking imaging [STI]) enable measurement of tissue velocity and deformation in one or two dimensions, which provide high-quality, precise, and objective information regarding regional and/or global myocardial function in real time, decrease the subjectivity of the interpretation, and increase the diagnostic accuracy.

Myocardial Structure and Motion

Myocardial fibers are organized in layers, forming a leftward helix in subepicardium, which transitions to a rightward helix in subendocardium (Figure 12-23). Because LV muscle volume remains constant during the cardiac cycle, this myocardial fiber arrangement results in longitudinal (along the major axis) and circumferential (tangent to

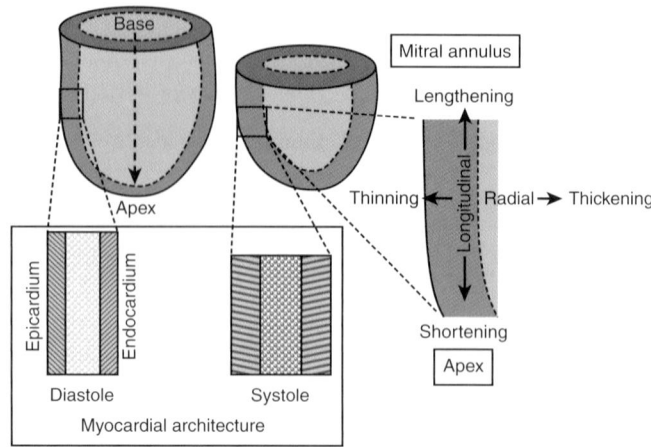

Figure 12-23 Myocardial architecture consists of helical (left-handed in epicardium and right-handed in endocardium) and circumferential (in midmyocardium) layers of myocardial fibers. This fiber arrangement results in longitudinal (mitral annulus to apex), radial (epicardium to endocardium), and circumferential (tangentially to epicardium) motions during systole and diastole. TEE, transesophageal echocardiogram.

the periphery) thinning and radial (along the minor axis) thickening during systole, with opposite directed changes in diastole.[112]

This 3D global cardiac motion cannot be appreciated during conventional TEE imaging, in which only radial motion (inward endocardial excursion and myocardial thickening in ME or TG views), related to midmyocardium function, is evaluated. Longitudinal (ME views) and circumferential motion (TG views) are difficult to evaluate. However, both radial and longitudinal motions are important. In systole, radial thickening predominates; 40% radial thickening is accompanied by 14% longitudinal shortening.[104] On the other, the first myocardial layer affected by ischemia is the subendocardium, which provides for longitudinal motion.[113] The subjective evaluation of regional LV motion is also limited during conventional TEE because the passive motion of a noncontracting segment, due to tethering to adjacent segments, cannot be reliably excluded. Many of these limitations can be overcome by assessing myocardial deformation (strain).

Deformation

Myocardial strain (S or ε) is the (systolic) deformation of a myocardial fiber, normalized to its original length:

$$S = \frac{L_1 - L_0}{L_0} \bullet 100 (\%)$$

where L_0 is the baseline (end-diastolic) length, and L_1 is the end-systolic length.[105]

By definition, strain is positive when the systolic dimension increases (the myocardial fiber lengthens or thickens) and negative when the systolic dimension decreases (the myocardial fiber shortens or thins). Therefore, radial thickening is associated with positive strain ($L_1 > L_0$), whereas longitudinal shortening and circumferential thinning are associated with negative strain ($L_1 < L_0$). Radial strain relates to motion from the endocardium to the epicardium; circumferential strain relates to motion along the circumference (curvature) of the left ventricle; and longitudinal strain relates to motion from the base to the LV apex.

Echocardiographically measured strain is measured in relation to time (t) and is called *Lagrangian* strain: (t) = [L(t) − L(t₀)]/L(t₀), where L(t₀) is the end-diastolic shape. For a 2D object, there is normal deformation (the motion is normal to the borders of the object and occurs along both the x-axis and y-axis) and shear deformation (motion occurs parallel to the borders of the object). For a 3D object, such as a myocardial segment, there are three *normal* strains (along the x-, y-, z-axes), and six *shear* strains (along the combinations of the different axes).[114] Because fiber contraction causes myocardial deformation, strain is a measure of myocardial contractile function. Echocardiographic deformation can be measured from velocity gradient using DTI[115] (or non-Doppler tracking of speckles [STI]).[116]

Strain rate (SR) reflects how fast regional myocardial deformation (strain) occurs, that is, strain rate expresses the speed of deformation:

$$SR = S/t (\%/sec)$$

where t is the time duration of this deformation (Figure 12-24).

Echocardiographic strain measurements with either technique have been validated against sonomicrometry[116,117] or magnetic resonance[118,119] imaging (MRI), with r values of 0.96 for strain and 0.94 for strain rate.[120] For normal myocardium, strain rate reflects regional contractile function because it is being relatively independent of HR, whereas systolic strain reflects changes in SV.[121,122] Evaluated with DTI or tagged cardiac MRI, LV regional strains increased from base to apex and from endocardium to epicardium.[114,123,124] Normal values are −16% to −24% (longitudinal strain), +48% (radial strain), and −20% (circumferential strain).[125-127] Some have found significantly greater strain values in women than in men.[128] Longitudinal right ventricular strain and strain rate values are inhomogeneous and greater than those of the left ventricle.[127] Strain and strain rate offer complementary information, and both should be measured and evaluated. For example, prolonged contraction may yield normal strain despite low strain rate. Consequently, strain rate is considered more sensitive than strain in revealing myocardial disease.

Strain rate showed good correlation with +dP/dt during isovolumic contraction (r = 0.74) and with −dP/dt during isovolumic relaxation (r = 0.67).[129] Strain is load dependent[117,128] and is not less load-insensitive than EF, FS, and other traditional indices of systolic function. For example, acute hypovolemia induced by withdrawal of 500 mL blood from healthy subjects led to decreased longitudinal DTI strain (−28% ± 8% to −21% ± 4%), whereas strain rate remained unchanged (−1.5 ± 0.35/sec to −1.4 ± 0.4/sec).[130] Similarly, STI strain is preload and afterload dependent; longitudinal strain decreased after hemodialysis in patients with end-stage renal disease (−18.4% ± 2.9% to −16.9% ± 3.2%),[131] and radial strain increased immediately after surgery after AV

replacement for AS (from 22.7% ± 2% to 23.7% ± 1.8%) and decreased (23.1% ± 3.5% to 21% ± 3.8%) after valve replacement for aortic regurgitation (AR).[132] However, others have shown that longitudinal DTI strain (recorded in healthy subjects) remained unchanged during preload manipulation (baseline −18% ± 3%, increased preload with Trendelenburg −18% ± 3%, reduced preload with venodilator −17% ± 3%), whereas myocardial velocities were affected.[133] Discrepancies in the previous findings are explained by study design, techniques used for strain measurement, and degrees of preload manipulation. However, it would be "safer" not to consider strain as a load-independent parameter of systolic function.

Principles of Doppler Tissue Imaging and Doppler Strain

As discussed earlier, a shift in frequency is caused when transmitted ultrasound is reflected off a moving target (Doppler effect). In conventional echocardiography, Doppler algorithms are set up to interrogate returning signals from the blood pool only using high gain settings (to amplify the low-amplitude signal of the fast moving blood), and a high-pass filter (to reject the "noise" generated by the slow-moving myocardium). Modification of these filter settings (reduction of gain amplification and bypass of the high-pass wall filter) will reject data from moving blood and permit recording of the myocardial motion signal, which is stronger (approximately 40 dB higher amplitude) but slower (<25 cm/sec), respectively, thus enabling DTI and measurement of strain.[134] The principles of DTI, together with applications and limitations, have been reviewed recently and are partially summarized in the Diastolic Function section later in this chapter.[135]

For DTI strain, color DTI is obtained as in conventional CFD, with a color sector positioned over the myocardial wall of interest. The mean myocardial velocities are computed using autocorrelation analysis, displayed in blue if directed away from and in red if directed toward the transducer, and are superimposed on a grayscale 2D tomographic view (Figure 12-25A).[136] While in color DTI mode, placement of a sample volume (see later step-by-step explanation) over the myocardial area of interest (see Figure 12-25B) will calculate the deformation parameters strain rate (SR; see Figure 12-25C) and strain (see Figure 12-25D) from within this sample volume:

$$SR = (V_2 - V_1)/\Delta x \approx (\Delta V)/L_0 \approx (\Delta L/\Delta t)/L_0) \approx (\Delta L/L_0)/\Delta t \approx S/\Delta t$$

Strain is derived by temporal integration of strain rate.

Strain rate and strain can resolve tethering to a functioning neighboring segment that causes a segment with impaired function to give the false impression of contraction. This can be graphically simulated by the example of a towed car; although the engine of the towed car is not functioning, the car has velocity. When no velocity gradient exists within the interrogated segment, there will be no deformation and strain rate (and strain) will be zero.

Strain and strain rate calculated from myocardial velocity gradients have been validated over a wide range of strain values using sonomicrometry in animals[117,137] and 3D tagged MRI in humans.[118,138] However, systolic strain correlates with MRI better in healthy than diseased individuals.[139] DTI strain and strain rate are strong noninvasive indices of LV contractility[122]; DTI strain and strain rate increased with dobutamine, decreased with esmolol, and correlated well with peak LV elastance in experimental settings.

DTI strain is time consuming, technically demanding, and does have important limitations. Reverberation or dropout artifacts from neighboring structures can affect the measured velocity gradient and interfere with calculation of deformation parameters. Most important, DTI strain is a Doppler technique and can display deformation along a single dimension only, that of the ultrasound plane. Therefore, the displayed value (strain rate and strain) may not relate to the true (longitudinal, radial, or circumferential) deformation. In ME views, when the ultrasound beam is parallel to the myocardial wall, the actual (longitudinal) velocity can be accurately measured, but the velocity of radial (transverse) deformation will be zero because radial motion will be perpendicular to the ultrasound beam. With any angle deviation

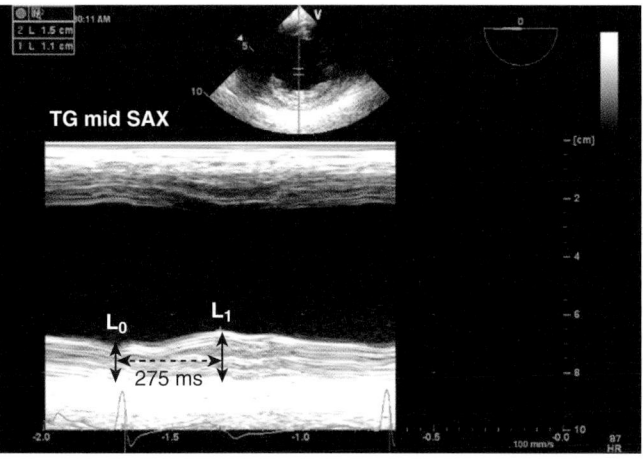

Strain = $\frac{L_1 - L_0}{L_0}$ = $\frac{1.5 - 1.1}{1.1}$ = 36%

Strain rate = $\frac{Strain}{\Delta t}$ = $\frac{36}{275}$ = 0.13/s

Figure 12-24 Illustrative example of estimation of strain and strain rate of midinferior and midanterior left ventricular segments using M-mode. L_0, end-diastolic length; L_1, end-systolic length; Δt, systolic time interval. SAX, short axis; TG, transgastric.

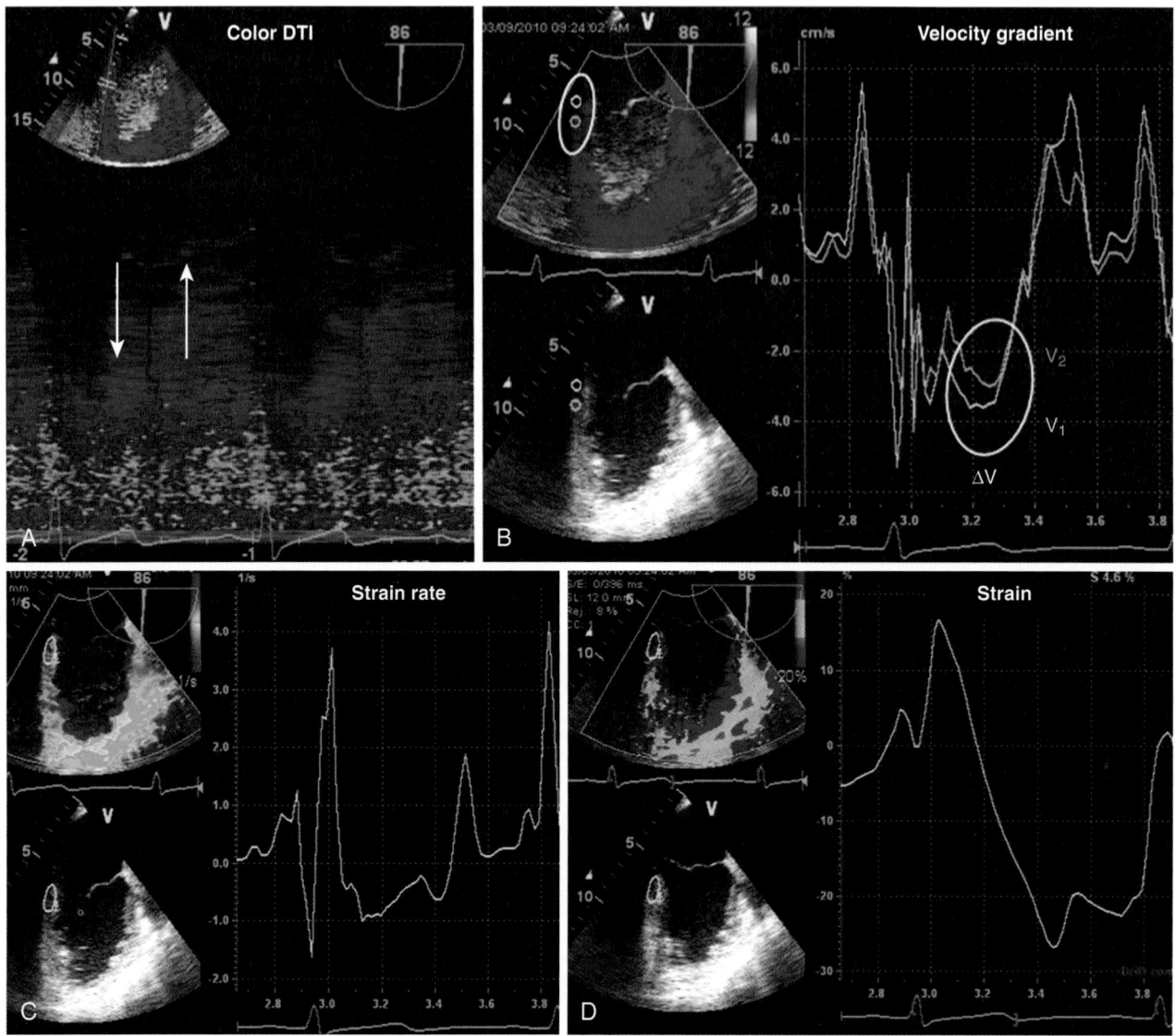

Figure 12-25 **Doppler strain and strain rate.** *A,* Activation of Doppler tissue imaging (DTI) function allows imaging of myocardial velocities in color, here with M-mode (from the inferior wall in a midesophageal two-chamber view). The velocities are directed away from the transducer in systole (and colored blue) and toward the transducer in diastole (and colored red). *B,* Spectral display of myocardial velocities from within sample volumes (insert panel at left) demonstrates a velocity gradient (ΔV). Basal (V_1) velocity is greater than apical (V_2) as the inferior wall shortens along its long axis. *C,* The velocity gradient (ΔV) of these points is used to calculate strain rate (SR). *D,* Integration of SR over time (Δt) derives strain.

from 0 degrees, the contribution of radial deformation to the measured velocity increases.[140] As a result, when using TEE, longitudinal strain and strain rate should be recorded only from ME views, and radial strain and strain rate from TG views. Furthermore, if the angle between the Doppler and motion plane is greater than 20 degrees, the true myocardial velocity gradient (and the calculated strain and strain rate) will be underestimated.[137] At an angle of 45 degrees, the measured DTI strain is zero.[117] This becomes more problematic in the presence of RWMAs.[141] Because of this angle dependency, DTI should be used primarily to assess longitudinal deformation parameters.

Step-by-Step Guide on How to Obtain Doppler Strain
The echocardiographic system must have a preset function to image and measure tissue velocity to obtain Doppler strain parameters. Of importance is optimal quality of 2D imaging and clear distinction between blood pool and myocardium (this may be facilitated by using second harmonic imaging, if available). High frame rates are required (usually >100 frames/sec) to show the subtle changes in myocardial velocity. This is accomplished by narrowing the sector width over the

myocardial wall of interest. Optimal ECG tracings with clear definition of QRS and P are essential, as well as PW or CW Doppler of transmitral and aortic flows (for timing of onset and end of systole). These temporal recordings should be concurrent with strain data acquisition.

First, DTI should be activated.[135] The TEE probe then is manipulated in such a way that myocardial motion and ultrasound planes are parallel to each other (or at an angle ≤ 20 degrees). The examination sequence should be standardized and the views labeled because the narrow sector removes neighboring structures used for identification. An adequate Nyquist limit is chosen, usually about ±20 cm/sec, to avoid aliasing while increasing spatial and temporal resolution. Next, the sector width and depth are optimized. The operator has two options: either a conventional sector width, which enables side-by-side comparison of diametrically opposite segments/walls, or a narrow sector (with the option of shallow depth), which maximizes the frame rate (DTI strain is optimal at >180 frames/sec). The ventilator may be switched off during acquisition of images, which are then reviewed and digitally stored. At least three beats (in sinus rhythm) or up to eight beats (in arrhythmia) should be captured and digitally stored.[142] TEE images used for Doppler strain are the three standard ME views (for LAX myocardial deformation) and the basal and mid-TG and mid-SAX views. Selection of these tomographic planes is dictated by the requirement for parallel orientation between the motion plane under examination and ultrasound direction (as described earlier). Addition of an M-mode line to the color DTI velocities will display a vertical line of color tissue velocity pattern along the M-mode beam with good temporal resolution (see Figure 12-25A).[143]

Further analysis is performed either on the initial echocardiographic system or on a dedicated workstation. Currently, Doppler strain techniques are proprietary software and analyze digitally stored images from the same system only. An appropriately sized sample volume (6 × 10 mm) is placed on the desired LV region, keeping in mind that larger sample volumes result in "smoothing" of the strain signals, whereas at the same time, temporal and spatial resolution decrease. The size of the sample volume determines the length (L_o) over which the velocity gradient is calculated. To keep the ROI within the myocardial borders, L_o is typically 10 mm for longitudinal data sets and 5 mm for radial data sets.[144] "Drift compensation" is a default setting that corrects for drift (i.e., when myocardium does not return to its original length at end-diastole) in the strain curves but can introduce error in the evaluations and should be taken into account as well. Because strain is the temporal integral of strain rate, strain is a "smoother" curve than strain rate. The strain rate curve should be inspected because a noisy strain rate curve indicates suboptimal tracking of the ROI and drift; if this is the case, it is better to reposition the sample volume.

The sample volumes are placed along the length of the myocardial wall (basal, mid, and apical segments) toward the endocardial surface (ME views) or in the middle of the myocardium (TG views) and should "track" (travel with) the segment throughout the cardiac cycle. The operator should verify that this happens by scrolling frame by frame and observing the concurrent motion of the sample volume with the myocardial segment. From each sample volume, strain rate, strain, and timing of peak values with respect to QRS are calculated (Figure 12-26). The reproducibility of strain measurements is reported to be less than 15%.[142] The suggested measurements and calculations are shown in Table 12-8.

Principles of Speckle-Tracking Imaging and 2D Strain
Interactions of ultrasound with myocardium result in reflection and scattering. These interactions generate a finely gray-shaded, speckled pattern. This speckled pattern is unique for each myocardial region and relatively stable throughout the cardiac cycle. The speckles function as acoustic markers; they are equally distributed within the myocardium and change their position from frame to frame in accordance with the surrounding myocardial deformation/tissue motion. In STI, the speckles within a predefined ROI are followed automatically frame by frame, and the change in their geometric position (which corresponds to local tissue movement) is used to extract strain, strain rate, velocity, and displacement. Because these acoustic markers can be followed in any direction, STI is a non-Doppler, angle-independent technique for calculation of cardiac deformation along two dimensions. Therefore, radial and longitudinal deformation can be measured in the ME views, and radial and circumferential deformation in the TG SAX views.[140]

Although considered as the only scientifically sound methodology for measuring cardiac deformation,[141] this non-Doppler technique also has limitations: (1) decreased sensitivity because of applied smoothing; (2) incorrect calculation of deformation, which is produced by erroneous tracking of stationary reverberations (when tissue moves, the speckle interference pattern may not move in exact accordance with tissue motion)[143]; (3) the necessity of clear visualization of the endocardial border for reliable radial and transverse tracking; and (4) undersampling in tachycardia because the optimal frame rate should be less

TABLE 12-8	Strain Echocardiography Measurements and Calculations
End-diastole	R wave of electrocardiogram
End-systole	Aortic valve closure (AVC)
End-systolic strain (S_{SYS})	Magnitude of systolic deformation between end-diastole and at end-systole (AVC)
Peak strain (S_{PEAK})	Maximum systolic deformation over a mean RR interval • Lowest value for longitudinal or circumferential strain • Highest value for radial strain
Postsystolic strain (S_{PS} or PSS)	The difference between S_{PEAK} and S_{SYS} $S_{PS} = S_{PEAK} - S_{SYS}$
Postsystolic strain index (PSI)	Represents the relative amount of ischemia-related segment thickening or shortening, found to occur after AVC $PSI = S_{PS}/S_{PEAK} = (S_{PEAK} - S_{SYS})/S_{PEAK}$ $S_{ps} - S_{es}/S_{es}$
Systolic strain rate (SR_{peak})	Maximum SR before end-systole
Peak systolic strain rate (SR_{peak})	Maximum SR
Rotation	Base rotates clockwise (initial, early systolic rotation is counterclockwise): (+)ve ° values Apex rotates counterclockwise (initial, early systolic rotation is clockwise): (−)ve ° values
Torsion	Basal rotation−apical rotation

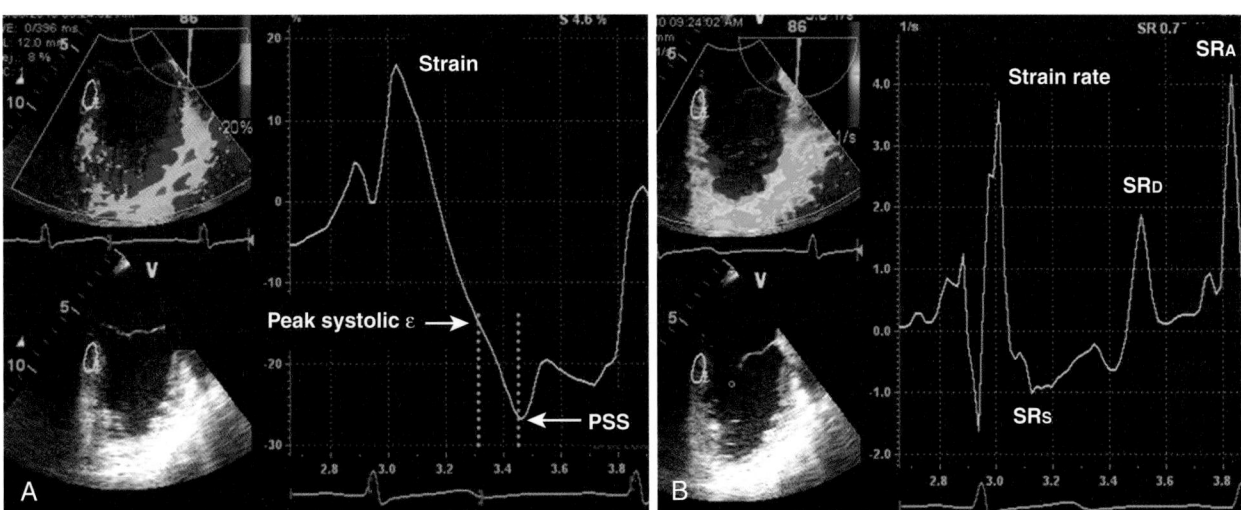

Figure 12-26 Measurement in Doppler strain echocardiography includes: **(A)** peak systolic (SR_S), early diastolic (SR_D) and late diastolic (SR_A) strain rate (SR); and **(B)** end-systolic strain (ε). Strain recorded after aortic valve closure (AVC) is called *postsystolic strain* (PSS).

than 100 frames/sec.[140] Equally important, STI algorithms require that the entire myocardium is visualized throughout the cardiac cycle. Echo dropout and mitral annulus calcification attenuate myocardial appearance in the TG or ME views, respectively, and do not allow adequate tracking of echocardiographic speckles.

Shear Strain and Torsion

The myocardial architecture of the epicardial and endocardial fibers will produce shear strain during the cardiac cycle (deformation parallel to the reference plane as the myocardial layers slide on each other; see Figure 12-23). This results in the base and the apex of the heart rotating in opposite directions. From a TEE perspective, the base rotates clockwise (preceded by an early systolic counterclockwise rotation because of earlier activation of subendocardial fibers) and the apex counterclockwise (preceded by an early systolic clockwise rotation). Torsion of the ventricle is the difference in apical and basal rotation, similar to wringing a towel dry.[104] As a result, during the cardiac cycle, there is a systolic twist and an early diastolic untwist of the left ventricle along its long axis because of opposite-directed apical and basal rotations. Rotation angles and torsion can be measured with STI,[145,146] and measurements correlate well with sonomicrometry and tagged MRI. Because basal and apical rotations are in opposite directions, somewhere between them there exists a level (the "equator") where rotation changes from one direction to the other.[146]

LV torsion occurs mainly by the counterclockwise apical rotation. Torsion is considered the mechanical link between systolic and diastolic function: systolic twisting stores elastic energy, which, released during the isovolumic phase of diastole, produces untwisting, generates intraventricular pressure gradients, and allows LV filling to proceed at low filling pressure.[104] During systole in healthy subjects, LV torsion increases and LV volume decreases; however, the relation between rapid untwisting (uncoiling) and increasing volume is nonlinear during diastole. Initiation of untwisting is an early and key mechanism that promotes early diastolic relaxation and early diastolic filling, possibly more important than recoil of systolic basal descent.[147]

LV torsion is preload dependent and increases with inotropy.[148] Approximately 40% of LV untwisting occurs during the isovolumic relaxation period, reaching a maximum just after MV opening, when approximately 20% of the SV had entered the left ventricle. By the peak of transmitral early filling (E wave), approximately 80% to 90% of untwisting is completed and essentially finished by the end of transmitral filling E wave, with the subsequent LV volume increase because of expansion in the short and long axes. LV systolic torsion and rapid untwisting increase significantly with exercise, storing additional potential energy that is released as diastolic suction increases. That is why the heart can increase the diastolic filling rate despite the shortened diastolic period during tachycardia. Patients with hypertrophic cardiomyopathy showed delayed untwisting that was not significantly augmented with exercise.[149] This explains the inability of patients to increase filling during exercise without a significant increase in left atrial pressure (LAP). The magnitude of torsion depends critically on the measurement level relative to LV base or other reference point. A limitation of STI in recording torsion is the in-out motion of the image plane as the left ventricle moves along its longitudinal axis. Selection of reproducible anatomic landmarks is important for measuring (and reporting) reproducible values. At the basal level, the fibrous mitral ring is used for orientation and reproducible image planes are easier to obtain. For apical recordings, the image plane should be just basal to the level with luminal closure at end-systole (there should be a recognizable apical cavity at end-systole).

Step-by-Step Guide on How to Perform Speckle Tracking Imaging

The technique of non-Doppler strain analysis has been described for ambulatory cardiac patients.[140,150] As compared with DTI, STI is less demanding and is closer to standard imaging (no Doppler is required and is performed at normal frame rate). The steps to perform STI in the anesthetized cardiac surgical patient are similar and are described in detail later. For the time being, analysis and measurements of 2D speckle strain parameters are possible off-line only, in a dedicated workstation (EchoPAC; GE Vingmed, Holton, Norway). As of this time, analysis is possible only on digitally acquired and stored images of the same vendor (there is no "cross talk" between systems from different vendors).

The operator starts by acquiring 2DE images of the left ventricle, which are digitally stored. Three ME views (4-chamber, 2-chamber, and LAX) and three TG views (basal, mid, and apical) are acquired with a frame rate between 40 and 80 per second, with adequate sector width and depth to image both endocardium and epicardium. In the anesthetized patient, it is better to stop ventilating to avoid image translation. Equally important is to acquire optimal quality 2D images and eliminate any myocardial areas with echo "dropout" (no speckles, no analysis). Timing of systole is based on the ECG-R wave, and end-systole is defined using M-mode tracings of the AV or PW Doppler of the trans-AV flow. This interval is used by the software to define the systolic time; therefore, it is practical to initiate postprocessing in an ME LAX view, in which the AV is seen, and then move to the other ME and TG views. In addition, it is important to acquire images rapidly and ensure that heart rate (and rhythm), as well as hemodynamics, remain stable. Otherwise, the systolic interval needs to be redefined before each strain analysis.

In each LV view stored, the operator manually traces the LV endocardium in a systolic frame, where it is best defined/imaged. Based on this initial endocardial tracing, the software generates an ROI, which encompasses the entire thickness of the cardiac wall between the LV epicardium and endocardium. This ROI may be adjusted manually by the operator so that the inner border is tracing the endocardium and the ROI "covers" the entire myocardium throughout the cardiac cycle. After approval of the software-generated myocardial wall delineation, speckle tracking analysis is done from within this region for one cardiac cycle at a time. In each view the LV myocardium is automatically divided into six segments, and the tracking quality is scored as either acceptable or unacceptable. If more than two segments have unacceptable quality, redefinition of the ROI or choosing a different beat should be done. Most of the time, the more important reasons for unacceptable segments are myocardial dropout and poor-quality 2D imaging; neither can be corrected postprocessing.

If tracking quality is acceptable, the operator approves the sampled segments and the software provides various deformation parameters for each segment: strain, strain rate, velocity, displacement, and rotation (torsion).[140,151] Examples of non-Doppler strain measurements are seen in Figure 12-27. Because acquisition of 2D images (in the ME and TG views) is standard procedure during a comprehensive TEE examination, appropriately stored, good-quality 2D images can be analyzed off-line (provided that the analysis system is of the same manufacturer) and provide STI parameters.

A three-click method (Automated Function Imaging [AFI]), whereby the operator "anchors" three points, at each side of the mitral annulus and at the apex of the left ventricle (in the ME views), further simplifies the process of tracking and analyzing peak systolic strain based on 2D strain. The computerized assessment is able to present the data in parametric (color), anatomic M-mode, strain curves, and "bull's-eye" displays. The usefulness of Automated Function Imaging is that deformation data are produced in an effortless manner and are comprehended more easily by an inexperienced operator.

The differences between Doppler and non-Doppler strain measurements are summarized in Table 12-9.[140] Deformation values are shown in Table 12-10.[152]

Correlation of Strain between Doppler Tissue Imaging and Speckle Tracking Imaging

If either DTI or STI measures deformation accurately, the respective strain values should correlate and give identical values. In 30 patients without AMI, longitudinal strain values differed only by 0.6% ± 6.0% (r = 0.53; P < 0.001), and radial strain values differed by 1.8% ± 13.4% (r = 0.46; P < 0.001).[138] Using receiver operating characteristic curves, STI showed greater area under the curve to discriminate among dysfunctional segments than DTI strain. Similarly, DTI and STI values were identical in healthy subjects, as well as in patients with cardiomyopathy.[120,123,125,127]

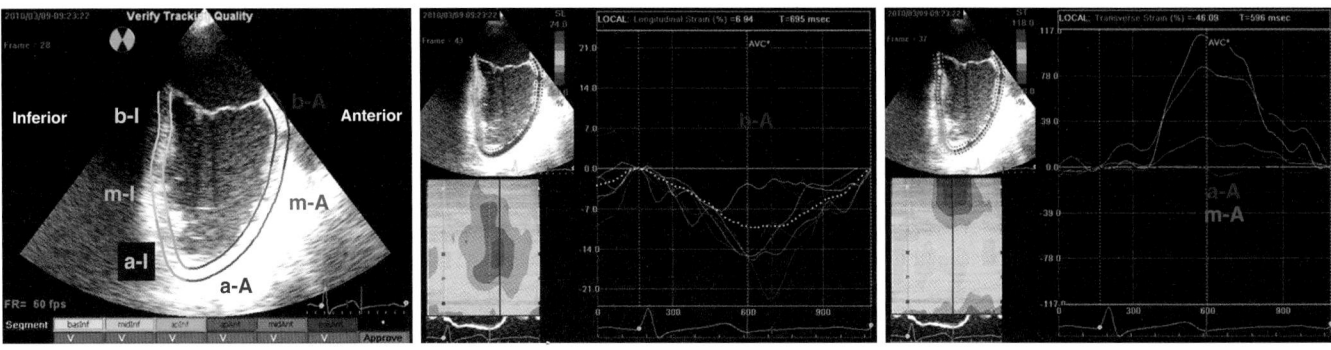

Figure 12-27 Speckle tissue imaging (STI). Longitudinal strain *(A)* and transverse strain *(B)* from a midesophageal four-chamber left ventricular view. *White dotted line* represents the global (average) longitudinal strain. Each myocardial segment is color coded. Longitudinal strain is abnormal in basal inferolateral (b-IL) segment (longitudinal expansion). Transverse strain is normal in only basal and midinferoseptal (IS) segments (transverse thickening). Circumferential *(C)* and radial *(D)* strain from a transgastric midpapillary short-axis view of the left ventricle. *White dotted line* represents the global (average) circumferential strain. Deformation is uniform (as compared with *A* and *B*). b-A, basal anterior; a-A, apical anterior; a-I, apical inferior; b-I, basal inferior; m-A, midanterior; m-I, midinferior.

The diagnostic ability of STI (performed with TTE) in patients undergoing dobutamine stress testing was less in the right and left circumflex territory than in the anterior circulation.[153] Contrary to DTI, STI depends on image quality. Poor imaging will result in decreased speckled appearance and poor tracking of the myocardium.

TABLE 12-9	Strain Echocardiography: Imaging Modalities	
	Doppler Tissue Imaging	*Speckle Tracking Imaging*
Technique	Manipulation of Doppler signal • Elimination of wall filter • Low-gain amplification Strain is calculated from velocity gradients, measured against a fixed reference (transducer)	Tracking of acoustic markers • Gray speckles within myocardium are tracked frame by frame Strain is directly measured from tracking of acoustic markers (speckles)
Display	Color map (±M-mode) PW at a specific space (regional values only)	Color map Spectral display (regional and global values)
Measurements	From color map (off-line): • Strain rate • Strain (Lagrangian) • Velocity (mean) • Displacement From PW (real-time): • Velocity (peak) • Displacement	• Strain rate • Strain (Lagrangian) • Velocity • Displacement • Torsion
Limitations	Only deformation parallel to ultrasound beam is measured Affected by translation and tethering Requires high frame rate	Requires lower frame rate (time between collection of consecutive image frames ≥ 10 milliseconds)—interpretation may be more reliable if tissue contains some stronger scattering structures Off-line implementation (not real time) Different image resolution in axial and lateral beam directions (long vs. radial in midesophageal and radial vs. circumferential in transgastric views) Dependent on optimal imaging Basal motion through image plane may result in poor spatial resolution

PW, pulsed wave.

Right Ventricular Function. Assessment of RV function is important; however, the complex geometric shape and thin wall structure of the right ventricle do not allow quantification with conventional 2D and M-mode techniques. In the experimental setting, systolic strain values obtained by DTI, in either inflow or outflow tract, were found to be comparable with those obtained by sonomicrometry (a method by which the actual length change is measured), whatever the RV loading conditions were.[154] RV longitudinal function is dominant over SAX function; and RV inflow tract, represented by the basal RV free wall, is the major contributor in global RV systolic and diastolic function. Therefore, measurement of longitudinal RV inflow deformation[127] offers valuable insights to global RV function. DTI longitudinal strain measurements showed an insignificant decline with age (average value of 31%, in 54 healthy adults).[155] In laboratory experiments with opened pericardium, increased afterload after PA constriction resulted in a shift of myocardial shortening from early-mid to end-systole or even diastole (postsystolic shortening [PSS]), whereas a reduction in preload caused by inferior vena cava occlusion induced earlier systolic shortening.[154] However, in healthy ambulatory subjects, DTI strain of RV inflow (recorded from the basal segment, lateral to the tricuspid annulus) did not change with preload or afterload increase.[156] DTI and STI RV peak systolic strain values correlate well ($r = 0.73$), with DTI values always being greater, overestimating peak systolic strain rate by 0.64%.[157] The correlation for strain rate was better ($r = 0.90$).

Deformation in the Operating Room. DTI strain is a sensitive means for detecting and localizing myocardial ischemia, as opposed to myocardial velocities. Intraoperative TEE measurements of DTI strain are comparable with transthoracic assessment, and pericardiotomy does not affect them.[158] As is expected, Doppler strain measurements are not easily obtained in the radial direction because of Doppler angle and translation cardiac motion.[159] DTI strain is better suited for the study of longitudinal cardiac deformation. DTI strain was found to be superior to myocardial velocity measurements in detecting and assessing regional myocardial ischemia during off-pump LAD revascularization. DTI strain demonstrated systolic lengthening of the apical septum and reduced longitudinal shortening of the midseptum during interrupted LAD flow. These changes occurred with concomitant deterioration of wall motion and were confined to the LAD territory, whereas there were no changes in the basal septum, supplied by the right coronary artery.[160] At the same time, DTI velocities remained unchanged in the apical septum during interrupted LAD flow, probably explained by traction from the basal segments.

Rotation and Twist. Apical rotation (12.2 ± 3.8 degrees) represents the dominant contribution to LV twist (73% ± 15%) and reflects LV twist over a wide range of hemodynamic conditions, making it a noninvasive, feasible clinical index of LV twist.[148] Estimation of LV

TABLE 12-10	Deformation Values				
References	*Strain Mode*				*Clinical Point*
Reisner, 2004[126]	STI	$n = 12$ global longitudinal S = −24.1% ± 2.9% global longitudinal SR = −1.02 ± 0.09/sec	$n = 27$ post-MI global longitudinal S = −14.7% ± 5.1% global longitudinal SR = −0.57 ± 0.23/s	WMS correlated well with global longitudinal S and SR	Cut-off: global longitudinal S < −21% global longitudinal SR < −0.9/sec for detection of post-MI patients
Jamal, 2002[322]	DTI	$n = 14$ *Regional longitudinal S* basal: −18% ± 5% mid: −21% ± 8% apex: −20% ± 9% *Regional longitudinal SR* basal: −1.1 ± 0.4/sec mid: −1.3 ± 0.5/sec apex: −1.3 ± 0.3/sec	$n = 40$ post-MI *Regional longitudinal S* (WMS = 2) basal: −10% ± 6% mid: −12% ± 6% apex: −11% ± 9% *Regional longitudinal SR* basal: −0.7 ± 0.3/s mid: −0.8 ± 0.4/sec apex: −0.8 ± 0.5/s Regional S (WMS = 3) basal: −4% ± 4% mid: −7% ± 6% apex: −6% ± 6% Regional SR basal: −0.4 ± 0.2/sec mid: −0.6 ± 0.3/sec apex: −0.6 ± 0.4/sec		Cutoff: S < −13% SR < −0.8/sec for infarcted segments
Serri, 2006[123]	DTI	$n = 45$ longitudinal S −19.12% ± 3.39%			
	STI	$n = 45$ longitudinal S −18.92% ± 2.19%			
Bogaert, 2001[114]	MRI tagged	$n = 87$ longitudinal S −17% Radial S 38% Circumferential S −40%			
Kowalski, 2001[127]	DTI	$n = 40$ longitudinal S −20% longitudinal SR −1.5–2.0/sec Radial S 46% Radial SR 3/sec			Higher long S and SR for RV wall Inhomogeneous values for RV
Hurlburt, 2007[128]	STI	$n = 60$ longitudinal S = −18.4% ± 4% (male) −20.8% ± 4.3% (female) circumferential S = −20.9% ± 4.3% (male) −25.4% ± 6.3% (female) radial S = 35% ± 10.2% (male) 40% ± 15.6% (female)			
Andersen, 2004[133]	DTI	$n = 32$ longitudinal S = −17.93% ± 2.65%			
Abali, 2005[130]	DTI	$n = 101$ longitudinal S = −28% ± 8% longitudinal SR = −1.5 ± 0.35/sec			
Zhang, 2005[328]	DTI	$n = 720$ segments longitudinal SR = −1.58 ± 0.38/sec			
Kukulski, 2003[319]	DTI	$n = 20$ longitudinal S = −18.9% ± 3.7% radial S = 25% ± 14%			
Andersen, 2003[124]	DTI	$n = 55$ Mean longitudinal SR = −1.5 ± 0.3/sec	Basal longitudinal SR −1.8 ± 0.6/sec Midlongitudinal SR −1.4 ± 0.3/sec Apical longitudinal SR −1.4 ± 0.3/sec		
Simmons, 2002[158]	DTI	$n = 13$ (septum) longitudinal S = −0.17% ± 0.04% $n = 11$ (inferior) longitudinal S = −0.13% ± 0.04%			
Mizuguchi, 2008[330]	STI	$n = 30$ longitudinal S = −22% ± 2.1% radial S = 73.2% ± 10.5% circumferential S = 22.1% ± 3.4% Tor = 19.3 ± 7.2 degrees			

TABLE 12-10	Deformation Values—Cont'd			
References	*Strain Mode*			*Clinical Point*
Helle-Valle, 2005[146]	STI	$n = 29$ Basal rotation 4.6 ± 1.3 degrees Apical rotation $-10.9 \pm 3.3°$ Torsion -14.5 ± 3.2 degrees		
Opdahl, 2008[148]	STI	$n = 18$ Basal rotation -5.9 ± 1.3 degrees Apical rotation 12.2 ± 3.8 degrees Torsion 17.8 ± 3.7 degrees	$N = 9$ (EF > 50%) Basal rotation -6 ± 3 degrees Apical rotation 13.6 ± 2.1 degrees Torsion 19.1 ± 4.1 degrees	$N = 18$ (EF < 50%) Basal rotation -4.8 ± 2.9 degrees Apical rotation 7.6 ± 3 degrees Torsion 11.6 ± 3.9 degrees
Takeuchi, 2007[162]	STI	$N = 15$ Radial $S_{base} = 52.8\% \pm 11.5\%$ Radial $S_{apex} = 26.5\% \pm 13.5\%$ Circumferential $S_{base} = -16.2\% \pm 3.4\%$ Circumferential $S_{apex} = -20.6\% \pm 3.3\%$ Torsion $= 9.3 \pm 3.6$ degrees	WMI = 16 (EF > 45%) Radial $S_{base} = 35.8\% \pm 10.7\%$ Radial $S_{apex} = 16.5\% \pm 9\%$ Circumferential $S_{base} = -13.7\%$ $\pm 4\%$ Circumferential $S_{apex} = -13.5\%$ $\pm 4.1\%$ Torsion $= 9.8 \pm 4$ degrees	WMI = 14 (EF < 45%) Radial $S_{base} = 27.4\% \pm 10.3\%$ Radial $S_{apex} = 12.8\% \pm 5.4\%$ Circumferential $S_{base} = -10.7\% \pm 5.1\%$ Circumferential $S_{apex} = -7.3\% \pm 2.6\%$ Torsion $= 5.6 \pm 2.6$ degrees
Teske, 2008[157]	DTI	$n = 22$ RV longitudinal S $= -30\% \pm 7.6\%$ RV longitudinal SR $= -1.77 \pm 0.55$/sec	STI RV longitudinal S $= -29.4 \pm 5.6$ RV longitudinal SR $= -1.75 \pm$ 0.55	
Chow, 2008[152]	STI	$n = 27$ RV global longitudinal S $= 26.3\% \pm$ 2.9% RV global longitudinal SR $= 1.33 \pm$ 0.23/sec		

DTI, Doppler tissue imaging; MI, myocardial infarction; RV, right ventricle; S, strain; SR, strain rate; STI, speckle tracking imaging; WMS, wall motion score.

twist from apical rotation eliminates the requirement of two separate recordings, one for the base and one for the apex, and possible calculation problem because of beat-to-beat variation in rotation, as well as the move-through of the LV image plane. In patients with chronic ischemia but preserved LVEF, rotation and twist were similar to healthy subjects; but in those with depressed LVEF, apical rotation and twist were reduced.[148]

In patients with diastolic dysfunction (DTI E′ < 8 cm/sec), peak LV twist is increased in early-stage diastolic dysfunction, mainly because of more vigorous and increased LV apical rotation.[161] It currently is unknown whether the mechanism of LV twisting and untwisting is independent of the underlying myocardial relaxation in patients with diastolic heart failure, or whether it is dependent on filling pressure (decreased twist with increased filling pressure).[161]

Systolic twist was depressed and diastolic untwisting prolonged in patients with anterior wall myocardial infarction (MI) and abnormal LV systolic function. These abnormalities were related to reduced apical rotation and associated with the reduction of apical circumferential strain.[162] In contrast, systolic twist was maintained in patients with anterior wall MI and LVEF greater than 45%. This is a result of the mild reduction of circumferential strain in the apex that may affect LV twist behavior in a mild manner.

Ventricular Synchronization

In the normal heart, electrical activation of the ventricles occurs after atrial contraction, spreads quickly (within 40 milliseconds) in both ventricles via conduction through the Purkinje fibers, and is associated with synchronous regional mechanical contraction of both ventricles. In mechanical dyssynchrony, there is delay in activation of the ventricles (interventricular dyssynchrony), or there is delay within the different LV segments or regions (intraventricular dyssynchrony; Figure 12-28). Typically, there is a prolonged QRS complex on the surface ECG. A classic type of dyssynchrony is left bundle branch block, where there is early electrical activation of the interventricular septum and late

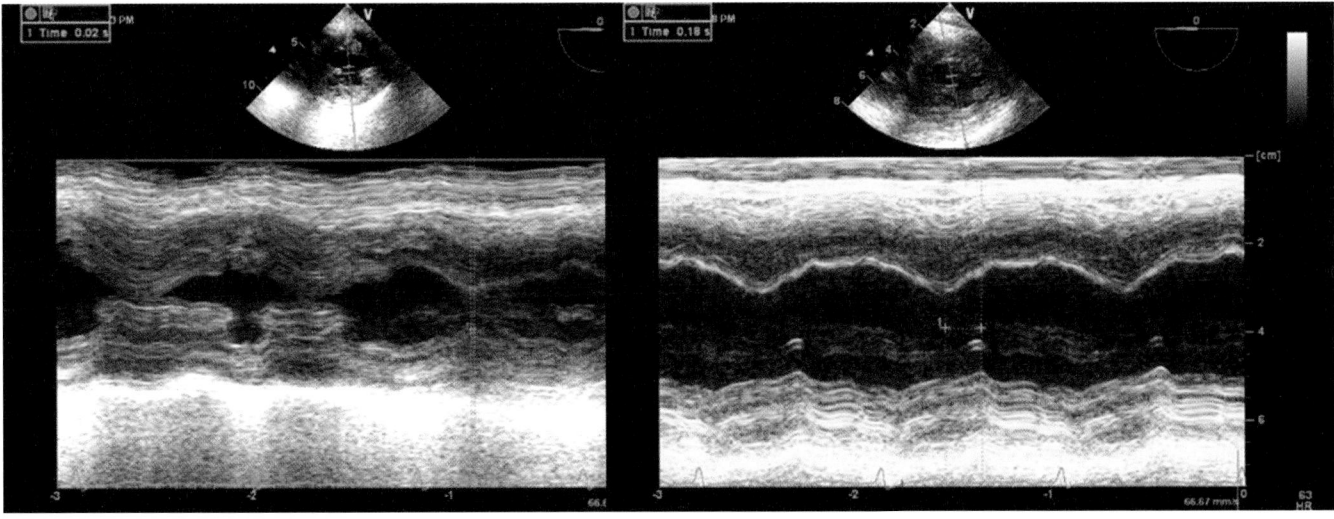

Figure 12-28   **NS figure dyssynchrony.** *Left,* Interventricular delay: 20 milliseconds. *Right,* Interventricular delay: 180 milliseconds.

activation of the inferolateral LV segments. The early septal contraction causes inferolateral stretching and late inferolateral contraction producing septal stretching. That is, one wall exerts forces on the contralateral wall and results in abnormal systolic performance, because the early septal contraction does not contribute to ejection because it occurs when LV pressure is low. Therefore, dyssynchrony is not innocuous, produces progressive dilation and distortion of the left ventricle, disrupts MV geometry, and results in inefficient LV systolic performance, increased LVESV, and wall stress, delayed relaxation, and mitral regurgitation. LV dyssynchrony has emerged as an important concept in patients with congestive heart failure. It is present in a significant proportion of patients with heart failure with left bundle branch block and in patients with normal QRS duration. Presence of LV dyssynchrony has been used to predict response to cardiac resynchronization treatment (CRT) in patients with end-stage heart failure.

CRT (by biventricular pacing) results in reverse remodeling, where LV size and function progressively improve over time, with better results in nonischemic patients,[163] and reduces mitral regurgitation by improving temporal coordination of mechanical activation of the papillary muscles.[164] CRT is indicated for patients with severe heart failure (NYHA Class III or IV), widened QRS greater than 120 milliseconds, and LVEF less than 35%. However, mechanical dyssynchrony may also exist in patients with depressed LV function and a narrow QRS. As a result, 25% to 35% of patients undergoing CRT fail to improve, and this may be because of widened QRS being a suboptimal marker for dyssynchrony. Additional factors associated with lack of response to CRT are ischemic disease with scar tissue that prohibits reverse remodeling, subsequent MI after CRT, or suboptimal lead placement.

Optimization of the techniques used to detect dyssynchrony is important to identify those patients who will respond to CRT because it appears that patients with minimal or no dyssynchrony have a lower probability of response and a poor prognosis after CRT.

Different echocardiographic modes have been used to detect dyssynchrony[165]:

1. M-mode with the cursor across the septal and inferolateral (posterior) segments. A delay between the opposing segments peak systolic excursion, usually longer than 130 milliseconds, was found to be fairly predictive for response to CRT (defined as >15% decrease in LVESV and improvement in clinical outcome).[166] However, because of unsatisfactory reproducibility[167] and lack of clear definition of systolic excursion of both septal and posterior walls, M-mode measurements (which are a single-dimensional assessment of LV dyssynchrony) are supplemental means to other echocardiographic modes, such as DTI.

2. DTI of longitudinal myocardial velocities has been the principal method in recent studies and the preferred echocardiographic approach. With color DTI, the direction of motion is color-coded and is used to identify the transition from inward to outward motion in opposing LV segments. Placement of sample volumes in basal, septal, and lateral LV segments produces a spectral display of mean myocardial velocities. The time delay between systolic myocardial excursion is measured (two-site method), and peak systolic delay longer than 65 milliseconds is predictive of clinical response to CRT and reverse remodeling.[168] Subsequent investigators used four or six basal segments as well. A "dyssynchrony index" is the standard deviation of the 12-segment times to peak regional myocardial systolic velocity; greater than 32/6 milliseconds has been proposed to be the best predictor of response to CRT.[169] An automated color-coding of time-to-peak systolic velocity termed *tissue synchronization imaging* has also been developed. Myocardial systolic velocity spectra can be produced by real-time PW DTI. However, the technique is considered time consuming and susceptible to artifacts because of breathing, patient movement, and translation. The major limitation of DTI techniques is that they cannot differentiate a passively moving segment because of tethering from an actively contracting one.

3. Cardiac deformation (stain) can differentiate active myocardial contraction or deformation from passive motion because of translation or tethering and has also been used to study dyssynchrony.[170] Longitudinal (the systolic deformation as imaged in the ME views) or radial (representing radial thickening as seen in TG views) strain can be challenging because it is affected by increased Doppler angle, whereas reproducibility of measurements is limited by the poor signal-to-noise ratio. Some believe that DTI velocities are far better than strain parameters in detecting dyssynchrony amenable to CRT.[171] Deformation studied with speckle-tracking imaging is a newer modality, which promises to bypass the limitations of DTI deformation.[172] Radial synchrony by STI is independent of clinical and echocardiographic parameters.[173]

4. The full-volume mode is capable of capturing the entire left ventricle in four beats.[174] With the use of integrated software programs, a 3D model of the left ventricle can be created within minutes, allowing the imager to view the 3D dynamics of the entire ventricle, including the timing of regional wall motion independently of its direction (Figure 12-29). Consequently, 3DE is considered an alternative approach to TDI for the quantification of LV dyssynchrony, showing good correlation against phase analysis of gated SPECT images.[175,176] Regional wall motion patterns can be visualized and quantified with semiautomatic contour tracing algorithms.[177] Its major limitation stems from the relatively low frame rate.

Optimal AV delay is defined as the one allowing completion of the atrial contribution to diastolic filling resulting in the most favorable preload before ventricular contraction. A too-short AV delay will interrupt the late diastolic wave (A), whereas a too-long AV delay will result in suboptimal LV preload. Despite these concerns, LV resynchronization is by far more important.[178]

Diastolic Function

Evaluation of diastolic function requires the assessment of the LV pressure-volume relation during diastolic filling. This relation can only be measured hemodynamically. Echocardiographic assessment of diastolic function attempts to evaluate diastolic filling by evaluating patterns and time of flow, such as from the LA into the left ventricle or pulmonary veins into the LA. The main determination of flow is the pressure differences in the two chambers.[179] The early diastolic pressure difference between the LA and the left ventricle mainly reflects the rate of LV relaxation. Thus, if filling is delayed, impaired relaxation usually is present. It is important to remember that other factors, such as chamber and myocardial compliance, LV loading conditions, ventricular interaction, and pericardial constraint, also can influence rates of LV filling. Diastolic function may be evaluated using left atrial size, Doppler analysis of MV inflow and pulmonary vein flow, color M-mode propagation velocities, and tissue Doppler analysis of the MV annulus.[180–182]

Indices for Evaluation
Left Atrial Size
Left atrial size is most accurately measured in the two- and four-chamber views.[100] It should be noted that although the Doppler velocity and time-interval measurement reflect filling pressures at the time of analysis, left atrial size measurements reflect cumulative effects over time.[182] Left atrial enlargement may occur in the absence of diastolic dysfunction. If left atrial enlargement is present, this measurement must be used in conjunction with other indices of LV diastolic function to interpret its significance.

Transmitral Doppler Analysis
Transmitral Doppler spectrum may be measured using PW Doppler. Typically, the PW Doppler gate is positioned at the tip of the MV leaflets in an ME four-chamber view.[182] Normally, transmitral spectrum consists of an early diastolic phase (E-wave) and a late diastolic component associated with atrial contraction (A-wave; Figure 12-30*A*). The velocity sweep speeds of 25 to 50 mm/sec should be used initially to evaluate respiratory variations in flow, as may be observed with pulmonary or pericardial disease, after which it may be increased to

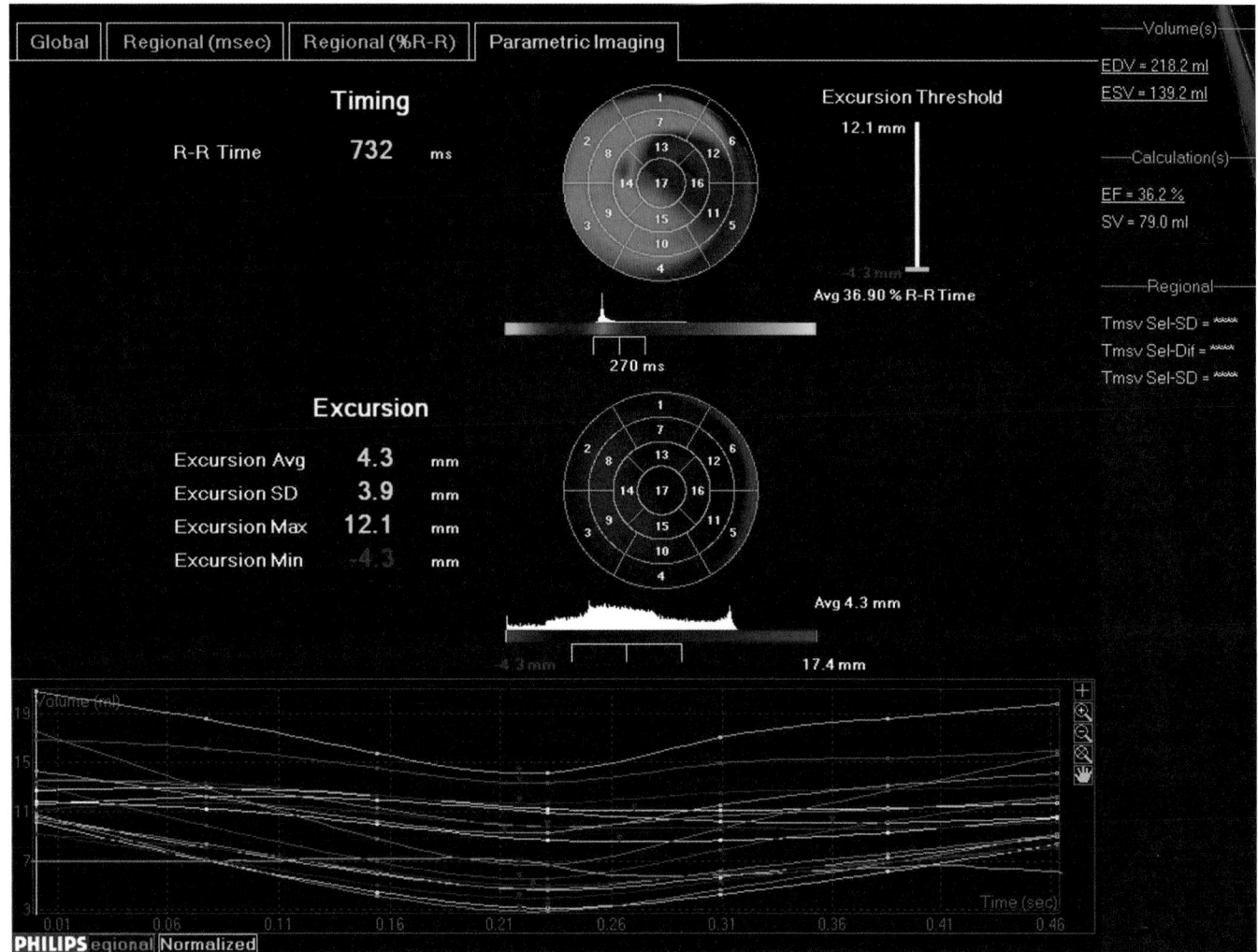

Figure 12-29 Parametric imaging of the left ventricle. Lateral wall shows severe timing delay in contraction, but only mild decrease in excursion. This technology can be helpful in optimizing ventricular synchrony.

100 mm/sec. The peak E- and A-wave velocities, A-wave duration, and E-wave deceleration time (DT) should be determined. The E-wave DT is measured from the peak of the E-wave until the actual or extrapolated intersection with zero. In addition, the isovolemic relaxation time (IVRT) may be measured by placing a CW cursor in the LVOT to simultaneously measure aortic ejection and ventricular inflow. Normal values are listed in Table 12-11. Generally, with increasing age, there is a decrease in E-wave velocity and E/A ratio and an increase in A-wave velocity and DT.

Mitral E-wave velocities are primarily determined by early diastolic LA-LV pressure gradient, which is primarily influenced by both left atrial preload and LV relaxation.[183] The A-wave velocity is affected by LV compliance and left atrial contractile function.[182] Finally, the E-wave DT is influenced by LV relaxation, LV diastolic pressures after MV opening, and LV compliance. With normal diastolic function, the E/A MV inflow ratio is between 0.8 and 1.5, with an E-wave DT of greater than 140 milliseconds. With impaired relaxation, there is an increase in the A-wave velocity and the E/A ratio becomes less than 0.8 (see Figure 12-30B). The E-wave DT is usually longer than 200 milliseconds. Further worsening in diastolic function results in increases in LAP. This increased LAP increases the E-wave velocity. This increased E-wave velocity results in a "pseudonormalization" of the E/A ratio (see Figure 12-30C). Further progression to restrictive cardiomyopathy results in the rapid increase in ventricular pressure during early

diastole with resultant shortened early diastolic filling. This is characterized by an E/A wave ratio greater than 1.5 and an E-wave DT less than 140 milliseconds (see Figure 12-30D).

Pulmonary Venous Flow Analysis

The pulmonary veins may be imaged from a number of views, as described earlier. The location of the vein may be optimized by CFD. Ideally, a 2- to 3-mm PW Doppler sample volume is placed more than 0.5 cm into the pulmonary vein, ensuring that the direction of pulmonary blood flow is parallel to the Doppler beam. The normal pulmonary venous tracing consists of a large positive systolic wave (i.e., flow toward the LA), a smaller diastolic wave, and a negative atrial wave (Figure 12-31). The systolic wave may have both an S1 and S2 component. The S1 component is associated with a "suction" effect of left atrial relaxation, whereas the S2 component is related to the pushing of blood by the right ventricle across the pulmonary circulation.[184] The peak systolic (S) and diastolic (D) velocities should be measured, as well as the atrial reversal (Ar) velocity and duration. If both S1 and S2 components of the pulmonary systolic flows are present, the S2 velocity should be used for calculations because S1 is related to atrial relaxation. After measurements of the transmitral Doppler spectrum, the difference between the Ar duration and A-wave duration should be calculated. The atrial systole component of the pulmonary venous flow (i.e., Ar) velocity usually is less than 35 cm/sec, and its duration is usually less than the transmitral E-wave duration.

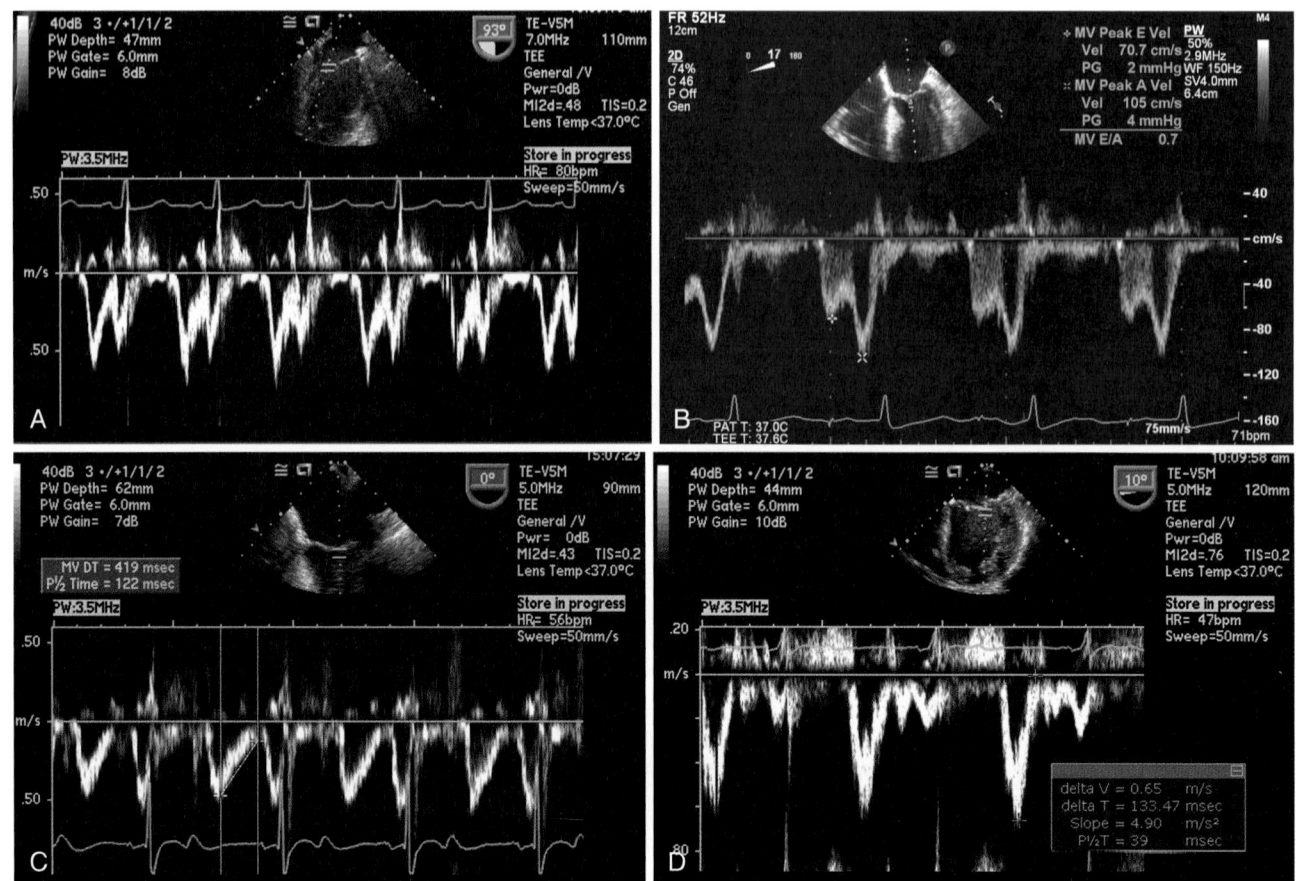

Figure 12-30 **Transmitral flow and diastolic dysfunction.** *A,* Normal transmitral spectrum consists of an early diastolic phase (E wave) and a late diastolic component associated with atrial contraction (A wave). The E-wave velocity is usually larger than the A-wave velocity. *B,* Delayed relaxation. With delayed relaxation, the A wave becomes smaller than the E wave. *C,* Pseudonormalization. With worsening diastolic dysfunction, left atrial pressure increases with a concomitant increase in the E-wave velocity. Although there is an increase in the E-wave deceleration time, differentiation of the pseudonormalization pattern from normal is dependent on additional indices of diastolic function. *D,* With the restrictive pattern, the E wave becomes dominant with a rapid deceleration time.

TABLE 12-11	Normal Values for Doppler Diastolic Measurements			
	Age (yr)			
Measurement	*16–20*	*21–40*	*41–60*	*>60*
IVRT (msec)	50 ± 9 (32–68)	67 ± 8 (51–83)	74 ± 7 (60–88)	87 ± 7 (73–101)
E/A ratio	1.88 ± 0.45 (0.98–2.78)	1.53 ± 0.40 (0.73–2.33)	1.28 ± 0.25 (0.78–1.78)	0.96 ± 0.18 (0.6–1.32)
DT (msec)	142 ± 19 (104–180)	166 ± 14 (138–194)	181 ± 19 (143–219)	200 ± 29 (142–258)
A duration (msec)	113 ± 17 (79–147)	127 ± 13 (101–153)	133 ± 13 (107–159)	138 ± 19 (100–176)
PV S/D ratio	0.82 ± 0.18 (0.46–1.18)	0.98 ± 0.32 (0.34–1.62)	1.21 ± 0.2 (0.81–1.61)	1.39 ± 0.47 (0.45–2.33)
PV Ar (cm/sec)	16 ± 10 (1–36)	21 ± 8 (5–37)	23 ± 3 (17–29)	25 ± 9 (11–39)
PV Ar duration (msec)	66 ± 39 (1–144)	96 ± 33 (30–162)	112 ± 15 (82–142)	113 ± 30 (53–173)
Septal e' (cm/sec)	14.9 ± 2.4 (10.1–19.7)	15.5 ± 2.7 (10.1–20.9)	12.2 ± 2.3 (7.6–16.8)	10.4 ± 2.1 (6.2–14.6)
Septal e'/a' ratio	2.4*	1.6 ± 0.5 (0.6–2.6)	1.1 ± 0.3 (0.5–1.7)	0.85 ± 0.2 (0.45–1.25)
Lateral e' (cm/sec)	20.6 ± 3.8 (13–28.2)	19.8 ± 2.9 (14–25.6)	16.1 ± 2.3 (11.5–20.7)	12.9 ± 3.5 (5.9–19.9)
Lateral e'/a' ratio	3.1*	1.9 ± 0.6 (0.7–3.1)	1.5 ± 0.5 (0.5–2.5)	0.9 ± 0.4 (0.1–1.7)

Data expressed as mean ± standard deviation (SD; 95% confidence intervals).
*SD not available.
Ar, atrial reversal; DT, deceleration time; IVRT, isovolemic relaxation time; PV, pulmonic valve; S/D, systolic/diastolic.
Adapted from Nagueh SF, Appleton CP, Gillebert TC, et al: Recommendations for the evaluation of left ventricular diastolic function by echocardiography, *J Am Soc Echocardiogr* 22:107–133, 2009; Klein AL, Burstow DJ, Tajik AJ, et al: Effects of age on left ventricular dimensions and filling dynamics in 117 normal persons, *Mayo Clin Proc* 69:212–224, 1994.

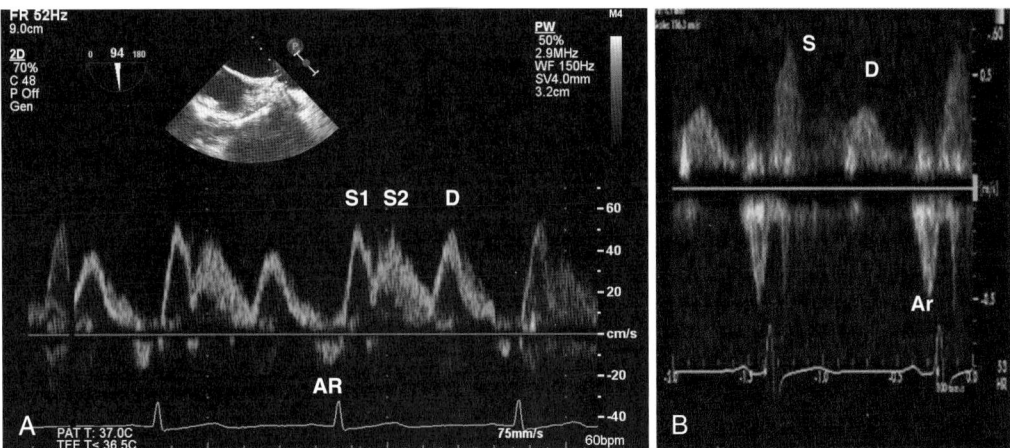

Figure 12-31 **Pulmonary venous tracing.** *A,* The normal pulmonary venous tracing is characterized by flow into the left atrium (toward the transducer) during both systole *(S)* and diastole *(D)* with a small flow reversal during atrial systole. The systolic component, which occurs immediately after the QRS complex, consists of both of an S1 and S2 component. The S1 component represents the suction effect during atrial relaxation, whereas the S2 component represents flow as a result of right ventricular systole. Flow during diastole *(D)* is normally less than systolic flow. Atrial contraction produces an atrial reversal wave *(Ar)* immediately before ventricular systole. *B,* With worsening left ventricular diastolic function, there is an increase in Ar velocity and duration. There is a markedly increased pulmonary venous Ar velocity at 50 cm/sec and its prolonged duration at greater than 200 milliseconds in comparison with mitral A (late diastolic) velocity. *(B, From Nagueh SF, Appleton CP, Gillebert TC, Marino PN, Oh JK, Smiseth OA, Waggoner AD, Flachskampf FA, Pellikka PA, Evangelista A.et al: Recommendations for the evaluation of left ventricular diastolic function by echocardiography.* J Am Soc Echocardiogr *22:107–133, 2009.)*

As Nagueh et al[182] summarized, "S1 velocity primarily is influenced by changes in LAP and left atrial contraction and relaxation, whereas S2 is related to SV and PW propagation in the pulmonary tree. D velocity is influenced by changes in LV filling and compliance and changes in parallel with mitral E-wave velocity. Pulmonary venous Ar velocity and duration are influenced by LV late diastolic pressures, atrial preload, and left atrial contractility. A decrease in left atrial compliance and an increase in LAP decrease the S velocity and increase the D velocity, resulting in an S/D ratio less than 1, a systolic filling fraction less than 40%, and a shortening of the DT of D velocity, usually less than 150 milliseconds. With increased left ventricular end-diastolic pressure (LVEDP), Ar velocity and duration increase, as well as the time difference between Ar duration and mitral A-wave duration." Increases in LAP result in a blunting of the systolic component of pulmonary venous flow compared with diastolic pulmonary venous flow. With greater increases in LVEDP, the Ar velocity exceeds 35 cm/sec and the duration becomes greater than 30 milliseconds compared with the transmitral E-wave duration (see Figure 12-31*B*).

Color M-Mode Flow Propagation Velocity (V$_p$)

Mitral-apical propagation velocity may be measured using color M-mode imaging. A clear view of LV inflow is obtained. CFD mapping is superimposed on the LV inflow, and the color mapping is adjusted to a displayed and aliased signal in the center of the ventricular inflow.[185] The M-mode scan line is displayed extending through the MV leaflet opening to the LV apex. V$_p$ is determined by measuring the slope of the aliasing velocity from the mitral inflow to approximately 4 cm into the LV cavity during early systole (Figure 12-32*A*). A V$_p$ greater than 50 cm/sec is considered normal.[182] This early filling wave is driven by the pressure gradient between the LV base and apex, which represents a suction force attributed to LV restoring forces and relaxation. A decrease in V$_p$ serves as a semiquantitative marker of LV diastolic dysfunction (see Figure 12-32*B*). In most cases of diastolic dysfunction, other indices of diastolic function are present; if these indices are inconclusive, Vp may provide useful information concerning estimation of LVEDP.

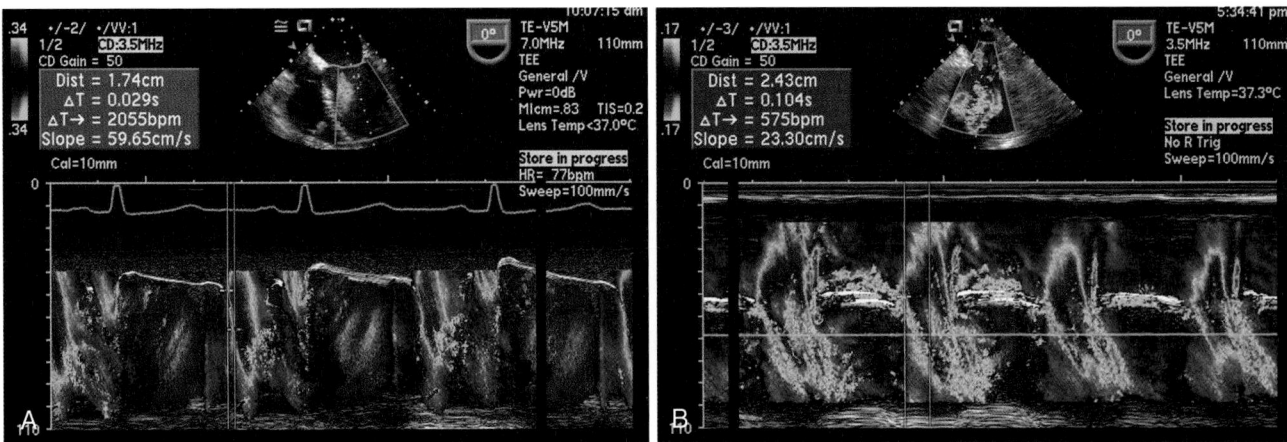

Figure 12-32 **Color M-mode propagation velocity.** *A,* Normal. The color M-mode slope of the left ventricular inflow is greater than 50 cm/sec. *B,* With decreased diastolic function, there is a decrease in the M-mode propagation slope.

Tissue Doppler

Spectral Doppler usually is used to determine blood-flow velocities. Because these velocities are relatively high and the amplitude of the Doppler signal is low, high-amplitude/low-velocity ultrasound signals usually are ignored. In contrast, during tissue Doppler examination, the primary interest is in the high-amplitude/low-velocity ultrasound signals created by the myocardium; low-amplitude/high-velocity signals are ignored. DTI of the MV annulus may be used to judge diastolic function.[186] Most modern ultrasound machines have presets optimized for tissue Doppler analysis to include the high-amplitude/low-velocity signals that normally are excluded. The sample volume should be positioned with 1 cm of the septal and lateral annular insertion points and should cover the longitudinal excursion of the mitral annulus in both systole and diastole.[182] Normally, this DTI wave consists of two diastolic components: one in early diastole (e') and one in late diastole (a'; Figure 12-33). Measurements should be taken at both points and the results averaged. The septal e' wave generally is lower than the lateral e'-wave velocity. The peak e' and a' velocities should be determined, and the e'/a' ratios, as well as the E/e' ratios, should be calculated. These two signals are in the opposite direction of MV inflow. The major determinants of e' velocity are LV relaxation, preload, systolic function, and LV minimal pressure. These indices may not be accurate with heavy annular calcification, mitral stenosis (MS), prosthetic MVs or annuli, or constrictive pericarditis. Because preload has minimal effect on e' velocity, the E/e' ratio is useful to correct for E-wave velocities in the presence of diastolic dysfunction. Normal values for these parameters are listed in Table 12-11. Septal E/e' ratios less than 8 and septal e' velocities greater than 8 cm/sec usually indicate normal LV filling pressures, whereas septal E/e' ratios greater than 16 and septal e' velocities less than 8 cm/sec (lateral e' velocity < 8.5 cm) usually indicate increased LV filling pressures.[180,182]

Classification of Diastolic Dysfunction

There are three primary stages of diastolic dysfunction: impaired relaxation, pseudonormalization, and restrictive cardiomyopathy, which may be classified using the indices presented (Figure 12-34).[182] In patients with mild diastolic dysfunction (impaired relaxation), the mitral E/A ratio is less than 0.8, DT is more than 200 milliseconds, IVRT is 100 milliseconds or longer, systolic is greater than diastolic pulmonary venous flow, annular e' velocity is less than 8 cm/sec, and the E/e' ratio is less than 8. In most of these cases, the LAP is not increased. With the progression to moderate diastolic dysfunction, there are mild-to-moderate increases in LV filling pressures. With these increases in LAP, the early diastolic LA-LV pressure gradient increases, which results in a pseudonormalization of the E/A ratio (0.8 to 1.5). This ratio may decrease by more than 50% with Valsalva. Other supporting data for the diagnosis of moderate diastolic dysfunction include an increase of the E/e' ratio to 9 to 12, e' less than 8 cm/sec, a pulmonary venous A$_r$ velocity greater than 30 cm/sec, diastolic pulmonary venous blood flow

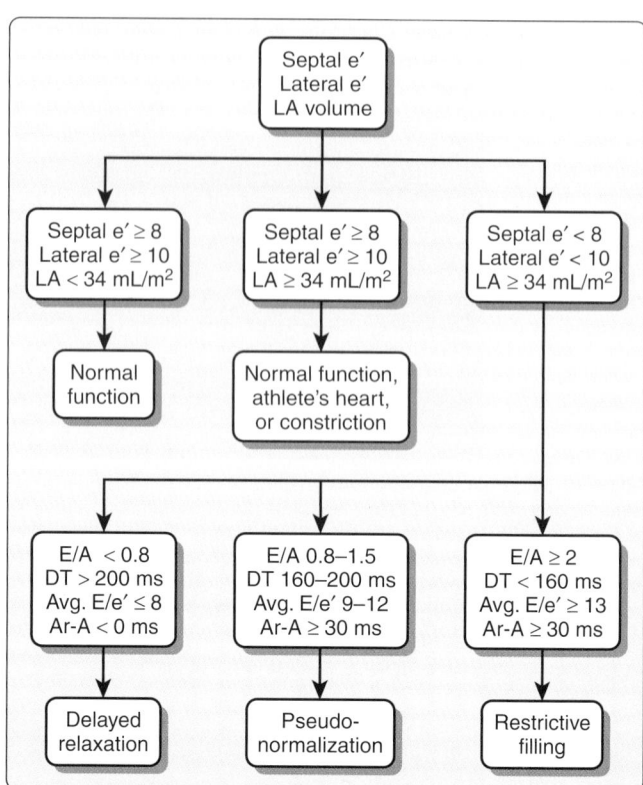

Figure 12-34 **Classification of diastolic dysfunction.** A, late diastolic transmitral velocity; Ar-A, difference between pulmonary venous atrial reversal duration and transmitral A wave duration; DT, E-wave deceleration time; E, early diastolic transmitral velocity; e', early diastolic tissue Doppler velocity; LA, left atrial.

velocity greater than systolic, and A$_r$-A duration 30 milliseconds or longer. Finally, severe diastolic dysfunction (restrictive LV filling) may be diagnosed with E/A ratio of 2 or more, DT less than 160 milliseconds, IVRT 60 milliseconds or less, pulmonary venous systolic filling fraction 40% or less of the diastolic fraction, mitral A-flow duration shorter than the Ar duration, and average E/e' ratio greater than 13 (or septal E/e' ≥ 15 and lateral E/e' > 12).

Intravascular Pressures

Various echocardiographic techniques have been used to gauge intracardiac or intravascular pressures. Based on the Doppler shift principle,

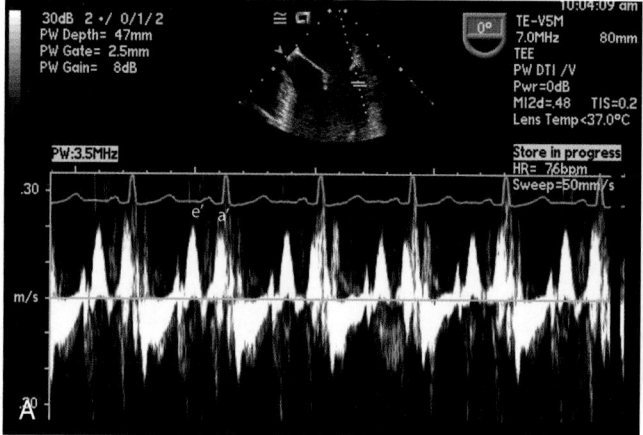

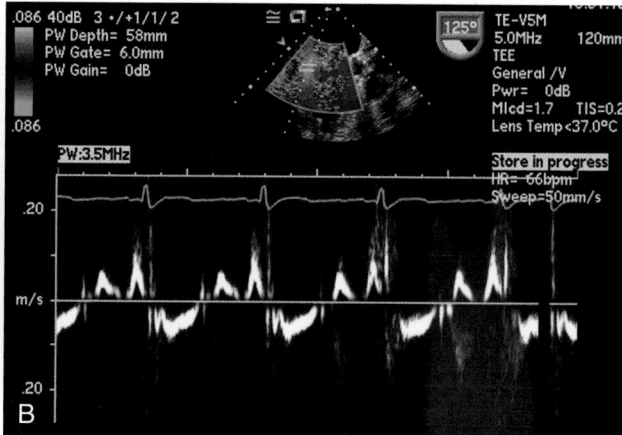

Figure 12-33 **Tissue Doppler measurements.** A, Normal tissue Doppler spectrum. e' is both greater than a' and more than 8 cm/sec. B, With worsening left ventricular diastolic function, there is a decrease in e' velocity.

blood-flow velocity can be used to determine pressure gradients. The modified Bernoulli equation describes the relation between pressure gradients and blood-flow velocities. When flow acceleration and viscous friction variables of blood are ignored and flow velocity proximal to a fixed obstruction is significantly less than flow velocity after the obstruction, the following formula applies:

$$P_1 - P_2 = 4(V)^2$$

where $P_1 - P_2$ is the pressure gradient across an obstruction, and V is the velocity distal to the obstruction. With this formula, the pressure gradient across a fixed orifice can be calculated.

Determination of Intravascular Pressures

The velocity of a regurgitant valve is a direct application of pressure gradient calculations because it represents the pressure decline across that valve, and, therefore, can be used to calculate intracardiac pressure. For example, tricuspid regurgitation (TR) velocity reflects systolic pressure differences between the right ventricle and RA. RV systolic pressure can be obtained by adding RA pressure (estimated or measured) to $4(TR velocity)^2$. In the absence of RVOT obstruction, PA systolic pressure will be the same as right ventricular end-systolic pressure (RVESP). For example,

If TR velocity(TR VEL) = 3.8 m/sec and right atrial

pressure(RAP) = 10 mm Hg,

then

$$RVESP = (TR VEL)^2 \times 4 + RAP$$

$$4(3.8)^2 = 58 mm Hg + 10 mm Hg$$

$$RVESP = PA systolic = 68 mm Hg$$

Similarly, pulmonary regurgitation (PR) velocity represents the diastolic pressure difference between the PA and the right ventricle. Therefore, $PAEDP = RVEDP + 4(PR end–diastolic velocity)^2$. Note that RVEDP is equal to RAP (estimated or measured). Mitral regurgitation (MR) velocity represents the systolic pressure difference between the left ventricle and the LA. In patients without LVOT obstruction, systolic pressure essentially is equal to LV systolic pressure; therefore, LAP is equal to SBP $- 4(MR)^2$. Finally, aortic regurgitation (AR) velocity reflects the diastolic pressure gradient between the aorta and the left ventricle. Note also that LVEDP can be estimated by various diastolic filling patterns from mitral and pulmonary venous flow velocity patterns. In summary,

$$PAP systolic = RVESP = 4(TR)^2 + RAP$$

$$PAP diastolic = 4(PR)^2 + RAP$$

$$LAP = SBP - 4(MR)^2$$

$$LVEDP = DBP - 4(AR)^2$$

where PAP represents pulmonary artery pressure, RAP is right atrial pressure, SBP represents systolic blood pressure, and DBP is diastolic blood pressure. Stevenson[187] compared six different echocardiographic techniques to measure PA pressure. When compared with direct measurements, some of these techniques yielded highly accurate correlations ($r = 0.97$), but they were not always applicable in all patients.

▓ Cardiac Output

M-Mode Echocardiographic Measurement

Early in the development of echocardiography, Feigenbaum et al[188] compared echocardiographic and angiographic volumes in an attempt to show that M-mode echo measurements were related to actual ventricular size. They cubed single M-mode echocardiographic dimensions

and correlated them with their angiographic equivalents. Although reasonably good correlations were obtained, they never intended to use M-mode ventricular diameters for the actual clinical measurements of ventricular volumes.

Two-Dimensional Echocardiographic Measurement

SV is calculated as the difference between end-diastolic volume (EDV) and end-systolic volume (ESV). The ASE has recommended that the diastolic dimension coincide with the Q wave on the ECG. The end-systolic dimension is best measured at the time of the peak downward motion of the posterior endocardium. When TEE was utilized to obtain ventricular dimensions, correlations between echo and indicator dilution varied from $r = 0.72$ in patients undergoing cardiac surgery to $r = 0.97$ in critically ill patients.[189] In patients undergoing CABG, SV was derived from 2D SAX views using echocardiography.[190] Comparisons of echo-derived cardiac index with simultaneous thermodilution-derived cardiac index yielded a correlation coefficient of 0.80 (see Chapter 14).

Doppler Measurements

Flow across the orifice is equal to the product of the cross-sectional area (CSA) of the orifice and the sum of the flow velocities. Because flow velocity is not constant throughout a flow cycle, the sum of all of the flow velocities during the entire ejection period is integrated to measure total flow.[191,192] This summation of flow velocities in a given period is called the *velocity–time integral* (VTI). The VTI is represented by the area enclosed within the baseline and spectral Doppler signal. In essence, the VTI is the area under the curve of the Doppler signal and represents the distance transversed by an object during a given period. Once VTI is determined, then SV and CO can be calculated:

$$SV = CSA \times VTI$$

$$CO = SV \times HR$$

In using these equations, there are a number of assumptions, including: (1) laminar blood flow in the area interrogated; (2) a flat or blunt flow velocity profile, such that the flow across the entire CSA interrogated is relatively uniform; and (3) Doppler angle of incidence between the Doppler beam and the main direction of blood flow is less than 20 degrees, so the underestimation of the flow velocity is less than 6%.

A number of Doppler methods have been attempted. Probably the most popular and accepted utilize the LVOT. Other methods using the mitral, tricuspid, and pulmonic orifices have been attempted with variable results. Their respective accuracy is dependent on the angle between the insonated Doppler signal and blood flow. It should be noted, however, that the major determinant of variability in estimating SV by the use of any technique is the accurate measurements of the CSA. The CSA for a circular orifice such as the LVOT is:

$$CSA = \pi(D/2)^2$$

where D represents the diameter obtained by 2D imaging. Therefore, any error in diameter measurement would be squared in the final results. A number of methods have been suggested for measuring the diameter of the AV orifice. In the absence of AV disease, the diameter at the level of the aortic root either at the level of the sinuses of Valsalva or immediately above them has been used to define the aortic orifice area. However, in the presence of AS, the aortic orifice area should be measured at the level of the LVOT, immediately underneath the AV insertion. If the LVOT diameter is used as the aortic CSA to obtain determinations of CO, changes in the diameter of the aortic root will be minimized throughout the cardiac cycle (systole vs. diastole).

A second source of variability in measuring aortic flow involves the proper recording of reproducible Doppler signals. If the LVOT is chosen as the CSA, the VTI should be obtained from the Doppler signal at this level. For this purpose, the systolic forward flow must be obtained from either a deep TG or TG LAX view. The sample volume of the pulsed Doppler should be placed in the high portion of the LVOT *exactly* at the same level where the diameter was measured. Occasionally, the Doppler signal is difficult to obtain and the morphology of the spectrum may be similar to a triangle with a spike at the peak velocity rather than a round "bell-shape" flow signal. Under such circumstances, it is inappropriate to estimate the VTI because underestimations or overestimations are likely to result. If attention is given to proper recording techniques, the interobserver variability in measuring the aortic VTI in healthy subjects should be less than 5%.

When the results of various studies are compared, it is important to know the method of calculating the VTI and the CSA, as well as where the Doppler sampling volume was located. Because PW Doppler provides a spectral display of instantaneous velocities, mean velocities or velocity modes are utilized for the integration of flow velocity. The measurement of the mitral orifice diameter probably should be repeated at various cosines. It has been well established that the size of the mitral orifice varies with varying flows. The importance of the sample volume location has been demonstrated in several studies.[133] The SV is underestimated when the sampling volume is placed at the mitral leaflet tips and overestimated when placed at the mitral annulus.

Using TEE, Roewer et al[193] calculated SV in 27 surgical patients. A comparison of Doppler-determined CO values with those obtained by thermodilution yielded an excellent correlation ($r = 0.95$). LaMantia et al,[194] who performed a similar study in 13 cardiac surgical patients, found only a modest correlation ($r = 0.68$). Other investigations have used PA Doppler flow velocity integrals and estimations of the vessel area to perform off-line calculations of SV and CO.[195] Muhiudeen et al[196] found that transmitral Doppler CO did not correlate with that obtained by thermodilution and PA Doppler CO correlated only weakly ($r = 0.65$) with that obtained by thermodilution. They concluded that transesophageal Doppler has significant limitations at the off-line monitor of CO. In contrast, Savino et al[195] found good agreement and correlation ($r = 0.93$) between transesophageal PA Doppler and thermodilution CO. They were, however, unable to visualize the main PA in 24% of patients. In addition, the method was tedious and not suitable for online analysis with current equipment and software.

In 50 cardiac surgery patients, CO obtained by thermodilution was compared with deep TG PW Doppler through the LVOT.[197] Of these patients, seven were excluded from analysis because Doppler measurements could not be obtained. Good correlation in measurements was obtained with a bias of 0.015 L/min with 29% error. The authors estimated that these Doppler estimates of CO were 92% sensitive and 71% specific for detecting more than 10% change in cardiac output.

The use of 3DE may increase the accuracy of CO measurements. Because geometric variability is more easily compensated in these measurements, ESV and EDV may be calculated and CO may be determined. Culp et al[198] compared 3DE determinations of CO with thermodilution during the prebypass period in 20 patients undergoing cardiac surgery. In their study, the mean bias was 0.27 L/min with a ±35% limit of agreement. They observed a good correlation between these two measurements; however, there were significant bias and wide limits of agreements between the measurements. Off-line analysis of 3DE images may be used to estimate CO. In a study of 40 patients undergoing heart transplantation, 3DE reconstruction of LVEDV and LVESV were estimated, allowing for calculation of SV and CO.[199] These CO measurements were correlated closely with compared thermodilution-derived measures, with a mean bias of 0.06 L/min and a standard deviation of 0.4 L/min. Notably, however, each measurement required approximately 3 minutes per case and poor image quality precluded analysis in four patients. Transthoracic 3DE determination of SV was highly correlated to catheterization data.[200] These 3D datasets tended to underestimate the SV by 7.5 mL, or 17%.

As described earlier, homogenous laminar flow and a cylindrical outlet are assumed during Doppler measurements. This, unfortunately, may not be the case. Three-dimensional color-Doppler echocardiography may be used to more accurately define the CSA of either the LVOT or MV, as well as more accurately describe the blood flow through these areas. In 3D color Doppler determination of CO, multiple 2DE slices with their associated Doppler data are obtained through a particular surface. Flow data may be computed using Gaussian control surface theory.[201] Gaussian theory states that for a curved surface, the flow passing through the surface is equal to the sum of all velocity components normal to the surface (Figure 12-35).

In a group of 47 postcardiac transplantation patients, CO was determined by thermodilution, as well as 2D and 3D Doppler echocardiography through both the LVOT and the mitral value.[202] The 3D measurement provided a lower bias and narrower limits of agreement

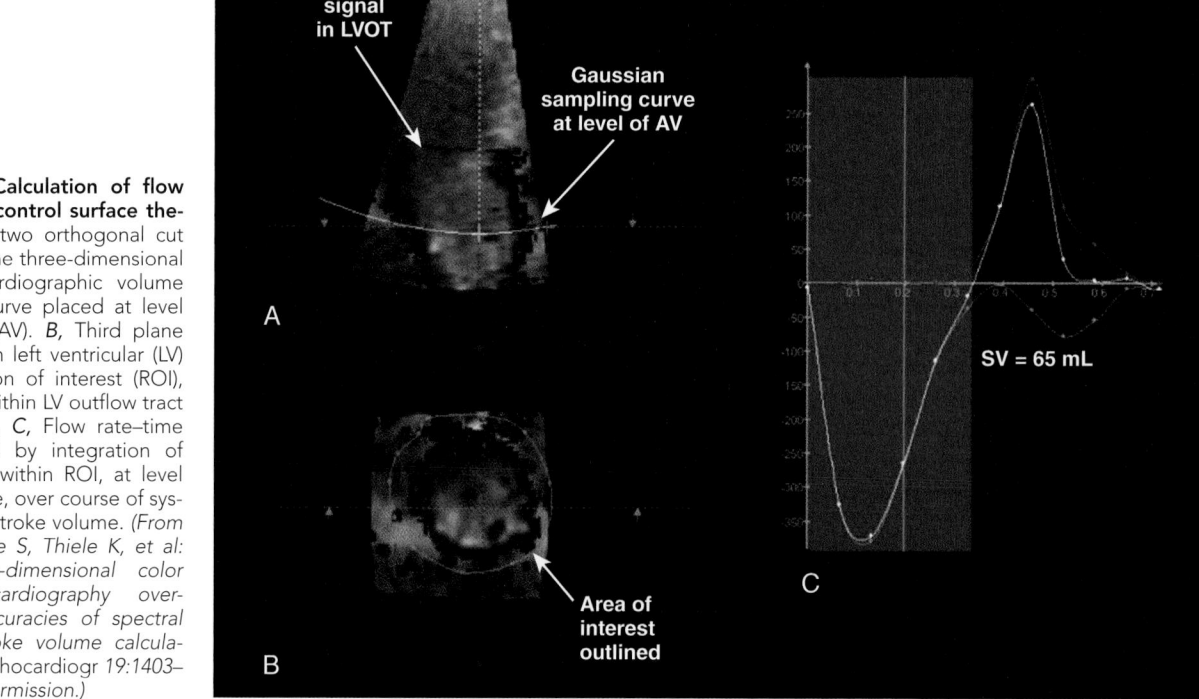

Figure 12-35 Calculation of flow using Gaussian control surface theory. *A,* One of two orthogonal cut planes of real-time three-dimensional Doppler echocardiographic volume with sampling curve placed at level of aortic valve (AV). *B,* Third plane as if viewed from left ventricular (LV) cavity, with region of interest (ROI), Doppler signal within LV outflow tract (LVOT), outlined. *C,* Flow rate–time curve generated by integration of Doppler signals within ROI, at level of sampling curve, over course of systole (green). SV, stroke volume. *(From Pemberton J, Ge S, Thiele K, et al: Real-time three-dimensional color Doppler echocardiography overcomes the inaccuracies of spectral Doppler for stroke volume calculation. J Am Soc Echocardiogr 19:1403–1410, 2006, by permission.)*

both in the LVOT measurements (−1.84 ± 16.8 vs. −8.6 ± 36.2 mL) and in the MV inflow position (−0.2 ± 15.6 vs. 10.0 ± 26 mL).

Assessment of Preload

End-Diastolic Dimensions

Whereas in conventional hemodynamics, preload often is estimated by measuring left-heart filling pressures (pulmonary capillary wedge pressure [PCWP], LAP, or LVEDP), in echocardiography, it can be determined by measuring LV end-diastolic dimensions or calculating LVEDPs. In M-mode echocardiography, a single ventricular diameter is obtained, whereas in 2DE, one or multiple tomographic cuts are recorded. It has been proposed that end-diastolic dimensions provide a better index of preload than the PCWP. When PCWP and EDV, derived from SAX areas at the level of the papillary muscles, were compared as predictors of cardiac index in patients undergoing CABG surgery, a strong correlation was observed between end-diastolic area (EDA) or EDV and cardiac index, whereas no significant correlation was found between PCWP and cardiac index.[203] Konstadt et al[204] compared TEE SAX images with images generated directly from the cardiac surface during cardiac surgery. There was a close correlation between EDA and end-systolic areas and area EFs derived from the two methods ($r = 0.88$ and 0.94).

In a study of 32 patients during cardiovascular surgery, Beaupre et al[205] provided evidence for the clinical value of intraoperative TEE for monitoring LV SAX dimension (preload) changes. They compared SAX area changes with simultaneous PCWP changes obtained from PA catheters. Their results showed that estimates of SV derived from SAX area changes were consistent with thermodilution data in 91% of patients. In contrast, EDA changes correlated with PCWP changes in only 23% of patients. Because LV compliance changes dramatically during cardiovascular surgery, PCWP is an inadequate guide to LV preload.

Clements et al[206] studied 14 patients during resection of abdominal aortic aneurysms. At multiple times during surgery, echocardiograms and first-pass radionuclide studies were recorded simultaneously. The correlation between echocardiographic and radionuclide estimates was excellent; however, virtually no correlation was seen between estimates

from either of these techniques and PA pressures. Thus, TEE (but not the pulmonary artery catheter [PAC]) provides the anesthesiologist with a direct, quantitative method to assess LV preload and ejection. However, if severe RWMAs are present, information from a single cross section may not be adequate for estimating these parameters.

TEE is often, for practical reasons, limited to a single SAX view at the level of the papillary muscles. Some evidence suggests that SAX EDAs measured at this level correlate reasonably well with measurements obtained by on-heart echocardiography and with EDVs measured simultaneously using radionuclides. However, Urbanowicz et al's[207] findings were in disagreement with these conclusions. Using a combined radionuclide and thermodilution technique, these investigators found that the correlation coefficient between the LVEDA by TEE and the LVEDV was only 0.74. In addition, they noted discordant changes in four of nine patients. Overall, it has been shown that despite variable loading conditions, changes in LV SAX area reflect changes in LV pressure or compliance factors. There are two main echocardiographic signs of decreased preload. First, decrease in EDA ($<5.5\,\text{cm}^2/\text{m}^2$) invariably reflects hypovolemia. It is, however, difficult to set an upper limit of EDA below which hypovolemia can be confirmed. This is particularly true in patients with impaired contractility in whom a compensatory baseline increase in preload makes the echocardiographic diagnosis of hypovolemia difficult. The second sign is obliteration of the end-systolic area ("the kissing ventricle sign") that accompanies the decrease in EDA in severe hypovolemia.

Geometric assumptions applied to the LV allow estimation of volumetric measurements based on 2D measurements. Although in the elliptically shaped "normal" left ventricle these approximations provide the imager with an acceptable approximation of LV volumes, this no longer holds true for the "pathologic" ventricle. Unfortunately, patients with impaired ventricular function (in whom EF is of great interest) are precisely the ones with altered geometry. In addition, the placement of the 2D plane can be subject to positioning errors that may lead to chamber foreshortening, which even in a normally configured left ventricle can lead to measurement errors. Studies comparing LV volumes and mass measured by 3DE, 2DE, and MRI, which is the gold standard, showed significantly better correlation between 3DE and MRI than between 2DE and MRI (Figure 12-36).[208–210]

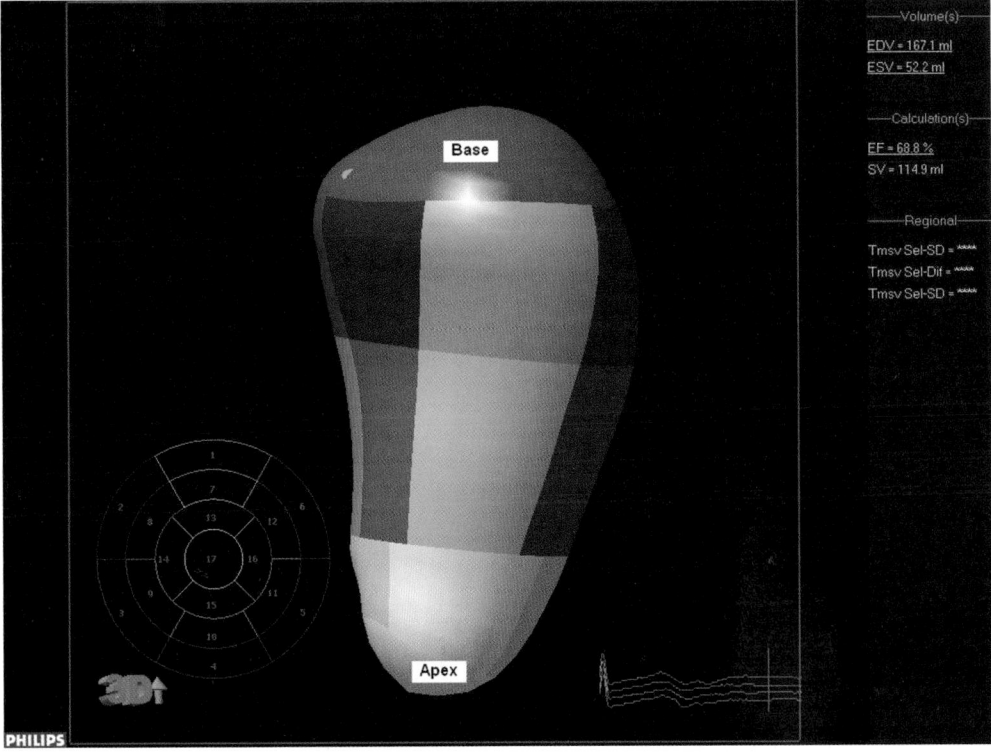

Figure 12-36 Model of left ventricle created from full-volume data set. The model represents a cast of the left ventricular cavity providing the echocardiographer both end-systolic and end-diastolic volumes.

Jenkins et al[211] compared LV measurements obtained by 2DE and 3DE with MRI-derived measurements in 110 patients. 3D measurements were performed both online using tracing and off-line using edge detection. They found that although all echocardiographic measurements underestimated LV volumes, the EF estimates were similar. The correlation between MRI and online 3DE was better than 2DE; however, the off-line 3DE provided the best correlation with MRI-derived volumes.

Left Atrial Pressure

The indices used to estimate LAP are discussed in detail in the earlier section describing the evaluation of diastolic dysfunction. The current recommendation suggests different algorithms for the evaluation of LAP based on EF.[182] These recommendations are summarized in Figures 12-37 and 12-38. Mitral inflow patterns may be used with reasonable accuracy to estimate LAP in patients with depressed EFs. If the E/A ratio is less than 1 and the E wave is 50 cm/sec or less, LAP probably is normal; if E/A pressure is greater than 2 and the DT is less than 150 millisecond, the LAP probably is increased. In the intermediate E/A ratios or a high E-wave velocity, other indices must be considered as well. Signs consistent with normal LAP include E/e′ less than 8, E/Vp less than 1.4, pulmonary venous systolic pressure greater than diastolic velocity, Ar-A less than 0 milliseconds, and systolic PA pressure less than 30 mm Hg. However, if E/e′ is more than 15, E/Vp is 2.5 or more, pulmonary venous systolic is less than diastolic velocity, Ar-A is greater than 30 milliseconds, and systolic PA pressure is greater than 35 mm Hg, increased LAP should be suspected.

With normal EF, the primary measurement to be considered is the E/e′ ratio (see Figure 12-38). If the septal, lateral, or average E/e′ is less than or equal to 8, then the LAP is normal.[212] If the septal E/e′ is greater than or equal to 15, lateral E/e′ is 12 or more, or the average E/e′ is greater than or equal to 13, then the LAP is considered increased. For intermediate values of E/e′ ratio, other factors associated with diastolic function must be considered. Left atrial volume greater than 34 mL/m², Ar-A duration

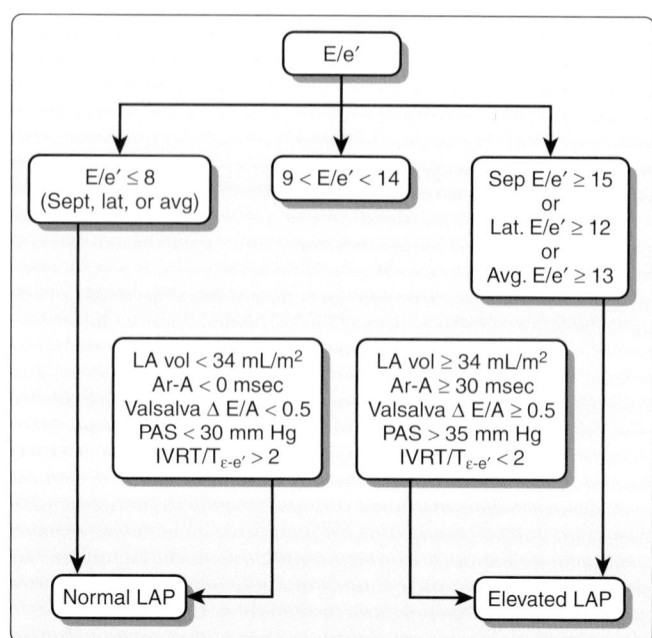

Figure 12-38 **Evaluation of left atrial pressure (LAP) in normal ejection fraction.** A, late diastolic transmitral velocity; Ar-A, difference between pulmonary venous atrial reversal duration and transmitral A wave duration; DT, E-wave deceleration time; E, early diastolic transmitral velocity; e′, early diastolic tissue Doppler velocity; IVRT, isovolemic relaxation time; LA, left atrial; lat, lateral; PAS, pulmonary artery systolic pressure; Sept, septal.

longer than 30 milliseconds, PA systolic pressure greater than 35 mm Hg, and the ratio of the IVRT/T$_{E-e'}$ less than 2 (which is defined as the time difference between the QRS to E-wave interval and the QRS to e′) are supportive of increased LAP. If more than one of these conditions is present, a conclusion of greater LAP may be made with greater confidence. Left atrial volume less than 34 mL/m₂, Ar-A duration less than 0 milliseconds, PA systolic pressure less than 30 mm Hg, or the ratio of the IVRT/T$_{E-e'}$ greater than 2 are supportive of normal LAP.

Valvular Evaluation

Aortic Valve Evaluation

Two-dimensional TEE interrogation provides information on valve area, leaflet structure, and mobility. The valve is composed of three fibrous cusps (right, left, and noncoronary) attached to the root of the aorta. Each cusp has a nodule, the noduli Arantii, in the center of the free edge at the point of contact of the three cusps. The spaces between the attachments of the cusps are the commissures, and the circumferential connection of these commissures is the sinotubular junction. The aortic wall bulge behind each cusp is known as the sinus of Valsalva. The sinotubular junction, the sinuses of Valsalva, the valve cusps, the junction of the AV with the ventricular septum, and anterior MV leaflet comprise the AV complex. The aortic ring is at the level of the ventricular septum and is the lowest and narrowest point of this complex. The three leaflets of the AV are easily visualized, and vegetations or calcifications can be identified on basal transverse imaging or longitudinal imaging.

Aortic Stenosis

AS may be caused by congenital unicuspid, bicuspid, tricuspid, or quadricuspid valves; rheumatic fever; or degenerative calcification of the valve in the elderly.[213,214] Valvular AS is characterized by thickened, echogenic, calcified, immobile leaflets and usually is associated with concentric LV hypertrophy and a dilated aortic root (Figure 12-39). The valve leaflets may be domed during systole; this finding is sufficient for a diagnosis of AS[215] (see Chapter 19).

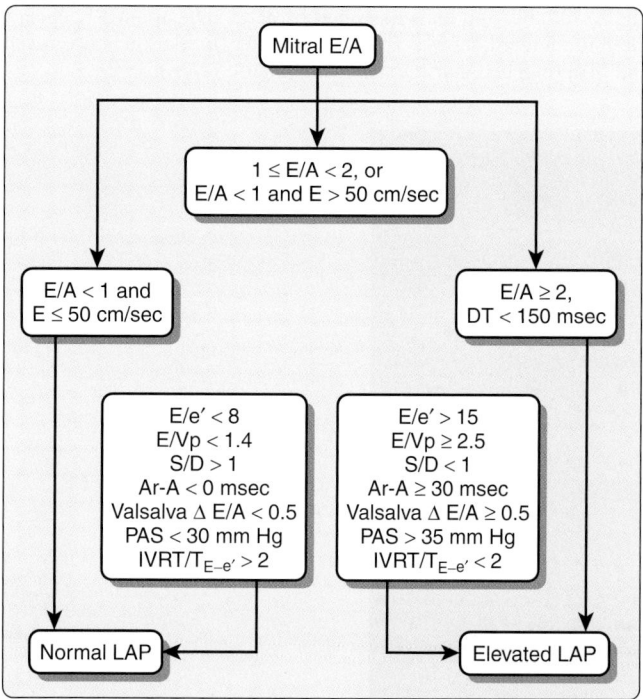

Figure 12-37 **Evaluation of left atrial pressure (LAP) with depressed ejection fraction.** A, late diastolic transmitral velocity; Ar-A, difference between pulmonary venous atrial reversal duration and transmitral A wave duration; D, diastolic pulmonary venous velocity; DT, E-wave deceleration time; E, early diastolic transmitral velocity; e′, early diastolic tissue Doppler velocity; IVRT, isovolemic relaxation time; S, systolic pulmonary venous velocity.

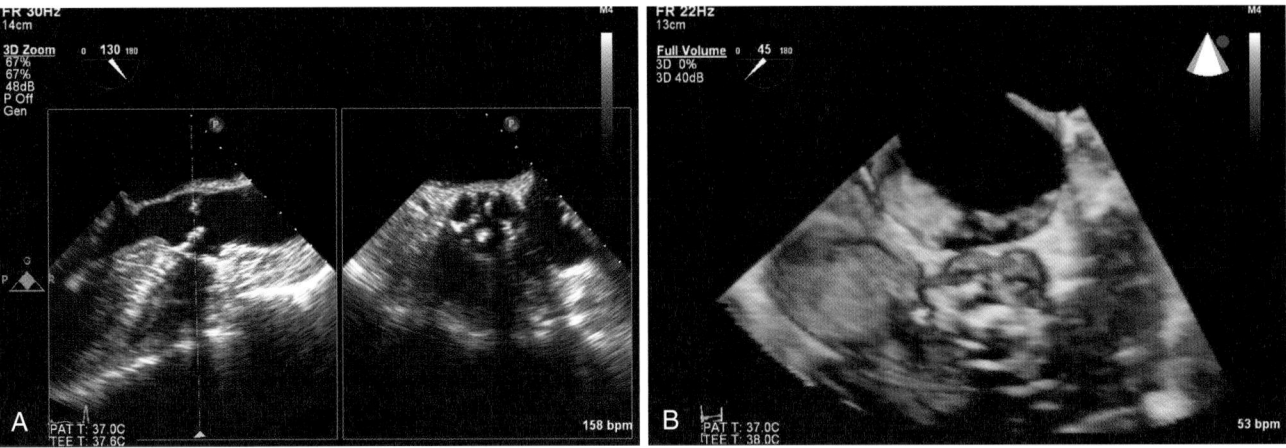

Figure 12-39 Aortic stenosis. *A,* Both midesophageal aortic valve (AV) long-axis and short-axis views are presented. The AV is stenotic, thickened, and calcific with significant valvular restriction. *B,* Three-dimensional reconstruction. The AV is viewed from the ascending aorta.

TABLE 12-12	Summary of Aortic Stenosis			
	Aortic Sclerosis	Mild	Moderate	Severe
Aortic jet velocity (m/sec)	≤2.5	2.6–2.9	3.0–4.0	>4.0
Mean gradient (mm Hg)		<20	20–40	>40
Aortic valve area (cm²)		>1.5	1.0–1.5	<1.0

Adapted from Baumgartner H, Hung J, Bermejo J, et al: Echocardiographic assessment of valve stenosis: EAE/ASE recommendations for clinical practice. *J Am Soc Echocardiogr* 22:1–23, 2009.

The quantification of AS is summarized in Table 12-12. Aortic valve area (AVA) may be measured by planimetry (Figure 12-40).[216] A cross-sectional view of the AV orifice may be obtained by using the ME AV SAX view, which corresponds well to measurements of AVA obtained by transthoracic echocardiography and cardiac catheterization, assuming the degree of calcification is not severe. The severity of AS may be quantified using CW Doppler echocardiography (Figure 12-41).[217] The evaluation of severity, however, may be limited by difficulty aligning the ultrasonic beam with the direction of blood flow through the LVOT. This limitation may be overcome by using either a deep TG or TG LAX view. Because severe stenosis limits AV opening, the imaging of the actual AV orifice may be challenging. Superimposition of a CFD spectrum over the calcific AV may guide accurate CW cursor placement. Normal Doppler signals

across the AV have a velocity less than 1.5 m/sec and have peak signals during early systole. With worsening AS, the flow velocity increases and the peak signal is later in systole. These high velocities will limit the use of PW Doppler and necessitate the use of either CW or high-pulse-repetition frequency Doppler.

The higher velocity central jet is characterized by a high-pitched audio sound, as well as a fine feathery appearance on the Doppler signal; this usually is less dense than the thicker parajets that are distal to the valve. Peak and mean transvalvular gradients may be calculated using the peak and mean velocities of the signals, respectively. Peak gradients measured by Doppler ultrasonography tend to be higher than those measured in the cardiac catheterization laboratory because Doppler-determined peak gradients are instantaneous, whereas those reported by the cardiac catheterization laboratory are peak-to-peak systolic pressure differences. In addition, Doppler determinations of peak gradient may overestimate gradient because of pressure recovery effects. As blood flows past a stenotic AV, the potential energy of the high-pressure left ventricle is converted into kinetic energy; there is a decrease in pressure with an associated increase in velocity. Distal to the orifice, flow decelerates again with both conversion of this loss of kinetic energy into heat, as well as a reconversion of some kinetic energy into potential energy with a corresponding *increase* in pressure. This increase in pressure distal to the stenosis is the pressure recovery effect.[218] Although usually minor, these differences in the observed gradient become more significant with a small aorta and moderate AS.[219]

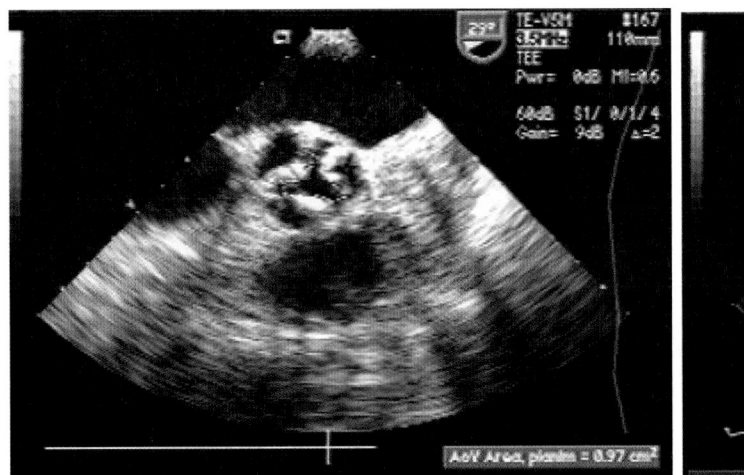
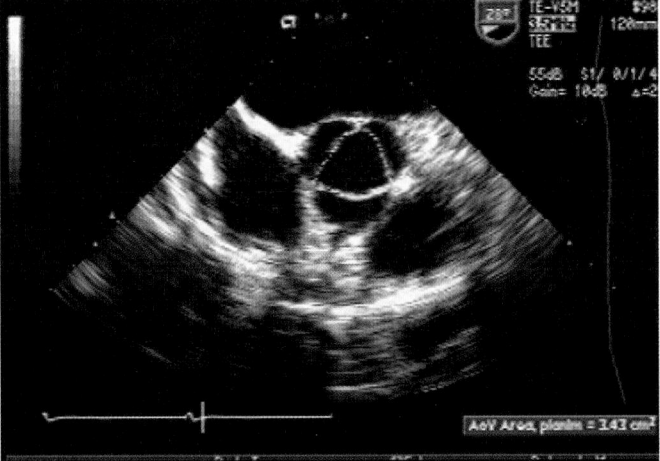

Figure 12-40 Aortic valve stenosis by planimetry. *Right,* Normal aortic valve. *Left,* Aortic valve with stenosis. Because there is not significant calcification of the valve, planimetry may be used.

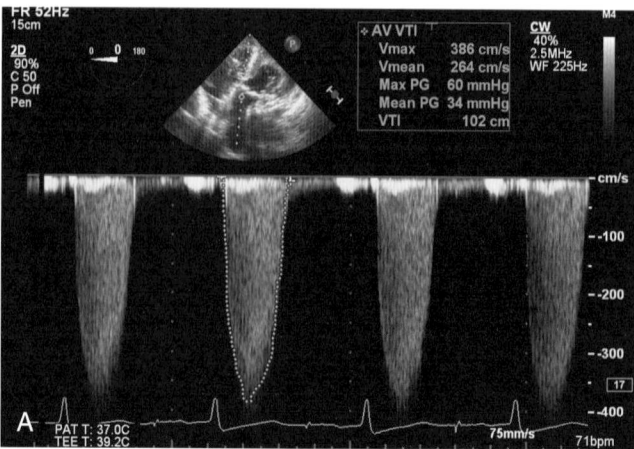

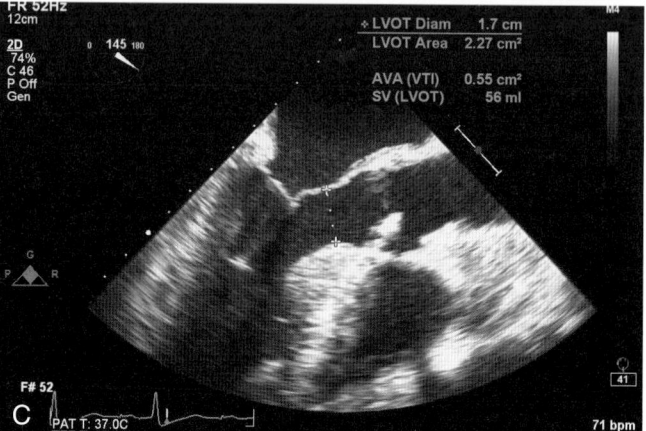

Figure 12-41 Determination of severity of aortic stenosis. *A,* Doppler spectrum through a stenotic aortic valve (AV). A continuous-wave (CW) Doppler curser is placed across the left ventricular outflow tract (LVOT) and AV in this deep transgastric view. A high-velocity jet is appreciated, which is consistent with severe aortic stenosis. *B,* Pulse-wave Doppler through the LVOT. *C,* Measurement of diameter of LVOT. The aortic valve area (AVA) may be calculated using the continuity equation. PW, pulse wave; SV, stroke volume; VTI, velocity-time integral.

LV dysfunction may either underestimate the severity of AS if gradients are used or may overestimate the severity if AVA is used (see later for measurements of AVA). LV dysfunction may severely decrease the rate of outflow through the left ventricle and AV. If resistance through the AV is constant, the pressure gradient generated across the AV is directly related to the CO: A low CO is associated with a low pressure gradient across the AV. Stated differently, a given severity of AS will result in a higher gradient across the AV with normal ventricular function compared with a lower gradient with decreasing ventricular function. The evaluation of AV gradient must be considered in the context of LV function. Although measurements of AVA factor CO in the measurement, AVA may nonetheless vary with flow rates.[220] Although this effect is not clinically significant with normal LV function, it becomes more pronounced with LV dysfunction because a minimum blood flow is required to maximally open the AV. Differentiation between severe AS with resultant LV systolic dysfunction from moderate AS with another cause of LV dysfunction may be made with dobutamine stress testing. The former state will not result in changes in AVA with improved cardiac function, whereas the latter will result in a significant increase in AVA with improved function.

Alternatively, AVA may be calculated using the continuity equation by comparing blood flow through the LVOT with blood through the AV. As discussed in more detail earlier, SV may be estimated by multiplying the CSA of a particular orifice by the VTI over one cardiac cycle through that orifice. The continuity equation states that the calculated SV should be equal independent of the site where it is measured: What goes in must come out. When estimating the severity of AS, SV through the LVOT and the AV is usually measured. The Doppler spectrum of the AV and LVOT is displayed using either a deep TG or TG LAX view using continuous and PW Doppler, respectively. The VTI through each of these structures is calculated. The diameter of the LVOT is measured in a ME LAX view. Remember,

$$SV = CSA * VTI$$

where the continuity equation states:

$$SV_{LVOT} = SV_{AV}$$

Substituting the SV equation into the continuity equation,

$$CSA_{LVOT} * VTI_{LVOT} = CSA_{AV} * VTI_{AV}$$

Rearranging the terms,

$$CSA_{AV} = CSA_{LVOT} * VTI_{LVOT} / VTI_{AV}$$

Because the LVOT is essentially cylindrical, the CSA_{LVOT} may be estimated by

$$CSA_{LVOT} = \pi(radius_{LVOT})^2$$

Because CSA_{LVOT}, VTI_{LVOT}, and VTI_{AV} are known, the CSA_{AV} or AVA may be calculated.

Multiple sources of error may affect the calculation of AVA using the continuity equation.[221] LVOT measurements may vary from 5% to 8%; therefore, when it is squared in the continuity equation, this may become a large source of error. Because the accuracy of the SV measurement through the LVOT assumes laminar flow, any sources of turbulence will affect results. In the presence of aortic insufficiency, the required high systolic velocities may result in a skewed velocity profile.

Although multiplane TEE planimetric estimations of AVA may be flawed by heavy aortic valvular calcification, measurements using the continuity equation are accurate compared with Gorlin-derived values.[222,223] In a study using TEE, Stoddard et al[224] reported good correlation between AVA measurements using the continuity equation and planimetry; however, they reported a steep learning curve for the acquisition of a suitable TG LAX view that adequately aligns flow through the AV with the ultrasound beam.

AS severity should be described by maximum velocity, mean gradient, and AVA. Aortic velocity allows classification of stenosis as mild (2.6 to 2.9 m/sec), moderate (3.0 to 4.0 m/sec), or severe (>4 m/sec).[221] Normal AVA is 3.0 to 4.0 cm². AVA consistent with mild AS is greater than 1.5 cm². An AVA of 1.0 to 1.5 cm² is consistent with moderate AS, and an area less than 1 cm² is consistent with severe disease.[221,225]

Aortic Regurgitation

AR may be caused by annular dilation, destruction of the annular support, or pathology of the aortic valvular cusps. Regurgitation secondary to annular dilation is characterized by a dilated aortic root, AV leaflets of normal appearance, and a centrally directed retrograde flow through the LVOT. Valvular lesions that may result in AR include leaflet vegetations and calcifications, perforation, or prolapse. These lesions may be seen on transverse imaging across the AV. Signs that may be associated with AR include high-frequency diastolic fluttering of the MV, premature closing of the MV, or reverse doming of the MV.[226,227]

Leaflet movement (excessive, restricted, or normal), origin of jet (central or peripheral), and direction of regurgitant jet (eccentric or central) should be determined to provide insight into the underlying pathology.[228] Bicuspid valve and TV prolapse are associated with excessive valve mobility and eccentric jet direction and origin. Annular dilation, rheumatic disease, sclerosis, and perforation are associated with normal or reduced cusp mobility and a central jet.

Physiologic changes that alter the estimated severity of AR include aortic diastolic pressure, LVEDP, heart rate, and LV compliance.[229] The severity of AR may be underestimated in the presence of eccentrically directed jets. In addition, several technical factors affect perceived severity of regurgitation as well, including severe malalignment of ultrasonic planes with blood flow, the presence of a prosthetic MV interfering with ultrasound penetration, gain settings, and PRF.

CFD traditionally has been the major method of assessing the severity of valvular regurgitation (Figure 12-42). In addition to providing the regurgitant jet area, the origin and width of the jet and the spatial orientation should be carefully defined. These parameters are dependent on technical factors. The severity of the regurgitant jet may be overestimated if the gain is too high or the Nyquist limits are too low. Ideally, these Nyquist limits should provide an aliasing velocity of approximately 50 to 60 cm/sec and a color gain that just eliminates the random color speckle from nonmoving regions.[230] Furthermore, excessive degradation of frame rate may be encountered if the CFD field is too large.

The criteria for qualitative grading of AR are summarized in Table 12-13. Aortic regurgitant flow through the outflow tract is characteristically a

TABLE 12-13	Quantification of Aortic Regurgitation			
	Mild	**Moderate**		**Severe**
	1+	*2+*	*3+*	*4+*
Left atrial size	Normal	Normal or dilated		Usually dilated
Aortic cusps	Normal or abnormal	Normal or abnormal		Abnormal/ flail or wide coaptation defect
Jet width in LVOT*	Small in central jets	Intermediate		Large in central jets; variable in eccentric jets
Continuous-wave jet density	Incomplete or faint	Dense		Dense
Jet deceleration rate (pressure half-time, msec)	Slow > 500	Medium 200–500		Steep < 200
Vena contracta width (cm)*	<0.3	0.3–0.60		≥0.6
Jet width/LVOT width (%)*	<25	25–45	46–64	≥65
Jet CSA/LVOT CSA (%)*	<5	5–20	21–59	≥60
Regurgitant orifice area (cm²)	<0.10	0.10–0.19	0.20–0.29	≥0.30
Regurgitant volume (mL/beat)	<30	30–44	45–59	≥60
Regurgitant fraction (%)	<30	30–39	40–49	≥50

*At Nyquist limits of 50 to 60 cm/sec.
CSA, cross-sectional area; LVOT, left ventricular outflow tract.
Adapted from Zoghbi WA, Enriquez-Sarano M, Foster E, et al: Recommendations for evaluation of the severity of native valvular regurgitation with two-dimensional and Doppler echocardiography. J Am Soc Echocardiogr 16:777–802, 2003.

high-velocity, turbulent jet extending through the LVOT and LV during diastole. The severity of AR may be assessed by examining the area, width, and distal extent of the jet by CFD measurements. Unfortunately, determination of the severity of AR by measurements of regurgitant jet areas alone has been questioned and probably is useful only for distinguishing mild from severe regurgitation.[231] A more accurate determination of AR may be made by examination of the ratio of the proximal jet width within the LVOT to the outflow tract width (w_J/w_{LVOT}).[232,233] A w_J/w_{LVOT} value of 0.25 discriminates mild from moderate regurgitation, and a value of 0.65 discriminates moderate from severe regurgitation.[230]

The vena contracta is the narrowest portion of a regurgitant jet that usually occurs at or immediately upstream from the valve. It usually is characterized by high-velocity, laminar flow and is slightly smaller than the regurgitant orifice.[230] A vena contracta diameter less than 0.3 cm is consistent with mild AR, and a diameter greater than 0.6 cm is consistent with severe aortic insufficiency. It should be noted, however, that jet shape may influence the estimation of the severity of regurgitation. An eccentric jet may be confined to a wall of the LVOT and, thus, may appear very narrow, underestimating the severity of regurgitation. Similarly, central jets may expand fully in the LVOT and may overestimate the severity of regurgitation.

Doppler characteristics of the regurgitant flow may be used to estimate the degree of AR (Figure 12-43). A very faint signal density is associated with mild AR, whereas a denser signal may represent more retrograde flow. In addition, the pressure half-time or slope of the AR jet may be determined. A normally functioning AV will maintain a large gradient during diastole between the aorta and the left ventricle. With a small degree of AR, there will be a small volume of blood entering the left ventricle through the AV, resulting in a slow increase in LV pressure during diastole. Doppler measurements will show a regurgitant flow of high velocity, which is maintained during most of diastole

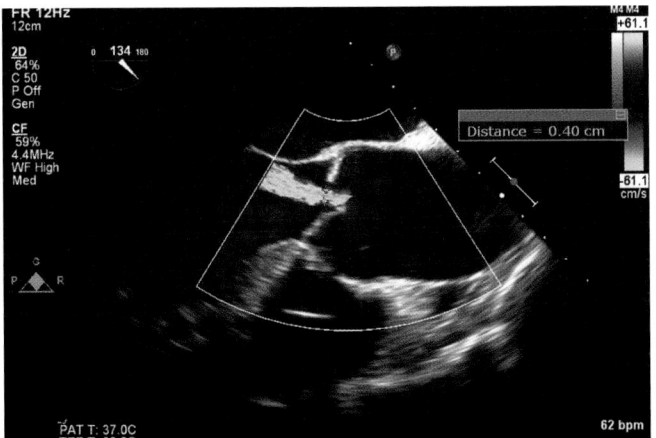

Figure 12-42 **Color-flow Doppler spectrum of a regurgitant aortic valve.** Midesophageal aortic valve long-axis view. An aortic regurgitant jet is visualized in the left ventricular outflow tract. The vena contract is less than 3 mm, which is consistent with mild regurgitation.

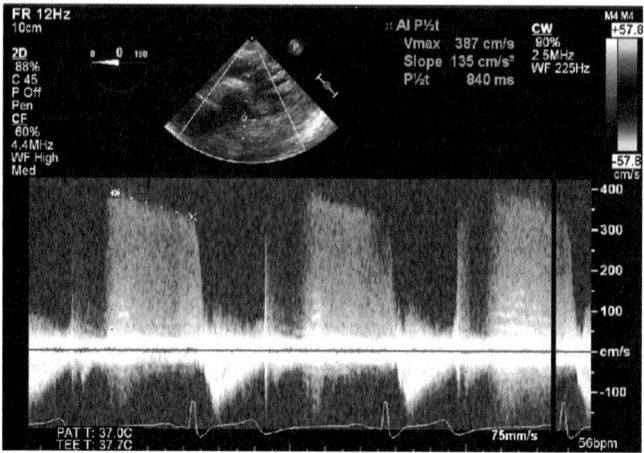

Figure 12-43 Continuous-wave (CW) Doppler determination of aortic regurgitation severity. Continuous retrograde flow from the aorta into the left ventricle through a regurgitant aortic valve may be demonstrated with CW Doppler. In this example, the flow velocity mildly degrades during diastole, yielding a shallow slope. This low slope value is consistent with mild aortic insufficiency.

(corresponding to a long pressure half-time). As aortic regurgitant flow becomes more severe, there is a more rapid equilibration between aortic and LV diastolic pressure, with the nadir of the gradient at end-diastole. As pressures equilibrate, driving pressure across the AV decreases and Doppler-derived AR velocities decrease over the diastolic period. This pattern of AR flow is characterized by a short pressure half-time.

Pressure half-time measurements have been validated as a measure of AR.[234] A pressure half-time of less than 200 milliseconds is consistent with severe AR, whereas a pressure half-time of greater than 500 milliseconds is consistent with mild AR.[230] The accuracy of this technique may be influenced by physiologic variables.[235] A greater systemic vascular resistance increases the rate of decline, whereas reduced ventricular compliance will increase the rate of intraventricular pressure rise, which will also affect the diastolic slope without affecting valvular competence. In a given patient, however, pharmacologic manipulation of afterload or inotropy may result in changes in AR slopes and pressure half-times that are contradictory to other measures of regurgitation.

Proximal isovelocity surface area measurements (PISA) and flow convergence are usually secondary techniques for the evaluation of the severity of AR; their calculation is discussed in more detail in the Mitral Regurgitation section later in this chapter. PISA provides accurate quantification of the severity of AR.[236] Furthermore, aortic diastolic flow reversal may provide an indication of the severity of regurgitation. With increasing AR, both the duration and velocity of the flow velocity increase; holodiastolic reversal is consistent with at least moderate AR.[237] Finally, the SV calculation through the LVOT may be compared with either the MV or pulmonary valve, assuming there is no more than minimal regurgitation of these latter valves. The difference in SV will be equal to the regurgitant volume.

Mitral Valve Evaluation

The mitral valve consists of two leaflets, chordae tendineae, two papillary muscles, and a valve annulus. The anterior leaflet is larger than the posterior and is semicircular; however, the posterior MV leaflet has a longer circumferential attachment to the MV annulus.[238] The posterior valve leaflet may be divided into three scallops: lateral (P1), middle (P2), and medial (P3). The leaflets are connected to each other at junctures of continuous leaflet tissue called the *anterolateral* and *posteromedial commissures*. Primary, secondary, and tertiary chordal structures arise from the papillary muscle, subdividing as they extend and attaching to the free edge and several millimeters from the margin on the ventricular surface of both the anterior and posterior valve leaflets.[239] The annulus of the MV primarily supports the posterior MV leaflet, whereas the anterior MV leaflet is continuous with the membranous ventricular septum, AV, and aorta.

Mitral Stenosis

The most common cause of MS is rheumatic heart disease; other causes are congenital valvular stenosis, vegetations and calcifications of the leaflets, parachute MV, and annular calcification. In addition to structural valvular abnormalities, MS may be caused by nonvalvular causative factors such as intra-atrial masses (myxomas or thrombus) or extrinsic constrictive lesions.[240,241] Generally, MS is characterized by restricted leaflet movement, a reduced orifice, and diastolic doming (Figure 12-44).[242] The diastolic doming occurs when the MV is unable to accommodate all the blood flowing from the LA into the ventricle, so the body of the leaflets separates more than the edges. In rheumatic disease, calcification of the valvular and subvalvular apparatus, as well as thickening, deformation, and fusion of the valvular leaflets at the anterolateral and posteromedial commissures, produce a characteristic fish-mouth-shaped orifice.[243] Other characteristics that may be associated with chronic obstruction to left atrial outflow include an enlarged LA, spontaneous echo contrast or smoke (which is related to low-velocity blood flow with subsequent rouleaux formation by red blood cells[244]), thrombus formation, and RV dilation.

The leaflets, annulus, chordae, and papillary muscles may be assessed in the ME four-chamber, commissural, two-chamber, and LAX views.

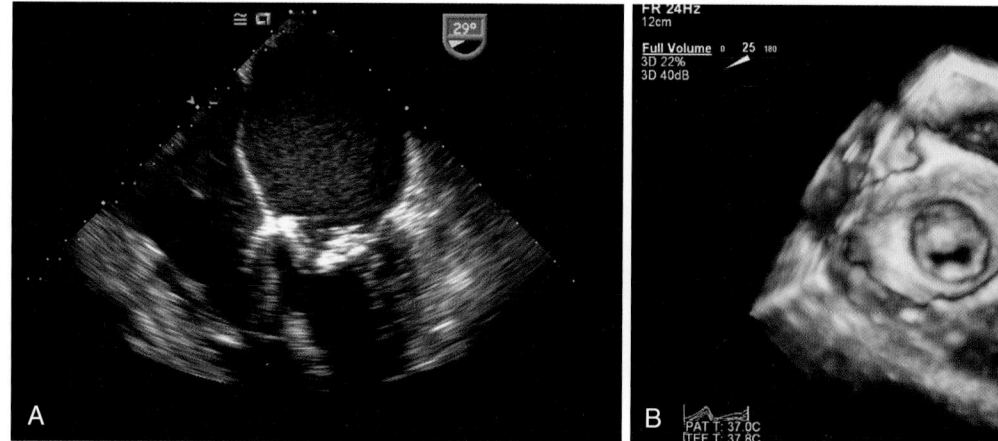
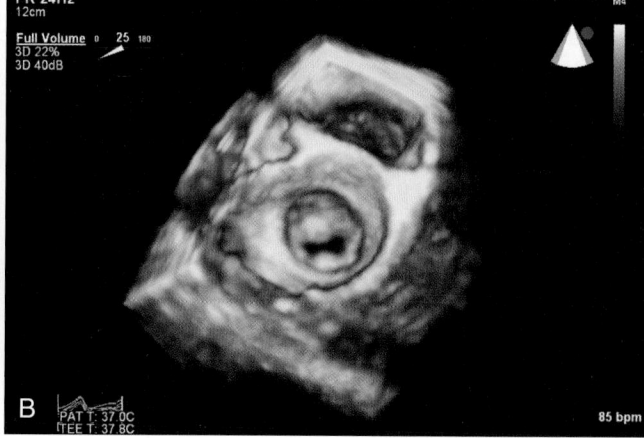

Figure 12-44 Mitral stenosis. *A,* Midesophageal four-chamber view. The mitral valve is severely stenotic with severe calcification of the annulus and leaflets, which is associated with severe left atrial dilation. *B,* Three-dimensional reconstruction in another patient with rheumatic heart disease. There is significant commissural fusion with severe leaflet restriction.

If there is significant annular calcification, the TG views may be necessary to assess the subvalvular apparatus. Because of the propensity for thrombus formation, the entire LA and appendage should be carefully interrogated for thrombus.

Because planimetry of the MV orifice is not influenced by assumptions of flow conditions, ventricular compliance, or associated valvular lesions, its use is the reference standard for the evaluation of mitral valve area (MVA) in MS.[221] This orifice opening is best visualized in the TG basal SAX view and is measured best in mid-diastole. Although at times technically difficult, care should be taken to image the orifice at the leaflet tips. Severe calcification of the MV may interfere with MVA determination, and in patients with significant subvalvular stenosis, underestimation of the degree of hemodynamic compromise may occur when determining MVA by planimetry.[215]

Doppler Assessment of Mitral Valvular Stenosis

A transmitral Doppler spectrum is measured along the axis of transmitral blood flow, which usually may be obtained in an ME four- or two-chamber view (Figure 12-45). Transmitral valve flow is characterized by two peaked waves of flow away from the transducer. The first wave (E) represents early diastolic filling, whereas the second wave (A) represents atrial systole. Transvalvular gradient may be estimated using the modified Bernoulli equation[245]: pressure gradient = $4 \times \text{velocity}^2$. Because peak gradient is heavily influenced by left atrial compliance and ventricular diastolic function, the mean gradient is the relevant clinical measurement.[221] The values obtained through this method have high correlation with those obtained using a transseptal puncture during cardiac catheterization.[246] The high velocities that may occur with MS limit the use of PW Doppler echocardiography; CW Doppler echocardiography should be utilized.

Normally, with MV opening during early diastole, there is a torrential increase in transmitral flow, which rapidly decreases to zero during diastasis when the left atrial and LV pressures equilibrate. With MS, a gradient between the left atrium and ventricle may be maintained for a longer period. This sustained pressure differential maintains flow between the atrium and ventricle, decreasing the slope of this early transmitral flow. The rate of decline of the E-wave velocity may be described by its pressure half-time, which is the time interval from the peak E-wave velocity to the time when the E-wave velocity has declined to half of its corresponding peak pressure value. The pressure half-time is inversely proportional to the MVA[247];

$$\text{Mitral valve area} = 220/\text{pressure half-time}$$

The E-wave may have a bimodal characteristic, with an initial rapid decline in transmitral velocity in early diastole compared with the latter aspect of diastole. In these cases, this latter gentler slope should be measured. The advantage of this technique is that it is independent of valvular geometry. This formula assumes that the MV is at least mildly stenotic. The presence of either mitral regurgitation or AR will decrease the accuracy of pressure half-time measurements for the determination of MS.[248] If there is associated AR, care should be taken that the aortic regurgitant jet is not included in the transmitral flow measurement.[249] Inadvertent inclusion of this AR flow may result in a false increase of transmitral velocity, as well as a false decrease in pressure half-time.[250] Alternatively, AR may result in a rapid increase in diastolic LV pressures, thus decreasing transmitral flow velocity. The continuity equation, using either the LVOT or the PA and PISA method (discussed later), may be used as secondary methods for the evaluation of the severity of MS.

The assessment of the severity of MS is summarized in Table 12-14. The mean transmitral gradient and the MVA as determined by the pressure half-time are the major measurements to be considered; however, planimetry may be used if there is discrepancy between these two measures.[221] Determination of the severity of MS by PISA or the continuity equation should not be considered as primary indices for evaluation.

Mitral Regurgitation

Mitral regurgitation may be caused by disorders of any component of the MV apparatus, specifically, the annulus, the leaflets and chordae, or papillary muscles. The mechanism of mitral regurgitation frequently is described using the Carpentier classification, which is summarized in Table 12-15 and Figure 12-46.[251] The classification is based on leaflet movement. Type I is associated with normal leaflet movement (Figure 12-47A, B). The cause of the mitral regurgitation may be secondary to annular dilation with poor leaflet coaptation or may be caused by a leaflet cleft or perforation. Type II is associated with excessive leaflet movement or prolapse (see Figure 12-47C, D). Most commonly, this type of regurgitation is caused by chordal rupture. Type III is subdivided into types IIIa and IIIb. Type IIIa is restricted leaflet motion both during systole and diastole (see Figure 12-47E, F). This type of mitral regurgitation usually is caused by processes of the leaflets themselves that interfere with normal leaflet function, such as rheumatic MV disease. Type IIIb is restricted leaflet motion during systole (see Figure 12-47G, H). The leaflets themselves usually are anatomically normal; however, substantial chordal tethering may interfere with complete valvular closure during diastole. This type of mitral regurgitation commonly occurs with LV dilation, which commonly results in restriction of P2 and P3.

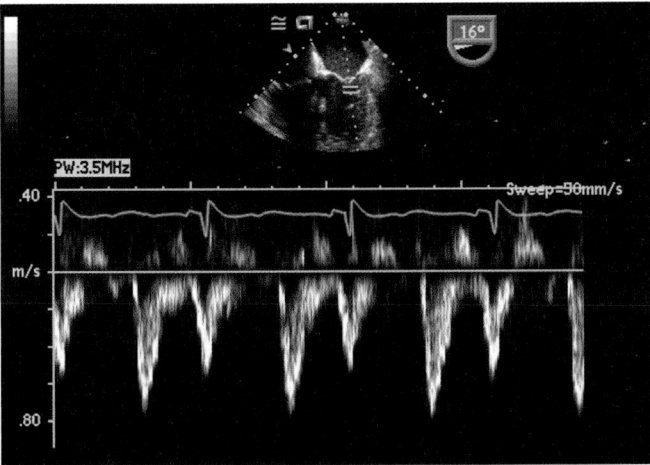
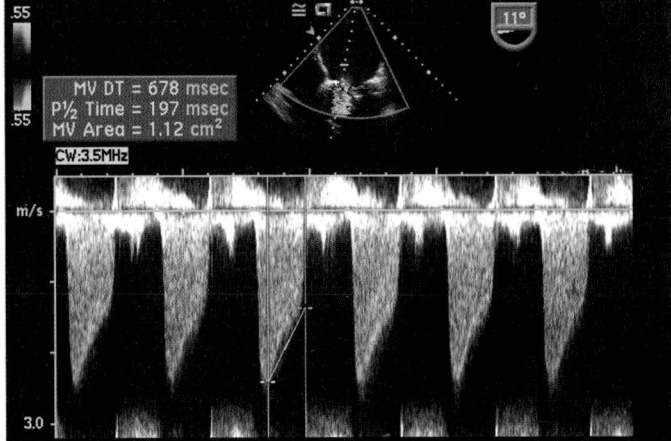

Figure 12-45 Transmitral Doppler spectrum. *Left,* Normal transmitral Doppler flow measured using pulse-wave Doppler. A clean envelope is visualized with E-wave velocity greater than the A-wave velocity. Both waves have velocities less than 1 m/sec with a normal deceleration time. *Right,* Transmitral flow in the presence of mitral stenosis. Because of the high gradient, continuous-wave Doppler was used. High-velocity gradients may be appreciated, and a longer pressure half-time is consistent with significant mitral stenosis.

TABLE 12-14 **Quantification of Mitral Stenosis**

	Mild	Moderate	Severe
Valve area (cm²)	>1.5	1.0–1.5	>1.5
Mean gradient (mm Hg)	<5	5–10	>10

Adapted from Baumgartner H, Hung J, Bermejo J, et al: Echocardiographic assessment of valve stenosis: EAE/ASE recommendations for clinical practice. *J Am Soc Echocardiogr* 22:1–23, 2009.

TABLE 12-15 **Carpentier Classification of Mitral Regurgitation**

	Leaflet Motion	Causative Factors
Type I	Normal	Annular dilation Leaflet perforation
Type II	Excessive (prolapsed)	Chordal elongation or rupture Papillary muscle elongation or rupture
Type IIIa	Restricted leaflet motion during systole and diastole	Leaflet and chordal thickening, e.g., rheumatic heart disease
Type IIIb	Restricted leaflet motion during systole	Left ventricular enlargement

From Carpentier A: Cardiac valve surgery-the "French correction." *J Thorac Cardiovasc Surg* 86:323–337, 1983.

With chronic mitral regurgitation, the annulus and atrium dilate and the annulus loses its normal elliptical shape, becoming more circular.[252] Annular dilation, in turn, leads to poor leaflet coaptation and worsening of valve incompetence. Although increased left atrial and ventricular dimensions may suggest severe mitral regurgitation, smaller dimensions do not exclude the diagnosis.[253] Elongated chords may produce prolapse of one or both attached leaflets; if only one leaflet is affected, leaflet malalignment may occur during systole. Excessively mobile structures near the leaflet tips during diastole may represent elongated chords or ruptured minor chords. These structures do not prolapse into the atrium during systole. In contrast, ruptured major chords are identified as thin structures with a fluttering appearance in the atrium during systole and are associated with marked prolapse of the affected leaflet; in this instance, the valve is said to be "flail." A flail leaflet generally points in the direction of the LA, and this directionality of leaflet pointing is the principal criterion for distinguishing a flailed leaflet from severe valvular prolapse.[254,255] Flail leaflets most commonly are caused by ruptured chordae and less commonly by papillary muscle rupture.

Regurgitation also may be caused by papillary muscle infarction in association with infarction of the adjacent LV myocardium because of a lack of the normal tethering function performed by these structures. When the adjacent segment is aneurysmal, the dyskinetic wall motion may prevent proper coaptation of the valve by restricting the normal movement of the mitral leaflets during systole.[256] Prior infarctions may

be indicated by thinning of the myocardium, atresia of the papillary muscles, and dyskinetic wall segments. Atretic papillary muscles are identified by their diminutive size and increased echocardiographic density on SAX imaging. This shrinkage in papillary muscle size may result in retraction of chordae and subsequent mitral regurgitation. Papillary muscle rupture typically appears as a mass (papillary muscle head) that prolapses into the LA during systole and is connected to the leaflet only by its attached chords. In addition to these structural abnormalities, mitral regurgitation is suggested by LV volume overload, a dilated hypercontractile left ventricle, a high EF, and systolic expansion of the LV.[257]

In patients with recent endocarditis, vegetations may be attached to the leaflets or chords. With rheumatic valve disease, thickening and/or calcification of the leaflets, restriction of leaflets, and a variable degree of shortening and thickening of the subvalvular apparatus may be identified. Ischemic mitral regurgitation usually is from LV remodeling and enlargement after prior MI. Myxomatous degeneration produces ballooning and scalloping of the valve leaflets, as well as localized areas of thinning and thickening, which can be seen echocardiographically.

Qualitative Grading Using Color-Flow Doppler

The diagnosis of mitral regurgitation is made primarily by the use of color-flow mapping. Because flow is best detected when it is parallel to the ultrasonic beam and because some mitral regurgitation jets may be thin and eccentric, multiple views of the LA should be interrogated for evidence of mitral regurgitation. It is important to remember that the regurgitant flow disturbances are 3D velocity fields with complex geometry, which must be sampled from multiple imaging planes to provide an accurate estimate of the maximal spatial extent of the CFD signal. It is common to detect trivial degrees of mitral regurgitation that extend just superior and posterior to the MV leaflet. Mitral regurgitation is detected more frequently by TEE compared with transthoracic imaging, and the degree of regurgitation is often graded as being more severe using TEE.[258,259]

Eccentric jet direction provides corroborative evidence of structural leaflet abnormalities, which may include leaflet prolapse, chordal elongation, chordal rupture, or papillary muscle rupture (Figure 12-48). For example, a jet that is directed laterally along the posterior wall of the LA is associated with anterior leaflet prolapse. Similarly, a jet that is directed medially behind the anterior mitral leaflet is associated with prolapse of the posterior leaflet.

Atrioventricular valve regurgitation is graded semiquantitatively on a scale of 0 to 4+, where 0 is no regurgitation, 1+ is mild, 2+ is moderate, 3+ is moderate-severe, and 4+ is severe regurgitation; the grading is summarized in Table 12-16. The most common method of grading the severity of mitral regurgitation is CFD mapping of the LA. With the Nyquist limits set at 50 to 60 cm/sec, jet areas less than 4 cm² or 20% of the left atrial size are usually classified as mild, whereas jets greater than 10 cm² or 40% of the atrial volume are classified as severe.[230] The area of the Doppler jet may be influenced by technical factors such as gain setting, carrier frequency of the transducer, imaging of low-velocity flows, differentiation of regurgitant

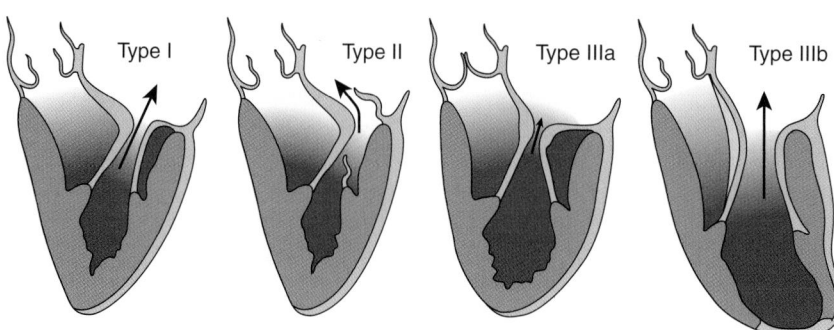

Figure 12-46 Schematic representation of Carpentier classification of mitral regurgitation. *(From Adams D: Available at: mitralvalverepair.org. Accessed March 17, 2010.)*

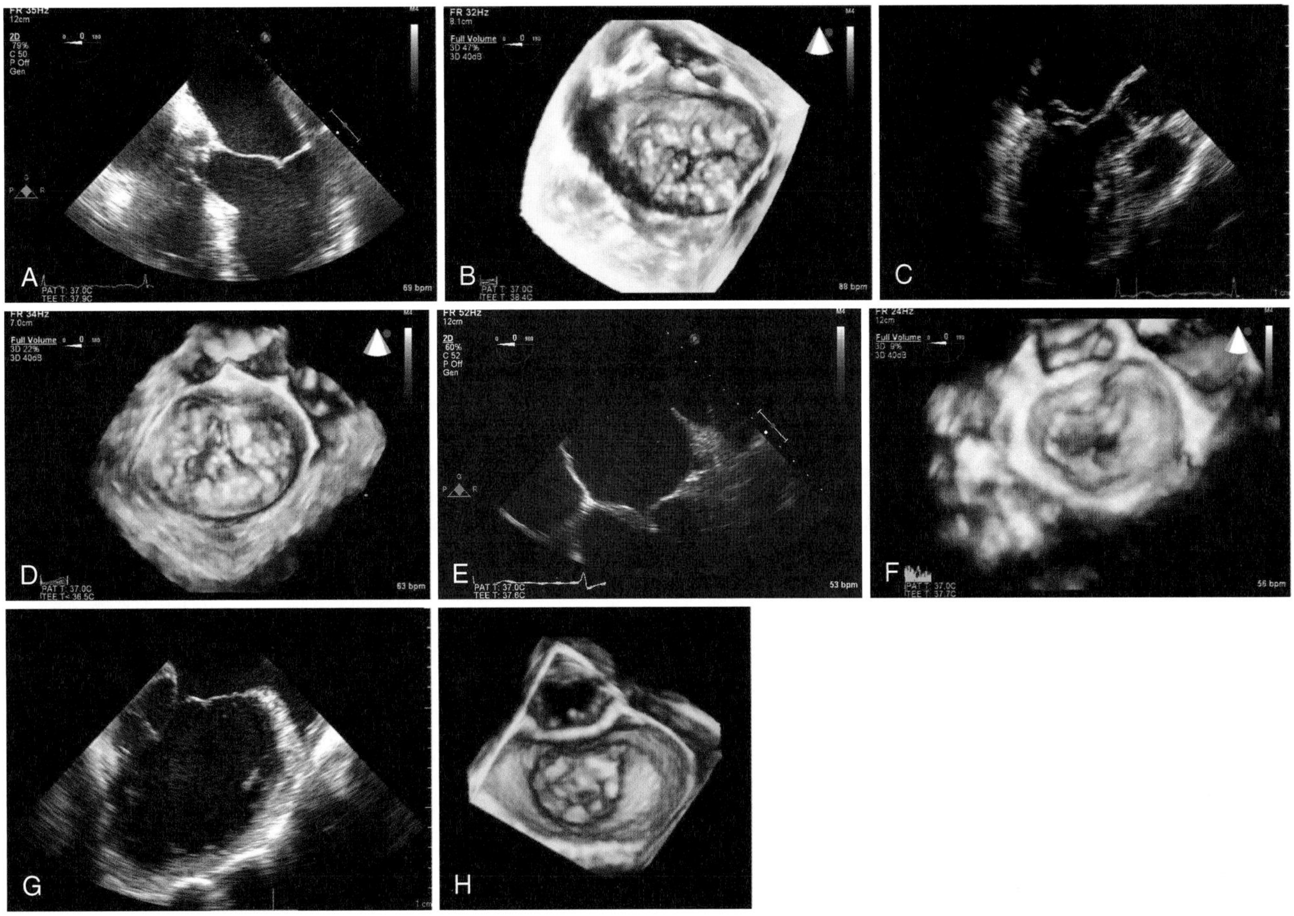

Figure 12-47 **Carpentier classification of mitral regurgitation.** *A* and *B,* Midesophageal four-chamber and three-dimensional reconstruction. With type I mechanism, the mitral valve leaflets coapt at the plane of the mitral valve; however, because of the large annular diameter, there is poor leaflet coaptation. The three-dimensional reconstruction clearly demonstrates a large cleft in the posterior leaflet between P1 and P2. *C* and *D,* Midesophageal long-axis and three-dimensional reconstruction. Type II mechanism: Flailed P2 segment. *E* and *F,* Type IIIa: Midesophageal four-chamber and three-dimensional reconstruction. Rheumatic heart disease results in restricted leaflet motion during both systole and diastole. *G* and *H,* Type IIIb: Midesophageal two-chamber and three-dimensional reconstruction. Ventricular dilation results in tethering of the P2 and P3 component of the posterior leaflet with result restriction of leaflet motion during systole.

from displacement flow, complexities in jet geometry such as multiple jets and vortex flow, temporal variation of jet size during systole, and differences between machines in color-Doppler display.[260] In addition, jet direction should be considered when grading regurgitation because eccentric jets that cling to the atrial wall (Coanda effect) have a smaller area than central (free) jets with similar regurgitant volumes and regurgitant fractions.[261-263] An alternative method of grading mitral regurgitation is based on the vena contracta width.[264] A vena contracta width less than 0.3 cm is associated with mild mitral regurgitation, whereas a width greater than 0.7 cm is associated with severe mitral regurgitation.[230]

CW Doppler integration may also be used in the assessment of the severity of mitral regurgitation.[265] A peak velocity that occurs during early systole and is directed toward the LA can be appreciated with mitral regurgitation, and the intensity of this recording may be proportional to the severity of regurgitation.[266] A dense full signal is associated with severe mitral regurgitation, whereas an incomplete and faint signal is associated with less severe regurgitation.

Pulmonary Vein Flow Pattern. Pulmonary vein flow imaged by TEE provides useful information regarding regurgitant severity.[267] Normally, pulmonary venous flow consists of a phase of retrograde flow during atrial systole and two phases of antegrade flow during ventricular systole and diastole (Figure 12-49). Because systolic pulmonary venous flow is driven by right ventricular systole, systolic antegrade pulmonary venous flow usually is greater than diastolic antegrade pulmonary venous flow. With mitral regurgitation, there is increased LAP during ventricular systole, which may either reduce antegrade systolic pulmonary venous flow or cause reversal of systolic flow in cases of severe regurgitation.

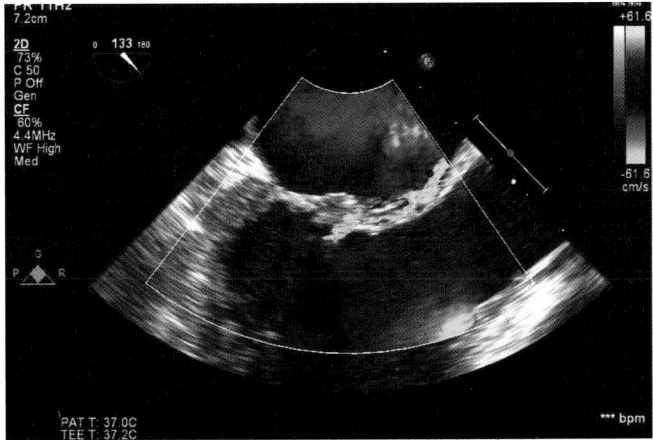

Figure 12-48 **Eccentric mitral valve regurgitant jet.** An eccentric mitral regurgitant jet is seen being directed anteriorly. If the area alone of the jet is used to estimate the degree of regurgitation, the severity of regurgitation will be underestimated.

TABLE 12-16	Summary of Mitral Regurgitation			
	Mild	**Moderate**		**Severe**
	1+	*2+*	*3+*	*4+*
Left atrial size	Normal	Normal or dilated		Usually dilated
Color-flow jet area*	Small central jet (<4 cm² or <20% LA area)			Large central jet (>10 cm² or >40% LA) or variable-sized wall impinging jet
Pulmonary venous flow	Systolic dominance	Systolic blunting		Systolic flow reversal
Continuous-wave jet contour	Parabolic	Usually parabolic		Early peaking triangular
Continuous-wave jet density	Incomplete or faint	Dense		Dense
Vena contracta width (cm)	<0.3	0.3–0.69		≥0.7
Regurgitant orifice area (cm²)	<0.20	0.20–0.29	0.30–0.39	≥0.40

*At Nyquist limits of 50–60 cm/sec.

Adapted from Zoghbi WA, Enriquez-Sarano M, Foster E, et al: Recommendations for evaluation of the severity of native valvular regurgitation with two-dimensional and Doppler echocardiography. *J Am Soc Echocardiogr* 16:777–802, 2003.

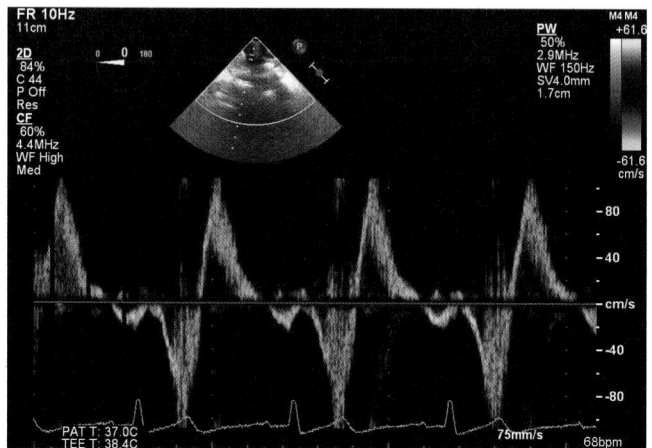

Figure 12-49 Pulmonary venous flow with severe mitral regurgitation. The systolic component of the pulmonary venous tracing, which occurs immediately after the QRS wave, indicates flow away from the left atrium (away from the transducer). This pulmonary systolic venous reversal is consistent with severe mitral regurgitation.

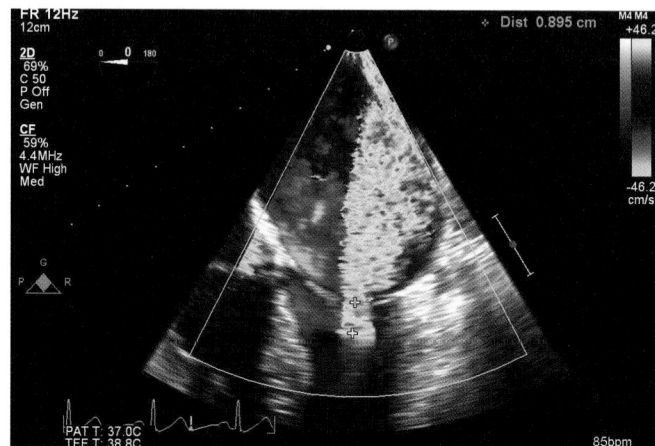

Figure 12-50 Determination of mitral regurgitation by proximal isovelocity surface area. Assuming normal hemodynamics, you may estimate the regurgitant orifice area of the mitral regurgitant volume. The Nyquist limit should be set for approximately 40 cm/sec, and the radius of the proximal isovelocity surface area (PISA) shell in centimeters *(r)* is measured. The regurgitant orifice area (ROA) in square millimeters (mm²) is approximately equal to $r^2/2$. In this case, the PISA radius is approximately 0.9 cm, which would yield an ROA of approximately 0.4 mm².

It is important to interrogate both right and left pulmonary veins. With eccentric jets, flow reversal may be more prominent in the pulmonary veins toward which the jet is directed; however, central mitral regurgitation also may result in discordant pulmonary venous flow patterns.[268] Although discordant flow primarily occurs with eccentric mitral regurgitant jets with systolic reversal primarily in the right upper pulmonary vein, some patients with central regurgitation also may have discordant pulmonary venous flows.

Proximal Isovelocity Surface Area. In addition to these previously discussed indices of mitral regurgitation, regurgitant flow convergence and flow volume may be used to assess the degree of regurgitation (Figure 12-50).[269] Quantification of mitral regurgitation by PISA assumes that as blood flows toward a regurgitant lesion, flow converges radially. This convergence occurs along increasing isovelocity hemispheres converging on the regurgitant lesion. Color Doppler may be used to identify these hemispheres of increasing velocity proximal to the lesion (identified by aliasing), and flow may be determined. Before performing the PISA calculations, a well-defined hemisphere must be imaged. This may be performed by either reducing the Nyquist limits or by shifting the CFD mapping baseline toward the direction of flow. The flow through this well-defined hemisphere is:

$$\text{Flow} = (\text{surface area of the hemisphere}) \times (\text{velocity at the hemisphere})$$

$$\text{If surface area hemisphere} = 2\pi r^2$$

where *r* is the radius of the hemispheric spheres,

$$\text{then flow hemisphere is} = 2\pi r^2 v_n$$

where v_n is the Nyquist limit.

Because flow through these isovelocity spheres equals flow through the regurgitant lesion,

$$2\pi r^2 v_n = \text{ROA } V_o$$

where ROA is the area of the regurgitant orifice area, and V_o is the maximal regurgitant velocity. Solving for ROA yields:

$$\text{ROA} = 2\pi r^2 v_n / V_o$$

Because the regurgitant volume is equal to the area of the regurgitant lesion multiplied by the VTI of the regurgitant velocity (VTI_{regurg}),

$$\text{Regurgitant volume} = \text{VTI}_{regurg}(\text{ROA}) = \text{VTI}_{regurg}(2\pi r^2 v_n / V_o)$$

If the base of the hemisphere is not flat (i.e., 180 degrees), then a correction for wall constraint should be performed by multiplying by the ratio of the adjacent angle formed by the wall and 180 degrees.[230]

The PISA method of determining mitral regurgitation is time-consuming; however, it has been validated as a method of identifying patients with severe mitral regurgitation.[270] Generally, it is most accurate for a central jet compared with an eccentric one. Because the hemispheric radius is squared, care must be taken to ensure and measure a well-defined shell. If the Nyquist limits are set for 40 cm/sec and assuming that the patient has "normal" systolic blood pressures (the difference between the systolic LV pressure and LAP is approximately 100 mm Hg), the calculation of ROA may be estimated to be:[271]

$$ROA = r^2/2$$

where r is the radius of the PISA shell in centimeters.

Tricuspid Valve

The TV consists of three leaflets, an annular ring, chordae tendineae, and multiple papillary muscles.[272] The anterior leaflet is usually the largest, followed by the posterior and septal leaflets. Chordae arise from a large single papillary muscle, double or multiple septal papillary muscles, and several small posterior papillary muscles, attached to the corresponding walls of the right ventricle.

Intrinsic structural abnormalities of the TV that can be well characterized by TEE include rheumatic tricuspid stenosis, carcinoid involvement of the TV, TV prolapse, flail TV, Ebstein's anomaly, and tricuspid endocarditis. Rheumatic involvement of the TV, which is typically seen with concomitant MV involvement, is characterized by thickening of the leaflets (particularly at their coaptation surfaces), fusion of the commissures, and shortening of the chordal structures, resulting in restricted leaflet motion.[273] Carcinoid syndrome results in a diffuse thickening of the TV (and PV) and endocardial thickening of right-heart structures, which may result in restricted TV motion (mixed stenosis and regurgitation) of the TV.[274] The bulky and redundant tricuspid leaflet tissue seen in TV prolapse is associated with billowing of leaflet tissue superior to the tricuspid annular plane into the RA. In patients with an overtly flail TV, the disrupted leaflet tissue wildly prolapses into the RA, exhibiting high-frequency systolic vibrations. Destructive processes such as infective endocarditis, valve trauma induced by inadvertent endomyocardial biopsy of the tricuspid apparatus, and spontaneous rupture of chordae may all result in a partially flail TV apparatus.

Supravalvular, valvular, or subvalvular restriction may cause tricuspid stenosis. The most common cause of tricuspid stenosis is rheumatic heart disease, whereas less common causes include carcinoid syndrome and endomyocardial fibrosis. Tricuspid stenosis is characterized by a domed thickened valve with restricted movement. TR may be secondary to annular or RV dilation, pathology of the leaflets, or subvalvular apparatus. CW Doppler measurements of the inflow velocities across the TV can be used to estimate the mean diastolic TV gradient with the modified Bernoulli equation.[275] Optimal alignment of the Doppler cursor parallel to tricuspid inflow can be difficult to achieve from TEE imaging windows. Often alignment can be achieved, however, by positioning the probe deep within the stomach such that the RV apex is imaged at the top of the sector scan. Alternatively, probe positioning at more rostral levels can display the TV adjacent to a basal SAX view of the AV (multiplane crystal orientation 25 to 30 degrees), which may be suitable for CW Doppler interrogation.

Evaluation of the severity of TR frequently is required in patients with severe MV disease, severe LV systolic dysfunction and secondary right-heart failure, or RV dysfunction caused by long-standing pulmonary hypertension. The quantification of TR is summarized in Table 12-17. The severity of TR can be estimated by the apparent size (area in a given imaging plane, volume reconstructed in 3D) of the color-flow disturbance of TR relative to RA size.[276] A central jet area of less than 5 cm² is consistent with mild regurgitation, whereas a jet area greater than 10 cm² is consistent with severe regurgitation.[230] A vena contracta width greater than 0.7 cm is consistent with severe regurgitation.[277] The apparent severity of TR is exquisitely sensitive to right-heart loading conditions. Thus, during the intraoperative evaluation of TR, PA and RA pressures should be kept near levels observed in the awake resting state. The hepatic veins can be interrogated from deep gastric positioning of the TEE probe to further assist the evaluation of the hemodynamic significance of TR. The presence of blunted systolic hepatic vein flow is associated with moderate regurgitation, and retrograde systolic flow is associated with hemodynamically severe TR.

Myocardial Ischemia Monitoring

Regional Wall Motion and Systolic Wall Thickness

Echocardiography has been used for decades in assessing RWMAs associated with myocardial ischemia.[278] The ability to reliably detect RWMAs is clinically relevant because of its diagnostic and therapeutic implications. Consequently, it is important to note that RWMAs detected by TEE always must be interpreted within the clinical context because not every RWMA is diagnostic for myocardial ischemia. Myocarditis, ventricular pacing, and bundle branch blocks can lead to wall motion abnormalities that potentially can lead to mismanagement of the patient.

When describing RWMAs, common classifications should be used to describe the anatomic localization and degree of dysfunction so that communication is possible between echocardiographer and nonechocardiographer, as well as documentation of ongoing disease course. A 16-segment model of the left ventricle has been published by the ASE (see Figure 12-20).[279] This model subdivides the left ventricle into three zones (basal, mid, and apical). The basal (segments 1 to 6) and midventricular zones (segments 7 to 12) are further subdivided into six segments each, whereas the apical zone consists of only four (segments 13 to 16). Another model published by the American Heart Association Writing Group on Myocardial Segmentation and Registration for Cardiac Imaging has added a 17th segment to the model. The 17th segment represents the apical cap of the previously described 16-segment model.[92]

By understanding coronary anatomy, the echocardiographer can make assumptions regarding localization of a potential coronary artery lesion based on the region of abnormal wall motion. Using the ASE

TABLE 12-17	Quantification of Tricuspid Regurgitation		
	Mild	*Moderate*	*Severe*
Right atrial size	Normal	Normal or dilated	Usually dilated
Tricuspid valve leaflets	Usually normal	Normal or abnormal	Abnormal/flail or wide coaptation defect
Jet area – central jets (cm²)*	<5	5–10	>10
Continuous-wave jet density	Soft and parabolic	Dense, variable contour	Dense, triangular with early peaking
Vena contracta width (cm)*	Not defined	Not defined, but <0.7	>0.7
PISA radius (cm)*	≤0.5	0.6–0.9	>0.9
Hepatic vein flow	Systolic dominance	Systolic blunting	Systolic reversal

*At Nyquist limits of 50–60.
PISA, proximal isovelocity surface area.
Adapted from Zoghbi WA, Enriquez-Sarano M, Foster E, et al: Recommendations for evaluation of the severity of native valvular regurgitation with two-dimensional and Doppler echocardiography. *J Am Soc Echocardiogr* 16:777–802, 2003.

model, the segments 1, 2, 7, 13, 14, and 17 are in the distribution territory of the LAD artery. Segments 5, 6, 11, 12, and 16 are associated with the circumflex artery, and segments 3, 4, 9, 10, and 15 belong to the right coronary artery. This segmental distribution can be variable among patients because of the variability of the coronary arteries. In addition to defining a system that defines anatomic segments of the left ventricle, it is important to grade segment thickening and excursion.

Wall Motion

The simplest assessment of wall motion is performed by "eyeballing" the motion of the individual segments of the left ventricle as described earlier in the ASE model. This qualitative assessment is classified as being either normal, hypokinetic, akinetic, dyskinetic, or aneurysmal. Subsequently, a numeric score of 1 to 5 can be assigned. A wall motion index can be derived by dividing the total score by the number of segments observed. A score of 1 would represent a normal ventricle; the higher the score, the more abnormal the ventricle. This score can be used to predict outcome after cardiac surgery and risk-stratify patients for adverse cardiac events.[280-282]

In addition to movement, the normal myocardium thickens during systole. Wall thickening can be assessed qualitatively, or it can be quantitatively evaluated by calculating systolic wall thickening from the following equation:

$$PSWT = SWT - DWT/SWT \times 100$$

where PSWT = percentage of systolic wall thickening; SWT = end-systolic wall thickening; and DWT = end-diastolic wall thickening. The degree of thickening also can be used to assess overall function of the observed segment. A thickening greater than 30% is normal, 10% to 30% represents mild hypokinesia, 0% to 10% is severe hypokinesia, no thickening is akinesia, and if the segment bulges during systole, dyskinesia would be present.

Diagnosis of Ischemia

The precise sequence of functional changes that occur in the myocardium after interruption of flow has been studied in models of acute ischemia, including percutaneous transluminal coronary angioplasty.[283-285] Abnormalities in diastolic function usually precede abnormal changes in systolic function. Normal function is critical for LV filling and is dependent on ventricular relaxation, compliance, and atrial contraction. Diastolic ventricular function can be assessed by monitoring the rate of filling associated with changes in the chamber dimensions (see earlier). Regional systolic function can be estimated by echocardiographic determination of wall thickening and wall motion during systole in both LAX and SAX views of the ventricle. The SAX view of the left ventricle at the papillary muscle level displays myocardium perfused by the three main coronary arteries and is, therefore, very useful. However, because the SAX view does not image the ventricular apex, and this is a common location of ischemia, the LAX and longitudinal ventricular views are also clinically important.[286]

Although wall thickening is probably a more specific marker of ischemia than wall motion, its measurement requires visualization of the epicardium, which is not always possible. Alternatively, by observing the movement of the endocardium toward the center of the cavity during systole, systolic wall motion can almost always be assessed. As the myocardial oxygen supply/demand balance worsens, graded systolic wall motion abnormalities progress from mild hypokinesia to severe hypokinesia, akinesia, and finally, dyskinesia.[287] Normal contraction is defined as greater than 30% shortening of the radius from the center to the endocardial border. Mild hypokinesia refers to inward contraction that is slower and less vigorous than normal during systole, with radial shortening of 10% to 30%. Severe hypokinesia is defined as less than 10% radial shortening. The precise distinction between varying degrees of hypokinesia can be difficult. Akinesia refers to the absence of wall motion or no inward movement of the endocardium during systole. Dyskinesia refers to paradoxic wall motion or movement outward during ventricular systole (see Chapter 18). These measurements of regional wall motion obviously are based on the determination of

the center of the ventricular cavity. Unfortunately, because of cardiac translation, this center may move during the cardiac cycle. Two reference systems have been used: fixed reference and floating reference. Because of its relative simplicity and the fact that in most situations the impact of translation is minimal, the fixed-reference system generally is used. In conditions of significant translation, such as after CPB, the more cumbersome floating system may be more appropriate.[288]

Relation to Other Monitors

Clinical studies have indicated that RWMAs occur earlier and are a more sensitive indicator of myocardial ischemia than the abnormal changes detected with an ECG or PAC.[289-295] In one study, 30 patients undergoing percutaneous transluminal coronary angioplasty were simultaneously monitored with 12-lead ECGs and echocardiography.[292] All the patients had isolated obstructive lesions in their LAD coronary arteries, stable angina, normal baseline ECGs, normal baseline myocardial function with no prior history of infarction, and no angiographic evidence of collateralization. In the study, all patients experienced development of RWMAs approximately 10 seconds after coronary artery occlusion. Electrocardiographic changes occurred in 27 of 30 patients approximately 22 seconds after coronary occlusion.

Smith et al[291] evaluated 50 patients at high risk for myocardial ischemia during peripheral vascular or cardiac surgery with TEE and a multilead ECG. In their study, 6 patients had repolarization changes diagnostic of ischemia and 24 had new evidence of RWMAs. ECG repolarization changes always were accompanied by a corresponding RWMA. In 50% of the patients who experienced ST-segment changes, the RWMAs had occurred minutes before. Three patients with evidence of new RWMAs developed perioperative MIs; however, only one patient of the three had evidence of ST-segment changes.

The value of PCWP monitoring for ischemia also has been compared with changes in regional LV function assessed with TEE. In one study, PCWP, 12-lead ECG, and LV wall motion were evaluated in 98 patients before CABG at predetermined intervals.[293] Myocardial ischemia was diagnosed by TEE in 14 patients. In 10 of the 14 patients, ischemia was associated with repolarization changes on the ECG. An increase of at least 3 mm Hg in PCWP was tested as an indicator for ischemia and was sensitive only 33% of the time, with a positive predictive value of only 16%. Overall, most studies indicate that the sensitivity of wall motion analysis for detection of myocardial ischemia generally is superior to that of the ECG or PCWP (see Chapters 14 and 18).

Limitations

Although TEE appears to have many advantages over traditional intraoperative monitors of myocardial ischemia, there remain potential limitations as well. The most obvious limitation of TEE monitoring is the fact that ischemia cannot be detected during critical periods, such as induction, laryngoscopy, intubation, emergence, and extubation. In addition, the adequacy of RWMA analysis may be influenced by artifact.[296] The ultrasound system itself or the particular tangential section being imaged can produce artifacts.

The septum, in particular, must be given special consideration with respect to wall motion and wall thickness assessment.[296,297] The septum is composed of two parts: the lower muscular portion and the basal membranous portion. The basal septum does not exhibit the same degree of contraction as the lower muscular part. At the most superior basal portion, the septum is attached to the aortic outflow tract. Its movement at this level is normally paradoxic during ventricular systole. The septum is also a unique region of the left ventricle because it is a region of the right ventricle as well, and is, therefore, influenced by forces from both ventricles. In addition, sternotomy, pericardiotomy, and CPB have been found to alter the translational and rotational motion of the heart within the chest, which may cause changes in ventricular septal motion.[297]

For these reasons, use of a floating reference system in the intraoperative period is recommended. Consequently, the exact imaging plane for wall motion assessment is critical. The SAX view of the left ventricle at the level of the midpapillary muscles is used to ensure constant internal landmarks as reference (anterior and posterior papillary muscles) and to ensure monitoring of the muscular septal region. It must be recognized that, although myocardial blood flow from the coronary arteries is best represented at the SAX midpapillary muscle level, there may be other myocardial regions that are underperfused and not adequately represented in one echocardiographic imaging plane.[298] One solution to this problem is to frequently reposition the probe to view other cross sections of the heart.

Another potential problem of RWMA assessment is evaluation of the uncoordinated contraction that occurs as a result of a bundle branch block or ventricular pacing. In these situations, the system used to assess RWMAs must compensate for global motion of the heart (usually done with a floating frame of reference) and evaluate not only regional endocardial wall motion but also myocardial thickening.

Not all RWMAs are indicative of myocardial ischemia or infarction. Clearly, under normal conditions, all hearts do not contract in a homogenous and consistent manner.[299] It is reasonable to assume, however, that most of the time an acute change in the regional contraction pattern of the heart during surgery is likely attributable to myocardial ischemia. An important exception to this rule may apply in models of acute coronary artery occlusion. In these models, it has been established that myocardial function becomes abnormal in the center of an ischemic zone, but it is also true that the myocardial regions adjacent to the ischemic zones become dysfunctional as well. Several studies have reported that the total area of dysfunctional myocardium commonly exceeds the area of ischemic or infarcted myocardium.[300,301] The impairment of function in nonischemic tissue has been thought to be caused by a "tethering effect" (Figure 12-51). Tethering, or the attachment of noncontracting tissue that is normally perfused, probably accounts for the consistent overestimation of infarct size by echocardiography when compared with postmortem studies.[302]

Another limitation of RWMA analysis during surgery is that it does not differentiate stunned or hibernating myocardium from acute ischemia, nor does it differentiate the cause of ischemia between increased oxygen demand and decreased oxygen supply.[303] Finally, it should be noted that areas of previous ischemia or scarring may become unmasked by changes in afterload and appear as new RWMAs.[304] This is particularly important in vascular surgery, in which major abrupt changes in afterload occur.

Outcome Significance

Data regarding the significance of intraoperative detection of RWMAs suggest that transient abnormalities unaccompanied by hemodynamic or ECG evidence of ischemia may not represent significant myocardial ischemia and usually are not associated with postoperative morbidity.[305] Hypokinetic myocardial segments appear to be associated with minimal perfusion defects compared with the significant perfusion defects that accompany akinetic or dyskinetic segments. Hence, hypokinesia may be a less predictive marker for postoperative morbidity.[291,306,307]

Intraoperative detection of new or worsened and persistent RWMAs during peripheral vascular surgery has been reported to be associated with postoperative cardiac morbidity by several investigators. The occurrence of new RWMAs during vascular surgery appears to be common; however, most of the time, they are transient and clinically insignificant[305–307] New RWMAs that are recognized to persist until the conclusion of surgery, in contrast, imply acute perioperative MI. Intraoperative RWMAs, therefore, may be spurious, reversible with or without treatment, or irreversible. The former may be associated with clinically insignificant, short periods of ischemia, whereas the latter are associated with significant ischemia or infarction.[291,306,307]

Intraoperative TEE has helped predict the results of CABG surgery. After CABG to previously dysfunctional segments, immediate improvement of regional myocardial function (which is sustained) has been demonstrated.[308,309] In addition, prebypass compensatory hypercontracting segments have been reported to revert toward normal immediately after successful CABG.[310] Persistent RWMAs after CABG appear to be related to adverse clinical outcomes, and lack of evidence of RWMAs after CABG has been shown to be associated with a postoperative course without cardiac morbidity.[303]

Stress Echocardiography

Dynamic imaging with *stress echocardiography* was first introduced in the late 1970s and has more recently been rigorously evaluated as a method to better distinguish viable from nonviable myocardium (see Chapter 2). Stress echocardiography uses mechanical, pharmacologic, or other stresses to the heart to achieve predetermined peak stress levels. Since the 1990s, stress echocardiography has emerged as a safe and sensitive method for the detection of CAD and a cost-efficient alternative to scintigraphy. Reversible RWMAs caused by transient myocardial ischemia are the hallmark of atherosclerotic CAD. Among the means for initiating the stress response are exercise, atrial pacing, intravenous dipyridamole, adenosine, and dobutamine. Exercise and dobutamine cause myocardial ischemia through marked increases in heart rate, systolic blood pressure, and contractility. Dipyridamole-induced ischemia, in contrast, is mainly caused by blood flow maldistribution, with a reduction in subendocardial flow in the regions of myocardium supplied by a stenotic coronary artery. Because dipyridamole predominantly affects the supply part of the supply/demand ratio, flow maldistribution may not be severe enough to always induce endocardial ischemia. It is not surprising that sensitivity is greater for detecting ischemic heart disease with exercise followed by dobutamine, whereas specificity is greater with dipyridamole echocardiography. The application of stress echocardiography for assessment of perioperative cardiac risk in patients undergoing major vascular surgery has been investigated and shown to be a safe and cost-efficient method for identifying patients at high and low risk for perioperative cardiac events. Srinivas et al's[311] meta-analysis has determined that its positive predictive value compares favorably with dipyridamole-thallium, Holter ECG, and radionuclide ventriculography for perioperative risk stratification.

A transient imbalance between oxygen supply and demand leads to ischemia. Signs of diastolic dysfunction followed by RWMAs occur before ECG changes and the clinical symptom of pain. Consequently, echocardiography is a useful tool because both diastolic dysfunction

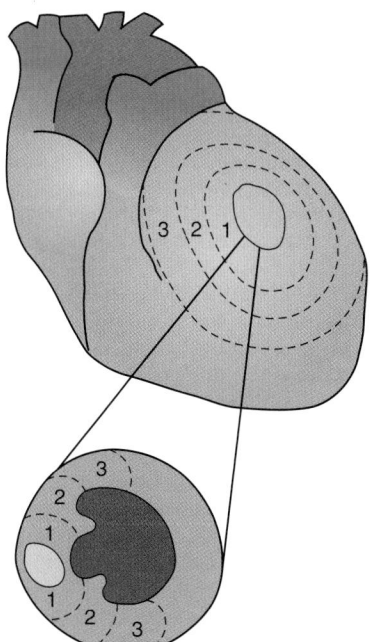

Figure 12-51   Tethering effect. Myocardial function becomes abnormal in the center of an ischemic zone, as well as in regions adjacent to the ischemic zone. Attachment of noncontracting tissue (the central zone) mechanically impairs contraction in normally perfused adjacent tissue (zones 1 through 3).

and RWMAs readily can be diagnosed. Because metabolic balance of the myocardium is a dynamic phenomenon, stress testing frequently is used to increase oxygen consumption. Although, historically, bicycle or treadmill testing has been used to provoke RWMAs, these modes of stress can only be performed in patients able to exercise, requiring rapid acquisition of sonographic images. Consequently, pharmacologically induced stress often is preferred. Dobutamine is the preferred agent because the effects seen on RWMAs are more pronounced when compared with adenosine or dipyridamole.

The test is performed by infusion of dobutamine and increasing the dosage every 3 minutes based on a preset protocol (5, 10, 20, 30, 40 μg/kg/min). The goal is to increase heart rate and metabolic demand, thus provoking RWMAs that can be visualized echocardiographically. The test is stopped if target heart rate is achieved ([220 − age] × 0.85); ST depression is greater than 2 mm; and there is significant tachyarrhythmia, symptomatic severe hypotension, and blood pressure greater than 240 mm Hg systolic or 140 mm Hg diastolic. Serious side effects are rare (1:1000 patients).[312] The accuracy of dobutamine stress echocardiography consistently is reported to be good, with sensitivity and specificity averaging 82% and 81%, respectively.[313] These results are comparable with perfusion imaging and superior to exercise ECG. As with other forms of stress testing, the higher the degree of vascular disease (one- vs. three-vessel disease), the more accurate the test.[314]

Doppler Tissue Imaging– and Speckle Tracking Imaging–Derived Strain

DTI-derived strain accurately measures cardiac deformation,[118] is sensitive to early ischemia,[315] and is useful in assessing myocardial viability after MI, better than DTI velocities or visual wall motion scoring.[316] DTI-derived strain in remote from ischemic regions will remain normal, contrary to spectral DTI velocities, which are affected because of tethering.[117,137]

Acute regional ischemia causes a rapid decrease in segmental contraction during systolic ejection, with the magnitude of regional shortening/thickening reduction in proportion to myocardial blood flow reduction. After systole, myocardial relaxation is delayed as postsystolic shortening (PSS)/thickening occurs.

DTI strain may be an important supplement to visual assessment of regional LV dysfunction. DTI strain and strain rate are more direct measures of regional function than tissue velocities, which are influenced by contractile function of other myocardial regions because of tethering.[117] In 17 patients with LAD disease (>75% obstruction), and normal baseline EF and wall motion score (WMS), DTI strain detected systolic longitudinal expansion in apical segments (baseline −17.7% ± 7.2% vs. 7.5% ± 6.5%) or reduced compression in midseptal segments (baseline −21.8% ± 8.2% vs. −13.1% ± 4.1%) in nearly all patients during balloon occlusion of the LAD. Segments not supplied by the LAD did not exhibit any strain changes. DTI strain was more sensitive than DTI velocities in detecting regional ischemia; the latter revealed longitudinal expansion in only two thirds of the involved segments.[317]

DTI strain indices differentiate acutely ischemic myocardium from normal and dysfunctional myocardium, even in segments that appear visually normal. An acute reduction in regional myocardial blood flow induces a local contractile dysfunction within seconds, which alters the regional deformation pattern. Consequently, during systole, the radial thickening and circumferential/longitudinal shortening of the ischemic segment are decreased. In addition, the segmental relaxation is considerably impaired during the ischemic insult, and the physiologic early diastolic radial thinning and circumferential/longitudinal lengthening are replaced by ongoing post-systolic thickening and shortening, respectively. Such consistent changes in early diastolic deformation have been proposed as an early marker of regional ischemia.

Postsystolic deformation (or PSS) is an important feature of ischemic myocardium. When associated with systolic hypokinesis or akinesis, it indicates actively contracting, potentially viable myocardium. In view of the findings from experimental and clinical studies, PSS should

be considered an expression of myocardial asynchrony. A segment that does not deform during contraction, when LV pressure increases, but does so when LV pressure decreases markedly during isovolumic relaxation, is not likely to be passive. DTI can quantify PSS. In an experimental setting, PSS was recorded during moderate (hypokinetic or akinetic myocardium), as well as severe, ischemia (dyskinetic myocardium).[318] During a 50% reduction of LAD flow, hypokinesis was accompanied by decreased longitudinal DTI systolic strain (from −12.3% ± 1.1% to −6.6% ± 1.3%) and substantial PSS (from 0.9% ± 0.2% to 5.1% ± 0.9%). Concurrent LV pressure-segment length and LV stress-segment length loop analysis indicated that PSS was active. Superimposed afterload augments those changes in a manner similar to LAD occlusion; in both cases, dyskinesis accompanied even more marked PSS.[318]

In a population of 90 consecutive patients with CAD who underwent percutaneous transluminal coronary angioplasty of a coronary artery with more than 90% obstruction, the baseline strain values in the at-risk segments (which had normal WMSs) were similar to those observed in control patients (radial: 49% ± 6.9% vs. 56.3% ± 11.7%; longitudinal: −21.2% ± 4.5% vs. −23.3% ± 4.7%). At-risk segments with abnormal WMSs had decreased strain values (radial: 21.9% ± 11%; longitudinal: −5.2% ± 4.5%) and increased postsystolic deformation (radial: 0.18 ± 0.14; longitudinal: 0.32 ± 0.26) as compared with normal and at-risk segments with normal WMS. Coronary occlusion resulted in a 50% reduction of radial and longitudinal strain, which peaked early in diastole, and increased postsystolic deformation in all at-risk segments (irrespective of WMS). These changes were reversible, and after 2 minutes of coronary reperfusion, segmental deformation parameters returned to the preocclusion state. Neighboring segments did not exhibit any changes, and presence of collaterals diminished the occlusion-associated strain parameter changes (less postsystolic strain).[319] DTI myocardial velocities changed during coronary occlusion only in segments with abnormal baseline function and had lower diagnostic accuracy when compared with strain.[320]

In the clinical setting, RWMAs may not be detected by DTI myocardial velocities because of tethering and translational effects. Only strain and strain rate offer quantitative and objective parameters indicating ischemia. As observed during dobutamine-exercise testing, DTI strain decreased and PSS markedly increased during ischemia, whereas DTI myocardial velocities did not reveal any changes.[321]

Using STI, global longitudinal strain less than −21% (normal: −24.1% ± 2.9%) and strain rate less than −0.9/sec (normal: −1.02 ± 0.09/sec) had good sensitivity and specificity (92% and 89%, and 92% and 96%, respectively) for detection of post-MI patients, with a good linear correlation with WMS index.[126] STI-derived circumferential and radial strain are sensitive to acute reduction of myocardial perfusion. During balloon occlusion, there were significant decreases in circumferential strain (baseline −18.5% ± 7.2% to −10.5% ± 3.8%) and radial strain (baseline 46.5% ± 19.4% to 35.7% ± 20.8%), as well as prolongation of the time to peak circumferential and radial strain.[151]

Longitudinal deformation parameters are potentially superior to visual WMS in identification and quantification of subtle ischemia-induced changes in regional contractility. When DTI strain parameters were correlated with the coronary angiogram, systolic strain and strain rate were significantly reduced in normokinetic segments supplied by a stenosed coronary artery (>70%), but not in normokinetic segments supplied by a coronary artery without significant lumen narrowing.[322] When compared with myocardial velocities, systolic strain and strain rate differentiated abnormal from normal contracting segments. Infarct-involved segments were differentiated from normal myocardium using cutoff values of less than −13% for strain and less than −0.8/sec for strain rate.[322]

DTI radial strain rate agrees well with wall motion and is reduced more in hypokinetic and akinetic segments (0.6 ± 0.5/sec and 0.008 ± 0.3/sec, respectively) than in normokinetic segments (2 ± 0.6/sec). Strain rate reflects changes in WMS induced by dobutamine challenge; it increased in those segments that revealed augmented wall motion (from 2 ± 0.7/sec to 4.7 ± 1.7/sec) and decreased in those segments that showed deteriorating or unchanged wall motion (from 2.1 ± 1 to 1.7 ± 0.8/sec).[323]

Radial and circumferential STI strain enable distinction among normokinetic, hypokinetic, and akinetic segments at rest (defined by cardiac MRI), in a highly reproducible manner and with small intraobserver and interobserver variability (5.3% ± 2.6% and 8.4% ± 3.7%, respectively).[324] A cutoff value of radial strain less than 29% defined hypokinetic from normokinetic segments with sensitivity and specificity of 83%, and a cutoff value of radial strain less than 21% akinetic from hypokinetic segments with sensitivity of 83% and specificity of 94%.

Similar discriminatory ability of STI radial strain was found when transmurality of MI was analyzed using contrast-enhanced cardiac MRI. Radial strain decreased significantly with increased relative hyperenhancement: 27.7% ± 8% (normal segments) versus 20.5% ± 9.7% (nontransmural infarction segments) versus 11.6% ± 8.5% (transmural infarction segments). Nontransmural infarction was distinguished from transmural infarction segments by radial strain cutoff value greater than 16.5%.[325]

In an experimental model of acute LAD ischemia/reperfusion, extent of infarct correlated well with radial and circumferential STI strain. Myocardial segments with more than 50% area of infarct (verified by postmortem histology) had lower end-systolic radial and circumferential strain and longer time to peak strain versus areas with 50% or less or no infarct. End-systolic radial strain less than 2% had 88% sensitivity and 95% specificity for detecting infarcted area larger than 50%.[326]

The use of STI strain for combined assessment of LAX and SAX cardiac function may allow differentiation of transmurality of chronic infarction and, therefore, overcome DTI strain, which is angle limited and can evaluate only longitudinal function reliably. In subendocardial infarction, STI radial strain (32.4% ± 20%) and circumferential strain (−15.4% ± 6.9%) are preserved, whereas longitudinal strain is reduced (−13.2% ± 5.6%). In contrast, in transmural infarcts, both SAX and LAX STI strain are significantly reduced (cutoff value for circumferential strain < −13.6%, sensitivity 73%, specificity 72%).[327]

Accurate identification of infarcted, nonviable myocardium from viable, hypokinetic segments has important clinical implications; revascularization benefits only patients with a sufficient amount of viable myocardium, whereas it is unlikely to benefit those with transmural MI. In post-MI patients, and in contrast with DTI myocardial velocities, longitudinal DTI strain rates of transmural infarcted segments (−0.51 ± 0.17/sec) were significantly decreased when compared with nontransmural (−1.06 ± 0.29/sec), subendocardial (−1.21 ± 0.41/sec) and normal segments (−1.58 ± 0.38/sec). Strain rates also were significantly reduced in subendocardial infarction compared with normal segments. A cutoff value of strain rate greater than −0.59/sec identified transmural from nontransmural and subendocardial MI, and a cutoff value of −0.98/sec > strain rate > −1.26/sec identified a subendocardial infarction from normal segments.[328]

STI radial strain is able to identify myocardial dysfunction and predict recovery of function using a cutoff value of peak radial strain greater than 17.2%. Segments that failed to recover had lower peak radial strain (15.2% ± 7.5%) than those that showed functional improvement after surgical or percutaneous revascularization (22.6% ± 6.3%). This predictive value (sensitivity of 70.2% and specificity of 85.1%) was similar to that of hyperenhancement by contrast-enhanced MRI.[329]

Among patients with cardiovascular risk factors but no overt cardiac disease, longitudinal strain and strain rate are decreased, and circumferential strain is increased in those with apparently normal mitral inflow velocities (E/A > 1). This may imply that LV systolic function and filling are compensated by circumferential shortening at ventricular systole.[330]

Ischemia-Related Diagnoses

Currently, echocardiography is widely used in patients with ischemic heart disease for characterization of cardiac anatomy, as well as for analysis of intracardiac flow velocities by Doppler echocardiographic modalities. Two-dimensional TEE has been shown to greatly enhance the diagnostic potential for detecting life-threatening sequelae of MI, such as a ruptured ventricular septum or ruptured papillary muscles.[331,332] It also has been recognized that TEE may enable the identification of subtle, but potentially significant, problems that complicate the management of ischemic heart disease, such as anomalous coronary artery origins[333] and atrial infarction. In addition, it is important to note that the assessment of right– and left–heart function can be accomplished with intraoperative echocardiography. The assessment of right– and left–heart damage during intraoperative ischemia monitoring is essential because the presence of RV dysfunction may be a limiting factor and, thus, influence perioperative treatment strategies[334,335] (see Chapters 24 and 34).

Pericardial Disease

The pericardium is a two-layered structure reflecting from a visceral layer to a parietal layer approximately 1 to 2 cm distal to the origin of the great vessels and around the pulmonary veins. Under normal circumstances, 5 to 10 mL fluid is contained within the pericardial sack, allowing for practically frictionless motion of the heart during the cardiac cycle. The parietal layer of the pericardium is rich on collagen fibers, making it a low-compliance structure confining the volume of the four cardiac chambers. In other words, a volume increase of one chamber requires a reduction of volume within another. Likewise, if an increase in volume is seen within the pericardial sack, a reduction of chamber volumes must occur.

Pericardial Effusion

Under normal circumstances, the echocardiographer is unable to visualize the fluid film between the two layers. Under pathologic conditions, fluid accumulation can occur, resulting in the development of a pericardial effusion. Typical causative factors leading to pericardial effusions are listed in Table 12-18.

Most echocardiographers use a qualitative grading system to characterize the quantity of the pericardial effusion present (minimal, small, moderate, or large). A quantitative score that can be utilized measures the diameter of the effusion in two dimensions (Table 12-19). In addition, the effusion can either encompass the entire heart (free) or be loculated. Free effusions typically are seen in medical conditions leading to pericardial effusions, whereas loculated effusions are seen after surgery or inflammatory processes. It is important that the echocardiographer pay attention to the anatomic relation of the effusion. A loculated effusion found primarily at the inferior aspect of the heart can lead to inadvertent injury of the right ventricle if a subxiphoidal approach is chosen for drainage. For the novice echocardiographer, it can be difficult to differentiate a left-sided pleural effusion from a pericardial effusion. A good clue is to identify the descending thoracic aorta. Because the reflection of the pericardium is typically anterior to the descending thoracic aorta, pericardial effusions generally are seen anterior and to the right of the aorta.

Cardiac Tamponade

Cardiac tamponade and pericardial effusion are not synonymous. A pericardial effusion is an anatomic diagnosis that may or may not

TABLE 12-18	Causes of Pericardial Effusions					
Idiopathic	*Infections*	*Inflammatory*	*Postmyocardial Infarction*	*Systemic Disease*	*Malignancy*	*Miscellaneous*
Acute	Viral	Lupus	Dressler	Uremia	Direct	After trauma
Chronic	Bacterial	Rheumatoid arthritis	Acute after transmural infarct	Cirrhosis	Lymphatic obstruction	After surgery
	Fungal			Hypothyroidism		Congestive heart failure

TABLE 12-19	Severity of Pericardial Effusions	
Diameter of Effusion		**Severity**
0–0.5 cm		Mild
0.6–2 cm		Moderate
>2.1 cm		Severe

TABLE 12-20	Differentiation of Constrictive Pericarditis from Restrictive Cardiomyopathy	
Variable	**Restriction**	**Constriction**
Septal motion	Normal	Respiratory shift
Mitral E/A ratio	> 1.5	> 1.5
Mitral deceleration time (msec)	< 160	< 160
Mitral inflow respiratory variation	Absent	Usually present
Hepatic vein Doppler	Inspiratory diastolic flow reversal	Expiratory diastolic flow reversal
Mitral septal annular e′	Usually < 7 cm/sec	Usually > 7 cm/sec
Mitral lateral annular e′	Greater than septal e′	Less than septal e′
Ventricular septal strain	Reduced	Usually normal

From Nagueh SF, Appleton CP, Gillebert TC, et al: Recommendations for the evaluation of left ventricular diastolic function by echocardiography. *J Am Soc Echocardiogr* 22:107–133, 2009.

lead to hemodynamic alterations. Because of the histologic structure of the pericardium characterized by a thick fibrous tissue, a constraint is exerted on the cardiac chambers within the thorax. Rapid fluid accumulation leads to a sharp increase in pressure within the pericardial sac because of its low compliance. On the other hand, slow accumulation of fluid can go undetected for long periods of time, resulting in volumes exceeding 1 L (see Chapter 22).

Under normal circumstances, respiratory variation of arterial pressure is less than 10 mm Hg. During mechanical ventilation, inspiratory positive pressure leads to impeded right-sided filling of the heart. The increase in intrathoracic pressure reduces the capacity of the pulmonary veins and augments the filling of the left side of the heart. During expiration, the exact opposite occurs. As the pressure increases within the pericardial sac, the total blood volume within the heart becomes limited, leading to an exaggerated response to the respiratory cycle. If the intrapericardial fluid is not relieved, an equalization will occur among diastolic pressures within the heart. Echocardiographically, this can be identified as an RV collapse during diastole, as well as an RA collapse during systole. More subtle signs of pericardial tamponade can be detected with Doppler-based modalities. A respiratory variation of more than 30% in peak transmitral or trans-TV flow velocity represents a typical finding. This can be achieved by positioning the PW gate just at the leaflet tips of the MV or TV. Although frequently a large pericardial effusion is associated with pericardial tamponade, other causes also can be responsible for respiratory variation in transvalvular flow velocities (e.g., high airway pressures, hematoma). The echocardiographic differentiation between a constrictive pericardial physiology and restrictive disease is summarized in Table 12-20.

FUTURE TECHNOLOGIES

Although much intraoperative echocardiographic research has been directed toward estimating pressures (e.g., PCWP) and flow (e.g., CO) to replace catheter-based techniques, new innovative technologies are exploring means of providing information distinct from and complementary to the traditional measurement of global cardiac hemodynamics and performance. Novel information can be extracted from the complex image analysis of the Doppler and echocardiographic signals to provide quantitative measures of endocardial position and excursion, intramyocardial velocity of shortening, and 3D reconstruction of cardiac anatomy. These techniques are currently in evolution and will need to undergo technical refinement before they become routine during intraoperative evaluation. There is the opportunity for clinical investigation to define the physiologic significance of the data derived by these techniques in the complex and dynamic intraoperative environment. These techniques can analyze common pathophysiologic problems encountered in the operating room in novel ways to shed new insights on clinical decision making. Although it is unlikely that these echocardiographic techniques will supplant traditional monitoring techniques, when used in concert with a comprehensive hemodynamic assessment of cardiac loading conditions and intracardiac blood flow, important information about global cardiac performance, regional diastolic and systolic function, and complex 3D relationships is likely to emerge. For instance, although existing techniques permit reasonable assessment of overall LV systolic function by EF and SV calculations, there may be ways of evaluating LV myocardial shortening in relation to systolic wall stress for specific layers of the myocardium, which may define the mechanisms of impaired systolic contraction; specific spatial or temporal contraction patterns may distinguish myocardial stunning, hibernating myocardium, myocardial edema, myocardial inflammation, or postcardioplegic myocardial dysfunction. These are unrealized potential applications that will provide the stimulus for future investigation and development of new echocardiographic technologies.

REFERENCES

1. Hendee WR, Ritenour ER: *Medical imaging physics,* ed 4, New York, 2002, Wiley-Liss.
2. Hangiandreou NJ: AAPM/RSNA physics tutorial for residents: Topics in US. B-mode US: Basic concepts and new technology, *Radiographics* 23:1019–1033, 2003.
3. Kerut EK, McIlwain EF, Plotnick GD: *Handbook of echo-Doppler interpretation,* ed 2, Elmsford, NY, 2004, Blackwell Futura.
4. Thomas JD, Rubin DN: Tissue harmonic imaging: Why does it work? *J Am Soc Echocardiogr* 11:803–808, 1998.
5. Hatle L, Angelsen B: *Doppler ultrasound in cardiology,* ed 2, Philadelphia, 1984, Lea & Febiger.
6. Kisslo J, Adams D, Mark DB: *Basic Doppler echocardiography,* New York, 1986, Churchill Livingstone.
7. Evans DH, McDicken WN, Skidmore R, et al: *Doppler ultrasound: Physics instrumentation and clinical applications,* New York, 1989, John Wiley & Sons.
8. Kisslo J, Adams DB, Belkin RN: *Doppler color–flow imaging,* New York, 1988, Churchill Livingstone.
9. Vegas A, Meineri M: Three-dimensional transesophageal echocardiography is a major advance for intraoperative clinical management of patients undergoing cardiac surgery, *Anesth Analg* 110:1548–1573, 2010.
10. Dekker DL, Piziali RL, Dong E Jr: A system for ultrasonically imaging the human heart in three dimensions, *Comput Biomed Res* 7:544–553, 1974.
11. De Simone R, Glombitza G, Vahl CF, et al: Three-dimensional color Doppler: A clinical study in patients with mitral regurgitation, *J Am Coll Cardiol* 33:1646–1654, 1999.
12. Coisne D, Erwan D, Christiaens L, et al: Quantitative assessment of regurgitant flow with total digital three-dimensional reconstruction of color Doppler flow in the convergent region: In vitro validation, *J Am Soc Echocardiogr* 15:233–240, 2002.
13. Samad BA, Alam M, Jensen-Urstad K: Prognostic impact of right ventricular involvement as assessed by tricuspid annular motion in patients with acute myocardial infarction, *Am J Cardiol* 90:778e81, 2002.
14. Sugeng L, Mor-Avi V, Weinert L, et al: Multimodality comparison of quantitative volumetric analysis of the right ventricle, *JACC Cardiovasc Imaging* 3:10–18, 2010.
15. Gramiak R, Shah PM, Kramer DH: Ultrasound cardiography: Contrast studies in anatomy and function, *Radiology* 92:939–948, 1969.
16. Serwer GA, Armstrong BE, Anderson PA, et al: Use of ventricular septal defects, *Circulation* 58:327–336, 1978.
17. Melzer RS, Hoogenhuyze DV, Serruys PW: Diagnosis of tricuspid regurgitation by contrast echocardiography, *Circulation* 63:1093, 1981.
18. Roelandt J: Contrast echocardiography, *Ultrasound Med Biol* 8:471–492, 1982.
19. Armstong WF, West SR, Mueller TM, et al: Assessment of location and size of myocardial infarction abnormalities with contrast-enhanced echocardiography, *J Am Coll Cardiol* 2:63–69, 1983.
20. DeMaria A, Bommer W, Kuan OL, et al: *In vivo* correlation of thermodilution cardiac output and video-densitometry indicator-dilution curves obtained from contrast two-dimensional echocardiograms, *J Am Coll Cardiol* 3:999–1004, 1984.
21. Goldman ME, Mindich BP, Teicholz LE, et al: Intraoperative contrast echocardiography to evaluate mitral valve operations, *J Am Coll Cardiol* 4:1035–1040, 1984.
22. Raisinghani A, DeMaria AN: Physical principles of microbubble ultrasound contrast agents, *Am J Cardiol* 90:3J–7J, 2002.
23. Frinkin PJA, Bouakaz A, Kirkhorn J, et al: Ultrasound contrast imaging: Current and new potential methods, *Ultrasound Med Biol* 26:965–975, 2000.
24. Stewart MJ: Contrast echocardiography, *Heart* 89:342–348, 2003.
25. Kaul S: Instrumentation for contrast echocardiography: Technology and techniques, *Am J Cardiol* 18:8J–14J, 2002.
26. Miller AP, Nanda NC: Contrast echocardiography: New agents, *Ultrasound Med Biol* 30:425–434, 2004.
27. Mulvagh SL, Rakowski H, Vannan MA, et al: American Society of Echocardiography Consensus Statement on the Clinical Applications of Ultrasonic Contrast Agents in Echocardiography, *J Am Soc Echocardiogr* 21:1179–1201, 2008.
28. Ward RP, Collins KA, Balasia B, et al: Harmonic imaging for endocardial visualization and myocardial contrast echocardiography during transesophageal echocardiography, *J Am Soc Echocardiogr* 17:10–14, 2004.

29. Masugata H, Yukiiri K, Takagi Y, et al: Potential pitfalls of visualization of myocardial perfusion by myocardial contrast echocardiography with harmonic gray scale B-mode and power Doppler imaging, *Int J Cardiovasc Imaging* 20:117–125, 2004.
30. Skyba DM, Price RJ, Linka AZ, et al: Direct in vivo visualization of intravascular destruction of microbubbles by ultrasound and its local effects on tissue, *Circulation* 98:290–293, 1998.
31. van Der Wouw PA, Brauns AC, Bailey SE, et al: Premature ventricular contractions during triggered imaging with ultrasound contrast, *J Am Soc Echocardiogr* 13:288–294, 2000.
32. Raisinghani A, Wei KS, Crouse L, et al: Myocardial contrast echocardiography (MCE) with triggered ultrasound does not cause premature ventricular complexes: Evidence from PB127 MCE studies, *J Am Soc Echocardiogr* 16:1037–1042, 2003.
33. Dolan MS, Riad K, El-Shafei A, et al: Effect of intravenous contrast for left ventricular opacification and border definition on sensitivity and specificity of dobutamine stress echocardiography compared with coronary angiography in technically difficult patients, *Am Heart J* 142:908–915, 2001.
34. Cohen JL, Cheirif J, Segar DS, et al: Improved left ventricular endocardial border delineation and opacification with Optison (FS069), a new echocardiographic contrast agent: Results of a phase III multicenter trial, *J Am Coll Cardiol* 32:746–752, 1998.
35. Thomson HL, Basmadjian AJ, Rainbird AJ, et al: Contrast echocardiography improves the accuracy and reproducibility of left ventricular remodeling measurements: A prospective, randomly assigned, blinded study, *J Am Coll Cardiol* 38:867–875, 2001.
36. Plana JC, Mikati IA, Dokainish H, et al: A randomized cross-over study for evaluation of the effect of image optimization with contrast on the diagnostic accuracy of dobutamine echocardiography in coronary artery disease: The OPTIMIZE trial, *JACC Cardiovasc Imaging* 1:145–152, 2008.
37. Yu EH, Sloggett CE, Iwanochko RM, et al: Feasibility and accuracy of left ventricular volumes and ejection fraction determination by fundamental, tissue harmonic, and intravenous contrast imaging in difficult-to-image patients, *J Am Soc Echocardiogr* 13:216–224, 2000.
38. Nakatani S, Imanishi T, Terasawa A, et al: Clinical application of transpulmonary contrast-enhanced Doppler technique in the assessment of severity of aortic stenosis, *J Am Coll Cardiol* 20:973–978, 1992.
39. Lindner JR, Wei K, Kaul S: Imaging of myocardial perfusion with SonoVue® in patients with a prior myocardial infarction, *Echocardiography* 16:753–760, 1999.
40. Palmieri V, Arezzi E, Pezzullo S, et al: Inter- and intra-study reproducibility of contrast echocardiography for assessment of interventricular septal wall perfusion rate in humans, *Eur J Echocardiogr* 5:367–374, 2004.
41. Moir S, Haluska BA, Jenkins C, et al: Incremental benefit of myocardial contrast to combined dipyridamole-exercise stress echocardiography for the assessment of coronary artery disease, *Circulation* 110:1108–1113, 2004.
42. Senior R, Lepper W, Pasquet A, et al: Myocardial perfusion assessment in patients with medium probability of coronary artery disease and no prior myocardial infarction: Comparison of myocardial contrast echocardiography with 99mTc single-photon emission computed tomography, *Am Heart J* 147:1100–1105, 2004.
43. Peltier M, Vancraeynest D, Pasquet A, et al: Assessment of the physiologic significance of coronary disease with dipyridamole real-time myocardial contrast echocardiography. Comparison with technetium-99m sestamibi single-photon emission computed tomography and quantitative coronary angiography, *J Am Coll Cardiol* 43:257–264, 2004.
44. Janardhanan R, Swinburn JM, Greaves K, et al: Usefulness of myocardial contrast echocardiography using low-power continuous imaging early after acute myocardial infarction to predict late functional left ventricular recovery, *Am J Cardiol* 92:493–497, 2003.
45. Janardhanan R, Burden L, Senior R: Usefulness of myocardial contrast echocardiography in predicting collateral blood flow in the presence of a persistently occluded acute myocardial infarction-related coronary artery, *Am J Cardiol* 93:1207–1211, 2004.
46. Balcells E, Powers ER, Lepper W, et al: Detection of myocardial viability by contrast echocardiography in acute infarction predicts recovery of resting function and contractile reserve, *J Am Coll Cardiol* 41:827–833, 2003.
47. Korosoglou G, Hansen A, Hoffend J, et al: Comparison of real-time myocardial contrast echocardiography for the assessment of myocardial viability with fluorodeoxyglucose-18 positron emission tomography and dobutamine stress echocardiography, *Am J Cardiol* 94:570–576, 2004.
48. Fukuda S, Hozumi T, Muro T, et al: Quantitative intravenous myocardial contrast echocardiography predicts recovery of left ventricular function after revascularization in chronic coronary artery disease, *Echocardiography* 21:119–124, 2004.
49. Sable C: Digital echocardiography and telemedicine applications in pediatric cardiology, *Pediatr Cardiol* 23:358–369, 2002.
50. Thomas JD, Adams DB, Devries S, et al: Digital Echocardiography Committee of the American Society of Echocardiography. Guidelines and Recommendations for Digital Echocardiography: A report from the Digital Echocardiography Committee of the American Society of Echocardiography, *J Am Soc Echocardiogr* 18:287–297, 2005.
51. Thomas JD, Greenberg NL, Garcia MJ: Digital Echocardiography 2002: Now is the time, *J Am Soc Echocardiogr* 15:831–838, 2002.
52. Mathewson JW, Dyar D, Jones FD, et al: Conversion to digital technology improves efficiency in the pediatric echocardiography laboratory, *J Am Soc Echocardiogr* 15:1515–1522, 2002.
53. Haluska B, Wahi S, Mayer-Sabik E, et al: Accuracy and cost- and time-effectiveness of digital clip versus videotape interpretation of echocardiograms in patients with valvular disease, *J Am Soc Echocardiogr* 14:292–298, 2001.
54. Shah DJ, Diluzio S, Ambardekar AV, et al: Evaluation of valvular regurgitation severity using digital acquisition of echocardiographic images, *J Am Soc Echocardiogr* 15:241–246, 2002.
55. Garcia MJ, Thomas JD, Greenberg N, et al: Comparison of MPEG-1 digital videotape with digitized sVHS videotape for quantitative echocardiographic measurements, *J Am Soc Echocardiogr* 14: 114–121, 2001.
56. Segar DS, Skolnick D, Sawada SG, et al: A comparison of the interpretation of digitized and videotape recorded echocardiograms, *J Am Soc Echocardiogr* 12:714–719, 1999.
57. Soble JS, Yurow G, Brar R, et al: Comparison of MPEG digital video with super VHS tape for diagnostic echocardiographic readings, *J Am Soc Echocardiogr* 11:819–825, 1998.
58. Harris KM, Schum KR, Knickelbine T, et al: Comparison of diagnostic quality of motion picture experts group–2 digital video with super VHS videotape for echocardiographic imaging, *J Am Soc Echocardiogr* 16:880–883, 2003.
59. Frankewitsch T, Söhnlein S, Müller M, et al: Computed quality assessment of MPEG4-compressed DICOM video data. In Engelbrecht R, et al, editors: *Connecting medical informatics and bio-informatics*, Amsterdam, 2005, IOS Press, pp 447–452.
60. Graham RNJ, Perriss RW, Scarsbrook AF: DICOM demystified: A review of digital file formats and their use in radiological practice, *Clin Radiol* 60:1133–1140, 2005.
61. Shanewise JS, Cheung AT, Aronson S, et al: ASE/SCA guidelines for performing a comprehensive intraoperative multiplane transesophageal echocardiography examination: Recommendations of the American Society of Echocardiography Council for Intraoperative Echocardiography and the Society of Cardiovascular Anesthesiologists Task Force for Certification in Perioperative Transesophageal Echocardiography, *Anesth Analg* 89:870–884, 1999.
62. Hisanaga K, Hisanaga A, Nagata K, et al: A new transesophageal real–time two–dimensional echocardiographic system using a flexible tube and its clinical application, *Proc Jpn J Med Ultrasonogr* 32:43, 1977.
63. Matsumoto M, Oka Y, Strom J, et al: Application of transesophageal echocardiography to continuous intraoperative monitoring of left ventricular performance, *Am J Cardiol* 46:95, 1980.
64. Schluter M, Langenstein B, Polster J, et al: Transesophageal cross–sectional echocardiography with a phased array transducer system. Technique and initial clinical results, *Br Heart Jr* 48:68, 1982.
65. Urbanowicz JH, Kernoff RS, Oppenheim G, et al: Transesophageal echocardiography and its potential for esophageal damage, *Anesthesiology* 72:40, 1990.
66. O'Shea JP, Southern JF, D'Ambra MN, et al: Effects of prolonged transesophageal echocardiographic imaging and probe manipulation on the esophagus—an echocardiographic–pathologic study, *J Am Coll Cardiol* 17:1426, 1991.
67. Min JK, Spencer KT, Furlong KT, et al: Clinical features of complications from transesophageal echocardiography: A single-center case series of 10,000 consecutive examinations, *J Am Soc Echocardiogr* 18:925–929, 2005.
68. Kallmeyer IJ, Collard CD, Fox JA, et al: The safety of intraoperative transesophageal echocardiography: A case series of 7200 cardiac surgical patients, *Anesth Analg* 92:1126–1130, 2001.
69. Piercy M, McNicol L, Dinh DT, et al: Major complications related to the use of transesophageal echocardiography in cardiac surgery, *J Cardiothorac Vasc Anesth* 23:62–65, 2009.
70. Everett ED, Hirschman JV: Transient bacteremia and endocarditis prophylaxis, *Medicine* 56:61, 1977.
71. Botoman VA, Surawicz CM: Bacteremia with gastrointestinal endoscopic procedures, *Gastrointest Endosc* 32:342, 1986.
72. Nikutta P, Mantey–Stiers F, Becht I, et al: Risk of bacteremia induced by transesophageal echocardiography: Analysis of 100 consecutive procedures, *J Am Soc Echocardiogr* 5:168, 1992.
73. Melendez LJ, Kwan–Leung C, Cheung PK, et al: Incidence of bacteremia in transesophageal echocardiography: A prospective study of 140 consecutive patients, *J Am Coll Cardiol* 18:1650, 1991.
74. Steckelberg JM, Khandheria BK, Anhalt JP, et al: Prospective evaluation of the risk of bacteremia associated with transesophageal echocardiography, *Circulation* 84:177, 1991.
75. Dajani AS, Bisno AAL, Chung KJ, et al: Prevention of bacterial endocarditis, *JAMA* 264:2919, 1990.
76. Cucchiara RF, Nugent M, Seward JB, et al: Air embolism in upright neurosurgical patients: Detection and localization by two–dimensional transesophageal echocardiography, *Anesthesiology* 60:353, 1984.
77. Humphrey LS: Esophageal stethoscope loss complicating transesophageal echocardiography, *J Cardiothorac Anesth* 3:356, 1988.
78. Ellis JE, Lichtor JL, Feinstein SB, et al: Right heart dysfunction, pulmonary embolism, and paradoxical embolization during liver transplantation, *Anesth Analg* 68:777, 1989.
79. Suriani RJ, Cutrone A, Feierman D, et al: Intraoperative transesophageal echocardiography during liver transplantation, *J Cardiothorac Vasc Anesth* 10:699–707, 1996.
80. Kaplan JA: Monitoring technology: Advances and restraints, *J Cardiothorac Anesth* 3:257, 1989.
81. Pearlman AS, Gardin JM, Martin RP, et al: Guidelines for physician training in transesophageal echocardiography: Recommendations of the American Society of Echocardiography, *J Am Soc Echocardiogr* 5:187–194, 1992.
82. Popp RL, Williams SV, et al: ACP/ACC/AHA Task Force on Clinical Privileges in Cardiology: Clinical competence in adult echocardiography, *J Am Coll Cardiol* 15:1465–1468, 1990.
83. Pearlman AS, Gardin JM, Martin RP, et al: Guidelines for optimal physician training in echocardiography. Recommendations of the American Society of Echocardiography Committee for Physician Training in Echocardiography, *Am J Cardiol* 60:158–163, 1987.
84. Thys DM, Abel M, Botlen B, et al: Practice parameters for intraoperative echocardiography, *Anesthesiology* 84:986–1006, 1996.
85. Practice Guidelines for Perioperative Transesophageal Echocardiography: An updated report by the ASA and SCA Task Force on TEE, *Anesthesiology* 112:1084–1096, 2010.
86. Calahan MK, Foster E: Training in transesophageal echocardiography: In the lab or on the job? *Anesth Analg* 81:217–218, 1995.
87. Savage RM, et al: Educational program for intraoperative transesophageal echocardiography, *Anesth Analg* 81:399–403, 1995.
88. Rafferty T, LaMantia KR, Davis E, et al: Quality assurance for intraoperative transesophageal echocardiography monitoring: A report of 836 procedures, *Anesth Analg* 76:228–232, 1993.
89. Minhaj M, Patel K, Muzic D, et al: The effect of routine intraoperative transesophageal echocardiography on surgical management, *J Cardiothorac Vasc Anesth* 21:800–804, 2007.
90. Eltzschig HK, Rosenberger P, Löffler M, et al: Impact of intraoperative transesophageal echocardiography on surgical decisions in 12,566 patients undergoing cardiac surgery, *Ann Thorac Surg* 85:845–852, 2008.
91. Shanewise J, Cheung A, Aronson S, et al: ASE/SCA Guidelines for Performing a Comprehensive Intraoperative Multiplane Transesophageal Echocardiography Examination: Recommendations of the American Society of Echocardiography Council for Intraoperative Echocardiography and the Society of Cardiovascular Anesthesiologists Task Force for Certification in Perioperative Transesophageal Echocardiography, *Anesth Analg* 89:870–884, 1999.
92. Cerqueira M, Weissman NJ, Dilsizian V, et al: Standardized myocardial segmentation and nomenclature for tomographic imaging of the heart: A statement for healthcare professionals from the Cardiac Imaging Committee of the Council on Clinical Cardiology of the American Heart Association, *J Am Soc Echocardiogr* 5:463–467, 2002.
93. Konstadt SN, Reich DL, Quintana C, et al: The ascending aorta: How much does transesophageal echocardiography see? *Anesth Analg* 78:240–244, 1994.
94. Konstadt SN, Reich DL, Kahn R, et al: Transesophageal echocardiography can be used to screen for ascending aortic atherosclerosis, *Anesth Analg* 81:225–228, 1995.
95. Djaiani G, Ali M, Borger MA, et al: Epiaortic scanning modifies planned intraoperative surgical management but not cerebral embolic load during coronary artery bypass surgery, *Anesth Analg* 106:1611–1618, 2008.
96. Glas KE, Swaminathan M, Reeves ST, et al: Guidelines for the performance of a comprehensive intraoperative epiaortic ultrasonographic examination: Recommendations of the American Society of Echocardiography and the Society of Cardiovascular Anesthesiologists; endorsed by the Society of Thoracic Surgeons. Council for Intraoperative Echocardiography of the American Society of Echocardiography; Society of Cardiovascular Anesthesiologists; Society of Thoracic Surgeons, *Anesth Analg* 106:1376–1384, 2008.
97. Katz ES, Tunick PA, Rusinek H, et al: Protruding aortic atheromas predict stroke in elderly patients undergoing cardiopulmonary bypass: Experience with intraoperative transesophageal echocardiography, *J Am Coll Cardiol* 20:70–77, 1992.
98. London MJ: Assessment of left ventricular global systolic function by transesophageal echocardiography, *Ann Card Anaesth* 9:157–163, 2006.
99. Bergquist BD, Leung JM, Bellows WH: Transesophageal echocardiography in myocardial revascularization: I. Accuracy of intraoperative real-time interpretation, *Anesth Analg* 82:1132–1138, 1996.
100. Lang RM, Bierig M, Devereux R, et al: Recommendations for chamber quantification: A report from the American Society of Echocardiography's Guidelines and Standards Committee and the Chamber Quantification Group, developed in conjunction with the European Association of Echocardiography, a branch of the European Society of Cardiology, *J Am Soc Echocardiogr* 18:1440–1463, 2005.
101. Quinones MA, Otto CM, Stoddard M, et al: Recommendations for quantification of Doppler echocardiography: A report from the Doppler quantification task force of the nomenclature and standards committee of the American Society of Echocardiography, *J Am Soc Echocardiogr* 15: 167–184, 2002.

102. Marwick TH: Techniques for comprehensive two dimensional echocardiographic assessment of left ventricular systolic function, *Heart* 89(Suppl III):iii2–iii8, 2003.
103. Chen C, Rodriguez L, Guerrero JL, et al: Noninvasive estimation of the instantaneous first derivative of left ventricular pressure using continuous-wave pressure echocardiography, *Circulation* 83:2101–2110, 1991.
104. Thomas JD, Popovic ZB: Assessment of left ventricular function by cardiac ultrasound, *J Am Coll Cardiol* 48:2012–2025, 2006.
105. Marwick TH: Measurements of strain and strain rate by echocardiography. Ready for prime time? *J Am Coll Cardiol* 47:1313–1327, 2006.
106. Lewis RP, Rittgers SE, Forester WF, et al: A critical review of the systolic time intervals, *Circulation* 56:146, 1977.
107. Weissler AM: Systolic time intervals, *N Engl J Med* 296:321, 1977.
108. Noble MIM, Trenchard D, Guz A: Left ventricular ejection in conscious dogs: 1. Measurement and significance of the maximum acceleration of blood from the left ventricle, *Circ Res* 19:139, 1966.
109. Bennett ED, Else W, Miller GAH, et al: Maximum acceleration of blood from the left ventricle in patients with ischaemic heart disease, *Clin Sci Mol Med* 46:49, 1974.
110. Sabbah HN, Khaja F, Brymer JF, et al: Noninvasive evaluation of left ventricular performance based on peak aortic blood acceleration measured with a continuous-wave Doppler velocity meter, *Circulation* 74:323, 1986.
111. Mehta N, Bennett DE: Impaired left ventricular function in acute myocardial infarction assessed by Doppler measurement of ascending aortic blood velocity and maximum acceleration, *Am J Cardiol* 57:1052, 1986.
112. Sengupta PP, Korinek J, Belohlavek M, et al: Left ventricular structure and function. Basic science for cardiac imaging, *J Am Coll Cardiol* 48:1988–2001, 2006.
113. Gallagher KP, Matsuzaki M, Koziol JA, et al: Regional myocardial perfusion and wall thickening during ischemia in conscious dogs, *Am J Physiol* 247:H727–H738, 1984.
114. Bogaert J, Rademakers F: Regional nonuniformity of normal adult human left ventricle, *Am J Physiol Heart Circ Physiol* 280:H610–H620, 2001.
115. Marwick TH: Clinical applications of tissue Doppler imaging: A promise fulfilled, *Heart* 89:1377–1378, 2003.
116. Korinek J, Wang J, Sengupta PP, et al: Two-dimensional strain—a Doppler-independent ultrasound method for quantification or regional deformation: Validation in vitro and in vivo, *J Am Soc Echocardiogr* 18:1247–1253, 2005.
117. Urheim S, Edvardsen T, Torp H, et al: Myocardial strain by Doppler echocardiography. Validation of a new method to quantify regional myocardial function, *Circulation* 102:1158–1164, 2000.
118. Edvardsen T, Gerber BL, Garot J, et al: Quantitative assessment of intrinsic regional myocardial deformation by Doppler strain rate echocardiography in humans: Validation against three-dimensional tagged magnetic resonance imaging, *Circulation* 106:50–56, 2002.
119. Amundsen BH, Helle-Valle T, Edvardsen T, et al: Noninvasive myocardial strain measurement by speckle tracking echocardiography. Validation against sonomicrometry and tagged magnetic resonance imaging, *J Am Coll Cardiol* 47:789–793, 2006.
120. Modesto KM, Cauduro S, Dispenzieri A, et al: Two-dimensional acoustic pattern derived strain parameters closely correlate with one-dimensional tissue Doppler derived strain measurements, *Eur J Echocardiogr* 7:315–321, 2006.
121. Weidemann F, Jamal F, Sutherland GR, et al: Myocardial function defined by strain rate and strain during alterations in inotropic states and heart rate, *Am J Physiol Heart Circ Physiol* 283:H792–H799, 2002.
122. Greenberg NL, Firstenberg MS, Castro PL, et al: Doppler-derived myocardial systolic strain is a strong index of left ventricular contractility, *Circulation* 105:99–105, 2002.
123. Serri K, Reant P, Lafitte M, et al: Global and regional myocardial function quantification by two-dimensional strain. Application in hypertrophic cardiomyopathy, *J Am Coll Cardiol* 47:1175–1181, 2006.
124. Andersen NH, Poulsen SH: Evaluation of the longitudinal contraction of the left ventricle in normal subjects by Doppler tissue tracking and strain rate, *J Am Soc Echocardiogr* 16:716–723, 2003.
125. Leitman M, Lysyanski P, Sidenko S, et al: Two-dimensional strain—a novel software for real-time quantitative echocardiographic assessment of myocardial function, *J Am Soc Echocardiogr* 17:1021–1029, 2004.
126. Reisner SA, Lysyanski P, Agmon Y, et al: Global longitudinal strain: A novel index of left ventricular systolic function, *J Am Soc Echocardiogr* 17:630–633, 2004.
127. Kowalski M, Kukulski T, Jamal F, et al: Can natural strain and strain rate quantify regional myocardial deformation? A study in healthy subjects, *Ultrasound Med Biol* 27:1087–1097, 2001.
128. Hurlburt HM, Aurigemma GP, Hill JC, et al: Direct ultasound measurement of longitudinal, circumferential, and radial strain using 2-dimensional strain imaging in normal adults, *Echocardiography* 24:723–731, 2007.
129. Hashimoto I, Li X, Hejmadi Bhat A, et al: Myocardial strain rate is a superior method for evaluation of left ventricular subendocardial function compared with tissue Doppler imaging, *J Am Coll Cardiol* 42:1574–1583, 2003.
130. Abali G, Tokgozoglu L, Ozcebe OI, et al: Which Doppler parameters are load independent? A study in normal volunteers after blood donation, *J Am Soc Echocardiogr* 18:1260–1265, 2005.
131. Choi J-O, Shin D-H, Cho SW, et al: Effect of preload on left ventricular longitudinal strain by 2D speckle tracking, *Echocardiography* 25:873–879, 2008.
132. Becker M, Kramann R, Dohmen G, et al: Impact of left ventricular loading conditions on myocardial deformation parameters: Analysis of early and late changes of myocardial deformation parameters after aortic valve replacement, *J Am Soc Echocardiogr* 20:681–689, 2007.
133. Andersen NH, Terkelsen CJ, Sloth E, et al: Influence of preload alterations on parameters of systolic left ventricular long-axis function: A Doppler tissue study, *J Am Soc Echocardiogr* 17:941–947, 2004.
134. Waggoner AD, Bierig SM: Tissue Doppler imaging: A useful echocardiographic method for the cardiac sonographer to assess systolic and diastolic ventricular function, *J Am Soc Echocardiogr* 14:1143–1152, 2001.
135. Skubas NJ: Intraoperative Doppler tissue imaging is a valuable addition to cardiac anesthesiologists' armamentarium: A core review, *Anesth Analg* 108:48–66, 2009.
136. Wilkenshoff UM, Sovany A, Wigström L, et al: Regional mean systolic myocardial velocity estimation by real-time color Doppler myocardial imaging: A new technique for quantifying regional systolic function, *J Am Soc Echocardiogr* 11:684–692, 1998.
137. Skulstad H, Urheim S, Edvardsen T, et al: Grading of myocardial dysfunction by tissue Doppler echocardiography. A comparison between velocity, displacement, and strain imaging in acute ischemia, *J Am Coll Cardiol* 47:1672–1682, 2006.
138. Cho G-Y, Chan J, Leano R, et al: Comparison of two-dimensional speckle and tissue velocity based strain and validation with harmonic phase magnetic resonance imaging, *Am J Cardiol* 97:1661–1666, 2006.
139. Herbots L, Maes F, D'hooge J, et al: Quantifying myocardial deformation throughout the cardiac cycle: A comparison of ultrasound strain rate, grey-scale M-mode and magnetic resonance imaging, *Ultrasound Med Biol* 30:591–598, 2004.
140. Teske AJ, De Boeck BWL, Melman PG, et al: Echocardiographic quantification of myocardial function using tissue deformation imaging, a guide to image acquisition and analysis using tissue Doppler and speckle tracking, *Cardiovasc Ultrasound* 5:27, 2007.
141. Thomas G: Tissue Doppler echocardiography—a case of right tool, wrong use, *Cardiovasc Ultrasound* 2:12, 2004.
142. Gilman G, Khanderia BK, Hagen ME, et al: Strain and strain rate: A step-by-step approach to image and data acquisition, *J Am Soc Echocardiogr* 17:1001–1020, 2004.
143. Sutherland GR, Bijnens B, McDicken WN: Tissue Doppler echocardiography. Historical perspectives and technological considerations, *Echocardiography* 16:445–453, 1999.
144. D'hooge J, Bijnens B, Thoen J, et al: Echocardiographic strain and strain-rate imaging: A new tool to study regional myocardial function, *IEEE Trans Med Imag* 9:1030, 2002.
145. Notomi Y, Lysyanski P, Setser RM, et al: Measurement of ventricular torsion by two-dimensional ultrasound speckle tracking imaging, *J Am Coll Cardiol* 45:2034–2041, 2005.
146. Helle-Valle T, Crosby J, Edvardsen T, et al: New noninvasive method for assessment of left ventricular rotation: Speckle tracking echocardiography, *Circulation* 112:3149–3156, 2005.
147. Foster E, Lease KE: New untwist on diastole. What goes around comes back, *J Am Coll Cardiol* 113:2477–2479, 2006.
148. Opdahl A, Helle-Valle T, Remme EW, et al: Apical rotation by speckle tracking echocardiography: A simplified bedside index of left ventricular twist, *J Am Soc Echocardiogr* 21:1121–1128, 2008.
149. Notomi Y, Martin-Miklovic MG, Oryszak SJ, et al: Enhanced ventricular untwisting during exercise. A mechanistic manifestation of elastic recoil described by Doppler tissue imaging, *J Am Coll Cardiol* 113:2524–2533, 2006.
150. Perk G, Tunick PA, Kronzon I: Non-Doppler two-dimensional strain imaging by echocardiography-from technical considerations to clinical applications, *J Am Soc Echocardiogr* 20:234–243, 2007.
151. Winter R, Jussila R, Nowak J, et al: Speckle tracking echocardiography is a sensitive tool for the detection of myocardial ischemia: A pilot study from the catheterization laboratory during percutaneous coronary intervention, *J Am Soc Echocardiogr* 20:974–981, 2007.
152. Chow P-C, Liang X-C, Cheung EWY, et al: Novel two-dimensional global longitudinal strain and strain rate imaging for assessment of systemic right ventricular function, *Heart* 94:855–859, 2008.
153. Hanekom L, Cho G-Y, Leano R, et al: Comparison of two-dimensional speckle and tissue Doppler strain measurement during dobutamine stress echocardiography: An angiographic correlation, *Eur Heart J* 28:1765–1772, 2007.
154. Jamal F, Bergerot C, Argaud L, et al: Longitudinal strain quantitates regional right ventricular contractile function, *Am J Physiol Heart Circ Physiol* 285:2842–2847, 2003.
155. Kjaergaard J, Sogaard P, Hassager C: Quantitative echocardiographic analysis of the right ventricle in healthy individuals, *J Am Soc Echocardiogr* 19:1365–1372, 2006.
156. Kjaergaard J, Snyder EM, Hassager C, et al: Impact of preload and afterload on global and regional right ventricular function and pressure: A quantitative echocardiography study, *J Am Soc Echocardiogr* 19:515–521, 2006.
157. Teske AJ, De Boeck BWL, Olimulder M, et al: Echocardiographic assessment of regional right ventricular function: A head-to-head comparison between 2-dimensional and tissue Doppler-derived strain analysis, *J Am Soc Echocardiogr* 21:275–283, 2008.
158. Simmons LA, Weidemann F, Sutherland GR, et al: Doppler tissue velocity, strain, and strain rate imaging with transesophageal echocardiography in the operating room: A feasibility study, *J Am Soc Echocardiogr* 15:768–776, 2002.
159. Norrild K, Pedersen TF, Sloth E: Transesophageal tissue Doppler echocardiography for evaluation of myocardial function during aortic valve replacement, *J Cardiothorac Vasc Anesth* 21:367–370, 2007.
160. Skulstad H, Andersen K, Edvardsen T, et al: Detection of ischemia and new insight into left ventricular physiology by strain Doppler and tissue velocity imaging: Assessment during coronary bypass operation of the beating heart, *J Am Soc Echocardiogr* 17:1225–1233, 2004.
161. Park SJ, Miyazaki C, Bruce CJ, et al: Left ventricular torsion by two-dimensional speckle tracking echocardiography in patients with diastolic dysfunction and normal ejection fraction, *J Am Soc Echocardiogr* 21:1129–1137, 2008.
162. Takeuchi M, Nishikage T, Nakai H, et al: The assessment of left ventricular twist in anterior wall myocardial infarction using two-dimensional speckle tracking imaging, *J Am Soc Echocardiogr* 20:36–44, 2007.
163. St John Sutton M, Plappert T, Hilpisch KE, et al: Sustained reverse left ventricular structural remodeling with cardiac resynchronization at one year is a function of etiology: Quantitative Doppler Echocardiographic Evidence From the Multicenter InSync Randomized Clinical Evaluation (MIRACLE), *Circulation* 113:266–272, 2006.
164. Kanzaki H, Bazaz R, Schawrtzman D, et al: A mechanism for immediate reduction in mitral regurgitation after cardiac resynchronization therapy. Insights from mechanical activation strain mapping, *J Am Coll Cardiol* 44:1619–1625, 2004.
165. Gorcsan J 3rd, Abraham T, Agler DA, et al: Echocardiography for cardiac resynchronization therapy: Recommendations for performance and reporting—a report from the American Society of Echocardiography Dyssynchrony Writing Group endorsed by the Heart Rhythm Society, *J Am Soc Echocardiogr* 21:191–213, 2008.
166. Pitzalis MV, Iacoviello M, Romito R, et al: Ventricular asynchrony predicts a better outcome in patients with chronic heart failure receiving cardiac resynchronization therapy, *J Am Coll Cardiol* 45:65–69, 2005.
167. Marcus GM, Rose E, Viloria EM, et al: Septal to posterior wall motion delay fails to predict reverse remodeling or clinical improvement in patients undergoing cardiac resynchronization therapy, *J Am Coll Cardiol* 46:2208–2214, 2005.
168. Bax JJ, Bleeker GB, Marwick TH, et al: Left ventricular dyssynchrony predicts response and prognosis after cardiac resynchronization therapy, *J Am Coll Cardiol* 44:1834–1840, 2004.
169. Yu C-M, Lin H, Zhang Q, et al: High prevalence of left ventricular systolic and diastolic asynchrony in patients with congestive heart failure and normal QRS duration, *Heart* 89:54–60, 2003.
170. Breithardt OA, Stellbrink C, Herbots L, et al: Cardiac resynchronization therapy can reverse abnormal myocardial strain distribution in patients with heart failure and left bundle branch block, *J Am Coll Cardiol* 42:486–494, 2003.
171. Yu C-M, Zhang Q, Chan Y-S, et al: Tissue Doppler velocity is superior to displacement and strain mapping in predicting left ventricular reverse remodelling response after cardiac resynchronization therapy, *Heart* 92:1452–1456, 2006.
172. Suffoletto MS, Dohi K, Cannesson M, et al: Novel speckle-tracking radial strain from routine black-and-white echocardiographic images to quantify dyssynchrony and predict response to cardiac resynchronization therapy, *Circulation* 113:960–968, 2006.
173. Ng AC, Tran DT, Newman M, et al: Left ventricular longitudinal and radial synchrony and their determinants in healthy subjects, *J Am Soc Echocardiogr* 21:1042–1048, 2008.
174. Kapetanakis S, Kearney MT, Siva A, et al: Real-time three-dimensional echocardiography: A novel technique to quantify global left ventricular mechanical dyssynchrony, *Circulation* 112:992–1000, 2005.
175. Gorcsan J III, Abraham T, Agler DA, et al: Echocardiography for cardiac resynchronization therapy: Recommendations for performance and reporting—a report from the American Society of Echocardiography Dyssynchrony Writing Group endorsed by the Heart Rhythm Society, *J Am Soc Echocardiogr* 21:191–213, 2008.
176. Marsan NA, Henneman MM, Chen J, et al: Real-time three-dimensional echocardiography as a novel approach to quantify left ventricular dyssynchrony: A comparison study with phase analysis of gated myocardial perfusion single photon emission computed tomography, *J Am Soc Echocardiogr* 21:801–807, 2008.

177. Kapetanakis S, Kearney MT, Siva A, et al: Real-time three-dimensional echocardiography: A novel technique to quantify global left ventricular mechanical dyssynchrony, *Circulation* 112:992–1000, 2005.
178. Auricchio A, Stellbrink C, Block M, et al: Effect of pacing chamber and atrioventricular delay on acute systolic function of paced patients with congestive heart failure, *Circulation* 99:2993–3001, 1999.
179. Rakowski H, Appleton C, Chan K, et al: Canadian consensus recommendations for the measurement and reporting of diastolic dysfunction by echocardiography, *J Am Soc Echocardiogr* 9:736–760, 1996.
180. Khouri SJ, Maly GT, Suh DD, et al: A practical approach to the echocardiographic evaluation of diastolic function, *J Am Soc Echocardiogr* 17:290–297, 2004.
181. Redfield MM, Jacobsen SJ, Burnett JC Jr, et al: Burden of systolic and diastolic ventricular dysfunction in the community: Appreciating the scope of the heart failure epidemic, *JAMA* 289:194–202, 2003.
182. Nagueh SF, Appleton CP, Gillebert TC, et al: Recommendations for the evaluation of left ventricular diastolic function by echocardiography, *J Am Soc Echocardiogr* 22:107–133, 2009.
183. Appleton CP, Hatle LK, Popp RL: Relation of transmitral flow velocity patterns to left ventricular diastolic function: New insights from a combined hemodynamic and Doppler echocardiographic study, *J Am Coll Cardiol* 12:426–440, 1988.
184. Smiseth OA, Thompson CR, Lohavanichbutr K, et al: The pulmonary venous systolic flow pulse—its origin and relationship to left atrial pressure, *J Am Coll Cardiol* 34:802–809, 1999.
185. De Meya S, De Sutterb J, Vierendeelsa J, et al: Diastolic filling and pressure imaging: Taking advantage of the information in a colour M-mode Doppler image, *Eur J Echocardiogr* 2:219–233, 2001.
186. Ommen SR, Nishimura RA: A clinical approach to the assessment of left ventricular diastolic function by Doppler echocardiography: Update 2003, *Heart* 89(Suppl III):iii18–iii23, 2003.
187. Stevenson JG: Comparison of several noninvasive methods for estimation of pulmonary artery pressure, *J Am Soc Echocardiogr* 2:157, 1989.
188. Feigenbaum H, Popp RL, Wolfe SB, et al: Ultrasound measurements of the left ventricle: A correlative study with angiocardiography, *Arch Intern Med* 129:461, 1972.
189. Terai C, Venishi M, Sugimoto H, et al: Transesophageal echocardiographic dimensional analysis of four cardiac chambers during positive end–expiratory pressure, *Anesthesiology* 63:640, 1985.
190. Stauffer JC, Mueller X, Homsi L, et al: Echocardiographic determination of ejection fraction with various methods: Comparison with contrast angiography, *J Am Soc Echocardiogr* 3:7–I, 1990.
191. Fisher DC, Sahn DJ, Allen HD, et al: The mitral valve orifice method for noninvasive two-dimensional echo Doppler determinations of cardiac output, *Circulation* 67:872, 1983.
192. Lewis JF, Kuo LC, Nelson JG, et al: Pulsed Doppler echocardiographic determination of stroke volume and cardiac output: Clinical validation of two new methods using the apical window, *Circulation* 70:425, 1984.
193. Roewer N, Bednarz F, Dziadka A, et al: Intraoperative cardiac output determination from transmitral and pulmonary blood flow measurements using transesophageal pulsed Doppler, *J Cardiothorac Anesth* 1:418, 1987.
194. LaMantia K, Harris S, Mortimore K, et al: Transesophageal pulse–wave Doppler assessment of cardiac output, *Anesthesiology* 69:A1, 1988.
195. Savino JS, Troianos CA, Aukburg S, et al: Measurement of pulmonary blood flow with two–dimensional echocardiography and Doppler echocardiography, *Anesthesiology* 75:445, 1991.
196. Muhiudeen IA, Kuecherer HF, Lee E, et al: Intraoperative estimation of cardiac output by transesophageal pulsed Doppler echocardiography, *Anesthesiology* 74:9, 1991.
197. Parra V, Fita G, Rovira I, et al: Transoesophageal echocardiography accurately detects cardiac output variation: A prospective comparison with thermodilution in cardiac surgery, *Eur J Anaesthesiol* 25:135–143, 2008.
198. Culp WC Jr, Ball TR, Burnett CJ: Validation and feasibility of intraoperative three-dimensional transesophageal echocardiographic cardiac output, *Anesth Analg* 105:1219–1223, 2007.
199. Hoole SP, Boyd J, Ninios V, et al: Measurement of cardiac output by real-time 3D echocardiography in patients undergoing assessment for cardiac transplantation, *Eur J Echocardiogr* 9:334–337, 2008.
200. Fleming SM, Cumberledge B, Kiesewetter C, et al: Usefulness of real-time three-dimensional echocardiography for reliable measurement of cardiac output in patients with ischemic or idiopathic dilated cardiomyopathy, *Am J Cardiol* 95:308–310, 2005.
201. Pemberton J, Ge S, Thiele K, et al: Real-time three-dimensional color Doppler echocardiography Overcomes the inaccuracies of spectral Doppler for stroke volume calculation, *J Am Soc Echocardiogr* 19:1403–1410, 2006.
202. Lodato JA, Weinert L, Baumann R, et al: Use of 3-dimensional color Doppler echocardiography to measure stroke volume in human beings: Comparison with thermodilution, *J Am Soc Echocardiogr* 20:103–112, 2007.
203. Thys DM, Hillel Z, Goldman ME, et al: A comparison of hemodynamic indices by invasive monitoring and two-dimensional echocardiography, *Anesthesiology* 67:630, 1987.
204. Konstadt SN, Thys D, Mindich BP, et al: Validation of quantitative intraoperative transesophageal echocardiography, *Anesthesiology* 65:418, 1986.
205. Beaupre PN, Kremer PF, Cahalan MK, et al: Intraoperative changes in left ventricular segmental wall motion by transesophageal two-dimensional echocardiography, *Am Heart J* 107:1021–1023, 1984.
206. Clements FM, Harpole D, Quill T, et al: Simultaneous measurements of cardiac volumes, areas and ejection fractions by transesophageal echocardiography and first–pass radionuclide angiography, *Anesthesiology* 69:A4, 1988.
207. Urbanowicz JH, Shaaban MJ, Cohen NH, et al: Comparison of transesophageal echocardiographic and scintigraphic estimates of left ventricular end-diastolic volume index and ejection fraction in patients following coronary artery bypass grafting, *Anesthesiology* 72:607, 1990.
208. Gopal AS, Schnellbaecher MJ, Shen Z, et al: Freehand three-dimensional echocardiography for determination of left ventricular volume and mass in patients with abnormal ventricles: Comparison with magnetic resonance imaging, *J Am Soc Echocardiogr* 10:853e61, 1997.
209. Takeuchi M, Nishikage T, Mor-Avi V, et al: Measurement of left ventricular mass by real-time three-dimensional echocardiography: Validation against magnetic resonance and comparison with two-dimensional and M-mode measurements, *J Am Soc Echocardiogr* 21:1001–1005, 2008.
210. Mor-Avi V, Sugeng L, Lang RM: Three-dimensional adult echocardiography: Where the hidden dimension helps, *Curr Cardiol Rep* 10:218–225, 2008.
211. Jenkins C, Chan J, Hanekom L, et al: Accuracy and feasibility of online 3-dimensional echocardiography for measurement of left ventricular parameters, *J Am Soc Echocardiogr* 19:1119–1128, 2006.
212. Rivas-Gotz C, Manolios M, Thohan V, et al: Impact of left ventricular ejection fraction on estimation of left ventricular filling pressures using tissue Doppler and flow propagation velocity, *Am J Cardiol* 91:780–784, 2003.
213. Carabello BA: Clinical practice. Aortic stenosis, *N Engl J Med* 346:677–682, 2002.
214. Rapaport E, Rackley CE, Cohn LH: Aortic valve disease. In Schlant RC, Alexander RW, O'Rourke RA, et al, editors: *Hurst's the heart: Arteries and veins*, New York, 1994, McGraw Hill.
215. Feigenbaum H: Acquired valvular heart disease. In *Echocardiography*, Philadelphia, 1994, Lea & Febiger, pp 239–349.
216. Stoddard MF, Arce J, Liddell NE, et al: Two dimensional transesophageal echocardiographic determination of aortic valve area in adults with aortic stenosis, *Am Heart J* 122:1415, 1991.
217. Otto CM: Valvular aortic stenosis: Disease severity and timing of intervention, *J Am Coll Cardiol* 47:2141–2151, 2006.
218. Cape EG, Jones M, Yamada I, et al: Turbulent/viscous interactions control Doppler/catheter pressure discrepancies in aortic stenosis. The role of the Reynolds number, *Circulation* 94:2975, 1996.
219. Niederberger J, Schima H, Maurer G, et al: Importance of pressure recovery for the assessment of aortic stenosis by Doppler ultrasound. Role of aortic size, aortic valve area, and direction of the stenotic jet in vitro, *Circulation* 15:1934, 1996.
220. Lancellotti P, Lebois F, Simon M, et al: Prognostic importance of quantitative exercise Doppler echocardiography in asymptomatic valvular aortic stenosis, *Circulation* 112(Suppl 9):I377–I382, 2005.
221. Baumgartner H, Hung J, Bermejo J, et al: Echocardiographic assessment of valve stenosis: EAE/ASE recommendations for clinical practice, *J Am Soc Echocardiogr* 22:1–23, 2009.
222. Cormier B, Iung B, Porte JM, et al: Value of multiplane transesophageal echocardiography in determining aortic valve area in aortic stenosis, *Am J Cardiol* 15:882, 1996.
223. Hoffmann R, Flachskampf FA, Hanrath P: Planimetry of orifice area in aortic stenosis using multiplane transesophageal echocardiography, *J Am Coll Cardiol* 22:529, 1993.
224. Stoddard MF, Hammons RT, Longaker RA: Doppler transesophageal echo-cardiographic determination of aortic valve area in adults with aortic stenosis, *Am Heart J* 132:337, 1996.
225. Bonow RO, Carabello BA, Chatterjee K, et al: Focused update incorporated into the ACC/AHA 2006 guidelines for the management of patients with valvular heart disease: A report of the American College of Cardiology/American Heart Association Task Force on Practice Guidelines, *Circulation* 118:e523–e661, 2008.
226. Roberson WS, Stewart J, Armstrong WF, et al: Reverse doming of the anterior mitral leaflet with severe aortic regurgitation, *J Am Coll Cardiol* 3:431, 1984.
227. Ambrose JA, Meller J, Teichholz LE, et al: Premature closure of the mitral valve: Echocardiographic clue for the diagnosis of aortic dissection, *Chest* 73:121, 1978.
228. Cohen GI, Duffy CI, Klein AL, et al: Color Doppler and two dimensional echocardiographic determination of the mechanism of aortic regurgitation with surgical correlation, *J Am Soc Echocardiogr* 9:508, 1996.
229. Perry GJ, Helmcke F, Nanda NC, et al: Evaluation of aortic insufficiency by Doppler color flow mapping, *J Am Coll Cardiol* 9:952–959, 1987.
230. Zoghbi WA, Enriquez-Sarano M, Foster E, et al: Recommendations for evaluation of the severity of native valvular regurgitation with two-dimensional and Doppler echocardiography, *J Am Soc Echocardiogr* 16:777–802, 2003.
231. Reimold SC, Thomas JD, Lee RT: Relationship between Doppler color flow variables and invasively determined jet variables in patients with aortic regurgitation, *J Am Coll Cardiol* 20:1143, 1992.
232. Ishii M, Jones M, Shiota T, et al: Evaluation of eccentric aortic regurgitation by color Doppler jet and color Doppler-imaged vena contracta measurements: An animal study of quantified aortic regurgitation, *Am Heart J* 132:796, 1996.
233. Dolan MS, Castello R, St Vrain JA, et al: Quantification of aortic regurgitation by Doppler echocardiography: A practical approach, *Am Heart J* 129:1014, 1995.
234. Grayburn PA, Handshoe R, Smith MD, et al: Quantitative assessment of the hemodynamic consequences of aortic regurgitation by means of continuous wave Doppler recordings, *J Am Coll Cardiol* 8:1341–1347, 1986.
235. Griffin BP, Flachskampf FA, Siu S, et al: The effects of regurgitant orifice size, chamber compliance, and systemic vascular resistance on aortic regurgitant velocity slope and pressure half-time, *Am Heart J* 122:1049, 1991.
236. Tribouilloy CM, Enriquez-Sarano M, Fett SL, et al: Application of the proximal flow convergence method to calculate the effective regurgitant orifice area in aortic regurgitation, *J Am Coll Cardiol* 32:1032–1039, 1998.
237. Touche T, Prasquier R, Nitenberg A, et al: Assessment and follow-up of patients with aortic regurgitation by an updated Doppler echocardiographic measurement of the regurgitant fraction in the aortic arch, *Circulation* 72:819–824, 1985.
238. Ranganathan N, Lam JHC, Wigle ED, et al: Morphology of the human mitral valve: II. The valve leaflets, *Circulation* 41:459–467, 1970.
239. Perloff JK, Roberts WC: The mitral apparatus: Functional anatomy of mitral regurgitation, *Circulation* 46:227–239, 1972.
240. Hammer WJ, Roberts WC, deLeon AC Jr: Mitral stenosis secondary to combined massive mitral annular calcific deposits and small, hypertrophied left ventricles: Hemodynamic documentation in four patients, *Am J Med* 64:371–376, 1978.
241. Pai RG, Tarazi R, Wong S: Constrictive pericarditis causing extrinsic mitral stenosis and a left heart mass, *Clin Cardiol* 19:517, 1996.
242. Felner JM, Martin RP: The echocardiogram. In Schlant RC, Alexander RW, O'Rourke RA, et al: *Hurst's the heart: Arteries and veins*, New York, 1994, McGraw Hill, pp 375–422.
243. Roberts WE: Morphological features of the normal and abnormal mitral valve, *Am J Cardiol* 51: 1005–1028, 1983.
244. Chen YT, Kan MN, Chen JS, et al: Contributing factors to formation of left atrial spontaneous echo contrast in mitral valvular disease, *J Ultrasound Med* 9:151–155, 1990.
245. Currie PJ, Seward JB, Reeder GS, et al: Continuous-wave Doppler echocardiographic assessment of severity of calcific aortic stenosis: A simultaneous Doppler-catheter correlative study in 100 adult patients, *Circulation* 71:1162, 1985.
246. Nishimura RA, Rihal CS, Tajik AJ, et al: Accurate measurement of the transmitral gradient in patients with mitral stenosis: A simultaneous catheterization and Doppler echocardiographic study, *J Am Coll Cardiol* 24:152–158, 1994.
247. Gorcsan J, Kenny WM, Diana P: Transesophageal continuous–wave Doppler to evaluate mitral prosthetic stenosis, *Am Heart J* 121:911, 1991.
248. Chang KC, Chiang CW, Kuo CT, et al: Effect of mitral regurgitation and aortic regurgitation on Doppler-derived mitral orifice area in patients with mitral stenosis, *Chang Keng I Hsueh* 16:217, 1993.
249. Moro E, Nicolosi GL, Zanuttini D, et al: Influence of aortic regurgitation on the assessment of the pressure half-time and derived mitral-valve area in patients with mitral stenosis, *Eur Heart J* 9:1010–1017, 1988.
250. Flachskampf FA, Weyman AE, Gillam L, et al: Aortic regurgitation shortens Doppler pressure half-time in mitral stenosis: Clinical evidence, in vitro simulation, and theoretic analysis, *J Am Coll Cardiol* 16:396, 1990.
251. Carpentier A: Cardiac valve surgery-the "French correction", *J Thorac Cardiovasc Surg* 86:323–337, 1983.
252. Ormiston JA, Shah PM, Tei C, et al: Size and motion of the mitral valve annulus in man, *Circulation* 64:113, 1981.
253. Burwash IG, Blackmore GL, Koilpillai CJ: Usefulness of left atrial and left ventricular chamber sizes as predictors of the severity of mitral regurgitation, *Am J Cardiol* 15:774, 1992.
254. Mintz GS, Kotler MN, Segal BL, et al: Two dimensional echocardiographic recognition of ruptured chordae tendineae, *Circulation* 57:244, 1978.
255. Ogawa S, Mardelli TJ, Hubbard FE: The role of cross-sectional echocardiography in the diagnosis of flail mitral leaflet, *Clin Cardiol* 1:85, 1978.
256. Carpentier A, Loulmet D, Deloche A, et al: Surgical anatomy and management of ischemic mitral valve incompetence, *Circulation* 76(Suppl IV):IV- 446, 1987.
257. Felner JM, Williams BR: Noninvasive evaluation of left ventricular overload and cardiac function, *Prac Cardiol* 5:158–196, 1979.
258. Smith MD, Harrison MOR, Pinton R, et al: Regurgitant jet size by transesophageal compared with transthoracic Doppler color flow imaging, *Circulation* 83:79–86, 1991.

259. Smith MD, Cassidy J, Gurley JC, et al: Echo Doppler evaluation of patients with acute mitral regurgitation: Superiority of transesophageal echocardiography with color flow imaging, *Am Heart J* 129:967, 1995.
260. Stevenson JG: Two dimensional color Doppler estimation of the severity of atrioventricular valve regurgitation: Important effects of instrument gain settings, pulse repetition frequency, and carrier frequency, *J Am Soc Echocardiolgr* 2:1, 1989.
261. Omoto R, Ky S, Matsumura M, et al: Evaluation of biplane color Doppler transesophageal echocardiography in 200 consecutive patients, *Circulation* 85:1237, 1992.
262. Sadoshima J, Koyanagi S, Sugimachi M, et al: Evaluation of the severity of mitral regurgitation by transesophageal Doppler flow echocardiography, *Am Heart J* 123:1245, 1992.
263. Chen C, Thomas JD, Anconina J, et al: Impact of impinging wall jet on color Doppler quantification of mitral regurgitation, *Circulation* 84:712, 1991.
264. Tribouilloy CB, Shen WF, Quere JP, et al: Assessment of severity of mitral regurgitation by measuring regurgitant jet width at its origin with transesophageal Doppler color flow imaging, *Circulation* 85:1248–1253, 1992.
265. Kisanuki A, Tei C, Minagoe S, et al: Continuous wave Doppler echocardiographic evaluations of the severity of mitral regurgitation, *J Cardiol* 19:831, 1989.
266. Utsunomiya T, Patel D, Doshi R, et al: Can signal intensity of the continuous wave Doppler regurgitant jet estimate severity of mitral regurgitation? *Am Heart J* 19:831, 1992.
267. Klein AL, Obarski TP, Stewart WJ, et al: Transesophageal Doppler echocardiography of pulmonary venous flow: A new marker of mitral regurgitation severity, *J Am Coll Cardiol* 18:518, 1991.
268. Mark JB, Ahmed SU, Kluger R, et al: Influence of jet direction on pulmonary vein flow patterns in severe mitral regurgitation, *Anesth Analg* 80:486, 1995.
269. Enriquez-Sarano FA, Miller SN, Hayes KR, et al: Effective mitral regurgitant orifice area: Clinical use and pitfalls of the proximal isovelocity surface area method, *J Am Coll Cardiol* 25:703–709, 1995.
270. Xie G, Berk MR, Hixson CS, et al: Quantification of mitral regurgitant volume by the color Doppler proximal isovelocity surface area method: a clinical study, *J Am Soc Echocardiogr* 8:48, 1995.
271. Lambert AS: Proximal isovelocity surface area should be routinely measured in evaluating mitral regurgitation: A core review, *Anesth Analg* 105:940–943, 2007.
272. Silver MD, Lam JHC, Ranganathan N, et al: Morphology of the human tricuspid valve, *Circulation* 43:333–348, 1971.
273. Guyer DE, et al: Comparison of the echocardiographic and hemodynamic diagnosis of rheumatic tricuspid stenosis, *J Am Coll Cardiol* 3:1135, 1984.
274. Lundin L, Landelius J, Andrea B, et al: Transesophaeal echocardiography improves the diagnostic value of cardiac ultrasound in patients with carcinoid heart disease, *Br Heart J* 64:190–194, 1990.
275. Perez JE, Ludbrook PA, Ahumada GG: Usefullness of Doppler echocardiography in detecting tricuspid valve stenosis, *Am J Cardiol* 55:601, 1985.
276. Miyatake K, et al: Evaluation of tricuspid regurgitation by pulsed Doppler and two dimensional echocardiography, *Circulation* 66:777, 1982.
277. Tribouilloy CM, Enriquez-Sarano M, Bailey KR, et al: Quantification of tricuspid regurgitation by measuring the width of the vena contracta with Doppler color flow imaging: A clinical study, *J Am Coll Cardiol* 36:472–478, 2000.
278. Nixon JV, Brown CN, Smitherman TC: Identification of transient and persistent segmental wall motion abnormalities in patients with unstable angina by two-dimensional echocardiography, *Circulation* 65:1497–1503, 1982.
279. Schiller NB, Shah PM, Crawford M, et al: Recommendations for quantitation of the left ventricle by two-dimensional echocardiography. American Society of Echocardiography Committee on Standards, Subcommittee on Quantitation of Two-Dimensional Echocardiograms, *J Am Soc Echocardiogr* 2:358e67, 1989.
280. Nath S, Haines DE, Kron IL, et al: Regional wall motion analysis predicts survival and functional outcome after subendocardial resection in patients with prior anterior myocardial infarction, *Circulation* 88:70–76, 1993.
281. Nath S, DeLacey WA, Haines DE, et al: Use of a regional wall motion score to enhance risk stratification of patients receiving an implantable cardioverter-defibrillator, *J Am Coll Cardiol* 22:1093–1099, 1993.
282. Kapetanopoulos A, Ahlberg AW, Taub CC, et al: Regional wall-motion abnormalities on post-stress electrocardiographic-gated technetium-99m sestamibi single-photon emission computed tomography imaging predict cardiac events, *J Nucl Cardiol* 14:810–817, 2007.
283. Massre BM, Botvinick EH, Brundage BH, et al: Relationship of regional myocardial perfusion to segmental wall motion: A physiological basis for understanding the presence of reversibility of asynergy, *Circulation* 58:1154, 1978.
284. Alam M, Khaja F, Brymer J, et al: Echocardiographic evaluation of left ventricular function during coronary angioplasty, *Am J Cardiol* 57:20, 1986.
285. Labovitz AJ, Lewen MK, Kern M, et al: Evaluation of left ventricular systolic and diastolic dysfunction during transient myocardial ischemia by angioplasty, *J Am Coll Cardiol* 10:748, 1988.
286. Shah PM, Shunei K, Matsumura M, et al: Utility of biplane transesophageal echocardiography in left ventricular wall motion analysis, *J Cardiothorac Vasc Anesth* 5:316, 1991.
287. Pandian NG, Kerber RE: Two-dimensional echocardiography in experimental coronary stenosis. I. Sensitivity and specificity in detecting transient myocardial dyskinesis: Comparison with sonomicrometers, *Circulation* 66:597, 1982.
288. Thys DM: The intraoperative assessment of regional myocardial performance: Is the cart before the horse? *J Cardiothorac Anesth* 1:273, 1987.
289. Battler A, Forelicher VF, Gallagher KT, et al: Dissociation between regional myocardial dysfunction and ECG changes during ischemia in the conscious dog, *Circulation* 62:735, 1980.
290. Tomoike H, Franklin D, Ross J Jr: Detection of myocardial ischemia by regional dysfunction during and after rapid pacing in conscious dogs, *Circulation* 58:48, 1978.
291. Smith JS, Cahalan MK, Benefiel DJ, et al: Intraoperative detection of myocardial ischemia in high-risk patients: Electrocardiography versus two–dimensional transesophageal echocardiography, *Circulation* 72:1015, 1985.
292. Wohlgelernter D, Jaffe CC, Cabin HS, et al: Silent ischemia during coronary occlusion produced by balloon inflation: Relation to regional myocardial dysfunction, *J Am Coll Cardiol* 10:491, 1987.
293. VanDaele ME, Sutherland GR, Mitchell MM, et al: Do changes in pulmonary capillary wedge pressure adequately reflect myocardial ischemia during anesthesia? *Circulation* 81:865, 1990.
294. Leung JM, O'Kelley B, Browner WS, et al: Prognostic importance of postbypass regional wall motion abnormalities in patients undergoing coronary artery bypass graft surgery, *Anesthesiology* 71:16, 1989.
295. Leung JM, O'Kelley BF, Mangano DT: Relationship of regional wall motion abnormalities to hemodynamic indices of myocardial supply and demand in patients undergoing CABG surgery, *Anesthesiology* 73:802, 1990.
296. Clements FM, de Bruijn NP: Perioperative evaluation of regional wall motion by transesophageal two–dimensional echocardiography, *Anesth Analg* 66:249, 1987.
297. Lehman KG, Korrester AL, MacKenzie WB, et al: Onset of altered intraventricular septal motion during cardiac surgery, *Circulation* 82:1325, 1990.
298. Chung F, Seyone C, Rakowski H: Transesophageal echocardiography may fail to diagnose perioperative myocardial infarction, *Can J Anaesth* 38:98, 1991.
299. Pandian NG, Skorton DJ, Collins SM, et al: Heterogeneity of left ventricular segmental wall motion thickening and excursion in 2–dimensional echocardiograms of normal human subjects, *Am J Cardiol* 51:1667, 1983.
300. Liberman AN, Weiss JL, Judutt BD, et al: Two–dimensional echocardiography and infarct size: Relationship of regional wall motion and thickening to the extent of myocardial infarction in the dog, *Circulation* 63:739, 1981.
301. Luma JAC, Becker LA, Melin JA, et al: Impaired thickening of non–ischemic myocardium during acute regional ischemia in the dog, *Circulation* 71:1048, 1985.
302. Force T, Kemper A, Perkins L, et al: Overestimation of infarct size by quantitative two–dimensional echocardiography: The role of tethering and of analytic procedures, *Circulation* 73:1360, 1986.
303. Braunwald E, Kloner RA: The stunned myocardium: Prolonged, postischemic ventricular dysfunction, *Circulation* 66:1146, 1982.
304. Buffington CW, Coyle RJ: Altered load dependence of postischemic myocardium, *Anesthesiology* 75:464, 1991.
305. London MJ, Tubau JF, Wong MG, et al: The "natural history" of segmental wall motion abnormalities in patients undergoing noncardiac surgery, *Anesthesiology* 73:644, 1990.
306. Roizen MF, Beaupre PN, Alpert RA, et al: Monitoring with two–dimensional transesophageal echocardiography. Comparison of myocardial function in patients undergoing supraceliac, suprarenal-infraceliac, or infrarenal aortic occlusion, *J Vasc Surg* 2:300, 1984.
307. Gewertz BL, Kremser PC, Zarins CK, et al: Transesophageal echocardiographic monitoring of myocardial ischemia during vascular surgery, *J Vasc Surg* 5:607, 1987.
308. Topol EJ, Weiss JL, Guzman PA, et al: Immediate improvement of dysfunctional myocardial segments after coronary revascularization: Detection by intraoperative transesophageal echocardiography, *J Am Coll Cardiol* 4:1123, 1984.
309. Koolen JJ, Visser CA, Van Wezel HB, et al: Influence of coronary artery bypass surgery on regional left ventricular wall motion: An intraoperative two-dimensional transesophageal echocardiography study, *J Cardiovasc Anesth* 1:276, 1987.
310. Voci P, Billotta F, Aronson S, et al: Changes in myocardial segmental wall motion, systolic wall thickening, and ejection fraction immediately following CABG: An echocardiographic analysis comparing dysfunctional and normal myocardium, *J Am Soc Echocardiogr* 4:289, 1991.
311. Srinivas M, Roizen MF, Barnard J, et al: Relative effectiveness of four preoperative tests to predict adverse cardiac outcomes following vascular surgery: A metaanalysis, *Anesth Analg* 79:422–433, 1994.
312. Picano E, Mathias W Jr, Pingitore A, et al: Safety and tolerability of dobutamine-atropine stress echocardiography: A prospective, multicentre study. Echo Dobutamine International Cooperative Study Group, *Lancet* 344:1190–1192, 1994.
313. Picano E, Bedetti G, Varga A, et al: The comparable diagnostic accuracies of dobutamine-stress and dipyridamole-stress echocardiographies: A meta-analysis, *Coron Artery Dis* 11:151–159, 2000.
314. Sawada SG, Segar DS, Ryan T, et al: Echocardiographic detection of coronary artery disease during dobutamine infusion, *Circulation* 83:1605–1614, 1991.
315. Voigt J-U, Exner B, Schmiedehausen K, et al: Strain-rate imaging during dobutamine stress echocardiography provides objective evidence of inducible ischemia, *Circulation* 107:2120–2126, 2003.
316. Hoffmann R, Altiok E, Nowak B, et al: Strain rate measurement by Doppler echocardiography allows improved assessment of myocardial viability in patients with depressed left ventricular function, *J Am Coll Cardiol* 39:443–449, 2002.
317. Edvardsen T, Skulstad H, Aakhus S, et al: Regional myocardial systolic function during acute myocardial ischemia assessed by strain Doppler echocardiography, *J Am Coll Cardiol* 37:726–730, 2001.
318. Skulstad H, Edvardsen T, Urheim S, et al: Postsystolic shortening in ischemic myocardium. Active contraction or passive recoil? *Circulation* 106:718–724, 2002.
319. Kukulski T, Jamal F, Herbots L, et al: Identification of acutely ischemic myocardium using ultrasonic strain measurements. A clinical study in patients undergoing coronary angioplasty, *J Am Coll Cardiol* 41:810–819, 2003.
320. Kukulski T, Jamal F, D'hooge J, et al: Acute changes in systolic and diastolic events during clinical coronary angioplasty: A comparison of regional velocity, strain rate, and strain measurement, *J Am Soc Echocardiogr* 15:1–12, 2002.
321. Voigt J-U, Nixdorff U, Bogdan R, et al: Comparison of deformation imaging and velocity imaging for detecting regional inducible ischaemia during dobutamine stress echocardiography, *Eur Heart J* 25:1517–1525, 2004.
322. Jamal F, Kukulski T, Sutherland GR, et al: Can changes in systolic longitudinal deformation quantify regional myocardial function after an acute infarction? An ultrasonic strain rate and strain study, *J Am Soc Echocardiogr* 15:723–730, 2002.
323. Nakatani S, Stugaard M, Hanatani A, et al: Quantitative assessment of short axis wall motion using myocardial strain rate imaging, *Echocardiography* 20:145–149, 2003.
324. Becker M, Bilke E, Kuehl H, et al: Analysis of myocardial deformation based on pixel tracking in two dimensional echocardiographic images enables quantitative assessment of regional left ventricular function, *Heart* 92:1102–1108, 2006.
325. Becker M, Hoffmann R, Kuehl H, et al: Analysis of myocardial deformation based on ultrasonic pixel tracking to determine transmurality in chronic myocardial infarction, *Eur Heart J* 27:2560–2566, 2006.
326. Migrino RQ, Zhu X, Pajewski N, et al: Assessment of segmental myocardial viability using regional 2-dimensional strain echocardiography, *J Am Soc Echocardiogr* 20:342–351, 2007.
327. Chan J, Hanekom L, Wong C, et al: Differentiation of subendocardial and transmural infarction using two-dimensional strain rate imaging to assess short-axis and long-axis myocardial function, *J Am Coll Cardiol* 48:2026–2033, 2006.
328. Zhang Y, Chan AKY, Yu C-M, et al: Strain rate imaging differentiates transmural from non-transmural myocardial infarction, *J Am Coll Cardiol* 46:864–871, 2005.
329. Becker M, Lenzen A, Ocklenburg C, et al: Myocardial deformation imaging based on ultrasonic pixel tracking to identify reversible myocardial dysfunction, *J Am Coll Cardiol* 51:1473–1481, 2008.
330. Mizuguchi Y, Oishi Y, Miyoshi H, et al: The functional role of longitudinal, circumferential, and radial myocardial deformation for regulating the early impairment of left ventricular contraction and relaxation in patients with cardiovascular risk factors: A study with two-dimensional strain imaging, *J Am Soc Echocardiogr* 21:1138–1144, 2008.
331. Koenig K, Kasper W, Hofman T, et al: Transesophageal echocardiography for diagnosis of rupture of the ventricular septum or left ventricular papillary muscle during acute myocardial infarction, *Am J Cardiol* 59:362, 1987.
332. Patel AM, Miller FA, Khandheria BK, et al: Role of TEE in the diagnosis of papillary muscle rupture secondary to myocardial function, *Am Heart J* 118:1330, 1989.
333. Garther NS, Rogan KM, Stajduhar K, et al: Anomalous origin and course of coronary arteries in adults: Identification and improved imaging utilizing transesophageal echocardiography, *Am Heart J* 122:69, 75, 1991.
334. Dell Italia LJ, Starling MR, Blumhardt R, et al: Comparative effects of volume loading, dobutamine, and nitroprusside in patients with predominant right ventricular function, *Circulation* 72:1327, 1985.
335. Vitanen A, Salmenpera M, Heinonen S: Right ventricular response to hypercarbia after cardiac surgery, *Anethesiology* 73:393, 1990.
336. Klein AL, Burstow DJ, Tajik AJ, et al: Effects of age on left ventricular dimensions and filling dynamics in 117 normal persons, *Mayo Clin Proc* 69:212–224, 1994.

13

Decision Making and Perioperative Transesophageal Echocardiography

STUART J. WEISS, MD, PHD | JOSEPH S. SAVINO, MD

KEY POINTS

1. The first step in decision making is to "frame" the problem by defining the parameters, priorities, and pertinent criteria.
2. The second step is the directed acquisition of data, "data collection," that includes all pertinent information, regardless of whether it is confirmatory or contradictory. The supplemental information from the preoperative evaluation should always be taken into consideration.
3. A comprehensive systematic transesophageal echocardiography examination permits the acquisition and interpretation of both qualitative and quantitative echocardiographic data for most cardiovascular diseases. The greatest risk and source of error are that of omission or misinterpretation leading to mismanagement.
4. The decision regarding patient management of a specific anatomic abnormality should be an evidence-based approach reflecting the severity of the lesion, coexisting factors, patient's wishes, and the current literature.
5. Intraoperative findings should be objectively and effectively characterized and discussed with the pertinent clinicians, surgeon, or cardiologist and the patient's family.
6. The decision and recommendations should be formally communicated through a reporting document that is accessible to other healthcare providers.
7. A systematic process for learning from the results of past decisions (quality improvement program) and continued education are critical for the future success of any intraoperative transesophageal echocardiography program.

"In the affair of so much importance, wherein you ask my advice, I cannot make for want of sufficient premises advise you what to determine, but if it please I will tell you how."

—Benjamin Franklin

All too often in medicine, critical decisions are made without the benefit of a thorough consideration of data, evidence, and framework. The paucity of clinical outcomes research in echocardiography, especially in the perioperative period, dampens the prospects for evidence-based decision making. In the absence of evidence-directed practice, decision making typically is based on anecdote, clinical impression, and tradition, with little effort devoted to the process of reaching an intelligent conclusion. The quantity of information is increasingly abundant in medicine, and the operating room is no exception. Its acquisition, interpretation, and application for decision making can be cumbersome, distracting, and misguided. In the era of increasing information, there is an imperative to develop a systematic process of handling data streams, organizing ideas and thoughts, defining and prioritizing problems, and effecting care through a well-thought-out decision. A formalized approach to the acquisition of data and decision making (Figure 13-1) enhances the quality of the intraoperative echocardiogram, its interpretation, and the

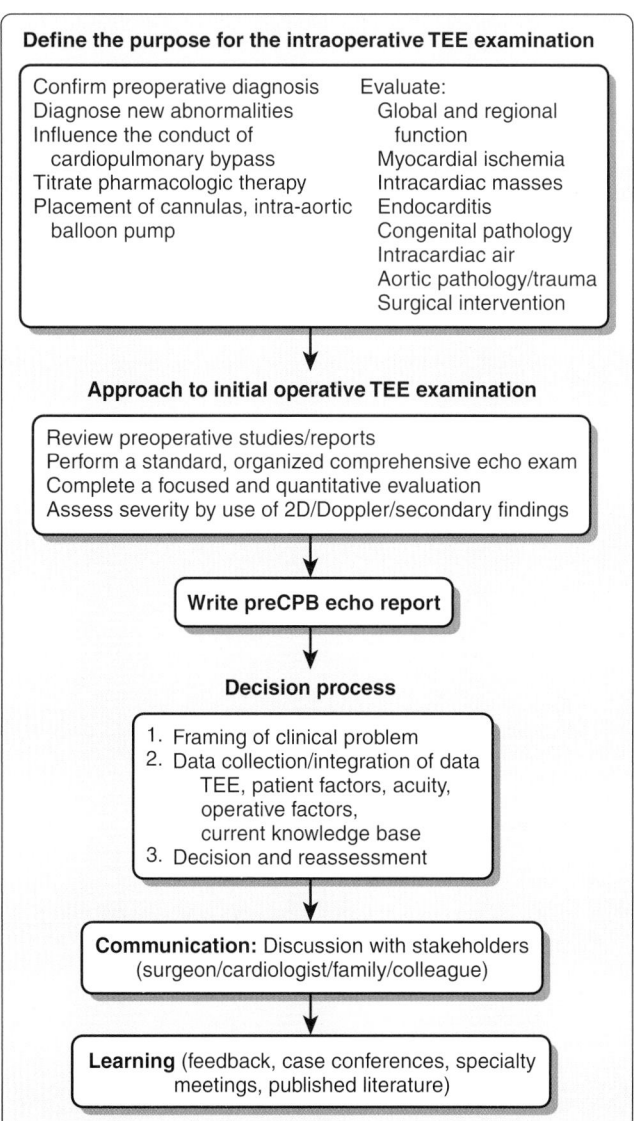

Define the purpose for the intraoperative TEE examination

Confirm preoperative diagnosis	Evaluate:
Diagnose new abnormalities	Global and regional
Influence the conduct of	function
cardiopulmonary bypass	Myocardial ischemia
Titrate pharmacologic therapy	Intracardiac masses
Placement of cannulas, intra-aortic	Endocarditis
balloon pump	Congenital pathology
	Intracardiac air
	Aortic pathology/trauma
	Surgical intervention

Approach to initial operative TEE examination

Review preoperative studies/reports
Perform a standard, organized comprehensive echo exam
Complete a focused and quantitative evaluation
Assess severity by use of 2D/Doppler/secondary findings

Write preCPB echo report

Decision process

1. Framing of clinical problem
2. Data collection/integration of data
   TEE, patient factors, acuity,
   operative factors,
   current knowledge base
3. Decision and reassessment

Communication: Discussion with stakeholders (surgeon/cardiologist/family/colleague)

Learning (feedback, case conferences, specialty meetings, published literature)

Figure 13-1 **An algorithm for the decision-making process.** CPB, cardiopulmonary bypass; TEE, transesophageal echocardiography.

confidence with which the findings are communicated to other members of the operative and nonoperative teams. Poor decisions are not made by the physician with bad intentions. Poor decisions are more commonly the result of individuals relying on limited medical knowledge (a database typically defined by the narrow bounds of their profession), narrow framing, and false or tenuous anchors. The echocardiographer who is overly confident in the abilities of his or her surgical counterpart may be falsely anchored to the prior performances of the surgeon, with little or no reliance on a formalized decision-making process. The lack of a structured paradigm for decision making is most worrisome when clinicians with lesser ability or experience are making the decisions. The least accomplished clinicians often have the most inflated estimate of their own abilities, thus lending themselves to the vulnerabilities of limited skills plus lack of a decision-making process.[1]

The intraoperative consultant in echocardiography is confronted with multiple channels of information (Boxes 13-1, 13-2, and 13-3). The broad database that is required to formulate an intelligent decision includes provider- and patient-specific data. Patient-specific data include history and demographics, preoperative diagnostic examinations, admitting diagnosis and comorbidities, the patient's wishes, recommendations of referring physicians, and intraoperative data. Intraoperative data include hemodynamic data, visual inspection, surgical

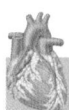

BOX 13-1. PATIENT HISTORY AND PHYSICAL SIGNS

- Symptoms
  - Shortness of breath
  - New York Heart Association classification for heart failure
  - Level of activity
  - Functional disability
  - Age
- Signs: vital signs, rales, peripheral edema, peripheral circulation
- Cardiac and noncardiac comorbidities, including esophageal disease
- Patient preferences (e.g., Jehovah's Witness, long-term anticoagulation)

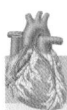

BOX 13-2. PATIENT DATA

- Intraoperative transesophageal echocardiography
- Left ventricle: systolic/diastolic function, ejection fraction, chamber size, wall thickness, regional wall motion
- Valvular function: pathology, severity, location, vena contracta, annular size, size of donor chamber, pressure gradient, flow-velocity profiles
- Cardiac catheterization
- Chest radiographs, electrocardiogram, blood tests, radionucleotide studies, positron-emission tomography scans, stress test, transthoracic echocardiography
- Hemodynamics
- Surgical inspection of the pathology

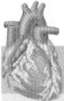

BOX 13-3. OPERATIVE FACTORS

- Complexity of planned surgery (e.g., redo sternotomy, prior valve repair, infectious process)
- Alternatives to the planned surgery
- Anticipated risk for a failed intervention
- Alternatives if original procedure is unsuccessful
- Equipment availability (ventricular assist device [VAD] backup, special retractors, specific valves, homografts, etc.)
- Expertise and experience of the operating team

input, and the transesophageal echocardiographic (TEE) examination. A systematic TEE examination of the heart and great vessels permits the acquisition and interpretation of qualitative and quantitative echocardiographic data applied to intraoperative decision making. The provider-specific data are composed of an accumulated database of knowledge acquired from training, experience, and continuous medical education. Expertise is gained from experience and enhances the repertoire of experiences from which a practitioner can draw but does not alter the cognitive engine and does not immunize the practitioner from errors in decision making. Intuition and experience are not reliable predictors of success. Learning through methods of trial and error and self-education by exploratory problem solving have little role in the arena of cardiac surgery. Heuristic methods of decision making often create a systematic and predictable bias. It is acceptable to be wrong. It is unacceptable to be consistently wrong in the same direction. A structured process of assessing all the data and weighing various alternatives (cognitive engine) will enable the physician to formulate a concise, organized approach to problem solving, communicating the findings and management alternatives.

Decision making can be encumbered by cognitive and emotional attachments that limit clinicians' intellectual flexibility. Poor problem solving and poor outcome can follow a single poor decision of great magnitude. However, the "creep effect" of a series of small poor decisions can insidiously lead to a poor outcome. The adherence to a poor course of action because of an attachment to the original decision is common in medicine. "The escalating commitment to a losing course of action often begins with small steps" (Roch Parayre, MBA, personal communication). In the perioperative setting, this process is most vivid in the care of critically ill patients with little or no hope for survival. Continued commitment of resources and intervention often contribute to patient discomfort and cost without benefit in quality of life or longevity. The prior commitment of resources often encourages further commitment and investment in a losing cause. The echocardiographic decisions during surgery may become part of an intraoperative sequence of diagnostic and therapeutic interventions in which the best course of action is a complete reversal in direction. Repeated attempts at repairing a mitral valve (MV) may follow an initial unsuccessful repair. The decision to replace the valve instead of repairing it often is not considered until late in the course. Repeated intervals of cardiopulmonary bypass (CPB) and aortic cross-clamping are not without their complications and associated morbidities. It often is difficult to retain an open mind and to consider alternative diagnoses or therapeutic alternatives. Effective decision-makers are able, if necessary, to abandon the original decision to repair an MV and move toward valve replacement.

An intraoperative TEE examination can correct preoperative inaccuracies in diagnosis or detect occult disease. With increasing emphasis on decreasing preoperative testing, avoiding redundant testing, and decreasing costs, accurate diagnoses of disease may not occur until the time of surgery. The increased reliance on the intraoperative TEE is fiscally wise but places greater responsibility and impact on the intraoperative echocardiographer. The detection of occult disease not appreciated during the preoperative evaluation often impacts operative management. It is necessary to reframe a problem when the data acquired reveal new insights. For example, the detection of mobile atheroma in the ascending aorta may influence positioning of an aortic infusion cannula or cross-clamp, hence changing circulatory management and the operation.[2–4] A change in clinical management in respect to otherwise asymptomatic and silent findings is often controversial. The change in the operation has typically not been discussed with the patient, as the findings were unanticipated. The intraoperative diagnosis of moderate aortic valve regurgitation (AR) that was not detected before surgery will create a clinical challenge for the surgical team regarding administration of cardioplegia and the decision whether to replace the aortic valve (AV). Hence, the decision to proceed with an unplanned aortic valve replacement (AVR) relies on the ability of the echocardiographer to establish the diagnosis and mechanism of valvular pathology, define the pertinent factors that sway the decision (preoperative symptoms of congestive heart failure [CHF], ventricular size and function, pulmonary hypertension), and communicate with the surgeon and the other pertinent stakeholders. It is important to realize that the decision to recommend AVR to a patient is not often guided by the degree of AR but rather by the degree of corresponding ventricular dilatation and dysfunction. The finding of moderate AR with normal ventricular systolic function and chamber size, normal left atrial pressure, and no preoperative history of CHF may sway the operative team to proceed with the originally planned surgery and to treat the occult finding medically with postoperative afterload reduction and follow-up serial echocardiograms. In contrast, in a patient with otherwise unexplained shortness of breath, pulmonary hypertension, and a dilated left ventricle (LV), the presence of moderate AR typically leads to AVR. The introduction of new findings to the operative team warrants a "time-out" approach to determine the impact of the findings on the intraoperative care.

CASE STUDY: STENOSIS WITHOUT STENOSIS

A patient with a history of syncope was scheduled for an AVR for the presumptive diagnosis of aortic stenosis (AS) based on a transthoracic echocardiogram (TTE) showing a sclerotic AV, an LV-to-aorta pressure gradient of 100 mm Hg, and severe left ventricular hypertrophy. The intraoperative TEE confirmed the preoperative findings but added new information. Inspection of the valve revealed a mobile but sclerotic three-cusp AV with a valve area of $1.1\,cm^2$. The left ventricular outflow tract (LVOT) contained an obstructing membrane that contributed to the "apparent" transvalvular pressure gradient. The surgeon, confronted with information that significantly altered the operative plan, called for an intraoperative "time-out" and contacted the referring cardiologist who performed the original echocardiogram. After discussion among the referring cardiologist, the intraoperative echocardiographer, and the cardiac surgeon, the patient underwent an AVR and surgical excision of the obstructing membrane in the outflow tract.

If a suggestion by the echocardiographer for a proposed course of action is rejected or modified, it is counterproductive to interpret the disagreement as a personal rejection. The echocardiographer is a consultant who performs, analyzes, and interprets findings in an objective manner. The final decision and ultimate responsibility for the operative plan typically lie with the attending cardiac surgeon, although this may be institution dependent.

Decision-Making Process

The process of decision making is, in essence, "deciding how to decide."[5] What is the primary issue that needs to be addressed? What are the pitfalls in the decision? What are the consequences of the decision? What tools and resources does the decision maker require? What information is needed to make an informed decision? Is there evidence to support one decision over another? How much time does the decision-maker need to make the decision? Rarely is there a valid reason for not taking enough time to make a well-thought-out decision, even in the high-productivity, high-throughput environment of the operating room. Does the decision-maker need help? The authors have applied the methods of Russo and Schoemaker[5] to decision making in medicine:

1. *Framing:* Framing defines the question and the factors that influence or sway the decision maker. Framing sets the vantage point of the decision maker and defines the boundaries, parameters, and priorities. By framing a question in the early stages of problem solving, it permits focus and bounded rationality. However, the price of focusing on a specific issue may be loss of peripheral vision. Adopting a narrowed vantage point can inadvertently impose significant bias and limitation. The decision should be addressed from a variety of vantage points so that all aspects of the decision can be considered.

   Failure to work beyond a single conceptual frame can lead to difficulties in communication among the different participants of the care team. In the setting of a complex MV repair, the intraoperative echocardiographer often is focused on performance of the TEE,

successful remedy of hemodynamic disturbances, surgical intervention, and documentation. If the echocardiographer is also the anesthesiologist, his or her frame is broadened to include patient safety and comfort, vigilance, and maintaining body homeostasis. The surgeon's frame includes his or her ability and limitations in achieving a competent surgical repair, alternatives in surgical management, and the covenant with the patient and family regarding surgical management (e.g., repair vs. replacement, bioprosthesis vs. mechanical prosthesis), patient overall outcome, and his or her reputation as a surgeon. The patient's vantage point may differ from those of the operative team. The patient wants the mitral regurgitation (MR) to be fixed, for the symptoms to be resolved, to return to a "normal routine," for the remedy to be long-lasting, and to be able to ride a Harley Davidson, which he or she would otherwise have to forfeit if he or she was taking lifelong warfarin (Coumadin). Hence, as a decision maker, broadening the understanding of the issues and consideration of multiple frames will account for the interests of multiple parties.

2. *Data collection:* Data collection is aimed at reducing uncertainty. Uncertainty is never eliminated and, hence, needs to be managed. The perioperative echocardiographer manages uncertainty not through pinpoint predictions but by uncertainty estimates. It is imperative in the decision-making process to systematically identify the causes that could lead to decision failure and to quantify the likelihood of such causes occurring. A dilated mitral annulus with a flail middle scallop of the posterior leaflet and two ruptured chordae are associated with a high rate of successful surgical repair. However, factors that are likely to affect this outcome include the technical ability of the surgeon, a parameter that is difficult to estimate and creates uncertainty in the expected outcome.

   The data should include echocardiographic and nonechocardiographic data (see Boxes 13-1 through 13-3). The importance and impact of TEE decisions have been generally recognized and accepted. The ability to make an appropriate decision is predicated on a comprehensive examination. Confirmatory information is useful, as is contradictory information. The process of decision making also includes defining what information "not to collect." Collecting as much data as possible typically leads to confusion and loss of direction in the reasoning process. A common hazard for the echocardiographer is the performance of an abridged examination because of either increased clinical demands or reliance on a preoperative examination. The conclusions drawn from an intraoperative examination and associated decisions should not be hurried and should be based on all aspects of the examination. Although physical injury from the TEE examination is a serious matter, the greatest risk of TEE is that of errors of omission or misinterpretation, leading to mismanagement and poor outcome.[6–11]

BOX 13-4. DECISION PROCESS

Projecting the impact of:
- Progression of disease
- Risk for redo surgery
- Short- and long-term outcomes
- Associated risks (e.g., anticoagulation)
- Size mismatch of prosthesis
- Effect of prolonged cardiopulmonary bypass on immediate postoperative outcome

Does the decision account for:
- Inconsistencies (among two-dimensional/Doppler/patient symptoms/preoperative evaluation)
- Plausibility of alternate explanation
- Alternate therapy
- Current literature
- Preoperative evaluations
- Patient factors (age, cardiac status, ability to tolerate anticoagulation, etc.)

3. *Decision and implementation:* A clinical decision is made based on the integration of knowledge, framing, and information (Box 13-4). Primary knowledge is "knowing what you know" and "knowing what you do not know," with the latter prompting a practitioner to seek assistance. Second-order knowledge is "not knowing what you do not know"; hence diagnoses are missed rather than misinterpreted. The broader the repertoire of primary knowledge, the more informed is the decision maker and the more reliable is the decision.

The echocardiographer is an intraoperative consultant who generates vital information that has a direct impact on intraoperative care and decision making. As consultants, suggestions and recommendations are offered, but rarely does the echocardiographer dictate the management to the operative team. The decision/recommendation is shared with the stakeholders (surgeons, perfusionists, nurses, referring cardiologists, postoperative intensivists, family and patient) and is communicated verbally and by written report. Decisions often are accompanied by discussion and sometimes persuasion. Making a sound decision concerning the surgical approach to an anatomic problem can benefit the patient only if it is effectively communicated to the operating surgeon. However, clinical judgment must take into account the skill set of the operative team and the pitfalls associated with each intervention. Persuading a surgeon to proceed with a complex reconstruction may appear to be the appropriate course of action according to an echocardiographer, but it may be the wrong thing to do if the surgeon is unfamiliar with the recommended repair (i.e., poor framing).

4. *Learning from knowledge to wisdom:* A systematic process for learning from the results of past decisions is designed to increase the decision maker's primary knowledge base and defines an effective clinical quality improvement program. The ability to achieve success or failure may depend on the ability of the decision maker to learn from past decisions and the decisions of others.[5] A fund of knowledge gained through training, continuous medical education, readings, and the performance of echocardiograms on a regular basis maintain the skills of the echocardiographer. Although it is often difficult to obtain feedback regarding the impact of decisions on long-term outcome, the increment in effort to seek such insight always renders the echocardiographer more prepared for the next clinical scenario that shares common cardiovascular themes (wisdom). Feedback can be sought from a variety of sources: surgeon, cardiologist, outpatient echocardiography data files, among others. Participation in quality improvement forums with cardiovascular anesthesiologists, cardiologists, and cardiac surgeons who tend to follow the patients longitudinally is a useful learning tool.

Although all four processes above are important, the initial framing of the problem prompts the subsequent steps of data collection, conclusion, and learning. Framing begins by articulating a question. By addressing the problem in terms of a specific question, a clinical situation is framed in a more manageable context. A framing strategy can be an effective method to rationally limit decision options and form the basis of communication.

Performance of the decision maker is judged based on final outcome. However, decision making should be based on the information the decision maker had at the time of the decision. A significant limitation of measuring performance during uncertainty is that it is often judged, not by the decision-making process, but by single case results. If the decision is followed by a good outcome, the decision maker often is applauded with little regard to the ability to reach an intelligent conclusion. A poor outcome does not necessarily imply a poor process or poor decision. High-risk surgery leads to poor outcomes in many cases despite robust decisions. In medicine, this often leads to individuals being reluctant to make any decision at all, knowing that a poor outcome is likely and that it will be linked to their decision making. The reality of performance assessment is that even if the decision to proceed with therapy is substantiated, a poor outcome often will reflect negatively on the abilities of the echocardiographer, anesthesiologist, surgeon, and the operative team. Conversely, a good outcome does not imply a good process or a good decision.[5] The surgeon's decision to perform a posterior sliding mitral valvuloplasty and quadrilateral resection of the posterior leaflet based on a dilated mitral annulus with normal leaflet motion as defined by TEE may result in a technically competent MV repair and good long-term results. The decision to perform a posterior sliding valvuloplasty may or may not have been a wise decision. Equally good results may have occurred with the insertion of an annular ring without leaflet resection. The measure of an outcome by recording a metric is a valid assessment of quality only if the metric is a function of the actions of the provider.[12] The outcome cannot be random; otherwise, there is no basis for estimating quality.

CASE STUDY: THE REGURGITANT CARPENTER

A 48-year-old asymptomatic woman presented for elective MV repair secondary to mitral regurgitation. She was otherwise healthy, except for mild pulmonary hypertension and rapidly increasing left ventricular dimensions. The woman was a union carpenter and absolutely refused to be subjected to lifelong anticoagulation. Physical examination was notable for a loud holosystolic murmur from the apex to the axilla. The lungs were clear. Baseline electrocardiogram (ECG) was normal, as were all laboratory blood tests. Preoperative chest wall echocardiogram demonstrated severe mitral regurgitation, no segmental wall motion abnormalities (SWMAs), and a flail MV. Intraoperatively, after induction of general anesthesia and tracheal intubation, the TEE was performed and demonstrated a severely dilated left atrium (LA), dilated LV, flail and thickened middle scallop of the posterior leaflet with multiple ruptured primary and secondary chordae to all scallops of the posterior leaflet, prolapse of the anterior leaflet, and a small perforation. The short-axis and bicommissural views of the MV suggested three regurgitant orifices. The surgeon was experienced in complex mitral repairs, with extensive experience in repairing myxomatous valves and chordal transfer. Consultation between the surgeon and the echocardiographer resulted in the surgeon proceeding with an MV repair, resection of excessive leaflet tissue of the posterior leaflet, chordal transfer from the anterior leaflet, and patch closure of the perforation, plus a mitral annular ring. Separation from CPB was facilitated with epinephrine, but the postrepair TEE demonstrated residual moderate central mitral regurgitation and residual anterior leaflet prolapse. No systolic anterior motion (SAM) of the MV was evident. No gradient existed between the LV and the aorta. CPB was reinstituted. The surgeon elected to replace the MV with a pericardial bioprosthesis, despite the patient's young age. The patient required the transfusion of blood, plasma, and platelets, as well as return to the operating room on the evening of surgery because of mediastinal bleeding. The patient emerged from the anesthetic and surgery on postoperative day 1 edematous and confused. Heart function showed a cardiac index of 2.4 L/min/m², mild pulmonary hypertension, and bounding peripheral pulses. Neurologic function recovered fully before discharge on postoperative day 7. Was the initial decision to repair the MV a sound decision? Do the poor initial results of the operation suggest the decision was a poor one? Would it have been wise to attempt a second repair after failing the initial attempt? Was the better decision to proceed directly to an MV replacement, decreasing the CPB and aortic cross-clamp times?

INTRAOPERATIVE TRANSESOPHAGEAL ECHOCARDIOGRAPHY: INDICATIONS

The first decision by the echocardiographer is whether TEE is indicated. Application of intraoperative TEE in the care of the patient with mitral disease is widely accepted. Even in this area, however, there is a paucity of data supporting an improved outcome for intraoperative patients cared for with TEE compared with no TEE. The decision to perform TEE during cardiac surgery is substantiated by practice expectations and consensus opinion. In an attempt to develop an evidence-based approach to this expanding technology, the American Society of Anesthesiologists (ASA) and the Society of Cardiovascular Anesthesiologists (SCA) cosponsored a task force to develop guidelines for defining the indications for perioperative TEE. Despite the scarcity of outcome data to support the application of TEE in the perioperative period, TEE had rapidly been adopted by cardiac surgeons and cardiac anesthesiologists as a routine monitoring and diagnostic modality during cardiac surgery. In 1996, the task force published their guidelines, designed to establish the scientific merit of TEE and justification of its use in defined patient cohorts.[13] The indications were grouped into three categories based on the strength of the supporting evidence/expert opinion that TEE improves outcome (Box 13-5). Category I indications suggested strong evidence/expert opinion that TEE was useful in improving clinical outcome. Category II indications suggested there was weak evidence/expert opinion that TEE improves outcome in these settings. Category III indications suggested there was little or no scientific merit or expert support for the application of TEE in these settings (see Chapters 12 and 41). These guidelines were further updated in 2010 to include virtually all adult cardiac surgery (Box 13-6).[14]

TEE is not without its serious complications. The risks of intraoperative TEE include physical injury to the mouth, dentition, and esophagus, plus the misinterpretation of a finding leading to mismanagement. When making the decision of whether to perform an intraoperative TEE, the physician should consider the cumulative effects of the indications and risks. A TEE should not be performed if the appropriate equipment, safety precautions, and skilled examiners are not available.

Population-based management decisions are driven by clinical trials, cost-effectiveness analysis, and resource allocation. However, few physicians take care of populations. Most physicians care for individuals.

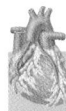

BOX 13-5. INDICATIONS FOR THE USE OF TRANSESOPHAGEAL ECHOCARDIOGRAPHY

Category I
- Heart valve repair
- Congenital heart surgery
- Hypertrophic obstructive cardiomyopathy
- Endocarditis
- Acute aortic dissection
- Acute, unstable aortic aneurysm
- Aortic valve function in the setting of aortic dissection
- Traumatic thoracic aortic disruption
- Pericardial tamponade

Category II
- Myocardial ischemia and coronary artery disease
- Increased risk for hemodynamic disturbances
- Heart valve replacement
- Aneurysms of the heart
- Intracardiac masses
- Intracardiac foreign bodies
- Air emboli
- Intracardiac thrombi
- Massive pulmonary emboli
- Traumatic cardiac injury
- Chronic aortic dissection
- Chronic aortic aneurysm
- Detection of aortic atheromatous disease as a source of emboli
- Evaluating the effectiveness of pericardiectomies
- Heart-lung transplantation
- Mechanical circulatory support

Category III
- Other cardiomyopathy
- Emboli during orthopedic procedures
- Uncomplicated pericarditis
- Pleuropulmonary disease
- Placement of intra-aortic balloon pump, pulmonary artery catheter
- Monitoring the administration of cardioplegia

Modified from the Practice guidelines for perioperative transesophageal echocardiography. A report by the American Society of Anesthesiologists and the Society of Cardiovascular Anesthesiologists Task Force on Transesophageal Echocardiography. *Anesthesiology* 84:986, 1996.

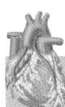

BOX 13-6. 2010 UPDATED RECOMMENDATIONS FOR TRANSESOPHAGEAL ECHOCARDIOGRAPHY

Cardiac and Thoracic Aortic Surgery
- *All* adult open-heart (e.g., valves) and thoracic aortic surgical procedures
- Consider in coronary artery bypass grafting surgery
- Transcatheter intracardiac procedures

Critical Care
- When diagnostic information that is expected to alter management cannot be obtained by transthoracic echocardiography or other modalities

Modified from Practice guidelines for perioperative transesophageal echocardiography: An updated report by the American Society of Anesthesiologists and the Society of Cardiovascular Anesthesiologists Task Force on Transesophageal Echocardiography. *Anesthesiology* 112:1084, 2010.

Evidence-based practice paradigms based on "population medicine" define the most effective management scheme for groups of patient cohorts but not every patient. Individual patient decisions by physicians are not always based on evidence. It is not uncommon to make these decisions based on "What would I do if it were my mother?" with the premise that more information is better. Should every patient undergoing repair of an abdominal aortic aneurysm have a dipyridamole or dobutamine stress test? The evidence does not support their use. Nonetheless, the practice in many centers is to obtain a nuclear stress test before major vascular surgery, even if the patient is asymptomatic. Should every patient undergoing cardiac surgery have an intraoperative TEE? The answer is unknown. Despite the reassurances provided by large clinical trials, practitioners do not consistently adhere to their recommendations and often rely on tradition, anecdote, and impression in their decision making.

The anchor to a "last case" experience creates bias and is all too prevalent in medicine; the experience from the previous case dictates the decision making on the subsequent one. If physicians are to remain the dispensers of medical care and resources, then they need to be cognizant of the effects of their decisions on all patients, not just the one lying on the operating room table. It is inappropriate to accrue healthcare costs without evidence that such financial investment provides any healthcare benefit. Unfortunately, the risk of uncertainty and medicolegal liability results in more testing than often is indicated.

INTRAOPERATIVE TRANSESOPHAGEAL ECHOCARDIOGRAPHY: PERFORMANCE OF THE INTRAOPERATIVE EXAMINATION

A detailed consideration of the TEE data precedes decision making. It takes time to consider all variables and make a decision in the operative environment. Hasty decisions because of perceived time pressures may unduly introduce misconceptions or surgical bias. It typically is more detrimental to keep changing or retracting diagnoses and recommendations than it is to take a few extra minutes to assemble the facts and present a concise, coherent assessment and plan.

The ability to render a sound conclusion often is predicated on the performance of a complete and quantitative echocardiographic examination. Incomplete and qualitative assessments may be subject to missed or inaccurate diagnoses. The complete TEE examination has been described through a consensus opinion.[15] The exact sequence of the comprehensive examination is less important than is adherence to it. A common practice is to perform a targeted examination, followed by the complete sequenced examination. This method allows for capture of the most important information should the patient become unstable and need rapid initiation of CPB before completion of the sequence of images that constitute the comprehensive TEE. The "soft" interpretation of "mild-to-moderate" is not always avoidable. The ability to "nail down" a diagnosis and establish a quantifiable measure of dysfunction allows for serial follow-up and comparison before and after treatment. The imperative for quantitative measures is directed at producing reproducible conclusions and trackable results.

Aliasing of color-flow Doppler in the LVOT is sensitive for detection of outflow obstruction but lacks specificity. Altered loading conditions, contractility, obstructive myopathy, and systolic anterior mitral motion may produce similar color Doppler findings. Spectral Doppler offers distinct advantages to color Doppler by measuring gradients and analysis of blood-flow velocity profiles, rendering the interpretation of abnormal flow patterns and pressure gradients more reliable and quantifiable. A similar approach is applied to assess abnormal blood-flow velocities across the MV (see Chapter 12).

Time permitting, the echocardiographer is encouraged to document in writing the prebypass TEE findings at the time they are discovered. It is acceptable to document a finding only to discover later that there is poor agreement with the surgical findings. This practice fosters learning and a systematic process. The process of writing a report ensures a formalized approach to evaluating the TEE.

▧ Cardiac Function and Regional Wall Motion Abnormalities

Framing

Ventricular function is a predictor of outcome after cardiac surgery and a predictor of long-term outcome in patients with cardiovascular disease. Patients with compensated CHF may have severely decreased ejection fraction (EF) with minimal symptoms. Regional ventricular dysfunction most commonly is caused by myocardial ischemia or infarction. Hence there is an imperative to detect ventricular dysfunction and institute treatment in an attempt to prevent acute or long-term consequences.

Is ventricular function normal or abnormal? Is the abnormal function global or regional? What is the coronary distribution that relates to an SWMA? Is the ventricle big or small? Is the myocardium thinned or hypertrophied? Is the abnormal function new or old? Does the medical or surgical intervention improve or decrease ventricular function?

Data Collection

Left ventricular systolic function is assessed echocardiographically based on regional and global wall motion. Methods of assessment include changes in regional wall thickness, radial shortening with endocardial excursion, fractional area change (FAC), and systolic apical displacement of the mitral annulus. Off-line measurements of EF can be calculated using Simpson's rule. However, the EF most commonly is estimated online from the four-chamber, two-chamber, and short-axis images of the LV. Other measures include end-diastolic area (EDA), end-systolic area (ESA), and, most recently, three-dimensional analysis.

Regional assessment provides an index of myocardial well-being that can be linked to coronary anatomy and blood flow. Although the measurement of coronary blood flow is not achieved by TEE, the perfusion beds and corresponding myocardium for the left anterior descending, left circumflex, and right coronary arteries are relatively distinct and can be scrutinized by TEE using multiplane imaging. The transgastric and long-axis imaging views of the LV are the most widely used for evaluating wall motion abnormalities. Digital archival systems have gained popularity for their ability to capture a single cardiac cycle that can then be examined more closely as a continuous cine loop. Cine loops also can permit side-by-side display of images obtained under varying conditions (e.g., prebypass and postbypass). Regional myocardial ischemia produces focal changes in the corresponding ventricular walls before changes occur on the ECG.[16] Changes progress from normal wall motion to hypokinesis or akinesis. Dyskinesis, thinning, and calcification of the myocardium suggest a nonacute process, likely a prior infarction.

Assessment of right ventricular systolic function is more problematic because it is less quantifiable. The crescent-shaped right ventricle (RV) is not amenable to quantitative measures of differences in chamber size during the cardiac cycle. Characterization of the RV is accomplished by comparing the size of the right ventricular chamber with that of the LV and assessing the relative contractile function of the right ventricular free wall and that of the interventricular septum.

Ventricular failure can be caused by diastolic dysfunction: the compromised ability of the ventricle to accommodate diastolic filling. Diastolic dysfunction is assessed echocardiographically by examining volumetric filling of the ventricle at the mitral or tricuspid valves and annular excursion. Normal diastolic filling is biphasic with an early (passive) component that exceeds the late (active) inflow velocities. Abnormalities of ventricular filling (e.g., impaired ventricular relaxation, restriction, constriction) produce characteristic changes in the spectral recordings of Doppler inflow velocities. Abnormalities of diastolic function can lend insight into the mechanisms of circulatory instability (see Chapter 12).

Discussion

Preexisting ventricular dysfunction suggests increased risk for surgery and poorer long-term outcome. The presence of such ventricular dysfunction may deteriorate intraoperatively, requiring the need for marked pharmacologic or mechanical support. A patient with a preoperative EF of 10% scheduled for coronary artery bypass grafting (CABG) and MV repair is at increased risk for intraoperative ischemia, acute heart failure, and difficulty maintaining hemodynamic stability during the immediate postbypass period. Anticipating such problems, consider placement of an intra-aortic balloon pump or femoral arterial catheter during the prebypass period (Figure 13-2). The same patient is likely to benefit from the administration of inotropic agents (see Chapter 32).

A marked decrement or unexpected decrease in global cardiac function after release of the aortic cross-clamp can be caused by poor myocardial preservation during cross-clamping or distention of the heart during bypass. The risk for such incidents can be reduced by the monitoring of the electrical activity of the heart and pulmonary artery pressures, as well as for distention of the RV and LV. Effective venting of the heart is often difficult to discern by visual inspection alone, especially with the use of minimally invasive surgery through small incisions. TEE imaging can diagnose ventricular distention produced by AV insufficiency.

Not all preexisting SWMAs benefit from coronary revascularization. Regions of akinesia and dyskinesia usually are the result of a myocardial infarction and may reflect nonviable myocardium, although "hibernating" myocardium is possible. Hypokinetic segments generally are viable and may represent active ischemia.[17] Preoperative positron emission tomographic scanning can detect hibernating myocardium and may be cost-effective to guide CABG.[18-20] The detection of hibernating myocardium in an area of chronic ischemia and regional hypokinesis will direct the surgeon to revascularize the corresponding stenosed coronary artery. In contrast, an occluded coronary artery with downstream infarction may not benefit from revascularization because contractile function may be irreversibly lost. However, in this latter scenario, revascularization postinfarction may provide some benefit in decreasing the risk for ventricular aneurysm formation.[21]

Diastolic dysfunction is associated with significant increases in mortality during long-term follow-up.[22] Characterization of abnormalities of diastolic function lends insight into the mechanisms of circulatory instability and hypotension. Severe left ventricular hypertrophy with a noncompliant LV and hyperdynamic systolic function may produce severe heart failure if adequate loading is not achieved. Hemodynamic indices obtained from a pulmonary artery catheter (PAC) may be misleading. The findings of a small left ventricular chamber size, blunted transmitral filling velocities, and an increased FAC demonstrate the cause of the hypotension. The decision to administer volume may be appropriate despite the increased pulmonary artery pressures.

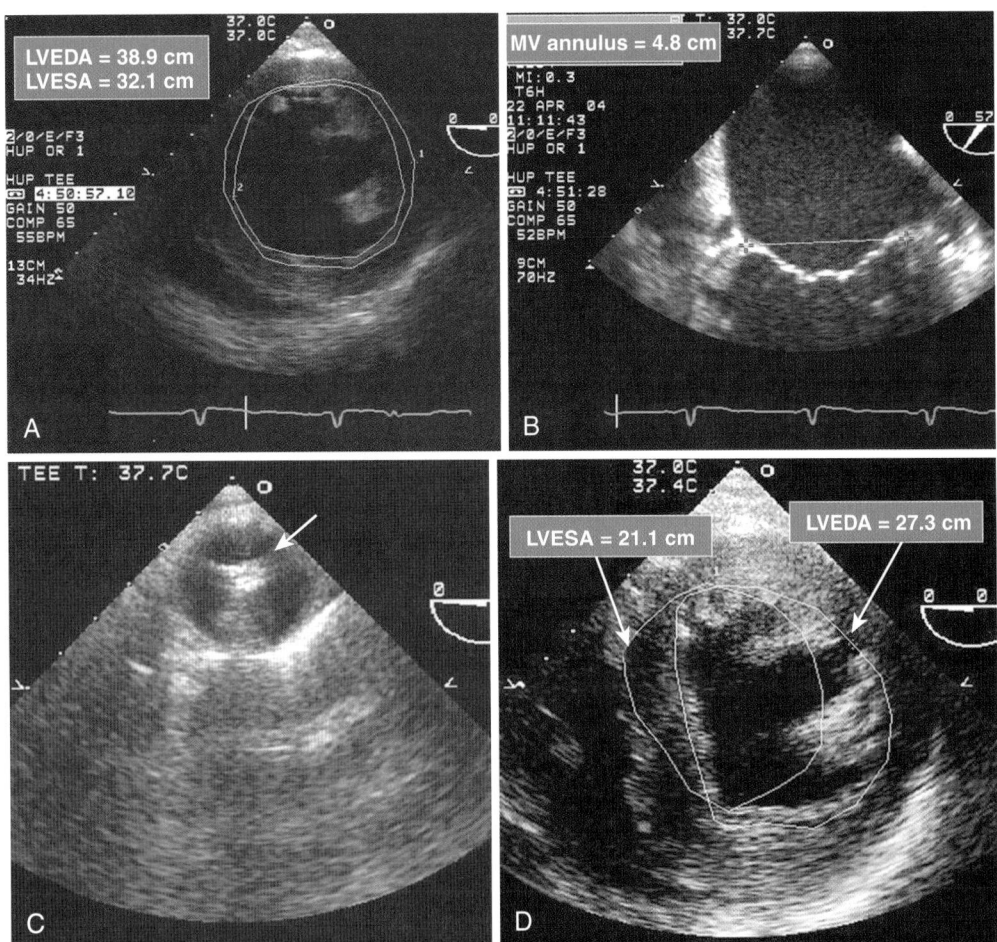

Figure 13-2 The prebypass transesophageal echocardiography (TEE) examination may have predictive value for postbypass circulatory management. A 63-year-old woman with a medical history of hypertension, congestive heart failure, pulmonary edema, dilated cardiomyopathy, diabetes, and obesity was scheduled for coronary artery bypass grafting (CABG) and mitral valve (MV) repair. The preoperative evaluation documented moderate-to-severe mitral regurgitation (MR) with reversal of systolic pulmonary vein blood flow velocity. The prebypass TEE midesophageal four-chamber view showed a markedly dilated left ventricle (LV) and mildly dilated right ventricle (RV) with mildly decreased global dysfunction (A). The transgastric view was characterized by severe global dysfunction and an LV end-diastolic diameter of 6.6 cm (A). The fractional area change (FAC) was 17% [FAC = (left ventricular end-diastolic area [LVEDA] – left ventricular end-systolic area [LVESA])/LVEDA × 100]. Revascularization alone was unlikely to significantly improve MV function. The midesophageal bicommissural view of the MV (B) demonstrated marked dilation of the MV annulus (major axis = 4.8 cm) and tethering of the leaflets below the valve plane that was caused by LV chamber dilation. A femoral arterial line was inserted for monitoring of central aortic pressure and/or possibly placing an intra-aortic balloon pump for moderate MR. The patient underwent a CABG × 3 and MV annuloplasty for moderate MR. The separation from bypass was difficult, requiring milrinone, epinephrine, vasopressin, and placement of an intra-aortic balloon pump. TEE, which was used to initially confirm the location of the femoral guidewire (C), was later used to position the balloon pump just downstream to the left subclavian artery. Worsening of RV function that was characterized by increased central venous pressure, new-onset tricuspid regurgitation, and a hypokinetic RV can be appreciated by ventricular septal flattening and dilation of the RV (D). The LV ejection fraction did not decrease as might be expected; after correcting MR, the FAC improved slightly from 17% to 22% after bypass. Cardiac function continued to improve, and the counterpulsation device was removed without complication on the first day after surgery. The infusions of milrinone and epinephrine were continued for several days.

If the intraoperative examination reveals new ventricular dysfunction, the intraoperative team must determine the cause and severity and then plan a treatment. Other causes of SWMAs such as conduction abnormalities (left bundle branch block or ventricular pacing) can be difficult to distinguish. Is the decrement in function potentially reversible with conservative therapy, or should additional intervention be considered? Treatment of myocardial ischemia may include optimizing hemodynamics; administering anticoagulants, nitrates, calcium channel blockers, or β-blockers; inserting an intra-aortic balloon pump; or instituting CPB and coronary revascularization. The presence of new-onset SWMAs after separation from CPB is worrisome for myocardial ischemia. Even the patient without coronary artery disease (CAD) remains at risk because of hypotension, a shower of air or debris into the coronary circulation, or coronary spasm. The patient with CAD

undergoing CABG may have all the above risks, technical difficulties at the anastomotic site, injury to the native coronary artery (e.g., stitch caught the back wall or occlusion of the circumflex artery during MV surgery), or occlusion of the coronary graft by thrombosis or aortic dissection. The coronary arteries, grafts, and anastomoses should be carefully inspected for patency and flow. Graft patency in the operating room is difficult to determine. Techniques include manual stripping and refill, measuring coronary flow by handheld Doppler, or administration of echo contrast agents (see Chapter 12). Hybrid operating rooms have been increasing in number with the intent of providing advanced imaging of the coronary circulation at the time of surgery.[23] A new SWMA in the distribution of a new coronary graft can prompt the decision-making strategies listed in Table 13-1 (see Chapters 18, 32, and 34).

TABLE 13-1	Management Strategies for New-Onset Myocardial Ischemia after Bypass	
Diagnosis	*Plausible Treatment*	
Coronary graft occlusion	Revise coronary graft	
Coronary air emboli	Increase coronary perfusion pressure, administer coronary dilators	
Coronary calcium/atheroma emboli	Support circulation	
Dissection of the aortic root	Repair dissection	
Coronary spasm	Administer coronary dilators	

Transesophageal Echocardiography as a Rescue Device: Management of Marked Hemodynamic Instability

Framing

There are many instances during the perioperative period when the patient may exhibit progressive, unremitting hemodynamic deterioration or acute cardiovascular collapse. Echocardiography offers a versatile modality to quickly and accurately diagnose the cause of hypotension and develop management strategies.

The echocardiographer may be summoned to evaluate an unstable patient in the operating room, intensive care unit, or emergency department with little or no preceding knowledge of the patient. Typically, there will be no consent for the TEE procedure; occasionally, a family member may be available to provide consent on the patient's behalf. TEE may need to be postponed in the trauma patient with suspected cervical spine injury or esophageal injury. The trauma patient with an unstable cervical spine is at increased risk for spinal cord injury with passive movement of the head and neck. Until the cervical spine has been documented to be stable, TEE should be avoided and TTE is the alternative. The risk for further esophageal injury in patients with a penetrating trauma poses an additional challenge. Esophagoscopy before TEE is performed in patients with suspected esophageal injury. However, delay in diagnosis is not without cost. Time must be used efficiently because permanent vital organ injury relates to the magnitude and duration of hypotension and malperfusion. A number of issues should be considered to guide the discussion and development of rational management strategies.

What is the cause of the hypotension? Does the cardiac or vascular pathology detected by TEE explain the decrease in blood pressure? Is the heart big or small? Is it full or empty? What is the global function of both ventricles? Are there SWMAs? Is there fluid in the pericardium? Is the observed decrease in cardiac function the primary cause, or is it a consequence of the decreased blood pressure? Is this event related to the patient's medical history or current operative procedure? What specific parameters of the ventricle may help explain the current episode of hypotension? What interventions or therapy can be performed to improve hemodynamics? Once therapy is initiated, what index or parameter should be monitored to guide management?

Data Collection

Clinicians must not underestimate the importance of medical history, chief complaint, and operative course when attempting to discern the causes of hemodynamic instability in the acute setting. Important hemodynamic indices include heart rhythm, rate, blood pressure, concentration of exhaled carbon dioxide, and central venous or pulmonary artery pressure, if available. Echocardiography can be used to develop a rational approach based on the critical factors of cardiac performance. The determinants of cardiac performance include stroke volume (SV) and heart rate (HR), as elucidated by the following equation: $CO = SV \times HR$, where CO represents cardiac output. The three components of SV that can be affected are preload, afterload, and myocardial contractility. Although quantitative analysis is possible, qualitative online analysis generally will yield sufficient information to form the basis of initial therapeutic intervention. Preload of the ventricle can be determined

by assessing EDA, afterload can be estimated by assessing the ESA, and contractility can be estimated by the velocity of circumferential shortening, FAC, or EF. Mechanical causes of hypotension must be considered (e.g., pericardial effusion).

Discussion

Initial inspection determines heart size and overall contractile function of both ventricles. Estimates of EDA and EF of the LV provide an index of ventricular load and global function. Attention to both right and left ventricular size and function helps distinguish between different inciting events.

The common causes of intraoperative or perioperative hypotension include intravascular hypovolemia, myocardial ischemia, myocardial infarction, and systemic vasodilatation, either pathologic from infection or inflammation, or iatrogenic from drug administration (e.g., vancomycin). Mechanical causes of hypotension typically are related to compressive forces impairing the heart's ability to fill or eject (e.g., pericardial fluid, tension pneumothorax). The MV is inspected for incompetence. Acute mitral regurgitation is rare in the absence of myocardial ischemia or infarction. A diagnosis of dynamic LVOT obstruction, an uncommon cause during the perioperative period, is difficult to establish in the absence of more invasive monitoring such as TEE (Figure 13-3). Systemic hypotension with a dilated RV and a small, underfilled LV implies either primary right ventricular failure (e.g., myocardial ischemia or infarction in the distribution of the right coronary artery) or secondary right ventricular failure from acute increases in pulmonary vascular resistance (e.g., pulmonary embolus [Figure 13-4], pneumothorax, or protamine reaction).

Decreased systemic vascular resistance during sepsis or a systemic inflammatory reaction is associated with decreased ESA and increased ventricular contractility (increased velocity of circumferential shortening), with concomitant increases in the EF and FAC. The increase in cardiac performance can be quantified by measuring the cardiac output (CO). In cases of hypotension associated with a markedly increased CO, the treatment of choice would be the administration of a vasopressor, such as phenylephrine or vasopressin. If decreased systemic vascular resistance and CO are present, administration of a positive inotrope having vasopressor actions, such as epinephrine or norepinephrine, might be more appropriate.

The distribution of the right coronary arterial system of most patients (right dominant system) includes the RV and the posterior descending coronary artery, which provides blood supply to the inferior and inferoseptal walls of the LV. Acute right ventricular dysfunction is not uncommon after the release of the aortic cross-clamp. Preservation of the RV is less reliable compared with the LV because of its exposure to ambient room temperature and variability in its coronary circulation. Open-chamber procedures increase the risk for right ventricular dysfunction because of retained intracardiac air. In the supine patient, the right coronary ostium is located in the least-dependent portion of the aortic root, predisposing it for the embolization of air bubbles. Air embolization to the right coronary artery produces acute ST-segment changes, marked global right ventricular dysfunction, and SWMAs of the inferior wall of the LV (Figure 13-5). Conservative treatment includes increasing the blood pressure to promote coronary perfusion while continuing CPB.

Pericardial Effusion and Tamponade

Framing

Small effusions are common after cardiac surgery, especially after removal of chest tubes. In isolation, pericardial effusion may not require surgical intervention. Cardiac tamponade occurs when the pressure exerted by the presence of a pericardial effusion (or any structure adjacent to the heart) compresses the heart, limits diastolic filling of any of the chambers of the heart, and impairs CO. Cardiac tamponade is an emergency, necessitating immediate diagnosis and intervention.

Is a pericardial effusion present? If so, does it contribute to cardiac dysfunction and the patient's present hemodynamic distress? What is

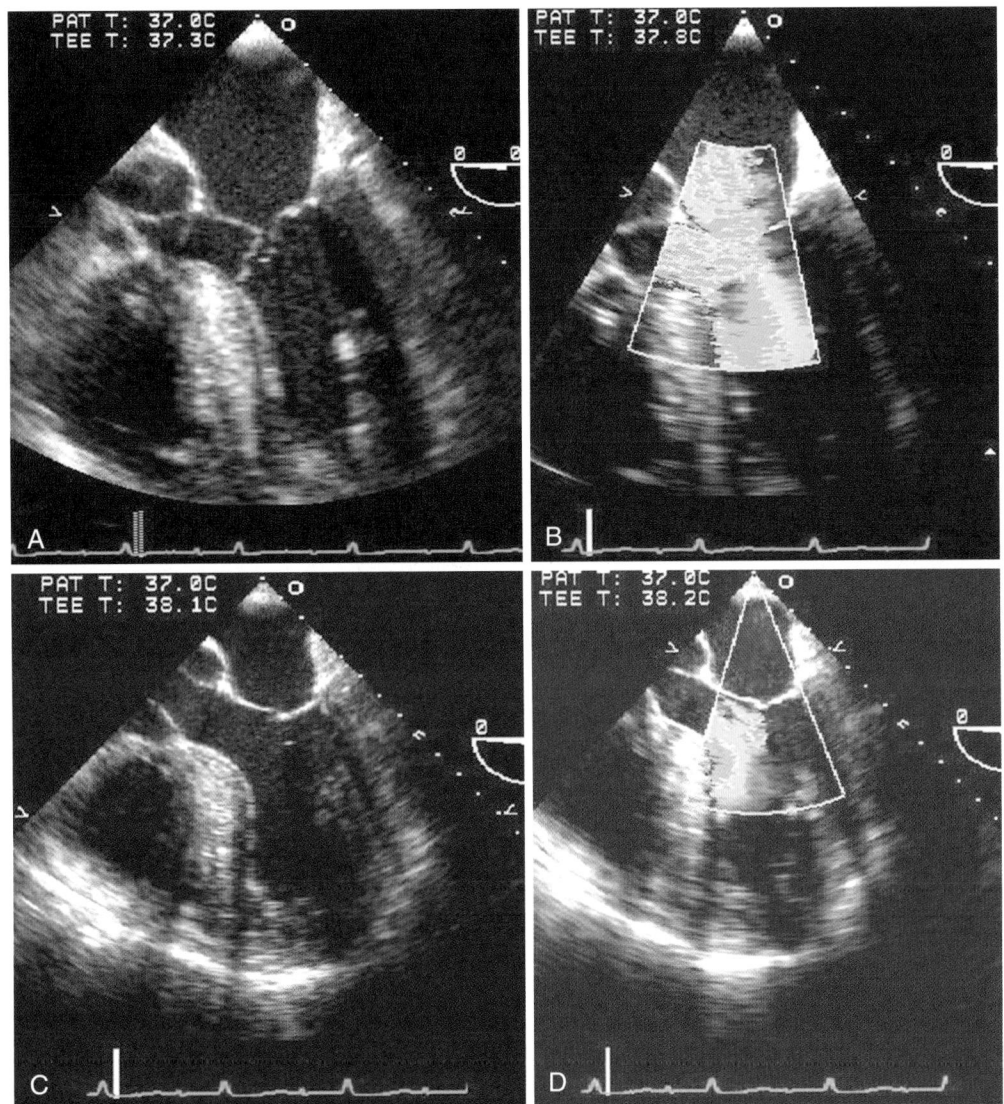

Figure 13-3 **Acute intraoperative hemodynamic deterioration.** A 65-year-old man with a medical history of hypertension, sleep apnea, and smoking was scheduled for resection of colon cancer. During the bowel resection, the patient had a profound episode of hypotension and new-onset hypoxia. Although the patient's hemodynamic condition initially improved after administration of phenylephrine and ephedrine, the patient became more hypotensive and hypoxic with evidence of pulmonary edema. Transesophageal echocardiography (TEE) was requested and was emergently placed to diagnose the cause of cardiovascular collapse and guide management. The midesophageal four-chamber view showed a moderately hypertrophied left ventricle (A). Left ventricular (LV) systole was associated with displacement of the mitral leaflet and chordae down into the outflow tract. The resulting defect in leaflet coaptation of the mitral valve (MV) and abnormal chordal position that was noted in A were associated with overwhelming mitral regurgitation (MR) and LV outflow tract obstruction. B, Administration of inotropes (epinephrine and ephedrine) was discontinued; the management strategy was changed to volume resuscitation and pressor administration. The hemodynamics normalized and the examination was repeated 10 minutes later (C, D). Displacement of the mitral leaflet and chordae had resolved together with the findings of MR and outflow tract obstruction. The patient was believed to have experienced a profound acute decline in the systemic vascular resistance in response to the release of vasoactive substances during bowel manipulation. The initial exacerbation of the hemodynamics was created by the relative hypovolemia and use of inotrope, leading to dynamic LV outflow tract obstruction. The concomitant episodes of hypoxia and pulmonary edema, which were attributed to the severe MR and increased left atrial pressures, resolved with the decrease in MR. The application of TEE was critical in making the correct diagnosis, altering management strategies, and initiating the appropriate therapy.

the cause of the effusion (acute or chronic)? Is the pericardial effusion the sequelae of another cardiovascular event or process (i.e., aortic dissection or cardiac catheterization)? Are there invaginations of the free walls of the right atrium (RA), RV, or LA? Is the effusion free flowing or loculated? Where is it located? Is echocardiographic assessment consistent with tamponade? What is the coagulation status?

Data Collection

Echocardiography is the standard modality for diagnosis of pericardial fluid. However, the diagnosis of cardiac tamponade is a clinical diagnosis based on hemodynamics and the patient's condition. Low CO,

hypotension, equalization of pressures, and high venous pressures are all signs of cardiac tamponade. Echo findings consistent with tamponade include presence of pericardial fluid, compression of the atria, compression of the RV, and loss of normal respiratory variability of ventricular inflow velocities.

The TEE examination quickly determines whether pericardial effusion is present, the location of the effusion (loculated, free-flowing), and impact on chamber filling. Location of the effusion is paramount should pericardiocentesis be deemed necessary for acute decompression. Right atrial and right ventricular collapse are the most sensitive signs of increased pericardial pressure. The effusion need not be a

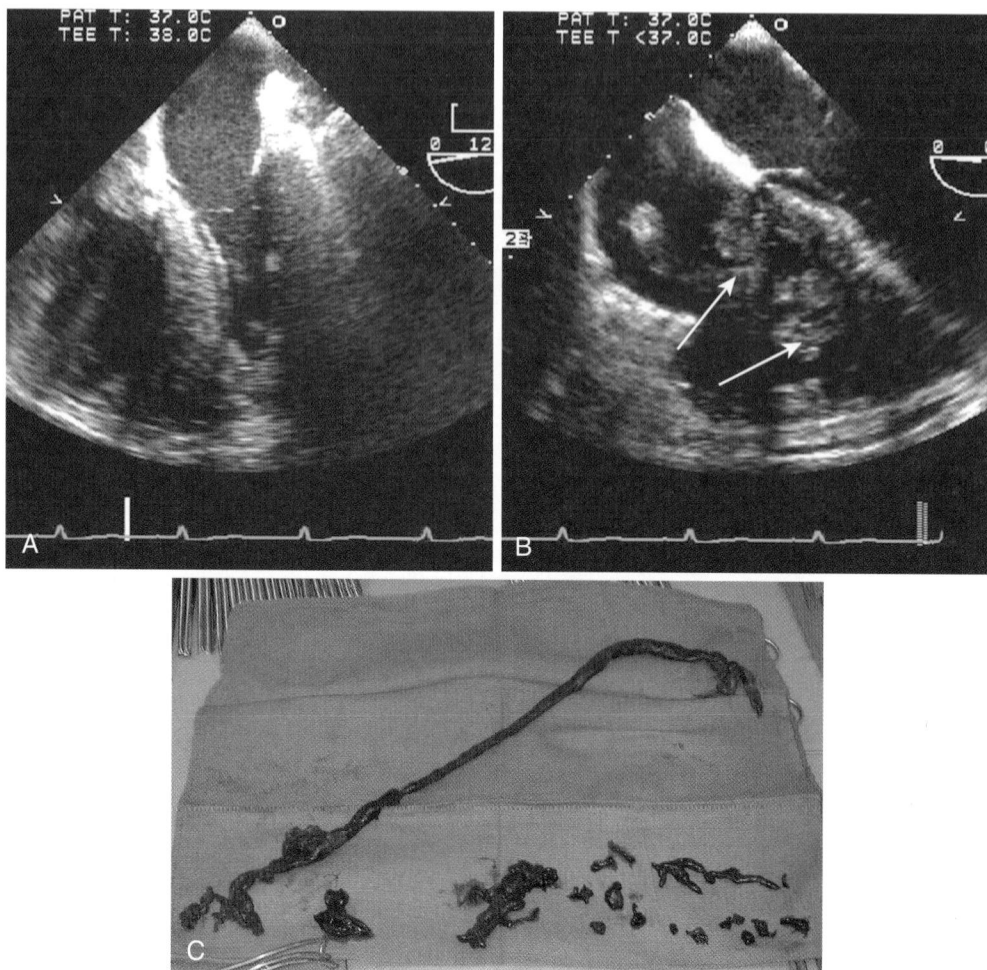

Figure 13-4 **Progressive hypoxia and hypotension after cardiac surgery.** A 58-year-old morbidly obese patient with a medical history of hypertension, diabetes, and smoking had recently undergone coronary artery bypass grafting × 3. Five days after surgery, the patient experienced development of new-onset atrial fibrillation together with progressive hypoxia and hypotension requiring readmission to the intensive care unit. The patient's condition continued to deteriorate and required tracheal intubation, ventilator support, and infusions of vasoactive agents. Transesophageal echocardiography (TEE) was performed to evaluate cardiac function and rule out a pericardial effusion. The midesophageal four-chamber view (A) showed a dilated right ventricle (RV) coincident with a relatively underfilled left ventricle (LV) and abnormal positioning of the ventricular septum. The displacement of the septum into the LV was consistent with RV dysfunction and RV volume overload. Inspection of the right heart revealed a dilated hypokinetic RV and a serpiginous density that extended from the right atrium into the RV (B). The thrombus appeared to be entangled in the chordal structure of the tricuspid valve. Although no thrombus was noted in the pulmonary arteries, the diagnosis of pulmonary embolism was made and the patient underwent an emergent embolectomy. A right atriotomy was performed and a 64-cm thrombus was extracted from the RV together with additional clots from both the right and left pulmonary arteries (C). The postbypass TEE documented improved right ventricular function and filling of the LV. TEE was critical in making the diagnosis and the decisions to institute and guide therapy.

large circumferential effusion to significantly impact cardiac function. Postcardiotomy pericardial clot may be smaller and more compartmentalized than a chronic circumferential effusion that may be free flowing. Interpreting the clinical significance on cardiac hemodynamics may be complicated by factors such as lability of hemodynamics, decreased intravascular volume, depressed cardiac function, mechanical ventilation and pulmonary dysfunction, soft-tissue changes, and chest tubes that obstruct some of the echocardiographic windows. Doppler is used as a complementary method of demonstrating the hemodynamic derangements of tamponade and to determine the clinical significance of an effusion. The echocardiographer should interrogate the phasic respiratory variation of blood flow through the tricuspid valve and MV. Although not specific for tamponade, the changes in respiratory variation of inflow velocity are the hallmark of increased pericardial pressure. Significant respiratory variation of blood inflow velocities also may be seen in constrictive pericarditis or conditions associated with changes in intrathoracic pressure, such as increased work of breathing, asthma, or positive-pressure ventilation, and may be exacerbated

in patients on positive end-expiratory pressure. Other important data pertaining to the cause and possible intervention include coagulation status.

Discussion

The American College of Cardiology/American Heart Association/American Society of Echocardiography (ACC/AHA/ASE) Task Force assigned a Class I recommendation to the use of echocardiography in patients with suspected bleeding in the pericardial space. Echocardiography is portable, quick, and noninvasive, yet it is a sensitive and specific modality for the detection and impact of a pericardial effusion. Pericardial effusions can be diagnosed and cardiovascular effects determined by TTE or TEE. However, during the postcardiac surgery period, the presence of positive-pressure ventilation, chest tubes, and bandages may severely limit the capability of TTE to assess fluid in the pericardium.

The effusion need not be a large circumferential effusion to significantly affect heart function. Loculated effusion may impinge only on

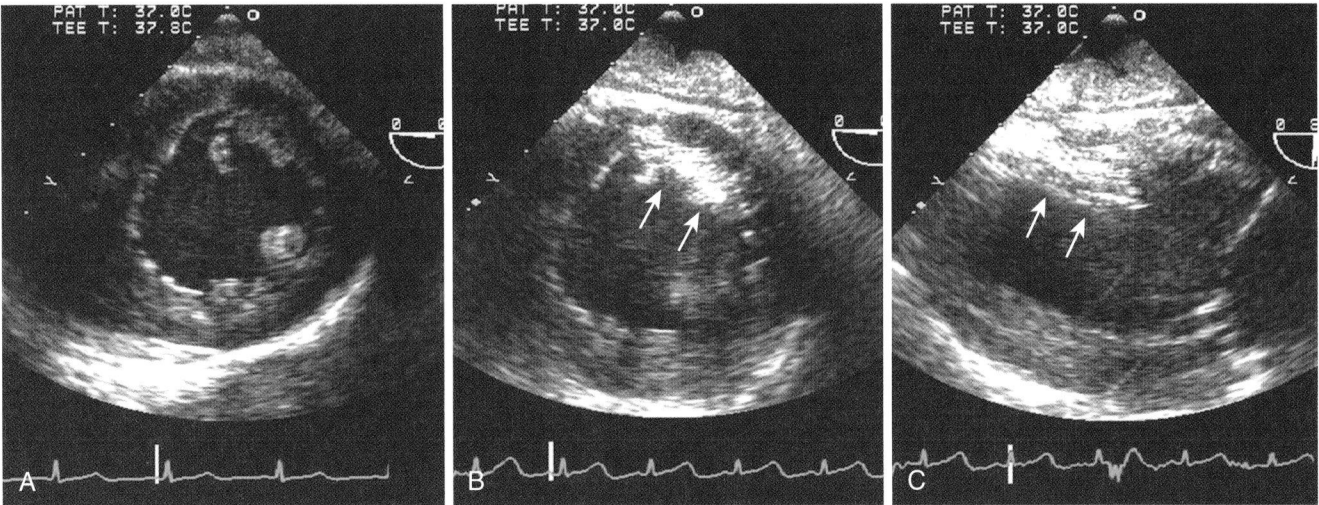

Figure 13-5   Air embolism after open-chamber procedure. A 57-year-old patient underwent surgical intervention to treat severe mitral regurgitation (MR) and two-vessel coronary artery disease. After performing the mitral valve (MV) repair, the right superior pulmonary vein vent catheter was advanced through the mitral valve to facilitate deairing. The patient was positioned in Trendelenburg and the aortic cross-clamp removed. After ventricular ejection, the left atrium and ventricle (LV) were relatively clear of air and the left atrial vent was removed. An aortic vent that had previously served as the cardioplegia cannula was used to vent the residual air from the ascending aorta. The patient was separated from bypass in normal sinus rhythm and maintained good hemodynamics. The initial postbypass transesophageal echocardiogram (TEE) showed normal ventricular function and filling (A). Shortly after starting administration of protamine, the blood pressure decreased and the electrocardiogram demonstrated ST-segment changes consistent with ischemia. The protamine administration was stopped, and vasopressors and inotropes were quickly administered. The TEE documented reduced cardiac function in the right ventricle and hypokinesis in the inferior and inferoseptal walls of the LV. The transgastric short- and long-axis views of the LV (B, C) showed that the myocardium in the distribution of the right coronary artery, as designated by the *arrows*, was characterized by increased echogenicity. Note the significantly elevated ST segments observed in B and C compared with the baseline (A). The absence of pulmonary hypertension and adequate diastolic filling of the LV supported a diagnosis other than acute anaphylactic protamine response or pulmonary embolism. The most likely culprit was air embolization causing transient myocardial ischemia. Air bubbles that migrated from the LV chamber embolized into the ostium of the right coronary artery, which lies at the most anterior aspect of the sinus of Valsalva. TEE served a crucial role in quickly evaluating and diagnosing the cause of hypotension. The hemodynamics, which were temporarily supported by boluses of vasopressors and inotropes, stabilized, and the protamine dose was completed. The patient was transferred to the intensive care unit without any further incident.

the LA and may not be discernible by the traditional acoustic windows used by TTE. A hemodynamically significant localized hematoma compressing only the LA may not produce right atrial and right ventricular collapse, or the constellation of equalization of pressures. Small effusions are common after cardiac surgery, especially after removal of chest tubes, and in heart transplant recipients in whom there is a mismatch between heart size and pericardial cradle. The presence of a pericardial effusion in the nonpostcardiotomy patient must lead to a search for the cause of the effusion. Pericardial effusion mandates close scrutiny of the aortic root for possible aortic dissection. Pericardial effusion in a trauma patient is worrisome for cardiac rupture, ventricular contusion, or foreign body injury.

Acute cardiac tamponade in the nonpostcardiotomy patient can develop after introduction of as little as 60 to 100 mL blood. Causes might include type A aortic dissection, myocardial infarction with rupture, acute pericarditis, bleeding from malignancy, myocardial contusion, or myocardial perforation from penetrating trauma. These life-threatening conditions may present with hypotension, tachycardia, plethora, and jugular venous distention. Other classic findings include narrowed pulse pressure, pulsus paradoxus, widening of the mediastinum on chest radiography, and electrical alternans on the ECG. Treatment is immediate decrease in pericardial pressure that could be accomplished through the removal of a relatively small volume of fluid. This temporizing measure can be life-saving until more definitive therapy is instituted.

Not all pericardial effusions require immediate intervention. Development of cardiac tamponade is related to the rate of accumulation of pericardial fluid and the capacity for the pericardium to stretch and accommodate fluid. Chronic pericardial effusions, which occur in cases of malignancy, uremia, connective tissue disease, Dressler syndrome, and postinfection pericarditis, uncommonly require emergent intervention. Acute pericardial effusions that occur postcardiotomy are

usually more ominous and often result in hemodynamic compromise, requiring treatment (see Chapters 22 and 34).

Hemodynamics may improve temporarily with the administration of volume, altering intrathoracic pressure (decreasing peak inflation pressure), but still may require drainage of the effusion. Chronic malignant effusions will improve after pericardiocentesis but often require a pericardial window for more definitive therapy. Effusions resulting from acute aortic syndromes or cardiac trauma require timely surgical intervention. Postcardiac surgery patients may require urgent re-exploration for evacuation of pericardial hematoma and to address the cause of continued bleeding. If hemodynamics improve after sternotomy but minimal clot is found, the physiologic tamponade may be related to generalized tissue edema and pulmonary dysfunction. In cases of poor cardiac function, the sternal incision may need to remain open and covered with a sterile dressing until edema recedes and cardiac function improves.

Management of Ischemic Mitral Regurgitation

Framing

Ischemic heart disease is the most common cause of mitral insufficiency in the United States. Mechanisms of valve incompetence are varied and include annular dilatation, papillary muscle dysfunction from active ischemia or infarction, papillary muscle rupture, or ventricular remodeling from scar, often leading to a tethering effect of the subvalvular apparatus. Mitral regurgitation leads to pulmonary hypertension, pulmonary vascular congestion, and pulmonary edema with functional disability. Ventricular function deteriorates as the LV becomes volume overloaded with corresponding chamber dilation. Left untreated, severe mitral regurgitation from ischemic heart disease has a poor prognosis, hence the imperative for diagnosis and treatment.[24-26] Less certain is the impact of lesser degrees of mitral insufficiency on functional status and long-term morbidity and mortality. Patients presenting for CABG often have concomitant mitral regurgitation of a mild or moderate degree. The intraoperative team is confronted with the decision whether to surgically address the MV during the coronary operation.

Does mitral regurgitation warrant mitral surgery? What is the mechanism of the regurgitation? What are the grade and chronicity of the mitral regurgitation? Is the mitral regurgitation likely to improve by coronary revascularization alone?

Data Collection

Pertinent data, including preoperative functional status and evaluation, need to be considered to appropriately interpret and place the intraoperative data in context. The preoperative echocardiogram and ventriculogram need to be reviewed. The intraoperative hemodynamic data are coupled with TEE information to complete the dataset needed to move forward with the decision-making process. The severity of mitral regurgitation on TEE is measured by the vena contracta, maximum area of the regurgitant jet, regurgitant orifice area, and pulmonary vein blood-flow velocities. Valvular disease causes changes in other cardiac structures. Chronic mitral regurgitation may be associated with a dilated LA, pulmonary hypertension, and right ventricular dysfunction. Wall motion assessment and the ECG are used for detecting reversible myocardial dysfunction that may benefit from revascularization. The hemodynamic and TEE data are coupled with provocative testing of the MV in an attempt to emulate the working conditions of the MV in an awake, unanesthetized state. It is not uncommon that preoperative mild-to-moderate mitral regurgitation with a structurally normal valve totally resolves under the unloading conditions of general anesthesia.[27-29]

Discussion

Most cases of ischemic mitral regurgitation are categorized as "functional" rather than structural. In a study of 482 patients with ischemic mitral regurgitation, 76% had functional ischemic mitral regurgitation, compared with 24% having significant papillary muscle dysfunction.[30] The mechanism of ischemic mitral regurgitation is attributed to annular dilatation, secondary to left ventricular enlargement and regional left ventricular remodeling with papillary muscle displacement, causing apical tethering and restricted systolic leaflet motion.[31] The importance of local left ventricular remodeling with papillary muscle displacement as a mechanism for ischemic mitral regurgitation has been reproduced in an animal model.[32]

The mitral regurgitation is prioritized in accordance with the principal diagnosis (e.g., CAD), comorbidities, functional disability, and short- and long-term outcome. Ischemic mitral regurgitation is quantified and the mechanism of valve dysfunction is defined. Intraoperative mitral regurgitation is compared with preoperative findings. Discrepancies between the preoperative and intraoperative assessment of the valve may reflect the pressure and volume unloading effects of general anesthesia. In patients with functional ischemic 1 to 2+ mitral regurgitation, the MV often is not repaired or replaced. However, the need for surgical intervention in patients with 2+ mitral regurgitation under anesthesia remains a point of debate and has not been definitively answered by prospective studies. MV surgery typically is recommended to improve functional status and long-term outcome for patients with 3+ ischemic mitral regurgitation or greater.[30] Ignoring significant ischemic mitral regurgitation at the time of CABG can limit the functional benefit derived from surgery.

The risks to the patient of not surgically altering the MV and anticipated residual regurgitation are weighted against the risk for atriotomy, mitral surgery, extending CPB and aortic cross-clamp times, and the likelihood that the CABG surgery will be successful at decreasing the severity of mitral regurgitation. Added risk includes commitment to a mechanical prosthesis should a reparative procedure prove

unsuccessful. Mitral regurgitation caused by acute ischemia may resolve after restoration of coronary blood flow (Figure 13-6). The reversibility of the regurgitation is difficult to predict: Factors supporting reversibility (and, hence, no immediate need to surgically address the valve) include a structurally normal MV, normal left atrial and left ventricular dimensions, including the mitral annulus, and SWMAs associated with transient regurgitation and pulmonary edema. Revascularization of the culprit myocardium with improvement in regional function may be all that is necessary to restore normal mitral coaptation.[33,34] Myocardial infarction with a fixed wall-motion defect or aneurysm, chronically dilated left-sided heart chambers, dilated annulus, or other structural abnormalities that are not reversible (ruptured papillary muscle or chordae, leaflet prolapse, leaflet perforation) suggest myocardial revascularization is unlikely to correct the valvular incompetence.

The decision whether to proceed with mitral surgery in the setting of ischemic heart disease is institution and surgeon dependent. Centers may elect to surgically address any degree of mitral regurgitation detected during the preoperative or intraoperative work-up of a patient scheduled for CABG surgery. Less aggressive sites elect to proceed with coronary revascularization, followed by repeat scrutiny of the ventricular wall motion and MV. If revascularization has not corrected the mitral regurgitation, the surgeon proceeds with CPB and mitral surgery. With the advent of off-pump coronary artery bypass surgery, this process has gained another level of complexity because decisions to proceed with mitral repair will commit the patient to CPB. Off-pump mitral surgical procedures may be possible in the near future. A device that decreases the minor annular axis by adjusting the length of an artificial subvalvular chord that spans the ventricle between anterior and posterior epicardial pads has been used to treat functional mitral regurgitation.[35,36] Likewise, percutaneous endovascular procedures to "clip" the free edges of the anterior and posterior mitral leaflets akin to the Alfieri surgical technique are aimed at noninvasively improving leaflet coaptation.[37,38] Short- and long-term outcome data regarding such investigational techniques remain forthcoming (see Chapters 3, 18, 19, 26, and 27).

◼ Myxomatous Degeneration of the Mitral Valve and Mitral Regurgitation

Framing

Myxomatous degeneration of the MV is a common cause of mitral regurgitation. Patients often are young and otherwise quite healthy. The diagnosis is commonly established before surgery, and patients are scheduled for elective surgery unless acute leaflet or chordal rupture leads to acute pulmonary edema and emergency surgery. The decisions to be addressed in this setting include: Can the surgeon perform the MV repair to address the mitral regurgitation, or is valve replacement necessary? What does the surgeon need to know to assess the possibility of repair and how to accomplish it? What are the possible complications of MV repair? Is the MV repair acceptable?

Data Collection

The surgeon cannot rely on visual inspection of the native MV in the flaccid arrested heart to discern the mechanism of mitral regurgitation. Unless the patient had a preoperative TEE as part of the preoperative evaluation, the intraoperative study often is critical in assisting the surgeon to plan the appropriate surgical correction.

The intraoperative TEE examination targets the mitral regurgitation, LA, LV, and RV. Two-dimensional and color-flow Doppler remain the standard, although increasing application of three-dimensional echo has targeted mitral surgery as a niche. Three-dimensional echo has made significant advances in miniaturization, speed of data processing, and user interfaces. In the past, it was a technology seeking an application. Mitral surgery for myxomatous disease appears to be one of its prime applications. Myxomatous mitral regurgitation typically is amenable to valve repair. Typical findings of myxomatous valves include excessive leaflet motion, redundant leaflet tissue, and a dilated mitral

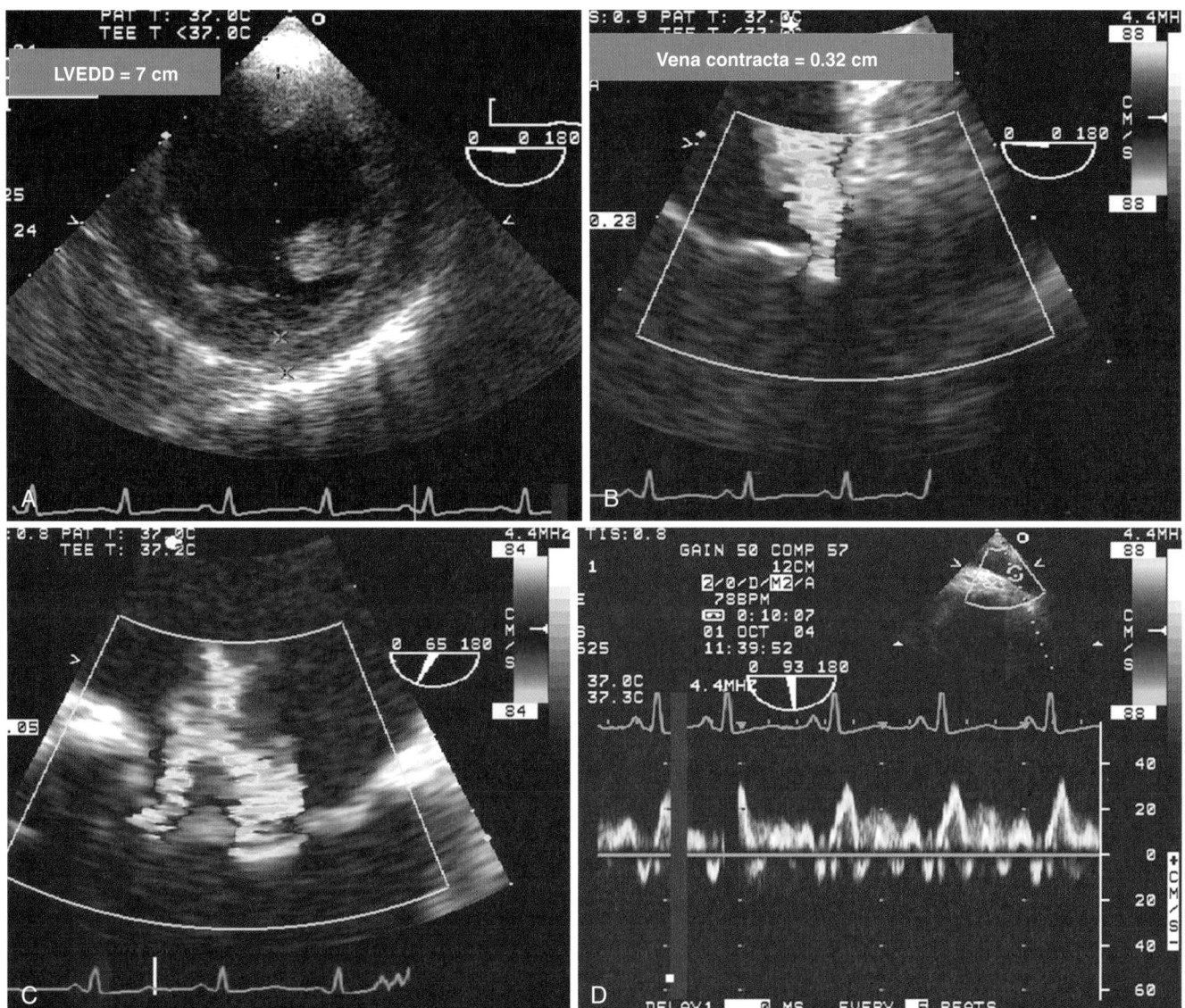

Figure 13-6   Evaluation of mitral regurgitation (MR) in a patient undergoing coronary artery bypass grafting. A 63-year-old man was scheduled to undergo off-pump coronary artery revascularization. The patient had a history of progressive congestive heart failure without evidence of acute pulmonary edema. The physical examination was significant for diffuse laterally displaced point of maximum impulse (PMI) and a systolic murmur at the apex that radiated to the axilla. The patient received an intraoperative transesophageal echocardiography (TEE) examination to evaluate the severity of MR. The left ventricle (LV) was significantly dilated with an LV end-diastolic dimension of 7 cm (A) and had depressed systolic function with an estimated ejection fraction of 40%. The MR was characterized by color-flow Doppler imaging to be a central jet of mild-to-moderate severity. The grading of MR was based on the area of the regurgitant jet and the vena contracta (B) viewed in a bicommissural view. The pathogenesis of MR was believed to be functional and resulted from restricted leaflet mobility caused by the dilated LV. The coaptation of the anterior and posterior leaflets was below the valve plane (C). The absence of reversal of pulmonary vein blood flow measured in the left lower pulmonary vein (C) supported the assessment of moderate MR. Because the annulus was not significantly dilated (the minor axis measured 2.97 cm) and the MR graded as only mild to moderate, the surgeon proceeded with his initial plan of off-pump coronary artery bypass grafting. The MR decreased immediately after revascularization, and the patient's symptoms were expected to further improve with afterload reduction.

annulus. Leaflets commonly prolapse into a dilated LA, the degree of which is based on the chronicity of the illness. Chordal rupture is common and leads to flail leaflets and severe mitral regurgitation. The imperative is to be exact in the descriptive anatomy of the MV. The accepted nomenclature of the anatomy of the MV is stated in a consensus guideline.[15] The locus of flailed scallops or leaflets and regurgitant orifice, the width of the anterior and posterior leaflets, the bisecting widths of the mitral annulus (minor and major axes), the locus of a perforation, severity of annular calcification (less common in isolated ischemic or myxomatous disease), and the size of the LA all contribute significantly to the planned repair. The findings of long and redundant anterior and posterior leaflets increase the risk for postoperative SAM

of the MV. Maslow et al[39] examined the predictors of LVOT obstruction after MV repair. In this study of patients who were undergoing repair for myxomatous valve disease, 11 of 33 patients experienced development of SAM and outflow tract obstruction. The major predictive factors were smaller anteroposterior length ratio (annulus to coaptation; 0.99 vs. 1.95) and short distance from septum to MV coaptation point (2.53 vs. 3.00 cm). The surgeon may elect to perform a posterior sliding valvuloplasty to move the point of coaptation laterally, thereby decreasing the risk for outflow obstruction and mitral incompetence associated with SAM.

Although assessment of valvular incompetence is made and the need for repair/replacement generally is decided before surgery, the severity and pathogenesis of mitral regurgitation should again be determined intraoperatively. The severity of mitral regurgitation can be quite variable and depend on the hemodynamic loading conditions and its pathogenesis. Discrepancies between preoperative and intraoperative assessment of mitral regurgitation are less likely in patients with structural abnormalities (e.g., ruptured chordae or leaflet perforation) of their MVs, in contrast with patients with functional mitral regurgitation (e.g., ischemic mitral regurgitation).

The repaired MV is scrutinized closely, with the ventricular vent removed at the discontinuation of CPB under typical loading conditions. The systolic and diastolic functions of the valve are examined for residual regurgitation, stenosis, and the presence of outflow tract obstruction. The postbypass examination is critical for determining the acceptability of the repair or guiding the subsequent revision, should the initial repair be unacceptable. Systolic valve dysfunction after repair typically produces residual mitral regurgitation. Residual mitral regurgitation after mitral repair is not uncommon and may not necessitate revision if the grade is trace or mild. Diastolic mitral function is ascertained by Doppler flow measurements across the mitral orifice to provide assurance that the repaired valve has not been rendered stenotic. Peak transvalvular blood-flow velocities and pressure half-times are measured to calculate valve gradients and valve areas.

Discussion

There is a growing imperative to repair instead of replace myxomatous MVs. The intraoperative echocardiographer soon becomes familiar with the abilities and limitations of his or her surgical counterparts. Outcomes may be quite dependent on the ability of the individual surgeon, more so than in valve replacement surgery. Hence it may be prudent to track short-term (intraoperative) results of these operations because outcomes may be less defined by national databases and more so by individual provider. In general, the likelihood of a successful repair is based on the severity and extent of involvement of the mitral leaflets. Isolated prolapse of the middle scallop of the posterior mitral leaflet associated with eccentric mitral regurgitation that overrides an otherwise normal anterior leaflet is associated with a high success rate. However, cases of extensive leaflet degeneration with bileaflet prolapse, multiple chordal ruptures from both leaflets, leaflet destruction from preceding endocarditis, two or more regurgitant orifices, and extensive calcification are associated with a significantly lower success rate for repair.[40] Many patients leave the operating room with a prosthetic MVR with preservation of the subchordal apparatus with excellent long-term results. Retention of the subvalvular apparatus preserves longitudinal shortening of the LV and decreases the incidence of HF in the long term.[41,42] In a comparative study, the EF of patients without chordal transfer decreased 24% after surgery compared with patients having chordal transfer who maintained preoperative function.[42]

Some degree of residual mitral regurgitation after repair is common. Most surgeons will not accept residual mitral regurgitation of 2+ or greater and will readdress the valve surgically. Assessment of valve function postbypass under unloaded conditions (decreased afterload with relative hypovolemia) may erroneously predict mitral regurgitation in the long term or under provoked conditions of exercise. Hypotension with decreased left ventricular contractility and chamber dilatation often responds to inotropic agents with improved coronary perfusion and decreased mitral regurgitation.

The mechanism of the failed repair is paramount to the decision process and treatment. Residual mild regurgitation associated with persistent leaflet prolapse may warrant further leaflet resection. Mild residual regurgitation in the setting of a "normal" MV may sway the surgeon to accept it. The presence of a central jet of mitral regurgitation may require resizing (smaller) or considering an edge-to-edge repair (i.e., Alfieri). The decision of re-repair or valve replacement often is a difficult one, weighing the balance between the risks for reoperation versus the risk for residual mitral regurgitation. The final decision of what is acceptable residual valvular regurgitation is patient specific (e.g., age, anticipated level of activity, ability to tolerate a return to CPB).

The finding of LVOT obstruction caused by SAM after mitral repair often is caused by the displacement of leaflet coaptation toward the septum, resulting in the anterior leaflet to paradoxically move into the LV, rather than toward the LA late in systole (Figure 13-7).[43] Displacing the anterior leaflet into the LVOT during ventricular ejection (Venturi effect) produces outflow tract obstruction, early closure of the AV, and mitral regurgitation. The incidence of postoperative SAM and the need to revise the surgical repair have decreased as understanding of the predisposing factors and management strategies has improved. SAM may be intermittent and dependent on loading conditions. If possible, patients should be examined after adequate volume resuscitation and with minimal inotropic support. Most cases of SAM resolve with conservative measures including β-blockade, vasoconstriction, and fluid administration. In a single-center retrospective study of 2076 patients who underwent MV repair, the incidence rate of intraoperative SAM was 8.4% (174 cases).[44] Revision of repair or valve replacement related to SAM during initial operation was undertaken in only two patients. However, in the case of persistent severe SAM with a high LV-to-aorta gradient, returning to CPB and revising the mitral repair (e.g., posterior sliding mitral valvuloplasty to "slide" the locus of coaptation laterally), performing an edge-to-edge repair or possibly replacing the MV should be considered. Patients who transiently demonstrate SAM or turbulence in the outflow tract in the operating room may be at increased risk during the immediate postoperative period (see Figure 13-3). An important role of the clinical echocardiographer is to recognize potentially important findings that may have an impact on subsequent patient care and long-term follow up (see Chapters 12, 19, and 22).

Occult Congenital Abnormalities: Persistent Left-Sided Superior Vena Cava

Framing

The finding of a persistent left-sided superior vena cava (SVC) is not a common incidental finding, but its diagnosis has important implications for the conduct of circulatory management during CPB.

What echocardiographic findings suggest persistent left-sided SVC? What confirmatory test can be performed? Does the finding of an anomalous left-sided SVC have implications for the conduct of CPB?

Data Collection

The echocardiographer should suspect a persistent left-sided SVC if the coronary sinus is significantly dilated or if significant difficulty was encountered while attempting to place a pulmonary artery catheter (PAC). Because the differential diagnosis of a dilated coronary sinus includes pathology associated with increased right-sided pressures, confirmation should be obtained by injecting agitated saline contrast into an intravenous catheter in the left arm. In the case of a persistent left-sided SVC, opacification of the coronary sinus occurs before that of the RA or RV (Figure 13-8). Once the diagnosis is confirmed, the echocardiographer should look for other associated congenital anomalies, including atrial septal defects (ASDs) or an unroofed coronary sinus with communication between the coronary sinus and the floor of the LA.

Discussion

Left-sided SVC is the consequence of arrested embryologic development that results in the left brachiocephalic vein emptying into the coronary sinus with subsequent flow into the right atrial return of blood. As a consequence, cannulation of the coronary sinus with administration of retrograde cardioplegia will be ineffective at providing cardiac protection during cardiac arrest. Once the diagnosis is confirmed, the surgeon is informed to modify the conduct of cardiac protection during CPB. If TEE is unable to confirm the diagnosis (absence of venous access in the left arm to inject contrast), the surgeon can confirm its presence by direct inspection.

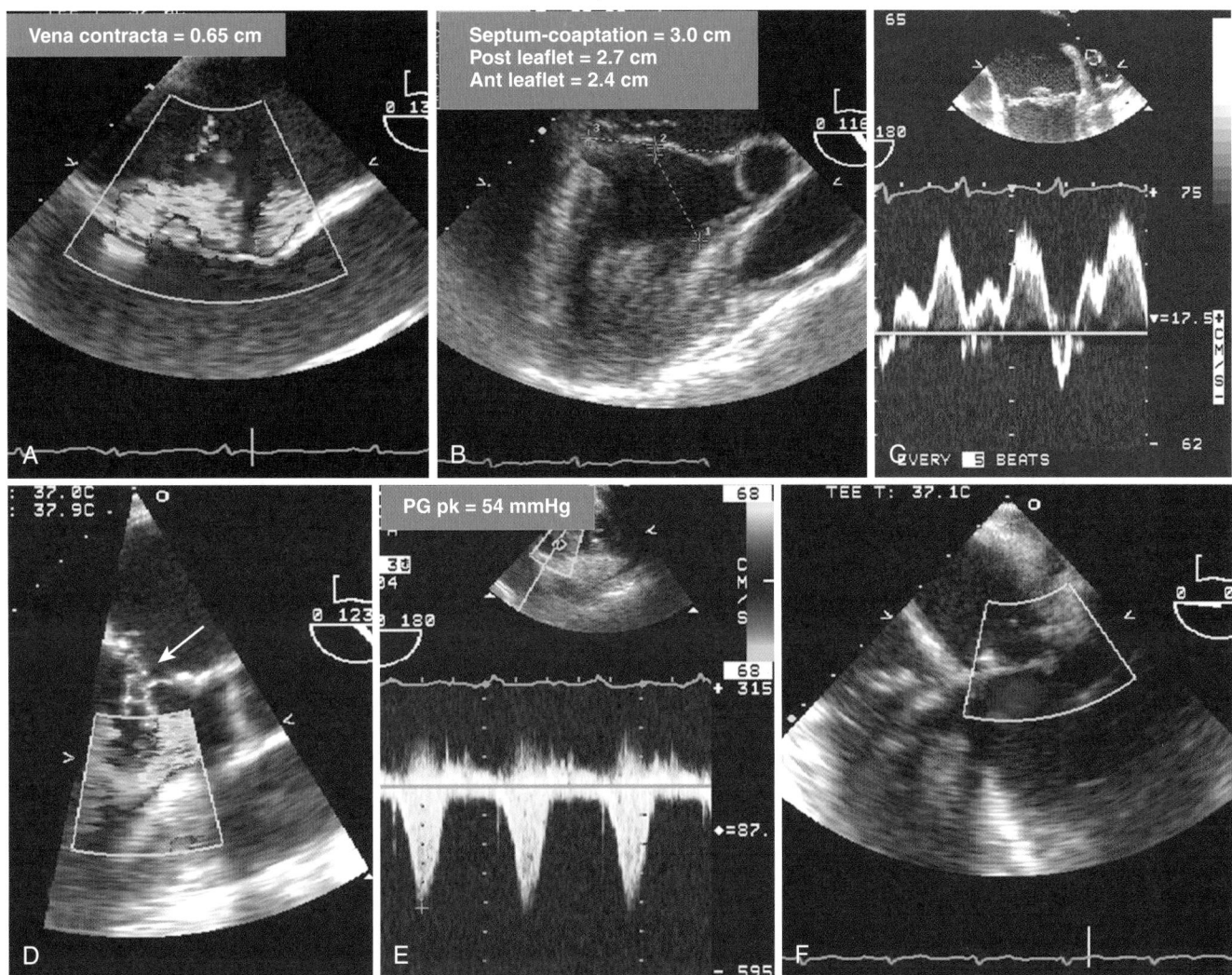

Figure 13-7   Complex mitral valve (MV) replacement/repair revision. A 58-year-old woman with severe mitral regurgitation (MR) and a history of congestive heart failure, pulmonary edema, and hypertension was scheduled for surgical repair of mitral insufficiency. The prebypass transesophageal echocardiogram (TEE) characterized the MV as having severe MR with mildly thickened, myxomatous leaflets and several ruptured chordae. The markedly dilated annulus was consistent with the chronic disease process. Prolapse of the posterior leaflet resulted in the MR jet overriding the anterior leaflet *(A)*. Although the distance from the septum to the coaptation point of the MV was greater than the value cited by Maslow as predictive of postbypass SAM, the ratio of the length of the anterior and posterior leaflets (0.89) suggested a risk for LV outflow obstruction *(B)*.[39] The midesophageal long-axis view demonstrates several ruptured chordae *(B)* that resulted in MR having a vena contracta of 0.65 cm. Blunting of the systolic component of pulmonary vein blood flow velocity corroborated the diagnosis of significant MR *(C)*. The surgeon performed a quadrangular resection of the posterior leaflet and secured the annulus with a No. 30 Physio ring. The postbypass imaging of the midesophageal long-axis view demonstrated a coaptation defect, designated by the *arrow*, and nonlaminar flow in the LV outflow tract *(D)*. Shift of the coaptation point medially created laxity of the redundant chordae that were drawn into the outflow tract by systolic LV ejection *(D)*. The outflow tract obstruction was characterized by a pressure gradient of 54 mm Hg as determined by continuous-wave Doppler through the outflow tract using the transgastric long-axis view *(E)*. Neither the MR nor the outflow tract obstruction was effectively addressed by volume loading and decreasing the inotropic support. Circulatory bypass was reinstituted, and the surgeon revised the previous repair by further resecting the posterior leaflet and enlarging the annular ring to a No. 34. The patient was successfully separated from bypass using minimal support and had resolution of LV outflow tract obstruction, return of normal hemodynamics, and reduction of MR to trace severity *(F)*.

Occult Congenital Abnormalities: Atrial Septal Defects and Patent Foramen Ovale

Framing

Incidental detection of an ASD or a patent foramen ovale (PFO) is a common occurrence. The clinical implications of an intracardiac defect are shunting, stroke, headaches, pulmonary hypertension, right ventricular dysfunction, and paradoxic embolization. If transseptal flow is present, it is generally from left to right, because left atrial pressure is generally greater throughout the cardiac cycle. Bidirectional flow is possible with transient increases of right atrial pressure that

can be observed during normal respiratory maneuvers (i.e., Valsalva, coughing, and physical straining).[45] Routine physical activities associated with a Valsalva maneuver include heavy physical activity, *lifting heavy objects*, defecation, or vigorous coughing.[46] Although uncommon, right-to-left shunting can produce episodes of relative hypoxia and paradoxic embolization. TEE is an extremely sensitive technique to detect an ASD or a PFO.[47] ASD or PFO is generally well tolerated and often remains asymptomatic into adulthood; hence their detection often is incidental during a routine intraoperative TEE examination.

What type of ASD is present: primum, secundum, sinus venosus, or PFO? What is the size of the defect? Does the defect produce transseptal blood flow? What is the shunt fraction: Q_s/Q_t? Does the patient

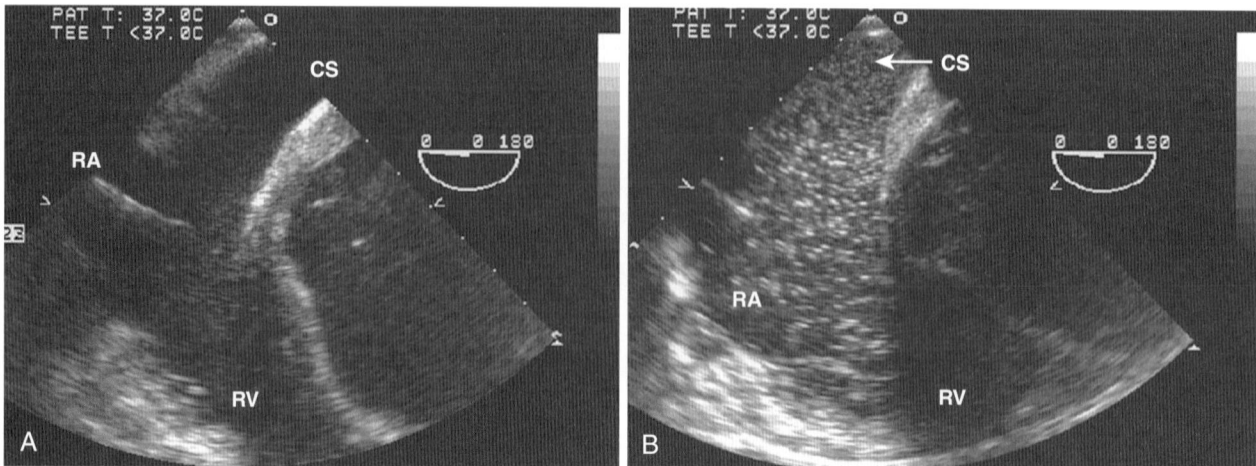

Figure 13-8 **Detection of occult persistent left superior vena cava alters circulatory management.** A 57-year-old patient was scheduled to undergo an aortic valve replacement for severe aortic stenosis. The intraoperative transesophageal echocardiography examination documented a bicuspid aortic valve (AV) with a dilated aortic root and ascending aorta, preserved left ventricular (LV) systolic function, moderate LV hypertrophy, and dilated coronary sinus (CS) (A). The diagnosis of persistent left superior vena cava was considered. An agitated mixture of saline, blood, and air was injected into the intravenous access in the left arm, and the diagnosis was confirmed when the coronary sinus was opacified before the right atrium (RA) and ventricle (RV). The diagnosis of a persistent left superior vena cava altered conduct of bypass by negating the standard use of retrograde cardioplegia and by relying solely on antegrade cardioplegia.

have any symptoms such as CHF, increased shortness of breath, history of stroke or transient ischemic attack, or refractory hypoxia? What is the pulmonary artery pressure and right ventricular function? Does the patient have any associated congenital abnormalities, such as a cleft MV with a primum ASD? Does the surgery as initially planned require the use of CPB? If so, was single or bicaval cannulation planned? Does the interatrial defect need to be closed?

Data Collection

The application of two-dimensional echocardiography, color-flow Doppler imaging, and contrast administration in the midesophageal four-chamber and midesophageal bicaval views provide for high sensitivity of detection and diagnosis of ASDs and PFOs. The clinical implication of these findings is determined by the type of pathology. The PFO may be detected in about 25% of adults; it occurs when the secundum septum fails to close or is stretched open because of elevated pressures in the LA (Figure 13-9). Ostium secundums, which account for 70% of ASDs, are located in the area of the foramen ovale. The cause of this lesion is attributed to poor growth of the secundum septum or excessive absorption of the primum septum. MV prolapse is present in up to 70% of patients with this abnormality and may be related to a change in the left ventricular geometry resulting from right ventricular

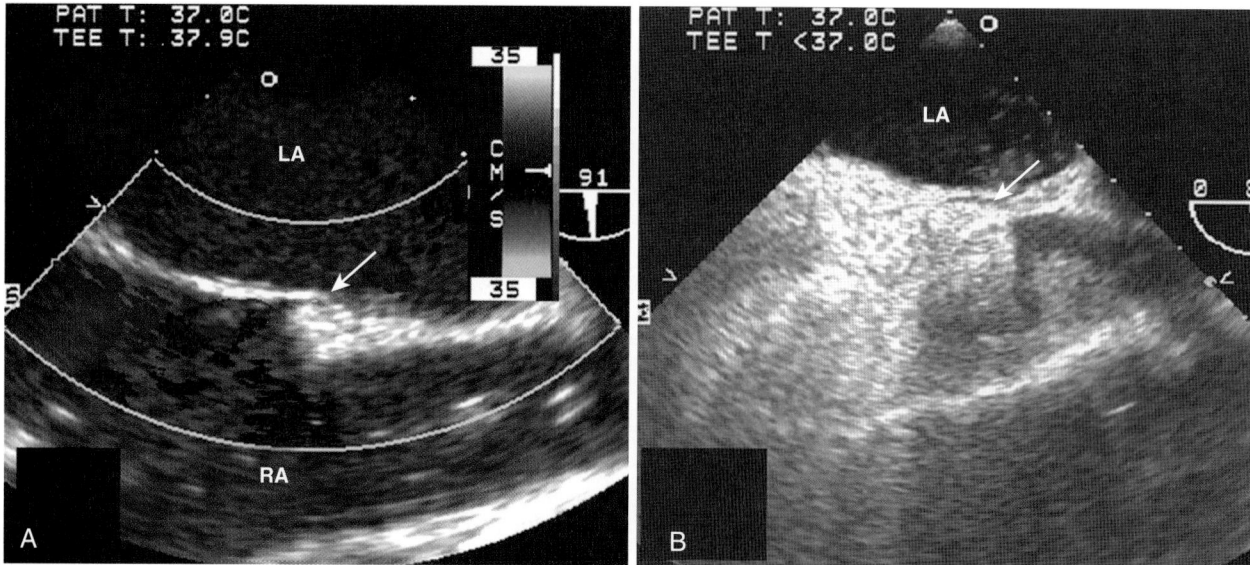

Figure 13-9 **Detection of a patent foramen ovale in a patient undergoing cardiac surgery.** A 68-year-old patient was undergoing two-vessel off-pump coronary artery bypass grafting (OPCAB). In addition to coronary artery disease, the patient had a medical history of hypertension, non–insulin-dependent diabetes, and a stroke of unknown cause. The intraoperative transesophageal echocardiographic (TEE) examination that included an inspection of the interatrial septum in the midesophageal four-chamber and bicaval imaging planes showed a new finding of an aneurysmal interatrial septum with a patent foramen ovale (PFO, arrow). Color-flow Doppler showed minimal shunt flow from the left atrium (LA) to the right atrium (RA). The presence of the PFO, which was initially diagnosed by color-flow Doppler imaging (A), was confirmed by the transient flow of injected contrast (arrow) into the LA (B), after it was injected into the venous circulation. A provocative maneuver such as Valsalva transiently increases RA pressure more than that of the LA, increasing the sensitivity of PFO detection.[47] Because of the patient's history of a cryptogenic stroke, the surgical plan and circulatory management were altered. The patient was fully heparinized and circulation supported by an extracorporeal pump, while the CABG was performed and the PFO was closed.

volume overload. The primum ASD develops when the septum fails to fuse with the endocardial cushion at the base of the interatrial septum. A primum ASD commonly is associated with cleft anterior leaflet of the MV and mitral regurgitation. The tricuspid valve also may be abnormal. The final type of ASD is a sinus venosus defect, which comprises only 10% of ASDs. It commonly is associated with abnormal insertion of the pulmonary veins into the RA or SVC.

Discussion

In general, patients benefit from ASD closure. Although often asymptomatic, ASDs may present with atrial arrhythmias, heart murmur, abnormal ECG, dyspnea, cerebrovascular injury or stroke, or migraine headaches. Medical management and surgical closure of secundum ASDs were compared in randomized trials; surgical closure was associated with significantly decreased morbidity and mortality.[48] However, there are little data concerning treatment strategies and outcomes for the occult ASD or PFO detected intraoperatively. In the absence of recognized consensus guidelines, the decision to proceed with definitive closure should be based on the following factors: history of neurologic event without a definite cause, recurrent stroke while receiving anticoagulation, significant shunting through the defect, previous episode of hypoxia that may be related to intracardiac shunting, right ventricular dysfunction, or previous paradoxic embolism. Detection of a primum or sinus venosus defect requires a more involved surgical procedure, and associated anomalies must be addressed. Alternatives to operative closure are increasing as transvenous percutaneous closure devices become increasingly applicable. Transvenous catheter–based closure of an ASD by interventional cardiologists can be performed only on a secundum ASD or PFO

(Figure 13-10). Approximately 30% of secundum ASDs are amenable to percutaneous closure.[49] The technique optimally requires a defect with limited size and a rim of tissue surrounding the defect of at least 5 mm to prevent obstruction of the coronary sinus or impingement of the AV (see Chapters 3 and 20).

A PFO is the most common congenital finding and usually is asymptomatic. However, a number of studies have found an increased prevalence of PFO and atrial septal aneurysms in patients having cryptogenic strokes (i.e., no identified cardioembolic or large vessel source).[50–56] Atrial septal aneurysm is a congenital outpouching of the interatrial septum at the fossa ovalis and is strongly associated with PFOs.[50,51,53] The occurrence of atrial septal aneurysms detected by echocardiography is about 10% in the general population and up to 28% in patients with a history of stroke or transient ischemic episode.[52–54,57] A meta-analysis of these case-control studies found that PFO, atrial septal aneurysms, or both were significantly associated with ischemic stroke in patients younger than 55 years.[58] However, the relation between septal pathology and neurologic events in patients older than 55 is less clear. The data on treating patients with atrial septal abnormalities for either primary or secondary prevention of stroke are limited. The Patent Foramen Ovale in Cryptogenic Stroke Study and a meta-analysis by Oregera found that warfarin treatment was superior to other antiplatelet therapy and comparable with surgical PFO closure for the prevention of recurrent cerebral events.[59] Chronic anticoagulation is associated with complications. The decision regarding closure of an incidental PFO considers the presence of right ventricular dysfunction that may increase the risk for right-to-left transatrial blood flow and cryptogenic stroke. Clinical practices typically are based on individual surgical preferences. A survey of cardiothoracic surgeons in the United States noted a high degree of variability in management

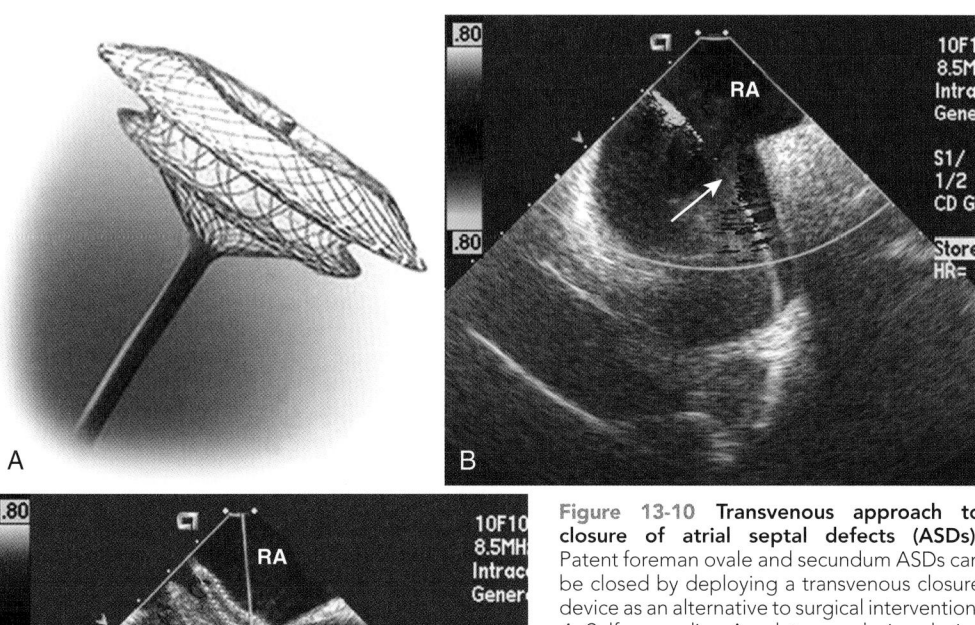

Figure 13-10 Transvenous approach to closure of atrial septal defects (ASDs). Patent foreman ovale and secundum ASDs can be closed by deploying a transvenous closure device as an alternative to surgical intervention. *A,* Self-expanding Amplatzer occlusion device (AGA Medical Corporation, Plymouth, MN) that is made from wires tightly woven into two interconnected disks. The device is deployed from the femoral vein and positioned using transesophageal echocardiography (TEE) or intravascular ultrasound. *B,* Color-flow Doppler image from an intravascular ultrasound that shows the deployment catheter as it enters through the right atrium (RA) and spans the secundum ASD. *C,* Color-flow Doppler ultrasound image showing the Amplatzer *(arrowhead)* in position across the interatrial septum, preventing shunt flow across the ASD.

of intraoperatively discovered PFO.[60] During planned on-pump CABG surgery, 27.9% of responders stated they always closed intraoperatively discovered PFOs, whereas 10.3% did not. Only 11% of surgeons converted a planned off-pump procedure to an on-pump procedure to close the defect, but the rate of closure increased to 96% if the patient had a history of possible paradoxic embolism. A single-institution retrospective study of 2277 patients from 1995 to 2006 confirmed that incidental detection of PFO is common, and that repair was not associated with a survival benefit. The authors found that propensity modeling of the data detected an increased incidence of postoperative stroke in patients having PFO repair. Several case reports describe postoperative complications related to hypoxia and neurologic events in patients with persistent PFOs.[60–63]

The benefit of aggressive management of a PFO in the absence of other interatrial septal abnormalities is less clear than ASD closure and is more controversial. Sometimes surgical intervention requires a significant alteration of the surgical plan and, therefore, may significantly increase operative risk. In cases in which PFO detection occurs during off-pump coronary artery bypass, surgical intervention necessitates marked changes in the conduct of both the operation and circulatory management. The off-pump coronary artery bypass patient with a small PFO typically will remain untreated. In the absence of recognized consensus guidelines, the decision to proceed with definitive closure should be based on the following factors: history of neurologic event without a definite cause, recurrent stroke while receiving anticoagulation, significant shunting through the defect, previous episode of hypoxia that may be related to intracardiac shunting, right ventricular dysfunction, or previous paradoxical embolism.

Management of Previously Undiagnosed Aortic Valve Disease

Framing

A relatively common clinical scenario for the echocardiographer is to assess the significance of previously unrecognized AV pathology. This discussion has pertinence for the echocardiographer faced with the new diagnosis of a bicuspid valve, AS, or AR.

What are the symptoms that brought the patient to medical attention? What is the patient's baseline function? What is the anatomy of the AV? What is the severity of AR or AS? How do the intraoperative findings of AV disease differ from the preoperative assessment? Would surgical repair or replacement of the AV benefit the patient's short- or long-term outcome? What is the planned procedure, and how would the risks be changed if the procedure was altered to address the new finding? Does another healthcare provider need to be involved in the decision whether to surgically address the valve? Is the pathology of the AV significant enough to require surgical intervention at this time?

Data Collection and Characterization of the Aortic Valve

Multiplane TEE permits an accurate assessment of AV area, valvular pathology, severity of regurgitation and stenosis, and detection of secondary cardiac changes. In the case of AS, the severity of valvular dysfunction is determined by measuring the transvalvular pressure gradient, calculating the AV area using the continuity equation, and by planimetry of the AV systolic orifice. Planimetry of the AV orifice with TEE is more closely correlated with the catheterization-determined valve area (using the Gorlin formula) than the value derived from TTE ($r = 0.91$ vs. 0.84).[64] The severity of AR by TEE generally is graded with color-flow Doppler imaging with measurement of the width of the regurgitant jet relative to the width of the LVOT. TEE is sensitive to even the most trivial amount of AR. Jet areas measured by TEE tend to be larger, and their severity is graded as greater compared with AR assessed by TTE.[65] Determining the clinical significance of AR typically requires assessment of more than just regurgitant grade, although severe 4+ AR is never left unaddressed. A more challenging decision is

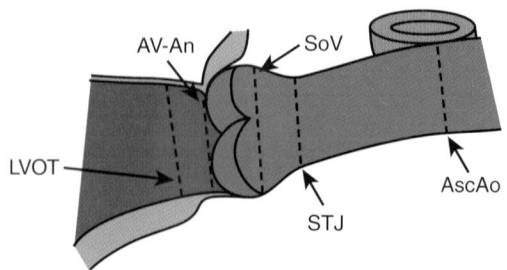

Figure 13-11   Anatomy of the aortic root. This schematic figure of the aortic valve in long axis shows the components of the aortic root, which include sinotubular junction (STJ), sinus of Valsalva (SoV), and the annulus of the aortic valve (AV-An). AscAo, ascending aorta; LVOT, left ventricular outflow tract.

whether to surgically address lesser degrees of AR in patients requiring cardiac surgery for another reason (see Chapters 3, 19, and 21).

The cause and extent of AV disease can be delineated best by TEE, as shown in Figure 13-11. The relatively high resolution of the AV and associated structures in the near field of the midesophageal short- and longitudinal-axis views permits an accurate assessment of the severity and mechanism of valvular disease. The aortic leaflets should be inspected in the midesophageal long-axis view for the presence of vegetations, perforation, restriction, thickening/calcification, malcoaptation, and leaflet prolapse. The presence of subvalvular disease, such as a discrete fibrous subaortic membrane, also can be reliably excluded. The ascending aorta from the valve to the right pulmonary artery also should be viewed in long axis. This view is usually optimal for examining associated pathology of the aortic root and ascending aorta (e.g., aortoannular ectasia, bicuspid valve, type A aortic dissection).

AS is caused by calcification of the AV and rheumatic heart disease. Bicuspid AVs are at greater risk compared with the general population. AS produces a systolic pressure gradient between the LV and aorta. Secondary findings are dependent on where the patient's condition is along the natural course of the disease. Secondary findings often contribute to the decision-making process because they infer the effects or consequences of the disease. AS is commonly associated with left ventricular hypertrophy and abnormal filling of the LV. The diastolic function is often impaired due to a thickened, noncompliant LV. Hence, MV and pulmonary vein blood flow velocities would demonstrate a blunted passive filling phase of the ventricle. Systolic function often is normal or hyperdynamic. The left ventricular chamber size is normal or small. However, longstanding AS results in progressive ventricular systolic dysfunction and heart failure. The LV becomes dilated with compromised contractile function. As the ventricle fails, CO decreases with a resultant decrease in trans-AV pressure gradient. Hence, the pressure gradient across an AV may be misleading as a measure for severity of AS.

Bicuspid Aortic Valve

A bicuspid AV is at increased risk for degeneration and calcification, leading to AR and calcific AS. Bicuspid AVs predispose for ascending aortic and arch aneurysm formation and are associated with increased incidences of aortic coarctation and ASD. The diagnosis of bicuspid AV prompts the echocardiographer to search for other commonly associated findings. The presence of isolated asymptomatic bicuspid AV without AS or AR does not mandate corrective surgery.

Bicuspid AVs are common in the general population, with an estimated incidence rate between 0.9% and 2.25%. The natural history of bicuspid valves is variable. Patients can go late into adulthood without AV or aortic disease. Bicuspid AVs can function without major hemodynamic abnormality well into the seventh decade of life.[66] In contrast, a significant percentage of patients experience progressive dilatation of the aortic root, producing AR, or premature calcification of the valve, producing AS.[67–71] For patients in their fourth decade of life, the predominant lesion at surgery is AR. With increasing age, the predominant lesion associated with bicuspid AVs becomes AS.[72] The architectural makeup of the wall of the aorta is abnormal in patients with a bicuspid AV, predisposing for aneurysm formation.[73–76] The decision-making process in regard to surgical correction of a bicuspid AV must account for the size of the aortic root and the likelihood the patient will return for aortic root surgery in the not-too-distant future. The rate of ascending aortic dilatation in patients with a bicuspid AV may be as high as 0.9 mm/year.[77] Even though patients with a bicuspid AV are at increased risk for cardiac surgery at a later time in life, surgical intervention is not recommended for a bicuspid AV in the absence of aortic root aneurysm, AS, or AR. A normally functioning bicuspid AV may have a longer duration than a bioprosthetic artificial valve. Some centers in North America have adopted a more aggressive stance toward repairing a mildly dilated ascending aorta (≥4-cm diameter) because of the increased risk for acute aortic dissection and ruptures.[78]

The majority of young patients with a bicuspid AV have a regurgitant lesion. If found as an incidental finding, valvular dysfunction is usually minimal and patients do not have a significantly increased risk for heart failure and death. Although AVR is associated with a low risk for mortality, the lifelong cumulative risk for valve replacement is not insignificant. Mechanical heart valves are associated with low but significant rates of valve thrombosis, thromboembolism, and hemorrhagic complications from lifelong anticoagulation. Biologic prosthetic valves are limited by degeneration of the bioprosthetic material. The use of a homograft or pulmonary autograft provides alternatives for patients who do not want to be or are at high risk for anticoagulation. Bicuspid AVs that can be rendered competent and nonstenotic may be "repaired" in the setting of surgery for aortic dissection or aneurysm. Reconstruction of an isolated, severely regurgitant bicuspid AV has been attempted and described[79–82] but is not in the mainstream of cardiac surgery in the United States because of the risk for recurrent AR. Surgical advances of AV repair have raised the hope of increased valve longevity that rivals or exceeds that of a biologic prosthesis (see Chapter 19).

Natural Course of Aortic Stenosis

The natural course of AS in the adult begins with a prolonged asymptomatic period associated with minimal mortality. Progression of the disease is manifested by a reduction in the valve area and an increase in the transvalvular systolic pressure gradient. The progression is quite variable, exhibiting a decrease in effective valve area ranging from approximately 0.1 to 0.3 cm²/year. AV calcification, as depicted by echocardiography, has been suggested to be an independent predictor of outcome. Patients with no or mild valvular calcification, compared with those with moderate or severe calcification, had significantly increased rates of event-free survival at 1 and 4 years (92% vs. 60% and 75% vs. 20%, respectively).[83] Decisions regarding valve replacement for mild or moderate AV disease in the setting of cardiac surgery for another cause are complicated by the variability in the natural progression of the disease. The pathogenesis of AS is an active process having many similarities to the progression of atherosclerosis.[84] AV calcification is not a random degenerative process but an actively regulated disease associated with hypercholesterolemia, inflammation, and osteoblast activity. More aggressive medical control of these processes might be expected to have a positive impact on outcome by retarding the degenerative process. Statin therapy has been proposed to slow the progression of disease.[85] The definitive evidence that such therapies attenuate the progress of AV stenosis remains unclear but should be forthcoming. If the progression of AV stenosis can be attenuated, the need for AVRs would decrease significantly (see Chapter 19).

Assessment of Mild and Moderate Aortic Stenosis

The intraoperative management of mild-to-moderate AS at the time of cardiac surgery remains controversial. A patient arrives in the operating room scheduled for a CABG but is discovered also to have mild or moderate AS that was unappreciated before surgery. The operative team must decide whether to surgically address the AV. The ACC/AHA Task Force recommends valve replacement at the time of coronary surgery if the asymptomatic patient has severe AS but acknowledges there are limited data to support intervention in the case of mild or moderate AS. It is in this exact scenario that the rate of progression of AS is of value, but it is rarely obtainable. A rapidly calcifying valve in a young patient that is becoming rapidly stenotic would sway the operative team to perform an AVR. A combined double cardiac procedure (CABG/AVR) increases the initial perioperative risk, as well as those risks associated with long-term prosthetic valve implantation. A delay in AVR and commitment to a second cardiac operation in the future subjects the patient to the risk for a redo sternotomy in the setting of patent coronary grafts and its associated morbidities. If the AV is not operated on during the initial presentation for CABG, the development of symptomatic AS may be quite delayed or may not happen.

A review of 1,344,100 patients in the national database of the Society of Thoracic Surgeons having CABG, CABG/AVR, or AVR alone culminated in a decision paradigm recommendation.[86] The study assumed rates of AV disease progression (pressure gradient of 5 mm Hg/yr), valve-related morbidity, and age-adjusted mortality rates that were obtained from published reports. The authors proposed three factors in the consideration of CABG or AVR/CABG: age (life expectancy), peak pressure gradient, and rate of progression of the AS (if known). Because the latter is difficult to discern, the analysis assumed an average rate of disease progression and recommended patients should undergo AVR/CABG when the pressure gradient exceeds 30 mm Hg. The threshold (AS pressure gradient) to perform both procedures is increased for patients older than 70 years because the reduced life expectancy diminishes the likelihood that they will become symptomatic from the AV disease. Whether to perform a concomitant AVR at the time of revascularization was also addressed by Rahimtoola,[87] who advocated a less aggressive approach. One problem with both studies is that they analyzed the transvalvular pressure gradient, which may be a misleading measure of the degree of stenosis of the AV because its value is dependent on CO. A low CO and flow rate will produce a low transvalvular pressure gradient, even in the setting of a severely stenotic AV. However, in the setting of preserved ventricular systolic function and mild or moderate AS, a pressure gradient is a useful metric. The variable rate of disease progression and the controversy regarding the indications for "prophylactic" AVR preclude a simple algorithm for dealing with this patient cohort. Increased age, lack of symptoms, minimal left ventricular hypertrophy, a valve area suggesting milder disease, and a pressure gradient less than 30 mm Hg would sway the decision not to replace the AV. In an asymptomatic young patient, a severely calcified valve, bicuspid valve, and left ventricular hypertrophy in the setting of moderate stenosis, as well as a pressure gradient greater than 30 mm Hg would suggest that an AVR might be beneficial in the long term. The considerations regarding the progression of AS and need for a subsequent, highly invasive redo surgery on older and presumably more ill patients must be reconsidered in the advent of the emerging technologies of the transcatheter AVR. Initial results seem promising; there is no evidence of early stenosis or prosthetic valve dysfunction. It often is useful to include the patient's primary cardiologist and family in the decision-making process.

Assessment of Low-Pressure Gradient Aortic Stenosis

Patients with left ventricular dysfunction and decreased CO in the setting of AS often present with only modest transvalvular pressure gradients(< 30 mm Hg). Distinguishing patients with a low CO and severe AS from patients with mild-to-moderate AS can be challenging (Figure 13-12). The standard for assessing severity of AS is AV area, typically calculated using either a continuity method or by planimetry. Patients with low-gradient AS with severe left ventricular dysfunction who received an AVR had improved survival and functional status compared with patients who did not have a valve replacement.[88–90]

A low-pressure gradient related to left ventricular dysfunction may not open the AV to its maximum capacity. Dobutamine challenge in a patient with low-pressure gradient AS can be useful in establishing true

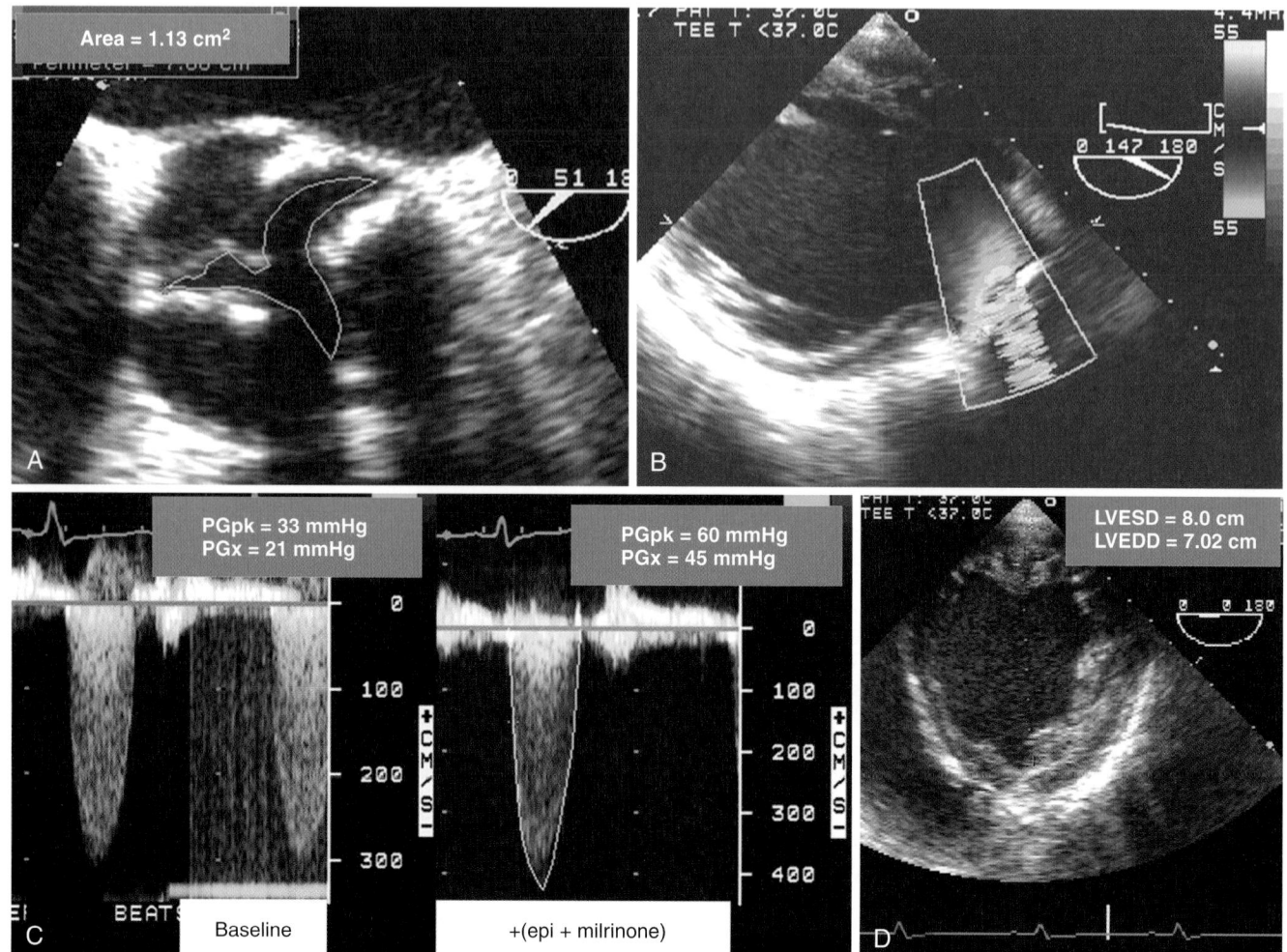

Figure 13-12   **Low-pressure gradient severe aortic stenosis.** A 76-year-old cachectic man was scheduled to undergo corrective surgery for severe mitral regurgitation (MR) and possibly clinically significant aortic stenosis (AS). The midesophageal short-axis view of the aortic valve (AV) showed a highly calcified trileaflet valve with restricted mobility (A). The measurement of AV area, 1.13 cm², which was obtained by planimetry, was believed to underestimate the severity of AS because of the shadowing artifacts related to the severity of calcification. The transgastric long axis of the left ventricle was obtained (B), and the velocity profiles of blood flow within the left ventricular (LV) outflow tract and the AV were measured. Although the patient had a diagnosis of severe AS, the maximal and mean pressure gradients were 33 and 21 mm Hg, respectively (C). The area of the AV was calculated to be 0.83 cm² using the continuity equation. The LV function was characterized by a severe dilated cardiomyopathy with an ejection fraction of 8%, LV end-systolic dimension (LVESD) of 7 cm, and LV end-diastolic dimension (LVEDD) of 8 cm (D). The diagnosis of low-pressure gradient AS was considered, and infusions of epinephrine and milrinone were started. Cardiac performance improved from 2.4 to 4.5 L/min, and the pressured gradients increased to 60 mm Hg, peak, and 41 mm Hg, mean (C). Although the calculated valve area that was recorded under conditions of inotrope support slightly increased to 0.9 cm², transesophageal echocardiography (TEE) clarified that the marked increase in the pressure gradient was consistent with a diagnosis of low-gradient AS and confirmed the presence of cardiac reserve.

AV area. The ability to distinguish between true AV stenosis and a state of "pseudostenosis" relies on characteristic changes in hemodynamic and structural measurements in response to the augmented CO. The test is not usually performed in the operative setting but rather as a preoperative evaluation. The increase in calculated AV area is related to the increase in the CO and is attributed to partial reversal of primary cardiac dysfunction.[91–94] If dobutamine improves CO and increases AV area, it is likely the baseline calculations overestimated the severity of the AS. The dobutamine challenge is conducted as follows: patients with low-gradient AS receive intravenous dobutamine at 5 μg/kg/min with stepwise increases in dose.[92] Patients may exhibit a significant increase in AV area (0.8 to 1.1 cm²) and a decline in valve resistance after dobutamine challenge. Patients with fixed, high-grade AS would demonstrate no change in valve area and an increase in valve resistance. The 2003 ACC/AHA/ASE Task Force gave a Class IIb recommendation (usefulness/efficacy is less well-established by evidence/opinion) for the use of dobutamine echocardiography in the evaluation of patients with low-gradient AS and ventricular dysfunction.[95] In addition to its

role in distinguishing between true stenosis and pseudostenosis, low-dose dobutamine echocardiography is helpful in risk-stratifying of patients with severe true AS. Patients with augmented contractile function after dobutamine administration have an improved outcome after surgery.[96,97]

Aortic Regurgitation: Natural Course and Management

Many elderly patients undergoing cardiac surgery will have some degree of AR. In most cases, the patients are asymptomatic and the severity is graded as trace to mild. The presence of AR has implications regarding the conduct of circulatory management, administration of cardioplegia, management of hemodynamics, and possible alteration of the surgical plan. The presence of AR obligates the echocardiographer to monitor for distention of the LV during CPB and cardiac arrest, as well as during the administration of antegrade cardioplegia. On release of the aortic cross-clamp, the heart may not instantaneously revert to an organized rhythm, precluding ejection of LV blood and predisposing for ventricular distention. The latter is particularly problematic in the setting of AR. The decision whether to surgically address the valvular dysfunction should not be based on left ventricular distention during CPB but considered in the context of the dataset that includes the natural history of AR in adults, established guidelines, and published outcomes, in addition to individual patient variables as previously described.

Chronic AR generally evolves in a slow and insidious manner with a very low morbidity during a long asymptomatic phase. Some patients with mild AR may remain asymptomatic for decades. Others exhibit progressive worsening of the regurgitant lesion and develop left ventricular systolic dysfunction, leading eventually to heart failure. Evaluation of left ventricular size and function is important because of the poor correlation between symptoms and severity of cardiac pathology. The nature of the transition between the compensated and uncompensated periods is poorly understood. Clinicians should be reluctant to consider valve replacement in an asymptomatic patient with preserved left ventricular function (Figure 13-13). Early surgery exposes the patient to perioperative mortality and morbidity, as well as to the long-term complications of a prosthetic valve. Guidelines for AV surgery in patients

with AR were published in 1998 by the ACC/AHA Task Force and in 2002 by the Working Group on Valvular Heart Disease of the European Society of Cardiology.[98,99] AVR is clearly indicated for symptomatic patients with chronic AR and left ventricular dysfunction. However, the decision to perform valve replacement is less apparent for asymptomatic patients. The published recommendations suggest serial examinations to detect the progression of left ventricular dysfunction. In a strategy similar to that applied for patients with low-gradient AS, the induction of stress exercise testing may be helpful for assessing functional capacity and timing of surgery. However, intraoperative detection of occult AR does not provide for the luxury of serial examinations.

The intraoperative decision for asymptomatic patients should be based on the severity of AR and the presence of left ventricular dysfunction. Patients with a left ventricular end-systolic dimension less than 50 mm would be expected to remain asymptomatic for the next few years; the risk for development of symptoms or left ventricular dysfunction would range from 1% to 2% per year to as high as 6% per year.[100,101] However, the yearly rate of becoming symptomatic or developing significant left ventricular dysfunction increases to greater than 20% when the left ventricular end-systolic dimension exceeds 50 mm.[100,102]

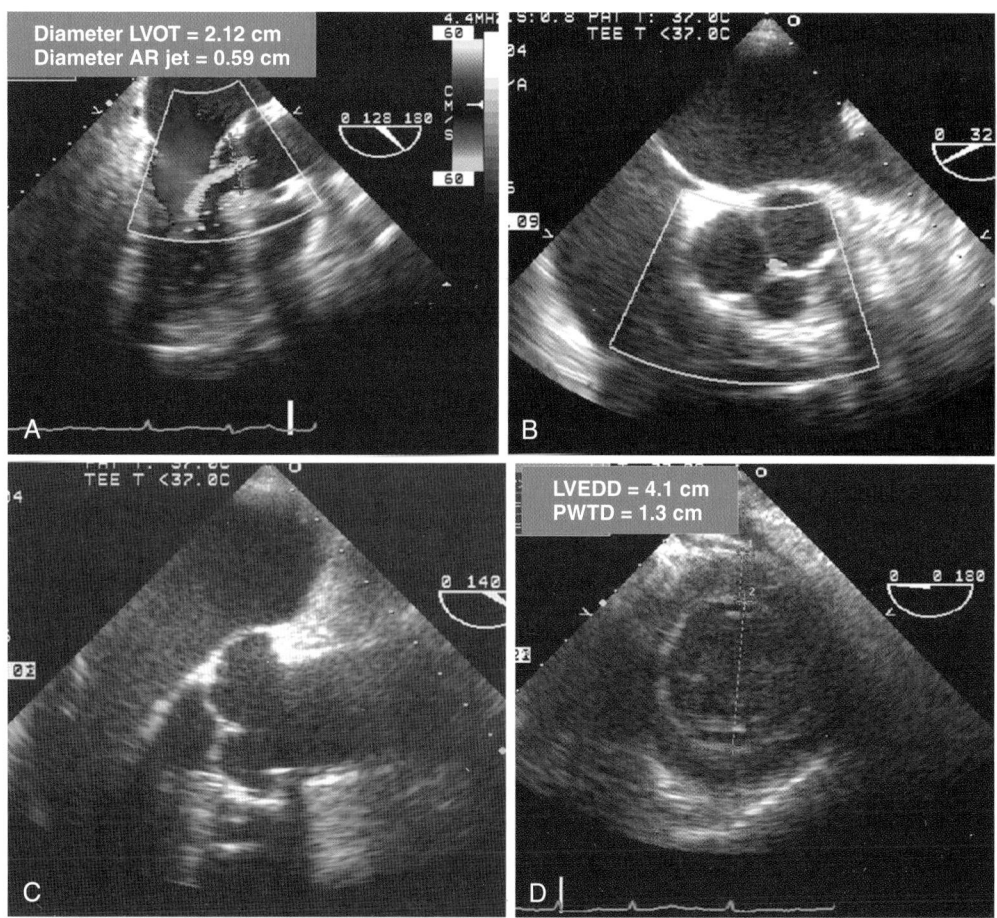

Figure 13-13 **Detection of occult aortic regurgitation (AR) during nonvalvular cardiac surgery.** A 66-year-old woman was scheduled to undergo coronary artery bypass grafting using extracorporeal circulatory support. An intraoperative transesophageal echocardiography (TEE) examination diagnosed presence of a central AR jet that extended halfway into the left ventricle (LV). The severity of AR, which was graded as mild, was based on assessing the retrograde flow in the LV outflow tract (LVOT) using color-flow Doppler imaging in midesophageal long-axis plane. The severity of AR is determined by comparing the width of the AR jet, 0.59 cm, with the diameter of the LVOT, 2.12 cm; the ratio of 0.28 is graded as mild (A). The anatomy of the valve was that of a normal trileaflet structure with mildly thickened leaflets (A, B). No leaflet prolapse, vegetations, or annular/root dilation was present. In addition, no significant aortic stenosis was detected by Doppler or calcification of the leaflets. LV chamber size was normal, LV end-diastolic dimension (LVEDD) was 4.14 cm, and presence of LV hypertrophy was consistent with hypertension (C). Because the severity of AR was not clinically significant and it was not expected to markedly increase, surgical intervention to the aortic valve was deferred. However, the diagnosis of AR altered circulatory management by increasing the vigilance of the echocardiographer to monitor LV chamber size during antegrade cardioplegia and initiating supplemental retrograde cardioplegia. PWTD, pulse-wave tissue Doppler.

■ Choice of Surgical Intervention

Framing

Once the decision to surgically intervene has been established, the echocardiographer can have a valuable role in assisting the surgeon in formulating and implementing the intended change of plans for surgical management.

What information would be required for the surgeon to determine whether surgical valve repair or valve replacement is more appropriate? Is the choice of surgical intervention limited by surgical experience or prosthesis availability? What type of valve prosthesis is most appropriate for this patient in these circumstances? What size of valve prosthesis can be inserted? Is pathology of the aortic root or ascending aorta present? Could valve replacement have unintended consequences that could be prevented or detected and treated? Does "pressure recovery" play an important role in estimating valve stenosis using a transvalvular gradient Doppler methodology?

Data Collection

The choice of specific intervention, whether to repair or to replace the valve, will depend on pathology of the diseased valve, experience of the surgical team, and discussion between the surgeon and the cardiologist, in addition to patient variables. The echocardiographer can best contribute to the surgeon's understanding of the pathogenesis of AV disease by assessing function and structure in the short- and long-axis imaging planes. The surgeon is provided with a complete anatomic echocardiographic assessment of the AV and root, including dimensions of the annulus, sinus of Valsalva and sinotubular junction, leaflet anatomy, primary mechanism of regurgitation, and severity of thickening/calcification.

Discussion

The development of reparative procedures for the AV has lagged behind those implemented for the MV or for the development of prosthetic devices. Some of the major factors are the apparently irreversible changes produced by calcification of the cusps, the retraction of cusp tissue in AR, and the lack of durable biologic material suitable for supplementing the valvular apparatus. It is unlikely that surgical repair of stenotic and highly calcified valves will achieve much success within the near future. However, aortic valvular repair has been successfully applied for the resuspension of the AV to correct acute AR resulting from an aortic dissection. Yacoub, Cohn, and others reported improved short- and long-term results for minimizing residual AR and freedom from reoperation.[103-105]

A diseased valve characterized by thickened, calcified leaflets and having restricted mobility is not a candidate for valve repair and would require valve replacement. Alternatively, remodeling of the aortic root and AV to improve the geometry of the tricuspid AV has been used successfully in cases of acute type A aortic dissection. In addition, a select cohort of patients having AR as the primary valvular diagnosis may be candidates for surgical repair. In the case of bicuspid AVs or isolated AR, successful repair of the AV was more likely when the anatomy demonstrated left coronary/right coronary cusp fusion and when the primary mechanism of AR was leaflet prolapse or commissural separation, compared with poor leaflet coaptation of a "central defect."[103] Although a complete review of the technical aspects and controversy of AV-sparing surgeries are beyond the scope of this chapter, it should be noted that aortic dilatation has a negative prognostic implication for successful long-term outcome. A more detailed discussion of surgical repair of the AV can be found in Chapter 19 and in literature reviews.[104,105]

Valve repair and replacement surgery for patients having symptomatic valve disease have been heralded as significant successes. Advances in surgical technique and perioperative care have enabled the morbidity and mortality of valve replacement to decrease despite the increasing proportion of high-risk patients. The choice of prosthetic heart valve replacement generally is based on patient age, size, and wishes[106] (Figure 13-14). A joint decision with the patient, the cardiologist, and the cardiac surgeon is indicated before surgery.

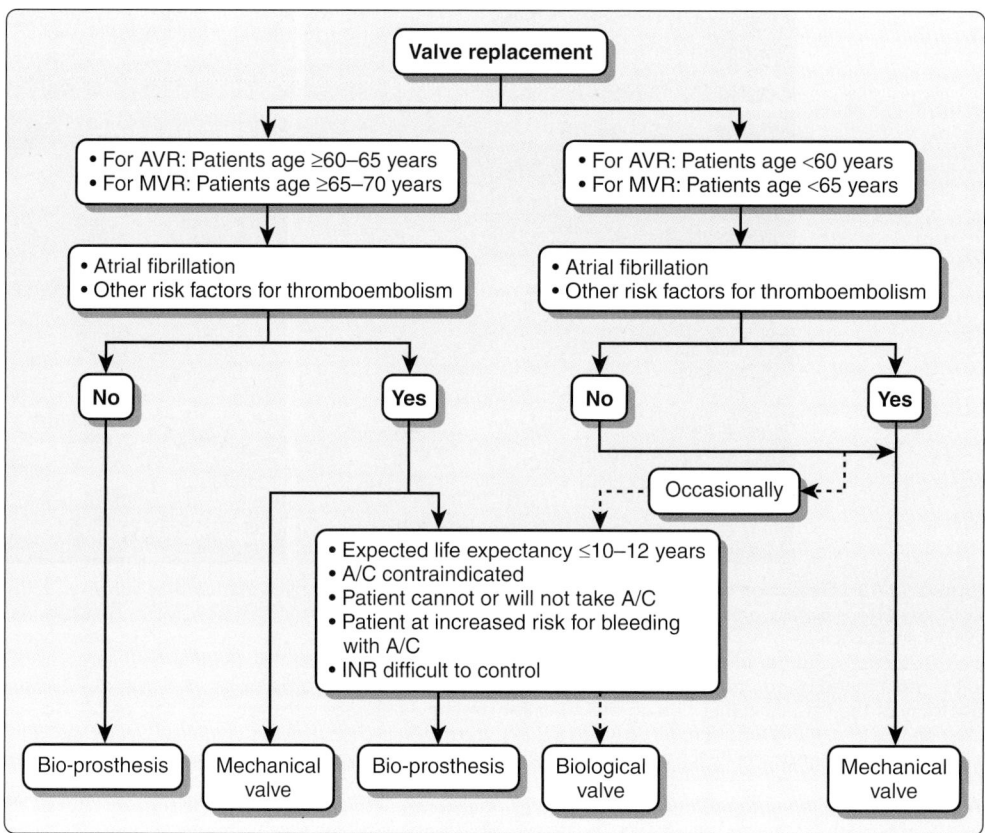

Figure 13-14 Algorithm for choice of prosthetic heart valve. A/C, anticoagulation; AVR, aortic valve replacement; INR, international normalized ratio; MVR, mitral valve replacement. *(Redrawn from Rahimtoola SH: Choice of prosthetic heart valve for adult patients. J Am Coll Cardiol 41:893, 2003, Figure 8.)*

Compared with nature's own heart valves, prosthetic valves are relatively stenotic. Prosthetic valves are sized based on their external diameter, even though their transvalvular gradient reflects the internal diameter and orifice size. Each valve has an "effective orifice area" (EOA) that is based on in vitro studies performed by the manufacturer. The clinical importance of the disparity between prosthesis annular size and EOA becomes evident when relatively small prosthetic valves are inserted into comparatively large patients. Prosthetic valve/patient mismatch results when transvalvular flow through a prosthetic valve is limited and produces clinically significant stenosis (Figure 13-15). The increase in transvalvular blood-flow velocity necessary to accommodate and sustain an acceptable SV in a large patient with a prosthetic AV can produce surprisingly high transvalvular pressure gradients.

An objective of valve replacement surgery is to provide the patient with the largest EOA. Prosthetic valve mismatch is more likely to occur in older patients, those with increased body surface area (BSA), smaller prosthetic valve size, and preoperative diagnosis of valvular stenosis.[107] The incidence of AV mismatch increases with prosthetic annular size less than 21 mm. In larger patients, mismatch can occur in patients receiving prosthetic AVs greater than 21 mm because dominant factors in determining the pressure gradient are the SV and CO, which are related to body size and level of activity. The association of mismatch with stenotic native AVs is a result of calcified native valves, a calcified annulus, and a smaller annular size. The treatment of AS through AVR in the setting of preserved ventricular systolic function may result in dramatic increases in SV and CO. The resultant increase in

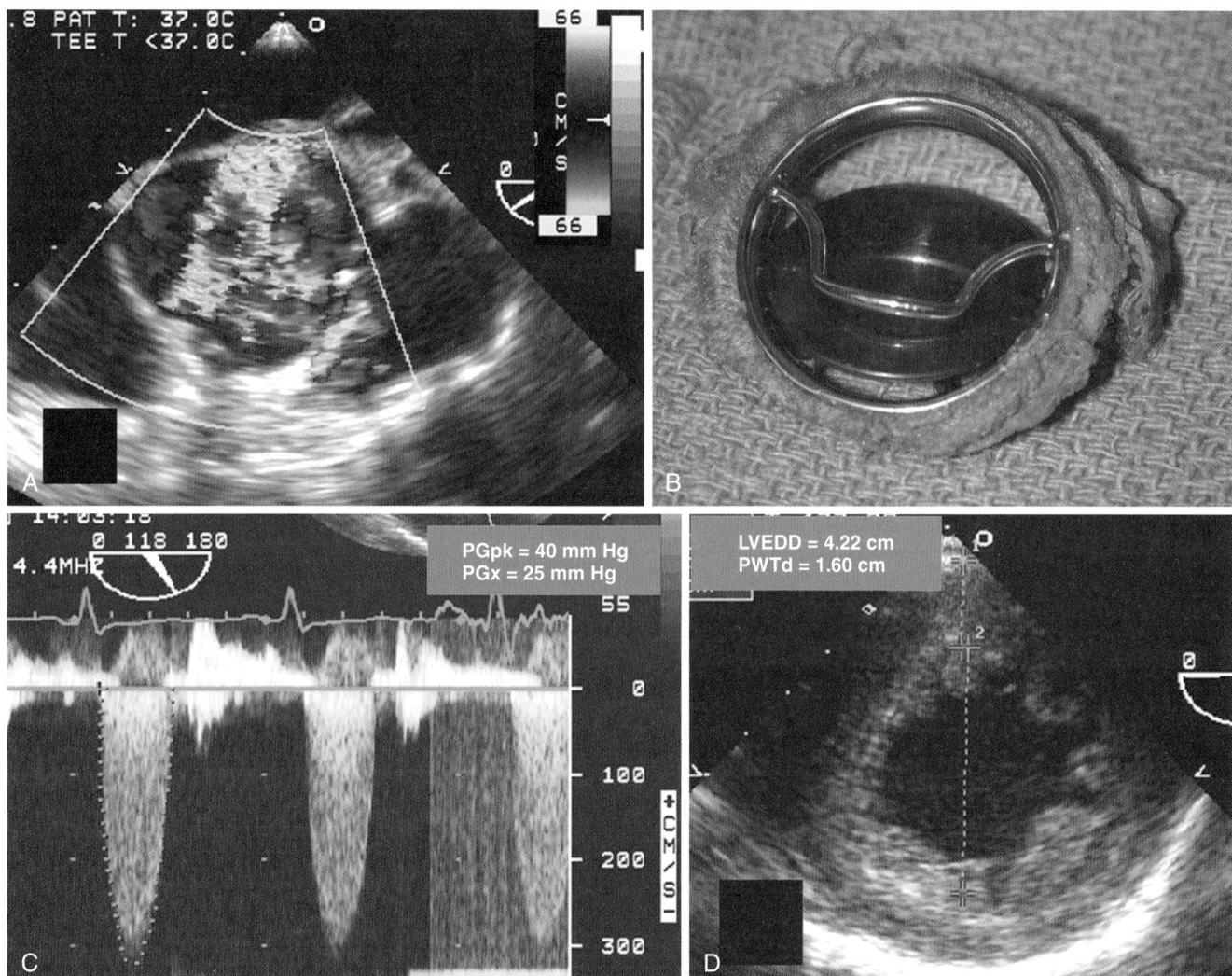

Figure 13-15 **Detection of a significant transvalvular pressure gradient across a previously implanted prosthetic aortic valve (AV).** Patient who underwent a previous AV replacement (AVR) was now scheduled for coronary artery bypass grafting and possible AVR for aortic stenosis. The preoperative evaluation included an echocardiogram that demonstrated a small paravalvular leak and blood cultures that were negative. *A,* Color-flow Doppler image of the AV in midesophageal short-axis imaging plane that shows turbid flow from the orifice of the 19-mm Bjork–Shiley mechanical valve. The aortic annulus and other valves were inspected for evidence of active infection or abscess, but none was found. The clinical decision was to replace the AV or repair the paravalvular leak. The prosthetic valve appeared to be functioning normally aside from a small paravalvular leak. The intraoperative transesophageal echocardiographic (TEE) examination documented preserved left ventricular (LV) systolic function and significant LV hypertrophy with a posterior wall thickness of 1.6 cm. Examination of the mechanical prosthetic valve showed a well-seated valve with a small paravalvular leak at the fibromuscular continuity and the absence of any abscess or vegetations *(B).* Although the valve appeared to be functioning normally, the transvalvular pressure gradient was 40 mm Hg in the absence of any outflow tract obstruction *(C, D).* The presence of a significant gradient in a normally functioning valve and presence of significant LV hypertrophy raised the possibility of valve mismatch; the small paravalvular leak was determined not to significantly contribute to the transvalvular gradient. The patient was an active 64-year-old man who weighed 98 kg and had a body surface area of 2.2 mm². The presence of a significant transvalvular gradient across an apparently normally functioning valve in a large patient supported the diagnosis of prosthetic valve mismatch. The patient underwent a root replacement (No. 23) and had a transvalvular pressure gradient of 14 mm Hg. LVEDD, LV end-diastolic dimension; PWTD, pulse-wave tissue Doppler.

transvalvular flow produces a large transprosthetic pressure gradient. In contrast, valvular insufficiency is usually associated with annular dilatation and decreased systolic function. Hence patients with annuloectasia often receive larger prosthetic valves, and functional AS after AVR rarely is a problem.

Increased postoperative transvalvular gradients have been implicated in increasing long-term morbidity and mortality.[108–110] The short-term clinical significance of prosthetic valve size mismatch is controversial and may be associated with immediate postoperative risk for cardiovascular complications and mortality. Controversy stems, in part, from studies with limited sample populations and the failure to normalize specific valvular EOA to a metric of patient size. Nonetheless, the concept of prosthetic valve mismatch adversely affecting outcome is generally accepted. The long-term risk for prosthetic valve mismatch is inability to restore or improve functional capacity. A consequence of an increased residual transvalvular pressure gradient is to prevent or attenuate regression of left ventricular hypertrophy.[111] Left ventricular hypertrophy is associated with diastolic dysfunction, decreased exercise capacity, and is a predictor of increased mortality. Significant differences in regression of left ventricular hypertrophy occur in patients who received prosthetic AVs larger than 21 mm (−21%) compared with patients with prosthetic valves that were less than 21 mm (−8%).[111,112] Hence it would be expected that a corresponding difference in functional capacity would parallel these differences in hypertrophy regression. A decreased indexed EOA (EOA/BSA = cm^2/m^2) was an independent predictor of long-term morbidity after aortic and MV replacement.[113]

In general, an indexed EOA for a prosthetic AV should be greater than 0.85 cm^2/m^2.[113] For a similar external rim size, the EOA can vary considerably between mechanical and bioprosthetic AVs and by manufacturer. Bioprosthetic valves tend to have a significantly larger EOA compared with mechanical valves. Biologic aortic roots have even larger EOAs. If the anatomy of the aortic root precludes implantation of a suitably sized prosthesis, the surgeon may perform a supra-annular implantation, allowing the placement of a larger valve. Alternatively, creation of a larger EOA may require enlargement of the aortic root, a biologic aortic root, a pulmonic valve autograft (Ross procedure), or implantation of a stentless valve (see Chapters 19 and 21).

Aortic Valve: Concomitant Mitral Regurgitation

Framing

Valvular diseases do not often occur in isolation. Other anatomic structures may be influenced, either by the same pathophysiology or as a secondary consequence of the primary valvular lesion. Mitral insufficiency is a common finding, occurring in about two thirds of the patients having significant AS.[114] Patients presenting for AVR commonly have mitral regurgitation and pose the question of whether to repair or replace the MV in addition to the AV (Figure 13-16). Such an undertaking is not without risk. Patients undergoing double-valve replacement have increased mortality compared with isolated AVR.

Should moderate mitral regurgitation be surgically addressed in patients undergoing AVR for AS? Does the severity of mitral regurgitation regress after AVR? Does the presence of AR in patients with severe AS alter the expected prognosis of the regression of mitral regurgitation after AVR? Can it be predicted which cohort of patients with AS would benefit from concomitant MV repair? In which patient cohort would the mitral regurgitation be expected to regress with the unloading effects of replacing a stenotic AV?

Data Collection

The most important data for these decisions are the grade of mitral regurgitation, AV area, anatomy of the MV, and cause of mitral regurgitation (i.e., rheumatic disease, ischemic, myxomatous degeneration). Patients are likely to have the signs and symptoms of AS and mitral regurgitation and pulmonary hypertension. The grade of mitral

regurgitation is often not evident until a TEE is performed and may be underestimated by a preoperative transthoracic examination. An enlarged LA suggests the mitral regurgitation is not acute.

Discussion

Mitral regurgitation is a maladaptive consequence of increasing AS. More significant mitral regurgitation is associated with greater trans-AV pressure gradients, as well as more progressive dilatation and worsening systolic function.[115,116] If MV anatomy is markedly abnormal and the severity of regurgitation is severe, the decision is relatively obvious: MV repair or replacement at the time of AVR. If the MV is anatomically normal (no leaflet prolapse, no perforation, no rheumatic changes) and the regurgitation is trace or mild, the decision is also relatively obvious: Correct the AS and do not surgically address the MV. In the setting of rheumatic AS, it is common to have other valves involved in the disease process. Hence mitral calcification, thickening, and leaflet fusion are common in patients with rheumatic AS. The MV is rarely replaced based on anatomic abnormality alone in the absence of significant stenosis or regurgitation.

The more controversial decision is whether to surgically address the MV that has mild-to-moderate regurgitation when a patient presents for AVR for AS. There is neither an absolute answer nor consensus. The uncertainty of the decision is based on the unpredictability of the residual mitral regurgitation after the AV is replaced. If the grade of mitral regurgitation of moderate or severe were expected to be reduced to mild, the operative team might elect not to operate on the MV. A confounding factor is the grade of mitral regurgitation during general anesthesia may be underestimated and not reflect the grade during the awake or exercising state. Furthermore, the lasting effects of replacing an AV in the setting of mitral regurgitation are not established immediately after CPB. The heart undergoes significant changes after AVR for AS, including changes in pressure-volume relations of the LV, transmitral pressure gradients, and left ventricular remodeling.

Mitral regurgitation with an anatomically normal MV is referred to as "functional mitral regurgitation." Increased left ventricular afterload, driving pressure, and left ventricular remodeling have been implicated in the development of functional mitral regurgitation in patients with severe AS. The natural history and clinical impact of mild-to-moderate mitral regurgitation in patients undergoing AVR for AS suggest that concurrent MV surgery may not be warranted in all cases. In the cohort of patients with functional mitral regurgitation and severe AS, the decrease in mitral regurgitation after AVR alone was variable; between 39% and 90% of patients having moderate mitral regurgitation experienced a regression in its severity after AVR.[117–122] In general, patients with functional mitral regurgitation of moderate grade had significant improvement (decrease) in the mitral regurgitation after AVR, suggesting that leaving the MV alone in this setting is not unreasonable. Conversely, a significant number of patients, between 8% and 64%, had either no change or an increase in mitral regurgitation severity. In a study of 196 patients who had concomitant mitral regurgitation, Moazami et al[121] noted a decrease in 3-year survival for those patients whose moderate-to-severe mitral regurgitation persisted after AVR and recommended surgical intervention for this cohort of patients.

In general, functional mitral regurgitation of moderate severity usually will regress at least one grade after AVR for severe AS (see Figure 13-16). Mild-to-moderate mitral regurgitation that improves after AVR for AS seems to be a lasting phenomenon.[117] Unfortunately, there has been little control for the severity of concurrent AR, which is a common finding associated with AS. Although the physiologic load of patients with combined AS and AR is different, the particular pathology of the AV did not affect regression of mitral regurgitation after AVR.[121] Harris et al[120] ascribed the decrease in the severity of mitral regurgitation after AVR to several anatomic changes: decreases in mitral annular area, left atrial size, and left ventricular length. Together with the decrease in driving pressure that occurs with resolution of AS, all three of these anatomic changes alter the architecture of the MV and ventricle and contribute to decreasing functional mitral regurgitation. The greater

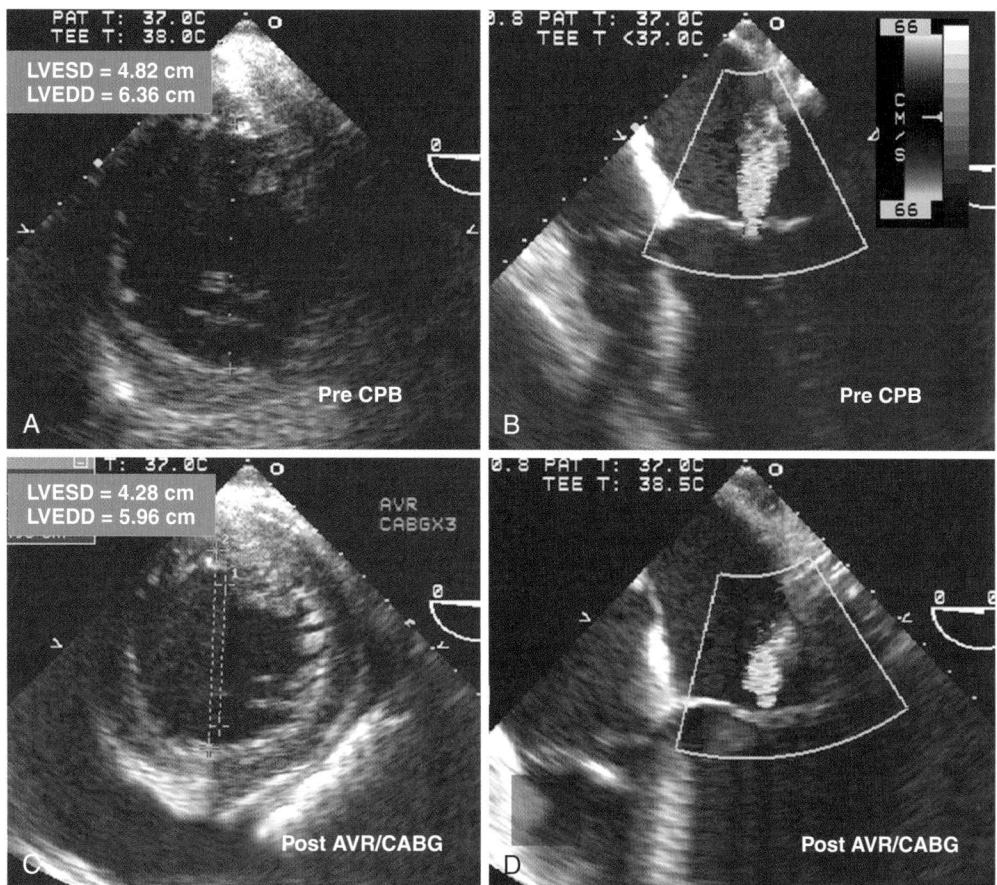

Figure 13-16 **Management of concurrent mitral regurgitation (MR) in a patient undergoing aortic valve replacement (AVR) for aortic stenosis (AS).** The patient is a 70-year-old who underwent an AVR for critical AS. The patient had history of hypertension, moderate MR, congestive failure, and episodes of shortness of breath. Left ventricular (LV) function was moderately depressed and the chamber size was dilated (LV end-diastolic dimension [LVEDD] = 6.36 cm) (A). B, The patient had a central jet of MR that was graded as mild; the annulus was mildly dilated, and the pathology of the leaflets and apparatus was only mildly thickened. The pulmonary vein blood flow showed minimal blunting of the systolic component, consistent with increased left atrial pressures but not clinically significant MR. The discrepancy in the severity of MR between the preoperative study and intraoperative transesophageal echocardiogram (TEE) reflects the effect of general anesthesia on loading conditions. After reviewing the prebypass TEE examination and the patient's history, it was decided to perform only an AVR. A bioprosthetic valve was chosen by the surgeon because of the patient's age, thus eliminating the requirement for anticoagulation. Because the MR was believed to be more functional, the replacement of the severely stenotic AV, the major pathologic lesion, was anticipated to decrease MR over time. The choice of implanting a No. 23 pericardial prosthetic valve was based on the annular size that was measured before initiation of bypass. The postbypass TEE examination documented that the gradient across the AV decreased from 74 to 18 mm Hg and cardiac function (C) and MR (D) improved after AVR. CABG, coronary artery bypass grafting; CPB, cardiopulmonary bypass.

the decrease in systolic area and increase in FAC of the LV after AVR, the greater is the reduction in postoperative mitral regurgitation.[120]

It is difficult to define the negative predictors for the regression of mitral regurgitation after AVR. The presence of valvular abnormalities, such as rheumatic leaflet thickening, calcification or prolapse (i.e., myxomatous degeneration), and chordal pathology that could contribute to a "nonfunctional" cause of mitral regurgitation would most likely persist. Mitral annular calcification is a potential complicating factor and its impact is unclear. Annular calcification would be expected to impede the reduction in MV area that normally occurs during systole. This reduction appears to be important in the mechanism of mitral regurgitation reduction after AVR for AS. Likewise, mitral annular calcification renders mitral surgery more difficult and the implantation of a mitral prosthesis more problematic, likely increasing the risk for paravalvular leak and AV groove disruption. Many patients with severe AS have a calcified AV with concomitant MV annular calcification. Mitral annular calcifications may be predictive of fixed mitral regurgitation after AVR.[123] An enlarged left atrium (>5 m) has been reported to be a significant predictor of persistent mitral regurgitation after AVR.[124] Other factors to consider include presence of CHF, CAD, pulmonary hypertension, and atrial fibrillation. Ischemic mitral regurgitation may improve after revascularization as a more favorable balance of myocardial oxygen supply/demand is produced after AVR.[118] "Functional" mitral regurgitation of moderate-to-severe grade that is not operated on during AVR may remain unchanged after AVR and require reinstitution of CPB for MV surgery. In the absence of more predictable criteria to define this group, patients with moderate-to-severe mitral regurgitation caused by intrinsic valvular pathology should be considered for surgical intervention. Reports suggest that AVR combined with MV repair can be accomplished with excellent long-term results and minimal effect on mortality.[118]

Ascending Aorta, a Source of Embolization

Framing

The most disabling complication after cardiac surgery is stroke. Major focal and nonfocal neurologic deficits, cognitive decline, and coma after surgery are common. The pathogenesis of cerebral damage is multifactorial, with embolism considered a major contributor. Other factors include hypotension, low flow, reperfusion injury, and inflammation.

Embolic events are strongly associated with the severity of atherosclerotic disease, characterized by plaque thickness of greater than 4 mm, ulcerated plaques, and mobile protruding plaques in the aorta.[125,126] The severity of atherosclerosis of the descending aorta, as determined by TEE, is a significant risk factor and an independent predictor of adverse cardiac and neurologic outcome in patients undergoing CABG.[127] Surgical manipulation of the thoracic aorta may liberate debris from diseased aortic tissue. The process of microembolization has been detected by transcranial Doppler during aortic cannulation, application and removal of the aortic cross-clamp, commencement of CPB, and initiation of ventricular ejection. The clinical consequence of distal embolization is dependent on the number, composition (e.g., air bubbles, fat particles, platelet aggregates, and calcium deposits), size, and location of the emboli (see Chapters 12, 16, 18, 19, 21, 28, and 36).

Is the patient at increased risk for postoperative neurologic dysfunction? Would epiaortic ultrasound or TEE improve detection of significant atheromatous disease? What modifications to the conduct of the general anesthesia, monitoring, CPB, or cardiac surgery could be implemented in a risk-reduction effort? Is epiaortic scanning necessary?

Data Collection

TEE imaging of the anterior wall of the ascending aorta is limited by far-field imaging resolution and its juxtaposition to air in the open chest. Imaging of the mid and distal ascending aorta by TEE is limited by the interposition of the airway with the esophagus and aorta. Epiaortic ultrasound can provide high-definition imaging of these otherwise hidden portions of the aorta. Epiaortic scanning offers higher sensitivity for detection of atheroma of the ascending aorta, as compared with TEE, especially in the mid and distal segments.[3,128] The descending aorta is immediately adjacent to the esophagus and easily imaged using conventional TEE. A common practice is the interrogation of the descending thoracic aorta for high-grade atheroma. In the absence of atheromatous disease in the descending aorta, the ascending aorta and locus of aortic cannulation are significantly less likely to have high-grade disease. If the descending aorta contains high-grade or mobile atheroma, it may be prudent to examine the ascending aorta with epiaortic scanning for potential sites for aortic cannulation and clamping (Figure 13-17).

Discussion

Historically, surgeons palpate the ascending aorta to determine the extent of intraluminal atherosclerotic disease in an effort to choose an appropriate location for cannulation, cross-clamping, and proximal graft anastomosis. However, palpation is a notoriously poor predictor of atheromatous disease.[129-131] The occurrence of atheroma in the ascending aorta of cardiac surgery patients may be as high as 60% to 90%.[130,132] Advanced age, hypertension, and diabetes are risk factors for atheromatous disease of the aorta and stroke after cardiac surgery.[3,133] The information provided by ultrasound imaging of the aorta defines the location and severity of atheromatous disease, which can guide the surgeon to more strategically choose the cannulation, cross-clamp, and anastomotic sites.

Possible modifications to the conduct of cardiac surgery and CPB include (1) altering the site of cannulation, (2) aborting CPB altogether and performing the CABG surgery as an off-bypass procedure, (3) performing the surgery on a fibrillating heart without aortic cross-clamping, (4) performing aortic atherectomy or replacement of the ascending aorta, or (5) attempting a "no-touch" technique using deep hypothermic circulatory arrest. Epiaortic scanning combined with modification of surgery techniques in patients undergoing CABG decreased the number of emboli as detected by transcranial Doppler and significantly reduced neurologic behavioral changes at 1 week and 1 month after surgery.[134] Modifications in the methods used in CABG revascularization, including the avoidance of proximal aortic graft anastomoses after detection of atheroma by echocardiography, resulted in a lower incidence of late neurologic complications.[2]

The application of epiaortic scanning for all patients undergoing cardiac surgery is controversial. Epiaortic scanning takes time and expertise

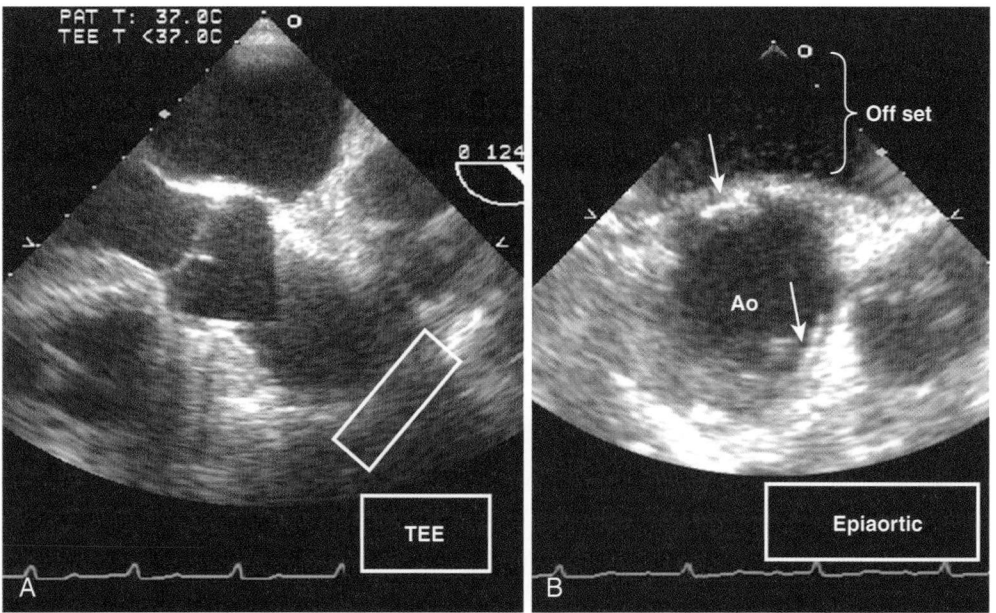

Figure 13-17 **Detection of atheromatous plaque by epiaortic ultrasound.** A 67-year-old patient was scheduled to undergo coronary artery bypass grafting × 3. The transesophageal echocardiographic (TEE) examination was performed to evaluate the mitral valve for mitral regurgitation that might necessitate surgical intervention. Routine examination of the descending thoracic aorta detected severe atherosclerotic disease characterized by several ulcerated areas and plaques with a thickness of 4 mm. Because the severity of atherosclerotic disease in the descending aorta predicts significant disease in the ascending aorta,[127] examination of the ascending aorta was attempted. TEE examination of the ascending aorta at the site of aortic cross-clamp and cannulation *(white rectangle)* was limited by resolution in the far field and interposition of the trachea *(A)*. A handheld probe that was placed in a sterile sleeve was used to examine the aorta *(B)*. The bottom of the sleeve was filled with saline as an offset to better image the anterior surface of the aorta (Ao). Several calcified plaques *(arrows)* were detected. Based on findings of the epiaortic scanning, the surgeon modified the site of cannulation and used a single cross-clamp technique to avoid a second clamping of the aorta during the proximal anastomosis.

in its interpretation and poses the potential risk for wound contamination. There are insufficient data to support its use in all cardiac patients, although high-risk patients (advanced age, diabetes, hypertension) are the most likely to benefit.[135,136] As the profile of patients undergoing cardiac surgery ages, they have a greater incidence of atherosclerosis of the aorta and the presence of concomitant risk factors for postoperative complications. Echocardiographers working in the operating room need the skill set to interrogate the aorta by handheld ultrasound and the ability to guide the surgeon in performing the examination. It could be potentially life-saving in high-risk patients. A diagnostic scan of the ascending aorta and arch to evaluate the location of possible cannulation and clamp sites can be performed in several minutes. Standardized approaches to a comprehensive organized intraoperative epiaortic and epicardial examination are useful guides.[137]

Intracardiac Clot, Calcium, and Air

Framing

The incidence of postoperative neurologic dysfunction is greater in patients undergoing open cardiac procedures. The sources of microemboli include atheroma, calcified debris, tissue, and entrapped air. The particulate matter can embolize to the coronary circulation (see Figure 13-5), causing acute right ventricular or left ventricular dysfunction; to the cerebral circulation, producing postoperative neurologic deficits; and/or to distal vital organs.[138–140]

Which patients are at risk for embolization from an intracardiac or aortic source? What are the echocardiographic characteristics that define this high-risk population? What techniques can be applied to detect intracardiac or aortic sources of emboli? Are any anesthetic or surgical interventions useful in decreasing the risk for embolic stroke during cardiac surgery?

Data Collection

TEE data collection is focused on intracardiac air, thrombus, calcium, or other particulate matter that is at high risk for embolization (e.g., endocarditis). Cardiac ultrasound is highly sensitive in the detection of intracardiac air. The American Society of Anesthesiologists/Society of Cardiovascular Anesthesiologists Task Force suggested the detection of air emboli during cardiotomy, heart transplant operations, and upright neurosurgical procedures to be classified as IIa indication for perioperative TEE. Classification IIa suggests a condition in which the existing evidence/opinion was in favor of the application of the technology. Entrapped air appears as bright, highly reflective particles that produce a shadowing artifact when the air coalesces. When performing de-airing maneuvers before release of the aortic cross-clamp and separation from CPB, the patients are placed in Trendelenburg position. In addition, an ascending aortic vent can be placed to aspirate the debris/air that was not removed by the left ventricular vent.

Discussion

The surgical team can perform several maneuvers to reduce sources of embolization that originate with open-chamber cardiac procedures. Placement of a drainage cannula in the LV via the right superior pulmonary vein can aspirate much of the debris that is suspended in solution. A small vent cannula in the anterior portion of the proximal ascending aorta often is inserted to aspirate gas bubbles or debris as they are ejected by left ventricular contraction. The heart is agitated by the surgeon in an attempt to eject the left ventricular debris or air while the "protective" aortic root vent continues to aspirate. The agitation often results in the release of pockets of air that may reside at the left atrial appendage, interatrial septum, and apex of the LV or are entrapped in the chordal structures or ventricular muscles of the heart. There is no consensus regarding when to terminate the de-airing process and separate from CPB. Not until some degree of pulmonary blood flow is restored is it possible to eliminate most of the retained intracardiac air. The aortic root vent often is left on continual aspiration even after CPB, with judicious volume replenishment through other sources.

The aortic root vent should be discontinued before the administration of protamine. Although there is a paucity of evidence to support improved outcome, TEE is commonly used in the detection of retained air and the monitoring of the de-airing procedures. The effectiveness of de-airing can be tracked qualitatively. The relation between degree of "echo contrast" and actual quantity of air is unknown.

Aortic Pathology and Transesophageal Echocardiography

Framing

The utility of TEE has expanded beyond simply examining cardiac performance and pathology. TEE is well suited as a quick, highly sensitive, and specific tool to detect the presence of aortic pathology and some of its life-threatening sequelae. The detection and differentiation of true aneurysms and pseudoaneurysms, aortic dissections and transections, intraluminal atherosclerotic disease, and abnormalities of the aortic root are often the challenge of the intraoperative team (see Chapter 21).

What are the limitations of TEE for evaluation of the thoracic aorta? Is TEE the most appropriate diagnostic test to evaluate aortic pathology in the elective and emergency patient? Does the acuity of the patient preclude other imaging modalities, such as magnetic resonance imaging (MRI) or computed tomographic (CT) scanning? What are the quantitative measures that impact surgical management of aortic dissection, aortic aneurysms, aortic root disease, and aortic transection? What information can the echocardiographer provide the surgeon to assist in formulating a management strategy? What degree of aortic dilatation is sufficient to necessitate replacement? What is the risk of not replacing an aneurysmal aorta?

Data Collection

Data acquired in the assessment of the patient with aortic disease include a targeted history for evidence of malperfusion or vital organ injury (e.g., stroke) and examination of blood pressure and pulse in each of the extremities, carotid arteries, and abdominal aorta. A history of chest or back pain is common with aortic dissection or aneurysm, with tearing of the aorta and its adventitia. Increasing shortness of breath may occur with AR, heart failure, or a left pleural effusion. Patients may present with hoarseness related to recurrent laryngeal nerve damage causing vocal cord dysfunction. The preoperative blood work may detect renal insufficiency with an increased blood creatinine concentration. The chest radiograph often shows a widened mediastinum or calcification of the thoracic aorta. The TEE data are aimed at dimensional and anatomic assessment of the aortic root, ascending arch, and descending aorta. The echocardiographer measures and reports the size of the aortic annulus, sinus of Valsalva, sinotubular junction, and ascending aorta (see Figure 13-11). Left ventricular hypertrophy may suggest long-lasting hypertension. A dilated LV may accompany chronic AR. Dilatation of the aortic root is common in the setting of AS and AR. Patients with a congenital predisposition for aortic aneurysm, such as Marfan syndrome or bicuspid AV, often develop a dilated and aneurysmal ascending aorta. Epiaortic scanning increases the sensitivity of detecting abnormalities of the ascending aorta because it is in the far field from a TEE window and may be hidden by the interposition of the trachea and left mainstem bronchus, which obstruct the distal half of the ascending aorta.[128]

Discussion

The echocardiographer may determine the definitive diagnosis and the extent of the disease. The information contributes to the decision of surgical management.

Aneurysm rupture occurred at a stunningly high frequency of 32% to 68% in patients with thoracic aortic aneurysms managed by conservative medical treatment and accounted for 32% to 47% of deaths. The one-, three-, and five-year survival of unoperated thoracic aneurysms was 65%, 36%, and 20%, respectively.[141–143] The risk for aortic rupture is a function of the size and rate of growth of the aneurysm. The risk for rupture for aneurysms less than 40, 40 to 59, and greater than 60 mm was 0%, 16%, and 31%, respectively.[144] The diameter of aneurysms tends to grow at a rate of approximately 5 mm/year. However, the rate of aneurysm expansion is variable. In general, the change in diameter of thoracic aortic aneurysms is a function of the initial diameter and increases more quickly in larger aneurysms.

Surgical intervention is a consideration for patients with an aneurysm of the aorta that is greater than 5 cm, accelerated rate of growth of the aneurysm, or the patient has a collagen vascular disease, such as Marfan syndrome. The incidence and progression of disease in the ascending aorta and arch after previous sternotomy have not been reported. The scarring and connective tissue growth around the mediastinal structures (aortic root, ascending aorta, and arch) after previous heart surgery would not be expected to alter the rate of aneurysm enlargement. However, it may change the pattern of rupture, likely decreasing the risk for frank rupture into a risk for a contained rupture. No consensus exists regarding management of cardiac patients having an incidental finding of an ascending aorta greater than 4 cm in diameter. The decision to pursue surgical intervention at the time of surgery depends on the pathogenesis of the disease, presence of symptoms, age of the patient, progression, and other operative and patient factors. A young patient with a 4.5-cm ascending aorta that is thinned and is associated with a bicuspid AV is more likely to undergo a root replacement and ascending aorta graft compared with an elderly patient with a similar aortic diameter who is undergoing CABG and whose aortic size has remained stable over the previous decade. Surgical replacement of the ascending aorta and arch is complex, requiring specialized surgical training. Significant modification of the initial surgical procedure may increase the risk for perioperative complications and potentially jeopardize the success of the originally planned operation. Extensive ascending aortic surgery involving the arch vessels requires hypothermic circulatory arrest followed by controlled exsanguination to allow for visualization of the operative field.

Disease of the AV often is accompanied by abnormalities of the thoracic aorta. Aortic root dilatation may require ascending aortic replacement. The decision is based on size of the aortic root diameter and presence of abnormalities of the aortic wall, such as thrombus, dissection, or focal aneurysm. There are no strict guidelines that dictate practice. The surgeon might choose to replace the entire root or just the AV and ascending aorta, sparing the sinuses of Valsalva. The Wheat procedure is a replacement of the AV and ascending aorta, while preserving the native sinuses of Valsalva and coronary ostia. Alternatively, in the setting of a dilated or aneurysmal sinus, the surgeon may elect to replace the entire aortic root. Choice of implanting a biologic root or composite AVR is a surgical decision based on many of the factors presented in Table 13-1. Implantation of a root or composite graft necessitates reattachment of the coronary arteries, increasing the risk for postoperative bleeding and coronary ischemia.[145] Despite a history of normal coronary arteries, the close scrutiny of regional wall motion after bypass is aimed at detecting newly created abnormalities of coronary blood flow. Air into the coronary circulation or compromise of coronary blood flow through the newly constructed coronary buttons may produce severe myocardial dysfunction and SWMAs within the specific coronary vascular distribution. Kinking of the coronaries or stenosis at the ostia often produce transmural ischemia that is not subtle. Enlargement of the sinus segment may facilitate coronary anastomoses. A prosthetic graft with an enlarged area to mimic the sinus of Valsalva has been developed. Enlargement of the sinus segment may facilitate coronary anastomoses and, thus, may decrease the risk for such complications, but this remains to be proved.

No consensus guidelines exist on the specific dimensions of the aortic root beyond which a root replacement is deemed necessary. However, distortion of the root producing severe AR or disruption in its integrity requires surgical attention. The echocardiographer reports the size of the aortic annulus, sinus of Valsalva, sinotubular junction, and ascending aorta (see Figure 13-11). These measurements are obtained using the AV long-axis view. The short- and longitudinal-axis views from

TEE can define the severity and mechanism of AR, as well as the success of AV repair. Patients scheduled for aorta surgery with an intrinsically normal AV with AR caused by a correctable aortic lesion (incomplete leaflet closure, leaflet prolapse, or dissection flap prolapse) can undergo AV repair.[104,146] In contrast, valvular pathology that includes connective tissue degeneration (Marfan or bicuspid valve), aortitis, or severe calcification would most likely require valve replacement. Surgical management is dependent on the skill set of the surgeon and individual patient factors.

Acute Aortic Syndromes

Framing

The unstable patient with suspected acute aortic disease or injury is often the most challenging of TEE cases. Few more crucially important decisions are posed to the intraoperative echocardiographer than to quickly and accurately diagnose the nature and extent of acute aortic injury. Hypotension and respiratory distress may prevent a complete and comprehensive evaluation before surgery (Figure 13-18). History often is unobtainable. The echocardiographer becomes a detective. Clues are quickly gathered from the available clinical presentation, history, and associated physical findings. The TEE is often the only modality used to establish the diagnosis and define the surgical plan.

CASE STUDY: "WHAT INCISION DO I NEED TO MAKE? HURRY PLEASE, THE PATIENT IS DYING!"

It is midnight on a gloomy rainy night. The hospital helicopter calls in "… young women, unrestrained driver, deceleration injury, steering wheel impact, chest contusion, unconscious, hypotensive. She is intubated with bilateral breath sounds. Her blood pressure is 70/40 mm Hg with a heart rate of 125 beats/min and sinus tachycardia. She is being fluid resuscitated and being transported directly to the cardiac operating room." The patient is too unstable for MRI or CT scanning. The patient arrives in the operating room with a portable chest radiograph obtained as she was whisked through the emergency department, showing a widened mediastinum. The vital signs have not changed except that she is receiving dopamine at 10 μg/kg/min. Pulses are palpable in the groin and the neck. The patient is transferred to the operating room table and everyone turns to the anesthesiologist-echocardiographer for guidance. The attending surgeon asks, "I need to know whether this is an anterior injury with heart contusion, injury to the ascending aorta, tamponade with blood in the pericardium, or is this a transected aorta at the isthmus or arch, or is this a nonoperable injury?" The former will require a sternotomy. A transection of the descending aorta or isthmus will require a left thoracotomy. "If we make the incorrect decision, the patient will surely die." The patient is stabilized in the operating room and the TEE probe is inserted. TEE reveals no blood in the pericardium, an intact aortic root with no evidence of type A dissection, a step-up in the intima at the site of the left subclavian artery, and a small left pleural effusion. The patient is positioned in the left lateral decubitus position and surgery proceeds to save a young life.

The sensitivity and specificity of TEE to detect and diagnose injury or disease of the thoracic aorta are significantly better than the sensitivity and specificity of TTE, and are comparable with CT scan and MRI.[147,148] TEE provides information regarding cardiac performance and the presence of other critically important sequelae that may be important in determining the approach and timing for surgical intervention. Hence TEE is indicated even if MRI or CT scanning has confirmed the diagnosis.

Can consent be obtained from the patient or family members? In these emergency circumstances, it may be more prudent to proceed with the TEE examination rather than delaying diagnosis and treatment in an attempt to find family members. What is the differential diagnosis of a widened mediastinum? How does TEE discriminate the

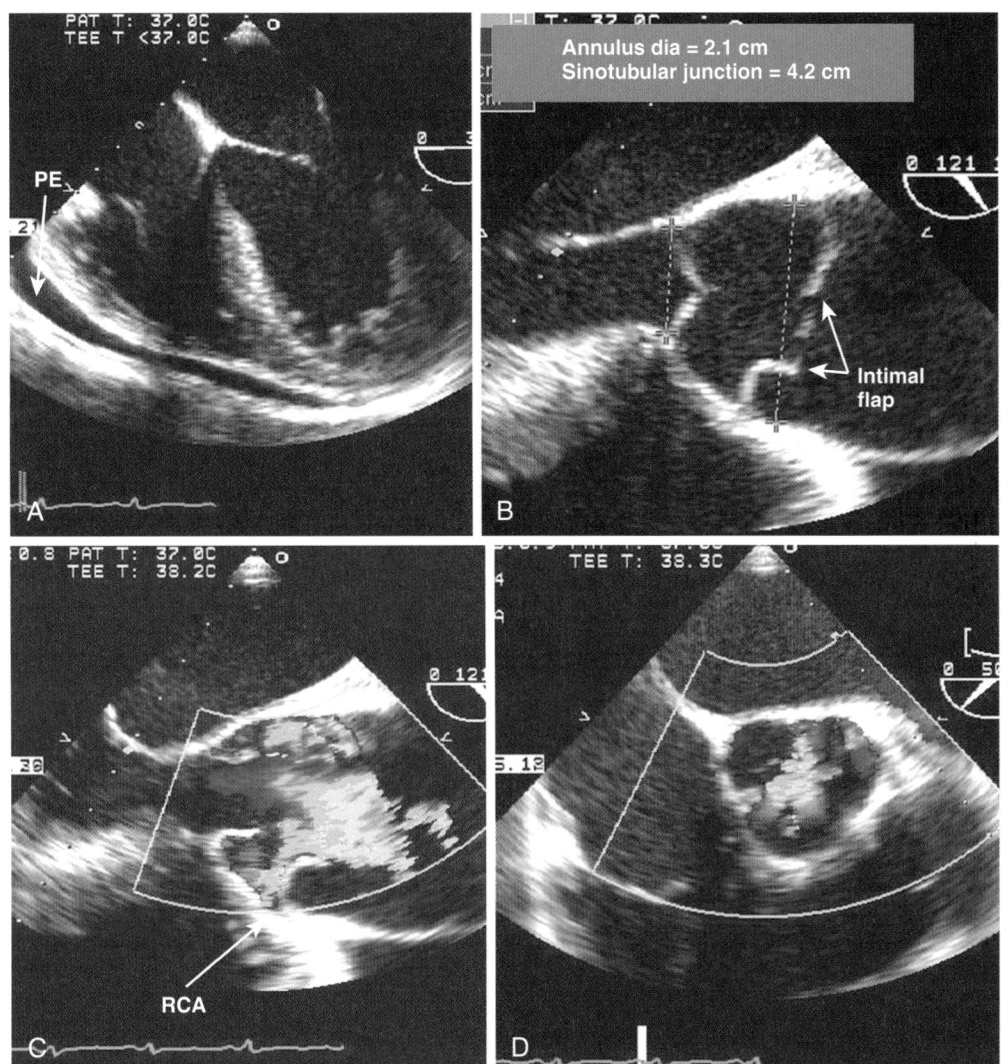

Figure 13-18 **Acute aortic syndrome as the cause of hemodynamic compromise.** A 62-year-old previously healthy, unrestrained driver had a motor vehicle accident. On arrival to the emergency department, the patient was hypotensive (blood pressure = 90/45) and tachycardic (heart rate = 120). He described an episode of loss of consciousness that was associated with severe chest pain but could not recall if the syncopal episode preceded the accident. The chest radiograph was significant for several fractured ribs, widened mediastinum, and a pleural effusion. The patient became progressively more unstable and was transferred to the operating room to perform diagnostic transesophageal echocardiography (TEE) and definitive surgical procedure if necessary. The echocardiographer performed a quick transthoracic echocardiographic examination that confirmed the presence of pericardial effusion with findings that were consistent for tamponade. After fluid resuscitation and induction of anesthesia, a TEE examination was performed. The midesophageal four-chamber view showed presence of a pericardial effusion (PE) that compromised right atrial filling (A). The midesophageal long-axis view of the aortic valve showed a type A dissection that was characterized by intimal flaps within the aortic root and that extended distally into the descending thoracic aorta. B, The annulus of the aortic valve was of normal size, but the sinus and root were markedly enlarged (diameter of sinotubular junction = 4.22 cm). The dissection extended into the noncoronary and right coronary sinus segments, narrowing blood flow at the coronary ostia (C, arrow). Although the electrocardiogram did not show acute ischemia, the right ventricular function and inferior wall of the left ventricle were mildly hypokinetic. Although an effaced aortic root, ascending aortic aneurysm, and acute dissection in this age group are suggestive of congenital bicuspid valve, the short-axis view of the aortic valve (D) showed a trileaflet valve with a coaptation defect with aortic insufficiency at the noncoronary cusp. The surgeon resuspended the aortic valve and replaced the ascending aorta and hemiarch with a tube graft. The valve repair was successful with only +1 aortic insufficiency and cardiac return to normal after surgery. RCA, right coronary artery.

different causes of a widened mediastinum? Is the TEE performed in the awake distressed patient, or is the TEE done under more controlled conditions of an anesthetized, intubated patient? Is there a risk for cervical spine injury? Is there a risk for esophageal injury? Can insertion of the TEE probe further compromise the patency of mediastinal structures? Is there fluid in the pericardium? What is the biventricular function? Is there myocardial rupture? Is there aortic rupture? Is the thoracic aorta intact? Is there an intimal flap and a dissection? Is there a transection? Is there a pleural or periaortic effusion/hematoma? Is there an intramural hematoma (IMH)? What factors determine the urgency of intervention and strategies for management?

Data Collection

Because the diagnosis and cause for instability are not established, the entire mediastinum, including the left pleural space, is interrogated before definitive therapy is initiated. Rarely is there not enough time to do a complete TEE examination. The operative team can often proceed with confidence in the management of these critically ill patients with only TEE to guide the treatment. The primary event in aortic dissection is a tear and separation of the aortic intima. It is uncertain whether the inciting event is a primary rupture of the intima with secondary dissection of the media or hemorrhage within the media and subsequent rupture of the overlying intima. Systolic ejection forces blood into the aortic media through a tear that leads to the separation of the intima from the surrounding media, creating a false lumen. Blood flow may exist in both the false and true lumens through communicating fenestrations. Aortic dissections are classified by one of two anatomic schemes (the DeBakey and Stanford classifications). Transection is diagnosed through the detection of para-aortic hematoma near the isthmus and a "step-up" in the internal media wall (see Chapter 21).

Discussion

Acute dissections (Stanford type A or DeBakey type I or type II) involving the ascending aorta or arch are considered acute surgical emergencies. In contrast, dissections confined to the descending aorta (distal to the left subclavian artery; Stanford type B or DeBakey type III) are treated medically unless the patient demonstrates proximal extension, hemorrhage, or malperfusion. From the International Registry of Acute Aortic Dissection, 73% of the 384 patients with type B dissections were managed medically; in-hospital mortality rate was 10%.[149] The long-term survival rate after applying medical therapy was approximately 60% to 80% at 4 to 5 years[149-152] and approximately 40% to 45% at 10 years.[151,152] Survival was best in patients with noncommunicating and retrograde dissections.[153] From the International Registry of Acute Aortic Dissection, in-hospital mortality rate for surgical patients was significantly greater (32%).[149] The increased rate of mortality for surgically treated patients likely was influenced by selecting a cohort of patients with more advanced disease and complicated course (malperfusion, leakage, extension). The overall reported short- and long-term outcomes were similar for medically treated patients with type B dissections.[152] Of 142 patients with type B aortic dissections, there was a trend toward lower mortality with medical therapy compared with surgical treatment at 1 year (15% vs. 33%). Both groups had similar survival rates at 5 and 10 years (60% and 35%).[152]

Endovascular stent grafting for descending thoracic aortic dissections is gaining momentum as a less invasive alternative to surgery in stable patients with type B dissections.[154,155] The stent graft is positioned to cover the intimal flap and seal the entry site of the dissection, resulting in thrombosis of the false lumen. In one non-randomized evaluation of 24 consecutive patients with a subacute or chronic thoracic type B dissection, there was no morbidity (paraplegia, stroke, embolization, malperfusion syndrome, or infection) or mortality with stent grafting.[154] In contrast, surgical intervention was associated with a 33% mortality rate and a 42% incidence rate of adverse events within a 12-month period. Other studies are promising but less positive.[156] In a series of 19 patients with acute dissections (15 type B and 4 type A dissections), the major morbidity rate was 21% (small-bowel and renal infarction and lower extremity ischemia) and 30-day mortality rate was 16%. However, there were no additional deaths or instances of aneurysm/aortic rupture during the subsequent 13-month follow-up period.

Ascending aortic dissections (involving the aortic root, ascending aorta, or arch) are acute surgical emergencies because of the high risk for a life-threatening complication such as AR, cardiac tamponade, myocardial infarction, rupture, and stroke. The mortality rate is as high as 1% to 2% per hour early after symptom onset.[157] Neither acute myocardial ischemia nor cerebral infarction should contraindicate urgent intervention. Although patients with stroke in progress may be at increased risk for hemorrhagic cerebral infarction because of intraoperative anticoagulation, leading to hemorrhagic stroke, the authors have seen several patients who experienced dramatic neurologic recovery. Operative mortality for ascending aortic dissections at experienced centers varied from 7% to 36%, well below the greater than 50% mortality with medical therapy.[150,157-164]

Traumatic aortic rupture is a life-threatening vascular injury that often results in lethal hemorrhage. In a multicenter trial of 274 patients, the overall mortality rate reached 31%, with 63% of deaths attributable to aortic rupture.[165] Aortic transection and rupture usually occurred at the aortic isthmus (between the left subclavian and the first intercostal arteries) and resulted from shear forces generated by unrestrained frontal collisions.[166] Although aortography had been considered the gold standard for the diagnosis of transection, TEE and contrast-enhanced spiral CT and MRI are currently favored, especially for patients with renal insufficiency.[167-171] Intravascular ultrasonography has been proposed as a potential diagnostic tool for the identification of limited aortic injuries.[172] Traumatic aortic rupture needs to be distinguished from an aortic dissection. Imaging of a dissected aorta typically reveals true and false lumens at multiple levels. The focal aortic injury of aortic transection is quite localized and may be overlooked when performing a cursory examination. A second potential diagnostic problem is that protuberant atherosclerotic changes of the aorta may be difficult to differentiate from partial aortic tears. The thick and irregular intraluminal flap, which corresponds to disruption of both intimal and medial aortic layers, can be imaged in both the short- and long-axis planes in the vicinity of the isthmus. In the longitudinal view, the medial flap is nearly perpendicular to the aortic wall because traumatic lesions are usually confined within a few centimeters distal to the left subclavian. The formation of a localized contained rupture of the false aneurysm is common.[168,173] Color-flow Doppler imaging and spectral Doppler can be used to detect turbulence associated with nonlaminar flow at the aortic defect and the presence of a pressure gradient. Traditional treatment includes immediate surgical invention using a right lateral decubitus approach and resection of the aorta with insertion of a tube graft. Deployment of endovascular stent grafts has been successful. Two series that included a total of 16 patients having aortic transection reported successful repair with no mortality or serious morbidity.[174,175] However, the application of this device under such conditions poses a high risk for left subclavian malperfusion and paraplegia.[176] The decision regarding appropriate management and time course of therapy will depend on the technical availability and expertise within the institution and the forthcoming results of clinical trials that use newer, less invasive technologies.

▣ Intramural Hematoma

Framing

The presence of an IMH is a subtle finding that may be missed when evaluating the thoracic aorta for a dissection or rupture. IMH is distinct from a classic aortic dissection but has been considered by some as being a variant.[177]

What are the characteristics of an IMH? What are the common findings and symptoms at presentation? What, if any, is the clinical significance of this pathologic finding? Does location influence the choice of medical or surgical approach? What are the prognostic indicators of progression?

Data Collection

Aortic IMH is often considered a variant of an aortic dissection.[177] Although many of the patients may present with chest or back pain, many of the associated sequelae, such as pericardial or pleural effusions, stroke, and myocardial infarction, are absent.[179-180] It is characterized by the absence of a detectable intimal tear. The hematoma probably is produced by a hemorrhage of the vaso vasorum into the aortic wall. In a meta-analysis, acute aortic IMH was most often associated with long-standing hypertension; traumatic cause was also a significant factor for 6% of cases.[178] In the meta-analysis of 143 cases, 81% were diagnosed by CT, and the remaining patients by MRI, TEE, or both.[178] The sensitivity and specificity of TEE to detect an IMH were reported to be 100% and 91%, respectively.[180] The diagnosis is characterized by the absence of a dissecting flap or intimal disruption with specific regional thickening of the aortic wall of greater than 7 mm in a crescent or circular shape. On MRI or CT, this crescent-shaped or circular area in the aortic wall demonstrates high attenuation that does not enhance with contrast.[181] Although IMHs can be detected in any portion of the aorta, the location appears to be a factor in its cause and prognosis. The ascending aorta, which was involved in 33% to 57% of cases, appeared to represent the early stage of a classic dissection,[178,179,181–183] whereas traumatic IMHs typically involved the descending thoracic aorta.[182]

Discussion

Acute management is similar to that of a classic aortic dissection. In the meta-analysis of 143 patients with aortic IMH, lesions of the ascending aorta were associated with a lower early mortality with surgical intervention than medical treatment (14% vs. 36%); lesions of the descending aorta had a similar mortality with medical or surgical therapy (14% vs. 20%).[178] The force of left ventricular systolic blood pressure, the driving force for disease progression, is reduced by the administration of β-blockers. Patients with an IMH in the descending thoracic aorta should be medically treated using β-blockers. Management of patients having IMH of the ascending aorta is controversial. A comprehensive evidence-based approach is not practical at present. Research publications have been limited to case reports, single-institutional series, multicenter registries, and meta-analyses. The experience seems to vary between the Asian centers (Japan and Korean), which have more success with medical management, and the Western centers (European and American), which have advocated a more aggressive surgical management. In a recent single-institutional study from Korea of 357 patients having acute aortic syndrome, 101 patients had IMH, 16% of whom were unstable receiving surgery and the rest were medically treated.[183]

Of the patients who initially received medical management, the aortic pathology progressed in 37% of patients, lending to delayed surgery or death. Prognostic factors of impending deterioration include IMH greater than 15 mm or increased aortic diameter. The difference in response to management strategies also may reflect population genetics, comorbid diseases (atherosclerosis, hypertension, environmental factors), or experience in accurately diagnosing this variant. The periaortic thickness of IMH, which can be small and subtle, may be underdiagnosed in the West.[184] The risk for sudden deterioration and death related to pursuing medical management must be balanced by the potential morbidity/mortality of surgery. In a center having low surgical mortality, a surgical approach might be favored. A high-risk patient at a surgical center of lesser experience may consider aggressive medical management.

In conclusion, the intraoperative echocardiographer is confronted with a broad array of diseases that require on-site decision making in the perioperative setting. The key ingredients to sound decision making are a broad fund of knowledge (database), a systematic approach with attention to all vantage points and frames, and identifying, addressing, and prioritizing the pertinent questions.

"Plans are nothing ... Planning is everything."

—Dwight Eisenhower

REFERENCES

1. Kruger J, Dunning D: Unskilled and unaware of it: How difficulties in recognizing one's own incompetence lead to inflated self-assessments, *J Person Soc Psychol* 77:1121, 1999.
2. Royse AG, Royse CF, Ajani AE, et al: Reduced neuropsychological dysfunction using epiaortic echocardiography and the exclusive Y graft, *Ann Thorac Surg* 69:1431, 2000.
3. Sylivris S, Calafiore P, Matalanis G, et al: The intraoperative assessment of ascending aortic atheroma: Epiaortic imaging is superior to both transesophageal echocardiography and direct palpation, *J Cardiothorac Vasc Anesth* 11:704, 1997.
4. Ura M, Sakata R, Nakayama Y, et al: Extracorporeal circulation before and after ultrasonographic evaluation of the ascending aorta, *Ann Thorac Surg* 67:478, 1999.
5. Russo JE, Schoemaker PJH: *The power of frames, winning decisions*, New York, 2002, Doubleday.
6. Kallmeyer IJ, Collard CD, Fox JA, et al: The safety of intraoperative transesophageal echocardiography: A case series of 7200 cardiac surgical patients, *Anesth Analg* 92:1126, 2001.
7. MacGregor DA, Zvara DA, Treadway RM Jr, et al: Late presentation of esophageal injury after transesophageal echocardiography, *Anesth Analg* 99:41, 2004.
8. Olenchock SA Jr, Lukaszczyk JJ, Reed J III, Theman TE: Splenic injury after intraoperative transesophageal echocardiography, *Ann Thorac Surg* 72:2141, 2001.
9. Pong MW, Lin SM, Kao SC, et al: Unusual cause of esophageal perforation during intraoperative transesophageal echocardiography monitoring for cardiac surgery—a case report, *Acta Anaesthesiol* 41:155, 2003.
10. Savino JS, Hanson CW III, Bigelow DC, et al: Oropharyngeal injury after transesophageal echocardiography, *J Cardiothorac Vasc Anesth* 8:76, 1994.
11. Venticinque SG, Kashyap VS, O'Connell RJ: Chemical burn injury secondary to intraoperative transesophageal echocardiography, *Anesth Analg* 97:1260, 2003.
12. Silber JH: Using outcomes analysis to assess quality of care: Applications for cardiovascular surgery, outcome measurements. In Tuman KJ, editor: *Cardiovascular medicine*, Philadelphia, 1999, Lippincott Williams & Wilkins, p 1.
13. Practice guidelines for perioperative transesophageal echocardiography. A report by the American Society of Anesthesiologists and the Society of Cardiovascular Anesthesiologists Task Force on Transesophageal Echocardiography, *Anesthesiology* 84:986, 1996.
14. Practice guidelines for perioperative transesophageal echocardiography: An updated report by the American Society of Anesthesiologists and the Society of Cardiovascular Anesthesiologists Task Force on Transesophageal Echocardiography, *Anesthesiology* 112:1084, 2010.
15. Shanewise JS, Cheung AT, Aronson S, et al: ASE/SCA guidelines for performing a comprehensive intraoperative multiplane transesophageal echocardiography examination: Recommendations of the American Society of Echocardiography Council for Intraoperative Echocardiography and the Society of Cardiovascular Anesthesiologists Task Force for Certification in Perioperative Transesophageal Echocardiography, *Anesth Analg* 89:870, 1999.
16. Battler A, Froelicher VF, Gallagher KP, et al: Dissociation between regional myocardial dysfunction and ECG changes during ischemia in the conscious dog, *Circulation* 62:735, 1980.
17. Foster E, O'Kelly B, LaPidus A, et al: Segmental analysis of resting echocardiographic function and stress scintigraphic perfusion: Implications for myocardial viability, *Am Heart J* 129:7, 1995.
18. Jacklin PB, Barrington SF, Roxburgh JC, et al: Cost-effectiveness of preoperative positron emission tomography in ischemic heart disease, *Ann Thorac Surg* 73:1403, 2002.
19. Landoni C, Lucignani G, Paolini G, et al: Assessment of CABG-related risk in patients with CAD and LVD. Contribution of PET with [18F]FDG to the assessment of myocardial viability, *J Cardiovasc Surg (Torino)* 40:363, 1999.
20. Kozman H, Cook JR, Wiseman AH, et al: Presence of angiographic coronary collaterals predicts myocardial recovery after coronary bypass surgery in patients with severe left ventricular dysfunction, *Circulation* 98:II–57, 1998.
21. Premaratne S, Razzuk A, Koduru S, et al: Incidence of postinfarction aneurysm within one month of infarct: Experience with 16 patients in Hawaii, *J Cardiovasc Surg* 40:473, 1999.
22. Redfield MM, Jacobsen SJ, Burnett JCJ, et al: Burden of systolic and diastolic ventricular dysfunction in the community: Appreciating the scope of the heart failure epidemic, *JAMA* 289:194, 2003.
23. Nollert G, Wich S: Planning a cardiovascular hybrid operating room: The technical point of view, *Heart Surg Forum* 12:E125, 2009.
24. Grigioni F, Enriquez-Sarano M, Zehr KJ, et al: Ischemic mitral regurgitation: Long-term outcome and prognostic implications with quantitative Doppler assessment, *Circulation* 103:1759, 2001.
25. Feinberg MS, Schwammenthal E, Shlizerman L, et al: Prognostic significance of mild mitral regurgitation by color Doppler echocardiography in acute myocardial infarction, *Am J Cardiol* 86:903, 2000.
26. Grossi EA, Goldberg JD, LaPietra A, et al: Ischemic mitral valve reconstruction and replacement: Comparison of long-term survival and complications, *J Thorac Cardiovasc Surg* 122:1107, 2001.
27. Bach DS, Deeb GM, Bolling SF: Accuracy of intraoperative transesophageal echocardiography for estimating the severity of functional mitral regurgitation, *Am J Cardiol* 76:508, 1995.
28. Choi H, Lee K, Lee H, et al: Quantification of mitral regurgitation using proximal isovelocity surface area method in dogs, *J Vet Sci* 5:163, 2004.
29. Grewal KS, Malkowski MJ, Piracha AR, et al: Effect of general anesthesia on the severity of mitral regurgitation by transesophageal echocardiography, *Am J Cardiol* 85:199, 2000.
30. Gillinov AM, Wierup PN, Blackstone EH, et al: Is repair preferable to replacement for ischemic mitral regurgitation? *J Thorac Cardiovasc Surg* 122:1125, 2001.
31. Yiu SF, Enriquez-Sarano M, Tribouilloy C, et al: Determinants of the degree of functional mitral regurgitation in patients with systolic left ventricular dysfunction: A quantitative clinical study, *Circulation* 102:1400, 2000.
32. Gorman JH III, Gorman RC, Jackson BM, et al: Annuloplasty ring selection for chronic ischemic mitral regurgitation: Lessons from the ovine model, *Ann Thorac Surg* 76:1556, 2003.
33. Guy TS, Moainie SL, Gorman JH III, et al: Prevention of ischemic mitral regurgitation does not influence the outcome of remodeling after posterolateral myocardial infarction, *J Am Coll Cardiol* 43:377, 2004.
34. Miller DC: Ischemic mitral regurgitation redux—to repair or to replace? *J Thorac Cardiovasc Surg* 122:1059, 2001.
35. Inoue M, McCarthy PM, Popovic ZB, et al: Mitral valve repair without cardiopulmonary bypass or atriotomy using the Coapsys device: Device design and implantation procedure in canine functional mitral regurgitation model, *Heart Surg Forum* 7:E117, 2004.
36. Fukamachi K, Popovic ZB, Inoue M, et al: Changes in mitral annular and left ventricular dimensions and left ventricular pressure-volume relations after off-pump treatment of mitral regurgitation with the Coapsys device, *Eur J Cardiothorac Surg* 25:352, 2004.
37. Fann JI, St Goar FG, Komtebedde J, et al: Beating heart catheter-based edge-to-edge mitral valve procedure in a porcine model: Efficacy and healing response, *Circulation* 110:988, 2004.
38. Condado JA, Velez-Gimon M: Catheter-based approach to mitral regurgitation, *J Interv Cardiol* 16:523, 2003.
39. Maslow AD, Regan MM, Haering JM, et al: Echocardiographic predictors of left ventricular outflow tract obstruction and systolic anterior motion of the mitral valve after mitral valve reconstruction for myxomatous valve disease, *J Am Coll Cardiol* 34:2096, 1999.
40. Hellemans IM, Pieper EG, Ravelli AC, et al: Prediction of surgical strategy in mitral valve regurgitation based on echocardiography. Interuniversity Cardiology Institute of the Netherlands, *Am J Cardiol* 79:334, 1997.
41. Lee EM, Shapiro LM, Wells FC: Superiority of mitral valve repair in surgery for degenerative mitral regurgitation, *Eur Heart J* 18:655, 1997.
42. Rozich JD, Carabello BA, Usher BW, et al: Mitral valve replacement with and without chordal preservation in patients with chronic mitral regurgitation. Mechanisms for differences in postoperative ejection performance, *Circulation* 86:1718, 1992.
43. Charls LM: SAM—systolic anterior motion of the anterior mitral valve leaflet postsurgical mitral valve repair, *Heart Lung* 32:402, 2003.
44. Brown ML, Abel MD, Click RL, et al: Systolic anterior motion after mitral valve repair: Is surgical intervention necessary? *J Thorac Cardiovasc Surg* 133:136, 2007.
45. Movsowitz C, Podolsky LA, Meyerowitz CB, et al: Patent foramen ovale: A nonfunctional embryological remnant or a potential cause of significant pathology? *J Am Soc Echocardiogr* 5:259, 1992.
46. Langholz D, Louie EK, Konstadt SN, et al: Transesophageal echocardiographic demonstration of distinct mechanisms for right to left shunting across a patent foramen ovale in the absence of pulmonary hypertension, *J Am Coll Cardiol* 18:1112, 1991.
47. Augoustides JG, Weiss SJ, Weiner J, et al: Diagnosis of patent foramen ovale with multiplane transesophageal echocardiography in adult cardiac surgical patients, *J Cardiothorac Vasc Anesth* 18:725, 2004.
48. Attie F, Rosas M, Granados N, et al: Surgical treatment for secundum atrial septal defects in patients >40 years old. A randomized clinical trial, *J Am Coll Cardiol* 38:2035, 2001.

49. Ferreira SM, Ho SY, Anderson RH: Morphological study of defects of the atrial septum within the oval fossa: Implications for transcatheter closure of left-to-right shunt, *Br Heart J* 67:316, 1992.
50. Mugge A, Daniel WG, Angermann C, et al: Atrial septal aneurysm in adult patients. A multicenter study using transthoracic and transesophageal echocardiography, *Circulation* 91:2785, 1995.
51. Belkin RN, Kisslo J: Atrial septal aneurysm: Recognition and clinical relevance, *Am Heart J* 120:948, 1990.
52. Cabanes L, Mas JL, Cohen A, et al: Atrial septal aneurysm and patent foramen ovale as risk factors for cryptogenic stroke in patients less than 55 years of age. A study using transesophageal echocardiography, *Stroke* 24:1865, 1993.
53. Mattioli AV, Aquilina M, Oldani A, et al: Atrial septal aneurysm as a cardioembolic source in adult patients with stroke and normal carotid arteries. A multicentre study, *Eur Heart J* 22:261, 2001.
54. Agmon Y, Khandheria BK, Meissner I, et al: Frequency of atrial septal aneurysms in patients with cerebral ischemic events, *Circulation* 99:1942, 1999.
55. Pearson AC, Nagelhout D, Castello R, et al: Atrial septal aneurysm and stroke: A transesophageal echocardiographic study, *J Am Coll Cardiol* 18:1223, 1991.
56. Lechat P, Mas JL, Lascault G, et al: Prevalence of patent foramen ovale in patients with stroke, *N Engl J Med* 318:1148, 1988.
57. Burger AJ, Sherman HB, Charlamb MJ: Low incidence of embolic strokes with atrial septal aneurysms: A prospective, long-term study, *Am Heart J* 139:149, 2000.
58. Overell JR, Bone I, Lees KR: Interatrial septal abnormalities and stroke: A meta-analysis of case-control studies, *Neurology* 55:1172, 2000.
59. Orgera MA, O'Malley PG, Taylor AJ: Secondary prevention of cerebral ischemia in patent foramen ovale: Systematic review and meta-analysis, *South Med J* 94:699, 2001.
60. Sukernik MR, Goswami S, Frumento RJ, et al: National survey regarding the management of an intraoperatively diagnosed patent foramen ovale during coronary artery bypass graft surgery, *J Cardiothorac Vasc Anesth* 19:150, 2005.
61. Kollar A, Reames MK, Coyle JP: Patent foramen ovale and pulmonary embolism. An underestimated co-morbidity following cardiac surgery, *J Cardiovasc Surg (Torino)* 39:355, 1998.
62. Yasu T, Fujii M, Saito M: Long-term follow-up of an interatrial right-to-left shunt that appeared after cardiac surgery—evaluation by transesophageal Doppler echocardiography, *Jpn Circ J* 60:70, 1996.
63. Akhter M, Lajos TZ: Pitfalls of undetected patent foramen ovale in off-pump cases, *Ann Thorac Surg* 67:546, 1999.
64. Stoddard MF, Arce J, Liddell NE, et al: Two-dimensional transesophageal echocardiographic determination of aortic valve area in adults with aortic stenosis, *Am Heart J* 122:1415, 1991.
65. Smith MD, Harrison MR, Pinton R, et al: Regurgitant jet size by transesophageal compared with transthoracic Doppler color flow imaging, *Circulation* 83:79, 1991.
66. Fenoglio JJ Jr, McAllister HA Jr, DeCastro CM, et al: Congenital bicuspid aortic valve after age 20, *Am J Cardiol* 39:164, 1977.
67. Osler W: The bicuspid condition of the aortic valves, *Trans Assoc Am Physicians* 1:185, 1886.
68. Grant RT, Wood JE Jr, Jones TD: Heart valve irregularities in relation to subacute bacterial endocarditis, *Heart* 14:247, 1928.
69. Keith JD: Bicuspid aortic valve. In Keith JD, Rowe RD, Vlad P, editors: *Heart disease in infancy and childhood*, London, 1978, MacMillan, p 728.
70. Roberts WC: The congenitally bicuspid aortic valve. A study of 85 autopsy cases, *Am J Cardiol* 26:72, 1970.
71. Larson EW, Edwards WD: Risk factors for aortic dissection: A necropsy study of 161 cases, *Am J Cardiol* 53:849, 1984.
72. Novaro GM, Tiong IY, Pearce GL, et al: Features and predictors of ascending aortic dilatation in association with a congenital bicuspid aortic valve, *Am J Cardiol* 92:99, 2003.
73. Borger MA, Preston M, Ivanov J, et al: Should the ascending aorta be replaced more frequently in patients with bicuspid aortic valve disease? *J Thorac Cardiovasc Surg* 128:677, 2004.
74. Olearchyk AS: Congenital bicuspid aortic valve and an aneurysm of the ascending aorta, *J Card Surg* 19:462, 2004.
75. Olearchyk AS: Congenital bicuspid aortic valve disease with an aneurysm of the ascending aorta in adults: Vertical reduction aortoplasty with distal external synthetic wrapping, *J Card Surg* 19:144, 2004.
76. Fedak PW, de Sa MP, Verma S, et al: Vascular matrix remodeling in patients with bicuspid aortic valve malformations: Implications for aortic dilatation, *J Thorac Cardiovasc Surg* 126:797, 2003.
77. Ferencik M, Pape LA: Changes in size of ascending aorta and aortic valve function with time in patients with congenitally bicuspid aortic valves, *Am J Cardiol* 92:43, 2003.
78. Borger MA, Preston M, Ivanov J, et al: Should the ascending aorta be replaced more frequently in patients with bicuspid aortic valve disease? *J Thorac Cardiovasc Surg* 128:677, 2004.
79. Cosgrove DM, Rosenkranz ER, Hendren WG, et al: Valvuloplasty for aortic insufficiency, *J Thorac Cardiovasc Surg* 102:571, 1991.
80. Haydar HS, He GW, Hovaguimian H, et al: Valve repair for aortic insufficiency: Surgical classification and techniques, *Eur J Cardiothorac Surg* 11:258, 1997.
81. Moidl R, Moritz A, Simon P, et al: Echocardiographic results after repair of incompetent bicuspid aortic valves, *Ann Thorac Surg* 60:669, 1995.
82. Casselman FP, Gillinov AM, Akhrass R, et al: Intermediate-term durability of bicuspid aortic valve repair for prolapsing leaflet, *Eur J Cardiothorac Surg* 15:302, 1999.
83. Rosenhek R, Binder T, Porenta G, et al: Predictors of outcome in severe, asymptomatic aortic stenosis, *N Engl J Med* 343:611, 2000.
84. Rajamannan NM, Subramaniam M, Springett M, et al: Atorvastatin inhibits hypercholesterolemia-induced cellular proliferation and bone matrix production in the rabbit aortic valve, *Circulation* 105:2660, 2002.
85. Bellamy MF, Pellikka PA, Klarich KW, et al: Association of cholesterol levels, hydroxymethylglutaryl coenzyme-A reductase inhibitor treatment, and progression of aortic stenosis in the community, *J Am Coll Cardiol* 40:1723, 2002.
86. Smith WT, Ferguson TB Jr, Ryan T, et al: Should coronary artery bypass graft surgery patients with mild or moderate aortic stenosis undergo concomitant aortic valve replacement? A decision analysis approach to the surgical dilemma, *J Am Coll Cardiol* 44:1241, 2004.
87. Rahimtoola SH: "Prophylactic" valve replacement for mild aortic valve disease at time of surgery for other cardiovascular disease? *J Am Coll Cardiol* 33:2009, 1999.
88. Pereira JJ, Lauer MS, Bashir M, et al: Survival after aortic valve replacement for severe aortic stenosis with low transvalvular gradients and severe left ventricular dysfunction, *J Am Coll Cardiol* 39:1356, 2002.
89. Brogan WC III, Grayburn PA, Lange RA, Hillis LD: Prognosis after valve replacement in patients with severe aortic stenosis and a low transvalvular pressure gradient, *J Am Coll Cardiol* 21:1657, 1993.
90. Connolly HM, Oh JK, Schaff HV, et al: Severe aortic stenosis with low transvalvular gradient and severe left ventricular dysfunction: Result of aortic valve replacement in 52 patients, *Circulation* 101:1940, 2000.
91. Ford LE, Feldman T, Chiu YC, Carroll JD: Hemodynamic resistance as a measure of functional impairment in aortic valvular stenosis, *Circ Res* 66:1, 1990.
92. deFilippi CR, Willett DL, Brickner ME, et al: Usefulness of dobutamine echocardiography in distinguishing severe from nonsevere valvular aortic stenosis in patients with depressed left ventricular function and low transvalvular gradients, *Am J Cardiol* 75:191, 1995.
93. Bermejo J, Garcia-Fernandez MA, Torrecilla EG, et al: Effects of dobutamine on Doppler echocardiographic indexes of aortic stenosis, *J Am Coll Cardiol* 28:1206, 1996.
94. Lin SS, Roger VL, Pascoe R, et al: Dobutamine stress Doppler hemodynamics in patients with aortic stenosis: Feasibility, safety, and surgical correlations, *Am Heart J* 136:1010, 1998.
95. Cheitlin MD, Armstrong WF, Aurigemma GP, et al: ACC/AHA/ASE 2003 guideline update for the clinical application of echocardiography—summary article: A report of the American College of Cardiology/American Heart Association Task Force on Practice Guidelines (ACC/AHA/ASE Committee to Update the 1997 Guidelines for the Clinical Application of Echocardiography), *J Am Coll Cardiol* 42:954, 2003.
96. Nishimura RA, Grantham JA, Connolly HM, et al: Low-output, low-gradient aortic stenosis in patients with depressed left ventricular systolic function: The clinical utility of the dobutamine challenge in the catheterization laboratory, *Circulation* 106:809, 2002.
97. Monin JL, Quere JP, Monchi M, et al: Low-gradient aortic stenosis: Operative risk stratification and predictors for long-term outcome: A multicenter study using dobutamine stress hemodynamics, *Circulation* 108:319, 2003.
98. ACC/AHA guidelines for the management of patients with valvular heart disease. A report of the American College of Cardiology/American Heart Association. Task Force on Practice Guidelines (Committee on Management of Patients with Valvular Heart Disease), *J Am Coll Cardiol* 32:1486, 1998.
99. Lung B, Gohlke-Barwolf C, Tornos P, et al: Recommendations on the management of the asymptomatic patient with valvular heart disease, *Eur Heart J* 23:1252, 2002.
100. Bonow RO, Rosing DR, McIntosh CL, et al: The natural history of asymptomatic patients with aortic regurgitation and normal left ventricular function, *Circulation* 68:509, 1983.
101. Bonow RO, Lakatos E, Maron BJ, Epstein SE: Serial long-term assessment of the natural history of asymptomatic patients with chronic aortic regurgitation and normal left ventricular systolic function, *Circulation* 84:1625, 1991.
102. Henry WL, Bonow RO, Rosing DR, Epstein SE: Observations on the optimum time for operative intervention for aortic regurgitation. II. Serial echocardiographic evaluation of asymptomatic patients, *Circulation* 61:484, 1980.
103. Nash PJ, Vitvitsky E, Cosgrove DM, et al: Echocardiographic predictors of aortic valve repair in patients with bicuspid valves and aortic regurgitation, *J Am Coll Cardiol* 41:516, 2003.
104. Yacoub MH, Cohn LH: Novel approaches to cardiac valve repair: From structure to function: Part II, *Circulation* 109:1064, 2004.
105. Carr JA, Savage EB: Aortic valve repair for aortic insufficiency in adults: A contemporary review and comparison with replacement techniques, *Eur J Cardiothorac Surg* 25:6, 2004.
106. Rahimtoola SH: Choice of prosthetic heart valve for adult patients, *J Am Coll Cardiol* 41:893, 2003.
107. Girard SE, Miller FA Jr, Orszulak TA, et al: Reoperation for prosthetic aortic valve obstruction in the era of echocardiography: Trends in diagnostic testing and comparison with surgical findings, *J Am Coll Cardiol* 37:579, 2001.
108. Rao V, Jamieson WR, Ivanov J, et al: Prosthesis-patient mismatch affects survival after aortic valve replacement, *Circulation* 102:III–5, 2000.
109. He GW, Grunkemeier GL, Gately HL, et al: Up to thirty-year survival after aortic valve replacement in the small aortic root, *Ann Thorac Surg* 59:1056, 1995.
110. Yazdanbakhsh AP, van den Brink RB, Dekker E, de Mol BA: Small valve area index: Its influence on early mortality after mitral valve replacement, *Eur J Cardiothorac Surg* 17:222, 2000.
111. Barner HB, Labovitz AJ, Fiore AC: Prosthetic valves for the small aortic root, *J Card Surg* 9:154, 1994.
112. Gonzalez-Juanatey JR, Garcia-Acuna JM, Vega FM, et al: Influence of the size of aortic valve prostheses on hemodynamics and change in left ventricular mass: Implications for the surgical management of aortic stenosis, *J Thorac Cardiovasc Surg* 112:273, 1996.
113. Pibarot P, Dumesnil JG: Hemodynamic and clinical impact of prosthesis-patient mismatch in the aortic valve position and its prevention, *J Am Coll Cardiol* 36:1131, 2000.
114. Come PC, Riley MF, Ferguson JF, et al: Prediction of severity of aortic stenosis: Accuracy of multiple noninvasive parameters, *Am J Med* 85:29, 1988.
115. Palta S, Gill KS, Pai RG: Role of inadequate adaptive left ventricular hypertrophy in the genesis of mitral regurgitation in patients with severe aortic stenosis: Implications for its prevention, *J Heart Valve Dis* 12:601, 2003.
116. Brener SJ, Duffy CI, Thomas JD, Stewart WJ: Progression of aortic stenosis in 394 patients: Relation to changes in myocardial and mitral valve dysfunction, *J Am Coll Cardiol* 25:305, 1995.
117. Absil B, Dagenais F, Mathieu P, et al: Does moderate mitral regurgitation impact early or mid-term clinical outcome in patients undergoing isolated aortic valve replacement for aortic stenosis? *Eur J Cardiothorac Surg* 24:217, 2003.
118. Christenson JT, Jordan B, Bloch A, Schmuziger M: Should a regurgitant mitral valve be replaced simultaneously with a stenotic aortic valve? *Tex Heart Inst J* 27:350, 2000.
119. Goland S, Loutaty G, Arditi A, et al: Improvement in mitral regurgitation after aortic valve replacement, *Isr Med Assoc J* 5:12, 2003.
120. Harris KM, Malenka DJ, Haney MF, et al: Improvement in mitral regurgitation after aortic valve replacement, *Am J Cardiol* 80:741, 1997.
121. Moazami N, Diodato MD, Moon MR, et al: Does functional mitral regurgitation improve with isolated aortic valve replacement? *J Card Surg* 19:444, 2004.
122. Tunick PA, Gindea A, Kronzon I: Effect of aortic valve replacement for aortic stenosis on severity of mitral regurgitation, *Am J Cardiol* 65:1219, 1990.
123. Tassan-Mangina S, Metz D, Nazeyllas P, et al: Factors determining early improvement in mitral regurgitation after aortic valve replacement for aortic valve stenosis: A transthoracic and transesophageal prospective study, *Clin Cardiol* 26:127, 2003.
124. Ruel M, Kapila V, Price J, et al: Natural history and predictors of outcome in patients with concomitant functional mitral regurgitation at the time of aortic valve replacement, *Circulation* 114(Suppl 1):I541, 2006.
125. Amarenco P, Cohen A, Tzourio C, et al: Atherosclerotic disease of the aortic arch and the risk of ischemic stroke, *N Engl J Med* 331:1474, 1994.
126. Davila-Roman VG, Barzilai B, Wareing TH, et al: Atherosclerosis of the ascending aorta. Prevalence and role as an independent predictor of cerebrovascular events in cardiac patients, *Stroke* 25:2010, 1994.
127. Hartman GS, Yao FS, Bruefach M III, et al: Severity of aortic atheromatous disease diagnosed by transesophageal echocardiography predicts stroke and other outcomes associated with coronary artery surgery: A prospective study, *Anesth Analg* 83:701, 1996.
128. Konstadt SN, Reich DL, Quintana C, Levy M: The ascending aorta: How much does transesophageal echocardiography see? *Anesth Analg* 78:240, 1994.
129. Katz ES, Tunick PA, Rusinek H, et al: Protruding aortic atheromas predict stroke in elderly patients undergoing cardiopulmonary bypass: Experience with intraoperative transesophageal echocardiography, *J Am Coll Cardiol* 20:70, 1992.
130. Marshall WG Jr, Barzilai B, Kouchoukos NT, Saffitz J: Intraoperative ultrasonic imaging of the ascending aorta, *Ann Thorac Surg* 48:339, 1989.
131. Hosoda Y, Watanabe M, Hirooka Y, et al: Significance of atherosclerotic changes of the ascending aorta during coronary bypass surgery with intraoperative detection by echography, *J Cardiovasc Surg (Torino)* 32:301, 1991.

132. Ohteki H, Itoh T, Natsuaki M, et al: Intraoperative ultrasonic imaging of the ascending aorta in ischemic heart disease, *Ann Thorac Surg* 50:539, 1990.
133. Davila-Roman VG, Barzilai B, Wareing TH, et al: Intraoperative ultrasonographic evaluation of the ascending aorta in 100 consecutive patients undergoing cardiac surgery, *Circulation* 84:III–47, 1991.
134. Hammon JW Jr, Stump DA, Kon ND, et al: Risk factors and solutions for the development of neurobehavioral changes after coronary artery bypass grafting, *Ann Thorac Surg* 63:1613, 1997.
135. Wilson MJ, Boyd SY, Lisagor PG, et al: Ascending aortic atheroma assessed intraoperatively by epiaortic and transesophageal echocardiography, *Ann Thorac Surg* 70:25, 2000.
136. Konstadt SN, Reich DL, Kahn R, Viggiani RF: Transesophageal echocardiography can be used to screen for ascending aortic atherosclerosis, *Anesth Analg* 81:225, 1995.
137. Eltzschig HK, Kallmeyer IJ, Mihaljevic T, et al: A practical approach to a comprehensive epicardial and epiaortic echocardiographic examination, *J Cardiothorac Vasc Anesth* 17:422, 2003.
138. Chandraratna A, Ashmeg A, Pasha HC: Detection of intracoronary air embolism by echocardiography, *J Am Soc Echocardiogr* 15:1015, 2002.
139. Baker RC, Graham AN, Phillips AS, Campalani G: An unusual iatrogenic cause of right coronary air embolism, *Ann Thorac Surg* 68:575, 1999.
140. Ohnishi Y, Uchida O, Hayashi Y, et al: [Relationship between retained microbubbles and neuropsychologic alterations after cardiac operation], *Masui* 44:1327, 1995.
141. Bickerstaff LK, Pairolero PC, Hollier LH, et al: Thoracic aortic aneurysms: A population-based study, *Surgery* 92:1103, 1982.
142. Pressler V, McNamara JJ: Thoracic aortic aneurysm: Natural history and treatment, *J Thorac Cardiovasc Surg* 79:489, 1980.
143. Crawford ES, DeNatale RW: Thoracoabdominal aortic aneurysm: Observations regarding the natural course of the disease, *J Vasc Surg* 3:578, 1986.
144. Clouse WD, Hallett JW Jr, Schaff HV, et al: Improved prognosis of thoracic aortic aneurysms: A population-based study, *JAMA* 280:1926, 1998.
145. Sioris T, David TE, Ivanov J, et al: Clinical outcomes after separate and composite replacement of the aortic valve and ascending aorta, *J Thorac Cardiovasc Surg* 128:260, 2004.
146. Feindel CM, David TE: Aortic valve sparing operations: Basic concepts, *Int J Cardiol* 97:61, 2004.
147. Nienaber CA, von Kodolitsch Y, Nicolas V, et al: The diagnosis of thoracic aortic dissection by noninvasive imaging procedures, *N Engl J Med* 328:1, 1993.
148. Roudaut RP, Billes MA, Gosse P, et al: Accuracy of M-mode and two-dimensional echocardiography in the diagnosis of aortic dissection: An experience with 128 cases, *Clin Cardiol* 11:553, 1988.
149. Suzuki T, Mehta RH, Ince H, et al: Clinical profiles and outcomes of acute type B aortic dissection in the current era: Lessons from the International Registry of Aortic Dissection (IRAD), *Circulation* 108(Suppl II):II–312, 2003.
150. Doroghazi RM, Slater EE, DeSanctis RW, et al: Long-term survival of patients with treated aortic dissection, *J Am Coll Cardiol* 3:1026, 1984.
151. Bernard Y, Zimmermann H, Chocron S, et al: False lumen patency as a predictor of late outcome in aortic dissection, *Am J Cardiol* 87:1378, 2001.
152. Umana JP, Lai DT, Mitchell RS, et al: Is medical therapy still the optimal treatment strategy for patients with acute type B aortic dissections? *J Thorac Cardiovasc Surg* 124:896, 2002.
153. Erbel R, Oelert H, Meyer J, et al: Effect of medical and surgical therapy on aortic dissection evaluated by transesophageal echocardiography. Implications for prognosis and therapy. The European Cooperative Study Group on Echocardiography, *Circulation* 87:1604, 1993.
154. Nienaber CA, Fattori R, Lund G, et al: Nonsurgical reconstruction of thoracic aortic dissection by stent-graft placement, *N Engl J Med* 340:1539, 1999.
155. Nienaber CA, Eagle KA: Aortic dissection: New frontiers in diagnosis and management: Part II: Therapeutic management and follow-up, *Circulation* 108:772, 2003.
156. Dake MD, Kato N, Mitchell RS, et al: Endovascular stent-graft placement for the treatment of acute aortic dissection, *N Engl J Med* 340:1546, 1999.
157. Nienaber CA, Eagle KA: Aortic dissection: New frontiers in diagnosis and management: Part I: From etiology to diagnostic strategies, *Circulation* 108:628, 2003.
158. Mehta RH, Suzuki T, Hagan PG, et al: Predicting death in patients with acute type A aortic dissection, *Circulation* 105:200, 2002.
159. Miller DC, Mitchell RS, Oyer PE, et al: Independent determinants of operative mortality for patients with aortic dissections, *Circulation* 70:I–153, 1984.
160. Haverich A, Miller DC, Scott WC, et al: Acute and chronic aortic dissections—determinants of long-term outcome for operative survivors, *Circulation* 72:II–22, 1985.
161. Pansini S, Gagliardotto PV, Pompei E, et al: Early and late risk factors in surgical treatment of acute type A aortic dissection, *Ann Thorac Surg* 66:779, 1998.
162. Sabik JF, Lytle BW, Blackstone EH, et al: Long-term effectiveness of operations for ascending aortic dissections, *J Thorac Cardiovasc Surg* 119:946, 2000.
163. Kawahito K, Adachi H, Yamaguchi A, Ino T: Preoperative risk factors for hospital mortality in acute type A aortic dissection, *Ann Thorac Surg* 71:1239, 2001.
164. Lai DT, Robbins RC, Mitchell RS, et al: Does profound hypothermic circulatory arrest improve survival in patients with acute type A aortic dissection? *Circulation* 106:I–218, 2002.
165. Fabian TC, Richardson JD, Croce MA, et al: Prospective study of blunt aortic injury: Multicenter Trial of the American Association for the Surgery of Trauma, *J Trauma* 42:374, 1997.
166. Fisher RG, Hadlock F: Laceration of the thoracic aorta and brachiocephalic arteries by blunt trauma. Report of 54 cases and review of the literature, *Radiol Clin North Am* 19:91, 1981.
167. Ben Menachem Y: Assessment of blunt aortic-brachiocephalic trauma: Should angiography be supplanted by transesophageal echocardiography? *J Trauma* 42:969, 1997.
168. Vignon P, Lang RM: Use of transesophageal echocardiography for the assessment of traumatic aortic injuries, *Echocardiography* 16:207, 1999.
169. Goarin JP, Cluzel P, Gosgnach M, et al: Evaluation of transesophageal echocardiography for diagnosis of traumatic aortic injury, *Anesthesiology* 93:1373, 2000.
170. Vignon P, Boncoeur MP, Francois B, et al: Comparison of multiplane transesophageal echocardiography and contrast-enhanced helical CT in the diagnosis of blunt traumatic cardiovascular injuries, *Anesthesiology* 94:615, 2001.
171. Patel NH, Stephens KE Jr, Mirvis SE, et al: Imaging of acute thoracic aortic injury due to blunt trauma: A review, *Radiology* 209:335, 1998.
172. Malhotra AK, Fabian TC, Croce MA, et al: Minimal aortic injury: A lesion associated with advancing diagnostic techniques, *J Trauma* 51:1042, 2001.
173. Goarin JP, Catoire P, Jacquens Y, et al: Use of transesophageal echocardiography for diagnosis of traumatic aortic injury, *Chest* 112:71, 1997.
174. Ott MC, Stewart TC, Lawlor DK, et al: Management of blunt thoracic aortic injuries: Endovascular stents versus open repair, *J Trauma* 56:565, 2004.
175. Scheinert D, Krankenberg H, Schmidt A, et al: Endoluminal stent-graft placement for acute rupture of the descending thoracic aorta, *Eur Heart J* 25:694, 2004.
176. Lorenzen HP, Geist V, Hartmann F, et al: Endovascular stent-graft implantation in acute traumatic aortic dissection with contained rupture and hemorrhagic shock, *Z Kardiol* 93:317, 2004.
177. Svensson LG, Labib SB, Eisenhauer AC, Butterly JR: Intimal tear without hematoma: An important variant of aortic dissection that can elude current imaging techniques, *Circulation* 99:1331, 1999.
178. Maraj R, Rerkpattanapipat P, Jacobs LE, et al: Meta-analysis of 143 reported cases of aortic intramural hematoma, *Am J Cardiol* 86:664, 2000.
179. Moizumi Y, Komatsu T, Motoyoshi N, Tabayashi K: Clinical features and long-term outcome of type A and type B intramural hematoma of the aorta, *J Thorac Cardiovasc Surg* 127:421, 2004.
180. Kang DH, Song JK, Song MG, et al: Clinical and echocardiographic outcomes of aortic intramural hemorrhage compared with acute aortic dissection, *Am J Cardiol* 81:202, 1998.
181. Song JK, Kim HS, Song JM, et al: Outcomes of medically treated patients with aortic intramural hematoma, *Am J Med* 113:181, 2002.
182. Vilacosta I, San Roman JA, Ferreiros J, et al: Natural history and serial morphology of aortic intramural hematoma: A novel variant of aortic dissection, *Am Heart J* 134:495, 1997.
183. Song JK, Yim JH, Ahn JM, et al: Outcomes of patients with acute type A aortic intramural hematoma, *Circulation* 120:2046, 2009.
184. Evangelista A, Eagle KA: Is the optimal management of acute type A aortic intramural hematoma evolving? *Circulation* 120:2029, 2009.

14

Monitoring of the Heart and Vascular System

DAVID L. REICH, MD | ALEXANDER J.C. MITTNACHT, MD |
GERARD R. MANECKE, JR., MD | JOEL A. KAPLAN, MD, CPE, FACC

KEY POINTS

1. Patients with severe cardiovascular disease and those undergoing surgery associated with rapid hemodynamic changes should be adequately monitored at all times.
2. Adequate monitoring is based on specific patient, surgical, and environmental factors.
3. Standard monitoring for cardiac surgery patients includes invasive blood pressure, electrocardiography, central venous pressure, transesophageal echocardiography, urine output, temperature, capnometry, pulse oximetry, and intermittent blood gas analysis.
4. Additional monitors used in specific patients includes a pulmonary artery catheter, left atrial pressure, cardiac outputs, or central nervous system monitoring such as the bispectral index (BIS), regional oxygen saturation, or cerebrospinal fluid pressure.
5. The American Society of Anesthesiologists has published recommendations for use of pulmonary artery catheters.
6. The Society of Cardiovascular Anesthesiologists and the American Society of Echocardiography have published recommendations for intraoperative transesophageal echocardiography (covered in Chapter 12).
7. Evidence-based data on the relation of monitoring to clinical outcomes in cardiac anesthesia are hard to obtain because of difficulties in conducting large prospective trials.
8. Minimally invasive and noninvasive techniques for hemodynamic assessment continue to be developed, with increasing functionality and accuracy. They will likely play an expanded role in the care of cardiac surgery patients.

HEMODYNAMIC MONITORING

For patients with severe cardiovascular disease and those undergoing surgery associated with rapid hemodynamic changes, adequate hemodynamic monitoring should be available at all times. With the ability to measure and record almost all vital physiologic parameters, the development of acute hemodynamic changes may be observed and corrective action may be taken in an attempt to correct adverse hemodynamics and improve outcome. Although outcome changes are difficult to prove, it is a reasonable assumption that appropriate hemodynamic

monitoring should reduce the incidence of major cardiovascular complications. This is based on the presumption that the data obtained from these monitors are interpreted correctly and that therapeutic decisions are implemented in a timely fashion.

Many devices are available to monitor the cardiovascular system. These devices range from those that are completely noninvasive, such as the blood pressure (BP) cuff and electrocardiogram (ECG), to those that are extremely invasive, such as the pulmonary artery catheter (PAC). To make the best use of invasive monitoring, the potential benefits to be gained from the information must outweigh the potential complications. In many critically ill patients, the benefit obtained does outweigh the risks, which explains the widespread use of invasive monitoring. Transesophageal echocardiography (TEE), a minimally invasive technology, provides extensive hemodynamic data and other diagnostic information and is described in detail in Chapters 11 to 13. Standard monitoring for cardiac surgical patients includes BP, ECG, central venous pressure (CVP), TEE, urine output, temperature, capnometry, pulse oximetry, and intermittent arterial blood gas analysis (Box 14-1). The next tier of monitoring includes PACs with thermodilution cardiac output (CO), other CO monitors, indices of tissue oxygen transport, and cerebral monitoring (cerebral oximetry and processed electroencephalography; Box 14-2). Rarely, left atrial pressure (LAP) catheters may still be utilized. The interpretation of these complex data requires an astute clinician who is aware of the patient's overall condition and the limitations of the monitors.

ARTERIAL PRESSURE MONITORING

BP monitoring is the most commonly used method of assessing the cardiovascular system. The magnitude of the BP is directly related to the CO and the systemic vascular resistance (SVR). This is conceptually similar to Ohm's law of electricity (voltage = current × resistance), in which BP is analogous to voltage, CO to current flow, and SVR to resistance. An increase in the BP may reflect an increase in CO or SVR, or both. Although BP is one of the easiest cardiovascular variables to measure, it gives only indirect information about the patient's cardiovascular status.

Mean arterial pressure (MAP) is probably the most useful parameter to measure in assessing organ perfusion, except for the heart, in which the diastolic blood pressure (DBP) is the most important. MAP is measured directly by integrating the arterial waveform tracing over time, or using the formula: MAP = (SBP + [2×DBP])/3, in which SBP is systolic blood pressure. The pulse pressure is the difference between SBP and DBP.

Anesthesia for cardiac surgery frequently is complicated by rapid and sudden changes in the BP because of several factors, including direct compression of the heart, impaired venous return because of retraction and cannulation of the vena cavae and aorta, arrhythmias from mechanical stimulation of the heart, and manipulations that may impair right ventricular (RV) outflow and pulmonary venous return. Sudden losses of significant amounts of blood may induce hypovolemia at almost any time. The cardiac surgical population also includes many patients with labile hypertension and atherosclerotic heart disease. A safe and reliable method of measuring acute changes in the BP is required during cardiac surgery with cardiopulmonary bypass (CPB).

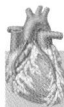

BOX 14-1. STANDARD MONITORING FOR CARDIAC SURGICAL PATIENTS

- (Invasive) blood pressure
- Electrocardiogram
- Pulse oximetry
- Capnometry
- Temperature
- Central venous pressure
- Transesophageal echocardiography
- Urine output
- Intermittent arterial blood gas analysis

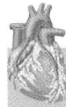

BOX 14-2. EXTENDED MONITORING FOR PATIENTS BASED ON CASE-SPECIFIC FACTORS

- Pulmonary artery catheter
- Cardiac output measurements
- Processed electroencephalography (e.g., bispectral index)
- Cerebral oximetry
- Tissue oxygenation monitoring
- Spinal drain (intrathecal) pressure

Numerous methods of noninvasive BP measurement are clinically available.[1,2] Nevertheless, most of these require the detection of flow past an occlusive cuff, and none generates an arterial waveform suitable for cardiac surgery. Continuous BP monitoring with noninvasive devices is feasible during anesthesia, but these devices have not proved to be suitable for cardiac surgery.[3,4] Intra-arterial monitoring provides a continuous, beat-to-beat indication of the arterial pressure and waveform, and having an indwelling arterial catheter enables frequent sampling of arterial blood for laboratory analyses. Direct intra-arterial monitoring remains the gold standard for cardiac surgical procedures.

The arterial waveform tracing can provide information beyond timely BP measurements. For example, the slope of the arterial upstroke correlates with the derivative of pressure over time, dP/dt, and gives an indirect estimate of myocardial contractility. This is not specific information because an increase in SVR alone also will result in an increase in the slope of the upstroke. The arterial waveform also can present a visual estimate of the hemodynamic consequences of arrhythmias, and the arterial pulse contour can be used to estimate stroke volume (SV) and CO. Hypovolemia is suggested when the arterial pressure shows large SBP variations during the respiratory cycle in the mechanically ventilated patient.[5,6] Coriat et al[7] found that TEE-derived left ventricular (LV) dimensions at end-diastole correlated well with the magnitude of SBP decrease during inspiration.

General Principles

The arterial pressure waveform ideally is measured in the ascending aorta. The pressure measured in the more peripheral arteries is different from the central aortic pressure because the arterial waveform becomes progressively more distorted as the signal is transmitted down the arterial system. The high-frequency components, such as the dicrotic notch, disappear, the systolic peak increases, the diastolic trough decreases, and there is a transmission delay. These changes are caused by decreased arterial compliance in the periphery and reflection and resonance of pressure waves in the arterial tree.[8] This effect is most pronounced in the dorsalis pedis artery, in which the SBP may be 10 to 20 mm Hg greater, and the DBP 10 to 20 mm Hg lower than in the central aorta (Figure 14-1).[9] Despite this distortion, the MAP measured in the peripheral arteries should be similar to the central aortic pressure under normal circumstances. However, this may not be the case after CPB.[10,11]

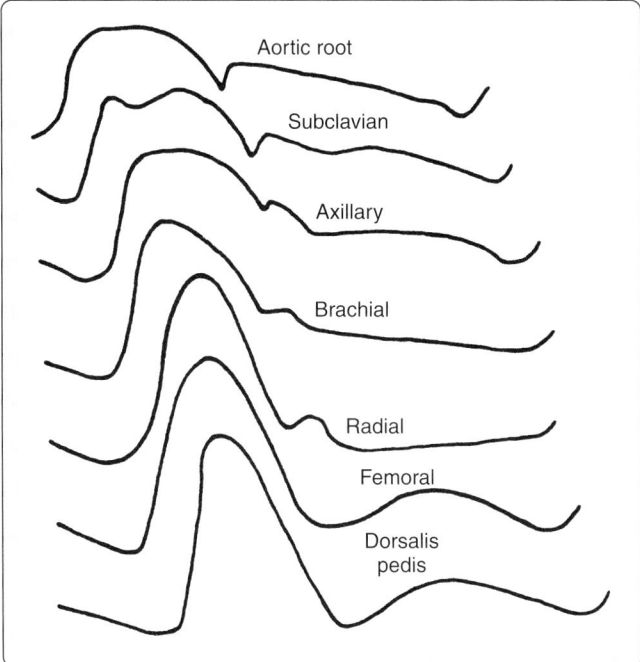

Figure 14-1 The waveform of the arterial pressure changes markedly according to the site of the intra-arterial catheter. These changes are shown as a progression from central monitoring *(top)* through peripheral monitoring *(bottom)*. These changes are thought to be caused by forward wave propagation and wave reflection. In the periphery, systolic pressure is greater, diastolic pressure is lower, and mean pressure is minimally lower. *(Modified from Bedford RF: Invasive blood pressure monitoring. In Blitt CD [ed]: Monitoring in anesthesia and critical care. New York: Churchill Livingstone, 1985, p 505.)*

Pressure waves in the arterial (or venous) tree represent the transmission of forces generated in the cardiac chambers. Measurement of these forces requires their transmission to a device that converts mechanical energy into electronic signals. The components of a system for intravascular pressure measurement include an intravascular catheter, fluid-filled tubing and connections, an electromechanical transducer, an electronic analyzer, and electronic storage and display systems.

Components of a Pressure Measurement System

Intravascular Catheters

For arterial pressure measurements, short, narrow catheters are recommended (20 gauge or smaller) because they have favorable dynamic response characteristics and are less thrombogenic than larger catheters.[12] Catheters made from Teflon are most widely used because they are softer and less thrombogenic, but they are prone to kinking. An artifact associated with intra-arterial catheters has been designated *end-pressure artifact*.[13] When flowing blood comes to a sudden halt at the tip of the catheter, it is estimated that an added pressure of 2 to 10 mm Hg results. Conversely, clot formation on the catheter tip will overdamp the system and narrow the pulse pressure.

Coupling System

The coupling system usually consists of pressure tubing, stopcocks, and a continuous flushing device. This is the major source of distortion of arterial pressure tracings. Hunziker[14] studied the damping coefficients and natural frequencies of various coupling systems. All systems were severely underdamped, and most led to systematic overestimation of the systolic arterial pressure.

Transducers

The function of transducers is to convert mechanical forces into electrical current or voltage. Over the years, this has been achieved by several different mechanisms, but today most transducers are of the resistance type. Pairs of resistors are incorporated into a circuit on the arms of a Wheatstone bridge type of electrical circuit. Most modern disposable transducers have a silicone diaphragm into which resistive elements have been etched. The manufacturers have adopted an output standard of 5 μV per volt excitation per 1 mm Hg so that, theoretically, any transducer can be used with any monitor.[15] The dynamic response of bare transducers is usually in the 100- to 500-Hz range. Modern disposable transducers have eliminated many of the difficulties that used to require frequent recalibration because of drifting of the zero point. The major practical problem remaining with transducer systems is improper zeroing relative to the patient.

Analysis and Display Systems

Most modern equipment designed to analyze and display pressure information consists of a computerized system that handles several tasks. These include the acquisition and display of pressure signals; the derivation of numerical values for systolic, diastolic, and mean pressures; alarm functions; internal data storage; automated data transfer to an anesthesia information management system; trend displays; and printing functions. The algorithms used to analyze the pressure information and to provide numerical data vary among manufacturers. Venous pressures, as well as arterial pressures, to a lesser degree, are significantly affected by respiratory fluctuations.[16] Most display systems average hemodynamic parameters over several cardiac cycles to minimize the effects of respiratory variability.

Flush Systems

The arterial catheter should be kept patent with a continuous infusion of normal saline solution (1 to 3 mL/hr). The infusion minimizes thrombus formation and helps prolong the usefulness of the catheter.[17] Heparin is no longer routinely recommended as an additive to flush solutions because of the risk for heparin-induced thrombocytopenia in susceptible patients.

Characteristics of a Pressure Measurement System

The dynamic response of a pressure measurement system is characterized by its natural frequency and its damping.[18] These concepts are best understood by snapping the end of a transducer-tubing assembly with a finger. The waveform on the monitor demonstrates rapid oscillations above and below the baseline (the natural frequency), which quickly decays to a straight line because of friction in the system (damping). The peaks and troughs of an arterial pressure waveform will be amplified if the transducer-tubing-catheter assembly has a natural frequency that lies close to the frequencies of the underlying sine waves of an arterial pressure waveform (typically < 20 Hz). This is commonly known as *ringing* or *resonance* of the system (Figure 14-2). For an arterial pressure monitoring system to remain accurate at greater heart rates (HRs), its natural frequency should, therefore, be higher, typically more than 24 Hz.[16] In practical terms, longer transducer tubing reduces the natural frequency of the system and tends to amplify the height of the SBP (peak) and the depth of the DBP (trough) values.[17,18] Boutros and Albert[19] demonstrated that, by changing the length of low-compliance (rigid) tubing from 6 inches to 5 feet, the natural frequency decreased from 34 to 7 Hz. As a result of the reduced natural frequency, the SBP measured with the longer tubing exceeded reference pressures by 17.3%.

Damping is the tendency of factors such as friction, compliant (soft) tubing, and air bubbles to absorb energy and decrease the amplitude of peaks and troughs in the waveform. The optimal degree

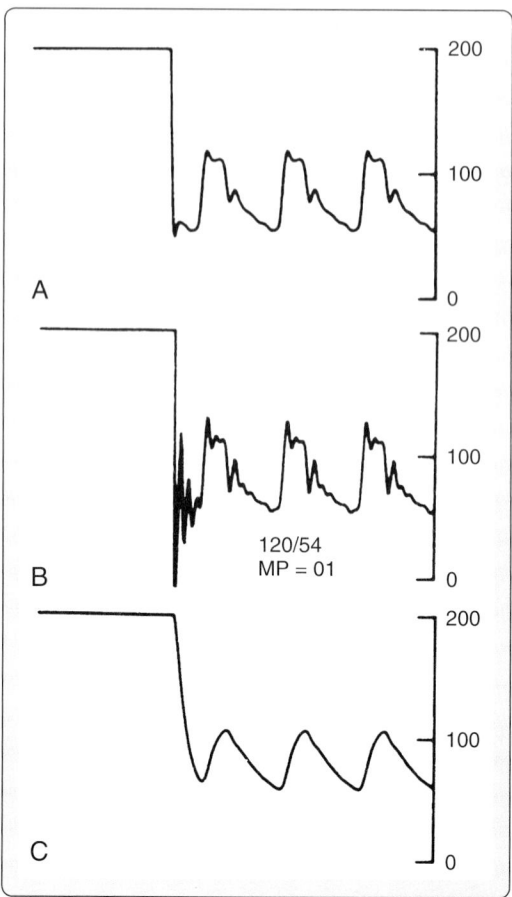

Figure 14-2 The fast-flush test demonstrates the harmonic characteristics of a pressure monitoring system (i.e., transducer, fluid-filled tubing, and intra-arterial catheter). In an optimally damped system (*A*), the pressure waveform returns to baseline after only one oscillation. In an underdamped system (*B*), the pressure waveform oscillates above and below the baseline several times. In an overdamped system (*C*), the pressure waveform returns to the baseline slowly with no oscillations. (*Adapted from Gibbs NC, Gardner RM: Dynamics of invasive pressure monitoring systems: Clinical and laboratory evaluation. Heart Lung 17:43, 1988.*)

of damping is that which counterbalances the distorting effects of transducer-tubing systems with lower natural frequencies. This is difficult to achieve. The damping of a clinical pressure measurement system can be assessed by observing the response to a rapid high-pressure flush of the transducer-tubing-catheter system (see Figure 14-2). In a system with a low damping coefficient, a fast-flush test results in several oscillations above and below the baseline before the pressure becomes constant. In an adequately damped system, the baseline is reached after one oscillation, whereas in an overdamped system, the baseline is reached after a delay and without oscillations.[20-23]

The formulas for calculating the natural frequency and damping coefficient are as follows:

$$\text{Natural frequency}: f_n = \frac{d}{8}\sqrt{\frac{3}{\pi L \rho V_d}}$$

$$\text{Damping coefficient}: \zeta \frac{16\eta}{d^3}\sqrt{\frac{3LV_d}{\pi \rho}}$$

where d = tubing diameter; L = tubing length; ρ = density of the fluid; V_d = transducer fluid volume displacement; and n = viscosity of the fluid.

Arterial Cannulation Sites

Factors that influence the site of arterial cannulation include the location of surgery, the possible compromise of arterial flow because of patient positioning or surgical manipulations, and any history of ischemia or prior surgery on the limb to be cannulated. Another factor that may influence the cannulation site is the presence of a proximal arterial cutdown. The proximal cutdown may cause damped waveforms or falsely low BP readings because of stenosis or vascular thrombosis. Surgeons may use the axillary artery as the site of cannulation for CPB in patients who require anterograde selective cerebral perfusion or with a severely diseased ascending aorta.[24–26] Depending on the surgical technique, possible complications associated with axillary (CPB) cannulation include distal limb ischemia (direct axillary artery CPB cannulation) or limb overcirculation with systemic hypoperfusion (axillary side graft anastomosis with graft cannulation).[27] Most clinicians would choose to monitor the arterial pressure in the contralateral upper extremity, but some have also advocated additional monitoring of the radial artery on the ipsilateral side to detect overcirculation to the arm and to intervene accordingly. Patients presenting for reoperation who have had prior axillary artery cannulation may have some degree of stenosis at the old cannulation site. Sites generally chosen for arterial cannulation are discussed in the following paragraphs.

Radial and Ulnar Arteries

The radial artery is the most commonly used artery for continuous BP monitoring because it is easy to cannulate with a short (20-gauge) catheter and readily accessible during surgery. The collateral circulation is usually adequate and easy to check. It is advisable to assess the adequacy of the collateral circulation and the absence of proximal obstructions before cannulating the radial artery for monitoring purposes.

The ulnar artery provides most blood flow to the hand in about 90% of patients.[28] The radial and ulnar arteries are connected by a palmar arch, which provides collateral flow to the hand in the event of radial artery occlusion. Palm[29] showed that if there is adequate ulnar collateral flow, circulatory perfusion pressure to the fingers is adequate after radial arterial catheterization. Some clinicians perform the Allen test before radial artery cannulation to assess the adequacy of collateral circulation to the hand.

The Allen test is performed by compressing the radial and ulnar arteries and exercising the hand until it is pale. The ulnar artery is then released (with the hand open loosely), and the time until the hand regains its normal color is noted.[30] With a normal collateral circulation, the color returns to the hand in about 5 seconds. If, however, the hand takes longer than 15 seconds to return to its normal color, cannulation of the radial artery on that side is controversial. The hand may remain pale if the fingers are hyperextended or widely spread apart, even in the presence of a normal collateral circulation.[31] Variations on the Allen test include using a Doppler probe or pulse oximeter to document collateral flow.[32–34] If the Allen test demonstrates that the hand depends on the radial artery for adequate filling, and other cannulation sites are not available, the ulnar artery may be selected.[35]

The predictive value of the Allen test has been challenged. In a large series of children in whom radial arterial catheterization was performed without preliminary Allen tests, there was an absence of complications.[36] Slogoff et al[37] cannulated the radial artery in 16 adult patients with poor ulnar collateral circulation (assessed using the Allen test) without any complications. An incidence of zero in a study sample of only 16 patients, however, does not guarantee that the true incidence of the complication is negligible. In contrast, Mangano and Hickey[38] reported a case of hand ischemia requiring amputation in a patient with a normal preoperative result for the Allen test. Thus, the predictive value of the Allen test is questionable. Alternatively, pulse oximetry or plethysmography can be used to assess patency of the collateral arteries of the hand. Barbeau et al[39] compared the modified Allen test with pulse oximetry and plethysmography in 1010 consecutive patients undergoing percutaneous radial artery cannulation for cardiac catheterization. Pulse oximetry and plethysmography were more sensitive

than the Allen test for detecting inadequate collateral blood supply, and only 1.5% of patients were not suitable for radial artery cannulation.

Another infrequently used method of radial arterial catheterization involves percutaneous insertion of a long catheter to obtain a central aortic tracing of arterial pressure.[40] No complications were attributed to these catheters in a series of patients.[41] The advantage of a central arterial tracing is the increased accuracy compared with radial arterial pressure in patients with low-flow states or after CPB.[42,43] Although reasons for the difference between central and peripheral measurements of BP are not entirely clear, after CPB, they are transiently present in 17% to 40% of patients in several studies.[11,44–46] Kanazawa et al[47] suggested that a decrease in the arterial elasticity is responsible for instances in which lower radial artery pressures (compared with aortic pressures) are observed after CPB. When the palpated central aortic pressure is high despite a low radial arterial BP value, the central aortic pressure also may be temporarily monitored using a needle attached to pressure tubing placed in the aorta by the surgeon until the problem resolves. Alternatively, a femoral arterial catheter may be inserted.

Chest wall retractors that are used during internal mammary artery dissection may impede radial arterial pressure monitoring in cardiothoracic procedures in some patients. The arm on the affected side may have diminished perfusion during extreme retraction of the chest wall. If the left internal mammary artery is used during myocardial revascularization, the right radial artery could be monitored to avoid this problem. Alternatively, a noninvasive BP cuff on the right side could be used to confirm the accuracy of the radial artery tracing during periods of chest wall retraction.

Monitoring of the radial artery distal to a brachial arterial cutdown site is not recommended. Acute thrombosis or residual stenosis of the brachial artery will lead to falsely low radial arterial pressure readings.[19] Other considerations related to the choice of a radial arterial monitoring site include prior surgery of the hand, selection of the nondominant hand, and the preferences of the surgeons and anesthesiologists.

Brachial and Axillary Arteries

The brachial artery lies medial to the bicipital tendon in the antecubital fossa, in close proximity to the median nerve. Brachial artery pressure tracings resemble those in the femoral artery, with less systolic augmentation than radial artery tracings.[48] Brachial arterial pressures were found to more accurately reflect central aortic pressures than radial arterial pressures before and after CPB.[49] The complications from percutaneous brachial artery catheter monitoring are fewer than those after brachial artery cutdown for cardiac catheterization.[50] A few series of patients with perioperative brachial arterial monitoring have documented the relative safety of this technique.[11,42,50] Armstrong et al[51] published data on 1326 patients with peripheral vascular disease undergoing angiography with percutaneous brachial artery access and found an overall complication rate of 1.28% with a greater risk for thrombosis in female patients. There is little or no collateral flow to the hand if brachial artery occlusion occurs, however. Most clinicians, therefore, choose other sites, if possible.

The axillary artery is normally cannulated by the Seldinger technique near the junction of the deltoid and pectoral muscles. This has been recommended for long-term catheterization in the intensive care unit (ICU) and in patients with peripheral vascular disease.[52,53] Because the tip of the 15- to 20-cm catheter may lie within the aortic arch, the use of the left axillary artery is recommended to minimize the risk for cerebral embolization during flushing. Lateral decubitus positioning or adduction of the arm occasionally results in kinking of axillary catheters with damping of the pressure waveform. Arterial pressures measured in the axillary artery (by radial artery cannulation with long catheters) more closely reflect central aortic BP than brachial arterial BP measurements.[45]

Femoral Artery

The femoral artery may be cannulated for monitoring purposes and typically provides a more reliable central arterial pressure after discontinuation of CPB. Scheer et al[54] have reviewed the literature on peripheral artery cannulation for hemodynamic monitoring, including 3899 femoral artery cannulations. Temporary occlusion was found in 10 patients (1.45%), whereas serious ischemic complications requiring extremity amputation were reported in 3 patients (0.18%). Other complications that were summarized from the published data were pseudoaneurysm formation (0.3%), sepsis (0.44%), local infection (0.78%), bleeding (1.58%), and hematoma (6.1%). Based on the reviewed literature, they concluded that using the femoral artery for hemodynamic monitoring purposes was safer than radial artery cannulation. Older literature stated that the femoral area was intrinsically dirty, and that catheter sepsis and mortality were significantly increased compared with other monitoring sites. This could not be confirmed in the more recent literature.[55,56]

In patients undergoing thoracic aortic surgery, distal aortic perfusion (using partial CPB, left-heart bypass, or a heparinized shunt) may be performed during aortic cross-clamping to preserve spinal cord and visceral organ blood flow. In these situations, it is useful to measure the distal aortic pressure at the femoral artery or a branch vessel (i.e., dorsalis pedis or posterior tibial artery) to optimize the distal perfusion pressure (see Chapter 21). In repairs of aortic coarctation, simultaneous femoral and radial arterial monitoring may help determine the adequacy of the surgical repair by documenting the pressure gradient after the repair. It is necessary to consult with the surgeon before cannulating the femoral vessels because these vessels may be used for extracorporeal perfusion or placement of an intra-aortic balloon pump during the surgical procedure.

Dorsalis Pedis and Posterior Tibial Arteries

The two main arteries to the foot are the dorsalis pedis artery and the posterior tibial artery, which form an arterial arch on the foot that is similar to the one formed by the radial and ulnar arteries in the hand. The dorsalis pedis or posterior tibial arteries are reasonable alternatives to radial arterial catheterization. The SBP is usually 10 to 20 mm Hg greater in the dorsalis pedis artery than in the radial or brachial arteries, whereas the diastolic pressure is 15 to 20 mm Hg lower (see Figure 14-1).[57] The dorsalis pedis is a relatively small artery that may be cannulated when other sites are not available, but the vessel may not be palpable or present in 5% to 12% of patients.[58] The incidence rate of failed cannulation is up to 20%, and the incidence rate of thrombotic occlusion is about 8%, because of the small size of the artery.[59] A modified Allen test may be performed by blanching the great toe during compression of the dorsalis pedis and posterior tibial arteries, and then releasing the pressure over the posterior tibial artery. These vessels should not be used in patients with severe peripheral vascular disease from diabetes mellitus or other causes.

Indications

The indications for invasive arterial monitoring are provided in Box 14-3.

Contraindications

The contraindications to arterial cannulation include local infection, coagulopathy, proximal obstruction, vaso-occlusive disorders, and surgical considerations.

Local Infection

Placement of an arterial catheter through infected tissues is likely to result in catheter sepsis. If signs of infection develop at an existing arterial cannulation site, the catheter must be removed. A separate cannulation site should be found. Strict aseptic technique is necessary during the insertion and maintenance of arterial cannulas.

Coagulopathy

Coagulopathy is a relative contraindication because it may result in hematoma formation during arterial cannulation. It is more difficult to apply direct arterial pressure with failed attempts or when the catheter is

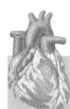

BOX 14-3. INDICATIONS FOR INTRA-ARTERIAL MONITORING

- Major surgical procedures involving large fluid shifts or blood loss
- Surgery requiring cardiopulmonary bypass
- Surgery of the aorta
- Patients with pulmonary disease requiring frequent arterial blood gases
- Patients with recent myocardial infarctions, unstable angina, or severe coronary artery disease
- Patients with decreased left ventricular function (congestive heart failure) or significant valvular heart disease
- Patients in hypovolemic, cardiogenic, or septic shock, or with multiple organ failure
- Procedures involving the use of deliberate hypotension or deliberate hypothermia
- Massive trauma cases
- Patients with right-heart failure, chronic obstructive pulmonary disease, pulmonary hypertension, or pulmonary embolism
- Patients requiring inotropes or intra-aortic balloon counterpulsation
- Patients with electrolyte or metabolic disturbances requiring frequent blood samples
- Inability to measure arterial pressure noninvasively (e.g., morbid obesity)

removed when using more central cannulation sites. In anticoagulated patients, it is therefore recommended that more peripheral arterial cannulation sites be considered when this form of monitoring is required.

Proximal Obstruction

Anatomic factors may lead to intra-arterial pressure readings that markedly underestimate the central aortic pressure. The thoracic outlet syndrome and congenital anomalies of the aortic arch vessels will obstruct flow to the upper extremities. Aortic coarctation will diminish flow to the lower extremities. Arterial pressure distal to a previous arterial cutdown or cannulation site may be lower than the central aortic pressure because of arterial stenosis at the site of the prior intervention.

Raynaud Syndrome and Buerger Disease

Radial and brachial arterial cannulations are contraindicated in patients with a history of Raynaud syndrome or Buerger disease (i.e., thromboangiitis obliterans). This is especially important in the perioperative setting because hypothermia of the hand is the main trigger for vasospastic attacks in Raynaud syndrome.[60] It is recommended that large arteries, such as the femoral or axillary, be used for intra-arterial monitoring if indicated in patients with either of these diseases.

Surgical Considerations

Several surgical maneuvers may interfere with intra-arterial monitoring. During mediastinoscopy, the scope intermittently compresses the innominate artery against the manubrium. In this situation, accurate systemic arterial pressure monitoring may be affected if a right-sided upper extremity arterial cannula is used. Regardless of which side is chosen for arterial cannulation, a pulse oximeter probe should be placed on the opposite hand. In case a left-sided arterial catheter is chosen, accurate systemic pressure readings can be monitored and compression of the innominate artery detected by a diminished pulse oximetry signal. Depending on the surgeon's and/or anesthesiologist's preference, this setup can be reversed.

The lateral decubitus position may compromise flow to the downward arm if an axillary roll is not properly positioned. In this situation, the damping may be prolonged. Nevertheless, during descending thoracic aortic aneurysm repairs, the right radial, brachial, or axillary artery should be monitored because the left subclavian artery may be occluded during various phases of the procedure.

◼ Insertion Techniques

Direct Cannulation

Proper technique is helpful in obtaining a high degree of success in arterial catheterization. The wrist is often placed in a dorsiflexed position on an armboard over a pack of gauze and immobilized in a supinated position. Overextension of the wrist should be avoided because this flattens and decreases the cross-sectional area of the radial artery[61] and may cause median nerve damage by stretching the nerve over the wrist. A 20-gauge or smaller, 3- to 5-cm, nontapered Teflon catheter over needle is used to make the puncture. If a syringe is used, the plunger may be removed to allow free flow of blood to detect when the artery has been punctured. The angle between the needle and the skin should be shallow (≤30 degrees), and the needle should be advanced parallel to the course of the artery. When the artery is entered, the angle between the needle and skin is reduced to 10 degrees, the needle is advanced another 1 to 2 mm to ensure that the tip of the catheter also lies within the lumen of the vessel, and the outer catheter is then threaded off the needle while watching that blood continues to flow out of the needle hub (Figure 14-3).

Transfixation

If blood ceases flowing while the needle is being advanced, the needle has penetrated the back wall of the vessel. In this technique, the artery has been transfixed by passage of the catheter-over-needle assembly "through-and-through" the artery. The needle is then completely withdrawn. As the catheter is slowly withdrawn, pulsatile blood flow emerges from the catheter when its tip is within the lumen of the artery. The catheter is then slowly advanced into the artery. A guidewire may be helpful at this point if the catheter does not advance easily into the artery. Alternatively, the catheter-over-needle assembly may be withdrawn slowly as one unit until flow of blood has returned. As soon as this occurs, the needle and catheter are most likely in the lumen of the artery and the catheter may be gently threaded off the needle into the artery.

Seldinger Technique

The artery is localized with a needle, and a guidewire is passed through the needle into the artery. A catheter is then passed over the guidewire into the artery. Alternatively, a catheter-over-needle assembly may be inserted in the artery in a through-and-through fashion, the needle withdrawn, and the wire passed through the catheter after pulsatile flow is encountered. It is important when using this technique to avoid withdrawal of guidewires through needles to prevent shearing of the wire and embolization. Mangar et al[62] showed that when using the direct or modified Seldinger technique compared with a direct-cannulation method, the success rate of arterial catheter placement increased from 62% to 82%.

Doppler-Assisted Technique

The artery is localized using a Doppler flow probe. The direction of insertion of the percutaneous catheter is guided by the acoustic Doppler signal.[63,64] This may be especially useful in small children and infants. In adults, this may be helpful when palpation of the artery is difficult, such as in obese patients requiring femoral arterial cannulation. With the more widespread availability of two-dimensional and color-Doppler ultrasonic devices, the acoustic Doppler-assisted method is used much less frequently.

Two-Dimensional Ultrasound-Assisted Method

The Doppler-assisted techniques have been supplanted in clinical practice by two-dimensional (2D) ultrasonic methods. Levin et al[65] randomized patients in a prospective study to ultrasound-guided (UG) radial artery cannulation versus a classic palpation technique. The use of ultrasound (US) resulted in a greater success rate on the first attempt, and fewer subsequent attempts were required to place the arterial catheter. The overall time for catheter placement was not significantly different between the two groups (trend for shorter overall time in UG group). In a similar study, Shiver et al[66] randomized patients in the emergency department to UG versus traditional palpation technique radial artery catheter placement. Patients in the UG group required a significantly shorter time (107 vs. 314 seconds; $P = 0.0004$), fewer placement attempts (1.2 vs. 2.2; $P = 0.001$), and fewer sites required for successful arterial catheter placement. The use of US in guiding arterial catheter placement is easy to learn when proper training in this technique is provided. There is, however, a significant learning curve, and studies reporting on the success rate of UG arterial cannulation compared with a traditional palpation technique have to be interpreted accordingly. Ganesh et al,[67] for example, did not find a significant difference in the time and attempts required in a pediatric patient population randomized to palpation versus UG radial artery catheter placement. None of the designated operators, however, had significant experience with this technique, with 19 of 20 pediatric subspecialty trainees and/or fully trained consultant anesthesiologists reporting experience with fewer than 5 cases. Figure 14-4 shows a proper full-sterile setup for UG arterial cannulation. Figure 14-5 demonstrates the "triangulation" technique typically applied with UG venous or arterial cannulation, or both. The US imaging plane and the needle plane can

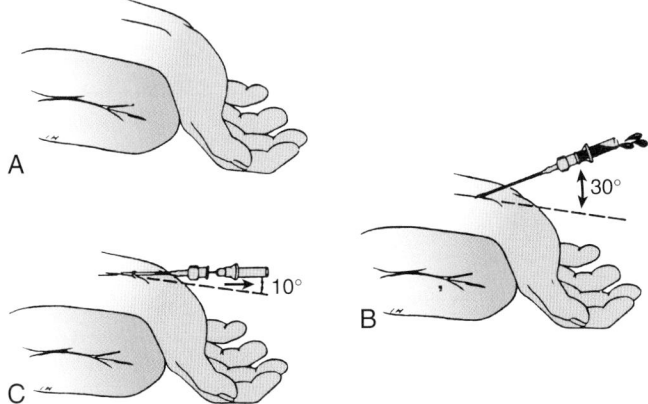

Figure 14-3 **The direct-cannulation technique for the radial artery.** *A,* The wrist is dorsiflexed over a towel or a small pack of gauze and loosely taped to a stable surface such as an armboard. *B,* The artery is directly cannulated at a 30- to 40-degree angle to the plane of the wrist. Arterial blood flows steadily into the "flashback" chamber. *C,* The catheter-over-needle assembly is lowered until the angle is approximately 10 degrees to the plane of the wrist. The entire assembly is advanced another 1 to 2 mm, until the tip of the catheter lies within the lumen of the artery. The catheter is then advanced into the artery completely while the needle is held motionless. *(From Lake CL: Cardiovascular anesthesia. New York: Springer-Verlag, 1985, p 54.)*

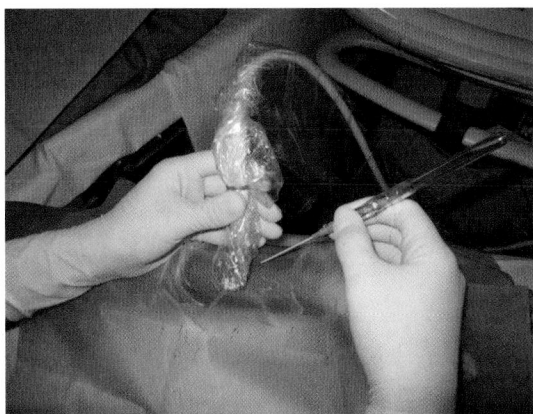

Figure 14-4 Demonstration of aseptic technique for ultrasonic guidance of radial artery cannulation.

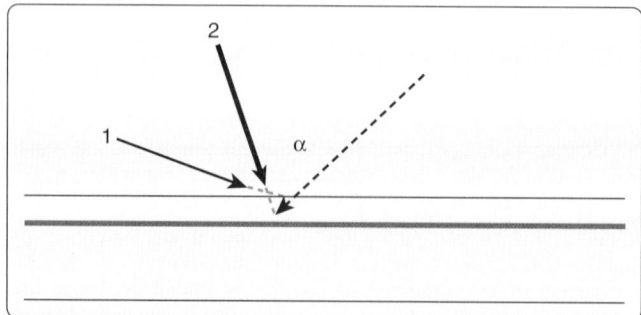

Figure 14-5 Demonstration of the "triangulation" technique typically applied with ultrasound-guided venous and/or arterial cannulation in the transverse imaging approach. The echo imaging plane and the needle plane can be viewed as the two sides of a triangle that should meet/intersect at the depth of the structure (e.g., radial artery [red line]) for which cannulation is attempted. The experienced operator will change the angle (α) between the two planes (ultrasound and needle) and the distance (needle insertion site vs. imaging plane) depending on the depth of the structure. The echo plane has to be further adjusted from needle entry through the skin to the perforation of the vessel to follow the needle tip in the transverse approach (vessel viewed in short axis). A greater angle is used (echo plane angled toward the skin [1]) to visualize the needle tip after it penetrates the skin, and then a more perpendicular angle relative to the skin is applied to see the needle tip entering the vessel lumen (2).

be viewed as the two sides of a triangle that should meet/intersect at the depth of the structure (e.g., radial artery) for which cannulation is attempted. The experienced operator will change the angle between the two planes (US and needle) and the distance (needle insertion site vs. imaging plane) depending on the depth of the structure. The US plane has to be adjusted further from needle entry through the skin to the perforation of the vessel to follow the needle tip in the transverse approach (vessel viewed in short axis). Figures 14-6 and 14-7 show typical US images obtained during short-axis (transverse) cannulation. Note the anatomic variation with a large (A1) radial artery next to a smaller size artery (A2) positioned laterally.

If a longitudinal ("in-plane") approach is chosen (i.e., the vessel viewed in its long axis), the needle tip can be followed more easily as it is advanced; however, structures adjacent to the US plane (lateral to the vessel) cannot be viewed simultaneously. For this reason, most practitioners prefer the transverse approach. Figure 14-8 shows the arterial catheter entering the radial artery using the longitudinal (in-plane)

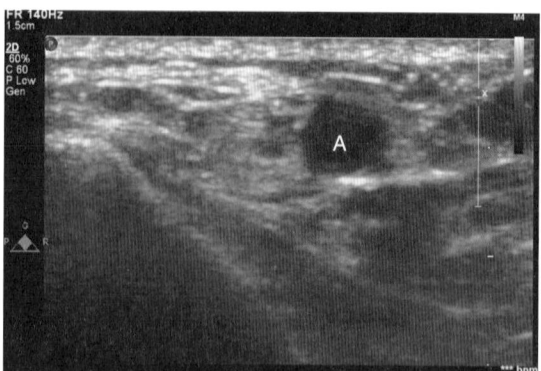

Figure 14-7 A typical ultrasound image during short-axis (transverse) cannulation.

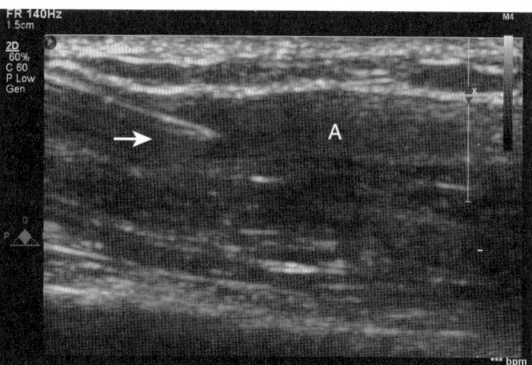

Figure 14-8 A catheter entering the radial artery using the longitudinal (in-plane) approach.

approach. Aseptic technique, including sterile sheaths, should always be used during UG of intra-arterial catheter placement to prevent catheter-related infections. A high-frequency linear array ultrasonic transducer (8 to 12 MHz) is optimal for UG arterial catheter placement because higher frequencies are needed for high-resolution imaging of the near field. Box 14-4 summarizes potential benefits and concerns related to UG arterial catheter placement.

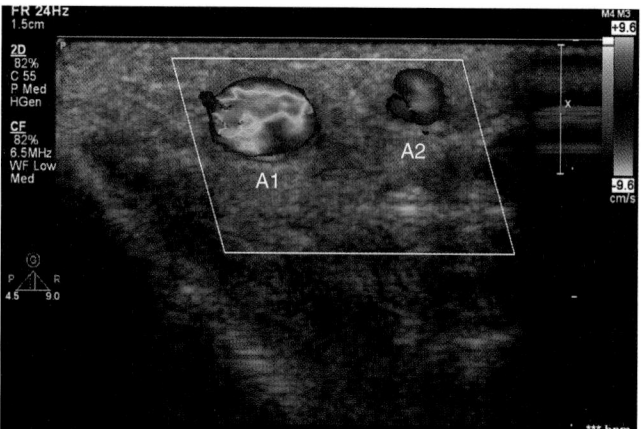

Figure 14-6 A typical ultrasound image with color Doppler during short-axis (transverse) cannulation. Note the anatomic variation with a large (A1) radial artery next to a smaller size artery (A2) positioned laterally.

BOX 14-4. ULTRASOUND-GUIDED ARTERIAL CANNULATION

Benefits
- Greater success rate on first attempt
- Fewer overall attempts
- Increased patient comfort (fewer attempts)
- Fewer complications (e.g., anticoagulated patients)
- Demonstration of vessel patency, anatomic variants
- Low or nonpulsatile flow (e.g., nonpulsatile assist devices, extracorporeal membrane oxygenation [ECMO], shock)
- Nonpalpable or weakly palpable pulses (e.g., peripheral edema, hematoma)
- Emergency access (e.g., catheter placement during resuscitation)

Concerns
- Risk for catheter-related infections if poor aseptic technique is applied
- Additional training required
- Costs involved with equipment required

Surgical Cutdown

An incision is made in the skin overlying the artery, and the surrounding tissues are dissected away from the arterial wall. Proximal and distal ligatures are passed around the artery to control blood loss but are not tied down. Under direct vision, the artery is cannulated with a catheter-over-needle assembly. Alternatively, a small incision is made in the arterial wall to facilitate passage of the catheter.

Complications

Infection

One potential complication that is common to all forms of invasive monitoring is infection from indwelling catheters. Indwelling percutaneous catheters can become infected because of insertion through an infected skin site, poor aseptic technique during insertion or maintenance, sepsis with seeding of the catheter, and prolonged duration of cannulation with colonization by skin flora. Historically, factors that were associated with catheter infection included nondisposable transducer domes, dextrose flush solutions, contaminated blood gas syringes, and duration of insertion.[68–71] In contrast with central venous catheterization, published data on vascular catheter infections did not find that full sterile barriers during arterial catheter placement reduced the risk for infection.[72,73] Nevertheless, these data do not exempt the practitioner from using strict aseptic technique. Guidelines for the prevention of intravascular catheter-related infections have been published by the Hospital Infection Control Practices Advisory Committee and the Centers for Disease Control and Prevention.[74]

It is still common practice to remove percutaneous catheters when vascular catheter infection is suspected. This concept has been challenged, and a watchful waiting strategy has been advocated until a catheter-related bloodstream infection has been confirmed instead of immediate removal of the catheter.[75] Whenever infection at the cannulation site or a catheter-related bloodstream infection is confirmed, the catheter should be removed. The catheter is a foreign body that cannot be sterilized with antibiotic therapy. Lymphangitic streaks or cellulitis may occur as a result of catheter infection. These problems require systemic antibiotic therapy.[76]

Hemorrhage

The use of an intra-arterial catheter carries the potential risk for major blood loss or exsanguination if the catheter or tubing assembly becomes disconnected. The use of Luer-Lok (instead of tapered) connections and monitors with low-pressure alarms should decrease the risk for this complication.[77] Stopcocks are an additional source of occult hemorrhage because of the potential for loose connections or inadvertent changes in the position of the control lever that would open the system to the atmosphere.

Thrombosis and Distal Ischemia

Thrombosis of the radial artery after cannulation has been extensively studied. Temporary arterial occlusion is the most commonly reported complication after radial artery cannulation.[54] Factors that correlate with an increased incidence of thrombosis include prolonged duration of cannulation,[78] larger catheters,[79] and smaller radial artery size (i.e., a greater proportion of the artery is occupied by the catheter).[80] The incidence of thrombosis is not affected by the technique of cannulation[81] but is reduced with aspirin pretreatment.[82]

The association between radial artery thrombosis and ischemia of the hand is less certain. An abnormal result for Allen test was not associated with hand complications after radial artery cannulation.[37] Despite the widespread use of radial artery cannulation, hand complications are rarely reported. Temporary occlusion after arterial cannulation is usually benign. Nevertheless, serious ischemic complications have been reported that required the amputation of a digit or extremity.[83–85] In the experience of Slogoff et al,[37] most ischemic complications occurred in

patients who had had multiple embolic phenomena from other sources or were on high-dose vasopressor therapy with resultant ischemia in multiple extremities.

The hand should be examined at regular intervals in patients with axillary, brachial, radial, or ulnar arterial catheters. Because thrombosis may appear several days after the catheter has been removed, examinations should be continued through the postoperative period. Although recanalization of the thrombosed artery can be expected in an average of 13 days, the collateral blood flow may be inadequate during this period.[12] Any evidence of hand ischemia should be investigated and treated promptly to prevent morbidity.[86]

The treatment plan should involve consultation with a vascular, hand, or plastic surgeon. Traditionally, treatment for arterial occlusion or thrombosis with adequate collateral flow has been conservative. However, fibrinolytic agents (e.g., streptokinase), stellate ganglion blockade, and surgical intervention are modalities that should be considered.

Skin Necrosis

Volar proximal skin necrosis has been reported in patients after radial arterial cannulation.[87,88] This has led to full-thickness skin loss over the volar aspect of the forearm. The skin necrosis is presumably caused by thrombosis of the radial artery with proximal propagation of the thrombosis to involve the cutaneous branches of the radial artery.

Embolization

Particulate matter or air that is flushed forcefully into an arterial catheter can move proximally, as well as distally, within the artery. Cerebral embolization is most likely from axillary cannulation sites but is also possible with brachial and radial artery catheters.[89,90] Emboli from the right arm are more likely to reach the cerebral circulation than those from the left arm because of the usual anatomy and direction of blood flow in the aortic arch. Other factors that influence the likelihood of cerebral embolization include the volume of flush solution, the rapidity of the injection, and the proximity of the intraluminal end of the catheter to the central circulation.[89,91,92]

Hematoma and Neurologic Injury

Hematoma formation may occur at any arterial puncture or cannulation site and is particularly common with a coagulopathy. Hematoma formation should be prevented by the application of direct pressure after arterial punctures and, if possible, the correction of any underlying coagulopathy. Posterior puncture/tear of the femoral or iliac arteries can produce massive bleeding into the retroperitoneal area.[93] Surgical consultation should be obtained if massive hematoma formation develops.

Nerve damage is possible if the nerve and artery lie in a fibrous sheath (e.g., the brachial plexus) or in a limited tissue compartment (e.g., the forearm).[94] Direct nerve injuries may also occur from needle trauma during attempts at arterial cannulation. The median nerve is in close proximity to the brachial artery, and the axillary artery lies within the brachial plexus sheath.

Late Vascular Complications

Incomplete disruption of the wall of an artery may eventually result in pseudoaneurysm formation.[95] The wall of the pseudoaneurysm is composed of fibrous tissue that continues to expand. If the pseudoaneurysm ruptures into a vein or if both a vein and artery are injured simultaneously, an arteriovenous fistula may result. Nonsurgical treatment options for the repair of pseudoaneurysms after arterial cannulation have been described and may replace surgery that is usually performed to treat this complication.[96]

Inaccurate Pressure Measurements

Despite the great advantages of intra-arterial monitoring, it does not always give accurate BP values. The monitoring system may be incorrectly zeroed and calibrated, or the transducers may not be at the appropriate level. The waveform will be damped if the catheter is kinked or partially thrombosed. In vasoconstricted patients, those in hypovolemic shock, and during the post-CPB period, the brachial and radial artery pressures may be significantly lower than the true central aortic pressure. Another possible cause of inaccurate measurements is unsuspected arterial stenosis proximal to the monitored artery, as occurs with thoracic outlet syndrome and subclavian stenosis. Unsuspected Raynaud syndrome also can yield unreliable BP readings from peripheral arteries.

CENTRAL VENOUS PRESSURE MONITORING

CVP catheters are used to measure the filling pressure of the right ventricle, give an estimate of the intravascular volume status, and assess RV function. For accurate pressure measurement, the distal end of the catheter must lie within one of the large intrathoracic veins or the right atrium (RA). In any pressure monitoring system, it is necessary to have a reproducible landmark (such as the midaxillary line) as a zero reference. Frequent changes in patient positioning without proper leveling of the transducers relative to the patient's left atrium (LA) produce proportionately larger errors compared with arterial pressure monitoring.

The normal CVP waveform consists of three upward deflections (A, C, and V waves) and two downward deflections (X and Y descents; Figure 14-9). The A wave is produced by right atrial contraction and occurs just after the P wave on the ECG. The C wave occurs because of the isovolumic ventricular contraction, forcing the tricuspid valve (TV) to bulge upward into the RA. The pressure within the RA then decreases as the TV is pulled away from the atrium during RV ejection, forming the X descent. Right atrial filling continues during late ventricular systole, forming the V wave. The Y descent occurs when the TV opens and blood from the RA empties rapidly into the right ventricle during early diastole.[97]

The CVP waveform may be useful in the diagnosis of pathologic cardiac conditions. For example, onset of an irregular rhythm and loss of the A wave suggest atrial flutter or fibrillation. Cannon A waves

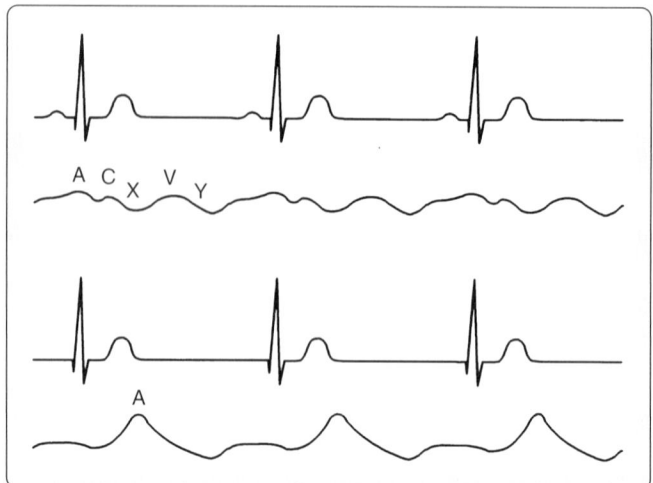

Figure 14-10 The relation of the central venous pressure (CVP) tracing to the electrocardiogram (ECG) during junctional (atrioventricular nodal) rhythm. The contraction of the atrium against the closed tricuspid valve results in the cannon A waves; notice that the P wave is hidden within the QRS complex of the ECG.

occur as the RA contracts against a closed TV, as occurs in junctional (atrioventricular nodal) rhythm, complete heart block, and ventricular arrhythmias (Figure 14-10). This is clinically relevant because nodal rhythms are frequently seen during anesthesia and may produce hypotension because of a decrease in SV. Cannon A waves may also be present when there is increased resistance to RA emptying, as in tricuspid stenosis, RV hypertrophy, pulmonary stenosis, or pulmonary hypertension. Early systolic or holosystolic "cannon V waves" (or C-V waves) occur if there is a significant degree of tricuspid regurgitation (TR). Large V waves may also appear later in systole if the ventricle becomes noncompliant because of ischemia or RV failure. A comprehensive review of CVP waveform analysis in various pathophysiologic states has been published by Mark.[98]

Pericardial constriction produces characteristic waveforms in the CVP tracing (Figure 14-11). There is a decrease in venous return because of the inability of the heart chambers to dilate because of the constriction. This causes prominent A and V waves and steep X and Y descents (creating an M configuration) resembling that seen with diseases that cause decreased RV compliance. Egress of blood from the RA to the right ventricle is initially rapid during early diastolic filling of the right ventricle (creating a steep Y descent) but is short-lived and abruptly halted by the restrictive, noncompliant right ventricle. The right atrial pressure then increases rapidly and reaches a plateau until the end of the A wave, at the end of diastole. This portion of the waveform is analogous to the ventricular diastolic dip-and-plateau sign.[98] With pericardial tamponade, the X descent is steep, but the Y descent is not present because early diastolic runoff is impaired by the pericardial fluid collection.

The CVP is a useful monitor if the factors affecting it are recognized and its limitations are understood. The CVP reflects the patient's blood volume, venous tone, and RV performance. Following serial measurements (trends) is more useful than individual numbers. The response of the CVP to a volume infusion is a useful test. Thromboses of the vena cavae and alterations of intrathoracic pressure, such as those induced by positive end-expiratory pressure (PEEP), also affect measurement of the CVP.[99] Many peaks and troughs in the CVP waveform are created artifactually from the transducer-tubing monitoring system. Tachycardia produces blending of the waveforms, especially the A and C waves.

The CVP does not give a direct indication of left-heart filling pressure, but it may be used as an estimate of left-sided pressures in patients with good LV function. Mangano[100] showed a good correlation between

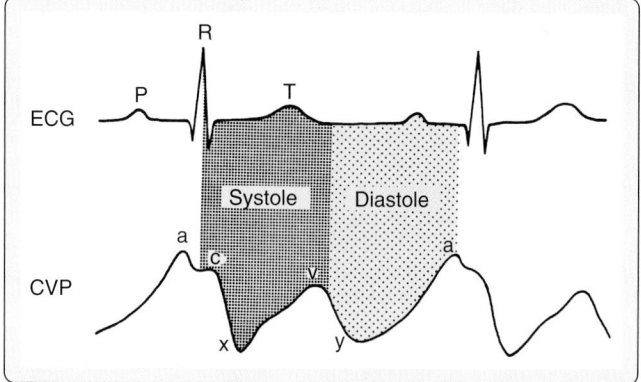

Figure 14-9 Relation of the central venous pressure (CVP) tracing to the electrocardiogram (ECG) in normal sinus rhythm. The normal CVP waveform consists of three upward deflections (A, C, and V waves) and two downward deflections (X and Y descents). The A wave is produced by right atrial contraction and occurs just after the P wave on the ECG. The C wave occurs because of the isovolumic ventricular contraction forcing the tricuspid valve to bulge upward into the right atrium (RA). The pressure within the RA then decreases as the tricuspid valve is pulled away from the atrium during right ventricular ejection, forming the X descent. The RA continues to fill during late ventricular systole, forming the V wave. The Y descent occurs when the tricuspid valve opens and blood from the RA empties rapidly into the RV during early diastole. *(Adapted from Mark JB: Central venous pressure monitoring: Clinical insights beyond the numbers. J Cardiothorac Vasc Anesth 5:163, 1991.)*

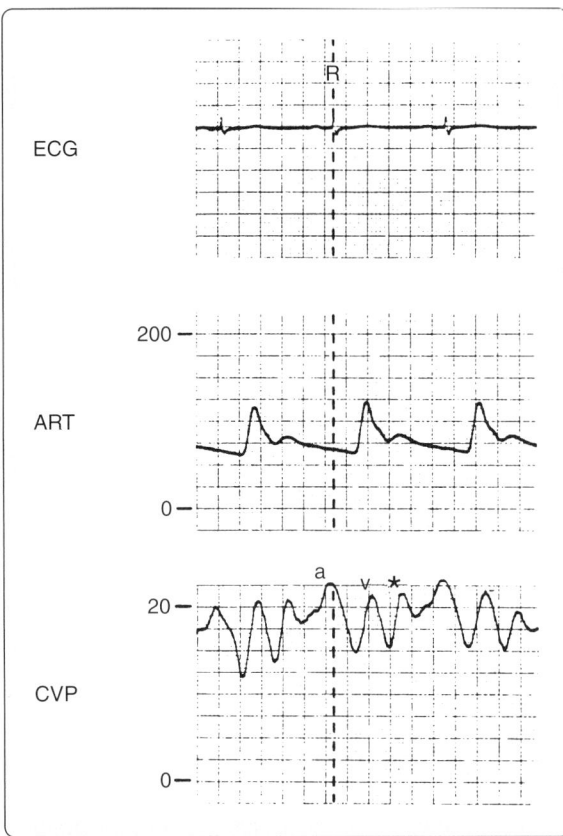

Figure 14-11 Central venous pressure (CVP) waveform during pericardial constriction. There is a characteristic M configuration with prominent A and V waves, accompanied by steep X and Y descents. An additional wave *(asterisk)* is present because of impairment of ventricular filling by the rigid pericardial shell. ART, arterial pressure; ECG, electrocardiogram. *(Adapted from Mark JB: Central venous pressure monitoring: Clinical insights beyond the numbers. J Cardiothorac Vasc Anesth 5:163, 1991.)*

the CVP and left-sided filling pressures during a change in volume status in patients with coronary artery disease and left ventricular ejection fraction greater than 0.4. Later studies have not replicated these results, demonstrating weak relations between the CVP and measures of LV preload.[101–104]

Techniques and Insertion Sites

Percutaneous central venous cannulation may be accomplished by catheter-through-needle, catheter-over-needle, or catheter-over-wire (Seldinger) techniques. The considerations for selecting the site of cannulation include the experience of the operator, ease of access, anatomic anomalies, and the ability of the patient to tolerate the position required for catheter insertion.

Internal Jugular Vein

Cannulation of the internal jugular vein (IJV) was first described by English et al[105] in 1969. Its popularity among anesthesiologists has steadily increased since that time. Advantages of this technique include the high success rate as a result of the relatively predictable relation of the anatomic structures; a short, straight course to the RA that almost always assures RA or superior vena cava (SVC) localization of the catheter tip; easy access from the head of the operating room table; and fewer complications than with subclavian vein catheterization. The IJV is located under the medial border of the lateral head of the sternocleidomastoid (SCM) muscle (Figure 14-12). The carotid artery is usually deep and medial to the IJV. The right IJV is preferred because this vein takes the straightest course into the SVC, the right cupola of the lung may be lower than the left, and the thoracic duct is on the left side.[106]

The preferred *middle approach* to the right IJV is shown in Figure 14-13. Trendelenburg position is typically chosen to distend the IJV; however, this position can be complicated by hypoxemia in cardiac surgical patients breathing room air, and nasal oxygen may ameliorate this problem. Trendelenburg position is not necessary when venous distention is present in the supine position as occurs in patients with a high CVP or right-sided heart failure. The head is then turned toward the contralateral side, and the fingers of the left hand are used to palpate the two heads of the SCM muscle and the carotid pulse.

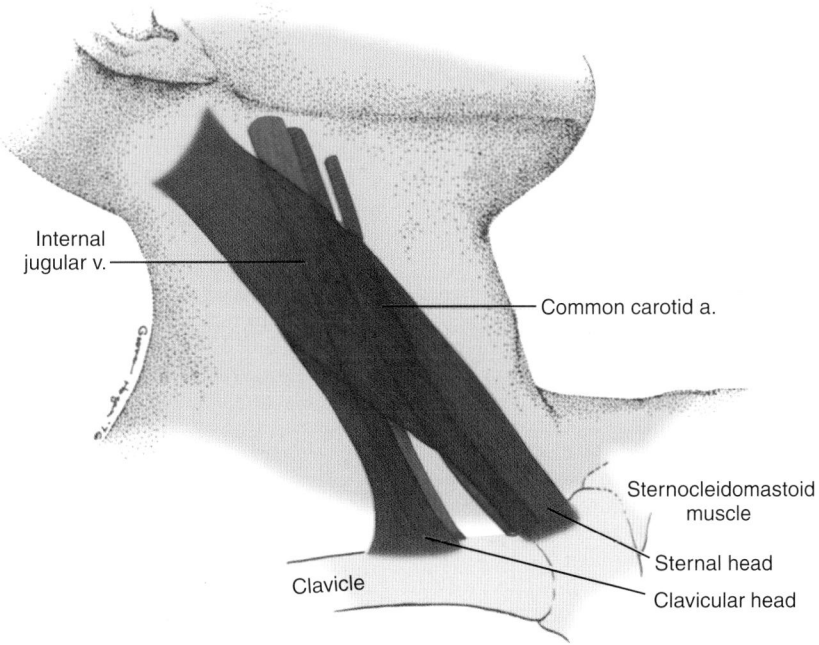

Figure 14-12 The internal jugular vein (v.) is usually located deep to the medial border of the lateral head of the sternocleidomastoid muscle, just lateral to the carotid pulse. a., artery.

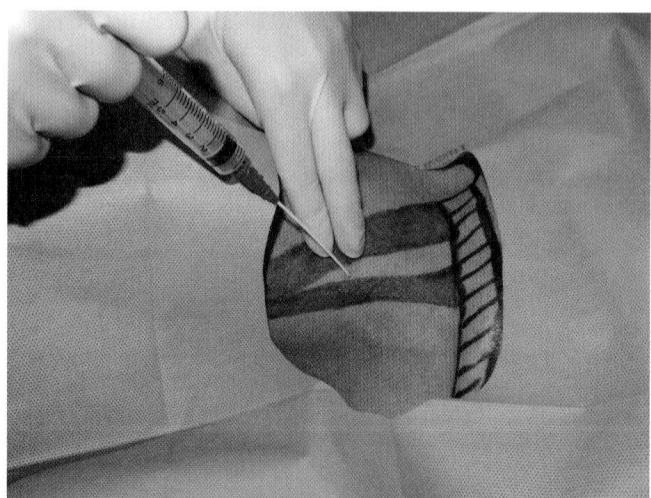

Figure 14-13   Preferred middle approach to the right internal jugular vein. The needle enters the skin at the apex of the triangle formed by the sternal and clavicular heads of the sternocleidomastoid muscle. The needle is held at a 30- to 45-degree angle to the skin and directed toward the ipsilateral nipple.

These fingers then hold the skin stable over the underlying structures while local anesthetic is infiltrated into the skin and subcutaneous tissues. A 22-gauge "finder" needle is placed at the apex of the triangle formed by the two heads of the SCM muscle at a 45-degree angle to the skin and directed toward the ipsilateral nipple. If venous blood return is not obtained, the needle is withdrawn to the subcutaneous tissue and then passed in a more lateral or medial direction until the vein is located. This small needle reduces the risk for consequences related to inadvertent carotid arterial puncture and tissue trauma if localization of the vein is difficult. When venous blood is aspirated through the "finder" needle, the syringe and needle are withdrawn, leaving a small trail of blood on the drape to indicate the direction of the vein. Alternatively, the needle and syringe can be fixated and used as an identifying needle. Then, a syringe attached to an 18-gauge intravenous catheter-over-needle is inserted in an identical fashion. When venous return is present, the whole assembly is lowered to prevent the needle from going through the posterior wall of the central vein and advanced an additional 1 to 2 mm until the tip of the catheter is within the lumen of the vein. The catheter is then threaded into the vein. The correct intravenous catheter position should be confirmed before placing a large-bore introducer sheath. It has been recommended to attach the cannula to a transducer by sterile tubing to observe the pressure waveform.[107,108] In a prospective study of 1284 patients, Jobes et al[109] diagnosed 10 episodes of arterial catheterization by this technique of pressure monitoring not recognized by other signs. Another option is to attach the cannula to sterile tubing and allow blood to flow retrograde into the tubing.[110] The tubing is then held upright as a venous manometer, and the height of the blood column is observed. If the catheter is in a vein, it will stop rising at a level consistent with the CVP and demonstrate respiratory variation. The blood column also can be aspirated to the top of the tubing and then observed as it drops down to the CVP level, demonstrating it is in a vein and not an artery. Maintaining proper aseptic technique is crucial to prevent catheter-related infections, and all-inclusive kits that include manometry tubing are available commercially. Despite its reported use in the past, color comparison and observation of nonpulsatile flow are notoriously inaccurate methods of determining that the catheter is not in the carotid artery. A guidewire is then passed through the 18-gauge catheter, and the catheter is exchanged for the wire. If a TEE probe has been previously inserted, proper intravenous position can further be confirmed by imaging the guidewire in the SVC and RA. The use of more than one technique to confirm the venous location of the guidewire may provide additional reassurance of correct placement

before cannulation of the vein with a larger catheter or introducer. Once it is certain that the guidewire is in the venous circulation, the CVP catheter is passed over it and the wire is removed.

Many other approaches to the right IJV have been described.[111] An anterior (high) approach to the IJV is performed at the level of the laryngeal cartilage. The needle enters the skin at the medial border of the SCM muscle and is directed lateral to the carotid artery pulse. The posterior approach to the IJV is performed near the intersection of the external jugular vein (EJV) and the lateral border of the SCM muscle. The needle is directed along the posterior surface of the SCM muscle toward the sternal notch. In this technique, the needle is aimed in the direction of the carotid artery, and the incidence of carotid artery puncture therefore may be greater. These alternative approaches are less successful and produce more complications than the standard middle approach in the experience of most clinicians.

Ultrasonic Guidance of Internal Jugular Vein Cannulation
Clinical Evidence for Ultrasound-Guided Internal Jugular Vein Cannulation

US increasingly has been used for central venous access, in particular, to guide IJV cannulation and to define the anatomic variations of the IJV.[112] There is now evidence that using US to guide central venous cannulation increases success rate and helps prevent complications and, thus, ultimately may help improve patient outcome. Troianos et al[113] compared UG IJV cannulation with a traditional landmark technique. Fewer attempts to successful cannulation were required, and the rate of complications such as carotid artery puncture was decreased in the UG group. More recent prospective studies confirmed these findings. Serafimidis et al,[114] in a prospective observational study, compared UG IJV cannulation with a landmark technique (347 patients vs. 204 patients, respectively). UG cannulation had a greater success rate, required fewer attempts, took less time, and had fewer complications. Further evidence comes from several published meta-analyses comparing the UG versus traditional IJV landmark techniques.[115,116] Overall, most studies have demonstrated that 2D UG IJV cannulation has a greater success rate on the first attempt and fewer complications.[117–121] Those findings also were confirmed in pediatric patients.[122–127] Only one study reported that UG IJV cannulation in children was less successful, had a greater incidence of arterial puncture, and that there was no time difference compared with the landmark method.[128]

Box 14-5 lists some of the recognized benefits and concerns of UG central venous cannulation. Circumstances in which ultrasonic guidance of IJV cannulation can be particularly advantageous include patients with difficult neck anatomy (e.g., short neck, obesity), prior neck surgery, anticoagulated patients, and infants.

BOX 14-5. ULTRASOUND-GUIDED CENTRAL VENOUS CANNULATION

Benefits
- Greater success rate on first attempt
- Fewer overall attempts
- Facilitates access with difficult neck anatomy (obesity, prior surgery)
- Fewer complications (e.g., carotid artery puncture, anticoagulated patients)
- Demonstration of vessel patency, anatomic variants
- Relatively inexpensive technology

Concerns
- Training personnel to maintain aseptic technique when using sterile probe sheaths
- Additional training required
- Lack of observation of surface anatomy
- Potential loss of landmark-guided skills when needed for emergency central venous catheterization

Technical Aspects

US has provided more precise data regarding the structural relation between the IJV and the carotid artery (see Figure 14-12). Troianos et al[129] found that, in more than 54% of patients, more than 75% of the IJV overlies the carotid artery. Patients who were older than 60 years were more likely to have this type of anatomy. Figure 14-14 shows the anatomic relation between the IJV and the carotid artery in two patients. In pediatric patients, Alderson et al[130] found that the carotid artery coursed directly posterior to the IJV in 10% of patients. Sulek et al[131] observed that there was greater overlap of the IJV and the carotid artery when the head is rotated 80 degrees compared with head rotation of only 0 to 40 degrees. The data from 2 and 4 cm above the clavicle did not differ, and the percentage overlap was larger on the left side of the neck compared with the right. Excessive rotation of the head of the patient toward the contralateral side may distort the normal anatomy in a manner that increases the risk for inadvertent carotid artery puncture. US has also been used to demonstrate that the Valsalva maneuver increases IJV cross-sectional area by approximately 25%, and that the Trendelenburg position increases it by approximately 37%.[132] Parry[133] showed that maximal right IJV diameter can be achieved by placing the patient in 15-degree Trendelenburg position, slightly elevating the head with a small pillow, keeping the head close to midline, and releasing the pressure administered to palpate the carotid artery before IJV cannulation. Box 14-6 summarizes some of the positional considerations in UG IJV cannulation.

For central venous catheterization, full aseptic technique is mandatory. After patient positioning and sterile preparation of the neck, a full-body sterile drape is applied and the probe is covered in a sterile sheath. Figure 14-15 demonstrates proper sterile technique and positioning of the US probe. A triangulation technique, as described earlier, is typically used. Although the long-axis (in-plane) approach allows better visualization of the true needle tip throughout the insertion and vessel penetration, the simultaneous display of IJV and its relation to the carotid artery is lost. In addition, the size of the US probe in patients with shorter neck anatomy often does not provide adequate room for an in-plane approach to the IJV. Most practitioners, therefore, choose the short-axis (out-of-plane) approach to UG IJV cannulation. The most important aspect of imaging a needle out of plane is avoiding

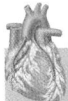

BOX 14-6. POSITIONAL CONSIDERATIONS IN ULTRASOUND-GUIDED RIGHT INTERNAL JUGULAR VENOUS CANNULATION

- Slight Trendelenburg position
- Head turned slightly away from cannulation side (turning too far may flatten IJV and rotate IJV above carotid artery)
- Overextension of head should be avoided, mild head elevation can be advantageous (overextension flattens IJV)
- Release of palpating finger pressure before puncture (avoid compression of IJV)
- Ultrasound probe should scan the course of the IJV to find best cannulation site (large IJV diameter and least overlap with carotid artery)

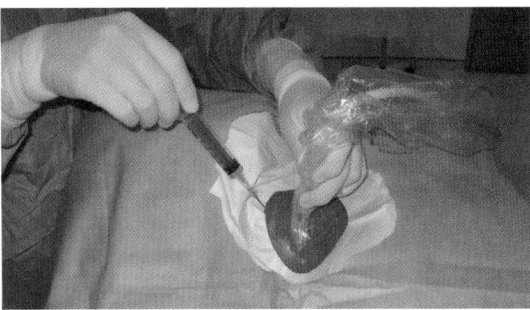

Figure 14-15 Demonstration of aseptic technique and positioning of the ultrasonic probe for internal jugular vein cannulation.

the mistake of visualizing the needle shaft rather than the needle tip. Otherwise, the needle tip could be in a structure not being imaged, such as the carotid artery and pleura. With experience, the practitioner will be able to follow the true needle tip as it enters the IJV. Additional favorable signs are indentation of the anterior wall of

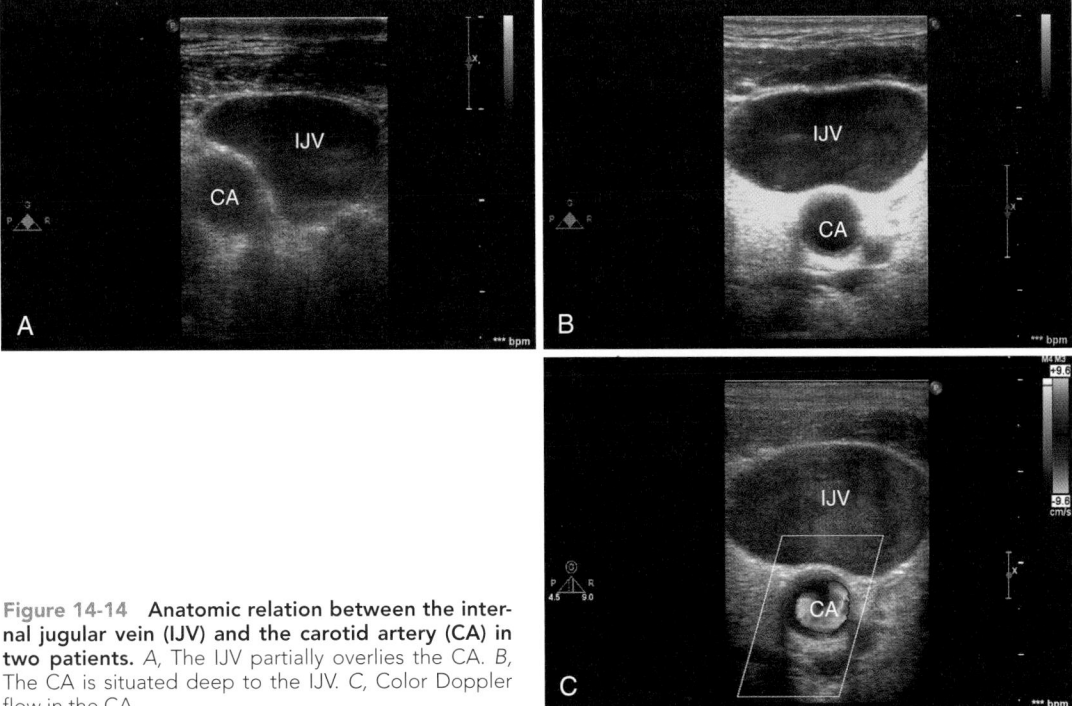

Figure 14-14 **Anatomic relation between the internal jugular vein (IJV) and the carotid artery (CA) in two patients.** *A,* The IJV partially overlies the CA. *B,* The CA is situated deep to the IJV. *C,* Color Doppler flow in the CA.

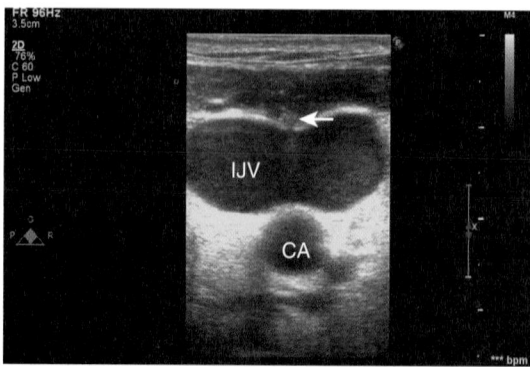

Figure 14-16 The thin-walled internal jugular vein (IJV) is compressed by the advancing needle *(arrow)* during IJV cannulation. CA, carotid artery.

the IJV as the needle tip encounters the vessel wall. Figure 14-16 demonstrates the thin-walled IJV as it is indented by the advancing needle tip. It is important to realize that UG IJV cannulation has reduced, but not eliminated, inadvertent carotid arterial cannulation, and that the insertion of large catheters into the carotid artery with US guidance has been reported.[134-138] Venous cannulation always should be confirmed before vessel dilation or insertion of the large-bore catheter/introducer sheath.[108] As noted earlier, manometry, pressure transduction, blood gas analysis, or guidewire visualization using fluoroscopy or TEE imaging of the guidewire in the SVC or RA (Figure 14-17) are all reasonable methods of assuring venous cannulation before inserting a large-bore sheath.

Current Recommendations

Ultrasonic guidance is not yet the standard of care for IJV cannulation.[139,140] Several national medical agencies have released recommendations, however, that strongly support the use of UG IJV cannulation. The Agency for Healthcare Research and Quality in the United States lists UG central catheter placement as 1 of 11 patient safety practices with the greatest strength of evidence supporting its use to improve patient outcome.[141] The National Institute of Clinical Excellence in the United Kingdom[142] also recommends UG IJV cannulation for children and adults. The availability of US equipment[143] and the associated costs of required hardware and training have been raised as reasons for lack of universal adoption of this technique. This is despite the fact that UG central catheter placement is easily accomplished, with evidence of improved patient outcomes. There is also some evidence that the use of UG central catheter placement is cost-effective even when initial hardware purchase and training are taken into consideration.[144]

External Jugular Vein

Although the EJV is another means of reaching the central circulation, the success rate with this approach is lower because of the tortuous path

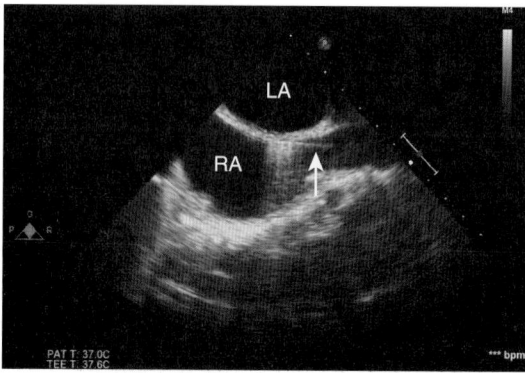

Figure 14-17 Position of the guidewire in the right atrium (RA) confirms that central venous cannulation was achieved in the midesophageal bicaval view. LA, left atrium.

followed by the vein. A valve is usually present at the point where the EJV perforates the fascia to join with the subclavian vein. One study, however, reported a success rate of 90% using a J-wire to manipulate past obstructions into the central circulation.[145] The main advantage of this technique is that there is no need to advance a needle into the deeper structures of the neck.

For this approach, the patient is placed supine or in the Trendelenburg position until the EJV becomes distended. The vein is then cannulated with an intravenous catheter. A guidewire with curved tip (i.e., J-wire) is passed through the cannula and manipulated into the central circulation. The curved tip is necessary to negotiate the tortuous course between the EJV and the SVC. Manipulation of the shoulder and rotation of the guidewire between the operator's fingers may be useful maneuvers when difficulty is encountered in passing the wire into the SVC.

Subclavian Vein

The subclavian vein is readily accessible from supraclavicular or infraclavicular approaches and has long been used for central venous access.[146] The success rate is greater than the EJV approach but lower than the right IJV approach. Cannulation of the subclavian vein is associated with a greater incidence of complications than the IJV approach, especially pneumothorax. Other complications associated with subclavian vein cannulation are arterial punctures, misplacement of the catheter tip, aortic injury, cardiac tamponade, mediastinal hematoma, and hemothorax.[147,148] This may be the cannulation site of choice, however, when CVP monitoring is indicated in patients undergoing carotid artery surgery. It is also useful for parenteral nutrition or for prolonged CVP access because the site is easier to maintain and well tolerated by patients.

The *infraclavicular approach* is performed with the patient supine or in the Trendelenburg position with a folded sheet between the scapulae and the shoulder lowered[149] (Figure 14-18). The head is turned to the contralateral side. A thin-walled needle or intravenous catheter is inserted 1 cm below the midpoint of the clavicle and advanced toward the suprasternal notch under the posterior surface of the clavicle. When a free flow of venous blood is obtained, the guidewire is passed into the subclavian vessel and is exchanged for a CVP catheter.

The *supraclavicular approach* is performed with the patient in the Trendelenburg position with the head turned away from the side of the insertion. This is usually not performed on the left side because of

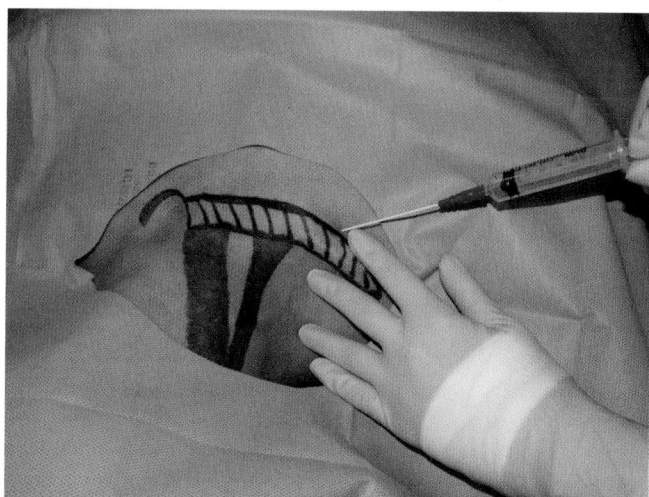

Figure 14-18 **Infraclavicular approach to the right subclavian vein.** The patient is positioned with a rolled towel between the scapulae to increase the distance between the clavicle and the first rib. The needle enters the skin 1 cm inferior to the midpoint of the clavicle and is directed underneath the clavicle toward the sternal notch. If the needle is directed too far posteriorly, the pleura may be punctured, resulting in a pneumothorax.

the risk for an injury to the thoracic duct. The finder needle is inserted at the lateral border of the SCM at the point of insertion into the clavicle. The needle is directed to bisect the angle between the SCM and the clavicle, about 15 to 20 degrees posteriorly. The vessel is very superficial (about 1 to 2 cm) and lies close to the innominate artery and the pleura.

Antecubital Veins

Another route for CVP monitoring is through the basilic or cephalic veins. The advantages of this approach are the low likelihood of complications and the ease of access intraoperatively, if the arm is exposed. The major disadvantage is that it is often difficult to assure placement of the catheter in a central vein. Studies have indicated that blind advancement will result in central venous cannulation in 59% to 75% of attempts.[150,151] Chest radiographs are usually necessary to confirm that the tip of the catheter has been appropriately placed, and this involves some time delay. Exact positioning of the catheter tip is crucial because movement of the arm will result in significant catheter migration and could cause cardiac tamponade.[152–154] Unsuccessful attempts result most frequently from failure to pass the catheter past the shoulder or cannulation of the ipsilateral IJV. Turning the head to the ipsilateral side may help prevent IJV placement of the catheter.[155]

Artru et al[156] reported a high success rate (92%) for the placement of multiorificed catheters from the antecubital veins using intravascular electrocardiography. These catheters are positioned at the SVC-RA junction and are used for the aspiration of air emboli in neurosurgical patients. Because of problems inherent with intravascular electrocardiography, Mongan et al[157] described a method for transducing the pressure waveform and identifying the point at which the catheter tip entered the right ventricle. They then calculated the distance required to withdraw the catheters to the SVC-RA junction (for three different types of air embolism-aspirating catheters). Others have used TEE to assist in the correct placement of these types of catheters.[158] Even though peripherally placed central venous catheters avoid the placement of needles into deep venous structures, there are still significant risks associated with their use.[159–162]

Femoral Vein

The femoral vein is rarely cannulated in the adult patient for intraoperative monitoring purposes. However, cannulation of this vein is technically simple and the success rate is high. Cannulation of the vessel should be done about 1 to 2 cm below the inguinal ligament. The vein typically lies medial to the artery. The older literature reported a high rate of catheter sepsis and thrombophlebitis with this approach. Although the incidence of complications is likely reduced with aseptic technique, disposable catheter kits, and improved catheter technology, femoral catheterization is not recommended in elective central venous catheterization when other sites are practical as part of multidisciplinary efforts to reduce central catheter-associated bloodstream infections.[163–165] In patients with SVC obstruction, the femoral vein is necessary for intravenous access and to obtain a true CVP measurement. The catheter should be long enough so that the tip lies within the mediastinal portion of the inferior vena cava.

▨ Indications

CVP monitoring is often performed to obtain an indication of intravascular volume status. The accuracy and reliability of CVP monitoring depend on many factors, including the functional status of the right and left ventricles, the presence of pulmonary disease, and ventilatory factors, such as PEEP. The CVP may reflect left-heart filling pressures, but only in patients with good LV function. Perioperative indications for the insertion of a central venous catheter are listed in Box 14-7.

The CVP should be monitored in all patients during CPB. When the catheter tip is in the SVC, it indicates right atrial pressure and cerebral venous pressure. Significant increases in CVP can produce critical decreases in cerebral perfusion pressure. This is occasionally caused

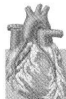

BOX 14-7. INDICATIONS FOR CENTRAL VENOUS CATHETER PLACEMENT

- Major operative procedures involving large fluid shifts or blood loss in patients with good heart function
- Intravascular volume assessment when urine output is not reliable or unavailable (e.g., renal failure)
- Major trauma
- Surgical procedures with a high risk for air embolism, such as sitting-position craniotomies in which the central venous pressure catheter may be used to aspirate intracardiac air
- Frequent venous blood sampling
- Venous access for vasoactive or irritating drugs
- Chronic drug administration
- Inadequate peripheral intravenous access
- Rapid infusion of intravenous fluids (using large cannulae)
- Total parenteral nutrition

by a malpositioned SVC cannula during CPB and must be corrected immediately by the surgeon to avoid cerebral edema and poor cerebral perfusion. Artifactually increased CVP readings can be seen with bicaval CPB venous cannulation (tip of CVP or PAC compressed next to fixated SVC cannula), and/or excessive vacuum use on CPB. In those instances, the pressure transducer should be connected to the most proximal catheter tip such as the introducer side-port instead.

▨ Contraindications

Absolute Contraindications

The SVC syndrome is a contraindication to placing a CVP catheter in the jugular veins, subclavian veins, or the upper extremities. Venous pressures in the head and upper extremities are increased by the SVC obstruction and do not reflect right atrial pressure. Medications that are administered into the obstructed venous circulation reach the central circulation by collateral vessels in a delayed fashion. Rapid fluid administration into the obstructed venous circulation may exacerbate the increased venous pressures and cause more pronounced edema. The mild SVC syndrome seen with some ascending aortic aneurysms, however, does not represent a contraindication to central venous cannulation of the upper body.

Relative Contraindications

Coagulopathies predispose to hemorrhagic complications of CVP placement, such as airway obstruction from a neck hematoma, hemothorax, or hematoma collection with subsequent infection. Newly inserted pacemaker and/or implantable cardioverter/defibrillator wires may be dislodged during the insertion of CVP catheters. This could result in severe arrhythmias, especially if the patient is pacemaker dependent. In general, it is preferable to wait 4 to 6 weeks before placing a central catheter in a patient with newly inserted pacemaker/defibrillator wires.

▨ Complications

The complications of central venous cannulation can be divided into three categories: complications of vascular access, complications of catheter insertion, or complications of catheter presence. These are summarized in Box 14-8, and specific information regarding several of the complications is detailed in this section.

Inadvertent arterial puncture during central venous cannulation is not uncommon.[166,167] The two main reasons why this phenomenon occurs are that all veins commonly used for cannulation lie in close proximity to arteries (except the EJV and cephalic) and that the venous anatomy is quite variable. Localized hematoma formation is the usual consequence. This may be minimized if a small-gauge needle is initially used to localize the vein or ultrasonic guidance is used.

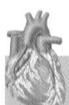

BOX 14-8. COMPLICATIONS OF CENTRAL VENOUS CATHETERIZATION

Complications of Central Venous Access and Cannulation
- Arterial puncture with hematoma
- Arteriovenous fistula
- Hemothorax
- Chylothorax
- Pneumothorax
- Nerve injury
- Brachial plexus injury
- Stellate ganglion injury (Horner syndrome)
- Air embolus
- Catheter or wire shearing
- Right atrial or right ventricular perforation

Complications of Catheter Presence
- Thrombosis, thromboembolism
- Infection, sepsis, endocarditis
- Arrhythmias
- Hydrothorax

If the arterial puncture is large, direct pressure may be difficult to apply secondary to the location of the artery. If the patient has a coagulopathy, a massive hematoma may form. In the neck, this may lead to airway obstruction requiring urgent tracheal intubation. In the arm or leg, venous obstruction may occur. If the artery is cannulated with a large-bore catheter, a surgical consultation may be required before its removal. Reports about successful percutaneous repair of inadvertent arterial injuries after central venous cannulation have been published.[168,169]

Arteriovenous fistulas from the carotid artery to the IJV also have been reported after central venous cannulation.[170,171] Hemothorax may occur if the subclavian artery is lacerated during cannulation attempts. Symptoms of hypovolemia may predominate because of the large capacity of the pleural cavity.[172]

Injury to the thoracic duct resulting in chylothorax has been reported after left IJV and left subclavian vein cannulation.[173,174] Fear of this complication is one of the major reasons for selecting right-sided IJV and subclavian approaches for central venous cannulation. This is a serious problem that may require surgical treatment.[175]

If the pleural cavity is entered and lung tissue is punctured during a cannulation attempt, a pneumothorax may result. Tension pneumothorax is possible if air continues to accumulate because of a "ball-valve" effect. Pneumothorax is most common with subclavian punctures and occurs only rarely with IJV cannulation.[176,177]

The brachial plexus, stellate ganglion, and phrenic nerve all lie in close proximity to the IJV. These structures may be injured during cannulation attempts. Paresthesias of the brachial plexus are not uncommon during attempts to localize the IJV. Direct needle trauma is the most likely cause of paresthesias or motor deficits, and this risk is somewhat increased by the long-beveled needles used for vascular access.[178,179] Transient deficits may result from the deposition of local anesthetic in the brachial plexus, stellate ganglion, or cervical plexus. A large hematoma or pseudoaneurysm could result in nerve injury after an inadvertent arterial puncture.[180] Horner's syndrome has also been reported after IJV cannulation.[181]

Venous air embolism is a potentially fatal complication that can occur when there is negative pressure in the venous system. Paradoxic embolization is a risk if there is a patent foramen ovale or another intracardiac defect, such as an atrial or ventricular septal defect. During central venous cannulation, air embolism usually can be prevented with positional maneuvers, such as the Trendelenburg position, which increase the venous pressure in the vessel. Once the CVP catheter has been placed, it is important to assure that the catheter is firmly attached to its connecting tubing. Air embolism may even occur after the catheter has been removed, if the subcutaneous tract persists.[182]

The diagnosis of venous air embolism is likely when there is a sudden onset of tachycardia associated with pulmonary hypertension and systemic hypotension. A new murmur may be heard because of turbulent flow in the RV outflow tract. 2D echocardiography (transesophageal or transthoracic) and precordial Doppler probe monitoring are highly sensitive methods of detecting air embolism. Venous air embolism is most effectively treated by aspirating the air by a catheter positioned at the SVC-RA junction. An older (and probably less effective) method involves turning the patient to the left lateral decubitus position to move the embolus out of the RV outflow tract.

Catheter or guidewire fragments may be sheared off by the inserting needle and embolize to the right heart and pulmonary circulation when catheter-through-needle or Seldinger-type cannulation kits are used. It is also possible to lose a guidewire within the patient by not withdrawing a sufficient length of the wire to grasp it at the external end before inserting the catheter.[183] The catheter fragment position within the right-sided circulation will determine whether surgery or percutaneous transvenous techniques are necessary for its removal.[184]

These problems can almost always be avoided using proper technique. A catheter must never be withdrawn through the inserting needle. Reinsertion of needles into standard (catheter-over-needle) intravenous cannulae cannot be recommended but should certainly never be performed if the cannula is kinked or resistance is encountered. Similarly, guidewires should not be inserted through cannulae if blood return is not present or forcefully inserted if resistance is encountered. In addition, guidewires should not be withdrawn through inserting needles. During unsuccessful catheterization, the needle and catheter or needle and guidewire must be withdrawn simultaneously.

If right atrial or RV perforation occurs during central venous cannulation, pericardial effusion or tamponade may result. The likelihood of this complication is increased when inflexible guidewires, long dilators, or catheters are used. This complication also has been reported with the use of an indwelling polyethylene catheter.[185] In an in vitro model, Gravenstein et al[186] evaluated the perforating aspects of central venous catheters. An angle of incidence less than 40 degrees, single-orifice catheters, polyurethane catheters, silicone rubber, and pigtail-tip catheters all significantly decreased the risk for perforation compared with conventional catheters.

Oropello et al[187] suggested that the dilators used in many of the central venous catheter kits may be a major cause of vessel perforation. They believe that the dilator may bend the guidewire, creating its own path, causing it to perforate a vessel wall. Several kits have dilators that are much longer than the catheters, and they constitute a further risk factor for possible perforation of the heart or vessels.

The physiology of fluid accumulation in the pericardial sac is such that sudden cardiovascular collapse occurs once a critical volume has been reached. This is explained by the compliance curve of the normal pericardium. The curve is flat until the critical volume is reached and then rises steeply with any further increment in volume. If pericardial tamponade is imminent, immediate pericardiocentesis is indicated. A long needle attached to a syringe is directed through the skin at the junction of the xiphoid process and the sternum on the left side, and directed toward the left shoulder. The needle is advanced while suction is maintained with the syringe until free-flowing blood is obtained. US guidance is often used. An ECG electrode can show an injury current (e.g., ST-segment elevation) when the needle is in contact with the myocardium. Withdrawal of small volumes of blood results in marked hemodynamic improvement because of the nature of pericardial compliance (see Chapter 22).

If the catheter tip is placed extravascularly in the pleural cavity or erodes into this position, the fluid that is infused into the catheter will accumulate in the pleural cavity (hydrothorax). The diagnosis is made by auscultation, percussion, and radiography of the chest. A pleurocentesis or thoracostomy (chest) tube might be necessary, and surgical consultation may be required.

Transient atrial and ventricular arrhythmias commonly occur as the guidewire is passed into the RA or right ventricle during central venous cannulation using the Seldinger technique. This most likely results from the relatively inflexible guidewire causing extrasystoles as it contacts the endocardium. Ventricular fibrillation during guidewire insertion has been reported.[188] The same investigators reported a 70% reduction in the incidence of arrhythmias when guidewire insertion was limited to 22 cm.

There are also reports of complete heart block caused by guidewire insertion during central venous cannulation.[189] These cases can be successfully managed using a temporary transvenous or external pacemaker. This complication previously has been reported with pulmonary artery catheterization. The problem most likely resulted from excessive insertion of the guidewire, with impingement of the wire in the region of the right bundle branch. It is recommended that the length of guidewire insertion be limited to the length necessary to reach the SVC-RA junction to avoid these complications. It is also imperative to monitor the patient appropriately (e.g., ECG and pulse monitoring), and to have resuscitative drugs and equipment immediately available when performing central venous catheterization.

Strict aseptic technique is required to minimize catheter-related infections. Full barrier precautions during insertion of central venous catheters have been shown to decrease the incidence of catheter-related infections.[74,190] Subcutaneous tunneling of central venous catheters inserted into the internal jugular and femoral veins,[191,192] antiseptic barrier-protected hub for central venous catheters,[193] and antiseptic/antibiotic-impregnated short-term central venous catheters[194,195] have been shown to reduce catheter-related infections.[196] It is well established that 2% chlorhexidine is now the standard skin preparation for skin antisepsis (except in neonates and infants) and is associated with a reduced risk for catheter-related infections, despite studies suggesting that povidone-iodine solution was equally effective.[197–200] Hospital policies differ with respect to the permissible duration of catheterization at particular sites, but routine replacement of central venous catheters to prevent catheter-related infections is not recommended.[201,202]

PULMONARY ARTERIAL PRESSURE MONITORING

The introduction of the flow-directed PAC was a quantum advance in the monitoring of patients in the perioperative period. Since the 1970s, its use has increased the amount of diagnostic information that can be obtained at the bedside to guide treatment in critically ill patients.[203] It is impressive to observe large changes in the pulmonary artery pressure (PAP) and PCWP with almost no reflection in the CVP. Connors et al[204] prospectively analyzed 62 consecutive pulmonary artery catheterizations. They found that less than half of a group of clinicians correctly predicted the PCWP or CO, and more than 50% made at least one change in therapy based on data from the PAC. Waller and Kaplan[205] demonstrated that a group of experienced cardiac anesthesiologists and surgeons who were blinded to the information from the PAC during coronary artery bypass grafting (CABG) surgery were unaware of any problem during 65% of severe hemodynamic abnormalities. Similarly, Iberti and Fisher[206] showed that ICU physicians were unable to accurately predict hemodynamic data on clinical grounds, and that 60% made at least one change in therapy and 33% changed their diagnosis based on PAC data. These data are impressive, but the clinical significance of these changes has been questioned because the weight of evidence-based medicine on the subject does not support improvements in outcome related to PAC monitoring.

In 1996, Connors et al[207] published the results of a large, prospective cohort study with data collected from five U.S. teaching hospitals between 1989 and 1994. They enrolled 5735 critically ill adult patients in ICU settings and found that right-heart catheterization was associated with increased mortality in this patient population. In the wake of this publication and the increasing evidence from further studies, most of which confirmed those findings, the use of the PAC has significantly decreased. Between 1993 and 2004, PAC use in the United States decreased by 65% for all medical admissions.[208] The most significant

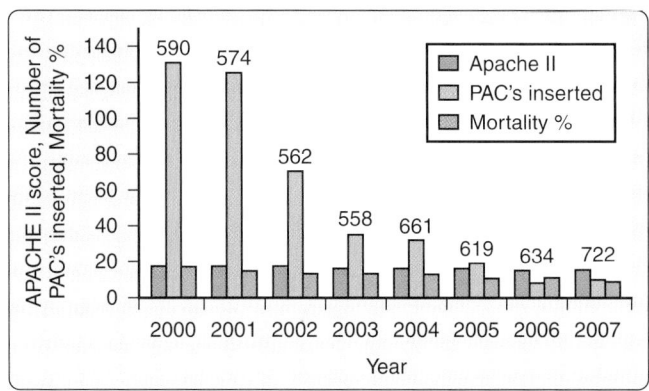

Figure 14-19 Annual decrease in pulmonary artery catheter (PAC) use with stable risk scoring and mildly decreased mortality in one intensive care unit over an 8-year period. *(From Leibowitz AB, Oropello JM: The pulmonary artery in anesthesia practice in 2007: An historical overview with emphasis on the past 6 years, Semin Cardiothorac Vasc Anesth 11:162–176, 2007, by permission.)*

decrease in PAC use was documented in patients with acute myocardial infarction, whereas those patients diagnosed with septicemia show the least decline in use. These findings were almost identical to the surgical patient population, in which the PAC use decreased by 63% in the same observed period. In another retrospective analysis, PAC use in patients hospitalized with acute coronary syndromes decreased from 5.4% in 2000 to 3.0% in 2007.[209] Leibowitz and Orapello[210] published data on PAC use in patients admitted to a surgical ICU (approximately 600 perioperative patients admitted per year) over an 8-year period. The number of PACs inserted decreased significantly from 23% of all admissions having a PAC inserted in 2000 to less than 2% in 2006. The patient risk profile (Acute Physiology and Chronic Health Evaluation [APACHE] II score) did not change, whereas hospital and ICU mortality in that patient population was slightly reduced in the observed period (Figure 14-19).

The incidence of right-heart (PAC) catheterization is highly variable among hospitals and within hospitals, according to service. Nevertheless, with the high incidence of multisystem organ dysfunction in cardiac surgical patients, PAC monitoring is likely to remain a prominent aspect of hemodynamic monitoring in many cardiac surgical centers for the foreseeable future. An understanding of the potential benefits and pitfalls of pulmonary artery catheterization is therefore essential for anesthesiologists.

▣ Technical Aspects of Pulmonary Artery Catheter Use

Considerations for the insertion site of a PAC are the same as for CVP catheters. The right IJV approach remains the technique of choice because of the direct path between this vessel and the RA. The placement of PACs through subclavian vein introducers may be complicated by kinking of the catheter when the sternum is retracted during cardiothoracic surgery. Forty-five percent of PACs placed through subclavian catheters became kinked and remained permanently nonfunctional after sternal retraction.[211]

Passage of the PAC from the vessel introducer to the PA can be accomplished by monitoring the pressure waveform from the distal port of the catheter or under fluoroscopic guidance. Waveform monitoring is the more common technique for perioperative right-heart catheterization. First, the catheter must be advanced through the vessel introducer (15 to 20 cm) before inflating the balloon. The inflation of the balloon facilitates further advancement of the catheter through the RA and right ventricle (RV) into the pulmonary artery (PA). Normal intracardiac pressures are listed in Table 14-1. The pressure waveforms seen during advancement of the PAC are shown in Figure 14-20.

TABLE 14-1	Normal Intracardiac Pressures	
Location	*Mean (mm Hg)*	*Range (mm Hg)*
Right atrium	5	1–10
Right ventricle	25/5	15–30/0–8
Pulmonary arterial systolic/diastolic	23/9	15–30/5–15
Mean pulmonary arterial	15	10–20
Pulmonary capillary wedge pressure	10	5–15
Left atrial pressure	8	4–12
Left ventricular end-diastolic pressure	8	4–12
Left ventricular systolic pressure	130	90–140

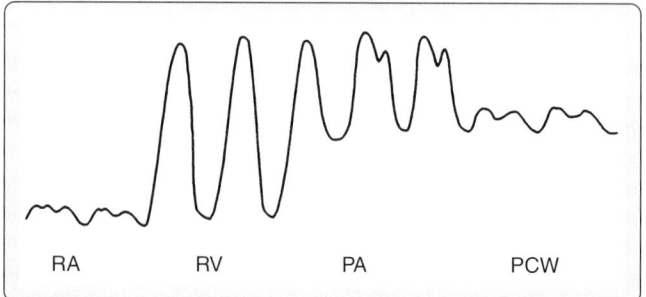

RA   RV   PA   PCW

Figure 14-20 The waveforms encountered during the flotation of a pulmonary artery catheter from the venous circulation to the pulmonary capillary wedge (PCW) position. Notice the sudden increase in systolic pressure as the catheter enters the right ventricle (RV), the sudden increase in diastolic pressure as the catheter enters the pulmonary artery (PA), and the decrease in mean pressure as the catheter reaches the PCW position. RA, right atrium.

In patients with prior TV ring annuloplasty, significant TR, and tricuspid stenosis, advancing the catheter past the TV may be cumbersome or even impossible. Catheter manipulation and positional changes may be useful. Trendelenburg positioning places the RV more superior to the RA and thus may aid in advancing the PAC past the TV. TEE guidance can prove invaluable in these cases. The experienced echocardiographer can assist in guiding the catheter tip toward the TV orifice by directing catheter and positional manipulations. The RA waveform is seen until the catheter tip crosses the TV and enters the RV. In the RV, there is a sudden increase in systolic pressure but little change in diastolic pressure compared with the RA tracing. Arrhythmias, particularly premature ventricular complexes, usually occur at this point but almost always resolve without treatment once the catheter tip has crossed the pulmonary valve. The catheter is advanced through the RV toward the pulmonary artery. Reverse Trendelenburg and right lateral tilt minimize arrhythmias and facilitate catheter passage through the RV outflow tract and pulmonary valve into the PA.[212]

As the catheter crosses the pulmonary valve, a dicrotic notch appears in the pressure waveform and there is a sudden increase in diastolic pressure. The PCWP tracing is obtained by advancing the catheter approximately 3 to 5 cm farther until there is a change in the waveform associated with a decline in the measured mean pressure. Deflation of the balloon results in reappearance of the pulmonary artery waveform and an increase in the mean pressure value. With the right IJV approach, the RA is entered at 25 to 35 cm, the RV at 35 to 45 cm, the PA at 45 to 55 cm, and the PCWP at 50 to 60 cm in most patients.

If the catheter does not enter the PA by 60 cm (from the RIJ approach), the balloon should be deflated and the catheter should be withdrawn into the RA. Further attempts can then be made to advance the catheter into proper position using the techniques described earlier. Excessive coiling of the catheter in the RA or RV should be avoided to prevent catheter knotting. The balloon should

be inflated only for short periods to measure the PCWP. The PA waveform should be monitored continually to be certain that the catheter does not advance into a constant wedge position because this may lead to PA rupture or pulmonary infarction. The PAC is covered by a sterile sheath that must be secured at both ends to prevent contamination of the external portion of the catheter. Not infrequently, the PAC must be withdrawn a short distance because the catheter softens and advances more peripherally into the PA over time. The PAC must frequently be withdrawn on CPB because of the decreased size of the heart causing the same effect.

The PCWP waveform is analogous to the CVP waveform described previously. The A, C, and V waves seen when the PAC balloon is inflated (pulmonary capillary wedge position) are similarly timed in the cardiac cycle. Large V waves can be seen on the PCWP waveform during mitral regurgitation, LV diastolic noncompliance, and episodes of myocardial ischemia.[213] They also are seen on the PA waveform (PAC not wedged) as large ("giant") V waves that occur slightly later than the typical upstroke on the PA tracing.[214] The V waves cause the PA waveform to become wider and to lose the dicrotic notch (Figure 14-21). The cause of large V waves during myocardial ischemia is probably a decrease in diastolic ventricular compliance and/or mitral regurgitation induced by ischemic papillary muscle dysfunction. In this instance, the V waves may occur earlier during the onset of the C wave (seen with onset of ventricular contraction) and are termed *C-V waves*. As mentioned earlier, V waves frequently are seen without ischemia, and the diagnostic value of V waves is, therefore, limited, especially in the era of TEE.[215,216]

Specific information that can be gathered with the PAC and the quantitative measurements of cardiovascular and pulmonary function that can be derived from this information are listed in Tables 14-2 and 14-3. One of the main reasons that clinicians measure PCWP and pulmonary artery diastolic pressure is that these parameters are estimates of LAP, which is an estimate of left ventricular end-diastolic pressure (LVEDP). LVEDP is an index of left ventricular end-diastolic volume (LVEDV), which correlates well with left ventricular preload.[217] The relation between LVEDP and LVEDV is described by the left ventricular compliance curve. This nonlinear curve is affected by many factors, such as ventricular hypertrophy and myocardial ischemia.[218–220] The relation of these parameters is diagrammed in Figure 14-22.

The PCWP and pulmonary artery diastolic pressures will not accurately reflect LVEDP in the presence of incorrect position of the PAC catheter tip, pulmonary vascular disease, high levels of PEEP, or mitral valvular disease. The patency of vascular channels between the distal

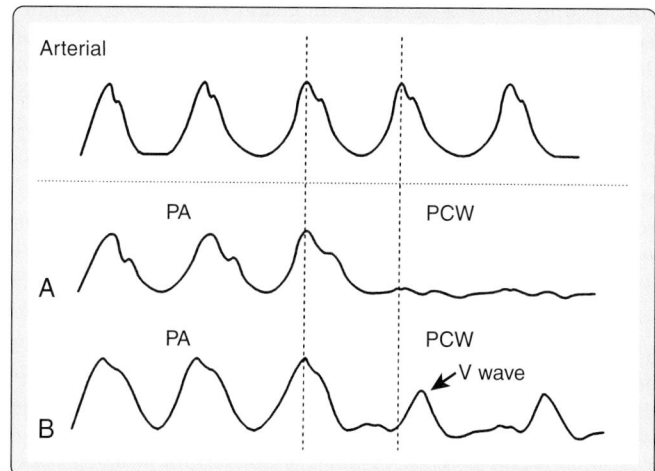

Arterial

A   PA   PCW

B   PA   PCW   ← V wave

Figure 14-21 The relation of the systemic arterial waveform, the pulmonary arterial (PA) waveform, and the pulmonary capillary wedge (PCW) waveform in the normal situation (*A*) and in the presence of V waves (*B*). Note the widening of the PA waveform and the loss of the dicrotic notch in the presence of V waves. Also note that the peak of the V wave occurs after the peak of the systemic arterial waveform.

TABLE 14-2	Derived Hemodynamic Parameters	
Formula		*Normal Values*
Cardiac index CI = CO/BSA		2.8–4.2 L/min/m²
Stroke volume SV = CO*1000/HR		50–110 mL (per beat)
Stroke index SI = SV/BSA		30–65 mL/beat/m²
Left ventricular stroke work index LVSWI = 1.36*(MAP − PCWP)*SI/100		45–60 gram-meters/m²
Right ventricular stroke work index RVSWI = 1.36*(MPAP − CVP)*SI/100		5–10 gram-meters/m²
Systemic vascular resistance SVR = (MAP − CVP)*80/CO		900–1400 dynes.sec.cm⁻⁵
Systemic vascular resistance index SVRI = (MAP − CVP)*80/CI		1500–2400 dynes.sec.cm⁻⁵/m²
Pulmonary vascular resistance PVR = (MPAP − PCWP)*80/CO		150–250 dynes.sec.cm⁻⁵
Pulmonary vascular resistance index PVRI = (MPAP − PCWP)*80/CI		250–400 dynes.sec.cm⁻⁵/m²

BSA, body surface area; CI, cardiac index; CO, cardiac output; CVP, central venous pressure; HR, heart rate; LVSWI, left ventricular stroke work index; MAP, mean arterial pressure; PAP, pulmonary arterial pressure; PCWP, pulmonary capillary wedge pressure; PVR, pulmonary vascular resistance; PVRI, pulmonary vascular resistance index; RVSWI, right ventricular stroke work index; SI, stroke index; SV, stroke volume; SVR, systemic vascular resistance; SVRI, systemic vascular resistance index.

TABLE 14-3	Oxygen Delivery Parameters	
Formula		*Normal Values*
Arterial O₂ content Cao₂ = (1.39*Hb*Sao₂) + (0.0031*Pao₂)		18–20 mL/dL
Mixed venous O₂ content Cvo₂ = 1.39*Hb*Svo₂ + 0.0031*Pvo₂		13–16 mL/dL
Arteriovenous O₂ content difference avdo₂ = Cao₂ − Cvo₂		4–5.5 mL/dL
Pulmonary capillary O₂ content Cco₂ = 1.39*Hb*Sco₂ + 0.0031*Pco₂		19–21 mL/dL
Pulmonary shunt fraction Qs/Qt = 100*(Cco₂ − Cao₂)/(Cco₂ − Cvo₂)		2–8%
O₂ delivery DO₂ = 10*CO*Cao₂		800–1100 mL/min
O₂ consumption Vo₂ = 10*CO*(Cao₂ − Cvo₂)		150–300 mL/min

Hb, hemoglobin; Pco₂, pulmonary capillary oxygen tension; Pvo₂, venous oxygen tension; Sco₂, pulmonary capillary oxygen saturation; Svo₂, venous oxygen saturation.
From McGrath R: Invasive bedside hemodynamic monitoring. *Prog Cardiovasc Dis* 29:129, 1986.

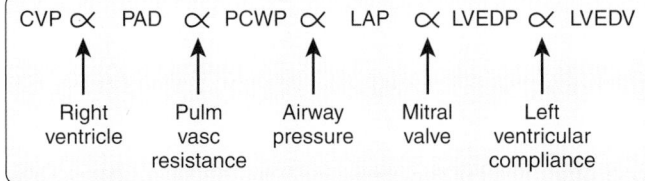

Figure 14-22 The left ventricular end-diastolic volume (LVEDV) is related to the left ventricular end-diastolic pressure (LVEDP) by the left ventricular compliance. The LVEDP is related to the left atrial pressure (LAP) by the diastolic pressure gradient across the mitral valve. The pulmonary capillary wedge pressure (PCWP) is related to the LAP by the pulmonary capillary resistance. The pulmonary artery diastolic pressure (PAD) is an estimate of the PCWP. The central venous pressure (CVP) will reflect the PAD if right ventricular function is normal.

port of the PAC and the LA is necessary to ensure a close relation between the PCWP and LAP. This condition is met only in the dependent portions of the lung (West's zone III), in which the pulmonary venous pressure exceeds the alveolar pressure.[221] Otherwise, the PCWP will reflect the alveolar pressure, not the LAP. Because PEEP decreases

the size of West's zone III, it has been shown to adversely affect the correlation between the PCWP and LAP, especially in the patient with hypovolemia.[222–224] Nevertheless, the correlation of PCWP and LAP could be maintained in the presence of PEEP by placing the catheter tip below the LA.[222,225]

The acute respiratory distress syndrome (ARDS) seems to prevent the transmission of increased alveolar pressure to the pulmonary interstitium. This preserves the relation between the PCWP and LAP even when PEEP levels up to 20 cm H₂O are applied.[226] Determination of the PCWP in patients on positive pressure ventilation, and especially those treated with high levels of PEEP, is particularly difficult. The most important concept is that PCWP should always be determined at end-expiration; this is the case in spontaneously breathing patients and those on mechanical ventilation. In patients on high levels of PEEP, it is not clear what percentage of the increased intrathoracic pressure is actually transmitted to the catheter tip, and furthermore, how that pressure reflects the true intravascular filling pressure and, by extension, estimation of the LVEDV. Temporary removal of high levels of PEEP (e.g., >10 mm Hg) is discouraged because rapid reduction in the functional residual capacity (FRC) and associated lung atelectasis might have acute adverse respiratory consequences.

Significant valvular disease greatly increases the difficulty in correctly interpreting the PCWP. The presence of large V waves in the PCWP tracing of patients with mitral regurgitation leads to an overestimation of the LVEDP.[227] In patients with mitral stenosis, PCWP will be increased despite decreased LV preload (LVEDV), and using the PCWP instead of the LAP to assess the transmitral gradient has been shown to overestimate the severity of mitral stenosis.[228] However, when the PCWP was adjusted for the time delay through the pulmonary vasculature, the mean LAP and mean PCWP correlated well in another study.[229] Significant aortic regurgitation will lead to premature MV closure and, thus, LVEDV will be underestimated. It has been demonstrated that there is a significant positive gradient between the PCWP and the LAP in the initial hour after CPB.[230] Box 14-9 is a summary of conditions that may alter the relation between the PCWP and the LVEDP. Special-purpose PACs for continuous CO, continuous mixed venous oximetry (Svo₂), pacing, and thermodilution right ventricular ejection fraction are also available and are described later.

Clinical Efficacy of Pulmonary Artery Catheter Use

Several large studies have addressed the controversies regarding the indications, risks, and benefits associated with PAC monitoring after the publication of Connor's findings[207] that PAC use may be harmful.

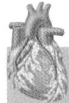

BOX 14-9. CONDITIONS RESULTING IN DISCREPANCIES BETWEEN PULMONARY CAPILLARY WEDGE PRESSURE AND LEFT VENTRICULAR END-DIASTOLIC PRESSURE

PCWP > LVEDP
- Positive-pressure ventilation
- Positive end-expiratory pressure
- Increased intrathoracic pressure
- Non–West lung zone III pulmonary artery catheter placement
- Chronic obstructive pulmonary disease
- Increased pulmonary vascular resistance
- Left atrial myxoma
- Mitral valve disease (e.g., stenosis, regurgitation)

PCWP < LVEDP
- Noncompliant left ventricle (e.g., ischemia, hypertrophy)
- Aortic regurgitation (premature closure of the mitral valve)

LVEDP, left ventricular end-diastolic pressure; PCWP, pulmonary capillary wedge pressure.

Adapted from Tuman KJ, Carrol CC, Ivankovich AD: Pitfalls in interpretation of pulmonary artery catheter data. *Cardiothorac Vasc Anesth Update* 2:1, 1991.

However, as more studies have been published, there is convincing evidence that PACs have little positive impact on patient outcomes.[231–234] Adjusting for the severity of illness, Murdoch et al[235] found that the use of the PAC in ICU patients was safe, but no beneficial effect was demonstrated. In 2001, Polanczyk et al[236] published the results of an observational study on 4059 patients undergoing major elective noncardiac surgical procedures, examining the relation between PACs and postoperative cardiac complications. Right-heart catheterization was associated with an increased incidence of major postoperative cardiac events. Barone et al's[237] meta-analysis asserted that only four prospective studies were adequately randomized, and that the use of the PAC did not improve outcome in vascular surgery patients. Rhodes et al's[238] prospective, randomized study found no significant difference in mortality in critically ill patients treated with or without the use of a PAC.

Sandham et al[239] reported a prospective, randomized, controlled outcome study of 1994 high-risk patients (American Society of Anesthesiologists [ASA] III or IV) scheduled for major surgery followed by ICU stay who were managed with or without the use of a PAC. No benefit to therapy directed by PAC compared with standard care (without the use of PAC) was found, with a greater risk for adverse events in the PAC group. Yu et al[240] performed a prospective cohort study of the relation between PAC use and outcome in 1010 patients with severe sepsis. PAC monitoring did not improve outcome in this patient population. Outcomes of patients with shock and ARDS also were not affected by PAC placement in a multicenter, randomized, controlled trial.[241] Sakr et al looked at outcomes related to PAC use in 3147 adult patients admitted to an ICU; this was a subanalysis of a large, multicenter, prospective, observational study designed to evaluate the epidemiology of sepsis in European countries.[242] After propensity score matching, there was no significant difference in outcome with or without PAC placement. Interestingly, significant differences in PAC use were reported between the various participating countries.

The ESCAPE trial (Evaluation Study of Congestive heart failure And Pulmonary artery catheterization Effectiveness)[243] included patients with symptoms of severe heart failure. This multicenter, randomized, controlled trial enrolled 433 patients at 26 sites but had no specific treatment algorithm. However, the use of inotropes was discouraged, and investigators were asked to follow national guidelines for treatment of heart failure, which promote the use of diuretics and vasodilators. The target in both groups was improvement of clinical symptoms of heart failure. In the PAC group, there was an additional target of a PCWP of 15 mm Hg and a CVP of 8 mm Hg. Overall, mortality did not differ between groups; however, more adverse events were recorded in the PAC group. Exercise and quality-of-life measures improved in both groups, and the investigators reported a statistically insignificant trend toward greater improvement with PAC use.

The PAC-Man study was a randomized, controlled trial that enrolled 1041 patients from 65 ICUs throughout the United Kingdom.[244] Patients were randomly assigned to management with or without PAC placement. Treatment in both arms of the study was at the discretion of the treating clinician. Neither benefit nor harm related to PAC use was found. Two randomized, controlled studies did not show improved patient outcomes with PAC use in patients with ARDS.[241,245] Randomized trials including patients with acute myocardial infarction also seemed to confirm these data.[246,247] Cohen et al[248] retrospectively studied 26,437 patients with acute coronary syndromes. A PAC was inserted in 2.8% of patients. In the United States, patients were 3.8 times more likely to have a PAC placed than non-US patients. After adjustment for confounding factors, PAC use was associated with a 2.6-fold increase in hospital mortality. The subset of patients who experienced development of cardiogenic shock had similar outcomes both with and without PAC use.

Schwann et al[249] retrospectively assessed the outcome of 2685 patients undergoing CABG in whom the decision to place a PAC was based on patient characteristics and risk factors. Using a highly selective strategy, they used no PAC in the majority of cases (91%) and the outcomes were comparable. In another retrospective trial, Ramsey et al[250] found that PACs in elective CABG surgery were associated with increased in-hospital mortality, longer lengths of stay, and greater

total costs. This effect was more pronounced in those hospital settings with low overall PAC use. Resano et al[251] looked at PAC use compared with CVP monitoring in patients undergoing off-pump coronary artery bypass surgery and found no difference in outcome. In a prospective, observational study, Djaiani et al[252] observed 200 consecutive patients undergoing CABG surgery where PACs were placed, but the numerical data other than CVP were blinded to the surgeon and anesthesiologist. Patients were managed as per routine, and data could be unblinded if required clinically. Twenty three percent of patients required unblinding of data; within this subgroup, preliminary diagnosis was confirmed in 14% and treatment was modified in 9%. The patients in the unblinded group went on to experience further morbidity. The investigators concluded that placement of a PAC can be safely delayed until the clinical need arises either intraoperatively or in the ICU.

A major issue with PAC outcome studies is the clinical setting, specifically operating room versus ICU. Haupt et al[253] observed that patients in the ICU might have diseases too far advanced to make invasive hemodynamic monitoring useful. Older studies that had reported improved outcome used invasive hemodynamic monitoring to optimize oxygen delivery in the perioperative period.[254–257] In their meta-analysis, Heyland et al[258] similarly argued that "maximizing oxygen delivery" in the perioperative setting (i.e., before the onset of irreversible organ damage) is more effective in comparison with the chronic ICU setting. Based on the intention-to-treat analysis of patients with preoperative PAC placement, they reported improved survival. Chittock et al[259] demonstrated that severity of illness may play an important role in defining subgroups of patients who may benefit from PAC monitoring. Of 7310 critically ill adult patients admitted to the ICU, those with APACHE II scores greater than 31 showed decreased mortality with PAC monitoring, whereas patients with lower APACHE II scores had increased mortality. Another meta-analysis by Ivanov et al[260] showed a significant reduction in morbidity when PAC-guided strategies were applied. In a prospective, randomized trial, Pölönen et al[261] applied goal-directed, PAC-guided therapy aimed to maintain a mixed venous saturation greater than 70% and blood lactate less than 2 mmol/L in patients after cardiac surgery. Using this strategy, they found that increasing oxygen delivery in the immediate postoperative period shortened hospital stay and decreased morbidity. In a retrospective database analysis (National Trauma Data Bank, 53,312 patients enrolled) of trauma patients admitted to an ICU, severely injured and older patients had decreased mortality associated with PAC use.[262]

There may be various explanations as to why most findings do not favor PAC use. Placing a PAC is a highly invasive procedure. Vascular structures are accessed with large-bore introducer sheaths with all the possible complications listed. Most importantly, even in the best of all circumstances, with uncomplicated PAC placement and correct data collection and interpretation, it has to be recognized that a PAC is only a monitoring tool. As such, a change in patient outcome cannot be expected unless the treatment that is initiated based on the PAC measurements improves patient outcome. In some of the most critically ill patients, such as those with sepsis, ARDS, or massive trauma, mortality remains high despite efforts to find new treatment strategies. Furthermore, diagnoses often can be made on clinical grounds only, and treatment strategies once thought to improve patient outcome actually may be harmful.

Despite the large number of studies regarding PACs and outcome, flaws in study design and insufficient statistical power are still an issue. The most common design flaws are a lack of therapeutic protocols or treatment algorithms and inadequate randomization, which introduce observer bias.[263] Physician knowledge is another confounding variable, as demonstrated in a multicenter study that indicated competency in interpreting PAC-derived data was lacking in many individuals and depended on such factors as the level of training and the frequency of use.[264] In one study, 47% of physicians could not correctly determine the PCWP to within 5 mm Hg.[265]

In summary, there are no convincing data showing improved outcomes in patients undergoing cardiac surgery with PAC placement compared with CVP monitoring alone.[266] The perioperative literature on the subject suggests that PAC use in patients undergoing low-risk cardiac surgery may be harmful.[267] Clinical evidence gained from the majority of well-designed, prospective studies indicates that patients undergoing low-risk cardiac surgery can be managed safely without PAC placement. Many clinicians, however, still consider high-risk cardiac surgery and, in particular, patients with right-heart failure or pulmonary hypertension to be indications for PAC placement.

Indications

In a global sense, the indications for using a PAC are assessing volume status, measuring CO, measuring Svo_2, and deriving hemodynamic parameters. In 2003, the ASA Task Force on Pulmonary Artery Catheterization published updated practice guidelines for pulmonary artery catheterization (http://www.asahq.org/publicationsAnd-Services/pulm_artery.pdf).[268] These guidelines emphasized that the patient, surgery, and practice setting had to be considered when deciding on the use of a PAC. Generally, the routine use of PACs is indicated in high-risk patients (e.g., ASA IV or V) and high-risk procedures (e.g., where large fluid changes or hemodynamic disturbances are expected). The practice setting is important because there is evidence that inadequate training or experience may increase the risk for perioperative complications associated with the use of a PAC. It is recommended that the routine use of a PAC should be confined to centers with adequate training and experience in the perioperative management of patients with PACs (Box 14-10). The authors of this chapter have composed a list of possible procedural indications (Box 14-11).

Historically, the use of the PAC contributed to the understanding and care of patients with cardiac disease. The risks associated with perioperative PAC monitoring, however, seem to outweigh the benefits in low-to-moderate risk patients, whereas high-risk patients undergoing major surgery may benefit from right-heart catheterization.

Contraindications

Contraindications to pulmonary artery catheterization are summarized in Box 14-12.

Absolute Contraindications

Contraindications to the use of a PAC include tricuspid or pulmonic valvular stenosis. It is unlikely that a PAC would be able to cross a stenotic valve, and it might worsen the obstruction to flow if it did. Friable right atrial or RV masses (i.e., tumor or thrombus) are absolute contraindications. The catheter may dislodge a portion of the mass, causing pulmonary or paradoxic embolization. In patients with tetralogy of Fallot, the RV outflow tract is hypersensitive. A PAC could induce a hypercyanotic episode ("tet spell") by eliciting spasm of the RV infundibulum.

Relative Contraindications

Use of a PAC may be contraindicated in patients with severe arrhythmias. Transient atrial and ventricular arrhythmias are common during PAC placement. The risk for inducing an arrhythmia in a patient prone to malignant arrhythmias must be weighed against the potential benefits of the information gained from PAC monitoring. Appropriate preparations must be undertaken for administration of antiarrhythmic drugs and cardiopulmonary resuscitation, as well as electrical cardioversion, defibrillation, or pacing, if required.

Coagulopathy may be a relative contraindication to the use of a PAC. This is related to the potential complications of obtaining central venous access in the patient with a coagulopathy. The risk for inducing endobronchial hemorrhage with inadvertent migration of the PAC or prolonged balloon inflation may be increased.

Newly inserted pacemaker wires may be a contraindication because they may be displaced by the PAC during insertion or withdrawal. In approximately 4 to 6 weeks, the pacemaker wires become firmly embedded in the endocardium and wire displacement becomes less likely.

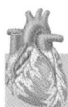

BOX 14-10. AMERICAN SOCIETY OF ANESTHESIOLOGIST PRACTICE GUIDELINES FOR PULMONARY ARTERY CATHETER USE

Opinions
- PA catheterization provides new information that may change therapy, with poor clinical evidence of its effect on clinical outcome or mortality.
- There is no evidence from large, controlled studies that preoperative PA catheterization improves outcome regarding hemodynamic optimization.
- Perioperative PAC monitoring of hemodynamic parameters leading to goal-directed therapy has produced inconsistent data in multiple studies and clinical scenarios.
- Having immediate access to PAC data allows important preemptive measures for selected subgroups of patients who encounter hemodynamic disturbances that require immediate and precise decisions about fluid management and drug treatment.
- Experience and understanding are the major determinants of PAC effectiveness.
- PA catheterization is inappropriate as routine practice in surgical patients and should be limited to cases in which the anticipated benefits of catheterization outweigh the potential risks.
- PA catheterization can be harmful.

Recommendations
- The appropriateness of PA catheterization depends on a combination of patient-, surgery-, and practice setting–related factors.
- Perioperative PA catheterization should be considered in patients who present with significant organ dysfunction or major comorbidity that pose an increased risk for hemodynamic disturbances or instability (e.g., ASA IV or V patients).
- Perioperative PA catheterization in surgical settings should be considered based on the hemodynamic risk of the individual case rather than generalized surgical setting-related recommendations. High-risk surgical procedures are those in which large fluid changes or hemodynamic disturbances can be anticipated and those that are associated with a high risk for morbidity and mortality.
- Because of the risk for complications from PA catheterization, the procedure should not be performed by clinicians or nursing staff, or done in practice settings in which competency in safe insertion, accurate interpretation of results, and appropriate catheter maintenance cannot be guaranteed.
- Routine PA catheterization is not recommended when the patient, procedure, or practice setting poses a low or moderate risk for hemodynamic changes.

ASA, American Society of Anesthesiologists; PA, pulmonary artery; PAC, pulmonary artery catheter.
From American Society of Anesthesiologists: *Practice guidelines for pulmonary artery catheterization.* Accessed November 11, 2010: http://journals.lww.com/anesthesiology/fulltext/2003/10000/Practice_Guidelines_for_Preoperative.36aspx.

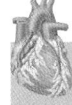

BOX 14-11. POSSIBLE CLINICAL INDICATIONS FOR PULMONARY ARTERY CATHETER MONITORING

Major procedures involving large fluid shifts or blood loss in patients with:
- Right-heart failure, pulmonary hypertension
- Severe left-heart failure not responsive to therapy
- Cardiogenic or septic shock, or with multiple-organ failure
- Hemodynamic instability requiring inotropes or intra-aortic balloon counterpulsation
- Surgery of the aorta requiring suprarenal cross-clamping
- Hepatic transplantation
- Orthotopic heart transplantation

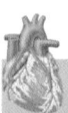

BOX 14-12. CONTRAINDICATIONS FOR PULMONARY ARTERY CATHETERIZATION

Absolute Contraindications
- Tricuspid or pulmonary stenosis
- Right atrial or right ventricular mass
- Tetralogy of Fallot

Relative Contraindications
- Severe arrhythmias
- Coagulopathy
- Newly inserted pacemaker wires

Complications

The complications associated with PAC placement include almost all of those detailed in the section on CVP placement. Additional complications that are unique to the PAC are detailed in the following subsections. The ASA Task Force on Pulmonary Artery Catheterization concluded that serious complications caused by PAC catheterization occur in 0.1% to 0.5% of patients monitored with a PAC.[268] Greater estimates are found in the literature and probably represent different patient populations, hospital settings, level of experience with PAC management, and other factors.[269]

Arrhythmias

The most common complications associated with PAC insertion are transient arrhythmias, especially premature ventricular contractions.[270] However, fatal arrhythmias have rarely been reported.[271,272] Intravenous lidocaine has been used in attempts to suppress these arrhythmias, with mixed results.[273,274] However, a positional maneuver entailing 5-degree head-up and right lateral tilt was associated with a statistically significant decrease in malignant arrhythmias (compared with the Trendelenburg position) during PAC insertion.[212]

Complete Heart Block

Complete heart block may develop during PA catheterization in patients with preexisting left bundle branch block (LBBB).[275–277] This potentially fatal complication is most likely due to electrical irritability from the PAC tip causing transient right bundle branch block (RBBB) as it passes through the RV outflow tract. The incidence rate of development of RBBB was 3% in a prospective series of patients undergoing PA catheterization.[278] However, none of the patients with preexisting LBBB developed complete heart block in that series. In another study of 47 patients with LBBB, complete heart block occurred in two patients with recent-onset LBBB.[279] It is imperative to have an external pacemaker immediately available or to use a pacing PAC when placing a PAC in patients with LBBB.

Endobronchial Hemorrhage

Numerous cases of iatrogenic rupture of the PA have been recorded in the medical literature.[280] The incidence rate of PAC-induced endobronchial hemorrhage is 0.064% to 0.20%.[270] Hannan et al[281] reported a 46% mortality rate in a review of 28 cases of PAC-induced endobronchial hemorrhage, but the mortality rate was 75% in anticoagulated patients. From these reports, several risk factors have emerged: advanced age, female sex, pulmonary hypertension, mitral stenosis, coagulopathy, distal placement of the catheter, and balloon hyperinflation. Balloon inflation in distal pulmonary arteries is probably accountable for most episodes of PA rupture because of the high pressures generated by the balloon.[282] Hypothermic CPB also may increase risk because of distal migration of the catheter tip with movement of the heart and hardening of the PAC.[283,284] It is now common practice to pull the PAC back approximately 3 to 5 cm when CPB is instituted.

It is important to consider the cause of the hemorrhage when forming a therapeutic plan. If the hemorrhage is minimal and a coagulopathy coexists, correction of the coagulopathy may be the only necessary therapy. Protection of the uninvolved lung is of prime importance. Tilting the patient toward the affected side, placement of a double-lumen endotracheal tube, and other lung-separation maneuvers should protect the contralateral lung.[285] Strategies proposed to stop the hemorrhage include the application of PEEP, placement of bronchial blockers, and pulmonary resection.[286] The clinician is obviously at a disadvantage unless the site of hemorrhage is known. A chest radiograph will usually indicate the general location of the lesion. Although the cause of endobronchial hemorrhage may be unclear, the bleeding site must be unequivocally located before surgical treatment is attempted. A small amount of radiographic contrast dye may help to pinpoint the lesion if active hemorrhage is present. In severe hemorrhage and with recurrent bleeding, transcatheter coil embolization has been used. This may emerge as the preferred treatment method.[287,288]

Pulmonary Infarction

Pulmonary infarction is a rare complication of PAC monitoring. An early report suggested that there was a 7.2% incidence rate of pulmonary infarction with PAC use.[289] However, continuously monitoring the PA waveform and keeping the balloon deflated when not determining the PCWP (to prevent inadvertent wedging of the catheter) were not standard practice at that time. Distal migration of PACs may also occur intraoperatively because of the action of the right ventricle, uncoiling of the catheter, and softening of the catheter over time. Inadvertent catheter wedging occurs during CPB because of the diminished RV chamber size and retraction of the heart to perform the operation. Embolization of thrombus formed on a PAC also could result in pulmonary infarction.

Catheter Knotting and Entrapment

Knotting of a PAC usually occurs as a result of coiling of the catheter within the right ventricle. Insertion of an appropriately sized guidewire under fluoroscopic guidance may aid in unknotting the catheter.[290] Alternatively, the knot may be tightened and withdrawn percutaneously along with the introducer if no intracardiac structures are entangled.[291] If cardiac structures, such as the papillary muscles, are entangled in the knotted catheter, then surgical intervention may be required.[292,293] Sutures placed in the heart may inadvertently entrap the PAC. Reports of such cases and the details of the percutaneous removal have been described.[294]

Valvular Damage

Withdrawal of the catheter with the balloon inflated may result in injury to the tricuspid[295] or pulmonary valves.[296] Placement of the PAC with the balloon deflated may increase the risk for passing the catheter between the chordae tendineae.[297] Septic endocarditis has also resulted from an indwelling PAC.[298,299]

Thrombocytopenia

Mild thrombocytopenia has been reported in dogs and humans with indwelling PACs.[300] This probably results from increased platelet consumption. Heparin-coated PACs can trigger heparin-induced thrombocytopenia, which has been reported in cardiac surgical patients (see Chapter 31).[301]

Thrombus Formation

The PAC is a foreign body that may serve as a nidus for thrombus formation. The thrombogenicity of PACs seems to have been reduced for up to 72 hours after insertion by the introduction of heparin-bonded PACs.[302,303] High-dose aprotinin therapy may lead to thrombus formation on PACs despite heparin bonding.[304] This phenomenon also has been reported with ε-aminocaproic acid therapy.[305] TEE can be an invaluable tool for detecting and monitoring this relatively rare complication.[306]

Incorrect Placement

The catheter may pass through an interatrial or interventricular communication into the left side of the heart. It is then possible for the catheter to enter the aorta through the LV outflow tract. A similar complication has been reported in which the catheter crossed a surgically repaired tear in the SVC into the left side of the heart.[307] This complication should be recognized by the similarity between the PA and systemic arterial waveforms. In a case report of a patient with an ascending aortic aneurysm, compression of the SVC by the aneurysm led to traumatic placement of the PAC directly into the pulmonary vein.[308]

Hypotension secondary to balloon inflation has been reported in a patient after a pneumonectomy in whom the balloon obstructed the pulmonary circulation.[309] Venous cannula obstruction has occurred in patients during CPB.[310–312] The temporal association with the abrupt loss of venous return and the negative pressure recorded on the distal lumen tracing are important indicators that this may be occurring. This stresses the importance of monitoring the pressure waveforms during CPB. Coronary sinus obstruction also has been reported from a PAC.[313] Placement of the PAC in the liver has been described; the wedged hepatic venous pressures may mimic the PAP waveform.[314] TEE has proved invaluable for confirming the proper placement of PACs. In many cases, TEE has detected incorrect placement and complications resulting from PACs.[306,308]

Balloon Rupture

Balloon rupture is not uncommon when the PAC has been left in place for several days or when the balloon is inflated with more than 1.5 mL of air. Small volumes of air injected into the PA are of little consequence, and balloon rupture is apparent if the injected air cannot be withdrawn. In patients with right-to-left shunts, carbon dioxide may be used for inflation. Great care must be taken not to rupture the balloon in these patients, with the attendant possibility of paradoxic gas embolization to the systemic circulation.

Ventricular Perforation

RV perforation is a rare complication with a balloon-tipped catheter, but it has been reported in the literature.[315]

Erroneous Interpretation of Data

Malfunctions of the catheter and balloon can lead to spurious numbers for the PCWP and incorrect treatment of the patient. Shin et al[316] reported the problem of eccentric inflation of the balloon, with the catheter tip impinging on the PA wall. Several reviews have pointed out many of the problems with clinical use of the PAC.[213,218–220,317] These problems include errors in interpretation because of ventilation modes (Figure 14-23), compliance changes, ventricular interdependence, and associated technical problems.

"Catheter whip" is an artifact that is associated with long catheters, such as PACs. Because the tip moves within the bloodstream of the cardiac chambers and great vessels, the fluid contained within the catheter is accelerated. This can produce superimposed pressure waves of 10 mm Hg in either direction.

SPECIAL-PURPOSE PULMONARY ARTERY CATHETERS

Pacing Pulmonary Artery Catheters

Electrode PACs, as well as pacing wire catheters, are available commercially. The possible indications for placement of a pacing PAC are shown in Box 14-13.

Electrode Catheters

A multipurpose PAC contains five electrodes for bipolar atrial, ventricular, or atrioventricular sequential pacing. The intraoperative success rates for atrial, ventricular, and atrioventricular sequential capture

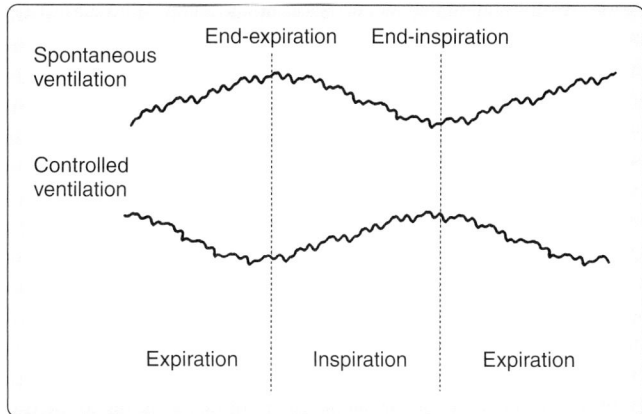

Figure 14-23 Respiratory variation of the pulmonary capillary wedge pressure waveform during spontaneous and mechanical ventilation. Inspiration is marked by negative mediastinal pressure in the spontaneously breathing patient and by positive mediastinal pressure in the mechanically ventilated patient.

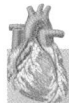

BOX 14-13. INDICATIONS FOR PERIOPERATIVE PLACEMENT OF PACING PULMONARY ARTERY CATHETERS

- Sinus node dysfunction or symptomatic bradycardia
- Second-degree (Mobitz II) atrioventricular block
- Complete (third-degree) atrioventricular block
- Digitalis toxicity
- Need for atrioventricular sequential pacing
- Left bundle branch block

have been reported as 80%, 93%, and 73%, respectively.[318] Electrode detachment has been reported as a complication.[319] Recently, Levin et al reported use of the pacing PAC to assist management during minimally invasive cardiac surgery.[320]

Pacing Wire Catheters

The Paceport and A-V Paceport PACs (Baxter Edwards) have lumina for the introduction of a ventricular wire, or both atrial and ventricular wires for temporary transvenous pacing. The success rate for ventricular pacing capture was 96% for the Paceport.[321] The success rates for atrial and ventricular pacing capture before CPB were 98% and 100%, respectively, in a study of the A-V Paceport.[322] The actual use and indications for placement of pacing PAC in a series of cardiac surgery patients has been published (Table 14-4).[323]

Mixed Venous Oxygen Saturation Catheters

Monitoring the Svo$_2$ is a means of providing a global estimation of the adequacy of oxygen delivery relative to the needs of the various tissues. The formula for Svo$_2$ calculation can be derived by modifying the Fick equation and assuming that the effect of dissolved oxygen in the blood is negligible:

$$SvO_2 = SaO_2 - \frac{\dot{V}O_2}{CO \bullet 1.34 \bullet Hb}$$

A decrease in the Svo$_2$ can indicate one of the following situations: decreased CO; increased oxygen consumption; decreased arterial oxygen saturation; or decreased hemoglobin (Hb) concentration. Blood is aspirated from the distal port of the PAC slowly to measure Svo$_2$, so as not to contaminate the sample with oxygenated alveolar blood.

TABLE 14-4	Use of Pacing Pulmonary Artery Catheters According to the Presence or Absence of Different Indications				
Indication	Indication Present*	Indication Present/Pacing PAC Used† (%)	Indication Absent*	Indication Absent/Pacing PAC Used† (%)	P
Sinus node dysfunction	24	6 (25.0)	576	32 (5.5)	0.002
First-degree AV block	52	1 (1.9)	548	37 (6.7)	0.24
Second-degree AV block	1	1 (100)			
Complete AV block	15	5 (33.3)	585	33 (5.6)	0.001
LBBB	41	5 (12.1)	559	33 (5.9)	0.17
RBBB	32	0 (0)	568	38 (6.6)	0.25
LAH	17	1 (5.8)	583	37 (6.3)	1.0
RBBB and LAH	5	0 (0)	595	38 (6.3)	1.0
Reoperation/with other indications present	61	14 (23.0)	539	24 (4.4)	<0.001
Reoperation/no other indications present	51	1 (1.9)	549	37 (6.7)	0.24
Aortic stenosis	88	11 (12.0)	512	27 (5.2)	0.02
Mitral stenosis	17	1 (5.8)	583	37 (6.3)	1.0
Aortic insufficiency	40	9 (22.5)	560	29 (5.1)	<0.001
Mitral regurgitation	65	7 (10.7)	535	31 (5.7)	0.17

*Total number of patients.
†Total number and percentage of patients with or without each indication.
AV, atrioventricular; LAH, left anterior block; LBBB, left bundle branch block; PAC, pulmonary artery catheter; RBBB, right bundle branch block.
From Risk SC, Brandon D, D'Ambra MN, et al: Indications for the use of pacing pulmonary artery catheters in cardiac surgery. *J Cardiothorac Vasc Anesth* 6:275, 1992.

The addition of fiberoptic bundles to PACs has enabled the continuous monitoring of Svo_2 using reflectance spectrophotometry. The catheter is connected to a device that includes a light-emitting diode and a sensor to detect the light returning from the pulmonary artery. Svo_2 is calculated from the differential absorption of various wavelengths of light by the saturated and desaturated hemoglobin.[324]

If it is assumed that there is constant oxygen consumption and arterial oxygen content, changes in Svo_2 should reflect changes in CO. Several investigators have come to the conclusion that it provides a valuable measure of CO during surgery.[325,326] The Svo_2 has been shown to correlate with cardiac index during CABG surgery when oxygen consumption is constant,[325] but not to correlate with the cardiac index when oxygen consumption is changing, such as during shivering after anesthesia.[327] The usefulness of the catheter may primarily be its ability to continuously monitor the balance between oxygen delivery and consumption.[328-331] Severe deterioration in the condition of critically ill patients, however, was often not predicted by changes in Svo_2.[332-334] London et al[335] published a prospective, multicenter, observational study in which continuous monitoring of Svo_2 was compared with standard PAC monitoring in 3265 cardiac surgical patients. They failed to show any improved outcome associated with the use of continuous Svo_2 catheters and only a small reduction in resource use.

Continuous monitoring of Svo_2 has been complicated by artifacts because of the vessel wall and clot formation on the catheter with loss of light intensity. Varying hematocrit may also introduce error, but not with all systems.[336] The values obtained with various fiberoptic catheter systems showed good agreement with in vitro (co-oximetry) Svo_2 measurements.[337-340]

CARDIAC OUTPUT MONITORING

The CO is the amount of blood delivered to the tissues by the heart each minute. It is a measurement that reflects the status of the entire circulatory system, not just the heart, because it is governed by autoregulation from the tissues. The CO is equal to the product of the SV and the heart rate (HR). Preload, afterload, HR, and contractility are the major determinants of the CO. The measurement of CO is of particular interest in patients with cardiac disease. This section describes methods of CO monitoring including thermodilution CO derived from the PAC.

▣ Fick Method

The Fick equation is derived from the concept that oxygen consumed by the tissues per unit time is equal to the amount of oxygen extracted per unit time from the circulation. The oxygen extracted from the circulation is the product of the arteriovenous oxygen content difference and the CO:

$$VO_2 = (CaO_2 - CvO_2) \times CO$$

Rearranging the equation, CO is calculated using the following formula:

$$CO = \frac{Vo_2}{(CaO_2 - CvO_2)}$$

in which CO is the cardiac output, Vo_2 is the oxygen consumption, CaO_2 is the arterial oxygen content, and CvO_2 is the mixed venous oxygen content.

In the direct Fick method, oxygen consumption is measured by indirect calorimetry using algorithms based on inspired and expired oxygen concentrations and volumes. Oxygen consumption can be calculated when the rate of fresh gas flow, respiratory rate, and change of oxygen concentration are known. Arterial oxygen content is measured from an arterial blood sample, and mixed venous oxygen content can be obtained from the PAC. Because of technical difficulties, oxygen consumption in pediatric patients is commonly estimated using the formulas of LaFarge and Miettinen[341] with the use of sex, HR, and age as variables. Oxygen consumption and arteriovenous oxygen content differences must be measured at steady state because the Fick principle is valid only when tissue oxygen uptake equals lung oxygen uptake.

The accuracy and reproducibility of the direct Fick CO technique have been determined in a variety of animal and human experiments. They usually have been found to be high.[342] The major limitations of the direct Fick technique are related to errors in sampling and analysis, difficulty in obtaining oxygen uptake continuously in the operating room, the presence of bulky equipment surrounding the endotracheal tube, or the inability to maintain steady-state hemodynamic and respiratory conditions.[343,344]

Some of these problems have been overcome with the introduction of metabolic modules for the measurement of oxygen consumption that are incorporated into the patient monitoring system and that do not depend on collecting gases in bulky sample chambers.[345] No flow or volume transducers are incorporated into these systems. Instead, continuous measurement of expiratory carbon dioxide concentrations in a constant flow allows for the calculation of the amount of carbon dioxide eliminated by the patient. This method is referred to as the "modified carbon dioxide Fick method." Inspiratory and expiratory oxygen and carbon dioxide concentrations are measured to obtain the respiratory quotient (RQ value), which is then used to derive oxygen consumption.

In the indirect Fick method of calculating CO, expired gases such as carbon dioxide (intermittent partial rebreathing of carbon dioxide) or acetylene replace oxygen consumption in the Fick equation.[346] Substituting CO_2 production for oxygen consumption, capnographic measurement of CO_2 concentrations may be used to provide a noninvasive Fick estimate of CO. The rebreathing technique is used to estimate mixed venous P_{CO_2}. In the clinical setting, patients are sedated and mechanically ventilated, and capnometry equipment is attached to a processor that calculates CO.[347] Studies comparing the CO_2 rebreathing method with standard measures of CO have yielded conflicting results.[348-352] Binder et al[353] studied postoperative cardiac surgical patients. They compared the CO_2 method with the thermodilution method and showed a good correlation. In contrast, van Heerden et al,[354] using a different device, found that CO measurements in cardiac surgery patients were overestimated using the CO_2 rebreathing technique.

Indicator Dilution

The indicator dilution method is based on the observation that, for a known amount of indicator introduced at one point in the circulation, the same amount of indicator should be detectable at a downstream point. The amount of indicator detected at the downstream point is equal to the product of CO and the change in indicator concentration over time. CO is calculated using the Stewart–Hamilton equation:

$$CO = I \times 60 \div \int C\, dt$$

in which I is amount of indicator injected, and $\int C\, dt$ is the integral of indicator concentration over time (60 converts seconds to minutes).

Cold saline (i.e., thermodilution) or lithium ions are used as indicators, whereas dye (e.g., indocyanine green) or radioisotopes are rarely used in current practice.[355] Blood flow is directly proportional to the amount of the indicator delivered and inversely proportional to the amount of indicator that is present at a sampling site distal to the injection site.

Thermodilution

Intermittent Thermodilution Cardiac Output
The thermodilution method, using the PAC, is the most commonly used method for invasively measuring CO in the clinical setting. With this technique, multiple COs can be obtained at frequent intervals using an inert indicator and without blood withdrawal. A bolus of cold fluid is injected into the RA, and the resulting temperature change is detected by the thermistor in the pulmonary artery.[203,356] When a thermal indicator is used, the modified Stewart–Hamilton equation is used to calculate CO:

$$CO = \frac{V(T_B - T_I) \times K_1 \times K_2}{\int_0^\infty \Delta T_B(t)dt}$$

in which CO is the cardiac output (L/min), V is the volume of injectate (mL), T_B is the initial blood temperature (°C), T_I is the initial injectate temperature (°C), K_1 is the density factor, K_2 is the computation constant, and $\int_0^\infty \Delta T_B(t)dt$ is the integral of blood temperature change over time.

A computer that integrates the area under the temperature versus time curve is used to perform the calculation. CO is inversely proportional to the area under the curve.

Accuracy
Salgado and Galetti[357] discovered that thermodilution CO was 2.9% greater than the true flows. Bilfinger et al[358] found that the average

difference between the thermodilution measurements and the reference values were 7% to 8% with room-temperature injectate and 11% to 13% with ice-cold saline injectate. Under strictly controlled in vitro conditions, the accuracy of the thermodilution CO technique varied from ±7% to ±13%.

When thermodilution measurements were compared with the direct Fick method, correlation coefficients of 0.96 were obtained in two studies.[359,360] Pelletier compared total electromagnetic flow, including coronary blood flow, with thermodilution CO in dogs.[361] He observed that, on average, thermodilution overestimated total aortic flow by ±3% compared with electromagnetic flow, whether iced or room-temperature injectate was used.

When CO measurements were compared using the thermodilution and indocyanine green methods, the results varied among various studies, with some investigators finding excellent correlations over a wide range of outputs, whereas others observed that thermodilution systematically overestimated dye dilution CO.[362-364]

The temperature-versus-time curve is the crux of this technique, and any circumstances that affect it have consequences for the accuracy of the CO measurement. Specifically, anything that results in less "cold" reaching the thermistor, more "cold" reaching the thermistor, or an unstable temperature baseline will adversely affect the accuracy of the technique. Less "cold" reaching the thermistor would result in overestimation of the CO. This could be caused by a smaller amount of indicator, indicator that is too warm, a thrombus on the thermistor, or partial "wedging" of the catheter. Conversely, underestimation of the CO will occur if excessive volume of injectate, or injectate that is too cold, is used to perform the measurement. Intracardiac shunts have unpredictable effects that depend on the anatomy and physiology of individual patients. In patients with large left-to-right shunts, PAC-derived thermodilution CO is not recommended for accurate CO measurement. Surprisingly, however, in one report, large left-to-right shunts were found not to adversely affect the measurement of systemic CO.[365] Box 14-14 lists common errors in PAC thermodilution CO measurements.

Wetzel and Latson[366] observed variations of up to 80% in measured CO when the rate of administration of intravenous crystalloid infusions caused fluctuations in baseline blood temperature. The rapid temperature decrease seen after weaning from hypothermic CPB has been shown to result in the underestimation of CO by 0.6 to 2.0 L/min.[367] In that study, the temperature decrease after CPB was 0.14°C/min. Latson et al[368] also found that the normal changes in the PA that occur with each respiratory cycle appear to be exaggerated in the early phase after hypothermic CPB. This may cause peak-to-peak errors in estimation of intermittent CO of up to 50% if initiated at different times during the ventilatory cycle. This effect was significantly decreased with thermal

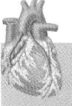

BOX 14-14. COMMON ERRORS IN PULMONARY ARTERY CATHETER THERMODILUTION CARDIAC OUTPUT MEASUREMENTS

Underestimation of True CO
- Injectate volume > programmed volume (typically 10 mL)
- Large amounts of fluid administered simultaneous to CO measurement (rapid infusions should be stopped)
- Injectate colder than measured temperature injectate (e.g., injectate temperature probe next to heat-emitting hardware instead of injectate fluid)

Overestimation of True CO
- Injectate volume < programmed volume
- Injectate warmer than measured temperature injectate

Other Considerations
- Surgical manipulation of the heart
- Fluid administration from aortic CPB cannula
- Arrhythmias

CO, cardiac output; CPB, cardiopulmonary bypass.

equilibration, approximately 30 minutes after CPB. This problem is less prevalent currently because hypothermic CPB is used less commonly.

TR generally has been considered as a source of error in thermodilution CO determinations. The scientific data, however, are contradictory. Some experimental reports indicate that TR does not impair the accuracy of thermodilution CO when compared with the Fick method[369] and electromagnetic flow probes.[370,371] In contrast, Heerdt et al[372] reported that thermodilution CO had wide variability in the direction and magnitude of error compared with Doppler and electromagnetic CO in a single patient with acute TR. The severity of TR also seems to be important in determining its effect on CO measurements by thermodilution, with underestimation of CO occurring in the presence of more severe TR.[373]

Slowing of the HR has been described as a side effect of rapid injection of cold injectate into the heart.[374] In a prospective study, Harris et al[375] observed that with the use of iced injectate, a decrease in HR of more than 10% occurred in 22% of the determinations. Nishikawa and Dohi[376] reported that HR slowing was more likely in patients with a low cardiac index, low mean PAP, and high SVR.

Precision

In vivo reproducibility can be assessed by obtaining a large number of thermodilution COs and calculating their standard deviation. Hoel[377] postulated that a true CO could be measured by calculating the average of an infinite number of thermal injections. Using probability calculus, he found that with two injections there was only a 50% probability of being within 5% of the true CO. With three injections, there was an 89% probability of being within 10% of the true CO. In an attempt to better delineate the reproducibility of the technique, Stetz et al[378] reviewed 14 publications on the use of thermodilution in clinical practice. They concluded that with the use of commercial thermodilution devices, a minimal difference of 12% to 15% (average, 13%) between determinations was required for statistical significance, provided that each determination was obtained by averaging three measurements.

A few studies also have evaluated the effects of the timing of the injection in the respiratory cycle on the reproducibility of thermodilution CO. In mechanically ventilated dogs, Snyder and Powner[379] observed that CO variations were present in each respiratory cycle and were usually greater than 10%. Stevens et al[380] studied the effects of the respiratory cycle on thermodilution CO in critically ill patients. They confirmed that injections at specific times in the respiratory cycle resulted in less variability but possibly decreased accuracy. They nevertheless concluded that, in clinical practice, the improvement in reproducibility was more important than the decrease in accuracy.

The effects of injectate volume and temperature on the variability of thermodilution CO have also been studied in critically ill patients.[381] Six combinations of injectate volume (3, 5, and 10 mL) and temperature (iced and room temperature) were studied in 18 adult, intubated patients. The best reproducibility was obtained with 10-mL injections at 0°C or room temperature.

In summary, the precision of the thermodilution CO technique is not very good, but it can be improved by ensuring that, for each determination, the rate and duration of the injection are kept as constant as possible.[382] Whenever possible, 10-mL volumes of injectate should be used, and the timing of the injection in the respiratory cycle should be the same. However, if injection is always at the same point in the respiratory cycle, some loss in accuracy is to be expected.

Continuous Thermodilution Cardiac Output

Pulmonary arterial catheters with the ability to measure CO continuously were introduced into clinical practice in the 1990s. The method that has gained the most clinical use functions by mildly heating the blood—originally using a "pseudorandom stochastic" fashion. In vitro and in vivo studies have shown that good correlations exist between this method and other measures of CO.[383–388] Unfortunately, the correlation with CO measurements using the intermittent thermodilution method is inconsistent.[389,390]

Bottiger et al[391] found that there was a poor correlation between intermittent and continuous thermodilution CO ($r = 0.273$) in the first

45 minutes after CPB. In contrast, there was an excellent correlation between intermittent and continuous CO measurements obtained in more physiologically stable periods. Perhaps the reason for this observation lies in the unstable thermal baseline after hypothermic CPB that was described in the previous section.

The routine use of continuous CO catheters in cardiac surgery patients has not been shown to improve outcome, and these catheters are more expensive than standard PACs. Bolus thermodilution CO still holds its place as the gold standard of CO measurements in the clinical setting. Even though its accuracy is adversely affected by imprecise technique, it introduces extra intravenous volume and the measurements are more labor intensive. Continuous CO catheters partially alleviate these problems and provide a continuous CO trend.[392] However, there is insufficient evidence to support their routine use in cardiac surgery patients.

Dye Dilution

The indicator dilution method using indocyanine green dye had been the most popular technique of CO measurement before the introduction of the thermodilution method. The dye was injected into a central vein and continuously sampled from arterial blood and passed through a densitometer to measure the change in indicator concentration over time. A computer calculated the area under the dye concentration curve by integration of the dye concentrations over time and computed CO. After completion of the CO determination, the sampled blood was returned to the patient. Recirculation of the indicator distorted the primary time-concentration curve, and the buildup of indicator in the blood resulted in high background concentrations, which limited the total number of measurements that could be obtained.

Intracardiac shunting could be diagnosed by alterations of the dye dilution curve. Left-to-right shunts produce a decrease in the peak concentration of the dye, a prolonged disappearance time, and absence of the recirculation peak. In contrast, right-to-left shunts produce an early-appearing hump on the dye dilution curve.

The introduction of lithium chloride as the indicator has led to a renaissance of the indicator dilution technique for the measurement of CO.[355,393–395] A lithium chloride solution is injected through a central venous catheter, and a lithium-selective electrode (that is connected to a standard intra-arterial cannula) measures plasma lithium concentrations. Only intra-arterial and central venous catheters are required. The Lithium Dilution CO system (LiDCO, Lake Villa, IL) requires only a peripheral venous catheter for injection of small doses of lithium and an arterial catheter equipped with a blood withdrawal system and lithium sensor. Agreement with PAC thermodilution is acceptable in most clinical settings.[396] This system also includes a continuous CO calculation capability based on the arterial pulse wave that must be calibrated to the lithium dilution value.

Transpulmonary Thermodilution

Using the same principle as PAC thermodilution, transpulmonary thermodilution (PiCCO; Philips Medical, Andover, MA) involves administration of cold injectate into a central vein, with the temperature change curve generated from a thermistor-containing central arterial catheter (femoral or axillary). Studies have indicated close agreement with PAC thermodilution.[39–41] In addition to providing CO measurements, the system provides estimates of global end-diastolic volume and extravascular lung water. Current systems are equipped with a continuous CO based on the arterial pulse wave that must be calibrated to the thermodilution value. The system should be calibrated frequently when rapid changes in vascular tone occur.[42]

ALTERNATIVE TECHNIQUES FOR ASSESSING CARDIAC OUTPUT

The development of clinically useful techniques to measure CO and assess volume status that do not require PA catheterization is flourishing. Numerous technologies based on platforms such as indicator dilution (lithium), US, arterial waveform analysis, and electrical bio-impedance are commercially available. Some of the more promising technologies are reviewed here, as are the "pros and cons" of using them for cardiac surgery patients.

Cardiac Output Measurements Using Ultrasound Technology

Measurements of SV and CO can be accomplished using various echocardiographic techniques. Early attempts were made using M-mode echocardiographic dimensions and results were promising.[397,398] 2D echocardiography measurements depend on adequate imaging and calculate volume dimensions from 2D data using a geometric assumption of chamber size and shape. With the introduction of 3D echocardiography, it should be possible to overcome some of the problems encountered with this mathematical approach and to determine and visualize true chamber size.[399] A different technique uses Doppler echocardiography to determine CO. Unlike 2D echocardiography-derived CO measurements, Doppler echocardiography is less dependent on geometric assumptions (see Chapter 12).

Doppler Ultrasound

US can be used for the measurement of CO based on the Doppler principle. Information on blood flow is obtained by applying Doppler frequency shift analysis to echoes reflected by the moving red blood cells. Blood flow velocity, direction, and acceleration can be instantaneously determined. From this information, SV and CO are calculated using the following formula:

$$SV = VTI \times CSA$$

in which VTI is the Doppler velocity-time integral (i.e., area under the Doppler spectral display curve), and CSA is the cross-sectional area at the site of flow measurement. The SV is then multiplied by HR to calculate the CO.

Blood flow in the human heart can be described by the continuity equation, which states that the flow measured at one CSA of the heart is equal to the flow measured at another cross section (as long as there is no intracardiac shunt). Theoretically, CO may be measured at all anatomic sites in which a CSA is determined and a Doppler beam positioned. Depending on the velocity being measured, pulsed-wave Doppler or continuous-wave Doppler technology is applied. The US signals can be transmitted and detected using transthoracic, transesophageal (TEE), suprasternal, or transtracheal transducers. With intraoperative TEE, CO measurements can be made at the aortic,[400,401] pulmonary artery,[402,403] or mitral valve positions,[404] with the former two being the more common. The degree of accuracy in comparative studies has been promising.[405-413] Technical limitations include the quality of the imaging, the accuracy of the valve or outflow tract area calculations, and the degree of alignment between the US beam and the direction of blood flow. Because the CSA is determined from 2D images, converting measurements of the radius to calculate area leads to exponential increases in any errors. Calculation of the CSA at the mitral valve site gives various results because the orifice is not constant throughout the cardiac cycle. The Doppler beam must be as parallel to the blood flow as possible. Angles larger than 30 degrees between the US beam and the direction of blood flow lead to increased error, despite angle-correction algorithms. The accurate measurement of CO using TEE can be time and labor intensive; it is best to obtain multiple measurements of both CSA and Doppler flow. For this reason, it is not commonly used as a primary means of assessing CO intraoperatively, but rather as a backup method when thermodilution is unavailable or when calculation of intracardiac shunt is desired (compare the CO measurements from the PA and left ventricular outflow tract).

Dedicated, automated systems are available for measuring CO continuously using Doppler technology (transesophageal Doppler). Recent meta-analyses indicate that they are generally accurate and can trend CO well.[414] These systems have a narrow, flexible probe placed in the esophagus, with the Doppler beam aimed posteriorly, toward the descending aorta. The CSA of the aorta can either be measured or assumed, and the SV is calculated from the product of the VTI and the aortic CSA. Possible sources of inaccuracy are errors in the measurement or assumption of the aortic CSA and malpositioning of the probe. These factors were mentioned as probable contributors to inaccuracies both during and after cardiac surgery.[415] Also, the device detects blood flow only to the lower part of the body (descending aorta). If the relation between upper and lower body blood flow changes, inaccuracies may develop. An example of this phenomenon is increasing P_{CO_2} resulting in increased cerebral blood flow, and thus underestimation of the global CO by transesophageal Doppler.[416]

Although these devices can be useful for monitoring CO in the critically ill[417] and managing fluid administration during major surgery ("goal-directed therapy"),[418] their use in cardiac anesthesia is limited because of the ever-increasing popularity and wider utility of TEE.

Two-Dimensional Echocardiography

Two-dimensional echocardiography allows for the calculation of CO using the following formula:

$$CO = (EDV - ESV) \times HR$$

in which EDV is the end-diastolic volume, ESV is the end-systolic volume, and HR is the heart rate. 2D echo-derived LV volume and CO determinations are based on geometric assumptions of chamber size and shape (i.e., Simpson's rule method). Reliable estimation of CO depends on adequate imaging that allows for exact tracing of the endocardial border. The echo-derived cardiac index shows a good correlation with the simultaneously measured value using the standard thermodilution method (see Chapter 12).[419-421]

Automated Border Detection

Automated border detection (ABD) is an endocardial tracking algorithm superimposed on B-mode 2D images. It is commercially available on some TEE machines and allows for semiautomated measurement of LV areas. The blood–endocardial interface is detected and displayed continuously. End-diastolic area, end-systolic area, and fractional area of contraction are displayed. Computer processing of the 2D data (using a single-plane modification of Simpson's rule) allows for an estimation of LV volumes and EF.[422,423] Validation studies comparing ABD with conductance catheter volume measurement or thermodilution showed promising results.[424-428] Absolute measurements of LV dimensions tend to be systematically underestimated by ABD techniques; however, ABD might still be useful for detecting CO trends rather than absolute values.[429] Several difficulties must be overcome. Signal quality depends on high-quality 2D echocardiographic images; a region of interest needs to be defined manually by the user; and endocardial image dropout requires repetitive readjustments by the user to optimize the image using power settings, gain adjustments, and probe manipulation. For those reasons, ABD is typically not clinically useful in the cardiac surgery operative setting.

Three-Dimensional Echocardiographic Cardiac Output

Eventually, 3D echocardiography will result in a major advance in minimally invasive CO monitoring. Calculations of 3D images require sequential acquisition of 2D echocardiographic data from multiple imaging planes. Early results of 3D evaluation of the heart were promising,[430-433] and advances in processor speed and echocardiographic technology have already helped to overcome some of the problems of this technology. Good correlation and accuracy could be demonstrated when 3D echocardiographic estimates of volumetric measures were compared with established methods.[434-436]

Cardiac Output Derived from Arterial Pulse Waves

A number of systems are now available that estimate CO using characteristics of the arterial pulse as transduced from an arterial catheter. It has long been known that pulsatility in the arterial tree is proportional to SV: the greater the SV, the greater the amplitude of the resulting pressure wave. This proportionality can be exploited if a proportionality constant (K), based on the resistance and compliance of the vessels, is known:

$$SV = (K)(P)$$

where K is the proportionality constant, and P is an index of pulsatility. Pulsatility is easily assessed using parameters such as area under the pressure wave, area under the systolic portion of the wave, or standard deviation of the wave. Deriving K is a more complex issue. A common approach has been to first measure the SV by another method (e.g., lithium dilution, transpulmonary thermodilution), measure the pulsatility, and then solve for the K value:

$$K = SV/P$$

The K value can subsequently be used to calculate SV continuously from the pulsatility of the wave. LiDCOplus (LiDCO Ltd, Lake Villa, IL, USA) and PiCCOplus (PULSION Medical Inc., Irring, TX, USA) both use this approach with success. A concern has been reported, however: If the PiCCOplus system is not recalibrated when changes occur in the resistance and/or compliance of the vascular tree, the SV calculation will be inaccurate.[437]

Another recently developed method does not require calibration, but rather calculates K from patient demographics (age, height, weight, sex) and characteristics of the arterial wave such as MAP, skewness, and kurtosis (Vigileo/FloTrac; Edwards Lifesciences, Irvine, CA).[438] This promising system is accurate under most steady-state conditions,[439] but like the calibrated systems, it has been suggested that rapid changes in vascular tone may lead to inaccuracies. In one study, acute changes in vascular tone resulting from vasopressor administration or sternotomy resulted in discrepancies between the FloTrac/Vigileo (fast-reacting) and continuous thermodilution CO (slow-reacting) systems.[440,441] Also, because pulse contour systems rely on an arterial wave that is purely reflective of the net forward SV, situations in which the arterial wave is distorted, either by artifact or a physiologic phenomenon (intra-aortic balloon counterpulsation, aortic regurgitation), will lead to inaccuracies.[442]

An added benefit of the arterial wave–based systems is that they all provide calculation of dynamic parameters: stroke volume variation, pulse pressure variation, or both. It has long been known that SV, and thus BP, varies with ventilation,[443] and this variation is exaggerated when cardiac filling is impaired (e.g., hypovolemia, constrictive pericarditis, cardiac tamponade). This variation can now be quantified continuously, offering a new method to predict fluid responsiveness.[444,445] The application of dynamic parameters during cardiac surgery may be limited because they are blunted when the chest is open, but they can be used after surgery as an aid in fluid therapy and diagnosis of hemodynamic instability. Specifically, they can help to differentiate between cardiac failure (low stroke volume variation) and hypovolemia (high stroke volume variation).

The future of the application of arterial-based CO systems for cardiac surgery is uncertain. Advantages include the minimally invasive nature (LiDCO and FloTrac), but possible disadvantages include ongoing concerns about accuracy under certain circumstances and the lack of invasive data such as PAP. With time, these systems will become increasingly accurate and powerful, becoming progressively more useful in the perioperative period for cardiac surgical patients.

Cardiac Output Derived from Bioimpedance

With advances in hardware and software technology, the past few years have seen a resurgence in interest in using changes in thoracic electrical impedance to estimate CO. Bioimpedance CO is based on the principle that cyclical increases in blood volume in the great vessels, as well as alignment of red blood cells in the thoracic aorta resulting from increased velocity, cause concomitant decreases in the electrical impedance in the chest. An alternating current of low amplitude is introduced and simultaneously sensed by electrodes placed around the neck, and laterally on the thorax, or abdomen to measure thoracic electrical bioimpedance. Changes in thoracic bioimpedance are induced by ventilation and pulsatile blood flow, and processing of the signal results in a characteristic impedance (Z) waveform. For measurement of SV, only the cardiac-induced pulsatile component of the total change in electrical impedance is analyzed (dZ/dt), as the respiratory component is filtered out.

Although accuracy concerns persist, correlation of the latest generations of these systems with PAC thermodilution has improved relative to earlier models, both for postoperative cardiac surgical patients,[446] and intraoperative patients with their chests open.[447] Recently, a bioimpedance monitor with electrodes mounted on a specially manufactured endotracheal tube has been introduced. Preliminary studies of its accuracy are encouraging.[448,449]

Alternative, less invasive means of determining CO continue to develop and will play an expanding role in the perioperative care of cardiac surgical patients. Characteristics of alternative methods of CO measurement are presented in Table 14-5.

Right Ventricular Ejection Fraction and End-Diastolic Volume

Using rapid-response thermistors that are incorporated into PACs, it is possible to determine the right ventricular ejection fraction from the exponential decay of the thermodilution curve. End-diastolic temperature points in the thermodilution curve are identified using the R-wave signal from an ECG input.[450,451] From these data, SV, RV end-diastolic volume, and RV end-systolic volume may be calculated. Assumptions that are essential to the accuracy of the technique include a regular RR interval, "instantaneous" mixing of the injectate or thermal heat signal with the RV blood, and absence of TR. The use of this type of monitoring could be justified in patients with severe RV dysfunction caused by myocardial infarction, right-sided coronary artery disease, pulmonary hypertension, left-sided heart failure, or intrinsic pulmonary disease. The accuracy of this technique has been questioned, however,[452,453] and right ventricular ejection fraction catheters are rarely used, especially with TEE becoming more prevalent in the OR setting.

LEFT ATRIAL PRESSURE MONITORING

Left atrial pressure monitoring is an invasive technique in which a catheter is placed by the surgeon into the right superior pulmonary vein (usually) and advanced into the LA. A Teflon-pledgetted purse-string stitch is placed around the catheter to provide a surface for clotting on removal of the catheter. The catheter is brought out through the skin in the subxiphoid region and is sutured in place. It is important to maintain positive airway pressure or distend the LA in some other way during insertion of the catheter to prevent air entry into the pulmonary vein and the left side of the heart.

The LAP is an extremely informative monitor, but it also requires extreme caution. The possibility of air embolism to the coronary or cerebral circulations is always present. This problem exists on insertion and during its continued use postoperatively in the ICU. There is also the risk for clot formation on the catheter and subsequent embolization when the catheter is flushed or removed; therefore, a continuous flushing system is

TABLE 14-5	Alternative Means of Determining Cardiac Output and Representative Commercially Available Systems				
Technology	Examples of Devices Available	Accuracy vs. PAC	Potential Sources of Inaccuracy	Potential for Cardiac Surgery, Advantages	
TEE Doppler	Standard TEE	++++	Doppler beam misalignment Inaccurate 2D cross-sectional area measurement	+++ Minimally invasive Potentially very accurate Access to right and left side for shunt determination	
TED Doppler	Cardio Q (Deltex)	+++	Doppler beam misalignment Inaccurate aortic cross-sectional area Distribution of blood flow, lower vs. upper body	+ Minimally invasive May be used after surgery	
TEE 2D	Standard TEE	+++	Exceptions to Simpson rule (ventricular aneurysm) Measurement of LV area	+ Minimally invasive	
Indicator dilution (lithium)	LiDCO	++++	Technical error, muscle relaxants, ingestion of lithium medication	+ Minimally invasive May be used after surgery	
Transpulmonary Thermodilution	PiCCO (Pulsion)	++++	Technical error, thermal changes in chest	+++ Global end-diastolic volume Extravascular lung water	
Arterial pulse wave	LidCO Plus PiCCO Plus (Pulsion) FloTrac (Edwards)	+++ +++	Arterial wave artifact Intra-aortic balloon Aortic regurgitation Rapid changes in vascular tone	+++ Minimally invasive Continuous Dynamic parameters provided FloTrac simpler to use and may track vascular tone changes better: does not require calibration	
Bioimpedance, Velocimetry	ICON (Cardiotronic) BioZ (Sonosite) ECOM (Conmed)	++	Ventilation pattern Lung water, opening and closing of chest	++ Noninvasive Continuous Technology improving	

Assessments at the time of writing, based on available literature and experience.

++++ very high; +++ high; ++ medium; + low; LV, left ventricular; PAC, pulmonary artery catheter; TED, transesophageal Doppler; TEE, transesophageal echocardiography.

Cardio Q (Deltex Medical, SC, Inc, Greenville, SC, USA); LiDCO (LiDCO Ltd, Lake Villa, IL, USA); PiCCO (PULSION Medical Inc, Irving, TX, USA); FloTrac (Edwards Lifesciences Corp, Irvine, CA, USA); ICON (Cardiotronic Inc, LaJolla, CA, USA); BioZ (Sonosite, Bothell, WA, USA); ECOM (Conmed Corp, Utica, NY, USA)

necessary to avoid thrombus formation on the catheter tip in the postoperative period. After surgery, there is also the risk for bleeding when the LAP catheter is removed. It therefore should be removed while the chest tubes are still in place to diagnose and treat this problem. Other reported complications include catheter retention and prosthetic valve entrapment.[454]

LAP monitoring is usually restricted to use in patients in whom PCWP determinations have been unsuccessful, are impractical, or are known to be inaccurate (e.g., in patients with pulmonary vascular disease or in small children). The catheter may also be used to infuse inotropic agents selectively to the systemic circulation to minimize the effects on the pulmonary circulation. This was more important before therapies that selectively treat pulmonary vasoconstriction were available.

ANALYSIS AND INTERPRETATION OF HEMODYNAMIC DATA

The information provided by hemodynamic monitoring permits the calculation of various derived parameters that assist in evaluating patients clinically. The formulas, normal values, and units for the calculation of various hemodynamic parameters are presented in Tables 14-2 and 14-3. These parameters include the SVR, pulmonary vascular resistance (PVR), SV, left ventricular stroke work, and right ventricular stroke work. As an example of information that may be obtained, graphs of PCWP versus SV can be constructed for individual patients; these "Starling curves" provide insight into the contractile state of the heart. Although these parameters are easily derived using the standard formulas, many modern monitors perform these calculations. The various hemodynamic parameters may be normalized by indexing them to body surface area to compare data among patients of different body weights and types.

Systemic and Pulmonary Vascular Resistances

SVR represents an estimation of the afterload of the left ventricle. Afterload is roughly defined as the force that impedes or opposes ventricular contraction (see Chapter 5). Greater SVR results in increased LV

systolic wall stress. This has clinical significance because LV wall stress is one of the major determinants of myocardial oxygen consumption. Increases in wall stress have been observed in patients with LV enlargement caused by systemic hypertension, aortic stenosis, and aortic regurgitation.[455]

Clinically, calculations of SVR are used to assess the response to inotropic, vasodilator, and vasoconstrictive agents. For example, a patient who is hypotensive despite a high normal CO has a low SVR. The SVR is calculated and then therapy is instituted (e.g., a vasoconstrictor). A repeat calculation of the SVR enables the clinician to titrate the therapy to the appropriate end point. Despite this common use in the operating room and ICU setting, there is good evidence that SVR is not an accurate indicator of true afterload.[456] Nevertheless, SVR currently remains the most useful clinical technique for measuring afterload.

PVR remains the traditional measure of afterload of the right ventricle. This is also a flawed assumption because the recruitable nature of the pulmonary vasculature violates the assumptions of the PVR formula.[457] As the PAP increases, the pulmonary vasculature distends (increasing the size of West's zone III of the lung).[458] The net gain in the cross-sectional area of the pulmonary vasculature results in a decrease in the measured PVR. Systolic PAP may provide a better estimation of RV afterload. PVR and PAP do provide some clinically useful information regarding the pulmonary vasculature and are readily available in patients with PACs. The PVR should be used in conjunction with other hemodynamic data to assess the response of the pulmonary vasculature to pharmacologic therapy and physiologic changes (see Chapter 5).

Frank-Starling Relations

Myocardial function depends on the contractile state and the preload of the ventricle (sarcomere length at end-diastole). The relation between the ventricular preload and myocardial work (ventricular stroke work) is the Frank-Starling relation. The slope of the curve indicates the contractile state of the myocardium (Figure 14-24). For clinical purposes, it is usually not feasible to measure actual end-diastolic volumes (can be estimated with TEE), and approximations of end-diastolic pressure,

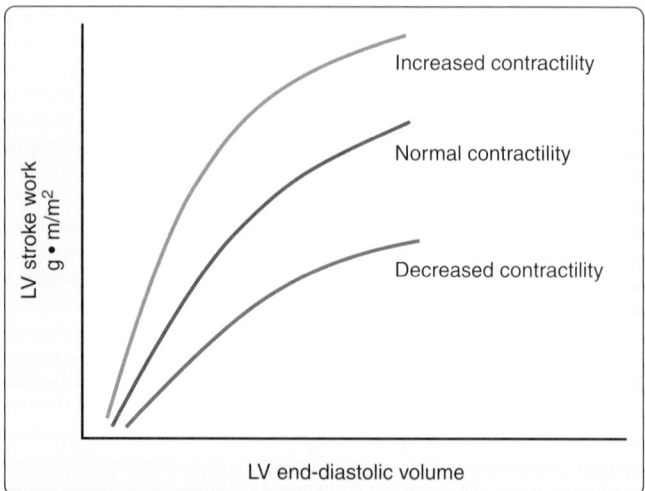

Figure 14-24 The graph of left ventricular (LV) stroke work versus LV preload (i.e., end-diastolic volume) is known as the Frank-Starling relation. Shifting of the curve upward and to the left represents increased contractility. Shifting of the curve downward and to the right represents decreased contractility. Alterations in afterload significantly affect the curve.

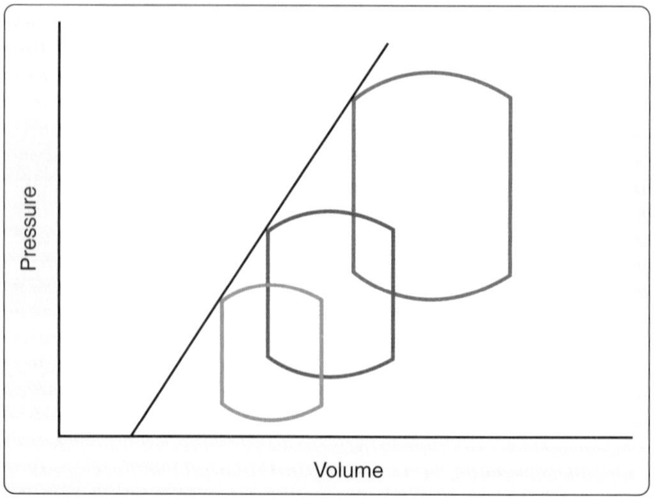

Figure 14-25 The end-systolic pressure-volume relation, also known as end-systolic elastance, is the line connecting the end-systolic points of multiple pressure-volume loops that are obtained at various preloads. An increased slope (i.e., steeper line) represents increased contractility, and a decreased slope represents decreased contractility. This measurement is relatively insensitive to variations in afterload.

such as the PCWP or LAP, are often substituted. This introduces error because the relation between end-diastolic pressure and volume is usually nonlinear (as described by the diastolic ventricular compliance curve) and is dynamic. The Frank-Starling relation is extremely sensitive to changes in afterload. Patients with LV or RV dysfunction may have severe decrements in SV with increased SVR or PVR, respectively.

End-Systolic Elastance and Pressure-Volume Loops

An important limitation of isovolumic and ejection phase indices of contractility (e.g., the Frank-Starling relationship) is their significant sensitivity to ventricular loading conditions. The use of load-independent indices has been explored to overcome this shortcoming. One such index is the LV end-systolic pressure-volume relation, also known as *end-systolic elastance*.[459] To measure this, multiple end-systolic pressures and volumes need to be measured during rapid and, preferably, pronounced alterations in LV preload (e.g., inferior vena cava occlusion). On a pressure-volume diagram, points defined by the end-systolic pressures and volumes of the several contractions will be positioned on a single line. The slope of this line is relatively independent of loading conditions and proportional to contractility; the steeper the slope, the greater the contractility (Figure 14-25; see Chapter 5).

The intraoperative determination of contractility by this technique has been hampered by difficulties in obtaining accurate ventricular volumes and pressures. Continuous LV pressure-volume loops may be displayed during cardiac surgery using LV conductance and micromanometry catheters that are introduced through the pulmonary veins.[460] End-systolic pressure-volume relation is still not a practical or routine means of assessing LV contractility in the clinical setting.

PULSE OXIMETRY

Pulse oximetry is probably one of the most important advances in anesthesia monitoring technology and has been accepted as an intraoperative monitoring standard. This is reflected in current practice parameters and recommendations for perioperative anesthetic monitoring published by the American Society of Anesthesiologists.[461] The results of outcome studies of pulse oximetry have been inconsistent, and the numbers of patients who would have to be studied in prospective, well-controlled

trials to show a change in outcome are prohibitively large.[462–464] In a recently published meta-analysis of controlled trials (Cochrane Central Register of Controlled Trials, searched time period 1956–2009) with a total of 22,992 patients included in the analysis, using pulse oximetry in the perioperative setting reduced the incidence of hypoxemia in the operating room, as well as in the recovery room.[465] Postoperative cognitive function, however, was not influenced by pulse oximetry monitoring. Postoperative complications (cardiovascular, respiratory, neurologic, and infectious) did not differ between patients monitored with or without pulse oximetry.

The advantages and limitations of the technique merit discussion to prevent misinterpretation of data provided by pulse oximetry devices. The absorbance spectra of oxyhemoglobin and reduced hemoglobin differ significantly. Oxyhemoglobin absorbs most infrared light (940 nm) and transmits most red light (660 nm). This may be remembered by considering that the red appearance of oxyhemoglobin would not be possible if it did not reflect (or transmit) red light. Reduced hemoglobin absorbs more red light (and appears blue) and transmits infrared light. The pulse oximeter uses this principle to determine the relative concentration of oxyhemoglobin in the blood.

Several things in addition to arterial blood also absorb red and infrared light in the tissues. These include capillary blood, venous blood, soft tissue, skin, and bone. All of these, however, absorb red and infrared light at a constant rate. The absorbance of the two waveforms of light increases as arterial blood rushes into the tissue during each cardiac cycle. It is this pulsatile component of the light absorbance that the pulse oximeter uses to calculate the arterial oxygen concentration. Many things interfere with the accuracy of pulse oximetry. Some of these include diminished tissue perfusion (e.g., limb ischemia, hypothermia, vasoconstricting drugs), ambient light, intravenous dyes, carboxyhemoglobin, and methemoglobin.[466]

As the signal strength of the pulse decreases in relation to the continuous absorption of the tissues, the ratio of absorbance of red-to-infrared light approaches unity. This would normally correlate with a saturation rate of 85%. It is important to regard a poor plethysmography tracing with a saturation rate of 85% as possibly representing artifact and to confirm the result with an independent technique.

In the lateral decubitus position, the downward hand may give a less reliable reading because of diminished tissue perfusion. It could be argued that this might serve as a good sign of improper axillary padding. However, the information provided by pulse oximetry is probably too important to lose intermittently during the operative procedure.

Another problem in cardiac procedures is that the plethysmography tracing often decreases in amplitude over the course of the procedure until the signal-to-noise ratio is too low for accurate oximetry. This is most likely due to hypothermia of the digits but also may be related to positioning, hypovolemia, high catecholamine levels, and extremes of age. It has been demonstrated that a digital perfusion pressure of 13 mm Hg and temperature of 24°C are the minimum requirements for accurate pulse oximetry readings before and after CPB.[467]

Reich et al[468] showed that there is a very high incidence of pulse oximetry failure in the cardiac surgery setting. The overall incidence rate of cases that had at least one continuous gap of 10 minutes or more in pulse oximetry data was 31%. The independent preoperative predictors of pulse oximetry data failure included ASA physical status III, IV, or V, and cardiac surgery. Intraoperative hypothermia, hypotension and hypertension, and duration of procedure also were independent risk factors.

Electrocautery also interferes with pulse oximetry. The electromagnetic field from the cautery device induces electrical current in the wires that connect to the pulse oximetry probe. These create a very high degree of electrical noise and may disrupt the oximetry reading.

The main disadvantage of pulse oximetry is that the Pao$_2$ must decline to less than 100 mm Hg before the device will begin to detect any change, and less than 60 mm Hg before rapid changes will occur. Thus, the device is not sensitive to changes in PaO$_2$ over wide ranges that are of clinical significance.

OXYGEN TRANSPORT CALCULATIONS

The ultimate purpose of circulation is the delivery of oxygen to the tissues. Oxygen is bound to hemoglobin and is also dissolved in the plasma (to a much smaller extent). If the hemoglobin concentration, arterial and mixed venous blood gases, and CO are available, then oxygen transport calculations may be performed. This can then allow for optimization of these parameters to improve delivery and uptake of the proper amount of oxygen to the tissues. These calculations are shown in Table 14-3.

▨ Monitoring Coronary Perfusion

The coronary perfusion pressure (CPP) is usually defined as the aortic diastolic blood pressure (DAP) minus the LVEDP:

$$CPP = DAP - LVEDP$$

Elevation of the LVEDP will decrease the gradient of blood flow to the vulnerable subendocardial tissue during diastole, as will a decrease in the DBP.[469] If coronary artery disease is present, significant stenosis will decrease the coronary artery DBP well below the aortic DBP, and elevation of LVEDP can seriously jeopardize the subendocardium.[470] An increase in the LVEDP is detrimental in two ways: decreased coronary blood flow and increased myocardial oxygen demand (Mvo$_2$), which explain the severe ischemia seen with overdistention of the left ventricle. Tachycardia is also extremely detrimental because it decreases

coronary filling time and increases oxygen demand. Subendocardial ischemia is commonly produced by a combination of tachycardia and increased LVEDP (see Chapters 6 and 18).

▨ Cerebral Oximetry

Near-infrared spectroscopy technology has been used to monitor cerebral oxygenation noninvasively, and these data may be predictive of adverse neurologic outcomes. Murkin et al[471] monitored near-infrared spectroscopy and targeted therapy to optimize cerebral tissue oxygen saturation (Scto$_2$) in patients undergoing CABG. They found that a composite measure of postoperative organ dysfunction was substantially improved in the treatment group where goal-directed therapy aimed to maintain the Scto$_2$ values within 25% of the preinduction baseline.[471] More recently developed Scto$_2$ technology using a four-wavelength interrogation of brain tissue has been validated as a monitor of absolute Scto$_2$.[472] A potential advantage of absolute brain tissue oxygenation is that threshold values may be more strongly associated with adverse outcomes than trends. Using that technology, Fischer et al's[473] recent investigation demonstrated that decreased Scto$_2$ values were associated with the major complications of prolonged postoperative mechanical ventilation and prolonged ICU and hospital length of stay in thoracic aortic arch surgical repairs. Both the nadir of Scto$_2$ and the integral of low Scto$_2$ over time were associated with severe adverse outcomes. Each additional decade of life was associated with greater risk for adverse outcomes.[473]

Slater et al[474] found that patients with prolonged low Scto$_2$ undergoing CABG had a greater incidence of early postoperative neurocognitive dysfunction and prolonged hospital length of stay (see Chapters 16 and 36). Casati et al[475] showed a shorter length of postanesthesia care unit and hospital length of stay in abdominal surgery when patients were actively treated to maintain Scto$_2$ greater than 75% of the baseline values using a preset algorithm.

In cardiac surgery, Scto$_2$ monitoring may be an index of overall organ perfusion and injury. Various investigators' findings that Scto$_2$ data predicted patient outcomes suggest that future studies may identify target Scto$_2$ values that should be maintained in different clinical settings.

SUMMARY

The choice of appropriate monitoring is a difficult task. Despite many years of clinical experience, there are no convincing outcome data that demonstrate the superiority of more invasive versus less invasive monitoring techniques. Therefore, the clinician must make a rational decision based on the following conditions:

- The patient's underlying medical diseases
- The degree of hemodynamic compromise, myocardial ischemia risk, and fluid shift likely to result from the proposed surgery
- The effects of the anesthetic drugs and techniques on the patient's cardiovascular system
- The skills of the practitioner and his or her understanding of the risks, benefits, and alternatives to the different types of hemodynamic monitoring
- The integration of data from hemodynamic monitoring and TEE in the perioperative period

REFERENCES

1. O'Brien E, Waeber B, Parati G, et al: Blood pressure measuring devices: Recommendations of the European Society of Hypertension, *BMJ* 322:531, 2001.
2. Jones DW, Appel LJ, Sheps SG, et al: Measuring blood pressure accurately: New and persistent challenges, *JAMA* 289:1027, 2003.
3. Parati G, Ongaro G, Bilo G, et al: Non-invasive beat-to-beat blood pressure monitoring: New developments, *Blood Press Monit* 8:31, 2003.
4. Belani K, Ozaki M, Hynson J, et al: A new noninvasive method to measure blood pressure: Results of a multicenter trial, *Anesthesiology* 91:686, 1999.
5. Dorje P, Tremper K: Systolic pressure variation: A dynamic measure of the adequacy of intravascular volume, *Semin Anesth Periop Med Pain* 24:147–153, 2005.
6. Gunn SR, Pinsky MR: Implications of arterial pressure variation in patients in the intensive care unit, *Curr Opin Crit Care* 7:212, 2001.
7. Coriat P, Vrillon M, Perel A, et al: A comparison of systolic blood pressure variations and echocardiographic estimates of end-diastolic left ventricular size in patients after aortic surgery, *Anesth Analg* 78:56, 1994.
8. Remington JW: Contour changes of the aortic pulse during propagation, *Am J Physiol* 199:331, 1960.
9. Husum B, Palm T, Eriksen J: Percutaneous cannulation of the dorsalis pedis artery, *Br J Anaesth* 51:1055, 1979.
10. Carmona MJ, Barboza Junior LC, Buscatti RY, et al: Evaluation of the aorta-to-radial artery pressure gradient in patients undergoing surgery with cardiopulmonary bypass, *Rev Bras Anestesiol* 57:618–629, 2007.
11. Gravlee GP, Wong AB, Adkins TG, et al: A comparison of radial, brachial, and aortic pressures after cardiopulmonary bypass, *J Cardiothorac Anesth* 3:20–26, 1989.
12. Kim JM, Arakawa K, Bliss J: Arterial cannulation: Factors in the development of occlusion, *Anesth Analg* 54:836, 1975.

13. Grossman W, Baim DS: *Cardiac Catheterization, Angiography, and Intervention*, ed 6, Baltimore, 2000, Lippincott Williams & Wilkins.
14. Hunziker P: Accuracy and dynamic response of disposable pressure transducer-tubing systems, *Can J Anaesth* 34:409, 1987.
15. Hill DW: *Physics Applied to Anesthesia*, ed 4, London, 1980, Butterworth.
16. Gorback MS: Considerations in the interpretation of systemic pressure monitoring. In Lumb PD, Bryan-Brown CW, editors: *Complications in Critical Care Medicine*, Chicago, 1988, Year Book, p 296.
17. Todorovic M, Jensen EW, Thogersen C: Evaluation of dynamic performance in liquid-filled catheter systems for measuring invasive blood pressure, *Int J Clin Monit Comput* 13:173, 1996.
18. Heimann PA, Murray WB: Construction and use of catheter-manometer systems, *J Clin Monit* 9:45, 1993.
19. Boutros A, Albert S: Effect of the dynamic response of transducer-tubing system on accuracy of direct blood pressure measurement in patients, *Crit Care Med* 11:124, 1983.
20. Kleinman B, Frey K, Stevens R: The fast-flush test—is the clinical comparison equivalent to its in vitro simulation? *J Clin Monit Comput* 14:485, 1998.
21. Kleinman B, Powell S, Kumar P, et al: The fast-flush test measures the dynamic response of the entire blood pressure monitoring system, *Anesthesiology* 77:1215, 1992.
22. Schwid HA: Frequency response evaluation of radial artery catheter-manometer systems: Sinusoidal frequency analysis versus flush method, *J Clin Monit* 4:181, 1988.
23. Gibbs NC, Gardner RM: Dynamics of invasive pressure monitoring systems: Clinical and laboratory evaluation, *Heart Lung* 17:43, 1988.
24. Shimazaki Y, Watanabe T, Takahashi T, et al: Minimized mortality and neurological complications in surgery for chronic arch aneurysm: Axillary artery cannulation, selective cerebral perfusion, and replacement of the ascending and total arch aorta, *J Card Surg* 19:338, 2004.
25. Strauch JT, Spielvogel D, Lauten A, et al: Axillary artery cannulation: Routine use in ascending aorta and aortic arch replacement, *Ann Thorac Surg* 78:103, 2004.
26. Sinclair MC, Singer RL, Manley NJ, et al: Cannulation of the axillary artery for cardiopulmonary bypass: Safeguards and pitfalls, *Ann Thorac Surg* 75:931, 2003.
27. Shekar PS, Ehsan A, Gilfeather MS, et al: Arterial pressure monitoring during cardiopulmonary bypass using axillary arterial cannulation, *J Cardiothorac Vasc Anesth* 19:665–666, 2005.
28. Mozersky DJ, Buckley CJ, Hagood C, et al: Ultrasonic evaluation of the palmar circulation, *Am J Surg* 126:810, 1973.
29. Palm T: Evaluation of peripheral arterial pressure in the thumb following radial artery cannulation, *Br J Anaesth* 49:819, 1977.
30. Allen EV: Thromboangiitis obliterans: Methods of diagnosis of chronic occlusive arterial lesions distal to the wrist with illustrated cases, *Am J Med Sci* 178:237, 1929.
31. Greenhow DE: Incorrect performance of Allen's test: Ulnar artery flow erroneously presumed inadequate, *Anesthesiology* 37:356, 1972.
32. Brodsky JB: A simple method to determine patency of the ulnar artery intraoperatively prior to radial artery cannulation, *Anesthesiology* 42:626, 1975.
33. Nowak GS, Moorthy SS, McNiece WL: Use of pulse oximetry for assessment of collateral arterial flow, *Anesthesiology* 64:527, 1986.
34. Castella X: A practical way of performing Allen's test to assess palmar collateral circulation, *Anesth Analg* 77:1085, 1993.
35. Kahler AC, Mirza F: Alternative arterial catheterization site using the ulnar artery in critically ill pediatric patients, *Pediatr Crit Care Med* 3:370, 2002.
36. Marshall AG, Erwin DC, Wyse RKH, et al: Percutaneous arterial cannulation in children, *Anaesthesia* 39:27, 1984.
37. Slogoff S, Keats AS, Arlund C: On the safety of radial artery cannulation, *Anesthesiology* 59:42, 1983.
38. Mangano DT, Hickey RF: Ischemic injury following uncomplicated radial artery catheterization, *Anesth Analg* 58:55, 1979.
39. Barbeau GR, Arsenault F, Dugas L, et al: Evaluation of the ulnopalmar arterial arches with pulse oximetry and plethysmography: Comparison with the Allen's test in 1010 patients, *Am Heart J* 147:489, 2004.
40. Gardner RM, Schwartz R, Wong HC, et al: Percutaneous indwelling radial artery catheters for monitoring cardiovascular function, *N Engl J Med* 290:1227, 1974.
41. Rulf ENR, Mitchell MM, Prakash O: Measurement of arterial pressure after cardiopulmonary bypass with a long radial artery catheter, *J Cardiothorac Anesth* 4:19, 1990.
42. VanBeck JO, White RD, Abenstein JP, et al: Comparison of axillary artery or brachial artery pressure with aortic pressure after cardiopulmonary bypass using a long radial artery catheter, *J Cardiothorac Vasc Anesth* 7:312, 1993.
43. Stern DH, Gerson JL, Allen FB, et al: Can we trust the direct radial artery pressure immediately after cardiopulmonary bypass? *Anesthesiology* 62:557, 1985.
44. Mohr R, Lavee J, Goor DA: Inaccuracy of radial artery pressure measurement after cardiac operations, *J Thorac Cardiovasc Surg* 94:286, 1987.
45. VanBeck J, White R, Abenstein J, et al: Comparison of axillary artery or brachial artery pressure with aortic pressure after cardiopulmonary bypass using a long radial artery catheter, *J Cardiothorac Vasc Anesth* 7:312, 1993.
46. Rich G, Lubanski R, McLoughlin T: Differences between aortic and radial artery pressure associated with cardiopulmonary bypass, *Anesthesiology* 77:63, 1992.
47. Kanazawa M, Fukuyama H, Kinefuchi Y, et al: Relationship between aortic-to-radial arterial pressure gradient after cardiopulmonary bypass and changes in arterial elasticity, *Anesthesiology* 99:48, 2003.
48. Pascarelli EF, Bertrand CA: Comparison of blood pressures in the arms and legs, *N Engl J Med* 270:693, 1964.
49. Bazaral MG, Welch M, Golding LAR, et al: Comparison of brachial and radial arterial pressure monitoring in patients undergoing coronary artery bypass surgery, *Anesthesiology* 73:38, 1990.
50. Barnes RW, Foster E, Jansen GA, et al: Safety of brachial artery catheters as monitors in the intensive care unit—prospective evaluation with the Doppler ultrasonic velocity detector, *Anesthesiology* 44:260, 1976.
51. Armstrong PJ, Han DC, Baxter JA, et al: Complication rates of percutaneous brachial artery access in peripheral vascular angiography, *Ann Vasc Surg* 17:107, 2003.
52. Gurman GM, Kriemerman S: Cannulation of big arteries in critically ill patients, *Crit Care Med* 13:217, 1985.
53. Yacoub OF, Bacaling JH, Kelly M: Monitoring of axillary arterial pressure in a patient with Buerger's disease requiring clipping of an intracranial aneurysm, *Br J Anaesth* 59:1056, 1987.
54. Scheer B, Perel A, Pfeiffer UJ: Clinical review: Complications and risk factors of peripheral arterial catheters used for haemodynamic monitoring in anaesthesia and intensive care medicine, *Crit Care* 6:199, 2002.
55. Frezza EE, Mezghebe H: Indications and complications of arterial catheter use in surgical or medical intensive care units: Analysis of 4932 patients, *Am Surg* 64:127, 1998.
56. Haddad F, Zeeni C, El Rassi I, et al: Can femoral artery pressure monitoring be used routinely in cardiac surgery? *J Cardiothorac Vasc Anesth* 22:418–422, 2008.
57. Johnstone RE, Greenhow DE: Catheterization of the dorsalis pedis artery, *Anesthesiology* 39:654, 1973.
58. Barnhorst BA, Boener HB: Prevalence of generally absent pedal pulses, *N Engl J Med* 278:264, 1968.
59. Youngberg JA, Miller ED: Evaluation of percutaneous cannulations of the dorsalis pedis artery, *Anesthesiology* 44:80, 1976.
60. Porter JM: Raynaud's syndrome. In Sabiston DC, editor: *Textbook of Surgery*, Philadelphia, 1985, WB Saunders Company, pp 1925–1932.
61. Schwemmer U, Arzet HA, Trautner H, et al: Ultrasound-guided arterial cannulation in infants improves success rate, *Eur J Anaesthesiol* 23:476–480, 2006.
62. Mangar D, Thrush D, Connell G, et al: Direct or modified Seldinger guidewire-directed technique for arterial catheter insertion, *Anesth Analg* 76:714, 1993.
63. Fukutome T, Kojiro M, Tanigawa K, et al: Doppler-guided "percutaneous" radial artery cannulation in small children, *Anesthesiology* 69:434, 1988.
64. Morray JP, Brandford GH, Barnes LF, et al: Doppler-assisted radial artery cannulation in infants and children, *Anesth Analg* 63:346, 1984.
65. Levin PH, Sheinin O, Gozal Y: Use of ultrasound guidance in the insertion of radial artery catheters, *Crit Care Med* 31:481–484, 2003.
66. Shiver S, Blaivas M, Lyon M: A prospective comparison of ultrasound-guided and blindly placed radial arterial catheters, *Acad Emerg Med* 13:1275–1279, 2006.
67. Ganesh A, Kaye R, Cahill AM, et al: Evaluation of ultrasound-guided radial artery cannulation in children, *Pediatr Crit Care Med* 10:45–48, 2009.
68. Band JD, Maki DG: Infection caused by arterial catheters used for hemodynamic monitoring, *Am J Med* 67:735, 1979.
69. Shinozaki T, Deane R, Mazuzan JE, et al: Bacterial contamination of arterial lines: A prospective study, *JAMA* 249:223, 1983.
70. Weinstein RA, Stamm WE, Kramer L: Pressure monitoring devices: Overlooked sources of nosocomial infection, *JAMA* 236:936, 1976.
71. Stamm WE, Colella JJ, Anderson RL, et al: Indwelling arterial catheters as a source of nosocomial bacteremia, *N Engl J Med* 292:1099, 1975.
72. Rijnders BJ, Van Wijngaerden E, Wilmer A, et al: Use of full sterile barrier precautions during insertion of arterial catheters: A randomized trial, *Clin Infect Dis* 36:743, 2003.
73. Sherertz RJ: Update on vascular catheter infections, *Curr Opin Infect Dis* 17:303, 2004.
74. O'Grady NP, Alexander M, Dellinger EP, et al: Guidelines for the prevention of intravascular catheter-related infections. Centers for Disease Control and Prevention, *MMWR Recomm Rep* 51(RR-10):1, 2002.
75. Rijnders BJ, Peetermans WE, Verwaest C: Watchful waiting versus immediate catheter removal in ICU patients with suspected catheter-related infection: A randomized trial, *Intensive Care Med* 30:1073, 2004.
76. Mermel LA, Farr BM, Sherertz RJ, et al: Guidelines for the management of intravascular catheter-related infections, *Clin Infect Dis* 32:1249, 2001.
77. Pierson DJ, Hudson LD: Monitoring hemodynamics in the critically ill, *Med Clin North Am* 67:1343, 1983.
78. Bedford RF, Wollman H: Complications of percutaneous radial artery cannulation: An objective prospective study in man, *Anesthesiology* 38:228, 1973.
79. Bedford RF: Radial arterial function following percutaneous cannulation with 18- and 20-gauge catheters, *Anesthesiology* 47:37, 1977.
80. Bedford RF: Wrist circumference predicts the risk of radial arterial occlusion after cannulation, *Anesthesiology* 48:377, 1978.
81. Jones RM, Hill AB, Nahrwold ML, et al: The effect of method of radial artery cannulation on postcannulation blood flow and thrombus formation, *Anesthesiology* 55:76, 1981.
82. Bedford RF, Ashford TP: Aspirin pretreatment prevents post-cannulation radial artery thrombosis, *Anesthesiology* 51:176, 1979.
83. Wong AY, O'Regan AM: Gangrene of digits associated with radial artery cannulation, *Anaesthesia* 58:1034, 2003.
84. Green JA, Tonkin MA: Ischaemia of the hand in infants following radial or ulnar artery catheterisation, *Hand Surg* 4:151, 1999.
85. Bright E, Baines DB, French BG, et al: Upper limb amputation following radial artery cannulation, *Anaesth Intensive Care* 21:351, 1993.
86. Vender JS, Watts RD: Differential diagnosis of hand ischemia in the presence of an arterial cannula, *Anesth Analg* 61:465, 1982.
87. Goldstein RD, Gordon MJV: Volar proximal skin necrosis after radial artery cannulation, *N Y State J Med* 90:375, 1990.
88. Wyatt R, Glaves I, Cooper DJ: Proximal skin necrosis after radial artery cannulation, *Lancet* 1:1135, 1974.
89. Lowenstein E, Little JW, Lo HH: Prevention of cerebral embolization from flushing radial artery cannulae, *N Engl J Med* 285:1414, 1971.
90. Chang C, Dughi J, Shitabata P, et al: Air embolism and the radial arterial line, *Crit Care Med* 16:141, 1988.
91. Weiss M, Balmer C, Cornelius A, et al: Arterial fast bolus flush systems used routinely in neonates and infants cause retrograde embolization of flush solution into the central arterial and cerebral circulation, *Can J Anaesth* 50:386–391, 2003.
92. Murphy GS, Szokol JW, Marymont JH, et al: Retrograde blood flow in the brachial and axillary arteries during routine radial arterial catheter flushing, *Anesthesiology* 105:492–497, 2006.
93. Zavela NG, Gravlee GP, Bewckart DH, et al: Unusual cause of hypotension after cardiopulmonary bypass, *J Cardiothorac Vasc Anesth* 10:553, 1996.
94. Qvist J, Peterfreund R, Perlmutter G: Transient compartment syndrome of the forearm after attempted radial artery cannulation, *Anesth Analg* 83:183, 1996.
95. Edwards DP, Clarke MD, Barker P: Acute presentation of bilateral radial artery pseudoaneurysms following arterial cannulation, *Eur J Vasc Endovasc Surg* 17:456, 1999.
96. Knight CG, Healy DA, Thomas RL: Femoral artery pseudoaneurysms: Risk factors, prevalence, and treatment options, *Ann Vasc Surg* 17:503, 2003.
97. O'Rourke RA, Silverman ME, Shaver J: The history, physical examination, and cardiac auscultation. In Fuster V, Alexander RW, O'Rourke RA, et al: *The Heart*, ed 11 New York, 2004, McGraw-Hill, pp 217–294.
98. Mark JB: Central venous pressure monitoring: Clinical insights beyond the numbers, *J Cardiothorac Anesth* 5:163, 1991.
99. Luecke T, Roth H, Herrmann P, et al: Assessment of cardiac preload and left ventricular function under increasing levels of positive end-expiratory pressure, *Intensive Care Med* 30:119, 2004.
100. Mangano DT: Monitoring pulmonary arterial pressure in coronary artery disease, *Anesthesiology* 53:364, 1980.
101. Kumar A, Anel R, Bunnell E, et al: Pulmonary artery occlusion pressure and central venous pressure fail to predict ventricular filling volume, cardiac performance, or the response to volume infusion in normal subjects, *Crit Care Med* 32:691, 2004.
102. Buhre W, Weyland A, Schorn B, et al: Changes in central venous pressure and pulmonary capillary wedge pressure do not indicate changes in right and left heart volume in patients undergoing coronary artery bypass surgery, *Eur J Anaesthesiol* 16:11, 1999.
103. Godje O, Peyerl M, Seebauer T, et al: Central venous pressure, pulmonary capillary wedge pressure and intrathoracic blood volumes as preload indicators in cardiac surgery patients, *Eur J Cardiothorac Surg* 13:533, 1998.

104. Lichtwarck-Aschoff M, Beale R, Pfeiffer UJ: Central venous pressure, pulmonary artery occlusion pressure, intrathoracic blood volume, and right ventricular end-diastolic volume as indicators of cardiac preload, *J Crit Care* 11:180, 1996.
105. English IC, Frew RM, Pigott JF, et al: Percutaneous catheterization of the internal jugular vein, *Anesthesia* 24:521, 1969.
106. Muralidhar K: Left internal versus right internal jugular vein access to central venous circulation using the Seldinger technique, *J Cardiothorac Anesth* 9:115, 1995.
107. Leibowitz AB, Rozner MA: PRO: Manometry should routinely be used during central venous catheterization, *Anesth Analg* 109:3–5, 2009.
108. Ezaru CS, Mangione MP, Oravitz TM, et al: Eliminating arterial injury during central venous catheterization using manometry, *Anesth Analg* 109:130–134, 2009.
109. Jobes DR, Schwartz AJ, Greenhow DE, et al: Safer jugular vein cannulation: Recognition of arterial puncture, *Anesthesiology* 59:353, 1983.
110. Fabian JA, Jesudian MC: A simple method for improving the safety of percutaneous cannulation of the internal jugular vein, *Anesth Analg* 64:1032, 1985.
111. Petty C: Alternate methods of internal jugular venipuncture for monitoring central venous pressure, *Anesth Analg* 54:157, 1975.
112. Denys BG, Uretsky BF: Anatomical variations of internal jugular vein location: Impact on central venous access, *Crit Care Med* 19:1516, 1991.
113. Troianos CA, Jobes DR, Ellison N: Ultrasound-guided cannulation of the internal jugular vein: A prospective, randomized study, *Anesth Analg* 72:823, 1991.
114. Serafimidis K, Sakorafas GH, Konstantoudakis G, et al: Ultrasound-guided catheterization of the internal jugular vein in oncologic patients; comparison with the classical landmark technique: A prospective study, *Int J Surg* 7:526–528, 2009.
115. Randolph AG, Cook DJ, Gonzales CA, et al: Ultrasound guidance for placement of central venous catheters: A meta-analysis of the literature, *Crit Care Med* 24:2053, 1996.
116. Hind D, Calvert N, McWilliams R, et al: Ultrasonic locating devices for central venous cannulation: Meta-analysis, *BMJ* 327:361, 2003.
117. Karakitsos D, Labropoulos N, De Groot E, et al: Real-time ultrasound-guided catheterization of the internal jugular vein: A prospective comparison with the landmark technique in critical care patients, *Crit Care* 10:R162, 2006.
118. Leung J, Duffy M, Finckh A: Real-time ultrasonographically-guided internal jugular vein catheterization in the emergency department increases success rates and reduces complications: A randomized, prospective study, *Ann Emerg Med* 48:540–547, 2006.
119. Gratz I, Ashar M, Kidwell P, et al: Doppler-guided cannulation of the internal jugular vein: A prospective, randomized trial, *J Clin Monit* 10:185, 1994.
120. Riopelle J, Ruiz D, Hunt J, et al: Circumferential adjustment of ultrasound probe position to determine the optimal approach to the internal jugular vein: A noninvasive geometric study in adults, *Anesth Analg* 101:924, 2005Erratum in *Anesth Analg* 100:512, 2005.
121. Denys BG, Uretsky BF, Reddy PS: Ultrasound assisted cannulation of the internal jugular vein. A prospective comparison to the external landmark-guided technique, *Circulation* 87:1557, 1993.
122. Xiao W, Yan F, Ji H, et al: A randomized study of a new landmark-guided vs traditional para-carotid approach in internal jugular venous cannulation in infants, *Paediatr Anaesth* 19:481–486, 2009.
123. Froehlich CD, Rigby MR, Rosenberg ES, et al: Ultrasound-guided central venous catheter placement decreases complications and decreases placement attempts compared with the landmark technique in patients in a pediatric intensive care unit, *Crit Care Med* 37:1090–1096, 2009.
124. Asheim P, Mostad U, Aadahl P: Ultrasound-guided central venous cannulation in infants and children, *Acta Anaesthesiol Scand* 46:390, 2002.
125. Liberman L, Hordof AJ, Hsu DT, et al: Ultrasound-assisted cannulation of the right internal jugular vein during electrophysiologic studies in children, *J Interv Card Electrophysiol* 5:177, 2001.
126. Verghese ST, McGill WA, Patel RI, et al: Ultrasound-guided internal jugular venous cannulation in infants: A prospective comparison with the traditional palpation method, *Anesthesiology* 91:71, 1999.
127. Verghese ST, McGill WA, Patel RI, et al: Comparison of three techniques for internal jugular vein cannulation in infants, *Paediatr Anaesth* 10:505, 2000.
128. Grebenik CR, Boyce A, Sinclair ME, et al: NICE guidelines for central venous catheterization in children. Is the evidence base sufficient? *Br J Anaesth* 92:827, 2004.
129. Troianos CA, Kuwik R, Pasqual J, et al: Internal jugular vein and carotid artery anatomic relation as determined by ultrasonography, *Anesthesiology* 85:43, 1996.
130. Alderson PJ, Burrows FA, Stemp LI, et al: Use of ultrasound to evaluate internal jugular vein anatomy and to facilitate central venous cannulation of paediatric patients, *Br J Anaesth* 70:145, 1993.
131. Sulek CA, Gravenstein N, Blackshear RH, et al: Head rotation during internal jugular vein cannulation and the risk of carotid artery puncture, *Anesth Analg* 82:125, 1996.
132. Mallory DL, Showker T, Evans G, et al: Effects of clinical maneuvers on sonographically determined internal jugular vein size during venous cannulation, *Crit Care Med* 18:1269, 1990.
133. Parry G: Trendelenburg position, head elevation and a midline position optimize right internal jugular vein diameter, *Can J Anaesth* 51:379, 2004.
134. Parsons AJ, Alfa J: Carotid dissection: A complication of internal jugular vein cannulation with the use of ultrasound, *Anesth Analg* 109:135–136, 2009.
135. Stone MB, Hern HG: Inadvertent carotid artery cannulation during ultrasound guided central venous catheterization, *Ann Emerg Med* 49:720, 2007.
136. Mittnacht AJ: Ultrasound-guided central venous cannulation: False sense of security, *Anesth Analg* 109:2029, 2009.
137. Augoustides JG, Horak J, Ochroch EA, et al: A randomized controlled trial of real-time needle-guided ultrasound for internal jugular venous cannulation in a large university department, *J Cardiothorac Vasc Anesth* 19:310–315, 2005.
138. Blaivas M, Adhikari S: An unseen danger: Frequency of posterior vessel wall penetration by needles during attempts to place internal jugular vein central catheters using ultrasound guidance, *Crit Care Med* 37:2345–2349, 2009.
139. Augoustides JGT, Cheung AT: Pro: Ultrasound should be the standard of care for central catheter insertion, *J Cardiothorac Vasc Anesth* 23:720–724, 2009.
140. Hessel I.I.E.A.: Con: We should not enforce the use of ultrasound as a standard of care for obtaining central venous access, *J Cardiothorac Vasc Anesth* 23:725–728, 2009.
141. Making health care safer: A critical analysis of patient safety practices, *Evid Rep Technol Assess* 43:1–668, 2001.
142. The clinical effectiveness and cost effectiveness of ultrasound locating devices for the placement of central venous lines (technology appraisal report #49), Accessed November 11, 2010: http://guidance.nice.org.UK/TA69/Guidance/pdf/English.
143. Bailey PL, Glance LG, Eaton MP, et al: A survey of the use of ultrasound during central venous catheterization, *Anesth Analg* 104:491–497, 2007.
144. Calvert N, Hind D, McWilliams R, et al: Ultrasound for central venous cannulation: Economic evaluation of cost-effectiveness, *Anaesthesia* 59:1116–1120, 2004.
145. Blitt CD, Wright WA, Petty WC, et al: Cardiovascular catheterization via the external jugular vein: A technique employing the J-wire, *JAMA* 229:817, 1974.
146. Defalque RJ: Subclavian venipuncture: A review, *Anesth Analg* 47:677, 1968.
147. Lefrant JY, Muller L, De La Coussaye JE, et al: Risk factors of failure and immediate complication of subclavian vein catheterization in critically ill patients, *Intensive Care Med* 28:1036, 2002.
148. Fangio P, Mourgeon E, Romelaer A, et al: Aortic injury and cardiac tamponade as a complication of subclavian venous catheterization, *Anesthesiology* 96:1520, 2002.
149. Kitagawa N, Oda M, Totoki T, et al: Proper shoulder position for subclavian venipuncture, *Anesthesiology* 101:1306–1312, 2004.
150. Kellner GA, Smart JF: Percutaneous placement of catheters to monitor "central venous pressure", *Anesthesiology* 36:515, 1972.
151. Webre DR, Arens JF: Use of cephalic and basilic veins for introduction of cardiovascular catheters, *Anesthesiology* 38:389, 1973.
152. Nadroo AM, Lin J, Green RS, et al: Death as a complication of peripherally inserted central catheters in neonates, *J Pediatr* 138:599, 2001.
153. Nadroo AM, Glass RB, Lin J, et al: Changes in upper extremity position cause migration of peripherally inserted central catheters in neonates, *Pediatrics* 110:131, 2002.
154. Loewenthal MR, Dobson PM, Starkey RE, et al: The peripherally inserted central catheter (PICC): A prospective study of its natural history after cubital fossa insertion, *Anaesth Intensive Care* 30:21, 2002.
155. Burgess GE, Marino RJ, Peuler MJ: Effect of head position on the location of venous catheters inserted via the basilic vein, *Anesthesiology* 46:212, 1977.
156. Artru AA, Colley PS: Placement of multiorificed CVP catheters via antecubital veins using intravascular electrocardiography, *Anesthesiology* 69:132, 1988.
157. Mongan P, Peterson R, Culling R: Pressure monitoring can accurately position catheters for air embolism aspiration, *J Clin Monit* 8:121, 1992.
158. Roth S, Aronson S: Placement of a right atrial air aspiration catheter guided by transesophageal echocardiography, *Anesthesiology* 83:1359, 1995.
159. Kumar M, Amin M: The peripherally inserted central venous catheter: Friend or foe? *Int J Oral Maxillofac Surg* 33:201, 2004.
160. Parikh S, Narayanan V: Misplaced peripherally inserted central catheter: An unusual cause of stroke, *Pediatr Neurol* 30:210, 2004.
161. Pettit J: Assessment of infants with peripherally inserted central catheters. Part 1. Detecting the most frequently occurring complications, *Adv Neonatal Care* 2:304, 2002.
162. Smith JR, Friedell ML, Cheatham ML, et al: Peripherally inserted central catheters revisited, *Am J Surg* 176:208, 1998.
163. Bansmer G, Keith D, Tesluk H: Complications following the use of indwelling catheters of the inferior vena cava, *JAMA* 167:1606, 1958.
164. Durbec O, Viviand X, Potie F, et al: A prospective evaluation of the use of femoral venous catheters in critically ill adults, *Crit Care Med* 25:1986, 1997.
165. Pawar M, Mehta Y, Kapoor P, et al: Central venous catheter-related bloodstream infections: Incidence, risk factors, outcome, and associated pathogens, *J Cardiothorac Vasc Anesth* 18:304, 2004.
166. Applebaum RM, Adelman MA, Kanschuger MS, et al: Transesophageal echocardiographic identification of a retrograde dissection of the ascending aorta caused by inadvertent cannulation of the common carotid artery, *J Am Soc Echocardiogr* 10:749, 1997.
167. Eckhardt W, Iaconetti D, Kwon J, et al: Inadvertent carotid artery cannulation during pulmonary artery catheter insertion, *J Cardiothorac Vasc Anesth* 10:283, 1996.
168. Fraizer MC, Chu WW, Gudjonsson T, et al: Use of a percutaneous vascular suture device for closure of an inadvertent subclavian artery puncture, *Catheter Cardiovasc Interv* 59:369, 2003.
169. Berlet MH, Steffen D, Shaughness G, et al: Closure using a surgical closure device of inadvertent subclavian artery punctures during central venous catheter placement, *Cardiovasc Intervent Radiol* 24:122, 2001.
170. Gobiel F, Couture P, Girard D, et al: Carotid artery-internal jugular fistula: Another complication following pulmonary artery catheterization via the internal jugular venous route, *Anesthesiology* 80:230, 1994.
171. Robinson R, Errett L: Arteriovenous fistula following percutaneous internal jugular vein cannulation: A report of carotid artery-to-internal jugular vein fistula, *J Cardiothorac Anesth* 2:488, 1988.
172. Kim J, Ahn W, Bahk JH: Hemomediastinum resulting from subclavian artery laceration during internal jugular catheterization, *Anesth Analg* 97:1257, 2003.
173. Kwon SS, Falk A, Mitty HA: Thoracic duct injury associated with left internal jugular vein catheterization: Anatomic considerations, *J Vasc Interv Radiol* 13:337, 2002.
174. Khalil DG, Parker FB, Mukherjee N, et al: Thoracic duct injury: A complication of jugular vein catheterization, *JAMA* 221:908, 1972.
175. Teba L, Dedhia HV, Bowen R, et al: Chylothorax review, *Crit Care Med* 13:49, 1985.
176. Cook TL, Deuker CW: Tension pneumothorax following internal jugular cannulation and general anesthesia, *Anesthesiology* 45:554, 1976.
177. Plewa MC, Ledrick D, Sferra JJ: Delayed tension pneumothorax complicating central venous catheterization and positive-pressure ventilation, *Am J Emerg Med* 13:532, 1995.
178. Porzionato A, Montisci M, Manani G: Brachial plexus injury following subclavian vein catheterization: A case report, *J Clin Anesth* 15:582, 2003.
179. Selander D, Dhuner K-G, Lundborg G: Peripheral nerve injury due to injection needles used for regional anesthesia. An experimental study of the acute effects of needlepoint trauma, *Acta Anaesth Scand* 21:182, 1977.
180. Nakayama M, Fulita S, Kawamata M, et al: Traumatic aneurysm of the internal jugular vein causing vagal nerve palsy: A rare complication of percutaneous catheterization, *Anesth Analg* 78:598, 1994.
181. Parikh RD: Horner's syndrome: A complication of percutaneous catheterization of the internal jugular vein, *Anaesthesia* 27:327, 1972.
182. Turnage WS, Harper JV: Venous air embolism occurring after removal of a central venous catheter, *Anesth Analg* 72:559, 1991.
183. Akazawa S, Nakaigawa Y, Hotta K: Unrecognized migration of an entire guidewire on insertion of a central venous catheter into the cardiovascular system, *Anesthesiology* 84:241, 1996.
184. Smyth NPD, Rogers JB: Transvenous removal of catheter emboli from the heart and great veins by endoscopic forceps, *Ann Thorac Surg* 11:403, 1971.
185. Friedman BA, Jergeleit HC: Perforation of atrium by polyethylene central venous catheter, *JAMA* 203:1141, 1968.
186. Gravenstein N, Blackshear R: In vitro evaluation of relative perforating potential of central venous catheters: Comparison of materials, selected models, number of lumens, and angles of incidence to simulated membrane, *J Clin Monit* 7:2, 1991.
187. Oropello J, Leibowitz A, Manasia A, et al: Dilator-associated complications of central venous catheter insertion: Possible mechanisms of injury and suggestions, *J Cardiothorac Vasc Anesth* 10:634, 1996.
188. Royster RL, Johnston WE, Gravlee GP, et al: Arrhythmias during venous cannulation prior to pulmonary artery catheter insertion, *Anesth Analg* 64:1214, 1985.
189. Eissa NT, Kvetan V: Guidewire as a cause of complete heart block in patients with preexisting left bundle-branch block, *Anesthesiology* 73:772, 1990.
190. Hu KK, Lipsky BA, Veenstra DL, et al: Using maximal sterile barriers to prevent central venous catheter-related infection: A systematic evidence-based review, *Am J Infect Control* 32:142, 2004.
191. Timsit JF, Sebille V, Farkas JC, et al: Effect of subcutaneous tunneling on internal jugular catheter-related sepsis in critically ill patients: A prospective randomized multicenter study, *JAMA* 276:1416, 1996.
192. Timsit JF, Bruneel F, Cheval C, et al: Use of tunneled femoral catheters to prevent catheter-related infection. A randomized, controlled trial, *Ann Intern Med* 130:729, 1999.

193. Leon C, Alvarez-Lerma F, Ruiz-Santana S, et al: Antiseptic chamber-containing hub reduces central venous catheter-related infection: A prospective, randomized study, *Crit Care Med* 31:1318, 2003.

194. Veenstra DL, Saint S, Saha S, et al: Efficacy of antiseptic-impregnated central venous catheters in preventing catheter-related bloodstream infection: A meta-analysis, *JAMA* 281:261, 1999.

195. McGee D, Gould M: Preventing complications of central venous catheterization, *N Engl J Med* 348:1123, 2003.

196. Cicalini S, Palmieri F, Petrosillo N: Clinical review: New technologies for prevention of intravascular catheter-related infections, *Crit Care* 8:157, 2004.

197. Maki DG, Ringer M, Alvarado CJ: Prospective randomised trial of povidone-iodine, alcohol, and chlorhexidine for prevention of infection associated with central venous and arterial catheters, *Lancet* 338:339, 1991.

198. Mimoz O, Pieroni L, Lawrence C, et al: Prospective, randomized trial of two antiseptic solutions for prevention of central venous or arterial catheter colonization and infection in intensive care unit patients, *Crit Care Med* 24:1818, 1996.

199. Chaiyakunapruk N, Veenstra DL, Lipsky BA, et al: Chlorhexidine compared with povidone-iodine solution for vascular catheter-site care: A meta-analysis, *Ann Intern Med* 136:792, 2002.

200. Humar A, Ostromecki A, Direnfeld J, et al: Prospective randomized trial of 10% povidone-iodine versus 0.5% tincture of chlorhexidine as cutaneous antisepsis for prevention of central venous catheter infection, *Clin Infect Dis* 31:1001, 2000.

201. Mermel LA: Prevention of intravascular catheter-related infections, *Ann Intern Med* 132:391, 2000.

202. Polderman KH, Girbes AR: Central venous catheter use. Part 2. Infectious complications, *Intensive Care Med* 28:18, 2002.

203. Swan HJC, Ganz W, Forrester JS, et al: Catheterization of the heart in man with the use of a flow-directed balloon-tipped catheter, *N Engl J Med* 283:447, 1970.

204. Connors AF, McCaffree DR, Gray BA: Evaluation of right-heart catheterization in the critically ill patient, *N Engl J Med* 308:263, 1983.

205. Waller JL, Johnson SP, Kaplan JA: Usefulness of pulmonary artery catheters during aortocoronary bypass surgery, *Anesth Analg* 61:221, 1982.

206. Iberti T, Fisher CJ: A prospective study on the use of the pulmonary artery catheter in a medical intensive care unit—Its effect on diagnosis and therapy, *Crit Care Med* 11:238, 1983.

207. Connors AF, Speroff T, Dawson NV, et al: The effectiveness of right-heart catheterization in the initial care of critically ill patients, *JAMA* 276:889, 1996.

208. Wiener RS, Welch HG: Trends in use of the pulmonary artery catheter in the United States, 1993-2004, *JAMA* 298:423–429, 2007.

209. Ruisi CP, Goldberg RJ, Kennelly BM, et al: Pulmonary artery catheterization in patients with acute coronary syndrome, *Am Heart J* 158:170–176, 2009.

210. Leibowitz AB, Oropello JM: The pulmonary artery in anesthesia practice in 2007: An historical overview with emphasis on the past 6 years, *Semin Cardiothorac Vasc Anesth* 11:162–176, 2007.

211. Mantia AM, Robinson JN, Lolley DM, et al: Sternal retraction and pulmonary artery catheter compromise, *J Cardiothorac Anesth* 2:430, 1988.

212. Keusch DJ, Winters S, Thys DM: The patient's position influences the incidence of dysrhythmias during pulmonary artery catheterization, *Anesthesiology* 70:582, 1989.

213. Schmitt EA, Brantigan CO: Common artifacts of pulmonary artery pressures: Recognition and interpretation, *J Clin Monit* 2:44, 1986.

214. Moore RA, Neary MJ, Gallagher HD, et al: Determination of the pulmonary capillary wedge position in patients with giant left atrial V waves, *J Cardiothorac Anesth* 1:108, 1987.

215. Haggmark S, Hohner P, Ostman M, et al: Comparison of hemodynamic, electrocardiographic, mechanical, and metabolic indicators of intraoperative myocardial ischemia in vascular surgical patients with coronary artery disease, *Anesthesiology* 70:19, 1989.

216. van Daele ME, Sutherland GR, Mitchell MM, et al: Do changes in pulmonary capillary wedge pressure adequately reflect myocardial ischemia during anesthesia? *Circulation* 81:865, 1990.

217. Lappas D, Lell WA, Gabel JC, et al: Indirect measurement of left atrial pressure in surgical patients—pulmonary capillary wedge and pulmonary artery diastolic pressures compared with left atrial pressure, *Anesthesiology* 38:394, 1973.

218. Raper R, Sibbald WJ: Misled by the wedge? *Chest* 89:427, 1986.

219. Nadeau S, Noble WH: Misinterpretation of pressure measurements from the pulmonary artery catheter, *Can Anaesth Soc J* 33:352, 1986.

220. Tuman KJ, Carroll G, Ivankovich AD: Pitfalls in interpretation of pulmonary artery catheter data, *J Cardiothorac Anesth* 3:625, 1989.

221. West JB: *Ventilation/Blood Flow and Gas Exchange*, ed 4, Oxford, 1970, Blackwell Scientific Publications.

222. Shasby DM, Dauber IM, Pfister S, et al: Swan-Ganz catheter location and left atrial pressure determine the accuracy of the wedge pressure when positive end-expiratory pressure is used, *Chest* 80:666, 1980.

223. Lorzman J, Powers SR, Older T, et al: Correlation of pulmonary wedge and left atrial pressure: A study in the patient receiving positive end-expiratory pressure ventilation, *Arch Surg* 109:270, 1974.

224. Kane PB, Askanazi J, Neville JF Jr, et al: Artifacts in the measurement of pulmonary artery wedge pressure, *Crit Care Med* 6:36, 1978.

225. Rajacich N, Burchard KW, Hasan FM, et al: Central venous pressure and pulmonary capillary wedge pressure as estimates of left atrial pressure: Effects of positive end-expiratory pressure and catheter tip malposition, *Crit Care Med* 17:7, 1989.

226. Teboul J-L, Zapol WM, Brun-Buisson C, et al: A comparison of pulmonary artery occlusion pressure and left ventricular end-diastolic pressure during mechanical ventilation with PEEP in patients with severe ARDS, *Anesthesiology* 70:261, 1989.

227. Haskell RJ, French WJ: Accuracy of left atrial and pulmonary artery wedge pressure in pure mitral regurgitation in predicting left ventricular end-diastolic pressure, *Am J Cardiol* 61:136, 1988.

228. Hildick-Smith DJ, Walsh JT, Shapiro LM: Pulmonary capillary wedge pressure in mitral stenosis accurately reflects mean left atrial pressure but overestimates transmitral gradient, *Am J Cardiol* 85:512, 2000.

229. Lange RA, Moore DM, Cigarroa RG, et al: Use of pulmonary capillary wedge pressure to assess severity of mitral stenosis: Is true left atrial pressure needed in this condition? *J Am Coll Cardiol* 13:825, 1989.

230. Entress JJ, Dhamee S, Olund T, et al: Pulmonary artery occlusion pressure is not accurate immediately after CPB, *J Cardiothorac Anesth* 4:558, 1990.

231. Shah MR, Hasselblad V, Stevenson LW, et al: Impact of the pulmonary artery catheter in critically ill patients, *JAMA* 294:1664–1670, 2005.

232. Afessa B, Spencer S, Khan W, et al: Association of pulmonary artery catheter use with in-hospital mortality, *Crit Care Med* 29:1145–1148, 2001.

233. Gattinoni L, Brazzi L, Pelosi P, et al: A trial of goal-oriented hemodynamic therapy in critically ill patients, *N Engl J Med* 333:1025–1032, 1995.

234. Taylor RW: Controversies in pulmonary artery catheterization, *New Horizons* 5:173–296, 1997.

235. Murdoch SD, Cohen AT, Bellamy MC: Pulmonary artery catheterization and mortality in critically ill patients, *Br J Anaesth* 85:611, 2000.

236. Polanczyk CA, Rohde LE, Goldman L, et al: Right-heart catheterization and cardiac complications in patients undergoing noncardiac surgery: An observational study, *JAMA* 286:309, 2001.

237. Barone JE, Tucker JB, Rassias D, et al: Routine perioperative pulmonary artery catheterization has no effect on rate of complications in vascular surgery: A meta-analysis, *Am Surg* 67:674, 2001.

238. Rhodes A, Cusack RJ, Newman PJ, et al: A randomised, controlled trial of the pulmonary artery catheter in critically ill patients, *Intensive Care Med* 28:256, 2002.

239. Sandham JD, Hull RD, Brant RF, et al: A randomized, controlled trial of the use of pulmonary artery catheters in high-risk surgical patients, *N Engl J Med* 348:5, 2003.

240. Yu DT, Platt R, Lanken PN, et al: Relationship of pulmonary artery catheter use to mortality and resource utilization in patients with severe sepsis, *Crit Care Med* 31:2734, 2003.

241. Richard C, Warszawski J, Anguel N, et al: Early use of the pulmonary artery catheter and outcomes in patients with shock and acute respiratory distress syndrome: A randomized controlled trial, *JAMA* 290:2713, 2003.

242. Sakr Y, Vincent JL, Reinhard K, et al: Use of the pulmonary artery catheter is not associated with worse outcome in the ICU, *Chest* 128:2722–2731, 2005.

243. Binanay C, Califf RM, Hasselblad V, et al: Evaluation study of congestive heart failure and pulmonary artery catheterization effectiveness: The ESCAPE trial, *JAMA* 294:1625–1633, 2005.

244. Harvey S, Harrison DA, Singer M, et al: Assessment of the clinical effectiveness of pulmonary artery catheters in management of patients in intensive care (PAC-Man): A randomised controlled trial, *Lancet* 366:472–477, 2005.

245. Wheeler AP, Bernard GR, Thompson BT, et al: Pulmonary-artery versus central venous catheter to guide treatment of acute lung injury. National Heart, Lung, and Blood Institute Acute Respiratory Distress Syndrome (ARDS) Clinical Trials Network, *N Engl J Med* 354:2213–2224, 2006.

246. Guyatt GOntario Intensive Care Group: A randomised control trial of right heart catheterization in critically ill patients, *J Intensive Care Med* 6:91–95, 1991.

247. Gore JM, Goldberg RJ, Spodick DH, et al: A community-wide assessment of the use of pulmonary artery catheters in patients with acute myocardial infarctions, *Chest* 92:721–727, 1987.

248. Cohen MG, Kelly RV, Kong DF, et al: Pulmonary artery catheterization in acute coronary syndromes: Insights from the GUSTO IIb and GUSTO III trials, *Am J Med* 118:482–488, 2005.

249. Schwann TA, Zacharias A, Riordan CJ, et al: Safe, highly selective use of pulmonary artery catheters in coronary artery bypass grafting: An objective patient selection method, *Ann Thorac Surg* 73:1394–1401, 2002.

250. Ramsey SD, Saint S, Sullivan SD, et al: Clinical and economic effects of pulmonary artery catheterization in nonemergent coronary artery bypass graft surgery, *J Cardiothorac Vasc Anesth* 14:113–118, 2000.

251. Resano FG, Kapetanakis EI, Hill PC, et al: Clinical outcomes of low-risk patients undergoing beating-heart surgery with or without pulmonary artery catheterization, *J Cardiothorac Vasc Anesth* 20:300–306, 2006.

252. Djaiani G, Karski J, Yudin M, et al: Clinical outcomes in patients undergoing elective coronary artery bypass graft surgery with and without utilization of pulmonary artery catheter-generated data, *J Cardiothorac Vasc Anesth* 20:307–310, 2006.

253. Haupt M, Shoemaker W, Haddy F, et al: Correspondence: Goal-oriented hemodynamic therapy, *N Engl J Med* 334:799, 1996.

254. Shoemaker WC, Appel PL, Kram HB, et al: Prospective trial of supranormal values of survivors as therapeutic goals in high-risk surgical patients, *Chest* 94:1176, 1988.

255. Boyd O, Grounds RM, Bennett ED: The beneficial effect of supranormalization of oxygen delivery with dopexamine hydrochloride on perioperative mortality, *JAMA* 270:2699, 1993.

256. Rao TLK, Jacobs KH, El-Etr AA: Reinfarction following anesthesia in patients with myocardial infarction, *Anesthesiology* 59:499, 1983.

257. Moore CH, Lombardo TR, Allums JA, et al: Left main coronary artery stenosis: Hemodynamic monitoring to reduce mortality, *Ann Thorac Surg* 26:445, 1978.

258. Heyland DK, Cook DL, King D, et al: Maximizing oxygen delivery in critically ill patients: A methodologic appraisal of the evidence, *Crit Care Med* 24:517, 1996.

259. Chittock DR, Dhingra VK, Ronco JJ, et al: Severity of illness and risk of death associated with pulmonary artery catheter use, *Crit Care Med* 32:911, 2004.

260. Ivanov R, Allen J, Calvin JE: The incidence of major morbidity in critically ill patients managed with pulmonary artery catheters: A meta-analysis, *Crit Care Med* 28:615, 2000.

261. Pölönen P, Ruokonen E, Hippeläinen M, et al: A prospective, randomized study of goal-oriented hemodynamic therapy in cardiac surgical patients, *Anesth Analg* 90:1052–1059, 2000.

262. Friese RS, Shafi S, Gentilello LM: Pulmonary artery catheter use is associated with reduced mortality in severely injured patients: A National Trauma Data Bank analysis of 53.312 patients, *Crit Care Med* 34:1597–1601, 2006.

263. Sandham JD: Pulmonary artery catheter use—refining the question, *Crit Care Med* 32:1070, 2004.

264. Gnaegi A, Feihl F, Perret C: Intensive care physicians' insufficient knowledge of right-heart catheterization at the bedside: Time to act? *Crit Care Med* 25:213, 1997.

265. Iberti TJ, Fischer EP, Leibowitz AB, et al: A multicenter study of physicians' knowledge of the pulmonary artery catheter, *JAMA* 264:2928, 1990.

266. Tuman KJ, McCarthy RJ, Spless BD, et al: Effect of pulmonary artery catheterization on outcome in patients undergoing coronary artery surgery, *Anesthesiology* 70:199–206, 1989.

267. Steward RD, Psyhojos T, Lahey SJ, et al: Central venous catheter use in low-risk coronary artery bypass grafting, *Ann Thorac Surg* 66:1306–1311, 1998.

268. American Society of Anesthesiologists Task Force on Pulmonary Artery Catheterization: Practice guidelines for pulmonary artery catheterization: An updated report by the American Society of Anesthesiologists Task Force on Pulmonary Artery Catheterization, *Anesthesiology* 99:988, 2003.

269. Poses RM, McClish DK, Smith WR, et al: Physicians' judgments of the risks of cardiac procedures. Differences between cardiologists and other internists, *Med Care* 35:603, 1997.

270. Shah KB, Rao TLK, Laughlin S, et al: A review of pulmonary artery catheterization in 6245 patients, *Anesthesiology* 61:271, 1984.

271. Lopez-Sendon J, Lopez de Sa E, Gonzalez Maqueda I, et al: Right ventricular infarction as a risk factor for ventricular fibrillation during pulmonary artery catheterization using Swan-Ganz catheters, *Am Heart J* 119:207, 1990.

272. Spring CL, Pozen RG, Rozanski JJ, et al: Advanced ventricular arrhythmias during bedside pulmonary artery catheterization, *Am J Med* 72:203, 1982.

273. Salmenperä M, Peltola K, Rosenberg P: Does prophylactic lidocaine control cardiac arrhythmias associated with pulmonary artery catheterization? *Anesthesiology* 56:210, 1982.

274. Shaw TJI: The Swan-Ganz pulmonary artery catheter. Incidence of complications with particular reference to ventricular dysrhythmias and their prevention, *Anaesthesia* 34:651, 1979.

275. Patil AR: Risk of right bundle-branch block and complete heart block during pulmonary artery catheterization, *Crit Care Med* 18:122, 1990.

276. Abernathy WS: Complete heart block caused by a Swan-Ganz catheter, *Chest* 65:349, 1974.

277. Thomson IR, Dalton BC, Lappas DG, et al: Right bundle-branch block and complete heart block caused by the Swan-Ganz catheter, *Anesthesiology* 51:359, 1979.

278. Sprung CL, Elser B, Schein RMH, et al: Risk of right bundle-branch block and complete heart block during pulmonary artery catheterization, *Crit Care Med* 17:1, 1989.

279. Morris D, Mulvihill D, Lew WYW: Risk of developing complete heart block during bedside pulmonary artery catheterization in patients with left bundle-branch block, *Arch Intern Med* 147:1987, 2005.

280. McDaniel DD, Stone JG, Faltas AN, et al: Catheter-induced pulmonary artery hemorrhage, *J Thoracic Cardiovasc Surg* 82:1, 1981.

281. Hannan AT, Brown M, Bigman O: Pulmonary artery catheter-induced hemorrhage, *Chest* 85:128, 1984.

282. Durbin CG: The range of pulmonary artery catheter balloon inflation pressures, *J Cardiothorac Anesth* 4:39, 1990.

283. Dhamee MS, Pattison CZ: Pulmonary artery rupture during cardiopulmonary bypass, *J Cardiothorac Anesth* 1:51, 1987.

284. Cohen JA, Blackshear RH, Gravenstein N, et al: Increased pulmonary artery perforating potential of pulmonary artery catheters during hypothermia, *J Cardiothorac Vasc Anesth* 5:234, 1991.

285. Stein JM, Lisbon A: Pulmonary hemorrhage from pulmonary artery catheterization treated with endobronchial intubation, *Anesthesiology* 55:698, 1981.

286. Purut CM, Scott SM, Parham JV, et al: Intraoperative management of severe endobronchial hemorrhage, *Ann Thorac Surg* 51:304, 1991.

287. Laureys M, Golzarian J, Antoine M, et al: Coil embolization treatment for perioperative pulmonary artery rupture related to Swan-Ganz catheter placement, *Cardiovasc Intervent Radiol* 27:407, 2004.

288. Abreu AR, Campos MA, Krieger BP: Pulmonary artery rupture induced by a pulmonary artery catheter: A case report and review of the literature, *J Intensive Care Med* 19:291, 2004.

289. Foote GA, Schabel SI, Hodges M: Pulmonary complications of the flow-directed balloon-tipped catheter, *N Engl J Med* 290:927, 1974.

290. Mond HG, Clark DW, Nesbitt SJ, et al: A technique for unknotting an intracardiac flow-directed balloon catheter, *Chest* 67:731, 1975.

291. England MR, Murphy MC: A knotty problem, *J Cardiothorac Vasc Anesth* 11:682, 1997.

292. Georghiou GP, Vidne BA, Raanani E: Knotting of a pulmonary artery catheter in the superior vena cava: Surgical removal and a word of caution, *Heart* 90:e28, 2004.

293. Arnaout S, Diab K, Al-Kutoubi A, et al: Rupture of the chordae of the tricuspid valve after knotting of the pulmonary artery catheter, *Chest* 120:1742, 2001.

294. Lazzam C, Sanborn TA, Christian F: Ventricular entrapment of a Swan-Ganz catheter: A technique for nonsurgical removal, *J Am Coll Cardiol* 13:1422, 1989.

295. Boscoe MJ, deLange S: Damage to the tricuspid valve with a Swan-Ganz catheter, *BMJ* 283:346, 1981.

296. O'Toole JD, Wurtzbacher JJ, Wearner NE, et al: Pulmonary valve injury and insufficiency during pulmonary artery catheterization, *N Engl J Med* 301:1167, 1979.

297. Kainuma M, Yamada M, Miyake T: Pulmonary artery catheter passing between the chordae tendineae of the tricuspid valve (correspondence), *Anesthesiology* 83:1130, 1995.

298. Rowley KM, Clubb KS, Smith GJ, et al: Right-sided infective endocarditis as a consequence of flow-directed pulmonary artery catheterization. A clinicopathological study of 55 autopsied patients, *N Engl J Med* 311:1152, 1984.

299. Greene JF Jr, Fitzwater JE, Clemmer TP: Septic endocarditis and indwelling pulmonary artery catheters, *JAMA* 233:891, 1975.

300. Kim YL, Richman KA, Marshall BE: Thrombocytopenia associated with Swan-Ganz catheterization in patients, *Anesthesiology* 53:261, 1980.

301. Moberg PQ, Geary VM, Sheikh FM: Heparin-induced thrombocytopenia: A possible complication of heparin-coated pulmonary artery catheters, *J Cardiothorac Anesth* 4:226, 1990.

302. Hofbauer R, Moser D, Kaye AD, et al: Thrombus formation on the balloon of heparin-bonded pulmonary artery catheters: An ultrastructural scanning electron microscope study, *Crit Care Med* 28:727, 2000.

303. Mangano DT: Heparin bonding and long-term protection against thrombogenesis, *N Engl J Med* 307:894, 1982.

304. Böhrer H, Fleischer F, Lang J, et al: Early formation of thrombi on pulmonary artery catheters in cardiac surgical patients receiving high-dose aprotinin, *J Cardiothorac Anesth* 4:222, 1990.

305. Dentz M, Slaughter T, Mark JB: Early thrombus formation on heparin-bonded pulmonary artery catheters in patients receiving epsilon aminocaproic acid (case reports), *Anesthesiology* 82:583, 1995.

306. Martins P, Driessen J, Vandekerckhove Y, et al: Transesophageal echocardiography detection of a right atrial thrombus around a pulmonary artery catheter, *Anesth Analg* 75:847, 1992.

307. Allyn J, Lichtenstein A, Koski G, et al: Inadvertent passage of a pulmonary artery catheter from the superior vena cava through the left atrium and left ventricle into the aorta, *Anesthesiology* 70:1019, 1989.

308. Saad R, Loubser P, Rokey R: Intraoperative transesophageal and contrast echocardiographic detection of an unusual complication associated with a misplaced pulmonary artery catheter, *J Cardiothorac Vasc Anesth* 10:247, 1996.

309. Willis C, Wight D, Zidulka A: Hypotension secondary to balloon inflation of a pulmonary artery catheter, *Crit Care Med* 12:915, 1984.

310. Gilbert T, Scherlis M, Fiocco M, et al: Pulmonary artery catheter migration causing venous cannula obstruction during cardiopulmonary bypass, *Anesthesiology* 82:596, 1995.

311. Meluch A, Karis JH: Obstruction of venous return by a pulmonary artery catheter during cardiopulmonary bypass, *Anesth Analg* 70:121, 1990.

312. Oyarzun JR, Donahoo JS, McCormick JR, et al: Venous cannula obstruction by Swan-Ganz catheter during cardiopulmonary bypass, *Ann Thorac Surg* 62:266, 1996.

313. Kozlowski JH: Inadvertent coronary sinus occlusion by a pulmonary artery catheter, *Crit Care Med* 14:649, 1986.

314. Tewari P, Kumar M, Kaushik S: Pulmonary artery catheter misplaced in liver, *J Cardiothorac Vasc Anesth* 9:482, 1995.

315. Karakaya D, Baris S, Tur A: Pulmonary artery catheter-induced right ventricular perforation during coronary artery bypass surgery, *Br J Anaesth* 82:953, 1999.

316. Shin B, McAslan TC, Ayella RJ: Problems with measurements using the Swan-Ganz catheter, *Anesthesiology* 43:474, 1975.

317. Kaufman B: Pitfalls of central hemodynamic monitoring, *Resident Staff Physician* 30:27, 1992.

318. Zaidan J, Freniere S: Use of a pacing pulmonary artery catheter during cardiac surgery, *Ann Thorac Surg* 35:633, 1983.

319. Macander PJ, Kuhnlein JL, Buiteweg J, et al: Electrode detachment: A complication of the indwelling pacing Swan-Ganz catheter, *N Engl J Med* 314:1711, 1986.

320. Levin R, Leacche M, Petracek M, et al: Extending the use of the pacing pulmonary artery catheter for safe minimally invasive cardiac surgery, *J Cardiothorac Vasc Anesth* 24:568–573, 2010.

321. Mora CT, Seltzer JL, McNulty SE: Evaluation of a new design pulmonary artery catheter for intraoperative ventricular pacing, *J Cardiothorac Anesth* 2:303–308, 1988.

322. Trankina MF, White RD: Perioperative cardiac pacing using an atrioventricular pacing pulmonary artery catheter, *J Cardiothorac Anesth* 3:154–162, 1989.

323. Risk SC, Brandon D, D'Ambra MN, et al: Indications for the use of pacing pulmonary artery catheters in cardiac surgery, *J Cardiothorac Vasc Anesth* 6:275–280, 1992.

324. Krouskop RW, Cabatu EE, Chelliah BP, et al: Accuracy and clinical utility of an oxygen saturation catheter, *Crit Care Med* 11:744, 1983.

325. Waller JL, Kaplan JA, Bauman DI, et al: Clinical evaluation of a new fiberoptic catheter oximeter during cardiac surgery, *Anesth Analg* 61:676, 1982.

326. Norwood SH, Nelson LD: Continuous monitoring of mixed venous oxygen saturation during aortofemoral bypass grafting, *Am Surg* 52:114, 1986.

327. Guffin A, Girard D, Kaplan JA: Shivering following cardiac surgery: Hemodynamic changes and reversal, *J Cardiothorac Anesth* 1:24, 1987.

328. Heiselman D, Jones J, Cannon L: Continuous monitoring of mixed venous oxygen saturation in septic shock, *J Clin Monit* 2:237, 1986.

329. Nelson LD: Continuous venous oximetry in surgical patients, *Ann Surg* 203:329, 1986.

330. Thys DM, Cohen E, Eisenkraft JB: Mixed venous oxygen saturation during thoracic anesthesia, *Anesthesiology* 69:1005, 1988.

331. Linton D, Gilon D: Advances in noninvasive cardiac output monitoring, *Ann Card Anaesth* 5:141, 2002.

332. Boutrous AR, Lee C: Value of continuous monitoring of mixed venous blood oxygen saturation in the management of critically ill patients, *Crit Care Med* 14:132, 1986.

333. Jastremski MS, Chelluri L, Beney K, et al: Analysis of the effects of continuous on-line monitoring of mixed venous oxygen saturation on patient outcome and cost-effectiveness, *Crit Care Med* 17:148, 1989.

334. Pearson KS, Gomez MN, Moyers JR, et al: A cost/benefit analysis of randomized invasive monitoring for patients undergoing cardiac surgery, *Anesth Analg* 69:336, 1989.

335. London MJ, Moritz TE, Henderson WG, et al: Standard versus fiberoptic pulmonary artery catheterization for cardiac surgery in the Department of Veterans Affairs: A prospective, observational, multicenter analysis, *Anesthesiology* 96:860, 2002.

336. Woerkens EC, Trouwborst A, Tenbrinck R: Accuracy of a mixed venous saturation catheter during acutely induced changes in hematocrit in humans, *Crit Care Med* 19:1025, 1991.

337. Reinhart K, Kuhn HJ, Hartog C, et al: Continuous central venous and pulmonary artery oxygen saturation monitoring in the critically ill, *Intensive Care Med* 30:1572, 2004.

338. Scuderi P, MacGregor D, Bowton D, et al: A laboratory comparison of three pulmonary artery oximetry catheters, *Anesthesiology* 81:245, 1994.

339. Pond CG, Blessios G, Bowlin J, et al: Perioperative evaluation of a new mixed venous oxygen saturation catheter in cardiac surgical patients, *J Cardiothorac Vasc* 6:280, 1992.

340. Armaganidis A, Dhainaut JF, Billard JL, et al: Accuracy assessment for three fiberoptic pulmonary artery catheters for Svo₂ monitoring, *Intensive Care Med* 20:484, 1994.

341. LaFarge CG, Miettinen OS: The estimation of oxygen consumption, *Cardiovasc Res* 4:23, 1970.

342. Wood EH, Bowers D, Shepherd JT, et al: O₂ content of mixed venous blood in man during various phases of the respiratory and cardiac output cycles in relation to possible errors in measurement of cardiac output by conventional applications of the Fick method, *J Appl Physiol* 215:605, 1968.

343. Grossman W: Fick oxygen method. In *Cardiac Catheterization and Angiography*, ed 3, Philadelphia, 1986, Lea & Febiger, pp 105.

344. Guyton AC: The Fick principle. In Guyton AC, Jones CE, Coleman TG, editors: *Circulatory Physiology: Cardiac Output and Its Regulation*, ed 2, Philadelphia, 1973, WB Saunders Company, pp 21.

345. Tissot S, Delafosse B, Bertrand O, et al: Clinical validation of the Deltatrac monitoring system in mechanically ventilated patients, *Intensive Care Med* 21:149, 1995.

346. Johnson BD, Beck KC, Proctor DN, et al: Cardiac output during exercise by the open circuit acetylene washing method: Comparison with direct Fick, *J Appl Physiol* 88:1650, 2000.

347. Jaffe MB: Partial CO₂ rebreathing cardiac output: Operating principles of the NICOTM system, *J Clin Monit* 15:387, 1999.

348. Rocco M, Spadetta G, Morelli A, et al: A comparative evaluation of thermodilution and partial CO₂ rebreathing techniques for cardiac output assessment in critically ill patients during assisted ventilation, *Intensive Care Med* 30:82, 2004.

349. Nilsson LB, Eldrup N, Berthelsen PG: Lack of agreement between thermodilution and carbon dioxide-rebreathing cardiac output, *Acta Anaesthesiol Scand* 45:680, 2001.

350. Arnold JH, Stenz RI, Grenier B, et al: Noninvasive determination of cardiac output in a model of acute lung injury, *Crit Care Med* 25:864, 1997.

351. Russell AE, Smith SA, West MJ, et al: Automated non-invasive measurements of cardiac output by the carbon dioxide rebreathing method: Comparisons with dye dilution and thermodilution, *Br Heart J* 63:195, 1990.

352. Arnold JH, Stenz RI, Thompson JE, et al: Noninvasive determination of cardiac output using single-breath CO₂ analysis, *Crit Care Med* 24:1701, 1996.

353. Binder JC, Parkin WG: Non-invasive cardiac output determination: Comparison of a new partial-rebreathing technique with thermodilution, *Anaesth Intensive Care* 29:19, 2001.

354. van Heerden PV, Baker S, Lim SI, et al: Clinical evaluation of the non-invasive cardiac output (NICO) monitor in the intensive care unit, *Anaesth Intensive Care* 28:427, 2000.

355. Kurita T, Morita K, Kato S, et al: Comparison of the accuracy of the lithium dilution technique with the thermodilution technique for measurement of cardiac output, *Br J Anaesth* 79:770, 1997.

356. Forrester JS, Ganz W, Diamond G, et al: Thermodilution cardiac output determination with a single flow-directed catheter, *Am Heart J* 83:306, 1972.

357. Salgado CR, Galletti PM: In vitro evaluation of the thermodilution technique for the measurement of ventricular stroke volume and end-diastolic volume, *Cardiologia* 49:65, 1966.

358. Bilfinger TV, Lin CY, Anagnostopoulos CE: In vitro determinations of accuracy of cardiac output measurements by thermal dilution, *J Surg Res* 33:409, 1982.

359. Goodyer AVN, Huvos A, Eckhardt WF, et al: Thermal dilution curves in the intact animal, *Circ Res* 7:432, 1959.

360. Pavek K, Lindquist O, Arfors KE: Validity of thermodilution method for measurement of cardiac output in pulmonary oedema, *Cardiovasc Res* 7:419, 1973.

361. Pelletier C: Cardiac output measurement by thermodilution, *Can J Surg* 22:347, 1979.

362. Runciman WB, Ilsley AH, Roberts JG: Thermodilution cardiac output—a systematic error, *Anaesth Intensive Care* 9:135, 1981.

363. Sorensen MB, Bille-Brahe NE, Engell HC: Cardiac output measurement by thermodilution, *Ann Surg* 183:67, 1976.

364. Weisel RD, Berger RL, Hechtman HB, et al: Measurement of cardiac output by thermodilution, *N Engl J Med* 292:682, 1975.

365. Pearl RG, Siegel LC: Thermodilution cardiac output measurement with a large left-to-right shunt, *J Clin Monit* 7:146, 1991.

366. Wetzel RC, Latson TW: Major errors in thermodilution cardiac output measurement during rapid volume infusion, *Anesthesiology* 62:684, 1985.

367. Bazaral M, Petre J, Novoa R: Errors in thermodilution cardiac output measurements caused by rapid pulmonary artery temperature decreases after cardiopulmonary bypass, *Anesthesiology* 77:31, 1992.

368. Latson TW, Whitten CW, O'Flaherty D, et al: Ventilation, thermal noise, and errors in cardiac output measurements after cardiopulmonary bypass, *Anesthesiology* 79:1233, 1993.

369. Hamilton MA, Stevenson LW, Woo M, et al: Effect of tricuspid regurgitation on the reliability of the thermodilution cardiac output in congestive heart failure, *Am J Cardiol* 64:945, 1989.

370. Buffington CW, Nystrom EUM: Neither the accuracy nor the precision of thermal dilution cardiac output measurements is altered by acute tricuspid regurgitation in pigs, *Anesth Analg* 98:884, 2004.

371. Kashtan HI, Maitland A, Salerno TA, et al: Effects of tricuspid regurgitation on thermodilution cardiac output: Studies in an animal model, *Can J Anaesth* 34:246, 1987.

372. Heerdt PM, Pond CB, Blessios GA, et al: Inaccuracy of cardiac output by thermodilution during acute tricuspid regurgitation, *Ann Thorac Surg* 53:706, 1992.

373. Balik M, Pachl J, Hendl J, et al: Effect of the degree of tricuspid regurgitation on cardiac output measurements by thermodilution, *Intensive Care Med* 28:1117, 2002.

374. Nishikawa T, Dohi S: Slowing of heart rate during cardiac output measurement by thermodilution, *Anesthesiology* 57:538, 1982.

375. Harris AP, Miller CF, Beattie C, et al: The slowing of sinus rhythm during thermodilution cardiac output determination and the effect of altering injectate temperature, *Anesthesiology* 63:540, 1985.

376. Nishikawa T, Dohi S: Hemodynamic status susceptible to slowing of heart rate during thermodilution cardiac output determination in anesthetized patients, *Crit Care Med* 18:841, 1990.

377. Hoel BL: Some aspects of the clinical use of thermodilution in measuring cardiac output, *Scand J Clin Lab Invest* 38:383, 1978.
378. Stetz CW, Miller RG, Kelly GE, et al: Reliability of the thermodilution method in the determination of cardiac output in clinical practice, *Am Rev Respir Dis* 126:1001, 1982.
379. Snyder JV, Powner DJ: Effects of mechanical ventilation on the measurement of the cardiac output by thermodilution, *Crit Care Med* 10:677, 1982.
380. Stevens JH, Raffin TA, Mihm FG, et al: Thermodilution cardiac output measurement: Effects of the respiratory cycle on its reproducibility, *JAMA* 253:2240, 1985.
381. Pearl RG, Rosenthal MH, Nieson L, et al: Effect of injectate volume and temperature on thermodilution cardiac output determination, *Anesthesiology* 64:798, 1986.
382. Nelson LD, Houtchens BA: Automatic versus manual injections for thermodilution cardiac output determinations, *Crit Care Med* 10:190, 1982.
383. Neto EP, Piriou V, Durand PG, et al: Comparison of the two semicontinuous cardiac output pulmonary artery catheters after valvular surgery, *Crit Care Med* 27:2694, 1999.
384. Jacquet L, Hanique G, Glorieux D, et al: Analysis of the accuracy of continuous thermodilution cardiac output measurement. Comparison with intermittent thermodilution and Fick cardiac output measurements, *Intensive Care Med* 22:1125, 1996.
385. Jakobsen CJ, Melsen NC, Andresen EB: Continuous cardiac output measurements in the perioperative period, *Acta Anaesthesiol Scand* 39:485, 1995.
386. Mihaljevic T, von Segesser LK, Tonz M, et al: Continuous thermodilution measurements of cardiac output: In-vitro and in-vivo evaluation, *Thorac Cardiovasc Surg* 42:32, 1994.
387. Hogue CW, Rosenbloom M, McCawley C, et al: Comparison of cardiac output measurements by continuous thermodilution with electromagnetometry in adult cardiac surgical patients, *J Cardiothorac Vasc Anesth* 8:631, 1994.
388. Zollner C, Polasek J, Kilger E, et al: Evaluation of a new continuous thermodilution cardiac output monitor in cardiac surgical patients: A prospective criterion standard study, *Crit Care Med* 27:293, 1999.
389. Zollner C, Goetz AE, Weis M, et al: Continuous cardiac output measurements do not agree with conventional bolus thermodilution cardiac output determination, *Can J Anaesth* 48:1143, 2001.
390. Leather HA, Vuylsteke A, Bert C, et al: Evaluation of a new continuous cardiac output monitor in off-pump coronary artery surgery, *Anaesthesia* 59:385, 2004.
391. Bottiger BW, Rauch H, Bohrer H, et al: Continuous versus intermittent cardiac output measurement in cardiac surgical patients undergoing hypothermic cardiopulmonary bypass, *J Cardiothorac Vasc Anesth* 9:405, 1995.
392. Medin DL, Brown DT, Wesley R: Validation of continuous thermodilution cardiac output in critically ill patients with analysis of systematic errors, *J Crit Care* 13:184, 1998.
393. Linton RA, Band DM, Haire KM: A new method of measuring cardiac output in man using lithium dilution, *Br J Anaesth* 71:262, 1993.
394. Linton R, Band D, O'Brian T, et al: Lithium dilution cardiac output measurement: A comparison with thermodilution, *Crit Care Med* 25:1767, 1997.
395. Garcia-Rodriguez C, Pittman J, Cassell CH, et al: Lithium dilution cardiac output measurement: A clinical assessment of central venous and peripheral venous indicator injection, *Crit Care Med* 30:2199, 2002.
396. Costa MG, Della Rocca G, Chiarandini P, et al: Continuous and intermittent cardiac output measurement in hyperdynamic conditions: Pulmonary artery catheter vs. lithium dilution technique, *Intensive Care Med* 34:257–263, 2008.
397. Feigenbaum H, Popp RL, Wolfe SB, et al: Ultrasound measurements of the left ventricle: A correlative study with angiocardiography, *Ann Intern Med* 129:461, 1972.
398. Kronik G, Slany J, Moslacher H: Comparative value of eight M-mode echocardiographic formulas for determining left ventricular stroke volume, *Circulation* 60:1308, 1979.
399. Nosir YF, Fioretti PM, Vletter WB, et al: Accurate measurement of left ventricular ejection fraction by three-dimensional echocardiography. A comparison with radionuclide angiography, *Circulation* 94:460, 1996.
400. Katz WE, Gasior TA, Quinland JJ, et al: Transgastric continuous wave Doppler to determine cardiac output, *Am J Cardiol* 71:853, 1993.
401. Darmon PL, Hillel Z, Mogtabar A, et al: Cardiac output by transesophageal echocardiography using continuous wave Doppler across the aortic valve, *Anesthesiology* 80:796, 1994.
402. Roewer N, Bednarz F, Schulte am Esch J: Continuous measurement of intracardiac and pulmonary blood flow velocities with transesophageal pulsed Doppler echocardiography: Technique and initial clinical experience, *J Cardiothorac Anesth* 1:418, 1987.
403. Muhiudeen IA, Kuecherer HF, Lee E, et al: Intraoperative estimation of cardiac output by transesophageal pulsed Doppler echocardiography, *Anesthesiology* 74:9, 1991.
404. Pu M, Griffin BP, Vandervoort PM, et al: Intraoperative validation of mitral inflow determination by transesophageal echocardiography: Comparison of single-plane, biplane and thermodilution techniques, *J Am Coll Cardiol* 26:1047, 1995.
405. Estagnasie P, Djedaini K, Mier L, et al: Measurement of cardiac output by transesophageal echocardiography in mechanically ventilated patients. Comparison with thermodilution, *Intensive Care Med* 23:753, 1997.
406. Perrino AC Jr, Harris SN, Luther MA: Intraoperative determination of cardiac output using multiplane transesophageal echocardiography: A comparison to thermodilution, *Anesthesiology* 89:350, 1998.
407. Dabaghi SF, Rokey R, Rivera J, et al: Comparison of echocardiographic assessment of cardiac hemodynamics in the intensive care unit with right-sided cardiac catheterization, *Am J Cardiol* 76:392, 1995.
408. Roewer N, Bednarz F, Dziadka A, et al: Intraoperative cardiac output determination from transmitral and pulmonary blood flow measurements using transesophageal pulsed Doppler, *J Cardiothorac Anesth* 1:418, 1987.
409. Savino JS, Trolanos CA, Aukburg S, et al: Measurement of pulmonary blood flow with two-dimensional echocardiography and Doppler echocardiography, *Anesthesiology* 75:445, 1991.
410. Miller WE, Richards KL, Crawford MH: Accuracy of mitral Doppler echocardiographic cardiac output determinations in adults, *Am Heart J* 119:905, 1990.
411. Maslow A, Communale M, Haering M, et al: Pulsed-wave Doppler measurements of cardiac output from the right ventricular outflow tract, *Anesth Analg* 83:466, 1996.
412. Hillel Z, Thys DM, Keene D, et al: A method to improve the accuracy of esophageal Doppler cardiac output determinations, *Anesthesiology* 71:A386, 1989.
413. Siegel LC, Shafer SL, Martinez GM, et al: Simultaneous measurements of cardiac output by thermodilution, esophageal Doppler, and electrical impedance on anesthetized patients, *J Cardiothorac Anesth* 2:590, 1989.
414. Laupland KB, Bands CJ: Utility of esophageal Doppler as a minimally invasive hemodynamic monitor: A review, *Can J Anaesth* 49:393–401, 2002.
415. Sharma J, Bhise M, Singh A, et al: Hemodynamic measurements after cardiac surgery: Transesophageal Doppler versus pulmonary artery catheter, *J Cardiothorac Vasc Anesth* 19:746–750, 2005.
416. Sawai T, Nohmi T, Ohnishi Y, et al: Cardiac output measurement using the transesophageal Doppler method is less accurate than the thermodilution method when changing PaCO2, *Anesth Analg* 101:1597–1601, 2005.
417. Dark PM, Singer M: The validity of trans-esophageal Doppler ultrasonography as a measure of cardiac output in critically ill adults, *Intensive Care Med* 30:2060–2066, 2004.
418. Gan TJ, Soppitt A, Maroof M, et al: Goal-directed intraoperative fluid administration reduces length of hospital stay after major surgery, *Anesthesiology* 97:820–826, 2002.
419. Liu N, Darmon PL, Saada M, et al: Comparison between radionuclide ejection fraction and fractional area changes derived from transesophageal echocardiography using automated border detection, *Anesthesiology* 85:468–474, 1996.
420. Ryan T, Burwash I, Lu J, et al: The agreement between ventricular volumes and ejection fraction by transesophageal echocardiography or a combined radionuclear and thermodilution technique in patients after coronary artery surgery, *J Cardiothorac Vasc Anesth* 10:323–328, 1996.
421. Urbanowicz JH, Shaaban MJ, Cohen NH, et al: Comparison of transesophageal echocardiographic and scintigraphic estimates of left ventricular end-diastolic volume index and ejection fraction in patients following coronary artery bypass grafting, *Anesthesiology* 72:607–612, 1990.
422. Goens MB, Martin GR: Acoustic quantification: A new tool for diagnostic echocardiography, *Curr Opin Cardiol* 11:52–60, 1996.
423. Perez JE, Miller JG, Holland MR, et al: Ultrasonic tissue characterization: Integrated backscatter imaging for detecting myocardial structural properties and on-line quantitation of cardiac function, *Am J Card Imaging* 8:106–112, 1994.
424. Gorcsan J 3rd, Denault A, Mandarino WA, et al: Left ventricular pressure-volume relations with transesophageal echocardiographic automated border detection: Comparison with conductance-catheter technique, *Am Heart J* 131:544–552, 1996.
425. Gorcsan J 3rd, Morita S, Mandarino WA, et al: Two-dimensional echocardiographic automated border detection accurately reflects changes in left ventricular volume, *J Am Soc Echocardiogr* 6:482–489, 1993.
426. Morrissey RL, Siu SC, Guerrero JL, et al: Automated assessment of ventricular volume and function by echocardiography: Validation of automated border detection, *J Am Soc Echocardiogr* 7:107–115, 1994.
427. Pinto FJ, Siegel LC, Chenzbraun A, et al: On-line estimation of cardiac output with a new automated border detection system using transesophageal echocardiography: A preliminary comparison with thermodilution, *J Cardiothorac Vasc Anesth* 8:625–630, 1994.
428. Tardif JC, Cao QL, Pandian NG, et al: Determination of cardiac output using acoustic quantification in critically ill patients, *Am J Cardiol* 74:810–813, 1994.
429. Katz WE, Gasior TA, Reddy SC, et al: Utility and limitations of biplane transesophageal echocardiographic automated border detection for estimation of left ventricular stroke volume and cardiac output, *Am Heart J* 128:389–396, 1994.
430. Kuhl HP, Franke A, Janssens U, et al: Three-dimensional echocardiographic determination of left ventricular volumes and function by multiplane transesophageal transducer: Dynamic in vitro validation and in vivo comparison with angiography and thermodilution, *J Am Soc Echocardiogr* 11:1113–1124, 1998.
431. Lee D, Fuisz AR, Fan PH, et al: Real-time 3-dimensional echocardiographic evaluation of left ventricular volume: Correlation with magnetic resonance imaging—a validation study, *J Am Soc Echocardiogr* 14:1001–1009, 2001.
432. Pandian NG, Roelandt J, Nanda NC, et al: Dynamic three-dimensional echocardiography: Methods and clinical potential, *Echocardiography* 11:237–259, 1994.
433. Panza JA: Real-time three-dimensional echocardiography: An overview, *Int J Cardiovasc Imaging* 17:227–235, 2001.
434. Arai K, Hozumi T, Matsumura Y, et al: Accuracy of measurement of left ventricular volume and ejection fraction by new real-time three-dimensional echocardiography in patients with wall motion abnormalities secondary to myocardial infarction, *Am J Cardiol* 94:552–558, 2004.
435. Jenkins C, Bricknell K, Hanekom L, et al: Reproducibility and accuracy of echocardiographic measurements of left ventricular parameters using real-time three-dimensional echocardiography, *J Am Coll Cardiol* 44:878–886, 2004.
436. Kawai J, Tanabe K, Morioka S, et al: Rapid freehand scanning three-dimensional echocardiography: Accurate measurement of left ventricular volumes and ejection fraction compared with quantitative gated scintigraphy, *J Am Soc Echocardiogr* 16:110–115, 2003.
437. Bein B, Meybohm P, Cavus E, et al: The reliability of pulse contour-derived cardiac output during hemorrhage and after vasopressor administration, *Anesth Analg* 105:107–113, 2007.
438. Pratt B, Roteliuk L, Hatib F, et al: Calculating arterial pressure-based cardiac output using a novel measurement and analysis method, *Biomed Instrum Technol* 41:403–411, 2007.
439. Mayer J, Boldt J, Poland R, et al: Continuous arterial pressure waveform-based cardiac output using the FloTrac/Vigileo: A review and meta-analysis, *J Cardiothorac Vasc Anesth* 23:401–406, 2009.
440. Manecke GR Jr: Cardiac output from the arterial catheter: Deceptively simple, *J Cardiothorac Vasc Anesth* 21:629–631, 2007.
441. Lorsomradee S, Cromheecke S, De Hert SG: Uncalibrated arterial pulse contour analysis versus continuous thermodilution technique: Effects of alterations in arterial waveform, *J Cardiothorac Vasc Anesth* 21:636–643, 2007.
442. Breukers RM, Sepehrkhouy S, Spiegelenberg SR, et al: Cardiac output measured by a new arterial pressure waveform analysis method without calibration compared with thermodilution after cardiac surgery, *J Cardiothorac Vasc Anesth* 21:632–635, 2007.
443. Michard F: Changes in arterial pressure during mechanical ventilation, *Anesthesiology 103:419–428* 449–455, 2005.
444. Michard F, Boussat S, Chemla D, et al: Relation between respiratory changes in arterial pulse pressure and fluid responsiveness in septic patients with acute circulatory failure, *Am J Respir Crit Care Med* 162:134–138, 2000.
445. Cannesson M, Musard H, Desebbe O, et al: The ability of stroke volume variations obtained with Vigileo/FloTrac system to monitor fluid responsiveness in mechanically ventilated patients, *Anesth Analg* 108:513–517, 2009.
446. Gujjar AR, Muralidhar K, Banakal S, et al: Non-invasive cardiac output by transthoracic electrical bioimpedence in post-cardiac surgery patients: Comparison with thermodilution method, *J Clin Monit Comput* 22:175–180, 2008.
447. Spiess BD, Patel MA, Soltow LO, et al: Comparison of bioimpedance versus thermodilution cardiac output during cardiac surgery: Evaluation of a second-generation bioimpedance device, *J Cardiothorac Vasc Anesth* 15:567–573, 2001.
448. Wallace AW, Salahieh A, Lawrence A, et al: Endotracheal cardiac output monitor, *Anesthesiology* 92:178–189, 2000.
449. Wallace AWGeneva B, Davis BS: In *Clinical Evaluation of the Endotracheal Cardiac Output Monitor (ECOM) in cardiac surgery patients*, ASA 2009 Annual Meeting, 2009, p A739. http://www.asaabstracts.com.
450. Kay HR, Afshari M, Barash P, et al: Measurement of ejection fraction by thermal dilution techniques, *J Surg Res* 34:337–346, 1983.
451. Spinale FG, Zellner JL, Mukherjee R, et al: Placement considerations for measuring thermodilution right ventricular ejection fraction, *Crit Care Med* 19:417–421, 1991.
452. Hein M, Roehl A, Baumert J, et al: Continuous right ventricular volumetry by fast-response thermodilution during right ventricular ischemia: Head-to-head comparison with conductance catheter measurements, *Crit care Med* 37:2962–2967, 2009.
453. Leibowitz AB: Pulmonary artery catheter determined right ventricular ejection fraction and right ventricular end-diastolic volume: Another case of "The Emperor Has No Clothes", *Crit Care Med* 37:2992, 2009.
454. Carvalho R, Loures D, Brofman P, et al: Left atrial catheter complications, *J Thorac Cardiovasc Surg* 92:162, 1986.
455. Bashore T: Afterload reduction in chronic aortic regurgitation: It sure seems like a good idea, *J Am Coll Cardiol* 45:1031, 2005.

456. Lang RM, Borow KM, Neumann A, et al: Systemic vascular resistance: An unreliable index of left ventricular afterload, *Circulation* 74:1114, 1986.
457. Gorback MS: Problems associated with the determination of pulmonary vascular resistance, *J Clin Monit* 6:118, 1990.
458. West JB: Recruitment in networks of pulmonary capillaries, *J Appl Physiol* 39:976, 1975.
459. Suga H, Sagawa K: Instantaneous pressure-volume relationships and their ratio in the excised, supported canine left ventricle, *Circ Res* 35:117, 1974.
460. Schreuder JJ, Biervliet JD, van der Velde ET, et al: Systolic and diastolic pressure-volume relationships during cardiac surgery, *J Cardiothorac Vasc Anesth* 5:539, 1991.
461. American Society of Anesthesiologists: Standards for basic anesthetic monitoring, Available at: http://www.asahq.org/publicationsAndServices/standards/02.pdf Accessed September 23, 2005.
462. Pedersen T, Petersen P, Moller AM: Pulse oximetry for perioperative monitoring, *Cochrane Database Syst Rev* 2:2001 CD002013.
463. Moller JT, Pedersen T, Rasmussen LS, et al: Randomized evaluation of pulse oximetry in 20,802 patients. I. Design, demography, pulse oximetry failure rate, and overall complication rate, *Anesthesiology* 78:436, 1993.
464. Moller JT, Johannessen NW, Espersen K, et al: Randomized evaluation of pulse oximetry in 20,802 patients. II. Perioperative events and postoperative complications, *Anesthesiology* 78:445, 1993.
465. Pedersen T, Moller AM, Hovhannisyan K: Pulse oximetry for perioperative monitoring, *Cochrane Database Syst Rev* 7:2009 CD002013.
466. Tremper KK, Barker SJ: Pulse oximetry, *Anesthesiology* 70:98, 1989.
467. Pälve H, Vuori A: Minimum pulse pressure and peripheral temperature needed for pulse oximetry during cardiac surgery with cardiopulmonary bypass, *J Cardiothorac Vasc Anesth* 5:327, 1991.
468. Reich DL, Timcenko A, Bodian CA, et al: Predictors of pulse oximetry failure, *Anesthesiology* 84:859, 1996.
469. Gamble WJ, LaFarge CG, Fyler DC, et al: Regional coronary venous oxygen saturation and myocardial oxygen tension following abrupt changes in ventricular pressure in the isolated dog heart, *Circ Res* 34:672, 1974.
470. Hoffman JIE, Buckberg GD: Regional myocardial ischemia: Causes, prediction and prevention, *Vasc Surg* 8:115, 1974.
471. Murkin JM, Adams SJ, Novick RJ, et al: Monitoring brain oxygen saturation during coronary bypass surgery: A randomized, prospective study, *Anesth Analg* 104:51–58, 2007.
472. CASMED: Web site: www.casmed.com.
473. Fischer GW, Lin HM, Virol M, et al: Noninvasive cerebral oxygenation may predict outcome in patients undergoing aortic oral surgery. *J Thorac Cardiovasc Surg,* 2010, Epub ahead.
474. Slater JP, Guarino T, Stack J, et al: Cerebral oxygen desaturation predicts cognitive decline and longer hospital stay after cardiac surgery, *Ann Thorac Surg* 87:36–44, 2009.
475. Casati A, Fanelli G, Pietropaoli P, et al: Continuous monitoring of cerebral oxygen saturation in elderly patients undergoing major abdominal surgery minimizes brain exposure to potential hypoxia, *Anesth Analg* 101:740–747, 2005.

15

Electrocardiographic Monitoring

SHAMSUDDIN AKHTAR, MBBS | VERONICA MATEI, MD | MARTIN J. LONDON, MD |
PAUL G. BARASH, MD

KEY POINTS

1. The electrocardiogram (ECG) reflects differences in transmembrane voltages in myocardial cells that occur during depolarization and repolarization within each cycle.
2. Processing of the ECG occurs in a series of steps.
3. Where and how ECG electrodes are placed on the body are critical determinants of the morphology of the ECG signal.
4. ECG signals must be amplified and filtered before display.
5. The ST segment is the most important portion of the QRS complex for evaluating ischemia.
6. How accurately the clinician places ECG leads on the patient's torso is probably the single most important factor influencing clinical utility of the ECG.
7. Use of inferior leads (II, III, aVF) allows superior discrimination of P-wave morphology, facilitating visual diagnosis of arrhythmias and conduction disorders.

As late as 1970, the electrocardiographic monitor was not considered an integral part of monitoring strategies in the perioperative period. As a matter of fact, luminaries in the specialty regarded the use of ECG monitoring as "questionable value because of possible iatrogenic problems." Concern also was expressed that anesthesiologists' attention would be diverted from the patient.[1] Currently, monitoring the ECG is a fundamental standard of monitoring of the American Society of Anesthesiologists.[2] Despite the introduction of more sophisticated cardiovascular monitors such as the pulmonary artery catheter and echocardiography, the electrocardiogram (ECG; coupled with blood pressure measurement) serves as the foundation for guiding cardiovascular therapeutic interventions in the majority of anesthetics.[3] It is indispensable for diagnosing arrhythmias, acute coronary syndromes, electrolyte abnormalities, (particularly of serum potassium and calcium), and some forms of genetically mediated electrical or structural cardiac abnormalities (e.g., Brugada syndrome; Table 15-1).[4]

One of the most important changes in electrocardiography that has occurred recently is the widespread use of computerized systems for recording ECGs. Bedside units are capable of recording diagnostic quality 12-lead ECGs that can be transmitted over a hospital network, for storage and retrieval. Most of the ECGs in the United States are recorded by digital, automated devices, equipped with software, which can measure ECG intervals and amplitudes and provide a virtually instantaneous interpretation. However, different automated systems may have different technical specifications that can result in significant differences in the measurement of amplitudes, intervals, and diagnostic statements.[5,6] The diagnostic specificity and sensitivity of the ECG to

diagnose a particular abnormality also are not consistent. For example, finite limits are defined by the relation between sensitivity and specificity (usually inversely related) for detecting obstructive coronary artery disease (CAD). During exercise testing, the 12-lead ECG has a mean sensitivity of only 68% and a specificity of 77%.[7,8] The resting 12-lead ECG is even less sensitive and specific.[8] More complex ECG modalities are likely to improve its utility in the future (high-frequency QRS signal averaging). In this chapter, the theory and the operating characteristics of ECG hardware used in the perioperative period are presented to facilitate proper use and interpretation of monitoring data.

HISTORICAL PERSPECTIVE

An extensive review of the history of electrocardiography is beyond the scope of this chapter. However, several excellent reviews were published in honor of the centennial of the first recording of the human ECG.[9–14] Willem Einthoven is universally considered the father of electrocardiography (for which he won the 1924 Nobel Prize for Medicine/Physiology). Many of the basic clinical abnormalities in electrocardiography were first described using the string galvanometer (e.g., bundle branch block, delta waves, ST-T changes with angina). It was used until the 1930s, when it was replaced by a system using vacuum tube amplifiers and a cathode ray oscilloscope. With advancements in electrical engineering technology, the devices became more compact, portable, and user friendly. In the 1950s, a portable direct-writing ECG cart was introduced. The first analog-to-digital (A/D) conversion systems for the ECG were introduced in the early 1960s, although their off-line use was impractical and restricted until the late 1970s. In the 1980s, microcomputer technology became widely available and is now standard for all diagnostic and monitoring systems. Further improvements in hardware and software design led to the development of automated ST-analysis algorithms and their use in routine clinical practice.

BASIC ELECTROPHYSIOLOGY AND ELECTRICAL ANATOMY OF THE HEART

The ECG is the final result of a complex series of physiologic and technologic processes.[15] Physiologically, the ECG reflects differences in transmembrane voltages in myocardial cells that occur during depolarization and repolarization within each cycle. Ionic currents are generated because of ionic fluxes across cell membranes in myocardial

TABLE 15-1	Basic Clinical Information Available from Electrocardiography

Anatomy or Morphology
- Infection
- Ischemia
- Hypertrophy

Physiology
- Automaticity
- Arrhythmogenicity
- Conduction
- Ischemia
- Autonomic tone
- Electrolyte abnormalities
- Drug toxicity or effect

452

cells during depolarization and repolarization. The cardiac cells are contiguous and electrically connected by ion channels (gap junctions), which allows the ion current to pass through the cells and spread depolarization.[16] Thus, the membrane potential changes in the heart can be considered a single depolarization that propagates through the whole heart, assuming different forms along the way.[16] The pattern and sequence of depolarization that occur in the heart are depicted in Figure 15-1. There are many different types and subtypes of ion channels that are involved in the synchronized generation of electrical activity in the heart. Of note are the sodium, potassium, calcium, and chloride channels.[15–17] Detailed discussion of these channels is beyond the scope of this chapter.

At any point in time, the electrical activity of the heart is composed of differently directed electrical forces. However, these currents are synchronized by cardiac activation and recovery sequences to generate a cardiac electrical field in and around the heart that varies with time during the cardiac cycle. This cardiac electrical field passes through various internal structures such as lungs, blood, and skeletal muscles. The currents reaching the skin are then detected by the electrodes that are placed in specific locations on the body and uniquely configured to produce different ECG patterns or waveforms. Direction and strength of a lead vector depend on the geometry of the body and on the varying electric impedances of the tissues in the torso.[18,19] As expected, placement of electrodes on the torso is distinct from direct placement on the heart because the localized signal strength that occurs with direct electrode contact is markedly attenuated and altered by torso inhomogeneities, which include thoracic tissue boundaries and variations in impedance. The standard 12-lead ECG records potential differences (represented as change of voltage over time) between prescribed sites on the body surface that vary during the cardiac cycle.[4]

The first deflection noted on the ECG is caused by atrial depolarization and is called the *P wave*. Although the depolarization of the sinoatrial node precedes the atrial depolarization (see Figure 15-1), the potential from these pacemaker cells are too small to be detected on the surface ECG. The width of the P wave reflects the time taken for the wave of depolarization to spread over both the right and left atria. In comparison with the ventricular action potential, the atrial action potential is narrower and has a less prominent plateau. The duration of atrial contraction is, thus, shorter, which permits another action potential to occur sooner and makes atria prone to a very high rate (atrial flutter). The repolarization atrial wave rarely is seen in a normal ECG because it is buried in the much larger QRS wave.

The ECG returns to its baseline between the end of atrial depolarization and the commencement of the QRS complex, which is the start of the QRS ventricular depolarization. This interval is called the *PR interval*. Though this period may seem electrically silent, it is a time of significant electrical activity. During this period, the wave of depolarization that started in the sinoatrial node is propagated through the AV node, the AV bundle, right and left bundle branches, and Purkinje fibers (see Figure 15-1).

The QRS complex is generated by potential differences that originate from the rapid depolarization of the ventricular myocardium (phase 0). The duration of the QRS complex (ventricular depolarization) is similar to that of the P wave (atrial depolarization). However, the amplitude of the QRS complex is significantly greater than that of P wave because the ventricular mass is much larger than that of the atria. The duration of the QRS complex can be increased when conduction through one of the bundle branches is blocked or a ventricle is depolarized by an ectopic focus that depolarizes one of the ventricles sooner than the other.

The QRS wave is followed by a period when the ECG returns to the baseline and is called the *ST segment*. It is a time when the ventricle is completely depolarized and is represented by phase 2 of the action potential (see Figure 15-1). Even though the ventricles are depolarized, the ECG does not record any positive or negative waveforms because the whole ventricles are depolarized and there is no potential difference between sites. The ECG does not measure absolute levels of membrane potential but only records the potential differences.[15] The same explanation also holds true for the T-P segment, which represents a time when the ventricles are fully repolarized; hence no significant potential difference is recorded on a surface ECG.

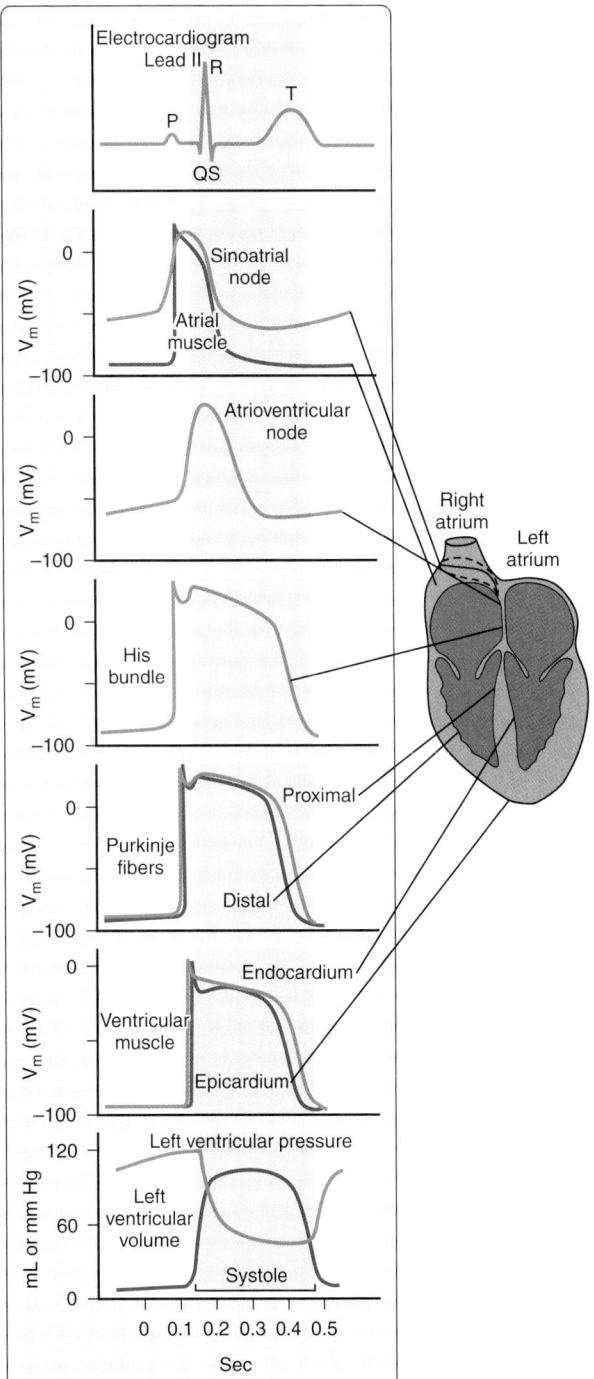

Figure 15-1 The action potential of an automatic cell such as the sinoatrial node differs from that of the ventricular muscle cell in that the cell slowly depolarizes spontaneously during phase 4. The inward current (I_f) is responsible for diastolic depolarization. The action potential in a Purkinje cell has the most rapid rate of depolarization, 400 to 800 V/sec. When the cell is stimulated, an action potential occurs because of a rapid influx of sodium ions (inward current) into the cell (phase 0). Phase 1 includes a notch caused by the "early outward current" (I_{to}), which is a transient K efflux, probably activated by an intracellular calcium increase. Phase 2 is the plateau of the action potential resulting principally from calcium entry (inward currents I_{CaL} and I_{CaT}) through the slow channel of the cell membrane. During phase 3, repolarization of the cell occurs (outward current IK1), whereas during phase 4, the sodium entering during phase 0 is actively pumped out of the cell. In a ventricular muscle cell, unlike the automatic cells, there is no spontaneous phase 4 depolarization. *(From Lynch C, Lake CL: Cardiovascular anatomy and physiology. In Youngberg J, Lake C, Roizen M et al (eds): Cardiac, Vascular, and Thoracic Anesthesia. Philadelphia: Churchill Livingstone, 2000, p 87.)*

A T wave is generated by repolarization of the ventricles. Repolarization proceeds slowly, is not due to a propagated wave, and hence the T wave is broad and of longer duration. It is influenced by many local factors.

The time between the onset of the QRS complex and the end of the T wave is called the *QT interval* and gives a useful measure of ventricular action potential duration. Measurement of this interval can be used to evaluate for certain diseases or effects of certain medication on ventricular repolarization. QT prolongation is important clinically because delayed repolarization is a substrate for arrhythmias and sudden death.

Sometimes small undulations can be seen after T waves but before P waves. These are called *U waves* and are thought to be generated by M cells, which are specialized midmyocardial cells with prolonged action potentials.[15]

TECHNICAL ASPECTS OF THE ELECTROCARDIOGRAM

Most clinicians assume that the ECG is a relatively simple technical device. However, an extensive amount of advanced electrical theory underlies both the recording and display of the ECG signal. Digital signal processing (DSP) is now used universally, and the average ECG unit incorporates several microprocessors. Anesthesiologists should familiarize themselves with the theory behind ECG acquisition to maximize rational clinical application and appreciate its clinical limitations. In this section, the basics of electrocardiography are presented, briefly considering the major components that are involved in the faithful rendition of the surface ECG, working from the skin and electrodes progressively to the final output on the screen. The reader is referred to a number of technical reviews for more detail.[4,5,12,20–23]

Processing of the ECG occurs in a series of steps as shown in Figure 15-2.[4] These steps include (1) signal acquisition, including filtering; (2) data transformation, or rendition of data for further processing, including finding the complexes, classification of the complexes into "dominant" and "nondominant" (ectopic) types, and formation of an average or median complex for each lead; (3) waveform recognition, which is the process for identification of the onset and offset of the diagnostic waves; (4) feature extraction, which is the measurement of intervals and amplitudes; and (5) for the bedside 12-lead ECG machines, diagnostic classification.[4] Diagnostic classification may be heuristic (i.e., deterministic, or based on experience-based rules) or statistical in approach.[24]

◼ Signal Acquisition and Power Spectrum of the Electrocardiogram

It is relevant to consider an electrocardiographic signal in terms of its amplitude (or voltage) and its frequency components (generally called its *phase*) to appreciate ECG signal acquisition. Voltage considerations differ depending on the signal source. Surface recording involves amplification of smaller voltages (on the order of 1 mV) than recording sites closer to the heart beneath the electrically resistant layers of the skin (e.g., endocardial, esophageal, and intratracheal leads). The "power spectrum" of the ECG (Figure 15-3) is derived by Fourier transformation, in which a periodic waveform is mathematically decomposed to its harmonic components (sine waves of various amplitudes and frequencies). The fundamental frequency for the QRS complex at the body surface is approximately 10 Hz, and most of the diagnostic information is contained below 100 Hz in adults. Spectra representing some of the major sources of artifact must be eliminated during the processing and amplification of the QRS complex.[22] The frequency of each of these components can be equated to the slope of the component signal.[6] The R wave with its steep slope is a high-frequency component (100 Hz), whereas P and T waves have lesser slopes and are lower in frequency (1 to 2 Hz). The ST segment has the lowest frequency, not much different from the "underlying" electrical (i.e., isoelectric) baseline of

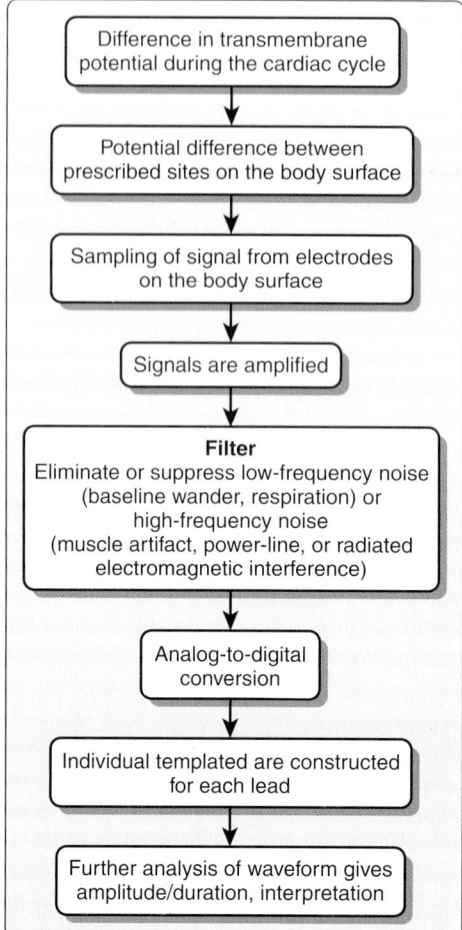

Figure 15-2 Schematic representation of the processes resulting in recording of the electrocardiogram.

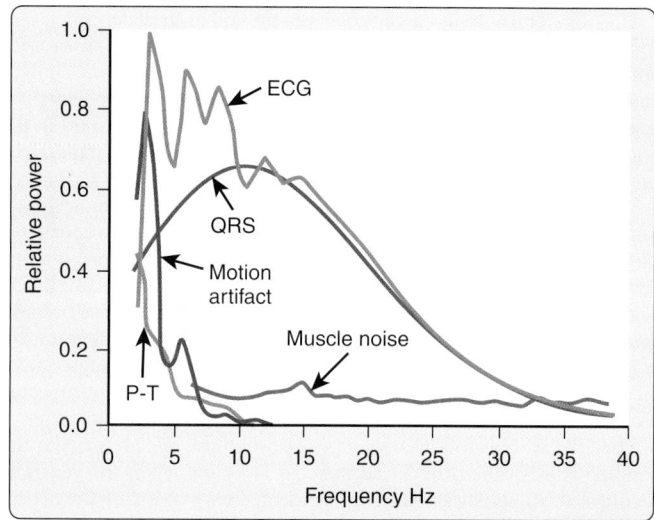

Figure 15-3 The typical power spectrum of the electrocardiogram (ECG) signal (obtained during ambulatory monitoring), including its subcomponents and common artifacts (i.e., motion and muscle noise). The power of the P and T waves (PT) is low frequency, and the QRS complex is concentrated in the midfrequency range, although residual power extends up to 100 Hz. (*From Thakor NV: From Holter monitors to automatic defibrillators: Developments in ambulatory arrhythmia monitoring. IEEE Trans Biomed Eng 31:770, 1984.*)

TABLE 15-2	Range of Signal Frequencies Included in Different Phases of Processing in an Electrocardiographic Monitor	
Processing	Frequency Range	
Display	0.5 (or 0.05)–40 Hz	
QRS detection	5–30 Hz	
Arrhythmia detection	0.05–60 Hz	
ST-segment monitoring	0.05–60 Hz	
Pacemaker detection	1.5–5 kHz	

the ECG. Before the introduction of DSP, accurately displaying the ST segment presented significant technical problems, particularly in operating room and intensive care unit bedside monitoring units. Although the overall frequency spectrum of the QRS complex does not appear to exceed 40 Hz, many components of the QRS complex, particularly the R wave, can exceed 100 Hz. The American Heart Association (AHA) recommends a bandwidth of 0.05 to 100 Hz for monitoring and detection of myocardial ischemia.[4] Very-high-frequency signals of particular clinical significance are pacemaker spikes. Their short duration and high amplitude present technical challenges for proper recognition and rejection to allow accurate determination of the heart rate. The frequencies of greatest importance for optimal ECG processing are presented in Table 15-2.[5]

Digital Signal Processing of the Electrocardiogram

Computerized ECG processing has been adapted to all major clinical applications of the ECG. The earliest application of A/D signal processing occurred during exercise tolerance testing, when significant motion artifact and electromyographic noise make acquisition of a "clean" ECG signal difficult. Outside of the exercise treadmill laboratory, computer processing allows automated analysis of the diagnostic 12-lead ECG.[25] The reader is referred elsewhere for more detailed discussions of this technology, and to the reports of the scientific council of the AHA on standardization and specifications for automated ECG and bedside monitors.[4,25-28]

Processing of the ECG signal by a digital electrocardiograph involves initial sampling of the signal from electrodes on the body surface. Nearly all current-generation ECG machines convert the analog ECG signal to digital form before further processing. The foundation of DSP is the A/D converter, which samples the incoming "continuous" analog signal (characterized by variable amplitude or voltage over time) at a very rapid rate, converting the sampled voltage into binary numbers, each of which has a precise time index or sequence. Greater sampling rates ($\geq$ 10,000 to 15,000/sec), which are typically less than 0.5 millisecond in duration help detect pacemaker output reliably. Several technical recommendations regarding low-frequency filtering and high-frequency filtering recently have been published by the AHA.[4]

Formation of a Representative Single-Lead Complex

After A/D conversion, the resultant data bits are inspected by a microprocessor using some form of mathematical construct to determine where reference points ("fiducial points") are located. A common method locates the point of most rapid change in amplitude (located on the downslope of the R wave). This process characterizes the baseline QRS complex (QRS recognition), providing a "template" on which subsequent beats are overlaid (beat alignment) and averaged (signal averaging). This not only allows visual display of the QRS complex and quantification of its components, but eliminates random electrical noise and wide-complex beats that fail to meet criteria established by the fiducial points.

QRS waveform amplitudes and durations are subject to beat-to-beat variability and to respiratory variability between beats. Digital ECGs

can adjust for respiratory variability and decrease beat-to-beat noise to improve the measurement precision in individual leads by forming a representative complex for each lead. Signal averaging is a critical component of this process. Noise is reduced using this technique proportionate by the square root of the number of beats averaged.[4] Thus, a 10-fold reduction in noise is accomplished by averaging only 100 beats. Automated measurements are made from these representative templates, not from measurement of individual complexes. Average complex templates are formed from the average amplitude of each digital sampling point for selected complexes. Median complex templates are formed from the median amplitude at each digital sampling point. As a result, measurement accuracy is strongly dependent on the fidelity with which representative templates are formed. Because of the proprietary nature of this technology (the specific algorithms used are patented), the method used may vary by manufacturer. Consequently, the processed QRS complexes may vary in the "quality" of representation (i.e., if noise or aberrant beats are averaged into the complex, it will vary from the raw analog complex). The averaging process involves comparison of the voltages at a particular time point between the incoming complex and the template. Although the easiest method is to use the mean difference between voltages to update the "template," the most accurate method is to use the median (because it is less affected by outliers, such as aberrant beats or other signals that have escaped QRS matching)[4] (Figure 15-4).

A feature incorporated into most monitors is a visual trend line from which deviations in the position of the ST segment can be rapidly detected, which can aid online detection of ischemia. In addition, nearly all monitors display on-screen numerical values for the position of the ST segment used for ischemia detection (generally 60 to 80 milliseconds after the J point), although the specific fiducial point (based on heart rate) used usually can be adjusted by the clinician (Figure 15-5).

History and Description of the 12-Lead System

Where and how ECG electrodes are placed on the body are critical determinants of the morphology of the ECG signal. Lead systems have been developed based on theoretical considerations and references to anatomic landmarks that facilitate consistency between individuals (e.g., standard 12-lead system). Einthoven established electrocardiography using three extremities as references: the left arm, right arm, and left leg. He recorded the difference in potential between the left arm and right arm (lead I), between the left leg and right arm (lead II), and between the left leg and left arm (lead III) (Figure 15-6). Because the signals recorded were differences between two electrodes, these leads were called *bipolar*. The right leg served only as a reference electrode. Because Kirchoff's loop equation states that the sum of the three voltage differential pairs must equal zero, the sum of leads I and III must equal lead II.[21] The positive or negative polarity of each of the limbs was chosen by Einthoven to result in positive deflections of most of the waveforms and has no innate physiologic significance. He postulated that the three limbs defined an imaginary equilateral triangle with the heart at its center. Wilson refined and introduced the precordial leads into clinical practice. To implement these leads, he postulated a mechanism whereby the absolute level of electrical potential could be measured at the site of the exploring precordial electrode (the positive electrode). A negative pole with zero potential was formed by joining the three limb electrodes in a resistive network in which equally weighted signals cancel each other out. He called this the "central terminal," and in a fashion similar to Einthoven's vector concepts, he postulated it was located at the electrical center of the heart, representing the mean electrical potential of the body throughout the cardiac cycle. He described three additional limb leads (aVL, aVR, and aVF; Figure 15-7). These leads measured new vectors of activation, and in this way, the hexaxial reference system for determination of electrical axis was established. He subsequently introduced the six unipolar precordial V leads in 1935 (see Figure 15-6).[29] Six electrodes are placed on the chest in the following

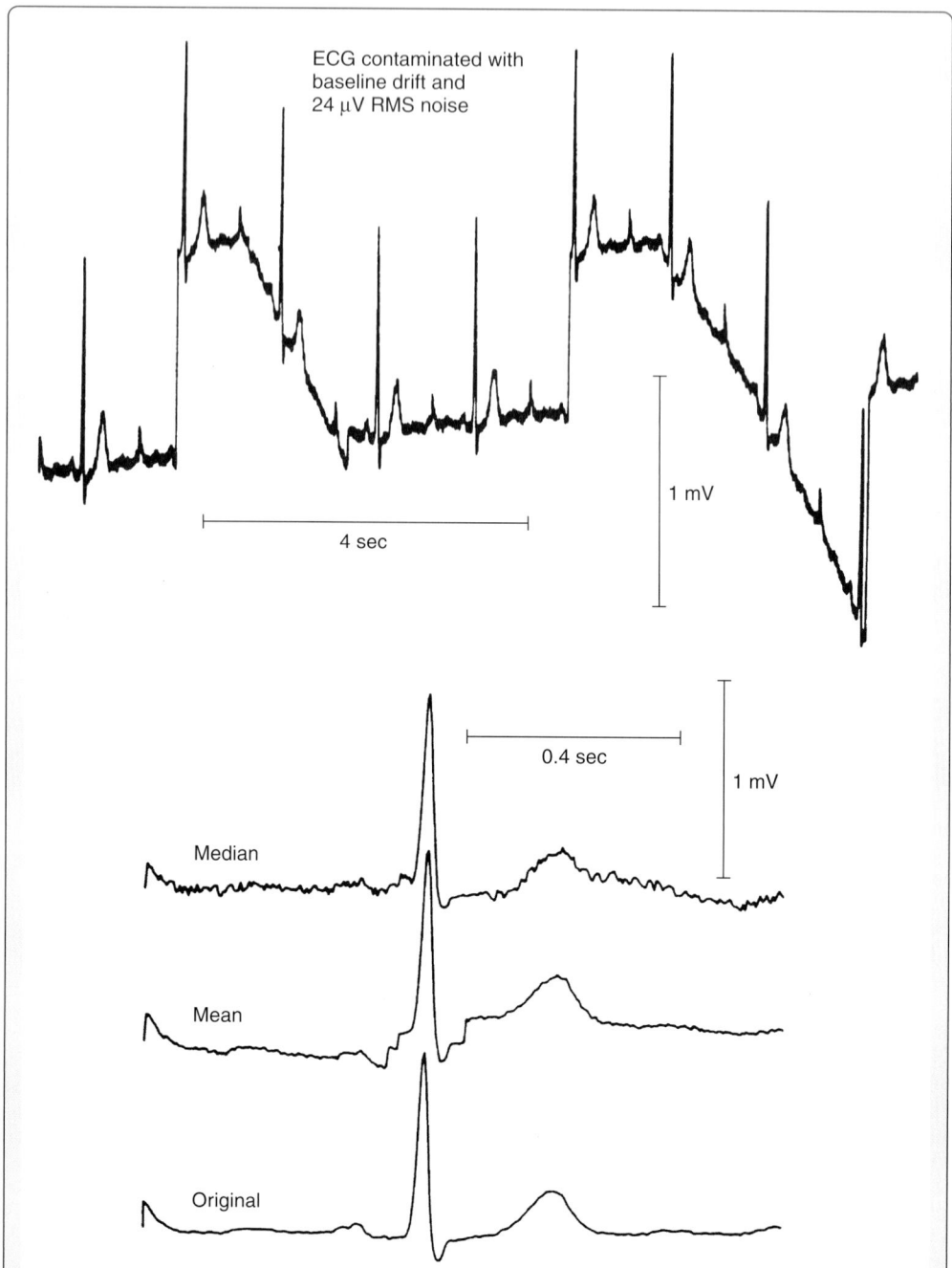

ECG contaminated with baseline drift and 24 µV RMS noise

4 sec

1 mV

0.4 sec

1 mV

Median

Mean

Original

Figure 15-4 Effects of averaging techniques on resolution of an electrocardiographic signal heavily contaminated with baseline and electrical noise. Despite a greater degree of baseline and electrical noise, median averaging results in a more accurate rendition of the original signal. Notice the abnormal J-point elevation in the mean averaged complex. ECG, electrocardiogram; RMS, root mean square. *(From Froelicher VF: Special methods: Computerized exercise ECG analysis. In Exercise and the Heart. Chicago: Year Book Medical Publishers, 1987, p 36.)*

locations: V_1, fourth intercostal space at the right sternal border; V_2, fourth intercostal space at the left sternal border; V_3, midway between V_2 and V_4; V_4, fifth intercostal space in the midclavicular line; V_5, in the horizontal plane of V_4 at the anterior axillary line, or if the anterior axillary line is ambiguous, midway between V_4 and V_6; and V_6, in the horizontal plane of V_4 at the midaxillary line[4] (see Figure 15-6).

Clinical application of the unipolar limb leads was limited because of their significantly smaller amplitude relative to the bipolar limb leads from which they were derived. They were not clinically applied until Goldberger augmented their amplitude (by a factor of 1.5) by severing the connection between the central terminal and the lead extremity being studied (which he called "augmented limb leads") in 1942. The limb leads, the precordial leads, and the augmented unipolar limb leads form what was accepted by the AHA as the conventional 12-lead ECG system.[30] Einthoven's law indicates that any one of the standard limb leads can be mathematically derived from the other two

limb leads. Therefore, the "standard" 12-lead ECG actually contains eight independent pieces of information: two measured potential differences from which the four remaining limb leads can be calculated and the six independent precordial leads.[4] In essence, all leads are effectively "bipolar," and the differentiation between "bipolar" and "unipolar" in the description of the standard limb leads, the augmented limb leads, and the precordial leads is discouraged in the most recent statement by the AHA.[4]

Technical Aspects of Electrode Placement

Monitoring electrodes preferentially should be placed directly over bony prominences of the torso (e.g., clavicular heads, iliac prominences) to minimize excursion of the electrode during respiration, which can cause baseline wander. Electrode impedance must be optimized to avoid loss and alteration of the signal. Skin impedance can

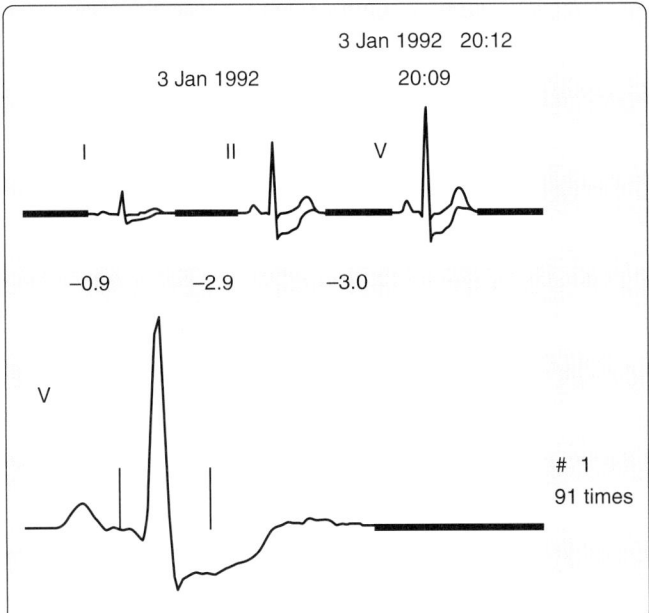

3 Jan 1992   20:12

3 Jan 1992   20:09

I   II   V

−0.9   −2.9   −3.0

V

1
91 times

Figure 15-5   The graphic output of the ST-adjustment window from a Marquette Electronics Series 7010 monitor (Milwaukee, WI) ST-segment analyzer. This software allows trending and display of three leads (i.e., I, II, and any single V lead). In this window, the initial complex ("learned" when the program was activated) is displayed together with the current complex. Two complexes are superimposed with different intensities to facilitate comparison. ST analysis is performed automatically at 80 milliseconds after the J point, although the user can manually adjust this. The number of QRS complexes that are input to the monitor is displayed. *(From Reich DL, Mittnacht A, London M, Kaplan J: Monitoring of the heart and vascular system. In Kaplan JA, et al (eds): Kaplan's Cardiac Anesthesia, 5th ed. Philadelphia: Saunders/Elsevier, 2006.)*

be reduced by a factor of 10 to 100 by removing a portion of the stratum corneum (e.g., gentle abrasion with a dry gauze pad resulting in a minor amount of surface erythema). Optimal impedance is 5000 ohms or less. The electrode may be covered with a watertight dressing to prevent surgical scrub solutions from undermining electrode contact.

Intrinsic and Extrinsic Electrocardiogram Artifact

Skin Impedance

Motion artifact and "baseline wander" result from several causes. Intrinsic to the body are electrical potentials generated by the skin.[31] Skin impedance has been shown to vary at different skin sites.

Electrodes

Direct current (DC) potentials actually are stored by the electrode itself (i.e., offset potentials), varying with the type of electrode used. A striking example of an offset potential is the transient obliteration of the ECG that occurs immediately after electrical defibrillation. Poor electrode contact enhances pickup of alternating current power-line interference (60-Hz signals).

Motor Activity

Another major physiologic source of artifact is electromyographic noise produced by motor activity, either voluntary (i.e., during treadmill testing or ambulatory ST-segment monitoring) or involuntary (i.e., shivering or Parkinsonian tremor). Electromyographic noise is similar in amplitude to the ECG but is generally of considerably higher frequency. Because it is a random signal, in contrast with the regular repetitive ECG, it is amenable to significant attenuation using routine DSP techniques (Figure 15-8).[32]

Extrinsic

There are also extrinsic or nonphysiologic causes of artifact. An important one is called *common-mode rejection*. The ECG signal is recorded as the difference in potential between two electrodes and is technically a differential signal. The body is not at absolute ground potential, which is why the right leg lead is used as a reference electrode.[22] This higher potential (over that of an absolute ground to earth) is called *common-mode potential* because it is common to both electrode inputs to the differential amplifier used to amplify the ECG signal. Common-mode potential must be rejected or it may alter the ECG signal.

Electrical Power-line Interference

Electrical power-line interference (60 Hz) is a common environmental problem. Power lines and other electrical devices radiate energy

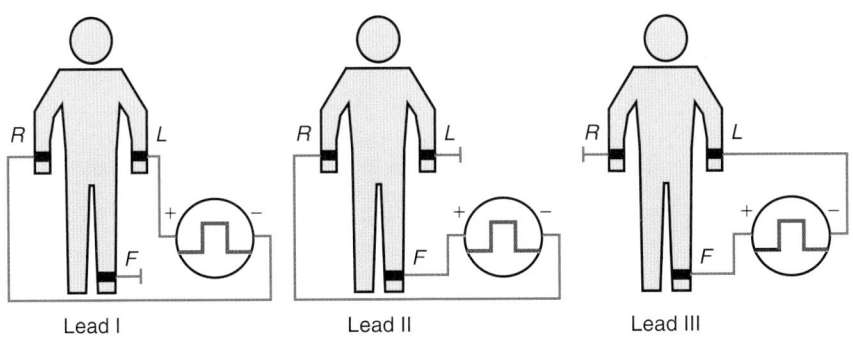

Lead I   Lead II   Lead III

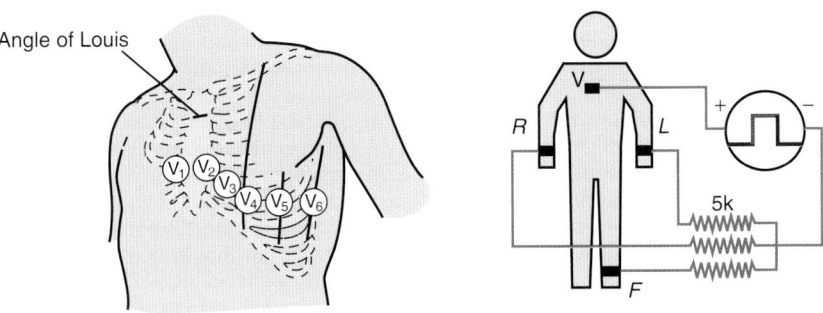

Angle of Louis

V₁ V₂ V₃ V₄ V₅ V₆

V

R   L

5k

F

Figure 15-6 *Top,* Electrode connections for recording the three standard limb leads I, II, and III. R, L, and F indicate locations of electrodes on the right arm, the left arm, and the left foot, respectively. *Bottom,* Electrode locations and electrical connections for recording a precordial lead. *Left,* The positions of the exploring electrode (V) for the six precordial leads. *Right,* Connections to form the Wilson central terminal for recording a precordial (V) lead. *(Reprinted from Mirvis DM, Goldberger AL: Electrocardiography. In Bonow RO, Mann DL, Zipes DP, Libby P (eds): Braunwald's Heart Disease: A Textbook of Cardiovascular Medicine, 8th ed. Philadelphia: Saunders/Elsevier, p.153, 2008.)*

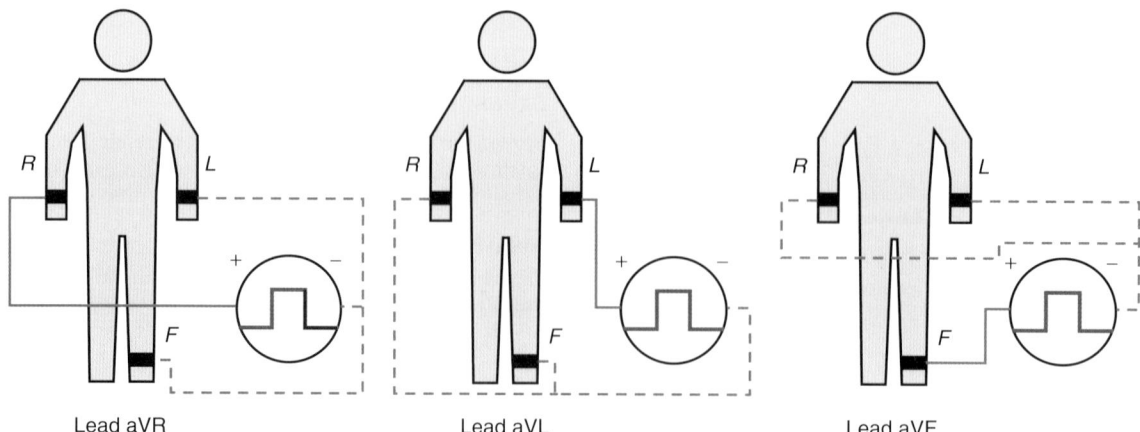

Lead aVR   Lead aVL   Lead aVF

Figure 15-7 Electrode locations and electrical connections for recording the three augmented limb leads aVR, aVL, and aVF. *Dashed lines* indicate connections to generate the reference electrode potential. *(Reprinted from Mirvis DM, Goldberger AL: Electrocardiography. In Bonow RO, Mann DL, Zipes DP, Libby P (eds): Braunwald's Heart Disease: A Textbook of Cardiovascular Medicine, 8th ed. Philadelphia: Saunders/Elsevier, p. 153, 2008.)*

Figure 15-8 Reduction of muscle artifact (simulated) by digital signal processing using signal averaging (PC2 Bedside Monitor; Spacelabs Healthcare, Redmond, WA). *Top,* The initial learned complex (i.e., dominant) on the left is followed by real-time complexes. *Bottom,* Median complexes are smoothed by signal processing. Notice that the ST segment position is isoelectric in the normal complex, but it does vary in accuracy with this degree of noise. The degree of noise reduction is proportional to the square root of the number of beats averaged. *(From Reich DL, Mittnacht A, London M, Kaplan J: Monitoring of the heart and vascular system. In Kaplan JA, et al (eds): Kaplan's Cardiac Anesthesia, 5th ed. Philadelphia: Saunders/Elsevier, 2006.)*

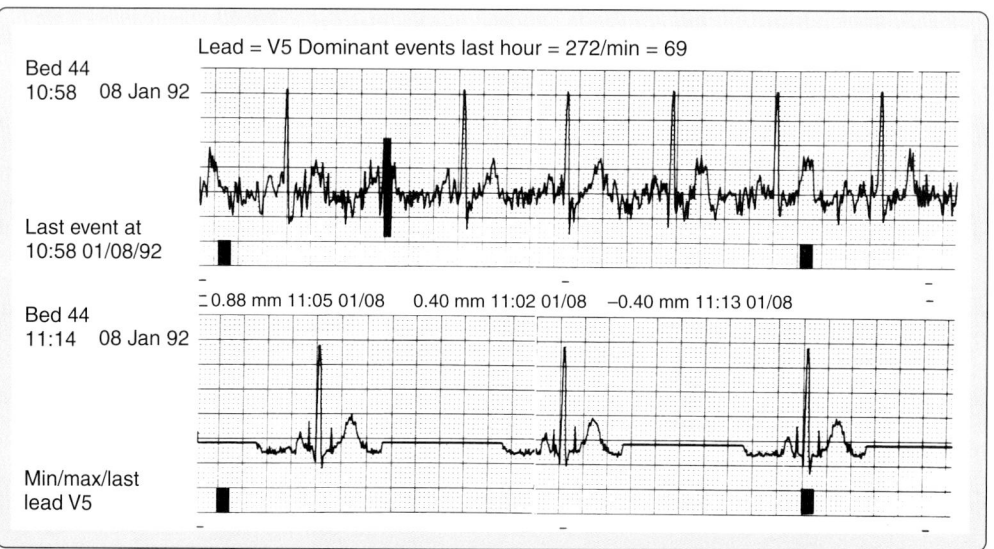

that can enter the monitor by poor electrode contact or cracked or poorly shielded lead cables. Interference can also be induced electromagnetically as these signals radiate through the loop formed by the body, lead cables, and monitor.[31] This type of interference can be reduced by twisting the lead cables together (reducing the loop area) or by minimizing the distance between the lead cables. In newer diagnostic ECG machines, A/D signal conversion occurs in an acquisition module close to the patient, which effectively reduces the length of the lead cables and the amount of signal induction possible. A line frequency "notch" filter is often used to remove 60-Hz noise. Other means of mathematical manipulation and processing also can remove 60-Hz noise.[33]

Electrocautery

Electrocautery units generate radiofrequency currents at very high frequencies (800 to 2000 kHz) and high voltages (1 kV, which is 100 times greater than the ECG signal). Older units used a modulation frequency of 60 Hz, which spread substantial electrical noise into the QRS frequency range of the ECG signal. Newer units use a modulation frequency of 20 kHz, minimizing this problem.[5] To minimize electrocautery artifact, place the right leg reference electrode as close as possible to the return plate and plug the ECG monitor into a different power outlet from the electrosurgical unit.

Clinical Sources of Artifact

Clinical devices with which the patient is in physical contact, particularly via plastic tubing, may at times cause clinically significant ECG artifact.[34–37] Although the exact mechanism is uncertain, two leading explanations are either a piezoelectric effect caused by mechanical deformation of the plastic or buildup of static electricity between two dissimilar materials, especially those in motion (as in the case of cardiopulmonary bypass [CPB] tubing and the roller pump head described later). In this scenario, the electricity generated in the pump flows into the patient via the tubing and is picked up by the electrodes. This artifact is not related to the electricity used to power the CPB pump because it has been reproduced by manually turning the pump heads.

Although ECG interference during CPB has been recognized for many years, Khambatta et al[36] were the first to document it in the literature. It is manifested by marked irregularity of the baseline, similar to ventricular fibrillation, with a frequency of 1 to 4 Hz and a peak amplitude up to 5 mV. Uncorrected, it may make effective diagnosis of arrhythmias and conduction disturbances difficult (Figure 15-9), especially during the critical period of weaning from CPB, and make accurate determination of asystolic arrest from the cardioplegia difficult. This artifact is more common in the winter than summer (56% vs. 13% of patients), with low relative humidity (45% to 48% or less), and

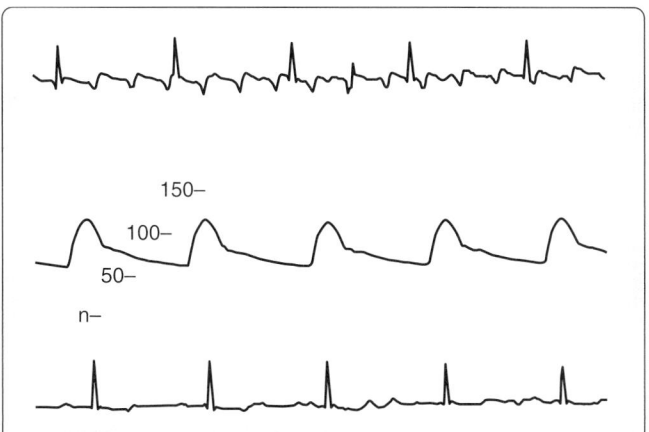

Figure 15-9 Baseline artifact simulates atrial flutter in a cannulated patient *(top)*, with stable arterial pressure *(middle)* just before institution of full cardiopulmonary bypass, similar to that described by Kleinman et al.[37] The "pseudoflutter waves" are corrected by application of the grounding cable *(bottom). (From London MJ, Kaplan JA: Advances in electrocardiographic monitoring. In Kaplan JA, et al (eds): Cardiac Anesthesia, 4th ed. Philadelphia: Saunders/Elsevier, 1999.)*

with room temperature less than 18° C to 20° C. Accumulation of static electricity is assumed to be the major causative factor, and the authors recommended maintaining ambient temperature above 20° C.

ECG artifact often mimics arrhythmias, primarily atrial, because the baseline artifact may resemble flutter waves or atrial fibrillation. Kleinman et al[37] (see earlier pump artifact) reported the commonly observed "atrial flutter" artifact (see Figure 15-9). Baseline artifact simulating flutter waves at 300 per minute occurred on an operating room monitor. The waves were observed to precisely track the pump head speed, disappearing when the pump was turned off. The artifact appears to have been caused by poor ECG electrode contact because the authors were able to produce it by undermining an ECG electrode with liquids. They pointed out that poor application of only one electrode can markedly impair the common-mode rejection capabilities of the ECG differential amplifier. This type of artifact also has been reported during noncardiac surgery.[34] Other clinical devices associated with ECG interference, albeit rarely, include infusion pumps and blood warmers. Isolated power supply line isolation monitors have also been associated with 60-Hz interference. This can be diagnosed by removing the line isolation monitor fuses to see whether the artifact disappears.[38]

Frequency Response of Electrocardiographic Monitors: Monitoring and Diagnostic Modes

ECG signals must be amplified and filtered before display. Each must be amplified equally to reproduce the component frequencies accurately. The monitor must have a "flat amplitude response" over the wide range of frequencies present. Similarly, because the slight delay in a signal as it passes through a filter or amplifier may vary in duration with different frequencies, all frequencies must be delayed equally. This is termed *linear phase response*. If the response is nonlinear, various components may appear temporally distorted (called *phase shift*). Given the importance of the ECG in diagnosing myocardial ischemia, it is important to realize that "significant" ST-segment depression or elevation can occur solely as a result of improper signal filtering in 12-lead ECG machines and bedside or ambulatory ST-segment monitors.[39-43] This artifact was a particular problem before the introduction of DSP. The AHA Committee on Electrocardiography Standardization has addressed specific frequency requirements for monitoring in this setting.[6,26]

Nonlinear frequency response in the low-frequency range (0.5 Hz) can cause artifactual ST depression, whereas phase delay in this range can

cause ST-segment elevation.[6] The AHA recommends a bandwidth from 0.05 to 100 Hz (at 3 dB).[30] Although a completely linear response is desirable, with analog filters, it is not generally possible. Because greater baseline noise is present when a 0.05-Hz cutoff is used, the 0.5-Hz cutoff often is used to display a more stable signal. This commonly is referred to as "monitoring mode," and use of a 0.05-Hz low-frequency cutoff is known as "diagnostic mode."[44] The difference in ST-segment morphology at various low-frequency cutoffs is illustrated in Figure 15-10. Because most newer monitors use signal averaging techniques that effectively eliminate most artifact even in the diagnostic mode, the clinician can usually (and should) avoid using the monitoring mode, whenever possible.

High-frequency response is of less importance clinically because the ST segment and T wave reside in the low-frequency spectrum. However, at the commonly used high-frequency cutoff of 40 Hz, the amplitude of the R and S waves may diminish significantly, making it difficult

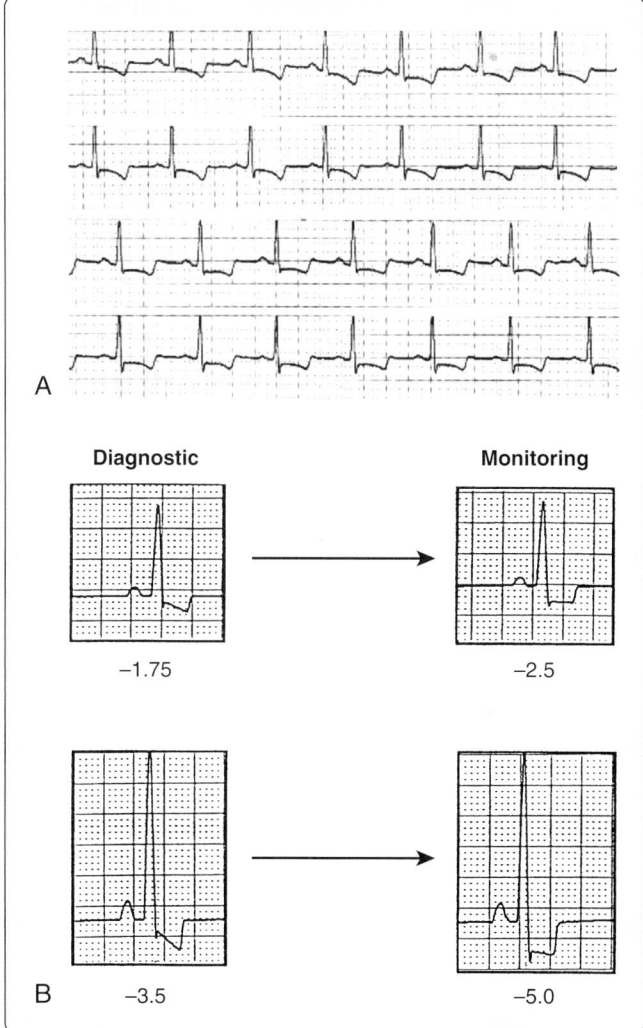

Figure 15-10 *A*, Monitoring versus diagnostic mode in leads II *(top trace)* and V5 *(bottom trace)* in a patient undergoing coronary artery bypass grafting. Notice the straightening of the baseline with use of the monitoring mode, which is most notable in lead II. The degree of the PR and ST segments is exaggerated in both leads. *B*, Effects of monitoring mode on ST-segment depth and morphology are illustrated using a digital electrocardiographic simulator. A SpaceLabs PC2 monitor (Redmond, WA) was switched from monitoring (0.5 to 40 Hz) to diagnostic mode (0.05 to 70 Hz). Notice the increase in the depth of ST-segment depression and the alteration of slope in both leads. *(From London MJ: Ischemia monitoring: ST segment analysis versus TEE. In Kaplan JA [ed]: Cardiothoracic and Vascular Anesthesia Update, vol. 3. Philadelphia: WB Saunders, 1993, pp 1–20.)*

to diagnose ventricular hypertrophy.[40,45] Significant reduction in QRS amplitude may occur in the following circumstances: major decreases in LV function, obesity, pericardial and pleural effusions, anasarca, and infiltrative or restrictive cardiac diseases.[46,47]

Tsuda et al[48] studied changes in R-wave amplitude in V_5 throughout the intraoperative period in 35 patients undergoing CABG or valve replacement. Amplitude was reduced by 50% to 60% before institution of CPB. CABG patients had a slower recovery of R-wave amplitude. Marked reduction and failure of recovery of R-wave amplitudes occurred in patients who died perioperatively, a finding often observed clinically but not previously documented in the literature. Crescenzi et al[49] have extended these observations by comparing R-wave amplitude in leads V_4 and V_5 in patients undergoing CABG with ($n = 35$) or without CPB ($n = 35$). A control group of patients undergoing mitral valve repair ($n = 31$) without CAD was included. A lack of change of amplitude in the R wave was found in the off-pump cases in contrast with reductions of R-wave amplitude in patients undergoing CABG or mitral valve surgery with CPB. Although biochemical markers of cardiac damage were significantly lower in the off-pump CABG group, no significant correlation was observed between alteration of R-wave amplitude and biochemical marker levels. It does not appear that fluid shifts or weight changes were considered in this analysis, factors that are more likely with the use of CPB. Larger sample sizes and more detailed analyses are required to better refine any potential clinically useful applications of QRS amplitude changes.

ELECTROCARDIOGRAPHIC CHANGES WITH MYOCARDIAL ISCHEMIA

Detection of Myocardial Ischemia

The ST segment is the most important portion of the QRS complex for evaluating ischemia.[50,51] It may come as a surprise that there are no gold standard criteria for the ECG diagnosis of myocardial ischemia.

Many anesthesiologists, when evaluating an ECG for signs of ischemia, look for signs of repolarization or ST-segment abnormalities. There are also many other signs of myocardial ischemia that may be evidenced in the ECG. These include T-wave inversion, QRS and T-wave axis alterations, R- or U-wave changes, and the development of previously undocumented arrhythmias or ventricular ectopy.[10] None of these, however, is as specific for ischemia as ST-segment depression or elevation.

The origin of the ST segment, at the J point, is easy to locate. However, J-point termination, which is generally accepted as the beginning of any change of slope of the T wave, is more difficult to determine. In normal individuals, there may be no discernible ST segment as the T wave starts with a steady slope from the J point, especially at rapid heart rates. The TP segment has been used as the isoelectric baseline from which changes in the ST segment are evaluated, but with tachycardia, this segment is eliminated, and during exercise testing, the PR segment is used. The PR segment is used in all ST-segment analyzers.

Repolarization of the ventricle proceeds from the epicardium to the endocardium, opposite to the vector of depolarization. The ST segment reflects the midportion, or phase 2, of repolarization during which there is little change in electrical potential.[52] It is usually isoelectric. Ischemia causes a loss of intracellular potassium, resulting in a current of injury. The electrophysiologic mechanism accounting for ST-segment shifts (elevation or depression) remains controversial. The two major theories are based on a loss of resting potential as current flows from the uninjured to the injured area (i.e., diastolic current) and on a true change in phase 2 potential as current flows from the injured to the uninjured area (i.e., systolic current; Figure 15-11). With subendocardial injury, the ST segment is depressed in the surface leads. With epicardial or transmural injury, the ST segment is elevated (Figure 15-12). When a lead is placed directly on the endocardium, opposite patterns are recorded.

With myocardial ischemia, repolarization is affected, resulting in downsloping or horizontal ST-segment depression. Various local effects and differences in vectors during repolarization result in different

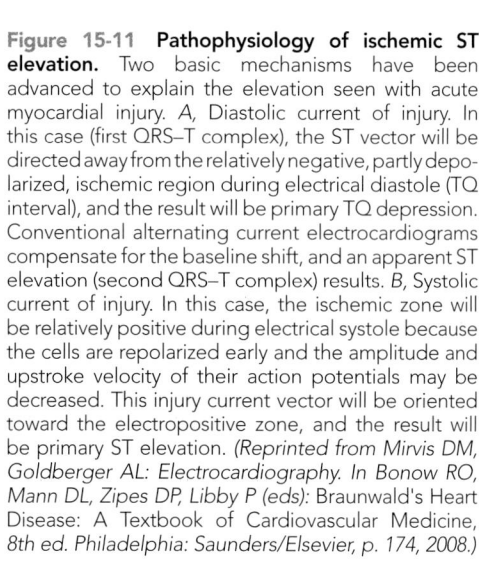

Figure 15-11 Pathophysiology of ischemic ST elevation. Two basic mechanisms have been advanced to explain the elevation seen with acute myocardial injury. *A*, Diastolic current of injury. In this case (first QRS–T complex), the ST vector will be directed away from the relatively negative, partly depolarized, ischemic region during electrical diastole (TQ interval), and the result will be primary TQ depression. Conventional alternating current electrocardiograms compensate for the baseline shift, and an apparent ST elevation (second QRS–T complex) results. *B*, Systolic current of injury. In this case, the ischemic zone will be relatively positive during electrical systole because the cells are repolarized early and the amplitude and upstroke velocity of their action potentials may be decreased. This injury current vector will be oriented toward the electropositive zone, and the result will be primary ST elevation. *(Reprinted from Mirvis DM, Goldberger AL: Electrocardiography. In Bonow RO, Mann DL, Zipes DP, Libby P (eds): Braunwald's Heart Disease: A Textbook of Cardiovascular Medicine, 8th ed. Philadelphia: Saunders/Elsevier, p. 174, 2008.)*

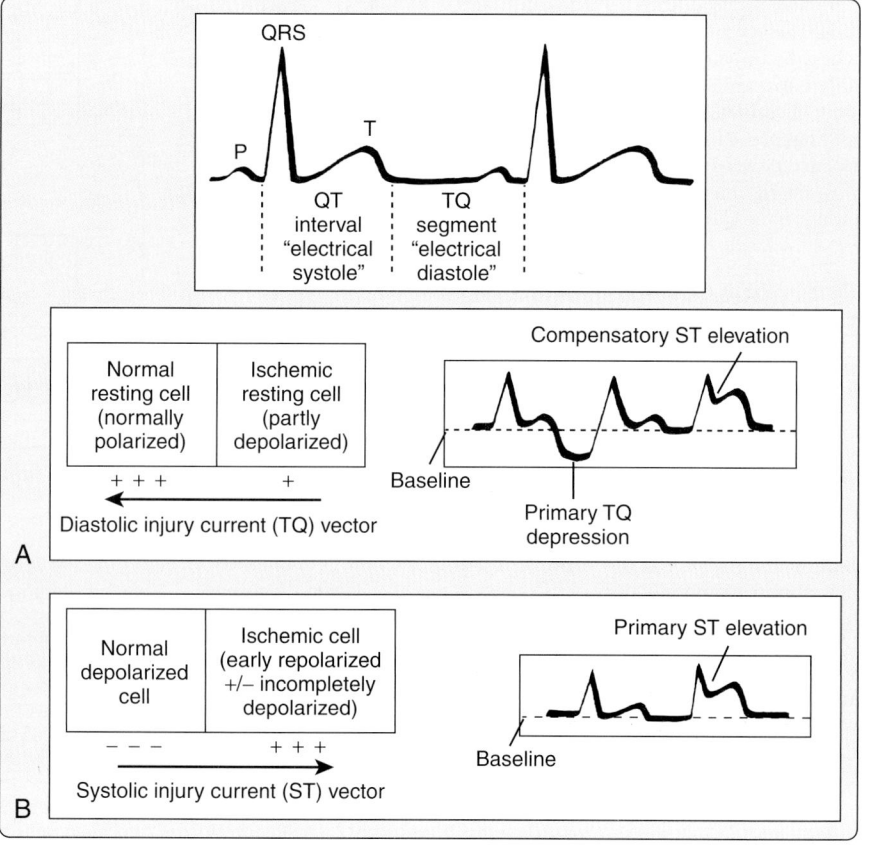

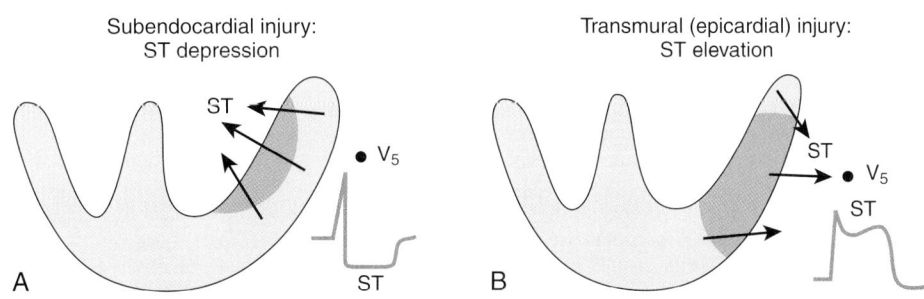

Figure 15-12 **Current of injury patterns with acute ischemia.** *A,* With predominant subendocardial ischemia, the resultant ST vector is directed toward the inner layer of the affected ventricle and the ventricular cavity. Overlying leads, therefore, record ST depression. *B,* With ischemia involving the outer ventricular layer (transmural or epicardial injury), the ST vector is directed outward. Overlying leads record ST elevation. Reciprocal ST depression can appear in contralateral leads. *(Reprinted from Mirvis DM, Goldberger AL: Electrocardiography. In Bonow RO, Mann DL, Zipes DP, Libby P (eds):* Braunwald's Heart Disease: A Textbook of Cardiovascular Medicine, *8th ed. Philadelphia: Saunders/Elsevier, p. 174, 2008.)*

ST morphologies that are recorded by the different leads. It generally is accepted that ST changes in multiple leads are associated with more severe degrees of CAD.

The classic criterion for ischemia is 0.1 mV (1 mm) of ST-segment depression measured 60 to 80 milliseconds after the J point (Figure 15-13).[50,51] The slope of the segment must be horizontal or downsloping. Downsloping depression may be associated with a greater number of diseased vessels and a worse prognosis than horizontal depression. Slowly upsloping depression with a slope of 1 mV/sec or less is also used but is considered less sensitive and specific (and difficult to assess clinically). The magnitude of ST-segment depression is related directly to the height of the associated R wave. Given that R waves are highest in the lateral precordium and lowest in the inferior regions, some have proposed "normalizing" ST depression for this variable.[53] However, this is controversial and not practical clinically. Nonspecific ST-segment depression can be related to drug use, particularly digoxin.[54] Interpretation of ST-segment changes in patients with LV hypertrophy is particularly controversial given the tall R-wave baseline, J-point depression, and steep slope of the ST segment. Although a number of studies have excluded such patients, others (including those using other modalities or epidemiologic studies) observed that LV hypertrophy is a highly significant predictor of adverse cardiac outcome.[55]

The criteria for myocardial ischemia with ST-segment elevation (0.1 mV in two contiguous leads) are used in conjunction with clinical symptoms or elevation of biochemical markers to diagnose acute coronary syndromes. It usually results from transmural ischemia, but it may potentially represent a reciprocal change in a lead oriented opposite to the primary vector with subendocardial ischemia (as may be seen in the reverse situation).[56,57] Perioperative ambulatory monitoring

studies also have included more than 0.2 mV in any single lead as a criterion, but ST elevation rarely is reported in the setting of noncardiac surgery. It is commonly observed, however, during weaning from CPB in cardiac surgery and during CABG surgery (on- and off-pump) with interruption of coronary flow in a native or graft vessel. ST elevation in a Q-wave lead should not be analyzed for acute ischemia, although it may indicate the presence of a ventricular aneurysm.

Despite the clinical focus on the ST segment for monitoring, the earliest ECG change at the onset of transmural ischemia is the almost immediate onset of tall and peaked (i.e., hyperacute) T waves, a so-called primary change. This phase is often transient. A significant increase in R-wave amplitude may also occur at this time.[58] T-wave inversions (symmetrical inversion) commonly accompany transmural ST-segment elevation changes, although most T-wave inversions or flattening observed perioperatively is nonspecific, resulting from transient alterations of repolarization because of changes in electrolytes, sympathetic tone, and other noncardiac factors.

Although repolarization changes (e.g., ST-T wave) are the focus of ischemia detection, computerized ECG analysis using signal averaging techniques has well-documented changes in depolarization with ischemia manifested by reduction in high-frequency components of the QRS complex (150 to 250 Hz). Such changes are not visible on the standard ECG, as they are in the range of only 10 to 20 mV, and are measured quantitatively using the root mean square (RMS) value (calculated by squaring the amplitude of each sample, determining the means of the squares, and then the square root of that mean value). Absolute changes in the RMS value greater than 0.6 mV or relative changes of more than 20% are considered clinically significant. This effect is likely due to slowing of conduction velocity in the ischemic

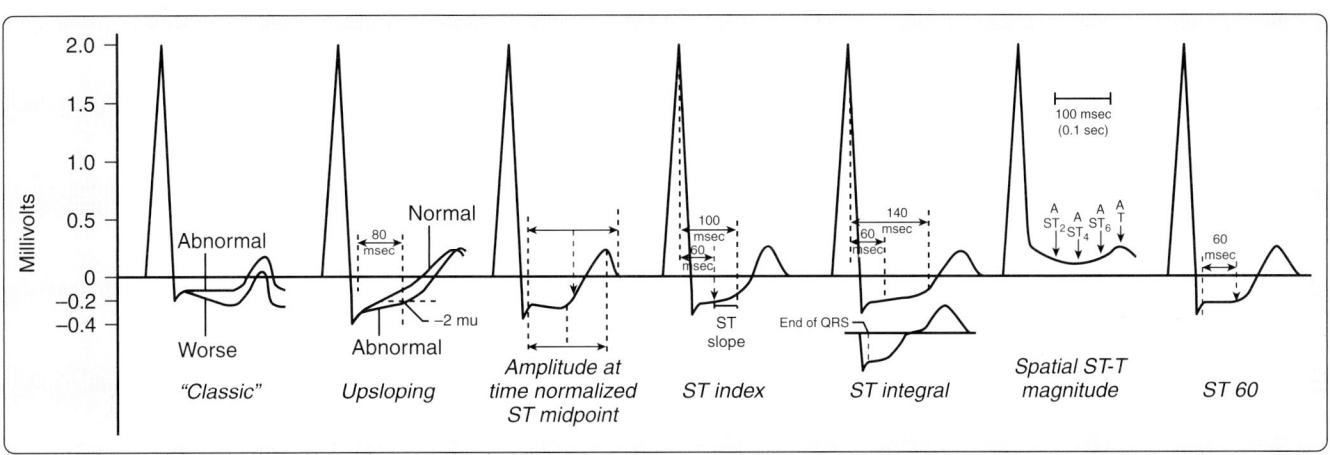

Figure 15-13 A variety of criteria for ischemic ST-segment changes has been proposed, including "classic" visual criteria and computer-derived indices. *(From Froelicher VF: Interpretation of specific exercise test responses. In* Exercise and the Heart. *Chicago: Year Book Medical Publishers, 1987, p 81.)*

region.[59] One study documented higher sensitivity of this approach compared with 12-lead ST-segment analysis in the detection of acute coronary occlusion during percutaneous transluminal coronary angioplasty.[60] The overall sensitivity was 88%, compared with 71% using ST-segment elevation criteria, or 79% by combining ST-segment elevation and depression. Its greatest value was in the detection of circumflex and right coronary artery occlusions.

Although this technology has been applied in several studies of patients undergoing cardiac surgery, all compared preoperative data with late (>1 week) postoperative data. Matsushita et al,[61] however, described its perioperative use in 70 patients undergoing CABG or valve surgery, evaluating RMS values 1 to 2 hours after removal of the aortic crossclamp. Dividing patients into quartiles of RMS values, they observed that decreases in cardiac index correlated significantly with progressive reductions in RMS, use of inotropes, and longer crossclamp times. At a threshold of 35% of preoperative values, a low cardiac output syndrome was more common. They hypothesized that the increase in intracellular calcium with ischemia is the common thread linking changes in conduction velocity with function. They recommended more common use of this technology because it is performed using an orthogonal lead set, which avoids the surgical field, is nearly real-time in nature, and extends the connection between ECG-derived parameters and cardiac function. Although intriguing, further studies from other groups clearly are required. It is unlikely this will be used commonly in the near future given the expense of replacing or upgrading existing equipment, but it remains a fertile topic for research.

Anatomic Localization of Ischemia with the Electrocardiogram

As noted earlier, ST-segment depression is a common manifestation of subendocardial ischemia. From a practical clinical standpoint, it has a single major strength and limitation. Its strength is that it is almost always present in one or more of the anterolateral precordial leads (V_4 through V_6).[62] However, it fails to "localize" the offending coronary lesion and has little relation to underlying segmental asynergy.[63,64]

In contrast, ST elevation correlates well with segmental asynergy and localizes the offending lesion relatively well.[63,65] Reciprocal ST-segment depression often is present in one or more of the other 12 leads. In patients with angiographically documented single-vessel disease, ST elevations (as well as Q waves or inverted T waves) in leads I, aVL, or V_1 through V_4 are closely correlated with disease of the left anterior descending artery, whereas similar findings in leads II, III, and aVF indicate disease of the right coronary or left circumflex arteries (surprisingly, the latter two cannot be differentiated by ECG criteria).[65] A multivariate analysis suggested that ST-segment elevation, abnormal Q waves, and inverted T waves in leads I and aVL (with normal V_1 and V_6) can be used to differentiate isolated first diagonal branch occlusion from the more ominous proximal left anterior descending artery occlusion.[66]

Berry et al[64] demonstrated the insensitivity of surface leads relative to a unipolar intracoronary lead (the distal end of a guidewire across a coronary stenosis) for evaluating ischemia in certain regions of the heart during percutaneous transluminal coronary angioplasty. Occlusion of the left circumflex artery resulted in ST elevation in only 32% of patients on the surface ECG, primarily in the inferior leads (83%) or in V_5 or V_6 (33%).

Clinical Lead Systems for Detecting Ischemia

Early clinical reports of intraoperative monitoring using the V_5 lead in high-risk patients were based on observations during exercise testing, in which bipolar configurations of V_5 demonstrated high sensitivity for myocardial ischemia detection (up to 90%). Subsequent studies using 12-lead monitoring (torso mounted for stability during exercise) confirmed the sensitivity of the lateral precordial leads.[67,68] Some studies,

however, reported higher sensitivity for leads V_4 or V_6 compared with V_5, followed by the inferior leads (in which most false-positive responses were reported).[62,69-74]

The factors responsible for precipitating ischemia during exercise testing and surgical settings may differ. For example, during exercise stress testing, most ischemia is demand related; whereas in the perioperative period, a larger proportion may be related to reduced oxygen supply. The most sensitive leads during exercise testing, however, are useful in the perioperative setting.

Given the relatively low sensitivity and specificity of the ECG, radionuclide and echocardiographic imaging now are used routinely in addition to the ECG in cardiac evaluations, but they are not practical in most perioperative settings. Other infrequently used parameters, such as R-wave amplitude and various patterns of heart rate change (e.g., heart rate recovery after exercise, heart rate change related to the slope of the ST segment), have been proposed as more sensitive means of detecting ischemia, compared with isolated ST-segment depression.

With the widespread growth of percutaneous coronary intervention for acute myocardial infarction and unstable angina in the 1990s, a number of investigators have reported on the use of continuous ECG monitoring (3 or 12 leads) in this setting. These observations have extended the classic teaching regarding localization of sites of coronary artery occlusion. Horacek and Wagner[75] reviewed the complexities and controversies regarding vessel-specific ECG responses to acute myocardial ischemia in detail. In general, ST-segment elevation in leads V_2 and V_3 is most sensitive for occlusion of the left anterior descending coronary artery, and leads III and aVF are most sensitive for the right coronary artery. In contrast, circumflex occlusion results in variable responses, with primary elevation in the posterior precordial leads V_7 through V_9 (which are rarely monitored clinically), and reciprocal ST-segment depression in the standard precordial leads (V_2 or V_3).[76,77] For transmural ischemia, sensitivity is highest in the anterior rather than the lateral precordial leads. An international multidisciplinary working group specifically recommended continuous monitoring of leads III, V_3, and V_5 for all acute coronary syndrome patients.[78]

Intraoperative Lead Systems

Detection of perioperative myocardial ischemia is an integral part of clinical monitoring and guides therapy (e.g., perioperative β-blockade). Many studies have demonstrated associations of perioperative ischemia with adverse cardiac outcomes in adults undergoing a variety of cardiac and noncardiac surgical procedures, particularly major vascular surgery.[79-82] Perhaps the bigger challenge is interpreting minor ST-segment changes in the context of the overall risk profile of the patient to avoid costly diagnostic tests being performed inappropriately. Studies document that transient myocardial ischemia occurs in the absence of significant CAD in unexpected patients, such as parturients, particularly with significant hemodynamic stress or hemorrhage.[83] Although the precise cause of such changes is uncertain, significant troponin release has been documented in these patients, confirming the suspicion that these ECG changes are true ischemic responses (probably related to subendocardial ischemia caused by global hypoperfusion).

How accurately the clinician places ECG leads on the patient's torso is probably the single most important factor influencing clinical utility of the ECG. Placement of the limb leads almost anywhere on the torso at, or near the origin of, the arms allows accurate rendition of lead II because both electrodes are farther than 12 cm from the heart (a distance considered to be the electrical infinity value beyond which amplitude of the QRS complex is unchanged).[84]

The cardiac anesthesiologist encounters a variety of ECG changes consistent with or pathognomonic for myocardial ischemia or infarction at many phases of the perioperative period in patients undergoing cardiac surgery. In the majority of these patients (i.e., those with known CAD), the sensitivity and specificity of the major signs described later are high, and few false-positive or -negative changes are encountered. However, the abnormal physiology of CPB, including acute changes in temperature, electrolyte concentrations, catecholamine levels, and so

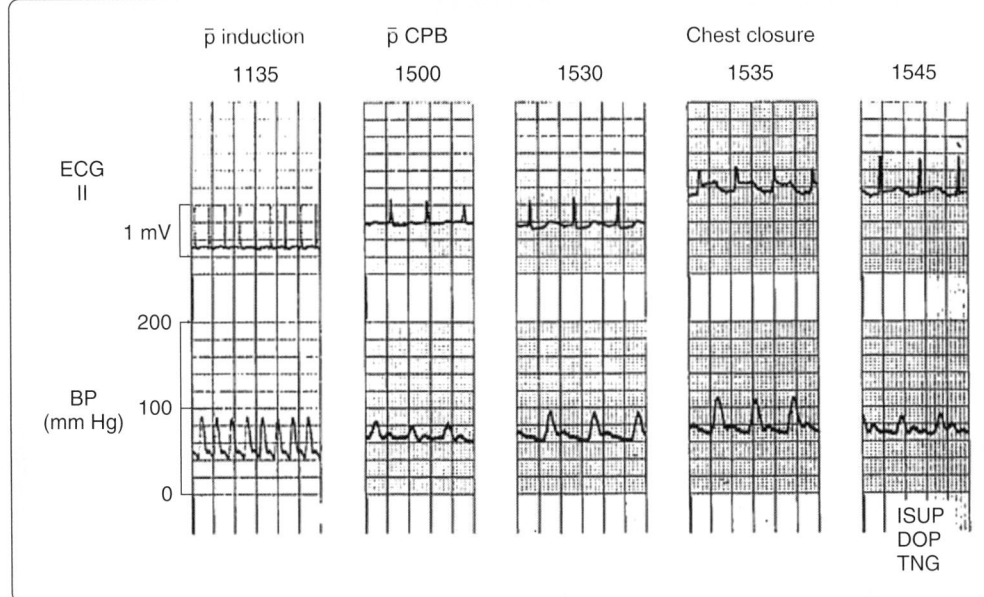

on, can significantly influence sensitivity and specificity. In addition, patients undergoing valve replacement, even those without coronary artery lesions, can develop significant subendocardial and transmural ischemia (e.g., coronary artery embolus of valve calcification, vegetations, or air). Even neonates can experience development of myocardial ischemia[85] (Figure 15-14).

Detecting and recognizing the clinical significance of various ECG signs of ischemia or infarction can enhance patient care acutely, as in emergency treatment of coronary artery spasm or air embolus, or by alerting the surgeon that myocardial revascularization may have been inadequate. This may lead to re-exploration of a saphenous vein or internal mammary artery anastomosis, especially if the TEE data support the diagnosis of ischemia. The early reports of Kaplan[87] and Dalton,[86] recommending routine intraoperative monitoring of V_5 in high-risk patients, cited exercise tolerance tests as the source of their recommendations (see Chapter 18). Subsequently, the recommended leads for intraoperative monitoring, based on several clinical studies, do not differ substantially from those used during exercise testing, although considerable controversy as to the optimal leads persists in both clinical settings. The coronary care unit's use of continuous ECG monitoring has received increasing attention.[88] A clinical study using continuous, computerized 12-lead ECG analysis in a mixed cohort (for vascular and other noncardiac procedures) by London et al[89] reported that almost 90% of responses involved ST-segment depression alone (75% in V_5 and 61% in V_4). In approximately 70% of patients, significant changes were observed in multiple leads. The sensitivity of each of the 12 leads in that study is shown in Figure 15-15. When considered in combination (as occurs clinically), the use of leads V_4 and V_5 increased sensitivity to 90%, whereas sensitivity for the standard clinical combination of leads II and V_5 was only 80%. Use of leads V_2 through V_5 and lead II captured all episodes (Table 15-3). A larger clinical study by Landesberg et al[90] of patients undergoing vascular surgery, using a longer period of monitoring (up to 72 hours) with more specific criteria for ischemia (>10-minute duration of episode), extended these observations. They reported that V_3 was most sensitive for ischemia (87%) followed by V_4 (79%), whereas V_5 alone was only 66% sensitive (Figure 15-16).[90] In the subgroup of patients in whom prolonged ischemic episodes ultimately culminated in infarction, V_4 was most sensitive (83%). In this study, all myocardial infarctions were non–Q-wave events detected by troponin elevation. Use of two precordial leads detected 97% to 100% of changes. Based on analysis of the resting isoelectric levels of each of the 12 leads (a unique component of this study), it was recommended that V_4 was the best single choice for monitoring of a single precordial

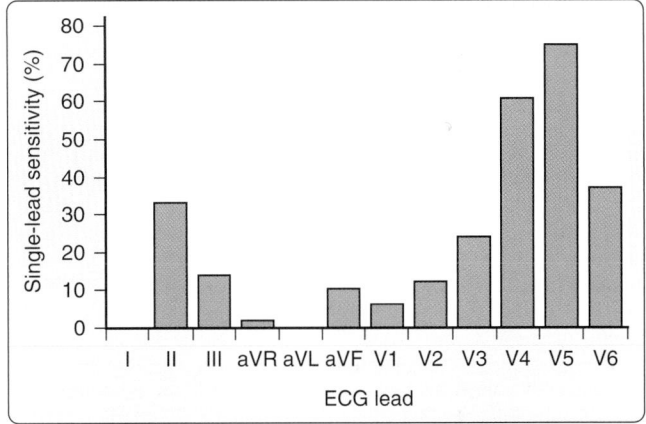

Figure 15-15 Single-lead sensitivity for the intraoperative detection of ischemia based on 51 episodes detected in 25 patients undergoing noncardiac surgery. Sensitivity was calculated by dividing the number of episodes detected in that lead by the total number of episodes. Sensitivity was greatest in lead V5, and the lateral leads (I, aVL) were insensitive. *(From London MJ, Hollenberg M, Wong MG, et al: Intraoperative myocardial ischemia: Localization by continuous 12-lead electrocardiography. Anesthesiology 69:232, 1988.)*

TABLE 15-3	Sensitivity for Different Electrocardiographic Lead Combinations		
Number of Leads	**Combination**	**Sensitivity (%)**
1 lead	II	33
	V4	61
	V5	75
2 leads	II/V5	80
	II/V4	82
	V4/V5	90
3 leads	V3/V4/V5	94
	II/V4/V5	96
4 leads	II/V2-V5	100

Data from London MJ, Hollenberg M, Wong MG, et al: Intraoperative myocardial ischemia: Localization by continuous 12-lead electrocardiography. *Anesthesiology* 69:232, 1988.

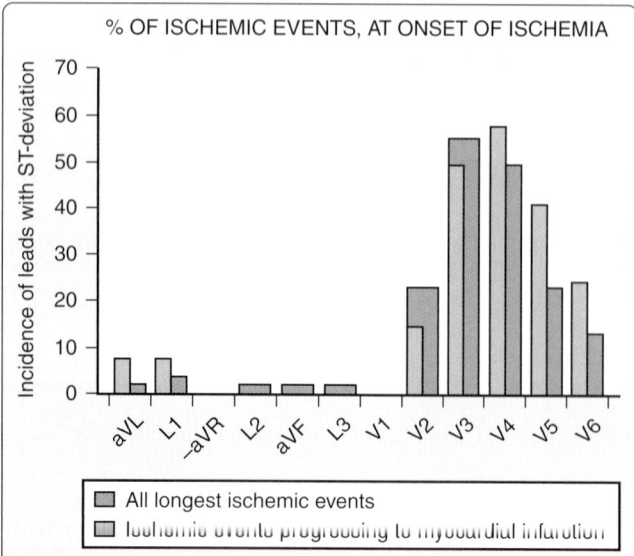

Figure 15-16 Histogram showing the incidence in which prolonged ischemia was first noted by each lead at the onset of ischemia in all 38 longest ischemic events and in the 12 ischemic events that progressed to myocardial infarction. *(From Landesberg G, Mosseri M, Wolf Y, et al: Perioperative myocardial ischemia and infarction: Identification by continuous 12-lead electrocardiogram with online ST-segment monitoring.* Anesthesiology 96:264–270, 2002.)

lead, because it was most likely to be isoelectric relative to the resting 12-lead preoperative ECG. In contrast, the baseline ST segment was more likely above isoelectric in V_1 through V_3 and below isoelectric in V_5 and V_6. Surprisingly, no episodes of ST elevation occurred in this study, as opposed to 12% in the earlier study of London et al,[89] in which such changes were detected in inferior and anteroseptal precordial leads. Martinez et al[91] evaluated a cohort of vascular surgical patients monitored in the intensive care unit for the first postoperative day with continuous 12-lead monitoring using a threshold of 20 minutes for an ischemic episode. Eleven percent of 149 patients met criteria, with ST depression in 71% and ST elevation alone in 18% (12% had both). Most changes were detected in V_2 (53%) and V_3 (65%). Using the standard two-lead system (II and V_5), only 41% of episodes would have been detected. Although these studies clearly support the value of precordial monitoring in patients at risk for subendocardial ischemia, clinicians must be vigilant for the rare patient with acute Q-wave infarction (most commonly in the inferior leads). The studies previously cited have all been conducted in patients undergoing noncardiac surgery because it is not practical to conduct such studies in those with open chests or extensive surgical dressings in the precordial region. There is no reason, however, to assume that there would be any significant differences in the cardiac patient. Sudden episodes of acute

transmural ischemia (associated with ST-segment elevation) are much more likely in this setting from acute ischemia/infarction (e.g., thrombotic occlusion) or surgery-induced reductions in coronary blood flow. The use of multiple precordial leads, although appealing, is not likely to become common clinical practice because of the limitations of existing monitors (and cables). Even if such equipment were available, it is likely that considerable resistance would occur from practitioners because of the extra effort associated with this approach. Perhaps, in the future, when lower cost wireless technologies are perfected, this approach may become a clinical reality.

Abnormalities in T-wave morphology are probably the most common perioperative ECG abnormality in the general surgical population. Breslow et al[92] noted new T-wave abnormalities within 1 hour after surgery in 18% of an unselected surgical population of 394 patients (excluding cardiac and neurosurgery). About two thirds of the changes were limited to T wave flattening, and the remainder had new inversions. The incidence was no different between patients with known CAD and those without. Out of a battery of variables, the only one statistically associated with T-wave abnormalities was intraabdominal surgery. Importantly, the ECG changes were not associated with any clinical morbidity. This study illustrates the known relation of T wave changes with a variety of autonomic stimuli, including changes in serum glucose, increased catecholamines, acute hyperventilation, and upper gastrointestinal disease. Similar analyses in patients undergoing cardiac surgery are not available, and the specificity of the response would be expected to be much lower.

ELECTROCARDIOGRAPHIC CHANGES WITH MEDICATIONS, ELECTROLYTES, AND PACEMAKERS

Use of inferior leads (II, III, aVF) allows superior discrimination of P-wave morphology, facilitating visual diagnosis of arrhythmias and conduction disorders. Although esophageal (and even intracardiac) leads allow the greatest sensitivity in detecting P waves, these rarely are used clinically. Nevertheless, they should be kept in mind for difficult diagnoses. With the increasing use of implantable defibrillators and automatic external defibrillators to treat ventricular fibrillation and ventricular tachycardia, there is considerable interest in the refinement of arrhythmia detection algorithms and their validation.[93] As expected, the accuracy of the devices for detecting ventricular arrhythmias is high, but is much lower for detecting atrial arrhythmias. In the settings of critical care and ambulatory monitoring, a variety of artifacts are common causes of false-positive responses.[93] Detection of pacemaker spikes may be complicated by very-low-amplitude signals related to bipolar pacing leads, amplitude varying with respiration, and total-body fluid accumulation.[93,94] Most critical care and ambulatory monitors incorporate pacemaker spike enhancement for small high-frequency signals (typically 5 to 500 mV with 0.5- to 2-millisecond pulse duration) to facilitate recognition. However, this can lead to artifact if there is high-frequency noise within the lead system.

References

1. Munson ES: Reports of scientific meetings, *Anesthesiology* 32:178–180, 1970.
2. American Society of Anesthesiologists: *Standards for Basic Anesthetic Monitoring*, 2005, pp 1–3.
3. Hurst JW: The renaissance of clinical electrocardiography, *Heart Dis Stroke* 2:290–295, 1993.
4. Kligfield P, Gettes LS, Bailey JJ, et al: Recommendations for the standardization and interpretation of the electrocardiogram: Part I: The electrocardiogram and its technology: A scientific statement from the American Heart Association Electrocardiography and Arrhythmias Committee, Council on Clinical Cardiology; the American College of Cardiology Foundation; and the Heart Rhythm Society: Endorsed by the International Society for Computerized Electrocardiology, *Circulation* 115:1306–1324, 2007.
5. Weinfurt PT: Electrocardiographic monitoring: An overview, *J Clin Monit* 6:132–138, 1990.
6. Tayler DI, Vincent R: Artefactual ST segment abnormalities due to electrocardiograph design, *Br Heart J* 54:121–128, 1985.
7. Stern S: Angina pectoris without chest pain: Clinical implications of silent ischemia, *Circulation* 106:1906–1908, 2002.
8. Fleisher LA, Beckman JA, Brown KA, et al: ACC/AHA 2007 Guidelines on Perioperative Cardiovascular Evaluation and Care for Noncardiac Surgery: Executive Summary: A Report of the American College of Cardiology/American Heart Association Task Force on Practice Guidelines, *Circulation* 116:1971–1996, 2007.
9. Cooper JK: Electrocardiography 100 years ago. Origins, pioneers, and contributors, *N Engl J Med* 315:461–464, 1986.
10. Fisch C: Evolution of the clinical electrocardiogram, *J Am Coll Cardiol* 14:1127–1138, 1989.
11. Krikler DM: The QRS complex, *Ann N Y Acad Sci* 601:24–30, 1990.
12. Rowlandson I: Computerized electrocardiography. A historical perspective, *Ann N Y Acad Sci* 601:343–352, 1990.
13. Fye WB: A history of the origin, evolution, and impact of electrocardiography, *Am J Cardiol* 73:937–949, 1994.
14. Hurst JW: Naming of the waves in the ECG, with a brief account of their genesis, *Circulation* 98:1937–1942, 1998.
15. Katz AM: *The Electrocardiogram, Physiology of the Heart*, Philadelphia, 2006, Lippincott Williams & Wilkins, pp 427–461.

16. Lynch C: Cellular electrophysiology of the heart. In Lynch C, editor: *Clinical Cardiac Electrophysiology*, Philadelphia, 1994, JB Lippincott Company, pp 1–52.
17. Rubart M, Zipes DP: Genesis of cardiac arrhythmias: Electrophysiological considerations. In Libby P, Bonow RO, Mann DL, Zipes DP, editors: *Brawnwald's Heart Disease*, Philadelphia, 2008, Saunders Elsevier, pp 727–762.
18. Burger HC: Heart-vector and leads, *Br Heart J* 8:157–161, 1946.
19. Burger HC, Van Milaan JB: Heart-vector and leads; geometrical representation, *Br Heart J* 10:229–233, 1948.
20. Carim HM: Bioelectrodes. In Webster JG, editor: *Encyclopedia of Medical Devices and Instrumentation*, New York, 1988, John Wiley & Sons, pp 195–224.
21. Plonsey R: Electrocardiography. In Webster JG, editor: *Encyclopedia of Medical Devices and Instrumentation*, New York, 1988, John Wiley & Sons, pp 1017–1040.
22. Thakor NV: Electrocardiographic monitors. In Webster JG, editor: *Encyclopedia of Medical Devices and Instrumentation*, New York, 1988, John Wiley & Sons, pp 1002–1017.
23. Thakor NV: Computers in electrocardiography. In Webster JG, editor: *Encyclopedia of Medical Devices and Instrumentation*, New York, 1988, John Wiley & Sons, pp 1040–1061.
24. Kors JA, van Bemmel JH: Classification methods for computerized interpretation of the electrocardiogram, *Methods Inf Med* 29:330–336, 1990.
25. Sheffield LT: Computer-aided electrocardiography, *J Am Coll Cardiol* 10:448–455, 1987.
26. Mirvis DM, Berson AS, Goldberger AL, et al: Instrumentation and practice standards for electrocardiographic monitoring in special care units. A report for health professionals by a Task Force of the Council on Clinical Cardiology, American Heart Association, *Circulation* 79:464–471, 1989.
27. Watanabe K, Bhargava V, Froelicher V: Computer analysis of the exercise ECG: A review, *Prog Cardiovasc Dis* 22:423–446, 1980.
28. Bhargava V, Watanabe K, Froelicher VF: Progress in computer analysis of the exercise electrocardiogram, *Am J Cardiol* 47:1143–1151, 1981.
29. Kossmann CE: Unipolar electrocardiography of Wilson: A half century later, *Am Heart J* 110:901–904, 1985.
30. Pipberger HV, ArzBaecher RC, Golberger AL: Recommendations for standardization of leads and of specifications for instruments in electrocardiography and vectorcardiography. Report of the Committee on Electrocardiography, American Heart Association, *Circulation* 52:1975.
31. Gardner RM, Hollingsworth KW: Optimizing the electrocardiogram and pressure monitoring, *Crit Care Med* 14:651–658, 1986.
32. de Pinto V: Filters for the reduction of baseline wander and muscle artifact in the ECG, *J Electrocardiol* 25(Suppl):40–48, 1992.
33. Levkov C, Mihov G, Ivanov R, et al: Removal of power-line interference from the ECG: A review of the subtraction procedure, *Biomed Eng Online* 4:50, 2005.
34. Lampert BA, Sundstrom FD: ECG artifact simulating supraventricular tachycardia during automated percutaneous lumbar discectomy, *Anesth Analg* 67:1096–1098, 1988.
35. Paulsen AW, Pritchard DG: ECG artifact produced by crystalloid administration through blood/fluid warming sets, *Anesthesiology* 69:803–804, 1988.
36. Khambatta HJ, Stone JG, Wald A, Mongero LB: Electrocardiographic artifacts during cardiopulmonary bypass, *Anesth Analg* 71:88–91, 1990.
37. Kleinman B, Shah K, Belusko R, Blakeman B: Electrocardiographic artifact caused by extracorporeal roller pump, *J Clin Monit* 6:258–259, 1990.
38. Marsh R: ECG artifact in the OR, *Health Devices* 20:140–141, 1991.
39. Berson AS, Pipberger HV: The low-frequency response of electrocardiographs, a frequent source of recording errors, *Am Heart J* 71:779–789, 1966.
40. Meyer JL: Some instrument induced errors in the electrocardiogram, *JAMA* 201:351–356, 1967.
41. Bragg-Remschel DA, Anderson CM, Winkle RA: Frequency response characteristics of ambulatory ECG monitoring systems and their implications for ST segment analysis, *Am Heart J* 103:20–31, 1982.
42. Bragg Remschel D: Silent myocardial ischemia. Problems with ST segment analysis in ambulatory ECG monitoring systems. In Rutishauser W, Roskamm H, editors: *Silent Myocardial Ischemia*, Berlin, 1984, Springer Verlag, pp 90–99.
43. Bailey JJ, Berson AS, Garson A Jr, et al: Recommendations for standardization and specifications in automated electrocardiography: Bandwidth and digital signal processing. A report for health professionals by an ad hoc writing group of the Committee on Electrocardiography and Cardiac Electrophysiology of the Council on Clinical Cardiology, American Heart Association, *Circulation* 81:730–739, 1990.
44. London MJ: Ischemia monitoring: ST segment analysis versus TEE. In Kaplan JA, editor: *Cardiothoracic and Vascular Anesthesia Update*, Philadelphia, 1993, WB Saunders Company, pp 1–18.
45. Garson A Jr: Clinically significant differences between the "old" analog and the "new" digital electrocardiograms, *Am Heart J* 114:194–197, 1987.
46. Madias JE, Bazaz R, Agarwal H, et al: Anasarca-mediated attenuation of the amplitude of electrocardiogram complexes: A description of a heretofore unrecognized phenomenon, *J Am Coll Cardiol* 38:756–764, 2001.
47. Madias JE: Recognizing the link between peripheral edema and voltage attenuation of QRS complexes: Implications for the critical care patient, *Chest* 124:2041–2044, 2003.
48. Tsuda H, Tobata H, Watanabe S, et al: QRS complex changes in the V_5 ECG lead during cardiac surgery, *J Cardiothorac Vasc Anesth* 6:658–662, 1992.
49. Crescenzi G, Scandroglio AM, Pappalardo F, et al: ECG changes after CABG: The role of the surgical technique, *J Cardiothorac Vasc Anesth* 18:38–42, 2004.
50. Fletcher GF, Froelicher VF, Hartley LH, et al: Exercise standards. A statement for health professionals from the American Heart Association, *Circulation* 82:2286–2322, 1990.
51. Froelicher VF: Interpretation of specific exercise test responses. In *Exercise and the Heart*, Chicago, 1987, Year Book Medical Publishers, pp 81–145.
52. Castellanos A, Interian A, Myerburg R: The resting electrocardiogram. In Fuster V, Alexander R, O'Rourke R, editors: *The Heart*, ed 11 New York, 2004, McGraw-Hill, pp 295–324.
53. Hollenberg M, Go M Jr, Massie BM, et al: Influence of R-wave amplitude on exercise-induced ST depression: Need for a "gain factor" correction when interpreting stress electrocardiograms, *Am J Cardiol* 56:13–17, 1985.
54. Goldberger AL: Electrocardiogram in coronary artery disease: Limitations in sensitivity. In *Myocardial Infarction: Electrocardiographic Differential Diagnosis*, St. Louis, 1984, CV Mosby, pp 303–308.
55. Hollenberg M, Mangano DT, Browner WS, et al: Predictors of postoperative myocardial ischemia in patients undergoing noncardiac surgery. The Study of Perioperative Ischemia Research Group, *JAMA* 268:205–209, 1992.
56. Croft CH, Woodward W, Nicod P, et al: Clinical implications of anterior S-T segment depression in patients with acute inferior myocardial infarction, *Am J Cardiol* 50:428–436, 1982.
57. Mirvis DM: Physiologic bases for anterior ST segment depression in patients with acute inferior wall myocardial infarction, *Am Heart J* 116:1308–1322, 1988.
58. Brody DA: A theoretical analysis of intracavitary blood mass influence on the heart-lead relationship, *Circ Res* 4:731–738, 1956.
59. Abboud S, Berenfeld O, Sadeh D: Simulation of high-resolution QRS complex using a ventricular model with a fractal conduction system. Effects of ischemia on high-frequency QRS potentials, *Circ Res* 68:1751–1760, 1991.
60. Pettersson J, Pahlm O, Carro E, et al: Changes in high-frequency QRS components are more sensitive than ST-segment deviation for detecting acute coronary artery occlusion, *J Am Coll Cardiol* 36: 1827–1834, 2000.
61. Matsushita S, Sakakibara Y, Imazuru T, et al: High-frequency QRS potentials as a marker of myocardial dysfunction after cardiac surgery, *Ann Thorac Surg* 77:1293–1297, 2004.
62. Chaitman BR, Hanson JS: Comparative sensitivity and specificity of exercise electrocardiographic lead systems, *Am J Cardiol* 47:1335–1349, 1981.
63. Bar FW, Brugada P, Dassen WR, et al: Prognostic value of Q waves, R/S ratio, loss of R wave voltage, ST-T segment abnormalities, electrical axis, low voltage and notching: Correlation of electrocardiogram and left ventriculogram, *J Am Coll Cardiol* 4:17–27, 1984.
64. Berry C, Zalewski A, Kovach R, et al: Surface electrocardiogram in the detection of transmural myocardial ischemia during coronary artery occlusion, *Am J Cardiol* 63:21–26, 1989.
65. Fuchs RM, Achuff SC, Grunwald L, et al: Electrocardiographic localization of coronary artery narrowings: Studies during myocardial ischemia and infarction in patients with one-vessel disease, *Circulation* 66:1168–1176, 1982.
66. Iwasaki K, Kusachi S, Kita T, Taniguchi G: Prediction of isolated first diagonal branch occlusion by 12-lead electrocardiography: ST segment shift in leads I and aVL, *J Am Coll Cardiol* 23:1557–1561, 1994.
67. Blackburn H, Katigbak R: What electrocardiographic leads to take after exercise? *Am Heart J* 67: 184–185, 1964.
68. Mason RE, Likar I: A new system of multiple-lead exercise electrocardiography, *Am Heart J* 71: 196–205, 1966.
69. Mason RE, Likar I, Biern RO, Ross RS: Multiple-lead exercise electrocardiography. Experience in 107 normal subjects and 67 patients with angina pectoris, and comparison with coronary cinearteriography in 84 patients, *Circulation* 36:517–525, 1967.
70. Tubau JF, Chaitman BR, Bourassa MG, Waters DD: Detection of multivessel coronary disease after myocardial infarction using exercise stress testing and multiple ECG lead systems, *Circulation* 61:44–52, 1980.
71. Koppes G, McKiernan T, Bassan M, Froelicher VF: Treadmill exercise testing. Part I, *Curr Probl Cardiol* 2:1–44, 1977.
72. Chaitman BR, Bourassa MG, Wagniart P, et al: Improved efficiency of treadmill exercise testing using a multiple lead ECG system and basic hemodynamic exercise response, *Circulation* 57:71–79, 1978.
73. Miller TD, Desser KB, Lawson M: How many electrocardiographic leads are required for exercise treadmill tests? *J Electrocardiol* 20:131–137, 1987.
74. Chaitman BR: The changing role of the exercise electrocardiogram as a diagnostic and prognostic test for chronic ischemic heart disease, *J Am Coll Cardiol* 8:1195–1210, 1986.
75. Horacek BM, Wagner GS: Electrocardiographic ST-segment changes during acute myocardial ischemia, *Card Electrophysiol Rev* 6:196–203, 2002.
76. Carley SD: Beyond the 12 lead: Review of the use of additional leads for the early electrocardiographic diagnosis of acute myocardial infarction, *Emerg Med (Fremantle)* 15:143–154, 2003.
77. Zimetbaum PJ, Josephson ME: Use of the electrocardiogram in acute myocardial infarction, *N Engl J Med* 348:933–940, 2003.
78. Drew BJ, Krucoff MW: Multilead ST-segment monitoring in patients with acute coronary syndromes: A consensus statement for healthcare professionals. ST- Segment Monitoring Practice Guideline International Working Group, *Am J Crit Care* 8:372–386, 1999 quiz 387–388.
79. Mangano DT, Browner WS, Hollenberg M, et al: Association of perioperative myocardial ischemia with cardiac morbidity and mortality in men undergoing noncardiac surgery. The Study of Perioperative Ischemia Research Group, *N Engl J Med* 323:1781–1788, 1990.
80. London MJT: The significance of perioperative ischemia in vascular surgery. In *Anesthesia Update. Cardiothoracic and Vascular Anesthesia*, Philadelphia, 1993, WB Saunders Company, pp 1–18.
81. Slogoff S, Keats AS: Randomized trial of primary anesthetic agents on outcome of coronary artery bypass operations, *Anesthesiology* 70:179–188, 1989.
82. London MJ: Perioperative myocardial ischemia in patients undergoing myocardial revascularization, *Curr Opin Anesthesiol* 6:98, 1993.
83. Karpati PC, Rossignol M, Pirot M, et al: High incidence of myocardial ischemia during postpartum hemorrhage, *Anesthesiology* 100:30–36, 2004 discussion 5A.
84. Constant J: Learning electrocardiography, Boston: Little, 1981, Brown and Company.
85. Bell C, Rimar S, Barash P: Intraoperative ST-segment changes consistent with myocardial ischemia in the neonate: A report of three cases, *Anesthesiology* 71:601–604, 1989.
86. Dalton B: A precordial ECG lead for chest operations, *Anesth Analg* 55:740–741, 1976.
87. Kaplan JA, King SB 3rd: The precordial electrocardiographic lead (V5) in patients who have coronary-artery disease, *Anesthesiology* 45:570–574, 1976.
88. London MJ: Multilead precordial ST-segment monitoring: "The next generation?", *Anesthesiology* 96:259–261, 2002.
89. London MJ, Hollenberg M, Wong MG, et al: Intraoperative myocardial ischemia: Localization by continuous 12-lead electrocardiography, *Anesthesiology* 69:232–241, 1988.
90. Landesberg G, Mosseri M, Wolf Y, et al: Perioperative myocardial ischemia and infarction: Identification by continuous 12-lead electrocardiogram with online ST-segment monitoring, *Anesthesiology* 96:264–270, 2002.
91. Martinez EA, Kim LJ, Faraday N, et al: Sensitivity of routine intensive care unit surveillance for detecting myocardial ischemia, *Crit Care Med* 31:2302–2308, 2003.
92. Breslow MJ, Miller CF, Parker SD, et al: Changes in T-wave morphology following anesthesia and surgery: A common recovery-room phenomenon, *Anesthesiology* 64:398–402, 1986.
93. Balaji S, Ellenby M, McNames J, Goldstein B: Update on intensive care ECG and cardiac event monitoring, *Card Electrophysiol Rev* 6:190–195, 2002.
94. Madias JE: Decrease/disappearance of pacemaker stimulus "spikes" due to anasarca: Further proof that the mechanism of attenuation of ECG voltage with anasarca is extracardiac in origin, *Ann Noninvasive Electrocardiol* 9:243–251, 2004.

16 Central Nervous System Monitoring

HARVEY L. EDMONDS, JR., PHD

KEY POINTS

1. Cardiac surgery–associated brain injury is common, multifactorial, and often preventable.
2. Electroencephalography can detect both cerebral ischemia/hypoxia and seizures and can measure hypnotic effect.
3. Middle-latency auditory-evoked potentials objectively document inadequate hypnosis.
4. Brainstem auditory-evoked potentials measure the effects of cooling and rewarming on deep brain structures.
5. Somatosensory-evoked potentials may detect developing injury in cortical and subcortical brain structures and peripheral nerves.
6. Transcranial electric motor-evoked potentials monitor function of the descending motor pathways.
7. Transcranial Doppler ultrasound assesses the direction and character of blood flow through large intracranial arteries and identifies microemboli.
8. Cerebral oximetry, using spatially resolved transcranial near-infrared spectroscopy, provides a continuous measure of change in the balance of cerebral oxygen supply and demand.
9. Used in concert, these technologies can reduce the incidence of brain injury and ensure the adequacy of hypnosis.

Many important new developments in neuromonitoring have occurred since the previous edition of this textbook went to press. First, professional society practice guidelines have been published for electroencephalographic (EEG), auditory- (AEPs), and somatosensory-evoked potentials (SSEPs), and transcranial Doppler (TCD) surgical monitoring. Second, randomized clinical trials have proved the clinical benefit of EEG and cerebral oximetry monitoring. Third, motor-evoked potential (MEP) monitoring has received U.S. Food and Drug Administration (FDA) clearance and has become a valuable tool to protect descending motor pathways in the brain and spinal cord. In this new edition, each of these developments is discussed, as well as many new studies extending the clinical value of perioperative neuromonitoring for cardiothoracic and vascular surgery.

Nearly half of the 1 million patients undergoing cardiac surgery each year worldwide will likely experience persistent cognitive decline.[1] The direct annual cost to U.S. insurers for brain injury from just one type of cardiac surgery, myocardial revascularization, is estimated at $4 billion.[2] Furthermore, the same processes that injure the central nervous system (CNS) also appear to cause dysfunction of other vital organs.

Thus, there are enormous clinical and economic incentives to improve CNS protection during cardiac surgery.

Historically, there has been little enthusiasm for neurophysiologic monitoring during cardiac surgery because of the presumed key role of macroembolization. It is widely assumed that most brain injuries during adult cardiac surgery result from cerebral embolization of atheromatous or calcified material dislodged from sclerotic blood vessels during their manipulation. Until the introduction of myocardial revascularization without cardiopulmonary bypass (CPB) or aortic clamp application, these injuries often have been viewed as unavoidable and untreatable.

Technical developments have begun to alter this perception. First, CNS injuries still occur despite reductions in aortic manipulation with the new approaches to coronary artery bypass and aortic surgery.[3] Second, neurophysiologic studies have implicated hypoperfusion and dysoxygenation as major causative factors in CNS injury[4,5] (Box 16-1). Because these functional disturbances are often detectable and correctable, there is an impetus to examine the role of neurophysiologic monitoring in CNS protection (see Chapter 36).

Cardiac anesthesia provider familiarity with neuromonitoring is becoming increasingly important. The introduction of compact and simplified monitors of brain electrical activity, blood flow velocity, and oxygenation promises to integrate these devices and their information into cardiac anesthetic management. The goal of this chapter is to highlight the practical issues involved with these emerging neuromonitoring technologies. This emphasis on practicality limits discussion to FDA-approved devices.

ELECTROENCEPHALOGRAPHY

EEG monitoring for ischemia detection has been performed since the first CPB procedures, but this long experience is not broad.[6] In contrast with its widespread use during carotid endarterectomy, EEG monitoring for cardiac surgery is performed primarily in academic centers or those specializing in pediatric surgery. Limited use appears to have several causes.

First, small, practical, and affordable EEG monitors have only recently become available. For example, using a book-sized box of electronics and a notebook computer, it is now possible to concurrently display multichannel conventional and processed EEG, as well as bilateral TCD ultrasonic spectra and cerebral oxygen saturation. All of the resulting data can be easily transmitted over high-speed data lines for Web-based consultation or archival or post hoc analysis.

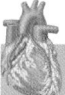

BOX 16-1. FACTORS CONTRIBUTING TO BRAIN INJURY DURING CARDIAC SURGERY

- Atheromatous emboli from aorta manipulation
- Lipid microemboli from recirculation of unwashed cardiotomy suction
- Gaseous microemboli from air leakage and cavitation
- Cerebral hypoperfusion or hyperperfusion
- Cerebral hyperthermia
- Cerebral dysoxygenation

Second, the traditional diagnostic approach to EEG analysis depended on complex pattern recognition of 16-channel analog waveforms to identify focal ischemic changes.[7] This analytic format necessitated extensive training and constant vigilance. As a result, cardiac surgery EEG monitoring directly by anesthesia providers has often been viewed as impractical. However, Craft et al[8] and Edmonds et al[9] have shown that a four-channel recording, which included bilateral activity from both the anterior and posterior circulation, was effective in identifying focal ischemia. In addition, computerized processing of EEG signals provides simplified trend displays that have helped to overcome many of the earlier complexities.

Third, EEG analysis during cardiac surgery was often confounded by anesthetics, hypothermia, and roller-pump artifacts.[10] Fortunately, these technical problems have now been overcome in the following ways: (1) elimination or replacement of the troublesome roller pumps with centrifugal pumps, (2) routine use of mild hypothermic or normothermic bypass, and (3) adoption of fast-track anesthesia protocols that avoid marked EEG suppression.

Physiologic Basis of Electroencephalography

EEG-directed interventions designed to correct cerebral hypoperfusion during cardiac surgery require an appreciation of the underlying neurophysiologic substrate. Scalp-recorded EEG signals reflect the temporal and spatial summation of long-lasting (10 to 100 milliseconds) postsynaptic potentials that arise from columnar cortical pyramidal neurons (Figure 16-1). These potentials are produced by dipoles distributed over soma-dendritic surfaces. Pyramidal neurons have a long, vertically oriented, apical dendrite and shorter basal dendrites radiating from the soma base. Near-synchronous excitation (or inhibition) of neighboring dendritic membranes produces large-amplitude spatially summating vertical dipoles, whereas radial current layers are generated in the somatic region. Simultaneous current generation in the two regions may appear to be self-canceling at distant surface electrodes. In addition, traditional EEG depicts only voltage change, not absolute voltage. Thus, sustained high-frequency neuronal activity may result in a large but nonvarying surface voltage deviation that would be invisible to the conventional EEG. These important EEG characteristics should be appreciated when interpreting low-amplitude signals; they do not necessarily indicate synaptic quiescence.

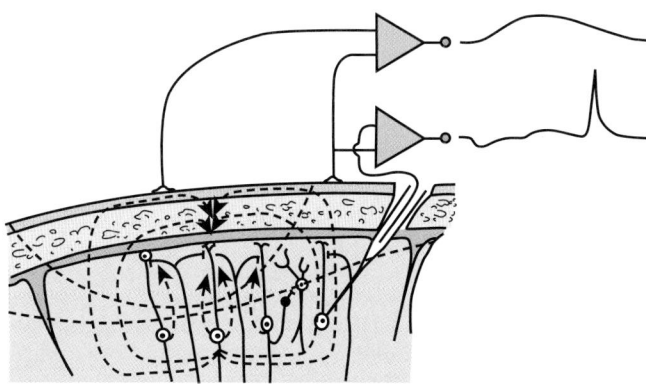

Figure 16-1 Production of electroencephalographic (EEG) waves. Scalp electrodes record potential differences that are caused by postsynaptic potentials in the cell membrane of cortical neurons. The *closed loops of the lighter dashed lines* represent the summation of extracellular currents produced by the postsynaptic potentials. *Open segments of the heavier dashed lines* connect all points having the same voltage level. The two scalp electrodes record changes in the voltage difference over time (top trace at upper right). The bottom trace from a microelectrode inserted in a single cortical neuron has little direct relation to the summated EEG wave. *(Modified from Fisch BJ: EEG primer, 3rd ed. New York: Elsevier, 1999, p 6.)*

EEG rhythms represent regularly recurring waveforms of similar shape and duration. These signal oscillations depend on the synchronous excitation of a neuronal population. The descriptive nature of conventional EEG characterizes the oscillations (measured in cycles per second [cps] or Hertz [Hz]) as sinusoids that were classified according to their amplitude and frequency. The terminology used to describe the frequency bands of the most common oscillatory patterns is illustrated (Figure 16-2). In addition, a high-frequency (25 to 55 Hz) gamma band is recognized (Box 16-2).

EEG oscillatory patterns are functional manifestations of specific intraneuronal networks. The extent of cortical processing among neighboring neuronal columns influences the extent of scalp-recorded EEG waveform synchronization and is not necessarily dependent on the subcortically mediated arousal level. At a high level of cortical processing, each neuronal palisade may function in relative independence. The resultant EEG signal will be of low amplitude, representing the distance-weighted average of many desynchronized micropotentials. The large number of small potentials is reflected in an EEG pattern characterized by a high dominant frequency (13- to 24-Hz beta waves). Such a pattern may be seen during very different vigilance states, such as awake, mentally alert (see Figure 16-2, top trace) versus rapid eye movement (REM; i.e., dream) sleep (see Figure 16-2, bottom trace). Partial cortical columnar synchronization develops with a reduction in information processing, resulting in higher amplitude and lower frequency EEG oscillations associated with a relaxed, drowsy state (see Figure 16-2; 8- to

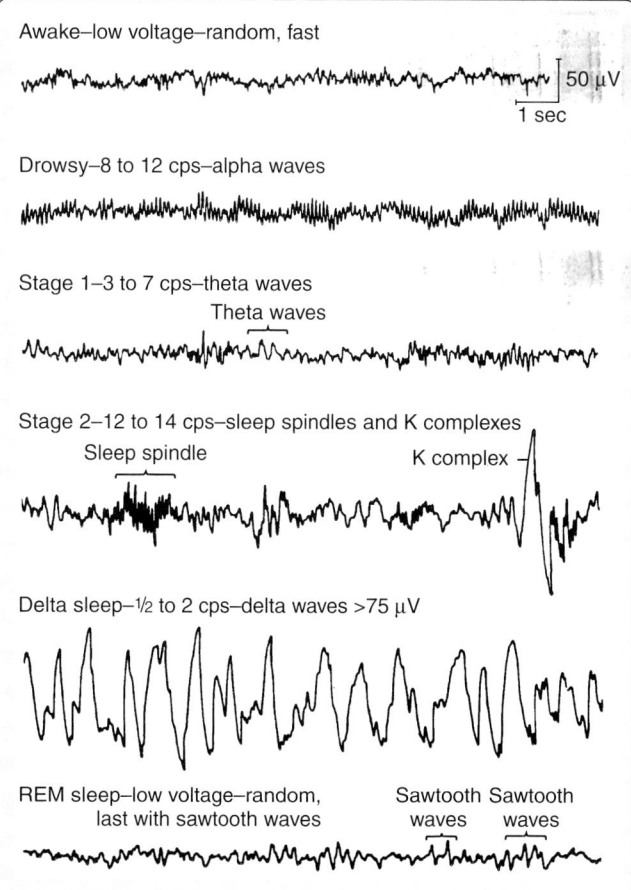

Figure 16-2 The specific electroencephalographic (EEG) characteristics of the different stages of the human sleep-wakefulness cycle are shown. Note the appearance of the four most common frequency bands from the lowest frequency delta, through theta and alpha to high-frequency beta. An even higher gamma frequency band (25 to 55 cycles/sec [cps]) is also described. REM, rapid eye movement. *(Modified from Yli-Hankala A [ed]: Handbook of four-channel EEG in anesthesia and critical care, Helsinki, Finland: GE Medical, Datex-Ohmeda Division, 2004, p 5.)*

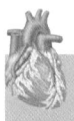

BOX 16-2. ELECTROENCEPHALOGRAPHIC FREQUENCY BANDS

Delta	0.5 to 2 Hz
Theta	3 to 7 Hz
Alpha	8 to 12 Hz
Beta	13 to 24 Hz
Gamma	25 to 55 Hz

12-Hz alpha rhythm). Progressive suppression is associated with lower frequency 3- to 7-Hz theta waves. Minimal processing leads to the very-high-amplitude, low-frequency hypersynchronous 0.5- to 2-Hz delta waves seen during the low vigilance states of deep coma, deepest sleep, hypoxia, ischemia, and some forms of surgical anesthesia.

Synchronization of cortical columns is influenced by subcortical structures, including the thalamus (Figure 16-3) and reticular activating system (Figure 16-4). Reticular inhibition can block the passage of sensory information to the cortex that is routed through thalamic relays. This state of functional deafferentation results in unconsciousness, an essential component of both natural sleep and surgical anesthesia.[11] However, the individual components of a modern balanced anesthetic

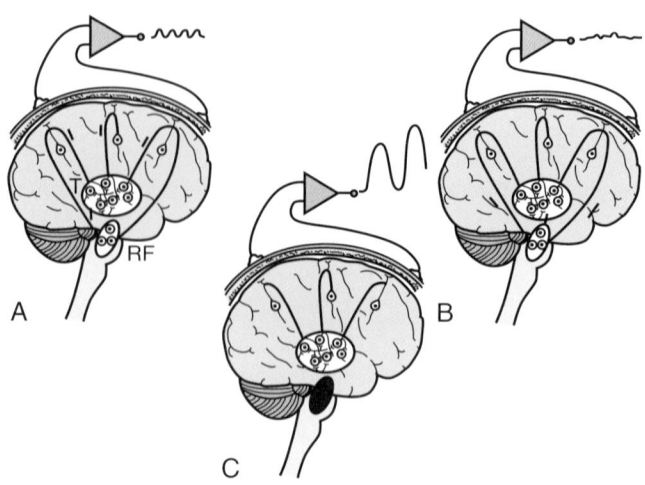

Figure 16-4 **Diagrams depict the role of the mesencephalic reticular formation (RF) in the generation of rhythmical electroencephalographic (EEG) activity.** *A,* In the absence of strong RF input, the thalamic pacemaker cells produce rhythmical EEG activity. *B,* RF activation sends inhibitory signals to the thalamus, suppressing rhythmic EEG and leading to a desynchronized pattern. *C,* In contrast, anesthetic or hypnotic RF suppression augments cortical EEG rhythms. *(Modified from Fisch BJ: EEG primer, 3rd ed. New York: Elsevier, 1999, p 12.)*

technique may differentially affect the separate control mechanisms for sensory processing and vigilance. Thus, an EEG pattern suggestive of a low vigilance state (i.e., surgical hypnosis) does not necessarily guarantee the absence of subcortical (i.e., unconscious) sensory perception (i.e., reflexive response to painful stimuli).[12] Furthermore, because the neuronal basis for the EEG is primarily of cortical origin, it is not surprising that many univariate (i.e., single-variable) EEG amplitude or frequency descriptors are only weakly correlated with clinical measures of anesthetic effect or developing pathology involving primarily or exclusively subcortical structures.

Practical Considerations of Electroencephalographic Recording and Signal Processing

This section describes practical issues involved in the conversion of these tiny potentials into interpretable EEG displays. The process begins with choice of scalp electrodes (subdermal needle, metallic disk, or silver-silver chloride gel self-adhesive patch) and their location. All three electrode types provide high-quality signals. Single-use sterile needle electrodes are easy to apply but are invasive, relatively expensive, and not well tolerated by conscious patients. Reusable disk electrodes, held in place with conductive gel, gel-free self-abrading plastic retainers, or built into a nylon mesh cap, may be used on conscious patients and are the least costly option. Adhesive patch electrodes are generally used only on glabrous skin and have a cost midway between the other options.

Standardized electrode placement is based on the International 10-20 System (Figure 16-5). It permits uniform spacing of electrodes, independent of head circumference, in scalp regions known to correlate with specific areas of cerebral cortex. Four anatomic landmarks are used: the nasion, inion, and preauricular points. Electrodes are located at 10% or 20% segments of the distance between two of these landmarks. The alphanumeric label for each site uses an initial uppercase letter to signify the skull region (i.e., frontal, central, temporal, parietal, occipital, auricular, and mastoid). Second and sometimes third letters, in lowercase, further delineate position (e.g., "p" represents frontal pole, whereas "z" indicates zero or midline). Subscript numbers represent left (odd) or right (even) and specific hemispheric location, with the lowest numbers closest to midline. The prime notation (′) is used to signify specialized locations designed for certain evoked potential

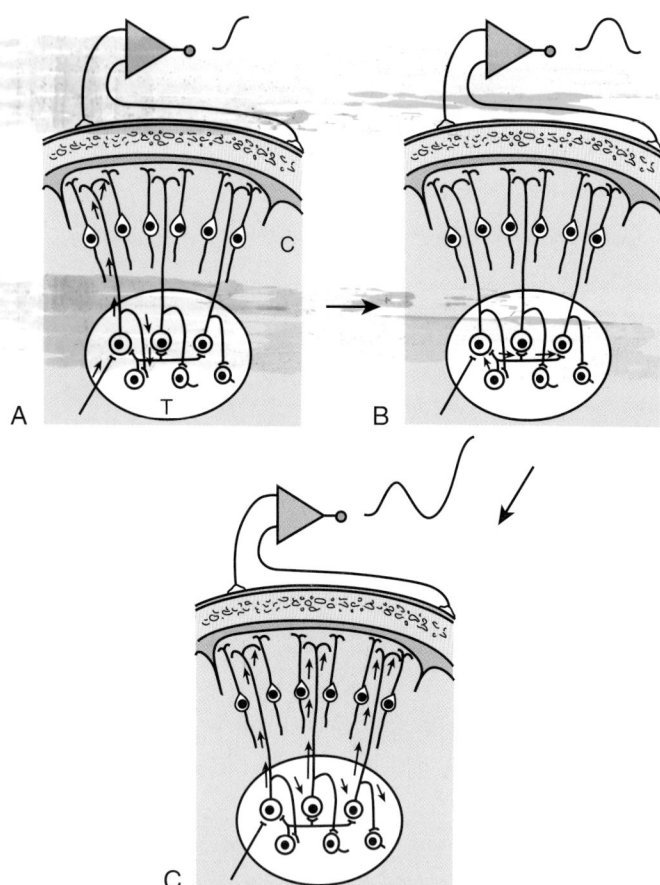

Figure 16-3 **Steps involved in the production of rhythmic electroencephalographic (EEG) activity.** *A,* Initiation of an EEG wave results from afferent excitation of a thalamocortical relay neuron (TCR) in the thalamus (T) and subsequent simultaneous transmission to a cortical and inhibitory thalamic interneuron. *B,* Output from the thalamic inhibitory interneuron suppresses neighboring TCR neurons, leading to the termination of the first EEG wave. *C,* After the inhibitory phase, additional TCR depolarization produces another EEG wave. *(Modified from Fisch BJ: EEG primer, 3rd ed. New York: Elsevier, 1999, p 10.)*

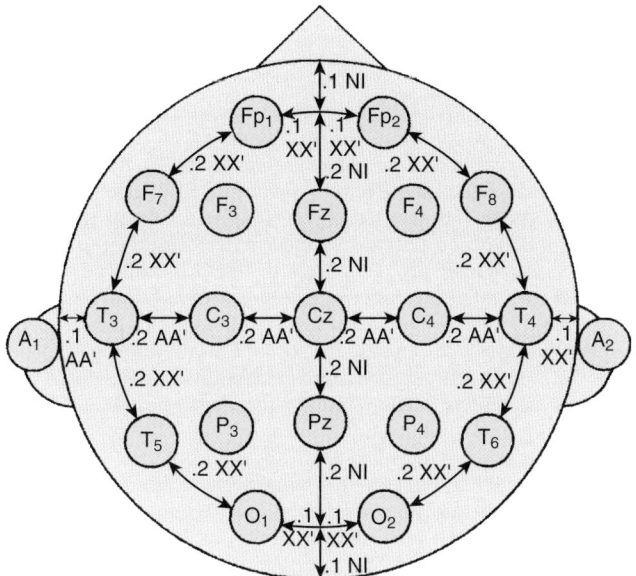

Figure 16-5 The position of the electrodes in the International 10-20 System according to scalp measurements. The sagittal hemicircumference (labeled AA') is measured from the root of one zygoma (just anterior to the ear) to the other, across the vertex. The third measurement is the ipsilateral hemicircumference (XX') measured from a point 10% of the coronal hemicircumference above the zygoma. Through these intersecting lines all of the scalp electrodes may be located, except frontal (F3, F4) and parietal (P3, P4). The frontal and parietal electrodes are placed along the frontal or parietal coronal line midway between the middle electrode and the electrode marked in the circumferential ring.

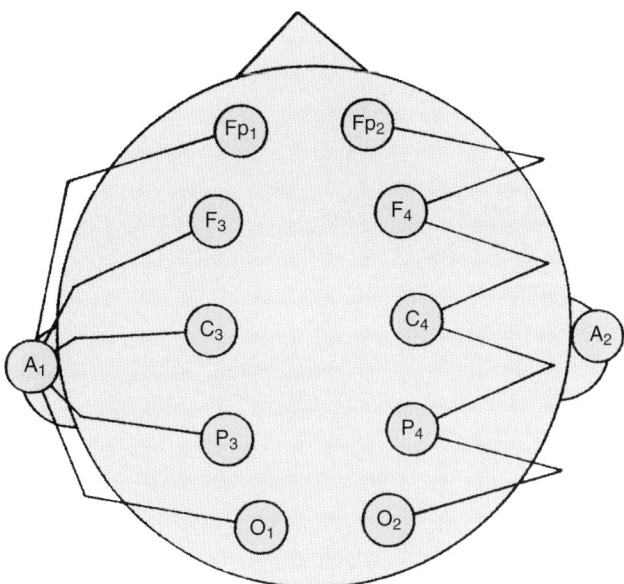

Figure 16-6 **Bipolar and common reference montages.** The left parasagittal electrodes are connected in a common reference montage using the left earlobe (A₁) as the common reference electrode. Five channels are recorded, each of them between the parasagittal electrode and the ear electrode. Differences among these channels represent differences in cerebral activity among the various parasagittal electrodes because each channel is recorded as the difference between the activity at the parasagittal electrode and the activity at the ear electrode. For comparison, the right parasagittal electrodes are connected in a bipolar chain. In this configuration, only four channels of electroencephalographic data are recorded. Each channel of data represents the electrical difference between the two electrodes.

applications (e.g., C_3' and C_4' represent 2 cm posterior to C_3 and C_4, directly over upper limb sensory cortex).

The differential amplifiers used in EEG recording measure the voltage difference between two inputs. By convention, a negative voltage at input 1 relative to input 2 results in an upward deflection of the tracing. With a referential arrangement (montage) of recording channel selections (Figure 16-6, left), the input 2 connections from a series of channels are connected to a single electrode, whereas input 1 electrode connections all differ. Alternatively, in bipolar recordings, a common reference is not used (see Figure 16-6, right).

Although an array of scalp electrodes theoretically permits many possible montages to be used, the capability to quickly change montage varies greatly among different EEG monitors. This ability to quickly change recording montage may be important in the detection and characterization of both focal and diffuse abnormalities. With a referential montage (Figure 16-7), the transient will be distorted if the reference lies within the transient electric field. Alternatively, with a bipolar montage, the potential may actually disappear because of in-phase cancellation.

Montage choice also influences susceptibility to artifact. For example, millivolt ECG potentials may contaminate the thousand-fold smaller EEG signal. Contamination is often problematic with an ear or mastoid reference montage but may be invisible with an anterior-to-posterior bipolar montage (Figure 16-8). The extreme lateral placement of ear or mastoid references maximizes contamination by the perpendicularly oriented high-voltage dipole generated by the heart.

The frequency range involved in production of the EEG waveform is termed its *bandwidth*. The upper and lower bandwidth boundaries are controlled by filters that reject frequencies above and below the EEG bandwidth. Both the appearance of the unprocessed EEG waveform and the value of univariate numeric EEG descriptors such as the mean frequency may be heavily influenced by signal bandwidth. The same cerebral biopotential recorded by different EEG devices may result in dissimilar waveforms and numeric values.

Modern EEG monitors use digital microprocessors to analyze the amplified analog biopotentials. Yet, analog-to-digital conversion imposes limitations on signal processing. Digitization converts a continuously varying biopotential into a series (i.e., sample) of discrete quantal values. At least two samples per period are required to minimize conversion inaccuracies. Sampling (Nyquist) frequency must be greater than twice the highest frequency of interest. For example, with an EEG bandwidth of 50 Hz, the minimum acceptable sampling frequency is 100 Hz (e.g., 10-millisecond sampling interval). Aliasing, the counting of high-frequency signals as low-frequency input, may occur if the complex biopotential contains frequencies above the Nyquist frequency. Therefore, most EEG monitors contain antialiasing filters that sharply attenuate waveform components above the Nyquist frequency. The details of filtering further add to the manufacturer-specific characteristics of processed EEG.

The continuous analog signal is also simplified into a (usually) discontinuous set of segments of a fixed duration (i.e., epoch). Window functions can minimize, but not totally eliminate, digital distortion produced by the abrupt truncation of a continuously varying waveform. These window functions are numerical series containing the same number of elements as the epoch. Their purpose is to reduce the value of epoch terminal elements. In addition to windowing, commercial EEG analyzers often use another form of signal conditioning called *whitening*. The energy content of the EEG is not uniform at all frequencies, but instead is heavily skewed to the lower range. Whitening mathematically alters the momentary frequency–amplitude relations to achieve nearly equal energy per octave and may improve pattern recognition in processed waveforms. Antialiasing, windowing, and whitening may vary not only among different devices but among software versions used with a single device. The user should be aware that a standard unprocessed analog EEG signal may generate digitally processed displays and numeric descriptors that are unique for each monitor design and software version.

BIPOLAR RECORDING

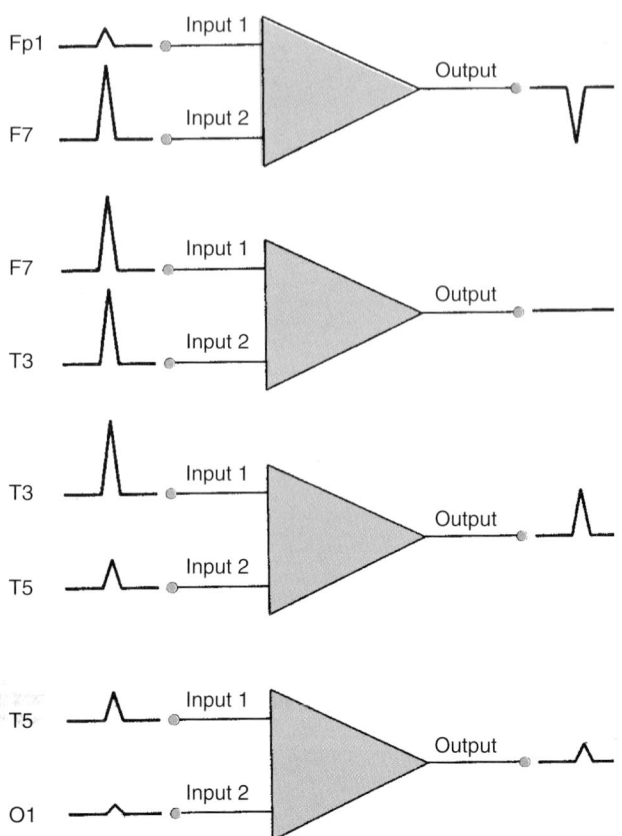

Figure 16-7 Accurate characterization of focal abnormalities requires that one of the amplifier's inputs be outside the field distribution of the transient. If both inputs lie within the transient field, the signal may become invisible because of in-phase cancellation. (*Modified from Goldenshohn ES, Legatt AD, Koszer S, et al [eds]: Goldensohn's EEG interpretation, 2nd ed. Armonk, NY: Futura Publishing, 1999, p 16.*)

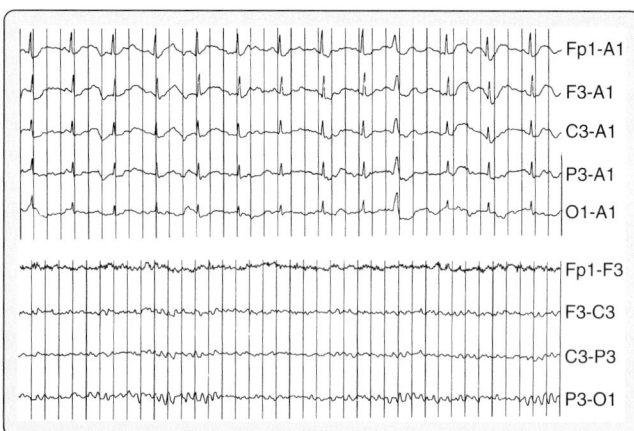

Figure 16-8 Ear-reference montages are particularly susceptible to electrocardiographic (ECG) artifact because their dipoles are oriented transversely to the prominent electrocardiac vector. In contrast, the anterior-posterior orientation of bipolar temporal chain scalp dipoles is oriented in parallel with the powerful cardiac vector. As a result, such montages are relatively immune from ECG artifact. (*Modified from Goldenshohn ES, Legatt AD, Koszer S, et al [eds]: Goldensohn's EEG interpretation, 2nd ed. Armonk, NY: Futura Publishing, 1999, p 72.*)

▣ Display of Electroencephalographic Information

Time-Domain Analysis

Traditional display of the EEG is a graph of biopotential voltage (y-axis) as a function of time and, consequently, is described as a time-domain process. The objective of a diagnostic EEG is to identify the most likely cause of a detected abnormality at one moment in time. Typically, a diagnostic EEG is obtained under controlled conditions, using precisely defined protocols. Recorded EEG appearance is visually compared with reference patterns. Interpretation is based on recognition of unique waveform patterns that are pathognomonic for specific clinical conditions.[13] In contrast, the goal of EEG monitoring is to identify clinically important change from an individualized baseline. Unlike diagnostic EEG interpretation, monitoring requires immediate assessment of continuously fluctuating signals in an electronically hostile, complex, and poorly controlled recording environment. Therefore, of necessity, interpretation relies less on pattern recognition and more on statistical characterization of change. Simple numerical descriptors thus may appropriately form an integral part of EEG monitoring.

Both EEG diagnostic and monitoring interpretations are based, in part, on the "Law of the EEG" (Box 16-3). It states that amplitude and dominant frequency are inversely related. As described earlier, synchronously generated postsynaptic potentials may produce large-amplitude biopotentials. However, long membrane time constants limit the number of changes that may occur per second (e.g., high amplitude, low frequency). Conversely, summation of spatially distributed asynchronous potentials results in EEG signals of low amplitude but relatively high frequency. Thus, the inverse relation between amplitude and frequency generally is maintained during unchanging cerebral metabolic states. Parallel increases in both may occur in some hypermetabolic states such as seizure activity, whereas decreases may be seen in hypometabolic states such as hypothermia. In the absence of these influences, simultaneous decreases in both amplitude and frequency may indicate ischemia or anoxia (Figure 16-9), whereas a parallel increase may be artifact (Figure 16-10).

BOX 16-3. LAW OF THE ELECTROENCEPHALOGRAM

- In the absence of pathology, electroencephalographic amplitude and frequency are inversely related.
- Simultaneous decrease may indicate ischemia, anoxia, or excessive hypnosis.
- Simultaneous increase may indicate seizure or artifact.

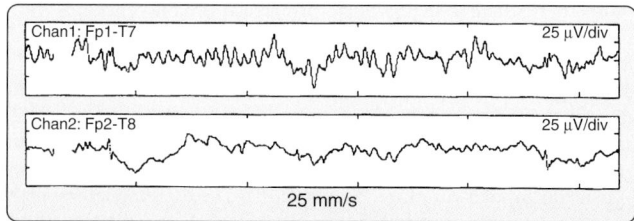

Figure 16-9 This two-channel electroencephalographic recording was made immediately after induction of anesthesia, before head repositioning for insertion of a central venous catheter. Anesthetic induction apparently uncovered a preexisting asymmetry that was not evident in the waking electroencephalogram. Although the patient had a history of an earlier mild cerebrovascular accident and transient ischemic attacks, he appeared neurologically normal at preoperative assessment. (*Modified from Yli-Hankala A [ed]: Handbook of four-channel EEG in anesthesia and critical care. Helsinki, Finland: GE Medical, Datex-Ohmeda Division, 2004, p 31.*)

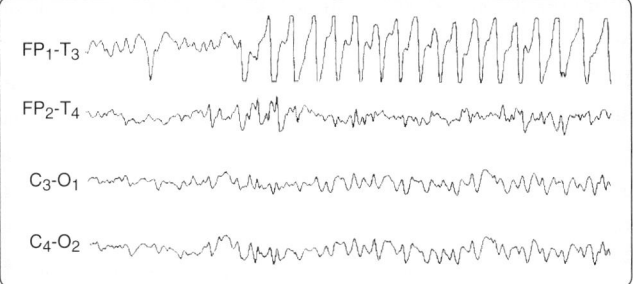

Figure 16-10 The large-amplitude 2-Hz triangular waves in the left frontotemporal derivation (top trace) are the result of temporalis muscle activation with a nerve stimulator. Current spread from the stimulating to the electroencephalographic recording electrodes may be minimized with use of the appropriate facial nerve stimulation site at the jaw angle. *(Modified from Yli-Hankala A [ed]: Handbook of four-channel EEG in anesthesia and critical care. Helsinki, Finland: GE Medical, Datex-Ohmeda Division, 2004, p 18.)*

Time-domain analysis of traditional electroencephalography uses linear amplitude voltage and time scales. The amplitude range of EEG signals is quite large (several hundred microvolts), and univariate statistical measures of its central tendency and dispersion may contain clinically useful information.[14] Furthermore, amplitude variation may present clinically significant changes in reactivity that can be obscured by frequency-domain analysis.[15] Advances in the technology of EEG amplitude integration have prompted a resurgent interest in this attractively simple approach, particularly in pediatrics.[16]

Frequency-Domain Analysis

An alternative method, frequency-domain analysis, is exemplified by the prismatic decomposition of white light into its component frequencies (i.e., color spectrum). As the basis of spectral analysis, the Fourier theorem states that a periodic function can be represented, in part, by a sinusoid at the fundamental frequency and an infinite series of integer multiples (i.e., harmonics). The Fourier function at a specific frequency equals the amplitude and phase angle of the associated sinusoid. Graphs of amplitude and phase angle as functions of frequency are called *Fourier spectra* (i.e., spectral analysis). The EEG amplitude spectral scale (Figure 16-11) squares voltage values to eliminate troublesome negative values. Squaring changes the unit of amplitude measure from microvolts to either picowatts (pW) or nanowatts (nW). However, a power amplitude scale tends to overemphasize large-amplitude changes. Clinically important changes in lower amplitude components that are readily discernible in the linearly scaled unprocessed EEG waveform may become invisible in power spectral displays.

Simplification of the large amount of spectral information generally has been achieved through the use of univariate numeric descriptors. Most commonly, the power contained in a specified traditional EEG

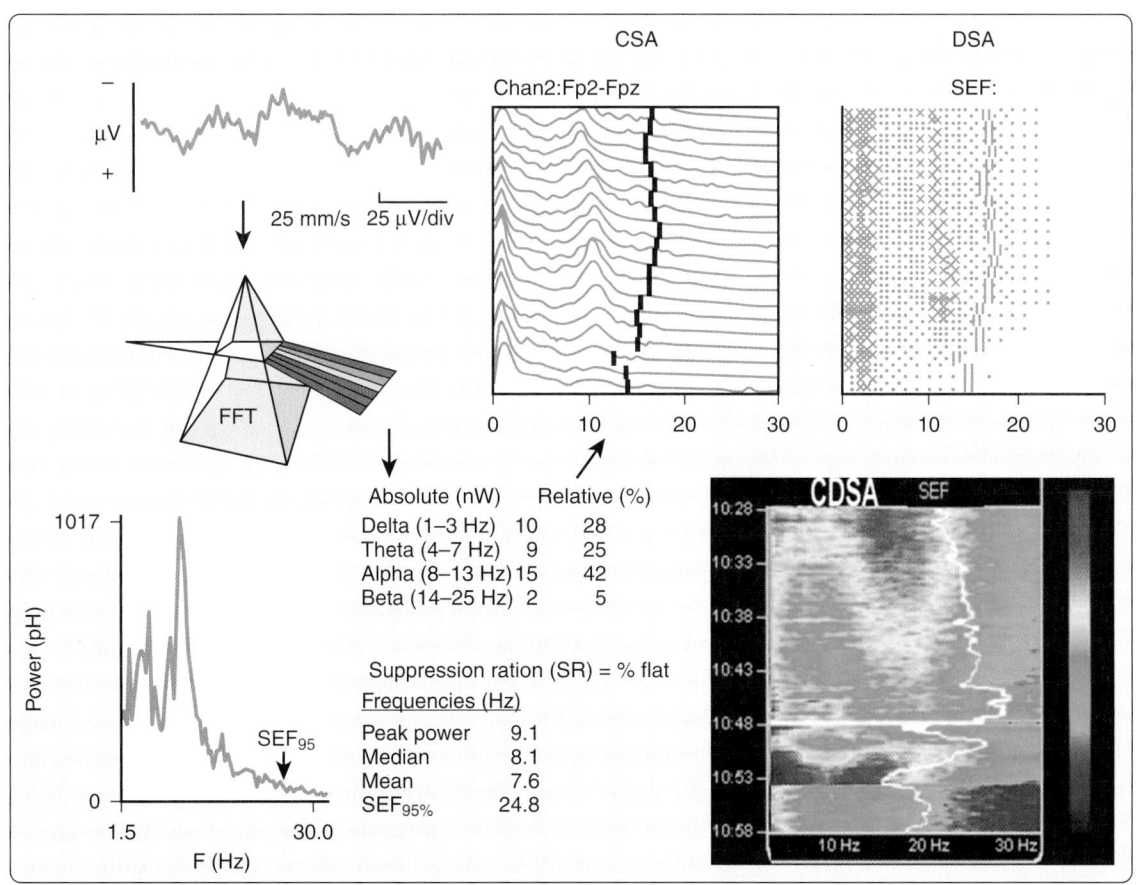

Figure 16-11 The traditional analog electroencephalographic (EEG) signal shown in the upper left is a time-domain graph of scalp-recorded amplitude (μV) as a function of time. Digitized EEG segments (epochs) are computer-processed using the fast Fourier transform (FFT), which, like a prism, decomposes a complex electromagnetic signal into a series of sinusoids, each with a discrete frequency. The instantaneous relation is then graphically depicted by the power spectrum (bottom left), a frequency-domain plot of power (μV² or pW) as a function of frequency. The spectral edge frequency (SEF) defines the signal amplitude upper boundary. The three-dimensional compressed spectral array (CSA) plots successive power spectra with time on the z-axis (upper middle). The density spectral array (upper right) improves data compression by using dot-density to represent signal amplitude (i.e., power). Amplitude resolution is improved through color coding in the color density spectral array (CDSA) shown at bottom right. SEF is shown as the *white vertical line*. Note the EEG suppression at the bottom of each spectral trend.

frequency band (delta, theta, alpha, or beta) is calculated in absolute, relative, or normalized terms. Relative amplitude represents the fraction of total power contained in a specified frequency band (relative delta power = delta [−0.5 to 2 Hz] power/total [0.5 to 55 Hz] power). Normalization equalizes the total power of successive epochs to that of some arbitrary reference before the calculation of relative power (the delta power is described as *Z*-score change from a previous individualized baseline). The latter two derived measures are particularly useful in minimizing misinterpretation of spectral changes. For example, during the production of hypothermia, absolute delta power declines in parallel with cerebral metabolism, whereas the fraction of the total power in the delta band remains unchanged. In this circumstance, exclusive focus on absolute delta power may lead to the erroneous conclusion that the hypnotic state is decreasing.

The most widely used univariate frequency descriptors (Box 16-4) are (1) peak power frequency (the single frequency of the spectrum that contains the highest amplitude), (2) median power frequency (frequency below which 50% of the spectral power occurs), (3) mean spectral frequency (sum of power contained at each frequency of the spectrum times its frequency divided by the total power), (4) spectral edge frequency (SEF; frequency below which a predetermined fraction, usually 95%, of the spectral power occurs), and (5) suppression ratio (SR; percentage of flatline EEG contained within sampled epochs). The performance of two descriptors in characterizing clinically important EEG changes is compared (Figure 16-12). Note that at anesthetic induction, the large transient decrease in SEF and reciprocal SR increase. However, later transient SR increases signifying marked EEG suppression were not detected by SEF, apparently because of low-level radiofrequency contamination.

Pronk[17] evaluated computer-processed univariate descriptors of EEG changes occurring before, during, and after CPB. Mean spectral frequency alone was sufficient to adequately describe all EEG changes except those occurring at very low amplitudes. Addition of a single-amplitude factor improved agreement with visual interpretation to 90%. Further factor addition did not improve agreement.

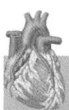

BOX 16-4. COMMON UNIVARIATE ELECTROENCEPHALOGRAPHIC DESCRIPTORS DETECTING ISCHEMIA

- Total power
- Peak power frequency
- Mean frequency
- Median frequency
- 95% spectral edge frequency
- Suppression ratio

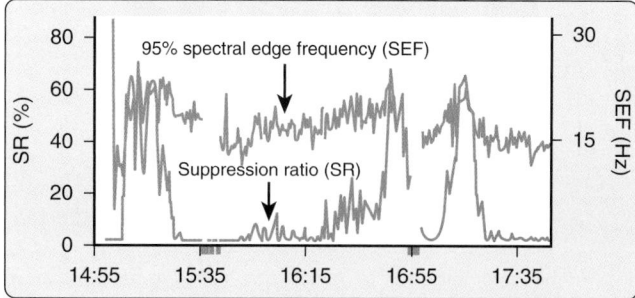

Figure 16-12 Certain univariate electroencephalographic (EEG) descriptors are particularly susceptible to the confounding influence of electronic interference. Note the peak in the suppression ratio (SR) trend at 17:00, correctly identifying marked EEG suppression. In contrast, the spectral edge frequency remains unchanged because of the presence of low-intensity electronic noise.

Multivariate (i.e., composed of several variables) descriptors have been developed to improve simple numeric characterization of clinically important EEG changes. With this approach, algorithms are used to generate a single number that represents the pattern of amplitude-frequency-phase relations occurring in a single epoch. Several commercially available monitors provide unitless numbers that have been transformed to arbitrary (i.e., 0 to 100) scales. Each monitor provides a different probability estimate of patient response to verbal instruction. Current monitors designed for use by anesthesia providers are listed in Box 16-5. BIS-XP, NT, PSI, and SNAP II are rule-based proprietary indices empirically derived from patient data. In contrast, CSI uses a fuzzy logic-based algorithm, whereas state entropy (SE) applies standard entropy equations to EEG analysis. Each product is designed to require the use of proprietary self-adhesive forehead sensors. Collectively, these products are now in widespread use as objective measures of hypnotic effect.

These hypnotic indices appear to provide clinically useful information. However, their fundamental differences may result in distinctly unique performances. Close agreement among these measures should not be expected. Thus, it is inappropriate and unjustified to apply clinical evidence of improved outcome obtained with one of these measures to a competing index. To date, adequately powered, prospective, randomized evidence of a statistically significant (i.e., 82%) reduction in risk for intraoperative awareness in adult noncardiac surgery has been achieved only with BIS-XP.[24] A recent meta-analysis review of the extensive peer-reviewed BIS literature concluded that "BIS could reduce the incidence of perioperative recall in surgical patients with high risk of awareness."[25] In addition, the review authors opined that anesthesia guided by BIS monitoring could decrease anesthetic consumption and enhance recovery from relatively deep anesthesia. These findings suggest that prevention of intraoperative awareness may represent only the tip of the iceberg of potential clinical and economic benefit to be derived from routine quantitative EEG perioperative monitoring.

Scalp-recorded cerebral biopotentials are complex physiologic signals representing the algebraic summation of voltage changes produced from cortical synaptic activity (i.e., EEG), upper facial muscle activity (i.e., facial electromyogram [fEMG]), and eye movement (i.e., electro-oculogram [EOG]). During consciousness and light sedation, high-frequency gamma power (i.e., 25 to 55 Hz) is a mixture of EEG and subcortically influenced facial electromyogram. Muscle activity makes a larger contribution because of the closer proximity of signal generators to the recording electrodes. Hypnotics and analgesics typically suppress both cerebral and muscle activities, resulting in reduced gamma power. Because the upper facial muscles are relatively insensitive to moderate

BOX 16-5. COMMERCIAL MULTIVARIATE QUANTITATIVE ELECTROENCEPHALOGRAPHIC DESCRIPTORS OF HYPNOTIC EFFECT

Acronym	Index Name	Mode	Mounting	Manufacturer
BIS-XP[18]	Bispectral	Bilateral	Pole-mounted	Covidien/Aspect Medical Systems, Boulder, CO
CSI[19]	Cerebral state	Unilateral	Handheld	Danmeter A/S, Odense, Denmark
NT[20]	Narcotrend	Bilateral	Shelf-mounted	MonitorTechnik, Bad Bramstedt, Germany
PSI[21]	Patient state	Bilateral	Pole-mounted	Hospira, Dallas, TX
SE[22]	State entropy	Unilateral	Monitor-based	GE Healthcare/DATEX-Ohmeda, Helsinki, Finland
SNAP II[23]	SNAP II	Unilateral	Handheld	Stryker Instruments, Kalamazoo, MI

neuromuscular blockade, they may remain reactive to noxious stimuli.[26] Nociception results in sudden gamma power increase, independent of activity in the lower frequency classical EEG bands.

The EEG analyzers just described either provide separate quantitative estimates of the high-frequency information or incorporate it into the hypnotic index. For example, the Datex-Ohmeda Entropy Module separately analyzes the 32- to 47-Hz band and terms the signal "response entropy." Addition of response entropy to the lower frequency SE is claimed by the manufacturer to facilitate distinction between changes in hypnosis and analgesia, although supporting evidence for this proposition awaits carefully designed and adequately powered randomized, prospective studies. EEG suppression decreases both entropy indices because noise-free flatline EEG segments are generally thought to have near-zero entropy. However, during cardiac surgery, EEG signals that appear to be totally suppressed may be associated with paradoxically very high entropy values. To minimize this problem, SE uses a special algorithm that assigns zero entropy to totally suppressed EEG epochs.

In addition to the quantitative EEG numeric indices, many monitors also display pseudo-three-dimensional plots of successive power spectra as a function of time. This frequency-domain approach was originated by Joy[27] and popularized by Bickford, who coined the term *compressed spectral array* (CSA).[28] Popularity stems, in part, from enormous data compression. For example, the essential information contained in a 4-hour traditional EEG recording consuming more than 1000 pages of unprocessed waveforms can be displayed in CSA format on a single page.

With CSA (see Figure 16-11), successive power spectra of brief (2- to 60-second) EEG epochs are displayed as smoothed histograms of amplitude as a function of frequency. Spectral compression is achieved by partially overlaying successive spectra, with time represented on the z-axis. Hidden-line suppression improves clarity by avoiding overlap of successive traces. Although the display is esthetically attractive, it has limitations. The extent of data loss caused by spectral overlapping depends on the nonstandard axial rotation that varies among EEG monitors. More important, epoch duration and the frequency with which each is measured (i.e., update rate) may critically affect the presentation of clinically important change. For example, there are three distinctly different burst-suppression CSA patterns: high-amplitude bursts, flat line, or a combination of the two.[29]

Fleming and Smith[30] designed an alternative to the CSA display to reduce data loss. Density-modulated spectral array (DSA) uses a two-dimensional monochrome dot matrix plot of time as a function of frequency (see Figure 16-11). The density of dots indicates the amplitude at a particular time-frequency intersection (e.g., an intense large spot indicates high amplitude). Clinically significant shifts in frequency may be detected earlier and more easily than with CSA. However, the resolution of amplitude changes is reduced. Therefore, the color density-modulated spectral array (CDSA) has been developed to enhance amplitude resolution (see Figure 16-11). The CSA, DSA, and CDSA displays are not well-suited for the detection of nonstationary or transient phenomena like burst-suppression or epileptiform activity.

In summary, a quick assessment of EEG change in either the time or frequency domain focuses on the following: (1) maximal peak-to-peak amplitude, (2) relation of maximal amplitude to dominant frequency, (3) amplitude and frequency variability, and (4) new or growing asymmetry between homotopic (i.e., same position on each cerebral hemisphere) EEG derivations. These objectives are generally best achieved through the viewing of both unprocessed and processed displays with a clear understanding of the characteristics and limitations of each (Box 16-6).

Electroencephalography for Injury Prevention during Cardiac Surgery

Since 2005, a great deal of new information has become available on the rationale for perioperative EEG monitoring. The American Society of Neurophysiologic Monitoring has just published its EEG practice guideline.[31] It describes the technical features and limitations of current EEG monitors and the available approaches to injury prevention. In addition, a new compendium has described the process of EEG monitoring in detail,[32,33] and special journal issues have been devoted specifically to cardiac surgery applications.[34,35]

The physiologic basis for EEG monitoring is the normally tight coupling among cerebral cortical synaptic activity, metabolism, and blood flow. Such coupling is necessary because of the large energy requirements of interneuronal communication. Indeed, at least 60% of neuronal oxygen and glucose is consumed in the processes of synaptic and axonal transmission, whereas the remainder is used to maintain cellular integrity. Neurons rapidly adjust their signaling capabilities to conserve vital energy stores. Even a slight new imbalance between supply and consumption of energy substrates is manifested by altered synaptic activity. The EEG provides a sensitive measure of this synaptic change and represents an early warning of developing injury. Identification and correction of the physiologic imbalance may then avert serious injury. It must be emphasized that EEG alterations signify imbalance, not necessarily injury. For example, using functional brain imaging with fluorodeoxyglucose, Alkire[36] demonstrated EEG relative alpha power to be linearly related to cerebral metabolism during propofol and isoflurane anesthesia. In this case, the synaptic depression manifested by the reduction in high-frequency activity signified anesthetic effect, not ischemia.

Furthermore, because clinically apparent neurologic injury often involves subcortical circuits and structures invisible to the EEG, an expectation of perfect agreement between specific EEG change and neurologic outcome is unwarranted. Imbalance in neuronal homeostasis may lead to either enhanced or diminished excitability. The majority of cortical neurons are small interneurons involved in maintenance of inhibitory tone. Their limited capacity for ionic buffering and energy storage makes them especially susceptible to imbalance. Early signs of energy deficiency may paradoxically result in EEG signs of excitation caused by disinhibition.[37] Conversely, with inadequate analgesia, intense sensory stimuli may result in a paradoxically depressed EEG activity resembling ischemia[38] (Box 16-7).

Although the EEG is a very sensitive indicator of cerebrocortical synaptic depression, possibly signifying cerebral ischemia or hypoxia, it is not specific. EEG suppression may also be the result of cooling or hypnotic agents. Fortunately, the time course of EEG suppression and information available from other monitors usually permit distinction between potentially harmful (e.g., ischemia) and harmless (e.g., hypothermia) causes. The following clinical situations provide the rationale for routine EEG monitoring during cardiac surgery: documentation of preexisting abnormalities, hypnotic adequacy, perfusion, cooling, rewarming, and seizure detection.

Documentation of Preexisting Electroencephalographic Abnormalities

Because there is a high likelihood of latent cerebrovascular disease in many older cardiac surgery patients, it is essential to examine the

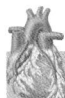

BOX 16-6. MEASURES THAT DEFINE ELECTROENCEPHALOGRAPHIC CHANGES

- Maximum peak-to-peak amplitude (or total power)
- Relation of maximum amplitude to dominant frequency
- Amplitude and frequency variability
- Right-left symmetry

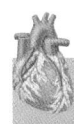

BOX 16-7. IMPORTANT CONSIDERATIONS DURING ELECTROENCEPHALOGRAPHIC INTERPRETATION

- Electroencephalographic (EEG) change signifies imbalance, not necessarily injury.
- The EEG is sensitive to imbalance but not specific for its cause.
- EEG prediction of neurologic outcome is good but not perfect.

waking EEG for signs of marked asymmetry before the induction of anesthesia. This serves to alert the anesthesia provider to the patient's increased vulnerability and to document the previously unappreciated risk.

Objective Measurement of Hypnotic Effect

Recording the transition from wakefulness to unresponsiveness permits detection of unusual sensitivity or resistance to general anesthetics (Figure 16-13). Such information is vital during fast-track anesthesia protocols to avoid excessive or inadequate anesthesia. Although no available neurophysiologic monitoring modality is an infallible predictor of anesthetic inadequacy, characteristic changes in the EEG frequency pattern provide an easily recognized warning of potential patient awareness. EEG detection of excessive or inadequate hypnosis during cardiac surgery may be aided by the multivariate EEG descriptors.

Head Position

Because of the diffuse nature of atherosclerotic vascular disease, many elderly patients are at increased risk for positional focal or regional cerebral ischemia that may occur before incision. Head rotation for surgical positioning or insertion of a pulmonary artery catheter may compress a vital carotid or vertebral artery. Such ischemia is generally identified by marked depression in the affected frontotemporal EEG derivation (see Figure 16-13).

Vascular Obstruction and Flow Misdirection

Manipulation or torsion of the aorta or vena cava may result in regional or global cerebral ischemia. During CPB, the aortic cannula can misdirect either cardiac or pump flow away from one or more head vessels while leaving the radial artery pressure unaltered. Alternatively, a malpositioned venous cannula may impair return from the head without noticeable change in central venous pressure or return flow to the venous reservoir.[39] Resulting intracranial hypertension leads to ischemic depression of the EEG (Figure 16-14).

Nonpulsatile Perfusion

Nonpulsatile perfusion used with CPB and some new left ventricular assist devices may result in microcirculatory collapse in susceptible regions of the cerebral cortex despite "acceptable" radial artery pressures. EEG-guided increases in arterial pressure, circulating volume, or both may be necessary to restore perfusion in the microvasculature.

Hemodilution

Hemodilution is used to improve vital organ perfusion by reducing viscosity. However, it may cause inadequate delivery of oxygenated hemoglobin to a high-demand brain, even though hematocrit and systemic venous oxygen saturation are within normal limits.[40] EEG deterioration may thus serve as an objective indicator for transfusion.

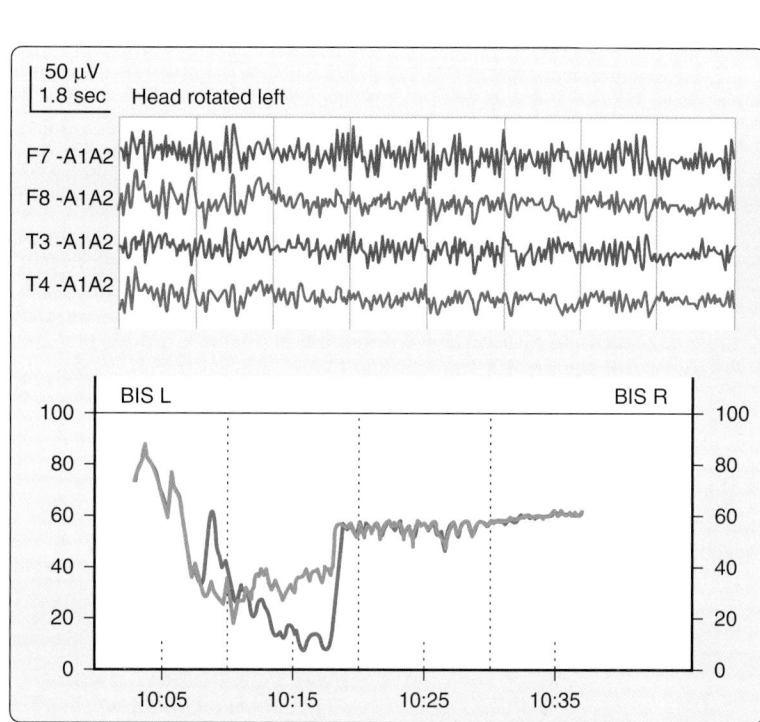
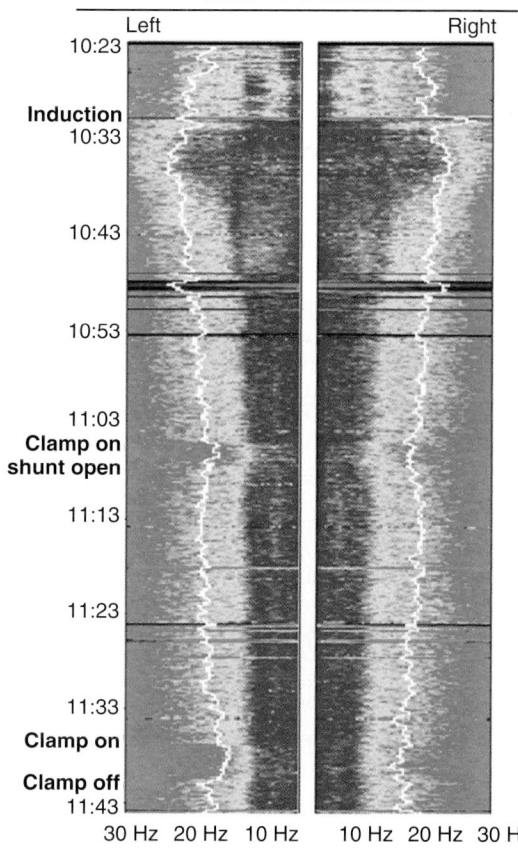

Figure 16-13   The panels containing unprocessed bilateral electroencephalogram (EEG; top left) and bispectral index (BIS) trend (bottom left) illustrate right hemisphere (red) EEG high-frequency loss after head rotation after anesthetic induction. The right panel bilateral color density spectral array (CDSA) trend depicts global power increase (i.e., high-amplitude, low-frequency waves) during anesthetic induction and later left hemisphere high-frequency loss associated with placement of a left common carotid clamp. Note prompt return of the high-frequency activity with insertion of an intravascular shunt. The EEG return documented proper shunt function, whereas maintenance of the high-frequency activity established that blood pressure was sufficient to prevent cerebral cortical hypoperfusion. *(Courtesy of Covidien/Aspect Medical Systems, Inc.)*

Figure 16-14 Insertion of a 14-French venous cannula in this pediatric patient during repair of an atrial septal defect caused a sudden diffuse electroencephalographic (EEG) slowing. The heart rate and blood pressure remained unchanged, although the central venous pressure increased from 6 to 45 mm Hg. Cannula repositioning restored both the former EEG pattern and central venous pressure. SVC, superior vena cava. *(Modified from Rodriguez RA, Cornel G, Semelhago L, et al: Cerebral effects in superior vena caval obstruction: The role of brain monitoring. Ann Thorac Surg 65:1820, 1997.)*

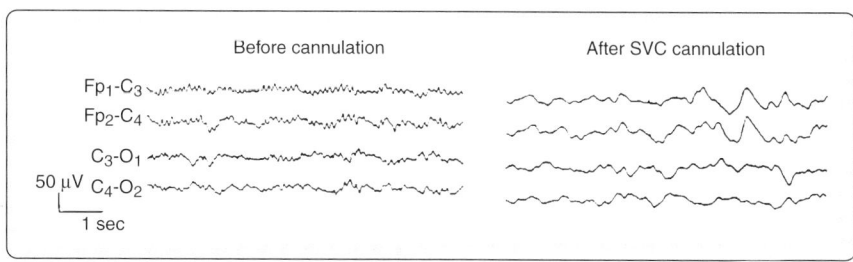

Hypocarbia and Hypercarbia

Cerebral arteries normally constrict in response to decreased carbon dioxide tension or hydrogen ion concentration. With reactive arteries, hypocarbia may lead to cerebral ischemia because flow is reduced 4%/mm Hg [CO_2]. In this circumstance, return to normocarbia can markedly improve cerebral perfusion.[41] Conversely, hypercarbia may steal blood from the dilated vessels of an already underperfused region, resulting in focal EEG slowing. This circumstance may be exacerbated by the use of volatile anesthetics causing cerebral vasodilation.

Cooling

During cardiac surgery requiring deep hypothermic circulatory arrest, the EEG provides an effective method for assessing the effects of cooling. Optimal brain temperature may be viewed as a balance between decreased cerebral oxygen consumption and increased risk for coagulopathy. Actual brain temperature cannot be measured directly and appears to be influenced by many variables including the rate of cooling, as well as acid-base and anesthetic management. The EEG is often used to assess the functional consequences of brain cooling because a flat line pattern signifies cortical synaptic quiescence. The wide interpatient variation in flat line temperature is the rationale for EEG guidance of the cooling process.[34] Alternative use of a fixed temperature criterion increases the risks for both excessive and inadequate brain cooling.

As nasopharyngeal or tympanic temperature decreases (Figure 16-15), there is a gradual loss of absolute spectral power across all frequency bands.[34] Although the reversible decreases in absolute spectral

band power are quite large, computing these changes as relative spectral band power minimizes them suggesting that initial brain cooling exerts a similar decrease in spectral power across all frequency bands and cortical regions.[42] Cooling below 28°C leads to progressive slowing of the residual EEG until the EEG waveform becomes a flat line.

Rewarming

After circulatory arrest, the EEG documents the recovery of synaptic function during rewarming. However, rapid rewarming may result in cerebral ischemia because of cold-triggered vasoparesis, which uncouples cerebral blood flow and metabolism. In this case, rewarming-induced increase in metabolic demand may outpace the lagging delivery of essential nutrients.[43] This situation is indicated by a loss of EEG high-frequency activity accompanying the increase in cranial temperature. Although the practice is controversial, administration of a metabolic suppressant drug such as propofol, dosed to EEG burst suppression, may facilitate balancing cerebral perfusion with metabolic demand.[44]

Myocardial Revascularization without Extracorporeal Support

Avoidance of CPB during myocardial revascularization may protect patients from the many potential hazards of this nonphysiologic insult.[45] EEG stability during beating-heart coronary revascularization is often observed, despite transient hypotension and bradycardia. Nevertheless, some surgeons believe that neuromonitoring is mandatory because the combination of controlled hypotension and vascular torsion can suddenly disrupt cerebral perfusion. In the absence of the neuroprotective effects of mild hypothermia, even relatively brief episodes of cerebral ischemia may result in injury.

Seizure Detection

Certain anesthetics and adjuvants such as etomidate, sevoflurane, and the opioid analgesics may produce seizure-like EEG activity, although the clinical manifestations may be obscured by neuromuscular blockade (Figure 16-16).[46–48] The consequences of this anesthetic-induced seizure-like activity have not been established in adults. However, seizures may be deleterious to the developing brain. Bellinger et al[49] showed that perioperative EEG seizure activity in infant cardiac surgery patients was associated with a 10-point decline in expected IQ when subsequently measured in the patients' fifth year after surgery (Box 16-8).

AUDITORY-EVOKED POTENTIALS

Important new literature on the intraoperative use of auditory-evoked potentials (AEPs) includes the publication of a professional society practice guideline,[50] a neuromonitoring textbook,[51] and a special journal issue on cardiac surgery neuromonitoring.[52]

AEPs assess specific areas of the brainstem, midbrain, and auditory cortices. Because of their simplicity, objectivity, and reproducibility, AEPs are suitable for monitoring patients during cardiovascular surgery. Specific applications of AEP monitoring in this environment are the assessment of temperature effects on brainstem function and evaluation of hypnotic effect. Direct involvement of cardiac anesthesia

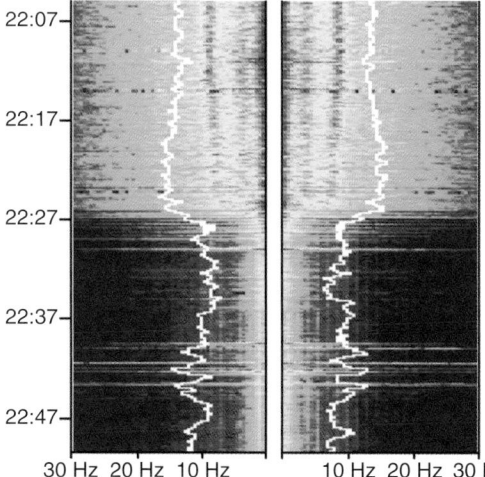

Figure 16-15 Progressive temperature-related electroencephalographic (EEG) suppression is shown in this bilateral color density spectral array (CDSA) display. Following the onset of cooling at 22:07, note the gradual decline in the power of the 9-Hz *(orange)* frequency band. Establishment of moderately deep hypothermia at 22:27 results in near-total EEG suppression. The spectral edge frequency *(white vertical lines)* does not fall to baseline because of the presence of background electrical contamination of the EEG signal. *(Courtesy of Covidien/Aspect Medical Systems, Inc.)*

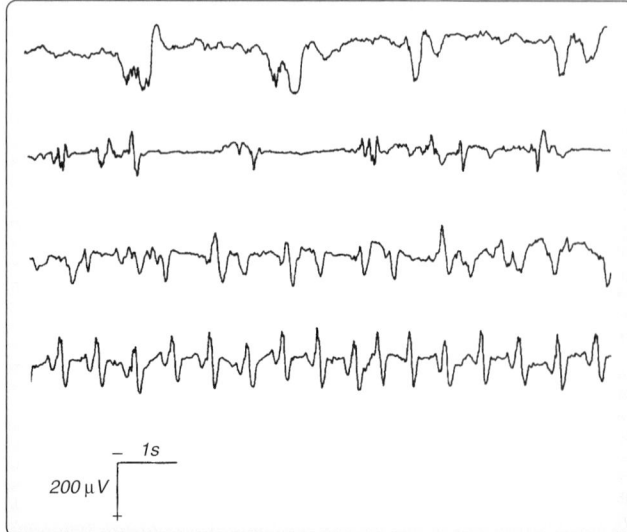

Figure 16-16 These epileptiform electroencephalographic (EEG) patterns are associated with mask induction of sevoflurane in adults. The patterns include: (1) slow delta monophasic activity with spikes, (2) burst suppression with spikes, (3) polyspikes, and (4) rhythmic polyspikes. *(Modified from Yli-Hankala A, Vakkuri A, Sarkela M, et al: Epileptiform EEG during induction of anesthesia with sevoflurane mask.* Anesthesiology 91:1596, 1999.)

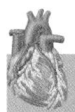

BOX 16-8. IMPORTANT IMBALANCES IDENTIFIED WITH ELECTROENCEPHALOGRAM

- Preexisting electroencephalographic abnormality
- Hypnotic effect
- Head malposition
- Hypocarbia-induced cerebral ischemia
- Malperfusion syndrome
- Need for blood replacement
- Optimal cooling and rewarming technique
- Seizures

providers with AEP monitoring is likely to increase after the introduction of EEG/AEP modules designed for use with available operating room physiologic monitors.

Acoustic stimuli trigger a neural response integrated by a synchronized neuronal depolarization that travels from the auditory nerve to the cerebral cortex. Scalp-recorded signals, obtained from electrodes located at the vertex and earlobe, contain both the AEPs and other unrelated EEG and EMG activity. Extraction of the relatively low-amplitude AEPs from the larger amplitude background activity requires signal-averaging techniques.[52] Because the AEP character remains constant for each stimulus repetition, averaging of many repetitions suppresses the inconstant background. For the AEP sensory stimulus, acoustic clicks are the most commonly used.[52] These broadband signals are generated by unidirectional rectangular short pulses (40 to 500 microseconds) with frequency spectra below 10 KHz.

The AEPs comprise a series of biopotentials generated at all levels of the auditory system in response to an acoustic stimulus (Figure 16-17). A dozen peaks have been identified within the first 100 milliseconds after stimulus onset using scalp electrodes.[52] Each peak is described by its poststimulus latency and peak-to-peak amplitude. AEPs are commonly classified as early or middle-latency potentials.[52] Figure 16-18 is a schematic representation of the AEPs most commonly used for surgical monitoring. Early AEPs are generated from the auditory nerve and the brainstem and include a series of wavelets recorded within the first 10 milliseconds poststimulus. These evoked responses have

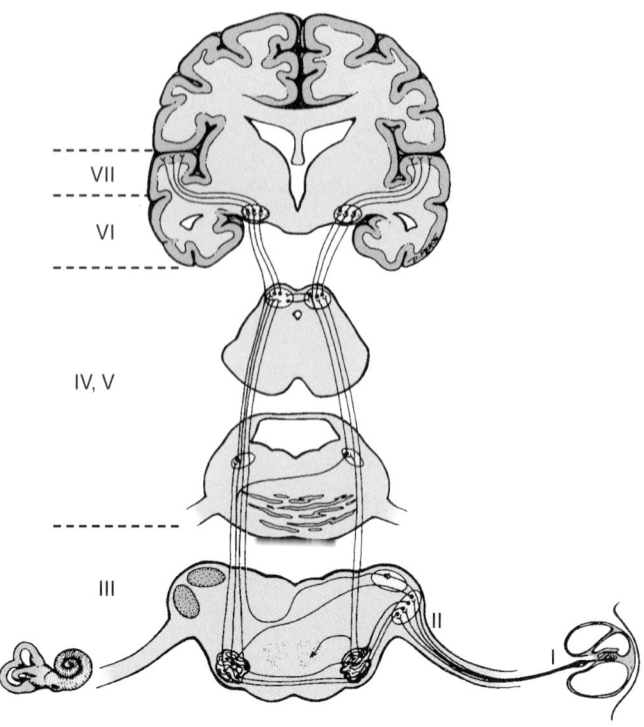

Figure 16-17 Putative sites at which the brainstem auditory-evoked potential is generated include the cochlear nerve, cochlear nucleus, trapezoid complex, lateral lemniscus, inferior colliculus, medial geniculate nucleus, and auditory radiations. Wave I is generated in the distal cochlear nerve near the spiral ganglion, and wave II is generated in the proximal cochlear nerve near the brainstem. All other waveforms are generated in multiple brainstem sites and do not bear a one-to-one relation to any particular structures, although the later waveforms do tend to be generated in more rostral sites. *(Modified from Friedman WA, et al: Advances in anesthesia. Chicago: Yearbook Medical Publishers, 1989, p 244.)*

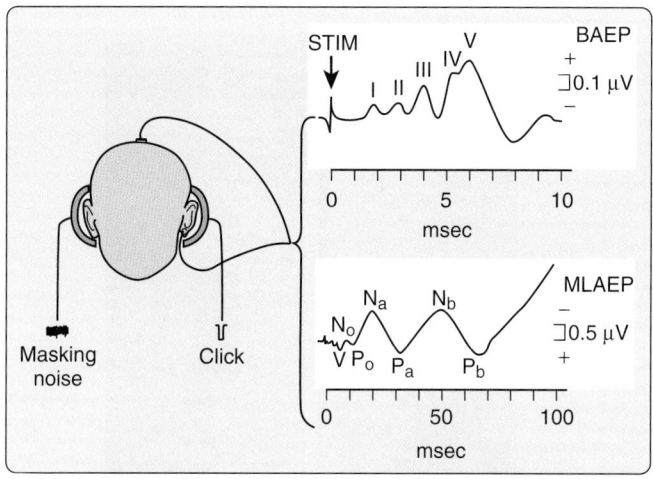

Figure 16-18 Schematic diagram of brainstem (BAEP) and middle-latency (MLAEP) auditory-evoked potential production. Stimulation of one ear and recording between the ipsilateral earlobe and vertex produce sequences of peaks that can be displayed at two different recording speeds and gain settings. Recording with a short 10-millisecond time base at a high gain reveals the first five peaks that comprise the BAEP. With a longer 100-millisecond time base and lower gain, the MLAEP peaks become evident. By a rather confusing convention, BAEP peaks represent positive deflections, whereas MLAEP peaks indicate negative deflections. *(Modified from Spehlmann R: Evoked potential primer. Boston: Butterworth, 1985, p 196.)*

been designated brainstem auditory-evoked potentials (BAEPs). Seven waves (I to VII) characterize the adult BAEP. Peaks I and II are generally thought to originate from the distal and proximal parts of the eighth nerve, and peak III arises from the cochlear nucleus. Peak IV sources include the superior olivary complex, cochlear nucleus, and nucleus of the lateral lemniscus. Peak V contributors seem to include both the lateral lemniscus and inferior colliculus. Peak VI and VII origins are not well defined but may arise from the medial geniculate body and the acoustic radiations. BAEPs are useful in assessing brainstem and subcortical function during surgery, in part because of their relative resistance to the suppressant effects of most anesthetics.[53]

The middle-latency auditory-evoked potentials (MLAEPs), with poststimulus latencies between 10 and 100 milliseconds, are generated in the midbrain and primary auditory cortex.[52] In an awake adult subject, the MLAEPs usually consist of three main peaks: Na, Pa, and Nb, with respective latencies near 15, 28, and 40 milliseconds (see Figure 16-18). Children under general anesthesia commonly display the trimodal configuration of the adult MLAEP waveform (Na, Pa, Nb waves), although neonates may exhibit only a small Pa wave.[54] Many agents with hypnotic effects prolong the latency and suppress the amplitude of Pa and Nb in a concentration-dependent manner.[55] It appears that the latency and amplitude changes allow reliable detection of consciousness and nociception during cardiac surgery.[55] In addition, parallel monitoring of MLAEP and quantitative EEG descriptors (i.e., BIS) may permit distinction between the hypnotic and antinociceptive anesthetic components.[55] This approach has also been used successfully in pediatric cardiac surgery patients to objectively assess postoperative sedation.[56]

Amplitude and latency from each of the primary MLAEP components have been integrated into a proprietary autoregressive linear function (A-Line; Danmeter A/S, Odense, Denmark) to facilitate continuous perioperative monitoring.[57] Subsequently, this metric was expanded to the A-Line Autoregressive Index (AAI), which included the quantitative EEG descriptors percentage burst suppression and β ratio (i.e., percentage of total EEG power contained in the high-frequency β frequency band).[58]

Part of the benefit of AEPs to cardiac surgery derives from their temperature sensitivity because cooling slows both axonal conduction and synaptic transmission. During cooling, the BAEP wave V Q_{10} (ratio of two values separated by 10°C) is 2.2.[59] A decrease of tympanic or nasopharyngeal temperature from 35°C to 25°C doubles wave V latency. Further cooling will eventually suppress waves III to V completely, signifying the virtual elimination of synaptic transmission within the brainstem auditory circuits. BAEPs document complete deep hypothermic electrocerebral silence before temporary circulatory arrest.[59]

The critical protective action of hypothermia on the brain cannot be accurately assessed by thermometry because of marked individual differences in thermal compartmentation throughout the body.[60] Even within the brain, cooling technique (e.g., rapid vs. slow, alpha-stat vs. pH-stat acid-base balance, α-adrenergic blockade vs. none) may result in substantial thermal inhomogeneity within the cerebrum.[59–61] Therefore, hypothermia-induced electrocortical silence (i.e., flat EEG) does not necessarily indicate cessation of synaptic activity within deep brain structures. The high metabolic rates of some of these structures (e.g., basal ganglia and inferior colliculus) render them particularly vulnerable to ischemic injury.[61] EEG quiescence plus a loss of BAEP waves III to V (Figure 16-19) ensure thorough cooling of the brain core. This approach appears to offer an optimal neuroprotective environment during temporary cessation of cerebral perfusion (Box 16-9).

▥ Somatosensory-Evoked Potentials

Somatosensory-evoked potentials (SSEPs) are briefly addressed here, in part, because of recent developments including: (1) a professional society surgical monitoring practice guideline,[62] (2) neuromonitoring textbook descriptions,[63–65] and (3) a special journal issue devoted to cardiac surgery neuromonitoring.[66] Like AEPs, SSEPs provide an objective

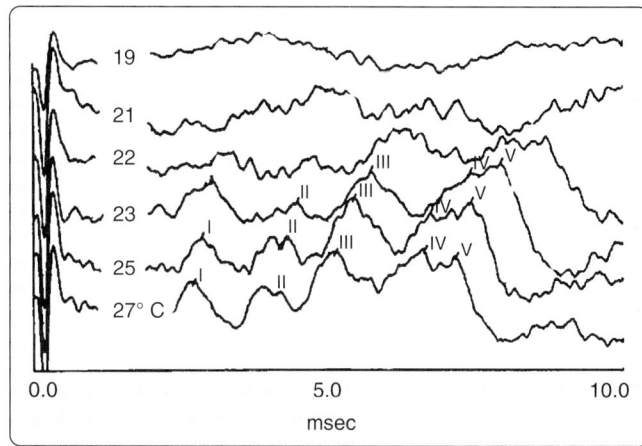

Figure 16-19 During repair of an aortic arch aneurysm, slow cooling resulted in a gradual loss of brainstem auditory-evoked potentials, progressing cephalad to caudad. Loss of wave III and later components ensured a cold-induced cessation of synaptic activity within the entire cerebrum. The global cessation indicated maximal neuroprotection during circulatory arrest. *(Modified from Yli-Hankala A [ed]: Handbook of four-channel EEG in anesthesia and critical care. Helsinki, Finland: GE Medical, Datex-Ohmeda Division, 2004, p 45.)*

BOX 16-9. AUDITORY-EVOKED POTENTIALS

- Brainstem auditory-evoked potentials measure temperature effects on brain core.
- Middle latency auditory-evoked potentials document inadequate hypnotic levels.

measure of ascending sensory pathway function. Figure 16-20A illustrates the key neural structures involved in a prominent upper limb sensory pathway suitable for cardiac surgery neuromonitoring.

Peripheral Nerve Injury Detection

During cardiothoracic or vascular surgery, improper patient positioning or sternal retraction can lead to injury, respectively, of the ulnar nerve[67] and brachial plexus.[68] Unfortunately, the standard recording electrode configuration illustrated in Figure 16-20A does not permit distinction of ulnar injury from plexopathy.[66] For this purpose, additional recording sites above the elbow or adjacent to the axilla should be used.[66] Lorenzini and Poterack[69] proposed SSEP noteworthy change criteria that appear to minimize the incidence of false-positive and false-negative responses. In the absence of marked body temperature change, these criteria are either a 60% amplitude reduction or 10% latency increase in the peripheral nerve components of the SSEP response.

Cerebral Ischemia Detection

In contrast with the typically robust subcortical N13 response, during cardiac or vascular surgery many factors other than ischemia may influence the SSEP N20 cortical response. These include anesthetic effects, body temperature, acid-base management, arterial blood oxygen-carrying capacity and blood pulsatility.[70] Therefore, traditional criteria for new cortical SSEP abnormality (Figure 16-21) long-established for other types of surgery (50% amplitude reduction and 20% increase in N13-N20 interpeak latency)[64] may result in an unacceptably high incidence of false-positive results. To overcome this problem, Astarci et al[71] proposed a more rigorous criterion of total N20 loss. A recent SSEP study during carotid endarterectomy supports this approach.[72]

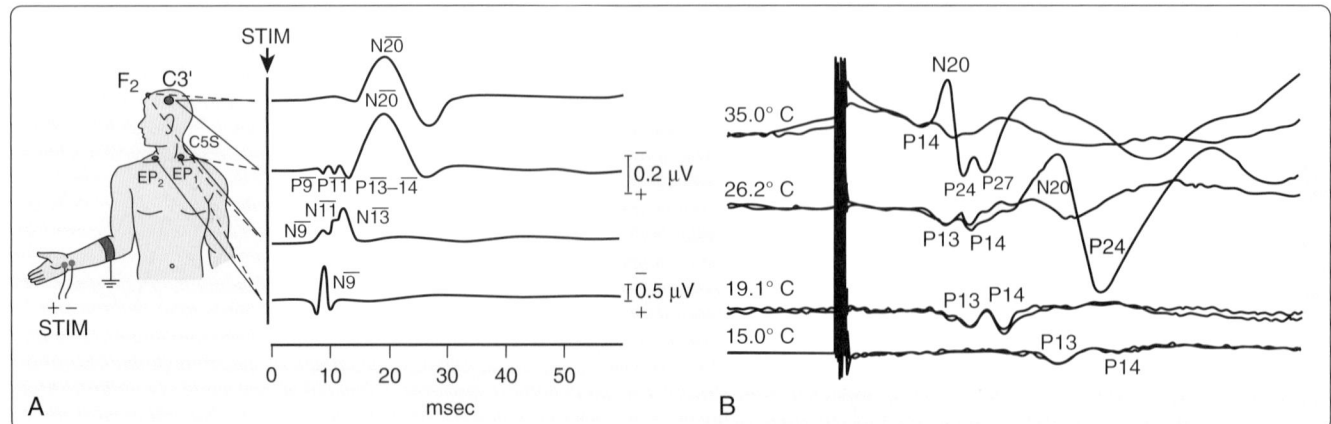

Figure 16-20   *A,* The waveforms show ascending responses to median nerve electrical stimulation. With the aid of noncephalic reference electrodes, the N9 clavicular (Erb's point) potential reflects signal passage through the brachial plexus, whereas the N13 potential represents activation of the cervical/brainstem lemniscal structures. Signals passing through the cortical radiations and sensory cortex result in the N20 potential when recorded between a scalp active electrode and cephalic reference. *B,* Each pair of upper-limb somatosensory-evoked potential (SSEP) waveforms is created by the superimposition of parietal recordings ipsilateral and contralateral to single-limb median nerve stimulation. *Shaded area* represents signal generated within the cortical mantle. Cooling to 26.2°C increases the latency of both subcortical and cortical waveform components, resulting in the emergence of a second (i.e., P13) brainstem potential. Although deep hypothermia at 19.1°C suppressed cortical activity, brainstem P13 and P14 responsiveness persists. *(A, From Misulis KE, Fakhoury T: Spehlmann's evoked potential primer, 3rd ed. Boston: Butterworth-Heinemann, 2001, p. 98; B, modified from Nuwer MR [ed]: Handbook of clinical neurophysiology, vol 8. New York: Elsevier, 2008, p. 834.)*

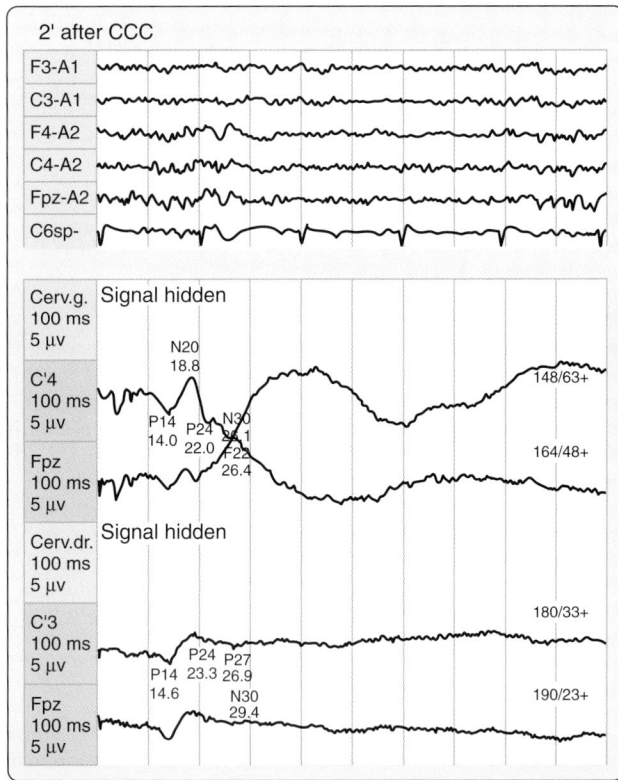

Figure 16-21   The upper traces represent normothermic, bihemispheric, anesthesia-suppressed electroencephalographic activity derived from scalp (Fpz, F3, F4, C3, and C4), cervical spine (C6sp), and earlobe (A1 and A2) recorded 2 minutes after left common carotid clamping (CCC). The lower traces represent contemporaneous bihemispheric upper-limb somatosensory-evoked potential (SSEP) responses. Electrophysiologic evidence of left hemispheric hypoperfusion is suggested only by the suppressed SSEP N20 component amplitude. *(Modified from Nuwer MR [ed]: Handbook of clinical neurophysiology, vol 8. New York: Elsevier, 2008, p. 787.)*

Brain Thermometer

Cooling prolongs SSEP peak and interpeak latencies and suppresses amplitude of predominantly the cortical response (see Figure 16-20B). However, because subcortical SSEP responses involve far fewer synapses than EEG, they often persist when cortical neuronal activity is totally cold-suppressed. Thus, detection of cerebral ischemia via SSEP can be achieved during EEG quiescence (Figure 16-22). In addition, the differential effect of cooling on the cortical and subcortical SSEP components can be used to identify the patient-specific nasopharyngeal or tympanic temperature suitable for the optimal cooling strategy for hypothermic brain protection.[66] For example, Guérit et al[73] found that there were no neurologic complications in a group of patients who underwent deep hypothermic circulatory arrest guided by abolition of the subcortical SSEP response. In contrast, patients who exhibited SSEP loss because of non–temperature-related causes experienced postoperative neurologic sequelae.

Motor-Evoked Potentials

The U.S. Food and Drug Administration recently cleared transcranial high-intensity electric stimulators for clinical use. By relying on the delivery of a rapid stimulus pulse train, it is now possible to continuously monitor the integrity of descending motor pathways using transcranial electric motor-evoked potentials (MEPs).[74-77] The most frequent application of this emerging monitoring modality for cardiothoracic surgery currently is during open surgical or endovascular repair of the descending aorta.[78,79] There remains a critical need for improved spinal cord protection because, even with modern cord preservation techniques, the 16% infarction rate during type I and II aneurysm repairs in patients without potential benefit of MEP monitoring remains disturbingly high.[80]

The neurophysiologic basis for the MEP is illustrated in Figure 16-23. Individual high-intensity transcranial stimuli depolarize cortical motor neurons directly in the axon hillock region or indirectly via activation of interneurons. Synaptic transmission of individual impulses to segmental α-motor neurons lowers the postsynaptic membrane potential but is often insufficient to initiate cell firing. Instead, this goal is achieved through use of a pulse train that triggers lower motor neuron discharge via temporal summation of individual subthreshold responses.

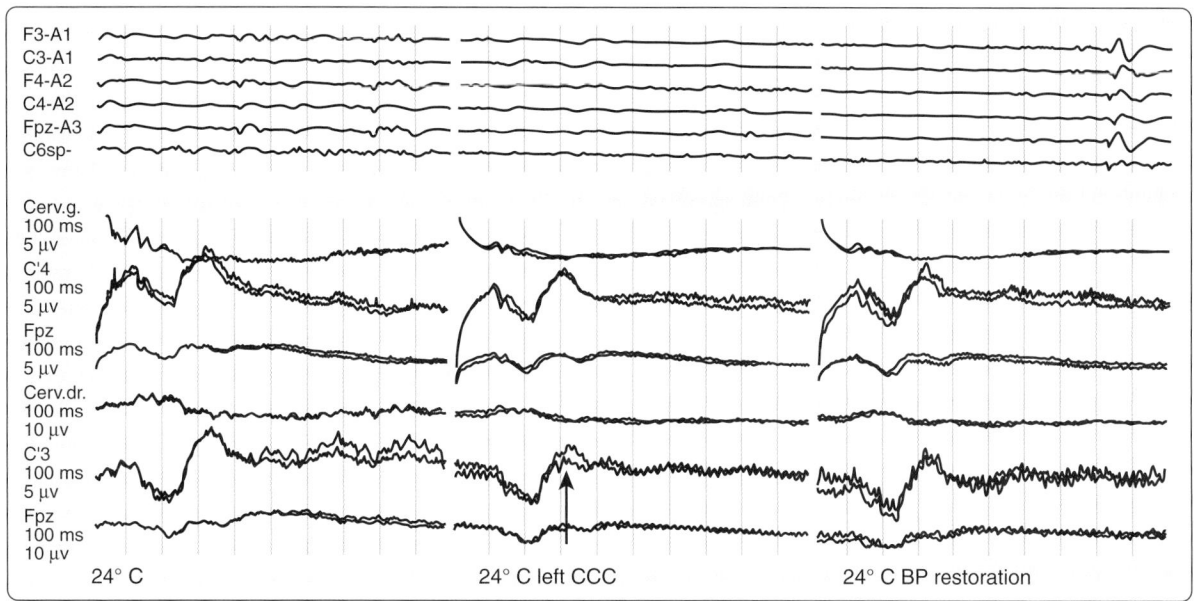

Figure 16-22 The upper traces represent bihemispheric, cold-suppressed electroencephalographic (EEG) activity derived from scalp (Fpz, F3, F4, C3, and C4), cervical spine (C6sp), and earlobe (A1, A2, and linked A3) recorded at 24°C. The lower traces represent contemporaneous bihemispheric upper-limb somatosensory-evoked potential (SSEP) responses. *Arrow* points to left hemispheric N20 suppression accompanying left common carotid clamping (CCC). Blood pressure increase restored the N20 amplitude. Note that this regional cerebral hypoperfusion was not apparent in the hypothermia-suppressed EEG recording. *(Modified from Nuwer MR [ed]: Handbook of clinical neurophysiology, vol 8. New York: Elsevier, 2008, p. 835.)*

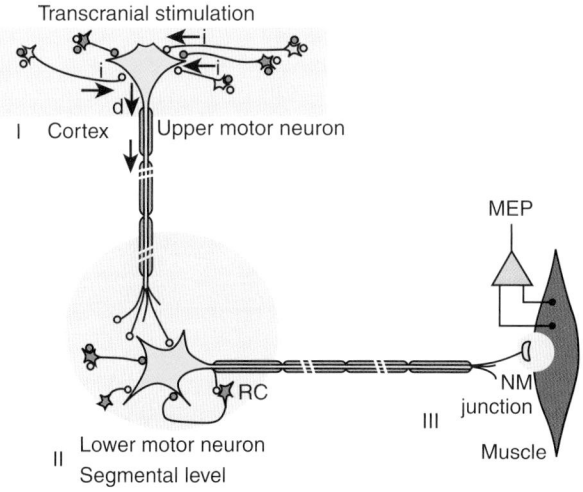

Figure 16-23 High-intensity transcranial electric or magnetic stimulation results in direct *(d)* activation of upper motor neurons. In addition, indirect motor neuron activation *(i)* results from transcranial activation of horizontally oriented excitatory (light) and inhibitory (dark) neuronal axons. Descending motor potentials are conducted unidirectionally through the corticospinal, rubrospinal, tectospinal, vestibulospinal, and cerebellospinal tracts to lower (alpha) motor neurons in the lateral and anterior spinal cord. In the absence of complete pharmacologic neuromuscular (NM) blockade, alpha motor neuron action potentials then produce muscle fiber contraction that is recorded by electromyography (EMG). MEP, motor-evoked potential; RC, Reushaw cell-mediated recurrent inhibition *(Modified from Nuwer MR [ed]: Handbook of clinical neurophysiology, vol 8, New York: Elsevier, 2008, p. 219.)*

Precise placement of subdermal stimulating electrodes (Figure 16-24*A*) is important because of its influence on motor pathway activation. The transcranial electric current generated from closely spaced electrodes depolarizes a discrete cortical region that may control only a restricted muscle group. In contrast, current produced using wide electrode separation bypasses the anesthetic-susceptible cortical neurons.

This results in direct depolarization of descending motor tracts that affect both upper and lower limb muscles (see Figure 16-24*B*). Even though lower limb MEPs are necessary to document the functional integrity of motor pathways in the thoracolumbar spinal cord, upper limb recording is also important. The upper limb responses identify generalized MEP suppression. Its causes include anesthetic-induced synaptic inhibition, hypocapnia, and hypothermia, as well as position-related ischemia involving cerebral and/or upper limb motor pathways (Figure 16-25). The effects of anesthetics on evoked potentials are summarized in Box 16-10. In additional to these generalized effects, it also should be appreciated that volatile anesthetics suppress both cortical and spinal cord motor neurons. Thus, their use should be avoided or minimized during attempted MEP monitoring.[81]

In contrast with AEP and SSEP, the large amplitude of MEP EMG responses obviates the need for signal averaging. However, the inherent variability of these individual responses (see Figure 16-25) means that precise measurement of peak amplitude and latency are more difficult to achieve than with the more stable averaged sensory-evoked potentials. Nevertheless, Kawanishi et al[82] found 100% sensitivity and 98% specificity for MEP detection of motor pathway dysfunction. Their criterion for noteworthy change was a persistent 25% peak-to-peak amplitude decline. Correct interpretation of MEP amplitude change requires precise monitoring and control of neuromuscular blockade. Information on the extent of neuromuscular blockade obtained from evoked EMG train-of-four responses in both upper and lower limb muscles bilaterally helps guide relaxant administration and detects limb ischemia.[83]

Although MEP monitoring is technically challenging and places additional burdens on anesthesia providers, the effort seems worthwhile. Even though large-sample, prospective, randomized outcome studies are lacking, there are many small-sample prospective or retrospective studies demonstrating benefit. For example, Etz et al[84] obtained an impressively low 2% neurodeficit incidence in 100 descending aorta surgical repairs, 73% of which were high-risk Crawford type I or II aneurysms. Current opinion on the value of MEP monitoring for this application is reflected by MacDonald and Dong's[79] recent review, which states: "There is now strong evidence that … MEP monitoring positively impacts descending aortic aneurysm surgery outcome when used to guide aggressive intervention."

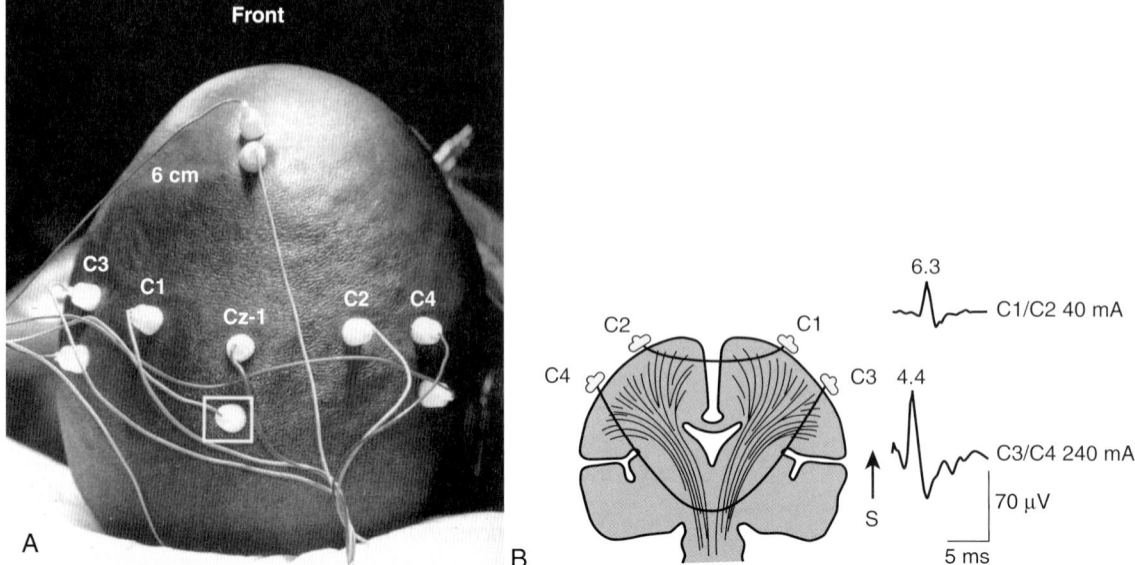

Figure 16-24 *A,* Placement of transdermal electrodes for generation of motor-evoked potential (MEP) by electrical stimulation. *B,* Transcranial electric current paths are shown following cortical (C1/C2) and subcortical (C3/C4) stimulation. The direct MEP responses were obtained from an electrode placed adjacent to exposed upper thoracic spinal cord. Note the large 240-mA current required for subcortical stimulation and the shorter latency between the stimulus (S) and C3/C4 response because of the reduced distance between stimulating and recording electrodes. *(Modified from Nuwer MR [ed]: Handbook of clinical neurophysiology, vol 8. New York: Elsevier, 2008, pp. 236–237.)*

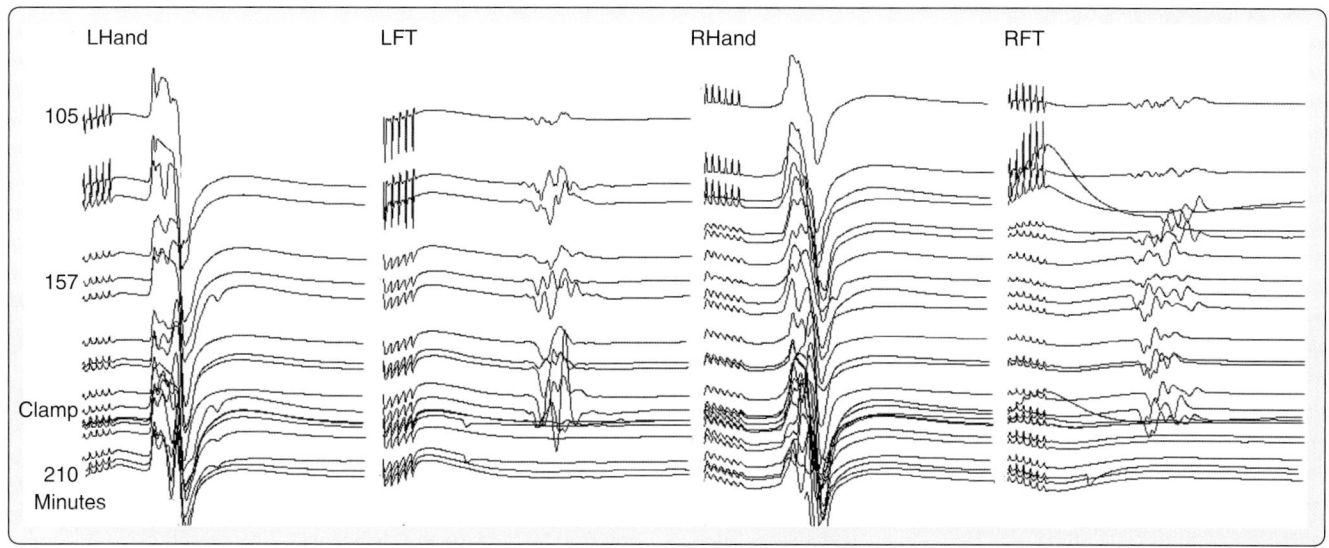

Figure 16-25 Changes are shown in upper (left hand [LHand] and right hand [RHand]) and lower (left foot [LFT] and right foot [RFT]) limb motor-evoked potential (MEP) responses to clamping of the descending aorta during surgical repair of a thoracoabdominal aneurysm. Note the bilateral loss of low-limb MEP with clamp application. MEP monitoring helped guide management of left heart bypass and reimplantation of the superior mesenteric and renal arteries into the aortic graft.

TRANSCRANIAL DOPPLER ULTRASOUND

Ultrasound Technology

Ultrasonic probes of a clinical TCD sonograph contain an electrically activated piezoelectric crystal that transmits low-power 1- to 2-MHz acoustic vibrations (i.e., insonation) through the thinnest portion of temporal bone (i.e., acoustic window) into brain tissue. Blood constituents (predominantly erythrocytes), contained in large arteries and veins, reflect these ultrasonic waves back to the probe, which also serves as a receiver. Because of laminar blood flow, erythrocytes traveling in the central region of a large blood vessel move with greater velocity than those near the vessel wall (Figure 16-26). Thus, within each vascular segment (i.e., sample volume), a series of echoes associated with varying velocities is created. The frequency differences between the insonation signal and each echo in the series are proportional to the associated velocity, and this velocity is determined from the Doppler equation (see Figure 16-26). Although several large intracranial arteries may be insonated through the temporal window, the middle cerebral artery is generally monitored during cardiac surgery because it carries approximately 40% of the hemispheric blood flow.

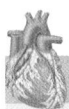

BOX 16-10. ANESTHETIC* EFFECTS ON SENSORY- AND MOTOR-EVOKED RESPONSES

		Cortical		Cortical
Pharmacologic Class	Agent	SSEP	AEP	MEP
Nonspecific inhibitor	Isoflurane	Suppression	Suppression	Suppression
	Sevoflurane	Suppression	Suppression	Suppression
	Desflurane	Suppression	Suppression	Suppression
	Barbiturates	Suppression	Suppression	Suppression
GABA-specific agonist	Propofol	Slight suppression	Suppression	Slight suppression
	Etomidate	Slight increase	Suppression	Slight suppression
α_2-Adrenergic agonist	Clonidine	Slight suppression	?	Slight suppression
	Dexmedetomidine	Slight suppression	?	Slight suppression
N-methyl-d-aspartate antagonist	Nitrous oxide	Suppression	Minimal effect	Suppression
	Ketamine	Increase	Minimal effect	Slight suppression
	Xenon	Slight suppression	Slight suppression	Slight suppression

*1 MAC-equivalent dose. (MAC, minimum alveolar concentration.)

Modified from Sloan TB, et al: Anesthetic effects on evoked potentials. In Nuwer MR [ed]: Handbook of clinical neurophysiology, vol 8: Intraoperative monitoring of neural function. New York: Elsevier, 2008, pp 94–126, by permission.

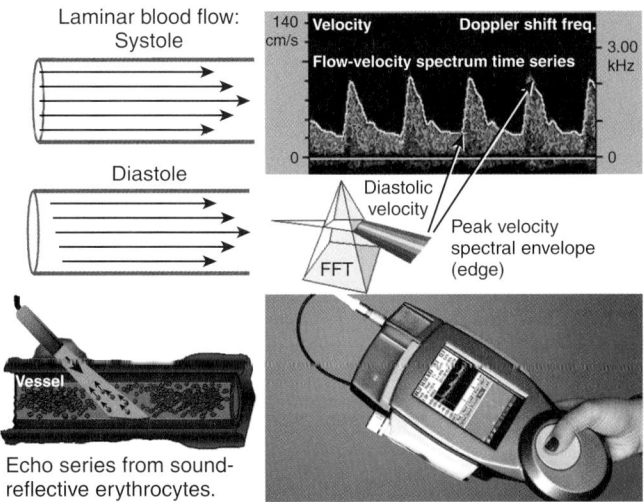

Figure 16-26 Large-vessel laminar flow results in a cross-sectional series of erythrocyte velocities, with the lowest values nearest the vessel wall. Ultrasonic vessel insonation produces a series of erythrocyte echoes. The frequency differences (i.e., Doppler-shift frequencies) between the insonating signal and its echoes are proportional to erythrocyte velocity and flow direction. Fast Fourier transform (FFT) analysis of this complex echo produces an instantaneous power spectrum analogous to that used in electroencephalographic analysis. The time series of successive Doppler-shift spectra (top right) resembles an arterial pressure waveform but represents fluctuating erythrocyte velocities during each cardiac cycle. Some modern transcranial Doppler sonographs are small enough to be handheld or incorporated into multimodal neurophysiologic signal analyzers. (Image of the 500P Pocket Transcranial Doppler is courtesy of Multigon Industries, Inc., Yonkers, NY.)

Pulsed-Wave Spectral Display

Pulsed-wave Doppler samples the ultrasonic echoes at a user-selected distance (i.e., single gate) below the scalp. The frequency composition of these Doppler-shifted echoes is analyzed by Fourier analysis, the same technique used to quantify EEG frequency patterns (see Figure 16-26). The analysis produces a momentary amplitude spectrum displayed as a function of blood flow velocity (e.g., Doppler-shift frequency). This relation is mapped as one vertical strip in the spectrogram display (see Figure 16-26, upper right). Amplitude at each frequency is expressed as log change (i.e., dB) from the background composed of random echoes. The momentary analysis is repeated 100 times a second to produce a scrolling spectrogram of time-related changes in flow velocity.

Signal amplitude at each frequency shift–time intersection is indicated by monochromatic dot density or color coding. The maximum velocity, the upper edge (envelope) of the velocity spectrum (analogous to the EEG SEF), represents the maximum Doppler shift (erythrocyte velocity) in the vessel center. Peak systolic and end-diastolic velocities are derived from this spectral edge. Intensity-weighted mean velocity is calculated by weighted averaging of the intensity of all Doppler spectral signals in a vessel cross section. Sampling echoes at multiple loci (multigating) produces spectrograms for each of the different probe-to-sample site distances (Figure 16-27).

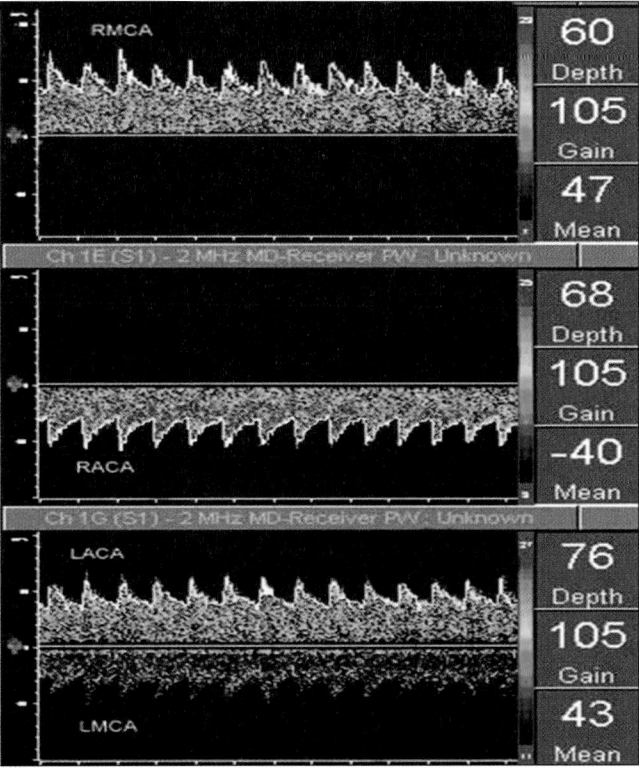

Figure 16-27 Multigating of pulsed-wave Doppler signals permits simultaneous display of echo spectra generated at several different intracranial loci. LACA, left anterior cerebral artery; LMCA, left middle cerebral artery; RACA, right anterior cerebral artery; RMCA, right middle cerebral artery.

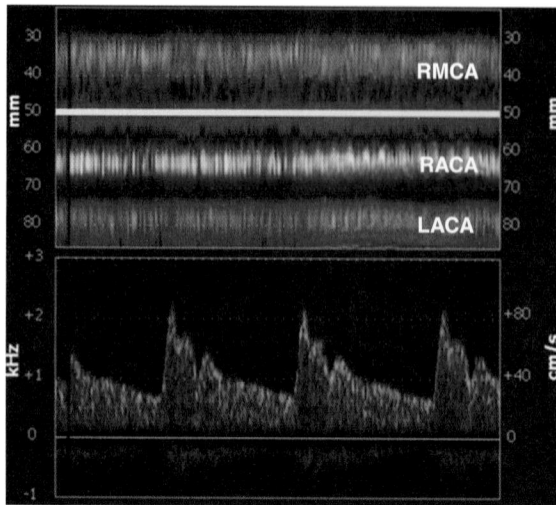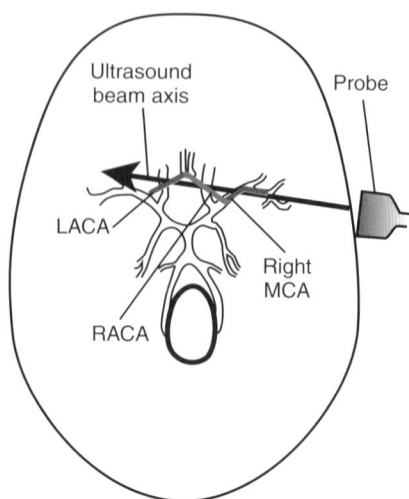

Figure 16-28 The transcranial Doppler (TCD) continuous-wave M-mode (top left) and pulsed-wave spectral (bottom left) displays are compared. The horizontal bands of the M-mode display represent a series of Doppler-shift echoes. Signals in the 30- to 50-mm-depth range (top red band) represent flow in the right middle cerebral artery (MCA) ipsilateral to the ultrasonic probe. Red color signifies flow directed toward the probe (right). Echoes arising between 55 and 70 mm from the probe emanate from the ipsilateral anterior cerebral artery (ACA). They are shown in the middle blue band of the M-mode display. Signals in the 72- to 85-mm range arise from the contralateral ACA with flow directed toward the probe (lower red band). The M-mode yellow line at a depth of 50 mm indicates the measurement site for the TCD frequency spectral display shown at the bottom left. *(Courtesy of Dr. Mark Moehring, Spencer Technologies, Seattle, WA.)*

Power M-Mode Doppler Display

An alternative method for processing pulsed-wave Doppler echoes is nonspectral power M-mode Doppler (PMD; Figure 16-28). Unlike the series of spectra generated with multigating, PMD creates one image with each depth represented by a plot of signal amplitude (i.e., power) and depth as functions of time. A color scale signifies flow direction (red is flow directed toward the probe; blue is flow away from the probe), whereas color intensity is directly related to signal power.

Embolus Detection

Erythrocytes (approximately 5 million/mL) are the most acoustically reflective, nonpathologic blood elements (i.e., high acoustic impedance). However, gaseous and particulate emboli are better reflectors of sound than erythrocytes. The presence of high-intensity transient signals (HITSs) within either the PMD or spectral TCD display may signify the presence of an embolus.[85,86] Because a gaseous or particulate embolus cannot simultaneously appear at all distances from the probe, either PMD or a multigated spectral display may be used to distinguish them from acoustic artifact (tapping on the ultrasonic probe produces a high-intensity transient acoustic artifact at all distances).

Figure 16-29 illustrates the appearance of HITSs in the two TCD display formats. The bottom spectral displays are generated from a small vascular segment at a distance of 50 ± 3 mm (6-mm sample volume) from the probe surface. The midpoint of the spectral sample is indicated on the top PMD displays as a light horizontal line at a 50-mm depth. An embolic track labeled "a" is a single embolus that is shown in the top PMD display moving toward the probe (i.e., decreasing distance from the probe face over time). Embolic tracks "b" and "d" display the characteristic "lambda" acoustic signature in the spectral display. The PMD shows that this pattern is due to embolus direction reversal within the spectral sample volume. The true behavior of the spectrally paradoxical track "c" (start and end points of the single acoustic signature are not connected) becomes clear in the PMD view. Track "c" direction reversal is invisible on the spectral display because it occurs outside the sampling region. Currently available spectral or PMD TCD monitors can determine neither the size nor composition of emboliform material responsible for HITSs. TCD devices designed for surgical monitoring typically provide a semiquantitative estimate of aggregate HITSs, irrespective of their origin (Box 16-11).

Intervention Threshold

Because erythrocyte velocity and flow may be differentially influenced by vessel diameter,[87] blood viscosity,[88,89] and pH,[89] as well as temperature,[89] TCD does not provide a reliable measure of cerebral blood flow. However, in the absence of hemodilution, *change* in TCD velocity does correlate closely with *change* in blood flow.[87] Sudden large changes in velocity or direction are readily detected by continuous TCD monitoring. The clinical significance of velocity changes has been assessed in conscious patients during implantable cardioverter-defibrillator and tilt-table testing.[90,91] In both circumstances, clinical evidence of cerebral hypoperfusion was accompanied by a mean velocity decline of greater than 60% and absent diastolic velocity. During nonpulsatile CPB, the ischemia threshold appears to be an 80% decrease below the preincision baseline.[92]

In general, reduction of flow velocity indicating severe ischemia is associated with profound depression of EEG activity.[92] However, with adequate leptomeningeal collateral flow, cerebral function may remain unchanged in the presence of a severely decreased or absent middle cerebral artery flow velocity.[93] Together, these findings form the rationale for a TCD-based intervention threshold. During cardiac surgery, mean velocity reductions of greater than 80% or velocity loss during diastole suggest clinically significant cerebral hypoperfusion.

Clinical Basis for Intervention

Before Cardiopulmonary Bypass

TCD provides cerebral hemodynamic information for the timely detection and correction of perfusion abnormalities that may occur *before* the onset of CPB. Vascular torsion during neck extension or axial head rotation may result in regional cerebral hypoperfusion detectable by TCD.[94] Cerebral blood flow obstruction may also be detected by TCD during endovascular repair of aortic dissection.[95] Excessive hyperventilation may result in inadvertent cerebral ischemia because blood flow declines by 4%/mm Hg $Paco_2$ in normally reactive cerebral arteries.[87] Cerebral dysautoregulation is often seen in hypertensive and diabetic patients.[96] This abnormality may result in pressure-dependent brain perfusion and place the patient at risk for ischemic brain injury during even moderate hypotension. TCD may be used to identify pressure dependency and facilitate appropriate individualization of acceptable perfusion pressure.[97] In addition, TCD has been used to identify the optimal aortic cannulation site.[98] For example, Mullges et al[99] observed

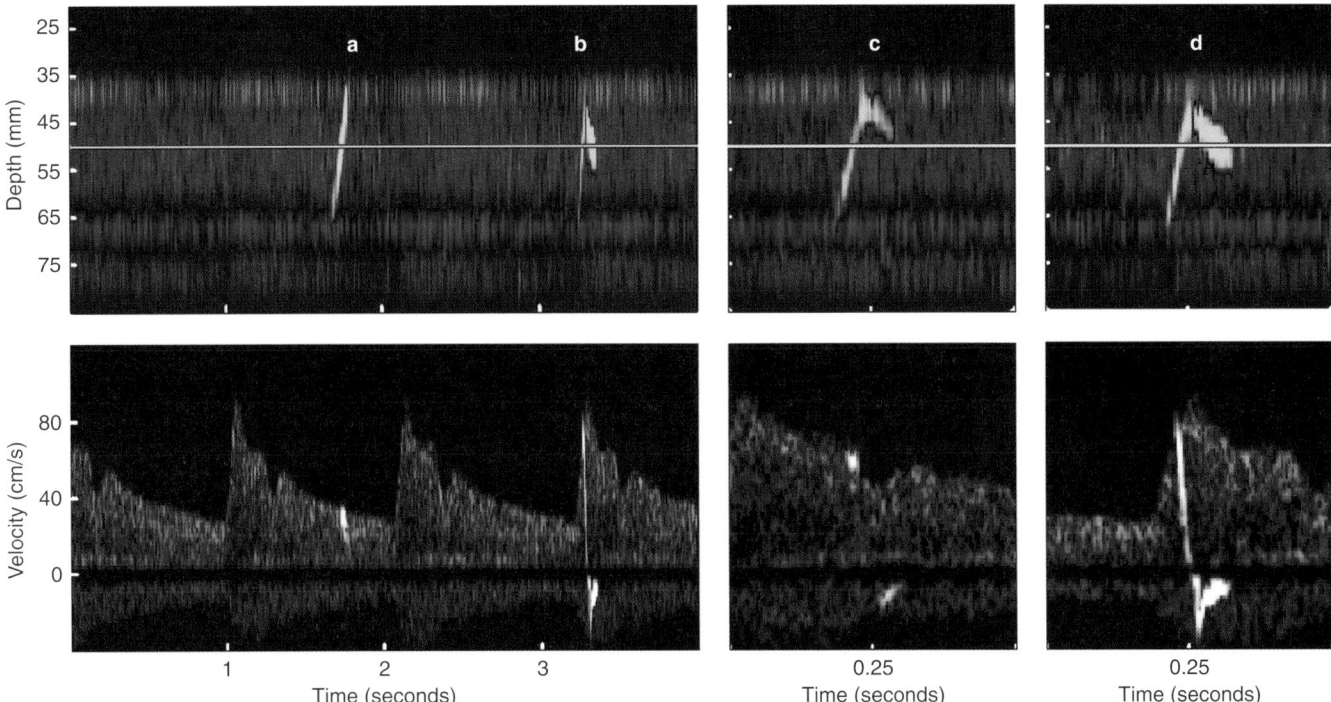

Figure 16-29 The appearance of emboliform high-intensity transient signals (HITSs) is compared using the M-mode and frequency spectral displays. *White horizontal line* at a depth of 50 mm depicts the site of the spectral measurement along the axis of the vessel. HIT$_a$ *(white transient)* represents linear migration of an embolus in the M2 segment of the ipsilateral middle cerebral artery. A single HIT *(white dot)* is noted on the spectral display as the embolus passes through the 50-mm measurement site. In contrast, emboli in the remaining panels suddenly change direction as they pass into a smaller branch vessel. HIT$_b$ and HIT$_d$ direction changes are noted on the spectral displays as the characteristic "lambda" sign. However, the HIT$_c$ behavior is misidentified as two emboli because the direction change occurs outside the spectral sample volume. *(Courtesy of Dr. Mark Moehring, Spencer Technologies, Seattle, WA.)*

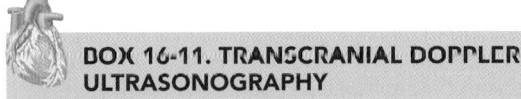

BOX 16-11. TRANSCRANIAL DOPPLER ULTRASONOGRAPHY

- Detects change in intracranial blood flow
- Detects emboli—particulate or gaseous

that the mean aggregate middle cerebral artery embolic load was significantly lower with a distal arch cannulation compared with the traditional ascending aorta site. These results are consistent with the studies using epiaortic ultrasound. Detection of malpositioned aortic or superior vena caval perfusion cannula is rapidly achieved with TCD monitoring.[100] In the former case, the malposition results in a sudden profound decrease in the peak systolic velocity (Figure 16-30), whereas in the latter, diastolic velocity is compromised (Figure 16-31).

During Cardiopulmonary Bypass

TCD is the only available method to continuously assess changes in cerebral hemodynamics associated with CPB. Despite the confounding influences of hemodilution, altered acid-base management, and cooling on absolute flow velocity, TCD nevertheless indicates the presence and direction of cerebral blood flow. A sudden large decrease, increase, or asymmetry indicates, respectively, inadvertent occlusion of a great vessel, hyperperfusion of a single cranial artery, or misdirection of aortic cannula flow (Figure 16-32).

During surgical repair of the aortic arch, TCD documents cerebral artery flow direction during attempts at supplemental retrograde (Figure 16-33) or antegrade (Figure 16-34) cerebral perfusion during systemic circulatory arrest.[101,102] Because peak velocity changes in large basal cerebral arteries are directly related to peak flow changes, TCD may aid in the determination of safe upper and lower limits for pump flow and perfusion pressure.[103] Deep cooling and circulatory arrest may

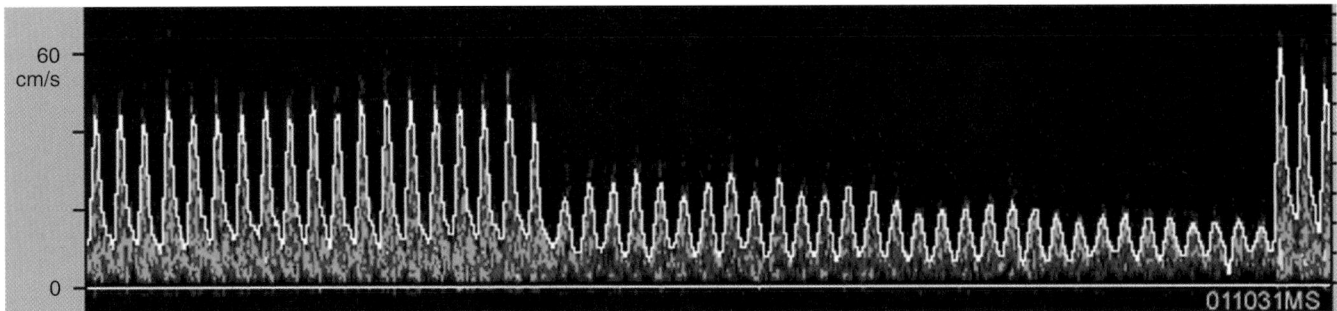

Figure 16-30 Malposition of an aortic perfusion cannula before the onset of cardiopulmonary bypass was identified on its insertion by the sudden large decrease in peak systolic velocity. Repositioning led to a prompt recovery of cerebral perfusion.

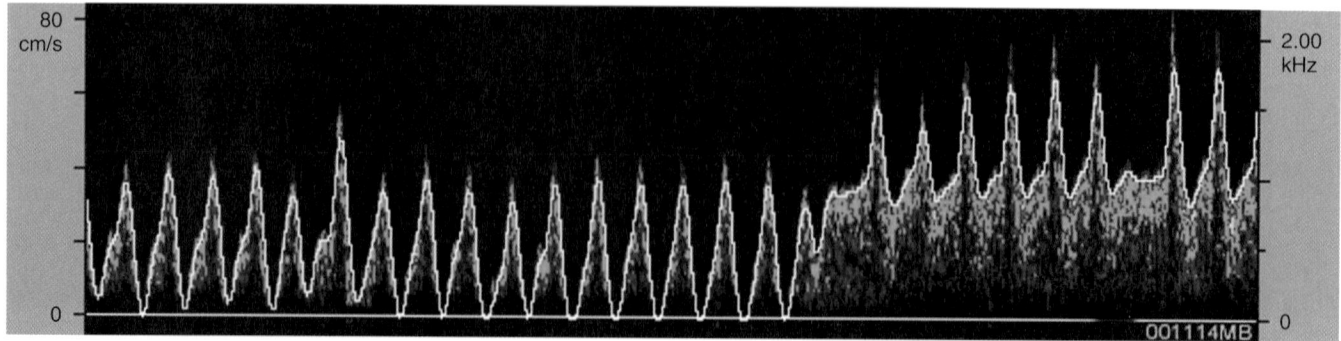

Figure 16-31 Malposition of a superior vena cava perfusion cannula before the onset of cardiopulmonary bypass was identified shortly after its insertion by the loss of end-diastolic velocity. Repositioning led to a prompt recovery of cerebral perfusion.

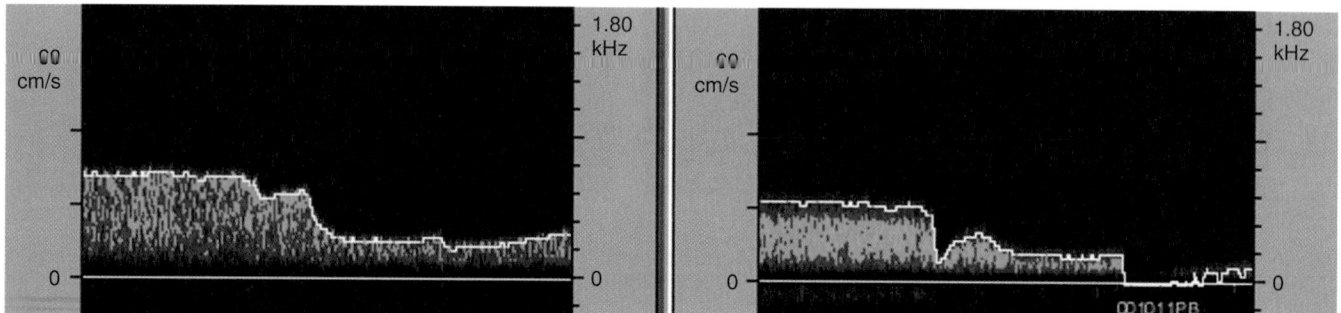

Figure 16-32 During total cardiopulmonary bypass with nonpulsatile perfusion, cerebral malperfusion was identified by asymmetric left/right hemisphere velocity decline. A slight change in the position of the aortic perfusion cannula corrected the problem.

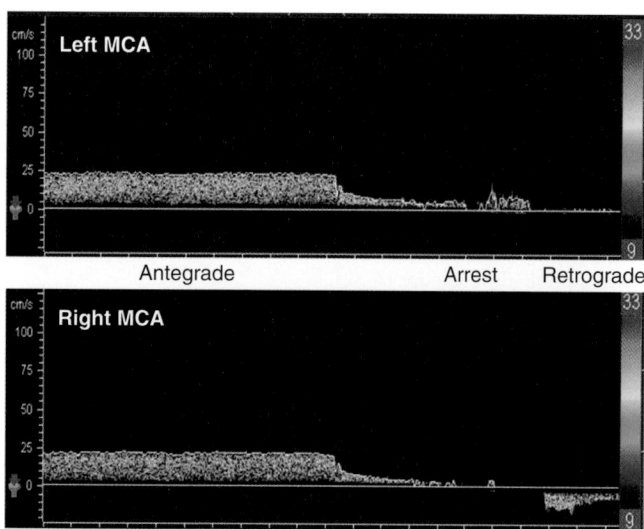

Figure 16-33 These two transcranial Doppler (TCD) frequency spectral displays show changes in left (top) and right (bottom) middle cerebral artery (MCA) flow velocity during attempted retrograde cerebral perfusion via the superior vena cava with carotid drainage. Spectral patterns above the zero-velocity baselines indicate antegrade blood flow directed toward the ultrasound probe.

produce a transient cerebral vasoparesis and result in uncoupling of cerebral blood flow and metabolism.[102] TCD identifies this phenomenon as an unchanging flow velocity during rewarming. Emboli detection by TCD can improve surgical and perfusion technique, as well as facilitate correction of technical problems such as an air leak[104–106] (see Figure 16-34 and Box 16-12).

Transcranial Doppler Clinical Benefit

A practice guideline for TCD perioperative monitoring has just been jointly published by the American Society of Neurophysiologic Monitoring and the American Society of Neuroimaging.[107] In addition, evidenced-based medicine now supports the use of TCD monitoring during cardiovascular surgery.[108,109] For example, the results of a randomized, prospective investigation demonstrated that TCD monitoring during acute aortic dissection repair reduced the incidence of transient neurologic deficit from 52% to 15%. This reduction was achieved, in part, through TCD-directed changes in perfusion cannula placement (29% of cases) and adjustments in the management of retrograde cerebral perfusion (79% of cases).[110] Prospective studies have also demonstrated the clinical utility of direct cerebral perfusion measurement. Although vasoconstrictors reliably increase arterial blood pressure, they may not alter cerebral perfusion pressure.[111] Similarly, nitrate vasodilators typically reduce arterial blood pressure, whereas cerebral perfusion pressure may remain unaltered[87] or may actually increase.[111] In the absence of cerebral perfusion monitoring, blood pressure management can easily result in adverse consequences to the brain.

JUGULAR BULB OXIMETRY

Oximeter catheters transmitting three wavelengths of light are inserted into the cerebral venous circulation to directly and continuously measure cerebral venous oxygen saturation ($Sjvo_2$). Commercially available devices are modifications of the catheter oximeter originally developed for the pulmonary circulation. External preinsertion calibration of the catheter and documentation of catheter position in the jugular bulb are required for accurate measurements. In vivo calibrations against co-oximeter samples can also be performed. Reflected light signals are averaged, filtered, and displayed. Conditions affecting the accuracy of these measurements include catheter kinking, blood flow around the

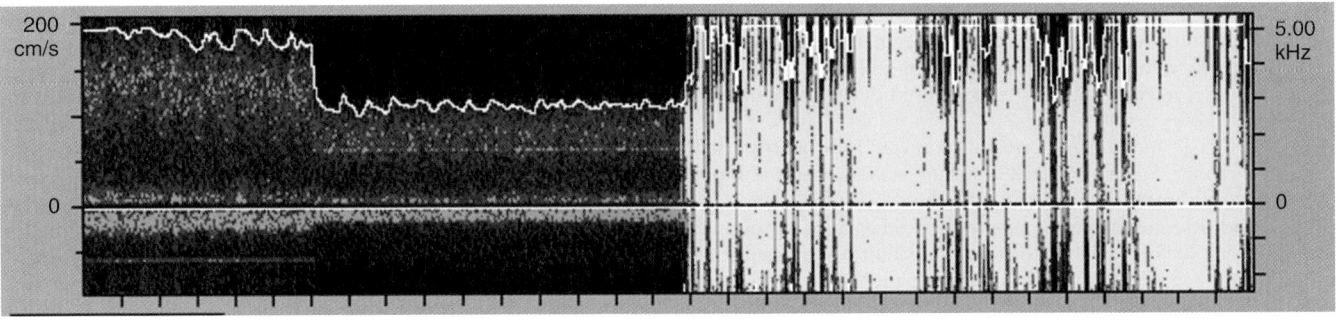

Figure 16-34 Hyperperfusion of the right middle cerebral artery was identified by transcranial Doppler during attempted supplemental antegrade cerebral perfusion during total circulatory arrest. Repositioning of the right axillary perfusion cannula led to a reduction in velocity followed shortly thereafter by the accidental introduction of a small amount of air. The leak was quickly identified and corrected.

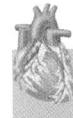

BOX 16-12. IMPORTANT IMBALANCES IDENTIFIED BY TRANSCRANIAL DOPPLER ULTRASONOGRAPHY

- Preexisting cerebral hemodynamic abnormalities
- Head malposition
- Hypocarbia-induced ischemia
- Appropriate aortic cannulation site
- Perfusion cannula malposition
- Malperfusion syndrome
- Successful supplementary cerebral perfusion during circulatory arrest
- Flow-metabolism uncoupling

catheter, changes in hematocrit, fibrin deposition on the catheter, and changes in temperature.

The normal $Sjvo_2$ range is widely assumed to be between 60% and 70%.[112] However, a recent study using radiographically confirmed catheter placement observed a much wider 45% to 70% range in healthy subjects.[113] Furthermore, the 95% confidence interval of the low threshold was 37% to 53%. Thus, some healthy individuals had $Sjvo_2$ values less than 35%.

There are two major limitations of the technology. First, $Sjvo_2$ represents a global measure of venous drainage from unspecified cranial compartments. Because cerebral and extracranial venous anatomy are notoriously varied, clinical interpretation of measured change is a major challenge. The difficulty is exemplified by the study of Mutch et al,[114] who used both $Sjvo_2$ and T2*-weighted magnetic resonance imaging to measure oxyhemoglobin and deoxyhemoglobin in a porcine model of CPB. Imaging demonstrated substantial hypoxic regions within the cerebral parenchyma that were invisible to the global jugular oxygen saturation measurement. Second, accurate measurement using jugular oximetry requires continuous adequate flow past the catheter. Low- or no-flow states such as profound hypoperfusion or complete ischemia render $Sjvo_2$ unreliable.[115] Despite these limitations, the global measure of brain oxygen balance has been used successfully as a transfusion trigger[116] and to document the deleterious effect of even modest cerebral hyperthermia.[117] In addition, $Sjvo_2$ monitoring determined that, compared with traditional myocardial revascularization, the "off-pump" procedure was associated with a two-fold increase in the incidence of noteworthy oxygen desaturation.[118]

CEREBRAL OXIMETRY

Near-Infrared Technology

Because the human skull is translucent to infrared light, intracranial intravascular regional hemoglobin oxygen saturation (rSo_2) may be measured noninvasively with transcranial near-infrared spectroscopy (NIRS). An infrared light source contained in a self-adhesive patch affixed to glabrous skin of the scalp transmits photons through underlying tissues to the outer layers of the cerebral cortex. Adjacent sensors separate photons reflected from the skin, muscle, skull, and dura from those of the brain tissue (Figure 16-35). NIRS measures all hemoglobin, pulsatile and nonpulsatile, in a mixed microvascular bed composed of gas-exchanging vessels with a diameter less than 100 μm.[119] The measurement is thought to reflect approximately 75% venous blood.[119] This ratio remains nearly constant in normoxia, hypoxia, and

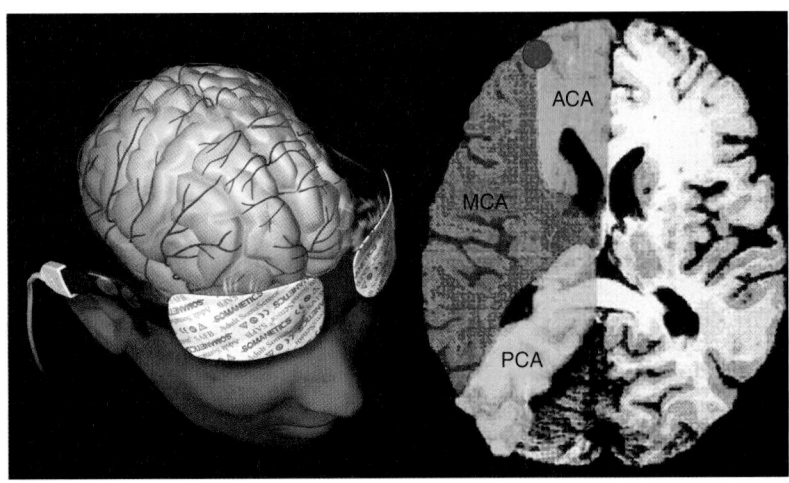

Figure 16-35 The frontal cortex anterior–middle cerebral artery watershed region may be sampled bilaterally by cerebral oximeter sensors located on the forehead above each eye. The diagram at right illustrates the anterior (green) and middle cerebral artery (pink) flow distributions and the approximate size and location of the oximetric sampling region (red dot). ACA, anterior cerebral artery; MCA, middle cerebral artery; PCA, posterior cerebral artery. (Courtesy of Somanetics Corporation, Troy, MI.)

hypocapnia.[119] Cerebral oximetry appears to both reliably quantify change from an individualized baseline and offer an objective measure of regional hypoperfusion.[120,121] Unlike pulse and jugular bulb oximetry, respectively, cerebral oximetry may be used during nonpulsatile CPB and circulatory arrest.

Similar to TCD monitoring, cerebral oximetry is primarily used to quantify change. Substantial NIRS intersubject baseline variability precludes establishment of an absolute threshold value for tissue ischemia.[122] An adverse shift in oxygen supply-demand balance is indicated by a decreasing oxyhemoglobin fraction. The clinical significance of the decline has been determined in conscious patients during G-force studies with high-speed centrifugation, implantable cardioverter/defibrillator testing, tilt-table testing, carotid artery occlusion, and intracranial artery balloon occlusion.[91,92,123,124] In each setting, a decline of greater than 20% was associated with syncope or signs of focal cerebral ischemia. The magnitude and duration of cerebral dysoxygenation are associated with hospital cost-driver increase, as well as the incidence and severity of adverse clinical outcome.[125–136]

The first commercial device to receive FDA clearance for continuous measurement of rSo_2 was the single-channel INVOS 3100 cerebral oximeter (Somanetics Corporation, Troy, MI). The latest model 5100 is a four-channel device that is cleared for continuous measurement of cerebral and somatic tissue oxygenation in patients larger than 2.5 kg. It uses two wavelengths of infrared light generated by broad bandwidth light-emitting diodes. Some investigators have expressed theoretical concern that the fixed 25:75 arterial/venous oxygen saturation ratio used by the INVOS device does not accurately represent the inevitable fluctuations in the actual arterial-venous volume relation.[137,138] However, experimental data demonstrate that rSo_2 is insensitive to substantial change in this ratio.[139,140] Through a process termed *spatial resolution,* INVOS uses multipoint extracranial and intracranial measurements to suppress the influences of extracranial hemoglobin absorption and intersubject variation in intracranial photon scatter. Independent studies have shown that the source of the resultant rSo_2 metric is approximately 85% intracranial[119] (Figure 16-36, left panel).

Three other cerebral oximeters have recently received FDA clearance. The CAS Medical (Branford, CT) Fore-Sight also uses two infrared sensors.[141] The proximal sensor is positioned very near the light source to detect exclusively extracranial photon migration. Photons detected

by the distal sensor arise from both extracranial and intracranial tissues (see Figure 16-36, right panel). Cerebral saturation is determined from the proximal-distal differential signal. Although this approach appears to suppress extracranial contamination, the single-point intracranial measurement may be influenced by individual variations in intracranial photon scatter. The manufacturer claims that photon scatter variation is mitigated by the use of four narrow-bandwidth laser-generated infrared wavelengths. There are as yet no peer-reviewed articles to substantiate this claim or that compare Fore-Sight performance with other cerebral oximeters, but several abstracts are available.[142,143]

The OrNim (Los Gatos, CA) CerOx measures brain or peripheral tissue regional oxygen saturation using a combination of multiple wavelength near-infrared light and phase-modulated ultrasound. Information on the manufacturer's website is insufficient to permit a valid comparison with other devices. There are as yet no peer-reviewed articles that characterize its performance.

Nonin (Minneapolis, MN) manufactures the EquanOX 7600 cerebral oximeter. It relies on dual light-emitting diode light sources and three wavelengths of infrared light. Infrared light source-sensor separation appears to be similar to the Somanetics INVOS 5100. Currently, only one abstract is available that describes device performance.[144]

Most articles describing clinical experience with FDA-cleared tissue oximetry have used the Somanetics rSo_2 metric. Unless otherwise indicated, subsequent discussion refers to the use of this saturation measure. Until more information becomes available, it would be imprudent to assume that tissue oxygen saturation values obtained with one brand of tissue oximeter are interchangeable with those from another.[145] Objective performance comparison is difficult because of the lack of a universally accepted direct reference standard measure of regional brain oxygen saturation.

Technologic Limitations

The technical limitations of cerebral oximetry primarily involve factors that influence photon migration. Sensor placement is currently limited to glabrous skin (e.g., forehead) lateral to the midline. Such placement prevents monitoring the critical posterior watershed at the juncture of the anterior, middle, and posterior cerebral arteries (see Figure 16-35). Dark hair and the follicles of dark hair absorb near-infrared light and can substantially reduce the signal-to-noise ratio. Thus, de Letter et al,[146] using a parietotemporal placement in head-shaved neurosurgical patients, failed to obtain saturation values in 18% of their patients. Weak signals may also result from hematoma or sensor placement over a venous sinus.[147] In either case, the large hemoglobin volume acts as a photon sink. Conversely, recording failures may arise from excessively large signals, such as those produced by a skull defect.[148]

Validation

The rSo_2 value has been validated from arterial and jugular bulb oxygen saturation measurements in pediatric and adult subjects.[149,150] In these studies, hypoxemia involving cerebral tissue proximate to the sensors was consistently detected by this technology. Except during ischemia and CPB, $Sjvo_2$ and rSo_2 generally correlate in the midrange saturation, although discrepancies may appear at the extremes.[151] The validity of rSo_2 also has been assessed by comparison with direct microprobe measurement of brain tissue oxygen partial pressure (tPo_2). Reasonable agreement between these two measures has been found in neurosurgical patients.[152,153]

Controversies

As with most new technologies, the emergence of cerebral and regional tissue oximetry has spawned controversy. Fortunately, a recent series of Pro and Con articles has addressed the major clinical concerns.[138,154–156] These issues are discussed later in the Intervention Rationale section.

Perhaps the most puzzling controversy involves the unqualified insistence by skeptics that multiple positive, large-scale prospective,

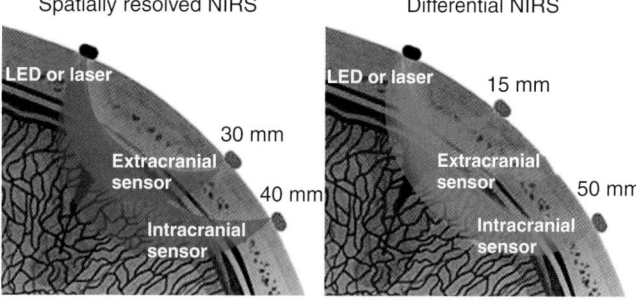

Figure 16-36   The mean photon path traveling through the adult cranium from an infrared source to sensors on neighboring scalp is banana shaped. With spatially resolved near-infrared spectroscopy (NIRS), both sensors are sufficiently distant from the light source to ensure that the mean photon paths of both signals pass intracranially (left). Two-point extracranial and intracranial measurement permits suppression of both the extracranial signal and interpatient variance in intracranial photon scatter. The resultant cerebral oxygen saturation measurement appears to be about 85% intracranial.[119] In contrast, differential NIRS uses a sensor placed very near the light source to record exclusively extracranial signal and another more distant sensor for intracranial measurement (right). Single-point subtraction suppresses extracranial signal but not intersubject variation in photon scatter. This second goal is claimed to be achieved through the use of additional wavelengths of infrared light.[141] LED, light-emitting diode. *(Left, Courtesy of Somanetics Corporation, Troy, MI.)*

randomized outcome trials must precede routine use of regional tissue oximetry during cardiac and major vascular surgery.[122,138,154] Such insistence is eminently reasonable for monitoring modalities that (1) pose a risk of injury; (2) are very expensive; or (3) have a difficult learning curve or require extensive, specialized training. Because regional tissue oximetry meets none of these criteria, the reason for this insistence is less clear.

The pulse oximetry precedent seems relevant to this controversy. In 1989, the American Society of Anesthesiologists House of Delegates mandated that pulse oximetry be used in every surgery involving general or regional anesthesia. The goal of the mandate was to reduce the probable risk of rare injury. No large-scale prospective, randomized trial preceded the mandate. Interestingly, the later trial involving more than 20,000 patients failed to detect an improved outcome in the pulse oximeter cohort.[157] In the accompanying editorial, Eichhorn[158] justified the earlier pulse oximeter mandate on the sensible grounds that "it is reasonable to be influenced and accept more indirect indications when considering the complex multivariate epidemiologic investigations dealing with anesthetic outcome."

Recently, Vohra et al[159] applied Eichhorn's reasoning to their conclusion of a 488-article cardiac surgery cerebral oximetry literature review. They stated, "Clinical benefit and lack of use-associated risk of injury at a modest expense support the use of rSo$_2$ monitoring *routinely* in patients undergoing cardiac surgery." Estimates of the extent of rSo$_2$ monitoring made in 2007 indicate that the technology is utilized in two thirds of pediatric[126] and one third of adult[125] U.S. cardiac centers. On the basis of these adoption rates and now-extensive evidence of rSo$_2$ clinical benefit including three positive prospective, randomized trials,[129–131] Murkin[128] suggests that the controversy has evolved to "standard of care for routine CPB vs. evolving standard for selective cerebral perfusion."

Normative Values

Kishi et al[160] examined surgical patient demographic influences on rSo$_2$. The measure appeared to be independent of weight, height, head size, or sex, although it was negatively correlated with age and positively correlated with hemoglobin concentration. Values were also affected as the sensor was moved laterally from the recommended position above the eye. In contrast, it is worth considering that the apparent age influence on rSo$_2$ may reflect advancing pathology in older patients.

Development of local physiologic norms is a common practice in neurophysiology units. Following this practice, in 1000 elective adult cardiac surgery patients (age range, 21 to 91; female sex, 32%), this author has determined a preprocedure rSo$_2$ value of 67 ± 10 scale units.[139] This value is significantly less than the 71 ± 6 previously reported for healthy volunteers (age range, 20 to 36).[150] The mean and median left-right difference for the cardiac surgery patients was zero, and only 5% of the differences were greater than 10. Only 5% of the rSo$_2$ baseline values were less than 50 or above 80. Thus, from a statistical perspective, a preinduction baseline rSo$_2$ value in adult elective cardiac surgery patients is abnormal if it is either outside the range of 50 to 80 or there is a right-left difference of greater than 10%. Normative data obtained with a differential spectrometer in 33 adult cardiac patients resulted in a similar mean saturation of 70% ± 4%.[143] The smaller variance is a likely result of the small sample size.

Intervention Threshold

Brain rSo$_2$ values less than or equal to 50 scale units appear to represent an increased risk for hypoxic injury.[134,136,161–165] In addition, numerous studies have observed clinical signs of cerebral hypoxia or adverse outcome, or both, after rSo$_2$ declines more than 20% below baseline.[123–133,166–170] Recently, a detailed cardiac surgery intervention algorithm based on this criterion has been proposed by Denault et al.[171] Current intervention strategy incorporates both concepts (Box 16-13). Thus, for most patients with awake baseline rSo$_2$ values greater than 50, intervention is triggered with a decline of more than 20%.

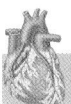

Alternatively, for individuals with a baseline of 50 or less, the objective is to maintain this abnormally low value throughout the perioperative period, using the tactics described in the Denault algorithm. With rSo$_2$ asymmetry, each cerebral hemisphere is managed independently. In this circumstance, the 20% criterion applies to a hemispheric baseline rSo$_2$ greater than 50, whereas the baseline maintenance criterion applies to hemispheric values of 50 or less. This approach to rSo$_2$ asymmetry is consistent with radiographic studies demonstrating a high incidence of clinically silent intracranial vascular disease before adult cardiac surgery.[172,173]

Intervention Rationale

Baseline rSo$_2$

Surgical cerebral oximetric monitoring should be initiated immediately after patient entry to the operating room. Self-adhesive patches containing the infrared light source with shallow (proximate) and deep (distant) sensors are fixed on the forehead on both sides of the midline. The initial objective is the establishment of a reference baseline before preoxygenation and anesthetic induction (Figure 16-37).

A high cerebral metabolic demand for oxygen may result in abnormally low rSo$_2$ values despite normal pulse oximetry readings. For example, the cerebral oximeter detected oxygen imbalance during high-altitude trekking that was unrecognized by pulse oximetry.[174] Similarly, patients in heart failure often have preoperative baseline values far below the normative range.[175–178] Abnormally high rSo$_2$ values may signify a silent infarction because injured or dead neurons consume little oxygen. Abnormal (>10 scale units) right-left rSo$_2$ may be caused by unrecognized carotid or intracranial arterial stenosis, intracranial space-occupying lesion, old infarction, skull defect, or extracranial sources such as a hemangioma, sinusitis, or artifactual

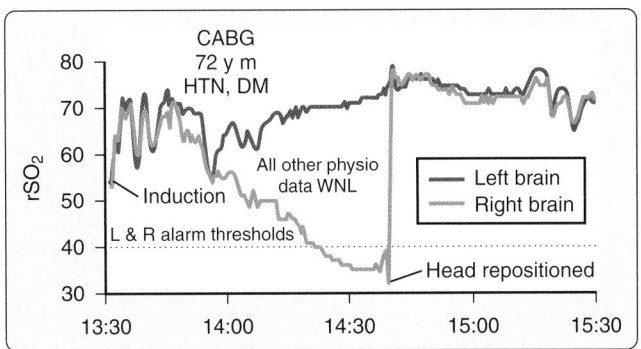

Figure 16-37 Right and left regional oxygen saturations (rSo$_2$) were symmetric and within normal limits (WNL) before anesthetic induction. Symmetric postinduction increase suggested intact CO_2 reactivity of the cerebral arterioles. Patient positioning resulted in a transient left hemisphere rSo$_2$ decline, whereas the right hemisphere decline was persistent and severe. Because all other physiologic signals were WNL, a patient malposition was suspected. Adjustment of the shoulder roll and head repositioning to correct a neck extension immediately resolved the regional desaturation. CABG, coronary artery bypass graft; DM, diabetes mellitus; HTN, hypertension.

interference from an infrared-emitting device.[179-182] An asymmetry or abnormal rSo_2 baseline, high or low, alerts the operative team to the increased potential for cerebral oxygen imbalance during surgical challenge.

Developing rSo_2 Asymmetry

A new asymmetry, signifying cerebral dysoxygenation, may develop quickly during anesthetic induction, pulmonary artery catheter insertion, or final patient positioning. During head positioning, an asymmetric rSo_2 decrease warns of developing regional cerebral hypoperfusion that otherwise may remain unrecognized.[139,155,183] Axial head rotation displaces the lateral mass of the contralateral atlas forward behind the internal carotid artery, just below its entrance into the carotid canal at the skull base. If this process is prolonged or if the artery is adherent to adjacent tissue, it can be compressed from behind, resulting in decreased flow.[184-186] Furthermore, volatile anesthetics may interfere with the regulatory mechanisms that normally maintain effective cerebral perfusion bilaterally during head rotation in conscious patients.[187]

The cerebral oximeter has detected potentially catastrophic cerebral desaturation because of great vessel torsion during cardiac manipulation.[188-192] Desaturation often appears to be the result of compromised venous return. Particularly in pediatric cardiac operations and in myocardial revascularization without CPB, cardiac manipulation may produce sudden large rSo_2 decreases without any appreciable change in mean arterial pressure (MAP) or arterial oxygen saturation.

Numerous reports have described rSo_2 detection of perfusion cannulae malposition[193-195] or regional malperfusion development during surgery involving the aortic arch or great vessels.[194-204] Malperfusion-related cerebral ischemia may be identified by EEG or SSEP, but these signals are susceptible to compromise by electrocautery, deep anesthesia, and hypothermia.[205] Similarly, TCD signals are susceptible to radiofrequency, acoustic, and movement artifact. Cerebral oximetry is also used during extracorporeal membrane oxygenation to detect regional deficiencies in brain perfusion associated with carotid cannulation.[206]

rSo_2 Responsiveness to CO_2

Induction of anesthesia and its attendant apnea during tracheal intubation often transiently alter the brain oxygen supply-demand relation. Hypnotic agents may transiently suppress cerebral metabolism more than blood flow; resulting relative hyperperfusion leads to an rSo_2 increase.[207] With normally reactive cerebral arterioles, ventilation disruption and CO_2 accumulation during tracheal intubation further increase rSo_2 as a result of the increased delivery of hyperoxygenated blood to a metabolically suppressed brain. Under these circumstances, even mild hypercapnia augments cerebral perfusion and oxygenation through local vasodilation.[208-211] Several investigators have demonstrated an rSo_2 increase (see Figure 16-37) associated with hypercapnia.[139,140,150,171]

Absence of rSo_2 increase with increasing arterial CO_2 tension suggests impairment of both CO_2 reactivity and cerebral autoregulation. Asymmetry warns of a potential vasculopathy (e.g., intracranial stenosis or silent infarction) and may prompt alterations in anesthetic and perfusion management to maintain cerebral perfusion in both hemispheres.[211]

Acid-base management during CPB remains controversial, particularly during deep cooling. Some propose that the greater CO_2 tension afforded by pH-stat acid-base management results in fewer neurologic complications.[212] Vijay et al[213] observed that during adult near-normothermic myocardial revascularization, vasopressor-induced perfusion pressure increases alone were sometimes inadequate to correct decreased rSo_2 occurring during CPB. In this situation, judiciously applied permissive hypercapnia often was effective in restoring rSo_2 to baseline.

Despite these seeming benefits, hypercapnia has potentially deleterious effects. Hypercapnia-induced cardiac output and heart rate also

increase myocardial oxygen demand, whereas cerebral vasodilation may exacerbate preexisting intracranial hypertension. Cerebral oximetry provides a convenient method to document appropriate bihemispheric CO_2 reactivity. In addition, continuous measurement of brain oxygen saturation permits CO_2 titration to achieve optimal tissue perfusion at the lowest risk.[214-216]

rSo_2 as a Transfusion Trigger

Two important determinants of tissue oxygenation are hemoglobin availability and plasma volume.[217,218] Madl et al[219] examined the relation between hemoglobin and rSo_2 in patients with septic shock. If a low hemoglobin (<8.5 mg/dL) was associated with an rSo_2 less than the normative range (i.e., <60%), transfusion consistently increased both variables. However, transfusion had no effect on rSo_2 values greater than 65%. Blas et al[220] described profound desaturation accompanying hemodilution with all other physiologic measures within normal limits. Brain saturation responded immediately to 2 units of packed red cells in this patient with bilateral carotid artery occlusions.

Due to the apparent association between rSo_2 and hemoglobin, transient brain oxygen desaturation is to be expected at the onset of CPB because the pump prime solution briefly displaces hemoglobin in the cerebral circulation. Vijay et al[221] demonstrated that the magnitude of this transient desaturation was related directly to the volume of crystalloid prime. Use of a blood prime in the arterial limb of the perfusion circuit appears to eliminate the transient rSo_2 decline accompanying CPB onset.[222] The hemoglobin influence on rSo_2 is the basis for use of cerebral oximetry as both a transfusion trigger[223] and a strategy to reduce or completely avoid administration of homologous blood.[224,225]

rSo_2 and Blood Volume

Tissue oximetry has been used to visualize the effect of volume expansion on cerebral perfusion during tilt-table diagnostic testing for syncope.[226] An rSo_2 sensor was placed on the gastrocnemius muscle to measure upright tilt-induced desaturation resulting from lower limb venous pooling. In susceptible patients, extensive pooling resulted in cerebral dysoxygenation and syncope. Crystalloid volume expansion reduced lower limb hemoglobin sequestration and prevented syncope. This same concept may be applied to cardiac surgery. Vasopressor ineffectiveness in the correction of an rSo_2 decline may indicate compromised microcirculatory gas exchange because of hypovolemia. In this circumstance, low rSo_2 values often respond to volume augmentation.

rSo_2 and Autoregulation

Numerous studies have concluded that cerebral autoregulation remains intact during cardiac operations, both before and during CPB. Although this conclusion may be correct for large groups of patients, it does not necessarily apply to each individual. Cerebral oximetry can identify the lower limit of autoregulation, the point at which brain blood flow and tissue oxygenation become pressure dependent.[139,227] The independence of MAP and cerebral oxygen saturation establishes intact cerebral autoregulation.[228,229]

Figure 16-38 illustrates the use of rSo_2 measurement in the determination of the lower autoregulatory limit. The rSo_2-versus-MAP relation in the top graph depicts intact autoregulation. The rSo_2 values remain independent of MAP over a wide pressure range. The bottom graph, generated later the same day in the same operating room by the same surgical team, depicts dysautoregulation because rSo_2 declines each time MAP declines to less than 80 mm Hg. Examination of MAP-rSo_2 relations from a large series of cardiac operations resulted in two findings.[230] First, the lower limit of autoregulation varies widely among patients, from a MAP of less than 40 to more than 100 mm Hg. Second, a substantial proportion of cardiac patients do not, in fact, maintain autoregulation throughout the entirety of the operation. These observations illustrate the potential benefit of continuously monitoring the adequacy of cerebral perfusion during cardiovascular surgery.

The driving force for hemoglobin through the gas-exchanging microvasculature is not arterial pressure per se, but the arterial-venous

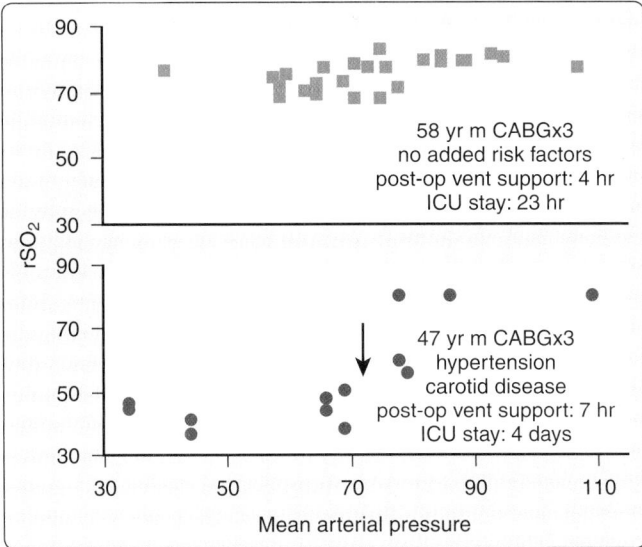

Figure 16-38 Relation between regional oxygen saturation (rSo$_2$) and mean arterial pressure during cardiopulmonary bypass is depicted. Each symbol represents a single point paired measurement obtained at 5-minute intervals. *Top,* Intact cerebral autoregulation with clear independence of rSo$_2$ and mean arterial pressure (MAP) over a wide range. The patient's outcome was uneventful. In contrast, the *bottom panel* depicts dysautoregulation with the classic appearance of a vascular waterfall. Each time the MAP declined to less than 80 mm Hg, a marked rSo$_2$ decrease occurred, indicating that the cerebral perfusion pressure had declined to less than the lower limit of autoregulation. Presumably, as a result of suboptimal cerebral perfusion, the patient experienced a prolonged recovery complicated by delirium. CABG, coronary artery bypass graft; ICU, intensive care unit.

pressure difference. Factors that increase cerebral venous pressure will compromise oxygen delivery, even if the arterial pressure remains in the normally acceptable range. It is most useful to examine a trend of the relation between rSo$_2$ and cerebral perfusion pressure (MAP − [the higher of central venous or intracranial pressure]).

Vasoactive drugs may have distinctly different effects on cerebral and systemic perfusion. These disparate pharmacologic actions further confound cerebral perfusion estimates on the basis of systemic blood pressure. Both vasodilators and vasoconstrictors may disrupt the expected brain blood flow-systemic blood pressure relation. Vasodilator nitrates may increase cerebral rSo$_2$ whereas systemic blood pressure is unchanged or declines.[231,232] Conversely, vasoconstrictors may increase cerebral rSo$_2$ only when MAP is below the lower limit of autoregulation.[233]

rSo$_2$ and Brain Temperature

Temperature has important effects on tissue oxygenation.[234] Because standard temperature monitoring during CPB does not accurately characterize the efficacy of brain cooling, cerebral oximetry may facilitate management of hypothermic neuroprotection.[235–238] In theory, temperature with CPB and alpha-stat acid-base management results in a linear decrease in cerebral blood flow and an exponential decline in metabolic rate.[239] Consequently, predicted "luxury" flow should ensure adequate cerebral oxygenation during cooling. However, Daubeney et al[151] demonstrated that other variables were also involved in the maintenance of adequate tissue oxygenation during deep hypothermia in pediatric patients. The rSo$_2$ at a 20°C target cooling temperature varied inversely with the cooling rate by the equation: rSo$_2$ = −20.5 (cooling rate, °C/min) + 97.4. In addition, they found that the rate of desaturation during total circulatory arrest was a function of the nasopharyngeal temperature at arrest onset, described by the equation: desaturation rate = 0.19 (nasopharyngeal temp, °C) − 2.5. At 20°C, the mean desaturation rate was 0.25% min, although decay was not linear. At temperatures slightly greater than 20°C (21°C to 26°C), desaturation

rate increased nearly 10-fold (2.0%/min). In normothermic infants, transient disruption of cerebral perfusion resulted in another 10-fold increase (i.e., ≈20% min) in the rate of desaturation.[240] The desaturation rates in hypothermic pediatric patients are somewhat less than those reported in adults.[215,216,238,241]

Deep hypothermia may also produce transient cerebral vasoparesis.[239,242] Consequently, rewarming may result in desaturation as the temperature-induced increase in cerebral metabolism is unsupported by adequate flow increase. Daubeney et al[188] described an inverse relation between rSo$_2$ and nasopharyngeal temperature during rewarming in pediatric patients, given by the equation: rSo$_2$ = −2.9 (nasopharyngeal temp) + 148. Liu et al[207] observed similar cerebral desaturation during rewarming in adult cardiac surgery patients. Small perfusion deficits decreased rSo$_2$ as oxygen extraction is increased to meet rising demand. When the oxygen extractive capacity is exceeded, functional compromise will be manifested by EEG or evoked potential abnormalities.[243]

rSo$_2$ Guides Supplemental Cerebral Perfusion

Several studies have demonstrated that rSo$_2$-guided retrograde cerebral perfusion may extend the "safe time" for hypothermic circulatory arrest during adult aortic arch reconstruction.[101,244,245] Blas et al[220] reported on the use of cerebral oximetry for detection of a superior vena cava cannula malposition during retrograde cerebral perfusion.

Higami et al[246] found rapid desaturation with total circulatory arrest, slow continual desaturation with retrograde cerebral perfusion, and no desaturation with supplemental antegrade cerebral perfusion (Figure 16-39). There was a high incidence of neurologic deficit in patients whose saturation declined more than 30% below the conscious baseline. Subsequently, many studies have found cerebral oximetry to be a useful guide for the management of regional low-flow perfusion and selective antegrade cerebral perfusion.[247–259]

rSo$_2$ Improves Systemic Hypoxemia Detection

The high oxygen demand of the brain means that signs of developing hypoxemia may first appear in regional cerebral measurements. Several reports have noted rSo$_2$ to decline earlier than Spo$_2$ at the onset of hypoxia.[260,261] Furthermore, continuous cerebral rSo$_2$ monitoring has provided the first indication of impaired oxygen delivery during nonpulsatile CPB.[262,263]

rSo$_2$ Facilitates Regional Tissue Hypoxia Detection

In 2004, Edmonds et al[264] reported on simultaneous brain and perivertebral rSo$_2$ monitoring during thoracoabdominal aneurysm repair.

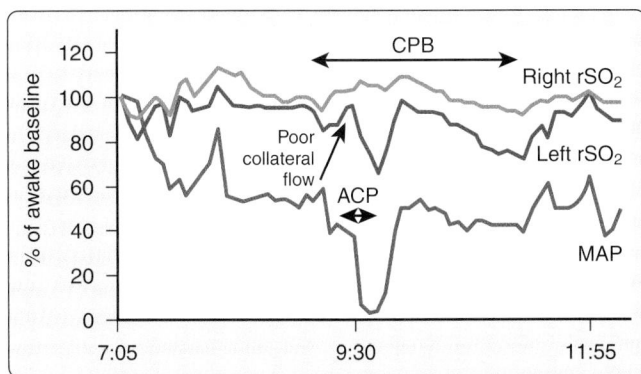

Figure 16-39 Cerebral oximetry provides continuous objective assessment of supplemental antegrade cerebral perfusion (ACP) during deep hypothermic systemic circulatory arrest. In this case, a single perfusion cannula for ACP was located in the right axillary artery. The stable regional oxygen saturation (rSo$_2$) value in the right hemisphere and falling rSo$_2$ in the left hemisphere document that ACP was only partially successful. Had a longer arrest period been anticipated, this information would have prompted the surgeon to perfuse through the left carotid as well. CPB, cardiopulmonary bypass; MAP, mean arterial pressure.

Desaturation occurring below the level of the aortic cross-clamp was interpreted as hypoperfusion within the extensive vertebrovenous plexus.[265] This preliminary observation was subsequently confirmed in a laboratory investigation using human adult-size swine[266] and a clinical study in pediatric aortic coarctation repair.[267] Now many reports document the value of multisite tissue oximetry.[268–276] Hepatic, perirenal, and splanchnic tissue perfusion have been successfully assessed in neonates, whereas limb perfusion monitoring has been achieved in both pediatric and adult cardiac surgery and intensive care patients. Harel et al[277] used strain-gauge and radionuclide plethysmography to validate the latter application of tissue oximetry.

rSo₂ and Anesthetic Adequacy

Another important determinant of tissue oxygenation is pain-induced stress.[278] With inadequate hypnosis or analgesia, pain-induced stress may result in cerebral oxygen consumption exceeding delivery and decreasing rSo_2. Hypnosis and analgesia monitoring by EEG and facial electromyogram can facilitate the prompt identification and correction of this source of cerebral dysoxygenation (Box 16-14).

Until recently, the inability to integrate neuromonitoring information from different modalities (Box 16-15) into a unified display has inhibited clinical studies using a multimodality approach in cardiac surgery. As a result, currently only three outcome studies have examined the impact of multimodality neuromonitoring using a combination of EEG, TCD, and cerebral oximetry. The study involving pediatric cardiac patients noted significant reductions in both neurologic complications and hospital cost in the neuromonitored cohort.[279] Both adult cardiac surgery studies[280,281] found a 2.7-day reduction in length of stay associated with multimodality neuromonitoring. Edmonds's[280] study also noted an 11% reduction in hospital expenses. In addition to the substantial reductions in hospital stay, charges, and neurologic complications, the results suggested possible benefit to other vital organ systems. This finding is not unexpected because the same processes that injure the brain may also injure other organs.[131,140] Future studies of neuromonitoring efficacy should not overlook these important accessory benefits. In addition, Lozano and Mossad[282] reviewed studies of neuromonitoring during pediatric cardiac surgery and showed that the monitoring was associated with enhanced outcomes (see Box 16-15).

The recent technologic developments address this limitation. New analysis and display systems (Figures 16-40*A* and *B*) can integrate multimodality neurophysiologic information, additional physiologic signals from anesthesia or critical care monitors, and information from ventilators, infusion pumps, and so forth into single, unified displays.

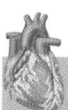

BOX 16-14. CLINICAL APPLICATIONS OF REGIONAL TISSUE OXIMETRY

- Detection of preexisting tissue oxygen imbalance
- Identification of new position-related perfusion asymmetry
- Documentation of cerebral arterial CO_2 reactivity and autoregulation
- Determination of need for blood replacement
- Objective assessment of volume status
- Detection of perfusion cannula malposition
- Detection of malperfusion syndrome
- Optimization of normothermic and hypothermic acid-base management
- Guidance of supplementary cerebral perfusion during systemic circulatory arrest

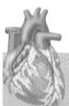

BOX 16-15. MULTIMODALITY NEUROMONITORING FOR CARDIAC SURGERY

Modality	Function
Electroencephalography	Cortical synaptic activity
Brainstem auditory-evoked potentials	Cochlear, auditory nerve, and brainstem auditory pathway function
Middle-latency auditory-evoked potentials function	Subcortical-cortical afferent auditory pathway
Somatosensory-evoked potentials	Peripheral nerve, spinal cord, and brain somatosensory afferent pathway function
Transcranial motor-evoked potentials	Cortical, subcortical, spinal cord, and peripheral nerve efferent motor pathway function
Transcranial Doppler ultrasonography	Cerebral blood flow change and emboli detection
Tissue oximetry	Regional tissue oxygen balance

SUMMARY

SSEPs assess function of the afferent somatosensory pathways, whereas transcranial electric MEPs monitor neural transmission through efferent motor pathways. Integrity and function of the subcortical and cortical portions of the afferent auditory pathway may be monitored, respectively, by BAEPs and MLAEPs. The EEG is an exquisitely sensitive measure of cerebral cortical synaptic function. Modern display and numeric trending techniques make it practical for the cardiac anesthesia provider to monitor multichannel EEG and evoked potentials. The EEG aids rapid detection of cerebral ischemia/hypoxia and seizure activity. Both EEG and MLAEPs quantify hypnotic adequacy, whereas the MLAEP and upper facial EMG may aid in assessment of nociception. EEG, SSEPs, and BAEPs offer simple measures of effective brain cooling. However, despite their sensitivity, EEG and evoked potential information is not specific. The cause of detected synaptic suppression must be determined by other techniques. Among these is TCD ultrasound, which continuously characterizes brain blood flow changes. In addition, TCD detects cerebral microemboli, regardless of their source or composition. Vital cerebral hemodynamic imbalance can be detected by TCD, but it offers no direct information on neuronal metabolism. This essential element is provided by cerebral oximetry, which describes changes in the regional balance of oxygen supply and demand. Recent application of this technology to noncerebral tissue has further expanded opportunity for the detection of regional tissue hypoxia. Thus, collectively, these monitoring modalities function "hand-in-glove." Newly developed, integrated, multimodality displays facilitate identification of physiologic imbalance, its causes, and the patient's response to corrective action. The risks of neuromonitoring are minimal, the costs modest, and the clinical and economic benefits substantial; cardiac surgery neuromonitoring is an established and expanding reality.

Disclosure

H.L.E. is a member of the Covidien speakers' bureau.

Acknowledgment

I am grateful for the editorial assistance of my wife, Jeanne.

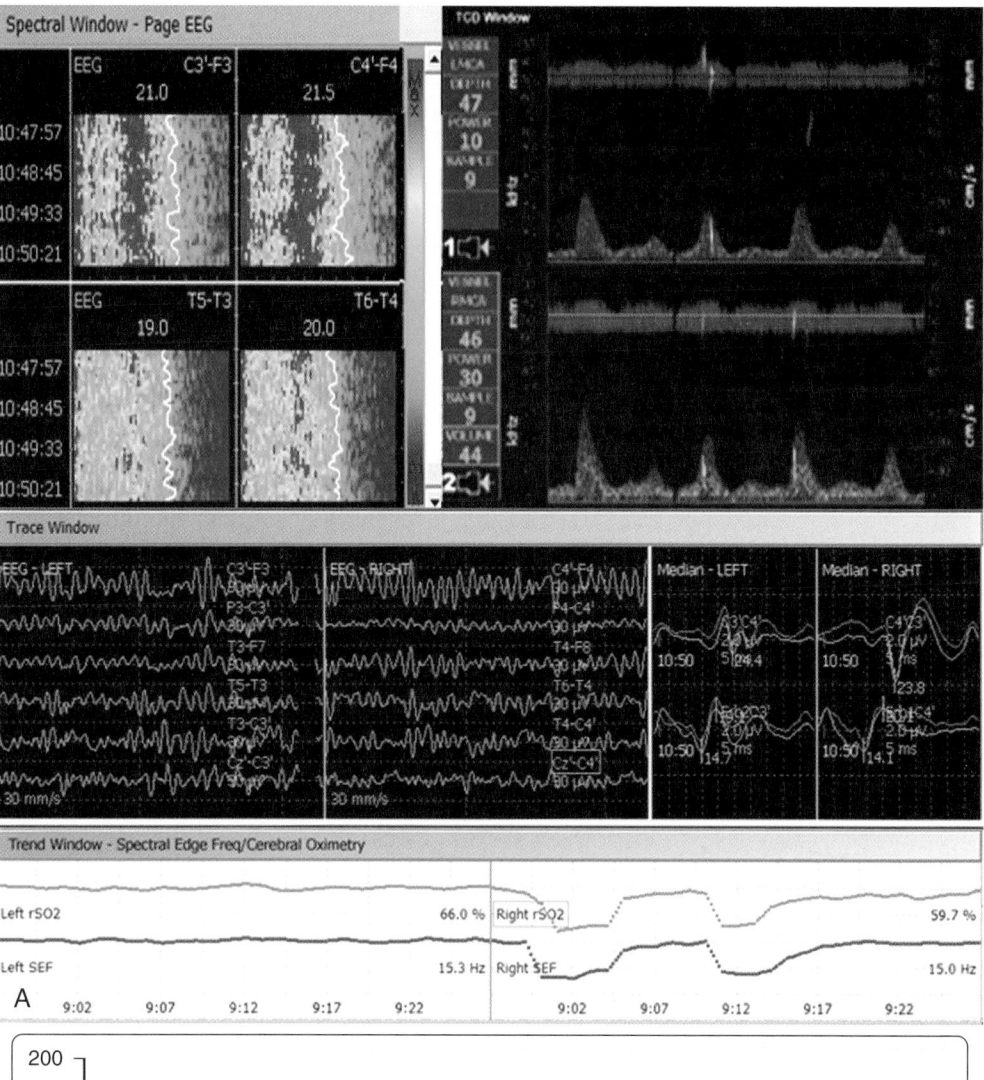

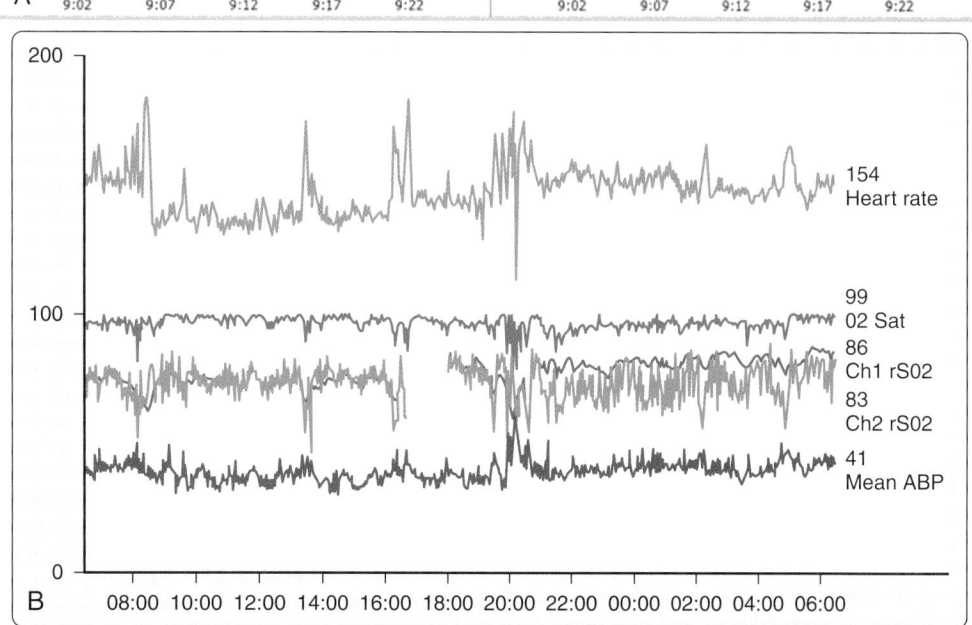

Figure 16-40 *A,* Multimodality neuromonitoring signals may be viewed on a single computer screen. In this case, the bilateral information includes: (1) a color density spectral array electroencephalographic (EEG) trend (top left), (2) traditional EEG (middle left), (3) EEG spectral edge frequency (SEF) and brain regional oxygen saturation (rSo$_2$) trends (bottom left), (4) upper limb somatosensory-evoked potentials to median nerve stimulation (middle right), and (5) transcranial Doppler (TCD) M-mode and frequency spectral displays (top right). *B,* Other multimodality analysis and display systems permit integration of information from many different physiologic monitors, ventilators, infusion pumps, and so on, into a unified, single time-base display. For example, this new FDA-approved system illustrates the integration of bilateral cerebral oximetry data with key physiologic signals from a neonatal critical care monitor. *(A, Courtesy of Axon Systems, Hauppauge, NY; the Vital Synch™ display is courtesy of Somanetics Corporation and was modified with permission.)*

REFERENCES

1. Newman MF, Kirchner JL, Phillips-Bute B, et al: Longitudinal assessment of neurocognitive function after coronary artery bypass surgery, *N Engl J Med* 344:395, 2001.
2. Roach GW, Kanchuger M, Mangano CM, et al: Adverse cerebral outcomes after coronary bypass surgery, *N Engl J Med* 335:1857, 1996.
3. Kilo J, Dzerny M, Gorlitzer M, et al: Cardiopulmonary bypass affects cognitive brain function after coronary artery bypass grafting, *Ann Thorac Surg* 72:1926, 2001.
4. Edmonds HL Jr, Rodriguez RA, Audenaert SM, et al: The role of neuromonitoring in cardiovascular surgery, *J Cardiothorac Vasc Anesth* 10:15, 1996.
5. Edmonds HL Jr: Detection and treatment of cerebral hypoxia are key to avoiding intraoperative brain injuries, *J Clin Monit Comput* 16:69, 2000.
6. Theye RA, Patrick RT, Kirklin JW: The electroencephalogram in patients undergoing open intracardiac operations with the aid of extracorporeal circulation, *J Thorac Surg* 34:709, 1957.
7. Blume WT, Sharbrough FW: EEG monitoring during carotid endarterectomy and open heart surgery. In Niedermeyer E, Lopes Da Silva F, editors: *Electroencephalography*, ed 4, Philadelphia, Lippincott Williams & Wilkins, 1999, pp 797–808.
8. Craft RM, Losasso TJ, Perkins WJ, et al: EEG monitoring or cerebral ischemia during carotid endarterectomy: How much is enough? *Anesthesiology* 81(3A):A214, 1994 (abstract).
9. Edmonds HL Jr, Sehic A, Gruenthal M: Comparison of 2-, 4- and 16-channel EEG for detection of cerebral ischemia, *Anesthesiology* 97(3A):A–305, 2002 (abstract).
10. Levy WJ: Monitoring of the electroencephalogram during cardiopulmonary bypass. Know when to say when, *Anesthesiology* 76:876, 1992.
11. Timofeev I, Contreras D, Steriade M: Synaptic responsiveness of cortical and thalamic neurons during various phases of slow sleep oscillation in cat, *J Neurophysiol (Lond)* 494:265, 1996.
12. Stockard J, Bickford RG: The neurophysiology of anaesthesia. In Gordon E, editor: *A basis and practice of neuroanaesthesia*, Amsterdam, 1975, Excerpta Medica, pp 3–46.
13. Sharbrough FW: Nonspecific abnormal EEG patterns. In Niedermeyer E, Lopes da Silva F, editors: *Electroencephalography*, ed 4, Philadelphia, Lippincott Williams & Wilkins, 1999, pp 215–234.
14. Goldstein L: Psychotropic drug-induced EEG changes as revealed by the amplitude integration method, *Mod Probl Pharmacopsychiatr* 8:131, 1974.
15. Prior PM, Maynard DE, Sheaff PC, et al: Monitoring cerebral function: Clinical experience with a new device for continuous recording of electrical activity of the brain, *Br Med J* 2:215, 1971.
16. Hellström-Westas L, de Vries LD, Rosén I: *An atlas of amplitude-integrated EEGs in the newborn*, Boca Raton, FL, Parthenon, 2003.
17. Pronk RAF: *EEG processing in cardiac surgery*, Utrecht, Institute of Medical Physics TNO, 1982.
18. Rampil I: EEG processing and the bispectral index, *Anesthesiology* 89:815, 1998.
19. Hoymork SC, Hval K, Jensen EW, et al: Can the cerebral state monitor replace the bispectral index in monitoring hypnotic effect during propofol/remifentanil anaesthesia? *Acta Anaesthesiol Scand* 51:210, 2007.
20. Russell IF: The Narcotrend 'depth of anaesthesia' monitor cannot reliably detect consciousness during general anaesthesia: An investigation using the isolated forearm technique, *Br J Anaesth* 96:346, 2006.
21. Drover D, Ortega H: Patient state index, *Best Pract Res Clin Anaesth* 20:121, 2006.
22. Viertiö-Oja H, Maja V, Särkelä M, et al: Description of the Entropy™ algorithm as applied in the Datex-Omeda S/5™ Entropy Module, *Acta Anaesthesiol Scand* 48:154, 2004.
23. Wong CA, Fragen RJ, Fitzgerald P, et al: A comparison of the SNAP II and BIS XP indices during sevoflurane and nitrous oxide anaesthesia at 1 and 1.5 MAC and at awakening, *Br J Anaesth* 97:181, 2006.
24. Myles PS, Leslie K, McNeil J, et al: Bispectral index monitoring to prevent awareness during anaesthesia. The B-Aware randomized controlled trial, *Lancet* 363:1757, 2004.
25. Punjasawadwong Y, Boonjeungmonkol N, Phongchiewboon A: Bispectral index for improving anaesthetic delivery and postoperative recovery, *Cochrane Database Syst Rev* 4: CD003843, 2007
26. Paloheimo M: Quantitative surface electromyography (qEMG): Applications in anaesthesiology and critical care, *Acta Anaesthesiol Scand Suppl* 93:1, 1990.
27. Joy RM: Spectral analysis of long EEG samples for comparative purposes, *Neuropharmacology* 10:471, 1971 (abstract).
28. Myers RR, Stockard JJ, Fleming NI, et al: The use of on-line telephonic computer analysis of the EEG in anaesthesia, *Br J Anaesth* 45:664, 1973.
29. Pichylmayr I, Lips U: EEG monitoring in anesthesiology and intensive care, *Neuropsychobiology* 10:239, 1983.
30. Fleming RA, Smith NT: An inexpensive device for analyzing and monitoring the electroencephalogram, *Anesthesiology* 50:456, 1979.
31. Isley MR, Edmonds HL Jr, Stecker M: Guidelines for intraoperative neuromonitoring using raw (analog or digital waveforms) and quantitative electroencephalography: A position statement by the American Society of Neurophysiological Monitoring, *J Clin Monit Comput* 23:369–390, 2009.
32. Van Huffelen AC: Electroencephalography used in monitoring neural function during surgery. In Nuwer MR, editor: *Handbook of clinical neurophysiology*, vol 8, Intraoperative monitoring of neural function, New York, Elsevier, 2008, pp 128–140.
33. Jäntti V, Sloan TB: EEG and anesthetic effects. In Nuwer MR, editor: *Handbook of clinical neurophysiology*, vol 8, Intraoperative monitoring of neural function, New York, Elsevier, 2008, pp 94–127.
34. Gugino LD, Aglio LS, Yli-Hankala A: Monitoring the electroencephalogram during bypass procedures, *Semin Cardiothorac Vasc Anesth* 8:61, 2004.
35. Williams GD, Ramamoorthy C: Brain monitoring and protection during pediatric cardiac surgery, *Semin Cardiothorac Vasc Anesth* 11:23, 2007.
36. Alkire MT: Quantitative EEG correlation with brain glucose metabolic rate during anesthesia in volunteers, *Anesthesiology* 89:323, 1998.
37. Gusev EI, Fedin Al, Erokhin OY, et al: Compressed spectral analysis of the EEG in patients with acute cerebrovascular disturbance, *Neurosci Behav Physiol* 15:144, 1985.
38. Oda Y, Tanaka K, Matsuura T, et al: Nitrous oxide induced paradoxical electroencephalographic changes after tracheal intubation during isoflurane and sevoflurane anesthesia, *Anesth Analg* 102:1094, 2006.
39. Rodriguez RA, Cornel G, Semelhago L, et al: Cerebral effects in superior vena caval obstruction: The role of brain monitoring, *Ann Thorac Surg* 64:1820, 1997.
40. Orth VH, Rehm M, Thiel M, et al: First clinical implications of perioperative red cell volume measurement with a nonradioactive marker, *Anesth Analg* 87:1234, 1998.
41. Hanel F, von Knobelsdorff G, Werner C, et al: Hypercapnia prevents jugular bulb desaturation during rewarming from hypothermic cardiopulmonary bypass, *Anesthesiology* 89:19, 1998.
42. Gugino LD, Chabot RJ, Aglio LS, et al: QEEG changes during cardiopulmonary bypass: Relationship to postoperative neuropsychological function, *Clin Electroencephalogr* 30:53, 1999.
43. Croughwell ND, Newman MF, Blumenthal JA, et al: Jugular bulb saturation and cognitive dysfunction after cardiopulmonary bypass, *Ann Thorac Surg* 58:1702, 1994.
44. Ederberg S, Westerlind A, Houltz E, et al: The effects of propofol on cerebral blood flow velocity and cerebral oxygen extraction during cardiopulmonary bypass, *Anesth Analg* 86:1201, 1998.
45. BhaskerRao B, VanHimbergen D, Edmonds HL Jr, et al: Evidence for improved cerebral function after minimally invasive bypass surgery, *J Card Surg* 13:27, 1998.
46. Reddy RV, Moorthy SS, Dierdorf SF, et al: Excitatory effects and electroencephalographic correlation of etomidate, thiopental, methohexital and propofol, *Anesth Analg* 77:1008, 1993.
47. Yli-Hankala A, Vakkuri A, Sarkela M, et al: Epileptiform EEG during induction of anesthesia with sevoflurane mask, *Anesthesiology* 91:1596, 1999.
48. Kearse LA Jr, Koski G, Husain MV, et al: Epileptiform activity during opioid anesthesia, *Electroencephalogr Clin Neurophysiol* 87:374, 1993.
49. Bellinger DC, Wypij D, Kuban KC, et al: Developmental and neurological status of children at 4 years of age after heart surgery with hypothermic circulatory arrest or low-flow cardiopulmonary bypass, *Circulation* 100:526, 1999.
50. Martin WH, Stecker MM: ASNM position statement: Intraoperative monitoring of auditory-evoked potentials, *J Clin Monit Comput* 22:75, 2008.
51. Legatt AD: BAEPs in surgery. In Nuwer MR, editor: *Handbook of clinical neurophysiology*, vol 8, Intraoperative monitoring of neural function, New York, Elsevier, 2008, pp 334–349.
52. Rodriguez RA: Human auditory evoked potentials in the assessment of brain function during major cardiovascular surgery, *Semin Cardiothorac Vasc Anesth* 8:85, 2004.
53. Thornton C: Evoked potentials in anaesthesia, *Eur J Anaesth* 8:89, 1991.
54. Kraus N, Smith DI, Reed NL: Auditory middle latency responses in children: Effects of age and diagnostic category, *Electroencephalogr Clin Neurophysiol* 62:343, 1985.
55. Musialowicz T, Niskanen M, Yppärilä-Wolters H, et al: Auditory-evoked potentials in bispectral index-guided anaesthesia for cardiac surgery, *Eur J Anaesth* 24:571, 2007.
56. Lamas A, López-Herce J, Sancho L, et al: Assessment of the level of sedation in children after cardiac surgery, *Ann Thorac Surg* 88:144, 2009.
57. Struys M, Jensen EW, Smith W, et al: Performance of the ARX-derived auditory evoked potential index as an indicator of anesthetic depth, *Anesthesiology* 96:803, 2002.
58. Bonhomme V, Llabres V, Dewandre P-Y, et al: Combined use of bispectral index and A-Line autoregressive index to assess the anti-nociceptive component of balanced anesthesia during lumbar arthrodesis, *Br J Anaesth* 93:353, 2006.
59. Rodriguez RA, Audenaert SM, Austin EH: Auditory evoked responses in children during hypothermic cardiopulmonary bypass, *J Clin Neurophysiol* 12:168, 1995.
60. Stone JG, Young WL, Smith CR, et al: Do standard monitoring sites reflect true brain temperature when profound hypothermia is rapidly induced and reversed? *Anesthesiology* 82:344, 1995.
61. Duebener LF, Hagino I, Sakamoto T, et al: Effects of pH management during deep hypothermic bypass on cerebral microcirculation: Alpha-stat versus pH-stat, *Circulation* 106(12 Suppl I):I–103, 2002.
62. Toleikis JR: Intraoperative monitoring using somatosensory evoked potentials: A position statement by the American Society of Neurophysiological Monitoring, *J Clin Monit Comput* 19:241, 2005.
63. Nuwer MR, Packwood JW: Somatosensory evoked potential monitoring with scalp and cervical recording. Nuwer MR, editor: *Handbook of clinical neurophysiology*, vol 8, Intraoperative monitoring of neural function, New York, Elsevier, 2008, pp 180–189.
64. Guérit J-M: Intraoperative monitoring during carotid endarterectomy. In Nuwer MR, editor: *Handbook of clinical neurophysiology*, vol 8, Intraoperative monitoring of neural function, New York, Elsevier, 2008, pp 776–790.
65. Guérit J-M: Intraoperative monitoring during cardiac surgery. In Nuwer MR, editor: *Handbook of clinical neurophysiology*, vol 8, Intraoperative monitoring of neural function, New York, Elsevier, 2008, pp 829–839.
66. Stecker MM: Evoked potentials during cardiac and major vascular operations, *Semin Cardiothorac Vasc Anesth* 8:101, 2004.
67. Cassells CD, Lindsey RW, Ebersole J, et al: Ulnar neuropathy after median sternotomy, *Clin Orthop Relat Res* 291:259, 1993.
68. Seal D, Galaton J, Coupland SG, et al: Somatosensory evoked potential monitoring during cardiac surgery: An examination of brachial plexus dysfunction, *J Cardiothorac Vasc Anesth* 11:187, 1997.
69. Lorenzini NA, Poterack KA: Somatosensory evoked potentials are not a sensitive indicator of potential positioning injury in the prone patient, *J Clin Monit Comput* 12:171, 1996.
70. Ostry S, Stejskal L, Kramer F, et al: Hypercapnia impact on vascular and neuronal reactivity, *Zent Neurochir* 68:59, 2007.
71. Astarci P, Guérit J-M, Robert A, et al: Stump pressure and somatosensory evoked potentials for predicting the use of shunt during carotid surgery, *Ann Vasc Surg* 21:312, 2007.
72. Moritz S, Kasprzak P, Arit M, et al: A comparison of transcranial Doppler sonography, near-infrared spectroscopy, stump pressure and somatosensory evoked potentials, *Anesthesiology* 107:563, 2007.
73. Guérit JM, Verhelst R, Rubay J, et al: The use of somatosensory evoked potentials to determine the optimal degree of hypothermia during circulatory arrest, *J Card Surg* 9:596, 1994.
74. Journee HL: Motor EP physiology, risks and specific anesthetic effects. In Nuwer MR, editor: *Handbook of clinical neurophysiology*, vol 8, Intraoperative monitoring of neural function, New York, Elsevier, 2008, pp 218–234.
75. Deletis V, Sala F: Corticospinal tract monitoring with D- and I-waves from the spinal cord and muscle MEPs from limb muscles. In Nuwer MR, editor: *Handbook of clinical neurophysiology*, vol 8, Intraoperative monitoring of neural function, New York, Elsevier, 2008, pp 235–251.
76. Burke D: Recording MEPs to transcranial electrical stimulation and SEPs to peripheral nerve stimulation simultaneously from the spinal cord. In Nuwer MR, editor: *Handbook of clinical neurophysiology*, vol 8, Intraoperative monitoring of neural function, New York, Elsevier, 2008, pp 252–259.
77. Mendiratta A, Emerson RG: Transcranial electrical MEP with muscle recording. In Nuwer MR, editor: *Handbook of clinical neurophysiology*, vol 8, Intraoperative monitoring of neural function, New York, Elsevier, 2008, pp 260–272.
78. Sloan TB: Electrophysiologic monitoring during surgery to repair the thoracoabdominal aorta, *Semin Cardiothorac Vasc Anesth* 8:113, 2004.
79. MacDonald DB, Dong CCJ: Spinal cord monitoring during descending aortic procedures. In Nuwer MR, editor: *Handbook of clinical neurophysiology*, vol 8, Intraoperative monitoring of neural function, New York, Elsevier, 2008, pp 815–828.
80. Webb TH, Williams GM: Thoracoabdominal aneurysm repair, *Cardiovasc Surg* 7:573, 1999.
81. Chen Z: The effects of isoflurane and propofol on intraoperative neurophysiologic monitoring during spinal surgery, *J Clin Monit Comput* 18:303–308, 2004.
82. Kawanishi Y, Munakata H, Matsumori M, et al: Usefulness of transcranial motor evoked potentials during thoracoabdominal aortic surgery, *Ann Thorac Surg* 83:456, 2007.
83. Sloan TB, Jäntti V: Anesthetic effects on evoked potentials. In Nuwer MR, editor: *Handbook of clinical neurophysiology*, vol 8, Intraoperative monitoring of neural function, New York, Elsevier, 2008, pp 94–126.
84. Etz CD, Halstead JC, Spielvogel D, et al: Thoracic and thoracoabdominal aneurysm repair: Is reimplantation of spinal cord arteries a waste of time? *Ann Thorac Surg* 82:1670, 2006.
85. Georgiadis D, Siebler M: Detection of microembolic signals with transcranial Doppler ultrasound, *Front Neurol Neurosci* 21:194–205, 2006.
86. Nitzöld A, Khattab A, Eggers J: Microemboli in aortic valve replacement, *Exp Rev Cardiovasc Therap* 4:853, 2006.
87. Zuj KA, Greaves DK, Hughson RL: WISE-2005: Reduced cerebral blood flow velocity with nitroglycerin—comparison with common carotid artery blood flow, *J Gravit Physiol* 14:P65, 2007.
88. Rudolph JL, Sorond FA, Pochay VE, et al: Cerebral hemodynamics during coronary artery bypass graft surgery: The effect of carotid stenosis, *Ultrasound Med Biol* 35:1235, 2009.
89. Polito A, Ricci Z, Di Chiara L, et al: Cerebral blood flow during cardiopulmonary bypass in pediatric cardiac surgery: The role of transcranial Doppler—a systematic review of the literature, *Cardiovasc Ultrasound* 4:47, 2006.

90. Singer I, Edmonds HL Jr: Changes in cerebral perfusion during third-generation implantable cardioverter-defibrillator testing, *Am Heart J* 127:1052, 1994.
91. Edmonds HL Jr, Singer I, Sehic A, et al: Multimodality neuromonitoring for neurocardiology, *J Interv Cardiol* 11:197, 1998.
92. Edmonds HL Jr: Protective effect of neuromonitoring during cardiac surgery, *Ann N Y Acad Sci* 1053:12, 2005.
93. McCarthy RJ, McCabe AE, Walker R, et al: The value of transcranial Doppler in predicting cerebral ischaemia during carotid endarterectomy, *Eur J Vasc Endovasc Surg* 21:408, 2001.
94. Chuang WC, Short JH, McKinney AM, et al: Reversible left hemisphere ischemia secondary to carotid compression in Eagle Syndrome: Surgical and CT angiographic correlation, *Am J Neuroradiol* 28:143, 2007.
95. Khoynezhad A, Kruse MJ, Donayre CE, et al: Use of transcranial Doppler ultrasound in endovascular repair of a Type B aortic dissection, *Ann Thorac Surg* 86:289, 2008.
96. Petrica L, Petrica M, Vlad A, et al: Cerebrovascular reactivity is impaired in patients with non-insulin-dependent diabetes mellitus and microangiopathy, *Wien Klin Wochenschrift* 119:365, 2007.
97. Panerai R: Transcranial Doppler for evaluation of cerebral autoregulation, *Clin Autonom Res* 19:197, 2009.
98. Borger MA, Taylor RL, Weisel RD, et al: Decreased cerebral emboli during distal aortic arch cannulation: A randomized clinical trial, *J Thorac Cardiovasc Surg* 118:740, 1999.
99. Mullges W, Franke D, Reents W, et al: Brain microembolic counts during extracorporeal circulation depend on aortic cannula position, *Ultrasound Med Biol* 27:933, 2001.
100. Rodriguez RA, Cornel G, Semelhago L, et al: Cerebral effects in superior vena caval cannula obstruction: The role of brain monitoring, *Ann Thorac Surg* 64:1820, 1997.
101. Ganzel BL, Edmonds HL Jr, Pank JR, et al: Neurophysiological monitoring to assure delivery of retrograde cerebral perfusion, *J Thorac Cardiovasc Surg* 113:748, 1997.
102. Gugino LD, Aglio LS, Edmonds HL Jr: Neurophysiological monitoring in vascular surgery, *Bailliere's Clin Anaesth* 14:17, 2000.
103. Jones TJ, Deal DD, Vernon JC, et al: How effective are cardiopulmonary bypass circuits at removing gaseous microemboli? *J Extra Corpor Technol* 34:151, 2002.
104. Yeh TJ Jr, Austin EH III, Sehic A, et al: Role of neuromonitoring in the detection and correction of cerebral air embolism, *J Thorac Cardiovasc Surg* 126:589, 2003.
105. Edmonds HL Jr: Emboli and renal dysfunction in CABG patients, *J Cardiothorac Vasc Anesth* 18:545, 2004 (editorial).
106. Shen Q, Stuart J, Venkatesh B, et al: Interobserver variability of the transcranial Doppler ultrasound technique. Impact of lack of practice on the accuracy of measurement, *J Clin Monit Comput* 15:179, 1999.
107. Edmonds HL Jr, Isley MR, Sloan T, et al: American Society of Neurophysiologic Monitoring (ASNM) & American Society of Neuroimaging (ASN) joint guidelines for transcranial Doppler (TCD) ultrasonic monitoring, *J Neuroimaging* (in press). DOI:10.1111j. 1552-6569. 2010. 00471.
108. Doblar DD: Intraoperative transcranial ultrasonic monitoring for cardiac and vascular surgery, *Semin Cardiothorac Vasc Anesth* 8:127, 2010.
109. Edmonds HL Jr: Monitoring of cerebral perfusion with transcranial Doppler ultrasound. In Nuwer MR, editor: *Handbook of clinical neurophysiology*, vol 8, Intraoperative monitoring of neural function, New York, Elsevier, 2008, pp 909–923.
110. Estrera AL, Garami Z, Miller CC III, et al: Cerebral monitoring with transcranial Doppler ultrasonography improves neurologic outcome during repairs of acute type A aortic dissection, *J Thorac Cardiovasc Surg* 129:277, 2005.
111. Moppett IK, Sherman RW, Wild MJ, et al: Effects of norepinephrine and glyceryl trinitrate on cerebral haemodynamics: Transcranial Doppler study in health volunteers, *Br J Anaesth* 100:240, 2008.
112. Bhatia A, Gupta AK: Neuromonitoring in the intensive care unit. II. Cerebral oxygenation monitoring and microdialysis, *Intensive Care Med* 19:97, 2007.
113. Chieregato A, Calzolari F, Frasforini G, et al: Normal jugular bulb saturation, *J Neurol Neurosurg Psychiatry* 74:784, 2003.
114. Mutch WAC, Ryner LN, Kozlowski P, et al: Cerebral hypoxia during cardiopulmonary bypass: A magnetic resonance imaging study, *Ann Thorac Surg* 64:695, 1997.
115. deVries JW, Visser GH, Bakker PFA: Neuromonitoring in defibrillation threshold testing. A comparison between near-infrared spectroscopy and jugular bulb oximetry, *J Clin Monit Comput* 13:303, 1997.
116. Vallet B: Physiologic transfusion triggers, *Best Pract Res Clin Anaesth* 21:173, 2007.
117. Shaaban AM, Harmer M, Kirkham F: Cardiopulmonary bypass temperature and brain function, *Anaesth* 60:365, 2005.
118. Diephuis JC, Moons KG, Nierich AN, et al: Jugular bulb desaturation during coronary artery surgery: A comparison of off-pump and on-pump procedures, *Br J Anaesth* 94:715, 2005.
119. Ferari M, Mottola L, Quaresima V: Principles, techniques and limitations of near-infrared spectroscopy, *Can J Appl Physiol* 29:463, 2004.
120. Kurth CD, Steven JM, Benaron D, et al: Near-infrared monitoring of the cerebral circulation, *J Clin Monit Comput* 9:163, 1993.
121. Stingele R, Schnippering H, Keller E, et al: Transcranial oximetry using fast near-infrared spectroscopy can detect failure of collateral blood supply in humans, *Comp Biochem Physiol A Mol Integr Physiol* 134:534, 2003.
122. Hirsch JC, Charpie JR, Ohye RG, et al: Near-infrared spectroscopy: What we know and what we need to know—a systematic review of the congenital heart disease literature, *J Thorac Caradiovasc Surg* 137:154, 2009.
123. Chelette TL, Albery WB, Esken RL, et al: Female exposure to high G: Performance of simulated flight after 24 hours of sleep deprivation, *Aviat Space Environ Med* 69:862, 1998.
124. Mortiz S, Kasprzak P, Arlt M, et al: Accuracy of cerebral monitoring in detecting cerebral ischemia during carotid endarterectomy, *Anesthesiology* 107:563, 2007.
125. Griepp RB: Panel discussion: Session II—aortic arch, *Ann Thorac Surg* 83:S824, 2007.
126. Wernovsky G, Ghanayem N, Ohye RC, et al: Hypoplastic left heart syndrome: Consensus and controversies in 2007, *Cardiol Young* 17:75, 2007.
127. Goldman SM, Sutter FP, Wertan MAC, et al: Outcome improvement and cost reduction in an increasingly morbid cardiac surgery population, *Semin Cardiothorac Vasc Anesth* 10:171, 2006.
128. Murkin JM: NIRS: A standard of care for CPB vs. an evolving standard for selective cerebral perfusion? *J Extra Corpor Technol* 41:P11, 2009.
129. Casati A, Fanelli G, Pietropaoli P, et al: Continuous monitoring of cerebral oxygen saturation in elderly patients undergoing major abdominal surgery minimizes brain exposure to potential hypoxia, *Anesth Analg* 101:740, 2005.
130. Baker RA, Knight JL: The OXICAB Trial: Cerebral oximetry in adult cardiac surgical patients, *J Extra Corpor Technol* 8:77, 2006 (abstract).
131. Murkin JM, Adams SJ, Novick RJ, et al: Monitoring brain oxygen saturation during coronary bypass surgery: A randomized, prospective study, *Anesth Analg* 104:51, 2007.
132. Schön J, Serien V, Hanke T, et al: Cerebral oxygen saturation monitoring in on-pump cardiac surgery—a 1 year experience, *Appl Cardiopulm Pathophysiol* 13:243, 2009.
133. Heringlake M, Serien V, Heinze H, et al: Cerebral oxygenation monitoring in patients undergoing deep hypothermic circulatory arrest for cardiothoracic surgery, *Appl Cardiopulm Pathophysiol* 11:45, 2007.
134. Hong SW, Shim JK, Choi YS, et al: Prediction of cognitive dysfunction and patients' outcome following valvular heart surgery and the role of cerebral oximetry, *Eur J Cardiothorac Surg* 33:560, 2008.
135. Schön J, Serien V, Heinze H, et al: Association between cerebral desaturation and an increased risk of stroke in patients undergoing deep hypothermic circulatory arrest for cardiothoracic surgery, *Appl Cardiopulm Pathphysiol* 13:201, 2009.
136. Slater JP, Guarino T, Stack J, et al: Cerebral oxygen desaturation predicts cognitive decline and longer hospital stay after cardiac surgery, *Ann Thorac Surg* 87:36, 2009.
137. Pattinson KTS, Imray CHE, Wright AD: What does cerebral oximetry measure? *Br J Anaesth* 94:863, 2005.
138. Davies LK, Janelle GM: Con: All cardiac surgical patients should have intraoperative cerebral oxygenation monitoring, *J Cardiothorac Vasc Anesth* 20:450, 2006.
139. Edmonds HL Jr, Ganzel BL, Austin EH 3rd: Cerebral oximetry for cardiac and vascular surgery, *Semin Cardiothorac Vasc Anesth* 8:147, 2004.
140. Murkin JM, Arango M: Near-infrared spectroscopy as an index of brain and tissue oxygenation, *Br J Anaesth* 103(BJA/PGA Suppl):i3, 2009.
141. Fischer GW: Recent advances in application of cerebral oximetry in adult cardiovascular surgery, *Semin Cardiothorac Vasc Anesth* 12:60, 2008.
142. MacLeod DB, Ikeda K, Keifer J, et al: Validation of the CAS adult cerebral oximeter during hypoxia in healthy volunteers, *Anesth Analg* 102:S162, 2006 (abstract).
143. MacLeod DB, Ideda K, Vacchiano C: Simultaneous comparison of FORE-SIGHT & INVOS cerebral oximeters to jugular bulb and arterial co-oximetry measures in healthy volunteers, *Anesth Analg* 108:SCA56, 2009 (abstract).
144. MacLeod DB, Ikeda K, Vacchiano C: Validation of the Nonin's dual emitter cerebral oximeter during oxygen desaturation in healthy adults, *Anesthesiology* 111:A1021, 2009 (abstract).
145. Gagnon RE, Macnab AJ, Gagnon FA, et al: Comparison of two spatially resolved NIRS oxygenation indices, *J Clin Monit Comput* 17:385, 2002.
146. de Letter J, Sie HT, Moll F, et al: Transcranial cerebral oximetry during carotid endarterectomy: Agreement between frontal and lateral probe measurements as compared with an electroencephalogram, *Cardiovasc Surg* 6:373, 1998.
147. Gopinath SP, Robertson CS, Grossman RG, et al: Near-infrared spectroscopic localization of intracranial hematomas, *J Neurosurg* 79:43, 1993.
148. Sehic A, Thomas MH: Cerebral oximetry during carotid endarterectomy: Signal failure resulting from large frontal sinus defect, *J Cardiothorac Vasc Anesth* 13:444, 2000.
149. Pigula FA, Siewers RD, Nemoto E: Hypothermic cardiopulmonary bypass alters oxygen/glucose uptake in the pediatric brain, *J Thorac Cardiovasc Surg* 121:366, 2001.
150. Kim MB, Ward DS, Cartwright CR: Estimation of jugular venous O_2 saturation from cerebral oximetry or arterial O_2 saturation during isocapnic hypoxia, *J Clin Monit* 16:191, 2000.
151. Daubeney PE, Pilkington SN, Janke E: Cerebral oxygenation measured by near-infrared spectroscopy: Comparison with jugular bulb oximetry, *Ann Thorac Surg* 61:930, 1996.
152. Holzschuh M, Woertgen C, Metz C: Dynamic changes of cerebral oxygenation measured by brain tissue oxygen pressure and near-infrared spectroscopy, *Neurol Res* 19:246, 1997.
153. Brawanski A, Faltermeier R, Rothoerl RD: Comparison of near-infrared spectroscopy and tissue Po_2 time series in patients after head injury and aneurysmal subarachnoid hemorrhage, *J Cereb Blood Flow Metab* 22:605, 2002.
154. Muehlschlegel S, Lobato EG: Con: All cardiac surgical patients should have intraoperative cerebral oxygenation monitoring, *J Cardiothorac Vasc Anesth* 20:613, 2006.
155. Edmonds HL Jr: Pro: All cardiac surgical patients should have intraoperative cerebral oxygenation monitoring, *J Cardiothorac Vasc Anesth* 20:445, 2006.
156. Hoffman GM: Pro: Near-infrared spectroscopy should be used for all cardiopulmonary bypass, *J Cardiothorac Vasc Anesth* 20:606, 2006.
157. Moller JT, Johannessen NW, Espersen K, et al: Randomized evaluation of pulse oximetry in 20,802 patients. II. Perioperative events and postoperative complications, *Anesthesiology* 78:445, 1993.
158. Eichhorn JH: Pulse oximetry as a standard of practice in anesthesia, *Anesthesiology* 78:423, 1993 (editorial).
159. Vohra HA, Modi A, Ohri SK: Does use of intra-operative cerebral regional oxygen saturation monitoring during cardiac surgery lead to improved clinical outcomes? *Interact Cardiovasc Thorac Surg* 9:318, 2009.
160. Kishi K, Kawaguchi M, Yoshitani K: Influence of patient variables and sensor location on regional cerebral oxygen saturation measured by INVOS 4100 near-infrared spectrometer, *J Neurosurg Anesth* 15:302, 2003.
161. Cho H, Nemoto E, Yonas H: Cerebral monitoring by means of oximetry and somatosensory evoked potentials during carotid endarterectomy, *J Neurosurg* 89:533, 1998.
162. Monk TG, Reno KA, Olsen BS, et al: Postoperative cognitive dysfunction is associated with cerebral oxygen desaturations, *Anesthesiology* 93:A167, 2000 (abstract).
163. Bhasker Rao B, Van Himbergen D, Jaber S, et al: Evidence for improved cerebral function after minimally invasive bypass surgery, *J Cardiac Surg* 13:27, 1998.
164. Yao FSF, Tseng CC, Trifiletti RR, et al: Low preoperative cerebral oxygen saturation is associated with postoperative frontal lobe and cognitive dysfunction and prolonged ICU and hospital stays, *Anesth Analg* 90:SCA30, 2000 (abstract).
165. Edmonds HL Jr, Austin EH 3rd, Seremet V, et al: Cost-benefit analysis of neuromonitoring for pediatric cardiac surgery, *Anesth Analg* 84:SCA22, 1997 (abstract).
166. Singer I, Dawn B, Edmonds HL Jr: Syncope is predicted by neuromonitoring in patients with ICDs, *PACE Pacing Clin Electrocardiol* 21(pt II):216, 1998.
167. Rodriguez-Nuñez A, Couceiro J, Alonso C: Cerebral oxygenation in children with syncope during head-upright tilt test, *Pediatr Cardiol* 18:406, 1997.
168. Tripp LD, Chelette T, Savul S: Female exposure to high G: Effects of simulated combat sorties on cerebral and arterial O_2 saturation, *Aviat Space Environ Med* 69:869, 1998.
169. Roberts KW, Crnkowic AP, Linneman LJ: Near-infrared spectroscopy detects critical cerebral hypoxia during carotid endarterectomy in awake patients, *Anesthesiology* 89(3A):A934, 1998 (abstract).
170. Samra SK, Dy EA, Welch K: Evaluation of a cerebral oximeter as a monitor of cerebral ischemia during carotid endarterectomy, *Anesthesiology* 93:964, 2000.
171. Denault A, Deschamps A, Murkin JM: A proposed algorithm for the intraoperative use of cerebral near-infrared spectroscopy, *Semin Cardiothorac Vasc Anesth* 11:274, 2007.
172. Hall RA, Fordyce DJ, Lee ME, et al: Brain SPECT imaging and neuropsychological testing in coronary artery bypass patients, *Ann Thorac Surg* 68:2082, 1999.
173. Nakamura Y, Kawachi K, Imagawa H, et al: The prevalence and severity of cerebrovascular disease in patients undergoing cardiovascular surgery, *Ann Thorac Cardiovasc Surg* 10:81, 2004.
174. Hadolt I, Litscher G: Noninvasive assessment of cerebral oxygenation during high altitude trekking in the Nepal Himalayas (2850-5600 m), *Neurol Res* 25:183, 2003.
175. Madsen PL, Nielsen HB, Christiansen P: Well-being and cerebral oxygen saturation during acute heart failure in humans, *Clin Physiol* 20:158, 2000.
176. Paquet C, Deschamps A, Denault AY, et al: Baseline regional cerebral oxygen saturation correlates with left ventricular systolic and diastolic function, *J Cardiothorac Vasc Anesth* 22:840, 2008.
177. Skhirtladze K, Birkenberg B, Mora B, et al: Cerebral desaturation during cardiac arrest: Its relation to arrest duration and left ventricular pump function, *Crit Care Med* 37:471, 2009.
178. Fenton KN, Freeman K, Glogowski K, et al: The significance of baseline cerebral oxygen saturation in children undergoing congenital heart surgery, *Am J Surg* 190:260, 2005.
179. Konishi A, Kikuchi K: Significance of regional cerebral oxygen saturation (rSo_2) during open heart surgery, *J Clin Anesth Jpn* 19:1759, 1995.

180. Nemoto E, Yonas H, Kassam A: Clinical experience with cerebral oximetry in stroke and cardiac arrest, *Crit Care Med* 28:1052, 2000.
181. Sehic A, Thomas MH: Cerebral oximetry during carotid endarterectomy: Signal failure resulting from large frontal sinus defect, *J Cardiothorac Vasc Anesth* 13:244, 2000.
182. Bar-Yosef S, Sanders EG, Grocott HP: Asymmetric cerebral near-infrared oximetric measurements during cardiac surgery, *J Cardiothorac Vasc Anesth* 17:773, 2003.
183. Fuchs G, Schwarz G, Kulier A: The influence of positioning on spectroscopic measurements of brain oxygenation, *J Neurosurg Anesthesiol* 12:75, 2000.
184. Boldrey E, Maass L, Miller ER: Role of atlantoid compression in etiology of internal carotid thrombosis, *J Neurosurg* 13:127, 1956.
185. Hardesty WH, Roberts S, Toole JF: Studies of carotid artery blood flow in man, *N Engl J Med* 263:944, 1960.
186. Toole JF, Tucker SH: Influence of head position upon cerebral circulation, *Arch Neurol* 2:616, 1960.
187. Lanier WL: Cerebral perfusion: Err on the side of caution, *Anesthesia Patient Safety Foundation Newsletter* 24:1, 2009.
188. Daubeney PEF, Smith DC, Pilkington SN: Cerebral oxygenation during paediatric cardiac surgery: Identification of vulnerable periods using near-infrared spectroscopy, *Eur J Cardiothorac Surg* 13:370, 1998.
189. Aavramides EJ, Murkin JM: The effect of surgical dislocation of the heart on cerebral blood flow in the presence of a single, two-state venous cannula during cardiopulmonary bypass, *Can J Anaesth* 43:A36, 1996 (abstract).
190. Paton B, Pearcy WC, Swan H: The importance of the electroencephalogram during cardiac surgery with particular reference to superior vena caval obstruction, *Surg Gynecol Obstet* 111:197, 1960.
191. Sakamoto T, Duebener LF, Laussen PC, et al: Cerebral ischemia caused by obstructed superior vena cava cannula is detected by near-infrared spectroscopy, *J Cardiothorac Vasc Anesth* 18:293, 2004.
192. Han S-H, Kim C-S, Lim C, et al: Obstruction of the superior vena cava cannula detected by desaturation of the cerebral oximeter, *J Cardiothorac Vasc Anesth* 19:420, 2005.
193. Gottlieb EA, Frazer CD Jr, Andropoulos DB, et al: Bilateral monitoring of cerebral oxygen saturation results in recognition of aortic cannula malposition during pediatric congenital heart surgery, *Paediatr Anaesth* 16:787, 2006.
194. Scholl FG, Webb D, Christian K, et al: Rapid diagnosis of cannula migration by cerebral oximetry in neonatal arch repair, *Ann Thorac Surg* 82:325, 2006.
195. Tirotta CF: Near-infrared spectroscopy for real-time cerebral/somatic oxygen monitoring, *Pediatr Anesth* 19:4, 2006.
196. Fukada J, Morishita K, Kawaharada N: Isolated cerebral perfusion for intraoperative cerebral malperfusion in type A aortic dissection, *Ann Thorac Surg* 75:266, 2003.
197. Joshi RK, Motta P, Horibe M, et al: Monitoring cerebral oxygenation in a pediatric patient undergoing surgery for vascular ring, *Paediatr Anaesth* 16:178, 2006.
198. Polito A, Ricci Z, DiChiara L, et al: Bilateral cerebral near-infrared spectroscopy monitoring during surgery for neonatal coarctation of the aorta, *Paediatr Anaesth* 17:906, 2007.
199. Schwartz JM, Vricella LA, Jeffries MA, et al: Cerebral oximetry guides treatment during Blalock-Taussig shunt procedure, *J Cardiothorac Vasc Anesth* 22:95, 2007.
200. Farouk A, Karimi M, Henderson M, et al: Cerebral regional oxygenation during aortic coarctation repair in pediatric population, *Eur J Cardiothorac Surg* 3:26, 2008.
201. Sakaguchi G, Komiya T, Tamura N, et al: Cerebral malperfusion in acute type A dissection: Direct innominate artery cannulation, *J Thorac Cardiovasc Surg* 129:1190, 2005.
202. Totaro P, Argano V: Innovative technique to treat acute cerebral and peripheral malperfusion during type A aortic dissection repair, *Interact Cardiovasc Thorac Surg* 7:133, 2008.
203. Khaladj N, Shrestha M, Peterss S, et al: Ascending aortic cannulation in acute aortic dissection type A: the Hannover experience, *Eur J Cardiothorac Surg* 34:792, 2008.
204. Yamashiro S, Kuniyoski Y, Arakaki K, et al: Intraoperative retrograde type I aortic dissection in a patient with chronic type IIIb dissecting aneurysm, *Interact Cardiovasc Thorac Surg* 8:283, 2009.
205. Borst HC, Laas J, Heinemann M: Type A aortic dissection: Diagnosis and management of malperfusion phenomena, *Semin Thorac Cardiovasc Surg* 3:238, 1991.
206. DuPlessis AJ: Near-infrared spectroscopy for the in vivo study of cerebral hemodynamics and oxygenation, *Curr Opin Pediatr* 7:632–639, 1995.
207. Liu R, Sun D, Hang Y, et al: Evaluation of cerebral oxygen balance by cerebral oximeter and transcranial Doppler during hypothermic cardiopulmonary bypass, *Anesthesiology* 89:A309, 1998 (abstract).
208. Kontos H: Regulation of cerebral circulation, *Ann Rev Physiol* 43:397, 1989.
209. Mandai K, Seuyoshi K, Fukunaga R, et al: Evaluation of cerebral vasoreactivity by three-dimensional time-of-flight magnetic resonance angiography, *Stroke* 25:1897, 1994.
210. Hosada K: Comparison of conventional region of interest and statistical mapping method in brain single-photon emission computed tomography for prediction of hyperperfusion after carotid endarterectomy, *Neurosurgery* 57:32, 2005.
211. Last D, de Bazelaire C, Alsop DC, et al: Global and regional effects of Type 2 diabetes on brain tissue volumes and cerebral vasoreactivity, *Diabetes Care* 30:1193, 2007.
212. Du Plessis AJ, Jonas RA, Wypij D: Perioperative effects of alpha-stat versus pH-stat strategies for deep hypothermic cardiopulmonary bypass in infants, *J Thorac Cardiovasc Surg* 114:991, 1997.
213. Vijay V, McCusker K, Stasko A, et al: Cerebral oximetry-directed permissive hypercapnia enhances cerebral perfusion during CPB for heart failure surgery, *Heart Surg Forum* 6:205, 2003.
214. Hoffman GM: Neurologic monitoring on cardiopulmonary bypass: What are we obligated to do? *Ann Thorac Surg* 81:S2373, 2006.
215. Baraka A, Naufal M, El-Khatib M: Cerebral oximetry during deep hypothermic circulatory arrest, *J Cardiothorac Vasc Anesth* 22:173, 2007.
216. Tobias JD, Russo P, Russo J: Changes in near-infrared spectroscopy during deep hypothermic circulatory arrest, *Ann Card Anaesth* 12:17, 2009.
217. Gosain A, Rabin J, Reymond JP: Tissue oxygen tension and other indicators of blood loss or organ perfusion during graded hemorrhage, *Surgery* 109:523, 1991.
218. Arkilic CF, Akça O, Taguchi M: Temperature monitoring and management during neuraxial anesthesia: An observational study, *Anesth Analg* 91:662, 2000.
219. Madl C, Eisenhuber E, Kramer L, et al: Impact of different hemoglobin levels on regional cerebral oxygen saturation, cerebral extraction of oxygen and sensory evoked potentials in septic shock, *Crit Care Med* 25(Suppl):4, 1997.
220. Blas M, Sulek C, Martin T: Use of near-infrared spectroscopy to monitor cerebral oxygenation during coronary artery bypass surgery in a patient with bilateral internal carotid artery occlusion, *J Cardiothorac Vasc Anesth* 6:732, 1999.
221. Vijay V, McCusker K, Stasko A, et al: Cerebral oximetry-based comparison of cerebral perfusion with standard versus condensed extracorporeal circuits in adult cardiac surgery, *Heart Surg Forum* 6:201, 2003.
222. McCusker K, Chalafant A, de Foe G, et al: Influence of hematocrit and pump prime on cerebral oxygen saturation in on-pump revascularization, *Perfusion* 21:149, 2006.
223. Torella F, Haynes SL, McCollum CN: Cerebral and peripheral oxygen saturation during red cell transfusion, *J Surg Res* 110:217, 2003.
224. Miyhaji K, Kohira S, Miyamoto T, et al: Pediatric cardiac surgery without homologous blood transfusion, using a miniaturized bypass system in infants with lower body weight, *J Thorac Cardiovasc Surg* 134:284, 2007.
225. Ging AL, St. Onge JR, Fitgerald DC, et al: Bloodless cardiac surgery and the pediatric patient: A case study, *Perfusion* 23:131, 2008.
226. Villafane J, Edmonds HL Jr: Volume expansion prevents tilt-induced syncope, *Cardiol Young* 11(Suppl 1):1168, 2001 (abstract).
227. Olsen KS, Svendsen B, Larsen FS: Validation of transcranial near-infrared spectroscopy for evaluation of cerebral blood flow autoregulation, *J Neurosurg Anesthesiol* 8:280, 1996.
228. Jalowiecki P, Plóro A, Dzlurdzlk P: Regional cerebral oxygenation monitoring in children undergoing elective scoliosis surgery with controlled urapidil-induced hypotension, *Med Sci Monit* 4:987, 1998.
229. Brady KM, Lee JK, Kibler KK, et al: Continuous time-domain analysis of cerebrovascular autoregulation using near-infrared spectroscopy, *Stroke* 38:2818, 2007.
230. Edmonds HL Jr, Thomas MH, Ganzel BL, et al: Effect of volatile anesthetics on cerebral autoregulation during cardiopulmonary bypass, *Anesthesiology* 95:A306, 2001 (abstract).
231. Aron JH, Fink GW, Swartz MF, et al: Cerebral oxygen desaturation after cardiopulmonary bypass in a patient with Raynaud's phenomenon detected by near-infrared cerebral oximetry, *Anesth Analg* 104:1034, 2007.
232. Piquette D, Deschamps A, Bélisle S, et al: Effect of intravenous nitroglycerin on cerebral saturation in high-risk cardiac surgery, *Can J Anesth* 54:718, 2007.
233. Yao F-SF, Ho C-YA, Tseng C-CA, et al: The divergent effects of phenylephrine on cerebral oxygen saturation, *Anesthesiology* 96:A157, 2002 (abstract).
234. Plattner O, Semsroth M, Sessler DI: Lack of nonshivering thermogenesis in infants anesthetized with fentanyl and propofol, *Anesthesiology* 86:772, 1997.
235. Kern FH, Jonas RA, Mayer JE: Temperature monitoring during CPB in infants: Does it predict efficient brain cooling? *Ann Thorac Surg* 54:749, 1992.
236. Wardle SP, Yoxall CW, Weindling AM: Cerebral oxygenation during cardiopulmonary bypass, *Arch Dis Child* 78:26, 1998.
237. Baraka A, Naufal M, El-Khatib M: Correlation between cerebral and mixed venous oxygen saturation during moderate versus tepid hypothermic hemodiluted cardiopulmonary bypass, *J Cardiothorac Vasc Anesth* 20:819, 2006.
238. Leyvi G, Bello R, Wasnick J, et al: Assessment of cerebral oxygen balance during deep hypothermic circulatory arrest by continuous jugular bulb venous saturation and near-infrared spectroscopy, *J Cardiothorac Vasc Anesth* 20:826, 2006.
239. Greeley WJ, Kern FH, Mault JR: Mechanisms of injury and methods of protection of the brain during cardiac surgery in neonates and infants, *Cardiol Young* 3:317, 1993.
240. deVries JW, Hoorntje T, Bakker PFA: Cerebral oxygen saturation monitoring in an infant undergoing ICD implantation, *J Cardiothorac Vasc Anesth* 12:442, 1998.
241. Dullenkopf A, Frey B, Baenziger O: Measurement of cerebral oxygenation in anaesthetized children using the INVOS 5100 cerebral oximeter, *Pediatr Anaesth* 13:384, 2003.
242. Manecke GR, Nieman JD, Phillips P: Deep hypothermia alters the vascular response to thiopental, *Anesthesiology* 96(3A):A169, 2002 (abstract).
243. Jones TH, Morawetz RB, Crowell RM: Threshold of focal cerebral ischemia in awake monkeys, *J Neurosurg* 54:773, 1981.
244. Deeb GM, Jenkins E, Bolling SF: Retrograde cerebral perfusion during hypothermic circulatory arrest reduces neurologic morbidity, *J Thorac Cardiovasc Surg* 109:259, 1995.
245. Estrera AL, Miller CC, Lee T-Y, et al: Ascending and transverse aortic arch repair, *Circulation* 118:S160, 2008.
246. Higami T, Kozawa S, Asada T: Retrograde cerebral perfusion versus selective cerebral perfusion as evaluated by cerebral oxygen saturation during aortic arch reconstruction, *Ann Thorac Surg* 67:1091, 1999.
247. Pigula FA, Nemoto EM, Griffith BP: Regional low-flow perfusion provides cerebral circulatory support during neonatal aortic arch reconstruction, *J Thorac Cardiovasc Surg* 199:331, 2000.
248. Hofer A, Haizinger B, Geiselseder G, et al: Monitoring of selective antegrade cerebral perfusion using near-infrared spectroscopy in neonatal aortic arch surgery, *Eur J Anaesth* 22:293, 2005.
249. Olsson C, Thelin S: Antegrade cerebral perfusion with a simplified technique: Unilateral versus bilateral perfusion, *Ann Thorac Surg* 81:868, 2006.
250. Olsson C, Thelin S: Regional cerebral saturation monitoring with near-infrared spectroscopy during selective antegrade cerebral perfusion: Diagnostic performance and relationship to postoperative stroke, *J Thorac Cardiovasc Surg* 131:371, 2006.
251. Cheng H-W, Chang H-H, Chen Y-J, et al: Clinical value of application of cerebral oximetry in total replacement of the aortic arch and concomitant vessels, *Acta Anaesthesiol Taiwan* 46:178, 2008.
252. De Paulis R, Salica A, Maselli D, et al: Initial experience of an arterial shunt for bilateral antegrade cerebral perfusion during hypothermic circulatory arrest, *Ann Thorac Surg* 85:624, 2008.
253. Fraser CD, Andropoulos DB: Principles of antegrade cerebral perfusion during arch reconstruction in newborns/infants, *Semin Thorac Cardiovasc Surg Pediatr Card Surg Annu* 11:61, 2008.
254. Göbölös L, Philipp A, Foltan M, et al: Surgical management for Stanford type A aortic dissection: Direct cannulation of real lumen at the level of the Botallo's ligament by Seldinger technique, *Interact Cardiovasc Thorac Surg* 7:107, 2008.
255. Kouchoukos NT, Masetti P, Mauney MC, et al: One-stage repair of extensive chronic aortic dissection using the arch-first technique and bilateral anterior thoracotomy, *Ann Thorac Surg* 86:1502, 2008.
256. Osborne-Bossert C, Fitzgerald D, Speir A, et al: Delivery of antegrade cerebral perfusion during descending aortic reconstruction: A case report, *Perfusion* 23:135, 2008.
257. Rubio A, Hakami L, Münch F, et al: Noninvasive control of adequate cerebral oxygenation during low-flow antegrade selective cerebral perfusion on adults and infants in the aortic arch surgery, *J Card Surg* 23:474, 2008.
258. Thompson B, Tsui SSL, Dunning J, et al: Pulmonary endarterectomy is possible and effective without the use of complete circulatory arrest—the UK experience in over 150 patients, *Eur J Cardiothorac Surg* 33:157, 2008.
259. Salazar J, Coleman R, Griffith S, et al: Brain preservation with selective cerebral perfusion for operations requiring circulatory arrest: Protection at 25° C is similar to 18° C with shorter operating times, *Eur J Cardiothorac Surg* 36:524, 2009.
260. Tobias JD: Cerebral oximetry monitoring provides early warning of hypercyanotic spells in an infant with Tetralogy of Fallot, *J Intensive Care Med* 22:118, 2007.
261. Tobias JD: Cerebral oximetry monitoring with near-infrared spectroscopy detects alterations in oxygenation before pulse oximetry, *J Intensive Care Med* 23:384, 2008.
262. Prabhune A, Sehic A, Spence PA, et al: Cerebral oximetry provides early warning of oxygen delivery failure during cardiopulmonary bypass, *J Cardiothorac Vasc Anesth* 16:204, 2002.
263. Webb DP, Deegan RJ, Greelish JP, et al: Oxygenation failure during cardiopulmonary bypass prompts new safety algorithm and training initiative, *J Extra Corpor Technol* 39:188, 2007.
264. Edmonds HL Jr, Ganzel BL: Spinal oximetry for ischemia detection during thoracoabdominal aneurysm repair, *Anesth Analg* 98:SCA72, 2004 (abstract).
265. Tobinick E: The cerebrospinal venous system: Anatomy, physiology, and clinical implications, *MedGenMed* 8:53, 2006.
266. LeMaire SA, Ochoa LN, Conklin LD, et al: Transcutaneous near-infrared spectroscopy for detection of regional spinal ischemia during intercostal artery ligation: Preliminary experimental results, *J Thorac Cardiovasc Surg* 132:1150, 2006.
267. Berens RJ, Stuth EA, Robertson FA, et al: Near-infrared spectroscopy monitoring during pediatric aortic coarctation repair, *Pediatr Anaesth* 16:777, 2006.
268. Ing RJ, Fischer S, Shipton S, et al: Regional cerebral oxygenation monitoring—intraoperative management in a patient with severe left ventricular dysfunction, *S Afr Med J* 96:1266, 2006.

269. Meier SD, Eble BK, Stapleton GE, et al: Mesenteric oxyhemoglobin desaturation improves with patent ductus arteriosus ligation, *J Perinatol* 26:562, 2006.

270. Felix D, Munro HM, DeCampli WM: Near-infrared spectroscopy used to detect preoperative aortic obstruction, *Paediatr Anaesth* 17:598, 2007.

271. Rossi M, Tirotta CF, Lagueruela RG, et al: Diminished Blalock-Taussig shunt flow detected by cerebral oximetry, *Paediatr Anaesth* 17:72, 2007.

272. Chakravarti S, Srivastava S, Mittnacht AJC: Near-infrared spectroscopy (NIRS) in children, *Semin Cardiothorac Vasc Anesth* 12:70, 2008.

273. Li J, Zhang G, Holtby H, et al: Carbon dioxide—a complex gas in a complex circulation: Its effects on systemic hemodynamics and oxygen transport, cerebra, and splanchnic circulation in neonates after the Norwood procedure, *J Thorac Cardiovasc Surg* 136:1207, 2008.

274. Tamariz-Gruz O, Palacios-Macedo A, Bouchan-Ramirez Y, et al: Post-operative heart failure management. Report from a case that consisted of correcting the Taussig-Bing disease using an arterial switch. Emphasis on the use of pediatric levosimendan and neural splanchnic monitoring, *Revista Mexicana de Anesthes* 31:20, 2008.

275. Horvath R, Shore S, Schultz SE, et al: Cerebral and somatic oxygen saturation decrease after delayed sternal closure in children after cardiac surgery, *J Thorac Cardiovasc Surg* 139:894–900, 2010.

276. White MC, Edgell D, Li J, et al: The relationship between cerebral and somatic oxygenation and superior and inferior vena cava flow, arterial oxygenation and pressure in infants during cardiopulmonary bypass, *Anaesthesia* 64:251, 2009.

277. Harel F, Denault A, Ngo Q, et al: Near-infrared spectroscopy to monitor peripheral blood flow perfusion, *J Clin Monit Comp* 22:37, 2008.

278. Akça O, Melischek M, Scheck T: Postoperative pain and subcutaneous oxygen tension, *Lancet* 354:41, 1999.

279. Austin EH 3rd, Edmonds HL Jr, Seremet V, et al: Benefit of neuromonitoring for pediatric cardiac surgery, *J Thorac Cardiovasc Surg* 114:707, 1997.

280. Edmonds HL Jr: Protective effect of neuromonitoring during cardiac surgery, *Ann N Y Acad Sci* 1053:12, 2005.

281. Laschinger J, Razumovsky AY, Stierer KA, et al: Cardiac surgery: Value of neuromonitoring, *Heart Surg Forum* 6:204, 2003.

282. Lozano S, Mossad E: Cerebral function monitors during pediatric cardiac surgery: Can they make a difference? *J Cardiothorac Vasc Anesth* 18:645, 2004.

17 Coagulation Monitoring

LINDA SHORE-LESSERSON, MD | LIZA J. ENRIQUEZ, MD

KEY POINTS

1. Monitoring the effect of heparin is done using the activated coagulation time (ACT), a functional test of heparin anticoagulation. The ACT is susceptible to prolongation because of hypothermia and hemodilution and to reduction because of platelet activation or thrombocytopathy.

2. Heparin resistance can be congenital or acquired. Pretreatment heparin exposure predisposes a patient to altered heparin responsiveness because of antithrombin III (AT III) depletion, platelet activation, or activation of extrinsic coagulation.

3. Heparin-induced thrombocytopenia (HIT) type I is benign and is a normal aggregation response of platelets to heparin. HIT type II is an abnormal immunologic response to the heparin/platelet factor 4 complex and is sometimes associated with overt thrombosis.

4. Protamine neutralization of heparin can be associated with "protamine reactions," which include vasodilatory hypotension, anaphylactoid reactions, and pulmonary hypertensive crises (types 1, 2, and 3, respectively).

5. Before considering a transfusion of plasma, it is important to document that the effect of heparin has been neutralized. This can be done using a heparinase-neutralized test or a protamine-neutralized test.

6. Point-of-care tests are available for use in transfusion algorithms that can measure coagulation factor activity (normalized ratio, activated partial thromboplastin time) and platelet function.

7. Fibrinolysis is common after cardiopulmonary bypass when antifibrinolytic therapy is not used.

8. New thrombin inhibitor drugs are available for anticoagulation in patients who cannot receive heparin. These can be monitored using the ecarin clotting time or a modified ACT. Bivalirudin and hirudin are the two direct thrombin inhibitors that have been used most often in cardiac surgery.

9. Platelet dysfunction is the most common reason for bleeding after cardiopulmonary bypass. Point-of-care tests can be used to measure specific aspects of platelet function.

10. The degree of platelet inhibition as measured by standard or point-of-care instruments has been shown to correlate with decreased ischemic outcomes after coronary intervention. However, cardiac surgical patients who are receiving antiplatelet medication are at increased risk for postoperative bleeding.

Cardiac surgery is an area in which coagulation monitoring has vital applications. Cardiopulmonary bypass (CPB) procedures could not be performed without an effective method of preventing blood from clotting in the extracorporeal circuit. In the early part of the 20th century, heparin was discovered to have anticoagulant properties; it remains the anticoagulant most commonly used during CPB. Reversal of heparin effect is most frequently performed using protamine, although a number of different pharmacologic agents and reversal techniques can be used.

CPB itself induces a "whole-body inflammatory response" because of contact of blood and cellular elements with the extracorporeal circuit. The resultant alterations include leukocyte activation, release of inflammatory mediators, free radical formation, complement activation, kallikrein release, platelet activation, and stimulation of the coagulation and fibrinolytic cascades. This complex interplay of systems induces a coagulopathy characterized by microvascular coagulation, platelet dysfunction, and enhanced fibrinolysis.[1,2] The homeostatic perturbations incurred during CPB are a major cause for the postbypass coagulopathy that is seen even after the effects of heparin are reversed with protamine.

The need to monitor anticoagulation during and after surgery is the reason that the cardiac surgical arena has evolved into a major site for the evaluation and use of hemostasis monitors. The rapid and accurate identification of abnormal hemostasis has been the major impetus toward the development of point-of-care tests that can be performed at the bedside or in the operating room. The detection and treatment of specific coagulation disorders in a timely and cost-efficient manner are major goals in hemostasis monitoring for the cardiac surgical patient. This chapter discusses the mechanisms of normal coagulation and how they are affected by CPB. The latter portion discusses the laboratory and point-of-care tests available for monitoring the coagulation system. A comprehensive overview of hemostasis, transfusion medicine, and the management of coagulopathy and bleeding disorders after CPB is provided in Chapters 30 and 31.

HEMOSTASIS

Hemostasis is the body's normal response to vascular injury and involves a complex interplay of systems within the body that helps to seal the endovascular defect and prevent exsanguination. The three major components of hemostasis include the vascular endothelium; the platelets, which constitute primary hemostasis; and the coagulation cascade glycoproteins (GPs), which constitute secondary hemostasis. Fibrinolysis is the normal physiologic response to clot formation, which ensures that coagulation remains localized to the area of vascular injury.

▩ Anticoagulation for Cardiopulmonary Bypass

The safe conduct of CPB could not be accomplished without anticoagulation of blood in preparation for its contact with the extracorporeal circuit. An ideal anticoagulant should be easy to administer, rapid in onset, titratable, predictable, measurable in a timely fashion, and reversible. Heparin use during CPB has continued until the present time, most likely because of its rapid onset, ease of measurement, and ease of reversibility. Decades of the use of heparin are either a testimonial to its effectiveness or demonstrative of the inability to find a more suitable alternative.

Heparin acts as an antithrombin III (AT III) agonist and accelerates AT III binding to thrombin.[3–5] In the absence of AT III, heparin is clinically ineffective as an anticoagulant; adequate AT III activity is necessary in patients about to undergo heparinization for cardiac surgical procedures.[6–9]

MONITORING HEPARIN EFFECT

Cardiac surgery had been performed for decades using empiric heparin dosing in the form of a bolus and subsequent interval dosing. Empiric dosing continued because of the lack of an easily applicable bedside test to monitor the anticoagulant effects of heparin. Many assays are available to measure the response to the heparin dose given to institute extracorporeal circulation. These tests are in the form of functional tests of anticoagulation or quantitative measures of the level of circulating heparin. The anticoagulant effect of heparin can be monitored using a variety of different techniques.

The first clotting time to be used to measure heparin's effect was the whole-blood clotting time (WBCT) or the Lee–White WBCT. This simply requires whole blood to be placed in a glass tube, maintained at 37°C, and manually tilted until blood fluidity is no longer detected. This test fell out of favor for monitoring the cardiac surgical patient because it was so labor intensive and required the undivided attention of the person performing the test for periods up to 30 minutes. Although the glass surface of the test tube acts as an activator of factor XII, the heparin doses used for cardiac surgery prolong the WBCT to such a profound degree that the test is impractical as a monitor of the effect of heparin during cardiac surgery.[10] To speed the clotting time so that the test was appropriate for clinical use, activators were added to the test tubes, and the activated coagulation time (ACT) was introduced into practice.[11]

▩ Activated Coagulation Time

The ACT was first introduced by Hattersley in 1966 and is still the most widely used monitor of heparin effect during cardiac surgery. Whole blood is added to a test tube containing an activator, diatomaceous earth (celite) or kaolin. The presence of activator augments the contact activation phase of coagulation, which stimulates the intrinsic coagulation pathway. ACT can be performed manually, whereby the operator measures the time interval from when blood is injected into the test tube to when clot is seen along the sides of the tube. More commonly, the ACT is automated as it is in the Hemochron and Hemotec systems. In the automated system, the test tube is placed in a device that warms the sample to 37°C. The Hemochron device (International Technidyne, Edison, NJ) rotates the test tube, which contains celite activator and a small iron cylinder, to which 2 mL whole blood is added. Before clot forms, the cylinder rolls along the bottom of the rotating test tube. When clot forms, the cylinder is pulled away from a magnetic detector, interrupts a magnetic field, and signals the end of the clotting time. Normal ACT values range from 80 to 120 seconds. The Hemochron ACT also can be performed using kaolin as the activator in a similar manner (Figure 17-1).

The Hemotec ACT device (Medtronic Hemotec, Parker, CO) is a cartridge with two chambers that contain kaolin activator and is housed in a heat block. Blood (0.4 mL) is placed into each chamber, and a

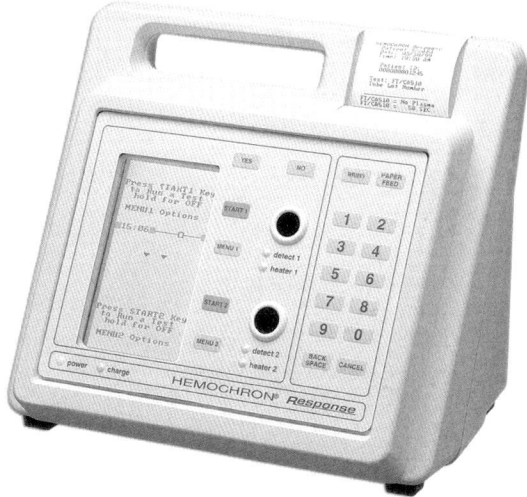

Figure 17-1 The Hemochron Response is a dual-chamber point-of-care coagulation monitor that is capable of measuring clotting times that are compatible with Hemochron technology. This system has software capability for calculation, data management, and storage of results. (*Courtesy of International Technidyne, Edison, NJ.*)

daisy-shaped plunger is raised and passively falls into the chamber. The formation of clot will slow the rate of descent of the plunger, and this decrease in velocity of the plunger is detected by a photo-optical system that signals the end of the ACT test. The Hemochron and Hemotec ACTs have been compared in a number of investigations and have been found to differ significantly at low heparin concentrations.[12] However, differences in heparin concentration, activator concentration, and the measurement technique make comparison of these tests difficult and have led to the realization that the Hemochron ACT result and the Hemotec ACT result are not interchangeable. In adult patients given 300 U/kg heparin for CPB, the Hemochron and Hemotec (Hepcon) ACTs were both therapeutic at all time points; however, at two points, the Hemochron ACT was statistically longer[13] (Figure 17-2). This difference was even more pronounced in pediatric patients, who have greater heparin consumption rates (Figure 17-3). The apparent "overestimation" of ACT by the Hemochron device during hypothermic CPB may be because of the different volumes of blood that each assay warms to 37°C.

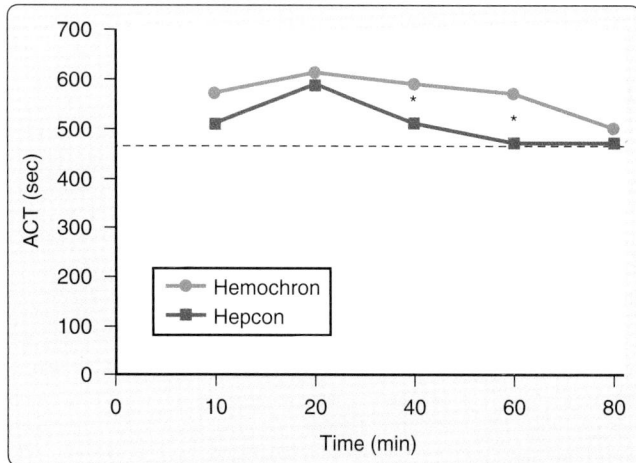

Figure 17-2 The Hemochron (*circles*) and Hemotec (Hepcon; *squares*) activated coagulation time (ACT) values in 20 adults at five time points during cardiopulmonary bypass (CPB). At 40 and 80 minutes on CPB, the Hemochron ACT was significantly greater. *$P < 0.01$. (*From Horkay F, Martin P, Rajah SM, Walker DR: Response to heparinization in adults and children undergoing cardiac operations. Ann Thorac Surg 53:822–826, 1992, by permission of Society of Thoracic Surgeons.*)

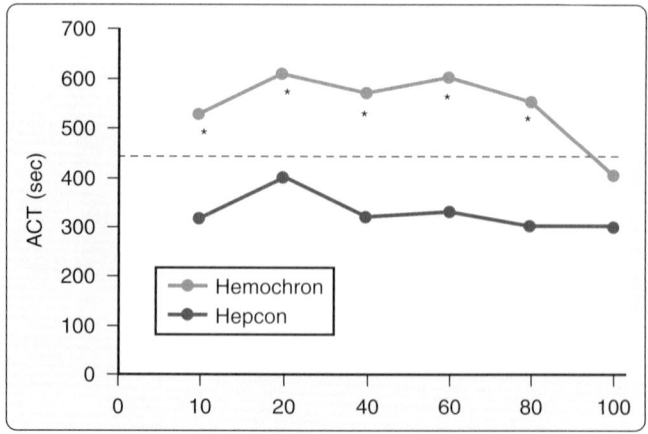

Figure 17-3   The Hemochron (*circles*) and Hemotec (Hepcon; *squares*) activated coagulation time (ACT) values in 22 pediatric patients at six time points during cardiopulmonary bypass (CPB). Hemochron ACT was significantly greater than Hemotec ACT at five time points. *$P < 0.01$. (*From Horkay F, Martin P, Rajah SM, Walker DR: Response to heparinization in adults and children undergoing cardiac operations. Ann Thorac Surg 53:822–826, 1992, by permission of Society of Thoracic Surgeons.*)

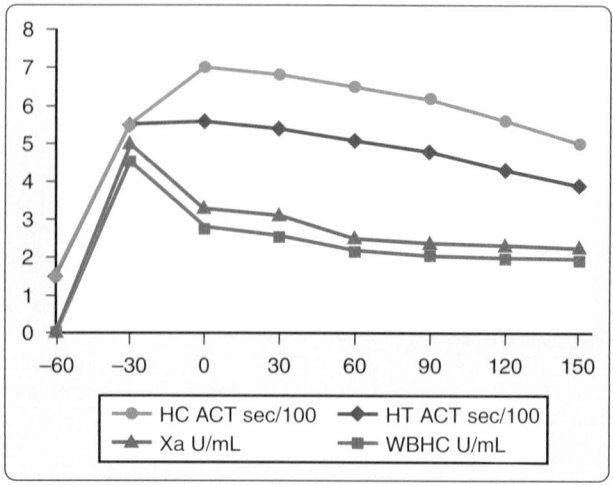

Figure 17-4   Anticoagulation measured at baseline (−60 minutes), heparinization (−30 minutes), and six time points after institution of cardiopulmonary bypass (CPB). Note the close correlation between the anti–factor Xa (Xa; *triangles*) activity and whole blood heparin concentration (WBHC; *squares*), which does not parallel the change in Hemochron (HC ACT; *circles*) or Hemotec activated coagulation time (HT ACT; *diamonds*). (*Modified from Despotis GJ, Summerfield AL, Joist JH: Comparison of activated coagulation time and whole blood heparin measurements with laboratory plasma anti-Xa heparin concentration in patients having cardiac operations. J Thorac Cardiovasc Surg 108:1076–1082, 1994.*)

The ACT test can be modified by the addition of heparinase. With this modification, the coagulation status of the patient can be monitored during CPB while the anticoagulant effects of heparin are eliminated. Because this test is a side-by-side comparison of the untreated ACT to the heparinase ACT, it also has the advantage of being a rapid test for the assessment of a circulating heparin-like substance or for residual heparinization after CPB.[14]

With the introduction of ACT monitoring into the cardiac surgical arena, clinicians have been able to more accurately titrate heparin and protamine dosages.[11,15] As a result, many investigators report reductions in blood loss and transfusion requirements, although many of these studies used retrospective analyses.[16] The improvements in postoperative hemostasis documented with ACT monitoring are potentially attributable to better intraoperative suppression of microvascular coagulation and improved monitoring of heparin reversal with protamine.[17]

ACT monitoring of heparinization is not without pitfalls, and its use has been criticized because of the extreme variability of the ACT and the absence of a correlation with plasma heparin levels (Figure 17-4). Many factors have been suggested to alter the ACT, and these factors are prevalent during cardiac surgical procedures. When the extracorporeal circuit prime is added to the patient's blood volume, hemodilution occurs and may theoretically increase ACT. Evidence suggests that this degree of hemodilution alone is not enough to actually alter ACT. Hypothermia increases ACT in a "dose-related" fashion. It has been shown by Culliford et al[18] that, although hemodilution and hypothermia significantly increase the ACT of a heparinized blood sample, similar increases do not occur in the absence of added heparin. The effects of platelet alterations are a bit more problematic. At mild-to-moderate degrees of thrombocytopenia, the baseline and heparinized ACT are not affected. It is not until platelet counts are reduced to less than 30,000 to 50,000/μL that ACT may be prolonged.[19] Patients treated with platelet inhibitors such as prostacyclin, aspirin, or platelet-membrane-receptor antagonists have a prolonged heparinized ACT compared with patients not treated with platelet inhibitors.[20] This ACT prolongation is not related exclusively to decreased levels of platelet factor 4 (PF4) (PF4 is a heparin-neutralizing substance) because it also occurs when blood is anticoagulated with substances that are not neutralized by PF4. Platelet lysis, however, significantly shortens the ACT because of the release of PF4 and other platelet membrane components, which may have heparin-neutralizing activities.[21] Gravlee et al[22]

showed that anesthesia and surgery decrease the ACT and create a hypercoagulable state, possibly by creating a thromboplastic response or through activation of platelets.

During CPB, heparin decay varies substantially and its measurement is problematic because hemodilution and hypothermia alter the metabolism of heparin. In a CPB study, Mabry et al[23] found that the consumption of heparin varied from 0.01 to 3.86 U/kg/min and there was no correlation between the initial sensitivity to heparin and the rate of heparin decay.[23] In the pediatric population, the consumption of heparin is increased to more than that of adult levels. The heparin administration protocol for pediatric patients undergoing CPB should account for a large volume of distribution, increased consumption, and a shorter elimination half-life. In monitoring the effects of heparin in pediatric patients, the minimum acceptable ACT value should be increased or an additional monitor should be used. The discrepancy between the Hemochron ACT and the Hemotec ACT that is demonstrated in Figure 17-2 is even more pronounced in pediatric patients (see Figure 17-3). Some investigators recommend the maintenance of heparin concentrations in addition to ACT during pediatric congenital heart surgery to ensure that optimal anticoagulation is being achieved.[24,25]

Cascade POC (Point of Care) System

A completely different technology for measuring the effect of heparin is used by the Cascade POC analyzer (Helena, Beaumont, TX; Formerly Rapid Point Coagulation Analyzer Bayer Diagnostics, Tarrytown, NY). This test system contains disposable cards with celite activator for the measurement of heparin activity. This variation of the ACT is called the "heparin management test" (HMT). This card contains paramagnetic iron oxide particles that move in response to an oscillating magnetic field within the device. When clot formation occurs, movement of the iron oxide particles is decreased and the end of the test is signaled. This system is capable of measuring prothrombin time (PT) and activated partial thromboplastin time (aPTT), which is discussed later. The suitability of this platform for the monitoring of ACT during cardiac surgery has been demonstrated in a variety of clinical studies.[26,27] Suitability for monitoring heparinization in the interventional cardiology laboratory also has been reported. HMT correlates well with anti-Xa heparin activity in CPB patients and is less variable than standard ACT measures. In a comparison with ACT, the coefficients of variation were similar between the tests at baseline but were three times greater for the ACT during heparinization. This degree of agreement with plasma anti-Xa measurements has not been demonstrated universally when studying blood from patients undergoing CPB.[28]

Heparin Resistance

Heparin resistance is documented by an inability to increase the ACT of blood to expected levels despite an adequate dose and plasma concentration of heparin. In many clinical situations, especially when heparin desensitization or a heparin inhibitor is suspected, heparin resistance can be treated by administering increased doses of heparin in a competitive fashion. If an adequately prolonged clotting time is ultimately achieved using greater than expected doses of heparin, a better term than heparin resistance would be heparin tachyphylaxis of "altered heparin responsiveness." During cardiac surgical procedures, the belief that a safe minimum ACT value of 300 to 400 seconds is required for CPB is based on a few clinical studies and a relative paucity of scientific data. However, inability to attain this degree of anticoagulation in the heparin-resistant patient engenders the fear among cardiac surgical providers that the patient will experience a microvascular consumptive coagulopathy or that clots will form in the extracorporeal circuit. This potential for fibrin formation in the extracorporeal circuit was reported by Young et al,[29] who found increased production of fibrin monomer and consumption of fibrinogen and platelets in six of nine rhesus monkeys when the ACT declined to less than 400 seconds. However, Metz and Keats[30] reported no adverse effects of thrombosis or excessive bleeding in 51 patients undergoing CPB whose ACT was less than 400 seconds. In a porcine model, the group whose ACT was maintained between 250 and 300 seconds did not have excessive consumption of coagulation factors, increases in fibrin monomer formation, or changes in oxygenator performance compared with the group whose ACT was maintained at greater than 450 seconds.[31]

Many clinical conditions are associated with heparin resistance.[32] Sepsis, liver disease, and pharmacologic agents represent just a few[33,34] (Table 17-1). Many investigators have documented decreased levels of AT III secondary to heparin pretreatment,[35] whereas others have not found decreased AT III levels.[36] Esposito et al[37] measured coagulation factor levels in patients receiving preoperative heparin infusions and

BOX 17-1. HEPARIN RESISTANCE

- It is primarily caused by antithrombin (AT) III deficiency in pediatric patients.
- It is multifactorial in adult cardiac surgical patients.
- The critical activated coagulation time value necessary in patients who demonstrate acquired heparin resistance is not yet determined.
- Heparin resistance also can be a sign of heparin-induced thrombocytopenia.

found that a lower baseline ACT was the only risk factor for predicting heparin resistance compared with patients not receiving preoperative heparin.

Patients receiving preoperative heparin therapy traditionally require larger heparin doses to achieve a given level of anticoagulation when that anticoagulation is measured by the ACT. Presumably, this "heparin resistance" is due to deficiencies in the level or activity of AT III.[34,37–40] Other possible causes include enhanced factor VIII activity and platelet dysfunction causing a decrease in ACT response to heparin. Levy et al[40] have shown that the in vitro addition of AT III enhances the ACT response to heparin. Lemmer and Despotis[39] demonstrated that this heparin resistance, as measured by the ACT, does not correlate with preoperative AT III levels. It is unclear that these patients have increased heparin requirements during CPB because the ideal ACT and monitoring techniques have yet to be elucidated. Nicholson et al[41] demonstrated that the temporal courses of ACT and AT III concentration do not parallel each other, further suggesting that AT III depletion is not the sole cause of heparin resistance during CPB. Lower ACTs (lower than 480s) were tolerated in this study with no adverse outcome. AT III concentrate is available as a heat-treated human product or in recombinant form and represents a reasonable method of treating patients with documented AT III deficiency (Box 17-1). Heparin responsiveness in the form of increased ACT levels is documented both in vitro and in vivo when heparin-resistant patients are treated with AT III.

In a multicenter, randomized, placebo-controlled trial using 75 U/kg recombinant AT III, AT III–treated patients received less FFP to augment ACT levels and also had evidence of less hemostatic activation while on CPB.[42] There was a trend toward increased blood loss in the AT III group, which is potentially a dose effect that requires further investigation.[43,44]

Heparin-Induced Thrombocytopenia

The syndrome known as heparin-induced thrombocytopenia (HIT) develops in anywhere from 5% to 28% of patients receiving heparin. HIT is commonly categorized into two subtypes. Type I is characterized by a mild decrease in platelet count and is the result of the proaggregatory effects of heparin on platelets. Type II (hereafter referred to as HIT) is considerably more severe, most often occurs after more than 5 days of heparin administration (average onset time, 9 days), and is mediated by antibody binding to the complex formed between heparin and PF4. Associated immune-mediated endothelial injury and complement activation cause platelets to adhere, aggregate, and form platelet clots, or "white clots." Among patients developing HIT, the incidence of thrombotic complications approximates 20%, which, in turn, may carry a mortality rate as high as 40%. Demonstration of heparin-induced proaggregation of platelets confirms the diagnosis of HIT. This can be accomplished with a heparin-induced serotonin release assay or a specific heparin-induced platelet activation assay. A highly specific enzyme-linked immunosorbent assay for the heparin/PF4 complex has been developed and has been used to delineate the course of IgG and IgM antibody responses in patients exposed to unfractionated heparin during cardiac surgery. Bedside antibody tests are being developed that may speed the diagnosis of this condition.

TABLE 17-1	Disease States Associated with Heparin Resistance
Disease State	**Comment**
Newborn	Decreased AT III levels until 6 months of age
Venous thromboembolism	May have increased factor VIII level
	Accelerated clearance of heparin
Pulmonary embolism	Accelerated clearance of heparin
Congenital AT III deficiency	40% to 60% of normal AT III concentration
Type I	Reduced synthesis of normal/abnormal AT III
Type II	Molecular defect within the AT III molecule
Acquired AT III deficiency	< 25% of normal AT III concentration
Preeclampsia	Levels unchanged in normal pregnancy
Cirrhosis	Decreased protein synthesis
Nephrotic syndrome	Increased urinary excretion of AT III
DIC	Increased consumption of AT III
Heparin pretreatment	85% of normal AT III concentration because of accelerated clearance
Estrogen therapy	
Cytotoxic drug therapy (L-asparaginase)	Decreased protein synthesis

ATIII, antithrombin III; DIC, disseminated intravascular coagulation.

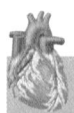

BOX 17-2. HEPARIN-INDUCED THROMBOCYTOPENIA

- The immunologic form is mediated by an antibody to the heparin/platelet factor 4 complex.
- This disease has variable penetrance even in the same individual.
- There is an associated 30% risk for thrombosis.
- Thrombosis carries a 50% mortality rate.

The risks and appropriate courses of action in patients with HIT are unclear because the antibodies associated with HIT often become undetectable several weeks after discontinuing heparin. Also, the clinical syndrome does not always recur on re-exposure to heparin and sometimes resolves despite continued drug therapy. Many patients never develop thrombosis and disseminated intravascular coagulation despite positive laboratory testing. HIT possibly should be considered in the differential diagnosis of intraoperative heparin resistance in patients receiving preoperative heparin therapy.

The options for treating these patients are few. If the clinician has the luxury of being able to discontinue heparin for a few weeks, often the antibody disappears and allows a brief period of heparinization for CPB without complication.[45,46] Changing the tissue source of heparin was an option when bovine heparin was predominantly in use. Some types of low-molecular-weight heparin have been administered to patients with HIT, but reactivity of the particular low-molecular-weight heparin with the patient's platelets should be confirmed in vitro. Supplementing heparin administration with pharmacologic platelet inhibition using prostacyclin, iloprost, aspirin, or aspirin and dipyridamole have been reported, all with favorable outcomes. The use of tirofiban with unfractionated heparin has been used in this clinical circumstance. Plasmapheresis may be used to reduce antibody levels. The use of heparin could be avoided altogether through anticoagulation with direct thrombin inhibitors such as argatroban, hirudin, or bivalirudin. These thrombin inhibitors have become standard of care in the management of the patient with HIT (Box 17-2). Bivalirudin has been studied in multicenter trials in HIT patients who must undergo CPB.[47] Monitoring the direct thrombin inhibitors during CPB is discussed later in this chapter.

■ Measurement of Heparin Sensitivity

Even in the absence of heparin resistance, patient response to an intravenous bolus of heparin is extremely variable.[48] The variability stems from different concentrations of various endogenous heparin-binding proteins such as vitronectin and PF4. This variability exists whether measuring heparin concentration or the ACT; however, variability seems to be greater when measuring the ACT. Because of the large interpatient variation in heparin responsiveness and the potential for heparin resistance, it is critical that a functional monitor of heparin anticoagulation (with or without a measure of heparin concentration) be used in the cardiac surgical patient. Bull et al[49] documented a threefold range of ACT response to a 200-U/kg heparin dose and similar discrepancy in heparin decay rates and, thus, recommended the use of individual patient dose–response curves to determine the optimal heparin dose. This is the concept on which point-of-care individual heparin dose–response (HDR) tests are based.

An HDR curve can be generated manually using the baseline ACT and the ACT response to an in vivo or in vitro dose of heparin. Extrapolation to the desired ACT provides the additional heparin dose required for that ACT. Once the actual ACT response to the heparin dose is plotted, further dose–response calculations are made based on the average of the target ACT and the actual ACT (Figure 17-5). This methodology was first described by Bull et al[49] and forms the scientific basis for the automated dose–response systems manufactured by Hemochron and Hemotec. The Hemochron RxDx system uses the heparin-response test,

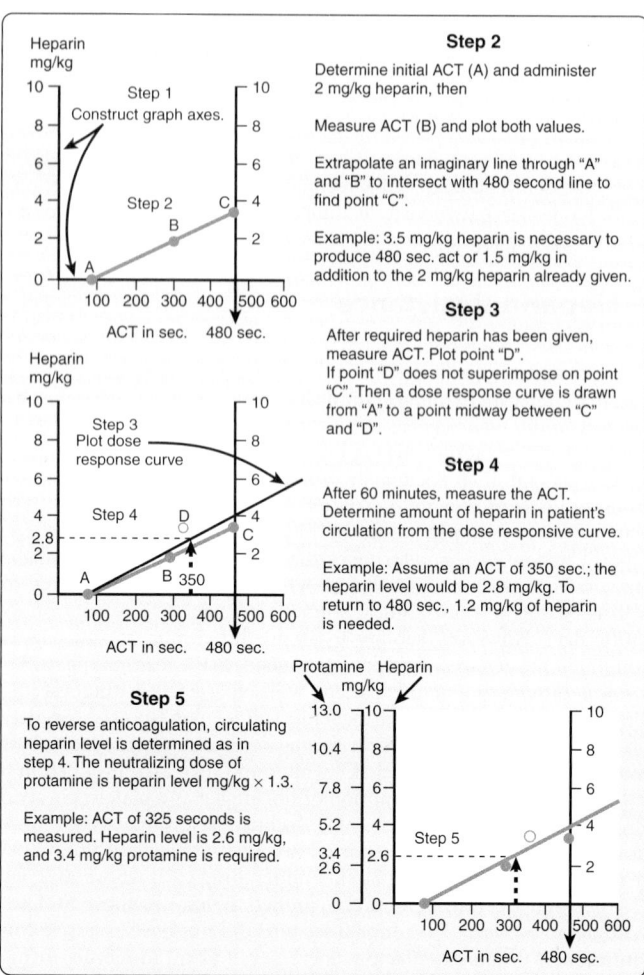

Figure 17-5 **Construction of a dose–response curve for heparin.** ACT, activated coagulation time. *(From Bull BS, Huse WM, Brauer FS, et al: Heparin therapy during extracorporeal circulation: II. The use of a dose-response curve to individualize heparin and protamine dosage. J Thorac Cardiovasc Surg 69:685–689, 1975.)*

which is an ACT with a known quantity of in vitro heparin (3 IU/mL). A dose–response curve is generated that enables calculation of the heparin dose required to attain the target ACT using an algorithm that incorporates the patient's baseline ACT, estimated blood volume, and heparin-response test. The patient's heparin sensitivity can be calculated in seconds per international units per milliliter (sec/IU/mL) by dividing the heparin-response test by 3 IU/mL.

The RxDx system also provides an individualized protamine dose using the protamine-response test (PRT). This is an ACT with one of two specific quantities of protamine, depending on the amount of circulating heparin suspected (2 or 3 IU/mL). The protamine dose needed to return the ACT to baseline can be calculated on the basis of a protamine–response curve using the patient's heparinized ACT, the PRT, and an estimate of the patient's blood volume. Jobes et al[50] reported that the heparin dose directed by the RxDx system resulted in ACT values far greater than the target ACT. In their patients, in vivo heparin sensitivity was higher than in vitro sensitivity. RxDx also resulted in lower protamine doses, lower postoperative mediastinal tube losses, and reduced transfusion requirements compared with a ratio-based system of heparin/protamine administration. In a larger study that standardized the treatment of heparin rebound, the reduced protamine dose was confirmed; however, the reductions in bleeding were not substantiated.[51] The use of a protamine dose–response curve has been shown to successfully reduce the protamine dose in vascular surgery compared with standard weight-based protamine dosing.[52]

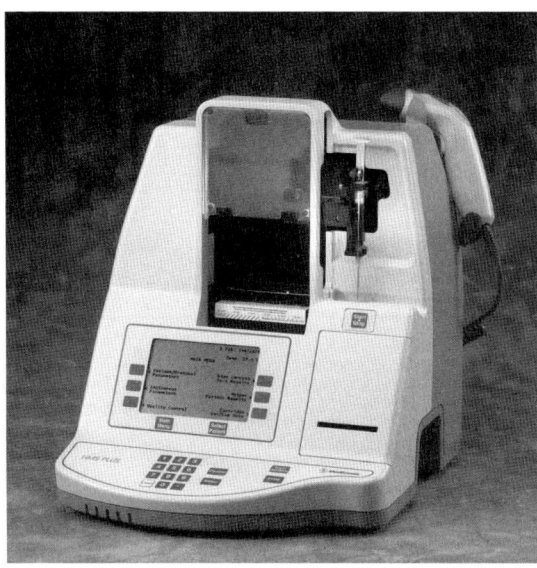

Figure 17-6 The HMS heparin management system has an automated dispenser that places the appropriate volume of whole blood into each chamber of the test cartridge. A variety of assays can be performed in this instrument, depending on the cartridge used. *(Courtesy of Medtronic, Parker, CO.)*

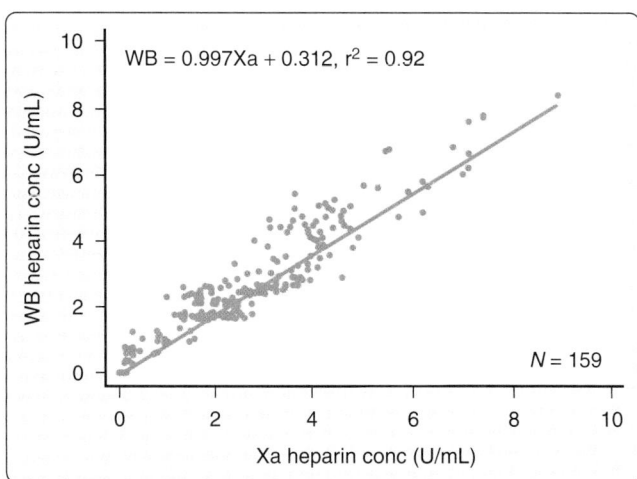

Figure 17-7 There is a strong linear relation between whole-blood heparin concentration (WB heparin conc) and the anti-Xa plasma heparin concentration (Xa heparin conc). WB heparin conc was measured using the Hepcon protamine titration assay and was corrected for hematocrit value. The Xa heparin conc was measured in plasma using a substrate assay. *(From Despotis GJ, Summerfield AL, Joist JH: Comparison of activated coagulation time and whole blood heparin measurements with laboratory plasma anti-Xa heparin concentration in patients having cardiac operations. J Thorac Cardiovasc Surg 108:1076–1082, 1994.)*

The Hepcon HMS system uses the HDR cartridge in the Hepcon instrument (Figure 17-6). Each cartridge houses six chambers. Chambers 1 and 2 contain heparin at a concentration of 2.5 IU/mL, chambers 3 and 4 contain heparin at a concentration of 1.5 IU/mL, and chambers 5 and 6 do not contain heparin. Once information regarding patient weight, height, and CPB prime volume is entered, the information that can be obtained from this test includes the baseline ACT (chambers 5 and 6) and an HDR slope. The dose–response slope, which is the increase in ACT from 1.5 to 2.5 IU/mL heparin, is extrapolated to the desired target ACT or target heparin concentration and the heparin dose is calculated.[32,53]

Heparin Concentration

Proponents of ACT measurement to guide anticoagulation for CPB argue that a functional assessment of the anticoagulant effect of heparin is mandatory and that the variability in ACT represents a true variability in the coagulation status of the patient. Opponents argue that during CPB, the sensitivity of the ACT to heparin is altered and ACT does not correlate with heparin concentration or with anti–factor Xa activity measurement. Heparin concentration can be measured using the Hepcon HMS system (Medtronic Hemotec), which uses an automated protamine titration technique. With a cartridge with four or six chambers containing tissue thromboplastin and a series of known protamine concentrations, 0.2 mL whole blood is automatically dispensed into the chambers. The first channel to clot is the channel whose protamine concentration most accurately neutralizes the heparin without a heparin or a protamine excess. Because protamine neutralizes heparin in the ratio of 1 mg protamine per 100 units heparin, the concentration of heparin in the blood sample can be calculated. A cartridge that monitors heparin concentration over a wide range can be used first, followed by another cartridge that can measure heparin concentrations within a more narrow range. The maintenance of a stable heparin concentration rather than a specific ACT level usually results in greater doses of heparin being administered because the hemodilution and hypothermia on CPB increase the sensitivity of the ACT to heparin. The measure of heparin concentration has been shown to correlate more closely with anti–factor Xa activity measurements than the ACT during CPB[54] (Figure 17-7), although the precision and bias of the test may not prove to be acceptable for exclusive use clinically (Figure 17-8).

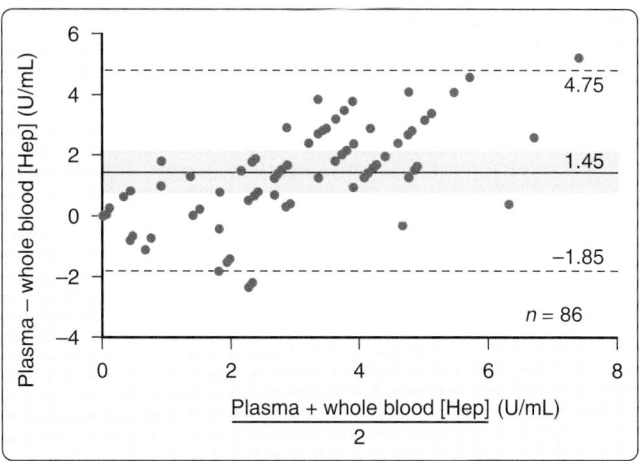

Figure 17-8 A Bland–Altman plot analyzing the limits of agreement between the whole-blood heparin concentration and the plasma anti-Xa heparin concentration. The bias (1.45) and two standard deviations are determined to be the limits of agreement. Note that the limits of agreement do not lie within the predetermined acceptable difference between the tests. *(From Hardy J-F, Belisle S, Robitaille D, et al: Measurement of heparin concentration in whole blood with the Hepcon/HMS device does not agree with laboratory determination of plasma heparin concentration using a chromogenic substrate for activated factor X. J Thorac Cardiovasc Surg 112:154–161, 1996.)*

In a small, prospective, randomized study comparing ACT and heparin concentration monitoring, Gravlee et al[55] demonstrated increased mediastinal tube drainage after surgery in the heparin concentration group, a finding that was initially attributed to greater total heparin doses. However, heparin rebound was not systematically assessed. In a follow-up study, the authors found a greater incidence of heparin rebound in the heparin concentration group, which, when treated, resulted in no difference in bleeding between the ACT and heparin concentration groups.[56] In a prospective, randomized trial, Despotis et al[57] demonstrated that by using a transfusion algorithm in association with Hepcon-based heparin management, chest tube drainage

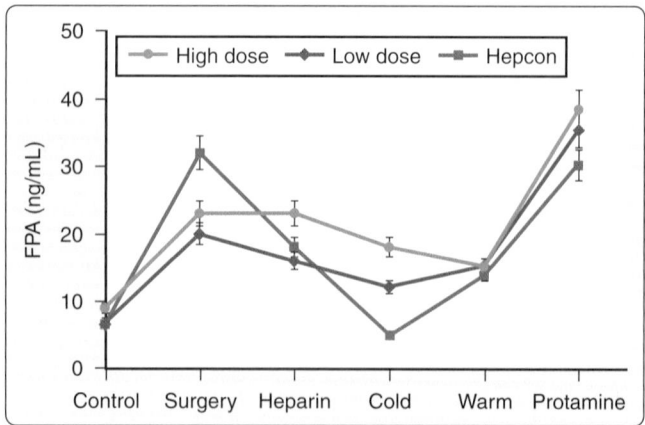

Figure 17-9 Fibrinopeptide A (FPA) levels during cardiopulmonary bypass (CPB) were measured in three groups of patients before anesthetic induction (Control), after heparin administration (Heparin), at lowest temperature on CPB (Cold), at esophageal temperature > 36°C (Warm), and 5 minutes after completion of the protamine dose (Protamine). Group 1, patients receiving heparin 300 IU/kg with activated coagulation time (ACT) heparin management; group 2, patients receiving heparin 250 IU/kg with ACT management; group 3, patients receiving 350 to 400 IU/kg with Hepcon heparin management. There were no differences in FPA levels among groups except during cold CPB group 3 versus group 1, P < 0.05. *(From Gravlee GP, Haddon WS, Rothberger HK, et al: Heparin dosing and monitoring for cardiopulmonary bypass. A comparison of techniques with measurement of subclinical plasma coagulation.* J Thorac Cardiovasc Surg 99:518–527, 1990.)

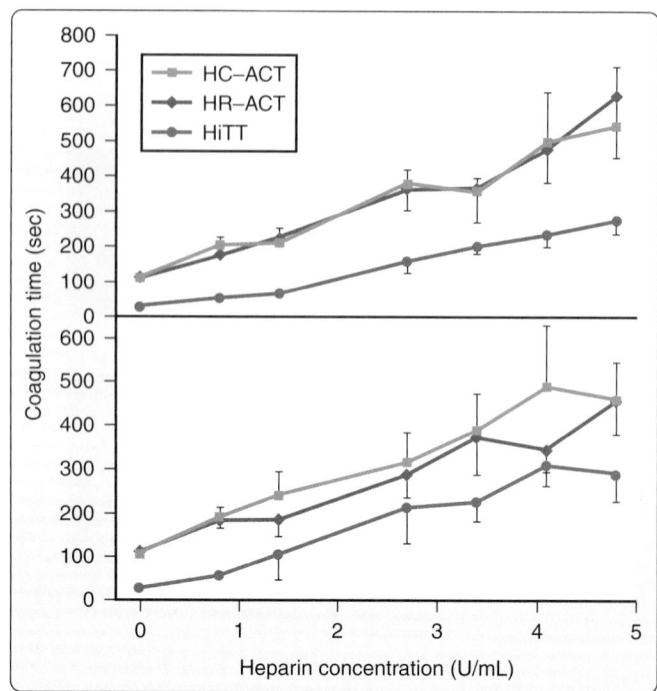

Figure 17-10 Hemochron ACT (HC-ACT; *squares*), Hepcon ACT (HR-ACT; *diamonds*), and high-dose thrombin time (HiTT; *circles*) at different in vitro heparin concentrations. The relationship is linear in each group. *(From Wang J-S, Lin C-Y, Karp RB: Comparison of high-dose thrombin time with activated clotting time for monitoring of anticoagulant effects of heparin in cardiac surgical patients.* Anesth Analg 79: 9–13, 1994.)

was minimally reduced and transfusion of non–red blood cell products could be significantly reduced relative to a group of patients who had ACT-based heparin management. They attributed their results to better preservation of the coagulation system by high heparin doses because the doses of heparin administered in the Hepcon group were nearly twice the doses used in the ACT management group. However, Gravlee et al[55] were unable to confirm suppression of ongoing coagulation using Hepcon CPB management. With the exception of during cold CPB, fibrinopeptide A (FPA) levels in patients who had heparin concentration monitoring were virtually indistinguishable from those in patients who had ACT monitoring (Figure 17-9). The Hepcon, however, remains one of the more sensitive tests for detecting residual heparinization after protamine reversal because the heparin concentration can be measured by protamine titration to levels as low as 0.4 IU/mL (see Monitoring for Heparin Rebound section later in this chapter).

Other tests that have been used to measure the heparin concentration include polybrene titration (functions similarly to protamine titration) and factor Xa inhibition. The latter requires plasma separation and is not practical for intraoperative monitoring. A modification of the thrombin time (TT) can be useful in monitoring heparin levels. One application would be an assay in which a known quantity of thrombin is added to patient blood or plasma. When mixed with a fibrin product, cleavage of the fibrin product can be measured fluorometrically. Only thrombin not bound by the heparin–AT III complex is available to cleave fibrin, thus yielding an indirect measure of heparin concentration.

High-Dose Thrombin Time

A functional test of heparin-induced anticoagulation that correlates well with heparin levels is the high-dose thrombin time (HiTT; International Technidyne, Edison, NJ). The TT is a clotting time that measures the conversion of fibrinogen to fibrin by thrombin. The TT is prolonged by the presence of heparin and by hypofibrinogenemias or dysfibrinogenemias. Because the TT is sensitive to very low

levels of heparin, a high dose of thrombin is necessary in the TT to accurately assay the high doses of heparin used for CPB. The HiTT is performed by adding whole blood to a prewarmed, prehydrated test tube that contains a lyophilized thrombin preparation. After the addition of 1.5 mL blood, the tube is inserted into a Hemochron well and the time to clot formation is measured. In vitro assays indicate that HiTT is equivalent to the ACT in evaluation of the anticoagulant effects of heparin at heparin concentrations in the range of 0 to 4.8 IU/mL (Figure 17-10). Unlike ACT, HiTT is not altered by hemodilution and hypothermia, and has been shown to correlate better with heparin concentration than the ACT during CPB.[58] While on CPB, heparin concentration and HiTT decrease, whereas the Hemochron and the Hepcon ACT increase (Figure 17-11). Another potential advantage of HiTT monitoring is for patients receiving aprotinin therapy. In the presence of heparin, aprotinin augments the celite ACT,[59] possibly because its kallikrein-inhibiting capacity prolongs activation of the intrinsic coagulation pathway by XIIa. This should not be interpreted to represent enhanced anticoagulation. The kaolin ACT is less affected by aprotinin therapy than the celite ACT, perhaps because kaolin, unlike celite, activates the intrinsic pathway by stimulation of factor XI directly.[60] Others have suggested that kaolin binds to aprotinin and reduces the anticoagulant effect of aprotinin in vitro. However, the heparinized kaolin ACT is still somewhat prolonged in the presence of aprotinin. HiTT is not affected by aprotinin therapy and can be used as a measure of heparinization for CPB patients receiving aprotinin therapy.[59] The high-dose thromboplastin time is another measure of anticoagulation that is not affected by aprotinin therapy.[61] The high-dose thromboplastin time is a WBCT in which celite is replaced by 0.3 mL of rabbit brain thromboplastin to which 1.2 mL blood is added. This test measures the time to coagulation via activation of the extrinsic pathway. This pathway of coagulation is also stimulated during pericardiotomy because of the rich thromboplastin environment of the pericardial cavity.

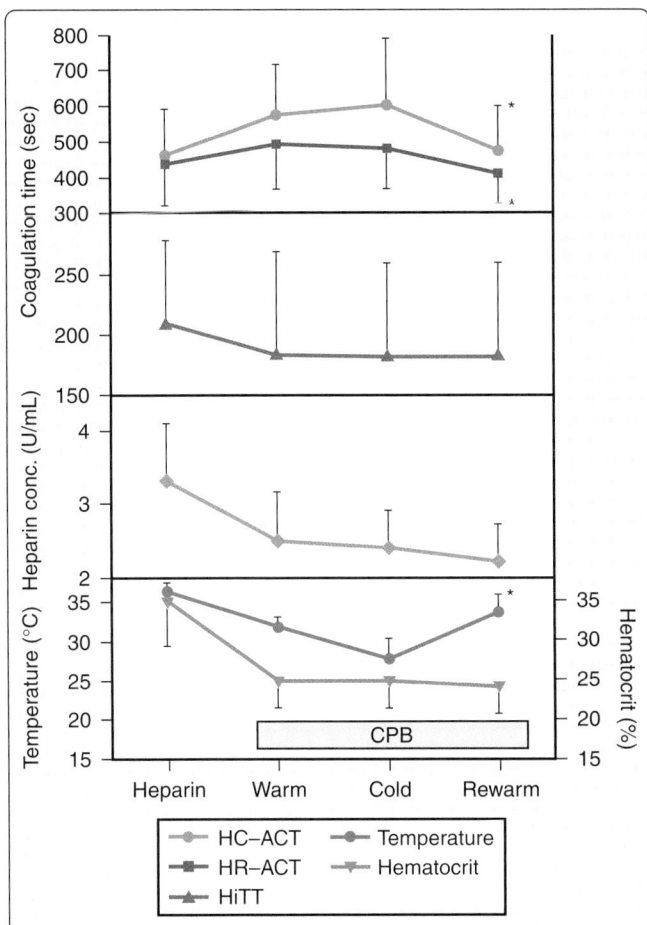

Figure 17-11 Changes over time in the Hemochron ACT (HC-ACT; *light circles*), Hepcon ACT (HR-ACT; *squares*), and high-dose thrombin time (HiTT; *upward triangles*) in cardiac surgical patients. HiTT is unaffected by the changes in temperature (*dark circles*) and hematocrit (*downward triangles*) during cardiopulmonary bypass (CPB). The HC-ACT and HR-ACT increase with the initiation of CPB and the heparin concentration and HiTT decrease. *Significant difference from previous time point (P < 0.05). (*From Wang J-S, Lin C-Y, Karp RB: Comparison of high-dose thrombin time with activated clotting time for monitoring of anticoagulant effects of heparin in cardiac surgical patients. Anesth Analg 79:9–13, 1994.)*

HEPARIN NEUTRALIZATION

Protamine Effects on Coagulation Monitoring

Reversal of heparin-induced anticoagulation is most frequently performed with protamine. Biologically, protamine binds to positively charged groups such as phosphate groups and may have important properties in angiogenesis and immune function. Different successful dosing plans have been proposed.[62,63] The recommended dose of protamine for heparin reversal is 1 to 1.3 mg protamine per 100 units heparin; however, this dose often results in a protamine excess.

Protamine injection causes adverse hemodynamic effects.[64] Protamine reactions have been classified into three types.[65] The most common of these reactions is the type I reaction characterized by hypotension. Type II (immunologic) reactions are categorized as IIA (anaphylaxis), IIB (anaphylactoid), and IIC (noncardiogenic pulmonary edema). Type III reactions are heralded by hypotension and catastrophic pulmonary hypertension leading to right-heart failure.[33,52,66]

In addition to hemodynamic sequelae, protamine has adverse effects on coagulation.[67] Large doses prolong the WBCT and the ACT, possibly

via thrombin inhibition.[68] In animals and in humans, protamine has been associated with thrombocytopenia, likely because of activation of the complement cascade.[64] The anticoagulant effect of protamine also may be caused by inhibition of platelet aggregation, alteration in the platelet surface membrane, or depression of the platelet response to various agonists.[68–70] These alterations in platelet function result from the presence of the heparin–protamine complex, not protamine alone. Protamine–heparin complexes activate AT III in vitro and result in complement activation. The anticoagulant effects of free protamine occur when protamine is given in doses in excess of those used clinically; however, the risk of free protamine being the cause of a hemostatic defect is small, given the rapid clearance of protamine relative to heparin.

Monitoring for Heparin Rebound

The phenomenon referred to as heparin rebound describes the reestablishment of a heparinized state after heparin has been neutralized with protamine. Various explanations for heparin rebound have been proposed.[9,56,71,72] The most commonly postulated is that rapid distribution and clearance of protamine occur shortly after protamine administration, leaving unbound heparin remaining after protamine clearance. Furthermore, endogenous heparin antagonists have an even shorter life span than protamine and are eliminated rapidly, resulting in free heparin concentrations. Also possible is the release of heparin from tissues considered heparin storage sites (endothelium, connective tissues). Endothelial cells bind and depolymerize heparin via PF4. Uptake into the cells of the reticuloendothelial system, vascular smooth muscle, and extracellular fluid may account for the storage of heparin that contributes to reactivation of heparin anticoagulation, referred to as heparin rebound.[9]

Residual low levels of heparin can be detected by sensitive heparin concentration monitoring in the first hour after protamine reversal and can be present for up to 6 hours after surgery. Gravlee et al's[56] study suggests that without careful monitoring for heparin rebound in the postoperative period, increased bleeding as a result of heparin rebound may occur, specifically when greater doses of heparin have been administered. Monitoring for heparin rebound can be accomplished using tests that are sensitive to low levels of circulating heparin.[52,57,73,74] These tests are also useful monitors for confirmation of heparin neutralization at the conclusion of CPB (see later).

Heparin Neutralization Monitors

To administer the appropriate dose of protamine at the conclusion of CPB, it would be ideal to measure the concentration of heparin present and give the dose of protamine necessary to neutralize only the circulating heparin. As a result of heparin metabolism and elimination, which vary considerably among individuals, the dose of protamine required to reverse a given dose of heparin decreases over time. Furthermore, protamine antagonizes the anti-IIa effects of heparin more effectively than the anti-Xa effects and, thus, varies in its potency depending on the source of heparin and its anti-IIa properties. Administration of a large fixed dose of protamine or a dose based on the total heparin dose given is no longer the standard of care and may result in an increased incidence of protamine-related adverse effects. An optimal dose of protamine is desired because unneutralized heparin results in clinical bleeding and an excess of protamine may produce an undesired coagulopathy. The use of individualized protamine dose–response curves uniformly results in a reduced protamine dose and has been shown to reduce postoperative bleeding.[49,73] One such dose–response test, the Hemochron PRT test, is an ACT performed on a heparinized blood sample that contains a known quantity of protamine. With knowledge of the ACT, PRT, and the estimated blood volume of the patient, the protamine dose needed to neutralize the existing heparin level can be extrapolated. The Hepcon instrument also has a PRT, which is

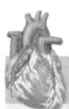

the protamine titration assay. The chamber that clots first contains the dose of protamine that most closely approximates the circulating dose of heparin. The protamine dose required for its neutralization is calculated on the basis of a specified heparin/protamine dose ratio by measuring the circulating heparin level.

At the levels of heparinization needed for cardiac surgery, tests that are sensitive to heparin become unclottable. ACT is relatively insensitive to heparin and is ideal for monitoring anticoagulation at high heparin levels but is too insensitive to accurately diagnose incomplete heparin neutralization. Reiner et al[75] showed that ACT had a high predictive value for adequate anticoagulation (confirmed by laboratory aPTT) when longer than 225 seconds but was poorly predictive for inadequate anticoagulation when shorter than 225 seconds. The low levels of heparin present when heparin is incompletely neutralized are best measured by other more sensitive tests of heparin-induced anticoagulation, such as heparin concentration, aPTT, and TT. Thus, after CPB, confirmation of return to the unanticoagulated state should be performed with a sensitive test for heparin anticoagulation[76–79] (Box 17-3).

Thrombin Time

TT is the time it takes for the conversion of fibrinogen to fibrin clot when blood or plasma is exposed to thrombin. Fibrin strands form in seconds. Detection of fibrin formation using standard laboratory equipment involves incubation of the blood or plasma sample within the chamber in which an optical or electrical probe sits. A detector senses either movement of the probe or the creation of an electrical field (electrical detection) because of fibrin formation and hence signals the end of the test. Hemochron manufactures a point-of-care TT test that uses a lyophilized preparation of thrombin in a Hemochron test tube to which 1 mL blood is added. Identification of fibrin formation in a Hemochron machine uses the standard Hemochron technology described previously with the ACT. The manufacturer suggests that the normal TT is 39 to 53 seconds for whole blood and 43 to 68 seconds for citrated blood. Because the TT specifically measures the activity of thrombin, it is very sensitive to heparin-induced enhancement of AT III activity. It is a useful test in the post-CPB period for differentiating the cause of bleeding when both PT and aPTT are prolonged because it excludes the intrinsic and extrinsic coagulation pathway limbs and evaluates the conversion of factor I to Ia. The TT is increased in the presence of heparin, hypofibrinogenemia, dysfibrinogenemia, amyloidosis, or antibodies to thrombin.[80] The TT is also increased in the presence of fibrin degradation products if the systemic fibrinogen concentration is low.

The TT is an appropriate laboratory test for monitoring the degree of fibrinolytic activity in patients receiving thrombolytic therapy. Measurements of the quantity of fibrinogen, plasminogen, or plasma proteins generated during fibrinolysis are difficult to interpret and yield no prognostic information for dose adjustments. Thrombolytic agents activate the fibrinolytic system to generate plasmin, which then causes clot dissolution and decreases the quantities of fibrinogen and fibrin. This effect can be monitored using the TT. The TT should be measured at baseline (before institution of fibrinolytic therapy) and 3 to 4 hours after therapy is initiated. If it is prolonged by 1.5 to 5 times the baseline value, therapy should be considered effective. If the TT is prolonged by greater than seven times the baseline value, an increased risk for bleeding is incurred; if the TT is not prolonged at all, therapy has failed to activate fibrinolysis.

Bedside Tests of Heparin Neutralization

Hepcon measures heparin concentration via a protamine titration assay. Cartridges with varying ranges of protamine concentration are available for use. The cartridge with the lower concentration of protamine in the titration is useful for the detection of residual circulating heparin and is sensitive to levels of heparin as low as 0.2 IU/mL. Whole-blood PT and aPTT assays are sensitive to deficiencies in coagulation factors and overly sensitive to low levels of heparin (aPTT); they lack specificity in assessing residual heparinization. The heparin-neutralized thrombin time (HNTT) is a TT assay with a small dose of protamine sufficient to neutralize 1.5 IU/mL heparin. Because the TT is increased in the presence of heparin, hypofibrinogenemia, or dysfibrinogenemia, HNTT and TT should be performed together to discriminate among these three causes. A normal HNTT in the presence of an increased TT virtually confirms residual heparin effect and would indicate the need for protamine administration. If HNTT is prolonged as well as the TT, the cause of bleeding may be attributed either to a fibrinogen problem or to a concentration of heparin greater than that which could be neutralized by the HNTT. In one study comparing bedside monitors of anticoagulation, the TT-HNTT difference bore a significant correlation with the aPTT increase. Using the line of best fit, aPTT elevation of 1.5 times the control corresponded to a 31-second difference in the TT and HNTT, indicating a convenient threshold value of TT-HNTT for the administration of protamine.[80]

Platelet Factor 4

A component of the alpha granule of platelets, PF4 binds to and inactivates heparin. The physiologic role of PF4 is that at the site of vascular injury, PF4 is released from platelets, binds heparin (or heparin-like compounds), and promotes thrombin and clot formation. PF4 adequately neutralizes heparin inhibition of factors Xa and IIa and may be superior to protamine in neutralizing anti-Xa effects. Animal data suggest that PF4 is devoid of the adverse hemodynamic effects seen with protamine and that it may be able to be infused more rapidly.[81,82] Heparin reversal has been documented by WBCT, ACT, and heparin concentration at a PF4 concentration of 40 U/mL, approximately twice the reversal dose of protamine.[74] Levy et al[83] subsequently found the reversal dose of PF4 to be approximately 60 U/mL and documented similar ACT and viscoelastic measurements of clot formation compared with protamine.

Heparinase

Heparinase (Neutralase I) is an enzyme that specifically degrades heparin by catalyzing cleavage of the saccharide bonds found in the heparin molecule. As demonstrated by the ACT, heparinase in a dose of 5 mg/kg has been shown to successfully neutralize heparin effects in healthy volunteers and in patients who have undergone CPB. A dose of 7 mg/kg has been demonstrated to be even more efficacious in returning ACT to baseline values. Doses sufficient to neutralize a dose of 300 IU/kg of heparin had no significant hemodynamic effects in a canine model.[84] Investigators have not found any platelet-depressive effects of heparinase in contrast with the well-documented platelet dysfunction associated with protamine therapy.[69] Return to the unanticoagulated state after the use of heparinase has been confirmed using ACT monitoring or heparin concentration monitoring.

TESTS OF COAGULATION

Standard tests of coagulation, the PT and the aPTT, are performed on plasma to which the anticoagulant citrate has been added. Because these tests are performed on plasma, they require centrifugation of blood and generally are not feasible for use at the bedside. The aPTT tests the integrity of the intrinsic and the final coagulation pathways and is more sensitive to low levels of heparin than the ACT. Factors IX and X are most sensitive to heparin effects, and thus the aPTT will be prolonged even at very low heparin levels. The test uses a phospholipid substance to simulate the interaction of the platelet membrane in activating factor XII. (Thromboplastin is a tissue extract containing tissue factor and phospholipid. The term *partial thromboplastin* refers to the use of the phospholipid portion only.) The aPTT is prolonged in the presence of deficiencies of factors XII, XI, IX, and VIII, HMWK (high molecular weight kininogen), and kallikrein. The aPTT reaction is considerably slower than the PT, and an activator such as celite or kaolin is added to the assay to speed activation of factor XII. After incubation of citrated plasma with phospholipid and activator, calcium is added and the time to clot formation is measured. Normal aPTT is 28 to 32 seconds, which often is expressed as a ratio with a control plasma sample from the same laboratory. This is important because partial thromboplastin reagents have different sensitivities to heparin, and many have nonlinear responses to heparin in various concentration ranges.

PT measures the integrity of the extrinsic and common coagulation pathways. PT will be prolonged in the presence of factor VII deficiency, warfarin sodium (Coumadin) therapy, or vitamin K deficiency. Large doses of heparin also prolong the PT because of inactivation of factor II. The addition of thromboplastin to citrated plasma results in activation of extrinsic coagulation. After a 3-minute incubation and recalcification, the time to clot formation is measured and is recorded as the PT. Normal PT is 12 to 14 seconds; however, because of differences in the quality and lot of the thromboplastin used, absolute PT values are not standardized and are difficult to compare across different testing centers. The international normalized ratio (INR) has been adopted as the standard for coagulation monitoring. The INR is an internationally standardized laboratory value that is the ratio of the patient's PT to the result that would have been obtained if the International Reference Preparation had been used instead of the laboratory reagents. Each laboratory uses reagents with a specific sensitivity (International Sensitivity Index [ISI]) relative to the International Reference Preparation. The ISI of a particular set of reagents is provided by each manufacturer so that the INR can be reported.

Bedside Tests of Coagulation

PT and aPTT tests performed on whole blood are available for use in the operating room or at the bedside. The Hemochron PT test tube contains acetone-dried rabbit brain thromboplastin to which 2 mL whole blood is added and the tube is inserted into a standard Hemochron machine. Normal values range from 50 to 72 seconds and are automatically converted by a computer to the plasma-equivalent PT and INR. Hemochron aPTT contains kaolin activator and a platelet factor substitute and is performed similarly to the PT. The aPTT is sensitive to heparin concentrations as low as 0.2 U/mL and displays a linear relation with heparin concentration up to 1.5 U/mL.

The former Thrombolytic Assessment System (TAS; Pharmanetics, Raleigh, NC), now the Cascade POC (Helena, Beaumont, TX), which was previously discussed for its ability to measure heparin via the HMT, also measures PT and aPTT. The sample is added to a cartridge containing paramagnetic iron oxide particles, which oscillate in a magnetic field as described. Specific activating reagents are used for each analyte. The analytes used include rabbit brain thromboplastin for the PT, aluminum magnesium silicate for aPTT, and celite for HMT. The blood moves by capillary action and mixes with paramagnetic iron oxide particles and reagent within the testing chamber. The decreased movement of the particles is detected optically as the sample clots, and the resultant time is displayed in seconds and as INRs for PT.

The CoaguChekProDM (Roche Diagnostics, Mannheim, Germany), former CoaguChek-plus, and formerly Ciba Corning Biotrack 512 coagulation monitor for evaluating bedside PT and aPTT, uses 0.1 mL whole blood placed into a disposable plastic cartridge for either PT or aPTT. The sample is drawn by capillary action into a heated chamber where exposure to reagents occurs. The PT uses rabbit brain thromboplastin. The aPTT uses soybean phosphatide as the platelet substitute and bovine brain sulfatide as the activator. From the reaction chamber, blood traverses a reaction path where clot formation is detected by a laser optical system. The resulting time to clot formation is converted to a ratio of the control value by a microprocessor that has control values encoded.

Many investigators have studied the former Ciba Corning Biotrack system for monitoring anticoagulation in different clinical scenarios. For patients receiving oral anticoagulant therapy, the Biotrack 512 monitor has been found to be suitable for monitoring PT and INR. Reiner et al[75] compared the bedside Biotrack aPTT with the laboratory aPTT and heparin level in patients receiving therapeutic heparinization after interventional cardiac catheterization. The authors found a strong correlation ($r = 0.89$) between the Biotrack aPTT and the aPTT from the hospital laboratory. The correlation between Biotrack aPTT and heparin level was not strong, probably because of the many other factors such as heparin neutralization and clearance that affect the heparin concentration in vivo.[85] Another study in patients receiving heparin compared the Ciba Corning Biotrack aPTT assay with standard laboratory aPTT and documented that Biotrack was less sensitive to heparin than the laboratory aPTT; however, the correlation coefficient of these two tests was $r = 0.82$.[86] In patients on warfarin therapy, the Biotrack aPTT was more sensitive than the laboratory aPTT and yielded consistently greater results for aPTT value. In another study in patients being anticoagulated for nonsurgical applications, the bedside aPTT was similar to the standard aPTT in its prediction of treatment in simple therapeutic algorithms. However, in more complex clinical situations, there was less agreement between the bedside aPTT and laboratory aPTT.[87]

In a comparison of bedside coagulation monitors after cardiac surgical procedures, Reich et al[80] documented acceptable accuracy and precision levels for Hemochron and Ciba Corning Biotrack PT in comparison with standard laboratory plasma PT, making them potentially valuable for use in the perioperative period. Neither Hemochron nor Ciba Corning aPTT reached this level of clinical competence compared with standard laboratory tests. Others have documented that this monitor seems to be more precise for PT than for aPTT.[88] Because of rapid turnaround times, these point-of-care coagulation monitors may be useful in predicting patients who will bleed after cardiac surgery[89] and have also been used successfully in transfusion algorithms to decrease the number of allogeneic blood products given to cardiac surgical patients.[90,91]

Measures of Fibrin Formation

The "Tenase complex" is the group of factors and cofactors that includes Xa, platelet-bound factor Va, platelet factor 3, and Ca^{2+}. All adhere on the platelet surface and catalyze the cleavage of prothrombin (factor II) to thrombin (factor IIa). Thrombin then catalyzes the cleavage of fibrinogen to form fibrin monomer and fibrinopeptide A and fibrinopeptide B. These end products of fibrinogen cleavage are commonly measured serum markers that help to quantify the degree of coagulation that occurs in certain experimental or clinical situations.

One such experimental situation is the use of heparin-bonded extracorporeal circuits during CPB with the expectation that thrombin activation and fibrin formation will be minimized. Coating of the extracorporeal circuit with the heparin ligand makes the circuit more biocompatible such that the inflammatory response elicited is diminished or nonexistent. Heparin-bonded circuits have been extensively studied and considered advantageous because of their ability to reduce the inflammatory response to CPB. Human studies reveal decreases in enzymes that mark leukocyte activation, thus showing a reduction in the whole-body inflammatory response similar to that seen with leukocyte-depletion techniques.[92–94]

Further enhancements in biocompatibility include less leukocyte activation and preserved platelet function. Reductions in thrombin generation have been difficult to document.[95] The increases in the fibrinogen fragment F1.2 and in D-dimer levels when heparin-coated circuits are used are similar to those seen when uncoated circuits are used.[96,97] Human studies have documented less bleeding and reduced transfusion requirements with the use of a heparin-coated extracorporeal circulation when these circuits are used in conjunction with a reduced systemic heparin dose.[98,99] In this circumstance, markers of thrombin generation are increased even greater than those in patients in whom full-dose heparin and uncoated circuits are used. In fact, increases are seen in fibrinopeptide A, prothrombin fragment F1.2, thrombin–antithrombin III complexes, D-dimers, and plasminogen activators during CPB and after protamine administration regardless of whether heparin-coated circuits are used and regardless of heparin dose.[100] Despite this, the use of reduced heparin doses and coated circuitry has resulted in diminished transfusion requirements and reduced chest tube drainage volumes without evidence of complications.[97,101] Because microvascular coagulation is not fully inhibited, the use of a reduced dose of heparin cannot be systematically advocated and should be implemented with caution.

Fibrinogen Level

Fibrinogen concentration is traditionally measured using either clottable protein methods, end-point detection techniques, or immunochemical tests. Of the former, the most commonly used fibrinogen assay relies on the method of Clauss. This method involves a 10-fold dilution of plasma, which ensures that fibrinogen is the rate-limiting step in clot formation. Subsequently, an excess of thrombin is added to the sample and the time to clot formation is measured. The clotting time is inversely related to the fibrinogen concentration. Because this assay relies on detection of actual clot, it can be affected by fibrin degradation products, polymerization inhibitors, or other inhibitors of fibrin formation. Because of the thrombin excess, small clinical concentrations of heparin do not affect fibrinogen determination according to the Clauss technique.

A whole-blood point-of-care fibrinogen assay is available using the Hemochron system. The specific test tube contains a lyophilized preparation of human thrombin, snake venom extract, protamine, buffers, and calcium stabilizers. The test tube is incubated with 1.5 mL distilled water and heated in the Hemochron instrument for 3 minutes. Whole blood is placed into a diluent vial, where it is 50% diluted, and from this vial, 0.5 mL diluted whole blood is placed into the specific fibrinogen test tube. The clotting time is measured using standard Hemochron technology as described previously. The fibrinogen concentration is determined by comparison with a standard curve for this test. Normal fibrinogen concentration of 180 to 220 mg/dL correlates with a clotting time of 54 ± 2.5 seconds. Fibrinogen deficiency of 50 to 75 mg/dL correlates with a clotting time of 150 ± 9.0 seconds.

Unlike the method of Clauss, the end-point detection assays rely on the detection of changes in turbidity of plasma when clot is formed. This technique does not require the maintenance of a stable cross-linked fibrin product and, therefore, does not report underestimated fibrinogen measurements because of the presence of inhibitors. Immunochemical measures of fibrinogen concentration are a direct and accurate measurement technique; however, they are expensive and time consuming and require specialized laboratory facilities.

MONITORING FIBRINOLYSIS

Fibrinolysis, the dissolution of fibrin, is the normal modifier of hemostasis that ensures that coagulation does not proceed unchecked. It occurs in the vicinity of a clot and dissolves clot when local endothelial healing occurs. Fibrinolysis is mediated by the serine protease plasmin, which is the product of the cleavage of plasminogen by tissue plasminogen activator (tPA). Fibrinolysis is a normal phenomenon in response to clot formation; when it occurs systemically, it represents a pathologic condition.

Fibrinolysis can be primary or secondary. Primary fibrinolysis occurs when fibrinolytic activators are released or produced in excess and does not represent a response to the coagulation process. Examples of primary fibrinolysis include the release of plasminogen activators during liver transplantation surgery and the exogenous administration of fibrinolytic agents such as streptokinase. During primary fibrinolysis, plasmin cleaves fibrinogen, yielding fibrinogen degradation products. These end products can be measured using immunologic techniques.

When fibrinolysis is a result of enhanced activation of the coagulation system, secondary fibrinolysis ensues. A well-known extreme form of secondary fibrinolysis is seen during disseminated intravascular coagulation, when both systemic coagulation and fibrinolysis are occurring in excess. During CPB, fibrinolysis is most likely secondary to the microvascular coagulation that is occurring despite attempts at suppression using high doses of heparin.[102,103]

The identification of fibrinolysis can be accomplished through either direct measurement of the clot lysis time (manual or viscoelastic tests) or measurement of the end-products of fibrin degradation. The manual clot lysis time simply involves the placement of whole blood into a test tube. This blood clots in a matter of minutes. Visual inspection determines the end point for observation of clot lysis, and this time period is the clot lysis time. This technique is considerably time consuming and requires constant observation by the person performing the test.

Viscoelastic Tests

Viscoelastic tests measure the unique properties of the clot as it is forming, organizing, strengthening, and lysing. As a result, fibrinolysis determination by this methodology requires that time elapse during which clot formation is occurring. It is subsequent to clot formation and platelet-fibrin linkages that clot lysis parameters can be measured. For this reason, viscoelastic tests often require longer than 1 hour to detect the initiation of fibrinolysis; however, if fibrinolysis is enhanced, results often can be obtained in 30 minutes.

End Products of Fibrin Degradation

Other methods for quantifying fibrinolysis include measurement of the end products of fibrin degradation. Fibrin degradation products are the result of the cleavage of fibrin monomers and polymers and can be measured using a latex agglutination assay. When plasmin cleaves cross-linked fibrin, dimeric units are formed that comprise one D-domain from each of two adjacent fibrin units. These "D-dimers" are frequently measured by researchers in clinical and laboratory investigations. They are measured by either enzyme-linked immunosorbent assays or latex agglutination techniques and, thus, are not available for on-site use. Controversy still exists regarding whether D-dimer level or fibrin degradation products are the most sensitive test for detecting fibrinolysis, but most agree that the presence of D-dimers is the most specific for cross-linked fibrin degradation.[104]

MONITORING THE THROMBIN INHIBITORS

A new class of drugs, the selective thrombin inhibitors, is a viable alternative to heparin anticoagulation for CPB. These agents include hirudin, argatroban, and other experimental agents. A major advantage of these agents over heparin is that they are able to effectively inhibit clot-bound thrombin in an AT III–independent fashion.[105] The platelet thrombin receptor is believed to be the focus of thrombin's procoagulant effects in states of thrombosis such as after coronary artery angioplasty. Because surface-bound thrombin is more effectively suppressed, thrombin generation can be reduced at lower levels of systemic anticoagulation than are achieved during anticoagulation by the heparin–AT III complex. This translates into less bleeding despite the lack of a clinically useful antidote for the thrombin antagonists.[106,107] Thrombin antagonists are also not susceptible to neutralization by PF4 and, thus, are not neutralized at endothelial sites where activated platelets reside. They are also useful in patients with HIT in whom the administration of heparin and subsequent antibody-induced platelet aggregation would be dangerous.[108] The lack of a potent antidote (such as protamine) and a prolonged duration of action are the major reasons that hirudin and other thrombin inhibitors have not found widespread clinical acceptance for use in CPB procedures (see Chapter 31).

Hirudin

Hirudin, a coagulation inhibitor isolated from the salivary glands of the medicinal leech *(Hirudo medicinalis)*, is a potent inhibitor of thrombin that, unlike heparin, acts independently of AT III and inhibits clot-bound thrombin, as well as fluid-phase thrombin. Hirudin does not require a cofactor and is not susceptible to neutralization by PF4. This would seem to be beneficial in patients in whom platelet activation and thrombosis are potential problems. Recombinant hirudin was administered as a 0.25-mg/kg bolus and an infusion to maintain the hirudin concentration at 2.5 µg/mL, as determined by the ecarin clotting time in studies by Koster et al.[109–117] The ecarin clotting time, modified for use in the Cascade POC analyzer, has been used in large series of patients with HIT.[109–114] Compared with standard treatment with heparin or low-molecular-weight heparins, recombinant hirudin–treated patients maintained platelet counts and hemoglobin levels, and had few bleeding complications, if renal function was normal.[115,116] Hirudin is a small molecule (molecular weight, 7 kDa) that is eliminated by the kidney and is easily hemofiltered at the end of CPB.[117] In patients with abnormal renal function, bivalirudin is preferable to hirudin. An alternative treatment in this setting would be administration of unfractionated heparin with a platelet antagonist, such as tirofiban, to prevent the hyperaggregability of platelets that occurs in patients with HIT.[116]

Bivalirudin

Bivalirudin is a small 20-amino acid molecule with a plasma half-life of 24 minutes. It is a synthetic derivative of hirudin and thus acts as a direct thrombin inhibitor. Bivalirudin binds to both the catalytic binding site and the anion-binding exosite on fluid-phase and clot-bound thrombin. The part of the molecule that binds to thrombin is actually cleaved by thrombin itself, so the elimination of bivalirudin activity is independent of specific organ metabolism. Bivalirudin has been used successfully as an anticoagulant in interventional cardiology procedures as a replacement for heparin therapy. In fact, in interventional cardiology, bivalirudin has been associated with less bleeding and equivalent ischemic outcomes compared with heparin plus a platelet inhibitor.[118] This may be the result of bivalirudin being both an antithrombin anticoagulant and an antithrombin at the level of the platelet. Merry et al[119] showed equivalence with regard to bleeding outcomes and an improvement in graft flow after off-pump cardiac surgery when bivalirudin was used (0.75-mg/kg bolus, 1.75-mg/kg/hr infusion). Case reports confirm the safety of bivalirudin use during CPB.[120–122] Multicenter clinical trials comparing bivalirudin with heparin in off-pump surgery[123] and in CPB[124] demonstrated "noninferiority" of bivalirudin. Efficacy of anticoagulation and markers of blood loss were similar in the two groups, suggesting that bivalirudin can be a safe and effective anticoagulant in CPB. These multicenter trials used the ACT as the monitor of anticoagulant activity during surgery, but ideal monitoring is performed using the ecarin clotting time, as seen with hirudin.[125] The ecarin clotting time has a closer correlation with anti-IIa activity and plasma drug levels than does the ACT. For this reason, standard ACT monitoring during antithrombin therapy is not preferred if ecarin clotting time can be measured. A plasma-modified ACT can be used to more accurately assay the anticoagulant effects of the thrombin inhibitor drugs than ACT. This test requires the addition of exogenous plasma and, thus, is not readily available as a point-of-care assay.[126]

BOX 17-4. THROMBIN INHIBITORS

- These anticoagulant drugs are superior to heparin.
- They inhibit both clot-bound and soluble thrombin.
- They do not require a cofactor, activate platelets, or cause immunogenicity.
- Heparin remains an attractive drug because of its long history of safe use and the fact that it has a specific drug antidote, protamine.
- These drugs include hirudin, argatroban, and bivalirudin.

The anticoagulant effects of the thrombin antagonists can be monitored using the ACT, aPTT, or the TT. The bleeding time also may be prolonged. In a canine CPB model, dogs receiving a synthetic thrombin inhibitor had less postoperative blood loss and greater platelet counts than those receiving heparin; however, those who received a large dose of the thrombin inhibitor still had ACT increases at 2 hours after CPB.[127] There were no differences in hemodynamics noted in the groups.

Bivalirudin has been compared favorably with heparin in patients undergoing coronary angioplasty for unstable angina.[128] The half-life of aPTT prolongation is approximately 40 minutes, and reductions in formation of fibrinopeptide A are evidence of thrombin inhibition and fibrinogen preservation. Careful monitoring should be used because there may be a rebound prothrombotic state after cessation of therapy, which could lead to recurrence of anginal symptoms (Box 17-4).

EVALUATION OF A PROLONGED ACTIVATED PARTIAL THROMBOPLASTIN TIME

The first step in evaluation of a prolonged aPTT is the elimination of heparin contamination as a cause of the elevation. Other potential causes of an elevated aPTT are the presence of factor deficiencies or inhibitors of coagulation. Factor deficiencies can be ruled out by mixing studies in which patient plasma is mixed with an equal volume of plasma derived from healthy volunteers. The test results should return to normal if a deficiency is present because mixing with normal plasma yields greater than the required concentrations of coagulation proteins for adequate clotting. If an inhibitor is present, mixing studies will not return the aPTT to normal values.

Inhibitors of factors VIII and IX and the "lupus anticoagulants" are the most common inhibitors encountered. The lupus anticoagulants are antiphospholipid antibodies that react with the phospholipid surfaces required for coagulation, thus the prolongation of the clotting time. In patients who do not have systemic lupus, this syndrome is referred to as primary antiphospholipid syndrome. Testing for this inhibitor has been performed using the aPTT or a dilute viper venom time. The latter consists of activation of factor X by venom and measurement of the clotting time, which will be prolonged if an inhibitor is present. Immunologic assays for anticardiolipin antibodies are available. Patient serum is incubated with solid-phase cardiolipin and bound immunoglobulin is measured.

MONITORING PLATELET FUNCTION

Circulating platelets adhere to the endothelium via platelet surface receptors that bind exposed collagen and become activated. This initiates platelet activation because collagen is a potent platelet activator. The unstimulated platelet, which is discoid in shape, undergoes a conformational change when activated. The activated platelet is spherical, extrudes pseudopodia, and expresses an increased number of activated surface receptors that can be measured to quantify the degree of platelet reactivity. The intensity of this platelet activation occurs in proportion to the quantity and nature of the platelet stimulus and increases in a graded fashion with increasing concentrations of agonists. The glycoprotein (GP) IIb/IIIa receptor is the primary receptor responsible for fibrinogen binding and the formation of the platelet plug.

▣ Platelet Count

Numerous events occur during cardiac surgical procedures that predispose patients to platelet-related hemostasis defects. The two major categories are thrombocytopenia and qualitative platelet defects. Thrombocytopenia commonly occurs during cardiac surgery as a result of hemodilution, sequestration, and destruction by nonendothelial surfaces. Platelet counts commonly decline to 100,000/μL or slightly less; however, the final platelet count is greatly dependent on the starting value and the duration of platelet destructive interventions (i.e., CPB).[129] Between 10,000/μL and 100,000/μL, bleeding time decreases directly; however, at platelet counts greater than 50,000/μL, neither the bleeding time nor platelet count has any correlation with postoperative bleeding in cardiac surgical patients. In contrast, platelet size or mean platelet volume does have some correlation with hemostatic function. Larger, younger platelets are more hemostatically active than smaller ones.[130,131] Mean platelet volume multiplied by the platelet count gives an estimation of overall platelet mass and is referred to as the "plateletcrit." It is important to appreciate the inverse relation between platelet volume and platelet count when using a measure such as the plateletcrit to assess the viability of the existing platelet population. Because the mean platelet volume is dependent on the method of specimen collection, the anticoagulant used, and temperature of the storage conditions, its reproducibility is dependent on standardized laboratory procedures.

Qualitative platelet defects occur more commonly than thrombocytopenia during CPB procedures. The range of possible causes of platelet dysfunction includes traumatic extracorporeal techniques, pharmacologic therapy, hypothermia, and fibrinolysis; the hemostatic insult increases with the duration of time spent on CPB.[132] The use of bubble oxygenators, noncoated extracorporeal circulation, and cardiotomy suctioning may cause platelets to become activated, initiate the release reaction, and partly deplete platelets of the contents of their alpha granules. Many of these changes are only transiently associated with CPB. Khuri et al[133] characterized the hematologic changes associated with CPB in a group of 85 patients. Whereas the platelet count declines and reaches a plateau at 2 hours after CPB, mean platelet volume reaches its nadir at 2 hours after CPB and then begins to increase during the ensuing 72 hours[131,133] (Figures 17-12 and 17-13). The relative thrombocytopenia seen up to 72 hours after cardiac surgery is not

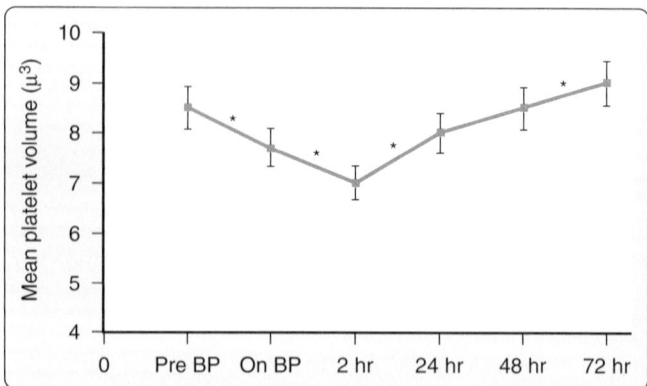

Figure 17-13   Changes in mean platelet volume (MPV) in patients undergoing cardiopulmonary bypass (CPB). Note that the decrease in MPV that occurs during CPB returns to and exceeds baseline values at 24 hours after surgery. *P < 0.05 change from previous value. *(From Khuri SF, Wolfe JA, Josa M, et al: Hematologic changes during and after cardiopulmonary bypass and their relationship to the bleeding time and nonsurgical blood loss. J Thorac Cardiovasc Surg 104:94–107, 1992.)*

consistently associated with a bleeding diathesis. Similarly, the clotting proteins fibrinogen, factor VIII–von Willebrand factor, and factor VIII-C also increase to levels greater than baseline in the 2 to 72 hours after CPB (Figure 17-14).

Large doses of heparin have been shown to reduce the ability of the platelets to aggregate and to reduce clot strength.[68] This effect is not reversed when protamine is administered; however, it may be mitigated by the prophylactic administration of aprotinin.[134,135] The adverse effects of heparin on platelet function may be because of its ability to inhibit the formation of thrombin, the most potent in vivo platelet activator.[136] However, heparin also activates the fibrinolytic system, a system that, through plasmin and other activators, has the ability to depress platelet function through other mechanisms. In an extracorporeal baboon model, intravenous heparin

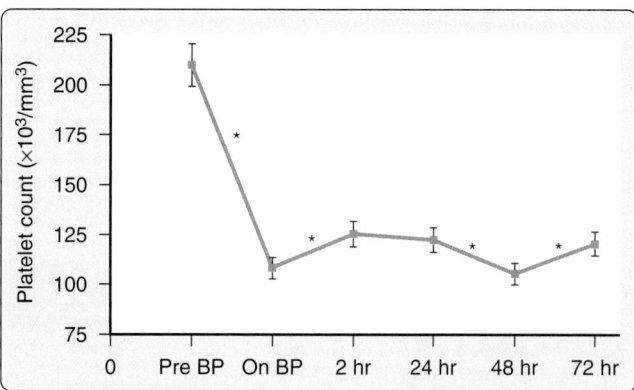

Figure 17-12   **Platelet count changes in patients undergoing cardiopulmonary bypass (CPB).** Significant decrease in platelet count occurs on initiation of CPB and remains until at least 72 hours after surgery. *P < 0.05 change from previous value. *(From Khuri SF, Wolfe JA, Josa M, et al: Hematologic changes during and after cardiopulmonary bypass and their relationship to the bleeding time and nonsurgical blood loss. J Thorac Cardiovasc Surg 104:94–107, 1992.)*

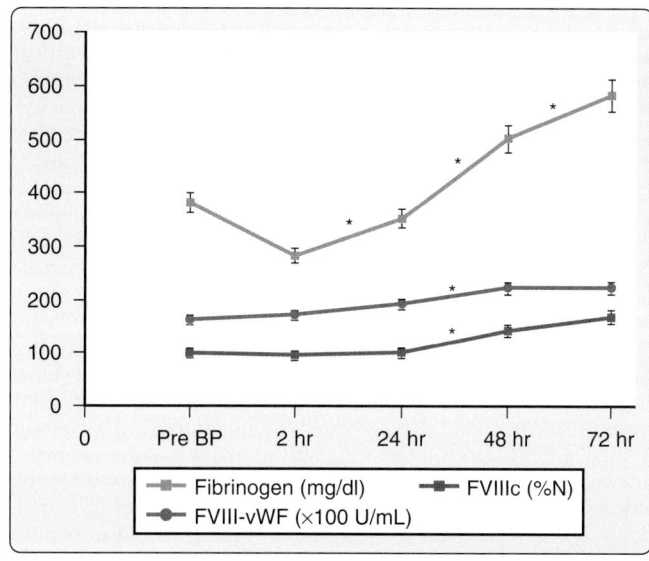

Figure 17-14   Fibrinogen values *(light squares)* decrease during cardiopulmonary bypass (CPB). All three clotting proteins increase to more than baseline levels in the 24 to 72 hours after CPB. *P < 0.05 change from previous value. Pre BP, prebypass; FVIIIc, factor VIIIc *(dark squares)*; FVIII-vWF, factor VIII–von Willebrand factor *(circles)*. *(From Khuri SF, Wolfe JA, Josa M, et al: Hematologic changes during and after cardiopulmonary bypass and their relationship to the bleeding time and nonsurgical blood loss. J Thorac Cardiovasc Surg 104:94–107, 1992.)*

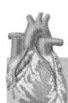

BOX 17-5. PLATELET FUNCTION

- The measure of platelet count does not correlate with bleeding after cardiac surgery.
- Patients frequently have extreme degrees of thrombocytopenia but do not bleed because they have adequate platelet function.
- It is the measure of platelet function that correlates temporally with the bleeding course seen after cardiac surgery.
- The thromboelastogram maximal amplitude, mean platelet volume, and other functional platelet tests are useful in transfusion algorithms.

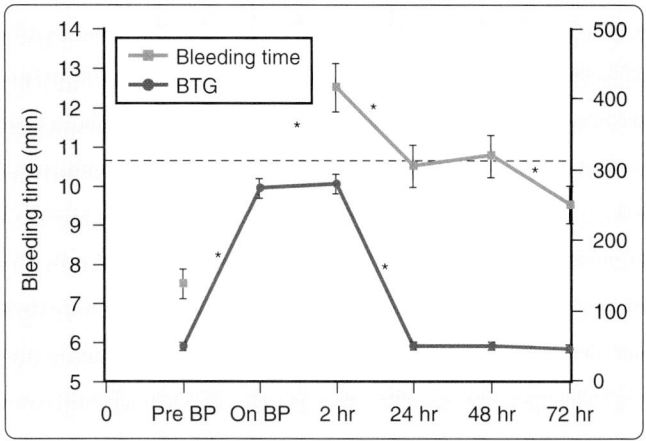

Figure 17-15 Bleeding time *(squares)* increases on cardiopulmonary bypass (CPB) and remains increased until at least 72 hours after surgery. However, platelet activation is maximal during CPB. The increase in b-thromboglobulin (BTG; *circles*), indicating platelet activation, occurs on initiation of CPB and returns to baseline by 24 hours afterward. *$P < 0.05$ change from previous value. *(From Khuri SF, Wolfe JA, Josa M, et al: Hematologic changes during and after cardiopulmonary bypass and their relationship to the bleeding time and nonsurgical blood loss. J Thorac Cardiovasc Surg 104:94–107, 1992.)*

administration resulted in increases in plasmin activity, in the quantity of immunoreactive plasmin light chain, and in immunoreactive fibrinogen fragment E.[1,137] In addition, various degrees of fibrinolysis occur after CPB. Circulating plasmin causes dissolution of the GP Ib platelet receptor and decreases the adhesiveness of platelets. Because fibrinolysis is partly responsible for the platelet dysfunction seen after heparin administration and CPB, the efficacy of antifibrinolytic agents as hemostatic drugs can be better appreciated. In addition to reducing platelet adhesiveness to von Willebrand factor, the fibrin degradation products formed depress platelet responsiveness to agonists.[138,139]

Protamine–heparin complexes and protamine alone also contribute to platelet depression after CPB. Mild-to-moderate degrees of hypothermia are associated with reversible degrees of platelet activation and platelet dysfunction,[140] which may be partly mitigated by the use of aprotinin therapy.[141] Overall, the potential coagulation benefits of normothermic CPB compared with hypothermic CPB require further study in well-conducted randomized trials (Box 17-5).

Bleeding Time

The bleeding time is performed by creating a skin incision and measuring the time to clot formation via the platelet plug. The Ivy bleeding time is performed on the volar surface of the forearm above which a cuff is inflated to 40 mm Hg (above venous pressure). Two parallel incisions are made using a template, and the incisions are blotted with filter paper every 30 seconds until no further bleeding occurs. The time from incision to cessation of blood seepage is the template bleeding time. The Duke bleeding time is performed on the earlobe and has advantages for cardiac surgery because the earlobe is more accessible and less likely to be subjected to the peripheral vasoconstriction seen after hypothermia. However, because neither the width/depth of the incision nor the venous pressure can be controlled in the Duke bleeding time, the Ivy bleeding time is considered the superior test. Normal bleeding time is 4 to 10 minutes.

Numerous prospective blinded investigations have confirmed that bleeding time has little or no value in predicting excessive hemorrhage after cardiac surgery.[142,143] Even in patients receiving therapeutic doses of aspirin, an increase in bleeding time does not necessarily translate to an increase in mediastinal tube drainage or transfusions if reinfusion and blood conservation techniques are used aggressively. There is substantial evidence that platelet-directed therapy in the form of platelet transfusions or desmopressin acetate shortens a prolonged bleeding time in patients with clinical hemorrhage.[144,145] In a study of 85 patients undergoing CPB, Khuri et al[133] demonstrated that bleeding time becomes abnormally increased during CPB and does not return to baseline even by 72 hours after surgery, whereas markers of platelet activation return to baseline by 24 hours after surgery (Figure 17-15). Because the bleeding time does not follow the temporal course of postoperative coagulopathy, the bleeding time may be a nonspecific and impractical test for detecting an existing platelet defect but may be suitable for following patient response to platelet-directed therapies.

Aggregometry

Activated platelets undergo aggregation, which is initially a reversible process. Activation also induces the release of substances from alpha and dense platelet granules and platelet lysosomes. Because platelet granules contain many platelet agonists, the release of granular contents further stimulates platelet activation and is responsible for the secondary phase of platelet aggregation. This secondary phase of platelet aggregation is dependent on the release of thromboxane and other substances from the platelet granules, is an energy-consuming process, and is irreversible (Table 17-2).

Aggregometry is a useful research tool for measuring platelet responsiveness to a variety of different agonists. The end result, platelet aggregation, is an objective measure of platelet activation. Platelet aggregometry uses a photo-optical instrument to measure light transmittance through a sample of whole-blood or platelet-rich plasma. Platelet-rich plasma undergoes a decrease in light transmittance on the early phase of platelet activation because of the change in platelet shape from discoid to spherical. When exposed to a platelet agonist such as thrombin, adenosine diphosphate (ADP), epinephrine, collagen, or ristocetin, the initial reversible aggregation phase results in increased light transmittance because of the platelet aggregates that decrease the turbidity of the sample. The larger the platelet aggregates, the greater is the transmittance of light. In the absence of further activation, disaggregation occurs and the plasma sample becomes turbid. However, when the platelet release reaction occurs, thromboxane and other activators

TABLE 17-2	Platelet Adhesion and Aggregation		
Ligand	*Receptor*	*Properties*
Collagen	GP Ia/IIa, GP IIb/IIIa, GP IV	Adhesion, aggregation, secretion
Thrombospondin	GP IV, $\alpha_v\beta_3$	Adhesion, antiadhesion
vWF	GP Ib/IX, GP IIb/IIIa	Adhesion
Fibrinogen	GP IIb/IIIa	Aggregation
Laminin	GP Ic/IIa	Attachment
Vitronectin	$\alpha_v\beta_3$, GP IIb/IIIa	$\alpha_v\beta_3$ = vitronectin receptor
Fibronectin	GP Ic/IIa, GP IIb/IIIa	Attachment, spreading

GP, glycoprotein; vWF, von Willebrand factor.

are released from the platelet alpha granules and the phase of secondary, or irreversible, aggregation occurs. This results in a further increase in light transmittance.

Defects in platelet aggregation can be seen in patients with storage pool deficiency, Bernard–Soulier syndrome, or Glanzmann's thrombasthenia and in patients taking salicylates. Impaired platelet aggregation has been demonstrated to occur after extracorporeal circulation, but investigators have had difficulty showing a correlation between impaired aggregation and clinical bleeding.[146,147] One ex vivo study demonstrated a significant correlation between platelet aggregation and 3-hour postoperative bleeding; however, correlations were greatest when preoperative aggregometry was performed using whole-blood samples and when postoperative measurements were performed using platelet-rich plasma.[147] The assessment of the platelet defect induced by aspirin consumption is more sensitive when whole-blood aggregometry is performed. The extreme sensitivity of this assay to minor defects in platelet function has resulted in a high negative predictive value but a rather low positive predictive value for bleeding. Its inability to be performed easily in the clinical arena has designated platelet aggregometry as strictly a research tool with occasional clinical applications.

Platelet-Mediated Force Transduction

An instrument that measures the force developed by platelets during clot retraction has been shown to be directly related to platelet concentration and function[148] (Hemodyne). The apparatus consists of a cup and a parallel upper plate. The cup is filled with blood or the platelet-containing solution, and the upper plate is lowered onto the clotting solution. Clot forms and adheres to the outer edges of the cup and to the plate above. A thin layer of oil is deposited onto the surfaces that are exposed to air. The upper plate is coupled to a displacement transducer that translates displacement caused by platelet retraction into a force. Normal values for platelet force development have been suggested by the investigators.[70] The antiplatelet effects of heparin have been evaluated using this force retractometer. Using this instrument, investigators have shown that high heparin concentrations completely abolish platelet force generation.[68] Furthermore, the concentration of protamine required to reverse the anticoagulant effects of heparin is not sufficient to reverse these antiplatelet effects. The antiplatelet effects of protamine alone also have been evaluated using this monitor.

Fluorescence Flow Cytometry

The introduction of fluorescence flow cytometry into the clinical laboratory has provided a sensitive and specific means for assessing causes of platelet dysfunction. Disadvantages of the in vitro assays, such as shear-induced stress and clot retraction measurements, are that they represent nonspecific markers of platelet defects. The measure of specific serum markers of platelet activation, such as b-thromboglobulin and PF4, can be performed; however, plasma collection techniques for these tests are cumbersome, and the assays are often affected by other metabolic functions. Aggregometry is only a semiquantitative process and requires a high concentration of platelets for its optimal performance.

Flow cytometry is ideal for the detection of low concentrations of specific proteins within a large population of cells. These proteins either may be static portions of the platelet surface or dynamic products of platelet activation. The platelet release reaction enables specific integrin proteins, which are a part of the platelet alpha granule membrane, to incorporate themselves into the platelet surface membrane through a mechanism analogous to exocytosis. A portion of the GP IIb/IIIa receptor is also a protein of the alpha granule membrane that becomes exposed on the surface membrane of the platelet in response to platelet activation. Flow cytometry allows for the detection and quantification of many of these surface membrane constituents as a result of immunofluorescent innovations.[149]

Flow cytometry techniques have been enhanced by the development of specific monoclonal antibodies, which recognize antigens on the platelet (or white blood cell) surface. Antibodies developed are

TABLE 17-3	Monoclonal Antibodies to Platelet Antigens	
Antibody Binding Site (Other Name)	**Antibodies Available**	**Requirement for Binding/Functional Activity**
GP Ib (CD42b)	AP-1; 6D1	von Willebrand receptor; platelet adhesion
GP IX	FMC25	Platelet adhesion to endothelium
GP IIb/IIIa complex ($\alpha IIB\beta_3$, CD41)	7E3; 10E5; 4F10; A2A9	Fibrinogen receptor; platelet aggregation
GP IIb/IIIa ($\alpha IIB\beta_3$, CD41a)	PAC1	Active conformation of GP IIb/IIIa only
Fibrinogen	2G5; 9F9	Receptor-induced changes because of bound fibrinogen
GP IIb heavy chain of GP IIb/IIIa	P2; PMI-1	Ligand-induced changes in GP IIb
IIIa portion of GP IIb/IIIa (CD61)	AP6; Ab15; Y2/51	Receptor bound by fibrinogen
GMP140 (CD62P, P-selectin)	S12; KC4; VH10	alpha granule membrane protein, mediates platelet–leukocyte interactions
LAMP-1 (CD63)	CLB-gran/12; H5G11	Lysosome membrane protein, expressed after platelet secretion
40-kDa protein	D495	Dense granule membrane protein
Thrombospondin	P8	Bound thrombospondin
Factor VIIIa light chain	1B3	Present on a procoagulant surface
Factor Va light chain	V237	Present on a procoagulant surface

GMP, granule membrane protein; GP, glycoprotein; LAMP, lysosme membrane protein.

so specific that different ligand binding sites can be measured on the same GP IIb/IIIa molecule that characterizes different phases of receptor activation. Some of the epitopes for which monoclonal antibodies have been developed include PADGEM and GMP-140 (markers of platelet activation), the activated GP IIb/IIIa complex, and the GP Ib receptor.[150–152] A large number of monoclonal antibodies are available for identification of specific platelet ligand-binding sites (Table 17-3). Antibodies that bind specifically to activated platelets but minimally to unstimulated platelets are referred to as "activation dependent." In utilizing activation-dependent monoclonal antibodies, flow cytometry measures the platelet reactivity or response to the addition of platelet agonists. The technique of flow cytometry can be performed using whole blood or platelet-rich plasma. The fluorescent-labeled monoclonal antibody directed against a specific platelet membrane protein is quantified by the flow cytometer, which is an instrument equipped with a laser or a light source of a specific excitation wavelength. Light scatter data are collected that help to differentiate platelets from other cellular particles. Fluorescent antibody detection is expressed as percentage of the total number of particles or as fluorescence intensity.

The ability to specifically identify platelet defects by fluorescence flow cytometry has greatly aided in the characterization of hematologic disease states such as the Bernard–Soulier syndrome and Glanzmann's thrombasthenia.[153,154] In the cardiac surgical arena, flow cytometry has aided in diagnosing the disorders of platelet function induced by CPB and protamine administration.[69,140,155,156] Kestin et al[136] used flow cytometric techniques to study the effects of CPB on the in vivo time-dependent upregulation of P-selectin in blood emerging from a bleeding wound. They showed that P-selectin expression is depressed after heparinization and during CPB, and recovers at approximately 2 hours after the conclusion of CPB. In contrast, in vitro activation of CPB blood with the platelet agonist phorbol myristate acetate did not reveal this depression of P-selectin expression at any time point. Using another platelet activator (thrombin-receptor agonist peptide) and flow cytometry, others did not demonstrate depression of P-selectin expression early in CPB but did so after 90 minutes of CPB and after protamine administration.[157]

Much uncertainty still exists regarding GP Ib receptor modulation in response to CPB. Using flow cytometry, George et al[149] found a modest reduction in platelet surface GP Ib during CPB. However, a subsequent study by van Oeveren et al,[2] confirming a reduction in GP Ib, subjected the platelets to centrifugation and processing techniques that might have induced in vitro artifactual platelet activation. Kestin et al[136] used monoclonal antibodies to many epitopes expressed on GP Ib and concluded that expression of this receptor is not reduced during CPB.

As a result of the many monoclonal antibodies directed at specific epitopes on the GP IIb/IIIa receptor, investigations into the dynamics of this receptor during CPB have yielded variable results. Some studies have confirmed modest reductions in the expression of GP IIb/IIIa, although not all have used whole-blood techniques. Rinder et al,[155] using a whole-blood technique, demonstrated a small decrease in GP IIb/IIIa expression. Monoclonal antibodies are available that bind to the GP IIb/IIIa fibrinogen binding site, and others are available that recognize receptor-bound fibrinogen. Flow cytometric techniques also have helped to characterize the mechanisms of action of several pharmacologic agents that have shown hemostatic potential in the perioperative period.[69]

BEDSIDE PLATELET FUNCTION TESTING

Viscoelastic Tests: Thromboelastography and Sonoclot

It was the late 19th century when investigators first began to explore the possibility that viscoelastic tests of blood might yield information regarding coagulation status. The changes that occur in the viscosity of blood as it clots could be studied and measured, and this information would reflect certain aspects of coagulation function. During the early part of the 20th century, many primitive viscometers were developed that used the basic mechanisms and principles on which modern viscoelastic tests are based.

Thromboelastography

The coaguloviscometers that were developed in the 1920s formed the basis of viscoelastic coagulation testing that is now known as thromboelastography. Thromboelastography in its current form was developed by Hartert in 1948 and has been used in many different clinical scenarios to diagnose coagulation abnormalities.[158–160] Although not yet truly portable, the thromboelastograph (TEG; Haemoscope, Niles, IL [now Haemonetics, Braintree, MA]) can be performed "onsite" either in the operating room or in a laboratory and provides a rapid whole-blood analysis that yields information about clot formation and clot dissolution (Table 17-4). Within minutes, information is obtained regarding the integrity of the coagulation cascade, platelet function, platelet–fibrin interactions, and fibrinolysis. The principle is as follows:

Whole blood (0.36 mL) is placed into a plastic cuvette into which a plastic pin is suspended; this plastic pin is attached to a torsion wire that is coupled to an amplifier and recorded; a thin layer of oil is added to the surface of the blood to prevent drying of the specimen; and the cuvette oscillates through an arc of 4 degrees, 45 minutes at 37°C. When the blood is liquid, movement of the cuvette does not affect the pin. However, as clot begins to form, the pin becomes coupled to the motion of the cuvette and the torsion wire generates a signal that is recorded. The recorded tracing can be stored by computer, and the parameters of interest are calculated using a simple software package. Alternatively, the tracing can be generated online with a recording speed of 2 mm/min. The tracing generated has a characteristic conformation that is the signature of the TEG (Figure 17-16).

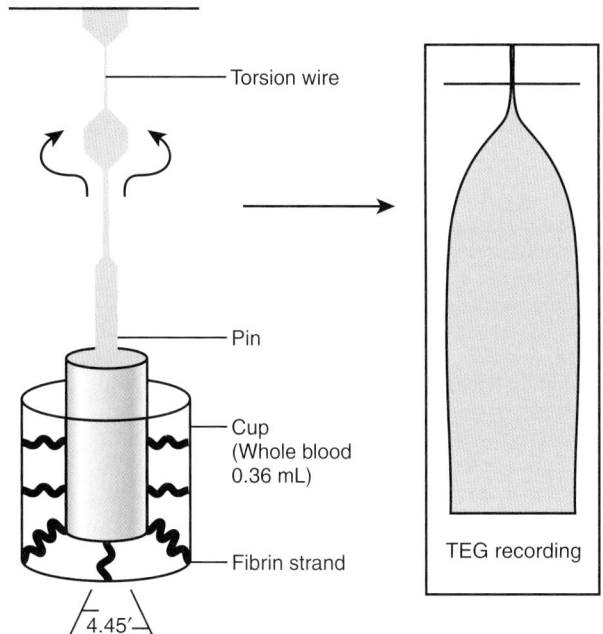

Figure 17-16 **Schematic diagram of the thromboelastograph (TEG) instrumentation *(left)* and a sample tracing *(right).*** A whole-blood sample is placed into the cup into which a plastic pin is suspended. This plastic pin is attached to a torsion wire that is coupled to an amplifier and recorder. *(From Mallett SV, Cox DJA: Thromboelastography. Br J Anaesth 69:307–313, 1992.)*

TABLE 17-4	Mechanisms of Point-of-Care Platelet Function Monitors		
Instrument	*Mechanism*	*Platelet Agonist*	*Clinical Utility*
Thromboelastograph[160]	Viscoelastic	Thrombin (native), ADP, arachidonic acid	Post-CPB, liver transplant, pediatric, obstetrics, drug efficacy
Sonoclot[167]	Viscoelastic	Thrombin (native)	Post-CPB, liver transplant
ROTEM[161]	Viscoelastic	Thrombin (native)	Post-CPB, transfusion algorithm
Hemostatus[144]	ACT reduction	PAF	Post-CPB, DDAVP, transfusion algorithm
PlateletWorks[196]	Platelet count ratio	ADP, collagen	Post-CPB, drug therapy
PFA-100[197]	In vitro bleeding time	ADP, epinephrine	vWD, congenital disorder, aspirin therapy, post-CPB
VerifyNow[198]	Agglutination	TRAP, ADP	GP IIb/IIIa receptor blockade therapy, drug therapy, post-CPB
Clot Signature Analyzer[199]	Shear-induced in vitro bleeding time	Collagen (one channel only)	Post-CPB, drug effects
Whole-blood aggregometry[147]	Electrical impedance	Multiple	Post-CPB
Impact Cone and Plate(let) analyzer[203]	Shear-induced platelet function	None	Post-CPB, congenital disorder, drug effects
Multiplate analyzer[210]	Electrical impedance	ADP, arachidonic acid, collagen, ristocetin, TRAP-6	Drug therapy, congenital disorder, post-CPB

ACT, activated clotting time; ADP, adenosine diphosphate; CPB, cardiopulmonary bypass; DDAVP, desmopressin; GP, glycoprotein; PAF, platelet-activating factor; TRAP, thrombin receptor agonist peptide; VWD, von Willebrand disease.

The specific parameters measured by the TEG include the reaction time (R value), coagulation time (K value), "a" angle, maximal amplitude (MA), amplitude 60 minutes after the maximal amplitude (A60), and clot lysis indices at 30 and 60 minutes after MA (LY30 and LY60, respectively). The reaction time, R, represents the time for initial fibrin formation and is a measure of the intrinsic coagulation pathway, the extrinsic coagulation pathway, and the final common pathway. R is measured from the start of the bioassay until fibrin begins to form, and the amplitude of the tracing is 2 mm. Normal values vary depending on the type of activator used, range from 7 to 14 minutes using celite activator, and are as short as 1 to 3 minutes using tissue factor activator. The K value is a measure of the speed of clot formation and is measured from the end of the R time to the time that the amplitude reaches 20 mm. Normal values (3 to 6 minutes) also vary with the type of activators used. The a angle, another index of speed of clot formation, is the angle formed between the horizontal axis of the tracing and the tangent to the tracing at 20-mm amplitude. Alpha values normally range from 45 to 55 degrees. Because both the K value and the a angle are measures of the speed of clot strengthening, each is improved by high levels of functional fibrinogen. MA (normal is 50 to 60 mm) is an index of clot strength as determined by platelet function, the cross-linkage of fibrin, and the interactions of platelets with polymerizing fibrin. The peak strength of the clot, or the shear elastic modulus "G," has a curvilinear relation with MA and is defined as $G = (5000 \bullet MA)/(96 - MA)$. The percentage reduction in MA after 30 minutes reflects the fibrinolytic activity present and normally is not more than 7.5%.

Characteristic TEG tracings can be recognized to be indicative of particular coagulation defects. A prolonged R value indicates a deficiency in coagulation factor activity or level and is seen typically in patients with liver disease and in patients on anticoagulants such as Coumadin or heparin. MA and a angle are reduced in states associated with platelet dysfunction or thrombocytopenia and are reduced even further in the presence of a fibrinogen defect. LY30, or the lysis index at 30 minutes after MA, is increased in conjunction with fibrinolysis. These particular signature tracings are depicted in Figure 17-17.

TEG is a useful tool for diagnosing and treating perioperative coagulopathy in patients undergoing cardiac surgical procedures because of a variety of potential coagulation defects that may exist.[159] Within 15 to 30 minutes, on-site information is available regarding the integrity of the coagulation system, the platelet function, fibrinogen function, and fibrinolysis.[160,161] With the addition of heparinase, TEG can be performed during CPB and can provide valuable and timely information regarding coagulation status.[162] Because TEG is a viscoelastic test and evaluates whole-blood hemostasis interactions, it is suggested that TEG is a more accurate predictor of postoperative hemorrhage than routine coagulation tests that analyze individual components of the hemostasis system. A number of clinical trials have confirmed that, in cardiac

surgical patients, TEG has a greater predictive value and greater specificity than routine coagulation tests for diagnosing patients known as "bleeders."[163] Tuman et al[160] studied 42 patients, of whom 9 were classified as bleeders. A routine coagulation screen consisting of ACT, PT, aPTT, and platelet count had only a 33% accuracy for predicting bleeding, whereas TEG and Sonoclot (Sienco, Morrison, CO; another viscoelastic test) had 88% and 74% accuracy, respectively. Mongan and Hosking[164] also found that TEG abnormalities predict postoperative bleeding, and using TEG parameters, they also were able to identify a population of patients who respond to therapy with desmopressin acetate. In a prospective study of 16-hour postoperative blood loss, Gravlee et al[165] reported on 897 cardiac surgical patients in whom routine coagulation tests were measured immediately on heparin reversal in the operating room. The weak correlations and poor predictive values of these tests confirm that these tests perform poorly as predictors of bleeding. TEG was not studied in this trial.

In a large, retrospective evaluation in more than 1000 patients, Spiess et al[166] found that the institution of a transfusion algorithm using TEG resulted in a significant reduction in the incidence of mediastinal exploration and in the rate of transfusion of allogeneic blood products. Because of its ease of use and application at the bedside, TEG has been used in many research settings to assess drug effects on platelet function and clot strength.[167,168] Information from the TEG also has been used to guide clinical decision making during orthotopic liver transplantation, obstetric procedures, and vascular surgical procedures.[168–171]

■ Thromboelastography Modifications

Thromboelastography was originally performed using recalcified citrated whole blood or celite activator. The addition of recombinant human tissue factor as an activator can be used to accelerate the rate of thrombin formation and, thus, the formation of fibrin.[172] This serves to shorten the time required for development of the MA. Because the MA primarily is reflective of clot strength and platelet function, this information can be obtained more quickly with tissue factor enhancement. The recombinant tissue factor is a thromboplastin agent and is available from a number of manufacturers.

An application of thromboelastography in the clinical arena is its use in monitoring GP IIb/IIIa-receptor blockade and ADP-receptor blockade in patients treated with specific antiplatelet agents. TEG with tissue factor acceleration speeds the appearance of MA and is accurate for monitoring the platelet inhibition by large concentrations of GP IIb/IIIa-receptor blockers. Using this technique with platelet-rich plasma, researchers have used the reduction of the MA as an index of platelet inhibition by GP IIb/IIIa-receptor blockers in the catheterization laboratory.[171] Comparison with the baseline MA yields a relative measure of the degree of platelet inhibition. Thrombin-receptor agonist peptide (TRAP)–induced aggregation correlates strongly with the TEG values measured in this fashion.[171]

Because the MA is a function of the platelet–fibrinogen interaction, a reduction in the MA can be accomplished by the addition of potent GP IIb/IIIa-receptor blockade to the assay. The resultant MA, in the presence of excessively high GP IIb/IIIa-receptor blockade, primarily is due to the fibrinogen concentration and the strength of fibrin alone. This value (called Ma_f) correlates strongly with plasma fibrinogen concentration.[173,174]

The thienopyridine ADP-receptor blockers, clopidogrel and ticlopidine, are widely used in cardiovascular medicine. The ability to measure the platelet defect induced by these drugs is difficult unless sophisticated laboratory techniques such as ADP-aggregometry are used. Aggregometry yields accurate results; however, it is not readily available in the perioperative period as a point-of-care test. Native TEG analysis does not measure the thienopyridine-induced platelet defect because the formation of thrombin in the assay has an overwhelming effect on the development of the TEG MA. A modification of the TEG removes thrombin from the assay and studies a nonthrombin clot, strengthened by the addition of ADP. Figure 17-18 depicts the different signature TEG tracings that are used to calculate the platelet

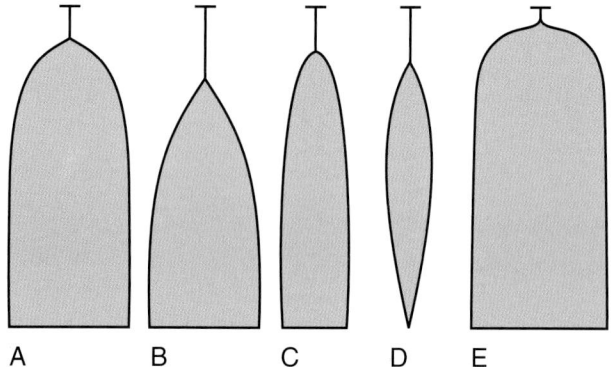

Figure 17-17 **Signature thromboelastograph tracings.** Tracing identification from left to right: *(A)* normal; *(B)* coagulation factor deficiency; *(C)* platelet dysfunction or deficiency; *(D)* fibrinolysis; *(E)* hypercoagulability. *(From Mallett SV, Cox DJA: Thromboelastography. Br J Anaesth 69:307–313, 1992.)*

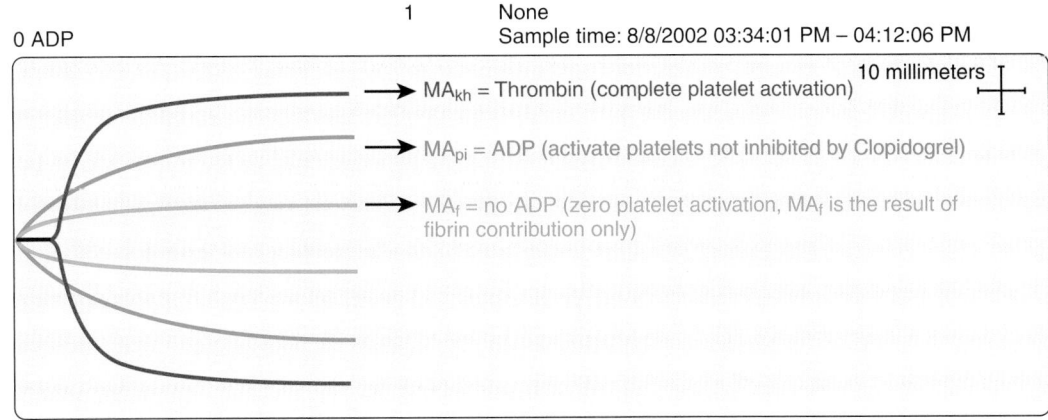

0 ADP

1

None
Sample time: 8/8/2002 03:34:01 PM – 04:12:06 PM

10 millimeters

MA_{kh} = Thrombin (complete platelet activation)

MA_{pi} = ADP (activate platelets not inhibited by Clopidogrel)

MA_f = no ADP (zero platelet activation, MA_f is the result of fibrin contribution only)

Figure 17-18 Thromboelastograph tracings using the modification to measure platelet inhibition by the thienopyridine drugs clopidogrel or ticlopidine. The measurements made are the maximal amplitude allowing thrombin activation of platelets (MA_{kh}; red). This is the standard kaolin-activated MA. Also measured are the maximal amplitude measuring only the fibrinogen component of MA (MA_f; blue). using a fibrinogen activator, and the maximal amplitude measuring the platelet contribution to MA by platelets able to be activated by adenosine diphosphate (ADP; MA_{pi}; green). This is using a fibrinogen activator plus ADP. Only platelets that are responsive to ADP will contribute to the MA_{pi}.

contribution to MA when a platelet inhibitor is present. This assay was specifically created to measure the platelet inhibition by ADP antagonists such as clopidogrel and is referred to as the "platelet mapping assay." The MA_{kh} is the maximal activation of platelets and fibrin, and is the largest amplitude that can be achieved. The MA_f is the maximal amplitude that is obtained when a thrombin-depleted fibrin clot is formed without a platelet contribution. The MA_{pi} is the MA_f contribution plus the platelet contribution. MA_{pi} is created by adding an activator such as ADP to the MA_f assay (for clopidogrel testing). Only platelets that can be activated by ADP contribute to the MA_{pi}. The following formula calculates the percentage reduction in platelet activity using this assay:

$$1 - [(MA_{pi} - MA_f)/(MA_{kh} - MA_f)] \times 100\%$$

Clopidogrel, ticlopidine, and even aspirin inhibition now can be studied at the point-of-care using this modification.[175,176]

Sonoclot

Another test of viscoelastic properties of blood is the Sonoclot. In 1975, von Kaulla introduced the Sonoclot (Sienco, Wheat Ridge, CO) which is a coagulation analyzer that measures the changing impedance on an ultrasonic probe that is immersed in a coagulating blood sample.[177] The machine consists of a plastic disposable probe mounted on an ultrasonic transducer that vibrates vertically at 200 Hz. The probe is immersed to a standard depth into 0.4 mL whole blood or plasma. The fluid exerts a force, or resistance, on the probe, which does not allow it to vibrate freely, and when the sample begins to clot, fibrin strands form on the tip of the probe and further increase the resistance. The electronic mechanism that drives the probe's vibration also acts as a transducer, measures the impedance to vibration, and, subsequently, converts it to a signal on paper. This signature of the Sonoclot reflects coagulation in real time, from the start of fibrin formation, to fibrin cross-linkage, platelet-mediated clot strengthening, and, eventually, to clot retraction and fibrinolysis.

Immersion of the probe into the blood sample causes an initial increase in the signal because of the increased impedance to vibration by fluid relative to air. The onset time is the time for initial fibrin formation and is defined as the time taken to reach an amplitude of 1 mm. This time also has been referred to as the "SonACT" (Figure 17-19). Further increase in the signal occurs because of an increased rate of fibrinogen conversion to fibrin. The rate of rise of this first peak (R1) is expressed as the percentage of the peak amplitude per unit time (normal values, 18% to 45%). After R1, there is a shoulder or a dip before the rise in amplitude that characterizes R2. This shoulder is a result of

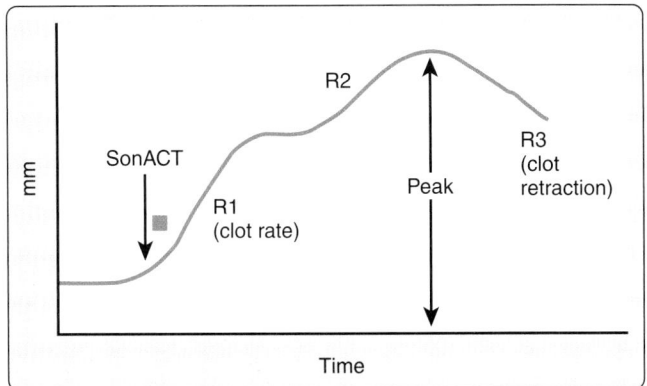

Figure 17-19 Normal Sonoclot tracing. *(From Hett DA, Walker D, Pilkington SN, Smith DC: Sonoclot analysis. Br J Anaesth 75:771–776, 1995, by permission of BMJ Publishing Group.)*

the action of platelets and fibrin in producing clot retraction. As the clot retracts from the walls of the cuvette, the impedance to vibration briefly decreases. As fibrinogen converts to fibrin and fibrin polymerizes, the speed of clot formation and the platelet–fibrin interactions are reflected by the slope R2, the second wave. In the presence of greater concentrations of fibrinogen, a larger clot mass is represented by a greater amplitude of the R2 wave because of a greater impedance to vibration. The amplitude of the peak of R2 is therefore related to the concentration of normal functional fibrinogen. The subsequent downward slope, R3, occurs as a result of platelet-mediated clot retraction that causes plasma expulsion and clot size diminution, and thus a lower impedance. The magnitude of the R3 drop is reflective of platelet number and function. Figure 17-19 demonstrates the normal Sonoclot tracing. Figure 17-20 depicts a tracing in a patient with dysfunctional or deficient fibrinogen levels. When fibrinolysis occurs, the signal decreases even further to baseline values. The time for fibrinolysis to occur varies with each sample and usually is seen on Sonoclot analysis only if a patient has accelerated fibrinolysis.

Sonoclot and TEG have been studied in the surgical arena because of their ability to measure viscoelastic properties of coagulation and their on-site applications. Tuman et al[160] found an accuracy of 74% using Sonoclot and an accuracy of 88% using TEG to predict bleeding after cardiac surgery. The reason that viscoelastic tests have been able to predict bleeding so successfully probably relates to their ability to measure platelet function, a major determinant of postoperative

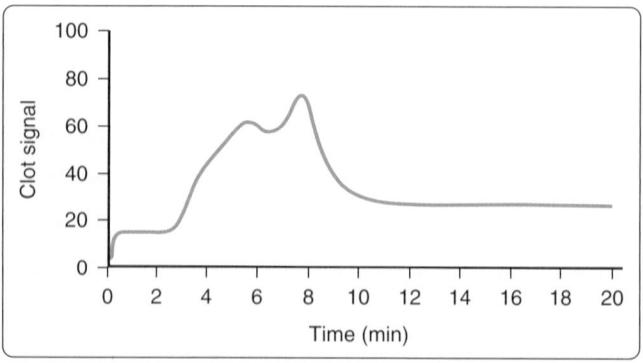

Figure 17-20 Sonoclot tracing in a patient with fibrinogen deficiency. In the presence of lower concentrations of fibrinogen, a smaller clot mass is represented by a smaller amplitude of the R2 wave because of less impedance to vibration. The amplitude of the peak of R2 is therefore directly related to the concentration of normal functional fibrinogen. *(From Hett DA, Walker D, Pilkington SN, Smith DC: Sonoclot analysis.* Br J Anaesth *75:771–776, 1995, by permission of BMJ Publishing Group.)*

hemostasis.[178] Significant correlations have been documented between specific Sonoclot parameters and platelet count and coagulation factor assays. This reproducibility has allowed the use of Sonoclot to also predict and successfully treat coagulation abnormalities in patients undergoing liver transplantation.[179] Like the TEG, Sonoclot is also useful in the diagnosis of hypercoagulable states.[180]

A direct comparison of TEG with Sonoclot is not likely to reveal a significant advantage of one test over the other because both tests measure the dynamic process of hemostasis by transducing the impedance changes that occur as blood clots. Both tests are easy to perform, can be performed on whole blood, and can be conveniently located in the operating room. Tuman et al[160] did not document a statistical difference between these two tests in clinical accuracy; however, they did show the viscoelastic tests to be superior to routine plasma coagulation testing. Sonoclot may provide coagulation information earlier because the initial deflection occurs when the first fibrin strands are forming. However, both TEG and Sonoclot accurately reflect the platelet–fibrin interactions required for clot formation.

ROTEM (Rotational Thrombelastometry)

The ROTEM gives a viscoelastic measurement of clot strength in whole blood (Pentapharm, Munich, Germany). A small amount of blood and coagulation activators is added to a disposable cuvette that is then placed in a heated cuvette holder. A disposable pin (sensor) that is fixed on the tip of a rotating shaft is lowered into the whole-blood sample. The loss of elasticity on clotting of the sample leads to changes in the rotation of the shaft that is detected by the reflection of light on a small mirror attached to the shaft. A detector records the axis rotation over time, and this rotation is translated into a graph or thromboelastogram.[160,161]

The main descriptive parameters associated with ROTEM are the following:
- Clotting time: corresponding to the time in seconds from the beginning of the reaction to an increase in amplitude of the tracing of 2 mm; it represents the initiation of clotting, thrombin formation, and start of clot polymerization
- Clotting formation time: the time in seconds between an increase in amplitude from 2 to 20 mm; this identifies the fibrin polymerization and stabilization of the clot with platelets and factor XIII
- Maximum clot firmness: the maximum amplitude in millimeters reached in the tracing that correlates with platelet count, platelet function, and with the concentration of fibrinogen
- Alpha (a) angle: the tangent to the clotting curve through the 2-mm point

- Maximum lysis: the ratio of the lowest amplitude after reaching the maximum clot firmness to the maximum clot firmness
- Maximum velocity (maxVel): the maximum of the first derivative of the clot curve
- Time to maximum velocity (t-maxVel): the time from the start of the reaction until maximum velocity is reached
- Area under curve: defined as the area under the velocity curve, that is, the area under the first derivative curve ending at a time point that corresponds to maximum clot firmness

ROTEM is approved for use in coagulation monitoring in Europe, and its use and familiarity are highest there. Spalding et al's[161] recent study has shown that implementation of ROTEM-guided coagulation management is useful in the choice of an appropriate therapeutic option in the bleeding patient. This reduces costs by avoiding administration of costly component therapy such as fresh-frozen plasma, cryoprecipitate, platelet concentrates, or antifibrinolytic agents. Its use in cardiac surgery and in transfusion algorithms is likely to be similar to that of TEG. ROTEM is currently seeking approval as a coagulation monitoring device from the Food and Drug Administration in the United States.

Tests of Platelet Response to Agonists

HemoSTATUS

Despite the introduction of numerous point-of-care coagulation analyzers that allow for rapid determination of a patient's coagulation status, the qualitative measure of platelet function, at the bedside, remains an elusive challenge. HemoSTATUS (Medtronic, Parker, CO) is a point-of-care platelet function assay that used the Hepcon HMS monitoring system to measure platelet reactivity. A six-channel cartridge measures the heparinized kaolin-activated ACT without platelet activator (channels 1 and 2) and with incrementally increasing doses of platelet-activating factor [PAF] (channels 3 to 6). The ACT of the PAF-activated channels will be shortened because of the ability of activated platelets to speed coagulation. The respective doses of PAF in channels 3 through 6 are 1.25, 6.25, 12.5, and 150 nmol/L. For each of channels 3 through 6, the degree of shortening of the ACT as a ratio to the ACT without PAF is the "clot ratio" and is calculated as $1 - (ACT_{activated}/ACT_{control})$. The "maximal" clot ratio is the clot ratio for channel 6 that was derived using blood from healthy volunteers (Figure 17-21). A comparison of the patient clot ratio to the maximal clot ratio (derived from normal volunteers) yields a comparative

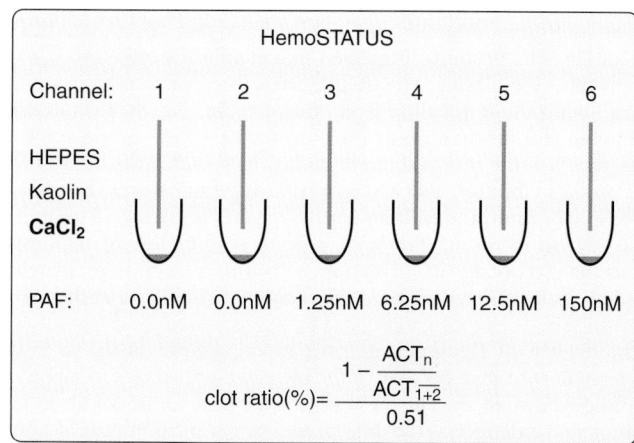

Figure 17-21 Schematic diagram of the HemoSTATUS measurement of platelet function. A specific cartridge placed into a Hepcon machine measures the reduction in the activated clotting time as a result of the addition of increasing amounts of platelet-activating factor (PAF). *ACT,* activated coagulation time; ACT_n, ACT of selected channel number; ACT_{1+2}, ACT average of channels 1 and 2.

measure of platelet function, termed the "percentage of maximal platelet function."

The potential ability to measure the qualitative function of platelets using a point-of-care assay provides innumerable advantages for clinicians caring for cardiac surgical patients. Platelet dysfunction is one of the more common hemostasis defects incurred during CPB, yet it is difficult to specifically measure platelet function rapidly and at the bedside. Viscoelastic tests conveniently measure platelet function, but their use in transfusion algorithms is limited by a lack of specificity to the measure of platelet dysfunction. Transfusion algorithms like the one published by Despotis et al,[91] which have been suggested to result in reduced transfusions in cardiac surgical patients, have incorporated only the measure of platelet number because the on-site ability to measure platelet function has been so elusive. Inclusion of a measure of platelet function into a transfusion algorithm potentially would reduce allogeneic transfusions even further.

An initial investigation of HemoSTATUS in cardiac surgical patients was performed by Despotis et al.[144] The authors studied 150 patients and conducted multivariate analyses to evaluate the relation between postoperative blood loss and multiple demographic, operative, and hemostatic measurements. They demonstrated a significant correlation between HemoSTATUS measurements on arrival in the intensive care unit and 4-hour postoperative mediastinal tube drainage ($r = -0.85$, channel 5; $r = -0.82$, channel 6). The accuracy of a number of hemostasis assays was measured using receiver operating characteristic curves for the detection of excessive mediastinal tube drainage. The highest predictability for bleeding was found in both the channel 5 clot ratio and the bleeding time. The PT, aPTT, and platelet count had much lower predictive value. HemoSTATUS-derived clot ratios also had the capability to detect enhanced platelet function after the administration of pharmacologic platelet therapy (desmopressin acetate) and after the transfusion of platelet concentrates. Subsequent investigations in cardiac surgical patients have confirmed a significant yet weak correlation of HemoSTATUS with postoperative bleeding, but have not found this test to be superior to TEG or routine coagulation tests in its predictive value.[163]

Validation studies have been performed to compare the assessment of platelet reactivity using HemoSTATUS with that measured by fluorescence flow cytometry. The percentage reduction in platelet function at multiple time points during cardiac surgery was compared using the two methodologies using each patient's baseline platelet function as the control. Both tests reflected a similar degree of platelet dysfunction at the time points 90 minutes into CPB, after protamine, and at intensive care unit arrival. Differences in the type of assay and the type of platelet activators used (thrombin peptide vs. PAF) may have accounted for the inability of the tests to correlate with each other at all of the time points studied.[157] This POC platelet function assay is no longer supported commercially, nor available.

Other Agonist-Activated Platelet Function Tests

VerifyNow (formerly marketed as Ultegra; Accumetrics, San Diego, CA) is a point-of-care monitor designed specifically to measure the platelet response to a TRAP. This technology was approved by the U.S. Food and Drug Administration for use as a platelet function assay. In whole blood, it measures TRAP activation-induced platelet agglutination of fibrinogen-coated beads using an optical detection system. After anticoagulated whole blood is added to the mixing chamber, the platelets become activated if they are responsive to the agonist. The activated GP IIB/IIIa receptors on the platelets bind to adjacent platelets via the fibrinogen on the beads and cause agglutination of the blood and the beads. Light transmittance through the chamber is measured and increases as agglutination increases, much like standard aggregometry. Antithrombotic drug effects cause a diminished agglutination (measured by light transmittance); thus, the degree of platelet inhibition can be quantified. Direct pharmacologic blockade of GP IIB/IIIa receptors with a GP IIb/IIIa antagonist is detected with high accuracy using this device and TRAP agonist. VerifyNow has been especially useful in accurately measuring receptor inhibition

in the invasive cardiology patients receiving GP IIb/IIIa–inhibiting drugs.[181–183] More recent cartridges using arachidonic acid as the agonist have been developed that can accurately assess aspirin-induced platelet dysfunction. Through inhibition of arachidonic acid, indirect prevention of GP IIb/IIIa expression is accomplished. The antiplatelet effects of the drug clopidogrel also can be measured using a VerifyNow cartridge that incorporates ADP as the agonist.[184] Each of these drug effects can be measured using the appropriate cartridge of the VerifyNow device.[185]

The Hemostatometer has been renamed the Clot Signature Analyzer (CSA; Xylum, Scarsdale, NY). Whole blood is maintained under a constant driving pressure of 60 mm Hg as it is forced out into a synthetic vessel. The pressure distally in the vessel is monitored. The tubing of this synthetic vessel is perforated, and the distal pressure decline is measured. The time to restoration of this distal pressure will be a function of development of a platelet plug. Thus, the time for initial closure is a measure of platelet function. A subsequent time is measured, and that is the time to complete pressure loss caused by complete vessel occlusion. This clot is the result of coagulation and clot formation, and the time to the second pressure decline is reflective of coagulation function. Another chamber of this device contains a collagen-coated fibril on which platelets adhere and form a plug. A similar pressure measurement technique indicates the formation of a platelet thrombus. This point-of-care assay has been used to measure platelet reactivity in high-risk patients with atherosclerotic coronary artery disease.[186–188] However, in cardiac surgical patients, preoperative platelet reactivity did not have predictive accuracy for bleeding.[189] Data evaluating the Clot Signature Analyzer in the postoperative period to predict bleeding are lacking.

The Platelet Function Analyzer (PFA-100; Dade Behring, Miami, FL) is a monitor of platelet adhesive capacity that is currently approved by the U.S. Food and Drug Administration and is valuable in its diagnostic abilities to identify drug-induced platelet abnormalities, platelet dysfunction of von Willebrand disease, and other acquired and congenital platelet defects.[190,191] The test is conducted as a modified in vitro bleeding time. Whole blood is drawn through a chamber by vacuum and is perfused across an aperture in a collagen membrane coated with an agonist (epinephrine or ADP). Platelet adhesion and formation of aggregates seal the aperture, thus indicating the "closure time" measured by the PFA-100.[192,193] In cardiac surgical patients, the preoperative PFA-100 closure time significantly correlated with postoperative blood loss ($r = 0.41$; $P = 0.022$).[194] However, preliminary evidence with post-CPB sampling and with in vitro addition of GP IIb/IIIa–inhibiting drugs suggests that these closure times may exceed those measurable using standard testing with the PFA-100.[195]

"Platelet Works" (Helena Laboratories, Beaumont, TX) is a test that uses the principle of the platelet count ratio to assess platelet reactivity. The instrument is a Coulter counter that measures the platelet count in a standard EDTA-containing tube. Platelet count also is measured in tubes containing the platelet agonist ristocetin, ADP, epinephrine, collagen, or thrombin. Addition of blood to these agonist tubes causes platelets to activate, adhere to the tube, and effectively be eliminated from the platelet count. The ratio of the activated platelet count to the nonactivated platelet count is a function of the reactivity of the platelets. Early investigation in cardiac surgical patients indicated that this assay is useful in providing a platelet count, and that it is capable of measuring the platelet dysfunction that accompanies CPB[196] (Box 17-6). Even more essential is the need to measure the antiplatelet effects of the oral antithrombotic agents used to treat cardiovascular patients with intracoronary stents. The point-of-care tests that are being promulgated currently are those that can monitor the effects of drugs like clopidogrel, prasugrel, and aspirin.[197–199]

Impact Cone and Plate(let) Analyzer (CPA; DiaMed Cressier, Switzerland)

In the Impact cone and plate(let) analyzer, whole blood is exposed to uniform shear by the spinning of a cone in a standardized cup. This

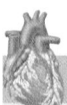

BOX 17-6. PLATELET FUNCTION TESTS

- The appropriate test to measure platelet function depends on the suspected platelet defect.
- The thromboelastograph and the Hemostatus are useful to measure the post-CPB platelet defect. VerifyNow is useful to measure the effects of GP IIb/IIIa-receptor-blocker therapy.
- The PFA-100 is useful to measure the effects of aspirin on platelet adhesion.
- It is important to understand the platelet defect being sought to accurately use the proper test.

allows for platelet function testing under conditions that mimic physiologic blood flow, thus achieving the most accurate pattern of platelet function. After automated staining, platelet adhesion to the cup is evaluated by image analysis software. The test yields two parameters: average size and surface coverage, which determine platelet function in terms of adhesion and aggregation. These values constitute a general platelet function parameter. This device identifies both congenital and acquired platelet defects, as well as the effects of antiplatelet drugs including GP IIb/IIIa antagonists, aspirin, and clopidogrel.[200–203] Recent studies suggest the Impact cone and plate(let) analyzer appears to be a useful tool for testing perioperative platelet function and may help in predicting postoperative blood loss.[204] Widespread experience with this instrument is limited because it has only recently become commercially available.

Multiplate Analyzer (Dynabyte Medical, Munich, Germany)

Multiplate analyzer is a test of platelet function in whole blood using impedance aggregometry.[205,206] First introduced in 2005, it is one of the most widely applied platelet aggregometers in Europe today. The analysis is performed in a single-use test cell, which incorporates a magnetic stirrer, as well as two independent impedance sensors. Activated platelets adhere and aggregate on the electrodes and, thus, enhance the electrical resistance between them. Typically, 300 µL buffered citrated blood is added to 300 µL isotonic saline and then analyzed. The device provides five channels for parallel determinations, as well as automatic analysis, calibration, and documentation using an integrated computer system. Several specific test reagents are available for stimulation of different receptors or activation of signal transduction pathways of platelets to detect changes induced

by drugs, as well as by acquired or hereditary platelet disorders. After an incubation time of 3 minutes, the selected agonist solution is added and the increase in electrical impedance is recorded continuously for 6 minutes. The resistance change is transformed to arbitrary aggregation units (AUs) and plotted against time. The area under the aggregation curve is used to quantify the aggregation response and is expressed in units (1 unit corresponds with 10 AU/min). The mean values of the two independent determinations are expressed as the area under the curve of the aggregation tracing (Figure 17-22). The system has a high sensitivity for antiplatelet drugs (aspirin, clopidogrel, prasugrel, IIbIIIa-antagonists).[207] Studies also have shown that Multiplate analysis is predictive for transfusion requirements in cardiac surgery[205,206,208–210] and can be predictive of thromboembolism in stent patients who are nonresponsive to platelet inhibitors.[211] This device is not currently available in the United States.

SUMMARY

It is essential to understand the complex array of hemostatic insults that occur as a result of extracorporeal circulation before selecting an appropriate coagulation or hemostasis monitor during cardiac surgery. Preoperative, intraoperative, and postoperative testing may be mandated for patients in whom a coagulation defect may predispose to serious degrees of postoperative coagulopathy. Even in hemostatically normal individuals, CPB induces a heparin effect, platelet dysfunction, fibrinolysis, and coagulation factor defects for which there are many clinical laboratory tests available for accurate diagnoses. With the increase in prescriptions of antithrombotic platelet inhibitors, the hemostatic defect after CPB is even more pronounced. This chapter has introduced the basic principles of hemostasis and the utility of many commonly used monitors for detecting disorders of the coagulation cascade, platelet function, and fibrinolysis. In addition, an increased emphasis on health care economics has created a milieu in which patients have a rapid transit time through the cardiac operating room with minimal exposure to allogeneic blood products. Prophylactic measures such as heparin-bonded circuitry and antifibrinolytics have reduced the actual incidence of microvascular bleeding in this population. However, when microvascular bleeding does occur, rapid diagnosis and therapeutic intervention are made possible by point-of-care hemostasis testing, which can take place directly in the operating room. If on-site testing is not available or does not provide sufficient timely information regarding the patient's coagulation defect, transfusion therapy for cardiac surgical patients will remain indiscriminate and empiric at best.

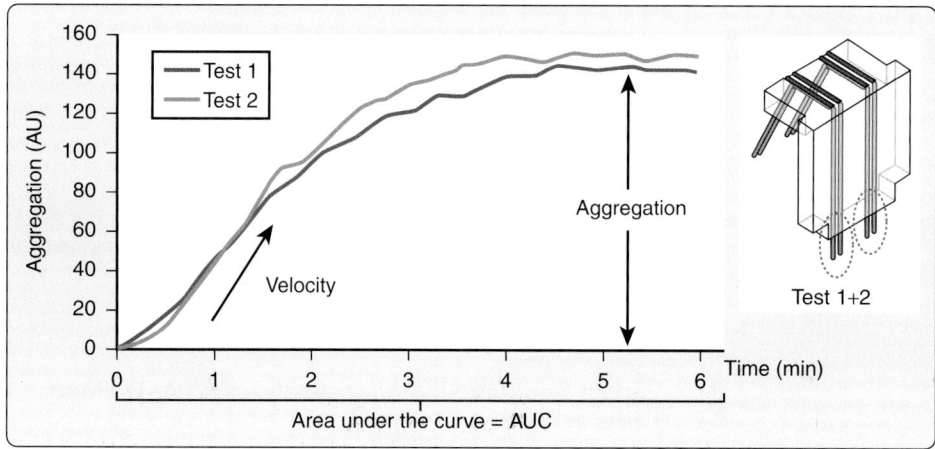

Figure 17-22 Multiplate tracing: The attachment of platelets onto the Multiplate sensors generates an increase in impedance that is transformed into arbitrary aggregation units (AU) and plotted against time. During a measurement period of 6 minutes, the parameters calculated by the software are the mean values of the two curves. *(From http://www.multiplate.net)*

REFERENCES

1. Khuri SF, Valeri CR, Loscalzo J, et al: Heparin causes platelet dysfunction and induces fibrinolysis before cardiopulmonary bypass, *Ann Thorac Surg* 60:1008, 1995.
2. van Oeveren W, Harder MP, Roozendaal KJ, et al: Aprotinin protects platelets against the initial effect of cardiopulmonary bypass, *J Thorac Cardiovasc Surg* 99:788, discussion 796, 1990.
3. Marciniak E: Physiology of antithrombin III, *Ric Clin Lab* 14:475, 1984.
4. Marciniak E, Gora-Maslak G: Enhancement by heparin of thrombin-induced antithrombin III proteolysis: Its relation to the molecular weight and anticoagulant activity of heparin, *Thromb Res* 28:411, 1982.
5. Marciniak E, Romond EH: Catabolism and distribution of functionally heterogeneous human antithrombin III, *J Lab Clin Med* 109:89, 1987.
6. Marciniak E: Thrombin-induced proteolysis of human antithrombin III: An outstanding contribution of heparin, *Br J Haematol* 48:325, 1981.
7. Hashimoto K, Yamagishi M, Sasaki T, et al: Heparin and antithrombin III levels during cardiopulmonary bypass: Correlation with subclinical plasma coagulation, *Ann Thorac Surg* 58:799, discussion 804, 1994.
8. Heller EL, Paul L: Anticoagulation management in a patient with an acquired antithrombin III deficiency, *J Extra Corpor Technol* 33:245, 2001.
9. Teoh KH, Young E, Bradley CA, Hirsh J: Heparin binding proteins. Contribution to heparin rebound after cardiopulmonary bypass, *Circulation* 88:II–420, 1993.
10. Jaberi M, Bell WR, Benson DW: Control of heparin therapy in open-heart surgery, *J Thorac Cardiovasc Surg* 67:133, 1974.
11. Roth JA, Cukingnan RA, Scott CR: Use of activated coagulation time to monitor heparin during cardiac surgery, *Ann Thorac Surg* 28:69, 1979.
12. Reich DL, Zahl K, Perucho MH, Thys DM: An evaluation of two activated clotting time monitors during cardiac surgery, *J Clin Monit* 8:33, 1992.
13. Horkay F, Martin P, Rajah SM, Walker DR: Response to heparinization in adults and children undergoing cardiac operations, *Ann Thorac Surg* 53:822, 1992.
14. Despotis GJ, Summerfield AL, Joist JH, et al: In vitro reversal of heparin effect with heparinase: Evaluation with whole blood prothrombin time and activated partial thromboplastin time in cardiac surgical patients, *Anesth Analg* 79:670, 1994.
15. Jobes DR, Schwartz AJ, Ellison N, et al: Monitoring heparin anticoagulation and its neutralization, *Ann Thorac Surg* 31:161, 1981.
16. Niinikoski J, Laato M, Laaksonen V, et al: Use of activated clotting time to monitor anticoagulation during cardiac surgery, *Scand J Thorac Cardiovasc Surg* 18:57, 1984.
17. Babka R, Colby C, El-Etr A, Pifarre R: Monitoring of intraoperative heparinization and blood loss following cardiopulmonary bypass surgery, *J Thorac Cardiovasc Surg* 73:780, 1977.
18. Culliford AT, Gitel SN, Starr N, et al: Lack of correlation between activated clotting time and plasma heparin during cardiopulmonary bypass, *Ann Surg* 193:105, 1981.
19. Ammar T, Fisher CF, Sarier K, Coller BS: The effects of thrombocytopenia on the activated coagulation time, *Anesth Analg* 83:1185, 1996.
20. Ammar T, Scudder LE, Coller BS: In vitro effects of the platelet glycoprotein IIb/IIIa receptor antagonist c7E3 Fab on the activated clotting time, *Circulation* 95:614, 1997.
21. Bode AP, Lust RM: Masking of heparin activity in the activated coagulation time (ACT) by platelet procoagulant activity, *Thromb Res* 73:285, 1994.
22. Gravlee GP, Whitaker CL, Mark LJ, et al: Baseline activated coagulation time should be measured after surgical incision, *Anesth Analg* 71:549, 1990.
23. Mabry CD, Read RC, Thompson BW, et al: Identification of heparin resistance during cardiac and vascular surgery, *Arch Surg* 114:129, 1979.
24. Andrew M, Ofosu F, Schmidt B, et al: Heparin clearance and ex vivo recovery in newborn piglets and adult pigs, *Thromb Res* 52:517, 1988.
25. Andrew M, MacIntyre B, MacMillan J, et al: Heparin therapy during cardiopulmonary bypass in children requires ongoing quality control, *Thromb Haemost* 70:937, 1993.
26. Papaconstantinou C, Radegran K: Use of the activated coagulation time in cardiac surgery. Effects on heparin-protamine dosages and bleeding, *Scand J Thorac Cardiovasc Surg* 15:213–215, 1981.
27. Roth JA, Cukingnan RA, Scott CR: Use of activated coagulation time to monitor heparin during cardiac surgery, *Ann Thorac Surg* 28:69–72, 1979.
28. Flom-Halvorsen HI, Ovrum E, Abdelnoor M, et al: Assessment of heparin anticoagulation: Comparison of two commercially available methods, *Ann Thorac Surg* 67:1012–1016, discussion 6–7, 1999.
29. Young JA, Kisker CT, Doty DB: Adequate anticoagulation during cardiopulmonary bypass determined by activated clotting time and the appearance of fibrin monomer, *Ann Thorac Surg* 26:231, 1978.
30. Metz S, Keats AS: Low activated coagulation time during cardiopulmonary bypass does not increase postoperative bleeding, *Ann Thorac Surg* 49:440, 1990.
31. Cardoso PF, Yamazaki F, Keshavjee S, et al: A reevaluation of heparin requirements for cardiopulmonary bypass, *J Thorac Cardiovasc Surg* 101:153, 1991.
32. Gravlee GP, Brauer SD, Roy RC, et al: Predicting the pharmacodynamics of heparin: A clinical evaluation of the Hepcon System 4, *J Cardiothorac Anesth* 1:379, 1987.
33. Utley JR: Pathophysiology of cardiopulmonary bypass: current issues, *J Card Surg* 5:177, 1990.
34. Young E, Prins M, Levine MN, Hirsh J: Heparin binding to plasma proteins, an important mechanism for heparin resistance, *Thromb Haemost* 67:639, 1992.
35. Marciniak E, Gockerman JP: Heparin-induced decrease in circulating antithrombin-III, *Lancet* 2:581, 1977.
36. Linden MD, Schneider M, Baker S, et al: Decreased concentration of antithrombin after preoperative therapeutic heparin does not cause heparin resistance during cardiopulmonary bypass, *J Cardiothorac Vasc Anesth* 18:131, 2004.
37. Esposito RA, Culliford AT, Colvin SB, et al: Heparin resistance during cardiopulmonary bypass. The role of heparin pretreatment, *J Thorac Cardiovasc Surg* 85:346, 1983.
38. Kanbak M: The treatment of heparin resistance with antithrombin III in cardiac surgery, *Can J Anaesth* 46:581, 1999.
39. Lemmer JH Jr, Despotis GJ: Antithrombin III concentrate to treat heparin resistance in patients undergoing cardiac surgery, *J Thorac Cardiovasc Surg* 123:213, 2002.
40. Levy JH, Montes F, Szlam F, Hillyer CD: The in vitro effects of antithrombin III on the activated coagulation time in patients on heparin therapy, *Anesth Analg* 90:1076, 2000.
41. Nicholson SC, Keeling DM, Sinclair ME, Evans RD: Heparin pretreatment does not alter heparin requirements during cardiopulmonary bypass, *Br J Anaesth* 87:844, 2001.
42. Avidan MS, Levy JH, van Aken H, et al: Recombinant human antithrombin III restores heparin responsiveness and decreases activation of coagulation in heparin-resistant patients during cardiopulmonary bypass, *J Thorac Cardiovasc Surg* 130:107–113, 2005.
43. Avidan MS, Levy JH, Scholz J, et al: A phase III, double-blind, placebo-controlled, multicenter study on the efficacy of recombinant human antithrombin in heparin-resistant patients scheduled to undergo cardiac surgery necessitating cardiopulmonary bypass, *Anesthesiology* 102:276–284, 2005.
44. Lobato RL, Despotis GJ, Levy JH, et al: Anticoagulation management during cardiopulmonary bypass: A survey of 54 North American institutions, *J Thorac Cardiovasc Surg* 139:1665–1666, 2010.
45. Warkentin TE, Kelton JG: Temporal aspects of heparin-induced thrombocytopenia, *N Engl J Med* 344:1286–1292, 2001.
46. Warkentin TE, Greinacher A: Heparin-induced thrombocytopenia and cardiac surgery, *Ann Thorac Surg* 76:638, 2003.
47. Koster A, Dyke CM, Aldea G, et al: Bivalirudin during cardiopulmonary bypass in patients with previous or acute heparin-induced thrombocytopenia and heparin antibodies: Results of the CHOOSE-ON trial, *Ann Thorac Surg* 83:572–577, 2007.
48. Mabry CD, Thompson BW, Read RC: Activated clotting time (ACT) monitoring of intraoperative heparinization in peripheral vascular surgery, *Am J Surg* 138:894, 1979.
49. Bull BS, Huse WM, Brauer FS, Korpman RA: Heparin therapy during extracorporeal circulation. II. The use of a dose-response curve to individualize heparin and protamine dosage, *J Thorac Cardiovasc Surg* 69:685, 1975.
50. Jobes DR, Aitken GL, Shaffer GW: Increased accuracy and precision of heparin and protamine dosing reduces blood loss and transfusion in patients undergoing primary cardiac operations, *J Thorac Cardiovasc Surg* 110:36, 1995.
51. Shore-Lesserson L, Reich DL, DePerio M: Heparin and protamine titration do not improve haemostasis in cardiac surgical patients, *Can J Anaesth* 45:10, 1998.
52. Szalados JE, Ouriel K, Shapiro JR: Use of the activated coagulation time and heparin dose-response curve for the determination of protamine dosage in vascular surgery, *J Cardiothorac Vasc Anesth* 8:515, 1994.
53. Despotis GJ, Levine V, Joiner-Maier D, Joist JH: A comparison between continuous infusion versus standard bolus administration of heparin based on monitoring in cardiac surgery, *Blood Coagul Fibrinolysis* 8:419, 1997.
54. Despotis GJ, Summerfield AL, Joist JH, et al: Comparison of activated coagulation time and whole blood heparin measurements with laboratory plasma anti-Xa heparin concentration in patients having cardiac operations, *J Thorac Cardiovasc Surg* 108:1076, 1994.
55. Gravlee GP, Haddon WS, Rothberger HK, et al: Heparin dosing and monitoring for cardiopulmonary bypass. A comparison of techniques with measurement of subclinical plasma coagulation, *J Thorac Cardiovasc Surg* 99:518, 1990.
56. Gravlee GP, Rogers AT, Dudas LM, et al: Heparin management protocol for cardiopulmonary bypass influences postoperative heparin rebound but not bleeding, *Anesthesiology* 76:393, 1992.
57. Despotis GJ, Joist JH, Hogue CW Jr, et al: The impact of heparin concentration and activated clotting time monitoring on blood conservation. A prospective, randomized evaluation in patients undergoing cardiac operation, *J Thorac Cardiovasc Surg* 110:46, 1995.
58. Wang JS, Lin CY, Karp RB: Comparison of high-dose thrombin time with activated clotting time for monitoring of anticoagulant effects of heparin in cardiac surgical patients, *Anesth Analg* 79:9, 1994.
59. Wang JS, Lin CY, Hung WT, Karp RB: Monitoring of heparin-induced anticoagulation with kaolin-activated clotting time in cardiac surgical patients treated with aprotinin, *Anesthesiology* 77:1080, 1992.
60. Dietrich W, Dilthey G, Spannagl M, et al: Influence of high-dose aprotinin on anticoagulation, heparin requirement, and celite- and kaolin-activated clotting time in heparin-pretreated patients undergoing open-heart surgery. A double-blind, placebo-controlled study, *Anesthesiology* 83:679, discussion 29A 1995.
61. Tabuchi N, Njo TL, Tigchelaar I, et al: Monitoring of anticoagulation in aprotinin-treated patients during heart operation, *Ann Thorac Surg* 58:774, 1994.
62. Dercksen SJ, Linssen GH: Monitoring of blood coagulation in open heart surgery. II. Use of individualized dosages of heparin and protamine controlled by activated coagulation times, *Acta Anaesthesiol Belg* 31:121, 1980.
63. Dercksen SJ, Linssen GH: Monitoring of blood coagulation in open heart surgery. I. Effects of conventional dosages of heparin and protamine, *Acta Anaesthesiol Belg* 31:113, 1980.
64. Ellison N, Jobes DR, Schwartz AJ: Implications of anticoagulant therapy, *Int Anesthesiol Clin* 20:121, 1982.
65. Jobes DR: Safety issues in heparin and protamine administration for extracorporeal circulation, *J Cardiothorac Vasc Anesth* 12:17, 1998.
66. Habazettl H, Conzen PF, Vollmar B, et al: Effect of leukopenia on pulmonary hypertension after heparin-protamine in pigs, *J Appl Physiol* 73:44, 1992.
67. Warkentin TE, Crowther MA: Reversing anticoagulants both old and new, *Can J Anaesth* 49:S11, 2002.
68. Carr ME Jr, Carr SL: At high heparin concentrations, protamine concentrations which reverse heparin anticoagulant effects are insufficient to reverse heparin anti-platelet effects, *Thromb Res* 75:617, 1994.
69. Ammar T, Fisher CF: The effects of heparinase 1 and protamine on platelet reactivity, *Anesthesiology* 86:1382, 1997.
70. Carr ME Jr: Measurement of platelet force: The Hemodyne hemostasis analyzer, *Clin Lab Manage Rev* 9:312, 1995.
71. Martin P, Horkay F, Gupta NK, et al: Heparin rebound phenomenon—much ado about nothing? *Blood Coagul Fibrinolysis* 3:187, 1992.
72. Jobes DR, Schwartz AJ, Ellison N: Heparin rebound (letter), *J Thorac Cardiovasc Surg* 82:940, 1981.
73. LaDuca FM, Zucker ML, Walker CE: Assessing heparin neutralization following cardiac surgery: Sensitivity of thrombin time-based assays versus protamine titration methods, *Perfusion* 14:181, 1999.
74. Ohata T, Sawa Y, Ohtake S, et al: Clinical role of blood heparin level monitoring during open heart surgery, *Jpn J Thorac Cardiovasc Surg* 47:600, 1999.
75. Reiner JS, Coyne KS, Lundergan CF, Ross AM: Bedside monitoring of heparin therapy: Comparison of activated clotting time to activated partial thromboplastin time, *Cathet Cardiovasc Diagn* 32:49, 1994.
76. D'Ambra M: Restoration of the normal coagulation process: Advances in therapies to antagonize heparin, *J Cardiovasc Pharmacol* 27:S58, 1996.
77. Martindale SJ, Shayevitz JR, D'Errico C: The activated coagulation time: Suitability for monitoring heparin effect and neutralization during pediatric cardiac surgery, *J Cardiothorac Vasc Anesth* 10:458, 1996.
78. Moriau M, Masure R, Hurlet A, et al: Haemostasis disorders in open heart surgery with extracorporeal circulation. Importance of the platelet function and the heparin neutralization, *Vox Sang* 32:41, 1977.
79. Shigeta O, Kojima H, Hiramatsu Y, et al: Low-dose protamine based on heparin-protamine titration method reduces platelet dysfunction after cardiopulmonary bypass, *J Thorac Cardiovasc Surg* 118:354, 1999.
80. Reich DL, Yanakakis MJ, Vela-Cantos FP, et al: Comparison of bedside coagulation monitoring tests with standard laboratory tests in patients after cardiac surgery, *Anesth Analg* 77:673, 1993.
81. Williams RD, D'Ambra MN, Maione TE, et al: Recombinant platelet factor 4 reversal of heparin in human cardiopulmonary bypass blood, *J Thorac Cardiovasc Surg* 108:975, 1994.
82. Cook JJ, Niewiarowski S, Yan Z, et al: Platelet factor 4 efficiently reverses heparin anticoagulation in the rat without adverse effects of heparin-protamine complexes, *Circulation* 85:1102, 1992.
83. Levy JH, Cormack JG, Morales A: Heparin neutralization by recombinant platelet factor 4 and protamine, *Anesth Analg* 81:35, 1995.
84. Michelsen LG, Kikura M, Levy JH, et al: Heparinase I (Neutralase) reversal of systemic anticoagulation, *Anesthesiology* 85:339, 1996.
85. Bain B, Forster T, Sleigh B: Heparin and the activated partial thromboplastin time—a difference between the in-vitro and in-vivo effects and implications for the therapeutic range, *Am J Clin Pathol* 74:668, 1980.

86. Ray MJ, Carroll PA, Just SJ, et al: The effect of oral anticoagulant therapy on APTT results from a bedside coagulation monitor, *J Clin Monit* 10:97, 1994.

87. Werner M, Gallagher JV, Ballo MS, Karcher DS: Effect of analytic uncertainty of conventional and point-of-care assays of activated partial thromboplastin time on clinical decisions in heparin therapy, *Am J Clin Pathol* 102:237, 1994.

88. Samama CM, Quezada R, Riou B, et al: Intraoperative measurement of activated partial thromboplastin time and prothrombin time with a new compact monitor, *Acta Anaesthesiol Scand* 38:232, 1994.

89. Nuttall GA, Oliver WC, Beynen FM, et al: Determination of normal versus abnormal activated partial thromboplastin time and prothrombin time after cardiopulmonary bypass, *J Cardiothorac Vasc Anesth* 9:355, 1995.

90. Despotis GJ, Santoro SA, Spitznagel E, et al: Prospective evaluation and clinical utility of on-site monitoring of coagulation in patients undergoing cardiac operation, *J Thorac Cardiovasc Surg* 107:271, 1994.

91. Despotis GJ, Grishaber JE, Goodnough LT: The effect of an intraoperative treatment algorithm on physicians' transfusion practice in cardiac surgery, *Transfusion* 34:290, 1994.

92. Borowiec J, Bagge L, Saldeen T, Thelin S: Biocompatibility reflected by haemostasis variables during cardiopulmonary bypass using heparin-coated circuits, *Thorac Cardiovasc Surg* 45:163, 1997.

93. Jansen PG, te Velthuis H, Huybregts RA, et al: Reduced complement activation and improved postoperative performance after cardiopulmonary bypass with heparin-coated circuits, *J Thorac Cardiovasc Surg* 110:829, 1995.

94. Gu YJ, Boonstra PW, Rijnsburger AA, et al: Cardiopulmonary bypass circuit treated with surface-modifying additives: A clinical evaluation of blood compatibility, *Ann Thorac Surg* 65:1342, 1998.

95. Gorman RC, Ziats N, Rao AK, et al: Surface-bound heparin fails to reduce thrombin formation during clinical cardiopulmonary bypass, *J Thorac Cardiovasc Surg* 111:1, discussion 11, 1996.

96. Baufreton C, Jansen PG, Le Besnerais P, et al: Heparin coating with aprotinin reduces blood activation during coronary artery operations, *Ann Thorac Surg* 63:50, 1997.

97. Ovrum E, Holen EA, Tangen G, et al: Completely heparinized cardiopulmonary bypass and reduced systemic heparin: Clinical and hemostatic effects, *Ann Thorac Surg* 60:365, 1995.

98. Aldea GS, Doursounian M, O'Gara P, et al: Heparin-bonded circuits with a reduced anticoagulation protocol in primary CABG: A prospective, randomized study, *Ann Thorac Surg* 62:410, 1996.

99. Weiss BM, von Segesser LK, Turina MI, et al: Perioperative course and recovery after heparin-coated cardiopulmonary bypass: Low-dose versus high-dose heparin management, *J Cardiothorac Vasc Anesth* 10:464, 1996.

100. Kuitunen AH, Heikkila LJ, Salmenpera MT: Cardiopulmonary bypass with heparin-coated circuits and reduced systemic anticoagulation, *Ann Thorac Surg* 63:438, 1997.

101. Ovrum E, Brosstad F, Am Holen E, et al: Effects on coagulation and fibrinolysis with reduced versus full systemic heparinization and heparin-coated cardiopulmonary bypass, *Circulation* 92:2579, 1995.

102. Muller N, Popov-Cenic S, Buttner W, et al: Studies of fibrinolytic and coagulation factors during open heart surgery. II. Postoperative bleeding tendency and changes in the coagulation system, *Thromb Res* 7:589, 1975.

103. Umlas J: Fibrinolysis and disseminated intravascular coagulation in open heart surgery, *Transfusion* 16:460, 1976.

104. Whitten CW, Greilich PE, Ivy R, et al: D-dimer formation during cardiac and noncardiac thoracic surgery, *Anesth Analg* 88:1226, 1999.

105. Weitz J, Klement P: Bivalirudin as an alternative anticoagulant to heparin in cardiopulmonary bypass: Data from a porcine model (abstract), *Anesthesiology* 99:A, 2003.

106. Lincoff AM, Bittl JA, Kleiman NS, et al: Comparison of bivalirudin versus heparin during percutaneous coronary intervention (the Randomized Evaluation of PCI Linking Angiomax to Reduced Clinical Events [REPLACE] trial), *Am J Cardiol* 93:1092, 2004.

107. Merry AF: Bivalirudin, blood loss, and graft patency in coronary artery bypass surgery, *Semin Thromb Hemost* 30:337, 2004.

108. Greinacher A: The use of direct thrombin inhibitors in cardiovascular surgery in patients with heparin-induced thrombocytopenia, *Semin Thromb Hemost* 30:315, 2004.

109. Koster A, Kuppe H, Hetzer R, et al: Emergent cardiopulmonary bypass in five patients with heparin-induced thrombocytopenia type II employing recombinant hirudin, *Anesthesiology* 89:777, 1998.

110. Koster A, Crystal GJ, Kuppe H, Mertzlufft F: Acute heparin-induced thrombocytopenia type II during cardiopulmonary bypass, *J Cardiothorac Vasc Anesth* 14:300, 2000.

111. Koster A, Hansen R, Kuppe H, et al: Recombinant hirudin as an alternative for anticoagulation during cardiopulmonary bypass in patients with heparin-induced thrombocytopenia type II: A 1-year experience in 57 patients, *J Cardiothorac Vasc Anesth* 14:243, 2000.

112. Koster A, Loebe M, Hansen R, et al: A quick assay for monitoring recombinant hirudin during cardiopulmonary bypass in patients with heparin-induced thrombocytopenia type II: Adaptation of the ecarin clotting time to the act II device, *J Thorac Cardiovasc Surg* 119:1278, 2000.

113. Koster A, Kuppe H, Crystal GJ, Mertzlufft F: Cardiovascular surgery without cardiopulmonary bypass in patients with heparin-induced thrombocytopenia type II using anticoagulation with recombinant hirudin, *Anesth Analg* 90:292, 2000.

114. Koster A, Hansen R, Grauhan O, et al: Hirudin monitoring using the TAS ecarin clotting time in patients with heparin-induced thrombocytopenia type II, *J Cardiothorac Vasc Anesth* 14:249, 2000.

115. Koster A, Pasic M, Bauer M, et al: Hirudin as anticoagulant for cardiopulmonary bypass: Importance of preoperative renal function, *Ann Thorac Surg* 69:37, 2000.

116. Koster A, Loebe M, Mertzlufft F, et al: Cardiopulmonary bypass in a patient with heparin induced thrombocytopenia II and impaired renal function using heparin and the platelet GP IIb/IIIa inhibitor tirofiban as anticoagulant, *Ann Thorac Surg* 70:2160, 2000.

117. Koster A, Merkle F, Hansen R, et al: Elimination of recombinant hirudin by modified ultrafiltration during simulated cardiopulmonary bypass: Assessment of different filter systems, *Anesth Analg* 91:265, 2000.

118. Maroo A, Lincoff AM: Bivalirudin in PCI: An overview of the REPLACE Trial, *Semin Thromb Hemost* 30:329, 2004.

119. Merry AF, Raudkivi PJ, Middleton NG, et al: Bivalirudin versus heparin and protamine in off-pump coronary artery bypass surgery, *Ann Thorac Surg* 77:925, 2004.

120. Davis Z, Anderson R, Short D, et al: Favorable outcome with bivalirudin anticoagulation during cardiopulmonary bypass, *Ann Thorac Surg* 75:264, 2003.

121. Gordon G, Rastegar H, Schumann R, et al: Successful use of bivalirudin for cardiopulmonary bypass in a patient with heparin-induced thrombocytopenia, *J Cardiothorac Vasc Anesth* 17:632, 2003.

122. Vasquez JC, Vichiendilokkul A, Mahmood S, Baciewicz FA Jr: Anticoagulation with bivalirudin during cardiopulmonary bypass in cardiac surgery, *Ann Thorac Surg* 74:2177, 2002.

123. Smedira NG, Dyke CM, Koster A, et al: Anticoagulation with bivalirudin for off-pump coronary artery bypass grafting: The results of the EVOLUTION-OFF study, *J Thorac Cardiovasc Surg* 131:686–692, 2006.

124. Dyke CM, Smedira NG, Koster A, et al: A comparison of bivalirudin to heparin with protamine reversal in patients undergoing cardiac surgery with cardiopulmonary bypass: The EVOLUTION-ON study, *J Thorac Cardiovasc Surg* 131:533–539, 2006.

125. Koster A, Spiess B, Chew DP, et al: Effectiveness of bivalirudin as a replacement for heparin during cardiopulmonary bypass in patients undergoing coronary artery bypass grafting, *Am J Cardiol* 93:356, 2004.

126. McDonald SB, Kattapurum BM, Saleem R, et al: Monitoring hirudin anticoagulation in two patients undergoing cardiac surgery with a plasma-modified act method, *Anesthesiology* 97:509–512, 2002.

127. Chomiak PN, Walenga JM, Koza MJ, et al: Investigation of a thrombin inhibitor peptide as an alternative to heparin in cardiopulmonary bypass surgery, *Circulation* 88:II–407, 1993.

128. Bittl JA, Strony J, Brinker JA, et al: Treatment with bivalirudin (Hirulog) as compared with heparin during coronary angioplasty for unstable or postinfarction angina. Hirulog Angioplasty Study Investigators, *N Engl J Med* 333:764, 1995.

129. Zilla P, Fasol R, Deutsch M, et al: Whole blood aggregometry and platelet adenine nucleotides during cardiac surgery, *Scand J Thorac Cardiovasc Surg* 22:165, 1988.

130. Halbmayer WM, Haushofer A, Radek J, et al: Platelet size, fibrinogen and lipoprotein(a) in coronary heart disease, *Coron Artery Dis* 6:397, 1995.

131. Boldt J, Zickmann B, Benson M, et al: Does platelet size correlate with function in patients undergoing cardiac surgery? *Intensive Care Med* 19:44, 1993.

132. Despotis GJ, Filos KS, Zoys TN, et al: Factors associated with excessive postoperative blood loss and hemostatic transfusion requirements: A multivariate analysis in cardiac surgical patients, *Anesth Analg* 82:13, 1996.

133. Khuri SF, Wolfe JA, Josa M, et al: Hematologic changes during and after cardiopulmonary bypass and their relationship to the bleeding time and nonsurgical blood loss, *J Thorac Cardiovasc Surg* 104:94, 1992.

134. Bertolino G, Locatelli A, Noris P, et al: Platelet composition and function in patients undergoing cardiopulmonary bypass for heart surgery, *Haematologica* 81:116, 1996.

135. Boldt J, Schindler E, Knothe C, et al: Does aprotinin influence endothelial-associated coagulation in cardiac surgery? *J Cardiothorac Vasc Anesth* 8:527, 1994.

136. Kestin AS, Valeri CR, Khuri SF, et al: The platelet function defect of cardiopulmonary bypass, *Blood* 82:107, 1993.

137. Upchurch GR, Valeri CR, Khuri SF, et al: Effect of heparin on fibrinolytic activity and platelet function in vivo, *Am J Physiol* 271:H528, 1996.

138. Adelman B, Michelson AD, Loscalzo J, et al: Plasmin effect on platelet glycoprotein Ib- von Willebrand factor interactions, *Blood* 65:32, 1985.

139. Adelman B, Michelson AD, Greenberg J, Handin RI: Proteolysis of platelet glycoprotein Ib by plasmin is facilitated by plasmin lysine-binding regions, *Blood* 68:1280, 1986.

140. Michelson AD, MacGregor H, Barnard MR, et al: Reversible inhibition of human platelet activation by hypothermia in vivo and in vitro, *Thromb Haemost* 71:633, 1994.

141. Boldt J, Zickmann B, Czeke A, et al: Blood conservation techniques and platelet function in cardiac surgery, *Anesthesiology* 75:426, 1991.

142. Burns ER, Billett HH, Frater RW, Sisto DA: The preoperative bleeding time as a predictor of postoperative hemorrhage after cardiopulmonary bypass, *J Thorac Cardiovasc Surg* 92:310, 1986.

143. Burns ER, Lawrence C: Bleeding time. A guide to its diagnostic and clinical utility, *Arch Pathol Lab Med* 113:1219, 1989.

144. Despotis GJ, Levine V, Filos KS, et al: Evaluation of a new point-of-care test that measures PAF-mediated acceleration of coagulation in cardiac surgical patients, *Anesthesiology* 85:1311, 1996.

145. Despotis GJ, Levine V, Saleem R, et al: Use of point-of-care test in identification of patients who can benefit from desmopressin during cardiac surgery: A randomized controlled trial, *Lancet* 354:106, 1999.

146. Mohr R, Martinowitz U, Lavee J, et al: The hemostatic effect of transfusing fresh whole blood versus platelet concentrates after cardiac operations, *J Thorac Cardiovasc Surg* 96:530, 1988.

147. Ray MJ, Hawson GA, Just SJ, et al: Relationship of platelet aggregation to bleeding after cardiopulmonary bypass, *Ann Thorac Surg* 57:981, 1994.

148. Carr ME Jr: In vitro assessment of platelet function, *Transfus Med Rev* 11:106, 1997.

149. George JN, Pickett EB, Saucerman S, et al: Platelet surface glycoproteins. Studies on resting and activated platelets and platelet membrane microparticles in normal subjects, and observations in patients during adult respiratory distress syndrome and cardiac surgery, *Clin Invest* 78:340, 1986.

150. Adelman B, Michelson AD, Handin RI, Ault KA: Evaluation of platelet glycoprotein Ib by fluorescence flow cytometry, *Blood* 66:423, 1985.

151. Michelson AD, Barnard MR: Thrombin-induced changes in platelet membrane glycoproteins Ib, IX, and IIb-IIIa complex, *Blood* 70:1673, 1987.

152. Nieuwenhuis HK, van Oosterhout JJ, Rozemuller E, et al: Studies with a monoclonal antibody against activated platelets: Evidence that a secreted 53,000-molecular weight lysosome-like granule protein is exposed on the surface of activated platelets in the circulation, *Blood* 70:838, 1987.

153. Michelson AD: Flow cytometric analysis of platelet surface glycoproteins: Phenotypically distinct subpopulations of platelets in children with chronic myeloid leukemia, *J Lab Clin Med* 110:346, 1987.

154. LaRosa CA, Rohrer MJ, Benoit SE, et al: Neutrophil cathepsin G modulates the platelet surface expression of the glycoprotein (GP) Ib-IX complex by proteolysis of the von Willebrand factor binding site on GPIb alpha and by a cytoskeletal-mediated redistribution of the remainder of the complex, *Blood* 84:158, 1994.

155. Rinder CS, Mathew JP, Rinder HM, et al: Modulation of platelet surface adhesion receptors during cardiopulmonary bypass, *Anesthesiology* 75:563, 1991.

156. Sloand JA, Sloand EM: Studies on platelet membrane glycoproteins and platelet function during hemodialysis, *J Am Soc Nephrol* 8:799, 1997.

157. Shore-Lesserson L, Ammar T, DePerio M, et al: Platelet-activated clotting time does not measure platelet reactivity during cardiac surgery, *Anesthesiology* 91:362, 1999.

158. Miller BE, Mochizuki T, Levy JH, et al: Predicting and treating coagulopathies after cardiopulmonary bypass in children, *Anesth Analg* 85:1196, 1997.

159. Spiess BD: Thromboelastography and cardiopulmonary bypass, *Semin Thromb Hemost* 21:27, 1995.

160. Tuman KJ, Spiess BD, McCarthy RJ, Ivankovich AD: Comparison of viscoelastic measures of coagulation after cardiopulmonary bypass, *Anesth Analg* 69:69, 1989.

161. Spalding GJ, Hartrumpf M, Sierig T, et al: Cost reduction of perioperative coagulation management in cardiac surgery: Value of "bedside" thrombelastography (ROTEM), *Eur J Cardiothorac Surg* 31:1052–1057, 2007.

162. Tuman KJ, McCarthy RJ, Djuric M, et al: Evaluation of coagulation during cardiopulmonary bypass with a heparinase-modified thromboelastographic assay, *J Cardiothorac Vasc Anesth* 8:144, 1994.

163. Ereth MH, Nuttall GA, Klindworth JT, et al: Does the platelet-activated clotting test (HemoSTATUS) predict blood loss and platelet dysfunction associated with cardiopulmonary bypass? *Anesth Analg* 85:259, 1997.

164. Mongan PD, Hosking MP: The role of desmopressin acetate in patients undergoing coronary artery bypass surgery. A controlled clinical trial with thromboelastographic risk stratification, *Anesthesiology* 77:38, 1992.

165. Gravlee GP, Arora S, Lavender SW, et al: Predictive value of blood clotting tests in cardiac surgical patients, *Ann Thorac Surg* 58:216, 1994.

166. Spiess BD, Gillies BS, Chandler W, Verrier E: Changes in transfusion therapy and reexploration rate after institution of a blood management program in cardiac surgical patients, *J Cardiothorac Vasc Anesth* 9:168, 1995.

167. Whitten CW, Allison PM, Latson TW, et al: Evaluation of laboratory coagulation and lytic parameters resulting from autologous whole blood transfusion during primary aortocoronary artery bypass grafting, *J Clin Anesth* 8:229, 1996.

168. Greilich PE, Alving BM, O'Neill KL, et al: A modified thromboelastographic method for monitoring c7E3 Fab in heparinized patients, *Anesth Analg* 84:31, 1997.
169. Kang YG, Martin DJ, Marquez J, et al: Intraoperative changes in blood coagulation and thromboelastographic monitoring in liver transplantation, *Anesth Analg* 64:888, 1985.
170. Martin LK, Kang Y, De Wolf AM: Coagulation changes immediately following liver graft reperfusion, *Transplant Proc* 23:1946, 1991.
171. Khurana S, Mattson JC, Westley S, et al: Monitoring platelet glycoprotein IIb/IIIa-fibrin interaction with tissue factor-activated thromboelastography, *J Lab Clin Med* 130:401, 1997.
172. Shore-Lesserson L, Manspeizer HE, DePerio M, et al: Thromboelastography-guided transfusion algorithm reduces transfusions in complex cardiac surgery, *Anesth Analg* 88:312, 1999.
173. Gottumukkala VN, Sharma SK, Philip J: Assessing platelet and fibrinogen contribution to clot strength using modified thromboelastography in pregnant women, *Anesth Analg* 89:1453, 1999.
174. Greilich PE, Alving BM, Longnecker D, et al: Near-site monitoring of the antiplatelet drug abciximab using the Hemodyne analyzer and modified thromboelastograph, *J Cardiothorac Vasc Anesth* 13:58, 1999.
175. Craft RM, Chavez JJ, Bresee SJ, et al: A novel modification of the Thromboelastograph assay, isolating platelet function, correlates with optical platelet aggregation, *J Lab Clin Med* 143:301, 2004.
176. Shore-Lesserson L, Fischer G, Sanders J, et al: Clopidogrel induces a platelet aggregation defect that is partially mitigated by ex-vivo addition of aprotinin, *Anesthesiology* 101:A, 2004.
177. Hett D.A., Walker D, Pilkington SN, Smith DC: Sonoclot analysis, *Br J Anaesth* 75:771, 1995.
178. Stern MP, DeVos-Doyle K, Viguera MG, Lajos TZ: Evaluation of post-cardiopulmonary bypass Sonoclot signatures in patients taking nonsteroidal anti-inflammatory drugs, *J Cardiothorac Anesth* 3:730, 1989.
179. Chapin JW, Becker GL, Hulbert BJ, et al: Comparison of Thromboelastograph and Sonoclot coagulation analyzers for assessing coagulation status during orthotopic liver transplantation, *Transplant Proc* 21:3539, 1989.
180. Peck SD: Evaluation of the in vitro detection of the hypercoagulable state using the thrombin generation test and plasma clot impedance test, *Thromb Haemost* 42:764, 1979.
181. Smith JW, Steinhubl SR, Lincoff AM, et al: Rapid platelet-function assay: An automated and quantitative cartridge-based method, *Circulation* 99:620, 1999.
182. Coller BS, Lang D, Scudder LE: Rapid and simple platelet function assay to assess glycoprotein IIb/IIIa receptor blockade, *Circulation* 95:860, 1997.
183. Coller BS, Folts JD, Scudder LE, Smith SR: Antithrombotic effect of a monoclonal antibody to the platelet glycoprotein IIb/IIIa receptor in an experimental animal model, *Blood* 68:783, 1986.
184. Paniccia R, Antonucci E, Gori AM, et al: Different methodologies for evaluating the effect of clopidogrel on platelet function in high-risk coronary artery disease patients, *J Thromb Haemost* 5:1835–1838, 2007.
185. van Werkum JW, Harmsze AM, Elsenberg EH, et al: The use of the VerifyNow system to monitor antiplatelet therapy: A review of the current evidence, *Platelets* 19:479–488, 2008.
186. Ikarugi H, Taka T, Nakajima S, et al: Norepinephrine, but not epinephrine, enhances platelet reactivity and coagulation after exercise in humans, *J Appl Physiol* 86:133, 1999.
187. John LC, Rees GM, Kovacs IB: Inhibition of platelet function by heparin. An etiologic factor in postbypass hemorrhage, *J Thorac Cardiovasc Surg* 105:816, 1993.
188. Kovacs IB, Mayou SC, Kirby JD: Infusion of a stable prostacyclin analogue, iloprost, to patients with peripheral vascular disease: Lack of antiplatelet effect but risk of thromboembolism, *Am J Med* 90:41, 1991.
189. Ratnatunga CP, Rees GM, Kovacs IB: Preoperative hemostatic activity and excessive bleeding after cardiopulmonary bypass, *Ann Thorac Surg* 52:250, 1991.
190. Bock M, De Haan J, Beck KH, et al: Standardization of the PFA-100 (R) platelet function test in 105 mmol/L buffered citrate: Effect of gender, smoking, and oral contraceptives, *Br J Haematol* 106:898, 1999.
191. Escolar G, Cases A, Vinas M, et al: Evaluation of acquired platelet dysfunctions in uremic and cirrhotic patients using the platelet function analyzer (PFA-100): Influence of hematocrit elevation, *Haematologica* 84:614, 1999.
192. Kundu SK, Heilmann EJ, Sio R, et al: Description of an in vitro platelet function analyzer—PFA-100, *Semin Thromb Hemost* 21:106, 1995.
193. Mammen EF, Comp PC, Gosselin R, et al: PFA-100 system: A new method for assessment of platelet dysfunction, *Semin Thromb Hemost* 24:195, 1998.
194. Wahba A, Sander S, Birnbaum DE: Are in-vitro platelet function tests useful in predicting blood loss following open heart surgery? *Thorac Cardiovasc Surg* 46:228, 1998.
195. Nuttall G, Oliver WC Jr, Ereth MH, et al: The PFA 100, correlation with platelet aggregometry with GP IIB/IIIA receptor antagonists (abstract), *Anesthesiology* 91:A518, 1999.
196. Carville DG, Schleckser PA, Guyer KE, et al: Whole blood platelet function assay on the ICHOR point-of-care hematology analyzer, *J Extra Corpor Technol* 30:171, 1998.
197. Slaughter TF, Sreeram G, Sharma AD, et al: Reversible shear-mediated platelet dysfunction during cardiac surgery as assessed by the PFA-100 platelet function analyzer, *Blood Coagul Fibrinolysis* 12:85, 2001.
198. Steinhubl SR, Talley JD, Braden GA, et al: Point-of-care measured platelet inhibition correlates with a reduced risk of an adverse cardiac event after percutaneous coronary intervention: Results of the GOLD (AU-Assessing Ultegra) multicenter study, *Circulation* 103:2572, 2001.
199. Kenet G, Lubetsky A, Shenkman B, et al: Utility of whole blood hemostatometry using the clot signature analyzer for assessment of hemostasis in cardiac surgery, *Anesthesiology* 96:1115, 2002.
200. Kenet G, Lubetsky A, Shenkman B, et al: Cone and platelet analyser (CPA): A new test for the prediction of bleeding among thrombocytopenic patients, *Br J Haematol* 101:255–259, 1998.
201. Varon D, Lashevski I, Brenner B, et al: Cone and plate(let) analyzer: Monitoring glycoprotein IIb/IIIa antagonists and von Willebrand disease replacement therapy by testing platelet disposition under flow conditions, *Am Heart J* 135(5 Pt 2 Su):S187–S193, 1998.
202. Shenkman B, Schneiderman J, Tamarin I, et al: Testing the effect of GPIIb-IIIa antagonist in patients undergoing carotid stenting: Correlation between standard aggregometry, flow cytometry and the cone and plate(let) analyzer (CPA) methods, *Thromb Res* 102:311–317, 2001.
203. Savion N, Varon D: Impact-the cona and plate(let) analyzer: Testing platelet function and anti-platelet drug response, *Pathophysiol Haemost Thromb* 35:83–88, 2006.
204. Gerrah R, Brill A, Tshori S, et al: Using cone and plate(let) analyzer to predict bleeding in cardiac surgery, *Asian Cardiovasc Thorac Ann* 14:310–315, 2006.
205. Rahe-Meyer N, Winterhalter M, Boden A, et al: Platelet concentrates transfusion in cardiac surgery and platelet function assessment by multiple electrode aggregometry, *Acta Anaesthesiol Scand* 53:168–175, 2009.
206. Rahe-Meyer N, Winterhalter M, Hartmann J, et al: An evaluation of cyclooxygenase-1 inhibition before coronary artery surgery: Aggregometry versus patient self-reporting, *Anesth Analg* 107:1791–1797, 2008.
207. Velik-Salchner C, Maier S, Innerhofer P, et al: Point-of-care whole blood impedance aggregometry versus classical light transmission aggregometry for detecting aspirin and clopidogrel: The results of a pilot study, *Anesth Analg* 107:1798–1806, 2008.
208. Velik-Salchner C, Maier S, Innerhofer P, et al: An assessment of cardiopulmonary bypass-induced changes in platelet function using whole blood and classical light transmission aggregometry: The results of a pilot study, *Anesth Analg* 108:1747–1754, 2009.
209. Mengistu AM, Röhm KD, Boldt J, et al: The influence of aprotinin and tranexamic acid on platelet function and postoperative blood loss in cardiac surgery, *Anesth Analg* 107:391–397, 2008.
210. Mengistu AM, Wolf MW, Boldt J, et al: Evaluation of a new platelet function analyzer in cardiac surgery: A comparison of modified thromboelastography and whole-blood aggregometry, *J Cardiothorac Vasc Anesth* 22:40–46, 2008.
211. Sibbing D, Braun S, Morath T, et al: Platelet reactivity after clopidogrel treatment assessed with point-of-care analysis and early drug-eluting stent thrombosis, *J Am Coll Cardiol* 53:849–856, 2009.

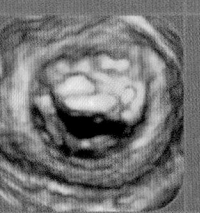

Anesthesia and Transesophageal Echocardiography for Cardiac Surgery

18

Anesthesia for Myocardial Revascularization

ALEXANDER J.C. MITTNACHT, MD | MENACHEM WEINER, MD | MARTIN J. LONDON, MD |
JOEL A. KAPLAN, MD, CPE, FACC

KEY POINTS

1. The risk profile of the average patient presenting for coronary artery bypass grafting (CABG) has increased with greater numbers of patients with triple-vessel disease, poor targets, reduced ventricular function, and reoperations.
2. Preoperative ordering of premedication should include careful consideration of all of the patient's relevant antihypertensive, antianginal, and other medications.
3. Preexisting abnormalities of ventricular function, wall motion, and ischemic mitral regurgitation, together with long ischemic time during cardiopulmonary bypass, are predictors of difficulty in weaning and postoperative low cardiac output states.
4. Possible indications for pulmonary artery catheter use in cardiac surgery patients are those with pulmonary hypertension, right-heart failure, or severely impaired ventricular function who require postoperative cardiac output monitoring.
5. The days of high-dose opioid anesthesia for CABG are over, with nearly universal adoption of fast-tracking programs aimed at early extubation with reduced intensive care unit and hospital stay.
6. All contemporary inhalation agents have been shown to have potent preconditioning effects, and randomized trials have demonstrated reductions in postoperative troponin release and improved ventricular function relative to exclusively intravenous techniques.
7. The role of the postconditioning effect of inhalation agents is also starting to be elucidated.
8. The risk for intraoperative recall is increased in all cardiac surgical procedures, although its incidence has declined substantially with the increased continuous use of inhalation anesthetics.
9. Developments in stabilization devices for off-pump CABG surgery have helped to establish this approach for myocardial revascularization. Despite apparent advantages compared with conventional CABG surgery, large prospective studies have yet to prove better outcome.

The role of the anesthesiologist in the perioperative care of patients presenting for myocardial revascularization continues to evolve. The anesthesiologist has to be well versed not only in a safe anesthesia technique, but in all areas of perioperative management in patients with coronary artery disease (CAD). This includes advances in pharmacologic risk reduction, new surgical techniques, and anesthetic management including monitoring techniques aiming to improve patient outcome. The overall number of patients presenting for coronary artery bypass graft (CABG) surgery has declined, mainly because of the growth of percutaneous coronary interventions (PCIs). Ischemic heart disease still accounts for approximately 1 of every 6 deaths in the United States. For 2010, it is estimated that 785,000 Americans will have a new heart attack, and every minute someone will die of it.[1] Those patients who are not eligible for PCIs typically have an increased risk for perioperative morbidity and mortality and depend more than ever on optimal anesthetic management. This chapter provides a sequential approach to the major management issues faced by the practitioner who provides anesthesia for patients presenting for CABG surgery with cardiopulmonary bypass (CPB) or for off-pump coronary artery bypass (OPCAB) procedures.

EPIDEMIOLOGY

In 2010, it is estimated that 1 in 3 Americans in the United States have one or more types of cardiovascular disease, with CAD estimated to occur in 17,600,000 individuals in the United States. The total direct and indirect cost of all cardiovascular disease and stroke in the United States for 2010 is estimated to be $503.2 billion. Ischemic heart disease constituted 13.8% of the conditions of all Medicare beneficiaries in 2004; this number increased to 39.1% when only patients in the top 5% for all expenditures were considered.[1] According to the same source, the number of cardiac catheterizations decreased slightly from 1996 to 2006 (Figure 18-1). There were 1,115,000 cardiac catheterizations performed in 2006, with 1,313,000 PCIs performed the same year.

Although precise data on the annual number of CABG and PCI procedures performed are not available, estimates based on sampling of large administrative and clinical databases, together with publications from discrete health care systems, have been used to derive strong estimates.[2–4] The most widely cited data for nonfederal institutions in the United States are obtained from the U.S. Department of Health and Human Services National Hospital Discharge Survey.[5] The latest data available estimated that, in 2006, 253,000 patients underwent a total of 448,000 CABG procedures.

PATHOPHYSIOLOGY OF CORONARY ARTERY DISEASE

Anatomy

The anesthesiologist should be familiar with coronary anatomy if only to interpret the significance of angiographic findings. An extensive review of cardiac anatomy can be found in reference cardiology or cardiac surgery texts.[6,7] The following is an abbreviated description of the epicardial coronary anatomy. The coronary circulation and common sites for placement of distal anastomoses during CABG are shown in Figures 18-2 to 18-4.

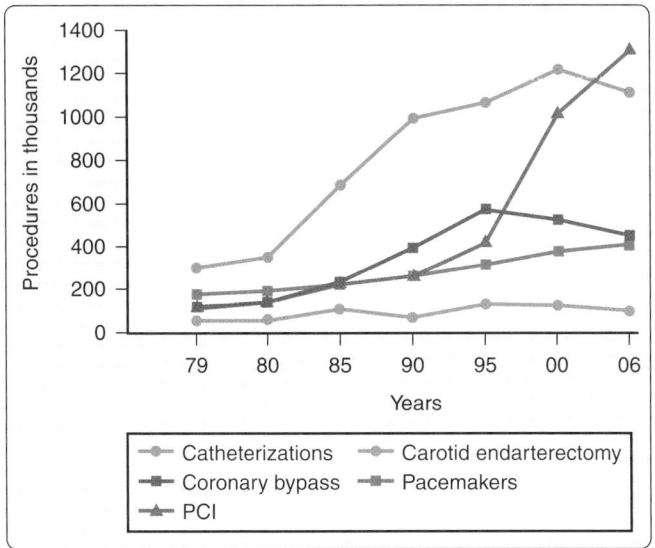

Figure 18-1 Trends in cardiovascular inpatient operations and procedures in the United States from 1979 to 2006. PCI, percutaneous coronary intervention. *(Source: National Health Data System, National Center for Health Statistics, and National Heart, Lung and Blood Institute; from the American Heart Association Committee and Stroke Statistics Subcommittee: Heart disease and stroke statistics 2010 update. Circulation 121:e1–e170, 2010, Chart 19.2.)*

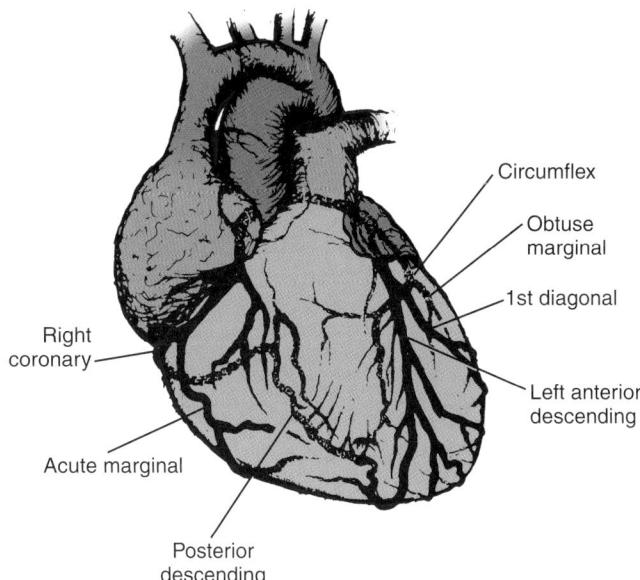

Figure 18-3 Ten-degree right anterior oblique angiographic view of the heart, which best shows the left main coronary artery dividing into the circumflex and left anterior descending arteries. *Lines* indicate common sites of distal vein graft anastomoses. *(Adapted from Stiles QR, Tucker BL, Lindesmith GG, et al: Myocardial revascularization: a surgical atlas. Boston: Little, Brown, 1976.)*

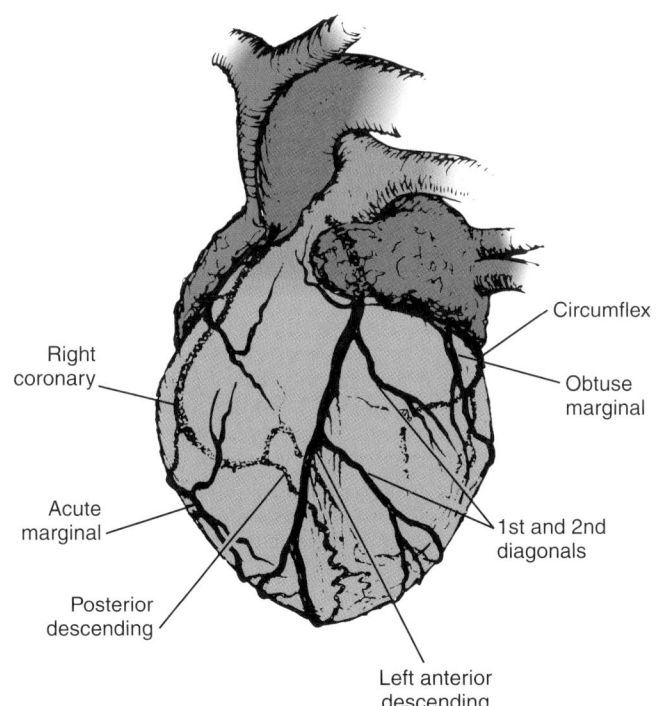

Figure 18-2 Thirty-degree left anterior oblique angiographic view of the heart, which best shows the right coronary artery. *Lines* indicate common sites of distal vein graft anastomoses. *(From Stiles QR, Tucker BL, Lindesmith GG, et al: Myocardial Revascularization: A Surgical Atlas. Boston: Little, Brown, 1976.)*

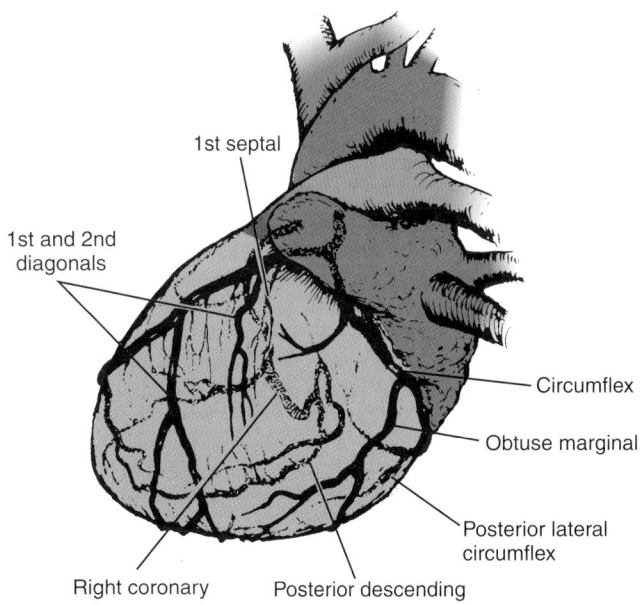

Figure 18-4 Seventy-five-degree left anterior oblique angiographic view of the heart, which best shows branches of the left anterior descending and circumflex coronary arteries. *(Adapted from Stiles QR, Tucker BL, Lindesmith GG, et al: Myocardial revascularization: a surgical atlas. Boston: Little, Brown, 1976.)*

The right coronary artery (RCA) arises from the right sinus of Valsalva and is best seen in the left anterior oblique view on coronary cineangiography (see Figure 18-2). It passes anteriorly for the first few millimeters, then follows the right atrioventricular groove, and curves posteriorly within the groove to reach the crux of the heart, the area

where the interventricular septum (IVS) meets the atrioventricular groove. In 84% of cases, it terminates as the posterior descending artery (PDA), which is its most important branch, being the sole supply to the posterior-superior IVS. Other important branches are those to the sinus node in 60% of patients and the atrioventricular node in approximately 85% of patients. Anatomists consider the RCA to be dominant when it crosses the crux of the heart and continues in the atrioventricular groove regardless of the origin of the PDA. Angiographers, however, ascribe dominance to the artery, right coronary or left coronary (circumflex [Cx]), that creates the PDA.

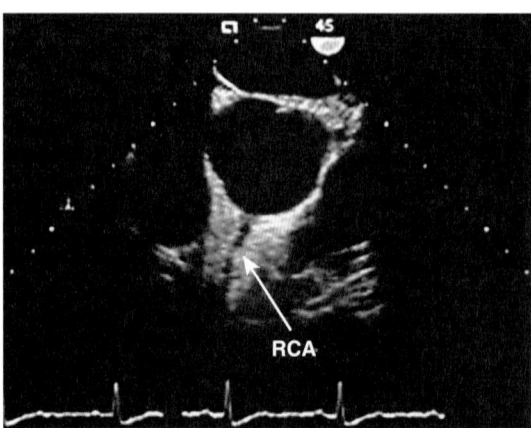

Figure 18-5 The vertical and superior orientation of the right coronary artery arising from the aortic root is identified by transesophageal echocardiography (TEE). The TEE transducer in the esophagus is on the top of the screen, and the patient's chest wall is on the bottom. Retained air preferentially enters the right coronary artery (RCA), which may cause inferior ischemia, depending on the amount of air and the coronary perfusion pressure. Increase of perfusion pressure using phenylephrine is often used to treat coronary air embolus. The left main artery (not visible) arises at approximately 3 o'clock on this image. *(Courtesy of Martin J. London, MD, University of California, San Francisco, CA)*

The vertical and superior orientation of the RCA ostium allows easy passage of air bubbles during aortic cannulation, CPB, or open valve surgery. In sufficient concentration (e.g., coronary air embolus), myocardial ischemia involving the inferior LV wall segments and the right ventricle (RV) may occur (Figure 18-5). In contrast, the near-perpendicular orientation of the left main coronary ostium makes air embolization much less common.

The left coronary artery arises from the left sinus of Valsalva as the left main coronary artery. This is best seen in a shallow right anterior oblique projection (see Figure 18-3). The left main coronary artery courses anteriorly and to the left, where it divides in a space between the aorta and pulmonary artery. Its branches are the left anterior descending (LAD) and Cx arteries. The LAD passes along the anterior intraventricular groove. It may reach only two thirds of the distance to the apex or extend around the apex to the diaphragmatic portion of the left ventricle. Major branches of the LAD are the diagonal branches, which supply the free wall of the left ventricle, and septal branches, which course posteriorly to supply the major portion of the IVS. Although there may be many diagonal and septal branches, the first diagonal and first septal branches serve as important landmarks in the descriptions of lesions of the LAD (see Figure 18-4).

The Cx arises at a sharp angle from the left main coronary artery and courses toward the crux of the heart in the atrioventricular groove. When the Cx gives rise to the PDA, the circulation is left dominant, and the left coronary circulation supplies the entire IVS and the atrioventricular node. In approximately 40% of patients, the Cx supplies the branch to the SA node. Up to four obtuse marginal arteries arise from the Cx and supply the lateral wall of the left ventricle (see Figure 18-4). All of the previously described epicardial branches create small vessels that supply the outer third of the myocardium and penetrating vessels that anastomose with the subendocardial plexus. This capillary plexus is unique in that it functions as an end-arterial system. Each epicardial arteriole supplies a capillary plexus that forms an end loop rather than anastomosing with an adjacent capillary from another epicardial artery.[8] Significant collateral circulation does not exist at the microcirculatory level. This capillary anatomy explains the distinct areas of myocardial ischemia or infarction that can be related to disease in a discrete epicardial artery (see Chapters 3 and 6).

CAD most commonly affects the epicardial muscular arteries with rare intramyocardial lesions (with the exception of the transplanted

heart). However, severe disorders of the microcirculation and primary impairment of coronary vascular reserve in normal coronary arteries have been described, especially in diabetics, female patients, and those with variant angina.[9-11] Atherosclerosis in all organs is most common at the outer edges of vessel bifurcations because in these regions blood flow is slower and changes direction during the cardiac cycle, resulting in less net shear stress (i.e., frictional force per unit area) than in other regions with more steady blood flow and higher shear stress.[12] Low shear stress has been shown to stimulate an atherogenic phenotype in the endothelium. Epicardial lesions can be single but are more often multiple. A combined lesion of the RCA and both branches of the left coronary artery is referred to as triple-vessel disease. The left coronary artery supplies the thickest portions of the LV, at least the exterior two thirds of the IVS, and the greater part of the atria. Most bypass grafts are done on the left coronary system.

Venous drainage of the myocardium is primarily to the coronary sinus, which drains 96% of the LV free wall and septum, and the remainder of the venous return goes directly into the right atrium.[7] A small fraction may enter other cardiac chambers directly through the anterior-sinusoidal, anterior-luminal, and thebesian veins.[13]

Myocardial Ischemia and Infarction

In patients with CAD, myocardial ischemia usually results from increases in myocardial oxygen demand that exceed the capacity of the stenosed coronary arteries to increase their oxygen supply (Figure 18-6). However, the determinants of myocardial oxygen balance are complex, and alterations may have several effects. For example, an increase in blood pressure (i.e., increased afterload) increases wall tension and oxygen demand while also increasing coronary blood flow (CBF). Myocardial ischemia may occur without changes in systemic hemodynamics and in awake patients may occur in the absence of chest pain (i.e., silent ischemia), particularly in patients with diabetes.

In atherosclerotic heart disease, the fundamental lesion is an intimal lipid plaque that causes chronic stenosis and episodic thrombosis, occurring most often in an epicardial coronary artery (Figure 18-7), thereby reducing myocardial blood supply. Characteristics of the vulnerable plaque include high lipid content, a thin fibrous cap, a reduced number of smooth muscle cells, and increased macrophage activity.[14] The lipid core is the most thrombogenic component of the plaque.

Fuster et al[15] described five phases in the progression of CAD by plaque morphology. Phase 1 is a small plaque present in many people younger than 30 years and usually progresses very slowly, depending on the presence of risk factors associated with CAD (i.e., increased low-density lipoprotein cholesterol). Phase 2 is a plaque with a high lipid content that has the potential to rupture. If it ruptures, it will lead to thrombosis and increased stenosis (phase 5), possibly producing unstable angina or an acute coronary syndrome. The phase 2 plaque usually does not rupture; it instead progresses into phases 3 and 4, with enlargement and fibrous tissue organization, which ultimately may produce an occlusive plaque at phase 5.

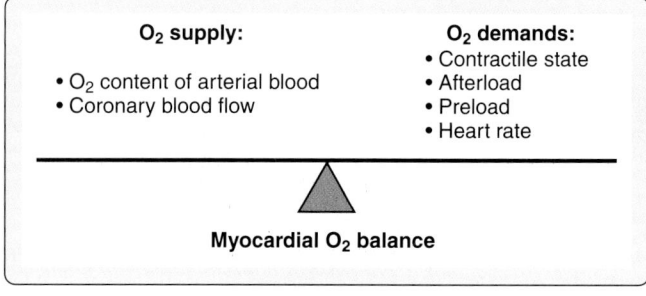

Figure 18-6 Factors determining myocardial oxygen supply and demand.

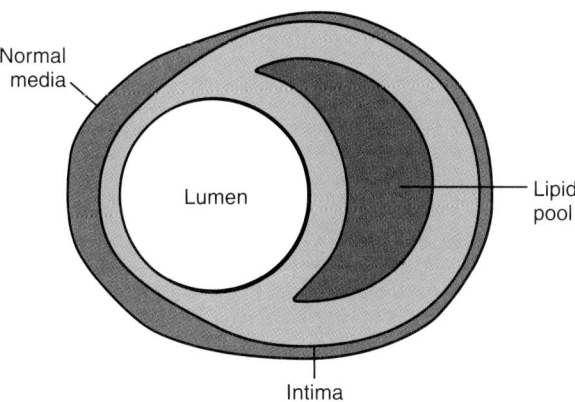

Normal media

Lumen

Lipid pool

Intima

Figure 18-7 Lipoid plaque lesion of a coronary artery. *(From Davies MJ: A macro and micro view of coronary vascular insult in ischemic heart disease. Circulation 82(Suppl II):II-38, 1990, by permission of American Heart Association.)*

Acute coronary syndrome is produced by a sudden decrease in CBF. In unstable angina, a relatively small fissure in a plaque may produce a temporary thrombotic occlusion of a vessel.[16] Release of vasoactive substances from platelets and white blood cells, as well as dysfunction of the endothelium, may lead to vasoconstriction and reduction of CBF.[17,18] Reduced vasoconstriction, spontaneous thrombolysis, or the opening of collateral channels may limit the duration of myocardial ischemia. A larger plaque disruption and prolonged thrombosis will produce a Q-wave infarction with transmural myocardial necrosis. The potential lesions seen with plaque fissure are shown in Figure 18-8. Several studies have found that the coronary artery responsible for an acute infarction is often only moderately obstructed.[19,20] It is the extent of plaque rupture and thrombosis that determines the size and extent of an infarction, rather than the degree of stenosis. Patients with severely obstructed coronary arteries often have extensive collateral circulations that protect them from infarction. Similar findings have been reported in patients developing postoperative myocardial infarction after noncardiac surgery.[21–23]

The physiology of the coronary circulation is reviewed in Chapter 6. CBF in the normal individual is independent of perfusion pressure, but it is related to tissue oxygen demand.[7] This phenomenon is referred to as *autoregulation*. Autoregulation affects all layers of the ventricular wall,

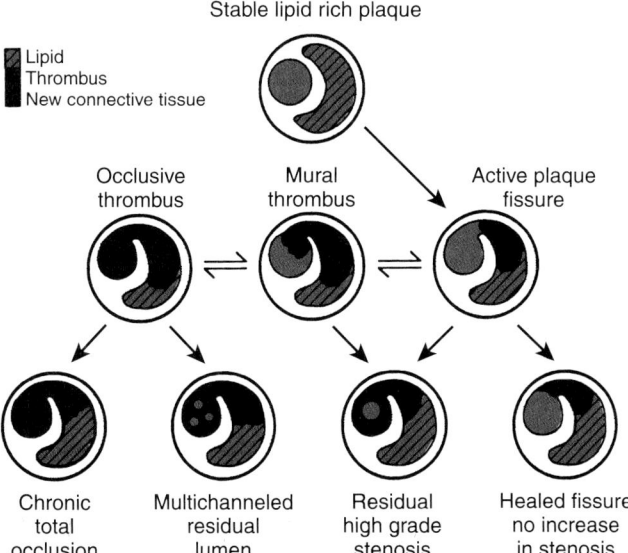

Figure 18-8 Possible outcomes of intimal plaque rupture. *(From Davies MJ: A macro and micro view of coronary vascular insult in ischemic heart disease. Circulation 82(Suppl II):II-38, 1990, by permission of American Heart Association.)*

maintaining essentially equal flows from the epicardium to the endocardium.[24,25] The difference between autoregulated flow and maximal flow constitutes the coronary vascular reserve. As an obstruction of a coronary artery increases in size, dilation of the capillary bed occurs, with maintenance of adequate blood supply as the result. Coronary flow reserve, however, is diminished and eventually exhausted, and autoregulation begins to fail. Autoregulatory failure is loss of metabolic control of CBF and the sole dependence on pressure gradients to determine flow. Autoregulation fails first in the subendocardium, where blood flow fails to match demand, resulting in subendocardial ischemia and dysfunction.[11,26]

Autoregulation is pressure dependent, in that as perfusion pressure declines below a critical value, autoregulation begins to fail. In conscious animals, the pressure at which autoregulation begins to fail is very low (mean arterial pressure [MAP] of 38 to 40 mm Hg).[27] Because CBF reserve is diminished in CAD, the pressure at which subendocardial autoregulation fails is increased. Heart rate (HR) also appears to have an effect on autoregulation. In an unanesthetized animal model, when the HR was doubled, the perfusion pressure that produced failure of subendocardial autoregulation was increased from a mean of 38 mm Hg at the normal HR to a mean of 61 mm Hg at the doubled rate.[28] This pressure is not that much less than normal perfusion pressures. This effect of HR on subendocardial autoregulation is related to the increased myocardial oxygen consumption and flow caused by tachycardia and to the reduction in diastolic time and, therefore, perfusion. The net effect is a reduction in coronary vascular reserve and earlier failure of autoregulation, with resultant subendocardial ischemia. Tachycardia, because of its effects on demand and supply (reduction in diastolic perfusion time), is especially deleterious in the presence of CAD, in which perfusion pressures beyond an epicardial arterial obstruction are unknown.[29] Avoidance of hypotension and tachycardia has been the basic tenet of anesthetic practice in patients with CAD for many years.

A coronary arterial stenosis may be rigid or, more commonly (70%), compliant in nature.[30] When the pressure in the coronary circulation distal to a fixed stenosis is decreased, flow across the stenotic area decreases. Conversely, when the pressure distal to a compliant obstruction is increased, flow across the lesion is increased.[31] The clinical implication is that decreased blood pressure to an area of myocardium supplied by a vessel with a variable stenosis will decrease blood supply to the myocardium by two mechanisms: loss of collateral flow and decreased flow across the compliant stenosis. Collateral vessels exist in normal hearts, but in the presence of CAD, they are increased in size and number.[32] When a coronary vessel has a high-grade stenosis, the microvasculature distal to it may be maximally dilated even at rest and subject to ischemia. Collaterals may develop between this ischemic zone and an adjacent nonischemic area supplied by a different vessel. When vasodilation of the microcirculation is induced by exercise or drugs, perfusion of the ischemic bed by the collateral circulation may be decreased or cut off, particularly when the collateral vessels are poorly developed, because these present a greater degree of resistance than collaterals that are well developed. When vasodilation occurs in the nonischemic bed, pressure within it is decreased, and flow across collateral vessels with high resistance is reduced. An increase in myocardial blood flow in one region that reduces flow in another is referred to as a coronary steal.[33] In experimental models, a partial lesion of the epicardial artery supplying the collateral vessel is required to produce a coronary steal.[34] This anatomic configuration, called *steal-prone anatomy*, occurred in 23% of patients with symptomatic CAD in one large registry of coronary angiograms.[35]

The hallmark symptom of myocardial ischemia is pain. It has been found, however, that significant ischemia may occur without pain ("silent ischemia").[36,37] Early research using ambulatory electrocardiographic (ECG) monitoring reported that these silent episodes were frequent and occurred at lower HRs and activity levels when compared with exercise stress test data for the same individuals.[38] Silent ischemic episodes are not considered to be an electrical anomaly but are due to myocardial perfusion impairment resulting in reduced regional function.[39] A study of patients presenting for elective CABG confirmed these findings in the perioperative period: 42% of 50 patients studied had ischemic episodes before surgery, 87% of these episodes were clinically silent, and few were precipitated by adverse hemodynamics.[40] In summary, there is no doubt that primary reductions in myocardial oxygen supply because of hypotension, anemia, or coronary vasoconstriction are important mechanisms in the development of ischemia, particularly in the perioperative period.

RISK ASSESSMENT IN PATIENTS SCHEDULED FOR CORONARY ARTERY BYPASS GRAFTING SURGERY

Operative mortality (usually defined as death within 30 days of surgery), as expected, varies widely with patient risk, acuity, and previous cardiac surgery. On average, however, it appears that mortality has declined progressively despite increases in patient risk (Figure 18-9).[41] The rapid growth of PCI has led to the perception of a shunting of healthier patients away from CABG, leaving a greater percentage of older and sicker patients not studied in the original CABG efficacy trials (e.g., the seminal coronary artery surgery study [CASS] trial excluded patients with ejection fractions [EFs] less than 35%). Publications since 1980 addressing whether patients presenting for CABG are sicker or at greater risk than they were previously have uniformly answered this affirmatively, noting older patients, worse ventricular function, and more emergent cases.[41] Despite these findings, however, operative mortality continues to decline. Davierwala et al[42] observed that LV dysfunction and reoperative status have decreased in significance as predictors of mortality in a large cohort of Canadian patients, whereas emergency surgery has increased in importance in predicting adverse outcome.

Preoperative risk assessment for patients undergoing CABG has evolved dramatically since 1990, driven by a variety of diverse factors. Institution of a federally mandated accounting of surgical outcomes for cardiac surgery in the Department of Veterans Affairs in the 1970s led to the establishment of what is considered the first large-scale, multicenter surgical outcomes database applying rigorous statistical methodology for comparing outcomes between centers.[43,44] This group and others have pioneered methodology for adjusting for different severities of illness between patients (i.e., risk adjustment) using multiple preoperative and perioperative variables thought to be of intrinsic value (usually by expert consensus) that easily could be captured and have high consistency of definition. Entering these variables into logistic regression models of mortality (considering all of the patients operated on in the particular time frame in which the variables were collected) allows determination of an "expected" mortality based on coefficients of the regression equation most correlated with outcome. By simple comparison of the "observed" to "expected" (i.e., the value calculated by entering a unique patient's coefficients into the general population mortality model)

mortality ratio (O/E ratio), hospitals in a particular system can be ranked from best (low O/E ratio) to worst (high O/E ratio).[45] However, as observed by a variety of experts, caution is advised in use of such adjectives given inherent assumptions and controversies in the statistical approaches for determining thresholds for "quality" and problems in "gaming" of the system by exploiting variables with imprecise definitions.[46]

Nonetheless, this methodology and its variants have been adopted widely by many organizations as a measure of quality of care.[47] The Society of Thoracic Surgeons (STS) instituted a voluntary clinical database system with this approach in the early 1990s, which has continued to grow rapidly as cardiac surgical groups are increasingly interested in benchmarking their practices against others.[48,49] Many states have established and maintain risk-adjusted mandatory reporting systems for hospital and individual surgeon performance.[50] A natural offshoot of this approach has been the exploration of surgeon and hospital volumes as predictors of outcome, a topic that has generated substantial controversy in the literature given conflicting findings (i.e., low-volume centers in which "high-volume" surgeons operate appear to do as well as high-volume centers, and low-risk patients do better relative to high-risk patients at high-volume centers).[51,52] This is a hotly contested topic given the high stakes involved in federal and private sector initiatives to regionalize cardiac surgery care into "centers of excellence."[53] The EuroSCORE scoring system is based on outcomes in 128 centers in 8 European countries and has received increasing attention. It appears to compare favorably with the STS model in North American patients.[54,55] It is freely accessible by means of an interactive Web-based calculator (www.euroscore.org) and is decidedly simpler and faster to use than the STS's scoring system, which is now also freely accessible to the public (http://www.sts.org/sections/stsnationaldatabase/riskcalculator/index.html).

Given the mass of literature on this topic and the large number of risk models available, some of which are easily calculated (e.g., a simple additive score), whereas others require manipulation of a logistic regression equation on an advanced calculator or microcomputer, considerable debate exists about how they are best applied. The American College of Cardiology/American Heart Association CABG guidelines group accords a Class IIa recommendation (level of evidence C) to their use for predicting hospital mortality.[56] However, they caution that risk scores should be individually calibrated for regional mortality rates (a difficult task) and updated periodically to maintain accuracy (many have not been, with the exception of the Department of Veterans Affairs program and the STS).

Table 18-1 presents an evaluation of the importance of risk factors in several major risk models and large-scale outcome analyses grouped by the classification that Jones et al[57-63] advocated.

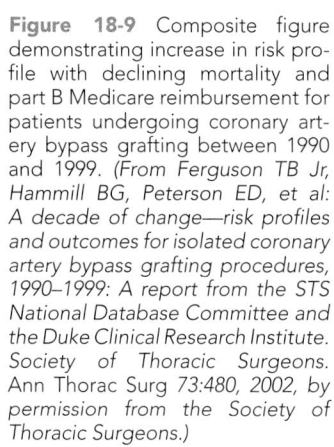
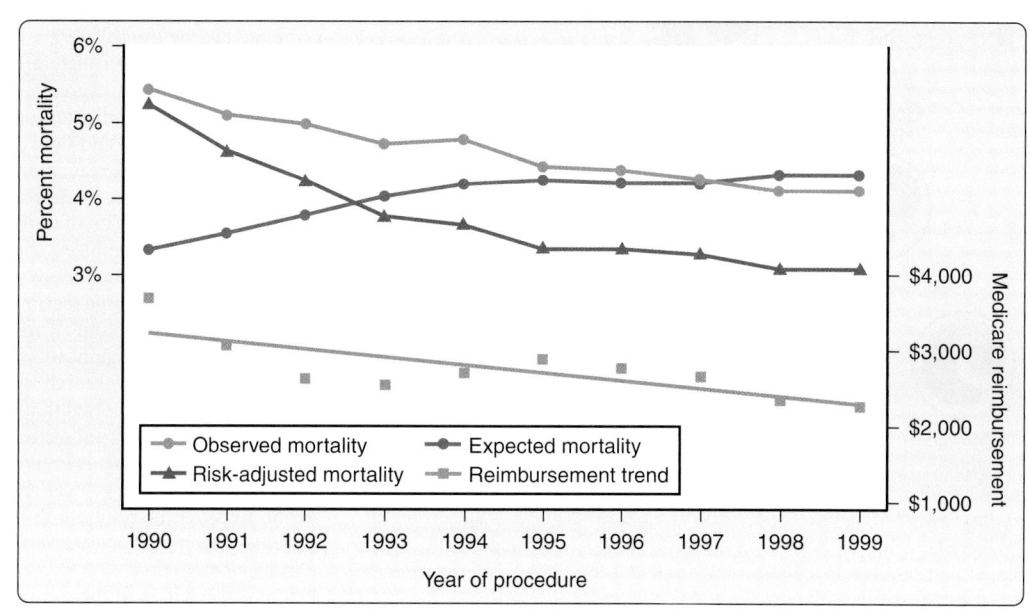

Figure 18-9 Composite figure demonstrating increase in risk profile with declining mortality and part B Medicare reimbursement for patients undergoing coronary artery bypass grafting between 1990 and 1999. (*From Ferguson TB Jr, Hammill BG, Peterson ED, et al: A decade of change—risk profiles and outcomes for isolated coronary artery bypass grafting procedures, 1990–1999: A report from the STS National Database Committee and the Duke Clinical Research Institute. Society of Thoracic Surgeons. Ann Thorac Surg 73:480, 2002, by permission from the Society of Thoracic Surgeons.*)

TABLE 18-1   Preoperative Risk Stratification Based on Clinical Databases

Variables	Society of Thoracic Surgeons[49]	Department of Veterans Affairs[58]	EuroSCORE[63]	New York State[60]	Cleveland Clinic[62]	HCA, Inc.[4]
				Clinical Databases		
Risk Equation Units	OR (95% CI)	OR	Additive score	OR (95% CI)	Additive Score	OR (95% CI)
Core Variables						
Acuity (stability)	Status: urgent or emergent = 1.96 (1.88–2.05); shock = 2.04 (1.90–2.19); IABP = 1.46 (1.37–1.55)	IABP = 1.7	Score 3 for critical preoperative state = V. tach, V. fib, CPR, IABP, inotropes, or acute renal failure; score 2 for emergency	IABP = 1.39 (1.15–1.69); disaster = 3.98 (31.2–5.08)	Score 6 for emergency	Cardiogenic shock = 8.35 (6.79–10.27); acute MI = 1.80 (1.38–1.84); IABP = 5.26 (4.57–6.05)
Prior cardiac surgery	First = 2.76 (2.62–2.91); multiple = 4.19 (3.61–4.86)	2.1	Score 3	3.73 (3.29–4.24)	Score 3	1.8 (1.34–2.43)
Age	1.05 (1.05–1.05)	1.5 (per 10 yr)	Score 1 per 5 yr over 60	1.05 (1.03–1.07) for >70 yr	Score 2 for age < 75 yr; score 1 for age 65–74 yr	1.04 (1.04–1.05)
Ejection fraction	EF < 50% = 0.98 (0.98–0.98)	Cardiomegaly = 1.5	Score 1 for EF = 30–50%; score 3 for <30%	<20% = 4.06 (3.16–5.21); 20–29% = 2.12 (1.89–2.58); 30–39% = 1.63 (1.43–1.86)	Score 3 for severe left ventricular dysfunction	NA
Sex	Male = 0.84 (0.80–0.98)	Female = 2.6	Score 1 for female	Female = 1.52 (1.36–1.69)	NA	Male = 0.71 (0.63–0.80)
Diseased vessels	Triple vessel = 1.21 (1.17–1.26)	NA	NA	NA	NA	Multivessel intervention = 0.64 (0.50–0.82)
Diseased left main	1.18 (1.14–1.24)	NA	NA	1.43 (1.23–1.67)	NA	NA
Level 1 Variables						
Creatinine	Renal failure/dialysis = 1.88 (1.80–1.96)	1.5–3.0 mg/dL = 1.6; >3.0 = 2.6	Score 2 for >100µmol/L	Dialysis = 2.80 (2.26–3.46)	Score 4 for >1.9mg/dL; score 1 for 1.6–1.8 mg/dL	Hemodialysis = 1.05 (10.56–16.13); chronic renal failure = NS
Cardiovascular disease	1.10 (1.04–1.17)	1.3			Score 1	
Myocardial infarction	1.18 (1.16–1.21)	>7 days before surgery = 1.2; <7 days before surgery = 2.1	Score 2 for <90 days before surgery	<7 days before surgery = 1.69 (1.45–1.97)	NA	0.80 (0.65–0.97)
Congestive heart failure	NS; NYHA Class IV = 1.15 (1.10–1.20)	NYHA Class II = 1.5; III = 1.5; IV = 2.3		1.77 (1.53–2.04)	NA	NA
Peripheral vascular disease	PVD/CVD = 1.29 (1.25–1.34)	1.4	Score 2 for carotid, aortic, or lower extremity disease		Score 2 for prior vascular surgery	1.21 (1.03–1.43); AAA = 2.47 (1.79–3.40)
PTCA current admission	<6 hr before surgery = 1.32 (1.18–1.48)	NA	NA	NA	NA	Thrombolytics = 0.42 (0.18–0.96); use of GPIIB/IIIa = 0.47 (0.30–0.71)
Arrhythmia	NA	1.3	Score 3 for critical preoperative state = V. tach, V. fib, CPR, IABP, inotropes, or acute renal failure; score 2 for emergency	NA	NA	NA
COPD	1.41 (1.36–1.48)	Resting ST depression = 1.4; CSS grade II = 1.0; III = 1.0; IV = 1.4	Score 1 for long-term use of bronchodilator or steroids	1.36 (1.20–1.54)	Score 2 on medication	1.41 (1.23–1.61)

Continued

TABLE 18-1 Preoperative Risk Stratification Based on Clinical Databases—Cont'd

Variables	Clinical Databases					
	Society of Thoracic Surgeons[49]	Department of Veterans Affairs[58]	EuroSCORE[63]	New York State[60]	Cleveland Clinic[62]	HCA, Inc.[4]
Risk Equation Units	OR (95% CI)	OR	Additive score	OR (95% CI)	Additive Score	OR (95% CI)
Angina	NA	NA	Score 3 for unstable angina	Unstable angina = 1.42 (1.27–1.60)	NA	NA
Mitral regurgitation	MR = 1.22 (1.17–1.28); aortic stenosis = 1.40 (1.21–1.61)	NA	NA	NA	Score 3	Valve disease = 1.03 (1.08–1.56)
Diabetes	IDDM = 1.50 (1.42–1.58); oral therapy = 1.15 (1.09–1.21)	NA	NA	1.50 (1.34–1.67)	Score 1 on any medication	IDDM, NIDDM = NS
Weight/height	BSA = 0.91 (0.89–0.93)	NA	NA	Morbid obesity = 1.49 (1.20–1.84)	Score 1 for <65 kg	NA
Level 2 Variables						
Smoking	NS	NA	NA	NA	NA	NA
Hypertension	1.12 (1.08–1.17)	NA	NA	NA	NA	0.82 (0.72–0.93)
Liver disease	NA	NA	NA	NA	NA	10.00 (6.83–14.63)
Malignancy	NA	NA	NA	NA	NA	NA
Immunosuppression	1.75 (1.57–1.95)	NA	NA	NA	NA	NA
Prior PTCA	NA	NA	NA	NA	NA	NS
Race	Black = 1.34 (1.23–1.45)	NA	NA	NA	NA	NA
Miscellaneous Features						
Hypercholesterolemia	0.82 (0.79–0.86)					
Neurologic dysfunction			Score 2			
Active endocarditis			Score 3			
Other procedure			Score 2 for other procedure; score 3 for surgery on thoracic aorta			
Postinfarct septal rupture			Score 4			
Pulmonary hypertension			Score 2 for syst. PA > 60 mm Hg			
Anemia					Score 2 for hematocrit <34%	

AAA, abdominal aortic aneurysm; BSA, body surface area; CCS, Canadian Cardiovascular Society grade scale for angina; CI, confidence interval; COPD, chronic obstructive pulmonary disease; CPR, cardiopulmonary resuscitation; CVD, cardiovascular disease; EF, ejection fraction; GP, glycoprotein; IABP, intra-aortic balloon pump; IDDM, insulin-dependent diabetes mellitus; MI, myocardial infarction; MR, mitral regurgitation; NA, not available; NS, not significant; NIDDM, non–insulin-dependent diabetes mellitus; NYHA, New York Heart Association; OR, odds ratio; PTCA, percutaneous transluminal coronary angioplasty; PVD, peripheral vascular disease; syst PA, systolic pulmonary artery pressure; V. fib, ventricular fibrillation; V. tach, ventricular tachycardia.

Adapted from Jones RH, Hannan EL, Hammermeister KE, et al: Identification of preoperative variables needed for risk adjustment of short-term mortality after coronary artery bypass graft surgery. The Working Group Panel on the Cooperative CABG Database Project. J Am Coll Cardiol 28:1478, 1996.

The major database models only predict perioperative mortality (usually defined as death within 30 days of surgery, although some use any death directly related to a perioperative complication regardless of the time interval, a factor further complicating comparison of models). As such, these models are often of less practical importance to the cardiac anesthesiologist. Predicting which patients are most likely to be difficult to wean from CPB because of development of a low cardiac output syndrome (LCOS) in the operating room or early postoperative period, or who may acquire postoperative complications, is of greater interest to the anesthesiologist. Despite publication of several studies, difficulty in standardization of what constitutes difficult weaning or LCOS has limited generalization of findings. However, given that most CABG mortality is related to difficulty in revascularization and/or myocardial protection, the risk factors are quite similar to those reported for overall mortality.[64,65] An analysis of 1009 patients undergoing CABG at Duke University, all of whom were monitored with transesophageal echocardiography (TEE), found six independent predictors of inotrope support, which was required in 39% of the cohort during weaning from CPB (Table 18-2 and Figure 18-10[66]; see Box 18-1).

The introduction and rapid growth of OPCAB have complicated matters because large-scale, well-calibrated outcome models are not yet available for this procedure. Initial publications have addressed this topic.[67,68]

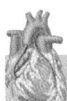

BOX 18-1. PREOPERATIVE EVALUATION AND MANAGEMENT

Preoperative "high-risk" cardiac characteristics and major comorbidities
1. Cardiac history and presenting symptoms:
   Acute unstable angina, acute myocardial infarction, uncompensated congestive heart failure, cardiogenic shock
2. Coronary artery anatomy:
   Left main high-grade lesion, triple-vessel disease, proximal left anterior descending artery lesions
3. Ventricular function:
   Ejection fraction < 30% (normal > 55%)
4. Valvular and structural anatomy and function:
   Concurrent aortic stenosis, acute mitral regurgitation, acute aortic insufficiency, ventricular septal defect
5. Electrocardiogram:
   Signs of acute or ongoing ischemia, left bundle branch block (potential complete heart block with passage of pulmonary artery catheter)
6. Chest radiograph, chest computed tomography scan:
   Pericardial effusion or tamponade, aortic calcification (inability to cross-clamp aorta, "porcelain aorta")
7. Carotid and cerebrovascular disease:
   High-grade occlusive carotid disease
8. Peripheral vascular disease (PVD):
   Significant PVD in descending aorta (intra-aortic balloon pump contraindicated)

TABLE 18-2 Multivariate Predictors of Inotrope Use

Variable	Parameter Estimate	OR (95% CI)	P
Intercept	−3.2827		
Cross-clamp time (min)	0.0133	1.013 (1.008–1.019)	<0.001
WMSI	1.4389	4.216 (2.438–7.292)	<0.001
Reoperation	0.8562	2.375 (1.083–5.212)	<0.001
CABG + MVRR	1.2829	3.607 (1.376–9.456)	0.009
Moderate/ severe MR	0.4144	2.277 (1.169–4.435)	0.016
LVEF < 35%	0.8654	2.376 (1.303–4.332)	0.005

CABG, coronary artery bypass grafting; CI, confidence interval; LVEF, left ventricular ejection fraction; MR, mitral regurgitation; MVRR, mitral valve repair or replacement; OR, odds ratio; WMSI, wall motion score index.
From McKinlay KH, Schinderle DB, Swaminathan M, et al: Predictors of inotrope use during separation from cardiopulmonary bypass. J Cardiothorac Vasc Anesth 18:404, 2004.

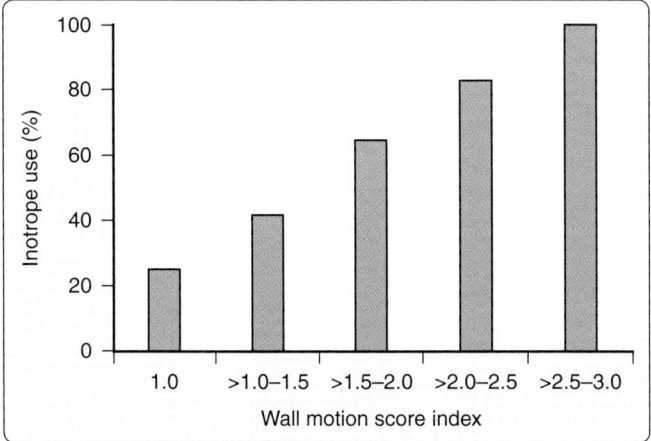

Figure 18-10 Correlation of degree of wall motion abnormalities before cardiopulmonary bypass (CPB) as reflected by an increasing wall motion score index associated with a greater use of inotropes during weaning from CPB. *(From McKinlay KH, Schinderle DB, Swaminathan M, et al: Predictors of inotrope use during separation from cardiopulmonary bypass. J Cardiothorac Vasc Anesth 18:404, 2004.)*

Considerable data have been reported on the potential impact of various anesthetic techniques on outcomes, particularly effects on pre-CPB myocardial ischemia and postoperative myocardial infarction. However, much of these data suffer from inadequate statistical power, use of single centers, and difficulties in standardization of definitions or reporting of *surrogate* (otherwise called *soft*) outcomes. Earlier reports supported a lack of effect of the anesthetic technique, suggesting that hemodynamic control was more important (e.g., "It's not what you use, but how you use it."), particularly for prevention of ischemia.[69,70] However, newer data support various degrees of efficacy with different approaches for preserving ventricular function with volatile anesthetics on weaning from CPB,[71,72] or high sympathetic blockade relative to intravenous techniques.[73] Some of these have been linked to improved recovery or shorter lengths of stay. However, the advantages appear to be modest, and demonstration of overt reductions in serious morbidity or mortality in large-scale, multicenter cohorts has not yet been reported. Similar data suggest that although use of a specific anesthetic agent (e.g., opioid or neuromuscular agent) may facilitate earlier extubation, the small magnitude of effect in most instances does not appear to reduce overall length of hospital stay, have significant effects on recovery, or substantially reduce cost.[74,75] Nonetheless, nearly all anesthesiologists continue to strive for the "perfect technique."

Several publications have attempted to more precisely delineate the association of perioperative hemodynamics with outcomes in larger cohorts of patients than have been previously reported in the older randomized trials of anesthetic techniques. Reich et al[76] merged computerized anesthesia record data from 2149 CABG patients (with CPB) at two New York hospitals from 1993 to 1995 with outcome data from the state's mandatory reporting database. Four independent predictors of mortality were identified: high mean pulmonary arterial pressure (PAP) before CPB (>30 mm Hg; odds ratio [OR] = 2.1), low MAP during CPB (40 to 49 mm Hg; OR =1.3), tachycardia (HR > 120 beats/min; OR = 3.1), and high diastolic PAP (>20 mmHg; OR =1.2) after CPB. The investigators observed that three of the four are markers of severe LV dysfunction.

Morbidity and mortality also are influenced by events in the operating room, including time on CPB and aortic cross-clamping, adequacy of revascularization, and complications such as cardiovascular decompensation or bleeding. Reevaluation of the patient's risk can be performed on arrival in the intensive care unit (ICU) at the start of the postoperative period. The APACHE (Acute Physiology and Chronic Health Evaluation) III system has been modified for CABG patients, and Becker et al[77] found that predictors of outcome included the risk score, age, reoperative status, and number of grafts. Higgins et al[78] devised the Cleveland Clinic ICU admission score, which includes preoperative and physiologic factors present on admission to the ICU. Morbidity rate was 3% with scores of 5 or less, and the rate increased to 83% with scores greater than 20.

The SYNTAX (Synergy between PCI with TAXUS drug-eluting stent and cardiac surgery) trial, a prospective, randomized, multicenter trial, originally was designed to evaluate current practice patterns and to evaluate optimal revascularization strategies in patients with three-vessel and left main CAD in Europe and the United States.[79] For the purpose of risk stratification in this trial, the SYNTAX score was developed, characterizing the complexity of coronary pathology. The SYNTAX score is based on already existing classifications and takes number, location, complexity, and functional impact of the coronary lesions into consideration.[80] Patients with more complex disease and potentially worse prognosis have greater SYNTAX scores. The initial analysis showed that there was no difference in outcome (major adverse cardiovascular and cerebrovascular events) among patients randomized to surgery between those who had low, intermediate, and high scores (major adverse, cardiovascular, and cerebrovascular events 14.4%, 11.7%, 10.7%, respectively).[81] In the patients randomized to PCI, however, the SYNTAX score was able to predict adverse outcome between the earlier mentioned risk groups at 12 months (13.5%, 16.6%, 23.3%, respectively). Based on these findings, it was concluded that patients with a low-risk SYNTAX score constellation of three-vessel and/or left main disease can be treated with surgery, PCI, or both, whereas intermediate-and high-risk groups should be referred for surgery. Further analysis of the SYNTAX trial and associated risk score will be performed at medium and long-term time points.

ANESTHESIA FOR CORONARY ARTERY BYPASS GRAFTING

The practitioner providing anesthetic care for patients presenting for coronary revascularization has to implement an anesthetic plan that takes patient and surgery specific factors into consideration but should also include the most recent recommendations and guidelines regarding the perioperative care of patients with CAD. Fast-track management including early extubation strategies (commonly interpreted as extubation within 8 hours after surgery) is frequently performed in many centers in the United States. However, it may not always be suitable for the increasing number of very-high-risk patients seen in the operating room. OPCAB is routinely performed in some centers and mostly linked to individual surgeon's preferences, although rarely performed in other institutions. Minimally invasive and robotic-assisted CABG surgery adds to the variety of scenarios that have to be considered in the anesthetic plan.

▓ Role of Central Neuraxial Blockade

A wide variety of techniques have been used for anesthetic induction and maintenance for CABG. A balanced general anesthetic, however, is still the most commonly used anesthetic technique in patients undergoing CABG surgery. Nevertheless, the interest in the use of thoracic epidural anesthesia (TEA) for cardiac surgery has increased steadily since 1990. It has been long appreciated that thoracic sympathectomy has favorable effects on the heart and coronary circulation.[82] Its coronary vasodilating effects have been well documented, and it has been used to treat unstable angina for many years, albeit infrequently because of logistics and the contemporary standard of use of potent antiplatelet agents. There has been increased interest in TEA including

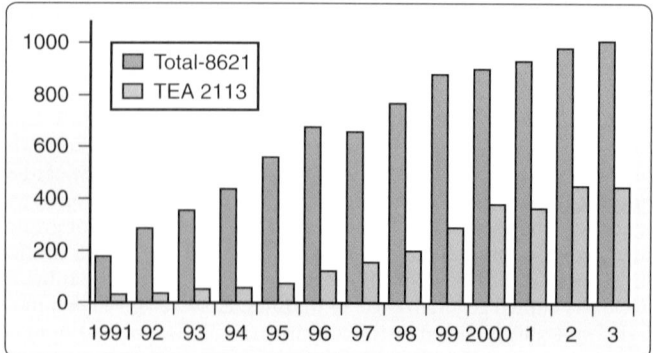

Figure 18-11 Frequency of use of thoracic epidural anesthesia (TEA) at a single center over the past 13 years (total of 2013 patients). All catheters were placed the day before surgery between C7 and T3. Dural puncture occurred in 0.9%, and temporary neurologic deficits occurred in 0.2%. No permanent deficits occurred. (*From Chakravarthy M, Thimmangowda P, Krishnamurthy J, et al: Thoracic epidural anesthesia in cardiac surgical patients: A prospective audit of 2,113 cases.* J Cardiothorac Vasc Anesth 19:44, 2005.)

reports of using chronically implanted, patient-controlled catheters[83–87] and its use as a supplement to general anesthesia for cardiac surgery, particularly in Europe and Asia (Figure 18-11).[88–90]

In the United States, medicolegal concerns about the rare but real danger of a devastating neurologic injury (see later) and the substantial logistic issues regarding placement the night before surgery (most patients presenting for nonemergent CABG surgery in the United States are day of admission), increased time to place relative to inducing general anesthesia, and the potential for cancellation of a case in the event of a bloody tap during epidural catheter placement are major limiting factors. The advent of fast-tracking could be considered a potential driving force (e.g., ability to extubate faster and have a more comfortable patient with TEA), although most evidence suggests that a wide variety of techniques can be used effectively to facilitate early extubation, and that the cardioprotective effects of volatile agents may be as effective as the beneficial effects of thoracic sympathectomy.

TEA in conscious patients appears to be increasingly used for OPCAB or minimally invasive direct coronary artery bypass approaches with recent reports from diverse settings (e.g., Canada, Germany, Turkey, India), and has been designated as conscious OPCAB.[91–96] Although most reports were of relatively small patient cohorts (15 to 30), Karagoz et al[97] described 137 patients, of whom 97% were successfully managed. In the reported series, most grafts were single-vessel left internal mammary artery (LIMA)-to-LAD grafts, although two-vessel and even a small group of three-vessel procedures were performed successfully. In most series, 2% to 3% of catheters were unable to be placed in potential candidates, and 2% to 3% of patients were converted to general anesthesia because of a large pneumothorax or incomplete analgesia. Patients were fast-tracked, an ICU stay was not used, and some were discharged from the hospital the day of surgery. Patient acceptance appeared to be quite high. No complications related to TEA were observed. This is clearly an area of growing interest and one that has potential advantages, particularly for countries with different health care systems, resource constraints, and sociocultural differences.

Given the fact that most conscious OPCABs are performed mostly for single-vessel LAD lesions, the sophistication and aggressiveness of the interventional cardiologists at a particular institution are major variables. Noiseux et al[98] recently published a series of 15 patients undergoing conscious OPCAB surgery combining a high TEA with a femoral nerve block for venous graft harvesting. Three patients needed conversion to general anesthesia. The authors concluded that even though this technique is feasible, technical limitations still exist that need to be overcome.

When neuraxial techniques are compared with general anesthesia alone, or as a combined technique, no significant difference in measured major outcome parameters such as perioperative mortality and major morbidity were found in most studies.[99-101] Differences in minor outcome findings such as quality of analgesia and time to extubation were reported in others. In a prospective study, Scott et al[102] randomized 420 patients undergoing CABG surgery under general anesthesia to either TEA or intravenous narcotic analgesia. No neurologic complications were associated with TEA. Many of the examined outcome parameters such as time to extubation, pulmonary function, atrial fibrillation, and renal function were significantly better in the TEA group. However, this study was widely criticized for design flaws that may have impacted the reported findings.

Priestley et al[103] consequently conducted another prospective, randomized study and did not find improved pulmonary or cardiac function with TEA or decreased length of hospital stay, despite improved analgesia and earlier extubation. In 2006, Hansdottir et al[104] randomized patients who all had a general anesthesia for cardiac surgery to either TEA (inserted before surgery) or intravenous morphine for postoperative analgesia. Again, even though time to extubation was shorter in the TEA group, none of the other examined outcome parameters was significantly different between the two groups. The authors concluded that TEA combined with general anesthesia offers no major advantage when compared with general anesthesia alone. Bracco et al[105] found fewer postoperative complications such as delirium, pneumonia, acute renal failure, and myocardial function in patients undergoing cardiac surgery who had TEA in addition to general anesthesia, compared with general anesthesia alone. Based on shorter ICU and mechanical ventilator times in patients with TEA, they calculated $8800 cost savings per person if TEA was used. A recently published randomized trial in obese patients (body mass index > 30 kg/m^2) undergoing OPCAB surgery showed better analgesia, improved lung function tests, and shorter time to extubation and length of ICU stay in patients who had TEA in addition to general anesthesia.[106] Liu et al[107] reported a meta-analysis of 15 randomized trials of TEA in 1178 patients. In contrast with an earlier mixed meta-analysis (i.e., cardiac and noncardiac surgery, observational and randomized),[108] there were no effects on postoperative myocardial infarction or mortality. However, significant favorable effects were observed for arrhythmias, pulmonary complications, time to extubation, and reduction in visual analog pain scales.

In a propensity-matched, retrospective study, Salvi et al[109] compared high TEA combined with general anesthesia with a total intravenous anesthesia technique (without TEA) in 1473 patients undergoing CABG surgery. There were no major differences in measured early outcome parameters (postoperative mortality, myocardial infarction, stroke, acute renal failure, ICU stay) between the two techniques. Patients with high TEA had shorter time to extubation.

The potential advantages of TEA on cardiac function were investigated specifically in the following studies. Berendes et al[110] reported improved regional LV function (by wall motion score index) with lower troponin I and atrial and brain natriuretic peptide levels. However, the control for this study was a total intravenous anesthetic technique, and it is unclear whether a volatile anesthetic would have similar effects, as demonstrated by several investigators. In a prospective, controlled study, Barrington et al[111] randomized 120 patients to general anesthesia with or without high TEA. Even though postoperative analgesia was improved in the TEA group and led to earlier extubation, there was no significant difference seen with troponin levels between the two groups. Crescenzi et al[112] evaluated the effect of TEA on N-terminal-protein-B-natriuretic peptide levels in elderly patients undergoing CABG surgery. TEA, in addition to general anesthesia, significantly attenuated N-terminal-protein-B-natriuretic peptide release. Lee et al[113] addressed a slightly different question, using total spinal sympathectomy (bupivacaine, 37.5 mg) before induction of general anesthesia. Patients randomized to bupivacaine had less β-receptor dysfunction in response to CPB of more than 1 hour, with lower catecholamine levels, a greater cardiac index, and a lower pulmonary vascular resistance index in the post-CPB period.

Safety concerns are a major consideration in use of neuraxial techniques in patients undergoing cardiac surgery given chronic use of antiplatelet agents, use of systemic anticoagulation and platelet inhibition for acute therapy of unstable angina, and high-dose systemic anticoagulation and potential coagulopathy induced by CPB. The true incidence of serious complications (particularly epidural hematoma) is unknown. The most recent and widely quoted estimation of the risk for epidural hematoma with TEA in patients undergoing cardiac surgery is 1 in 12,000, with 95% confidence intervals of 1:2,100 to 1:68,000, and 1 in 1000 with 99% confidence.[114] Intrathecal risks from a different older source of risk assessment are quoted as 1 in 3610 and 1 in 2400, respectively.[115] Even when under-reporting of such complications is assumed,[116] there is increasing evidence that neuraxial anesthesia can be performed safely even in patients undergoing cardiac surgery with full heparinization.

Chakravarthy et al[117] presented an audit of 2113 cardiac surgery TEA cases over a 13-year period with no permanent neurologic deficits, a 0.9% dural puncture rate, and 0.2% transient neurologic deficits. Jack et al published their experience of thoracic epidural catheter placement in 2837 patients undergoing cardiac surgery.[118] No epidural hematoma was seen in this series. Similar results were reported by Royse et al,[119] who reviewed 874 cardiac surgery cases involving epidural anesthesia over a 7-year period with no complications attributable to epidural catheter use. Pastor et al[120] reported 714 uneventful cases over a 7-year period, emphasizing their use of safety guidelines in which antiplatelet drugs were discontinued 7 days before surgery, and routine coagulation tests and neurologic examinations were performed after surgery.

Careful attention to the most recent guidelines on neuraxial anesthesia in the setting of anticoagulant and antiplatelet agents is of paramount importance. The American Society of Regional Anesthesia and Pain Medicine published Consensus Statements on Neuraxial Anesthesia and Anticoagulation.[121] These include recommendations for appropriate withdrawal of anticoagulant and antiplatelet therapy before neuraxial anesthesia (these recommendations can be found online at: www.asra.com). Chaney[122] also has published an extensive review on the use of intrathecal and epidural anesthesia and analgesia for patients undergoing cardiac surgery.

In summary, it seems that neuraxial techniques offer mostly theoretic benefits. Relevant outcome parameters, such as major morbidity and mortality, are minimally affected by the anesthetic technique chosen, but probably depend more on patient-related factors and the quality of surgical intervention.

Premedication

The concept of "premedication" has been evolving beyond the traditional ordering of sedative-hypnotics or related agents to reduce patient anxiety and promote amnesia. The cardiac anesthesiologist must be familiar with the potential benefits of administering (or hazards of not administering) a variety of medications including antianginal medications, β-blockers, and antiplatelet drugs. The anesthesiologist, in concert with the surgeon, cardiologist, and other consultants, may impact directly patient outcome, as well as provide anxiolysis, amnesia, and analgesia in the early intraoperative period.

Anxiolysis, Amnesia, and Analgesia

The purposes of premedication are to pharmacologically reduce apprehension and fear, to provide analgesia for potentially painful events before induction (e.g., vascular cannulation), and to produce some degree of amnesia. In patients with CAD, premedication may help prevent preoperative anginal episodes that are relatively commonly observed and may be elicited by tachycardia caused by anxiety or painful stimuli, or both. Regardless of the drugs used, the clinician should be prepared to give intravenous drugs (e.g., short-acting benzodiazepines) when the patient arrives in the preoperative area. All patients should receive supplemental oxygen after premedication and be monitored with pulse oximetry, ECG, and noninvasive blood pressure.

The sedative and anesthetic-sparing actions of α_2-adrenergic agonists (e.g., clonidine, dexmedetomidine) have been evaluated for their efficacy in several studies of CABG patients alone or in combination with a benzodiazepine.[123-125] The use of α_2-adrenergic agonists reduced stress response and anesthetic requirements compared with conventional regimens. A meta-analysis reported reductions in mortality and postoperative myocardial infarction with their use in cardiac surgery (started before surgery and often continuing until CPB).[126] Nevertheless, some of the hemodynamic side effects of α_2-agonists warrant caution in certain patient populations. Decreased HR, MAP, cardiac output (CO), contractility, and transiently increased systemic vascular resistance (SVR) seen with the less-selective α_2-blocker clonidine, as well as an increased risk for hypotension during anesthesia induction, have been reported in general and cardiac surgery patients who were premedicated with α_2-agonists.[127,128] Consequently, α_2-agonists should be used with caution in patients with preexisting severe bradycardia, conduction problems such as second- or third-degree heart block, hypovolemia, or hypotension.

Management of Antianginal and Antihypertensive Medications

The use of β-blocking agents in patients with poor ventricular function has been evaluated. Contrary to earlier reports,[129] Kaplan et al[130,131] reported in the mid-1970s and long before the ongoing discussion of perioperative β-blockade in noncardiac surgical patients that it was safe to continue β-blockade in patients presenting for cardiac and noncardiac surgery. Slogoff et al[132] performed a randomized trial evaluating the safety of administration of propranolol within 12 hours of surgery. Based on a significantly greater increase in the incidence of pre-CPB ischemia in patients withdrawn from propranolol (within 24 to 72 hours), they also recommended continuation of therapy up until the time of surgery. Further work by these and other investigators in the 1980s documented the efficacy of β-blocker continuation through CABG surgery with regard to reducing pre-CPB ischemia and their superior efficacy over the increasingly popular calcium channel blockers[133,134] (Box 18-2).

The earlier mentioned studies were instrumental in laying the groundwork for the subsequent noncardiac surgery studies in the late 1980s.[135-137] They led to the contemporary randomized trials of Poldermans et al[138] and Mangano et al,[139] which rallied support for routine perioperative β-blocker use; and the most recent conclusions drawn from the POISE trial[140] that questioned parts of this practice. These trials resulted in the latest recommendations of β-blockade in patients undergoing noncardiac surgery.[141] There is little doubt that β-blockers are beneficial for most CABG patients, particularly if HR is increased. When acutely administered in adequate dose, they significantly reduce myocardial oxygen demand and the incidence of atrial and ventricular arrhythmias. Several observational studies have documented associations of β-blocker therapy with reduction in perioperative mortality in CABG patients.[142,143] The largest of these by Ferguson et al[144] considered 629,877 patients in the STS database (1996 to 1999) in which a modest but statistically significant reduction in 30-day risk-adjusted mortality was reported. This treatment effect was observed in many high-risk subgroups, although a trend toward increased mortality was seen in patients with EF less than 30%. In a meta-analysis, Wiesbauer et al[145] found that perioperative β-blockers reduced perioperative arrhythmias after cardiac surgery, but they had no effect on myocardial infarction or mortality. Considerable efforts are being expended by major organizations (STS, American College of Cardiology) in increasing compliance with existing guidelines for use of β-blockers at the time of hospital discharge (together with use of aspirin, statins, and angiotensin-converting enzyme [ACE] inhibitors).[146,147]

An increasing number of patients are presenting for CABG surgery while being treated with platelet inhibitors. Aspirin is a well-recognized component of primary and secondary prevention strategies for all patients with ischemic heart disease.[148,149] Treatment with clopidogrel is required for coronary artery stent placement, has been shown to improve outcome, and is now recommended in combination with aspirin after acute coronary syndrome.[150,151] Antiplatelet therapy is also used after CABG to reduce ischemic complications. Aspirin (and other platelet inhibitors such as dipyridamole) have long been recognized to

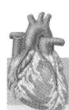

BOX 18-2. PREOPERATIVE MEDICATION MANAGEMENT

1. β-Adrenergic blockers: Should be continued perioperatively in patients already on β-blocker therapy. Consider β-blockers in high-risk patients with heart rate greater than 60 beats/min (contraindications: hypotension, third-degree heart block, bronchospasm).
2. Statins: Should be continued perioperatively in patients already on statin therapy. Consider statins in all patients with CAD because of emerging data that the complex effects of statins, including lipid-stabilizing effects and anti-inflammatory properties, improve outcome, including in patients undergoing CABG surgery.
3. Calcium channel blockers: Should be continued perioperatively; greater incidence of heart block or need for pacing.
4. Angiotensin-converting enzyme inhibitor: Perioperative use controversial; possible increased risk for hypotension during induction, vasoplegic syndrome, and mortality.
5. Diuretics: No firm recommendations; ensure adequate serum potassium levels.
6. Aspirin: Strong data to suggest that aspirin should be continued in high-risk patients despite slightly increased risk for bleeding (beneficial for early and late graft patency and mortality).
7. Antiplatelet agents such as glycoprotein IIb/IIIa inhibitors: Associated with increased risk for bleeding. Recommendations to hold 5 days before surgery. However, in high-risk patients and/or after drug-eluting stents, recommendations may change and glycoprotein IIb/IIab inhibitors may even be continued perioperatively despite increased risk for bleeding (always consult with surgeon).
8. Heparin: Regimen is often surgeon specific. Usually discontinued 4 hours before for stable patients, continued up to and through

pre-CPB period for critical left main disease or acutely unstable angina patients.
9. Oral hypoglycemic agents: Data suggest that oral antidiabetic drugs may abolish the preconditioning effect of potent inhalation anesthetics. No firm recommendations; consider holding administration. However, glucose control has to be ensured.
10. Antibiotic prophylaxis: Optimal timing and weight adjustment (especially important with antibiotics that have slow tissue penetration, e.g., vancomycin). Typically, second-generation cephalosporin such as cephazolin (1 to 2 g intravenously [IV]) or cefuroxime (1.5 g IV) administered 30 to 60 minutes before incision; vancomycin (15 mg/kg) administered as slow infusion to avoid hypotension and flushing (because slow tissue penetration infusion should be completed 30 minutes before skin incision). Consider clindamycin (600 to 900 mg IV) for penicillin or cephalosporin allergy; adjust as appropriate for renal failure. Repeat cefazolin every 4 hours, cefuroxime every 3 to 4 hours, vancomycin every 6 to 12 hours (except in patients with renal impairment), and clindamycin every 3 to 6 hours.
11. Anxiolytic or analgesic premedication: Consider short-acting benzodiazepine (e.g., midazolam) orally or IV after insertion of an intravenous catheter (supplemental nasal oxygen to avoid desaturation and ischemia).
12. Preoperative (time 6 to 8 hours) insertion of epidural catheter: Controversial, may reduce stress response, preserve adrenoreceptor function, and decrease time to extubation, pulmonary complications, and pain scores.

have strong efficacy in the prevention of early graft thrombosis after CABG.[152] Mangano et al,[153] in a large observational analysis, reported substantial reduction in overall mortality rate (1.3% vs. 4.0%) and ischemic complications of the heart, brain, kidneys, and gastrointestinal tract in 5065 patients at 70 hospitals when aspirin was administered within 48 hours after surgery.

The combination of aspirin and clopidogrel after CABG may be even more effective.[154] However, great controversy exists in regard to preoperative antiplatelet therapy. The risk for hemorrhagic complications needs to be weighed against the potential benefits of antiplatelet therapy. In a recent meta-analysis, patients receiving aspirin immediately before surgery had more mediastinal bleeding and received more blood products.[155] Several retrospective studies have reported that CABG surgery in patients receiving clopidogrel is associated with increased bleeding and transfusion requirements.[156] Filsoufi et al[157] also reported longer ICU and hospital length of stay (LOS) and increased all-cause morbidity and mortality in clopidogrel-treated patients. In a multicenter, retrospective study, Berger et al[158] reported that clopidogrel-treated patients were at increased risk for reoperation, major bleeding, and increased LOS.

Recent guidelines from the American College of Chest Physicians on antithrombotic and thrombolytic therapies recommend institution of aspirin within 6 hours after CABG surgery over continuation of preoperative therapy (level of evidence IIa).[159] In those with ongoing bleeding, it should be administered as soon as possible thereafter. In those allergic to aspirin, clopidogrel should be used instead. Low-dose aspirin should be continued indefinitely. They further recommend the use of clopidogrel in addition to aspirin for 9 to 12 months after CABG after a non–ST-elevation acute coronary syndrome. The STS has released formal practice guidelines on this topic. In high-risk patients (those with unstable angina or recent myocardial infarction) requiring urgent or emergent CABG, aspirin should be continued until the time of surgery (Class IIa recommendation) unless they are in an "aspirin-sensitive high-risk subgroup" (i.e., those on other antiplatelets or anticoagulants, or those who have platelet abnormalities). For elective patients in whom active platelet aggregation is less likely to be a critical factor in precipitating ischemia, they recommend discontinuation of aspirin for 3 to 5 days before surgery to reduce transfusion requirements (Class IIa), with reinstitution in the early postoperative period (Class I).[160] The American College of Chest Physicians practice guidelines, as well as the American Heart Association/American College of Cardiology guidelines, also suggest discontinuing clopidogrel 5 days before CABG surgery in patients who received clopidogrel for acute coronary syndrome if clinical circumstances allow.[159,161]

The efficacy of calcium channel antagonists with regard to their anti-ischemic properties in patients undergoing CABG is a controversial topic. Early observational studies suggest they were ineffective, particularly relative to β-blockers.[162,163] Subsequently, there was even less enthusiasm for their use given concerns in the mid-1990s of excess mortality with shorter-acting preparations (in particular, nifedipine, which was thought to cause reflex adrenergic activation because of abrupt vasodilation with each dose).[164] Two meta-analyses evaluating their efficacy in noncardiac surgery produced conflicting information.[165,166] However, one meta-analysis and a large observational cohort study with propensity matching adjustment suggest they are effective in reducing mortality in CABG patients.[167,168] For patients taking them chronically, it appears prudent to continue them perioperatively. Caution is advised with concurrent administration of nondihydropyridine drugs (diltiazem) and β-blockers, although the risk (purported to be possible precipitation of advanced degrees of atrioventricular block) appears to be minor, based on a lack of problems in a reported large cohort of thoracotomy patients in whom this was done frequently.[169] A new issue recently has been raised as well, which will require further investigation. A recent observational study concluded that calcium channel blockers decrease clopidogrel-mediated platelet inhibition, the latter playing a crucial role in the management of CAD.[170]

ACE inhibitors and 3-hydroxy-3-methylglutaryl coenzyme A reductase inhibitors (statins) currently are receiving special attention as agents because of a variety of important "pleiotropic" effects (e.g., effects independent of their primary antihypertensive or lipid-lowering actions, respectively).[171–173] Potent anti-inflammatory and antithrombotic effects and beneficial effects on endothelial function have been reported for both agents, as well as less clear effects on angiogenesis.[174,175] Both agents commonly are administered acutely during PCI,[176–178] and have direct effects on platelet aggregation and plasminogen activator inhibitors.[173,179] Statins have been reported to reduce circulating levels of adhesion molecules, which have been implicated in endothelial dysfunction after CPB (Figure 18-12).[180–182] Statins also have been shown to attenuate myocardial reperfusion injury after cardiac surgery.[183] ACE inhibitors are widely considered to be vasculoprotective, particularly with regard to ventricular remodeling after acute myocardial infarction, and they appear to reduce damage after ischemic reperfusion (likely related to reduction in ischemia-induced vasoconstriction and reduction in leukocyte adhesion).[184] Several investigators have published retrospective studies with similar reports of the efficacy of statins to reduce the short-and long-term mortality of CABG patients.[185–189] In a large meta-analysis evaluating the impact of preoperative statin use on adverse clinical outcomes after cardiac surgery, Liakopoulos et al[190] reported that preoperative statin use significantly reduced all-cause mortality after surgery. Statins also have been found in retrospective studies to decrease the need for postoperative renal replacement therapy,[191] possibly a reflection of their anti-inflammatory properties, with conflicting results regarding a reduction in acute renal dysfunction.[192,193] In addition, statins have been shown to decrease the incidence of atrial fibrillation after cardiac surgery.[194] The current American College of Cardiology/American Heart Association guidelines on perioperative cardiovascular evaluation and care for noncardiac surgery patients recommend the continuation of statins in patients currently on them and the consideration of starting statins in patients with clinical risk factors.[195] Most clinicians continue them routinely (albeit orally only, so there is usually a short withdrawal period after surgery). Postoperative withdrawal of statin treatment is independently associated with increased hospital mortality after CABG.[196]

Fewer studies have been performed on ACE inhibitors. The QUO VADIS (QUinapril on Vascular Ace and Determinants of Ischemia) study[197] showed a significant reduction in ischemic events in patients on ACE inhibitors before CABG. ACE inhibitor therapy before CABG

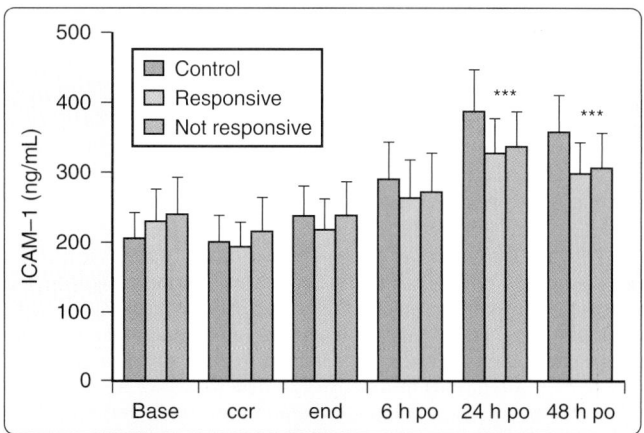

Figure 18-12 Bar graph of the mean values of circulating intercellular adhesion molecule-1 (ICAM-1), a glycoprotein circulating adhesion molecule expressed by endothelial cells in response to inflammation. Levels in response to cardiopulmonary bypass are shown for 15 control subjects, 15 patients on simvastatin with good control of cholesterol (i.e., responsive), and 15 patients on the drug but with poor control (i.e., not responsive) of cholesterol. Statin patients had lower ICAM-1 levels at 24 and 48 hours after surgery (***, statistically significant), suggesting possible anti-inflammatory properties. Base, baseline; ccr, cross-clamp release; end, end of cardiopulmonary bypass; po, postoperative period. (*From Chello M, Carassiti M, Agro F, et al: Simvastatin blunts the increase of circulating adhesion molecules after coronary artery bypass surgery with cardiopulmonary bypass. J Cardiothorac Vasc Anesth 18:605, 2004.*)

has also been associated with a reduced risk for acute kidney injury[198] and may be effective in the prevention of new-onset atrial fibrillation.[199] ACE inhibitors, however, also have been associated with greater degrees of hypotension during induction or even profound degrees of vasodilation (vasoplegic syndrome) during CPB and weaning because of their vasodilatory effects.[200–208] In a large, retrospective, observational study on more than 10,000 patients undergoing CABG surgery, preoperative ACE inhibitor therapy was associated with an increased incidence of perioperative hypotension and ACE inhibitor therapy was found to be an independent predictor of mortality, need for inotropic support, postoperative renal dysfunction, and new-onset postoperative atrial fibrillation.[209] Another concern expressed by Lazar[210] was in relation to potential antagonism between ACE inhibitors and aspirin because ACE inhibitors increase prostaglandin levels, whereas aspirin inhibits them. Despite strongly promoting their perioperative use, he advised they be withheld for 24 to 48 hours before surgery if possible and restarted after surgery after reinstitution of β-blockade (assuming systolic blood pressure > 100 mm Hg). They are otherwise contraindicated with renal insufficiency, and their adverse effect of cough can be detrimental to sternal stability in the early postoperative period. At this point, further studies are needed to make recommendations about the perioperative use and/or continuation of ACE inhibitors and their effect on outcome parameters in patients undergoing CABG surgery.

Monitoring

Electrocardiogram

On arrival in the operating room, the patient undergoing CABG should have routine monitors placed, including pulse oximetry, noninvasive blood pressure (BP), and the ECG. A five-lead system is standard in patients undergoing cardiac surgery. Monitoring leads V_5 and II allows for the detection of 90% of ischemic episodes, as well as monitoring the rhythm to diagnose various atrial and ventricular arrhythmias. The ECG detection of myocardial ischemia is reviewed in Chapter 15 (Box 18-3).

Arterial Pressure Monitoring

The radial artery usually is cannulated for BP monitoring during CABG. Choosing the best site for radial artery cannulation depends on surgery-specific considerations, as well as institutional and practitioner preferences. Surgical technique such as radial artery harvesting or axillary CPB cannulation may influence the site chosen for invasive arterial pressure monitoring. With modern sternal retractors, blunting of the arterial pressure tracing on the ipsilateral side of internal mammary artery (IMA) dissection is not typically seen. Some practitioners use bilateral arterial cannulation or choose a more central artery such as the axillary or femoral artery to ensure accurate pressure readings after CPB. Radial arterial pressures have been shown to be inaccurate immediately after hypothermic CPB. Substantial reductions in radial arterial versus aortic pressure have been reported in several clinical investigations, often requiring 20 to 60 minutes after CPB to resolve.[211–215] Alterations in forearm vascular resistance (decrease) are believed to be responsible for this common phenomenon. This problem can be overcome by temporarily transducing the arterial pressure directly from the aorta (by a needle or a cardioplegia cannula).

Central Venous Cannulation

The placement of a central venous pressure (CVP) catheter routinely is performed in cardiac anesthesia both for pressure measurement and for infusing vasoactive drugs. Some centers routinely place two catheters (a large introducer and a smaller CVP catheter) in the central circulation to facilitate volume infusion and vasoactive or inotropic drug administration. Increasingly, ultrasound guidance is used for placement, although there remains controversy in the literature regarding whether it is a standard of care[216–218] (see Chapter 14).

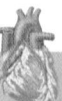

BOX 18-3. INTRAOPERATIVE MONITORING FOR MYOCARDIAL REVASCULARIZATION

1. Electrocardiogram: V_3 to V_5 most sensitive for ischemia; lead II for inferior ischemia and rhythm monitoring.
2. Arterial blood pressure: Continuous invasive arterial blood pressure monitoring and blood gas sampling via indwelling arterial catheter. (Consider site of radial artery harvesting, reoperation, bilateral radial artery monitoring for axillary CPB cannulation, femoral artery cannulation for emergency intraaortic balloon pump [IABP] insertion, and more central arterial cannulation [axillary, femoral] for more accurate readings after discontinuation of cardiopulmonary bypass [CPB]).
3. Pulmonary artery catheter (PAC): No evidence of improved outcome with PAC use. Treatment guidance in conjunction with transesophageal echocardiography (TEE) monitoring and for postoperative care in the intensive care unit, particularly in patients with severely reduced ventricular function and patients with pulmonary hypertension.
4. TEE: Used in many centers for coronary artery bypass graft (CABG) surgery. Use in CABG and off-pump coronary artery bypass (OPCAB) surgery is now recommended. TEE can assist in pre-CPB evaluation of cardiac function, associated valvular lesions including functional mitral regurgitation, evaluation of atheromatous plaques in the aorta (site of cannulation and aortic cross-clamping, possible no-touch technique), detection of patent foramen ovale, persistent left superior vena cava (retrograde cardioplegia problematic), CPB cannulation including retrograde cardioplegia cannula positioning, aortic cannula positioning and associated complications such as iatrogenic aortic dissection and cannula positioning, volume status, ventricular function and response to inotropic agents, de-airing after release of aortic cross-clamp and during weaning off CPB).
5. Neurophysiologic monitoring: Increasing evidence suggests that cerebral oximetry aids in detecting catastrophic events, pending data from large prospective studies regarding outcome.
6. Temperature monitoring: Bladder or esophageal (core temperature) and nasopharyngeal or tympanic (brain temperature) are recommended for all CPB cases to minimize temperature gradients and cerebral hyperthermia during rewarming. For OPCABs, bladder temperature only is sufficient.
7. Foley placement for all patients.

Pulmonary Artery Catheterization

The use of PAC in medical and surgical settings has declined steadily, mostly because of the increasing amount of data from large randomized studies showing that major clinical outcomes (particularly mortality) are not changed by PAC use and that adverse effects of PAC monitoring have to be considered. This includes surgery for myocardial revascularization and in the ICU setting, suggesting that despite the substantial amount of physiologic information obtained, patient outcome is independent of PAC use. Tuman et al,[219] in a prospective observational study, examined the effect of the PAC on outcome in 1094 patients undergoing CABG surgery. Although no direct data on LV function were provided, there was no difference in the incidence of LV dysfunction between the group treated with a CVP versus the group treated with a PAC. In this study, the investigators could not demonstrate that a PAC had any effect on outcome; however, 7% of the patients initially assigned to CVP monitoring subsequently required a PAC for management.

Several other reports have focused exclusively on PAC use in CABG surgery. Stewart et al[220] reported a retrospective analysis of 312 patients undergoing CABG (in 1996) who were believed to be low risk and suitable for CVP monitoring alone. Of these, 32% had a PAC placed and received greater volumes of fluid, gained more weight, and had longer times to extubation. Ramsey et al[221] retrospectively analyzed a

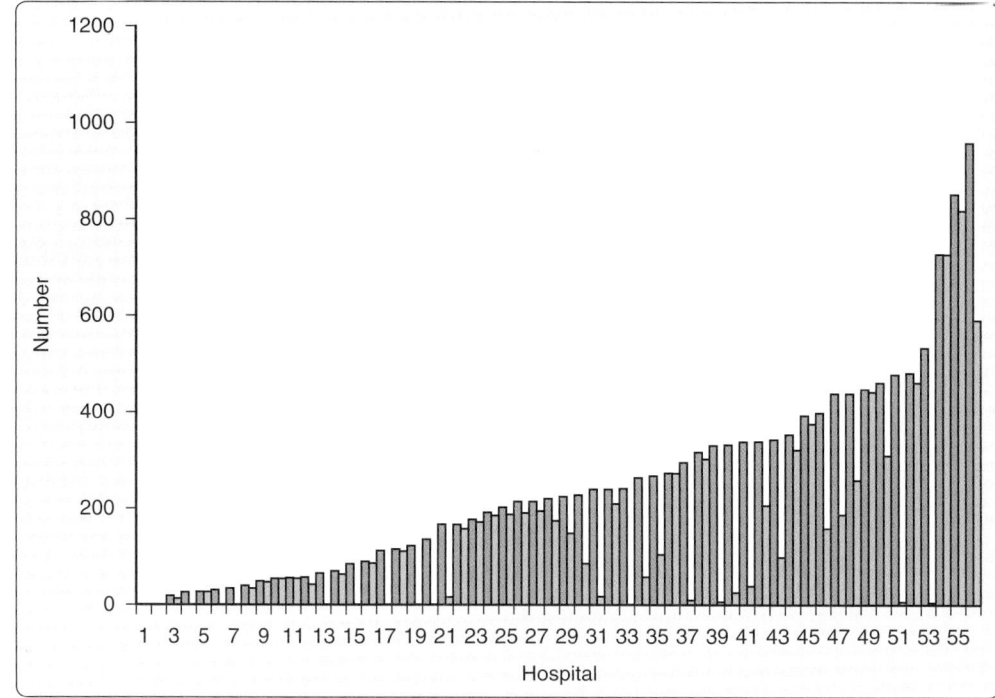

Figure 18-13 Variation in the use of pulmonary artery catheter (PAC) for elective coronary artery bypass grafting (CABG) in 13,907 patients at 56 community-based hospitals in 26 states in 1997, with data obtained from an administrative health outcomes benchmarking database. PAC was used in 58% and was associated with greater risk of in-hospital mortality, particularly in hospitals with the lowest use of PAC, hospital length of stay, and costs. *Purple bars* indicate the total number of CABG cases; *gray bars* indicate the number of patients with PAC. *(From Ramsay SD, Saint S, Sullivan SD, et al: Clinical and economic effects of pulmonary artery catheterization in nonemergent coronary artery bypass graft surgery. J Cardiothorac Vasc Anesth 14:113, 2000.)*

commercial health care outcomes benchmarking database with 13,907 patients undergoing nonemergent CABG in 56 hospitals (Figure 18-13). Patients who had a PAC placed for perioperative monitoring (58% of the patients) were found to have a greater risk for mortality after risk adjustment (relative risk = 2.1), longer lengths of stay, and higher total costs, particularly in the hospitals with low rates of PAC use. Schwann et al[222] retrospectively analyzed 2685 consecutive CABG patients at a single private center (1994 to 1998) in which PAC use was "highly selective" (i.e., used in only 9% based on consideration of multiple cardiac risk factors). Of these PACs, 6.6% were planned, with the remainder placed after surgery in response to adverse intraoperative events. Multivariate analysis revealed EF, STS risk score, use of IABP, congestive heart failure, redo operation, and New York Heart Association Class IV to be independent predictors of PAC use. Based on their reported overall mortality rate (2.3%), it appears as if this highly selective approach was safe, although these data cannot necessarily be generalizable outside this particular center given multiple other process variables involved in providing care for these patients. London et al[223] documented the high rate of PAC use based on analysis of 3256 CABG patients included in a larger multicenter, observational study in patients undergoing cardiac surgery in the Department of Veterans Affairs (1994 to 1996). More than 95% of all cases were monitored with a PAC, and 49% of these used the more expensive mixed venous oxygen saturation catheter. Use of this catheter was clearly center specific, and with the exception of a small reduction in number of postoperative arterial blood gas and thermodilution CO measurements, it was not associated with improvement in outcome over the routine PAC.

Based on the existing literature, it is not possible to give precise criteria for PAC use in CABG surgery (see Chapter 14). The greater the patient risk (based primarily on established preoperative clinical predictors), the more favorable is the risk/benefit ratio. Risk factors include significant impairment of ventricular function (EF < 30%), and patients with known pulmonary hypertension and/or right-heart failure. Some authors have advocated a wait-and-see approach. In a prospective observational study, Djaiani et al[224] showed the safety and usefulness of delaying the insertion of a PAC until the clinical need arises in the operating room or in the ICU after CABG surgery.

Although most of the recent clinical reports of patients undergoing OPCAB have used and many recommend the use of a PAC, it is not possible to give firm recommendations on this because of the lack of evidence-based data. In a retrospective study, Resano et al[225] did not find significant differences in mortality, conversion to on-pump procedure, or inotropic drug use between the group treated with a CVP versus the group treated with a PAC.

Many of the complications reported with PAC use are related to large-bore catheter central vein cannulation. With the increasing use of intraoperative TEE monitoring, PAC use may decrease even more. For a more detailed review of PAC use, see Chapter 14.

Transesophageal Echocardiography

The ASA, together with the Society of Cardiovascular Anesthesiologists, developed practice guidelines in 1996 to provide recommendations for the perioperative use of TEE.[226] These guidelines were updated recently,[227] and the routine use of TEE is now recommended for all cardiac or thoracic aortic surgery, which includes most patients undergoing CABG or OPCAB surgery, or both. The ASA Task Force thereby acknowledged the increasing evidence that TEE can provide important information that may impact perioperative anesthetic and surgical management and, possibly, patient outcome.

TEE is highly sensitive but not specific for myocardial ischemia.[228,229] It is appreciated that the earliest signs of myocardial ischemia include diastolic dysfunction followed by systolic regional wall motion abnormalities (RWMAs), which occur within seconds of acute coronary occlusion. New RWMAs detected in the intraoperative period, however, frequently may occur because of nonischemic causes such as changes in loading conditions, alteration in electrical conduction in the heart, post-CPB pacing, myocardial stunning caused by ischemia before or during weaning from CPB, or poor myocardial preservation. Worsening of RWMAs after CABG surgery is associated with an increased risk for long-term adverse cardiac morbidity and has been suggested as a prognostic indicator of adverse cardiovascular outcome.[230] The transgastric short-axis midpapillary muscle view, commonly used because of its inclusion of myocardium supplied by the three major coronary arteries, may entirely miss RWMAs occurring in the basal or apical portions of the heart. A comprehensive TEE examination recommended by the American Society of Echocardiography/Society of Cardiovascular Anesthesiologists Task Force before and after

CPB or after completion of revascularization in OPCAB is, therefore, recommended.[231] TEE is not perfect for ischemia monitoring because all wall segments would have to be monitored continuously in real-time and compared with preoperative findings.

A wide variety of uses aside from detection of ischemia are well documented for TEE. TEE can assist in the pre-CPB evaluation of cardiac function, associated valvular lesions including functional mitral regurgitation, evaluation of atheromatous plaques in the aorta (site of cannulation and aortic cross-clamping, possible no-touch technique), detection of a patent foramen ovale, and persistent left superior vena cava (retrograde cardioplegia problematic). CPB cannulation including retrograde cardioplegia cannula positioning, aortic cannula positioning and associated complications such as iatrogenic aortic dissection and positioning in the left subclavian artery, verification of PAC location, volume status, ventricular function and response to inotropic agents, and de-airing after release of the aortic cross-clamp can also be evaluated by TEE.

A new and exciting application of perioperative TEE is now emerging. The conventional method for analyzing regional myocardial function is by visual assessment of inward radial motion and wall thickening from two-dimensional (2D) echocardiographic images. Precise and reproducible quantitative assessment is much more appealing. Early attempts at using Doppler-based techniques for this purpose have been limited by angle-dependency and artifacts.[232,233] A novel quantitative approach is speckle tracking. It uses 2D images and analyzes the movement of stable acoustic markers (speckles) between frames.[234] Kukucka et al[235] demonstrated the feasibility of intraoperative determination of speckle tracking–derived strain from TEE images and correlated it with visual assessment of RWMA. They showed that it had better interobserver agreement than visually obtained data, allowed for determination of radial and longitudinal RWMAs, and that strain analysis and not visually obtained semiquantitative assessment of wall motion detected differences between normally perfused and ischemic segments (see Chapter 12).

The use of perioperative TEE in patients undergoing cardiac surgery is increasing, and it will be interesting to see how this trend develops with the newly adopted ASA guidelines on the perioperative use of TEE in patients undergoing cardiac surgery. Morewood et al[236] obtained more than 1800 survey responses from members of the Society of Cardiovascular Anesthesiologists in 2000. Of approximately 1500 clinicians involved in CABG, only 11% reported never using TEE, but more than 30% used it frequently or always. This number is probably greater today because of the growth of OPCAB and ongoing popularity of the technology. A variety of observational studies since 1990 have supported the efficacy of this technique, although in the absence of a true randomized, controlled trial, it is impossible to conclusively prove the efficacy of intraoperative TEE on patient outcome parameters such as perioperative morbidity and mortality.[237–239] Proper education and certification are critical, and guidelines about training requirements and certification have been published[240,241] (see Chapter 41). The clinician must realize that there are serious complications that can and do occur (albeit rarely) with the intraoperative use of TEE and that a strong association between esophageal dysmotility and aspiration, particularly in elderly patients, has been suggested in several observational reports.[242–247]

Cerebral Oximetry

Cerebral oximetry monitoring, a continuous, noninvasive monitor of regional cerebral oxygen saturation, is being used increasingly during cardiac surgery. The technologic background of near-infrared spectroscopy technology has been reviewed in detail elsewhere (see Chapter 16).[248] The main principles on which near-infrared spectroscopy devices rely are the facts that most biologic tissues, other than hemoglobin and cytochrome oxidase, are relatively transparent to infrared light in the range closest to the visual spectrum (700 to 1000 nm) and that the absorbance spectrum of hemoglobin depends on its oxygenation status (deoxygenated hemoglobin absorbs more red light and less infrared light than oxygenated hemoglobin). Regardless of the manufacturer, all devices emit light at wavelengths within the earlier

mentioned spectrum and analyze photons returning to the transducer. The source of the light signal(s) (laser vs. diode), number of wavelengths used, and distance of the emitting light source to the receiving sensors vary among the manufacturers. Because the change in intensity of the reflected light is dependent on the oxyhemoglobin/deoxyhemoglobin ratio, oxyhemoglobin saturation can be derived.[249] Because the greatest contribution to a tissue's absorption spectrum is from blood contained within venules and veins (approximately 3:1 ratio of venous to arterial blood), these devices provide a venous weighted value.[250] In comparison, pulse oximetry provides measurement of an arterial oxygen saturation reflecting oxygen supply to tissue. Therefore, near-infrared spectroscopy technology is considered complementary to pulse oximetry. Unlike pulse oximetry that requires pulsatile flow, tissue oximetry does not and is, therefore, ideal in low-flow conditions such as LCOS and/or nonpulsatile CPB or cardiocirculatory assist devices.

The use of cerebral oximetry has been suggested for cardiac surgical patients for several reasons. It is unique in its ability to continuously monitor regional tissue oxygenation even in the LCOS and nonpulsatile flow, the latter commonly seen during CPB. Multiple case reports have demonstrated that cerebral oximetry can provide early warning signs for detecting catastrophic events otherwise not detected by other monitoring devices such as pulse oximetry.[251] In addition, the cerebral cortex can be seen as an index organ. Although autoregulatory mechanisms have to be considered, low cerebral tissue oxygenation correlates with measures of systemic oxygen delivery and consumption.[252] Postoperative cognitive dysfunction is still one of the most frequently reported complications after cardiac surgery. It is likely multifactorial in origin, but embolization and hypoperfusion of the brain are two of the most frequently cited causative factors.[253] Although cerebral oximetry, because of its localized area of interrogation, may not detect even massive particulate emboli to the brain resulting in catastrophic neurologic adverse outcomes such as stroke, these events fortunately are rare, with rates of 1% to 3% reported in the literature (see Chapter 36).[254]

Many studies have estimated the incidence of neurocognitive dysfunction after cardiac surgery to be greater than 50%.[255] There are emerging data that a correlation exists between cerebral oxygen desaturations (measured with cerebral oximetry) and cognitive dysfunction in CABG patients.[256,257] There has been an ongoing debate, however, about the clinical value of near-infrared spectroscopy monitoring as a trend monitor only or as a noninvasive tool that allows clinical decision making based on adequate correlation with absolute measurements. There still need to be data from large, randomized, controlled studies with clearly defined treatment protocols and outcome measures to demonstrate that interventions based on cerebral oximetry readings can improve neurologic outcome in CABG patients.[258] Two prospective trials in CABG patients that fit those criteria have been published to date. Slater et al[257] randomized 265 CABG patients to a blinded control group or an unblinded intervention group. There were no statistically significant differences in cognitive decline and major postoperative complications (cerebrovascular accident, myocardial infarction, renal insufficiency, reoperation for bleeding) between the two study groups, a result the authors attributed to poor compliance with the treatment protocol. In the multivariate analysis, however, prolonged rSo_2 desaturation was an independent risk factor for postoperative cognitive decline regardless of the assigned study group. Murkin et al,[259] in a similar study, demonstrated that treatment of cerebral oxygen desaturations improved outcome in patients undergoing CABG surgery. They randomized 200 patients undergoing CABG surgery to either an intervention group in which cerebral tissue desaturation was linked to a treatment intervention protocol attempting to correct those readings back to baseline values or a control group in which cerebral oximetry readings were blinded to the practitioner. The hypothesis was that most of the interventions to optimize cerebral oxygen saturation would influence systemic perfusion as well. There was no difference in the overall incidence of adverse complications; however, significantly more patients in the control group had major organ morbidity or mortality such as death, ventilation longer than 48 hours, stroke, myocardial infarction, and return for re-exploration. The results of both studies clearly demonstrated that further studies are needed to determine whether postoperative cognitive dysfunction can be reduced by treatment of intraoperative cerebral oxygen desaturations, as well as to define a clear threshold below which the risk for postoperative cognitive dysfunction is increased.

Induction and Maintenance of General Anesthesia

Induction of anesthesia should take place in a calm and relaxed manner, preferably in a quiet operating room. Attention should be paid to the ambient room temperature or warm blankets placed on the patient because entry into an excessively cold operating room can elicit an unwanted sympathetic response with increases in blood pressure and HR increasing oxygen demand. Allaying the patient's anxiety with premedication and calm, reassuring verbal interaction is also critical. Preoxygenation should be used and invasive continuous blood pressure monitoring should be in place before induction.

The main considerations in choosing an induction technique for patients undergoing CABG are LV function and coronary pathology. In addition, limiting the amount of opioids and/or the use of short-acting drugs is encouraged in patients eligible for fast-tracking and early extubation. With modern cardioplegia techniques and assuming an uneventful intraoperative course, cardiac function typically is well preserved and patients usually can be extubated within 2 to 4 hours after surgery if attention is paid to adequate rewarming and postoperative analgesia and if high doses of respiratory depressant anesthetics (particularly opioids and benzodiazepines) have been avoided.

It is evident that no single approach to anesthesia for CABG procedures is suitable for all patients. Most hypnotics, opioids, and volatile agents have been used in different combinations for the induction and maintenance of anesthesia, with good results in the hands of experienced clinicians (Box 18-4).

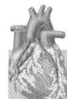

BOX 18-4. GENERAL CONSIDERATIONS FOR ANESTHESIA INDUCTION AND MAINTENANCE IN PATIENTS UNDERGOING MYOCARDIAL REVASCULARIZATION

1. Anesthetic induction with tight control of hemodynamic parameters (avoid tachycardia, hypotension), particularly in patients with left main disease
2. Fast-track anesthetic protocols aiming for early extubation favored in most patients (restrict a high-dose opioid technique for patients at very high risk who do not tolerate inhalation anesthetics)
3. Given the increasing evidence for preconditioning effects, a potent volatile agent should be part of the anesthetic regimen; avoid nitrous oxide because of the possibility of expanding gaseous emboli
4. Maintain coronary perfusion pressure without increasing myocardial oxygen demand (phenylephrine, nitroglycerin, avoid tachycardia)
5. Antifibrinolytic therapy (epsilon aminocaproic acid or tranexamic acid) except in off-pump coronary artery bypass (OPCAB) patients; aprotinin is no longer available in the United States
6. Low tidal volume mechanical ventilation to facilitate LIMA dissection
7. Heparin usually is administered before clamping of the LIMA pedicle to avoid thrombosis; papaverine often is injected retrograde into the LIMA by the surgeon, which occasionally causes hypotension
8. Heparin administration, 300 to 400 IU/kg, or as calculated by heparin titration (Hepcon) in coronary artery bypass grafting (CABG) patients with cardiopulmonary bypass (CPB); activated coagulation time between 450 and 500 seconds is required for institution of CPB

Anesthetic Agents

Considerations for choice of induction agent in the patient undergoing CABG are based on theoretic and practical clinical considerations. Hypertension and tachycardia are most commonly seen in patients with normal ventricular function, a history of arterial hypertension, and left ventricular hypertrophy. They should be avoided, as well as hypotension and excessive myocardial depression, in a patient with depressed ventricular function or with severe flow-dependent stenoses (e.g., left main or proximal LAD disease, coexisting severe valvular stenosis). The cardiac effects of each of the commonly used induction agents have been investigated over many years, sometimes with conflicting results. Increasing sophistication of experimental preparations and measurements is providing new information. Unraveling the direct versus indirect effects of a particular drug on the heart and circulation is complex because overall effects are based on contractility, vascular tone, and response of the autonomic nervous system and baroreceptors. Closely related to this are the details of the animal preparation (e.g., species, acute vs. chronic preparation, open vs. closed chest) or the clinical setting (e.g., type and speed of induction, use of concurrent β-blockers, or other antihypertensives, sophistication of cardiac monitoring) in which the drug is being investigated. Rarely is one drug used exclusively (particularly in this setting in which opioids, volatile agents, and benzodiazepines are often used simultaneously). All of the drugs usually are titrated to effect.

Thiopental had been used for decades for induction in this setting; however, it is rarely used nowadays. Its predominant hemodynamic effects include reductions in MAP and CO accompanied by a modest increase in HR. These are believed to result from a combination of direct myocardial depression, venodilation, and a decrease in central sympathetic outflow. In isolated muscle, whole-animal,[260] and clinical studies (including use of load-independent measures of contractility),[261,262] it generally is reported to have greater negative inotropic effects than propofol. A greater degree of vasodilation with propofol also may account for less depression of CO.[263,264] A study of isolated human atrial muscle from CABG patients reported no effect of propofol, midazolam, and etomidate on contractility in contrast with strong effects for thiopental and, paradoxically, slight negative effects for ketamine.[265] However, a sheep preparation, in which "site-directed" coronary arterial injection was used to isolate direct cardiac effects using doses small enough to preclude indirect effects from recirculated drug in the central nervous system, reported similar direct cardiac depressant effects for thiopental and propofol (including the thiopental enantiomer and racemate).[266] Despite these findings and its use in epidemiologic studies of anesthetic techniques for CABG,[267] the use of thiopental in most centers has declined substantially in favor of propofol. Adverse effects on airway resistance, a greater propensity to elicit bronchospasm, and a greater association with postoperative nausea and vomiting are other potential factors (see Chapter 9).

Administration of *ketamine* generally is associated with increases in HR and MAP through indirect central and peripheral sympathetic stimulation (e.g., inhibition of neuronal reuptake of catecholamines). In states associated with depletion of catecholamines and in isolated preparations, ketamine appears to have direct negative inotropic and vasodilating effects,[265,268] and it may have a negative lusitropic effect decreasing diastolic compliance.[269] In a double-blind, randomized, controlled trial, Zilberstein et al[270] documented a potent anti-inflammatory effect (i.e., suppression of increases in superoxide anion production after CPB) with a very small dose of ketamine (0.25 mg/kg) that persisted for several days after surgery. Ketamine is used relatively infrequently in CABG patients and is reserved primarily for induction in those with severe reduction of EF.

Etomidate appears to have minimal or no direct negative inotropic effects or sympathomimetic effects.[271,272] In an isolated rabbit heart preparation, Komai et al[273] demonstrated that at very high concentrations, etomidate inhibited the influx of extracellular calcium but had no effect on availability of intracellular calcium required for excitation-contraction coupling. It is known to inhibit adrenal mitochondrial hydroxylase activity, resulting in reduced steroido-genesis even after a single bolus dose, although the studies are con-flicting.[274,275] Its use for induction in cardiac patients with impaired ventricular function is common. Myoclonic jerking can be observed in the absence of muscle relaxation. The use in patients with normal ventricular function should be carefully considered because blunt-ing of the adrenergic response to intubation is poor and may result in hypertension and tachycardia, particularly with the low-dose opioid techniques used today. Greater associations with postoperative nausea and vomiting are other potential adverse effects seen with etomidate administration.

The clinical effects of *propofol* are, in general, similar to those of thio-pental. However, it has numerous advantages over thiopental based on its predictable pharmacokinetics and dynamics.[276,277] It often is used for sedation after CABG surgery,[278] although with the recent approval of dexmedetomidine for this indication,[279] its use may decline. Its iso-lated effects on contractility are controversial, with conflicting findings depending on the model used. A sophisticated analysis of its effects in CABG patients using TEE assessment of preload-adjusted maximal power, a load-independent measure of contractility, at four different plasma concentrations (0.6 to 2.6 mg/mL) found no direct effect on contractility, although it lowered preload and afterload.[280] It previously was evaluated in numerous clinical studies for induction and main-tenance with an opioid (most commonly sufentanil) compared with a volatile-opioid combination for CABG in patients with normal and depressed EF. These studies reported minimal differences in hemo-dynamics or in the incidence of myocardial ischemia.[281–286] However, more sophisticated and larger contemporary studies closely evaluating ventricular function on weaning from CPB and perioperative release of biomarkers of ischemia consistently reported better myocardial pro-tective properties with the use of volatile agents over a total intrave-nous anesthetic technique with propofol. This is apparently related to anesthetic preconditioning and postconditioning effects of volatile agents (see Chapter 9). Propofol has been reported to have strong free radical scavenging properties that in one CABG study appeared to have attenuated myocardial lipid peroxidation in atrial tissue biopsies.[287] In addition, propofol may have cardioprotective properties. The PRO-TECT II (PROpofol cardioproTECTion for type II diabetics) study is investigating whether high-dose propofol can confer cardioprotection to diabetics, a population that may not benefit as much from inhala-tion anesthetics.[288]

Benzodiazepines commonly are used in combination with a nar-cotic to induce anesthesia for CABG. In most settings, midazolam has replaced diazepam, given its numerous advantages (particularly water solubility, a shorter half-life, and absence of metabolites capable of accumulation, prolonging the sedative effects).[289] Stanley et al[290,291] and Liu et al[292] were among the first to report on the addition of diaz-epam to high-dose morphine and, shortly thereafter, fentanyl anes-thesia for CABG. They reported a mild-to-moderate reduction in CO (approximately 20% relative to opioid alone, with the greatest decrease in the fentanyl group). These studies suggested that diazepam should not be used, particularly in patients with impaired ventricular func-tion. However, with the realization that breakthrough adrenergic responses, as well as a substantial incidence of anesthetic recall with fentanyl alone, can occur, supplementation with diazepam or midazo-lam quickly grew in popularity together with high-dose opioids in the early to mid-1980s.

Numerous clinical series of widely different sizes and designs, report-ing on the efficacy of diazepam or, more commonly, midazolam used with high-dose opioids, were subsequently published.[293–304] Moderate degrees of hypotension were reported in most studies, primarily attrib-uted to a reduction in SVR (or from the effects of the high-dose opioid itself given the potent bradycardic effects of high-dose sufentanil). With rare exception, most investigators considered it safe and effective.[305]

There has been relatively little research on the direct cardiac effects of midazolam. Messina et al[306] reported a clinical study of 40 CABG patients in whom 0.1 mg/kg midazolam was administered after induc-tion and intubation with thiopental, fentanyl, and pancuronium.

Contractility was depressed by midazolam, although afterload was reduced simultaneously, resulting in no net change in cardiac index. Patients with depressed baseline EF had lower indices of contractility at baseline but a similar magnitude of change. This study provided clini-cal confirmation of the safety of midazolam in clinical practice, par-ticularly given its experimental design. Most clinicians have reduced dosing of midazolam to the range used in the latter study. Midazolam is used widely because of clinicians concerns regarding recall. However, with the use of continuous volatile anesthesia and availability of conve-nient neuromonitoring techniques, it should no longer be considered a necessity, particularly with use of small amounts as a component of the premedication.

High-dose opioid anesthesia was introduced into cardiac surgery by Lowenstein et al[307] in 1969, in an attempt to provide safe anesthesia without myocardial depression in patients with severe valvular heart disease and compromised cardiac function. Although this revolution-ized anesthesia for patients with cardiac dysfunction, it was apparent that morphine had several disadvantages: vasodilation from hista-mine release, increased requirements for fluids and vasoconstrictors, and prolonged respiratory depression. When morphine was given to patients with normal LV function, with most patients undergoing CABG particularly in the previous decades, dramatic hemodynamic responses occurred with surgical stress and amnesia could not be guar-anteed; the anesthesia often was inadequate. Despite these well-known adverse effects, morphine has regained attention because of its possibly unique cardioprotective and anti-inflammatory properties.[308,309]

In the late 1970s, Stanley and collaborators first reported on the use of high doses of the synthetic opioid fentanyl for CABG, with and without supplemental benzodiazepines.[310–312] Clinicians worldwide who perceived the lack of histamine release to be a favorable property rapidly adopted it into their clinical practice.[313–319] However, it was rec-ognized early on that recall still could be a problem.[320] Reports on the use of the more potent sufentanil appeared at the same time as fenta-nyl, although most studies were not reported until the late 1980s.[321–330] It, too, was widely adopted, although there was concern over its potent bradycardic effects at high dosages, particularly when administered with nonvagolytic muscle relaxants.[331,332]

In the mid-1990s, remifentanil was introduced. Fueled by intense interest in fast-tracking (being promoted in the same time frame), it has been intensively investigated.[333–342] Careful planning with regard to when it is terminated and adequate continuation of pain control is required. The combination with neuraxial anesthetics also has been advocated.[343] There have been reports of greater degrees of hypotension compared with fentanyl or sufentanil.[344,345] Remifentanil infusion was found to attenuate the perioperative endocrine stress response as com-pared with fentanyl boluses as an adjunct to inhalation anesthesia.[346]

Based on computer modeling and clinical data, sufentanil appears to have the most favorable characteristics for continuous infusion with very predictable termination of effect.[347,348] This characteristic was believed to be particularly important in the early 1990s when early postoperative suppression of ischemia by "intensive analgesia" was proposed as an important treatment goal just before the widespread interest in fast-tracking.[349] The substantially greater costs of sufentanil (than fentanyl) and the apparent aversion of many cardiac anesthesiol-ogists to use continuous anesthetic infusions have limited its use. Most evidence suggests that despite documented associations of sufentanil use with shorter times to extubation, overall costs and hospital lengths of stay are unaffected relative to fentanyl.[350–352] Nonetheless, it remains popular with many clinicians, many of whom infuse it continuously during surgery.

These drugs are pure opioid agonists, and none provides com-plete anesthesia as defined by predictable dose–response relations for suppression of the stress response and release of endogenous catecholamines (particularly norepinephrine), even with high serum concentrations.[353–355] Hypertension and tachycardia commonly have been reported in response to induction/intubation and surgical stim-uli (particularly with sternotomy) in older studies of high-dose opi-oid anesthesia with fentanyl or sufentanil.[356,357] Figures 18-14 and 18-15

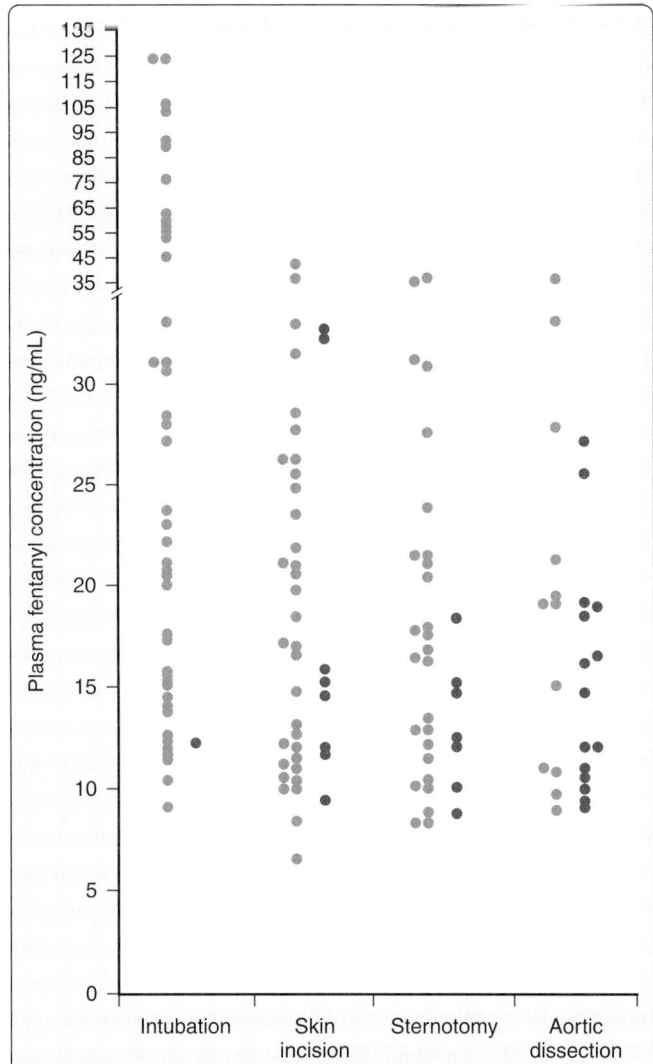

Figure 18-14 The plasma fentanyl concentration and number of patients with a hypertensive response at each event studied. *Purple circles indicate hypertensive status; green circles indicate normotensive status. (From Wynands JE, Townsend GE, Wong P, et al: Blood pressure response and plasma fentanyl concentrations during high and very high-dose fentanyl anesthesia for coronary artery surgery. Anesth Analg 62:661, 1983.)*

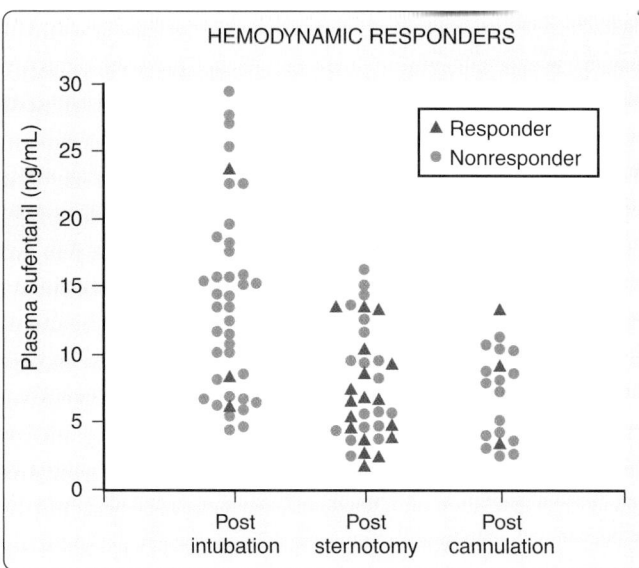

Figure 18-15 The graph plots patients with a hemodynamic response and the plasma sufentanil concentration at that time, as well as the sufentanil concentrations for the nonresponders. Therapy was initiated at the time of the initial response, and no further data points were included for those patients. *(From Philbin DM, Rosow CE, Schneider RC, et al: Fentanyl and sufentanil anesthesia revisited: How much is enough? Anesthesiology 73:5, 1990.)*

demonstrate this lack of association of serum levels with hemodynamic responses. The seminal study of Philbin et al[358] (see Figure 18-15) investigated the relation between opioid dose and hemodynamic effect with fentanyl or sufentanil in a randomized study of CABG patients. Forty premedicated patients were allocated to receive fentanyl (50 or 100 μg/kg) or sufentanil (10, 20, or 30 μg/kg) in bolus dosing with 100% oxygen and the relaxant metocurine, with an additional 40 patients randomized to sufentanil bolus dosing (10, 20, or 40 μg/kg, followed by continuous infusions). Plasma opioid (only for sufentanil in the bolus/continuous infusion groups) and catecholamine concentrations were obtained after intubation and after sternotomy. A hemodynamic response was defined as a 15% or greater increase in systolic blood pressure (HRs were not reported), and a hormonal response was a 50% or greater increase from control. For both opioids, the frequency of hemodynamic responders (33% to 60%) was similar between all fentanyl and sufentanil bolus groups. In the sufentanil infusion groups, the plasma concentrations were consistent and dose related, with wide spreads between the groups. Twenty-four of the 40 patients were hemodynamic responders (with 18 occurring with sternotomy),

and the frequency of response was unrelated to plasma sufentanil levels. Although this study had design flaws (e.g., small sample sizes and lack of power analyses, lack of reporting of actual hemodynamics), it is widely quoted to support the contention that even high-dose opioids alone provide incomplete anesthesia. Despite this, "narcotic anesthesia" was for many years considered synonymous with a "cardiac anesthetic" that should be used in all patients with CAD. It is only recently that this erroneous association is being laid to rest as volatile-based fast-tracking techniques have become standard of care in most patients undergoing myocardial revascularization.

The usual practice to provide complete anesthesia is to supplement opioids with inhaled or other intravenous agents. This permits a reduction in the total dose of opioid and, particularly with volatile agents, more rapid return of respiratory drive, facilitating early extubation. Thomson et al[359] have incorporated this approach and extended the concepts investigated by Philbin and Roscow[360] in a small but sophisticated study of CABG patients whereby specific effect site concentrations of fentanyl or sufentanil were targeted by using a computer-assisted infusion pump. Three targeted concentrations for each opioid were evaluated: sufentanil 0.4, 0.8, and 1.2 ng/mL and fentanyl 5, 10, and 15 ng/mL and the end-tidal concentration of isoflurane required to control MAP and HR in the prebypass period by predetermined criteria were monitored. The sufentanil subgroups required approximately 1.9, 3.1, and 4.9 μg/kg, and fentanyl subgroups received 18.8, 33.9, and 50.4 μg/kg in this period. The average end-tidal concentration of isoflurane was significantly greater between the low and medium/high groups, with no difference between medium and high groups. Most of the responses were increases in MAP (incidentally, the prime focus of Philbin and Roscow's[360] study). Regression analysis revealed significant correlations between serum opioid concentrations and isoflurane concentrations at most of the time points sampled in the pre-CPB period. By inspecting plots of the data pairs, they were able to ascertain the inflection point at which the isoflurane concentration began to increase rapidly, indicating poor control of hemodynamics by the respective opioid. For sufentanil, this was 0.71 ± 0.13 ng/mL, and for fentanyl, it was 7.3 ± 1.1 ng/mL. Given the use for fast-tracking with approximate ranges of 20 μg/kg for fentanyl and 3 μg/kg for sufentanil for the entire case, it is unlikely these concentrations will be obtained. However, reliance on volatile anesthesia, benzodiazepines, propofol, or dexmedetomidine infusion can provide hemodynamic control. The level of preexisting β-blockade and/or calcium channel-blockade and the type of muscle relaxant used influence each patient's response.

Neuromuscular Blocking Agents

All of the available neuromuscular blocking agents have been used to produce adequate intubating conditions and relaxation during CABG surgery (Table 18-3). Murphy et al[361] conducted a national survey of more than 400 active members of the Society of Cardiovascular Anesthesiologists evaluating their neuromuscular blocking drug of choice in the cardiac surgical setting. Despite availability of newer short-acting neuromuscular blocking agents, pancuronium was still used in most patients undergoing on-pump and off-pump cardiac surgical procedures 10 years ago. Traditionally, pancuronium had been advocated for use with high-dose narcotic techniques, because it offset opioid-induced bradycardia. However, it has long been recognized that clinically significant tachycardia resulting in myocardial ischemia could occur during induction of anesthesia with high-dose fentanyl and pancuronium.[362] With the increasing popularity of fast-track cardiac surgery, early extubation is now most desirable, and the longer duration of action of pancuronium is a potential disadvantage. Several studies have compared the durations of action of pancuronium and rocuronium in patients undergoing cardiac surgery. Irrespective of a single intubating dose or a continuous infusion, patients receiving rocuronium had significantly less residual neuromuscular blockade[363] and shorter time to extubation.[364,365]

When continuous infusions of rocuronium and cisatracurium were compared in prolonged surgical procedures, recovery to 75% of the train of four was faster in patients receiving cisatracurium.[366] Reich et al[367] compared neuromuscular transmission recovery times in pediatric cardiac patients receiving cisatracurium or vecuronium infusions in the ICU setting. Cisatracurium was associated with significantly faster spontaneous recovery of neuromuscular function. Especially in fast-track cardiac surgery, shorter-acting neuromuscular blocking agents such as cisatracurium or rocuronium are recommended to avoid residual paralysis and to allow for early extubation and ICU discharge. Neuromuscular transmission monitoring to assess for residual blockade and use of pharmacologic reversal is advisable, especially if a fast-track anesthesia technique is used.[368,369] In patients with a potentially difficult airway or emergency patients who are not NPO, succinylcholine is still the agent of choice.

Additional considerations are warranted in patients with underlying comorbidities such as chronic renal failure, which may alter pharmacokinetics. When magnesium is administered to cardiac surgical patients for prophylaxis of perioperative arrhythmias, blockade from nondepolarizing neuromuscular blocking agents may be significantly prolonged.[370] There remains the question whether continuous neuromuscular blockade for cardiac surgery really is necessary. Gueret et al[371] showed that a single intubating dose of atracurium or cisatracurium provided adequate paralysis and surgical conditions leading to quicker neuromuscular blockade recovery in cardiac surgical patients.

Advocates of this technique also point to potential advantages with regard to prevention of recall (as indicated by patient movement). However, potential disadvantages include the possibility of greater oxygen demand and consumption, or movement during surgery.

α₂-Agonists: Dexmedetomidine

The intraoperative use of α_2-agonists can be a useful adjunct, given their sedative, analgesic, and hemodynamic-stabilizing properties. α_2-Agonists prevent hypertension and tachycardia during intubation, surgical stimulation, and emergence from anesthesia, and decrease plasma catecholamine levels.[372–375] Jalonen et al,[376] in a randomized, double-blind study, administered dexmedetomidine or placebo to CABG patients starting before induction (50 ng/kg/min for 30 minutes) and continued until the end of surgery (7 ng/kg/min). Patients receiving dexmedetomidine had significantly lower plasma norepinephrine levels and more stable hemodynamics (less increase in MAP and HR during induction, less intraoperative variability of systolic arterial pressure). Dexmedetomidine administration was associated with decreased incidences of intraoperative (5% vs. 32%) and postoperative (4% vs. 40%) tachycardia when compared with placebo. Patients who received dexmedetomidine also were less likely to receive β-blocker therapy for tachycardia. Despite the findings before and after CPB, a greater incidence of hypotension (MAP < 30 mm Hg) was seen during CPB (22% vs. 0% patients, dexmedetomidine vs. placebo). These data demonstrate that dexmedetomidine is effective in attenuating sympathetic responses, although this effect may predispose patients toward hypotension.

Because of the decreased oxygen demand and HR seen with dexmedetomidine administration, it may be beneficial during OPCAB. Nevertheless, in a small series of OPCAB patients, hypotension (12 mm Hg below baseline) occurred shortly after its administration during rewarming in the ICU, prompting the study authors to recommend volume loading and normothermia before its use.[377] Experimental data demonstrated a decrease in the inflammatory response to endotoxin-induced shock in a rat model.[378]

Inhalation Anesthetics and Myocardial Protection

There is steadily increasing evidence from laboratory and clinical studies that inhalation anesthetic agents have favorable properties in patients undergoing CABG surgery, particularly in comparison with total intravenous anesthetic approaches. Concurrent with the now routine use of fast-track anesthesia techniques, there has been a major resurgence in their use as the primary anesthetic in patients undergoing cardiac surgery. Inhalation anesthetics are thought to protect the myocardium against ischemia by their ability to elicit protective cellular responses that are seen with ischemic preconditioning. The latter has been shown to reduce myocardial infarction size after periods of ischemia,[379] protect the heart against postischemic LV dysfunction,[380] and reduce the incidence of arrhythmias after cardiac surgery.[381]

Murry et al[382] first showed that brief periods of ischemia before 40 minutes of coronary artery occlusion significantly reduced infarction

TABLE 18-3	Nondepolarizing Neuromuscular Blocking Agents Commonly Used in Cardiac Anesthesia				
Relaxant	*Intubating Dose (mg/kg)*	*Maintenance*	*Clinical Duration (min)*	*Hemodynamic Effects*	*Special Considerations*
Pancuronium	0.08–0.12	0.01 mg/kg q20–60 min	60–120	Vagolytic ++ at clinical dosages, releases norepinephrine	Reduce dose or avoid completely in renal insufficiency
Vecuronium	0.08–0.2	0.8–2 μg/kg/hr	45–90	Insignificant	Accumulation of active metabolite with long-term use
Cisatracurium	0.15–0.2	1–2 μg/kg/min	40–75	Insignificant	Hoffman elimination
Rocuronium	0.4–1.0	0.01 mg/kg/min	35–75	Mildly vagolytic (high dosage)	No active metabolites

size after myocardial reperfusion. Exposing the myocardium to short periods of ischemia followed by reperfusion is called *ischemic preconditioning*. These brief periods of ischemia initiate signaling pathways that render the myocardium resistant to subsequent prolonged periods of ischemia (i.e., memory effect).[383] After a short ischemic period (i.e., preconditioning signal), the myocardium is rendered more resistant to prolonged ischemia when the subsequent ischemic event occurs within a certain time window. This may occur in two distinct phases as early preconditioning (about 2 hours) and delayed or late preconditioning (24 to 72 hours), although not all stimuli elicit both responses. Even though multiple approaches are used to protect the heart during CPB (e.g., blood cardioplegia, topical hypothermia, pharmacologic additives), aortic cross-clamping defines a period of myocardial ischemia that often results in transient or prolonged dysfunction after reperfusion.[384,385] Brief periods of aortic cross-clamping with consequent reperfusion intervals before a period of ventricular fibrillation have been shown to preserve adenosine triphosphate (ATP) content, decrease markers of ischemia such as troponin I, and improve cardiac function in patients undergoing CABG.[386–389] However, this approach is controversial and cumbersome because an ischemic episode may reduce cardiac reserves and exacerbate symptoms.[390] In addition, the accomplishment of brief periods of ischemia by short cross-clamping of an atherosclerotic aorta may result in embolism formation and endothelial damage, thereby increasing mortality.[391] Interestingly, this protection is now believed to be conferred even when the brief period of ischemia is applied to organs or tissues remote from the heart (remote preconditioning), thus improving its applicability.[392–396]

Pharmacologic interventions have been sought that mimic ischemic preconditioning. There is increasing evidence that aside from potent volatile anesthetics, opioids and, in particular, morphine trigger preconditioning.[397,398] Other intravenous anesthetics such as etomidate and ketamine do not appear to have the same cardioprotective properties.[399,400] Pharmacologic preconditioning and ischemic preconditioning initiate similar pathways that protect the myocardial cell against ischemic damage.

The pathways associated with myocardial preconditioning involve a variety of triggering stimuli, mediators, receptors, and effectors.[401] It is thought that activation of sarcolemmal and mitochondrial K_{ATP} channels play a pivotal role in the preconditioning process.[402] Opening of these channels protects the myocardium by preventing cytosolic and mitochondrial Ca^{2+} overload. The exact mechanisms of preconditioning are still actively under investigation. After the administration of a preconditioning signal such as ischemia, inhalation anesthetics including the noble gases, morphine, bradykinin, or nitroglycerin (NTG), membrane-bound receptors (adenosine A_1, adrenergic, bradykinin, muscarinic, delta-1 opioid) coupled to inhibitory G proteins are activated.[403–408] Consequently, products of intracellular transduction pathways (e.g., protein kinase C [PKC], tyrosine kinases, MAP kinases) mediate the opening and stabilization of ATP-sensitive mitochondrial K_{ATP} channels, the effectors thought to be mainly responsible for the preconditioning phenomenon.[409,410] Increased formation of nitric oxide (NO),[411,412] free oxygen radicals,[413] and enzymes such as cyclooxygenase-2[414] are also involved in the preconditioning process. The role of NO recently was confirmed by Smul et al using a rabbit model.[415] The delayed phase of myocardial protection, which may last well beyond the documented 24 to 72 hours, probably is based on transcriptional changes of protective proteins,[416,417] which may explain the gap of time between early and late preconditioning.[418] Inhalation anesthetics also preserve cardiac function after reperfusion and decrease ischemia-induced intracoronary adhesion of polymorphonuclear neutrophils and platelets.[419–423]

Initially, most data were based on in vitro studies or from data obtained during PCIs. Whether these results could be generalized to cardiac surgery remained questionable. Multiple studies now have investigated anesthetic preconditioning in the cardiac surgery setting and its impact on outcome parameters. Belhomme et al[424] exposed patients to 5 minutes of preconditioning with a 2.5 minimum alveolar concentration of isoflurane after the onset of CPB but before aortic cross-clamping. Troponin I and creatine kinase (CK)-MB

levels were not significantly different from those of the control group. Nevertheless, patients who were exposed to isoflurane had increased activity of 5-nucleotidase, a marker for protein kinase C activation, which is early evidence of preconditioning pathway activation similar to the in vitro findings. Penta de Peppo et al[425] reported on myocardial function and the preconditioning effects of enflurane in patients undergoing CABG surgery. Myocardial function was assessed using the end-systolic pressure-area relation, a relatively load-independent index of myocardial contractility. Although the number of patients studied was small, myocardial function was better preserved in patients who were exposed to enflurane before cardioplegic arrest.

Julier et al,[426] in a double-blinded, placebo-controlled, multicenter study, reported on the effect of sevoflurane preconditioning on biochemical markers for myocardial and renal dysfunction in patients undergoing CABG surgery. Patients who had sevoflurane preconditioning during the first 10 minutes of CPB had lower levels of biochemical markers of myocardial and renal impairment. Brain natriuretic peptide level as an indicator of myocardial dysfunction was significantly decreased in the sevoflurane group. Conzen et al[427] studied randomized patients undergoing OPCAB surgery with a propofol infusion versus a continuous inhalation-based anesthetic technique with sevoflurane. Patients in the sevoflurane group had significantly lower troponin I levels, as well as better LV function. Nader et al[428] added vaporized sevoflurane (2%) versus oxygen alone to a cold blood cardioplegia solution in a small randomized trial of patients undergoing CABG surgery. Markers of the inflammatory response (i.e., neutrophil β-integrins, tumor necrosis factor-α, and interleukin-6) were lower, and cardiac function (i.e., stroke work index and wall motion analysis) was better preserved in the sevoflurane group (Figure 18-16). Table 18-4 summarizes the results of the randomized, prospective clinical studies.[429–440]

Whether these biochemical markers of improved cardiac outcome actually translate into reduced mortality or improved long-term outcome remains a matter of debate.[441] Garcia et al[435] reported on the results of a prospective, randomized study of the effect of sevoflurane preconditioning (10 minutes before aortic cross-clamping) on late

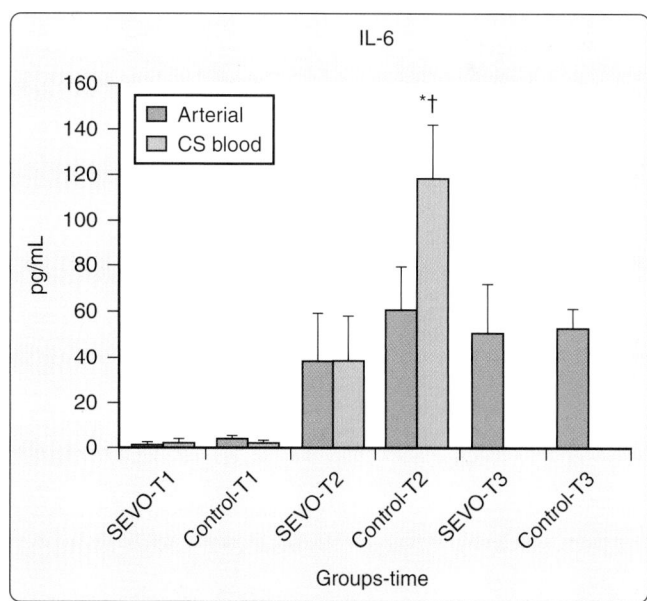

Figure 18-16 Blunting of increase of interleukin-6 (IL-6) levels in response to cardiopulmonary bypass (CPB) in patients receiving 2% sevoflurane (SEVO) added to the cardioplegia solution (1.4 ± 1.2 to 38.2 ± 21.6 pg/mL vs. 4.1 ± 1.4 to 118.2 ± 23.5 pg/mL; $P < 0.05$). Levels were similar by 6 hours after CPB. CS, coronary sinus; T1, baseline; T2, after separation from CPB; T3, 6 hours after separation from CPB. *†, statistically significant. *(From Nader ND, Li CM, Khadra WZ, et al: Anesthetic myocardial protection with sevoflurane. J Cardiothorac Vasc Anesth 18:269, 2004.)*

TABLE 18-4 Clinical Studies of Volatile Agent Preconditioning for Coronary Artery Bypass Grafting

Study	Drugs, Route	N	End Points	Results	Comments
Belhomme, 1999[424]	ISO (2.5 MAC on CPB) for 5 min before AoX vs. case-matched controls; TIVA propofol-opioid base anesthetic	18	A. CK-MB/Trop I	0	
			B. Ecto-5′-nucleotidase	1 (increase activity)	Marker of protein kinase C activation
Penta de Peppo, 1999[425]	ENF (0.5–2.0%) to reduce SPB by 25% 5 min before AoX vs. control; TIVA propofol-opioid base anesthetic	16	A. CK-MB/Trop I	0	
			B. CI	0	
			C. LV contractility	1 (preserved)	Pressure-area loops measured by TEE
Tomai, 1999[439]	ISO before AoX	40	A. CK-MB/Trop I	0	Significant only with preoperative EF < 50%
Haroun-Bizri, 2001[440]	ISO (≈1 MAC) before CPB vs. control; TIVA propofol-opioid base anesthetic	49	A. CI	1 (higher in ISO)	
			B. ST-segment changes	1 (less in ISO)	
De Hert, 2002[429]	SEVO continuous (0.5–2%) vs. PROP; remifentanil in both	20	A. Trop I	1 (lower in SEVO)	
			B. LV systolic/diastolic function (LVP parameters pre/post leg elevation)	1 (preserved in SEVO)	
Julier, 2003[426]	SEVO (2 MAC) vaporized on CPB for 10 min before AoX vs. control; TIVA propofol-opioid base anesthetic	72	A. CK-MB/Trop T/Holter ST segments	0	
			B. Brain natriuretic peptide	1 (lower in SEVO)	Marker of contractile dysfunction
			C. Protein kinase C translocation	1 (greater in SEVO)	Immunohistologic analysis from atrial tissue
			D. Plasma cystatin C	1 (lower in SEVO)	Marker of renal dysfunction
Conzen, 2003[427]	SEVO (≈1 MAC) continuous vs. PROP (OPCAB); sufentanil base in both	20	A. CK-MB	0	
			B. Trop I	1 (lower in SEVO)	
			C. CI	1 (higher in SEVO)	
De Hert, 2003[431]	SEVO (0.5–2%), DES (1–4%), PROP (2–4 µg/mL target concentration); high-risk elderly patients	45	A. Trop I	1 (high in PROP)	Cohort: age > 70 yr, EF < 50% with impaired length-dependent regulation of myocardial function
			B. LV systolic/diastolic function (LVP parameters pre/post leg elevation)	1 (preserved in SEVO, DES)	
De Hert, 2004[430]	SEVO (0.5–2%), DES (1–4%), MIDAZ (0.5–1.5 µg/kg/min), PROP (2 µg/mL target concentration); remifentanil base anesthetic	320	A. Trop I	1 (lower in SEVO, DES)	
			B. LOS in ICU or hospital	1 (less in SEVO, DES)	
			C. Inotrope use	1 (less in SEVO, DES)	
			D. LV function	1 (preserved in SEVO, DES)	
De Hert, 2004[432]	SEVO pre-CPB vs. SEVO post-CPB vs. SEVO-continuous vs. PROP alone; TIVA propofol-opioid base anesthetic	200	A. Trop I	1 (lower in SEVO continuous)	
			B. LOS in ICU	1 (less in SEVO continuous)	
			C. Inotrope use	1 (less in SEVO continuous)	
			D. LV systolic/diastolic function (LVP parameters pre/post leg elevation)	1 (better preserved in SEVO esp. continuous)	

TABLE 18-4	Clinical Studies of Volatile Agent Preconditioning for Coronary Artery Bypass Grafting—Cont'd					
Study	*Drugs, Route*	*N*	*End Points*	*Results*	*Comments*	
Nader, 2004[428]	SEVO, placebo (2% SEVO vaporized in cardioplegia); TIVA propofol-opioid base anesthetic	21	A. LV function (TEE, LVSWI)	↑ (better preserved in SEVO)		
			B. Inflammatory response (neutrophil β-integrins, tumor necrosis factor, interleukin-6)	↓ (lower in SEVO)		
Garcia, 2005[435]	12-mo follow-up of Julier et al's[426] cohort	72	A. Endothelial function (transcript levels of PECAM-1, catalase, heat shock protein)	↑ (better with SEVO)	PECAM-1 levels lower in SEVO, may have role in transition of coronary plaques to unstable state	
			B. Late cardiac events (6–12 months)	↓ (lower with SEVO)	3% vs. 17% for composite outcome ($P = 0.04$); peak perioperative BNP and Trop I greater in patients with events; no deaths	

AoX, aortic cross-clamping; BNP, brain natriuretic peptide; CI, confidence interval; CK-MB, isoenzyme of creatine kinase with muscle and brain subunits; CPB, cardiopulmonary bypass; DES, desflurane; EF, ejection fraction; ENF, enflurane; ICU, intensive care unit; ISO, isoflurane; LOS, length of stay; LV, left ventricular; LVP, left ventricular pressure; LVSWI, left ventricular stroke work index; MAC, minimum alveolar concentration; MIDAZ, midazolam; OPCAB, off-pump coronary artery bypass grafting; PECAM-1, platelet–endothelial cell adhesion molecule-1; PROP, propofol; SEVO, sevoflurane; SPB, systolic blood pressure; TEE, transesophageal echocardiography; TIVA, total intravenous anesthetic; Trop I, troponin I.

cardiac events. Coronary artery reocclusion, congestive heart failure, and cardiac death were assessed at 6 and 12 months after surgery. Preconditioning with sevoflurane significantly reduced the incidence of late cardiac events. In a prospective, randomized, nonblinded study, De Hert et al[442] compared the inhalation anesthetics desflurane and sevoflurane with an intravenous anesthetic technique with a continuous propofol infusion in high-risk patients undergoing CABG surgery. In the volatile anesthetic group, myocardial function was better preserved, troponin I levels were lower, and ICU and hospital LOS were shorter compared with propofol or midazolam-based anesthetic regimens in this setting.[443] Guarrancino et al[444] showed that a desflurane-based anesthetic resulted in reduced troponin I release, inotropic drug use, and number of patients requiring prolonged hospitalization compared with a propofol-based technique in off-pump CABG.

Three recent meta-analyses examined preconditioning and mortality or long-term outcome in patients undergoing cardiac surgery. In a meta-analysis that included only studies with sevoflurane and desflurane, Landoni et al[445] showed a reduction in mortality and the incidence of myocardial infarction after cardiac surgery. In two other meta-analyses that also included isoflurane, no such benefit was seen.[446,447] Data from a retrospective Danish database multicenter analysis including 10,535 patients did not show any difference in overall postoperative mortality or myocardial infarction between propofol and sevoflurane-based anesthesia.[448] To further investigate these controversial findings, Bignami et al[449] conducted a longitudinal survey among 64 Italian cardiac surgical centers to study the correlation between the use of volatile anesthetics and 30-day mortality in CABG surgery. The results showed that risk-adjusted 30-day mortality was significantly reduced when volatile agents were used during cardiac surgery, especially when there was prolonged use of these agents. Interestingly, the most consistent results were found when isoflurane was used. In a recent multicenter trial comparing desflurane or sevoflurane with propofol-based anesthesia, De Hert et al[450] were unable to find a difference in troponin release but did show that the use of inhalation anesthetics reduced hospital LOS and patients in the inhalation anesthetic group had a lower 1-year mortality.

The optimal timing and duration of inhalation anesthetic administration are still under investigation.[451-454] Whereas some of the studies use brief periods of anesthetic preconditioning before aortic cross-clamping, others have reported on use of volatile anesthetics throughout the operative period. The older studies using brief periods of preconditioning showed improved cardiac function, although markers of myocardial injury such as CK-MB or troponin I often were not significantly different from the control group. De Hert et al[455] showed

that the best results for myocardial protection were achieved when sevoflurane was administered throughout the intraoperative period and not just immediately before the planned myocardial ischemic event. Most similarly designed studies have confirmed those findings. Bein et al,[456] however, found that myocardial cell damage and dysfunction were lower in patients who received sevoflurane in an interrupted manner. Frassdorf et al[457] also demonstrated that preconditioning-related myocardial protection was superior with multiple periods of sevoflurane administration applied rather than one short period. When sevoflurane was added to the anesthesia regimen after the coronary anastomoses were completed, myocardial recovery was faster compared with a propofol-based anesthetic technique. Nevertheless, patients who received sevoflurane during the entire procedure had the lowest troponin I levels, and the stroke volume changed the least compared with baseline levels.[455] Most data available to date suggest not limiting the use of inhalation anesthetics to brief periods, but rather to use prolonged administration.

Research on pharmacologic preconditioning is not restricted only to inhalation anesthetics. There is increasing evidence that a variety of drugs that are administered perioperatively have cardioprotective properties involving preconditioning pathways. Besides inhalation anesthetics, opioids (delta-opioid receptor), adenosine (adenosine A$_1$ receptor), and bradykinin have been investigated for their preconditioning effects, with variable results.[458-461]

During cardiac surgery, several of the known preconditioning triggering agents may be used and appear to be additive or synergistic in effect. Toller et al[462] reported that the administration of sevoflurane and mechanical ischemic preconditioning reduced infarction size significantly compared with either stimulus alone. Ludwig et al[463] demonstrated the additive effect of isoflurane and morphine on the reduction of infarction size. There are still insufficient data on how the potential beneficial effect of potent inhalation anesthetics differs between OPCAB and on-pump CABG patients, with some preliminary data that OPCAB patients may benefit more.[464]

Several clinical factors appear to impair the protective effects of preconditioning. Two groups of patients, diabetic and female patients, appear to have attenuated responses to mechanical preconditioning signals (during PCI).[465] Intraoperative hyperglycemia blocks the preconditioning effect, although this effect may be reversed by N-acetylcysteine, an oxygen radical scavenger.[466-470]

The role of postconditioning is now also starting to be elucidated. Prompt treatment of myocardial ischemia is essential for limiting myocardial damage. However, the damage to the myocardium is not only a result of the ischemic time but of the reperfusion itself. Brief episodes of ischemia/reperfusion applied during the first few minutes of reperfusion after a prolonged ischemia have been shown to decrease myocardial infarct size to the same extent as that induced by ischemic preconditioning.[471,472] It is thought that mitochondrial K_{ATP} channels, NO, and protein kinase C play important roles in postconditioning as well.[473] Protein kinase C is one of a larger group of kinases labeled "reperfusion injury salvage kinases" that play a role in postconditioning.[474–476] The beneficial effects of ischemic postconditioning also have been shown in humans during coronary angioplasty for acute myocardial infarction.[477,478] As in preconditioning, postconditioning also has been found to work when applied remotely.[479] Inhalation anesthetics also may be effective in blunting the deleterious effects of postischemic reperfusion injury and the inflammatory response syndrome after cardiac surgery.[480,481] Thus far, most data about anesthetic postconditioning have been gathered from studies in animals and in vitro isolated human myocardium. Postconditioning has been shown to improve contractile function[482] and attenuate postischemic arrhythmias.[483] Recent data further suggest that the protective properties of potent inhalation anesthetics may not be restricted only to the myocardium but extend to other organ systems.[484–487]

In summary, there is increasing evidence suggesting that potent inhalation anesthetics should be part of the anesthetic regimen in patients undergoing cardiac surgery, particularly in patients undergoing CABG, OPCAB, and/or patients at high risk for ischemic events.[488]

Intraoperative Awareness and Recall

Intraoperative awareness (i.e., recall), usually defined as postoperative memory for intraoperative events, is an infrequent but well-recognized phenomenon during general anesthesia. Awareness, a conscious subjective experience (i.e., implicit memory), may be much more frequent than conscious recall (i.e., explicit memory) of intraoperative events.[489] In a prospective, nonrandomized, descriptive cohort study of more than 19,000 patients undergoing surgery with general anesthesia at seven academic medical centers in the United States, awareness with explicit recall occurred in 0.13% of the cases.[490] Patients undergoing cardiac surgery always have been considered to be at increased risk because of anesthetic regimens intentionally devoid of cardiodepressant inhalation anesthetics (before the era of improved myocardial preservation and fast-tracking) and because of frequent periods of light anesthesia in the presence of hemodynamic instability resulting from surgical manipulation of the heart and great vessels, depressed contractility after CPB, or bleeding. The published incidence rate of awareness in patients undergoing cardiac surgery is significantly greater than that reported for general surgery, with older reports of up to 23%.[491] However, the introduction of fast-track anesthesia techniques and the more frequent use of inhalation agents have helped to reduce the risk for intraoperative awareness for this type of surgery. Ranta et al[492] found definite intraoperative awareness with recall in 0.5% of patients undergoing cardiac surgery under general anesthesia, with various anesthesia regimens using inhalation or total intravenous anesthetic techniques. Greater doses of benzodiazepines, such as midazolam, resulted in a lower incidence of awareness. Phillips et al[493] interviewed 700 patients after cardiac surgery with CPB and found that 8 patients (1.8%) reported intraoperative recall regardless of whether benzodiazepines or inhalation agents were used. Fast-track anesthesia techniques typically combine low-dose narcotics with short-acting anesthetics such as inhalation agents or propofol infusions. Dowd et al[494] reported a low incidence rate (0.3%) of intraoperative awareness with this technique, attributing it to the continuous administration of volatile anesthetics or propofol.

Measures to prevent intraoperative awareness typically are based on anesthetic regimens that interfere with memory processing, such as the use of inhalation anesthetics and benzodiazepines. However, the anesthesia technique does not always correlate with the incidence of intraoperative awareness. In a large series of more than 11,000 patients undergoing general anesthesia, 18 cases of recall occurred (0.18%), but the analysis suggested that this number could not have been reduced

with monitoring of end-tidal anesthetic gas concentrations or more frequent use of preoperatively administered benzodiazepines.[495] Efforts to determine time periods that are prone to awareness or recall usually are based on physiologic or hemodynamic parameters that indicate light anesthesia, such as tachycardia, arterial hypertension, or patient movement. Nevertheless, Kerssens et al[496] showed that hemodynamic variables were poor predictors of intraoperative awareness, although these parameters were able to differentiate between patients with or without *conscious* recall. In contrast, electroencephalogram-derived parameters were highly significant predictors of intraoperative awareness but were not able to detect patients with conscious recall.

Consequently, if hemodynamic parameters or measures of anesthetic concentrations are insufficient in preventing intraoperative awareness, the question arises whether monitoring neurophysiologic parameters such as processed electroencephalographic data decreases the incidence of intraoperative awareness or recall (see Chapter 16). Neurophysiologic monitoring is usually based on fast Fourier transformation and bispectral analysis of one-channel electroencephalographic data obtained from electrodes on the patient's forehead. Several devices have been approved by the U.S. Food and Drug Administration (FDA).[497–500] Two large studies showed a significant reduction in awareness under general anesthesia when the Bispectral Index (BIS) was monitored. Myles et al[501] studied 2463 patients considered to be at high risk for awareness in a prospective, randomized, double-blinded, multicenter trial with 45% undergoing high-risk cardiac surgery or OPCAB. Patients were randomized to BIS-guided or routine anesthesia care. BIS monitoring reduced the risk rate for awareness by 82%, although the absolute number of confirmed events was small (2 vs. 11). In patients undergoing cardiac surgery, three events occurred (two routine, one BIS). "Possible" awareness events (not confirmed by the end-point committee) occurred irrespective of the use of BIS monitoring. Ekman et al,[502] in a large, nonrandomized, historically controlled study, also showed a significantly reduced incidence rate of intraoperative awareness (0.04% vs. 0.18%) in the BIS monitored patients. However, in a small series of patients, Barr et al[503] found no correlation between bispectral electroencephalographic analysis of anesthesia depth and conscious recall in patients undergoing cardiac surgery. This was attributed to exclusive use of midazolam and fentanyl.

Besides monitoring anesthetic depth, neurophysiologic monitoring also may help to decrease the incidence of hemodynamic disturbances, may guide titration of anesthetic agents to their effective dose, and may be associated with improved patient satisfaction.[504,505] In clinical experience, the use of BIS monitoring has been helpful in more accurately gauging the need for reinstitution of volatile anesthesia after weaning from CPB. In this potentially unstable period with a depressed myocardium or untoward responses to protamine, this can be an important factor. Often the BIS remains in the low range for the first 15 to 30 minutes after weaning, especially in older patients with longer pump times. It also is helpful to ensure adequacy of burst suppression for hypothermic circulatory arrest.

In summary, published data appear to indicate that despite a substantial reduction in awareness resulting from a shift to greater use of volatile anesthetics, patients undergoing cardiac surgery are still at risk for intraoperative awareness or recall. Neurophysiologic monitoring decreases the incidence of these events, but given the low incidence, a large number of patients have to be monitored to prevent one case of intraoperative awareness. The implications of intraoperative awareness or conscious recall are not yet fully understood. These events may be unrecognized or not necessarily experienced as unpleasant,[506] but they also may lead to severe posttraumatic stress disorders with chronic health impairment.[507]

Myocardial Ischemia in Patients Undergoing Revascularization Surgery

Incidence

In addition to providing anesthesia, a major concern of the anesthesiologist is the prevention and treatment of myocardial ischemia. Numerous laboratory and clinical studies have examined the incidence of myocardial ischemia in the perioperative period, as it relates to the administration of anesthetic drugs. Although the incidence rate of pre-bypass ischemia in patients appears to be between 10% and 50%, it is not at all clear that the anesthetic drug combination per se is a determinant of this incidence. Several studies have addressed whether the anesthetic technique (e.g., fast-track or early extubation, high thoracic epidural) is related to perioperative morbidity and myocardial ischemic events. An extensive meta-analysis of more than 30 randomized, controlled trials of patients undergoing cardiac surgery showed no difference in the relative risk of postoperative myocardial ischemia when early extubation protocols were compared with conventional extubation management.[508]

Hemodynamic Changes Related to Myocardial Ischemia

Besides ECG abnormalities, some hemodynamic changes should alert the anesthesiologist to the possibility of intraoperative myocardial ischemia. The association of tachycardia with hypotension or increased LV filling pressure, both of which reduce coronary perfusion pressure [CPP], is a particularly undesirable combination, jeopardizing the oxygen supply-demand relation. Figure 18-17 demonstrates how hypertension in the absence of tachycardia, in response to surgical stress (skin incision), can be associated with pulmonary hypertension, increased PCWP, and prominent A and V waves on the PCWP waveform.[509] Although ECG changes occurred later, the early hemodynamic abnormalities almost certainly were the result of ischemic LV dysfunction. Treatment included deepening anesthesia and administering an NTG infusion.

LV diastolic dysfunction detected with TEE is one of the earliest changes identified after coronary artery occlusion, and it often precedes the development of abnormal systolic function. RWMAs also have been described as early signs of ischemia. They occur within seconds of inadequate blood flow or oxygen supply. RWMAs detected by TEE have been shown to be a more sensitive method of detecting myocardial ischemia in patients undergoing CABG, compared with ST-segment changes.[510] Myocardial ischemia or repositioning the heart during OPCAB can be the cause of a sudden onset of mitral regurgitation or worsening of preexisting mitral regurgitation, both of which can be detected with TEE monitoring (see Chapter 12).

Intraoperative Treatment of Myocardial Ischemia

Close attention to hemodynamic control and rapid treatment of abnormalities are fundamental principles of the intraoperative management of the patient with CAD. If there is a hemodynamic abnormality that is temporally related to the onset of ischemia, it should be treated accordingly. Hemodynamic treatment to ensure an adequate CPP (diastolic blood pressure minus left ventricular end-diastolic pressure [LVEDP]) should be a priority, as should control of HR, the single most important treatable determinant of myocardial oxygen consumption. Table 18-5 summarizes the treatment of acute perioperative myocardial ischemia. The earliest objective evidence of successful treatment of ischemia may be the return to normal of the PAP and the PCWP waveforms. In the following section, some of the routinely used pharmacologic interventions for intraoperative myocardial ischemia are discussed.

Intravenous Nitroglycerin

Since the introduction in 1976 by Kaplan et al[511] of the V_5 lead to diagnose myocardial ischemia, and intravenous NTG to treat it,[512] NTG has been one of the mainstays in the treatment of perioperative myocardial ischemia. Intravenous NTG acts immediately to reduce LV preload and wall tension, primarily by decreasing venous tone in lower doses. In larger doses, it also may decrease arterial resistance and epicardial coronary arterial resistance.[513,514] NTG has been shown to consistently decrease LV filling pressures, systemic BP, and myocardial oxygen consumption and to improve LV performance in patients with severe dysfunction.[515] It is most effective in treating acute myocardial ischemia with ventricular dysfunction accompanied by sudden increases in LVEDV, LVEDP, and PAP. These increases in LV preload and wall tension further exacerbate perfusion deficits to the ischemic subendocardium and usually respond immediately to NTG (Figure 18-18).

Before surgery, NTG often is used to treat patients with unstable angina or ischemic mitral regurgitation and limit the size of an evolving myocardial infarction, reduce associated complications, and reverse RWMAs.[516,517] In the pre-CPB period and during OPCAB, NTG is used to treat signs of ischemia such as ST-segment depression, hypertension uncontrolled by the anesthetic medication, ventricular dysfunction, or coronary artery spasm (Box 18-5). During CPB, NTG can be used to control the MAP with a time to onset of effect ranging from 4.1 ± 0.8 to 7.8 ± 2.8 minutes at doses of 1.7 ± 0.3 to 2.9 ± 0.7 μg/kg/min.[518] However, NTG is not always effective in controlling MAP during CPB (approximately 60% of patients respond) because of alterations of the pharmacokinetics and pharmacodynamics of the drug with CPB. Factors contributing to the reduction of its effectiveness include adsorption to the plastic in the CPB system, alterations in regional blood flow, hemodilution, and hypothermia. Booth et al[519] have shown that different oxygenators and filters sequester up to 90%

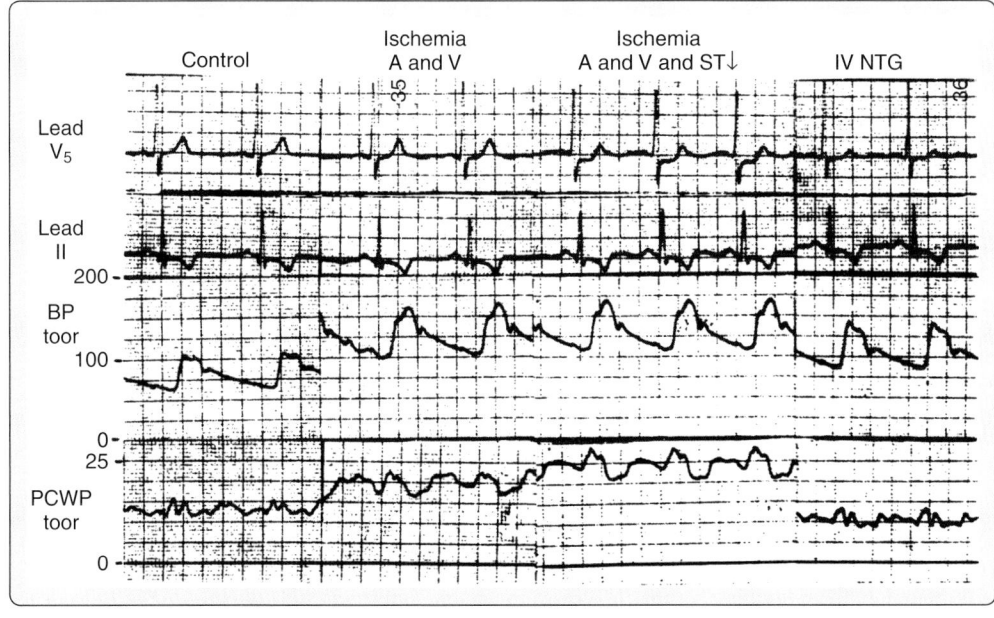

Figure 18-17 Nitroglycerin (NTG) relieved postintubation intraoperative myocardial ischemia, as evidenced by large V waves in the pulmonary capillary wedge pressure (PCWP) tracing and then by ST-segment depression. BP, blood pressure. *(From Kaplan JA, Wells PH: Early diagnosis of myocardial ischemia using the pulmonary arterial catheter. Anesth Analg 60:789, 1981.)*

TABLE 18-5	Acute Treatments for Suspected Intraoperative Myocardial Ischemia	
Associated Hemodynamic Finding	Therapy	Dosage
Hypertension, tachycardia*	Deepen anesthesia	
	IV β-blockade	Esmolol, 20–100 mg, +50–200 µg/kg/min PRN
		Metoprolol, 0.5–2.5 mg
		Labetalol, 2.5–10 mg
	IV nitroglycerin	Nitroglycerin, 33–330 µg/min†
Normotension, tachycardia*	Ensure adequate anesthesia, change anesthetic regimen	
	IV β-blockade	β-blockade, as above
Hypertension, normal heart rate	Deepen anesthesia	
	IV nitroglycerin or nicardipine	Nicardipine, 1–5 mg, +1–10 µg/kg/min
		Nitroglycerin, as above
Hypotension, tachycardia*	IV α-agonist	Phenylephrine, 25–100 µg
		Norepinephrine, 2–4 µg
	Alter anesthetic regimen (e.g., lighten)	
	IV nitroglycerin when normotensive	Nitroglycerin, as above
Hypotension, bradycardia	Lighten anesthesia	
	IV ephedrine	Ephedrine, 5–10 mg
	IV epinephrine	Epinephrine, 4–8 µg
	IV atropine	Atropine, 0.3–0.6 mg
	IV nitroglycerin when normotensive	Nitroglycerin, as above
Hypotension, normal heart rate	IV α-agonist/ephedrine	α-Agonist, as above
	IV epinephrine	Epinephrine, as above
	Alter anesthesia (e.g., lighten)	
	IV nitroglycerin when normotensive	Nitroglycerin, as above
No abnormality	IV nitroglycerin	Nitroglycerin, as above
	IV nicardipine	Nicardipine, as above

Ensure adequacy of oxygenation, ventilation, and intravascular volume status, and consider surgical factors, such as manipulation of heart or coronary grafts.

IV, intravenous; PRN, as needed.

*Tachyarrhythmias (e.g., paroxysmal atrial tachycardia, atrial fibrillation) should be treated directly with synchronized cardioversion or specific pharmacologic agents.

†Bolus doses (25–50 µg) and high infusion rate may be required initially.

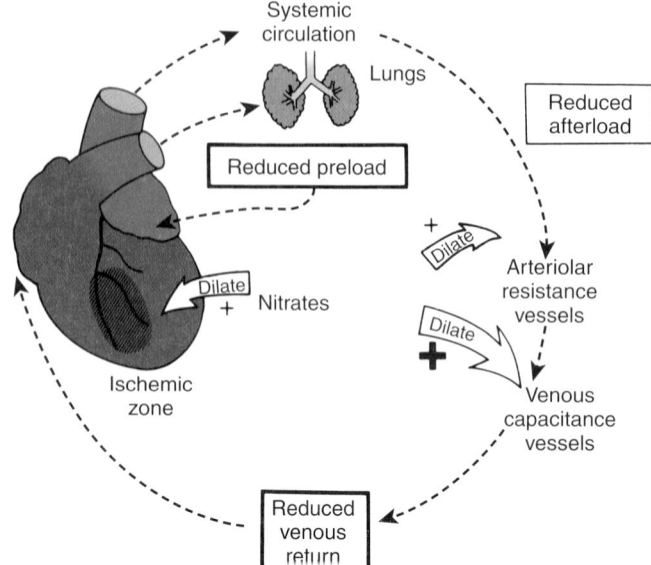

Figure 18-18 The effects of nitrates on the circulation include prominent venodilation and reduction of preload. Afterload is decreased because of mild arteriolar dilatation. Coronary dilation also occurs to benefit the ischemic myocardium. *(From Opie LH: Drugs and the heart. II. Nitrates. Lancet 1:750, 1980.)*

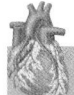

BOX 18-5.   INTRAOPERATIVE USE OF INTRAVENOUS NITROGLYCERIN

Hypertension > 20% above control values
Pulmonary capillary wedge pressure > 18 to 20 mm Hg
AC and V waves > 20 mm Hg
ST changes > 1 mm
New regional wall motion abnormalities on transesophageal echocardiography
Acute right ventricular or left ventricular dysfunction
Coronary artery spasm

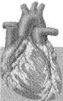

BOX 18-6.   USES OF INTRAVENOUS NITROGLYCERIN ON TERMINATION OF CARDIOPULMONARY BYPASS

- Increased pulmonary capillary wedge pressure
- Increased systemic vascular resistance or pulmonary vascular resistance
- Incomplete revascularization
- Ischemia
- Intraoperative myocardial infarction
- Coronary artery spasm
- Infusion of oxygenator reservoir volume

of circulating NTG during CPB. After revascularization, NTG is used to treat residual ischemia or coronary artery spasm and reduce preload and afterload. It may be combined with vasopressors (e.g., phenylephrine) to increase the CPP when treating coronary air embolism (Box 18-6).

Studies of the prophylactic role of NTG in preventing perioperative myocardial ischemia have shown mixed results, with most studies showing no effects of NTG infusions on the incidence of perioperative myocardial ischemic events.[520–522] In a prospective, double-blinded, placebo-controlled study, Zvara et al[523] randomized patients undergoing CABG surgery using a fast-track anesthesia technique to 2 µg/kg/min NTG or placebo starting before induction and continuing until 6 hours after extubation in the ICU. They found a similar incidence, severity of symptoms, and duration of myocardial ischemia, regardless of whether the patients received NTG or placebo (37% vs. 35%, respectively). Even though there were more patients in the placebo group with positive enzymes and ECG signs of myocardial infarction, these findings

were not statistically significant. Similarly, in a prospective, randomized, controlled study, 0.5 to 1 µg/kg/min NTG administered after aortic cross-clamp release in patients undergoing CABG surgery did not decrease the incidence of postoperative myocardial ischemia.[524]

Intravenous NTG has been compared with other vasodilators such as nitroprusside and the calcium channel blockers during CABG and in other clinical situations. Kaplan and Jones[525] demonstrated that NTG was preferable to nitroprusside during CABG. Both drugs were shown to control intraoperative hypertension and to decrease myocardial oxygen consumption; however, NTG improved ischemic changes on the ECG, but nitroprusside did not. The lack of improvement in the ischemic ST segments with nitroprusside was thought to result from a decrease in CPP or the production of an intracoronary steal. When NTG was compared with calcium channel blockers in patients undergoing CABG surgery, the results depended on the class of calcium channel blocker, the usage of arterial conduits, and the administered doses.

Calcium Channel Antagonists

The calcium antagonists are a structurally diverse group of drugs that inhibit the passage of calcium through the slow channels of the cell membrane. These agents collectively relax arterial smooth muscle, with little effect on most venous beds. Despite areas of commonality, however, the calcium antagonists differ in their actions and hemodynamic effects. For example, nifedipine acts primarily on vascular smooth muscle, with little effect on the atrioventricular node. In contrast, verapamil acts mainly on the cardiac conduction system and has less effect on vascular smooth muscle and the myocardium. Neither diltiazem nor verapamil has been found to significantly increase CBF or to consistently decrease coronary vascular resistance. Verapamil and diltiazem have been shown to produce significant hemodynamic changes with myocardial depression and conduction disturbances during anesthesia.[526,527] This limits their use in the treatment of perioperative myocardial ischemia. Nevertheless, the perioperative use of nicardipine and recent studies with clevidipine showing a reduced incidence of cardiac events in patients who received calcium antagonists during cardiac surgery have led to an increased interest in this diverse group of drugs in patients presenting for CABG or OPCAB surgery.[528,529]

Calcium antagonists have been found to be cardioprotective against reperfusion injury. This is due to their energy-saving actions of negative inotropy and chronotropy. These antagonists also have been shown to reduce reperfusion arrhythmias and attenuate myocardial stunning. In a review of methods to reduce ischemia during OPCAB, Kwak[530] included the calcium antagonists along with newer drugs such as NO-releasing agents, free radical scavengers, and Na^+/H^+ exchange inhibitors in the management of ischemia/reperfusion injury.

Nicardipine is a short-acting dihydropyridine calcium antagonist similar to nifedipine, but possessing a tertiary amine structure in the ester side chain. Nicardipine is stable as a parenteral solution and, therefore, can be administered intravenously.[531] It has highly specific modes of action, which include coronary antispasmodic and vasodilatory effects and systemic vasodilation. Among the calcium antagonists, nicardipine is unique in its consistent augmentation of CBF and its ability to induce potent and more selective vasodilator responses in the coronary bed than in the systemic vascular bed. Other important hemodynamic effects include reductions in BP and SVR, and increases in myocardial contractility and CO.[532,533] Nicardipine also produces minimal myocardial depression and significant improvement in diastolic function in patients with ischemic heart disease.[534,535] Intravenous doses of 5 to 10 mg of nicardipine administered to patients with CAD produce therapeutic plasma levels. Plasma concentrations decline in a biphasic manner, with an initial half-life of 14 minutes and a terminal half-life of 4.75 hours.[536] Clearance of nicardipine results mainly from its metabolism by the liver, and excretion is primarily through bile and the feces. It undergoes rapid and extensive first-pass hepatic metabolism with the production of inactive metabolites.

The rapid onset and cessation of action of nicardipine make it an attractive drug for the perioperative management of hypertension or myocardial ischemia.[537] It has been administered to control hemodynamics during and after vascular surgery and CABG. Begon et al[538] demonstrated that 5 mg of nicardipine was effective in treating intraoperative hypertension. The MAP decreased by 35%, with the peak onset of action in 6 minutes and duration of action of 45 minutes. Van Wezel et al[539] used a 3 to 12 μg/kg/min infusion of nicardipine and compared it with a 1 to 3 μg/kg/min infusion of nitroprusside.

Both drugs were found to be equally effective in controlling BP; however, there was a 24% incidence rate of ST-segment depression in the nitroprusside group versus 9% in the nicardipine group. Van Wezel et al[540] also compared intravenous NTG with intravenous administration of verapamil or nifedipine in patients undergoing CABG. NTG was found to be the drug of choice because it controlled BP while not producing as much tachycardia (as nifedipine) or myocardial depression and conduction blockade (seen with verapamil). Apostolidou et al[541] randomized patients undergoing CABG surgery with CPB to nicardipine (0.7 to 1.4 μg/kg/min), NTG (0.5 to 1 μg/kg/min), or placebo. Immediately after coronary revascularization (after aortic cross-clamp release until end of surgery), there were significantly fewer episodes of myocardial ischemia in the nicardipine group (0% vs. 10% vs. 24%, respectively). During the following postoperative period, there was no difference regarding myocardial ischemia among the drug groups. Apart from preventing myocardial ischemia, nicardipine effectively controls arterial hypertension in the postoperative period.[542,543] From these studies, nicardipine appears to offer significant advantages over other drugs such as nitroprusside in the intraoperative and postoperative management of hypertension and myocardial ischemia after CABG surgery.

More recently, clevidipine has been introduced for the treatment of perioperative hypertension.[544] Clevidipine is an ultrashort-acting intravenously administered dihydropyridine calcium channel blocker. Clevidipine acts as an arterial-selective vasodilator, and its action is rapidly terminated by blood and tissue esterases. In a randomized, double-blinded, placebo-controlled multicenter trial in patients undergoing cardiac surgery, clevidipine effectively reduced arterial blood pressure.[545] The Evaluation of Clevidipine In the Perioperative Treatment of Hypertension (ECLIPSE) trial compared clevidipine with NTG, sodium nitroprusside, and nicardipine for acute hypertension treatment in cardiac surgery patients.[546] Clevidipine effectively maintained the arterial blood pressure within a prespecified range. Compared with nitroprusside, clevidipine-treated patients had a significantly reduced mortality ($P = 0.04$).

Esmolol

Hypertension, tachycardia, arrhythmias, and myocardial ischemia from sympathetic stimulation are common occurrences in the perioperative period. Despite the benefits of early use of β-blockers in the treatment of myocardial ischemia, the relatively long half-life and prolonged duration of action of previously available β-blockers have limited their usefulness during surgery and the immediate postoperative period.[547] The introduction of esmolol, an ultrashort-acting cardioselective $β_1$-blocker with a half-life of 9 minutes because of rapid esterase metabolism, provides a β-blocker that is extremely useful in the perioperative period. Esmolol has been shown to be effective in treating patients with acute unstable angina or during acute coronary occlusion. A mean esmolol dose of 17 ± 16 mg/min, with a range of 8 to 24 mg/min, was found to be effective in alleviating chest pain while increasing CO in patients with unstable angina.[548] LV diastolic function was shown to improve with β-blockade. Kirshenbaum et al[549] showed that esmolol was effective in treating acute myocardial ischemia even in patients with poor LV function (increased PCWP of 15 to 25 mm Hg). Esmolol was infused in these patients in doses up to 300 μg/kg/min and produced decreases in HR, BP, and CI. However, the PCWP was not significantly altered by the drug infusion. These results suggested that even in the presence of moderate LV dysfunction, esmolol can safely reduce BP and HR in patients with acute myocardial ischemia. During percutaneous transluminal coronary angioplasty, esmolol also was found to reduce the amount of ST-segment elevation and the onset of RWMAs.[550] Esmolol has been used during CABG in a prophylactic manner to prevent hypertension, tachycardia, and myocardial ischemia.[551] Before the introduction of newer stabilizing mechanical devices, it had been used frequently during OPCAB procedures to slow the HR during the surgical procedure. Esmolol also has been used to treat intraoperative hypertension, tachycardia, and myocardial ischemia. Bolus doses of 1.5 mg/kg have been found to be effective in treating ST-segment changes in patients with CAD.[552] More commonly, a smaller bolus dose is used and is combined with an infusion of esmolol. Bolus doses ranging from 0.5 to 1.0 mg/kg have been used, followed by infusions of 50 to 300 µg/kg/min.[553] These doses have been found to effectively treat increases in HR that occur during surgery and to block the β-adrenergic effects of catecholamines associated with surgical stress. In patients with poor LV function, doses as small as 20 mg have been found to be effective.

Weaning Patients from Cardiopulmonary Bypass after Coronary Revascularization

Chapter 32 provides a detailed discussion about the various predictors and techniques of weaning a patient successfully from CPB. Some factors and concerns are more specific to patients undergoing myocardial revascularization. Obviously, a good surgical technique, not only in the quality of anastomoses, but in preserving the heart during aortic cross-clamping, is key to cardiac function immediately after separation from CPB. The administration of cardioplegia can be problematic in patients with CAD, and various techniques are used including a combination of antegrade and retrograde cardioplegia. In patients with normal preoperative function, minimal, if any, inotropic support is usually required. In patients with impaired ventricular function, TEE evaluation immediately before weaning off CPB can provide invaluable information in choosing an inotropic or vasoconstrictive agent. In patients who present to the operating room with an IABP inserted, this support typically is continued into the postoperative period. In patients with poor ventricular function, the insertion of an IABP to support ventricular function during weaning from CPB can be helpful.[554,555]

Immediate Postoperative Period

Sedation

Patients usually are sedated to facilitate transport to the ICU and in the immediate postoperative period until extubation criteria are fulfilled. α₂-Adrenergic receptor agonists such as dexmedetomidine, as well as propofol, are intravenously administered agents with favorable properties in this setting.

α_2-Adrenergic receptor agonists have unique properties (Box 18-7) that explain their increasing use in cardiac surgical patients. Although the FDA approved clonidine in 1974, it was available only as an oral formulation in the United States, limiting its widespread use. In 1999, the FDA approved dexmedetomidine for continuous (up to 24 hours) intravenous sedation in the ICU setting. It is seeing increasing use in the operating room and ICU settings. Dexmedetomidine is a more selective α_2-adrenoceptor agonist than clonidine (approximately eight times greater). It exhibits both central sympatholytic and peripheral vasoconstrictive effects. Intravenous infusion of dexmedetomidine (0.2 to 0.7 µg/kg/hr) causes transient increases of MAP and SVR because

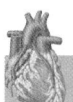

BOX 18-7. α_2-AGONIST PROPERTIES

- Sedation
- Anxiolysis
- Analgesia
- Hemodynamic stability
- Central sympatholytic effect
- Decreased blood pressure and heart rate
- Decreased perioperative oxygen consumption
- Decreased plasma catecholamine levels
- Decreased incidence of tachyarrhythmias
- Facilitation of diuresis
- Prevention of histamine-induced bronchoconstriction
- Treatment and prevention of postoperative shivering
- Treatment and prevention of postoperative delirium
- Blunting of withdrawal symptoms in drug and alcohol addicts
- Possible inhibition of inflammatory response

of stimulation of α- and β₂-adrenergic receptors in vascular smooth muscle. This is followed by decreases in MAP, HR, SV, CO, and plasma catecholamine levels.[556,557] Greater doses of dexmedetomidine result in more profound sedation and analgesia with a persistent increase in MAP, SVR, and PAP.[558]

There are limited data from animal studies demonstrating potential coronary vasoconstrictive and cardiodepressant effects.[559–562] However, coronary vasoconstriction was seen mainly with bolus doses of 10 µg/kg and greater. At the recommended loading doses (0.5 to 2 µg/kg) and maintenance (0.2 to 0.7 µg/kg/hr), dexmedetomidine most likely has a favorable effect on myocardial perfusion.[563] Roekaerts et al[564,565] showed an increase in endocardial-to-epicardial blood flow ratio in the postischemic myocardium, with an overall reduction of myocardial oxygen demand after experimentally induced myocardial ischemia in dogs. As expected, the greatest reduction in oxygen demand is seen when baseline HR and arterial BP are increased. Intravenous dexmedetomidine exhibits a rapid distribution phase with a distribution half-life of about 6 minutes. Dexmedetomidine shows high protein binding (94%) and undergoes extensive biotransformation in the liver with direct glucuronidation and cytochrome P450–mediated metabolism. Although dexmedetomidine mainly is excreted renally (95%), no dose adjustments are necessary in patients with renal insufficiency, although slightly prolonged sedation should be expected.[566] Severe hepatic impairment may necessitate a dose reduction.

Dexmedetomidine may be a useful agent in the early postoperative period because its sedative properties are associated with minimal respiratory depression and, in this regard, appear to mimic natural sleep patterns.[567] When administered continuously in postsurgical patients, it caused no statistical differences in respiratory rate, oxygen saturation, arterial pH, and arterial carbon dioxide tension when compared with placebo.[568] These patients usually were effectively sedated but still arousable and cooperative to verbal stimulation.[569] Because of its analgesic properties, it significantly reduced additional opioid analgesia requirements in mechanically ventilated patients in the ICU.[570–572] The α_2-agonists have been used successfully in patients with postoperative delirium and withdrawal symptoms in alcohol or drug addicts, and they are associated with a low rate of shivering.[573,574]

Propofol has been used extensively intraoperatively, as well as for sedation in the ICU. Several studies compared propofol and dexmedetomidine in the postoperative period after surgery. Venn et al[575] randomized a small number of patients to propofol versus dexmedetomidine sedation in the immediate postoperative period. Dexmedetomidine reduced the requirement for opioid analgesia, but importantly for patients after myocardial revascularization, it reduced HR more than propofol, whereas the arterial blood pressure did not differ between the two groups. In a multicenter, randomized study, Herr et al[576] compared a dexmedetomidine-based sedation regimen with propofol sedation after CABG in the ICU. Although there were no differences in time to extubation, the investigators found a significantly reduced need for additional analgesics (i.e., propofol-sedated patients required four times the mean dose of morphine), antiemetics and diuretics and had fewer episodes of tachyarrhythmias requiring β-blockade (ventricular tachycardia in 5% of the propofol-sedated group vs. none in the dexmedetomidine group). In this study, however, hypotension was more common in the dexmedetomidine group compared with the propofol-sedated patients (24% vs. 16%; Figure 18-19). Approximately 25% of the dexmedetomidine-associated hypotension occurred in the first hour of the study (starting at sternal closure), particularly during or within 10 minutes after the loading infusion of 1 µg/kg. The combination of reduction of preload during sternal closure and the loading dose would seem to indicate this was not the optimal manner in which to use this agent. Loading doses are infrequently administered in today's clinical practice to avoid hypotension seen with a large loading dose of dexmedetomidine, but a continuous maintenance dose started earlier to achieve appropriate plasma levels at the time of patient transfer from the operating room.

With regard to patient satisfaction, insufficient data are available to clearly favor one of the two agents. Corbett et al[577] randomized 89 adult

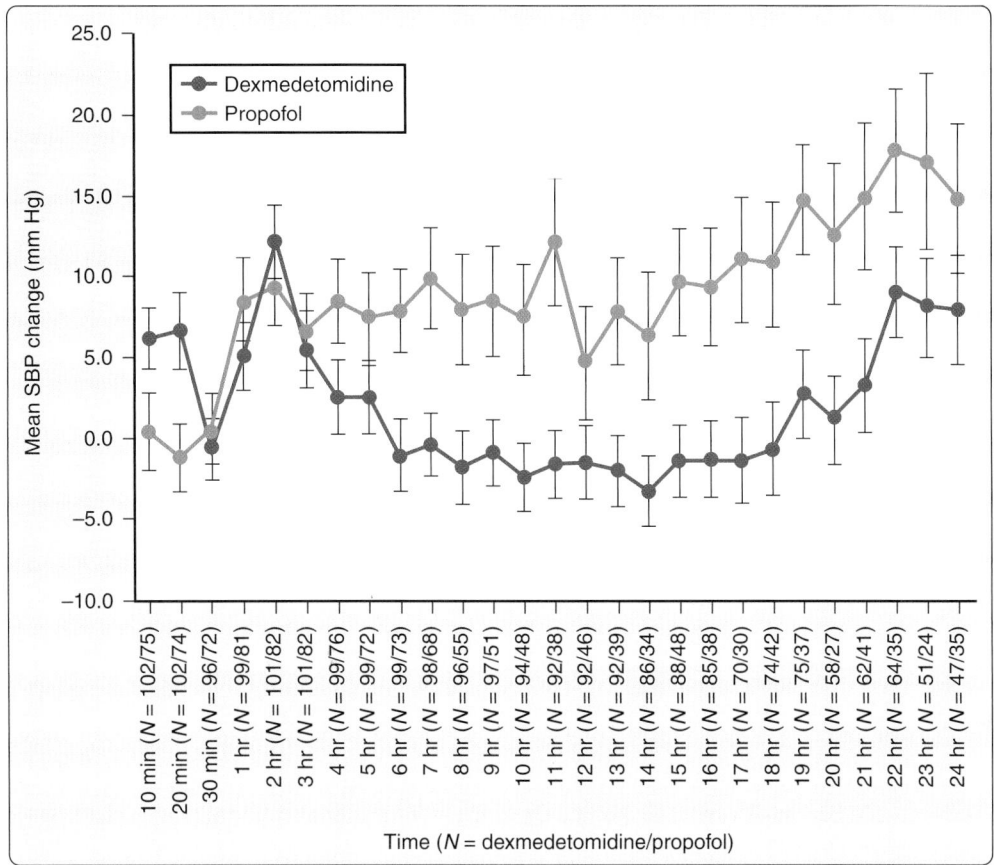

Figure 18-19 Changes from baseline in systolic blood pressure (SBP) between coronary artery bypass grafting (CABG) patients sedated with dexmedetomidine or propofol. The baseline is mean systolic pressure for each treatment group just before sternal closure. Numbers of patients receiving each drug (x-axis) declines progressively as they are extubated after surgery. *(From Herr DL, Sum-Ping ST, England M: ICU sedation after coronary artery bypass graft surgery: Dexmedetomidine-based versus propofol-based sedation regimens. J Cardiothorac Vasc Anesth 17:576, 2003.)*

patients after CABG surgery to either dexmedetomidine or propofol. Patients were interviewed regarding awareness, recall, generalized comfort, level of pain, ability to interact with healthcare providers and family, feelings of agitation and anxiety, ability to sleep and rest, and overall satisfaction with ICU stay. The level of awareness and additional morphine and midazolam requirements did not differ between the groups. Patients favored propofol to sleep and rest, there were more patient discomfort and pain in the dexmedetomidine group, and the authors concluded that dexmedetomidine did not offer any advantages over propofol for short-term sedation after CABG surgery. The increased incidence of pain in the dexmedetomidine group is surprising, and most studies show reduced opioid requirements with α_2-adrenoceptor agonists. Barletta et al[578] compared propofol and dexmedetomidine after CABG and/or valve surgery in a fast-track recovery room setting. Patients (*n* = 100) were matched according to surgery type and left ventricular function. Dexmedetomidine resulted in lower opioid requirements, but this did not result in shorter duration of mechanical ventilation, improved quality of sedation, or rate of adverse events.

In summary, even though there are theoretic advantages to using dexmedetomidine for sedation after CABG surgery, no clear benefits have been documented for either drug, and sedation-related costs are greater with dexmedetomidine administration.

Coronary Artery and Arterial Conduit Spasm

Since 1981, when Buxton et al[579] first reported coronary artery spasm immediately after CABG, there have been numerous descriptions of this problem. Spasm usually has been associated with profound ST-segment elevation on the ECG, hypotension, severe dysfunction of the ventricles, and myocardial irritability. Many hypotheses have been put forward to explain the origin of coronary artery spasm; some of the mechanisms that may play a role are demonstrated in Figure 18-20.[580] The mechanism of postoperative spasm may or may not be the same as that underlying Prinzmetal's variant angina, but the same stimuli seem to be present and therapy is usually effective with a wide range of vasodilators such as NTG, calcium channel blockers, milrinone, or combinations of NTG and calcium channel blockers in both situations. Arterial grafts such as the LIMA, and particularly radial artery grafts, are prone to spasm after revascularization, and its prevention and recognition are crucial to prevent serious complications.[581] He et al[582] tested the reactivity of ring segments of human IMAs in organ baths to various constrictor and dilator agents. It was found that thromboxane was the most potent IMA constrictor, followed by norepinephrine, serotonin, phenylephrine, and potassium chloride. NTG, NO, papaverine, and the calcium channel blockers nifedipine, verapamil, and diltiazem, as well as milrinone, all produced relaxation. In a similar study, Mussa et al[583] observed the vasodilating properties of topically applied phenoxybenzamine. It prevented vasoconstriction with a long-lasting effect (>5 hours) in response to various vasoconstrictors, followed by verapamil/NTG (5 hours) and papaverine (1 hour). In vivo, for prophylaxis of IMA spasm, the calcium antagonists, especially diltiazem, were thought to be as useful as NTG.[584–586]

Nevertheless, prevention and treatment of arterial conduit spasm with diltiazem may cause serious adverse effects such as low CO or conduction abnormalities. Diltiazem is a more expensive drug compared with NTG. Shapira et al[587] showed in vitro (radial artery, IMA, saphenous vein) and in vivo (radial artery) that NTG was a superior vasodilator compared with diltiazem. The same investigators monitored patients undergoing

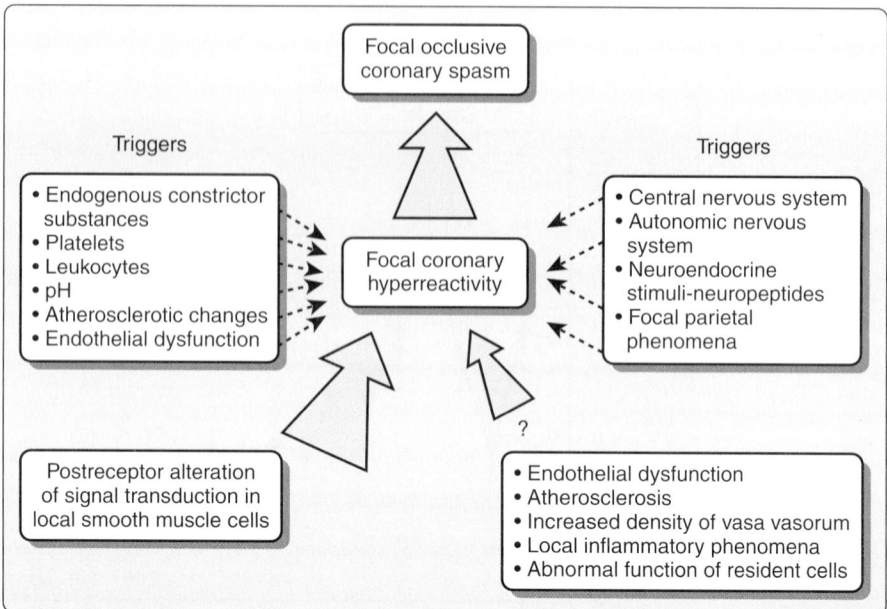

Figure 18-20 Schematic representation of the pathogenesis of coronary artery spasm.

CABG surgery using radial artery grafts who were randomized to receive NTG or diltiazem intravenously after induction of anesthesia followed by an NTG patch or oral diltiazem after surgery for 6 months. There was no significant difference in outcome (morbidity, myocardial infarction, CK-MB) between the two groups. Nevertheless, the 6-month diltiazem treatment was associated with 16-fold greater costs and significantly more patients requiring cardiac pacing compared with NTG (28% vs. 13%, respectively).[588] In a double-blind, randomized study, Mollhoff et al[589] compared milrinone (0.375 μg/kg/min) with nifedipine (0.2 μg/kg/min) in patients with impaired LV function undergoing CABG surgery. ST changes after revascularization (including the use of the IMA graft) indicative of myocardial ischemia occurred in 33.3% of the milrinone group compared with 86.6% in the nifedipine group. Biochemical markers of myocardial damage (CK-MB and troponin I) after 24 hours were significantly greater in the nifedipine group.

Fast-Track Management for Coronary Artery Bypass Grafting Surgery

Efforts to reduce resource consumption for patients undergoing CABG have received considerable attention by a variety of interested payers since the 1990s. With the changing pattern of reimbursement based on the ever-escalating costs of health care, payers have drastically reduced incentives to expend unnecessary resources, with hospitals and clinicians attempting to minimize consumption yet maintain patient safety. The financial pressures are illustrated by the observation that Medicare costs for CABG increased from $2.8 billion in 1990 to $7.3 billion in 1997, whereas case volume increased only 40% during that period. In 1990, Krohn et al[590] reported a study of 240 patients undergoing CABG at a private southern California hospital between 1984 and 1986, describing a clinical pathway emphasizing early extubation, rapid mobilization, intraoperative fluid restriction, and steroid administration. This program was associated with a median postoperative LOS of 4 days and in-hospital mortality rate of only 2%. This program itself was forged out of intense economic competition with the first major incursion of managed care into this area's competitive market. This particular pathway is widely recognized as the first formal report of what is now called *fast-tracking* for cardiac surgery. In a similar time frame, reports from the financially constrained U.K. health care system, in which formal ICU care was "bypassed" based primarily on rapid early extubation (with apparent success), appeared.[591,592] The publicity associated with these reports contributed to Medicare's interest in cost reduction, leading to the Medicare Participating Heart Bypass Center Demonstration

conducted between 1991 and 1996, in which seven participating hospitals agreed to a single sharply discounted rate for CABG (in return for preferential market share, a concept that ultimately has not materialized).[593] Over the 5-year period, it is estimated that $50.3 million dollars were saved. In their summary report, reduction of cost and LOS by retooling processes of care is emphasized (and reducing time to extubation was considered a key factor). In the participating centers, LOS, together with mortality, declined annually despite increased severity of case mix. Observational data by Engelman et al,[594,595] from the Baystate Medical Center of a large case series of fast-track patients, generated additional widespread publicity in the surgical community (particularly among members of the influential Society of Thoracic Surgery).

Although the fast-track clinical pathway encompasses a variety of perioperative (and after-hospital discharge) management strategies, early extubation is the one that has received perhaps the greatest attention (Box 18-8) (see Chapter 33). Because it is a simple, continuous variable (e.g., hours to extubation), it is one that many observational reports, a smaller number of randomized, controlled trials, and meta-analyses have reported to be safe and effective.[596,597] Early extubation is acknowledged as a key component of the fast-track clinical pathway and one that was considered perhaps the most radical change in practice during the peak

BOX 18-8. PERIOPERATIVE GOALS OF FAST-TRACK MANAGEMENT

- Preoperative education
- Same-day admission whenever possible
- Anesthetic technique tailored to early extubation and effective early postoperative analgesia
- Flexibility in the use of recovery areas (e.g., use of postanesthesia care unit instead of an intensive care unit)
- Early extubation incorporating nurse- or respiratory therapist–driven protocols for stable patients
- Early mobilization and removal of catheters, tubes, and similar devices
- Early intensive care unit and hospital discharge for patients meeting criteria
- Early follow-up (e.g., telephone, office visits) after hospital discharge
- Formalized clinical pathway and interdisciplinary continuous quality improvement strategies

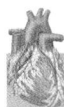

BOX 18-9. SUGGESTED CRITERIA FOR EARLY EXTUBATION

Systemic
1. Body temperature stable and > 36° C or < 38° C
2. Arterial pH > 7.30

Cardiovascular
1. Stable hemodynamics on minimal or decreasing doses of inotrope or vasodilator therapy; cardiac index > 2.0 L/min/m², stable SvO_2, minimal base deficit
2. Stable cardiac rhythm or good response to pacing

Respiratory
1. Spontaneous respiratory rate > 10 to 12 and < 25 to 30, vital capacity > 10 mL/kg, maximal negative inspiratory force > –20 cm H_2O with minimal respiratory support (e.g., low levels of continuous positive airways pressure, pressure support)
2. Adequate arterial blood gases: PaO_2 > 70 to 80 mm Hg (Fio_2 = 0.4 to 0.5), $PaCO_2$ < 40 to 45 mm Hg
3. Chest radiograph without major abnormalities (e.g., minimal atelectasis)

Renal
1. Adequate urine output (non–dialysis-dependent patients), stable electrolytes, and input/output values for patients on preoperative dialysis

Neurologic
1. Awake, alert, cooperative, moving all extremities
2. Adequate motor strength (e.g., hand grip); if not, consider relaxant reversal, especially for patients receiving pancuronium

Surgical
1. Adequate hemostasis with decreasing or stable mediastinal drainage

of scrutiny of the fast-track pathway (middle to late 1990s; Box 18-9). Reports of prolonged ventilatory management after cardiac surgery first appeared in the late 1950s (for valve surgery as CABG was not yet performed), and those from the 1960s (including the first reports of CABG patients) strongly advocated its routine use.[598] This was further emphasized with the adoption of high-dose morphine and, subsequently, fentanyl and sufentanil, at the end of that decade.[599,600]

As early as 1974, the first reports advocating early extubation, primarily by greater reliance on volatile anesthesia, appeared.[601] In 1980, Quasha et al[602] reported the first small, randomized, controlled trial enrolling CABG patients ($n = 38$), in which 89% were extubated in less than 8 hours. Ramsay et al[603] reported a small, randomized, controlled trial ($n = 20$) in which opioid reversal with nalbuphine was used. However, this resulted in an unacceptable increase in postoperative pain. The larger and more rigorous randomized, controlled trial reported by Cheng et al[604] in 1996 ($n = 100$), in which mean time to extubation was 4.1 hours, generally is recognized as the most influential of the contemporary studies of early extubation. Since 1995, reports of successful use of fast-tracking in a variety of patient populations have been reported, including academic,[605,606] private,[607–611] elderly,[612–614] rural settings, and Veterans Affairs patients[615,616] from the United States and many other countries. It now is used as a quality improvement marker in many healthcare systems.[617–619] In some of these, alterations of the traditional models of ICU care have been adopted, although many use routine ICU models, just with shorter stays. It has been clearly pointed out that the ability to maximize the potential of early extubation with regard to saving money and reducing LOS involves close coordination of a particular center's staffing (particularly nursing), which often is not efficient and in many centers remains so.[620,621] Despite these issues, average LOS for CABG has declined substantially (see Chapters 33 and 35).

Based on accumulated data from randomized, controlled trials, the first meta-analyses of early extubation were reported. Myles et al[622] reviewed studies in which fast-tracking was defined as use of reduced opioid dosing (fentanyl ≤ 20 μg/kg) with stated intention to attempt extubation in less than 10 hours after surgery. They identified 10 trials ($n = 1800$), with most involving CABG patients, from 1989 to 2002. As expected, fast-track groups had shorter times to extubation (by 8.1 hours), with no significant differences in major morbidity or mortality and only one instance of reintubation. ICU LOS was reduced by 5.4 hours, although hospital LOS was not shortened.

Hawkes et al[623] reported a meta-analysis from the U.K.-based Cochrane Collaboration. These investigators considered only randomized, controlled trials in which time to extubation was defined as within 8 hours and which specifically evaluated mortality (in ICU, 30 days, and up to 1 year), incidence of postoperative myocardial ischemia (e.g., biomarkers, ECG), and pulmonary outcomes (e.g., reintubation, respiratory dysfunction). Secondary outcomes of ICU and hospital LOS were analyzed. Given their more stringent requirements and predetermined hypotheses for testing, they found only six studies ($n = 871$)[624–629] meeting criteria, and almost half of the patients were from a single study (Reyes et al[628]). That study is unusual because both treatment groups received high-dose fentanyl, in contrast with all other studies of fast-tracking in which opioid doses were deliberately lower. However, exclusion of this study did not alter the findings. Three of the studies excluded patients older than 70 to 75 years, and 144 patients did not undergo CABG (i.e., had valve-only or other cardiac surgery). Most cases were elective (24 urgent or emergent), and all studies excluded patients "at high risk," although the criteria varied among the studies. This analysis also included the "old" study of Quasha et al,[630] which is clearly from a different generation with regard to contemporary processes of care (but is numerically small). Because not all of the studies reported on the specific outcomes of interest, the number of studies for each analysis varied from one to six. With regard to mortality, ICU (four studies) and 30-day mortality (two studies) were no different. One-year mortality was assessed in only one study (no difference). The incidence of postoperative myocardial ischemia (six studies) was not different (although methods for detection of this diagnosis varied). The incidence of early reintubation (1.6%) within 24 hours (four studies) was no different, with two studies having none. Late reintubation after 24 hours (three studies) was no different, with two studies having none and one study having a rate of 1.5%. Consideration of respiratory outcomes was not possible because of variable methodology. Atelectasis did not appear to vary among groups. With regard to secondary outcomes, ICU LOS (four studies) was significantly reduced by 7 hours and hospital LOS (two studies) was significantly reduced by 1.1 days. The study authors described several important issues. No studies have been properly statistically powered to determine whether outcome rates are equivalent, only whether there was no difference. This is a subtle point, but statistical methodology for this requires much larger sample sizes. They also observed that early extubation has become routine clinical practice and further research is needed to evaluate the impact of very early extubation on pain control, stress modification, and long-term outcome (Table 18-6).

It can be seen that the fast-track knowledge base is incomplete with regard to defining all patient subgroups (e.g., who is at high risk for early extubation) despite meta-analyses because these studies cannot always accurately risk-adjust the patient groups. For the anesthesiologist, reintubation is of particular interest. London et al[631] summarized the data and observed that although the rate of early reintubation is very low with fast-track management, the frequency of later reintubation is substantial in many series (up to 6.6%). In a series of Veterans Affairs patients, a group that most clinicians consider to be at high risk for adverse respiratory outcomes because of the high prevalence of chronic obstructive pulmonary disease and smoking, only 1 of 304 fast-track patients was reintubated emergently, but 5% went on to later reintubation.[632] More research is needed to clearly define who is at risk, although female sex and longer periods of initial ventilation (no fast-tracking) have been reported as risk factors.[633,634]

TABLE 18-6 Contemporary Randomized, Controlled Trials of Fast-Tracking in Cardiac Surgery

Study	Inclusion Criteria	Anesthesia	N	Time to Extubation (hr)	Extubated (%)	Reintubation (%)	SICU LOS	Mortality (%)	Comments
Cheng, 1996[64]	Elective CABG, age < 75 yr, first case								
	Early	Fent, Prop, Iso	60	4.1 ± 1.1*	85	1.6	42 ± 12*	0	ICU stats "by criteria"
	Conventional	Fent, Midaz, Iso	60	18.9 ± 1.4	85	0	57 ± 29	5	
Myles, 1997[65]	Elective CABG; low/medium-risk patients								
	Early	Fent (15 µg/kg), Prop	58	9.1 median*	100	NR	22 median	NR	
	Conventional	Enf, Fent (31 µg/kg), Midaz	66	12.3 median	100	NR	22 median	NR	
Reyes, 1997[62]	Low- or intermediate-risk patients; all CABG or valve	All with "high-dose fentanyl", Benzo induction							
	Early	Fent (65 µg/kg)	201	10 median*	60	6.5†	27 median*	9.0	
	Conventional	Fent (67 µg/kg)	203	21 median	74	3.5	44 median	7.4	
Berry, 1998[626]	Elective CABG, low/medium-risk patients								No intent to treat, primary study of ischemia
	Early	Fent (15 µg/kg), Iso	50 (43 analyzed)	1.8 median‡	94	NR	NR	0	No differences in indices of ischemia, including Holter ST
	Conventional	Fent (50 µg/kg), Iso	48 (42 analyzed)	12.6 median	100	NR	NR	2%	
Michalopoulos, 1998[627]	Elective CABG; age < 70 yr, low/medium-risk patients								
	Early	Fent (15–20 µg/kg), Iso or Halo or Prop, Midaz	72	6.3 ± 0.7*	100	0	17 ± 1.3*	0	
	Conventional	Fent (50 µg/kg), Iso or Halo, Midaz	72	11.6 ± 1.3	100	0	22 ± 1.2	0	
Silbert, 1998[62]	Elective CABG; low-risk patients								No intent to treat
	Early	Fent (15 µg/kg), Prop	50 (38 analyzed)	4.0 median*	100	0	NR	2% (of 50)	
	Conventional	Fent (50 µg/kg), Midaz, Prop	50 (42 analyzed)	7.0 median	100	0	NR	2% (of 50)	

Benzo, benzodiazepine; CABG, coronary artery bypass grafting; Enf, enflurane; Fent, fentanyl; Halo, halothane; ICU, intensive care unit; Iso, isoflurane; LOS, length of stay; Midaz, midazolam; NR, not reported; Prop, propofol; SICU, surgical intensive care unit.

*$P \leq 0.05$ between early and conventional groups.
†$P < 0.04$, worse in early group.
‡Statistic not reported.

Despite gaps in knowledge, it is clear that various centers (most often related to a single surgeon with a large-volume practice) have adopted aggressive fast-track programs. Walji et al[635] coined the term *ultrafast-tracking* to describe their practice, reporting a 56% hospital discharge rate by postoperative day 4 (of 258 patients) and 23% discharge by postoperative day 2 (although the readmission rate was 3.9%, albeit with no early mortality). Perhaps most impressive is Ovrum et al's report[636] from Norway on a cohort of 5658 CABG patients, 99% of whom were extubated by 5 hours (median, 1.5 hours), with a 1.1% reintubation rate. More than 99% of patients were transferred to the ward the next morning, and a similar percentage was walking outdoors by postoperative day 7. An impressive in-hospital mortality rate of only 0.4% was reported. Precise time of discharge was not reported, and the study authors observed that readmission (with the exception of deep sternal infections) was not tracked (as it occurred at other hospitals). With the exception of a low incidence of redo patients (1.8%, who are said to have similar times to extubation), the cohort appears similar in risk to U.S. centers (with IMA grafting in 99% and a median of four distal anastomoses). As expected, CPB time was short (median, 55 minutes). With regard to anesthetic management, low-dose diazepam or midazolam (0 to 0.2 mg/kg), fentanyl (4 to 8 µg/kg), pancuronium, isoflurane, or nitrous oxide was used. A PAC was used only in cases of severe cardiac decompensation (precise figure not given, but only 2% received prolonged inotropes or IABP therapy), and TEE was never used. Both reports made the point that their on-pump results were equal to, or even better than, results of many off-pump studies. It will be interesting to see whether with ongoing adoption of OPCAB that these results can be improved further. The lack of advanced monitoring in the Ovrum series would appear to put pressure on academic anesthesia to continue to rigorously explore the efficacy of advanced monitoring for CABG.

CORONARY ARTERY BYPASS GRAFTING WITHOUT CARDIOPULMONARY BYPASS

Introduction and Surgical Considerations

Although the term *off-pump coronary artery bypass* (OPCAB) encompasses a range of surgical approaches (based on the degree of invasiveness encompassing full, limited, or no sternotomy), the technique that is most commonly performed is OPCAB with a full sternotomy. The precise number of such procedures performed remains in the 20% to 30% range. Surgeons appear to adopt it either enthusiastically or not at all. Although the literature base (incorporating a large number of observational series and a smaller number of true randomized, controlled trials) is increasing rapidly, the final word about difference in outcome and which patients may benefit from an OPCAB technique is still years away (given several large ongoing randomized, controlled trials).[637-639] The clinician will immediately notice that the pace and tempo of anesthetic management differs substantially from that of conventional CABG. The focused involvement of the anesthesiologist is perhaps more important in OPCAB than during on-pump CABG, especially in cases where immediate extubation is planned in the operating room.[640]

Although OPCAB is perceived as a contemporary development, surgery on the beating heart was first performed in the 1950s and early 1960s, preceding the widespread use of CPB-based CABG because of the slower development and application of CPB techniques in the late 1960s. In the late 1980s and early 1990s, introduction of the short-acting β-blocker esmolol led some surgeons to "experiment" with OPCAB (on the LAD) by reducing the HR. However, it was not until the mid- to late 1990s when surgical researchers developed efficient mechanical stabilizer devices that minimized motion around the anastomosis site (independent of HR) that this technique became widespread. The ability to expose the posterior surface of the heart to access the posterior descending and the Cx vessels using suction devices usually placed on the apex of the heart, pericardial retraction sutures, slings, or other techniques, without producing major hemodynamic compromise, was

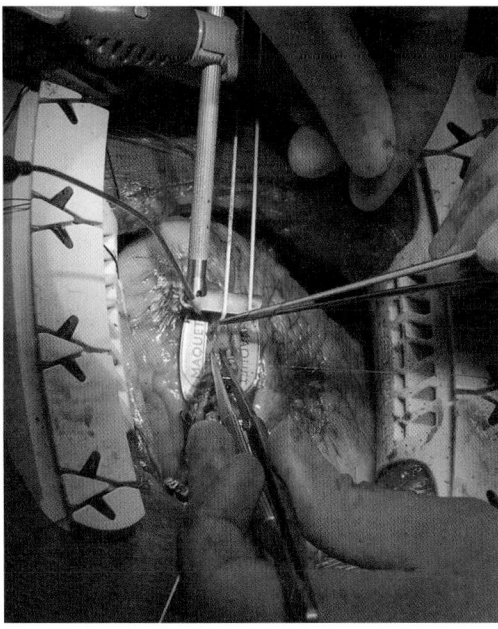

Figure 18-21 Left anterior descending (LAD) artery anastomosis during off-pump coronary artery bypass grafting using a left internal mammary artery (LIMA) graft. The view is from the head of the patient. The Maquet mechanical stabilizer (MAQUET, Wayne, NJ) is in place together with vascular snare sutures used to transiently occlude the artery. The LIMA is being anastomosed to the LAD, assisted by use of pressurized and heavily humidified carbon dioxide ("mister blower" metal cannula) to facilitate visualization of the vessel lumen. (*Courtesy of Alexander Mittnacht, MD, Mount Sinai School of Medicine, New York, NY*)

critical for multivessel application of this technique. This commonly is referred to as *verticalization*, in contrast with *displacement* for the LAD and diagonal anastomoses (Figures 18-21 to 18-23).

OPCAB extends the range of surgeon-induced hemodynamic changes the anesthesiologist encounters relative to routine CABG. The skilled cardiac anesthesiologist must be able to anticipate and communicate with the surgeon to minimize the adverse impact of these changes on the heart and other important organs. The surgical manipulations involve a variety of geometric distortions of cardiac anatomy (e.g., compression of the RV[641] and, to a lesser degree, some distortion of the mitral valve annulus[642]). The magnitude of distortion varies with the patient's individual anatomy (most notably the size and shape of their right and left ventricles), the skill of the surgeon in placement of stabilizer devices, use of "deep" pericardial stay sutures (which facilitate forward superior apical displacement for LAD anastomosis), and manipulation of the pleural space (e.g., right pleural incision to create space for the compressed RV). With a skilled surgeon, the changes usually are modest or easily treated with the Trendelenburg position, use of vasoconstrictors or inotropes, and judicious volume expansion. However, severe changes because of acute ischemia, mitral regurgitation, or unrecognized right ventricular compression may occur, necessitating emergent conversion to CPB.

Cardiovascular Effects of Off-Pump CABG

Evaluation of the hemodynamic consequences of OPCAB involves the two independent variables of distortion of the right or left atria and ventricles by stabilizer and suspension devices, and the effects of myocardial ischemia induced by vessel occlusion during anastomosis. Grundeman et al[641] have investigated hemodynamics, CBF, and echocardiographic changes with use of the suction cup Octopus stabilizer systems (Medtronic, Minneapolis, MN) during verticalization to 90 degrees and anterior displacement of the posterior wall (as would be used to access Cx vessels during OPCAB) in an anesthetized and

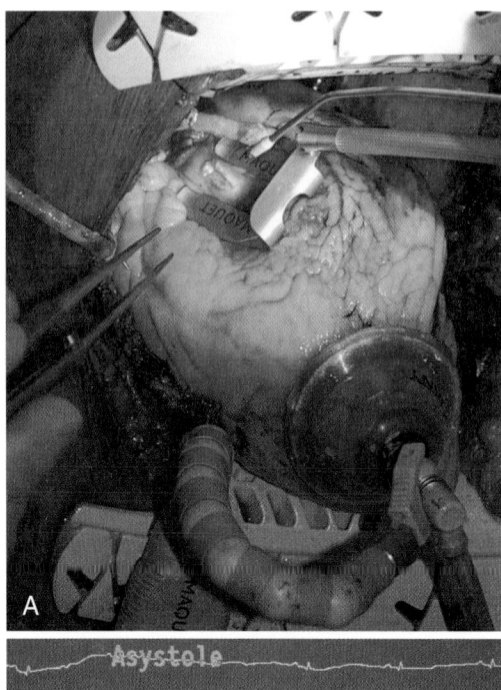

B

Figure 18-22 *A*, Image depicting posterior descending artery (PDA) anastomosis during off-pump coronary artery bypass grafting using a saphenous vein graft. The view is from the head of the patient. The Maquet access device (MAQUET, Wayne, NJ) uses suction to position the heart (verticalization) for easy access to the inferior surface of the left ventricle. The stabilizer is in place, and the anastomosis to the PDA is being performed. *B*, Image depicts characteristic electrocardiographic (ECG) tracing during verticalization of the heart to facilitate exposure of the PDA for anastomosis during off-pump coronary artery bypass grafting. Heart manipulations modify the positional relation between the heart and surface electrodes. Therefore, the shape of the tracing is altered and the amplitude is reduced. The low-voltage ECG is interpreted by the device as asystole, an audible alarm sounds, and the practitioner is alerted with "Asystole" next to the ECG tracing. *(Courtesy of Alexander Mittnacht, MD, Mount Sinai School of Medicine, New York, NY.)*

β-blocked pig model. With the stabilizer alone, they found significant reductions in SV (44% reduction), CO (32%), MAP (26%), and HR (26%) that were corrected with 20% head-down tilt. They also evaluated CBF in the three major coronary distributions using flow probes.[643] With a 42% decrease in CO, coronary flow was reduced in all three distributions, with the greatest decline in the Cx distribution (50%). However, with Trendelenburg position, the changes largely were ameliorated. Placement of an omniplane TEE probe between the two arms of the Octopus stabilizer demonstrated substantial compression of the RV, with a decrease in diastolic cross-sectional area of 62%, but the LV area declined by only 20% (Figure 18-24). No valvular incompetence was observed, and institution of right-heart CPB restored all hemodynamic parameters; LV bypass had only marginal effects. This documents the importance of compression of the thin-walled, low-pressure RV in hemodynamic compromise during OPCAB. They also reported on use of the Starfish apical suction device (Medtronic, Minneapolis, MN) using this pig model.[644,645] They observed substantially fewer hemodynamic changes, with only a 6% reduction in SV and 5% reduction in MAP, no reduction in coronary flows, and approximately 30% increases in RVEDPs and LVEDPs. With institution of Trendelenburg position, mild overshoot in SV and MAP occurred, with greater increases in RVEDP and LVEDP, suggesting that this maneuver is not required. Using a sheep model, Porat et al[646] demonstrated significant hemodynamic benefits using a right-heart internal cannula system that

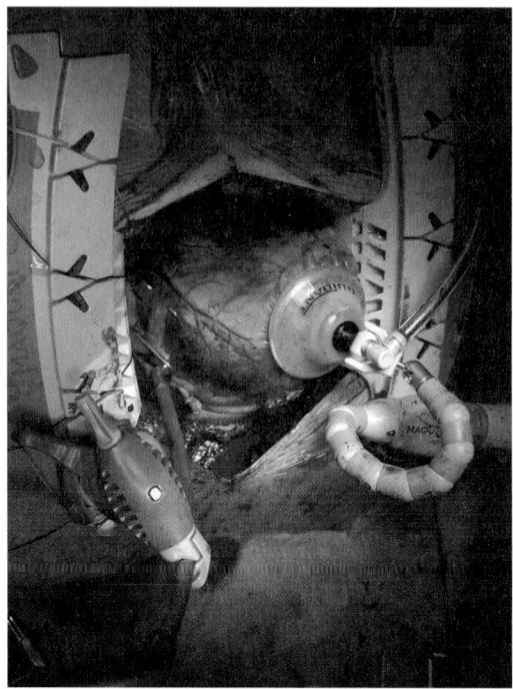

Figure 18-23 Image depicting the first obtuse marginal (OM1) anastomosis during off-pump coronary artery bypass grafting using a saphenous vein graft. View is from the head of the patient. The previously completed left internal mammary artery to left anterior descending anastomosis is seen. The Maquet access device (MAQUET, Wayne, NJ) uses suction to position the heart (verticalization) for easy access to the circumflex coronary artery system. *(Courtesy of Alexander Mittnacht, MD, Mount Sinai School of Medicine, New York, NY.)*

expels blood from the right atrium into the pulmonary artery, bypassing the compressed RV (increasing CO and MAP with reduction in CVP by 49%).

Human Clinical Data

Hemodynamic effects in human clinical series have been reported primarily using routine monitoring (e.g., PAC, TEE, Svo$_2$), although several have used more sophisticated methods (RVEF, pressure-volume loops).[647,648] Most of the data have been obtained from patients with normal or only mildly depressed ventricular function without significant valvular disease. Mathison et al[649] measured RVEDPs and LVEDPs in 44 patients (i.e., using catheters inserted through the pulmonary veins, as is done for LV venting, and by pulling back the PAC during measurements for the RV). They evaluated the effects of displacement with the Octopus stabilizer in Trendelenburg position. RVEDP increased in each position, with the greatest increase with exposure of the Cx vessels (Figue 18-25). This position was associated with the greatest deterioration of SV (approximately 29% vs. 22% for PDA and 18% for LAD). When comparing patients with EFs of more than or less than 40%, there were nonsignificant trends toward greater reductions in MAP and CO with lower EF. TEE, used in 31 patients, revealed moderate-to-severe biventricular compression with CX and PDA positioning. Nierich et al[650] reported on use of the Octopus stabilizer in a larger cohort (*n* = 150 patients, including 54 patients with anterolateral thoracotomy exposure undergoing LAD or diagonal anastomosis only). Although only routine hemodynamics was presented, this study also evaluated hemodynamic effects during the actual surgical anastomotic period. Stroke volume decreased 6% with LAD, 14% with RCA, and 21% with obtuse marginal anastomoses. Trendelenburg position was required in only 50% of LAD anastomoses, increasing to 100% with obtuse marginal anastomosis. Dopamine was used in only 5% of LAD anastomoses, increasing to 30% with obtuse marginal anastomoses (Figure 18-26).

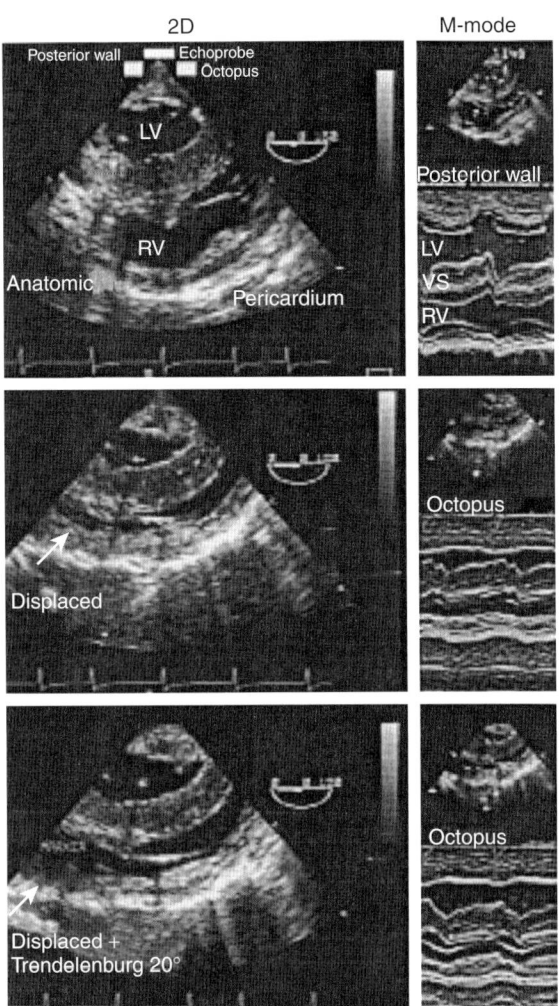

2D   M-mode

Figure 18-24 Alteration in right ventricular (RV) and left ventricular (LV) chamber sizes with verticalization of the heart and subsequent Trendelenburg positioning in a porcine open chest model obtained from a transesophageal echocardiographic probe placed between the two arms of a stabilizer device on the posterior wall. Two-dimensional *(left)* and M-mode images *(right)* are displayed. *(From Grunderman PF, Borst C, Verlaan CW, et al: Exposure of circumflex branches in the tilted, beating porcine heart: Echocardiographic evidence of right ventricular deformation and the effect of right or left heart bypass. J Thorac Cardiovasc Surg 118:316, 1999.)*

Mishra et al[651] have reported large-scale, prospective observational data on patients undergoing OPCAB at a tertiary center in New Delhi. TEE and PAC were used in all patients and approximately 40% were considered high risk. In contrast with some of the smaller studies mentioned earlier, the degree of hemodynamic compromise was greater. In their first report of 500 patients, verticalization for exposure of the posterior wall was associated with a reduction in MAP by 18%, increase in CVP by 66%, reduction in SV by 36%, and CI by 45%. New RWMAs were common (60%), and global function decreased in a similar proportion. Their practice involved use of inotropes during this period (79% vs. 22% for the anterior wall). However, only 11% required IABP, and 0.7% required CPB; in-hospital mortality rate was 1.2%. They reported on predictors of need for IABP or conversion to CPB in an additional 500 patients (4.8% of patients). On multivariate analysis, an EF less than 25%, myocardial infarction within the prior month, congestive heart failure, and preoperative hemodynamic instability (the latter was only marginally significant) were identified. The in-hospital mortality rate for the latter 500 patients was only 0.8%.

Specific Anesthetic Considerations in Patients Undergoing Off-Pump Coronary Artery Bypass

The anesthesia technique in patients undergoing OPCAB surgery does not differ much from on pump coronary artery surgery (Box 18-10). The anesthesia technique should be tailored to the individual patient and, among other factors, also depends on the indication for OPCAB surgery. Patients with advanced age, significant ascending aortic disease, poor LV function, and multiple comorbidities may be scheduled for OPCAB surgery to avoid aortic cross-clamping, and a single LIMA-to-LAD anastomosis is performed. These patients may not be ideal for ultra-fast-track anesthesia. If the surgeon routinely performs OPCAB revascularization, early ICU and hospital discharge is frequently a goal associated with OPCAB surgery,[652,653] particularly in patients with adequate LV function. Consequently, fast-tracking with or without a neuraxial anesthesia technique is being used frequently. A neuraxial technique often is administered for postoperative analgesia or as the primary anesthetic technique, or both. A challenge during OPCAB surgery can be the hemodynamic changes encountered during positioning of the heart. Pulmonary artery and PCWP, as well as CVP, typically are increased during this phase; the occurrence of large v-waves should alert the practitioner to acute ischemia, mitral regurgitation, or both. Wall motion abnormalities and acute significant mitral regurgitation frequently are seen on TEE. Exacerbation or new onset of mitral regurgitation may be related to structural changes from positioning the heart and/or stabilizer application, or from ischemia.[654,655]

Hemodynamic compromise during OPCAB surgery can be managed with Trendelenburg position, volume administration, and temporary vasoconstrictor administration to maintain CPP during distal anastomosis. Opening of the right pleural space may accommodate the RV, relieving the compression with hemodynamic improvement. Maintaining the CPP is critical during distal coronary anastomosis. Depending on the severity of the lesion and the degree of collateralization, ischemia and RWMAs can be seen. In poorly collateralized vessels, severe hemodynamic compromise may result from clamping the target vessel. Vasoconstrictor and volume therapy are preferred with inotrope use only with severe hemodynamic compromise. In the setting of ongoing ischemia, the greater increase in oxygen demand with inotropes may place the patient at substantial risk for myocardial injury. In the setting of significant mitral regurgitation not responsive to anti-ischemic treatment, however, further increasing the afterload may worsen the clinical picture. Positive inotropic medications are then temporarily indicated if the surgeon cannot correct the position of the heart during critical phases of surgical anastomosis. The surgeon may or may not place temporary intracoronary shunts to allow distal coronary perfusion. However, there are controversial data and opinions whether shunts have a clinical benefit in providing myocardial protection or rather cause endothelial damage.[656–658]

CPB should always be immediately available during OPCAB in case the hemodynamic situation cannot be managed pharmacologically. A lower arterial blood pressure typically is preferred during the proximal (aortic) anastomosis to avoid complications seen with partial aortic clamping (aortic side-clamp). Automated suture devices also are being used, as well as techniques that eliminate any aortic cross-clamp.[659–661] Regardless of the specific technique/device used, the MAP should be kept around 60 mm Hg during this phase. Vasodilators such as NTG are frequently administered and titrated to achieve this goal. Because CPB with a heat exchanger is not available for maintaining a certain target temperature, patients are at increased risk for hypothermia during OPCAB surgery. This is particularly problematic if fast-tracking with early extubation is the goal. The room temperature should be adjusted accordingly, as well as patient warming devices applied.

Anticoagulation in patients undergoing OPCAB surgery is an area of controversy and always should be discussed with the surgeon before anesthesia induction. Some surgeons prefer low-dose heparinization

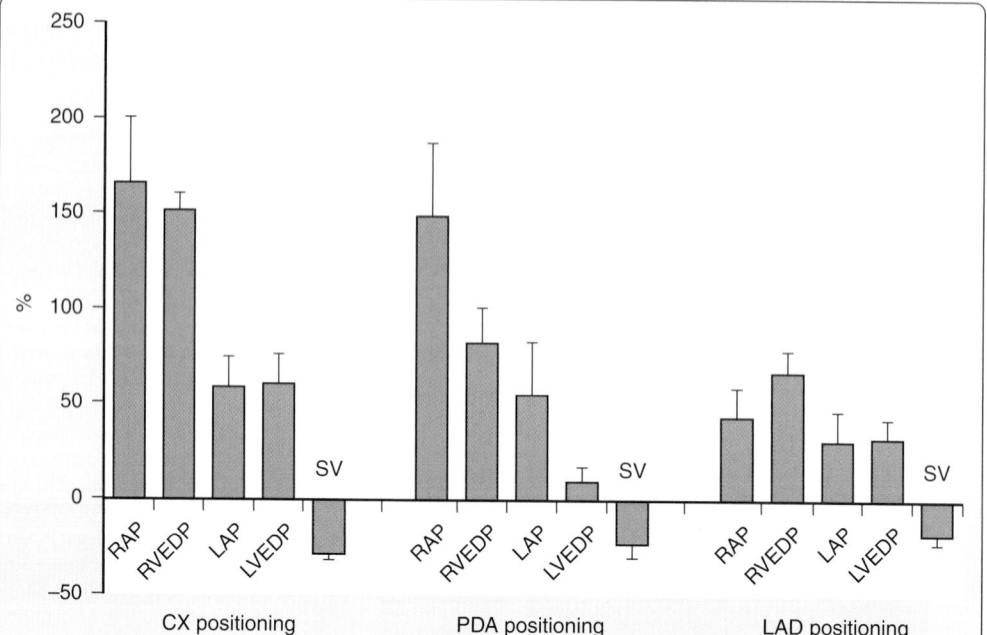

Figure 18-25 Hemodynamic changes (mean ± standard error) with off-pump coronary artery bypass (OPCAB) grafting and cardiac positioning with application of the stabilizer in 44 patients. CX, circumflex artery; LAD, left anterior descending artery; LAP, left atrial pressure; LVEDP, left ventricular end-diastolic pressure; PDA, posterior descending artery; RAP, right atrial pressure; RVEDP, right ventricular end-diastolic pressure; SV, stroke volume. *(From Mathison M, Edgerton JR, Horswell JL, et al: Analysis of hemodynamic changes during beating heart surgical procedures. Ann Thorac Surg 70:1355, 2000, by permission of the Society of Thoracic Surgeons.)*

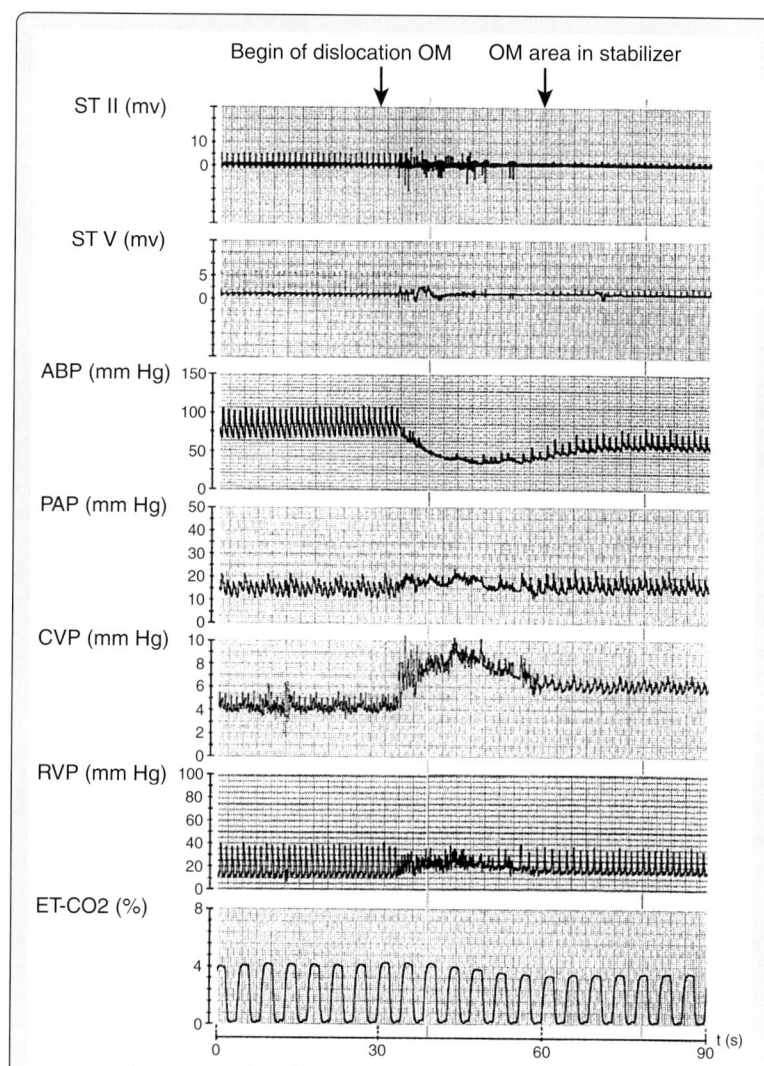

Figure 18-26 Acute hemodynamic alterations during verticalization and placement of a stabilizer in an actual patient demonstrating reduction in electrocardiographic voltage, wedging of the pulmonary artery catheter, decrease of end-tidal carbon dioxide (ET-CO$_2$), and increase in central venous pressure (CVP). Changes partially resolve after stabilizer placement. ABP, arterial blood pressure; OM, obtuse marginal arteries; RVP, right ventricular pressure. *(From Nierich AP, Diephuis J, Jansen EW, et al: Heart displacement during off-pump CABG: How well is it tolerated? Ann Thorac Surg 70:466, 2000, by permission of the Society of Thoracic Surgeons.)*

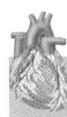

> **BOX 18-10. ANESTHETIC CONSIDERATIONS FOR OFF-PUMP CORONARY ARTERY BYPASS SURGERY**
>
> 1. Standard monitoring including invasive arterial blood pressure monitoring and central venous access.
> 2. A pulmonary artery catheter (PAC) currently is inserted in most patients undergoing OPCAB surgery.
> 3. Unless there are contraindications, transesophageal echocardiography (TEE) is recommended in all patients undergoing OPCAB surgery.
> 4. The use of warming devices to maintain normothermia is recommended.
> 5. Dosing of heparin for OPCAB cases is controversial, with centers using full- or low-dose regimens.
> 6. Fast-tracking, including early extubation, is often a goal in OPCAB surgery.
> 7. A neuraxial anesthesia technique may be used for postoperative analgesia and/or as the primary anesthetic technique. Potent antiplatelet regimens frequently are administered in these patients, however, and neuraxial techniques have to be planned accordingly and may even be contraindicated.
> 8. Hemodynamic compromise may be seen with positioning of the heart and/or stabilizer application. Positional maneuvers, volume administration, and vasoactive medications are used to maintain hemodynamic stability. Cardiopulmonary bypass always should be immediately available.

(e.g., 100 to 200 U/kg heparin) with a target activated coagulation time of 250 to 300 seconds, whereas others may choose full heparinization (e.g., 300 U/kg) during the procedure. The activated coagulation time is measured every 30 minutes and heparin administered accordingly to maintain the target activated coagulation time. Patients who are immobilized, undergoing major surgery, are hypercoagulable and at increased risk for thrombotic events. The major concern in OPCAB surgery is early graft occlusion with potentially catastrophic consequences including sudden cardiac death after revascularization. For that reason, some surgeons continue antiplatelet medications until the day of surgery, and newer, more potent drugs such as clopidogrel may be reinstituted immediately after the procedure. When planning the anesthesia technique, it is, therefore, important to follow current recommendations for neuraxial catheter placement in patients on anticoagulant medications. A neuraxial technique may not be feasible or may even be contraindicated.

Outcomes in Off-Pump Coronary Artery Bypass Grafting

Several investigators and working groups have comprehensively reviewed outcomes in patients undergoing OPCAB.[662,663] Raja and Dreyfus[664] have reviewed observational and randomized trials, scoring efficacy of OPCAB by levels of literature evidence on outcomes related to various organ systems and processes of care. Although this grading must be considered informal (given lack of a formal consensus panel of experts), it mirrors results obtained from a meta-analysis of randomized trials by Cheng et al.[637] These investigators analyzed 37 randomized trials of 3369 patients with comparable treatment groups with the exception of a marginal difference in number of grafts performed (2.6 OPCAB vs. 2.8 CABG). All but one of the studies *specifically* excluded "high-risk" patients. Although various definitions were used, most excluded patients with low EF, redo procedures, and renal failure, and several studies excluded patients with diseased Cx vessels. As expected, not all studies reported on all outcomes. The investigators found no significant differences in 30-day or 1- to 2-year mortality, myocardial infarction, stroke (30 day and 1 to 2 years), renal dysfunction, need for IABP, wound infection, or reoperation for bleeding or

reintervention (for ischemia). OPCAB was associated with significant reductions in atrial fibrillation (OR – 0.58), numbers of patients transfused (OR = 0.43), respiratory infections (OR – 0.41), need for inotropes (OR = 0.48), duration of ventilation (weighted mean difference of 3.4 hours), ICU LOS (weighted mean difference of 0.3 day), and hospital LOS (weighted mean difference of 1.0 day). Changes in neurocognitive dysfunction were not different in the immediate postoperative period; they were significantly improved at 2 to 6 months (OR = 0.57), but there were no differences seen at 12 months. The critical issue of graft patency was addressed in only four studies, and these varied substantially with regard to when this was assessed (3 months in two and 12 months in two). Only one study reported a difference (reduction in Cx patency with OPCAB). Because of the small numbers of patients, the overall data for this category were considered inadequate for meta-analysis.

Four randomized, controlled trials have analyzed quality of life. Various methods precluded inclusion in the meta-analysis, but it generally appears there is little difference between operations. Of the 20 trials reporting conversion rates, 8% of OPCAB patients required conversion to CABG, whereas only 1.7% were converted from CABG to OPCAB. The conversion rate for OPCAB in these low- to medium-risk patients is substantial and would be expected to be even greater in higher-risk patients with greater disease burdens, more complex lesions, or impaired ventricular function in whom tolerance of stabilization and verticalization may be less. The anesthesiologist must be prepared for rapid institution of CPB at all times. This comprehensive analysis suggested that for every 1000 patients undergoing OPCAB, 91 fewer patients would experience development of atrial fibrillation, 143 fewer would require transfusion, 83 fewer would require inotropes, 53 fewer would acquire respiratory infections, 100 fewer would have cognitive dysfunction at 2 to 6 months after surgery, and there would be 300 fewer ICU days and 1000 fewer hospital days. The neutral findings regarding stroke, renal failure, myocardial infarction, and mortality are surprising but may be found to be different in higher-risk patients once additional data are accumulated in high-risk trials.

A working group of the American Heart Association's Council on Cardiovascular Surgery and Anesthesia analyzed the current literature and several small meta-analyses, but not that of Cheng et al discussed earlier.[637] In an informal manner, they concluded that OPCAB probably is associated with less bleeding, less renal dysfunction, less short-term neurocognitive dysfunction (especially in patients with calcified aortas), and shorter hospital LOS. However, they also observed that it is more technically demanding, has a greater "learning curve," and may be associated with lower rates of long-term graft patency.[666] Perhaps related to the greater technical demands, surgeons appear to place fewer grafts relative to on-pump CABG, and incomplete revascularization could influence long-term outcomes. They emphasize the ongoing need for large-scale, randomized study data.

The fact that OPCAB surgery is technically more demanding and requires a significant learning curve was highlighted recently when Shroyer et al[667] published the results of their prospective randomized study on on-pump versus off-pump CABG surgery in the *New England Journal of Medicine,* with significant media attention. The authors reported worse composite outcomes and poorer graft patency in the off-pump group. This study was criticized, however, for inadequate surgeon experience with off-pump technique (only a minimum of 20 cases experience was required for study participation), a conversion rate to on-pump of 12.4% (<1% with experienced surgeons[668]) with associated higher mortality,[669] and a greater rate of incomplete revascularization in the OPCAB group. In addition, the 2203 patients were almost exclusively male (female patients are higher-risk patients who have been shown to benefit from OPCAB[670]). When patients who were converted to on-pump were excluded from the analysis, there was no significant difference in 1-year primary end-point outcome.

Puskas et al[671] recently reviewed 12,812 CABG patients (1997 to 2006) and compared in-hospital major adverse events and long-term survival after off-pump (OPCAB) versus on-pump CABG surgery. Long-term (10-year follow-up) outcome did not differ significantly between on-pump and off-pump patients. OPCAB was associated with significant reductions in short-term outcomes such as operative mortality, stroke, and major adverse cardiac events. Further data analysis showed that short-term outcome (operative mortality) did not differ between the two groups in patients at low risk (STS predicted risk for mortality), whereas lower mortality was found for OPCAB surgery in high-risk patients.[672] Female sex was associated with greater rates of death, stroke, myocardial infarction, and other major adverse cardiac events. Women undergoing OPCAB surgery had a lower mortality compared with on-pump CABG.

In summary, there are now increasing data showing that OPCAB surgery can be performed safely and may benefit certain patient populations. Remaining concerns are incomplete revascularization, especially in patients with poor targets, and the significant learning curve and surgeon experience required. Patient selection is critical in obtaining good results. With ongoing technologic advances, it is likely this approach will continue to expand in numbers of patients and surgical complexity.

MINIMALLY INVASIVE CORONARY ARTERY SURGERY

Minimally invasive direct coronary artery bypass (MIDCAB) surgery was first reported in 1967 with a limited left thoracotomy and LIMA-to-LAD graft on a beating heart.[673] In the more than four decades that have passed since the publication of this case series, coronary artery surgery via a midline sternotomy has become the most commonly used approach for surgical coronary artery revascularization. Especially in the earlier years of cardiac surgery, this involved a large midline incision with associated complications such as wound infection and brachial plexus injury. Less-invasive techniques were sought and developed with the goal of avoiding such complications, faster patient recovery, earlier hospital discharge, and improved patient satisfaction (e.g., cosmetically more appealing incision). Some of the following terminology is a sample of what is commonly being used to describe the various surgical approaches.

The original term MIDCAB refers to LIMA takedown and anastomosis to the LAD via a small anterior thoracotomy (Figure 18-27).[674–676] This can be performed off-pump or on-pump with femoral CPB cannulation. Thoracoscopic and robotic techniques have been developed to avoid chest wall retraction and associated complications.[677–679] Because of limited access to the coronary artery system using this approach, this procedure is often combined with percutaneous revascularization using coronary stents (hybrid procedures) (see Chapter 26).[680]

Totally endoscopic coronary revascularization describes complete surgical revascularization via small chest wall incisions using thoracoscopic instruments and a robot to access coronary lesions that are

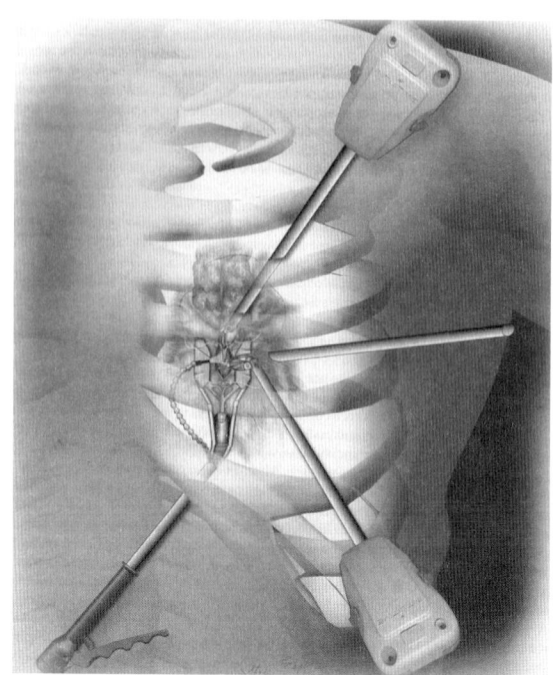

Figure 18-28 Totally endoscopic coronary artery revascularization on the beating heart: The stabilizer is inserted through a subxiphoid incision.

not in close proximity to the chest wall incision (Figure 18-28).[681] This can be performed with or without CPB, the latter called *beating heart totally endoscopic coronary revascularization.*[682] Finally, endoscopically-assisted CABG has been developed to avoid the high costs associated with robotic use.[683] In place of expensive robotic equipment, endoscopically-assisted CABG uses a thoracoscope and nondisposable instruments to harvest the LIMA. The coronary anastomosis is performed on a beating heart. The advantages, as well as problems, encountered with the earlier mentioned various minimally invasive techniques go beyond the scope of this text and have been published extensively elsewhere. Proper patient selection and experience of the surgeon are crucial in obtaining good results.[684] The following paragraphs describe specific anesthetic considerations for patients presenting for minimally invasive coronary artery surgery.

Most minimally invasive coronary artery surgery techniques are technically more demanding and require the surgical team, together with the anesthesiologist, to plan the exact approach including the type and location of surgical incision, on-pump versus off-pump, patient access during surgery (especially in robotic surgery), and goal of fast-tracking including early extubation and adequate pain relief. Although a fast-track anesthesia technique often is preferred, anesthesia induction and maintenance do not differ from a midline sternotomy approach (Box 18-11). One important difference is the requirement for lung deflation on the side of surgical incision during a beating heart minimal thoracotomy or thoracoscopy approach. Lung separation techniques, including a double-lumen tube and bronchial blockers with a standard endotracheal tube, have been described.[685–687] Alternatively, jet ventilation has been reported to facilitate surgical access.[688] An additional challenge compared with thoracic surgery with one-lung ventilation is the thoracic insufflation of CO_2, which is required for intrathoracic surgical instrument manipulation and access to surgical anastomosis on the heart, and its hemodynamic consequences. The insufflation pressures are typically kept below 10 to 15 mm Hg; nevertheless, significant increases in CVP and PAP typically are noted.[689–691] RWMAs have been described with thoracic insufflation,[692] as well as decreased CO at greater insufflation pressures.[693] Fluid is administered to counteract some of these intrathoracic positive-pressure–related changes but is limited by the surgeon often requesting a relatively underfilled

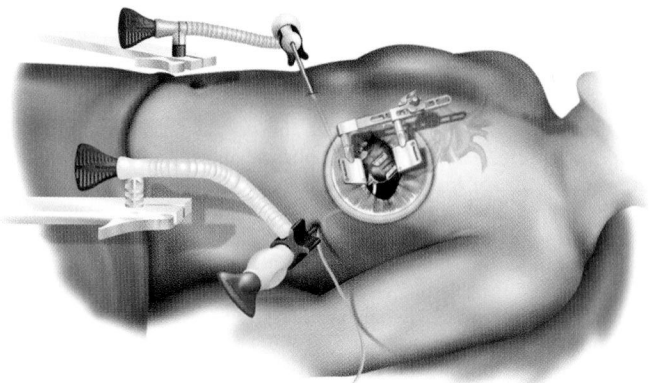

Figure 18-27 Stabilization of the left anterior descending artery with a commercial retractor during small thoracotomy revascularization (MICS CABG illustration: Octopus® Neuro Stabilizer and Starfish® NS Heart Positioner, Meditronic, Inc., Minneapolis, MN.)

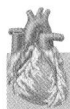

BOX 18-11. ANESTHETIC CONSIDERATIONS FOR MINIMALLY INVASIVE CORONARY ARTERY SURGERY

1. Fast-track anesthesia technique including adequate postoperative pain management.
2. Intraoperative monitoring should include central venous access, invasive arterial pressure monitoring, transesophageal echocardiography (TEE), and in more complex multivessel coronary artery revascularization, benefits of pulmonary artery catheter (PAC) monitoring may outweigh risks (no data available).
3. Defibrillator pads are mandatory and need to be placed with regard to the exact location of surgical incision.
4. Lung separation may be required if the procedure is performed off-pump.
5. Intrathoracic CO_2 insufflation can cause hemodynamic changes and needs to be monitored carefully.
6. Frequently, hemodynamic changes need to be counteracted with positional maneuvers, volume administration, and inotropic and/or vasoconstrictive support.
7. In prolonged procedures, measurements of adequate body perfusion and oxygen balance should be performed frequently.
8. Emergency conversion to on-pump procedure and/or emergency sternotomy may be required.

heart to facilitate surgical anastomosis. Vasoconstrictor (e.g., norepinephrine, vasopressin) agents, as well as drugs with more pronounced positive inotropic effects (e.g., dobutamine, epinephrine, milrinone, dopamine), are frequently added to maintain hemodynamic stability. Urine output, plasma lactate, and Svo_2 should be monitored frequently, especially during long procedures. If hemodynamic stability cannot be maintained, or in the setting of acute hemodynamic compromise including uncontrolled surgical bleeding, the use of femoral-femoral CPB cannulation and prompt initiation of CPB can be lifesaving. Any otherwise unexplained increase in end-tidal CO_2 should alert the practitioner to increased CO_2 absorption from the positive pressure thoracic insufflation. Sudden decreases in end-tidal CO_2 have been described with positive pressure CO_2 insufflation in different settings and, if encountered, should alert the practitioner to possible massive CO_2 embolization.[694,695]

Because of the hemodynamic changes associated with thoracic inflation and prolonged one-lung ventilation in these often long surgical cases, adequate monitoring of hemodynamic, as well as oxygenation parameters, is considered prudent.[696] TEE is recommended, and even though outcome data are lacking, a PAC catheter is inserted in the majority of cases, especially if more than a single-vessel LIMA anastomosis is planned. Complete minimally invasive revascularization in multivessel CAD can be time-consuming, and some centers routinely monitor Svo_2 and CO continuously with specific PACs for early detection of LCOS and decreased tissue perfusion. Access to the heart is limited, and defibrillator pads have to be placed before the patient is positioned and draped. This is further complicated by interference with surgical instruments and left chest wall incisions, and the defibrillator pad position may have to be modified accordingly. Because possible advantages often cited are early patient mobilization and hospital discharge, fast-track anesthesia is often part of the perioperative management strategy. It has long been recognized that a midline sternotomy is less painful for most patients compared with even a small thorascopic incision with chest wall retraction. Adequate pain management is, therefore, mandatory in achieving fast-tracking goals in these patients.[697] Nerve blocks including intercostal blocks or thoracic paravertebral blocks can smooth the transition into the postoperative period.

CONCLUSIONS

Anesthesia for myocardial revascularization continues to evolve rapidly, with advances in surgical approach and technique, anesthetic pharmacology, and monitoring technologies, as well as basic science, clinical, and epidemiologic research. Considerable healthcare resources are consumed by revascularization procedures relative to other medical therapies. Yet, an urgent need exists to better control hospital costs and LOS. Since the 1990s, major changes in practice have occurred with high-dose opioid-benzodiazepine anesthesia being replaced by fast-tracking with volatile anesthesia and early extubation. This has been followed by an increase in OPCAB and minimally invasive revascularization procedures in a variety of forms with which fast-track anesthesia appears well suited. The once routinely used PAC is now used less commonly, but TEE use continues to increase, with its strong emphasis in training programs and by organizations such as the Society of Cardiovascular Anesthesiologists. Regional anesthesia for CABG and OPCAB has enjoyed a resurgence in interest, although use of thoracic epidurals in the United States remains low. Anesthesiologists increasingly are involved in perioperative issues before and after surgery with active surgical and hybrid operating teams. Cardiac anesthesiologists will continue to see sicker and more interesting cases, and the well-prepared and engaged anesthesiologist will be a strong component of successful surgical interventions for many years to come.

 ## Case 1

Acute LAD Rupture during Percutaneous Coronary Angioplasty

Framing

A 58-year-old man presented to the emergency room with severe chest pain radiating to his left arm. It was not relieved by nitroglycerin. His past medical history included hypertension, diabetes mellitus type 2, and chronic renal insufficiency. An EKG performed in the emergency room demonstrated ST-elevation in the anterior leads, V2-V4. The patient was taken to the cardiac catheterization laboratory for revascularization. Coronary angiography demonstrated almost complete occlusion of the proximal left anterior descending coronary artery (LAD). An attempt was made to perform a percutaneous coronary angioplasty including intracoronary stent placement at the site of the LAD blockage. During the course of the procedure the patient's condition suddenly deteriorated and an acute LAD rupture was noted. A pericardial drain and an intraaortic balloon pump (IABP) were placed. The patient was rushed to the operating room with ongoing mechanical and pharmacological resuscitation. Emergency cardiopulmonary bypass (CPB) was established via the femoral vein and artery, and emergency coronary artery bypass graft (CABG) performed. The patient was successfully weaned from CPB and was transferred to the intensive care unit from where he was discharged later without any apparent neurological sequelae.

Data Collection and Interpretation

Regional wall motion abnormalities (RWMAs) are typically seen during myocardial ischemia. It has been demonstrated that these changes in regional myocardial function correlate with specific coronary perfusion defects, can be seen shortly after the onset of ischemia, and may occur even before any ECG changes are noticed. Echocardiographic criteria that describe cardiac function and in particular myocardial wall motion have been established and are usually reported as wall motion inward (radial shortening) and thickening during systole. Normal myocardial thickening during contraction is defined as greater than 30%, with less than 10% being the cut-off for severe. Intraoperatively, transesophageal echocardiography (TEE) can be used to assess global cardiac function as well as RWMA and monitor for new onset RWMAs as an early sign of myocardial ischemia. In the presented case, acute dissection of the LAD was accompanied by severe hemodynamic compromise. The initial TEE images obtained after the patient was transferred to the OR can be seen in Video 1. The transgastric midpapillary short-axis view is usually recommended for myocardial ischemia monitoring because wall segments supplied by all three main coronary arteries are displayed. This patient shows RWMAs in the LAD distribution area with akinesis of the anteroseptal and midpapillary segments. Further TEE views are shown demonstrating RWMAs in the whole LAD distribution, including more basal and apical anterior segments. Following coronary revascularization and discontinuation from CPB, the anterior wall segments are still severely hypokinetic.

Conclusion

Intraoperative TEE monitoring can help detect myocardial ischemia by monitoring for new-onset RWMAs. TEE can guide therapeutic decisions and response to treatment, and may therefore have prognostic implications in patients undergoing surgery for myocardial revascularization.

Case 2

Patient Presenting for OPCAB Surgery with Poor Ventricular Function

Framing

A 72-year-old female presented with three-vessel coronary artery disease (CAD) for off-pump coronary artery bypass grafting (OPCAB). Aside from her coronary artery disease, she had a 30-pack/year history of cigarette smoking, chronic obstructive pulmonary disease (COPD), arterial hypertension, diabetes mellitus type 2, and chronic renal insufficiency. Her preoperative cardiac catheterization report showed three-vessel CAD, no significant left main disease, moderately depressed LV function with an EF estimated to be 30%, and mildly elevated left ventricular end-diastolic pressure. The patient had been referred for coronary artery revascularization and scheduled for OPCAB surgery. After uneventful anesthesia induction, a transesophageal echocardiography (TEE) probe was inserted for intraoperative hemodynamic monitoring. A total of three venous grafts and a left internal mammary graft to the left anterior descending (LAD) artery were performed. The patient was transferred to the intensive care unit, from which she was discharged later without any apparent neurological sequelae.

Data Collection and Interpretation

TEE is recommended for all cardiac surgery cases, including OPCAB surgery. Although positional maneuvers during the various anastomoses can interfere with optimal imaging of the heart, TEE can still provide invaluable information, including volume status, global function and new onset regional wall motion abnormalities, new onset mitral regurgitation, and response to therapeutic interventions. In the presented case, the initial TEE images obtained after general anesthesia had been induced and an endotracheal tube had been inserted, which can be seen in Video 2. The transgastric midpapillary short-axis view is usually recommended for myocardial ischemia and hemodynamic monitoring because wall segments supplied by all three main coronary arteries are displayed and loading conditions can be easily estimated. Video 2 shows severe RWMAs in the LAD as well as right coronary artery (RCA) distribution area, with akinesis of the inferior, anteroseptal, and anterior midpapillary segments. The overall cardiac function was moderate-to-severely depressed. Cardiac output was determined with a thermodilution technique (pulmonary artery catheter) and measured as a cardiac index of 1.4 L/min/m². The surgeon requested a continuous intravenous infusion of milrinone (0.35 mcg/kg/min), which resulted in improved cardiac output. Systemic arterial pressure was maintained with a continuous norepinephrine infusion (0.03 mcg/kg/min). Fluid was administered to compensate for surgical blood loss and guided mostly by TEE estimates of left ventricular end-diastolic area. Intracardiac pressure readings during patient positioning (e.g., Trendelenburg) and vertical displacement of the heart during posterior-

descending coronary artery anastomosis did not correlate well with TEE findings. Following coronary artery revascularization, significantly improved global and regional wall motion function can be seen on TEE examination.

Conclusion

Intraoperative TEE monitoring is recommended in patients presenting for OPCAB surgery. TEE can guide therapeutic decisions and response to treatment, and therefore may have prognostic implications in patients undergoing surgery for myocardial revascularization.

Case 3

Patient Presenting for CABG Surgery with a History of Myocardial Infarction with Residual Left Ventricular Myocardial Aneurysm

Framing

A 47-year-old male was referred for coronary artery bypass grafting (CABG) surgery. He had a history of myocardial infarction 2 years prior for which he underwent percutaneous coronary intervention with multiple intracoronary stents. His other past medical history included insulin-dependent diabetes, poorly controlled arterial hypertension, and obesity. On follow-up cardiac catheterization in-stent stenosis was found, in addition to aneurysmal appearance of the left ventricle at the site of the original myocardial infarction. The overall ventricular function was reported to be mildly depressed. The patient was referred for further surgical management, including CABG surgery and possible aneurysmectomy. After uneventful anesthesia induction, a transesophageal echocardiography (TEE) probe was inserted for intraoperative hemodynamic monitoring and assessment of ventricular function. A total of 4 venous grafts as well as left internal mammary graft to left anterior descending (LAD) artery were performed. The patient was successfully weaned off cardiopulmonary bypass on minimal inotropic support (3 mcg/kg/min dobutamine) and transferred to the intensive care unit, from which she was discharged later without any apparent neurological sequelae.

Data Collection and Interpretation

TEE is recommended for all cardiac surgery cases including CABG surgery. TEE can provide invaluable information, including volume status, global function and new onset regional wall motion abnormalities, new onset mitral regurgitation, and response to therapeutic interventions. In the presented case, the initial TEE images obtained after general anesthesia had been induced and an endotracheal tube had been inserted can be seen in Video 3. The transgastric midpapillary short-axis view usually is recommended for myocardial ischemia and hemodynamic monitoring because wall segments supplied by all three main coronary arteries are displayed, and loading conditions can be easily estimated. Video 3 shows mildly depressed LV function in the transgastric midpapillary short-axis view. The midpapillary anterior myocardium seems thinned out. Additional views include the transgastric 2-chamber view and the transgastric long-axis view. The full extent of the left ventricular myocardial aneurysm can now be appreciated. Although the basal segments are spared, the myocardium is aneurysmal and thinned out, particularly starting in the midpapillary anterior and anteroseptal wall segments extending towards the apex. The aneurysmal wall is akinetic without thickening or radial shortening. No thrombus can be seen and the surgeon decided to proceed without aneurysmectomy.

Conclusion

Intraoperative TEE monitoring is recommended in all patients presenting for cardiac surgery. TEE can guide therapeutic decisions and response to treatment, and therefore may have prognostic implications in patients undergoing surgery for myocardial revascularization.

REFERENCES

1. The American Heart Association Committee and Stroke Statistics Subcommittee: Heart disease and stroke statistics 2010 update, *Circulation* 121:e1–e170, 2010.
2. American Heart Association: *Heart disease and stroke statistics—2004 update*, Dallas, TX, 2004, American Heart Association.
3. Maynard C, Sales AE: Changes in the use of coronary artery revascularization procedures in the Department of Veterans Affairs, the National Hospital Discharge Survey, and the Nationwide Inpatient Sample, 1991–1999, *BMC Health Serv Res* 3:12, 2003.
4. Mack MJ, Brown PP, Kugelmass AD, et al: Current status and outcomes of coronary revascularization 1999 to 2002: 148,396 surgical and percutaneous procedures, *Ann Thorac Surg* 77:761, 2004.
5. DeFrances C, Hall M: *National Hospital Discharge Survey, Advance Data from Vital and Health Statistics (Publication no. 342)*, Hyattsville, MD, 2004, National Center for Health Statistics.
6. Nakagawa Y, Nakagawa K, Sdringola S, et al: A precise, three-dimensional atlas of myocardial perfusion correlated with coronary arteriographic anatomy, *J Nucl Cardiol* 8:580, 2001.
7. Wei K, Kaul S: The coronary microcirculation in health and disease, *Cardiol Clin* 22:221, 2004.
8. Factor SM, Okun EM, Minase T, et al: The microcirculation of the human heart: End-capillary loops with discrete perfusion fields, *Circulation* 66:1241, 1982.
9. Panting JR, Gatehouse PD, Yang GZ, et al: Abnormal subendocardial perfusion in cardiac syndrome X detected by cardiovascular magnetic resonance imaging, *N Engl J Med* 346:1948, 2002.
10. Egashira K, Inou T, Hirooka Y, et al: Evidence of impaired endothelium-dependent coronary vasodilatation in patients with angina pectoris and normal coronary angiograms, *N Engl J Med* 328:1659, 1993.
11. Rajappan K, Rimoldi OE, Dutka DP, et al: Mechanisms of coronary microcirculatory dysfunction in patients with aortic stenosis and angiographically normal coronary arteries, *Circulation* 105:470, 2002.
12. Malek AM, Alper SL, Izumo S: Hemodynamic shear stress and its role in atherosclerosis, *JAMA* 282:2035, 1999.
13. Tian G, Dai G, Xiang B, et al: Effect on myocardial perfusion of simultaneous delivery of cardioplegic solution through a single coronary artery and the coronary sinus, *J Thorac Cardiovasc Surg* 122:1004, 2001.
14. Virmani R, Burke AP, Farb A, et al: Pathology of the unstable plaque, *Prog Cardiovasc Dis* 44:349, 2002.
15. Fuster V, Moreno PR, Fayad ZA, et al: Atherothrombosis and high-risk plaque, *J Am Coll Cardiol* 46:937, 2005.
16. Yeghiazarians Y, Braunstein JB, Askari A, et al: Unstable angina pectoris, *N Engl J Med* 342:101, 2000.
17. Virmani R, Burke AP, Farb A, et al: Pathology of the unstable plaque, *Prog Cardiovasc Dis* 44:349, 2002.
18. Shah PK: Pathophysiology of coronary thrombosis: Role of plaque rupture and plaque erosion, *Prog Cardiovasc Dis* 44:357, 2002.
19. Naghavi M, Libby P, Falk E, et al: From vulnerable plaque to vulnerable patient: A call for new definitions and risk assessment strategies. Part II, *Circulation* 108:1772, 2003.
20. Naghavi M, Libby P, Falk E, et al: From vulnerable plaque to vulnerable patient: A call for new definitions and risk assessment strategies. Part I, *Circulation* 108:1664, 2003.
21. Dawood MM, Gutpa DK, Southern J, et al: Pathology of fatal perioperative myocardial infarction: Implications regarding pathophysiology and prevention, *Int J Cardiol* 57:37, 1996.
22. Cohen MC, Aretz TH: Histological analysis of coronary artery lesions in fatal postoperative myocardial infarction, *Cardiovasc Pathol* 8:133, 1999.
23. Ellis SG, Hertzer NR, Young JR, et al: Angiographic correlates of cardiac death and myocardial infarction complicating major nonthoracic vascular surgery, *Am J Cardiol* 77:1126, 1996.
24. Hoffman JI: Maximal coronary flow and the concept of coronary vascular reserve, *Circulation* 70:153, 1984.
25. DeFily DV, Chilian WM: Coronary microcirculation: Autoregulation and metabolic control, *Basic Res Cardiol* 90:112, 1995.
26. Hoffman JIE: Transmural myocardial perfusion, *Prog Cardiovasc Dis* 29:429, 1987.
27. Canty JM Jr: Coronary pressure-function and steady-state pressure-flow relations during autoregulation in the unanesthetized dog, *Circ Res* 63:821, 1988.
28. Hoffman JI: Autoregulation and heart rate, *Circulation* 82:1880, 1990.
29. Boudoulas H, Lewis RP, Rittgers SE, et al: Increased diastolic time: A possible important factor in the beneficial effect of propranolol in patients with coronary artery disease, *J Cardiovasc Pharmacol* 1:503, 1979.
30. Schwartz JS: Effect of distal coronary pressure on rigid and compliant coronary stenoses, *Am J Physiol* 245:H1054, 1983.
31. Brown BG, Bolson EL, Dodge HT: Dynamic mechanisms in human coronary stenosis, *Circulation* 70:917, 1984.
32. Gregg DE, Patterson RE: Functional importance of the coronary collaterals, *N Engl J Med* 303:1404, 1980.
33. Bache RJ, Dymek DJ: Local and regional regulation of coronary vascular tone, *Prog Cardiovasc Dis* 24:191, 1981.
34. Becker LC: Conditions for vasodilator-induced coronary steal in experimental myocardial ischemia, *Circulation* 57:1103, 1978.
35. Buffington CW, Davis KB, Gillispie S, et al: The prevalence of steal-prone coronary anatomy in patients with coronary artery disease: An analysis of the Coronary Artery Surgery Study Registry, *Anesthesiology* 69:721, 1988.
36. Cohn PF: Prognosis in exercise-induced silent myocardial ischemia and implications for screening asymptomatic populations, *Prog Cardiovasc Dis* 34:399, 1992.
37. Deanfield JE, Maseri A, Selwyn AP, et al: Myocardial ischaemia during daily life in patients with stable angina: Its relation to symptoms and heart rate changes, *Lancet* 2:753, 1983.
38. Chierchia S, Gallino A, Smith G, et al: Role of heart rate in pathophysiology of chronic stable angina, *Lancet* 2:1353, 1984.
39. Chierchia S, Lazzari M, Freedman B, et al: Impairment of myocardial perfusion and function during painless myocardial ischemia, *J Am Coll Cardiol* 1:924, 1983.
40. Knight AA, Hollenberg M, London MJ, et al: Perioperative myocardial ischemia: Importance of the preoperative ischemic pattern, *Anesthesiology* 68:681, 1988.
41. Ferguson TB Jr, Hammill BG, Peterson ED, et al: A decade of change—risk profiles and outcomes for isolated coronary artery bypass grafting procedures, 1990–1999: A report from the STS National Database Committee and the Duke Clinical Research Institute. Society of Thoracic Surgeons, *Ann Thorac Surg* 73:480–489, 2002.
42. Davierwala PM, Maganti M, Yau TM: Decreasing significance of left ventricular dysfunction and reoperative surgery in predicting coronary artery bypass grafting-associated mortality: A twelve-year study, *J Thorac Cardiovasc Surg* 126:1335, 2003.
43. Grover FL, Shroyer AL, Hammermeister KE: Calculating risk and outcome: The Veterans Affairs database, *Ann Thorac Surg* 62:S6, 1996.
44. Grover FL, Cleveland JC Jr, Shroyer LW: Quality improvement in cardiac care, *Arch Surg* 137:28, 2002.
45. Daley J, Henderson WG, Khuri SF: Risk-adjusted surgical outcomes, *Annu Rev Med* 52:275, 2001.
46. Shahian DM, Normand SL, Torchiana DF, et al: Cardiac surgery report cards: Comprehensive review and statistical critique, *Ann Thorac Surg* 72:2155, 2001.
47. Shahian DM, Blackstone EH, Edwards FH, et al: Cardiac surgery risk models: A position article, *Ann Thorac Surg* 78:1868, 2004.
48. Grover FL: The Society of Thoracic Surgeons National Database: Current status and future directions, *Ann Thorac Surg* 68:367, 1999.
49. Shroyer AL, Coombs LP, Peterson ED, et al: The Society of Thoracic Surgeons: 30 day operative mortality and morbidity risk models, *Ann Thorac Surg* 75:1856, 2003.
50. Hannan EL, Kilburn H Jr, O'Donnell JF, et al: Adult open heart surgery in New York State. An analysis of risk factors and hospital mortality rates, *JAMA* 264:2768, 1990.
51. Peterson ED, Coombs LP, DeLong ER, et al: Procedural volume as a marker of quality for CABG surgery, *JAMA* 291:195, 2004.
52. Glance LG, Dick AW, Mukamel DB, et al: Is the hospital volume-mortality relationship in coronary artery bypass surgery the same for low-risk versus high-risk patients? *Ann Thorac Surg* 76:1155, 2003.
53. Vaughan-Sarrazin MS, Hannan EL, Gormley CJ, et al: Mortality in Medicare beneficiaries following coronary artery bypass graft surgery in states with and without certificate of need regulation, *JAMA* 288:1859, 2002.
54. Roques F, Nashef SA, Michel P, et al: Risk factors and outcome in European cardiac surgery: Analysis of the EuroSCORE multinational database of 19030 patients, *Eur J Cardiothorac Surg* 15:816, 1999.
55. Nashef SA, Roques F, Hammill BG, et al: Validation of European System for Cardiac Operative Risk Evaluation (EuroSCORE) in North American cardiac surgery, *Eur J Cardiothorac Surg* 22:101, 2002.
56. Eagle KA, Guyton RA, Davidoff R, et al: ACC/AHA 2004 Guideline Update for Coronary Artery Bypass Graft Surgery: Summary Article: A Report of the American College of Cardiology/American Heart Association Task Force on Practice Guidelines (Committee to update the 1999 Guidelines for Coronary Artery Bypass Graft Surgery), *Circulation* 110:1168–1176, 2004.
57. Mack MJ, Brown PP, Kugelmass AD, et al: Current status and outcomes of coronary revascularization 1999 to 2002: 148,396 surgical and percutaneous procedures, *Ann Thorac Surg* 77:761, 2004.
58. Grover FL, Cleveland JC Jr, Shroyer LW: Quality improvement in cardiac care, *Arch Surg* 137:28, 2002.
59. Shroyer AL, Coombs LP, Peterson ED, et al: The Society of Thoracic Surgeons: 30-day operative mortality and morbidity risk models, *Ann Thorac Surg* 75:1856, 2003.
60. Hannan EL, Kilburn H Jr, Racz M, et al: Improving the outcomes of coronary artery bypass surgery in New York State, *JAMA* 271:761, 1994.
61. Jones RH, Hannan EL, Hammermeister KE, et al: Identification of preoperative variables needed for risk adjustment of short-term mortality after coronary artery bypass graft surgery. The Working Group Panel on the Cooperative CABG Database Project, *J Am Coll Cardiol* 28:1478, 1996.
62. Higgins TL, Estafanous FG, Loop FD, et al: Stratification of morbidity and mortality outcome by preoperative risk factors in coronary artery bypass patients. A clinical severity score [published erratum appears in JAMA 268:1860, 1992], *JAMA* 267:2344, 1992.
63. Nashef SA, Roques F, Michel P, et al: European system for cardiac operative risk evaluation (EuroSCORE), *Eur J Cardiothorac Surg* 16:9, 1999.
64. Rao V, Ivanov J, Weisel RD, et al: Predictors of low cardiac output syndrome after coronary artery bypass, *J Thorac Cardiovasc Surg* 112:38, 1996.
65. Ferraris VA, Ferraris SP: Risk factors for postoperative morbidity, *J Thorac Cardiovasc Surg* 111:731, 1996.
66. McKinlay KH, Schinderle DB, Swaminathan M, et al: Predictors of inotrope use during separation from cardiopulmonary bypass, *J Cardiothorac Vasc Anesth* 18:404, 2004.
67. Plomondon ME, Cleveland JC, Ludwig ST, et al: Off-pump coronary artery bypass is associated with improved risk-adjusted outcomes, *Ann Thorac Surg* 72:114, 2001.
68. Wu Y, Grunkemeier GL, Handy JR Jr: Coronary artery bypass grafting: Are risk models developed from on-pump surgery valid for off-pump surgery? *J Thorac Cardiovasc Surg* 127:174, 2004.
69. Slogoff S, Keats AS: Randomized trial of primary anesthetic agents on outcome of coronary artery bypass operations, *Anesthesiology* 70:179, 1989.
70. Tuman KJ, McCarthy RJ, Spiess BD, et al: Does choice of anesthetic agent significantly affect outcome after coronary artery surgery? *Anesthesiology* 70:189, 1989.
71. De Hert SG, Van der Linden PJ, Cromheecke S, et al: Choice of primary anesthetic regimen can influence intensive care unit length of stay after coronary surgery with cardiopulmonary bypass, *Anesthesiology* 101:9, 2004.
72. De Hert SG, Cromheecke S, ten Broecke PW, et al: Effects of propofol, desflurane, and sevoflurane on recovery of myocardial function after coronary surgery in elderly high-risk patients, *Anesthesiology* 99:314, 2003.
73. Berendes E, Schmidt C, Van Aken H, et al: Reversible cardiac sympathectomy by high thoracic epidural anesthesia improves regional left ventricular function in patients undergoing coronary artery bypass grafting: A randomized trial, *Arch Surg* 138:1283, 2003.
74. Butterworth J, James R, Prielipp RC, et al: Do shorter-acting neuromuscular blocking drugs or opioids associate with reduced intensive care unit or hospital lengths of stay after coronary artery bypass grafting? CABG Clinical Benchmarking Data Base Participants, *Anesthesiology* 88:1437, 1998.
75. London MJ, Shroyer AL, Coll JR, et al: Early extubation following cardiac surgery in a veterans population, *Anesthesiology* 88:1447, 1998.
76. Reich DL, Bodian CA, Krol M, et al: Intraoperative hemodynamic predictors of mortality, stroke, and myocardial infarction after coronary artery bypass surgery, *Anesth Analg* 89:814, 1999.
77. Becker RB, Zimmerman JE, Knaus WA, et al: The use of APACHE III to evaluate ICU length of stay, resource use, and mortality after coronary artery by-pass surgery, *J Cardiovasc Surg (Torino)* 36:1, 1995.
78. Higgins TL, Estafanous FG, Loop FD, et al: ICU admission score for predicting morbidity and mortality risk after coronary artery bypass grafting, *Ann Thorac Surg* 64:1050, 1997.
79. Kappetein AP, Dawkins KD, Mohr FW, et al: Current percutaneous coronary intervention and coronary artery bypass grafting practices for three-vessel and left main coronary artery disease. Insights from the SYNTAX run-in phase, *Eur J Cardiothorac Surg* 29:486–491, 2006.
80. Sianos G, Morel MA, Kappetein AP, et al: The SYNTAX score: An angiographic tool grading the complexity of coronary artery disease, *EuroIntervention* 1:219–227, 2005.
81. Serruys PW, Onumo Y, Garg S, et al: Assessment of the SYNTAX score in the Syntax study, *EuroIntervention* 5:50–56, 2009.
82. Meissner A, Rolf N, Van Aken H: Thoracic epidural anesthesia and the patient with heart disease: Benefits, risks, and controversies, *Anesth Analg* 85:517, 1997.
83. Blomberg S, Curelaru I, Emanuelsson H, et al: Thoracic epidural anaesthesia in patients with unstable angina pectoris, *Eur Heart J* 10:437, 1989.
84. Gramling-Babb P, Miller MJ, Reeves ST, et al: Treatment of medically and surgically refractory angina pectoris with high thoracic epidural analgesia: Initial clinical experience, *Am Heart J* 133:648, 1997.
85. Olausson K, Magnusdottir H, Lurje L, et al: Anti-ischemic and anti-anginal effects of thoracic epidural anesthesia versus those of conventional medical therapy in the treatment of severe refractory unstable angina pectoris, *Circulation* 96:2178, 1997.

86. Overdyk FJ, Gramling-Babb PM, Handy JR Jr, et al: Thoracic epidural anesthesia as the last option for treating angina in a patient before coronary artery bypass surgery, *Anesth Analg* 84:213, 1997.
87. Gramling-Babb PM, Zile MR, Reeves ST: Preliminary report on high thoracic epidural analgesia: Relationship between its therapeutic effects and myocardial blood flow as assessed by stress thallium distribution, *J Cardiothorac Vasc Anesth* 14:657, 2000.
88. Liem TH, Booij LH, Hasenbos MA, et al: Coronary artery bypass grafting using two different anesthetic techniques. Part I. Hemodynamic results, *J Cardiothorac Vasc Anesth* 6:148, 1992.
89. Liem TH, Hasenbos MA, Booij LH, et al: Coronary artery bypass grafting using two different anesthetic techniques. Part 2. Postoperative outcome, *J Cardiothorac Vasc Anesth* 6:156, 1992.
90. Liem TH, Booij LH, Gielen MJ, et al: Coronary artery bypass grafting using two different anesthetic techniques. Part 3. Adrenergic responses, *J Cardiothorac Vasc Anesth* 6:162, 1992.
91. Aybek T, Kessler P, Khan MF, et al: Operative techniques in awake coronary artery bypass grafting, *J Thorac Cardiovasc Surg* 125:1394, 2003.
92. Aybek T, Kessler P, Dogan S, et al: Awake coronary artery bypass grafting: Utopia or reality? *Ann Thorac Surg* 75:1165, 2003.
93. Chakravarthy M, Jawali V, Patil TA, et al: High thoracic epidural anesthesia as the sole anesthetic for performing multiple grafts in off-pump coronary artery bypass surgery, *J Cardiothorac Vasc Anesth* 17:160, 2003.
94. Kessler P, Neidhart G, Bremerich DH, et al: High thoracic epidural anesthesia for coronary artery bypass grafting using two different surgical approaches in conscious patients, *Anesth Analg* 95:791, 2002.
95. Meininger D, Neidhart G, Bremerich DH, et al: Coronary artery bypass grafting via sternotomy in conscious patients, *World J Surg* 27:534, 2003.
96. Watanabe G, Yamaguchi S, Tomiya S, Ohtake H: Awake subxyphoid minimally invasive direct coronary artery bypass grafting yielded minimum invasive cardiac surgery for high risk patients, *Interact Cardiovasc Thorac Surg* 7:910–912, 2008.
97. Karagoz HY, Kurtoglu M, Bakkaloglu B, et al: Coronary artery bypass grafting in the awake patient: Three years' experience in 137 patients, *J Thorac Cardiovasc Surg* 125:1401, 2003.
98. Hemmerling TM, Prieto I, Bracco D, et al: Coronary artery bypass grafting in the awake patient combining high thoracic epidural and femoral nerve block: First series of 15 patients, *Br J Anaesth* 100:184–189, 2008.
99. Slogoff S, Keats AS: Randomized trial of primary anesthetic agents on outcome of coronary artery bypass operations, *Anesthesiology* 70:179, 1989.
100. Tuman KJ, McCarthy RJ, Spiess BD, et al: Does choice of anesthetic agent significantly affect outcome after coronary artery surgery? *Anesthesiology* 70:189, 1989.
101. Royse C, Royse A, Soeding P, et al: Prospective randomized trial of high thoracic epidural analgesia for coronary artery bypass surgery, *Ann Thorac Surg* 75:93–100, 2003.
102. Scott NB, Turfrey DJ, Ray DAA, et al: A prospective randomized study of the potential benefits of thoracic epidural anesthesia and analgesia in patients undergoing coronary artery bypass grafting, *Anesth Analg* 93:528–535, 2001.
103. Priestley MC, Cope L, Halliwell R, et al: Thoracic epidural anesthesia for cardiac surgery: The effect on tracheal intubation time and length of hospital stay, *Anesth Analg* 94:275–282, 2002.
104. Hansdottir V, Philip J, Olsen MF, et al: Thoracic epidural versus intravenous patient-controlled analgesia after cardiac surgery, *Anesthesiology* 104:142–151, 2006.
105. Bracco D, Noiseux N, Dubois MJ, et al: Epidural anesthesia improves outcome and resource use in cardiac surgery: A single-center study of a 1293-patient cohort, *Heart Surg Forum* 10:E449–E458, 2007.
106. Sharma M, Mehta Y, Sawhney R, et al: Thoracic epidural analgesia in obese patients with body mass index of more than 30 kg/m^2 for off pump coronary bypass surgery, *Ann Card Anaesth* 13:28–33, 2010.
107. Liu SS, Block BM, Wu CL: Effects of perioperative central neuraxial analgesia on outcome after coronary artery bypass surgery: A meta-analysis, *Anesthesiology* 101:153, 2004.
108. Beattie WS, Badner NH, Choi P: Epidural analgesia reduces postoperative myocardial infarction: A meta-analysis, *Anesth Analg* 93:853, 2001.
109. Salvi L, Parolari A, Veglia F, et al: High thoracic epidural anesthesia in coronary artery bypass surgery: A propensity-matched study, *J Cardiothorac Vasc Anesth* 21:810–815, 2007.
110. Berendes E, Schmidt C, Van Aken H, et al: Reversible cardiac sympathectomy by high thoracic epidural anesthesia improves regional left ventricular function in patients undergoing coronary artery bypass grafting: A randomized trial, *Arch Surg* 138:1283, 2003.
111. Barrington MJ, Kluger R, Watson R, et al: Epidural anesthesia for coronary artery bypass surgery compared with general anesthesia alone does not reduce biochemical markers of myocardial damage, *Anesth Analg* 100:921–928, 2005.
112. Crescenzi G, Landoni G, Monaco F, et al: Epidural anesthesia in elderly patients undergoing coronary artery bypass graft surgery, *J Cardiothorac Vasc Anesth* 23:807–812, 2009.
113. Lee TW, Grocott HP, Schwinn D, et al: High spinal anesthesia for cardiac surgery: Effects on beta-adrenergic receptor function, stress response, and hemodynamics, *Anesthesiology* 98:499, 2003.
114. Bracco D, Hemmerling T: Epidural analgesia in cardiac surgery: An updated risk assessment, *Heart Surg Forum* 10:E334–E337, 2007.
115. Ho AM, Chung DC, Joynt GM: Neuraxial blockade and hematoma in cardiac surgery: Estimating the risk of a rare adverse event that has not (yet) occurred, *Chest* 117:551, 2000.
116. Rosen DA, Hawkinberry DW 2nd, Rosen KR, et al: An epidural hematoma in an adolescent patient after cardiac surgery, *Anesth Analg* 98:966–969, 2004.
117. Chakravarthy M, Thimmangowda P, Krishnamurthy J, et al: Thoracic epidural anesthesia in cardiac surgical patients: A prospective audit of 2,113 cases, *J Cardiothorac Vasc Anesth* 19:44, 2005.
118. Jack ES, Scott NB: The risk of vertebral canal complications in 2837 cardiac surgery patients with thoracic epidurals, *Acta Anaesthesiol Scand* 51:722–725, 2006.
119. Royse CF, Soeding PF, Royse AG: High thoracic epidural analgesia for cardiac surgery: An audit of 874 cases, *Anaesth Intensive Care* 35:374–377, 2007.
120. Pastor MC, Sanchez MJ, Casas MA, et al: Thoracic epidural analgesia in coronary artery bypass graft surgery: Seven years' experience, *J Cardiothorac Vasc Anesth* 17:154, 2003.
121. Horlocker TT, Wedel DJ, Benzon H, et al: Regional anesthesia in the anticoagulated patient: Defining the risks (The second ASRA Consensus Conference on Neuraxial Anesthesia and Anticoagulation), *Reg Anesth Pain Med* 28:172–197, 2003.
122. Chaney MA: Intrathecal and epidural anesthesia and analgesia for cardiac surgery, *Anesth Analg* 102:45–64, 2006.
123. Thomson IR, Peterson MD, Hudson RJ: A comparison of clonidine with conventional preanesthetic medication in patients undergoing coronary artery bypass grafting, *Anesth Analg* 87:292, 1998.
124. Howie MB, Hiestand DC, Jopling MW, et al: Effect of oral clonidine premedication on anesthetic requirement, hormonal response, hemodynamics, and recovery in coronary artery bypass graft surgery patients, *J Clin Anesth* 8:263, 1996.
125. Jalonen J, Hynynen M, Kuitunen A, et al: Dexmedetomidine as an anesthetic adjunct in coronary artery bypass grafting, *Anesthesiology* 86:331, 1997.
126. Wijeysundera DN, Naik JS, Beattie WS: Alpha-2 adrenergic agonists to prevent perioperative cardiovascular complications: A meta-analysis, *Am J Med* 114:742, 2003.
127. Dorman BH, Zucker JR, Verrier ED, et al: Clonidine improves perioperative myocardial ischemia, reduces anesthetic requirement, and alters hemodynamic parameters in patients undergoing coronary artery bypass surgery, *J Cardiothorac Vasc Anesth* 7:386, 1993.
128. Scheinin H, Jaakola ML, Sjovall S, et al: Intramuscular dexmedetomidine as premedication for general anesthesia. A comparative multicenter study, *Anesthesiology* 78:1065, 1993.
129. Viljoen J, Estafanous F, Kellner G: Propranolol and cardiac surgery, *J Thorac Cardiovasc Surg* 64:826, 1972.
130. Kaplan JA, Dunbar RW, Bland JW, et al: Propranolol and cardiac surgery: A problem for the anesthesiologist? *Anesth Analg* 54:571, 1975.
131. Kaplan JA, Dunbar RW: Propranolol and surgical anesthesia, *Anesth Analg* 55:1, 1976.
132. Slogoff S, Keats AS, Ott E: Preoperative propranolol therapy and aortocoronary bypass operation, *JAMA* 240:1487, 1978.
133. Slogoff S, Keats AS: Does chronic treatment with calcium entry blocking drugs reduce perioperative myocardial ischemia? *Anesthesiology* 68:676, 1988.
134. Chung F, Houston PL, Cheng DC, et al: Calcium channel blockade does not offer adequate protection from perioperative myocardial ischemia, *Anesthesiology* 69:343, 1988.
135. Pasternack PF, Imparato AM, Baumann FG, et al: The hemodynamics of beta-blockade in patients undergoing abdominal aortic aneurysm repair, *Circulation* 76:III1, 1987.
136. Stone JG, Foëx P, Sear JW, et al: Myocardial ischemia in untreated hypertensive patients: Effect of a single small oral dose of a beta-adrenergic blocking agent, *Anesthesiology* 68:495, 1988.
137. Stone JG, Foëx P, Sear JW, et al: Risk of myocardial ischaemia during anaesthesia in treated and untreated hypertensive patients, *Br J Anaesth* 61:675, 1988.
138. Poldermans D, Boersma E, Bax JJ, et al: The effect of bisoprolol on perioperative mortality and myocardial infarction in high-risk patients undergoing vascular surgery, *N Engl J Med* 341:1789, 1999.
139. Mangano DT, Layug EL, Wallace A, et al: Effect of atenolol on mortality and cardiovascular morbidity after noncardiac surgery, *N Engl J Med* 335:1713, 1996.
140. Poise Study Group: Effects of extended release metoprolol succinate in patients undergoing non-cardiac surgery (POISE trial): A randomized controlled trial, *Lancet* 31:1839, 2008.
141. Fleisher LA, Beckman JA, Brown KA, et al: ACC/AHA 2007 guidelines on perioperative cardiovascular evaluation and care for noncardiac surgery. A report of the American College of Cardiology/American Heart Association task force on practice guidelines, *Circulation* 116:e418, 2007.
142. Weightman WM, Gibbs NM, Sheminant MR, et al: Drug therapy before coronary artery surgery: Nitrates are independent predictors of mortality and beta-adrenergic blockers predict survival, *Anesth Analg* 88:286, 1999.
143. ten Broecke PW, De Hert SG, Mertens E, et al: Effect of preoperative beta-blockade on perioperative mortality in coronary surgery, *Br J Anaesth* 90:27, 2003.
144. Ferguson TB Jr, Coombs LP, Peterson ED: Preoperative beta-blocker use and mortality and morbidity following CABG surgery in North America, *JAMA* 287:2221, 2002.
145. Wiesbauer F, Schlager O, Domanovits H, et al: Perioperative beta-blockers for preventing surgery related mortality and morbidity: A systematic review and meta-analysis, *Anesth Analg* 104:27, 2007.
146. Denton TA, Fonarow GC, LaBresh KA, et al: Secondary prevention after coronary bypass: The American Heart Association "Get with the Guidelines" program, *Ann Thorac Surg* 75:758, 2003.
147. Ferguson TB Jr, Peterson ED, Coombs LP, et al: Use of continuous quality improvement to increase use of process measures in patients undergoing coronary artery bypass graft surgery: A randomized controlled trial, *JAMA* 290:49, 2003.
148. Denton TA, Fonarow GC, LaBresh KA, et al: Secondary prevention after coronary bypass: The American Heart Association "Get with the Guidelines" program, *Ann Thorac Surg* 75:758, 2003.
149. Berger JS, Brown DL, Becker RC: Low-dose aspirin in patients with stable cardiovascular disease: A meta-analysis, *Am J Med* 121:43, 2008.
150. Yusuf S, Zhao F, Mehta SR, et al: Effects of clopidogrel in addition to aspirin in patients with acute coronary syndromes without ST-segment elevation, *N Engl J Med* 345:494, 2001.
151. Becker RC, Meade TW, Berger PB, et al: The primary and secondary prevention of coronary artery disease: American College of Chest Physicians evidence-based clinical practice guidelines (8th edition), *Chest* 133:776S,, 2008.
152. Chesebro JH, Clements IP, Fuster V, et al: A platelet-inhibitor-drug trial in coronary-artery bypass operations: Benefit of perioperative dipyridamole and aspirin therapy on early postoperative vein-graft patency, *N Engl J Med* 307:73, 1982.
153. Mangano DT: Aspirin and mortality from coronary bypass surgery, *N Engl J Med* 347:1309, 2002.
154. Fox KA, Mehta SR, Peters R, et al: Benefits and risks of the combination of clopidogrel and aspirin in patients undergoing surgical revascularization for non-ST-elevation acute coronary syndrome: The Clopidogrel in Unstable Angina to prevent Recurrent ischemic events (CURE) trial, *Circulation* 110:1202, 2004.
155. Sun JC, Whitlock R, Cheng J, et al: The effect of pre-operative aspirin on bleeding, transfusion, myocardial infarction, and mortality in coronary artery bypass surgery: A systematic review of randomized and observational studies, *Eur Heart J* 29:1057, 2008.
156. Mehta RH, Roe MT, Mulgund J, et al: Acute clopidogrel use and outcomes in patients with non-ST-segment elevation acute coronary syndromes undergoing coronary artery bypass surgery, *J Am Coll Cardiol* 48:281, 2006.
157. Filsoufi F, Rahmanian PB, Castillo JG, et al: Clopidogrel treatment before coronary artery bypass graft surgery increases post-operative morbidity and blood product requirements, *J Cardiothorac Vasc Anesth* 22:60, 2008.
158. Berger JS, Frye CB, Harshaw Q, et al: Impact of clopidogrel in patients with acute coronary syndromes requiring coronary artery bypass surgery: A multi-center analysis, *J Am Coll Cardiol* 52:1693, 2008.
159. Becker RC, Meade TW, Berger PB, et al: The primary and secondary prevention of coronary artery disease: American College of Chest Physicians evidence-based clinical practice guidelines (8th edition), *Chest* 133:776S, 2008.
160. Ferraris VA, Ferraris SP, Moliterno DJ, et al: The Society of Thoracic Surgeons practice guideline series: Aspirin and other antiplatelet agents during operative coronary revascularization (executive summary), *Ann Thorac Surg* 79:1454, 2005.
161. Eagle KA, Guyton RA, Davidoff R, et al: ACC/AHA 2004 guideline update for coronary artery bypass graft surgery: A report of the American College of Cardiology/American Heart Association Task Force on Practice Guidelines (Committee to Update the 1999 Guidelines for Coronary Artery Bypass Graft Surgery), *Circulation* 110:e340, 2004.
162. Slogoff S, Keats AS: Does chronic treatment with calcium entry blocking drugs reduce perioperative myocardial ischemia? *Anesthesiology* 68:676, 1988.
163. Chung F, Houston PL, Cheng DC, et al: Calcium channel blockade does not offer adequate protection from perioperative myocardial ischemia, *Anesthesiology* 69:343, 1988.
164. Opie LH, Yusuf S, Kubler W: Current status of safety and efficacy of calcium channel blockers in cardiovascular diseases: A critical analysis based on 100 studies, *Prog Cardiovasc Dis* 43:171, 2000.
165. Stevens RD, Burri H, Tramer MR: Pharmacologic myocardial protection in patients undergoing noncardiac surgery: A quantitative systematic review, *Anesth Analg* 97:623, 2003.
166. Wijeysundera DN, Beattie WS: Calcium channel blockers for reducing cardiac morbidity after noncardiac surgery: A meta-analysis, *Anesth Analg* 97:634, 2003.
167. Wijeysundera DN, Beattie WS, Rao V, et al: Calcium antagonists are associated with reduced mortality after cardiac surgery: A propensity analysis, *J Thorac Cardiovasc Surg* 127:755, 2004.
168. Wijeysundera DN, Beattie WS, Rao V, et al: Calcium antagonists reduce cardiovascular complications after cardiac surgery: A meta-analysis, *J Am Coll Cardiol* 41:1496, 2003.
169. Amar D, Roistacher N, Rusch VW, et al: Effects of diltiazem prophylaxis on the incidence and clinical outcome of atrial arrhythmias after thoracic surgery, *J Thorac Cardiovasc Surg* 120:790, 2000.

170. Gremmel T, Steiner S, Seidinger D, et al: Calcium channel blockers decrease clopidogrel-mediated platelet inhibition, *Heart* 96:186–189, 2010.
171. Halcox JP, Deanfield JE: Beyond the laboratory: Clinical implications for statin pleiotropy, *Circulation* 109:II42, 2004.
172. Lazar HL: Role of angiotensin-converting enzyme inhibitors in the coronary artery bypass patient, *Ann Thorac Surg* 79:1081, 2005.
173. Le Manach Y, Coriat P, Collard CD, et al: Statin therapy within the perioperative period, *Anesthesiology* 108:1141, 2008.
174. Ray KK, Cannon CP: The potential relevance of the multiple lipid-independent (pleiotropic) effects of statins in the management of acute coronary syndromes, *J Am Coll Cardiol* 46:1425, 2005.
175. Lazar HL: Role of angiotensin-converting enzyme inhibitors in the coronary artery bypass patient, *Ann Thorac Surg* 79:1081, 2005.
176. Chan AW, Bhatt DL, Chew DP, et al: Early and sustained survival benefit associated with statin therapy at the time of percutaneous coronary intervention, *Circulation* 105:691, 2002.
177. Chan AW, Bhatt DL, Chew DP, et al: Relation of inflammation and benefit of statins after percutaneous coronary interventions, *Circulation* 107:1750, 2003.
178. Patti G, Pasceri V, Colonna G, et al: Atorvastatin preteatment improves outcomes in patients with acute coronary syndromes undergoing early percutaneous coronary intervention: Results of the ARMYDA-ACS randomized trial, *J Am Coll Cardiol* 49:1272, 2007.
179. Pretorius M, Murphey LJ, McFarlane JA, et al: Angiotensin-converting enzyme inhibition alters the fibrinolytic response to cardiopulmonary bypass, *Circulation* 108:3079, 2003.
180. Chello M, Mastroroberto P, Patti G, et al: Simvastatin attenuates leucocyte-endothelial interactions after coronary revascularisation with cardiopulmonary bypass, *Heart* 89:538, 2003.
181. Chello M, Carassiti M, Agro F, et al: Simvastatin blunts the increase of circulating adhesion molecules after coronary artery bypass surgery with cardiopulmonary bypass, *J Cardiothorac Vasc Anesth* 18:605, 2004.
182. Chello M, Patti G, Candura D, et al: Effects of atorvastatin on systemic inflammatory response after coronary bypass surgery, *Crit Care Med* 34:660, 2006.
183. Lazar HL, Bao Y, Zhang Y, et al: Pretreatment with statins enhances myocardial protection during coronary revascularization, *J Thorac Cardiovasc Surg* 125:1037, 2003.
184. Lazar HL: Role of angiotensin-converting enzyme inhibitors in the coronary artery bypass patient, *Ann Thorac Surg* 79:1081, 2005.
185. Dotani MI, Morise AP, Haque R, et al: Association between short-term simvastatin therapy before coronary artery bypass grafting and postoperative myocardial blood flow as assessed by positron emission tomography, *Am J Cardiol* 91:1107, 2003.
186. Pan W, Pintar T, Anton J, et al: Statins are associated with a reduced incidence of perioperative mortality after coronary artery bypass graft surgery, *Circulation* 110:II45, 2004.
187. Collard CD, Body SC, Shernan SK, et al: Preoperative statin therapy is associated with reduced cardiac mortality after coronary artery bypass graft surgery, *J Thorac Cardiovasc Surg* 132:392–400, 2006.
188. Liakopoulos OJ, Choi YH, Kuhn EW, et al: Statins for prevention of atrial fibrillation after cardiac surgery: A systemic literature review, *J Thorac Cardiovasc Surg* 138:678, 2009.
189. Tabata M, Khalpey Z, Cohn LH, et al: Effect of preoperative statins in patients without coronary artery disease who undergo cardiac surgery, *J Thorac Cardiovasc Surg* 136:1510, 2008.
190. Liakopoulos OJ, Choi YH, Haldenwang PL, et al: Impact of preoperative statin therapy on adverse postoperative outcomes in patients undergoing cardiac surgery: A meta-analysis of over 30,000 patients, *Eur Heart J* 29:1548, 2008.
191. Huffmyer JL, Mauermann WJ, Thiele RH, et al: Preoperative statin administration is associated with lower mortality and decreased need for postoperative hemodialysis in patients undergoing coronary artery bypass graft surgery, *J Cardiothorac Vasc Anesth* 23:468, 2009.
192. Pan W, Pintar T, Anton J, et al: Statins are associated with a reduced incidence of perioperative mortality after coronary artery bypass graft surgery, *Circulation* 110:II45, 2004.
193. Tabata M, Khalpey Z, Pirundini PA, et al: Renoprotective effect of preoperative statins in coronary artery bypass grafting, *Am J Cardiol* 100:442, 2007.
194. Patti G, Chello M, Candura D, et al: Randomized trial of atorvastatin for reduction of post-operative atrial fibrillation in patients undergoing cardiac surgery: Results of the ARMYDA-3 (Atorvastatin for Reduction of MYocardial Dysrhythmia After cardiac surgery) study, *Circulation* 114:1455, 2006.
195. Fleisher LA, Beckman JA, Brown KA, et al: ACC/AHA 2007 guidelines on perioperative cardiovascular evaluation and care for noncardiac surgery. A report of the American College of Cardiology/American Heart Association task force on practice guidelines, *Circulation* 116:e418, 2007.
196. Collard CD, Body SC, Shernan SK, et al: Preoperative statin therapy is associated with reduced cardiac mortality after coronary artery bypass graft surgery, *J Thorac Cardiovasc Surg* 132:392–400, 2006.
197. Oosterga M, Voors AA, Pinto YM, et al: Effects of quinapril on clinical outcome after coronary artery bypass grafting (The QUO VADIS Study). QUinapril on Vascular Ace and Determinants of Ischemia, *Am J Cardiol* 87:542, 2001.
198. Benedetto U, Sciarretta S, Roscitano A, et al: Preoperative angiotensin-converting inhibitors and acute kidney injury after coronary artery bypass grafting, *Ann Thorac Surg* 86:1160, 2008.
199. Dabrowski R, Sosnowski C, Jankowska A, et al: ACE inhibitor therapy: Possible effective prevention of new-onset atrial fibrillation following cardiac surgery, *Cardiol J* 14:274, 2007.
200. Coriat P, Richer C, Douraki T, et al: Influence of chronic angiotensin-converting enzyme inhibition on anesthetic induction, *Anesthesiology* 81:299, 1994.
201. Tuman KJ, McCarthy RJ, O'Connor CJ, et al: Angiotensin-converting enzyme inhibitors increase vasoconstrictor requirements after cardiopulmonary bypass, *Anesth Analg* 80:473, 1995.
202. Brabant SM, Bertrand M, Eyraud D, et al: The hemodynamic effects of anesthetic induction in vascular surgical patients chronically treated with angiotensin II receptor antagonists, *Anesth Analg* 89:1388, 1999.
203. Pigott DW, Nagle C, Allman K, et al: Effect of omitting regular ACE inhibitor medication before cardiac surgery on haemodynamic variables and vasoactive drug requirements, *Br J Anaesth* 83:715, 1999.
204. Bertrand M, Godet G, Meersschaert K, et al: Should the angiotensin II antagonists be discontinued before surgery? *Anesth Analg* 92:26, 2001.
205. Meersschaert K, Brun L, Gourdin M, et al: Terlipressin-ephedrine versus ephedrine to treat hypotension at the induction of anesthesia in patients chronically treated with angiotensin converting-enzyme inhibitors: A prospective, randomized, double-blinded, crossover study, *Anesth Analg* 94:835, 2002.
206. Tuman KJ, McCarthy RJ, O'Connor CJ, et al: Angiotensin-converting enzyme inhibitors increase vasoconstrictor requirements after cardiopulmonary bypass, *Anesth Analg* 80:473, 1995.
207. Levin M, Lin HM, Castillo JG, et al: Early on-cardiopulmonary bypass hypotention and other factors associated with vasoplegic syndrome, *Circulation* 120:1664, 2009.
208. Deakin CD, Dalrymple-Hay MJ, Jones P, et al: Effects of angiotensin converting enzyme inhibition on systemic vascular resistance and vasoconstrictor requirements during hypothermic cardiopulmonary bypass, *Eur J Cardiothorac Surg* 26:387, 2003.
209. Miceli A, Capoun R, Fino C, et al: Effects of angiotensin-converting enzyme inhibitor therapy on clinical outcome in patients undergoing coronary artery bypass grafting, *J Am Coll Cardiol* 54:1778–1784, 2009.
210. Lazar HL: Role of angiotensin-converting enzyme inhibitors in the coronary artery bypass patient, *Ann Thorac Surg* 79:1081, 2005.
211. Rich GF, Lubanski RE Jr, McLoughlin TM: Differences between aortic and radial artery pressure associated with cardiopulmonary bypass, *Anesthesiology* 77:63, 1992.
212. Thrush DN, Steighner ML, Rasanen J, et al: Blood pressure after cardiopulmonary bypass: Which technique is accurate? *J Cardiothorac Vasc Anesth* 8:269, 1994.
213. Dorman T, Breslow MJ, Lipsett PA, et al: Radial artery pressure monitoring underestimates central arterial pressure during vasopressor therapy in critically ill surgical patients, *Crit Care Med* 26:1646, 1998.
214. Chauhan S, Saxena N, Mehrotra S, et al: Femoral artery pressures are more reliable than radial artery pressures on initiation of cardiopulmonary bypass, *J Cardiothorac Vasc Anesth* 14:274, 2000.
215. Kanazawa M, Fukuyama H, Kinefuchi Y, et al: Relationship between aortic-to-radial arterial pressure gradient after cardiopulmonary bypass and changes in arterial elasticity, *Anesthesiology* 99:48, 2003.
216. McGee DC, Gould MK: Preventing complications of central venous catheterization, *N Engl J Med* 348:1123, 2003.
217. Augoustides JGT, Cheung AT: Pro: Ultrasound should be the standard of care for central catheter insertion, *J Cardiothorac Vasc Anesth* 23:720–724, 2009.
218. Hessel I.I.E.A.: Con: We should not enforce the use of ultrasound as a standard of care for obtaining central venous access, *J Cardiothorac Vasc Anesth* 23:725–728, 2009.
219. Tuman KJ, McCarthy RJ, Spiess BD, et al: Effect of pulmonary artery catheterization on outcome in patients undergoing coronary artery surgery, *Anesthesiology* 70:199, 1989.
220. Stewart RD, Psyhojos T, Lahey SJ, et al: Central venous catheter use in low-risk coronary artery bypass grafting, *Ann Thorac Surg* 66:1306, 1998.
221. Ramsey SD, Saint S, Sullivan SD, et al: Clinical and economic effects of pulmonary artery catheterization in nonemergent coronary artery bypass graft surgery, *J Cardiothorac Vasc Anesth* 14:113, 2000.
222. Schwann TA, Zacharias A, Riordan CJ, et al: Safe, highly selective use of pulmonary artery catheters in coronary artery bypass grafting: An objective patient selection method, *Ann Thorac Surg* 73:1394, 2002.
223. London MJ, Moritz TE, Henderson WG, et al: Standard versus fiberoptic pulmonary artery catheterization for cardiac surgery in the Department of Veterans Affairs: A prospective, observational, multicenter analysis, *Anesthesiology* 96:860, 2002.
224. Djaiani G, Karski J, Yudin M, et al: Clinical outcomes in patients undergoing elective coronary artery bypass graft surgery with and without utilization of pulmonary artery catheter-generated data, *J Cardiothorac Vasc Anesth* 20:307, 2006.
225. Resano FG, Kapetanakis EI, Hill PC, et al: Clinical outcomes of low-risk patients undergoing beating heart surgery with or without pulmonary artery catheterization, *J Cardiothorac Vasc Anesth* 20:300, 2006.
226. Anonymous Practice guidelines for perioperative transesophageal echocardiography. A report by the American Society of Anesthesiologists and the Society of Cardiovascular Anesthesiologists Task Force on Transesophageal Echocardiography, *Anesthesiology* 84:986, 1996.
227. Thys DM, Abel MD, Brooker RF, et al: For the Task Force on Perioperative Transesophageal Echocardiography: Practice guidelines for perioperative transesophageal echocardiography, *Anesthesiology* 112:1084, 2010.
228. Comunale ME, Body SC, Ley C, et al: The concordance of intraoperative left ventricular wall-motion abnormalities and electrocardiographic S-T segment changes: Association with outcome after coronary revascularization. Multicenter Study of Perioperative Ischemia (McSPI) Research Group, *Anesthesiology* 88:945, 1998.
229. Skidmore KL, London MJ: Myocardial ischemia. Monitoring to diagnose ischemia: How do I monitor therapy? *Anesthesiol Clin North Am* 19:651, 2001.
230. Swaminathan M, Morris RW, De Meyts DD, et al: Deterioration of regional wall motion immediately after coronary artery bypass graft surgery is associated with long-term major adverse cardiac events, *Anesthesiology* 107:739–745, 2007.
231. Shanewise JS, Cheung AT, Aronson S, et al: ASE/SCA guidelines for performing a comprehensive intraoperative multiplane transesophageal echocardiography examination: Recommendations of the American Society of Echocardiography Council for Intraoperative Echocardiography and the Society of Cardiovascular Anesthesiologists Task Force for Certification in Perioperative Transesophageal Echocardiography, *Anesth Analg* 89:870, 1999.
232. Sutherland GR, Di Salvo G, Claus P, et al: Strain and strain rate imaging: A new clinical approach to quantifying regional myocardial function, *J Am Soc Echocardiogr* 17:788, 2004.
233. Simmons LA, Weidemann F, Sutherland GR, et al: Doppler tissue velocity, strain, and strain rate imaging with transesophageal echocardiography in the operating room: A feasibility study, *J Am Soc Echocardiogr* 15:768, 2002.
234. Leitman M, Lysyansky P, Sidenko S, et al: Two-dimensional strain: A novel software for real time quantitative echocardographic assessment of myocardial function, *J Am Soc Echocardiogr* 17:1021, 2004.
235. Kukucka M, Nasseri B, Tscherkaschin A, et al: The feasibility of speckle tracking for intraoperative assessment of regional myocardial function by transesophageal echocardiography, *J Cardiothorac Vasc Anesth* 23:462, 2009.
236. Morewood GH, Gallagher ME, Gaughan JP, et al: Current practice patterns for adult perioperative transesophageal echocardiography in the United States, *Anesthesiology* 95:1507, 2001.
237. Kato M, Nakashima Y, Levine J, et al: Does transesophageal echocardiography improve postoperative outcome in patients undergoing coronary artery bypass surgery? *J Cardiothorac Vasc Anesth* 7:285, 1993.
238. Bergquist BD, Leung JM, Bellows WH: Transesophageal echocardiography in myocardial revascularization: I. Accuracy of intraoperative real-time interpretation, *Anesth Analg* 82:1132, 1996.
239. Bergquist BD, Bellows WH, Leung JM: Transesophageal echocardiography in myocardial revascularization. II. Influence on intraoperative decision making, *Anesth Analg* 82:1139, 1996.
240. Jacka MJ, Cohen MM, To T, et al: The use of and preferences for the transesophageal echocardiogram and pulmonary artery catheter among cardiovascular anesthesiologists, *Anesth Analg* 94:1065, 2002.
241. Cahalan MK, Stewart W, Pearlman A, et al: American Society of Echocardiography and Society of Cardiovascular Anesthesiologists task force guidelines for training in perioperative echocardiography, *J Am Soc Echocardiogr* 15:647, 2002.
242. Hogue CWJ, Lappas GD, Creswell LL, et al: Swallowing dysfunction after cardiac operations. Associated adverse outcomes and risk factors including intraoperative transesophageal echocardiography, *J Thorac Cardiovasc Surg* 110:517, 1995.
243. Brinkman WT, Shanewise JS, Clements SD, et al: Transesophageal echocardiography: Not an innocuous procedure, *Ann Thorac Surg* 72:1725, 2001.
244. Han YY, Cheng YJ, Liao WW, et al: Delayed diagnosis of esophageal perforation following intraoperative transesophageal echocardiography during valvular replacement—a case report, *Acta Anaesthesiol Sin* 41:81, 2003.
245. Lecharny JB, Philip I, Depoix JP: Oesophagotracheal perforation after intraoperative transoesphageal echocardiography in cardiac surgery, *Br J Anaesth* 88:592, 2002.
246. Massey SR, Pitsis A, Mehta D, et al: Oesophageal perforation following perioperative transoesophageal echocardiography, *Br J Anaesth* 84:643, 2000.
247. Zalunardo MP, Bimmler D, Grob UC, et al: Late oesophageal perforation after intraoperative transoesophageal echocardiography, *Br J Anaesth* 88:595, 2002.
248. Fischer GW: Recent advances in application of cerebral oximetry in adult cardiovascular surgery, *Semin Cardiothorac Vasc Anesth* 12:60–69, 2008.
249. Wahr JA, Tremper KK, Samra S, Delpy DT: Near-infrared spectroscopy: Theory and applications, *J Cardiothorac Vasc Anesth* 10:406–418, 1996.

250. Watzman HM, Kurth CD, Montenegro LM, et al: Arterial and venous contributions to near-infrared cerebral oximetry, *Anesthesiology* 93:947–953, 2000.
251. Fischer GW, Stone ME: Cerebral air embolism recognized by cerebral oximetry, *Semin Cardiothorac Vasc Anesth* 13:56, 2009.
252. Murkin JM, Arango M: Near-infrared spectroscopy as an index of brain and tissue oxygenation, *Br J Anaesth* 103(Suppl 1):i3–i13, 2009.
253. Diegeler A, Hisch R, Schneider F, et al: Neuromonitoring and neurocognitive outcome in off-pump versus conventional coronary bypass operation, *Ann Thorac Surg* 69:1162, 2000.
254. Filsoufi F, Rahmanian PB, Castillo JG, et al: Incidence, imaging analysis, and early and late outcomes of stroke after cardiac valve operation, *Am J Cardiol* 101:1472, 2008.
255. Zimpfer D, Czerny M, Vogt F, et al: Neurocognitive deficit following coronary artery bypass grafting: A prospective study of surgical patients and nonsurgical controls, *Ann Thorac Surg* 78:513, 2004.
256. Yao FF, Tseng CA, Ho CA, et al: Cerebral oxygen desaturations is associated with early postoperative neuropsychological dysfunction in patients undergoing cardiac surgery, *J Cardiothorac Vasc Anesth* 18:552, 2004.
257. Slater JP, Guarino T, Stack J, et al: Cerebral oxygen desaturations predicts cognitive decline and longer hospital stay after cardiac surgery, *Ann Thorac Surg* 87:36, 2009.
258. Edmonds HL, Jr: 2010 standards of care for central nervous system monitoring during cardiac surgery, *J Cardiothorac Vasc Anesth* 24:541–543, 2010.
259. Murkin JM, Adams SJ, Novick RJ, et al: Monitoring brain oxygen saturation during coronary bypass surgery: A randomized, prospective study, *Anesth Analg* 104:51, 2007.
260. De Hert SG, Vermeyen KM, Adriaensen HF: Influence of thiopental, etomidate, and propofol on regional myocardial function in the normal and acute ischemic heart segment in dogs, *Anesth Analg* 70:600, 1990.
261. Mulier JP: Cardiodynamic effects of propofol in comparison to thiopental. Use of the end-systolic pressure-volume relationship and arterial elastance, *Anesth Analg* 76:677, 1993.
262. Mulier JP, Wouters PF, Van Aken H, et al: Cardiodynamic effects of propofol in comparison with thiopental: Assessment with a transesophageal echocardiographic approach, *Anesth Analg* 72:28, 1991.
263. Rouby JJ, Andreev A, Leger P, et al: Peripheral vascular effects of thiopental and propofol in humans with artificial hearts, *Anesthesiology* 75:32, 1991.
264. Gauss A, Heinrich H, Wilder-Smith OH: Echocardiographic assessment of the haemodynamic effects of propofol: A comparison with etomidate and thiopentone, *Anaesthesia* 46:99, 1991.
265. Gelissen HP, Epema AH, Henning RH, et al: Inotropic effects of propofol, thiopental, midazolam, etomidate, and ketamine on isolated human atrial muscle, *Anesthesiology* 84:397, 1996.
266. Mather LE, Duke CC, Ladd LA, et al: Direct cardiac effects of coronary site-directed thiopental and its enantiomers: A comparison to propofol in conscious sheep, *Anesthesiology* 101:354, 2004.
267. Tuman KJ, McCarthy RJ, Spiess BD, et al: Does choice of anesthetic agent significantly affect outcome after coronary artery surgery? *Anesthesiology* 70:189, 1989.
268. Pagel PS, Kampine JP, Schmeling WT, et al: Ketamine depresses myocardial contractility as evaluated by the preload recruitable stroke work relationship in chronically instrumented dogs with autonomic nervous system blockade, *Anesthesiology* 76:564, 1992.
269. Pagel PS, Schmeling WT, Kampine JP, et al: Alteration of canine left ventricular diastolic function by intravenous anesthetics in vivo. Ketamine and propofol, *Anesthesiology* 76:419, 1992.
270. Zilberstein G, Levy R, Rachinsky M, et al: Ketamine attenuates neutrophil activation after cardiopulmonary bypass, *Anesth Analg* 95:531, 2002.
271. De Hert SG, Vermeyen KM, Adriaensen HF: Influence of thiopental, etomidate, and propofol on regional myocardial function in the normal and acute ischemic heart segment in dogs, *Anesth Analg* 70:600, 1990.
272. Gelissen HP, Epema AH, Henning RH, et al: Inotropic effects of propofol, thiopental, midazolam, etomidate, and ketamine on isolated human atrial muscle, *Anesthesiology* 84:397, 1996.
273. Komai H, DeWitt DE, Rusy BF: Negative inotropic effect of etomidate in rabbit papillary muscle, *Anesth Analg* 64:400, 1985.
274. Donmez A, Kaya H, Haberal A, et al: The effect of etomidate induction on plasma cortisol levels in children undergoing cardiac surgery, *J Cardiothorac Vasc Anesth* 12:182, 1998.
275. Jackson WL Jr: Should we use etomidate as an induction agent for endotracheal intubation in patients with septic shock? A critical appraisal, *Chest* 127:1031, 2005.
276. Shafer SL: Advances in propofol pharmacokinetics and pharmacodynamics, *J Clin Anesth* 5:14S, 1993.
277. Barr J, Egan TD, Sandoval NF, et al: Propofol dosing regimens for ICU sedation based upon an integrated pharmacokinetic-pharmacodynamic model, *Anesthesiology* 95:324, 2001.
278. Hall RI, MacLaren C, Smith MS, et al: Light versus heavy sedation after cardiac surgery: Myocardial ischemia and the stress response, *Anesth Analg* 85:971, 1997.
279. Herr DL, Sum-Ping ST, England M: ICU sedation after coronary artery bypass graft surgery: Dexmedetomidine-based versus propofol-based sedation regimens, *J Cardiothorac Vasc Anesth* 17:576, 2003.
280. Schmidt C, Roosens C, Struys M, et al: Contractility in humans after coronary artery surgery, *Anesthesiology* 91:58, 1999.
281. Bell J, Sartain J, Wilkinson GA, et al: Propofol and fentanyl anaesthesia for patients with low cardiac output state undergoing cardiac surgery: Comparison with high-dose fentanyl anaesthesia, *Br J Anaesth* 73:162, 1994.
282. Hall RI, Murphy JT, Moffitt EA, et al: A comparison of the myocardial metabolic and haemodynamic changes produced by propofol-sufentanil and enflurane-sufentanil anaesthesia for patients having coronary artery bypass graft surgery, *Can J Anaesth* 38:996, 1991.
283. Hall RI, Murphy JT, Landymore R, et al: Myocardial metabolic and hemodynamic changes during propofol anesthesia for cardiac surgery in patients with reduced ventricular function, *Anesth Analg* 77:680, 1993.
284. Jain U, Body SC, Bellows W, et al: Multicenter study of target-controlled infusion of propofol-sufentanil or sufentanil-midazolam for coronary artery bypass graft surgery. Multicenter Study of Perioperative Ischemia (McSPI) Research Group, *Anesthesiology* 85:522, 1996.
285. Engoren MC, Kraras C, Garzia F: Propofol-based versus fentanyl-isoflurane-based anesthesia for cardiac surgery, *J Cardiothorac Vasc Anesth* 12:177, 1998.
286. Sorbara C, Pittarello D, Rizzoli G, et al: Propofol-fentanyl versus isoflurane-fentanyl anesthesia for coronary artery bypass grafting: Effect on myocardial contractility and peripheral hemodynamics, *J Cardiothorac Vasc Anesth* 9:18, 1995.
287. Sayin MM, Ozatamer O, Tasoz R, et al: Propofol attenuates myocardial lipid peroxidation during coronary artery bypass grafting surgery, *Br J Anaesth* 89:242, 2002.
288. Ansley DM, Raedschelders K, Chen DYY, et al: Rationale, design, and baseline characteristics of the PRO-TECT II study: PROpofol cardioproTECTion for type II diabetics. A randomized, controlled trial of high dose propofol versus isoflurane preconditioning in patients undergoing on-pump coronary artery bypass graft surgery, *Contemp Clin Trials* 30:380, 2009.
289. Brown CR, Sarnquist FH, Canup CA, et al: Clinical, electroencephalographic, and pharmacokinetic studies of a water-soluble benzodiazepine, midazolam maleate, *Anesthesiology* 50:467, 1979.
290. Stanley TH, Bennett GM, Loeser EA, et al: Cardiovascular effects of diazepam and droperidol during morphine anesthesia, *Anesthesiology* 44:255, 1976.
291. Stanley TH, Webster LR: Anesthetic requirements and cardiovascular effects of fentanyl-oxygen and fentanyl-diazepam-oxygen anesthesia in man, *Anesth Analg* 57:411, 1978.
292. Liu WS, Bidwai AV, Stanley TH, et al: The cardiovascular effects of diazepam and of diazepam and pancuronium during fentanyl and oxygen anaesthesia, *Can Anaesth Soc J* 23:395, 1976.
293. Slogoff S, Keats AS: Randomized trial of primary anesthetic agents on outcome of coronary artery bypass operations, *Anesthesiology* 70:179, 1989.
294. Raza SM, Masters RW, Zsigmond EK: Haemodynamic stability with midazolam-ketamine-sufentanil analgesia in cardiac surgical patients, *Can J Anaesth* 36:617, 1989.
295. Gordon AR, O'Connor JP, Ralley FE, et al: Midazolam-ketamine vs sufentanil for rapid sequence induction of anaesthesia for CABG surgery, *Can J Anaesth* 37:S43, 1990.
296. Samuelson PN, Reves JG, Kouchoukos NT, et al: Hemodynamic responses to anesthetic induction with midazolam or diazepam in patients with ischemic heart disease, *Anesth Analg* 60:802, 1981.
297. Schulte-Sasse U, Hess W, Tarnow J: Haemodynamic responses to induction of anaesthesia using midazolam in cardiac surgical patients, *Br J Anaesth* 54:1053, 1982.
298. Heikkila H, Jalonen J, Arola M, et al: Midazolam as adjunct to high-dose fentanyl anaesthesia for coronary artery bypass grafting operation, *Acta Anaesthesiol Scand* 28:683, 1984.
299. Kawar P, Carson IW, Clarke RS, et al: Haemodynamic changes during induction of anaesthesia with midazolam and diazepam (Valium) in patients undergoing coronary artery bypass surgery, *Anaesthesia* 40:767, 1985.
300. Raza SM, Zsigmond EK, Barabas E: Midazolam causes no adverse hemodynamic effects in cardiac patients, *Clin Ther* 10:40, 1987.
301. Raza SM, Masters RW, Vasireddy AR, et al: Haemodynamic stability with midazolam-sufentanil analgesia in cardiac surgical patients, *Can J Anaesth* 35:518, 1988.
302. Tuman KJ, McCarthy RJ, el-Ganzouri AR, et al: Sufentanil-midazolam anesthesia for coronary artery surgery, *J Cardiothorac Anesth* 4:308, 1990.
303. van der Maaten JM, Epema AH, Huet RC, et al: The effect of midazolam at two plasma concentrations of hemodynamics and sufentanil requirement in coronary artery surgery, *J Cardiothorac Vasc Anesth* 10:356, 1996.
304. Driessen JJ, Giart M: Comparison of isoflurane and midazolam as hypnotic supplementation to moderately high-dose fentanyl during coronary artery bypass grafting: Effects on systemic hemodynamics and early postoperative recovery profile, *J Cardiothorac Vasc Anesth* 11:740, 1997.
305. Heikkila H, Jalonen J, Arola M, et al: Midazolam as adjunct to high-dose fentanyl anaesthesia for coronary artery bypass grafting operation, *Acta Anaesthesiol Scand* 28:683, 1984.
306. Messina AG, Paranicas M, Yao FS, et al: The effect of midazolam on left ventricular pump performance and contractility in anesthetized patients with coronary artery disease: Effect of preoperative ejection fraction, *Anesth Analg* 81:793, 1995.
307. Lowenstein E, Hallowell P, Levine FH, et al: Cardiovascular response to large doses of intravenous morphine in man, *N Engl J Med* 281:1389, 1969.
308. Murphy GS, Szokol JW, Marymont JH, et al: The effects of morphine and fentanyl on the inflammatory response to cardiopulmonary bypass in patients undergoing elective coronary artery bypass graft surgery, *Anesth Analg* 104:1334–1342, 2007.
309. Murphy GS, Szokol JW, Marymont JH, et al: Morphine-based cardiac anesthesia provides superior early recovery compared with fentanyl in elective cardiac surgery patients, *Anesth Analg* 109:311–319, 2009.
310. Stanley TH, Webster LR: Anesthetic requirements and cardiovascular effects of fentanyl-oxygen and fentanyl-diazepam-oxygen anesthesia in man, *Anesth Analg* 57:411, 1978.
311. Liu WS, Bidwai AV, Stanley TH, et al: The cardiovascular effects of diazepam and of diazepam and pancuronium during fentanyl and oxygen anaesthesia, *Can Anaesth Soc J* 23:395, 1976.
312. Lunn JK, Stanley TH, Eisele J, et al: High dose fentanyl anesthesia for coronary artery surgery: Plasma fentanyl concentrations and influence of nitrous oxide on cardiovascular responses, *Anesth Analg* 58:390, 1979.
313. Tomicheck RC, Rosow CE, Philbin DM, et al: Diazepam-fentanyl interaction—hemodynamic and hormonal effects in coronary artery surgery, *Anesth Analg* 62:881, 1983.
314. Bovill JG, Sebel PS: Pharmacokinetics of high-dose fentanyl. A study in patients undergoing cardiac surgery, *Br J Anaesth* 52:795, 1980.
315. Prakash O, Verdouw PD, de Jong JW, et al: Haemodynamic and biochemical variables after induction of anaesthesia with fentanyl and nitrous oxide in patients undergoing coronary artery by-pass surgery, *Can Anaesth Soc J* 27:223, 1980.
316. Sebel PS, Bovill JG, Schellekens AP, et al: Hormonal responses to high-dose fentanyl anaesthesia. A study in patients undergoing cardiac surgery, *Br J Anaesth* 53:941, 1981.
317. Waller JL, Hug CC Jr, Nagle DM, et al: Hemodynamic changes during fentanyl—oxygen anesthesia for aortocoronary bypass operation, *Anesthesiology* 55:212, 1981.
318. Walsh ES, Paterson JL, O'Riordan JB, et al: Effect of high-dose fentanyl anaesthesia on the metabolic and endocrine response to cardiac surgery, *Br J Anaesth* 53:1155, 1981.
319. Sonntag H, Larsen R, Hilfiker O, et al: Myocardial blood flow and oxygen consumption during high-dose fentanyl anesthesia in patients with coronary artery disease, *Anesthesiology* 56:417, 1982.
320. Hilgenberg JC: Intraoperative awareness during high-dose fentanyl—oxygen anesthesia, *Anesthesiology* 54:341, 1981.
321. Raza SM, Masters RW, Zsigmond EK: Haemodynamic stability with midazolam-ketamine-sufentanil analgesia in cardiac surgical patients, *Can J Anaesth* 36:617, 1989.
322. Raza SM, Masters RW, Vasireddy AR, et al: Haemodynamic stability with midazolam-sufentanil analgesia in cardiac surgical patients, *Can J Anaesth* 35:518, 1988.
323. Tuman KJ, McCarthy RJ, el-Ganzouri AR, et al: Sufentanil-midazolam anesthesia for coronary artery surgery, *J Cardiothorac Anesth* 4:308, 1990.
324. Dubois-Primo J, Dewachter B, Massaut J: Analgesic anesthesia with fentanyl (F) and sufentanil (SF) in coronary surgery. A double blind study, *Acta Anaesthesiol Belg* 30:113, 1979.
325. de Lange S, Boscoe MJ, Stanley TH, et al: Antidiuretic and growth hormone responses during coronary artery surgery with sufentanil-oxygen and alfentanil-oxygen anesthesia in man, *Anesth Analg* 61:434, 1982.
326. de Lange S, Boscoe MJ, Stanley TH, et al: Comparison of sufentanil—O_2 and fentanyl—O_2 for coronary artery surgery, *Anesthesiology* 56:112, 1982.
327. Bovill JG, Sebel PS, Fiolet JW, et al: The influence of sufentanil on endocrine and metabolic responses to cardiac surgery, *Anesth Analg* 62:391, 1983.
328. O'Young J, Mastrocostopoulos G, Hilgenberg A, et al: Myocardial circulatory and metabolic effects of isoflurane and sufentanil during coronary artery surgery, *Anesthesiology* 66:653, 1987.
329. Thomson IR, Hudson RJ, Rosenbloom M, et al: A randomized double-blind comparison of fentanyl and sufentanil anaesthesia for coronary artery surgery, *Can J Anaesth* 34:227, 1987.
330. Helman JD, Leung JM, Bellows WH, et al: The risk of myocardial ischemia in patients receiving desflurane versus sufentanil anesthesia for coronary artery bypass graft surgery. The S.P.I. Research Group, *Anesthesiology* 77:47, 1992.
331. Spiess BD, Sathoff RH, El-Ganzouri ARS, et al: High-dose sufentanil: Four cases of sudden hypotension on induction, *Anesth Analg* 65:703, 1986.
332. Starr NJ, Sethna DH, Estafanous FG: Bradycardia and asystole following the administration of sufentanil with vecuronium, *Anesthesiology* 64:521, 1986.
333. Egan TD, Lemmens HJ, Fiset P, et al: The pharmacokinetics of the new short-acting opioid remifentanil (GI87084B) in healthy adult male volunteers, *Anesthesiology* 79:881, 1993.
334. Latham P, Zarate E, White PF, et al: Fast-track cardiac anesthesia: A comparison of remifentanil plus intrathecal morphine with sufentanil in a desflurane-based anesthetic, *J Cardiothorac Vasc Anesth* 14:645, 2000.

335. Olivier P, Sirieix D, Dassier P, et al: Continuous infusion of remifentanil and target-controlled infusion of propofol for patients undergoing cardiac surgery: A new approach for scheduled early extubation, *J Cardiothorac Vasc Anesth* 14:29, 2000.
336. Cheng DC, Newman MF, Duke P, et al: The efficacy and resource utilization of remifentanil and fentanyl in fast-track coronary artery bypass graft surgery: A prospective randomized, double-blinded controlled, multi-center trial, *Anesth Analg* 92:1094, 2001.
337. Engoren M, Luther G, Fenn-Buderer N: A comparison of fentanyl, sufentanil, and remifentanil for fast-track cardiac anesthesia, *Anesth Analg* 93:859, 2001.
338. Howie MB, Cheng D, Newman MF, et al: A randomized double-blinded multicenter comparison of remifentanil versus fentanyl when combined with isoflurane/propofol for early extubation in coronary artery bypass graft surgery, *Anesth Analg* 92:1084, 2001.
339. Mollhoff T, Herregods L, Moerman A, et al: Comparative efficacy and safety of remifentanil and fentanyl in 'fast track' coronary artery bypass graft surgery: A randomized, double-blind study, *Br J Anaesth* 87:718, 2001.
340. Myles PS, Hunt JO, Fletcher H, et al: Remifentanil, fentanyl, and cardiac surgery: A double-blinded, randomized, controlled trial of costs and outcomes, *Anesth Analg* 95:805, 2002.
341. Reddy P, Feret BM, Kulicki L, et al: Cost analysis of fentanyl and remifentanil in coronary artery bypass graft surgery without cardiopulmonary bypass, *J Clin Pharm Ther* 27:127, 2002.
342. Winterhalter M, Brandl K, Rahe-Meyer N, et al: Endocrine stress response and inflammatory activation during CABG surgery. A randomized trial comparing remifentanyl infusion to intermittent fentanyl, *Eur J Anaesthesiol* 25:326, 2008.
343. Lena P, Balarac N, Lena D, et al: Fast-track anesthesia with remifentanyl and spinal analgesia for cardiac surgery: The effect on pain control and quality of recovery, *J Cardiothorac Vasc Anesth* 22:536, 2008.
344. Elliott P, O'Hare R, Bill KM, et al: Severe cardiovascular depression with remifentanil, *Anesth Analg* 91:58, 2000.
345. Pleym H, Stenseth R, Wiseth R, et al: Supplemental remifentanil during coronary artery bypass grafting is followed by a transient postoperative cardiac depression, *Acta Anaesthesiol Scand* 48:1155, 2004.
346. Winterhalter M, Brandl K, Rahe-Meyer N, et al: Endocrine stress response and inflammatory activation during CABG surgery. A randomized trial comparing remifentanyl infusion to intermittent fentanyl, *Eur J Anaesthesiol* 25:326, 2008.
347. Shafer SL, Varvel JR: Pharmacokinetics, pharmacodynamics, and rational opioid selection, *Anesthesiology* 74:53, 1991.
348. Ethuin F, Boudaoud S, Leblanc I, et al: Pharmacokinetics of long-term sufentanil infusion for sedation in ICU patients, *Intensive Care Med* 29:1916, 2003.
349. Mangano DT, Siliciano D, Hollenberg M, et al: Postoperative myocardial ischemia. Therapeutic trials using intensive analgesia following surgery, *Anesthesiology* 76:342, 1992.
350. Butterworth J, James R, Prielipp RC, et al: Do shorter-acting neuromuscular blocking drugs or opioids associate with reduced intensive care unit or hospital lengths of stay after coronary artery bypass grafting? CABG Clinical Benchmarking Data Base Participants, *Anesthesiology* 88:1437, 1998.
351. Sanford TJ, Smith NT, Dec-Silver H, et al: A comparison of morphine, fentanyl, and sufentanil anesthesia for cardiac surgery: Induction, emergence, and extubation, *Anesth Analg* 65:259, 1986.
352. London MJ, Shroyer ALW, Grover FL: Fast tracking into the new millennium: An evolving paradigm, *Anesthesiology* 91:936, 1999.
353. Wynands JE, Townsend GE, Wong P, et al: Blood pressure response and plasma fentanyl concentrations during high- and very-high-dose fentanyl anesthesia for coronary artery surgery, *Anesth Analg* 62:661, 1983.
354. Lacoumenta S, Yeo TH, Paterson JL, et al: Hormonal and metabolic responses to cardiac surgery with sufentanil-oxygen anaesthesia, *Acta Anaesthesiol Scand* 31:258, 1987.
355. Thomson IR, Hudson RJ, Rosenbloom M, et al: Catecholamine responses to anesthetic induction with fentanyl and sufentanil, *J Cardiothorac Anesth* 2:18, 1988.
356. Sonntag H, Larsen R, Hilfiker O, et al: Myocardial blood flow and oxygen consumption during high-dose fentanyl anesthesia in patients with coronary artery disease, *Anesthesiology* 56:417, 1982.
357. Sonntag H, Stephan H, Lange H, et al: Sufentanil does not block sympathetic responses to surgical stimuli in patients having coronary artery revascularization surgery, *Anesth Analg* 68:584, 1989.
358. Philbin DM, Rosow CE, Schneider RC, et al: Fentanyl and sufentanil anesthesia revisited: How much is enough? *Anesthesiology* 73:5, 1990.
359. Thomson IR, Henderson BT, Singh K, et al: Concentration-response relationships for fentanyl and sufentanil in patients undergoing coronary artery bypass grafting, *Anesthesiology* 89:852, 1998.
360. Philbin DM, Rosow CE: Fentanyl and sufentanil anesthesia revisited, *J Cardiothorac Vasc Anesth* 5:651–652, 1991.
361. Murphy GS, Szokol JW, Vender JS, et al: The use of neuromuscular blocking drugs in adult cardiac surgery: Results of a national postal survey, *Anesth Analg* 95:1534, 2002.
362. O'Connor JP, Ramsay JG, Wynands JE, et al: The incidence of myocardial ischemia during anesthesia for coronary artery bypass surgery in patients receiving pancuronium or vecuronium, *Anesthesiology* 70:230, 1989.
363. McEwin L, Merrick PM, Bevan DR: Residual neuromuscular blockade after cardiac surgery: Pancuronium vs rocuronium, *Can J Anaesth* 44:891, 1997.
364. Murphy GS, Szokol JW, Marymont JH, et al: Impact of shorter-acting neuromuscular blocking agents on fast-track recovery of the cardiac surgical patient, *Anesthesiology* 96:600, 2002.
365. Thomas R, Smith D, Strike P: Prospective randomised double-blind comparative study of rocuronium and pancuronium in adult patients scheduled for elective 'fast-track' cardiac surgery involving hypothermic cardiopulmonary bypass, *Anaesthesia* 58:265, 2003.
366. Jellish WS, Brody M, Sawicki K, et al: Recovery from neuromuscular blockade after either bolus and prolonged infusions of cisatracurium or rocuronium using either isoflurane or propofol-based anesthetics, *Anesth Analg* 91:1250, 2000.
367. Reich DL, Hollinger I, Harrington DJ, et al: Comparison of cisatracurium and vecuronium by infusion in neonates and small infants after congenital heart surgery, *Anesthesiology* 101:1122, 2004.
368. Murphy GS, Szokol JW, Marymont JH, et al: Recovery of neuromuscular function after cardiac surgery: Pancuronium versus rocuronium, *Anesth Analg* 96:1301, 2003.
369. Cammu G, De Keersmaecker K, Casselman F, et al: Implications of the use of neuromuscular transmission monitoring on immediate postoperative extubation in off-pump coronary artery bypass surgery, *Eur J Anaesthesiol* 20:884, 2003.
370. Pinard AM, Donati F, Martineau R, et al: Magnesium potentiates neuromuscular blockade with cisatracurium during cardiac surgery, *Can J Anaesth* 50:172, 2003.
371. Gueret G, Rossignol B, Kiss G, et al: Is muscle relaxant necessary for cardiac surgery? *Anesth Analg* 99:1330, 2004.
372. Menda F, Köner O, Sayin M, et al: Dexmedetomidine as an adjunct to anesthetic induction to attenuate hemodynamic response to endotracheal intubation in patients undergoing fast-track CABG, *Ann Card Anaesth* 13:16–21, 2010.
373. Talke P, Chen R, Thomas B, et al: The hemodynamic and adrenergic effects of perioperative dexmedetomidine infusion after vascular surgery, *Anesth Analg* 90:834, 2000.
374. Hogue CW Jr, Talke P, Stein PK, et al: Autonomic nervous system responses during sedative infusions of dexmedetomidine, *Anesthesiology* 97:592, 2002.
375. Lawrence CJ, De Lange S: Effects of a single pre-operative dexmedetomidine dose on isoflurane requirements and peri-operative haemodynamic stability, *Anaesthesia* 52:736, 1997.
376. Jalonen J, Hynynen M, Kuitunen A, et al: Dexmedetomidine as an anesthetic adjunct in coronary artery bypass grafting, *Anesthesiology* 86:331, 1997.
377. Ruesch S, Levy JH: Treatment of persistent tachycardia with dexmedetomidine during off-pump cardiac surgery, *Anesth Analg* 95:316, 2002.
378. Taniguchi T, Kidani Y, Kanakura H, et al: Effects of dexmedetomidine on mortality rate and inflammatory responses to endotoxin-induced shock in rats, *Crit Care Med* 32:1322, 2004.
379. Cope DK, Impastato WK, Cohen MV, et al: Volatile anesthetics protect the ischemic rabbit myocardium from infarction, *Anesthesiology* 86:699, 1997.
380. De Hert SG, ten Broecke PW, Mertens E, et al: Sevoflurane but not propofol preserves myocardial function in coronary surgery patients, *Anesthesiology* 97:42, 2002.
381. Wu ZK, Iivainen T, Pehkonen E, et al: Arrhythmias in off-pump coronary artery bypass grafting and the antiarrhythmic effect of regional ischemic preconditioning, *J Cardiothorac Vasc Anesth* 17:459, 2003.
382. Murry CE, Jennings RB, Reimer KA: Preconditioning with ischemia: A delay of lethal cell injury in ischemic myocardium, *Circulation* 74:1124, 1986.
383. Zaugg M, Lucchinetti E, Uecker M, et al: Anaesthetics and cardiac preconditioning. Part I. Signalling and cytoprotective mechanisms, *Br J Anaesth* 91:551, 2003.
384. Stein KL, Breisblatt W, Wolfe C, et al: Depression and recovery of right ventricular function after cardiopulmonary bypass, *Crit Care Med* 18:1197, 1990.
385. Breisblatt WM, Stein KL, Wolfe CJ, et al: Acute myocardial dysfunction and recovery: A common occurrence after coronary bypass surgery, *J Am Coll Cardiol* 15:1261, 1990.
386. Illes RW, Swoyer KD: Prospective, randomized clinical study of ischemic preconditioning as an adjunct to intermittent cold blood cardioplegia, *Ann Thorac Surg* 65:748, 1998.
387. Jenkins DP, Pugsley WB, Alkhulaifi AM, et al: Ischaemic preconditioning reduces troponin T release in patients undergoing coronary artery bypass surgery, *Heart* 77:314, 1997.
388. Laurikka J, Wu ZK, Iisalo P, et al: Regional ischemic preconditioning enhances myocardial performance in off-pump coronary artery bypass grafting, *Chest* 121:1183, 2002.
389. Baldwin D, Chandrashekhar Y, McFalls E, et al: Ischemic preconditioning prior to aortic cross-clamping protects high-energy phosphate levels, glucose uptake, and myocyte contractility, *J Surg Res* 105:153, 2002.
390. Landoni G, Fochi O, Tritapepe L, et al: Cardiac protection by volatile anesthetics. A review, *Minerva Anestesiol* 75:269, 2009.
391. Piriou V, Chiari P: Con: Ischemic preconditioning is not necessary because volatile agents can accomplish it, *J Cardiothorac Vasc Anesth* 18:803, 2004.
392. Hausenloy DJ, Yellon DM: Remote ischaemic preconditioning: Underlying mechanisms and clinical application, *Cardiovasc Res* 79:377, 2008.
393. Kharbanda RK, Nielsen TT, Redington AN: Translation of remote ischaemic preconditioning into clinical practice, *Lancet* 374:1557, 2009.
394. Takagi H, Manabe H, Kawai N, et al: Review and meta-analysis of randomized controlled clinical trials of remote ischemic preconditioning in cardiovascular surgery, *Am J Cardiol* 102:1487, 2008.
395. Venugopal V, Hausenloy DJ, Ludman A, et al: Remote ischaemic preconditioning reduces myocardial injury in patients undergoing cardiac surgery with cold-blood cardioplegia: A randomised controlled trial, *Heart* 95:1567, 2009.
396. Hoole SP, Heck PM, Sharples L, et al: Cardiac Remote Ischemic Preconditioning in Coronary Stenting (CRISP Stent) Study: A prospective, randomized control trial, *Circulation* 119:820, 2009.
397. Ludwig LM, Patel HH, Gross GJ, et al: Morphine enhances pharmacological preconditioning by isoflurane: Role of mitochondrial K(ATP) channels and opioid receptors, *Anesthesiology* 98:705, 2003.
398. Bolling SF, Badhwar V, Schwartz CF, et al: Opioids confer myocardial tolerance to ischemia: Interaction of delta opioid agonists and antagonists, *J Thorac Cardiovasc Surg* 122:476, 2001.
399. Zaugg M, Lucchinetti E, Spahn DR, et al: Differential effects of anesthetics on mitochondrial K(ATP) channel activity and cardiomyocyte protection, *Anesthesiology* 97:15, 2002.
400. Smul TM, Lange M, Redel A, et al: Propofol blocks desflurane-induced preconditioning, but not ischemic-induced preconditioning, *Anesthesiology* 103:A462, 2005.
401. Tanaka K, Ludwig LM, Kersten JR, et al: Mechanisms of cardioprotection by volatile anesthetics, *Anesthesiology* 100:707, 2004.
402. Riess ML, Stowe DF, Warltier DC: Cardiac pharmacological preconditioning with volatile anesthetics: From bench to bedside? *Am J Physiol Heart Circ Physiol* 286:H1603, 2004.
403. Kudo M, Wang Y, Xu M, et al: Adenosine A(1) receptor mediates late preconditioning via activation of PKC-delta signaling pathway, *Am J Physiol Heart Circ Physiol* 283:H296, 2002.
404. Zhao TC, Hines DS, Kukreja RC: Adenosine-induced late pre-conditioning in mouse hearts: Role of p38 MAP kinase and mitochondrial K(ATP) channels, *Am J Physiol Heart Circ Physiol* 280:H1278, 2001.
405. Leesar MA, Stoddard MF, Dawn B, et al: Delayed preconditioning-mimetic action of nitroglycerin in patients undergoing coronary angioplasty, *Circulation* 103:2935, 2001.
406. Leesar MA, Stoddard MF, Manchikalapudi S, et al: Bradykinin-induced preconditioning in patients undergoing coronary angioplasty, *J Am Coll Cardiol* 34:639, 1999.
407. Cohen MV, Yang XM, Liu GS, et al: Acetylcholine, bradykinin, opioids, and phenylephrine, but not adenosine, trigger preconditioning by generating free radicals and opening mitochondrial K(ATP) channels, *Circ Res* 89:273, 2001.
408. Pagel PS: Remote exposure to xenon produces delayed preconditioning against myocardial infarction in vivo: Additional evidence that noble gases are not biologically inert, *Anesth Analg* 107:1768, 2008.
409. Wolfrum S, Schneider K, Heidbreder M, et al: Remote preconditioning protects the heart by activating myocardial PKCepsilon-isoform, *Cardiovasc Res* 55:583, 2002.
410. da Silva R, Grampp T, Pasch T, et al: Differential activation of mitogen-activated protein kinases in ischemic and anesthetic preconditioning, *Anesthesiology* 100:59, 2004.
411. Laude K, Favre J, Thuillez C, et al: NO produced by endothelial NO synthase is a mediator of delayed preconditioning-induced endothelial protection, *Am J Physiol Heart Circ Physiol* 284:H2053, 2003.
412. Bell RM, Yellon DM: The contribution of endothelial nitric oxide synthase to early ischaemic preconditioning: The lowering of the preconditioning threshold. An investigation in eNOS knockout mice, *Cardiovasc Res* 52:274, 2001.
413. Tanaka K, Ludwig LM, Kersten JR, et al: Mechanisms of cardioprotection by volatile anesthetics, *Anesthesiology* 100:707, 2004.
414. Alcindor D, Krolikowski JG, Pagel PS, et al: Cyclooxygenase-2 mediates ischemic, anesthetic, and pharmacologic preconditioning in vivo, *Anesthesiology* 100:547, 2004.
415. Smul TM, Lange M, Redel A, et al: Desflurane-induced cardioprotection against ischemia-reperfusion injury depends on timing, *J Cardiothorac Vasc Anesth* 23:607, 2009.
416. Rizvi A, Tang XL, Qiu YM, et al: Increased protein synthesis is necessary for the development of late preconditioning against myocardial stunning, *Am J Physiol Heart Circ Physiol* 46:H874, 1999.
417. Zaugg M, Schaub MC: Signaling and cellular mechanisms in cardiac protection by ischemic and pharmacological preconditioning, *J Muscle Res Cell Motil* 24:219, 2003.
418. Frassdorf J, De Hert S, Schlack W: Anaesthesia and myocardial ischaemia/reperfusion injury, *Br J Anaesth* 103:89, 2009.
419. Kowalski C, Zahler S, Becker BF, et al: Halothane, isoflurane, and sevoflurane reduce postischemic adhesion of neutrophils in the coronary system, *Anesthesiology* 86:188, 1997.

420. Heindl B, Becker BF, Zahler S, et al: Volatile anaesthetics reduce adhesion of blood platelets under low-flow conditions in the coronary system of isolated guinea pig hearts, *Acta Anaesthesiol Scand* 42:995, 1998.
421. Heindl B, Reichle FM, Zahler S, et al: Sevoflurane and isoflurane protect the reperfused guinea pig heart by reducing postischemic adhesion of polymorphonuclear neutrophils, *Anesthesiology* 91:521, 1999.
422. Heindl B, Conzen PF, Becker BF: The volatile anesthetic sevoflurane mitigates cardiodepressive effects of platelets in reperfused hearts, *Basic Res Cardiol* 94:102, 1999.
423. Hu G, Salem MR, Crystal GJ: Isoflurane and sevoflurane precondition against neutrophil-induced contractile dysfunction in isolated rat hearts, *Anesthesiology* 100:489, 2004.
424. Belhomme D, Peynet J, Louzy M, et al: Evidence for preconditioning by isoflurane in coronary artery bypass graft surgery, *Circulation* 100:II340, 1999.
425. Penta de Peppo A, Polisca P, Tomai F, et al: Recovery of LV contractility in man is enhanced by preischemic administration of enflurane, *Ann Thorac Surg* 68:112, 1999.
426. Julier K, da Silva R, Garcia C, et al: Preconditioning by sevoflurane decreases biochemical markers for myocardial and renal dysfunction in coronary artery bypass graft surgery: A double-blinded, placebo-controlled, multicenter study, *Anesthesiology* 98:1315, 2003.
427. Conzen PF, Fischer S, Detter C, et al: Sevoflurane provides greater protection of the myocardium than propofol in patients undergoing off-pump coronary artery bypass surgery, *Anesthesiology* 99:826, 2003.
428. Nader ND, Li CM, Khadra WZ, et al: Anesthetic myocardial protection with sevoflurane, *J Cardiothorac Vasc Anesth* 18:269, 2004.
429. De Hert SG, ten Broecke PW, Mertens E, et al: Sevoflurane but not propofol preserves myocardial function in coronary surgery patients, *Anesthesiology* 97:42, 2002.
430. De Hert SG, Van der Linden PJ, Cromheecke S, et al: Choice of primary anesthetic regimen can influence intensive care unit length of stay after coronary surgery with cardiopulmonary bypass, *Anesthesiology* 101:9, 2004.
431. De Hert SG, Cromheecke S, ten Broecke PW, et al: Effects of propofol, desflurane, and sevoflurane on recovery of myocardial function after coronary surgery in elderly high-risk patients, *Anesthesiology* 99:314, 2003.
432. De Hert SG, Van der Linden PJ, Cromheecke S, et al: Cardioprotective properties of sevoflurane in patients undergoing coronary surgery with cardiopulmonary bypass are related to the modalities of its administration, *Anesthesiology* 101:299, 2004.
433. Conzen PF, Fischer S, Detter C, et al: Sevoflurane provides greater protection of the myocardium than propofol in patients undergoing off-pump coronary artery bypass surgery, *Anesthesiology* 99:826, 2003.
434. Julier K, da Silva R, Garcia C, et al: Preconditioning by sevoflurane decreases biochemical markers for myocardial and renal dysfunction in coronary artery bypass graft surgery: A double-blinded, placebo-controlled, multicenter study, *Anesthesiology* 98:1315, 2003.
435. Garcia C, Julier K, Bestmann L, et al: Preconditioning with sevoflurane decreases PECAM-1 expression and improves one-year cardiovascular outcome in coronary artery bypass graft surgery, *Br J Anaesth* 94:159–165, 2005.
436. Belhomme D, Peynet J, Louzy M, et al: Evidence for preconditioning by isoflurane in coronary artery bypass graft surgery, *Circulation* 100:II340, 1999.
437. Penta de Peppo A, Polisca P, Tomai F, et al: Recovery of LV contractility in man is enhanced by preischemic administration of enflurane, *Ann Thorac Surg* 68:112, 1999.
438. Nader ND, Li CM, Khadra WZ, et al: Anesthetic myocardial protection with sevoflurane, *J Cardiothorac Vasc Anesth* 18:269, 2004.
439. Tomai F, De Paulis R, Penta de Peppo A, et al: Beneficial impact of isoflurane during coronary bypass surgery on troponin I release, *G Ital Cardiol* 29:1007, 1999.
440. Haroun-Bizri S, Khoury SS, Chehab IR, et al: Does isoflurane optimize myocardial protection during cardiopulmonary bypass? *J Cardiothorac Vasc Anesth* 15:418, 2001.
441. Pagel PS: Cardioprotection by volatile anesthetics: Established scientific principle or lingering clinical uncertainity? *J Cardiothorac Vasc Anesth* 23:589–543, 2009.
442. De Hert SG, Cromheecke S, ten Broecke PW, et al: Effects of propofol, desflurane, and sevoflurane on recovery of myocardial function after coronary surgery in elderly high-risk patients, *Anesthesiology* 99:314, 2003.
443. De Hert SG, Van der Linden PJ, Cromheecke S, et al: Choice of primary anesthetic regimen can influence intensive care unit length of stay after coronary surgery with cardiopulmonary bypass, *Anesthesiology* 101:9, 2004.
444. Guarrancino F, Landoni G, Tritapepe L, et al: Myocardial damage prevented by volatile anesthetics: A multicenter randomized controlled study, *J Cardiothorac Vasc Anesth* 20:477, 2006.
445. Landoni G, Biondi-Zoccai GG, Zangrillo A, et al: Desflurane and sevoflurane in cardiac surgery: A meta-analysis of randomized clinical trials, *J Cardiothorac Vasc Anesth* 21:502, 2007.
446. Symons JA, Myles PS: Myocardial protection with volatile anesthetic agents during coronary artery bypass surgery: A meta-analysis, *Br J Anaesth* 97:127, 2006.
447. Yu CH, Beattie WS: The effects of volatile anesthetics on cardiac ischemic complications and mortality in CABG: A meta analysis, *Can J Anaesth* 53:906, 2006.
448. Jakobsen CJ, Berg H, Hindsholm KB, et al: The influence of propofol versus sevoflurane anesthesia on outcome in 10,535 cardiac surgical procedures, *J Cardiothorac Vasc Anesth* 21:664, 2007.
449. Bignami E, Biondi-Zoccai GG, Landoni G, et al: Volatile anesthetics reduce mortality in cardiac surgery, *J Cardiothorac Vasc Anesth* 23:594, 2009.
450. De Hert S, Vlasselaers D, Barbe R, et al: A comparison of volatile and non volatile agents for cardioprotection during on-pump coronary surgery, *Anaesthesia* 64:953, 2009.
451. Kehl F, Krolikowski JG, Mraovic B, et al: Is isoflurane-induced preconditioning dose related? *Anesthesiology* 96:675, 2002.
452. Riess ML, Kevin LG, Camara AK, et al: Dual exposure to sevoflurane improves anesthetic preconditioning in intact hearts, *Anesthesiology* 100:569, 2004.
453. Frassdorf J, Borowski A, Ebel D, et al: Impact of preconditioning protocol on anesthetic-induced cardioprotection in patients having coronary artery bypass surgery, *J Thorac Cardiovasc Surg* 137:1436, 2009.
454. Bein B, Renner J, Caliebe D, et al: The effects of interrupted or continuous administration of sevoflurane on preconditioning before cardio-pulmonary bypass in coronary artery surgery: Comparison with continuous propofol, *Anaesthesia* 63:1046, 2008.
455. De Hert SG, Van der Linden PJ, Cromheecke S, et al: Cardioprotective properties of sevoflurane in patients undergoing coronary surgery with cardiopulmonary bypass are related to the modalities of its administration, *Anesthesiology* 101:299, 2004.
456. Bein B, Renner J, Caliebe D, et al: The effects of interrupted or continuous administration of sevoflurane on preconditioning before cardio-pulmonary bypass in coronary artery surgery: Comparison with continuous propofol, *Anaesthesia* 63:1046, 2008.
457. Frassdorf J, Borowski A, Ebel D, et al: Impact of preconditioning protocol on anesthetic-induced cardioprotection in patients having coronary artery bypass surgery, *J Thorac Cardiovasc Surg* 137:1436, 2009.
458. Ludwig LM, Patel HH, Gross GJ, et al: Morphine enhances pharmacological preconditioning by isoflurane: Role of mitochondrial K(ATP) channels and opioid receptors, *Anesthesiology* 98:705, 2003.
459. Bolling SF, Badhwar V, Schwartz CF, et al: Opioids confer myocardial tolerance to ischemia: Interaction of delta opioid agonists and antagonists, *J Thorac Cardiovasc Surg* 122:476, 2001.
460. Wei M, Wang X, Kuukasjarvi P, et al: Bradykinin preconditioning in coronary artery bypass grafting, *Ann Thorac Surg* 78:492, 2004.
461. Muraki S, Morris CD, Budde JM, et al: Experimental off-pump coronary artery revascularization with adenosine-enhanced reperfusion, *J Thorac Cardiovasc Surg* 121:570, 2001.
462. Toller WG, Kersten JR, Pagel PS, et al: Sevoflurane reduces myocardial infarct size and decreases the time threshold for ischemic preconditioning in dogs, *Anesthesiology* 91:1437, 1999.
463. Ludwig LM, Patel HH, Gross GJ, et al: Morphine enhances pharmacological preconditioning by isoflurane: Role of mitochondrial K(ATP) channels and opioid receptors, *Anesthesiology* 98:705, 2003.
464. Ghosh S, Galinanes M: Protection of the human heart with ischemic preconditioning during cardiac surgery: Role of cardiopulmonary bypass, *J Thorac Cardiovasc Surg* 126:133, 2003.
465. Laskey WK, Beach D: Frequency and clinical significance of ischemic preconditioning during percutaneous coronary intervention, *J Am Coll Cardiol* 42:998, 2003.
466. Kersten JR, Schmeling TJ, Orth KG, et al: Acute hyperglycemia abolishes ischemic preconditioning in vivo, *Am J Physiol* 275:H721, 1998.
467. Kehl F, Krolikowski JG, Mraovic B, et al: Hyperglycemia prevents isoflurane-induced preconditioning against myocardial infarction, *Anesthesiology* 96:183, 2002.
468. Kehl F, Krolikowski JG, Weihrauch D, et al: N-acetylcysteine restores isoflurane-induced preconditioning against myocardial infarction during hyperglycemia, *Anesthesiology* 98:1384, 2003.
469. Kersten JR, Toller WG, Gross ER, et al: Diabetes abolishes ischemic preconditioning: Role of glucose, insulin, and osmolality, *Am J Physiol Heart Circ Physiol* 278:H1218, 2000.
470. Zaugg M, Lucchinetti E, Spahn DR, et al: Differential effects of anesthetics on mitochondrial K(ATP) channel activity and cardiomyocyte protection, *Anesthesiology* 97:15, 2002.
471. Zhao ZQ, Corvera JS Halkos ME, et al: Inhibition of myocardial injury by ischemic PostC during reprofusion: Comparision with ischemic preconditioning, *Am J Physiol Heart Cerc Physiol* 285:H579, 2003.
472. Lie RH, Hasenkam JM, Nielsen TT, et al: Post-conditioning reduces infarct size in an open-chest porcine acute ischmia-reperfusion model, *Acta Anaesthesiol Scand* 52:1188, 2008.
473. Penna c., Rastaldo R, Mancardi D, et al: Post-conditioning induced cardioprotection requires signaling through a redox-sensitive mechanism, mitochondrial ATP-sensitive K+ channel and protein kinase C activation, *Basic Res Cardiol* 101:180, 2006.
474. Frassdorf J, De Hert S, Schlack W: Anaesthesia and myocardial ischaemia/reperfusion injury, *Br J Anaesth* 103:89, 2009.
475. Kaur S, Jaggi AS, Singh N: Molecular aspects of ischaemic postconditioning, *Fundam Clin Pharmacol* 23:521, 2009.
476. Penna C, Mancardi D, Raimondo S, et al: The paradigm of postconditioning to protect the heart, *J Cell Mol Med* 12:435, 2008.
477. Staat P, Rioufol G, Piot C, et al: PostC the human heart, *Circulation* 112:2143, 2005.
478. Ma XJ, Zhang X, Li C, et al: Effect of PostC on coronary blood flow velocity and endothelial function and LV recovery after myocardial infarction, *J Interv Cardiol* 19:367, 2006.
479. Gritsopoulos G, Iliodromitis EK, Zoga A, et al: Remote postconditioning is more potent than classic postconditioning in reducing the infarct size in anesthetized rabbits, *Cardiovasc Drugs Ther* 23:193, 2009.
480. El Azab SR, Rosseel PM, De Lange JJ, et al: Effect of sevoflurane on the ex vivo secretion of TNF-alpha during and after coronary artery bypass surgery, *Eur J Anaesthesiol* 20:380, 2003.
481. De Hert SG, Preckel B, Hollman MW, Schlack WS: Drugs mediating myocardial protection, *Eur J Anaesthesiol* 26:985, 2009.
482. Bopassa JC, Ferrera R, Gateau-Roesch O, et al: PI3-kinase regulates the mitochondrial transition pore in controlled reperfusion and PostC, *Cardiovasc Res* 69:178, 2006.
483. Kloner RA, Dow J, Bhandari A: PostC markedly attenuates ventricular arrhythmias after ischemia-reperfusion, *J Cardiovasc Pharmacol Ther* 11:55, 2006.
484. Adamczyk S, Robin E, Simerabet M, et al: Sevoflurane pre- and post-conditioning protect the brain via the mitochondrial K ATP channel, *Br J Anaesth* 104:191–200, 2010.
485. De Hert SG, Preckel B, Schlack WS: Update on inhalational anaesthetics, *Curr Opin Anaesthesiol* 22:491, 2009.
486. Eberlin KR, McCormack MC, Nguyen JT, et al: Ischemic preconditioning of skeletal muscle mitigates remote injury and mortality, *J Surg Res* 148:24, 2008.
487. Vianna PT, Castiglia YM, Braz JR, et al: Remifentanil, isoflurane, and preconditioning attenuate renal ischemia/reperfusion injury in rats, *Transplant Proc* 41:4080–4082, 2009.
488. Zaugg M, Lucchinetti E, Garcia C, et al: Anaesthetics and cardiac preconditioning. Part II. Clinical implications, *Br J Anaesth* 91:566, 2003.
489. Adams DC, Hilton HJ, Madigan JD, et al: Evidence for unconscious memory processing during elective cardiac surgery, *Circulation* 98:II289, 1998.
490. Sebel PS, Bowdle TA, Ghoneim MM, et al: The incidence of awareness during anesthesia: A multicenter United States study, *Anesth Analg* 99:833, 2004.
491. Goldmann L, Shah MV, Hebden MW: Memory of cardiac anaesthesia. Psychological sequelae in cardiac patients of intra-operative suggestion and operating room conversation, *Anaesthesia* 42:596, 1987.
492. Ranta SO, Herranen P, Hynynen M: Patients' conscious recollections from cardiac anesthesia, *J Cardiothorac Vasc Anesth* 16:426, 2002.
493. Phillips AA, McLean RF, Devitt JH, et al: Recall of intraoperative events after general anaesthesia and cardiopulmonary bypass, *Can J Anaesth* 40:922, 1993.
494. Dowd NP, Cheng DC, Karski JM, et al: Intraoperative awareness in fast-track cardiac anesthesia, *Anesthesiology* 89:1068, 1998.
495. Sandin RH, Enlund G, Samuelsson P, et al: Awareness during anaesthesia: A prospective case study, *Lancet* 355:707, 2000.
496. Kerssens C, Klein J, Bonke B: Awareness: Monitoring versus remembering what happened, *Anesthesiology* 99:570, 2003.
497. White PF, Tang J, Ma H, et al: Is the patient state analyzer with the PSArray2 a cost-effective alternative to the Bispectral Index monitor during the perioperative period? *Anesth Analg* 99:1429, 2004.
498. Bauer M, Wilhelm W, Kraemer T, et al: Impact of Bispectral Index monitoring on stress response and propofol consumption in patients undergoing coronary artery bypass surgery, *Anesthesiology* 101:1096, 2004.
499. Schmidt GN, Bischoff P, Standl T, et al: SNAP index and Bispectral Index during different states of propofol/remifentanil anaesthesia, *Anaesthesia* 60:228, 2005.
500. Ellerkmann RK, Liermann VM, Alves TM, et al: Spectral entropy and Bispectral Index as measures of the electroencephalographic effects of sevoflurane, *Anesthesiology* 101:1275, 2004.
501. Myles PS, Leslie K, McNeil J, et al: Bispectral Index monitoring to prevent awareness during anaesthesia: The B-Aware randomised controlled trial, *Lancet* 363:1757, 2004.
502. Ekman A, Lindholm ML, Lennmarken C, et al: Reduction in the incidence of awareness using BIS monitoring, *Acta Anaesthesiol Scand* 48:20, 2004.
503. Barr G, Anderson RE, Samuelsson S, et al: Fentanyl and midazolam anaesthesia for coronary bypass surgery: A clinical study of bispectral electroencephalogram analysis, drug concentrations and recall, *Br J Anaesth* 84:749, 2000.
504. Forestier F, Hirschi M, Rouget P, et al: Propofol and sufentanil titration with the Bispectral Index to provide anesthesia for coronary artery surgery, *Anesthesiology* 99:334, 2003.

505. Lehmann A, Karzau J, Boldt J, et al: Bispectral Index-guided anesthesia in patients undergoing aortocoronary bypass grafting, *Anesth Analg* 96:336, 2003.
506. Ranta SO, Laurila R, Saario J, et al: Awareness with recall during general anesthesia: Incidence and risk factors, *Anesth Analg* 86:1084, 1998.
507. Lennmarken C, Bildfors K, Enlund G, et al: Victims of awareness, *Acta Anaesthesiol Scand* 46:229, 2002.
508. Hawkes CA, Dhileepan S, Foxcroft D: Early extubation for adult cardiac surgical patients, *Cochrane Database Syst Rev* 4:CD003587, 2003.
509. Kaplan JA, Wells PH: Early diagnosis of myocardial ischemia using the pulmonary arterial catheter, *Anesth Analg* 60:789, 1981.
510. Comunale ME, Body SC, Ley C, et al: The concordance of intraoperative left ventricular wall-motion abnormalities and electrocardiographic S-T segment changes: Association with outcome after coronary revascularization. Multicenter Study of Perioperative Ischemia (McSPI) Research Group, *Anesthesiology* 88:945, 1998.
511. Kaplan JA, King SB 3rd: The precordial electrocardiographic lead (V5) in patients who have coronary-artery disease, *Anesthesiology* 45:570, 1976.
512. Kaplan JA, Dunbar RW, Jones EL: Nitroglycerin infusion during coronary-artery surgery, *Anesthesiology* 45:14, 1976.
513. Kaplan JA, Jones EL: Vasodilator therapy during coronary artery surgery. Comparison of nitroglycerin and nitroprusside, *J Thorac Cardiovasc Surg* 77:301, 1979.
514. Parker JD, Parker JO: Nitrate therapy for stable angina pectoris, *N Engl J Med* 338:520, 1998.
515. Kelly RA, Han X: Nitrovasodilators have (small) direct effects on cardiac contractility: Is this important? *Circulation* 96:2493, 1997.
516. Jugdutt BI, Warnica JW: Intravenous nitroglycerin therapy to limit myocardial infarct size, expansion, and complications. Effect of timing, dosage, and infarct location, *Circulation* 79:1151, 1989. Erratum in.*Circulation* 78:906, 1988.
517. Fujita M, Yamanishi K, Hirai T, et al: Significance of collateral circulation in reversible left ventricular asynergy by nitroglycerin in patients with relatively recent myocardial infarction, *Am Heart J* 120:521, 1990.
518. Townsend GE, Wynands JE, Whalley DG, et al: A profile of intravenous nitroglycerin use in cardiopulmonary bypass surgery, *Can Anaesth Soc J* 30:142, 1983.
519. Booth BP, Henderson M, Milne B, et al: Sequestration of glyceryl trinitrate (nitroglycerin) by cardiopulmonary bypass oxygenators, *Anesth Analg* 72:493, 1991.
520. Gallagher JD, Moore RA, Jose AB, et al: Prophylactic nitroglycerin infusions during coronary artery bypass surgery, *Anesthesiology* 64:785, 1986.
521. Lell W, Johnson P, Plagenhoef J, et al: The effect of prophylactic nitroglycerin infusion on the incidence of regional wall-motion abnormalities and ST segment changes in patients undergoing coronary artery bypass surgery, *J Card Surg* 8(Suppl):228, 1993.
522. Thomson IR, Mutch WA, Culligan JD: Failure of intravenous nitroglycerin to prevent intraoperative myocardial ischemia during fentanyl-pancuronium anesthesia, *Anesthesiology* 61:385, 1984.
523. Zvara DA, Groban L, Rogers AT, et al: Prophylactic nitroglycerin did not reduce myocardial ischemia during accelerated recovery management of coronary artery bypass graft surgery patients, *J Cardiothorac Vasc Anesth* 14:571, 2000.
524. Apostolidou IA, Despotis GJ, Hogue CW Jr, et al: Antiischemic effects of nicardipine and nitroglycerin after coronary artery bypass grafting, *Ann Thorac Surg* 67:417, 1999.
525. Kaplan JA, Jones EL: Vasodilator therapy during coronary artery surgery. Comparison of nitroglycerin and nitroprusside, *J Thorac Cardiovasc Surg* 77:301, 1979.
526. Kates RA, Kaplan JA: Cardiovascular responses to verapamil during coronary artery bypass graft surgery, *Anesth Analg* 62:821, 1983.
527. Griffin RM, Dimich I, Jurado R, Kaplan JA: Haemodynamic effects of diltiazem during fentanyl-nitrous oxide anaesthesia. An in vivo study in the dog, *Br J Anaesth* 60:655, 1988.
528. Wijeysundera DN, Beattie WS, Rao V, Karski J: Calcium antagonists reduce cardiovascular complications after cardiac surgery: A meta-analysis, *J Am Coll Cardiol* 41:1496, 2003.
529. Wijeysundera DN, Beattie WS, Rao V, et al: Calcium antagonists are associated with reduced mortality after cardiac surgery: A propensity analysis, *J Thorac Cardiovasc Surg* 127:755, 2004.
530. Kwak YL: Reduction of ischemia during off-pump coronary artery bypass graft surgery, *J Cardiothorac Vasc Anesth* 19:667, 2005.
531. Turlapaty P, Vary R, Kaplan JA: Nicardipine, a new intravenous calcium antagonist: A review of its pharmacology, pharmacokinetics, and perioperative applications, *J Cardiothorac Anesth* 3:344, 1989.
532. Parmley W: New calcium antagonists: Relevance of vasoselectivity, *Am Heart J* 120(Pt 1):1408, 1990.
533. Pepine CJ, Lambert CR: Effects of nicardipine on coronary blood flow, *Am Heart J* 116(Pt 1):248, 1988.
534. Ogawa T, Sekiguchi T, Ishii M, et al: Acute effects of intravenous nicardipine on hemodynamics and cardiac function in patients with a healed myocardial infarction and no evidence of congestive heart failure, *Am J Cardiol* 68:301, 1991.
535. Aroney CN, Semigran MJ, Dec GW: Left ventricular diastolic function in patients with left ventricular systolic dysfunction due to coronary artery disease and effect of nicardipine, *Am J Cardiol* 67:823, 1991.
536. Turlapaty P, Vary R, Kaplan JA: Nicardipine, a new intravenous calcium antagonist: A review of its pharmacology, pharmacokinetics, and perioperative applications, *J Cardiothorac Anesth* 3:344, 1989.
537. Kaplan JA: Clinical considerations for the use of intravenous nicardipine in the treatment of postoperative hypertension, *Am Heart J* 119:443, 1990.
538. Begon C, Dartayet B, Edouard A, et al: Intravenous nicardipine for treatment of intraoperative hypertension during abdominal surgery, *J Cardiothorac Anesth* 3:706, 1984.
539. Van Wezel HB, Koolen JJ, Visser CA, et al: The efficacy of nicardipine and nitroprusside in preventing poststernotomy hypertension, *J Cardiothorac Anesth* 3:700, 1989.
540. Van Wezel HB, Bovill JG, Schuller J, et al: Comparison of nitroglycerin, verapamil and nifedipine in the management of arterial pressure during coronary artery surgery, *Br J Anaesth* 58:267, 1986.
541. Apostolidou IA, Despotis GJ, Hogue CW Jr, et al: Antiischemic effects of nicardipine and nitroglycerin after coronary artery bypass grafting, *Ann Thorac Surg* 67:417, 1999.
542. Kwak YL, Oh YJ, Bang SO: Comparison of the effects of nicardipine and sodium nitroprusside for control of increased blood pressure after coronary artery bypass graft surgery, *J Int Med Res* 32:342, 2004.
543. Halpern NA, Goldberg M, Neely C, et al: Postoperative hypertension: A multicenter, prospective, randomized comparison between intravenous nicardipine and sodium nitroprusside, *Crit Care Med* 20:1637, 1992.
544. Kenyon KW: Clevidipine: An ultra short-acting calcium channel antagonist for acute hypertension, *Ann Pharmacother* 43:1258–1265, 2009.
545. Levy JH, Mancao MY, Gitter R, et al: Clevidipine effectively and rapidly controls blood pressure preoperatively in cardiac surgery patients: The results of the randomized, placebo-controlled efficacy study of clevidipine assessing its preoperative antihypertensive effect in cardiac surgery-1, *Anesth Analg* 105:918–925, 2007.
546. Aronson S, Dyke CM, Stierer KA, et al: The ECLIPSE trials: Comparative studies of clevidipine to nitroglycerin, sodium nitroprusside, and nicardipine for acute hypertension treatment in cardiac surgery patients, *Anesth Analg* 107:1110–1121, 2008.
547. Kaplan JA: Role of ultrashort-acting beta-blockers in the perioperative period, *J Cardiothorac Anesth* 2:683, 1988.
548. Barth C, Ojile M, Pearson AC, Labovitz AJ: Ultra short-acting intravenous beta-adrenergic blockade as add on therapy in acute unstable angina, *Am Heart J* 121(Pt 1):782, 1991.
549. Kirshenbaum JM, Kloner RF, McGowan N, Antman EM: Use of an ultrashort-acting beta-receptor blocker (esmolol) in patients with acute myocardial ischemia and relative contraindications to beta-blockade therapy, *J Am Coll Cardiol* 12:773, 1988.
550. Labovitz AJ, Barth C, Castello R, et al: Attenuation of myocardial ischemia during coronary occlusion by ultrashort-acting beta-adrenergic blockade, *Am Heart J* 121:1347, 1991.
551. Nicolson SC, Jobes DR, Quinlan JJ: Cardiovascular effects of esmolol in patients anesthetized with sufentanil-pancuronium for myocardial revascularization, *J Cardiothorac Anesth* 4(Suppl 2):55, 1990.
552. Girard D, Shulman BJ, Thys DM, et al: The safety and efficacy of esmolol during myocardial revascularization, *Anesthesiology* 65:157, 1986.
553. Reves JG, Croughwell NC, Hawkins E, et al: Esmolol for treatment of intraoperative tachycardia and/or hypertension in patients having cardiac operations. Bolus loading technique, *J Thorac Cardiovasc Surg* 100:221, 1990.
554. Dyub AM, Whitlock RP, Abouzahr LL, et al: Preoperative intra-aortic balloon pump in patients undergoing coronary bypass surgery: A systematic review and meta-analysis, *J Card Surg* 23:79–86, 2008.
555. The current practice of intr-aortic balloon counterpulsation: Results from the Benchmark Registry, *J Am Coll Cardiol* 38:1456–1462, 2001.
556. Bloor BC, Ward DS, Belleville JP, et al: Effects of intravenous dexmedetomidine in humans. II. Hemodynamic changes, *Anesthesiology* 77:1134, 1992.
557. Talke P, Richardson CA, Scheinin M, et al: Postoperative pharmacokinetics and sympatholytic effects of dexmedetomidine, *Anesth Analg* 85:1136, 1997.
558. Ebert TJ, Hall JE, Barney JA, et al: The effects of increasing plasma concentrations of dexmedetomidine in humans, *Anesthesiology* 93:382, 2000.
559. Flacke WE, Flacke JW, Bloor BC, et al: Effects of dexmedetomidine on systemic and coronary hemodynamics in the anesthetized dog, *J Cardiothorac Vasc Anesth* 7:41, 1993.
560. Coughlan MG, Lee JG, Bosnjak ZJ, et al: Direct coronary and cerebral vascular responses to dexmedetomidine. Significance of endogenous nitric oxide synthesis, *Anesthesiology* 77:998, 1992.
561. Talke P, Lobo E, Brown R: Systemically administered alpha2-agonist-induced peripheral vasoconstriction in humans, *Anesthesiology* 99:65, 2003.
562. Jalonen J, Hynynen M, Kuitunen A, et al: Dexmedetomidine as an anesthetic adjunct in coronary artery bypass grafting, *Anesthesiology* 86:331, 1997.
563. Lawrence CJ, Prinzen FW, de Lange S: The effect of dexmedetomidine on the balance of myocardial energy requirement and oxygen supply and demand, *Anesth Analg* 82:544, 1996.
564. Roekaerts PM, Prinzen FW, de Lange S: Coronary vascular effects of dexmedetomidine during reactive hyperemia in the anesthetized dog, *J Cardiothorac Vasc Anesth* 10:619, 1996.
565. Roekaerts PM, Prinzen FW, De Lange S: Beneficial effects of dexmedetomidine on ischaemic myocardium of anaesthetized dogs, *Br J Anaesth* 77:427, 1996.
566. De Wolf AM, Fragen RJ, Avram MJ, et al: The pharmacokinetics of dexmedetomidine in volunteers with severe renal impairment, *Anesth Analg* 93:1205, 2001.
567. Hsu YW, Cortinez LI, Robertson KM, et al: Dexmedetomidine pharmacodynamics. Part I. Crossover comparison of the respiratory effects of dexmedetomidine and remifentanil in healthy volunteers, *Anesthesiology* 101:1066, 2004.
568. Venn RM, Hell J, Grounds RM: Respiratory effects of dexmedetomidine in the surgical patient requiring intensive care, *Crit Care* 4:302, 2000.
569. Venn RM, Grounds RM: Comparison between dexmedetomidine and propofol for sedation in the intensive care unit: Patient and clinician perceptions, *Br J Anaesth* 87:684, 2001.
570. Martin E, Ramsay G, Mantz J, et al: The role of the alpha2-adrenoceptor agonist dexmedetomidine in postsurgical sedation in the intensive care unit, *J Intensive Care Med* 18:29, 2003.
571. Triltsch AE, Welte M, von Homeyer P, et al: Bispectral index guided sedation with dexmedetomidine in intensive care: A prospective, randomized, double blind, placebo-controlled phase II study, *Crit Care Med* 30:1007, 2002.
572. Arain SR, Ruehlow RM, Uhrich TD, et al: The efficacy of dexmedetomidine versus morphine for postoperative analgesia after major inpatient surgery, *Anesth Analg* 98:153, 2004.
573. Dobrydnjov I, Axelsson K, Berggren L, et al: Intrathecal and oral clonidine as prophylaxis for postoperative alcohol withdrawal syndrome: A randomized double-blinded study, *Anesth Analg* 98:738, 2004.
574. Kranke P, Eberhart LH, Roewer N, et al: Single-dose parenteral pharmacological interventions for the prevention of postoperative shivering: A quantitative systematic review of randomized controlled trials, *Anesth Analg* 99:718, 2004.
575. Venn RM, Grounds RM: Comparison between dexmedetomidine and propofol for sedation in the intensive care unit: Patient and clinician perceptions, *Br J Anaesth* 87:684–690, 2001.
576. Herr DL, Sum-Ping ST, England M: ICU sedation after coronary artery bypass graft surgery: Dexmedetomidine-based versus propofol-based sedation regimens, *J Cardiothorac Vasc Anesth* 17:576, 2003.
577. Corbett SM, Rebuck JA, Greene CM, et al: Dexmedetomidine does not improve patient satisfaction when compared with propofol during mechanical ventilation, *Crit Care Med* 33:940–945, 2005.
578. Barletta JF, Miedema SL, Wiseman D, et al: Impact of dexmedetomidine on analgesic requirements in patients after cardiac surgery in a fast-track recovery room setting, *Pharmacotherapy* 29:1427–1432, 2009.
579. Buxton AE, Goldberg S, Harken A, et al: Coronary-artery spasm immediately after myocardial revascularization: Recognition and management, *N Engl J Med* 304:1249, 1981.
580. Kaski JC: Mechanisms of coronary artery spasm, *Trends Cardiovasc Med* 1:289, 1991.
581. Apostolidou IA, Skubas NJ, Despotis GJ, et al: Occurrence of myocardial ischemia immediately after coronary revascularization using radial arterial conduits, *J Cardiothorac Vasc Anesth* 15:433, 2001.
582. He GW, Rosenfeldt FL, Buxton BF, Angus JA: Reactivity of human isolated internal mammary artery to constrictor and dilator agents. Implications for treatment of internal mammary artery spasm, *Circulation* 80(Suppl I):I141, 1989.
583. Mussa S, Guzik TJ, Black E, et al: Comparative efficacies and durations of action of phenoxybenzamine, verapamil/nitroglycerin solution, and papaverine as topical antispasmodics for radial artery coronary bypass grafting, *J Thorac Cardiovasc Surg* 126:1798, 2003.
584. He GW, Buxton BF, Rosenfeldt FL, et al: Pharmacologic dilatation of the internal mammary artery during coronary bypass grafting, *J Thorac Cardiovasc Surg* 107:1440, 1994.
585. Jett GK, Guyton RA, Hatcher CR, Abel PW: Inhibition of human internal mammary artery contractions. An in vitro study of vasodilators, *J Thorac Cardiovasc Surg* 104:977, 1992.
586. Du ZY, Buxton BF, Woodman OL: Tolerance to glyceryl trinitrate in isolated human internal mammary arteries, *J Thorac Cardiovasc Surg* 104:1280, 1992.
587. Shapira OM, Xu A, Vita JA, et al: Nitroglycerin is superior to diltiazem as a coronary bypass conduit vasodilator, *J Thorac Cardiovasc Surg* 117:906, 1999.
588. Shapira OM, Alkon JD, Macron DS, et al: Nitroglycerin is preferable to diltiazem for prevention of coronary bypass conduit spasm, *Ann Thorac Surg* 70:883, 2000, discussion 888.
589. Mollhoff T, Schmidt C, Van Aken H, et al: Myocardial ischaemia in patients with impaired left ventricular function undergoing coronary artery bypass grafting—milrinone versus nifedipine, *Eur J Anaesthesiol* 19:796, 2002.

590. Krohn BG, Kay JH, Mendez MA, et al: Rapid sustained recovery after cardiac operations, *J Thorac Cardiovasc Surg* 100:194, 1990.
591. Chong JL, Pillai R, Fisher A, et al: Cardiac surgery: Moving away from intensive care, *Br Heart J* 68:430, 1992.
592. Chong JL, Grebenik C, Sinclair M, et al: The effect of a cardiac surgical recovery area on the timing of extubation, *J Cardiothorac Vasc Anesth* 7:137, 1993.
593. Cromwell J, Dayhoff DA, McCall NT, et al: *Medicare participating heart bypass center demonstration (extramural research report)*, 1998, Health Care Financing Administration. Health Economics Research, Inc.
594. Engelman RM, Rousou JA, Flack JE 3rd, et al: Fast-track recovery of the coronary bypass patient, *Ann Thorac Surg* 58:1742, 1994.
595. Engelman RM: Fast-track recovery in the elderly patient, *Ann Thorac Surg* 63:606, 1997.
596. Myles PS, Daly DJ, Djaiani G, et al: A systematic review of the safety and effectiveness of fast-track cardiac anesthesia, *Anesthesiology* 99:982, 2003.
597. Hawkes CA, Dhileepan S, Foxcroft D: Early extubation for adult cardiac surgical patients, *Cochrane Database Syst Rev* 4: CD003587, 2003.
598. Lefemine AA, Harken DE: Postoperative care following open-heart operations: Routine use of controlled ventilation, *J Thorac Cardiovasc Surg* 52:207, 1966.
599. Lowenstein E, Hallowell P, Levine FH, et al: Cardiovascular response to large doses of intravenous morphine in man, *N Engl J Med* 281:1389, 1969.
600. Stanley TH, Webster LR: Anesthetic requirements and cardiovascular effects of fentanyl-oxygen and fentanyl-diazepam-oxygen anesthesia in man, *Anesth Analg* 57:411, 1978.
601. Midell AI, Skinner DB, DeBoer A, et al: A review of pulmonary problems following valve replacement in 100 consecutive patients, *Ann Thorac Surg* 18:219, 1974.
602. Quasha AL, Loeber N, Feeley TW, et al: Postoperative respiratory care: A controlled trial of early and late extubation following coronary-artery bypass grafting, *Anesthesiology* 52:135, 1980.
603. Ramsay JG, Higgs BD, Wynands JE, et al: Early extubation after high-dose fentanyl anaesthesia for aortocoronary bypass surgery: Reversal of respiratory depression with low-dose nalbuphine, *Can Anaesth Soc J* 32:597, 1985.
604. Cheng DC, Karski J, Peniston C, et al: Morbidity outcome in early versus conventional tracheal extubation after coronary artery bypass grafting: A prospective randomized controlled trial, *J Thorac Cardiovasc Surg* 112:755, 1996.
605. Butterworth J, James R, Prielipp RC, et al: Do shorter-acting neuromuscular blocking drugs or opioids associate with reduced intensive care unit or hospital lengths of stay after coronary artery bypass grafting? CABG Clinical Benchmarking Data Base Participants, *Anesthesiology* 88:1437, 1998.
606. Butterworth J, James R, Prielipp R, et al: Female gender associates with increased duration of intubation and length of stay after coronary artery surgery. CABG Clinical Benchmarking Database Participants, *Anesthesiology* 92:414, 2000.
607. Engoren M, Luther G, Fenn-Buderer N: A comparison of fentanyl, sufentanil, and remifentanil for fast-track cardiac anesthesia, *Anesth Analg* 93:859, 2001.
608. Arom KV, Emery RW, Petersen RJ, et al: Cost-effectiveness and predictors of early extubation, *Ann Thorac Surg* 60:127, 1995.
609. Arom KV, Emery RW, Petersen RJ, et al: Patient characteristics, safety, and benefits of same-day admission for coronary artery bypass grafting, *Ann Thorac Surg* 61:1136, 1996.
610. Habib RH, Zacharias A, Engoren M: Determinants of prolonged mechanical ventilation after coronary artery bypass grafting, *Ann Thorac Surg* 62:1164, 1996.
611. Walji S, Peterson RJ, Neis P, et al: Ultra-fast track hospital discharge using conventional cardiac surgical techniques, *Ann Thorac Surg* 67:363, 1999.
612. Ott RA, Gutfinger DE, Miller MP, et al: Rapid recovery after coronary artery bypass grafting: Is the elderly patient eligible? *Ann Thorac Surg* 63:634, 1997.
613. Ott RA, Gutfinger DE, Miller M, et al: Rapid recovery of octogenarians following coronary artery bypass grafting, *J Card Surg* 12:309, 1997.
614. Lee JH, Graber R, Popple CG, et al: Safety and efficacy of early extubation of elderly coronary artery bypass surgery patients, *J Cardiothorac Vasc Anesth* 12:381, 1998.
615. London MJ, Shroyer AL, Coll JR, et al: Early extubation following cardiac surgery in a veterans population, *Anesthesiology* 88:1447, 1998.
616. London MJ, Shroyer AL, Jernigan V, et al: Fast-track cardiac surgery in a Department of Veterans Affairs patient population, *Ann Thorac Surg* 64:134, 1997.
617. Holman WL, Sansom M, Kiefe CI, et al: Alabama coronary artery bypass grafting project: Results from phase II of a statewide quality improvement initiative, *Ann Surg* 239:99, 2004.
618. Butterworth J, James R, Prielipp RC, et al: Do shorter-acting neuromuscular blocking drugs or opioids associate with reduced intensive care unit or hospital lengths of stay after coronary artery bypass grafting? CABG Clinical Benchmarking Data Base Participants, *Anesthesiology* 88:1437, 1998.
619. Butterworth J, James R, Prielipp R, et al: Female gender associates with increased duration of intubation and length of stay after coronary artery surgery. CABG Clinical Benchmarking Database Participants, *Anesthesiology* 92:414, 2000.
620. Dexter F, Macario A, Dexter EU: Computer simulation of changes in nursing productivity from early tracheal extubation of coronary artery bypass graft patients, *J Clin Anesth* 10:593, 1998.
621. Cheng DC: Fast track cardiac surgery pathways: Early extubation, process of care, and cost containment, *Anesthesiology* 88:1429, 1998.
622. Myles PS, Daly DJ, Djaiani G, et al: A systematic review of the safety and effectiveness of fast-track cardiac anesthesia, *Anesthesiology* 99:982, 2003.
623. Hawkes CA, Dhileepan S, Foxcroft D: Early extubation for adult cardiac surgical patients, *Cochrane Database Syst Rev* 4:CD003587, 2003.
624. Quasha AL, Loeber N, Feeley TW, et al: Postoperative respiratory care: A controlled trial of early and late extubation following coronary-artery bypass grafting, *Anesthesiology* 52:135, 1980.
625. Cheng DC, Karski J, Peniston C, et al: Morbidity outcome in early versus conventional tracheal extubation after coronary artery bypass grafting: A prospective randomized controlled trial, *J Thorac Cardiovasc Surg* 112:755, 1996.
626. Berry PD, Thomas SD, Mahon SP, et al: Myocardial ischaemia after coronary artery bypass grafting: Early vs late extubation, *Br J Anaesth* 80:20, 1998.
627. Michalopoulos A, Nikolaides A, Antzaka C, et al: Change in anaesthesia practice and postoperative sedation shortens ICU and hospital length of stay following coronary artery bypass surgery, *Respir Med* 92:1066, 1998.
628. Reyes A, Vega G, Blancas R, et al: Early vs conventional extubation after cardiac surgery with cardiopulmonary bypass, *Chest* 112:193, 1997.
629. Silbert BS, Santamaria JD, O'Brien JL, et al: Early extubation following coronary artery bypass surgery: A prospective randomized controlled trial. The Fast Track Cardiac Care Team, *Chest* 113:1481, 1998.
630. Quasha AL, Loeber N, Feeley TW, et al: Postoperative respiratory care: A controlled trial of early and late extubation following coronary-artery bypass grafting, *Anesthesiology* 52:135, 1980.
631. London MJ, Shroyer ALW, Grover FL: Fast tracking into the new millennium: An evolving paradigm, *Anesthesiology* 91:936, 1999.
632. London MJ, Shroyer AL, Jernigan V, et al: Fast-track cardiac surgery in a Department of Veterans Affairs patient population, *Ann Thorac Surg* 64:134, 1997.
633. Butterworth J, James R, Prielipp R, et al: Female gender associates with increased duration of intubation and length of stay after coronary artery surgery. CABG Clinical Benchmarking Database Participants, *Anesthesiology* 92:414, 2000.
634. Engoren M, Buderer NF, Zacharias A, et al: Variables predicting reintubation after cardiac surgical procedures, *Ann Thorac Surg* 67:661, 1999.
635. Walji S, Peterson RJ, Neis P, et al: Ultra-fast track hospital discharge using conventional cardiac surgical techniques, *Ann Thorac Surg* 67:363, 1999.
636. Ovrum E, Tangen G, Schiott C, et al: Rapid recovery protocol applied to 5,658 consecutive "on-pump" coronary bypass patients, *Ann Thorac Surg* 70:2000, 2008.
637. Cheng DC, Bainbridge D, Martin JE, et al: Does off-pump coronary artery bypass reduce mortality, morbidity, and resource utilization when compared with conventional coronary artery bypass? A meta-analysis of randomized trials, *Anesthesiology* 102:188, 2005.
638. Raja SG, Dreyfus GD: Off-pump coronary artery bypass surgery: To do or not to do? Current best available evidence, *J Cardiothorac Vasc Anesth* 18:486, 2004.
639. Sellke FW, DiMaio JM, Caplan LR, et al: Comparing on-pump and off-pump coronary artery bypass grafting: Numerous studies but few conclusions: A scientific statement from the American Heart Association council on cardiovascular surgery and anesthesia in collaboration with the interdisciplinary working group on quality of care and outcomes research, *Circulation* 111:2858, 2005.
640. Chamchad D, Horrow JC, Nachamchik L, et al: The impact of immediate extubation in the operating room on intensive care and hospital lengths of stay, *J Cardiothorac Vasc Anesth* 24:780–784, 2010.
641. Grundeman PF, Borst C, Verlaan CW, et al: Exposure of circumflex branches in the tilted, beating porcine heart: Echocardiographic evidence of right ventricular deformation and the effect of right or left heart bypass, *J Thorac Cardiovasc Surg* 118:316, 1999.
642. George SJ, Al-Ruzzeh S, Amrani M: Mitral annulus distortion during beating heart surgery: A potential cause for hemodynamic disturbance—a three-dimensional echocardiography reconstruction study, *Ann Thorac Surg* 73:1424, 2002.
643. Grundeman PF, Borst C, van Herwaarden JA, et al: Vertical displacement of the beating heart by the octopus tissue stabilizer: Influence on coronary flow, *Ann Thorac Surg* 65:1348, 1998.
644. Grundeman PF, Budde R, Beck HM, et al: Endoscopic exposure and stabilization of posterior and inferior branches using the endo-starfish cardiac positioner and the endo-octopus stabilizer for closed-chest beating heart multivessel CABG: Hemodynamic changes in the pig, *Circulation* 108(Suppl 1):II34, 2003.
645. Grundeman PF, Verlaan CW, van Boven WJ, et al: Ninety-degree anterior cardiac displacement in off-pump coronary artery bypass grafting: The Starfish cardiac positioner preserves stroke volume and arterial pressure, *Ann Thorac Surg* 78:679, 2004.
646. Porat E, Sharony R, Ivry S, et al: Hemodynamic changes and right heart support during vertical displacement of the beating heart, *Ann Thorac Surg* 69:1188, 2000.
647. Kwak YL, Oh YJ, Jung SM, et al: Change in right ventricular function during off-pump coronary artery bypass graft surgery, *Eur J Cardiothorac Surg* 25:572, 2004.
648. Biswas S, Clements F, Diodato L, et al: Changes in systolic and diastolic function during multivessel off-pump coronary bypass grafting, *Eur J Cardiothorac Surg* 20:913, 2001.
649. Mathison M, Edgerton JR, Horswell JL, et al: Analysis of hemodynamic changes during beating heart surgical procedures, *Ann Thorac Surg* 70:1355, 2000.
650. Nierich AP, Diephuis J, Jansen EW, et al: Heart displacement during off-pump CABG: How well is it tolerated? *Ann Thorac Surg* 70:466, 2000.
651. Mishra M, Shrivastava S, Dhar A, et al: A prospective evaluation of hemodynamic instability during off-pump coronary artery bypass surgery, *J Cardiothorac Vasc Anesth* 17:452, 2003.
652. Lee JH, Capdeville M, Marsh D, et al: Earlier recovery with beating-heart surgery: A comparison of 300 patients undergoing conventional versus off-pump coronary artery bypass graft surgery, *J Cardiothorac Vasc Anesth* 16:139, 2002.
653. Djaiani GN, Ali M, Heinrich L, et al: Ultra-fast-track anesthesia technique facilitates operating room extubation in patients undergoing off-pump coronary revscularization surgery, *J Cardiothorac Vasc Anesth* 15:152, 2001.
654. George SJ, Al-Ruzzeh S, Amrani M: Mitral annulus distorsion during beating heart surgery: A potential cause for hemodynamic disturbance—a three dimensional echocardiography reconstruction study, *Ann Thorac Surg* 73:1424, 2002.
655. Kinjo S, Tokumine J, Sugahara K, et al: Unexpected hemodynamic deterioration and mitral regurgitation due to a tissue stabilizer during left anterior descending coronary anastomosis in off-pump coronary artery bypass graft surgery, *Ann Thorac Cardiovasc Surg* 11:324, 2005.
656. Hangler H, Mueller L, Ruttmann E, et al: Shunt or snare: Coronary endothelial damage due to hemostatic devices for beating heart coronary surgery, *Ann Thorac Surg* 86:1873–1877, 2008.
657. Collison SP, Agarwal A, Trehan N: Controversies in the use of intraluminal shunts during off-pump coronary artery bypass grafting surgery, *Ann Thorac Surg* 82:1559–1566, 2006.
658. Demaria AG, Malo O, Carrier M, Perrault LP: Influence of intracoronary shunt size on coronary endothelial function during off-pump coronary artery bypass, *Interact Cardiovasc Thorac Surg* 2:281–286, 2003.
659. Biancari F, Mosorin M, Lahtinen J, et al: Results with the Heartstring anastomotic device in patients with diseased ascending aorta, *Scand Cardiovasc J* 40:238–239, 2006.
660. Douglas JM Jr, Spaniol SE: A multimodal approach to the prevention of postoperative stroke in patients undergoing coronary artery bypass surgery, *Am J Surg* 197:587–590, 2009.
661. Athanasiou T, Ashrafian H, Krasopoulos G, et al: Clampless arterial coronary artery bypass grafting with the use of magnetic coupling devices, *Heart Surg Forum* 9:E607–E611, 2006.
662. Puskas JD, Williams WH, Mahoney EM, et al: Off-pump vs conventional coronary artery bypass grafting: Early and 1-year graft patency, cost, and quality of life outcomes. A randomized trial, *JAMA* 291:1841, 2004.
663. Sellke FW, DiMaio JM, Caplan LR, et al: Comparing on-pump and off-pump coronary artery bypass grafting: Numerous studies but few conclusions: A scientific statement from the American Heart Association council on cardiovascular surgery and anesthesia in collaboration with the interdisciplinary working group on quality of care and outcomes research, *Circulation* 111:2858, 2005.
664. Raja SG, Dreyfus GD: Off-pump coronary artery bypass surgery: To do or not to do? Current best available evidence, *J Cardiothorac Vasc Anesth* 18:486, 2004.
665. Myles PS, Buckland MR, Weeks AM, et al: Hemodynamic effect, myocardial ischemia, and timing of tracheal extubation with propofol-based anesthesia for cardia surgery, *Anesth Analg* 84:12, 1997.
666. Song HK, Peterson RJ, Sharoni E, et al: Safe evolution towards routine off-pump coronary bypass: Negotiating the learning curve, *Eur J Cardiothorac Surg* 24:947–952, 2003.
667. Shroyer AL, Grover FL, Hatler B, et al for the Veteran Affairs Randomized On/Off Bypass (ROOBY) Study Group: On-pump versus off-pump coronary-artery bypass surgery, *N Engl J Med* 361:1827–1837, 2009.
668. Reeves BC, Ascione R, Caputo M, et al: Morbidity and mortality following acute conversion from off-pump to on-pump coronary surgery, *Eur J Cardiothorac Surg* 29:941–947, 2006.
669. Jin R, Hiratzka LF, Grunkemeier GL, et al: Aborted off-pump coronary artery bypass patients have much worse outcomes than on-pump or successful off-pump patients, *Circulation* 112:I332–I337, 2005.
670. Puskas JD, Kilgo PD, Kutner M, et al: Off-pump techniques disproportionally benefit women and narrow the gender disparity in outcomes after coronary artery surgery bypass surgery, *Circulation* 116:I192–I199, 2007.
671. Puskas JD, Kilgo PD, Lattouf OM, et al: Off-pump coronary bypass provides reduced mortality and morbidity and equivalent 10-year survival, *Ann Thorac Surg* 86:1139–1146, 2008.
672. Puskas JD, Thourani VH, Kilgo P, et al: Off-pump coronary artery bypass disproportionally benefits high-risk patients, *Ann Thorac Surg* 88:1142–1147, 2009.

673. Kolessov VL: Mammary artery-coronary anastomoses as a method of treatment for angina pectoris, *J Thorac Cardiothorac Surg* 54:535–544, 1967.

674. Thiele H, Neumann-Schniedewind P, Jacobs S, et al: Randomized comparison of minimally invasive direct coronary artery bypass surgery versus sirolimus-eluting stenting in isolated proximal left anterior descending coronary artery stenosis, *J Am Coll Cardiol* 53:2324–2331, 2009.

675. Kofidis T, Emmert MY, Paeschke HG, et al: Long-term follow-up after minimal invasive direct coronary artery bypass grafting procedure: A multi-factorial retrospective analysis at 1000 patient-years, *Interact Cardiovasc Thorac Surg* 9:990–994, 2009.

676. Jaffery Z, Kowalski M, Weaver WD, et al: A meta-analysis of randomized control trials comparing minimally invasive direct coronary bypass grafting versus percutaneous coronary intervention for stenosis of the proximal left anterior descending artery, *Eur J Cardiothorac Surg* 31:691–697, 2007.

677. Loulmet D, Carpentier A, d'Attellis N, et al: Endoscopic coronary artery bypass grafting with the aid of robotic assisted instruments, *J Thorac Cardiovasc Surg* 118:4–10, 1999.

678. Bonaros N, Schachner T, Wiedemann D, et al: Quality of life improvement after robotically assisted coronary artery bypass grafting, *Cardiology* 114:59–66, 2009.

679. Turner WF Jr, Sloan JH: Robotic-assisted coronary artery bypass on a beating heart: Initial experience and implications for the future, *Ann Thorac Surg* 82:790–794, 2006.

680. Bonatti J, Schachner T, Bonaros N, et al: Simultaneous hybrid coronary revascularization using totally endoscopic left internal mammary artery bypass grafting and placement of rapamycin eluting stents in the same interventional session. The COMBINATION pilot study, *Cardiology* 110:92–95, 2008.

681. Bonatti J, Schachner T, Bonaros N, et al: Robotic totally endoscopic double-vessel bypass grafting: A further step toward closed-chest surgical treatment of multivessel coronary artery disease, *Heart Surg Forum* 10:E239–E242, 2007.

682. Nishida S, Watanabe G, Ishikawa N, et al: Beating-heart totally endoscopic coronary artery bypass grafting: Report of a case, *Surg Today* 40:57–59, 2010.

683. Vassiliades TA Jr, Reddy VS, Puskas JD, Guyton RA: Long-term results of the endoscopic atraumatic coronary artery bypass, *Ann Thorac Surg* 83:979–984, 2007.

684. Argenziano M, Katz M, Bonatti J, et al: Results of the prospective multicenter trial of robotically assisted totally endoscopic coronary artery bypass grafting, *Ann Thorac Surg* 81:1666–1675, 2006.

685. Campos JH: An update on bronchial blockers during lung separation techniques in adults, *Anesth Analg* 97:1266–1274, 2003.

686. Cohen E: Pro: The new bronchial blockers are preferable to double-lumen tubes for lung isolation, *J Cardiothorac Vasc Anesth* 22:920–924, 2008.

687. Slinger P: Con: The new bronchial blockers are not preferable to double-lumen tubes for lung isolation, *J Cardiothorac Vasc Anesth* 22:925–929, 2008.

688. Ender J, Brodowsky M, Falk V, et al: High-frequency jet ventilation as an alternative method compared to conventional one-lung ventilation using double-lumen tubes: A study of 40 patients undergoing minimally invasive coronary artery bypass graft surgery, *J Cardiothorac Vasc Anesth* 24:602–607, 2010.

689. Ohtsuka T, Imanaka K, Endoh M, et al: Hemodynamic effects of carbon dioxide insufflation under single-lung ventilation during thoracoscopy, *Ann Thorac Surg* 68:29–32, 1999.

690. Byhahn C, Mierdl S, Meininger D, et al: Hemodynamics and gas exchange during carbon dioxide insufflation for totally endoscopic coronary artery bypass grafting, *Ann Thorac Surg* 71:1496–1501, 2001.

691. Wolfer RS, Krasna MJ, Hasnain JU, et al: Hemodynamic effects of carbon dioxide insufflation during thoracoscopy, *Ann Thorac Surg* 58:404–408, 1994.

692. Mierdl S, Byhahn C, Lischke V, et al: Segmental myocardial wall motion during minimally invasive coronary arery bypass grafting using open and endoscopic surgical techniques, *Anesth Analg* 100:306–314, 2005.

693. Brock H, Rieger R, Gabriel C, et al: Haemodynamic changes during thoracoscopic surgery. The effects of one-lung ventilation compared with carbon dioxide insufflation, *Anaesthesia* 55:10–16, 2000.

694. Lin SM, Chang WK, Tsao WM, et al: Carbon dioxide embolism diagnosed by transesophageal echocardiography during endoscopic vein harvesting for coronary artery bypass grafting, *Anesth Analg* 96:683–685, 2003.

695. Kypson AP, Greenville NC: Sudden cardiac arrest after coronary artery bypass grafting as a result of massive carbon dioxide embolism, *J Thorac Cardiovasc Surg* 130:936–937, 2005.

696. Ceballos A, Chaney MA, LeVan PT, et al: Robotically assisted cardiac surgery, *J Cardiothorac Vasc Anesth* 23:407–416, 2009.

697. Mehta Y, Arora D, Sharma KK, et al: Comparison of continuous thoracic epidural and paravertebral block for postoperative analgesia after robotic-assisted coronary artery bypass surgery, *Ann Card Anaesth* 11:91–96, 2008.

19

Valvular Heart Disease
Replacement and Repair

DAVID J. COOK, MD | PHILIPPE R. HOUSMANS, MD, PHD | KENT H. REHFELDT, MD

KEY POINTS

1. Although various valvular lesions generate different physiologic changes, all valvular heart disease is characterized by abnormalities of ventricular loading.
2. The left ventricle normally compensates for increases in afterload by increases in preload. This increase in end-diastolic fiber stretch or radius further increases wall tension in accordance with Laplace's law, resulting in a reciprocal decline in myocardial fiber shortening. The stroke volume is maintained because the contractile force is augmented at the higher preload level.
3. Factors that influence heart function include afterload stress, preload reserve, ventricular compliance, contractility, and the existence of pathology such as valve lesions, aortic stenosis, and hypertrophy.
4. Treatment modalities for hypertrophic obstructive cardiomyopathy, a relatively common genetic malformation of the heart, include β-adrenoceptor antagonists, calcium channel blockers, and myectomy of the septum. Newer approaches include dual-chamber pacing and septal reduction (ablation) therapy with ethanol.
5. The severity and duration of symptoms of aortic regurgitation may correlate poorly with the degree of hemodynamic and contractile impairment, delaying surgical treatment while patients are undergoing progressive deterioration.
6. Mitral regurgitation causes left ventricular volume overload. Treatment depends on the underlying mechanism and includes early reperfusion therapy, angiotensin-converting enzyme inhibitors, and surgical repair or replacement of the mitral valve.
7. Rheumatic disease and congenital abnormalities of the mitral valve are the main causes of mitral stenosis, a slowly progressive disease. Surgical treatment options include closed and open commissurotomy and percutaneous mitral commissurotomy.
8. Most tricuspid surgery occurs in the context of significant aortic or mitral disease, and anesthetic management primarily is determined by the left-sided valve lesion.
9. Innovations in surgical valve repair include aortic valve repair and closed- and open-chamber procedures for mitral regurgitation.

In many ways, surgery for coronary artery disease (CAD) has matured, and although there will continue to be incremental advances like off-pump surgery, anastomotic connectors, and endoscopic vein harvest, coronary artery surgery may have seen its best days, in no small part because of advances in interventional cardiology. The same has not been true of valve surgery. At surgical institutions where valve surgery is well represented, surgical volumes are stable. This reflects the aging of the population and the lesser impact of cardiologic interventions on the valvular heart disease (VHD) process.

From the standpoint of anesthetic care, valve surgery also is usually very different from coronary artery bypass grafting (CABG). Chronically, over the natural history of VHD, the physiology changes markedly; and acutely in the operating room, physiologic conditions and hemodynamics are quite dynamic and are readily influenced by anesthetic interventions. It also is true that, for some types of valve lesions, it can be relatively difficult to predict before surgery how the heart will respond to the altered loading conditions associated with valve repair or replacement.

It is essential to understand the natural history of each of the major adult acquired valve defects and how the pathophysiology evolves. Clinicians must also understand surgical decision making for valve repair or replacement because a valve operated on at the appropriate stage of its natural history will have a good and more predictable outcome in contrast with a heart operated on at a later stage in which the perioperative result can be quite poor. Because the pathophysiology is dynamic and differs importantly between valve lesions, understanding the physiology and the natural history of the individual valve defects is the foundation of developing an anesthetic plan that will include differing requirements for preload, pacing rate and rhythm, use of inotropes (or negative inotropes), as well as vasodilators or vasoconstrictors to alter loading conditions.

Although valvular lesions impose differing physiologic changes, a unifying concept is that all VHD is characterized by abnormalities of ventricular loading. The status of the ventricle changes over time as both ventricular function and the valvular defect itself are influenced by the progression of either volume or pressure overload. As such, the clinical status of patients with VHD can be complex and dynamic. It is possible to have clinical decompensation in the context of normal ventricular contractility, or ventricular decompensation performance with normal ejection indices. In other words, the altered loading conditions characteristic of VHD may result in a divergence between the function of the heart as a systolic pump and the intrinsic inotropic state of the myocardium. This divergence between cardiac performance and inotropy occurs as a result of compensatory physiologic mechanisms that are specific to each of the ventricular loading abnormalities.

In analyzing the physiologic response of the left ventricle (LV) to a variety of abnormal loading conditions, it is useful to consider the concepts of afterload mismatch and preload reserve.[1] These concepts frame discussions of the pathophysiology of the individual valvular lesions. Another set of physiologic concepts essential to understanding VHD and its evolution are pressure-volume loops and the linear end-systolic pressure-volume relation (ESPVR). The former provides a graphic analysis of ventricular pressure-volume relations in a single beat, whereas the latter is a method for quantifying the intrinsic contractility of the myocardium over multiple contractions and is relatively independent of changes in loading conditions (see Chapters 5, 12, 13 and 14).

PATHOPHYSIOLOGY

Pressure-Volume Loops

The pressure and volume changes that occur during a normal cardiac cycle are depicted in Figure 19-1. A pressure-volume loop is generated when ventricular volumes are plotted against simultaneously occurring ventricular pressures for a single contraction (Figure 19-2). Familiarity with this graphic analysis of cardiac function, the normal pressure-volume loop of the LV, provides a basis for appreciating a load-insensitive index of contractility, the ESPVR. Phase 1 in Figure 19-2 shows ventricular filling and represents the loading of the heart before contraction (i.e., preload). During early and middle diastole, filling of the ventricle is rapid, depending on the pressure gradient between the left atrium and the LV. In late diastole, the left atrium

contracts (*a* wave), which results in the final left ventricular end-diastolic volume (LVEDV) and pressure (LVEDP). Atrial contraction in the normal heart accounts for 15% to 20% of ventricular filling. The normal ventricle accommodates large changes in ventricular volume with only a small change in ventricular diastolic pressure.

Ventricular systole occurs in two stages: the isovolumic and ejection phases. During isovolumic, or isometric, systole (phase 2 of the cardiac cycle), intraventricular pressure increases dramatically. However, there is little or no concurrent decrease in ventricular volume because the aortic valve is still closed. Phase 3 is the systolic ejection period. When intraventricular pressure exceeds aortic pressure, the aortic valve opens and ejection begins. At the end of phase 3, the aortic valve closes. This point is the end-systolic pressure-volume coordinate, which may uniquely reflect the cardiac inotropic state.

Afterload Stress and Preload Reserve

Figure 19-3 shows the response of the LV to changes in afterload, with preload held constant, in the context of the pressure-volume loops from single contractions. These curves are constructed experimentally by infusing a pure α-adrenergic agonist while simultaneously measuring the corresponding end-systolic volumes (ESVs). The resultant curves describe the diastolic pressure-volume relation (ventricular compliance) and the linear ESPVR at a given level of myocardial contractility. Each counterclockwise loop represents a cardiac cycle. The stroke volume (SV) progressively decreases as the impedance to ejection increases from beats 1 to 3. This pattern continues until beat 4, when the peak ventricular systolic pressure fails to open the aortic valve and only isovolumic contraction ensues.[1] This inverse relation

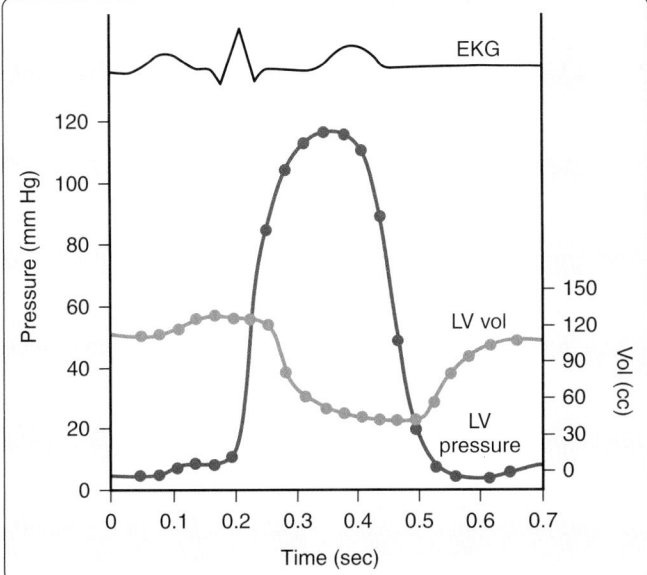

Figure 19-1 Simultaneous left ventricular (LV) volume and pressure during one cardiac cycle. EKG, electrocardiogram. (*From Barash PG, Kopriva DJ: Cardiac pump function and how to monitor it. In Thomas SJ [ed]:* Manual of cardiac anesthesia. *New York: Churchill Livingstone, 1984, p 1.*)

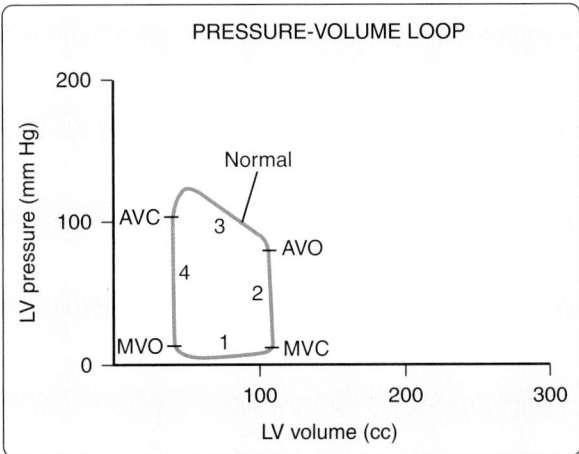

Figure 19-2 An idealized pressure-volume loop for a single cardiac cycle. AVC, aortic valve closure; AVD, aortic valve opening; LV, left ventricular; MVC, mitral valve closure; MVD, mitral valve opening. (*From Jackson JM, Thomas SJ, Lowenstein E: Anesthetic management of patients with valvular heart disease.* Semin Anesth *1:239, 1982.*)

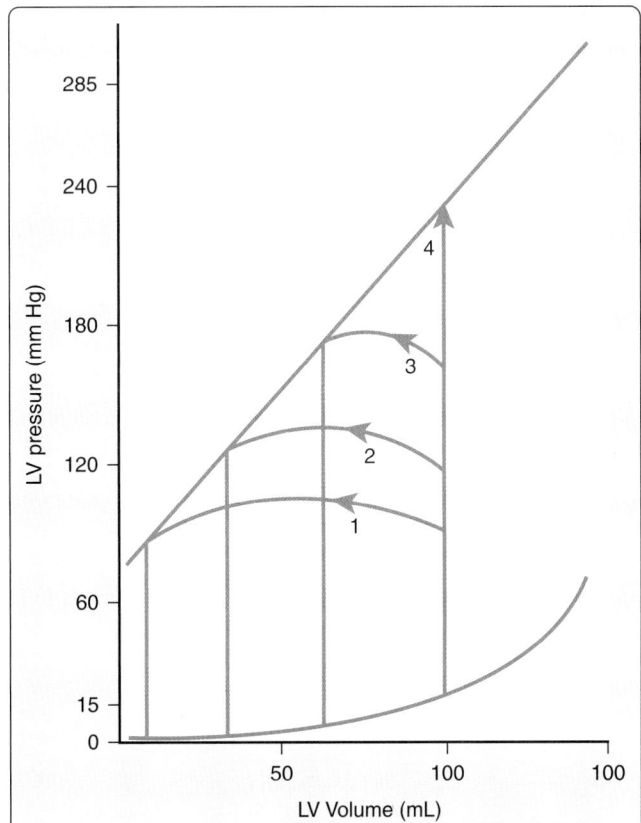

Figure 19-3 Pressure-volume loops illustrating the response of the left ventricle (LV) to progressive increases in afterload when the preload is artificially held constant. (*From Ross J Jr: Afterload mismatch in aortic and mitral valve disease: Implications for surgical therapy.* J Am Coll Cardiol *5:811, 1985.*)

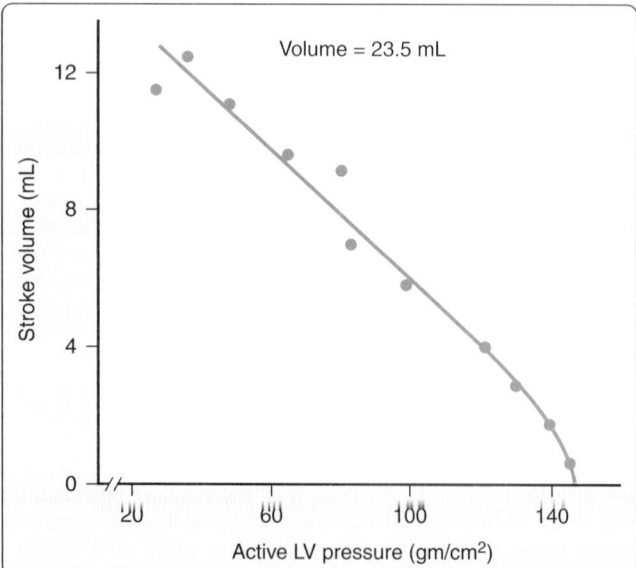

Figure 19-4 Plot of left ventricular (LV) stroke volume versus LV systolic pressure when the ventricle's end-diastolic volume is held constant (the inverse force-velocity relation). *(From Burns JW, Covell JW, Ross J Jr: Mechanics of isotonic left ventricular contractions. Am J Physiol 224:725, 1973.)*

law, resulting in a reciprocal decline in myocardial fiber shortening (i.e., inverse force-velocity relation). Despite this relative decline in fiber shortening, the SV is maintained because contractile force is augmented at the higher preload (i.e., Starling or length-active tension effect). This increased contractility at higher LVEDVs may be mediated by an increased sensitivity to the inotropic effects of extracellular calcium at longer muscle lengths.[7-9]

Use of this "preload reserve" allows the LV to maintain its SV in the face of an afterload stress,[1] as shown in Figure 19-6.[1] The increase in afterload (beat 2) elicits a compensatory increase in end-diastolic volume (EDV; beat 3), preserving SV at the higher afterload. However, when the ventricle reaches the limit of its preload reserve, it overdistends, and preload behaves as if it were fixed. SV then decreases with further increases in the systolic pressure (afterload mismatch; beat 4), a clinical corollary of the inverse force-velocity relation.

between afterload and SV (inverse force-velocity relation) also was documented experimentally in a canine preparation in which the LVEDV was held constant (Figure 19-4).[2] In the intact heart, afterload is a function of ventricular size and arterial pressure.[3] Its pivotal role in cardiovascular regulation is summarized in Figure 19-5. Afterload is defined as the tension, or force per unit of cross-sectional area, in the ventricular wall during ejection.[4] Laplace's law provides a mathematical expression for the wall tension[5] (in which P is the intraventricular pressure) developed in a spherical chamber of radius, R, and wall thickness, h:

$$\text{Wall tension} = P \times R/2h$$

This means that ventricular afterload, a function of the constantly changing intraventricular pressure and radius, varies continuously during systole. It is extremely difficult to precisely quantify afterload in the clinical setting, and commonly used approximations such as blood pressure or systemic vascular resistance (SVR) are inherently misleading because they fail to reflect instantaneous pressure-volume variations. Left ventricular size or preload is a determinant of the SV and afterload.[6] Normally, the LV compensates for increases in afterload by increases in preload. This increase in end-diastolic fiber stretch or radius further increases wall tension in accordance with Laplace's

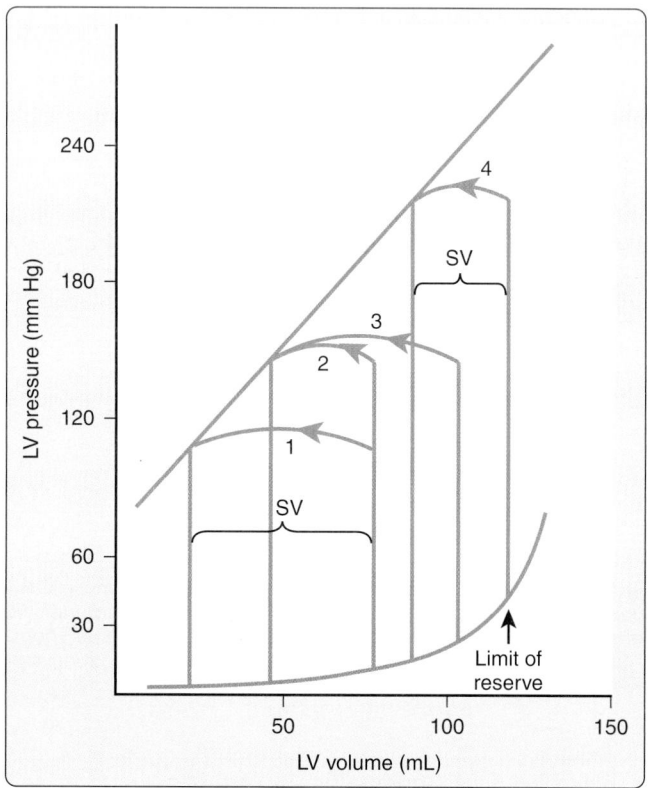

Figure 19-6 Pressure-volume loops illustrating the concept of preload reserve. An increase in afterload elicits a compensatory increase in left ventricular (LV) end-diastolic volume such that stroke volume (SV) is maintained at the higher afterload. *(From Ross J Jr: Afterload mismatch in aortic and mitral valve disease: Implications for surgical therapy. J Am Coll Cardiol 5:811, 1985.)*

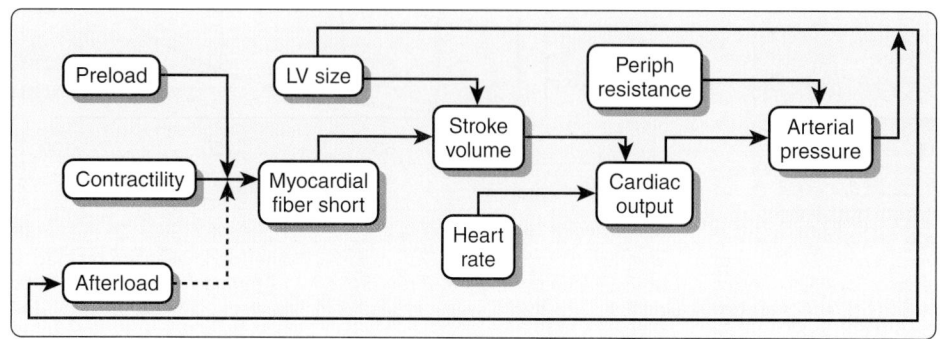

Figure 19-5 **Role of afterload in cardiac regulation.** LV, left ventricular; Periph, peripheral. *(From Braunwald E: Regulation of the circulation. N Engl J Med 290:1124, 1974.)*

Ventricular Compliance

Translating this physiologic analysis to the clinical setting is complicated by a number of practical constraints. One of the most important is the inconstant relation between LVEDV and LVEDP. The diastolic pressure-volume relation for the normal mammalian LV is a curvilinear function (Figure 19-7).[3,10] The slope of this curve (i.e., ratio of change in volume to change in pressure during diastole) is the ventricular compliance (dV/dP). Although the normal ventricle is extremely compliant in the physiologic range, the instantaneous compliance decreases with increments in diastolic filling. This progressively increasing slope of the pressure-volume curve becomes evident at the extremes of ventricular volume, in which succeeding increments in volume result in exponentially greater increases in end-diastolic pressure (EDP). Patients with acute aortic regurgitation (AR) experience the hemodynamic consequences of this phenomenon. The catastrophic increases in ventricular filling pressure reflect the absolute magnitude of the volume overload and are a corollary of a precipitously declining compliance relation.

These hemodynamic manifestations of acute shifts up and down a single compliance curve must be distinguished from chronic, pathologic alterations in ventricular compliance, which produce actual shifts of the entire curve relating diastolic pressure and volume. For example, in animal models of chronic volume overload, the entire pressure-volume curve is shifted to the right, such that substantial increases in ventricular volume are tolerated with relatively little change in EDP (Figure 19-8).[11] In this example, the slope of the new pressure-volume curve (i.e., compliance) is decreased. Similarly, time-dependent, rightward shifts of the entire pressure-volume relation have been shown to occur in patients with severe ventricular volume overload resulting from chronic AR.[12] In these examples, the development of a new relation between pressure and volume may reflect the physiologic process of *creep*, the time-dependent change in size or the dimension of tissue maintained at a constant level of stress.[4]

Myocardial wall thickness is an important determinant of diastolic compliance. In clinical settings of chronic pressure overload (e.g., aortic stenosis [AS], chronic hypertension), diastolic compliance and ventricular wall thickness have been shown to be linearly and inversely related (Figure 19-9).[13] This may explain why the normal, thinner-walled right ventricle (RV) is more compliant than the normal LV, even though the ventricles share similar qualities of intrinsic myocardial stiffness.[3,14] This association between pathologic hypertrophy of the ventricle and deterioration in its diastolic compliance is a well-documented but poorly understood phenomenon.

It has become customary to characterize diastolic function in certain disease states as normal or abnormal, such as diastolic dysfunction or diastolic failure.[15,16] The latter condition is a distinct pathophysiologic entity that results from an increased resistance to ventricular filling and leads to an inappropriate upward shift of the diastolic pressure-volume relation.[17] For example, diastolic dysfunction is seen in ischemic cardiomyopathy, particularly when combined with pressure overload hypertrophy.[18]

In certain diseases, these primary derangements of diastolic function may predominate over abnormalities of diastolic function associated with ventricular hypertrophy. For example, in hypertrophic cardiomyopathy (HCM), the impaired ventricular relaxation inherent in the myopathic process appears to play the greater role in the observed abnormalities of diastolic filling because the diastolic dysfunction is often disproportionate to the degree of ventricular hypertrophy.[19,20] The effects of pathologic hypertrophy on diastolic compliance and ventricular relaxation are complex and are considered in more detail later in the Aortic Stenosis and Hypertrophic Cardiomyopathy sections.

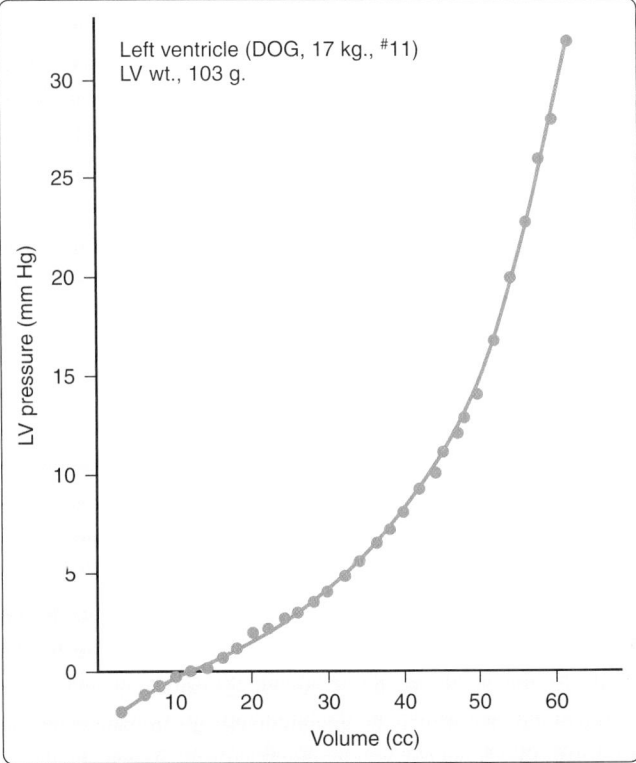

Figure 19-7 **The normal diastolic pressure-volume relation.** LV, left ventricular. *(From Spotnitz HM, Sonnenblick EH, Spiro D: Relation of ultrastructure to function in the intact heart: Sarcomere structure relative to pressure-volume curves of the intact left ventricles of dog and cat. Circ Res 18:49, 1966.)*

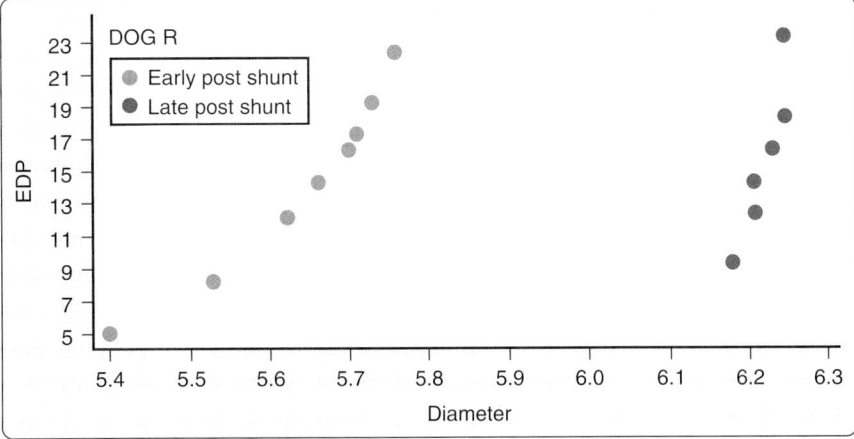

Figure 19-8 Relations between left ventricular end-diastolic pressure (EDP) and volume (diameter) in an animal studied early *(light circles)* and late *(dark circles)* after the production of chronic volume overloading (arteriovenous fistula). *(From McCullagh WH, Covell JW, Ross J Jr: Left ventricular dilation and diastolic compliance changes during chronic volume overloading. Circulation 45:943, 1972.)*

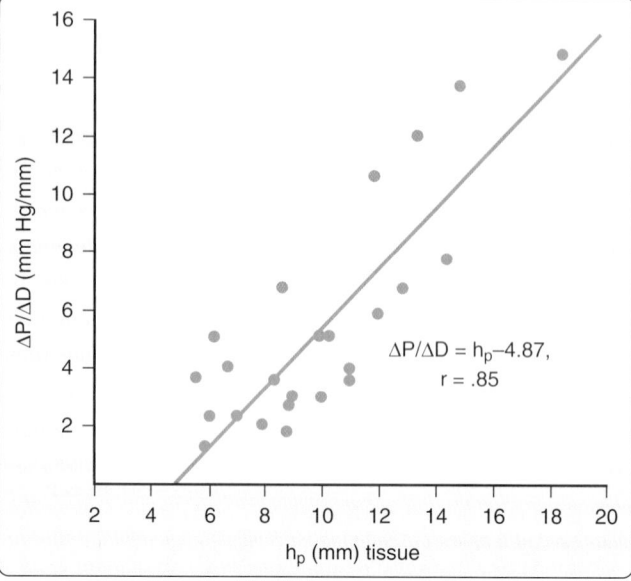

Figure 19-9 Relation between chamber stiffness (ΔP/ΔD, the inverse of compliance) and ventricular wall thickness. *(From Grossman W, McLaurin P, Moos SP, et al: Wall thickness and diastolic properties of the left ventricle. Circulation 49:129, 1974.)*

Filling of one ventricle or changes in its configuration or compliance properties can significantly alter the diastolic pressure-volume characteristics of the other ventricle.[21,22] Progressive increases in right ventricular filling shift the left ventricular compliance curve up and to the left. This effect is greatest at high right ventricular filling pressures and is accentuated by the presence of the pericardium.[23] With severe right ventricular distention, the interventricular septum encroaches on the LV. This encroachment reduces the size of the LV and alters its geometric configuration such that its compliance declines.[21] As a result, left ventricular filling pressures may fail to reflect even directional changes in left ventricular size.[24]

Contractility

Myocardial contractility can be defined as the ability of the heart to generate force at a given preload.[25] Although most clinicians and researchers seem to be comfortable with their intuitive notions of the cardiac inotropic state, the search for a consensus on a quantitative yardstick of ventricular inotropy has proved to be elusive. Its accurate and reproducible measurement is of more than theoretic interest because the contractile function of the heart is a key determinant of prognosis for most cardiac diseases, and it is especially important in critical decisions regarding the timing of surgical correction in patients with VHD.

Historically, methods of assessing myocardial contractility have been divided into two groups, based on analysis of the isovolumetric or the ejection phase of cardiac contraction.[4] Details of their clinical determination and relative reproducibility are beyond the scope of this discussion, but more information can be found in several excellent reviews,[4,26,27] as well as in Chapters 5 and 14. The isovolumetric indices include measurements such as maximal velocity of myocardial fiber shortening (V_{max}), peak pressure development (dP/dt), and peak dP/dt measured at an instantaneous pressure (dP/dt/P). Although relatively insensitive to loading conditions, these tests poorly reflect basal levels of contractility and are unreliable for comparing contractility among patients or assessing directional changes in contractility in an individual patient over time.[26]

Ejection phase indices, such as the ejection fraction (EF), are determined, in part, by the intrinsic inotropic state and can be used to define basal levels of contractility.[26] Such measurements are extremely useful in evaluating ventricular function in patients with CAD or other

conditions that do not significantly alter ventricular loading conditions.[28] Ejection phase indices are understandably popular because they are readily available, and they are the most widely used clinical measures of left ventricular function. However, these indices are directly proportional to preload, vary inversely with ventricular afterload, and are accordingly unreliable for assessing contractile performance in patients with most forms of VHD.

The use of the pressure-volume diagram and analysis of the ESPVR allow a more precise appreciation of left ventricular contractility, which is independent of preload.[29] The extent of myocardial shortening, and therefore of end-systolic fiber length, is a direct function of afterload (i.e., inverse force-velocity relation), and myocardial contractility can be evaluated by making use of this fundamental property. In most instances, end-systolic pressure (ESP) can be substituted for afterload. Only with pathologic degrees of ventricular hypertrophy is there a major divergence between ESP and afterload. This means that for any level of contractility, the ESV to which a ventricle contracts is a linearly increasing function of ESP. A stronger ventricle contracts to a smaller ESV (i.e., empties more completely) at any given level of ventricular afterload. Changes in the inotropic state also can be viewed in the context of the idealized pressure-volume loop. Positive inotropic interventions shift the curve up and to the left, increasing the work that can be performed at any given EDV (preload). Conversely, negative inotropic interventions shift the curve down and to the right[30] (Figure 19-10; see Chapters 5 and 14). These load-independent indices of contractility are largely research tools, but in the future, it may be possible to construct pressure-volume loops and quantify ESPVRs in real time with echocardiographic equipment featuring automated border detection[31] (see Chapter 12).

Clinical studies of patients with relatively normal loading conditions have shown that variations in the ESV reliably correlate with changes in ejection phase indices (Figure 19-11).[32] The ESPVR represents an index of contractility that depends on systolic ventricular pressure (i.e., afterload) but is independent of end-diastolic length (i.e., preload).[28,33,34] Pressure-volume loops also provide a framework for considering the interactions between systolic (inotropic) and diastolic (lusitropic) function. Although the preload (i.e., EDV) is an independent determinant of SV, because of the circular nature of blood flow, the SV ultimately determines venous return and the resultant preload for the next cardiac cycle.[30] The "inotropically determined" ESV is the other element besides the venous return that contributes to the EDV. Just as the ESPVR uniquely describes systolic function, the end-diastolic pressure-volume relation is a manifestation of the intrinsic relaxation (lusitropic) properties of the ventricle. Positive lusitropic interventions facilitate ventricular filling and shift the end-diastolic pressure-volume relation down and to the right, and a negative lusitropic intervention shifts it up and to the left (Figure 19-12).

AORTIC STENOSIS

Clinical Features and Natural History

Aortic stenosis (AS) is the most common cardiac valve lesion in the United States. Approximately 1% to 2% of the population is born with a bicuspid aortic valve, which is prone to stenosis with aging, and the population is aging. Clinically significant aortic valve stenosis is present in 2% of unselected individuals older than 65 years, and in 5.5% of those older than 85 years.[35] Incipient aortic valve stenosis with calcification and stiffening is observed in 50% of people in the 75 to 80 age group and in up to 75% in those older than 85 years. Bicuspid aortic valve is a common congenital cardiac abnormality, occurring in approximately 1% of the population.[36] The heritability coefficient is estimated at 89%, suggesting that the bicuspid aortic valve is almost entirely genetic in nature.[37] It is a risk factor for premature AS and ascending aortic aneurysms. The ascending aorta in bicuspid valvular disease has the same histopathologic features as Marfan syndrome, such as medial degeneration, decreased fibrillin-1, and enhanced matrix metalloproteinase activity in the aortic wall. Recent data from the International Registry

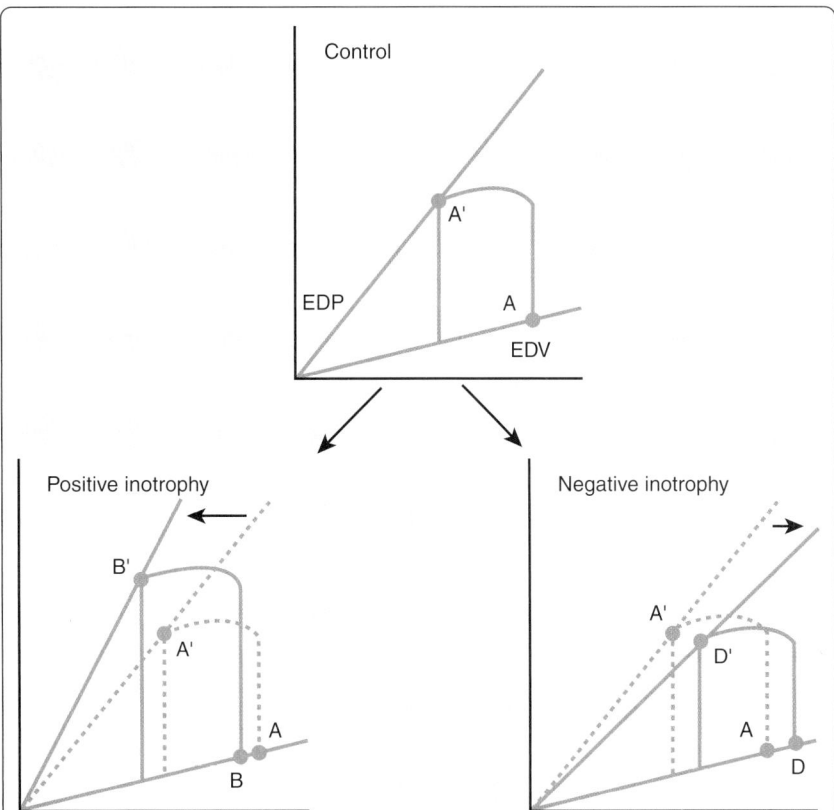

Figure 19-10 A positive inotropic intervention increases the heart's ability to do work at a given end-diastolic volume (EDV) and pressure (EDP). As shown in this example, increased inotropy need not imply an increased stroke volume (SV); however, the latter is maintained despite a greater peak systolic pressure, producing the upward and leftward shift of the end-systolic pressure-volume point. Negative inotropy shifts the end-systolic pressure-volume point down and to the right. The SV is unchanged, but the end-diastolic and end-systolic volumes are increased, and the peak systolic pressure achieved is reduced. *(From Katz AM: Influence of altered inotropy and lusitropy on ventricular pressure-volume loops. J Am Coll Cardiol 11:438, 1988.)*

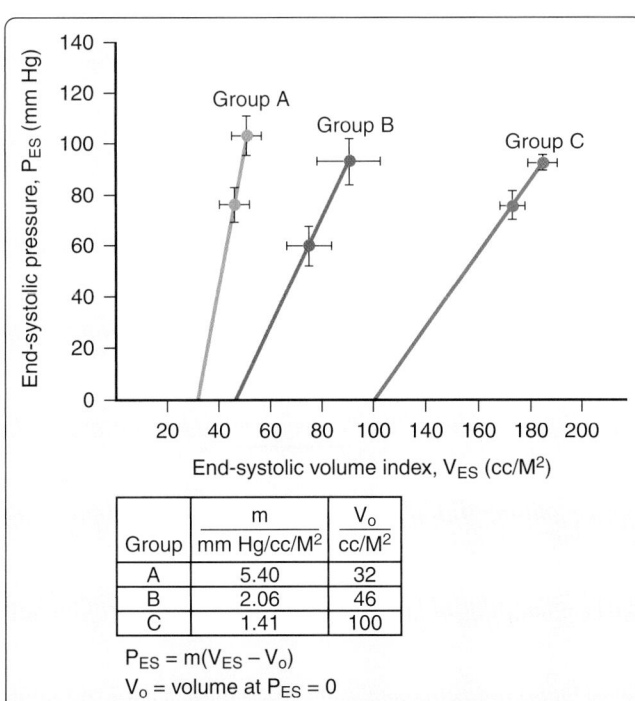

Group	m (mm Hg/cc/M²)	V_o (cc/M²)
A	5.40	32
B	2.06	46
C	1.41	100

$$P_{ES} = m(V_{ES} - V_o)$$
$$V_o = \text{volume at } P_{ES} = 0$$

Figure 19-11 Average values of end-systolic pressure versus end-systolic volume (at two levels of afterload) plotted for groups (A, B, and C) with different contractile performance as evaluated by ejection fraction (A > 0.6; B = 0.41 to 0.59; C < 0.4). The end-systolic volume point correlates inversely with contractility. *(From Grossman W, Braunwald E, Mann T, et al: Contractile state of the left ventricle in man as evaluated from end-systolic pressure-volume relations. Circulation 56:845, 1977.)*

of Acute Aortic Dissection demonstrate that patients with bicuspid aortic valve have a 6.14% lifetime risk rate of aortic dissection (nine times that of the general population), compared with 40% for patients with Marfan syndrome. Yet, bicuspid aortic valvular disease is a hundred times more common than Marfan syndrome and is, therefore, responsible for a larger number of aortic dissections.[36] Calcific AS has several features in common with CAD. Both conditions are more common in men, older people, and patients with hypercholesterolemia, and both result, in part, from an active inflammatory process. There is clinical evidence of an atherosclerotic hypothesis for the cellular mechanism of aortic valve stenosis. There is a clear association between clinical risk factors for atherosclerosis and the development of AS: increased lipoprotein levels, increased low-density lipoprotein (LDL) cholesterol, cigarette smoking, hypertension, diabetes mellitus, increased serum calcium and creatinine levels, and male sex.[38] Homozygous familial hypercholesterolemia produces a severe form of AS in children.[39] The early lesion of aortic valve sclerosis may be associated with CAD and vascular atherosclerosis. The extent of aortic valve calcification was observed as an important predictor of poor outcome in patients with AS.[40] These and other studies suggest that aortic valve calcification is an inflammatory process promoted by atherosclerotic risk factors.

The early lesion of AS resembles that of the initial plaque of CAD, and there is a close correlation between calcification found in coronary arteries and the amount of calcification found in the aortic valve. Pathologic studies of aortic valves revealed the presence of LDL, suggesting a common cellular mechanism for the genesis of valvular and vascular atherosclerotic disease.[38] Degenerative lesions on aortic valves contain an inflammatory infiltrate of nonfoam cells and foam cell macrophages, T lymphocytes, and other inflammatory cells. Lipid is accumulated in the fibrosa immediately below the endothelium layer on the aortic side of the valve. LDL- and apolipoprotein E–containing lipoproteins are present as well. Little is known about the synthesis of bone matrix proteins in calcific aortic valve stenosis. The calcifications

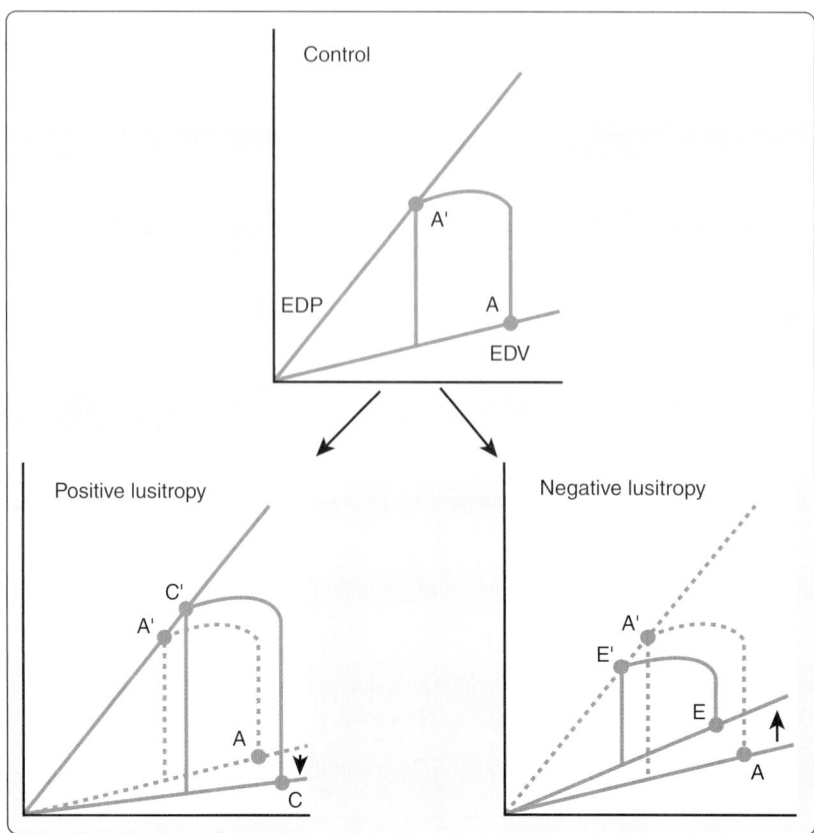

Figure 19-12 Positive lusitropic interventions enhance diastolic filling, shifting the end-diastolic pressure-volume point down and to the right. A negative lusitropic intervention shifts the end-diastolic pressure-volume point up and to the left. EDP, end-diastolic pressure; EDV, end-diastolic volume. *(From Katz AM: Influence of altered inotropy and lusitropy on ventricular pressure-volume loops. J Am Coll Cardiol 11:438, 1988.)*

are composed of hydroxyapatite on a matrix of collagen, osteopontin, and other bone matrix proteins.

A potential mechanism for this cellular inflammation process involves the combination of macrophages, LDL, and the secretion by macrophages of transforming growth factor-β and platelet-derived growth factor to stimulate the conversion of valvular fibroblast cells into osteoblasts that produce bone proteins.[38] Most surprising are the findings that 3-hydroxy-3-methylglutaryl coenzyme A reductase inhibitors (e.g., statins) retard the progression of CAD and AS.[41,42] The odds ratio of AS progression was 0.46 in 38 treated patients compared with 118 untreated patients.[43] Other studies have shown similar results, and it is possible that therapy with statins or other drugs may be used to block or slow the progression of valve lesions in the future.[38,44] In addition to recruitment of inflammatory cells and lipid accumulation into valves, calcification is a prominent feature that contributes to leaflet thickness and rigidity. Early development of aortic valve calcification may be related to vitamin D–receptor genotypes or mutations in the *Notch* gene.[35] Calcification is an active process that includes osteopontin, osteonectin, osteocalcin, and other bone morphogenic proteins that regulate calcification and ossification. Active osteoblastic bone formation and osteoclastic bone resorption occur in stenotic valves. Increased fibroblasts produce collagen, leading to fibrosis. Concomitant elastin degradation also contributes to valve stiffening. Whereas normal valves are avascular, microvessels form in thickened stenotic valves, assuring the continued supply of inflammatory cells and lipids. Recent advances in genetic epidemiology have demonstrated a strong inheritability of bicuspid aortic valve with three loci on chromosomes 18q, 5q, and 13q, which likely contain genes responsible for bicuspid aortic valve.[37] The mode of inheritance of other valvular diseases is unclear. No inheritability or inheritance studies have been reported for calcific aortic valve disease. In smaller genetic studies, a small number of candidate genes such as *VDR, APOE, APOB, IL-10,* and *ESR1* have been identified as

possibly playing a role in aortic valve disease. A recent breakthrough in the genetics of aortic valve disease was the identification of the Notch1 signaling pathway, involved in embryonic patterning, and that is highly expressed within the developing embryonic aortic valve. Notch1 is a repressor of Runx2, a critical regulator of osteoblast development. This supports the concept that a developmental program might be reactivated in disease processes.[37]

The rate of progression is, on average, a decrease in aortic valve area (AVA) of 0.1 cm²/year, and the peak instantaneous gradient increases by 10 mm Hg/year.[45] The rate of progression of AS in men older than 60 is faster than in women, and it is faster in women older than 75 than in women 60 to 74 years old.[46] Treatment with hemodialysis, the use of calcium supplements, and increased serum creatinine levels correlated with rapid progression of AS.[47] Plasma brain natriuretic peptide, produced to a large extent by the ventricles, and the N-terminal part of the propeptide may serve as early markers of left ventricular hypertrophy (LVH), whereas atrial natriuretic peptide and the N-terminal part of the propeptide reflect atrial pressure increase.[48] Repeated measurements of this marker may reflect information on the stage of AS and its hemodynamic impact.[49]

Angina, syncope, and congestive heart failure (CHF) are the classic symptoms of the disease, and their appearance is of serious prognostic significance because postmortem studies indicate that symptomatic AS is associated with a life expectancy of only 2 to 5 years.[50–52] These early natural history studies were completed before the availability of cardiac catheterization studies, and some patients, although symptomatic, may have had objectively less severe degrees of stenosis. The "hemodynamically insignificant murmur of aortic stenosis" seen so often in cardiologic consultations does not portend such dire consequences, although it is sometimes difficult to correlate AS severity with clinical symptoms. There is evidence that patients with moderate AS (i.e., valve areas of 0.7 to 1.2 cm²) are also at increased risk for the development of complications, with the appearance of symptoms further increasing their risk.[53] According to recent American College of Cardiology (ACC) and American Heart Association (AHA) guidelines, peak velocity greater than 4 m/sec, a mean gradient greater than 40 mm Hg, and a valve area less than 1.0 cm[2] are considered hemodynamically severe AS.[54] Aortic valve surgery should be performed promptly in symptomatic patients. In asymptomatic patients, high aortic valve calcium content and a positive exercise test are features that suggest a benefit from early aortic valve replacement (AVR).

An interesting question is whether the natural history of AS has changed significantly in recent years.[55] The question is prompted by two trends. The first, at least in North America, is related to the steadily diminishing number of patients with rheumatic disease. Today, AS is essentially the bicuspid, the calcific, or what has been traditionally referred to as the senile variety. The second trend is related to the senile attribution. People are living longer, particularly those with heart disease. The typical patient with AS is older and much more likely to have other significant medical problems, including major coexisting cardiac disease, most often CAD.

Angina is a frequent and classic symptom of the disease, occurring in approximately two thirds of patients with critical AS, and about half of symptomatic patients are found to have anatomically significant CAD.[56–58] However, a controversy persists about the incidence of CAD in patients with AS who do not have angina, and the controversy probably reflects this underlying sense of a change in the natural history of the disease. Some studies report that the absence of angina virtually excludes the possibility of atherosclerotic heart disease.[59,60] In contrast, a 25% incidence rate of angiographically significant (> 70% obstruction) coronary occlusions was described in angina-free patients, most of whom had single-vessel disease.[61] However, a much larger study found that 14% of patients with triple-vessel or left main CAD and AS presented without angina.[62] Underscoring the continued lack of a consensus on this topic is the finding of a review that the reported incidence rates of significant CAD in asymptomatic patients range from 0% to 33%.[63] Identification of asymptomatic patients is important because although coexistent, untreated (i.e., unbypassed) CAD has a detrimental effect on early and late survival after AVR, concomitant CABG with AVR does not increase perioperative mortality.[64–67] It appears that a substantial number of patients with coexisting CAD may have symptoms other than chest pain.[68] However, there do not appear to be other significant differences in the clinical or hemodynamic findings between patients with normal coronary arteries and those with coexistent coronary stenoses.

If the traditional natural history of AS is perhaps more ominous in the elderly patient with likely coexistent CAD, is there any rationale for prophylactic AVR? With steady improvement in surgical results, this question has been raised, although rigorous studies still suggest that asymptomatic patients with hemodynamically significant disease face a very low risk for sudden death before the onset of symptoms.[69–71] As if by way of settling this particular question, an editorial by Braunwald[72] stated that there was no role for prophylactic AVR, and that "operative treatment is the most common cause of sudden death in asymptomatic patients with aortic stenosis." These patients warrant careful follow-up, and the case against prophylactic surgical intervention is further supported by studies showing that ventricular function is preserved and myocardial hypertrophy regresses after successful valve replacement.[73–75]

It is probably never too late to operate on patients with symptomatic AS.[76,77] First, unlike AR, most symptomatic patients undergo valve replacement when left ventricular function is still normal. Second, even when impaired left ventricular function develops in AS, the relief of pressure overload almost always restores normal function or at least produces considerable improvement. Morbidity rates, mortality rates, and clinical results are favorable even in the oldest surgical candidates.[78,79] Recent advances in operative techniques and perioperative management have contributed to excellent results after AVR in patients 80 years of age or older, with minimal incremental postoperative morbidity.[80] The principal postoperative complication is respiratory failure.

The preoperative assessment of AS with Doppler echocardiography includes measurement of the AVA and the transvalvular pressure gradient.[81,82] The latter is calculated from the Doppler-quantified transvalvular velocity of blood flow, which is increased in the presence of AS. This maximal velocity (v) is then inserted into the modified Bernoulli equation to determine the pressure gradient (PG) between the LV and the aorta (see Figure 19-2):

$$PG = P(\text{left ventricle}) - P(\text{aorta}) = 4(v^2)$$

The *pressure gradient* is the maximal difference between the LV and aortic pressures that occurs during ventricular systole.[83,84] This maximal instantaneous gradient is not the same as the peak-to-peak gradient determined by cardiac catheterization. The peak-to-peak gradient is determined by separate measurements of events that are not synchronous in real time. Of more practical interest is the fact that the best estimate of obstruction severity, as determined from pressure data alone, is the mean systolic gradient, which is calculated online by Doppler equipment[85] (see Chapters 3 and 12).

The Doppler-calculated gradient is subject to the same flow limitation as invasively calculated gradients. Best understood by considering the extreme, this means that a patient with true end-stage AS would exhibit a relatively low calculated gradient because of minimal flow across a critically narrowed valve. In part because of this flow dependency, pressure gradients determined invasively or by Doppler echocardiography correctly classify AS severity in less than 50% of cases compared with estimates of AVA.[86] However, the latter also can be determined by Doppler echocardiographic techniques. The preferred method requires only two Doppler-generated velocities: those proximal and those distal to the stenotic valve. These values are inserted into the continuity equation, which relates the respective velocities and cross-sectional areas proximal and distal to a stenotic area (see Figure 19-3). Specifically, the equation states:

$$V\text{max} \times AVA = \text{area}(LVOT) \times V(LVOT)$$

in which AVA is the aortic valve area, V is the volume, and LVOT is the left ventricular outflow tract. Several studies have demonstrated the reliability of these Doppler-determined valve areas.[83–86]

Although advances in Doppler technology allow completely noninvasive evaluation of a large number of patients, coronary angiography is probably indicated in all patients older than 50 years who are demonstrated to have significant AS. Angiography and, if indicated, CABG may improve the long-term outlook for patients with CAD who undergo AVR.[62] Angiography also can identify a smaller number of patients whose CAD alone would warrant CABG.

Pathophysiology

The normal AVA is 2.6 to 3.5 cm[2], with hemodynamically significant obstruction usually occurring at cross-sectional valve areas of 1 cm[2] or less. Generally accepted criteria for critical outflow obstruction include a systolic pressure gradient greater than 50 mm Hg, with a normal cardiac output, and an AVA of less than 0.4 cm[2]. In view of the ominous natural history of severe AS (AVA < 0.7 cm[2]),[55,87] symptomatic patients with this degree of AS are generally referred for immediate AVR.[88] The Hakki equation is a simplification of the Gorlin equation to calculate the AVA based on the cardiac output (CO) and the peak pressure gradient (PG) across the valve.

$$\text{Valve area} = \frac{CO}{\sqrt{(PG)}}$$

An obvious corollary of the previously described relation is that "minimal" pressure gradients may actually reflect critical degrees of outflow obstruction when the CO is significantly reduced (i.e., the generation of a pressure gradient requires some finite amount of flow). Clinicians have long recognized this phenomenon as a "paradoxic" decline in the intensity of the murmur (i.e., minimal transvalvular flow) as the AS worsens.

Stenosis at the level of the aortic valve results in a pressure gradient from the LV to the aorta. The intracavitary systolic pressure generated to overcome this stenosis directly increases myocardial wall tension in accordance with Laplace's law:

$$\text{Wall tension} = P \times R/2h$$

in which P is the intraventricular pressure, R is the inner radius, and h is the wall thickness.

This increase of wall tension is believed to be the direct stimulus for the further parallel replication of sarcomeres, which produces the concentrically hypertrophied ventricle characteristic of chronic pressure overload.[89,90] The consequences of this LVH include alterations in diastolic compliance, potential imbalances in the myocardial oxygen supply and demand relationship, and possible deterioration of the intrinsic contractile performance of the myocardium.

Figure 19-13 shows a typical pressure-volume loop for a patient with AS. Two differences from the normal curve are immediately apparent. First, the peak pressure generated during systole is much greater because of the high transvalvular pressure gradient. Second, the slope of the diastolic limb is steeper, reflecting the reduced left ventricular diastolic compliance that is associated with the increase in chamber thickness.[13] Clinically, this means that small changes in diastolic volume produce relatively large increases in ventricular filling pressure.

This increased chamber stiffness places a premium on the contribution of atrial systole to ventricular filling, which in patients with AS may account for up to 40% of the LVEDV, rather than the 15% to 20% characteristic of the normal LV. Echocardiographic and radionuclide studies have documented that diastolic filling and ventricular relaxation are abnormal in patients with hypertrophy from a variety of causes, with significant prolongation of the isovolumic relaxation period being the most characteristic finding.[91–94] This necessarily compromises the duration and amount of filling achieved during the early rapid diastolic filling phase and increases the relative contribution of atrial contraction to overall diastolic filling (Figure 19-14). A much greater mean left atrial (LA) pressure is necessary to distend the LV in the absence of the sinus mechanism. One treatment of junctional rhythm is volume infusion.

The systolic limb of the pressure-volume loop shows preservation of pump function, as evidenced by maintenance of the SV and EF (see Figure 19-13). It is likely that use of preload reserve and adequate LVH are the principal compensatory mechanisms that maintain forward flow. Clinical studies have confirmed that ejection performance is

preserved at the expense of myocardial hypertrophy, and the adequacy of the hypertrophic response has been related to the degree to which it achieves normalization of wall stress, in accordance with the Laplace relation.[95–97] LVH can be viewed as a compensatory physiologic response that completes a negative feedback loop (Figure 19-15). It is possible, however, that severe afterload stress and proportionately massive LVH could decrease subendocardial perfusion and superimpose a component of ischemic contractile dysfunction.

In patients with AS, LVH develops as a result of the increase in pressure load. The development of LVH and its regression after therapeutic interventions are accompanied by changes in the cardiac extracellular matrix guided by an increase in *ECM1* gene expression during LVH and complete regression after complete correction.[98]

Systemic hypertension and AS represent an increase in afterload to the LV, and each contributes to left ventricular remodeling and LVH. In a large series of 193 patients with AS, 62 of whom were hypertensive, symptoms manifested with larger AVAs and lower stroke work loss.[99] Patterns of left ventricular remodeling (i.e., concentric vs. eccentric remodeling and hypertrophy) were not different between hypertensive and normotensive patients. Left ventricular mass decreased by 23% 1 year after AVR, back into the normal range, in patients with normal preoperative ventricular function; diastolic function improved concomitantly. Improvements in myocardial blood flow and coronary vasodilator reserve after AVRs result from reduced extravascular compression and increased diastolic perfusion time.[100–102]

Ejection phase indices of contractile function are abnormal in many patients with AS.[103,104] However, indices of contractile function, which are exquisitely sensitive to afterload, are inherently unreliable for quantitating the inotropic state in a disease such as AS, in which the essence of the hemodynamic insult is the severely increased ventricular afterload. This in no way excludes the possibility that a subset of patients also may experience some intrinsic depression of myocardial contractility. For example, patients with AS may be particularly at risk for superimposed, ischemic ventricular dysfunction, but this possibility can be assessed only by the application of load-insensitive measurements of contractile function.

In most patients, however, load-insensitive indices of contractility (i.e., end-systolic stress-diameter determinations) are virtually identical before and after the development of hypertrophy, suggesting that the increase in chamber thickness compensates for the afterload stress, and myocardial contractility is, therefore, normal, albeit appropriate for the higher afterload. Figure 19-16 illustrates the adaptation of the LV to chronic pressure overload. Figure 19-16*A* shows the pressure-volume relation before (loop A) and after (loop B) the development of concentric hypertrophy. The linear ESPVR is shifted up and to the left after concentric hypertrophy occurs. However, the ESPVR may not be as accurate or load insensitive in assessing contractility at the extremes of afterload. Figure 19-16*B* shows normalization of this apparently supranormal contractility, when wall stress (rather than pressure) is used as a more exact measure of ventricular afterload. Concentric hypertrophy normalizes wall stress, and contractility remains unchanged. A decline in any index of myocardial contractility in patients with AS may represent relatively inadequate hypertrophy for the degree of wall stress, some intrinsic depression of contractility, or a combination of these two factors.[56,105,106] The fact that most patients have normal contractility is the reason for the usually favorable response to AVR.

In AS, signs and symptoms of CHF usually develop when preload reserve is exhausted, not because contractility is intrinsically or permanently impaired. This contrasts with mitral and AR, in which irreversible myocardial dysfunction may develop before the onset of significant symptoms. An important exception is the patient with AS whose symptoms of CHF occur in the setting of associated mitral regurgitation. The latter may accompany hypertrophy-induced left ventricular chamber or mitral annular enlargement. Mitral regurgitation in patients with AS is often referred to as *functional* as opposed to anatomic mitral insufficiency. The implication is that with relief of the high intracavitary systolic pressure, the mitral regurgitation will largely resolve, given

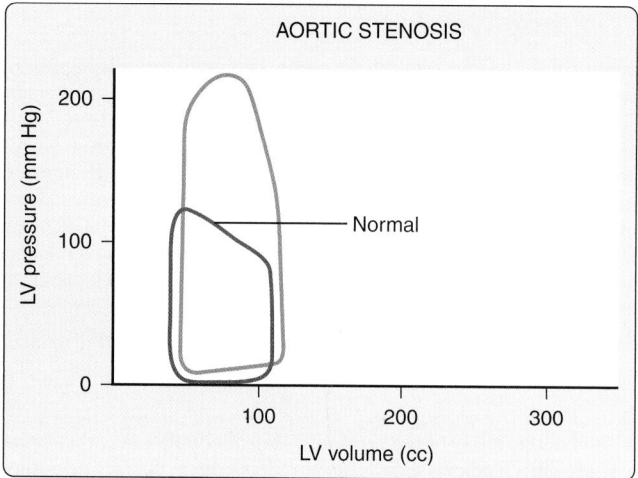

Figure 19-13 Pressure-volume loop in aortic stenosis. LV, left ventricular. *(From Jackson JM, Thomas SJ, Lowenstein E: Anesthetic management of patients with valvular heart disease. Semin Anesth 1:239, 1982.)*

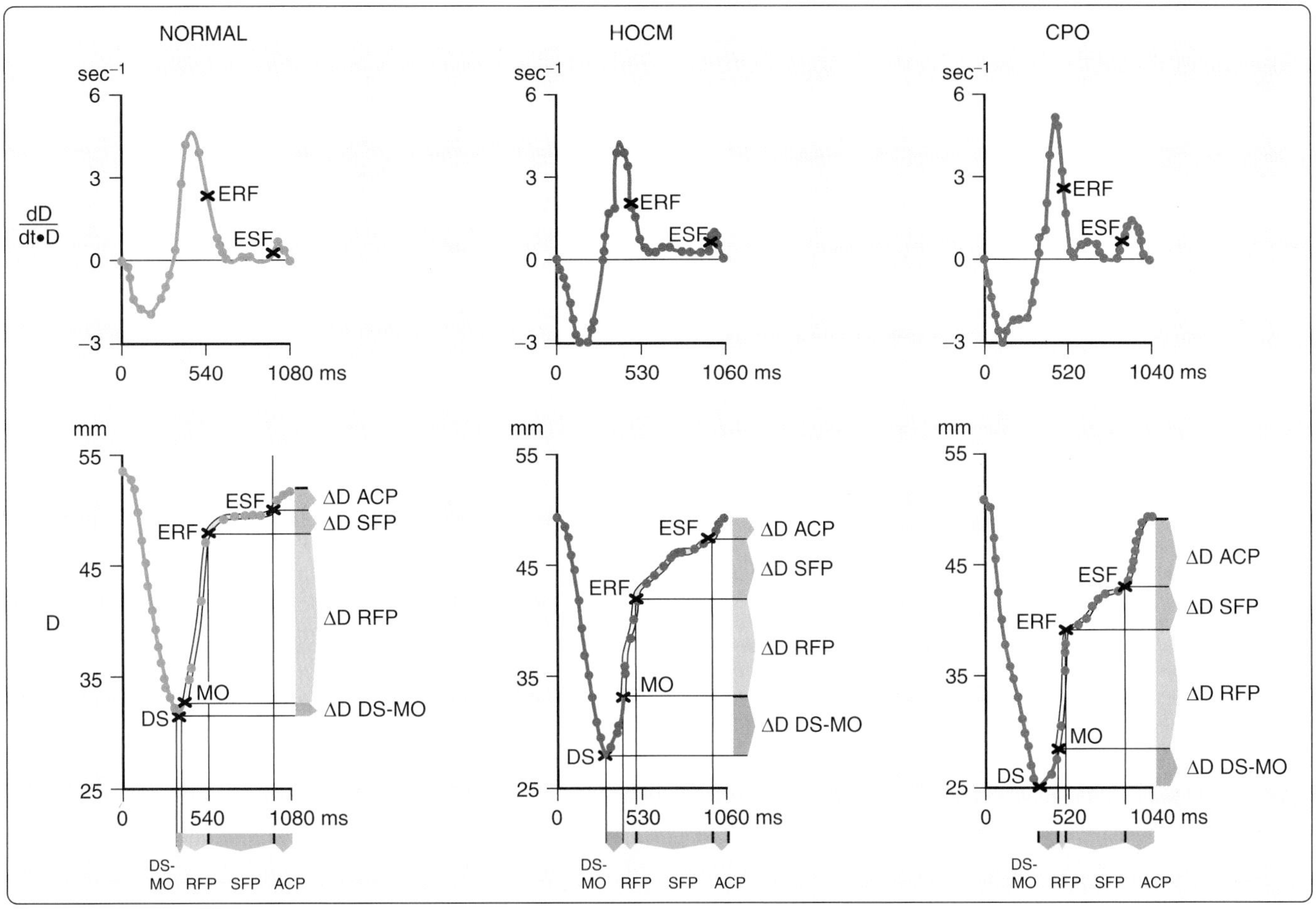

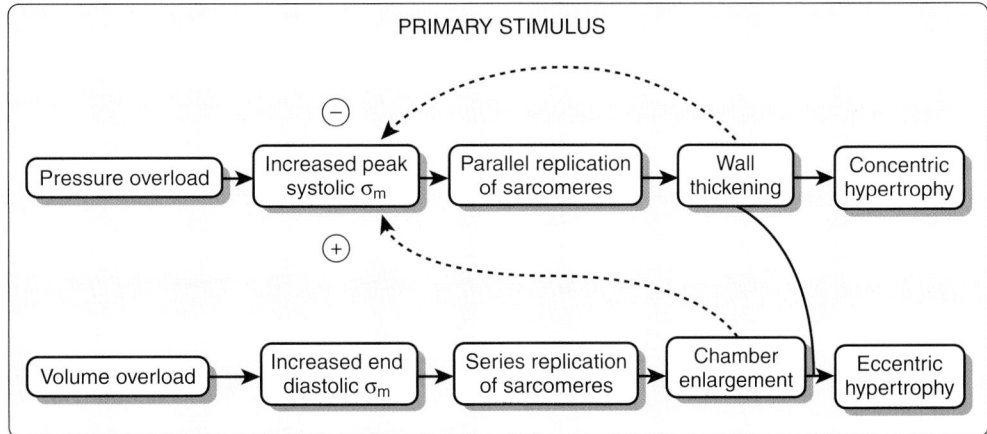

Figure 19-14 Computer-generated echograms of left ventricular (LV) cavity size in healthy subjects and patients with ventricular hypertrophy (i.e., hypertrophic obstructive cardiomyopathy [HOCM] or chronic pressure overload [CPO]). Top panels show the rate of ventricular dimensional change. In the bottom panels, for patients with both forms of hypertrophy, the mitral valve opening (MO) with regard to end-systolic LV dimension (DS) is delayed, and the dimensional change during this interval (ΔD DS-MO) is abnormally large. The duration of the rapid-filling phase (RFP) and the volume change during this interval (ΔD RFP) are correspondingly reduced. This is followed by a large dimensional increase during the atrial contraction phase (ΔD ACP) in the patient with chronic pressure overload; ERF, endpoint of rapid filling phase; ESF, endpoint of slow filling phase; SFP, slow filling phase. *(From Hanrath P, Mathey DG, Siegert R, et al: Left ventricular relaxation and filling pattern in different forms of left ventricular hypertrophy: An echocardiographic study. Am J Cardiol 45:15, 1980.)*

Figure 19-15 The increased peak systolic wall stress resulting from chronic pressure overload directly stimulates concentric ventricular hypertrophy, which tends to counteract or "normalize" the increased ventricular wall stress. *(From Grossman W, Jones D, McLaurin LP: Wall stress and patterns of hypertrophy in the human left ventricle. J Clin Invest 56:56, 1975.)*

an anatomically normal mitral valve. It is not uncommon for grade 2 or 3 mitral regurgitation to be significantly reduced after AVR.

More commonly, intrinsic contractility is preserved, and the major threat to the hypertrophied ventricle is its exquisite sensitivity to ischemia. Ventricular hypertrophy directly increases basal myocardial oxygen demand (Mvo$_2$). The other major determinants of overall Mvo$_2$ are heart rate, contractility, and, most important, wall tension. Increases in the latter occur as a direct consequence of Laplace's law in patients with relatively inadequate hypertrophy. The possibility of ischemic contractile dysfunction in the inadequately hypertrophied

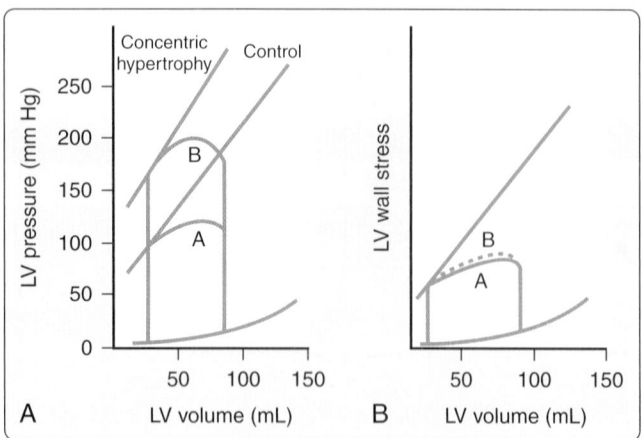

Figure 19-16 **Adaptation to pressure overload.** *A,* Pressure-volume curves and the linear end systolic pressure-volume relation before and after the development of concentric hypertrophy. After hypertrophy, the end-systolic pressure-volume relation is shifted upward and to the left (i.e., apparent supranormal contractility). *B,* The same relationships are plotted as wall stress-volume loops. The loops before and after concentric hypertrophy are essentially the same, reaching the identical end-systolic wall stress-volume point (i.e., contractility unchanged). *(From Ross J Jr: Afterload mismatch in aortic and mitral valve disease: Implications for surgical therapy. J Am Coll Cardiol 5:811, 1985.)*

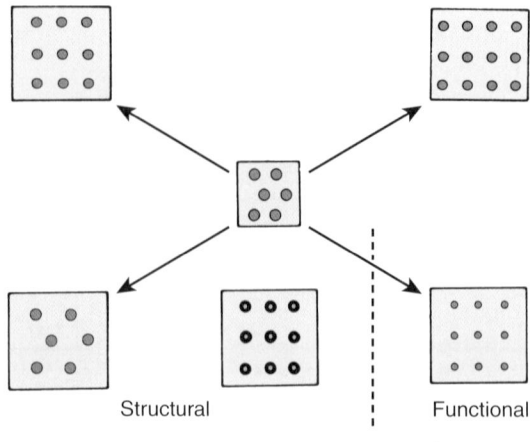

a. ↑ Systolic compression

b. ↑ Vasomotor tone

Figure 19-17 **Possible coronary circulatory changes accompanying ventricular hypertrophy.** The size of the box indicates myocardial mass, and the area of *circles* indicates the cross-sectional area of coronary vasculature. The relation may be normal, as illustrated by top left box, when growth of the coronary bed has kept pace with ventricular hypertrophy. Experimental data support two possible anatomic derangements: inadequate growth of structurally normal vessels (bottom left) or appropriate growth of abnormally thickened resistance vessels whose luminal area is accordingly compromised. *(From Marcus ML: Effects of cardiac hypertrophy on the coronary circulation. In Marcus ML [ed]: The coronary circulation in health and disease. New York: McGraw-Hill, 1983.)*

ventricle arises from increases in wall tension, which directly parallels the imbalance between the increased peak systolic pressure and the degree of mural hypertrophy. Although there is considerable evidence for "supply-side" abnormalities in the myocardial supply and demand relation in patients with AS, clinical data also support increased Mvo_2 as important in the genesis of myocardial ischemia.

On the supply side, the greater LVEDP of the poorly compliant ventricle inevitably narrows the diastolic coronary perfusion pressure (CPP) gradient. With severe outflow obstruction, decreases in SV and resultant systemic hypotension may critically compromise coronary perfusion. A vicious cycle may develop because ischemia-induced abnormalities of diastolic relaxation can aggravate the compliance problem and further narrow the CPP gradient.[107] This sets the stage for ischemic contractile dysfunction, additional decreases in SV, and worsening hypotension.

Cardiac hypertrophy also is associated with structural abnormalities of the coronary circulation (Figure 19-17).[108,109] Animal models have documented that epicardial coronary vessels do not enlarge proportionately when the LV is subjected to a chronic pressure load.[110,111] LVH accompanying chronic hypertension is associated with an increased wall lumen ratio of the coronary arterioles, a change that limits vessel dilation and augments active constriction.[112,113] Animal models of pressure-induced myocardial hypertrophy also have shown a decrease in the capillary density of about 20% to 30%.[108,110,112–116] There is considerable evidence that in LVH caused by pressure overload, a reduction in the coronary vascular reserve may underlie episodes of myocardial ischemia[117,118] (see Chapter 6).

Echocardiographic and hemodynamic assessments of the myocardial oxygen supply and demand ratio are not significantly different in the presence or absence of angina in patients with AS.[119] However, considerable data indicate that dynamic factors relative to oxygen supply may be crucial to the pathogenesis of angina in these patients.[120] Several clinical studies have documented a decrease in coronary vascular reserve in adult and pediatric patients with significant LVH or right ventricular hypertrophy (RVH).[121–123] It is further postulated that repeated episodes of subendocardial ischemia may contribute to the development of subendocardial fibrosis, a component of ischemic contractile dysfunction.[108]

It is possible that myocardial ischemia underlies the impaired ventricular relaxation that has been documented in patients with

myocardial hypertrophy because of a variety of causes.[91,93,94] Prolongation of ventricular relaxation and resultant diastolic dysfunction (i.e., poor compliance) are probably universal features of myocardial ischemia in a variety of clinical settings.[124–128] Experimental data suggest that ischemia-induced impairment of calcium sequestration by the sarcoplasmic reticulum may underlie the increased diastolic chamber stiffness.[129] Prevention of ischemia-induced myoplasmic calcium overload may be the mechanism by which the calcium channel blockers are able to improve diastolic dysfunction in patients with CAD.[130] These drugs also ameliorate ventricular relaxation and diastolic filling in patients with HCM, although the mechanism of action is controversial.[91,131–133] The absence of diastolic filling abnormalities in patients with physiologic, as opposed to pathologic, hypertrophy also may reflect the relative likelihood of ischemia in the two conditions.[134–136]

In summary, the pathophysiologic response to chronic pressure overload is a complex one characterized by unique interaction among the divergent effects of hypertrophy on systolic and diastolic function. Mural thickening enhances systolic performance, maximizing the mechanical work performed while minimizing its metabolic cost. The price of this systolic efficiency is relatively inadequate growth of the coronary microcirculation, which contributes to relaxation abnormalities, diastolic dysfunction, and the potential for superimposition of ischemia-induced abnormalities of systolic dysfunction (Table 19-1).[137] The potentially deleterious effects of LVH cannot be overemphasized. Even in the absence of AS, in which LVH can be viewed as a compensatory and potentially beneficial pathophysiologic response, LVH has been found to have an independent adverse effect on survival.[138,139]

TABLE 19-1	Pressure-Overload Hypertrophy	
Beneficial Aspects	*Detrimental Aspects*
Increases ventricular work	Decreases ventricular diastolic distensibility
Normalizes wall stress	Impairs ventricular relaxation
Normalizes systolic shortening	Impairs coronary vasodilator reserve, leading to subendocardial ischemia

From Lorell BH, Grossman W: Cardiac hypertrophy: The consequences for diastole. *J Am Coll Cardiol* 9:1189, 1987.

Difficulty of Low-Gradient, Low-Output Aortic Stenosis

A subset of patients with severe AS, left ventricular dysfunction, and low transvalvular gradient suffers a high operative mortality rate and poor prognosis.[140] It is difficult to assess accurately the AVA in this low-flow, low-gradient AS because the calculated valve area is proportional to forward SV and because the Gorlin constant varies in low-flow states. Some patients with low-flow, low-gradient AS have a decreased AVA as a result of inadequate forward SV rather than anatomic stenosis. Surgical therapy is unlikely to benefit these patients because the underlying pathology is a weakly contractile myocardium. However, patients with severe anatomic AS may benefit from valve replacement despite the increased operative risk associated with the low-flow, low-gradient hemodynamic state.[140] Guidelines from the ACC and AHA call for a dobutamine echocardiography evaluation to distinguish patients with fixed anatomic AS from those with flow-dependent AS with left ventricular dysfunction.[141] Low-flow, low-gradient AS is defined as a mean gradient of less than 30 mm Hg and a calculated AVA less than 1.0 cm^2.

Dobutamine echocardiography revealed three basic response patterns—fixed AS, relative AS, and absence of contractile reserve—in an initial study by deFilippi et al.[142] In a series of 45 patients with low-flow, low-gradient AS, the 30-day operative mortality rate was 8% for patients with contractile reserve and 50% for those without contractile reserve.[143] Dobutamine challenges during cardiac catheterization provided unique insights into low-flow, low-gradient AS, and the details are summarized in Figure 19-18.[144] In Figure 19-18A, the transvalvular gradient and cardiac output increased, and the valve area did not change. Patients represented in Figure 19-18B increased their CO with little or no change in gradient, and the calculated valve area increased slightly. This group still benefited from surgery. The third group of patients had no contractile reserve because CO did not increase with dobutamine, and the transvalvular gradient decreased (see Figure 19-18C). Dobutamine infusion in the cardiac catheterization laboratory appears to be helpful in identifying patients with low-flow, low-gradient AS who have a truly fixed anatomic stenosis that may benefit from valve replacement. The findings of these studies also emphasize that contractile reserve is an important prognostic indicator in these patients and dobutamine challenge may help select patients for valve replacement. It appears that patients with contractile reserve and fixed AS have a relatively good prognosis with valve replacement. Left ventricular contractile reserve appears to be a critical variable for prognosis. Recent studies have focused on AS with low transvalvular gradients and normal ventricular EF. The pathophysiology of the low transvalvular gradient has been explained by decreased EDV caused by excessive ventricular hypertrophy accompanied by increased SVR. In a recent series of patients with severe AS (AVA < 0.8 cm^2) with ventricular dysfunction (EF < 35%) and/or a low transvalvular gradient (< 30 mm Hg), mortality predictors were advanced age, low EF, renal insufficiency, and lack of AR. Regardless of ventricular function, patients who underwent AVR had a significantly better survival.[36]

Developments in the Hemodynamic Management of Critical Aortic Stenosis Patients

The use of vasodilators is traditionally contraindicated in patients with severe AS because cardiac output is relatively fixed across a narrowed orifice. Vasodilation reduces SVR without any possibility for a compensatory increase in CO and severe hypotension would typically result. This traditional paradigm recently was re-examined in patients with fixed, severe AS (area < 1.0 cm^2) and left ventricular dysfunction (EF < 0.35).[145] Nitroprusside was carefully titrated to maintain a mean arterial pressure of more than 60 mm Hg with concomitant hemodynamic monitoring. The cardiac index increased over 24 hours from a mean of 1.60 to 2.52 L/min/m^2 with no changes in heart rate and mean arterial pressure (Figure 19-19). The pulmonary capillary wedge pressure (PCWP) and SVR decreased, whereas SV increased.

It appears that this treatment is effective to alleviate to some extent the left ventricular dysfunction component of the complete syndrome. Left ventricular dysfunction benefits derived from unloading and careful titration of the nitroprusside most likely allowed SVR to decrease without changes in mean arterial pressure. This titrated unloading may benefit patients with severe AS and left ventricular dysfunction, and it may serve as a temporary bridge to AVR or oral vasodilator therapy.[145] It is unclear whether treatment with positive inotropic agents would produce similar effects with fewer risks. Adequate treatment of patients with AS, a depressed EF, and a low transvalvular gradient continues to pose a diagnostic and therapeutic challenge.[146] The use of nitroprusside in AS in the absence of ventricular dysfunction may not be as effective and even be deleterious because of the prompt decrease in preload by nitroprusside.

Timing of Intervention

In asymptomatic patients with AS, it appears to be relatively safe to delay surgery until symptoms develop, but outcomes vary widely. The presence of moderate or severe valvular calcification along with a rapid increase in aortic-jet velocity identify patients with a very poor prognosis. These patients should be considered for early valve replacement rather than delaying until symptoms develop.[40]

Echocardiography and exercise testing may identify asymptomatic patients who are likely to benefit from surgery.[147] In a study of 58 asymptomatic patients, 21 had symptoms for the first time during exercise testing.[148] Guidelines for AVR in patients with AS are shown in Table 19-2.

Functional outcome after AVR in patients older than 80 years is excellent, operative risk is limited, and late survival rates are good.[149] In patients with severe left ventricular dysfunction and low transvalvular mean gradient, operative mortality is increased, but AVR was associated with improved functional status.[150] Postoperative survival was best in younger patients and with larger prosthetic valves, whereas medium-term survival was related to improved postoperative functional class.[150]

Anesthetic Considerations

The described pathophysiologic principles dictate that anesthetic management be based on the avoidance of systemic hypotension, maintenance of sinus rhythm and an adequate intravascular volume, and awareness of the potential for myocardial ischemia (Box 19-1). In the absence of CHF, adequate premedication may reduce the likelihood of undue preoperative excitement, tachycardia, and the resultant potential for exacerbating myocardial ischemia and the transvalvular pressure gradient. In patients with truly critical outflow tract obstruction, however, heavy premedication with an exaggerated venodilatory response can reduce the appropriately increased LVEDV (and LVEDP) needed to overcome the systolic pressure gradient. In these patients, in particular, the additional precaution of administering supplementary oxygen may provide worthwhile insurance against the possibility of a similarly pronounced response to the sedative effects of the premedicant.

Intraoperative monitoring should include a standard five-lead electrocardiographic (ECG) system, including a V$_5$ lead, because of the LV's vulnerability to ischemia. A practical constraint in terms of interpretation is that these patients usually exhibit ECG changes because of preoperative LVH. The associated ST-segment abnormalities (i.e., strain pattern) may be indistinguishable from or at least very similar to those of myocardial ischemia, making the intraoperative interpretation difficult. Lead II and possibly an esophageal ECG should be readily obtainable because they may be useful for assessing the P-wave changes in the event of supraventricular arrhythmias (see Chapter 25).

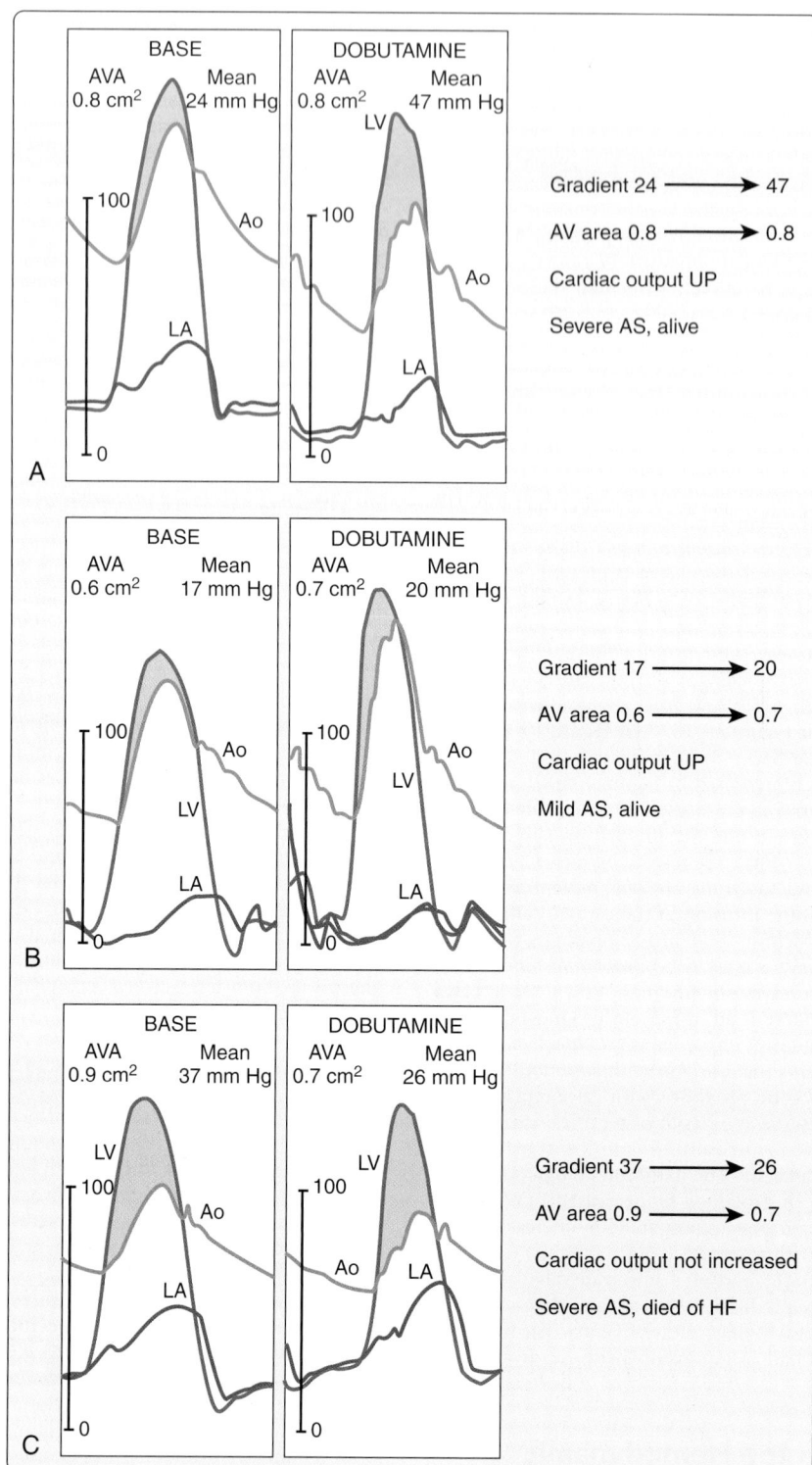

Figure 19-18 **Hemodynamic tracings from three patients representing three different responses to dobutamine.** Ao, aorta; AS, aortic stenosis; AV, aortic valve; AVA, aortic valve area; HF, heart failure; LA, left atrium; LV, left ventricle. *(Adapted from Nishimura RA, Grantham JA, Connolly HM, et al: Low-output, low-gradient aortic stenosis in patients with depressed left ventricular systolic function: The clinical utility of the dobutamine challenge in the catheterization laboratory. Circulation 106:809, 2002.)*

Hemodynamic monitoring is controversial, and few prospective data are available on which to base an enlightened clinical decision. The central venous pressure (CVP) is a particularly poor estimate of left ventricular filling when left ventricular compliance is reduced. A normal CVP can significantly underestimate the LVEDP or PCWP. The principal risks, although minimal, of using a pulmonary artery catheter (PAC) in the patient with AS are arrhythmia-induced

hypotension and ischemia. Loss of synchronous atrial contraction or a supraventricular tachyarrhythmia can compromise diastolic filling of the poorly compliant LV, resulting in hypotension and the potential for rapid hemodynamic deterioration. The threat of catheter-induced arrhythmias is significant for the patient with AS. However, accepting a low-normal CVP as evidence of good ventricular function can lead to similarly catastrophic underfilling of the LV on the basis of insufficient

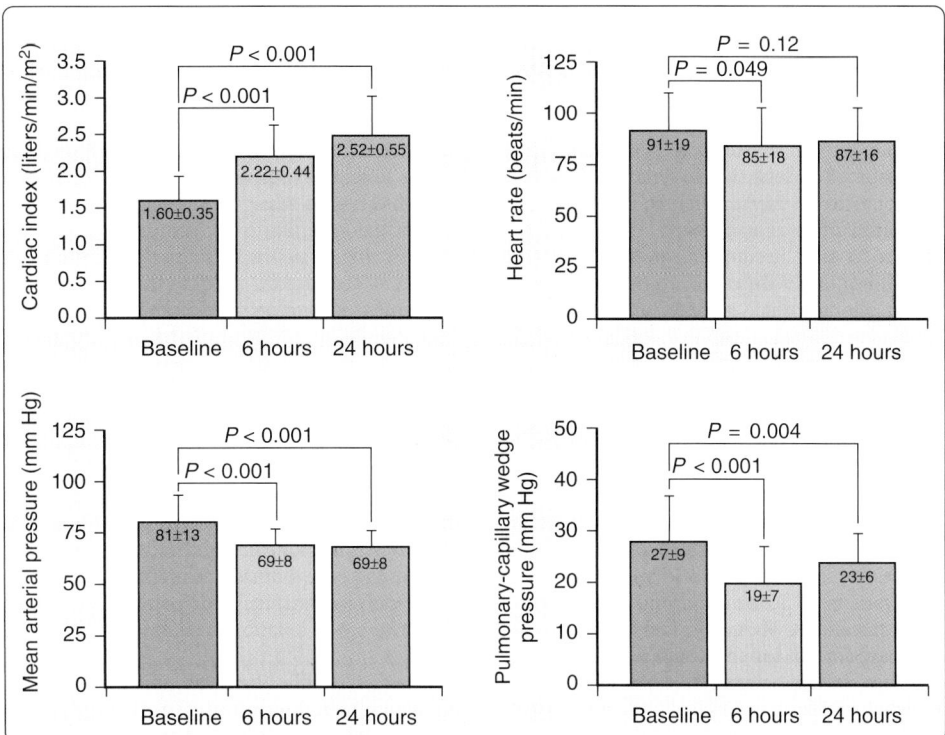

Figure 19-19 Changes in cardiac index, heart rate, mean arterial pressure, and pulmonary-capillary wedge pressure during titration with nitroprusside over 24 hours in patients with severe aortic stenosis and left ventricular dysfunction. (*Adapted from Khot UN, Novaro GM, Popovic ZB, et al: Nitroprusside in critically ill patients with left ventricular dysfunction and aortic stenosis. N Engl J Med 348:1756, 2003.*)

replenishment of surgical blood loss. To some extent, even the PCWP can underestimate the LVEDP (and LVEDV) when ventricular compliance is markedly reduced. Placement of a PAC also allows for measurement of CO, derived hemodynamic parameters, mixed venous oxygen saturation (Svo$_2$), and possible transvenous pacing (see Chapter 14).

Intraoperative fluid management should be aimed at maintaining appropriately increased left-sided filling pressures. This is one reason why many clinicians believe that the PAC is worth its small arrhythmogenic risk. Keeping up with intravascular volume losses is particularly important in noncardiovascular surgery, in which the shorter duration of the operation may make an inhalation or potentially vasodilating regional anesthetic preferable to a narcotic technique.

Patients with symptomatic AS are usually encountered only in the setting of cardiovascular surgery because of their ominous prognosis

without AVR. Few studies have specifically addressed the response of these patients to the standard intravenous and inhalation induction agents; however, the responses to narcotic[151,152] and nonnarcotic[153,154] intravenous agents are apparently not dissimilar from those of patients with other forms of VHD. The principal benefit of a narcotic induction is the assurance of an adequate depth of anesthesia during intubation, which reliably blunts potentially deleterious reflex sympathetic responses capable of precipitating tachycardia and ischemia.

Many clinicians also prefer a pure narcotic technique for maintenance. The negative inotropy of the inhalation anesthetics is a theoretical disadvantage for a myocardium faced with the challenge of overcoming outflow tract obstruction. A more clinically relevant drawback may be the increased risk for arrhythmia-induced hypotension, particularly that associated with nodal rhythm and resultant loss of the atrium's critical contribution to filling of the hypertrophied ventricle[155,156] (see Chapter 9).

Occasionally, surgical stimulation elicits a hypertensive response despite the impedance posed by the stenotic valve and a seemingly adequate depth of narcotic anesthesia. In such patients, a judicious trial of low concentrations of an inhalation agent, used purely for control of hypertension, may prove efficacious. The ability to concurrently monitor CO is useful in this situation. The temptation to control intraoperative hypertension with vasodilators should be resisted in most cases. Given the risk for ischemia, nitroglycerin seems to be a particularly attractive drug. Its effectiveness in relieving subendocardial ischemia in patients

TABLE 19–2	Recommendations for the Use of Aortic Valve Replacement in Patients with Aortic Stenosis	
Replacement Indicated	*Replacement Possibly Indicated*	
Patients with severe aortic stenosis and any of its classic symptoms (e.g., angina, syncope, dyspnea)	Patients with moderate aortic stenosis who require coronary artery bypass surgery or surgery on the aorta or heart valves	
Patients with severe aortic stenosis who are undergoing coronary artery bypass surgery	Asymptomatic patients with severe aortic stenosis and at least one of the following: ejection fraction of no more than 0.50, hemodynamic instability during exercise (e.g., hypotension), ventricular tachycardia; not indicated to prevent sudden death in asymptomatic patients who have none of the findings listed	
Patients with severe aortic stenosis who are undergoing surgery on the aorta or other heart valves		

Adapted from the American Heart Association website (www.americanheart.org).

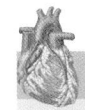

BOX 19-1. AORTIC STENOSIS

Preload: increased
Afterload: increased
Goal: sinus rhythm
Avoid: hypotension, tachycardia, bradycardia

with AS is controversial[157,158]; however, there is always the risk for even transient episodes of "overshoot." The hypertrophied ventricle's critical dependence on an adequate CPP may be unforgiving of even a momentary dip in the systemic arterial pressure.

Intraoperative hypotension, regardless of the primary cause, should be treated immediately and aggressively with a direct α-adrenergic agonist such as phenylephrine.[159] The goal should be to immediately restore the CPP and then to address the underlying problem (e.g., hypovolemia, arrhythmia). After the arterial pressure responds, treatment of the precipitating event should be equally aggressive, but rapid transfusion or cardioversion should not delay the administration of a direct-acting vasoconstrictor. Patients with severe AS in whom objective signs of myocardial ischemia persist despite restoration of the blood pressure should be treated extremely aggressively. This may mean the immediate use of an inotropic agent or simply accelerating the institution of cardiopulmonary bypass (CPB).

Intraoperative myocardial ischemic injury in the patient with AS has been appreciated for some time, and there are several theories regarding its pathogenesis. The potential vulnerability of the hypertrophied myocardium to ischemic damage was initially speculated on by cardiac surgeons who described the phenomenon of irreversible ischemic contracture—what they called the *stone heart*—occurring after AVR in a group of patients with severe LVH.[160] The anatomic and hemodynamic bases for an unfavorable myocardial oxygen supply and demand relation have already been considered, but the possibility that these patients might be experiencing prebypass ischemic injury remains a plausible, although unproven, hypothesis.

Most attention has been focused on the potential for irreversible cellular damage occurring during the period of ischemic cardiac arrest. Although there is a consensus that improved myocardial preservation has been crucial in reducing the mortality rate after CABG, there is evidence that current cardioplegic techniques may provide suboptimal protection for patients with VHD.[161,162] Specifically, there is ultrastructural evidence (e.g., intracellular or mitochondrial edema) suggesting that the hypertrophied myocardium is uniquely susceptible to ischemic damage during the aortic cross-clamp interval, despite the presumed protection. Although these changes are observed in patients whose clinical course is seemingly unremarkable, such ischemic cellular damage also may underlie the frequent occurrence of postoperative low-output syndromes and the greater mortality rates associated with valvular operations.[163]

Although a detailed consideration of myocardial preservation is beyond the scope of this chapter (see Chapters 28 and 29), certain aspects are peculiar to the operative management of patients with AS, and it is likely that improved cardioplegic techniques will play an important role in reducing operative morbidity and mortality rates. Because the operation requires an ascending aortotomy, many surgeons routinely use direct coronary ostial cannulation for the delivery of the cardioplegic solution. Problems associated with this approach are uncommon but include the inherent hazard of injury to the coronary ostia; cannula-induced late stenosis of the left main coronary artery also has been described.[164] Coronary ostial delivery requires interrupting the surgical procedure for subsequent reinfusions of the cardioplegic solution. These problems are obviated by the use of cardioplegia delivery by the coronary sinus. The retrograde technique commonly is used in conjunction with an initial dose of antegrade cardioplegia; the latter provides for a more immediate electromechanical arrest.[165–167]

Noncardiac Surgery in the Patient with Aortic Stenosis

Patients with AS who undergo noncardiac surgery were identified by Goldman et al[148] as being at increased risk for cardiac complications, including myocardial infarction, CHF, and supraventricular tachyarrhythmias. Likewise, the ACC Task Force on perioperative evaluation of the cardiac patient identified patients with severe or symptomatic AS as being at increased risk for serious perioperative cardiac morbidity.[168]

It stated that symptomatic stenotic lesions are associated with the risk for perioperative severe CHF or shock and often require percutaneous valvotomy or valve replacement before noncardiac surgery to reduce cardiac risk. With the overall aging of the surgical population and given a peak incidence of significant AS in the fifth and sixth decades, it is likely that these patients will be encountered with increasing frequency in the setting of noncardiac surgery. Given the natural history of the disease and following the conservative ACC guidelines cited previously, one approach is to recommend immediate but elective AVR to all AS patients, before any noncardiac procedures. Although there is a rationale for this "shotgun" solution, a variety of ethical, practical, and economic constraints argue for a more selective approach.

A common clinical problem is the elderly, asymptomatic patient, with a harsh systolic ejection murmur, who is scheduled for noncardiac surgery. Risk assessment for the asymptomatic patient is challenging because the prognosis in the absence of AVR may be quite benign. However, symptoms correlate poorly with AS severity, which may by itself portend a more ominous natural history. In these patients, the use of a two-dimensional (2D) Doppler echocardiographic examination allows for the noninvasive assessment of the severity of stenosis[57] and for some quantification of contractile function (see Chapters 1, 2, and 12). Patients with moderate AS have a greater short-term incidence of cardiovascular complications, and this risk is further increased by the presence of symptoms or objective evidence of contractile impairment.[53] Armed with the echocardiographic evaluation (e.g., stenosis severity, contractile state), the clinician can make an initial assessment of relative risk. Depending on the overall clinical picture, some of these patients may warrant immediate elective AVR, whereas in others, it may be more appropriate to proceed with the noncardiac operation, with hemodynamic monitoring as dictated by the echocardiographic data and the nature of the surgery. A reality of the clinical setting is that the overall picture often seems to dictate that the anesthesiologist should proceed with the originally planned operation, albeit at increased risk for perioperative cardiac morbidity.

HYPERTROPHIC CARDIOMYOPATHY

Hypertrophic Obstructive Cardiomyopathy

Hypertrophic obstructive cardiomyopathy is a relatively common genetic malformation of the heart with a prevalence of approximately 1 in 500 (see Chapter 22). The hypertrophy initially develops in the septum and extends to the free walls, often giving a picture of concentric hypertrophy. Asymmetric septal hypertrophy leads to a variable pressure gradient between the apical left ventricular chamber and the LVOT. The LVOT obstruction leads to increases in left ventricular pressure, which fuels a vicious cycle of further hypertrophy and increased LVOT obstruction.[169] Various treatment modalities include β-adrenoceptor antagonists, calcium channel blockers, and surgical myectomy of the septum. For more than 40 years, the traditional standard treatment has been the ventricular septal myotomy-myomectomy of Morrow, in which a small amount of muscle from the subaortic septum is resected.[170] Two new treatment modalities have gained popularity in recent years: dual-chamber pacing and septal reduction (ablation) therapy with ethanol.

Dual-chamber DDD pacing is based on the observation that excitation of the septum of the LV contracts it away from the apposing wall, which may reduce the LVOT gradient. The precise mechanism by which dual-chamber pacing decreases LVOT gradient or improves symptoms is uncertain. Possible mechanisms are asynchronous ventricular activation, paradoxic septal wall motion, a negative inotropic effect, an increase in ESV, decreased systolic anterior leaflet motion, altered myocardial perfusion, and regression of LVH.[171] The AV interval must be sufficiently short to guarantee early right ventricular apical activation without conduction through the His-Purkinje system. Although some studies have shown a decrease in the LVOT gradient of 25%, there are still variable results with respect to improvements in exercise capacity and symptoms.[171–174]

Patients with severe, drug-resistant symptoms of CHF, angina, or syncope are considered for nonsurgical septal reduction therapy. In one series, patients with a resting gradient of more than 40 mm Hg or a dobutamine-induced gradient of more than 60 mm Hg were included.[175] After coronary angiography to exclude significant CAD and after placement of temporary pacing wires, the LVOT gradient was measured at rest and during various interventions (e.g., Valsalva, postextrasystolic, isoproterenol, amyl nitrite). The coronary septal branches were cannulated with a small balloon-equipped catheter. The balloon was inflated to prevent overflow or spillage into the left anterior descending coronary artery. Depending on the septal branch size and area of septal hypertrophy, a dose of 2 to 5 mL ethanol was injected slowly through the balloon catheter lumen. The LVOT gradient decreased immediately in 85% to 90% of patients.[171] Further decreases in gradient were reported after 6 months.[171] The septal muscle mass was not decreased adequately through alcohol injections at the time of the intervention, but ventricular remodeling continued and led to sustained symptomatic improvement, most dramatically over the first 3 to 6 months.[169] Exercise tolerance increased as well, but atrioventricular block, right bundle branch block, and left bundle branch block were frequent adverse consequences. Permanent heart blocks still occurred in 5% to 10% of cases.[176]

Clinical Features and Natural History

HCM is an uncommon familial disorder in which there is pronounced hypertrophy of histologically abnormal sarcomeres with characteristically disproportionate involvement of the interventricular septum.[177–179] This disease has numerous pathologic and pathophysiologic features, which vary in their relative predominance in individual patients. A variety of other names have been applied to the disorder, including asymmetric septal hypertrophy, muscular subaortic stenosis, and idiopathic hypertrophic subaortic stenosis, with each emphasizing some aspect of the disease that may or may not be a prominent feature of its presentation in an individual patient. The cause and exact pattern of inheritance of the disease remain unknown, although it appears to be an autosomal dominant trait expressed with a high degree of penetrance[179–181] (see Chapter 22).

Patients vary widely in their clinical presentation. The contribution of echocardiography to the diagnosis has unquestionably increased the number of asymptomatic patients who carry the diagnosis. Most patients with HCM are asymptomatic and have been seen by the echocardiographer because of relatives having clinical disease. Follow-up remains an important problem for cardiologists because sudden death or cardiac arrest may occur as the presenting symptom in slightly more than half of previously asymptomatic patients.[182]

Less dramatic frequently presenting complaints include dyspnea, angina, and syncope.[179] The clinical picture is often similar to valvular AS. The symptoms may share a similar pathophysiologic basis (e.g., poor diastolic compliance) in the two conditions. The prognostic implications of clinical disease, however, are less certain for patients with HCM. Although cardiac arrest may be an unheralded event, other patients may have a stable pattern of angina or intermittent syncopal episodes for many years.[183] Palpitations also are frequently described and may be related to a variety of underlying arrhythmias. Of patients studied with continuous ambulatory monitoring, ventricular arrhythmias occur in more than 75%, supraventricular tachycardias in 25%, and atrial fibrillation (AF) in 5% to 10%.[184–186] The latter often precipitates clinical deterioration because of the dependence of the noncompliant LV on atrial systole for its filling.[187]

The natural history of patients with HCM also is extremely variable. These patients are all at risk for sudden death, although those with a family history of this problem form an especially high-risk group.[188] Unfortunately, younger and previously asymptomatic patients with minimal subaortic gradients also may be at greater risk for sudden death because of their more frequent and vigorous physical activity.[182,189] It is

unknown whether vigorous physical activity in patients with HCM is an independent risk factor for sudden death, but this disease is the most frequent autopsy finding in previously healthy competitive athletes who die suddenly.[190]

Although patients referred to diagnostic centers for evaluation of HCM are usually young-to-middle-aged persons, a syndrome with similar clinical and echocardiographic findings has been identified in the elderly.[93] Echocardiographically, these patients exhibit a similarly thickened and hypercontractile LV. Their most common symptoms are those of CHF and are thought to reflect severe reductions in the ventricular diastolic compliance. As in younger patients with classic HCM, there is marked systolic anterior motion (SAM) of the mitral apparatus. However, in HCM of the elderly, the SAM is seemingly caused or at least accentuated by a severe degree of mitral annular calcification, which results in a particularly small LVOT.[191] Previously asymptomatic, these patients often experience the onset of progressively severe symptoms in the sixth decade of life, and the response to medical therapy, usually calcium channel-blocking drugs, has been poor.[191] This lack of improvement with medical therapy may reflect the fact that mitral annular calcification plays a key role in producing a truly physical (i.e., less dynamic) subaortic obstruction. This also would explain the female predominance of the disease because mitral annular calcification is more common in elderly women. It is unclear whether this represents a true variant of classic HCM with late onset or it is perhaps etiologically linked to long-standing systemic hypertension, with secondary, unexplained, disproportionate involvement of the interventricular septum.[93]

Pathophysiology

In HCM, the principal pathophysiologic abnormality is myocardial hypertrophy. The hypertrophy is a primary event in these patients and occurs independently of outflow tract obstruction. Unlike in AS, the hypertrophy begets the pressure gradient, not the other way around. Histologically, the hypertrophy consists of myocardial fiber disarray, and, anatomically, there is usually disproportionate enlargement of the interventricular septum.[192]

Controversy exists concerning the intrinsic contractile strength of the myocardium in patients with HCM. Several studies have demonstrated normal or supranormal indices of systolic function in patients with this disease.[193–195] Left ventricular ejection is rapid, with 80% of the SV being ejected very early during systole.[193,196] This is true regardless of the presence, temporal location during systole, or magnitude of outflow tract obstruction. However, studies have shown that end-systolic stress is significantly reduced in relation to ESV (Figure 19-20).[197,198] Reiteration of the Laplace formula for wall stress, P × R/2h, shows that, in HCM, the degree of primary hypertrophy (i.e., with increased wall thickness [h]) should minimize instantaneous left ventricular afterload. As a result, there is preservation, perhaps even elevation, of afterload-sensitive indices of systolic function, such as the EF.[199] Myocardial hypertrophy, particularly to the extent that it accentuates subaortic obstruction, increases the ESPVR, widening the divergence between it and the more accurate (load-insensitive) ratio of end-systolic wall stress to ESV. High peak systolic pressures (i.e., subaortic obstruction), elevation of ejection phase indices, and low ESV (i.e., minimal afterload) may reflect uncontrolled hypertrophy of an abnormal and perhaps intrinsically depressed myocardium. Whether overall contractility is normal, supranormal, or impaired in a given patient, it is likely that there will be regional differences in a ventricle's contractile function, which correlate with the histologic heterogeneity so characteristic of this disease.[200]

A consensus exists that the disease is characterized by a wide spectrum of the severity of obstruction. It is totally absent in some patients, may be variable in others, or may be critically severe. Its most distinctive qualities are its dynamic nature (depending on contractile state and loading conditions), its timing (begins early, peaks variably), and its subaortic location.[193,201] Those accepting the phenomenon of physical subaortic obstruction believe that it arises from the hypertrophied

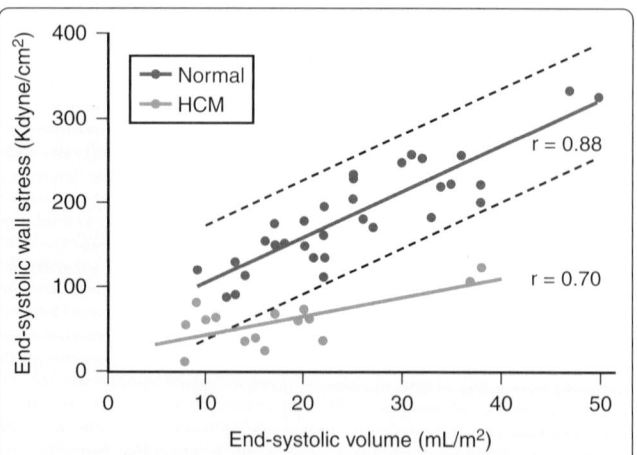

Figure 19-20 End-systolic stress versus end-systolic volume in healthy subjects *(dark circles)* and in patients with hypertrophic cardiomyopathy (HCM; *light circles); dashed lines* indicate the 95% confidence limit. Stress-volume data for most patients with HCM are located downward and to the right of the confidence band (i.e., decreased end-systolic stress related to volume), which is indicative of intrinsically depressed myocardial contractility. *(From Pouleur H, Rousseau MF, van Eyll C, et al: Force-velocity-length relations in hypertrophic cardiomyopathy: Evidence of normal or depressed myocardial contractility. Am J Cardiol 52:813, 1983.)*

septum's encroachment on the systolic outflow tract, which is bounded anteriorly by the interventricular septum and posteriorly by the anterior leaflet of the mitral valve. In most patients with obstruction, exaggerated anterior (i.e., toward the septum) motion of the anterior mitral valve leaflet during systole accentuates the obstruction.[202] The cause of this SAM is unclear. One possibility is that the mitral valve is pulled toward the septum by contraction of the papillary muscles, whose orientation is abnormal because of the hypertrophic process.[203] Another theory is that vigorous contraction of the hypertrophied septum results in rapid acceleration of the blood through a simultaneously narrowed outflow tract. This could generate hydraulic forces consistent with a Venturi effect, whereby the anterior leaflet of the mitral valve would be drawn close to or within actual contact with the interventricular septum[204] (Figure 19-21). This means that after the obstruction is

triggered, the mitral valve leaflet is forced against the septum by the pressure difference across the orifice. However, the pressure difference further decreases orifice size and further increases the pressure difference in a time-dependent amplifying feedback loop.[205] This analysis also is consistent with observations that the measured gradient is directly correlated with the duration of mitral-septal contact. Although still controversial,[206–208] there appears to be good correlation between the degree of SAM and the magnitude of the pressure gradient.[209,210] The SAM-septal contact also underlies the severe subaortic obstruction characteristic of HCM of the elderly, although the narrowing usually is more severe and the contribution of septal movement toward the mitral valve is usually greater.[191]

The timing of SAM-septal contact also is important because the magnitude of the subaortic gradient is proportional to the fraction of forward flow ejected in the presence of anatomic obstruction.[211] In general, large gradients occur as a result of early and prolonged SAM-septal contact, and small gradients arise from delayed and brief SAM-septal contact.[204,209] In studies of patients with various degrees of subaortic obstruction, the proportion of flow ejected in the presence of a gradient has varied between 30% and 70%.[209,212,213] Patients with evidence of systolic obstruction at rest have the longest intervals of systolic contact between the anterior leaflet of the mitral valve and the septum.[214] However, if SAM-septal contact is restricted to late systole, a pressure gradient may occur on the basis of "cavity obliteration" in the absence of any functional obstruction to blood flow.[215,216] In such patients, 95% of the SV may be ejected by the halfway point in systole, when SAM-septal contact is just beginning.[193,209] Despite its seemingly critical role in producing outflow tract obstruction, SAM of the mitral valve is not a specific finding for HCM, and it may occur in patients with HCM who do not have obstruction.[206,207,214]

In addition to SAM, approximately two thirds of patients exhibit a constellation of structural malformations of the mitral valve.[217] These malformations include increased leaflet area and elongation of the leaflets or anomalous papillary muscle insertion directly into the anterior mitral valve leaflet. HCM is not a disease process confined to cardiac muscle alone because these anatomic abnormalities of the mitral valve are unlikely to be acquired or secondary to mechanical factors.

Three basic mechanisms—increased contractility, decreased afterload, and decreased preload—exacerbate the degree of SAM-septal contact and produce the dynamic obstruction characteristic of patients with HCM. The common pathway is a reduction in ventricular volume (actively by increased contractility, directly or reflexly in response to vasodilation, or passively by reduced preload), which increases the proximity of the anterior mitral valve leaflet to the hypertrophied septum.[179,183,218] Factors that usually impair contractile performance, such as myocardial depression, systemic vasoconstriction, and ventricular overdistention, characteristically improve systolic function in patients with HCM and outflow tract obstruction. Diagnostically, these paradoxes are exploited by quantifying the degree of subaortic obstruction after isoproterenol (e.g., increased inotropy, tachycardia, and decreased volume) and the Valsalva maneuver (e.g., decreased venous return and ventricular volume), both of which reliably elicit increases in the pressure gradient. In the operating room, catheter-induced ectopy or premature ventricular contractions resulting from cardiac manipulation also may transiently exacerbate the gradient by increased inotropy from postextrasystolic potentiation. Therapeutically, volume loading, myocardial depression, and vasoconstriction should minimize obstruction and augment forward flow.

Patients with HCM demonstrate critical derangements in diastolic function, which, although in some ways more subtle than the unique phenomenon of subaortic obstruction, may contribute equally to the challenge posed.[219–222] These abnormalities include prolongation of the isovolumic relaxation time (i.e., aortic valve closure to mitral valve opening) and reduction in the peak velocity of left ventricular filling.[91,195] Diastolic dysfunction exhibits the same heterogeneity characteristic of its systolic function, probably because its underlying cause is intrinsic to the primary myopathic process and not merely secondary to the associated chamber hypertrophy.[223] Accordingly, diastolic

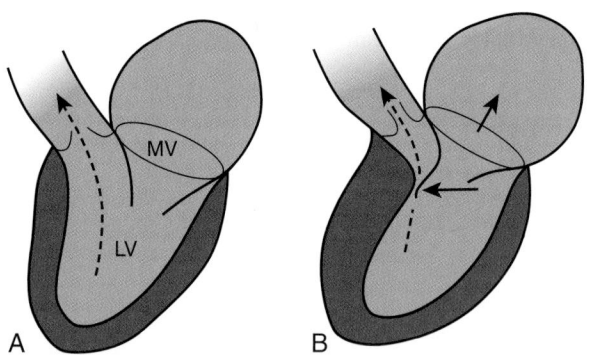

Figure 19-21 **Proposed mechanism of systolic anterior motion in hypertrophic cardiomyopathy.** *A,* Normally, blood is ejected from the left ventricle (LV) through an unimpeded outflow tract. *B,* Thickening of the ventricular septum results in a restricted outflow tract, and this obstruction causes the blood to be ejected at a higher velocity, closer to the area of the anterior mitral valve (MV) leaflet. As a result of its proximity to this high-velocity fluid path, the anterior MV leaflet is drawn toward the hypertrophied septum by a Venturi effect *(arrow). (From Wigle ED, Sasson Z, Henderson MA, et al: Hypertrophic cardiomyopathy: The importance of the site and the extent of hypertrophy. A review. Prog Cardiovasc Dis 28:1, 1985.)*

filling abnormalities in HCM are largely independent of the magnitude of LVH and are seen even in patients with only mild, localized hypertrophy.[20]

Poor diastolic compliance is the most clinically apparent manifestation of the relaxation abnormalities. Left ventricular filling pressures are markedly increased despite enhanced systolic ejection and the normal or subnormal EDV. This reduced ventricular volume re-emphasizes the pivotal role played by the hypertrophied but intrinsically depressed myocardium. Reductions in afterload, mediated by hypertrophy, support the ventricle's systolic performance, resulting in increased emptying and a small diastolic volume. However, hypertrophy also impairs relaxation, resulting in poor diastolic compliance and an increased ventricular filling pressure. The key point is that the high filling pressure does not reflect distention of a failing ventricle, even though stress-volume relations suggest that its contractility is intrinsically depressed (Figure 19-22 and Table 19-3). This disease is characterized by systolic and diastolic dysfunction.

As in patients with valvular AS, relatively high filling pressures reflect the LVEDV (i.e., degree of preload reserve) needed to overcome the outflow obstruction. Intervention with vasodilators is, therefore, inappropriate. The poor ventricular compliance also means that patients with HCM depend on a large intravascular volume and the maintenance of sinus rhythm for adequate diastolic filling. The atrial contribution to ventricular filling is even more important in HCM than in valvular AS, and it may approach 75% of total SV.[132]

Another similarity between HCM and valvular AS is that the combination of myocardial hypertrophy, with or without LVOT obstruction, may precipitate imbalances in the myocardial oxygen supply and demand relation. Angina-like discomfort is one of the classic symptoms of patients with HCM, and its pathogenesis has been attributed to increases in Mvo$_2$, specifically the increased overall muscle mass and the high systolic wall tension generated by the ventricle's ejection against the dynamic subaortic obstruction. However, as in patients with AS, there is also evidence of a compromise in myocardial oxygen supply.[224,225] Patients with HCM suffer from several types of hypertrophy-related abnormalities of the coronary circulation; some are common to other conditions associated with pathologic hypertrophy (e.g., AS), and others are apparently unique to this distinctive form of hypertrophy.[226] A reduced capillary density in the hypertrophied myocardium prevents flow from increasing in proportion to the increase in myocardial mass.[227] It also is possible that there are primary HCM-associated abnormalities of the coronary

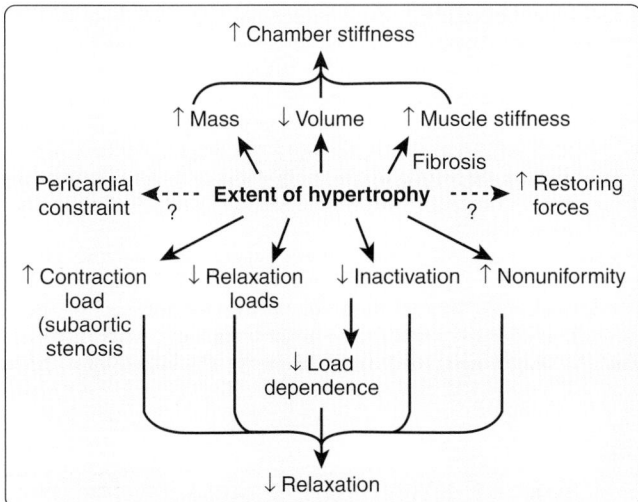

Figure 19-22 Proposed interactions between myocardial hypertrophy and other related properties of ventricular function. (*From Wigle ED, Sasson Z, Henderson MA, et al: Hypertrophic cardiomyopathy: The importance of the site and the extent of hypertrophy. A review.* Prog Cardiovasc Dis *28:1, 1985.*)

TABLE 19-3	Factors That Affect Left Ventricular Diastolic Filling in Hypertrophic Cardiomyopathy

Chamber stiffness*
Relaxation
  Loads
    Contraction load
      Subaortic stenosis
    Relaxation loads
      Late-systolic loading
      End-systolic deformation (restoring forces)
      Coronary filling
      Ventricular filling
  Inactivation
    Myoplasmic calcium overload
      Primary
      Ischemic
  Nonuniformity of load and inactivation in space and time†
Pericardial constraints and ventricular interaction
Effect of extent of hypertrophy on the preceding factors

*Chamber stiffness = Myocardial mass × Myocardial stiffness/Ventricular volume.
†Nonuniformity of contraction and relaxation.
From Wigel ED, Wilansky S: Diastolic dysfunction in hypertrophic cardiomyopathy. *Heart Fail* 3:85, 1987.

circulation that are unrelated to myocardial hypertrophy.[228] In addition to these coronary circulatory abnormalities, there is evidence of a metabolic derangement in the hypertrophied interventricular septum, whereby there is a decreased use of adequately delivered metabolic substrates.[225]

The reduction in coronary vascular reserve is similar to that observed in patients with valvular AS, in whom Mvo$_2$ may be presumed to be uniformly increased.[118] However, angina also occurs in patients with HCM in the absence of subaortic obstruction. Although basal Mvo$_2$ is increased in proportion to the increased muscle mass, it is particularly interesting that clinical studies support a greater pathogenetic role for coronary circulatory abnormalities in producing ischemia in patients with nonobstructive hypertrophy.[229]

Hemodynamic derangements peculiar to the disease may aggravate the ventricle's anatomic vulnerability to ischemia. The increased LVEDP for any LVEDV (i.e., poor compliance) inevitably narrows the diastolic CPP gradient. This may precipitate subendocardial ischemia in some patients with HCM, particularly those faced with the increased oxygen demand of overcoming late-systolic obstruction.[219] There is evidence that hypertrophy-induced myocardial ischemia may underlie the diastolic dysfunction characteristic of HCM.[230] As in patients with valvular AS, ischemia-induced abnormalities of diastolic calcium sequestration may further exacerbate relaxation abnormalities, initiating a vicious cycle (Figure 19-23).[107,122,137,160,161,231]

β-Blockers and calcium channel blockers form the basis of medical therapy for HCM. β-Blockade is most useful for preventing sympathetically mediated increases in the subaortic gradient and for the prevention of tachyarrhythmias, which also can exacerbate outflow obstruction. Disopyramide also has been used to reduce contractility and for its antiarrhythmic properties.[232] Calcium channel blockers often prove clinically effective in patients with HCM regardless of the presence or absence of systolic obstruction.[233] The mechanism of action involves improvement in diastolic relaxation, allowing an increase in LVEDV at a relatively lower LVEDP. The negative inotropy may attenuate the subaortic pressure gradient; however, in selected patients, the gradient may worsen because of pronounced and unpredictable degrees of vasodilation.[234,235]

Surgery—a septal myotomy or partial myomectomy by the aortic approach—is reserved for those patients who remain symptomatic despite maximal pharmacologic therapy. In a long-term retrospective study, the cumulative survival rate was significantly better in surgically than in pharmacologically treated patients.[236] However, it is quite likely that pharmacologic therapy may be more appropriate for the patient

CONTROL OF [Ca++] IN MYOCARDIUM

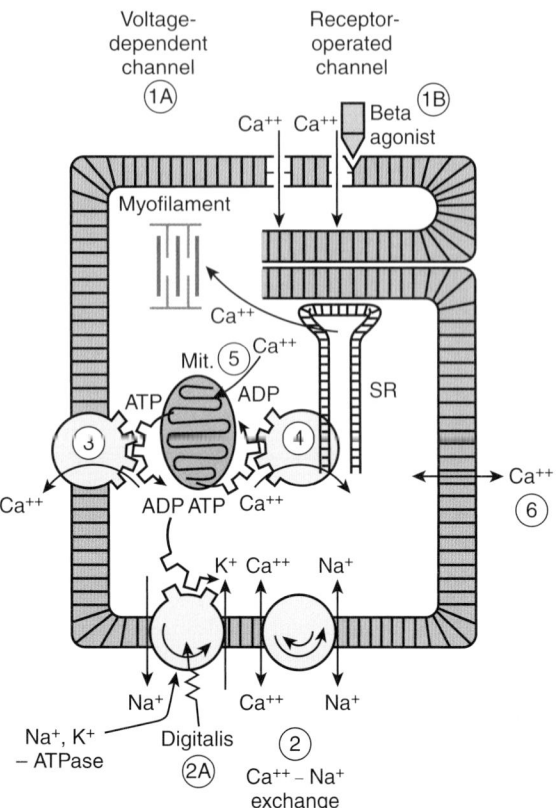

Figure 19-23 Regulation of cytoplasmic calcium. The diastolic extrusion of calcium from the myofilaments occurs at several sites. At two of the most important sites, energy (adenosine triphosphate [ATP]) is required for the active reuptake of calcium by the sarcolemma (3) and the sarcoplasmic reticulum (SR; 4). ADP, adenosine diphosphate. (*From Braunwald E: Mechanisms of action of calcium channel blocking agents. N Engl J Med 307:1618, 1982.*)

with a dynamic component to their degree of subaortic obstruction.[237] Further improvement in the clinical outcome of surgically treated patients may be achieved with the addition of verapamil, presumably reflecting a two-pronged attack on the systolic (myomectomy) and diastolic (verapamil) components of the disease. Enthusiasm continues for the therapeutic use of dual-chamber pacing in this disease, with some patients demonstrating reductions in their subaortic gradients.[171–174,238,239] It was not an option for patients in AF.

Myomectomy usually results in significant symptomatic improvement, together with a reduction in the subaortic gradient.[240] The intraoperative guidance and evaluation of the surgical result by an experienced echocardiographer are essential for the success of this procedure.[241–243] In successful cases, the postmyomectomy study will show dramatic septal thinning, widening of the LVOT, and resolution of SAM and the LVOT color mosaic.

As in any disease with diverse diagnostic criteria, it is difficult to compare mortality rates among various series, but perioperative mortality rates for isolated septal myomectomy are less than 2%, although operative risks are greater when combined with other procedures.[244,245] However, clinical studies of predominantly elderly patients reported mortality rates in excess of 15%. Complications other than heart block are infrequent, although more than one third of patients will experience new, clinically insignificant AR.[246] It is unclear whether this new AR poses a long-term risk for these patients from the standpoint of CHF, but it probably warrants the continued use of endocarditis prophylaxis.

Anesthetic Considerations

Priorities in anesthetic management are to avoid aggravating the subaortic obstruction while remaining aware of the derangements in diastolic function that may be somewhat less amenable to direct pharmacologic manipulation (Box 19-2). It is, therefore, necessary to maintain an appropriate intravascular volume while avoiding direct or reflex increases in contractility or heart rate. The latter goals can be achieved with a deep level of general anesthesia (GA) and the associated direct myocardial depression. Regardless of the specific technique, the preservation of an adequate CPP, using vasoconstrictors rather than inotropes, is necessary to avoid myocardial ischemia. Heavy premedication is advisable with a view to avoiding anxiety-induced tachycardia or a reduction in ventricular filling. Chronic β-blockade or calcium-channel blockade, or both, should be continued up to and including the day of surgery. These medications should be restarted immediately after surgery, particularly in those patients undergoing noncardiac surgery.

Intraoperative monitoring should include an ECG system with the capability of monitoring a V_5 lead and each of the six limb leads. Inspection of lead II may be helpful in the accurate diagnosis of supraventricular and junctional tachyarrhythmias, which may precipitate catastrophic hemodynamic deterioration because of the potential for inadequate ventricular filling resulting from the reduction in diastolic time or loss of the atrial contribution to ventricular filling. The latter may be crucial in patients with significantly reduced diastolic compliance.[132] Abnormal Q waves have been described on the electrocardiograms in 20% to 50% of patients with HCM.[179] These waves should not raise concern about a previous myocardial infarction; instead, they probably represent accentuation of normal septal depolarization or delay in depolarization of electrophysiologically abnormal cells.[247] Some patients exhibit a short PR interval with initial slurring of the QRS complex, and they may be at increased risk for supraventricular tachyarrhythmias on the basis of preexcitation.[248] Although the specific predisposing factors are unknown, patients with HCM are at increased risk for any type of arrhythmia in the operative setting.[249]

Given the pronounced abnormalities in left ventricular diastolic compliance, the CVP is likely to be an inaccurate guide to changes in left ventricular volume. However, a CVP catheter is extremely useful for the prompt administration of vasoactive drugs if they become necessary. As in valvular AS, the information provided by insertion of a PAC is worth the small arrhythmogenic risk. The potential for hypovolemia-induced exacerbation of outflow tract obstruction makes it crucial that the clinician have an accurate gauge of intravascular filling. The reduced diastolic compliance means that the PCWP will overestimate the patient's true volume status, and a reasonable clinical objective is to maintain the PCWP in the high-normal to elevated range. A PAC with pacing capability is ideal because atrial overdrive pacing can effect immediate hemodynamic improvement in the event of episodes of junctional rhythm (see Chapters 14, 22, and 25). The absolute requirement of these patients for an adequate preload cannot be overemphasized because even abrupt positioning changes have resulted in acute hemodynamic deterioration, including acute pulmonary edema.[250]

Intraoperative arrhythmias require aggressive therapy. During cardiac surgery, insertion of the venous cannulae may precipitate atrial arrhythmias. Because the resultant hypotension may be severe, the surgeon should cannulate the aorta before any atrial manipulations. Supraventricular or junctional tachyarrhythmias may require

BOX 19-2. HYPERTROPHIC CARDIOMYOPATHY

Preload: increased
Afterload: increased
Goal: myocardial depression
Avoid: tachycardia, inotropes, vasodilators

immediate cardioversion if they precipitate catastrophic degrees of hypotension. Although verapamil is one drug of choice for paroxysmal atrial and junctional tachycardia, it has the potential of disastrously worsening the LVOT obstruction if it elicits excessive vasodilation or if it is used in the setting of severe hypotension.[235] Cardioversion is preferable when the mean arterial pressure is already very low; the concurrent administration of phenylephrine also is advisable. This drug is almost always a low-risk, high-yield choice for the hypotensive patient with HCM. It augments perfusion, may ameliorate the pressure gradient, and often elicits a potentially beneficial vagal reflex when used to treat tachyarrhythmia-induced hypotension.

The inhalation anesthetics commonly are used for patients with HCM. Their dose-dependent myocardial depression is ideal because negative inotropy reduces the degree of SAM-septal contact, which results in LVOT obstruction. Hypotension is almost always the result of underlying hypovolemia, which is potentially exacerbated by anesthetic-induced vasodilation. Inotropes, β-adrenergic agonists, and calcium are all contraindicated because they worsen the systolic obstruction and perpetuate the hypotension. In most cases, a beneficial response can be obtained with aggressive replenishment of intravascular volume and concurrent infusion of phenylephrine.

Several investigators have suggested that regional anesthesia, with its potential for accentuating peripheral vasodilation, may be relatively contraindicated in the management of patients with HCM.[251,252] The theoretic constraints are similar to those for patients with valvular AS, and the same clinical caveats apply. If the vascular system is kept appropriately full and "tight" with vasopressors, it is reasonable to consider these techniques in the light of other clinical advantages they might offer the patient. Catheter techniques (e.g., continuous spinals, epidurals) may be preferable to the bolus administration of local anesthetics to achieve a finer degree of control of the anesthetic level.[253] There unquestionably is the potential for a cascade of iatrogenic complications if sympatholytic hypotension is treated in a knee-jerk fashion with ephedrine, epinephrine, or a variety of other equally contraindicated β-adrenergic agonists.

Although echocardiography has undoubtedly contributed to an increased frequency of diagnosis of this disease, an occasional patient escapes detection by ultrasound examination in the course of the preoperative workup. When other objective data, including the physical examination, ECG results, and chest radiograph, show only nonspecific abnormalities, it is easy to disregard vague or atypical complaints of chest pain, presyncope, and dyspnea. This is particularly true when the symptoms might reasonably be attributed to the primary condition that brought the patient to surgery (e.g., CABG).[254] Other identifiable populations are said to be at high risk for occult HCM. HCM of the elderly already has been discussed, and probably only a fraction of such patients arrive in the operating room with such a formal diagnosis. However, it is not uncommon for the anesthesiologist to encounter an elderly patient with long-standing systemic hypertension and unexplained episodes of pulmonary congestion for whom the primary physician has prescribed a digitalis preparation. Anesthesiologists occasionally may be presented with the opportunity to diagnose unsuspected HCM or one of its variants. Intraoperative events that could conceivably provoke or accentuate physiologic manifestations of the disease include hypovolemia, tachycardia, spontaneous or "manipulative" ectopy, and paradoxic responses to vasoactive drugs (e.g., inotropes, vasodilators, and vasoconstrictors) or anesthetic agents.[254,255] Clues such as these allow the experienced and astute clinician to recognize the phenomenon of dynamic subaortic obstruction when it occurs in less obvious clinical settings.

AORTIC REGURGITATION

Clinical Features and Natural History

AR may result from an abnormality of the valve itself, from bicuspid anatomy, have a rheumatic or infectious origin, or occur in association with any condition producing dilation of the aortic root and leaflet

separation. Nonrheumatic valvular diseases commonly resulting in AR include infective endocarditis, trauma, and connective tissue disorders such as Marfan syndrome or cystic medionecrosis of the aortic valve.[56] Aortic dissection from trauma, hypertension, or chronic degenerative processes also can result in dilatation of the root and functional incompetence (see Chapter 21).

The natural history of chronic AR is that of a long asymptomatic interval during which the valvular incompetence and secondary ventricular enlargement become progressively more severe.[3,141] When symptoms do appear, they are usually those of CHF, and chest pain, if it occurs, is often nonexertional in origin. The life expectancy for patients with significant disease has historically been about 9 years, and in contrast with AS, the onset of symptoms because of AR does not portend an immediately ominous prognosis.[256,257] In the absence of surgery, early recognition of AR and chronic use of vasodilators appear to be prolonging life span in this patient population.[141,258]

A relatively unique and problematic feature of chronic AR is that the severity of symptoms and their duration may correlate poorly with the degree of hemodynamic and contractile impairment.[141,259] The issue in surgical decision making is that many patients can remain asymptomatic, during which time they are undergoing progressive deterioration in their myocardial contractility. Noninvasive diagnostic studies (e.g., radionuclide cineangiography and 2D and Doppler echocardiographic assessment of response to pharmacologic afterload stress) may facilitate the detection of early derangements in contractile function in relatively asymptomatic patients.[260–262] These findings are important to the cardiologist when considering surgical referral (see Chapters 1 to 3) because patients with depressed preoperative left ventricular function have a greater perioperative mortality rate and are at increased risk for persistent postoperative heart failure (HF).[96,263,264]

As in acute mitral regurgitation, the physiology of acute AR is quite different from chronic AR. Common causes include endocarditis, trauma, and acute aortic dissection. Because of a lack of chronic compensation, these patients usually present with pulmonary edema and HF refractory to optimal medical therapy. These patients are often hypotensive and clinically appear to be on the verge of cardiovascular collapse.

Pathophysiology

Left ventricular volume overload is the pathognomonic feature of chronic AR. The degree of volume overload is determined by the magnitude of the regurgitant flow, which is related to the size of the regurgitant orifice, the aorta-ventricular pressure gradient, and the diastolic time. It has been suggested that the size of the regurgitant aortic orifice is constant and independent of changes in loading conditions.[265] However, in other valvular lesions (e.g., AS, mitral regurgitation), the orifice size is not constant and is dependent on the hemodynamic state. There is some evidence, in an experimental model of acute AR, that the regurgitant orifice area can change with increases or decreases in the transvalvular pressure gradient.[266] When AR occurs in the absence of valvular fibrosis or calcification (valve elasticity is preserved), reduction of regurgitant area may be one of the mechanisms of the beneficial effect of afterload reduction.

The hemodynamic effects of changes in heart rate are also less straightforward than might be assumed.[267] Theoretically, tachycardia should maximize net forward flow by shortening the regurgitant diastolic time interval. This hypothesis, first offered by Corrigan in 1832, may be the pathophysiologic basis for the seemingly paradoxic observation that patients with AR may tolerate exercise despite having symptoms of pulmonary congestion at rest. Sympathetically mediated vasodilation, increased inotropy, and tachycardia may contribute to the increased CO achieved during isometric exercise in patients with AR.[268] Chronically, similar, reflex-induced hemodynamic changes may contribute to the beneficial effects of arteriolar dilators.[269] The peripheral vasculature directly affects regurgitant volume through reflex changes in heart rate; it also can alter volume loading by effects on the diastolic time. It plays a key role in the overall pathophysiology of AR[270,271] (Figure 19-24).

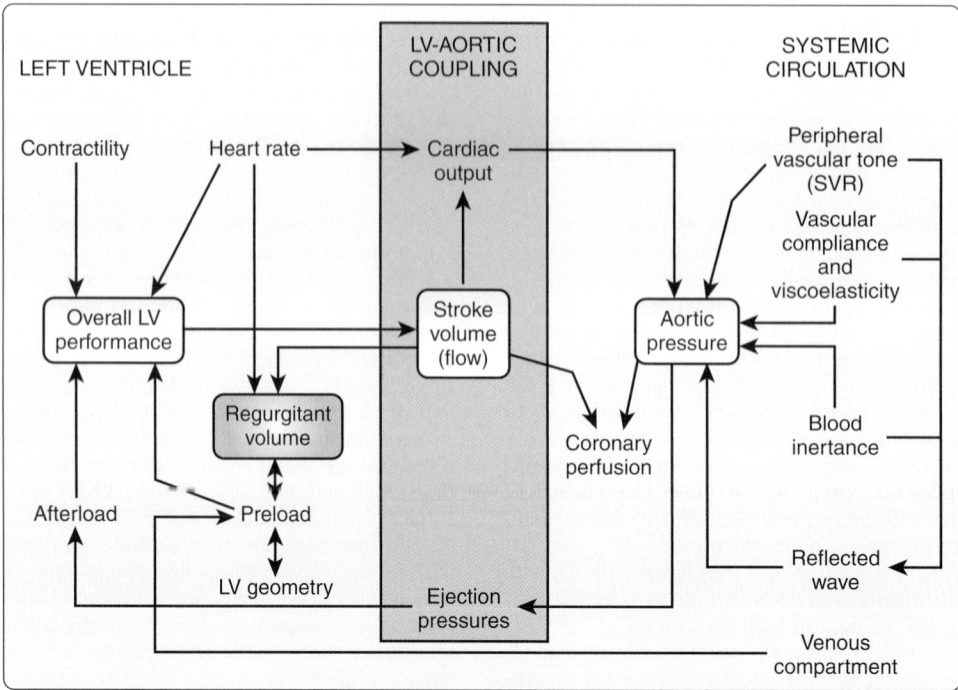

Figure 19-24 The peripheral circulation plays a pivotal role in supporting left ventricular (LV) performance in the face of chronic volume overloading. *(From Borow KM, Marcus RH: Aortic regurgitation: The need for an integrated physiologic approach.* J Am Coll Cardiol *17:898, 1991.)*

Despite these observations, the beneficial effects of shortened diastolic time alone may be less clear-cut. Angiographic study of subjects with chronic AR has shown that pacing-induced tachycardia can decrease the SV, LVEDV, and LVEDP and can increase cardiac output,[272] but that the ratio of the regurgitant volume to the total SV may remain unchanged. This occurs because tachycardia shortens the diastolic period per stroke, but increases the number of strokes per minute, leaving the net diastolic time per minute relatively unchanged. Similar observation has been made with radionuclide studies that demonstrated that tachycardia can increase CO and decrease LVEDV; however, pulmonary arterial pressure (PAP) and PCWP may not change with increasing heart rate.[273] This divergence between the effects of tachycardia on left ventricular volume (decreased) and filling pressures (unchanged) may reflect the pronounced rightward shift of the left ventricular pressure-volume loop that is characteristic of long-standing AR.

Chronically, AR results in a state of left ventricular volume and pressure overload. Progressive volume overloading from AR increases end-diastolic wall tension (i.e., ventricular afterload) and stimulates the serial replication of sarcomeres, producing a pattern of eccentric ventricular hypertrophy.[97,264] This dilation of the ventricle, in accordance with Laplace's law, also increases the systolic wall tension, stimulating some concentric hypertrophy. The result is normalization of the ratio of ventricular wall thickness to cavitary radius.[97] This process of eccentric hypertrophy results in the greatest absolute degrees of cardiomegaly seen in valve disease. EDV may be three to four times normal, and very high cardiac outputs can be sustained.[274]

Figure 19-25 shows the pressure-volume loops for acute and chronic AR. In the chronic form, the diastolic pressure-volume curve is shifted far to the right. This permits a tremendous increase in LVEDV with minimal change in filling pressure, a property frequently described as high diastolic compliance.[274] However, animal models of chronic left ventricular volume overloading instead suggest that the entire diastolic pressure-volume curve is shifted to the right (see Figure 19-8).[11] This accounts for the apparent paradox of high ventricular volumes at relatively low filling pressures.

The parallel shifts of the entire curve relating diastolic pressure and volume are a manifestation of the physiologic process known as "creep."[4] This refers to the time-dependent increase in dimension that occurs as a result of an applied stress—in this case, volume overload. Because of this chronic adaptation, left ventricular filling pressures are in the low-to-normal range and are relatively insensitive to changes in intravascular volume. This is not true of greater filling pressures, for which increases are a reliable guide to volume overload and ventricular distention.

Because the increase in preload is compensated for by ventricular hypertrophy, CO is maintained by the Frank-Starling mechanism, and cardiac failure is not seen. This is true despite probable decreases in contractility.[258] There is virtually no isovolumic diastolic phase because the ventricle is filling throughout diastole. The isovolumic phase of systole also is brief because of the low aortic diastolic pressure. This minimal impedance to the forward ejection of a large SV allows for the performance of maximal myocardial work at a minimum of oxygen consumption. Eventually, however, progressive volume overload increases ventricular EDV to the point that compensatory hypertrophy is no longer sufficient to compensate, and a decline in systolic function occurs. As systolic function declines, end-systolic dimension increases further, left ventricular wall stress increases, and left ventricular function is further compromised by the excessive ventricular afterload. At this point, the decline of ventricular function is progressive and can be quite rapid. As is shown in Figure 19-26A, in the patient with compensated AR, the eccentrically dilated ventricle maintains its SV and EF by using preload reserve; wall stress is only slightly increased. In Figure 19-26B, the limit of preload reserve has been reached and ventricular dysfunction has shifted the end-systolic wall stress relation to the right. As a result of the higher wall stress, the SV and EF inevitably decline. In patients in whom the EF has become less than 25% or the end-systolic diameter larger than 60 mm, irreversible myocardial changes are likely to have occurred.[141]

The primary determinants of Mvo_2—contractility and wall tension—usually are not significantly increased with chronic AR, although calculated myocardial work may be twice normal. Actual Mvo_2 may be only minimally increased because the greater proportion of myocardial work is spent in the energy-efficient process of fiber shortening, with little increase occurring in oxygen-consuming tension development[275] (see Figure 19-26).

Despite the relatively normal Mvo_2, angina can occur in one third of patients with severe AR, even in the absence of CAD.[276] Patients

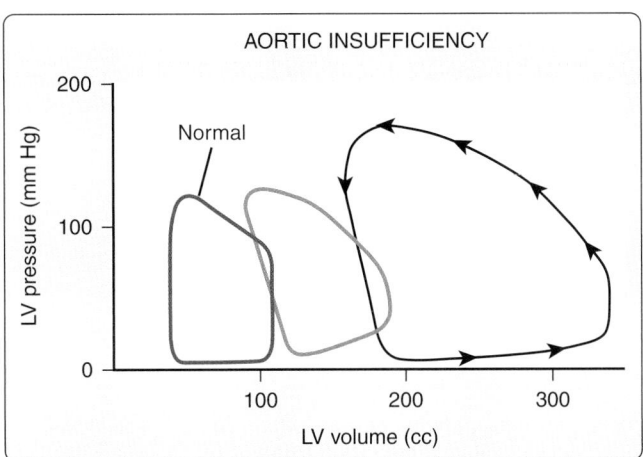

Figure 19-25 **Pressure-volume loop in aortic regurgitation (AR).** Acute AR (middle loop); chronic AR (right loop). LV, left ventricular. *(Adapted from Jackson JM, Thomas SJ, Lowenstein E: Anesthetic management of patients with valvular heart disease. Semin Anesth 1:239, 1982.)*

It also is important to remember that intraoperatively, patients with chronic AR may be at risk for acute ischemia with episodes of significant bradycardia. As bradycardia prolongs diastolic time, it increases regurgitant flow, and left ventricular diastolic pressure and wall tension increase rapidly. Simultaneously, the CPP is decreased as aortic runoff occurs during diastole and diastolic ventricular pressure is increased.[281] Under these conditions, myocardial perfusion pressure may be insufficient. Clinically, very rapid decompensation can occur. The ischemic ventricle can dilate rapidly such that progressively increased end-systolic dimensions are seen, and ischemia and ventricular failure become a positive feedback loop.

Surgical Decision Making

From the discussion of the pathophysiology of chronic AR, it is evident that an accurate assessment of contractility is crucial to surgical decision making, because the clinical history may be an unreliable index of ventricular function. It is not uncommon for asymptomatic patients to have ventricular dysfunction, whereas symptomatic patients may be free of even modest myocardial depression. A variety of prognostic indicators have been used to identify early ventricular dysfunction as a trigger for surgical intervention. Clinical status, such as exercise capacity and New York Heart Association (NYHA) class, and noninvasive and invasive laboratory tests have been used. Hemodynamic parameters such as the end-systolic stress-volume relation and estimates of the left ventricular contractile state have been evaluated as predictors of worsening left ventricular function.

Although ejection phase indices (e.g., EF) are most familiar to anesthesiologists, they are inherently unreliable for quantifying ventricular function in the setting of chronic volume overloading, because the Starling mechanism continues to support increases in the SV long after the onset of intrinsic myocardial depression. Left ventricular dilation, compensatory hypertrophy, and minimal afterload may normalize the EF, even though contractility is significantly depressed.[258] Preload can be exquisitely sensitive to changes in heart rate and systemic vascular tone. Ventricular performance, therefore, may not be adequately reflected by the EF.[282,283] The often-reported regurgitant volume or regurgitant fraction are similarly rate and load dependent, and they may correlate poorly with the underlying inotropic state.[284]

A variety of end-systolic indices have been examined in chronic AR, and these provide a more load-independent assessment of the inotropic state. Although the left ventricular end-systolic volume (LVESV) is preload independent, it does vary with myocardial contractility and

with chronic AR may be at risk for myocardial ischemia caused by hypertrophy-induced abnormalities of the coronary circulation. The increase in total myocardial mass can increase baseline Mvo$_2$, and there is evidence that total coronary blood flow, although increased, fails to keep pace with the increase in myocardial mass. Evidence suggests that the insidious development of contractile dysfunction may, in part, have an ischemic basis.[277]

Despite these rather favorable considerations in terms of myocardial energetics, an increase in Mvo$_2$ may pose a threat to the patient with chronic AR because of decreased coronary vascular reserve.[278] Although this phenomenon has been more thoroughly documented in patients with chronic pressure-induced hypertrophy, some studies indicate that the coronary vascular reserve is similarly compromised in patients with left ventricular volume overload.[279,280] The process of hypertrophy may be a double-edged sword from the standpoint of the myocardial oxygen balance. Hypertrophy minimizes oxygen consumption as measured by wall stress, but increases basal Mvo$_2$ and may elicit derangements in the quality or quantity of the coronary vasculature.

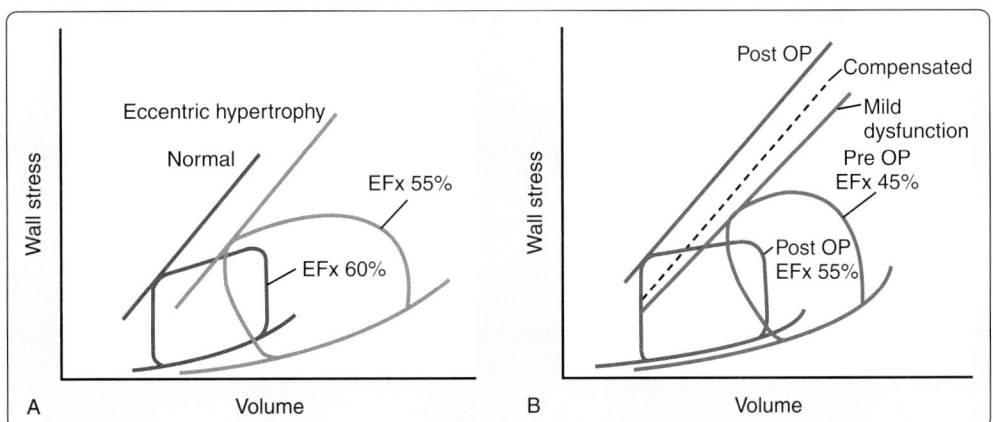

Figure 19-26 **Adaptation to volume overload.** *A,* Stress-volume curves and the linear end-systolic stress-volume relationship are shifted to the right in compensated aortic regurgitation compared with normal. The stroke volume and ejection fraction (EFx) are maintained despite slightly increased systolic wall stress. *B,* The same associations in a hypothetical patient with mild left ventricular dysfunction as evidenced by rightward shift of the end-systolic wall stress-volume relationship. Exhaustion of preload reserve causes wall stress to increase, resulting in reciprocal declines in the stroke volume and the ejection fraction. Valve replacement corrects afterload mismatch, allowing the end-diastolic and end-systolic volume relations to shift to the left. Lower wall stress allows the ejection fraction to return to normal. Post OP, postoperative; Pre OP, preoperative. *(From Ross J Jr: Afterload mismatch in aortic and mitral valve disease: Implications for surgical therapy. J Am Coll Cardiol 5:811, 1985.)*

afterload. An increased ESV may reflect a depressed inotropic state, or it may increase because of an increased left ventricular afterload resulting from increased chamber size or pressure.[282] There also is evidence that the relative load independence of the LVESV is limited when ventricular hypertrophy is primarily eccentric.[25] However, with long-standing volume overload, virtually all studies have found that an increased end-systolic dimension correlates with a poor prognosis and a significantly depressed contractile state.[261,285]

When valve surgery is performed after ventricular decompensation has occurred, the immediate and long-term results are marginal. Much of the increased mortality is a function of postoperative deaths from HF.[264,286] When valve surgery occurs before significant ventricular decompensation, ventricular recovery is remarkable, with remodeling and a reduction in left ventricular size beginning as early as 2 weeks after surgery.[141,264] Because delays in surgical intervention can be catastrophic and because the response to surgery is so good, there is evidence of a shift toward earlier valve replacement, and surgery in relatively asymptomatic patients has been advocated.[264] Based on review of the published literature, the ACC and the AHA have provided practice guidelines for surgical intervention in chronic AR.[141] Valve surgery is recommended for asymptomatic patients with left ventricular systolic dysfunction. Surgery also should be considered if ventricular dilation has occurred in the asymptomatic patient, even if the EF is normal. In patients who are symptomatic but have normal ventricular function, the ACC and AHA recommend further evaluation for an unrelated cause and observation. In these cases, serial echocardiographic assessment is appropriate. Symptomatic patients with left ventricular dysfunction should undergo surgery.[13]

Acute Aortic Regurgitation

In acute AR, sudden diastolic volume overload of a nonadapted LV results in a precipitous increase in the EDP because the ventricle is operating on the steepest portion of the diastolic pressure-volume curve (see Figure 19-25).[287] In severe acute AR, the LVEDP can equilibrate with aortic diastolic pressure and exceed the LA pressure in late diastole. This may be sufficient to cause closure of the mitral valve before atrial systole.[288] This is an important echocardiographic finding indicative of severe AR.[289] Although this phenomenon initially shields the pulmonary capillaries from the full force of the dramatically increased LVEDP, the protection may be short-lived.[290] Severe left ventricular distention often follows and produces mitral annular enlargement and functional mitral regurgitation.

The inevitable decline in SV in acute decompensating AR elicits a reflex sympathetic response so that tachycardia and a high SVR are common. Moderate tachycardia beneficially shortens the regurgitant time without reducing the transmitral filling volume.[291] Vasoconstriction, however, preserves CPP at the expense of increasing the aorta-ventricular gradient and regurgitation.

As may be expected, patients with acute AR may be at greater risk for myocardial ischemia. As with chronic AR and bradycardia, coronary perfusion may be compromised by the combination of a low diastolic arterial pressure and the precipitously increased LVEDP. This narrowing of CPP may be so severe that the phasic epicardial blood flow may change to a predominantly systolic pattern with severe acute AR.[292] Dissection of the coronary ostia is rare but frequently causes fatality in patients with acute AR. In addition to the structural impediment to myocardial oxygen delivery, catastrophic hypotension and high LVEDP combine to cause accentuated ischemia and ventricular dilation. Immediate surgical correction is the only hope for salvaging these patients, who often prove refractory to inotropes and vasodilators. Attempts at stabilizing the ischemic component of their injury with the intra-aortic balloon are usually contraindicated because augmenting the diastolic pressure worsens regurgitation.

Acute AR most commonly is due to infective endocarditis or aortic dissection, and intraoperative transesophageal echocardiography (TEE) has assumed increasing importance both in diagnosis of acute AR and in decisions regarding its surgical management.[293] Transesophageal echocardiographic studies are highly sensitive and specific for the diagnosis of infective endocarditis, and are significantly more sensitive than transthoracic echocardiography.[294] TEE has been shown to be particularly useful in the diagnosis of abscesses associated with endocarditis,[295] and may detect previously unsuspected abnormalities (Roger Click, MD, Mayo Clinic, personal communication). Although an area of active investigation, there is currently no completely satisfactory noninvasive method for quantifying the severity of AR. Premature closure of the mitral valve, determination of the pressure half-time of AR, and color-flow estimation of both the regurgitant jet's width and its size in relation to the LVOT are commonly described techniques.[296–298] (Refer to Chapters 12 and 13 for further discussion.)

Anesthetic Considerations

Intraoperative monitoring should include an ECG system with the capability of monitoring a lateral precordial lead because ischemia is a potential hazard (Box 19-3). For most valvular procedures, a PAC provides useful information. A PAC allows determination of basal filling pressures and cardiac output, which is particularly useful in chronic AR given the potential unreliability of the clinical history and EF. Equally important is the ability to accurately monitor ventricular preload and CO response to pharmacologic interventions. The aggressive use of vasodilators often is appropriate therapy perioperatively for the failing ventricle, but their use can compromise the preload to which the ventricle has chronically adjusted. Concurrent preload augmentation, guided by the pulmonary artery diastolic pressure or PCWP, may be crucial to optimize CO when afterload is pharmacologically manipulated[299–301] (see Chapters 10, 12 to 14, 32, and 34). The other requirement for a PAC is to allow for pacing when it is anticipated. The deleterious effects of significant bradycardia in AR have been described. In patients who arrive in the operating room with heart rates less than 70 beats/min or in patients for whom rapid epicardial pacing may be difficult to establish (e.g., redo operations), placement of a pacing wire probably is indicated. Typically, only a ventricular wire would be appropriate; it is more reliable than atrial pacing, and in AR, the atrial contribution to ventricular diastolic volume usually is not essential. Capturing the ventricle with a PAC-based, transvenous wire can be difficult because of the very large ventricular cavity size in patients with chronic AR.

Because patients with AR may differ widely in their degree of myocardial dysfunction, anesthetic management must be appropriately individualized. For cardiac or noncardiac surgery, the hemodynamic goals are a mild tachycardia, a positive inotropic state, and a controlled reduction in SVR. For cardiac surgery, dopamine or dobutamine, pancuronium, ketamine, and nitroprusside infusions are excellent choices. For the patient with acute AR, the goals are the same, but urgency must be stressed. It is essential to try to rapidly reduce end-diastolic and end-systolic ventricular volumes with the very aggressive use of inotropes (e.g., epinephrine) and vasodilators. There is sometimes concern that inotropes may exacerbate the root dissection in acute AR by increasing the shear force on the aortic wall. Despite this theoretic concern, positive inotropes should not be withheld from the patient who deteriorates in the operating room because they may provide the precious additional minutes of hemodynamic stability needed to get on CPB. In acute and chronic forms of AR, serial measurements of CO can indicate that ventricular size and CO have been optimized, regardless of the systemic pressure. TEE also is useful to look at ventricular size, but probably maximizing CO under these conditions gets closer to the

BOX 19-3. AORTIC REGURGITATION

Preload: increased
Afterload: decreased
Goal: augmentation of forward flow
Avoid: bradycardia

therapeutic goal than looking at ventricular size alone. With acute AR and premature closure of the mitral valve, PAPs may grossly underestimate the LVEDP, which continues to increase under the influence of the diastolic regurgitant jet from the aorta. For noncardiac surgery in the patient with AR, there are advantages to epidural or other regional techniques when appropriate. Epidural anesthesia usually is preferable to spinal techniques in which more precipitous declines in SVR can occur.

Predicting the response of the patient with AR to anesthetic interventions can be difficult if the contractile state of the ventricle is unknown. Although reductions in functional status or EF are broad indicators of poorer outcomes, examining the medical history for *serial* measurements of EF or ventricular ESVs may be most useful. Because patients with chronic AR are subject to a rapid, self-perpetuating decline in ventricular performance, demonstration of recent decreases in EF or increases in ventricular size may be the best indicators of a challenging intraoperative course.

A few other practical points bear comment in surgery for AR. The early and late phases of CPB can be a real problem in AR, particularly in redo operations. Before cross-clamp placement, the ventricle is at risk for distention if it is not ejecting or being vented. If the ventricle dilates with AR during CPB, the intraventricular pressures may equilibrate with the aortic root pressures. Under these conditions, there is no coronary perfusion, and the ventricle may dilate rapidly and become profoundly ischemic. This can occur before cross-clamp placement with bradycardia, ventricular fibrillation, tachycardia, or even with a rapid supraventricular rhythm that compromises organized mechanical activity. Correcting the rhythm, pacing, cross-clamping the aorta, or venting the ventricle addresses this problem. This also can occur in cardiac surgery for conditions other than AR. In patients with unknown or uncorrected AR, removal of the cross-clamp causes the same ventricular dilation and ischemia if a rhythm and ejection are not rapidly established. Ventricular venting or pacing may be essential until an organized, mechanically efficient rhythm is established. This problem must be considered in patients referred for CABG alone, in those with mild or moderate AR not having AVR, and in patients in whom intraoperative TEE is not used.

MITRAL REGURGITATION

Clinical Features and Natural History

Unlike mitral stenosis (MS), which is almost always the result of rheumatic valve disease, mitral regurgitation may result from a variety of disease processes that affect the valve leaflets, the chordae tendineae, the papillary muscles, the valve annulus, or the LV. Mitral regurgitation can be classified as organic or functional. Organic mitral regurgitation describes diseases that result in distortion, disruption, or destruction of the mitral leaflets or chordal structures. In Western countries, degenerative processes that lead to leaflet prolapse with or without chordal rupture represent the most common cause of mitral regurgitation.[300] Other causes of organic mitral regurgitation include infective endocarditis, mitral annular calcification, rheumatic valve disease, and connective tissue disorders such as Marfan or Ehlers-Danlos syndrome. Much less common causes of organic mitral regurgitation include congenital mitral valve clefts, diet-drug or ergotamine toxicity, and carcinoid valve disease with metabolically active pulmonary tumors or right-to-left intracardiac shunting.[302] Mitral valve prolapse (MVP) is a common (2.4%) disorder with a strong hereditary component. Several genes play a pivotal role in heart valve formation, including calcineurin, Wnt/beta-catenin signaling, fibroblast growth factor 4 (FGF-4), the homeobox gene *Sox4,* and the downstream modulator of transforming growth factor-β superfamily signaling Smad6. Genotypic linkage was found to chromosomes 11, 13, and 16. The recent finding of a mutation in familial mitral valve prolapse not related to connective tissue syndromes, an X-linked filament A mutation, suggests that mitral valve prolapse may be the final common outcome of multiple genetic defects.

Functional mitral regurgitation describes cases in which mitral regurgitation occurs despite structurally normal leaflets and chordae tendineae. Resulting from altered function or geometry of the LV or mitral annulus, functional mitral regurgitation often occurs in the setting of ischemic heart disease, and the term *ischemic mitral regurgitation* is sometimes used interchangeably with *functional mitral regurgitation.* However, the functional form can occur in patients without demonstrable CAD, such as those with idiopathic dilated cardiomyopathy and mitral annular dilatation. The term *ischemic mitral regurgitation* probably best applies to functional cases with a known ischemic cause. Rupture of a papillary muscle with acute, severe mitral regurgitation is somewhat more difficult to classify. Although usually a sequela of acute myocardial infarction (AMI) with normal leaflets and chordae, there is an obvious anatomic disruption of the mitral apparatus.

Because it can be caused by a wide variety of disease processes, the natural history of mitral regurgitation is quite variable.[302] Even among patients with acute-onset disease, the clinical course depends on the mechanism of regurgitation and the response to treatment. For instance, patients with acute, severe mitral regurgitation caused by a ruptured papillary muscle have a dismal outcome without surgery.[302] However, the clinical course of acute mitral regurgitation caused by endocarditis could be favorable if the patient responds well to antibiotic therapy.[302] Although those with chronic mitral regurgitation usually enter an initial, often asymptomatic, compensated phase, the time course for progression to left ventricular dysfunction and symptomatic HF is unpredictable.[302] The literature reflects the wide variability in the natural history of mitral regurgitation, with published 5-year survival rates for patients with mitral regurgitation of 27% to 97%.[303] Selection bias, small study populations, and poorly defined degrees of mitral regurgitation likely explain these discrepancies.[304] Later studies better define the clinical course of certain subgroups of patients with mitral regurgitation. For instance, Ling et al[305] examined the natural history of patients with mitral regurgitation because of flail leaflets. Among this select group, the investigators observed an excess annual mortality rate of 6.3% with a combined rate of death or surgery of 90% within a 10-year period.[305] Patients with flail mitral valve leaflets also experience an increased risk for sudden death.[306] Grigioni et al[306] reported a 1.8% per year rate of sudden death among patients with flail mitral leaflets who were being medically managed. The rate of sudden death diminished after surgical intervention in this population.[306]

The application of quantitative Doppler echocardiography to the prospective study of mitral regurgitation has allowed researchers to document the progressive nature of this condition. Enriquez-Sarano et al[307] found that, on average, the regurgitant volume increases 7.5 mL and the effective regurgitant orifice increases 5.9 mm² each year. However, as with the natural history of mitral regurgitation in general, there was significant variability in the rate of progression among patients. Rapid progression of its severity occurred among patients who developed flail leaflets, but mitral regurgitation regressed in 11% of those studied.[307]

Pathophysiology

Mitral regurgitation causes left ventricular volume overload. The regurgitant volume combines with the normal LA volume and returns to the LV during each diastolic period. This increased preload leads to increased sarcomere stretch and, in the initial phases of the disease process, augmentation of left ventricular ejection performance by the Frank-Starling mechanism. Systolic ejection into the relatively low-pressure left atrium further enhances the contractile appearance of the LV.

The presentation of patients with mitral regurgitation varies depending on the pathophysiology of the specific condition, which is affected by the mechanism, severity, and acuity of the mitral regurgitation. In cases of acute, severe mitral regurgitation, such as in patients with a ruptured papillary muscle after AMI, the sudden increase in preload enhances left ventricular contractility by the Frank-Starling mechanism. Despite the increased preload, left ventricular size initially is normal. Normal left ventricular size combined with the ability to eject into a low-pressure circuit (i.e., the left atrium) results in decreased afterload in the acute setting. The measured LVEF in cases of sudden, severe mitral regurgitation may approach 75%, although forward SV is reduced.[302] However, because the left atrium has not yet dilated in response to the large regurgitant volume, LA pressure increases acutely and may lead to pulmonary vascular congestion, pulmonary edema, and dyspnea.[302]

Many patients with mitral regurgitation, particularly those whose valvular incompetence develops more slowly, may enter a chronic, compensated phase. In this phase, chronic volume overload triggers left ventricular cavity enlargement by promoting eccentric hypertrophy (see Figure 19-15). Increased preload continues to augment left ventricular systolic performance. At the same time, the left atrium dilates in response to the ongoing regurgitant volume. Although LA dilatation maintains a low-pressure circuit that facilitates left ventricular systolic ejection, the increased radius of the left ventricular cavity leads to increased wall tension according to the law of Laplace, which was given earlier.

Unlike the case of sudden, acute mitral regurgitation, which is characterized by normal left ventricular size and reduced afterload, afterload remains in the normal range in the chronic, compensated phase of mitral regurgitation.[308] The changes seen in chronic, compensated mitral regurgitation are represented graphically in Figure 19-27. The isovolumic contraction phase is shortened as the blood is ejected into the low-pressure left atrium early in the cycle of ventricular systole. Because the dilated, compliant LV accepts increased diastolic volumes at low or normal filling pressures, some physicians believe that left ventricular diastolic function is enhanced in patients with chronic mitral regurgitation.[308] Whereas dilatation of the left heart chambers permits left ventricular filling at low or normal pressures, chamber enlargement progressively dilates the mitral annulus, potentially increasing the effective regurgitant orifice and regurgitant volume over time. Patients may tolerate the phase of chronic, compensated mitral regurgitation for many years because increased preload maintains left ventricular ejection performance. If symptoms develop during this time, they often are related to diminished forward CO because the regurgitant fraction may exceed 50%. Rather than dyspnea or signs of pulmonary congestion, fatigue and weakness predominate.

With the eventual decline in left ventricular systolic function, patients enter a decompensated phase. Progressive left ventricular dilatation increases wall stress and afterload, causing further deterioration in

left ventricular performance,[302] mitral annular dilatation, and worsening of the mitral regurgitation. Left ventricular end-systolic pressure increases. The increased left ventricular filling pressures result in increase of LA pressures and, given time, pulmonary vascular congestion, pulmonary hypertension, and right ventricular dysfunction. In addition to fatigue and weakness, patients with decompensated, chronic mitral regurgitation also may report dyspnea and orthopnea. It is difficult to predict when a patient with mitral regurgitation is likely to decompensate clinically. The progression of disease in any given patient depends on the underlying cause of mitral regurgitation, its severity, the response of the LV to volume overload, and possibly the effect of medical management.[302,309]

Assessment of left ventricular function in patients with mitral regurgitation is controversial but critically important for clinical decision making.[303] As in AR, the altered loading conditions that characterize mitral regurgitation confound traditional, load-dependent measures of left ventricular systolic function such as EF. Although numerous methods of assessing left ventricular function have been proposed, no consensus exists.[303] Despite its limitations, EF remains the most studied variable of left ventricular function in patients with mitral regurgitation and the most predictive of clinical outcome. For instance, preoperative EF is the most important prognostic factor for long-term survival after surgery for mitral regurgitation.[310] Preoperative EF also predicts postoperative EF and the occurrence of CHF after the surgical correction of mitral regurgitation.[311,312] Because of the combination of increased preload and the ability to eject into the low-pressure left atrium, a normally functioning LV should display an increased EF in the presence of significant mitral regurgitation. Conversely, an EF considered normal in a patient with competent valves may represent diminished left ventricular function in the setting of mitral regurgitation. In patients with severe mitral regurgitation, an EF in the range of 50% to 60% likely represents significant left ventricular dysfunction and is itself an indication for surgery.[141] Enriquez-Sarano et al[310] reported that the postoperative survival after mitral repair or replacement declines after the preoperative EF decreases to less than 60%.

A number of studies provide insight into the origin of left ventricular dysfunction in the setting of mitral regurgitation. In animal models of the disease, myocardial mass accumulates mainly through a decrease in the natural degradation of cellular elements, rather than by an increased rate of protein synthesis.[313–315] In contrast, myocardial protein synthesis increases within hours of the creation of simulated AS and left ventricular pressure overload.[316] Histologic preparations from animals with experimental mitral regurgitation and left ventricular dysfunction also show a 35% reduction in contractile elements within individual myocytes.[317] Examination of pressure-volume loops from patients with AS and mitral regurgitation is also insightful (see Figures 19-13 and 19-27). If the area contained within each loop is examined, it can be seen that this area, or stroke work, is similar for the two disease states. However, patients with AS generally display a greater degree of myocardial hypertrophy when compared with patients suffering from mitral regurgitation. Stroke work per gram of myocardium is greater in patients with mitral regurgitation, a finding that also may explain left ventricular dysfunction in this patient population.[308]

Ischemic Mitral Regurgitation

Ischemic mitral regurgitation (IMR) represents mitral regurgitation occurring in the setting of ischemic heart disease in patients without significant abnormalities of the valve leaflets or chordal structures. Some clinicians use the terms *ischemic mitral regurgitation* and *functional mitral regurgitation* interchangeably. However, IMR more accurately describes those cases of functional mitral regurgitation that occur in the setting of CAD. Papillary muscle rupture, which is almost always a sequela of AMI, also may be classified as IMR, although a clear organic defect of the mitral apparatus exists.

Clinicians increasingly are recognizing the importance of IMR because it is quite common. The incidence rate of mitral regurgitation

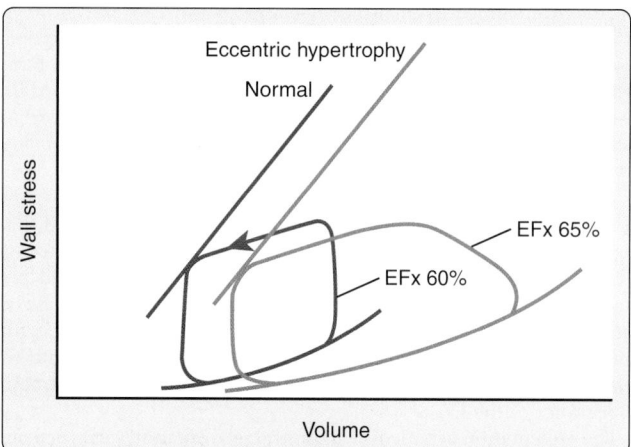

Figure 19-27 Volume overload with mitral regurgitation (MR). As in volume overloading from aortic regurgitation, wall stress-volume loops of the eccentrically hypertrophied left ventricle are shifted to the right. However, in chronic MR, retrograde ejection into the low-pressure left atrium minimizes ventricular wall stress, supporting the ejection fraction (EFx). *(From Ross J Jr: Afterload mismatch in aortic and mitral valve disease: Implications for surgical therapy. J Am Coll Cardiol 5:811, 1985.)*

after AMI as detected by echocardiography ranges from 39% to 73%.[309] Echocardiographic studies also demonstrate that in 13% to 29% of cases, the IMR is at least moderate in severity.[309] The presence of IMR also portends a worse clinical outcome. For instance, patients with IMR after AMI experience a twofold to sixfold increase in cardiovascular mortality in the first year after the ischemic event.[318] Patients with severe IMR have a 1-year mortality rate that approaches 50%.[319] However, in evaluating patients with mitral regurgitation presumed to be of ischemic origin, clinicians should attempt to identify the severity of the regurgitation, the time of onset, and the likely mechanism of valvular incompetence, because these factors influence prognosis and treatment. For instance, patients with mild IMR in the early phase of an AMI rarely experience hemodynamic sequelae from this mitral leakage, whereas those with ischemic rupture of a papillary muscle often present with acute CHF and have a poor prognosis without surgical intervention.

Investigators have identified certain patient characteristics associated with an increased incidence of IMR. For instance, patients with advanced age, inferior or posterior AMI, spherical left ventricular geometry, and multiple-vessel CAD tend to display greater rates of IMR.[309,320] Other factors associated with increased rates of IMR include LA enlargement, mitral annular dilatation, and decreased EF.[309] Frank rupture of a papillary muscle, which occurs in 1% of AMI cases, usually involves the posteromedial papillary muscle because its blood supply is derived from a single coronary artery.

The understanding of the pathophysiologic basis of IMR continues to evolve. Early investigators proposed ischemic papillary muscle dysfunction as a primary cause of IMR.[321–323] Later studies indicated that isolated ischemia of one or both papillary muscles does not cause significant mitral regurgitation.[324–327] Instead, ischemia of the papillary muscle and the adjacent myocardium is necessary to produce IMR.[309,324,326,327] Myocardial ischemia may result in focal or global left ventricular bulging and, with time, ventricular remodeling to a more spherical shape. Such geometric changes cause outward migration of the papillary muscles. The finding most strongly correlated with chronic IMR is outward papillary muscle displacement.[309,328] When the papillary muscles are displaced outward, the point of mitral leaflet coaptation moves apically and away from the mitral annulus, resulting in the appearance of valve tenting. Besides outward bulging of the LV, scarring and retraction of the papillary muscles also may produce mitral leaflet tethering, with the net effect of incomplete leaflet coaptation and valvular incompetence. Some investigators believe that papillary muscle dysfunction may reduce the degree of IMR in certain patients.[329,330] Komeda et al[330] suggested that reduced contractility of the papillary muscles may counteract the tethering effect of ischemic myocardium, thereby allowing leaflet coaptation to occur closer to the mitral annulus. An additional potential mechanism of IMR is decreased contractility of the posterior mitral annulus. During systole, annular contraction reduces the mitral orifice area by 25%.[331–333] Because the anterior portion of the mitral annulus is more fibrous, posterior annular contraction plays a greater role in reducing the size of the mitral orifice. Loss of posterior annular contraction may contribute to mitral regurgitation in the setting of myocardial ischemia.

The clinical approach to IMR depends on its underlying mechanism. Timely surgical intervention often is warranted in cases of papillary muscle rupture. For patients with an intact mitral apparatus who present with IMR in the setting of AMI, early reperfusion therapy improves regional and global left ventricular function, reduces ventricular dilatation, and decreases the likelihood of adverse remodeling and associated papillary muscle displacement.[329,334–337] The resultant improvements in ventricular function and geometry combine to reduce the incidence of IMR. Clinicians often prescribe angiotensin-converting enzyme inhibitors to patients with ischemic heart disease. Chronic angiotensin-converting enzyme inhibitor therapy may decrease the incidence and severity of IMR by preventing left ventricular remodeling, although data to support this theory are lacking.[329]

Assessment of Mitral Regurgitation

Clinicians may suspect mitral regurgitation on the basis of current symptoms, medical history, or findings on physical examination. Echocardiography with the capability of 2D and Doppler (including color-flow) imaging represents the diagnostic modality of choice for the assessment of mitral regurgitation. Transthoracic echocardiogram (TTE) is readily available in most areas, is noninvasive, and provides detailed information about the mechanism of mitral regurgitation, its severity, and its impact on cardiac chamber size and function. Additional information available from TTE includes calculation of right ventricular systolic pressure based on the peak velocity of the tricuspid regurgitant signal and an estimate of right atrial pressure. Whenever possible, echocardiographers should attempt to provide a quantitative assessment of mitral regurgitation severity. Techniques that allow the determination of effective regurgitant orifice, regurgitant volume, or regurgitant fraction include the proximal isovelocity surface area (PISA) method and the continuity equation. Other echocardiographic findings such as pulmonary vein systolic flow reversals suggest severe mitral regurgitation, and they should be reported if present. Assessment of the size of the regurgitant jet in the left atrium may provide a gross estimation of mitral regurgitation severity but is limited by factors such as LA size and pressure, machine settings such as color-flow gain and aliasing velocity, and the orientation of the regurgitant jet itself. Eccentric regurgitant jets propagating along the wall of the left atrium often appear smaller than a centrally directed jet of equivalent severity. When transthoracic echocardiography is suboptimal, patients may be referred for TEE. Because of the proximity of the transducer to the mitral valve, TEE often produces superior images of the mitral valve. When performing intraoperative TEE examinations, anesthesiologists should recall that altered loading conditions, such as anesthetic-induced decreases in SVR, might favor forward cardiac output and diminish the observed amount of mitral regurgitation. More detailed discussions of the echocardiographic evaluation of the mitral valve are presented in Chapters 1, 2, 12 and 13.

Cardiac catheterization with left ventriculography may also be used to evaluate mitral regurgitation. This invasive procedure often is reserved for cases in which the echocardiographic data are suboptimal, conflicting, or discordant with the clinical findings.[302] Assessment of severity by ventriculography requires analysis of the amount of contrast material that enters the left atrium after injection into the LV. However, the amount of contrast material appearing in the left atrium depends on the severity of mitral regurgitation and on the volume of the left atrium, the catheter position, and the rate of contrast injection.[302] Right-heart catheterization may or may not demonstrate the presence of v waves in patients with significant mitral regurgitation. A high degree of LA compliance makes the appearance of prominent v waves less likely (see Chapter 3).

Other diagnostic tests commonly obtained in patients with mitral regurgitation include an electrocardiogram and chest radiograph. ECG findings such as AF, LA enlargement, and ST-segment abnormalities may be observed in patients with mitral regurgitation, but they are not specific.[301] Similarly, chest radiographs may identify enlargement of the left heart chambers and pulmonary vascular congestion, but such findings are not specific for mitral regurgitation.

Surgical Decision Making

Just as progress in the understanding of the pathophysiology of mitral regurgitation has evolved, so too has the surgical approach to this disease process. A high operative mortality associated with the surgical correction of mitral regurgitation in the 1980s led many clinicians to manage patients conservatively.[303,304,338] Because favorable loading conditions and high LA compliance allow even patients with significant mitral regurgitation to remain asymptomatic for long periods, it is likely that many patients did not undergo surgery until the onset of disabling symptoms. Studies show that more severe preoperative symptoms are associated with a lower EF and a greater incidence of postoperative CHF.[304,311,312] Historically, poor outcomes after surgery for mitral regurgitation might have occurred because clinicians did not appreciate the true degree of left ventricular dysfunction at the time of surgery in symptomatic patients. An EF of less than 60% in the setting of severe mitral regurgitation represents significant left ventricular dysfunction and predicts a worse outcome with surgery or medical management.[305,310] Surgical techniques common in the 1980s probably also contributed to unfavorable postoperative outcomes. For instance, although the mechanisms are incompletely understood, resection of the subvalvular apparatus contributes to decreased left ventricular systolic performance after mitral replacement.[339]

In part because of improved surgical techniques, the operative mortality rate for patients with organic mitral regurgitation who are younger than 75 years is about 1% in some centers.[310] Besides preservation of the subvalvular apparatus, valve repair represents another surgical technique associated with improved postoperative outcome.[304,340] Although not applicable to all patients, such as those with advanced rheumatic disease, the popularity of valve repairs continues to grow. Studies indicate numerous benefits associated with mitral repair. For instance, after accounting for baseline characteristics, patients who undergo mitral repair instead of replacement experience lower operative mortality and better long-term survival, largely because of improved postoperative left ventricular function.[304,340] The survival benefit that accompanies valve repair also is observed among patients undergoing combined valve and CABG surgery.[340] Valve repair does not increase the likelihood of reoperation when compared with replacement.[340] Although originally used most often for posterior leaflet disease, surgeons now routinely repair anterior mitral leaflets with good success.[341] When repairing anterior leaflet prolapse, surgeons may insert artificial chordae.[342,343] The approach to flail or prolapsing posterior mitral leaflet segments often involves resection of a portion of the leaflet.[343] In addition to resecting a portion of the leaflet and plicating the redundant tissue, an annuloplasty ring often is placed to reduce mitral orifice size and return the annulus to a more anatomic shape.[343] Some surgeons favor a flexible, partial, posterior annuloplasty band, which may allow improved systolic contraction of the posterior annulus and better postoperative left ventricular function.[332,343,344]

Timely and appropriate surgical referral helps improve the perioperative outcome of patients with mitral regurgitation. To appropriately refer patients for surgery, clinicians should have an understanding of the factors that influence surgical risk in this population.[303] The factors that correlated best with increased operative risk in patients with significant mitral regurgitation included age older than 75, severe preoperative symptoms of CHF, and concomitant CAD.[310,345,346] Even though they represent a high-risk group, patients with severe mitral regurgitation and symptoms of HF should still be referred for surgery, because valve repair or replacement offers a survival advantage compared with medical management.[303,305] Similarly, although perioperative risk remains increased, patients with evidence of left ventricular dysfunction, such as an EF less than 60% or an end-systolic left ventricular diameter greater than 45 mm, should be referred for surgery to prevent further, possibly irreversible deterioration in ventricular performance.[141,303] Asymptomatic patients without evidence of left ventricular dysfunction also should be considered for surgery if conditions such as AF, ventricular tachycardia, or pulmonary hypertension are identified or the effective regurgitant orifice is greater than 40 mm.[2,141,303] Institutional experience, particularly with techniques such as valve repair, is an important consideration for clinicians contemplating early surgical referral.[303]

Minimally Invasive Mitral Valve Surgery

Beginning in the mid-1990s, several groups adopted a minimally invasive approach to mitral valve repair.[347,348] Typically performed via lower ministernotomies or right parasternal incisions, aortic cannulation for CPB was accomplished via the chest. The venous cannula was placed either via the femoral vein[347] or the right atrium.[348] Standard surgical repair techniques were utilized. In reporting a series of 707 minimally invasive mitral valve repairs, McClure et al[347] noted an operative mortality rate of 0.4% and an incidence rate of stroke of 2%. Failed repair necessitating reoperation occurred in 4.8% of cases, with long-term follow-up demonstrating 83% survival beyond 11 years. When compared with conventional sternotomy for mitral repair, these authors also noted reductions in hospital length of stay, aortic cross-clamp time, and total CPB time in their minimally invasive cases.[347,349] Additional benefits of these minimally invasive approaches were reported by Svensson et al.[348] From a cohort of patients who underwent minimally invasive mitral repair between 1995 and 2004, the authors selected 590 cases that were matched using propensity scores with 590 patients who received mitral repair via conventional sternotomy. This study demonstrated improved pain scores and FEV$_1$ (forced expiratory volume in 1 second), together with reductions in perioperative bleeding and transfusion requirements in the minimally invasive group. Procedural success was not reduced by the adoption of a minimally invasive approach, and in fact, there was a trend toward fewer patients with 3+ or 4+ residual mitral regurgitation at 1- and 5-year follow-up in this cohort.

The trend toward even less invasive mitral repair continued in the late 1990s with the advent of thoracoscopic and robotic-assisted procedures. In 1996, Carpentier[350] performed the first video-assisted mitral valve repair via a minithoracotomy with fibrillatory arrest. The era of robotic-assisted mitral repair began the following year when Mohr[351] used a voice-controlled robotic arm or AESOP (automated endoscopic system for optimal positioning) to provide thoracoscopic visualization of the mitral valve during a repair that was accomplished through a 4-cm right thoracotomy. Then, in 1998, Carpentier used a prototype robotic system (da Vinci; Intuitive Surgical, Mountain View, CA) to perform a mitral repair.[352] Although approved 2 years earlier for general laparoscopic surgery, the da Vinci system was given FDA approval for mitral valve surgery in the United States in 2002.[353] Since that time, there has been a rapid increase in literature reports related to robotic-assisted cardiac surgery. In fact, within a 6-year period, more than 200 articles were published related to robotic-assisted cardiac surgery, including 60 from a single author.[354] Several centers have published series of more than 100 robotic cases.[355–357]

Currently, the concept of minimally invasive mitral surgery generally refers to valve repairs accomplished via a 3- or 4-cm right inframammary incision in the fourth or fifth intercostal space (Figure 19-28). Several additional, 1-cm incisions surround the primary incision and facilitate placement of robotic arms or other thoracoscopic instruments. The arterial cannula for CPB is inserted in the femoral artery (Figure 19-29). Venous cannulation is also accomplished via the femoral route using TEE guidance (Figure 19-30). Supplementary venous drainage is used in some centers by inserting either a 15 to 17 French right internal jugular vein cannula or specialized PAC with multiple end holes that drains to the venous reservoir during CPB. Cardioplegia may be given either antegrade into the aortic root or retrograde via the coronary sinus. Surgeons typically administer antegrade cardioplegia by

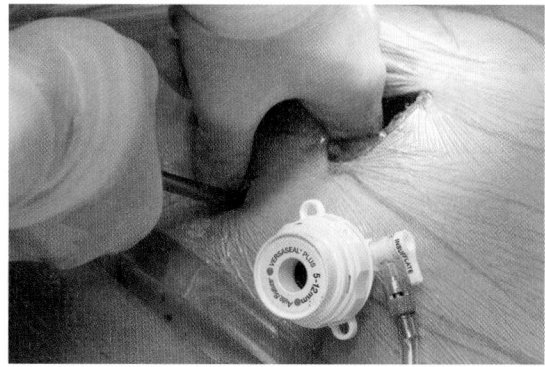

Figure 19-28 Close-up view of the chest incisions for a robotic-assisted mitral valve repair. The surgeon has inserted his left index finger into the 4-cm primary incision located in the fourth intercostal space.

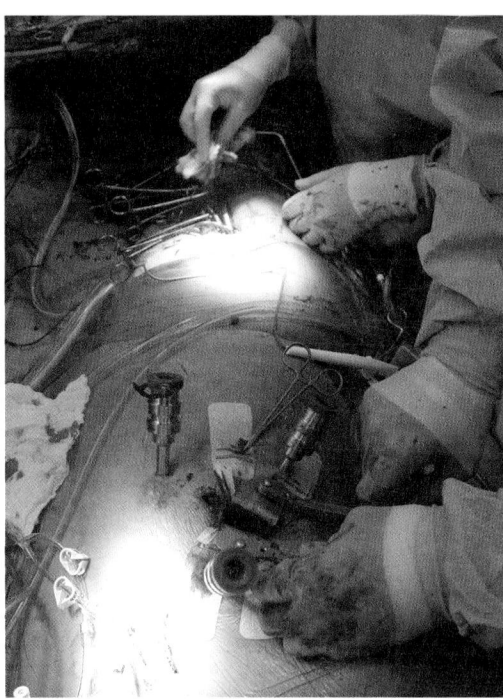

Figure 19-29 Intraoperative photograph taken from near the patient's head before robotic-assisted mitral valve repair. Femoral cannulation for cardiopulmonary bypass has been completed (top). The primary surgical incision and working ports are also shown (bottom).

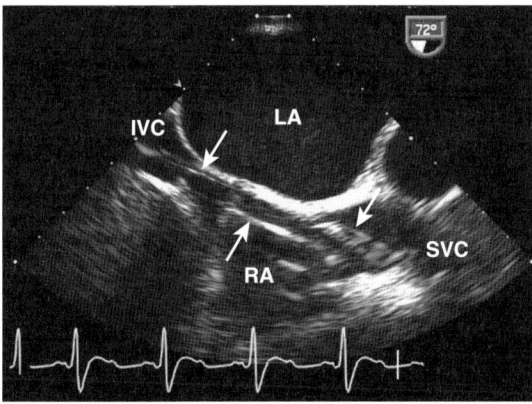

Figure 19-30 Midesophageal, bicaval, transesophageal echocardiogram demonstrating the venous cannula (*arrows*), which has been passed through the inferior vena cava (IVC), across the right atrium (RA), and into the superior vena cava (SVC). The left atrium (LA) is visualized at the top of the image.

one of two methods. The first involves the placement of a catheter tip into the ascending aorta through a right parasternal stab incision under thoracoscopic vision. This method is similar to standard antegrade cardioplegia administration in median sternotomy cases. A long-shafted aortic cross-clamp placed through a stab incision in the right lateral chest wall is used to occlude the aorta distal to the cardioplegia cannula. The second method of antegrade cardioplegia administration utilizes a specialized endoaortic cannula inserted via the femoral artery. A balloon near the distal end of this cannula is positioned in the ascending aorta using TEE guidance. Inflation of the balloon occludes the ascending aorta while antegrade cardioplegia delivery commences at the distal tip of the device. Although the choice of antegrade cardioplegia system varies between surgeons and institutions, use of the endoaortic clamp and cardioplegia delivery system have been associated with increased

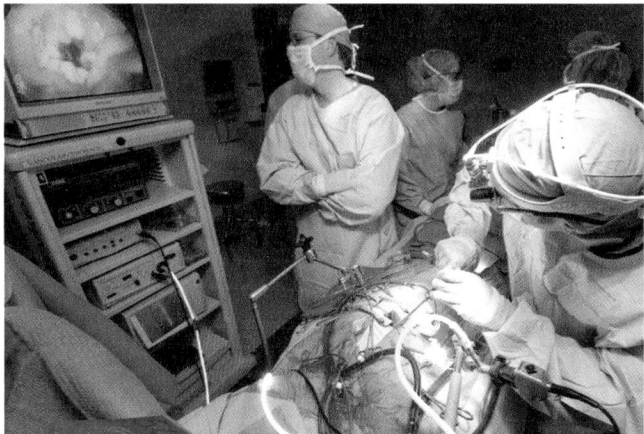

Figure 19-31 **Minimally invasive thoracoscopic mitral valve repair.** The surgeon (right) is repairing the mitral valve via a right minithoracotomy using long-shafted instruments. A thoracoscopic view of the mitral valve can be seen on the television monitor (left).

morbidity, cost, and cross-clamp times.[358] Retrograde cardioplegia may be given, if desired, by means of a coronary sinus catheter that has been percutaneously placed via the right internal jugular vein. When using a right minithoracotomy approach, the actual repair may be performed using long-handled, thoracoscopic instruments (Figure 19-31) or robotic assistance. Though referred to as "robotic," systems such as the da Vinci are probably more appropriately described as telemanipulators. As such, these devices receive direct input from the hands and feet of the surgeon who is seated at a remote console and translate these motions to end-effectors within the chest of the patient (Figure 19-32). Proponents of robotic-assisted mitral repair cite a number of advantages of this approach compared with minimally invasive thoracoscopic surgery.[353] When seated at the remote console of a robotic device, the surgeon has near-stereoscopic vision compared with viewing a 2D image on a television screen. In addition, robotic devices provide motion scaling and tremor filtration to smooth movements. Because the robotic arms have articulating "wrists" at their distal ends, the surgeon can achieve 7 degrees of freedom of movement within the chest, similar to open surgery. By comparison, long-handled thoracoscopic instruments, which are often oriented nearly parallel to one another, afford only 4 degrees of freedom. Both thoracoscopic and robotic-assisted approaches utilize the same operative techniques as standard open repairs. Thus, techniques such as leaflet resection, chordal insertion or transfer, sliding plasties, edge-to-edge repair, and annuloplasty band insertion may be used by experienced surgeons.

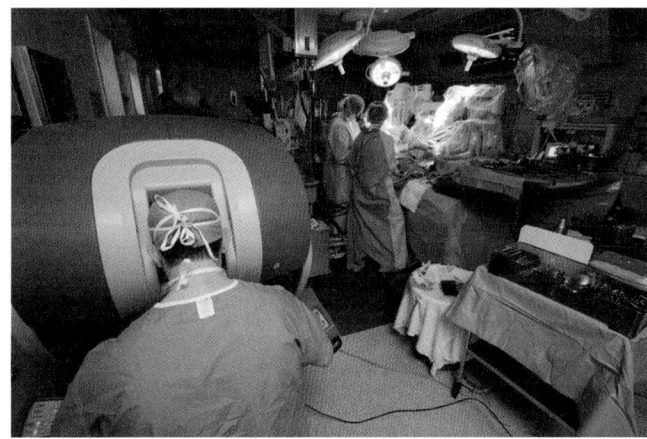

Figure 19-32 **Robotic-assisted mitral valve repair.** The surgeon (lower left) controls the robotic arms while seated at a console remote from the patient.

The procedural success and operative mortality of robotic-assisted mitral repair in larger series appear relatively comparable with traditional surgical approaches. In reporting their first 300 robotic-assisted mitral repairs, Chitwood et al[355] noted a 30-day mortality of 0.7% with a stroke rate of 0.7%. Mean CPB time was 159 minutes with a mean aortic cross-clamp time of 122 minutes. Eighty-nine concomitant procedures were performed, such as the Maze procedure and closure of atrial level shunts. At a mean follow-up of 815 days, 93% of patients were found to have residual mitral regurgitation that ranged from none to mild. Technical failure, such as annuloplasty band dehiscence, led to reoperation in 3.3% of cases. Hospital length of stay averaged 5.2 days. Cheng et al[356] recently described the outcomes of their first 120 robotic-assisted mitral repair cases. Similar to Chitwood et al,[355] Cheng et al[356] reported a 30-day mortality rate of less than 1%. Mean CPB time was 157 minutes with a mean aortic cross-clamp time of 117 minutes. Fifty-three concomitant procedures were performed in these patients. Failed repair necessitating reoperation was encountered in 5% of cases. Citing a procedural learning curve, the authors noted that all failed repairs occurred within the first 74 cases. Average hospital length of stay was 6.3 days.

Just as catheter-based techniques have been developed to treat valvular AS, efforts also are under way to develop catheter-based interventions for mitral regurgitation. Currently, the two primary percutaneous techniques under investigation involve edge-to-edge repair and annuloplasty band insertion.[359] The edge-to-edge repair, popularized in open mitral operations by Alfieri, uses a percutaneously delivered clip to secure the anterior leaflet to the posterior leaflet, thereby creating a double-orifice mitral valve. Although several proprietary devices are under development by different manufacturers, the MitraClip (Evalve, Menlo Park, CA) is currently the subject of investigation in the phase II multicenter EVEREST II (Endovascular Valve Edge-to-edge Repair Study) trial.[360]

Although transventricular devices are under investigation, the most popular approach to percutaneous mitral annuloplasty relies on the anatomic proximity of the coronary sinus to the posterior mitral annulus. Tension applied to a device anchored in the coronary sinus has effectively limited mitral annular size both in animal models and early human experience.[360]

Anesthetic Considerations

Patients who present to the operating room with mitral regurgitation may differ significantly with respect to duration of disease, symptoms, hemodynamic stability, ventricular function, and involvement of the right heart and pulmonary circulation (Box 19-4). For instance, a patient with severe mitral regurgitation caused by acute papillary muscle rupture may enter the operating room in cardiogenic shock with pulmonary congestion requiring intra-aortic balloon pump augmentation. Another patient with a newly diagnosed flail posterior mitral leaflet may enter the surgical suite with relatively preserved left ventricular function and no symptoms whatsoever. In the latter patient, the compliance of the left atrium may have prevented pulmonary vascular congestion, pulmonary hypertension, and right ventricular dysfunction. Despite the differences in presentation, the general management goals remain similar and include maintenance of forward cardiac output and reduction in the mitral regurgitant fraction. The anesthesiologist also must seek to optimize right ventricular function, in part by avoiding increases in pulmonary vascular congestion and pulmonary hypertension. Various degrees of intervention are needed

to achieve these hemodynamic management goals, depending on the patient's presentation.

Information obtained during the preoperative interview and examination provides the anesthesiologist with important insight into the patient's degree of hemodynamic compromise. For example, a patient who reports dyspnea at rest or with minimal activity may have significant pulmonary vascular congestion and possibly compromised right ventricular function. This information combined with the estimated pulmonary artery systolic pressure derived from the preoperative TTE report helps the anesthesiologist prepare for potential right-heart dysfunction intraoperatively. In such a patient, the anesthesiologist avoids heavy premedication with its attendant risk for obtundation, hypoventilation, and further increase of PAPs. Auscultation of the heart may reveal rhythm disturbances such as AF and the systolic murmur of mitral regurgitation. Clinicians should recall, however, that in cases of acute, severe mitral regurgitation, a significant increase in LA pressure decreases the systolic pressure gradient between the left heart chambers, and the murmur of mitral regurgitation may be diminished or even absent.[302]

Invasive hemodynamic monitoring provides the anesthesiologist with a wealth of important information. Arterial catheters are essential for monitoring beat-to-beat changes in blood pressure that occur in response to a variety of surgical and anesthetic manipulations. PACs facilitate many aspects of intraoperative patient management. Intraoperative use of a PAC allows the anesthesiologist to more carefully optimize left-sided filling pressures. Although the PCWP and pulmonary artery diastolic pressure depend on LA and left ventricular compliance and filling, examination of intraoperative trends in these variables enhances the ability of the anesthesiologist to provide appropriate levels of preload while avoiding volume overload. Periodic determination of cardiac output allows a more objective assessment of the patient's response to interventions such as fluid administration or inotropic infusion. The presence or size of a v wave on a PCWP tracing does not reliably correlate with the severity of mitral regurgitation, because this finding depends on LA compliance. Just as in the management of patients with aortic valvular regurgitation, another benefit of PAC insertion is the ability to introduce a ventricular pacing wire to rapidly counteract hemodynamically significant bradycardia. In patients with right ventricular compromise, monitoring trends in the CVP recording also may be helpful. Tricuspid regurgitation (TR) detected through analysis of the CVP tracing may suggest right ventricular dilatation, which may be caused by pulmonary hypertension.[361]

Intraoperative TEE provides invaluable information during the surgical correction of mitral regurgitation. It reliably identifies the mechanism of mitral regurgitation, thereby guiding the surgical approach,[362] and it objectively demonstrates the size and function of the cardiac chambers. TEE can readily identify the cause of hemodynamic derangements, facilitating proper intervention. For instance, the appearance of SAM of the mitral apparatus immediately after valve repair allows the anesthesiologist to intervene with volume infusion and medications such as esmolol or phenylephrine as appropriate. In rare circumstances when hemodynamically significant SAM persists despite these interventions, the surgeon may elect to further repair or even replace the mitral valve. TEE also identifies concomitant pathology that may warrant surgical attention, such as atrial level shunts and additional valve disease (see Chapters 12 and 13).

During minimally invasive and robotic-assisted mitral valve surgery, intraoperative TEE is essential. The use of a right minithoracotomy for these procedures precludes bypass cannulation via the chest. Instead, femoral arterial and venous cannulation are selected, with or without supplementary venous drainage from the superior vena cava or pulmonary artery. Real-time TEE imaging typically guides cannulation for CPB. If an endoaortic balloon clamp is used, the echocardiographer ensures that the balloon is correctly positioned in the ascending aorta. If a transthoracic aortic cross-clamp is chosen, the aortic cannula inserted into the femoral artery generally is not visualized with TEE. However, confirmation of guidewire placement in the descending aorta may be requested to exclude accidental passage into the

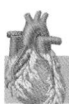

BOX 19-4. MITRAL REGURGITATION

Preload: increased
Afterload: decreased
Goal: mild tachycardia, vasodilation
Avoid: myocardial depression

contralateral iliac artery. The desired position of the tip of the femoral venous cannula is variable; some prefer the tip within the superior vena cava, whereas others select the right atrium or inferior vena cava-right atrial junction. Whatever the chosen position for the venous cannula, TEE imaging can identify a malpositioned cannula or guidewire (Figure 19-33). Tamponade after perforation of the LA appendage by a guidewire that was placed across a patent foramen ovale has been reported.[363] TEE also is invaluable during the percutaneous placement of coronary sinus catheters for retrograde cardioplegia delivery (Figure 19-34A and B). Patients who may benefit from retrograde cardioplegia, such as those with significant AR, may be identified by the intraoperative echocardiographer.

In addition to specific TEE considerations related to cannulation procedures, the selection of a minimally invasive or robotic-assisted approach to mitral repair necessitates other changes in anesthetic management. Though not universally used, one-lung ventilation is preferred in many centers. This may be achieved by the usual methods, such as a double-lumen endotracheal tube or bronchial blocker. Impaired oxygenation is not uncommon when one-lung ventilation is used during the termination of CPB during these procedures.[364] The delivery of cardioplegia requires special attention from both the surgical and anesthesia teams. If an endoaortic balloon clamp system is used, one or more methods should be used to verify its position. In addition to

TEE, some centers place arterial catheters in both the right and left radial arteries; dampening of the right radial arterial waveform could signify balloon migration toward the innominate artery. If retrograde cardioplegia is administered via a percutaneously placed catheter, its position should be well documented by TEE, with or without fluoroscopy. Coronary sinus pressure should be monitored at baseline, during balloon inflation, and during cardioplegia administration. External patches for defibrillation are generally applied before patient positioning. A multimodal approach to analgesia may facilitate early extubation in these patients. Some centers include a regional technique such as intrathecal opioids or paravertebral blocks as part of the anesthetic plan.

The intraoperative management of patients with mitral regurgitation before the institution of CPB focuses on optimizing forward cardiac output, minimizing the mitral regurgitant volume, and preventing deleterious increases in PAPs. Maintaining adequate left ventricular preload is essential. An enlarged LV that operates on a higher portion of the Frank-Starling curve requires adequate filling. At the same time, excessive volume administration is to be avoided because it may cause unwanted dilatation of the mitral annulus and worsening of the mitral regurgitation. Excessive fluid administration may precipitate right ventricular failure in patients with pulmonary vascular congestion and pulmonary hypertension. Optimization of preload is aided by analysis of data obtained from PAC measurements and TEE images. Because significant left ventricular dysfunction is present in many patients with mitral regurgitation, anesthesiologists often select specific induction and maintenance regimens to avoid further depressing left ventricular function. For this reason, large doses of narcotics have been popular in the past.[151,152] Other researchers have shown that smaller doses of narcotics combined with vasodilating inhalation anesthetics also produce acceptable intraoperative hemodynamics.[365,366] By reducing the amount of narcotics administered, the addition of a vasodilating inhalation agent to the anesthetic regimen may allow for faster extubation of the trachea after surgery. With the current trend toward early referral of asymptomatic patients for mitral repair, anesthetic regimens that reduce the duration of postoperative mechanical ventilation may be advantageous.

In patients with severe left ventricular dysfunction, infusions of inotropic medications such as dopamine, dobutamine, or even epinephrine may be required to maintain an adequate cardiac output. Phosphodiesterase inhibitors such as milrinone also may augment systolic ventricular performance and reduce pulmonary and peripheral vascular resistances. By reducing pulmonary and

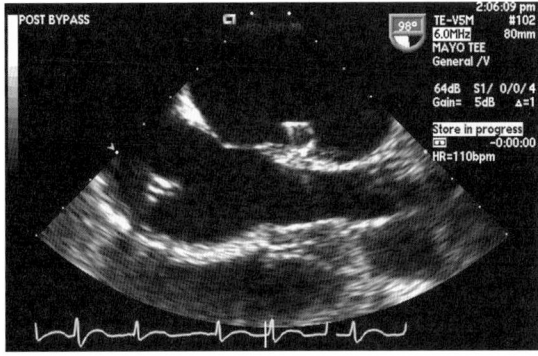

Figure 19-33 Midesophageal, bicaval, transesophageal echocardiogram demonstrating the J-tipped guidewire for the femoral venous cannula crossing a patent foramen ovale.

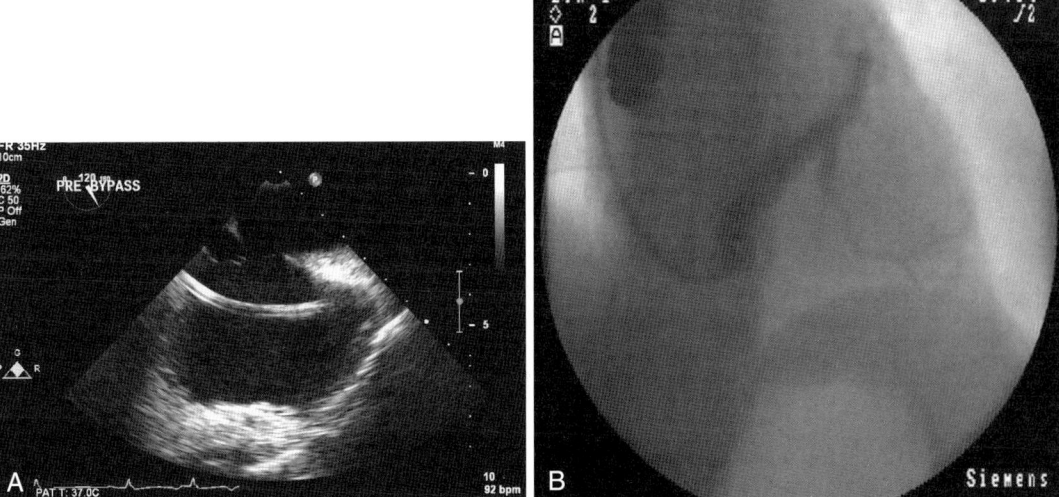

Figure 19-34 *A,* Modified midesophageal, bicaval, transesophageal echocardiogram demonstrating a percutaneously placed coronary sinus catheter entering the coronary sinus (left side). *B,* Intraoperative fluoroscopic image taken after contrast injection into the distal tip of a correctly placed coronary sinus catheter.

peripheral vascular resistance, forward cardiac output is facilitated. Nitroglycerin and sodium nitroprusside represent two additional options for reducing the impedance to ventricular ejection. If patients prove refractory to inotropic and vasodilator therapy, insertion of an intra-aortic balloon pump should be strongly considered (see Chapters 10, 13, 27, 32, and 34).

Manipulation of the heart rate may be necessary in some patients to optimize hemodynamics. Bradycardia generally should be avoided because slower heart rates allow for larger filling volumes, potentially resulting in left ventricular distention and mitral annular dilatation. Regurgitant volumes may increase at slower heart rates. Slightly increased heart rates, especially when combined with increased left ventricular contractility, favor a smaller mitral annular area and may decrease the regurgitant fraction. Sinus rhythm and preserved atrial contraction are less important in patients with mitral regurgitation compared with patients with stenotic valves. Mitral annular dilatation accompanies most cases of long-standing mitral regurgitation. Patients with pure mitral regurgitation generally have no impedance to left ventricular filling, and AF usually is better tolerated than in patients with stenotic lesions.

Because severe mitral regurgitation may result in pulmonary hypertension and right ventricular dysfunction, anesthesiologists should tailor their intraoperative management strategies accordingly. Hypercapnia, hypoxia, and acidosis increase PAPs and should be avoided. Mild hyperventilation may be beneficial in some patients. The effect of nitrous oxide on pulmonary vascular resistance (PVR) and pulmonary hypertension is controversial. Some studies show no change in PVR when administered to anesthetized patients with CAD or VHD.[367–369] Other studies in patients with MS demonstrate an increase in PVR after nitrous oxide administration, and in vitro evidence suggests that nitrous oxide increases norepinephrine release from the pulmonary artery.[370–372]

Patients with severe right ventricular dysfunction after CPB can prove exceptionally difficult to manage. Besides avoiding the factors known to increase PVR, only a few options exist for these patients. Inotropic agents with vasodilating properties such as dobutamine, isoproterenol, and milrinone augment right ventricular systolic performance and decrease PVR, but their use often is confounded by systemic hypotension. Prostaglandin E_1 (PGE$_1$) reliably reduces PVR and undergoes extensive first-pass metabolism in the pulmonary circulation.[373,374] Although PGE$_1$ reduces PAPs after CPB, systemic hypotension requiring infusions of vasoconstrictors through an LA catheter also has occurred.[375–378] Inhaled nitric oxide represents another alternative available for the treatment of right ventricular failure in the setting of pulmonary hypertension. Nitric oxide reliably relaxes the pulmonary vasculature and is then immediately bound to hemoglobin and inactivated. Studies indicate that systemic hypotension during nitric oxide therapy is unlikely.[379,380] (See Chapter 24.)

Left ventricular dysfunction also may contribute to post-CPB hemodynamic instability. With mitral competence restored, the low-pressure outlet for left ventricular ejection is removed. The enlarged LV must then eject entirely into the aorta. Because left ventricular enlargement leads to increased wall stress, a condition of increased afterload often exists after CPB. At the same time, the preload augmentation inherent to mitral regurgitation is removed. It is, therefore, not surprising that the systolic performance of the LV often declines after surgical correction of mitral regurgitation. Treatment options in the immediate post-CPB period include inotropic and vasodilator therapy and, if necessary, intra-aortic balloon pump augmentation.

MITRAL STENOSIS

Clinical Features and Natural History

Clinically significant MS in adult patients usually is a result of rheumatic disease. Congenital abnormalities of the mitral valve represent a rare cause of MS in younger patients. Other uncommon conditions that do not directly involve the mitral valve apparatus but may limit left

ventricular inflow and simulate the clinical findings of MS include cor triatriatum, large LA neoplasms, and pulmonary vein obstruction.[381]

A decades-long asymptomatic period characterizes the initial phase of rheumatic MS. Symptoms rarely appear until the normal mitral valve area of 4 to 6 cm^2 (Figure 19-35) has been reduced to 2.5 cm^2 or less.[382] When the mitral valve area reaches 1.5 to 2.5 cm^2, symptoms usually occur only in association with exercise or other conditions such as fever, pregnancy, or AF, that lead to increases in heart rate or cardiac output.[383,384] After the mitral valve area decreases to less than 1.5 cm^2, symptoms may develop at rest. Some patients are able to remain asymptomatic for long periods by gradually reducing their level of activity.[381] Patients with MS commonly report dyspnea as their initial symptom, a finding reflective of increased LA pressure and pulmonary congestion. In addition to dyspnea, patients may report palpitations that signal the onset of AF. Systemic thromboembolization occurs in 10% to 20% of patients with MS and does not appear to be correlated with the mitral valve area or LA size.[383] Chest pain that simulates angina is present in a small number of patients with MS and may result from RVH rather than CAD.[383]

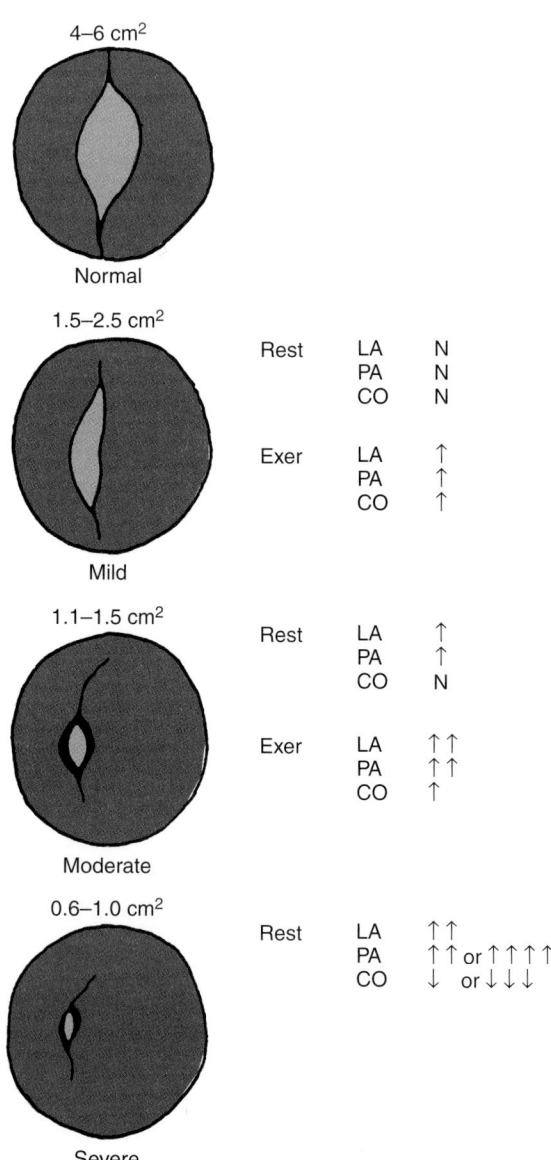

Figure 19-35   Hemodynamic changes with progressive narrowing of the mitral valve. CO, cardiac output; LA, left atrium; PA, pulmonary artery. (*From Rapaport E: Natural history of aortic and mitral valve disease. Am J Cardiol 35:221, 1971.*)

There has been a change in the typical age of presentation of patients with MS.[383] Previously, patients, often women, presented with MS while in their 20s and 30s.[383,385,386] Since the early 1990s, perhaps because of more slowly progressive disease in the United States, patients have been presenting in their 40s and 50s.[383,387,388] After symptoms develop, MS remains a slow, progressive disease. Often, patients live 10 to 20 years with mild symptoms, such as dyspnea with exercise, before disabling NYHA Class III and IV symptoms develop. The symptomatic state of the patient predicts the clinical outcome. For instance, the 10-year survival rate of patients with mild symptoms approaches 80%, but the 10-year survival rate of patients with disabling symptoms is only 15% without surgery.[383,388–390]

Pathophysiology

Rheumatic MS results in valve leaflet thickening and fusion of the commissures. Later in the disease process, leaflet calcification and subvalvular chordal fusion may occur.[383] These changes combine to reduce the effective mitral valve area and limit diastolic flow into the LV. As a result of the fixed obstruction to left ventricular inflow, LA pressures increase. Elevated LA pressures limit pulmonary venous drainage and result in increased PAPs.[310] Over time, pulmonary arteriolar hypertrophy develops in response to chronically increased pulmonary vascular pressures.[311] Pulmonary hypertension may trigger increases in RVEDV and RVEDP, and in some patients, signs of right ventricular failure such as ascites or peripheral edema may appear.[385,386] LA enlargement is an almost-universal finding in patients with established MS and is a risk factor for the development of AF.

Patients with MS tolerate tachycardia particularly poorly. Left ventricular inflow, already limited by a mechanically abnormal valve, is further compromised by the disproportionate decline in the diastolic period that accompanies tachycardia. The flow rate across the stenotic valve must increase to maintain left ventricular filling in a shorter diastolic period. Because the valve area remains constant, the pressure gradient between the LA and LV increases by the square of the increase in the flow rate, according to the Gorlin formula, in which PG is the transvalvular pressure gradient:

$$\text{Valve area} = \text{Transvalvular flow rate}/\text{Constant} \times \sqrt{PG}$$

Tachycardia necessitates a significant increase in the transvalvular pressure gradient and may precipitate feelings of breathlessness in awake patients. In patients with AF, it is the increased ventricular rate that is most deleterious, rather than the loss of atrial contraction.[312] Although coordinated atrial activity is always preferable, the primary goal in treating patients with MS and AF should be control of the ventricular rate.

MS results in diminished left ventricular preload reserve. As seen in the pressure-volume loop in Figure 19-36, LVEDV and LVEDP are reduced with an accompanying decline in SV. Controversy exists, however, regarding the contractile state of the LV in these patients. Gash et al[391] reported that almost one third of their study population of patients with MS had an EF less than 50%. Limited preload may contribute to a reduced EF in some of these patients. However, the observation that left ventricular contractile impairment persists after surgery in some patients suggests that other causes of left ventricular dysfunction may exist. Rheumatic myocarditis has been reported, although its role in producing left ventricular contractile dysfunction is uncertain.[391] Other investigators have described posterobasal regional wall motion abnormalities, perhaps a consequence of thickening and calcification of the mitral apparatus.[314,315] Vasoconstriction occurring in response to diminished CO also may impair left ventricular ejection.[392] Afterload also may be increased because of inadequate myocardial wall thickness.[391] The lack of adequate wall thickness leads to elevations in wall stress in accordance with the law of Laplace.

In addition to abnormalities in systolic function, patients with MS may have impaired diastolic function. MS creates an obvious impairment of left ventricular diastolic filling. However, the intrinsic

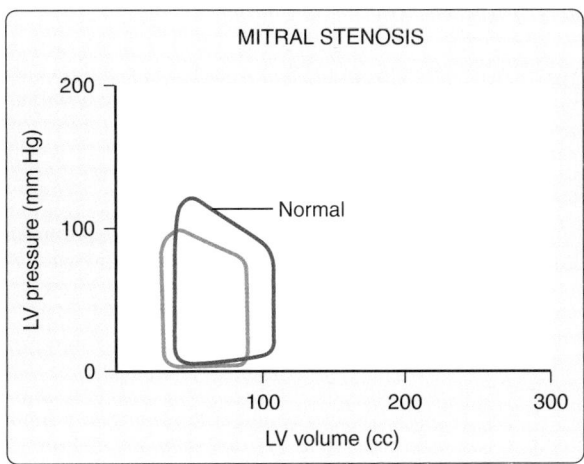

Figure 19-36 **Pressure-volume loop in mitral stenosis.** LV, left ventricular. *(From Jackson JM, Thomas SJ, Lowenstein E: Anesthetic management of patients with valvular heart disease. Semin Anesth 1:239, 1982.)*

compliance of the LV also may be reduced by the rheumatic disease process. Using conductance catheter and micromanometer techniques, Liu et al[393] discovered decreased left ventricular compliance in a group of patients with MS scheduled for mitral balloon valvuloplasty. On repeat measurements taken immediately after valvuloplasty, the investigators observed a significant increase in left ventricular compliance. Because the increase in compliance occurred immediately after valvuloplasty, the physicians hypothesized that the changes associated with rheumatic MS create an internal constraint that limits left ventricular compliance.

Assessment of Mitral Stenosis

As for patients with mitral regurgitation, echocardiography represents the diagnostic modality of choice for patients with suspected MS.[381,394,395] Two-dimensional and Doppler echocardiographic techniques are able to accurately and noninvasively measure the transvalvular pressure gradient and mitral valve area. Because the pressure gradient varies with the flow rate and diastolic period, the assessment of MS severity ideally should be based on the measured or calculated mitral valve area.[381] Echocardiographic methods used to obtain mitral valve area include the pressure half-time technique, the continuity equation, planimetry of the valve orifice, and PISA analysis. Other invaluable information obtained during an echocardiographic study includes the size and function of the ventricle and an estimation of the PAP.

Exercise echocardiography can be used when the patient's symptoms and the resting echocardiographic data are discordant.[394] In such cases, echocardiography may be performed while the patient exercises on a supine bicycle. If during exercise the transmitral gradient or PAP increases significantly, MS is the likely cause of the patient's symptoms.[394]

With the accuracy and widespread use of echocardiography, cardiac catheterization and invasive measurements of hemodynamics are almost never necessary.[383,395] Even patients referred for preoperative coronary angiography need not undergo invasive hemodynamic studies at the time of catheterization if adequate echocardiographic data already have been obtained.[395] Catheter-based hemodynamic assessments are reserved for situations in which echocardiographic studies are suboptimal or conflict with the clinical picture because invasive mitral valve hemodynamic studies are complex and limited.[383] For instance, a transseptal puncture is required to measure the LA-to-LV pressure gradient directly and entails risks such as tamponade, aortic injury, and heart block.[383] If the PCWP is used in place of direct LA pressure measurements, the gradient derived is less accurate than that obtained with Doppler echocardiography.[319]

Similar to patients with mitral regurgitation, nonspecific findings commonly are seen on electrocardiograms and chest radiographs in patients with MS. Potential ECG findings include AF and LA enlargement. Radiographs may also reveal LA enlargement and pulmonary vascular congestion.

Surgical Decision Making

Appropriate referral of patients for surgical intervention requires integration of clinical and echocardiographic data. Patients presenting with severe symptoms (i.e., NYHA Class III and IV) should be immediately referred for surgery because their outcome is poor if treated medically.[313,383] Patients with only mild MS and few or no symptoms may be managed conservatively with periodic evaluation. Patients who are asymptomatic but have moderate MS (i.e., mitral valve area between 1.0 and 1.5 cm²) require careful assessment. If significant pulmonary hypertension (i.e., pulmonary artery systolic pressure > 50 mm Hg) is present, surgical intervention should be considered.[313] Intervention also may be indicated if a patient becomes symptomatic or PAPs increase significantly during exercise testing.[383]

The surgical options for treating MS continue to evolve. Closed commissurotomy, in which the surgeon fractures fused mitral commissures, was first performed in the 1920s. It became popular in the 1940s and still is used to treat MS in developing countries.[394] With the advent of CPB in the 1950s, techniques of open commissurotomy developed, allowing the surgeon to directly inspect the valve before splitting the commissures.[394] The common goals of closed and open mitral commissurotomy include increasing the effective mitral valve area and decreasing the LA-to-LV pressure gradient, with a resultant relief in the patient's symptoms.

Percutaneous mitral commissurotomy (PMC) allows a less invasive, catheter-based approach to MS. First reported by Inoue in 1984,[396] clinicians worldwide perform PMC more than 10,000 times each year.[397] The technique of PMC involves directing a balloon-tipped catheter across the stenotic mitral valve. Specifically designed balloons allow sequential inflation of the distal and proximal portions of the balloon, ensuring correct positioning across the mitral valve before the middle portion of the device is inflated to split the fused commissures.[398] Patient selection for PMC requires careful echocardiographic evaluation. Echocardiographic grading scales have been developed to evaluate mitral leaflet mobility, thickness, calcification, and subvalvular fusion.[399] Patients who score favorably on such echocardiographic assessments (i.e., adequate leaflet mobility with little calcification) may be referred for PMC. Success rates for PMC are similar to those achieved with surgical commissurotomy, and most patients experience a doubling in the effective mitral valve area.[394] An increase in the amount of mitral regurgitation represents the most common complication associated with PMC.[394]

Not all patients are candidates for surgical commissurotomy or PMC. For instance, those with heavily calcified valves or significant mitral regurgitation are likely to experience suboptimal results after commissurotomy. Mitral valve anatomy unsuitable for PMC is more commonly encountered in Western countries, where patients with MS typically present at an older average age.[397] Mitral valve replacement commonly is recommended for these patients. The risk for mitral valve replacement depends on patient characteristics such as age, functional status, and other comorbid conditions.[394] Surgical risk in younger patients with few coexisting medical problems generally is less than 5%. Conversely, surgical risk in elderly patients with severe symptoms related to MS and multiple comorbidities may be 10% to 20%.[394]

Anesthetic Considerations

Several important goals should guide the anesthetic management of patients with significant MS. First, the anesthesiologist should seek to prevent tachycardia and treat it promptly if it develops in the perioperative period (Box 19-5). Maintenance of left ventricular preload without exacerbation of pulmonary vascular congestion represents a

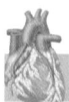

BOX 19-5. MITRAL STENOSIS

Preload: normal or increased
Afterload: normal
Goal: controlled ventricular response
Avoid: tachycardia, pulmonary vasoconstriction

second management goal. Third, anesthesiologists should avoid factors that aggravate pulmonary hypertension and impair right ventricular function.

Prevention and treatment of tachycardia are central to the perioperative management of these patients. Tachycardia shortens the diastolic filling period. An elevation in transvalvular flow rate is required with a resultant increase in the LA-to-LV pressure gradient to maintain left ventricular preload with a shortened diastolic period. Avoidance of tachycardia begins in the preoperative period. Anxiety-induced tachycardia may be treated with small doses of narcotics or benzodiazepines. However, excessive sedation is counterproductive because sedative-induced hypoventilation can result in hypoxemia or hypercarbia, potentially aggravating a patient's underlying pulmonary hypertension, and because large doses of premedication can jeopardize the patient's already limited left ventricular preload. Appropriate monitoring and supplemental oxygen therapy should be considered for patients receiving preoperative narcotics or benzodiazepines. Medications taken by the patient before surgery to control heart rate, such as digitalis, β-blockers, calcium-receptor antagonists, or amiodarone, should be continued in the perioperative period. Additional doses of β-blockers and calcium-receptor antagonists may be required intraoperatively, particularly to control the ventricular rate in patients with AF. Control of the ventricular rate remains the primary goal in managing patients with AF, although cardioversion should not be withheld from patients with atrial tachyarrhythmias who become hemodynamically unstable. Narcotic-based anesthetics often are helpful in avoiding intraoperative tachycardia. However, clinicians should realize these patients may be receiving other vagotonic drugs, and that profound bradycardia is possible in response to large doses of narcotics.[326,327] The selection of a muscle relaxant such as pancuronium may help prevent the unwanted bradycardia associated with high-dose narcotics.

Maintenance of preload is another important goal for managing patients who have a fixed obstruction to left ventricular filling. Appropriate replacement of blood loss and prevention of excessive anesthetic-induced venodilation help preserve hemodynamic stability intraoperatively. Invasive hemodynamic monitoring allows the anesthesiologist to maintain adequate preload while avoiding excessive fluid administration that could aggravate pulmonary vascular congestion. Placement of an arterial catheter facilitates timely recognition of hemodynamic derangements. PACs can be invaluable in the management of patients with significant MS. Even though the PCWP overestimates left ventricular filling and the pulmonary artery diastolic pressure may not accurately reflect left-heart volume in patients with pulmonary hypertension, examination of trends and responses to intervention can be more readily assessed. Tachycardia increases the pressure gradient between the left atrium and LV. Increased heart rates widen the discrepancy between the PCWP and the true LVEDP. Despite these limitations, the PAC remains a useful monitoring tool, providing information on cardiac output and PAPs. As anesthesiologists gain an increasing appreciation for the role of intraoperative TEE, this powerful imaging modality will no doubt be used more frequently to assess ventricular filling and function.

Many patients with MS present with pulmonary hypertension. Anesthetic techniques that avoid increases in PVR are likely to benefit these patients and prevent additional right ventricular embarrassment. Meticulous attention to arterial blood gas results allows appropriate adjustment of ventilatory parameters. Vasodilator therapy in patients with pulmonary hypertension generally is ineffective because the venodilation produced further limits left ventricular filling and does not improve cardiac output. The only MS patients who may benefit from vasodilator therapy are those with concomitant mitral regurgitation, or those with severe pulmonary hypertension and right ventricular dysfunction in whom pulmonary vasodilation can facilitate transpulmonary blood flow and improve left ventricular filling.[325] The treatment of right ventricular dysfunction has been discussed in preceding sections.

TRICUSPID REGURGITATION

Clinical Features and Natural History

Surgical tricuspid disease is caused by a structural defect in the valve apparatus or is a functional lesion. Functional TR is far more common and usually results from right ventricular overload and tricuspid annular dilation. Left-sided valvular disease, usually mitral regurgitation, most commonly is responsible. Functional tricuspid incompetence also can result from MS, AR, or AS, or from isolated pulmonary hypertension. When mitral regurgitation is severe enough to warrant valve repair or replacement, TR may be present in 30% to 50% of patients.[400–402]

TR also may be caused by structural defects as in rheumatic valve disease, carcinoid syndrome, endocarditis, Epstein's anomaly, or trauma.[403,404] In rheumatic disease, histologic involvement of the tricuspid valve may occur in 46% of patients, but it is rarely clinically severe, and in these cases, the valve usually is also stenotic.[56,405] TR also has been described in association with CAD as a result of ischemia, infarction, or rupture of the right ventricular papillary muscles.[406]

Another cause of structural tricuspid valve defects may be occurring with increasing frequency. Although this has not been reported in the literature, at some institutions, such as that of the authors, there appears to be an increasing incidence of isolated tricuspid insufficiency related to long-standing transvenous pacemaker wires. Given the rapid escalation of the use of pacemakers and the aging of the population, this result is expected. This is occurring in the absence of endocarditis. The presence of the pacemaker wire tends to scar and tether one of the tricuspid leaflets. Historically, isolated tricuspid repair or replacement has been uncommon, but physicians may see more of this procedure for this reason.

Symptoms of isolated tricuspid insufficiency are usually minor in the absence of concurrent pulmonary hypertension. Intravenous drug abusers who experience development of tricuspid endocarditis are the classic example. In these patients, structural damage to the valve may be quite severe, but because they are free of other cardiac disease, they can tolerate complete excision of the tricuspid valve with few adverse effects.[407] Excision of the tricuspid valve in endocarditis has been common because of the undesirability of placing a valve prosthesis in a region of infection.[404] Surgical annuloplasty may be a better long-term option if the valve is structurally salvageable. Another factor that broadly favors tricuspid repair rather than replacement is the high incidence of thrombotic complications with a valve in this position. The lower pressure and flow state on the right side of the heart are responsible for this phenomenon. Increasingly, valve replacement in the tricuspid area is relegated to those patients who truly have unreconstructable rheumatic valve disease, totally destroyed tricuspid valves from endocarditis, or rare congenital lesions.[408–414] This is true because the literature shows improved longer-term outcomes with valve repair over replacement.[415]

In chronic TR caused by right ventricular dilation, the clinical scenario often is much different from that of isolated tricuspid disease. The major hemodynamic derangements are usually those of the associated mitral or aortic valve disease. The RV dilates in the face of the afterload stress from long-standing pulmonary hypertension, and the resultant increase in end-diastolic fiber stretch (i.e., preload reserve) promotes increases in SV mediated by the Starling mechanism. These increases are negated by a concurrently increasing right ventricular afterload, however, because of relatively inadequate RVH.[416] Regurgitation

through the tricuspid valve reduces right ventricular wall tension at the price of a decrease in effective forward SV.

An important corollary of right ventricular chamber enlargement is the possibility of a leftward shift of the interventricular septum and encroachment on the left ventricular cavity.[417] This phenomenon can reduce the left ventricular chamber size and the slope of the left ventricular diastolic pressure-volume curve, rendering the LV less compliant.[418–420] Septal encroachment may mask left ventricular underfilling by decreasing left ventricular compliance, thereby artificially increasing LVEDP. A failing right ventricular underloads the left side by reduced effective SV and anatomic (septal shift) mechanisms.

Right ventricular failure may be relatively mild early in the course of functional TR, but over time, the regurgitation will worsen, with further dilation leading to further right ventricular volume overload and chamber enlargement, which may worsen the tricuspid incompetence.[403] As in mitral regurgitation, the incompetent tricuspid valve serves as a pop-off circulation during right ventricular systole, and over time, the capacitance of the right atrium and vena cavae can increase dramatically. Untreated, this eventually leads to systemic venous congestion, hepatic congestion, severe peripheral edema, and ascites. Because tricuspid insufficiency in the absence of pulmonary hypertension is rare, it has been difficult to demonstrate that chronic volume overload and ventricular dilation result in right ventricular cardiomyopathy. However, when right ventricular volume overload occurs in the context of pulmonic valve insufficiency, right ventricular failure results from volume overload.[421] Clinical experience supports the presumption of right ventricular cardiomyopathy in severe TR as well. In late tricuspid insufficiency, right ventricular function can decline when tricuspid valve repair renders the valve competent.

Surgical Decision Making

In structural tricuspid insufficiency, the decision to repair or replace the valve is straightforward. The same cannot be said of functional TR. Because most functional cases are the consequence of left-sided valve lesions with right ventricular overload, the TR usually improves significantly after the aortic or mitral valve is repaired or replaced, typically at least one grade. It can be unclear in the operating room whether addition of a tricuspid procedure to the left-sided valve surgery is indicated. In this situation, intraoperative TEE plays an essential role. If the TR is severe in the pre-CPB assessment, tricuspid valve surgery is almost always performed.[400] However, the evidence is less clear when the regurgitation is graded as moderate. Some surgeons choose to repair the tricuspid with moderate regurgitation, but others advocate observation.[400,402,422] It is common with moderate or moderate-to-severe TR, in the context of left-sided valve surgery, to complete the left-sided procedure and then reassess the tricuspid valve with TEE when the heart is full and ejecting.[423,424] If the regurgitation remains more than moderate after the left-sided valve is fixed, many surgeons then do the tricuspid procedure. If the regurgitation is moderate or less, the appropriate surgical course may remain unclear. Some patients having left-sided valve procedures must return to the operating room in the future for tricuspid surgery, and data from the Mayo Clinic suggest that this problem may be increasing.[425] When this occurs, the morbidity and mortality rates are probably significantly increased over what would have been experienced were the tricuspid valve fixed at the time of the aortic or mitral valve procedure. Decision making in functional TR is made more complicated by the inability to rigorously quantify the severity of the regurgitation and right ventricular dysfunction.[425] When regurgitation is severe or mild, the assessment of the severity of TR is not critical to surgical decision making, but determinations from mild to moderate and moderate to severe are essential.

As with mitral regurgitation and the LV, the presence of significant TR makes right ventricular function difficult to assess because the regurgitant fraction leads to a falsely increased EF. In the absence of sophisticated echocardiographic assessments, such as determination of rate of right ventricular pressure increase with pulsed Doppler, it is common to look at enlarged right ventricular chamber size and any decrease in

RVEF as indicators of decompensation.[425,426] Clinical experience suggests that pulmonary hypertension also is likely to be a marker for right ventricular failure after tricuspid surgery, but studies of sufficient size are still lacking. Like assessment of right ventricular function, grading of severity of TR is at best semiquantitative. Color-flow mapping of the volume of the regurgitant jet within the right atrium is standard,[415] and this can be supplemented by looking for systolic flow reversal in the portal veins using pulsed-wave Doppler.[427] Even though the assessment of residual TR after left-sided valve surgery is important, the tricuspid valve is sometimes difficult to examine with TEE, and the presence of an aortic or, particularly, a mitral mechanical prosthesis makes this assessment more difficult.

Anesthetic Considerations

Because most tricuspid surgery occurs in the context of significant aortic or mitral disease, anesthetic management primarily is determined by the left-sided valve lesion. The exception to this is when significant pulmonary hypertension and right ventricular failure are present. Under these conditions, the primary impediment to hemodynamic stability after surgery will be right ventricular failure rather than the left-sided process.

If right ventricular dysfunction is predicted, it is useful to place a PAC, even if the tricuspid valve will be replaced. Even if the PAC has to be removed because of tricuspid valve replacement, it still can be helpful to obtain CO and PAPs before CPB to get insight into right ventricular function and anticipate the hemodynamic support that may be required. A PAC is also of greater use than a CVP alone because the CVP is a poor index of intravascular filling and the degree of TR. This is true because the atrium and vena cavae are highly compliant and will accept large regurgitant volumes with relatively little change in pressure. A PAC also is useful even if intraoperative TEE is used. As in aortic insufficiency with the LV, the RV in chronic TR is volume overloaded and dilated, and requires a large EDV to maintain forward flow. At the same time, because of the unreliability of the CVP as an indicator of filling, it is possible to volume overload patients with TR and right ventricular failure. Cardiac output in right ventricular failure often can be augmented with the use of vasodilators, and even though right ventricular dimensions can be followed intraoperatively with TEE, maximizing cardiac output (sometimes at the cost of systemic arterial pressure) is best done with serial CO measurements (as in AR). Whenever there is significant right ventricular distention, the possibility of septal shift and secondary deterioration of left ventricular diastolic compliance should be carefully considered. Echocardiography is uniquely helpful for this assessment.

The post-CPB management of the patient undergoing an isolated tricuspid valve procedure is usually straightforward. These patients usually do not have significant right ventricular failure or pulmonary hypertension and typically require only a brief period of CPB without aortic cross-clamping. A larger group of patients, particularly those with TR related to AS, typically come off CPB with little need for support of the RV. These patients often do well because the improvement in left ventricular function after AVR for AS is usually sufficient to reduce PAPs significantly and offload the right heart. When the left-sided valve surgery is for mitral disease, the improvement usually is not as marked, and greater degrees of inotropic support of the RV often are indicated. The combination of a phosphodiesterase inhibitor with a vasodilator and a catecholamine infusion is useful. Serial CO measurements to balance systemic pressure and right ventricular output and filling are critical.

A few other practical points on tricuspid valve repair and replacement should be made. First, because right-sided pressures can be chronically increased with TR, it is important to look for a patent foramen ovale and the potential for right-to-left shunting before initiation of CPB. Second, intravascular volume may be quite high in this patient population, and it is often practical to avoid red blood cell transfusion by hemofiltration during bypass. Third, if significant right ventricular dysfunction is present or there is peripheral edema or ascites, there is the potential for a coagulopathy related to liver congestion, and the patient should be managed accordingly. Fourth, it is important to ensure that central venous catheters, particularly PACs, are not entrapped in right atrial suture lines.

INNOVATIONS IN VALVE REPAIR

Interventional cardiology has had a significant impact on the volume of CABG, and it can be predicted that interventional cardiology will alter surgery for VHD over time. Multiple, less invasive approaches to mitral valve repair are in animal or clinical trials, and tremendous inroads have been made in percutaneous replacement of the aortic valve. Innovations in surgical valve repair also are being made. These include aortic valve repair, and closed- and open-chamber procedures for mitral regurgitation.

Aortic Valve Repair

Over the last several years there has been a major shift from valve replacement to valve repair in degenerative mitral valve disease. The same has not been true of the aortic valve, in part because the valve disease is different in the majority of patients, but also because the high flow and pressure conditions across the aortic valve make repair more prone to failure. That said, aortic valve repair is being increasingly done as an appropriate patient population is being defined. Although valve repair for AR has found broader use when regurgitation is associated with dissection or dilation of the aortic root,[428,429] isolated valve repair has been less common. A growing body of data suggests that aortic valve repair may offer advantages over valve replacement in younger individuals with AR secondary to bicuspid valves.[428,430] In contrast with AVR, this eliminates the need for anticoagulation for a mechanical valve and should delay the need for reoperation unlike if a tissue valve would have been placed. When regurgitation occurs with a bicuspid valve, the insufficiency usually is caused by retraction or prolapse, or both, of the conjoined cusp, and repair consists of triangular incision to shorten and elevate that cusp to improve apposition. Although very long-term follow-up has not been reported, in a large series from the Mayo Clinic, with a mean follow-up of 4.2 years, late failure of the repair requiring reoperation occurred in 14 of 160 consecutive patients, with most of that failure occurring from repairs done in the first decade of the 15-year experience.[428]

As a result of this experience, aortic valve repair is likely to find increasing application in this patient population. For this group, anesthetic management usually is straightforward, although the clinical indications for valve repair in AR are the same as those for valve replacement. The compelling issue for the anesthesiologist in these cases is echocardiographic assessment of the valve for suitability of repair and the adequacy of the repair after the procedure.

New Techniques for Mitral Valve Repair

Mitral regurgitation frequently is associated with CHF. In dilated and ischemic cardiomyopathy, enlargement of the mitral annulus results in a failure of coaptation of the mitral leaflets and valve incompetence. Although cardiac surgery is an effective treatment, morbidity with operation can be high. Three different approaches have been developed to address mitral regurgitation occurring in the absence of structural mitral pathology. These approaches address the failure of leaflet coaptation at either the level of the valve leaflets, the valve annulus, or by altering the anatomic relation of the septal and lateral walls of the LV.

Mitral Leaflet Repair

Alfieri and colleagues[431] showed that mitral regurgitation could be improved using an edge-to-edge technique in which mitral valve leaflets are brought together by a central suture. This approach led to a catheter-based technology, which, by apposing the edges of a regurgitant MV, results in edge-to-edge repair.

The MitraClip device (Evalve, Menlo Park, CA) consists of a catheter-mounted clip that is placed using a femoral venous and trans-septal approach.[432] Under general anesthesia (GA) with echocardiographic and fluoroscopic guidance, the clip is placed to achieve apposition of the central portion of the anterior and posterior leaflets. If the severity of mitral regurgitation is not reduced, the device can be opened and repositioned. Animal studies show incorporation of the device into the leaflets at 6 to 10 weeks with persistent coaptation.[432] The clinical trials of the Phase I EVEREST trial reported results for 6 months in a population of 27 patients.[433] Of 27 patients, 24 underwent clip placement, and of those, 6 needed open surgical repair, 3 (12.5%) had unresolved mitral regurgitation, and 3 had partial clip detachment for a total failure rate of 25% (Figure 19-37). Of the 18 remaining patients, 13 had ≤2+ mitral regurgitation at 6 months and 5 had ≥3+ mitral regurgitation.

The results of the EVEREST MitraClip trial do not compare favorably with surgery, in which results are much better. This conclusion is further supported because patient selection for the MitraClip trial included patients who would have had predictably good surgical results (56% P2 prolapse or flail and 40% bileaflet prolapse or flail). That said, there may still be a place for this technology in high-risk patients who are poor surgical candidates or as part of combined hybrid procedures (limited coronary revascularization plus MitraClip) when an improvement in functional status without a perfect surgical result may be appropriate (see Chapter 26).

The EVEREST 2 trial is an ongoing, multicenter trial directly comparing MitraClip results with surgical mitral repair in a 2:1 randomization. Results of that trial will add information about the clinical applicability of this technology.

Percutaneous Transvenous Mitral Annuloplasty

The second type of approach to functional mitral regurgitation is alteration of the mitral annulus, as might occur with a traditional open mitral repair; but with the percutaneous approach, the annulus

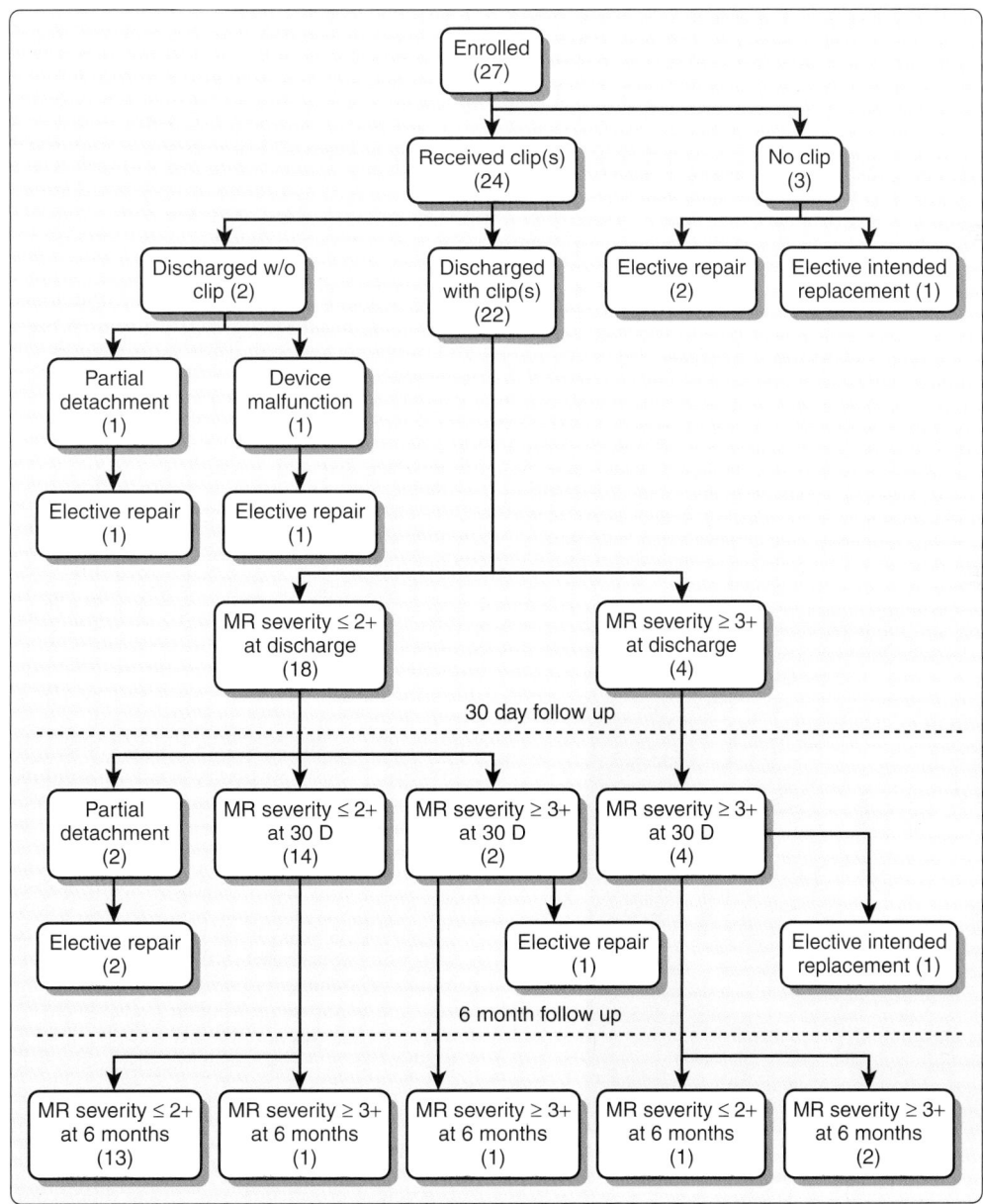

Figure 19-37 **Flow chart showing overall results for the 27 study patients.** MR, mitral regurgitation. *(From Webb JG, Harnek J, Munt BI, et al: Percutaneous transvenous mitral annuloplasty: Initial human experience with device implantation in the coronary sinus. Circulation 113:851–855, 2006.)*

is downsized by an extracardiac restraint.[434,435] With this technique, interventional cardiologists percutaneously thread a wire from the venous system into the right atrium and into the coronary sinus. The relation between the coronary sinus and posterior leaflet allows downsizing of the septal-lateral diameter from this position. Under echocardiographic guidance, tension is applied to cinch the mitral annulus smaller, and an anchor is deployed to maintain position. In animal trials in a sheep model, a significant reduction in mitral annular dimension was achieved and mitral regurgitation was eliminated in seven of nine animals.[434] Only trivial mitral regurgitation remained in the remaining two. In addition, PAPs were significantly reduced and CO increased (Figure 19-38).

Temporary[436] and permanent implantation of these devices in humans has been reported.[437] Differing designs are being investigated, but in the Edwards system, the implant is made up of three parts: a distal anchor seated in the great cardiac vein, a bridging section that applies anterior force to the posterior annulus, and a proximal anchor seated in the ostium of the coronary sinus. In a series of five patients with chronic, ischemic mitral regurgitation, the device was successfully placed in four patients.[437] At hospital discharge, three of four patients had a reduced mitral regurgitation grade (Figure 19-39). Follow-up continued for 180 days after implantation, but separation of the bridge portion of the device occurred in three patients at 22, 28, and 81 days. Although there were no adverse events associated with bridge separation, the feasibility trial was stopped. The authors acknowledge that results were inferior to surgical mitral repair and that technical success is limited by great variation in coronary venous anatomy.[437]

Altering Ventricular Anatomy to Reduce Mitral Regurgitation

The third approach to "closed" mitral valve repair consists of altering the geometry of the lateral and septal left ventricular walls to bring the valve leaflets together. The commercial Coapsys has entered clinical trials. This device consists of anterior and posterior epicardial pads connected by a cord. With an open chest, the cord is placed transventricularly in a subvalvular position, and the tension on the cord is adjusted before the opposing epicardial pad is fixed in place.[438] This effectively brings the ventricular walls together and in doing so improves leaflet coaptation. TEE is used to optimize cord length and pad positioning.

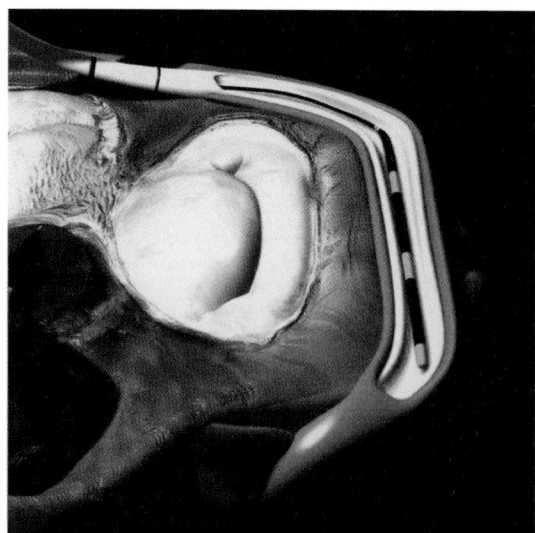

Figure 19-38 Effect of annuloplasty device on mitral annular geometry. The annuloplasty device decreases the distance between the anterior and posterior annulus, increasing leaflet coaptation. *(From Liddicoat JR, Mac Niell BD, Gillinov AM, et al: Percutaneous mitral valve repair: A feasibility study in a bovine model of acute ischemic mitral regurgitation. Catheter Cardiovasc Interv 60:411, 2003.)*

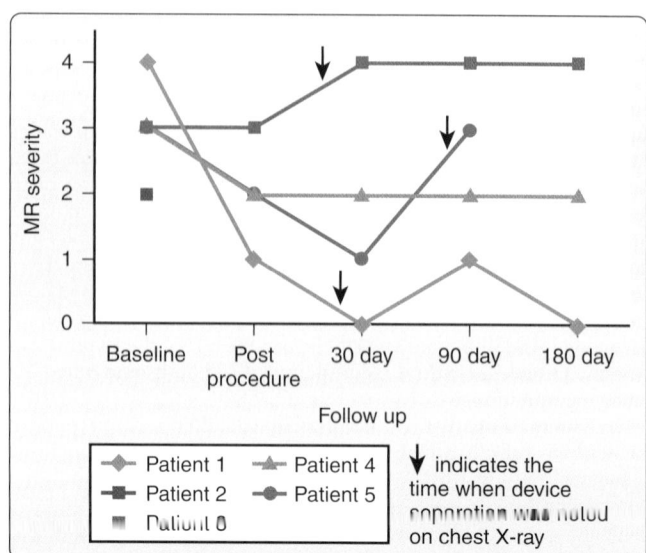

Figure 19-39 Mitral regurgitation (MR) grade as estimated by transthoracic color Doppler echocardiography versus days after device implantation. Note that no device was implanted in Patient 2, and that Patient 5 died before the 180-day follow-up. *(From Feldman T, Wasserman HS, Herrmann HC, et al: Percutaneous mitral valve repair using the edge-to-edge technique: Six-month results of the EVEREST Phase I Clinical Trial. J Am Coll Cardiol 46:2134–2140, 2005.)*

In contrast with the leaflet-based and annular-based approaches, the Coapsys approach is surgical, requiring an open chest but not CPB. The position of the epicardial vessels and the relation of the submitral apparatus could pose significant risk, but the device has been used successfully in animal models.

Percutaneous Valve Replacement

Although surgery, particularly for aortic valve disease, has expanded to include a much older population in recent years, there remains a subset of patients for whom cardiac surgery may entail unacceptable risks. For this population, less invasive techniques such as percutaneous valve replacement are being developed.

The first clinical percutaneous placement of an aortic valve was reported in 2002.[439] The second report[440] included six inoperable patients with severe AS and Class IV HF. This initial technique began with femoral vein catheterization, a trans-septal, transmitral approach, wherein a balloon-tipped catheter was placed antegrade across the stenotic aortic valve. After valvuloplasty, the aortic valve stent was seated at the native valve over a second balloon.[440] However, the technical complexity of this approach, and the potential for severe mitral regurgitation and hemodynamic collapse as large delivery catheters were placed across the mitral valve, contributed to its abandonment.[441]

Experience and technical refinement have led to the two current strategies for transcatheter AVR: (1) retrograde via the femoral artery advanced into the aorta and across the aortic valve; and (2) antegrade via limited thoracotomy, wherein a valve-loaded catheter punctures the left ventricular apex and the new valve is seated antegrade.

Covello et al[442] described management strategies and periprocedural outcomes in 18 patients in whom retrograde, percutaneous AVR was performed via the femoral artery, whereas the management of 100 patients who underwent successful transapical antegrade aortic prosthesis placement was reported by Fassl.[443] Although the technical aspects of prosthetic valve delivery differ, common themes emerge. These include the need for rigorous assessment of aortic leaflet, root and coronary ostial anatomy, a well-coordinated, multidisciplinary approach to patient evaluation and clinical management, the use of rapid ventricular pacing to diminish cardiac output during prosthesis deployment, and the potential for sudden hemodynamic collapse necessitating emergent intervention.

In Covello et al's[442] report of retrograde transfemoral AVR, GA was used early (14 patients); however, with experience, MAC was selected. This contrasts with the practice of anesthesiologists at other centers where relatively large numbers of transfemoral, retrograde AVR procedures are performed. The advantages of GA include patient immobility during rapid ventricular pacing, valvuloplasty, and prosthesis deployment. Furthermore, GA facilitates surgical repair of the femoral cannulation site, which may be required. In addition, the use of GA allows for prolonged TEE imaging and rapid intervention in the event that sternotomy or CPB should become an emergent necessity.

In that report of the transfemoral technique, prosthesis positioning, deployment, and the immediate postdeployment assessment of prosthetic function were guided fluoroscopically. This differs from the practice at many institutions, where TEE is performed frequently during the procedure to assess annular size, device positioning, and immediate postdeployment prosthesis function.

Covello et al[442] provide a brief overview of short-term outcome related to transfemoral AVR. Two of 18 patients required defibrillation during the procedure. The 30-day mortality rate was 0%. However, 3 of 18 patients died within 6 months because of conditions that were not directly related to the aortic valve. In addition, half the patients had mild-to-moderate residual paravalvular AR after the procedure.[442]

Transapical catheter-based AVR typically is selected because of vasculopathy, small or tortuous femoral and iliac vessels, or severe aortic atheromatous disease. After GA, typically in a hybrid operating suite, a small left anterior thoracotomy is made and the ventricular apex exposed. Stay sutures are placed, a needle is passed into the ventricular apex, and a wire is threaded across the aortic valve. Balloon aortoplasty is performed, and under a combination of fluoroscopic and echocardiographic guidance, the aortic valve is seated with deployment of a balloon (see Chapter 26).

Fassl et al[443] detailed the hemodynamic management of 100 patients undergoing transapical antegrade AVR. Rapid ventricular pacing facilitated valvuloplasty and subsequent prosthesis delivery by minimizing CO, thus diminishing the likelihood of device dislodgement at critical points in the procedure. In the first 10 patients, CPB was used electively to ensure the procedure feasibility. Thereafter, CPB was used in 10% of patients because of hemodynamic deterioration. Intra-aortic balloon pump augmentation was required in 5%, and one patient was placed on extracorporeal membrane oxygenation. Three patients required defibrillation during the procedure.

Although other outcome data such as mortality are omitted from that report,[443] a study by Walther et al,[444] from the same institution, offers insights. Of 50 patients described, 3 required emergent sternotomy for reasons of a proximally dislodged prosthesis, aortic dissection, and coronary occlusion. The 30-day survival rate in Walther's group was 92% with a 6-month survival rate of 74%. No deaths occurred because of prosthesis-related causes.

The suitability of the patient for catheter-based AVR and the choice of transfemoral or transapical approaches necessitate careful screening. Native aortic valve size, leaflet anatomy, and length and coronary ostial position are critical to valve selection, to reduce perivalvular leak, and to avoid compromising the coronary ostia at valve deployment. Second, both approaches share features such as the induction and maintenance of anesthesia in patients with severe AS. Third, several aspects of device deployment are similar regardless of the route of delivery. For instance, both transfemoral and transapical methods use rapid ventricular pacing during initial valvuloplasty and subsequent prosthesis deployment. Fourth, currently, applicability is limited because only three prosthesis sizes exist for transcatheter AVR. The prosthesis chosen is deliberately larger than predicted on the basis of annular size in an effort to achieve improved prosthesis seating and reduced paravalvular regurgitation. Finally, many of the

same periprocedural complications are possible regardless of delivery catheter insertion site. Ventricular fibrillation may ensue during rapid ventricular pacing, aortic dissection has been reported, obstruction of a coronary orifice by the prosthesis or displaced native valve tissue, and device embolization or dislodgement have been reported with both approaches.[444,445]

Questions remain regarding transcatheter AVR. The currently available prostheses consist of tissue leaflets mounted in an expandable metal stent, so questions remain related to the optimal use and duration of antiplatelet therapy for these patients. More importantly, the durability of the catheter-implanted aortic prosthesis is unknown.

Although pulmonic valve disease is much less common than aortic, progress in percutaneous pulmonic valve replacement also is undergoing investigation.[446] In a sheep model, Boudjemline et al[446] have implanted a pulmonary artery stent and valve using a percutaneous approach from the internal jugular vein. This has been done in both single- and two-staged approaches. One subgroup of animals underwent stent and valve insertion simultaneously, and in another group, the stent was placed in the first step and the valve was inserted into the stent 6 to 10 weeks later.

In 8 of 10 animals, the stent and graft were successfully implanted and there was no early or late stent migration. The two failures resulted from problems related to the anatomic relation between the tricuspid valve and the right ventricular outlet. The valves placed into the stent percutaneously were competent angiographically and hemodynamically at follow-up.

It is likely that many of these technologies will lead to expanded clinical trials and will demonstrate varying degrees of efficacy. That said, it is unclear what the long-term benefits of these less invasive interventions will be, or how they will compare with each other or with traditional surgical approaches. Some may find use in high-risk patients, as temporizing procedures, in place of reoperations, or in conjunction with percutaneous approaches for CAD. These technologies will get better and there will be pressure for clinical application. The most important considerations will be case selection and long-term follow-up of outcomes; otherwise, these innovations, and others like it, will add markedly to the burden of health care costs without clear social benefit.

▣ CASE STUDY 1—Transapical Aortic Valve Implantation

Framing

89-year-old gentleman with medical history significant for CABG × 4 eleven years previously. Recurrent CAD with recent bare metal stent (BMS) ×2 placement to the LIMA into the left anterior descending (LAD) artery at distal anastomosis 1 month prior. Dyspnea on exertion with mild chest tightness that goes away with rest.

Severe symptomatic AS, and **he does not wish to be considered for redo sternotomy.** The patient's femoral anatomy is not conducive to transfemoral transcutaneous aortic valve replacement; consider for transapical approach.

NYHA CLASS II HEART FAILURE.

His STS risk for mortality is 20.9%.

Medical/Surgical History Included

1. Severe AS with a valve area of 0.73, mild-moderate AR with a mean transaortic gradient of 44 mm Hg
2. CAD, status post-CABG ×4 eleven years ago
3. Bare metal stents (two): placement 1 month prior
4. Moderate mitral regurgitation
5. Atherosclerotic cerebrovascular disease, status postbilateral carotid endarterectomy, both 2 years prior
6. Mild pulmonary hypertension
7. Diabetes mellitus, type 2

8. Hypercholesterolemia
9. Hypertension
10. Chronic kidney disease
11. Peripheral vascular disease
12. Sleep apnea

His Current Medications Were

furosemide, 40 mg day,
glipizide, 10 mg BID,
hydralazine, 25 mg TID,
metoprolol, 25 mg BID,
nitroglycerin, [NITROQUICK], 0.4 mg PRN,
rosuvastatin, 20 mg, and
timolol, 0.5 % drops.
NO KNOWN MEDICATION ALLERGIES

Vital Signs Were

height 154.80 cm,
weight 61 kg,
BMI 25.5 kg/m²,
BSA 1.64 m²,
afebrile,
pulse 58/minute, and
BP 156/61 mm Hg.

CXR: Sternotomy. Prominent left nipple shadow. Fibrotic strands in the bases. Calcified granulomas. Surgical clips left side of the neck. Unchanged since previous x-ray.

ECG: VENTRICULAR RATE 56. Sinus bradycardia, left ventricular hypertrophy with secondary ST-T abnormalities. Cannot rule out anteroseptal infarct. No significant change was found.

Labs Included:

Hgb 12.8 g%,
platelets 164,000,
INR 1.0,
Na⁺ 136, K⁺ 4.0,
glucose 109 mg %, and
creatinine 2.2 mg/dL.

Data Collection and Interpretation
CT Chest, Abdomen, and Pelvis (without contrast)

The aortic annulus measures 33 mm. The left main-to-aortic valve annulus dimension was 18 mm. The diameter at the sinus of Valsalva was 35 mm. The sinotubular junction is 31 mm. The ascending aorta is 34 mm. The aortic arch was 24 mm. The aorta at the diaphragm was 24 mm. Extensive vascular disease including coronary artery calcifications. Extensive aortic valve and mitral annular calcifications.

Bilateral renal atrophy. Vascular dimensions are external dimensions as the lumens cannot be evaluated without contrast. The infrarenal aorta was 10 × 12 mm. The right common iliac was 10 × 11 mm. The right external iliac was 8 × 8 mm. The right common femoral was 5 × 6 mm. The left common iliac was 10 × 9 mm. The left external iliac was 9 × 9 mm, and the left common femoral was 5 × 5 mm.

Cardiac Catheterization/Percutaneous Transluminal Coronary Angioplasty Summary

The patient had a prior four-vessel bypass. Angiography showed patent vein grafts to both first and second OM and to the diagonal branch. The free left internal mammary artery graft to the LAD artery had severe disease. The patient's native right coronary artery had severe disease; however, this vessel could not be bypassed earlier when he had CABG surgery.

The patient also has chronic renal insufficiency limiting the possibility of multivessel percutaneous coronary intervention because of limitation in contrast load.

He had successful PTCA of the middle LAD artery and successful PTCA of the distal site of free internal mammary graft to the middle LAD artery.

Decision Making and Reassessment
Description of Operation

The patient underwent GA in the supine position. He was prepped and draped, and a left inframammary incision was made and the chest entered over the top of the fifth rib. Purse-string sutures were placed just lateral to the apex of the heart. Heparin was given and the ACT was maintained above 300 seconds. The apex of the heart was punctured with a needle and the wire advanced across the aortic valve under fluoroscopic guidance. A wire was advanced up into the proximal ascending aorta, and a 23-cm, 7-French sheath advanced across the aortic valve. The 7-French sheath was removed. The Ascendra sheath was inserted without difficulty. The balloon was advanced across the aortic valve. Rapid ventricular pacing was instituted and the balloon aortic valvuloplasty completed. The balloon was removed, but the patient remained hypotensive with increases in his PAPs refractory to escalating doses of epinephrine. The authors elected to proceed rapidly with placement of the valve.

Rapid ventricular pacing was instituted, and the valve was positioned perfectly. The balloon was deflated, rapid ventricular pacing was stopped, but the patient remained hypotensive. The Ascendra sheath and wire were removed, and TEE showed good valvular function with no significant AR. However, there was significant PAP elevation and right-heart function was poor by TEE, so the patient was prepared for femoral-femoral bypass.

A percutaneous arterial cannula was placed over a wire and the femoral artery was dilated without apparent difficulty, and a 15-French percutaneous arterial inflow cannula was placed. A 22-French percutaneous venous cannula was then inserted and CPB was initiated. During this time, the patient was hypotensive and required initiation of external cardiac massage. The patient had recurrent VF and was successfully defibrillated to a stable cardiac rhythm. The PAPs began to decline, and the heart function appeared to improve. However, the CPB circuit volume could not be maintained and a retrograde arteriogram identified extravasation of contrast at the bifurcation of the right common iliac artery. We then attempted to place an endograft. A balloon was inflated in the infrarenal aorta to achieve proximal control to come off CPB. The arterial inflow line was transferred to the venous line to continue to give blood. Limited angiography confirmed the disruption of the proximal right external iliac artery. Blood pressure could not be supported; the patient deteriorated and arrested. Despite cardiopulmonary resuscitation, the patient expired. (See Video 1.)

Discussion

This case illustrates nearly every major clinical point regarding the assessment and care of patients undergoing transapical AVR. There were clinical indications for a catheter-based approach. These included: (1) the patients' desire not to undergo an open-chest approach, (2) the history of prior multivessel CABG, and perioperative risk factors, including (3) advanced age, (4) diffuse vasculopathy, and (5) chronic renal insufficiency. Next, evaluation for a catheter-based approach demonstrated aortic valvular, sinus, and coronary anatomy suitable to catheter-based placement but severe iliac and femoral vasculopathy that excluded a transarterial approach.

A multidisciplinary approach to evaluation and preoperative optimization included participation of cardiac surgery, echocardiography, and interventional cardiology, anesthesiology, and radiology. The patient underwent cardiac catheterization and PTCA, as well as noncontrast CT, and surgery was scheduled a month later to allow renal recovery.

Case preparation involved scheduling more than a week in advance, conduct in a hybrid operating room, presence of interventional cardiology, cardiac and vascular surgery, CPB standby, and 1:1 coverage by a cardiovascular anesthesiologist. Surgically, the technical approach was exactly as planned; femoral vessels were "wired" in advance and, via a transapical approach, the valve was positioned without difficulty. However, the patient developed three complications relatively common with this technique in this population: (1) refractory hypotension after rapid ventricular pacing, (2) difficulty in establishing rapid CPB support because of the small size and calcification of femoral and iliac vessels (in spite of vessels being "wired" before), and (3) iliac artery disruption.

Although catheter-based AVR is less invasive than the open-chest approach, it probably requires more planning and complex assessment and coordination than conventional cardiac surgery. In addition, most of these patients have comorbid conditions that make them poor open surgical candidates, so untoward events during these techniques are life-threatening.

CASE STUDY 2

Robotic-Assisted Mitral Valve Repair

Framing

A 46-year-old woman presented with a 4-month history of decreasing tolerance for strenuous exercise. An advertising executive and amateur triathlete, she reported that increased fatigue currently prevented her from jogging more than 4 miles in a day. Evaluation by her physician revealed a new systolic murmur and she was referred for echocardiography. A TTE revealed a flail posterior mitral valve leaflet with an eccentric, anteromedially directed jet of severe mitral regurgitation. Reliable quantification of the regurgitant volume by PISA method was not possible. However, systolic flow reversals were noted during pulsed-wave Doppler examination of the right superior pulmonary vein. This study also demonstrated normal left ventricular dimensions in both systole and diastole with a calculated EF of 67%. The left atrium was mildly enlarged. In addition, the right-heart chambers were of normal size and the calculated right ventricular systolic pressure was 35 mm Hg. During an appointment with a cardiologist, surgical consultation for possible mitral valve repair was recommended. The patient was hesitant to pursue surgery for several reasons: she worried about missing work and being unable to drive during a multiweek postoperative convalescence, she was concerned about the cosmetic implications of a median sternotomy, and she was uncertain of her need for surgical intervention at this time because she experienced symptoms only with vigorous exercise.

Data Collection and Interpretation

Although visualization of the mitral valve is superior with TEE when compared with TTE, flail mitral leaflets often can be identified during transthoracic examinations. This patient had a flail leaflet that was likely secondary to chordal rupture. Although quantification of the mitral regurgitant volume or effective regurgitant orifice by PISA method was not possible during the TTE examination, the severity of the regurgitation was supported by the finding of systolic flow reversals in the right superior pulmonary vein. The right superior pulmonary vein is often the easiest pulmonary vein to visualize during TTE studies when using an apical four-chamber view. PISA analysis may be difficult in some patients with eccentrically directed regurgitant jets because of the difficulty in aligning the Doppler cursor with a significant portion of the regurgitant jet, with the resultant inability to measure the peak regurgitant velocity and obtain a complete regurgitant velocity-time integral. In addition to detecting severe, organic mitral regurgitation, other important information was obtained during the TTE examination. For example, there was no evidence of left ventricular enlargement, and the calculated EF was 67%. Mild LA enlargement was consistent with the reported 4-month history of symptoms; severe mitral regurgitation of longer duration might be expected to produce a greater degree of LA

dilation. A calculated right ventricular systolic pressure of 35 mm Hg likely corresponds to a mean PAP of less than 25 mm Hg, and thus does not indicate the presence of pulmonary hypertension.

If surgical intervention is anticipated, additional information would be sought. Confirmation of the mechanism of mitral regurgitation and thorough inspection for anterior leaflet pathology could be obtained by intraoperative TEE. The presence or absence of a patent foramen ovale could be determined by intraoperative TEE as well. The decision of whether to pursue preoperative coronary angiography in a 46-year-old, athletic woman would depend on the presence of other risk factors for premature CAD in this patient, as well as physician preference. The preoperative electrocardiogram would be examined for evidence of atrial tachyarrhythmias such as AF that might lead to consideration of additional surgical interventions such as the Maze procedure or exclusion of the LA appendage.

Decision Making and Reassessment

In deciding whether to proceed with surgery in this patient, a number of different factors must be considered. Her mitral regurgitation is organic in nature, and medical management is unlikely to prevent deleterious structural changes in the heart over time, such as left ventricular dilation. In fact, progression of the severity of mitral regurgitation can be expected in the absence of surgical intervention.[307] Furthermore, the presence of a flail mitral leaflet is associated with a small but defined increase in the annual risk for sudden cardiac death; that risk can be reduced by surgical repair.[306] Currently, the patient's LVEF is acceptable. Postponing surgery risks the development of left ventricular systolic dysfunction. A decline in EF to less than 60% is associated with reduced survival after mitral surgery.[310] All these factors combined with a procedural mortality rate of less than 1% in many centers argue for early elective mitral valve repair.

Concerns related to cosmetic outcome and delayed return to work may be addressed by offering the patient a minimally invasive surgical approach, with or without robotic assistance. A 4-cm incision in the right inframammary crease provides an excellent cosmetic result for many women. Also, minimally invasive techniques, including robotic-assisted surgery, have been associated with decreased postoperative pain scores, earlier hospital discharge, and earlier return to work.

The patient was referred to a surgeon who was experienced in robotic-assisted mitral valve repair. On the day of surgery, the anesthesiologist performed a series of right paravertebral injections before induction of anesthesia. One-lung ventilation was achieved by means of a double-lumen endotracheal tube. The intraoperative TEE confirmed the presence of a flail middle scallop of the posterior mitral leaflet with multiple ruptured chords (see Videos 2 and 3). No additional valvular pathology was noted and the atrial septum was intact. Cannulation for CPB, which was guided by intraoperative TEE, included femoral arterial and venous lines, as well as a 16-French superior vena cava cannula placed percutaneously via the right internal jugular vein. Cardioplegia was given antegrade via a catheter placed into the aorta via a right parasternal stab incision. Aortic cross-clamping was accomplished with a long-shafted clamp introducer through a stab incision in the right lateral chest wall. Mitral repair was performed with robotic assistance and consisted of a triangular resection of the middle scallop of the posterior mitral leaflet and insertion of a flexible posterior annuloplasty band. The patient was weaned from CPB without difficulty and extubated in the operating room at the conclusion of surgery. Her postoperative course was uneventful and she was discharged on the third postoperative day.

REFERENCES

1. Ross J Jr: Afterload mismatch in aortic and mitral valve disease: Implications for surgical therapy, *J Am Coll Cardiol* 5:811–826, 1985.
2. Burns JW, Covell JW, Ross J Jr: Mechanics of isotonic left ventricular contractions, *Am J Physiol* 224:725–732, 1973.
3. Braunwald ER: Contraction of the normal heart. In *Contraction of the normal heart*, ed 4, Philadelphia, 1992, WB Saunders.
4. Braunwald E, Ross J Jr, Sonnenblick EHR: *Mechanisms of contraction of the normal and failing heart*, Boston, 1976, Little, Brown.
5. Baudeer HSR: Contractile tension in the myocardium, *Am Heart J* 66:432, 1963.
6. Braunwald ER: Regulation of the circulation. I, *N Engl J Med* 290:1124–1129, 1974.
7. Jewell BRR: Activation of contraction in cardiac muscle, *Mayo Clin Proc* 57(Suppl):6–13, 1982.
8. Fabiato A, Fabiato FR: Dependence of calcium release, tension generation and restoring forces on sarcomere length in skinned cardiac cells, *Eur J Cardiol* 4(Suppl):13–27, 1976.
9. Gordon AM, Pollack GHR: Effects of calcium on the sarcomere length-tension relation in rat cardiac muscle. Implications for the Frank-Starling mechanism, *Circ Res* 47:610–619, 1980.
10. Grossman W, McLaurin LPR: Diastolic properties of the left ventricle, *Ann Intern Med* 84:316–326, 1976.
11. McCullagh WH, Covell JW, Ross J Jr: Left ventricular performance following correction of free aortic regurgitation, *Circulation* 45:943–951, 1972.
12. Gault JH, Covell JW, Braunwald E, et al: Left ventricular performance following correction of free aortic regurgitation, *Circulation* 42:773–780, 1970.
13. Grossman W, McLaurin LP, Moos SP, et al: Wall thickness and diastolic properties of the left ventricle, *Circulation* 49:129–135, 1974.

14. Leyton RA, Spotnitz HM, Sonnenblick EHR: Cardiac ultrastructure and function: Sarcomeres in the right ventricle, *Am J Physiol* 221:902–910, 1971.
15. Gaasch WHR: Diagnosis and treatment of heart failure based on left ventricular systolic or diastolic dysfunction, *JAMA* 271:1276–1280, 1994.
16. Little WC, Applegate RJR: Congestive heart failure: Systolic and diastolic function, *J Cardiothorac Vasc Anesth* 7:2–5, 1993.
17. Brutsaert DL, Sys SU, Gillebert TCR: Diastolic failure: Pathophysiology and therapeutic implications, [erratum appears in *J Am Coll Cardiol* 1993 Oct;22(4):1272]. *J Am Coll Cardiol*, 22:318–325, 1993.
18. Eberli FR, Apstein CS, Ngoy S, et al: Exacerbation of left ventricular ischemic diastolic dysfunction by pressure-overload hypertrophy. Modification by specific inhibition of cardiac angiotensin converting enzyme, *Circ Res* 70:931–943, 1992.
19. Spirito P, Maron BJR: Relation between extent of left ventricular hypertrophy and diastolic filling abnormalities in hypertrophic cardiomyopathy, *J Am Coll Cardiol* 15:808–813, 1990.
20. Wigle EDR: Impaired left ventricular relaxation in hypertrophic cardiomyopathy: Relation to extent of hypertrophy, *J Am Coll Cardiol* 15:814–815, 1990.
21. Bemis CE, Serur JR, Borkenhagen D, et al: Influence of right ventricular filling pressure on left ventricular pressure and dimension, *Circ Res* 34:498–504, 1974.
22. Glantz SA, Parmley WWR: Factors which affect the diastolic pressure-volume curve, *Circ Res* 42: 171–180, 1978.
23. Spadaro J, Bing OH, Gaasch WH, et al: Pericardial modulation of right and left ventricular diastolic interaction, *Circ Res* 48:233–238, 1981.
24. Santamore WP, Lynch PR, Meier G, et al: Myocardial interaction between the ventricles, *J Appl Physiol* 41:362–368, 1976.
25. Carabello BA: Ratio of end-systolic stress to end-systolic volume: Is it a useful clinical tool? *J Am Coll Cardiol* 14:496, 1989.
26. Braunwald ER: *Assessment of cardiac function: Assessment of cardiac function*, Philadelphia, 1992, WB Saunders Company.
27. Ross J Jr: Cardiac function and myocardial contractility: A perspective, *J Am Coll Cardiol* 1:52–62, 1983.
28. Carabello BA, Spann JF: The uses and limitations of end-systolic indexes of left ventricular function, *Circulation* 69:1058–1064, 1984.
29. Carabello BAR: Clinical assessment of systolic dysfunction, *ACC Curr J Rev* 1:25, 1994.
30. Katz AMR: Influence of altered inotropy and lusitropy on ventricular pressure-volume loops, *J Am Coll Cardiol* 11:438–445, 1988.
31. Gorcsan J 3rd, Romand JA, Mandarino WA, et al: Assessment of left ventricular performance by on-line pressure-area relations using echocardiographic automated border detection, *J Am Coll Cardiol* 23:242–252, 1994.
32. Grossman W, Braunwald E, Mann T, et al: Contractile state of the left ventricle in man as evaluated from end-systolic pressure-volume relations, *Circulation* 56:845–852, 1977.
33. Sagawa KR: The end-systolic pressure-volume relation of the ventricle: Definition, modifications and clinical use, *Am J Cardiol* 40:748, 1977.
34. Sagawa KR: End-systolic pressure/volume ratio: A new index of ventricular contractility, *Circulation* 63:1223, 1981.
35. Helske S, Kupari M, Lindstedt KA, et al: Aortic valve stenosis: An active atheroinflammatory process, *Curr Opin Lipidol* 18:483–491, 2007.
36. Augoustides JG, Wolfe Y, Walsh EK, et al: Recent advances in aortic valve disease: Highlights from a bicuspid aortic valve to transcatheter aortic valve replacement, *J Cardiothorac Vasc Anesth* 23: 569–576, 2009.
37. Bosse Y, Mathieu P, Pibarot P: Genomics: The next step to elucidate the etiology of calcific aortic valve stenosis, *J Am Coll Cardiol* 51:1327–1336, 2008.
38. Rajamannan NM, Gersh B, Bonow RO: Calcific aortic stenosis: From bench to the bedside—emerging clinical and cellular concepts, *Heart* 89:801–805, 2003.
39. Sprecher DL, Schaefer EJ, Kent KM, et al: Cardiovascular features of homozygous familial hypercholesterolemia: Analysis of 16 patients, *Am J Cardiol* 54:20–30, 1984.
40. Rosenhek R, Binder T, Porenta G, et al: Predictors of outcome in severe, asymptomatic aortic stenosis, *N Engl J Med* 343:611–617, 2000.
41. Carabello BA: Evaluation and management of patients with aortic stenosis, *Circulation* 105: 1746–1750, 2002.
42. Novaro GM, Tiong IY, Pearce GL, et al: Effect of hydroxymethylglutaryl coenzyme a reductase inhibitors on the progression of calcific aortic stenosis, *Circulation* 104:2205–2209, 2001.
43. Bellamy MF, Pellikka PA, Klarich KW, et al: Association of cholesterol levels, hydroxymethylglutaryl coenzyme-A reductase inhibitor treatment, and progression of aortic stenosis in the community, *J Am Coll Cardiol* 40:1723–1730, 2002.
44. Mitka M: Researchers probe aortic stenosis: An active, potentially treatable disease process? *JAMA* 289:2197–2198, 2003.
45. Otto CM, Burwash IG, Legget ME, et al: Prospective study of asymptomatic valvular aortic stenosis. Clinical, echocardiographic, and exercise predictors of outcome, *Circulation* 95:2262–2270, 1997.
46. Nassimiha D, Aronow WS, Ahn C, et al: Rate of progression of valvular aortic stenosis in patients > or = 60 years of age, *Am J Cardiol* 87:807–809, A9, 2001.
47. Wongpraparut N, Apiyasawat S, Crespo G, et al: Determinants of progression of aortic stenosis in patients aged > or =40 years, *Am J Cardiol* 89:350–352, 2002.
48. Qi W, Mathisen P, Kjekshus J, et al: Natriuretic peptides in patients with aortic stenosis, *Am Heart J* 142:725–732, 2001.
49. Gerber IL, Stewart RA, Legget ME, et al: Increased plasma natriuretic peptide levels reflect symptom onset in aortic stenosis, *Circulation* 107:1884–1890, 2003.
50. Ross J, Braunwald ER: The influence of corrective operations on the natural history of aortic stenosis, *Circulation* 37(Suppl 5):61, 1968.
51. Rotman M, Morris JJ Jr, Behar VS, et al: Aortic valvular disease. Comparison of types and their medical and surgical management, *Am J Med* 51:241–257, 1971.
52. Frank S, Johnson A, Ross J Jr: Natural history of valvular aortic stenosis, *Br Heart J* 35:41–46, 1973.
53. Kennedy KD, Nishimura RA, Holmes DR Jr, et al: Natural history of moderate aortic stenosis, *J Am Coll Cardiol* 17:313–319, 1991.
54. Chaliki HP, Brown ML, Sundt TM, et al: Timing of operation in asymptomatic severe aortic stenosis, *Expert Rev Cardiovasc Ther* 5:1065–1071, 2007.
55. Selzer AR: Changing aspects of the natural history of valvular aortic stenosis, *N Engl J Med* 317:91–98, 1987.
56. Bonow ROBE: *Valvular heart disease: Valvular heart disease*, Philadelphia, 2005, Elsevier, pp 1553–1632.
57. Berger M, Berdoff RL, Gallerstein PE, et al: Evaluation of aortic stenosis by continuous wave Doppler ultrasound, *J Am Coll Cardiol* 3:150–156, 1984.
58. Hakki AH, Kimbiris D, Iskandrian AS, et al: Angina pectoris and coronary artery disease in patients with severe aortic valvular disease, *Am Heart J* 100:441–449, 1980.
59. Graboys TB, Cohn PFR: The prevalence of angina pectoris and abnormal coronary arteriograms in severe aortic valvular disease, *Am Heart J* 93:683–686, 1977.
60. Bonchek LI, Anderson RP, Rosch J: Should coronary arteriography be performed routinely before valve replacement? *Am J Cardiol* 31:462–466, 1973.
61. Green SJ, Pizzarello RA, Padmanabhan VT, et al: Relation of angina pectoris to coronary artery disease in aortic valve stenosis, *Am J Cardiol* 55:1063–1065, 1985.

62. Mullany CJ, Elveback LR, Frye RL, et al: Coronary artery disease and its management: Influence on survival in patients undergoing aortic valve replacement, *J Am Coll Cardiol* 10:66–72, 1987.
63. Exadactylos N, Sugrue DD, Oakley CMR: Prevalence of coronary artery disease in patients with isolated aortic valve stenosis, *Br Heart J* 51:121–124, 1984.
64. Lytle BW, Cosgrove DM, Loop FD, et al: Replacement of aortic valve combined with myocardial revascularization: Determinants of early and late risk for 500 patients, 1967-1981, *Circulation* 68:1149–1162, 1983.
65. Magovern JA, Pennock JL, Campbell DB, et al: Aortic valve replacement and combined aortic valve replacement and coronary artery bypass grafting: Predicting high risk groups, *J Am Coll Cardiol* 9: 38–43, 1987.
66. Czer LS, Gray RJ, Stewart ME, et al: Reduction in sudden late death by concomitant revascularization with aortic valve replacement, *J Thorac Cardiovasc Surg* 95:390–401, 1988.
67. Lytle BW, Cosgrove DM, Gill CC, et al: Aortic valve replacement combined with myocardial revascularization. Late results and determinants of risk for 471 in-hospital survivors, *J Thorac Cardiovasc Surg* 95:402–414, 1988.
68. Lombard JT, Selzer AR: Valvular aortic stenosis. A clinical and hemodynamic profile of patients, *Ann Intern Med* 106:292–298, 1987.
69. Lund OR: Preoperative risk evaluation and stratification of long-term survival after valve replacement for aortic stenosis. Reasons for earlier operative intervention, *Circulation* 82:124–139, 1990.
70. Cheitlin MDR: Should an asymptomatic patient with hemodynamically severe aortic stenosis ever have aortic valve surgery? *Cardiol Rev* 1:344, 1993.
71. Pallikka PA, Nishimura RA, Bailey KR, et al: The natural history of adults with asymptomatic hemodynamically significant aortic stenosis, *J Am Coll Cardiol* 15:1012, 1990.
72. Braunwald ER: On the natural history of severe aortic stenosis, *J Am Coll Cardiol* 15:1018–1020, 1990.
73. Pantely G, Morton M, Rahimtoola SHR: Effects of successful, uncomplicated valve replacement on ventricular hypertrophy, volume, and performance in aortic stenosis and in aortic incompetence, *J Thorac Cardiovasc Surg* 75:383–391, 1978.
74. Kennedy JW, Doces J, Stewart DKR: Left ventricular function before and following aortic valve replacement, *Circulation* 56:944–950, 1977.
75. Schwarz F, Flameng W, Schaper J, et al: Myocardial structure and function in patients with aortic valve disease and their relation to postoperative results, *Am J Cardiol* 41:661–669, 1978.
76. Croke RP, Pifarre R, Sullivan H, et al: Reversal of advanced left ventricular dysfunction following aortic valve replacement for aortic stenosis, *Ann Thorac Surg* 24:38–43, 1977.
77. Smith N, McAnulty JH, Rahimtoola SHR: Severe aortic stenosis with impaired left ventricular function and clinical heart failure: Results of valve replacement, *Circulation* 58:255–264, 1978.
78. Peter M, Hoffmann A, Parker C, et al: Progression of aortic stenosis. Role of age and concomitant coronary artery disease, *Chest* 103:1715–1719, 1993.
79. Culliford AT, Galloway AC, Colvin SB, et al: Aortic valve replacement for aortic stenosis in persons aged 80 years and over, *Am J Cardiol* 67:1256–1260, 1991.
80. Filsoufi F, Rahmanian PB, Castillo JG, et al: Excellent early and late outcomes of aortic valve replacement in people aged 80 and older, *J Am Geriatr Soc* 56:255–261, 2008.
81. Yeager M, Yock PG, Popp RLR: Comparison of Doppler-derived pressure gradient to that determined at cardiac catheterization in adults with aortic valve stenosis: Implications for management, *Am J Cardiol* 57:644–648, 1986.
82. Tribouilloy C, Shen WF, Peltier M, et al: Quantitation of aortic valve area in aortic stenosis with multiplane transesophageal echocardiography: Comparison with monoplane transesophageal approach, *Am Heart J* 128:526–532, 1994.
83. Hegrenaes L, Hatle LR: Aortic stenosis in adults. Non-invasive estimation of pressure differences by continuous wave Doppler echocardiography, *Br Heart J* 54:396–404, 1985.
84. Hatle L, Angelsen BA, Tromsdal AR: Non-invasive assessment of aortic stenosis by Doppler ultrasound, *Br Heart J* 43:284–292, 1980.
85. Miller FA Jr: Aortic stenosis: Most cases no longer require invasive hemodynamic study, *J Am Coll Cardiol* 13:551–553, 1989.
86. Oh JK, Taliercio CP, Holmes DR Jr, et al: Prediction of the severity of aortic stenosis by Doppler aortic valve area determination: Prospective Doppler-catheterization correlation in 100 patients, *J Am Coll Cardiol* 11:1227–1234, 1988.
87. Chizner MA, Pearle DL, deLeon AC Jr: The natural history of aortic stenosis in adults, *Am Heart J* 99:419–424, 1980.
88. Schwarz F, Baumann P, Manthey J, et al: The effect of aortic valve replacement on survival, *Circulation* 66:1105–1110, 1982.
89. Hood WP Jr, Rackley CE, Rolett ELR: Wall stress in the normal and hypertrophied human left ventricle, *Am J Cardiol* 22:550–558, 1968.
90. Peterson MB, Lesch MR: Protein synthesis and amino acid transport in the isolated rabbit right ventricular muscle. Effect of isometric tension development, *Circ Res* 31:317–327, 1972.
91. Hanrath P, Mathey DG, Siegert R, et al: Left ventricular relaxation and filling pattern in different forms of left ventricular hypertrophy: An echocardiographic study, *Am J Cardiol* 45:15–23, 1980.
92. Betocchi S, Bonow RO, Bacharach SL, et al: Isovolumic relaxation period in hypertrophic cardiomyopathy: Assessment by radionuclide angiography, *J Am Coll Cardiol* 7:74–81, 1986.
93. Topol EJ, Traill TA, Fortuin NJR: Hypertensive hypertrophic cardiomyopathy of the elderly, *N Engl J Med* 312:277–283, 1985.
94. Sanderson JE, Traill TA, Sutton MG, et al: Left ventricular relaxation and filling in hypertrophic cardiomyopathy. An echocardiographic study, *Br Heart J* 40:596–601, 1978.
95. Huber D, Grimm J, Koch R, et al: Determinants of ejection performance in aortic stenosis, *Circulation* 64:126–134, 1981.
96. Henry WL, Bonow RO, Borer JS, et al: Evaluation of aortic valve replacement in patients with valvular aortic stenosis, *Circulation* 61:814–825, 1980.
97. Grossman W, Jones D, McLaurin LP: Wall stress and patterns of hypertrophy in the human left ventricle, *J Clin Invest* 56:56–64, 1975.
98. Walther T, Schubert A, Falk V, et al: Regression of left ventricular hypertrophy after surgical therapy for aortic stenosis is associated with changes in extracellular matrix gene expression, *Circulation* 104:I54–I58, 2001.
99. Antonini-Canterin F, Huang G, Cervesato E, et al: Symptomatic aortic stenosis: Does systemic hypertension play an additional role? *Hypertension* 41:1268–1272, 2003.
100. Kuhl HP, Franke A, Puschmann D, et al: Regression of left ventricular mass one year after aortic valve replacement for pure severe aortic stenosis, *Am J Cardiol* 89:408–413, 2002.
101. Ikonomidis I, Tsoukas A, Parthenakis F, et al: Four year follow up of aortic valve replacement for isolated aortic stenosis: A link between reduction in pressure overload, regression of left ventricular hypertrophy, and diastolic function, *Heart* 86:309–316, 2001.
102. Beyerbacht HP, Lamb HJ, van Der Laarse A, et al: Aortic valve replacement in patients with aortic valve stenosis improves myocardial metabolism and diastolic function, *Radiology* 219:637–643, 2001.
103. Liedtke AJ, Gentzler RD 2nd, Babb JD, et al: Determinants of cardiac performance in severe aortic stenosis, *Chest* 69:192–200, 1976.
104. Thompson R, Yacoub M, Ahmed M, et al: Influence of preoperative left ventricular function on results of homograft replacement of the aortic valve for aortic stenosis, *Am J Cardiol* 43:929–938, 1979.

105. Sasayama S, Franklin D, Ross JJR: Hyperfunction with normal inotropic state of the hypertrophied left ventricle, *Am J Physiol* 232:H418–H425, 1977.
106. Gunther S, Grossman WR: Determinants of ventricular function in pressure overload hypertrophy in man, *Circulation* 59:679, 1977.
107. Brutsaert DL, Rademakers FE, Sys SU: Triple control of relaxation: Implications in cardiac disease, *Circulation* 69:190–196, 1984.
108. Marcus MLR: *Effects of cardiac hypertrophy on the coronary circulation: Effects of cardiac hypertrophy on the coronary circulation*, New York, 1983, McGraw-Hill.
109. Tomanek RJR: Response of the coronary vasculature to myocardial hypertrophy, *J Am Coll Cardiol* 15:528–533, 1990.
110. Stack RS, Schirmer B, Greenfield JCR: Coronary artery luminal diameters in normal and hypertrophied canine ventricles (abstract), *Circulation* 62(Suppl III):III-64, 1980.
111. Alyono D, Anderson RW, Parrish DG, et al: Alterations of myocardial blood flow associated with experimental canine left ventricular hypertrophy secondary to valvular aortic stenosis, *Circ Res* 58:47–57, 1986.
112. Yamori Y, Mori C, Nishio T, et al: Cardiac hypertrophy in early hypertension, *Am J Cardiol* 44: 964–969, 1979.
113. Hallback-Nordlander M, Noresson E, Thoren PR: Hemodynamic consequences of left ventricular hypertrophy in spontaneously hypertensive rats, *Am J Cardiol* 44:986–993, 1979.
114. Hinquell L, Odoroff CL, Honig CRR: Intercapillary distance and capillary reserve in hypertrophied rat hearts beating in situ, *Circ Res* 41:400, 1979.
115. Murray PA, Baig H, Fishbein MC, et al: Effects of experimental right ventricular hypertrophy on myocardial blood flow in conscious dogs, *J Clin Invest* 64:421–427, 1979.
116. Rakusan KR: Quantitative morphology of capillaries of the heart. Number of capillaries in animal and human hearts under normal and pathological conditions, *Methods Achiev Exp Pathol* 5:272–286, 1971.
117. Opherk D, Mall G, Zebe H, et al: Reduction of coronary reserve: A mechanism for angina pectoris in patients with arterial hypertension and normal coronary arteries, *Circulation* 69:1–7, 1984.
118. Marcus ML, Doty DB, Hiratzka LF, et al: Decreased coronary reserve: A mechanism for angina pectoris in patients with aortic stenosis and normal coronary arteries, *N Engl J Med* 307:1362–1366, 1982.
119. Nadell R, DePace NL, Ren JF, et al: Myocardial oxygen supply/demand ratio in aortic stenosis: Hemodynamic and echocardiographic evaluation of patients with and without angina pectoris, *J Am Coll Cardiol* 2:258–262, 1983.
120. Marcus ML, White CWR: Coronary flow reserve in patients with normal coronary angiograms, *J Am Coll Cardiol* 6:1254, 1985.
121. Marcus ML, Doty DB, Hiratzka LFR: Impaired coronary reserve in children with cyanotic congenital heart disease, *Circulation* 64:32, 1981.
122. Brutsaert DL, Housmans PR, Goethals MAR: Dual control of relaxation. Its role in the ventricular function in the mammalian heart, *Circ Res* 47:637–652, 1980.
123. Brutsaert DL, Rademakers FE, Sys SU, et al: Analysis of relaxation in the evaluation of ventricular function of the heart, *Prog Cardiovasc Dis* 28:143–163, 1985.
124. Grossman WR: Why is left ventricular diastolic pressure increased during angina pectoris? *J Am Coll Cardiol* 5:607, 1985.
125. McLaurin LP, Rolett EL, Grossman WR: Impaired left ventricular relaxation during pacing-induced ischemia, *Am J Cardiol* 32:751–757, 1973.
126. Bourdillon PD, Lorell BH, Mirsky I, et al: Increased regional myocardial stiffness of the left ventricle during pacing-induced angina in man, *Circulation* 67:316–323, 1983.
127. Carroll JD, Hess OM, Hirzel HO, et al: Exercise-induced ischemia: The influence of altered relaxation on early diastolic pressures, *Circulation* 67:521–528, 1983.
128. Serruys PW, Wijns W, van den Brand M, et al: Left ventricular performance, regional blood flow, wall motion, and lactate metabolism during transluminal angioplasty, *Circulation* 70:25–36, 1984.
129. Paulus WJ, Serizawa T, Grossman WR: Altered left ventricular diastolic properties during pacing-induced ischemia in dogs with coronary stenoses. Potentiation by caffeine, *Circ Res* 50:218–227, 1982.
130. Lorell BH, Turi Z, Grossman WR: Modification of left ventricular response to pacing tachycardia in nifedipine in patients with coronary artery disease, *Am J Med* 71:667–675, 1981.
131. Bonow RO, Rosing DR, Bacharach SL, et al: Effects of verapamil on left ventricular systolic function and diastolic filling in patients with hypertrophic cardiomyopathy, *Circulation* 64:787–796, 1981.
132. Hanrath P, Mathey DG, Kremer P, et al: Effect of verapamil on left ventricular isovolumic relaxation time and regional left ventricular filling in hypertrophic cardiomyopathy, *Am J Cardiol* 45:1258–1264, 1980.
133. Brown RO, Rosing DR, Bacharach SLR: Left ventricular systolic function and diastolic filling in patients with hypertrophic cardiomyopathy, *Circulation* 62(Suppl III):III-317, 1980.
134. Colan SD, Sanders SP, MacPherson D, et al: Left ventricular diastolic function in elite athletes with physiologic cardiac hypertrophy, *J Am Coll Cardiol* 6:545–549, 1985.
135. Granger CB, Karimeddini MK, Smith VE, et al: Rapid ventricular filling in left ventricular hypertrophy: I. Physiologic hypertrophy, *J Am Coll Cardiol* 5:862–868, 1985.
136. Smith VE, Schulman P, Karimeddini MK, et al: Rapid ventricular filling in left ventricular hypertrophy: II. Pathologic hypertrophy, *J Am Coll Cardiol* 5:869–874, 1985.
137. Lorell BH, Grossman WR: Cardiac hypertrophy: The consequences for diastole, *J Am Coll Cardiol* 9:1189–1193, 1987.
138. Ghali JK, Liao Y, Simmons B, et al: The prognostic role of left ventricular hypertrophy in patients with or without coronary artery disease, *Ann Intern Med* 117:831–836, 1992.
139. Sullivan JM, Vander Zwaag RV, el-Zeky F, et al: Left ventricular hypertrophy: Effect on survival, *J Am Coll Cardiol* 22:508–513, 1993.
140. Grayburn PA, Eichhorn EJ: Dobutamine challenge for low-gradient aortic stenosis, *Circulation* 106:763–765, 2002.
141. Bonow RO, Carabello B, de Leon AC, et al: ACC/AHA Guidelines for the Management of Patients With Valvular Heart Disease. Executive Summary. A report of the American College of Cardiology/American Heart Association Task Force on Practice Guidelines (Committee on Management of Patients With Valvular Heart Disease), *J Heart Valve Dis* 7:672–707, 1998.
142. deFilippi CR, Willett DL, Brickner ME, et al: Usefulness of dobutamine echocardiography in distinguishing severe from nonsevere valvular aortic stenosis in patients with depressed left ventricular function and low transvalvular gradients, *Am J Cardiol* 75:191–194, 1995.
143. Monin JL, Monchi M, Gest V, et al: Aortic stenosis with severe left ventricular dysfunction and low transvalvular pressure gradients: Risk stratification by low-dose dobutamine echocardiography, *J Am Coll Cardiol* 37:2101–2107, 2001.
144. Nishimura RA, Grantham JA, Connolly HM, et al: Low-output, low-gradient aortic stenosis in patients with depressed left ventricular systolic function: The clinical utility of the dobutamine challenge in the catheterization laboratory, *Circulation* 106:809–813, 2002.
145. Khot UN, Novaro GM, Popovic ZB, et al: Nitroprusside in critically ill patients with left ventricular dysfunction and aortic stenosis, *N Engl J Med* 348:1756–1763, 2003.
146. Zile MR, Gaasch WH: Heart failure in aortic stenosis—improving diagnosis and treatment, *N Engl J Med* 348:1735–1736, 2003.
147. Carabello BA: Clinical practice. Aortic stenosis, *N Engl J Med* 346:677–682, 2002.
110. Goldman L, Caldera DL, Nussbaum SR, et al: Multifactorial index of cardiac risk in noncardiac surgical procedures, *N Engl J Med* 297:845–850, 1977.
149. Sundt TM, Bailey MS, Moon MR, et al: Quality of life after aortic valve replacement at the age of > 80 years, *Circulation* 102:III70–III74, 2000.
150. Connolly HM, Oh JK, Schaff HV, et al: Severe aortic stenosis with low transvalvular gradient and severe left ventricular dysfunction: Result of aortic valve replacement in 52 patients, *Circulation* 101:1940–1946, 2000.
151. Stanley TH, Webster LR: Anesthetic requirements and cardiovascular effects of fentanyl-oxygen and fentanyl-diazepam-oxygen anesthesia in man, *Anesth Analg* 57:411–416, 1978.
152. Bovill JG, Warren PJ, Schuller JL, et al: Comparison of fentanyl, sufentanil, and alfentanil anesthesia in patients undergoing valvular heart surgery, *Anesth Analg* 63:1081–1086, 1984.
153. Dhadphale PR, Jackson AP, Alseri SR: Comparison of anesthesia with diazepam and ketamine vs. morphine in patients undergoing heart-valve replacement, *Anesthesiology* 51:200–203, 1979.
154. Lindeburg T, Spotoft H, Bredgaard Sorensen M, et al: Cardiovascular effects of etomidate used for induction and in combination with fentanyl-pancuronium for maintenance of anaesthesia in patients with valvular heart disease, *Acta Anaesthesiol Scand* 26:205–208, 1982.
155. Atlee JL 3rd, Alexander SC: Halothane effects on conductivity of the AV node and His-Purkinje system in the dog, *Anesth Analg* 56:378–386, 1977.
156. Atlee JL 3rd, Rusy BF, Kreul JF, et al: Supraventricular excitability in dogs during anesthesia with halothane and enflurane, *Anesthesiology* 49:407–413, 1978.
157. Perloff JG, Ronan JA, deLeon AC Jr: The effect of nitroglycerin on left ventricular wall tension in fixed orifice aortic stenosis, *Circulation* 32:204, 1965.
158. Grose R, Nivapumin TR: Mechanisms of nitroglycerin action in valvular aortic stenosis, *Am J Cardiol* 44:1371, 1965.
159. Goertz AW, Lindner KH, Seefelder C, et al: Effect of phenylephrine bolus administration on global left ventricular function in patients with coronary artery disease and patients with valvular aortic stenosis, *Anesthesiology* 78:834–841, 1993.
160. Cooley DA, Reul GJ, Wukasch DCR: Ischemic contracture of the heart: "Stone heart", *Am J Cardiol* 29:575–577, 1972.
161. Buckberg GDR: Antegrade cardioplegia, retrograde cardioplegia, or both? *Ann Thorac Surg* 45: 589–590, 1988.
162. Kirklin JW, Conti VR, Blackstone EHR: Prevention of myocardial damage during cardiac operations, *N Engl J Med* 301:135–141, 1979.
163. Warner KG, Khuri SF, Kloner RA, et al: Structural and metabolic correlates of cell injury in the hypertrophied myocardium during valve replacement, *J Thorac Cardiovasc Surg* 93:741–754, 1987.
164. Menasche P, Piwnica AR: Cardioplegia by way of the coronary sinus for valvular and coronary surgery, *J Am Coll Cardiol* 18:628–636, 1991.
165. Partington MT, Acar C, Buckberg GD, et al: Studies of retrograde cardioplegia. II. Advantages of antegrade/retrograde cardioplegia to optimize distribution in jeopardized myocardium, *J Thorac Cardiovasc Surg* 97:613–622, 1989.
166. Buckberg GD, Beyersdorf F, Allen BSR: Integrated myocardial management in valvular heart disease, *J Heart Valve Dis* 4(Suppl 2):S198–S212, 1995, discussion S212–S213.
167. Menasche P, Tronc F, Nguyen A, et al: Retrograde warm blood cardioplegia preserves hypertrophied myocardium: A clinical study, *Ann Thorac Surg* 57:1429–1434, 1994, discussion 1434–1435.
168. ACC: Report of the American College of Cardiology/AHA task force on practice guidelines (Committee on perioperative cardiovascular evaluation for noncardiac surgery), *Anesth Analg* 82:854, 1996.
169. Roberts R, Sigwart U: New concepts in hypertrophic cardiomyopathies, part II, *Circulation* 104: 2249–2252, 2001.
170. Spencer WH 3rd, Roberts R: Alcohol septal ablation in hypertrophic obstructive cardiomyopathy: The need for a registry, *Circulation* 102:600–601, 2000.
171. Lakkis N: New treatment methods for patients with hypertrophic obstructive cardiomyopathy, *Curr Opin Cardiol* 15:172–177, 2000.
172. Nishimura RA, Trusty JM, Hayes DL, et al: Dual-chamber pacing for hypertrophic cardiomyopathy: A randomized, double-blind, crossover trial, *J Am Coll Cardiol* 29:435–441, 1997.
173. Maron BJ, Nishimura RA, McKenna WJ, et al: Assessment of permanent dual-chamber pacing as a treatment for drug-refractory symptomatic patients with obstructive hypertrophic cardiomyopathy. A randomized, double-blind, crossover study (M-PATHY), *Circulation* 99:2927–2933, 1999.
174. Erwin JP 3rd, Nishimura RA, Lloyd MA, et al: Dual chamber pacing for patients with hypertrophic obstructive cardiomyopathy: A clinical perspective in 2000, *Mayo Clin Proc* 75:173–180, 2000.
175. Lakkis NM, Nagueh SF, Kleiman NS, et al: Echocardiography-guided ethanol septal reduction for hypertrophic obstructive cardiomyopathy, *Circulation* 98:1750–1755, 1998.
176. Talreja DR, Nishimura RA, Edwards WD, et al: Alcohol septal ablation versus surgical septal myectomy: Comparison of effects on atrioventricular conduction tissue, *J Am Coll Cardiol* 44: 2329–2332, 2004.
177. Louie EK, Edwards LC 3rd: Hypertrophic cardiomyopathy, *Prog Cardiovasc Dis* 36:275–308, 1994.
178. Nishimura RA, Holmes DR Jr: Clinical practice. Hypertrophic obstructive cardiomyopathy, *N Engl J Med* 350:1320–1327, 2004.
179. Wynne J, Braunwald ER: The cardiomyopathies and myocarditides. In *The cardiomyopathies and myocarditides*, ed 2, Philadelphia, 1984, WB Saunders.
180. Ciro E, Nichols PF 3rd, Maron BJR: Heterogeneous morphologic expression of genetically transmitted hypertrophic cardiomyopathy. Two-dimensional echocardiographic analysis, *Circulation* 67:1227–1233, 1983.
181. Clark CE, Henry WL, Epstein SER: Familial prevalence and genetic transmission of idiopathic hypertrophic subaortic stenosis, *N Engl J Med* 289:709–714, 1973.
182. Maron BJ, Roberts WC, Edwards JE, et al: Sudden death in patients with hypertrophic cardiomyopathy: Characterization of 26 patients with functional limitation, *Am J Cardiol* 41:803–810, 1978.
183. Braunwald E, Lambrew CT, Rockoff SDR: Idiopathic hypertrophic subaortic stenosis, *Circulation* 29/30:IV–1, 1964.
184. McKenna WJ, Chetty S, Oakley CM, et al: Arrhythmia in hypertrophic cardiomyopathy: Exercise and 48 hour ambulatory electrocardiographic assessment with and without beta adrenergic blocking therapy, *Am J Cardiol* 45:1–5, 1980.
185. Savage DD, Seides SF, Maron BJ, et al: Prevalence of arrhythmias during 24-hour electrocardiographic monitoring and exercise testing in patients with obstructive and nonobstructive hypertrophic cardiomyopathy, *Circulation* 59:866–875, 1979.
186. McKenna WJ, England D, Doi YL, et al: Arrhythmia in hypertrophic cardiomyopathy. I: Influence on prognosis, *Br Heart J* 46:168–172, 1981.
187. Bonow RO, Frederick TM, Bacharach SL, et al: Atrial systole and left ventricular filling in hypertrophic cardiomyopathy: Effect of verapamil, *Am J Cardiol* 51:1386–1391, 1983.
188. Maron BJ, Lipson LC, Roberts WC, et al: "Malignant" hypertrophic cardiomyopathy: Identification of a subgroup of families with unusually frequent premature death, *Am J Cardiol* 41:1133–1140, 1978.
189. Maron BJ, Roberts WC, Epstein SER: Sudden death in hypertrophic cardiomyopathy: A profile of 78 patients, *Circulation* 65:1388–1394, 1982.
190. Maron BJ, Roberts WC, McAllister HA, et al: Sudden death in young athletes, *Circulation* 62:218–229, 1980.
191. Lewis JF, Maron BJR: Elderly patients with hypertrophic cardiomyopathy: A subset with distinctive left ventricular morphology and progressive clinical course late in life, *J Am Coll Cardiol* 13:36–45, 1989.

192. Wigle ED, Silver MDR: Myocardial fiber disarray and ventricular septal hypertrophy in asymmetrical hypertrophy of the heart, *Circulation* 58:398–402, 1978.
193. Murgo JP, Alter BR, Dorethy JF, et al: Dynamics of left ventricular ejection in obstructive and nonobstructive hypertrophic cardiomyopathy, *J Clin Invest* 66:1369–1382, 1980.
194. Pohost GM, Vignola PA, McKusick KE, et al: Hypertrophic cardiomyopathy. Evaluation by gated cardiac blood pool scanning, *Circulation* 55:92–99, 1977.
195. Sutton MG, Tajik AJ, Gibson DG, et al: Echocardiographic assessment of left ventricular filling and septal and posterior wall dynamics in idiopathic hypertrophic subaortic stenosis, *Circulation* 57: 512–520, 1978.
196. Wilson WS, Criley JM, Ross RSR: Dynamics of left ventricular emptying in hypertrophic subaortic stenosis. A cineangiographic and hemodynamic study, *Am Heart J* 73:4–16, 1967.
197. Pouleur H, Rousseau MF, van Eyll C, et al: Force-velocity-length relations in hypertrophic cardiomyopathy: Evidence of normal or depressed myocardial contractility, *Am J Cardiol* 52:813–817, 1983.
198. Hirota Y, Furubayashi K, Kaku K, et al: Hypertrophic nonobstructive cardiomyopathy: A precise assessment of hemodynamic characteristics and clinical implications, *Am J Cardiol* 50:990–997, 1982.
199. Cannon RO 3rd, Schenke WH, Bonow RO, et al: Left ventricular pulsus alternans in patients with hypertrophic cardiomyopathy and severe obstruction to left ventricular outflow, *Circulation* 73: 276–285, 1986.
200. Kramer CM, Reichek N, Ferrari VA, et al: Regional heterogeneity of function in hypertrophic cardiomyopathy, *Circulation* 90:186–194, 1994.
201. Morrow AG, Braunwald ER: Functional aortic stenosis: A malformation characterized by resistance to left ventricular outflow without anatomic obstruction, *Circulation* 20:181, 1959.
202. Henry WL, Clark CE, Glancy DL, et al: Echocardiographic measurement of the left ventricular outflow gradient in idiopathic hypertrophic subaortic stenosis, *N Engl J Med* 288:989–993, 1973.
203. Cape EG, Simons D, Jimoh A, et al: Chordal geometry determines the shape and extent of systolic anterior mitral motion: In vitro studies, *J Am Coll Cardiol* 13:1438–1448, 1989.
204. Wigle ED, Sasson Z, Henderson MA, et al: Hypertrophic cardiomyopathy. The importance of the site and the extent of hypertrophy. A review, *Prog Cardiovasc Dis* 28:1–83, 1985.
205. Sherrid MV, Chu CK, Delia E, et al: An echocardiographic study of the fluid mechanics of obstruction in hypertrophic cardiomyopathy, *J Am Coll Cardiol* 22:816–825, 1993.
206. King JF, DeMaria AN, Miller RRR: Markedly abnormal mitral valve motion without simultaneous intraventricular pressure gradient due to uneven mitral-septal contact in idiopathic hypertrophic subaortic stenosis, *Am J Cardiol* 50:360, 1982.
207. Rossen RM, Goodman DJ, Ingham RE, et al: Echocardiographic criteria in the diagnosis of idiopathic hypertrophic subaortic stenosis, *Circulation* 50:747–751, 1974.
208. Feizi O, Emanuel RR: Echocardiographic spectrum of hypertrophic cardiomyopathy, *Br Heart J* 37:1286–1302, 1975.
209. Pollick C, Rakowski H, Wigle EDR: Muscular subaortic stenosis: The quantitative relationship between systolic anterior motion and the pressure gradient, *Circulation* 69:43–49, 1984.
210. Lin CS, Chen KS, Lin MC, et al: The relationship between systolic anterior motion of the mitral valve and the left ventricular outflow tract Doppler in hypertrophic cardiomyopathy, *Am Heart J* 122: 1671–1682, 1991.
211. Levine RH, Weyman AER: Dynamic subaortic obstruction in hypertrophic cardiomyopathy: Criteria and controversy, *J Am Coll Cardiol* 6:15, 1985.
212. Ross J Jr, Braunwald E, Gault JH, et al: The mechanism of the intraventricular pressure gradient in idiopathic hypertrophic subaortic stenosis, *Circulation* 34:558–578, 1966.
213. Maron BJ, Gottdiener JS, Arce J, et al: Dynamic subaortic obstruction in hypertrophic cardiomyopathy: Analysis by pulsed Doppler echocardiography, *J Am Coll Cardiol* 6:1–18, 1985.
214. Gilbert BW, Pollick C, Adelman AG, et al: Hypertrophic cardiomyopathy: Subclassification by m mode echocardiography, *Am J Cardiol* 45:861–872, 1980.
215. Criley JM, Lewis KB, White RI Jr, et al: Pressure gradients without obstruction. A new concept of "hypertrophic subaortic stenosis", *Circulation* 32:881–887, 1965.
216. Criley JM, Siegel RJR: Has 'obstruction' hindered our understanding of hypertrophic cardiomyopathy? *Circulation* 72:1148–1154, 1985.
217. Klues HG, Maron BJ, Dollar AL, et al: Diversity of structural mitral valve alterations in hypertrophic cardiomyopathy, *Circulation* 85:1651–1660, 1992.
218. Glancy DL, Shepherd RL, Beiser D, et al: The dynamic nature of left ventricular outflow obstruction in idiopathic hypertrophic subaortic stenosis, *Ann Intern Med* 75:589–593, 1971.
219. Lorell BH, Paulus WJ, Grossman W, et al: Modification of abnormal left ventricular diastolic properties by nifedipine in patients with hypertrophic cardiomyopathy, *Circulation* 65:499–507, 1982.
220. Rosing DR, Epstein SER: Verapamil in the treatment of hypertrophic cardiomyopathy, *Ann Intern Med* 96:670–672, 1982.
221. Rosing DR, Kent KM, Borer JS, et al: Verapamil therapy: A new approach to the pharmacologic treatment of hypertrophic cardiomyopathy. I. Hemodynamic effects, *Circulation* 60:1201–1207, 1979.
222. TenCate FJ, Serruys PW, Mey S, et al: Effects of short-term administration of verapamil on left ventricular relaxation and filling dynamics measured by a combined hemodynamic-ultrasonic technique in patients with hypertrophic cardiomyopathy, *Circulation* 68:1274–1279, 1983.
223. Losi MA, Betocchi S, Grimaldi M, et al: Heterogeneity of left ventricular filling dynamics in hypertrophic cardiomyopathy, *Am J Cardiol* 73:987–990, 1994.
224. O'Gara PT, Bonow RO, Maron BJ, et al: Myocardial perfusion abnormalities in patients with hypertrophic cardiomyopathy: Assessment with thallium-201 emission computed tomography, *Circulation* 76:1214–1223, 1987.
225. Grover-McKay M, Schwaiger M, Krivokapich J, et al: Regional myocardial blood flow and metabolism at rest in mildly symptomatic patients with hypertrophic cardiomyopathy, *J Am Coll Cardiol* 13: 317–324, 1989.
226. Maron BJ, Wolfson JK, Epstein SE, et al: Intramural ("small vessel") coronary artery disease in hypertrophic cardiomyopathy, *J Am Coll Cardiol* 8:545–557, 1986.
227. Pasternac A, Noble J, Streulens Y, et al: Pathophysiology of chest pain in patients with cardiomyopathies and normal coronary arteries, *Circulation* 65:778–789, 1982.
228. Camici P, Chiriatti G, Lorenzoni R, et al: Coronary vasodilation is impaired in both hypertrophied and nonhypertrophied myocardium of patients with hypertrophic cardiomyopathy: A study with nitrogen-13 ammonia and positron emission tomography, *J Am Coll Cardiol* 17:879–886, 1991.
229. Cannon RO 3rd, Schenke WH, Maron BJ, et al: Differences in coronary flow and myocardial metabolism at rest and during pacing between patients with obstructive and patients with nonobstructive hypertrophic cardiomyopathy, *J Am Coll Cardiol* 10:53–62, 1987.
230. Hayashida W, Kumada T, Kohno F, et al: Left ventricular regional relaxation and its nonuniformity in hypertrophic nonobstructive cardiomyopathy, *Circulation* 84:1496–1504, 1991.
231. Miyamoto MI, Rockman HA, Guth BD, et al: Effect of alpha-adrenergic stimulation on regional contractile function and myocardial blood flow with and without ischemia, *Circulation* 84:1715–1724, 1991.
232. Pollick CR: Muscular subaortic stenosis: Hemodynamic and clinical improvement after disopyramide, *N Engl J Med* 307:997–999, 1982.
233. Chatterjee K, Raff G, Anderson D, et al: Hypertrophic cardiomyopathy—therapy with slow channel inhibiting agents, *Prog Cardiovasc Dis* 25:193–210, 1982.
234. Bonow RO, Ostrow HG, Rosing DR, et al: Effects of verapamil on left ventricular systolic and diastolic function in patients with hypertrophic cardiomyopathy: Pressure-volume analysis with a nonimaging scintillation probe, *Circulation* 68:1062–1073, 1983.
235. Epstein SE, Rosing DRR: Verapamil: Its potential for causing serious complications in patients with hypertrophic cardiomyopathy, *Circulation* 64:437–441, 1981.
236. Seiler C, Hess OM, Schoenbeck M, et al: Long-term follow-up of medical versus surgical therapy for hypertrophic cardiomyopathy: A retrospective study, *J Am Coll Cardiol* 17:634–642, 1991.
237. Chahine RAR: Surgical versus medical therapy of hypertrophic cardiomyopathy: Is the perspective changing? *J Am Coll Cardiol* 17:643–645, 1991.
238. Fananapazir L, Cannon RO 3rd, Tripodi D, et al: Impact of dual-chamber permanent pacing in patients with obstructive hypertrophic cardiomyopathy with symptoms refractory to verapamil and beta-adrenergic blocker therapy, *Circulation* 85:2149–2161, 1992.
239. Maron BJR: Appraisal of dual-chamber pacing therapy in hypertrophic cardiomyopathy: Too soon for a rush to judgment? *J Am Coll Cardiol* 27:431–432, 1996.
240. Williams WG, Wigle ED, Rakowski H, et al: Results of surgery for hypertrophic obstructive cardiomyopathy, *Circulation* 76:V104–V108, 1987.
241. Grigg LE, Wigle ED, Williams WG, et al: Transesophageal Doppler echocardiography in obstructive hypertrophic cardiomyopathy: Clarification of pathophysiology and importance in intraoperative decision making, *J Am Coll Cardiol* 20:42–52, 1992.
242. Joyce FS, Lever HM, Cosgrove DM 3rd: Treatment of hypertrophic cardiomyopathy by mitral valve repair and septal myectomy, *Ann Thorac Surg* 57:1025–1027, 1994.
243. Gilligan DM, Chan WL, Stewart R, et al: Cardiac responses assessed by echocardiography to changes in preload in hypertrophic cardiomyopathy, *Am J Cardiol* 73:312–315, 1994.
244. Cohn LH, Trehan H, Collins JJ Jr: Long-term follow-up of patients undergoing myotomy/myectomy for obstructive hypertrophic cardiomyopathy, *Am J Cardiol* 70:657–660, 1992.
245. ten Berg JM, Suttorp MJ, Knaepen PJ, et al: Hypertrophic obstructive cardiomyopathy. Initial results and long-term follow-up after Morrow septal myectomy, *Circulation* 90:1781–1785, 1994.
246. Sasson Z, Prieur T, Skrobik Y, et al: Aortic regurgitation: A common complication after surgery for hypertrophic obstructive cardiomyopathy, *J Am Coll Cardiol* 13:63–67, 1989.
247. Cosio FG, Moro C, Alonso M, et al: The Q waves hypertrophic cardiomyopathy: An electrophysiologic study, *N Engl J Med* 302:96–99, 1980.
248. Krikler DM, Davies MJ, Rowland E, et al: Sudden death in hypertrophic cardiomyopathy: Associated accessory atrioventricular pathways, *Br Heart J* 43:245–251, 1980.
249. Anderson KP, Stinson EB, Derby GC, et al: Vulnerability of patients with obstructive hypertrophic cardiomyopathy to ventricular arrhythmia induction in the operating room. Analysis of 17 patients, *Am J Cardiol* 51:811–816, 1983.
250. Wulfson HD, LaPorta RFR: Pulmonary oedema after lithotripsy in a patient with hypertrophic subaortic stenosis, *Can J Anaesth* 40:465–467, 1993.
251. Thompson RC, Liberthson RR, Lowenstein ER: Perioperative anesthetic risk of noncardiac surgery in hypertrophic obstructive cardiomyopathy, *JAMA* 254:2419–2421, 1985.
252. Loubser P, Suh K, Cohen SR: Adverse effects of spinal anesthesia in a patient with idiopathic hypertrophic subaortic stenosis, *Anesthesiology* 60:228–230, 1984.
253. Larson CP Jr: Use of spinal anesthesia in patients with idiopathic hypertrophic subaortic stenosis, *Anesthesiology* 61:229, 1984.
254. Pearson J, Reves JGR: Unusual cause of hypotension after coronary artery bypass grafting: Idiopathic hypertrophic subaortic stenosis, *Anesthesiology* 60:592–594, 1984.
255. Lanier W, Prough DSR: Intraoperative diagnosis of hypertrophic obstructive cardiomyopathy, *Anesthesiology* 60:61–63, 1984.
256. Smith HJ, Neutze JM, Roche AH, et al: The natural history of rheumatic aortic regurgitation and the indications for surgery, *Br Heart J* 38:147–154, 1976.
257. Goldschlager N, Pfeifer J, Cohn K, et al: The natural history of aortic regurgitation. A clinical and hemodynamic study, *Am J Med* 54:577–588, 1973.
258. Ishii K, Hirota Y, Suwa M, et al: Natural history and left ventricular response in chronic aortic regurgitation, *Am J Cardiol* 78:357–361, 1996.
259. Schwarz F, Flameng W, Langebartels F, et al: Impaired left ventricular function in chronic aortic valve disease: Survival and function after replacement by Bjork-Shiley prosthesis, *Circulation* 60:48–458, 1979.
260. Tam JW, Antecol D, Kim HH, et al: Low dose dobutamine echocardiography in the assessment of contractile reserve to predict the outcome of valve replacement for chronic aortic regurgitation, *Can J Cardiol* 15:73–79, 1999.
261. Padial LR, Oliver A, Vivaldi M, et al: Doppler echocardiographic assessment of progression of aortic regurgitation, *Am J Cardiol* 80:306–314, 1997.
262. Levine HJ, Gaasch WHR: Ratio of regurgitant volume to end-diastolic volume: A major determinant of ventricular response to surgical correction of chronic volume overload, *Am J Cardiol* 52: 406–410, 1983.
263. Bonow RO, Rosing DR, Kent KM, et al: Timing of operation for chronic aortic regurgitation, *Am J Cardiol* 50:325–336, 1982.
264. Green GR, Miller DC: Continuing dilemmas concerning aortic valve replacement in patients with advanced left ventricular systolic dysfunction, *J Heart Valve Dis* 6:562–579, 1997.
265. Eichorn EJ, Konstam MAR: *Quantitation of aortic regurgitation: Quantitation of aortic regurgitation*, Boston, 1988, Kluwer Academic, p 108.
266. Reimold SC, Byrne JG, Caguioa ES, et al: Load dependence of the effective regurgitant orifice area in a sheep model of aortic regurgitation, *J Am Coll Cardiol* 18:1085–1090, 1991.
267. Enriquez-Sarano M, Tajik AJ: Clinical practice. Aortic regurgitation, *N Engl J Med* 351:1539–1546, 2004.
268. Elkayam U, McKay CR, Weber L, et al: Favorable effects of hydralazine on the hemodynamic response to isometric exercise in chronic severe aortic regurgitation, *Am J Cardiol* 53:1603–1607, 1984.
269. Greenberg BH, DeMots H, Murphy E, et al: Mechanism for improved cardiac performance with arteriolar dilators in aortic insufficiency, *Circulation* 63:263–268, 1981.
270. Devlin WH, Petrusha J, Briesmiester K, et al: Impact of vascular adaptation to chronic aortic regurgitation on left ventricular performance, *Circulation* 99:1027–1033, 1999.
271. Borow KM, Marcus RH: Aortic regurgitation: The need for an integrated physiologic approach, *J Am Coll Cardiol* 17:898–900, 1991.
272. Judge TP, Kennedy JW, Bennett LJ, et al: Quantitative hemodynamic effects of heart rate in aortic regurgitation, *Circulation* 44:355–367, 1971.
273. Firth BG, Dehmer GJ, Nicod P, et al: Effect of increasing heart rate in patients with aortic regurgitation. Effect of incremental atrial pacing on scintigraphic, hemodynamic and thermodilution measurements, *Am J Cardiol* 49:1860–1867, 1982.
274. Dodge HT, Kennedy JW, Petersen JLR: Quantitative angiocardiographic methods in the evaluation of valvular heart disease, *Prog Cardiovasc Dis* 16:1–23, 1973.
275. Segal J, Harvey WP, Hufnagel C: A clinical study of one hundred cases of severe aortic insufficiency, *Am J Med* 21:200–210, 1956.
276. Johnson AE, Engler RL, LeWinger M: The medical and surgical management of patients with aortic valve disease. A symposium, *West J Med* 126:460, 1977.
277. Kawachi K, Kitamura S, Oyama C, et al: Relations of preoperative hemodynamics and coronary blood flow to improved left ventricular function after valve replacement for aortic regurgitation, *J Am Coll Cardiol* 11:925–929, 1988.

278. Eastham CL, Doty DB, Hiratzka LF: Volume-overload left ventricular hypertrophy impairs coronary reserve in humans, *Circulation* 64(Suppl IV):IV–26, 1981.
279. Strauer BE: Ventricular function and coronary hemodynamics in hypertensive heart disease, *Am J Cardiol* 44:999–1006, 1979.
280. Tauchert M, Hilger HH: *Application of the coronary reserve concept to the study of myocardial perfusion: Application of the coronary reserve concept to the study of myocardial perfusion*, Amsterdam, 1979, Elsevier/North-Holland, pp 141–167.
281. Braunwald E: *Valvular heart disease: Valvular heart disease*, Philadelphia, 1992, WB Saunders Company.
282. Borow KM: Surgical outcome in chronic aortic regurgitation: A physiologic framework for assessing preoperative predictors, *J Am Coll Cardiol* 10:1165–1170, 1987.
283. Gerson MC, Engel PJ, Mantil JC, et al: Effects of dynamic and isometric exercise on the radionuclide-determined regurgitant fraction in aortic insufficiency, *J Am Coll Cardiol* 3:98–106, 1984.
284. Huxley RL, Gaffney FA, Corbett JR, et al: Early detection of left ventricular dysfunction in chronic aortic regurgitation as assessed by contrast angiography, echocardiography, and rest and exercise scintigraphy, *Am J Cardiol* 51:1542–1550, 1983.
285. Tarasoutchi F, Grinberg M, Spina GS, et al: Ten-year clinical laboratory follow-up after application of a symptom-based therapeutic strategy to patients with severe chronic aortic regurgitation of predominant rheumatic etiology, *J Am Coll Cardiol* 41:1316–1324, 2003.
286. Verheul HA, van den Brink RB, Bouma BJ, et al: Analysis of risk factors for excess mortality after aortic valve replacement, *J Am Coll Cardiol* 26:1280–1286, 1995.
287. Welch GH Jr, Braunwald E, Sarnoff SJ: Hemodynamic effects of quantitatively varied experimental aortic regurgitation, *Circ Res* 5:546–551, 1957.
288. Mann T, McLaurin L, Grossman W, et al: Assessing the hemodynamic severity of acute aortic regurgitation due to infective endocarditis, *N Engl J Med* 293:108–113, 1975.
289. Botvinick EH, Schiller NB, Wickramasekaran R, et al: Echocardiographic demonstration of early mitral valve closure in severe aortic insufficiency. Its clinical implications, *Circulation* 51:836–847, 1975.
290. Wigle ED, Labrosse CJ: Sudden, severe aortic insufficiency, *Circulation* 32:708–720, 1965.
291. Laniado S, Yellin EL, Yoran C, et al: Physiologic mechanisms in aortic insufficiency. I. The effect of changing heart rate on flow dynamics. II. Determinants of Austin Flint murmur, *Circulation* 66:226–235, 1982.
292. Ardehali A, Segal J, Cheitlin MD: Coronary blood flow reserve in acute aortic regurgitation, *J Am Coll Cardiol* 25:1387–1392, 1995.
293. van Herwerden LA, Gussenhoven EJ, Roelandt JR, et al: Intraoperative two-dimensional echocardiography in complicated infective endocarditis of the aortic valve, *J Thorac Cardiovasc Surg* 93:587–591, 1987.
294. Shapiro SM, Bayer AS: Transesophageal and Doppler echocardiography in the diagnosis and management of infective endocarditis, *Chest* 100:1125–1130, 1991.
295. Daniel WG, Mugge A, Martin RP, et al: Improvement in the diagnosis of abscesses associated with endocarditis by transesophageal echocardiography, *N Engl J Med* 324:795–800, 1991.
296. Teague SM, Heinsimer JA, Anderson JL, et al: Quantification of aortic regurgitation utilizing continuous wave Doppler ultrasound, *J Am Coll Cardiol* 8:592–599, 1986.
297. Perry GJ, Helmcke F, Nanda NC, et al: Evaluation of aortic insufficiency by Doppler color flow mapping, *J Am Coll Cardiol* 9:952–959, 1987.
298. Oh JK, Hatle LK, Sinak LJ, et al: Characteristic Doppler echocardiographic pattern of mitral inflow velocity in severe aortic regurgitation, *J Am Coll Cardiol* 14:1712–1717, 1989.
299. Stone JG, Hoar PF, Khambatta HJ: Influence of volume loading on intraoperative hemodynamics and perioperative fluid retention in patients with valvular regurgitation undergoing prosthetic replacement, *Am J Cardiol* 52:530–533, 1983.
300. Stone JG, Hoar PF, Calabro JR, et al: Afterload reduction and preload augmentation improve the anesthetic management of patients with cardiac failure and valvular regurgitation, *Anesth Analg* 59:737–742, 1980.
301. Cohn JN, Franciosa JA: Vasodilator therapy of cardiac failure (parts 1 and 2), *N Engl J Med* 297:27–31, 254–258, 1977.
302. Karon BL, Enriquez-Sarano M: Valvular regurgitation. In *Valvular regurgitation*, ed 2, Philadelphia, 2000, Lippincott Williams & Wilkins, pp 303–330.
303. Enriquez-Sarano M, Avierinos JF, Messika-Zeitoun D, et al: Quantitative determinants of the outcome of asymptomatic mitral regurgitation, *N Engl J Med* 352:875–883, 2005.
304. Enriquez-Sarano M, Orszulak TA, Schaff HV, et al: Mitral regurgitation: A new clinical perspective, *Mayo Clin Proc* 72:1034–1043, 1997.
305. Ling LH, Enriquez-Sarano M, Seward JB, et al: Clinical outcome of mitral regurgitation due to flail leaflet, *N Engl J Med* 335:1417–1423, 1996.
306. Grigioni F, Enriquez-Sarano M, Ling LH, et al: Sudden death in mitral regurgitation due to flail leaflet, *J Am Coll Cardiol* 34:2078–2085, 1999.
307. Enriquez-Sarano M, Basmadjian AJ, Rossi A, et al: Progression of mitral regurgitation: A prospective Doppler echocardiographic study, *J Am Coll Cardiol* 34:1137–1144, 1999.
308. Carabello BA: The pathophysiology of mitral regurgitation, *J Heart Valve Dis* 9:600–608, 2000.
309. Otsuji Y, Handschumacher MD, Kisanuki A, et al: Functional mitral regurgitation, *Cardiologia* 43:1011–1016, 1998.
310. Enriquez-Sarano M, Tajik AJ, Schaff HV, et al: Echocardiographic prediction of survival after surgical correction of organic mitral regurgitation, *Circulation* 90:830–837, 1994.
311. Enriquez-Sarano M, Tajik AJ, Schaff HV, et al: Echocardiographic prediction of left ventricular function after correction of mitral regurgitation: Results and clinical implications, *J Am Coll Cardiol* 24:1536–1543, 1994.
312. Enriquez-Sarano M, Schaff HV, Orszulak TA, et al: Congestive heart failure after surgical correction of mitral regurgitation. A long-term study, *Circulation* 92:2496–2503, 1995.
313. Matsuo T, Carabello BA, Nagatomo Y, et al: Mechanisms of cardiac hypertrophy in canine volume overload, *Am J Physiol* 275:H65–H74, 1998.
314. Carabello BA, Nakano K, Corin W, et al: Left ventricular function in experimental volume overload hypertrophy, *Am J Physiol* 256:H974–H981, 1989.
315. Kleaveland JP, Kussmaul WG, Vinciguerra T, et al: Volume overload hypertrophy in a closed-chest model of mitral regurgitation, *Am J Physiol* 254:H1034–H1041, 1988.
316. Imamura T, McDermott PJ, Kent RL, et al: Acute changes in myosin heavy chain synthesis rate in pressure versus volume overload, *Circ Res* 75:418–425, 1994.
317. Urabe Y, Mann DL, Kent RL, et al: Cellular and ventricular contractile dysfunction in experimental canine mitral regurgitation, *Circ Res* 70:131–147, 1992.
318. Lehmann KG, Francis CK, Dodge HT: Mitral regurgitation in early myocardial infarction. Incidence, clinical detection, and prognostic implications. TIMI Study Group, *Ann Intern Med* 117:10–17, 1992.
319. Tcheng JE, Jackman JD Jr, Nelson CL, et al: Outcome of patients sustaining acute ischemic mitral regurgitation during myocardial infarction, *Ann Intern Med* 117:18–24, 1992.
320. Lamas GA, Mitchell GF, Flaker GC, et al: Clinical significance of mitral regurgitation after acute myocardial infarction. Survival and Ventricular Enlargement Investigators, *Circulation* 96:827–833, 1997.
321. Phillips JH, Burch GE, Depasquale NP: The syndrome of papillary muscle dysfunction. Its clinical recognition, *Ann Intern Med* 59:508–520, 1963.
322. Burch GE, DePasquale NP, Phillips JH: The syndrome of papillary muscle dysfunction, *Am Heart J* 75:399–415, 1968.
323. Burch GE, De Pasquale NP, Phillips JH: Clinical manifestations of papillary muscle dysfunction, *Arch Intern Med* 112:112–117, 1963.
324. Levine RA: Dynamic mitral regurgitation—more than meets the eye, *N Engl J Med* 351:1681–1684, 2004.
325. Kaul S, Spotnitz WD, Glasheen WP, et al: Mechanism of ischemic mitral regurgitation. An experimental evaluation, *Circulation* 84:2167–2180, 1991.
326. Mittal AK, Langston M Jr, Cohn KE, et al: Combined papillary muscle and left ventricular wall dysfunction as a cause of mitral regurgitation. An experimental study, *Circulation* 44:174–180, 1971.
327. Tsakiris AG, Rastelli GC, Amorim Dde S, et al: Effect of experimental papillary muscle damage on mitral valve closure in intact anesthetized dogs, *Mayo Clin Proc* 45:275–285, 1970.
328. Otsuji Y, Handschumacher MD, Schwammenthal E, et al: Insights from three-dimensional echocardiography into the mechanism of functional mitral regurgitation: Direct in vivo demonstration of altered leaflet tethering geometry, *Circulation* 96:1999–2008, 1997.
329. Birnbaum Y, Chamoun AJ, Conti VR, et al: Mitral regurgitation following acute myocardial infarction, *Coron Artery Dis* 13:337–344, 2002.
330. Komeda M, Glasson JR, MacIsaac A, et al: Systolic "dysfunction" of ischemic papillary muscle may serve as a compensatory mechanism for left ventricular wall motion abnormality (abstract), *Circulation* 92:I357, 1995.
331. Dent JM, Spotnitz WD, Kaul S: Echocardiographic evaluation of the mechanisms of ischemic mitral regurgitation, *Coron Artery Dis* 7:188–195, 1996.
332. Ormiston JA, Shah PM, Tei C, et al: Size and motion of the mitral valve annulus in man. I. A two-dimensional echocardiographic method and findings in normal subjects, *Circulation* 64:113–120, 1981.
333. Tsakiris AG, Von Bernuth G, Rastelli GC, et al: Size and motion of the mitral valve annulus in anesthetized intact dogs, *J Appl Physiol* 30:611–618, 1971.
334. Ma HH, Honma H, Munakata K, et al: Mitral insufficiency as a complication of acute myocardial infarction and left ventricular remodeling, *Jpn Circ J* 61:912–920, 1997.
335. Tenenbaum A, Leor J, Motro M, et al: Improved posterobasal segment function after thrombolysis is associated with decreased incidence of significant mitral regurgitation in a first inferior myocardial infarction, *J Am Coll Cardiol* 25:1558–1563, 1995.
336. Leor J, Feinberg MS, Vered Z, et al: Effect of thrombolytic therapy on the evolution of significant mitral regurgitation in patients with a first inferior myocardial infarction, *J Am Coll Cardiol* 21:1661–1666, 1993.
337. Kinn JW, O'Neill WW, Benzuly KH, et al: Primary angioplasty reduces risk of myocardial rupture compared to thrombolysis for acute myocardial infarction, *Cathet Cardiovasc Diagn* 42:151–157, 1997.
338. Scott WC, Miller DC, Haverich A, et al: Operative risk of mitral valve replacement: Discriminant analysis of 1329 procedures, *Circulation* 72:II108–II119, 1985.
339. Rozich JD, Carabello BA, Usher BW, et al: Mitral valve replacement with and without chordal preservation in patients with chronic mitral regurgitation. Mechanisms for differences in postoperative ejection performance, *Circulation* 86:1718–1726, 1992.
340. Enriquez-Sarano M, Schaff HV, Orszulak TA, et al: Valve repair improves the outcome of surgery for mitral regurgitation. A multivariate analysis, *Circulation* 91:1022–1028, 1995.
341. Mohty D, Orszulak TA, Schaff HV, et al: Very long-term survival and durability of mitral valve repair for mitral valve prolapse, *Circulation* 104:I1–I7, 2001.
342. David TE, Armstrong S, Sun Z: Replacement of chordae tendineae with Gore-Tex sutures: A ten-year experience, *J Heart Valve Dis* 5:352–355, 1996.
343. Pearson PJ, Schaff HV: Valve repair and choice of valves. *Valve repair and choice of valves*, ed 2, London, 2003, BMJ Books, pp 809–816.
344. David TE, Komeda M, Pollick C, et al: Mitral valve annuloplasty: The effect of the type on left ventricular function, *Ann Thorac Surg* 47:524–527, 1989, discussion 527–528.
345. Tribouilloy CM, Enriquez-Sarano M, Schaff HV, et al: Impact of preoperative symptoms on survival after surgical correction of organic mitral regurgitation: Rationale for optimizing surgical indications, *Circulation* 99:400–405, 1999.
346. Tribouilloy CM, Enriquez-Sarano M, Schaff HV, et al: Excess mortality due to coronary artery disease after valve surgery. Secular trends in valvular regurgitation and effect of internal mammary artery bypass, *Circulation* 98:II108–II115, 1998.
347. McClure RS, Cohn LH, Wiegerinck E, et al: Early and late outcomes in minimally invasive mitral valve repair: An eleven-year experience in 707 patients, *J Thorac Cardiovasc Surg* 137:70–75, 2009.
348. Svensson LG, Atik FA, Cosgrove DM, et al: Minimally invasive versus conventional mitral valve surgery: A propensity-matched comparison, *J Thorac Cardiovasc Surg* 139:926–932.e1-2, 2010.
349. Mihaljevic T, Cohn LH, Unic D, et al: One thousand minimally invasive valve operations: Early and late results, *Ann Surg* 240:529–534, 2004.
350. Carpentier A, Loulmet D, Carpentier A, et al: [Open heart operation under videosurgery and minithoracotomy. First case (mitral valvuloplasty) operated with success], *C R Acad Sci III* 319:219–223, 1996.
351. Mohr FW, Falk V, Diegeler A, et al: Minimally invasive port-access mitral valve surgery, *J Thorac Cardiovasc Surg* 115:567–574, 1998, discussion 574–576.
352. Carpentier A, Loulmet D, Aupecle B, et al: Computer assisted open heart surgery. First case operated on with success, *C R Acad Sci III* 321:437–442, 1998.
353. Palep JH: Robotic assisted minimally invasive surgery, *J Minim Access Surg* 5:1–7, 2009.
354. Robicsek F: Robotic cardiac surgery: Time told!, *J Thorac Cardiovasc Surg* 135:243–246, 2008.
355. Chitwood WR Jr, Rodriguez E, Chu MW, et al: Robotic mitral valve repairs in 300 patients: A single-center experience, *J Thorac Cardiovasc Surg* 136:436–441, 2008.
356. Cheng W, Fontana GP, DeRobertis MA, et al: Is robotic mitral valve repair a reproducible approach? *J Thorac Cardiovasc Surg* 139:628–633, 2010.
357. Deeba S, Aggarwal R, Sains P, et al: Cardiac robotics: A review and St. Mary's experience, *Int J Med Robot* 2:16–20, 2006.
358. Reichenspurner H, Detter C, Deuse T, et al: Video and robotic-assisted minimally invasive mitral valve surgery: A comparison of the Port-Access and transthoracic clamp techniques, *Ann Thorac Surg* 79:485–490, 2005, discussion 490–491.
359. Gillinov AM, Liddicoat JR: Percutaneous mitral valve repair, *Semin Thorac Cardiovasc Surg* 18:115–121, 2006.
360. Wong MC, Clark DJ, Horrigan MC, et al: Advances in percutaneous treatment for adult valvular heart disease, *Intern Med J* 39:465–474, 2009.
361. Grose R, Strain J, Yipintosoi T: Right ventricular function in valvular heart disease: Relation to pulmonary artery pressure, *J Am Coll Cardiol* 2:225–232, 1983.
362. Enriquez-Sarano M, Freeman WK, Tribouilloy CM, et al: Functional anatomy of mitral regurgitation: Accuracy and outcome implications of transesophageal echocardiography, *J Am Coll Cardiol* 34:1129–1136, 1999.
363. LeVan P, Stevenson J, Develi N, et al: Cardiovascular collapse after femoral venous cannula placement for robotic-assisted mitral valve repair and patent foramen ovale closure, *J Cardiothorac Vasc Anesth* 22:590–591, 2008.

364. Kottenberg-Assenmacher E, Kamler M, Peters J: Minimally invasive endoscopic port-access intracardiac surgery with one lung ventilation: Impact on gas exchange and anaesthesia resources, *Anaesthesia* 62:231–238, 2007.
365. Bastard OG, Carter JG, Moyers JR, et al: Circulatory effects of isoflurane in patients with ischemic heart disease: A comparison with halothane, *Anesth Analg* 63:635–639, 1984.
366. Smith JS, Cahalan MK, Benefiel DJ: Fentanyl versus fentanyl and isoflurane in patients with impaired left ventricular function, *Anesthesiology* 63:A18, 1985.
367. McCammon RL, Hilgenberg JC, Stoelting RK: Hemodynamic effects of diazepam and diazepam-nitrous oxide in patients with coronary artery disease, *Anesth Analg* 59:438–441, 1982.
368. Price HL, Cooperman LH, Warden JC, et al: Pulmonary hemodynamics during general anesthesia in man, *Anesthesiology* 30:629–636, 1969.
369. Stoelting RK, Reis RR, Longnecker DE: Hemodynamic responses to nitrous oxide-halothane and halothane in patients with valvular heart disease, *Anesthesiology* 37:430–435, 1972.
370. Schulte-Sasse U, Hess W, Tarnow J: Pulmonary vascular responses to nitrous oxide in patients with normal and high pulmonary vascular resistance, *Anesthesiology* 57:9–13, 1982.
371. Hilgenberg JC, McCammon RL, Stoelting RK: Pulmonary and systemic vascular responses to nitrous oxide in patients with mitral stenosis and pulmonary hypertension, *Anesth Analg* 59:323–326, 1980.
372. Rorie DK, Tyce GM, Sill JC: Nitrous oxide increases norepinephrine release from pulmonary artery, *Anesthesiology* 63:A89, 1985.
373. Hammond GL, Cronau LH, Whittaker D, et al: Fate of prostaglandins E(1) and A(1) in the human pulmonary circulation, *Surgery* 81:716–722, 1977.
374. Said SI: Pulmonary metabolism of prostaglandins and vasoactive peptides, *Ann Rev Physiol* 44: 257–268, 1982.
375. Mikawa K, Maekawa N, Goto R, et al: Use of prostaglandin E1 to treat peri-anaesthetic pulmonary hypertension associated with mitral valve disease, *J Intern Med Res* 21:161–164, 1993.
376. Kunimoto F, Arai K, Isa Y, et al: A comparative study of the vasodilator effects of prostaglandin E1 in patients with pulmonary hypertension after mitral valve replacement and with adult respiratory distress syndrome, *Anesth Analg* 85:507–513, 1997.
377. D'Ambra MN, LaRaia PJ, Philbin DM, et al: Prostaglandin E1. A new therapy for refractory right heart failure and pulmonary hypertension after mitral valve replacement, *J Thorac Cardiovasc Surg* 89:567–572, 1985.
378. Vincent JL, Carlier E, Pinsky MR, et al: Prostaglandin E1 infusion for right ventricular failure after cardiac transplantation, *J Thorac Cardiovasc Surg* 103:33–39, 1992.
379. Fullerton DA, Jones SD, Jaggers J, et al: Effective control of pulmonary vascular resistance with inhaled nitric oxide after cardiac operation, *J Thorac Cardiovasc Surg* 111:753–762, 1996, discussion 762–763.
380. Fullerton DA, McIntyre RC Jr: Inhaled nitric oxide: Therapeutic applications in cardiothoracic surgery, *Ann Thorac Surg* 61:1856–1864, 1996.
381. Nishimura RA: Valvular stenosis. In *Valvular stenosis*, ed 2, London, 2003, BMJ Books, pp 285–301.
382. Gorlin R, Gorlin SG: Hydraulic formula for calculation of the area of stenotic mitral valve, other cardiac valves and central circulatory shunts. I, *Am Heart J* 41:1–29, 1951.
383. Bruce CJ, Nishimura RA: Clinical assessment and management of mitral stenosis, *Cardiol Clin* 16:375–403, 1998.
384. Hugenholtz PG, Ryan TJ, Stein SW, et al: The spectrum of pure mitral stenosis. Hemodynamic studies in relation to clinical disability, *Am J Cardiol* 10:773–784, 1962.
385. Wood P: An appreciation of mitral stenosis. I. Clinical features, *Br Med J* 4870:1051–1063, 1954.
386. Wood P: An appreciation of mitral stenosis: II. Investigations and results, *Br Med J* 4871:1113–1124, 1954.
387. Carroll JD, Feldman T: Percutaneous mitral balloon valvotomy and the new demographics of mitral stenosis, *JAMA* 270:1731–1736, 1993.
388. Selzer A, Cohn KE: Natural history of mitral stenosis: A review, *Circulation* 45:878–890, 1972.
389. Rowe JC, Bland EF, Sprague HB, et al: The course of mitral stenosis without surgery: Ten- and twenty-year perspectives, *Ann Intern Med* 52:741–749, 1960.
390. Olesen KH: The natural history of 271 patients with mitral stenosis under medical treatment, *Br Heart J* 24:349–357, 1962.
391. Gash AK, Carabello BA, Cepin D, et al: Left ventricular ejection performance and systolic muscle function in patients with mitral stenosis, *Circulation* 67:148–154, 1983.
392. Carabello BA: Mitral valve disease: Indications for surgery. In *Mitral valve disease: Indications for surgery*, ed 2, London, 2003, BMJ Books, pp 758–766.
393. Liu CP, Ting CT, Yang TM, et al: Reduced left ventricular compliance in human mitral stenosis. Role of reversible internal constraint, *Circulation* 85:1447–1456, 1992.
394. Bruce CJ, Nishimura RA: Newer advances in the diagnosis and treatment of mitral stenosis, *Curr Probl Cardiol* 23:125–192, 1998.
395. Popovic AD, Stewart WJ: Echocardiographic evaluation of valvular stenosis: The gold standard for the next millennium? *Echocardiography* 18:59–63, 2001.
396. Inoue K, Owaki T, Nakamura T, et al: Clinical application of transvenous mitral commissurotomy by a new balloon catheter, *J Thorac Cardiovasc Surg* 87:394–402, 1984.
397. Iung B, Vahanian A: The long-term outcome of balloon valvuloplasty for mitral stenosis, *Curr Cardiol Rep* 4:118–124, 2002.
398. Nishimura RA, Holmes DR Jr, Reeder GS: Efficacy of percutaneous mitral balloon valvuloplasty with the inoue balloon, *Mayo Clin Proc* 66:276–282, 1991.
399. Abascal VM, Wilkins GT, Choong CY, et al: Mitral regurgitation after percutaneous balloon mitral valvuloplasty in adults: Evaluation by pulsed Doppler echocardiography, *J Am Coll Cardiol* 11: 257–263, 1988.
400. Mueller XM, Tevaearai HT, Stumpe F, et al: Tricuspid valve involvement in combined mitral and aortic valve surgery, *J Cardiovasc Surg* 42:443–449, 2001.
401. Cohn LHR: Tricuspid regurgitation secondary to mitral valve disease: When and how to repair, *J Card Surg* 9:237–241, 1994.
402. Katircioglu SF, Yamak B, Ulus AT, et al: Treatment of functional tricuspid regurgitation by bicuspidalization annuloplasty during mitral valve surgery, *J Heart Valve Dis* 6:631–635, 1997.
403. Messika-Zeitoun D, Thomson H, Bellamy M, et al: Medical and surgical outcome of tricuspid regurgitation caused by flail leaflets, *J Thorac Cardiovasc Surg* 128:296–302, 2004.
404. Sons H, Dausch W, Kuh JH: Tricuspid valve repair in right-sided endocarditis, *J Heart Valve Dis* 6:636–641, 1997.
405. Chopra P, Tandon HD: Pathology of chronic rheumatic heart disease with particular reference to tricuspid value involvement, *Acta Cardiol* 32:423–434, 1977.
406. Vatterott PJ, Nishimura RA, Gersh BJ, et al: Severe isolated tricuspid insufficiency in coronary artery disease, *Int J Cardiol* 14:295–301, 1987.
407. Arbulu A, Holmes RJ, Asfaw I: Tricuspid valvulectomy without replacement. Twenty years' experience, *J Thorac Cardiovasc Surg* 102:917–922, 1991.
408. Arbulu A, Asfaw I: Tricuspid valvulectomy without prosthetic replacement. Ten years of clinical experience, *J Thorac Cardiovasc Surg* 82:684–691, 1981.
409. Farid L, Dayem MK, Guindy R, et al: The importance of tricuspid valve structure and function in the surgical treatment of rheumatic mitral and aortic disease, *Eur Heart J* 13:366–372, 1992.
410. Gayet C, Pierre B, Delahaye JP, et al: Traumatic tricuspid insufficiency. An underdiagnosed disease, *Chest* 92:429–432, 1987.
411. Kaul TK, Ramsdale DR, Mercer JL: Functional tricuspid regurgitation following replacement of the mitral valve, *Int J Cardiol* 33:305–313, 1991.
412. McGrath LB, Gonzalez-Lavin L, Bailey BM, et al: Tricuspid valve operations in 530 patients. Twenty-five-year assessment of early and late phase events, *J Thorac Cardiovasc Surg* 99:124–133, 1990.
413. Morrison DA, Ovitt T, Hammermeister KE: Functional tricuspid regurgitation and right ventricular dysfunction in pulmonary hypertension, *Am J Cardiol* 62:108–112, 1988.
414. Mullany CJ, Gersh BJ, Orszulak TA, et al: Repair of tricuspid valve insufficiency in patients undergoing double (aortic and mitral) valve replacement. Perioperative mortality and long-term (1 to 20 years) follow-up in 109 patients, *J Thorac Cardiovasc Surg* 94:740–748, 1987.
415. Bajzer CT, Stewart WJ, Cosgrove DM, et al: Tricuspid valve surgery and intraoperative echocardiography: Factors affecting survival, clinical outcome, and echocardiographic success, *J Am Coll Cardiol* 32:1023–1031, 1998.
416. Iskandrian AS, Hakki AH, Ren JF, et al: Correlation among right ventricular preload, afterload and ejection fraction in mitral valve disease: Radionuclide, echocardiographic and hemodynamic evaluation, *J Am Coll Cardiol* 3:1403–1411, 1984.
417. Kerber RE, Dippel WF, Abboud FM: Abnormal motion of the interventricular septum in right ventricular volume overload. Experimental and clinical echocardiographic studies, *Circulation* 48:86–96, 1973.
418. Laver MB, Strauss HW, Pohost GM: Herbert Shubin Memorial Lecture. Right and left ventricular geometry: Adjustments during acute respiratory failure, *Crit Care Med* 7:509–519, 1979.
419. Ross J Jr: Acute displacement of the diastolic pressure-volume curve of the left ventricle: Role of the pericardium and the right ventricle, *Circulation* 59:32–37, 1979.
420. Taylor RR, Covell JW, Sonnenblick EH, et al: Dependence of ventricular distensibility on filling of the opposite ventricle, *Am J Physiol* 213:711–718, 1967.
421. Discigil B, Dearani JA, Puga FJ, et al: Late pulmonary valve replacement after repair of tetralogy of Fallot, *J Thorac Cardiovasc Surg* 121:344–351, 2001.
422. Shatapathy P, Aggarwal BK, Kamath SG: Tricuspid valve repair: A rational alternative, *J Heart Valve Dis* 9:276–282, 2000.
423. Wong M, Matsumura M, Kutsuzawa S, et al: The value of Doppler echocardiography in the treatment of tricuspid regurgitation in patients with mitral valve replacement. Perioperative and two-year postoperative findings, *J Thorac Cardiovasc Surg* 99:1003–1010, 1990.
424. Lambertz H, Minale C, Flachskampf FA, et al: Long-term follow-up after Carpentier tricuspid valvuloplasty, *Am Heart J* 117:615–622, 1989.
425. Staab ME, Nishimura RA, Dearani JA: Isolated tricuspid valve surgery for severe tricuspid regurgitation following prior left heart valve surgery: Analysis of outcome in 34 patients, *J Heart Valve Dis* 8:567–574, 1999.
426. Pai RG, Bansal RC, Shah PM: Determinants of the rate of right ventricular pressure rise by Doppler echocardiography: Potential value in the assessment of right ventricular function, *J Heart Valve Dis* 3:179–184, 1994.
427. Loperfido F, Lombardo A, Amico CM, et al: Doppler analysis of portal vein flow in tricuspid regurgitation, *J Heart Valve Dis* 2:174–182, 1993.
428. Minakata K, Schaff HV, Zehr KJ, et al: Is repair of aortic valve regurgitation a safe alternative to valve replacement? *J Thorac Cardiovasc Surg* 127:645–653, 2004.
429. Fraser CD Jr, Wang N, Mee RB, et al: Repair of insufficient bicuspid aortic valves, *Ann Thorac Surg* 58:386–390, 1994.
430. Casselman FP, Gillinov AM, Akhrass R, et al: Intermediate-term durability of bicuspid aortic valve repair for prolapsing leaflet, *Eur J Cardiothorac Surg* 15:302–308, 1999.
431. Fucci C, Sandrelli L, Pardini A, et al: Improved results with mitral valve repair using new surgical techniques, *Eur J Cardiothorac Surg* 9:621–626, 1995, discussion 626–627.
432. Block PC: Percutaneous mitral valve repair for mitral regurgitation, *J Int Cardiol* 16:93–96, 2003.
433. Feldman T, Wasserman HS, Herrmann HC, et al: Percutaneous mitral valve repair using the edge-to-edge technique: Six-month results of the EVEREST Phase I Clinical Trial, *J Am Coll Cardiol* 46: 2134–2140, 2005.
434. Kaye DM, Byrne M, Alferness C, et al: Feasibility and short-term efficacy of percutaneous mitral annular reduction for the therapy of heart failure-induced mitral regurgitation, *Circulation* 108: 1795–1797, 2003.
435. Liddicoat JR, Mac Neill BD, Gillinov AM, et al: Percutaneous mitral valve repair: A feasibility study in an ovine model of acute ischemic mitral regurgitation, *Catheter Cardiovasc Interv* 60:410–416, 2003.
436. Dubreuil O, Basmadjian A, Ducharme A, et al: Percutaneous mitral valve annuloplasty for ischemic mitral regurgitation: First in man experience with a temporary implant, *Catheter Cardiovasc Interv* 69:1053–1061, 2007.
437. Webb JG: Percutaneous aortic valve replacement, *Curr Cardiol Rep* 10:104–109, 2008.
438. Inoue M, McCarthy PM, Popovic ZB, et al: The Coapsys device to treat functional mitral regurgitation: In vivo long-term canine study, *J Thorac Cardiovasc Surg* 127:1068–1076, 2004 discussion, 1076–1077.
439. Cribier A, Eltchaninoff H, Bash A, et al: Percutaneous transcatheter implantation of an aortic valve prosthesis for calcific aortic stenosis: First human case description, *Circulation* 106:3006–3008, 2002.
440. Cribier A, Eltchaninoff H, Tron C, et al: Early experience with percutaneous transcatheter implantation of heart valve prosthesis for the treatment of end-stage inoperable patients with calcific aortic stenosis, *J Am Coll Cardiol* 43:698–703, 2004.
441. Cheung A, Ree R: Transcatheter aortic valve replacement, *Anesthesiol Clin* 26:465–479, 2008.
442. Covello RD, Maj G, Landoni G, et al: Anesthetic management of percutaneous aortic valve implantation: Focus on challenges encountered and proposed solutions, *J Cardiothorac Vasc Anesth* 23:280–285, 2009.
443. Fassl J, Walther T, Groesdonk HV, et al: Anesthesia management for transapical transcatheter aortic valve implantation: A case series, *J Cardiothorac Vasc Anesth* 23:286–291, 2009.
444. Walther T, Falk V, Kempfert J, et al: Transapical minimally invasive aortic valve implantation; the initial 50 patients, *Eur J Cardiothorac Surg* 33:983–988, 2008.
445. Webb JG, Harnek J, Munt BI, et al: Percutaneous transvenous mitral annuloplasty: Initial human experience with device implantation in the coronary sinus, *Circulation* 113:851–855, 2006.
446. Boudjemline Y, Agnoletti G, Bonnet D, et al: Percutaneous pulmonary valve replacement in a large right ventricular outflow tract: An experimental study, *J Am Coll Cardiol* 43:1082–1087, 2004.

20

Congenital Heart Disease in Adults

VICTOR C. BAUM, MD | DUNCAN G. DE SOUZA, MD, FRCPC

KEY POINTS

1. Because of surgical successes in treating congenital cardiac lesions, there are currently as many or more adults than children with congenital heart disease (CHD).
2. These patients may require cardiac surgical intervention for primary cardiac repair, repair after prior palliation, revision of repair because of failure or lack of growth of prosthetic material, or conversion of a suboptimal repair to a more modern operation.
3. These patients will be encountered by noncardiac anesthesiologists for a vast array of ailments and injuries requiring surgery.
4. If at all possible, noncardiac surgery on adult patients with moderate-to-complex CHD should be done at an adult congenital heart center with the consultation of an anesthesiologist experienced with adult CHD.
5. Delegation of one anesthesiologist as the liaison with the cardiology service for preoperative evaluation and triage of adult CHD patients will be helpful.
6. All relevant cardiac tests and evaluations should be reviewed in advance.
7. Sketching out the anatomy and path(s) of blood flow is often an easy and enlightening aid in simplifying apparently complex lesions.

Advances in perioperative care for children with congenital heart disease (CHD) over the past several decades has resulted in an ever-increasing number of these children reaching adulthood with their cardiac lesions palliated or repaired. The first article on adult CHD was published in 1973[1]; the field has grown such that there are now several texts devoted to it, and even a specialty society dedicated to it, the International Society for Adult Congenital Cardiac Disease (http://www.isaccd.org). There are estimated to be about 32,000 new cases of CHD each year in the United States and 1.5 million worldwide.[2] More than 85% of infants born with CHD are expected to grow to adulthood. It is estimated that there are more than 1,000,000 adults in the United States with CHD,[3] and this population is growing at approximately 5% per year; 55% of these adults remain at moderate-to-high risk, and more than 115,000 have complex disease.[4] The increasing survival of children with complex disease has shifted the spectrum of adults with CHD. Where once it was thought that adults represent milder degrees of disease, this is now changing.[3] Put another way, there are more adults than children with CHD and, in fact, as many adults as children have congenital cardiac defects considered severe.[5] As an

example to support the increased life expectancy of this patient group, the leading cause of mortality in adults with CHD in the United States is currently coronary artery disease.[6] These patients can be seen by anesthesiologists for primary cardiac repair, repair after a prior palliation, revision of repair because of failure or lack of growth of prosthetic material, or conversion of a suboptimal repair to a more modern operation (Box 20-1). In addition, these adults with CHD will be seen for all the other ailments of aging and trauma that require surgical intervention. Lastly, women of child-bearing age with CHD may become pregnant. They must cope with the added physiologic demands of pregnancy and will require analgesia for labor and anesthesia for Cesarean delivery. Although it has been suggested that teenagers and adults can have repair of congenital cardiac defects with morbidity and mortality approaching that of surgery done during childhood, these data are limited and may reflect only a relatively young and acyanotic sampling.[7] Other data suggest that, in general, adults older than 50 years represent an excessive proportion of the early postoperative mortality encountered, and the number of previous operations and cyanosis are both risk factors.[8] Risk factors for noncardiac surgery include heart failure, pulmonary hypertension, and cyanosis.[9]

Despite the fact that congenital cardiac disease carries implications for lifelong medical problems, a significant number of patients, even those with lesions deemed severe, will not have continuing cardiology follow-up, despite ongoing general medical care.[10] These patients bring with them anatomic and physiologic complexities of which physicians accustomed to caring for adults may be unaware, as well as medical problems associated with aging or pregnancy that might not be familiar to physicians used to caring for children. This problem has led to the establishment of the growing subspecialty of adult CHD. There have been two Bethesda conferences devoted to the issue, most recently in 2001[11]; and the American College of Cardiology reviewed the available evidence and published superb guidelines for the care of these patients in 2008.[12] It is important to note that most of the current recommendations are based on Level C evidence (only consensus opinion or case studies) because prospective studies and large registries of patient outcomes are rare. An informed anesthesiologist is a critical member of the team required to care optimally for these patients. A specific recommendation of that conference was that noncardiac surgery on adult patients with moderate-to-complex CHD be done at an adult congenital heart center (regional centers) with the consultation of an anesthesiologist experienced with adult CHD.[11,13] In fact, one of the founding fathers of the subspecialty wrote: "A cardiac anesthesiologist with experience in CHD is pivotal....The cardiac anesthesiologist and the attending cardiologist are more important than the noncardiac surgeon."[2] High-risk patients

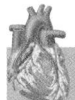

BOX 20-1. INDICATIONS FOR CARDIAC SURGERY IN ADULTS WITH CONGENITAL HEART DISEASE

- Primary repair
- Total correction after palliation
- Revision of total correction
- Conversion of suboptimal obsolescent operation into more modern repair

TABLE 20-1	Rhythm Disturbances in Adults with Congenital Heart Disease
Rhythm Disturbance	*Associated Lesions*
Tachycardias	
Wolff-Parkinson-White syndrome	Ebstein's anomaly
	Congenitally corrected transposition
Intra-atrial reentrant tachycardia (atrial flutter)	Postoperative Mustard
	Postoperative Senning
	Postoperative Fontan
	Tetralogy of Fallot
	Other
Atrial fibrillation	Mitral valve disease
	Aortic stenosis
	Tetralogy of Fallot
	Palliated single ventricle
Ventricular tachycardia	Tetralogy of Fallot
	Aortic stenosis
	Other
Bradycardias	
Sinus node dysfunction	Postoperative Mustard
	Postoperative Senning
	Postoperative Fontan
	Sinus venosus ASD
	Heterotaxy syndrome
Spontaneous AV block	AV septal defects
	Congenitally corrected transposition
Surgically induced AV block	VSD closure
	Subaortic stenosis relief
	AV valve replacement

ASD, atrial septal defect; AV, atrioventricular; VSD, ventricular.
(Reprinted from ACC/AHA 2008 guidelines for the management of adults with congenital heart disease: A report of the American College of Cardiology/American Heart Association Task Force on Practice Guidelines (Writing Committee to Develop Guidelines on the Management of Adults With Congenital Heart Disease). Developed in Collaboration with the American Society of Echocardiography, Heart Rhythm Society, International Society for Adult Congenital Heart Disease, Society for Cardiovascular Angiography and Interventions, and Society of Thoracic Surgeons. J Am Coll Cardiol 52:e143–e263, 2008.)

TABLE 20-2	Potential Noncardiac Organ Involvement in Patients with Congenital Heart Disease

Potential Respiratory Implications
Decreased compliance (with increased pulmonary blood flow or impediment to pulmonary venous drainage)
Compression of airways by large, hypertensive pulmonary arteries
Compression of bronchioles
Scoliosis
Hemoptysis (with end-stage Eisenmenger syndrome)
Phrenic nerve injury (prior thoracic surgery)
Recurrent laryngeal nerve injury (prior thoracic surgery; rarely from encroachment of cardiac structures)
Blunted ventilatory response to hypoxemia (with cyanosis)
Underestimation of $Paco_2$ by capnometry in cyanotic patients

Potential Hematologic Implications
Symptomatic hyperviscosity
Bleeding diathesis
Abnormal von Willebrand factor
Artifactually increased prothrombin/partial thromboplastin times with erythrocytic blood
Artifactual thrombocytopenia with erythrocytic blood
Gallstones

Potential Renal Implication
Hyperuricemia and arthralgias (with cyanosis)

Potential Neurologic Implications
Paradoxical emboli
Brain abscess (with right-to-left shunts)
Seizure (from old brain abscess focus)
Intrathoracic nerve injury (iatrogenic phrenic, recurrent laryngeal, or sympathetic trunk injury)

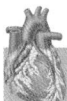

BOX 20-2. NONCARDIAC ORGAN SYSTEMS WITH POTENTIAL INVOLVEMENT BY LONGSTANDING CONGENITAL HEART DISEASE

- Pulmonary
- Hematologic
- Renal
- Neurologic
- Vasculature
- Genitourinary (pregnancy)
- Psychosocial

include, but are not limited to, those with Fontan physiology, cyanotic disease, severe pulmonary arterial hypertension, complex disease with residua such as heart failure, valve disease or the need for anticoagulation, or the potential for malignant arrhythmias (Table 20-1). Centers may find it helpful to delegate one attending anesthesiologist to be the liaison with the cardiology service to centralize preoperative evaluations and triage of patients to an anesthesiologist with specific expertise in managing patients with CHD, rather than random consultations with generalist anesthesiologists.

GENERAL NONCARDIAC ISSUES WITH LONGSTANDING CONGENITAL HEART DISEASE

A variety of organ systems can be affected by longstanding CHD; these are summarized in Table 20-2 and Box 20-2. Because congenital cardiac disease can be one manifestation of a multiorgan genetic or dysmorphic syndrome, all patients require a full review of systems and examination.

Pulmonary

Any lesion that results in either increased pulmonary blood flow or pulmonary venous obstruction can cause increased pulmonary interstitial fluid with decreased pulmonary compliance and increased work of breathing.[14] Patients with cyanotic heart disease have increased minute ventilation and maintain normocarbia.[15] These patients have a

normal ventilatory response to hypercapnia but a blunted response to hypoxemia that normalizes after corrective surgery and the establishment of normoxia.[16–18] End-tidal CO_2 underestimates arterial $Paco_2$ in cyanotic patients with decreased, normal, or even increased pulmonary blood flow.[19]

Although enlarged hypertensive pulmonary arteries or an enlarged left atrium can impinge on bronchi in children, this is rare in adults. Late-stage Eisenmenger syndrome can result in hemoptysis, and patients with Eisenmenger physiology and erythrocytosis can develop thrombosis of upper lobe pulmonary arteries.[20] Prior thoracic surgery could have injured the phrenic nerve with resultant diaphragmatic paresis or paralysis.

Scoliosis can occur in up to 19% of CHD patients, most commonly in cyanotic patients. It can also develop in adolescence, years after surgical resolution of cyanosis.[21] The relative contributions of cyanosis and congenital cardiovascular defects versus early lateral thoracotomy remain unclear: Scoliosis occurs more commonly with open surgical versus interventional techniques but is nevertheless increased over the general population in children with coarctation or patent ductus who had percutaneous rather than open interventions.[22] Scoliosis is rarely severe enough to impact respiratory function.

In an attempt to increase pulmonary blood flow, large collateral vessels originating from the aorta may have developed. These are sometimes embolized in the catheterization laboratory before thoracic surgery to prevent excessive intraoperative blood loss.

Hematologic

Hematologic manifestations of chronic CHD are primarily a consequence of longstanding cyanosis and incorporate abnormalities of both hemostasis and red cell regulation. Longstanding hypoxemia causes increased erythropoietin production in the kidney and resultant increased red cell mass. Because solely red cell production is affected, these patients are correctly referred to as erythrocytotic rather than polycythemic. There is, however, a fairly poor relation among oxygen saturation, red cell mass, and 2,3-diphosphoglycerate.[23] The oxygen-hemoglobin dissociation curve is normal or minimally shifted to the right. Most patients have established an equilibrium state at which they have a stable hematocrit and are iron replete. Some patients, however, develop excessive hematocrits and are iron deficient, causing a hyperviscous state. Iron-deficient red cells are less deformable and have been said to cause increased viscosity for the same hematocrit.[24] However, recently there is some conflicting evidence.[25] Symptoms of hyperviscosity are uncommon and typically develop only at hematocrits exceeding 65% provided the patient is iron replete. Iron deficiency also shifts the oxygen-hemoglobin dissociation curve to the right, decreasing oxygen affinity in the lungs.[26] Symptoms of hyperviscosity are listed in Box 20-3. Iron deficiency can be the result of misguided attempts to reduce the hematocrit by means of repeated phlebotomies.[27] The red cells in these patients may be hypochromic and microcytic despite the high hematocrit. Assessment of iron status is best done by measures of serum ferritin and transferrin rather than inferences from red cell indices.[27] Treatment with oral iron needs to be undertaken with care because rapid increases in hematocrit can result.

Symptomatic hyperviscosity is the indication for treatment to temporarily relieve symptoms. It is not indicated to treat otherwise asymptomatic increased hematocrits (generally hemoglobin > 20 and hematocrit > 65). Treatment is by means of a partial isovolumic exchange transfusion, and it is assumed that the increased hematocrit is not related to dehydration. Partial isovolumic exchange transfusion usually results in regression of symptoms within 24 hours. It is rare to require exchange of more than 1 unit of blood. Before surgery, phlebotomized blood can be banked for autologous perioperative retransfusion if required. Elective preoperative isovolumic exchange transfusion has decreased the incidence of hemorrhagic complications of surgery.[28,29]

Hyperviscosity and erythrocytosis can cause cerebral venous thrombosis in younger children, but it is not a problem in adults, regardless of the hematocrit.[20] Protracted preoperative fasts need to be avoided in erythrocytotic patients because they can be accompanied by rapid increases in the hematocrit.

Bleeding dyscrasias have been described in up to 20% of patients. A variety of clotting abnormalities have been described in association with cyanotic CHD, although none uniformly.[30] Bleeding dyscrasias are uncommon until the hematocrit exceeds 65%, although excessive surgical bleeding can occur at lower hematocrits. Generally, higher hematocrits are associated with a greater bleeding diathesis. Abnormalities of a variety of factors in both the intrinsic and extrinsic coagulation

BOX 20-3. SYMPTOMS OF HYPERVISCOSITY

- Headache
- Faintness, dizziness, light-headedness
- Blurred or double vision
- Fatigue
- Myalgias, muscle weakness
- Paresthesias of fingers, toes, or lips
- Depressed or dissociative mentation

pathways have been described inconsistently. Both cyanotic and acyanotic patients have been reported with deficiencies of the largest von Willebrand factor multimers, which have normalized after reparative surgery.[31] Fibrinolytic pathways are normal.[32]

The decreased plasma volume in erythrocytic blood can result in spuriously increased measures of the prothrombin and partial thromboplastin times, and the fixed amount of anticoagulant will be excessive because it presumes a normal plasma volume in the blood sample. Erythrocytic blood has more red cells and less plasma in the same volume. If informed in advance of a patient's hematocrit, the clinical laboratory can provide an appropriate sample tube. Normalizing to a hematocrit of 45%, the amount of citrate added to the tube can be calculated as follows:

$$mL\ citrate = (0.1 \times blood\ volume\ collected)$$
$$\times [(100 - patient's\ hematocrit)/55]$$

Platelet counts are typically normal or occasionally low, but bleeding is not due to thrombocytopenia. Platelets are reported per milliliter of blood, not milliliter of plasma. When corrected for the decreased plasma fraction in erythrocytic blood, the total plasma platelet count is closer to normal. That said, abnormalities in platelet function and life span have on occasion been reported.[33,34] Patients with low-pressure conduits (Fontan pathway) or synthetic vascular anastomoses are often maintained on antiplatelet drugs.

Cyanotic erythrocytotic patients have excessive hemoglobin turnover, and adults have an increased incidence of calcium bilirubinate gallstones. Biliary colic can develop years after cyanosis has been resolved by cardiac surgery.[20]

A variety of mechanical factors can also affect excessive surgical bleeding in cyanotic CHD patients. These factors include increased tissue capillary density, increased systemic venous pressure, aortopulmonary and transpleural collaterals that have developed to increase pulmonary blood flow, and prior thoracic surgery. Aprotinin and ε-aminocaproic acid improve postoperative hemostasis in patients with cyanotic CHD.[35] The results with tranexamic acid have been mixed.[36]

Renal

Some degree of renal insufficiency is not uncommon in adults with CHD, and the severity is a predictor of mortality. Moderate or severe renal dysfunction (estimated glomerular filtration rate < 60 mL/min/m²) carry a fivefold increased risk for death at 6-year follow-up compared with patients with normal glomerular filtration rate and a threefold increase over those with mild increases in glomerular filtration rate.[37] Renal dysfunction is particularly prevalent in cyanotic patients and those with poor cardiac function. Adult patients with cyanotic CHD can develop abnormal renal histology with hypercellular glomeruli and basement membrane thickening, focal interstitial fibrosis, tubular atrophy, and hyalinized afferent and efferent arterioles.[38] Cyanotic CHD is often accompanied by increases in plasma uric acid levels that are due to inappropriately low fractional uric acid excretion.[39] Decreased urate reabsorption is thought to result from renal hypoperfusion with a high filtration fraction. Despite the increased uric acid levels, urate stones and urate nephropathy are rare.[40] Although arthralgias are common, true gouty arthritis is less frequent than would be expected from the degree of hyperuricemia.[39] There appears to be an increased incidence of postcardiopulmonary bypass renal dysfunction in adults with longstanding cyanosis.[41]

Neurologic

Adults with persistent or potential intracardiac shunts remain at risk for paradoxic embolism. Paradoxical emboli can occur even through shunts that are predominantly left to right because during the cardiac cycle there can be small transient reversals of the shunt direction. It has been said that, unlike in children, adults with cyanotic CHD are not at risk for the development of cerebral thrombosis despite the hematocrit.[20,42] However, this assertion has been challenged by Ammash and Warnes,[43] who suggested an association of stroke not with red cell mass, but with iron deficiency and repeated venesection. Adults do, however, remain at risk for the development of brain abscess. A healed childhood brain abscess can provide the nidus for the development of seizures throughout life.

Prior thoracic surgery can result in permanent peripheral nerve damage. Surgery at the apices of the lungs is particularly associated with the risk for nerve damage. These operations would include Blalock–Taussig shunts, ligation of patent ductus arteriosus (PDA), banding of the pulmonary artery, and repair of aortic coarctation. Nerves that are susceptible to injury include the recurrent laryngeal nerve, the phrenic nerve, and the sympathetic chain. The incidence of migraine headaches is greater in adults with CHD compared with a control group with acquired heart disease (45% vs. 11%) and is increased in left-to-right, right-to-left, and no-shunt groups.[44]

Vasculature

Vessel abnormalities can be congenital or iatrogenic. They can affect the suitability of vessels for cannulation by the anesthesiologist or measurement of correct pressures. These abnormalities are described in Table 20-3.

Pregnancy

The physiologic changes of pregnancy, labor, and delivery can significantly alter the physiologic status of women with CHD. Several texts are available that specifically discuss issues of the pregnant woman with CHD in more detail than is possible here,[45–47] and there has been a recent review of generic cardiac surgery in the parturient.[48] Management and clinical outcomes during pregnancy and delivery for several cardiac lesions are included under the later discussions of those lesions.

Although cardiac complications, spontaneous abortions, premature delivery, thrombotic complications, peripartum endocarditis, and poor fetal outcomes can occur,[49] successful pregnancy to term with vaginal delivery is possible for most patients with congenital defects.[50] High-risk factors for mother and fetus are shown in Box 20-4. Eisenmenger

physiology is a particular risk factor. Up to 47% of cyanotic women have worsening of functional capacity during pregnancy.[51] Hematocrits greater than 44% are associated with birth weights in less than the 50th percentile, and fetal death is about 90% or more with hemoglobin levels greater than 18 gm/dL or oxygen saturation less than 85%, with most losses in the first trimester. The increases in stroke volume and cardiac output during pregnancy can stress an already pressure-overloaded ventricle. The decrease in systemic vascular resistance that accompanies pregnancy is better tolerated by women with regurgitant lesions and typically offsets the added insult of pregnancy-related hypervolemia. The decrease in systemic vascular resistance can, however, increase right-to-left shunting. Hypervolemia can be problematic in patients with poor ventricular function. Maternal cyanosis is associated with increased incidences of prematurity and intrauterine growth retardation. Profound cyanosis is associated with a high rate of spontaneous abortion.[52] Endocarditis prophylaxis is not currently recommended for vaginal deliveries.[53] The recurrence risk rate of any congenital cardiac defect in a newborn is 2.3% with one affected older sibling (any defect), 7.3% with two, 6.7% if the mother has a congenital cardiac defect, but only 2.1% if the father is affected.[2] However, it has become apparent that recurrence risk can be specific to the type of maternal defect and the underlying genetic basis. If possible, pregnancies in mothers with CHD should be managed in a high-risk obstetric center with cardiologists experienced with the care of adult CHD, and with early consultation with the obstetric anesthesia service. Women on long-term anticoagulation will likely need peripartum modifications, and postpartum thromboembolism is a potential significant problem.

Anesthesiologists will generally encounter pregnant patients well into the last trimester. Most of the major physiologic changes associated with pregnancy occur before the third trimester, and if the patients have maintained good functional status to this point, they will have declared themselves to be in a relatively low-risk group. Pregnancy is a stress test, and if they have successfully arrived at the mid-to-late third trimester, it is more likely that they will successfully tolerate delivery. Also, many high-risk women will have been counseled to avoid pregnancy. There is no *a priori* reason to favor an instrumented or Caesarean delivery over a vaginal one. This is an obstetric, not cardiologic decision. A functioning epidural makes uterine contractions easy to tolerate. Bearing down, associated with the second stage, requires close observation. The third stage can be accompanied by an autotransfusion of placental blood, or potentially with hypovolemia with uterine atony and hemorrhage Oxytocin will decrease systemic vascular resistance and increase heart rate and pulmonary vascular resistance. Methylergonovine will increase systemic vascular resistance. These rapid changes in loading conditions can be poorly tolerated in mothers with fixed cardiac output and pulmonary edema, or heart failure can develop.

Some mothers will be taking medications for their cardiac condition, including antiarrhythmics. In general, these are safe for the infant.[54] Exceptions include β-blockers that can interfere with fetal growth and the response of the fetus to the stress of labor, as well as amiodarone that can affect fetal thyroid function. Maternal cardioversion would appear to be safe for the fetus at all stages, because of the low intensity of the electrical field at the uterus. However, the fetus should be monitored throughout the procedure. Women with implanted internal defibrillators have carried successfully to term.[55] Should cardiopulmonary bypass (CPB) be required during pregnancy, it carries with it increased fetal risk, particularly if hypothermia is used.

TABLE 20-3	Potential Vascular Access Issues	
Vessel	**Possible Problem**
Femoral vein(s)	May have been ligated if cardiac catheterization was done by cutdown; large therapeutic catheters in infants often thrombose femoral veins
Inferior vena cava	Some lesions, particularly when associated with heterotaxy (polysplenia), have discontinuity of the inferior vena cava; will not be able to pass a catheter from the groin to the right atrium
Left subclavian and pedal arteries	Distal blood pressure will be low in the presence of coarctation of the aorta or after subclavian flap repair (subclavian artery only), and variably so if postoperative recoarctation; pulses can be absent or palpable with abnormal blood pressure
Subclavian artery	Blood pressure low with classic Blalock-Taussig shunt on that side, and variably so with modified Blalock-Taussig shunt
Right subclavian artery	Blood pressure artifactually high with supravalvular aortic stenosis (Coanda effect)
Superior vena cava	Risk for catheter-related thrombosis with Glenn operation

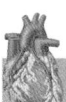

BOX 20-4. RISK FACTORS FOR PREGNANCY

- Pulmonary hypertension
- Depressed ventricular function
- Marfan syndrome with dilated aortic root
- Cyanosis
- Severe left-heart obstructive lesions
- Pressure (vs. volume) lesions

Psychosocial

Teenagers with CHD are certainly no different from other teenagers in that issues of denial, a sense of immortality, and risk-taking behavior can affect optimal care for these youngsters. Bodies that carry scars from prior surgery and physical limitations can complicate the body-conscious teenage years. Although most adolescents and adults with CHD function well, adults with CHD are less likely to be married or cohabitating and are more likely to be living with their parents.[56]

There are several series of adolescent and adult patients and psychosocial outcome, but there are no well-done controlled studies.[57-64] It has been suggested that depression is common and can exacerbate the clinical consequences of the cardiac defect.

Adolescent CHD patients have higher medical care expenses than the general population, and they can have difficulty in obtaining life and health insurance after they can no longer be covered under their parents' policies.[65-67] Life insurance is somewhat more available to adult CHD patients than in the past; however, policies vary widely among insurers.[68]

CARDIAC ISSUES

The basic hemodynamic effects of an anatomic cardiac lesion can be modified by time and by the superimposed effects of chronic cyanosis, pulmonary disease, or the effects of aging. Although surgical cure is the goal, true universal cure, without residua, sequelae, or complications, is uncommon on a population-wide basis. Exceptions include closure of a nonpulmonary hypertensive PDA or atrial septal defect (ASD), probably in childhood. Although there have been reports of series of surgeries on adults with CHD, the wide variety of defects and sequelae from prior surgery make generalizations difficult, if not impossible. Poor myocardial function can be inherent in the CHD but can also be affected by longstanding cyanosis or superimposed surgical injury, including inadequate intraoperative myocardial protection.[68,69] This is particularly true of adults who had their cardiac repair several decades ago when myocardial protection may not have been as good and when repair was undertaken at an older age. Postoperative arrhythmias are common, particularly when surgery entails long atrial suture lines, and the incidence of atrial arrhythmias increases with time, either as a primary sequela or as an indicator of diminished cardiac function.[70] Thrombi can be found in these atria precluding immediate cardioversion.[71] Bradyarrhythmias can be secondary to surgical injury to the sinus node or conducting tissue or can be a component of the cardiac defect.

The number of cardiac lesions and subtypes, together with the large number of contemporary and obsolescent palliative and corrective surgical procedures, make a complete discussion of all CHD impossible. The reader is referred to one of the current texts on pediatric cardiac anesthesia for more detailed descriptions of these lesions, the available surgical repairs, and the anesthetic implications during primary repair.[72,73] Some general perioperative guidelines to caring for these patients are offered in Table 20-4. This chapter provides a discussion of the more common and physiologically important defects that will be encountered in an adult CHD population. Defining outcome after CHD surgery is like trying to hit a continuously moving target. Both short-term and long-term results from older series can differ significantly from contemporary results.

Aortic Stenosis

Most aortic stenosis in adults is due to a congenitally bicuspid valve that does not become problematic until late middle age or later, although endocarditis risk is lifelong. Congenital aortic stenosis can, on some occasions, however, become severe enough to warrant surgical correction in adolescence or young adulthood, in addition to those severely affected valves that present in infancy. Once symptoms (angina, syncope, near-syncope, heart failure) develop, survival is markedly shortened. Median survival is 5 years after the development of angina, 3 years after syncope, and 2 years after heart failure.[74] Anesthetic management of aortic stenosis does not vary whether the stenosis is congenital (most common) or acquired (see Chapter 19).

Most mothers with aortic stenosis can successfully carry pregnancies to term and have vaginal deliveries. Severe stenosis (valve area < 1.0 cm^2) can result in clinical deterioration and maternal and fetal mortality. Hemodynamic monitoring during delivery with maintenance of adequate preload and avoidance of hypotension are critical. When surgical intervention is required during pregnancy, percutaneous balloon valvuloplasty appears to carry lower risk than open valvotomy.

TABLE 20-4	General Approach to Anesthesia for Patients with Congenital Heart Disease

General

The best care for both cardiac and noncardiac surgery in adult patients with CHD is afforded in a center with a multidisciplinary team experienced in the care of adults with CHD, and knowledgeable about both the anatomy and physiology of CHD and the manifestations and considerations specific to adults with CHD

Preoperative

Review most recent laboratory data, catheterization, and echocardiogram, and other imaging data; the most recent office letter from the cardiologist is often most helpful; obtain and review these in advance

Drawing a diagram of the heart with saturations, pressures, and direction of blood flow often clarifies complex and superficially unfamiliar anatomy and physiology

Avoid prolonged fast if patient is erythrocytotic to avoid hemoconcentration

No generalized contraindication to preoperative sedation

Intraoperative

Large-bore intravenous access for redo sternotomy and cyanotic patients (see Table 20-3 for vascular access considerations)

Avoid air bubbles in all intravenous catheters; there can be transient right-to-left shunting even in lesions with predominant left-to-right shunting (filters are available but will severely restrict ability to give volume and blood)

Apply external defibrillator pads for redo sternotomies and patients with poor cardiac function

Appropriate endocarditis prophylaxis (orally or intravenously before skin incision)[40]

Consider antifibrinolytic therapy, especially for patients with prior sternotomy

Transesophageal echocardiography for cardiac operations

Modulate pulmonary and systemic vascular resistances as appropriate pharmacologically and by modifications in ventilation

Postoperative

Appropriate pain control (cyanotic patients have normal ventilatory response to hypercarbia and narcotics)

Maintain hematocrit appropriate for arterial saturation

Maintain central venous and left atrial pressures appropriate for altered ventricular diastolic compliance or presence of beneficial atrial level shunting

Pao_2 may not increase significantly with the application of supplemental oxygen in the face of right-to-left shunting; similarly, neither will it decrease much with the withdrawal of oxygen (in the absence of lung pathology)

Aortopulmonary Shunts

Depending on their age, adult patients may have had one or more of several aortopulmonary shunts to palliate cyanosis during childhood. These are shown in Figure 20-1. Although life saving, there were considerable shortcomings of these shunts in the long term. All were inherently inefficient, as some of the oxygenated blood returning through the pulmonary veins to the left atrium and ventricle would then return to the lungs through the shunt, thus volume loading the ventricle. It was difficult to quantify the size of the earlier shunts such as the Waterston (side-to-side ascending aorta to right pulmonary artery) and Potts (side-to-side descending aorta to left pulmonary artery). If too small, the patient was left excessively cyanotic; if too large, there was pulmonary overcirculation with the risk for development of pulmonary vascular disease. The Waterston, in fact, could, on occasion, stream blood flow unequally, resulting in a hyperperfused, hypertensive ipsilateral (right) pulmonary artery and a hypoperfused contralateral (left) pulmonary artery. There were also surgical issues when complete repair became possible. Takedown of Waterston shunts often required a pulmonary arterioplasty to correct deformity of the pulmonary artery at the site of the anastomosis, and the posteriorly located Potts anastomoses could not be taken down from a median sternotomy. Patients with a classic Blalock–Taussig shunt almost always lack palpable pulses on the side of the shunt. Even if there is a palpable pulse (from collateral flow around the shoulder), blood pressure obtained from that arm will be artifactually low. Even after a modified Blalock–Taussig shunt (using a piece of Gore-Tex tubing instead of an end-to-side anastomosis of the subclavian and pulmonary arteries), there can be a blood pressure disparity between the arms. Preoperative blood pressure should be measured in both arms to ensure a valid measurement (Box 20-5).

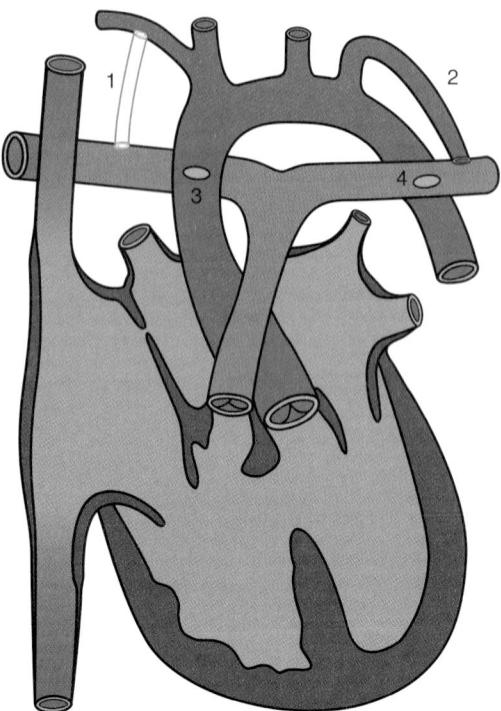

Figure 20-1 **Various aortopulmonary anastomoses.** The illustrated heart is one with tetralogy of Fallot. The anastomoses are: 1, modified Blalock-Taussig; 2, classic Blalock-Taussig; 3, Waterston (Waterston-Cooley); and 4, Potts. *(From Baum VC: The adult with congenital heart disease. J Cardiothorac Vasc Anesth 10:261, 1996.)*

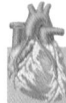

BOX 20-6. COMPLICATIONS OF ATRIAL SEPTAL DEFECT IN ADULTHOOD

- Paradoxical emboli
- Effort dyspnea
- Atrial tachyarrhythmias
- Right-sided failure with pregnancy
- Pulmonary hypertension
- ↑ Right-sided failure with ↓ left ventricular compliance with aging
- Mitral insufficiency

BOX 20-5. AORTOPULMONARY SHUNTS

Waterston	Ascending aorta→right pulmonary artery	No longer done
Potts	Descending aorta→left pulmonary artery	No longer done
Classic Blalock–Taussig	Subclavian artery→ipsilateral pulmonary artery	No longer done
Modified Blalock–Taussig	Gore-Tex tube subclavian artery→ipsilateral pulmonary artery	Current
Central shunt	Gore-Tex tube ascending aorta→main pulmonary artery	Current

Atrial Septal Defect and Partial Anomalous Pulmonary Venous Return

There are several anatomic types of ASD. The most common type, and if otherwise undefined the presumptive type, is the secundum type located in the midseptum. The primum type at the lower end of the atrial septum is a component of endocardial cushion defects, the most primitive of which is the common atrioventricular canal (see later). The sinus venosus type, high in the septum near the entry of the superior vena cava (SVC), is almost always associated with partial anomalous pulmonary venous return, most frequently drainage of the right upper pulmonary vein to the low SVC. An uncommon atrial septal–type defect is when blood passes from the left atrium to the right via an unroofed coronary sinus. For purposes of this section, only secundum defects are considered, although the natural histories of all of the defects are similar (Box 20-6).

Both the natural history and the postoperative outcome of ASDs and the physiologically related partial anomalous venous return are similar.[75–77] Because the symptoms and clinical findings of an ASD can be quite subtle and patients often remain asymptomatic until adulthood, ASDs represent approximately one third of all CHD discovered in adults. Although asymptomatic survival to adulthood is common, significant shunts ($\dot{Q}_p/\dot{Q}_s > 1.5:1$) will probably cause symptoms over time, and paradoxical emboli can occur through defects with smaller shunts. Surgical repair of restrictive lesions 5 mm or smaller in size does not impact the natural history. Thus, surgical closure of small lesions is not indicated in the absence of paradoxical emboli. Effort dyspnea occurs in 30% by the third decade, and atrial flutter or fibrillation in about 10% by age 40.[75] The avoidance of complications developing in adulthood provides the rationale for surgical repair of asymptomatic children. The mortality for a patient with an uncorrected ASD is 6% per year after 40 years of age, and essentially all patients older than 60 years are symptomatic.[75–77] Large, unrepaired defects can cause death from atrial tachyarrhythmias or right ventricular failure in 30- to 40-year-old patients.[78] With the decreased left ventricular diastolic compliance accompanying the systemic hypertension or coronary artery disease that is common with aging, left-to-right shunting increases with age. Pulmonary vascular disease typically does not develop until after the age of 40, unlike ventricular or ductal level shunts, which can lead to it in early childhood. Mitral insufficiency can be found in adult patients and is significant in about 15% of adult patients.[79] Paradoxical emboli remain a lifelong risk.

Late closure of the defect, after 5 years of age, has been associated with incomplete resolution of right ventricular dilation.[80] Left ventricular dysfunction has been reported in some patients having defect closure in adulthood, and closure, particularly in middle age, may not prevent the development of atrial tachyarrhythmias or stroke.[81–84] Survival of patients without pulmonary vascular disease has been reported to be best if operated on before 24 years of age, intermediate if operated on between 25 and 41 years of age, and worst if operated on thereafter.[84] However, more recent series have shown that even at ages older than 40, surgical repair provides an overall survival and complication-free benefit compared with medical management.[85] Surgical morbidity in these patients is primarily atrial fibrillation, atrial flutter, or junctional rhythm.[82] Current practice is to close these defects in adults in the catheterization laboratory via transvascular devices if anatomically practical (Figure 20-2). For example, there needs to be an adequate rim of septum around the defect to which the device can attach. Device closure is inappropriate if the defect is associated with anomalous pulmonary venous drainage. The indications for closure with a transvascular device are the same as for surgical closure.[86]

An otherwise uncomplicated secundum ASD, unlike most congenital cardiac defects, is not associated with an increased endocarditis risk.[87] Presumably, this is because the shunt, although potentially large, is low pressure and unassociated with jet lesions of the endocardium.

Although some discussion is given to onset times with intravenous or inhalation induction agents, clinical differences are hard to notice with modern low-solubility volatile agents. Thermodilution cardiac output reflects pulmonary blood flow, which will be in excess of systemic blood flow. Pulmonary arterial catheters are not routinely indicated. Patients

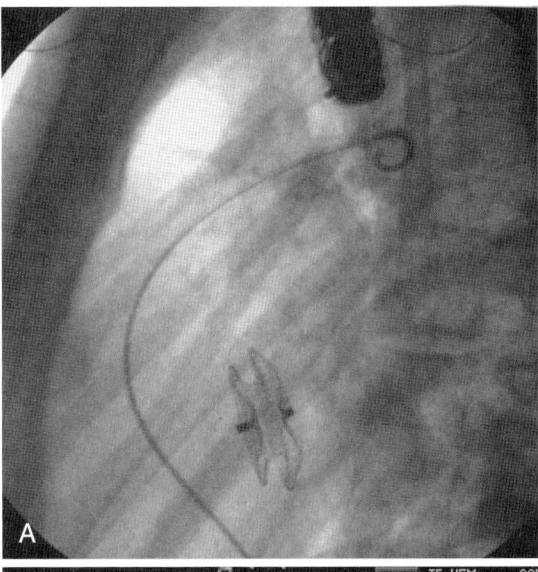

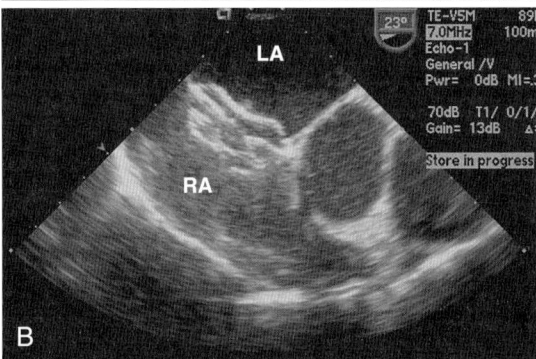

Figure 20-2 **Closure of an atrial septal defect in an adult with use of a transvascular device (the Amplatzer septal occluder).** *A,* Radiograph. *B,* Transesophageal echocardiogram. The device is clearly visualized spanning and occluding the atrial septal defect. LA, left atrium; RA, right atrium. *(Courtesy of Dr. Scott Lim.)*

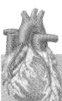

BOX 20-7. COMPLICATIONS OF AORTIC COARCTATION IN ADULTHOOD

- Left ventricular failure
- Premature coronary atherosclerosis
- Rupture of cerebral aneurysm
- Aneurysm at site of coarctation repair
- Complications of associated bicuspid aortic valve
- Exacerbation of hypertension during pregnancy

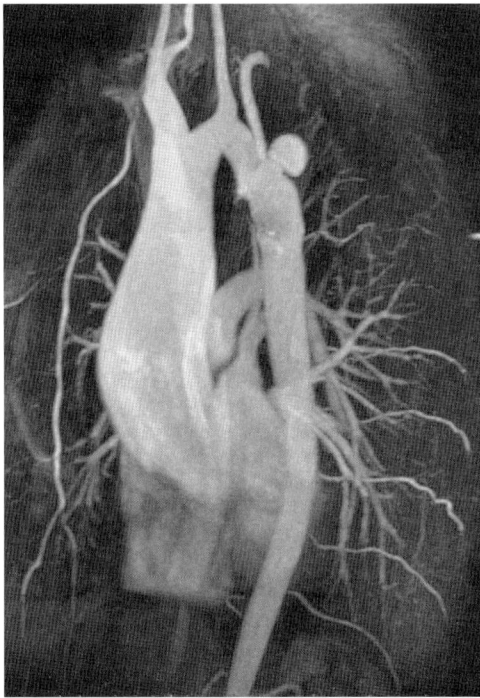

Figure 20-3 Magnetic resonance image of a 37-year-old man showing descending thoracic aortic pseudoaneurysm at the site of a coarctation that had been repaired years earlier. This patient also has a bicuspid aortic valve and an aneurysm of the ascending aorta that was later repaired. *(Courtesy of Dr. Christopher Kramer.)*

generally do tolerate any appropriate anesthetic; however, particular care should be taken in patients with pulmonary arterial hypertension or right-sided failure.

Most women with an ASD tolerate pregnancy well. However, the normal hypervolemia associated with pregnancy can result in heart failure in women with large defects. Hypovolemia accompanying delivery can result in right-to-left shunting through the defect, and there is a risk for pulmonary thromboembolism or paradoxical embolism.

Coarctation of the Aorta

Unrepaired coarctation of the aorta in the adult brings with it significant morbidity and mortality. Mortality rate is 25% by age 20, 50% by age 30, 75% by age 50, and 90% by age 60.[78,88–90] Left ventricular aneurysm, rupture of cerebral aneurysms, and dissection of a postcoarctation aneurysm all contribute to the excessive mortality. Left ventricular failure can occur in patients older than 40 with unrepaired lesions. If repair is not undertaken early, there is incremental risk for the development of premature coronary atherosclerosis. Even with surgery, coronary artery disease remains the leading cause of death 11 to 25 years after surgery.[91] Coarctation is accompanied by a bicuspid aortic valve in the majority of patients. Although endocarditis of this abnormal valve is a lifelong risk, these valves often do not become stenotic until middle age or later. Coarctation can also be associated with mitral valve abnormalities (Box 20-7).

Aneurysms at the site of coarctation repair can develop years later (Figure 20-3), and restenosis as well can develop in adolescence or

adulthood. Repair includes resection of the coarctation and end-to-end anastomosis. Because this sometimes resulted in recoarctation when done in infancy, for many years a common repair was the Waldhausen or subclavian flap operation, in which the left subclavian artery is ligated and the proximal segment opened and rotated as a flap to open the area of the coarctation. Aneurysms in the area of repair are a particular concern in adolescents and adults after coarctectomy. Persistent systemic hypertension is common after coarctation repair.[92] The risk for hypertension parallels the duration of unrepaired coarctation. Adult patients require continued periodic follow-up for hypertension. A pressure gradient of 20 mm Hg or more (less in the presence of extensive collaterals) is an indication for treatment.[93] Recoarctation can be treated surgically or by balloon angioplasty with stenting.[94] Surgical repair of recoarctation or aneurysm in adults is associated with increased mortality and can be associated with significant intraoperative bleeding because of previous scar or extensive collateral vessels. It requires lung isolation for optimal surgical exposure and placement of an arterial catheter in the right arm. Endovascular repair by ballooning/stenting has proved useful for these patients.[95,96]

Half of patients operated on after age 40 have persistent hypertension, and many of the remainder have an abnormal hypertensive response to surgery. Long-term survival is worse for patients having repair later in life. Patients older than 40 undergoing repair have a 15-year survival rate of only 50%.[91]

Blood pressure should be obtained in the right arm unless pressures in the left arm or legs are known to be unaffected by residual or recurrent coarctation. Postoperative hypertension is common after repair of coarctation and often requires treatment for some months. Postoperative ileus is also common, and patients should be maintained NPO for about 2 days.

Pregnancy can exacerbate preexisting hypertension in women with unrepaired lesions, increasing the risk for aortic dissection or rupture, heart failure, angina, and rupture of a circle of Willis aneurysm. Adequate blood pressure control during pregnancy is paramount in these women. Most aortic ruptures during pregnancy occur during labor and delivery. Presumably, epidural analgesia would moderate hypertension during delivery.

Congenitally Corrected Transposition of the Great Vessels (L-Transposition, Ventricular Inversion)

"Transposition" in this context refers solely to the fact that the aorta arises anterior to the pulmonary artery. It bears no reference to the origin of blood in the aorta or pulmonary artery, or to the ventricle of origin of those vessels. In L-transposition, as a consequence of the embryonic heart tube rotating to the left rather than to the right, the flow of blood is through normal vena cavae to the right atrium, through a mitral valve to a right-sided anatomic left ventricle, to the pulmonary artery, through the pulmonary circulation, to the left atrium, through a tricuspid valve to a left-sided anatomic right ventricle, and thence to the aorta (Figure 20-4) Although anatomically altered, the physiologic flow of blood is appropriate and there are no associated shunts. L-Transposition of the great arteries (L-TGA) is frequently associated with other cardiac lesions, most commonly a ventricular septal defect (VSD), subpulmonic stenosis, heart block, or systemic atrioventricular (tricuspid) valve regurgitation. In the absence of any of these associated cardiac defects, L-TGA will usually be asymptomatic through infancy and childhood. When L-transposition is an isolated lesion, most patients maintain normal biventricular function through early adulthood, and can attain a normal life span.

Systemic atrioventricular (tricuspid) valve insufficiency may not develop until later in life, resulting in approximately 60% of patients being diagnosed as adults.[97] Dysfunction of the right or systemic ventricle can develop with aging, and asymptomatic aging is relatively uncommon.[98] By age 45, heart failure will be present in 67% of those patients with associated lesions and 25% of those without.[99] These patients can be born with congenital heart block, which can progress in degree. Second- or third-degree heart block occurs at a rate of about 2% per year. More than 75% of patients develop some degree of heart block, although the intrinsic pacemaker remains above the His bundle with a narrow QRS complex. L-Transposition can be associated with an Ebstein-like deformity of the systemic atrioventricular (tricuspid) valve, and there can be a bundle of Kent causing the Wolff-Parkinson-White syndrome associated with that abnormal valve. There is a significant incidence of tricuspid valve insufficiency in the systemic ventricle, and this is greater still in patients with an Ebstein's deformity of the valve.[100] Anesthetic management depends on the presence of any associated lesions and the adequacy of right (systemic) ventricular function.

Although women generally do well with pregnancy,[101] the physiologic stresses of pregnancy and delivery can result in ventricular or valvular dysfunction, particularly with baseline dysfunction and/or an insufficient systemic atrioventricular valve; but even if these develop, pregnancy can be successfully managed.[101-104] The decrease in systemic vascular resistance associated with both pregnancy and neuraxial analgesia might be advantageous in women with tricuspid (systemic) valve insufficiency. The acute autotransfusion associated with delivery could potentially cause problems for women with existing diminished systemic ventricle function.

Ebstein's Anomaly of the Tricuspid Valve

Ebstein's anomaly, one of arrested or incomplete delamination of the embryonic tricuspid valve from the right ventricular myocardium, resulting in apically displaced valve tissue, is the most common cause of congenital tricuspid insufficiency. The septal leaflet tends to be the most dysplastic. The anterior leaflet tends to be large and redundant. The defect is associated with a patent foramen ovale or a secundum ASD. There is "atrialization" of part of the right ventricle. The displacement of the tricuspid valve toward the right ventricular apex results in a portion of the right ventricle being above the tricuspid valve and becoming functionally part of the right atrium. Apicalization of the tricuspid valve results in a portion of the heart above the valve having a ventricular intracardiac electrogram (it is ventricular myocardium) but atrial pressures (it lies above the tricuspid valve). The right atrium can be massively enlarged (Figure 20-5), and the right ventricle, lacking the inflow portion that is now part of the right atrium, is smaller than usual with varying degrees of pulmonic stenosis. Patients with L-transposition (see earlier) can have Ebstein's anomaly of a left-sided tricuspid valve.

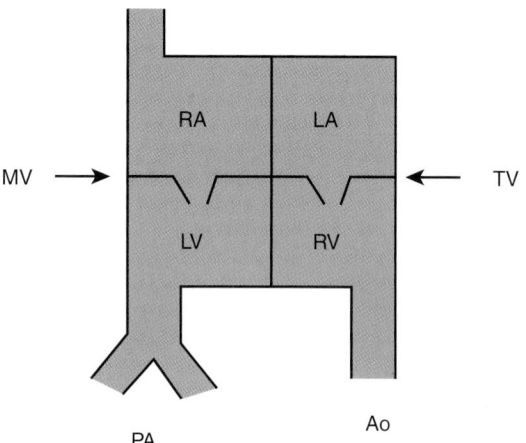

Figure 20-4 **Diagram of the anatomy of L-TGA.** Note that the atrioventricular valves are associated with the "usual" ventricle. Ao, aorta; LA, left atrium; LV, anatomic left ventricle; MV, mitral valve; PA, pulmonary artery; RA, right atrium; RV, anatomic right ventricle; TV, tricuspid valve.

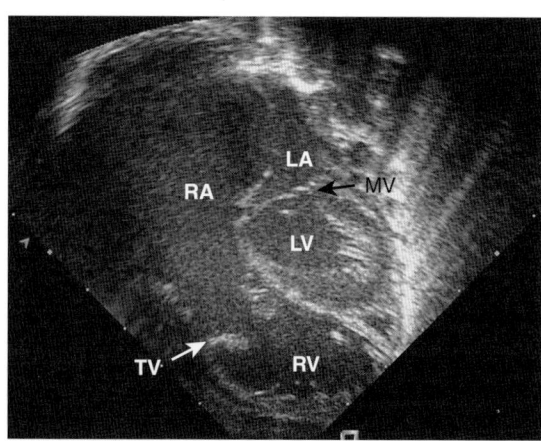

Figure 20-5 **Ebstein's anomaly of the tricuspid valve.** This echocardiogram shows the apically displaced redundant tricuspid valve tissue and a massively enlarged right atrium with bowing of the atrial septum to the left. LA, left atrium; LV, left ventricle; MV, mitral valve; RA, right atrium; RV, right ventricle; TV, tricuspid valve. *(From Baum VC: Abnormalities of the atrioventricular valves. In Lake CL, Booker P [eds]: Pediatric cardiac anesthesia, 4th ed. Philadelphia, 2004: Lippincott Williams & Wilkins.)*

Symptoms will vary based on the amount of displacement of the valve and the size of the smaller than normal right ventricle. Cyanosis from atrial-level right-to-left shunting can be a neonatal phenomenon, resolving with the normal postnatal decrease in pulmonary vascular resistance, only to recur in adolescence or adulthood. Very mild disease is quite compatible with asymptomatic survival into adulthood, although overall earlier reports suggested a mean age at death of about 20 years, with about one third dying before 10 years of age and only 15% survival rate by 60 years.[105–107] About half of patients experience development of arrhythmias, typically supraventricular tachyarrhythmias. Once symptoms develop, disability rapidly progresses.

Valve repair is currently the approach of choice, and only uncommonly will tricuspid valve replacement be required.[108] Additional intervention may be required for progressive insufficiency, stenosis, prosthetic valve failure, or valve replacement with growth. After valve replacement, up to 25% of patients experience development of high-grade atrioventricular block. Ebstein's valves are often associated with a right-sided bypass tract, causing Wolff-Parkinson-White syndrome. This is of concern because 25% to 30% of patients experience development of supraventricular tachyarrhythmias. The dilated right atrium is ready substrate for the development of atrial fibrillation. In addition to a decrease in cardiac performance, atrial fibrillation is also potentially dangerous in patients with underlying Wolff-Parkinson-White syndrome because very high atrial rates can be conducted to the ventricle through the bypass tract.

The major concerns when anesthetizing patients who have Ebstein's anomaly include decreased cardiac output, right-to-left atrial-level shunting with cyanosis, and the propensity for atrial tachyarrhythmias. The right atria of these patients are very sensitive, and arrhythmias are easily induced by catheters or guidewires passed into the right atrium or during surgical manipulation; arrhythmias remain a concern into the postoperative period. Supraventricular arrhythmias should be treated aggressively. If associated with significant hypotension, the arrhythmia needs to be electrically cardioverted.

In the absence of marked cyanosis, pregnancy and delivery are generally well tolerated. There is, however, an increased incidence of prematurity and fetal loss, and birth weights are lower in infants of cyanotic mothers,[109] as well as an increased incidence of CHD in the offspring.

Eisenmenger Syndrome

Eisenmenger described a particular type of large VSD with dextroposition of the aorta.[110] In a general way, the term *Eisenmenger syndrome* has come to describe the clinical setting in which a large left-to-right cardiac shunt results in the development of pulmonary vascular disease and has been the subject of recent reviews.[111] Although early on the pulmonary vasculature remains reactive, with continued insult, pulmonary hypertension becomes fixed and does not respond to pulmonary vasodilators. Ultimately, the level of pulmonary vascular resistance is so high that the shunt reverses and becomes right to left. Clinically, patients who are cyanotic from intracardiac right-to-left shunting are deemed to have Eisenmenger physiology even though their PVR may not yet truly be "fixed." This is the intermediate phase of the disease before progression to a truly fixed PVR. That is, at baseline they shunt right to left but may still retain some pulmonary vascular reactivity in the presence of vasodilating agents such as oxygen or nitric oxide. The degree of reactivity can be determined in the catheterization laboratory by measuring the pulmonary blood flow on room air, pure oxygen, and pure oxygen with nitric oxide added. The development of pulmonary vascular disease is dependent on shear rate. Lesions with high shear rates, such as a large VSD or a large PDA, can result in pulmonary hypertension in early childhood. Lesions such as an ASD with high pulmonary blood flow but low pressure may not result in pulmonary vascular disease until late middle age. Pulmonary vascular disease progression is also accelerated in patients living at high altitudes.

The most common presenting symptom is dyspnea on exertion. Additional symptoms include palpitations, edema, hemoptysis, syncope, hyperpnea, and of course, increasing cyanosis. Hepatic synthetic

function can be altered from the increased central venous pressure. There can be CNS symptoms from increased blood viscosity from the erythrocytosis associated with cyanosis. Right ventricular ischemia is a possibility. Patients may be on chronic therapy with drugs such as intravenous prostacyclin, an oral phosphodiesterase-5 inhibitor such as sildenafil (e.g., Revatio), or an oral endothelin receptor antagonist such as bosentan (e.g., Tracleer). Because of the risk for pulmonary thromboses,[112] patients may be on chronic anticoagulants.

Eisenmenger physiology is compatible with survival into adulthood.[113,114] However, reported rates of survival after diagnosis vary, probably based on the relatively long life expectancy and variability in the time of diagnosis. Cantor et al[115] reported median survival to 53 years but with wide variation. Saha et al[116] reported a survival rate of 80% at 10 years after diagnosis and 42% at 25 years. Oya et al,[117] however, reported survival rate of 77% at 5 years and 58% at 10 years. Syncope, increased central venous pressure, and arterial desaturation to less than 85% are all associated with poor short-term outcome.[113] Other factors associated with mortality include syncope, age at presentation, functional status, supraventricular arrhythmias, increased right atrial pressure, renal insufficiency, severe right ventricular dysfunction, and trisomy 21. Most deaths are sudden cardiac deaths. Other causes of death include heart failure, hemoptysis, brain abscess, thromboembolism, and complications of pregnancy and noncardiac surgery.[118] These patients face potentially significant perioperative risks. Findings of Eisenmenger syndrome are summarized in Table 20-5.

Surgical closure of cardiac defects with fixed pulmonary vascular hypertension is associated with very high mortality. Lung or heart-lung transplantation is a surgical alternative.[119] Although there are several surgical series reporting survival after heart-lung or single- or double-lung transplantation performed for primary pulmonary hypertension, it is unclear whether this cohort of patients is similar to patients with Eisenmenger physiology.

When noncardiac surgery is deemed essential and time permits, a preoperative cardiac catheterization may be helpful to determine the presence of pulmonary reactivity to oxygen or nitric oxide. Fixed pulmonary vascular resistance precludes rapid adaptation to perioperative hemodynamic changes. Changes in systemic vascular resistance are mirrored by changes in intracardiac shunting. A decrease in systemic vascular resistance is accompanied by increased right-to-left shunting and a decrease in systemic oxygen saturation. Systemic vasodilators, including regional anesthesia, need to be used with caution, and close assessment of intravascular volume is important. Epidural analgesia has been used successfully in patients with Eisenmenger physiology, but the local anesthetic needs to be delivered slowly and incrementally with close observation of blood pressure and oxygen saturation.[120] Postoperative postural hypotension can also increase the degree of right-to-left shunting, and these patients should change position slowly. All intravenous catheters need to be maintained free of air bubbles.

Placement of pulmonary artery catheters in these patients is problematic for a variety of reasons, and they are of less utility than might

TABLE 20-5	Findings in Eisenmenger Syndrome

- Physical examination: loud pulmonic component of the second heart sound, single or narrowly split second heart sound, Graham-Steell murmur of pulmonary insufficiency, pulmonic ejection sound ("click")
- Chest radiography: decreased peripheral pulmonary arterial markings with prominent central pulmonary vessels ("pruning")
- Electrocardiogram: right ventricular hypertrophy
- Impaired exercise tolerance
- Exertional dyspnea
- Palpitations (often caused by atrial fibrillation or flutter)
- Complications from erythrocytosis/hyperviscosity
- Hemoptysis from pulmonary infarction, rupture of pulmonary vessels, or aortopulmonary collateral vessels
- Complications from paradoxical embolization
- Syncope from inadequate cardiac output or arrhythmias
- Heart failure (usually end stage)

be expected. Pulmonary arterial hypertension is a risk factor for pulmonary artery rupture from a pulmonary artery catheter. Rupture is particularly worrisome in these cyanotic patients who can also have hemostatic deficits associated with erythrocytosis.[121] Abnormal intracardiac anatomy and right-to-left shunting can make successful passage into the pulmonary artery difficult without fluoroscopy. Relative resistances of the pulmonary and systemic beds are reflected in the systemic oxygen saturation, readily measured by pulse oximetry, so measures of pulmonary artery pressure are not required. In addition, in the presence of right-to-left shunting, thermodilution cardiac outputs do not accurately reflect systemic output. Thus, the value of pulmonary artery catheters in these patients is minimal at best, and they essentially are never indicated. The one potential exception is the patient with an ASD who is at risk for development of right ventricular failure if suprasystemic right ventricular pressure develops.[122]

Fixed pulmonary vascular resistance is, by definition, unresponsive to pharmacologic or physiologic manipulation, but as previously mentioned, only patients at the true end stage of disease have fixed PVR. Thus, the clinician must still avoid factors known to increase pulmonary vascular resistance, including cold, hypercarbia, acidosis, hypoxia, and α-adrenergic agonists. Although the last of these is commonly listed to be avoided, it seems that in the face of pulmonary vascular disease caused by intracardiac shunting, the systemic vasoconstrictive effects predominate and systemic oxygen saturation increases.

Nerve blocks offer an attractive alternative to general anesthesia if otherwise appropriate. If patients have general anesthesia, consideration should be given to postoperative observation in an intensive or intermediate care unit. Because of the increased perioperative risk, patients should be observed overnight, particularly if they have not had recent surgery or anesthesia, because their responses will be unknown. Ambulatory surgery is possible for patients having uncomplicated minor surgery with sedation or nerve block.

Pregnancy carries a very high mortality risk and risk for premature delivery. From 20% to 30% of pregnancies result in spontaneous abortions, and premature delivery occurs in about half.[123] At least half of newborns have intrauterine growth retardation. From 30% to 45% of all pregnancies end in maternal death intrapartum or during the first postpartum week, and successful first pregnancy does not preclude maternal death during a subsequent pregnancy.[124] The hemodynamic changes of both pregnancy and delivery increase maternal risk. Pulmonary microembolism and macroembolism have caused peripartum maternal deaths, even days after delivery. Factors that influence mortality include thromboembolism (44%), hypovolemia (26%), and preeclampsia (18%).[123,124] Mortality is similar with Cesarean section or vaginal delivery, and both are significantly greater than the mortality rate for spontaneous abortions. Pregnancy should be discouraged in these women. Women who do become pregnant should be closely monitored with arterial catheters during delivery. Epidural analgesia, delivered slowly and incrementally, can moderate many of the deleterious hemodynamic changes of active labor. Pulmonary arterial catheters are of little to no use during delivery. Prompt treatment of blood loss and hypotension during delivery is absolutely required. Postpartum observation should be in an intensive care setting. Pulmonary hypertension in pregnancy was reviewed in detail.[125,126]

Endocardial Cushion Defects (Atrioventricular Canal Defects)

The endocardial cushions are embryonic cardiac tissue that form the crux of the heart—the primum (lower) atrial septum, the posterior basal part of the ventricular septum, the septal leaflet of the tricuspid valve, and the anterior leaflet of the mitral valve. The endocardial cushion defects then consist of one or more of a primum ASD, inlet VSD, cleft septal leaflet of the tricuspid valve, and/or cleft anterior leaflet of the mitral valve. The most primitive form is the complete atrioventricular canal. In this defect, there is a single large atrioventricular valve with mitral and tricuspid components with large ASDs and VSDs. This

valve is usually "balanced." In the more complex, unbalanced defects, one component of the valve can be predominant, and this large valve is not centered over the ventricular septum, leading to underfilling of one of the ventricles. These defects can occur alone or can be part of more complex cardiac defects such as tetralogy of Fallot or single ventricle. Half of all children with Down syndrome have CHD; half of these children have an endocardial cushion defect. These lesions are marked by a typical electrocardiogram with first-degree block and a superior QRS axis with a counterclockwise QRS loop. Although adults with unrepaired complete atrioventricular canal will likely have developed inoperable pulmonary arterial hypertension, partial canal defects can sometimes be first diagnosed in adults and will be appropriate candidates for surgical repair. The atrioventricular node and bundle of His are displaced inferiorly, putting them at risk for surgical injury and the induction of heart block.

There is much subtlety required to construct two separate functional atrioventricular valves without residual stenosis or insufficiency of either component. Postoperative or residual mitral insufficiency is not uncommon, and 10% to 30% require repeat surgery.[127] The strongest predictor of postoperative mitral insufficiency is the degree of preoperative regurgitation of the common atrioventricular valve. Anesthesia for these patients depends on the degree of shunt, valve insufficiency, and pulmonary vascular disease.

Fontan Physiology

In 1968, performing the operation that now bears his name, Fontan and Baudet[128] proved that it was possible to deliver the entire systemic venous return to the lungs without the benefit of a ventricular pump. The Fontan operation was a landmark development in CHD because it established a "normal" series circulation in patients with a single ventricle. The price to be paid for a series circulation is the unique physiologic demand of passive pulmonary blood flow. Complications never envisioned at the time of the original operation have occurred, necessitating significant changes in operative technique. Fontan's original operation (Figure 20-6) was soon modified to an atriopulmonary connection[129] (Figure 20-7). The original strict eligibility criteria[130] have been liberalized, but patients meeting as many of the criteria as possible still have the best prognosis for good long-term survival. By the mid-1980s, it became clear that the success of Fontan circulation was based on an unobstructed pathway from systemic veins to pulmonary artery, a pulmonary vasculature that was free from anatomic distortion (from previous Blalock-Taussig shunt, for example), low PVR, and good ventricular function without significant atrioventricular valve regurgitation. The incorporation of the atrium in the Fontan pathway proved disappointing. The atrium lost its contractile function, providing no assistance to pulmonary blood flow and causing serious

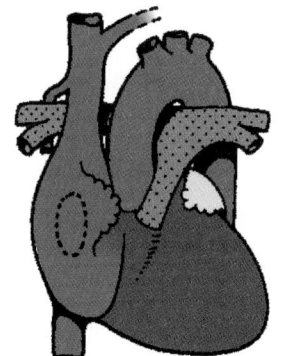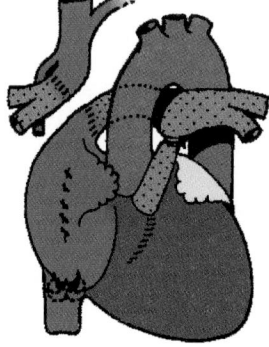

Figure 20-6 **The original Fontan operation.** Note the classic Glenn shunt connecting the superior vena cava to the right pulmonary artery and the homografts at the inferior vena cava-right atrial junction and connecting the right atrium to the left pulmonary artery. *(From Fontan F, Baudet E: Surgical repair of tricuspid atresia. Thorax 26:240, 1971.)*

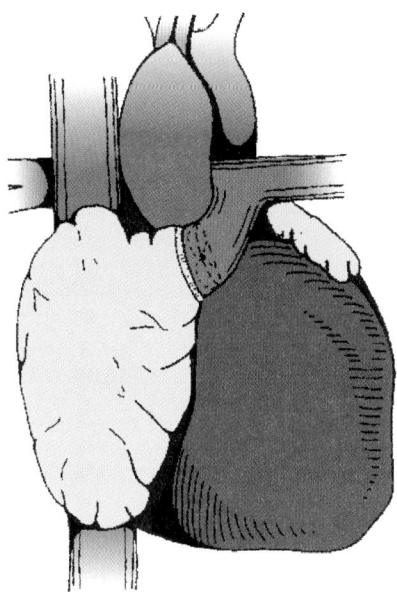

Figure 20-7 The atriopulmonary modification of the Fontan operation. *(From Kreutzer G, Galindez E, Bono H, et al: An operation for the correction of tricuspid atresia.* J Thorac Cardiovasc Surg 66:613, 1973.)

complications. Understanding these complications and how the Fontan operation has evolved is the key to managing these challenging patients whose complex CHD has been palliated, not cured.

Complications

The dilated, noncontractile atrium serves as a reservoir of blood and a ready source of thrombus.[131-133] Pulmonary embolization will impair the passive blood flow necessary for successful Fontan circulation. Atrial thrombus could embolize paradoxically through residual right-to-left shunts. Patients are also at risk for arterial thrombosis, secondary to a mild hypercoagulable state.[134,135] Given the morbidity associated with thromboembolism, it seems reasonable to prescribe aspirin therapy to all Fontan patients.[136] Those who display further potential for thrombosis such as low cardiac output state, atrial arrhythmia with significant atrial dilation, or marked venous hypertension may benefit from warfarin (Coumadin). Box 20-8 lists complications of the Fontan procedure.

Fontan patients show a steady increase in atrial tachyarrhythmias with an incidence of more than 50% at 20 years.[137] Changes in surgical technique evolved, in part, to decrease the rate of atrial arrhythmias. Although initial results were promising,[138] unfortunately, much of this benefit is lost with longer term follow-up.[139] Fontan surgical patients tolerate tachycardia poorly, and acute episodes usually require urgent treatment with medical therapy to control ventricular rate or cardioversion. Late-onset atrial tachyarrhythmias usually occur between 6 and 10 years after Fontan completion.[140] The most common tachyarrhythmia is right intra-atrial reentrant tachycardia. Over time, episodic attacks of tachycardia become more frequent. Frequently, atrial fibrillation occurs and the loss of atrioventricular synchrony results in decreased effort tolerance. The onset of atrial tachyarrhythmias mandates an evaluation of the Fontan pathway with attention turned to relieving

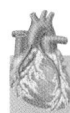

BOX 20-8. COMPLICATIONS OF FONTAN OPERATION

- Atrial thrombus
- Atrial arrhythmia (tachyarrhythmia or bradyarrhythmia)
- Ventricular dysfunction
- Chylothorax
- Protein-losing enteropathy

any significant obstructions. In the setting of passive pulmonary blood flow, even small gradients can be hemodynamically significant.[141] Therapies for chronic atrial arrhythmias consist of medication, catheter ablation, and surgery. Given the complex anatomy, dilated atrium and atrial scar with suture lines from prior surgeries, it is not surprising that atrial arrhythmias can become refractory to standard treatment in many patients. Catheter ablation typically has high initial success rates that are not maintained.[141]

Bradyarrhythmias, caused by sinus node ischemia, are common. In a large cohort of patients with atriopulmonary connections, the incidence rate of bradyarrhythmias requiring pacemakers was 13%.[142] Progressive fibrosis and scar around the sinus node, caused by prior surgical dissection, eventually leads to ischemia and clinical sinus node dysfunction. If accompanied by premature atrial contractions, sinus or junctional bradycardia can precipitate an intra-atrial reentry tachycardia. Thus, sinus node dysfunction also serves as a risk factor for the development of atrial tachyarrhythmias. Clinically significant bradyarrhythmias require pacing. Pacemakers pose special problems in the Fontan patient because the altered anatomy precludes transvenous placement. Thus, Fontan patients who require pacing end up with epicardial leads placed via repeat sternotomy with all the risks that entails. Even though atrioventricular synchrony can be achieved with pacing, it is still not as good as intrinsic sinus rhythm. The incidence of sinus node dysfunction is less with a cavopulmonary versus an atriopulmonary connection.[143] However, a clear benefit from an extracardiac connection (see later) when compared with the lateral tunnel approach has been difficult to prove.[144,145]

The last major complication of Fontan physiology is protein-losing enteropathy (PLE), a condition as confounding as it is serious. The incidence rate is quoted as high as 15%, but a large international multicenter study found a rate of 3.7%.[146] Clinically, there is an edematous state with ascites and pleural-pericardial effusions. Serum albumin is low and the diagnosis is confirmed by finding enteric protein loss with increased levels of stool α1 antitrypsin. Most ominously, PLE is accompanied by a 50% mortality rate 5 years from diagnosis despite treatment. It was believed that PLE constituted a straightforward situation of increased portal pressures secondary to central venous hypertension. Increased portal pressures lead to vascular congestion, lymphatic obstruction, and enteric protein loss from the gut. Unfortunately, there is not a good correlation between central venous pressures and PLE.[147] This has led to a broader understanding of PLE as a multifactorial phenomenon caused by reduced mesenteric perfusion,[147] chronic inflammation,[148] and enterocyte dysfunction.[149] Patients who present with PLE should have a complete hemodynamic evaluation. This is vital because interventions that improve cardiac output have proved successful in PLE. Any Fontan pathway obstruction should be treated and cardiac output optimized with medical therapy, fenestration, or pacing. In the absence of correctable obstructions, PLE portends a poor prognosis, despite surgery or cardiac transplantation.

The Modern Fontan Operation

The atriopulmonary connection proved an inefficient method of pulmonary blood flow. Colliding streams of blood from the SVC and inferior vena cava (IVC) resulted in energy loss and turbulence within the atrium.[150] The energy required to propel blood forward into the pulmonary vasculature was lost as blood swirled sluggishly in the dilated atrium (Figure 20-8). The modern Fontan operation is a total cavopulmonary connection (Figure 20-9). The "lateral tunnel Fontan" improved pulmonary blood flow, and only the lateral wall of the atrium was exposed to central venous hypertension. There was no dilated atrium to serve as a source of thrombus. The extensive atrial suture lines, however, remained a risk for arrhythmia. The "extracardiac Fontan" is a further modification of the total cavopulmonary connection. The "extracardiac Fontan" greatly reduces the number of atrial incisions and hopefully the long-term development of atrial arrhythmias. Has the modern Fontan improved outcomes? Reductions in arrhythmia and improvements in overall survival have been noted.[151]

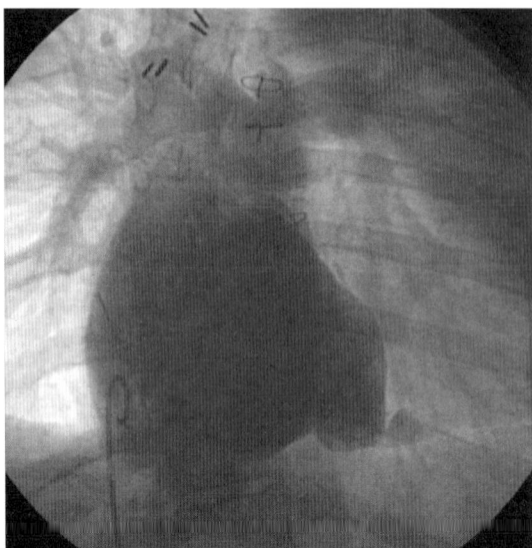

Figure 20-8 Injection of contrast into the inferior vena cava reveals a markedly dilated right atrium after an atriopulmonary Fontan operation.

Results for the extracardiac Fontan are even better than the lateral tunnel Fontan but are limited by the shorter duration of follow-up. It is not yet certain whether the development of long-term complications has been truly reduced or only delayed.

Preoperative Assessment

Patients with Fontan physiology are presenting in larger numbers for the entire array of noncardiac surgery including obstetric procedures. Preoperative assessment begins with a directed history, concentrating on functional status and the presence of major complications. Heightened suspicion is clearly needed for patients with atriopulmonary connections, as well as those with a systemic right ventricle. Patients with Fontan circulation have a low cardiac output state. This low output state exists despite the presence of good ventricular function, minimal atrioventricular valve regurgitation, and low PVR. A cohort of patients with an atriopulmonary Fontan performed at an older age showed striking reductions in anaerobic threshold (< 50% of control subjects), $\dot{V}O_2$ max (< 33% of control subjects), and systemic ejection fraction both at rest and exercise.[152] Further compounding the issue is that patients' self-assessment grossly overestimates their objective exercise

capacity.[153] This places the anesthesiologist in a considerable dilemma when faced with a Fontan patient who rates his or her functional status as "good." The authors believe that transthoracic echocardiography should be the initial preoperative investigation and is mandatory except in cases of very minor surgery. Further testing is guided by the results of the echocardiogram and in consultation with a cardiologist experienced in caring for adults with CHD. Normal ventricular function on an echocardiogram would stratify the patient as "low risk" only in the context of patients with Fontan circulation.

A term that should immediately get the attention of the anesthesiologist is "failing Fontan." The specific reason for failing may be different, but the common denominator in these patients is a marked limitation of functional status. They will manifest some combination of refractory arrhythmias, PLE, liver dysfunction, hypoxemia, or congestive heart failure. Although PLE always signifies a failing Fontan, the converse is not always true. That is, patients can have severely limited function with increased central venous pressures and even evidence of cirrhosis on liver biopsy without demonstrating PLE.[154] Patients with a "failing Fontan" require a search for correctable lesions.[155] First, any obstructions within the Fontan pathway should be treated, preferably with percutaneous techniques of dilation and stenting. Second, loss of sinus rhythm should be treated with pacing. If loss of sinus rhythm is accompanied by severe tachyarrhythmias, Fontan conversion surgery is indicated. Third, some patients develop collateral vessels. Aortopulmonary collaterals result in a progressive volume load on the single ventricle. Collaterals from the venous system to the systemic atrium or ventricle cause hypoxemia. In both cases, large collaterals should be coil occluded in the catheterization laboratory. Another option is the creation of a fenestration, which can improve cardiac output and lower central venous pressures but at the expense of a right-to-left shunt. Unfortunately, not all of these therapeutic options are indicated or successful in every patient. At this point, if no realistic hope of further improvement exists, the only option is cardiac transplantation.

The functional state of Fontan patients exists across a spectrum but generally falls into two groups. The first and largest group is those who report New York Heart Association Class I-II level of function but have been shown to possess much less cardiorespiratory reserve than age-matched two-ventricle control subjects. These patients will tolerate most surgical procedures with an acceptably low risk. The second group is smaller but consists of those patients who have manifested one of more of the "failing Fontan" criteria. Surgery in these patients carries much greater risk and should only be undertaken after careful consultation with physicians experienced in adult CHD. When it comes to a discussion of anesthetic technique, the same lessons learned in caring for patients with acquired coronary artery disease apply. That is, there is no right drug for these patients, nor is there a single "best" anesthetic

Figure 20-9 Two variations of the modern Fontan operation, the lateral tunnel and extracardiac operations. IVC, inferior vena cava; RA, right atrium; RPA, right pulmonary artery; SVC, superior vena cava. (From D'Udekem Y, Iyengar AJ, Cochrane AD, et al: The Fontan procedure: Contemporary techniques have improved long-term outcomes. Circulation 116:I157, 2007.)

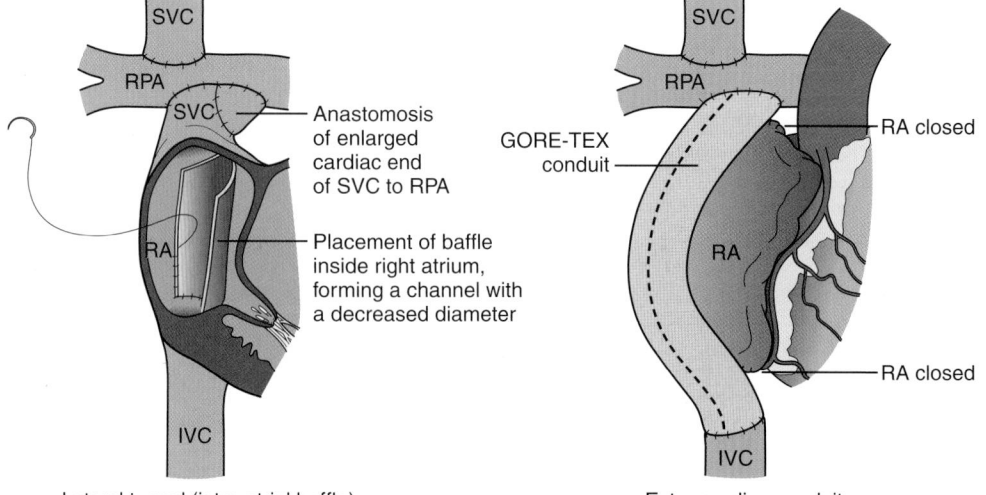

Lateral tunnel (intra-atrial baffle)

Extra-cardiac conduit

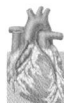

BOX 20-9. MANAGEMENT PRINCIPLES FOR PATIENTS WITH FONTAN PHYSIOLOGY

1. Maintenance of preload is essential. A prolonged NPO period without intravenous hydration should be avoided.
2. Regional and neuraxial techniques are attractive options, with appropriate attention to volume status. A neuraxial anesthetic is a poor choice if a high level of block is required. A slowly titrated epidural is preferable to a rapid-acting spinal anesthetic.
3. Airway management must be skilled to avoid hypercarbia and increases in pulmonary vascular resistance (PVR).
4. Adequate levels of anesthesia must be established before stimulating events such as laryngoscopy. A surge of catecholamines may precipitate dangerous tachycardia.
5. Spontaneous ventilation that augments pulmonary blood flow is desirable but must not be pursued at all costs. Spontaneous ventilation under deep levels of anesthesia will result in significant hypercarbia. The benefit of spontaneous ventilation may be negated by the increase in PVR secondary to hypercarbia.
6. A plan must be in place to treat tachyarrhythmias.
7. Patients with pacemakers must have the device interrogated before surgery and a plan developed to avoid potential interference from electrocautery, particularly if the patient is pacemaker dependent.
8. If large-volume shifts are anticipated, invasive monitoring with central lines and transesophageal echocardiography is recommended.
9. An appropriate plan for postoperative pain management should be established. The need for anticoagulation in many Fontan patients may preclude the use of epidural analgesia.
10. A cardiologist experienced in caring for patients with congenital heart disease should be involved perioperatively.

technique. Rather, the critical issue is to gain a clear and comprehensive understanding of the patient's pathophysiology. It is not the drugs used, but rather how they are used. Certain principles for patients with Fontan physiology are important and need to be stressed (Box 20-9).

Ventilatory Management

In an effort to minimize pulmonary vascular resistance, functional residual capacity should be maintained by the application of small amounts of positive end-expiratory pressure or continuous positive airway pressure, and excessive lung volumes should be avoided. Positive end-expiratory pressure or continuous positive airway pressure will not significantly impede cardiac output if less than 6 cm H_2O. Spontaneous ventilation has been assumed to be optimal for these patients to minimize intrathoracic pressure and encourage forward flow into the pulmonary circulation; but as discussed by Steven and McGowan,[156] hard evidence for this approach is mostly lacking.

Pregnancy

It was inevitable that as some of the female Fontan patients reached childbearing age they would become pregnant. Case reports first began appearing in 1989.[157,158] Unfortunately, the body of knowledge on this important subject consists primarily of more case reports with no large registry documenting outcomes. The physiologic changes of pregnancy are well-known and described in standard texts. Can a Fontan patient cope with the increased cardiovascular demands of pregnancy? The dilemma facing physicians caring for these patients is that Fontan patients are known to have decreased cardiac reserve, even those who report good functional status. Because pregnancy is a "stress test," who will pass this test and who will fail? The literature provides conflicting data. One series of 33 pregnancies found women tolerated pregnancy, labor, and delivery well, but there was an increased risk for spontaneous abortion.[50] More recently, a smaller series found

live birth pregnancies complicated by high rates of New York Heart Association class deterioration, atrial arrhythmia, prematurity, and intrauterine growth retardation.[49] What can be made of these reports? They suffer from the usual problems of retrospective review and self-reporting. However, they do provide clinicians with some reassuring information. First, pregnancy is usually undertaken only in those patients with relatively good functional status, thereby removing the highest-risk patients. Undoubtedly, most adult congenital cardiologists would counsel against pregnancy in any patient with evidence of a failing Fontan circulation. In patients with good functional status, pregnancy can be successfully carried to term, albeit with increased risk for miscarriage and premature delivery. A review of the case reports in the anesthetic literature shows that epidural analgesia is well tolerated and indeed recommended for the first stage of labor. The Caesarian section rate approaches 50%.[50] Neuraxial anesthesia for Caesarian section, in addition to its usual benefits, preserves spontaneous ventilation, which is desirable in Fontan patients. However, no increased risk from general anesthesia was identified. Perioperative complications are low, and peripartum cardiac decompensation is rare.

Fontan Conversion Surgery

There is now a large cohort of patients with atriopulmonary connections suffering from some degree of thrombosis, arrhythmia, PLE, or ventricular dysfunction. These patients are candidates for Fontan conversion surgery, which is the most commonly performed high-risk operation in the adult CHD population. Case reports and small case series began to appear in the literature in the mid-1990s. At that time, interest focused on the best indications for this major surgery, outcome predictors, and optimizing the surgical technique. There are now some answers to these important questions. It was believed that conversion of an atriopulmonary Fontan to the improved hemodynamics of the modern Fontan would relieve severe atrial arrhythmias. The profile of the early patient undergoing Fontan conversion surgery was one of refractory atrial arrhythmias and poor functional state.[159] Two general trends have been identified. First, in this very high risk group of patients, perioperative mortality was low. Second, arrhythmia control was much better in the group that underwent extracardiac connection with arrhythmia surgery. Conversion to extracardiac Fontan without an ablative procedure resulted in a high rate of arrhythmia recurrence. The largest experience came from Mavroudis,[160] whose preferred technique was conversion to an extracardiac Fontan with intraoperative electrophysiologic mapping, arrhythmia ablation, and pacemaker placement. The risk factors for death or transplantation were right or ambiguous ventricular morphology, PLE, atrioventricular valve regurgitation graded moderate or worse, and long CPB time.

These encouraging results give hope to the many patients with atriopulmonary connections and poor functional status. Patients should not have multiple failed attempts at arrhythmia ablation in the catheterization laboratory because of a fear that surgery is associated with an unacceptably high mortality. The ideal patient is one with refractory arrhythmia and poor functional status despite adequate ventricular function. The higher-risk groups of patients are those with significant ventricular dysfunction, atrioventricular valve regurgitation, or PLE. Fontan conversion surgery provides myriad challenges to the anesthesiologist. Before surgery, the important factors are the degree of arrhythmia control and the ventricular function. Most of the patients will be taking at least one antiarrhythmic drug. They may be in sinus rhythm, but it is more likely they have an atrial arrhythmia with some degree of ventricular rate control. They retain the ability to become tachycardic very easily. This is almost always associated with prompt hemodynamic deterioration. The underlying ventricular function may be poor because of longstanding arrhythmia, made worse by the negative inotropic effect of antiarrhythmic medications. Transcutaneous patches for cardioversion should be placed before induction. Intravenous induction can be prolonged because blood moves sluggishly through the greatly dilated atrium. Airway management needs to be prompt and skilled, as it does for all Fontan patients.

Once safely through induction and intubation, large-bore intravenous access must be established. This is usually not a problem because the central venous hypertension of Fontan patients creates dilated peripheral veins. Small central venous catheters are appropriate for delivering inotropic drugs and monitoring, but some centers will prefer to place transthoracic atrial lines and completely avoid central access for fear of thrombosis. Transesophageal echocardiography (TEE) is routinely used to assess volume status and ventricular function, as well as to exclude intracardiac thrombus. The repeat sternotomy, usually at least the third, can be especially bloody because of the increased central venous pressure. Maintenance of preload and the ability for large volume transfusion is required. Also, a plan should be worked out with the surgeon and perfusionist for emergency establishment of femoral bypass if necessary. Patients with pacemakers are vulnerable to electromagnetic interference because the repeat sternotomy requires extensive use of electrocautery in close proximity to the heart and pacemaker generator. If pacemaker dependent, consideration should be given to reprogram the device to an asynchronous mode. The ability to pace using transcutaneous patches is necessary. The prebypass period can obviously be one of high stress.

In preparation to separate from CPB, full recruitment of the lungs and modest hyperventilation with 100% oxygen are necessary to keep PVR as low as possible. Other factors that increase PVR such as acidosis and hypothermia must be corrected before separation from CPB. Fontan conversion is a lengthy surgery, and the long duration of CPB can precipitate a potent inflammatory response with release of numerous mediators that increase PVR. Milrinone's pulmonary vasodilating properties make it an attractive choice. Despite long CPB times for this type of surgery, aortic cross-clamp time usually is short. Thus, ventricular function after CPB is generally good but must be supported as necessary with inotropes to ensure that atrial and pulmonary venous pressures remain low. Last, aggressive management of coagulation is required, and in this regard there is no substitute for point-of-care testing to guide transfusion products.

Patent Ductus Arteriosus

Beyond the neonatal period, spontaneous closure of a PDA is uncommon. The risk for a longstanding moderate-to-large PDA is volume overloading of the left atrium and left ventricle with the risk for development of pulmonary vascular disease. The progression of pulmonary vascular disease is relatively accelerated when compared with patients with other types of right-to-left shunts. The development of pulmonary vascular disease is dependent on the volume and pressure of the right-to-left shunt. A PDA delivers blood at high shear stress (i.e., arterial pressure) to the pulmonary vasculature, and flow occurs continuously throughout the cardiac cycle. With time, the ductus can become calcified or aneurysmally dilated with a risk for rupture. Ductal calcification or aneurysm increases the risk for surgery, which rarely requires CPB.[161] Unrepaired, the natural history is for one third of patients to die of heart failure, pulmonary hypertension, or endocarditis by 40 years of age and two thirds by age 60.[162] Although small PDAs are of no hemodynamic consequence, even small PDAs carry relatively high endocarditis risk. Surgical closure should be considered for all adults with PDA, and transvascular closure by means of one of several devices is possible.[161] With calcification and friability of the ductus, if device closure is not practicable, it is possible to do a patch closure from inside the aorta or pulmonary artery.

Small PDAs do not carry a hemodynamic risk for pregnancy. The decrease in systemic vascular resistance accompanying pregnancy could lead to right-to-left shunting in a woman with a large PDA.

Pulmonary Valve Stenosis

Long-term asymptomatic survival is typical of patients, with the exception of neonates with critical stenosis.[163] There is a 94% survival rate 20 years after diagnosis, and adults generally do not require surgical intervention.[164] With aging, however, right ventricular fibrosis and

failure can develop, and this is the most common cause of death, usually in the fourth decade of life. Almost all patients who have relief of stenosis either surgically or by balloon valvuloplasty have normal right ventricular function after surgery. However, abnormal ventricular function may not resolve after late surgical correction. The development of isolated pulmonary valvular stenosis, even of a severe degree, is usually well tolerated during pregnancy, even in the face of the volume overload that accompanies it.[165]

In patients with significant right ventricular hypertension, right ventricular ischemia can occur if systemic hypotension and decreased coronary perfusion occur. This is manifest on the electrocardiogram. Coronary ischemia resolves if coronary perfusion pressure is increased, as with use of phenylephrine.

Single Ventricle

See the Fontan Physiology section earlier in this chapter for a detailed discussion.

Tetralogy of Fallot

As with many things in medicine, tetralogy of Fallot was first described by someone else—probably in 1673 by Stenson. The classic description of tetralogy of Fallot includes: (1) a large, nonrestrictive malaligned VSD, with (2) an overriding aorta, (3) infundibular pulmonic stenosis, and (4) consequent right ventricular hypertrophy, all derived from an embryonic anterocephalad deviation of the outlet septum. However, there is a spectrum of disease with more severe defects including stenosis of the pulmonary valve, stenosis of the pulmonary valve annulus, or stenosis and hypoplasia of the pulmonary arteries in the most severe cases. Pentalogy of Fallot refers to the addition of an ASD. With advances in genetics, up to one third or more of cases of tetralogy have been ascribed to one of several genetic abnormalities, including trisomy 21, the 22q11 microdeletion, the genes *NKX 2.5* and *FOG 2.4,* and others. Tetralogy of Fallot is the most common cyanotic lesion encountered in the adult population. Unrepaired or nonpalliated, approximately 25% of patients survive to adolescence, after which the mortality rate is 6.6% per year. Only 3% survive to age 40.[166] Unlike children, teenagers and adults with tetralogy do not develop "tet spells." Long-term survival with a good quality of life is expected after repair. The 32- to 36-year survival rate has been reported to be 85% to 86%, although symptoms, primarily arrhythmias and decreased exercise tolerance, occur in 10% to 15% at 20 years after the primary repair[167–170] (Box 20-10). In the past, most children with tetralogy were managed with a preliminary palliation with an aortopulmonary shunt such as a Blalock-Taussig, followed by complete correction. Essentially all patients would eventually have come for complete repair. Currently, most children are managed with a complete repair in infancy, without preceding palliation.

It is uncommon to encounter an adolescent or adult with unrepaired tetralogy. However, it can be encountered in immigrants or in patients whose anatomic variation was considered to be inoperable when they were children. In tetralogy, the right ventricle "sees" the obstruction from the pulmonic stenosis. Pulmonary vascular resistance is

BOX 20-10. RISK FACTORS FOR SUDDEN DEATH AFTER REPAIR OF TETRALOGY OF FALLOT

- Repair requiring ventriculotomy
- Older age at repair
- Severe left ventricular dysfunction
- Postoperative right ventricular hypertension (residual outflow tract obstruction)
- Wide-open pulmonary insufficiency
- Prolongation of the QRS

typically normal to low. Right-to-left shunting is caused by obstruction at the level of the right ventricular outflow tract and is unaffected by attempts at modulating pulmonary vascular resistance. Shunting is minimized, however, by pharmacologically increasing systemic vascular resistance. Increases in the inotropic state of the heart increase the dynamic obstruction at the right ventricular infundibulum and worsen right-to-left shunting. β-Blockers are often used to decrease inotropy. Although halothane was the historic anesthetic of choice in children with tetralogy because of its myocardial depressant effects and ability to maintain systemic vascular resistance, current practice is to use sevoflurane, without undue consequence from a reduction in systemic vascular resistance.[171] Anesthetic induction in adults can easily be achieved with any of the available agents, keeping in mind the principles of maintenance of systemic blood pressure, avoidance of hypovolemia, and preventing increases in inotropy.

Patients require closure of the VSD and resolution of the pulmonic stenosis. Although current practice is to repair the VSD through the right atrium in an effort to maintain competence of the pulmonary valve and limit any ventriculotomy, older patients will likely have had repair via a right ventriculotomy. A large right ventriculotomy increases the risks for arrhythmias and sudden death.[172] Patients who have had a right ventriculotomy will have an obligate right bundle branch block pattern on the electrocardiogram. However, unlike the more usual bundle branch block in adults, this represents disruption of the His-Purkinje system only in the right ventricular outflow, in the area of the right ventricular incision. Because most His-Purkinje conduction is intact, it does not carry increased risk for the development of complete heart block. These patients can have an abnormal response to exercise.

Some patients require repair of pulmonic stenosis by placement of a transannular patch, with obligate residual pulmonary insufficiency. Isolated mild-to-moderate pulmonary insufficiency is generally well tolerated, but in the long term, it can contribute to right ventricular dysfunction with a risk for ventricular tachycardia and sudden death. Patients requiring pulmonary valve replacement in their late teens or early 20s after a transannular patch in early childhood are a growing proportion of the adult CHD population. Atrial tachyarrhythmias occur in about one third of adults late after repair and can contribute to late morbidity.[173,174] The development of atrial flutter or atrial reentrant tachycardia is often a harbinger of hemodynamic compromise. The substrate is usually an atrial surgical scar and the trigger is atrial dilation, such as from tricuspid insufficiency with right ventricular dysfunction. The mechanism for the development of ventricular arrhythmias is presumably the same, namely, dilation superimposed on surgical scar.

In some cases, the right ventricular outflow tract patch needs to be extended onto the branch pulmonary arteries to relieve obstruction. Patients with abnormal coronary arteries may have required repair using a right ventricle-to-pulmonary artery conduit to avoid doing a right ventriculotomy in the area of the coronary artery. Repair at a younger age (< 12 years) results in better postoperative right ventricular function.[175] Because there is an unrestrictive VSD, in the unrepaired adult, systemic hypertension developing in adult life imposes an additional load on both ventricles, not just the left. The increase in systemic vascular resistance decreases right-to-left shunting and diminishes cyanosis but at the expense of right ventricular or biventricular failure.

Sudden death or ventricular tachycardia requiring treatment can occur in up to 5.5% of postoperative patients older than 30 years, often years after surgery.[168,169,176] The foci for these arrhythmias are typically in the right ventricular outflow tract in the area that has had surgery, and they can be ablated in the catheterization laboratory. Older age at repair, severe left ventricular dysfunction, postoperative right ventricular hypertension from residual or recurrent outflow tract obstruction, wide-open pulmonary insufficiency, and prolongation of the QRS (to > 180 milliseconds) are all predictors of sudden death.[172,177] Premature ventricular contractions and even nonsustained ventricular tachycardia are not rare but do not seem to be associated with sudden death, making appropriate treatment options difficult.[178] QRS

prolongation to longer than 180 milliseconds, although highly sensitive, has a low positive predictive value.[179] The impact of this risk factor in the current group of younger patients who have not had ventriculotomies is unclear because their initial postoperative QRS durations are shorter than in patients who had a right ventriculotomy.

Although for many years it was thought that moderate-to-severe pulmonary insufficiency in these patients was well tolerated, it has become apparent from a number of series that right ventricular dysfunction and both atrial and ventricular arrhythmias can be common long-term sequelae. For this reason, patients with symptomatic pulmonary insufficiency from a transannular patch or aneurysm formation at the site of a right ventricular outflow tract patch can require reoperation to replace a widely incompetent pulmonary valve with a bioprosthetic valve with or without a tricuspid annuloplasty.[180] Interestingly, the incidence of atrial arrhythmias may not be diminished when adult patients have a pulmonary valve placed, although the incidence of ventricular arrhythmias is decreased. Right ventricular dysfunction improves in a variable number of adults, suggesting that pulmonary valve placement be done sooner rather than later. The development of a pulmonary valve that can be delivered via a vascular catheter holds much promise.[181]

Additional possible late-term complications include residual VSD, patch dehiscence, progressive aortic insufficiency, left ventricular dysfunction from surgical injury to an anomalous coronary artery or longstanding preoperative cyanosis, and heart block from VSD closure (uncommon today). Because patients who have had repairs using a conduit require multiple sternotomies and the valved conduit tends to lie immediately behind and in close proximity to the sternum, sternotomy carries with it significant potential risk for laceration of the conduit. On occasion, the femoral vessels are cannulated for bypass before sternotomy.

Most adult patients require reoperation to repair the right ventricular outflow tract or to insert or replace a valve in the pulmonic position. Other reasons for reoperation include repair of an outflow tract aneurysm at the site of a patch, repair of a residual VSD, or repair of an incompetent tricuspid valve.[170] These patients often have diminished right ventricular diastolic compliance and require higher than normal central venous pressure. Postoperative management includes minimizing pulmonary vascular resistance and maintaining central venous pressure. Patients often require treatment postbypass with an inotrope and afterload reduction.[182]

Women with good surgical results without residual defects should tolerate pregnancy and delivery well with outcomes approximating those of the general population.[183] Women with uncorrected tetralogy, particularly those with significant cyanosis, have a high incidence of fetal loss (80% with hematocrit > 65%). The decline in systemic vascular resistance that accompanies pregnancy and delivery can worsen cyanosis, and the physiologic volume loading of pregnancy can exaggerate failure of both ventricles.

Transposition of the Great Arteries (D-Transposition)

In D-transposition of the great arteries, there is a discordant connection of the ventricles and the great arteries. The aorta (with the coronary arteries) arises from the right ventricle, and the pulmonary artery arises from the left ventricle. Thus, the two circulations are separate. Postnatal survival requires interchange of blood between the two circulations, typically via a patent foramen ovale and/or a PDA or VSD. With a 1-year mortality rate approximating 100%, all adults with D-transposition have had some type of surgical intervention. Older adults will have had atrial-type repairs (Mustard or Senning), whereas children born after the mid-1980s will have had repair by arterial switch (the Jatene operation). Some will also have had repair of D-transposition with a moderate-to-large VSD by means of a Rastelli operation (see later).

Atrial repairs function by redirecting systemic venous blood to the left ventricle (and thence to the transposed pulmonary artery)

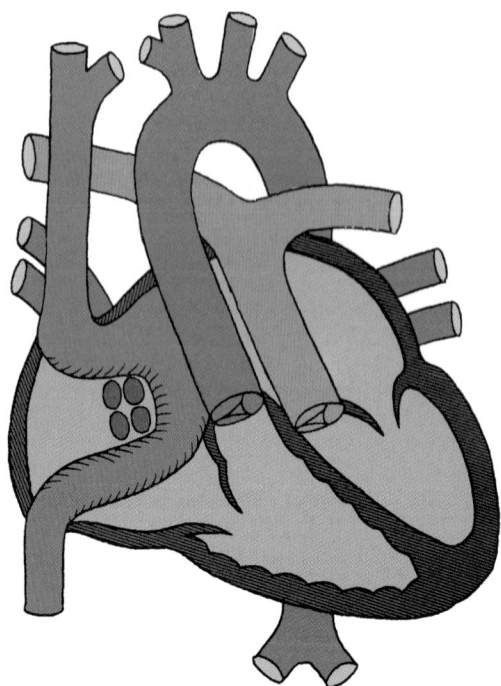

Figure 20-10 **The Mustard operation.** An intra-atrial baffle has directed vena caval blood across the excised atrial septum to the mitral valve and pulmonary venous blood to the tricuspid valve. The right ventricle remains as the systemic ventricle and the left ventricle as the subpulmonary ventricle. *(From Mullins C, Mayer D: Congenital heart disease. A diagrammatic atlas. New York: Wiley-Liss, 1988, by permission of Wiley-Liss, Inc., a subsidiary of John Wiley & Sons, Inc.)*

and pulmonary venous blood to the right ventricle (and thence to the aorta). The Mustard operation uses an intra-atrial conduit of native pericardium (Figure 20-10), whereas the Senning operation uses native atrial tissue to fashion the conduit. The arterial switch operation transposes transected aorta and pulmonary artery such that they now arise above the appropriate ventricle. This operation also requires transposing the coronary arteries from the aorta to the pulmonary root, which, after the procedure, becomes the aortic root. The Rastelli procedure closes the VSD on a bias such that the left ventricle empties into the aorta and connects the right ventricle to the pulmonary artery by means of a valved conduit.

Atrial repairs result in a systemic right ventricle, and these patients consistently have abnormal right ventricular function that can be progressive with a right ventricular ejection fraction of about 40%.[184] Mild tricuspid insufficiency is common, but severe tricuspid insufficiency suggests the development of severe right ventricular dysfunction. There is an 85% to 90% 10-year survival with these operations, but by 20 years, survival is less than 80%.[185–187] Over 25 years, about half experience development of moderate right ventricular dysfunction and one third experience development of severe tricuspid insufficiency.[185,186,188–190] Although it always remains abnormal, it has been suggested that earlier surgery minimizes right ventricular dysfunction.[191] Because of the incidence of right ventricular dysfunction, some patients with atrial repairs have been converted to an arterial switch, after preparation of the left ventricle by a pulmonary artery band to prepare it to tolerate systemic arterial pressure.[192]

Atrial repairs bring an incidence of late electrophysiologic sequelae including sinus node dysfunction (bradycardia), junctional escape rhythms, atrioventricular block, and supraventricular arrhythmias. Atrial flutter occurs in 20% of patients by age 20, with half having progressive sinus node dysfunction by that time.[185,189] On occasion, these tachyarrhythmias can result in sudden death, presumably from 1:1 conduction producing ventricular fibrillation.[185,193] The loss of sinus

rhythm in the face of right ventricular (the systemic ventricle) dysfunction can also contribute to late sudden death. The risk for late death after an atrial repair is almost three times greater if there is an associated VSD. The incidence of tachyarrhythmias does decrease, however, after the tenth postoperative year.

An arterial switch operation can be done after a failed atrial repair in adults, but the outcome is generally poor. It is suggested that younger patients do better.[194] Survival after an arterial switch operation, even early in the experience with this operation, is approximately 90% at 10 years.[195] Very-long-term outcome after the arterial switch procedure is still not known. It does appear that there is essentially no mortality after 5 years after surgery, and late surgical reintervention is mostly because of supravalvular pulmonic stenosis.[196] Although many of these children have abnormal resting myocardial perfusion, up to 9% can have evidence of exercise-induced myocardial ischemia.[197] The implication for the development of premature coronary artery disease in adulthood is not known, and there is also some concern about the ultimate function of the neoaortic valve. Patients who have had a Rastelli repair will require episodic reoperation for replacement of the prosthetic conduit valve.

After an atrial or a Rastelli repair, pregnancy and delivery are generally well tolerated, although right ventricular failure and deterioration in functional capacity can occur. There is an increased incidence of prematurity and small-for-date infants in these women.

Truncus Arteriosus

Truncus arteriosus derives from lack of septation of the embryonic truncus arteriosus into aortic and pulmonary artery components, resulting in a single great vessel, the aorta, arising from the heart with a truncal (semilunar) valve. The truncal valve is an amalgamation of the aortic and pulmonary valves, and therefore contains between three and six cusps. In addition, truncal valve insufficiency is a common finding with this morphologically abnormal valve. A large malalignment-type VSD allows filling from both ventricles. The pulmonary arteries arise from the ascending aorta. Although various types have been described depending on the exact anatomy of the pulmonary artery origin, there is really a spectrum of types I through III. Type IV, or pseudotruncus, describes the situation of pulmonary atresia with VSD and supply of the pulmonary arteries from large collaterals originating from the descending aorta. Repair is by closure of the VSD and connection of the right ventricle to the pulmonary artery (or pulmonary arteries) by a conduit containing a homograft valve.

Because of the very high risk for congestive heart failure followed by pulmonary vascular disease in childhood from high pulmonary blood flow from the aorta, essentially all patients who survive to adolescence have had surgical repair or will have inoperable pulmonary vascular disease. The rare exception is the patient with stenosis near the origin of the pulmonary arteries from the aorta. Patients with valved conduits placed in infancy and early childhood have requisite reoperations to replace the conduit with patient growth, even in the face of adequate valve function. Conduits placed in later childhood can suffice until adulthood. There can be ongoing problems with incompetence and stenosis of the truncal valve (postoperatively functioning as the aortic valve), and eventual dysfunction from stenosis and/or incompetence of the homograft conduit is routinely encountered, requiring replacement.[198,199] Because these patients require multiple sternotomies and the valved conduit tends to lie immediately behind and in close proximity to the sternum, sternotomy carries with it significant potential risk for laceration of the conduit. On occasion, the femoral vessels are cannulated for bypass before sternotomy.

Ventricular Septal Defects

The natural history of VSDs has been reviewed in detail.[163] More than 75% of small and moderate VSDs close spontaneously during childhood by a gradual ingrowth of surrounding septum. Of those that close spontaneously, almost all have closed by 10 years of age. Other mechanisms for natural closure include closure by tricuspid valve tissue, closure by prolapsed aortic leaflet, and closure by endocarditis. Some VSDs result in the development of aortic insufficiency in adults from prolapse of the aortic valve into the defect.[200] Although the risk for endocarditis is ongoing, there is no hemodynamic risk for a small VSD in the adult. If pulmonary vascular disease is present, it can progress if closure of a large VSD is delayed.

Although some studies have reported possible ventricular dysfunction years after surgical repair, these are older reports and patients were operated on later than by current standards.[201–203] It does appear, though, that the ventricle successfully remodels from chronic volume overload if surgical correction is done by 5 years of age and perhaps up to 10 to 12 years of age. Iatrogenic heart block is a possible surgical complication, but was much more common in the earlier days of cardiac surgery. Percutaneous closure devices for use with certain VSDs are available, but not currently for widespread commercial use.

Although some discussion is given to onset times with intravenous or inhalation induction agents, clinical differences are hard to notice with modern low-solubility volatile agents. Thermodilution cardiac output reflects pulmonary blood flow, which will be in excess of systemic blood flow. Pulmonary arterial catheters are not routinely indicated. In the patient with a moderate or large left-to-right shunt, low inspired oxygen and moderate hypercarbia avoid intraoperative decreases in pulmonary vascular resistance with pulmonary overcirculation and left ventricular dilation. However, unlike children, it would be rare to encounter adults with large left-to-right shunts. Adults with unrepaired lesions would have either small shunts or would have had large shunts that caused Eisenmenger physiology.

Pregnancy is well tolerated in the absence of preexisting heart failure or pulmonary hypertension. Pregnancy with a naturally or surgically closed defect carries with it no additional risk, in the absence of additional cardiac problems.

ECHO CASES

Case Study 1

Atrial Septal Defect

Framing

The different types of ASDs arise from problems that occur in the various embryologic structures that combine to form the atrial septum (Figure 20-11). The echocardiographer is required to know the different types of ASD and any associated cardiac defects that accompany each lesion. Secundum ASDs are by far the most common type and are rarely associated with other cardiac defects. Those lesions requiring intervention are usually treated with percutaneous device closure providing there is an adequate rim of surrounding atrial septum for the device to "grab on to." The echocardiographer is vital in helping the interventional cardiologist to "see" the atrium in three dimensions and guide placement of the device.

The primum ASD arises from an endocardial cushion defect. When combined with an inlet VSD, it becomes the atrial component of complete atrioventricular canal. As an isolated septal defect, a primum ASD is frequently associated with mitral regurgitation because of a cleft in the anterior leaflet of the mitral valve. Sinus venosus ASD occurs at the cavo-atrial junction, either superiorly or inferiorly. The superior sinus venosus ASD is usually accompanied by anomalous drainage of the right superior pulmonary vein to the SVC. The inferior sinus venosus ASD is strongly associated with anomalous drainage of the right inferior pulmonary vein to the IVC. These associated defects are crucial information for the echocardiographer to incorporate into the TEE examination.

Data Collection and Interpretation

The intraoperative TEE examination is focused on confirming the presumptive diagnosis of ASD and determining the presence of any other associated defects. The Society of Cardiovascular Anesthesiologists has published guidelines with 20 views that constitute a comprehensive

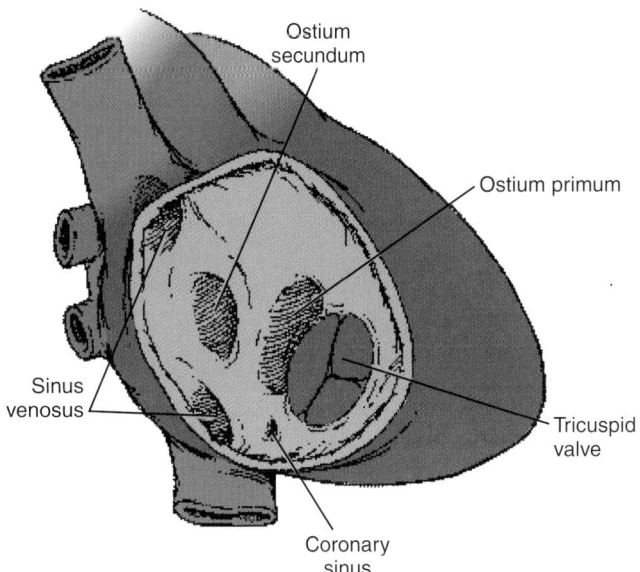

Figure 20-11 Types of atrial septal defects. *(From Nichols DG, Cameron DE, Greeley WG, et al [eds]: Critical heart disease in infants and children. St. Louis: Mosby, 1995.)*

intraoperative TEE examination.[204] When a more detailed examination of a specific cardiac structure is sought, we recommend focusing on the structure by using the zoom feature. The specific structure can then be carefully assessed by using the multiplane function to advance 15 to 30 degrees at a time until the structure has been visualized in multiple views from 0 to 180 degrees. In this example, the echocardiographer would focus on the atrial septum in the midesophageal four-chamber view at 0 degree and then slowly multiplane forward to 180 degrees, providing a comprehensive examination of the structure. The pulmonary veins can be difficult to identify, even for experienced echocardiographers. In the midesophageal four-chamber view with the multiplane angle at 0 degree, the ultrasound image is focused on the left atrium. The probe is then gently turned to the patient's left to identify the left-sided pulmonary veins and then to the right to identify the right-sided pulmonary veins. Visualizing two separate pulmonary veins from each side is challenging because they arrive at a confluence as they enter the left atrium. The use of color Doppler is often helpful to identify blood flowing within the pulmonary veins.

Decision Making and Interpretation

A patient was scheduled for surgical resection of an ASD. Preoperative transthoracic echocardiography confirmed a large secundum ASD with inferior extension toward the IVC (Figure 20-12). The size and inferior extension of the ASD precluded percutaneous device closure. The TEE examination confirmed the preoperative findings and demonstrated four pulmonary veins returning to the left atrium. The volume of left-to-right shunting was large (Figure 20-13). Right ventricular volume overload was present with significant right ventricular dilation (Figure 20-14). After closure of the ASD and separation from CPB, a residual ASD was seen at the inferior aspect of the ASD patch (Figure 20-15). Comparing Figures 20-13 and 20-15 demonstrates the echocardiographic difference in appearance between a high-volume, low-velocity shunt and a more restrictive, higher velocity shunt. The configuration of the TEE machine in the color Doppler mode identifies blood flow toward the transducer in red and blood flow away from the transducer in blue. There is also a threshold of velocity set, such that when blood flow exceeds the velocity threshold, speckling occurs. In Figure 20-13, there is a uniform blue color demonstrating a significant volume shunt. The absence of color speckling confirms low-velocity blood flow. Figure 20-15, taken after attempted repair of the ASD, shows a smaller blue area with orange speckling. The speckling confirms higher velocity blood

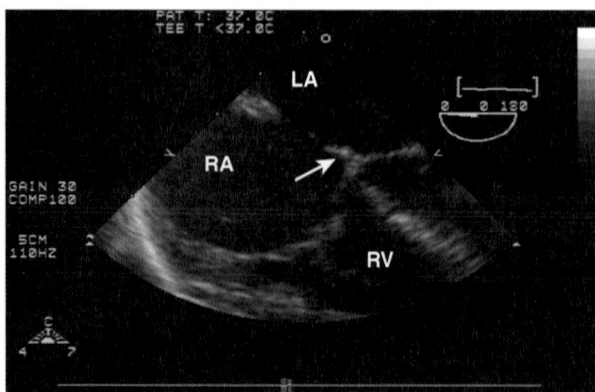

Figure 20-12 **Midesophageal four-chamber TEE view at 0 degree focusing on the atrial septum.** *There is a large secundum atrial septal defect (ASD) with only a small rim of inferior atrial septum (arrow). LA, left atrium; RA, right atrium; RV, right ventricle.*

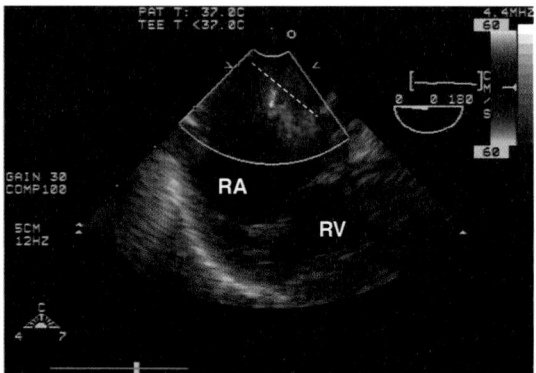

Figure 20-13 **Midesophageal four-chamber view at 0 degree with color-flow Doppler.** There is a large-volume left-to-right shunt (blue color) across the atrial septal defect (ASD). *Dashed line* represents the approximate location of the ASD. The uniform blue color confirms low-velocity flow through a large defect. RA, right atrium; RV, right ventricle.

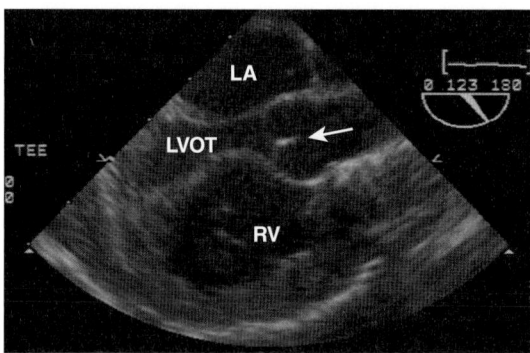

Figure 20-14 **Midesophageal aortic valve long-axis view at 123 degrees.** The aortic valve *(arrow)* is closed, signifying diastole. The atrial septal defect (ASD) has caused marked volume overload of the right ventricle (RV). During diastolic filling of the RV, the septum bulges into the left ventricle. LA, left atrium; LVOT, left ventricular outflow tract.

flow, which is to be expected because the residual defect is much smaller than the unrepaired ASD. Velocity increases as blood flows through a narrower orifice.

How is a residual septal defect assessed? The defect can be assessed qualitatively by examining the degree of shunt using color-flow Doppler. After attempted surgical repair it would be unusual to have a large residual septal defect. What other information can guide the surgeon

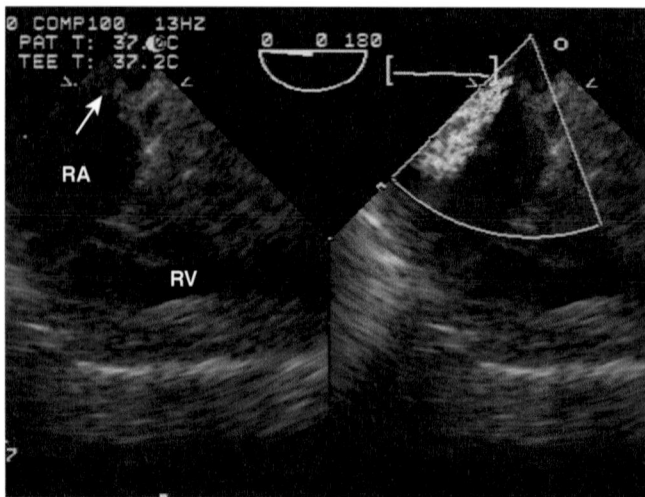

Figure 20-15 Side-by-side images in 2D (left image) and with color-flow Doppler (right image). In the 2D image, there is a possible inferior residual atrial septal defect (ASD; *arrow*). With color-flow Doppler, the residual ASD is clearly appreciated. The orange speckling superimposed on the blue color confirms high-velocity flow. RA, right atrium; RV, right ventricle.

in determining whether to return to CPB and attempt to close what appears to be a small residual defect? The residual defect results in a left-to-right shunt that allows the measurement of the "oxygen step up" between the SVC and pulmonary artery. To do this, the patient should be ventilated with room air. High levels of inspired oxygen result in left atrial blood having a high Pao_2, which causes an overestimation of the residual shunt. After a period of 5 minutes to allow equilibration, blood gas samples from the SVC and pulmonary artery were sent. The oxygenation saturation was 58% in the SVC and 72% in the pulmonary artery. Using a simple equation allows for an estimation of the ratio of pulmonary to systemic blood flow ($Q_p:Q_s$). The saturation at four anatomic locations is entered into the following equation. The oxygen saturations from the SVC and pulmonary artery are measured, the oxygen saturation for the aorta is taken from the peripheral pulse oximeter, and the oxygen saturation for the pulmonary vein is assumed to be 100%.

$$Q_p : Q_s = \frac{Aorta - SVC}{Pulmonary\,vein - Pulmonary\,artery}$$
$$= \frac{100 - 58}{100 - 72} = 1.5$$

The $Q_p:Q_s$ ratio of 1.5 was high enough that, if unrepaired, would likely leave the patient symptomatic from excessive pulmonary blood flow. Integrating the echocardiographic images with quantitative data estimating the degree of the shunt provided the surgeon with a sound justification to return to CPB and attempt to close the residual ASD. The echocardiographic images suggested it was unlikely the residual defect would close spontaneously. The decision to return to CPB and subject the heart to another period of aortic cross-clamping and ischemia can never be made lightly. It was the surgeon's opinion that the residual defect was not amenable to closure with a percutaneous device at some later date, and the patient's underlying heart function was good enough to withstand another period of ischemia and aortic cross-clamping.

After the second attempt at repair, the patient separated easily from CPB. The ASD patch appeared intact on TEE examination, but there was an unusual color-flow Doppler jet seen originating from the junction of the IVC and right atrium. What are the possible explanations? Could this simply be turbulence in the area of the ASD repair? The echocardiographer must now rely on knowledge of the lesion and the potential surgical complications associated with its repair. Figure 20-11 clearly demonstrates the close proximity of an inferior sinus venosus ASD to the IVC. A known, albeit rare, complication of inferior sinus venosus ASD repair is to suture the ASD patch from the IVC to the ASD, thus creating a path from the IVC to left atrium. This suspicion was bolstered by the fact the peripheral pulse oximeter reading varied between 85% and 88%. This was confirmed with an arterial blood gas. The presence of a right-to-left shunt demanded correction. The patient returned to CPB for a third time for takedown of the patch and closure of the ASD. Based on the two previous attempted repairs, the surgeon realized the secundum ASD might extend even farther into the sinus venosus region of the septum than previously imagined. The IVC venous cannula was repositioned more inferiorly, allowing greater exposure of the defect. After repair, the patient once again separated easily from CPB. The TEE examination confirmed the success of the repair with no residual shunting. This case well demonstrates the need for the intraoperative echocardiographer to be more than a "technician" and integrate supporting physiologic information with the TEE images.

Case Study 2

Anomalous Left Main Coronary Artery

Framing

Anomalous coronary arterial lesions comprise a spectrum of defects. In one variant, the left main coronary artery (LMCA) originates from the pulmonary artery. The clinical presentation is heart failure secondary to left ventricular ischemia and generally occurs in the first few months of life. A more insidious but also potentially lethal form of anomalous coronary arterial lesion is both coronary arteries arising from the aorta but from abnormal locations. Most well described is an anomalous LMCA that originates from the right coronary sinus. The LMCA may originate from a separate ostium or may share the same ostium as the right coronary artery (RCA) (Figure 20-16). As Figure 20-16 demonstrates, the path of the LMCA is abnormal. First, the LMCA travels within the wall of the aorta for a short distance before exiting onto the epicardial surface of the heart. This is known as an *intramural coronary artery*. The path of LMCA then follows a path between the aorta and pulmonary artery. The abnormal path of the anomalous LMCA explains why the clinical presentation is sudden death, most often during exercise. The increased blood flow caused by exercise results in dilation of both the aorta and pulmonary artery. This dilation can compress the LMCA between the aorta and pulmonary artery. Alternatively, if the LMCA is intramural, it may be compressed within the wall of the aorta. Either case leads to ischemia in the entire territory of the LMCA with sudden cardiac death. Tragically, an anomalous LMCA is often a postmortem finding after an unexplained sudden death in an otherwise healthy young person. For reasons that are unclear, patients rarely, if ever, develop exertional chest pain. Also, the amount of exertion that precipitates a cardiac event is not predictable. That is, the patient may have vigorously exercised in the past without a problem but suffers a cardiac event during more modest exertion. For these reasons, if a diagnosis of anomalous LMCA is made, surgery is indicated for the prevention of sudden cardiac death.

Data Collection and Interpretation

The diagnosis of LMCA is most often an incidental finding when echocardiography is done for other indications. Proving the absence of a structure is difficult because it may be present but not well visualized by the particular test being used. Echocardiography, either transthoracic or transesophageal, is not the recommended test for demonstrating the origins of the coronary arteries. Therefore, if the ostium of the LMCA is not seen with echocardiography, confirmatory testing is needed. Magnetic resonance imaging or computed tomography is both highly specific and sensitive in accurately diagnosing coronary artery anomalies.

The preferred surgical approach is to divide the LMCA from the right coronary sinus and reimplant it in its proper location. This requires mobilization of the LMCA to allow safe reimplantation on the left coronary sinus. An anomalous LMCA does not cause chronic ischemia. The TEE examination should demonstrate normal left ventricular function. The absence of the LMCA ostium may be noted, but even in patients with normal coronary anatomy, the ostia are frequently not well visualized.

Decision Making and Interpretation

During investigations for nonspecific chest pains, an otherwise healthy patient was discovered to have an anomalous LMCA and was scheduled for coronary reimplantation. After induction of anesthesia, the TEE probe was inserted that demonstrated normal left ventricular function and the LMCA originating from the right coronary cusp, sharing a common ostium with the RCA (Figure 20-17). After the aortic cross-clamping was applied and cardioplegia delivered, the heart was slow to arrest. The cardioplegia circuit was checked and found to be working properly. However, throughout the period of aortic cross-clamping, the heart frequently recovered electrical and mechanical activity before the next scheduled dose of cardioplegia. At the conclusion of the coronary reimplantation, the surgeon believed the myocardial preservation had been poor and the patient would likely need inotropic support. On attempted separation from CPB, the patient was hypotensive with poor myocardial function. What is the differential diagnosis of ventricular dysfunction after CPB? The electrocardiogram showed sinus tachycardia with nonspecific ST- changes in lead II and V_5. This was confirmed in other electrocardiogram leads. The question to be answered was whether ventricular dysfunction was caused by possible poor myocardial preservation or whether the LMCA reimplantation was unsuccessful. By visual inspection, the right ventricle was contracting well. There was no ST- elevation in lead II to suggest air embolus to the RCA. What is the preferred TEE view to assess ventricular function? The transgastric short-axis view at the midpapillary level is used routinely to assess preload, contractility, and regional wall motion abnormalities. Knowing the coronary artery that corresponds to the various left ventricular segments allows the echocardiographer to identify regional wall motions abnormalities caused by ischemia (Figure 20-18). The transgastric image showed marked left ventricular dilation with akinesis of the septal, anterior, lateral, and posterior walls. There was minimal decrease in left ventricular cavity size during systole (see Video 20-1, available online). The reimplanted LMCA could not

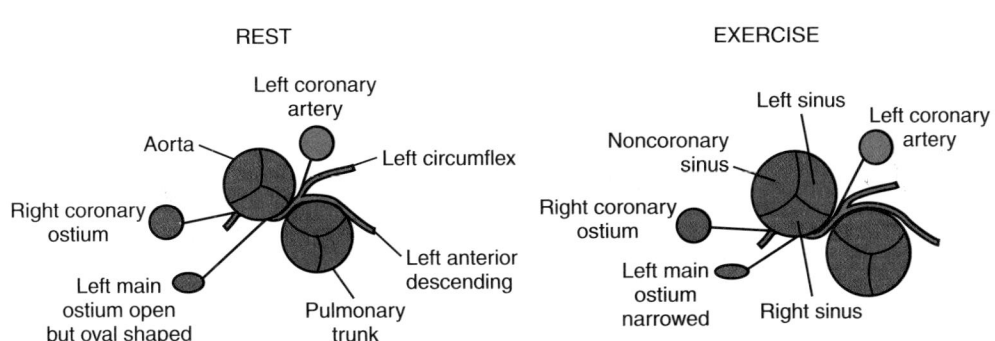

REST   EXERCISE

Figure 20-16 Anomalous left main coronary artery. Compression of the left main coronary artery occurs during exercise. *(From Basilico FC: Cardiovascular disease in athletes. Am J Sports Med 27:108–121, 1999.)*

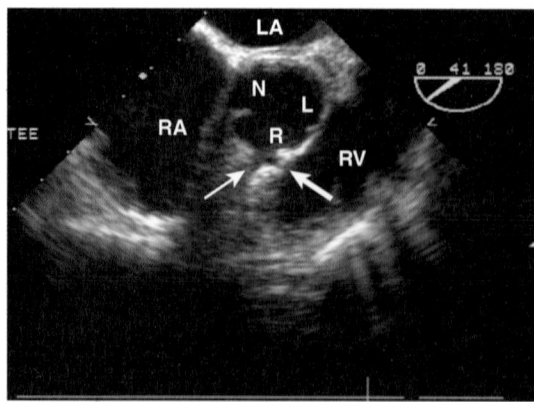

Figure 20-17   Midesophageal aortic valve short-axis view at 41 degrees. The left main coronary artery *(thick arrow)* and right coronary artery *(thin arrow)* both arise from a single ostium in the right coronary sinus. L, left coronary sinus; LA, left atrium; N, noncoronary sinus; R, right coronary sinus; RA, right atrium; RV, right ventricle.

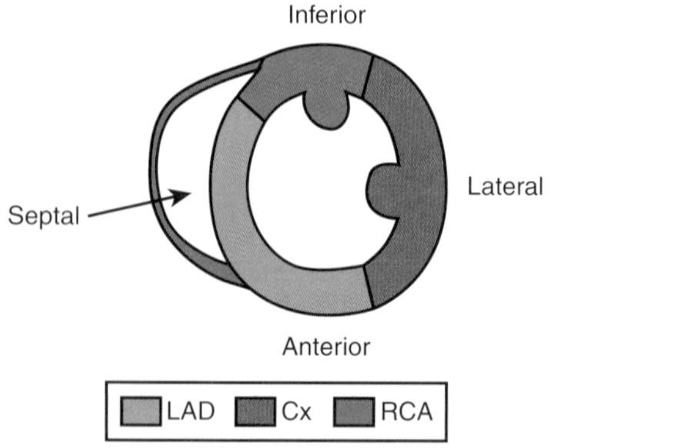

Figure 20-18   Regional left ventricular anatomy with the corresponding coronary artery distribution. Cx, circumflex artery; LAD, left anterior descending artery; RCA, right coronary artery. *(From Shanewise JS, Cheung AT, Aronson S, et al: ASE/SCA guidelines for performing a comprehensive intraoperative multiplane transesophageal echocardiography examination: Recommendations of the American Society of Echocardiography Council for Intraoperative Echocardiography and the Society of Cardiovascular Anesthesiologists Task Force for Certification in Perioperative Transesophageal Echocardiography.* Anesth Analg *89:870–884, 1999.)*

be seen originating from the left coronary sinus. Global ventricular dysfunction secondary to poor myocardial preservation was unlikely because right ventricular function was good. The inferior region of left ventricle, which is supplied by the RCA, had normal function. The findings of severe regional wall motion abnormalities in the distribution of the LMCA confirmed the suspicion of unsuccessful LMCA reimplantation. The extensive wall motion abnormalities suggested the patient had a left dominant coronary circulation. By inspection, the reimplanted LMCA appeared to be free of tension or kinking. After consultation with the surgeon and a description of the TEE findings, it was decided that a second attempt at LMCA reimplantation was likely to be successful.

A decision was made to perform a left internal mammary artery to proximal left anterior descending artery graft. It was hoped that a very proximal anastomosis to the left anterior descending would ensure flow into the circumflex artery as well. The patient separated easily from CPB. The TEE revealed normal left ventricular function with dramatic resolution of the previous regional wall motion abnormalities (see Video 20-2, available online). Specifically, the lateral and posterior

regions of the left ventricle had good function, which provided strong evidence that the left internal mammary artery to proximal left anterior descending graft was also perfusing the circumflex artery. Contrasting the two video images illustrates that the echocardiographic assessment of contractility is based on the degree of ventricular wall thickening during systole. In the first image, the ischemic regions (septal, anterior, lateral, posterior) of the left ventricle do not thicken during systole, but they do move because they are contiguous with the other regions that retain normal function. Although unlikely in this example because the findings are so dramatic, the novice echocardiographer can often confuse ventricular motion with contractility. After the left internal mammary artery to left anterior descending graft, the previously akinetic segments increase their wall thickness by more than 50% during systole. The significant reduction in left ventricular cavity size during systole denotes a normal ejection fraction.

References

1. Perloff JK: Pediatric congenital cardiac patient becomes a postoperative adult. The changing population of congenital heart disease, *Circulation* 47:606–619, 1973.
2. Perloff JK, Warnes CA: Challenges posed by adults with repaired congenital heart disease, *Circulation* 103:2637–2643, 2001.
3. Williams RG, Pearson GD, Barst RJ, et al: Report of the National Heart, Lung, and Blood Institute Working Group on research in adult congenital heart disease, *J Am Coll Cardiol* 47:701–707, 2006.
4. Warnes CA, Liberthson R, Danielson GK, et al: Task force 1: The changing profile of congenital heart disease in adult life, *J Am Coll Cardiol* 37:1170–1175, 2001.
5. Marelli AJ, Mackie AS, Ionescu-Ittu R, et al: Congenital heart disease in the general population: Changing prevalence and age distribution, *Circulation* 115:163–172, 2007.
6. Pillutla P, Shetty KD, Foster E: Mortality associated with adult congenital heart disease: Trends in the US population from 1979 to 2005, *Am Heart J* 158:874–879, 2009.
7. Andropoulos DB, Stayer SA, Skjonsby BS, et al: Anesthetic and perioperative outcome of teenagers and adults with congenital heart disease, *J Cardiothorac Vasc Anesth* 16:731–736, 2002.
8. Dore A, Glancy DL, Stone S, et al: Cardiac surgery for grown-up congenital heart patients: Survey of 307 consecutive operations from 1991 to 1994, *Am J Cardiol* 80:906–913, 1997.
9. Warnes CA: The adult with congenital heart disease: Born to be bad? *J Am Coll Cardiol* 46:1–8, 2005.
10. Mackie AS, Ionescu-Ittu R, Therrien J, et al: Children and adults with congenital heart disease lost to follow-up: Who and when? *Circulation* 120:302–309, 2009.
11. Webb GD, Williams RG: Care of the adult with congenital heart disease: Introduction, *J Am Coll Cardiol* 37:1166, 2001.
12. Warnes CA, Williams RG, Bashore TM, et al: ACC/AHA 2008 guidelines for the management of adults with congenital heart disease: A report of the American College of Cardiology/American Heart Association Task Force on Practice Guidelines (Writing Committee to Develop Guidelines on the Management of Adults with Congenital Heart Disease). Developed in Collaboration with the American Society of Echocardiography, Heart Rhythm Society, International Society for Adult Congenital Heart Disease, Society for Cardiovascular Angiography and Interventions, and Society of Thoracic Surgeons, *J Am Coll Cardiol* 52:e143–e263, 2008.
13. Landzberg MJ, Murphy DJ Jr, Davidson WR Jr, et al: Task force 4: Organization of delivery systems for adults with congenital heart disease, *J Am Coll Cardiol* 37:1187–1193, 2001.
14. Bancalari E, Jesse MJ, Gelband H, et al: Lung mechanics in congenital heart disease with increased and decreased pulmonary blood flow, *J Pediatr* 90:192–195, 1977.
15. Sietsema KE, Perloff JK: Cyanotic congenital heart disease: Dynamics of oxygen uptake and control of ventilation during exercise. In Perloff JK, Child JS, editors: *Congenital heart disease in adults*, Philadelphia, 1991, WB Saunders, pp 104–110.
16. Blesa MI, Lahiri S, Rashkind WJ, et al: Normalization of the blunted ventilatory response to acute hypoxia in congenital cyanotic heart disease, *N Engl J Med* 296:237–241, 1977.
17. Edelmann NH, Lahiri S, Braudo L, et al: The ventilatory response in cyanotic congenital heart disease, *N Engl J Med* 282:405–411, 1970.
18. Sorensen SC, Severinghaus JW: Respiratory insensitivity to acute hypoxia persisting after correction of tetralogy of Fallot, *J Appl Physiol* 25:221–223, 1968.
19. Burrows FA: Physiologic dead space, venous admixture, and the arterial to end-tidal carbon dioxide difference in infants and children undergoing cardiac surgery, *Anesthesiology* 70:219–225, 1989.
20. Perloff JK, Rosove MH, Child JS, et al: Adults with cyanotic congenital heart disease: Hematologic management, *Ann Intern Med* 109:406–413, 1988.
21. Kawakami N, Mimatsu K, Deguchi M, et al: Scoliosis and congenital heart disease, *Spine* 20:1252–1255, 1995.
22. Roclawski M, Sabiniewicz R, Potaz P, et al: Scoliosis in patients with aortic coarctation and patent ductus arteriosus: Does standard posterolateral thoracotomy play a role in the development of the lateral curve of the spine? *Pediatr Cardiol* 30:941–945, 2009.
23. Berman WJ, Wood SC, Yabek SM, et al: Systemic oxygen transport in patients with congenital heart disease, *Circulation* 75:360–368, 1987.
24. Linderkamp O, Klose HJ, Betke K, et al: Increased blood viscosity in patients with cyanotic congenital heart disease and iron deficiency, *J Pediatr* 95:567–569, 1979.
25. Broberg CS, Bax BE, Okonko DO, et al: Blood viscosity and its relationship to iron deficiency, symptoms, and exercise capacity in adults with cyanotic congenital heart disease, *J Am Coll Cardiol* 48:356–365, 2006.
26. Gidding SS, Stockman JA 3rd: Effect of iron deficiency on tissue oxygen delivery in cyanotic congenital heart disease, *Am J Cardiol* 61:605–607, 1988.
27. Spence MS, Balaratnam MS, Gatzoulis MA: Clinical update: Cyanotic adult congenital heart disease, *Lancet* 370:1530–1532, 2007.
28. Maurer HM, McCue CM, Robertson LW, et al: Correction of platelet dysfunction and bleeding in cyanotic congenital heart disease by simple red cell volume reduction, *Am J Cardiol* 35:831–835, 1975.
29. Wedemeyer AL, Lewis JH: Improvement in hemostasis following phlebotomy in cyanotic patients with heart disease, *J Pediatr* 83:46–50, 1973.
30. Tempe DK, Virmani S: Coagulation abnormalities in patients with cyanotic congenital heart disease, *J Cardiothorac Vasc Anesth* 16:752–765, 2002.
31. Weinstein M, Ware JA, Troll J, et al: Changes in von Willebrand factor during cardiac surgery: Effect of desmopressin acetate, *Blood* 71:1648–1655, 1988.

32. Rosove MH, Hocking WG, Harwig SS, et al: Studies of beta-thromboglobulin, platelet factor 4, and fibrinopeptide A in erythrocytosis due to cyanotic congenital heart disease, *Thromb Res* 29:225–235, 1983.
33. Waldman JD, Czapek EE, Paul MH, et al: Shortened platelet survival in cyanotic heart disease, *J Pediat* 87:77–79, 1975.
34. Ware JA, Reaves WH, Horak JK, et al: Defective platelet aggregation in patients undergoing surgical repair of cyanotic congenital heart disease, *Ann Thorac Surg* 36:289–294, 1983.
35. Chauhan S, Kumar BA, Rao BH, et al: Efficacy of aprotinin, epsilon aminocaproic acid, or combination in cyanotic heart disease, *Ann Thorac Surg* 70:1308–1312, 2000.
36. Levin E, Wu J, Devine DV, et al: Hemostatic parameters and platelet activation marker expression in cyanotic and acyanotic pediatric patients undergoing cardiac surgery in the presence of tranexamic acid, *Thromb Haemost* 83:54–59, 2000.
37. Dimopoulos K, Diller GP, Koltsida E, et al: Prevalence, predictors, and prognostic value of renal dysfunction in adults with congenital heart disease, *Circulation* 117:2320–2328, 2008.
38. Spear GS: The glomerular lesion of cyanotic congenital heart disease, *Johns Hopkins Med J* 140: 185–188, 1977.
39. Ross EA, Perloff JK, Danovitch GM, et al: Renal function and urate metabolism in late survivors with cyanotic congenital heart disease, *Circulation* 73:396–400, 1986.
40. Young D: Hyperuricemia in cyanotic congenital heart disease, *Am J Dis Child* 134:902–903, 1980.
41. Dittrich S, Kurschat K, Dahnert I, et al: Renal function after cardiopulmonary bypass surgery in cyanotic congenital heart disease, *Int J Cardiol* 73:173–179, 2000.
42. Perloff JK, Marelli AJ, Miner PD: Risk of stroke in adults with cyanotic congenital heart disease, *Circulation* 87:1954–1959, 1993.
43. Ammash N, Warnes CA: Cerebrovascular events in adult patients with cyanotic congenital heart disease, *J Am Coll Cardiol* 28:768–772, 1996.
44. Truong T, Slavin L, Kashani R, et al: Prevalence of migraine headaches in patients with congenital heart disease, *Am J Cardiol* 101:396–400, 2008.
45. Colman JM, Sermer M, Seaward G, et al: Congenital heart disease: Pathophysiology, clinical recognition, diagnosis, and management. In Wilansky S, Willerson JT, editors: Heart disease in women, New York, 2002, Churchill Livingstone, pp 443–455.
46. Gatzoulis M, Webb GD, Daubeney PEF: Diagnosis and management of adult congenital heart disease, Philadelphia, 2003, Churchill Livingstone.
47. Warnes CA, Elkayam U: Congenital heart disease and pregnancy. In Elkayam U, Gleicher N, editors: Cardiac problems in pregnancy, ed 3 New York, 1998, Wiley-Liss, pp 39–53.
48. Chandrasekhar S, Cook CR, Collard CD: Cardiac surgery in the parturient, *Anesth Analg* 108: 777–785, 2009.
49. Drenthen W, Pieper PG, Roos-Hesselink JW, et al: Pregnancy and delivery in women after Fontan palliation, *Heart* 92:1290–1294, 2006.
50. Canobbio MM, Mair DD, van der Velde M, et al: Pregnancy outcomes after the Fontan repair, *J Am Coll Cardiol* 28:763–767, 1996.
51. Shime J, Mocarski EJ, Hastings D, et al: Congenital heart disease in pregnancy: Short- and long-term implications, *Am J Obstet Gynecol* 156:313–322, 1987.
52. Presbitero P, Somerville J, Stone S, et al: Pregnancy in cyanotic congenital heart disease. Outcome of mother and fetus, *Circulation* 89:2673–2676, 1994.
53. Wilson W, Taubert KA, Gewitz M, et al: Prevention of infective endocarditis: Guidelines from the American Heart Association: A guideline from the American Heart Association Rheumatic Fever, Endocarditis, and Kawasaki Disease Committee, Council on Cardiovascular Disease in the Young, and the Council on Clinical Cardiology, Council on Cardiovascular Surgery and Anesthesia, and the Quality of Care and Outcomes Research Interdisciplinary Working Group, *Circulation* 116: 1736–1754, 2007.
54. Qasqas SA, McPherson C, Frishman WH, et al: Cardiovascular pharmacotherapeutic considerations during pregnancy and lactation, *Cardiol Rev* 12:240–261, 2004.
55. Natale A, Davidson T, Geiger MJ, et al: Implantable cardioverter-defibrillators and pregnancy: A safe combination? *Circulation* 96:2808–2812, 1997.
56. Foster E, Graham TP Jr, Driscoll DJ, et al: Task force 2: Special health care needs of adults with congenital heart disease, *J Am Coll Cardiol* 37:1176–1183, 2001.
57. Bromberg JI, Beasley PJ, D'Angelo EJ, et al: Depression and anxiety in adults with congenital heart disease: A pilot study, *Heart Lung* 32:105–110, 2003.
58. Cox D, Lewis G, Stuart G, et al: A cross-sectional study of the prevalence of psychopathology in adults with congenital heart disease, *J Psychosomat Res* 52:65–68, 2002.
59. Kamphuis M, Ottenkamp J, Vliegen HW, et al: Health related quality of life and health status in adult survivors with previously operated complex congenital heart disease, *Heart* 87:356–362, 2002.
60. Kamphuis M, Vogels T, Ottenkamp J, et al: Employment in adults with congenital heart disease, *Arch Pediatr Adolesc Med* 156:1143–1148, 2002.
61. Lane DA, Lip GY, Millane TA: Quality of life in adults with congenital heart disease, *Heart* 88:71–75, 2002.
62. Lip GY, Lane DA, Millane TA, et al: Psychological interventions for depression in adolescent and adult congenital heart disease, *Cochrane Database Syst Rev* 2003 CD004394.
63. van Rijen EH, Utens EM, Roos-Hesselink JW, et al: Psychosocial functioning of the adult with congenital heart disease: A 20-33 years follow-up, *Eur Heart J* 24:673–683, 2003.
64. Kovacs AH, Saidi AS, Kuhl EA, et al: Depression and anxiety in adult congenital heart disease: Predictors and prevalence, *Int J Cardiol* 137:158–164, 2009.
65. Moons P, Siebens K, De Geest S, et al: A pilot study of expenditures on, and utilization of resources in, health care in adults with congenital heart disease, *Cardiol Young* 11:301–313, 2001.
66. Skorton DJ, Garson A Jr, Allen HD, et al: Task force 5: Adults with congenital heart disease: Access to care, *J Am Coll Cardiol* 37:1193–1198, 2001.
67. Vonder Muhll I, Cumming G, Gatzoulis MA: Risky business: Insuring adults with congenital heart disease, *Eur Heart J* 24:1595–1600, 2003.
68. Truesdell SC, Clark EB: Health insurance status in a cohort of children and young adults with congenital cardiac diagnoses, *Circulation* 84(Suppl 2):II–386, 1991.
69. Graham TP Jr, Cordell GD, Bender HW: Ventricular function following surgery. In Kidd BS, Rowe RD, editors: The child with congenital heart disease after surgery, Mt. Kisco, NY, 1995, Futura Publishing Co.
70. Bouchardy J, Therrien J, Pilote L, et al: Atrial arrhythmias in adults with congenital heart disease, *Circulation* 120:1679–1686, 2009.
71. Feltes TF, Friedman RA: Transesophageal echocardiographic detection of atrial thrombi in patients with nonfibrillation atrial tachyarrhythmias and congenital heart disease, *J Am Coll Cardiol* 24: 1365–1370, 1994.
72. Andropoulos DB, Stayer SA, Russell IA: *Anesthesia for congenital heart disease*, Armonk, NY, 2004, Futura.
73. Lake CL, Booker PD: Pediatric cardiac anesthesia, Philadelphia, 2004, Lippincott-Williams & Wilkins.
74. Carabello BA, Carawford FAJ: Valvular heart disease, *N Engl J Med* 337:32–41, 1997.
75. Craig RJ, Selzer A: Natural history and prognosis of atrial septal defect, *Circulation* 37:805–815, 1968.
76. Markman P, Howitt G, Wade EG: Atrial septal defect in the middle-aged and elderly, *Q J Med* 34: 409–426, 1965.
77. Mattila S, Merikallio E, Tala P: ASD in patients over 40 years of age, *Scand J Thorac Cardiovasc Surg* 13:21–24, 1979.
78. Campbell M: Natural history of coarctation of the aorta, *Br Heart J* 32:633–640, 1970.
79. Boucher CA, Liberthson RR, Buckley MJ: Secundum atrial septal defect and significant mitral regurgitation: Incidence, management and morphologic basis, *Chest* 75:697–702, 1979.
80. Liberthson RR, Boucher CA, Strauss HW, et al: Right ventricular function in adult atrial septal defect. Preoperative and postoperative assessment and clinical implications, *Am J Cardiol* 47:56–60, 1981.
81. Davies H, Oliver GC, Rappoport WJ, et al: Abnormal left heart function after operation for atrial septal defect, *Br Heart J* 32:747–753, 1970.
82. Gatzoulis MA, Freeman MA, Siu SC, et al: Atrial arrhythmia after surgical closure of atrial septal defects in adults, *N Engl J Med* 340:839–846, 1999.
83. Konstantinides S, Geibel A, Olschewski M, et al: A comparison of surgical and medical therapy for atrial septal defect in adults, *N Engl J Med* 333:469–473, 1995.
84. Murphy JG, Gersh BJ, McGoon MD, et al: Long-term outcome after surgical repair of isolated atrial septal defect. Follow-up at 27 to 32 years, *N Engl J Med* 323:1645–1650, 1990.
85. Attie F, Rosas M, Granados N, et al: Surgical treatment for secundum atrial septal defects in patients > 40 years old. A randomized clinical trial, *J Am Coll Cardiol* 38:2035–2042, 2001.
86. Du ZD, Hijazi ZM, Kleinman CS, et al: Comparison between transcatheter and surgical closure of secundum atrial septal defect in children and adults: Results of a multicenter nonrandomized trial, *J Am Coll Cardiol* 39:1836–1844, 2002.
87. Dajani AS, Taubert KA, Wilson W, et al: Prevention of bacterial endocarditis. Recommendations by the American Heart Association, *JAMA* 277:1794–1801, 1997.
88. Abbott ME: Coarctation of the aorta of adult type: II. A statistical study and historical retrospect of 200 recorded cases with autopsy, of stenosis or obliteration of the descending arch in subjects above the age of two years, *Am Heart J* 3:392–421, 1928.
89. Mitchell SC, Korones SB, Berendes HW: Congenital heart disease in 56,109 births. Incidence and natural history, *Circulation* 43:323–332, 1971.
90. Reifenstein GH, Levine SA, Gross RE: Coarctation of the aorta: A review of 104 autopsied cases of the "adult type," 2 years of age or older, *Am Heart J* 33:146–168, 1947.
91. Maron BJ, Humphries JO, Rowe RD, et al: Prognosis of surgically corrected coarctation of the aorta. A 20-year postoperative appraisal, *Circulation* 47:119–126, 1973.
92. Clarkson PM, Nicholson MR, Barratt-Boyes BG, et al: Results after repair of coarctation of the aorta beyond infancy: A 10 to 28 year follow-up with particular reference to late systemic hypertension, *Am J Cardiol* 51:1481–1488, 1983.
93. Therrien J, Gatzoulis M, Graham T, et al: Canadian Cardiovascular Society Consensus Conference 2001 update: Recommendations for the Management of Adults with Congenital Heart Disease—Part II, *Can J Cardiol* 17:1029–1050, 2001.
94. Hamdan MA, Maheshwari S, Fahey JT, et al: Endovascular stents for coarctation of the aorta: Initial results and intermediate-term follow-up, *J Am Coll Cardiol* 38:1518–1523, 2001.
95. Golden AB, Hellenbrand WE: Coarctation of the aorta: Stenting in children and adults, *Catheter Cardiovasc Interv* 69:289–299, 2007.
96. Kutty S, Greenberg RK, Fletcher S, et al: Endovascular stent grafts for large thoracic aneurysms after coarctation repair, *Ann Thorac Surg* 85:1332–1338, 2008.
97. Beauchesne LM, Warnes CA, Connolly HM, et al: Outcome of the unoperated adult who presents with congenitally corrected transposition of the great arteries, *J Am Coll Cardiol* 40:285–290, 2002.
98. Graham TP Jr, Parrish MD, Boucek RJJ, et al: Assessment of ventricular size and function in congenitally corrected transposition of the great arteries, *Am J Cardiol* 51:244–251, 1983.
99. Graham TP Jr, Bernard YD, Mellen BG, et al: Long-term outcome in congenitally corrected transposition of the great arteries: A multi-institutional study, *J Am Coll Cardiol* 36:255–261, 2000.
100. Connelly MS, Robertson P, Liu P, et al: Congenitally corrected transposition of the great arteries in adults: Natural history, *Circulation* 90:I–51, 1994.
101. Connolly HM, Grogan M, Warnes CA: Pregnancy among women with congenitally corrected transposition of great arteries, *J Am Coll Cardiol* 33:1692–1695, 1999.
102. Arendt KW, Connolly HM, Warnes CA, et al: Anesthetic management of parturients with congenitally corrected transposition of the great arteries: Three cases and a review of the literature, *Anesth Analg* 107:1973–1977, 2008.
103. Cordone M, Wolfson A, Wolfson N, et al: Anesthetic management of labor in a patient with congenitally corrected transposition of the great arteries, *Int J Obstet Anesth* 17:57–60, 2008.
104. Therrien J, Barnes I, Somerville J: Outcome of pregnancy in patients with congenitally corrected transposition of the great arteries, *Am J Cardiol* 84:820–824, 1999.
105. Celermajer DS, Cullen S, Sullivan ID, et al: Outcome in neonates with Ebstein's anomaly, *J Am Coll Cardiol* 19:1041–1046, 1992.
106. Kumar AE, Fyler DC, Miettinen OS, et al: Ebstein's anomaly. Clinical profile and natural history, *Am J Cardiol* 28:84–95, 1971.
107. Spitaels SE: Ebstein's anomaly of the tricuspid valve complexities and strategies, *Cardiol Clin* 20: 431–439, 2002 vii.
108. Stulak JM, Dearani JA, Danielson GK: Surgical management of Ebstein's anomaly, *Semin Thorac Cardiovasc Surg Pediatr Card Surg Annu* 105–111, 2007.
109. Connolly HM, Warnes CA: Ebstein's anomaly: Outcome of pregnancy, *J Am Coll Cardiol* 23: 1194–1198, 1994.
110. Eisenmenger V: Die angeborenen Defects des Kammerscheidewand des Herzen, *Z Klin Med* 32(Suppl):1–28, 1897.
111. Diller GP, Gatzoulis MA: Pulmonary vascular disease in adults with congenital heart disease, *Circulation* 115:1039–1050, 2007.
112. Silversides CK, Granton JT, Konen E, et al: Pulmonary thrombosis in adults with Eisenmenger syndrome, *J Am Coll Cardiol* 42:1982–1987, 2003.
113. Vongpatanasin W, Brickner ME, Hillis LD, et al: The Eisenmenger syndrome in adults, *Ann Intern Med* 128:745–755, 1998.
114. Diller GP, Dimopoulos K, Broberg CS, et al: Presentation, survival prospects, and predictors of death in Eisenmenger syndrome: A combined retrospective and case-control study, *Eur Heart J* 27:1737–1742, 2006.
115. Cantor WJ, Harrison DA, Moussadji JS, et al: Determinants of survival and length of survival in adults with Eisenmenger syndrome, *Am J Cardiol* 84:677–681, 1999.
116. Saha A, Balakrishnan KG, Jaiswal PK, et al: Prognosis for patients with Eisenmenger syndrome of various aetiology, *Int J Cardiol* 45:199–207, 1994.
117. Oya H, Nagaya N, Uematsu M, et al: Poor prognosis and related factors in adults with Eisenmenger syndrome, *Am Heart J* 143:739–744, 2002.
118. Daliento L, Somerville J, Presbitero P, et al: Eisenmenger syndrome. Factors relating to deterioration and death, *Eur Heart J* 19:1845–1855, 1998.
119. Bando K, Armitage JM, Paradis IL, et al: Indications for and results of single, bilateral, and heart-lung transplantation for pulmonary hypertension, *J Thorac Cardiovasc Surg* 108:1056–1065, 1994.
120. Holzman RS, Nargozian CD, Marnach R, et al: Epidural anesthesia in patients with palliated cyanotic congenital heart disease, *J Cardiothorac Vasc Anesth* 6:340–343, 1992.
121. Devitt JH, Noble WH, Byrick RJ: A Swan-Ganz catheter related complication in a patient with Eisenmenger's syndrome, *Anesthesiology* 57:335–337, 1982.
122. Perloff JK: *The clinical recognition of congenital heart disease,* ed 3, Philadelphia, 1987, WB Saunders.

123. Avila WS, Grinberg M, Snitcowsky R, et al: Maternal and fetal outcome in pregnant women with Eisenmenger's syndrome, *Eur Heart J* 16:460–464, 1995.
124. Gleicher N, Midwall J, Hochberger D, et al: Eisenmenger's syndrome and pregnancy, *Obstet Gynecol Surv* 34:721–741, 1979.
125. Weiss BM, Hess OM: Pulmonary vascular disease and pregnancy: Current controversies, management strategies, and perspectives, *Eur Heart J* 21:104–115, 2000.
126. Weiss BM, Zemp L, Seifert B, et al: Outcome of pulmonary vascular disease in pregnancy: A systematic overview from 1978 through 1996, *J Am Coll Cardiol* 31:1650–1657, 1998.
127. Masuda M, Kado H, Kajihara N, et al: Early and late results of total correction of congenital cardiac anomalies in infancy, *Jpn J Thorac Cardiovasc Surg* 49:497–503, 2001.
128. Fontan F, Baudet E: Surgical repair of tricuspid atresia, *Thorax* 26:240–248, 1971.
129. Kreutzer G, Galindez E, Bono H, et al: An operation for the correction of tricuspid atresia, *J Thorac Cardiovasc Surg* 66:613–621, 1973.
130. Choussat, Fontan A, Besse P: Selection criteria for Fontan's procedure. In Anderson RH, Shinebourne EA, editors: *Pediatric cardiology*, Edinburgh, 1978, Churchill Livingstone.
131. Coon PD, Rychik J, Novello RT, et al: Thrombus formation after the Fontan operation, *Ann Thorac Surg* 71:1990–1994, 2001.
132. Monagle P, Karl TR: Thromboembolic problems after the Fontan operation, *Semin Thorac Cardiovasc Surg Pediatr Card Surg Annu* 5:36–47, 2002.
133. Varma C, Warr MR, Hendler AL, et al: Prevalence of "silent" pulmonary emboli in adults after the Fontan operation, *J Am Coll Cardiol* 41:2252–2258, 2003.
134. Cromme-Dijkhuis AH, Henkens CM, Bijleveld CM, et al: Coagulation factor abnormalities as possible thrombotic risk factors after Fontan operations, *Lancet* 336:1087–1090, 1990.
135. Odegard K, McGowan FXJ, Zurakowski D, et al: Procoagulant and anticoagulant factor abnormalities following the fontan procedure: Increased factor VIII may predispose to thrombosis, *J Thorac Cardiovasc Surg* 125:1260–1267, 2003.
136. Jacobs ML, Pourmoghadam KK, Geary EM, et al: Fontan's operation: Is aspirin enough? Is coumadin too much? *Ann Thorac Surg* 73:64–68, 2002.
137. Weipert J, Noebauer C, Schreiber C, et al: Occurrence and management of atrial arrhythmia after long-term Fontan circulation, *J Thorac Cardiovasc Surg* 127:457–464, 2004.
138. Gelatt M, Hamilton RM, McCrindle BW, et al: Risk factors for atrial tachyarrhythmias after the Fontan operation, *J Am Coll Cardiol* 24:1735–1741, 1994.
139. Durongpisitkul K, Porter CJ, Cetta F, et al: Predictors of early- and late-onset supraventricular tachyarrhythmias after Fontan operation, *Circulation* 98:1099–1107, 1998.
140. Kirsh JA, Walsh EP, Triedman JK: Prevalence of and risk factors for atrial fibrillation and intra-atrial reentrant tachycardia among patients with congenital heart disease, *Am J Cardiol* 90:338–340, 2002.
141. Deal BJ, Mavroudis C, Backer CL: Arrhythmia management in the Fontan patient, *Pediatr Cardiol* 28:448–456, 2007.
142. Driscoll DJ, Offord KP, Feldt RH, et al: Five- to fifteen-year follow-up after Fontan operation, *Circulation* 85:469–496, 1992.
143. Balaji S, Gewillig M, Bull C, et al: Arrhythmias after the Fontan procedure. Comparison of total cavopulmonary connection and atriopulmonary connection, *Circulation* 84:III162–III167, 1991.
144. Cohen MI, Bridges ND, Gaynor JW, et al: Modifications to the cavopulmonary anastomosis do not eliminate early sinus node dysfunction, *J Thorac Cardiovasc Surg* 120:891–900, 2000.
145. Giannico S, Hammad F, Amodeo A, et al: Clinical outcome of 193 extracardiac Fontan patients: The first 15 years, *J Am Coll Cardiol* 47:2065–2073, 2006.
146. Mertens L, Hagler DJ, Sauer U, et al: Protein-losing enteropathy after the Fontan operation: An international multicenter study. PLE study group, *J Thorac Cardiovasc Surg* 115:1063–1073, 1998.
147. Ostrow A, Freeze H, Rychik J: Protein-losing enteropathy after Fontan operation: Investigations into possible pathophysiologic mechanisms, *Ann Thorac Surg* 82:695–701, 2006.
148. Rychik J, Piccoli DA, Barber G: Usefulness of corticosteroid therapy for protein-losing enteropathy after the Fontan procedure, *Am J Cardiol* 68:819–821, 1991.
149. Donnelly JP, Rosenthal A, Castle VP, et al: Reversal of protein-losing enteropathy with heparin therapy in three patients with univentricular hearts and Fontan palliation, *J Pediatr* 130:474–478, 1997.
150. de Leval MR, Kilner P, Gewillig M, et al: Total cavopulmonary connection: A logical alternative to atriopulmonary connection for complex Fontan operations. Experimental studies and early clinical experience, *J Thorac Cardiovasc Surg* 96:682–695, 1988.
151. d'Udekem Y, Iyengar AJ, Cochrane AD, et al: The Fontan procedure: Contemporary techniques have improved long-term outcomes, *Circulation* 116:I157–I164, 2007.
152. Harrison DA, Liu P, Walters JE, et al: Cardiopulmonary function in adult patients late after Fontan repair, *J Am Coll Cardiol* 26:1016–1021, 1995.
153. Gratz A, Hess J, Hager A: Self-estimated physical functioning poorly predicts actual exercise capacity in adolescents and adults with congenital heart disease, *Eur Heart J* 30:497–504, 2009.
154. Kiesewetter CH, Sheron N, Vettukattill JJ, et al: Hepatic changes in the failing Fontan circulation, *Heart* 93:579–584, 2007.
155. Ghanayem NS, Berger S, Tweddell JS: Medical management of the failing Fontan, *Pediatr Cardiol* 28:465–471, 2007.
156. Steven JM, McGowan FX: Neuraxial blockade for pediatric cardiac surgery: Lessons yet to be learned, *Anesth Analg* 90:1011–1013, 2000.
157. Carp H, Jayaram A, Vadhera R, et al: Epidural anesthesia for cesarean delivery and vaginal birth after maternal Fontan repair: Report of two cases, *Anesth Analg* 78:1190–1192, 1994.
158. Fyfe DA, Gillette PC, Jones JS, et al: Successful pregnancy following modified Fontan procedure in a patient with tricuspid atresia and recurrent atrial flutter, *Am Heart J* 117:1387–1388, 1989.
159. Sheikh AM, Tang AT, Roman K, et al: The failing Fontan circulation: Successful conversion of atriopulmonary connections, *J Thorac Cardiovasc Surg* 128:60–66, 2004.
160. Mavroudis C, Deal BJ, Backer CL, et al: J. Maxwell Chamberlain Memorial Paper for congenital heart surgery. 111 Fontan conversions with arrhythmia surgery: Surgical lessons and outcomes, *Ann Thorac Surg* 84:1457–1465, 2007 discussion 65–66.
161. Fisher RG, Moodie DS, Sterba R, et al: Patent ductus arteriosus in adults—long-term follow-up: Nonsurgical versus surgical treatment, *J Am Coll Cardiol* 8:280–284, 1986.
162. Campbell M: Natural history of patent ductus arteriosus, *Br Heart J* 30:4–13, 1968.
163. O'Fallon WM, Weidman WH: Long-term follow-up of congenital aortic stenosis, pulmonary stenosis and ventricular septal defect, *Circulation* 87(Suppl I):I1–I126, 1993.
164. Hayes CJ, Gersony WM, Driscoll DJ, et al: Second natural history study of congenital heart defects. Results of treatment of patients with pulmonary valvar stenosis, *Circulation* 87:I28–I37, 1993.
165. Hameed AB, Goodwin TM, Elkayam U: Effect of pulmonary stenosis on pregnancy outcomes—a case-control study, *Am Heart J* 154:852–854, 2007.
166. Bertranou EG, Blackstone EH, Hazelrig JB, et al: Life expectancy without surgery in tetralogy of Fallot, *Am J Cardiol* 42:458–466, 1978.
167. Harrison DA, Harris L, Siu SC, et al: Sustained ventricular tachycardia in adult patients late after repair of tetralogy of Fallot, *J Am Coll Cardiol* 30:1368–1373, 1997.
168. Murphy JG, Gersh BJ, Mair DD, et al: Long-term outcome in patients undergoing surgical repair of tetralogy of Fallot, *N Engl J Med* 329:593–599, 1993.
169. Nollert G, Fischlein T, Bouterwek S, et al: Long-term survival in patients with repair of tetralogy of Fallot: 36-year follow-up of 490 survivors of the first year after surgical repair, *J Am Coll Cardiol* 30:1374–1383, 1997.
170. Oechslin EN, Harrison DA, Harris L, et al: Reoperation in adults with repair of tetralogy of Fallot: Indications and outcomes, *J Thorac Cardiovasc Surg* 118:245–251, 1999.
171. Russell IA, Miller Hance WC, Gregory G, et al: The safety and efficacy of sevoflurane anesthesia in infants and children with congenital heart disease, *Anesth Analg* 92:1152–1158, 2001.
172. Gatzoulis MA, Balaji S, Webber SA, et al: Risk factors for arrhythmia and sudden cardiac death late after repair of tetralogy of Fallot: A multicentre study, *Lancet* 356:975–981, 2000.
173. Harrison DA, Siu SC, Hussain F, et al: Sustained atrial arrhythmias in adults late after repair of tetralogy of Fallot, *Am J Cardiol* 87:584–588, 2001.
174. Roos-Hesselink J, Perlroth MG, McGhie J, et al: Atrial arrhythmias in adults after repair of tetralogy of Fallot. Correlations with clinical, exercise, and echocardiographic findings, *Circulation* 91:2214–2219, 1995.
175. Rammohan M, Airan B, Bhan A, et al: Total correction of tetralogy of Fallot in adults—surgical experience, *Int J Cardiol* 63:121–128, 1998.
176. Kavey RE, Blackman MS, Sondheimer HM: Incidence and severity of chronic ventricular dysrhythmias after repair of tetralogy of Fallot, *Am Heart J* 103:342–350, 1982.
177. Abd El Rahman MY, Abdul-Khaliq H, Vogel M, et al: Relation between right ventricular enlargement, QRS duration, and right ventricular function in patients with tetralogy of Fallot and pulmonary regurgitation after surgical repair, *Heart* 84:416–420, 2000.
178. Cullen S, Celermajer DS, Franklin RC, et al: Prognostic significance of ventricular arrhythmia after repair of tetralogy of Fallot: A 12-year prospective study, *J Am Coll Cardiol* 23:1151–1155, 1994.
179. Gatzoulis MA, Till JA, Somerville J, et al: Mechanoelectrical interaction in tetralogy of Fallot. QRS prolongation relates to right ventricular size and predicts malignant ventricular arrhythmias and sudden death, *Circulation* 92:231–237, 1995.
180. Discigil B, Dearani JA, Puga FJ, et al: Late pulmonary valve replacement after repair of tetralogy of Fallot, *J Thorac Cardiovasc Surg* 121:344, 2001.
181. Momenah TS, El Oakley R, Al Najashi K, et al: Extended application of percutaneous pulmonary valve implantation, *J Am Coll Cardiol* 53:1859–1863, 2009.
182. Heggie J, Poirer N, Williams RG, et al: Anesthetic considerations for adult cardiac surgery patients with congenital heart disease, *Semin Cardiothorac Vasc Anesth* 7:141–152, 2003.
183. Veldtman GR, Connolly HM, Grogan M, et al: Outcomes of pregnancy in women with tetralogy of Fallot, *J Am Coll Cardiol* 44:174–180, 2004.
184. Graham TP Jr: Ventricular performance in congenital heart disease, *Circulation* 84:2259–2274, 1991.
185. Gelatt M, Hamilton RM, McCrindle BW, et al: Arrhythmia and mortality after the Mustard procedure: A 30-year single-center experience, *J Am Coll Cardiol* 29:194–201, 1997.
186. Wilson NJ, Clarkson PM, Barratt-Boyes BG, et al: Long-term outcome after the mustard repair for simple transposition of the great arteries. 28-year follow-up, *J Am Coll Cardiol* 32:758–765, 1998.
187. Oechslin E, Jenni R: 40 years after the first atrial switch procedure in patients with transposition of the great arteries: Long-term results in Toronto and Zurich, *J Thorac Cardiovasc Surg* 48:233–237, 2000.
188. Myridakis DJ, Ehlers KH, Engle MA: Late follow-up after venous switch operation (Mustard procedure) for simple and complex transposition of the great arteries, *Am J Cardiol* 74:1030–1036, 1994.
189. Puley G, Siu S, Connelly M, et al: Arrhythmia and survival in patients > 18 years of age after the mustard procedure for complete transposition of the great arteries, *Am J Cardiol* 83:1080–1084, 1999.
190. Warnes CA, Somerville J: Transposition of the great arteries: Late results in adolescents and adults after the Mustard procedure, *Br Heart J* 58:148–155, 1987.
191. Graham TP Jr, Burger J, Bender HW, et al: Improved right ventricular function after intra-atrial repair of transposition of the great arteries, *Circulation* 72:II45–II51, 1985.
192. Cochrane AD, Karl TR, Mee RB: Staged conversion to arterial switch for late failure of the systemic right ventricle, *Ann Thorac Surg* 56:854–861, 1993.
193. Garson AJ: The emerging adult with arrhythmias after congenital heart disease: Management and financial health care policy, *Pacing Clin Electrophysiol* 13:951–954, 1990.
194. Mavroudis C, Backer CL: Arterial switch after failed atrial baffle procedures for transposition of the great arteries, *Ann Thorac Surg* 69:851–857, 2000.
195. Hutter PA, Kreb DL, Mantel SF, et al: Twenty-five years' experience with the arterial switch operation, *J Thorac Cardiovasc Surg* 124:790–797, 2002.
196. Losay J, Touchot A, Serraf A, et al: Late outcome after arterial switch operation for transposition of the great arteries, *Circulation* 104:I121–I126, 2001.
197. Mahle WT, McBride MG, Paridon SM: Exercise performance after the arterial switch operation for D-transposition of the great arteries, *Am J Cardiol* 87:753–758, 2001.
198. Rajasinghe HA, McElhinney DB, Reddy VM, et al: Long-term follow-up of truncus arteriosus repaired in infancy: A twenty-year experience, *J Thorac Cardiovasc Surg* 113:869–878, 1997.
199. Schreiber C, Eicken A, Balling G, et al: Single centre experience on primary correction of common arterial trunk: Overall survival and freedom from reoperation after more than 15 years, *Eur J Cardiothorac Surg* 18:68–73, 2000.
200. Wilson NJ, Neutze JM: Adult congenital heart disease: Principles and management guidelines: Part II, *Aust NZ J Med* 23:697–705, 1993.
201. Jarmakani JM, Graham TP Jr, Canent RV Jr, et al: The effect of corrective surgery on left heart volume and mass in children with ventricular septal defect, *Am J Cardiol* 27:254–258, 1971.
202. Jarmakani JM, Graham TPJ, Canent RVJ: Left ventricular contractile state in children with successfully corrected ventricular septal defect, *Circulation* 45(Suppl 1):102–110, 1972.
203. Maron BJ, Redwood DR, Hirshfeld JWJ, et al: Postoperative assessment of patients with ventricular septal defect and pulmonary hypertension. Response to intense upright exercise, *Circulation* 48:864–874, 1973.
204. Shanewise JS, Cheung AT, Aronson S, et al: ASE/SCA guidelines for performing a comprehensive intraoperative multiplane transesophageal echocardiography examination: Recommendations of the American Society of Echocardiography Council for Intraoperative Echocardiography and the Society of Cardiovascular Anesthesiologists Task Force for Certification in Perioperative Transesophageal Echocardiography, *Anesth Analg* 89:870–874, 1999.

21

Thoracic Aorta

JOHN G. AUGOUSTIDES, MD, FASE, FAHA | ENRIQUE J. PANTIN, MD | ALBERT T. CHEUNG, MD

KEY POINTS

1. Deliberate hypothermia is the most important therapeutic intervention to prevent cerebral ischemia during temporary interruption of cerebral perfusion during aortic arch reconstruction.
2. Selective antegrade cerebral perfusion should be considered if the anticipated duration of deep hypothermic circulatory arrest is longer than 30 to 45 minutes.
3. Early detection and interventions to increase spinal cord perfusion pressure are effective for the treatment of delayed-onset spinal cord ischemia after thoracic or thoracoabdominal aortic aneurysm repair.
4. Stanford type A aortic dissection involving the ascending aorta and aortic arch is a surgical emergency.
5. Stanford type B aortic dissection confined to the descending thoracic or abdominal aorta should be managed medically when possible.
6. Thoracic aortic aneurysms can cause compression of the trachea, left mainstem bronchus, right ventricular outflow tract, right pulmonary artery, or esophagus.
7. Intraoperative transesophageal echocardiography can be used to diagnose type A aortic dissection or traumatic aortic injuries that require emergency surgery.
8. Intraoperative transesophageal echocardiography and ultrasound imaging of the carotid arteries are useful for the diagnosis of aortic regurgitation, cardiac tamponade, myocardial ischemia, or cerebral malperfusion, complicating type A aortic dissection.
9. Severe atheromatous disease or thrombus in the thoracic or descending aorta is a risk factor for stroke.
10. Distal aortic perfusion pressure should be maintained to prevent spinal cord ischemia in patients with aortic coarctation.
11. Multidisciplinary guidelines for the diagnosis and management of thoracic aortic disease summarize the evidence and expert consensus for this challenging group of important diseases.

Thoracic aortic diseases typically require surgical intervention (Table 21-1). Acute aortic dissections, rupturing aortic aneurysms, and traumatic aortic injuries are surgical emergencies. Subacute aortic dissection and expanding aortic aneurysms require urgent surgical intervention. Stable thoracic or thoracoabdominal aortic aneurysms (TAAAs), aortic coarctation, or atheromatous disease causing embolization may be addressed surgically on an elective basis. The volume of thoracic aortic procedures has grown steadily because of factors such as increased public awareness, an aging population, earlier diagnosis, multiple advances in imaging, and advances in surgical techniques including endovascular stenting. Medical centers have emerged that specialize in thoracic aortic diseases, resulting in improved management and survival. This progress has created a set of patients who later require reoperation for long-term complications such as valve or graft failure, pseudoaneurysm at anastomotic sites, endocarditis, and/or progression of the original disease process into residual native aorta.

The anesthetic management of thoracic aortic diseases has unique considerations including the temporary interruption of blood flow, often resulting in ischemia of major organ systems. Critical components of anesthetic management include the maintenance of organ perfusion, the protection of vital organs during ischemia, and the monitoring and management of end-organ ischemia. As a result, the vigilant and skillful anesthesiologist contributes importantly to the overall success of these operations. The procedures performed by the thoracic aortic team for organ protection, such as partial left-heart bypass (PLHB) for distal aortic perfusion, cardiopulmonary bypass (CPB) with deep hypothermic circulatory arrest (DHCA), selective cerebral perfusion, and lumbar cerebrospinal fluid (CSF) drainage, are practiced routinely in no other area of medicine. The recently published multisociety guidelines represent a contemporary evidence-based, consensus-driven approach to thoracic aortic diseases. Their recommendations are referred to throughout this chapter, based on the well-known classification of recommendations and levels of evidence (Tables 21-2 and 21-3) by the American College of Cardiology (ACC) and American Heart Association (AHA).[1]

ANATOMY OF THE AORTA

The aorta is the large artery running from the aortic valve to the iliac bifurcation. It serves both as a conducting vessel and as a secondary passive pump because of its elastic recoil. During ventricular systole, the aortic lumen distends as it receives the entire stroke volume. In diastole, after aortic valve closure, the blood is propelled forward as a result of the aorta's elastic recoil. This pulse wave is transmitted distally at approximately 5 m/sec, exceeding the aortic blood flow velocity of 40 to 50 cm/sec. The aortic systolic blood pressure results from the summated effects of stroke volume, aortic compliance, and peripheral vascular resistance. Isolated systolic hypertension develops with aging as the aorta loses elasticity and cannot dampen the stroke volume.

During fetal development, the ductus arteriosus diverts blood from the pulmonary artery into the distal aortic arch. After birth, lung expansion and constriction of the ductus arteriosus because of increased blood oxygen content drives the blood from the pulmonary artery into the pulmonary circulation. Typically, the ductus arteriosus is functionally closed by 48 hours and is permanently

TABLE 21-1	Thoracic Aortic Diseases Amenable to Surgical Treatment

Aneurysm
Congenital or developmental
 Marfan syndrome, Ehlers–Danlos syndrome
Degenerative
 Cystic medial degeneration
 Annuloaortic ectasia
 Atherosclerotic
Traumatic
 Blunt and penetrating trauma
Inflammatory
 Takayasu's arteritis, Behçet syndrome, Kawasaki disease
Microvascular diseases (polyarteritis)
Infectious (mycotic)
 Bacterial, fungal, spirochetal, viral
Mechanical
 Poststenotic, associated with an arteriovenous fistula
 Anastomotic (postarteriotomy)
Pseudoaneurysm
Aortic dissection
 Stanford type A
 Stanford type B
Intramural hematoma
Penetrating atherosclerotic ulcer
Atherosclerotic disease
Traumatic aortic injury
Aortic coarctation

Data from Kouchoukos NT, Dougenis D: Surgery of the aorta. *N Engl J Med* 336:1876, 1997.

TABLE 21-2	Classification Scheme for Clinical Recommendations
Clinical Recommendations	**Definition of Recommendation Class**
Class I	The procedure/treatment should be performed (benefit far outweighs the risk).
Class IIa	It is reasonable to perform the procedure/treatment (benefit still clearly outweighs risk).
Class IIb	It is not unreasonable to perform the procedure/treatment (benefit probably outweighs the risk).
Class III	The procedure/treatment should not be performed as it is not helpful and may be harmful (risk may outweigh benefit).

Data from Hiratzka LF, Bakris GL, Beckman JA, et al: 2010 ACCF/AHA/AATS/ACR/ASA/SCA/SCAI/SIR/STS/SVM guidelines for the diagnosis and management of patients with thoracic aortic disease: Executive summary. A report of the American College of Cardiology Foundation, American Heart Association Task Force on Practice Guidelines, American Association for Thoracic Surgery, American College of Radiology, American Stroke Association, Society of Cardiovascular Anesthesiologists, Society for Cardiovascular Angiography and Interventions, and Society for Vascular Medicine. *Circulation* 121:e266–e369, 2010.

TABLE 21-3	Classification Scheme for Supporting Evidence for Clinical Recommendations
Supporting Evidence	**Estimate of Certainty**
Level A	Data derived from multiple randomized clinical trials (RCT) or meta-analysis.
Level B	Data derived from a single RCT or nonrandomized studies.
Level C	Only consensus opinions of experts, case studies, or standard of care.

Data from Hiratzka LF, Bakris GL, Beckman JA, et al: 2010 ACCF/AHA/AATS/ACR/ASA/SCA/SCAI/SIR/STS/SVM guidelines for the diagnosis and management of patients with thoracic aortic disease: Executive summary. A report of the American College of Cardiology Foundation, American Heart Association Task Force on Practice Guidelines, American Association for Thoracic Surgery, American College of Radiology, American Stroke Association, Society of Cardiovascular Anesthesiologists, Society for Cardiovascular Angiography and Interventions, and Society for Vascular Medicine. *Circulation* 121:e266–e369, 2010.

closed by 3 weeks after birth.[2] It subsequently fibroses to become the "ligamentum arteriosum." Occasionally, this process fails and the ductus arteriosus remains patent. Furthermore, occasionally a ductal diverticulum may persist and be confused in later life with an aortic injury during aortic imaging. The pathogenesis of aortic coarctation may be related to residual ductal tissue that narrows the aorta as it constricts.

The aortic wall has three layers: a thin intima or inner layer lined by endothelium, a thick media or middle layer, and a thin adventitia or outermost layer. The endothelium is in direct contact with blood, is easily traumatized, and is the site for atherosclerosis. The media comprises 80% of the aortic wall thickness and consists of spirally arranged intertwining layers of elastic tissue that provide the aorta's tensile strength and elasticity. The adventitia consists mainly of collagen and

contains the vasa vasorum that nourishes the outer half of the aortic wall. The fact that the vasa vasorum are absent in the infrarenal aorta may explain the frequency of infrarenal aortic aneurysms. These three aortic layers typically are indistinguishable by current clinical imaging techniques. Pathologic aortic processes can separate the aortic wall layers to make them evident on computed tomography (CT), magnetic resonance imaging (MRI), or transesophageal echocardiography (TEE).

The thoracic aorta comprises the ascending aorta, the aortic arch, and the descending aorta. The ascending aorta is about 9 cm long and comprises the aortic root and ascending aorta. The aorta begins at the aortic valve just to the right of midline at the left ventricular base. The aortic root and proximal ascending aorta lie within the pericardial sac. The aorta then travels superiorly and anteriorly to the left. It then turns posteriorly and continues to the left to the fourth thoracic vertebra. Thereafter, it travels inferiorly, initially anterior and to the left of the spine to cross the diaphragm, ending in front of the fourth lumbar vertebra. The aortic root includes the aortic valve annulus and the sinuses of Valsalva that terminate at the sinotubular junction. The origin of the innominate artery marks the end of the ascending aorta and the beginning of the aortic arch. The aortic arch lies within the superior mediastinum between the ascending and descending thoracic aorta. The aortic arch ends after the origin of the left subclavian artery. The aortic isthmus is the segment of aorta where the distal aortic arch becomes the descending thoracic aorta. At the aortic isthmus, the relatively mobile ascending aorta and arch join the descending thoracic aorta that is fixed to the posterior thoracic cage by pleural reflections, the intercostal arteries, the ligamentum arteriosum, and the left subclavian artery. As a result, the aortic isthmus is vulnerable to traumatic injury as it is subjected to high shear forces after blunt trauma or rapid deceleration. Furthermore, the aortic isthmus also is the most common site for aortic coarctation.

The coronary arteries are the first branches of the aorta. The aortic arch subsequently gives origin to the innominate, left carotid, and left subclavian arteries that supply the head, neck, and arms. The innominate artery (brachiocephalic trunk) is the first branch of the aortic arch, followed by the left common carotid artery, and, finally, the left subclavian artery. There are multiple aortic arch anatomic variations, including vascular rings, right-sided aortic arch, and branching anomalies. A right-sided aortic arch is found in about 0.1% of the population. A relatively common aortic arch branch anomaly with a 4% prevalence rate is an isolated left vertebral artery, so named because it arises directly from the aortic arch.[3]

The aortic arch also modulates blood pressure via baroreceptors within its outer wall. The aortic bodies are located inferior to the aortic arch. The aortic baroreceptors respond to a greater threshold pressure and thus are less sensitive when compared with the carotid sinus receptors. These receptors send impulses to the brainstem that interact with the medullary cardiovascular center for modulation of autonomic nervous system activity.[4]

GENERAL CONSIDERATIONS FOR THE PERIOPERATIVE CARE OF AORTIC SURGICAL PATIENTS

Patients undergoing thoracic aortic surgery share common considerations for the safe conduct of anesthesia and perioperative care that are addressed in this section (Table 21-4). The unique considerations and care that apply to specific diseases and procedures are addressed in subsequent sections devoted to their management.

Preanesthetic Assessment

The preanesthetic assessment of the thoracic aorta surgical patient ideally begins before admission to the operating room (OR). The first consideration is whether the planned procedure is emergent, urgent, or elective. For urgent or emergent operations, it is most efficient to assign team members specific tasks for rapid and comprehensive patient and OR preparation. For example, one team member can review the patient chart and diagnostic studies to formulate an anesthetic plan. A second team member can interview the patient and obtain informed consent. The remaining team members simultaneously can prepare the OR, apply physiologic monitors, secure intravascular access, and send laboratory specimens including blood for cross-matching.

The second consideration is to determine the aortic diagnosis because its extent and physiologic consequences dictate both anesthetic management and surgical approach. Aortic diseases proximal to the left carotid artery typically are approached via a median sternotomy, whereas aortic diseases distal to this point usually are approached via a left thoracotomy or thoracoabdominal incision. Although an aortic diagnosis often is established in advance, at times a definitive diagnosis must be verified after OR admission by direct review of diagnostic studies or by subsequent TEE. In every case, a review of the operative plan with the surgical team facilitates thorough anesthetic preparation. Direct review of adequate aortic diagnostic imaging studies not only verifies the operative diagnosis but also determines the surgical possibilities (ACC/AHA Class I recommendation; level of evidence C).[1] The anatomic details of an aortic disease permit the anesthesiologist to anticipate potential perioperative difficulties, including likely postoperative complications.

The systematic assessment of each organ system in the aortic surgical patient should focus on how it will affect the conduct of anesthesia and surgery. The baseline functional reserve of each organ system determines the likely perioperative complications and allows ranking of organ-protective strategies. It is reasonable to obtain further tests to quantitate the functional reserve of affected organ systems, for example, neurocognitive testing, brain imaging, noninvasive carotid artery imaging, pulmonary function testing, echocardiography, and cardiac catheterization (ACC/AHA Class IIa recommendation; level of evidence C).[1] For example, significant cerebrovascular disease affects blood pressure management to ensure adequate cerebral perfusion. Significant cardiac compromise typically increases the risks for heart failure, myocardial ischemia, and arrhythmias. Significant lung disease often is predictive for postoperative respiratory failure, pneumonia, or both. Significant renal insufficiency affects fluid management, triggers the avoidance of nephrotoxic drugs, and customizes the dosing of renally cleared drugs. Hepatic disease and hematologic dysfunction are risk factors for perioperative bleeding and transfusion. Severe aortic atheroma is a major risk factor for atheroembolism and consequent stroke and limb ischemia.

Because myocardial ischemia is an important predictor of perioperative outcome, it has featured prominently in the guidelines for thoracic aortic diseases. Patients with evidence of myocardial ischemia should undergo further evaluation to determine the extent and

TABLE 21-4	Anesthetic Considerations for the Care of Thoracic Aortic Surgical Patients
Preanesthetic Assessment	
Urgency of the operation (emergent, urgent, or elective)	
Pathology and anatomic extent of the disease	
Median sternotomy vs. thoracotomy vs. endovascular approach	
Mediastinal mass effect	
Airway compression or deviation	
Preexisting or Associated Medical Conditions	
Aortic valve disease	
Cardiac tamponade	
Coronary artery stenosis	
Cardiomyopathy	
Cerebrovascular disease	
Pulmonary disease	
Renal insufficiency	
Esophageal disease (contraindications to TEE)	
Coagulopathy	
Prior aortic operations	
Preoperative Medications	
Warfarin (Coumadin)	
Antiplatelet therapy	
Antihypertensive therapy	
Anesthetic Management	
Hemodynamic monitoring	
Proximal aortic pressure	
Distal aortic pressure	
Central venous pressure	
Pulmonary artery pressure and cardiac output	
TEE	
Neurophysiologic monitoring	
Electroencephalography	
Somatosensory-evoked potentials	
Motor-evoked potentials	
Jugular venous oxygen saturation	
Lumbar cerebrospinal fluid pressure	
Body temperature	
Single-lung ventilation for thoracotomy	
Double-lumen endobronchial tube	
Endobronchial blocker	
Potential for bleeding	
Large-bore intravenous access	
Blood product availability	
Antifibrinolytic therapy	
Antibiotic prophylaxis	
Postoperative Care Considerations and Complications	
Hypothermia	
Hypotension	
Hypertension	
Bleeding	
Spinal cord ischemia	
Stroke	
Renal insufficiency	
Respiratory insufficiency	
Phrenic nerve injury	
Diaphragmatic dysfunction	
Recurrent laryngeal nerve injury	
Pain management	

severity of coronary artery disease (CAD; ACC/AHA Class I recommendation; level of evidence C).[1] If significant CAD is responsible for an acute coronary syndrome, then coronary revascularization is indicated before or concomitant with the thoracic aortic procedure (ACC/AHA Class I recommendation; level of evidence C).[1] Concomitant coronary artery bypass grafting (CABG) is reasonable in patients who have not only stable but significant CAD, but who are also scheduled to undergo surgery for diseases of the ascending aorta or aortic arch, or both (ACC/AHA Class IIa recommendation; level of evidence C).[1] In contrast, the benefit of coronary revascularization is less clear in patients who have stable but significant CAD and who are scheduled to undergo surgical intervention for descending thoracic aortic disease (ACC/AHA Class IIb recommendation; level of evidence C).[1]

Preoperative Medications

Preoperative medications typically provide detailed information about concomitant medical conditions. As a general rule, all cardiac, pulmonary, and antiseizure medications should be continued up until the morning of surgery. Angiotensin-converting enzyme inhibitors and angiotensin-receptor blockers should be discontinued the day before surgery to minimize the risk for perioperative vasoplegia and adverse outcomes.[5,6] All oral hypoglycemic agents should be discontinued the night before surgery to avoid hypoglycemia. If possible, metformin should be discontinued the day before surgery to minimize the risks for severe lactic acidosis associated with exposure to iodinated contrast agents or perioperative hypovolemia. If a patient is receiving insulin, up to 50% of the typical morning dose should be given the day of surgery with subsequent close glucose monitoring. Warfarin (Coumadin) should be discontinued for approximately 5 days before surgery for full recovery of coagulation function as verified by a normalized international normalized ratio.[7] If this is not possible, then the patient should be admitted for heparinization until shortly before surgery. Patients chronically exposed to low-molecular-weight heparin, aspirin, adenosine diphosphate platelet-receptor inhibitors (clopidogrel and prasugrel), and platelet glycoprotein IIb/IIIa inhibitors (abciximab, eptifibatide, tirofiban) are typically at increased risk for perioperative bleeding. Optimally, aspirin and clopidogrel should be discontinued at least 5 to 7 days before surgery to allow adequate recovery of platelet function for perioperative hemostasis.[7]

Finally, the consequences for anesthetic procedures must be carefully considered. For example, coagulopathy caused by organ dysfunction or concomitant medication, or both, increases the risks for hemorrhagic complications associated with neuraxial techniques such as lumbar CSF drainage and epidural analgesia. Cervical spine or esophageal disease may prohibit the use of intraoperative TEE. Aortic pathologies may produce an intrathoracic mass effect to complicate tracheal intubation, selective lung ventilation, and/or hemodynamic stability after anesthetic induction.

Anesthetic Management

Overall, the anesthetic plan including techniques, drugs, and monitoring should be individualized to enhance the conduct of the procedure including perfusion technique, hemodynamic monitoring, and preservation of organ function (ACC/AHA Class I recommendation; level of evidence C).[1] Because thoracic aortic procedures may result in massive bleeding and cardiovascular collapse, it is essential to have immediate availability of packed red blood cells, large-bore vascular access, invasive blood pressure monitoring, and central venous access. Pulmonary artery catheterization assists in the management of cardiac dysfunction associated with CPB, DHCA, and PLHB. Intraoperative TEE is indicated in thoracic aortic procedures, including endovascular interventions, in which it assists in hemodynamic monitoring, procedural guidance, and endoleak detection (ACC/AHA Class IIa recommendation; level of evidence B).[1]

A rationale exists for choosing to cannulate the left or right radial artery for intra-arterial blood pressure monitoring. Right radial arterial pressure monitoring will often detect compromised flow into the innominate artery because of aortic cross-clamping too near its origin. Right radial arterial pressure monitoring makes sense in procedures that require clamping of the left subclavian artery. Left radial arterial pressure monitoring is indicated when selective antegrade cerebral perfusion (ACP) is planned via the right axillary artery. At times, bilateral radial arterial pressure monitoring may be required. Femoral arterial pressure monitoring allows the assessment of distal aortic perfusion in procedures with PLHB.

Large-bore peripheral intravenous cannulation (e.g., two 16-gauge catheters) secures vascular access for rapid intravascular volume expansion. Rapid transfusion is desirable via an intravenous set with a fluid warming device. Alternatively, large-bore central venous cannulation can be utilized for volume expansion. If a pulmonary artery catheter (PAC) is required, a second introducer sheath dedicated to volume expansion also can be placed in the same central vein. Central venous cannulation with ultrasound guidance often increases speed and safety, especially in emergencies.[8] Both a urinary and a nasopharyngeal temperature probe are required for monitoring the absolute temperature of the peripheral and core, as well as the rates of change during deliberate hypothermia and subsequent rewarming. The rectum is an alternative site for monitoring peripheral temperature, and the PAC can provide core temperature monitoring.

The induction of general anesthesia requires careful hemodynamic monitoring with anticipation of changes because of anesthetic drugs and tracheal intubation. Appropriate vasoactive drugs should be immediately available as required. Concomitant vasodilator infusions often are discontinued before anesthetic induction. Because etomidate does not attenuate sympathetic responses with no direct effects on myocardial contractility, it may be preferred in the setting of hemodynamic instability. Thereafter, titration of a narcotic such as fentanyl and a benzodiazepine such as midazolam will provide maintenance of general anesthesia. In elective cases, anesthetic induction can proceed with routine intravenous hypnotics, followed by narcotic titration for attenuation of the hypertensive responses to tracheal intubation and skin incision. Antibiotic therapy optimally should be completed in most cases at least 30 minutes before skin incision to achieve adequate bactericidal tissue levels.

General anesthetic maintenance is typically with a balanced technique, and neuromuscular blockade is achieved by titration of a nondepolarizing muscle relaxant. Anesthetics can be reduced during moderate hypothermia and then discontinued during deep hypothermia. With concomitant electroencephalographic (EEG) and/or somatosensory-evoked potential (SSEP) monitoring, anesthetic signal interference is minimized with the avoidance of barbiturates, bolus propofol, and doses of inhaled anesthetic greater than 0.5 minimum alveolar concentration. Propofol infusion, narcotics, and neuromuscular blocking drugs do not interfere with SSEP monitoring. With intraoperative motor-evoked potential (MEP) monitoring, high-quality signals are obtained when the anesthetic technique comprises total intravenous anesthesia with propofol and a narcotic such as remifentanil without neuromuscular blockade. Neuromonitoring (EEG, SSEP, MEP) in thoracic aortic procedures is not only compatible with contemporary anesthetic techniques but is also reasonable when the resulting data will guide perioperative management (ACC/AHA Class IIa recommendation; level of evidence B).[1] The decision to utilize this monitoring modality should be based on procedural urgency, institutional resources, patient needs, and planned operative technique (ACC/AHA Class IIa recommendation; level of evidence B).[1]

In most cases, the duration of general anesthesia continues for several hours after admission to the intensive care unit (ICU) to permit a controlled anesthetic emergence. If epidural analgesia is used intraoperatively, a dilute solution of local anesthetic and narcotic is preferred to minimize postoperative hypotension from a concomitant sympathectomy and to minimize motor blockade to permit serial neurologic assessment of lower extremity function. Neuraxial anesthetic techniques are not recommended in patients at risk for neuraxial hematoma in the setting of concomitant thienopyridine antiplatelet therapy, low-molecular-weight heparins, and clinically significant anticoagulation (ACC/AHA Class III recommendation; level of evidence C).[1,7]

The potential for significant bleeding and rapid transfusion is always relevant in thoracic aortic procedures. Consequently, it is prudent to have fresh frozen plasma and platelets available for ongoing replacement during massive red blood cell transfusion. The time delay associated with standard laboratory testing severely limits the intraoperative relevance of these data to guide transfusion. Strategies to decrease bleeding and transfusion in these procedures include timely preoperative cessation of anticoagulants and platelet blockers, antifibrinolytic therapy, intraoperative cell salvage, biologic glue, activated factor VII, and avoidance of perioperative hypertension. It is reasonable to have an institutional algorithmic approach to the management of bleeding and transfusion for thoracic aortic surgery (ACC/AHA Class IIa recommendation; level of evidence C).[1] This algorithm will depend significantly on institutional variations in point-of-care coagulation testing, blood component availability, and access to recombinant factor VII (ACC/AHA Class IIa recommendation; level of evidence C).[1]

The antifibrinolytic lysine analogs, ε-aminocaproic acid or tranexamic acid, are commonly utilized in thoracic aortic surgery with and without DHCA. The concerns with aprotinin are now historical because it was widely withdrawn from clinical practice after a large randomized trial demonstrated its significant mortality risk in the setting of high-risk cardiac surgery, including thoracic aortic surgery with DHCA.[9,10] Even more recently, high-dose tranexamic acid has been correlated with a significantly increased risk for seizures after cardiac surgery.[11,12] Based on the lessons from aprotinin, further adequately powered trials should examine the safety of lysine analogs in thoracic aortic surgery.[9–12] Recombinant activated factor VII is a synthetic agent that accelerates hemostasis by binding with tissue factor at the site of tissue injury. Although this agent has demonstrated efficacy for hemostatic rescue in massive bleeding during thoracic aortic surgery, recent meta-analysis suggest further study for adequate delineation of its perioperative safety.[13,14]

Postoperative Care

After completion of the operation, the patient should be transported directly from the OR to the ICU. The continuation of care from the OR to the ICU should be seamless and protocol based.[15] In the absence of complications, early anesthetic emergence is preferable for early assessment of neurologic function. If delayed anesthetic emergence is indicated, then sedation and analgesia can be provided. Common early complications include hypothermia, coagulopathy, delirium, stroke, hemodynamic lability, respiratory failure, metabolic disturbances, and renal failure. Frequent clinical and laboratory assessment are essential to manage this dynamic postoperative recovery, including the safe conduct of tracheal extubation. The management of blood glucose levels has been standardized with a recent guideline from the Society of Thoracic Surgeons (STS).[16] The chest roentgenogram allows confirmation of endotracheal tube and intravascular catheter position, as well as the diagnosis of acute intrathoracic pathologies. Antibiotic prophylaxis is continued for 48 hours after surgery to minimize surgical infection risk.

THORACIC AORTIC ANEURYSM

A thoracic aortic aneurysm is a permanent localized thoracic aortic dilatation that has at least a 50% diameter increase and three aortic wall layers.[1] Localized dilatation of the thoracic aorta less than 150% of normal is termed *ectasis*. Annuloaortic ectasia is defined as isolated dilatation of the ascending aorta, aortic root, and aortic valve annulus. Pseudoaneurysm or a false aneurysm is a localized dilation of the aorta that does not contain all three layers of the vessel wall and instead consists of connective tissue and clot. Pseudoaneurysms are caused by a contained rupture of the aorta or arise from intimal disruptions, penetrating atheromas, or partial dehiscence of the suture line at the site of a previous aortic prosthetic vascular graft.

Thoracic aortic aneurysms are common and are the 15th most common cause of death in people older than 65.[16] This disease process is virulent (Box 21-1) but indolent because it typically grows slowly at an approximate rate of 0.1 cm/yr.[16] The most common reason for more rapid degeneration is acute aortic dissection. Besides acquired risk factors such as hypertension, hypercholesterolemia, and smoking, current evidence points to the strong influence of genetic inheritance.[17,18] Genetic analysis suggests that thoracic aortic aneurysms divide into

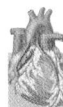

BOX 21-1. COMPLICATIONS OF THORACIC AORTIC ANEURYSMS

- Aortic rupture
- Aortic regurgitation
- Tracheobronchial and esophageal compression
- Right pulmonary artery or right ventricular outflow tract obstruction
- Systemic embolism from mural thrombus

two groups at the level of the ligamentum arteriosum. Above the ligamentum arteriosum, the disease is not related to typical arterial risk factors and has a smooth, noncalcified wall accompanied by no debris or clot. Below the ligamentum arteriosum, the disease process primarily is atherosclerotic, with an irregular calcified wall accompanied by copious debris and clot. This freedom from atheromatous disease in patients with thoracic aortic aneurysms of the ascending aorta has been called a "silver lining."[17] Inflammatory causes for thoracic aortic aneurysm include syphilis, mycotic aneurysm from endocarditis, giant-cell arteritis, and Takayasu arteritis.[1]

The aneurysm's location and extent determine the operative strategy and related perioperative complications. Aneurysms of the aortic root and/or ascending aorta commonly are associated with a bicuspid aortic valve.[19] Dilation of the aortic valve annulus, aortic root, and ascending aorta pulls the aortic leaflets apart and causes central aortic regurgitation (AR).[18] Aneurysms involving the aortic arch require temporary interruption of cerebral blood flow to accomplish the operative repair. Endovascular stent repair is an established therapy for aneurysms isolated to the descending thoracic aorta.[1,20] Repair of descending thoracic aortic aneurysms requires the sacrifice of multiple segmental intercostal artery branches that compromise spinal cord perfusion and results in a significant risk for postoperative paraplegia from spinal cord ischemia.[21]

The shape of thoracic aortic aneurysms can be described as either fusiform or saccular. Fusiform aneurysms are more common, associated with atherosclerotic or collagen vascular disease, and usually affect a longer segment of the aorta, producing a dilation of the entire circumference of the vessel wall. Saccular aneurysms are more localized, confined to an isolated segment of the aorta, and produce a localized outpouching of the vessel wall.

Thoracic aortic aneurysms mostly are asymptomatic and frequently are discovered incidentally.[1,17] Common symptoms of thoracic aortic aneurysm include chest and back pain caused by aneurysmal dissection, rupture, or bony erosion. The intrathoracic "mass effect" from a large thoracic aortic aneurysm can compress local structures to cause hoarseness (recurrent laryngeal nerve), dyspnea (trachea, mainstem bronchus, pulmonary artery), central venous hypertension (superior vena cava syndrome), and/or dysphagia (esophagus). Rupture of thoracic aortic aneurysms is a surgical emergency and is often accompanied with acute pain with or without hypotension. Although rupture of an ascending aortic aneurysm may cause cardiac tamponade, rupture in the descending thoracic aorta may cause hemothorax, aortobronchial fistula, or aortoesophageal fistula.

Diagnostic Imaging for Thoracic Aortic Aneurysms

The chest radiograph may suggest a thoracic aortic aneurysm with features such as a widened mediastinum, enlarged aortic knob, dilated descending thoracic aorta, aortic calcifications, leftward tracheal deviation, upward deviation of the left mainstem bronchus, and/or new left pleural effusion. Typically, transthoracic echocardiography can provide a reasonable examination of the thoracic aorta, although the acoustic windows are limited by the lungs. The contemporary imaging modalities of choice are CT, MRI, and TEE. Computed tomographic angiography (CTA) images the thoracic aorta during the arterial phase of an intravenous radiocontrast agent injection. It defines vascular anatomy and surrounding nonvascular structures. Aneurysm leak is detected as extravascular contrast extravasation. This imaging modality has multiple advantages such as high resolution, wide availability, rapid acquisition, imaging in patients with metallic implants, and generation of volumetric aortic images for stent design. Because CTA requires iodinated contrast agents, it carries a risk for contrast nephropathy that can be attenuated by administration of acetylcysteine and sodium bicarbonate.[22] (See Chapters 2 and 3.)

Contrast-enhanced magnetic resonance angiography with gadolinium also images the entire thoracic aorta in fine detail. Although the spatial resolution of magnetic resonance angiography is slightly inferior to CTA, it does allow for degrees of tissue and fluid characterization. The disadvantages of magnetic resonance angiography include its limited availability, lack of imaging in patients with metallic implants, imaging difficulty in the setting of continuous hemodynamic monitoring, and the time required for image acquisition. Its advantages are the avoidance of ionizing radiation and the lack of renal toxicity.[1,17]

TEE can image the thoracic aorta from the aortic valve to the distal ascending aorta and from the distal aortic arch to the proximal abdominal aorta. The distal ascending aorta and proximal aortic arch cannot be reliably imaged by TEE because the intervening trachea and left mainstem bronchus obstruct the acoustic window; this is known as the "blind spot" of TEE.[23] It is possible to overcome this blind spot with modalities such as imaging across the trachea temporarily filled with a saline-filled balloon (the A-view) and utilizing an expanded aortic view.[23,24] The advantages of TEE include its portability, its real-time interpretation, its compatibility at the bedside and in the OR, and its multiple imaging modalities for complete aortic and cardiac assessment. Its disadvantages include the requirement for sedation or general anesthesia and the risks for upper gastrointestinal injury.[25]

Surgical Considerations for Thoracic Aortic Aneurysms

Surgical repair aims to replace the aortic aneurysm with a tube graft to prevent further aneurysmal complications (Table 21-5). The first indication for thoracic aortic aneurysm resection is whenever the aneurysm is symptomatic regardless of size (ACC/AHA Class I recommendation; level of evidence C).[1,17] Symptoms often herald the onset of rupture or dissection and should be interpreted as an urgent indication for surgery. A symptomatic presentation occurs in about 5% of patients. Unfortunately, the first symptom in the remaining 95% of patients often is death.

The second indication for resection is aortic diameter. In the ascending aorta, a diameter of 6.0 cm is the critical hinge point after which the risk for aneurysm rupture increases exponentially. Consequently, surgical resection is recommended in the ascending aorta when the diameter reaches 5.5 cm (ACC/AHA Class I recommendation; level of evidence C).[1,17] In patients with genetically mediated aortopathies

TABLE 21-5	Indications for Surgical Repair of Thoracic Aortic Aneurysms	
Atherosclerotic aneurysm diameter		
Ascending aorta		≥5.5 cm
Descending aorta		≥6.5 cm
Marfan's or familial thoracic aneurysm diameter		
Ascending aorta		≥5.0 cm
Descending aorta		≥6.0 cm
Severe aortic regurgitation		
Aortoannular ectasia with aortic root aneurysm		
Rupture		
Refractory pain		

(Marfan syndrome, bicuspid aortic valve, familial thoracic aortic aneurysm or dissection; vascular Ehlers-Danlos syndrome; and Turner syndrome), surgical resection is recommended at a lower ascending aortic diameter of 5.0 cm (ACC/AHA Class I recommendation; level of evidence C).[1,17] Ascending aortic aneurysms with diameters less than 5.5 cm but with an annual growth rate in diameter greater than 0.5 cm/yr qualify for surgical resection (ACC/AHA Class I recommendation; level of evidence C).[1] It is reasonable to consider prophylactic replacement of the aortic root and ascending aorta in a woman with Marfan syndrome who is planning a pregnancy and who has an aortic root or ascending aortic diameter larger than 4.0 cm (ACC/AHA Class IIa recommendation; level of evidence C).[1] In adults with the aggressive aortopathy of the Loeys-Dietz syndrome, it is reasonable to consider proximal thoracic aortic repair when the internal aortic diameter exceeds 4.2 cm (ACC/AHA Class IIa recommendation; level of evidence C).[1,26] The ascending aortic aneurysm diameter also must be indexed to body size.[27] For example, if the maximal cross-sectional area of the aortic root or ascending aorta (in square centimeters) divided by the patient's height (in meters) exceeds a ratio of 10, then surgical repair is a reasonable option (ACC/AHA Class IIa recommendation; level of evidence C).[1] The rationale behind indexing the aortic dimensions to body size is that shorter adults dissect and rupture their aortas at smaller diameters.[1,27] Furthermore, those patients who are undergoing open aortic valve procedures and who have an aortic root or ascending aortic diameter larger than 4.5 cm should be considered for concomitant aortic replacement resection (ACC/AHA Class I recommendation; level of evidence C).[1]

The hinge point for rupture in the descending thoracic aorta is a diameter of 7.0 cm.[17] Consequently, surgical resection is recommended in thoracoabdominal aneurysms when the aortic diameter exceeds 6.0 cm or less when it is associated with a connective tissue disorder such as Marfan syndrome (ACC/AHA Class I recommendation; level of evidence C).[1] In patients who have aneurysmal degeneration of the descending thoracic aorta associated with prior dissection and/or a connective tissue disorder, surgical resection is recommended when the aortic diameter is more than 5.5 cm (ACC/AHA Class I recommendation; level of evidence B).[1] Patients with aneurysms of the descending thoracic aorta should be considered for thoracic endovascular aortic repair (TEVAR) when technically feasible (ACC/AHA Class I recommendation; Level of Evidence B).[1,20]

Aneurysms of the ascending aorta and aortic arch are approached from a median sternotomy incision. Standard CPB can be used for the repair of aneurysms limited to the aortic root and ascending aorta that do not extend into the aortic arch by cannulating the distal ascending aorta or proximal aortic arch and applying an aortic cross-clamp between the aortic cannula and the aneurysm. Aneurysms that involve the aortic arch require CPB with temporary interruption of cerebral perfusion (DHCA). Neuroprotection strategies in this setting include deep hypothermia, selective ACP, and retrograde cerebral perfusion (RCP). Aortic aneurysms of the descending thoracic aorta require lateral thoracotomy for surgical access. Aneurysmal resection requires cross-clamping with or without distal aortic perfusion.

Surgical Repair of Ascending Aortic and Arch Aneurysms

The type of surgical repair depends on aortic valve function and the aneurysm extent. Perioperative TEE can evaluate the aortic valve structure and function to guide and assess the surgical intervention (reimplantation, repair, replacement). Furthermore, TEE can assess the diameters of the aortic root, ascending aorta, and aortic arch to guide intervention. The most common aortic valve diseases associated with ascending aortic aneurysm are bicuspid aortic valve or AR caused by dilation of the aortic root (Figure 21-1). If the aortic valve and aortic root are normal, a simple tube graft can be used to replace the ascending aorta. If the aortic valve is diseased but the sinuses of Valsalva are normal, an aortic valve replacement combined with a tube graft for the

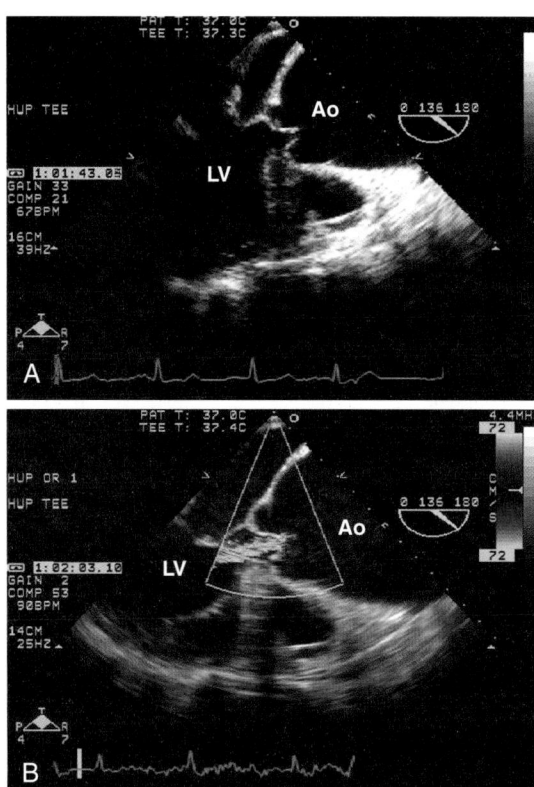

Figure 21-1 Transesophageal echocardiographic (TEE) midesophageal long-axis images of the aortic valve demonstrating aneurysmal dilation of the aortic root and ascending aorta (A). Doppler color-flow imaging (B) demonstrating severe aortic regurgitation caused by outward tethering of the aortic valve cusps by the aortic aneurysm. Ao, aorta; LV, left ventricle.

into the aortic branch vessels may require repair with branched or trifurcated tube grafts to permit separate anastomosis to the innominate, left carotid, and left subclavian arteries.[30] In patients with aortic arch aneurysms and concomitant severe comorbidity, recent guidelines support an endovascular repair technique (Class IIb recommendation; level of evidence C).[1,20] However, in patients who have aortic arch aneurysms and who have reasonable surgical risk, the recent guidelines advise against an endovascular repair technique (Class III recommendation; level of evidence A).[1,20]

Anesthetic Management for Ascending Aorta and Arch Aneurysms

The conduct of general anesthesia in this setting has specific concerns. The imaging studies should be reviewed for aneurysm compression of mediastinal structures such as the right pulmonary artery and left mainstem bronchus (Figure 21-6). Prevention of hypertension increases forward flow in AR and minimizes the risk for aneurysm rupture. A right radial arterial catheter is preferred for most cases. If arterial cannulation of the right axillary, subclavian, or innominate artery is planned for CPB and ACP, bilateral radial arterial catheters often are required to measure cerebral and systemic perfusion pressures. Nasopharyngeal, tympanic, and bladder temperatures are important for estimating brain and core temperatures for monitoring the conduct of DHCA. Monitoring of jugular bulb venous oxygen saturation and the EEG may reflect cerebral metabolic activity to guide the conduct of DHCA. Intraoperative TEE is essential to guide and assess the surgical interventions. In patients with AR, TEE can assist in the conduct of CPB by guiding placement of cannulae such as the retrograde cardioplegia cannula (coronary sinus) and by monitoring left ventricular (LV) volume to ensure that the LV drainage cannula keeps the ventricle collapsed. Intraoperative TEE is reasonable in thoracic aortic procedures, including endovascular interventions, in which it assists in hemodynamic monitoring, procedural guidance, and endoleak detection (ACC/AHA Class IIa recommendation; level of evidence B).[1]

Neuroprotection Strategies for Temporary Interruption of Cerebral Blood Flow

The risk for stroke is substantial during the cerebral ischemia that accompanies aortic arch reconstruction.[31] The first mechanism is cerebral ischemia due to hypoperfusion or temporary circulatory arrest during aortic arch repair. The second mechanism is cerebral ischemia due to embolization secondary to CPB and atheroma. Arterial emboli causes include air introduced into the circulation from open cardiac chambers, vascular cannulation sites, or arterial anastomosis. Atherosclerotic particulate debris may be released during clamping and unclamping of the aorta, the creation of anastomoses in the ascending aorta and aortic arch, or the excision of severely calcified and diseased cardiac valves. CPB may result in the microparticulate aggregates of platelets and fat. The turbulent high-velocity blood flow out of the aortic cannula used for CPB also may dislodge atherosclerotic debris within the aorta. Retrograde blood flow through a diseased descending thoracic aorta as a consequence of CPB conducted with femoral artery cannulation may cause retrograde cerebral embolization. For all these reasons, strategies to provide neurologic protection are essential in thoracic aortic operations (Box 21-2).

Deep Hypothermic Circulatory Arrest

The brain is exquisitely susceptible to ischemic injury within minutes after the onset of circulatory arrest because it has a high metabolic rate, continuous requirement for metabolic substrate, and limited reserves of high-energy phosphates. The physiologic basis for deep hypothermia as a neuroprotection strategy is to decrease cerebral metabolic rate

ascending aorta without need for reimplantation of the coronary arteries can be performed (Wheat procedure; Figure 21-2; ACC/AHA class I recommendation; level of evidence C).[1]

If disease also involves the aortic valve and the aortic root, the patient requires aortic root replacement and aortic valve intervention. If technically feasible, the aortic valve can be reimplanted with a modified David technique, which includes graft reconstruction of the aortic root with reimplantation of the coronary arteries (ACC/AHA Class I recommendation; level of evidence C).[1,28] If not feasible, aortic root replacement with a composite valve-graft conduit is indicated (Bentall procedure; Figure 21-3; ACC/AHA Class I recommendation; level of evidence C).[1] Aortic root replacement requires coronary reimplantation or aortocoronary bypass grafting (Cabrol technique; Figure 21-4).

Repairing aortic aneurysms that extend into or involve the aortic arch requires CPB with DHCA with or without perfusion adjuncts. For ascending aortic aneurysms that involve only the proximal aortic arch, partial arch replacement (hemiarch technique) is reasonable in which a tubular graft is interposed between the ascending aorta or aortic root and the underside of the aortic arch (ACC/AHA Class IIa recommendation; level of evidence B).[1] Ascending aorta with hemiarch reconstruction often is performed using DHCA with or without ACP/RCP to make the distal anastomosis feasible without cross-clamping ("open technique"). In patients who have isolated aortic arch aneurysms and who have a low operative risk, arch replacement is reasonable when the arch diameter exceeds 5.5 cm (ACC/AHA Class IIa recommendation; level of evidence B).[1] Total aortic arch replacement is reasonable in aneurysms that involve the entire arch (ACC/AHA Class IIa recommendation; level of evidence B).[1] Ascending aortic aneurysms that extend through the aortic arch into the descending aorta can be repaired with the "elephant trunk" technique (Figure 21-5; ACC/AHA Class IIa recommendation; level of evidence B).[1,29] Aortic arch aneurysms that extend

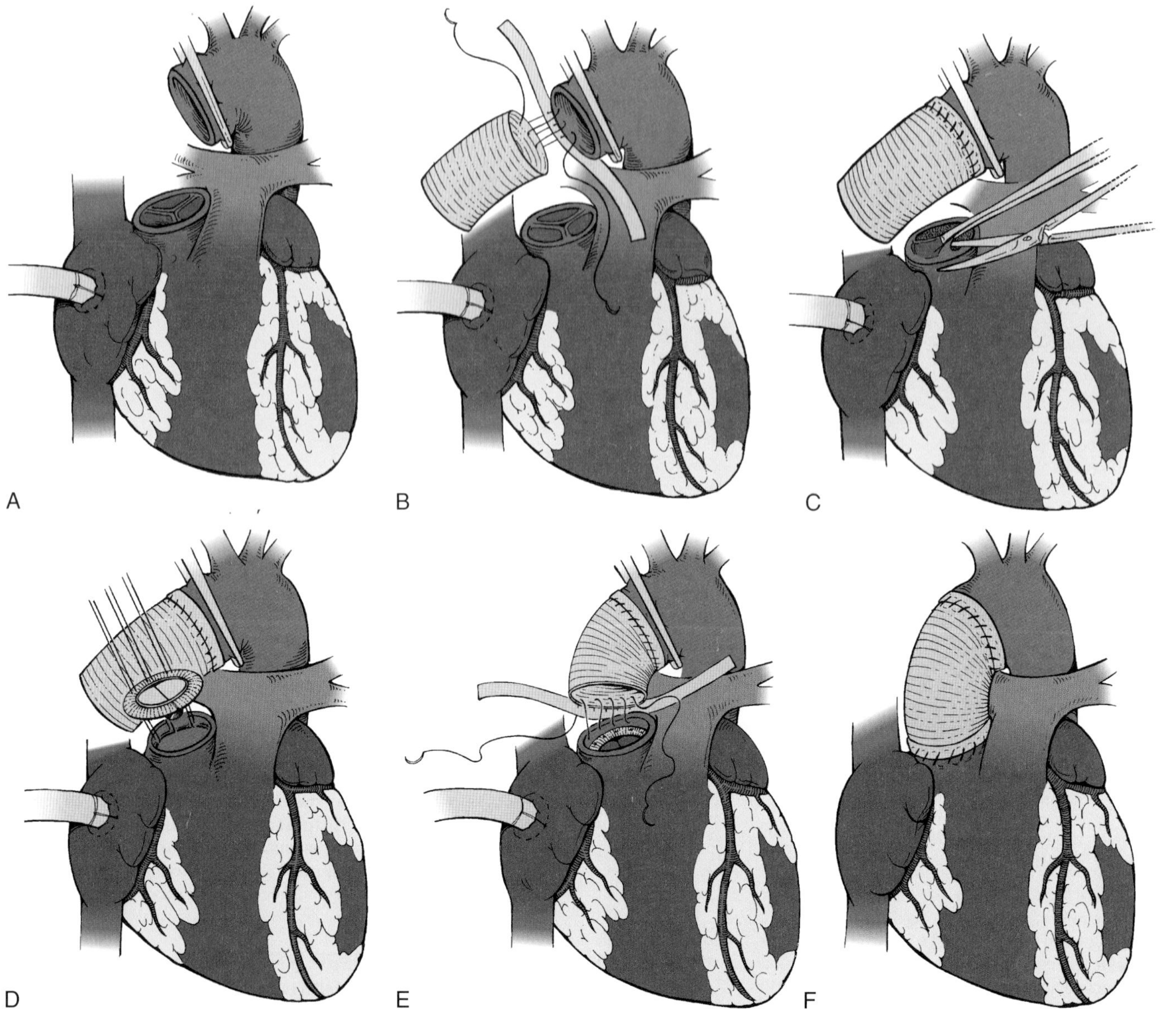

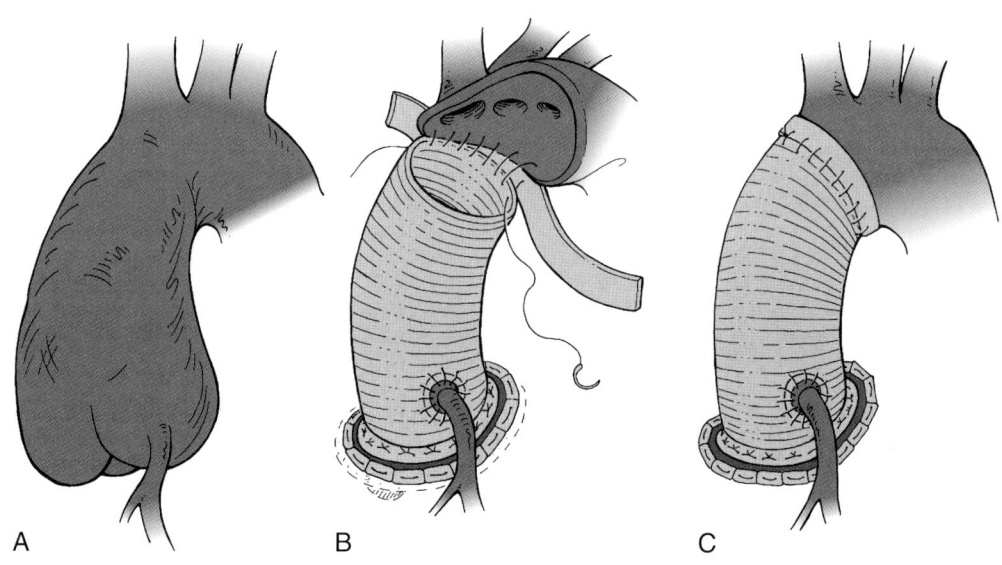

Figure 21-2 Replacement of the ascending aorta with a prosthetic tube graft for ascending aortic aneurysm or type A aortic dissection (A, B, F). In the presence of aortic valvular disease, the aortic valve can be replaced *(C–E)* or repaired (not shown). Extension of the aneurysm or dissection into the aortic arch may require replacement of part or all of the aortic arch with a prosthetic tube graft (not shown). A small rim of the native aortic root containing the right and left coronary ostia was left behind in this repair. *(Adapted from Downing SW, Kouchoukos NT: Ascending aortic aneurysm. In Edmunds LH [ed]:* Cardiac Surgery in the Adult. *New York, McGraw-Hill, 1997, p 1176, by permission.)*

Figure 21-3 Replacement of the entire aortic root with a composite valved conduit for ascending aortic aneurysm. The underside of the aortic arch was also incorporated into the prosthetic graft. The right and left coronary arteries were reimplanted into the graft (A–C). Alternatively, the aortic root can be replaced with a cryopreserved homograft or porcine bioprosthesis (not shown). *(Adapted from Griepp RB, Ergin A: Aneurysms of the aortic arch. In Edmunds LH [ed]:* Cardiac Surgery in the Adult. *New York, McGraw-Hill, 1997, p 1209, by permission.)*

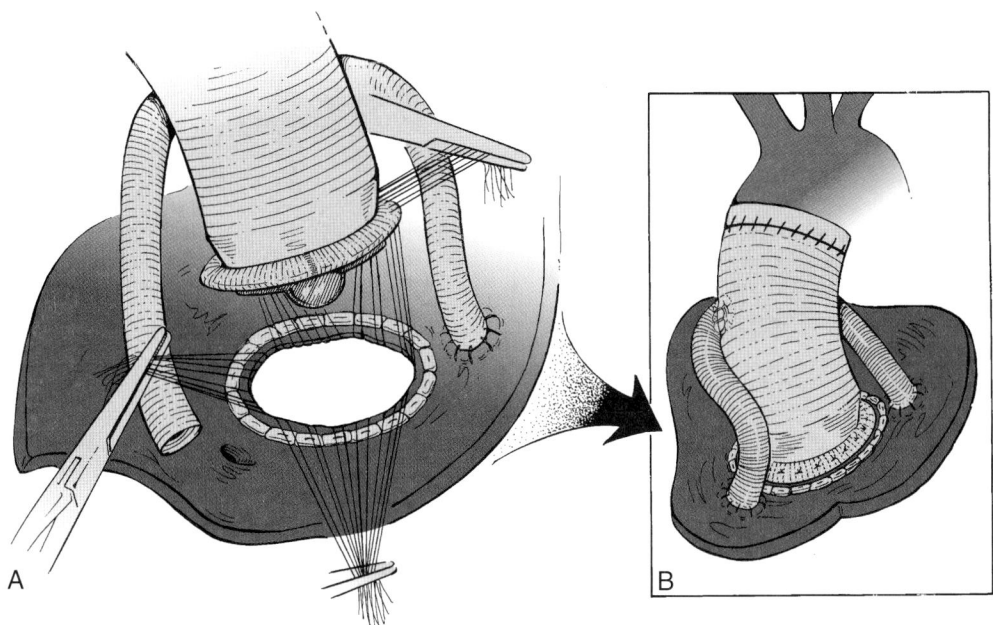

Figure 21-4 Replacement of the entire aortic root with a composite valved conduit for ascending aortic aneurysm combined with end-to-end anastomosis of the right and left coronary arteries to an 8-mm or 10-mm prosthetic tube graft that was then anastomosed to the aortic root **(A, B).** (*Adapted from Downing SW, Kouchoukos NT: Ascending aortic aneurysm. In Edmunds LH [ed]: Cardiac Surgery in the Adult. New York, McGraw-Hill, 1997, p 1181, by permission*).

and oxygen demands to increase the period that the brain can tolerate circulatory arrest.[32] Existing evidence indicates that autoregulation of cerebral blood flow is maintained during deliberate hypothermia with alpha-stat blood gas management without compromise of clinical outcome.[33] Direct measurement of cerebral metabolites and brainstem electrical activity in adults undergoing DHCA with RCP at 14°C indicated the onset of cerebral ischemia after only 18 to 20 minutes (Figure 21-7).[34] Despite this observation, the large body of experimental evidence and clinical experience with the deliberate hypothermia suggest that it is the single most important intervention for preventing neurologic injury in response to circulatory arrest.

Despite the proven efficacy of hypothermia for operations that require circulatory arrest, no consensus exists on an optimal protocol for the conduct of deliberate hypothermia for circulatory arrest. A strategy to protect the brain during aortic arch surgery must be a high priority in the perioperative management of these procedures to prevent stroke and optimize cognitive function (ACC/AHA Class I recommendation; level of evidence C).[1] Although the average nasopharyngeal temperature for DHCA may be about 18°C, the optimal temperature for DHCA has not been established.[31,32] A challenge in the selection of the ideal temperature for DHCA is the inability to directly measure the brain temperature. In an EEG-based approach to this question, the median nasopharyngeal temperature for electrocortical silence was 18°C, although a nasopharyngeal temperature of 12.5°C or cooling on CPB for at least 50 minutes achieved electrocortical silence in 99.5% of cases (Figure 21-8).[35] Although the EEG functions well as a physiologic end point for cerebral metabolic suppression during cooling for DHCA as part of an institutional protocol, its outcome benefit remains to be demonstrated in a randomized trial.[15,31,36] A jugular bulb venous oxygen saturation greater than 95% measured using an oximetric catheter represents an alternative physiologic end point to detect maximum cerebral metabolic suppression for DHCA.[37] It is important to note that deep hypothermia to a set temperature (mean = 19°C) as an end point for DHCA without EEG or jugular bulb venous oxygen saturation has been associated with excellent neurologic outcomes in recent series.[38,39] In addition to systemic hypothermia produced by extracorporeal circulation, topical hypothermia by packing the head in ice also has been incorporated in

leading institutional DHCA protocols to minimize passive warming of the head.[38,39] When providing topical hypothermia, care should be exercised to protect the eyes, nose, and ears from frostbite by protecting these vulnerable areas. Recent clinical studies support the practice of limiting the duration of straight DHCA to shorter than 45 minutes to avoid the associated significant increases in stroke and mortality risks.[31] The technique of DHCA alone is a reasonable approach for neuroprotection during aortic arch surgery in the setting of adequate institutional experience (ACC/AHA Class IIa recommendation; level of evidence B).[1]

The conduct of DHCA extends CPB duration with consequent risks for coagulopathy and embolization. Rewarming increases cerebral metabolic rate and can aggravate neuronal injury during ischemia/reperfusion. Consequently, it is important to rewarm gradually by maintaining a temperature gradient of no more than 10°C in the heat exchanger and avoiding cerebral hyperthermia (nasopharyngeal temperature > 37.5°C). The current guidelines advise against cerebral hyperthermia in aortic arch procedures (ACC/AHA Class III recommendation; level of evidence B).[1]

Retrograde Cerebral Perfusion

RCP is performed by infusing cold oxygenated blood into the superior vena cava cannula at a temperature of 8°C to 14°C via CPB (Figure 21-9). The internal jugular venous pressure is maintained at less than 25 mm Hg to prevent cerebral edema. Internal jugular venous pressure is measured from the introducer port of the internal jugular venous cannula at a site proximal to the superior vena cava perfusion cannula and zeroed at the level of the ear. The patient is positioned in 10 degrees of Trendelenburg to decrease the risk for cerebral air embolism and prevent trapping of air within the cerebral circulation in the presence of an open aortic arch. RCP flow rates of 200 to 600 mL/min usually can be achieved. The potential benefits of RCP include partial supply of cerebral metabolic substrate, cerebral embolic washout, and maintenance of cerebral hypothermia.[40] Although RCP has been associated with excellent clinical results in aortic arch repair, it has not become the standard technique for neuroprotection in DHCA.[15,41] A recent large, single-center study (1991–2007; N = 1107; RCP in 82%)

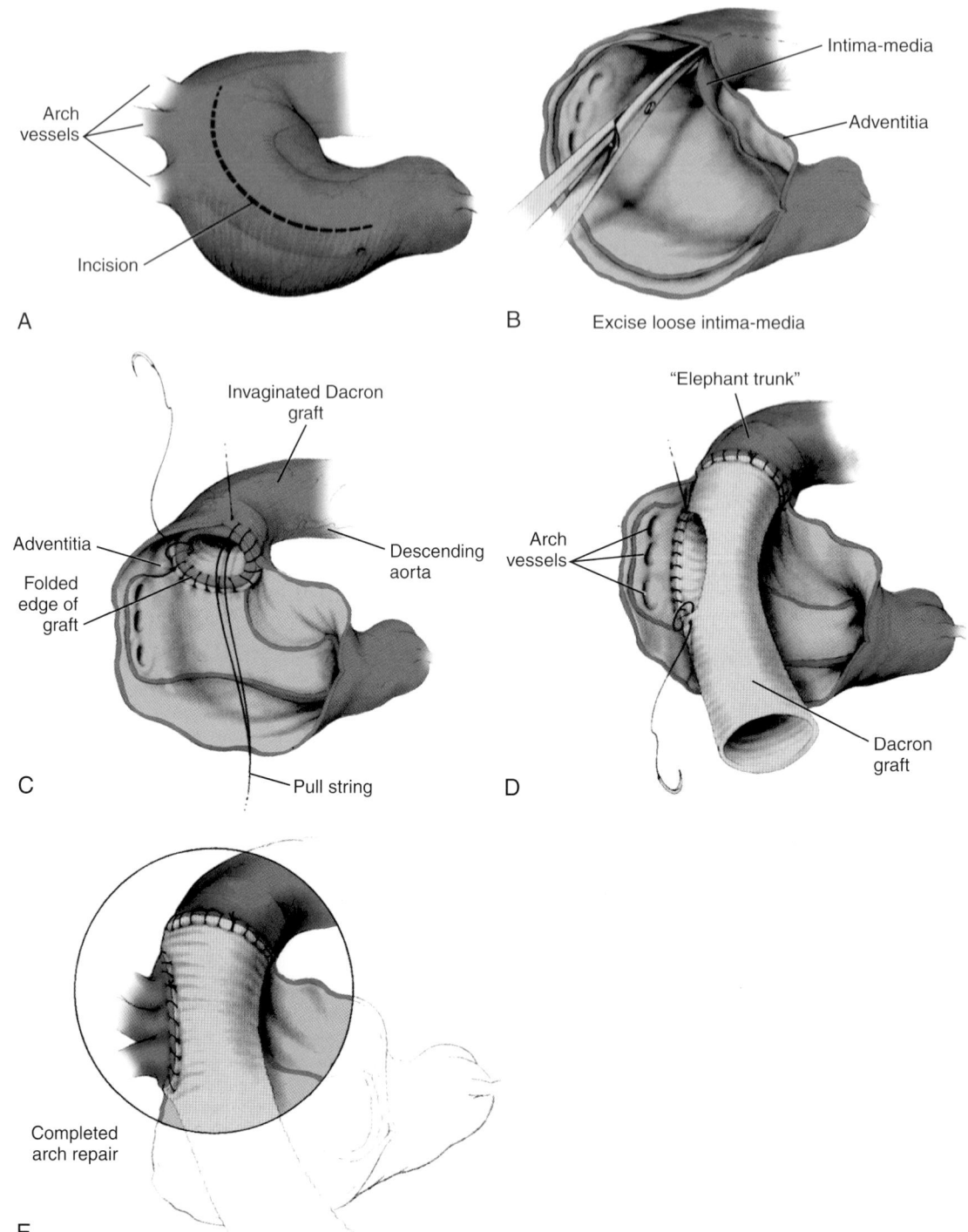

Figure 21-5 **Elephant trunk procedure for prosthetic graft replacement of the ascending aorta, aortic arch, and descending thoracic aorta.** The aortic aneurysm or dissection is opened its entire length and extended through the aortic arch (A, B). The prosthetic tube graft is implanted with its distal end extending into the descending thoracic aorta, "elephant trunk" (C, D). The graft is pulled back into the arch for implantation of the arch branch vessels and construction of the proximal anastomosis (D, E). In the second stage of the procedure, the descending thoracic aorta is replaced by constructing a proximal graft-to-graft anastomosis (not shown). *(From Doty DB: Aortic aneurysm. In Brown M, Baxter S [eds]: Cardiac Surgery: Operative technique. St. Louis, Mosby-Year Book, 1997, p 324.)*

evaluated the role of RCP in proximal thoracic aortic repair. The perioperative rates for mortality and stroke in this series were 10.4% and 2.8%, respectively. The application of RCP was significantly protective against mortality (odds ratio, 0.42; 95% confidence interval, 0.25-0.70; $P = 0.0009$) and stroke (odds ratio, 0.35; 95% confidence interval, 0.15-0.81; $P = 0.02$).[42] Despite the lack of randomized trials, RCP is safe and easily

implemented in aortic arch repair as an adjunct to maintain cerebral hypothermia, provide partial metabolic substrate delivery, and decrease the risk for cerebral embolization.[36–42] The technique of DHCA with RCP is a reasonable approach for neuroprotection during aortic arch surgery in the setting of adequate institutional experience (ACC/AHA Class IIa recommendation; level of evidence B).[1]

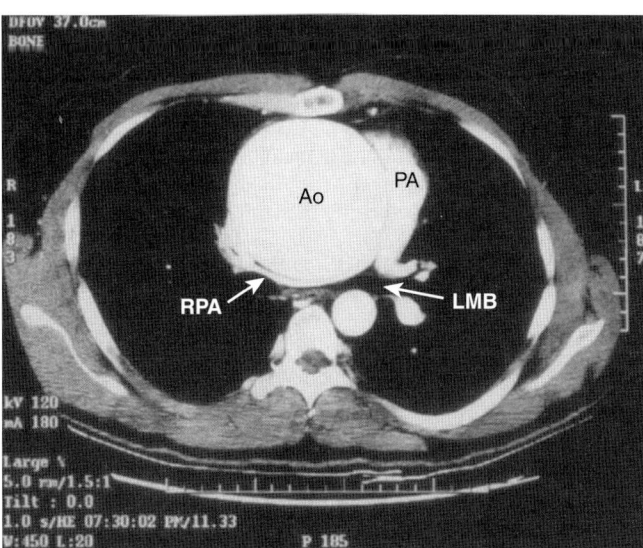

Figure 21-6 Computed tomographic angiogram of the chest demonstrating a large ascending aortic aneurysm (Ao) causing compression of the right pulmonary artery (RPA), distal trachea, and left main stem bronchus (LMB).

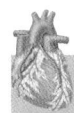

BOX 21-2. BRAIN PROTECTION FOR AORTIC ARCH RECONSTRUCTION

- Deep systemic hypothermia
- Topical cerebral cooling
- Retrograde cerebral perfusion
- Selective antegrade cerebral perfusion
- Cerebral hyperthermia prevention during rewarming

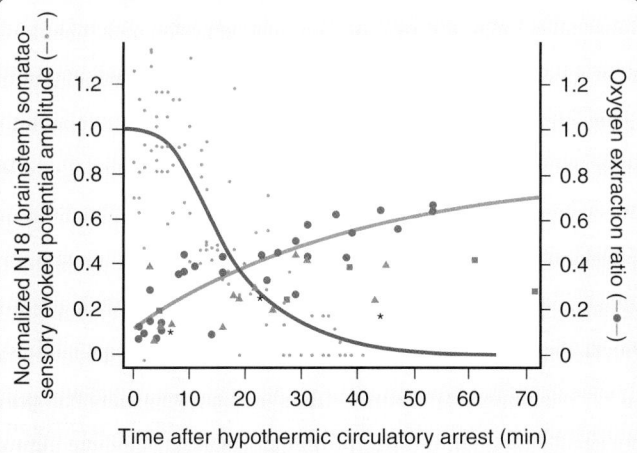

Figure 21-7 Changes in brainstem (N18) somatosensory-evoked potential amplitudes (dots) after initiation of deep hypothermic circulatory arrest with retrograde cerebral perfusion superimposed on the change in brain oxygen extraction ratio (OER) in patients without strokes (circles; n = 19), preoperative strokes (triangles; n = 4), intraoperative strokes (squares; n − 3), and both preoperative and intraoperative strokes (asterisks; n = 1). The N18 somatosensory-evoked potential decayed to half its original amplitude at 16 minutes after interruption of antegrade cerebral perfusion. The OER decreased to half its maximal value of 0.66 also at 16 minutes after interruption of antegrade cerebral perfusion. (Adapted from Cheung AT, Bavaria JE, Pochettino A, et al: Oxygen delivery during retrograde cerebral perfusion in humans. Anesth Analg 88:14, 1999.)

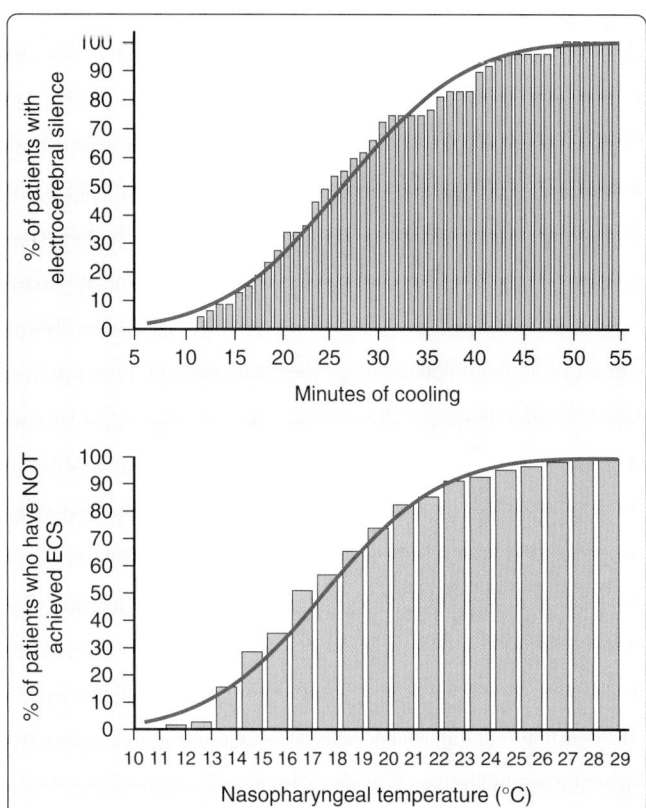

Figure 21-8 The relation between electroencephalographic activity to minutes of cooling (top) and nasopharyngeal temperature (bottom) before deep hypothermic circulatory arrest in 109 patients undergoing thoracic aortic operations requiring circulatory arrest. Electrocortical silence (ECS) was achieved by electroencephalogram (EEG) in all patients after 50 minutes of cooling or at a nasopharyngeal temperature of 12.5°C. At a nasopharyngeal temperature of 18°C, only 50% of patients had ECS by EEG. (Adapted from Stecker MM, Cheung AT, Pochettino A, et al: Deep hypothermic circulatory arrest: I. Effects of cooling on electroencephalogram and evoked potentials. Ann Thorac Surg 71:19, 2001, by permission of the Society of Thoracic Surgeons.)

Selective Antegrade Cerebral Perfusion

Selective ACP should be considered for aortic arch repairs longer than 45 minutes.[31] ACP typically is initiated during DHCA by selective cannulation of the right axillary artery, right subclavian artery, innominate artery, or left common carotid artery (Figure 21-10).[43] In transverse aortic arch reconstruction procedures, ACP can be accomplished by inserting individual perfusion cannulae into the open end of the aortic branch vessels after opening the aortic arch. After reattachment of the aortic arch branch vessels to the vascular graft, ACP can be provided through a separate arm of the vascular graft or by direct cannulation of the graft. A functional circle of Willis may provide contralateral brain perfusion during interruption of antegrade perfusion in the innominate, left carotid, or left subclavian arteries during construction of the vascular anastomoses. ACP with oxygenated blood at 10°C to 14°C at flow rates in the range of 250 to 1000 mL/min typically achieves a cerebral perfusion pressure in the range of 50 to 80 mm Hg.

Unilateral ACP via right axillary arterial cannulation is a popular technique for adult aortic repair.[43] This technique assumes an adequate circle of Willis; however, the anatomic completeness of the circle of Willis does not guarantee adequate cerebral cross-perfusion during aortic arch repair.[44,45] Consequently, it remains essential to monitor the contralateral hemisphere in unilateral ACP with modalities such as cerebral oximetry, carotid artery scanning, and transcranial Doppler.[46–48]

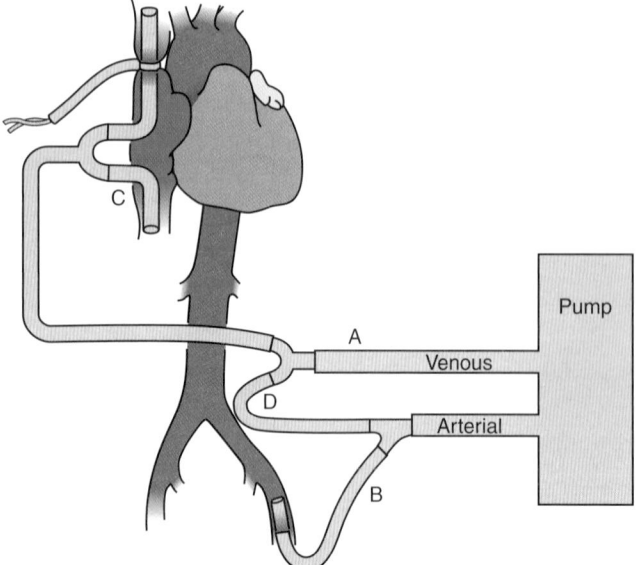

Figure 21-9 Extracorporeal perfusion circuit used to deliver retrograde cerebral perfusion. The bridge *(D)* is clamped during cardiopulmonary bypass. After initiation of deep hypothermic circulatory arrest, clamps are placed on the venous return line *(A)*, the proximal arterial cannula *(B)*, and inferior vena caval cannula *(C)*, and the bridge *(D)* is unclamped to permit retrograde perfusion into the superior vena cava. *(Adapted from Bavaria JE, Woo YJ, Hall RA, et al: Retrograde cerebral and distal aortic perfusion during ascending and thoracoabdominal aortic operations. Ann Thorac Surg 60:347, 1995, by permission of the Society of Thoracic Surgeons.)*

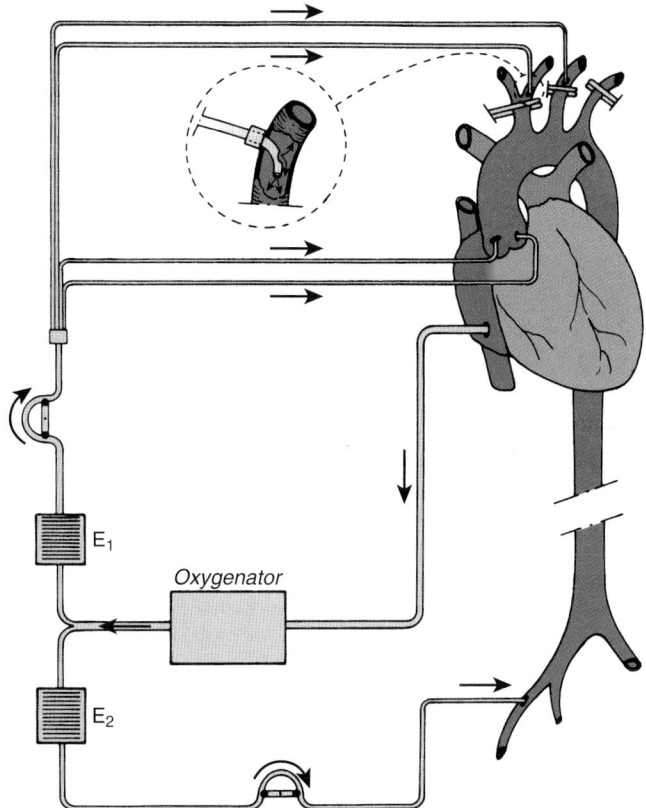

Figure 21-10 Extracorporeal perfusion circuit used for selective antegrade cerebral perfusion. After achieving deep hypothermia on cardiopulmonary bypass, individual cannulas are inserted into the coronary, innominate, and left carotid arteries for selective antegrade perfusion of the heart and brain. *(From Bachet J, Teodori G, Goudot B, et al: Replacement of the transverse aortic arch during emergency operations for type A acute aortic dissection. J Thorac Cardiovasc Surg 96:878, 1988.)*

Given that ACP may be unilateral or bilateral, there remains controversy about which ACP technique is superior.[49] A recent literature review combined 17 studies for a total sample size of 3548 patients; 83.1% with bilateral ACP and 16.9% with unilateral ACP.[50] Although the stroke rates were less than 5% regardless of technique, the period of safe ACP was significantly prolonged with bilateral ACP (86–164 minutes) compared with unilateral ACP (30–50 minutes). The evidence favors bilateral ACP in the setting of aortic arch repair times longer than 60 minutes.[50]

Pilot clinical series in adult aortic arch repair also have been undertaken in the setting of ACP with moderate hypothermic circulatory arrest (MHCA; systemic temperature = 25°C).[51,52] A large, single-center study (1999–2006; N = 501 [36.1% emergency cases]; median age, 64 years; 63.9% male sex) evaluated perioperative outcomes with this technique.[53] With a perioperative mortality rate of 11.6%, multivariate predictors for mortality included age and CPB time. The stroke rate was 9.6% with operative time and renal dysfunction as its multivariate predictors for stroke. The rate of temporary neurologic dysfunction was 13.4%, its multivariate predictors including MHCA duration (odds ratio, 1.015; $p = 0.01$). Although MHCA with cold ACP appears to be an adequate technique for adult aortic arch repair, its safety is limited in the settings of the elderly, multiple comorbidities, and extended operative time. The safety of aortic arch repair recently was further demonstrated with bilateral ACP and a greater mean MHCA temperature of 28°C (2002–2008; N = 229; mean age, 70.8 ± 9.7 years; 68.1% male sex).[54] Although MHCA with ACP appears to be a reasonable technique for adult aortic arch repair, its safety for ischemic protection of the spinal cord and kidney are still questioned.[55,56] The technique of DHCA with ACP is a reasonable approach for neuroprotection during aortic arch surgery in the setting of adequate institutional experience (ACC/AHA Class IIa recommendation; level of evidence B).[1]

Pharmacologic Neuroprotection Strategies for Deep Hypothermic Circulatory Arrest

There are no proven pharmacologic regimens that have demonstrated effectiveness for decreasing the risk or severity of neurologic injury in the setting of thoracic aortic operations.[36] The agents that have been reported in aortic arch series include thiopental, propofol, steroids, magnesium sulfate, and lidocaine.[15,32,57] Furthermore, there is considerable variation in practice with these agents in aortic arch repair.[57] In general, the existing evidence suggests that pharmacologic neuroprotection should be considered as a neuroprotective adjunct and not a substitute for hypothermia to protect against cerebral ischemia in the setting of hypoperfusion. The technique of DHCA with pharmacologic adjuncts is a reasonable approach for neuroprotection during aortic arch surgery in the setting of an institutional protocol and adequate institutional experience (ACC/AHA Class IIa recommendation; level of evidence B).[1]

Descending Thoracic and Thoracoabdominal Aortic Aneurysms

Surgical therapy for thoracic and TAAAs is to replace aneurysmal aorta with a prosthetic tube graft. Surgical access is via lateral thoracotomy or thoracoabdominal incision. Despite recent advances, major surgical challenges remain because the typical patient is elderly with multiple significant comorbidities (Table 21-6). The risks for spinal, mesenteric, renal, and lower extremity ischemia are significant due to thromboembolism, loss of collateral vascular networks, temporary interruption of blood flow, and reperfusion injury. The risks for wound dehiscence and respiratory failure remain significant because of the large incisions and diaphragmatic division, as well as injuries to the phrenic and recurrent laryngeal nerves. Consequently, TAAA repair is high risk (Table 21-7).[58]

Aneurysms of the descending thoracic aorta are classified by considering which third(s) of the descending thoracic aorta is (are) involved.[1] Extent A involves the proximal third, extent B involves the middle third, and extent C involves the distal third. If more than one third is involved,

TABLE 21-6 Preoperative Features in Patients with Thoracoabdominal Aortic Aneurysm (N = 1220)

Characteristic	No. of Patients (%)
Crawford extent	
Extent I	423 (34.7)
Extent II	371 (30.4)
Extent III	201 (16.5)
Extent IV	225 (18.4)
Acute dissection	46 (3.8)
Chronic dissection	272 (22.3)
Marfan syndrome	72 (5.9)
Symptomatic aneurysms	855 (70.1)
Acute presentation	112 (9.2)
Rupture	76 (6.2)
Preoperative paraplegia or paraparesis	16 (1.3)
Concurrent aneurysm	224 (18.4)
Prior aneurysm repair	502 (41.2)
Prior thoracic aortic aneurysm repair	281 (23.0)
Diabetes	69 (5.7)
Hypertension	940 (77.1)
Coronary artery disease	435 (35.7)
Prior coronary artery bypass or angioplasty	202 (16.6)
Cerebrovascular disease	135 (11.1)
Renal arterial occlusive disease	312 (25.6)
Renal insufficiency	151 (12.4)
Chronic obstructive lung disease	491 (40.3)
Peptic ulcer disease	83 (6.8)

Data from Coselli JS, LeMaire SA, Miller CC 3rd, et al: Mortality and paraplegia after thoracoabdominal aortic aneurysm repair: A risk factor analysis. *Ann Thorac Surg* 69:409, 2000.

TABLE 21-7 Clinical Outcomes of Thoracoabdominal Aortic Aneurysm (TAAA) Repair (United States: 1988–1998)

Complication	Intact TAAA (n = 1542)	Ruptured TAAA (n = 321)
Cardiac	14.8%	18.1%
Pulmonary	19.0%	12.7%
Hemorrhage	12.4%	10.9%
Acute renal failure	14.2%	28.0%
Paraplegia	—*	3.4%
Any complication	55.2%	51.7%
In-hospital mortality	22.3%	53.8%

*Incidence of paraplegia not reported.
TAAA, thoracoabdominal aortic aneurysm.
Data from Cowan JA, Dimick JB, Henke PK, et al: Surgical treatment of intact thoracoabdominal aortic aneurysms in the United States: Hospital and surgeon volume-related outcomes. J Vasc Surg 37:1169, 2003; and Cowan JA, Dimick JB, Wainess RM, et al: Ruptured thoracoabdominal aortic aneurysm treatment in the United States: 1988 to 1998. J Vasc Surg 38: 312, 2003.

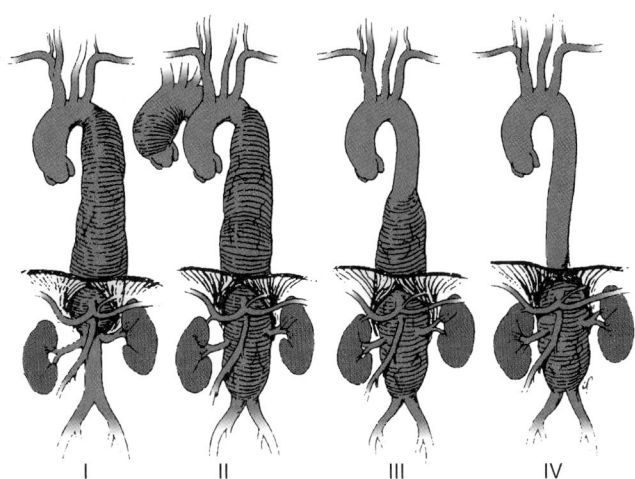

Figure 21-11 Crawford classification of thoracoabdominal aortic aneurysm extent. (*From Coselli JS: Descending thoracoabdominal aortic aneurysms. In Edmunds LH [ed]: Cardiac Surgery in the Adult. New York, McGraw-Hill, 1997, p 1232.*)

TABLE 21-8 Mortality and Paraplegia after Thoracoabdominal Aortic Aneurysm Repair (N = 1220)

TAAA Extent	No. of Patients	30-Day Mortality	Hospital Mortality	Paraplegia/ Paraparesis
I	400 (35.1%)	20 (5.0%)	30 (7.5%)	16 (4.1%)
II	343 (30.1%)	18 (5.2%)	29 (8.5%)	28 (8.2%)
III	184 (16.1%)	9 (4.9%)	9 (4.9%)	7 (3.8%)
IV	213 (18.7%)	7 (3.3%)	12 (5.6%)	3 (1.4%)

Data from Coselli JS, LeMaire SA, Miller CC 3rd, et al: Mortality and paraplegia after thoracoabdominal aortic aneurysm repair: A risk factor analysis. *Ann Thorac Surg* 69:409, 2000.

then the extent is classified according to which thirds are involved, for example, an aneurysm involving the proximal two-thirds is classified as extent AB. Essentially, multisegment aneurysms can be classified as proximal or distal because these extents influence the risk for spinal cord ischemia after surgical repair, whether open or endovascular.

Aneurysms of the thoracoabdominal aorta typically are defined by the Crawford classification (Figure 21-11). Extent I TAAA begins at the left subclavian artery and ends below the diaphragm, but above the renal arteries. Extent II TAAA involves the entire descending thoracic aorta and ends below the diaphragm at the aortic bifurcation. Extent III TAAA begins in the lower half of the descending thoracic aorta and ends below the diaphragm at the aortic bifurcation. Extent IV TAAA is confined to the entire abdominal aorta. If an extent I or extent II TAAA involves the distal aortic arch, its surgical replacement often requires DHCA for the proximal anastomosis. The Crawford classification stratifies operative risk and guides perioperative management (Table 21-8). Open repair of TAAA typically is accomplished by one of three major techniques; (1) aortic cross-clamping, (2) aortic cross-clamping with a Gott shunt, and (3) aortic cross-clamping with PLHB or partial CPB (Figure 21-12).

Simple Aortic Cross-Clamp Technique

Although this technique was developed by Crawford, its major disadvantage is the concomitant vital organ ischemia below the aortic clamp. Consequently, surgical speed is critical to achieve an ischemic time less than 30 minutes to limit the risk for vital organ dysfunction.[59] Its further disadvantages include proximal aortic hypertension, bleeding, and hemodynamic instability on reperfusion. Despite anesthetic interventions, this proximal aortic hypertension may induce LV ischemia.[60] Blood loss can be minimized with intraoperative red blood cell salvaging. Hemodynamic instability during reperfusion can be minimized with correction of metabolic acidosis, rapid intravascular volume expansion, vasopressor therapy, and/or gradual clamp release. Mild systemic hypothermia and selective spinal cooling protect against the ischemia associated with this technique.[61,62] Despite its physiologic consequences, this technique remains popular because it is simple and has proven clinical outcomes (Table 21-9).

Gott Shunt

The Gott shunt allows passive shunting of blood from the proximal to distal aorta during aortic cross-clamping for thoracic aortic repair (see Figure 21-12B).[63] Blood flow from the proximal to distal aorta through the Gott shunt depends on proximal aortic pressure, shunt length and diameter, and distal aortic pressure. Monitoring the femoral arterial pressure facilitates assessment of distal aortic perfusion and shunt flow. The advantages of the Gott shunt are its simplicity, its low cost, and its requirement for only partial anticoagulation. Its disadvantages include vessel injury, dislodgment, bleeding, and atheroembolism.

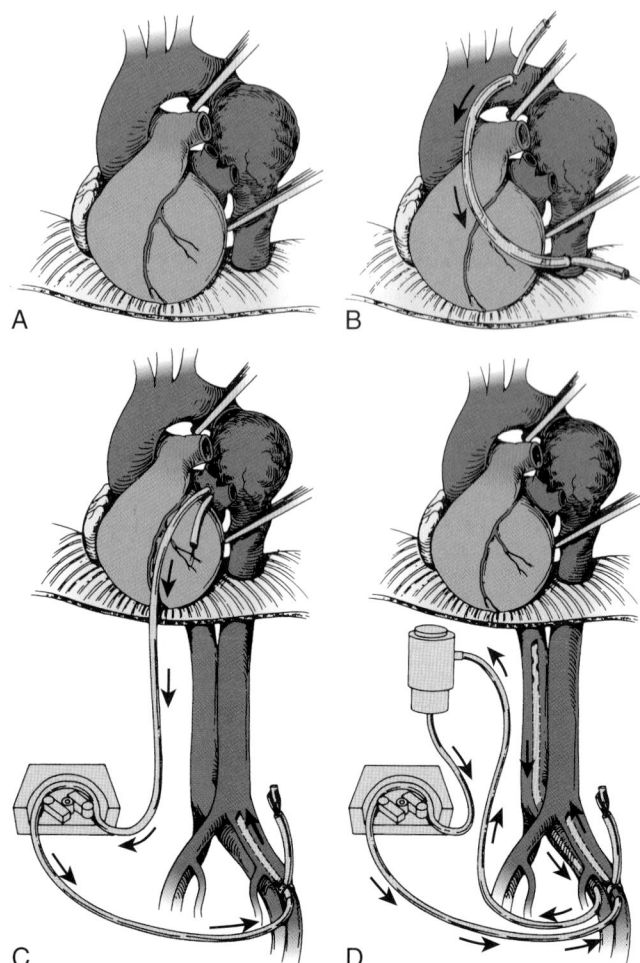

Figure 21-12   Operative techniques for repair of thoracic or thoracoabdominal aortic aneurysms. In the clamp-and-sew technique, the distal aorta is not perfused (A). Alternatively, distal aortic perfusion during repair can be provided by a passive Gott shunt (B), partial left heart bypass (C), or partial cardiopulmonary bypass (D). Deep hypothermic circulatory arrest may be necessary if the proximal cross-clamp cannot be safely applied in aneurysms extending into the distal aortic arch (not shown). *(From O'Connor CJ, Rothenberg DM: Anesthetic considerations for descending thoracic aortic surgery: Part II. J Cardiothorac Vasc Anesth 9:734, 1995.)*

TABLE 21-9	Advantages and Disadvantages of Distal Perfusion Techniques

Potential Advantages

Control of proximal hypertension

Decrease left ventricular afterload

Less hemodynamic perturbations with aortic clamping and unclamping

Decrease duration of mesenteric ischemia

Decrease risk for paraplegia from spinal cord ischemia

Ability to control systemic temperature with heat exchanger

Vascular access for rapid volume expansion

Ability to oxygenate blood with extracorporeal oxygenator

Capability to selectively perfuse mesenteric organs or aortic branch vessels

Maintain lower extremity SSEPs and MEPs for neurophysiologic monitoring

Potential Disadvantages

Require greater level of systemic anticoagulation

Increase risk for vascular injury at cannulation sites

Increase risk for thromboembolic events.

Require perfusion team

Need to monitor and control upper and lower body arterial pressure and flow

Increase technical complexity of operation

Partial Left-Heart Bypass

The control of both proximal and distal aortic perfusion during TAAA repair is achieved with PLHB. This technique requires left atrial cannulation, usually via a left pulmonary vein (see Figure 21-12C). Oxygenated blood from the left atrium flows through the CPB circuit into the distal aorta or a major branch via the arterial cannula.[61] The CPB circuit can include a heat exchanger, membrane oxygenator, and/or a venous reservoir. The degree of heparinization for PLHB is minimal with heparin-coated circuits without an oxygenator. Full systemic anticoagulation with ACT greater than 400 seconds is required for CPB circuits with membrane oxygenators and heat exchangers.[64] During PLHB, the proximal mean arterial pressure (MAP; radial artery) is generally maintained in the 80 to 90 mm Hg range. Flow rates in the range of 1.5 to 2.5 L/min typically maintain a distal aortic MAP in the 60 to 70 mm Hg range, monitored via a femoral arterial catheter.[64] Sequential advancement of the aortic cross-clamp during PLHB permits segmental aortic reconstruction with a decrease in end-organ ischemia. The advantages of PLHB include control of aortic pressures and systemic temperature, reliable distal aortic perfusion, and selective antegrade perfusion of important branch vessels (Figure 21-13).[61] Its disadvantages include increased expense, increased complexity, and requirement for systemic anticoagulation (see Table 21-9). An alternative technique uses partial CPB by femoral vein to femoral artery perfusion with or without an oxygenator. This can allow for distal perfusion without the need for cannulation of the heart or aorta. However, it does not offer the control that is achieved with proper PLHB.

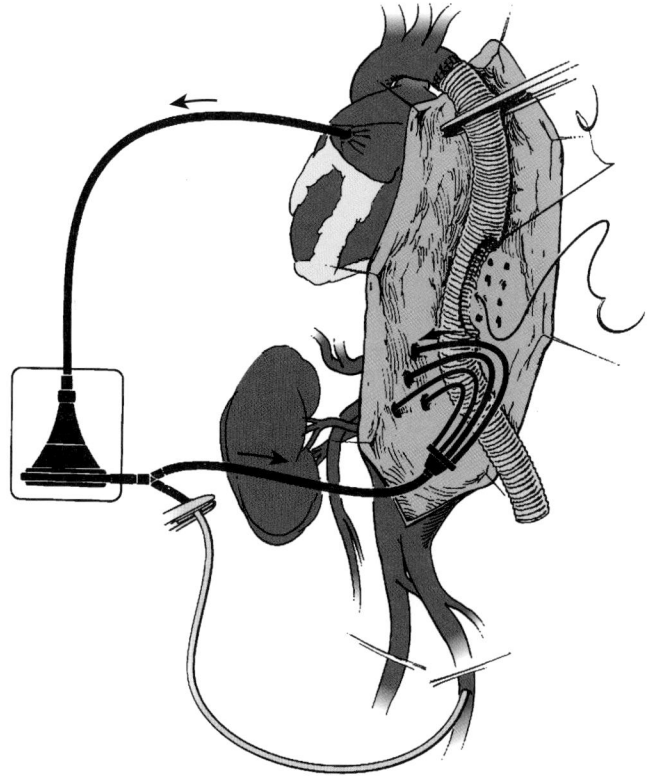

Figure 21-13 Extracorporeal perfusion circuit for repair of an extensive thoracoabdominal aortic aneurysm. Cannulation of the left atrium and femoral artery provides distal aortic perfusion by partial left heart bypass. Visceral perfusion can be provided by selective cannulation of the celiac, superior mesenteric, and renal arteries. *(Adapted from Coselli JS: Descending thoracoabdominal aortic aneurysms. In Edmunds LH [ed]: Cardiac Surgery in the Adult. New York, McGraw-Hill, 1997, p 1237.)*

Cardiopulmonary Bypass with Deep Hypothermic Circulatory Arrest

When a TAAA involves the distal aortic arch, CPB with DHCA is required to allow completion of the distal anastomosis. This technique has acceptable perioperative outcome for major reconstruction of the thoracoabdominal aorta because it also protects the spinal cord and mesenteric organs from ischemia.[65] If CPB with DHCA is planned for TAAA repair through a left thoracotomy incision, TEE should monitor for AR so that any LV distention with the onset of asystole during deliberate hypothermia can be managed with insertion of a drainage cannula. The disadvantages of CPB with DHCA include the limited safe period for DHCA, risk for stroke from retrograde aortic perfusion, increased CPB duration, and bleeding. For TAAA with extension into the distal aortic arch, a two-stage elephant-trunk procedure can be performed instead of using CPB with DHCA.[66] In the two-stage elephant-trunk procedure, the transverse aortic arch graft is performed first through a median sternotomy, leaving a short segment of graft extending into the descending aorta (see Figure 21-5). The second stage of the repair is performed through a left thoracotomy incision to access and anastomose the distal end of the transverse arch graft to the proximal end of the descending thoracic aortic graft. This two-stage repair avoids the need for retrograde CPB perfusion through the diseased descending thoracic aorta and decreases the risk for injury to the recurrent laryngeal nerve, esophagus, and pulmonary artery located in the proximity of the distal aortic arch.

Endovascular Stent Graft Repair of Thoracic Aortic Aneurysms

TEVAR was established for the management of thoracic aortic aneurysms and now has recent management guidelines.[20] Endovascular stent grafts are tube grafts reinforced by a wire frame that are collapsed within a catheter for delivery and deployment within the aortic lumen. The principle of TEVAR is that the deployed stent complex spans the length of diseased aorta to exclude blood flow into the aneurysm cavity. TEVAR requires a landing zone for each end of the tubular graft. Endoleak is defined as blood flow within the aneurysm but outside the endovascular graft (Table 21-10).

The current guidelines from the STS suggest TEVAR for aneurysms of the descending thoracic aorta when the aortic diameter is larger than 5.5 cm (Class IIa recommendation; level of evidence B, when the patient has significant comorbidity; Class IIb recommendation; level of evidence C, when the patient has no significant comorbidity).[20] When

the aortic diameter is less than 5.5 cm, the STS guidelines advise against TEVAR (Class III recommendation; level of evidence C).[20] In the setting of TAAA, the STS guidelines support TEVAR in patients with severe comorbidity (Class IIb recommendation; level of evidence C).[20] In patients with severe comorbidity and aortic arch aneurysm with distal extension, the STS guidelines support an endovascular repair technique (Class IIb recommendation; level of evidence C).[1,20] In patients who have reasonable surgical risk and who have aortic arch aneurysms with distal extension, the STS guidelines advise against an endovascular repair technique (Class III recommendation; level of evidence A).[1,20]

Endovascular stent graft repair for isolated descending thoracic aortic aneurysms with a proximal landing zone that involves the left subclavian artery can be accomplished using a two-stage procedure (Figure 21-14). In the first stage, the left subclavian artery can be

TABLE 21-10	Classification of Endoleaks	
Type	Cause of Perigraft Flow	Consequences and Therapeutic Strategy
I	Inadequate seal at proximal and/or distal landing zone	Systemic blood pressure is transmitted to aneurysm with risk for rupture: timely repair is indicated.
II	Retrograde flow from aortic branches into aneurysm	It may thrombose. If aneurysm is expanding, aortic branch embolization is indicated.
III	Structural failure of stent, e.g., perforations, fractures	Systemic blood pressure is transmitted to aneurysm with risk for rupture: timely repair is indicated.
IV	Stent graft fabric porosity	This usually occurs at implantation and disappears with anticoagulation reversal.
V	Aneurysm expansion without obvious endoleak ("endodistention")	The endovascular repair can be strengthened with a second stent.

Data from Hiratzka LF, Bakris GL, Beckman JA, et al: 2010 ACCF/AHA/AATS/ACR/ASA/SCA/SCAI/SIR/STS/SVM guidelines for the diagnosis and management of patients with thoracic aortic disease: Executive summary. A report of the American College of Cardiology Foundation, American Heart Association Task Force on Practice Guidelines, American Association for Thoracic Surgery, American College of Radiology, American Stroke Association, Society of Cardiovascular Anesthesiologists, Society for Cardiovascular Angiography and Interventions, and Society for Vascular Medicine. *Circulation* 121:e266–e369, 2010.

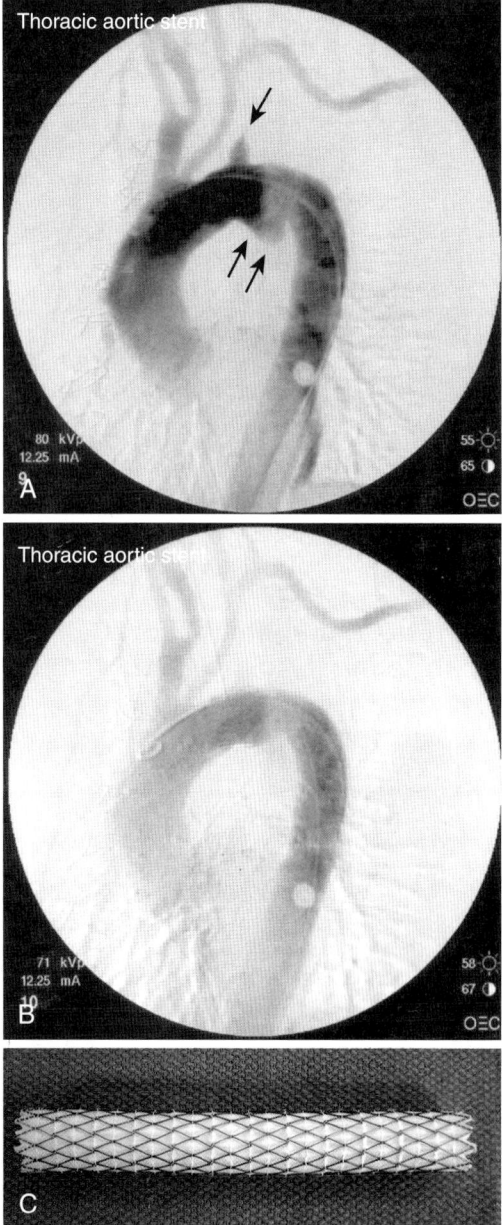

Figure 21-14 Intraoperative angiogram demonstrating an isolated saccular aneurysm *(double arrows)* of the thoracic aorta *(A)*. The left subclavian artery *(single arrow)* was previously divided and transposed onto the left carotid artery to create a proximal landing site for endovascular stent repair *(A)*. Intraoperative angiogram *(B)* after deployment of the endovascular stent graft *(C)* demonstrated exclusion of the aneurysm.

divided and anastomosed onto the left common carotid artery. This first stage of the procedure provides a proximal landing zone, allowing the deployment of the endovascular stent graft over the left subclavian artery branch in the distal aortic arch in the second stage of the procedure without compromising flow through the vessel. Multiple recent meta-analyses have demonstrated the outcome importance of not sacrificing the left subclavian artery during TEVAR to avoid the risks for stroke, paraplegia, and left upper extremity ischemia.[67–69] The recent guidelines from the Society of Vascular Surgery strongly support this principle but also recognize that in urgent TEVAR for life-threatening acute aortic syndromes, left subclavian artery coverage is unavoidable.[70]

There are currently two major options for endovascular TAAA repair, namely, total TEVAR and hybrid TEVAR. Total endovascular TAAA repair requires customized stents that preserve major aortic branches with fenestrations or side branches. Recent series have demonstrated the safety and efficacy of this TEVAR modality in high-risk TAAA patients.[71–73] In hybrid TAAA repair, the landing zone for the nonfenestrated endovascular graft is created by aortic debranching procedures, for example, the renal and mesenteric arteries are anastomosed to the iliac arteries. Recent multiple series and meta-analyses have demonstrated the safety and efficacy of this TEVAR modality in high-risk patients.[74–78] This hybrid approach also has been utilized in aortic arch reconstruction for high-risk patients with aortic arch aneurysms.[79] Furthermore, TEVAR recently has extended proximally for therapy of select aneurysms of the ascending aorta.[80,81] In summary, TEVAR for TAAA, whether wholly endovascular or hybrid, is in recent clinical development with an established niche in patients with excessive operative risk. It is likely that these technologies will mature further in the coming years. This maturation of TEVAR for diseases of the descending thoracic aorta likely will be rapid given that recent meta-analysis ($N = 5888$, 42 nonrandomized studies) demonstrated that TEVAR as compared with open aortic repair reduced perioperative mortality (odds ratio, 0.44; 95% confidence interval, 0.33–0.59), paraplegia (odds ratio, 0.42; 95% confidence interval, 0.28–0.63), pneumonia, cardiac complications, renal failure, bleeding, and transfusion, as well as length of hospital stay.[82]

Anesthetic Management for Thoracoabdominal Aortic Aneurysm Repair

The anesthetic management of patients undergoing TAAA repair often requires selective right lung ventilation in the setting of a major left thoracotomy and anesthetic interventions to prevent spinal cord ischemia. Right radial arterial pressure monitoring typically is preferred, especially if the aortic repair involves clamping the left subclavian artery or surgical endovascular access via the left brachial artery. Femoral arterial pressure monitoring is required when distal aortic perfusion is planned either with PLHB or a Gott shunt. Hemodynamic monitoring with a PAC usually is helpful for the management of the concomitant specialized perfusion techniques already discussed. The anesthetic plan must allow for spinal cord monitoring with SSEPs, MEPs, or both to account for decreases in renal function and include a plan for postoperative analgesia.

Lung Isolation Techniques

Selective ventilation of the right lung with concomitant left lung collapse during TAAA repair enhances surgical access and protects the right lung from left lung bleeding. Collapse of the left lung typically is achieved when the left main bronchus is intubated either with a double-lumen endobronchial tube (DLT) or a bronchial blocker. Routine fiberoptic bronchoscopic guidance guarantees the effectiveness of either technique. The increased length of the left mainstem bronchus facilitates placement of a left-sided DLT and subsequently anchors it during surgery. Endobronchial blockade is achieved with one of the following devices: the Arndt blocker, the Cohen blocker, or

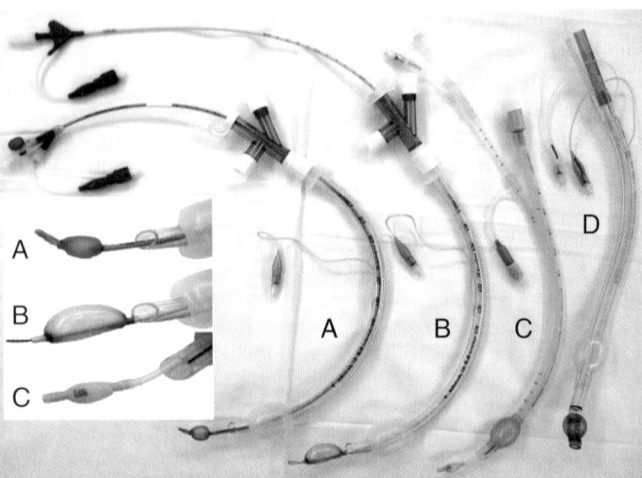

Figure 21-15 Single-lung ventilation for thoracic or thoracoabdominal aortic aneurysm repair requiring a left thoracotomy can be accomplished using a Cohen bronchial blocker inserted through a standard endotracheal tube (A), an Arndt wire-guided bronchial blocker inserted through a standard endotracheal tube (B), a Univent endotracheal tube with an integrated bronchial blocker (C), or a left-sided double-lumen endobronchial tube (D).

the Univent tube (Figure 21-15).[83] Wire-guided endobronchial blocking catheters permit the balloon-tipped catheter to be guided and positioned precisely in the left mainstem bronchus with a fiberoptic bronchoscope. The advantages of a left DLT include the ability to apply selective continuous positive airway pressure to the left lung. Its disadvantages include increased difficulty in difficult airways and bronchial injury in distorted endobronchial anatomy. The major advantage of endobronchial blockade is its compatibility with an existing standard 8.0-mm endotracheal tube. This is advantageous in emergencies and in difficult airways.[83] The disadvantages of endobronchial blockade include increased time for left-lung collapse and dislodgement during surgery. The majority of patients will require temporary postoperative mechanical ventilation, usually via a single-lumen endotracheal tube. ICU personnel often are unaccustomed to managing patients with DLTs with their risks for malposition, airway obstruction, and difficulty with airway secretions. Endotracheal tube exchange may be challenging if there is airway edema. An endotracheal tube exchange catheter in combination with direct laryngoscopy often facilitates safe endotracheal tube exchange.[84] It is recommended that in the setting of upper airway edema, DLTs are not routinely exchanged for single-lumen tubes (ACC/AHA Class III recommendation; level of evidence C).[1]

Paraplegia after Thoracoabdominal Aortic Aneurysm Repair

Paraplegia after TAAA repair is a devastating complication. The temporary interruption of distal aortic perfusion and sacrifice of spinal segmental arteries during TAAA repair are central events in the pathogenesis of spinal cord ischemia and paraplegia. There are multiple contributing factors (Table 21-11).[85] The typical level of spinal cord ischemia after TAAA is midthoracic and is associated with a high perioperative mortality. There are many management strategies for prevention of this devastating complication after TAAA (Table 21-12).[1,85]

The spinal cord arterial supply provides a partial explanation for the clinical features of paraplegia after TAAA repair (Figure 21-16).[85,86] The anterior spinal artery supplies the anterior two thirds of the spinal cord, and the posterior spinal arteries supply the posterior third.

TABLE 21-11	Factors That Contribute to Paraplegia after Thoracic or Thoracoabdominal Aortic Procedures

Thoracoabdominal aortic aneurysm extent
Hypotension or cardiogenic shock
Emergency surgery
Aortic rupture
Presence of aortic dissection
Duration of aortic cross-clamp
Sacrifice of intercostal or segmental artery branches
Prior thoracic or abdominal aortic aneurysm repair
Prior repair of type A aortic dissection
Occlusive peripheral vascular disease
Anemia

TABLE 21-12	Minimizing Paraplegic Risk after Thoracic or Thoracoabdominal Aortic Procedures

Minimize Aortic Cross-clamp Time
Distal aortic perfusion
Passive shunt (Gott)
Partial left heart bypass
Partial cardiopulmonary bypass
Deliberate Hypothermia
Mild-to-moderate systemic hypothermia (32°C to 35°C)
Deep hypothermic circulatory arrest (14°C to 18°C)
Selective spinal cord hypothermia (epidural cooling, 25°C)
Increase Spinal Cord Perfusion Pressure
Reimplantation of critical intercostal and segmental arterial branches
Lumbar cerebrospinal fluid (CSF) drainage (CSF pressure ≤ 10 mm Hg)
Arterial pressure augmentation (mean arterial pressure ≥ 85 mm Hg)
Intraoperative Monitoring of Lower Extremity Neurophysiologic Function
Somatosensory-evoked potentials
Motor-evoked potentials
Postoperative Neurologic Assessment for Early Detection of Delayed-Onset Paraplegia
Serial neurologic examinations
Pharmacologic Neuroprotection
Glucocorticoid
Barbiturate or central nervous system depressants
Magnesium sulfate
Mannitol
Naloxone
Lidocaine
Intrathecal papaverine

Branches from each vertebral artery join to form the anterior spinal artery that descends along the midline of the anterior surface of the spinal cord. The anterior spinal artery sometimes is discontinuous and fed in a variable extent by radicular arteries derived from ascending cervical, deep cervical, intercostal, lumbar, and sacral segmental arteries. The posterior spinal arteries also are derived from the vertebral arteries and receive collateral supply from posterior radicular arteries. The terminal cord segments are supplied by radicular arteries that arise from the internal iliac and sacral arterial network. The thoracolumbar spinal cord typically has multiple arterial sources with a clinical vulnerability to significant ischemia. In this watershed region, an important blood supply is derived from a large radicular artery (intercostal arteries T9-T12 in 75% of patients, T8-L3 in 15%, and L1-L2 in 10%).[87,88] This important artery is known as the arteria magna or the artery of Adamkiewicz. Ischemia in the anterior spinal artery territory classically causes motor paralysis with preservation of proprioception.[85] Clinical experience, however, has demonstrated that spinal cord ischemia after TAAA repair is variable, asymmetric, and can affect motor or sensory function, or both.[85,89]

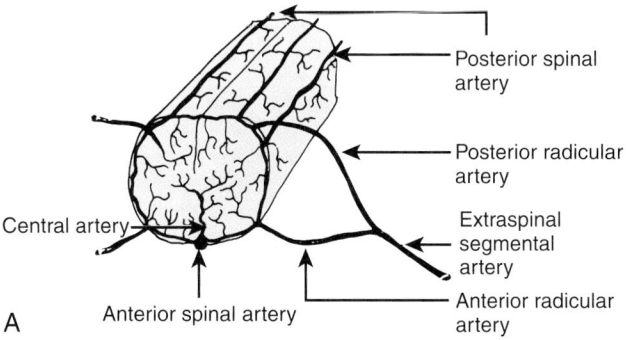

A

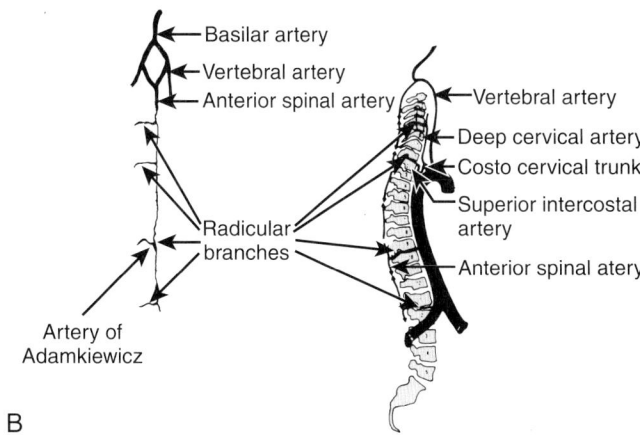

B

Figure 21-16 The arterial supply to the spinal cord is provided by the anterior spinal artery and paired posterior spinal arteries that branch off the vertebral arteries (A). Radicular arterial branches off the descending thoracic aorta provide collateral arterial supply to the anterior and posterior spinal arteries (B). The arteria magna or artery of Adamkiewicz refers to a large radicular branch located between the T9 and L2 vertebral levels that supplies the anterior spinal artery (B).

Paraplegia is defined as lower extremity motor weakness with muscle strength weaker than gravity. Paraparesis is defined as lower extremity weakness with muscle power that allows movement at least against gravity (Table 21-13).[89] Spinal cord ischemia may have an immediate onset, defined as lower extremity weakness on emergence from anesthesia within 24 hours of the procedure.[85,89] Delayed-onset spinal cord ischemia is defined as lower extremity weakness that follows a normal postoperative neurologic examination after emergence from anesthesia. In the largest series of TAAA repairs ever reported (N = 2286; 1986–2006), the incidence rate of symptomatic spinal cord ischemia

TABLE 21-13	Description of Lower Extremity Weakness Caused by Spinal Cord Ischemia	
Score	*Description*	
Paraplegia	**Paraplegia**	
0	No movement of lower extremity	
1	Minimal movement or flicker of lower extremity	
2	Movement of the lower extremity but not against resistance or gravity (e.g., bend knee, move leg)	
Paraparesis	**Paraparesis**	
3	Movement of the lower extremity against resistance and gravity but without ability to stand or walk	
4	Ability to stand and walk with assistance	

Data from Greenberg RK, Lu Q, Roselli E, et al: Contemporary analysis of descending thoracic and thoracoabdominal aneurysm repair: A comparison of endovascular and open techniques. *Circulation* 118:808, 2008.

was 3.8%, with 63% of these cases having an immediate onset and 37% a delayed onset.[61] Multiple series have indicated that delayed-onset spinal cord ischemia can present days, weeks, or even months after TAAA repair.[61,85,89,90]

Immediate-onset paraplegia likely is a consequence of spinal cord ischemia, leading to infarction that occurred during surgery. In contrast with delayed-onset paraplegia, recovery with intervention in immediate-onset paraplegia has not been consistently demonstrated. This lack of therapeutic response likely indicates that irreversible spinal cord injury has occurred. Consequently, strategies to prevent immediate-onset paraplegia are directed toward intraoperative spinal cord protection (Box 21-3). The objective of intraoperative spinal cord monitoring is to detect spinal cord ischemia for immediate intervention to improve spinal cord perfusion. Distal aortic perfusion maintains spinal cord function during aortic cross-clamping and improves the ability to monitor spinal cord integrity during surgery with SSEP or MEPs.

Delayed-onset paraplegia indicates that, although the spinal cord was protected intraoperatively, it remains vulnerable to ischemia after surgery. Although the causes of this syndrome are incompletely understood, it often is preceded by hypotension.[91] Strategies to minimize delayed-onset paraplegia concern the prevention of perioperative hypotension, early anesthetic emergence for early and subsequent serial neurologic assessment, and lumbar CSF drainage (Box 21-4). Given the catastrophic sequelae of permanent paraplegia after TAAA repair, all reasonable attempts to treat delayed-onset paraplegia can be justified.

Lumbar Cerebrospinal Fluid Drainage

Lumbar CSF drainage is a strongly recommended spinal cord protective strategy for TAAA repair (ACC/AHA Class I recommendation; level of evidence B).[1,92–95] The physiologic rationale is that reduction of CSF pressure improves spinal cord perfusion pressure (SCPP) and also may counter CSF pressure increases caused by aortic cross-clamping, reperfusion, increased central venous pressure, and/or spinal cord edema.[85] Lumbar CSF drainage is performed by the insertion of a silicon elastomer ventriculostomy catheter via a 14-gauge Tuohy needle at the L3-L4

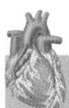

BOX 21-3. TECHNIQUES TO DECREASE THE RISK FOR INTRAOPERATIVE SPINAL CORD ISCHEMIA

- Mild systemic hypothermia
- Lumbar cerebrospinal fluid drainage
- Selective spinal cord cooling
- Distal aortic perfusion
- Minimizing the ischemic time
- Segmental aortic reconstruction
- Intercostal artery preservation
- Pharmacologic neuroprotection
- Intraoperative motor- or somatosensory-evoked potential monitoring
- Arterial pressure augmentation

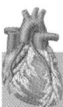

BOX 21-4. PREVENTION AND TREATMENT OF DELAYED-ONSET SPINAL CORD ISCHEMIA

- Maintain mean arterial pressure ≥ 85 mm Hg
- Serial neurologic assessment for lower extremity weakness or sensory loss
- Immediate treatment to augment spinal cord perfusion pressure
- Arterial pressure augmentation with vasopressor therapy
- Lumbar cerebrospinal fluid drainage
- Prevent hypotension

vertebral interspace. The catheter usually is advanced 10 to 15 cm into the subarachnoid space and securely fastened to the skin to prevent catheter movement while the patient is anticoagulated. The open end of the catheter is attached to a sterile reservoir, and CSF is drained when the lumbar CSF pressure exceeds 10 mm Hg. The lumbar CSF pressure is measured with a pressure transducer zero-referenced to the midline of the brain. Currently, the best strategy to manage a traumatic lumbar puncture or the drainage of blood-tinged CSF has not been determined.[96,97] The lumbar CSF drainage catheter is inserted before or at the time of surgery for CSF drainage up to the first 24 hours after surgery. The lumbar drainage catheter subsequently can be capped and left in place for the next 24 hours. It then can be removed, assuming a normal neurologic examination and adequate coagulation.

The complications of lumbar CSF drainage include neuraxial hematoma, catheter fracture, meningitis, intracranial hypotension, and spinal headache.[64,85] Neuraxial hemorrhage after lumbar drain insertion remains a risk in patients subsequently subjected to systemic anticoagulation for CPB. Despite this risk, the overall safety of this technique has been established in multiple case series.[64,85,98,99] Measures to minimize neuraxial hematoma include establishing normal coagulation for both CSF catheter insertion and removal, as well as allowing a few hours between its insertion and heparinization for CPB.[85,98] In two large contemporary series (combined $N = 2001$), the complication rate associated with CSF drainage for thoracic aortic repair was about 1% with no spinal hematomas. Both series identified excessive CSF drainage as a principal risk factor for intracranial hypotension and subsequent subdural hematoma and emphasized the outcome benefit associated with a limited CSF drainage protocol.[98,99] For routine use, CSF only should be drained, using a closed circuit reservoir, when the lumbar CSF pressure exceeds 10 mm Hg. Meningitis is characterized by high fever, altered mentation, and CSF pleocytosis often with bacteria. The risk for catheter fracture can be minimized by careful catheter removal.

Arterial Pressure Augmentation

The optimization of SCPP for spinal cord protection is recommended as part of an institutional perioperative protocol (ACC/AHA Class IIa recommendation; level of evidence B).[1] This recommendation also recognized the variety of suitable techniques such as maintenance of proximal aortic pressure and distal aortic perfusion with the caveat that technique selection often is a function of institutional experience.[1] In keeping with this recommendation are the principles of arterial pressure augmentation and CSF drainage for prevention and management of postoperative spinal cord ischemia (Figure 21-17).[90] Spinal cord ischemia after TAAA repair is more likely in the setting of hypotension because the spinal arterial collateral network has been reduced due to factors such as intercostal artery sacrifice.[91,100,101] Recent surgical techniques to preserve SCPP include selective intraoperative spinal cord perfusion and intercostal artery revascularization with interposition grafts.[102,103]

SCPP is estimated as the MAP minus the lumbar CSF pressure. In general, the SCPP should be maintained greater than 70 mm Hg after TAAA repair, that is, a MAP of 80 to 100 mm Hg.[85,90,100] Because spinal cord ischemia often involves the thoracolumbar cord, it often is accompanied by a significant sympathectomy known as spinal vasodilatory shock.[1,85,90] Early intervention to treat hypotension with vasopressor therapy may counter the autonomic nervous system dysfunction accompanying spinal cord ischemia and also augment SCPP. As in the treatment of neurogenic shock, high-dose vasopressor therapy with norepinephrine, phenylephrine, epinephrine, and/or vasopressin typically is required to restore systemic vascular resistance and spinal cord perfusion, with a MAP in the 80 to 100 mm Hg range.[90] Recovery from spinal cord ischemia often is heralded by recovery of systemic vascular tone and a decreasing vasopressor requirement. Therapeutic hypertension, as discussed here, for the management of spinal cord ischemia after TAAA must be weighed against the risks for arterial bleeding.

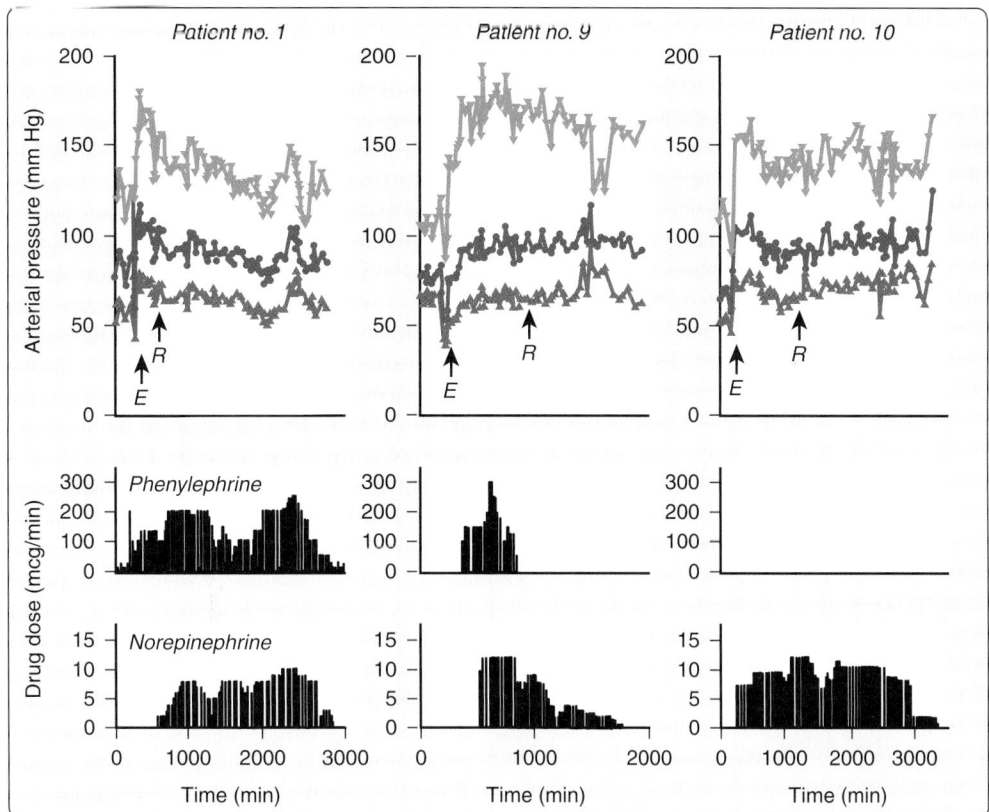

Figure 21-17   Systolic, mean, and diastolic blood pressures in the period surrounding the onset *(E)* and recovery *(R)* from delayed-onset paraplegia in three patients after thoracoabdominal aortic aneurysm repair. Autonomic nervous system dysfunction caused by spinal cord ischemia may have contributed to the decrease in arterial pressure during the events. Arterial pressures were augmented with vasopressor therapy *(bottom)*. Vasopressor requirements decreased after recovery from spinal cord ischemia. *(From Cheung AT, Weiss SJ, McGarvey ML, et al: Interventions for reversing delayed-onset postoperative paraplegia after thoracic aortic reconstruction. Ann Thorac Surg 74:417, 2002, by permission of the Society of Thoracic Surgeons.)*

Intraoperative Neurophysiologic Monitoring

Neurophysiologic monitoring of the spinal cord (SSEPs and/or MEPs) is recommended as a strategy for the diagnosis of spinal cord ischemia so as to allow immediate intraoperative neuroprotective interventions such as intercostal artery implantation, relative arterial hypertension, and CSF drainage (ACC/AHA Class IIb recommendation; level of evidence B).[1] This management strategy may prevent immediate-onset postoperative paraplegia. SSEP monitoring is performed by applying electrical stimuli to peripheral nerves and recording the evoked potential that is generated at the level of the peripheral nerves, spinal cord, brainstem, thalamus, and cerebral cortex.[104] Because SSEP monitors posterior spinal column integrity, MEPs have been advocated because they monitor the anterior spinal columns that are typically at risk during TAAA repair. MEP monitoring is performed by applying paired stimuli to the scalp and recording the evoked potential that is generated in the anterior tibialis muscle.[105,106] (See Chapter 16.)

Paraplegia caused by spinal cord ischemia significantly dampens lower extremity evoked potentials as compared with the upper extremity (Figure 21-18). Intraoperative comparison of upper and lower extremity evoked potentials distinguishes spinal cord ischemia from the generalized effects of anesthetics, hypothermia, and/or electrical interference. As discussed earlier, the anesthetic must be designed for minimal interference with the selected neuromonitoring strategy. Although SSEPs can reliably exclude spinal cord ischemia with a negative predictive value of 99.2%, their sensitivity for its detection is only 62.5%, with no clinically useful predictive value for delayed-onset paraplegia.[107] A recent study (*N* = 233) compared both MEPs and SSEPs for spinal cord monitoring in extensive descending thoracic and TAAA repairs.[108] Both monitoring modalities had a nearly 90% correlation

for spinal cord infarction (correlation statistic = 0.896; *P* < 0.0001), as well as a 98% negative predictive value for immediate-onset paraplegia. Furthermore, reversible changes in MEPs and SSEPs had no correlation with permanent paraplegia. In summary, despite the theoretic advantages of MEPs for monitoring the at-risk anterior spinal columns, in practice, this most recent data set suggests that SSEPs alone suffice for clinical purposes, and that MEPs did not add significantly to clinical management.[108] This assessment also is reflected in the neuromonitoring recommendations of the latest thoracic aortic disease guidelines.[1]

Spinal Cord Hypothermia

Although DHCA is effective, moderate systemic hypothermia is also reasonable for spinal cord protection during TAAA repair (ACC/AHA Class IIa recommendation; level of evidence B).[1] Furthermore, topical spinal cord hypothermia is possible with cold saline epidural infusion to avoid ischemia during TAAA repair.[109,110] Although clinical experience with this technique has been limited to a few institutions, it has demonstrated clinical benefit as part of a multimodal spinal protection protocol.[95,109,110] Epidural cooling is recommended as an adjunctive technique for spinal cord protection during major distal thoracic aortic reconstructions (ACC/AHA Class IIb recommendation; level of evidence B).[1] This technique may disseminate further, given its adjunctive benefit and the recent clinical development of a specialized countercurrent closed-lumen epidural catheter for epidural cooling during major distal aortic reconstructions.[111]

Pharmacologic Protection of the Spinal Cord

Pharmacologic spinal cord protection with agents such as high-dose systemic glucocorticoids, mannitol, intrathecal papaverine, and

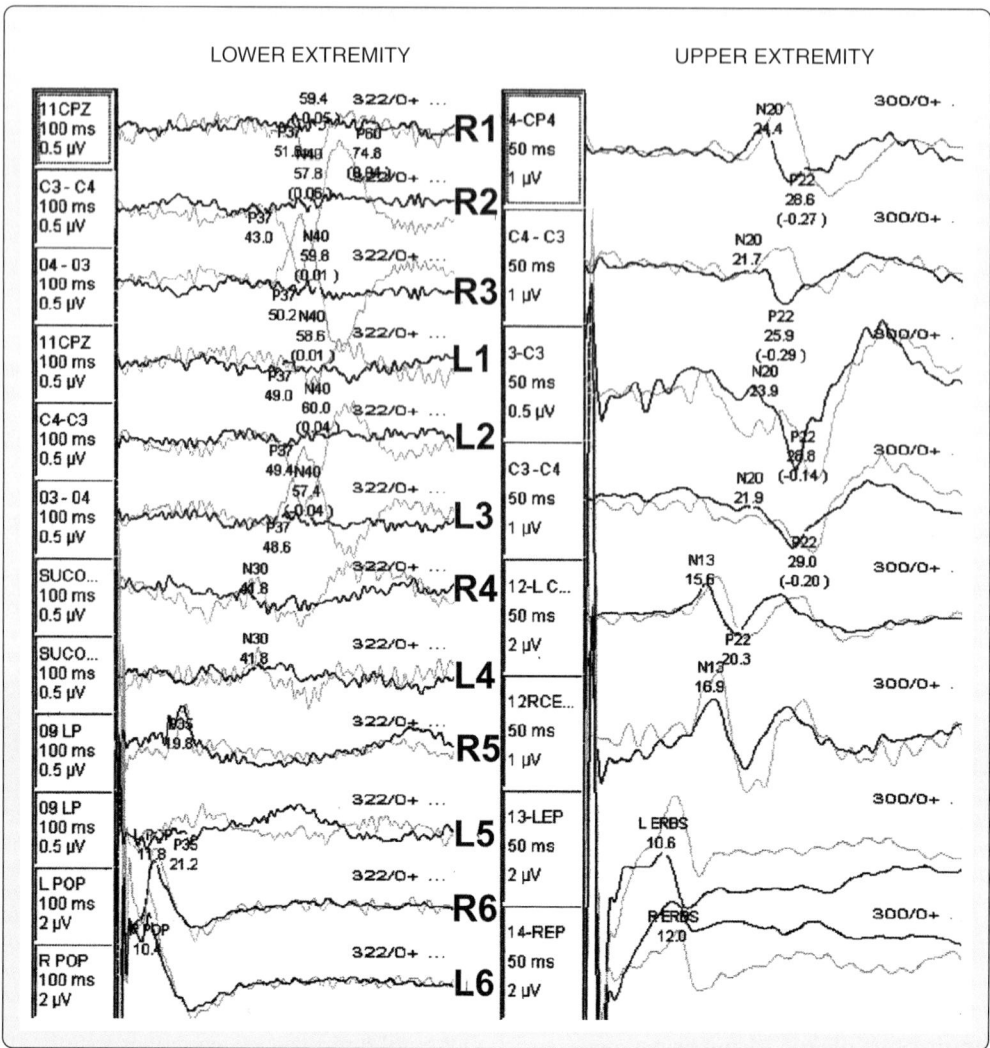

Figure 21-18 Intraoperative somatosensory-evoked potential (SSEP) recordings from the lower *(left)* and upper *(right)* extremities that demonstrated spinal cord ischemia during thoracoabdominal aortic aneurysm repair. Disappearance of SSEP signals from the right (R) and left (L) lower extremities recorded at the cortex (R1, R2, R3, L1, L2, L3) and spine (R4, L4) with preservation of SSEP signals from the lumbar plexus (R5, L5) and popliteal nerves (R6, L6) indicated the acute onset of spinal cord ischemia. Upper extremity SSEP signals were maintained during the episode. The *light gray tracings* were the baseline SSEP signals used for comparison.

anesthetic agents is recommended as an adjunctive technique in a multimodal neuroprotective protocol (ACC/AHA Class IIb recommendation; level of evidence B).[1,95] Additional neuroprotective agents that have been studied in this regard include lidocaine, naloxone, and magnesium.[95,112,113] Although there are multiple agents with potential benefit, only a few are utilized routinely in clinical practice.[112]

Renal Protection during Thoracoabdominal Aortic Aneurysm Repair

Even though there has been major progress in TAAA repair, renal dysfunction remains common and still independently predicts for adverse clinical outcomes.[61,114] The thoracic aortic guidelines recommend preoperative hydration and intraoperative mannitol administration as reasonable nephroprotective strategies in extensive distal open thoracic aortic repairs, including TAAA repair (ACC/AHA Class IIb recommendation; level of evidence C).[1] Furthermore, intraoperative cold renal perfusion with blood or crystalloid is recommended as a reasonable intraoperative nephroprotective strategy during TAAA repair (ACC/AHA Class IIb recommendation; level of evidence C).[1,115,116] The administration of furosemide, mannitol, or dopamine for the sole

purpose of renal preservation is not recommended in distal thoracic aortic repairs (ACC/AHA Class IIb recommendation; level of evidence B).[1] Rhabdomyolysis from lower extremity ischemia was recently identified as a mechanism for renal dysfunction after TAAA repair.[117–119] The maintenance of lower extremity perfusion bilaterally during distal aortic perfusion has been shown to ameliorate this rhabdomyolysis with a significant nephroprotective effect.

Postoperative Analgesia after Thoracoabdominal Aortic Aneurysm Repair

It is well recognized that the extensive thoracoabdominal incision is very painful. Because epidural analgesia has proved outcome utility in this type of extensive incision, it typically is part of the analgesic plan after TAAA repair.[120] The timing of epidural catheter placement and analgesia must take into account the perioperative anticoagulation status of the patient to minimize the risk for neuraxial hematoma.[7] Furthermore, the epidural analgesia regimen should be formulated for a predominantly sensory block to allow serial motor assessment of the lower extremities and to minimize systemic vasodilation from a sympathectomy. For example, bupivacaine, 0.05%, combined with fentanyl,

2 µg/mL, can be initiated at a basal rate of 4 to 8 mL/hr after the patient exhibits normal neurologic function.[90] Bolus administration of concentrated local anesthetic through the epidural catheter should be discouraged to avoid sympathetic blockade and associated hypotension. The epidural catheter can be inserted before surgery, at the time of surgery, or in the postoperative period.

Anesthetic Management for Thoracic Endovascular Aortic Repair

TEVAR has revolutionized the management of descending thoracic and TAAAs with significant clinical outcome benefit.[20,82] The anesthetic management is based on the principles of care for patients undergoing endovascular abdominal aortic repair, but with the additional concerns of spinal cord ischemia and stroke.[121] Typically, these patients undergo a balanced general anesthetic with invasive blood pressure monitoring and central venous access. The right radial artery is preferred for blood pressure monitoring, given that the left subclavian artery frequently may be covered and/or the left brachial artery may be accessed as part of the procedure.[67–70] PAC monitoring may be helpful in the setting of significant cardiac disease. TEE is reasonable in TEVAR in which it may assist in hemodynamic monitoring, procedural guidance, and endoleak detection (ACC/ACC Class IIa recommendation; level of evidence B).[1] As discussed earlier, if spinal cord monitoring is planned (SSEPs and/or MEPs), the anesthetic technique must be designed not to interfere with their signal quality.

The risk factors for stroke after TEVAR include a history of prior stroke, mobile aortic arch atheroma, and TEVAR of the proximal or entire descending thoracic aorta.[121,122] Therefore, the detection of mobile atheroma in the aortic arch is an important TEE finding in TEVAR because it predicts a greater stroke risk. The risk factors for spinal cord ischemia after TEVAR include perioperative hypotension (decreased SCPP), prior abdominal/descending thoracic aortic procedures (compromised spinal collateral arterial network), and coverage of the entire descending thoracic aorta (significant loss of intercostal arteries).[121,123] Consequently, indications for CSF lumbar drainage in TEVAR include planned extensive coverage of the descending thoracic aorta, history of prior abdominal/descending thoracic aortic procedures, and postoperative paraparesis/paraplegia despite relative hypertension.[121,123] Lumbar CSF drainage is a strongly recommended spinal cord protection strategy for TEVAR in patients with identified risk factors (ACC/AHA Class I recommendation; level of evidence B).[1,121–123]

AORTIC DISSECTION

Aortic dissection results from an intimal tear that exposes the media to the pulsatile force of blood within the aortic lumen (Figure 21-19).[1,124] Blood may exit the true aortic lumen and dissect the aortic wall to create a false lumen. The aortic dissection may remain localized at the primary entry site at the original intimal tear, or it may extend proximally, distally, or both. It also may extend into the aortic branch vessels to cause branch occlusion, or intima may shear at the site of branch vessels to result in intimal fenestrations. Propagation of the dissection into the aortic root can cause AR.[124] The weakened aortic wall often results in acute aortic dilation, which can progress to rupture resulting in pericardial tamponade, exsanguination, or both.

There are two generally accepted classifications of thoracic aortic dissections (Table 21-14).[1,124] The DeBakey scheme classifies aortic dissections into three groups (Figure 21-20). (See Videos on the website.) DeBakey type I dissections originate from a primary entry site in the ascending aorta and extend to involve the entire aorta. DeBakey type II dissections originate from a primary entry site in the ascending aorta and are confined to the ascending aorta. DeBakey type III dissections originate from a primary entry site in the descending thoracic aorta and are confined to the descending thoracic aorta distal to the origin of the left subclavian artery. DeBakey type III dissections also can be subdivided into subtype IIIA that are confined to the descending thoracic

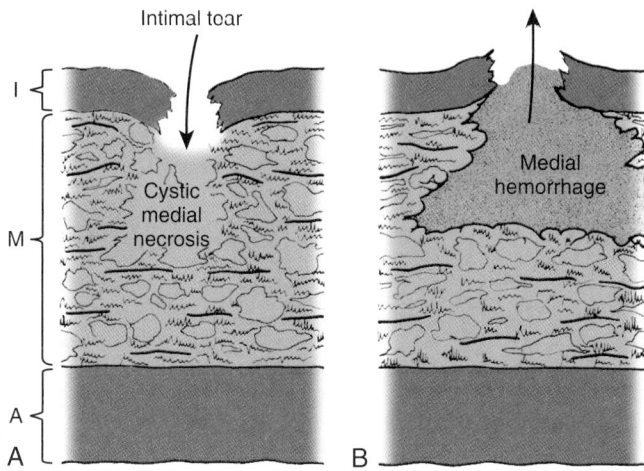

Figure 21-19 **A potential mechanism for aortic dissection is cystic medial necrosis** with an intimal tear allowing blood from the aortic lumen to enter the medial layer of the aorta *(M)*, leading to separation of the intima *(I)* from the adventitia *(A)*. *(From Eagle KA, De Sanctis RW: Diseases of the aorta. In Braunwald E [ed]: Heart disease, 4th ed. Philadelphia, 1992, WB Saunders, p 1528.)*

TABLE 21-14	Classification of Acute Aortic Dissection

DeBakey Classification

Type I: The entire aorta is involved (ascending, arch, and descending)

Type II: Confined to the ascending aorta

Type III: Intimal tear originating in the descending aorta with either distal or retrograde extension

Type IIIA: Intimal tear originating in the descending aorta with extension distally to the diaphragm or proximally into the aortic arch

Type IIIB: Intimal tear originating in the descending aorta with extension below the diaphragm or proximally into the aortic arch

Stanford Classification

Type A: Involvement of the ascending aorta or aortic arch regardless of the site of origin or distal extent

Type B: Confined to the descending aorta distal to the origin of the left subclavian artery

aorta above the diaphragm and subtype IIIB that extend below the diaphragm into the abdominal aorta. The Stanford scheme classifies aortic dissections into two groups (Figure 21-21). Stanford type A dissections are aortic dissections that involve the ascending aorta regardless of extent, origin, or entry sites. Stanford type B dissections are confined to the descending thoracic aorta distal to the origin of the left subclavian artery regardless of the extent or entry sites. (See Videos 1 and 2.)

Type A Aortic Dissection

Aortic dissections that involve the ascending aorta (Stanford type A) are considered surgical emergencies (Box 21-5) (ACC/AHA Class I recommendation; level of evidence B).[1] The mortality rate without emergency surgery is about 1% per hour for the first 48 hours, 60% by about 1 week, 74% by 2 weeks, and 91% by 6 months (Figure 21-22).[1,124,125] Immediate surgical intervention significantly improves the mortality rate (Table 21-15), especially in patients younger than 80 years.[1,124–126] The principal causes of mortality include rupture, cardiac tamponade, myocardial ischemia from coronary dissection, severe acute AR, stroke caused by brachiocephalic dissection, and malperfusion syndromes including renal failure, ischemic bowel, and limb ischemia (Table 21-16). The type of preoperative presentation in type A dissection significantly determines operative mortality, prompting a clinical classification developed at the University of

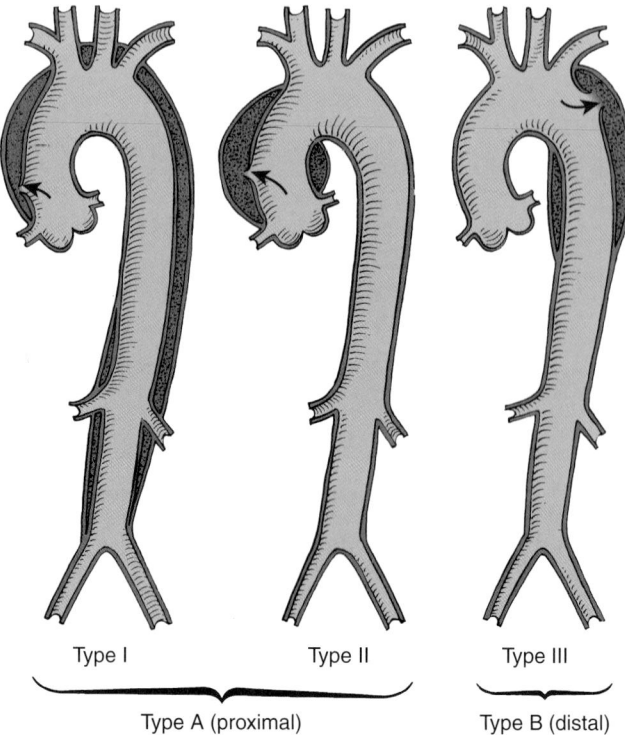

Figure 21-20   DeBakey classification of aortic dissections. Type I: intimal tear in the ascending aorta with extension of the dissection to the descending aorta. Type II: ascending intimal tear with dissection limited to the ascending aorta. Type III: intimal tear in the descending aorta with proximal extension of the dissection to involve the ascending aorta. Type IIIB: intimal tear in the descending aorta with dissection limited to the descending aorta. *(Reprinted from Larson EW, Edwards WD: Risk factors for aortic dissection: A necropsy study of 161 cases. Am J Cardiol 53:849, 1984, by permission of Excerpta Medica, Inc.)*

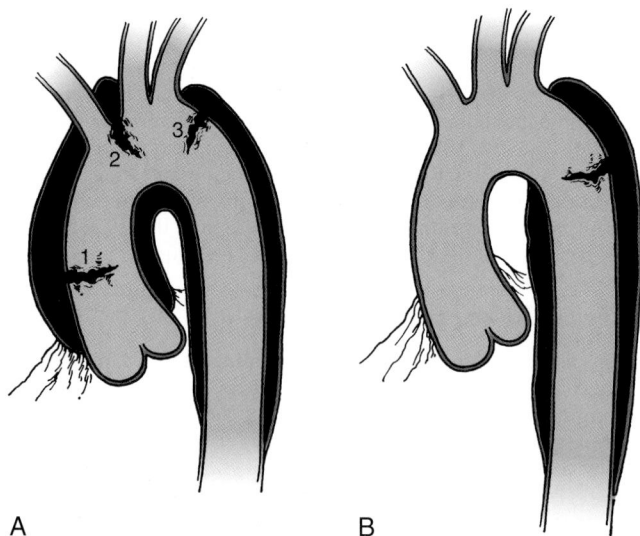

Figure 21-21   Stanford classification of aortic dissection. In type A aortic dissection, the ascending aorta is dissected regardless of the location or number of intimal tears *(A)*. In type B aortic dissection, the dissection is limited to the descending aorta *(B)* distal to the origin of the left subclavian artery. *(Reprinted from Daily PO, Trueblood HW, Stinson EB, et al: Management of acute aortic dissections. Ann Thorac Surg 10:237–247, 1970, by permission of Society of Thoracic Surgeons.)*

BOX 21-5. POTENTIAL COMPLICATIONS OF ACUTE TYPE A AORTIC DISSECTION

- Cardiac tamponade
- Aortic regurgitation
- Myocardial infarction
- Stroke
- Limb ischemia
- Mesenteric ischemia

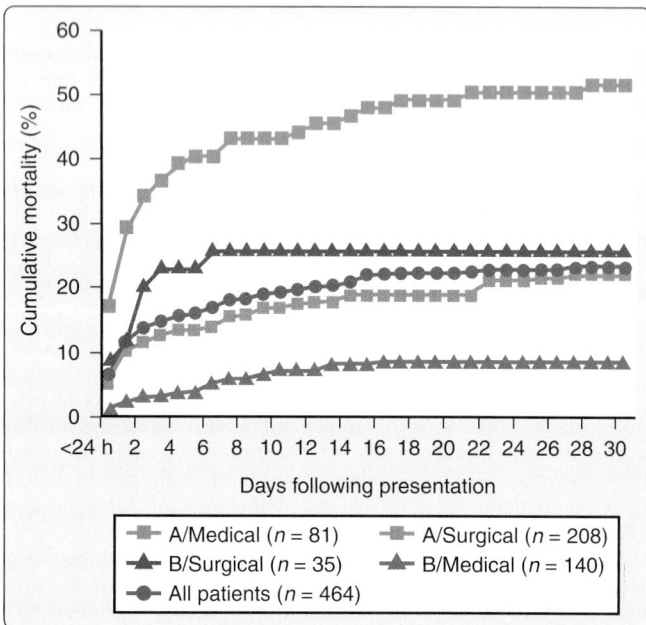

Figure 21-22   Thirty-day mortality in 464 patients from the International Registry of Aortic Dissection (IRAD) stratified by medical and surgical treatment in both type A and type B aortic dissection. *(From Nienaber CA, Eagle KA: Aortic dissection: New frontiers in diagnosis and management. Part I: From etiology to diagnostic strategies. Circulation 108:631, 2003.)*

TABLE 21-15	Mortality in Acute Aortic Dissection According to Dissection Type and Management	
Dissection Type	*N*	*Hospital Mortality (%)*
Stanford type A	289	101 (34.9)
Medical management	81	47 (58.0)
Surgical management	208	54 (26.0)
Stanford type B	175	26 (14.9)
Medical management	140	15 (10.7)
Surgical management	35	11 (31.4)

Data from Hagan PG, Nienaber CA, Isselbacher EM, et al: The International Registry of Acute Aortic Dissection (IRAD). New insights into an old disease. *JAMA* 283:897, 2000.

TABLE 21-16	Complications of Acute Stanford Type A Aortic Dissection (n = 513)	
Complications		*Percentage*
All neurologic defects		18.0
Coma/altered consciousness		14.0
Myocardial ischemia/infarction		10.0
Limb ischemia		10.0
Mesenteric ischemia/infarction		4.0
Acute renal failure		6.2
Hypotension		26.0
Cardiac tamponade		17.0
Mortality		30.0

Data from Bossone E, Rampoldi V, Nienaber CA, et al: Usefulness of pulse deficit to predict in-hospital complications and mortality in patients with acute type A aortic dissection. *Am J Cardiol* 89:851, 2002.

TABLE 21-17	Penn Classification of Ischemic Presentations in Acute Stanford Type A Aortic Dissection	
Type A Dissection Presentation	Definition	Mortality Rate
Penn presentation a Type Aa	Type A dissection with absence of ischemia	3.1%
Penn presentation b Type Ab	Type A dissection with branch vessel malperfusion producing clinical organ ischemia (e.g., stroke, renal failure, ischemic extremity, mesenteric ischemia)	25.6%
Penn presentation c Type Ac	Type A dissection with circulatory collapse (systolic blood pressure < 80 mm Hg and/or vasopressor therapy) with or without cardiac involvement	17.6%
Penn presentation b + c Type A b + c	Types Ab and Ac together	40%

Data from Augoustides JG, Geirsson A, Szeto W, et al: Observational study of mortality risk stratification by ischemic presentation in patients with acute type A aortic dissection: The Penn classification. *Nat Clin Pract Cardiovasc Med* 6:140, 2009

Pennsylvania (Penn classification: Table 21-17).[127] An aortic dissection less than 2 weeks old is classified as acute and older than 2 weeks is classified as chronic. This distinction is clinically important because after 2 weeks, mortality risk has plateaued and thus emergency surgery is not necessarily indicated.

Type B Aortic Dissection

Aortic dissections confined to the descending thoracic aorta (Stanford type B) should be managed medically unless there are life-threatening complications present such as malperfusion, aortic rupture, as well as severe pain and/or hypertension despite aggressive medical therapy (ACC/AHA Class I recommendation; level of evidence B).[1,124] Mortality with medical management in this type of aortic dissection is significantly lower than perioperative mortality (see Table 21-15).[1,124,125] The greater operative mortality is due to the severe complications of type B aortic dissection and the operation itself. TEVAR for the therapy of complicated acute type B dissection is highly recommended (STS guideline: Class I recommendation; level of evidence A).[1,20]

Aortic Intramural Hematoma

Aortic intramural hematoma (IMH) is a variant of the classic aortic dissection (Table 21-18).[1,124,125] IMH has no intimal flap with no obvious intimal tear on aortic imaging. This class of intimal tear comprises about 17% of all dissections, with a 30-day mortality rate of 24%: 36% in type A IMH and 12% with type B IMH ($P < 0.05$).[126] Surgical management of type A IMH reduces mortality rate by 61.1% (14% vs. 36%; $P = 0.02$). Medical management for type B IMH reduced mortality fourfold (8% vs. 33%; $P < 0.05$).[126] Surgical indications in type A IMH include ascending aortic diameter larger than 50 mm or

TABLE 21-18	Aortic Intramural Hematoma
Diagnostic Criteria	
Crescent-shaped or circumferential thickening of aortic wall	
Hematoma thickness > 7 mm	
No dissection flap	
No intimal tear	
No blood flow within hematoma	
Risk Factors for Mortality or Progression	
Ascending aorta or arch involvement (type A)	
Aortic diameter > 45 mm	
Hematoma thickness > 11 mm	

IMH thickness more than 12 mm. Surgical indications in type B IMH include rapid progression, rupture, or severe clinical symptoms despite aggressive medical therapy. It is, therefore, reasonable to manage IMH similar to classic aortic dissection in the corresponding thoracic aortic segment (ACC/AHA Class IIa recommendation; level of evidence C).[1] Although IMH may be caused by rupture of the vas vasorum in the aortic wall without intimal hematoma, there are frequently small intimal tears that are beyond the resolution of current aortic scanners and are only identifiable on close aortic inspection during surgery or autopsy.[1,127-130]

Clinical Diagnosis and Imaging Studies for Aortic Dissection

Aortic dissection is more common in men and has a peak incidence in later life.[1,124,125] It often has an earlier onset in the setting of Marfan syndrome, Ehlers-Danlos syndrome, Loeys-Dietz syndrome, bicuspid aortic valve, aortic coarctation, and familial aortic dissection.[1,124,125] It also is commonly associated with hypertension but less so with atherosclerosis.[17] Further predisposing factors include pregnancy, cocaine abuse, arteritis, aortic trauma, and aortic instrumentation.[1]

The pain of aortic dissection typically is severe, abrupt in onset, and has a ripping, tearing, or stabbing quality (ACC/AHA Class I recommendation; level of evidence B).[1] Highly suggestive physical findings include a pulse deficit, a systolic blood pressure limb differential greater than 20 mm Hg, focal neurologic deficit, and a new murmur of AR (ACC/AHA Class I recommendation; level of evidence B).[1] Besides a chest radiograph (ACC/AHA Class I recommendation; level of evidence C) and an electrocardiogram (ACC/AHA Class I recommendation; level of evidence B), urgent and definitive aortic imaging (TEE, CT, MRI) is strongly recommended in suspected aortic dissection (ACC/AHA Class I recommendation; level of evidence B).[1] A negative chest radiograph should not delay aortic imaging, especially in patients suspected of presenting with aortic dissection (ACC/AHA Class I recommendation; level of evidence B).[1] The selection of an aortic imaging modality should be guided by patient and institutional variables, including immediate test availability (ACC/AHA Class I recommendation; level of evidence C).[1] If initial aortic imaging is negative in the setting of high clinical suspicion for dissection, a second imaging study should be arranged (ACC/AHA Class I recommendation; level of evidence C).[1]

The most common imaging study is contrast-enhanced spiral CT or CTA because it is widely available. Typical findings in acute aortic dissection include an intimal flap, luminal displacement of intimal calcifications, and aortic dilation (Figure 21-23).[124,125] IMH appears as a crescent-shaped high-attenuation thickening of the aortic wall in noncontrast CT (Figure 21-24).[124,125] CT can demonstrate rupture, branch-vessel involvement, and false lumen extent. Although MRI has a near 100% sensitivity and specificity, and is widely available, it also takes significantly longer than CT (Figure 21-25).[1,124,125]

At experienced centers, TEE provides high-resolution aortic images with comparable sensitivity and specificity to MRI and CT.[1,124,125] Furthermore, TEE can look for complications by interrogating the aortic valve (AR severity and mechanism), assessing ventricular function including regional wall motion for coronary dissection, and diagnosing cardiac tamponade and pericardial effusion. Aortic dissection appears on TEE examination as an undulating intimal flap within the aorta separating a true and false lumen (Figure 21-26). It is sometimes difficult to distinguish the true lumen from the false lumen, but the true lumen tends to be smaller with pulsatile high-velocity flow in systole. Doppler color-flow imaging can detect flow communication between the true and false lumens at intimal tear sites. Aortic IMH appears as an echo-dense crescent-shaped thickening (>7 mm) of the aortic wall that may contain echolucent pockets of noncommunicating blood (see Figure 21-24). TEE also may distinguish clinical mimickers of aortic dissection and can assess the thoracic aortic anatomy in detail to guide surgical decision making.[131,132]

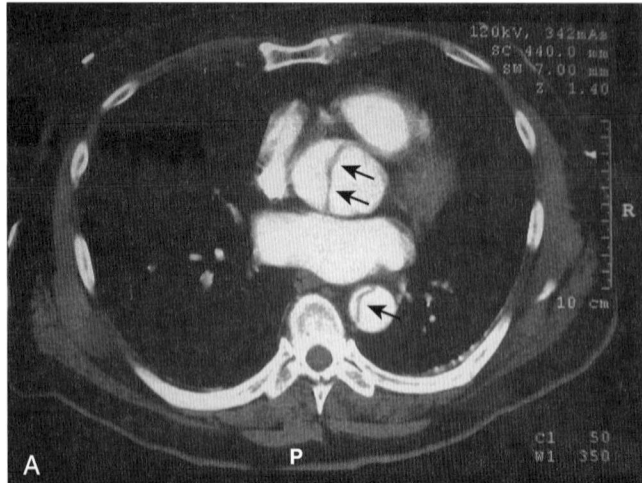

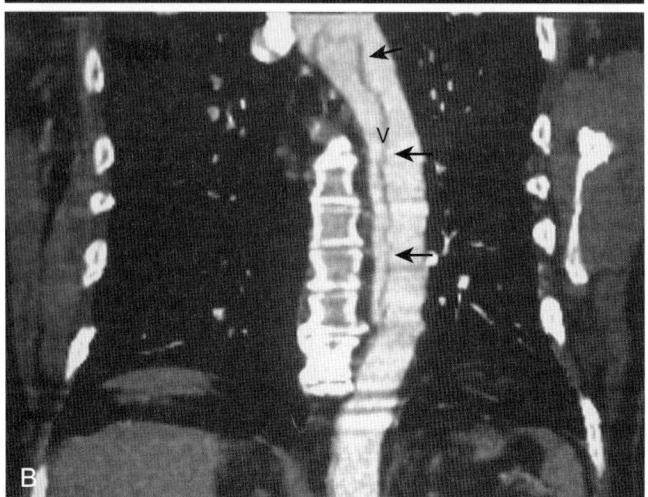

Figure 21-23 **Computed tomographic angiogram in a patient with a type A aortic dissection.** Axial images of the chest (*A*) demonstrated an intimal flap that extended from the ascending aorta (*double arrows*) into the descending thoracic aorta (*single arrow*). Sagittal reconstruction (*B*) demonstrated the presence of an intimal flap in the descending thoracic aorta (*single arrows*).

Anesthetic Management for Aortic Dissection

Acute aortic dissection is a medical emergency. Acute medical management is directed at treatment of pain and decreasing the arterial pressure with antihypertensive agents. Vasodilator therapy should be initiated to decrease wall stress with control of heart rate and blood pressure (ACC/AHA Class I recommendation; level of evidence C).[1] In the presence of acute AR, β-blockers should be used with caution because they block the compensatory tachycardia (ACC/AHA Class I recommendation; level of evidence C).[1] In the absence of contraindications, β-blockers should be titrated to a heart rate of 60 beats/min (ACC/AHA Class I recommendation; level of evidence C).[1] Esmolol is a particularly useful β-blocker because it has a short pharmacologic half-life and can be rapidly titrated. Esmolol can be administered as an initial bolus of 5 to 25 mg intravenously, followed by a continuous infusion of 25 to 300 μg/kg/min. In patients with β-blocker contraindications, heart rate control should be gained with titration of nondihydropyridine calcium channel blockers such as verapamil or diltiazem (ACC/AHA Class I recommendation; level of evidence C).[1] Alternatively, labetalol, a drug that has a 1:7 ratio of β-blocker to α-blocker activity, can be administered as a 20 to 80 mg intravenous bolus followed by an infusion at 0.5 to 2.0 mg/min. Metoprolol, a cardioselective β-blocker,

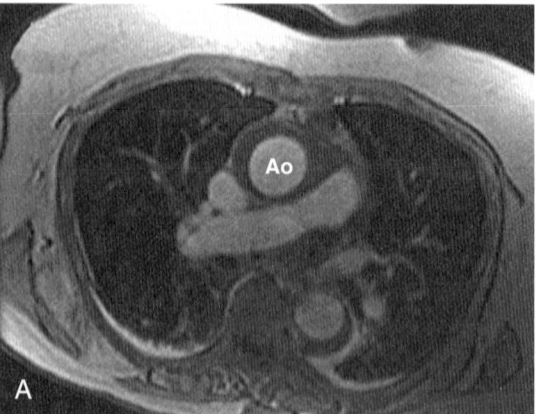

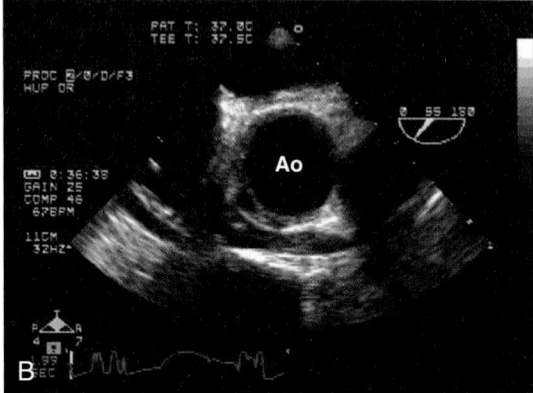

Figure 21-24 **Computed tomographic angiogram of the chest (*A*) and transesophageal echocardiographic upper esophageal short-axis images of the aorta (*B*)** demonstrating an aortic intramural hematoma that extended from the ascending aorta into the descending thoracic aorta. A crescent-shaped or circumferential thickening of the aortic wall is diagnostic for aortic intramural hematoma. Ao, aorta.

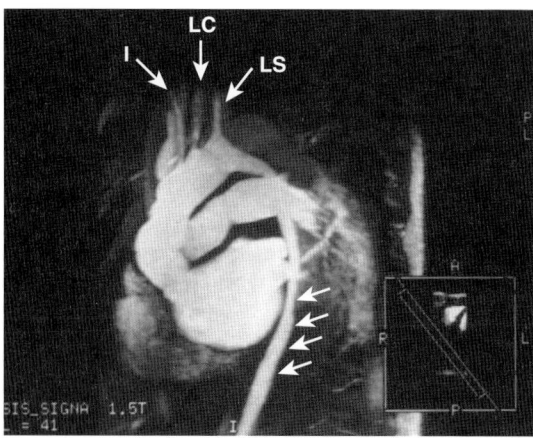

Figure 21-25 **Magnetic resonance imaging of the chest** with gadolinium contrast injection in a patient with a type A aortic dissection. The dissection extended into the innominate artery (*I*), left carotid artery (*LC*), left subclavian artery (*LS*), and into the descending aorta (*arrows*).

may be advantageous in patients with reactive airway disease who are sensitive to β-adrenergic antagonists. Metoprolol is administered at a dose of 5 to 15 mg intravenously every 4 to 6 hours. If the systolic blood pressure remains greater than 120 mm Hg with adequate heart rate control, then vasodilators (e.g., nitroprusside at a dosage of 0.5 to 2.0 μg/kg/min or nicardipine at a dose of 1 to 15 mg/hr) should be

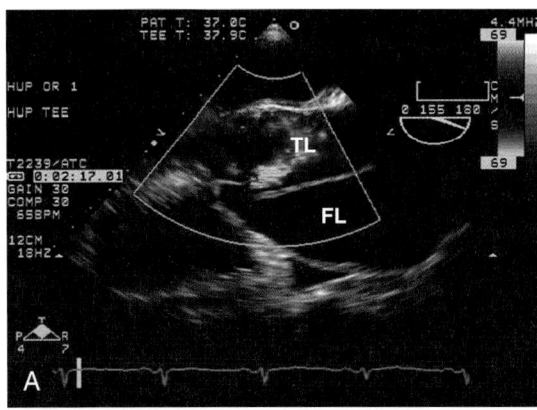

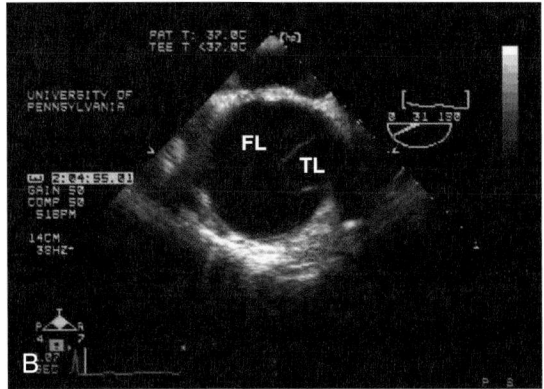

Figure 21-26   **Transesophageal echocardiographic midesophageal long-axis image of the aortic valve (A) and short-axis image of the ascending aorta (B) in a patient with a type A aortic dissection.** An intimal flap separating the true lumen *(TL)* of the aorta with the false lumen *(FL)* was demonstrated in the aortic root and ascending aorta. Extension of the dissection into the aortic root may cause aortic regurgitation or coronary insufficiency.

titrated for further reductions of blood pressure while still maintaining adequate vital organ perfusion (ACC/AHA Class I recommendation; level of evidence C).[1] Vasodilator therapy should not be initiated before heart rate control to avoid the associated reflex tachycardia that might aggravate the aortic dissection (ACC/AHA Class III recommendation; level of evidence C).[1]

In general, the anesthetic management of type A aortic dissection resembles the management of ascending aortic aneurysms that require DHCA. The anesthetic management of type B aortic dissections resembles the management of TAAA repair. Large-bore intravenous catheters are essential for intravenous medications and rapid volume expansion. A radial arterial catheter for invasive blood pressure monitoring is preferred over a femoral artery catheter to allow for CPB cannulation, depending on surgeon preference. If a pulse deficit is detected, the site for arterial pressure monitoring should be chosen to best represent the central aortic pressure. A central venous or PAC to monitor CVP, pulmonary artery pressure, and cardiac output is useful. TEE insertion is performed after anesthetic induction.

Critically unstable patients should be resuscitated by standard ACC/AHA guidelines or by securing the airway, providing mechanical ventilation, and administering drugs to support the circulation. Emergent TEE should follow to verify the diagnosis of type A aortic dissection and to detect cardiac tamponade, hypovolemia, AR, and/or heart failure. If TEE detects cardiac tamponade, immediate sternotomy with preparations to institute CPB via femoral artery cannulation should be performed. Opening the pericardium and relief of cardiac tamponade can be followed by hypertension causing aortic rupture.

The induction of general anesthesia in hemodynamically stable patients with aortic dissection should proceed in a cautious manner.

The dose of intravenous antihypertensive drugs may need to be reduced at the time of anesthetic induction to prevent severe hypotension when combined with anesthetic drugs. Hypotension also may occur on anesthetic induction in response to the attenuation of sympathetic nervous system tone or decreased cardiac preload caused by venodilation and positive pressure ventilation in patients with preexisting concentric left ventricular hypertrophy. The hypertensive response to endotracheal intubation, TEE probe insertion, and sternotomy should be anticipated and attenuated with narcotic analgesics.

Surgical Treatment of Stanford Type A Aortic Dissection

Surgical repair for type A aortic dissection requires resection of the proximal extent of the dissection. A partially dissected aortic root may be repaired with aortic valve resuspension. A destroyed aortic root must be replaced with a composite graft or a valve-sparing root replacement. In the setting of a DeBakey type II dissection, the entire dissected aorta merits replacement. CABG sometimes is necessary for aortic dissections that involve the coronary ostia. These surgical principles are all highly recommended (ACC/AHA Class III recommendation; level of evidence C).[1]

Although femoral arterial cannulation is popular for CPB, recent evidence suggests that it is associated with adverse clinical outcomes including death, stroke, and malperfusion syndromes.[133,134] Cannulation of the distal ascending aorta or the axillary artery (ideally with an end-to-end graft) has been associated with significantly enhanced clinical outcome as compared with standard femoral arterial cannulation.[133,134] It remains important to monitor cerebral perfusion throughout the operative procedure for detection and correction of acute malperfusion.[46–48]

In DeBakey type I dissections, the dissected descending thoracic aorta often undergoes aneurysmal degeneration and is responsible for significant aorta-related mortality in the long term.[135] Consequently, long-term outcomes after extensive type A dissection would be significantly improved if this distal aortic degeneration could be prevented.[135,136] Recent clinical series have demonstrated the efficacy and safety of anterograde stenting of the descending thoracic aorta during open aortic arch repair for DeBakey type 1 aortic dissection.[137–139] This technique is also known as the endovascular stented elephant-trunk technique or the frozen elephant-trunk technique. The long-term aneurysmal degeneration of the descending thoracic aorta is prevented by immediate stenting in the acute dissection phase; thus, favorable long-term aortic remodeling is facilitated.

Integrated Management of Stanford Type B Aortic Dissection

Uncomplicated type B aortic dissection currently has the best clinical outcome when managed medically.[20] Medical therapy for type B aortic dissection is directed at control of systemic hypertension to prevent aortic aneurysm formation, aortic rupture, and extension of the aortic aneurysm (ACC/AHA Class I recommendation; level of evidence C).[1] Combination therapy with a diuretic, β-blocker, angiotensin-converting enzyme inhibitor, or other antihypertensive agents usually is necessary to achieve and maintain blood pressure less than 130/80 mm Hg. All patients after repair of type A aortic dissection also should be managed aggressively with antihypertensive therapy because many are left with a residual distal aortic dissection after repair. Serial imaging of the aorta is necessary to detect expansion of the aortic lumen and aneurysm development that may warrant surgical correction.

In the presence of life-threatening complications, TEVAR has emerged as a preferred alternative therapy to surgery.[20,82,140,141] A recent landmark randomized trial demonstrated that, in the short term, TEVAR added no survival advantage over medical management for uncomplicated type B aortic dissection.[142] However, because TEVAR did improve aortic remodeling in this trial, further adequately powered trials are indicated to test whether this translates into better aortic outcomes.[143] Malperfusion syndromes associated with type B dissection also can be managed with intimal fenestration.[144]

PENETRATING ATHEROSCLEROTIC ULCER

Penetrating atherosclerotic ulcer describes an isolated disruption of the intimal layer of the aortic wall at the site of atheromatous disease (Figure 21-27).[1] This class of intimal tear may occur at any aortic locus but is most common in the descending thoracic aorta. It typically is associated with severe aortic atheroma in the elderly and penetrates through to the aortic adventitia.[1] It may have associated IMH or pseudoaneurysm.[145] Initial symptoms include chest and back pain similar to aortic dissection.[1] Diagnosis typically is made with contrast-enhanced CT.[146] Although patients may be managed medically, TEVAR has emerged as a major management strategy, especially in severely symptomatic or complicated presentations (STS Class IIa recommendation; level of evidence C).[20,147,148] Furthermore, in asymptomatic presentations of this intimal syndrome, TEVAR currently is not recommended (STS Class IIa recommendation; level of evidence C).[20]

TRAUMATIC AORTIC INJURY

The most common cause of traumatic aortic injury is blunt chest trauma or rapid deceleration injuries associated with motor vehicle accidents or falls. Although this injury may be fatal, the majority of patients have injuries in the region of the aortic isthmus.[149] Patients with traumatic aortic injury commonly will have associated significant injuries. TEE is helpful in the management of traumatic aortic injury because it is portable, is often available in the OR, provides a rapid diagnosis, and does not require aortic instrumentation or radiographic contrast injection. TEE also can detect cardiac tamponade, left pleural effusion, hypovolemia, ventricular dysfunction from myocardial contusion, or vascular injuries from penetrating chest wounds.[150] Its

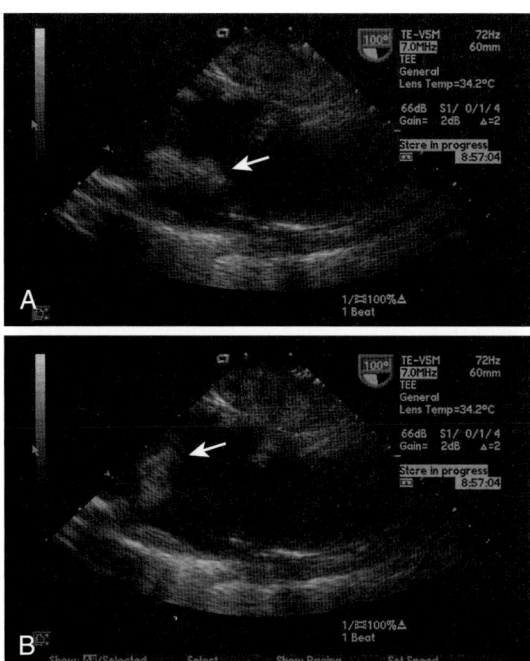

Figure 21-27 Transesophageal echocardiographic (TEE) long-axis images of the descending thoracic aorta demonstrating severe atherosclerotic disease with atheroma protruding into the vessel lumen. Images obtained in diastole (A) and in systole (B) demonstrated a large mobile atheroma (arrow) that may represent an atheromatous plaque that has ruptured and detached from the aortic wall.

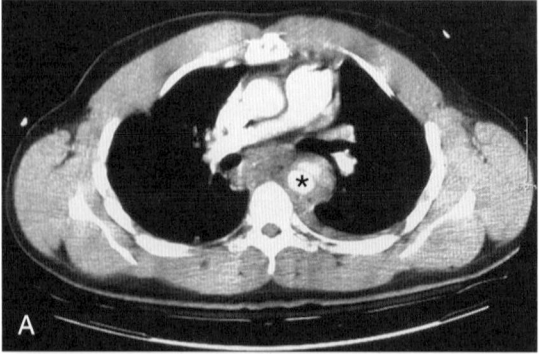

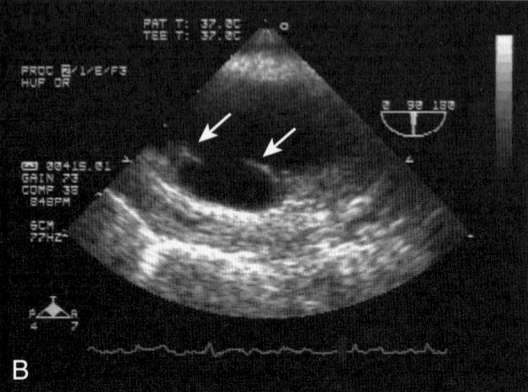

Figure 21-28 Computed tomographic angiogram of the chest (A) in a trauma patient who presented with a widened mediastinum on the chest roentgenogram demonstrating traumatic intimal disruption of the aorta in the region of the aortic isthmus (asterisk). Perivascular hematoma and extravasation of contrast agent into the mediastinum and left pleural cavity indicated a rupture of the descending aorta. Intraoperative transesophageal echocardiographic (TEE) long-axis image of the proximal descending thoracic aorta (B) demonstrated a thick mural flap (arrows) and surrounding hematoma at the site of the intimal disruption.

disadvantages include limited imaging in the setting of facial injuries, suspected cervical spine injuries, and lesions in the distal ascending aorta. The characteristic features of traumatic aortic injury detected by TEE are a mural flap at the site of intimal disruption and regional deformities of the aortic wall caused by the contained rupture (Figure 21-28). The mural flap commonly is limited to a 1- to 2-cm aortic segment located at the aortic isthmus just distal to the origin of the left subclavian artery. This mural flap usually is thick compared with the intimal flap seen in aortic dissection and is less mobile because it usually contains several layers of the vessel wall. Contrast-enhanced CT is frequently selected for aortic imaging because these patients typically require CT scanning as part of their initial diagnostic evaluation.[151]

Injuries to the ascending aorta or aortic arch typically require CPB with DHCA for repair. Injuries to the aortic isthmus can be repaired via a left thoracotomy. The descending thoracic aorta usually is repaired with an interposition graft with the aid of PLHB. The risk for perioperative spinal cord ischemia is minimal when distal aortic perfusion is provided (Table 21-19) because only a short segment of the thoracic aorta is replaced. Although open repair is possible, TEVAR has emerged as the preferred intervention whenever possible because of the well-documented outcome advantages (STS Class I recommendation; level of evidence B).[20,151–153]

AORTIC ATHEROMATOUS DISEASE

Severe aortic atheroma is a major risk factor for stroke.[1,20] Thoracic aortic replacement is indicated for serious embolism and to facilitate the conduct of concomitant cardiac procedures that require the

TABLE 21-19	Incidence of Postoperative Paraplegia after Surgical Repair of Traumatic Aortic Injury in Relation to Operative Technique	
Operative Technique	No. of Patients	Paraplegia (%)
Clamp and sew	73	16.4*†
Distal aortic perfusion	134	4.5
Gott shunt	4	0
Full CPB	22	4.5
Partial CPB	39	7.7
Centrifugal pump	69	2.9*

*$P < 0.004$, distal aortic perfusion vs. clamp and sew.
†$P < 0.01$, centrifugal pump vs. clamp and sew.
CPB, cardiopulmonary bypass.
Data from Fabian TC, Richardson JD, Croce MA, et al: Prospective study of blunt aortic injury: Multicenter trial of the American Association for the Surgery of Trauma. *J Trauma* 42:374, 1997.

safe cross-clamping of the aorta (see Figure 21-27). The anesthetic management of patients undergoing thoracic aortic reconstruction for atheromatous disease resembles the management of thoracic aortic aneurysms for corresponding aortic segments. Intraoperative epiaortic ultrasound imaging is superior to manual palpation or TEE for thoracic aortic atheroma.[154,155] The epiaortic ultrasound is important for selecting the optimal site for aortic cannulation for CPB or placement of the aortic cross-clamp to minimize atheroembolic events such as stroke.[154,155]

TAKAYASU ARTERITIS

Takayasu arteritis is a chronic vasculitis that affects primarily the thoracic aorta, its branches, and even the pulmonary artery (Figure 21-29).[1] Takayasu arteritis occurs most frequently in young Asian women and occurs worldwide. Its onset is insidious with the gradual development of vascular insufficiency. Dilation and aneurysm formation also may occur in diseased aortic segments. Diagnostic criteria include onset of disease at age younger than 40 years, claudication of the extremities, decreased brachial pulses, a systolic blood pressure differential of 10 mm Hg between the arms, subclavian or abdominal aortic bruits, and angiographic demonstration of narrowing of the aorta and/or its primary branches.[1]

Initial therapy consists of high-dose corticosteroids (ACC/AHA Class I recommendation; level of evidence B).[1] Elective revascularization should be postponed until the acute inflammatory state has been adequately treated (ACC/AHA Class I recommendation; level of evidence B).[1] Anesthetic management of Takayasu arteritis is complicated by limited sites for arterial blood pressure measurement. The femoral artery may be the only site for accurate measurement of central aortic pressure in patients with stenosis of both subclavian arteries.

AORTIC COARCTATION

Aortic coarctation is a common malformation that ranges from a discrete narrowing of the aorta to a long hypoplastic segment of the vessel to complete discontinuity of the aorta (Figure 21-30).[156] The site of coarctation can be variable but is typically juxtaductal in location, affecting the proximal descending thoracic aorta just distal to the origin of the left subclavian artery. The distal descending aorta often is hypoplastic in severe cases. Conditions associated with aortic coarctation include Turner syndrome, bicuspid aortic valve, ventricular septal defect, patent ductus arteriosus, and intracerebral aneurysm.[1,156]

Adults with coarctation may present with headache, epistaxis, heart failure, or lower extremity claudication. Its typical hemodynamic profile is upper extremity hypertension combined with lower extremity hypotension and weak pulses. If the origin of the left subclavian artery is distal to the coarctation, blood pressure in the arms also may be diminished. The chest radiograph often shows rib notching caused by the enlarged intercostal arteries that serve as collateral vessels to supply the lower body. The electrocardiogram often shows left ventricular hypertrophy. The diagnosis is confirmed by definitive aortic imaging. Cardiac catheterization, MRI, and echocardiography are useful to detect associated cardiac abnormalities (see Chapter 20).

Balloon angioplasty with stenting is the preferred treatment when coarctation is limited to a discrete segment of the aorta.[156,157] Although sedation often will suffice for the procedure, general anesthesia may be required when dilation of the coarctation is expected to be painful or when it is necessary to keep the patient immobile for the procedure. Complications of balloon angioplasty have included residual stenosis, recoarctation, paracoarctation aortic dissection or rupture, aortic aneurysm, and injury to the femoral artery. Aortic dissection or aneurysm at

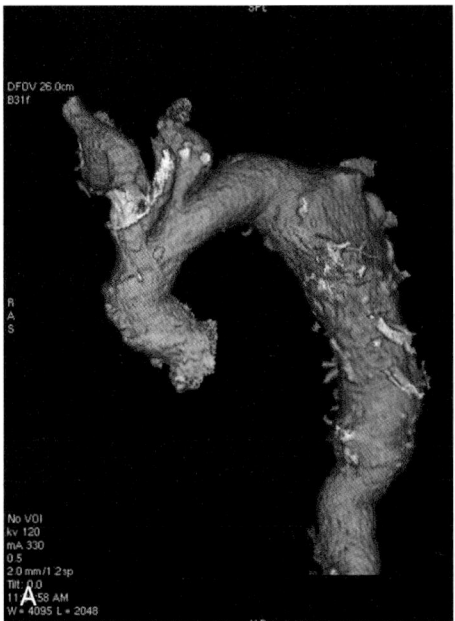
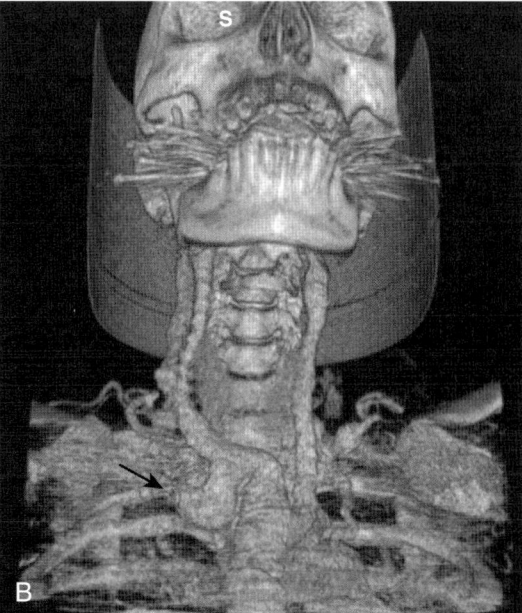

Figure 21-29 **Three-dimensional reconstruction from a computed tomographic angiogram of the aorta (A) and aortic arch branch vessels (B) from a patient with Takayasu arteritis.** The reconstructions demonstrated aneurysmal dilation of the descending thoracic aorta, proximal innominate artery, and both subclavian arteries. The left and right (arrow) subclavian arteries were occluded distal to the aneurysm.

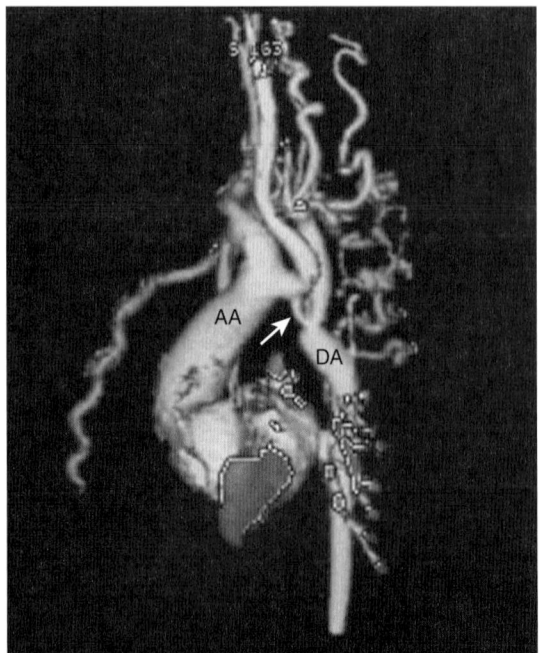

Figure 21-30 **Three-dimensional reconstruction from a computed tomographic angiogram of a patient with aortic coarctation.** In this patient, the site of coarctation was located between the left carotid and left subclavian arteries *(arrow)*. Repair was performed by construction of an extra-anatomic bypass graft between the ascending *(AA)* and descending *(DA)* thoracic aorta.

or near the angioplasty site may be a consequence of mechanical damage to the aortic wall or congenital defects of the aortic wall.

Operative repair in adults may involve interposition graft repair or extra-anatomic bypass grafting from the proximal aorta or left subclavian artery to the descending aorta. Extra-anatomic bypass is advantageous for reoperations or in adults when the distal aortic arch cannot be mobilized to perform an end-to-end anastomosis. Avoiding surgical dissection in the region of the distal aortic arch also decreases the risk for injury to the recurrent laryngeal and phrenic nerves. Although perioperative mortality is low, spinal cord ischemia is possible during repair if collateral circulation is inadequate or if distal aortic perfusion pressure is too low. Preventive strategies include intraoperative monitoring of distal aortic perfusion pressure, neuromonitoring with SSEPs and/or MEPs, deliberate hypothermia, and distal aortic perfusion with PLHB.[158] Postoperative hypertension after repair may require aggressive monitoring and management.

ILLUSTRATIVE TRANSESOPHAGEAL ECHOCARDIOGRAPHY CASES

Case Study 1

Thoracic Aortic Atheroma

A 78-year-old man with diabetes and hypertension presented for CABG for triple-vessel disease. He had severe peripheral vascular disease. After induction of general anesthesia, a TEE was performed.

Framing

Because this patient has advanced atherosclerosis with multiple risk factors, it is likely that his thoracic aorta will have extensive atheromatous disease. Thoracic aortic atheroma is a major risk factor for stroke, especially in the setting of intraoperative aortic manipulation and instrumentation. What is the surgical plan in this case: Is this CABG on-pump or off-pump? If there is significant aortic atheroma, then the ascending aortic manipulation associated with aortic cannulation and

cross-clamping for on-pump CABG would likely be associated with significant atheroembolism and a significant stroke risk. The cardiac surgeon requests an assessment of the atheroma burden in the thoracic aorta to guide the conduct of the CABG.

Questions

What is the extent of the thoracic aortic atheroma? Which aortic segments are involved? What is the severity of the aortic atheroma? Is there severe atheroma with a high embolic risk in the thoracic aortic segment involved in the planned procedure? In this case of planned CABG, the ascending aorta is the aortic segment of interest.

Data Collection

Severe thoracic aortic atheroma is characterized by atheroma protrusion larger than 5 mm into the aortic lumen or mobile atheroma, or both. Severe protruding and mobile atheroma, as depicted in Figures 21-31 to 21-35, disseminated throughout the descending thoracic aorta and aortic arch, make it likely that the ascending aorta also is involved with severe atheroma because advanced atheroma is a disseminated arterial process. The detection of severe thoracic aortic atheroma by TEE, therefore, represents a major opportunity to modify surgical decision making to minimize stroke risk in the setting of heavy aortic atheroma burden.

Discussion

In this CABG scenario, there are at least three broad options for minimizing aortic atheroembolism and stroke:

1. Guided by epiaortic scanning, manipulate the least-diseased ascending aortic segments and proceed with on-pump CABG.
2. Avoid ascending aortic manipulation and proceed with off-pump CABG with a no-touch aortic technique.
3. Cannulate the axillary artery for CPB and replace the severely diseased ascending aorta and proximal arch under DHCA. This would not only minimize the long-term stroke risk because of massive proximal aortic atheroma burden, but would allow completion of the CABG on-pump with minimal risk for cerebral atheroembolism.

In this case, after extensive discussion with the cardiac surgeon, the joint decision was to proceed with off-pump CABG, given the high likelihood of severe ascending aortic disease and the considerable experience of the surgeon with this off-pump CABG technique.

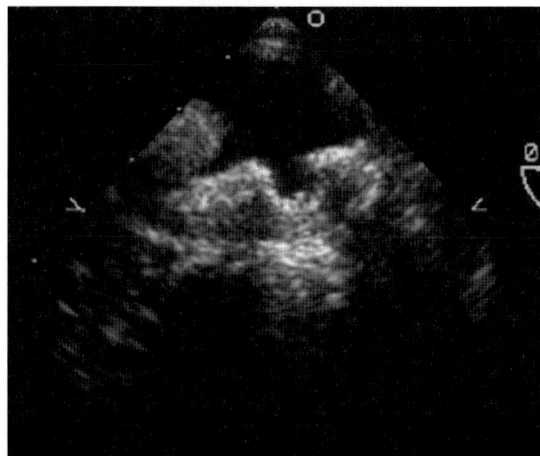

Figure 21-31 **Short-axis view of the descending thoracic aorta.** There is severe aortic atheroma greater than 5 mm in diameter. This large atheroma is sessile and does not appear to have any mobile components. There are no associated complications of aneurysm or dissection apparent on this view. This severe aortic atheroma predicts severe atheroma in the aortic arch and ascending aorta, as well as a high perioperative stroke risk associated with surgical aortic manipulation.

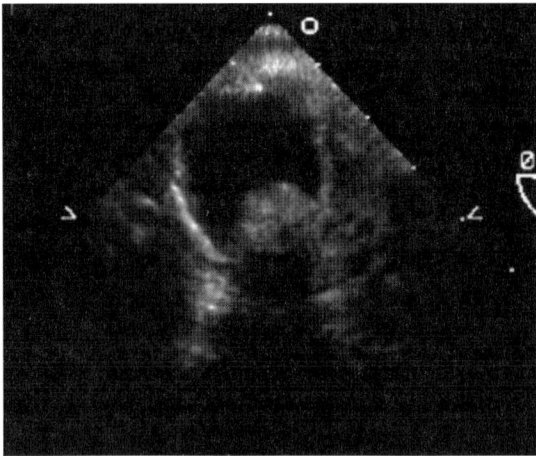

Figure 21-32 Short-axis view of the descending thoracic aorta. In this aortic segment, there is also severe sessile aortic atheroma with a diameter greater than 5 mm. Notice the variation in morphology as compared with another descending thoracic aortic segment, as in Figure 21-31. When severe atheroma are detected, it is important to comprehensively evaluate the entire thoracic aorta as in this patient. Multiple thoracic aortic views demonstrate severe aortic atheroma. It is clear that this patient has a severe atheroma burden based not only on the severity but also on the extent.

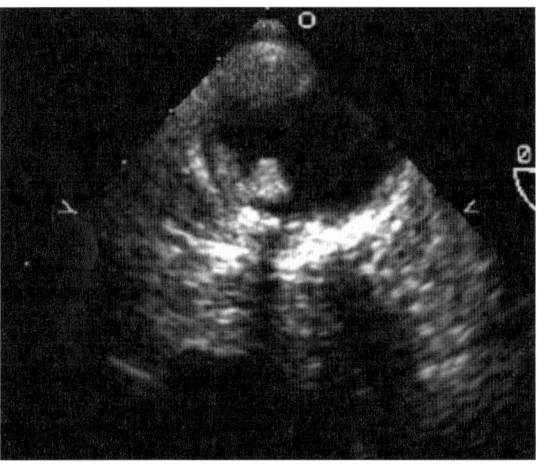

Figure 21-33 Short-axis view of the descending thoracic aorta. Again, there is severe aortic atheroma with variations in morphology. There is a pedunculated mobile atheroma that is at high risk for embolism downstream in the aorta. Taken together, Figures 21-31 through 21-33 show that this patient has a heavy atheroma burden throughout his descending thoracic aorta. Because atheroma is seldom a selective disease process, this atheroma burden is likely in the ascending aorta and aortic arch.

Severe aortic arch and descending thoracic aortic atheroma also are major risk factors for stroke after TEVAR, especially with lesions of the proximal descending thoracic aorta that necessitate hardware manipulation in the aortic arch with the associated risk for arch atheromatous cerebral embolism. This principle also is applicable to the stroke risk associated with transfemoral aortic valve implantation in which the hardware has to cross retrograde across the aortic arch to reach the aortic valve. In this scenario, the detection of severe mobile atheroma provides a strong rationale to proceed with transapical aortic valve implantation because the hardware would not cross the aortic arch but would proceed anterograde to the aortic valve through the left ventricular apex.

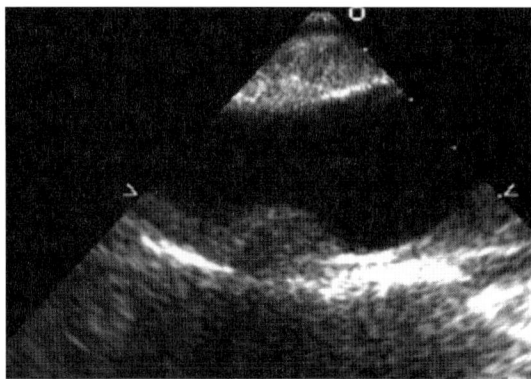

Figure 21-34 Long-axis view of the aortic arch. There is severe focal sessile aortic atheroma evident in this view. Notice that there is relative sparing of the surrounding intima. There is no evidence of penetrating atheromatous ulceration with associated aneurysm or intramural hematoma. This severe atheromatous disease present in the aortic arch is in keeping with the atheroma burden in the descending thoracic aorta. This patient has a high perioperative stroke risk that focuses attention on the conduct of the coronary artery surgery to minimize this risk.

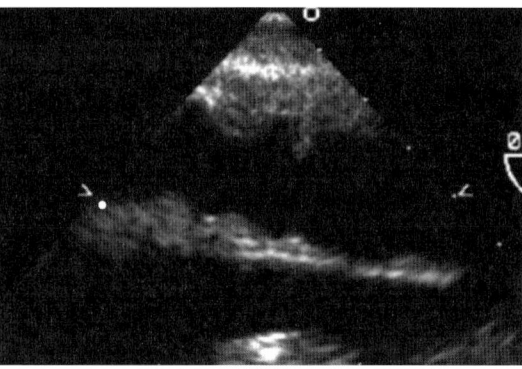

Figure 21-35 Long-axis view of the aortic arch. There is severe aortic atheroma not only because of a thickness greater than 5 mm but also because of the presence of a mobile pedunculated atheroma. These features further highlight the heavy atheroma burden of the aortic arch and the high stroke risk in this patient associated with on-pump coronary artery bypass grafting.

Severe atheroma of the aortic arch and distal thoracic aorta are important in procedures such as acute type A dissection in which femoral arterial cannulation commonly is performed for arterial access required for bypass. This cannulation strategy would carry a significant retrograde cerebral atheroembolic risk. The presence of severe atheroma as demonstrated by TEE provides a strong rationale to proceed with anterograde arterial flow via cannulation of the axillary artery. Furthermore, the atheroma burden of this patient also provides a strong rationale to avoid intra-aortic balloon counterpulsation. In summary, the assessment of thoracic aortic atheroma (extent, severity, embolic risk) should be related to the operative plan to minimize the risks for vital organ atheroembolism.

Case Study 2

Acute Thoracic Aortic Dissection

A 45-year-old man with known Marfan syndrome presented to the emergency department with severe acute tearing back pain. Physical signs suggestive of acute aortic dissection included a pulse deficit, severe jugular venous distention, and a new precordial murmur. His chest radiograph showed a widened mediastinum, and his electrocardiogram was consistent with sinus tachycardia with no acute ischemia. Because of severe hemodynamic instability, he was transferred emergently to the OR before definitive aortic imaging could be undertaken. After his resuscitation and anesthetic induction, a TEE was performed.

Framing

Because this patient has multiple highly suggestive features, there is a high pre-TEE probability of acute thoracic aortic dissection. Time matters here because the mortality rate is about 1% to 2% per hour. The diagnosis needs to be confirmed. The dissection extent should be characterized to guide definitive management. The known complications of acute aortic dissection should be assessed. The TEE examination serves multiple purposes including establishing the diagnosis, characterizing the full extent of the disease process, providing the data to guide operative decision making, and assessing the results of the surgical repair. The cardiac surgeon requests a comprehensive echocardiographic assessment to guide surgical management of this hemodynamic emergency.

Questions

Is there an intimal flap compatible with acute aortic dissection? Is it type A or type B aortic dissection? Are there associated complications of the dissection process? Is there a pericardial effusion with tamponade physiology? What is the status of biventricular function? Are there regional wall motion abnormalities compatible with dissection of a major coronary artery? If so, which coronary artery? Is CABG required? Is there AR? If so, what is the severity and mechanism? Can the native aortic valve be resuspended or is aortic valve replacement required? Can the aortic root be spared or is aortic root replacement required? Does the descending thoracic aorta require endovascular stenting?

Data Collection

There is type A dissection that requires surgical intervention (Figures 21-36 to 21-41). The aortic root is dilated and dissected. The ascending aorta is dilated and dissected with extension into the aortic arch and descending thoracic aorta (DeBakey I extent) (See Videos 3 and 4). Although there is severe AR, the mechanisms are intimal prolapse and

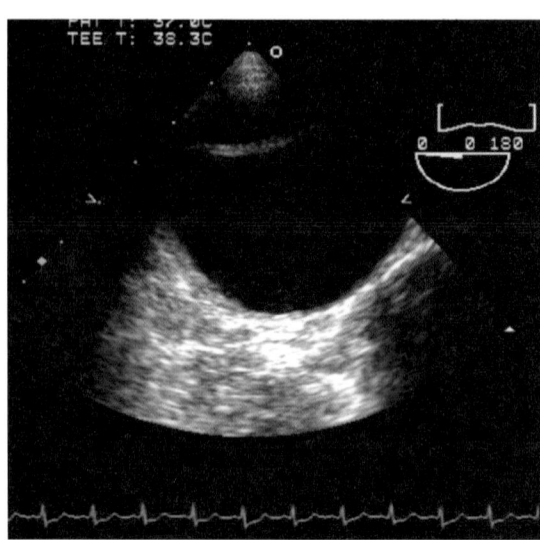

Figure 21-37 **Midesophageal short-axis view of the descending thoracic aorta (at zero degree of rotation).** An intimal dissection flap is evident. This view demonstrates that the extent of this type A dissection is compatible with a DeBakey type I aortic dissection. The descending thoracic aortic dissection can be addressed during open aortic arch repair with a thoracic endovascular aortic stent deployed anterograde through the open aortic arch. This is an example of the frozen elephant trunk technique, which is designed to improve long-term aortic remodeling and thus minimize the adverse outcomes associated with aneurysmal degeneration of the dissected descending thoracic aorta.

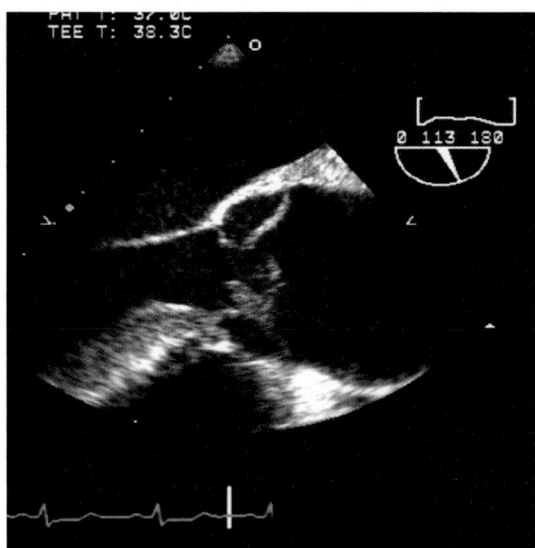

Figure 21-36 **Midesophageal long-axis view of the aortic valve and ascending aorta in systole before cardiopulmonary bypass (at 113 degrees of rotation).** There is an intimal dissection flap in the ascending aorta that not only has a large fenestration but is also prolapsing into the left ventricular outflow tract. This view confirms dissection proximal to the left subclavian artery (Stanford type A); thus, immediate surgical repair is indicated.

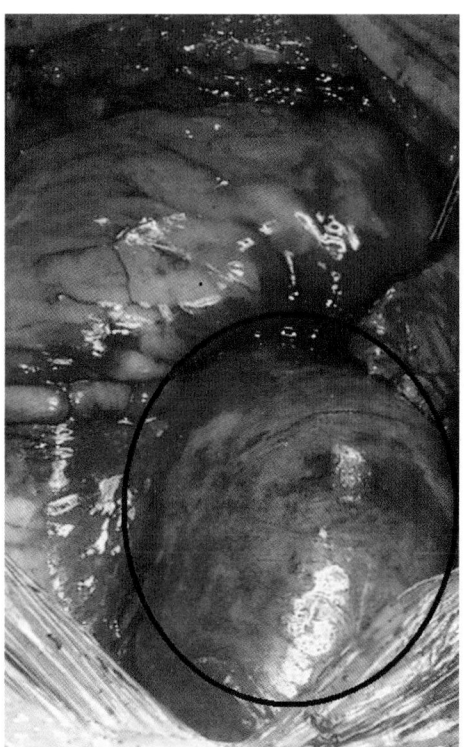

Figure 21-38 **Intraoperative photograph of the ascending aorta after sternotomy and pericardiotomy.** The ascending aorta is dissected: The wall is hemorrhagic and in places transparent through the adventitia (area indicated within the *black circle*). Aortic rupture was imminent in this case. The decision to operate emergently and proceed with proximal thoracic aortic replacement on cardiopulmonary bypass with deep hypothermic circulatory arrest was based on the transesophageal echocardiographic findings, as shown in Figures 21-36 and 21-37.

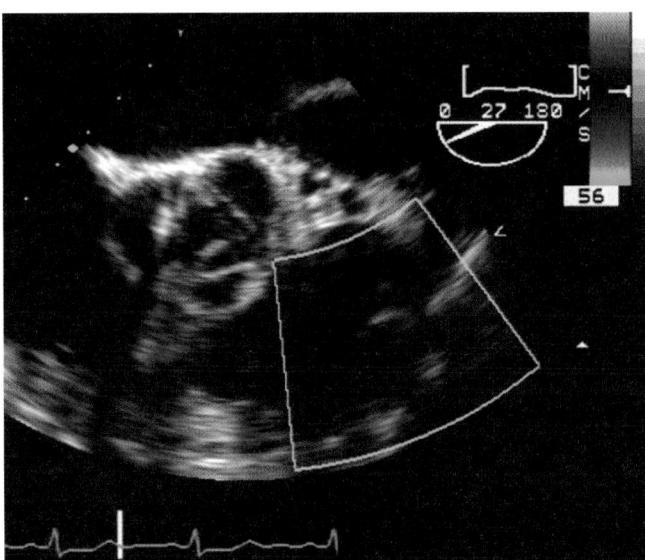

Figure 21-39   Midesophageal short-axis view of the aortic valve in diastole (at 27 degrees of rotation). The aortic leaflets appear normal. There is prolapse of the intimal dissection flap through the aortic valve, preventing diastolic coaptation and giving the appearance of a "double aortic valve." Severe aortic regurgitation results from this mechanism, as shown in Figure 21-41. This view also allows for assessment of right ventricular function, in particular, right ventricular hypokinesis caused by ischemia from right coronary dissection. Color-flow Doppler interrogation in this view shows trace pulmonic insufficiency, a common incidental finding. There is also a small pericardial collection evident: This is the residual from the hemopericardium that was drained at pericardiotomy. Before pericardiotomy, the hemopericardium was under tension and had resulted in severe cardiac tamponade.

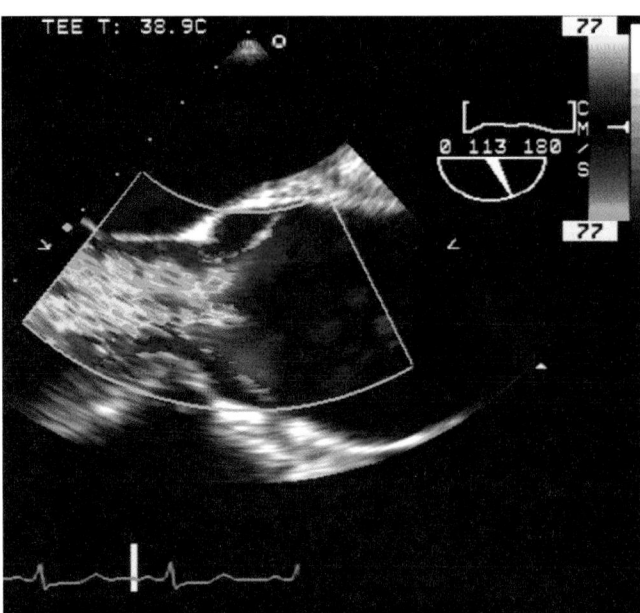

Figure 21-41   Midesophageal long-axis view of the aortic valve and ascending aorta in systole before cardiopulmonary bypass (at 113 degrees of rotation). Color-flow Doppler interrogation reveals severe aortic regurgitation, as the diastolic jet visualized by color Doppler imaging fills the entire left ventricular outflow tract. The mechanisms of this severe aortic regurgitation, namely, intimal prolapse and aortic root dilation, are more fully explained in Figures 21-39 and 21-40.

aortic root dilation without native aortic cusp destruction. There are no regional wall motion abnormalities to suggest myocardial ischemia from coronary dissection. There is a pericardial tamponade.

Discussion

In the emergency management of acute aortic dissection, the OR can function as a diagnostic suite where TEE is promptly performed after anesthetic induction, endotracheal intubation, and hemodynamic resuscitation. TEE is ideally suited for the fast-track management of this acute aortic syndrome. TEE offers near-100% sensitivity and specificity for the diagnosis and localization of aortic dissection. There are three possibilities in this diagnostic process: (1) surgery for type A dissection or complicated type B dissection; (2) medical therapy for uncomplicated type B dissection; and (3) there is no acute aortic syndrome, in which case, further diagnostic workup should proceed to identify and manage the cause.

In this case of type A dissection, the TEE examination not only provides the rationale for immediate surgical intervention but also guides the operative plan. The tense hemopericardium with clinical tamponade was managed with pericardiotomy; the immediate hemodynamic improvement and consequent hypertension were managed immediately to avoid aortic rupture. Because the AR was not related to native aortic cusp destruction, aortic valve resuspension was undertaken. The dissected aortic root was replaced and coronary reimplantation was by means of the button technique. The dissected ascending aorta and aortic arch were replaced. The aortic arch repair was with the hemiarch technique with DHCA. During the open aortic arch anastomosis, the dissected descending thoracic aorta was repaired by means of antero-grade deployment of an endovascular stent (frozen elephant-trunk technique). After separation from CPB, TEE demonstrated normal native aortic valve function, normal biventricular function with no regional wall motion abnormalities, and an endovascular stent in the descending thoracic aorta with no flow in the false lumen.

Acute type A dissection is a life-threatening surgical emergency. TEE is a standard of care in this acute aortic syndrome at all stages of its definitive management: prompt diagnosis, detection of complications, conduct of the operative repair, and acute evaluation of surgical results.

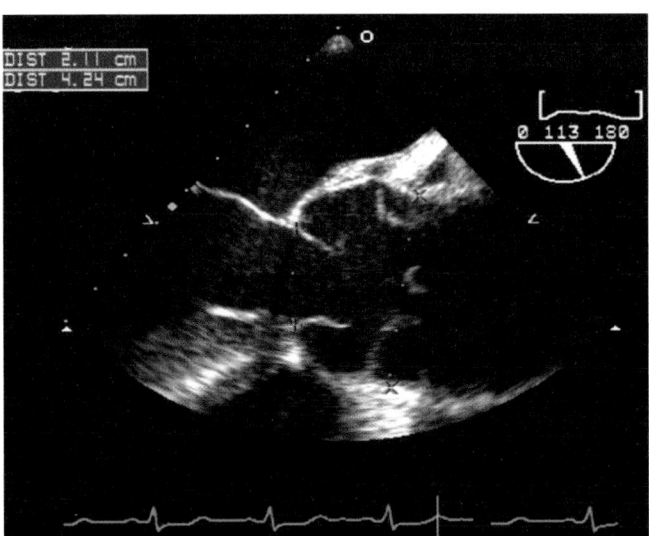

Figure 21-40   Midesophageal long-axis view of the aortic valve and ascending aorta in systole before cardiopulmonary bypass (at 113 degrees of rotation). An intimal dissection flap in the ascending aorta has a large fenestration. The sinotubular junction is splayed and dilated because of the dissection. This is a second mechanism for aortic regurgitation, as the dilated aortic root will result in diastolic aortic cusp separation. In this case, the intimal flap is also responsible for the severe aortic insufficiency, as shown in Figure 21-41.

Case Study 3
Thoracic Aortic Transection

A 42-year-old woman was involved in a motor vehicle accident. She was an unrestrained driver and sustained a side impact injury with no loss of consciousness. She had no significant medical history. She presented to the emergency department for evaluation. Her physical examination was within normal limits. Her chest radiograph showed a widened mediastinum. Although initially stable, the patient developed shock that was unresponsive to pressors and fluid resuscitation, and so the patient was emergently transferred to the OR for a diagnostic TEE and possible operative aortic repair. She underwent a TEE after induction of general anesthesia.

Framing

Because this patient likely has an acute aortic syndrome resulting from traumatic aortic transection, it is essential that TEE not only confirm the diagnosis but also fully characterize the aortic lesion. The location and extent of the aortic transection will determine the operative plan. The cardiac surgeon requests a detailed echocardiographic interrogation of the thoracic aorta to plan the surgical intervention. The surgeon asks whether the incision should be a sternotomy or left thoracotomy.

Clinical Questions

Is there a thoracic aortic transection? If so, what is the extent? Which thoracic aortic segments are involved? Is endovascular aortic repair possible? If not, should the surgeon expose the thoracic aorta via sternotomy or left thoracotomy? What perfusion techniques are required? Is full CPB with DHCA required? Is PLHB required?

Data Collection

The TEE examination confirms thoracic aortic transection localized to the aortic arch with brachiocephalic involvement (Figures 21-42 to 21-48). The ascending aorta and descending thoracic aorta, including the isthmus, are not involved. In other words, there is no extension either proximal or distal to the aortic arch. This transection and associated IMH involve most of the aortic arch. There is contained rupture of the aortic arch.

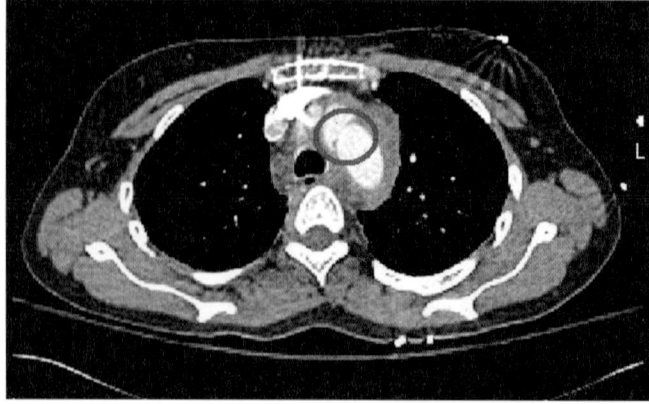

Figure 21-43 **Computed tomographic scan of the thoracic aorta done soon after hospital admission.** The aortic arch is circled in red. This aortic arch view shows aortic arch disruption compatible with a transection, given the history of a recent automobile accident.

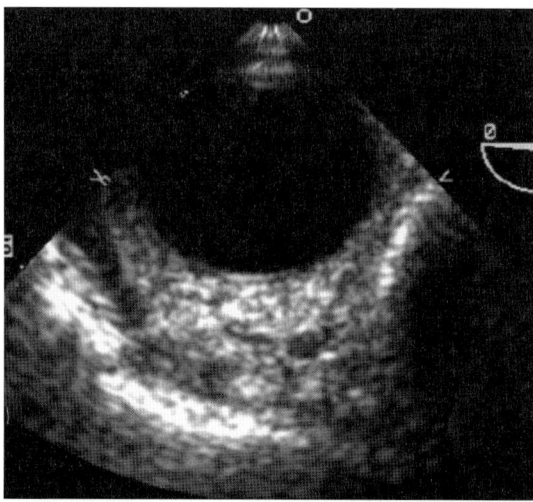

Figure 21-44 **Upper esophageal transesophageal echocardiographic short-axis view of the distal ascending aorta (at zero degree of rotation).** No intimal flap is compatible with dissection. However, there is extensive anterior intramural hematoma.

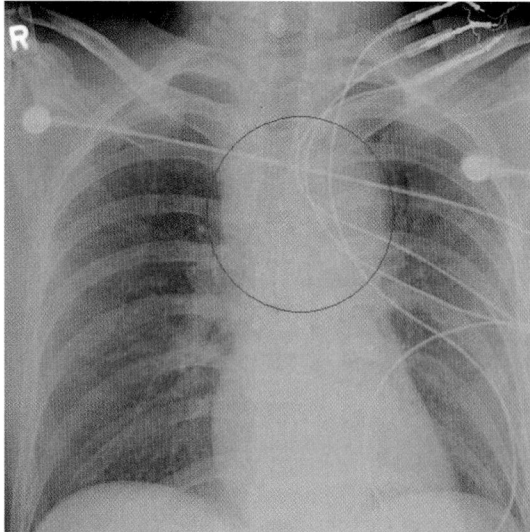

Figure 21-42 **Chest radiograph taken on hospital admission.** Note the widened mediastinum (area enclosed by the *red circle*). This finding is suggestive of a thoracic aortic syndrome. Although a chest radiograph may be suggestive, it is important to remember that a normal chest radiograph does not reliably rule out major thoracic aortic pathology.

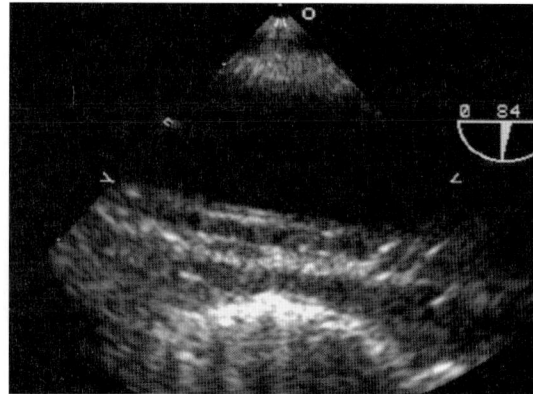

Figure 21-45 **Upper esophageal transesophageal echocardiographic (TEE) long-axis view of the midaortic arch (at 84 degrees of rotation).** There is no intimal flap compatible with dissection. There is extensive anterior intramural hematoma, as evidenced by the extensive anterior aortic wall thickening.

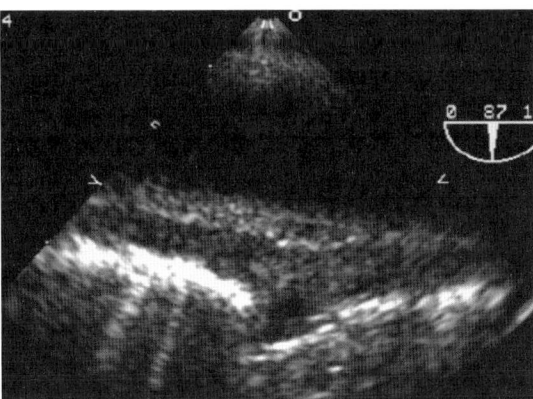

Figure 21-46 **Upper esophageal transesophageal echocardiographic (TEE) long-axis view of the midaortic arch (at 87 degrees of rotation).** There is extensive anterior intramural hematoma with a break in the aortic wall, compatible with a significant near-full thickness tear in the aortic arch. This view is diagnostic of focal traumatic transection of the aortic arch.

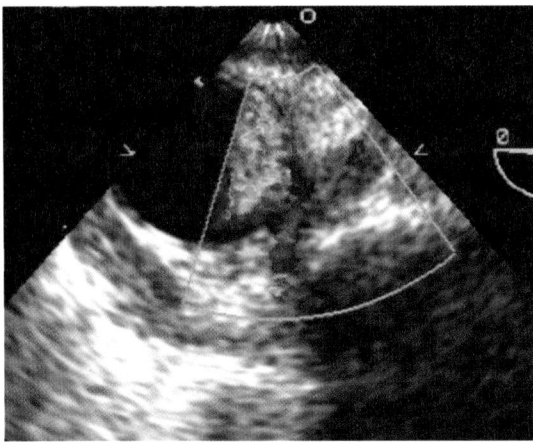

Figure 21-47 **Upper esophageal transesophageal echocardiographic (TEE) short-axis view of the distal aortic arch (at zero degree of rotation).** Color-flow Doppler interrogation in this view shows flow into the site of the arch transection. This flow is still contained by periaortic hematoma evident at this aortic level. The next step in the evolution of this pathology is free aortic rupture, a lethal event.

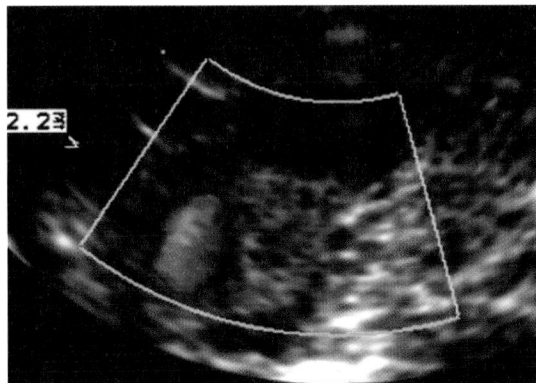

Figure 21-48 **Transcutaneous short-axis views of the right carotid artery and right internal jugular vein.** There is extensive hematoma around the lumen of the carotid artery. Color-flow Doppler interrogation of the carotid artery demonstrates intact flow. There is no obvious carotid dissection. These views indicate extension of the mural hematoma into the brachiocephalic vessels. Hence the brachiocephalic vessels at the level of the aortic arch may require reconstruction. These findings suggest a total aortic arch replacement with brachiocephalic reconstruction, a major surgical procedure.

Discussion

The TEE examination suggests that the aortic arch requires extensive acute repair. Although acute endovascular aortic arch repair may be possible in the future, acute total arch endovascular repair is not currently part of standard thoracic aortic endovascular intervention. The current endovascular technology still consists mainly of tubular components with no fenestrations or branches. Given that this is a young patient with minimal comorbidities, the thoracic aorta was accessed anteriorly via sternotomy, and a total aortic arch repair with CPB and DHCA was performed (Figures 21-49 and 21-50). If the patient was elderly with multiple comorbidities, a hybrid aortic arch repair might

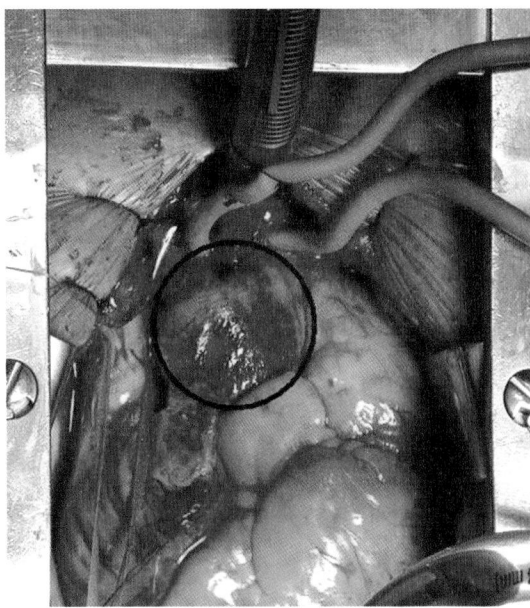

Figure 21-49 **Intraoperative photograph of the thoracic aorta after sternotomy.** There is extensive intramural hematoma evident in the proximal aortic arch (area enclosed by the *black circle*).

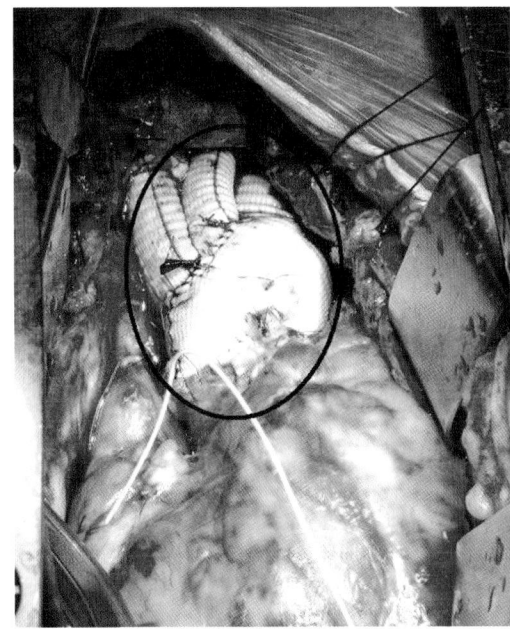

Figure 21-50 Intraoperative photograph of the aortic arch after cardiopulmonary bypass and deep hypothermic circulatory arrest (area enclosed by the black circle). The entire aortic arch has been replaced with a trifurcated prosthetic graft.

have been considered. In this procedure, the brachiocephalic arteries are transposed to the ascending aorta to create the landing zone for aortic arch stenting. This procedure is typically performed off-pump via sternotomy: Stent deployment can be anterograde through the ascending aorta or retrograde via the femoral artery.

This case of aortic arch transection is unusual. About 85% to 90% of aortic transactions occur at the aortic isthmus, just distal to the left subclavian artery. The remaining 10% occur in the reminder of the thoracic aorta, including the ascending aorta, the aortic arch, and the distal descending aorta. TEE clearly images the thoracic aortic segments where the overwhelming majority of aortic transections occur. The blind spot of TEE is the distal ascending aorta and proximal aortic arch, where transections are rare. Furthermore, in the setting of chest trauma, TEE also can evaluate the heart for evidence of further traumatic injury that may significantly affect perioperative management. Traumatic myocardial contusion may be evidenced by regional wall motion abnormalities that may be severe enough to mandate inotropic support. Traumatic hemopericardium with cardiac tamponade may require surgical drainage. The tricuspid valve also is at risk for traumatic rupture. Significant tricuspid regurgitation may mandate surgical repair or replacement.

In this case, TEE showed an acute aortic arch transection with extensive brachiocephalic vessel involvement. After total aortic arch replacement, the patient had an uncomplicated hospital course and a complete recovery.

Case Study 4

Bicuspid Aortic Valve

A 43-year-old man presented with progressive heart failure. His father had undergone aortic valve replacement at 50 years of age. His physical examination was compatible with advanced AR. Transthoracic echocardiography showed severe AR and a possible bicuspid valve. Coronary catheterization excluded significant CAD. He was referred for aortic valve surgery. The patient expressed a strong preference to avoid chronic anticoagulation after surgery. He requested aortic valve repair (see Chapter 19).

Framing

Because this patient has symptomatic AR, he has qualified for surgical intervention. In the setting of a bicuspid aortic valve and patient preference for valve repair, valve anatomy and the mechanism of AR strongly determine the feasibility of successful valve repair. Furthermore, because the bicuspid valve is associated with aortic dilation, the diameters of the aortic root and ascending aorta must be assessed for possible replacement at the time of surgery. The current thoracic aortic guidelines recommend consideration of proximal thoracic aortic replacement when the diameter exceeds 40 mm to avoid the future risks for rupture and dissection.

Questions

Is there a bicuspid valve? Is the valve calcified? Is there aortic stenosis? Is there AR? If so, what are the severity and mechanism of the AR? Is the valve anatomy compatible with successful valve repair? What are the aortic root diameters? What is the diameter of the ascending aorta? Is the proximal thoracic aorta dissected? Does the patient qualify for aortic root replacement? Does the patient qualify for ascending aortic replacement?

Data Collection

The aortic valve is bicuspid (Figures 21-51 to 21-58). There is no detectable aortic valve calcification and no aortic stenosis. There is severe eccentric AR because of anterior leaflet prolapse in the region of the raphe. Although mildly dilated, the aortic root does not qualify for replacement at this point. The ascending aorta is not dissected but has a diameter at the level of the pulmonary artery of 43 mm.

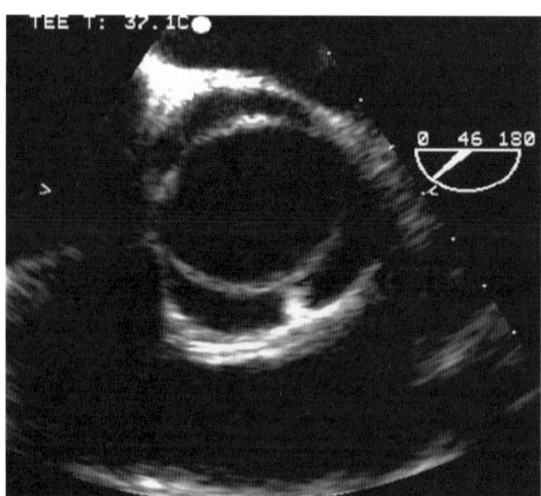

Figure 21-51 Midesophageal short-axis view of the aortic valve in systole (imaging angle of 46 degrees). The aortic valve is bicuspid with an anterior raphe evident. The aortic cusps appear normal. There is no restricted mobility evident in systole. The cross-sectional area of this bicuspid valve measured 3.2 cm^2. This was within the normal range even when indexed for body surface area.

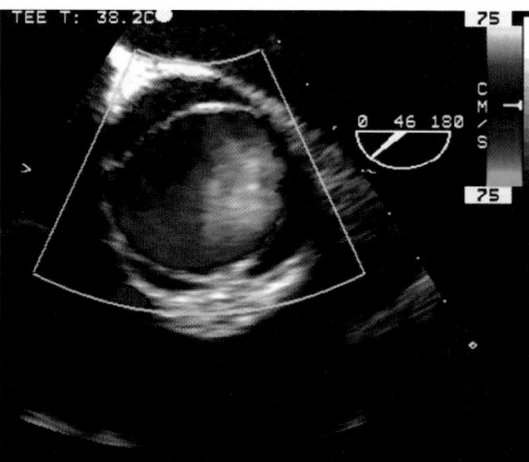

Figure 21-52 Midesophageal short-axis view of the aortic valve in systole (imaging angle of 46 degrees). Color-flow Doppler mapping shows laminar flow through the aortic valve consistent with an adequate valve area. There is no suggestion of aortic stenosis.

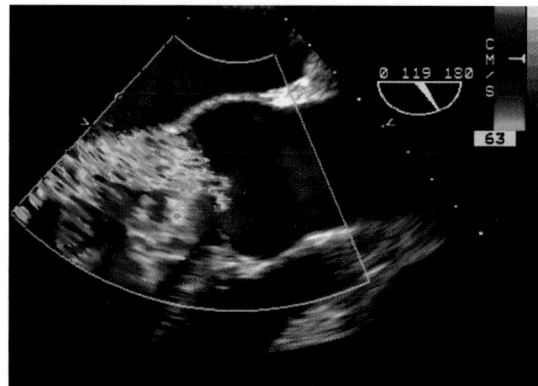

Figure 21-53 Midesophageal long-axis view of the aortic valve (imaging angle of 119 degrees). Color-flow Doppler imaging reveals severe aortic regurgitation. The jet of aortic regurgitation almost fills the entire left ventricular outflow tract. It is partly directed posteriorly toward the anterior mitral leaflet. This posterior eccentric flow may be caused by prolapse of the anterior aortic cusp or a perforation in the posterior cusp.

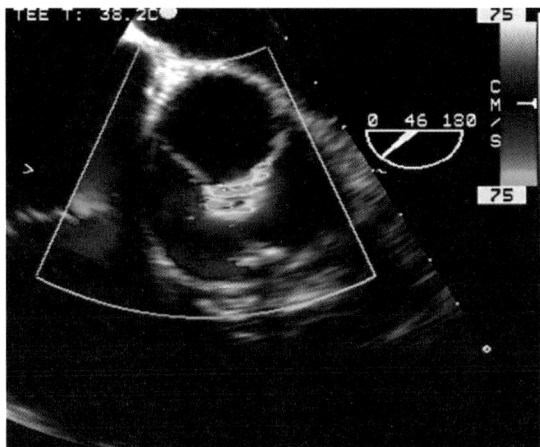

Figure 21-54 Midesophageal short-axis view of the aortic valve in diastole (imaging angle of 46 degrees). Color-flow Doppler imaging shows central commissural aortic regurgitation at the midpoint of the anterior cusp. This location of the regurgitation suggests focal prolapse of an aortic cusp. When considered together with the posterior eccentric flow evident in Figure 21-53, the mechanism for the aortic regurgitation in this case is focal prolapse of the anterior cusp in the region of the raphe. This identification of this focal mechanism suggests the possibility of a focal aortic valve repair.

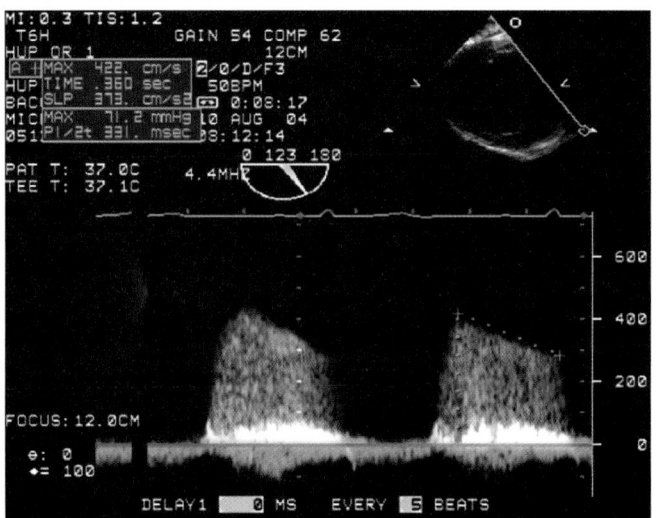

Figure 21-55 Transgastric long-axis view of the aortic valve (imaging angle of 123 degrees). Continuous-wave Doppler interrogation of the aortic valve shows significant aortic regurgitation (flow above the baseline). The pressure half-time has been quantified at 331 milliseconds, consistent with moderate aortic insufficiency. However, the final grading of the aortic insufficiency was severe when considered together with color-flow Doppler in Figure 21-53 and effects on the left ventricle in Figure 21-56. Because the jet of insufficiency is eccentric, it is possible to underestimate the peak diastolic velocity with continuous-wave Doppler. This is the probable explanation for the underestimation of the aortic regurgitation by the pressure half-time method. This underlines the importance of quantifying the valve lesion by multiple methods.

Discussion

Bicuspid aortic valve is common and is an established risk factor for ascending aortic aneurysm and type A aortic dissection. Although the anatomic orientation of bicuspid aortic cusps varies, the most common arrangement is anterior-posterior, as in this case. The anterior cusp has a raphe where the commissure between the right and left cusps would be in a tricuspid aortic valve. The anterior cusp usually is elongated and thus is prone to diastolic prolapse, as in this case.

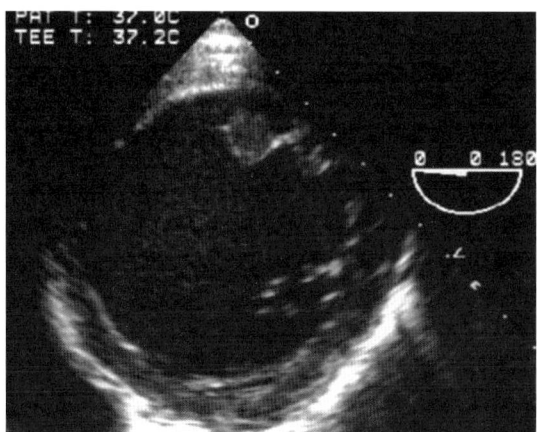

Figure 21-56 Transgastric midpapillary short-axis view of the left ventricle at end-diastole (imaging angle of zero degree). The left ventricle is severely dilated with an end-diastolic diameter of 6.5 cm. This is consistent with chronic severe aortic regurgitation.

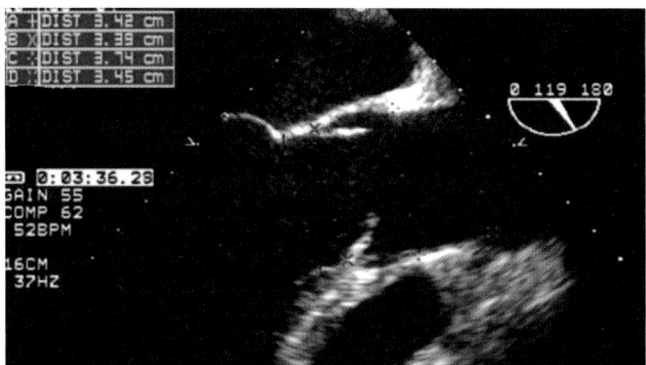

Figure 21-57 Midesophageal long-axis view of the aortic root (imaging angle of 119 degrees). The diameters of the left ventricular outflow tract (1), the aortic annulus (2), the sinuses of Valsalva (3), and the sinotubular junction (4) have been measured. These diameters are consistent with a mild degree of annular and root dilation, a common association with a bicuspid aortic valve. It is important that these diameters are accurately measured because excessive annuloaortic ectasia may dictate aortic root replacement with or without native aortic valve sparing.

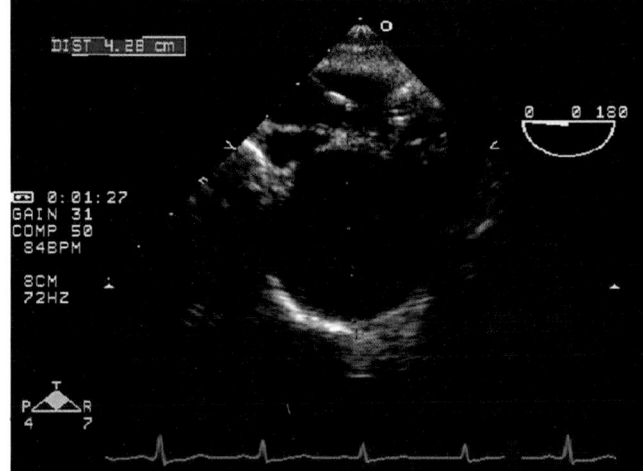

Figure 21-58 High esophageal transesophageal echocardiographic (TEE) short-axis view of the ascending aorta at the level of the pulmonary artery bifurcation (imaging angle of zero degrees). The diameter of the ascending aorta at this level is 4.3 cm.

The posterior cusp usually is normal. The TEE examination should focus on the anatomy, orientation, and mechanism of aortic insufficiency in bicuspid aortic valve cases. As in this case, the delineation of an otherwise competent aortic valve with focal prolapse merits strong consideration for repair. The ascending aorta and not the aortic root met criteria for aortic replacement in this young patient. The aortic arch also was mildly dilated.

In this case, surgical inspection of the aortic valve confirmed the TEE findings. The aortic root, although mildly dilated, did not merit intervention. The raphe of the anterior cusp was excised. The free prolapsing edge was excised in a triangular fashion as part of the anterior aortic leaflet valvuloplasty. The ascending aorta was replaced under DHCA with the addition of an aortic arch repair (hemiarch technique; DHCA time = 15 minutes). This complete resection of the ascending aorta was undertaken to avoid leaving the cross-clamped ascending aorta in situ because it was judged to be at a greater risk for future dissection. Furthermore, the aortic arch also was mildly dilated. This lower threshold for aggressive proximal thoracic aortic resection was undertaken because of the bicuspid aortic valve, the low operative risk of the patient, and the extensive experience of the thoracic aortic team. After separation from CPB, TEE demonstrated normal aortic valve function with no AR. There was no dissection in the residual native thoracic aorta. There was improved LV function. The patient had an uneventful recovery.

TEE provides important information in the planning of proximal thoracic aortic intervention in the setting of a bicuspid aortic valve. Thorough echocardiographic interrogation of the aortic valve, the aortic root, the ascending aorta, and aortic arch typically provides all the data required for operative decision making. The bicuspid aortic valve signals the presence of an abnormal proximal thoracic aorta that should be managed as carefully as the associated aortic valve dysfunction.

REFERENCES

1. Hiratzka LF, Bakris GL, Beckman JA, et al: ACCF/AHA/AATS/ACR/ASA/SCA/SCAI/SIR/STS/SVM guidelines for the diagnosis and management of patients with thoracic aortic disease: Executive summary. A report of the American College of Cardiology Foundation, American Heart Association Task Force on Practice Guidelines, American Association for Thoracic Surgery, American College of Radiology, American Stroke Association, Society of Cardiovascular Anesthesiologists, Society for Cardiovascular Angiography and Interventions, and Society for Vascular Medicine, *J Am Coll Cardiol* 55:1509, 2010.
2. Corbet AJ: Medical manipulation of the ductus arteriosus. In Garson A, Bricker T, Fisher D, Neish S, editors: *The Science and Practice of Pediatric Cardiology*, ed 2 Baltimore, 1997, Williams & Wilkins, pp 2489.
3. Kern MJ, Serota H, Callicoat P, et al: Use of coronary arteriography in the preoperative management of patients undergoing urgent repair of the thoracic aorta, *Am Heart J* 119:143, 1990.
4. Sanders JS, Ferguson DW, Mark AL: Arterial baroreflex control of sympathetic nerve activity during elevation of blood pressure in normal man: Dominance of aortic baroreflexes, *Circulation* 77:279, 1988.
5. Miceli A, Capoun R, Fino C, et al: Effects of angiotensin-converting enzyme inhibitor therapy on clinical outcome in patients undergoing coronary artery bypass grafting, *J Am Coll Cardiol* 54:1778, 2009.
6. Augoustides JG: Should all antihypertensive agents be continued before surgery? In Fleisher LA, editor: *Evidence-Based Practice of Anesthesiology*, ed 2 Philadelphia, 2009, Saunders Elsevier, p 49.
7. Horlocker TT, Wedel DJ, Rowlingson JC, et al: Regional anesthesia in the patient receiving antithrombotic or thrombolytic therapy, *Reg Anesth Pain Med* 35:64, 2010.
8. Augoustides JG, Cheung AT: Pro: Ultrasound should be the standard of care for central catheter insertion, *J Cardiothorac Vasc Anesth* 23:720, 2009.
9. Fergusson DA, Herbert PC, Mazer CD, et al: A comparison of aprotinin and lysine analogues in high-risk cardiac surgery, *N Engl J Med* 358:2319, 2008.
10. Augoustides JG: Aprotinin and renal dysfunction: What does history teach us? *Expert Opin Drug Saf* 8:5, 2009.
11. Hgaage DL, Bland JM: Lessons from aprotinin: Is the routine use and inconsistent dosing of tranexamic acid prudent? Meta-analysis of randomized and large matched observational studies, *Eur J Cardiothorac Surg* 37:1375–1383, 2010.
12. Murkin JM, Falter F, Granton J, et al: High-dose tranexamic acid is associated with nonischemic clinical seizures in cardiac surgical patients, *Anesth Analg* 110:350, 2010.
13. Tritapepe L, De Santis V, Vitale D, et al: Recombinant activated Factor VII for refractory bleeding after acute aortic dissection surgery: A propensity score analysis, *Crit Care Med* 35:1685, 2007.
14. Zangrillo A, Mizzi A, Biondi-Zoccai G, et al: Recombinant activated factor VII in cardiac surgery: A meta-analysis, *J Cardiothorac Vasc Anesth* 23:34, 2009.
15. Appoo JJ, Augoustides JG, Pochettino A, et al: Perioperative outcome in adults undergoing elective deep hypothermic circulatory arrest with retrograde cerebral perfusion in proximal aortic arch repair: Evaluation of protocol-based care, *J Cardiothorac Vasc Anesth* 20:3, 2009.
16. Lazar HL, McDonnell M, Chipkin SR, et al: The Society of Thoracic Surgeons practice guideline series: Blood glucose management during adult cardiac surgery, *Ann Thorac Surg* 87:663, 2009.
17. Elefteriades JA, Farkas EA: Thoracic aortic aneurysm, *J Am Coll Cardiol* 55:841, 2010.
18. Albornoz G, Coady MA, Roberts M, et al: Familial thoracic aortic aneurysms and dissections—incidence, modes of inheritance, and phenotypic patterns, *Ann Thorac Surg* 82:1400, 2006.
19. Augoustides JG, Wolfe Y, Walsh EK, et al: Recent advances in aortic valve disease: Highlights from a bicuspid aortic valve to transcatheter aortic valve replacement, *J Cardiothorac Vasc Anesth* 23:569, 2009.
20. Svensson LG, Kouchoukos NT, Miller DC, et al: Expert consensus document on the treatment of descending thoracic aortic disease using endovascular stent grafts, *Ann Thorac Surg* 85:S1, 2008.
21. Sinha A, Cheung AT: Spinal cord protection and thoracic aortic surgery, *Curr Opin Anaesthesiol* 23:195, 2010.
22. Brown JR, Block CA, Malenka DJ, et al: Sodium bicarbonate plus N-acetylcysteine prophylaxis: A meta-analysis, *JACC Cardiovasc Interv* 2:1116, 2009.
23. Mahajan A, Crowley R, Ho JK, et al: Imaging the ascending aorta and aortic arch using transesophageal echocardiography: The expanded aortic view, *Echocardiography* 25:408, 2008.
24. Nierich AP, van Zaane B, Buhre WF, et al: Visualization of the distal ascending aorta with A-mode transesophageal echocardiography, *J Cardiothorac Vasc Anesth* 22:766, 2008.
25. Augoustides JG, Hosalkar HH, Milas BL, et al: Upper gastrointestinal injuries related to perioperative transesophageal echocardiography: Index case, classification proposal, and call for a registry, *J Cardiothorac Vasc Anesth* 20:379, 2006.
26. Augoustides JG, Plappert T, Bavaria JE: Aortic decision-making in the Loeys-Dietz syndrome: Aortic root aneurysm and a normal-caliber ascending aorta and aortic arch, *J Thorac Cardiovasc Surg* 138:502, 2009.
27. Davies RR, Gallo A, Coady MA, et al: Novel measurement of relative aortic size predicts rupture of thoracic aortic aneurysms, *Ann Thorac Surg* 81:169, 2006.
28. Song HK, Bavaria JE, Kindem MW, et al: Surgical treatment of patients enrolled in the national registry of genetically triggered thoracic aortic conditions, *Ann Thorac Surg* 88:781, 2009.
29. Toda K, Taniguchi K, Masai T, et al: Arch aneurysm repair with long elephant trunk: A 10-year experience in 111 patients, *Ann Thorac Surg* 88:16, 2009.
30. Spielvogel D, Etz CD, Silovitz D, et al: Aortic arch replacement with a trifurcated graft, *Ann Thorac Surg* 83:S791, 2007.
31. Stein LH, Elefteriades JA: Protecting the brain during aortic surgery: An enduring debate with unanswered questions, *J Cardiothorac Vasc Anesth* 24:316–321, 2010.
32. Harrington DK, Fragomeni F, Bonser RS: Cerebral perfusion, *Ann Thorac Surg* 83:S799, 2007.
33. Abdul Aziz KA, Meduoye A: Is pH-stat or alpha-stat the best technique to follow in patients undergoing deep hypothermic circulatory arrest? *Interact Cardiovasc Thorac Surg* 10:271, 2010.
34. Cheung AT, Bavaria JE, Pochettino A, et al: Oxygen delivery during retrograde cerebral perfusion in humans, *Anesth Analg* 88:8, 1999.
35. Stecker MM, Cheung AT, Pochettino A, et al: Deep hypothermic circulatory arrest: I. Effects of cooling on electroencephalogram and evoked potentials, *Ann Thorac Surg* 71:14, 2001.
36. Shuhaiber JH: Evaluating the quality of trials of hypothermic circulatory arrest aortic surgery, *Asian Cardiovasc Thorac Ann* 15:449, 2007.
37. Reich DL, Horn M, Hossain S, et al: Using jugular bulb oxyhemoglobin saturation to guide onset of deep hypothermic circulatory arrest does not predict post-operative neuropsychological function, *Eur J Cardiothorac Surg* 25:401, 2004.
38. Percy A, Widman S, Rizzo JA, et al: Deep hypothermic circulatory arrest with high cognitive needs: Full preservation of cognitive abilities, *Ann Thorac Surg* 87:117, 2009.
39. Gega A, Rizzo JA, Johnson MH, et al: Straight deep hypothermic arrest: Experience in 394 patients supports its effectiveness as a sole means of brain preservation, *Ann Thorac Surg* 84:759, 2007.
40. Pochettino A, Cheung AT: Pro: Retrograde cerebral perfusion is useful for deep hypothermic circulatory arrest, *J Cardiothorac Vasc Anesth* 17:764, 2003.
41. Augoustides JG, Andritsos M: Innovations in aortic disease: The ascending aorta and aortic arch, *J Cardiothorac Vasc Anesth* 24:198–207, 2010.
42. Estrera AL, Miller CC, Lee TY, et al: Ascending and transverse aortic arch repair: The impact of retrograde cerebral perfusion, *Circulation* 118:S160, 2008.
43. Etz CD, Plestis KA, Kan FA, et al: Axillary cannulation significantly improves survival and neurologic outcome after atherosclerotic aneurysm repair of the aortic root and ascending aorta, *Ann Thorac Surg* 86:441, 2008.
44. Urbanski PP, Lenos A, Blume JC, et al: Does anatomical completeness of the circle of Willis correlate with sufficient cross-perfusion during unilateral cerebral perfusion, *Eur J Cardiothorac Surg* 33:402, 2008.
45. Morita S, Yasaka M, Yasumori K, et al: Transcranial Doppler study to assess intracranial arterial communication before aortic arch operation, *Ann Thorac Surg* 86:448, 2008.
46. Murkin JM: NIRS: A standard of care for CPB vs an evolving standard for selective cerebral perfusion? *J Extra Corpor Technol* 41:11, 2009.
47. Augoustides JG, Kohl BA, Harria H, et al: Color-flow Doppler recognition of intraoperative brachiocephalic malperfusion during operative repair of acute type A aortic dissection: Utility of transcutaneous carotid artery ultrasound scanning, *J Cardiothorac Vasc Anesth* 21:81, 2007.
48. Estrera AL, Garami Z, Miller CC, et al: Cerebral monitoring with transcranial Doppler ultrasonography improves neurologic outcome during repairs of acute type A aortic dissection, *J Thorac Cardiovasc Surg* 129:277, 2005.
49. Kazui T: Which is more appropriate as a cerebral protection method—unilateral or bilateral perfusion? *Eur J Cardiothorac Surg* 29:1039, 2006.
50. Malvindi PG, Scrascia G, Vitale N: Is unilateral antegrade cerebral perfusion equivalent to bilateral cerebral perfusion for patients undergoing aortic arch surgery? *Interact Cardiovasc Thorac Surg* 7:891, 2008.
51. Cook RC, Goa M, Macnab AJ, et al: Aortic arch reconstruction: Safety of moderate hypothermia and antegrade cerebral perfusion during systemic circulatory arrest, *J Card Surg* 21:158, 2006.
52. Kamiya H, Hagl C, Kropivnitskaya I, et al: The safety of moderate hypothermic lower body circulatory arrest with selective perfusion: A propensity score analysis, *J Thorac Cardiovasc Surg* 133:501, 2007.
53. Khaladji N, Shrestha M, Meck S, et al: Hypothermic circulatory arrest with selective antegrade cerebral perfusion in ascending and aortic arch surgery: A risk factor analysis for adverse outcome in 501 patients, *J Thorac Cardiovasc Surg* 135:908, 2008.
54. Minatoya K, Ogino H, Matsuda H, et al: Evolving selective cerebral perfusion for aortic arch replacement: High flow rate with moderate hypothermic circulatory arrest, *Ann Thorac Surg* 86:1827, 2008.
55. Etz CD, Luehr M, Kari FA, et al: Selective cerebral perfusion at 28 degrees C—is the spinal cord safe? *Eur J Cardiothoracic Surg* 36:946, 2009.
56. Ohno M, Omoto T, Fukuzumi M, et al: Hypothermic circulatory arrest: Renal protection by atrial natriuretic peptide, *Asian Cardioavsc Thorac Ann* 17:401, 2009.
57. Dewhurst AT, Moore SJ, Liban JB: Pharmacological agents as cerebral protectants during deep hypothermic circulatory arrest in adult thoracic aortic surgery: A survey of current practice, *Anaesthesia* 57:1016, 2002.
58. Cowan JA Jr, Dimick JB, Henke PK, et al: Surgical treatment of intact thoracoabdominal aortic aneurysms in the United States: Hospital and surgeon volume-related outcomes, *J Vasc Surg* 37:1169, 2003.
59. Livesay JJ, Cooley DA, Ventemiglia RA, et al: Surgical experience in descending thoracic aneurysmectomy with and without adjuncts to avoid ischemia, *Ann Thorac Surg* 39:37, 1985.

60. Roizen MF, Beaupre PN, Alpert RA, et al: Monitoring with two-dimensional transesophageal echocardiography: Comparison of myocardial function in patients undergoing supraceliac, suprarenal-infraceliac, or infrarenal aortic occlusion, *J Vasc Surg* 1:300, 1984.
61. Coselli JS, Bozinovski J, LeMaire SA: Open surgical repair of 2286 thoracoabdominal aortic aneurysms, *Ann Thorac Surg* 83:S862, 2007.
62. Tabayashi K, Motoyoshi N, Saiki Y, et al: Efficacy of perfusion cooling of the epidural space and cerebrospinal fluid drainage during repair of extent I and extent II thoracoabdominal aneurysms, *J Cardiovasc Surg (Torino)* 49:749, 2008.
63. Verdant A: Contemporary results of standard open repair of acute traumatic rupture of the thoracic aorta, *J Vasc Surg* 51:294, 2010.
64. Cheung AT, Pochettino A, Guvakov DV, et al: Safety of lumbar drains in thoracic aortic operations performed with extracorporeal circulation, *Ann Thorac Surg* 76:1190, 2003.
65. Kulik A, Castner CF, Kouchoukos NT: Replacement of the descending thoracic aorta: Contemporary outcomes using hypothermic circulatory arrest, *J Thorac Cardiovasc Surg* 139:249, 2010.
66. Etz CD, Plestis KA, Kari FA, et al: Staged repair of thoracic and thoracoabdominal aortic aneurysms using the elephant trunk technique: A consecutive series of 215 first stage and 120 complete repairs, *Eur J Cardiothorac Surg* 34:605, 2008.
67. Dunning J, Martin JE, Shennib H, et al: Is it safe to cover the left subclavian artery when placing an endovascular stent in the descending thoracic aorta? *Interact Cardiovasc Thorac Surg* 7:690, 2008.
68. Rizvi AZ, Murad MH, Fairman RM, et al: The effect of left subclavian artery coverage on morbidity and mortality in patients undergoing thoracic aortic interventions: A systematic review and meta-analysis, *J Vasc Surg* 50:1159, 2009.
69. Cooper DG, Walsh SR, Sadat U, et al: Neurological complications after left subclavian artery coverage during thoracic endovascular aortic repair: A systematic review and meta-analysis, *J Vasc Surg* 49:1594, 2009.
70. Matsumara JS, Lee WA, Mitchell RS, et al: The Society of Vascular Surgery practice guidelines: Management of the left subclavian artery with thoracic endovascular repair, *J Vasc Surg* 50:1155, 2009.
71. Gilling-Smith GL, McWilliams RG, Scurr JR, et al: Wholly endovascular repair of thoracoabdominal aneurysm, *Br J Surg* 95:703, 2008.
72. D'Elia P, Tyrrell M, Sobocinski J, et al: Endovascular thoracoabdominal aortic aneurysm repair: A literature review of early and mid-term results, *J Cardiovasc Surg (Torino)* 50:439, 2009.
73. Haulon S, D'Elia P, O'Brien N, et al: Endovascular repair of thoracoabdominal aortic aneurysms, *Eur J Vasc Endovasc Surg* 39:171, 2010.
74. Bakoyiannis C, Kalles V, Economopoulos K, et al: Hybrid procedures in the treatment of thoracoabdominal aortic aneurysms: A systematic review, *J Endovasc Ther* 16:443, 2009.
75. Drinkwater SL, Bockler D, Eckstein H, et al: The visceral hybrid repair of thoracoabdominal aortic aneurysms—a collaborative approach, *Eur J Vasc Endovasc Surg* 38:578, 2009.
76. Patel R, Conrad MF, Parachuri V, et al: Thoracoabdominal aneurysm repair: Hybrid versus open repair, *J Vasc Surg* 50:15, 2009.
77. Chiesa R, Tshiomba Y, Melissano G, et al: Is hybrid procedure the best treatment option for thoracoabdominal aortic aneurysm? *Eur J Vasc Endovasc Surg* 38:26, 2009.
78. Biasi L, Ali T, Loosemore T, et al: Hybrid repair of complex thoracoabdominal aortic aneurysms using applied endovascular strategies combined with visceral and renal revascularizations, *J Thorac Cardiovasc Surg* 138:133, 2009.
79. Szeto WY, Bavaria JE: Hybrid repair of aortic arch aneurysms: Combined open arch reconstruction and endovascular repair, *Semin Thorac cardiovasc Surg* 21:1347, 2009.
80. Szeto WY, Moser WG, Desai ND, et al: Transapical deployment of endovascular thoracic aortic stent graft for an ascending aortic pseudoaneurysm, *Ann Thorac Surg* 89:616, 2010.
81. Szeto Wy, Fairman RM, Acker MA, et al: Emergency endovascular deployment of stent graft in the ascending aorta for contained rupture of innominate artery pseudoaneurysm in a pediatric patient, *Ann Thorac Surg* 81:1872, 2006.
82. Cheng D, Martin J, Shennib H, et al: Endovascular aortic repair versus open surgical repair for descending thoracic aortic disease: A systematic review and meta-analysis of comparative studies, *J Am Coll Cardiol* 55:986, 2010.
83. Campos JH: Lung isolation techniques for patients with difficult airway, *Curr Opin Anesthesiol* 23:12, 2010.
84. Augoustides JG: Esophageal placement of an airway exchange catheter, *J Cardiothorac Vasc Anesth* 21:773, 2007.
85. Sinha AC, Cheung AT: Spinal cord protection and thoracic aortic surgery, *Curr Opin Anaesthesiol* 23:95, 2010.
86. Backes WH, Nijenhuis RJ, Mess WH, et al: Magnetic resonance angiography of collateral blood supply to spinal cord in thoracic and thoracoabdominal aortic aneurysm patients, *J Vasc Surg* 48:261, 2008.
87. Nojiri J, Matsumoto K, Kato A, et al: The Adamkiewicz artery: Demonstration by intra-arterial computed tomographic angiography, *Eur J Cardiothorac Surg* 31:249, 2007.
88. Boll DT, Bulow H, Blackham KA, et al: MDCT angiography of the spinal vasculature and the artery of Adamkiewicz, *AJR Am J Roentgenol* 187:1054, 2006.
89. Greenberg RK, Lu Q, Roselli E, et al: Contemporary analysis of descending thoracic and thoracoabdominal aneurysm repair: A comparison of endovascular and open techniques, *Circulation* 118:808, 2008.
90. Cheung AT, Weiss SJ, McGarvey ML, et al: Interventions for reversing delayed-onset postoperative paraplegia after thoracic aortic reconstruction, *Ann Thorac Surg* 74:413, 2002.
91. Kawanishi Y, Okada K, Matsumori M, et al: Influence of perioperative hemodynamics on spinal cord ischemia in thoracoabdominal aortic repair, *Ann Thorac Surg* 84:488, 2007.
92. Ling E, Arellano R: Systematic overview of the evidence supporting the use of cerebrospinal fluid drainage in thoracoabdominal aneurysm surgery for prevention of paraplegia, *Anesthesiology* 93:1115, 2000.
93. Khan SN, Stansby G: Cerebrospinal fluid drainage in thoracic and thoracoabdominal aneurysm surgery, *Cochrane Database Syst Rev* 1:CD003635, 2004.
94. Cina CS, Abouzahr L, Arena GO, et al: Cerebrospinal fluid drainage to prevent paraplegia during thoracic and thoracoabdominal aneurysm surgery: A systematic review and meta-analysis, *J Vasc Surg* 40:36, 2004.
95. Acher CW, Wynn M: A modern theory of paraplegia in the treatment of aneurysms of the thoracoabdominal aorta: An analysis of technique specific observed/expected ratios for paralysis, *J Vasc Surg* 49:1117, 2009.
96. Sethi M, Grigore AM, Davison JK: Pro: It is safe to proceed with thoracoabdominal aneurysm surgery after encountering a bloody tap during cerebrospinal fluid catheter placement, *J Cardiothorac Vasc Anesth* 20:269, 2006.
97. Wynn MM, Mittnacht A, Norris E: Con: Surgery should not proceed when a bloody tap occurs during spinal drain placement for elective thoracoabdominal aortic surgery, *J Cardiothorac Vasc Anesth* 20:273, 2006.
98. Estrera Al R, Sheinbaum, Miller CC III, et al: Cerebrospinal fluid drainage during thoracic aortic repair: Safety and current management, *Ann Thorac Surg* 88:9, 2009.
99. Wynn MM, Mell MW, Tefera G, et al: Complications of spinal fluid drainage in thoracoabdominal aortic aneurysm repair: A report of 486 patients treated from 1987 to 2008, *J Vasc Surg* 49:29, 2009.
100. Griepp RB, Griep EB: Spinal cord perfusion and protection during descending thoracic and thoracoabdominal aortic surgery: The collateral network concept, *Ann Thorac Surg* 83:S865, 2007.
101. Etz CD, Luehr M, Kari FA, et al: Paraplegia after extensive thoracic and thoracoabdominal aortic aneurysm repair: Does critical spinal cord ischemia occur postoperatively? *J Thorac Cardiovasc Surg* 135:324, 2008.
102. Woo EY, McGarvey M, Jackson BM, et al: Spinal cord ischemia may be reduced via a novel technique of intercostal artery revascularization during open thoracoabdominal aneurysm repair, *J Vasc Surg* 46:421, 2007.
103. Kawaharada N, Ito T, Koyanagi T, et al: Spinal cord protection with selective spinal perfusion during descending thoracic and thoracoabdominal aortic surgery, *Interact Cardiovasc Thorac Surg* 10:986–990, 2010 discussion 990–991.
104. McGarvey MI, Cheung AT, Szeto W, et al: management of neurologic complications of thoracic aortic surgery, *J Clin Neurophysiol* 24:336, 2007.
105. Jacobs MJ, Mess W, Mochtar B, et al: The value of motor evoked potentials in reducing paraplegia during thoracoabdominal aneurysm repair, *J Vasc Surg* 43:239, 2006.
106. Sloan TB, Jameson LC: Electrophysiologic monitoring during surgery to repair the thoracoabdominal aorta, *J Clin Neurophysiol* 24:316, 2007.
107. Achouh PE, Estrera AL, Miller CC III, et al: Role of somatosensory evoked potentials during thoracic and thoracoabdominal aneurysm repair, *Ann Thorac Surg* 84:782, 2007.
108. Keyhani K, Miller CC III, Estrera AL, et al: Analysis of motor and somatosensory evoked potentials during thoracic and thoracoabdominal aortic aneurysm repair, *J Vasc Surg* 49:36, 2009.
109. Motoyoshi N, Takahashi G, Sakurai M, et al: Safety and efficacy of epidural cooling for regional spinal cord hypothermia during thoracoabdominal aneurysm repair, *Eur J Cardiothorac Surg* 25:139, 2004.
110. Tabayashi K, Motoyoshi N, Saiki Y, et al: Efficacy of perfusion cooling of the epidural space and cerebrospinal fluid drainage during repair of extent I and II thoracoabdominal aortic aneurysm, *J Cardiovasc Surg (Torino)* 49:7499, 2008.
111. Shimizu H, Mori A, Yamada T, et al: Regional spinal cord cooling using a countercurrent closed-lumen epidural catheter, *Ann Thorac Surg* 89:1312, 2010.
112. Reece TB, Kern JA, Tribble CG, et al: The role of pharmacology in spinal cord protection during thoracic aortic reconstruction, *Semin Thorac Cardiovasc Surg* 15:365, 2003.
113. Kohno H, Ishida A, Imamaki M, et al: Efficacy and vasodilatory benefit of magnesium prophylaxis for protection against spinal cord ischemia, *Ann Vasc Surg* 21:352, 2007.
114. Hagiwari S, Saima S, Negishi K, et al: High incidence of renal failure in patients with aortic aneurysms, *Nephrol Dial Transplant* 22:1361, 2007.
115. Koksoy C, Lemaire SA, Curling PE, et al: Renal perfusion during thoracoabdominal aortic operations: Cold crystalloid is superior to normothermic blood, *Ann Thorac Surg* 73:730–738, 2002.
116. Lemaire SA, Jones MM, Conklin LD, et al: Randomized comparison of cold blood and cold crystalloid renal perfusion for renal protection during thoracoabdominal aortic aneurysm repair, *J Vasc Surg* 49:11, 2009.
117. Miller CC III, Villa MA, Sutton J, et al: Serum myoglobin and renal morbidity and mortality following thoracic and thoracoabdominal aortic repair: Does rhabdomyolysis play a role? *Eur J Endovasc Surg* 37:388, 2009.
118. Miller CC III, Villa MA, Achouch P, et al: Intraoperative skeletal muscle ischemia contributes to risk of renal dysfunction following thoracoabdominal aortic repair, *Eur J Cardiothorac Surg* 33:691, 2008.
119. Miller CC III, Grimm JC, Estrera AL, et al: Postoperative renal function preservation with nonischemic femoral arterial cannulation for thoracoabdominal aortic repair, *J Vasc Surg* 51:38, 2010.
120. Popping DM, Elia N, Marret E, et al: Protective effects of epidural analgesia on pulmonary complications after abdominal and thoracic surgery: A meta-analysis, *Arch Surg* 143:990, 2008.
121. Gutsche JT, Szeto W, Cheung AT: Endovascular stenting of thoracic aneurysm, *Anesthesiol Clin* 26:481, 2008.
122. Gutsche JT, Cheung AT, McGarvey ML, et al: Risk factors for perioperative stroke after thoracic endovascular aortic repair, *Ann Thorac Surg* 84:1195, 2007.
123. Cheung AT, Pochettino A, McGarvey ML, et al: Strategies to manage paraplegia risk after endovascular stent repair of descending thoracic aortic aneurysms, *Ann Thorac Surg* 80:1280–1288, 2005 discussion 1288–1289.
124. Golledge J, Eagle KA: Acute aortic dissection, *Lancet* 372:55, 2008.
125. Ramanath VS, Oti JK, Sundt TM 3rd, et al: Acute aortic syndromes and thoracic aortic aneurysm, *Mayo Clin Proc* 84:465, 2009.
126. Trimarchi S, Eagle KA, Nienaber CA, et al: Role of age in acute type A aortic dissection outcome: Report from the International Registry of Acute Aortic Dissection (IRAD), *J Thorac Cardiovasc Surg* 140:784, 2010.
127. Augoustides JG, Geirsson A, Szeto W, et al: Observational study of mortality risk stratification by ischemic presentation in patients with acute type A aortic dissection: The Penn classification, *Nat Clin Pract Cardiovasc Med* 6:140, 2009.
128. Attia R, Young C, Fallouh HB, et al: In patients with acute aortic intramural haematoma is open surgical repair superior to conservative management? *Interact Cardiovasc Thorac Surg* 9:868, 2009.
129. Park KHLim C, Chopi JH, et al: Prevalence of aortic intimal defect in surgically treated type A intramural hematoma, *Ann Thorac Surg* 86:1494, 2008.
130. Chao CP, Walker TG, Kalava SP, et al: Natural history and CT appearances of aortic intramural hematoma, *Radiographics* 29:791, 2009.
131. Augoustides JG, Floyd TF, Kolansky DM: Echocardiography in suspected acute type A aortic dissection: Detection and management of a false positive presentation, *J Cardiothorac Vasc Anesth* 20:912, 2006.
132. Augoustides JG, Harris H, Pochettino A: Direct innominate artery cannulation in acute type A dissection and severe aortic atheroma, *J Cardiothorac Vasc Anesth* 21:727, 2007.
133. Kamiya H, Kallenbach K, Halmer D, et al: Comparison of ascending aorta versus femoral artery cannulation for acute aortic dissection type A, *Circulation* 120:S282, 2009.
134. Tiwari KK, Murzi M, Bevilacqua S, et al: Which cannulation (ascending aortic cannulation or peripheral arterial cannulation) is better for acute type A aortic dissection surgery? *Interact Cardiovasc Thorac Surg* 10:797–802, 2010.
135. Geirsson A, Bavaria JE, Swarr D, et al: Fate of the residual distal and proximal aorta after acute type A dissection repair using a contemporary surgical reconstruction algorithm, *Ann Thorac Surg* 84:1955, 2007.
136. Schoder M, Lammer J, Czerny M: Endovascular aortic arch repair: Hopes and certainties, *Eur J Vasc Endovasc Surg* 38:255, 2009.
137. Pochettino A, Brinkman WT, Moeller P, et al: Antegrade thoracic stent grafting during repair of acute Debakey I dissection prevents development of thoracoabdominal aneurysms, *Ann Thorac Surg* 88:482, 2009.
138. Sun L, Oi R, Chang Q, et al: Surgery for acute type A dissection using total arch replacement combined with stented elephant trunk implantation: Experience in 107 patients, *J Thorac Cardiovasc Surg* 138:1358, 2009.
139. Tsagakis K, Kamler M, Kuehl H, et al: Avoidance of proximal endoleak using a hybrid stent graft in arch replacement and descending aorta stenting, *Ann Thorac Surg* 88:773, 2009.

140. Adams JD, Garcia LM, Kern JA: Endovascular repair of the thoracic aorta, *Surg Clin North Am* 89:895, 2009.
141. Szeto WY, McGarvey M, Pochettino A, et al: Results of a new surgical paradigm: Endovascular repair for acute complicated type B aortic dissection, *Ann Thorac Surg* 85:S1, 2008.
142. Nienaber CA, Rousseau H, Eggebrecht H, et al, for the INSTEAD Trial: Randomized comparison of strategies for type B dissection. The Investigation of Stent grafts In Aortic Dissection (INSTEAD) trial, *Circulation* 120:2519, 2009.
143. Tang DG, Dake MD: TEVAR for acute uncomplicated aortic dissection: Immediate repair vs medical therapy, *Semin Vasc Surg* 22:145, 2009.
144. Pradhan S, Elefteriades JA, Sumpio BE: Utility of the aortic fenestration technique in the management of acute aortic dissections, *Ann Thorac Cardiovasc Surg* 13:296, 2007.
145. Lee S, Cho SH: Huge ascending aortic pseudoaneurysm caused by penetrating atherosclerotic ulcer, *Circ Cardiovasc Imaging* 1:e19, 2008.
146. Yoo SM, Lee HY, White CS: MDCT evaluation of the acute aortic syndrome, *Radiol Clin North Am* 48:67, 2010.
147. Eggebrecht H, Plicht B, Kahlert P, et al: Intramural hematoma and penetrating ulcers: Indications to endovascular treatment, *Eur J Endovasc Surg* 38:659, 2009.
148. Brinster DR: Endovascular repair of the descending thoracic aorta for penetrating atherosclerotic ulcer disease, *J Card Surg* 24:203, 2009.
149. Steenburg SD, Ravenel JG, Ikonomidis JS, et al: Acute traumatic aortic injury: Imaging evaluation and management, *Radiology* 248:748, 2008.
150. Cinnella G, Dambrosio M, Brienza N, et al: Transesophageal echocardiography for diagnosis of traumatic aortic injury: An appraisal of the evidence, *J Trauma* 57:1246, 2004.
151. Demetriades D, Velmanos GC, Scalea TM, et al: Diagnosis and treatment of blunt thoracic injuries: changing perspectives, *J Trauma* 64:1415, 2008.
152. Akowuah E, Angelini G, Bryan AJ: Open versus endovascular repair of traumatic aortic rupture: A systematic review, *J Thorac Cardiovasc Surg* 138:768, 2009.
153. Barnard J, Humphreys J, Bittar MN: Endovascular versus open repair for blunt thoracic aortic injury, *Interact Cardiovasc Thorac Surg* 9:506, 2009.
154. Van Zaane B, Zuithoff NP, Reitsma JB, et al: Meta-analysis of the diagnostic accuracy of transesophageal echocardiography for assessment of atherosclerosis in the ascending aorta in patients undergoing cardiac surgery, *Acta Anesthesiol Scand* 52:1179, 2008.
155. Royse AG, Royse CF: Epiaortic ultrasound assessment of the aorta in cardiac surgery, *Best Practice Res Clin Anesthesiol* 23:335, 2009.
156. Siversides C, Kiess M, Beauchesne L, et al: Canadian Cardiovascular Society 2009 Consensus Conference on the management of adults with congenital heart disease: Outflow tract obstruction, coarctation of the aorta, tetralogy of Fallot, Ebstein anomaly and Marfan's syndrome, *Can J Cardiol* 26:80, 2010.
157. Wheatley GH 3rd, Koullias GJ, Rodrigues-Lopez JA, et al: Is endovascular repair the new gold standard for primary adult coarctation? *Eur J Cardiothorac Surg* 38:305–310, 2010.
158. Flore AC, Ruzmetov M, Johnson RG, et al: Selective use of left heart bypass for aortic coarctation, *Ann Thorac Surg* 89:851, 2010.

22

Uncommon Cardiac Diseases

WILLIAM C. OLIVER, JR., MD | **WILLIAM J. MAUERMANN, MD** | **GREGORY A. NUTTALL, MD**

KEY POINTS

1. Uncommon diseases and coexisting problems of patients undergoing cardiac surgery are covered with a general overview of the disease or condition followed by guidelines and considerations to facilitate anesthetic management.
2. Carcinoid heart disease, a serious condition that requires cardiac surgery, continues to undergo changes in the optimal anesthetic management.
3. Great advances in the management and outcome of surgery with hypertrophic cardiomyopathy are detailed in addition to updates on the pathophysiology and management of arrhythmogenic right ventricular cardiomyopathy.
4. Current approach to mitral valve prolapse and the range of clinical presentations from mitral valve prolapse syndrome to degenerative valve disease and severe mitral regurgitation is a common reason for cardiac surgery today.
5. The management of patent foramen ovale in both noncardiac and cardiac surgical situations is updated. The incidental patent foramen ovale found during cardiac surgery with echocardiography continues to evolve regarding closure.
6. The definitive approach to a patient with both carotid and coronary artery disease will require a large, multicenter, randomized trial; however, the many approaches to the surgical management of combined procedures are described.
7. Heart disease continues to be the leading cause of maternal and fetal death during pregnancy, so the important features of managing the pregnant patient who requires cardiopulmonary bypass and cardiac surgery is updated.
8. With newly developed therapies, the incubation time to development of acquired immunodeficiency syndrome after infection and life expectancy of those with human immunodeficiency virus have been extended, so the likelihood of cardiac surgery is greater; consequently, the rates of exposure, types of procedures, and the precautions of the individuals are addressed.
9. Individuals with chronic renal failure, not necessarily dialysis dependent before surgery, are more frequently undergoing cardiac surgery and likely to experience development of worsening renal function after cardiopulmonary bypass, so the identification of steps that may improve outcome are discussed.
10. Anesthetic concerns for patients with hematologic problems who undergo cardiac surgery are further complicated by the stress cardiopulmonary bypass places on coagulation and oxygen-carrying systems, and require special considerations and techniques.

Uncommon diseases and coexisting problems of patients undergoing cardiac surgery are reviewed in this chapter. Each subsection includes a general overview of the disease or condition and emphasizes anesthetic management, including relevant echocardiographic considerations of the coexistent disease in the setting of cardiac surgery. It is important that the anesthesiologist understand the pathology and pathophysiology of coexisting diseases, how they are affected by anesthesia, and how they affect the underlying cardiac problem.

CARDIAC TUMORS

Cardiac tumors increasingly are diagnosed before autopsy because of advancements in imaging, especially metastatic tumors of the heart and pericardium that account for a majority of cardiac tumors. Data pooled from 22 large autopsy series show the prevalence rate of adult primary cardiac tumors is 0.02% but causes considerable morbidity and mortality.[1] Primary cardiac tumors in adults are usually benign, with only 20% to 25% malignant.[2-5] Diagnosis can be elusive because these tumors may be associated with nonspecific symptoms mimicking other disease entities. Two-dimensional (2D) echocardiography (echo) modalities and magnetic resonance imaging (MRI) have allowed earlier, more frequent, and more complete assessment of cardiac tumors.[6,7] The advent of three-dimensional (3D) echo increases the confidence of the diagnosis of a cardiac mass by giving more detailed characterization of mass size, composition, location, and relation to other structures.[8]

Primary cardiac tumors may originate from any cardiac tissue. Myxoma is the most common cardiac neoplasm, accounting for nearly 50% of tumors in adults (Table 22-1). Less frequently observed benign tumors that may require surgery include rhabdomyoma, fibroma, papillary fibroelastoma, lipoma, and angioma. Malignant primary cardiac tumors include sarcomas that are 95% of these tumors, followed by lymphoma. Sarcomas include angiosarcoma, rhabdomyosarcoma, and acquired immunodeficiency syndrome (AIDS)–related sarcomas.[9] Rhabdomyosarcoma represents 20% of malignant neoplasms. Excision of these tumors seldom is curative, in part because of the delay in

TABLE 22-1	Benign Neoplasms of the Heart	
Neoplasms	*Incidence Rate in Adults (%)*
Myxoma	45
Lipoma	20
Papillary fibroelastoma	15
Angioma	5
Fibroma	3
Hemangioma	5
Rhabdomyoma	1
Teratoma	< 1

From Shapiro LM: Cardiac tumors: Diagnosis and management. *Heart* 85:218, 2001.

diagnosis caused by the nonspecific nature of the clinical symptoms. Surgery, radiation therapy, and chemotherapy may slow a tumor's encroachment on intracavitary spaces or relieve obstruction.

The incidence rate of metastatic cardiac tumors has increased from 0.2% to 10% as a result of improved survival.[10] Metastatic cardiac tumors are much more common than primary cardiac tumors. Adenocarcinomas of the lung and breast, lymphomas that are commonly associated with AIDS or transplant immunosuppression, and melanoma are the most frequent metastatic cardiac tumors.[11] Melanoma has a special tendency for metastasis to the heart and pericardium. However, metastasis of these tumors rarely is limited to the heart. The onset of arrhythmias or congestive heart failure (CHF) in patients with carcinomas suggests invasion of the myocardium by metastasis, but more than 90% of metastatic lesions to the heart are clinically silent.[4]

The most effective treatment of primary tumors generally is surgical resection, with 2% operative mortality. This is based on a recent retrospective study of 323 consecutive patients who underwent surgical resection of primary cardiac tumors over a period of 48 years in one institution.[12] Recurrence rate in these tumors varied between 3% and 13%, but appeared to be related to a biologic propensity rather than surgical technique, as was previously believed. The overall rate of tumor embolization was 25% compared with previous reports of 12% to 45%. Embolic complications were seen more often in patients with minimal or no symptoms than those with large tumors associated with hemodynamic changes. Papillary fibroelastoma and aortic valve tumors are most commonly preceded by an embolic event. Even patients who are diagnosed by embolic events benefit greatly from surgical resection with excellent short- and long-term survival that is comparable with a cohort of patients with tumors undergoing surgery for other reasons.[7] Orthotopic cardiac transplantation has been recommended for unresectable tumors,[13] but the benefit is indeterminate. Although more infrequent, the surgical risk and outcome for malignant compared with benign tumor resection are usually much worse,[2] especially in younger patients.[12]

Myxoma

Often a diagnostic challenge, myxoma, a benign, solitary neoplasm slowly proliferating, microscopically resembles an organized clot, which often obscures its identity as a primary cardiac tumor. The pedunculated mass is believed to arise from undifferentiated cells in the fossa ovalis and adjoining endocardium projecting into the left atrium (LA) and right atrium (RA) 75% and 20% of the time, respectively. However, myxomas appear in other locations of the heart, even occupying more than one chamber.[14] The undifferentiated cells of a myxoma develop along a variety of cell lines, accounting for the multiple presentations and pathologies observed.[15] Besides a variable amount of stroma, myxomas include hemorrhage, hemosiderin, thrombus, and calcium (Figure 22-1). Myxomas predominate in the 30- to 60-year-old age range, but any age group may be affected. More than 75% of the affected patients are women.[16] Although most cases occur sporadically, 7% to 10% of atrial myxomas will occur in a familial pattern with an autosomal dominant transmission pattern.[17]

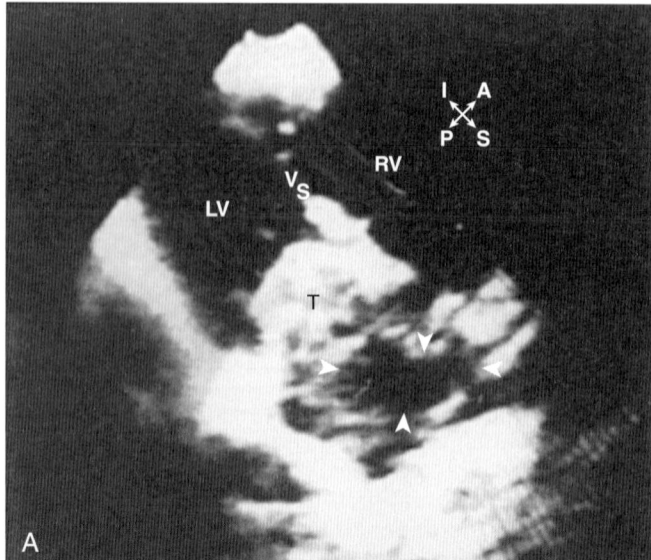

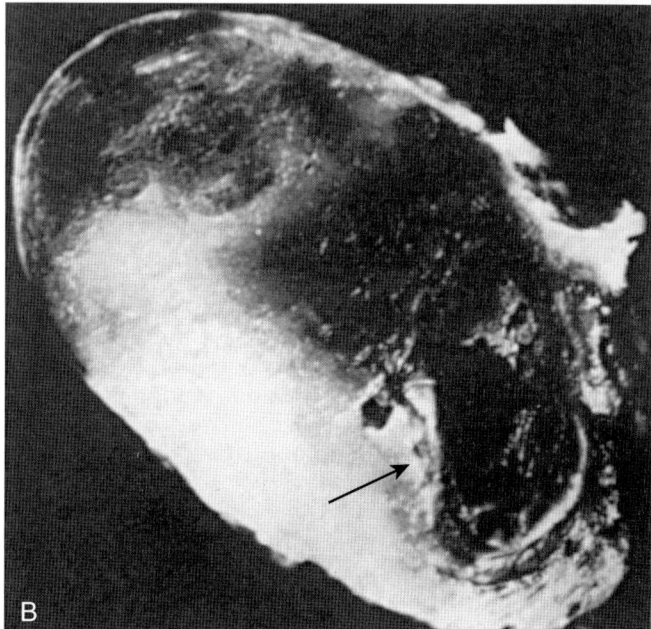

Figure 22-1 *A,* Parasternal long-axis view of large, firm left atrial myxoma remaining impacted in left atrium. Tumor *(T)* contains a central region of echolucency *(arrowheads)* that corresponds to an area of liquefaction. *B,* Cut section of gross specimen of myxoma. LV, left ventricle; RV, right ventricle; VS, ventricular septum. *(From Fyke FE III, Seward JB, Edwards WD, et al: Primary cardiac tumors: Experience with 30 consecutive patients since the introduction of two-dimensional echocardiography. J Am Coll Cardiol 5:1465, 1985, by permission of the American College of Cardiology.)*

Rarely discovered by incidental echo examination, myxomas may manifest a variety of symptoms. The classic triad includes embolism, intracardiac obstruction, and constitutional symptoms. Approximately 80%[14] of individuals will present with one component of the triad. Up to 10% may be asymptomatic even with mitral myxomas that arise from both atrial and ventricular sides of the anterior mitral leaflet.[18] The most common initial symptom, dyspnea on exertion,[16] reflects mitral valve obstruction usually present with left atrial myxomas (Figure 22-2). Because of the pedunculated nature of some myxomas, temporary obstruction of blood flow may cause hemolysis, hypotension, syncope, or sudden death. Other symptoms of mitral obstruction similar to mitral stenosis such as hemoptysis, systemic embolization,

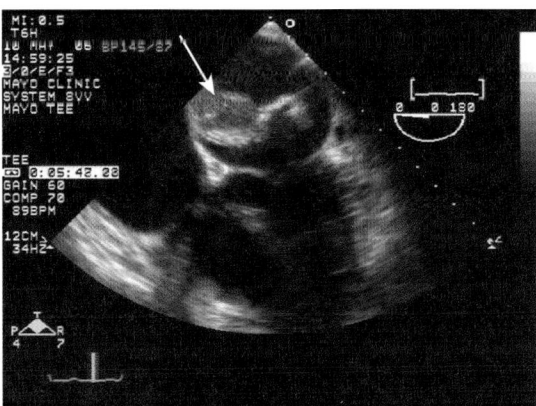

Figure 22-2 A large myxoma (arrow) is seen in the left atrium with its point of attachment at the interatrial septum. Note the irregular shape and nonhomogenous echogenicity of the tumor.

fever, and weight loss also may occur. If the tumor is obstructing the mitral valve, a "tumor plop" may be heard after the second heart sound on chest auscultation. The persistence of sinus rhythm in the presence of such symptoms may help distinguish atrial myxoma from mitral stenosis. Severe pulmonary artery hypertension (PAH) without significant mitral valve involvement suggests recurrent pulmonary emboli known to occur with a myxoma in the RA or right ventricle (RV). Occasionally, right-sided tumors may appear as cyanotic congenital heart lesions because of intracardiac shunting.[19]

Recurrent fragmentation and embolization of the gelatinous-like tumor usually appear with systemic manifestations and are characteristic of myxoma. It is the smaller myxoma in the LA that does not create hemodynamic complications, exists for years undiagnosed, and is more likely to cause embolization.[7] Cerebral aneurysms often exist in patients with recurrent systemic embolization from intracardiac myxoma probably secondary to damage by the systemic tumor emboli. The kidneys also are more susceptible to damage from myxoma emboli. Constitutional symptoms such as malaise, fever, and weight loss occur in about one third of patients, reflecting a possible autoimmune component but also delaying the diagnosis. Differential diagnosis includes endocarditis, connective tissue disorders, and malignancies. In general, the anatomic type of myxoma portends the clinical presentation. The solid, ovoid tumors are more often associated with CHF, whereas papillary myxomas present with cerebral embolization.[20] Tumor size does not correlate with symptoms.[16]

Findings on a chest roentgenogram of a myxoma may be absent in one third of patients. Calcification on the chest roentgenogram is more diagnostic of right atrial myxoma, but rarely presents in left atrial myxoma. Before the availability of echo, angiography was used to identify

all myxomas, but currently is probably only useful to determine coronary anatomy if considered necessary.[2] Computerized tomography (CT) and MRI can help delineate the extent of the tumor and its relations to surrounding cardiac and thoracic structures.[21] MRI is especially valuable in the diagnosis of myxoma when masses are equivocal or suboptimal by echo, or if the tumor is atypical in presentation.[14] Difficulty may arise in differentiating thrombus from myxoma because both are so heterogenous.

Transthoracic echocardiography (TTE) is excellent for identifying intracavitary tumors because it is noninvasive, identifies tumor type, and permits complete visualization of each cardiac chamber (see Figure 22-1).[22] It is the predominant imaging modality for screening.[2] Transesophageal echocardiography (TEE) increases the diagnostic potential, as the nature of the tumor according to location, dimensions, number of masses, and echogenic pattern is better identified.[23] Specifically, it yields morphologic detail in the evaluation of cardiac tumors, including points of tumor attachment and degree of mobility.

Myxomas have a typical echo appearance and often are irregular in shape with protruding fronds of tissue. There may be areas of calcification, and the echogenicity of the mass may not be homogenous.[24] The presence of a large mass in the LA with an attachment to the interatrial septum is highly suggestive of myxoma. However, it must be emphasized that echo cannot provide a tissue diagnosis. Rarely, thrombus can be attached to the atrial septum.[25] The degree of obstruction to ventricular filling caused by the tumor may be evaluated with Doppler echo (Figure 22-3). Qualitatively, color-Doppler imaging will show aliasing and flow acceleration through the atrioventricular valve when obstruction is present. Continuous-wave Doppler imaging is able to quantify the gradient between the atrium and ventricle. Before surgery, the goal of echo is to determine the site of tumor attachment, the absence of multiple masses, and to ensure that the tumor is not attached to the valve leaflets. If this cannot be accomplished with TTE, a TEE examination should be performed to aid in planning the surgical approach.

Currently, evaluation of cardiac tumors is a Class II indication for intraoperative TEE (supported by weaker evidence and expert opinion).[26] When the primary reason for cardiac surgery is removal of an intracardiac mass, an intraoperative TEE evaluation should take place before the surgical incision to ensure that the mass is still present and has not embolized out of the heart (or dissolved as in the case of intracardiac thrombus). In the case of myxoma, an intraoperative examination in the presence of the surgeon can aid in finalizing the surgical plan. After tumor removal, the goal of TEE is to ensure that all visible mass was removed and there was no damage to adjacent structures. Specifically, in the case of a myxoma attached to the atrial septum, it is important to ensure that there is no interatrial shunting after removal. If the tumor was attached to, or near, a valve apparatus, the examiner must determine that the valve is competent after tumor removal.

The first surgical resection of an atrial myxoma was performed in 1954. Subsequently, surgical resection has been recommended even

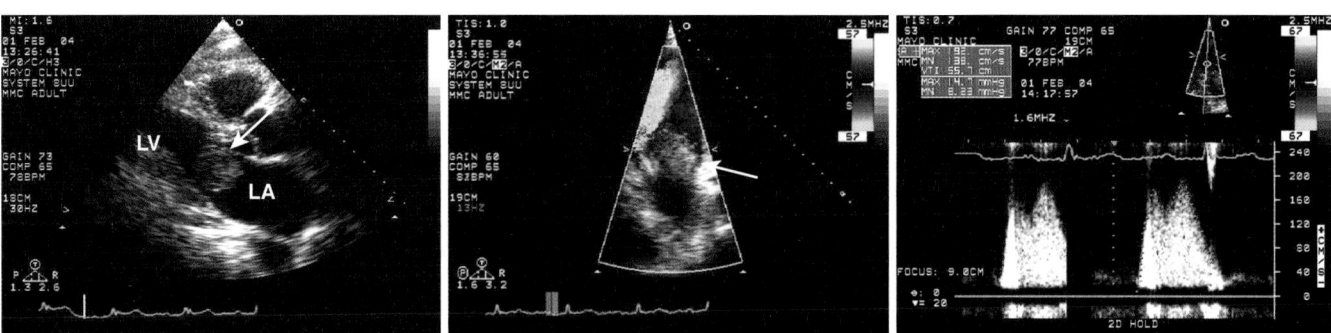

Figure 22-3 Left, A large left atrial myxoma (arrow) can be seen prolapsing through the mitral valve into the left ventricle during diastole. Middle, Color-Doppler imaging shows aliasing of flow indicating obstruction of left ventricular filling during diastole. Indeed, when a continuous-wave Doppler signal is placed through the mitral annulus, a gradient of 8 mm Hg is seen between the left atrium and ventricle. The obstruction to ventricular filling caused by the myxoma prolapse would be equivalent to moderate mitral valve stenosis. LA, left atrium; LV, left ventricle.

if the myxoma is discovered incidentally, mainly because the risk for embolization to the central nervous system may be 30% to 40%. Generally, the time interval between onset of symptoms and surgical resection is about 4 months, but surgery has been delayed for 10 years.[16] Surgery is associated with a mortality rate of 0% to 7%.[1,7] More importantly, it recently was documented for the first time that the long-term survival of an individual who underwent resection of myxoma was no different from an age- and sex-matched population.[12]

Anesthetic Considerations

Tumor location has a strong influence on anesthetic management. Left atrial myxomas most likely will cause mitral valve obstruction, often in conjunction with PAH and pulmonary venous hypertension. Anesthetic management will closely resemble a patient with mitral stenosis. In contrast, right atrial myxomas may produce signs of right-sided heart failure corresponding to tricuspid valve obstruction. Positioning of the patient for surgery must be carefully performed to detect severe restriction of venous return that may often be followed quickly with profound hypotension and arrhythmias. A large tumor increases the likelihood of hemodynamic instability, whereas a small tumor is associated with increased risk for embolization.[7] Perioperative arrhythmias, especially atrial fibrillation or flutter, may arise in 25% of these patients, requiring immediate treatment. Hemodynamic instability with low cardiac output (CO) and arrhythmias are common.

Consideration for not placing a pulmonary artery catheter (PAC), as well as avoiding the RA completely, should include the risk for tumor embolization. If the tumor is located in the RA, placement of central venous catheters in the subclavian or internal jugular vein under TEE guidance deserves consideration. If the wire or catheter is contacting the tumor, it should be pulled back from the RA to avoid embolizing parts of the tumor. After surgery, the patient must be observed closely for evidence of neurologic injury secondary to cerebral embolization and hemorrhage.

Median sternotomy is recommended for resection of atrial myxoma, although anterior thoracotomy may be used in some benign tumors,[2] as well as minimally invasive techniques. Femoral cannulation for initiation of cardiopulmonary bypass (CPB) may minimize the risk for dislodgment or fragmentation of the tumor. Subsequently, a venous cannula can be placed high in the superior vena cava because a biatrial approach to an atrial septal tumor is necessary. The most preferred surgical approach is the single atrial approach.[12] Moderate systemic hypothermia, deep topical cooling, and cardioplegic arrest are often used, whereas circulatory arrest is reserved for malignant tumors with significant extension. The heart should not eject during CPB, to minimize systemic embolization of tumor fragments. Electrically induced ventricular fibrillation has been used to prevent ejection of blood after initiation of CPB. Wide excision of the septal base of the myxoma with Dacron or pericardial patching of the resulting defect is the preferred operation.[27] Mitral valve replacement may be necessary in large tumors, ventricular side tumors, or tumors with other manifestations besides a propensity to embolize.[18] Less extensive operations risk a greater incidence of tumor recurrence because of incomplete tumor excision or a second tumor originating in susceptible atrial tissue. The recurrence rate after complete excision of a sporadic cardiac myxoma is less than 5%.[5] After surgery, the most common complication is a 25% incidence rate of transient arrhythmias, mostly supraventricular in nature.

▨ Other Benign Tumors

Papillomas (papillary fibroelastoma) are rare tumors but are the third most common primary cardiac tumor (after myxoma and fibroma).[5] Initially thought to be incidental findings during autopsies, today most are discovered in living patients.[28] Mostly singular (90%), 1 to 4 cm in size, highly papillary, pedunculated, and avascular, papillomas are covered by a single layer of endothelium containing fine elastic fibrils in a hyaline stroma. Macroscopically, they resemble sea anemones.

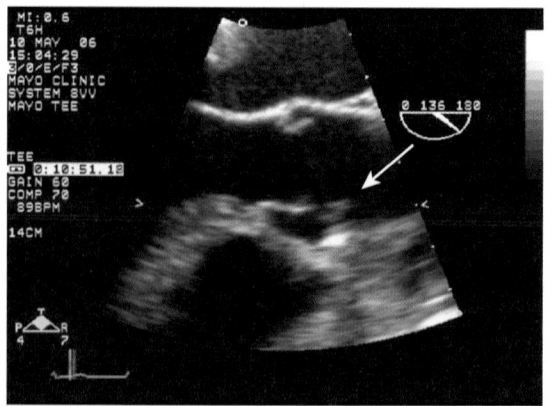

Figure 22-4   The typical appearance of a fibroelastoma (arrow) attached to what is likely the right coronary cusp of the aortic valve. This tumor is thin, and its motion is independent from that of the aortic leaflet.

They originate most commonly from valvular endocardium,[29] usually involving the ventricular surface of the aortic valve or the atrial surface of the mitral valve, but infrequently rendering the involved valve incompetent. They account for 75% of all primary cardiac valvular tumors.[12,30] Adults between the ages of 40 and 80 primarily are affected, with the mean age at the time of detection of 60 years.[5] Many patients are asymptomatic, so it is not surprising that 47% of these tumors are discovered incidentally during echo, catheterization, or even cardiac surgery. Echocardiographically, fibroelastomas have a typical appearance (Figure 22-4). They usually are small (mean size, 12 × 9 mm) and their motion is independent from that of the attached valve leaflet.[31] They may appear similar to vegetations seen in endocarditis, or they may be confused with Lambl's excrescences, which tend to be more nodular in appearance.

Currently, many tumors are found in a search to find the cause of embolic symptoms. These symptoms are most common when the aortic valve is involved. Previously believed to be harmless, postmortem studies have shown a high incidence of embolization to the cerebral and coronary circulations.[4] Not surprisingly, symptoms often are related to stroke or transient ischemic attack and myocardial infarction (MI). Although embolization may be a tumor, it may be a thrombus because tumors are excellent sites for thrombus formation.[5] It is important that the diagnosis is made because acute valvular dysfunction and even sudden death may occur.[29] Surgical resection is curative but may require valvular repair or replacement in one third of cases.[28] Recurrence is rare.

The incidence of cardiac lipomas[4] is similar to papillary fibroelastoma. They occur as intracavitary tumors, intramyocardial masses, and pericardial tumors. Histologically, they usually consist of encapsulated groups of mature fat cells. Patients with these tumors often are asymptomatic, but if they occur in an intracavitary location, they may resemble myxomas. An intramyocardial location may provoke arrhythmias and conduction abnormalities. Pericardial lipomas are associated with tamponade and cardiac compression. These tumors tend to enlarge over time, and when symptoms appear, surgical excision is required.

Rhabdomyomas are primarily childhood tumors (majority before 1 year of age) located intramyocardially, and arise from all areas of the heart and at multiple locations of the heart. Tuberous sclerosis often is associated with these tumors.[32] They represent 45% of all benign tumors of childhood, but only 1% of benign adult primary cardiac tumors.[4] As pedunculated masses, rhabdomyomas usually originate in the ventricle, leading to inflow and outflow ventricular obstruction, and on the atrioventricular valves.[5] Symptoms are caused by the obstruction of blood flow and arrhythmias, but life-threatening complications are rare. Although surgical resection may be necessary in 25% of cases, these tumors most often resolve spontaneously. Because of their space-occupying properties, rhabdomyomas may mimic other congenital defects such as left hypoplastic heart syndrome.

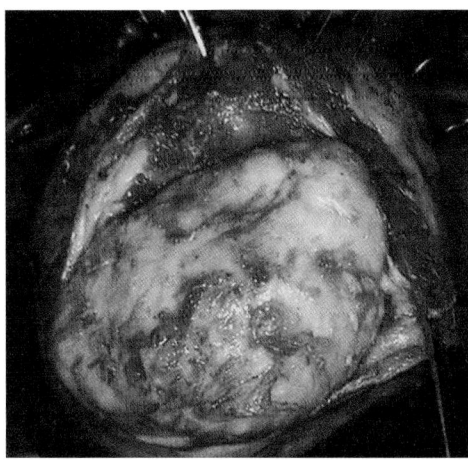

Figure 22-5 Dissection of ventricular fibroma (Patient 12; patient's head is at top). *(From Cho JM, Danielson GK, Puga FJ, et al: Surgical resection of ventricular cardiac fibromas: Early and late results, Ann Thorac Surg 76:1933, 2003, by permission.)*

Fibromas are connective tissue tumors found primarily in children, making up 15% of pediatric benign primary cardiac tumors.[4] They are usually solitary, located in the wall of the heart, and often involve the apical or septal areas of the left ventricle (LV) (Figure 22-5). Echocardiographically, fibromas tend to be well demarcated from the myocardium by calcifications (Figure 22-6).[33] These tumors frequently interfere with the conduction pathways. Ventricular arrhythmias are common, and ventricular tachycardia with sudden death is not infrequent. The tumor may occlude or displace the coronary arteries. Patients may present with CHF or angina. Surgical resection is favored even for asymptomatic patients in view of the risk for fatal ventricular arrhythmias.[34] Cardiac transplantation has been advocated for septal tumors that are unresectable; however, a subtotal resection achieves excellent late survival.

Two vascular tumors, angiomas and pheochromocytomas of the heart (paraganglioma), are rare. Angiomas are found in the interventricular septum, and their vascular nature makes surgery difficult. Primary cardiac pheochromocytomas are located along the atrioventricular groove near the epicardial arteries.[35] These tumors arise from neuroendocrine cells. Although cardiac pheochromocytomas became known based on symptoms related to catecholamine secretion, the symptoms are less dramatic than the corresponding adrenal tumors because norepinephrine is not converted to epinephrine in the cardiac tumors. Cardiac pheochromocytomas may go undiagnosed for years while undergoing exploratory laparotomy and multiple diagnostic tests before a cardiac location is considered. If these tumors are nonsecretors of catecholamines, often they are not detected until superior vena cava obstruction, pericardial effusion, or tamponade.[36] Fifty percent of these tumors are hereditary, such as in neurofibromatosis or Hippel-Lindau disease. Although surgical excision is curative, total excision may be difficult. Severe intraoperative bleeding is known to occur with these tumors.[35] Furthermore, clinicians should be prepared to treat these tumors as catecholamine-secreting tumors that may result in hemodynamic derangements during anesthesia with uncontrolled hypertension, pulmonary edema, and MI.[36] Current perioperative management for these tumors has been reviewed.[37]

Malignant Tumors

Approximately 25% of primary cardiac tumors are malignant,[5] and 95% of these are sarcomas. They are found infiltrating the RA and causing cavitary obstruction, but may have variable clinical presentations based on the location, causing diagnosis to be elusive. They usually occur between the ages of 30 and 50, preceded by vague symptoms such as dyspnea, but rapidly progressing to death. Angiosarcomas, the most common sarcoma,[4] are rapidly spreading vascular tumors that arise most often from the RA, appearing near the inferior vena cava with extension to the mediastinum. They occur most commonly in adults and male individuals.[5] Presenting symptoms include chest pain and dyspnea, progressive CHF, and bloody pericardial effusion.[9] There are two clinicopathologic forms of the tumor. The first type deposits small tumor in the pericardium or epicardium and is associated with skin lesions or risk factors for Kaposi sarcoma. The second involves large tumor in the RA. Treatment is palliative as the response to chemotherapy and radiation is poor. Resection may be possible, but survival is less than 2 years. Rhabdomyosarcomas are aggressive tumors that have cellular elements that resemble striated muscle. These tumors occur in both sexes equally. They may originate in any chamber of the heart, but in contrast with angiosarcomas, they rarely become diffusely involved with the pericardium. They are bulky and invasive, growing rapidly. Surgical resection is possible, but distant metastasis reduces the chances of success. Chemotherapy and radiation are ineffective.[5]

Echo tends to be less helpful in the management of these patients than it is in patients with benign tumors. It may reveal physiologic complications of the tumor such as cavitary obliteration or valvular regurgitation, and it is helpful in finding associated pericardial effusions and tamponade physiology. However, these tumors have complex anatomy, and the perimeters of the tumor, as well as their involvement in valve apparatuses and coronary anatomy, can be difficult to

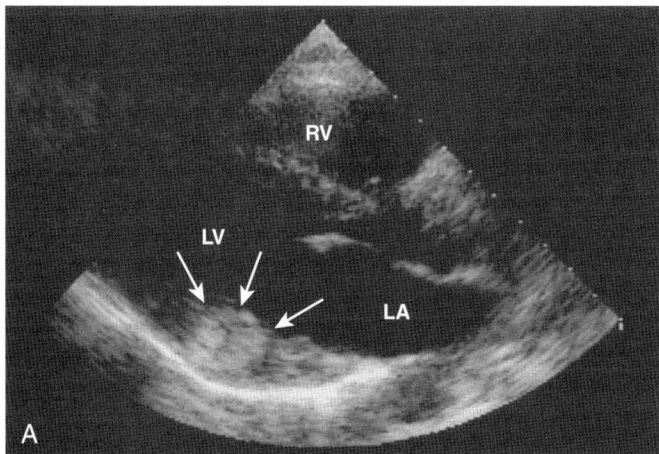

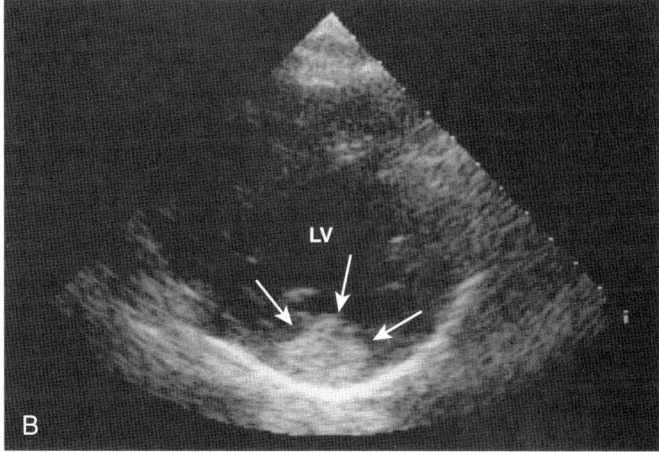

Figure 22-6 Transthoracic, parasternal long- *(A)* and short-axis *(B)* views of a left ventricular (LV) fibroma *(arrows)*. It is well circumscribed in the posterior free wall. It may cause ventricular arrhythmia, but it does not produce any hemodynamic abnormality. LA, left atrium; RV, right ventricle. *(Reprinted from Oh JK, Seward JB, Tajik AJ: The Echo Manual, 3rd ed. Philadelphia: Lippincott Williams & Wilkins, 2006, by permission.)*

determine even with TEE. In addition, echo does not image adjacent cardiac structures such as the lung and mediastinum in detail. When echo is combined with other imaging modalities such as CT and MRI, the clinician may obtain the anatomic information needed (from the CT or MRI), as well as the physiologic consequences (from echo).[24]

Other primary malignant tumors of the heart include malignant fibrous histiocytoma, fibrosarcomas, osteosarcoma, leiomyosarcoma (rarest malignant cardiac tumor), undifferentiated sarcoma, neurogenic sarcoma, and lymphomas. Primary cardiac lymphoma is defined as a non-Hodgkin lymphoma and accounts for about 1% of primary cardiac tumors.[38] The prevalence of these tumors has been increasing in part because of AIDS and early detection from imaging advancements such as echo. Lymphomas are generally large masses with extensive infiltration into adjacent areas of the heart from the point of tumor origin. These commonly are located in the RA and RV. These primary tumors are rare, representing less than 2% of all cardiac tumors.[39] Treatment involves a combination of chemotherapy and radiation, occasionally extending survival up to 5 years, but the median survival is 1 year. Malignant fibrous histiocytoma, in contrast with other sarcomas, generally is found in the LA. Despite resection, metastasis is common, as well as local recurrence. Surgical excision may be useful to alleviate symptoms but ultimately does not influence the poor survival.[40]

In general, malignant primary cardiac tumors may require a combination of surgery, radiation, and chemotherapy simply to limit cavitary obstruction to blood flow because of rapid growth and metastasis. Local recurrence is more likely to cause death than metastasis.[41] More aggressive approaches for malignant tumors with extensive local disease before metastasis include autotransplantation.[3] The heart is removed from the chest cavity and inverted to provide better exposure. Its value is still indeterminate, but no intraoperative deaths have occurred. Although still controversial, orthotopic heart transplantation may be considered for unresectable tumors that involve only the heart, but survival is not extended beyond 1 to 2 years.[2] The rate of intraoperative death with malignant tumor resection is seven times that of benign resection, and there is twice the morbidity rate.

Most cardiac tumors are rarely associated with airway problems.[42] Rather, the large pericardial effusions create significant hemodynamic instability and deterioration. Manipulation of these tumors also may exacerbate hemodynamics. If a large pericardial effusion is present before induction of anesthesia, it should be drained. Beyond the standard monitoring used for a cardiac surgical patient, the overall physical status and risk for embolization must be evaluated. Femoral arterial and central venous monitoring are recommended for patients with right atrial tumors. Sudden right-sided tumor embolization may be recognized based on an increased end-tidal carbon dioxide gradient. Left-sided embolization is difficult to assess during anesthesia.

Tumors with Systemic Cardiac Manifestations

Carcinoid tumors are metastasizing neuroendocrine tumors that arise primarily from the small bowel, occurring in 1 to 2 per 100,000 people in the population.[43] On diagnosis, 20% to 30% of individuals with carcinoid tumors present with carcinoid syndrome. It is characterized by episodic vasomotor symptoms, bronchospasm, hypotension, diarrhea, and right-sided heart disease attributed to release of serotonin, histamine, bradykinins, and prostaglandins often in response to manipulation or pharmacologic stimulation. Manifestations of carcinoid syndrome occur primarily in patients with liver metastasis and impair the ability of the liver to inactivate large amounts of vasoactive substances.

Initially described in 1952,[43] aspects of carcinoid heart disease may occur in 20% to 50% of patients with carcinoid syndrome.[44,45] Carcinoid heart disease may be the initial feature of metastatic carcinoid disease in 20% of patients. The prognosis has improved substantially since the early 1980s for individuals with malignant carcinoid tumors and carcinoid heart disease, but it still causes considerable morbidity and mortality. The median life expectancy is 5.9 years without carcinoid heart disease, but declines to 2.6 years if it is present.[45] Circulating serotonin levels had been found to be more than twice as high in persons with carcinoid syndrome who develop carcinoid heart disease,[46] but this is no longer true because most patients receive somatostatin analogs.[45]

Carcinoid heart disease characteristically involves tricuspid regurgitation and pulmonic stenosis and regurgitation resulting in severe right-heart failure (Figure 22-7). Tumor growth in the liver permits large amounts of tumor products to reach the RV without the benefit of first-pass metabolism. Carcinoid plaques composed of

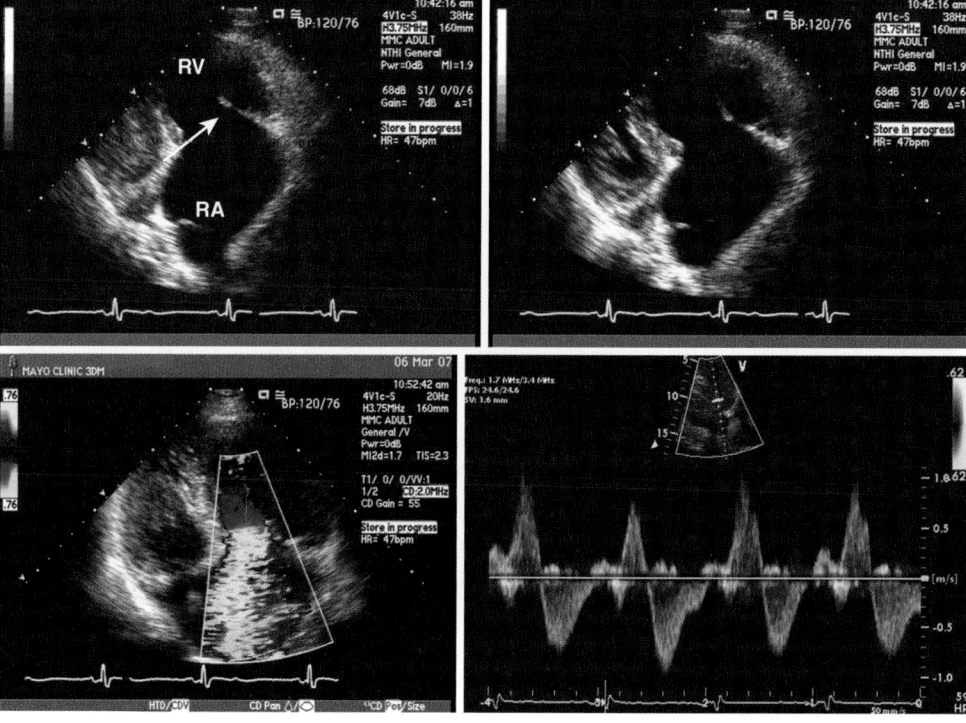

Figure 22-7 Transthoracic imaging using an apical view in a patient with carcinoid heart disease. The tricuspid valve *(arrow)* in both systole *(top left)* and diastole *(top right)*. Note the thickened tricuspid leaflets move little between systole and diastole, and there is an enormous coaptation defect during systole *(top left)*. Color-Doppler imaging *(bottom left)* reveals massive tricuspid regurgitation that fills the entire right atrium (RA), which is severely dilated. *Bottom right*, Continuous-wave Doppler imaging of the hepatic veins reveals systolic flow reversals (deflection of Doppler signal above the baseline during systole) indicative of severe tricuspid regurgitation. RV, right ventricle.

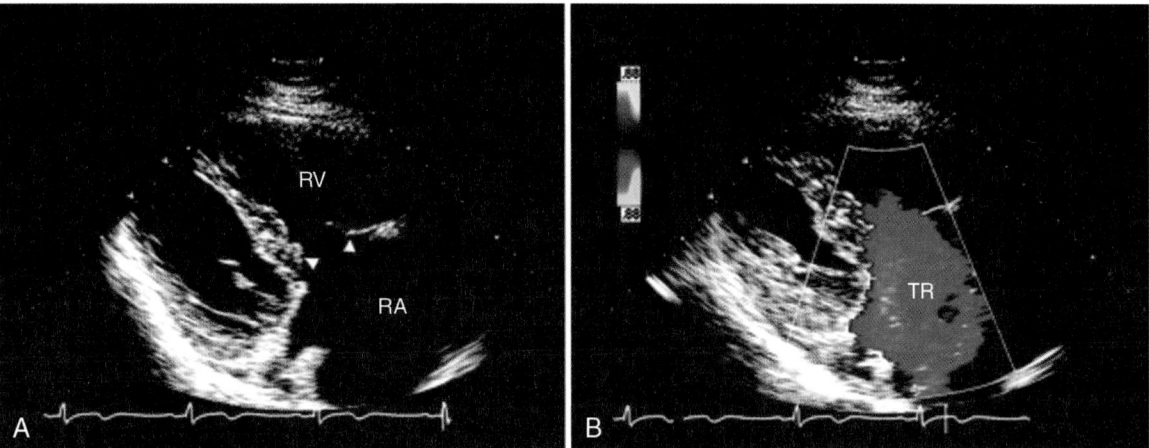

Figure 22-8 *A,* Two-dimensional echocardiographic systolic image (right ventricular inflow view) demonstrates thickened septal and anterior tricuspid valve leaflets *(arrowheads)* and enlargement of the right ventricle (RV) and right atrium (RA) in a patient with carcinoid heart disease. *B,* Color flow Doppler image demonstrates severe tricuspid regurgitation (TR) in the same patient. Note laminar color flow *(blue)* filling an enlarged right atrium. *(From Otto CM, Bonow RO (eds): Valvular Heart Disease: A Companion to Braunwald's Heart Disease, 3rd Edition. Philadelphia, Saunders/Elsevier, 2009, P. 339, whith permission.)*

myofibroblasts, collagen, and myxoid matrix[47] are deposited primarily on the tricuspid and pulmonary valves, bringing about immobility and thickening of the valve leaflets, causing the distinctive valvular changes (Figure 22-8). After surgery, 80% of tricuspid valves are observed to be incompetent, with only 20% stenotic, whereas the affected pulmonary valves tend to be equally divided between incompetence and stenosis.[47] The exact mechanism that causes valve injury is unknown, but high levels of serotonin sometimes are found in those patients with carcinoid heart disease.[43] Less than 10% of those with carcinoid heart disease have left-heart involvement, possibly because of inactivation of serotonin in the lungs,[48] but it may exist with the presence of a bronchial carcinoid or an interatrial shunt.

Echo features of carcinoid heart disease, particularly of the tricuspid valve, are practically diagnostic of the underlying disease process. The leaflets are thickened and retracted. The appearance of the tricuspid leaflets is often as if the leaflets were curled under (see Figure 22-7). The thickening and retraction result in a large coaptation defect and severe valvular regurgitation. The pulmonic valve may be difficult to image with TTE, but the midesophageal TEE view at 70 to 90 degrees often shows the valve well. With severe tricuspid regurgitation, the RV will dilate and abnormalities of ventricular septal motion may be noted. The thickness of the ventricular wall is usually normal. Doppler imaging of the hepatic veins will show systolic flow reversals consistent with severe tricuspid regurgitation. A careful search for a patent foramen ovale (PFO) should be undertaken because this has implications for left-sided valvular involvement.

Without treatment, median survival with carcinoid heart disease is 11 months.[43] A large percentage of patients with carcinoid heart disease are asymptomatic because the disease is mild. Early detection can affect prognosis as progression of cardiac disease, especially to right ventricular failure, increases mortality.[44] Treatment of the tumor and the malignant carcinoid syndrome does not result in regression of carcinoid heart disease.[45] Surgery to replace both tricuspid and pulmonary valve with either bioprosthetic or mechanical valve is the only viable therapeutic option.[49] The decision regarding mechanical or bioprosthetic valve(s) depends on individual risks and concerns.[43,50] The optimal timing to operate is uncertain, but consideration should be given when signs of right ventricular failure appear. Even after surgery, right ventricular dysfunction will persist. Perioperative mortality rate is less than 10%.[48]

Anesthetic Considerations

Patients who have carcinoid heart disease and require cardiac surgery pose an anesthetic challenge.[51–54] A carcinoid crisis with vasoactive mediator release is a life-threatening event that can be provoked by

stress, physical stimulation, anesthesia, catecholamines, long-acting opioids (meperidine, morphine), or histamine-releasing muscle relaxants (atracurium). Preoperative control of carcinoid activity is a critical aspect of perioperative management made considerably easier with the administration of octreotide, a synthetic analog of somatostatin that inhibits the vasoactive compounds that produce carcinoid syndrome. It reduces the occurrence of symptoms in more than 70% of patients. The longer half-life of octreotide than somatostatin allows subcutaneous injection of 150 µg three times daily to control symptoms. After surgery, intravenous octreotide (50 to 100 µg/hr) should be started 2 hours before surgery and continued for 48 hours after surgery. Additional intermittent intravenous doses of 50 to 200 µg are given to stop severe hypotension and prevent further carcinoid symptoms.[55] Anesthesiologists should be prepared to give large doses of octreotide (300 µg/hr) for stabilization during the intraoperative and postoperative periods. Atrial fibrillation is present in 18% of carcinoid patients, possibly because of the right-sided failure and chamber enlargement, as well as the proarrhythmic effects of seratonin.[56] Severe hyperglycemia may occur with octreotide because of its inhibition of insulin secretion, especially in combination with steroids, so glucose monitoring is recommended.[50]

Preoperative medication to reduce anxiety is strongly suggested for these patients.[51] Individuals with more active carcinoid disease experience greater reductions in systolic blood pressure with induction of anesthesia. Etomidate has been recommended for induction instead of thiopental (histamine-releasing) with short-acting opioids (fentanyl and sufentanil) and nonhistamine-releasing muscle relaxants.[50] Benzodiazepines are especially valuable for preoperative anxiety, as well as part of anesthetic maintenance. The standard low-to-moderate dose of fentanyl or sufentanil anesthetic with isoflurane is recommended with a nonhistamine-producing muscle relaxant.[57]

Sudden intraoperative hypotension should be regarded as carcinoid crisis and intravenous octreotide administered until hemodynamic stability returns. Careful attention should be paid to physiologic parameters such as airway pressures as early warning signs of impending carcinoid crisis and treated before onset of severe hypotension. Previously, certain catecholamines (epinephrine, norepinephrine, dopamine, and isoproterenol) were considered to provoke mediator release in carcinoid syndrome, but a recent retrospective study of 100 consecutive patients who underwent cardiac surgery with carcinoid heart disease did not show a significant increase in intraoperative octreotide need or mortality with the use of vasoactive medications.[54] The majority of patients in this study received vasopressor agents such as epinephrine, dopamine, and calcium. Because nearly 75% of these patients for cardiac surgery will be in New York Heart Association (NYHA) Class III and require multiple valve replacement, vasoactive medication should be administered according to hemodynamic indices. The safety of vasoactive medications in these patients with octreotide use has been confirmed in a subsequent study.[57] Low CO from right ventricular failure and hypotension from vasoplegia are common in the postbypass period, so identifying carcinoid crisis in such circumstances is problematic.

The use of an antifibrinolytic is routine in many centers to reduce blood loss and transfusion requirements associated with CPB and cardiac surgery.[58] Because patients with carcinoid heart disease often require surgery involving multiple valves in association with liver metastasis, coagulopathy and excessive hemorrhage after CPB are likely and considered one of the two major complications associated with surgery.[55,57] Weingarten et al[54] reported significant reductions in red blood cell (RBC) and non-RBC transfusions in patients undergoing cardiac surgery for carcinoid heart disease who received aprotinin compared with those who did not. Aprotinin use was not associated with a reduction in mortality. Aprotinin has the dual properties of antifibrinolysis and anti-inflammation compared with other popular synthetic antifibrinolytic agents (tranexamic acid and aminocaproic acid), but it is no longer available for administration. Synthetic antifibrinolytics appear safe for use in carcinoid heart disease.[57]

CARDIOMYOPATHY

Previously, the World Health Organization (WHO)/International Society of Cardiology defined cardiomyopathy as heart muscle disease of unknown cause, unlike heart muscle disease attributed to a specific cause or associated with a disease process. With more knowledge concerning pathogenesis and causative factors, the difference between cardiomyopathy and specific heart disease has become less distinct. Previously, cardiomyopathy was classified as dilated, hypertrophic, and restrictive. Over time, each classification has become a recognized clinical condition. In 1995, the WHO/International Society of Cardiology redefined the cardiomyopathies according to dominant pathophysiology or, if possible, by "etiologic/pathogenetic factors."[59] Cardiomyopathies are now defined as "diseases of the myocardium associated with cardiac dysfunction." The original cardiomyopathies classified as dilated cardiomyopathy (DCM), restrictive cardiomyopathy (RCM), and hypertrophic cardiomyopathy (HCM) were preserved, and arrhythmogenic right ventricular cardiomyopathy (ARVC) was added.

The annual incidence of cardiomyopathy in adults is 8.7 cases per 100,000 person-years.[60] Underlying causes of cardiomyopathies are different but carry some prognostic significance.[61] General characteristics of all four cardiomyopathies are displayed in Table 22-2. Reviews of the clinical, pathophysiologic, and therapeutic aspects of these cardiomyopathies

are available.[62–64] This section focuses on cardiomyopathy in relation to cardiac surgery, but it is relevant for the larger number of patients with a cardiomyopathy who undergo noncardiac surgery.

All the cardiomyopathies maintain some relation to genetic transmission. The genetics of these cardiomyopathies will not be addressed in detail, but this does not reflect a lack of importance. Genetic testing is advancing rapidly, with the ability to identify disease-causing mutations in those family members at risk but asymptomatic. The result is heightened clinical surveillance and, possibly, earlier intervention and prevention of the sequelae of the disease. More information is available in this review.[65]

Dilated Cardiomyopathy

Formerly referred to as congestive cardiomyopathy or idiopathic cardiomyopathy, DCM is by far the most common of the four cardiomyopathies in adults (60%). The term *idiopathic* has become less applicable to cardiomyopathies as developments in molecular biology and genetics have provided better insight into the pathogenesis of DCM. In the United States alone, nearly 550,000 individuals are newly diagnosed with CHF, whereas close to 4.6 million receive treatment for it. Even with current management, survival for adults at 1 and 5 years after diagnosis is 76% and 35%, respectively, representing a major health care concern.[66] Interestingly, diagnosis of DCM in asymptomatic patients occurs in 30% of patients with extended quality of life and survival if medical treatment is initiated.[67] This would suggest a less-advanced disease process and being more amenable to treatment. Nonischemic causes comprise 25% to 35% of adult patients with left ventricular dysfunction and CHF, of which DCM is a major component.[63]

DCM has diverse causes, such as viral, inflammatory, toxic, or familial/genetic. It is associated with many cardiac and systemic disorders that influence the prognosis. Approximately 1230 patients with cardiomyopathy were evaluated and grouped according to a specific cause.[61] Table 22-3 shows that 50% of patients had common causes for DCM, but 50% were characterized as idiopathic. Currently, there is a greater appreciation for the role of genetic and familial factors in the cause of DCM (Figure 22-9).[64,68,69] Between 10% and 35% of cases of DCM are familial with an autosomal dominant expression.[63] Incomplete penetrance may account for differences in disease severity and progression in familial DCM despite sharing identical mutations.[64] Similarities in clinical course that evoke a common set of molecular and cellular pathways may lead to better therapy in the future despite the many different causes of DCM.

DCM is characterized morphologically by enlargement of right and left ventricular cavities with hypertrophied muscle fibers without an appropriate increase in the ventricular septal or free wall thickness, giving an almost spherical shape to the heart. These hearts are two to three times larger than normal.[64] The valve leaflets may be normal,

TABLE 22-2	Characteristics of Cardiomyopathies			
Characteristics	*Hypertrophic Cardiomyopathy*	*Dilated Cardiomyopathy*	*Arrhythmogenic Right Ventricular Cardiomyopathy*	*Restrictive Cardiomyopathy*
Clinical				
Heart failure	Occasional (LV)	Frequent (LV or BV)	Frequent (RV)	Frequent (BV)
Arrhythmias	Atrial and ventricular arrhythmias	Atrial and ventricular arrhythmias, conduction defects	Ventricular tachycardia (RV), conduction defects	Atrial fibrillation
Sudden death	0.7–11% per year	Frequent (ND)	Frequent (ND)	1–5% per year
Hemodynamically				
Systolic function	Hyperdynamic, outflow tract obstruction (occasionally)	Reduced	Normal-reduced	Near normal
Diastolic function	Reduced	Reduced	Reduced	Severely reduced
Morphologic				
Cavity size				
Ventricle	Reduced (LV)	Enlarged (LV or BA)	Enlarged (RV)	Normal or reduced (BV)
Atrium	Normal-enlarged (LA)	Enlarged (LA or BA)	Enlarged (RV)	Enlarged (BA)
Wall thickness	Enlarged, asymmetric (LV)	Normal-reduced (LV or BV)	Normal-reduced (RV)	Normal (BV)

BA, both atria; BV, both ventricles; LA, left atrium; LV, left ventricle; ND, not determined; RA, right atrium; RV, right ventricle.
From Franz WM, Müller OJ, Katus HA: Cardiomyopathies: From genetics to the prospect of treatment. *Lancet* 358:1628, 2001.

TABLE 22-3	Common Clinicopathologic Diagnoses in 1230 Patients with Initially Unexplained Cardiomyopathy	
Diagnosis		*No. of Patients (%)*
Idiopathic dilated cardiomyopathy		616 (50)
Myocarditis		111 (9)
Ischemic cardiomyopathy		91 (7)
Infiltrative disease		59 (5)
Peripartum cardiomyopathy		51 (4)
Hypertension		49 (4)
Human immunodeficiency virus infection		45 (4)
Connective tissue disease		39 (3)
Substance abuse		37 (3)
Doxorubicin related		15 (1)
Other causes		111 (10)

From Wu LA, Lapeyre AC, Cooper LT: Current role of endomyocardial biopsy in the management of dilated cardiomyopathy and myocarditis. *Mayo Clin Proc* 76: 1030–1038, 2001.

yet dilation of the heart has been associated with a regurgitant lesion secondary to displacement of the papillary muscle. Histologic changes are nonspecific and not associated with positive immunohistochemical, ultrastructural, or microbiologic tests. Microscopically, instead of large losses of myocardium, there is patchy and diffuse loss of tissue with interstitial fibrosis and scarring, uncharacteristic of ischemic myocardium.[64] Degenerative changes are responsible for bundle branch block on the electrocardiogram (ECG).

With DCM, there is more impairment of systolic function even though diastolic function is affected. As contractile function diminishes, stroke volume initially is maintained by augmentation of end-diastolic volume. Despite a severely decreased ejection fraction, stroke volume may be almost normal. Eventually, increased wall stress caused by marked left ventricular dilation and normal or thin left ventricular wall thickness occurs.[63] Increasing left atrial size may indicate worsening diastolic dysfunction in these patients, contributing significantly to functional mitral regurgitation.[70] It is important to expand the diagnosis of mitral regurgitation with echo beyond the left ventricular

geometry and mitral orifice because contractility and dyssynchrony are essential for the correct diagnosis. Dilation, combined with valvular regurgitation, compromises the metabolic capabilities of heart muscle and produces overt circulatory failure. Compensatory mechanisms may allow symptoms of myocardial dysfunction to go unnoticed for an extended period. However, the onset of mitral regurgitation signals a poor prognosis as the ventricular function progressively worsens without intervention. The importance of corresponding neurohumoral influences, such as the renin-angiotensin system, on this pathologic process recently was appreciated as a major factor in the appearance of typical signs and symptoms of CHF and formation of therapeutic options (Figure 22-10).[71,72] Additional evidence of cytokine activity and endothelium dysfunction provide a complex interplay of forces leading to circulatory failure. The possibility of blocking this neurohumoral response of CHF pharmacologically has not been fully realized, as early trials have been disappointing.[73]

Although DCM occurs in children, its presentation is generally in the fourth and fifth decades of life.[64] The clinical picture of DCM typically includes signs and symptoms of CHF often corresponding to months of fatigue, weakness, and reduced exercise tolerance before diagnosis.[62] One-third of individuals report chest pain.[63] However, the first indication of DCM may be a stroke, arrhythmia, or even sudden death. Increasingly, individuals are presenting for routine medical screening to be informed of cardiomegaly on a routine chest roentgenogram. Symptoms may appear insidiously over a period of years or evolve rapidly after an unrelated illness. Physical signs of DCM, depending on the disease's progression, include pulsus alternans, jugular venous distention, murmurs of atrioventricular valvular regurgitation, tachycardia, and gallop heart sounds.

A chest roentgenogram demonstrates variable degrees of cardiomegaly and pulmonary venous congestion (Figure 22-11). An ECG may be surprisingly normal or depict low QRS voltage, abnormal axis, nonspecific ST-segment abnormalities, left ventricular hypertrophy, conduction defects, and evidence of atrial enlargement. Atrial fibrillation is common, and about one fourth of patients have nonsustained ventricular tachycardia.[62] Although the LV is affected, the RV may be spared in some patients, and this finding has been associated with

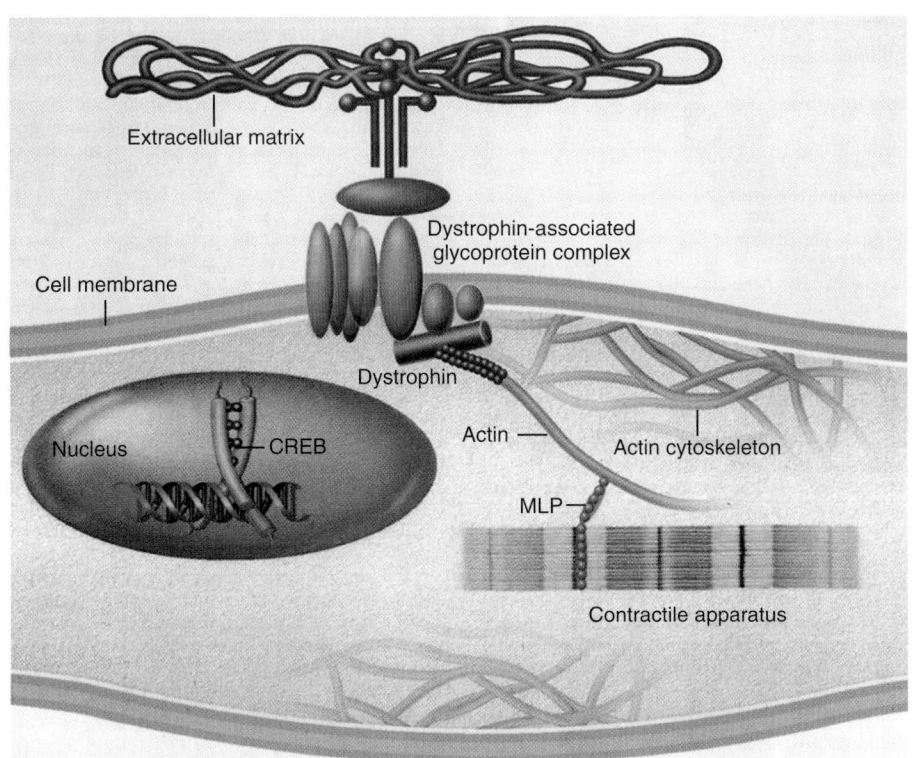

Figure 22-9 A cardiac myocyte and the molecules that have been implicated in dilated cardiomyopathy. CREB, cyclic AMP response element binding protein; MLP, muscle LIM protein. (*From Leiden JM: The genetics of dilated cardiomyopathy—emerging clues to the puzzle.* N Engl J Med *337:1080–1081, 1997, by permission.*)

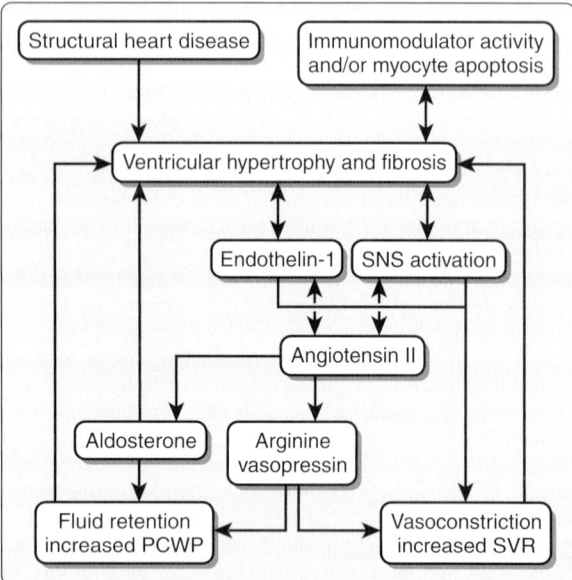

Figure 22-10 Impact of pathophysiologic mediators on hemodynamics in patients with heart failure. PCWP, pulmonary capillary wedge pressure; SNS, sympathetic nervous system; SVR, systemic vascular resistance. *(From McBride BF, White CM: Acute decompensated heart failure: A contemporary approach to pharmacotherapeutic management. Pharmacotherapy 23:1002, 2003, by permission.)*

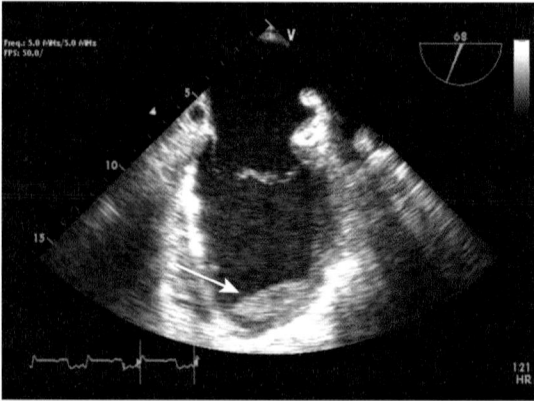

Figure 22-12 **Transesophageal echocardiogram, midesophageal, two-chamber view in a patient with dilated cardiomyopathy.** There is a large amount of the thrombus *(arrow)* seen in the apex of the left ventricle. In any patient with severe left ventricular dysfunction undergoing an echocardiographic examination, it is important to image the left ventricle as completely as possible to rule out the presence of thrombus.

improved survival.[74] Coronary catheterization usually reveals normal coronary vessels. Coronary angiography also will distinguish between ischemic and idiopathic DCM, a finding that has therapeutic and prognostic implications. An endomyocardial biopsy rarely is valuable to identify the cause of DCM but may be useful to rule out other pathologies with similar presentation to DCM.[64] The biopsy has no prognostic value or correlation with ventricular function.

Echo is extremely useful in the ambulatory management of patients with DCM. The characteristic 2D findings are a dilated LV with globally decreased systolic function. Indeed, all markers of systolic function (ejection fraction, fractional shortening, stroke volume, and CO) are uniformly decreased.[33] Other associated findings may include a dilated mitral annulus with incomplete mitral leaflet coaptation, dilated atria, right ventricular enlargement, and thrombus in the left ventricular apex (Figure 22-12). In some instances, regional wall motion abnormalities

will be present. Color Doppler imaging is useful in assessing the presence or absence of valvular regurgitation. Pulsed-wave and continuous-wave Doppler are used to quantify CO and evaluate filling pressures and pulmonary artery pressures. Well-compensated patients with DCM may have only mild impairment of diastolic function. As the disease progresses and patients become less well-compensated, the left ventricular diastolic filling pattern changes to that of restricted filling. Although systolic function may not change in these patients, the increased filling pressures associated with restrictive left ventricular filling will often worsen their CHF symptomatology.

Management of acute decompensated CHF continues to evolve, but the onset of overt CHF is a poor prognostic indicator for persons with DCM.[71] However, compared with ischemic CHF, patients with nonischemic DCM show greater improvement in symptoms, left ventricular function, and remodeling during more contemporary therapy than in the past.[75] Treatment revolves around management of symptoms and progression of DCM, whereas other measures are designed to prevent complications such as pulmonary thromboembolism and arrhythmias. The mainstay of therapy for DCM is vasodilators combined with digoxin and diuretics. All patients receive angiotensin-converting enzyme inhibitors to reduce symptoms, improve exercise tolerance, and reduce cardiovascular mortality without a direct myocardial effect.[62,76,77]

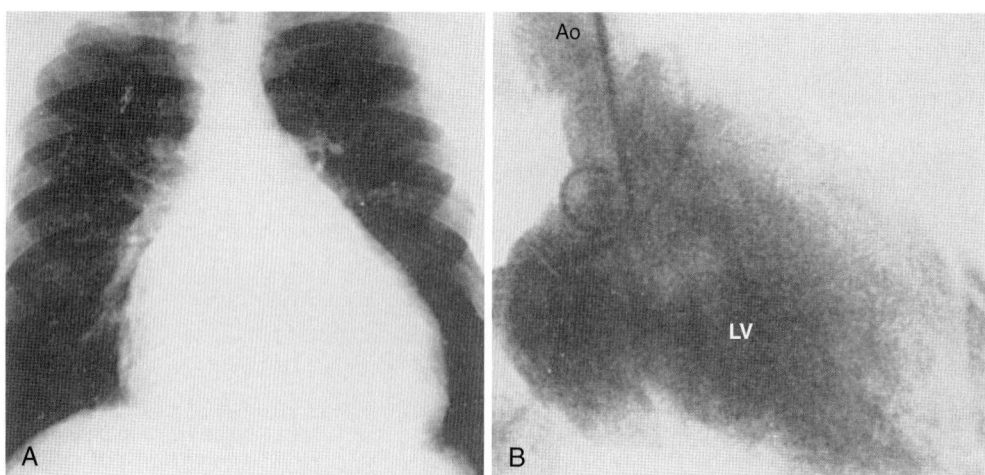

Figure 22-11 *A,* Chest radiograph showing marked cardiomegaly in a 28-year-old man with idiopathic dilated cardiomyopathy. Pulmonary vascularity is within normal limits. *B,* Left ventriculogram in systole shows marked dilatation. Ao, aorta; LV, left ventricle. *(From Stevenson, LW, Perloff JK: The dilated cardiomyopathies: Clinical aspects. Cardiol Clin 6:187, 1988, by permission.)*

Perhaps more important than the hemodynamic effects, angiotensin-converting enzyme inhibitors suppress ventricular remodeling and endothelial dysfunction, accounting for the improvement in mortality noted with this medication in DCM.[78] Other afterload-reducing agents, such as selective phosphodiesterase-3 inhibitors like milrinone, may improve quality of life but do not affect mortality, and thus are rarely administered in chronic situations. More recently, spironolactone has assumed a greater role in treatment as mortality rate was reduced by 30% from all causes in patients receiving standard angiotensin-converting enzyme inhibitors for DCM with the addition of spironolactone in a large, double-blind, randomized trial.[79] Although aldosterone increases sodium retention and reduces potassium loss, it also has been shown to cause myocardial and vascular fibrosis, impair baroreceptor function, and prevent catecholamine reuptake by the myocardium.

Until recently, β-blockers were contraindicated in DCM. In 1982, Bristow et al[80] found decreased catecholamine sensitivity and β-receptor density in the failing human myocardium, leading to loss of contractility. The association between excess sympathetic activity and the failing heart has been aptly demonstrated.[81] Recently, the dobutamine stress test has been shown to identify changes that reflect increased sympathetic stimulation in the ventricle of asymptomatic to mildly symptomatic patients with DCM.[82] This finding may aid in the initiation of β-blockers in patients with normal resting parameters. The use of β-blockers in DCM has not only provided symptomatic improvement, but also substantial reductions in sudden and progressive death with NYHA Class II and III heart failure.[83] This is especially significant because almost 50% of deaths are sudden.[84]

High-grade ventricular arrhythmias are common with DCM. Approximately 12% of all patients with DCM die suddenly,[85] but overall prediction of sudden death in an individual with DCM is poor.[84] Electrophysiologic (EP) testing has a poor negative predictive value that limits its usefulness. The best predictor of sudden death remains the degree of left ventricular dysfunction. Patients who have sustained ventricular tachycardia or out-of-hospital ventricular fibrillation are at increased risk for sudden death, but more than 70% of patients with DCM have nonsustained ventricular tachycardia during ambulatory monitoring.[77] Furthermore, the prognostic significance of ventricular arrhythmias and response to prophylactic antiarrhythmia therapy in patients with DCM are not well established.

Antiarrhythmic medications are hazardous in patients with poor ventricular function because of their negative inotropic and sometimes proarrhythmic properties. Antiarrhythmic therapy may only be considered in DCM if inducible ventricular tachycardia or symptomatic arrhythmias are present. Class I agents are not indicated because they clearly have demonstrated increased mortality in patients with advanced CHF.[62] Amiodarone is the preferred antiarrhythmic agent in DCM because its negative inotropic effect is less than other antiarrhythmic medications[84] and its proarrhythmic potential is lowest.[86] Counter to most trials of antiarrhythmic prophylaxis, results of a recent large multicenter trial of antiarrhythmic therapy in patients with CHF[86] demonstrated that amiodarone was associated with a significantly lower mortality rate of 38% compared with 62% without therapy in persons with a higher resting heart rate. Not withstanding these results, implantable defibrillators reduce the risk for sudden death, as well as reducing mortality.[84,85] Recent evidence has indicated that with previous cardiac arrest or sustained ventricular tachycardia, more benefit was gained from an implantable defibrillator.[87] This was based on a 27% reduction in the relative risk for death attributed to a 50% reduction in arrhythmia-related mortality compared with treatment with amiodarone (see Chapters 4, 10, and 25).

Other treatments for DCM include digoxin, which has been reaffirmed as clinically beneficial in two large trials of adults.[74] The risk for thromboembolic complications is significant in DCM for adults. Patients with moderate ventricular dilation and moderate-to-severe systolic dysfunction have intracavitary stasis and a decreased ejection of blood, so they are likely to receive anticoagulants if any history of stroke, atrial fibrillation, or evidence of intracardiac thrombus exists.

Patients who are resistant to pharmacologic therapy for CHF have received dual-chamber pacing, cardiomyoplasty, left ventricular assist devices, cardiac surgery (nontransplantation) and transplantation in recent years. Cardiac resynchronization therapy with dual ventricular pacing improves NYHA functional class and ejection fraction 6 months after implantation.[88] Placement of implantable left ventricular assist devices has enabled end-stage patients to reach transplantation or become destination therapy for those in whom transplantation is not an option.[89] If mitral regurgitation develops in patients with DCM, mitral valve repair or replacement is recommended. The surgery in this high-risk population is safe and improves NYHA classification and survival.[90] Transplantation can substantially prolong lives, with current survival at 15 years of 50% if younger than 55 years of age[91]; however, limited organ availability and drug-related morbidity for those with end-stage DCM looks to future improvements in assist devices and new surgical procedures to provide the best opportunity for increased survival. An example is a new surgical procedure called *surgical ventricular restoration* that may improve symptoms and cardiac status. It is performed with an arrested heart during CPB. Coronary artery bypass grafting (CABG) is first performed followed by ventriculotomy to insert the mannequin to reshape the ventricle (see Chapters 18 and 27).[92]

Anesthetic Considerations

The most common cardiac procedures for patients with DCM are correction of atrioventricular valve insufficiency, placement of an implantable cardioverter-defibrillator for refractory ventricular arrhythmias, and left ventricular assist device placement or allograft transplantation. Anesthetic management is formulated on afterload reduction, optimal preload, and minimal myocardial depression.

Individuals with DCM are extremely sensitive to cardiodepressant anesthetic drugs. Intravenously administered anesthetic agents such as fentanyl (30 μg/kg) provide excellent anesthesia and hemodynamics in patients with ejection fractions less than 30%[93] but contribute to prolonged respiratory depression delaying extubation. Shorter-acting narcotics such as remifentanil may be unsuitable for patients with poor left ventricular function undergoing cardiac surgery because of high incidences of bradycardia and severe hypotension.[94] A comparison of remifentanil-sevoflurane with fentanyl-etomidate-isoflurane found significantly greater reduction in mean arterial pressure and greater incidence of bradycardia with the remifentanil anesthetic.[95] Also, etomidate has been shown to have little effect on the contractility of the cardiac muscle in patients undergoing cardiac transplantation.[96] Ketamine has been recommended for induction in critically ill patients[97,98] because of its cardiovascular actions attributed mainly to a sympathomimetic effect from the central nervous system. Ketamine is a positive inotrope in the isolated rat papillary muscle and, more importantly, in a model of cardiomyopathic hamsters, did not display a negative inotropic effect.[99] This makes ketamine (less than 0.5 mg/kg) an excellent choice to use in combination with fentanyl for induction in patients with severe myocardial dysfunction secondary to cardiomyopathy. The use of propofol with cardiomyopathy may be a concern because cardiovascular depression has been observed possibly because of inhibition of sympathetic activity and a vasodilatory property. However, in a cardiomyopathic hamster model, there was no direct effect on myocardial contractility with propofol.[100] Caution is still prudent with propofol because of the indirect inhibitory effects of sympathetic activity that many patients with cardiomyopathy and reduced left ventricular function may depend on for hemodynamic stability.

Volatile agents have long been a concern in persons with failing hearts because of their known depressant effects on myocardial contractility. The effect of currently used volatile anesthetics on intrinsic myocardial contractility is difficult to project clinically. Animal data indicate halogenated volatile agents may have more profound negative inotropic effects in cardiomyopathic muscle than healthy cardiac muscle.[101] An anesthetic technique that minimizes myocardial depression is essential. There is little from a cardiovascular standpoint to support a selection of sevoflurane over isoflurane in adults.

Although the failing myocardium has been thought to be more sensitive to the depressant effects of volatile agents, there is no synergistic myocardial depression in the presence of moderate left ventricular dysfunction and volatile agents.[102] Desflurane, which possesses the lowest blood/gas partition coefficient of the volatile agents allowing rapid induction and emergence, would appear to have some theoretic benefit for early extubation in patients undergoing cardiac surgery. In healthy hamster papillary muscles, desflurane did not appear to have a negative inotropic effect; however, in cardiomyopathic papillary muscles, there was a profound negative inotropic effect.[103] On the other hand, sevoflurane and desflurane were shown not to adversely affect the ability of the LV to respond to increased work despite their negative inotropic properties in patients undergoing CPB and cardiac surgery.[104] Even with the limitations of generalizing findings of in vitro experiments to clinical situations, this difference of inotropic effect regarding healthy versus cardiomyopathic myocardium is an important distinction not present in all halogenated anesthetics and should be considered in patients with cardiomyopathy.

Invasive hemodynamic monitoring is indispensable with volatile agents and DCM. Of particular pertinence for anesthesiologists is that physical signs and symptoms of DCM may not accurately reflect physiologic parameters. Eighty percent of patients with pulmonary capillary wedge pressures greater than 25 mm Hg have no detectable rales.[105] The use of more aggressive monitoring will depend partially on the operation. Patients receiving implantable defibrillators usually have severely depressed left ventricular function but are routinely managed without a PAC. Echo also is useful for patients undergoing both cardiac and noncardiac surgery. For most cardiac surgical procedures (mitral valve surgery, left ventricular assist devices), echo is considered necessary to evaluate the results of the operation. In both cardiac and noncardiac surgery, echo can provide real-time data as to how interventions such as addition of inotropes or vasodilators change ventricular function and indirectly assess CO.

Hemodynamic instability that may occur with DCM can be lessened with a low dose of inotrope and vasodilator. Acute administration of inotropes, such as dobutamine, improves hemodynamics temporarily, but tolerance begins in 3 to 4 days.[77] Phosphodiesterase-3 inhibitors are useful if combined with another β-adrenergic agonist, such as milrinone and epinephrine, for short-term hemodynamic support. Afterload reduction in DCM is important because it improves regional and global indices of ventricular relaxation and ejection fraction during anesthesia when myocardial depression may be significant. It also may reduce valvular regurgitation and atrial volumes.[106] The use of levosimendan, an effective calcium-sensitizing agent with vasodilatory and inotropic features, may be an excellent agent to maintain hemodynamics because it also increases myocardial performance without major changes in the oxygen consumption or effects on the diastolic function.[107] Some patients with DCM may be chronically taking amiodarone, which has a negative inotropic effect that interacts with volatile agents to further reduce contractility and conduction, requiring careful titration of these anesthetic agents.[108] Arrhythmogenic factors such as hypokalemia, hypomagnesemia, and sympathetic activation should be monitored and corrected. Because of the structural nature of DCM, atrial fibrillation is likely to be present in 25% of cases. Patients with atrial fibrillation and DCM show significantly diminished myocardial perfusion and perfusion reserve compared with those in normal sinus rhythm.[109]

Hypertrophic Cardiomyopathy

Referred to as *idiopathic hypertrophic subaortic stenosis, hypertrophic obstructive cardiomyopathy,* and *asymmetric septal hypertrophy,* among other names, the accepted name is *hypertrophic cardiomyopathy* (HCM). It is the most common genetic cardiac disease with marked heterogeneity in clinical expression, pathophysiology, and prognosis. The overall prevalence rate for adults in the general population is 0.2%,[110] affecting men and women equally. The management continues to evolve with ever-increasing information discovered regarding HCM.

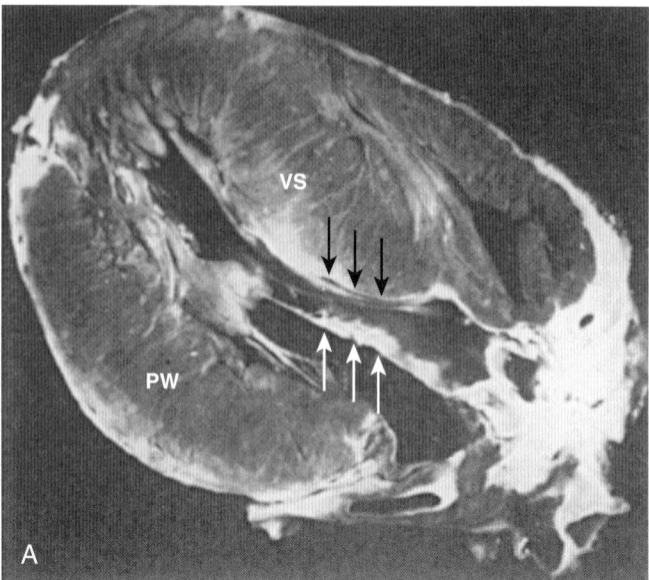

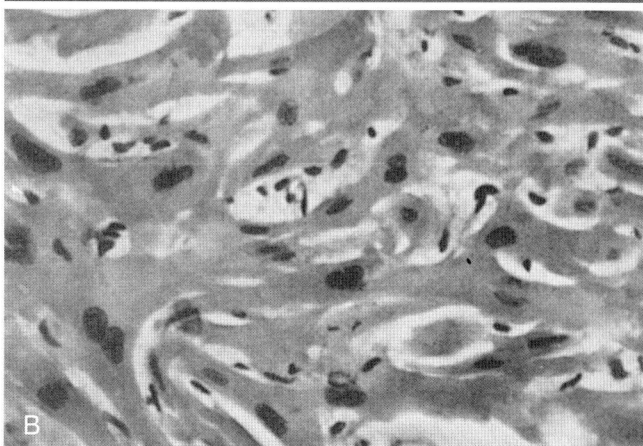

Figure 22-13 *A,* Hypertrophic cardiomyopathy (HCM) from the long-axis view. Ventricular cavity is small and has pronounced septal and posterior wall thickening. *Arrows* indicate narrowing of the left ventricular outflow tract caused by the thickened ventricular septum and anterior leaflet of the mitral valve. PW, posterior wall of the left ventricle; VS, ventricular septum. *B,* Photomicrograph of the myocardium in HCM. There are pronounced disarray and hypertrophy of the individual muscle fibers, resulting in a "whorling" appearance of the muscle fiber. Hematoxylin and eosin stain, original magnification ×165. (A, *From Edwards WD, Zakheim R, Mattioli L: Asymmetric septal hypertrophy in childhood: Unreliability of histologic criteria for differentiation of obstructive and nonobstructive forms. Hum Pathol 8:277, 1977, by permission; B, courtesy of William D. Edwards, MD; from Giuliani ER, Fuster V, Gersh BJ, et al: Cardiology: Fundamentals and Practice. St. Louis, Mosby, 1991, by permission of Mayo Foundation, by permission.)*

HCM is a primary myocardial abnormality with sarcomeric disarray and asymmetric left ventricular hypertrophy (Figure 22-13). The extent of sarcomeric disarray distinguishes HCM from other conditions.[59] The hypertrophied muscle is composed of muscle cells with bizarre shapes and multiple intercellular connections arranged in a chaotic pattern.[110] Increased connective tissue, combined with markedly disorganized and hypertrophied myocytes, contributes to the diastolic abnormalities of HCM that manifest as increased chamber stiffness, impaired and prolonged relaxation, and an unstable EP substrate that causes complex arrhythmias and sudden death. In contrast with the diastolic function, systolic function in HCM usually is normal or hyperdynamic, but eventually diminishes in the later stages of the disease.

Besides diastolic dysfunction, the other major abnormality and fundamental characteristic of HCM is myocardial hypertrophy unrelated to increased systemic vascular resistance (SVR). This nonuniform, asymmetric hypertrophy typically occurs in the basal anterior ventricular septum and anterior free wall, with a disproportionate increase in the thickness of the ventricular wall relative to the posterior free wall (Figure 22-13A). Less commonly, the hypertrophy occurs at the apex, lateral wall, or concentrically. The left ventricular wall thickness is the most extensive of all cardiac conditions.[110] Heart size may be deceptive because it may vary from normal to more than 100% enlarged. However, chamber enlargement is not responsible for the increase in ventricular mass but rather increases in wall thickness.

HCM is the most common genetic cardiovascular disease inherited in an autosomal dominant manner (1:500 of the general population).[59] It may be caused by mutations in any of 10 genes; however, 3 genes that encode proteins of the cardiac sarcomere predominate in frequency.[111] The similarity of the genes accounts for the many different expressions of HCM while resembling one disease entity. Patients without a family history of HCM may have sporadic gene mutations or simply a mild form of the disease. DNA analysis of mutant genes is the most definitive method to establish the diagnosis. The phenotype appears not only to depend on the mutation but also other modifier genes and environmental factors.[111,112] Not all patients who possess a gene for HCM will manifest clinical features of the disease, reflecting incomplete genetic expression.[110] A preclinical diagnosis in a patient without symptoms is possible with gene testing not routinely performed now or used to establish a treatment strategy.

HCM is unique for its range of clinical presentations from infancy to 90 years of age. Although major referral centers describe a disease with severe symptomatology, many elderly adults with mild-to-asymptomatic disease were unaccounted for, resulting in an actual annual mortality rate for HCM closer to 1% per year than previously reported to be 3% to 6% per year.[110] Even left ventricular outflow tract (LVOT) obstruction may be tolerated longer than initially believed. Most patients with HCM are asymptomatic or have mild symptoms that progress slowly or not at all.[63]

Symptoms of HCM are nonspecific and include chest pain, palpitations, dyspnea, and syncope. Dyspnea occurs in 90% of patients secondary to diastolic abnormalities that increase filling pressures causing pulmonary congestion. Syncope occurs in only 20% of patients, but 50% may have presyncopal symptoms. The physical examination is sometimes unreliable because classic physical findings are associated with LVOT obstruction that is not present in all patients; however, a recent study observed prospectively 320 patients with HCM and their gradients.[113] They found that 37% of patients had LVOT obstruction at rest and another 33% only with provocation. Symptoms usually appear in the second or third decade, but HCM is not a static disease, and left ventricular hypertrophy can occur at any age and increase or decrease dynamically throughout the person's life.[110] The ECG is abnormal in most individuals showing increased QRS voltage, ST-segment and T-wave abnormalities, QRS axis shift, and left ventricular hypertrophy with strain pattern. There is little correlation between ECG voltages and the degree of left ventricular hypertrophy.[110] A chest roentgenogram may show left atrial enlargement or be normal.

Echo is the modality of choice for the evaluation of HCM. Two-dimensional TTE usually allows the clinician to characterize the morphology of the disease and location of the hypertrophy. Doppler and color-flow imaging have typical appearances in HCM. Continuous-wave Doppler is used to quantify the gradient across the LVOT. The Doppler signal has a unique "dagger-shaped" appearance (Figure 22-14). The LVOT Doppler signal typically is obtained with an apical position of the transducer during TTE or from a deep transgastric view when TEE is utilized. If the LVOT gradient is less than expected, provocative maneuvers should be utilized in an effort to demonstrate an increased gradient. A Valsalva maneuver, by decreasing preload and ventricular filling, and inhalation of amyl nitrite are both noninvasive techniques that can be used in the conscious patient (see Figure 22-14). Mitral regurgitation usually accompanies LVOT obstruction when the obstruction

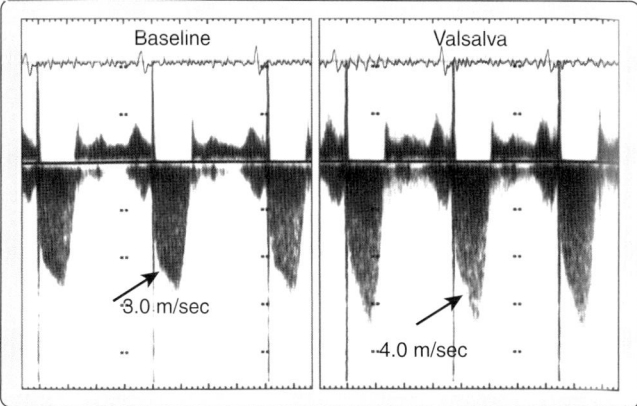

Figure 22-14 Continuous-wave Doppler spectra obtained from the apex demonstrating dynamic left ventricular outflow tract (LVOT) obstruction. Note the typical late-peaking configuration resembling a dagger or ski slope *(arrows)*. The baseline (left) velocity is 2.8 m/sec, corresponding to the peak LVOT of 31 mm Hg (4 × 2.8²). With the Valsalva maneuver (right), the velocity increased to 3.5 m/sec, corresponding to a gradient of 55 mm Hg. *(From Oh JK, Seward JB, Tajik AJ: The Echo Manual, 3rd ed. Philadelphia, 2006, Lippincott Williams & Wilkins, by permission.)*

is severe or symptomatic. The narrowing of the LVOT by septal hypertrophy necessitates an increase in flow velocity through the LVOT. This increase in flow velocity draws the anterior leaflet of the mitral valve into the LVOT, called the *Venturi effect.* The mitral leaflet and apparatus subsequently cause obstruction of flow through the LVOT, as well as mitral regurgitation. Temporally, mitral regurgitation occurs after LVOT obstruction: ejection → obstruction to left ventricular outflow → mitral regurgitation. The jet of mitral regurgitation typically is directed posterolaterally (Figure 22-15). It is important to note that if the mitral regurgitant jet is not posterolateral, there likely is another component to the mitral regurgitation such as mitral valve prolapse (MVP) or ruptured chordae. This has important ramifications in terms of planning a surgical repair. The diastolic filling pattern associated with HCM is that of severely impaired myocardial relaxation secondary to hypertrophy.[110]

Intraoperative TEE is essential in the care of patients undergoing septal myectomy.[114] Before incision, TEE can identify the location of hypertrophy in relation to the aortic annulus, as well as the thickness of the ventricular septum, which assists the surgeon in planning the location and depth of the myectomy. The mitral valve should be closely evaluated for abnormalities that may contribute to mitral regurgitation, particularly if the regurgitant jet is directed centrally or anterior. After the myectomy, TEE is used to assess the degree of residual mitral regurgitation and evidence of continued systolic anterior motion (SAM) and LVOT obstruction. The ventricular septum also must be closely evaluated for evidence of shunting via an iatrogenic ventricular septal defect (VSD). It is common to see small shunts into the area of the LVOT from transection of coronary vessels at the site of the myectomy (Figure 22-16). It is important that these are not confused with shunting from a VSD. When an iatrogenic VSD occurs, the expected shunt would be from the LV into the RV, as opposed to the flow observed into the LV from transection of septal coronary artery branches. In addition, shunting through a VSD would be expected to occur predominantly during systole, whereas flow into the LV from septal perforators is predominantly during diastole.

Angiography may show a left ventricular pressure gradient, decreased ventricular volume, and increased left ventricular end-diastolic pressure. Coronary artery diseases may be absent angiographically, but thallium redistribution scans demonstrate that HCM patients may experience myocardial ischemia often associated with atypical chest pain, not relieved with nitrates.[115] Blunted coronary perfusion despite angiographically normal coronary arteries is

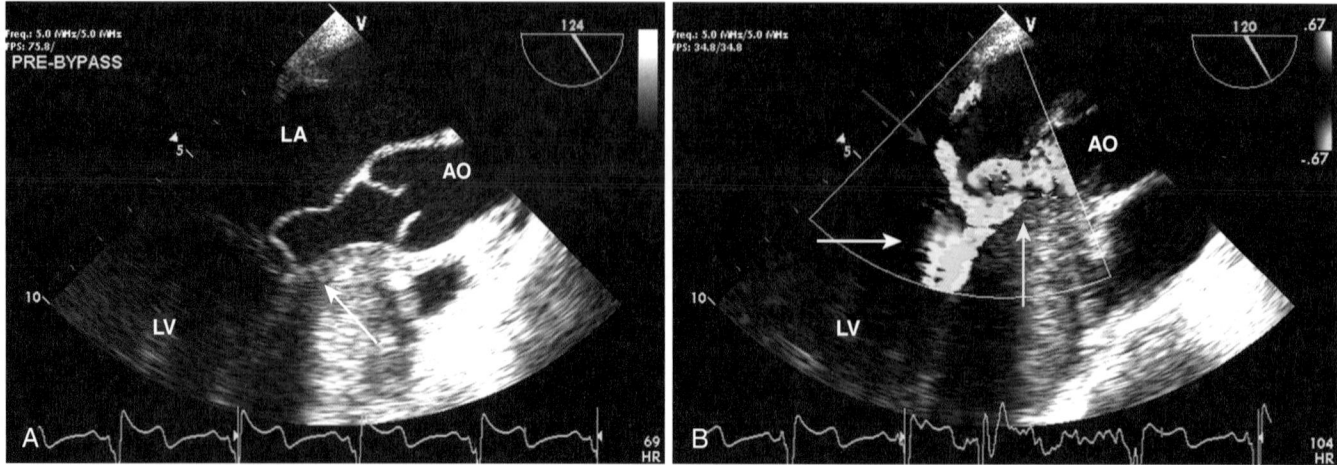

Figure 22-15 **Transesophageal long-axis view of the aortic valve and left ventricular outflow tract (LVOT) in a patient with hypertrophic obstructive cardiomyopathy (HCM).** *Left,* Two-dimensional image. The septum is thickened *(arrow).* The aortic valve is opening indicating systole, and both of the mitral valve leaflets have been drawn into the LVOT. Right, Classic color Doppler image of a patient with HCM is displayed. Aliasing of the Doppler spectra begins at the base of the heart, the site of the septal hypertrophy *(yellow arrow),* and becomes more severe in the LVOT *(white arrow).* The mitral regurgitation signal *(red arrow)* is directed posterolaterally. The three color signals form a Y shape. AO, aorta; LA, left atrium; LV, left ventricle.

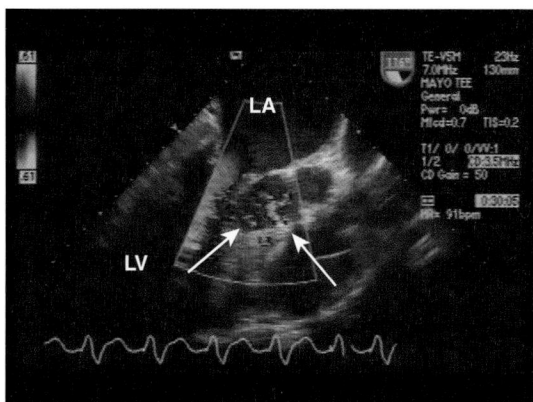

Figure 22-16 **Transesophageal image from a patient after a septal myectomy for hypertrophic obstructive cardiomyopathy.** The probe is in the midesophagus in a modified long-axis view. Color Doppler imaging reveals two jets of blood flow into the left ventricular outflow *(arrows)* tract from small coronary perforators that were transected during the myectomy. It is important that these jets of blood flow are not confused with a ventricular septal defect. LA, left atrium; LV left ventricle.

characteristic of a coronary microvascular dysfunction that increases the risk for ischemia, especially in the subendocardium. More recently, the degree of LVOT obstruction and wall stress were found to exacerbate microvascular dysfunction.[116] This may have implications for treatments that reduce left ventricular mass and wall stress instead of increasing diastolic filling time with medications such as β-blockers and calcium channel blockers, and partially explain the benefit of myectomy. Thallium abnormalities may represent relatively underperfused myocardium with abnormal intramyocardial coronary arteries that exist in patients with HCM. Abnormal coronary vasodilation in both nonhypertrophied and hypertrophied myocardium occur in HCM.[117] This suggests that impaired coronary vasodilation has a major role in the pathogenesis of HCM and is not secondary to only myocardial hypertrophy. However, a mismatch between myocardial oxygen demand resulting from systolic and diastolic abnormalities, increased ventricular mass, and coronary circulation may exacerbate myocardial ischemia. Thus, myocardial death and scarring may then serve as a substrate for ventricular tachycardia and fibrillation.[110]

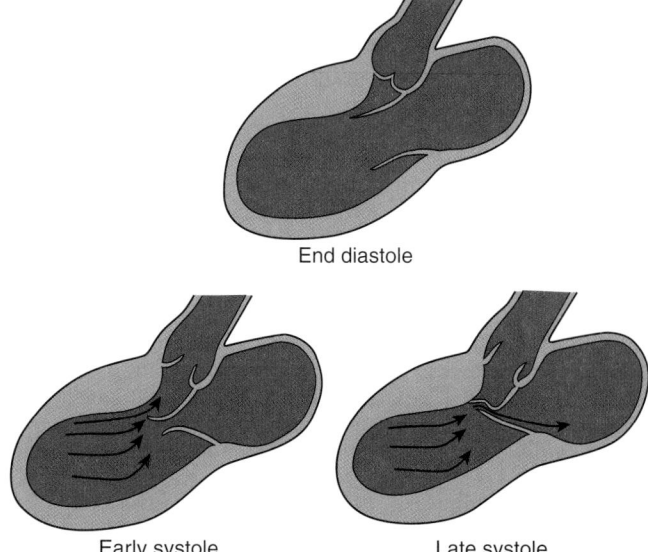

End diastole

Early systole   Late systole

Figure 22-17 Depiction of the modern concepts of the mechanism of left ventricular outflow tract obstruction in hypertrophic cardiomyopathy. In early systole (bottom left), abnormal flow around the hypertrophied septum pushes the mitral valve in the outflow tract and results in obstruction and mitral valve regurgitation (bottom right). *(From Ommen SR, Shah PM, Tajik AJ: Left ventricular outflow tract obstruction in hypertrophic cardiomyopathy: Past, present and future. Heart 94:1276–1281, 2008, by permission.)*

Two thirds of individuals with LVOT obstruction will become severely symptomatic, and there is a 10% mortality rate within 4 years of diagnosis. The LVOT is narrowed from septal hypertrophy and anterior displacement of the papillary muscles and mitral leaflets, creating a dynamic left ventricular outflow obstruction. Elongation of the mitral leaflets results in coaptation of the body of the leaflets instead of the tips. The part of the anterior leaflet distal to the coaptation is subjected to strong Venturi forces that provoke SAM, mitral septal contact, and ultimately, LVOT obstruction (Figure 22-17).[111] However, studies suggest that the mechanism of SAM is more complex. SAM can occur before the opening of the aortic valve and the generation of maximum Venturi effect because of the position of the mitral leaflets on the LVOT,

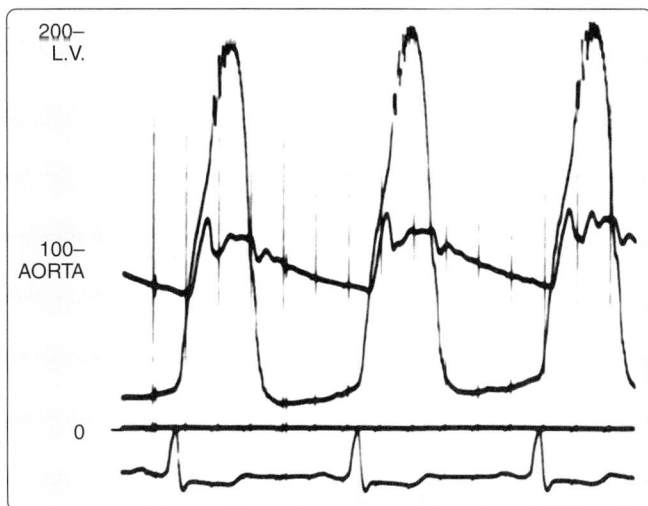

Figure 22-18 Simultaneous left ventricular (LV) and aortic pressure tracings from a patient with muscular subaortic stenosis (resting obstruction). *(From Wigle ED, Sasson Z, Henderson MA, et al: Hypertrophic cardiomyopathy: The importance of the site and extent of hypertrophy: A review. Prog Cardiovasc Dis 28:1, 1985, by permission.)*

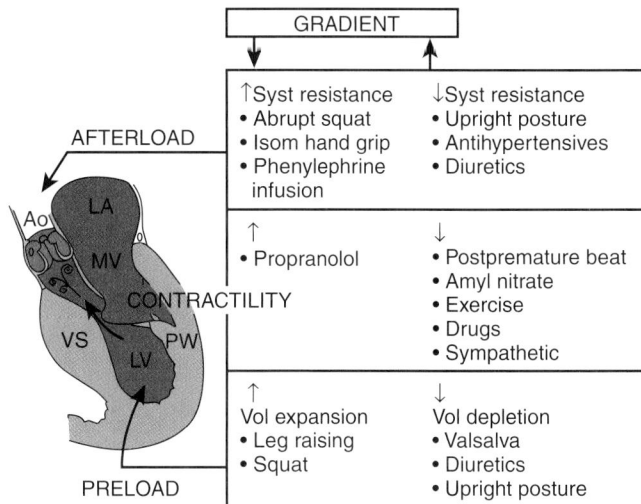

Figure 22-19 Interventions that change the outflow gradient in hypertrophic cardiomyopathy (HCM), with resultant change in intensity of the systolic murmur in HCM. Outflow gradient is affected by changes in afterload, preload, and contractility. Ao, aorta; LA, left atrium; LV, left ventricle; MV, mitral valve; PW, posterior wall; VS, ventricular septum. *(From Giuliani ER, Fuster V, Gersh BJ, et al: Cardiology: Fundamentals and Practice. St. Louis, Mosby, 1991, by permission of Mayo Foundation.)*

reflecting its importance in SAM compared with traditional explanations. Longitudinal flow in the ventricle may push the mitral valve into the LVOT.[118] SAM of the anterior leaflet also may cause mitral regurgitation that is unlike that seen with intrinsic structural abnormalities of the valve. The onset and duration of mitral leaflet-septal contact determine the magnitude of the gradient and the degree of mitral regurgitation. The pressure gradient between the aorta and LV (Figure 22-18) is worsened by decreased end-diastolic volume, increased contractility, or decreased aortic outflow resistance (Figure 22-19).[119] The cavity of the LV often is small in those with severe gradients (Figure 22-20).

Dynamic LVOT obstruction is not limited to HCM but may occur in cardiac tamponade or acute MI.[119] It may be seen in the immediate postoperative period after aortic valve replacement for aortic stenosis or mitral valve repair. Importantly, dynamic pressure gradients do not necessarily correlate with symptoms of HCM. Significant functional limitation, disability, and sudden death may all occur even with no gradient. However, gradients exceeding 30 mm Hg are usually of physiologic and

prognostic importance in HCM patients.[111] The severity of symptoms is not worse once a gradient exceeds 30 mm Hg. LVOT obstruction is an independent predictor of death in HCM.[120] Because LVOT obstruction is likely to be associated with increased wall stress, myocardial ischemia, cell death, and eventual fibrosis, treatment to relieve it is desirable.

The clinical course and treatment of HCM are best approached in relation to subgroups: sudden death, CHF, and atrial fibrillation with embolic stroke (Figure 22-21). Sudden death increases the annual mortality rate from 1% to 5% overall.[110] Often these patients are asymptomatic or mildly symptomatic and constitute a small part of the HCM population. Sudden death is not age restricted but occurs more commonly in younger individuals, frequently in association with physical exertion. HCM is the most common cause of sudden death in otherwise healthy young individuals, reaching up to 6% per year in those 20 to 30 years of age.[121] Risk stratification for sudden death is useful now that it has been found that ventricular tachycardia or ventricular

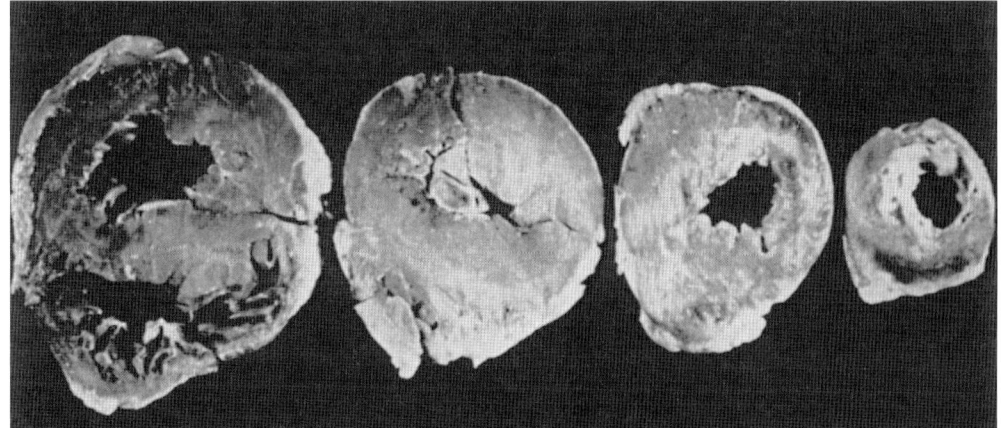

Figure 22-20 **Midventricular hypertrophy.** Cross-sectional slices of the heart from a patient who was shown, by hemodynamic, angiographic, and echocardiographic techniques, to have midventricular obstruction. The site of the obstruction was at the level of the papillary muscles, where there was massive hypertrophy (second slice from left). The slice at left is from the base of the heart, and the two slices at the right are from the apex. The apex of the left ventricle was the site of extensive myocardial infarction and aneurysm formation that was evidenced in life by a dyskinetic apical chamber on angiography and by persistent ST-segment elevation in leads V_4 to V_6 on the electrocardiogram. The coronary arteries revealed no significant luminal narrowings. The patient died of intractable ventricular arrhythmias. *(From Wigle ED, Rakowski H, Kimball BP, et al: Hypertrophic cardiomyopathy. Clinical spectrum and treatment. Circulation 92:1680, 1995, by permission.)*

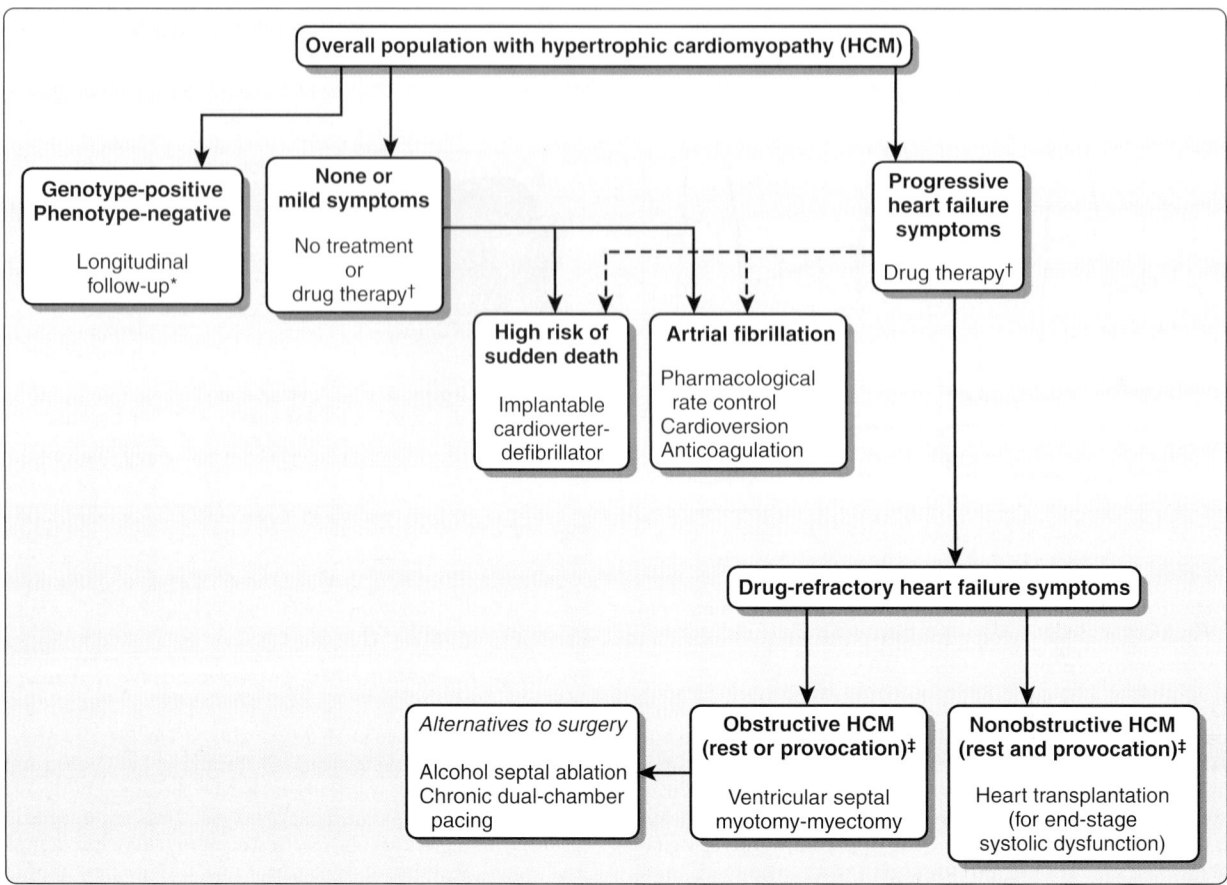

Figure 22-21 Hypertrophic cardiomyopathy (HCM) clinical subgroups are not necessarily mutually exclusive; overlap or progression from one subgroup to another may occur (*thin solid* and *dashed arrows*). Most patients with HCM who are at high risk for sudden death or who experience development of atrial fibrillation are initially in the "None or Mild Symptoms" clinical subgroup. *Asterisk* indicates that patients with a positive genotype and negative phenotype may subsequently show morphologic conversion to the HCM phenotype with left ventricular hypertrophy (usually in adolescence, but also in midlife or later). *Dagger* indicates that drug therapy may include β-blockers, calcium channel blockers (particularly verapamil), disopyramide, as well as diuretic agents. *Double dagger* indicates that for major interventions, obstructive HCM is generally regarded as a left ventricular outflow gradient of approximately 50 mm Hg at rest or with provocative maneuvers; in this context, nonobstructive HCM is regarded as a left ventricular outflow gradient of less than approximately 30 to 50 mm Hg at rest, as well as with provocative maneuvers. Width of the arrows from the overall HCM population represent the approximate relative proportion of patients with HCM within each major clinical subgroup. (*Originally adapted from Spirto et al: The management of hypertrophic cardiomyopathy.* N Engl J Med 336:775–785, 1997, *by permission of the Massachusetts Medical Society; reprinted with permission from Maron BJ: Hypertrophic cardiomyopathy: A systematic review* JAMA 287:1313, 2002.)

fibrillation is the culprit.[110,122] High-risk individuals are more likely to have these characteristics: diagnosis by 30 years of age, prior cardiac arrest, symptomatic ventricular tachycardia per Holter monitor, and family history of sudden death or syncope.[121] Additional risk factors include identification of a high-risk mutant gene, unexplained syncope, abnormal blood pressure with exercise, resting LVOT obstruction of 30 mm Hg or greater, atrial fibrillation, and even coronary artery disease.[111,121] Two or more risk factors are associated with a risk for sudden death of 4% to 5% per year.

The value of EP testing as it relates to prediction of sudden death is mixed.[111,123,124] Recently, routine risk stratification with EP testing was abandoned in HCM patients.[111] Extreme left ventricular wall thickness has been associated with greater incidence of spontaneous ventricular arrhythmias and sudden death. Myocardial ischemia also appears to be related to sudden death in younger patients.[125] In the future, genotyping may be able to reliably define the risk for sudden death, but currently there is no ability to screen patients to determine risk stratification with clinical gene tests for characteristics such as sudden death.[126] Septal myectomy reduces the risk for sudden death in patients compared with those with LVOT obstruction and no surgery and those with nonobstructive HCM. The mechanism for this improved survival is indeterminate.[127]

The only effective modality to prevent sudden death associated with HCM currently is the implantable cardioverter-defibrillator. Pharmacologic therapy for prevention of sudden death recently was shown to reduce symptoms but not risk for sudden death.[128] Symptomatic patients or those with a positive EP test appear to benefit from implantable cardioverter-defibrillator placement. A retrospective study found that 25% of high-risk cohorts required termination of lethal ventricular arrhythmias and 60% experienced some type of intervention by an implantable cardioverter-defibrillator.[122] The implantable cardioverter-defibrillator has been shown in a randomized, prospective trial to be superior to drug therapy.[129] However, a long-term follow-up of patients receiving implantable cardioverter-defibrillators for HCM has shown a worrisome rate of inappropriate (5.3%/year) versus appropriate (4%/year) shocks.[130] The overall incidence rate of device complications was concerning at 36% during a 5-year period. Even though the implantable cardioverter-defibrillator saves lives in high-risk patients, the risk for complications should factor into the decision to implant it. Amiodarone is no longer the first line of antiarrhythmic therapy for patients at risk for sudden death as previous studies were nonrandomized case studies.[63]

Another subgroup is patients with CHF who develop progressive symptoms with preserved systolic function but quickly advance to end-stage CHF with impaired systolic function.[111] Symptoms are primarily attributed to the diastolic abnormality; therefore, symptomatic relief is achieved by improving ventricular relaxation. Medications with negative inotropic effect generally are successful in relieving symptoms of exercise intolerance and dyspnea associated with CHF,[131] but symptoms may return in up to 60% of pharmacologically treated patients.[132] In general, β-blockers have been a mainstay of therapy for years in adults and are preferred over calcium channel blockers. High doses of β-blockers usually are needed for therapeutic value. Verapamil may be given if β-blockers are not tolerated or ineffective, but symptomatic improvement may be less than 50%.[132] The combination of β-blockers and calcium channel blockers has not proven beneficial. β-Blockers relieve symptoms of angina and dyspnea and improve exercise tolerance by limiting the gradient associated with exercise. The gradient is not reduced at rest by these medications.[111] Other beneficial effects of β-blockers include heart rate reduction, lower myocardial oxygen demand, and longer diastolic filling times, but diastolic function is neither improved nor is long-term survival prolonged. Verapamil improves diastolic function and ventricular relaxation, causing improved filling and decreased obstructive features in 50% of HCM patients. Patients with obstructive symptoms may worsen with calcium channel blockers that contain strong vasodilator properties. Disopyramide, a negative inotrope that alters calcium kinetics and produces a vasoconstrictor effect, has been recommended instead of calcium channel blockers in obstructive HCM.[111] Disopyramide is the most effective agent to reduce LVOT obstruction and gradient, as well as relieve symptoms.[133] Combined with β-blockers, disopyramide prolongs exercise times more successfully than verapamil.

Surgical correction of HCM is directed primarily at relieving symptoms of LVOT obstruction in the 5% of patients who are refractory to medication.[111] In general, these are individuals with subaortic gradients in excess of 50 mm Hg with or without provocation and frequently associated with severe CHF.[63,110] A myotomy-myectomy through a transaortic approach is the primary method used to relieve the obstruction (Figure 22-22). The muscle is excised from the proximal septum extending just beyond the mitral valve leaflets that widens the LVOT. Currently, the classic Morrow technique has been replaced by a more extensive resection that is described in more detail elsewhere.[133,134] This is a technically challenging operation because of the limited exposure and precise area to excise the muscle. It usually is reserved for centers with considerable experience with myectomy. When myectomy is successful, the LVOT is widened and SAM, mitral regurgitation, and outflow gradient are all decreased. Mitral valve repair or replacement has accompanied myectomy when there is coexistent primary mitral valve structural abnormalities, but mitral valve replacement is not indicated for treating LVOT obstruction alone.[118] If the valve is not repaired during myectomy, incomplete or temporary relief of obstruction may occur. Recently, Wan et al[135] described the use of mitral valve repair in those with LVOT obstruction and degenerative mitral valve disease. Mitral valve repair was effective compared with replacement with low early mortality and successful treatment of both obstruction and mitral valve regurgitation. Mitral valve replacement is rare.

Surgery provides persistent, long-lasting relief from symptoms that exceeds any form of current medical treatment.[131] Five years after myectomy, 85% of patients have improved enough to advance one NYHA functional class.[136] The concomitant reduction in left atrial size may partially account for the lower incidence of atrial fibrillation after myectomy.[111] Septal myectomy results in reduction in left ventricular mass that exceeds the myocardium resected over time, indicating a relief of the pressure overload.[137] Myectomy also is associated with a mortality rate of less than 1% in major institutions.[132] This low mortality rate is even more noteworthy because surgical patients usually have more severe disease than those treated medically. Long-term survival rates at 1, 5, and 10 years are 98%, 96%, and 83%, respectively. Surgical patients have an overall survival rate that is equivalent to the age- and sex-matched general population.[127] Complications of myectomy such

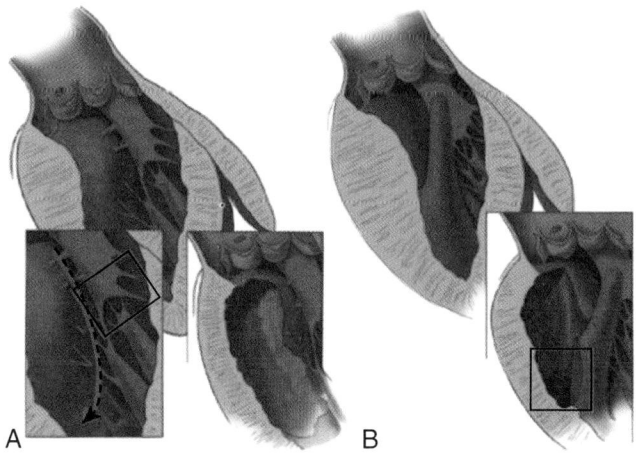

Figure 22-22 Two operative approaches for performing septal myectomy in obstructive hypertrophic cardiomyopathy. *A,* Typical outflow tract morphology with predominant basal septal hypertrophy and subaortic obstruction caused primarily by systolic anterior motion of the mitral valve. Endocardial thickening at the line of apposition of the anterior mitral leaflet to the septum (friction lesion) can be seen (right insert). A standard rectangular myectomy trough (Morrow procedure) is created from 1 cm below the aortic valve apically to a point beyond the line of mitral-septal contact and intraventricular obstruction, allowing relief of the outflow tract gradient and preservation of sinus rhythm (left insert). *B,* In the presence of muscular midcavity obstruction caused by anomalous papillary muscles with direct insertion into the mitral valve or to extensive diffuse septal hypertrophy extending to the bases of the papillary muscles, a much more substantial myectomy is performed by combining the standard operation with an extended midventricular resection. The apical portion of the myectomy trough is much wider and includes the distal third of the right side of the septum. *(From Dearani JA, Ommen SR, Gersh BJ, et al: Surgery insight: Septal myectomy for obstructive hypertrophic cardiomyopathy—the Mayo Clinic experience. Nat Clin Pract Cardiovasc Med 4:503–512, 2007, by permission.)*

as complete heart block or septal perforation (0% to 2%) are rare.[133] Similarly, recurrence of LVOT gradient or SAM requiring repeat myectomy is less than 2%.[118]

Surgery is not recommended for HCM without an obstructive component or if the individual is asymptomatic to mildly symptomatic for the following reasons: (1) Better survival with surgery versus medical therapy is not established; (2) operative mortality may exceed the risk of HCM in mildly affected patients; (3) LVOT obstruction may be compatible with longevity in selected individuals; and (4) no evidence exists that surgery halts the progression of HCM to end-stage.[111] End-stage patients with nonobstructive HCM who have severely reduced systolic function are effectively treated with heart transplantation with 7-year survival rate of 90% that compares equally to those with DCM who require transplantation.[138] Medical treatment for asymptomatic HCM patients is not clearly indicated.

Possible alternatives to surgery have included dual-chamber pacing and percutaneous alcohol septal ablation. Previously, atrioventricular sequential pacing had been shown to decrease subaortic gradients, possibly by causing abnormal septal motion, and thus was considered a possible treatment even though the mechanism has not been proved.[131] Pacing has become the most rigorously evaluated treatment of all therapies for HCM. A series of nonrandomized and randomized studies have shown reductions in the LVOT gradient and improvement in symptoms, but others have found no differences in gradient, NYHA class, quality-of-life score, exercise duration, or maximal oxygen uptake, reflecting a significant placebo effect.[139] Within groups, there appear to be responders, but no variables that identified these patients.[118] Consequently, the optimal use of pacing in HCM requires continued reevaluation.[131] When pacing was compared with surgical therapy, LVOT gradient was reduced to less than 20 mm Hg in only

26% of patients, compared with more than 90% of surgical patients,[118] creating drastically fewer indications for pacing. Furthermore, symptoms were improved in all patients with surgery compared with only 50% with pacing. The role of pacing has been relegated to one in which there are absolute contraindications to other therapies.

Septal ablation with alcohol is a nonsurgical myocardial reduction first attempted in 1994 based on interruption of blood supply to the interventricular septum, causing infarction. This resulted in reduced septal thickness and LVOT modeling with resolution of symptoms in HCM.[140] Alcohol is administered through an angioplasty balloon to the first major septal perforator of the left anterior descending coronary artery. The success rate has been good as indicated by a recent systematic review of ablation incorporating 42 studies and nearly 3000 patients.[141] The study showed effective gradient reduction and improvement in NYHA class comparable with myectomy 12 months after ablation. However, 20% of patients required a second procedure, and some even required myectomy after alcohol ablation. A retrospective review of 375 patients who underwent alcohol ablation identified 20 patients who underwent subsequent surgical myectomy for recurrent dynamic LVOT obstruction.[142] The surgery was successful in all of the failed ablation patients, indicating myectomy as rescue therapy for failed alcohol septal ablation. There is concern about the incidences of complications and mortality accompanying alcohol ablation. Annual mortality rate with alcohol septal ablation in the best centers in the United States is 2%, with Canada reporting 4% to 10%.[118] Besides mortality, the incidence of nonfatal complications is a concern compared with surgical myectomy. Heart block necessitating pacemaker placement has been reported in between 11% and 38% of patients.[143] The toxic effect of alcohol on both the coronary circulation and the myocardium has the potential to generate morbidity.[131]

Perhaps the greatest concern is that fewer surgeons are learning and performing myectomy because of the steep learning curve, but the relative ease of the septal ablation in comparison with myectomy has greatly increased the individuals performing ablation. Because the longest follow-up studies for alcohol ablation are 2 years, long-term benefit for this procedure is lacking. Retrospective studies do not permit any conclusion regarding the superiority of septal ablation with myectomy, so clinicians are awaiting a long-term comparative study to define its role in HCM. Because management of HCM continues to be made based on experience and consensus to a large degree, surgical myectomy remains the first option for HCM with ablation as an alternative, especially if serious comorbidity exists.[111] Treatment will continue to evolve as the proper patient selection and long-term effects are evaluated.

Anesthetic Considerations

Anesthetic management of individuals with HCM is based on similar principles for those having cardiac or noncardiac surgery. The characteristic diastolic dysfunction makes the heart sensitive to changes in volume, contractility, and SVR. Because of this diastolic dysfunction, an acute increase in the pulmonary artery pressure may warn of the rapid onset of pulmonary congestion and edema. If the patient has LVOT obstruction, anesthetic management should minimize or prevent any exacerbation of obstruction and the corresponding increase in the intraventricular gradient that will affect systolic blood pressure. Induction of anesthesia is a hazardous period because the preoperative fast will reduce preload combined with a rapid decline in the venous tone, provoking an increase in LVOT obstruction. Central venous pressure monitoring is recommended to optimize and maintain preload. Hypotension may be treated temporarily with positioning (Trendelenburg), volume replacement, and/or vasoconstriction. Vasoconstrictors rather than inotropes are preferred to maintain SVR.[144] Intravenously administered agents, such as narcotics, have been used successfully in HCM for induction of anesthesia. For shorter surgical procedures, propofol is popular, but its effect on hemodynamics has not been fully established. The systolic blood pressure often decreases significantly with propofol during induction of anesthesia.

The mechanism of this decline in blood pressure is not completely defined but is likely an interaction of baroreflex activity, direct peripheral vasodilation, blunting of the sympathetic nervous outflow, and possibly a decrease in the myocardial contractility.[145] An experimental hamster with HCM received propofol, and the myocardium was found to be unaffected compared with the healthy muscle.[100] In addition, a continuous propofol infusion has been used successfully in a patient with HCM for mitral valve replacement and myectomy.[144]

For anesthesia maintenance, the volatile agent, halothane, is advantageous because it decreases contractility and heart rate but rarely is used today. However, halothane, in comparison with enflurane and isoflurane, has the least effect on SVR and heart rate. The potential for severe myocardial depression with volatile agents in these patients is less than once believed. There is continuing evidence in hamster models with HCM that the negative inotropic effect in the affected myocardium compared with healthy myocardium is more severe with desflurane than either isoflurane or sevoflurane.[101,103] Vecuronium is the preferred muscle relaxant because it does not have histamine-releasing properties or hemodynamic effects.

Arrhythmias may complicate the anesthetic management of individuals with HCM. Ninety percent of adults with HCM have complex ventricular arrhythmias on Holter monitoring irrespective of whether HCM is obstructive or nonobstructive.[111] Nonsustained ventricular tachycardia occurs in 25% to 33% of patients, whereas sustained monomorphic ventricular tachycardia is rare.[146] Asymptomatic, nonsustained ventricular tachycardia tends to be benign.[122] Implantable cardioverter-defibrillators need to be temporarily suspended in patients before use of cautery in the operating room (see Chapter 25).

Besides ventricular arrhythmias, there is a 30% to 50% incidence rate of paroxysmal supraventricular tachycardia in these patients.[146] Atrial fibrillation is the most common supraventricular tachycardia, occurring in 25% of individuals.[110] New onset of atrial fibrillation is observed in 84% of patients who report worsening symptoms.[131] The combination of worsening symptoms and new onset of atrial fibrillation may rapidly deteriorate to CHF.[147] Prompt cardioversion may be necessary. Junctional rhythms also are poorly tolerated in HCM because of the loss of the atrial kick. Chronic atrial fibrillation can be controlled with β-blockers and verapamil, although this combination may be deleterious to some individuals with severe LVOT obstruction and CHF.[110] Amiodarone is especially effective in restoring normal sinus rhythm in HCM and reducing recurrences.

Restrictive Cardiomyopathy

RCM has included such entities as amyloidosis and eosinophilic endomyocardial disease. The 1995 WHO guidelines defined RCM as "restrictive filling and reduced diastolic volume of either or both ventricles with normal or near-normal systolic function and wall thickness."[59] Instead of being classified according to morphologic criteria, as are HCM and DCM, RCM is characterized by function. It may appear in the final stages of other cardiac conditions. Although a clinically challenging diagnosis to make, it is important to distinguish "restrictive" physiology from "constrictive" because management and treatment are decidedly different. Restrictive/constrictive physiology is not solely limited to RCM, but occurs in mitral stenosis, tricuspid stenosis, and aortic stenosis.

RCM is much less frequent than DCM or HCM.[148] It is classified as myocardial (infiltrative, noninfiltrative, and storage) or endomyocardial (Box 22-1) according to cause. The compliance of the "restrictive" myocardium is reduced by one of these processes: extracellular infiltration, intracellular accumulation of abnormal substances, inflammation, or endocardial disease.[148,149] Restrictive myocardial disorders are characteristically atypical in presentation and hemodynamics at times, complicating perioperative management. With idiopathic RCM, the cause is entirely unknown and lacks any identifiable histopathologic distinctiveness. Its occurrence is quite rare, with few actual series in adults.[150] More extensive reviews of the many types of RCM are available.[150–152]

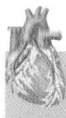

BOX 22-1. CLASSIFICATION OF TYPES OF RESTRICTIVE CARDIOMYOPATHY ACCORDING TO CAUSE

Myocardial
Noninfiltrative
  Idiopathic cardiomyopathy*
  Familial cardiomyopathy
  Hypertrophic cardiomyopathy
  Scleroderma
  Pseudoxanthoma elasticum
  Diabetic cardiomyopathy
Infiltrative
  Amyloidosis*
  Sarcoidosis*
  Gaucher disease
  Hurler disease
  Fatty infiltration
Storage diseases
  Hemochromatosis
  Fabry disease
  Glycogen storage disease

Endomyocardial
Endomyocardial fibrosis*
Hypereosinophilic syndrome
Carcinoid heart disease
Metastatic cancers
Radiation*
Toxic effects of anthracycline*
Drugs causing fibrous endocarditis (serotonin, methysergide, ergotamine, mercurial agents, busulfan)

*This condition is more likely than the others to be encountered in clinical practice.
From Kushwaha SS, Fallon JT, Fuster V: Medical progress: Restrictive cardiomyopathy. N Engl J Med 336:268, 1997.

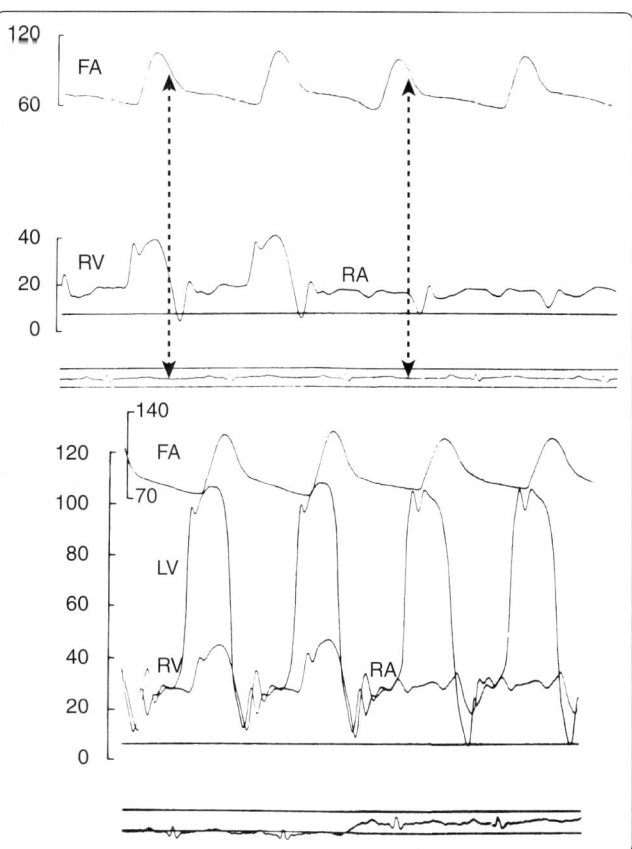

Figure 22-23 **Intracardiac pressure tracings from a patient with idiopathic primary restrictive cardiomyopathy.** *Top,* Right ventricular (RV) and right atrial (RA) tracings with a typical diastolic square-root configuration in the RV tracing and a prominent y descent in the early diastolic period of the right atrial tracing. *Bottom,* Simultaneous left ventricular (LV)-RV pressures and LV-RA pressures, showing a square-root configuration in the LV tracing and equalization of pressures during diastole in the three chambers. FA, femoral artery. *(From Giuliani ER, Fuster V, Gersh BJ, et al: Cardiology: Fundamentals and Practice. St. Louis, Mosby, 1991, by permission of Mayo Foundation.)*

Systolic function is minimally affected in RCM. Diastolic dysfunction is evident by abnormalities of ventricular relaxation and compliance. Impaired ventricular relaxation occurs before abnormal compliance. Poor compliance of the ventricle causes rapid filling in early diastole and the characteristic ventricular diastolic waveform of dip-and-plateau (square-root sign; Figure 22-23). However, the characteristic dip-and-plateau pattern may be absent in 50% of affected individuals because it depends on the degree of impaired ventricular relaxation and the level of atrial driving pressure.[151] The atrial pressure waveform will have the appearance of an M or W pattern because of the rapid y descent combined with a slightly greater x descent. The rapid y descent is due to the rapid early decline of the atrial pressure corresponding to the early diastolic ventricular filling. Filling early in diastole is accentuated and impeded during the rest of diastole because of reduced ventricular distensibility. Pressure in the ventricle increases precipitously in response to small volume. Once ventricular filling is restricted, the prognosis is much worse. Both ventricles appear thick with small cavities. In contrast, the corresponding atria appear dilated despite normal left ventricular volumes. Cardiomegaly or ventricular dilation should not exist. The left-sided pulmonary venous pressures usually exceed the right-sided venous pressures by 5 mm Hg. The pulmonary artery systolic pressure also may be increased to 50 mm Hg.

Because one or both ventricles may be involved, symptoms may predominate as right- or left-sided. The increased filling pressures that occur in early diastole of both ventricles lead to symptoms of right-sided failure manifested by increased venous pressures, peripheral edema, and ascites, or left-sided failure manifested by CHF, progressive dyspnea, and orthopnea. Both groups of symptoms may occur separately or simultaneously. Insidious onset of fatigue and exertional dyspnea are common. Symptoms and signs should be present without evidence of cardiomegaly. The jugular venous pulse fails to fall during inspiration and may even rise (Kussmaul's sign).[152] Pulsus paradoxus is infrequent and nonspecific. The liver may be enlarged and actually pulsatile. The chest roentgenogram is nondiagnostic. Pulmonary congestion and a normal or smaller than anticipated heart size suggest a diagnosis of RCM. Thromboembolic complications are common with the initial presentation of the disease. The ECG may reflect abnormalities of depolarization such as bundle branch block, low voltage, and QR or QS complexes, but these are not specific to RCM and rarely are useful to distinguish RCM from constrictive pericarditis (CP). ECG evidence of biatrial enlargement may be present.[149]

It is important to distinguish between RCM and CP because management of the two diseases is very different. Important distinguishing features of CP and RCM are listed in Table 22-4. Both conditions have rapid and early diastolic filling with increased filling pressures and normal filling volumes. In RCM, the impediment to filling is usually an infiltrative process involving the myocardium rather than the pericardium. Although not an absolute sign, the right ventricular and left ventricular end-diastolic pressures are increased and equal with constrictive physiology, whereas in RCM, end-diastolic pressure is usually 5 mm Hg greater on the left than on the right side because of the unequal compliance between the two ventricles.[150,153] Unfortunately, symptoms and physical signs do not reliably discriminate between RCM and CP.

Advances in echo and other noninvasive methods have been used to try to reliably discriminate between pericardial disease and RCM. The

TABLE 22-4	Differentiation of Pericardial Constriction versus Myocardial Restriction	
Characteristic	*Constrictive Pericarditis*	*Restrictive Cardiomyopathy*
Jugular venous waveform	Increased with less rapid *y*-descent	Increased with, more rapid *y*-descent Large A waves
LAP > RAP	Absent	Almost always
Auscultation	Early S_3 high pitched; no S_4	Late S_3 low pitched; S_4 in some cases
Mitral or tricuspid regurgitation	Frequently absent	Frequently present
Chest roentgenogram	Calcification of pericardium (20–30%)	Pericardial calcification rare
Heart size	Normal to increased	Normal to increased
Electrocardiogram	Conduction abnormalities rare	Conduction abnormalities common
Echocardiogram	Slight enlargement of atria	Major enlargement of atria
Right ventricular pressure waveform	Square-root pattern	Square-root pattern; dip-and-plateau often less prominent
Right and left heart diastolic pressures (mm Hg)	Within 5 of each other in almost all cases	Seldom within 5 of each other
Peak right ventricular systolic pressure (mm Hg)	Almost always < 60, sometimes < 40	Usually > 40 sometimes > 60
Discordant respiratory variation of peak ventricular systolic pressures	Right and left are out of phase with respiration	In phase
Paradoxical pulse	Often present	Rare
CT/MRI	Thickened pericardium	Rarely thickened pericardium
Endomyocardial biopsy	Normal or nonspecific changes	Nonspecific abnormalities

CT, computerized axial tomography; LAP, left atrial pressure; MRI, magnetic resonance imaging; RAP, right atrial pressure.
From Hancock EW: Cardiomyopathy: Differential diagnosis of restrictive cardiomyopathy and constrictive pericarditis. *Heart* 86:343–349, 2001; and Chatterjee K, Alpert J: Constrictive pericarditis and restrictive cardiomyopathy: Similarities and differences. *Heart Failure Monit* 3:118–126, 2003.

usual 2D echo findings are those of normal size, thickness, and preserved systolic function of the ventricles with enlargement of the atria (Figure 22-24). Classic Doppler findings are described in Table 22-5. Doppler findings may indicate the severity of RCM once the diagnosis is certain. Because the pericardium is responsible for CP and a noncompliant ventricle for RCM, some differences exist between RCM and CP regarding M-mode, 2D, and Doppler examinations.[154] A pericardial thickness of 3 mm measured by echo is indicative of CP. But overall, Doppler and echo have insufficient sensitivity and specificity to provide a *clinically* significant differentiation between RCM and CP. More recently, tissue Doppler imaging has demonstrated some success in providing differentiation between RCM and CP by measuring E velocity to determine ventricular relaxation with 89% sensitivity and 100% specificity.[155] Other noninvasive methods that may be helpful are the CT to determine the thickness of the pericardium and the MRI to diagnose infiltrative processes such as amyloidosis.[149]

Cardiac catheterization still is performed to differentiate between RCM and CP. During catheterization, increased left and right venous pressures with large A and V waves may be observed in RCM (see Figure 22-23). It is not uncommon to see right atrial pressures of 15 to 20 mm Hg. The ventricular pressure curve may display the diastolic dip-and-plateau pattern (square-root sign) as described previously. Recently, more advanced catheterization criteria for differentiation of RCM and CP have been devised.[156] This new measurement, systolic

area index, assesses the dynamic changes in ventricular pressure area during inspiration and expiration to distinguish CP from RCM. In CP, there is a dissociation between intrathoracic and intracardiac pressures that causes decreased filling in the LV during inspiration. The constricting pericardium also causes increased ventricular interaction so that the RV is better filled during inspiration. This new index has 97% sensitivity and 100% predictive accuracy in patients with documented CP compared with older catheterization indices that generated predictive accuracy for RCM and CP that was less than 75%.

Endomyocardial biopsy may differentiate RCM from CP. The biopsy in RCM rarely is normal compared with CP. Although a biopsy may identify specific causes of restrictive physiology,[148] more often, only patchy endocardial and interstitial fibrosis with some myofibril hypertrophy are found.[150,153] If biopsy or tests such as radionuclide angiography, Doppler, or echo do not identify either RCM or pericardial disease, exploratory surgery may be needed. Surgery is the most definitive method of differentiating RCM from CP, but the patient with RCM may not tolerate anesthesia and surgery well, so it is used sparingly.[157]

There is no specific treatment for RCM. Various regimens have been developed based on the specific cause of RCM[158] (Table 22-6). It is important to rule out the presence of extracardiac diseases that may hamper effective treatment of RCM before it becomes intractable. Diuretics often are administered to reduce pulmonary and venous congestion, but low CO with severe hypoperfusion is a risk. With the

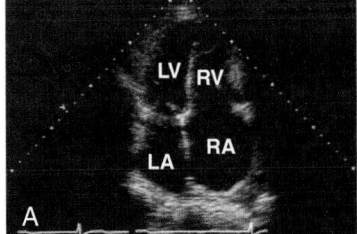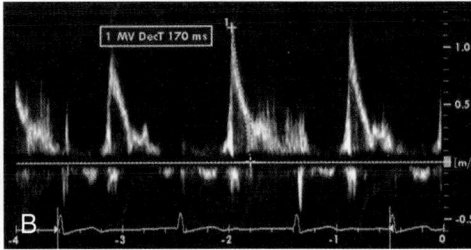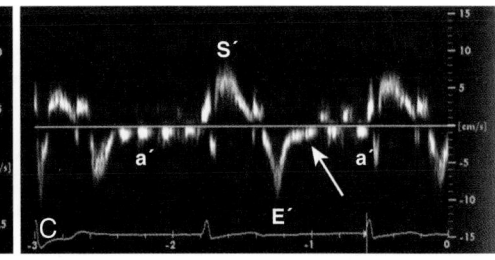

Figure 22-24   Apical four-chamber view of a typical case of restrictive cardiomyopathy with normal left ventricular (LA) size, normal LV ejection fraction, and marked biatrial enlargement. *B*, Patients with restrictive cardiomyopathy are frequently in atrial fibrillation. A mitral inflow pulsed-wave Doppler velocity recording shows a deceleration time (DecT) of 170 milliseconds and mild variation in E velocities. *C*, Mitral annulus tissue velocity recording demonstrating E′ of 8 cm/sec and delayed relaxation *(arrow)*, and a′ related to atrial fluttering or fibrillating motion. E′, mitral annulus early diastolic velocity; E/E′, 100/8 = 13, consistent with a mild increase in filling pressures; LA, left atrium; RA, right atrium; RV, right ventricle; S′, systolic velocity of the mitral annulus. *(From Oh JK, Seward JB, Tajik AJ: The Echo Manual, 3rd ed. Philadelphia, 2006, Lippincott Williams & Wilkins, by permission.)*

TABLE 22-5	Doppler and Echocardiographic Features Differentiating Restrictive Cardiomyopathy and Constrictive Pericarditis	
Modality	Restrictive Cardiomyopathy	Constrictive Pericarditis
M-mode	No septal notch	Septal notch
2D	No septal shudder	Septal shudder
Pulsed-wave mitral and tricuspid inflow	Less variation	Prominent respiratory variation (> 10%)
		Significant decrease in IVRT from inspiration to expiration (usually noted in the first beat after expiration)
Pulsed-wave pulmonary vein	Less variation	Significant increase (> 18%) in peak diastolic velocity from inspiration to expiration
	S/D ratio < 0.4	S/D ratio ≥ 0.65 in inspiration
Pulsed-wave hepatic veins		> 25% reduction in diastolic forward flow
		Prominent late diastolic flow reversal after the onset of expiration
RVSP	> 40 mm Hg	< 40 mm Hg
Tricuspid regurgitation	Less respiratory change	Marked inspiratory increase in peak velocity, time-velocity integral, and duration of jet
Tissue-Doppler mitral annulus	E′ < 8 cm/sec	E′ ≥ 8 cm/sec
	E/E′ > 15	E/E′ < 15
Color M-mode	Vp < 45 cm/sec	Vp ≥ 100 cm/sec

E′, early peak velocity; IVRT, isovolumic relation time; RVSP, right ventricular systolic pressure; S/D, systolic/diastolic; Vp, propagation velocity.
From Tam JW, Shaikh N, Sutherland E: Echocardiographic assessment of patients with hypertrophic and restrictive cardiomyopathy: imaging and echocardiography. *Curr Opin Cardiol* 17:474, 2002.

TABLE 22-6	Treatment Strategies in Restrictive Cardiomyopathy	
Etiology	Specific Symptom	Treatment
Idiopathic	To relieve congestion	Diuretics
	Control of heart rate	β-Blockers, amiodarone, heart rate regulating CCBs
	Atrial fibrillation:	
	to maintain sinus rhythm	Amiodarone, dofetilide
	paroxysmal or persistent	Long-term anticoagulation
	To control ventricular rate	β-Blockers, heart rate–regulating calcium channel blockers, amiodarone, digoxin, atrioventricular node ablation and pacemaker
	Atrioventricular block	Dual-chamber pacing
	To enhance myocardial relaxation	Calcium channel blockers (unproven), angiotensin inhibition (unproven)
	Refractory heart failure	Cardiac transplantation
Amyloidosis		Melphalan, prednisone, and colchicine; stem cell implant (under investigation); heart and liver transplant (in rare instances)
Hemochromatosis		Phlebotomy, desferrioxamine
Carcinoid heart disease		Somatostatin analogs; serotonin antagonists; valvuloplasty for severe tricuspid and pulmonary stenosis; valve replacement for severe tricuspid and pulmonary regurgitation
Sarcoidosis		Corticosteroids; pacemaker for heart block; implantable cardioverter defibrillator for ventricular arrhythmia; cardiac transplant for refractory heart failure
Eosinophilic endocarditis		Initial stage: corticosteroids, hydroxyurea, vincristine
Endomyocardial fibrosis		Endocardiectomy with repair or replacement of tricuspid and mitral valves

CCB, calcium channel blocker.
From Chatterjee K, Alpert J: Constrictive pericarditis and restrictive cardiomyopathy: Similarities and differences. *Heart Failure Mont* 3:125, 2003.

characteristic limited stroke volume, heart rate with atrial contraction is important to support CO. Enlarging atria may increase the risk for supraventricular arrhythmias. The lower CO and enlarging atria make chronic anticoagulation important in view of the risk for thrombin formation. A surgical option for RCM is rare with the exception of endomyocardial fibrosis with eosinophilic cardiomyopathy. The fibrotic endocardium may be excised in combination with mitral or tricuspid valve replacement.

Survival with RCM depends largely on the causative factor. True idiopathic RCM has a 5-year overall survival rate of 64%, but if increasing signs of pulmonary venous congestion appear, the prognosis worsens.[150] Transplantation is not always an option for adults with RCM because the processes responsible for RCM would invariably affect the newly transplanted heart.

Anesthetic Considerations

Adults with RCM rarely require cardiac surgery for reasons other than mitral or tricuspid valve replacement and transplantation.[159] Occasionally, anesthesia will be administered for a scheduled pericardiectomy only to discover RCM instead of CP. Despite essentially normal ventricular systolic function, the diastolic dysfunction and filling abnormalities result in a poor CO and systemic perfusion.[153] Aggressive preoperative diuretic therapy may contribute hypotension secondary to inadequate circulating blood volume. In contrast, pulmonary congestion resulting in increased airway pressures may impair oxygen delivery to the tissues.

Induction of anesthesia should avoid medications associated with decreased venous return, bradycardia, or myocardial depression. Fentanyl (30 μg/kg) or sufentanil (5 μg/kg) provides stable hemodynamics for induction and maintenance in patients with poor myocardial function. These anesthetics provide minimal hemodynamic fluctuation in patients undergoing cardiac surgery for valvular disease who have developed severe preexisting volume or pressure loads on the heart. Etomidate is an excellent alternative or adjuvant to fentanyl as an induction agent because it has minimal effect on contractility of the cardiac muscle as demonstrated in patients undergoing cardiac transplantation.[96] Similarly, ketamine has been advocated for induction in patients with cardiac tamponade or CP because sympathetic activity is preserved. Ketamine is an excellent choice to use with fentanyl for induction in patients with severe myocardial dysfunction and low

CO caused by cardiomyopathy. Concerns of exacerbating PAH with ketamine are unfounded if ventilation is maintained. Shorter-acting narcotics such as remifentanil may be unsuitable for patients with RCM because of a greater incidence of bradycardia and severe hypotension.[94] Fentanyl-etomidate-isoflurane has been shown superior to remifentanil-sevoflurane in terms of maintaining arterial pressure and heart rate.[95] Propofol may have no direct myocardial depression, but indirect inhibition of sympathetic activity and a vasodilatory property may cause hemodynamic instability in patients with RCM. Sevoflurane and desflurane are attractive agents for maintenance of anesthesia in this population because they have been shown not to adversely affect the ability of the LV to respond to increased work despite their negative inotropic properties.[104]

Invasive hemodynamic monitoring is important because both left and right filling pressures do not accurately reflect ventricular volumes, so small volume shifts may greatly impact CO. Inotropic support may be indicated to support hemodynamics because the risk for death from low CO is high. Despite chronic CHF, diuretics and vasodilators may be deleterious because greater filling pressures are needed to maintain CO. Some individuals may be sensitive to β-blockers and cardiac glycosides.[153] Patients may be chronically taking amiodarone, which has a negative inotropic effect that interacts with volatile agents to further reduce contractility and conduction, requiring careful titration of these anesthetic agents.[108]

Arrhythmogenic Right Ventricular Cardiomyopathy

Formerly called *arrhythmogenic right ventricular dysphasia*, arrhythmogenic right ventricular cardiomyopathy (ARVC) was defined by the 1995 WHO as "progressive fibrofatty replacement of right ventricular myocardium, initially with typical regional and later global right ventricular and some left ventricular involvement, with relative sparing of the septum."[59] Evidence of a more progressive involvement of not only the RV but LV with long-term follow-up convinced the WHO to classify ARVC as a "disease of the myocardium" that incorporates the many different clinical presentations and aspects of this condition.

ARVC is familial in 30% to 50% of cases, with primarily autosomal dominant inheritance with variable expressivity and reduced penetrance.[65] The incidence and prevalence are uncertain, but it usually appears during adolescence, though it may occur in younger individuals. It presents most commonly with the onset of arrhythmias ranging from premature ventricular contractions to ventricular fibrillation originating from the RV. The disease is now known to proceed through three phases: (1) concealed phase without symptoms but some EP changes that place patients at risk for sudden death; (2) overt arrhythmias; and (3) advanced stage with myocardial loss, biventricular involvement with CHF.[160] Diagnosis is rare in the early stages,[161] but not at autopsy.[162] Distinguishing symptoms may be missing when the structural and functional changes are present or absent in the RV.[163] Standard diagnostic criteria have continued to be revised.[164] Postmortem examination reveals diffuse or segmental loss of myocardium, primarily in the RV, replaced with fat and fibrous tissue, and right ventricular dilation and thinning of the wall (Figure 22-25). The diagnosis also includes the functional changes associated with the RV beyond the structural alterations. These changes are believed to occur by three possible mechanisms: myoblasts differentiate to adipoblasts, apoptosis, or inflammation.[161] An inflammatory process is evident within the myocardial tissue. The replacement of myocardium with fat and fibrous tissue creates an excellent environment for a fatal arrhythmia, possibly the first sign of ARVC.[160] Although considered a disease of the RV, left ventricular involvement also can occur and even precede RV presentation.[165] Sudden death occurs in up to 75% of patients, although it is difficult to accurately state in view of number of patients who go undiagnosed. Sudden death occurs most often

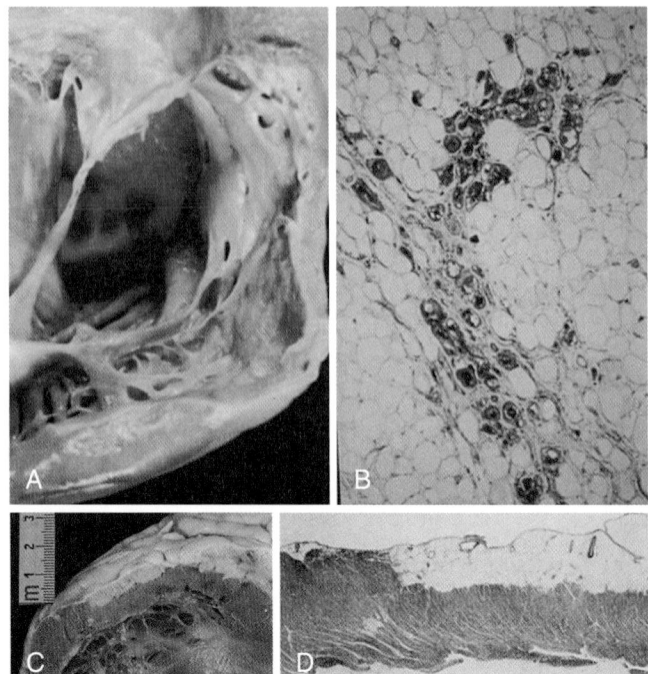

Figure 22-25 *A,* Gross view of the RV outflow tract showing severe transmural loss of the RV freewall and infundibular parchment-like aneurysm. *B,* Histologic view at high magnification of surviving degenerated RV myocytes in the setting of extensive fatty replacement and tiny interstitial fibrosis. *C,* Gross and *(D)* histologic sections of the anterior left ventricular wall showing striking subepicardial fatty infiltration and fibrosis. *(From Corrado D, Basso C, Thiene G, et al: Spectrum of clinicopathologic manifestations of arrhythmogenic right ventricular cardiomyopathy/dysplasia: A multicenter study. J Am Coll Cardiol 30;1517, 1997, by permission.)*

during sports-related exercise, primarily from ventricular tachycardia/fibrillation.[166] Although a rare disease, it accounts for 20% of sudden deaths in the young.[163]

The electrical instability characteristic of ARVC is not solely responsible for the natural history of the disease. Clinical presentation may range from asymptomatic myopathic involvement to overt clinical disease with diffuse biventricular involvement.[160,166] Progressive right and left ventricular dysfunction can be appreciated with serial echo examinations. Echo findings from 29 patients with ARVC have been described (Figure 22-26).[167] The systolic and diastolic right ventricular outflow tract dimensions were increased on 2D echo. Regional wall motion abnormalities of the RV were common, and more than half of patients had abnormal right ventricular systolic function. Right ventricular trabeculations were also commonly found. Although there are typical echo features in ARVC, the disease may present before the appearance of these morphologic features. Recently, it has been shown that significant ventricular mechanical dyssynchrony is present in 50% of patients.[168] This leads to a more dilated RV, as well as one with poorer function compared with those without it. Myocardial loss with progressive ventricular dysfunction progresses ultimately to CHF, accounting for 20% of deaths. End-stage ARVC may be difficult to distinguish from DCM because the extent of left ventricular involvement only recently has been appreciated.

Diagnosis is based on ECG, structure, genetic studies, and arrhythmias.[161] The characteristic ECG includes inverted T waves in the right precordial leads, QRS prolongation > 110 milliseconds, and extrasystoles with left bundle branch block. Diagnosis may depend on endomyocardial biopsy to reveal the distinctive changes of ARVC, yet is unrewarding if the biopsy is obtained from the septal area of the myocardium known for its lack of characteristic features.[63] A new immunohistochemical analysis of a biopsy sample has proved to be

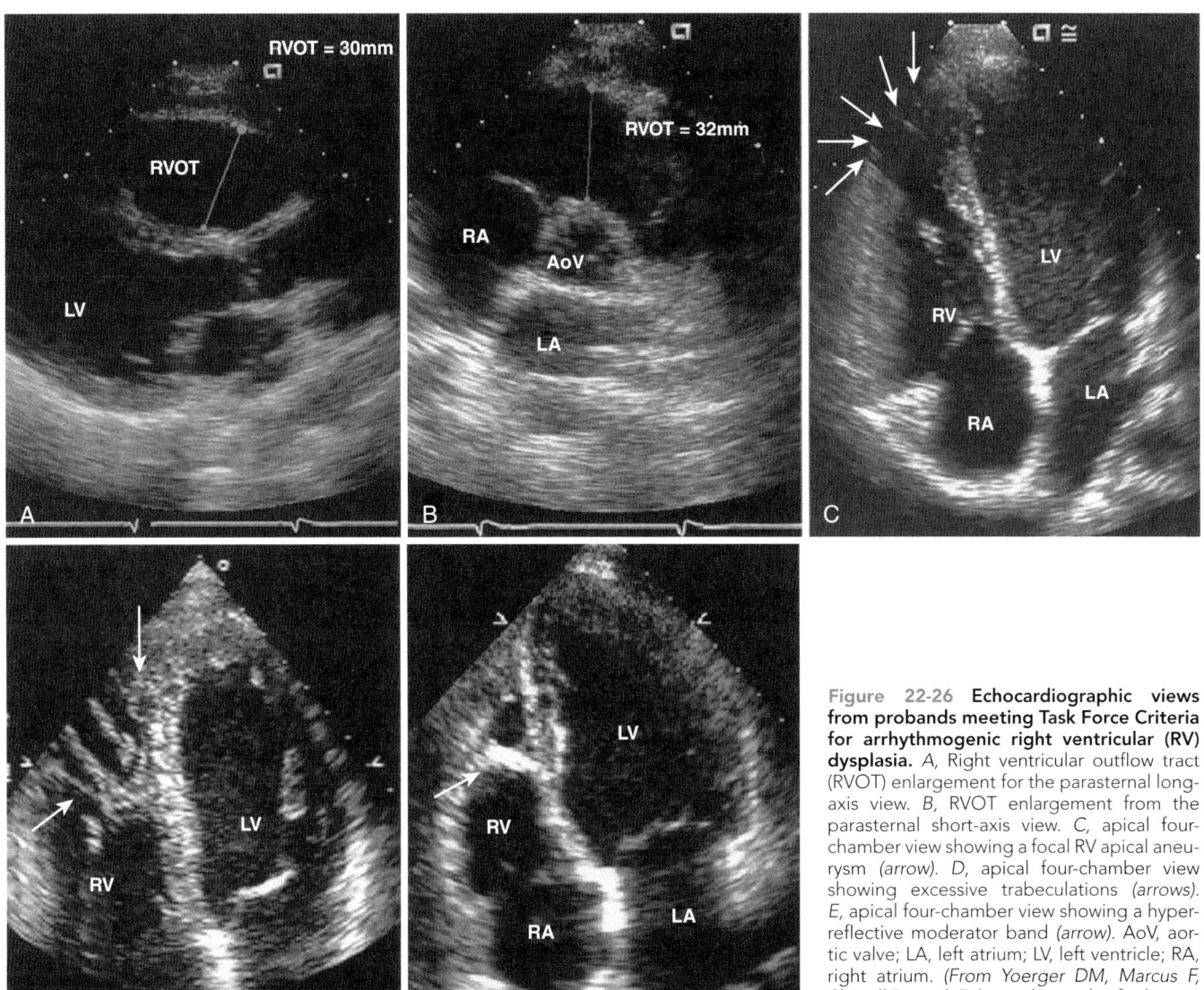

Figure 22-26 **Echocardiographic views from probands meeting Task Force Criteria for arrhythmogenic right ventricular (RV) dysplasia.** *A,* Right ventricular outflow tract (RVOT) enlargement for the parasternal long-axis view. *B,* RVOT enlargement from the parasternal short-axis view. *C,* apical four-chamber view showing a focal RV apical aneurysm *(arrow)*. *D,* apical four-chamber view showing excessive trabeculations *(arrows)*. *E,* apical four-chamber view showing a hyper-reflective moderator band *(arrow)*. AoV, aortic valve; LA, left atrium; LV, left ventricle; RA, right atrium. *(From Yoerger DM, Marcus F, Sherrill D, et al: Echocardiographic findings in patients meeting task force criteria for arrhenogenic right ventricular dysplasia. J Am Coll Cardiol 45:860–865, 2005, by permission.).*

highly sensitive and specific for the identification of ARVC.[169] The importance of this test is that it has been used to differentiate those patients in the early stages of the disease from the more advanced state. A prospective longitudinal study examined 108 newly diagnosed patients over a 2-year period and found that their clinical profile differed from the patient with the more advanced disease. This finding may offer some options for future treatments.[163]

Anesthetic Considerations

Two adolescents undergoing routine operations were reported to experience development of refractory arrhythmias and sudden death after general anesthesia.[162] Autopsy demonstrated typical features of ARVC. A family history of sudden death or syncope at an early age should heighten the awareness for diagnosis of ARVC and merits further evaluation.[161] During the course of ARVC, arrhythmias of both a supraventricular and ventricular nature may occur at any time. Because arrhythmias are more likely in the perioperative period, noxious stimuli, hypovolemia, hypercarbia, and light anesthesia must be minimized

intraoperatively and during recovery. However, general anesthesia alone does not appear to be arrhythmogenic. Houfani et al[162] reported that more than 200 patients with ARVC underwent general anesthesia without a single cardiac arrest. Anesthesia has been conducted successfully with propofol, midazolam, and alfentanil.[161] Acidosis may be especially detrimental because of its effect on arrhythmia generation and myocardial function.

Currently, there are no guidelines for arrhythmia prophylaxis. Amiodarone is the first line of antiarrhythmic medication during anesthesia. Empiric administration of antiarrhythmia agents is ineffective at preventing arrhythmias or sudden death in these patients.[166] Sotalol appears to be the only antiarrhythmic that may reduce arrhythmias. Placement of an implantable cardioverter-defibrillator is beneficial. Link et al[170] identified 12 patients with ARVC who had implantable cardioverter-defibrillators placed and determined 8 patients had appropriate discharges for ventricular tachycardia. Subsequently, it has been reported that placement of an implantable cardioverter-defibrillator is associated with an excellent prognosis in patients with ARVC.[160]

MITRAL VALVE PROLAPSE

MVP with severe mitral regurgitation is a common reason for cardiac surgery today. Knowledge about MVP has evolved greatly since the 1960s. Unrecognized as a part of the midsystolic click and systolic murmur known as Barlow disease until 1961, the finding of mitral regurgitation in 1963 by Barlow et al[171] in conjunction with the ballooning of the posterior mitral leaflet on angiography resulted in the condition called *Barlow syndrome* or *floppy-valve syndrome*. It was during this time that the true cause of MVP was understood to be a degenerative condition with myxoid found on histologic examination that caused thickening, elongation, and a change in the chords. With the advent of echo in 1970, eventually a diagnosis based on 3D echo parameters of the normal mitral valve was derived in 1987 for MVP.[172] In essence, only the valve that displayed prolapse in the long-axis view had "true" MVP.[173] This allowed the "true" prevalence of MVP to be determined, as well as the specific process associated with the corresponding mitral regurgitation. Carpentier was further able to differentiate the degenerative changes of MVP from another causative factor that did not cause billowing of the valve or excess tissue, now referred to as "fibroelastic deficiency."[174] Currently, MVP is known to be a structural and functional disorder affecting less than 1% of the population depending on accepted criteria for diagnosis.

MVP is a multifactorial valvular abnormality that may be caused by histologic abnormalities of the valve structure and surrounding structures of the myocardium.[175] It is most likely a genetically inherited disease, but the genetic defect has not been identified. Transmission appears to be in an autosomal dominant manner. As the most commonly diagnosed cardiac valve abnormality, it occurs in adults who are otherwise healthy or in association with many pathologic conditions and is equally distributed between men and women (Box 22-2).[175]

Mitral valve leaflets normally close just before ventricular systole, thus preventing regurgitation of blood into the LA. In patients with degenerative valve disease, there are two forms: Barlow disease and fibroelastic deficiency. Barlow disease is believed to result from myxomatous degeneration of the mitral valve, elongation and thinning of the chordae tendineae, and the presence of redundant and excessive valve tissue. The mechanism is unknown, but regulation of the extracellular matrix components appears to be a primary issue. Normal mitral valve leaflets may billow slightly with closure; but in MVP, redundant mitral leaflets prolapse into the LA during mid-to-late systole as the ventricle is emptied (Figure 22-27). Superior arching of the mitral leaflets above the level of the atrioventricular ring is diagnostic for MVP. Distortion or malfunction of any of the component structures of the mitral valve may cause prolapse and generate audible clicks or regurgitation associated with a murmur. If the chordae tendineae are lengthened, the valves may billow even more and progress to prolapse when valve leaflets fail to appose each other. The degree of these changes will determine the presence of mitral regurgitation. The degenerative valve changes that are responsible for progression from an asymptomatic state with murmurs and systolic clicks to dyspnea with severe mitral regurgitation occur over an average of 25 years.[176]

Another category of MVP that was first identified by Carpentier with no billowing or excess valve tissue was fibroelastic deficiency.[174] In this situation, the chords were thin and possibly ruptured, often involving a segment of the posterior leaflet. The mechanism is impaired connective tissue production caused by a deficiency of collagens, elastins, and proteoglycans, but the cause is unknown. The leaflet tissue is preserved. Unlike Barlow disease, symptoms generally arrive with chordal rupture, frequently with advancing age. This is a much less pronounced, generalized degeneration of the mitral valve than Barlow disease. Surgical repair also is less complex. Finally, even histologically normal mitral valves may prolapse.[175] Normal mitral valve function depends on a number of factors including the size of the LV and mitral leaflets. Changes in these components may cause "innocent" MVP.

There are no universal criteria for diagnosis of MVP. Physical diagnosis and echo are the requirements for diagnosis of MVP. Auscultatory criteria that are strictly applied are highly sensitive for the diagnosis but lack some specificity. Typical auscultatory features are midsystolic click and late-systolic murmur. The click is related to deceleration of blood on the undersurface of the valve prolapsing into the LA. The murmur is late, with progressively increasing regurgitation that results in a crescendo systolic murmur. Certain maneuvers aid with the auscultatory diagnosis of MVP such as Valsalva, squatting, or leg raises that change the left ventricular end-diastolic volume to move the timing of the click within systole.[175] Auscultatory findings may be absent despite echo determination of MVP. MVP is diagnosed more often now with 2D echo because recognition and assessment of the severity are superior. Given the saddle-shaped nature of the mitral annulus, the diagnosis of MVP is typically made from the parasternal long-axis view using TTE. MVP is defined as more than 2-mm displacement of one or both mitral leaflets into the LA during systole. If the mitral leaflets appear thickened or myxomatous, the diagnosis is

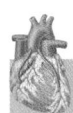

BOX 22-2. CONDITIONS ASSOCIATED WITH MITRAL VALVE PROLAPSE

Connective Tissue Disorders—Genetic
Mitral valve prolapse—isolated
Marfan syndrome
Ehlers-Danlos syndrome—types I, II, IV
Pseudoxanthoma elasticum
Osteogenesis imperfecta
Polycystic kidneys

Other Genetic Disorders
Duchenne muscular dystrophy
Myotonic dystrophy
Fragile X syndrome
Mucopolysaccharidoses

Acquired Collagen—Vascular Disorders
Systemic lupus erythematosus
Relapsing polychondritis
Rheumatic endocarditis
Polyarteritis nodosa

Other Associated Disorders
Atrial septal defect—secundum
Hypertrophic obstructive cardiomyopathy
Wolff-Parkinson-White syndrome
Papillary muscle dysfunction
    Ischemic heart disease
    Myocarditis
Cardiac trauma
Postmitral valve surgery
von Willebrand disease

From Robert A. O'Rourke (ed): *Current Problems in Cardiology.* 1991, p 333.

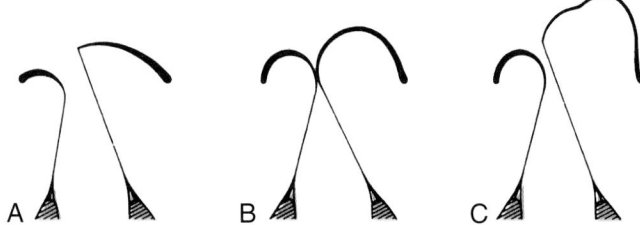

Figure 22-27 Diagrammatic representation of the functional pathology of the mitral valve mechanism. *A,* Mitral valve prolapse. Regurgitation is present. *B,* Billowing mitral valve without prolapse or regurgitation. *C,* Billowing and prolapsed mitral leaflets with regurgitation. *(From Barlow JB, Pocock WA: Mitral valve prolapse enigma—two decades later. Mod Concepts Cardiovasc Dis 53:13, 1984, by permission of American Heart Association.)*

more certain. Color Doppler and continuous-wave Doppler imaging can quantify the degree of mitral regurgitation when it is present.

Most patients with MVP are asymptomatic, but symptoms may range from mild to severe. Altered autonomic function, catecholamine responsiveness, or possibly a combination of the two may account for complaints of chest pain, fatigue, palpitations, dyspnea, dizziness, syncope, and panic attacks among others. These symptoms and some clinical findings of thin body type, low blood pressure, and ECG repolarization abnormalities have been associated with MVP and termed *MVP syndrome*.[175] However, controlled studies have identified palpitations as the only symptom linked to MVP. Nearly 50% of patients describe palpitations.[177] Neuropsychiatric symptoms are no longer considered a part of MVP. The possibility of a complex of unexplained cardiovascular symptoms associated with MVP has not been completely eliminated and may exist in a few patients. The cause may be abnormal autonomic activity that leads to symptoms of vasoconstriction, enhanced β-receptor activity, and decreased plasma volume; however, a relation with MVP remains undefined.

The prognosis for most MVP patients is excellent with a normal life expectancy.[175] Development of severe echo abnormalities is rare in patients with MVP. Although a benign course is typical for many patients with MVP, serious complications such as severe mitral regurgitation, infective endocarditis, sudden death, and cerebral ischemia may occur. The incidence rates of cardiovascular morbidity and mortality in MVP are just under 1% per year.[178] It is a subset of patients who appear to be at increased risk for serious complications that may be defined by echo and clinical findings. These risk factors vary from reduced left ventricular systolic function to valve thickening greater than 5 mm to others that have been described.[175]

Mitral regurgitation is the most serious complication associated with MVP. Severe mitral regurgitation develops in approximately 2% to 4% of patients with MVP, two thirds of whom are male.[177] Most patients will have mild-to-moderate mitral regurgitation that does not require surgery. MVP is the most common cause of severe mitral regurgitation, and its onset signals the need for therapeutic intervention. Irrespective of symptoms, the onset of severe mitral regurgitation can result in reduced life expectancy. Patients are usually younger than 60 years with Barlow's form of MVP and mitral regurgitation. Mitral regurgitation in Barlow disease is not caused by the billowing of the leaflet body but from the marginal prolapse (Figure 22-28).[174] The annulus is severely dilated. The posterior leaflet is affected more frequently than the anterior leaflet. Changes often are observed at the site of chordal insertion leading to rupture of the chordae and tethering of the valve leaflet. With the onset of severe mitral regurgitation, PAH, left atrial enlargement, and atrial fibrillation frequently emerge. Early repair is recommended to preserve left ventricular function and reduce the likelihood of atrial fibrillation.

The management of MVP and mitral regurgitation without symptoms continues to be reconsidered in terms of the timing for cardiac surgery, especially in view of the risk for mitral valve repair and the improved outcomes associated with earlier surgery. Without overt symptoms, the degree of ventricular dysfunction may be worsening, unknowingly placing the patient at increased risk for permanent dysfunction and worse surgical outcome.[175] Male individuals are three times more likely to require surgery than female individuals, even though there is no difference in the overall incidence of MVP between them. Noninvasive monitoring of mitral regurgitation and developing left ventricular dysfunction may help evaluate the optimal time for surgery. Flail mitral leaflet is an especially important risk for a poor surgical outcome if not addressed immediately.

Mitral valve repair is widely recommended for treatment of MVP compared with replacement. It provides long-term benefit with either causes of MVP and a low rate of recurrence.[179] Mitral valve repair confers a significantly improved operative survival, as well as 5- and 10-year survival, compared with mitral valve replacement.[180] The Cox maze procedure may be added to mitral valve repair safely to effectively reduce late complications of mitral valve disease.[181] Advantages of mitral valve repair compared with replacement include lower risks for thromboembolism, bleeding, and infectious endocarditis, temporary anticoagulation, and better ventricular function because the valve structure is preserved.[182] Most patients with degenerative mitral disease (90%)[183] are able to undergo repair with low morbidity and mortality with excellent long-term outcomes according to retrospective studies.[184] Recently, there has been a prospective, observational study of patients who underwent mitral valve repair or replacement for mitral regurgitation (ischemic and degenerative causes), and it found a statistically significant survival benefit in those who had repair.[185] Notably, repair of the valve returns the patient to a similar life expectancy with a comparable noncardiac surgical patient.

Posterior leaflet prolapse is the most common defect in mitral regurgitation.[175] The posterior leaflet repair is very low risk, but the bileaflet repair is more technically challenging, requiring more skill and advanced techniques. The anterior prolapse repair has a greater rate of reoperation and decreased survival.[184] Recently, the use of robotic technology has advanced to a point that allows safe and feasible mitral repair in these circumstances, although there is no long-term followup.[186] Surgical strategy does not involve annular plication and annuloplasty for annular dilation, but leaflet resection for excessive valve tissue to restore the normal valvular geometry (Figure 22-29). Once the repair is completed and the patient has separated from CPB, it is important to observe for SAM so it can be surgically corrected immediately. All valves cannot be successfully repaired, whereon 10% with prolapse of a degenerative mitral posterior leaflet require mitral valve replacement (see Chapter 19).

The association of arrhythmias and sudden death with MVP is a long-held observation. Premature atrial and ventricular beats, atrioventricular block, and supraventricular or ventricular tachyarrhythmias are common during ambulatory monitoring in adults with MVP.[187] The causes of these arrhythmias are multifactorial, probably combining an anatomic substrate with some form of dysautonomia.[188]

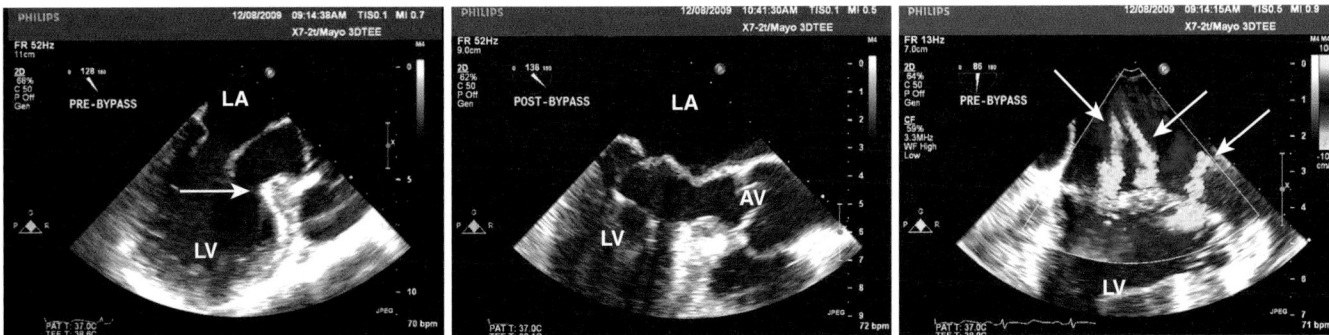

Figure 22-28 *Left,* Transesophageal long-axis view of the left ventricular (LV) outflow tract. Note the hypertrophy of the basal portion of the interventricular septum. *Middle,* Similar image during systole revealing bileaflet prolapse of the mitral valve. With color-Doppler imaging *(right),* at least three jets of mitral regurgitation *(arrows)* are noted. AV, aortic valve; LA, left atrium.

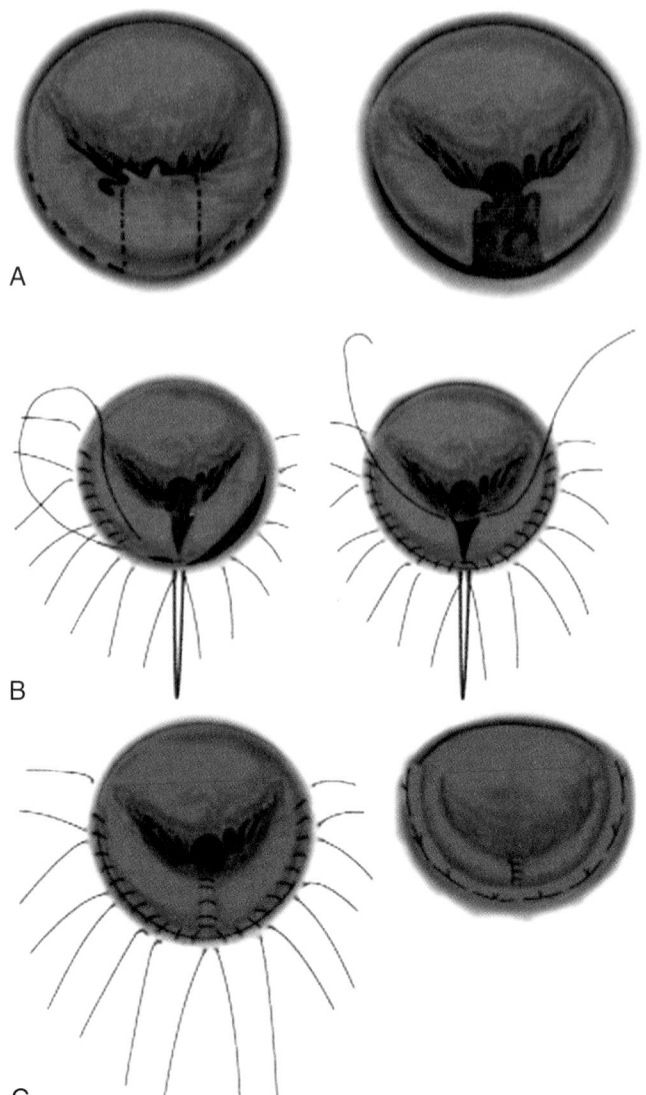

A

B

C

Figure 22-29 Mitral valve repair with sliding annuloplasty technique. *A,* Quadrangular section removed from the posterior leaflet, remainder of the leaflet freed from annulus. *B,* Middle scallop reapproximated and sliding repair undertaken by suturing posterior leaflet to the annulus, shortening the leaflet. *C,* Finally, annuloplasty band applied to reinforce the posterior valve. *(From Gillinov AM, Cosgrove DM 3rd, Shiota T, et al: Cosgrove-Edwards annuloplasty system: Midterm results. Ann Thorac Surg 69:717–72, 2000, by permission.)*

Mechanisms that have been proposed for arrhythmias include ventricular enlargement, hyperadrenergic states, electrolyte imbalances, and mechanical irritation of the ventricle because of traction of the chordae tendineae. Arrhythmias may be secondary to mitral regurgitation, not MVP. According to a study of individuals with nonischemic mitral regurgitation, complex arrhythmias were common and equally prevalent regardless of whether the patient had MVP.[189] Ventricular tachycardia occurred in 35% of those subjects with mitral regurgitation, in contrast with only 5% of participants with MVP alone. Similarly, the risk for sudden death for patients with MVP may be related to mitral regurgitation in view of a reduction in ventricular arrhythmias that occurred with mitral valve repair or replacement.

The occurrence of sudden death with MVP in adults has been debated for years. The risk is low, with an estimated yearly rate of 40 per 10,000, but this is twice the expected rate in the population.[175] Sudden death does occur within families of patients with MVP.[187] The ECG is abnormal in approximately two thirds of persons with MVP,

but ambulatory ECG monitoring does not show an excess of atrial or ventricular arrhythmias unless accompanied by severe mitral regurgitation.[175] EP testing has been unable to identify an arrhythmogenic focus or reliably identify those at increased risk, but it is useful in the pharmacologic management of patients with ongoing complex sustainable arrhythmias. Patients with severe mitral regurgitation, flail segment, and depressed LV appear to be at greater risk for sudden death. Prophylaxis has not averted sudden death in high-risk patients with severe mitral regurgitation. An implantable cardioverter-defibrillator is a consideration in patients with inducible ventricular tachycardia or ventricular fibrillation, but these patients are rare.[190] In general, most low-risk patients do not require treatment for either their symptoms or prevention of sudden death.

MVP has been reported to be associated with cerebral ischemic events, especially in the young. Mitral cusp elongation and expansion that occur with MVP may generate thrombus, vegetation, and calcification of the mitral valve. Mobile masses have been found in conjunction with cerebral events. However, a population-based cohort study involving 1079 patients found no difference in the incidence of strokes in patients younger than 45 years with MVP unless another cardiac disease process was present.[191] In contrast, a more recent study of individuals in Olmsted County of Rochester, Minnesota, found the incidence rate of stroke was 0.07%/year, almost twice the normal rate.[192] The strongest factors associated with increased risk in these patients with MVP included thick valves, mitral valve surgery, atrial fibrillation, and age (> 50 years). Factors that were independently associated with stroke were advanced age, coronary artery disease, CHF, and diabetes.

Bacterial endocarditis is an infrequent complication of MVP, but its incidence is three to eight times greater in these individuals than the general population.[177] Male patients are three times more likely to experience development of endocarditis. Current guidelines from the American Heart Association are specific and do not recommend antibiotic prophylaxis for individuals without a prosthetic cardiac valve, complex congenital heart disease, postcardiac transplant valvular lesions, or a history of bacterial endocarditis.[193] Patients with isolated clicks probably do not benefit from antibiotic prophylaxis, but cost-effectiveness with MVP has been proved nonetheless.[194] Patients at greater risk for development of endocarditis (previous bacterial endocarditis, systolic murmurs, thickened leaflets, or mitral regurgitation) should receive antibiotics before undergoing procedures commonly associated with bacteremia because the risk increases to about 0.05% per year.[175] The turbulent flow from the mitral regurgitation and the thickened valve tissue may cause the increased risk for infection. Patients who may require oral endotracheal intubation or fiberoptic bronchoscopy do not require antibiotic prophylaxis.[176] Unfortunately, as recommendations regarding antibiotic prophylaxis have continued to be modified over the years, there is still insufficient evidence to guide the physician on the issue of prophylaxis and MVP.

Anesthetic Considerations

It is important to understand the broad nature of the condition called MVP with respect to anesthetic considerations. Most individuals with MVP have an uncomplicated general anesthetic because they have MVP without serious complications, often referred to as "MVP syndrome." These patients are usually younger than 45 years, with few risk factors for anesthesia. Invasive monitoring usually is unnecessary. Patients may be taking β-blockers. Preoperative sedation is useful to suppress a possible increased sensitivity to catecholamines. Painful stimuli may exacerbate the autonomic system, possibly causing arrhythmias, although rarely malignant in nature. Significant decreases in left ventricular end-diastolic volume and SVR, or increased contractility and tachycardia should be minimized because MVP may be enhanced such that CO and coronary perfusion are decreased. Intraoperative arrhythmias usually resolve spontaneously or respond to standard therapy. If an arrhythmia occurs, adequate oxygenation should be confirmed and other causes of intraoperative arrhythmias investigated. If β-blockers are required perioperatively, esmolol will avoid the potential for prolonged blockade that might cause hemodynamically significant bradycardia.

Anticholinergic preoperative medications are best avoided despite an increased vagal tone in MVP. A moderate anesthetic depth is desirable to minimize catecholamine levels and potential arrhythmias. Ketamine or drugs that have sympathomimetic effects must be administered with caution. Volatile anesthetics sensitize the heart to catecholamines and, thus, potentially promote arrhythmias. Isoflurane is probably less sensitizing than halothane, but autonomic imbalance may actually be more important in arrhythmogenesis than any direct effect of volatile agents in patients with MVP. These patients with MVP syndrome have been shown to possess good left ventricular function if mitral regurgitation or coronary artery disease is absent[195]; therefore, myocardial depression from volatile agents will be well tolerated. Narcotics such as fentanyl will block sympathetic responses and promote hemodynamic stability; however, prolonged postoperative respiratory depression is a disadvantage with higher doses. Shorter-acting narcotics such as alfentanil and remifentanil, as well as other intravenous agents such as propofol, are available to facilitate rapid extubation.[196] Hypercapnia, hypoxia, and electrolyte disturbances increase ventricular excitability and should be corrected. If muscle relaxation is desired, vecuronium is an excellent choice because it does not cause tachycardia.

Patients with MVP who have mitral regurgitation or are at greater risk for complications warrant a different anesthetic approach compared with those with MVP syndrome. Patients with more severe forms of MVP may rapidly go into CHF unexpectedly and require cardiac surgery. The severity of mitral regurgitation will strongly influence anesthetic management. Routine monitoring for patients undergoing cardiac surgery should be utilized in these patients even if it is a noncardiac operation. Intraoperative TEE is placed after induction. Opioid agents provide excellent hemodynamic stability without depressing myocardial function.[93] Although avoidance of ketamine has been recommended by some for patients with MVP syndrome, dosing less than 0.5 mg/kg ketamine preserves hemodynamic stability in patients who are severely ill, especially used in combination with opioids such as fentanyl. Ketamine will better preserve sympathetic activity and blood pressure in hemodynamically compromised patients. More extensive review of anesthetic management of valvular disease is provided in Chapter 19.

Case Study 1

Mitral Valve Regurgitation and Septal Hypertrophy

The patient was an otherwise healthy 48-year-old woman referred for mitral valve surgery because of severe mitral regurgitation. She was thin and fit. Chest auscultation revealed regular rate and rhythm with a 3/6 systolic murmur. Her preoperative TTE was remarkable for bileaflet prolapse, and an left ventricular ejection fraction of 68%. The surgeon reviewed the TEE and noted that the basal ventricular septum appeared hypertrophied. The surgeon was experienced in complex valve repair and believed the valve was repairable but was concerned that the septal hypertrophy would result in significant postoperative SAM of the mitral leaflet. He requested further evaluation with TEE before CPB was initiated.

The prebypass TEE confirmed the TTE findings. The basal ventricular septum measured 21 mm (see Figure 22-28). At rest, there was no evidence of SAM or LVOT obstruction. It was decided to challenge the patient with isoproterenol. With 4 mg isoproterenol the heart rate increased from 70 to 135 beats/min, and the aortic blood pressure decreased from 126/52 to 77/45. Under these conditions, the TEE showed a significant amount of SAM and turbulent flow in the LVOT with obstruction (Figure 22-30). Needles placed in the aorta and LV were transduced and revealed a gradient across the LVOT of 67 mm Hg. Based on these findings, the surgical plan was altered.

CPB was instituted and the heart arrested. The aorta was opened and myectomy was performed through the aortic valve. The mitral valve was repaired with a posterior leaflet resection, and neochordae were placed to the anterior leaflet. The patient was weaned from CPB.

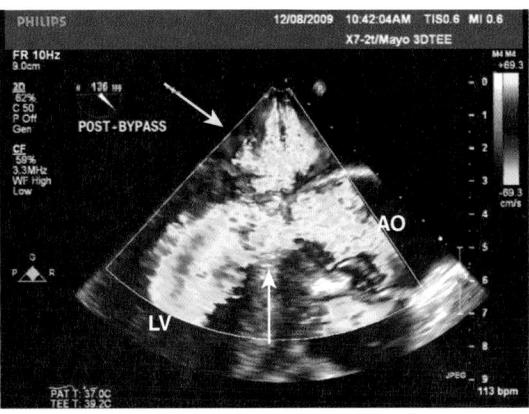

Figure 22-30 Midesophageal long-axis view of the left ventricular outflow tract (LVOT) after administration of isoproterenol. The heart rate has increased and the blood pressure has decreased. The mitral regurgitation (*yellow arrow*) has worsened, and now there is aliasing of the color-Doppler signal in the LVOT (*white arrow*) indicating turbulence of blood flow. AO, aorta; LV, left ventricle.

On TEE, a residual shelf of septal hypertrophy was seen. In addition, there was mild-to-moderate mitral regurgitation that was posteriorly directed and assumed because of tethering of the anterior leaflet by the neochordae. CPB was reinstituted; a second myectomy was performed and the neochordae removed. After weaning from CPB there was no mitral regurgitation and the ventricular septum appeared adequately myectomized. With an isoproterenol challenge achieving similar hemodynamics to those seen before CPB, there was no evidence of SAM or LVOT obstruction by TEE. There was no gradient when needles were placed in the aorta and LV. The patient had an uneventful postoperative course.

In this instance, TEE was absolutely essential in guiding this complex mitral repair. It was able to determine the hemodynamic significance of the septal hypertrophy, the inadequacy of the initial myectomy, and the need to release the neochordae to the anterior leaflet. An alternative operation would have been mitral valve replacement. However, under TEE guidance, the patient received a mitral valve repair, which is superior to replacement for the reasons indicated earlier.

PATENT FORAMEN OVALE

A patent foramen ovale (PFO) is the most common congenital anomaly. It was first recognized as a causal relation with stroke in 1877[197] and has since been proved one of the mechanisms of stroke.[198] Air, thrombus, or fat may travel from the RA to the LA into the systemic circulation, causing a paradoxic embolus that may affect cerebral or coronary circulations. For years, a PFO was identified in the catheterization laboratory, surgery, or autopsy. The advent of echo with its availability and diagnostic capability has increased considerably the number of PFOs that are identified inside the operating room and in the outpatient setting. The ability to so readily and safely close a PFO without surgery has created the need to develop guidelines to address the management of PFO.[199]

The foramen ovale is present during fetal circulation to direct better oxygenated blood from the umbilical veins through the Eustachian valve selectively into the LA. At birth, pulmonary vascular resistance declines dramatically, increasing left atrial blood return that increases the left atrial pressure more than the right atrial pressure, causing a functional closure of the foramen ovale. If the flaplike covering from the septum primum does not fuse with the septum secundum over a period of a year, there is anatomic failure of closure forming a PFO (Figure 22-31). Any condition that results in right atrial pressures exceeding left atrial pressures after birth causes a right-to-left shunt. A left-heart condition that results in left atrial pressures exceeding right atrial pressures causes

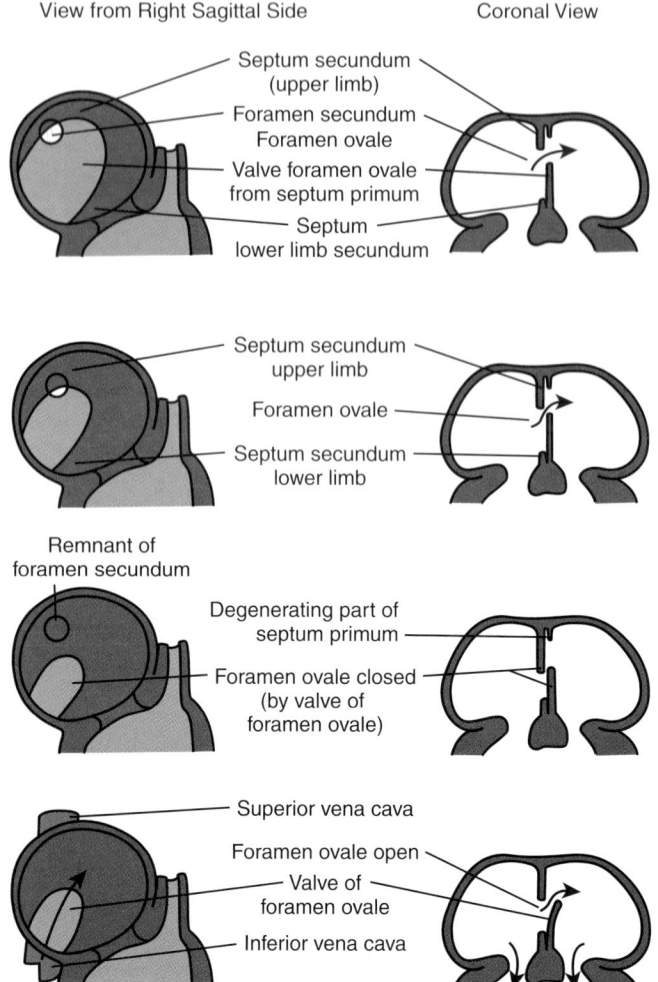

Figure 22-31 Embryologic development of the interatrial septum. (From Hara H, Virmani R, Ladich E, et al: Patent foramen ovale: current pathology, pathophysiology, and clinical status. J Am Coll Cardiol 46:1768–1776, 2005, by permission.)

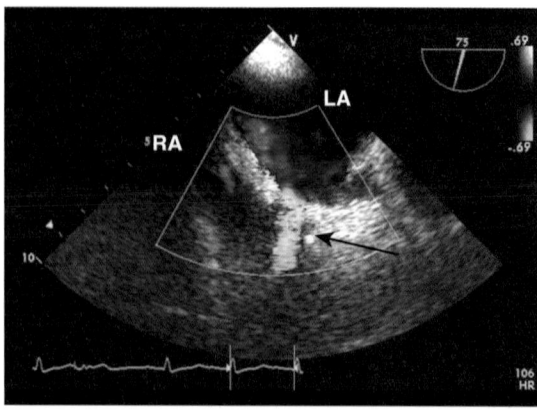

Figure 22-32 **Transesophageal image from the midesophagus at 75 degrees focusing on the interatrial septum.** Color-Doppler imaging readily reveals a moderate-sized shunt from the left atrium (LA) to the right atrium (RA) through a patent foramen ovale.

BOX 22-3. DISEASES AND RISKS ASSOCIATED WITH PATENT FORAMEN OVALE

Proved Causal Relation
Stroke
Transient ischemic attack
Myocardial infarction
Eye infarction
Visceral infarction
Arterial limb embolism
Economy class stroke syndrome
Platypnea orthodeoxia
Fat embolism in major orthopedic surgery
Air embolism in brain surgery in sitting position
Decompression illness

Presumed Causal Relation
Migraine (particularly with aura)
Transitory global amnesia
High-altitude pulmonary edema
Sleep apnea syndrome
Excessive snoring
Increased risk for systemic embolism in:
    Deep sea divers
    Brass musicians
    Glass blowers
    Professionals working in squatting position
    Supersonic jet pilots
    Astronauts

From Meier B: Catheter-based closure of the patent foramen ovale. *Circulation* 120:1837–1841, 2009, by permission.

a left-to-right shunt. An individual may remain asymptomatic for years with a PFO depending on the size of the shunt.

The incidence of PFO in the population has varied depending on the study and diagnostic technique. Hagen et al[200] reported a 27% incidence rate of PFO in nearly 1000 autopsies. This study is considered by many to be the definitive data on incidence of PFO. Subsequent studies involving various modes of echo have reported the incidence rate of PFO in the population to be between 3% and 45%.[201] A recent retrospective study reviewing more than 10 years of cardiac surgery in 13,000 patients reported an incidence rate of PFO as 17% with TEE.[202] TTE is now recognized as less sensitive than TEE, possibly accounting for such variation in previous studies regarding the incidence of PFO. TEE, with its higher image resolution than other methods and 100% sensitivity and specificity with autopsy findings, has become the gold standard for diagnosis of PFO (Figure 22-32).[201] Because TEE is more invasive, additional technical advances in both TEE and transcranial Doppler have improved their sensitivity, and when combined, they may be adequate for PFO screening purposes.[203]

Although a number of conditions are associated with PFO (Box 22-3) that may merit consideration for therapy, stroke receives the most attention. Approximately 700,000 strokes occur each year in the United States, with 20% considered cryptogenic. A PFO is present in 40% to 50% of those strokes.[204] In those individuals with a history of cerebral events, the prevalence rate of PFO ranges from 7% to 40% depending on the

diagnostic technique.[205] Several studies show a strong relation between cryptogenic stroke and PFO based on epidemiologic evidence,[198] but others dispute it. Petty et al[206] conducted a population-based study observing TEE in patients with cerebral ischemic events compared with control subjects who had TEE, but not for cerebral ischemic events, to eliminate bias present in other studies regarding PFO. They found that PFO was not an independent risk factor for stroke even when considering the size of the shunt. Although some recognize the PFO as an increased risk for cryptogenic stroke, it remains inconclusive.

The decision to close a PFO will include individual risk factors for stroke or other complications such as hypoxia that may occur with PFO. Paradoxical embolus is more common if atrial septal aneurysm, large Eustachian valve, migraines, and older age (≥ 50 years) are present.

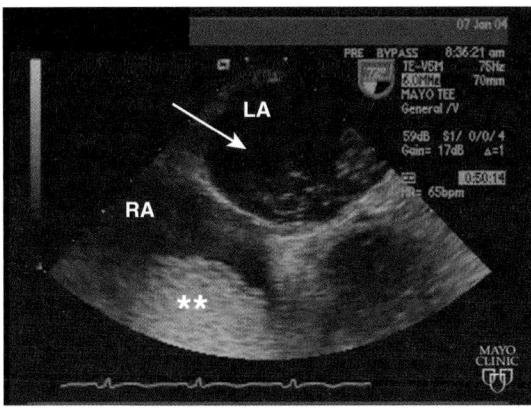

Figure 22-33 Transesophageal image from the midesophagus at 72 degrees focusing on the interatrial septum. Agitated saline (double asterisk) is being used for contrast and can be seen in the right atrium (RA). With the release of a Valsalva maneuver, the contrast is seen to enter the left atrium (LA) through a small patent foramen ovale.

Medium-to-large shunts in combination with any coagulation abnormalities are highly correlated with PFO and paradoxic embolus,[199] and thrombus has been identified at the atrial septum in association with cryptogenic stroke.[198] However, others found no relation to the size of the shunt with PFO and stroke.[206]

It is essential to perform a correct provocative measure to ensure right-to-left movement of air or contrast to diagnose a paradoxical embolus (Figure 22-33). Agitated saline directed through a central catheter with a Valsalva maneuver most commonly is used to confirm the diagnosis. The increased intrathoracic pressure from the Valsalva maneuver will lead to a temporary increased return of venous blood after the Valsalva has ended, so the right atrial pressure will exceed left atrial pressure briefly to allow contrast administered into the right internal jugular vein to pass to the LA.[203] False-negative results may occur if the left atrial pressure is very increased so that the provocative measure does not cause right-to-left shunting.

Management of a PFO is very dependent on the circumstances. Medical therapy basically consists of various anticoagulation regimens that may suffice for some; however, most observational and meta-analysis studies comparing medical therapy with percutaneous closure shows it to be inferior.[207] Percutaneous closure of the PFO is indicated especially in those patients with recurrent paradoxic emboli. There is a reduction in the incidence of stroke.[199] Another advantage over medical therapy is the lack of chronic anticoagulation.[198] There are no randomized, prospective trials comparing medical therapy with percutaneous PFO closure to sufficiently answer the question of superiority between options; however, in nonrandomized trials, short-term complications appear to slightly favor medical treatment over percutaneous closure.[207]

Closure of PFO is performed either surgically or percutaneously. Although available in the late 1980s, percutaneous closure of PFO really became popular in 1992 after a report describing successful closure of 36 PFOs in patients with known right-to-left shunt and presumed paradoxical emboli.[208] Percutaneous closure generally is performed in a catheterization laboratory with conscious sedation. Success rates (incidence of no residual shunting) have been good initially, but the methods used to evaluate success may have been flawed, accounting for the wide range of success rates between 50% and 100%.[205] Recently, using transcranial Doppler to assess PFO closure, researchers found 9% of patients to have significant shunting after only 1 year after percutaneous closure.[209] There are no data concerning the success rate of surgical compared with percutaneous closure. Although the percutaneous closure is being done routinely, complications occur in about 1.5% of cases. They include cardiac perforation, air embolism with placement, thrombus formation, and even death.[209]

Currently, it is rare to surgically close an isolated PFO, with the safety and availability of percutaneous closure. However, use of intraoperative TEE during cardiac operations has increased the number of incidentally diagnosed PFOs. A recent retrospective look at more than 10 years of cardiac operations in 13,000 patients found 17% of cases with PFO.[202] Looking at the incidence of PFO year by year from 1995 to 2010, the incidence remained relatively static each year; however, the percentage of PFOs that were closed surgically increased to a maximum of 39% over that period. Not only are more PFOs closed as a percentage, but more surgeons as a percentage are choosing to close them over time.[199] The causes for these trends are not certain, but a PFO diagnosed incidentally during surgery creates a dilemma for the surgeon. A majority of surgeons examine the circumstances, size of the PFO, and other criteria to decide on closure during the ongoing surgery.

The decision to close an incidental PFO during cardiac surgery is not always evident based on short- and long-term risk to the patient. Because the finding was incidental, recurrent paradoxic emboli and neurologic injury usually have not occurred. Certain conditions would almost mandate closure of the PFO, such as the insertion of a left ventricular assist device that would promote paradoxic embolus[203] or the onset of severe hypoxia because of increased right-sided pressures causing a large right-to-left shunt. Surgical PFO closure does not confer additional morbidity or mortality based on retrospective review of all surgical closure of isolated PFOs from one institution that demonstrated no mortality and minimal morbidity. Recent data have confirmed that adding PFO closure during cardiac surgery did not increase mortality.[202] Surgical PFO closure is done routinely through a sternotomy, but the use of new techniques of minimally invasive surgery also allow the incision to be a right thoracotomy. Closure requires CPB and cardioplegic arrest. Certain operations such as tricuspid or mitral valve repair or placement that include CPB and atriotomy require minimal deviation from the originally planned procedure to close the PFO and, thus, incur little risk. In contrast, CABG performed without CPB would entail the risk of going on CPB, aortic cross-clamping, and other complications associated with extracorporeal circulation. The decision to close the incidental PFO may depend on the long-term risk of not closing it.

Based on a survey of cardiac surgeons, 27.9% of respondents always closed PFOs if detected during CABG.[203] However, there really is no evidence to indicate all PFOs found incidentally during a cardiac operation merit closure.[202] A retrospective study looking at those with and without PFOs showed no differences between stroke, hospital and intensive care unit (ICU) duration, MI, and death when propensity matching was applied for the comparison.[202] Long-term follow-up for 10 years also did not demonstrate any difference between those who had PFOs and those without PFOs. Outcome for those who had PFOs repaired versus not repaired found no differences in outcome except for a slight but significantly increased incidence of stroke after surgery in the repaired group that could not be explained. Other than the concern for stroke, the risk for severe desaturation after surgery if there was no PFO closure was possible, but a case series of 11 off-pump CABG with incidental PFOs that were not closed showed no adverse problems perioperatively with desaturation.[210] A subset of patients may exist who do not behave well perioperatively with off-pump CABG because of a PFO.

Anesthesia

Anesthesia management for PFO closure percutaneously requires only conscious sedation in most patients. Anesthesia management for closure of an incidental PFO requires little deviation from the original anesthetic management of the scheduled original cardiac operation. However, once the PFO has been identified, there are some considerations specifically for a PFO.

Routine care for preventing venous air should be standard for cardiac surgery. Obviously, there is a great need to be diligent with the injection of medications to remove extraneous air from entering the venous system. It is important to appreciate the potential for paradoxic embolus with any patient who requires mechanical ventilation.

In situations in which the pulmonary vascular resistance may increase, such as during hypercapnia or with positive end-expiratory pressure greater than 15 mm Hg, the potential for right-to-left shunting is increased.[211] Choice of anesthetic seems to have little impact on management of PFO because the patients will tolerate most regimens.

Case Study 2

Incidental Patent Foramen Ovale Found during Coronary Artery Bypass Grafting Surgery

A 60-year-old man with a medical history of hypertension presented with angina on exertion. Specifically, he had bouts of recurring chest pain after jogging for 15 minutes on a treadmill. Previously, he had been able to jog for 30 minutes without difficulty. On physical examination, he appeared thin and fit. The heart was regular in rate and rhythm without a murmur, and the lungs were clear to auscultation. A stress echo was positive for ischemia and coronary angiography showed severe triple-vessel disease, so CABG was scheduled.

In the operating room, a TEE probe was placed for the purposes of monitoring ventricular function and evaluation of regional wall motion abnormalities. The prebypass examination revealed an ejection fraction of 65%, normal valves, and no regional wall motion abnormalities. The interatrial septum appeared redundant. Agitated saline was injected into the central line. After the release of sustained positive pressure ventilation, contrast was seen to enter the LA via a small PFO (see Figure 22-33). No shunt was detected by color-Doppler imaging.

The surgeon was informed of the previously undiagnosed PFO. A discussion ensued regarding the implications of repairing the PFO compared with leaving it undisturbed. The surgeon previously had not repaired a small PFO during CABG surgery, finding the patient had suffered a stroke, presumably because of a paradoxical embolism, 2 years later. Given the patient's young age and previous experience, the surgeon elected to repair the PFO that altered the surgical planning. The cannulation strategy was changed from a single right atrial venous cannula to bicaval cannulation. A right atriotomy was performed, and the PFO was closed with two stitches. The patient was easily weaned from CPB and had an uneventful postoperative course.

PULMONARY HEMORRHAGE

Pulmonary hemorrhage occurs in about 1.5% of patients with hemoptysis,[212] but mortality may reach 85%.[213] The definition of massive hemoptysis varies but commonly is characterized as more than 600 mL of expectorated blood over 24 hours or recurrent bleeding of greater than 100 mL per day for several days. Four hundred milliliters of blood in the alveolar space seriously impairs oxygenation. Pulmonary hemorrhage may stabilize only to worsen again without an obvious explanation reflecting its unpredictable nature. Notably, death is not attributable to hemodynamic instability with hemorrhage but to excessive blood in the alveoli that causes hypoventilation and refractory hypoxia. Moreover, one clot may obstruct an entire lobe of the lungs. Mortality is related to the amount of bleeding that occurs over time.[213,214] If more than 600 mL blood is lost over 16 hours, the mortality rate is 45%, whereas it is only 5% if blood loss totals 600 mL over 48 hours. A delay in initiating treatment because of difficulty in isolating the location of bleeding contributes greatly to the high mortality of pulmonary hemorrhage.

Hemoptysis may occur with various diseases and circumstances (Table 22-7). In the United States, chronic inflammatory lung disease and bronchogenic carcinoma are the most common causes of hemoptysis.[215] Of these causes, bronchitis (26%), lung cancer (23%), pneumonia (10%), and tuberculosis (8%) are most frequent. The inflammatory response is an important factor in the occurrence of bleeding.[216] The combination of chronic infection, inflammation, and vascular growth result in hypervascularization of the bronchial circulation that ultimately erodes into the alveoli.[217] Pulmonary hemorrhage also may result from vigorous suctioning of the lungs, surgery, and improper

TABLE 22-7	Causes of Massive Hemoptysis
Tracheobronchial disorders	
Amyloidosis	
Bronchial adenoma	
Bronchiectasis*	
Bronchogenic carcinoma	
Broncholithiasis	
Bronchovascular fistula	
Cystic fibrosis	
Foreign body aspiration	
Tracheobronchial trauma	
Cardiovascular disorders	
Congenital heart disease	
Mitral stenosis	
Pulmonary arteriovenous fistula	
Septic pulmonary emboli	
Ruptured thoracic aneurysm	
Arteriovenous malformation	
Localized parenchymal diseases	
Amebiasis	
Aspergilloma*	
Atypical mycobacterial infection*	
Coccidioidomycosis	
Lung abscess	
Mucormycosis	
Pulmonary tuberculosis*	
Diffuse parenchymal diseases	
Goodpasture syndrome	
Idiopathic pulmonary hemosiderosis	
Polyarteritis nodosa	
Systemic lupus erythematosus	
Wegener's granulomatosis	
Other	
Pulmonary artery rupture from a pulmonary artery catheter	
Iatrogenic (e.g., bronchoscopy, cardiac catheterization)	
Pulmonary hypertension	
Pulmonary edema	
Pulmonary infarction	

*Most common causes.
From Thompson AB, Tescheler H, Rennard SI: Pathogenesis, evaluation, and therapy for massive hemoptysis. *Clin Chest Med* 13:69, 1992.

positioning of a PAC.[218] Massive hemoptysis usually is an emergency because the underlying pulmonary disorder minimizes the patient's ability to tolerate it.

It is helpful to appreciate the anatomy of the pulmonary circulation to understand the pathogenesis of pulmonary hemorrhage. The lungs have a dual blood supply. The pulmonary arterial circuit is a high-flow, low-pressure circuit. The nutritive supply of the pulmonary structures is the bronchial arteries, which originate from the aorta. Bronchial arteries extend into many areas around the lymph nodes, esophagus, and lungs, ultimately penetrating the bronchial wall to supply the bronchial mucosa. The bronchial and pulmonary circulations anastomose at several locations. Massive pulmonary hemorrhage usually involves bleeding caused by disruption of the high-pressure bronchial circulation.[212] These high-pressure, tortuous bronchial arteries are found throughout the thoracic cage. They become dilated and rupture or erode or feed into the lower pressure pulmonary veins that may easily rupture. The bronchial circulation accounts for 98% of pulmonary hemorrhage, and the pulmonary circulation accounts for the remainder.[214]

Diagnosis of hemoptysis requires a few simple tests. Visual inspection usually can distinguish gastrointestinal bleeding from pulmonary hemorrhage. Hemoptysis often is bright red with some sputum. Hemoptysis caused by pulmonary artery rupture usually is copious (200 to 2000 mL).[218] Treatment begins with conservative management and simultaneous efforts to locate the bleeding site. A chest roentgenogram may reveal an infiltrate, but neither chest roentgenogram nor physical examination has been reliable in localizing the affected lung. Recently, better noninvasive technology such as the multidetector-row CT is capable of determining rapidly and accurately the site of bleeding.[215] Flexible bronchoscopy of the airways may be limited by severe bleeding that obscures the view and attempts should not persist, delaying other therapies. Rigid bronchoscopy is better suited for identification of bleeding during massive hemoptysis and the removal of any large clot that may be obstructing the airway. However, the view of the upper lobes is limited and requires general anesthesia. Instillation of epinephrine in the bronchi may facilitate better visualization by slowing the bleeding. Ultimately, angiography of the pulmonary and bronchial arteries may be necessary to localize the source of the bleeding.[213] Imaging for bronchial artery bleeding begins with a thoracic aortogram to localize all the main systemic arteries to the lungs that may be bronchial or nonbronchial. Once the feeding arteries are localized, selective bronchial arteriography is then used to identify the bleeding vessels.[219]

Therapeutic options for bleeding depend on the extent of bleeding. Conservative treatment may suffice. Once the bleeding patient has been placed in the ICU and antibiotics administered, flexible bronchoscopy may be able to identify the source of bleeding, as well as perform techniques to minimize hemorrhage such as epinephrine flush, cold-saline lavage, and possible balloon bronchial blockers to tamponade any bleeding.[220] Advancements in bronchoscopy have seen the successful use of topically applied agents consisting of oxidized regenerated cellulose mesh injected at the site of bleeding.[215] In addition, the use of topically applied factor VIIa (FVIIa) has been reported in massive hemolysis secondary to a medical cause, although its use in this manner is off-label.[217] FVIIa has been anecdotally reported beneficial with massive hemoptysis despite low platelet count, trauma, vasculitis, and bone marrow transplant. Other medications that have been recommended for increasing clotting to reduce bleeding are Premarin, desmopressin, vasopressin, and tranexamic acid.[221]

If bleeding continues to be heavy, a double-lumen endotracheal tube (ETT) is beneficial to isolate the bleeding from the unaffected lung, although placement may prove difficult in the midst of active bleeding. Misplacement of a double-lumen ETT occurs in 45% of patients after the initial attempt and 54% after patient positioning.[222] If the patient was anticoagulated, airway manipulation in connection with double-lumen ETT placement may incite further mucosal damage and bleeding. A Fogarty catheter, as described by Larson and Gasior,[223] may be passed within an existing ETT under bronchoscopic guidance to the affected bronchus, minimizing additional trauma to the airway caused by reintubation and protecting the uninvolved lung. The Univent ETT is an alternative to a double-lumen ETT but requires exchanging the existing ETT for the Univent tube. A single-lumen ETT should not be advanced into the right main bronchus if bleeding is believed to be in the right lung, because of the proximal location of the right upper lobe bronchus (see Chapter 24).

Continued bleeding after stabilization and conservative therapy necessitates bronchial artery embolization. First used in 1974 to stop massive hemoptysis,[219] it is considered the first-line therapy for massive hemoptysis. It may stop the bleeding 75% to 98% of the time, but 16% to 20% of patients will rebleed in the following year.[224-226] Bronchial artery embolization often is done simultaneously with the thoracic aortogram to identify the bleeding vessels. The offending vessels are injected with a form of polyvinyl alcohol particles, Gelfoam, and possibly dextran microspheres. A recent study found 88% of patients who underwent bronchial artery embolization had bleeding controlled immediately and another group of patients (81%) had bleeding stopped by 48 hours.[227] Bronchial artery embolization has greatly advanced the success of dealing with pulmonary hemorrhage. It may require more than one procedure to be effective. Immediate recurrence of hemoptysis after embolization may be because of arteries that were not identified and not embolized. Latent hemoptysis is due to recanalization or collateralization. Although it has proved effective, it is

not without complications, especially vascular complications such as coronary artery syndrome, spinal cord ischemia, and esophageal wall necrosis.[219]

The ability to use an array of treatment options in a multidisciplinary approach to this life-threatening condition will increase survival and reduce complications.[220] Efforts to control bleeding for at least 48 hours with nonsurgical alternatives before surgery have reduced surgical mortality and postoperative complications compared with earlier implementation of surgery for massive hemoptysis in the past. If bleeding continues unabated, exsanguination may be unavoidable, so surgery is the definitive treatment. A localized bleeding site and sufficient lung function are essential to determine before surgery because resection may extend to a pneumonectomy. Postoperative mortality rate varies tremendously from 1% to 50%.[212] Surgery is contraindicated in those with lung carcinoma invading the trachea, mediastinum, heart or great vessels, terminal malignancy, and progressive pulmonary fibrosis.

Introduction of the PAC enabled physicians to obtain CO, SVR, and estimates of left ventricular performance and to detect early myocardial ischemia perioperatively, greatly increasing their use. Unfortunately, with more use, a rare but often fatal cause of pulmonary hemorrhage, rupture of the pulmonary artery by the PAC in patients undergoing cardiac surgery, emerged.[218] The incidence rate ranges from 0.06% to 0.2% of cases, with a corresponding mortality rate of 45% to 64% and serious morbidity.[228] With respect to cardiac surgical patients, death may occur within minutes of pulmonary artery rupture or over a period of 1 to 14 days after surgery.[229] The diagnosis may be initially missed because patients may be asymptomatic or only mildly symptomatic. A small amount of hemoptysis may herald the onset of severe pulmonary hemorrhage.[230] If a patient is anticoagulated, bleeding may be profuse. Other signs of pulmonary artery rupture are hypotension, decreased arterial oxygenation, bronchospasm, pleural effusion, hemothorax, and pneumothorax. Pulmonary hemorrhage rarely occurs during cardiac surgery; however, when it does, it is life-threatening not only because of anticoagulation, but because of the severity of the patient's cardiovascular disease.

Certain factors predispose patients to pulmonary artery rupture such as age older than 60, anticoagulation, and distal migration of the PAC.[218] Although PAH often is present with pulmonary artery rupture, it is not a risk factor[229] but simply may promote distal migration of the PAC. Chronic PAH weakens the pulmonary artery and veins; thus, a patient's susceptibility to rupture is increased. The mechanism of pulmonary artery rupture is multifactorial, but the balloon of the catheter is instrumental.[231] Maximal pressures for balloon inflation are approximately 1700 mm Hg and easily reach 1000 mm Hg with the start of inflation. PACs that reside distally will reduce the inflation pressures necessary to rupture the pulmonary artery, particularly in the elderly. Distal migration of the PAC also occurs more easily in patients undergoing hypothermic CPB because hypothermia stiffens the PAC. Eccentric inflation of the PAC balloon contributes to pulmonary artery rupture, as evidenced in both cadavers and patients.[232] Inflation that distorts the balloon drives the catheter tip through the vessel wall (Figure 22-34). Manipulation of the heart also may perforate the pulmonary artery.

The extent of bleeding after pulmonary artery rupture will determine treatment. If rupture occurs during CPB, then it should be maintained to ensure adequate oxygenation and identify the site of rupture under controlled conditions. Mild bleeding may require positive end-expiratory pressure once anticoagulation is neutralized.[229,233] Similarly, the balloon of a PAC may tamponade a bleeding site in the bronchus. These preceding measures are meant to be only temporary until definitive treatment is instituted. If anticoagulation has been neutralized, blood loss of 1000 mL or more over 24 hours should merit consideration for early surgical intervention if the patient has the respiratory reserve to tolerate it.[213,214] If there is concern about tolerating surgery, treatment should progress to bronchial artery embolization and, ultimately, pulmonary lobectomy if bleeding is refractory.

To reduce the possibility of pulmonary artery rupture, placement or migration of a PAC distally in the pulmonary artery should be avoided. It is not advisable to advance the PAC more than 5 cm beyond the

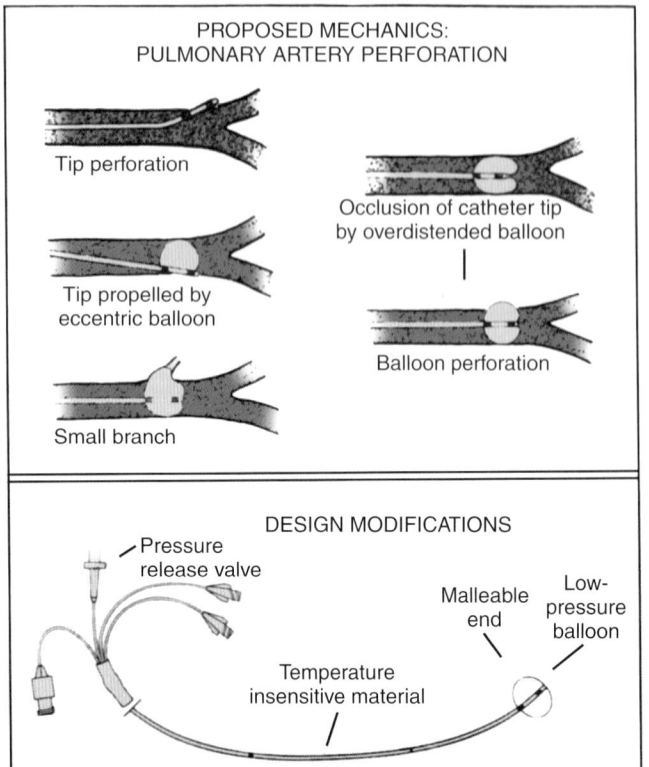

Figure 22-34   Possible mechanisms of pulmonary artery perforation with balloon-tipped flow-guided catheter. These problems require modifications in catheter design. *(Reprinted from Barash PG, Nardi D, Hammond G, et al: Catheter-induced pulmonary artery perforation: Mechanisms, management, and modifications. J Thorac Cardiovasc Surg 82:5, 1981.)*

pulmonary valve. The balloon should not be inflated against increased resistance, particularly if the patient is anticoagulated or after separation from CPB. The pulmonary artery waveform should always be carefully observed with inflation and deflation of the balloon. Retracting the PAC into the RV on the initiation of CPB or withdrawing the PAC 5 cm immediately before CPB is advisable.

PERICARDIAL HEART DISEASE

The pericardium is a two-layer sac that encloses the heart and the great vessels. Its inner layer is a serous membrane (visceral pericardium) covering the surface of the heart. Its outer layer is a fibrinous sac (parietal pericardium), which is attached to the great vessels, diaphragm, and sternum. The parietal pericardium is a stiff collagenous membrane that resists acute expansion. The space between the two layers is the pericardial space. The pericardial space normally contains up to 50 mL clear fluid that is an ultrafiltrate of plasma. It gradually can dilate to accept large volumes of fluid if slowly accumulated, but if accumulated rapidly will lead to cardiac tamponade. The two layers of the pericardium are joined at the level of the great vessels and at the central tendon of the diaphragm caudally, and a serous layer extends past these junctions to line the inside of the fibrinous sac (parietal pericardium). The vagus nerve, left recurrent laryngeal nerve, and esophageal plexus innervate the pericardium, together with sympathetic contributions from the stellate ganglion, first dorsal ganglion, and other ganglia. The lateral course of the phrenic nerve on either side of the heart is an important anatomic relation because this nerve is encapsulated in the pericardium and, thus, easily can be damaged during pericardiectomy (Figure 22-35). The pericardium is not essential for life, and pericardiectomy causes no apparent disability, but it has many subtle functions that are advantageous. Foremost, it acts to minimize torsion of the

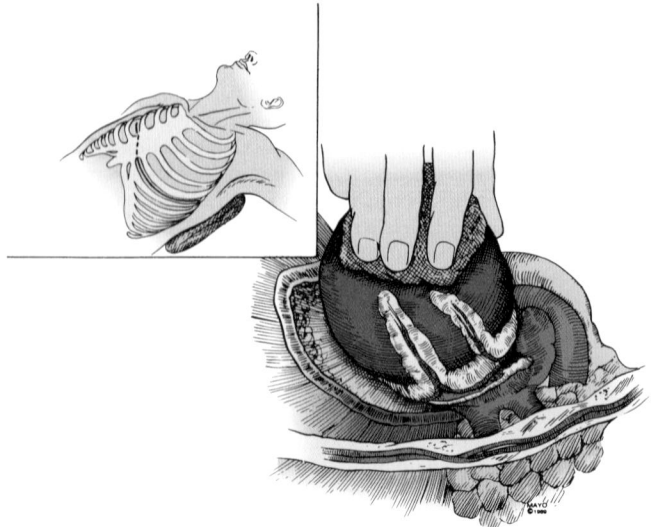

Figure 22-35   Approach for pericardiectomy through a fifth left intercostal space for anterolateral thoracotomy. The phrenic nerves are preserved on pedicles. The lateral course of the phrenic nerves and the pericardial attachment make the phrenic nerves easily damaged during removal of the pericardium. *(From Tuna IC, Danielson GK: Surgical management of pericardial disease. Cardiol Clin 8:683, 1990, by permission.)*

heart and reduce the friction from surrounding organs. Recently, it has been shown that the pericardium also has immunologic, vasomotor, paracrine, metabolic, and fibrinolytic activities.[234]

Acute Pericarditis

Acute pericarditis is common, but the actual incidence is unknown because it often goes unrecognized. It generally is self-limited, lasting 6 weeks. Acute pericarditis has many causes (Box 22-4); the most common is viral (30% to 50%).[235] Only 25% of cases have a defined cause, although this is improving.[236] Unfortunately, acute pericarditis resembles many other conditions. Anesthesiologists encounter patients with acute pericarditis in situations of malignancy, MI, postcardiotomy syndrome, uremia, or infection when surgery is required because symptoms are incapacitating and medical therapy has failed.

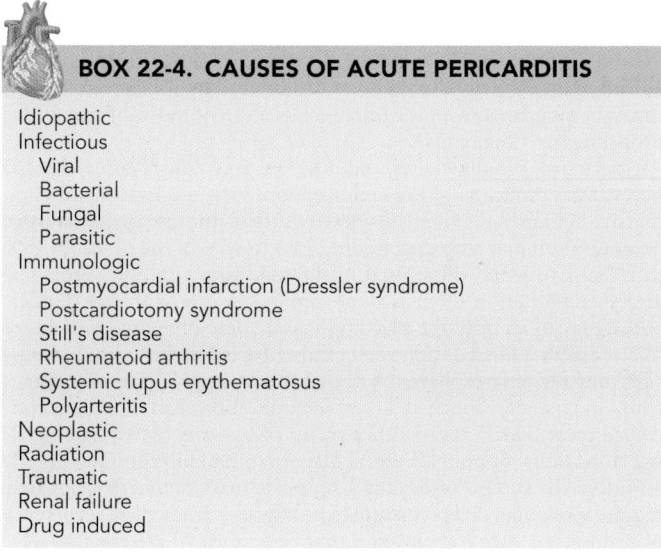

BOX 22-4.   CAUSES OF ACUTE PERICARDITIS

Idiopathic
Infectious
  Viral
  Bacterial
  Fungal
  Parasitic
Immunologic
  Postmyocardial infarction (Dressler syndrome)
  Postcardiotomy syndrome
  Still's disease
  Rheumatoid arthritis
  Systemic lupus erythematosus
  Polyarteritis
Neoplastic
Radiation
Traumatic
Renal failure
Drug induced

From Oakley CM: Myocarditis, pericarditis and other pericardial diseases. *Heart* 84:449–454, 2000.

Acute pericarditis is characterized by fibrin deposits localized on the pericardial surface. A serous effusion may accompany the fibrinous inflammation. Consequently, the mesothelial cell layer is replaced by a fibrin membrane that has white blood cells scattered throughout it. Pericardial fluid may suggest a bacterial, neoplastic, or viral and inflammatory cause.[235] Pericarditis occurs in about 20% of patients who suffer an MI, primarily within the first week.[237] A distinction is made between pericarditis that occurs during the first week and Dressler syndrome, which usually appears 2 to 3 months after an MI. With acute pericarditis, pleuritic chest pain is described in the center of the chest radiating to the back and left trapezius muscle. This pain is more continuous than the intermittent pain of myocardial ischemia. Some degree of dyspnea may be present with acute pericarditis. Occasionally, pericarditis may present as right-heart failure because large and rapid accumulations of pericardial fluid will increase intrapericardial pressure sufficiently to obstruct right ventricular filling through the superior and inferior vena cava, resulting in tamponade. Atrial arrhythmias also may occur.

In general, acute pericarditis can be differentiated from MI by measurement of serum cardiac enzymes, but myocardial enzymes are sometimes found in the serum of patients with pericarditis. It also is common to see the early onset of a low-grade fever that lasts for days to weeks and the presence of a friction rub after the onset of chest pain. Pericardial friction rub is pathognomonic of pericarditis but may be heard only intermittently. Early ECG changes typical of pericarditis are ST-segment elevation in 2 or 3 standard limb leads and in most of the precordial leads. ST-T wave elevation often is present but may be confused with MI (Figure 22-36). Acute pericarditis generally results in diffuse ST-T changes, whereas MI usually is associated with more localized ST-T changes. T-wave inversions follow the acute ST-segment abnormalities as pericarditis enters the subacute phase. Q waves usually do not appear during progression of ECG changes. The echo findings in a patient with suspected acute pericarditis are variable. There may be a pericardial effusion present, the pericardium may be thickened, or it may appear completely normal. If an effusion is present, tamponade physiology must be excluded. If the pericardium appears

thickened, additional evidence for constrictive physiology should be sought (see later). The chest roentgenogram may reveal a slightly enlarged cardiac silhouette with a pericardial effusion that indicates the effusion is at least 250 mL. A rapid accumulation of pericardial fluid may cause tamponade. Conversely, if it accumulates slowly, a liter or more of pericardial fluid may collect without symptoms of cardiac tamponade. Pericardial fluid also may be found with CHF, valvular disease, or endocarditis. Pericardiocentesis is performed in acute pericarditis, either to confirm the diagnosis or to relieve tamponade. It may be associated with serious complications, even cardiovascular collapse and shock. Echo should evaluate ventricular contractile function before pericardiocentesis. If repeated aspirations are required for relief of tamponade, pericardiectomy may be necessary.

Detection of myocardially directed serum antibodies in Dressler syndrome and in postpericardiotomy syndrome suggests that these syndromes are immune-related responses. Postpericardiotomy syndrome consists of acute nonspecific pericarditis that usually begins between 10 days and 3 months after cardiac surgery or trauma. In a prospective study of 944 adult patients who underwent cardiac surgery, the incidence rate of postpericardiotomy syndrome was 17.8%, although it has been reported as high as 50% of postoperative cardiac patients.[238]

Treatment of acute pericarditis consists of symptomatic relief and treating the underlying systemic illness. Symptomatic relief involves support, bed rest, and nonsteroidal anti-inflammatory agents for analgesia. Left stellate ganglion block has been used to relieve unremitting pain.

Constrictive Pericarditis

CP is a dense fusion of the parietal and visceral pericardium that limits diastolic filling of the heart irrespective of cause. The changes in the pericardium can be caused by scarring, induced by a single episode of acute pericarditis or by a prolonged exposure to a recurrent or chronic inflammatory process. CP is a progressive disease. Tuberculosis was a major cause of CP, but currently most cases (33%) are idiopathic.[239] The leading identifiable causes of CP are pericarditis, cardiac surgery,

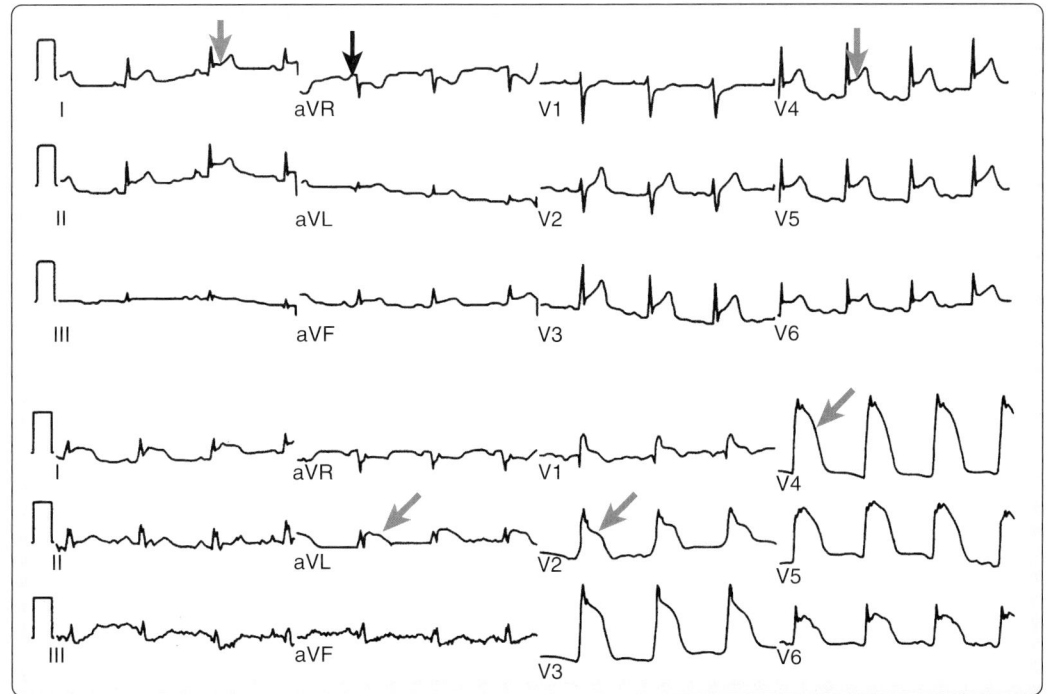

Figure 22-36 Acute pericarditis: Note the upward-concavity ST elevations in limb leads I, II, aVF, and aVL, and in precordial leads V_3, V_4, V_5, and V_6 (light arrows) and the PR-segment elevation in aVR (bold arrow). Acute myocardial infarction: Note the concavity-downward ST elevation in leads I, aVL, V_1, V_2, V_3, V_4, V_5, and V_6 (light arrows), indicating a large anterior myocardial infarction. (Aikat S, Ghaffari S: A review of pericardial diseases: Clinical, ECG and hemodynamic features and management. Cleve Clin J Med 67: 907, 2000, by permission.)

TABLE 22-8	Causes of Constrictive Pericarditis	
Cause	Percentage
Idiopathic pericarditis	40%
Post-CABG	30%
Tuberculosis	10%
Radiation induced	5%
Collagen vascular disease	5%
Others (malignancy, uremia, purulent)	5%

CABG, coronary artery bypass grafting.
From Kabbani SS, LeWinter MM: Diastolic heart failure, constrictive, restrictive and pericardial. *Cardiol Clin* 18:505, 2000.

and mediastinal irradiation in the developed world.[240] Table 22-8 lists some of the causes of chronic CP. Idiopathic, neoplastic, postirradiation, or uremic pericarditis account for most cases of CP that require surgery. Eighteen percent of pericardiectomies are attributed to previous cardiac surgery,[239] which may explain the increase in the number of cases of CP since the middle 1990s.[241]

CP clinically resembles the congestive states of myocardial and chronic liver disease.[234] The most frequent physical signs are jugular venous distention, hepatomegaly, and ascites suggestive of heart failure. Symptoms are nonspecific and progress over years unless the cause is radiation, cardiac surgery, or trauma that can instead develop over months. The normal filling phases of the jugular venous pulse are shown in Figure 22-37. Venous pressure waves in pericardial constriction are characterized by a prominent *y* descent. Kussmaul's sign (a paradoxical increase in venous pressure with inspiration) may be present. Systemic venous congestion accounts for some of the classic symptoms of CP such as hepatic congestion and peripheral edema.[151] A significant paradoxical pulse occurs in only one third of patients with chronic CP.

Characteristic ECG changes are P mitrale (broadened P wave), low QRS voltage, and T-wave inversion.[241] One fourth of patients have

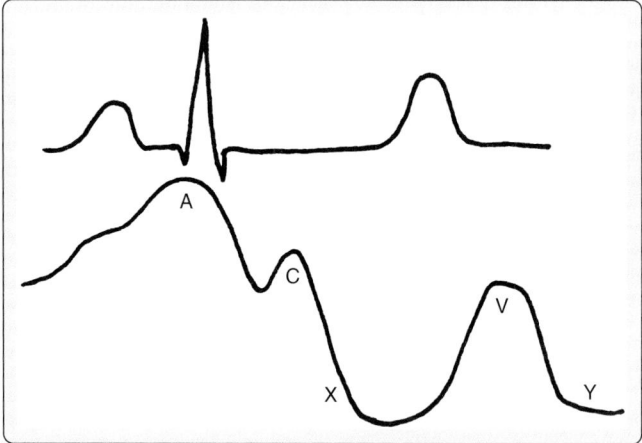

Figure 22-37 Schematic depiction of normal jugular venous pressure waves in relation to the electrocardiogram (ECG). The A wave is a result of atrial contraction; the prominent negative *x* descent occurs during ventricular systole and is a result of downward displacement of the base of the heart and tricuspid valve, as well as continued atrial relaxation. The small C wave, which interrupts the *x* descent, is probably caused by the bulging of the tricuspid valve into the right atrium. The V wave represents right atrial filling while the tricuspid valve is closed. Finally, the *y* descent occurs after opening of the tricuspid valve and during rapid inflow of blood from the right atrium into the ventricle. *(From Legler D: Uncommon diseases and cardiac anesthesia. In Kaplan JA [ed]: Cardiac Anesthesia, 2nd ed. Philadelphia, WB Saunders Company, 1987, p 785, by permission.)*

atrial fibrillation. Cardiomegaly on chest roentgenogram is nonspecific. Pericardial calcification sometimes is apparent in lateral chest roentgenograms (< 30%),[240] although less common than in the past because the incidence of tuberculosis has declined so greatly in developed nations. Although calcification is very specific for CP, it is not very sensitive. CT and MRI may demonstrate the typically thickened pericardium of CP; however, patients with surgically proven CP may have a normal-appearing pericardium with imaging tests in 28% of individuals.[156]

A comprehensive echo examination including 2D and Doppler imaging is an essential part of the diagnostic workup and often adequate for diagnosis. The 2D findings may include a thickened pericardium, abnormal motion of the ventricular septum, inferior vena cava dilation, and flattening of the left ventricular posterior wall during diastole.[33] A key diagnostic finding in constriction is ventricular interdependence. Diastolic filling of the ventricles is reliant on each other because the overall cardiac volume is fixed by the stiffened pericardium. With inspiration, intrathoracic pressure declines, as does the pressure in the pulmonary vasculature. The thickened pericardium prevents transmission of this pressure decrease to the ventricles. Thus, filling of the LV decreases just after inspiration because of the decline in pressure within the pulmonary vasculature. Because the interpericardial space is fixed, a decrease in filling pressure to the LV allows increased filling in the RV. The result is a shift in the ventricular septum into the LV during inspiration, as well as an increase in hepatic vein diastolic flow.[33] With expiration, intrathoracic pressure increases, the pressure in the pulmonary vasculature increases, and left ventricular filling is augmented with a shift of the ventricular septum into the RV during diastole. Right ventricular filling is now decreased because of the positive intrathoracic pressure, and flow reversals occur during diastole in the hepatic veins. When several cardiac cycles are viewed consecutively, the ventricular septum appears to "bounce" between the LV and RV.

Ideally, a respiratory variation of 25% or more in mitral inflow E velocity will accompany the diastolic flow reversals in the hepatic veins during expiration and support the diagnosis of pericardial constriction (Figure 22-38). However, this finding is present in only approximately 50% of patients with constriction.[242,243] More recently, tissue Doppler imaging of the mitral annulus has become a valuable tool in the diagnosis of constriction. In myocardial disease, such as RCM, relaxation is impaired and the mitral annular velocity is low (< 7 cm/sec).[33] However, in constriction, relaxation is normal or increased. This can be a valuable tool in differentiating between restrictive and constrictive disease, but there is no uniform acceptance of Doppler indices that differentiate CP from RCM.[234] Right and left cardiac catheterization are necessary to confirm hemodynamic abnormalities in cases that are seen with Doppler imaging.[151,241] Even with the Doppler echo, clinicians must be aware of the loading conditions and respiratory effort of the patient during the Doppler examination. Doppler features in CP have been more extensively reviewed.[151,156,240]

TEE is not tremendously helpful in patients presenting for pericardiectomy. When it is utilized, right ventricular function and degree of tricuspid regurgitation can be evaluated before and after the procedure. However, it is important to remember that the diagnosis of constriction relies on the Doppler findings in spontaneously breathing individuals. These findings have never been evaluated in patients undergoing positive-pressure ventilation, and the operating room is not the correct place to confirm or refute a suspected diagnosis of constriction.

The hemodynamic changes of CP are primarily related to the isolation of the cardiac chambers from respiratory effects on thoracic pressure and a fixed end-diastolic ventricular volume.[240] The pericardium limits the filling of the LV during inspiration, which leads to increased filling in the RV because the pericardium is so noncompliant. With expiration, the opposite is seen as the LV is overfilled and the RV is limited. Limitation of right ventricular diastolic filling occurs when the cardiac volume approximates the pericardial volume, usually in mid and late diastole characterized by the square-root or dip-and-plateau sign (Figure 22-39). Filling is limited by the noncompliant pericardium.

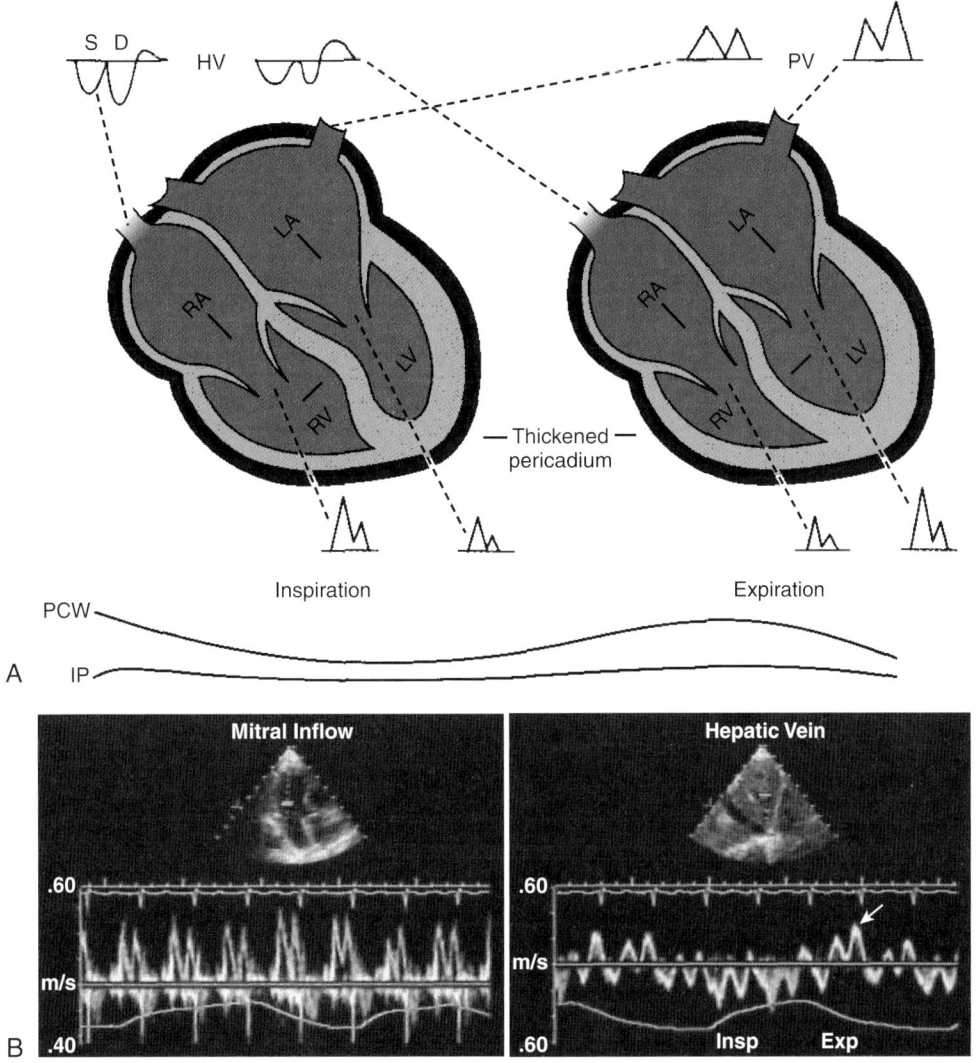

Figure 22-38 *A*, Diagram of a heart with a thickened pericardium to illustrate the respiratory variation in ventricular filling and the corresponding Doppler features of the mitral valve, tricuspid valve, pulmonary vein (PV), and hepatic vein (HV). These changes are related to discordant pressure changes in the vessels in the thorax, such as pulmonary capillary wedge pressure (PCWP) and intrapericardial (IP) and intracardiac pressures. *B*, Typical mitral inflow and hepatic vein pulsed-wave Doppler recordings in constrictive pericarditis together with simultaneous recording of respiration (bottom) (onset of inspiration at upward deflection and onset of expiration at downward deflection). *Left*, The first mitral inflow is at the onset of inspiration, and the fourth mitral inflow is soon after the onset of expiration. Mitral inflow E velocity is decreased with inspiration (first and sixth beats). *Right*, With expiration there is a marked diastolic flow reversal *(arrow)* in the hepatic vein (sixth beat soon after the downward deflection of the respirometer recording). *Hatched area under curve* indicates reversal of flow; *thicker arrows* denote greater filling; D, diastolic flow; exp, expiration; Insp, inspiration; LA, left atrium; LV, left ventricle; RA, right atrium; RV, right ventricle; S, systolic flow. *(From Oh JK, Seward JB, Tajik AJ:* The Echo Manual, *3rd ed. Philadelphia: Lippincott Williams & Wilkins, 2006, by permission.)*

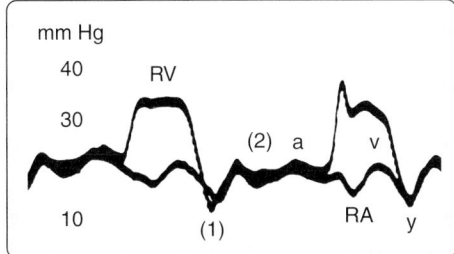

Figure 22-39 Right ventricular (RV) and right atrial (RA) pressure tracings recorded with a fluid-filled system from a patient with chronic constrictive pericarditis. *(From Shabetai R: Pathophysiology and differential diagnosis of restrictive cardiomyopathy.* Cardiovasc Clin *19:123, 1988, by permission.)*

The square-root sign occurs because the constricting pericardium is essentially part of the ventricular wall. When the ventricle contracts, the pericardium is deformed like a spring. As diastole begins, the spring is released and the ventricle fills rapidly, decreasing the ventricular pressure and creating the dip of the dip-and-plateau wave. As cardiac filling approaches the limit set by the fixed pericardium, the plateau of the ventricular filling curve arrives. There are marked increases of right atrial and left atrial and ventricular filling pressures. Pulmonary artery diastolic pressure, pulmonary capillary wedge pressure, and right atrial pressure are equal and elevated ("pressure plateau") in CP because of the limitation of the pericardium. Pulmonary artery systolic and right ventricular systolic pressures range from 35 to 45 mm Hg, although PAH is rare. Most importantly, the myocardium is unaffected in CP. The systolic and early diastolic functions are normal. Differences between CP and RCM have been reviewed previously.

Pericardiectomy is performed for recurrent pericardial effusion and CP. Pericardial dissection for effusive pericarditis is straightforward; however, pericardiectomy for CP is a surgical challenge with an operative mortality rate of 5.9% to 11.9%.[244] The 5-year survival rate is 78%.[157,245] The occurrence of tricuspid regurgitation may present similar to CP with signs of right-heart failure and volume overload. In fact, a recent review found one fifth of patients presenting to surgery for CP with significant tricuspid regurgitation.[244] Unfortunately, surgical treatment of tricuspid regurgitation with CP had no effect on long-term survival, but also did not increase the risk for surgery. The presence of tricuspid regurgitation may identify a subset of patients with CP who have more advanced disease and may need special attention during anesthetic management.

Persistent low CO immediately after pericardiectomy is the primary cause of morbidity and mortality, occurring in 14% to 28% of patients in the immediate postoperative period.[246] The pathophysiologic mechanism of early death after pericardiectomy remains unsolved. Examination of patients who had pericardiectomy for CP with preoperative cardiac catheterization utilizing a micromanometer catheter was performed recently.[246] The specialized catheter allowed nonejection indices of cardiac function to be obtained. The study compared patients with abnormalities with those with normal nonejection measurements. The most important finding was that a significant number of patients with CP had abnormal left ventricular contractility and relaxation abnormalities based on a high-fidelity manometer. More importantly, they incurred the greatest risk for operative and long-term mortality. This finding is in contrast with the accepted notion that the pericardium is the problem in these patients and the LV should be normal. Myocardial function is important as a determinant of outcome and even inotropic support. This is consistent with the clinical behavior of patients after pericardiectomy. Although patients with cardiac tamponade usually improve clinically once the pericardium is opened, improvement is not always apparent immediately after pericardiectomy. Instead, noticeable improvement in cardiac function may take weeks, but 90% of patients ultimately experience relief of symptoms with surgery.[239]

Median sternotomy provides excellent exposure and access for pericardiectomy, but thoracotomy in the left anterolateral position also is an option. Opinions vary regarding the extent of pericardial resection for alleviation of cardiac constriction and the need for CPB. Recently, total pericardiectomy was found to result in superior outcomes compared with partial pericardiectomy in a retrospective review.[247] Removal of adherent and scarred pericardium to release both the RV and LV involves extensive manipulation of the heart and hemodynamic instability. The decision to use CPB is influenced by the surgeon's confidence in being able to achieve complete pericardial excision with hemodynamic stability. More aggressive approaches to pericardiectomy with CPB have increased over the years as survival has improved, and the trend may continue.[244] However, good results have been reported with and without CPB.[247] The use of CPB entails full heparinization and may exacerbate blood loss from the many exposed cardiac surfaces. Furthermore, prolonged CPB in debilitated patients contributes to early mortality associated with pericardiectomy. An especially high-risk group of patients undergoing pericardiectomy are those with postradiation CP. They suffer not only from the effects of radiation on the myocardium that may create a more sustained restrictive effect even after pericardiectomy, but also from radiation injury to the lungs.[244]

Anesthetic Considerations

Anesthetic goals for managing patients with CP for pericardiectomy include minimizing bradycardia and myocardial depression, and minimizing decreases in afterload or preload. Monitoring considerations include arterial and central venous pressures. A femoral arterial catheter in patients with uremic pericarditis may preserve future potential arteriovenous fistula sites in the upper extremities. One groin site should be reserved for femoral cannulation if necessary to emergently initiate CPB. PAC monitoring is recommended because of the occurrence of low CO syndrome after surgery. Low CO syndrome develops in a subset of patients with CP irrespective of the approach or extent of pericardiectomy.[247] Low CO, hypotension, and arrhythmias (atrial and ventricular) are common during chest dissection. Because of limited ventricular diastolic filling, CO is rate dependent. If myocardial function or heart rate is depressed, β-agonists or pacing will improve CO. Catastrophic hemorrhage can occur suddenly if the atrium or ventricle is perforated, so sufficient venous access is imperative. Damage to coronary arteries also may occur during dissection, so careful monitoring of the ECG for signs of ischemia is prudent. Pericardiectomy via left anterior thoracotomy requires close monitoring of oxygenation because the left lung is severely compressed during dissection. Currently, the anesthetic technique is based on achieving early extubation similar to other cardiac surgical cases; however, patients who undergo pericardiectomy for CP may benefit from remaining intubated for at least 6 to 12 hours to assess bleeding and the possibility of low CO syndrome occurring.

▣ Cardiac Tamponade

Cardiac tamponade occurs in a variety of clinical situations, but most often in malignancies with medical patients and after pericardiocentesis.[248] It is a continuum of physiologic changes that necessitate rapid diagnosis and treatment. It may be easily missed in the early stages as the signs and symptoms are subtle until it is critical. Decompensated cardiac tamponade is an emergency that requires either immediate pericardiocentesis or surgery to maintain viability.

Tamponade exists when fluid accumulation in the pericardial sac increases to an intrapericardial pressure that limits filling of the heart. The rate of fluid accumulation is the critical factor rather than the absolute volume of fluid that creates the urgency of the condition. The suspicion for cardiac tamponade must exist to increase the chance for a good outcome. Mild tamponade often is asymptomatic. One of the reasons for greater delay in the appreciation of tamponade today than 10 years ago is the tendency of clinicians to overestimate the sensitivity of clinical signs such as hypotension, pulsus paradoxus, and jugular venous distention.[249] In several studies, dyspnea is the earliest and most sensitive symptom to indicate tamponade,[249] and severe tamponade is accompanied by both dyspnea and chest discomfort.[234] If an ECG is obtained, tamponade may show low-voltage QRS complexes, electrical alternans, and T-wave abnormalities (Figure 22-40).[250] Sinus rhythm usually is present in tamponade. The chest roentgenogram requires at least 200 mL fluid to accumulate in the pericardium before the silhouette, known as the "water-bottle" effect, is seen.[251] The classic diagnostic triad, known as Beck's triad, of acute tamponade consists of (1) decreasing arterial pressure; (2) increasing venous pressure; and (3) a small, quiet heart. It is observed in only 10% to 40% of patients.[251] Pulsus paradoxus may be present (Figure 22-41). It is a decline in systolic blood pressure of more than 12 mm Hg during inspiration caused by a reduced left ventricular stroke volume generated by increased filling of the right heart during inspiration. It is not sensitive or specific for tamponade because it may be present in those with obstructive pulmonary disease, right ventricular infarction, or CP. It may be absent if there is left ventricular dysfunction, positive-pressure breathing, atrial septal defect, or severe aortic regurgitation.

Hemodynamic monitoring may aid in the diagnosis of cardiac tamponade. As diastolic filling begins to disappear, the jugular venous pulse loses a prominent y descent. A prominent x descent remains by the decrease in intrapericardial pressure that occurs during ventricular ejection. Eventually, the pericardial pressure-volume curve becomes almost vertical, so any additional fluid greatly restricts cardiac filling and reduces diastolic compliance.[252] Ultimately, the right atrial pressure, pulmonary artery diastolic pressure, and pulmonary capillary wedge pressure equilibrate (Figure 22-42). Equilibration of these pressures (within 5 mm Hg of each other) merits immediate action to rule out acute tamponade. Echo is the current method of choice and most reliable noninvasive method to detect pericardial effusion and exclude tamponade.

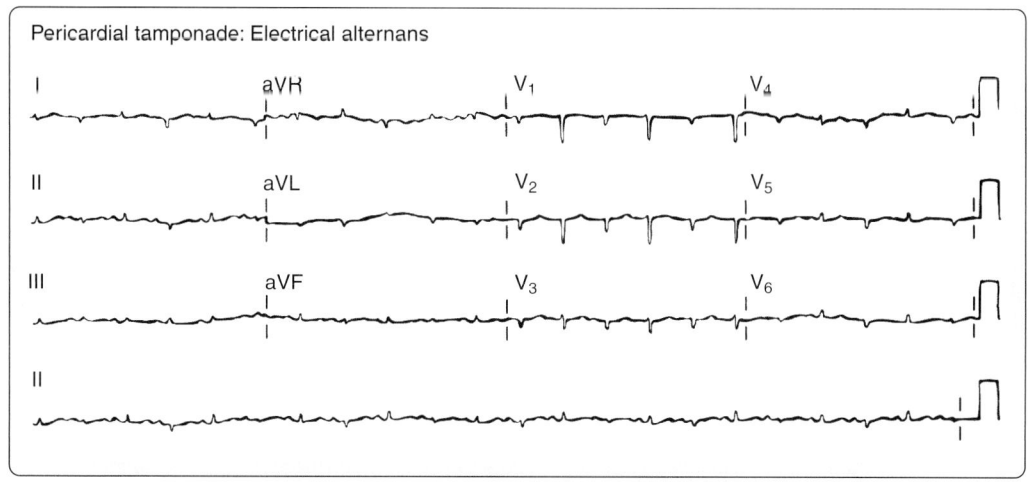

Figure 22-40 Electrical alternans in pericardial tamponade caused by the swinging of the heart within the pericardial space. *(From Aikat S, Ghaffari S: A review of pericardial diseases: Clinical, ECG and hemodynamic features and management.* Cleve Clin J Med *67:909, 2000, by permission; originally modified from Longo MJ, Jaffe CC: Images in clinical medicine electrical alternans.* N Engl J Med *341:2060, 1999, by permission.)*

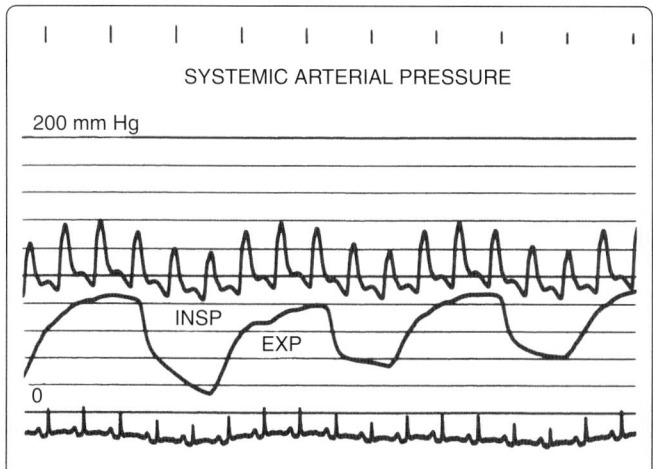

Figure 22-41 **Pulsus paradoxus.** During inspiration, arterial systolic pressure declines by more than 12 mm Hg. EXP, expiration; INSP, inspiration. *(From Reddy PS, Curtiss EI: Cardiac tamponade.* Cardiol Clin *8:627–637, 1990, by permission.)*

The major hemodynamic changes and compensatory mechanisms of tamponade are outlined in Figure 22-43. Increased intrapericardial pressure on the heart during the cardiac cycle except for ejection is responsible for the hemodynamic changes of cardiac tamponade. Hemodynamic manifestations are due mainly to atrial rather than ventricular compression. Initially, with mild tamponade, increased atrial and pericardial pressures limit diastolic filling. Even though the intracardiac pressures are increased with tamponade, the effective preload is greatly reduced, causing lower stroke volume and CO. Sympathetic reflexes are stimulated to increase heart rate and contractility to maintain CO.[241] The increasing right atrial pressure also reflexly stimulates tachycardia and peripheral vasoconstriction. Blood pressure is maintained by vasoconstriction, but CO begins to decline, as well as blood pressure, as pericardial fluid continues to increase. Once venous pressures are unable to increase to equal pericardial pressures, the decline in blood pressure is so precipitous that coronary perfusion pressure and blood flow cause ischemia, especially subendocardially.[252] This resembles hypovolemic shock and will respond to fluid resuscitation, initially further confusing the diagnosis, but deterioration will soon occur if tamponade is not treated and can become fatal.[234]

Echo features of tamponade have been reviewed.[241] Echo usually reveals an exaggerated motion of the heart within the pericardial sac

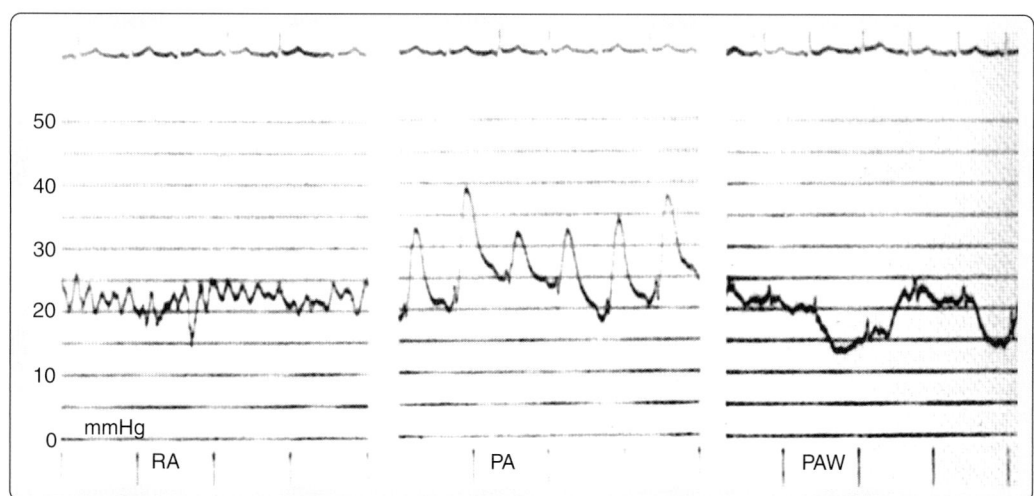

Figure 22-42 **Hemodynamic changes in cardiac tamponade.** Equilibration of right atrial (RA), pulmonary artery (PA) diastolic, and pulmonary artery wedge (PAW) pressures is demonstrated. *(From Temkin LP, Ewy GA: Cardiac catheterization. In Conahan TJ III [ed]: Cardiac Anesthesia.* Menlo Park, CA, 1982, Addison-Wesley, p 1.)*

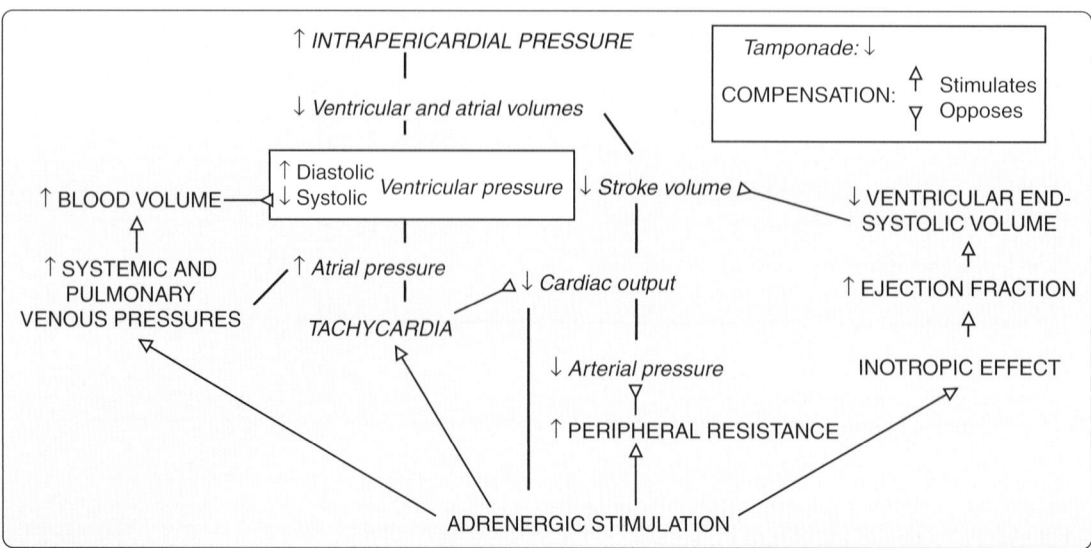

Figure 22-43 Cardiac tamponade. Relations among major hemodynamic events and major compensatory mechanisms. *Simple arrows* represent tamponade sequences; *pointed arrowheads* represent stimulatory compensatory action; *blunt arrowheads* represent oppositional compensatory actions. *(From Spokick DH: Pathophysiology of cardiac tamponade. Chest 113:1374, 1998, by permission; originally modified from Spodick DH: In: Spodick DH [ed]: The Pericardium: a Comprehensive Textbook. New York, 1997, Dekker, p 182.)*

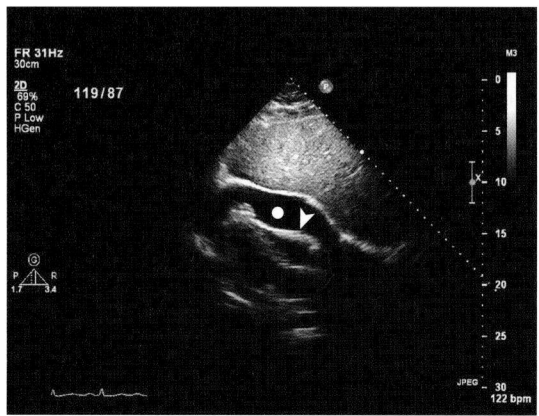

Figure 22-44 Cardiac tamponade. A subcostal transthoracic view with the liver seen at the apex of the image. The large echolucent space seen in the pericardium *(white dot)* is acute accumulation of fluid. Note the collapse of the right side of the heart *(arrowhead)* during diastole. This patient underwent urgent pericardiocentesis under the guidance of echocardiography.

in conjunction with atrial and ventricular collapse (Figure 22–44). Fluid accumulation greater than 25 mL will identify an echo-free space throughout the cardiac cycle.[33] Specific 2D echo findings that support cardiac tamponade include diastolic collapse of the RV, inversion of the RA during diastole, abnormal ventricular septal motion, and variation of ventricular size with the respiratory cycle.[253] Diastolic collapse of the right-sided chambers occurs because of pericardial pressure exceeding intracardiac pressure during diastole. Right atrial collapse is a specific finding during echo examination if it is present for more than one third of the cardiac cycle.

Normally, a decrease in intrathoracic pressure during inspiration is transmitted to the pulmonary vasculature, as well as the intrapericardial and intracardiac spaces. In tamponade, this decrease in pressure during inspiration does not occur within the pericardium because of the presence of fluid. Thus, the gradient for left-sided filling is decreased and the mitral inflow E velocity will decrease with inspiration. In addition, right and left ventricular filling display interdependence similar to that seen in pericardial constriction.

Bedside echo can be used to direct needle or catheter placement for pericardiocentesis. Indeed, in some centers, the bulk of pericardiocentesis is performed under echo guidance.[254] Removal of no more than 50 mL fluid may be therapeutic for severe tamponade because of the steepness of the pericardial pressure-volume curve. Typically, a pigtail catheter is left in the pericardial space for several days until drainage becomes minimal. Tamponade is a clinical diagnosis, so echo alone is not an indication for treatment. Failure to recognize the insidious nature of tamponade and anticipate the progression of hemodynamic changes may lead to delay in using echo to confirm the diagnosis and begin treatment. Examples include unstable hemodynamics that accompany a penetrating chest injury or an abrupt decrease in bleeding after cardiac surgery; both require rapid confirmation of tamponade and possibly emergency sternal opening.

Hemorrhagic tamponade in excessively bleeding patients after CPB is increasingly common and may be fatal. Depending on the diagnostic techniques, cardiac tamponade occurs in up to 8.8% of patients after cardiac surgery. However, almost 75% of postcardiac surgical tamponade occurs late (5 to 7 days), especially with patients who have undergone valve procedures in contrast with CABG.[255] The causes of early tamponade are attributed primarily to coagulopathy secondary to CPB, whereas the causes of late tamponade are multifactorial, with aspirin and anticoagulants increasing the risk for bleeding.[255] Persistent poor CO and hypotension with increased and equalized right atrial and left atrial pressures strongly suggest tamponade. However, the multitude of causes of hypotension in the postoperative cardiac surgical patient complicates the diagnosis of tamponade. The classic features of tamponade may be absent or blunted after surgery.[256] Arterial hypotension, pulsus paradoxus, and increased jugular venous pressures were absent in 30%, 40%, and 50%, respectively, in one series of cardiac surgical patients.[257] A delay in diagnosis contributes greatly to mortality in late cardiac tamponade.

With postoperative cardiac surgical patients, no one finding, hemodynamic, clinical, or echo, is sufficient to make a diagnosis of tamponade, but all require consideration together.[258] Although echo is capable of identifying the size of pericardial effusions after surgery, it does not necessarily reflect its likelihood to cause tamponade. Most patients after cardiac surgery will have evidence of pericardial effusions, but less than 1% will develop hemodynamically significant tamponade.[255] TTE may be unable to provide a complete examination in the postoperative cardiac surgical patient because of interference of chest tubes, patient positioning, and other factors, so TEE may be more effective. TTE may have 20% false-negatives compared with TEE, in part because of the formation of clot and thrombus in the pericardium that is difficult to differentiate with TTE but not TEE.

Pericardiocentesis is indicated for life threatening cardiac tamponade in conjunction with a fluid infusion to maintain filling pressures. Hemodynamics will improve immediately after pericardiocentesis. Although it does provide immediate relief of the symptoms of tamponade, definitive therapy requires drainage of the pericardial space. In contrast, after cardiac surgery, tamponade caused by hemorrhage requires immediate mediastinal exploration to determine bleeding site and stabilize hemodynamics. Major complications of pericardiocentesis include coronary laceration, cardiac puncture, and pneumothorax.

Anesthetic Considerations

Severe hypotension or cardiac arrest has followed induction of general anesthesia in patients with tamponade. The causes include additional myocardial depression, sympatholysis, decreased venous return, and changes in heart rate. Resuscitation requires immediate drainage of pericardial fluid. Pericardiotomy via a subxiphoid incision with only local anesthetic infiltration or light sedation is an option. If intrapericardial injury is confirmed, general anesthesia can be induced after decompression of the pericardial space.[259] Ketamine, 0.5 mg/kg, and 100% oxygen have been used with local anesthetic infiltration of the preexisting sternotomy to drain severe pericardial tamponade.[260] Spontaneous respiration instead of positive-pressure ventilation will support CO more effectively until tamponade is relieved. Correction of metabolic acidosis is mandatory. Volume expansion has been recommended for years and even recently, until more definitive treatment is available, but this is only evident in dogs.[261] A prospective study of patients with "medical" causes of cardiac tamponade had their hemodynamic response to a 500-mL bolus studied.[262] They found that volume infusion was not consistently associated with improved hemodynamics and should be directed toward patients with low blood pressure to achieve a favorable response. Catecholamine infusions or pacing may be used to avoid bradycardia. In a dog model of pericardial tamponade, dobutamine infusion delayed the onset of lactic acidosis by maintaining CO and tissue oxygen delivery.[263]

Case Study 3

Tamponade

A 65-year-old man with a history of chronic venous insufficiency was hospitalized for a venous stasis ulcer that ultimately required skin grafting. On the day of his planned discharge, he was found to have multiple pulmonary emboli and a large lower extremity deep venous thrombosis.

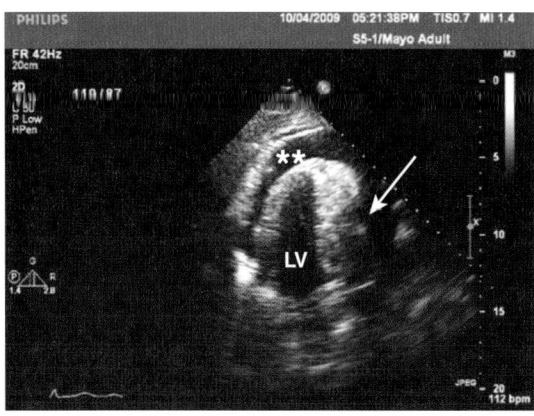

Figure 22-45 Transthoracic echocardiogram in parasternal four-chamber view. There is a large echo-lucency in the pericardium (double asterisk) indicating a large pericardial effusion. The right side of the heart completely collapses in diastole (arrow), indicating hemodynamically significant tamponade physiology. LV, left ventricle.

Anticoagulation was initiated, a filter was placed in the inferior vena cava, and lower extremity venous catheters were placed for catheter-directed thrombolytic therapy. Two days later, mechanical extraction of the lower extremity thrombus was undertaken without any known complications.

When he returned to his hospital room after the thrombus extraction, the patient quickly became hemodynamically unstable. He received fluid boluses and required intubation and mechanical ventilation for respiratory distress. Ultimately, he required a short period of CPR and epinephrine boluses. An emergent TTE revealed a large pericardial effusion (Figure 22-45).

Because of the urgency of the situation, a bedside pericardiocentesis was undertaken using echo guidance (Figure 22-46). A large amount of blood was removed from the pericardium and the effusion appeared to resolve (Figure 22-47). The patient's hemodynamics rapidly improved. He required a period of mechanical ventilation but was ultimately discharged from the hospital in good condition.

COMBINED CAROTID AND CORONARY ARTERY DISEASE

Patients with concomitant symptomatic coronary and carotid disease are few, but they comprise a much higher risk group than either group of patients with carotid or coronary disease alone.[264-266] CABG is proven

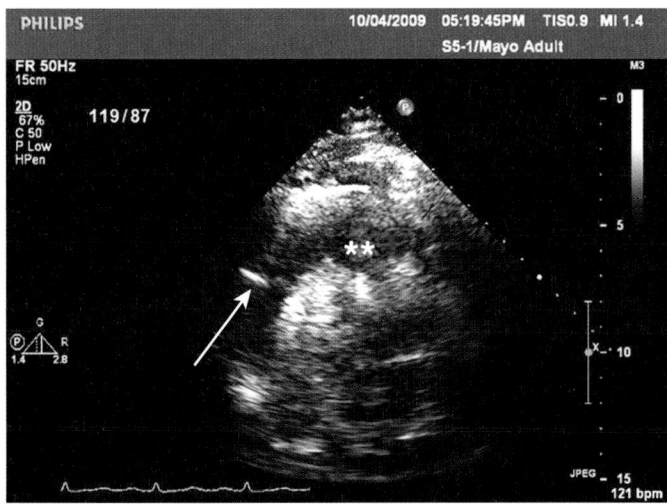
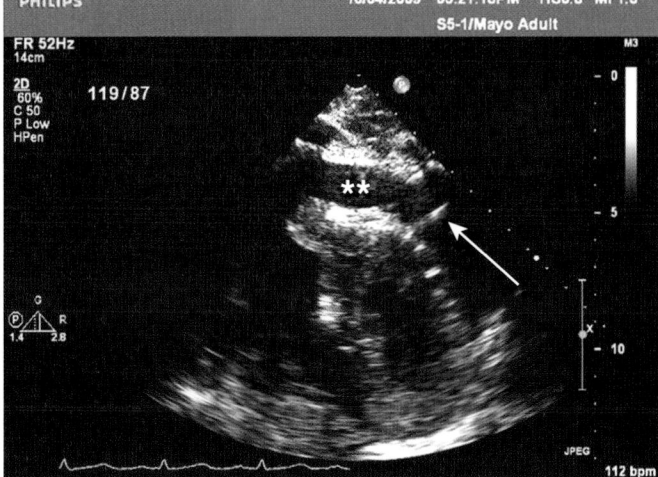

Figure 22-46   Two transthoracic echocardiograms; short-axis views of the heart showing a needle (arrows) advanced into the pericardial space (double asterisks) under echocardiographic guidance.

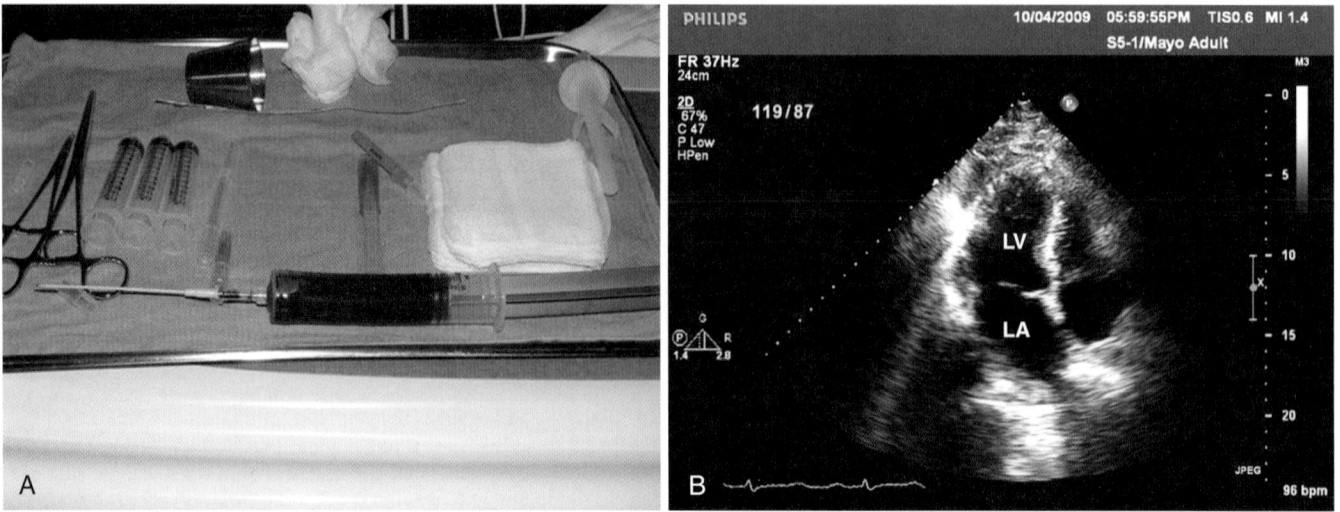

Figure 22-47 *A*, Photograph of the catheter and syringe used for the pericardiocentesis. *B*, Transthoracic echocardiogram; parasternal four-chamber view showing resolution of the pericardial effusion. The right side of the heart is now well filled in diastole. LA, left atrium; LV, left ventricle.

therapy for ischemic heart disease.[267] Advancements in myocardial preservation, CPB technology, and perioperative care over the last three decades have reduced morbidity and mortality associated with cardiac surgery. However, stroke remains the major noncardiac complication of CABG, impacting quality of life, economic well-being, and survival. Although the overall incidence of stroke associated with CABG is approximately 2%, the role of extracranial carotid disease in the occurrence of stroke remains indeterminate.

The combination of carotid endarterectomy (CEA) and CABG was first proposed by Bernhard et al[268] in 1972 to reduce morbidity and mortality from coexistent carotid and coronary disease. Renewed interest in this approach now stems from recent controlled trials that demonstrated the benefits of isolated CEA for both symptomatic and asymptomatic severe carotid stenosis.[269] During the time period from 2000 to the end of 2004, there were 27,084 combined CEA and CABG procedures performed according to the Nationwide Inpatient Sample database.[270] According to the same database, the proportion of combined CABG and CEA increased from 1.1% to 1.58% of all CABG performed from 1993 to 2002.[271] As the population ages, the number of patients with carotid bifurcation stenosis greater than 70% will continue to increase. The result is more patients with combined carotid and coronary disease,[269] but no consensus regarding their treatment. A large, multicenter, randomized trial will be necessary to resolve the management of these patients. Unfortunately, the complexities of such a study with the heterogeneity of patients, varying degrees of coronary and carotid disease, and differing institutional preferences for carotid revascularization decrease its likelihood.

Neurologic injury associated with CPB largely is embolic in origin,[272] causing cerebral hypoperfusion and ischemia. Emboli originate primarily from aortic cannulation, aortic cross-clamp release, and cardiac manipulation based on transcranial Doppler ultrasonography. Less common causes of cerebral emboli are left ventricular thrombus and air. However, the cause of stroke after CABG is multifactorial. Univariate analysis of systematic review of stroke associated with CABG has identified the following risk factors for stroke: carotid stenosis of 80% or more, carotid occlusion, prior stroke or transient ischemic attack, peripheral vascular disease, postinfarction angina, female sex, prolonged duration of CPB, age (older), previous CEA, diabetes, smoking, hypertension, left main disease, and carotid bruit.[273–275] Carotid bruits may be present in 9.93% of patients undergoing CABG and increase the risk for stroke by a factor of four. Differentiating significant stenosis by auscultation is unreliable.[276] Carotid bruits may be audible with minimal carotid stenosis and silent with a carotid lumen of 1 to 2 mm in diameter. The combination of ultrasonography of the

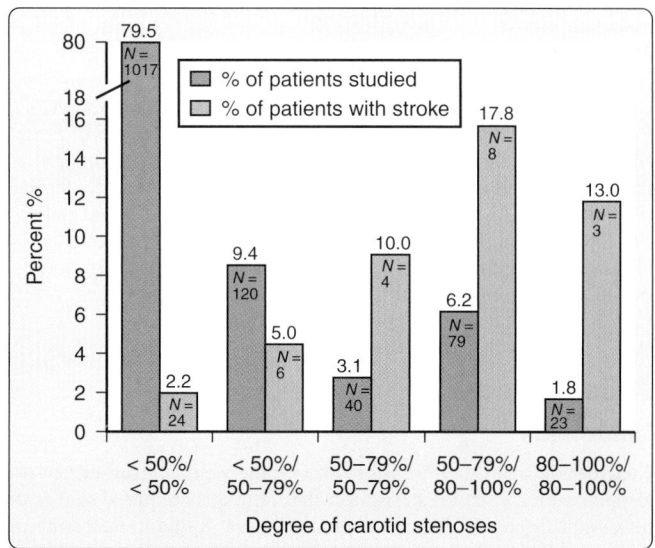

Figure 22-48 Prevalence of carotid stenoses in patients undergoing noninvasive carotid screening and occurrence of stroke by degree of carotid stenosis. *(From D'Agostino RS, Svensson, Neumann DJ, et al: Screening carotid ultrasonography and risk factors for stroke in coronary artery surgery patients. Ann Thoracic Surg 62:1714–1723, 1996, by permission.)*

carotid arteries and risk factors is very predictive of patients likely to have a stroke in association with CABG (Figure 22-48).

Carotid artery disease should be considered in all individuals with ischemic heart disease. Severe carotid disease increases the risk for stroke with CABG by a factor of four.[273] Early estimates of the incidence of hemodynamically significant carotid stenosis in patients needing CABG varied between 2% and 16%.[277] Faggioli et al[278] confirmed the occurrence of severe carotid disease, defined as carotid stenosis greater than 75%, in patients older than 60 years, to be 11% in patients who underwent CABG. More recently, noninvasive ultrasonography has shown the percentage of persons with severe carotid and coronary disease to be greater than in prior studies.[275] Patients undergoing CABG were prospectively evaluated for carotid disease with ultrasonography, and approximately 20% had significant carotid stenosis unilaterally or bilaterally. Large systematic reviews of stroke and CABG point to a relation between an increased incidence of stroke with higher degree of carotid stenosis.[273,279] The frequency of stroke with cardiac surgery was less than 2% in those with no carotid disease (0% to 49% stenosis), increased to 3% with asymptomatic disease (unilateral stenosis 50% to 99%), 5% in those with bilateral stenosis (50% to 99%), and 7% to 11% in those with carotid occlusion. These data would support the potential benefit of CEA in either a staged or combined manner with CABG to reduce the chance of stroke in these patients.

It generally is accepted that patients with symptomatic carotid disease undergoing CABG are at a significantly increased risk for stroke and merit revascularization of the carotid and coronary arteries as a combined or staged procedure.[275] However, the management of unilateral or bilateral *asymptomatic* carotid stenosis continues to evolve. Asymptomatic severe carotid stenosis is a risk for ipsilateral hemispheric stroke with cardiac surgery and CPB,[266,275,280] but identifying it in the asymptomatic patient hinders determination of this "true" risk assessment. This is important because, recently, isolated CEA was shown to reduce risk for stroke not only in patients with symptomatic carotid stenosis greater than 70%,[271] but also in asymptomatic patients with severe high-grade carotid stenosis.[269] With the incidence of neurologic injury ipsilateral to the carotid artery comprising 40% to 50% of strokes associated with cardiac surgery,[281] prophylactic measures to prevent strokes merit consideration.[270]

In most patients, the degree of either carotid or coronary disease will not limit the ability of the patient to undergo the higher priority operation, CEA or CABG, safely. In contrast, treatment options for those with active concomitant carotid disease and ischemic heart disease are a combined, synchronous, or staged approach. The staged approach does not include CEA and CABG in one anesthetic but two separate ones. Many surgeons support the combined CABG and CEA, whereas others believe the risk exceeds the benefit.[279,282]

The sequence of CEA and CABG is important regarding the outcome with either the combined or staged approach. In 1989, Hertzer et al[264] found a lower incidence of stroke if CEA was performed before rather than after CABG as a combined approach in one of the few randomized, prospective trials involving this issue. Since then, CEA commonly has been performed first. Rizzo et al[266] confirmed the benefit of performing CEA before CABG by reporting the risk for stroke may reach 14% if CABG is performed before CEA. More recently, a systematic review of synchronous and staged CEA and CABG operations demonstrated that reverse-staged procedures (CABG–CEA) were associated with the greatest ipsilateral and global stroke rate compared with staged or combined procedures performed with the CEA first.[279] Less than 10% of staged operations currently are performed as CABG – CEA.

The sequence of performing CEA – CABG is more common than the reverse order but is not without disadvantages. Myocardial morbidity may reach 20% if CEA is performed before CABG in a staged approach.[266] MI has been recognized for years as the major cause of mortality with isolated CEA. Surgically uncorrectable coronary disease may exist in 40% of those undergoing CEA.[277] CEA in patients with severe, symptomatic coronary disease has been associated with a 17% and 20% incidence rate of MI and mortality, respectively. Most importantly, 20% of the MIs accounted for 60% of deaths.[274] A recent systematic literature review of combined and staged CEA – CABG confirmed that the incidence of MI was greatest if the CEA performed before the CABG (6.5%) rather than after CABG (0.9%).[279] Differences in standards for reporting MI since the 1980s challenge the accuracy of the incidence of MI after CEA being 6.5%. Without well-defined cardiovascular risks for either the staged or combined approach, the correct decision for the patient is difficult.

The recommendation to perform a combined or staged CEA and CABG for those with concomitant carotid and coronary disease continues to evolve. In a prospective trial, Hertzer et al[264] found a lower incidence of perioperative stroke with combined rather than staged CABG and CEA. A comparative analysis of studies that included 50 patients or more who underwent CABG with unoperated major carotid disease found the risk for stroke averaged 5.5% for patients with unoperated carotid disease and CABG versus 3.1% for patients who underwent combined procedures. However, the role of carotid disease as a direct cause of perioperative stroke after isolated CABG is not always clear. It is relatively simple to diagnose the likely cause of a perioperative stroke associated with isolated CEA.

Individual studies involving concomitant carotid and coronary disease suffer from great variation in the definition of a stroke, selection bias, patient demographics, and surgical techniques that limit the widespread application of study recommendations. To make up for these deficiencies, large, systematic reviews of the studies have attempted to provide insight into the optimal practice for concomitant carotid and coronary artery disease. Recently, a review found no advantage in outcomes for staged or combined procedures.[279] Staged procedures had lower rates of stroke (2.7% vs. 4.6%) and death but were not statistically significant. Others have found combined surgery not only unnecessary but also potentially detrimental. Gerraty et al[282] prospectively studied a series of 358 patients undergoing peripheral vascular procedures or CABG who underwent ultrasonography before surgery. If the carotid stenosis was asymptomatic, the risk for stroke was so low that it did not merit prophylactic CEA. An audit of one institution's last 5 years with combined CEA-CABG for asymptomatic carotid stenosis (> 50%) found no perioperative strokes at 30 days after surgery in the 61 patients who had unilateral stenosis that were not revascularized. This led to an institutional halt to the performance of combined procedures.[281] Unfortunately, their studies can do no more than challenge the hypothesis that a combined or staged CEA-CABG will reduce the risk for stroke in asymptomatic, unilateral carotid disease.

A major concern for those who do not support the combined or staged approach for carotid and coronary disease is that some data demonstrate a stroke rate for combined CEA and CABG of approximately twice the stroke rate of each operation alone.[266] Safety of the combined CEA-CABG recently was evaluated in 277 patients (3.34%) with carotid stenosis greater than 70% unilaterally or bilaterally that underwent some form of combined CEA and CABG compared with a control of 8000 isolated CABGs.[283] There was no statistical difference in the mortality or incidence of stroke in those undergoing combined procedures compared with those undergoing CABG alone. The increased risk for stroke or even death found in some studies regarding combined CEA-CABG may be related to the overall severity of the atherosclerotic disease and likelihood of embolic plaque in the aorta in this particular population of patients. Ricotta et al[265] were able to define a stroke model through multivariate logistic regression analysis in patients undergoing CABG without carotid stenosis greater than 80%. The risk factors for stroke were age, CPB duration, aortoiliac disease, ECG evidence of left ventricular hypertrophy, and an extensively calcified aorta. Examination of patients who underwent combined CEA-CABG found them to have three of the four risk factors for postoperative stroke. Although the stroke rate for the combined group was 3.9% compared with 1.7% for control, it was not different from the expected stroke risk based on the inherent risk factors of the patients. It could be concluded that patients with combined disease are at greater risk for stroke not caused by the combination of CEA and CABG but from the individual preoperative risk factors. The high-grade carotid disease may be a marker for greater cardiovascular morbidity in these patients and less related directly to the carotid disease.

The risk for mortality and morbidity associated with combined CEA-CABG procedure also was compared with patients undergoing isolated CABG in New York State for control.[269] Surprisingly, once propensity scores could be matched between isolated CABG and combined CEA-CABG, no significant differences were found in occurrence of stroke, MI, or death between combined and isolated CABG. Another important factor in looking at patients for combined procedures is that, although as a group the mortality may be greater in the combined compared with isolated CABG, the risks for combined patients vary greatly within their own group.[283] In a comparison of isolated CABG with combined procedures, the stroke, mortality, and MI rates were very low in patients who had either unilateral or bilateral carotid stenosis, but those with previous stroke and more advanced age or contralateral internal carotid artery occlusion were at significantly greater risk for stroke, mortality, and MI compared with the other patients undergoing combined procedures. In conclusion, the intrinsic risk factors of patients who undergo combined procedures contribute more to postoperative stroke than the addition of CEA. The important issue is that the data indicate that combined procedures can be safely performed without increases in complications because of the combination of procedures.

The use of carotid artery stenting (CAS) has gained popularity in recent years as a substitute for CEA in a staged approach but currently represents only a small part of prophylactic carotid revascularization (3.3%) compared with CEA for patients scheduled for CABG.[270] In a comparison with combined CEA-CABG using a Nationwide Inpatient Sample database including 5 years of patients, the postoperative stroke rate for CAS-CABG was significantly less (2.4%) compared with CEA-CABG (3.9%; $P < 0.001$), but no difference in the incidence of death was found. It was significant that symptomatic patients undergoing both prophylactic procedures before cardiac surgery instead reported a fivefold increase in stroke associated with CAS-CABG versus CEA-CABG. When CAS was used as the only form of prophylactic treatment of carotid stenosis before CABG in 52 patients in a staged manner, the combination of minor stroke, major stroke, and death rate for this study was 19.2%.[284] Increased stroke rates with CAS-CABG may be because of inadequate anticoagulation without clopidogrel to minimize postoperative bleeding after CABG. CAS-CABG has been performed with acceptable stroke and death rates if the patient is neurologically asymptomatic; however, Timaran et al[270] found a fivefold increase in the risk for CAS with CABG compared with CEA for neurologically symptomatic patients.

A benefit of CAS is that myocardial events may occur less frequently than with CEA, perhaps because CAS can be performed with conscious sedation and is less invasive. A serious disadvantage with CAS is the need for multiple antiplatelet therapy and occasional hemodynamic depression associated with CAS that may limit its role in those with unstable coronary artery disease. Complications from stenting can be as high as 5.7%, and the delay in CABG may be responsible for deaths that occurred, so more frequent future use of CAS may depend on additional studies. It may be that CAS-CABG necessarily will be less risky if performed as a staged procedure instead of a combined one.

Anesthetic Considerations

Anesthetic management of patients with carotid and coronary disease must provide optimal conditions for the brain and myocardium. Beyond the routine monitoring for cardiac surgery, electroencephalography or other modalities to assess neurophysiologic integrity are useful but have a high false-positive rate. For the anesthesiologist, it is helpful to know that the majority of strokes cannot be ascribed to an adverse intraoperative event such as hypotension or low flow.[273] However, it is more difficult to differentiate a "true" stroke from other states of temporary neurologic impairment associated with CABG such as heavy sedation, residual muscle weakness from a paralyzing agent, or encephalopathy secondary to cerebral edema. By using general anesthesia for CEA, clinical methods to determine neurologic integrity, as well as treatment, are delayed. In contrast, use of mild sedation with local anesthesia for CEA has proved to be a more reliable means to detect intraluminal shunting during CEA than other measures of neurologic testing.[285] The sensitivity and specificity of CEA with local anesthesia to detect neurologic deficit have been established. The use of local anesthetic for CEA in the combined procedure has proved to be valuable in reducing exposure to anesthesia and reduction of shunt-related complications, allowing repair with less risk for damage.[286] The use of local anesthesia for the CEA instead of one continuous general anesthetic has become more popular in recent years. The added ability to identify the timing of the neurologic insult may prove valuable compared with general anesthesia. This is especially true because the neurologic examination in the conscious patient is more reliable than other methods such as stump pressure and electroencephalogram. However, anxiety and pain must be controlled to minimize myocardial ischemia during CEA with local anesthesia.

Mean arterial pressure should be maintained in the middle-to-upper-normal range without large increases in afterload or heart rate. Normocapnia is recommended. Techniques often used during anesthesia for cerebral protection such as barbiturates, inhalation anesthetics, benzodiazepines, or propofol to decrease cerebral metabolic rate have not been proved beneficial in clinical trials. Attempts to provide cerebral protection should not be used at the expense of myocardial perfusion and function. Usually, if the CEA is performed before CABG, the site of the CEA will be left open until cardiac surgery is completed to ensure that bleeding at the site of the CEA is minimal.

Early extubation is desirable to allow earlier neurologic evaluation in combined cases. Fast-track anesthetic management to achieve early extubation is routine. Prompt tracheal extubation after cardiac surgery with CPB may be accomplished with various anesthetic agents. Shorter-acting opioids have been characterized as achieving more rapid extubation than fentanyl.[287] However, Engoren et al[288] found no difference in the time to extubation with sufentanil or remifentanil compared with fentanyl, with the median time to extubation of 4.75, 3.90, and 2.78 hours, respectively. The combination of remifentanil and propofol was associated with mean extubation times of 163 minutes after arrival in the ICU.[289]

Extubation in the operating room is possible with high-thoracic epidural,[290] but early risks for hypothermia, bleeding, and hemodynamic instability may outweigh any benefit of prompt neurologic examination. Furthermore, the need for rapid institution of CPB during an awake CEA may prove challenging. Another possibility is the use of general anesthesia for the CEA followed by a wake-up test.[291] This would allow evaluation and treatment of any apparent neurologic injury before initiation of CPB. This approach may be more feasible in the lower risk CABG patient who is less likely to have more labile hemodynamics on waking. Aggressive vasoactive management frequently is required to treat hypertension and tachycardia resulting from reduced opioids. Shorter-acting muscle relaxants than pancuronium also have been considered to shorten duration of intubation; however, a large, multicenter trial of more than 1100 patients undergoing CABG did not demonstrate a difference in the duration of mechanical ventilation with either vecuronium or pancuronium in a fast-track anesthetic regimen.[287] After surgery, hypertension should be aggressively treated to avoid hyperperfusion syndromes leading to transient seizures or intracerebral hemorrhage and avoid exacerbating bleeding at the site of the CEA.

CORONARY ARTERIOVENOUS FISTULA

Coronary arteriovenous fistula is an abnormal communication between a coronary artery and another cardiac chamber or venous structure, bypassing the myocardial capillary network. Common sites include coronary sinus, cardiac vein, pulmonary artery, superior vena cava, pulmonary vein, or any one of the cardiac chambers. The incidence rate in the overall population is 0.002%.[292] Coronary artery fistula is the most common significant coronary artery anomaly and occurs in 0.3% to 0.8% of angiographic series.[293] Coronary arteriovenous fistula usually is congenital but also may occur from acquired (coronary atherosclerosis, Takayasu arteritis), traumatic, or iatrogenic causes. Interestingly, 10% to 30% of patients with coronary fistula may have another congenital anomaly such as tetralogy of Fallot, atrial septal defect, and partial anomalous pulmonary venous connection. It is not sex-specific. Most congenital arteriovenous fistulas (60%) involve the right coronary artery, are small, and have no clinical significance. The left coronary artery is the site of the fistula in 35% of cases, although more recent studies have suggested that asymptomatic coronary fistulae originate from the left coronary system.[294] Multiple coronary fistulae occur in 5% of patients.[295] The most common distal connection of the fistula with the right coronary artery is the RV, which represents 41% of the distal fistula sites. Low-pressure structures are the most common connections for coronary fistula, with left-sided connections occurring rarely.[292] Most fistulae are single connections. The most proximal part of the fistula does develop some aneurysmal dilation and is often up to three times the normal diameter of the coronary artery.[294]

The clinical importance generally is associated with adulthood in which larger fistulae cause significant left-to-right shunts and CHF. Fistulae that connect to the left side do not shunt but cause an effect similar to mitral regurgitation. However, it is rare to find the degree of shunting significant enough to see an oxygen step-up effect during right-sided catheterization. Fifty percent of patients with large fistulae experience development of complications.[292] The most common symptom is dyspnea, which occurs in 30% of patients. Most adults are thought to be asymptomatic, but more recent reports suggest that nearly 50% are symptomatic at the time of presentation. The average age of symptoms is 18 years. Other problems that may lead to the diagnosis are arrhythmias, infective endocarditis, and myocardial ischemia. Usually myocardial blood flow is not compromised because the shunt is so small, but coronary arteriovenous fistulae may cause angina pectoris by stealing blood from the normal coronary circulation. This situation is usually limited to exercise.[296] Additional complications of coronary fistulae such as thrombosis, embolization, PAH, aneurysmal dilation of the involved vessel, and even sudden death may occur in patients diagnosed at later ages. Coronary fistulae rarely lead to aneurysmal rupture. Coronary arteriovenous fistulae can occur after penetrating injury to the chest and present as pericardial tamponade.

A continuous murmur with diastolic accentuation suggests an arteriovenous fistula. The murmur is continuous in a crescendo-decrescendo manner that persists through both systole and diastole. The murmur does not peak at the second heart sound as most of the other continuous murmurs do. The site where the murmur is the loudest is the site of entry into the heart for the fistula. Discovery of a continuous murmur along the upper left sternal border after CABG is an indication for angiography to verify proper placement of a saphenous vein graft into a coronary artery. Angiography is useful to differentiate this condition from other causes of continuous murmurs, such as patent ductus arteriosus, VSD, and atrial septal defect. Many of these fistulae are found incidentally during angiography. If the coronary artery is significantly enlarged, echo may be diagnostic. TEE is useful to identify drainage sites of a coronary arteriovenous fistula. More recently, MRI and CT angiogram have contributed to the diagnostic process because, although angiography is the gold standard for imaging the coronary arteries, it may not provide the course and relation to other structures, as well as an MRI and CT angiogram.[293]

The majority of small symptomatic fistulae do not require intervention.[296] Often, with infants who do not demonstrate CHF, medical management may reduce symptoms. With growth, the size of the fistula and shunt will become smaller and less symptomatic. The natural history of these fistulae is variable. Spontaneous closure has been reported but is rare and mostly in infants.[292] In some asymptomatic patients, the size of the shunt may reach Q_p/Q_s of 1.5 but rarely more than 2, leading to severe fluid overload.

Management is controversial, in part because of treatment based on anecdotal reports or small case series. Some will start antiplatelet medication, but others oppose it.[292] Symptoms are the primary impetus for closure of the coronary fistula. Asymptomatic patients may be considered for treatment, but the concern is the possibility of future complications. Treatment options to close the fistula include the longstanding therapy of surgery or a variety of percutaneous techniques such as coils, balloons, double-umbrella devices, and vascular occlusion devices. With either technique, long-term follow-up of the patient is necessary because recanalization is possible.

Surgical treatment of coronary fistula with direct endocardial ligation has proved safe, with no morbidity or mortality, and effective, with excellent long-term results of 10 years without problems.[297] Fistulae can be closed either from external plication on a beating heart or from an intracardiac location using CPB. The distal end of the fistula is closed from within the recipient cavity during CPB to eliminate the fistulous tract.[298] Selected fistulae may be ligated without CPB. The use of coronary revascularization without CPB may be effective

to protect the myocardial territories subtended by the fistula.[296] In about 50% of cases, when fistulae are corrected with surgery, CPB is used.[294] Cardioplegic arrest may be difficult with aortic cross-clamping of the aorta, so the option for temporarily clamping the fistula is acceptable unless the fistula is calcified. Intraoperative TEE can localize fistulae, verify complete repair, and monitor ventricular function to avoid ischemic complications of ligation.[299] It is rare to encounter major problems with surgery for coronary fistulae, but MI, arrhythmias, and stroke occur.

The first successful transcatheter closure of a coronary fistula occurred in 1983.[293] This catheter-based technique of closing coronary fistulae has enjoyed good success. Although many techniques are available to close the fistula, most have been done with coils.[300] The use of the coils results in thrombosis of the fistula to the level of the first branch, reducing the left-to-right shunt and returning myocardial blood flow. This technique has compared favorably with the surgical option in terms of morbidity, mortality, and effectiveness.[293,294] Series have noted that leaks may develop from transcatheter closure in approximately 10% of patients.[294] Long-term follow-up has not been as rigorous or able to determine problems, but nearly half of these follow-ups are associated with persistent abnormalities.

Anesthetic Considerations

Anesthetic management of arteriovenous fistulae is similar to anesthetic management for CABG. ECG monitoring for detection of ischemic changes is invaluable for ligation of coronary arteriovenous fistulae. The use of echo is extremely valuable to determine myocardial ischemia, as well as the degree of shunt.

▣ Case Study 4

Coronary Artery Fistula

A 56-year-old woman with a history of hypertension presented with new-onset dyspnea on exertion. Her physical examination was unremarkable with the exception of a continuous, soft murmur heard on auscultation of the chest. A preoperative TTE revealed normal valves, normal ventricular function, and no regional wall motion abnormalities. There was an area of turbulent flow in the RV, raising concern for the presence of a right coronary artery fistula communicating with the RV. This finding was confirmed with a preoperative angiogram, and surgery was recommended. In the operating room, the site of communication between the fistula and the RV was identified with TEE. Using color-Doppler imaging, a site of turbulent flow was identified entering the RV. Turbulent flow also was seen outside of the ventricle, presumably occurring within the fistula. The surgeon placed a suture around the coronary fistula at its site of entrance to the RV. As the suture was tightened, the turbulent flow entering the RV was no longer seen on TEE. The result was considered acceptable and the surgeon proceeded to ligate the fistula. The right coronary artery was assumed to remain intact.

After a short period of observation, it was noted that the ST segments in the inferior leads had become elevated. Ischemia was considered but could not be confirmed as the source of mild ST elevation. When the heart was reimaged with TEE, right ventricular function was described as normal. However, there clearly were new regional wall motion abnormalities in the inferior wall of the LV. Given these new wall motion abnormalities combined with ST-segment elevation, it was believed that the right coronary artery had been compromised. CPB was instituted and a vein graft was placed from the aorta to the distal right coronary artery, followed by easy separation from CPB. Biventricular function was normal and the wall motion abnormalities were no longer present. The patient had an uncomplicated postoperative course.

In this case, TEE not only guided ligation of the fistula, but also confirmed damage to the coronary artery requiring CABG during the ongoing anesthetic and avoiding another separate procedure and anesthetic.

CARDIAC SURGERY DURING PREGNANCY

Heart disease is a major risk factor for maternal and fetal death during pregnancy, with an incidence rate of 1% to 3%.[301] It is the most common cause of nonobstetric mortality during pregnancy, accounting for 10% to 15% of maternal mortality. Although maternal cardiac disease represents only 15% of obstetric ICU admissions, it accounts for 50% of the obstetric ICU deaths.[302] Obstetric patients with heart disease are at great risk for serious complications because of hemodynamic changes associated with pregnancy and delivery. If cardiac surgery is required during or immediately after pregnancy, anesthetic management demands an appreciation for the many changes of pregnancy and their impact on the corresponding heart disease and well-being of the fetus.

Certain physiologic changes of pregnancy negatively impact the female patient with heart disease. Heart rate and stroke volume are each increased by 25% by the end of the second trimester. Early in the third trimester, intravascular volume has expanded by nearly 50%.[303] These three changes during pregnancy cause a 50% increase in CO that is aggravated by physiologic anemia and aortocaval compression. Labor contractions can rapidly increase the already increased CO. Such increases in blood volume and CO are especially difficult for a parturient with valvular heart disease. Increased CO will increase myocardial oxygen demand, exacerbating CHF, and low SVR will worsen coronary perfusion, causing myocardial ischemia. Low SVR also may compromise maternal pulmonary blood flow or alter shunt physiology with certain congenital heart defects. It is not uncommon to see a nonpregnant woman with well-compensated cardiac disease acutely or gradually decompensate as cardiac demands increase during pregnancy.

Cardiovascular morbidity and mortality strongly are associated with maternal functional status. Four major risk factors predict poor maternal outcomes according to a prospective evaluation of more than 600 pregnancies complicated by maternal cardiac disease: CHF, transient ischemic attacks, stroke, or arrhythmias; prepregnancy NYHA Class > 2; left-heart obstruction; and ejection fraction less than 40%.[302] The likelihood of complications increases to 75% if more than one risk factor is present. Most commonly, the complication takes the form of pulmonary edema or arrhythmias.

Rheumatic heart disease accounts for nearly 75% of maternal heart disease, but congenital heart disease continues to increase its share as more women with congenital heart disease are reaching childbearing years. Native valve disease and prosthetic valve dysfunction comprise most of the operations during pregnancy. Dissecting or traumatic rupture of the aorta, pulmonary embolism, closure of a PFO, and cardiac tumors comprise only a small percentage of cases.[304] Mitral valve disease is the most common valvular disorder that requires surgery in pregnancy. Chronic mitral or aortic regurgitation actually may be associated with a small symptomatic improvement secondary to the normal physiologic changes of pregnancy. In contrast, stenotic valvular lesions tolerate these changes poorly.[301] Aortic and mitral stenosis are common problems that may lead to hemodynamic deterioration, forcing emergency delivery before cardiac surgery. The most frequent indication for emergency cardiac surgery during pregnancy is decompensation from CHF because of mitral stenosis.[305] New onset of atrial fibrillation with mitral stenosis causing severe hypotension and decreased CO is one of the more common potentially life-threatening situations to the mother and fetus.

Because cardiac surgical morbidity and mortality are greater in the parturient than the nonpregnant patient undergoing the same cardiac operation, every effort is made to manage the patient without surgery. Extensive exposure to radiation may, however, limit therapeutic invasive catheterization procedures. If nonsurgical therapy is not feasible or conflicts with fetal interests, cardiac surgery and CPB are reasonable because delaying surgery until after delivery carries a greater maternal mortality risk than proceeding with surgery.[301] If the fetus is 24 weeks gestation, the obstetrician may perform a cesarean section just before CPB, because of the greater fetal mortality associated with cardiac surgery. Although general anesthesia is recommended for patients requiring cesarean section before CPB, volatile agents may induce uterine atony, resulting in serious bleeding; therefore, total intravenous anesthesia merits consideration.

Since 1958, when Leyse and colleagues described the first cardiac surgery requiring CPB in a pregnant patient, maternal morbidity has decreased from 5%[304,305] to less than 1%.[306] Fetal mortality remains high, ranging from 16% to 33%.[304,305,307] Unfortunately, fetal mortality is related to the use of CPB, duration of surgery, and hypothermia. The nonphysiologic nature of CPB combines with the changes of pregnancy for an uncertain response and tolerance by mother and fetus.

CPB exposes the fetus to many undesirable effects that may have unpredictable consequences. Initiation of CPB activates a whole-body inflammatory response,[308] with multiple effects on coagulation, autoregulation, release of vasoactive substances, hemodilution, and other physiologic processes that may adversely impact both the fetus and mother. Maternal blood pressure may decline immediately after or within 5 minutes of initiation of CPB, decreasing placental perfusion secondary to low SVR, hemodilution, and release of vasoactive agents.[305] Fetal heart rate variability often is lost, and fetal bradycardia (< 80 beats/min) also may occur at this time.[309] Because uterine blood flow is not autoregulated and relies on maternal blood flow, decreases of maternal blood pressure cause fetal hypoxia and bradycardia. Increasing CPB flows (> 2.5 L/m²/min) or perfusion pressure (> 70 mm Hg) will raise maternal blood flow and usually return the fetal heart rate to 120 beats/min.[310] A compensatory catecholamine-driven tachycardia (170 beats/min) may ensue that suggests an oxygen debt existed.[309] Nonetheless, increasing CPB flow and mean arterial pressure do not always correct fetal bradycardia, and if not, then other causes must be considered.

Problems with venous return or other mechanical aspects of extracorporeal circulation also may limit systemic flow, causing reduced placental perfusion. If acidosis persists throughout CPB, other factors may be responsible for it rather than low maternal blood pressure, such as maternal hypothermia, uterine contractions, or medications that are transferable to the fetus. Monitoring the fetal heart rate is important to assess fetal viability and subsequent therapeutic initiatives. Fetal monitoring reduces mortality partially by early recognition of problems.[305] Immediately after delivery, the CO increases suddenly because of mobilization of extracellular fluids and removal of aortocaval compression to greatly burden the diseased cardiovascular system.[301]

Hypothermia has been used for years in cardiac surgery but is not recommended for the pregnant patient. There are reports of fetal survival with maternal core temperatures of 23° C to 25° C, and fetal survival is even documented after 37 minutes of hypothermic (19° C) circulatory arrest.[311,312] However, when hypothermic versus normothermic CPB was examined retrospectively in 69 pregnant patients who underwent cardiac surgery during 1958 to 1992, hypothermia was associated with an embryo fetal mortality rate of 24% compared with 0% for normothermia (Table 22-9). The fetus appears to maintain autoregulation of the heart rate with mild hypothermia, but most functions are reduced with severe hypothermia.[309] Maternal mortality was not influenced by differences in CPB temperature.

Beyond the effect of hypothermia on acid-base status, coagulation, and arrhythmias, it may precipitate uterine contractions that limit placental perfusion and risk fetal ischemia and survival. The explanation for hypothermia-induced contractions may be related to the severe dilution that accompanies CPB and reduces progesterone levels, thus activating uterine contractions. Contractions are more likely to occur the older the gestational age of the fetus.[307,313] Accordingly, uterine monitoring is strongly recommended if CPB is required during pregnancy. If uterine contractions should begin during CPB, it is vitally important for fetal survival to stop them. Treatment includes ethanol infusion, magnesium sulfate, terbutaline, or ritodrine. Many of these tocolytic agents have potential side effects and toxicities that can be especially detrimental to patients with heart disease.[314] However, tocolytic agents may be necessary if the contractions are associated with marked fetal decelerations indicative of severe oxygen debt. Infants have died of protracted contractions.[315] Prophylactic measures to

TABLE 22-9	Fetal and Maternal Mortality and Morbidity after Cardiopulmonary Bypass				
Variable	No. of Patients	Embryofetal Mortality, n (%)	Maternal Mortality, n (%)	Embryofetal Morbidity, n (%)	Maternal Morbidity, n (%)
Total cases	69	14 (20.2)	2 (2.9)	5 (7.2)	3 (4.3)
1958–1974	29	9 (31.0)	2 (6.9)	1 (3.4)	0
1975–1991	40	5 (12.5)	0	4 (10.0)	3 (7.5)
< 15 wk	24	3 (12.5)	1 (4.2)	4 (16.6)	1 (4.2)
≥ 16 wk	41	9 (21.9)	0	1 (2.4)	2 (4.9)
Hypothermia (< 35°C)	25	6 (24.0)	0	4 (16.0)	1 (4.0)
Normothermia (≥ 36°C)	13	0	0	0	2 (15.3)

From Pomini F, Mercogliano D, Cavalletti C, et al: Cardiopulmonary bypass in pregnancy. *Ann Thorac Surg* 61:265, 1996.

prevent contractions, such as progesterone, have been of indeterminate value. Pulsatile CPB may lessen the risk for contractions as fewer premature contractions were noted, but the mechanism is unclear and has not gained popularity.[316]

As noted previously, the initiation of CPB is accompanied by moderate hemodilution. It has been recommended that the hematocrit remain greater than 28% to optimize oxygen-carrying capacity for mother and fetus.[301] The $Paco_2$ should be slightly hypercapnic because this increases uterine blood flow. Anticoagulation and its neutralization for CPB should be consistent with routine management for nonmaternal patients, as unfractionated heparin does not cross the placenta and can be used safely. Anticoagulation during pregnancy has been extensively reviewed.[317] A cesarean section has been advised for neonates with a gestational age of more than 28 weeks, immediately after heparinization and cannulation but before commencement of CPB,[318] because at 24 to 28 weeks, organogenesis is complete and neonates do well. If avoidance of CPB with the fetus is not possible, the appropriate management to achieve optimal outcome for the mother and fetus is not firmly established with prospective randomized trials.

Approximately 30 to 60 minutes after separation from CPB, the fetus experiences development of a severe and progressive respiratory acidosis.[309] Although correctable, hours later a more severe metabolic acidosis ensues with the potential for fetal death. It has been postulated that catecholamines and the fetal stress response may be responsible for poor CO secondary to significant vasoconstriction, reflected in a persistent acidosis.[307] The effects of vasopressors and inotropic agents on uterine blood flow in pregnant patients with cardiac disease are indeterminate. Angiotensin-converting enzyme inhibitors and angiotensin-converting enzyme receptor antagonists are contraindicated during pregnancy.[301] Current guidelines are based on animal data, not the intact human maternal-fetal unit. Uterine blood flow is directly proportional to mean perfusion pressure and inversely proportional to uterine vascular resistance. The uterine vascular bed is maximally dilated during pregnancy. Stimulation of α-adrenergic receptors increases uterine vascular resistance and potentially decreases uterine blood flow. However, improvements in maternal CO, blood pressure, and uterine blood flow by certain vasopressors may outweigh any detrimental effect on uterine vascular resistance. Ephedrine has been the vasopressor of choice for maternal hypotension for years. Ephedrine and phenylephrine are safe when treating maternal hypotension during cesarean section after spinal or epidural anesthesia.[319,320] In pregnant ewes, the effect of dopamine on uterine blood flow is mixed. Epinephrine has been associated with decreased uterine blood flow, although in one clinical report, an infusion of epinephrine improved maternal hemodynamics after CPB and resolved fetal bradycardia.[321] Overall, the use of these agents during CPB appears to have few negative effects.[309]

Anesthetic Considerations

Medications for anesthesia must be considered in the context of the maternal heart disease, influence of CPB, and effect on the fetus. Maternal safety must be ensured, as well as optimal fetal outcome. It is important to be aware of the safety of the more commonly used drugs in cardiac anesthesia during pregnancy. The risk for teratogenesis with a myriad of medications and exposures of the fetus during cardiac surgery and CPB is high, but most infants successfully have avoided these effects.[312,313] No anesthetic agent has been shown to be teratogenic in humans. Fetal teratogenicity is always a concern of anesthetic management, especially during the first trimester when fetal organogenesis occurs. Commonly used induction agents and sedatives, such as thiopental, ketamine, etomidate, propofol, midazolam, and diazepam, rapidly cross the placental barrier to the fetal circulation.[41,322–324] Animal studies show that halothane, enflurane, isoflurane, and sevoflurane appear to be safe anesthetics and lack teratogenic effects.[325,326] Despite concerns about the action of nitrous oxide on DNA synthesis, human and animal studies indicate that it is safe to use nitrous oxide for anesthesia during pregnancy. Fentanyl and sufentanil decrease beat-to-beat variability and may mask fetal distress but do not produce teratogenic effects. Both depolarizing and nondepolarizing muscle relaxants cross the placenta to different degrees. Pancuronium, atracurium, and pipecuronium have been administered either intramuscularly or intravenously directly to the human fetus in utero without apparent adverse sequelae.

Many medications administered during cardiac anesthesia do not provide anesthesia. β-Blockers such as propranolol, esmolol, and labetalol cross the placenta but appear safe for acute and chronic use.[327] Nitroprusside, nitroglycerin, and hydralazine appear to be safe for treating maternal hypertension. Nitroprusside rapidly crosses the placental membrane in pregnant ewes, but infusion rates of less than 2 μg/kg/min do not generate toxic levels of cyanide in fetal lambs.[318] Mannitol and furosemide cross the placenta and induce fetal diuresis but have no apparent adverse fetal consequences. Regional anesthesia carries considerable risk in view of the degree of anticoagulation necessary for CPB, although it has been used successfully.

A team approach with anesthesiologist, surgeon, neonatologist, and obstetrician is critical for the care of mother and fetus, especially if optimal management for the mother does not necessarily coincide with fetal interests. The decision to operate needs to be made in the context of the potential survivability of the fetus outside the uterus should delivery of the baby become probable.

RISKS OF HUMAN IMMUNODEFICIENCY VIRUS TRANSMISSION

In the United States, 1.2 million people are infected with human immunodeficiency virus (HIV), representing 2.5% of the global infections.[328] More than 50,000 new cases occur annually in the United States.[329] Concern exists among health care workers about the risk for infection with HIV. Only 57 cases of documented occupational HIV infection in health care workers in the United States have been reported between 1981 and 2001.[328] Cardiac surgery is one of the greatest risk settings for occupational HIV transmission because of the considerable blood exposure that often occurs with excessive bleeding after CPB. This risk is not expected to improve greatly in the foreseeable future. However, the pattern of HIV transmission is changing to include more heterosexual and progressively older individuals. New therapies and a delayed incubation time to development of AIDS after infection have extended life expectancy of those with HIV.[330] However, since the introduction of the highly active antiretroviral therapy, reduction in deaths has been slipping in response to potential resistance to combination drug therapies. Currently, the number of cases has stabilized in the United States. As patients with HIV live longer and reach ages when the likelihood of cardiac surgery is greater, the number of HIV patients who require cardiac surgery also will increase.

The risk for exposure to HIV for the health care worker continues to evolve. Earlier studies show transmission risks from patients were overall minimal. Henderson et al[331] prospectively studied 1344 healthcare workers over a 6-year period to assess the risk for HIV transmission during occupational activities. The authors combined data from multiple sources and stated, "The risk for HIV-1 transmission associated with percutaneous exposure to blood from an HIV-1 infected patient is approximately 0.3% per exposure." The risk after mucous membrane and cutaneous exposure to an HIV patient is 0.09%. Transmission of HIV has been reported after nonintact skin exposure, but the risk is less than mucous membrane transmission.[332] A Centers for Disease Control and Prevention prospective surveillance project found a 0.36% HIV seroconversion rate in health care workers who sustained percutaneous exposure to HIV-contaminated blood.[333] No seroconversions occurred in health care workers who had mucous membrane or cutaneous exposure to HIV-infected blood.

Rates of exposure are subject to the study methods, types of procedures, and the precautions of the individuals involved; consequently, the stated risk for transmission with a single exposure may be greater than initially suspected. Factors that have been identified to alter rate of conversion are a deep injury contact, injury by a device visibly contaminated with a patient's blood, or injury by a device placed in the artery or vein. These factors are associated with a higher titer of viral exposure, so the rate of conversion is greater than the rate of 0.5% noted previously.[334] The risk for transmission also is greater with exposure to a larger quantity of blood or an HIV-infected person with a terminal illness.[332] Rates of conversion in surgical settings are known to vary widely.[335] The specific occupational risk of blood-borne infections in the health care setting primarily depends on three factors: (1) the prevalence of infected patients within the patient population, (2) the probability of acquiring a specific infection after a single occupational exposure, and (3) the frequency of at-risk exposures.[330] In a study examining the risk for transmission of HIV by surgical subspecialties and occupation, cardiothoracic surgery had the greatest rate. The rate of mucocutaneous contamination by blood splashing during surgery has been estimated to be greater, approximately 50% for cardiothoracic surgery. It appears that almost 60% of exposures in cardiac surgery occur in the operating room, with suture representing one third of the contacts. However, HIV infection accounts for only 5% of these exposures compared with 78% for hepatitis C. Blood-to-hand contacts represent many of the exposures in the operating room for the cardiac surgical setting.[335] Contact of blood with the body increases the risk for infection dramatically as blood loss exceeds 500 mL.

The best way to prevent occupationally related HIV infection is to prevent exposure to HIV-contaminated bodily fluids, most notably blood. Greene et al,[336] using data confined to anesthesia personnel and obtained in 1991 to 1993, found that the majority of percutaneous injuries were from contaminated needles, usually hollow bore, and were preventable. Hollow-bore needles that have been used in venous or arterial puncture appear to have a greater incidence of HIV transmission than solid needles. Needleless or protected needle infusion devices and revised anesthesia practice protocols have reduced the incidence of percutaneous injuries.[337] All anesthesia personnel should routinely wear face shields or eye protection and gloves to prevent cutaneous and mucous membrane contamination.

The safety of blood transfusion regarding infection has been confirmed.[338] All donated blood undergoes HIV antibody screening, but a "window period" of approximately 22 days exists when antigen may exist in a donor's blood without antibody. As of 1995, there are only 29 documented cases of AIDS attributed to receiving HIV seronegative blood, although the actual number may be greater. Lackritz

et al[339] evaluated the American Red Cross blood system and estimated that 1 blood donation in 360,000 occurred during the "window period." Furthermore, 15% to 42% of this blood was discarded because of other laboratory abnormalities. They also estimated that 1 in 2,600,000 donations was HIV positive, but because of laboratory error it was missed. The American Red Cross defined the risk for the administration of HIV-infected blood as 1 in 450,000 to 660,000 donations. Extrapolating their data nationwide to all 12 million annual donations, approximately 18 to 27 HIV-infected donations are available for transfusion. Schreiber et al[340] estimated that 1 in 493,000 donated units of blood would result in HIV transmission. They also estimated the risks for transmitting human T-cell lymphotropic virus, hepatitis C virus, and hepatitis B virus to be 1 in 641,000, 1 in 103,000, and 1 in 63,000, respectively. Despite the appropriate concern about HIV transmission during blood transfusion, similar attention should be directed toward the transmission of hepatitis B and C.

The effectiveness of postexposure prophylaxis has been difficult to prove in view of the small number of exposures that prevent an adequate statistical analysis of the rate of seroconversion after contact. In case-controlled trials, zidovudine is the only drug that has been shown to reduce the rate of seroconversion.[341] Table 22-10 outlines the recommendations of the U.S. Public Health Service for postexposure prophylaxis. Postexposure chemoprophylaxis with two drugs is indicated when health care workers are at risk for acquiring HIV via percutaneous exposure. The two-drug combination of nucleoside reverse transcriptase inhibitor agents is recommended if significant exposure occurs. Possible combinations include zidovudine-lamivudine, lamivudine-stavudine, or didanosine-lamivudine.[332] A third drug is recommended if the risk is believed to be even greater or the HIV titer is higher in the exposure. Therapy should be initiated as soon as possible because there is a "window" before the systemic infection occurs. Earlier exposure to the antiretroviral therapy permits a better chance to preserve immune function and alter the course of the disease. Current recommendations suggest at least 1 to 2 hours from the time of exposure for initiation of prophylaxis to be successful, but this has not been proved. In some cases, prophylaxis has been successfully administered 36 hours after exposure.[337] It has been shown that those who are exposed to HIV through their occupation who do not seroconvert may still develop markers of T-cell–mediated response to the virus. However, the risk for this is lower if the exposed person has received antiretroviral prophylaxis.[337]

All patients at any stage of infection with HIV, even the "window of opportunity," are at risk for transmission.[342] To date, only 22 patients have had HIV seroconversion after prophylaxis, with 6 of those patients receiving combination therapy. Follow-up for the occurrence of side effects should start after 4 weeks and continue for at least 6 months after exposure.[337] Serologic testing for conversion should occur 6 weeks, 3 months, and 6 months from time of exposure. If hepatitis C was confirmed, testing for seroconversion should continue for another 12 months because of the effect of hepatitis C delaying HIV seroconversion. Zidovudine has potential complications, so its administration should be carefully considered because most exposures to HIV do not result in seroconversion. In addition, zidovudine has been associated with several failures and complications.[335]

With the recent rise of resistant strains, prophylaxis therapy for occupational exposure should involve investigation into the source of the exposure to carefully design the optimal regimen. It is critical to determine the HIV serology of the source for infection as soon as possible to minimize any exposure to prophylaxis if the source is found to be HIV negative. Prophylaxis is not indicated if the patient is negative for HIV. If there is delay in testing the infecting source, at least one dose of prophylactic agents should be administered.[329] The viral load for prophylaxis differs greatly if the donor is chronically infected and the postexposure prophylaxis will be influenced by it. The proper prophylaxis is important because incremental toxicity increases as the number of antiretroviral agents is increased.

Since new therapies for HIV have become more widespread,[343] patients undergoing cardiac surgery may be receiving these newer

Type of Exposure	Source Material*	Antiretroviral Prophylaxis†	Antiretroviral Regimen‡
Percutaneous	Blood§		
	Highest risk	Recommend	ZDV plus 3TC plus IDV
	Increased risk	Recommend	ZDV plus 3TC, ± IDV**
	No increased risk	Offer	ZDV plus 3TC
	Fluid containing visible blood, other potentially infectious fluid,¶ or tissue	Offer	ZDV plus 3TC
	Other body fluid (e.g., urine)	Not offer	
Mucous membrane	Blood	Offer	ZDV plus 3TC, ± ID**
	Fluid containing visible blood, other potentially infectious fluid,¶ or tissue	Offer	ZDV ± 3TC
	Other body fluid (e.g., urine)	Not offer	
Skin	Blood	Offer	ZDV plus 3TC, ± IDV**
Increased risk**	Fluid containing visible blood, other potentially infectious fluid,¶ or tissue	Offer	ZDV ± 3TC
	Other body fluid (e.g., urine)	Not offer	

*Any exposure to concentrated human immunodeficiency virus (HIV; e.g., in a research laboratory or production facility) is treated as percutaneous exposure to blood with greatest risk.
†Recommend: Postexposure prophylaxis (PEP) should be recommended to the exposed worker with counseling. Offer: PEP should be offered to the exposed worker with counseling. Not offer: PEP should not be offered because these are not occupational exposures to HIV.
‡Regimens: zidovudine (ZDV), 200 mg three times a day; lamivudine (3TC), 150 mg twice daily; indinavir (IDV), 800 mg three times a day (if IDV is not available, saquinavir may be used, 600 mg three times a day). Prophylaxis is given for 4 weeks. For full prescribing information, see package inserts.
§Highest risk: Both larger volume of blood (e.g., deep injury with large-diameter hollow needle previously in source patient's vein or artery, especially involving an injection of source patient's blood) and blood containing high titer of HIV (e.g., source with acute retroviral illness or end-stage AIDS; viral load measurement may be considered, but its use in relation to PEP has not been evaluated). Increased risk: Either exposure to larger volume of blood or blood with high titer of HIV. No increased risk: Neither exposure to larger volume of blood nor blood with high titer of HIV (e.g., solid suture needle injury from source patient with asymptomatic HIV infection).
**Possible toxicity of additional drug may not be warranted.
¶Includes semen; vaginal secretions; or cerebrospinal, synovial, pleural, peritoneal, pericardial, and amniotic fluids.
**For skin, risk is increased for exposures involving high titer of HIV; prolonged contact; and extensive area, or an area in which skin integrity is visibly compromised. For skin exposures without increased risk, the risk for drug toxicity outweighs the benefit of PEP.
From Cardo DM, Bell DM: Bloodborne pathogen transmission in health care workers. Infect Dis Clin North Am 11:341, 1997 (from Centers for Disease Control and Prevention: Update: Provisional public health service recommendations for chemoprophylaxis after occupational exposure to HIV. *MMWR Morb Mortal Wkly Rep* 45:468, 1996).

medications. Triple-drug therapy is now the standard of care. The complexity of medications that these patients may receive certainly increases the possibility of drug interactions. The nucleoside analog reverse transcriptase inhibitors are primarily secreted by the kidneys, so fewer drug interactions are likely. However, the non-nucleoside analog reverse transcriptase inhibitors and protease inhibitors are metabolized by the liver with the cytochrome P450 mechanism so that many drug interactions are possible, especially with anesthetic agents. Ritonavir, a potent protease inhibitor, can increase the blood concentration levels of amiodarone, midazolam, diazepam, and meperidine. Drug interactions should be considered if a patient is taking these medications and requires cardiac surgery.

RENAL INSUFFICIENCY AND CARDIAC SURGERY

In recent years, the number of individuals with chronic renal failure (CRF) undergoing cardiac surgery has increased to 2% to 3% of the cardiac surgical population.[344] Patients with CRF may not necessarily be dialysis dependent before surgery but are more likely to develop worsening renal function after CPB than those with normal preoperative renal function.[345] Morbidity and mortality are especially high in long-term dialysis patients undergoing cardiac surgery and CPB, ranging from 17% to 77% and 8% to 31%, respectively.[346] Because CRF accelerates the development of atherosclerosis, myocardial revascularization is common in these patients. Irrespective of whether the patient with CRF is dialysis dependent, this patient is an anesthetic challenge, especially in regard to fluid management, electrolyte status, and hemostasis. The ability to avoid dialysis in the patient with nondialysis-dependent CRF is important to hospital stay and long-term mortality. A collaborative effort by the cardiac surgeon, anesthesiologist, nephrologist, and cardiologist is instrumental in the care of these patients. Unfortunately, long-term survival is still appreciably diminished even with minimal perioperative morbidity.

Patients with CRF are more prone to fluid overload, hyponatremia, hyperkalemia, and metabolic acidosis. Optimal hemodynamic and fluid status before surgery are important. Hemodialysis should be strongly considered the day before surgery, especially in those who are strictly dialysis dependent. Chronic dialysis patients tend to arrive for surgery with worsened left ventricular function, possibly from inefficient waste and toxin removal. CHF can occur as a result of hypervolemia and poor left ventricular function manifesting as pulmonary edema and respiratory distress. Dialysis and medical therapy directed at improving cardiac function may be required to optimize the patient before surgery. Chronic medications should be carefully reviewed to ensure that certain medications were given, such as antihypertensive agents. The importance of preoperative preparation for patients with CRF is evident by the significantly higher mortality associated with urgent surgery.[344]

Perioperative mortality of patients with CRF undergoing cardiac surgery is associated with several risk factors. A preoperative creatinine concentration of 2.5 mg/dL is associated with greater mortality, even in those patients with nondialysis-dependent CRF.[346] Late mortality rates may range from 8.3% to 55% if dialysis is ongoing for more than 60 months.[344] Pulmonary dysfunction also increases the perioperative mortality of patients with CRF.

Patients with CRF differ from those with normal renal function in a variety of ways that influence anesthesia management. A normochromic, normocytic anemia is common, primarily because of decreased or absent erythropoietin secretion for which the kidney is the predominant source. Anemia now is treated with recombinant human erythropoietin therapy instead of blood. The cardiovascular benefits are especially noticeable with correction of anemia. However, treatment is costly and requires multiple injections weeks before surgery, which may not always be possible.

Efforts to find renoprotective agents for patients either at high risk for renal failure or those with CRF have been unfulfilling. Recently, a randomized, double-blind, prospective trial looking at the use of N-acetylcysteine for patients undergoing CPB with CRF found no difference in renal parameters.[347] N-acetylcysteine is an antioxidant and vasodilator with the ability to increase cyclic guanosine monophosphate and nitric oxide and has shown promise in contrast-related renal failure. Fenoldopam, a new dopamine-1 receptor agonist, was studied in patients undergoing CPB with preoperative creatinine levels greater than 1.5 mg/dL.[348] Subjects were given renal-dose dopamine or fenoldopam perioperatively. Postoperative parameters were improved only in those receiving fenoldopam, suggesting a renal-protective effect, but additional studies are needed. Mannitol and furosemide may also prevent early oliguric renal failure.[349]

Anesthetic Considerations

CRF affects dosing of medications that have a large volume of distribution. Decreased serum protein concentration diminishes plasma binding, leading to greater levels of free drug to bind with receptors. Many patients with CRF are hypoalbuminemic. In general, anesthetic induction agents and benzodiazepines are safe to use in patients with CRF. A once common induction agent, thiopental, is highly protein bound, so the dose would be reduced accordingly. Medications that rely totally on renal excretion have a limited role. Fentanyl and sufentanil may be more effective for pain management because excretion is not as renally dependent as morphine sulfate. Currently used volatile anesthetic agents rarely cause any additional renal dysfunction, even with underlying CRF, unless severely prolonged duration of anesthesia occurs. Muscle relaxants and agents for antagonism of muscle paralysis have varying degrees of renal excretion (Table 22-11).

A rapid-sequence induction with cricoid pressure is recommended in those with CRF in response to the likelihood of delayed gastric emptying. Significant extracellular volume contraction also may be present before induction of anesthesia because of a 6- to 8-hour fast before surgery and dialysis within 24 hours of surgery that may lead to hypotension on induction. Because fluid requirements usually are high with CPB, a PAC is especially useful to manage fluid administration. TEE may complement fluid management by assessment of left ventricular volume and function. Before the initiation of CPB, fluid administration should be limited, especially if the patient is dialysis dependent. In the nondialysis-dependent patient, fluid should be given to maintain adequate urine output but avoid excessive cardiovascular filling pressures that incite pulmonary edema. Fluids should not be restricted too aggressively because it may cause acute renal failure superimposed on CRF. Low-dose dopamine has been recommended for patients with CRF, but its value is indeterminate.

In general, CRF will worsen after CPB, in part because a combination of nonpulsatile flow, low renal perfusion, and hypothermia.[346] Studies remain mixed regarding the ability of pulsatile flow during CPB to preserve renal function compared with nonpulsatile CPB.[350] Renal perfusion is reduced as CPB is initiated, increasing the chance for ischemia

of the renal cortex. Mean arterial pressure should be kept greater than 80 mm Hg. The stress of surgery and hypothermia may impair autoregulation so that renal vasoconstriction reduces renal blood flow. The fluid required to initiate CPB may significantly reduce the hemoglobin (Hb) and oxygen-carrying capacity in view of the preexisting anemia of CRF without the addition of red blood cells (RBCs) to the priming volume or immediately on initiation of CPB. A hematocrit of 25% should be maintained during CPB.[346] Washed RBCs are recommended for RBC transfusion to lessen excessive potassium and glucose levels intraoperatively. Potassium plasma levels should be checked periodically. Patients with CRF often have glucose intolerance from an abnormal insulin response, so more frequent determination of serum glucose levels is advisable.

The anephric patient poorly tolerates post-CPB hypervolemia associated with prolonged duration of CPB. Dialysis can be performed during CPB and is technically easy and effective because small molecules (uremic solutes, electrolytes) are removed.[351] Instead of dialysis during CPB, hemofiltration (ultrafiltration) is performed more frequently, effectively clearing excess water without the hemodynamic instability of dialysis. Circulating blood passes through the hollow fibers of the hemoconcentrators, which have a smaller pore size than albumin (55,000 daltons) that remove water and solutes. These midsize molecules (inflammatory molecules) are small enough to pass through the pores to concentrate the blood. Potassium is eliminated, helping reduce excessive potassium concentration commonly associated with cardioplegia administration. Hemofiltration during CPB may not achieve a net reduction in the overall total fluid balance of the patient, in part because a minimum volume of fluid must be maintained in the venous reservoir of the extracorporeal circuit but may be associated with earlier extubation after CPB.[352]

Excessive bleeding after CPB is not uncommon in those with CRF, in part because of preoperative platelet dysfunction. Antifibrinolytic medications are pharmacologic measures used to successfully reduce excessive bleeding and transfusion requirements associated with cardiac surgery.[58] Tranexamic acid, an inexpensive, synthetic antifibrinolytic, is excreted primarily through the kidneys, so a dose reduction will be required based on the preoperative creatinine level. A newer dosing regimen has been developed based on levels of tranexamic acid.[353] Aprotinin, a serine protease inhibitor with anti-inflammatory and antifibrinolytic properties, is concentrated in the proximal renal tubules. Recently, aprotinin was found to triple the risk for renal failure with dialysis compared with tranexamic acid and aminocaproic acid in patients undergoing CABG in an observational study involving more than 4000 patients.[354] This was followed by a randomized double-blind trial of patients undergoing cardiac surgery with either aprotinin, aminocaproic acid, or tranexamic acid that was halted before completion of enrollment because of the increase in mortality with aprotinin compared with the other lysine analog antifibrinolytic agents.[355] Although this trial did not find a statistically significant increase in renal failure or the need for renal replacement therapy, there was an increase in the number of patients who had their creatinine double. Ultimately, the U.S. Food and Drug Administration has removed aprotinin from clinical use.

After surgery, if dialysis is required in patients with end-stage renal disease, the risk for dialysis dependence is greatly increased.[349] If the patient is dialysis-dependent before surgery, dialysis usually is resumed within 24 to 48 hours of surgery and then according to the patient's preoperative routine to optimize fluid, electrolyte, and metabolic status. Dialysis may be needed soon after return from the operating room if mobilization of fluids into the intravascular space causes CHF. Hemodialysis primarily corrects electrolyte imbalances and removes organic acids to correct metabolic acidosis. Dialysis may lessen the platelet dysfunction associated with uremia to minimize hemostatic abnormalities and excessive hemorrhage. Peritoneal dialysis may be preferable if the postoperative hemodynamic status of the patient is unstable. Peritoneal dialysis, compared with hemodialysis, is more convenient to administer and does not require the immediate support of a nephrologist. However, continuous renal replacement therapy can be

TABLE 22-11	Commonly Used Muscle Relaxants and Renal Failure	
Relaxant	Acceptable	Renal Excretion
Atracurium	Yes	< 5%
Curare	Yes, with caution	60%
Cis-atracurium	Yes	< 10%
Doxacurium	Yes, with caution	70%
Gallamine	No	100%
Metocurine	Yes	50%
Pancuronium	Yes, with caution	70%
Pipecuronium	Yes, with caution	70%
Vecuronium	Yes	30%
Rocuronium	Yes	9%*
Mivacurium	Yes	7%†
Succinylcholine	Yes, with normokalemia	0%

Prolonged neuromuscular blockade has been reported.
*Data from Khuenl-Brady K, Castagnoli KP, Canfell PC, et al: The neuromuscular blocking effects and pharmacokinetics of ORG 9426 and ORG 9616 in the cat. Anesthesiology 72:669–674, 1990.
†Data from Cook DR, Freeman JA, Lai AA, et al: Pharmacokinetics of mivacurium in normal patients and in those with hepatic or renal failure. Br J Anaesth 69:580–585, 1992.
Adapted from Barash PG, Cullen BF, Stoelting RK, et al: Clinical Anesthesia. Philadelphia, 1989, JB Lippincott Company and Miller RD, Savarese JJ, et al: Pharmacology of muscle relaxants and their antagonists. In Miller RD (ed): Anesthesia. New York, 1990, Churchill Livingstone, pp 389–436, by permission.

instituted intraoperatively and postoperatively to manage acute renal failure with volume overload and metabolic instability with excellent results in cardiac patients after CPB.[356] Continuous renal replacement therapy has become popular in cardiac surgical patients since 2000 because the bedside nurse can direct the degree of fluid pull in response to the patient's changing hemodynamic status. Between 0.7% and 1.4% of patients undergoing cardiac surgery may require this transient form of therapy for renal failure.

Patients with CRF are at high risk for morbidity and mortality with cardiac surgery involving CPB. Attention to the following aspects may improve outcome: (1) conditions that are associated with CRF that lead to complications such as platelet function, lung function, and anemia must be assessed; (2) adequate RBC mass must be provided; (3) fluid and electrolyte care are extremely important, particularly after CPB; (4) hemofiltration; (5) blood conservation techniques and treatment of coagulopathy; (6) judicious use of dialysis; and (7) scrutiny for infections that patients with CRF are more susceptible to develop.

HEMATOLOGIC PROBLEMS IN PATIENTS UNDERGOING CARDIAC SURGERY

Anesthetic concerns for patients with hematologic problems who undergo cardiac surgery are further complicated by the stress CPB places on coagulation and oxygen-carrying systems. Hemophilia, cold agglutinins (CAs), sickle cell disease (SCD), antithrombin (AT) deficiency, and von Willebrand disease (vWD) are a few of the hematologic disorders that may require special consideration if CPB is used. In general, a multidisciplinary approach, including individuals with expertise in these areas, is helpful in providing optimal care with such rare conditions.

Hemophilia

In the 1940s and 1950s, the coagulation factors that separated hemophilia A (factor VIII [FVIII] deficiency) from hemophilia B (factor IX [FIX] deficiency) were identified. Before that discovery, hemophilia was a debilitating disease with a life expectancy of less than 20 years. Subsequently, improvements in FVIII therapy prolonged life, but the early factor concentrates were not virally safe, so that 60% to 95% of individuals with hemophilia beyond 8 years of age were infected with hepatitis C virus,[357] and eventually two thirds of individuals with hemophilia became infected with HIV.[358] Although life expectancy decreased to younger than 40 years temporarily,[359] new FVIII replacement therapy such as recombinant FVIII (rFVIII) greatly reduced viral transmission. The result was more autonomy for patients with hemophilia but prolonged their life beyond 50 years, ensuring that they will more likely experience age-related disorders such as coronary artery disease.

Hemophilia A is the third most common X-linked disorder, occurring in 1 in 5000 male births.[357] Hemophilia B, also known as Christmas disease, is also an X-linked disorder with one fourth the incidence of hemophilia A. FVIII is instrumental for a normally functioning clotting cascade. With a half-life of only 8 to 12 hours, FVIII and FIXa accelerate activation of factor X. Hemophilia, in its severe form, is characterized by spontaneous bleeding in joints and muscles. Hemophilia A and B are similar in presentation, course, and treatment. Treatment of hemophilia A and B primarily depends on replacement of FVIII or FIX, respectively. Preparations of rFVIII, developed in the 1990s, effectively control 80% of bleeding episodes with a single dose. Viral contamination essentially has been eliminated, so the incidence of inhibitors is no more likely than plasma-derived factors. Cardiac operations require more intense hemostasis than most other surgical and nonsurgical situations. This is exacerbated by the stress on the coagulation system and increased risk for excessive bleeding associated with cardiac surgery.[360]

Specific challenges are involved in undergoing cardiac surgery and CPB with hemophilia. Management is derived from case reports and series without randomized, prospective trials. Relatively few institutions have experience in performing cardiac surgery in those with hemophilia, so there is limited systematic information regarding optimal perioperative care. However, a recent study indicated similar outcomes in patients undergoing CPB with or without hemophilia.[361]

Preoperative assessment of the cardiac surgical patient with hemophilia must determine the severity of the patient's hemophilia by history and laboratory tests because perioperative bleeding is related to the degree of factor deficiency. Factor deficiency in hemophilia may range from factor levels of 6% to 30% with occasional symptoms. A factor level less than 1% with easy bleeding could become severe during surgery if factor activity remains less than 1%. Most patients arrive for surgery with a FVIII or FIX activity less than 5%. Although a factor level near 50% of normal is regarded as adequate to achieve noncardiac surgical hemostasis; hemostatic demand and associated coagulation abnormalities[360] with cardiac surgery and CPB will require a greater FVIII level.

Before surgery, FVIII activity should be 80% to 100% for cardiac surgery. The amount of factor replacement is estimated from the total fluid volume of the extracorporeal circuit (priming volume), plasma volume, and the desired factor activity. If the preoperative FVIII or FIX level determination is recent (morning of surgery), this value may be acceptable for determination of FVIII and FIX replacement for initiation of CPB. Otherwise, FVIII and FIX levels should be obtained before initiation of CPB. Replacement of FVIII or FIX during CPB may be achieved by intermittent bolus or continuous infusions, but the optimal factor activity for CPB has not been established. Based on hemodilution that typically occurs during CPB, 30% to 50% FVIII or FIX levels would be consistent with other coagulation factors during this period, but FVIII levels are difficult to obtain during CPB secondary to the high heparin dosing required. Consequently, a bolus of FVIII or FIX before the initiation of CPB is a consideration.

The disadvantage of bolus administration of factor replacement is the resulting high peak levels, but it ensures that trough levels will be adequate for hemostasis. Continuous infusions may preserve FVIII levels at a constant "safe" level to minimize bleeding.[362] Currently, few forms of rFVIII can be used for continuous infusions because of product instability. Depending on the bolus dose of rFVIII (50 IU/kg), a continuous infusion of 4 IU/k/hr may be infused for 72 hours to maintain FVIII activity greater than 100%.[363] It still is important to obtain FVIII or FIX levels after heparin neutralization to guide factor replacement, in combination with attempts to obtain hemostasis after CPB. FVIII levels after heparin neutralization and after surgery should approach 100% to reduce the risk for excessive bleeding. FVIII levels are helpful every other day for a period of 1 to 2 weeks while the chest tubes remain.[364] FVIII levels will vary tremendously because no treatment provides a sustained FVIII level with the diverse individual requirements and consumption of FVIII among cardiac surgical patients. A platelet antagonist like aspirin may be recommended to prevent thrombosis because of the excessive levels of FVIII that may occur during bolus dosing.[361]

Antifibrinolytic therapy has been used in patients with hemophilia to inhibit the normal clot lysing process. A recent study has demonstrated a hemostatic benefit with tranexamic acid for cardiac surgery and CPB.[361] Antifibrinolytic agents, tranexamic acid and epsilon-aminocaproic acid, are used prophylactically to reduce blood loss and transfusion requirements in cardiac surgery involving CPB.[58] Another antifibrinolytic, aprotinin, has been removed from clinical use because of increased risk for death compared with the other lysine analog antifibrinolytic agents.[354,355] Antifibrinolytics routinely are stopped 2 hours after arrival in the ICU, but some benefit has been seen by extending the duration of administration.[361] Serial thromboelastograph is useful if antifibrinolytics are going to be administered for an extended duration, with close inspection for hypercoagulable changes in the thromboelastograph shape. Additional methods and techniques for blood conservation should be considered to reduce the risk for bleeding and transfusion with hemophilia.

1-Desamino-8-d-arginine vasopressin (DDAVP), a vasopressin analog, has been used successfully in mild-to-moderate hemophilia A to decrease intraoperative transfusion requirements.[357,365,366] A rapid increase in all components of FVIII occurs after DDAVP administration, but FVIII level will decline by 50% ten hours after administration. The response of DDAVP depends on the resting FVIII level and hemostatic demand. If the patient with hemophilia possesses 5% to 20% procoagulant activity, he or she is more likely to respond to DDAVP, in contrast with those with severe FVIII deficiencies who will not respond to DDAVP.[366] The peak effect occurs 1 hour after an intravenous dose of 0.3 µg/kg is given. DDAVP may be given at 12- to 24- hour intervals, but tachyphylaxis is possible after multiple doses.

Therapy for hemophilia B has changed significantly with the availability of a concentrated purified rFIX. rFIX is not exposed to human or animal protein. Previously, individuals with hemophilia B were treated with plasma-derived products called *prothrombin complex concentrates* that contain factors IX, X, II, and VII. These active complexes have resulted in fatal thrombotic reactions because these active complexes are not normally generated or regulated by the coagulation pathway. Circulating FIX levels will not increase as much as FVIII after transfusion because FIX is distributed in both intravascular and extravascular spaces, unlike FVIII, so that the calculated dose must be doubled.[367] FIX activity of approximately 50% is adequate to achieve hemostasis yet minimize the risk for thrombotic complications[368]; however, others have recommended higher dosing to achieve 100% activity.[367,369] Recently, FIX product has been used successfully for continuous infusion for replacement therapy during CPB and cardiac surgery.[369] Typically, rFIX is given as a bolus once daily for surgery. Continuous infusion of rFIX has been shown recently to be effective in providing conditions for optimal hemostasis for cardiac surgery with CPB, as well as in reducing the overall amount of concentrate administered.[369] Furthermore, the occurrence of inhibitors with rFIX is rare but must be evaluated before treatment. rFIX concentrate is not licensed yet in the United States for continuous infusion. Recommended levels for perioperative FIX levels have not been established for cardiac surgical patients despite multiple case reports of effective and safe use in cardiac surgical patients. More information about dosing of rFIX is available.[369]

Antibodies to FVIII or FIX may occur in patients with hemophilia who have received replacement therapy. The incidence of FVIII or FIX inhibitors is 18% to 52% and 2% to 16% of the hemophilia population, respectively.[370,371] Inhibitors occur more often in patients receiving the purest replacement factors, which is a major concern for future replacement therapy with purer products.[372] The strength of the immune response is instrumental in the development of inhibitors. For example, HIV-positive patients with hemophilia do not develop FVIII inhibitors. The inhibitor titer will characterize the patients as mild or high responders. High responders are at great risk because the anamnestic response may generate very high antibody titers that can render factor replacement therapy totally ineffective hemostatically.[373] The problem with patients who develop inhibitors and require surgery is the inability to predict hemostasis at any point of the hospitalization.

Cardiac surgery has been successfully performed in patients with FVIII inhibitors.[374] Patients with low antibody titers often tolerate conventional concentrate infusion but require greater and more frequent dosages for efficacy. The defect in the intrinsic coagulation pathway must be bypassed and prothrombin complex concentrates given that contain activated forms of factors VII, IX, and X and are largely successful in achieving hemostasis in the presence of FVIII and FIX inhibitors.[358] Recently, a new rFVIIa has become available.[375] FVIIa appears to bind to tissue factor on the surface of the activated platelet to form complexes at the site of injury. This activates other coagulation intrinsic and extrinsic factors and platelets. It causes generation of thrombin and fibrin to create hemostasis. It is infused as a bolus, 90 to 120 µg/kg, and repeated at 3-hour intervals to a maximum of four times. In more than 1900 surgical and nonsurgical bleeding episodes in more than 400 patients with hemophilia A or B, FVIIa has been shown to be safe with more than 103 major operations and excellent results in 80% of cases.[376] A randomized, controlled trial in cardiac surgery with FVIIa has been performed in adults without hemophilia and showed reductions in allogeneic transfusions.[377]

Particular caution must be taken in managing the airway in patients with hemophilia to avoid any trauma-induced bleeding. Nonsteroidal pain medications may be counterproductive in these patients because of the effect on platelet function. Strict asepsis must be maintained because the immune system of these patients may be weak and extremely susceptible to bacterial and viral infections.

von Willebrand Disease

vWD is the most commonly inherited hemostatic abnormality, with a prevalence rate in the general population of 0.8%.[378] It is an autosomal dominant bleeding disorder caused by a deficiency and/or abnormality of von Willebrand factor (vWF). An acquired form of vWD is associated with various disease states and medications.[379] The nomenclature of vWF and FVIII complex have been standardized to resolve past confusion (Table 22-12).

vWF is a large, adhesive glycoprotein that is produced by vascular endothelial cells and megakaryocytes. It is found in platelet α-granules, plasma, and subendothelium. It circulates in blood as an array of multimers of various sizes. Large multimers have more binding sites for platelets; therefore, they augment platelet adhesion and aggregation. Each vWF subunit has a site for a platelet receptor to bind and the extracellular matrix component of the vessel wall to attach.[380] vWF has two major hemostatic functions: (1) a carrier protein and stabilizer for FVIII, and (2) mediation of platelet adhesion to injured sites.[381] It plays a crucial role in mediating platelet adhesion, platelet aggregation, and clotting during high shear conditions.[382] Patients with vWD have abnormalities of both vWF and FVIII. vWD is classified into three major types and four subtypes: I, II, and III (Table 22-13).[383] Individuals with type 1 and 2

TABLE 22-12	Recommended Nomenclature of Factor VIII/Von Willebrand Factor Complex
Factor VIII	
Protein	VIII
Antigen	VIII:Ag
Function	VIII:C
von Willebrand Factor	
Protein	vWF
Antigen	vWF:Ag
Function	vWF:RCo*

*Although not measuring "true" von Willebrand factor (vWF) activity, ristocetin cofactor activity is used as a surrogate test for vWF activity in vitro. This activity depends on both vWF level and multimeric structure.
From Castaman G, Rodeghiero F: Current management of von Willebrand's disease. *Drugs* 50:602, 1995.

TABLE 22-13	Classification of Von Willebrand Disease	
*New**	*Old**	*Characteristics*
1	I platelet normal, I platelet low, 1A, I-1, I-2, I-3	Partial quantitative deficiency of vWF
2A		Qualitative variants with decreased platelet-dependent function that is associated with the absence of high-molecular-weight vWF multimers
2B		Qualitative variants with increased affinity for platelet GPIb
2M		Qualitative variants with decreased platelet dependent function that is not caused by the absence of high-molecular-weight vWF multimers
2N		Qualitative variants with markedly decreased affinity for factor VIII
3		Virtually a complete deficiency of vWF

GPIb, glycoprotein receptor Ib; vWF, von Willebrand factor.
*Data from Castaman G, Rodeghiero F: Current management of von Willebrand's disease. *Drugs* 50:602–614, 1995.

vWD comprise 70% and 20% of people with vWD, respectively.[384] Type 3 vWD represents only 10% of individuals and is autosomal recessive. Type 3 vWD individuals are severely affected and present in a similar manner to individuals with hemophilia who have a very low FVIII activity (1% to 4%).

Erik von Willebrand first identified the abnormal bleeding time (BT) that characterized vWD. The laboratory diagnosis of vWD is complex because of the broad phenotypes that exist. No single laboratory test is diagnostic for vWD. The BT is sensitive for vWD, but it is prolonged in only 50% of individuals with type 1 vWD. It is markedly prolonged in type 3 vWD. The activated partial thromboplastin time is usually prolonged, but it is not a good screening test for vWD because FVIII activity, which affects the activated partial thromboplastin time, varies greatly in vWD. The ristocetin cofactor assay vWF:ristocetin cofactor (RCo), also known as the vWF activity, is the most sensitive and specific test for vWD and the single best test to identify vWD (Table 22-14).[384] It measures the ability of vWF to bind to glycoprotein Ib platelet receptors. The vWF antigen test measures the quantity of vWF protein, not functional activity. vWF multimers can be visualized by electrophoresis and establish the type of vWD by their presence or absence. FVIII activity frequently is low in vWD. In mild cases of vWD, activated partial thromboplastin time, FVIII, and BT may be normal with only slight decreases in the RCo and vWF antigen.[385] Factors such as age, estrogen levels, adrenergic stimulus, and inflammation can directly affect vWF levels and complicate laboratory evidence of vWD.

A complete medical history is important to complement laboratory testing. Family history is a sensitive indicator of vWD. Individuals with vWD frequently describe bleeding that is more mucosal in origin (epistaxis) compared with people with hemophilia. Medical history is important because routine laboratory screening may fail to detect vWD. Unlike hemophilia, patients with mild vWD may go unnoticed for years with unremarkable bleeding patterns and rarely need long-term prophylaxis. Variant forms of vWD further increase the possibility of missing the diagnosis. If undiagnosed, surgical bleeding may be severe, particularly if combined with ingestion of antiplatelet medications. Aspirin and anti-inflammatory medication consumption should be identified before surgery. It is important to question the patient individually to determine the severity of bleeding, because even within a family and with similar laboratory tests, there can be major differences in the bleeding tendencies.[379] It is the severity of bleeding that usually determines replacement therapy, instead of DDAVP or the use of antifibrinolytics.[386]

Because vWF has a dual role in hemostasis, correction of platelet vessel-wall interaction and deficiency of FVIII must be achieved with a prophylaxis regimen to undergo cardiac surgery requiring CPB. Correction of vWF deficiency may be accomplished by either facilitating vWF release from in vivo storage sites or administering exogenous components. Each type of vWD requires a specific therapeutic approach. Preoperative FVIII or RCo levels are recommended to optimize hemostatic capability for surgery. FVIII levels should be obtained intraoperatively and then once per day after surgery. Both FVIII and vWF levels will decrease on initiation of CPB, but vWF will subsequently increase as it is released from storage pools.[382] BT rarely is used anymore to guide therapy because its correlation with surgical hemostasis is poor.[386] FVIII level and vWF should be normalized intraoperatively and 7 to 10 days after surgery to reach effective hemostasis.[387] The reliability of guides to dosing with vWD is poor, and the achievement of hemostasis should be the catalyst for additional therapy.

DDAVP is a synthetic analog of the natural hormone vasopressin without the pressor effect. It is the first choice for treatment in vWD, but not all types of vWD respond to it. It is effective in type 1 vWD.[388] It is ill-advised in type 2B vWD because thrombocytopenia may result. It is useless in type 3 vWD because there are no stores of vWF to release.[389] DDAVP does not directly cause release of FVIII/vWF from the endothelial cell but stimulates monocytes to produce a substance that releases vWF. A response to DDAVP should occur in 30 minutes, with a threefold to eightfold increase in FVIII and vWF that may persist 8 to 10 hours.[388] Hemostasis may require one or two doses of DDAVP at least 12 hours apart. It is readily available, inexpensive, and has minimal risk for patients but may be contraindicated in those with atherosclerosis, CHF, or require diuretic therapy.[390] DDAVP is effective given in an intravenous, intranasal, or subcutaneous manner, but the intranasal preparation lacks predictability and strength of the intravenous preparation.[384] Intravenous dosing (0.3 µg/kg) requires 20 to 30 minutes to avoid a decline in mean arterial pressure of 15% to 20%. Tachyphylaxis may occur, with a 30% decrease in the effectiveness of the second dose if DDAVP is given more than once in each 24-hour period. For a majority of patients with mild vWD, DDAVP is effective and avoids exposure to plasma products. Adverse effects of DDAVP include facial flushing, headache, and fluid retention with hyponatremia. Reports of increased thrombosis with DDAVP are anecdotal.

Blood products should not be administered to patients with vWD unless other treatment is ineffective or contraindicated. Plasma-derived factor concentrates are the current standard for replacement therapy if the patient is unresponsive to DDAVP.[390] Factor concentrates in the past were not always effective in vWD because VWF:RCo was low and many of the hemostatically active vWF multimers were absent so that FVIII levels were adequately replenished, but platelet function was impaired. These commercially available concentrates contain large amounts of both vWF and FVIII but differ in their purification and pathogen removal and inactivation techniques. Consequently, there is broad variation in the ratio of vWF and FVIII in the products and their multimer compositions that are so important for effective hemostasis. The various types of products and their dosing recently were reviewed.[386,387,390] In general, the dosing is 60 to 80 IU/kg for a bolus dose of the factor concentrate to maintain hemostasis. The safety of these purified plasma-derived factor concentrates regarding viral transmission has been shown to be excellent (Table 22-15). An especially good product that contains a ratio of vWF:FVIII (2.4) is Haemate P/Humate-P. Clinicians must be cautious of the ratio of vWF:FVIII in the product and the type of the vWD to correctly treat the patient. The definitive amount of vWF or FVIII that is required to control bleeding for the optimal care is indeterminate. Platelet infusions should be considered in patients with type 3 vWD if bleeding persists after administration of replacement concentrates.

Antifibrinolytic agents should be considered in patients with vWD to reduce clot lysis. Tranexamic acid is the most common agent utilized, whereas aprotinin is no longer available.[355] As in hemophilia, inhibitors can occur in vWD causing life-threatening bleeding. Prothrombin-complex concentrates have been used to treat bleeding, but there is a risk for inducing a prothrombotic state and thrombosis in cardiac patients with mechanical valves[391] (see Chapters 30 and 31).

Antithrombin

AT and protein C are two primary inhibitors of coagulation. A delicate balance exists between the procoagulant system and the inhibitors of coagulation (Table 22-16). AT is the most abundant and important of the coagulation pathway inhibitors. The impact of deficiencies of AT and advisability of restoration of normal levels continues to evolve with respect to cardiac surgery.

TABLE 22-14	Patterns of Von Willebrand Disease			
Type	RIPA	Ristocetin cofactor	vWF antigen	Factor VIII
1	D	D	D	D
2A	D	D or DD	D or N	N or D
2B	I	D	D or N	N or D
2M	D	D or DD	D	N or D
2N	D	D or DD	D	N or D
3	DD	DD	DD	DD

D, decreased; I, increased; N, normal; RIPA, ristocetin-induced platelet aggregation; vWF, von Willebrand factor.

TABLE 22-15	Proposed Dosing and Plasma Levels of Factor VIII Coagulant Activity and von Willebrand Factor Ristocetin Cofactor during Invasive Procedures and Surgery						
			Target Levels (IU mL^{-1})				
			Perioperative		Postoperative		
Type of Procedure	Loading dose FVIII:C/VWF:RCo (IU mL^{-1})	No. of Infusions per Day	FVIII:C	VWF:RCo	FVIII:C	VWF:RCo	
Major	0.5–1.0	1–2	1.0	1.0	0.5	0.5	
Minor	0.2–0.5	1	0.5	0.5	0.3	0.3	

Figures should be adjusted according to frequent clinical observations during and after the procedure. Concomitant treatment with tranexamic acid can usually be recommended.
FVIII:C, factor VIII coagulant activity; VWF:RCo, von Willebrand factor ristocetin cofactor activity.
Reprinted from Berntorp E: Prophylaxis in von Willebrand disease. *Haemophilia* 14:47–53, 2008, by permission.

TABLE 22-16	Balance That Normally Exists between Prothrombotic and Antithrombotic Forces within the Circulation
Prothrombotic Factors	**Antithrombotic Factors**
Thrombin	Antithrombin
Factor Xa	Protein C
Factor VIIa	Protein S
Tissue factor	Heparin cofactor II
Activated platelets	TFPI
Perturbed endothelial cells	Thrombomodulin
Others	APC cofactor 2
	Others

APC, activated protein C; TFPI, tissue factor protein inhibitor.
From Blajchman MA: An overview of the mechanism of action of antithrombin and its inherited deficiency states. *Blood Coagul Fibrinolysis* 5(Suppl 1):S5, 1994, by permission.

AT is an α_2-globulin that is produced primarily in the liver. It binds thrombin, as well as other serine proteases, factors IX, X, XI, and XII, kallikrein, and plasmin irreversibly, which neutralizes their activity. However, only inhibition of thrombin and factor Xa by AT has physiologic and clinical significance.[392] AT deficiency may occur as a congenital or acquired deficiency. Acquired deficiencies are secondary to increased AT consumption, loss of AT from the intravascular compartment (renal failure, nephrotic syndrome), or liver disease (cirrhosis). A normal AT level is 80% to 120%, with activity less than 50% considered clinically important.[393]

Congenital deficiency of AT is the prototypical, hypercoagulable state produced by an imbalance of coagulation and fibrinolytic factors (Box 22-5). The prevalence is 1 in 2000 to 5000 persons.[394] Congenital AT deficiency is separated into four types (I-IV) based on the quantitative and qualitative defects of the AT molecule. It is transmitted in an

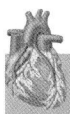

BOX 22-5. DISEASES OR SITUATIONS CAUSING INCREASED HEPARIN RESISTANCE

Infective endocarditis
Intra-aortic balloon counterpulsation
Hypereosinophilic syndrome
Oral contraceptives
Shock
Low-grade intravascular coagulation
Previous heparin therapy
Previous streptokinase
Presence of a clot within the body
Congenital antithrombin deficiency
Pregnancy
Neonatal respiratory distress syndrome
Increased platelet levels
Increased factor VIII levels
Secondary decrease in antithrombin levels
Ongoing clotting and utilization of heparin

From Anderson EF: Heparin resistance prior to cardiopulmonary bypass. *Anesthesiology* 64:504, 1986, by permission.

autosomal dominant pattern, with affected individuals typically maintaining 50% AT activity. If the levels decline to less than 50% activity, the risk for venous thrombosis is significant.[393] The only abnormal coagulation test associated with this condition is the assay for AT activity, which is diagnostic. Affected individuals may experience a thromboembolic event at an early age, but arterial thrombosis is encountered in less than 1% of persons.[395] The advisability of long-term anticoagulation is indeterminate in these individuals. Anticoagulation prophylaxis is recommended in cases in which the risk for thrombosis temporarily is increased, such as surgery.[396] The risk for thrombosis is greater in congenital forms than acquired forms of AT deficiency.[394,397]

In contrast with the rare case of congenital AT deficiency, acquired deficiencies of AT commonly are encountered in cardiac surgical patients. Anticoagulation with heparin for CPB depends on AT to inhibit clotting because heparin alone has no effect on coagulation. Heparin catalyzes AT inhibition of thrombin more than 1000-fold by binding to a lysine residue on AT and altering its conformation. Thrombin actually attacks AT, disabling it, but in the process attaches AT to thrombin, forming the AT and thrombin complex. This complex has no activity and rapidly is removed. Thirty percent of AT is consumed during this process, so AT levels are reduced temporarily. If AT levels are not restored, then a condition called *heparin resistance* may arise. The many causes of heparin resistance are listed in Box 22-5. Heparin resistance is defined as the failure of a specific heparin dose (300 to 400 U/kg) to prolong an activated coagulation time beyond 480 seconds in preparation for initiation of CPB. Failure to reach 480 seconds may be considered inadequate anticoagulation with risk for thrombus formation during CPB.

Heparin resistance is increasingly common in cardiac surgical practice today because heparin exposure before cardiac surgery is more common. Heparin resistance has been reported to occur in 3% to 13% of cardiac surgical patients. A recent randomized prospective study analyzing 2270 cardiac cases identified only 3.7% of patients to be heparin resistant.[398] It is uncommon to observe visible clot in the CPB circuit even with inadequate anticoagulation. However, inadequate anticoagulation during CPB will systematically activate the hemostatic and inflammatory systems generating thrombin, platelet and clotting factor consumption, and excessive fibrinolysis. This combination of physiologic processes places the patient at risk for both neurologic injury and excessive bleeding.

The importance of AT deficiency in heparin resistance has been demonstrated,[399,400] but it is not the only issue. Platelets, fibrin, vascular surfaces, and plasma proteins all interact to determine the anticoagulant effect of heparin. This is evident from a randomized, double-blind, placebo-controlled trial comparing treatments for heparin resistance.[399] Eleven patients remained heparin resistant despite FFP and AT administration. Similarly, adequate activated coagulation time values of 480 seconds were not achieved in 30% of patients even with 800 U/kg heparin.[401] Typically, with heparin resistance, 50% more heparin is given during CPB for anticoagulation. Unfortunately, aggressive heparin dosing in the midst of heparin resistance will further exacerbate a preoperative AT deficiency. On initiation of CPB, AT activity decreases by 25% to 50% secondary to dilution and elimination of the AT and thrombin complex.[394,397] Low levels of AT induce a prothrombotic environment conducive to thromboembolic behavior based partly on the occurrence of clotting in AT-deficient patients exposed to

CPB.[402] The mean baseline AT level of heparin-resistant patients is 56% ± 25%, which is consistent with previous studies.[398] AT levels may even decrease to less than 40% after deep hypothermic circulatory arrest and prolonged CPB compared with the average AT level identified as 82% before surgery in a recent trial.[403]

Heparin resistance was routinely treated with FFP for many years. However, a large disparity between AT levels after recombinant AT compared with FFP was noted in a prospective, randomized trial of recombinant AT or FFP for patients who were consistently defined as heparin resistant.[400] More recently, 2 units of FFP often failed to normalize AT levels in patients who were defined as heparin resistant.[404] A 75-μg/kg bolus dose of recombinant AT effectively has improved pre-CPB AT levels from 56% to 75% ± 31%.[398] The use of allogeneic blood products to treat AT deficiency should be discouraged.

In 1974, AT was isolated from human plasma and AT concentrates were discovered.[395] AT concentrate preparations are derived from human plasma pools but are subjected to fractionation procedures and heating to inactivate potential viral contaminants without reducing biologic activity.[397] Recombinant AT concentrates have been studied in cardiac surgical patients.[399,400,405] One bottle of AT is approximately 500 units and may be given over 10 to 20 minutes safely.[406] AT levels often are low before surgery for cardiac surgical patients, with a further decline because of CPB hemodilution and heparinization, leading to mean AT levels of 42% activity.[400] AT concentrates are beneficial in both hereditary and acquired AT deficiency.[394,395] The optimal AT level for CPB has not been defined, but a level greater than 80% is considered less likely to be associated with thrombus formation.

Inadequate anticoagulation during CPB will cause thrombin generation, leading to platelet activation and clotting factor consumption; however, definitive proof that AT supplementation will improve outcome is absent. AT supplementation has demonstrated reduced thrombin and fibrinolytic activity in patients undergoing CPB, based on statistically significant improvements in biochemical markers of hemostatic activation such as prothrombin fragment 1.2 concentrations, D-dimer concentration, and AT/thrombin complexes.[400,405,407] Unfortunately, clinical measures such as mediastinal chest tube drainage and transfusion requirements have been less consistent than biochemical measures.[397,398,400,405,407] Recently, AT supplementation was demonstrated to normalize thrombin generation with an in vitro preparation that used the plasma of five patients who had undergone prolonged CPB and deep hypothermic circulatory arrest to measure thrombin generation.[403] The addition of normal donor plasma or AT-deficient plasma to the test plasma resulted in excessive thrombin generation compared with control blood. It was only the pure AT concentrate that arrested thrombin formation, with the test plasma returning it to below baseline in the control plasma (Figure 22-49). Two studies have shown increased bleeding and transfusion requirements with AT levels less than 63%[408] and 58%.[401] However, to prove rare clinical end points with AT supplementation compared with placebo in prospective trials would be problematic.

The benefit of restoring AT levels may go beyond simple heparin responsiveness to an association with postoperative outcome. AT levels of 58% or less, obtained after cardiac surgery, in a prospective, observational study were found to be predictive of increased incidences of surgical reexploration, adverse neurologic outcome, thromboembolic events, and prolonged ICU duration.[401] Both duration of CPB and preoperative heparin use also were found to be associated with lower postoperative values of AT. Similarly, low preoperative AT levels were associated with lower postoperative AT levels, worse survival, and longer time to extubation, based on a retrospective analysis of cardiac surgical patients.[408] However, no conclusions can be made about AT supplementation until a prospective trial has been performed in

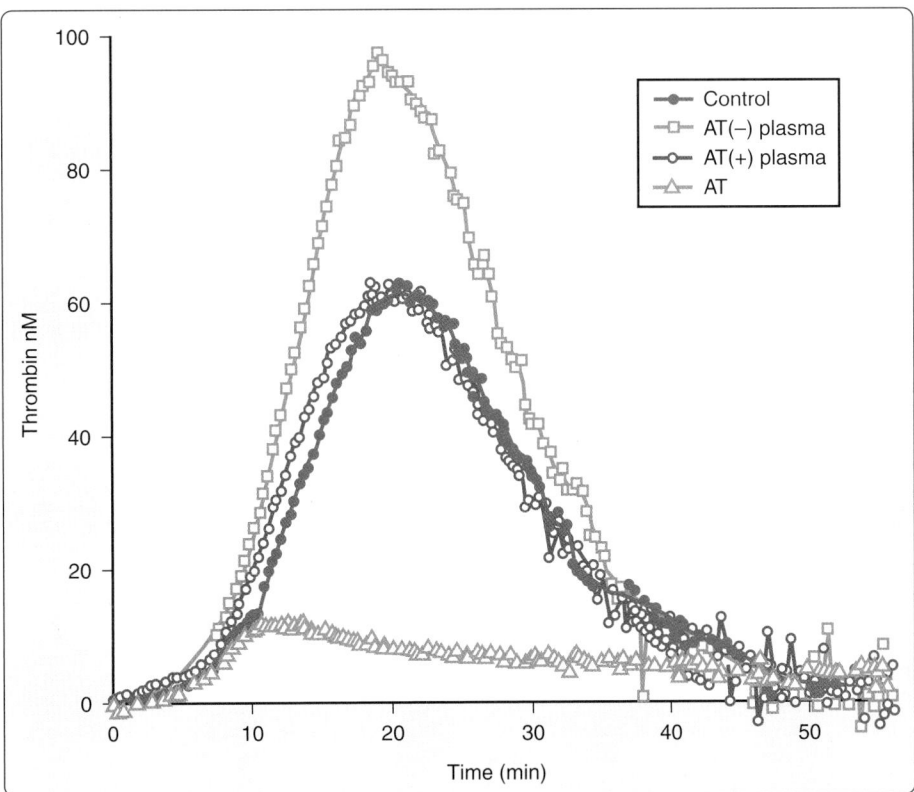

Figure 22-49 Thrombin generation in platelet-poor plasma after cardiopulmonary bypass (representative tracings of five experiments). *Filled circles* represent control (platelet-poor plasma only); *triangles* represent AT (platelet-poor plasma supplemented with antithrombin concentrate); *squares* represent AT(–) (platelet-poor plasma supplemented with antithrombin depleted plasma); *open circles* represent AT(+) (platelet-poor plasma supplemented with normal [non–AT-depleted] plasma). *(From Sniecinski R, Szlam F, Chen EP, et al: Antithrombin deficiency increases thrombin activity after prolonged cardiopulmonary bypass. Anesth Analg 106:713–718, 2008, by permission.)*

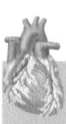

BOX 22-6. INDICATIONS FOR ANTITHROMBIN REPLACEMENT THERAPY

Approved Indications (clinical data suggest efficacy)
Congenital AT deficiency
Perioperative
Postsurgical prophylaxis for deep vein thrombosis
Acute thromboembolism
Pregnancy: delivery and abortion
Neonates with congenital AT deficiency*

Probable Indications (data suggest improvement in laboratory and clinical measures)
Neonates born to mothers with congenital AT deficiency or with strong family history of thrombosis
DIC caused by sepsis, trauma, burns, associated with pregnancy
Heparin resistance associated with low AT
Extracorporeal circulation (cardiopulmonary bypass, hemodialysis)
Hepatic artery thrombosis after OLT

Possible Indications (data suggest improvement in laboratory values without proven clinical efficacy)
VOD
OLT
LeVeen peritoneovenous shunt
Chronic hepatic insufficiency

Investigational Use
Nephrotic syndrome
AT deficiency because of gastrointestinal loss (inflammatory bowel disease, protein-losing enteropathy)
Pregnancy: preeclampsia, gestational hypertension, and acute fatty liver of pregnancy
Neonatal respiratory distress syndrome

AT, antithrombin; DIC, disseminated intravascular coagulation; OLT, orthotopic liver transplant; VOD, veno-occlusive disease.
From Bucur SZ, Levy JH, Despotis GJ, et al: Uses of antithrombin III concentrate in congenital and acquired deficiency states. *Transfusion* 38:482, 1998.

a blinded, randomized fashion to assess the value of AT. An excellent summary of trials evaluating the value of AT concentrate for prophylaxis regarding AT-deficient patients before surgery strongly recommended AT supplementation.[394] Other indications for AT are listed in Box 22-6. After surgery, AT levels will continue to decline at a rate dependent on the extent of tissue disruption and hemorrhage. The nadir occurs on the third day and preoperative levels return by the fifth day, so supplementation is not required after this time.

Cold Agglutinins

CAs are common but rarely clinically important. The incidence rate in cardiac surgical patients varies between 0.8% and 4%.[409] Often associated with lymphoreticular neoplasms, mycoplasma pneumonia, and infectious mononucleosis, they are IgM class autoantibodies directed against the RBC I-antigen or related antigens.[410] CAs form a complement antigen-antibody reaction on the surface of the RBC membrane that causes lysis. The degree of hemolysis is related to the circulating titer and thermal amplitude of the CAs.[411] Thermal amplitude, the blood temperature below which the CAs will react, is the key information to assign clinical relevance. The titer and thermal amplitude are determined at a range of temperatures in the serum by an indirect hemagglutination test. Most individuals have cold autoantibodies that react at 4° C but in very low titers. Accelerated destruction of RBCs occurs if the thermal amplitude is above 30° C. The more pathologic CAs have a higher thermal amplitude and higher titers at 30° C. From a pathologic standpoint, thermal amplitude is more important than titer. Pathologic CAs cause RBC clumping and vascular occlusion that injure the myocardium, liver, and kidney.[412] Microscopic RBC clumping may erroneously be attributed to other possibilities

during hypothermic CPB unless agglutination is observed. Some have reported visible agglutination in the cardioplegic line.[413] Increasing the temperature will rapidly inactivate CA.[414]

Blood banks routinely screen for the presence of autoantibodies at 37° C, but cold antibodies, only reactive at lower temperatures, are not detected. The significance of CA is determined by evaluating agglutination of RBCs in 20° C saline and 30° C albumin. If there is no agglutination, significant hemolysis is unlikely.[415] Before initiation of CPB, the titer and thermal amplitude of CA must be determined to avoid a temperature during CPB that would cause hemolysis. Intraoperatively, low-thermal-amplitude CA can be determined by mixing cold cardioplegia with some of the patient's blood to check for separation of cells. If there is concern about CA after routine testing, the sample also can be diluted to simulate CPB, cooled, and inspected for RBC agglutination. The occurrence of hemodilution commonly associated with CPB may weaken agglutination and hemolysis in a patient with high reactivity and titer of CA exposed to hypothermia.

Clinical suspicion is necessary to detect CA because there are many other explanations for hemolysis during CPB. Consequently, if CAs are suspected or identified before surgery, avoidance of hypothermia is the safest course. Despite normothermic CPB, cold cardioplegia may cause RBC agglutination in small myocardial vessels.[413] Evidence of CA also may manifest as incomplete cardioplegic delivery or high pressures in the CPB circuit.[416] Hypothermic myocardial protection has been used successfully in some patients with CA. A review of 832 patients scheduled to undergo surgery and CPB identified only seven cases of CA that were strongly positive at 4° C.[414] They concluded that asymptomatic patients with nonspecific, low-titer, and low-thermal-amplitude CAs may undergo hypothermia and CPB without serious detectable sequelae. However, the possibility of subtle end-organ damage exists.

If hypothermic CPB is necessary despite the presence of CA, the choices are preoperative plasmapheresis, hemodilution, and maintenance of CPB temperature above the CA thermal amplitude (Figure 22-50).[411,417] Cold cardioplegia may be used without first undergoing plasmapheresis if normothermic CPB is used and 37° C cardioplegic solution is injected before administration of 4° C cardioplegic solution, clearing all potentially reactive cells. The risk for hemolysis is still high in patients with high-thermal-amplitude CA. If CAs are particularly malignant, all the patient's blood from the venous reservoir is drained and discarded. It is replaced entirely by donor blood,[418] unfortunately exposing the patient to the risks of allogeneic blood products. Normothermic CPB and antegrade or retrograde warm blood cardioplegia may be the best option.[419] If CA should go undetected, postoperative end-organ damage or low CO may occur. Subsequently, plasma exchange, steroids, increased urine output, and maintenance of a good CO are recommended.[409]

All participants in the care of a patient with CA should be acutely aware of the potential risk to the patient of hypothermia. Anesthetic gases, intravenous fluids, blood, and plasma should be heated before administration to theses individuals. Operating room temperature should be warm. Washed RBCs may also be useful if transfusions of fresh components are necessary.[412]

Sickle Cell Disease

SCD is a heterogenous group of inherited disorders involving the sickle β-globin gene. Survival in SCD has improved because of early diagnosis, antibiotics, and supportive care; however, it remains an important health threat, particularly if major surgery is contemplated.[420] The median life expectancy in male and female African Americans with SCD is 42 and 48 years, respectively. Preparation and meticulous intraoperative care are imperative for the best results.

The β-globin gene has worldwide distribution but is found most often in West Central Africa. HbA and HbS genes have codominant expression, which allows both genes to be represented in the Hb molecule. One in 10 African Americans is a heterozygous carrier of the β-globin gene, referred to as sickle cell trait (AS), whereas the homozygous state, sickle cell anemia (SS), occurs in 1 of 400 African Americans.

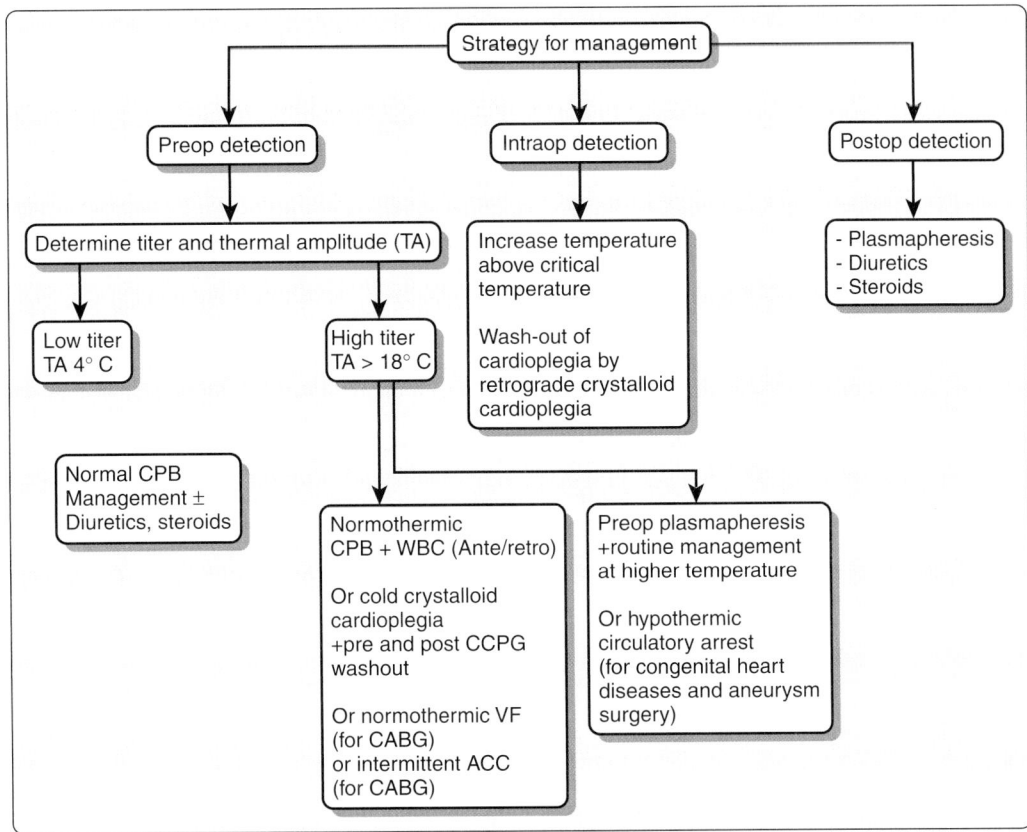

Figure 22-50 **Algorithm for CA management.** ACC, aortic cross-clamp; CABG, coronary artery bypass grafting; CCPG, cold crystalloid cardioplegia; CPB, cardiopulmonary bypass; Intraop, intraoperative; Postop, postoperative; Preop, preoperative; VF, ventricular fibrillation; WBC, warm blood cardioplegia. *(From Agarwal SK, Ghosh PK, Gupta D: Cardiac surgery and cold-reactive proteins. Ann Thorac Surg 60:1143, 1995, by permission.)*

The prevalence rate of SCD in African Americans is 0.2%. HbC disease (SC) occurs in approximately 2% of African Americans; SS accounts for 60% to 70% of SCD in the United States.

The β-globin gene has a mutation in the DNA that results in a substitution of the amino acid, valine, for glutamic acid in the β-globin chain that is responsible for normal Hb polymerization on deoxygenation. The mutated Hb molecule is less negatively charged than the normal Hb; therefore, as oxygen saturation approaches 85%, Hb tends to polymerize.[421] As the HbS comes out of solution and gels intracellularly, the RBC sickles (Figure 22-51). Sickling is a reversible change in the RBC shape. Desaturation is the primary stimulus for sickling. Besides desaturation, the risk for sickling is related to the amount of HbS in the RBC. AS individuals do not sickle until the oxygen saturation is less than 40% because their ratio of HbS to total Hb is low. Because SS and SC patients have significantly more HbS, they sickle at an oxygen saturation of 85%, typically the venous saturation. HbS is responsible for the major hallmarks of SCD: sickling, hemolytic anemia, and vaso-occlusive events.[420,422] Vaso-occlusive events are more likely because sickled RBCs have an increased affinity for the endothelial surface of blood vessels that markedly increases blood viscosity leading to stasis.[421,423] During a vaso-occlusive episode, the endothelium will produce activators such as endothelin that alter the endothelial surface and cause vasoconstriction and injury.

The clinical severity of SS, SC, and AS vary as a function of both inherited (thalassemia or fetal Hb) and acquired factors.[423] Patients with AS are asymptomatic unless they become profoundly hypoxic, acidotic, or hypothermic.[424] On the contrary, individuals with either SS or SC are chronically ill with a life-threatening illness. However, survival for individuals with SS is 95% at 20 years and even longer with SCD.[425] Individuals with SS usually are undersized, skeletally deformed because of bone marrow hyperplasia, and may be slightly jaundiced. They are chronically anemic with an Hb concentration often less than 8 g/dL.

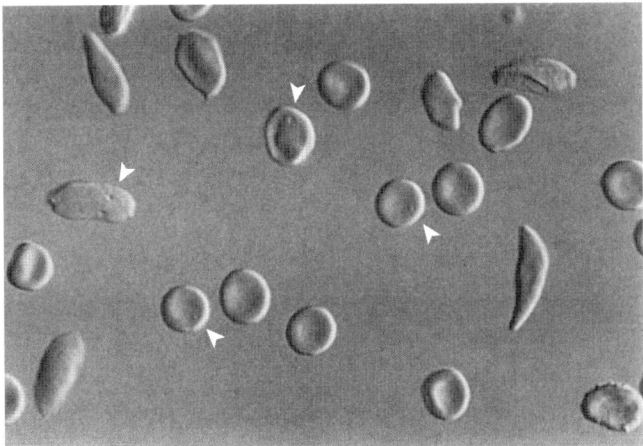

Figure 22-51 Use of the red cell pit count to assess splenic reticuloendothelial function. Erythrocytes from a child with sickle cell anemia were fixed in isotonic buffered glutaraldehyde and viewed by Nomarski differential interference contrast microscopy. The increased percentage of red cells with large endocytic vacuoles (pitted or pocked cells, *arrowheads*) indicates functional asplenia. *(From Lane PA: Sickle cell disease. Pediatr Clin North Am 43:639–644, 1996, by permission.)*

The RBCs are more fragile, with an RBC viability of 10% of normal accounting for chronic anemia. As a major site of sickling, the spleen eventually becomes nonfunctional; consequently, individuals with SS are extremely susceptible to infections, especially bacterial infections. Strict asepsis is important.

Three critical conditions may occur in those with SCD: painful crisis, aplastic crisis, and crisis affecting major organs. The painful crisis (sickle cell crisis) is a vaso-occlusive, infarctive process, resulting in tissue anoxia exemplified by pulmonary infarctions. Diagnosis is often one of exclusion. Vaso-occlusive crises primarily affect male patients 15 to 25 years of age. They are initiated by exertion, infection, dehydration, cold, acidosis, hypoxia, or vascular stasis.[426] The rheologic properties of the sickle RBCs combine with the tendency for adherence to the vessel wall to cause poor microvascular perfusion. Hydration with dextrose and water is important during a crisis so that free water may enter the cells to reduce the Hb concentration, but in this situation, blood transfusion is not helpful.[421] Aplastic crisis is much less common than painful crisis but is the most feared hematologic complication of SS. It is characterized by a precipitous decline in Hb secondary to hemolysis without the normal bone marrow response. In contrast with vaso-occlusive crisis, transfusion is not only helpful but essential. Aplastic crisis will last 7 to 10 days. Finally, various major organ systems such as the lungs (acute chest syndrome), spleen (splenic infarcts), kidneys, heart (myocardial dysfunction), and the central nervous system (stroke) are poorly perfused, causing permanent injury. Coronary artery occlusions are rare. Stroke is secondary to an intimal injury and thrombosis within the artery. Stroke occurs in about 8% of individuals with SS, and children are more likely affected. The lifetime chance of neurologic complications in those with SCD is 25%. Two thirds will have a subsequent stroke within 36 months.

Not all individuals with SCD have been identified before general anesthesia, and death has been the first manifestation of the disease.[427] Hb electrophoresis is the most accurate diagnostic test, but peripheral blood smears are not diagnostic. Hematologic consultation should be obtained in any person suspected to have SCD who is scheduled for any type of surgery or anesthesia. Patients with SS have been considered at increased risk for surgery, general anesthesia, and postoperative complications. Results from the Cooperative Study of SCD, which included 3765 SCD patients in 23 clinical centers across the United States, determined the overall mortality rate was 0.3%, with only 3 deaths related to anesthesia or surgery.[428] No deaths occurred in children younger than 14 years. Postoperative complications were variable and primarily related to the operative procedure. In spite of many different surgical procedures and anesthetics in this large multicenter study, there was a low mortality rate with few complications. Modern techniques and monitoring capabilities have enabled individuals with SCD to receive better care and outcome,[420] so surgery is a more viable option for consideration.

Before surgery, complete assessment of the cardiovascular system, specifically looking for myocardial ischemia, PAH,[429] and CHF is important in the individual anticipating cardiac surgery. It is estimated by echo that 20% to 30% of those with SCD have PAH, and its presence increases the risk for death. Problematically, autopsy series have shown that nearly one third of patients with SCD had pathologic evidence of PAH without a diagnosis. Until recently, PAH was thought to occur from a thrombotic or embolic cause, but now a precapillary form of PAH is evident.[429] Renal function is also likely to be abnormal.[430] Folic acid and careful intravenous hydration in the preoperative period reduce the risk for dehydration, hyperosmolality, and low urine output.[431] An increased incidence of pulmonary dysfunction in patients with SS increases the risk for hypoxia, so that preoperative sedation must be carefully titrated together with careful patient observation. The value of prophylactic antibiotics is indeterminate.

The role of preoperative transfusion in the management of patients with SS has been debated for years. The recommendation for preoperative RBC transfusion in patients with SS is based on a reduction in circulating concentration of HbS in an effort to improve oxygen-carrying capacity, suppress the erythropoietic drive, and shift the P_{50} to the left; nevertheless; the possibility of sickling is not eliminated.[423] A HbS less than 30% has been traditionally regarded as necessary for individuals to undergo surgery. A multicenter, randomized trial of 551 patients with SCD undergoing various noncardiac operations was conducted to verify this. Preoperative transfusion was designed with either a conservative or aggressive strategy to be evaluated according

to the incidence of perioperative complications.[432] The percentage of HbS in the patients managed conservatively was 60% compared with 30% for the aggressive strategy. The conservative strategy was associated with half as many transfusion-associated complications. This supports other work that found maintaining HbS at 50% instead of 30% was as effective in reducing the risk for stroke in nonsurgical situations.[433] For noncardiac surgery, there is growing evidence that dilution of sickle cells with transfusions should be limited,[428] and intraoperative transfusion should reflect standard transfusion guidelines.[420]

For initiation of CPB, 5% HbS often is recommended,[434] although an HbS of 30% appears suitable.[435] Currently, alternatives to allogeneic transfusion are few for CPB and cardiac surgery. Exchange transfusion has been used successfully to correct anemia before surgery with less risk of volume overload than simple transfusion.[436] It is important with the exchange transfusion for cardiac surgery to preserve the patient's platelets and plasma to be given after separation from CPB.[437] RBC transfusion alone increases blood viscosity more than exchange transfusion because a significant amount of HbS remains. There is concern that increased viscosity may temporarily negate an improvement in oxygen delivery corresponding to the presence of additional RBCs.[438] The lower blood viscosity and increased oxygen delivery to the tissues derived from the exchange transfusion probably are more efficient. Exchange transfusion has become routine before major surgery, but no prospective trials of exchange transfusion have been conducted to establish its value.

Anesthetic management of individuals with SCD has been reviewed.[424,431] The availability of blood must be established before any surgery because of the possibility of alloimmunization. The incidence of antibodies may approach 50%, with more than two thirds being Kell or Rh in SCD.[438] Antibodies may delay availability of blood and increase the chance of a delayed hemolytic transfusion reaction that can mimic a painful crisis. Therefore, any donor blood must be typed to ensure compatibility for ABO, Rh, and Kell antigens. Blood for transfusion should be less than 7 days old and warmed. Before induction of anesthesia, preoxygenation is essential. Maintenance of oxygenation throughout the operation is critical but in no way guarantees an uncomplicated course. Volatile agents are associated with less sickling.[423] Maintenance of perfusion to the major organs and peripherally is important to maintain normal acid-base status. The occurrence of hypotension is best treated initially with fluid administration to optimize volume status and avoid vasopressors. Renal dysfunction causes patients with SCD to concentrate urine poorly, so volume status is dynamic. Efforts should be made to maintain the patient normothermic. Intraoperative sickle crisis will occur sometimes despite the best care but poses a problem to diagnose during anesthesia. Signs of an intraoperative crisis include seizure, change in respiratory pattern, hypotension, or hematuria, but unfortunately are nonspecific and unreliable. Laboratory tests are not helpful either. Nothing pharmacologically, such as alkalinization of the blood or administration of urea, can reduce the tendency to sickle.[423]

CPB has been associated with significant morbidity and mortality in adults and children with SCD.[439] CPB imposes severe physiologic stresses such as low-flow states, circulatory arrest, aortic cross-clamping, mechanical destruction of blood elements, and protein denaturation that predispose the individual to a sickling crisis. There are no evidence-based guidelines for temperature, cardioplegia, priming solution, and transfusion practice during CPB.[440] The effect and safety of systemic and regional hypothermia (cardioplegia) in patients with SCD are indeterminate. In vitro, the solubility of deoxygenated HbS increases as the body temperature is decreased, which reduces sickling. However, decreased temperature increases blood viscosity. Viscosity increases by 30% when body temperature declines to 30° C.[431] The harmful effects of hypothermia may be primarily related to vasoconstriction and vascular stasis so that hypothermia may be tolerated if peripheral perfusion and oxygenation are good. Today, many patients undergo normothermic instead of hypothermic CPB because of advantages related to postoperative myocardial function.[441] Patients with either AS or SS have been cooled to 26° C or less without a sickling crisis, but partial or total exchange transfusion with a final HbS of 10% was performed in some of the patients.[440] Speculation is that because oxygenation during CPB is excellent during moderate hypothermia, sickling may be less common even without partial or full exchange transfusion.[422]

A reduction of HbS has been recommended before initiation of CPB. This can be accomplished by dilution with a nonsanguineous priming solution, a blood priming solution, cardioplegia, intravenous fluid, and simple transfusion or blood component sequestration. These measures decrease the percentage of HbS, but a significant number of RBCs remain at risk for sickling. Only a form of exchange transfusion removes sickled cells. Exchange transfusions are advisable if deliberate hypothermia is planned.[440] Automated RBC exchange can be done in the operating room or in the preoperative area. Intraoperative exchange can be performed more safely with the benefit of intraoperative monitoring to guide transfusion and avoid volume overload and possible cardiac decompensation in patients with serious cardiac conditions. In addition, with CPB, it is possible to drain blood from the CPB circuit. Another novel approach involves partial RBC removal with the autotransfusion device before CPB to decrease the percentage of HbS, followed by an acute one-volume whole-blood exchange during the initiation of CPB. The advantage is the procurement of a platelet-pheresed product with both techniques.[435] Another option is to use primarily allogeneic blood in the priming volume where, on initiation of CPB, venous blood is diverted to other reservoirs and the warmed blood in the priming volume reaches the patient, resulting in an HbS concentration less than 5%. The diverted blood may have the RBCs separated from the plasma and platelets and discarded while the remaining non-RBC components subsequently are infused. This process decreases blood product exposure and allows transfusion of normal donor blood. These techniques of blood component sequestration may eliminate the need for a hemapheresis procedure. It also can be used in patients with severe SCD who have a history of sickle crisis. Not everyone subscribes to the need for these measures with SCD. Metras et al[442] described 15 patients with SCD (13 with AS) who underwent cardiac surgery. None of the patients received preoperative exchange transfusions despite use of moderate hypothermia, aortic cross-clamping, and cold cardioplegia. There was no evidence of sickling or increased postoperative complications. The authors concluded that as long as hypoxia, acidosis, and dehydration are avoided, preoperative exchange transfusions or blood transfusions are not mandatory; however, they did not study the most severe cases of SCD (see Chapters 28 to 31).

The advisability of cell salvage techniques in SCD is questionable. Intraoperative autotransfusion has been condemned by those who claim an adverse effect on sickling, but it is supported by others.[443] The patient's percentage of HbS may influence how well intraoperative autotransfusion is tolerated. If intraoperative autotransfusion is used, recommendations are to exchange or transfuse to an HbS less than 40%, increase hematocrit to greater than 30%, and heparinize until harvesting. Solutions need a physiologic pH.[423]

Individuals with SCD are known to be at risk for a variety of thromboembolic complications such as stroke, MI, pulmonary embolism, and deep vein thrombosis. This may be important in terms of providing anticoagulation in patients for CPB. All aspects of hemostasis including platelet function, procoagulant proteins, anticoagulant proteins, and fibrinolytic systems are altered in the direction of procoagulation.[444] Chronic depletion of nitric oxide and arginine may also contribute to the hypercoagulable states in SCD. There is evidence that tissue factor expression on circulating endothelial cells may be abnormal, with a more procoagulant activity compared with individuals without SCD. There also is evidence of increased thrombin formation based on biochemical markers in SCD. Finally, some of the anticoagulant proteins such as proteins S and C are below normal levels. The impact on attempts to provide anticoagulation are not known, but it is important to carefully assess the procoagulant state of the patient

frequently during treatment of excessive bleeding to avoid increasing the risk for thrombotic complications after surgery. Empirical transfusion may lead to excess blood products after CPB, which may result in a procoagulant state, so algorithm-directed transfusion is advantageous.[445] The thromboelastogram especially is useful after CPB to determine whether the patient has developed a hypercoagulable state that may be detrimental to those with SCD (see Chapter 17).

In children undergoing CPB with SS, larger doses of fentanyl have been reported to attenuate stress during the surgery, especially intubation.[446] Also, nearly one third of SS patients will have PAH, and higher-dose fentanyl also will attenuate pulmonary vascular responses.[429] Early extubation after CABG has minimal risk (Box 22-7). However, it is important to review the patient's history regarding analgesia. Narcotic intolerance is common, so they may require more aggressive perioperative pain therapy.[447] Patients who return to surgery for any reason may be at increased risk for postoperative pneumonia. Acute chest syndrome may appear as pneumonia or mask true pneumonia. Acute chest syndrome has resulted in fatalities. Patients with AS are not at increased risk for postoperative complications.

ACKNOWLEDGMENTS

This chapter is dedicated to the memory of Dwight C. Legler, MD, who first authored this chapter. He is still sadly missed by all members of the Cardiovascular Division of the Department of Anesthesiology at the Mayo Clinic. Many thanks to Maria A. de Castro, MD, and Robert A. Strickland, MD, for their previous excellent contributions to this chapter.

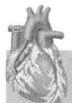

BOX 22-7. PROPOSED GUIDELINES FOR PERIOPERATIVE MANAGEMENT OF PATIENTS WITH SICKLE CELL DISORDERS UNDERGOING CORONARY ARTERY BYPASS GRAFTING SURGERY

Preoperative Period
Hb electrophoretic studies
Correction of any coexisting infection
Partial or complete exchange transfusions for patients with Hb SS
Light benzodiazepine premedication
Supplemental oxygen to avoid a decrease in oxygen saturation

Intraoperative Period
Preoxygenation for 3 to 5 minutes in all cases
Small dose of opioid and hypnotic induction
Inhaled or IV maintenance of anesthesia
Tepid or warm cardiopulmonary bypass
Mean pump flow > 50 mL $\cdot$ kg^{-1} $\cdot$ min^{-1}, perfusion pressure ≥ 60 mm Hg
Blood transfusion if hematocrit < 20%
Retransfusion of pump blood is not advisable

Postoperative Period
Early extubation within 2 to 6 hours
Maintenance of intravascular volume and body temperature
Avoidance of vasopressors is desirable
Early incentive spirometry
Multimodal approach to pain relief (opioids, NSAIDs, acetaminophen)
Warming blankets to maintain temperature ≥ 37° C
Shivering: meperidine, 10 to 25 mg IV
Routine antibiotic coverage for 2 days
Blood transfusion: Hb < 7.5 g/dL for those ≤ 70 years old; Hb < 8.5 g/dL for those > 70 years old
Close monitoring of oxygenation, perfusion, and acid-base indices for 12 to 24 hours

CABG, coronary artery bypass graft; Hb, hemoglobin; IV, intravenous; NSAID, nonsteroidal anti-inflammatory drug; SS, sickle cell anemia.
From Djaiani GN, Cheng DCH, Carroll JA, et al: Fast-track cardiac anesthesia in patients with sickle cell abnormalities. *Anesth Analg* 89:601, 1999.

REFERENCES

1. Reynen K: Frequency of primary tumors of the heart, *Am J Cardiol* 77:107, 1996.
2. Bakaeen FG, Reardon MJ, Coselli JS, et al: Surgical outcome in 85 patients with primary cardiac tumors, *Am J Surg* 186:641, 2003.
3. Reardon MJ, DeFelice CA, Sheinbaum R, et al: Cardiac autotransplant for surgical treatment of a malignant neoplasm, *Ann Thorac Surg* 67:1793, 1999.
4. Shapiro LM: Cardiac tumours: Diagnosis and management, *Heart* 85:218, 2001.
5. Maraj S, Pressman GS, Figueredo VM: Primary cardiac tumors, *Int J Cardiol* 133:152, 2009.
6. Borges AC, Witt C, Bartel T, et al: Preoperative two- and three-dimensional transesophageal echocardiographic assessment of heart tumors, *Ann Thorac Surg* 61:1163, 1996.
7. Elbardissi AW, Dearani JA, Daly RC, et al: Embolic potential of cardiac tumors and outcome after resection: A case-control study, *Stroke* 40:156, 2009.
8. Plana JC: Added value of real-time three-dimensional echocardiography in assessing cardiac masses, *Curr Cardiol Rep* 11:205, 2009.
9. Raaf HN, Raaf JH: Sarcomas related to the heart and vasculature, *Semin Surg Oncol* 10:374, 1994.
10. Wee JO, Sepic JD, Mihaljevic T, et al: Metastatic carcinoid tumor of the heart, *Ann Thorac Surg* 76:1721, 2003.
11. Klatt EC, Heitz DR: Cardiac metastases, *Cancer* 65:1456, 1990.
12. Elbardissi AW, Dearani JA, Daly RC, et al: Survival after resection of primary cardiac tumors: A 48-year experience, *Circulation* 118:S7, 2008.
13. Gowdamarajan A, Michler RE: Therapy for primary cardiac tumors: Is there a role for heart transplantation? *Curr Opin Cardiol* 15:121, 2000.
14. Grebenc ML, Rosado-de-Christenson ML, Green CE, et al: Cardiac myxoma: Imaging features in 83 patients, *Radiographics* 22:673, 2002.
15. Amano J, Kono T, Wada Y, et al: Cardiac myxoma: Its origin and tumor characteristics, *Ann Thorac Cardiovasc Surg* 9:215, 2003.
16. Pinede L, Duhaut P, Loire R: Clinical presentation of left atrial cardiac myxoma. A series of 112 consecutive cases, *Medicine* 80:159, 2001.
17. Percell RL Jr, Henning RJ, Siddique Patel M: Atrial myxoma: Case report and a review of the literature, *Heart Dis* 5:224, 2003.
18. Choi BW, Ryu SJ, Chang BC, et al: Myxoma attached to both atrial and ventricular sides of the mitral valve: Report of a case and review of 31 cases of mitral myxoma, *Int J Card Imaging* 17:411, 2001.
19. De Carli S, Sechi LA, Ciani R, et al: Right atrial myxoma with pulmonary embolism, *Cardiology* 84:368, 1994.
20. Shimono T, Makino S, Kanamori Y, et al: Left atrial myxomas. Using gross anatomic tumor types to determine clinical features and coronary angiographic findings, *Chest* 107:674, 1995.
21. Freedberg RS, Kronzon I, Rumancik WM, et al: The contribution of magnetic resonance imaging to the evaluation of intracardiac tumors diagnosed by echocardiography, *Circulation* 77:96, 1988.
22. Fyke FE 3rd, Seward JB, Edwards WD, et al: Primary cardiac tumors: Experience with 30 consecutive patients since the introduction of two-dimensional echocardiography, *J Am Coll Cardiol* 5:1465, 1985.
23. Padalino MA, Basso C, Moreolo GS, et al: Left atrial myxoma in a child: Case report and review of the literature, *Cardiovasc Pathol* 12:233, 2003.
24. Otto C: *Textbook of Clinical Echocardiography*, ed 3, Philadelphia, 2004, Saunders.
25. Colman T, de Ubago JL, Figueroa A, et al: Coronary arteriography and atrial thrombosis in mitral valve disease, *Am J Cardiol* 47:973, 1981.
26. Practice guidelines for perioperative transesophageal echocardiography: A report by the American Society of Anesthesiologists and the Society of Cardiovascular Anesthesiologists Task Force on Transesophageal Echocardiography, *Anesthesiology* 84:986, 1996.
27. Cooley DA: Surgical treatment of cardiac neoplasms: 32-year experience, *Thorac Cardiovasc Surg* 38(Suppl 2):176, 1990.
28. Gegouskov V, Kadner A, Engelberger L, et al: Papillary fibroelastoma of the heart, *Heart Surg Forum* 11:E333, 2008.
29. Koolbergen DR, Voigt P, Kolowca M, et al: Elective surgery for fibroelastoma of the aortic valve, *Ann Thorac Surg* 77:725, 2004.
30. Gowda RM, Khan IA, Nair CK, et al: Cardiac papillary fibroelastoma: A comprehensive analysis of 725 cases, *Am Heart J* 146:404, 2003.
31. Klarich KW, Enriquez-Sarano M, Gura GM, et al: Papillary fibroelastoma: Echocardiographic characteristics for diagnosis and pathologic correlation, *J Am Coll Cardiol* 30:784, 1997.
32. Nir A, Tajik AJ, Freeman WK, et al: Tuberous sclerosis and cardiac rhabdomyoma, *Am J Cardiol* 76:419, 1995.
33. Oh JK, Seward JB, Tajik AJ: *The Echo Manual*, ed 3, Philadelphia, 2006, Lippincott Williams & Wilkins.
34. Cho JM, Danielson GK, Puga FJ, et al: Surgical resection of ventricular cardiac fibromas: Early and late results, *Ann Thorac Surg* 76:1929, 2003.
35. Osranek M, Bursi F, Gura GM, et al: Echocardiographic features of pheochromocytoma of the heart, *Am J Cardiol* 91:640, 2003.
36. Soran PD, Akram S, Mihm F, et al: Unexpected findings during the anesthetic management of a patient with a cardiac paraganglioma, *J Cardiothorac Vasc Anesth* 22:570, 2008.
37. Van Braeckel P, Carlier S, Steelant PJ, et al: Perioperative management of phaeochromocytoma, *Acta Anaesthesiol Belg* 60:55, 2009.
38. Gowda RM, Khan IA: Clinical perspectives of primary cardiac lymphoma, *Angiology* 54:599, 2003.
39. Antoniades L, Eftychiou C, Petrou PM, et al: Primary cardiac lymphoma: Case report and brief review of the literature, *Echocardiography* 26:214, 2009.
40. Okamoto K, Kato S, Katsuki S, et al: Malignant fibrous histiocytoma of the heart: Case report and review of 46 cases in the literature, *Intern Med* 40:1222, 2001.
41. Bakke OM, Haram K, Lygre T, et al: Comparison of the placental transfer of thiopental and diazepam in caesarean section, *Eur J Clin Pharmacol* 21:221, 1981.
42. Kussman BD, Devavaram P, Hansen DD, et al: Anesthetic implications of primary cardiac tumors in infants and children, *J Cardiothorac Vasc Anesth* 16:582, 2002.
43. Bernheim AM, Connolly HM, Hobday TJ, et al: Carcinoid heart disease, *Prog Cardiovasc Dis* 49:439, 2007.
44. Bhattacharyya S, Toumpanakis C, Caplin ME, et al: Analysis of 150 patients with carcinoid syndrome seen in a single year at one institution in the first decade of the twenty-first century, *Am J Cardiol* 101:378, 2008.
45. Moller JE, Pellikka PA, Bernheim AM, et al: Prognosis of carcinoid heart disease: Analysis of 200 cases over two decades, *Circulation* 112:3320, 2005.
46. Robiolio PA, Rigolin VH, Wilson JS, et al: Carcinoid heart disease. Correlation of high serotonin levels with valvular abnormalities detected by cardiac catheterization and echocardiography, *Circulation* 92:790, 1995.
47. Simula DV, Edwards WD, Tazelaar HD, et al: Surgical pathology of carcinoid heart disease: A study of 139 valves from 75 patients spanning 20 years, *Mayo Clin Proc* 77:139, 2002.
48. Connolly HM: Carcinoid heart disease: medical and surgical considerations, *Cancer Control* 8:454, 2001.
49. Connolly HM, Schaff HV, Mullany CJ, et al: Carcinoid heart disease: Impact of pulmonary valve replacement in right ventricular function and remodeling, *Circulation* 106:I51, 2002.
50. Castillo JG, Filsoufi F, Rahmanian PB, et al: Early and late results of valvular surgery for carcinoid heart disease, *J Am Coll Cardiol* 51:1507, 2008.
51. Botero M, Fuchs R, Paulus DA, et al: Carcinoid heart disease: A case report and literature review, *J Clin Anesth* 14:57, 2002.
52. Neustein SM, Cohen E: Anesthesia for aortic and mitral valve replacement in a patient with carcinoid heart disease, *Anesthesiology* 82:1067, 1995.
53. Propst JW, Siegel LC, Stover EP: Anesthetic considerations for valve replacement surgery in a patient with carcinoid syndrome, *J Cardiothorac Vasc Anesth* 8:209, 1994.
54. Weingarten TN, Abel MD, Connolly HM, et al: Intraoperative management of patients with carcinoid heart disease having valvular surgery: A review of one hundred consecutive cases, *Anesth Analg* 105:1192, 2007.
55. Bhattacharyya S, Davar J, Dreyfus G, et al: Carcinoid heart disease, *Circulation* 116:2860, 2007.
56. Langer C, Piper C, Vogt J, et al: Atrial fibrillation in carcinoid heart disease: The role of serotonin. A review of the literature, *Clin Res Cardiol* 96:114, 2007.
57. Castillo JG, Filsoufi F, Adams DH, et al: Management of patients undergoing multivalvular surgery for carcinoid heart disease: The role of the anaesthetist, *Br J Anaesth* 101:618, 2008.
58. Ereth MH, Oliver WC Jr, Santrach PJ: Perioperative interventions to decrease transfusion of allogeneic blood products, *Mayo Clin Proc* 69:575, 1994.
59. Richardson P, McKenna W, Bristow M, et al: Report of the 1995 World Health Organization/International Society and Federation of Cardiology Task Force on the Definition and Classification of Cardiomyopathies, *Circulation* 93:841, 1996.
60. Codd MB, Sugrue DD, Gersh BJ, et al: Epidemiology of idiopathic dilated and hypertrophic cardiomyopathy. A population-based study in Olmsted County, Minnesota, 1975-1984, *Circulation* 80:564, 1989.
61. Felker GM, Thompson RE, Hare JM, et al: Underlying causes and long-term survival in patients with initially unexplained cardiomyopathy, *N Engl J Med* 342:1077, 2000.
62. Elliott P: Cardiomyopathy. Diagnosis and management of dilated cardiomyopathy, *Heart* 84:106, 2000.
63. Franz WM, Muller OJ, Katus HA: Cardiomyopathies: From genetics to the prospect of treatment, *Lancet* 358:1627, 2001.
64. Luk A, Ahn E, Soor GS, et al: Dilated cardiomyopathy: A review, *J Clin Pathol* 62:219, 2009.
65. Hershberger RE, Cowan J, Morales A, et al: Progress with genetic cardiomyopathies: Screening, counseling, and testing in dilated, hypertrophic, and arrhythmogenic right ventricular dysplasia/cardiomyopathy, *Circ Heart Fail* 2:253, 2009.
66. Givertz MM: Underlying causes and survival in patients with heart failure, *N Engl J Med* 342:1120, 2000.
67. Aleksova A, Sabbadini G, Merlo M, et al: Natural history of dilated cardiomyopathy: From asymptomatic left ventricular dysfunction to heart failure—a subgroup analysis from the Trieste Cardiomyopathy Registry, *J Cardiovasc Med* 10:699, 2009.
68. Bachinski LL, Roberts R: New theories. Causes of dilated cardiomyopathy, *Cardiol Clin* 16:603, 1998.
69. Leiden JM: The genetics of dilated cardiomyopathy—emerging clues to the puzzle, *N Engl J Med* 337:1080, 1997.
70. Park S-M, Park SW, Casaclang-Verzosa G, et al: Diastolic dysfunction and left atrial enlargement as contributing factors to functional mitral regurgitation in dilated cardiomyopathy: Data from the Acorn trial, *Am Heart J* 157:762.e3, 2009.
71. McBride BF, White CM: Acute decompensated heart failure: A contemporary approach to pharmacotherapeutic management, *Pharmacotherapy* 23:997, 2003.
72. Patterson JH, Adams KF Jr: Pathophysiology of heart failure: Changing perceptions, *Pharmacotherapy* 16:27S:1996.
73. Tang WH, Francis GS: Novel pharmacological treatments for heart failure, *Expert Opin Investig Drugs* 12:1791, 2003.
74. Siu SC, Sole MJ: Dilated cardiomyopathy, *Curr Opin Cardiol* 9:337, 1994.
75. Ng ACC, Sindone AP, Wong HSP, et al: Differences in management and outcome of ischemic and non-ischemic cardiomyopathy, *Int Cardiol* 129:198, 2008.
76. Koga Y, Toshima H, Tanaka M, et al: Therapeutic management of dilated cardiomyopathy, *Cardiovasc Drugs Ther* 8:83, 1994.
77. O'Connell JB, Moore CK, Waterer HC: Treatment of end stage dilated cardiomyopathy, *Br Heart J* 72(Suppl):S52, 1994.
78. De Keulenaer GW, Brutsaert DL: Dilated cardiomyopathy: Changing pathophysiological concepts and mechanisms of dysfunction, *J Card Surg* 14:64, 1999.
79. Pitt B, Zannad F, Remme WJ, et al: The effect of spironolactone on morbidity and mortality in patients with severe heart failure. Randomized Aldactone Evaluation Study Investigators, *N Engl J Med* 341:709, 1999.
80. Bristow MR, Ginsburg R, Minobe W, et al: Decreased catecholamine sensitivity and β-adrenergic receptor density in failing human hearts, *N Engl J Med* 307:205, 1982.
81. Waagstein F: The role of beta-blockers in dilated cardiomyopathy, *Curr Opin Cardiol* 10:322, 1995.
82. Kobayashi M, Izawa H, Cheng XW, et al: Dobutamine stress testing as a diagnostic tool for evaluation of myocardial contractile reserve in asymptomatic or mildly symptomatic patients with dilated cardiomyopathy, *JACC Cardiovasc Imaging* 1:718, 2008.
83. Anonymous: Effect of metoprolol CR/XL in chronic heart failure: Metoprolol CR/XL Randomised Intervention Trial in Congestive Heart Failure (MERIT-HF), *Lancet* 353:1999, 2001.
84. Borggrefe M, Block M, Breithardt G: Identification and management of the high risk patient with dilated cardiomyopathy, *Br Heart J* 72(Suppl):S42, 1994.
85. Brachmann J, Hilbel T, Grunig E, et al: Ventricular arrhythmias in dilated cardiomyopathy, *Pacing Clin Electrophysiol* 20:2714, 1997.
86. Nul DR, Doval HC, Grancelli HO, et al: Heart rate is a marker of amiodarone mortality reduction in severe heart failure. The GESICA-GEMA Investigators. Grupo de Estudio de la Sobrevida en la Insuficiencia Cardiaca en Argentina-Grupo de Estudios Multicentricos en Argentina, *J Am Coll Cardiol* 29:1199, 1997.
87. Connolly SJ, Hallstrom AP, Cappato R, et al: Meta-analysis of the implantable cardioverter defibrillator secondary prevention trials. AVID, CASH and CIDS studies. Antiarrhythmics vs Implantable Defibrillator study. Cardiac Arrest Study Hamburg. Canadian Implantable Defibrillator Study, *Eur Heart J* 21:2071, 2000.
88. Abraham WT: Cardiac resynchronization therapy for heart failure: Biventricular pacing and beyond, *Curr Opin Cardiol* 17:346, 2002.
89. Frazier OH, Rose EA, Oz MC, et al: Multicenter clinical evaluation of the HeartMate vented electric left ventricular assist system in patients awaiting heart transplantation, *J Thorac Cardiovasc Surg* 122:1186, 2001.
90. Romano MA, Bolling SF: Update on mitral repair in dilated cardiomyopathy, *J Card Surg* 19:396, 2004.
91. Tjang YS, van der Heijden G.J.M.G., Tenderich G, et al: Impact of recipient's age on heart transplantation outcome, *Ann Thorac Surg* 85:2051, 2008.
92. Di Donato M, Castelvecchio S, Kukulski T, et al: Surgical ventricular restoration: Left ventricular shape influence on cardiac function, clinical status, and survival, *Ann Thorac Surg* 87:455, 2009.

93. Wynands JE, Wong P, Whalley DG, et al: Oxygen-fentanyl anesthesia in patients with poor left ventricular function: Hemodynamics and plasma fentanyl concentrations, *Anesth Analg* 62:476, 1983.
94. Elliott P, O'Hare R, Bill KM, et al: Severe cardiovascular depression with remifentanil, *Anesth Analg* 91:58, 2000.
95. Wang JY, Winship SM, Thomas SD, et al: Induction of anaesthesia in patients with coronary artery disease: A comparison between sevoflurane-remifentanil and fentanyl-etomidate, *Anaesth Intensive Care* 27:363, 1999.
96. Sprung J, Ogletree-Hughes ML, Moravec CS: The effects of etomidate on the contractility of failing and nonfailing human heart muscle, *Anesth Analg* 91:68, 2000.
97. Stulz P, Schlapfer R, Feer R, et al: Decision making in the surgical treatment of massive pulmonary embolism, *Eur J Cardiothorac Surg* 8:188, 1994.
98. Syed MA, Masters RW, Zsigmond EK: Haemodynamic stability with midazolam-ketamine-sufentanil analgesia in cardiac surgical patients, *Can J Anaesth* 36:617, 1989.
99. Riou B, Viars P, Lecarpentier Y: Effects of ketamine on the cardiac papillary muscle of normal hamsters and those with cardiomyopathy, *Anesthesiology* 73:910, 1990.
100. Riou B, Lejay M, Lecarpentier Y, et al: Myocardial effects of propofol in hamsters with hypertrophic cardiomyopathy, *Anesthesiology* 82:566, 1995.
101. Vivien B, Hanouz JL, Gueugniaud PY, et al: Myocardial effects of halothane and isoflurane in hamsters with hypertrophic cardiomyopathy, *Anesthesiology* 87:1406, 1997.
102. Pagel PS, Lowe D, Hettrick DA, et al: Isoflurane, but not halothane improves indices of diastolic performance in dogs with rapid ventricular, pacing-induced cardiomyopathy, *Anesthesiology* 85:644, 1996.
103. Vivien B, Hanouz JL, Gueugniaud PY, et al: Myocardial effects of desflurane in hamsters with hypertrophic cardiomyopathy, *Anesthesiology* 89:1191, 1998.
104. De Hert SG, Van der Linden PJ, ten Broecke PW, et al: Effects of desflurane and sevoflurane on length-dependent regulation of myocardial function in coronary surgery patients, *Anesthesiology* 95:357, 2001.
105. Stevenson LW, Perloff JK: The dilated cardiomyopathies: Clinical aspects, *Cardiol Clin* 6:187, 1988.
106. Hamilton MA, Stevenson LW, Child JS, et al: Sustained reduction in valvular regurgitation and atrial volumes with tailored vasodilator therapy in advanced congestive heart failure secondary to dilated (ischemic or idiopathic) cardiomyopathy, *Am J Cardiol* 67:259, 1991.
107. Toller WG, Stranz C: Levosimendan, a new inotropic and vasodilator agent, *Anesthesiology* 104:556, 2006.
108. Rooney RT, Marijic J, Stommel KA, et al: Additive cardiac depression by volatile anesthetics in isolated hearts after chronic amiodarone treatment, *Anesth Analg* 80:917, 1995.
109. Range FT, Paul M, Schafers KP, et al: Myocardial perfusion in nonischemic dilated cardiomyopathy with and without atrial fibrillation, *J Nucl Med* 50:390, 2009.
110. Maron BJ: Hypertrophic cardiomyopathy: A systematic review, *JAMA* 287:1308, 2002.
111. Maron BJ, McKenna WJ, Danielson GK, et al: American College of Cardiology/European Society of Cardiology clinical expert consensus document on hypertrophic cardiomyopathy. A report of the American College of Cardiology Foundation Task Force on Clinical Expert Consensus Documents and the European Society of Cardiology Committee for Practice Guidelines, *J Am Coll Cardiol* 42:1687, 2003.
112. Roberts R, Sigwart U: New concepts in hypertrophic cardiomyopathies, part I, *Circulation* 104:2113, 2001.
113. Maron MS, Olivotto I, Zenovich AG, et al: Hypertrophic cardiomyopathy is predominantly a disease of left ventricular outflow tract obstruction, *Circulation* 114:2232, 2006.
114. Ommen SR, Park SH, Click RL, et al: Impact of intraoperative transesophageal echocardiography in the surgical management of hypertrophic cardiomyopathy, *Am J Cardiol* 90:1022, 2002.
115. Cannon RO 3rd, Dilsizian V, O'Gara PT, et al: Myocardial metabolic, hemodynamic, and electrocardiographic significance of reversible thallium-201 abnormalities in hypertrophic cardiomyopathy, *Circulation* 83:1660, 1991.
116. Knaapen P, Germans T, Camici PG, et al: Determinants of coronary microvascular dysfunction in symptomatic hypertrophic cardiomyopathy, *Am J Physiol Heart Circ Physiol* 294:H986, 2008.
117. Camici P, Chiriatti G, Lorenzoni R, et al: Coronary vasodilation is impaired in both hypertrophied and nonhypertrophied myocardium of patients with hypertrophic cardiomyopathy: A study with nitrogen-13 ammonia and positron emission tomography, *J Am Coll Cardiol* 17:879, 1991.
118. Ommen SR, Shah PM, Tajik AJ: Left ventricular outflow tract obstruction in hypertrophic cardiomyopathy: Past, present and future, *Heart* 94:1276, 2008.
119. Kern MJ, Deligonul U: Interpretation of cardiac pathophysiology from pressure waveform analysis: III. Intraventricular pressure gradients, *Cathet Cardiovasc Diagn* 22:145, 1991.
120. Maron MS, Olivotto I, Betocchi S, et al: Effect of left ventricular outflow tract obstruction on clinical outcome in hypertrophic cardiomyopathy, *N Engl J Med* 348:295, 2003.
121. Hagege AA, Desnos M: New trends in treatment of hypertrophic cardiomyopathy, *Arch Cardiovasc Dis* 102:441, 2009.
122. Maron BJ, Shen WK, Link MS, et al: Efficacy of implantable cardioverter-defibrillators for the prevention of sudden death in patients with hypertrophic cardiomyopathy, *N Engl J Med* 342:365, 2000.
123. Chang AC, McAreavey D, Fananapazir L: Identification of patients with hypertrophic cardiomyopathy at high risk for sudden death, *Curr Opin Cardiol* 10:9, 1995.
124. Maron BJ: Risk stratification and prevention of sudden death in hypertrophic cardiomyopathy, *Cardiol Rev* 10:173, 2002.
125. Dilsizian V, Bonow RO, Epstein SE, et al: Myocardial ischemia detected by thallium scintigraphy is frequently related to cardiac arrest and syncope in young patientss with hypertrophic cardiomyopathy, *J Am Coll Cardiol* 22:796, 1993.
126. Brown ML, Schaff HV: Surgical management of obstructive hypertrophic cardiomyopathy: The gold standard, *Expert Rev Cardiovasc Ther* 6:715, 2008.
127. Ommen SR, Maron BJ, Olivotto I, et al: Long term effects of surgical septal myectomy on survival in patients with obstructive hypertrophic cardiomyopathy, *J Am Coll Cardiol* 46:470, 2005.
128. Melacini P, Maron BJ, Bobbo F, et al: Evidence that pharmacological strategies lack efficacy for the prevention of sudden death in hypertrophic cardiomyopathy, *Heart* 93:708, 2007.
129. Anonymous: A comparison of antiarrhythmic-drug therapy with implantable defibrillators in patients resuscitated from near-fatal ventricular arrhythmias. The Antiarrhythmics versus Implantable Defibrillators (AVID) Investigators, *N Engl J Med* 337:1576, 1997.
130. Lin G, Nishimura RA, Gersh BJ, et al: Device complications and inappropriate implantable cardioverter defibrillator shocks in patients with hypertrophic cardiomyopathy, *Heart* 95:709, 2009.
131. Fifer MA, Vlahakes GJ: Management of symptoms in hypertrophic cardiomyopathy, *Circulation* 117:429, 2008.
132. Brown ML, Schaff HV: Surgical management of hypertrophic cardiomyopathy in 2007: What is new? *World J Surg* 32:350, 2008.
133. Sherrid MV, Chaudhry FA, Swistel DG: Obstructive hypertrophic cardiomyopathy: Echocardiography, pathophysiology, and the continuing evolution of surgery for obstruction, *Ann Thorac Surg* 75:620, 2003.
134. Minakata K, Dearani JA, Nishimura RA, et al: Extended septal myectomy for hypertrophic obstructive cardiomyopathy with anomalous mitral papillary muscles or chordae, *J Thorac Cardiovasc Surg* 127:481, 2004.
135. Wan CKN, Dearani JA, Sundt TM 3rd, et al: What is the best surgical treatment for obstructive hypertrophic cardiomyopathy and degenerative mitral regurgitation? *Ann Thorac Surg* 88:727, 2009.
136. Louie EK, Edwards LC III: Hypertrophic cardiomyopathy, *Prog Cardiovasc Dis* 36:275, 1994.
137. Deb SJ, Schaff HV, Dearani JA, et al: Septal myectomy results in regression of left ventricular hypertrophy in patients with hypertrophic obstructive cardiomyopathy, *Ann Thorac Surg* 78:2118 2004.
138. Biagini E, Spirito P, Leone O, et al: Heart transplantation in hypertrophic cardiomyopathy, *Am J Cardiol* 101:387, 2008.
139. Nishimura RA, Trusty JM, Hayes DL, et al: Dual-chamber pacing for hypertrophic cardiomyopathy: A randomized, double-blind, crossover trial, *J Am Coll Cardiol* 29:435, 1997.
140. Sigwart U: Non-surgical myocardial reduction for hypertrophic obstructive cardiomyopathy, *Lancet* 346:211, 1995.
141. Alam M, Dokainish H, Lakkis N: Alcohol septal ablation for hypertrophic obstructive cardiomyopathy: A systematic review of published studies, *J Interv Cardiol* 19:319, 2005.
142. Nagueh SF, Buergler JM, Quinones MA, et al: Outcome of surgical myectomy after unsuccessful alcohol septal ablation for the treatment of patients with hypertrophic obstructive cardiomyopathy, *J Am Coll Cardiol* 50:795, 2007.
143. Nishimura RA, Holmes DR Jr: Clinical practice. Hypertrophic obstructive cardiomyopathy, [erratum appears in *N Engl J Med* 2004 Sep 2;351(10):1038], *N Engl J Med* 350:1320, 2004.
144. Bell MD, Goodchild CS: Hypertrophic obstructive cardiomyopathy in combination with a prolapsing mitral valve. Anaesthesia for surgical correction with propofol, *Anaesthesia* 44:409, 1989.
145. Searle NR, Sahab P: Propofol in patients with cardiac disease, *Can J Anaesth* 40:730, 1993.
146. Stewart JT, McKenna WJ: Management of arrhythmias in hypertrophic cardiomyopathy, *Cardiovasc Drugs Ther* 8:95, 1994.
147. Wigle ED, Rakowski H, Kimball BP, et al: Hypertrophic cardiomyopathy. Clinical spectrum and treatment, *Circulation* 92:1680, 1995.
148. Stollberger C, Finsterer J: Extracardiac medical and neuromuscular implications in restrictive cardiomyopathy, *Clin Cardiol* 30:375, 2007.
149. Mogensen J, Arbustini E: Restrictive cardiomyopathy, *Curr Opin Cardiol* 24:214, 2009.
150. Ammash NM, Seward JB, Bailey KR, et al: Clinical profile and outcome of idiopathic restrictive cardiomyopathy, *Circulation* 101:2490, 2000.
151. Kabbani SS, LeWinter MM: Diastolic heart failure. Constrictive, restrictive, and pericardial, *Cardiol Clin* 18:501, 2000.
152. Kushwaha SS, Fallon JT, Fuster V: Restrictive cardiomyopathy, *N Engl J Med* 336:267, 1997.
153. Wilmshurst PT, Katritsis D: Restrictive cardiomyopathy, *Br Heart J* 63:323, 1990.
154. Tam JW, Shaikh N, Sutherland E: Echocardiographic assessment of patients with hypertrophic and restrictive cardiomyopathy: Imaging and echocardiography, *Curr Opin Cardiol* 17:470, 2002.
155. McCall R, Stoodley PW, Richards DAB, et al: Restrictive cardiomyopathy versus constrictive pericarditis: Making the distinction using tissue Doppler imaging, *Eur J Echocardiogr* 9:591, 2008.
156. Talreja DR, Nishimura RA, Oh JK, et al: Constrictive pericarditis in the modern era: Novel criteria for diagnosis in the cardiac catheterization laboratory, *J Am Coll Cardiol* 51:315, 2008.
157. Seifert FC, Miller DC, Oesterle SN, et al: Surgical treatment of constrictive pericarditis: Analysis of outcome diagnostic error, *Circulation* 72(Suppl 2):II–264, 1985.
158. Chatterjee K, Alpert J: Constrictive pericarditis and restrictive cardiomyopathy: Similarities and differences, *Heart Fail Monit* 3:118, 2003.
159. Metras D, Coulibaly AO, Ouattara K: Surgical treatment of endomyocardial fibrosis: Results in 55 patients, *Circulation* 72(Suppl II):II, 1985.
160. El Demellawy D, Nasr A, Aloawmi S: An updated review on the clinicopathologic aspects of arrhythmogenic right ventricular cardiomyopathy, *Am J Forensic Med Pathol* 30:78, 2009.
161. Fontaine G, Gallais Y, Fornes P, et al: Arrhythmogenic right ventricular dysplasia/cardiomyopathy, *Anesthesiology* 95:250, 2001.
162. Houfani B, Meyer P, Merckx J, et al: Postoperative sudden death in two adolescents with myelomeningocele and unrecognized arrhythmogenic right ventricular dysplasia, *Anesthesiology* 95:257, 2001.
163. Marcus FI, Zareba W, Calkins H, et al: Arrhythmogenic right ventricular cardiomyopathy/dysplasia clinical presentation and diagnostic evaluation: Results from the North American Multidisciplinary Study, *Heart Rhythm* 6:984, 2009.
164. Hamid MS, Norman M, Quraishi A, et al: Prospective evaluation of relatives for familial arrhythmogenic right ventricular cardiomyopathy/dysplasia reveals a need to broaden diagnostic criteria, *J Am Coll Cardiol* 40:1445, 2002.
165. Sen-Chowdhry S, Syrris P, Ward D, et al: Clinical and genetic characterization of families with arrhythmogenic right ventricular dysplasia/cardiomyopathy provides novel insights into patterns of disease expression, *Circulation* 115:1710, 2007.
166. Corrado D, Basso C, Thiene G, et al: Spectrum of clinicopathologic manifestations of arrhythmogenic right ventricular cardiomyopathy/dysplasia: A multicenter study, *J Am Coll Cardiol* 30:1512, 1997.
167. Yoerger DM, Marcus F, Sherrill D, et al: Echocardiographic findings in patients meeting task force criteria for arrhythmogenic right ventricular dysplasia: New insights from the multidisciplinary study of right ventricular dysplasia, *J Am Coll Cardiol* 45:860, 2005.
168. Tops LF, Prakasa K, Tandri H, et al: Prevalence and pathophysiologic attributes of ventricular dyssynchrony in arrhythmogenic right ventricular dysplasia/cardiomyopathy, *J Am Coll Cardiol* 54:445, 2009.
169. Asimaki A, Tandri H, Huang H, et al: A new diagnostic test for arrhythmogenic right ventricular cardiomyopathy, *N Engl J Med* 360:1075, 2009.
170. Link MS, Wang PJ, Haugh CJ, et al: Arrhythmogenic right ventricular dysplasia: Clinical results with implantable cardioverter defibrillators, *J Interv Card Electrophysiol* 1:41, 1997.
171. Barlow JB, Pocock WA: The significance of late systolic murmurs and mid-late systolic clicks, *Am Heart J* 66:443, 1963.
172. Weisse AB: Mitral valve prolapse: Now you see it; now you don't: Recalling the discovery, rise and decline of a diagnosis, *Am J Cardiol* 99:129, 2007.
173. Levine RA, Handschumacher MD, Sanfilippo AJ, et al: Three-dimensional echocardiographic reconstruction of the mitral valve, with implications for the diagnosis of mitral valve prolapse, *Circulation* 80:589, 1989.
174. Anyanwu AC, Adams DH: Etiologic classification of degenerative mitral valve disease: Barlow's disease and fibroelastic deficiency, *Semin Thorac Cardiovasc Surg* 19:90, 2007.
175. Hayek E, Gring CN, Griffin BP: Mitral valve prolapse, *Lancet* 365:507, 2005.
176. Hanson EW, Neerhut RK, Lynch C 3rd: Mitral valve prolapse, *Anesthesiology* 85:178, 1996.
177. Devereux RB: Recent developments in the diagnosis and management of mitral valve prolapse, *Curr Opin Cardiol* 10:107, 1995.
178. Zuppiroli A, Rinaldi M, Kramer-Fox R, et al: Natural history of mitral valve prolapse, *Am J Cardiol* 75:1028, 1995.
179. Flameng W, Meuris B, Herijgers P, et al: Durability of mitral valve repair in Barlow disease versus fibroelastic deficiency, *J Thorac Cardiovasc Surg* 135:274, 2008.
180. Enriquez-Sarano M, Schaff HV, Orszulak TA, et al: Valve repair improves the outcome of surgery for mitral regurgitation. A multivariate analysis, *Circulation* 91:1022, 1995.
181. Handa N, Schaff HV, Morris JJ, et al: Outcome of valve repair and the Cox maze procedure for mitral regurgitation and associated atrial fibrillation, *J Thorac Cardiovasc Surg* 118:628, 1999.

182. Sakamoto Y, Hashimoto K, Okuyama H, et al: Long-term assessment of mitral valve reconstruction with resection of the leaflets: Triangular and quadrangular resection, *Ann Thorac Surg* 79:475, 2005.
183. David TE, Ivanov J, Armstrong S, et al: Late outcomes of mitral valve repair for floppy valves: Implications for asymptomatic patients, *J Thorac Cardiovasc Surg* 125:1143, 2003.
184. Mohty D, Orszulak TA, Schaff HV, et al: Very long-term survival and durability of mitral valve repair for mitral valve prolapse, *Circulation* 104:I1, 2001.
185. Jokinen JJ, Hippelainen MJ, Pitkanen OA, et al: Mitral valve replacement versus repair: Propensity-adjusted survival and quality-of-life analysis, *Ann Thorac Surg* 84:451, 2007.
186. Rodriguez E, Nifong LW, Chu MWA, et al: Robotic mitral valve repair for anterior leaflet and bileaflet prolapse, *Ann Thorac Surg* 85:438, 2008.
187. Levy S: Arrhythmias in the mitral valve prolapse syndrome: Clinical significance and management, *Pacing Clin Electrophysiol* 15:1080, 1992.
188. Digeos-Hasnier S, Copie X, Paziaud O, et al: Abnormalities of ventricular repolarization in mitral valve prolapse, *Ann Noninvasive Electrocardiol* 10:297, 2005.
189. Kligfield P, Hochreiter C, Kramer H, et al: Complex arrhythmias in mitral regurgitation with and without mitral valve prolapse: Contrast to arrhythmias in mitral valve prolapse without mitral regurgitation, *Am J Cardiol* 55:1545, 1985.
190. Vohra J, Sathe S, Warren R, et al: Malignant ventricular arrhythmias in patients with mitral valve prolapse and mild mitral regurgitation, *Pacing Clin Electrophysiol* 16:387, 1993.
191. Orencia AJ, Petty GW, Khandheria BK, et al: Risk of stroke with mitral valve prolapse in population-based cohort study, *Stroke* 26:7, 1995.
192. Avierinos J-F, Brown RD, Foley DA, et al: Cerebral ischemic events after diagnosis of mitral valve prolapse: A community-based study of incidence and predictive factors, *Stroke* 34:1339, 2003.
193. Dhoble A, Vedre A, Abdelmoneim SS, et al: Prophylaxis to prevent infective endocarditis: To use or not to use? *Clin Cardiol* 32:429, 2009.
194. Devereux RB, Frary CJ, Kramer-Fox R, et al: Cost-effectiveness of infective endocarditis prophylaxis for mitral valve prolapse with or without a mitral regurgitant murmur, *Am J Cardiol* 74:1024, 1994.
195. Vavuranakis M, Kolibash AJ, Wooley CF, et al: Mitral valve prolapse: Left ventricular hemodynamics in patients with chest pain, dyspnea or both, *J Heart Valve Dis* 2:544, 1993.
196. Bacon R, Chandrasekan V, Haigh A, et al: Early extubation after open-heart surgery with total intravenous anaesthetic technique, *Lancet* 345:133, 1995.
197. Seiler C: How should we assess patent foramen ovale? *Heart* 90:1245, 2004.
198. Windecker S, Meier B: Is closure recommended for patent foramen ovale and cryptogenic stroke? Patent foramen ovale and cryptogenic stroke: To close or not to close? Closure: what else!, *Circulation* 118:1989, 2008.
199. Rigatelli G, Cardaioli P, Chinaglia M: Asymptomatic significant patent foramen ovale: Giving patent foramen ovale management back to the cardiologist, *Catheter Cardiovasc Interv* 71:573, 2008.
200. Hagen PT, Scholz DG, Edwards WD: Incidence and size of patent foramen ovale during the first 10 decades of life: An autopsy study of 965 normal hearts, *Mayo Clin Proc* 59:17, 1984.
201. Schneider B, Zienkiewicz T, Jansen V, et al: Diagnosis of patent foramen ovale by transesophageal echocardiography and correlation with autopsy findings, *Am J Cardiol* 77:1202, 1996.
202. Krasuski RA, Hart SA, Allen D, et al: Prevalence and repair of intraoperatively diagnosed patent foramen ovale and association with perioperative outcomes and long-term survival, *JAMA* 302:290, 2009.
203. Sukernik MR, Bennett-Guerrero E: The incidental finding of a patent foramen ovale during cardiac surgery: Should it always be repaired? A core review, *Anesth Analg* 105:602, 2007.
204. Argenziano M: PRO: The incidental finding of a patent foramen ovale during cardiac surgery: Should it always be repaired? *Anesth Analg* 105:611, 2007.
205. Meier B: Catheter-based closure of the patent foramen ovale, *Circulation* 120:1837, 2009.
206. Petty GW, Khandheria BK, Meissner I, et al: Population-based study of the relationship between patent foramen ovale and cerebrovascular ischemic events, *Mayo Clin Proc* 81:602, 2006.
207. Messe SR, Kasner SE: Is closure recommended for patent foramen ovale and cryptogenic stroke? Patent foramen ovale in cryptogenic stroke: Not to close, *Circulation* 118:1999, 2008.
208. Bridges ND, Hellenbrand W, Latson L, et al: Transcatheter closure of patent foramen ovale after presumed paradoxical embolism, *Circulation* 86:1902, 1992.
209. Anzola GP, Morandi E, Casilli F, et al: Does transcatheter closure of patent foramen ovale really "shut the door?" A prospective study with transcranial Doppler, *Stroke* 35:2140, 2004.
210. Sukernik MR, Mets B, Kachulis B, et al: The impact of newly diagnosed patent foramen ovale in patients undergoing off-pump coronary artery bypass grafting: Case series of eleven patients, *Anesth Analg* 95:1142, 2002.
211. Jaffe RA, Pinto FJ, Schnittger I, et al: Aspects of mechanical ventilation affecting interatrial shunt flow during general anesthesia, *Anesth Analg* 75:484, 1992.
212. Jean-Baptiste E: Clinical assessment and management of massive hemoptysis, *Crit Care Med* 28:1642, 2000.
213. Thompson AB, Teschler H, Rennard SI: Pathogenesis, evaluation, and therapy for massive hemoptysis, *Clin Chest Med* 13:69, 1992.
214. Cahill BC, Ingbar DH: Massive hemoptysis. Assessment and management, *Clin Chest Med* 15:147, 1994.
215. Fartoukh M, Parrot A, Khalil A: Aetiology, diagnosis and management of infective causes of severe haemoptysis in intensive care units, *Curr Opin Pulm Med* 14:195, 2008.
216. Knott-Craig CJ, Oostuizen JG, Rossouw G, et al: Management and prognosis of massive hemoptysis. Recent experience with 120 patients, *J Thorac Cardiovasc Surg* 105:394, 1993.
217. Lau EMT, Yozghatlian V, Kosky C, et al: Recombinant activated factor VII for massive hemoptysis in patients with cystic fibrosis, *Chest* 136:277, 2009.
218. Sekkal S, Cornu E, Christides C, et al: Swan-Ganz catheter induced pulmonary artery perforation during cardiac surgery concerning two cases, *J Cardiovasc Surg (Torino)* 37:313, 1996.
219. Lee EW, Grant JD, Loh CT, et al: Bronchial and pulmonary arterial and venous interventions, *Semin Respir Crit Care Med* 29:395, 2008.
220. Shigemura N, Wan IY, Yu SCH, et al: Multidisciplinary management of life-threatening massive hemoptysis: A 10-year experience, *Ann Thorac Surg* 87:849, 2009.
221. Stenbit A, Flume PA: Pulmonary complications in adult patients with cystic fibrosis, *Am J Med Sci* 335:55, 2008.
222. Klein U, Karzai W, Bloos F, et al: Role of fiberoptic bronchoscopy in conjunction with the use of double-lumen tubes for thoracic anesthesia: A prospective study, *Anesthesiology* 88:346, 1998.
223. Larson CE, Gasior TA: A device for endobronchial blocker placement during one lung anesthesia, *Anesth Analg* 71:311, 1990.
224. Cremaschi P, Nascimbene C, Vitulo P, et al: Therapeutic embolization of bronchial artery: A successful treatment in 209 cases of relapse hemoptysis, *Angiology* 44:295, 1993.
225. Efrati O, Harash O, Rivlin J, et al: Hemoptysis in Israeli CF patients—prevalence, treatment, and clinical characteristics, *J Cyst Fibros* 7:301, 2008.
226. Tan RT, McGahan JP, Link DP, et al: Bronchial artery embolisation in management of haemoptysis, *J Intervent Radiol* 6:67, 1991.
227. Swanson KL, Johnson CM, Prakash UBS, et al: Bronchial artery embolization: Experience with 54 patients, *Chest* 121:789, 2002.
228. Kearney TJ, Shabot MM: Pulmonary artery rupture associated with Swan-Ganz catheter, *Chest* 108:1349, 1995.
229. Muller BJ, Gallucci A: Pulmonary artery catheter induced pulmonary artery rupture in patients undergoing cardiac surgery, *Can Anaesth Soc J* 32:258, 1985.
230. Rosenbaum L, Rosenbaum SH, Askanazi J, et al: Small amounts of hemoptysis as an early warning sign of pulmonary artery rupture by a pulmonary arterial catheter, *Crit Care Med* 9:319, 1981.
231. Hardy J-F, Morissette M, Taillefer J, et al: Pathophysiology of rupture of the pulmonary artery by pulmonary artery balloon-tipped catheters, *Anesth Analg* 62:925, 1983.
232. Barash PG, Nardi D, Hammond G, et al: Catheter-induced pulmonary artery perforation: Mechanisms, management, and modifications, *J Thorac Cardiovasc Surg* 82:5, 1981.
233. Hasnain JU, Moulton AL: Life-threatening pulmonary artery perforation during cardiopulmonary bypass, *Crit Care Med* 14:748, 1986.
234. Hoit BD: Pericardial disease and pericardial tamponade, *Crit Care Med* 35:S355, 2007.
235. Maisch B, Ristic AD: The classification of pericardial disease in the age of modern medicine, *Curr Cardiol Rep* 4:13, 2002.
236. Aikat S, Ghaffari S: A review of pericardial diseases: clinical, ECG and hemodynamic features and management, *Cleve Clin J Med* 67:903, 2000.
237. Spodick DH: Pericarditis, pericardial effusion, cardiac tamponade, and constriction, *Crit Care Clin* 5:455, 1989.
238. Miller RH, Horneffer PJ, Gardner TJ, et al: The epidemiology of the postpericardiotomy syndrome: A common complication of cardiac surgery, *Am Heart J* 116:1323, 1988.
239. Ling LH, Oh JK, Schaff HV, et al: Constrictive pericarditis in the modern era: Evolving clinical spectrum and impact on outcome after pericardiectomy, *Circulation* 100:1380, 1999.
240. Dal-Bianco JP, Sengupta PP, Mookadam F, et al: Role of echocardiography in the diagnosis of constrictive pericarditis, *J Am Soc Echocardiogr* 22:24, 2009.
241. Asher CR, Klein AL: Diastolic heart failure: Restrictive cardiomyopathy, constrictive pericarditis, and cardiac tamponade: Clinical and echocardiographic evaluation, *Cardiol Rev* 10:218, 2002.
242. Ha JW, Oh JK, Ommen SR, et al: Diagnostic value of mitral annular velocity for constrictive pericarditis in the absence of respiratory variation in mitral inflow velocity, *J Am Soc Echocardiogr* 15:1468, 2002.
243. Ha JW, Ommen SR, Tajik AJ, et al: Differentiation of constrictive pericarditis from restrictive cardiomyopathy using mitral annular velocity by tissue Doppler echocardiography, *Am J Cardiol* 94:316, 2004.
244. Gongora E, Dearani JA, Orszulak TA, et al: Tricuspid regurgitation in patients undergoing pericardiectomy for constrictive pericarditis, *Ann Thorac Surg* 85:163, 2008.
245. Tuna IC, Danielson GK: Surgical management of pericardial disease, *Cardiol Clin* 8:683, 1990.
246. Ha J-W, Oh JK, Schaff HV, et al: Impact of left ventricular function on immediate and long-term outcomes after pericardiectomy in constrictive pericarditis, *J Thorac Cardiovasc Surg* 136:1136, 2008.
247. Chowdhury UK, Subramaniam GK, Kumar AS, et al: Pericardiectomy for constrictive pericarditis: A clinical, echocardiographic, and hemodynamic evaluation of two surgical techniques, *Ann Thorac Surg* 81:522, 2006.
248. Laham RJ, Cohen DJ, Kuntz RE, et al: Pericardial effusion in patients with cancer: Outcome with contemporary management stategies, *Heart* 75:67, 1996.
249. Gandhi S, Schneider A, Mohiuddin S, et al: Has the clinical presentation and clinician's index of suspicion of cardiac tamponade changed over the past decade? *Echocardiography* 25:237, 2008.
250. Shabetai R, Hurst JW, Schlant RC, et al: *The Heart, Arteries and Veins*, New York, 1990, McGraw-Hill.
251. Qureshi AC, Lindsay AC, Mensah K, et al: Tamponade and the rule of tens, *Lancet* 371:1810, 2008.
252. Spodick DH: Pathophysiology of cardiac tamponade, *Chest* 113:1372, 1998.
253. Armstrong WF, Schilt BF, Helper DJ, et al: Diastolic collapse of the right ventricle with cardiac tamponade: An echocardiographic study, *Circulation* 65:1491, 1982.
254. Tsang TS, Enriquez-Sarano M, Freeman WK, et al: Consecutive 1127 therapeutic echocardiographically guided pericardiocenteses: Clinical profile, practice patterns, and outcomes spanning 21 years, *Mayo Clin Proc* 77:429, 2002.
255. Kuvin JT, Harati NA, Pandian NG, et al: Postoperative cardiac tamponade in the modern surgical era, *Ann Thorac Surg* 74:1148, 2002.
256. Sangalli F, Colagrande L, Manetti B, et al: Hemodynamic instability after cardiac surgery: Transesophageal echocardiographic diagnosis of a localized pericardial tamponade, *J Cardiothorac Vasc Anesth* 19:775, 2005.
257. Ball JB, Morrison WL: Experience with cardiac tamponade following open heart surgery, *Heart Vessels* 11:39, 1996.
258. Imren Y, Tasoglu I, Oktar GL, et al: The importance of transesophageal echocardiography in diagnosis of pericardial tamponade after cardiac surgery, *J Card Surg* 23:450, 2008.
259. Johnson SB, Nielsen JL, Sako EY, et al: Penetrating intrapericardial wounds: Clinical experience with a surgical protocol, *Ann Thorac Surg* 60:117, 1995.
260. Kaplan JA, Bland JW Jr, Dunbar RW: The perioperative management of pericardial tamponade, *South Med J* 69:417, 1976.
261. Gascho JA, Martins JB, Marcus ML, et al: Effects of volume expansion and vasodilators in acute pericardial tamponade, *Am J Physiol* 240:H49, 1981.
262. Sagrista-Sauleda J, Angel J, Sambola A, et al: Hemodynamic effects of volume expansion in patients with cardiac tamponade, *Circulation* 117:1545, 2008.
263. Zhang H, Spapen H, Vincent JL: Effects of dobutamine and norepinephrine on oxygen availability in tamponade-induced stagnant hypoxia: A prospective, randomized, controlled study, *Crit Care Med* 22:299, 1994.
264. Hertzer NR, Loop FD, Beven EG, et al: Surgical staging for simultaneous coronary and carotid disease: A study including prospective randomization, *J Vasc Surg* 9:455, 1989.
265. Ricotta JJ, Char DJ, Cuadra SA, et al: Modeling stroke risk after coronary artery bypass and combined coronary artery bypass and carotid endarterectomy, *Stroke* 34:1212, 2003.
266. Rizzo RJ, Whittemore AD, Couper GS, et al: Combined carotid and coronary revascularization: The preferred approach to the severe vasculopath, *Ann Thorac Surg* 54:1099, 1992.
267. Yusuf S, Zucker D, Peduzzi P, et al: Effect of coronary artery bypass graft surgery on survival: Overview of 10-year results from randomised trials by the Coronary Artery Bypass Graft Surgery Trialists Collaboration [Erratum appears in *Lancet* 1994 Nov 19;344(8934):1446], *Lancet* 344:563, 1994.
268. Bernhard VM, Johnson WD, Peterson JJ: Carotid artery stenosis. Association with surgery for coronary artery disease, *Arch Surg* 105:837, 1972.
269. Ricotta JJ, Wall LP, Blackstone E: The influence of concurrent carotid endarterectomy on coronary bypass: A case-controlled study, *J Vasc Surg* 41:397, 2005.
270. Timaran CH, Rosero EB, Smith ST, et al: Trends and outcomes of concurrent carotid revascularization and coronary bypass, *J Vasc Surg* 48:355, 2008.
271. Dubinsky RM, Lai SM: Mortality from combined carotid endarterectomy and coronary artery bypass surgery in the US, *Neurology* 68:195, 2007.
272. Clark RE, Brillman J, Davis DA, et al: Microemboli during coronary artery bypass grafting: Genesis and effect on outcome, *J Thorac Cardiovasc Surg* 109:249, 1995.
273. Naylor AR, Mehta Z, Rothwell PM, et al: Carotid artery disease and stroke during coronary artery bypass: A critical review of the literature, *Eur J Vasc Endovasc Surg* 23:283, 2002.
274. Trachiotis GD, Pfister AJ: Management strategy for simultaneous carotid endarterectomy and coronary revascularization, *Ann Thorac Surg* 64:1013, 1997.
275. D'Agostino RS, Svensson LG, Neumann DJ, et al: Screening carotid ultrasonography and risk factors for stroke in coronary artery surgery patients, *Ann Thorac Surg* 62:1714, 1996.
276. Balderman SC, Gutierrez IZ, Makula P, et al: Noninvasive screening for asymptomatic carotid artery disease prior to cardiac operations: Experience with 500 patients, *J Thorac Cardiovasc Surg* 85:427, 1983.

277. Hertzer NR, Young JR, Beven EG, et al: Coronary angiography in 506 patients with extracranial cerebrovascular disease, *Arch Intern Med* 145:849, 1985.
278. Faggioli GL, Curl GR, Ricotta JJ: The role of carotid screening before coronary artery bypass, *J Vasc Surg* 12:724, 1990.
279. Naylor AR, Cuffe RL, Rothwell PM, et al: A systematic review of outcomes following staged and synchronous carotid endarterectomy and coronary artery bypass, *Eur J Vasc Endovasc Surg* 25:380, 2003.
280. Schwartz LB, Bridgman AH, Kieffer RW, et al: Asymptomatic carotid artery stenosis and stroke in patients undergoing cardiopulmonary bypass, *J Vasc Surg* 21:146, 1995.
281. Baiou D, Karageorge A, Spyt T, et al: Patients undergoing cardiac surgery with asymptomatic unilateral carotid stenoses have a low risk of peri-operative stroke, *Eur J Vasc Endovasc Surg* 38:556, 2009.
282. Gerraty RP, Gates PC, Doyle JC: Carotid stenosis and perioperative stroke risk in symptomatic and asymptomatic patients undergoing vascular or coronary surgery, *Stroke* 24:1115, 1993.
283. Kougias P, Kappa JR, Sewell DH, et al: Simultaneous carotid endarterectomy and coronary artery bypass grafting: Results in specific patient groups, *Ann Vasc Surg* 21:408, 2007.
284. Randall MS, McKevitt FM, Cleveland TJ, et al: Is there any benefit from staged carotid and coronary revascularization using carotid stents? A single-center experience highlights the need for a randomized controlled trial, *Stroke* 37:435, 2006.
285. Cinar B, Goksel OS, Karatepe C, et al: Is routine intravascular shunting necessary for carotid endarterectomy in patients with contralateral occlusion? A review of 5-year experience of carotid endarterectomy with local anaesthesia, *Eur J Vasc Endovasc Surg* 28:494, 2004.
286. Cinar B, Goksel OS, Kut S, et al: A modified combined approach to operative carotid and coronary artery disease: 82 cases in 8 years, *Heart Surg Forum* 8:E184, 2005.
287. Butterworth J, James R, Prielipp RC, et al: Do shorter-acting neuromuscular blocking drugs or opioids associate with reduced intensive care unit or hospital lengths of stay after coronary artery bypass grafting? CABG Clinical Benchmarking Data Base Participants, *Anesthesiology* 88:1437, 1998.
288. Engoren M, Luther G, Fenn-Buderer N: A comparison of fentanyl, sufentanil, and remifentanil for fast-track cardiac anesthesia, *Anesth Analg* 93:859, 2001.
289. Olivier P, Sirieix D, Dassier P, et al: Continuous infusion of remifentanil and target-controlled infusion of propofol for patients undergoing cardiac surgery: A new approach for scheduled early extubation, *J Cardiothorac Vasc Anesth* 14:29, 2000.
290. Royse CF, Royse AG, Soeding PF: Routine immediate extubation after cardiac operation: A review of our first 100 patients, *Ann Thorac Surg* 68:1326, 1999.
291. Turkoz A, Turkoz R, Gulcan O, et al: Wake-up test after carotid endarterectomy for combined carotid-coronary artery surgery: A case series, *J Cardiothorac Vasc Anesth* 21:540, 2007.
292. Luo L, Kebede S, Wu S, et al: Coronary artery fistulae, *Am J Med Sci* 332:79, 2006.
293. Gowda RM, Vasavada BC, Khan IA: Coronary artery fistulas: Clinical and therapeutic considerations, *Int J Cardiol* 107:7, 2006.
294. Latson LA: Coronary artery fistulas: How to manage them, *Catheter Cardiovasc Interv* 70:110, 2007.
295. Jung S-H, Cho W-C, Choo SJ, et al: Images in cardiovascular medicine. Multiple coronary arteriovenous fistulas to the coronary sinus with an unruptured coronary sinus aneurysm and restrictive coronary sinus opening to the right atrium, *Circulation* 120:1138, 2009.
296. Mahesh B, Navaratnarajah M, Mensah K, et al: Treatment of high-output coronary artery fistula by off-pump coronary artery bypass grafting and ligation of fistula, *Interact Cardiovasc Thorac Surg* 9:124, 2009.
297. Kamiya H, Yasuda T, Nagamine H, et al: Surgical treatment of congenital coronary artery fistulas: 27 years' experience and a review of the literature, *J Card Surg* 17:173, 2002.
298. Fernandes ED, Kadivar H, Hallman GL, et al: Congenital malformations of the coronary arteries: The Texas Heart Institute experience, *Ann Thorac Surg* 54:732, 1992.
299. Stevenson JG, Sorensen GK, Stamm SJ, et al: Intraoperative transesophageal echocardiography of coronary artery fistulas, *Ann Thorac Surg* 57:1217, 1994.
300. Kabbani Z, Garcia-Nielsen L, Lozano ML, et al: Coil embolization of coronary artery fistulas. A single-centre experience, *Cardiovasc Revasc Med* 9:14, 2008.
301. Chandrasekhar S, Cook CR, Collard CD: Cardiac surgery in the parturient, *Anesth Analg* 108:777, 2009.
302. Martin SR, Foley MR: Intensive care in obstetrics: An evidence-based review, *Am J Obstet Gynecol* 195:673, 2006.
303. Conklin KA, Chestnut DH: *Obstetric Anesthesia. Principles and Practice*, St. Louis, 1994, Mosby, p 17.
304. Weiss BM, von Segesser LK, Alon E, et al: Outcome of cardiovascular surgery and pregnancy: A systematic review of the period 1984-1996, *Am J Obstet Gynecol* 179:1643, 1998.
305. Mahli A, Izdes S, Coskun D: Cardiac operations during pregnancy: Review of factors influencing fetal outcome, *Ann Thorac Surg* 69:1622, 2000.
306. Gopal K, Hudson IM, Ludmir J, et al: Homograft aortic root replacement during pregnancy, *Ann Thorac Surg* 74:243, 2002.
307. Parry AJ, Westaby S: Cardiopulmonary bypass during pregnancy, *Ann Thorac Surg* 61:1865, 1996.
308. Laffey JG, Boylan JF, Cheng DC: The systemic inflammatory response to cardiac surgery: Implications for the anesthesiologist, *Anesthesiology* 97:215, 2002.
309. Pomini F, Mercogliano D, Cavalletti C, et al: Cardiopulmonary bypass in pregnancy, *Ann Thorac Surg* 61:259, 1996.
310. Lamb MP, Ross K, Johnstone AM, et al: Fetal heart monitoring during open heart surgery. Two case reports, *Br J Obstet Gynaecol* 88:669, 1981.
311. Buffolo E, Palma JH, Gomes WJ, et al: Successful use of deep hypothermic circulatory arrest in pregnancy, *Ann Thorac Surg* 58:1532, 1994.
312. Strickland RA, Oliver WC Jr, Chantigian RC, et al: Anesthesia, cardiopulmonary bypass, and the pregnant patient, *Mayo Clin Proc* 66:411, 1991.
313. Becker RM: Intracardiac surgery in pregnant women, *Ann Thorac Surg* 36:453, 1983.
314. Chambers CE, Clark SL: Cardiac surgery during pregnancy, *Clin Obstet Gynecol* 37:316, 1994.
315. Izquierdo LA, Kushnir O, Knieriem K, et al: Effect of mitral valve prosthetic surgery on the outcome of a growth-retarded fetus. A case report, *Am J Obstet Gynecol* 163:584, 1990.
316. Jahangiri M, Clarke J, Prefumo F, et al: Cardiac surgery during pregnancy: Pulsatile or nonpulsatile perfusion? *J Thorac Cardiovasc Surg* 126:894, 2003.
317. Oakley CM: Anticoagulation and pregnancy, *Eur Heart J* 16:1317, 1995.
318. Ellis SC, Wheeler AS, James FM III, et al: Fetal and maternal effects of sodium nitroprusside used to counteract hypertension in gravid ewes, *Am J Obstet Gynecol* 143:766, 1982.
319. Moran DH, Perillo M, LaPorta RF, et al: Phenylephrine in the prevention of hypotension following spinal anesthesia for cesarean delivery, *J Clin Anesth* 3:301, 1991.
320. Ramanathan S, Grant GJ: Vasopressor therapy for hypotension due to epidural anesthesia for cesarean section, *Acta Anaesthesiol Scand* 32:559, 1988.
321. Hood DD, Dewan DM, James FM III: Maternal and fetal effects of epinephrine in gravid ewes, *Anesthesiology* 64:610, 1986.
322. Bach V, Carl P, Ravlo O, et al: A randomized comparison between midazolam and thiopental for elective cesarean section anesthesia: III. Placental transfer and elimination in neonates, *Anesth Analg* 68:238, 1989.
323. Dailland P, Cockshott ID, Lirzin JD, et al: Intravenous propofol during Cesarean section: Placental transfer, concentrations in breast milk, and neonatal effects. A preliminary study, *Anesthesiology* 71:827, 1989.
324. Ellingson A, Haram K, Sagen N, et al: Transplacental passage of ketamine after intravenous administration, *Acta Anaesthesiol Scand* 21:41, 1977.
325. Mazze RI, Fujinaga M, Rice SA, et al: Reproductive and teratogenic effects of nitrous oxide, halothane, isoflurane, and enflurane in Sprague-Dawley rats, *Anesthesiology* 64:339, 1986.
326. O'Leary G, Bacon CL, Odumeru O, et al: Antiproliferative actions of inhalational anesthetics: Comparisons to the valproate teratogen, *Int J Dev Neurosci* 18:39, 2000.
327. Lowe SA, Rubin PC: The pharmacological management of hypertension in pregnancy, *J Hypertens* 10:201, 1992.
328. Hariri S, McKenna MT: Epidemiology of human immunodeficiency virus in the United States, *Clin Microbiol Rev* 20:478, 2007.
329. Landovitz RJ, Currier JS: Clinical practice. Postexposure prophylaxis for HIV infection, *N Engl J Med* 361:1768, 2009.
330. Puro V, De Carli G, Scognamiglio P, et al: Risk of HIV and other blood-borne infections in the cardiac setting: Patient-to-provider and provider-to-patient transmission, *Ann N Y Acad Sci* 946:291, 2001.
331. Henderson DK, Fahey BJ, Willy M, et al: Risk for occupational transmission of human immunodeficiency virus type 1 (HIV-1) associated with clincial exposures. A prospective evaluation, *Ann Intern Med* 113:740, 1990.
332. Saltzman DJ, Williams RA, Gelfand DV, et al: The surgeon and AIDS: Twenty years later, *Arch Surg* 140:961, 2005.
333. Tokars JI, Bell DM, Culver DH, et al: Percutaneous injuries during surgical procedures, *JAMA* 267:2899, 1992.
334. Centers for Disease Control and Prevention (CDC): Update: Provisional Public Health Service recommendations for chemoprophylaxis after occupational exposure to HIV, *MMWR Morb Mortal Wkly Rep* 45:468, 1996.
335. Cardo DM, Bell DM: Bloodborne pathogen transmission in health care workers. Risks and prevention strategies, *Infect Dis Clin North Am* 11:331, 1997.
336. Greene ES, Berry AJ, Arnold WP 3rd, et al: Percutaneous injuries in anesthesia personnel, *Anesth Analg* 83:273, 1996.
337. Medical Center Occupational Health S: HIV and AIDS in the workplace, *J Occup Environ Med* 51:243, 2009.
338. Sloand EM, Pitt E, Klein HG: Safety of the blood supply, *JAMA* 274:1368, 1995.
339. Lackritz EM, Satten GA, Aberle-Grasse J, et al: Estimated risk of transmission of the human immunodeficiency virus by screened blood in the United States, *N Engl J Med* 333:1721, 1995.
340. Schreiber GB, Busch MP, Kleinman SH, et al: The risk of transfusion-transmitted viral infections, *N Engl J Med* 334:1685, 1996.
341. Hovanessian HC: New developments in the treatment of HIV disease: An overview, *Ann Emerg Med* 33:546, 1999.
342. Ippolito G, Puro V, Heptonstall J, et al: Occupational human immunodeficiency virus infection in health care workers: Worldwide cases through September 1997, *Clin Infect Dis* 28:365, 1999.
343. Dunning J, Nelson M: Novel strategies to treat antiretroviral-naive HIV-infected patients, *J Antimicrob Chemother* 64:674, 2009.
344. Gelsomino S, Morocutti G, Masullo G, et al: Open heart surgery in patients with dialysis-dependent renal insufficiency, *J Card Surg* 16:400, 2001.
345. Provenchere S, Plantefeve G, Hufnagel G, et al: Renal dysfunction after cardiac surgery with normothermic cardiopulmonary bypass: Incidence, risk factors, and effect on clinical outcome, *Anesth Analg* 96:1258, 2003.
346. Durmaz I, Buket S, Atay Y, et al: Cardiac surgery with cardiopulmonary bypass in patients with chronic renal failure, *J Thorac Cardiovasc Surg* 118:306, 1999.
347. Ristikankare A, Kuitunen T, Kuitunen A, et al: Lack of renoprotective effect of i.v. N-acetylcysteine in patients with chronic renal failure undergoing cardiac surgery, *Br J Anaesth* 97:611, 2006.
348. Caimmi PP, Pagani L, Micalizzi E, et al: Fenoldopam for renal protection in patients undergoing cardiopulmonary bypass, *J Cardiothorac Vasc Anesth* 17:491, 2003.
349. Sutton RG: Renal considerations, dialysis, and ultrafiltration during cardiopulmonary bypass, *Int Anesthesiol Clin* 34:165, 1996.
350. Murphy GS, Hessel EA 2nd, Groom RC: Optimal perfusion during cardiopulmonary bypass: An evidence-based approach, *Anesth Analg* 108:1394, 2009.
351. Kubota T, Miyata A, Maeda A, et al: Continuous haemodiafiltration during and after cardiopulmonary bypass in renal failure patients, *Can J Anaesth* 44:1182, 1997.
352. Oliver WC Jr, Nuttall GA, Orszulak TA, et al: Hemofiltration but not steroids results in earlier tracheal extubation following cardiopulmonary bypass: A prospective, randomized double-blind trial, *Anesthesiology* 101:327, 2004.
353. Nuttall GA, Gutierrez MC, Dewey JD, et al: A preliminary study of a new tranexamic acid dosing schedule for cardiac surgery, *J Cardiothorac Vasc Anesth* 22:230, 2008.
354. Mangano DT, Tudor IC, Dietzel C, et al: The risk associated with aprotinin in cardiac surgery, *N Engl J Med* 354:353, 2006.
355. Fergusson DA, Hebert PC, Mazer CD, et al: A comparison of aprotinin and lysine analogues in high-risk cardiac surgery, *N Engl J Med* 358:2319, 2008.
356. Petroni KC, Cohen NH: Continuous renal replacement therapy: Anesthetic implications, *Anesth Analg* 94:1288, 2002.
357. DiMichele D: Hemophilia 1996. New approach to an old disease, *Pediatr Clin North Am* 43:709, 1996.
358. Mannucci PM: Hemophilia and related bleeding disorders: A story of dismay and success. (Lectures), *Hematology* 1, 2002.
359. Evatt BL: AIDS and hemophilia—current issues, *Thromb Haemost* 74:36, 1995.
360. Nuttall GA, Oliver WC, Jr, Ereth MH, et al: Coagulation tests predict bleeding after cardiopulmonary bypass, *J Cardiothorac Vasc Anesth* 11:815, 1997.
361. Tang M, Wierup P, Terp K, et al: Cardiac surgery in patients with haemophilia, *Haemophilia* 15:101, 2009.
362. Stieltjes N, Altisent C, Auerswald G, et al: Continuous infusion of B-domain deleted recombinant factor VIII (ReFacto) in patients with haemophilia A undergoing surgery: Clinical experience, *Haemophilia* 10:452, 2004.
363. Stine KC, Becton DL: Use of factor VIII replacement during open heart surgery in a patient with haemophilia A, *Haemophilia* 12:435, 2006.
364. Eren A, Friedl R, Hannekum A, et al: Cardiac surgery in a patient with haemophilia A, *Thorac Cardiovasc Surg* 54:212, 2006.
365. Mannucci PM, Cattaneo M: Desmopressin: A nontransfusional treatment of hemophilia and von Willebrand disease, *Haemostasis* 22:276, 1992.
366. Warrier AI, Lusher JM: DDAVP: A useful alternative to blood components in moderate hemophilia A and von Willebrand disease, *J Pediatr* 102:228, 1983.
367. Donahue BS, Emerson CW, Slaughter TF: Case 1—1999. Elective and emergency cardiac surgery on a patient with hemophilia B, *J Cardiothorac Vasc Anesth* 13:92, 1999.
368. Roskos RR, Gilchrist GS, Kazmier FJ, et al: Management of hemophilia A and B during surgical correction of transposition of great arteries, *Mayo Clin Proc* 58:182, 1983.
369. Krakow EF, Walker I, Lamy A, et al: Cardiac surgery in patients with haemophilia B: A case report and review of the literature, *Haemophilia* 15:108, 2009.
370. Mannucci PM: Modern treatment of hemophilia: From the shadows towards the light, *Thromb Haemost* 70:17, 1993.

371. Nilsson IM: The management of hemophilia patients with inhibitors, *Transfus Med Rev* 6:285, 1992.

372. Seremetis SV, Aledort LM: Congenital bleeding disorders. Rational treatment options, *Drugs* 45:541, 1993.

373. DiMichele DM, Lasak ME, Miller CH: A study of in vitro factor VIII recovery during the delivery of four ultra-pure factor VIII concentrate by continuous infusion, *Am J Hematol* 51:99, 1996.

374. Leggett PL, Doyle D, Smith WB, et al: Elective cardiac operation in a patient with severe hemophilia and acquired factor VIII antibodies, *J Thorac Cardiovasc Surg* 87:556, 1984.

375. Tagariello G, De Biasi E, Gajo GB, et al: Recombinant FVIIa (NovoSeven) continuous infusion and total hip replacement in patients with haemophilia and high titre of inhibitors to FVIII: Experience of two cases, *Haemophilia* 6:581, 2000.

376. Lusher J, Ingerslev J, Roberts H, et al: Clinical experience with recombinant factor VIIa, *Blood Coagul Fibrinolysis* 9:119, 1998.

377. Diprose P, Herbertson MJ, O'Shaughnessy D, et al: Activated recombinant factor VII after cardiopulmonary bypass reduces allogeneic transfusion in complex non-coronary cardiac surgery: Randomized double-blind placebo-controlled pilot study, *Br J Anaesth* 95:596, 2005.

378. Rodeghiero F, Castaman G, Dini E: Epidemiological investigation of the prevalence of von Willebrand's disease, *Blood* 69:454, 1987.

379. Rick ME: Diagnosis and management of von Willebrand's syndrome, *Med Clin North Am* 78:609, 1994.

380. Oliver WC, Jr, Nuttall GA, Pifarre R: *New Anticoagulants for the Cardiovascular Patient*, Philadelphia, 1997, Hanley and Belfus.

381. Sadler JE, Matsushita T, Dong Z, et al: Molecular mechanism and classification of von Willebrand disease, *Thromb Haemost* 74:161, 1995.

382. Perrin EJ, Ray MJ, Hawson GA: The role of von Willebrand factor in haemostasis and blood loss during and after cardiopulmonary bypass surgery, *Blood Coagul Fibrinolysis* 6:650, 1995.

383. Berntorp E: Plasma product treatment in various types of von Willebrand's disease, *Haemostasis* 24:289, 1994.

384. Castaman G, Rodeghiero F: Current management of von Willebrand's disease, *Drugs* 50:602, 1995.

385. Rick ME: Laboratory diagnosis of von Willebrand's disease, *Clin Lab Med* 14:781, 1994.

386. Berntorp E: Prophylaxis in von Willebrand disease, *Haemophilia* 14(Suppl 5):47, 2008.

387. Michiels JJ, van Vliet HHDM, Berneman Z, et al: Managing patients with von Willebrand disease type 1, 2 and 3 with desmopressin and von Willebrand factor-factor VIII concentrate in surgical settings, *Acta Haematol* 121:167, 2009.

388. Batlle J, Noya MS, Giangrande P, et al: Advances in the therapy of von Willebrand disease, *Haemophilia* 8:301, 2002.

389. Logan LJ: Treatment of von Willebrand's disease, *Hematol Oncol Clin North Am* 6:1079, 1992.

390. Auerswald G, Kreuz W: Haemate P/Humate-P for the treatment of von Willebrand disease: Considerations for use and clinical experience, *Haemophilia* 14(Suppl 5):39, 2008.

391. White R, Rushbrook J, McGoldrick J: The dangers of prothrombin complex concentrate administration after heart surgery, *Blood Coagul Fibrinolysis* 19:609, 2008.

392. Blajchman MA: An overview of the mechanism of action of antithrombin and its inherited deficiency states, *Blood Coagul Fibrinolysis* 5(Suppl I):S5, 1994.

393. Marciniak E, Farley CH, DeSimone PA: Familial thrombosis due to antithrombin III deficiency, *Blood* 43:219, 1974.

394. Bucur SZ, Levy JH, Despotis GJ, et al: Uses of antithrombin III concentrate in congenital and acquired deficiency states, *Transfusion* 30:481, 1990.

395. Hellstern P, Moberg U, Ekblad M, et al: In vitro characterization of antithrombin III concentrates—a single-blind study, *Haemostasis* 25:193, 1995.

396. Demers C, Ginsberg JS, Hirsh J, et al: Thrombosis in antithrombin-III-deficient persons. Report of a large kindred and literature review, *Ann Intern Med* 116:754, 1992.

397. Slaughter TF, Mark JB, El-Moalem H, et al: Hemostatic effects of antithrombin III supplementation during cardiac surgery: Results of a prospective randomized investigation, *Blood Coagul Fibrinolysis* 12:25, 2001.

398. Williams MR, D'Ambra AB, Beck JR, et al: A randomized trial of antithrombin concentrate for treatment of heparin resistance, *Ann Thorac Surg* 70:873, 2000.

399. Avidan MS, Levy JH, Scholz J, et al: A phase III, double-blind, placebo-controlled, multicenter study on the efficacy of recombinant human antithrombin in heparin-resistant patients scheduled to undergo cardiac surgery necessitating cardiopulmonary bypass, *Anesthesiology* 102:276, 2005.

400. Avidan MS, Levy JH, van Aken H, et al: Recombinant human antithrombin III restores heparin responsiveness and decreases activation of coagulation in heparin-resistant patients during cardiopulmonary bypass, *J Thorac Cardiovasc Surg* 130:107, 2005.

401. Ranucci M, Frigiola A, Menicanti L, et al: Postoperative antithrombin levels and outcome in cardiac operations, *Crit Care Med* 33:355, 2005.

402. Jackson MR, Olsen SB, Gomez ER, et al: Use of antithrombin III concentrates to correct antithrombin III deficiency during vascular surgery, *J Vasc Surg* 22:804, 1995.

403. Sniecinski RM, Szlam F, Chen EP, et al: Antithrombin deficiency increases thrombin activity after prolonged cardiopulmonary bypass, *Anesth Analg* 106:713, 2008.

404. Sniecinski RM, Chen EP, Tanaka KA: Reduced levels of fibrin (antithrombin I) and antithrombin III underlie coagulopathy following complex cardiac surgery, *Blood Coagul Fibrinolysis* 19:178, 2008.

405. Levy JH, Despotis GJ, Szlam F, et al: Recombinant human transgenic antithrombin in cardiac surgery: A dose-finding study, *Anesthesiology* 96:1095, 2002.

406. Lemmer JH Jr, Despotis GJ: Antithrombin III concentrate to treat heparin resistance in patients undergoing cardiac surgery, *J Thorac Cardiovasc Surg* 123:213, 2002.

407. Koster A, Chew D, Kuebler W, et al: High antithrombin III levels attenuate hemostatic activation and leukocyte activation during cardiopulmonary bypass, *J Thorac Cardiovasc Surg* 126:906, 2003.

408. Paparella D, Cappabianca G, Scrascia G, et al: Antithrombin after cardiac surgery: Implications on short and mid-term outcome, *J Thromb Thrombolysis* 27:105, 2009.

409. Agarwal SK, Ghosh PK, Gupta D: Cardiac surgery and cold-reactive proteins, *Ann Thorac Surg* 60:1143, 1995.

410. Williams AC: Cold agglutinins. Cause for concern? *Anaesthesia* 35:887, 1980.

411. Landymore R, Isom W, Barlam B: Management of patients with cold agglutinins who require open-heart surgery, *Can J Surg* 26:79, 1983.

412. Shahian DM, Wallach SR, Bern MM: Open heart surgery in patients with cold-reactive proteins, *Surg Clin North Am* 65:315, 1985.

413. Dake SB, Johnston MF, Brueggeman P, et al: Detection of cold hemagglutination in a blood cardioplegia unit before systemic cooling of a patient with unsuspected cold agglutinin disease, *Ann Thorac Surg* 47:914, 1989.

414. Moore RA, Geller EA, Mathews ES, et al: The effect of hypothermic cardiopulmonary bypass on patients with low-titer, nonspecific cold agglutinins, *Ann Thorac Surg* 37:233, 1984.

415. Leach AB, Van Hasselt GL, Edwards JC: Cold agglutinins and deep hypothermia, *Anaesthesia* 38:140, 1983.

416. Atkinson VP, Soeding P, Horne G, et al: Cold agglutinins in cardiac surgery: Management of myocardial protection and cardiopulmonary bypass, *Ann Thorac Surg* 85:310, 2008.

417. Klein HG, Faltz LL, McIntosh CL, et al: Surgical hypothermia in a patient with a cold agglutinin: Management by plasma exchange, *Transfusion* 20:354, 1980.

418. Lee MC, Chang CH, Hsieh MJ: Use of a total wash-out method in an open heart operation, *Ann Thorac Surg* 47:57, 1989.

419. Aoki A, Kay GL, Zubiate P, et al: Cardiac operation without hypothermia for the patient with cold agglutinin, *Chest* 104:1627, 1993.

420. Wayne AS, Kevy SVNathan DG: Transfusion management of sickle cell disease, *Blood* 81:1109, 1993.

421. Steingart R: Management of patients with sickle cell disease, *Med Clin North Am* 76:669, 1992.

422. Kingsley CP, Chronister T, Cohen DJ, et al: Anesthetic management of a patient with hemoglobin SS disease and mitral insufficiency for mitral valve repair, *J Cardiothorac Vasc Anesth* 10:419, 1996.

423. Scott-Conner CEH, Brunson CD: The pathophysiology of the sickle hemoglobinopathies and implications for perioperative management, *Am J Surg* 168:268, 1994.

424. Esseltine DW, Baxter MR, Bevan JC: Sickle cell states and the anaesthetist, *Can J Anaesth* 35:385, 1988.

425. Lane PA: Sickle cell disease, *Pediatr Clin North Am* 43:639, 1996.

426. Dorn-Beineke A, Frietsch T: Sickle cell disease—pathophysiology, clinical and diagnostic implications, *Clin Chem Lab Med* 40:1075, 2002.

427. Kalhan S, DeBoer G: Preoperative screening for sickle cell trait, *JAMA* 259:3558, 1988.

428. Koshy M, Weiner SJ, Miller ST, et al: Surgery and anesthesia in sickle cell disease. Cooperative Study of Sickle Cell Diseases, *Blood* 86:3676, 1995.

429. Benza RL: Pulmonary hypertension associated with sickle cell disease: Pathophysiology and rationale for treatment, *Lung* 186:247, 2008.

430. Gyasi HK, Zarroug AW, Matthew M, et al: Anaesthesia for renal transplantation in sickle cell disease, *Can J Anaesth* 37:778, 1990.

431. Dobson MB: Anesthesia for patients with hemoglobinopathies, *Int Anesthesiol Clin* 23:197, 1985.

432. Vichinsky EP, Haberkern CM, Neumayr L, et al: A comparison of conservative and aggressive transfusion regimens in the perioperative management of sickle cell disease. The Preoperative Transfusion in Sickle Cell Disease Study Group, *N Engl J Med* 333:206, 1995.

433. Cohen AR, Martin MB, Silber JH, et al: A modified transfusion program for prevention of stroke in sickle cell disease, *Blood* 79:1657, 1992.

434. Pagani FD, Polito RJ, Bolling SF: Mitral valve reconstruction in sickle cell disease, *Ann Thorac Surg* 61:1841, 1996.

435. Shulman G, McQuitty C, Vertrees RA, et al: Acute normovolemic red cell exchange for cardiopulmonary bypass in sickle cell disease, *Ann Thorac Surg* 65:1444, 1998.

436. Riethmuller R, Grundy EM, Radley-Smith R: Open heart surgery in a patient with homozygous sickle cell disease, *Anaesthesia* 37:324, 1982.

437. Bhatt K, Cherian S, Agarwal R, et al: Perioperative management of sickle cell disease in paediatric cardiac surgery, *Anaesth Intensive Care* 35:792, 2007.

438. Davies SC, Olatunji PO: Blood transfusion in sickle cell disease, *Vox Sang* 68:145, 1995.

439. Baxter MR, Bevan JC, Esseltine DW, et al: The management of two pediatric patients with sickle cell trait and sickle cell disease during cardiopulmonary bypass, *J Cardiothorac Anesth* 3:477, 1989.

440. Balasundaram S, Duran CG, al-Halees Z, et al: Cardiopulmonary bypass in sickle cell anaemia. Report of five cases, *J Cardiovasc Surg (Torino)* 32:271, 1991.

441. Lichtenstein SV, Ashe KA, el Dalati H, et al: Warm heart surgery, *Ann Thorac Surg* 101:269, 1991.

442. Metras D, Coulibaly AO, Ouattara K, et al: Open-heart surgery in sickle-cell haemoglobinopathies: Report of 15 cases, *Thorax* 37:486, 1982.

443. Brajtbord D, Johnson D, Ramay M: Use of the cell saver in patients with sickle cell trait, *Anesthesiology* 70:878, 1989.

444. Ataga KI, Key NS: Hypercoagulability in sickle cell disease: New approaches to an old problem, *Hematology* 91, 2007.

445. Nuttall GA, Oliver WC, Santrach PJ, et al: Efficacy of a simple intraoperative transfusion algorithm for nonerythrocyte component utilization after cardiopulmonary bypass, *Anesthesiology* 94:773, 2001.

446. Harban FMJ, Connor P, Crook R, et al: Cardiopulmonary bypass for surgical correction of congenital heart disease in children with sickle cell disease: A case series, *Anaesthesia* 63:648, 2008.

447. Geller AK, O'Connor MK: The sickle cell crisis: A dilemma in pain relief, *Mayo Clin Proc* 83:320, 2008.

Anesthesia for Heart, Lung, and Heart-Lung Transplantation

JOSEPH J. QUINLAN, MD | ANDREW W. MURRAY, MB, CHB | ALFONSO CASTA, MD

KEY POINTS

1. Cardiac denervation is an unavoidable consequence of heart transplantation and reinnervation is at best partial and incomplete.
2. Drugs acting directly on the heart are the drugs of choice for altering cardiac physiology after heart transplantation.
3. Allograft coronary vasculopathy remains the greatest threat to long-term survival after heart transplantation.
4. Broadening of donor criteria has decreased time to lung transplantation.
5. Air trapping in patients with severe obstructive lung disease may impair hemodynamics and require deliberate hypoventilation.
6. Newly transplanted lungs should be ventilated with a low tidal volume and inspiratory pressure, and as low an inspired oxygen concentration as can be tolerated.
7. Reperfusion injury is the most common cause of perioperative death.
8. The frequency of heart-lung transplantation has decreased as the frequency of lung transplantations has increased.

HEART TRANSPLANTATION

The history of heart transplantation spans almost a century. Canine heterotopic cardiac transplantation was first reported in 1905,[1] but such efforts were doomed by ignorance of the workings of the immune system (Box 23-1). Further research in the late 1950s and early 1960s set the stage for the first human cardiac transplant by Barnard in 1966.[2] However, there were few long-term survivors in this era because of continued deficiency in understanding and modulating the human immune system, and the procedure fell into general disfavor. Continued research at selected centers (such as Stanford University) and lessons learned from renal transplantation led to greater understanding of the technical issues and immunology required, and by the early 1980s, cardiac transplantation gained widespread acceptance as a realistic option for patients with end-stage cardiomyopathy.

Heart transplantation experienced explosive growth in the mid-to-late 1980s, but the annual number of heart transplants worldwide plateaued by the early 1990s at approximately 3500 per year.[3] The factor limiting continued growth has been a shortage of suitable donors. As of January 2010, there were slightly more than 3000 patients on the United Network for Organ Sharing (UNOS) cardiac transplant waiting list (includes all U.S. candidates), whereas only 2028 heart transplants were performed in the United States during the 2009 calendar year. The median waiting time for a cardiac graft varies widely according to blood type (approximately 52 days for type AB recipients in contrast with 242 days for type O recipients listed for the period 2003–2004). In aggregate, approximately 30% to 37% of those patients on the heart transplant list had spent more than a year waiting for a transplant during 2007.[4] Adult patients on the heart transplant waiting list are assigned a status of 1A, 1B, or 2. Status 1A patients require mechanical circulatory support, mechanical ventilation, high-dose or multiple inotropes, with continuous monitoring of left ventricular filling pressure. Status 1B patients require mechanical circulatory support beyond 30 days or inotropic support without continuous monitoring of left ventricular filling pressure. All other patients are classified as Status 2.[4] The most frequent recipient indications for adult heart transplantation remain either idiopathic or ischemic cardiomyopathy. Other less common diagnoses include viral cardiomyopathy, systemic diseases such as amyloidosis, and complex congenital heart disease (CHD).

The 1-year survival rate after heart transplantation has been reported to be 79%, with a subsequent mortality rate of approximately 4%/year.[3] There has been only slight improvement in the survival statistics over the past decade; the Organ Procurement and Transplant Network reports that the 1- and 3-year survival rates after heart transplantation for those transplanted in the United States during the period 1997–2004 was approximately 87% and 78%, respectively, at the time this chapter was written. One-year survival rate after repeat heart transplantation more than 6 months after the original procedure is slightly lower (63%) but substantially worse if performed within 6 months of the original grafting (39%).[3] Risk factors for increased mortality have been associated with recipient factors (prior transplantation, poor human leukocyte antigen matching, ventilator dependence, age, and race), medical center factors (volume of heart transplants performed, ischemic time), and donor factors (race, sex, age). Early deaths most frequently are due to graft failure, whereas intermediate-term deaths are caused by acute rejection or infection. Late deaths after heart transplantation most frequently are due to allograft vasculopathy, post-transplant lymphoproliferative disease or other malignancy, and chronic rejection (Box 23-1).

▣ Recipient Selection

Potential candidates for heart transplantation generally undergo a multidisciplinary evaluation including a complete history and physical examination, routine hematology, chemistries (to assess renal and hepatic function), viral serology, electrocardiography, chest radiography, pulmonary function tests, and right- and left-heart catheterization. Ambulatory electrocardiography, echocardiography, and nuclear gated scans are performed if necessary. The goals of this evaluation are to confirm a diagnosis of end-stage heart disease that is not amenable to other therapies and that will likely lead to death within 1 to 2 years, as well as to exclude extracardiac organ dysfunction that could lead to death soon after heart transplantation. Patients typically have New

737

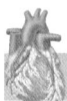

BOX 23-1. HEART TRANSPLANTATION

- Frequency of transplantation remains limited by donor supply.
- Pathophysiology before transplantation is primarily that of end-stage ventricular failure.
- Pathophysiology after transplantation reflects the effects of denervation.
- Allograft coronary vasculopathy is a frequent long-term complication.

York Heart Association Class IV symptoms and a left ventricular ejection fraction less than 20%. Although most centers eschew a strict age cutoff, the candidate should have a "physiologic" age younger than 60. Detecting pulmonary hypertension and determining whether it is due to fixed elevation of pulmonary vascular resistance (PVR) is crucial; early mortality because of graft failure is threefold greater in patients with increased PVR (transpulmonary gradient > 15 mm Hg or PVR > 5 dynes•sec•cm^{-5}).[5] If increased PVR is detected, a larger donor heart, a heterotopic heart transplant, or a heart–lung transplant may be more appropriate. Active infection and recent pulmonary thromboembolism with pulmonary infarction are additional contraindications to heart transplantation. The results of this extensive evaluation should be tabulated and available to the anesthesia team at all times because heart transplantation is an emergency procedure.

Donor Selection and Graft Harvest

Once a brain-dead donor has been identified, the accepting transplant center must further evaluate the suitability of the allograft. Centers generally prefer donors to be free of previous cardiac illness and younger than 35 years because the incidence of coronary artery disease markedly increases at older ages. However, the relative shortage of suitable cardiac donors has forced many transplant centers to consider older donors without risk factors and symptoms of coronary artery disease. If it is necessary and the services are available at the donor hospital, the heart can be further evaluated by echocardiography (for regional wall motion abnormalities) or coronary angiography, to complement standard palpation of the coronaries in the operating room. The absence of sepsis, prolonged cardiac arrest, severe chest trauma, and a high inotrope requirement also are important. The donor is matched to the prospective recipient for ABO blood-type compatibility and size (within 20%, especially if the recipient has high PVR); a cross-match is performed only if the recipient's preformed antibody screen is positive.

Donors can exhibit major hemodynamic and metabolic derangements that can adversely affect organ retrieval.[6] Most brain-dead donors will be hemodynamically unstable.[7] Reasons for such instability include hypovolemia (secondary to diuretics or diabetes insipidus), myocardial injury (possibly a result of "catecholamine storm" during periods of increased intracranial pressure), and inadequate sympathetic tone because of brainstem infarction. Donors often also have abnormalities of neuroendocrine function such as low T$_3$ and T$_4$ levels. Administration of T$_3$ to brain-dead animals improves ventricular function after transplantation[8]; T$_3$ administration has enabled decreases in inotropic support in some[9,10] but not all human studies.[11] Donor volume status should be assiduously monitored, and inotropic and vasopressor therapy should be guided by data from invasive monitors.

Donor cardiectomy is performed through a median sternotomy, usually simultaneously with recovery of other organs such as lungs, kidneys, and liver. Just before cardiac harvesting, the donor is heparinized and an intravenous cannula is placed in the ascending aorta for administration of conventional cardioplegia. The superior vena cava (SVC) is ligated and the inferior vena cava (IVC) transected to decompress the heart, simultaneous with the administration of cold hyperkalemic cardioplegia into the aortic root. The aorta is cross-clamped when the heart ceases to eject. The heart also is topically cooled with ice-cold saline. After arrest has been achieved, the pulmonary veins

are severed, the SVC is transected, the ascending aorta is divided just proximal to the innominate artery, and the pulmonary artery (PA) is transected at its bifurcation. The heart is then prepared for transport by placing it in a sterile plastic bag that is placed, in turn, in another bag filled with ice-cold saline, all of which are carried in an ice chest. Of all the regimens tested, conventional cardioplegia has proved most effective in maintaining cardiac performance.[12] The upper time limit for ex vivo storage of human hearts appears to be approximately 6 hours.[13]

Surgical Procedures

Orthotopic Heart Transplantation

Orthotopic heart transplantation is carried out via a median sternotomy, and the general approach is similar to that used for coronary revascularization or valve replacement. Frequently, patients will have undergone a prior median sternotomy; repeat sternotomy is cautiously performed using an oscillating saw. The groin should be prepped and draped to provide a rapid route for cannulation for cardiopulmonary bypass (CPB) if necessary. After the pericardium is opened, the aorta is cannulated as distally as possible and the IVC and SVC are individually cannulated via the high right atrium. Manipulation of the heart before institution of CPB is limited if thrombus is detected in the heart with transesophageal echocardiography (TEE; Figure 23-1). After initiation of CPB and cross-clamping of the aorta, the heart is arrested and excised (Figure 23-2). The aorta and PA are separated and divided just above the level of their respective valves, and the atria are transected at their grooves. A variant of this classic approach totally excises both atria, mandating bicaval anastomoses. This technique may reduce the incidence of atrial arrhythmias, better preserve atrial function by avoiding tricuspid regurgitation, and enhance cardiac output (CO) after transplantation.[14,15]

The donor graft then is implanted with every effort to maintain a cold tissue temperature, beginning with the left atrial (LA) anastomosis. If the foramen ovale is patent, it is sutured closed. The donor right atrium is opened by incising it from the IVC to the base of the right atrial (RA) appendage (to preserve the donor sinoatrial node), and the RA anastomosis is constructed. Alternatively, if the bicaval technique is used, individual IVC and SVC anastomoses are sewn. The donor and recipient pulmonary arteries are then brought together in an end-to-end manner, followed by the anastomosis of the donor to the recipient aorta. After removal of the aortic cross-clamp, the heart is de-aired

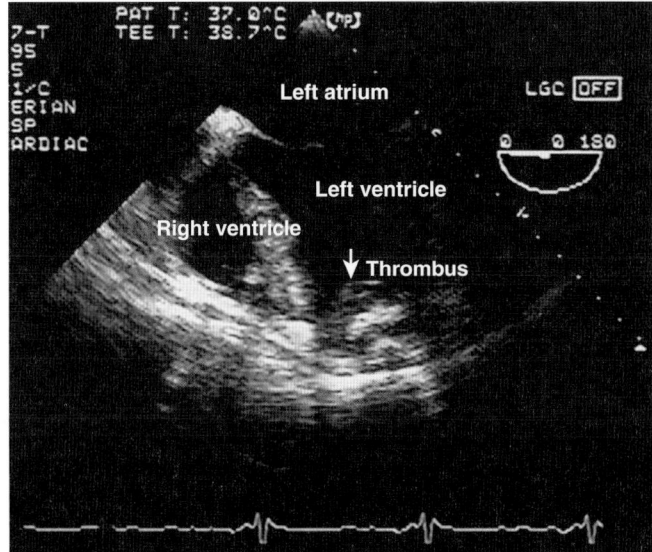

Figure 23-1 Transesophageal echocardiographic image of laminated intraventricular thrombus in the native left ventricular apex. If intracavitary thrombus is found, great caution is warranted during dissection before cardiopulmonary bypass to avoid systemic embolization.

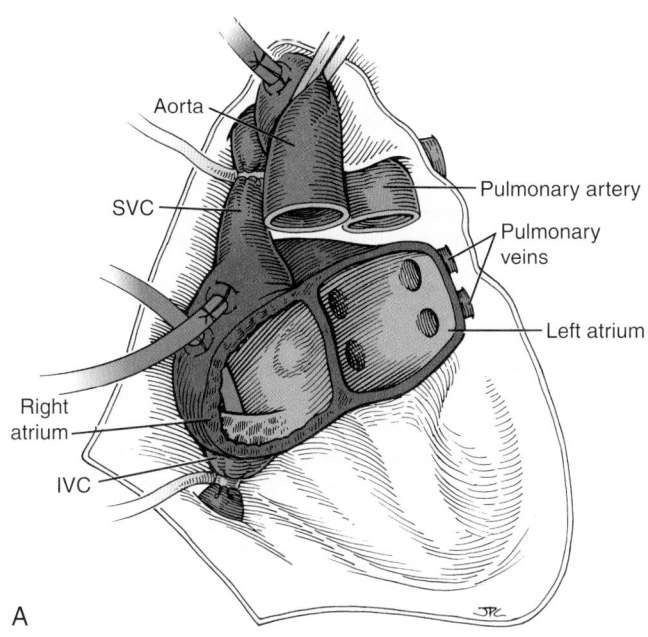

A

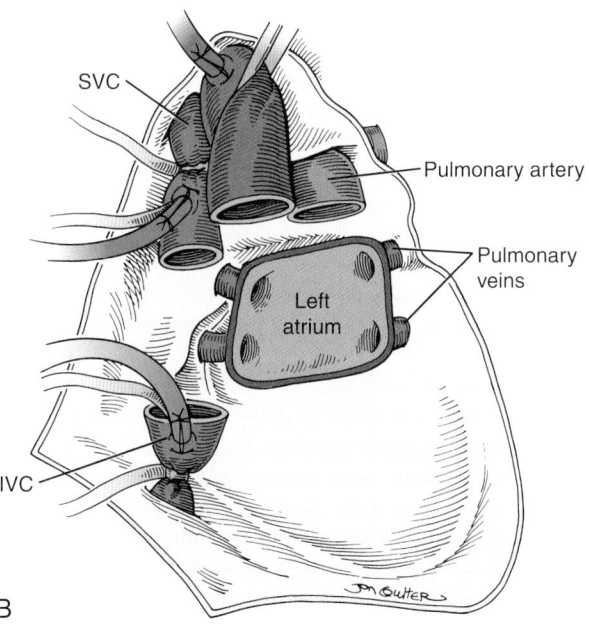

B

Figure 23-2 Mediastinum after excision of the heart but before allograft placement. Venous cannulas are present in the superior (SVC) and inferior vena cava (IVC), and the arterial cannula is present in the ascending aorta. *A,* Classic orthotopic technique. *B,* Bicaval anastomotic technique.

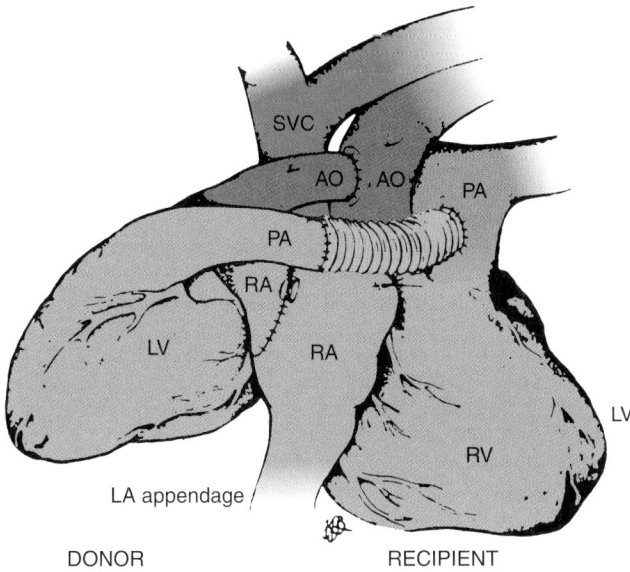

Figure 23-3 Placement of heterotopic graft in the right chest, with anastomoses to the corresponding native left (LA) and right atria (RA), ascending aorta (AO), and an interposition graft to the native pulmonary artery (PA). LV, left ventricle; RV, right ventricle; SVC, superior vena cava. *(From Cooper DKC, Lanza LP:* Heart Transplantation: The Present Status of Orthotopic and Heterotopic Heart Transplantation. *Lancaster, United Kingdom, MTP Press, 1984.)*

via a vent in the ascending aorta. Just before weaning from CPB, one of the venous cannulae is withdrawn into the right atrium and the other removed. The patient is then weaned from CPB in the usual manner. After hemostasis is achieved, mediastinal tubes are placed for drainage, the pericardium is left open, and the wound is closed in the standard fashion.

Heterotopic Heart Transplantation

Although orthotopic placement of the cardiac graft is optimal for most patients, certain recipients are not candidates for the orthotopic operation, and instead the graft is placed in the right chest and connected to the circulation in parallel with the recipient heart. The two primary indications for heterotopic placement are significant irreversible pulmonary hypertension and gross size mismatch between the donor

and recipient. Heterotopic placement may avoid the development of acute right ventricular (RV) failure in the unconditioned donor heart in the face of acutely increased RV afterload.

Donor harvesting for heterotopic placement is performed in the previously described manner, except that the azygos vein is ligated and divided to increase the length of the donor SVC; the PA is extensively dissected to provide the longest possible main and right PA; and the donor IVC and right pulmonary veins are oversewn, with the left pulmonary veins incised to create a single large orifice. The operation is performed via a median sternotomy in the recipient, but the right pleura is entered and excised. The recipient SVC is cannulated via the RA appendage, and the IVC via the lower right atrium. After arresting the recipient heart, the LA anastomosis is constructed by incising the recipient left atrium near the right superior pulmonary vein and extending this incision inferiorly, and then anastomosing the respective left atria. The recipient RA-SVC is then incised and anastomosed to the donor RA-SVC, after which the donor aorta is joined to the recipient aorta in an end-to-side manner. Finally, the donor PA is anastomosed to the recipient main PA in an end-to-side manner if it is sufficiently long; otherwise, they are joined via an interposed vascular graft (Figure 23-3).

Special Situations

Mechanical ventricular assist devices (see Chapters 27 and 32) have been used successfully to "bridge" patients who would otherwise die of acute heart failure awaiting transplantation.[16] The technique of transplantation is virtually identical in such patients to that for ordinary orthotopic transplantation. However, repeat sternotomy is obligatory. Placement of large-bore intravenous access is prudent because excessive hemorrhage can occur during the transplant procedure.

Rarely, patients will present for cardiac transplantation combined with transplantation of the liver.[17] The cardiac allograft usually is implanted first to better enable the patient to survive potential hemodynamic instability associated with reperfusion of the hepatic allograft. Large-bore intravenous access is mandatory. Conventional full heparinization protocols or low-dose heparin with heparin-bonded circuits may be used. A venous cannula can be left in the right atrium at the completion of the heart transplant procedure to serve as a return site for subsequent venovenous bypass during liver transplantation.

Pathophysiology before Transplantation

The pathophysiology of heart transplant candidates is predominantly end-stage cardiomyopathy. Normally, such patients will have both systolic dysfunction (characterized by decreased stroke volume and increased end-diastolic volume) and diastolic dysfunction, characterized by an increased intracardiac diastolic pressure. As compensatory mechanisms to maintain CO fail, the increased LV pressures lead to increases in pulmonary venous pressures and development of pulmonary vascular congestion and edema. A similar process occurs if RV failure also occurs. Autonomic sympathetic tone is increased in patients with heart failure, leading to generalized vasoconstriction, as well as salt and water retention. Vasoconstriction and ventricular dilation combine to substantially increase myocardial wall tension. Over time, the high levels of catecholamines lead to a decrease in the sensitivity of the heart and vasculature to these agents via a decrease in receptor density (i.e., "downregulation") and a decrease in myocardial norepinephrine stores.[18]

Therapy of heart failure seeks to reverse or antagonize these processes (see Chapters 10, 32, and 34). Almost all candidates will be maintained on diuretics; hypokalemia and hypomagnesemia secondary to urinary losses are likely, and the anesthesiologist must be alert to the possibility that a patient is hypovolemic from excessive diuresis. Another mainstay of therapy is vasodilators (such as nitrates, hydralazine, and angiotensin-converting enzyme inhibitors), which decrease the impedance to LV emptying and improve cardiac function and survival in patients with end-stage heart failure.[19,20] Paradoxically, slow incremental β-blockade with agents such as the β_1-antagonist metoprolol also can improve hemodynamics and exercise tolerance in some patients awaiting heart transplantation.[21] Patients who are symptomatic despite these measures often will require inotropic therapy. Digoxin is an effective but weak inotrope, and its use is limited by toxic side effects. Phosphodiesterase inhibitors such as amrinone, milrinone, and enoximone are efficacious, but chronic therapy is restricted by concerns about increased mortality in those receiving these agents.[22,23] Therefore, inotrope-dependent patients often are treated with intravenous infusions of β-adrenergic agonists such as dopamine or dobutamine. Patients refractory to even these measures may be supported with intra-aortic balloon counterpulsation, but its use is fraught with significant vascular complications and essentially immobilizes the patient. Many patients with low CO are maintained on anticoagulants such as warfarin to prevent pulmonary or systemic embolization, especially if they have atrial fibrillation.

Pathophysiology after Transplantation

The physiology of patients after heart transplantation is of interest not only to anesthesiologists in cardiac transplant centers but to the anesthesiology community at large because a substantial portion of these patients return for subsequent surgical procedures.[24,25]

Cardiac denervation is an unavoidable consequence of heart transplantation. Many long-term studies indicate that reinnervation is absent,[26,27] or at best partial or incomplete,[28] in humans. Denervation does not significantly change baseline cardiac function,[29,30] but it does substantially alter the cardiac response to demands for increased CO. Normally, increases in heart rate can rapidly increase CO, but this mechanism is not available to the transplanted heart. Heart rate increases only gradually with exercise, and this effect is mediated by circulating catecholamines.[26] Increases in CO in response to exercise are instead mostly mediated via an increase in stroke volume.[31] Therefore, maintenance of adequate preload in cardiac transplant recipients is crucial. Lack of parasympathetic innervation probably is responsible for the gradual decrease in heart rate after exercise seen in transplant recipients, rather than the usual sharp decline.

Denervation has important implications in the choice of pharmacologic agents used after cardiac transplantation. Drugs that act indirectly on the heart via either the sympathetic (ephedrine) or parasympathetic (atropine, pancuronium, edrophonium) nervous systems generally will be ineffective. Drugs with a mixture of direct and indirect effects will exhibit only their direct effects (leading to the absence of the normal increase in refractory period of the atrioventricular node with digoxin,[32] tachycardia with norepinephrine infusion, and bradycardia with neostigmine).[33] Thus, agents with direct cardiac effects (such as epinephrine or isoproterenol) are the drugs of choice for altering cardiac physiology after transplantation. However, the chronically high catecholamine levels found in cardiac transplant recipients may blunt the effect of α-adrenergic agents, as opposed to normal responses to β-adrenergic agents.[34]

Allograft coronary vasculopathy remains the greatest threat to long-term survival after heart transplantation. Allografts are prone to the accelerated development of an unusual form of coronary atherosclerosis that is characterized by circumferential, diffuse involvement of entire coronary arterial segments, as opposed to the conventional form of coronary atherosclerosis with focal plaques often found in eccentric positions in proximal coronary arteries.[35] The pathophysiologic basis of this process remains elusive, but it is likely due to an immune cell–mediated activation of vascular endothelial cells to upregulate the production of smooth muscle cell growth factors.[36] More than half of all heart transplant recipients have evidence of concentric atherosclerosis 3 years after transplant, and more than 80% at 5 years.[37] Because afferent cardiac reinnervation is rare, a substantial portion of recipients with accelerated vasculopathy will have silent ischemia.[38] Noninvasive methods of detecting coronary atherosclerosis are insensitive for detecting allograft vasculopathy.[39] Furthermore, coronary angiography often underestimates the severity of allograft atherosclerosis[40]; other diagnostic regimens such as intravascular ultrasound and dobutamine stress echocardiography may detect morphologic abnormalities or functional ischemia, respectively, in the absence of angiographically significant lesions.[35,40,41] Therefore, the anesthesiologist should assume that there is a substantial risk for coronary vasculopathy in any heart transplant recipient beyond the first 2 years, regardless of symptoms, the results of noninvasive testing, and even angiography.

Anesthetic Management

Preoperative Evaluation and Preparation

The preoperative period often is marked by severe time constraints because of the impending arrival of the donor heart. Nevertheless, a rapid history should screen for last oral intake, recent anticoagulant use, intercurrent deterioration of ventricular function, or change in anginal pattern; a physical examination should evaluate present volume status, and a laboratory review (if available) and a chest radiograph should detect the presence of renal, hepatic, or pulmonary dysfunction. Many hospitalized patients will be supported with inotropic infusions and/or an intra-aortic balloon pump, and the infusion rates and timing of the latter should be reviewed.

Equipment and drugs similar to those usually used for routine cases requiring CPB should be prepared. A β-agonist such as epinephrine should be readily available both in bolus form and as an infusion to rapidly treat ventricular failure; and an α-agonist such as phenylephrine or norepinephrine is useful to compensate for the vasodilatory effects of anesthetics because even small decreases in preload and afterload can lead to catastrophic changes in CO and coronary perfusion in these patients.

Placement of invasive monitoring before induction will facilitate rapid and accurate response to hemodynamic events during induction. In addition to standard noninvasive monitoring, an arterial catheter and a PA catheter (with a long sterile sheath to allow partial removal during graft implantation) are placed after judicious use of sedation and local anesthetics. Placing the arterial catheter in a central site rather than the radial artery will avoid the discrepancy between radial and central arterial pressure often seen after CPB, but it also may be necessary to cannulate a femoral artery for arterial inflow for CPB if there has been a prior sternotomy. Floating the PA catheter into correct position may be difficult because of cardiac chamber dilation and severe tricuspid regurgitation. Large-bore intravenous access is mandatory, especially if a sternotomy has been previously performed, in which case external defibrillator/pacing patches also may be useful. The overall hemodynamic "picture" should be evaluated and optimized insofar as possible just before induction. If the hemodynamics seem tenuous, then starting or increasing an inotrope infusion may be advisable.

Induction

Most patients presenting for heart transplantation will not be in a fasting state and should be considered to have a "full stomach." Therefore, the induction technique should aim to rapidly achieve control of the airway to prevent aspiration while avoiding myocardial depression. A regimen combining a short-acting hypnotic with minimal myocardial depression (etomidate, 0.3 mg/kg), a moderate dose of narcotic to blunt the tachycardic response to laryngoscopy and intubation (fentanyl, 10 μg/kg), and succinylcholine (1.5 mg/kg) is popular[42]; high-dose narcotic techniques with or without benzodiazepines also have been advocated.[43,44] Vasodilation should be countered with an α-agonist. Anesthesia can be maintained with additional narcotic and sedatives (benzodiazepines or scopolamine).[44,45]

Intraoperative Management

After induction, the stomach can be decompressed with an orogastric tube and a TEE probe introduced while the bladder is catheterized. A complete TEE examination often will reveal useful information not immediately available from other sources, such as the presence of cardiac thrombi (see Figure 23-1), ventricular volume and contractility, and atherosclerosis of the ascending aorta and aortic arch. Cross-matched blood should be immediately available once surgery commences, especially if the patient has had a previous sternotomy; patients not previously exposed to cytomegalovirus should receive blood from donors who are likewise cytomegalovirus negative. Sternotomy and cannulation for CPB are performed as indicated earlier. The period before CPB often is uneventful, apart from arrhythmias and slow recovery of coronary perfusion because of manipulation of the heart during dissection and cannulation. The PA catheter should be withdrawn from the right heart before completion of bicaval cannulation.

Once CPB is initiated, ventilation is discontinued and the absence of a thrill in the carotid arteries is documented. Most patients will have an excess of intravascular volume, and administration of a diuretic and/or the use of hemofiltration via the pump may be beneficial by increasing the hemoglobin concentration. A dose of glucocorticoid (methylprednisolone, 500 mg) is administered as the last anastomosis is being completed before release of the aortic cross-clamp to attenuate any hyperacute immune response. During the period of reperfusion an infusion of an inotrope is begun for both inotropy and chronotropy. TEE is used to monitor whether the cardiac chambers are adequately de-aired before weaning from CPB.

Weaning from bypass begins after ventilation is resumed and the cannula in the SVC is removed. The donor heart should be paced if bradycardia is present despite the inotropic infusion. Once the patient is separated from CPB, the PA catheter can be advanced into position. Patients with increased PVR are at risk for acute RV failure and may benefit from a pulmonary vasodilator such as prostaglandin E_1 (0.05 to 0.15 μg/kg/min).[46] Rarely, such patients will require support with a RV assist device.[47] TEE often will provide additional useful information about right- and left-heart function and volume, and document normal flow dynamics through the anastomoses. Unless a bicaval anastomosis was created, a ridge of redundant tissue will be evident in the left atrium and should not cause alarm (see Videos 1A and 1B, available online).

Protamine then is given to reverse heparin's effect after satisfactory weaning from CPB. Continued coagulopathy despite adequate protamine is common after heart transplantation, especially if there has been a prior sternotomy. Treatment is similar to that used for other postbypass coagulopathies: meticulous attention to surgical hemostasis, empiric administration of platelets, and subsequent addition of fresh-frozen plasma and cryoprecipitate guided by subsequent coagulation studies (see Chapters 17, 30 and 31). After adequate hemostasis is achieved, the wound is closed in standard fashion and the patient transported to the intensive care unit (ICU).

Postoperative Management and Complications

Management in the ICU after the conclusion of the procedure essentially is a continuation of the anesthetic management after CPB.[48] The electrocardiogram; arterial, central venous, and/or PA pressures; and arterial oxygen saturation are monitored continuously. Cardiac recipients will continue to require β-adrenergic infusions for chronotropy and inotropy for up to 3 to 4 days. Vasodilators may be necessary to control arterial hypertension and decrease impedance to LV ejection. Patients can be weaned from ventilatory support and extubated when the hemodynamics are stable and hemorrhage has ceased. The immunosuppressive regimen of choice (typically consisting of cyclosporine, azathioprine, and prednisone, or tacrolimus and prednisone) should be started after arrival in the ICU. Invasive monitoring can be withdrawn as the inotropic support is weaned, and mediastinal tubes removed after drainage subsides (usually after 24 hours). Patients usually can be discharged from the ICU after 2 or 3 days (see Chapters 33–35).

Early complications after heart transplantation include acute and hyperacute rejection, cardiac failure, systemic and pulmonary hypertension, cardiac arrhythmias, renal failure, and infection. Hyperacute rejection is an extremely rare but devastating syndrome mediated by preformed recipient cytotoxic antibodies against donor heart antigens. The donor heart immediately becomes cyanotic from microvascular thrombosis and ultimately ceases to contract.[49] This syndrome is lethal unless the patient can be supported mechanically until a suitable heart is found. Acute rejection is a constant threat in the early postoperative period and may present in many forms (e.g., low CO, arrhythmias). Acute rejection occurs most frequently during the initial 6 months after transplantation, so its presence is monitored by serial endomyocardial biopsies, with additional biopsies to evaluate any acute changes in clinical status. Detection of rejection mandates an aggressive increase in the level of immunosuppression, usually including pulses of glucocorticoid or a change from cyclosporine to tacrolimus. Low CO after transplantation may reflect a number of causative factors: hypovolemia, inadequate adrenergic stimulation, myocardial injury during harvesting, acute rejection, tamponade, or sepsis. Therapy should be guided by invasive monitoring, TEE, and endomyocardial biopsy. Systemic hypertension may be caused by pain, so adequate analgesia should be obtained before treating blood pressure with a vasodilator. Because fixed pulmonary hypertension will have been excluded during the recipient evaluation, pulmonary hypertension after heart transplantation usually will be transient and responsive to vasodilators such as prostaglandin E_1, nitrates, or hydralazine after either orthotopic or heterotopic placement.[50,51] Atrial and ventricular tachyarrhythmias are common after heart transplantation[52]; once rejection has been ruled out as a cause, antiarrhythmics are used for conversion or control (except those acting via indirect mechanisms such as digoxin, or those with negative inotropic properties such as β-blockers and calcium channel blockers). Almost all recipients will require either β-adrenergic agonists or pacing to increase heart rate in the immediate perioperative period, but 10% to 25% of recipients also will require permanent pacing.[53,54] Renal function often improves immediately after transplantation, but immunosuppressives such as cyclosporine and tacrolimus may impair renal function.[55,56] Finally, infection is a constant threat to immunosuppressed recipients. Bacterial pneumonia is frequent early in the postoperative period, with opportunistic viral and fungal infections becoming more common after the first several weeks (see Chapter 37).

▣ Pediatric Considerations

In the pediatric population, dilated cardiomyopathy and complex congenital heart defects are the primary indications for heart transplantation. Although the number of donors and recipients has remained stable in recent years, the overall survival has improved in children undergoing heart transplantation. Factors that contribute to this trend are enhanced preservation of the donor heart, improved selection of recipients and donors, and refinements in surgical techniques and immunosuppressive therapy.[57]

Cardiac transplantation is recommended when the child's expected survival is less than 1 year. In some centers, this therapy is offered as the primary intervention to the infant born with hypoplastic left-heart syndrome. The perioperative and intraoperative management of these infants undergoing heart transplant have been extensively reviewed.[58]

The preoperative assessment for heart transplantation in the patient with complex CHD might be more extensive depending on the heart defect and previous corrective or palliative procedures. Similar to the child with dilated cardiomyopathy, assessment of the indexed pulmonary vascular resistance (PVRI) is essential.[57] In adults, a PVRI greater than 5 units and a transpulmonary gradient greater than 15 mm Hg are contraindications for transplantation. In children, the acceptable PVRI is less than 10 units, but it is not unusual for a pediatric heart transplant candidate to have a PVRI greater than 10 units. In one pediatric cardiac center, 20% of the transplanted patients had PVRIs greater than 6 units. However, in the 6 to 10 unit range, the child is at risk for acute RV failure because the donor's right ventricle is thin walled and the myocardium has been ischemic. If the PVRI decreases significantly in the catheterization laboratory, with a trial of vasodilator testing, hyperventilation, 100% O_2, and nitric oxide, the candidate is acceptable for transplant. If the PVRI remains borderline, the candidate is admitted to the hospital for a 1- or 2-week trial with milrinone and dobutamine. If the PVRI then falls, transplantation is offered. These patients might benefit from pulmonary vasodilation therapy during weaning from CPB and in the ICU.

Another aspect to be emphasized in the pretransplant evaluation of these patients with complex CHD is the need for a detailed anatomic evaluation. It is not uncommon for this group of patients to have branch PA stenosis or discontinuous pulmonary arteries. Anomalies of systemic and pulmonary veins are associated with atrial isomerism, and different surgical techniques are needed to address these issues during transplantation. High-output failure may develop in the recipient with large aortopulmonary collaterals in the postoperative period. Although the donor ischemic time, ICU days, and total hospital days are prolonged in these patients, the outcome is comparable with the patient with dilated cardiomyopathy after heart transplantation.

Cardiac transplantation also is offered to patients with the so-called failed Fontan for physiologic repair of cardiac defects with single ventricle. They present with protein-losing enteropathy, chronic liver disease, and pulmonary arteriovenous malformations. These malformations may complicate the postoperative course. If they are large enough, moderate-to-severe hypoxemia may lead to primary graft failure. Small malformations may regress with time.

In some recipients, the circulation is supported by extracorporeal membrane oxygenation (ECMO) or a ventricular assist device before transplantation. Prolonged support is associated with bleeding, sepsis, and multiorgan dysfunction. It is not uncommon to list an infant who is on ECMO for heart transplant after a failed Norwood procedure. Transportation of this infant to the operating room can be quite complicated.

Besides determining the blood type (ABO), it is important to assess for the presence of antibodies against human histocompatability leukocyte antigen.[59] Antibodies against human histocompatability leukocyte antigen may have developed in the recipient who was exposed to blood products during palliation for complex CHD. Hyperacute rejection may lead to graft loss in the operating room in this setting. The risk for primary graft failure is greater if more than mild systolic dysfunction was present in the donor heart before transplantation. In pediatrics, the donor-recipient heart size matching in weight ranges between 80% and 300%. At surgery, the bicaval technique is preferred.

As in adults, sedation before surgery is provided with benzodiazepines or scopolamine. Full-stomach precautions generally are

taken. Induction of anesthesia is accomplished with etomidate (0.2 to 0.3 mg/kg), fentanyl, and a muscle relaxant (succinylcholine or a nondepolarizer). Titration to vital signs is important. Frequently, the groin vessels are exposed for urgent cannulation before sternotomy, and during this procedure fewer narcotics are required. If hemodynamics are adequate, a volatile agent can be used. An opioid with a benzodiazepine is used for maintenance of anesthesia. Recall of operative events has been documented in young adolescents. A PA catheter is useful in the older child, but just an RV catheter can be used when there are concerns about pulmonary hypertension.

LUNG TRANSPLANTATION

History and Epidemiology

Although the first human lung transplant was performed in 1963, surgical technical problems and inadequate preservation and immunosuppression regimens prevented widespread acceptance of this procedure until the mid-1980s (Box 23-2). Advances in these areas have since made lung transplantation a viable option for many patients with end-stage lung disease. For the period January 1, 1985, to June 30, 2008, a total of 29,732 lung transplants were reported to the Registry of the International Society for Heart and Lung Transplantation.[3] The frequency of both single- and double-lung transplants increased exponentially during the period up until 1993, with the sharpest growth in unilateral transplants. According to data collected by UNOS between 2000 and 2002, the annual frequency of lung transplantation has remained stagnant, with the total number still averaging in the vicinity of 1000. This is unchanged from the time between 1993 and 1995, when the numbers first leveled off. Further growth in lung transplantation is constrained by a shortage of donor organs, with demand for organs still vastly exceeding supply. This may potentially be exacerbated by data that were published in 2009, revealing that double-lung transplant afforded fewer hospitalizations and potentially better long-term survival.[60]

It is estimated that in excess of a million individuals with end-stage lung disease are potential recipients of lung transplants.[61] Some had hoped that non–heart-beating donors would provide an alternative source of organs, but this has not been the case. The Organ Procurement and Transplantation Network currently registers approximately 4000 patients for lung transplantation. This number does not accurately reflect the number of organs required because some patients will require bilateral lung transplantation. Average time to transplant increased to as much as 451 days in 1999; however, recently, that time has again decreased significantly. Currently, about one fourth of patients are transplanted within 251 days. Most of this improvement has been seen with recipients who are 50 years and older. One explanation for this may be increasing leniency in organ-selection criteria. This seems not to have been associated with increasing mortality rates. Mortality for patients on the waiting list also has continued to decline, from a 1993 high of close to 250 per 1000 patient-years to approximately 140 in 2002. Although some of this improvement may be ascribed to better medical management of patients on the waiting list, it is also likely due to broadened criteria for acceptance for transplantation and subsequent inclusion of patients with less severe illness.

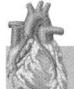

BOX 23-2. LUNG TRANSPLANTATION

- Broader donor criteria have decreased the time from listing to transplantation.
- Nitric oxide minimizes reperfusion injury.
- Donor lungs should be ventilated with a protective strategy (low inspired oxygen, low tidal volume/inspired pressure) after transplantation.

Increased experience with lung transplantation has been accompanied by a decrease in both operative and long-term mortality. For example, 30-day mortality rate for double-lung transplantation decreased from 44% in 1988 to 13.6% in 1991, whereas that for single-lung transplantation decreased from 22.7% to 12.6%.[62] As of the end of 2008, 3-year actuarial survival for recipients of both single- and double-lung transplants performed in the era 1992 to 1995 was approximately between 56% and 67% depending on recipient age percentage, which is a trend of continuing improvement of the periods preceding 2005.[3] Even better survival data have been reported from centers with extensive experience with these procedures (1-year survival rates of 82% for double-lung recipients and 90% for single-lung recipients).[63] Infection is the most frequent cause of death in the first year after transplant, but this is superseded in later years by bronchiolitis obliterans.[3] Notable is that 21% of all lung transplants were performed at 21 centers around the world averaging 50 procedures per year.[3]

Some of the most challenging patients are those with cystic fibrosis. The 1-year survival rate of 79% and 5-year survival rate of 57% after lung transplantation has shown that despite the high incidence of poor nutrition and the almost ubiquitous colonization by multidrug-resistant organisms, these patients can still successfully undergo lung transplantation with acceptable outcomes data.[64]

It is a sign of the maturity of lung transplantation procedures that survival data for "redo" lung transplantation also are becoming available. A late-1991 survey of centers reported that actuarial survival after redo transplantation was significantly worse than that of first-time recipients (e.g., 35% vs. > 75% at 1 year),[65] and subsequent data have confirmed this observation.[3] Infection and multiorgan failure before repeat transplant are associated with an almost uniformly fatal outcome. Subsequent data from UNOS, however, have shown an improvement, with the 1-year survival rate at 66.3% in the retransplant patients as compared with 83.8% in the primary transplant population. This is, however, significantly worse at 3 years, with repeat survival rate at 38.8% compared with 63.2%.

Recipient Selection

Because donor lungs are scarce, it is important to select those most likely to benefit from lung transplantation as recipients. In general, candidates should be terminally ill with end-stage lung disease (New York Heart Association Class III or IV, with a life expectancy of approximately 2 years), be psychologically stable, and be devoid of serious medical illness (especially extrapulmonary infection) compromising other organ systems. Patients already requiring mechanical ventilation are poor candidates, although lung transplantation can be successful in such a setting. Other factors such as advanced age, previous thoracic surgery or deformity, and steroid dependence may be regarded as relative contraindications by individual transplant centers. Hepatic disease solely caused by right-heart dysfunction should not preclude candidacy.

Potential recipients undergo a multidisciplinary assessment of their suitability, including pulmonary spirometry, radiography (plain film and chest CT scan), and echocardiography or multigated image acquisition scan. Patients older than 40 years and those with pulmonary hypertension usually undergo left-heart catheterization to exclude significant coronary atherosclerosis or an intracardiac shunt. TEE may yield data (e.g., unanticipated atrial septal defect) that will alter subsequent surgical approach in approximately one quarter of patients with severe pulmonary hypertension.[66] Candidates who are accepted often are placed on a physical conditioning regimen to reverse muscle atrophy and debilitation and kept within 20% of their ideal body weight. Because lung transplantation is an emergency procedure (limited by a lung preservation time of 6 to 8 hours),[67] results of this comprehensive evaluation should be readily available to the anesthesia team at all times. Weiss[68] published data in 2009 that supported the cautious transplantation of patients older than 60 years but recommended against transplantation of patients older than 70. Data from the same authors suggested that race-matching also provided a survival benefit that manifested itself in the first 2 years after transplant.[69]

Donor Selection and Graft Harvest

The ongoing shortage of suitable donor organs has led to a liberalization of selection criteria. Prospective lung donors who were cigarette smokers are no longer rejected simply based on a pack-year history. Computed tomography has been used to assess the structural integrity of the lung, particularly in donors who have suffered traumatic chest injury. Lungs that have contusion limited to less than 30% of a single lobe can be considered adequate.[70] Greater use also has been made of organs from older but otherwise healthy donors (55 to 60 years old), especially when the ischemic period will be short.[71] A clear chest radiograph, normal blood gas results, unremarkable findings on bronchoscopy, sputum stain, and direct intraoperative evaluation confirm satisfactory lung function. The lungs are matched to the recipient for ABO blood type and size (oversized lungs can result in severe atelectasis and compromise of venous return in the recipient, especially after double-lung transplantation). Donor serology and tracheal cultures will guide subsequent antibacterial and antiviral therapy in the recipient.

Most lung grafts are recovered during a multivisceral donor harvest procedure. The heart is removed as described for heart transplantation, using inflow occlusion and cardioplegic arrest, with division of the IVC and SVC, the aorta, and the main PA. Immediately after cross-clamping, the pulmonary vasculature is flushed with ice-cold preservative solution, which often contains prostaglandin E$_1$. This is believed to promote pulmonary vasodilation, which aids homogenous distribution of the preserving solution. Other additives that have been included are nitroglycerin and low-potassium 5% dextran. The left atrium is divided to leave an adequate LA cuff for both the heart graft and lung graft(s) with the pulmonary veins. After explantation, the lung also may be flushed to clear all pulmonary veins of any clots. After the lung is inflated, the trachea (or bronchus for an isolated lung) is clamped, divided, and stapled closed. Inflating the lung has been shown to increase cold ischemia tolerance of the donor organ. The lung graft is removed, bagged, and immersed in ice-cold saline for transport.

Surgical Procedures

Because of the relative shortage of lung donors, and the finding that recipients can gain significant exercise tolerance even with only one transplanted lung,[72] single-lung transplantation is the procedure of choice for all lung transplant candidates, except when leaving one of the recipient's lungs in place would predispose to complications. For example, the presence of lung disease associated with chronic infection (cystic fibrosis and severe bronchiectasis) mandates double-lung transplantation to prevent the recipient lung from acting as a reservoir of infection and subsequently cross-contaminating the allograft. Patients with severe air trapping may require double-lung transplantation if uncontrollable ventilation/perfusion mismatching will be likely after transplantation. Lobar transplantation into children and young adults from living-related donors is discussed separately later in this chapter.

Single-Lung Transplant

The choice of which lung to transplant is usually based on multiple factors, including avoidance of a prior operative site, preference for removing the native lung with the worst ventilation/perfusion ratio, and donor lung availability. The recipient is positioned for a posterolateral thoracotomy, with the ipsilateral groin prepped and exposed in case CPB becomes necessary. With the lung deflated, a pneumonectomy is performed, with special care to preserve as long a PA segment as possible. After removal of the diseased native lung, the allograft is positioned in the chest with precautions to maintain its cold tissue temperature. The bronchial anastomosis is performed first. A "telescoping" anastomosis is used if there is significant discrepancy in size between the donor and the recipient. The object of the technique is to minimize the chance of dehiscence. Although it was once common to wrap bronchial anastomoses with omentum, wrapping produces no added benefit when a telescoping anastomosis is performed. The PA is anastomosed next, and finally the pericardium is opened and the

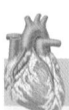

BOX 23-3. WARM PULMONOPLEGIA

Hematocrit 18 to 20, leukocyte-depleted
L-Glutamate
L-Aspartate
Adenosine
Lidocaine
Nitroglycerin
Verapamil
Dextrose
Insulin

allograft LA cuff containing the pulmonary venous orifices is anastomosed to the native left atrium. The pulmonary circuit is then flushed with blood and de-aired. The initial flush solution is usually cold (4° C) but is followed by a warm (37° C) flush. The warm flush usually is performed during final completion of the vascular anastomoses. The goal of the flushing is to achieve a controlled reperfusion.[73] The contents of this solution are listed in Box 23-3.

After glucocorticoid administration, the vascular clamps are removed, reperfusion is begun, and the lung reinflated with a series of ventilations to full functional residual capacity. After achieving adequate hemostasis and satisfactory blood gases, chest tubes are placed, the wound is closed, and the patient is transported to the ICU.

Double-Lung Transplant

Early attempts at double-lung transplantation using an en bloc technique via a median sternotomy were plagued by frequent postoperative airway dehiscence because of poor vascular supply of the tracheal anastomosis, by hemorrhage caused by extensive mediastinal dissection (which also resulted in cardiac denervation), by the requirement for complete CPB and cardioplegic arrest (to facilitate pulmonary arterial and venous anastomoses), and by poor access to the posterior mediastinum. The subsequent development of the bilateral sequential lung transplant technique via a "clamshell" thoracosternotomy (essentially two single-lung transplants performed in sequence) has avoided many of the problems inherent in the en bloc technique.[74,75] An alternative to using a clamshell incision in slender patients is an approach through two individual anterolateral thoracotomies. This results in a particularly pleasing cosmetic result in female patients because the scar falls in the breast crease. Use of CPB is optional, exposure of the posterior mediastinum is enhanced (improving hemostasis), and cardiac denervation usually can be avoided. Pleural scarring usually is extensive in patients with cystic fibrosis, and postoperative hemorrhage and coagulopathy are the rule if CPB is required. Transplantation of both lungs is performed in the supine position. The groin is prepped and exposed in case CPB is required. If a clamshell incision is utilized, the arms are padded and suspended over the head on an ether screen (Figure 23-4). In the slender patient whose anteroposterior chest dimensions are normal, the arms may be tucked at the patient's sides. Recipient pneumonectomy and implantation of the donor lung are performed sequentially on both lungs in essentially the same manner as described earlier for a single-lung transplant. The native lung with the worst function should be transplanted first. In patients whose indication for transplantation is suppurative disease, the pleural cavity is pulse-lavaged with antibiotic-containing solution that has been tailored to that patient's antimicrobial sensitivity profile. In addition to this, the anesthesiologist irrigates the trachea and bronchi with diluted iodophor solution before the donor lung is brought onto the surgical field.

Pathophysiology before Transplantation

Patients with highly compliant lungs and obstruction of expiratory airflow cannot completely exhale the delivered tidal volume, resulting in positive intrapleural pressure throughout the respiratory cycle

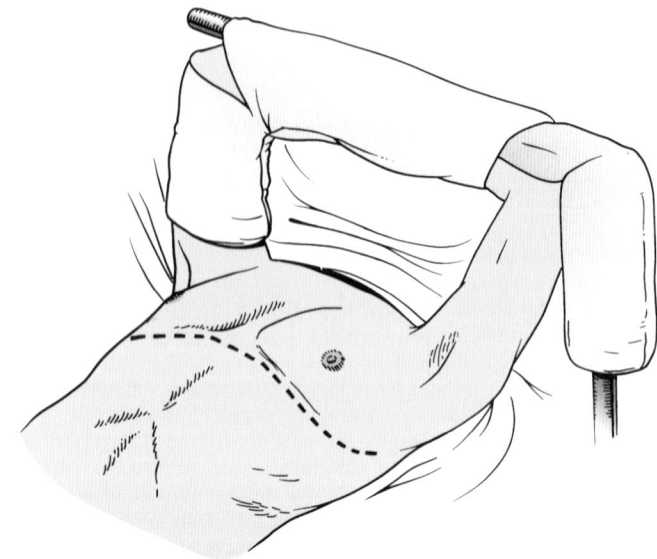

Figure 23-4 **Patient positioning for "clamshell" thoracosterno-tomy.** The arms are padded and suspended from an ether screen above the head of the patient. Path of surgical incision is shown with *dotted line. (From Firestone LL, Firestone S: Organ transplantation. In Miller RD [ed]: Anesthesia, 4th ed. New York: Churchill Livingstone, 1994, p 1981.)*

("auto-PEEP" [positive end-expiratory pressure] or "intrinsic PEEP"), which decreases venous return and causes hypotension.[76] The presence of auto-PEEP is highly negatively correlated with forced expiratory volume in 1 second (FEV_1; percentage predicted) and highly positively correlated with pulmonary flow resistance and resting hypercarbia.[77] Hyperinflation is a frequent complication of single-lung ventilation during lung transplantation in patients with obstructive lung disease. Hyperinflation-induced hemodynamic instability can be diagnosed by turning off the ventilator for 30 seconds and opening the breathing circuit to the atmosphere. If the blood pressure returns to its baseline value, hyperinflation is the underlying cause. Hyperinflation can be ameliorated with deliberate hypoventilation (decreasing both the tidal volume and rate).[78] Although this may result in profound hypercarbia, high carbon dioxide tensions are well tolerated in the absence of hypoxemia. PEEP also may decrease air trapping because it decreases expiratory resistance during controlled mechanical ventilation.[79] However, the application of PEEP requires close monitoring because if the level of extrinsic PEEP applied exceeds the level of auto-PEEP, further air trapping may result.

RV failure frequently is encountered in lung-transplant recipients with pulmonary hypertension because of chronically increased RV afterload. The response of the right ventricle to a chronic increase in afterload is to hypertrophy, but eventually this adaptive response is insufficient. As a result, RV stroke volume decreases and chamber dilation results. The following should be kept in mind when caring for patients with severe dysfunction (Box 23-4). First, increases in intrathoracic pressure may markedly increase PVR,[80] leading to frank RV failure in patients with chronic RV dysfunction. Changes in RV function may occur immediately after adding PEEP, increasing tidal volume, or decreasing expiratory time, and can have devastating consequences. In addition, although intravascular volume expansion in the presence of normal PVR increases CO, overzealous infusion in patients with increased PVR will increase RV end-diastolic pressure and RV wall stress, decreasing CO.[81] Inotropes with vasodilating properties (such as dobutamine or milrinone) often are a better choice than volume for augmenting CO in the setting of increased PVR. Furthermore, the right ventricle has a greater metabolic demand yet a lower coronary perfusion pressure than normal. RV performance can be augmented by improving RV coronary perfusion pressure with α-adrenergic

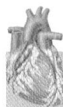

BOX 23-4. TREATMENT OF INTRAOPERATIVE RIGHT VENTRICULAR FAILURE

- Avoid large increases in intrathoracic pressure from:
  - Positive end-expiratory pressure (PEEP)
  - Large tidal volumes
  - Inadequate expiratory time
- Intravascular volume
  - Increase preload if pulmonary vascular resistance is normal
  - Rely on inotropes (dobutamine) if pulmonary vascular resistance is increased
- Maintain right ventricular coronary perfusion pressure with α-adrenergic agonists
- Cautious administration of pulmonary vasodilators (avoid systemic and gas exchange effects)
  - Prostaglandin E₁ (0.05 to 0.15 μg/kg/min)
  - Inhaled nitric oxide (20 to 40 ppm)

agents, provided these vasoconstrictors do not disproportionately increase PVR. This can sometimes be a better choice than augmenting the perfusion pressure with β-adrenergic agents because the oxygen supply is increased without a large increase in oxygen demand. Finally, vasodilators such as nitroprusside or prostaglandin E₁ may be effective in decreasing PVR and improving RV dysfunction early in the disease process, when only mild-to-moderate pulmonary hypertension is present. However, they are of notably limited value in the presence of severe, end-stage pulmonary hypertension. Systemic vasodilation and exacerbation of shunting often limit their use. Inhaled nitric oxide has shown promise as a means of acutely decreasing PVR without altering systemic hemodynamics both during the explantation phase and after lung transplantation.[82,83] Nitric oxide decreases both PA pressure and intrapulmonary shunting. Further, the combination of inhaled nitric oxide and aerosolized prostacyclin had a synergistic effect, without causing deleterious effects on the systemic perfusion pressure. The use of nitric oxide with or without inhaled prostacyclin may be helpful in avoiding CPB in patients having lung transplantation (see Chapters 10, 24, and 34).

Pathophysiology after Lung Transplantation

The implantation of the donor lung(s) causes marked alterations in recipient respiratory physiology. In single-lung recipients, the pattern of ventilation/perfusion matching depends on the original disease process. For example, with pulmonary fibrosis, blood flow and ventilation gradually divert to the transplanted lung, whereas in patients transplanted for diseases associated with pulmonary hypertension, blood flow is almost exclusively diverted to the transplanted lung, which still receives only half of the total ventilation.[84] In such patients the native lung represents mostly dead-pace ventilation. Transplantation results in obligatory sympathetic and parasympathetic denervation of the donor lung and, therefore, alters the physiologic responses of airway smooth muscle. Exaggerated bronchoconstrictive responses to the muscarinic agonist methacholine have been noted in some (but not all) studies of denervated lung recipients.[85,86] The mechanism of hyper-responsiveness may involve cholinergic synapses, inasmuch as they are the main mediators of bronchoconstriction. For example, electrical stimulation of transplanted bronchi (which activates cholinergic nerves) produces a hypercontractile response.[87] This suggests either enhanced release of acetylcholine from cholinergic nerve endings because of an increased responsiveness of parasympathetic nerves or else loss of inhibitory innervation. Such effects are unlikely to be postsynaptic in origin because the number and affinity of muscarinic cholinergic receptors on transplanted human bronchi are similar to controls.[88] Reinnervation during subsequent weeks

to months has been demonstrated in several animal models,[89,90] but there was no definitive evidence concerning reinnervation of transplanted human lungs until a small study was published in 2008 that showed return of cough reflex to noxious stimuli (distal to the anastomosis) within 12 months. The presence of nerve cells in the anastomoses of deceased patients also was noted.[91] Mucociliary function is transiently severely impaired after lung transplantation and remains depressed for up to a year after the procedure.[92] Thus, transplant recipients require particularly aggressive endotracheal suctioning to remove airway secretions.

Lung transplantation also profoundly alters the vascular system. The ischemia and reperfusion that are an obligatory part of the transplantation process damage endothelia. Cold ischemia alone decreases β-adrenergic cyclic adenosine monophosphate–mediated vascular relaxation by approximately 40%, and subsequent reperfusion produces even greater decreases in both cyclic guanosine monophosphate–mediated and β-adrenergic cyclic adenosine monophosphate–mediated pulmonary vascular smooth muscle relaxation.[93] Endothelial damage in the pulmonary allograft also results in "leaky" alveolar capillaries and the development of pulmonary edema. Pulmonary endothelial permeability is approximately three times greater in donor lungs than in healthy volunteers.[94] Regulation of pulmonary vasomotor tone solely by circulating humoral factors is another side effect of denervation. Changes in either the levels of circulating mediators or in the responsiveness of the pulmonary vasculature to such mediators may result in dramatic effects on the pulmonary vasculature. An example of the former is the finding that the potent vasoconstrictor endothelin is present at markedly increased levels (two to three times normal) immediately after transplantation and remains increased for up to a week thereafter.[95] Alterations in the response of denervated pulmonary vasculature to α₁-adrenergic agents[96] and prostaglandin E₁,[97] as well as a reduction in nitric oxide activity, also have been demonstrated in acutely denervated lung.[96] Dysfunctional responses to mediators may be exaggerated if CPB is required.[96] Pulmonary vacular resistance can be substantially decreased with the administration of inhaled nitric oxide after reperfusion. It remains unclear whether nitric oxide also ameliorates reperfusion injury. Several studies suggest that nitric oxide prevents or modulates reperfusion injury as measured by decreased lung water, lipid peroxidase activity, neutrophil aggregation in the graft, and decreased IL-6, IL-8, and IL-10.[98–101] However, a number of studies suggest that although nitric oxide has an effect on pulmonary hemodynamics, it does not ameliorate reperfusion injury.[102–104]

Aerosolized inhaled prostacyclin also decreases PVR after reperfusion and improves oxygenation without the added theoretic risk for worsening reperfusion injury.[105] Inhaled prostacyclin has approximately the same effectiveness as nitric oxide in treating lungs damaged by reperfusion injury and offers the added benefit of being cheaper.[106]

A number of other agents have shown promise in decreasing postreperfusion injury in animal studies. Tetrahydrobiopterin, an essential cofactor in the nitric oxide synthase pathway, decreased the intracellular water, myeloperoxidase activity, and lipid peroxidation, and increased cyclic guanosine monophosphate levels when given during reperfusion.[107] The administration of surfactant into the donor lung before harvest also appeared to ameliorate ischemia/reperfusion injury in pigs. There was a decrease in the PVR, less inflammatory cellular infiltrate, and an increase in nitric oxide levels in the group that received surfactant.[108]

Given these pathophysiologic derangements, it is not surprising that PVR increases in the transplanted lung.[109,110] However, what the clinician observes in the lung-transplant patient will depend on the severity of pulmonary vascular dysfunction present before surgery. PA pressures decrease dramatically during lung transplantation in patients who had pulmonary hypertension before transplantation[111] and remain so for weeks to months thereafter.[111–117] Concomitant with the decrease in PA pressure, there is an immediate decrease in RV size after lung transplantation in those patients with preexisting pulmonary hypertension, as well as a return to a more normal geometry of the interventricular septum.[111] Both of these effects are sustained over several weeks to months.[111-117] Although echocardiographic indices of RV function (RV fractional area change) have not shown a consistent improvement in the immediate post-transplant period,[111] several other studies have documented improvement in RV function during the first several months after lung transplantation.[111,112,114-117] One striking finding was that persistent depression of RV function (defined as baseline RV fractional area change of less than 30% with failure to increase after transplant by either at least 5% or by 20% of baseline) was statistically associated with death in the immediate perioperative period.[111]

Anesthetic Management

Preoperative Evaluation and Preparation

Immediate pretransplant re-evaluation pertinent to intraoperative management includes a history and physical examination to screen for intercurrent deterioration or additional abnormalities that affect anesthetic management. Particular attention should be given to recent physical status, especially when the transplant evaluation was performed more than 9 to 12 months previously. A decrease in the maximal level of physical activity from that at the time of initial evaluation can be a sign of progressive pulmonary disease or worsening RV function. Most patients are maintained on supplemental nasal oxygen yet are mildly hypoxemic. Patients who are bedridden, or who must pause between phrases or words while speaking, possess little functional reserve and are likely to exhibit hemodynamic instability during induction. The time and nature of the last oral intake should be determined to aid in deciding the appropriate method of securing the airway. The physical examination should focus on evaluation of the airway for ease of laryngoscopy and intubation, on the presence of any reversible pulmonary dysfunction such as bronchospasm, and on signs of cardiac failure. New laboratory data often are not available before the beginning of anesthesia care, but special attention should be directed to evaluation of the chest radiograph for signs of pneumothorax, effusion, or hyperinflation because they may affect subsequent management.

Equipment necessary for this procedure is analogous to that used in any procedure in which CPB and cardiac arrest are a real possibility. Special mandatory pieces of equipment include some method to isolate the ventilation to each lung; although bronchial blockers have their advocates, double-lumen endobronchial tubes offer the advantages of easy switching of the ventilated lung, suctioning of the nonventilated lung, and facile independent lung ventilation after surgery. A left-sided double-lumen endobronchial tube is suitable for virtually all lung transplant cases (even left-lung transplants; Figure 23-5).

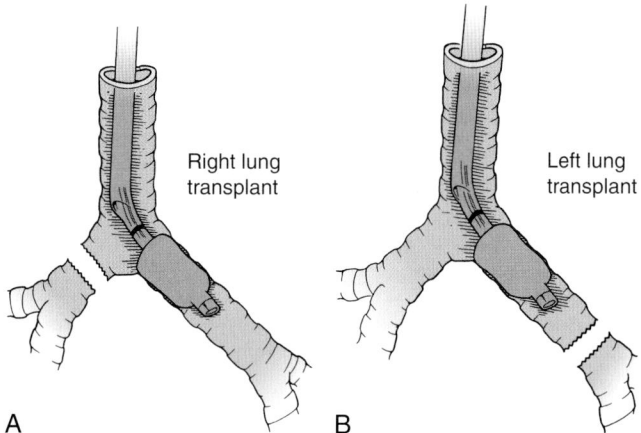

Figure 23-5   Left endobronchial tube during (A) right- and (B) left-lung transplantation. When the endobronchial tube is correctly positioned, either bronchus may be opened for anastomosis of the donor lung without compromising the surgical field or interfering with isolated lung ventilation.

Regardless of whether a bronchial blocker or double-lumen tube is used, a fiberoptic bronchoscope is absolutely required to rapidly and unambiguously verify correct tube positioning, evaluate bronchial anastomoses, and clear airway secretions. An adult-sized bronchoscope offers better field of vision and superior suctioning capability but can be used only with 41 or 39 French double-lumen tubes. A ventilator with low internal compliance is necessary to adequately ventilate the noncompliant lungs of recipients with restrictive lung disease or donor lungs suffering from reperfusion injury. The added capability of the ventilator to deliver pressure-controlled ventilation also is important, especially for the patients who have pulmonary fibrotic disease or reperfusion injury. Single-lung recipients with highly compliant lungs may require independent lung ventilation with a second ventilator after transplantation (discussed in detail later). A PA catheter capable of estimating right ventricular ejection fraction (RVEF) can be useful in diagnosing RV failure and its response to inotropes and vasodilators, as well as the response of the right ventricle to clamping of the PA. However, RVEF catheters are not accurate in the presence of significant tricuspid regurgitation or when malpositioned. Continuous mixed venous oximetry is beneficial in evaluating tissue oxygen delivery in patients subject to sudden, severe cardiac decompensation in the course of the operation, as well as the responses to therapy. A rapid-infusion system can be lifesaving in cases in which major hemorrhage occurs because of anastomotic leaks, inadequate surgical ligation of mediastinal collateral vessels, chest wall adhesions, or coagulopathy after CPB.

Induction of Anesthesia

Patients presenting for lung transplantation frequently arrive in the operating room area without premedication. Indeed, many will be admitted directly to the operating room from home. Because of the nature of the procedure planned, and many months on the transplant waiting list, these patients are often extremely anxious. Considering the risk for respiratory depression from sedatives in patients who are chronically hypoxic or hypercapnic, or both, only the most judicious use of intravenous benzodiazepines or narcotics is warranted. Assiduous administration of adequate local anesthesia during placement of invasive monitoring will also considerably improve conditions for both the patient and anesthesiologist. The standard noninvasive monitoring typical of cardiovascular procedures (two electrocardiogram leads including a precordial lead, blood pressure cuff, pulse oximetry, capnography, and temperature measurement) is used. Intravenous access sufficient to rapidly administer large volumes of fluid is required. Generally, two large-bore (16- or, preferably, 14-gauge catheters, or a 9 French introducer sheath) intravenous catheters are placed. Patients for bilateral sequential lung transplantation who will receive a "clamshell" thoracosternotomy (see Figure 23-4) should have intravenous catheters placed in the internal or external jugular veins, because peripherally placed intravenous catheters often are unreliable when the arms are bent at the elbow and suspended from the ether screen. An intra-arterial catheter is an absolute requirement for blood pressure monitoring and for obtaining specimens for arterial blood gases. Continuous monitoring via a fiberoptic electrode placed in the arterial catheter occasionally may be useful if this technology is available. The femoral artery should be avoided, if possible, because the groin may be needed as a site for cannulation for CPB. Although the radial or brachial artery may be used in single-lung transplantation patients, these sites are not optimal in those who will require CPB (e.g., en bloc double-lung transplants or patients with severe pulmonary hypertension) because the transduced pressure may inaccurately reflect central aortic pressure during and after CPB, as well as in patients undergoing a clamshell thoracosternotomy, because of the positioning of the arms. In the authors' institution, the majority of patients now have bilateral limited thoracotomies instead of the thoracosternotomy. An axillary arterial catheter may be useful in the latter situations because it provides a more accurate measure of central aortic pressure and allows sampling blood closer to that perfusing the brain. This may be important if partial CPB with a femoral arterial

Right lung transplant

Left lung transplant

A   B

cannula is used because differential perfusion of the upper and lower half of the body may result. A PA catheter is inserted via the internal or external jugular veins. A TEE probe is placed after the airway is secured. PA pressure monitoring is most useful in patients who have preexisting pulmonary hypertension, especially during induction and during initial one-lung ventilation (OLV) and PA clamping. Position of the PA catheter can be verified by TEE to ensure that it is residing in the main PA.

If the procedure is planned without CPB, care should be taken to ensure that the patient is kept at ideal physiologic temperature to minimize coagulopathy and increases in the Mvo_2. This can be achieved with a warming blanket on the bed, on the patient's head and arms, and on the legs below the knees. A fluid warmer is also useful in this regard.

Three main principles should guide the formulation of a plan for induction: (1) protection of the airway; (2) avoidance of myocardial depression and increases in RV afterload in patients with RV dysfunction; and (3) avoidance and recognition of lung hyperinflation in patients with increased lung compliance and expiratory airflow obstruction (Box 23-5). All lung transplants are done on an emergency basis, and the majority of patients will have recently had oral intake and must be considered to have "full stomachs." Because aspiration during induction would be catastrophic, every measure must be taken to protect the airway. Patients with known or suspected abnormalities of airway anatomy should be intubated awake after topical anesthesia is applied to the airway. Although a conventional rapid-sequence intravenous induction with a short-acting hypnotic (such as etomidate, 0.2 to 0.3 mg/kg), a small amount of narcotic (e.g., up to 10 μg/kg fentanyl), and succinylcholine usually will be tolerated, patients with severe RV dysfunction may exhibit profound hemodynamic instability in response to this induction regimen. For such patients, a more gradual induction is recommended, with greater reliance on high doses of narcotics and ventilation with continuous application of cricoid pressure. Patients with bullous disease or fibrotic lungs requiring high inflation pressures may develop a pneumothorax during initiation of positive-pressure ventilation. Acute reductions in Sao_2 accompanied by difficulty in ventilating the lungs and refractory hypotension should generate strong suspicions that a tension pneumothorax has developed. RV function can be impaired during induction by drug-induced myocardial depression, increases in afterload, or by ischemia secondary to acute RV dilation. Agents that act as myocardial depressants (such as thiopental) should be avoided in such patients. Increases in RV afterload can result from inadequate anesthesia, exacerbation of chronic hypoxemia and hypercarbia and metabolic acidosis, as well as increases in intrathoracic pressure because of positive-pressure ventilation. Systemic hypotension is poorly tolerated because increased RV end-diastolic pressure will diminish net RV coronary perfusion pressure. In addition, chronic increase of RV afterload increases the metabolic requirements of RV myocardium. Once the trachea is intubated and positive-pressure ventilation initiated, the avoidance of hyperinflation in patients with increased pulmonary compliance or bullous disease is crucial. Small tidal volumes, low respiratory rates, and inspiratory/expiratory (I:E) ratios should be used ("permissive hypercapnia"). If hemodynamic instability does occur with positive-pressure ventilation, the ventilator should be disconnected from the patient. If hyperinflation is the cause of hypotension, blood pressure will increase within 10 to 30 seconds of the onset of apnea. Ventilation then can be resumed at a tidal volume and/or rate compatible with hemodynamic stability.

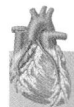

BOX 23-5. KEY PRINCIPLES OF ANESTHETIC INDUCTION FOR LUNG TRANSPLANTATION

- Secure the airway.
  - Intravenous rapid sequence induction versus gradual narcotic induction with continuous cricoid pressure
- Avoid myocardial depression and increases in right ventricular afterload.
- Avoid lung hyperinflation.

Anesthesia can be maintained using a variety of techniques. A moderate dose of narcotic (5 to 15 μg/kg fentanyl or the equivalent), combined with low doses of a potent inhalation anesthetic, offers the advantages of stable hemodynamics, a high inspired oxygen concentration, a rapidly titratable depth of anesthesia, and the possibility of extubation in the early postoperative period. Patients with severe RV dysfunction who cannot tolerate even low concentrations of inhalation anesthetics may require a pure narcotic technique. Nitrous oxide generally is not used because of the requirement for a high inspired oxygen concentration throughout the procedure and its possible deleterious effects if gaseous emboli or an occult pneumothorax is present.

Intraoperative Management

Institution of OLV occurs before hilar dissection and may compromise hemodynamics or gas exchange, or both (Box 23-6). Patients with diminished lung compliance often can tolerate OLV with normal tidal volumes and little change in hemodynamics. In contrast, patients with increased lung compliance and airway obstruction often will exhibit marked hemodynamic instability, unless the tidal volume is decreased and the expiratory time is increased. The magnitude of hypoxemia generally peaks about 20 minutes after beginning OLV. Hypoxemia during OLV may be treated with continuous positive airway pressure applied to the nonventilated lung,[118] PEEP to the ventilated lung, or both. Continuous positive airway pressure attempts to oxygenate the shunt fraction but may interfere with surgical exposure. PEEP attempts to minimize atelectasis in the ventilated lung, but may concomitantly increase shunt through the nonventilated lung. Definitive treatment of shunt in the nonventilated lung is provided by rapid isolation and clamping of the PA of the nonventilated lung. Pneumothorax on the nonoperative side may result during OLV if a large tidal volume is used.

PA clamping usually is well tolerated, except in the face of pulmonary hypertension with diminished RV reserve. If the degree of RV compromise is uncertain, a 5- to 10-minute trial of PA clamping is attempted; then the RV is evaluated by serial COs and RVEF measurements and inspection by TEE. A significant decrease in CO may predict patients who will require extracorporeal support.[119] Other indications for CPB in lung transplantation are listed in Box 23-7.[120]

Patients with severe pulmonary hypertension (greater than two thirds of systemic pressure) generally will be placed on CPB before PA

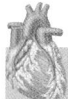

BOX 23-6. MANAGEMENT PRINCIPLES FOR ONE-LUNG VENTILATION DURING LUNG TRANSPLANTATION

- Tidal volume and respiratory rate
  - Maintain in patients with normal or decreased lung compliance (i.e., primary pulmonary hypertension, fibrosis)
  - Decrease both tidal volume and rate in patients with increased compliance (e.g., obstructive lung disease) to avoid hyperinflation ("permissive hypercapnia")
- Maintain oxygenation by:
  - 100% inspired oxygen
  - Applying CPAP (5 to 10 cm H_2O) to nonventilated lung
  - Adding PEEP (5 to 10 cm H_2O) to ventilated lung
  - Intermittent lung reinflation if necessary
  - Surgical ligation of the pulmonary artery of the nonventilated lung
- Be alert for development of pneumothorax on nonoperative side
  - Sharp decline in oxygen saturation, end-tidal carbon dioxide
  - Sharp increase in peak airway pressures
  - Increased risk with bullous lung disease
- Therapy
  - Relieve tension
  - Resume ventilation
  - Emergency cardiopulmonary bypass

CPAP, continuous positive airway pressure; PEEP, positive end-expiratory pressure.

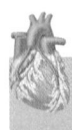

clamping. The intraoperative use of nitric oxide (20 to 40 parts per million [ppm]) may allow some procedures to proceed without the use of CPB.[121]

Lung transplantation usually can be performed without the aid of CPB; even during bilateral sequential lung transplantation, experienced teams utilize CPB for only about one quarter of patients.[122,123] Although CPB may provide stable hemodynamics, it is associated with an increased transfusion requirement.[78] In addition, graft function (as reflected by alveolar-arterial oxygen gradient) may be compromised,[124] endothelium-dependent cyclic guanosine monophosphate–mediated and β-adrenergic cyclic adenosine monophosphate–mediated pulmonary vascular relaxation may be impaired to a greater degree,[125] and a longer period of mechanical ventilation may be necessary.[122] Several exceptional circumstances require CPB: the presence of severe pulmonary hypertension because clamping of the PA will likely result in acute RV failure and "flooding" of the nonclamped lung, the repair of associated cardiac anomalies (e.g., patent foramen ovale, atrial or ventricular septal defects), treatment of severe hemodynamic or gas exchange instabilities, and living-related lobar transplantation. Hypercarbia generally is well tolerated and should not be considered a requirement for CPB per se.[78] Thus, the frequency of CPB will depend on recipient population factors such as prevalence of end-stage pulmonary vascular disease and associated cardiac anomalies.[126] The use of femoral venous and arterial cannulae for CPB during lung transplantation may lead to poor venous drainage and/or "differential perfusion" of the lower and upper body. Moreover, native pulmonary blood flow continues and may act as an intrapulmonary shunt during CPB. In this case, the cerebral vessels receive this desaturated blood, whereas the lower body is perfused with fully oxygenated blood from the CPB circuit. This effect is detectable by blood gas analysis of samples drawn from suitable arteries or by appropriately located pulse oximeter probes. Treatment includes conventional measures to increase venous return and augment bypass flow, or placing a venous cannula in the right atrium if this is feasible. The anesthesiologist also should maximize the inspired oxygen concentration and add PEEP to decrease intrapulmonary shunt. If all other measures fail, ventricular fibrillation can be induced using alternating current.[127]

ECMO also has been suggested as an alternative method of CPB during lung transplantation. It has been suggested that the use of ECMO with heparin-bonded circuits might improve the outcome of both single- and double-lung transplants by lessening the amount of pulmonary edema, especially in those patients who need CPB because of hemodynamic instability or who have primary pulmonary hypertension. An added benefit of this technique is that it clears the operative field of bypass cannulae, making left-sided transplant as unimpeded as right-sided transplant. There is no apparent increase in transfusion requirement.[128] Another added benefit of using ECMO in situ is that reperfusion of the lungs can be more easily controlled because the CO transiting the newly transplanted lung can be precisely controlled. This is especially the case for patients with advanced pulmonary hypertension.[129]

If CPB is used, weaning from circulatory support occurs when the graft anastomoses are complete. Ventilation is resumed with a lung protection strategy similar to that used in the ARDSnet (Acute Respiratory Distress Syndrome Network) trial.[71] This demonstrated that patients with decreased compliance related to acute respiratory

distress syndrome had a 22% decrease in mortality rate when applying tidal volumes of 6 mL/kg and a plateau pressure less than 30 cm H_2O.[71] Minimizing the inspired fraction of O_2 may help prevent generation of oxygen free radicals and modulate reperfusion injury. Fio_2 can be decreased to the minimum necessary to maintain the Spo_2 greater than 90%. Special attention should be directed to assessing and supporting RV function during this period, inasmuch as RV failure is the most frequent reason for failure to wean. Although the right ventricle often can be seen in the surgical field, TEE is more valuable for visualizing this structure's functional properties at this juncture. TEE also allows the evaluation of PA (see Video 2, available online) and pulmonary vein anastomoses. The PA diameter should be greater than 1 cm. Interrogating the pulmonary veins should demonstrate a two-dimensional diameter that is at least 0.5 cm with the presence of flow as measured by color-flow Doppler. In addition, pulse wave Doppler interrogation should yield flow rates less than 100 cm/sec to indicate adequacy of anastomosis. The operator must ensure that they align the Doppler beam angle with the pulmonary vein flow because misalignment may lead to underestimation of the true peak venous flow (see Video 3, available online). Care should be taken to measure these flow rates with both lungs being perfused because the measurements could be erroneous if measured with one PA clamped (Figure 23-6).[130,131] Inotropic support with dobutamine or epinephrine, as well as pulmonary vasodilation with nitroglycerin, nitroprusside, milrinone, or nitric oxide, may be necessary if RV dysfunction is evident. Milrinone has the advantage of providing both inotropic and vasodilatory effects; however, its administration can be complicated by significant systemic hypotension, necessitating the concomitant use of epinephrine or norepinephrine (see Chapters 10, 24, 27, 32, and 34).

Coagulopathy after weaning from CPB is common. The severity of coagulopathy may be worse after double- than single-lung transplantation, probably because of the more extensive dissection, presence of collaterals and scarring, and the longer duration of CPB. Factors under the anesthesiologist's control include incomplete reversal of heparin's effects, which should be assayed by the activated coagulation time. Similarly, preexisting deliberate anticoagulation (e.g., caused by warfarin) should be aggressively corrected with fresh-frozen plasma. Because platelet dysfunction is common after CPB, empiric administration is justified if coagulopathy persists. The thrombotic and fibrinolytic systems are activated during lung transplantation, especially if CPB is used, and although aprotinin can reduce this activation and perhaps reduce perioperative hemorrhage,[132–134] it has been withdrawn from production. The utility of ε-aminocaproic acid, tranexamic acid, and desmopressin (DDAVP) in replacing aprotinin in this setting remains unknown (see Chapter 31), although some preliminary data suggest that tranexamic acid may be similar in efficacy to aprotinin.

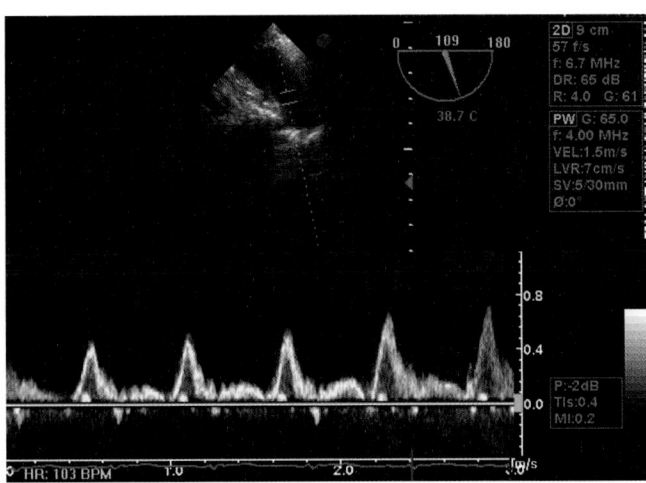

Figure 23-6 Pulsed-wave Doppler interrogation of the left superior pulmonary vein after lung transplantation.

Reperfusion without CPB often is accompanied by a mild-to-moderate decrease in systemic blood pressure, and occasionally is complicated by severe hypotension. This is usually the result of profound systemic vasodilation. The causative factor is unknown but may be caused by ionic loads such as potassium or additives such as prostaglandin E₁ in preservation solutions, or vasoactive substances generated during ischemia and reperfusion. This hypotension generally responds well to large doses of α-adrenergic agents and fortunately is short-lived. Agents of greatest use in this setting are norepinephrine and vasopressin. Ventilation is resumed with a lung protection strategy identical to that used when weaning from CPB.

Patients with preexisting increased lung compliance, as found in chronic obstructive pulmonary disease, can manifest great disparity in lung compliance after single-lung transplant. The donor lung usually will exhibit normal to decreased compliance, depending on the presence of reperfusion injury. This will result in relative hyperinflation of the native lung and underinflation with loss of functional residual capacity in the donor lung. Hyperinflation of the native lung may cause hemodynamic instability because of mediastinal shift, especially if PEEP is applied. Therefore, patients exhibiting signs of hyperinflation during OLV, which improves with deliberate hypoventilation, should be treated with independent lung ventilation after reperfusion. To accomplish this, the patient's postoperative ventilator is brought to the operating room while the donor lung is being implanted. When all anastomoses are completed, the donor lung is ventilated with a normal tidal volume (8 to 10 mL/kg) and rate, with PEEP initially applied at 10 cm H₂O. These settings can be adjusted according to blood gas analysis. Most gas exchange will take place in the donor lung. The native lung is ventilated with a low tidal volume (2 to 3 mL/kg) and a low rate (2 to 4/min) without PEEP. The objective is to prevent this lung from overinflating or developing a large shunt. Carbon dioxide exchange occurs predominantly in the donor lung.

Although some degree of pulmonary edema commonly is detected by chest radiograph after surgery, it is uncommon to encounter severe pulmonary edema in the operating room immediately after reperfusion of the graft. However, when it does occur, postreperfusion pulmonary edema can be dramatic and life-threatening. Copious pink frothy secretions may require almost constant suctioning to maintain a patent airway and may be accompanied by severe gas exchange and compliance abnormalities. Treatment includes high levels of PEEP using selective lung ventilation, diuresis, and volume restriction. Occasionally, patients may require support with ECMO for several days until reperfusion injury resolves; a high percentage of patients so treated ultimately survive.[135,136] Adequate analgesia is crucial for these patients to facilitate the earliest possible extubation, ambulation, and participation in spirometric exercises to enhance or preserve pulmonary function. Lumbar or thoracic epidural narcotic analgesia provides excellent analgesia while minimizing sedation. Epidural catheters can be placed before the procedure if time permits or after conclusion of the procedure. Placement of epidural catheter in cases in which a high expectation exists for the necessity of CPB remains a controversial topic. If CPB has been used or coagulopathy has developed, placement should be deferred until coagulation tests have normalized (see Chapter 38).

Fluid therapy also can impact the outcomes of lung transplantation as was demonstrated by McIlroy et al, who showed that the greater the amount of colloid (gelatin) that was used, the greater the A-a gradient, and the greater likelihood of delayed extubation. It was unclear, though, whether this effect extended to other colloids.[137]

Postoperative Management and Complications

Routine postoperative management of the lung transplant recipient continues many of the monitoring modes and therapies begun in the operating room. Positive-pressure ventilation is continued for at least several hours; if differential lung ventilation was used intraoperatively, this is continued in the early postoperative period. Because the lung graft is prone to the development of pulmonary edema because of preservation/reperfusion and the loss of lymphatic drainage, fluid

administration is minimized and diuresis encouraged when appropriate. When hemorrhage has ceased, the chest radiograph is clear, and the patient meets conventional extubation criteria, the endotracheal tube can be removed. Prophylactic antibacterial, antifungal, and antiviral therapy, as well as the immunosuppressive regimen of choice, are begun after arrival in the ICU.

Surgical technical complications are uncommon immediately after lung transplantation but may be associated with high morbidity.[138] Pulmonary venous obstruction usually presents as acute, persistent pulmonary edema of the transplanted lung.[139] Color-flow and Doppler TEE will show narrowed pulmonary venous orifices with turbulent, high-velocity flow and loss of the normal phasic waveform. PA anastomotic obstruction should be suspected if PA pressures fail to decrease after reperfusion of the lung graft. If the right PA is obstructed, this usually is evident on a TEE examination in the same way as for pulmonary venous obstruction; it is usually much more difficult to adequately inspect the left PA anastomosis with TEE, although some centers have reported a high success rate.[140] The diagnosis can be definitively made by measuring the pressure gradient across the anastomosis either by inserting needles on both sides of the anastomosis to transduce the respective pressures or by advancing the PA catheter across it. However, care should be taken not to measure this gradient while the contralateral PA is clamped, because the shunting of the entire CO through one lung will exaggerate the gradient present.[141] Angiography and perfusion scanning also are useful for making this diagnosis but are not immediately available in the operating room. Bronchial dehiscence or obstruction is extremely rare in the immediate perioperative period and can be evaluated by fiberoptic bronchoscopy.

Pneumothorax must be a constant concern for the anesthesiologist, especially involving the nonoperative side. Diagnosis of pneumothorax on the nonoperative side during a thoracotomy is extremely difficult. A sudden increase in inflation pressures with deterioration of gas exchange and possibly hypotension are characteristic. However, these same findings are possible with hyperinflation, mucous plugging, or malpositioning of the endobronchial tube. Transient cessation of ventilation and immediate fiberoptic bronchoscopy may rule out the former explanations, and the observation of an upward shift of the mediastinum in the surgical field may be observed in the presence of tension pneumothorax. If this diagnosis is strongly suspected, needle thoracostomy on the field may be lifesaving. Alternatively, the surgeon may be able to directly dissect across the mediastinum and decompress the nonoperative thorax, facilitating reinflation.

Tension pneumopericardium and postoperative hemothorax with complete ventilation/perfusion mismatch are other rare complications that have been reported after lung transplantation.[142,143] Patients with pulmonary hypertension and RV hypertrophy occasionally may develop dynamic RV outflow obstruction when transplantation acutely decreases RV afterload; the diagnosis can be confirmed using TEE.[144] Hyperacute rejection of a kind similar to that seen with heart transplantation has not been noted with lung transplantation.

The most common cause of death in the immediate perioperative period is graft dysfunction from reperfusion injury, which usually presents with hypoxemia, pulmonary infiltrates, poor lung compliance, pulmonary hypertension, and RV failure. If there are no technical reasons to account for pulmonary hypertension and RV failure, then graft dysfunction must be suspected. Unfortunately, few treatments will specifically ameliorate graft dysfunction and therapy is largely supportive. Vasodilator therapy to directly decrease PVR and, therefore, RV afterload may improve hemodynamics and, in some cases, may improve gas exchange. Both prostaglandin E₁ and nitrates can reverse severe hypoxemia and pulmonary hypertension after lung transplantation, and the latter attenuate the increase in transcription of vasoconstrictor genes (such as for endothelin and platelet-derived growth factor) induced by hypoxia.[145] Indeed, a "prophylactic" low-dose infusion of prostaglandin E₁ has been reported to preserve arterial oxygen tension without altering pulmonary hemodynamics in dogs after single-lung transplantation.[146] Improvement in pulmonary hemodynamics and gas exchange in patients with graft dysfunction also have been reported with the administration of nitric oxide.[82,147,148] Compared with historic control patients who developed graft dysfunction before the advent of nitric oxide, inhalation of nitric oxide decreased the duration of mechanical ventilation, frequency of airway complications, and mortality.[148] Improved hemodynamics and gas exchange may reflect the ability of nitric oxide to compensate for the decrease in endothelium-derived relaxant factor activity after transplantation. If nitric oxide has been used to control pulmonary hypertension after surgery, it should be weaned gradually to avoid any rebound pulmonary vasoconstriction.[149] Finally, ECMO may be used to support the patient until there is adequate recovery of pulmonary function.[135,136]

Infection is a constant threat in these immunosuppressed patients. Prophylactic antibiotic coverage is aimed at agents commonly causing nosocomial and aspiration pneumonias because these are common in donors. Coverage can be modified once culture results from the donor trachea are available. Patients with cystic fibrosis should receive antibiotics targeted at bacteria found in the native lungs before transplantation. Infection should be suspected as the cause of any infiltrate found on chest radiograph, especially if fever or leukocytosis develops, but distinguishing infection from reperfusion injury and rejection may be difficult. Diagnostic bronchoscopy and bronchoalveolar lavage are useful in defining therapy and differentiating infection from rejection,[150,151] but open-lung biopsy occasionally is necessary for definitive diagnosis. Patients who are seronegative to viral agents to which the donor was seropositive (e.g., cytomegalovirus) will require prophylactic antiviral therapy. Vadnerkar et al's[152] study showed that 43% of patients who had undetected mold infections at the time of transplant were at risk for very poor outcomes, with a mortality rate of 29%.

Rejection episodes are common and may occur as early as several days after transplantation. Rejection often presents as new infiltrates on chest radiograph in the setting of deteriorating gas exchange. Bronchoscopy with transbronchial biopsy helps to rule out other causes of deterioration and document acute changes consistent with rejection. Therapy for acute lung rejection consists of large pulses of steroids such as methylprednisolone or changing the immunosuppressive agents (cyclosporine to tacrolimus or vice versa). Expired nitric oxide has been shown to be an indicator of chronic rejection in post–lung-transplant patients. Measurements of expired nitric oxide have been shown to decrease with the switch of cyclosporine to tacrolimus, reflecting a decrease in the inflammation in the pulmonary mucosa.[153] Expired nitric oxide may be a useful tool to observe patients for the presence or change in chronic graft rejection.[154]

One of the most serious complications of lung transplantation occurs late. Bronchiolitis obliterans is a syndrome characterized by alloimmune injury leading to obstruction of small airways with fibrous scar.[155] Patients with bronchiolitis obliterans present with cough, progressive dyspnea, obstruction on flow spirometry, and interstitial infiltrates on chest radiograph. Therapy for this syndrome includes augmentation of immunosuppression,[156] cytolytic agents (which have been used with varying degrees of success),[157,158] or retransplantation in refractory cases.

Living-Related Lung Transplantation

The scarcity of suitable donor lungs has resulted in waiting times on transplant lists in excess of 2 years, during which time up to 30% of candidates succumb to their illness.[159] Living-related lung transplantation programs have developed to address the needs of lung transplant candidates with acute deterioration expected to preclude survival. Successful grafting of a single lobe for children with bronchopulmonary dysplasia or Eisenmenger syndrome, or two lobes for children and young adults with cystic fibrosis, has encouraged several centers to consider such procedures.[73,160] The anesthetic management issues related to such undertakings have been reviewed.[64] Donor candidates will have undergone a rigorous evaluation to ensure that there are no contraindications to lobe donation and that the donation is not being coerced. Donor lobectomy is performed via a standard posterolateral thoracotomy.[83] Of special note to the anesthesiologist during such procedures is the requirement for OLV to optimize surgical exposure, the

continuous infusion of prostaglandin E_1 to promote pulmonary vasodilation, and the administration of heparin and steroids just before lobe harvest. Anesthetic management of the recipient is identical to that for a standard lung transplant, except that the use of CPB is mandatory for bilateral lobar transplant.

Pediatric Considerations

The number of pediatric lung transplants has decreased since the late 1990s. Cystic fibrosis, CHD, and primary pulmonary hypertension are the main indications for lung transplantation in children.[161] In infants, CHD is the most common indication for lung transplantation, whereas cystic fibrosis is the most common vascular indication in adolescents. Because of the underlying pulmonary vascular disease or infectious process in these children, bilateral single-lung transplantation is the operation of choice. Single-lung transplantation is less commonly performed in this age group. Transplantation is recommended when the life expectancy of the child is 2 years or less.

Bilateral single-lung transplantation surgery is performed via a bilateral anterior thoracotomy with transverse division of the sternum ("clamshell" incision) with the patient lying supine.[162] Size disparities between the donor and recipient are not uncommon because of the limited donor pool. Accommodation of a large donor lung is achieved by parenchymal reduction. Placement of a small donor lung is facilitated by intraoperative and postoperative pulmonary arterial vasodilation with nitric oxide.

The average experience in pediatric lung transplantation is two to three patients per center per year.[163] The majority of these patients are scheduled as emergencies the day of transplantation. The family and patient usually are very anxious. Judicious premedication is given to the recipient before general anesthesia. Morbidity during induction of anesthesia is increased by hypoxemia, hypercapnia, and systemic hypotension in these critically ill patients.

After placement of routine monitors, anesthesia is induced with a hypnotic agent (e.g., etomidate), an opioid, and titration of an inhalation agent. A muscle relaxant is added to facilitate tracheal intubation. Cardiac arrest and circulatory collapse may occur after induction of anesthesia in the recipient with primary pulmonary hypertension and CHD with pulmonary hypertension.[164] An inhalation agent, additional opioid, benzodiazepines, and muscle relaxants are used throughout the procedure. A thickened hypertrophic right ventricle requires additional volume administration. Frequent endotracheal tube suctioning usually is required intraoperatively before transplantation in the recipient with cystic fibrosis.

In contrast with the adult population, CPB frequently is utilized during lung transplantation in children. Bronchial anastomosis is assessed by fiberoptic bronchoscopy. A PA catheter is advanced after unclamping of the PA.

Weaning from CPB is challenging and may be complicated by bleeding, reperfusion injury, pulmonary hypertension, and pulmonary edema. During weaning from bypass, the Fio_2 is decreased to prevent reperfusion injury. Moderate levels of PEEP are used to treat pulmonary edema. The patient is kept sedated and the trachea intubated. A thoracic epidural facilitates weaning from mechanical ventilation and extubation in the ICU. Low-dose dopamine enhances renal blood flow after CPB.

The immediate postoperative course can be complicated by graft failure or dysfunction and/or infection. After the first year, morbidity is increased by bronchiolitis obliterans, systemic hypertension, renal dysfunction, and diabetes mellitus.

HEART-LUNG TRANSPLANTATION
History and Epidemiology

The diminished frequency of heart-lung transplantation since 1990 reflects that it is being supplanted by lung transplantation. The number of heart-lung transplants worldwide peaked at 241 in 1989, and there has been a continual decline in subsequent years to approximately half that number.[3] Approximately only 173 heart-lung transplant candidates were registered with UNOS as of early March 2005, less than 5% of the number on the lung transplant list. The most common recipient indications remain primary pulmonary hypertension, CHD (including Eisenmenger syndrome), and cystic fibrosis.

One-year survival rate after heart-lung transplantation is 60%, significantly less than that for isolated heart or lung transplantation.[3] Mortality in subsequent years is approximately 4% per year, similar to that for heart transplantation. Risk factors for increased mortality after heart-lung transplant are recipient ventilator dependence, male recipient sex, and a donor age older than 40 years.[3] Early deaths are most often due to graft failure or hemorrhage, whereas midterm and late deaths primarily are due to infection and bronchiolitis obliterans, respectively. Repeat heart-lung transplant is a rare procedure and likely to remain so because the 1-year survival rate after repeat heart-lung transplant is dismal (28%).[3]

Recipient Selection

Candidates undergo an evaluation similar to that for lung transplant candidates. As more patients with pulmonary hypertension and cystic fibrosis are treated with isolated lung transplantation, it is likely that the indications for heart-lung transplantation will be limited to CHD with irreversible pulmonary hypertension that is not amenable to repair during simultaneous lung transplantation or diseases with both pulmonary hypertension and concomitant severe left ventricular dysfunction.

Donor Selection and Graft Harvest

Potential heart-lung donors must meet not only the criteria for heart donors but also those for lung donation, both described earlier in this chapter. Graft harvesting is carried out in a manner similar to that previously described for heart transplantation. After mobilization of the major vessels and trachea, cardiac arrest is induced with inflow occlusion and infusion of cold cardioplegia into the aortic root. After arrest, the PA is flushed with a cold preservative solution often containing prostaglandin E_1. The ascending aorta, SVC, and trachea are transected, and the heart-lung bloc removed after it is dissected free of the esophagus. The trachea is clamped and the graft immersed in cold solution before being bagged for transport.

Surgical Procedures

The operation generally is performed through a median sternotomy, but a clamshell thoracosternotomy also is an acceptable approach. Both pleurae are incised. Any pulmonary adhesions are taken down before anticoagulation for bypass. Cannulae for CPB are placed in a manner similar to that for heart transplantation. After the aorta is cross-clamped, the heart is excised in a manner similar to that for orthotopic heart transplant. Each lung is then individually removed, including its pulmonary veins. The airways are divided at the level of the respective main bronchi for bibronchial anastomoses. For a tracheal anastomosis, the trachea is freed to the level of the carina without stripping its blood supply and an anastomosis is constructed just above the level of the carina. The atrial anastomosis is performed in a manner similar to that for orthotopic heart transplantation, and, finally, the aorta is joined to the recipient aorta. After de-airing and reperfusion, the patient is weaned from CPB, hemostasis is achieved, and the wound is closed.

Pathophysiology before Transplantation

The pathophysiology of heart-lung transplant recipients combines the elements discussed earlier in this chapter. Patients usually will have end-stage biventricular failure with severe pulmonary hypertension. The cardiac anatomy may be characterized by complex congenital malformations. If obstruction of pulmonary airflow is present, there is a danger of hyperinflation after application of positive-pressure ventilation.

Pathophysiology after Transplantation

Like isolated heart recipients, heart-lung transplant recipients' physiology is characterized by cardiac denervation, transient cardiac ischemic insult during graft harvest, transport, and implantation, and long-term susceptibility to accelerated allograft vasculopathy and rejection. As is the case for lung recipients, heart-lung recipients have denervated pulmonary vascular and airway smooth muscle responses, transient pulmonary ischemic insult, altered pulmonary lymphatic drainage, and impaired mucociliary clearance.

Anesthetic Management

The anesthetic management of heart-lung transplantation more closely resembles that of heart than lung transplantation because the use of CPB is mandatory. After placement of invasive and noninvasive monitoring similar to that used for heart transplantation, anesthesia can be induced with any of the techniques previously described for heart and lung transplantation. Similar to lung transplantation, avoidance of myocardial depression, as well as protection and control of the airway are paramount. Although a double-lumen endotracheal tube is not mandatory, it will aid in exposure of the posterior mediastinum for hemostasis after weaning from CPB. Otherwise, anesthetic management before CPB is similar to that for heart transplantation.

A bolus of glucocorticoid (e.g., methylprednisolone, 500 mg) is given when the aortic cross-clamp is removed. After a period of reperfusion, an inotrope infusion is started and the heart is inspected with TEE for adequate de-airing. Ventilation is resumed with normal tidal volume and rate, along with the addition of PEEP (5 to 10 cm) before weaning from CPB. After successful weaning from CPBN, the PA catheter can be advanced into the PA again. Protamine then is administered to reverse heparin-induced anticoagulation. The inspired oxygen concentration often can be decreased to less toxic levels based on blood gas analysis.

Problems encountered after weaning from CPB are similar to those encountered after isolated heart or lung transplantation. Lung reperfusion injury and dysfunction may compromise gas exchange, so administration of crystalloid should be minimized. Occasionally, postreperfusion pulmonary edema may require support with high levels of PEEP and inspired oxygen in the operating room. Ventricular failure usually responds to an increase in β-adrenergic support. Unlike isolated heart or lung transplantation, frank RV failure is uncommon immediately after heart-lung transplantation unless lung preservation was grossly inadequate. Coagulopathy often is present after heart-lung transplant and should be aggressively treated with additional protamine (if indicated), platelets, and fresh-frozen plasma.

Postoperative Management and Complications

The principles of the immediate postoperative care of heart-lung transplant recipients are a combination of those of isolated heart and lung recipients. Invasive and noninvasive monitoring done in the operating room is continued. Inotropic support is continued in a manner similar to that for heart transplantation. Ventilatory support is similar to that after lung transplantation; the lowest acceptable inspired oxygen concentration is used to avoid oxygen toxicity, and the patient is weaned from the ventilator after hemodynamics have been stable for several hours, hemorrhage has ceased, and satisfactory gas exchange is present. Diuresis is encouraged. Finally, the immunosuppressive regimen of choice is begun. Barring any complications, the patient can be discharged from the ICU after several days.

Infection is a more frequent and serious complication in heart-lung recipients than in isolated heart recipients. Bacterial and fungal infections are especially common in the first month after transplantation, with viral and other pathogens (*Pneumocystis carinii* and *Nocardia*) occurring in subsequent months.[165]

Similar to isolated heart or lung transplants, rejection episodes are common early after heart-lung transplantation. Rejection may occur independently in either the heart or lung.[106] Therapy is similar to that for rejection of isolated heart or lung grafts.

Heart grafts in heart-lung blocs are prone to accelerated coronary vasculopathy in a manner similar to those of isolated heart grafts. As with lung transplantation, a feared late complication of heart-lung transplantation is bronchiolitis obliterans. Clinical presentation is similar to that seen with lung transplant patients. Approximately one third of heart-lung recipients develop this process. Anecdotal reports indicate that most affected patients also have accelerated coronary vasculopathy.

Pediatric Considerations

Although the number of heart-lung transplants performed worldwide has been decreasing since 1990, of the 49 cases performed in the United States in 1992, more than half were in children.[166] The overall decline has been attributed to earlier referral for isolated lung transplantation, before cor pulmonale becomes irreversible. However, there are still a number of uncorrectable types of CHD that inevitably lead to Eisenmenger syndrome in children; thus, the need for pediatric heart-lung transplantation will continue for the foreseeable future.[107,108]

The number of pediatric heart and lung transplantations continue to decrease.[167] Only 10 pediatric heart and lung transplants were performed in 2001 worldwide. Since 1990, the majority of recipients were adolescents. In this group of patients, cystic fibrosis and CHD were the main indications. Only 20% of the recipients are alive 10 years after the transplantation. Early mortality is caused by graft failure; after 1 year after transplantation, the cause is bronchiolitis obliterans. The lack of survival improvement in these patients calls for reassessment of heart and lung transplantation in children.

REFERENCES

1. Carrel A, Guthrie CC: The transplantation of veins and organs, *Am J Med* 1:1101, 1905.
2. Barnard CN: The operation. A human cardiac transplant: An interim report of a successful operation performed at Groote Schuur Hospital, Cape Town, *S Afr Med J* 41:1271–1274, 1967.
3. Hosenpud JD, Novick RJ, Bennett LE, et al: The Registry of the International Society for Heart and Lung Transplantation: Thirteenth Official Report, *J Heart Lung Transplant* 15:655, 1996.
4. Organ Procurement and Transplantation Network: OPTN 2008 Annual Report. Available at: http://optn.transplant.hrsa.gov/data/annualreport.asp.
5. Murali S, Kormos RL, Uretsky BF, et al: Preoperative pulmonary hemodynamics and early mortality after orthotopic cardiac transplantation: The Pittsburgh experience, *Am Heart J* 126:896, 1993.
6. Darby JM, Stein K, Grenvik A, et al: Approach to management of the heartbeating brain dead organ donor, *JAMA* 261:2222, 1989.
7. Nygaard CE, Townsend RN, Diamond DL: Organ donor management and organ outcome a 6 year review from a level 1 trauma center, *J Trauma* 30:728, 1990.
8. Votapka TV, Canvasser DA, Pennington DG, et al: Effect of triodothyronine on graft function in a model of heart transplantation, *Ann Thoracic Surg* 62:78, 1996.
9. Novitzky D: Transplantation, euthyroid sick syndrome, and triiodothyronine replacement, *J Heart Lung Transplant* 11:S196, 1992.
10. Novitzky D, Cooper DKC, Reichart B: Hemodynamic and metabolic responses to hormonal therapy in brian-dead potential organ donors, *Transplantation* 43:852, 1987.
11. Randell TT, Hockerstedt KA: Triiodothyronine treatment in brain-dead multiogran donors—a controlled study, *Transplantation* 54:736, 1992.
12. Hardesty RL, Griffith BP, Deep GM, et al: Improved cardiac function using cardioplegia during procurement and transplantation, *Transplant Proc* 15:1253, 1983.
13. Watson DC, Reitz BA, Baumgartner WA: Distant heart procurement for transplantation, *Surgery* 86:56, 1979.
14. Grant SCD, Khan MA, Yonan N, et al: Technique of anastomosis and incidence of atrial tachyarrythmias following heart transplantation, *Br Heart J* 71:40, 1994.
15. El-Gamel A, Deiraniya AK, Rahman AN, et al: Orthotopic heart transplantation hemodynamics: Does atrial preservation improve cardiac output after transplantation? *J Heart Lung Transplant* 15:564, 1996.
16. Mehta SM, Aufiero TX, Pae WE: Combined registry for the clinical use of mechanical ventricular assist pumps and the total artificial heart in conjunction with heart transplantation: Sixth official report, *J Heart Lung Transplant* 14:585, 1994.
17. Shaw BW Jr, Bahnson HT, Hardesty RL, et al: Combined transplantation of the heart and liver, *Ann Surg* 202:667, 1985.
18. Bristow MR, Ginsburg R, Minobe W, et al: Decreased catecholamine sensitivity and beta adrenergic receptor density in failing human hearts, *N Engl J Med* 307:205, 1982.
19. Cohn JN, Archibald DG, Ziesche S, et al: Effect of vasodilator therapy on mortality in chronic congestive heart failure, *N Engl J Med* 314:1547, 1986.
20. Anonymous: Effects of enalapril on mortality in severe congestive heart failure. Results of Cooperative North Scandinavian Enalapril Survival Study (Consensus), *N Engl J Med* 316:1429, 1987.
21. Kalman J, Buchholz C, Steinmetz M, et al: Safety and efficacy of beta-blockade in patients with chronic congestive heart failure awaiting transplantation, *J Heart Lung Transplant* 14:1212, 1995.
22. Remme WJ: Inodilator therapy for heart failure. Early, late or not at all? *Circulation* 87:IV97, 1993.
23. Packer M, Carver JR, Rodeheffer RJ, et al: Effect of oral milrinone on mortality in severe chronic heart failure, *N Engl J Med* 325:1468, 1991.
24. Steed DL, Brown B, Reilly JJ, et al: General surgical complications in heart and heart-lung transplantation, *Surgery* 98:739, 1985.
25. Isono SS, Woolson ST, Schurman DJ: Total joint arthroplasty for steroid-induced osteonecrosis in cardiac transplant patients, *Clin Orthop* 217:201, 1987.
26. Stinson EB, Griepp RB, Schroeder JS: Hemodynamic observations one and two years after cardiac transplantation in man, *Circulation* 45:1183, 1972.
27. Rowan RA, Billingham ME: Myocardial innervation in long-term heart transplant survivors: A quantitative ultrastructural survey, *J Heart Transplant* 7:448, 1988.
28. Wilson RF, Christensen BV, Olivari MT, et al: Evidence for structural sympathetic reinnervation after orthotopic cardiac transplantation in humans, *Circulation* 83:1210, 1991.
29. Stinson EB, Griepp RB, Clark DA, et al: Cardiac transplantation in man. VIII. Survival and function, *J Heart Transplant* 7:145, 1970.
30. Verani MS, George SE, Leon CA, et al: Systolic and diastolic ventricular performance at rest and during exercise in heart transplantation recipients, *J Heart Transplant* 7:145, 1988.
31. Kent KM, Cooper T: The denervated heart: A model for studying autonomic control of the heart, *N Engl J Med* 291:1017, 1974.
32. Goodman DJ, Rossen RM, Cannom DS, et al: Effect of digoxin on atrioventricular conduction. Studies in patients with and without cardiac autonomic innervation, *Circulation* 51:251, 1975.
33. Backman SB, Ralley FE, Fox GS: Neostigmine produces bradycardia in a heart transplant recipient, *Anesthesiology* 78:777, 1993.
34. Borow KM, Neumann A, Arensman FW, et al: Cardiac and peripheral vascular responses to adrenoceptor stimulation and blockade after cardiac transplantation, *J Am Coll Cardiol* 14:1229, 1989.
35. Tuzcu EM, DeFranco AC, Hobbs R, et al: Prevalence and distribution of transplant coronary artery disease, *J Heart Lung Transplant* 14:S202, 1995.
36. Hosenpud JD, Morris TE, Shipley GD, et al: Cardiac allograft vasculopathy transplantation, *Transplantation* 61:939, 1996.
37. Gao SZ, Hunt SA, Schroeder JS, et al: Early development of accelerated graft coronary artery disease: Risk factors and course, *J Am Coll Cardiol* 28:673, 1996.
38. Stark RP, McGinn AL, Wilson RF: Chest pain in cardiac-transplant recipients, *N Engl J Med* 324:1791, 1991.
39. Smart FW, Ballantyne CM, Cocanougher B, et al: Insensitivity of noninvasive test to detect coronary artery vasculopathy after heart transplant, *Am J Cardiol* 67:243, 1991.
40. St Goar FG, Pinto FJ, Alderman EL, et al: Intracoronary ultrasound in cardiac transplant recipients: In vivo evidence of angiographically silent intimal thickening, *Circulation* 85:979, 1992.
41. Akosah KO, Mohanty PK, Funai JT, et al: Noninvasive detection of transplant coronary artery disease by dobutamine stress echocardiography, *J Heart Lung Transplant* 13:1024, 1994.
42. Waterman PM, Bjerke R: Rapid-sequence induction technique in patients with severe ventricular dysfunction, *J Cardiothorac Anesth* 2:602, 1988.
43. Murkin JM, Moldenhauer CC, Hug CC Jr: High-dose fentanyl for rapid induction of anaesthesia in patients with coronary artery disease, *Can Anaesth Soc J* 32:320, 1985.
44. Hensley FA, Martin DE, Larach DR, et al: Anesthetic management for cardiac transplantation in North America, *J Cardiothorac Anesth* 1:429, 1987.
45. Berberich JJ, Fabian JA: A retrospective analysis of fentanyl and sufentanil for cardiac transplantation, *J Cardiothorac Anesth* 1:200, 1987.
46. Armitage JM, Hardesty RL, Griffith BP: An effective treatment of right heart failure after orthotopic heart transplantation, *J Heart Transplant* 6:348, 1987.
47. Fonger JD, Borkon AM, Baumgartner WA: Acute right ventricular failure following heart transplantation: Improvement with PGE1 and right ventricular assist, *J Heart Transplant* 5:317, 1986.
48. Stein KL, Armitage JM, Martich GD: Intensive care of the cardiac transplant recipient. In Ayres SM, Grenvik A, Holbrook PR, Shoemaker WC, editors: *Textbook of Critical Care*, ed 3. WB Saunders, 1995, p 1649.
49. Weil R III, Clarke DR, Iwaki Y, et al: Hyperacute rejection of a transplanted human heart, *Transplantation* 32:71, 1981.
50. Bhatia SJS, Kirshenbaum JM, Shemin RJ, et al: Time course of resolution of pulmonary hypertension and right ventricular remodeling after orthotopic cardiac transplantation, *Circulation* 76:819, 1987.
51. Villanueva FS, Murali S, Uretsky BF, et al: Resolution of severe pulmonary hypertension after heterotopic cardiac transplantation, *J Am Coll Cardiol* 14:1239, 1989.
52. Jacquet L, Ziady G, Stein K, et al: Cardiac rhythm disturbances early after orthotopic heart transplantation: Prevalence and clinical importance of the observed abnormalities, *J Am Coll Cardiol* 16:832, 1990.
53. Scott CD, Omar I, McComb JM, et al: Long-term pacing in heart transplant recipients is usually unnecessary, *Pacing Clin Electrophysiol* 14:1792, 1991.
54. Romhilt DW, Doyle M, Sagar KB, et al: Prevalence and significance of arrhythmias in long-term survivors of cardiac transplantation, *Circulation* 66:I219, 1982.
55. Chomette G, Auriol M, Beaufil H, et al: Morphology of cyclosporine nephrotoxicity in human heart transplant recipients, *J Heart Transplant* 5:273, 1986.
56. Platz KP, Mueller AR, Blumhardt G, et al: Nephrotoxicity following orthotopic liver transplantation. A comparison between cyclosporine and FK506, *Transplantation* 58:170, 1994.
57. Burch M, Aurora P: Current status of paediatric heart, lung, and heart-lung transplantation, *Arch Dis Child* 89:386–389, 2004.
58. Lillehei CW, Mayer JE Jr, Shamberger RC, et al: Pediatric lung transplantion and "Lessons from Green Surgery". *Ann Thoracic Surg* 68:S25–S27, 1999.
59. Spray TL, Bridges ND: Lung transplantation for pediatric pulmonary hypertension, *Prog Pediatr Cardiol* 12:319–325, 2001.
60. Weiss ES, Allen JG, Merlo CA, et al: Factors indicative of long-term survival after lung transplantation: A review of 836 10 year survivors, *J Heart Lung Transplant* 29:240–246, 2010.
61. Olson CM, editor: Diagnostic and therapeutic technology assessment: Lung transplantation, *JAMA* 269:931, 1993.
62. Kaye MP: The Registry of the International Society for Heart and Lung Transplantation: Ninth official report, *J Heart Lung Transplant* 11:599, 1992.
63. Trulock EP, Cooper JD, Kaiser LR, et al: The Washington University–Barnes Hospital experience with lung transplantation, *JAMA* 266:1943, 1991.
64. Quinlan JJ, Gasior TA, Firestone S, et al: Anesthesia for living-related (lobar) lung transplantation, *J Cardiothorac Vasc Anesth* 10:391, 1996.
65. Novick RJ, Kaye MP, Patterson GA, et al: Redo lung transplantation: A North American-European experience, *J Heart Lung Transplant* 12:5, 1993.
66. Gorcsan J III, Edward TD, Ziady GM, et al: Transesophageal echocardiography to evaluate patients with severe pulmonary hypertension for lung transplantation, *Ann Thoracic Surg* 59:717, 1995.
67. Hardesty RL, Aeba R, Armitage JM, et al: A clinical trial of University of Wisconsin solution for pulmonary preservation, *J Thorac Cardiovasc Surg* 105:660, 1993.

68. Weiss ES, Merlo CA, Shah AS: Impact of advanced age in lung transplantation: An analysis of United Network for Organ Sharing data, *J Am Coll Surg* 208:400–409, 2009.
69. Allen JG, Weiss ES, Merlo CA, et al: Impact of donor-recipient race matching on survival after Lung Transplantation: Analysis of over 11000 patients, *J Heart Lung Transplant* 28:1063–1071, 2009.
70. Gilbert S, Dauber J, Hattler B, et al: Lung and heart-lung transplantation at the University of Pittsburgh 1982–2002, *Clin Transpl* 253–261, 2002.
71. Brower RG, Matthay MA, Morris A, et al: Ventilation with lower tidal volumes as compared with traditional tidal volumes for acute lung injury and the acute respiratory distress syndrome. The Acute Respiratory Distress Syndrome Network, *N Engl J Med* 342:1301–1308, 2000.
72. Low DE, Trulock EP, Kaiser LR, et al: Morbidity, mortality, and early results of single versus bilateral lung transplantation for emphysema, *J Thorac Cardiovasc Surg* 103:1119, 1992.
73. Starnes VA, Barr ML, Cohen RG: Lobar transplantation: Indications, technique and outcome, *J Thorac Cardiovasc Surg* 108:403, 1994.
74. Kaiser LR, Pasque MK, Trulock EP, et al: Bilateral sequential lung transplantation: The procedure of choice for double-lung replacement, *Ann Thorac Surg* 52:438, 1991.
75. Bisson A, Bonnette P: A new technique for double-lung transplantation, *J Thorac Cardiovasc Surg* 103:40, 1992.
76. Pepe PE, Marini JJ: Occult positive end-expiratory pressure in mechanically ventilated patients with airflow obstruction. The Auto-PEEP effect, *Am Rev Respir Dis* 126:166, 1982.
77. Haluszka J, Chartrand DA, Grassino AE, et al: Intrinsic PEEP and arterial PCO2 in stable patients with chronic obstructive pulmonary disease, *Am Rev Respir Dis* 141:1194, 1990.
78. Quinlan JJ, Buffington CW: Deliberate hypoventilation in a patient with air trapping during lung transplantation, *Anesthesiology* 78:1177, 1993.
79. Smith TC, Marini JJ: Impact of PEEP on lung mechanics and work of breathing in severe airflow obstruction, *J Appl Physiol* 65:1488, 1988.
80. Biondi JW, Hines RL, Matthay RA: Comparative right ventricular function during assist control, intermittent mandatory and spontaneous ventilation, *Anesth Analg* 65:S18, 1986.
81. Prewitt R, Ghignone M: Treatment of right ventricular dysfunction in acute respiratory failure, *Crit Care Med* 5:346, 1983.
82. Adatia I, Lillehei C, Arnold JH, et al: Inhaled nitric oxide in the treatment of postoperative graft dysfunction after lung transplantation, *Ann Thoracic Surg* 57:1311, 1994.
83. Cohen RG, Barr ML, Schenkel FA, et al: Living-related donor lobectomy for bilateral lobar transplantation in patients with cystic fibrosis, *Ann Thorac Surg* 57:1423, 1994.
84. Kramer MR, Marshall SE, McDougall IR, et al: The distribution of ventilation and perfusion after single-lung transplantation in patients with pulmonary fibrosis and pulmonary hypertension, *Transplant Proc* 23:1215, 1991.
85. Maurer JR, McLean PA, Cooper JD, et al: Airway hyperactivity in patients undergoing lung and heart/lung transplantation, *Am Rev Respir Dis* 139:1038, 1989.
86. Herve P, Picard N, Le Roy Ladurie M, et al: Lack of bronchial hyperresponsiveness to methacholine and to isocapnic dry air hyperventilation in heart/lung and double-lung transplant recipients with normal lung histology, *Am Rev Respir Dis* 145:1503, 1992.
87. Tavakoli R, Buvry A, Le Gall G, et al: In vitro bronchial hyperresponsiveness after lung transplantation in the rat, *Am J Physiol* 262:L322, 1992.
88. Stretton CD, Mak JCW, Belvisi MG, et al: Cholinergic control of human airways in vitro following extrinsic denervation of the human respiratory tract by heart-lung transplantation, *Am Rev Respir Dis* 142:1030, 1990.
89. Takichi T, Maeda M, Shirakusa T, et al: Sympathetic reinnervation of unilaterally denervated rat lung, *Acta Physiol Scand* 154:43, 1995.
90. Clifford PS, Coon RL, Von Colditz JH, et al: Pulmonary denervation in the dog, *J Appl Physiol* 54:1451, 1983.
91. Duarte AG, Terminella L, Smith JT, et al: Restoration of cough reflex in lung transplant recipients, *Chest* 134:310–316, 2008.
92. Dolovich M, Rossman C, Chambers C: Muco-ciliary function in patients following single lung or lung/heart transplantation, *Am Rev Respir Dis* 135:A363, 1987.
93. Fullerton DA, Mitchell MB, McIntyre RC, et al: Cold ischemia and reperfusion each produce pulmonary vasomotor dysfunction in the transplanted lung, *J Thorac Cardiovasc Surg* 106:1213, 1993.
94. Hunter DN, Morgan CJ, Yacoub M, et al: Pulmonary endothelial permeability following lung transplantation, *Chest* 102:417, 1992.
95. Shennib H, Serrick C, Saleh D, et al: Plasma endothelin-1 levels in human lung transplant recipients, *J Cardiovasc Pharmacol* 26(Suppl 3):S516, 1995.
96. Flavahan NA, Aleskowitch TD, Murray PA: Endothelial and vascular smooth muscle responses are altered after left lung autotransplantation, *Am J Physiol* 266:H2026, 1994.
97. Kukkonen S, Heikkila L, Verkkala K, et al: Pulmonary vasodilatory properties of prostaglandin e1 are blunted after experimental single-lung transplantation, *J Heart Lung Transplant* 14:280, 1995.
98. Ueda K, Date H, Fujita T, et al: Effects of inhaled nitric oxide in a canine living-donor lobar lung transplant model, *Jpn J Thorac Cardiovasc Surg* 48:693–699, 2000.
99. Lang JD Jr, Leill W: Pro: Inhaled nitric oxide should be used routinely in patients undergoing lung transplantation, *J Cardiothorac Vasc Anesth* 15:785–789, 2001.
100. Karamasetty M, Klinger J: NO: More than just a vasodilator in lung transplantation, *Am J Respir Cell Mol Biol* 26:1–5, 2002.
101. Moreno I, Vicente R, Mir A, et al: Effects of inhaled nitric oxide on primary graft dysfunction in lung transplantation, *Transplant Proc* 41:2210–2212, 2009.
102. Meade MO, Granton J, Matte-Martyn A, et al: A randomized trial of inhaled nitric oxide to prevent ischemia reperfusion injury after lung transplantation, *Am J Respir Crit Care Med* 167:1483–1489, 2003.
103. Ardehali A, Laks H, Levine M, et al: A prospective trial of inhaled nitric oxide in clinical lung transplantation, *Transplantation* 72:112–115, 2001.
104. Botha P, Jeykanthan M, Rao JN, et al: Inhaled nitric oxide for modulation of ischemia-reperfusion injury in lung transplantation, *J Heart Lung Transplant* 26:1199–1205, 2007.
105. Royston D: High-dose aprotinin therapy: A review of the first five years' experience, *J Cardiothorac Vasc Anesth* 6:76, 1992.
106. Griffith BP, Hardesty RL, Trento A, et al: Asynchronous rejection of heart and lungs following cardiopulmonary transplantation, *Ann Thoracic Surg* 40:488, 1985.
107. Smyth RL, Scott JP, Whitehead B: Heart-lung transplantation in children, *Transplant Proc* 22:1470, 1990.
108. Starnes VA, Marshall SE, Lewiston NJ, et al: Heart-lung transplantation in infants, children and adolescents, *J Pediatr Surg* 26:434, 1991.
109. Corris PA, Odom NJ, Jackson G, et al: Reimplantation injury after lung transplantation in a rat model, *J Heart Transplant* 6:234, 1987.
110. Jones MT, Hsieh C, Yoshikawa K, et al: A new model for assessment of lung preservation, *J Thorac Cardiovasc Surg* 96:608, 1988.
111. Katz WE, Gasior TA, Quinlan JJ, et al: Immediate effects of lung transplantation on right ventricular morphology and function in patients with variable degrees of pulmonary hypertension, *J Am Coll Cardiol* 27:384, 1996.
112. Yeoh TK, Kramer MR, Marshall S, et al: Changes in cardiac morphology and function following single-lung transplantation, *Transplant Proc* 23:1226, 1991.
113. Frist WH, Lorenz CH, Walker ES, et al: MRI complements standard assessment of right ventricular function after lung transplantation, *Ann Thoracic Surg* 60:268, 1995.
114. Carere R, Patterson GA, Liu PP, et al: Right and left ventricular performance after single and double-lung transplantation, *J Thorac Cardiovasc Surg* 102:115, 1991.
115. Ritchie M, Waggoner AD, Davila-Roman VG, et al: Echocardiographic characterization of the improvement in right ventricular function in patients with severe pulmonary hypertension after single-line transplantation, *J Am Coll Card* 22:1170, 1993.
116. Scuderi LJ, Bailey SR, Calhoon JH, et al: Echocardiographic assessment of right and left ventricular function after single-line transplantation, *Am Heart J* 127:636, 1994.
117. Kramer MR, Valatine HA, Marshall SE, et al: Recovery of the right ventricle after single-lung transplantation in pulmonary hypertension, *Am J Cardiol* 73:494, 1994.
118. Benumof JL: *Anesthesia for Thoracic Surgery*, Philadelphia, 1987, WB Saunders.
119. Hirt SW, Haverich A, Wahlers T, et al: Predictive criteria for the need of extracorporeal circulation in single-lung transplantation, *Ann Thorac Surg* 54:676, 1992.
120. Chetham P: Anesthesia for heart or single or double lung transplantation, *J Card Surg* 15:167–174, 2000.
121. Myles PS, Venama H: Avoidance of cardiopulmonary bypass during bilateral sequential lung transplantation using inhaled nitric oxide, *J Cardiothorac Vasc Anesth* 9:571, 1995.
122. Myles PS, Weeks AM, Buckland MR, et al: Anesthesia for bilateral sequential lung transplantation: Experience of 64 cases, *J Cardiothorac Vasc Anesth* 11:177, 1997.
123. Triantafillou AN, Pasque MK, Huddleston CB, et al: Predictors, frequency, and indications for cardiopulmonary bypass during lung transplantation in adults, *Ann Thoracic Surg* 57:1248, 1994.
124. Aeba R, Griffith BP, Kormos RL, et al: Effect of cardiopulmonary bypass on early graft dysfunction in clinical lung transplantation, *Ann Thoracic Surg* 57:715, 1994.
125. Fullerton DA, McIntyre RCJ, Mitchell MB, et al: Lung transplantation with cardiopulmonary bypass exaggerates pulmonary vasomotor dysfunction in the transplanted lung, *J Thorac Cardiovasc Surg* 109:212, 1995.
126. Firestone L, Carrera J, Firestone S, et al: Single-lung transplants: Who needs bypass? *Anesthesiology* 79:A46, 1993.
127. Sekela ME, Noon GP, Holland VA, et al: Differential perfusion: Potential complication of femoral-femoral bypass during single lung transplantation, *J Heart Lung Transplant* 10:322, 1991.
128. Ko WJ, Chen YS, Lee YC: Replacing cardiopulmonary bypass with extracorporeal membrane oxygenation in lung transplantation operations, *Artif Organs* 25:607–612, 2001.
129. Pereszlenyi A, Lang G, Steltzer H, et al: Bilateral lung transplantation with intra and postoperatively prolonged ECMO support in patients with pulmonary hypertension, *Eur J Cardiothorac Surg* 21:858–863, 2002.
130. Michel-Cherqui M, Brusset A, Liu N, et al: Intraoperative transesophageal echocardiographic assessment of vascular anastomoses in lung transplantation. A report of 18 cases, *Chest* 111:1229–1235, 1997.
131. Hausmann D, Daniel WG, Mugge A: Imaging of pulmonary artery and vein anastomoses by transesophageal echocardiography after lung transplantation, *Circulation* 86(5 Suppl):II251–II258, 1992.
132. Royston D: Aprotinin therapy in heart and heart-lung transplantation, *J Heart Lung Transplant* 12:S19, 1993.
133. Gu YJ, de Haan J, Brenken UP, et al: Clotting and fibrinolytic disturbance during lung transplantation: Effect of low-dose aprotinin, *J Thorac Cardiovasc Surg* 112:599, 1996.
134. Jaquiss RD, Huddleston CB, Spray TL: Use of aprotinin in pediatric lung transplantation, *J Heart Lung Transplant* 14:302, 1995.
135. Zenati M, Pham SM, Keenan RJ, et al: Extracorporeal membrane oxygenation for lung transplant recipients with primary severe donor lung dysfunction, *Transpl Int* 9:227, 1996.
136. Glassman LR, Keenan RJ, Fabrizio MC, et al: Extracorporeal membrane oxygenation as an adjunct treatment for primary graft failure in adult lung transplant recipients, *J Thorac Cardiovasc Surg* 110:723, 1995.
137. McIlroy DR, Pilcher DV, Snell GI: Does anaesthetic management affect early outcomes after lung transplant? An exploratory analysis, *Br J Anesth* 102:506–514, 2009.
138. Leibowitz DW, Smith CR, Michler RE, et al: Incidence of pulmonary vein complications after lung transplantation: A prospective transesophageal echocardiographic study, *J Am Coll Cardiol* 24:671, 1994.
139. Malden ES, Kaiser LR, Gutierrez FR: Pulmonary vein obstruction following single-lung transplantation, *Chest* 102:671, 1992.
140. Hausmann D, Daniel WG, Mugge A, et al: Imaging of pulmonary artery and vein anastomoses by transesophageal echocardiography after lung transplantation, *Circulation* 86:II–251, 1992.
141. Despotis GJ, Karanikolas M, Triantafillou AN, et al: Pressure gradient across the pulmonary artery anastomosis during lung transplantation, *Ann Thorac Surg* 60:630, 1995.
142. Cohrane LJ, Mitchell ME, Raju S, et al: Tension pneumopericardium as a complication of single-lung transplantation, *Ann Thorac Surg* 50:808, 1990.
143. Jellinek H, Klepetko W, Hiesmayr M: Komplettes Ventilations/Perfusions Mibverhaltnis Nachy Einseitiger Lungentransplantation und Postoperativem Hamatothorax, *Anaesthetist* 41:134, 1992.
144. Gorcsan J III, Reddy SC, Armitage JM, et al: Acquired right ventricular outflow tract obstruction after lung transplantation: Diagnosis by transesophageal echocardiography, *Am Soc Echocardiogr* 6:324, 1993.
145. Mentzer SJ, Reilly JJ, DeCamp M, et al: Potential mechanism of vasomotor dysregulation after lung transplantation for primary pulmonary hypertension, *J Heart Lung Transplant* 14:387, 1995.
146. Aoe M, Trachiotis GD, Okabayashi K, et al: Administration of prostaglandin E1 after lung transplantation improves early graft function, *Ann Thorac Surg* 58:655, 1994.
147. MacDonald P, Mundy J, Rogers P, et al: Successful treatment of life-threatening acute reperfusion injury after lung transplantation with inhaled nitric oxide, *J Thorac Cardiovasc Surg* 110:861, 1995.
148. Date H, Triantafillou AN, Trulock EP, et al: Inhaled nitric oxide reduced human lung allograft dysfunction, *J Thorac Cardiovasc Surg* 111:913, 1996.
149. Lindberg L, Sjoberg T, Ingemansson R, et al: Inhalation of nitric oxide after lung transplantation, *Ann Thorac Surg* 61:956–962, 1996.
150. Scott JP, Fradet G, Smyth RL, et al: Prospective study of transbronchial biopsies in the management of heart-lung and single lung transplant patients, *J Heart Lung Transplant* 10:626, 1991.
151. Higgenbottam T, Stewart S, Penketh A, et al: Transbronchial lung biopsy for the diagnosis of rejection in heart-lung transplant patients, *Transplantation* 46:532, 1988.
152. Vadnerkar A, Clancy CJ, Celik U, et al: Impact of mold infection in explanted lungs on outcomes of lung transplantation, *Transplantation* 89:253–260, 2010.
153. Verleden G, Dupont L, Raemdonck DV, et al: Effect of switching from cyclosporine to tacrolimus on exhaled nitric oxide and pulmonary function in patients with chronic rejection after lung transplantation, *J Heart Lung Transplant* 22:908–913, 2002.
154. Gabbay E, Walters EH, Orsida B, et al: Post-lung transplant bronchiolitis obliterans syndrome (BOS) is characterized by increased exhaled nitric oxide levels and epithelial inducible nitric oxide synthetase, *Am J Respir Crit Care Med* 162:2182–2187, 2000.
155. Reichenspurner H, Girgis RE, Robbins RC, et al: Obliterative bronchiolitis after lung and heart-lung transplantation, *Ann Thorac Surg* 60:1845, 1995.
156. Allen MD, Burke CM, McGregor CGA, et al: Steroid-responsive bronchiolitis after human heart-lung transplantation, *J Thorac Cardiovasc Surg* 92:449, 1986.
157. Snell GI, Esmore DS, Williams TJ: Cytolytic therapy for the bronchiolitis obliterans syndrome complicating lung transplantation, *Chest* 109:874, 1996.

158. Kesten S, Rajagopalan N, Maurer J: Cytolytic therapy for the treatment of bronchiolitis obliterans syndrome following lung transplantation, *Transplantation* 61:427, 1996.

159. Paradis I, Manzetti J, Foust D: When to refer for lung transplantation? Characteristics of candidates who die vs. those who survive to receive a transplant, *Am Rev Respir Dis* 147:A597, 1993.

160. Starnes VA, Lewiston NJ, Luikart H, et al: Current trends in lung transplantation: Lobar transplantation and expanded use of single lungs, *J Thorac Cardiovasc Surg* 104:1060, 1992.

161. Webber SA: The current state of, and future prospects for, cardiac transplantation in children, *Cardiol Young* 13:64–83, 2003.

162. Quinlan JJ, Firestone S, Firestone LL: Anesthesia for heart, lung, and heart-lung transplantation. In Kaplan JA, Reich DL, Konstadt SN, eds. *Cardiac Anesthesia*. WB Saunders, Philadelphia, 1998.

163. Brawn WJ, Barron DJ: Management and outcome in hypoplastic left heart syndrome, *Curr Paediatr* 14:26–32, 2004.

164. Reddy SC, Webber SA: Pediatric heart and lung transplantation, *Indian J Pediatr* 70:19–25, 2003.

165. Kramer MR, Marshall SE, Starnes VA, et al: Infectious complications in heart-lung transplantation, *Arch Intern Med* 153:2010, 1993.

166. Bailey LL: Heart transplantation techniques in complex congenital heart disease, *J Heart Lung Transplant* 12:S168, 1993.

167. Boucek MM, Edwards LB, Keck BM, et al: The registry of the International Society for Heart and Lung Transplantation: Sixth official pediatric report 2003, *J Heart Lung Transplant* 22:636–652, 2003.

24

Pulmonary Thromboendarterectomy for Chronic Thromboembolic Pulmonary Hypertension

DALIA A. BANKS, MD | GERARD R. MANECKE, JR., MD | TIMOTHY M. MAUS, MD | KIM M. KERR, MD, FCCP | STUART W. JAMIESON, MB, FRCS

KEY POINTS

1. Incidence of thromboembolic disease is difficult to estimate because of the ambiguous symptoms and the public lack of awareness of the disorder, making clinical diagnosis difficult.

2. Chronic thromboembolic pulmonary hypertension (CTEPH) results from incomplete resolution of a pulmonary embolus (PE) or from recurrent pulmonary emboli. It is an underappreciated phenomenon.

3. Pulmonary thromboendarterectomy (PTE) is the safest, most effective treatment for patients with a history of CTEPH.

4. Patients typically present with progressive exertional dyspnea and exercise intolerance because of increased pulmonary vascular resistance (PVR), limiting cardiac output and increasing minute ventilation requirements because of increased alveolar dead space.

5. Assessment of surgical candidacy should be performed at centers with expertise in the diagnosis and management of CTEPH. Right-heart catheterization defines the severity of the pulmonary hypertension and degree of cardiac dysfunction.

6. Patients with preoperative PVRs greater than 1000 dynes·sec·cm^{-5} have been shown to have a greater operative mortality rate, but a markedly increased preoperative PVR does not exclude the patient from being a surgical candidate.

7. There are two specific complications to the PTE procedure: reperfusion pulmonary edema and persistent pulmonary hypertension.

8. In 2008, the Surgeon General called for action to reduce the incidence of deep venous thrombosis and PE in the United States and emphasized educating all Americans about this preventable disease. Furthermore, Medicare & Medicaid Services are moving aggressively to encourage greater patient safety for hospital-acquired "never events."

9. Size of the thromboembolus, together with release of vasoactive and bronchoactive agents, lead to deleterious ventilation/perfusion mismatching. Right ventricular failure will eventually impede left ventricular filling and decrease cardiac output.

10. A major goal of treatment after acute PE is the prevention of new thrombi and reducing the risk for death. Recurrence has a very high mortality rate.

11. Pulmonary arterial hypertension (PAH) is a disorder in which flow to the pulmonary arterial circulation is decreased, leading to increased vascular remodeling and proliferation resulting in increased PVR and ending with right-heart failure.

12. The goal for treatment in patients with PAH is geared toward improving symptoms and quality of life. Calcium channel blockers, prostaglandins, endothelin-receptor antagonists, and phosphodiesterase-5 inhibitors play a large role in the treatments of PAH.

Pulmonary arterial hypertension (PAH) resulting from chronic pulmonary embolism (PE) is a major cause of morbidity and mortality worldwide. It is much more common than generally appreciated and is certainly underdiagnosed. The incidence is difficult to estimate because of the uncertainty regarding the frequency of acute PE, as well as the percentage of patients in whom embolic residua fail to resolve. Chronic thromboembolic pulmonary hypertension (CTEPH) is a common variation of pulmonary hypertension. There are an estimated 2500 new cases in the United States,[1] or a calculated prevalence of about 3 of 100 cases of PE (20 per 1 million). Pulmonary thromboendarterectomy (PTE) is the curative procedure for CTEPH. Medical management provides only limited and temporary relief of symptoms. Lung transplantation is the only other therapy for patients with pulmonary hypertension and in some centers is still the surgical therapy of choice for patients with thromboembolic disease. Transplant surgery, however, is not a reasonable choice for CTEPH patients when taking into account the risk for death on the waiting list, shortage of organ supply, expense, the risk of immunosuppressive agents, risk for infection, and rejection. The mortality rate for lung transplant has been reported to be 20% including the waiting period versus 4% for PTE at the University of California San Diego (UCSD) Medical Center. Therefore, PTE remains the only permanent curative surgical therapy for patients with CTEPH. PTE historically is how the procedure has been known; however, other terms for the procedure that have been used interchangeably are *pulmonary artery endarterectomy* (PAE) or *pulmonary endarterectomy* (PEA). The success of the operation revolves around endarterectomy of the organized fibrous thrombus in the intimal and part of the medial layers of the pulmonary vascular tree. CTEPH results from obstruction of the pulmonary arteries by nonresolving thromboemboli causing increased pulmonary vascular resistance (PVR), right-heart failure, and death if left untreated. Distinguishing CTEPH from other forms of pulmonary hypertension is imperative because CTEPH is potentially curable with PTE. This chapter focuses on information about the clinical history, diagnostic workup, surgical approach, anesthesia, and postoperative care for patients with CTEPH undergoing PTE surgery. Acute PE and PAH also are discussed in this chapter, concluding with three cases demonstrating the application of intraoperative transesophageal echocardiography (TEE) in patients with CTEPH.

EPIDEMIOLOGY AND PATHOPHYSIOLOGY

Acute or recurrent PEs are thought to be the inciting event in the development of CTEPH. Incomplete resolution of the emboli followed by thrombus organization and fibrosis lead to partial or complete vessel obstruction. In addition, vascular remodeling in the distal pulmonary arteries (pulmonary arteriopathy) also may contribute to the increased PVR seen in CTEPH[1-3] and is the cause of residual pulmonary hypertension seen in some patients after otherwise successful PTE. Unresolved PEs in the proximal pulmonary arterial tree cause vascular obstruction by two ways: canalization of the clot leading to multiple small endothelized channels separated by bands and webs or fibrin clot organization; the other way is absent canalization leading to dense fibrous connective tissue completely occluding the arterial lumen.[4-6] This fibrous plug is firm and adherent to the arterial wall, and the challenge is to remove enough of the fibrous plug as one unit to reduce the vascular resistance without disrupting the arterial wall.

Generally, most patients with PE have complete resolution of the thromboembolic event. However, there is a small portion of patients in whom embolic resolution is incomplete, resulting in the development of CTEPH. The mechanism by which thromboembolic material remains unresolved and becomes incorporated in the pulmonary arterial wall is not exactly known. A variety of factors may play a role: The volume of the embolic substance may simply overwhelm the lytic system or total occlusion of a major arterial branch, preventing the lytic material from reaching and dissolving the embolus completely. The emboli may be made of substances such as well-organized fibrous thrombus, fat, or tumor that cannot be dissolved by normal mechanisms. Some patients may have tendencies for thrombus formation, a hypercoagulable state, or abnormal lytic mechanism. Rosenhek and colleagues[7] showed that subjects under normal physiologic conditions have greater levels of tissue plasminogen activator versus plasminogen activator inhibitor 1 expression in the PA compared with the aorta, leading to improved natural fibrinolysis. However, Olman et al[8] and Lang et al[9] were unable to demonstrate a reversal in the tissue plasminogen activator/plasminogen activator inhibitor 1 relation favoring incomplete thrombus resolution in patients with history of CTEPH.

CTEPH is a common, but under-recognized, cause of pulmonary hypertension, in which the actual incidence of CTEPH remains somewhat uncertain. Pengo et al[10] observed 223 patients for a median of 94.3 months after an acute PE event in which 3.8% of patients experienced development of symptomatic CTEPH. Ribeiro et al[11] examined echocardiograms in 278 patients surviving acute PE for 1 year and performed clinical follow-up for 5 years. Five percent of these patients experienced development of clinically significant CTEPH. Dentali et al[12] noted similar findings in 91 patients examined at 6 months after acute PE. Pulmonary hypertension associated with residual perfusion defects were identified in eight patients (8.8%), four of whom were symptomatic. Related factors that predispose patients to development of CTEPH remain unclear. It can be argued that unresolved thrombi with recurrent

asymptomatic PE may be the reason for the development of clinically significant CTEPH.[13] However, another possibility is based on clinical observation of patients with a history of PE who received anticoagulant therapy and still developed CTEPH. Pengo et al's[10] study identified a younger age at presentation, larger perfusion defects at diagnosis, idiopathic thromboembolic disease, and a history of multiple PE events as risk factors for development of CTEPH after an acute PE.

Bonderman et al[14] identified the following risk factors for CTEPH in a controlled retrospective cohort study: ventriculoatrial shunts, infected pacemakers, splenectomy, previous venous thromboembolism (VTE), recurrent VTE, blood group other than O, lupus anticoagulant/antiphospholipid antibodies, thyroid replacement therapy, and a history of malignancy. Despite being a risk factor for VTE, the prevalence of hereditary thrombophilic states (deficiencies of antithrombin III, protein C and protein S, and factor II and factor V Leiden mutations) is similar to that in normal control subjects or in patients with idiopathic pulmonary hypertension.[15] In contrast, lupus anticoagulant/antiphospholipid antibodies can be found in up to 21% of CTEPH patients,[15] and Bonderman et al[16] demonstrated increased levels of factor VIII in 41% of CTEPH patients. Finally, small, preliminary studies suggest that there may be structural and functional abnormalities of fibrinogen in CTEPH patients, perhaps conferring resistance to fibrinolysis.[17,18] Morris et al[17] reported a relative resistance of fibrin to plasmin-mediated lysis caused by an alteration in fibrin(ogen) structure affecting accessibility to plasmin cleavage sites in patients with CTEPH.

CLINICAL MANIFESTATIONS

The initial symptoms of CTEPH typically are progressive exertional dyspnea and exercise intolerance, nonspecific symptoms that often are attributed to more commonly occurring medical conditions such as obstructive lung disease, cardiac disease, obesity, or deconditioning. These symptoms are due to an increased PVR limiting cardiac output (CO) and increased minute ventilation requirements because of increased alveolar dead space.[1,3] Many patients have no history of a documented acute VTE, making the diagnosis even more challenging.[14,19,20] As the disease progresses and the right heart fails, patients may experience development of ascites, early satiety, epigastric or right upper quadrant fullness, edema, chest pain, and presyncope/syncope. Other symptoms reported include nonproductive cough, hemoptysis, and palpitations. Left vocal cord dysfunction and hoarseness may arise from compression of the left recurrent laryngeal nerve between the aorta and an enlarged left main PA. Early in the disease process, the physical examination may be normal or may reveal an accentuated pulmonic component of the second heart sound, but this can be easily overlooked.[1,3] Pulmonary flow murmurs are bruits heard over the lung fields and are caused by turbulent blood flow through partially occluded or recanalized thrombi. These flow murmurs are heard in 30% of CTEPH patients and are not found in idiopathic pulmonary hypertension.[21] Late in the disease process when right ventricular (RV) function fails to meet normal resting metabolic needs, patients start to experience exertion-related syncope and resting dyspnea. The nonspecific nature of these complaints is indisputably the reason that most patients with chronic thromboembolic events experience a delay in diagnosis or are improperly labeled with a different diagnosis. Furthermore, the fact that some patients do not report a history of PE or deep venous thrombosis (DVT) makes proper diagnosis challenging. The physical signs are far from uniform, and the physical examination may be surprisingly unrewarding if right-heart failure did not ensue, even in the presence of severe dyspnea. Physical findings of RV failure such as jugular venous distention, RV lift, fixed splitting of the second heart sound, murmur of tricuspid regurgitation (TR), RV gallop, hepatomegaly, ascites, and edema may appear with later stages of the disease.[1,3] Cyanosis, if present, may suggest right-to-left shunting through a patent foramen ovale (PFO) in patients with pulmonary hypertension. Pulmonary function tests often demonstrate minimal changes in lung volume and ventilation. Diffusing capacity often is reduced and may be the only abnormality on pulmonary function testing. Pulmonary arterial pressures are increased and are not infrequently suprasystemic. Resting COs and indices are lower than the reference range, and pulmonary arterial oxygen saturations are reduced. The majority of patients are hypoxic, with room-air arterial oxygen tension ranging between 50 and 83 mm Hg[22]; CO_2 tension is slightly reduced and is compensated for by reduced bicarbonate. Dead space ventilation is increased, together with moderate ventilation/perfusion mismatch, which correlates poorly with the degree of pulmonary vascular obstruction.[23]

Increased hematocrit with long-standing hypoxemia, abnormal liver function tests reflecting liver congestion from RV failure, and unexpected isolated prolongation of the activated partial thromboplastin time may indicate the presence of lupus anticoagulant or other antiphospholipid antibodies, or, more commonly, a normal prothrombin time and partial thromboplastin time are laboratory findings seen frequently in this patient population.

DIAGNOSTIC EVALUATION

Once the diagnosis of pulmonary vascular disease is entertained, the patient evaluation involves three goals: to establish the presence and severity of PAH, to determine the cause of the PAH, and if thromboembolic disease is present, to determine whether it is amenable to surgical correction. Standard diagnostic tests performed in the evaluation of dyspnea may be suggestive of pulmonary vascular disease.[1] Chest radiography may be normal in the early stages of disease, but with worsening PAH, dilation of the central pulmonary arteries and enlargement of the right atrium and ventricle can be seen (Figure 24-1). CTEPH patients also may have irregularly shaped and asymmetrically enlarged pulmonary vessels.[24] Electrocardiographic (ECG) findings such as right-axis deviation, right ventricular hypertrophy (RVH), right atrial enlargement, right bundle branch block, ST-segment abnormalities, and T-wave inversions in the precordial and inferior leads may be seen. Pulmonary function testing frequently is performed in the evaluation of dyspnea and is useful in excluding coexisting parenchymal lung disease. Normal lung volumes or mild to moderate restrictive defects because of parenchymal scarring from pulmonary infarction may be seen in CTEPH.[25] A mild-to-moderate reduction in single-breath diffusing capacity of carbon monoxide also may be present in CTEPH, but a severe reduction should stimulate further evaluation for an alternative pulmonary process disrupting the distal pulmonary vascular bed.[26] CTEPH patients may demonstrate a normal Pao[2] at rest but exhibit a decline with exertion. Hypoxemia at rest occurs in the setting of severe RV dysfunction or a right-to-left shunt, such as a PFO.[3]

Transthoracic echocardiography (TTE) frequently is the first study to suggest the presence of pulmonary hypertension. Depending on the severity of the disease, echocardiography may demonstrate right-heart chamber enlargement, abnormal RV function, TR, leftward displacement of the interventricular septum (IVS), decreased left ventricular size, and abnormal ventricular systolic and diastolic function.[27] PA systolic pressures can be estimated by Doppler evaluation of the tricuspid regurgitant envelope. Contrast injection may demonstrate a right-to-left shunt as a result of the increased right atrial pressures and a PFO. The echocardiogram is also useful in excluding left ventricular dysfunction, valvular disease, or congenital heart disease, which may cause pulmonary hypertension (see Chapters 1 and 2).

Radioisotopic ventilation-perfusion scanning is essential in distinguishing large-vessel occlusive disease from small-vessel pulmonary vascular disease (Figure 24-2). Patients with CTEPH invariably have one or more segmental or larger mismatched perfusion defects. This is in contrast to patients with idiopathic pulmonary arterial hypertension (IPAH) or other forms of small-vessel PAH in which the perfusion scans are normal or demonstrate subsegmental or mottled perfusion abnormalities.[28,29] Notably, the magnitude of perfusion defects often underestimates the degree of vascular obstruction in CTEPH. This is due to organization and recanalization of clot resulting in partial obstruction of pulmonary arteries that allows limited passage of radiolabeled aggregated albumin resulting in "gray zones" in areas of hypoperfused lung on perfusion scan.[30] Hence, even a single, mismatched, segmental perfusion abnormality should raise the question of CTEPH in a patient with pulmonary hypertension. Conversely, unmatched perfusion defects are not specific for thromboembolic disease because similar defects can be seen with pulmonary vascular tumors, large-vessel arteritis, extrinsic compression, and pulmonary veno-occlusive disease.[31,32] Consequently, further imaging is required. Contrast-enhanced chest computed tomography (CT) imaging is assuming an increasingly important role in the evaluation of thromboembolic disease. Although a negative CT scan does not rule out the diagnosis of CTEPH, when used in conjunction with ventilation/perfusion scanning, it may aid in making the diagnosis and determining operability in patients with CTEPH. CT findings in CTEPH include chronic thromboembolic material in the central pulmonary arteries, mosaic perfusion of the lung parenchyma, central PA enlargement, variability in the size and distribution of pulmonary arteries, right atrial and ventricular enlargement, and increased bronchial collateral arteries[33] (Figure 24-3). Chest CT scanning also is valuable in assessing the lung parenchyma in patients with coexistent emphysematous or fibrotic lung disease, as well as assessing patients who suffer

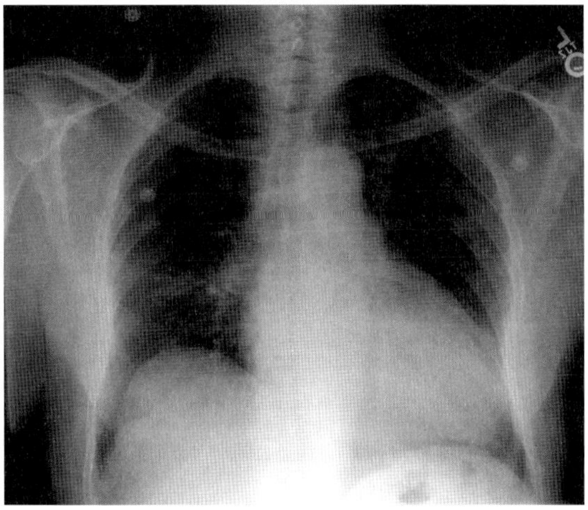

Figure 24-1 Chest radiograph demonstrating cardiomegaly and enlargement of the right pulmonary artery.

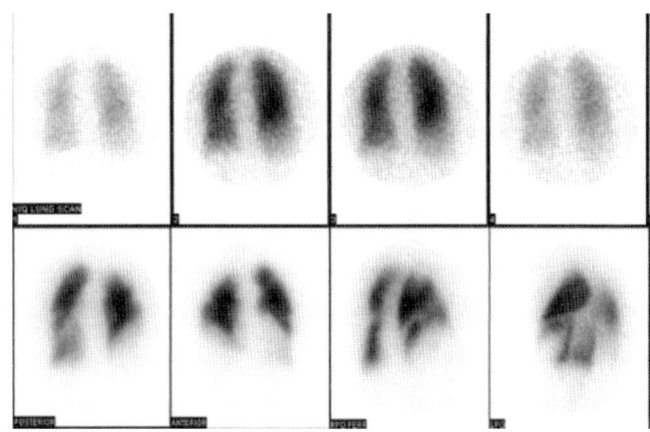

Figure 24-2 **Radioisotopic ventilation and perfusion scan.** The top row demonstrates ventilation wash-in, equilibrium, and wash-out of Xenon in the posterior view. There is some decreased ventilation of the right lower lobe corresponding to the elevated right hemidiaphragm in Figure 24-1. Perfusion images in multiple views are seen in the bottom row and demonstrate markedly diminished flow to the left lower lobe, lingula, right middle lobe, and right lower lobe.

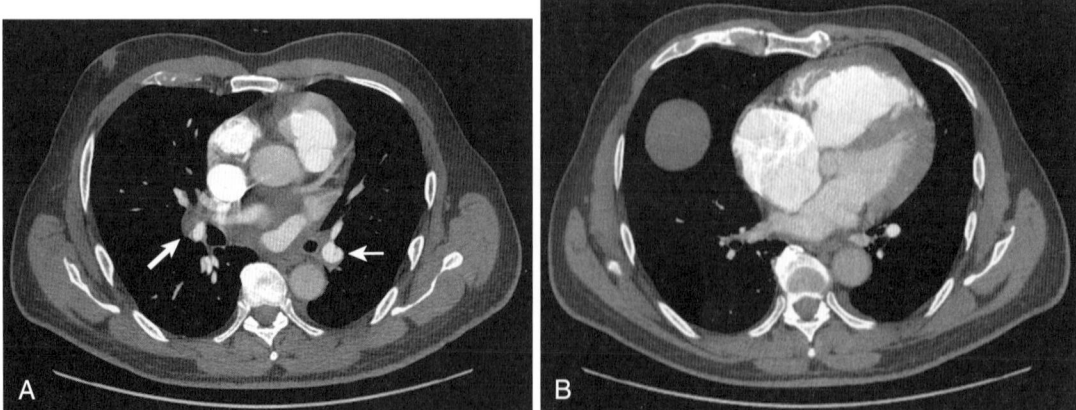

Figure 24-3 *A,* Computed tomographic angiogram of the same patient in Figure 24-2. Lining thrombus can be seen in the right interlobar artery *(thick arrow),* and a web is noted in the left descending pulmonary artery *(thin arrow). B,* Right atrial and ventricular enlargement in the same patient.

from other diseases that can obstruct central pulmonary arteries and mimic CTEPH, such as mediastinal fibrosis, tumors, lymphadenopathy, and arteritis.[1,3,34] Finally, the presence of lining thrombus in the central pulmonary arteries has been described in IPAH (previously referred to as primary pulmonary hypertension) and other end-stage lung disease.[35,36] The radioisotope perfusion scan is helpful in distinguishing such patients from CTEPH, which is essential because PTE carries substantial risk in these patients and is unlikely to result in hemodynamic benefit.[1,3] More recently, there is an increasing interest in the use of helical CT scanning,[37] single-photon emission CT-CT fusion imaging,[38] and magnetic resonance angiography[39] in the evaluation of CTEPH[40] patients, but further experience and research are needed.

Pulmonary angiography remains the gold standard in the evaluation of CTEPH and can be performed safely by experienced individuals, even in patients with severe hemodynamic impairment.[41] The angiographic appearance of chronic thromboembolic disease is distinctly different from that of acute PE because of the organization and recanalization that take place during partial embolic resolution. Characteristic angiographic findings in CTEPH include vascular webs or bandlike narrowings, intimal irregularities, pouch defects, abrupt narrowing of

vessels, and proximal obstruction of pulmonary arteries[5] (Figure 24-4). Biplane imaging is optimal in providing anatomic detail because lateral images provide better detail of lobar and segmental vessels that overlap on anteroposterior images.[1]

Cardiac catheterization may be performed at the time of pulmonary angiography. Right-heart catheterization defines the severity of the PAH and degree of cardiac dysfunction. Typically, the right atrial (RA), RV, PA, and pulmonary artery occlusion pressures (PAOP); CO; and mixed venous oxygen saturation (Svo_2) are measured. These hemodynamics are helpful in assessing risk of surgical intervention. Left-heart catheterization and coronary arteriography also are performed in patients at risk for coronary artery disease or in suspected left-heart dysfunction or valvular heart disease.[3] Ascertaining the differential diagnosis between PAH and distal and small vessel with thromboembolic disease remains a challenge in about 10% to 15% of cases. Usually, these patients will not have a clear history of thromboembolism. Pulmonary angioscopy often is helpful in such cases. The pulmonary angioscope is a fiberoptic bronchoscope 120 cm in length and 3 mm in external diameter. The distal tip can flex and extend, and it has a balloon that is then filled with CO_2 and pushed against the vessel wall,

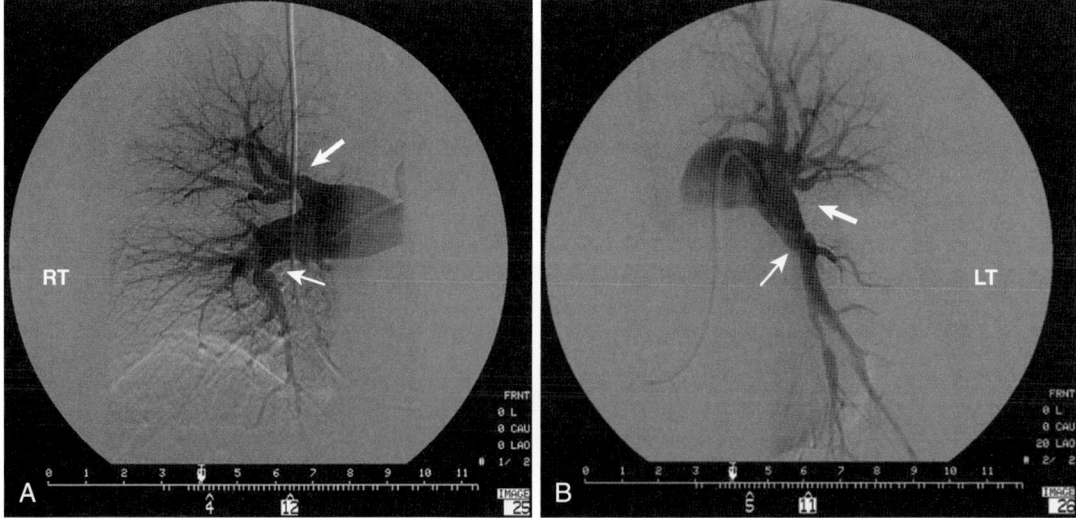

Figure 24-4 *A,* Right pulmonary angiogram in the same patient seen in previous figures demonstrates a pouch deformity in the right upper lobe *(thick arrow)* and abrupt narrowing of the descending pulmonary artery with proximal narrowing (bands) in the right middle and lower lobe vessels *(thin arrow). B,* Left pulmonary angiogram shows abrupt narrowing of the descending pulmonary artery with luminal irregularities *(thick arrow)* and occlusion of the lingula. A prominent band is seen in the descending artery *(thin arrow)* with areas of irregular narrowing of the basilar segments of the left lower lobe.

creating a bloodless field to better visualize the PA wall. This is easily accomplished through placement via a central venous catheter to gain access to the PA. The normal appearance of the vessel wall is of pink, white, smooth, and glistening material, whereas the classic appearance of chronic pulmonary thromboembolic disease by angioscopy consists of intimal thickening, irregularity, scarring, pitting, and the presence of pouches, bands, and webs across small vessels. These features are due to the organization of PE with recanalization and subsequent fibrosis. The bands and webs are thought to be the residue of the resolved thrombi occluding small and medium vessels and are important diagnostic findings.

OPERABILITY

Pulmonary endarterectomy offers the potential for cure and results in substantial improvement in hemodynamics, functional status, and long-term survival.[42–45] Assessment of surgical candidacy should be performed at centers with expertise in the diagnosis and management of CTEPH. To be considered surgical candidates, patients must have surgically accessible chronic thromboembolic disease (Box 24-1). The definition of "surgically accessible" will vary depending on the experience and skill of the surgeon. In addition to the location of chronic thrombi, the extent of vessel obstruction and its correlation to hemodynamic compromise are important in determining candidacy for surgery. Most patients presenting for this operation are within New York Heart Association Class III or IV. Age ranges from 7 to 85 years. Many patients (20%) have a PVR greater than 1000 dynes·sec·cm^{-5}, and it is not uncommon to have suprasystemic pulmonary artery pressures (PAPs).

The increase in PVR arises from not only central surgically accessible lesions but also distal, small-vessel arteriopathy. Patients with a significant component of small-vessel arteriopathy may not experience a significant decrease in PVR after PTE, leaving them at increased risk for short-and long-term consequences. Patients with a postoperative PVR greater than 500 dynes·sec·cm^{-5} have a perioperative mortality rate of 30%, compared with 1% in those with a postoperative PVR less than 500 dynes·sec·cm^{-5}.[19]

Several techniques are being studied to attempt to partition the upstream (thromboembolic disease) from downstream (arteriopathy) resistance, but they remain investigational.[46,47] Most patients who undergo PTE typically have PVRs greater than 300 dynes·sec·cm^{-5}, and most are in the range of 700 to 1100 dynes·sec·cm^{-5}. Surgery may be considered for patients with normal resting hemodynamics if they have significant obstruction of one main PA, those with a vigorous lifestyle who exhibit significant pulmonary hypertension with exercise, and those who are symptomatic from increased dead space ventilation.[3] Patients with preoperative PVRs greater than 1000 dynes·sec·cm^{-5} have been shown to have a greater operative mortality rate,[19] but a markedly increased preoperative PVR does not exclude the patient from being a surgical candidate. Comorbid diseases also must be assessed as part of the preoperative evaluation. Severe underlying parenchymal diseases, particularly involving regions of the lung that would be reperfused by PTE, are a contraindication to surgery.

MEDICAL TREATMENT OF CHRONIC THROMBOEMBOLIC PULMONARY HYPERTENSION

Untreated, CTEPH has a poor prognosis, with more than half of patients with mean pulmonary artery pressure (mPAP) of more than 50 mm Hg not surviving beyond 1 year after diagnosis.[48] Surgery is associated with increased survival rate, when significant reductions in pulmonary hemodynamics and PVR are achieved.[19] Despite the advances achieved by PTE, up to 50% of patients are judged inoperable and more than 10% of them experience persistent or recurrent PAH after PTE. Medical therapy may be beneficial for select patients with CTEPH. There are four different groups in whom medical therapy can be beneficial (Box 24-2): patients in whom comorbidities are so significant that surgery is contraindicated or because of personal choice they opt to not proceed with PTE surgery; and patients with severe PAH and RV failure who exhibit distal limited resectable chronic thrombus and are unlikely to benefit from PTE surgery. For those patients, medical therapy may be the only possibility, with lung transplant reserved for the most severely ill individuals. Another group is high-risk patients with extremely poor hemodynamics, which includes those with functional Class IV symptoms, mPAP greater than 50 mm Hg, cardiac index less than 2.0 L/min/m^2, and PVR greater than 1000 dynes·sec·cm^{-5}. For these patients, intravenous epoprostenol may be considered as a therapeutic bridge to PTE. Although this approach may improve surgical success, medical therapy should not significantly delay PTE. Patients with residual pathology after PTE (about 10%) should be considered for medical therapy.

Vasodilator therapy in select patients with CTEPH deserves further evaluation. Ono et al[49] evaluated the use of an oral prostacyclin analog, "beraprost," in a small number of patients with inoperable CTEPH together with conventional therapy compared with a matched group undergoing conventional therapy alone. Fifty percent of patients who received beraprost experienced functional improvement compared with no functional improvement in the group who received the conventional therapy alone. During the same time, modest declines in the mPAP and total pulmonary resistance were observed and, throughout follow-up, improved survivorship was seen in patients treated with beraprost. Bonderman et al[50] evaluated the use of bosentan, an endothelin-receptor antagonist, in 16 patients with inoperable CTEPH, showing an improvement in New York Heart Association functional status in 11 patients during a period of 6 months, a reduction in pro-brain natriuretic peptide levels, and an improvement in 6-minute walk (6MW) distance. The greatest results were observed in CTEPH patients who had undergone endarterectomy surgery. Sildenafil,[51] a phosphodiesterase-5 (PDE-5) inhibitor, has dual effects, increasing RV inotropy and decreasing RV afterload, and it may be more advantageous than

---

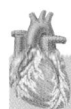

BOX 24-1. PATIENT SELECTION CRITERIA FOR PULMONARY THROMBOENDARTERECTOMY

- Presence of hemodynamically significant pulmonary vascular obstruction; PVR greater than 300 dynes·sec·cm^{-5}
- Most patients are New York Heart Association (NYHA) functional Class III or IV
- There must be no concurrent illnesses representing an immediate threat to life
- Patients must desire surgery based on dissatisfaction with their poor cardiorespiratory function or prognosis
- Patients must be willing to accept the mortality rate of the procedures, which is about 2.5% at UCSD

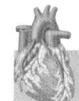

BOX 24-2. GROUPS TO CONSIDER FOR MEDICAL TREATMENT

1. Patients in whom comorbidities are so significant that surgery is contraindicated
2. Patients with severe pulmonary hypertension and right ventricular failure who exhibit distal limited resectable chronic thrombus and are unlikely to benefit from pulmonary thromboendarterectomy (PTE) surgery
3. Patients who have severe pulmonary hypertension and right heart failure, in whom medical therapy would be a "stabilizing bridge" to surgery
4. Patients with residual pulmonary hypertension after PTE surgery

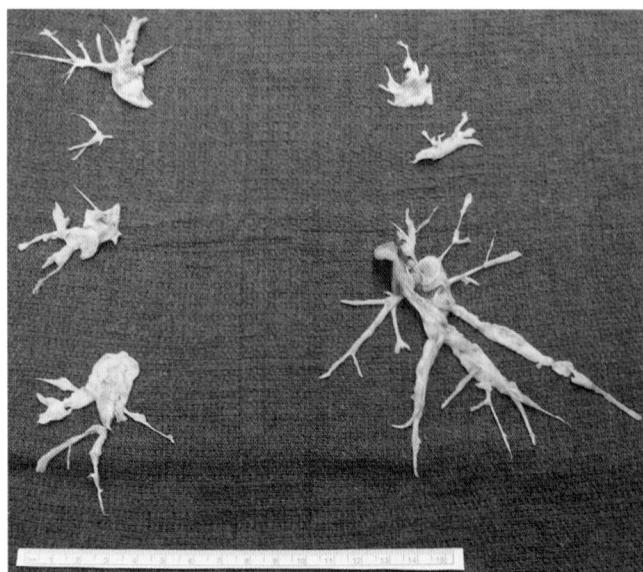

Figure 24-5   Surgical specimen obtained at pulmonary thromboendarterectomy from patient depicted in previous figures.

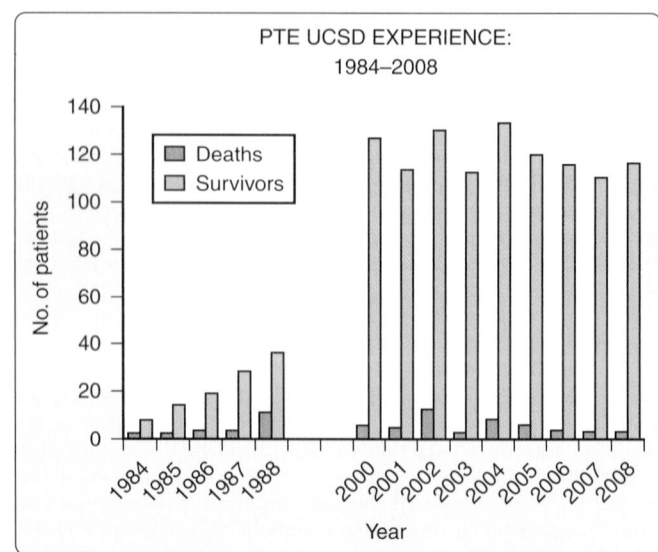

Figure 24-6   University of California San Diego (UCSD) experience from 1984 to 2008. PTE, pulmonary thromboendarterectomy.

drugs that affect only the PA. An expert consensus document released in 2009 recommended the use of either sildenafil or endothelin-receptor antagonists as first-line therapy in patients with PAH, with functional Class II or early Class III disease.[52] Alternative medical therapy includes prostacyclin analogs (e.g., iloprost, Flolan, Remodulin).[49,53] It is recommended that patients on a prostacyclin analog continue their medications before surgery and not discontinue them abruptly, because these medications can lead to severe rebound hypertension, resulting in catastrophic events.[54] Regarding patients presenting for surgery on epoprostenol or teprostenol infusions, it is recommended to discontinue the infusion during the prebypass period, and depending on the surgical results, it is either continued after bypass or after surgery in the intensive care unit (ICU). Further details of the pharmacotherapy for PAH are discussed in the Pulmonary Arterial Hypertension section later in this chapter.

The use of pulmonary vasodilator therapy as a bridge to PTE and its effects on postoperative outcome remain unknown and it should not delay surgical intervention. This is a mechanical condition that cannot be effectively treated by pharmacotherapy or angioplasty; it can only be removed by open operation. Figure 24-5 depicts the surgical specimen obtained at PTE from the patient depicted in the previous figures.

OPERATION

Historical Development

Chronic thromboembolic disease was not recognized as a distinct diagnostic entity until the late 1920s and has remained severely underdiagnosed since then. The first surgical attempt to remove the adherent thrombus from the pulmonary arterial wall was reported by Hurwitt et al in 1958.[55] This was the landmark operation that provided the distinction between an endarterectomy rather than an embolectomy as the surgical procedure of choice for chronic thromboembolic disease. In 1961 and 1962, systemic hypothermia and CPB standby were used to perform two successful endarterectomies. A historical review of the world's experience for PTE up to 1985 published by Chitwood et al[56] revealed an overall perioperative mortality rate of 22% in 85 patients who underwent surgical endarterectomy. Moser et al[23] published their experience of 42 patients with CTEPH who underwent PTE, with an in-hospital mortality rate of 16.6%. Of the 35 survivors (mean follow-up, 28 months), 16 had NYHA Class I disease, 18 Class II, and 1 Class III. PVR declined significantly after surgery

from 897 ± 352 to 278 ± 135 dynes·sec·cm^{-5}. This study confirmed the substantial improvements and functional ability experienced by these patients one year after surgery.[23] Nina Braunwald commenced the UCSD experience with this operation in 1970, which now totals more than 2400 cases. The first patient was a 67-year-old man who underwent the operation on July 14, 1970. Through a right lateral thoracotomy, a PTE was performed using CPB. The patient was discharged from the hospital and returned to full activity. A total of seven surgeons have been involved with the program since the beginning. Drs. Braunwald, Utley, Daily, and Dembitsky, who together performed 188 procedures between 1970 and 1989, made progressive modifications to the surgical technique, including the use of a median sternotomy and hypothermic circulatory arrest. Drs. Jamieson and Kapelanski performed more than 1400 cases from 1989 to early 2000. Recently, Dr. Jamieson, together with Dr. Michael Madani, has expanded the total number of cases to more than 2400. UCSD is the world's pioneer in PTE surgery, and most of the surgical experience in PTE to date has been reported from there; hence this section is based on their extensive experience (Figure 24-6).

Pulmonary Endarterectomy Procedure

There are several guiding principles for the pulmonary endarterectomy procedure. The endarterectomy must be bilateral because this is a bilateral disease in most patients, and for pulmonary hypertension to be a major factor, both pulmonary arteries must be substantially involved. A median sternotomy incision is made to treat both pulmonary arteries. Historically, there were many reports of unilateral operation, and, occasionally, this is still performed in inexperienced centers through a thoracotomy. However, the unilateral approach ignores the disease on the contralateral side, subjects the patient to hemodynamic jeopardy during the clamping of the PA, does not allow good visibility because of the continued presence of bronchial blood flow, and exposes the patient to a repeat operation on the contralateral side. In addition, collateral channels develop in chronic thrombotic hypertension not only through the bronchial arteries, but from diaphragmatic, intercostal, and pleural vessels. The dissection of the lung in the pleural space via a thoracotomy incision can, therefore, be extremely bloody. The median sternotomy incision, apart from providing bilateral access, avoids entry into the pleural cavities and allows the ready institution of CPB.

Cardiopulmonary bypass is essential to ensure cardiovascular stability when the operation is performed and to cool the patient to allow circulatory arrest. Excellent visibility is required, in a bloodless field, to define an adequate endarterectomy plane and to then follow the pulmonary endarterectomy specimen deep into the subsegmental vessels. Because of the copious bronchial blood flow usually present in these cases, periods of circulatory arrest are necessary to ensure perfect visibility. Again, there have been sporadic reports of the performance of this operation without circulatory arrest. However, it should be emphasized that although endarterectomy is possible without circulatory arrest, a complete endarterectomy is not. The authors always initiate the procedure without circulatory arrest, and a variable amount of dissection is possible before the circulation is stopped, but never complete dissection. The circulatory arrest periods are limited to 20 minutes, with restoration of flow between each arrest. With experience, the endarterectomy usually can be performed with a single period of circulatory arrest on each side. A true endarterectomy in the plane of the media must be accomplished. It is essential to appreciate that the removal of visible thrombus is largely incidental to this operation. Indeed, in most patients, no free thrombus is present, and on initial direct examination, the pulmonary vascular bed may appear normal. The early literature on this procedure indicates that thrombectomy was often performed without endarterectomy; in these cases, the PAPs did not improve, often with the resultant death of the patient. After a median sternotomy incision, the pericardium is incised longitudinally and attached to the wound edges. Typically, the right heart is enlarged, with a tense right atrium and a variable degree of TR. There is usually severe RVH, and with critical degrees of obstruction, the patient's condition may become unstable with the manipulation of the heart.

Anticoagulation is achieved with the use of beef-lung heparin sodium (400 U/kg, intravenously) administered to prolong the activated coagulation time beyond 400 seconds. Full CPB is instituted with high ascending aortic cannulation and two caval cannulae. These cannulae must be inserted into the superior and inferior vena cavae sufficiently to enable subsequent opening of the right atrium if necessary. The heart is emptied on CPB, and a temporary PA vent is placed in the midline of the main PA 1 cm distal to the pulmonary valve. This will mark the beginning of the left pulmonary arteriotomy.

When CPB is initiated, surface cooling with both the head jacket and the cooling blanket is begun. The blood is cooled with the pump-oxygenator. During cooling, a 10°C gradient between arterial blood and bladder or rectal temperature is maintained.[57] Cooling generally takes 45 minutes to an hour. When ventricular fibrillation occurs, an additional vent is placed in the left atrium through the right superior pulmonary vein. This prevents atrial and ventricular distention from the large amount of bronchial arterial blood flow that is common with these patients.

It is most convenient for the primary surgeon to stand initially on the patient's left side. During the cooling period, some preliminary dissection can be performed, with full mobilization of the right PA from the ascending aorta. The superior vena cava also is fully mobilized. The approach to the right PA is made medial, not lateral, to the superior vena cava. All dissection of the pulmonary arteries takes place intrapericardially, and neither pleural cavity should be entered. An incision then is made in the right PA from beneath the ascending aorta out under the superior vena cava and entering the lower lobe branch of the PA just after the take-off of the middle lobe artery. It is important that the incision stays in the center of the vessel and continues into the lower rather than the middle lobe artery.

Any loose thrombus, if present, is removed. This is necessary to obtain good visualization. It is most important to recognize, however, that, first, an embolectomy without subsequent endarterectomy is quite ineffective, and second, that in most patients with chronic thromboembolic hypertension, direct examination of the pulmonary vascular bed at operation generally shows no obvious embolic material. Therefore, to the inexperienced or cursory glance, the pulmonary vascular bed may well appear normal even in patients with severe chronic embolic pulmonary hypertension.

If the bronchial circulation is not excessive, the endarterectomy plane can be found during this early dissection. However, although a small amount of dissection can be performed before the initiation

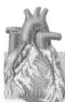

of circulatory arrest, it is unwise to proceed unless perfect visibility is obtained because the development of a correct plane is essential.

There are four broad types of pulmonary occlusive disease related to thrombus that can be appreciated, and the authors use the following classification[58,59] (Box 24-3):

Type I disease (approximately 10% of cases of thromboembolic pulmonary hypertension): Major vessel clot is present and readily visible on the opening of the pulmonary arteries (Figure 24-7). As mentioned earlier, all central thrombotic material has to be completely removed before the endarterectomy.

Type II disease (approximately 70% of cases): No major vessel thrombus can be appreciated (Figure 24-8). In these cases, only thickened intima can be seen, occasionally with webs, and the endarterectomy plane is raised in the main, lobar, or segmental vessels.

Type III disease (approximately 20% of cases): This type presents the most challenging surgical situation (Figure 24-9) because the disease is very distal and confined to the segmental and subsegmental branches. No occlusion of vessels can be seen initially. The endarterectomy plane must be raised carefully and painstakingly in each segmental and subsegmental branch. Type III disease is most often associated with presumed repetitive thrombi from indwelling catheters (such as pacemaker wires) or ventriculoatrial shunts.

Type IV disease does not represent primary thromboembolic pulmonary hypertension and is inoperable. In this entity, there is intrinsic small-vessel disease, although secondary thrombus may

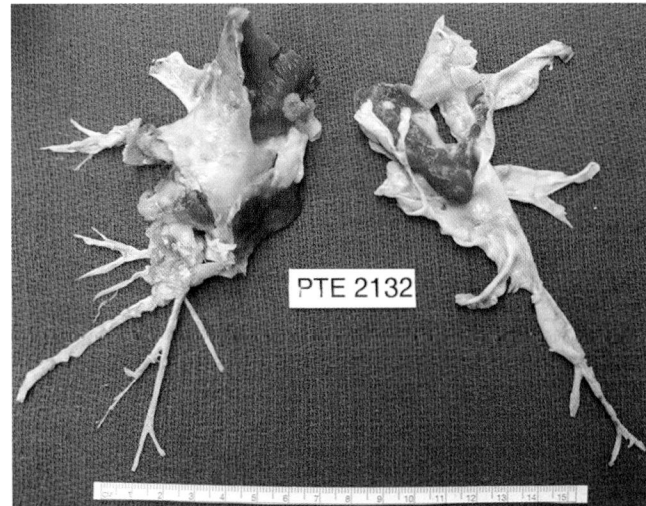

Figure 24-7 **A typical case of type 1 chronic thromboembolic pulmonary hypertension.** On opening the pulmonary artery major vessel, thrombus is encountered. This should be removed. However, the operation is an *endarterectomy* not an *embolectomy*, and from this illustration, it is obvious that removal of the thrombus without subsequent endarterectomy will be ineffective in restoring blood flow.

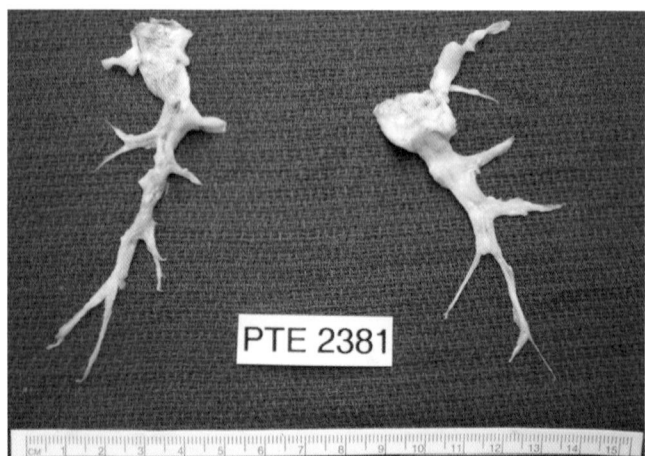

Figure 24-8 A typical case of type 2 chronic thromboembolic pulmonary hypertension. No major vessel thrombus is present, and the obstruction is caused by thickened intima and media of the pulmonary artery, representing unresolved thrombus that becomes incorporated into the vessel wall.

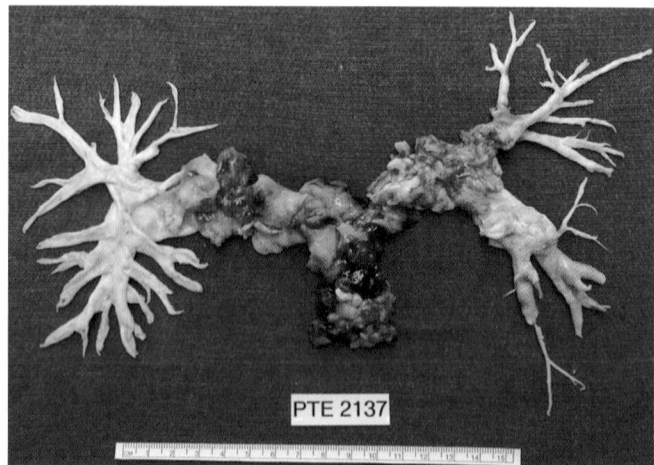

Figure 24-10 Occasionally, pulmonary artery tumors (sarcoma) mimic thromboembolic disease. The diagnosis often is made before surgery because of the presence of main pulmonary artery obstruction. The treatment, although palliative, is the same: pulmonary endarterectomy.

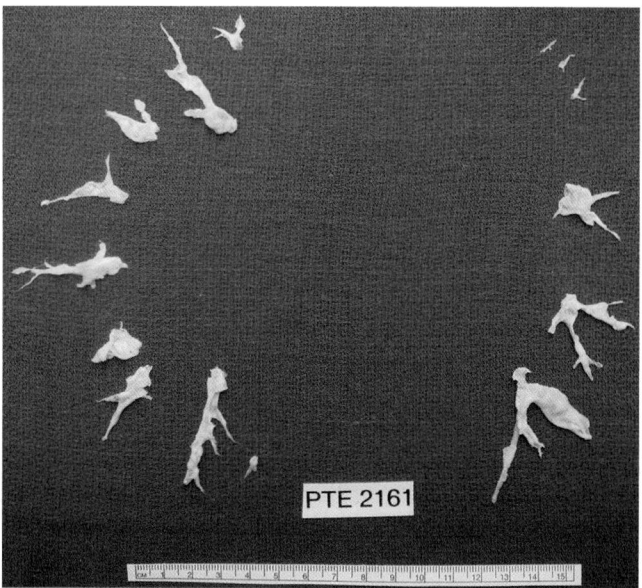

Figure 24-9 Type 3 chronic thromboembolic pulmonary hypertension. The plane is raised, and the endarterectomy is performed at each segmental and subsegmental level. This is the most difficult and time-consuming of the spectrum of disease, often associated with in-dwelling catheters, pacing wires, and atrioventricular shunts. With appropriate time and attention paid to removing all obstruction, good results can be obtained.

occur as a result of stasis. Small-vessel disease may be unrelated to thromboembolic events ("primary" pulmonary hypertension) or occur in relation to thromboembolic hypertension as a result of a high-flow or high-pressure state in previously unaffected vessels similar to the generation of Eisenmenger syndrome. The authors believe that there also may be sympathetic "cross talk" from an affected contralateral side or stenotic areas in the same lung. Figure 24-10 depicts a sarcoma removed from the PA.

When the patient's temperature reaches 20°C, the aorta is cross-clamped and a single dose of cold cardioplegic solution (1 L) is administered. Additional myocardial protection is obtained by the use of a cooling jacket. The entire procedure is performed with a single aortic cross-clamp period with no further administration of cardioplegic solution.

A modified cerebellar retractor is placed between the aorta and superior vena cava. When blood obscures direct vision of the pulmonary vascular bed, thiopental is administered (500 mg to 1 g) until the electroencephalogram becomes isoelectric. Circulatory arrest then is initiated, and the patient undergoes exsanguination. All monitoring catheters to the patient are turned off to prevent the aspiration of air. Snares are tightened around the cannulae in the superior and inferior vena cavae. It is rare that one 20-minute period for each side is exceeded. Although retrograde cerebral perfusion has been advocated for total circulatory arrest in other procedures, it is not helpful in this operation because it does not allow a completely bloodless field, and with the short arrest times that can be achieved with experience, it is not necessary (see Chapter 21).

Any residual loose, thrombotic debris encountered is removed. Then a microtome knife is used to develop the endarterectomy plane posteriorly because any inadvertent egress into this site could be repaired readily, or simply left alone. Dissection in the correct plane is critical because if the plane is too deep, the PA may perforate with fatal results; and if the dissection plane is not deep enough, inadequate amounts of the chronically thromboembolic material will be removed. The plane should only be sought in the diseased parts of the artery. This often requires the initial dissection to begin quite distally. When the proper plane is entered, the layer will strip easily, and the material left with the outer layers of the PA will appear somewhat yellow. The ideal layer is marked with a pearly white plane, which strips easily. There should be no residual yellow plaque. If the dissection is too deep, a reddish or pinkish color indicates the adventitia has been reached. A more superficial plane should be sought immediately.

Once the plane is correctly developed, a full-thickness layer is left in the region of the incision to ease subsequent repair. The endarterectomy then is performed with an eversion technique, using a specially developed dissection instrument ("Jamieson aspirator"; Fehling Corporation, Acworth, GA). Because the vessel is partly everted and subsegmental branches are being worked on, a perforation here will become completely inaccessible and invisible later. This is why absolute visualization in a completely bloodless field provided by circulatory arrest is essential. It is important that each subsegmental branch is followed and freed individually until it ends in a "tail," beyond which there is no further obstruction. Residual material should never be cut free; the entire specimen should "tail off" and come free spontaneously. Once the right-sided endarterectomy is completed, circulation is restarted, and the arteriotomy is repaired with a continuous 6—0 polypropylene suture. The hemostatic nature of this closure is aided by the nature of the initial dissection, with the full thickness of the PA being preserved immediately adjacent to the incision.

After the completion of the repair of the right arteriotomy, the surgeon moves to the patient's right side. The pulmonary vent catheter is withdrawn, and an arteriotomy is made from the site of the pulmonary vent hole laterally beneath the pericardial reflection, and again into the lower lobe, but avoiding entry into the left pleural space. Additional lateral dissection does not enhance intraluminal visibility, may endanger the left phrenic nerve, and makes subsequent repair of the left PA more difficult. There often is a lymphatic vessel encountered on the left PA at the level of the pericardial reflection, and it is wise to clip this prior to it being divided with the PA incision.

The left-sided dissection is virtually analogous in all respects to that accomplished on the right. By the time the circulation is arrested once more, it will have been reinitiated for at least 10 minutes, by which time the venous oxygen saturations are in excess of 90%. The duration of circulatory arrest intervals during the performance of the left-sided dissection is subject to the same restriction as the right.

After the completion of the endarterectomy, CPB is reinstituted and warming is commenced. Methylprednisolone (500 mg, intravenously) and mannitol (12.5 g, intravenously) are administered, and during warming a 10° C temperature gradient is maintained between the perfusate and body temperature, with a maximum perfusate temperature of 37° C. If the systemic vascular resistance (SVR) is high, nitroprusside is administered to promote vasodilatation and warming. The rewarming period generally takes approximately 90 to 120 minutes but varies according to the body mass of the patient.

When the left pulmonary arteriotomy has been repaired, the PA vent is replaced at the top of the incision. The right atrium is then opened and examined. Any intra-atrial communication is closed. Although tricuspid valve regurgitation is invariable in these patients and is often severe, tricuspid valve repair is not performed unless there is independent structural damage to the tricuspid valve itself. RV remodeling occurs within a few days, with the return of tricuspid competence. If other cardiac procedures are required, such as coronary artery or mitral or aortic valve surgery, these are conveniently performed during the systemic rewarming period. Myocardial cooling is discontinued once all cardiac procedures have been concluded. The left atrial vent is removed, and the vent site is repaired. All air is removed from the heart, and the aortic cross-clamp is removed. When the patient has rewarmed, CPB is discontinued. Dopamine is routinely administered at renal doses, and other inotropic agents and vasodilators are titrated as needed to sustain acceptable hemodynamics. The CO is generally high, with a low SVR. Temporary atrial and ventricular epicardial pacing wires are placed. Despite the duration of extracorporeal circulation, homeostasis is readily achieved, and blood products are generally unnecessary. Wound closure is routine. A vigorous diuresis is usual for the next few hours, also a result of the previous systemic hypothermia.

ANESTHETIC MANAGEMENT FOR PATIENTS UNDERGOING PULMONARY THROMBOENDARTERECTOMY

Preoperative Preparation

Patients are admitted before surgery for a full workup. Right-heart catheterization demonstrates the severity of pulmonary hypertension, typically with a PVR greater than 300 dynes·sec·cm^{-5} or more and mPAPs greater than 25 mm Hg. With disease awareness and more recognition of CTEPH surgical candidates, more advanced cases are presenting with PVRs well above 1000 dynes·sec·cm^{-5} and suprasystemic pulmonary hypertension. Hartz et al[60] found that a preoperative PVR greater than 1100 dynes·sec·cm^{-5} and an mPAP greater than 50 mm Hg predicted a higher operative mortality. In a recent report of 500 surgical patients by Jamieson et al,[19] a postoperative mortality rate of 10% was associated with a preoperative PVR above 1000 dynes·sec·cm^{-5}, compared with 1.3% in patients with a preoperative PVR less than 1000 dynes·sec·cm^{-5}.

The preoperative right-heart catheterization focuses on specific data: RA pressures, RV pressures, with RV diastolic pressures more than 14 mm Hg, suggesting RV failure, PAPs, and PVR. CO and index also provide an insight to RV dysfunction. Before surgery, all PTE patients undergo inferior vena caval filter placement to prevent future PE after the endarterectomy. Transthoracic echocardiogram is a valuable diagnostic tool for PAH to exclude primary pathology of the LV, valvular disease, or intracardiac shunting as the cause for the clinical presentation. Preoperative TTE evaluates right heart chamber enlargement and function, paradoxical interventricular septal motion, and intracardiac shunting, and identifies any thrombus in the RA or pulmonary arteries. All these data are critical to identify before proceeding with induction.

On the day of surgery, a large-bore peripheral intravenous catheter and a radial arterial catheter are placed before surgery. Benzodiazepines occasionally are administered as sedation but with extreme caution, with full monitoring, and preferably in the operating room. It should be individualized on a case-to-case basis, noting that anxiety and pain can increase PVR, whereas excessive sedation can cause hypercarbia and hypoxia, resulting in an increase in PVR.

Hemodynamic Consideration and Induction

The majority of patients with CTEPH presenting for PTE are without left ventricular pathology. Induction and decision making are, thus, centered on RV function. The right ventricle typically is hypertrophied and dilated, associated with a dilated right atrium. PTE patients have a relatively fixed PVR and concomitant RV dysfunction; therefore, any significant decrease in mean arterial pressure during induction may compromise RV perfusion, causing cardiovascular collapse and death. Maintenance of adequate SVR, adequate inotropic state, and normal sinus rhythm serve to preserve systemic hemodynamics, as well as RV coronary perfusion. Attempts to reduce PVR pharmacologically using nitroglycerin or nitroprusside should be avoided because they have minimal efficacy in treating the relatively fixed PVR and result in SVR reduction that compromises RV coronary perfusion and RV function, rapidly leading to hypotension and cardiovascular collapse. Hence administration of vasopressors, such as phenylephrine or vasopressin, is vital to maintain SVR and ensure adequate RV perfusion. Despite a relatively fixed PVR, attempts should be made to minimize conditions that increase PVR further such as avoiding episodes of hypoxia, hypercarbia, and acidosis, and any changes should be treated aggressively. The choice of anesthetic induction drugs depends on the degree of hemodynamic instability. Etomidate frequently is used because it maintains sympathetic tone and does not possess significant direct myocardial depressant effect. Succinylcholine or a rapid-sequence dose of rocuronium can be used to achieve a fast intubation environment and control of the airway. However, other nondepolarizing agents remain appropriate choices. It is recommended that titration of narcotics take effect after control of ventilation to avoid any chest rigidity and hypoventilation episodes, as well as any response to intubation. Inotropic support with an infusion of a catecholamine is used in patients who are at high risk for cardiovascular collapse (Box 24-4).

A pulmonary artery catheter (PAC) routinely is placed after induction rather than before because the hemodynamic status and goals are usually known. A PAC is vital to assess the impact of surgery on pulmonary vascular reactivity without delay. In addition, patients with advanced disease are unable to lie supine or in Trendelenburg position, which sometimes can lead to cardiorespiratory collapse. If the preoperative TTE reveals

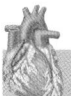

BOX 24-4. SIGNS OF IMPENDING COLLAPSE

- Right ventricular end-diastolic pressure > 14 mm Hg
- Severe tricuspid regurgitation
- Pulmonary vascular resistance > 1000 dynes·sec·cm^{-5}

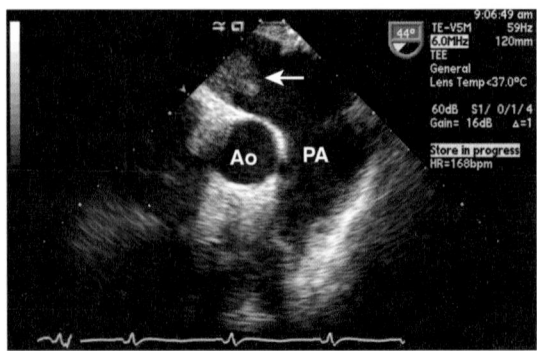

Figure 24-11 Midesophageal ascending aortic short-axis view in a patient with type I Jamieson chronic thromboembolic pulmonary hypertension disease. Note the dilated pulmonary artery, which is significantly larger than the ascending aorta. *Arrow* points to thrombus within the right pulmonary artery. Ao, ascending aorta; PA, main pulmonary artery.

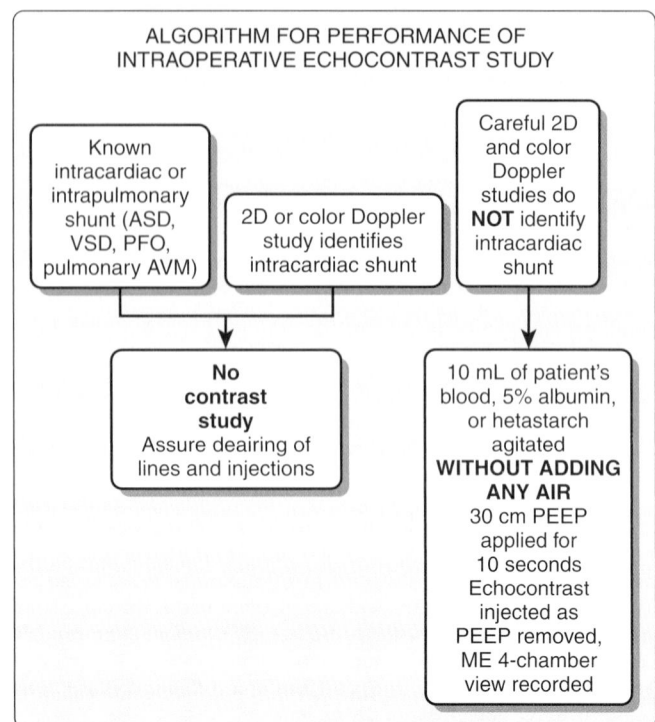

Figure 24-12 **Algorithm for performance of intraoperative echocontrast study for pulmonary thromboendarterectomy patients.** ASD, atrial septal defect; AVM, arteriovenous malformation; 2D, two-dimensional; ME, midesophageal; PEEP, positive end-expiratory pressure; PFO, patent foramen ovale; VSD, ventricular septal defect.

evidence of RA, RV, or main PA thrombi, TEE is performed immediately after induction and before placement of the PAC (Figure 24-11). In this instance, PAC placement is guided with TEE and the PAC is left in the superior vena cava (at 20 cm) until completion of the surgical procedure. PAC placement can be challenging because of the dilated right atrium and right ventricle, as well as significant TR. TEE guidance often assists in placement. Because all PTE patients undergo prolonged CPB and circulatory arrest, a femoral arterial catheter is placed after induction to monitor arterial pressure after CPB as a radial artery catheter significantly underestimates systemic arterial pressure with a gradient of as much as 20 mm Hg. This phenomenon has been observed by Mohr et al[61] and Baba et al[62]; they proposed redistribution of blood flow away from the extremity as the cause (see Chapter 14).

SEDLine brain-function monitoring (Hospira, Lake Forest, IL) is used to monitor brain function. A four-channel processed electroencephalograph monitor provides monitoring of the isoelectric electroencephalogram and confirmation of minimal oxygen utilization of the brain before circulatory arrest. It also serves as a monitor for the level of consciousness during the entire procedure. The INVOS system (Somanetics Corporation, Troy, MI) is utilized to monitor cerebral oximetry. The device represents a balance between oxygen delivery and consumption by the brain. In a retrospective study of more than 2000 patients, Goldman et al[63] confirmed that the institution of cerebral oximetry in their practice decreased the stroke rate in cardiac surgical patients. Yao et al[64] observed an association between cerebral desaturation and neurocognitive dysfunction in 101 patients undergoing cardiac surgery. They found that patients with a cerebral oxygen saturation of less than 40% for longer than 10 minutes had an increased incidence of neurocognitive dysfunction (see Chapter 16).

Temperature monitoring is achieved in several ways during PTE to allow accurate quantification of thermal gradients and to ensure even cooling and rewarming. Bladder temperature and rectal probes are used for core temperature estimation. A tympanic membrane probe is used for brain temperature estimation, and the PAC measures blood temperature.[65]

Acute normovolemic hemodilution often is used in the setting of an increased starting hematocrit without the presence of any concomitant cardiac disease. Typically, 1 to 2 units of whole-blood postinduction is removed, depending on the starting hematocrit, and replaced with colloid in a 1:1 ratio to maintain hemodynamic stability. Acute normovolemic hemodilution has added benefits for deep hypothermic circulatory arrest (DHCA) because it will help decrease blood viscosity, optimize capillary blood flow, and promote uniform cooling. Autologous whole blood is reinfused to the patient after protamine administration because it is rich in platelets and factors. Antifibrinolytics are not used routinely with PTE cases because patients are often inherently procoagulant.

TEE is used routinely in PTE patients to monitor hemodynamics, evaluate right and left ventricular function, identify any intracardiac thrombus or valvular pathology, and evaluate RV function and deair-

ing after bypass. A thorough intra-atrial septal evaluation, including a bubble study with a Valsalva maneuver, is performed to rule out a PFO (Figure 24-12; see Chapters 12 and 13).

PFO is present in 25% to 35% of PTE patients.[66] Most PFOs are repaired intraoperatively if detected by color-flow Doppler or with the use of an agitated saline test because some patients may experience high right-sided pressures after surgery. In such cases, hypoxemia will ensue because of right-to-left shunting. In rare instances when results of the operation are not favorable and severe right-sided pressures are expected, the PFO is left open as a "pop-off" to improve RV function and increase CO at the expense of some hypoxemia. It has been suggested that closure of a PFO can be detrimental to clinical status by reducing LV filling and increasing filling of the noncompliant right ventricle.[67]

Because all PTE patients undergo circulatory arrest, the head is wrapped in a cooling blanket. The head-wrap system (Polar Care; Breg, Vista, CA) is composed of two items: the "Polar Care 500" cooling device (cooling bucket, pump, pump bracket, and AC power transformer), which is reusable, and the actual "wrap," which is a one-time-use item. The "wrap" utilized was actually designed as a cold therapy pad for postoperative shoulder surgery, but it functions well as a head wrap (Figure 24-13). In a series of 55 patients in whom this device was used during circulatory arrest, they had a mean tympanic membrane temperature of 15.1° C.[19] It is the impression that the head wrap provides sufficient cooling to the brain, wraps the whole head, and is far easier to use than ice bags. So far it has been used in more than 2400 cases without any complication.

Initiation of Cardiopulmonary Bypass

The prebypass time is typically short unless concomitant CABG is planned. The bypass pump is primed with 1100 mL of plasmalyte A, 100 mL of 25% albumin, 5–12 mL (100 units/kg) of heparin, 12.5 grams of mannitol, and 1 ampule of bicarbonate. Methylprednisolone, 30 mg/kg max, is given; 3g shortly after

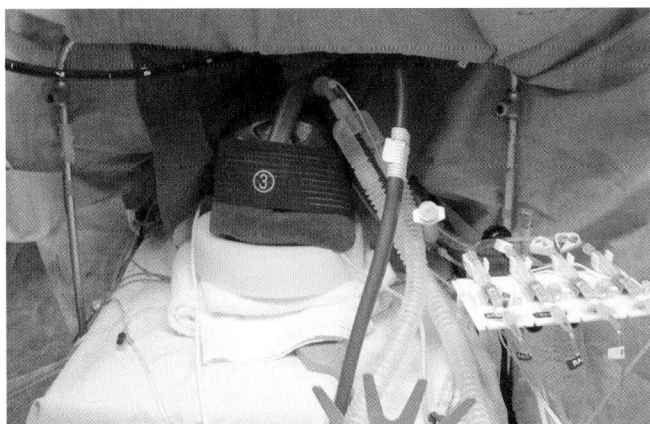

Figure 24-13 "Polar Care 500" head wrap used during circulatory arrest during pulmonary thromboendarterectomy procedures.

initiation of bypass and an additional 500 mg at rewarming. Methylprednisolone theoretically functions as a cell-membrane stabilizer and anti-inflammatory agent.[68] Cooling begins immediately after initiation of bypass, using CPB temperature adjustment and the cooling blankets present under the patient, together with the head wrap. Allowing appropriate time to cool and warm the patient in each direction using rectal, bladder, tympanic, PAC, and perfusate temperatures with appropriate thermal gradients ensures even and thorough cooling and warming, respectively.

Phenytoin, 15 mg/kg of propofol, is administered by the perfusionist shortly after initiation of CPB for prophylaxis of postoperative seizures after DHCA. Thiopental, 500 mg, or 2.5 mg/kg of propofol, is administered immediately before DHCA to provide cerebral protection because of dose-dependant reductions in both cerebral blood flow and cerebral metabolic rate.[69,70] Although no clear evidence supports the benefit of thiopental administration for DHCA and global cerebral ischemia,[71,72] it may be beneficial in focal ischemia because brain cooling may be uneven or incomplete, cerebral emboli may occur as PTE is an open procedure, and in case of sparse electroencephalographic activity, thiopental will abolish any residual activity. Interestingly, Harris et al[73] found that thiopental given during profound hypothermia was associated with a dose-related increase in mean arterial pressure of 32 ± 11 mm Hg ($P < 0.0001$), and flow may need to be decreased temporarily to prevent hypertension.

Several checklists need to be reviewed at the institution of circulatory arrest: The electroencephalograph must be isoelectric, tympanic membrane temperature 18°C or less, bladder/rectal temperatures ≤ 20°C, and all monitoring catheters to the patient turned off, decreasing the risk for entraining air into the vasculature during exsanguination.

Rewarming Phase and Separation from Bypass

The temperature goals during rewarming are never to exceed a 10°C gradient between blood and bladder/rectal temperatures, and never allow the perfusate temperature to be more than 37.5°C. Warming too quickly promotes systemic gas bubble formation, cerebral O_2 desaturation, and uneven warming, which can aggravate cerebral ischemia. The rewarming period can take up to 120 minutes to achieve a core temperature of 36.5°C, correlating closely to the patient's weight and systemic perfusion.

Separation from CPB follows the same guidelines as any other cardiac surgery requiring CPB, with a few minor exceptions. Communication with the surgeon is of paramount importance because surgical classification of the thromboembolic disease and how much organized clot was successfully removed will dictate how much inotropic and vasopressor support (if any) is needed to separate from bypass. Type I and type II Jamieson disease are likely to have improved hemodynamics with substantial reduction in PVR and improved RV function, which is revealed immediately postbypass with TEE[74] (Figure 24-14). Blanchard et al[75] demonstrated that the RV Tei index is abnormally increased in CTEPH patients and decreases substantially after PTE. Tei index is a useful parameter in estimating PVR independent of ventricular geometry, and it is monitored easily in CTEPH patients before and after PTE.

In contrast, with type III and IV Jamieson disease, the patient is less likely to have reduced PVR and improved RV function immediately after PTE because surgery is likely to be only partially successful at best. Anticipated need for more aggressive inotropic support (e.g., dopamine, 3 to 7 µg/kg/min, or epinephrine, 0.03 to 0.15 µg/kg/min), together with pulmonary vasodilators such as milrinone, inhaled prostacyclin, and nitric oxide (NO) usually are considered. NO frequently is used if surgery is partially successful because it exerts its effect on the pulmonary vasculature mediating vascular smooth muscle relaxation with minimal systemic effects. Atrial and ventricular epicardial pacing leads are placed routinely to improve RV and atrial function, together with moderate inotropic support to ensure adequate RV coronary perfusion. End-tidal carbon dioxide is a poor measure of ventilation adequacy in these patients both before and after CPB because dead space ventilation is an integral part of the disease process. The arterial-to-end-tidal carbon dioxide gradient will improve after successful surgery, but the response varies. Greater minute ventilation often is required to compensate for a metabolic acidosis that develops after prolonged periods of CPB, circulatory arrest, and hypothermia. Before separation from CPB, intracardiac air and right and left ventricular function are assessed with TEE. With successful operative results, immediate improvements of RV function with resolution of interventricular septal distortion and flattening are seen on intraoperative TEE. With the dramatic resolution of pulmonary hypertension after PTE, transmitral diastolic flow improves in a predictable manner. Not surprisingly, this correlates

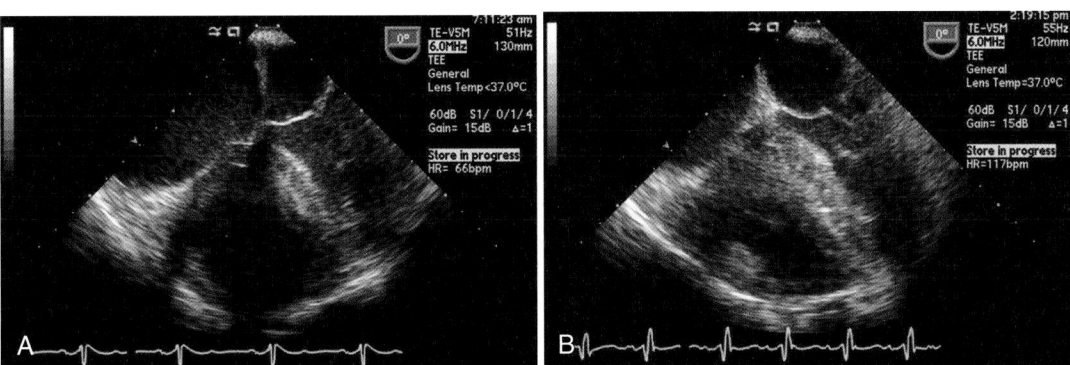

Figure 24-14 *A,* Midesophageal four-chamber view in a patient with chronic thromboembolic pulmonary hypertension going for pulmonary thromboendarterectomy (PTE; before picture). Note the severely dilated right atrium and right ventricle, with the interatrial septum bulging toward the left atrium. *B,* After PTE surgery, note the improvement in the right atrial and right ventricular size after successful PTE.

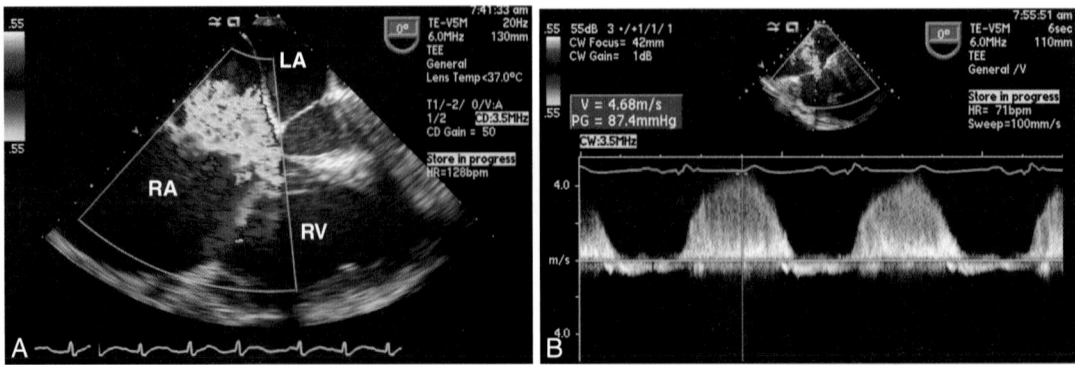

Figure 24-15 *A,* Modified midesophageal four-chamber view in a patient with chronic thromboembolic pulmonary hypertension (CTEPH) and severe tricuspid regurgitation. Note the severely dilated right atrium, right ventricle, and interatrial septum bulging toward the left atrium. The severely enlarged right heart often prevents proper midesophageal views, yielding difficulty in imaging the left heart. Severe tricuspid regurgitation often results from a dilated tricuspid annulus secondary to right ventricular dilation and may be confirmed via systolic flow reversal in the hepatic veins. *B,* Continuous-wave Doppler through a tricuspid regurgitant jet demonstrating severe pulmonary hypertension in a patient with CTEPH. LA, left atrium; RA, right atrium; RV, right ventricle.

with improvement in the CO and cardiac index.[76] Tricuspid annuloplasty rarely is performed, even if severe TR was documented before surgery, because tricuspid annular geometry is restored with remodeling of the right ventricle after PTE. Figure 24-15 demonstrates severe TR with color-flow and continuous-wave Doppler. It is of paramount importance that the anesthesiologist check the endotracheal tube before separation from CPB because the presence of frothy sputum or bleeding indicates either reperfusion pulmonary edema or airway bleeding, two of the most dreaded complications of the procedure.[77] Reperfusion pulmonary edema can start as early as a few hours after the endarterectomy, when the endotracheal tube is suctioned, and escalating amounts of positive end-expiratory pressure (PEEP) are applied.

If frank blood is seen in the endotracheal tube, this signifies a mechanical violation of the airway barrier and stems from a technical error during the operation. Bleeding and pulmonary edema can be distinguished by inspection of the endotracheal tube but may coexist. The two main goals for the treatment of these bleeding episodes are to prevent exsanguination and ensure adequate gas exchange. Management depends on the severity of the bleeding. Often, conservative management consisting of PEEP, topical vasoconstrictors, reversal of heparin, and correction of coagulopathies will reduce the bleeding. If bleeding is severe, resumption of CPB is indicated, and diagnostic fiberoptic bronchoscopy is used to evaluate the source of bleeding, as well as to help isolate the bleeding segment. A double-lumen tube is the best method for lung isolation, and differential ventilation and PEEP can be used effectively. The only caveat with a double-lumen tube is the difficulty in using a large bronchoscope that limits suctioning and diagnostic capabilities, and exchanging the tube can be risky. A Univent tube is an alternative to a double-lumen tube. Treatment options (e.g., lung isolation, PEEP, topical vasoconstrictors such as vasopressin, phenylephrine) depend on the severity of bleeding.[77] Risk factors for bleeding in these patients are difficult to identify before. They include the presence of friable vessels, residual pulmonary hypertension, spontaneous rupture, trauma, and a technically difficult procedure.

Pulmonary hemorrhage most likely manifests on reinstitution of pulmonary blood flow during weaning from CPB. Unfortunately, it is difficult to test the integrity of the PA during the endarterectomy because cardiac ejection of blood into the PA and appropriate systolic pressure are needed. The anesthesiologist involved with these procedures should be prepared to provide diagnostic and therapeutic maneuvers such as bronchial blockade, differential lung ventilation, endobronchial administration of vasoconstrictors, and pharmacologic control of residual pulmonary hypertension (Figure 24-16). Massive pulmonary hemorrhage after PTE, although a rare event, is the third most common cause for perioperative mortality in the PTE population, with residual pulmonary hypertension and reperfusion pulmonary edema as the leading two causes.

A portable transport ventilator is utilized for transport to the ICU for all PTE patients, not only to standardize ventilation but also to maintain PEEP. Propofol is used during transport and in the ICU for sedation for the first 24 hours; although within 1 to 2 hours after arrival in the ICU, the patients are allowed to awaken for a brief neurologic examination. Most patients are discharged from the ICU on the second or third postoperative day, with subsequent hospital discharge approximately 1 to 2 weeks after the operation.

Postoperative Period and Adverse Effects

The postoperative course frequently is complicated by prolonged mechanical ventilation, and patients may experience minimal improvement in symptoms after their surgery. Hepatic and renal insufficiency may complicate the perioperative period, but may improve with correction of pulmonary hypertension and RV failure. Advanced age and obesity increase perioperative risks but are not absolute contraindications to surgery. Coronary artery disease and valvular heart disease can be corrected at the time of PTE. Good postoperative management is essential for the success of this procedure. All patients remain intubated for at least 24 hours and require diuresis with the goal of reaching preoperative weight within 24 hours. Hematocrit level should be maintained between 28% and 30%.

Ventilation

A large tidal volume ventilation strategy initially is recommended. The rationale behind the larger tidal volume strategy than normally recommended is due to more occlusion on the right side of the lung and the lower lobes than the upper lobes; thus, blood flow after PTE is directed toward the lower lobes and the right lung. Adequate ventilation to both lower lobes is necessary to avoid the gas exchange consequences associated with areas of low ventilation/perfusion ratio or venous admixture. Efforts are made to facilitate extubation on postoperative day 1 because prolonged intubation impairs cough response, and PEEP can decrease right and left ventricular preload and CO. There are two specific complications to this procedure: reperfusion pulmonary edema and persistent pulmonary hypertension.

Reperfusion Pulmonary Edema

Most patients undergoing PTE will develop some degree of localized pulmonary edema or "reperfusion response."[78] Reperfusion response or reperfusion injury is a localized form of acute respiratory distress syndrome defined as a radiologic opacity seen in the areas of the lungs that underwent endarterectomy. It usually occurs within 24 to 72 hours, but in its most severe form, it is seen right after CPB separation after

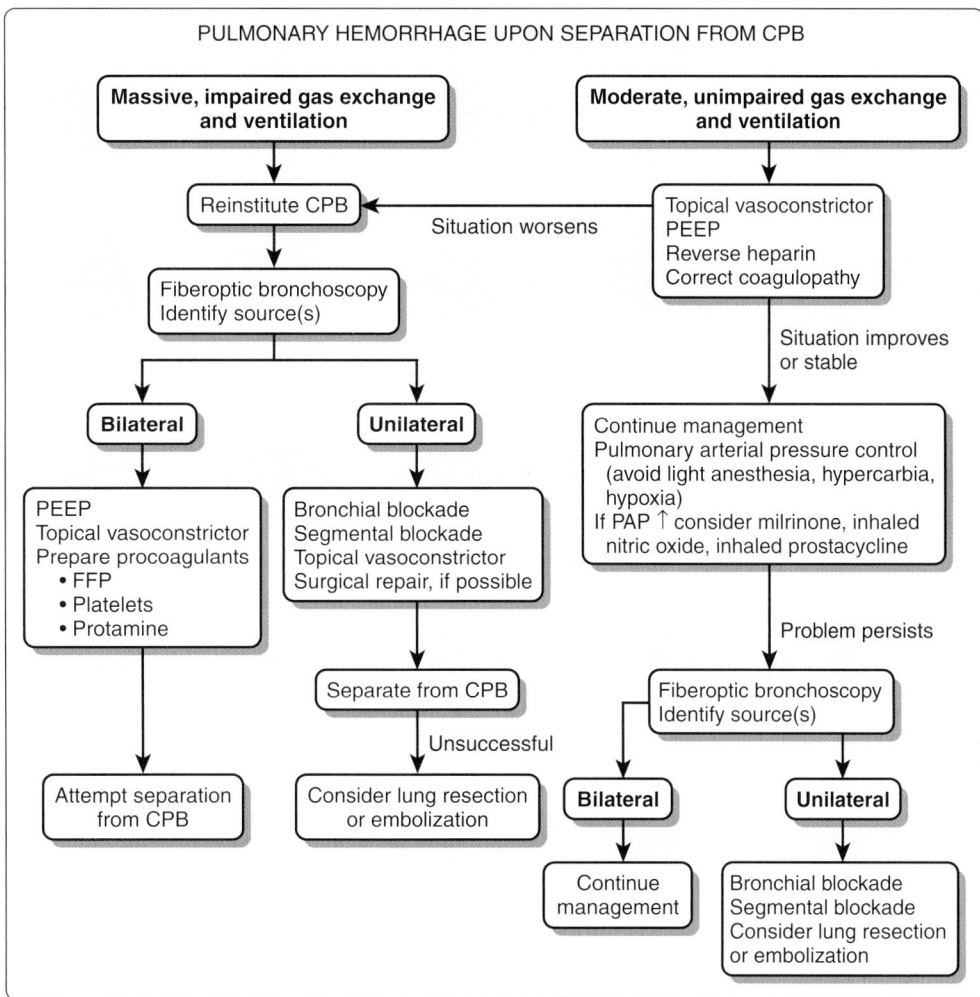

Figure 24-16 **General algorithm for management of postcardiopulmonary bypass hemorrhage.** CPB, cardiopulmonary bypass; FFP, fresh frozen plasma; PAP, pulmonary arterial pressure; PEEP, positive end-expiratory pressure.

the endarterectomy, presenting as profound desaturation. Mortality from clinically significant reperfusion injury is observed in less than 10% of patients. One common cause of the reperfusion pulmonary edema is persistent high PAPs after a thorough endarterectomy, with a large part of the pulmonary vascular bed affected by type IV disease. However, the reperfusion phenomenon may be seen in patients after a complete resolution of high PAPs. One theory of the cause is reactive hyperemia after restoration of blood flow to segments of the PA bed after periods of no flow. Other contributing factors may include pulmonary ischemia and conditions associated with high-permeability lung injury. The incidence of this complication is much less common now secondary to the large experience acquired over the past ten years, leading to more complete and expeditious endarterectomies.

Management of the "Reperfusion Response."
Aggressive measures should be taken to minimize the development of pulmonary edema with diuresis, maintenance of adequate hematocrit levels, and the early use of PEEP. Careful management of ventilation and fluid balance is required, and usually reperfusion pulmonary edema resolves. PEEP is initiated with a gradual transition from volume-limited to pressure-limited inverse ratio ventilation and the acceptance of moderate hypercapnia.[78] Inhaled NO at 20 to 40 parts per million (ppm) has been used occasionally to improve gas exchange. Extracorporeal perfusion support (extracorporeal membrane oxygenation or extracorporeal carbon dioxide removal) has been limited to patients with hemodynamic improvement who are suffering from significant reperfusion response.[79,80]

Persistent Pulmonary Hypertension

Persistent pulmonary hypertension is typically related to inadequate endarterectomy or surgically inaccessible disease (i.e., small-vessel vasculopathy). Most patients have a successful endarterectomy with immediate and sustained restoration of PAPs to normal levels. In a few patients, however, an immediate reduction of PVR is not achieved, but over the next few days, substantial reduction may occur because of the subsequent relaxation of small vessels and the resolution of intraoperative factors such as pulmonary edema. In such patients, it is not unusual to see a large PA pulse pressure and low diastolic pressure, indicating good runoff yet persistent pulmonary arterial inflexibility resulting in a high systolic pressure.

In rare instances when certain patients will unlikely survive waiting for a lung transplant donor, the surgeons will operate on them despite considerable risk. More than one third of perioperative deaths in the most recent 500 patients who were operated on in this institution were directly attributable to inadequate relief of PAH. This was a diagnostic rather than an operative technical problem. Pharmacologic attempts to reduce high residual PVR levels with sodium nitroprusside, epoprostenol, or inhaled NO generally are not effective. Mechanical circulatory support or extracorporeal membrane oxygenation use in these patients is not appropriate.[79,80]

Pulmonary Vascular Steal

Pulmonary arterial steal is a postoperative phenomenon in which blood flow is diverted from the previously well-perfused segments to the newly endarterectomized segments.[81] The steal entity was recognized when perfusion scans obtained after the operation showed regions of reduced perfusion suggestive of recurrent emboli.[81] Whether the cause is failure of autoregulation in the newly endarterectomized segments or secondary small-vessel changes in the previously open segments is not clear. Preferentially perfused areas may be the site of reperfusion response in patients with steal phenomena and residual hypertension, leading to severe hypoxia from areas that are not effectively contributing to oxygenation. However, long-term follow-up has documented a decrease in pulmonary vascular steal in the majority of patients, suggesting a remodeling process in the pulmonary vascular bed.[82]

Other Postoperative Complications

Delirium had a greater incidence in the early experience before 1990. A prospective study of 28 patients showed that 77% of patients who underwent PTE experienced delirium, with peak incidence at 72 hours after surgery.[83] Analysis attributed delirium to a circulatory arrest time greater than 55 minutes. The incidence rate declined to 11% and, in a recent cohort of 1000 patients, to 1.3%. More experience, expeditious operations resulting in shorter circulatory arrest time, and the use of a direct cooling jacket placed around the head have contributed to the substantial decline in neurologic complications. Postoperative confusion in PTE cases is now the same as with other cardiac surgery.

Pericardial effusion is another complication that has been reduced in frequency with experience. The cause is suspected to be due to lymphatic tissue dissection around the hilum, together with mobilization of the superior vena cava and reduction of cardiac size after the operation. Currently, with the practice of creating a posterior pericardial window or placing a posterior pericardial drain, this problem essentially has been eliminated.

Lastly, the incidence rate of atrial arrhythmias is 10% in PTE patients, which is no more common than that encountered in similar cardiac surgeries.

Postoperative Anticoagulation

Lifelong anticoagulation with warfarin is begun as soon as pacing wires and mediastinal drainage tubes are removed, with a target international normalized ratio of 2.5 to 3.5. Thromboembolic recurrence is rare in patients who have been maintained on adequate anticoagulation.

Pulmonary Thromboendarterectomy in Patients with Sickle Cell Disease

Management of patients with concomitant sickle cell disease and CTEPH presents unique challenges because treatment of CTEPH with PTE involves prolonged CPB, deep hypothermia, and intervals of circulatory arrest, all of which are factors that may promote sickling. There are reports of successful completion of PTE with resolution of pulmonary hypertension in two patients with sickle cell disease complicated with CTEPH.[84] Moser and Shea[85] and Collins and Orringer[86] confirmed the relation among pulmonary infarction, cor pulmonale, and sickle cell states. In addition, two studies by Sutton et al[87] and Simmons et al[88] reported 20% to 60% prevalence rates of pulmonary hypertension in sickle cell disease, respectively. With innovations in management of sickle cell patients and extended life expectancy, it might be expected to see more sickle cell patients present with CTEPH disease.

Previous reports of CPB in adults with sickle cell disease involved only patients undergoing valvular or septal repair.[89,90] In contrast, PTE patients require periods of deep hypothermia to 18°C to 20°C and circulatory arrest to allow for a bloodless field. Sickling and hemolysis during or after CPB have been repeatedly reported.[91,92] Stagnation of blood, deep hypothermia, anemia, and acidosis encountered during circulatory arrest are expected to increase the likelihood of sickling.[93]

"Prophylactic" exchange transfusion remains controversial. A multicenter trial comparing conservative exchange transfusion with an aggressive transfusion regimen in patients with sickle cell disease found that there was no difference and the conservative approach resulted in only half as many transfusion-associated complications.[94] Hypoxia has been recognized to potentially incite sickling because of increased viscosity from a deoxygenated form of sickle hemoglobin and sickle cell adhesion to endothelial cells. Particular attention should be paid to various hypoxic complications such as atelectasis and reperfusion pulmonary edema during the postoperative period, and oxygen saturation should be maintained at or greater than 95% throughout hospitalization.

In conclusion, patients with sickle cell disease presenting for PTE should undergo thorough preoperative evaluation to prepare them for surgery, with particular attention to correction of anemia, early screening for antibodies in blood typing, preoperative and intraoperative exchange transfusion, and avoidance of hypoxemia and acidosis during and after surgery.

Pulmonary Thromboendarterectomy in Patients with Heparin-Induced Thrombocytopenia

Management of CPB for patients with heparin-induced thrombocytopenia (HIT) undergoing PTE may be challenging. In these cases, alternative means of anticoagulation during CPB must be used. Three direct-thrombin inhibitors are available for alternative anticoagulant therapy, and their use is dependent on patient-specific factors (see Chapter 31).

There are reports of successful use of recombinant hirudin as an alternative anticoagulant to heparin in a patient with CTEPH and HIT undergoing PTE with circulatory arrest.[95] Hirudin, an anticoagulant naturally produced by the salivary gland of the medicinal leech, interacts with both the fibrinogen-binding and catalytic sites of thrombin, completely inhibiting all procoagulant actions of thrombin, including thrombin on fibrin lining the CPB circuit. It is metabolized through the kidney with a half-life of 80 minutes.[96] Argatroban is metabolized through the hepatobiliary system with a half-life of 40 to 50 minutes. Bivalirudin is a 20-amino acid synthetic peptide, which consists of two peptide fragments (connected by a tetraglycine spacer) that inhibit thrombin by specifically binding both to the active catalytic site and to the anion-binding exosite of thrombin. Its unique mechanism of action results in a predictable, consistent anticoagulant effect.[96] It directly inhibits thrombin; inhibits both clot-bound and circulating thrombin; is highly specific for thrombin, without binding to other plasma proteins; and binds reversibly, with a short half-life (25 minutes in patients with normal renal function). Clearance was reduced approximately 20% in patients with moderate and severe renal impairment (80% in dialysis-dependent patients). There is no reversal agent for bivalirudin. However, because of its short half-life and enzymatic elimination, it is considerably safer than other direct-thrombin inhibitors (argatroban, lepirudin).

Unfortunately, although the activated partial thromboplastin time is adequate to monitor hirudin when using small quantities as in an ICU setting, the activated partial thromboplastin time to hirudin relation flattens at the high concentrations required during CPB. Further, the activated coagulation time does not correlate well with hirudin levels, although it has been used for this purpose. Reliable results at this time only are obtained using the ecarin clotting time, which can be measured rapidly using whole blood. Because hypoprothrombinemia caused by hemodilution occurs on CPB, supplementation of normal human plasma to the blood is required for a reliable test.[97,98] Unfortunately, the ecarin clotting time is not readily available in the United States.

Bivalirudin use as an anticoagulant has been promising during both off- and on-pump cardiac surgery in patients with HIT; however, its safety in DHCA needs further evaluation. Stagnant blood should be avoided because local bivalirudin levels will decrease due to its metabolism by proteases in blood exposed to wound or foreign surfaces, leading to local clot formation.

The most common alternative strategy has involved the concomitant use of anticoagulation with unfractionated heparin (UFH), together with a platelet antagonist (iloprost, a prostacyclin analog, or tirofiban).[99] Another method used is epoprostenol (Flolan), a freeze-dried preparation of prostacyclin itself. Its very short half-life (6 minutes) requires continuous infusion, and its major downside is severe hypotension often requiring intraoperative vasopressors.[100] Systemic anticoagulation in patients with demonstrated or suspected type II HIT (HIT II), utilizing the GPIIb/IIIa inhibitor tirofiban (Aggrastat) and UFH, has been successful in the authors' experience. Tirofiban binds competitively to platelets' GPIIb/IIIa receptors and has a half-life of approximately 2 hours.[101–103] With greater than 80% blockage of GPIIb/IIIa receptors, systemic heparinization can be administered despite HIT and thrombosis. Ideally, tirofiban is administered before surgical incision and activation of platelets, and at least 15 minutes before systemic heparinization. A loading dose of 10 µg/kg is given to be followed with a continuous infusion at 0.15 µg/kg/min.[102,103] Once platelet inhibition is greater than 80%, systemic heparinization is administered at a dose of 400 IU/kg. Heparin concentration is monitored every 30 minutes. The tirofiban infusion is stopped 1 hour before cessation of CPB. In patients with compromised renal function, the level is reduced during the last hour with ultrafiltration. UFH is neutralized with protamine as usual, and donor platelets are transfused if necessary.[103] It is critical that exposure to heparin before and after bypass is avoided, as well as any heparin-treated components and monitoring catheters.

The University of California San Diego Experience

UCSD has been the pioneer in PTE surgery. Although this procedure is now performed at several major cardiovascular centers around the world, the reported world literature on this operation (exclusive of UCSD) is approximately 1500 cases. However, from 1970 to the present, more than 2400 PTE operations have been performed at UCSD. The perioperative mortality rate at UCSD has declined significantly from 16% in the 1980s to 2.5% in 2008, despite a patient population with greater risk factors (Figure 24-17). This certainly reflects the evolution and refinements in the surgical technique. Table 24-1 lists the experience for the last 1100 patients' hemodynamic improvement based on their thromboembolic disease classification after endarterectomy.[42]

The secret to the success of this procedure has been the close communication of multiple medical teams, including pulmonary medicine, anesthesiology, perfusion, and cardiac surgery. This operation has revolutionized the treatment of CTEPH, providing significant and permanent lifestyle improvements for patients.[104] The advantage of this procedure over lung transplant surgery, the only other alternative definitive treatment, includes a lower mortality rate, better survival, and avoidance of long-term immunosuppressive treatment and allograft rejection.

Between PTE becoming a safe and efficient treatment for CTEPH and an increased awareness of the disease, it is anticipated that surgical therapy will become the definitive treatment during earlier stages of the disease process. However, future studies in areas of CTEPH cause

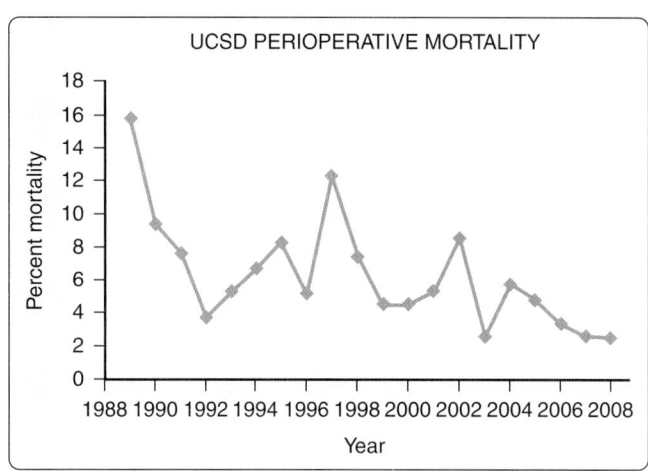

Figure 24-17 University of California at San Diego (UCSD) perioperative mortality from 1988 to 2008.

and complications such as reperfusion pulmonary edema and vascular steal are necessary. RV failure, cerebral protection, and persistent pulmonary edema also remain areas of future research.

ACUTE PULMONARY EMBOLISM

Epidemiology

Venous thromboembolism (VTE) is the term used to describe DVT and its complication, PE. Deep vein thrombosis originating in the lower extremities is the most common cause of PE, and it can present in a variety of ways from asymptomatic to massive PE.

Acute PE carries a high risk for morbidity and mortality both in the United States and worldwide. Actual incidence and mortality rates for PE are unknown secondary to the vague clinical presentation requiring a high index of suspicion for clinical diagnosis. The public has not been well-educated about PE; consequently, prompt diagnosis and early detection lags far behind the public awareness for a heart attack. One study estimated autopsy findings of unsuspected acute PE to be involved in 60% of patients who died in the hospital, and the diagnosis was missed in up to 70% of those cases.[105] The incidental finding of PE at autopsy is, surprisingly, common and does not seem to have changed over the past few decades. Aging accounts for the increasing numbers of VTE and PE. Therefore, with the average age of the U.S. population increasing and the total number of VTEs increasing per year, these result in the increased incidence of PE. Primary prevention becomes essential to improve survival and prevent complications by focusing on risk-factor modification, as well as appropriate prophylaxis of patients at risk.

TABLE 24-1	Thromboembolic Classification: Hemodynamic Results				
Variable	*All Patients* (n = 1100, 100%)	*Type 1* (n = 415, 37.7%)	*Type 2* (n = 469, 42.6%)	*Type 3* (n = 192, 17.5%)	*Type 4* (n = 24, 2.2%)
PVR (dynes·sec·cm⁻⁵)	859.4 ± 439.5	924.2 ± 450.4	799.9 ± 417.2	863.2 ± 454.6	884.6 ± 412.3
	290.4 ± 195.7	269.8 ± 176.6	270.5 ± 191.3	350.8 ± 183.3	595.2 ± 360.2
CO (L/min)	3.9 ± 1.3	3.7 ± 1.4	4.1 ± 1.3	4.0 ± 1.5	3.8 ± 1.2
	5.4 ± 1.5	5.5 ± 1.5	5.5 ± 1.5	5.2 ± 1.4	4.5 ± 1.1
Systolic PA pressure (mm Hg)	75.9 ± 18.6	76.8 ± 18.7	75.0 ± 19.5	75.8 ± 16.4	78.4 ± 15.6
	46.4 ± 16.6	4.4 ± 15.1	44.5 ± 15.0	52.7 ± 17.1	73.8 ± 32.1
Diastolic PA pressure (mm Hg)	28.5 ± 9.7	29.8 ± 9.6	27.3 ± 10.0	28.3 ± 8.8	32.3 ± 9.5
	18.5 ± 7.2	17.7 ± 6.5	17.9 ± 6.8	20.6 ± 79	27.3 ± 12.8
Mean PA pressure (mm Hg)	46.2 ± 11.3	47.0 ± 11.4	45.2 ± 11.6	46.5 ± 10.3	50.2 ± 10.5
	28.4 ± 9.6	27.2 ± 8.7	27.5 ± 9.1	31.8 ± 10.1	42.4 ± 15.5
Mortality (%)	52 (4.7)	16 (3.9)	22 (4.7)	12 (6.3)	4 (16.7)

University of California San Diego (UCSD) experience for the last 1100 patients whose hemodynamic improvements were based on their thromboembolic disease classification after endarterectomy. Data are shown as means ± standard deviation or number (percentage). Top numbers are preoperative values and bottom numbers are postoperative values obtained just before removal of the Swan–Ganz catheter.
CO, cardiac output; PA, pulmonary artery; PVR, pulmonary vascular resistance.
Reprinted from Thistlethwaite PA, Kaneko K, Madani MM, Jamieson SW: Technique and outcomes of pulmonary endarterectomy surgery. *Ann Thorac Cardiovasc Surg* 14:274, 2008.

The overall incidence of VTE has been relatively constant at about 100 per 10,000 since 1980[106,107] despite improved prophylaxis regimens and more widespread use of prophylaxis. In the United States alone, about 900,000 people will experience development of blood clots in the lungs or major veins annually; 400,000 cases have been attributed to nonfatal DVT, 200,000 cases to nonfatal PE, and 300,000 cases to fatal VTE. Community-acquired VTE accounted for approximately 300,000 cases, and hospital-acquired VTE was estimated at 600,000 cases.[108] More than two thirds of the 900,000 VTE events were related to hospital inpatients.[106] VTE poses a major national health problem of similar magnitude to other thrombotic diseases. Although recent studies estimate the incidence of VTE to be around 120 per 100,000, this incidence varies markedly depending on age and sex.[108,109] The incidence begins to increase dramatically around age 50; for octogenarians or older, the incidence can reach up to 1000 per 100,000. In patients younger than 15 years, the incidence decreases substantially to less than 1 per 100,000 person-years. Women of childbearing age and men older than 50 have a greater incidence of VTE.[109] The incidence of VTE also varies by race. Compared with whites, the incidence among African Americans is about 30% greater, whereas Asian and Native Americans have an incidence rate that is about 70% lower. The incidence among Hispanics lies somewhere in between whites and Asian Americans.[110,111] Thirty percent of patients who have a history of VTE will experience development of a second episode within the next 10 years; recurrence is greater within the first 2 years.[112,113] In the International Cooperative Pulmonary Embolism Registry (ICOPER), the overall mortality rate for all patients with PE during the first 3 months was 17.4%.[114] Although the in-hospital mortality rate increased to 31% in patients presenting with hemodynamic instability in the Management Strategies and Determinants of Outcome in Acute Pulmonary Embolism Trial (MAPPET),[115] the mortality rate directly credited to PE was 45% in the ICOPER[10] and in-hospital mortality was 91% in the MAPPET.[115] Thus, PE warrants recognition because it remains common, underdiagnosed, and often fatal. The post-thrombotic syndrome and CTEPH are long-term effects of VTE disease. Twelve percent of patients with post-thrombotic syndrome, also termed *venous-stasis syndrome*, had a history of DVT in the past,[116] and approximately 30% of patients with DVT will subsequently experience development of venous-stasis syndrome within the next 10 years.[117,118]

Pathophysiology

The initial description of the pathogenesis of DVT dates back to the 19th century, when pathologist Rudolf Virchow first described Virchow's triad: venous stasis, injury to the intima, and enhanced coagulation properties of the blood.[119] Although PE and DVT share a similar pathologic process, they are, in fact, two distinct entities.

Asymptomatic venous thrombus, originating primarily from proximal deep veins, is the source of PE in 80% of patients with documented PE. Figure 24-18 demonstrates the pathophysiology of PE. The potent fibrinolytic capacity of the lung dissolves most emboli spontaneously, rendering them clinically silent. The size of the thromboembolus and

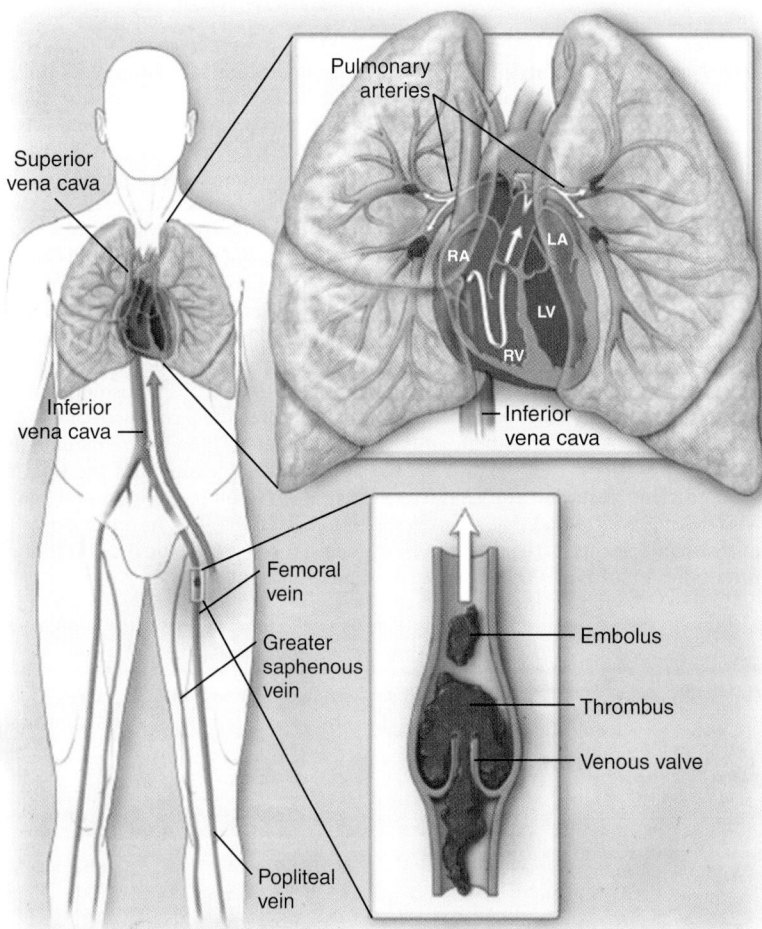

Figure 24-18 **Pathophysiology of pulmonary embolism.** Pulmonary embolism usually originates from the deep veins of the legs, most commonly the calf veins. These venous thrombi originate predominantly in venous valve pockets and at other sites of presumed venous stasis (bottom inset). If a clot propagates to the knee vein or above, or if it originates above the knee, the risk for embolism increases. Thromboemboli travel through the right side of the heart to reach the lungs. LA, left atrium; LV, left ventricle; RA, right atrium; RV, right ventricle. *(Reprinted from Tapson VF: Acute pulmonary embolism. N Engl J Med 358:1037, 2008, by permission of the Massachusetts Medical Society.)*

coexisting cardiopulmonary disease play important roles in the hemodynamic response and clinical presentation associated with PE. The most important cause of compromised physiology is anatomic obstruction combined with the release of vasoactive and bronchoactive agents such as serotonin from platelets, thrombin from plasma, and histamine from tissue leading to deleterious ventilation/perfusion mismatching.[120,121] As PVR increases, tension in the RV wall increases, leading to RV dilatation, dysfunction, annular dilation with TR, and ultimately, ischemia and RV failure. RV failure produces a decreased right-sided CO and ultimately impairs LV filling and output. In the first 12 to 48 hours after a PE, most patients maintain a normal systemic arterial pressure but later may abruptly develop persistent systemic arterial hypotension resistant to vasopressors. This leads to decreased RV stroke volume, CO, and hypotension. Clinically, patients may exhibit syncope or full cardiac arrest. Hypoxemia occurs because of ventilation/perfusion mismatch, leading to impaired pulmonary oxygen transfer. PE causes redistribution of blood flow so that some areas of the lung have a low ratio of ventilation to perfusion, whereas others have a high ratio of ventilation to perfusion. The failure of supplemental oxygen to correct arterial hypoxemia accompanying acute PE often reflects either shunting through a PFO as RA pressure exceeds LA pressure or intrapulmonary shunting. PEEP may worsen intracardiac shunting by compressing pulmonary vessels and increasing PVR. This further increases RA pressure, exacerbating the right-to-left intracardiac shunt. Total dead space increases because areas of the lung are ventilated despite decreased perfusion. This increased dead space impairs the efficient elimination of carbon dioxide. Despite the increased dead space, most patients with PE present with a lower-than-normal arterial Pco_2 with resultant respiratory alkalosis because of greater minute ventilation rate from stimulation of medullary chemoreceptors. Certain risk factors enhance the probability for development of acute DVT and, consequently, PE. Risk factors for VTE are listed in Table 24-2. Recent family-based studies indicate an increasing genetic predisposition to venous thrombosis with a high prevalence of mutant genes that increase susceptibility to thrombosis.[122–124] Protein C, protein S, and antithrombin deficiency are potent risk factors for VTE, although their incidence is rare. When combined with environmental risk factors such as oral contraceptives or pregnancy, they increase the risk for VTE substantially. These findings support the hypothesis that an acquired or inherited thrombophilia may actually predict who will experience development of symptomatic VTE.[125,126] Common risk factors for a clinically recognizable PE include advanced age, previous VTE, prolonged immobility or paralysis, malignancy, congestive heart failure, hospitalization for acute medical illness, nursing home confinement, prolonged mechanical ventilation, and surgery that involves extensive pelvic or abdominal dissection.[127,128] Obesity, cigarette smoking, and hypertension are the most common reversible risk factors

for PE. Age plays a factor in the incidence of VTE, both idiopathic and secondary, and might be attributable to the biology of aging rather than exposure to risks factors with natural aging.[127] Among women, use of oral contraceptives, obesity, pregnancy, the postpartum period, and hormone therapy are common risk factors.[128,129] Compared with community residents, hospitalized individuals are 100 times more likely to experience development of VTE and PE.[107] Immobility has been noted in more than 50% of patients within 3 months of a PE.

Clinical Presentation

Recognizing signs and symptoms of VTE may reduce diagnostic delays.[130,131] A high index of suspicion is necessary to diagnose PE because symptoms are nonspecific.[132] Leg pain, warmth, or swelling may indicate that a patient has DVT. Dyspnea or chest pain, both evolving gradually over a period of days to weeks and/or abrupt in onset, is suspicious of acute PE. Pleuritic chest pain and hemoptysis together with a pleural rub are characteristic of patients with pulmonary infarction. Enlarged neck veins, accentuated second heart sound, a right-sided gallop, and an RV lift are signs of right-sided strain because of pulmonary hypertension as a result of PE. Tachypnea and tachycardia are common but nonspecific findings.

Dyspnea is the most common symptom, occurring in 73% of patients with PE, followed by pleuritic chest pain (66%) and hemoptysis (13%).[130] Dyspnea, chest pain, or tachypnea occurs in 97% of documented cases. However, signs or symptoms of venous thrombosis in the lower extremities appear in less than 25% of patients with documented PE.[132] The multicenter study Prospective Investigation of Pulmonary Embolism Diagnosis (PIOPED) found that symptoms are as likely to be present in a patient with a negative angiogram as in a patient with a positive one.[133,134]

Diagnostic Approaches

Objective testing is necessary to exclude or to establish a diagnosis of PE, but some tests remain too insensitive and nonspecific. A large alveolar-to-arterial (A-a) oxygen gradient and respiratory alkalosis are common in PE, but an arterial oxygen partial pressure (Pao_2) greater than 80 mm Hg or a normal A-a oxygen gradient does not preclude PE.[131] A normal Pao_2 may occur in patients with PE who are able to hyperventilate. Similarly, a low Pao_2 is not diagnostic of PE; the PIOPED study showed that 74% of patients with PE had a Pao_2 less than 80 mm Hg.[132,135] Arterial blood gas results may be more helpful in assessing the severity of a PE than in diagnosing it. A chest roentgenogram may show atelectasis or pulmonary parenchymal abnormalities in two thirds of these individuals and be normal in another 15%.[130,136] Its primary value is to exclude other pulmonary conditions. Atelectasis, caused by loss of surfactant and alveolar hemorrhage, also may contribute to arterial hypoxemia. Classic electrocardiographic (ECG) findings of RV strain and S1Q3T3 are uncommon except with a massive embolus. Left-axis deviation occurs as often as right-axis deviation with PE. P pulmonale, RVH, right-axis deviation, or right bundle branch block was noted in only 6% of PIOPED patients.[137,138] The ECG primarily is useful to exclude conditions that may mimic PE such as myocardial infarction or pericarditis.[139] The D-dimer test (which measures plasma levels of a specific derivative of cross-linked fibrin) may be useful, although a positive study is nonspecific because it also may be positive in patients with cancer, trauma, myocardial infarction, and other inflammatory states.[140,141] The D-dimer is increased in almost all patients with PE because of endogenous, albeit ineffective, fibrinolysis, which causes plasmin to digest some of the fibrin clot and release D-dimers into the systemic circulation. In contrast, D-dimer enzyme-linked immunosorbent assay has been shown to have an excellent negative predictive value (99.6%) for acute PE.[142] In addition, the D-dimer/fibrinogen ratio of greater than 103 is highly specific for acute PE.[142] However, these findings do not pertain to inpatients suspected of PE. D-dimer testing is best considered together with clinical probability scores. Three scoring systems have been tested prospectively

TABLE 24-2	Risk Factors for Venous Thromboembolism	
Hereditary Factors	*Acquired Factors*
Antithrombin III deficiency	Reduced mobility
Protein C deficiency	Advanced age
Protein S deficiency	Cancer
Factor V Leiden	Acute medical illness
Activated protein C resistance without factor V Leiden	Major surgery
	Trauma
Prothrombin gene mutation	Spinal cord injury
Dysfibrinogenemia	Pregnancy and postpartum period
Plasminogen deficiency	Polycythemia vera
	Antiphospholipid antibody syndrome
	Oral contraceptives
	Hormone replacement therapy
	Heparins
	Chemotherapy
	Obesity
	Central venous catheterization
	Immobilizer or cast

and validated in large clinical trials: the Wells' score,[143–145] Geneva score,[145,146] and Pisa score.[147,148] All three scoring systems achieved reasonably good results in outpatients and emergency departments. Wells et al[143] developed a simple clinical model to predict the likelihood of PE and showed that managing patients for suspected PE on the basis of pretest probability (low, moderate, and high: 1.3%, 16.2%, and 37.5%, respectively) and D-dimer results were safe, with a decreased need for unnecessary diagnostic imaging. Their scoring system has been extensively validated (Table 24-3). The negative predictive value for the use of the clinical model combined with D-dimer testing in these patients was 99.5%.[143] In patients with a low or moderate pretest probability and a negative ELISA-based D-dimer, the likelihood of DVT and PE is low and precluded the need for specific imaging studies.[141,149] In contrast, in patients with a high pretest probability, imaging is the first step, not D-dimer testing.[150,151]

The most widely used technique to evaluate suspected PE is the radionucleide ventilation perfusion scan (and in some centers, the xenon lung scan). As a cornerstone for diagnosis of PE, it is least affected by preexisting cardiac or pulmonary disease. A negative scan essentially eliminates a PE, and a high-probability scan has a positive predictability of 85%.[133] However, only 13% of patients suspected of PE had a high-probability scan, and only 41% of suspected patients who had positive angiography had high-probability scans in the PIOPED study.[133] A corroborating clinical history increases the predictive ability of a lung scan.[136] A high-probability scan with low clinical suspicion was positive for PE in 56% of individuals. An intermediate scan was associated with a 30% likelihood of PE. Spiral CT scanning is gaining acceptance as the preferred imaging modality for acute PE.[152] It allows imaging of large areas of the chest, visualizing the PAs with one large breath. It has a sensitivity and specificity of 90% and 90%, respectively, which gives it positive and negative predictive values of 93% and 94%, respectively.[136] The accuracy of interpreting results depends on the generation of scanner that is used. First-generation scanners may fail to detect one third of PEs because they have 5-mm resolution, especially in the subsegmental pulmonary arteries. Third-generation scanners provide 1-mm resolution with a single breath-hold.[153] Spiral CT has become the first-line method for evaluating patients with suspected PE. DeMonaco et al[154] established that with the increasing use of spiral CT scans, the incidence of diagnosed PE is increasing but with lower severity of illness and lower mortality, suggestive of earlier diagnosis. In a retrospective review of 1500 consecutive patients suspected of acute PE, anticoagulation was withheld based on a negative spiral CT.[155]

Pulmonary angiography remains the gold standard because it detects approximately 98% of all clinically significant PE.[137,156] It may actually be underutilized because less than 15% of patients with nondiagnostic

ventilation-perfusion scans undergo angiography.[136] Angiography is a contributing factor in the death of less than 0.5% of patients.[157]

Ventilation-perfusion scanning is most likely to be diagnostic in the absence of cardiopulmonary disease, and a normal lung scan effectively rules out acute PE.[133] However, large trials have demonstrated that most patients with suspected embolism who underwent ventilation-perfusion scanning did not have any findings.

The PIOPED II trial compared the use of multidetector CT arteriography alone with its use in combination with CT venography for detecting suspected acute PE. Spiral CT arteriography sensitivity alone was 83%, whereas when combined with CT venography, the sensitivity increased to 90%, suggesting that a combined approach might facilitate clinical management, particularly for the treatment of inpatients with complex cases.[158,159] Figure 24-19 depicts a diagnostic algorithm for suspected acute PE.

Echocardiography is not recommended to definitively diagnose PE.[160] However, echocardiography has emerged as the principal tool to assess the risk for mortality during acute PE.[161] Patients fall into three categories: (1) low risk (no RV dysfunction), (2) submassive PE (RV dysfunction with preservation of systolic blood pressure), and (3) massive PE (RV dysfunction and shock) that carry an in-hospital mortality rate of less than 4%, 5% to 10%, and greater than 30%, respectively.[160] RV function is significant as an independent predictor of mortality.[162]

A PE may occur in all operative settings, but recognition may be difficult during general anesthesia.[163] The extensive pulmonary vascular network of the lung may be obliterated up to 50% by a clot, yet ventilation-perfusion matching could be minimally affected. Abrupt hemodynamic changes may appear with the onset of a PE. Meanwhile, other symptoms and signs of respiratory distress such as wheezing, cyanosis, hypoxemia, and hypocapnia may not occur under anesthesia. Capnography and pulse oximetry findings are nonspecific. Even if the patient is being monitored with a PAC, acute onset of PAH with a normal pulmonary capillary wedge pressure also may represent hypoxia, pneumothorax, pulmonary aspiration, vasoconstrictive medications, or air embolism.[164] Assessment of RV dysfunction with TEE better delineates PE and assesses and guides therapeutic measures.[160]

MASSIVE PULMONARY EMBOLISM

Massive PE represents 5% of cardiac arrests, with more than 60% of those noted to have pulseless electrical activity.[160] It is characterized as massive by the presence of arterial hypotension in addition to clinical signs of tissue hypoperfusion and hypoxia, inclusive of an altered level of consciousness, a urine output of less than 30 mL/hr, or cold and clammy extremities. Signs and symptoms include profound dyspnea at rest, cyanosis, tachycardia, and increased central venous pressure. Massive PE occurs with 50% or greater obstruction of pulmonary blood flow, leading to RV failure. On mechanical obstruction, humoral mediators are released, augmenting pulmonary vasoconstriction and PAH. This sudden increase in RV afterload results in RV dilation and dysfunction that displaces the interventricular septum (IVS), causing underfilling of the LV (Figure 24-20). Low CO and severe hypotension follow, ultimately leading to circulatory collapse and death.[165] Increased RV pressure also compresses the right coronary artery, causing RV ischemia and contributing to RV failure.[166] Mortality rate is 40% to 80% within 2 hours of the onset of a PE. Massive PE should be considered with the onset of unexplainable severe and sudden hypoxia or hypotension. The diagnosis is solidified if LV function is relatively maintained in the midst of profound RV dysfunction.[160] The differential diagnosis is cardiac tamponade, myocardial infarction, aortic dissection, and severe mitral regurgitation.[167] Interventions that improve RV function should receive priority because perfusion pressure to the right side is compromised.[166] It is controversial whether resuscitation should proceed with crystalloid versus vasopressor administration. Excessive fluid administration in the presence of RV dysfunction frequently exacerbates RV wall stress, intensifies RV ischemia, and causes further interventricular septal shift toward the left, which compromise

TABLE 24-3	Canadian Wells Prediction Score for Likelihood of Pulmonary Embolism	
Risk Factors		**Points**
DVT symptoms and signs		3.0
Different diagnosis less likely than PE		3.0
Heart rate > 100 beats/min		1.5
Immobilization or surgery in previous 4 weeks		1.5
Previous DVT or PE		1.5
Hemoptysis		1.0
Cancer		1.0
Clinical Probability		
Low: < 2.0		
Intermediate: 2.0–6.0		
High: > 6.0		

Canadian Wells clinical model to predict the likelihood of PE. Their scoring system has a maximum of 12.5 points based on 7 variables.

DVT, deep venous thrombosis; PE, pulmonary embolism.

Adapted from Chagnon I, Bounameaux H, Aujesky D, et al: Comparison of two clinical prediction rules and implicit assessment among patients with suspected pulmonary embolism, *Am J Med* 113:269–275, 2002.

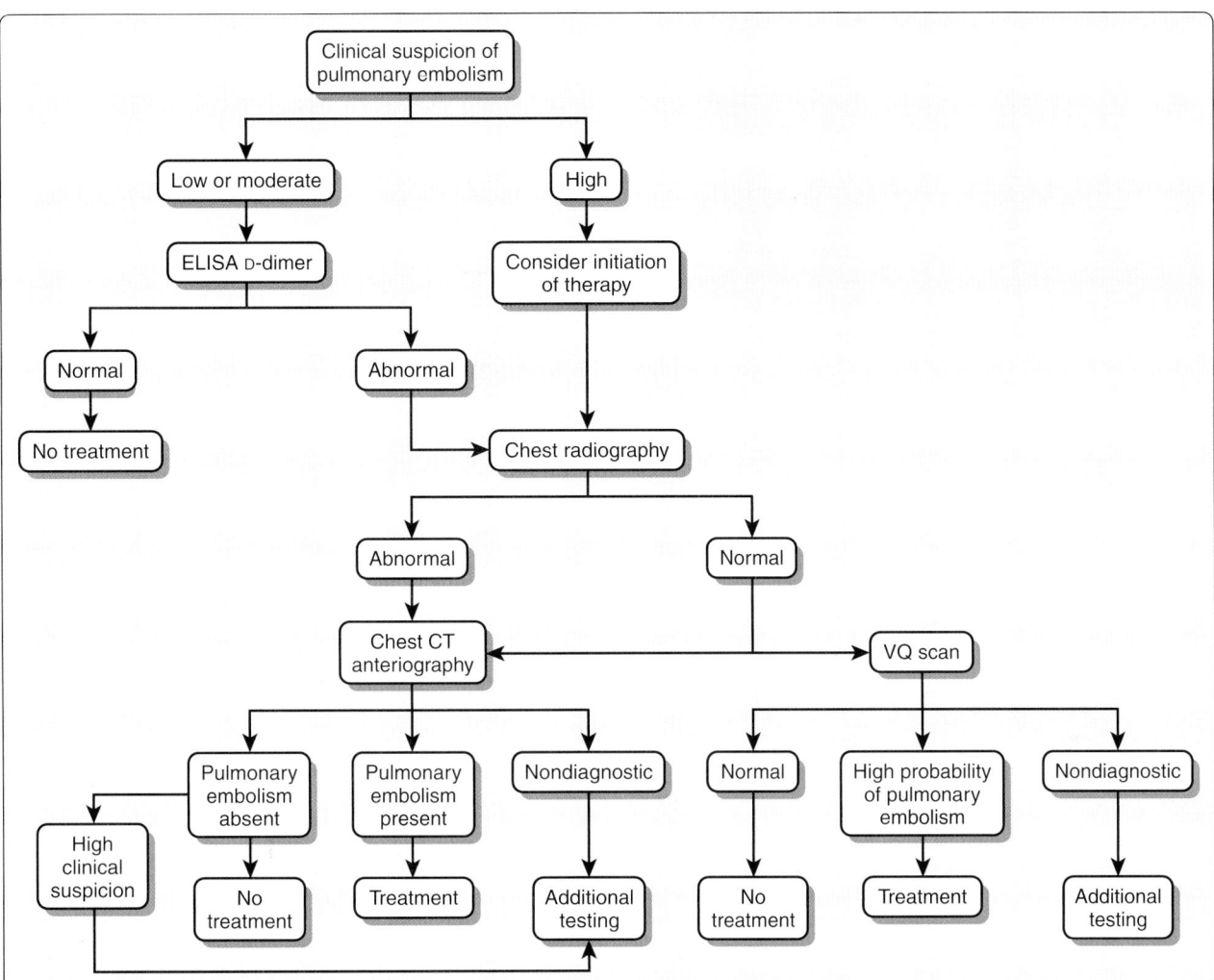

Figure 24-19 Diagnostic approach to suspected acute pulmonary embolism. The use of prediction rules and D-dimer testing may reduce the need for imaging. If the risk for bleeding is deemed to be low, initiation of therapy before a proven diagnosis of pulmonary embolism should be considered. At this juncture, the chest radiograph and other specific imaging may already be completed. A ventilation-perfusion (V/Q) scan is more likely to yield a diagnosis when there is no associated cardiopulmonary disease. A scan indicating a high probability of pulmonary embolism is confirmatory except when there has been a prior pulmonary embolism, in which case a previous V/Q scan may be useful in proving that defects are new. As with computed tomography arteriography (CTA), the approach to a nondiagnostic scan includes evaluation of clinical probability, as well as consideration of additional testing. Deep venous thrombosis discovered by leg ultrasonography, computed tomography (CT) venography, or magnetic resonance venography suggests concomitant pulmonary embolism. Standard pulmonary arteriography or venography is rarely necessary. Adding CT venography to CT arteriography enhances the overall sensitivity for detecting venous thromboembolism, although an excellent outcome has been demonstrated without additional testing when CTA is negative. With the use of CTA or CT venography, caution is advised when the creatinine level increases above 1.5 mg/dL; the patient's age relative to the creatinine clearance should be considered.[36] ELISA, enzyme-linked immunosorbent assay. *(Originally adapted from Tapson VF: Acute pulmonary embolism. N Engl J Med 358:1037, 2008, by permission of the Massachusetts Medical Society).*

LV compliance and filling, thereby reducing CO.[121] Epinephrine and dobutamine are first-line inotropic agents for patients in shock secondary to a PE. Both agents increase CO, but also increase PAP to a lesser extent, thus potentially decreasing PVR and decreasing the stress on the right ventricle. Norepinephrine is another vasoactive agent often used to achieve hemodynamic stability. Although isoproterenol is appealing because of its β-adrenergic properties and pulmonary vasodilatation, RV perfusion pressure may decline, worsening RV ischemia.[167]

Treatment Modalities

A major goal of treatment after acute PE is the prevention of new thrombi and reducing the risk for death. Recurrence of PE is a major risk and associated with a very high mortality. Frequently, the initial clot of a PE is small and symptoms are few or nonspecific, but a subsequent clot may significantly increase PVR and compromise hemodynamics

without a clear warning. Prevention of recurrence may include one or more of the following: anticoagulation, thrombolysis, mechanical interruption (vena caval filters), and embolectomy. Anticoagulation lessens morbidity, mortality, and recurrence of PE by addressing VTE.[168] Thus, as soon as massive PE is suspected or a patient has a high-probability ventilation-perfusion scan with strong clinical suspicion, anticoagulation is begun. Anticoagulation is initiated with a heparin bolus of 80 U/kg followed by a heparin infusion of 18 U/kg to maintain the activated partial thromboplastin time at 1.5 to 2 times control.[169] In the meantime, warfarin is initiated simultaneously with UFH or low-molecular-weight heparin (LMWH) until the international normalized ratio is in the therapeutic range (2.0 to 3.0) for 2 days. Subsequently, the oral anticoagulant is continued for at least 3 months. Several major trials compared the efficacy of LMWH with UFH in patients with DVT or PE.[170,171] LMWH was demonstrated to be as effective as UFH in preventing recurrence of DVT. LMWH has several advantages over

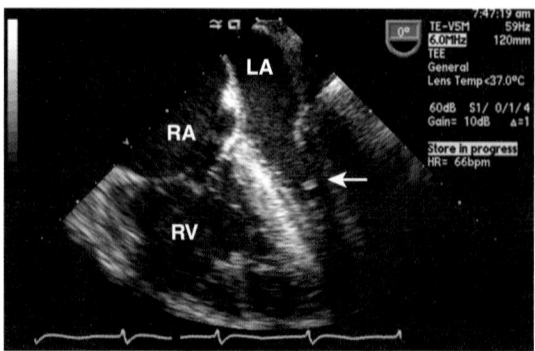

Figure 24-20 **Midesophageal four-chamber view in a patient with severe chronic thromboembolic pulmonary hypertension (CTEPH).** Note the dilated and hypertrophied right ventricle, which is significantly larger than the left ventricle, and the dilated right atrium with the interatrial septum bulging toward the left atrium. The arrow points to a vastly underfilled left ventricle. LA, left atrium; RA, right atrium; RV, right ventricle.

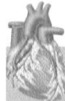

BOX 24-5. CONTRAINDICATIONS OF THROMBOLYTIC THERAPY

Absolute Contraindications
- Active internal bleeding
- Intracranial disease, e.g., neoplasms, arteriovenous malformation
- Recent (within 2 months) cerebrovascular accident or other active intracranial processes
- History of hemorrhagic stroke or stroke of unknown origin
- Bleeding disorder

Relative Contraindications
- Recent (< 10 days) major surgery
- Recent obstetric delivery
- Recent organ biopsy
- Gastrointestinal bleeding within 10 days
- Recent previous puncture of noncompressible vessels
- Recent serious trauma within 15 days
- Neurosurgery or ophthalmologic surgery within a month
- Severe hypertension (systolic > 180 mm Hg, diastolic > 110 mm Hg)
- Bacterial endocarditis
- Recent minor trauma including cardiopulmonary resuscitation
- High likelihood of left-heart thrombus (e.g., mitral stenosis with atrial fibrillation)
- Pregnancy
- Diabetic hemorrhagic retinopathy
- Platelet count < 100,000/mm³, prothrombin time < 50%

UFH—it does not require monitoring, has greater bioavailability, is more predictable, and is easier to use. In addition, LMWH is administered subcutaneously rather than as an intravenous infusion and has lower rates of HIT.[172,173] Tinzaparin and fondaparinux[172] are approved for use in acute PE, whereas enoxaparin is approved for treatment of DVT. Fondaparinux is contraindicated in patients with chronic renal insufficiency. Platelet count should be monitored in patients receiving LMWH or UFH for HIT. In cases in which patients develop HIT, alternative anticoagulation methods should be used such as direct thrombin inhibitors (e.g., argatroban, or lepirudin). If PE recurs during anticoagulation, a continuing predisposition to PE exists, or if there is a contraindication to anticoagulation, a Greenfield filter is placed transvenously in the inferior vena cava to prevent a fatal embolus. The inferior vena caval filter is effective in 98% of cases but does not provide absolute protection.[174]

With the advent of fibrinolytic agents that convert circulating plasminogen to plasmin, clots in the PAs may be lysed, thus removing or decreasing mechanical obstruction to pulmonary blood flow. This is referred to as thrombolytic therapy; however, there is no absolute indication for this therapy with PE. Thrombolytic therapy generally is considered if pulmonary blood flow is reduced by 40% to 50% with severe hypoxia or right-sided failure and/or deteriorating hemodynamics.[175] Successful thrombolysis may reverse right-sided heart failure. An overview of the five randomized, controlled trials that included patients with massive PE (shock or major disability) demonstrated a 50% reduction in the overall mortality of PE with thrombolytic therapy compared with heparin anticoagulation alone.[176] Thrombolytic therapy has been shown to produce more rapid (2 to 24 hours) clot lysis when compared with heparin alone based on angiography, perfusion scans, or echocardiography.

Thrombolytic agents now are recognized as superior to heparin therapy alone for correcting defects found on angiographic and perfusion scans, as well as for correcting hemodynamic abnormalities including RV dysfunction. Fewer complications and more rapid improvement occur with thrombolytic therapy than with heparin alone.[165,177] There is also a reduced incidence of recurrent PE compared with heparin therapy, in part because of a resolution of the probable underlying venous thrombus and less RV hypokinesis.[160] Nonetheless, anticoagulation with heparin should be started simultaneously with thrombolytic therapy. Based on RV dysfunction identified on echocardiography and impending right-sided heart failure, thrombolysis and anticoagulation together provide better results than anticoagulation alone.[178]

Streptokinase and urokinase are the most commonly used fibrinolytic agents. Because they are not fibrin specific, there is an increased risk for severe bleeding compared with heparin alone (22% vs. 12%, respectively).[176,179] The development of more specific thrombolytic

agents, such as recombinant tissue-type plasminogen activator, which preferentially activates plasminogen in the presence of fibrin, should lessen severe bleeding. Direct comparisons of recombinant tissue-type plasminogen activator and urokinase in two separate trials, however, found no statistically significant differences between the two fibrinolytic agents.[177]

Bleeding complications are more likely with thrombolysis than with heparin alone, particularly if the patient has undergone pulmonary angiography (Box 24-5). Specific thrombolytic agents, such as recombinant tissue-type plasminogen activator, appear to reduce bleeding complications. It is paramount to detect any neurologic deterioration in a patient receiving thrombolysis. Intracranial bleeding, the most feared complication, occurs in 1.9% of patients receiving thrombolysis[178] and represents a medical emergency. Bleeding can be treated with immediate transfusion of 10 units cryoprecipitate and 2 units fresh-frozen plasma.

Beyond thrombolysis, pulmonary embolectomy remains an option for massive PE if pharmacologic thrombolysis has been unsuccessful. Echocardiography is particularly valuable in the triage of patients to either thrombolysis, catheter embolectomy, or surgical embolectomy.[167,180] As previously noted, RV function after PE is a major determinant of outcome, so aggressive efforts to reverse RV dysfunction should be pursued early after the onset of PE. Multiple percutaneous techniques are available to treat massive PE including local catheter-directed thrombolytic therapy, thrombus aspiration with mechanical fragmentation techniques, and percutaneous mechanical thrombectomy.[177,181] The rationale for proximal clot dissolution is that the significantly greater cross-sectional area of the peripheral pulmonary arterioles than the central pulmonary arteries will permit the clot to travel distally and be tolerated far better hemodynamically than central PA obstruction. Catheter embolectomy reduces embolic load with suction of clot in the PA through a venotomy site, but mortality rate may reach 32%. Percutaneous mechanical thrombectomy uses a combination of devices to fragment the thrombus.[182] However, fragmentation of the embolus versus extraction can distribute the fragments more distally in the pulmonary circulation with subsequent pulmonary hypertension. Figure 24-21 depicts treatment algorithm for patients diagnosed with acute PE.

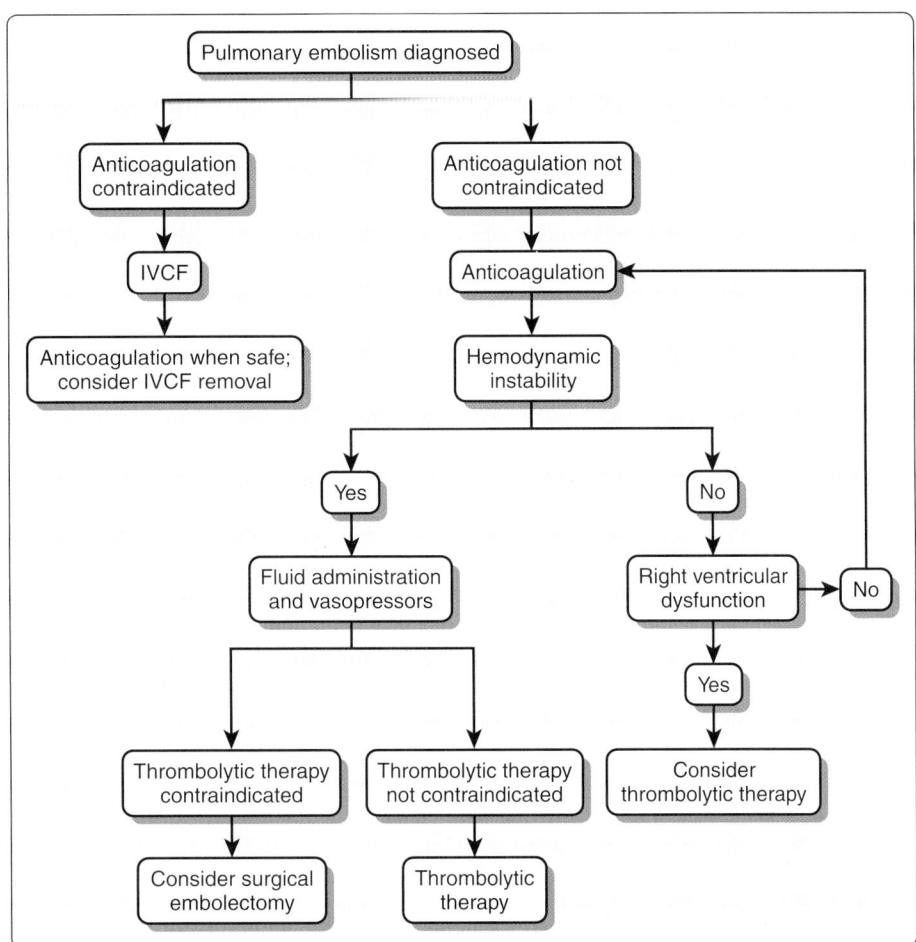

Figure 24-21 **Treatment approach of acute pulmonary embolism.** Low-molecular-weight heparin is preferable to unfractionated heparin in most settings. Use of an optional (retrievable) inferior vena caval filter (IVCF) offers the potential for removal when risk factors are deemed transient. Anticoagulation should be initiated when the risk for bleeding subsides. Although the clearest indication for thrombolytic therapy is hemodynamic instability with cardiogenic shock caused by acute pulmonary embolism, hypotension, particularly if refractory to initial supportive measures (e.g., cautious fluid administration), also merits consideration of this approach. Some clinicians consider right ventricular dysfunction to be an indication for thrombolysis, but no study has been large enough to prove that thrombolytic therapy reduces mortality in this setting or in the setting of severe hypoxemia and respiratory failure. Each case must be considered individually. Thrombolytic agents with shorter infusion times, such as tissue plasminogen activator (t-PA; 100 mg given intravenously over a period of 2 hours) have been recommended. Intracranial abnormalities are generally considered to be absolute contraindications. *(Originally adapted from Tapson VF: Acute pulmonary embolism. N Engl J Med 358:1037, 2008, by permission of the Massachusetts Medical Society.)*

■ Anesthesia Considerations for Pulmonary Embolectomy

The first surgical embolectomy was described by Trendelenburg in 1908, and until 1924 there were no reports of long-term survival after acute embolectomy. In 1958, 12 reports of survivors emerged in the European literature, including Steenberg et al[183] reporting the first survivor of the "Trendelenburg operation" in the United States. A significant milestone in the success of the embolectomy procedure was the introduction of CPB described by Cooley et al[184] in 1961 and by Sharp[185] in 1962. This procedure has been on the decline since the introduction of pulmonary thrombolysis. In general, it has been reserved for PE patients with refractory circulatory compromise, failed medical management, or contraindications to thrombolysis. Open pulmonary embolectomy before RV ischemia and cardiac arrest ensue is imperative for the favorable outcome of patients with massive acute PE.[186] Contraindication to thrombolysis accounts for more than one third of embolectomies.[177] The best surgical candidates are the ones with an accessible clot in the main PA or proximal right and left PA. More distal embolic disease results in less successful procedures. Patients with shock caused by RV failure had a mortality rate of 30%, whereas patients with an episode of cardiac arrest had a significant mortality rate of 70%.[121]

The overall mortality of pulmonary embolectomy varies between 20% and 90%.[187] Most patients awaiting embolectomy are in sustained, acute shock; up to two thirds require closed-chest massage.[188] Preoperative cardiac arrest increases operative mortality rate by more than 50%. Age older than 60 years and a long history of dyspnea also increase the mortality of embolectomy. Echocardiography and spiral CT have greatly decreased the time to surgery by enabling a rapid and reliable diagnosis to be made, which has improved not only initial survival rate of embolectomy but long-term survival.[186]

Induction of anesthesia is a critical period, especially in the presence of PE and RV dysfunction. Intraoperative monitoring should include an arterial catheter, ECG, pulse oximeter, capnograph, and CVP catheter or PAC. Large-bore intravenous catheters are necessary to ensure good venous access in case of massive pulmonary hemorrhage.[189] Frequently, an inotrope is required before or during induction to maintain perfusion pressure to the right heart. In cases of a massive PE in which 50% of the pulmonary blood flow is obstructed, a fixed CO makes them extremely susceptible to hemodynamic collapse. Some surgeons prefer cannulation of the femoral vessels before induction in preparation for immediate CPB in the setting of hemodynamic compromise. A right atrial pressure of 15 to 20 mm Hg usually is adequate; however, the RA pressure may be unreliable in the setting of RV failure.

It is imperative to avoid RV distention that inevitably worsens hemodynamics.[190] It is also extremely important to implement measures to decrease PVR, such as treating acidosis and maintaining hypocapnia, without excessively increasing airway pressure.

Induction methods should emphasize the importance of avoiding any situations that would lead to hypoxia, hypercarbia, or hypotension. Anesthetic agents that increase PVR must be used with caution in this setting. Furthermore, it should be emphasized that any decrease in the systemic blood pressure or increase in RV pressure will compromise the RV blood/oxygen supply. The hemodynamics of the patient primarily depends on the degree of pulmonary vascular obstruction. Dobutamine and epinephrine, when titrated to maintain a moderate blood pressure, improve ventricular performance, whereas PVR does not increase significantly.[190,191] Isoproterenol decreases PVR and is associated with arrhythmias, hypotension, and a worse outcome.[191]

TEE is used in all patients to exclude a PFO, atrial septal defect, or any visible thrombus in the right atrium, right ventricle, or main PA. The presence of a PFO or intracardiac thrombi alters the surgical procedure. The surgical approach is through a median sternotomy with cannulation for CPB accomplished after full heparinization. Typically, the patient is maintained normothermic, the aorta is not cross-clamped, and cardioplegia is not administered unless concomitant repair of a PFO is required. The main PA is approached through a longitudinal arteriotomy, and fresh clot is removed under direct vision.[192]

PULMONARY ARTERIAL HYPERTENSION

PAH is a disorder in which flow to the pulmonary arterial circulation is constrained, leading to increased vascular remodeling and proliferation, resulting in increased PVR and ending with right-heart failure. By definition, PAH constitutes an mPAP greater than 25 mm Hg at rest or more, a PVR greater than 300 dynes·sec·cm^{-5}, and a PAOP less than 15 mm Hg. Severe PAH is defined as an mPAP greater than 50 mm Hg and a PVR greater than 600 dynes·sec·cm^{-5}.

The World Health Organization recently revised the classification for PAH into the following groups:

I—includes idiopathic pulmonary arterial hypertension (IPAH), familial pulmonary arterial hypertension, and PAH associated with conditions such as connective tissue disorder, portal hypertension, pulmonary veno-occlusive disease, HIV, and anorexia

II—PAH with left-heart disease

III—PAH with lung diseases and/or hypoxemia

IV—PAH caused by chronic thromboembolic disease

V—miscellaneous[193]

Regardless of the primary pathologic mechanisms, once PAH exists, the effects on the right heart and pulmonary arteries are similar.

IPAH is a rare debilitating disorder, affecting the pulmonary vasculature, leading to PAH and, consequently, right-heart failure and death. It is identified when no cause for the PAH is established; diagnosis is often delayed an average of 2 years because of the nonspecific nature of the symptoms. In 1951, Dresdale et al[194] revealed the first antemortem pathologic findings for IPAH. They were consistent with prothrombotic diathesis, excessive endothelial proliferation, and antiapoptotic cells within the vascular lumen. The endothelium displays an imbalance between vasoconstrictors relative to vasodilators.[195,196]

"Plexogenic pulmonary arteriopathy" is the pathologic hallmark of primary pulmonary hypertension, and it reflects a dysregulation of phenotypically altered endothelial growth.[197–199] PAH is a panvasculopathy mostly affecting small and medium arterial vessels with a wide range of abnormalities, including intimal hyperplasia, medial hypertrophy, adventitial proliferation, and plexiform arteriopathy.

Epidemiology

The annual incidence of IAPH is roughly 6 per million, with 6% to 12% involving autosomal dominance inheritance. Women are two times more likely to experience development of PAH compared with men, with a mean age at diagnosis of 35 years and mean survival of 2.8 years if left untreated.[200–202]

The differences between the sexes are not well understood, though female predominance is not common before puberty. With better understanding of the PAH disease process, the 1-year survival rate for these patients increased from 68% in the 1980s to 85% current.[203,204] Familial PAH is as a result of a mutation in BMP-RII, an inherited autosomal dominant disease, with incomplete penetrance and genetic anticipation. It is found in up to 25% of patients with IPAH and in 15% of patients with PAH caused by anorexogenics.[205]

Pathogenesis

The pulmonary vasculature is a low-pressure, high-flow circuit balancing vasodilatation and constriction, leaning toward vasodilatation. The endothelium modulates vascular smooth muscle cell activity through the production of various vasodilators (prostacyclin and NO) and vasoconstrictors (thromboxane A_2 and endothelin). The endothelium of the lung is markedly different from endothelium of the systemic vasculature.[206] Although the stimuli that trigger primary PAH may differ, an undefined injury to the endothelium causes increased coagulation, proliferation, and vasoconstriction, which are instrumental in the development of PAH. The endothelium releases thromboxane A_2, a potent vasoconstrictor, cell proliferators, and powerful platelet activator, in addition to prostacyclin, a potent vasodilator and potent inhibitor of platelet aggregation.[207] Mediator imbalance results in pulmonary vasoconstriction that leads to the disordered endothelial cell proliferation in combination with proliferation of intimal cells that form the characteristic plexiform lesions (Figure 24-22). However, there is no specific histopathologic lesion that defines primary PAH. Evidence of proliferative and obliterative intimal lesions composed of myofibroblasts is found in the pulmonary arteries and arterioles from increased production of endothelial mediators. In addition, thickened arterial smooth muscle (isolated medial hypertrophy), destruction and fibrosis of vessel walls, and in situ thrombosis lead to stiffening of the arteries, contributing to greater vasoconstriction (see Figure 24-22). Eventually, the endothelial mediators that maintain the low-pressure, high-flow pulmonary circulation (NO, endothelium-derived hyperpolarizing factor, natriuretic peptides, adrenomedullin, and α_2-agonists) are lost, and PAP increases at rest and exercise. Regardless of the primary pathophysiologic pathways to PAH, a similar end point is reached.

Hypercoagulability is enhanced by increased platelet activity, increased levels of serotonin, plasminogen activator inhibitor, and fibrinopeptide A, together with a decrease in thrombomodulin levels.[208] Endothelin-1 (ET-1), a potent vasoconstrictor, was found in high levels in arterial plasma compared with venous plasma in IAPH, suggesting ET-1 may contribute to increased PVR in these patients.[209–211] IPAH has been associated with increased local expression of ET-1 in pulmonary vascular endothelial cells, contributing to the pathogenesis of PAH.[212] The inhibition of voltage-gated (Kv) channels raises the membrane potential, activating the voltage-gated L-type calcium channel, which increases the calcium levels leading to vasoconstriction and possibly initiating cell proliferation[213] (Figure 24-23).

Clinical Manifestation

Diagnosis of PAH often is significantly delayed because of the nonspecific symptoms that mimic known underlying pulmonary or cardiac disorders. Gradual onset of shortness of breath is the earliest symptom of PAH, reflecting an inability to increase CO in proportion to activity. Right-sided chest pain is prevalent in PAH despite normal coronary arteries, together with syncope, fatigue, and peripheral edema. Hemoptysis may occur as a result of rupture of dilated distended pulmonary vessels. The recurrent laryngeal nerve may be compressed by the enlarged PA, leading to hoarseness in these patients.

Physical examination focuses on signs of both PAH and RVH (Table 24-4). Accentuation of the pulmonic component of the second heart sound might be the only finding on physical examination and

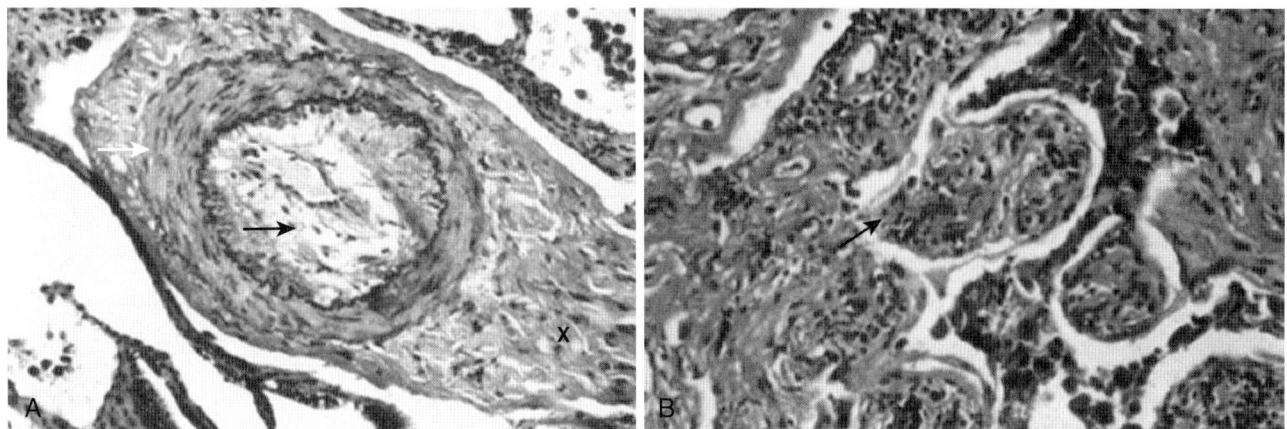

Figure 24-22   Characteristic lung pathology in primary pulmonary hypertension. *A,* Muscular pulmonary artery from a patient with primary pulmonary hypertension and medial hypertrophy *(white arrow),* luminal narrowing by intimal proliferation *(black arrow),* and proliferation of adventitia *(X).* *B,* Characteristic plexiform lesion from an obstructed muscular pulmonary artery *(arrow). (Reprinted from Gaine SP, Rubin LJ: Primary pulmonary hypertension. Lancet 352:721, 1998.)*

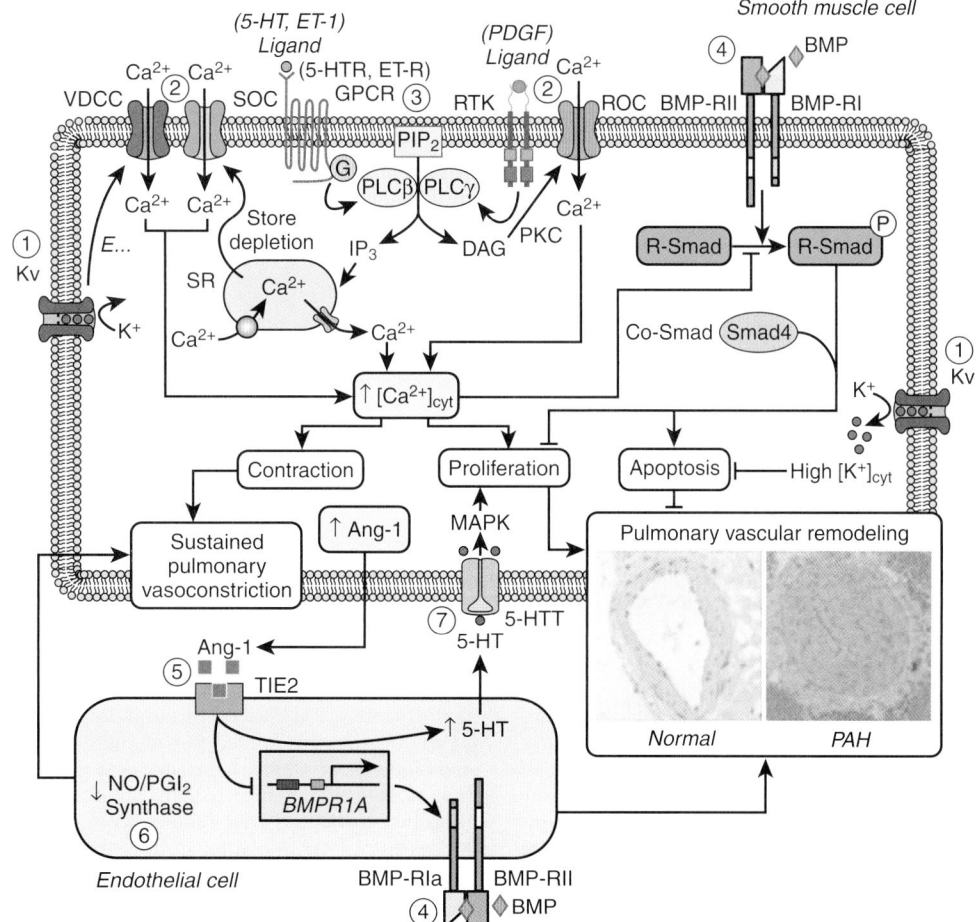

Figure 24-23   Schematic depicting the potential "hits" involved in the development of pulmonary arterial hypertension (PAH). An increase in [Ca^{2+}] cytosine (cyt) in pulmonary artery smooth muscles (PASMCs; caused by increased voltage-gated potassium channel (Kv) activity and membrane depolarization, which opens voltage-dependent calcium channels [VDCCs]; upregulated transient receptor potential channels (TRPCs) that participate in forming receptor- and store-operated calcium ion (Ca^{2+}) channels; and upregulated membrane receptors [e.g., serotonin, endothelin, or leukotriene receptors] and their downstream signaling cascades) causes pulmonary vasoconstriction, stimulates PASMC proliferation, and inhibits the bone morphogenetic protein (BMP) signaling pathway that leads to antiproliferative and proapoptotic effects on PASMCs. Dysfunction of BMP signaling because of BMP type II receptor (BMP-RII) mutation and BMP-RII/BMP-RI downregulation and inhibition of Kv channel function and expression attenuate PASMC apoptosis and promote PASMC proliferation. Increased angiopoietin (Ang-1) synthesis and release from PASMCs enhance 5-hydroxytryptamine (5-HT) production and downregulate BMP receptor IA (BMPR-IA) in pulmonary arterial endothelial cells (PAECs) and further enhance PASMC contraction and proliferation, whereas inhibited nitric oxide and prostacyclin synthesis in PAECs would attenuate the endothelium-derived relaxing effect on pulmonary arteries and promote sustained vasoconstriction and PASMC proliferation. Increased activity and expression of the 5-HT transporter (5-HTT) would serve as an additional pathway to stimulate PASMC growth via the mitogen-activated protein kinase (MAPK) pathway. 5-HTR, 5-hydroxytryptophan; AVD, apoptotic volume decrease; Co-Smad, common smad; DAG, diacylglycerol; Em, membrane potential; ET-1, endothelin-1; ET-R, endothelin receptor; GPCR, G protein-coupled receptor; IP$_3$, inositol 1,4,5-trisphosphate; K, potassium; NO/PGI$_2$, nitric oxide/prostacyclin; PDGF, platelet-derived growth factor; PIP$_2$, phosphatidylinositol biphosphate; PLC, phospholipase C; PKC, protein kinase C; ROC, receptor-operated calcium channel; R-Smad, receptor-activated smad signaling pathway; RTK, receptor tyrosine kinase; SOC, store-operated channel; SR, sarcoplasmic reticulum; TIE2, tyrosine-protein kinase receptor. *(Reprinted from McLaughlin VV, Archer SL, Badesch DB, et al: ACCF/AHA 2009 expert consensus document on pulmonary hypertension: A report of the American College of Cardiology Foundation Task Force on Expert Consensus Documents. J Am Coll Cardiol 53:1573, 2009, by permission of the American College of Cardiology Foundation and American Heart Association.)*

TABLE 24-4	Features of the Physical Examination Pertinent to the Evaluation of Pulmonary Hypertension
Sign	*Implication*
Physical Signs That Reflect Severity of PH	
Accentuated pulmonary component of S_2 (audible at apex in > 90%)	High pulmonary pressure increases force of pulmonic valve closure
Early systolic click	Sudden interruption of opening of pulmonary valve into high-pressure artery
Midsystolic ejection murmur	Turbulent transvalvular pulmonary outflow
Left parasternal lift	High right ventricular pressure and hypertrophy present
Right ventricular S_4 (in 38%)	High right ventricular pressure and hypertrophy present
Increased jugular "a" wave	Poor right ventricular compliance
Physical Signs That Suggest Moderate-to-Severe PH	
Moderate-to-severe PH	
Holosystolic murmur that increases with inspiration	Tricuspid regurgitation
Increased jugular v waves	
Pulsatile liver	
Diastolic murmur	Pulmonary regurgitation
Hepatojugular reflux	High central venous pressure
Advanced PH with right ventricular failure	
Right ventricular S_3 (in 23%)	Right ventricular dysfunction
Distention of jugular veins	Right ventricular dysfunction or tricuspid regurgitation or both
Hepatomegaly	Right ventricular dysfunction or tricuspid regurgitation or both
Peripheral edema (in 32%)	
Ascites	
Low blood pressure, diminished pulse pressure, cool extremities	Reduced cardiac output, peripheral vasoconstriction
Physical Signs That Suggest Possible Underlying Cause or Associations of PH	
Central cyanosis	Abnormal V/Q, intrapulmonary shunt, hypoxemia, pulmonary-to-systemic shunt
Clubbing	Congenital heart disease, pulmonary venopathy
Cardiac auscultatory findings, including systolic murmurs, diastolic murmurs, opening snap, and gallop	Congenital or acquired heart or valvular disease
Rales, dullness, or decreased breath sounds	Pulmonary congestion or effusion, or both
Fine rales, accessory muscle use, wheezing, protracted expiration, productive cough	Pulmonary parenchymal disease
Obesity, kyphoscoliosis, enlarged tonsils	Possible substrate for disordered ventilation
Sclerodactyly, arthritis, telangiectasia, Raynaud phenomenon, rash	Connective tissue disorder
Peripheral venous insufficiency or obstruction	Possible venous thrombosis
Venous stasis ulcers	Possible sickle cell disease
Pulmonary vascular bruits	Chronic thromboembolic PH
Splenomegaly, spider angiomata, palmar erythema, icterus, caput medusa, ascites	Portal hypertension

PH, pulmonary hypertension.
Reprinted from McLaughlin VV, Archer SL, Badesch DB, et al: ACCF/AHA 2009 expert consensus document on pulmonary hypertension: A report of the American College of Cardiology Foundation Task Force on Expert Consensus Documents. *J Am Coll Cardiol* 53:1573, 2009, by permission of the American College of Cardiology Foundation and American Heart Association.

easily is overlooked. Hepatomegaly and peripheral edema are signs of advanced PAH.

The first step in diagnosing PAH is recognition of patients at high risk for development of pulmonary vasculopathy, including those with genetic substrates, risk factors, or symptoms and physical examination findings suggestive of PAH. Chest radiograph and ECG may display markers indicative of PAH but are not very specific. Based on the history and physical examination, echocardiography is the most appropriate next step. The consensus was that no treatment should be initiated based on exercise-induced PAH alone. CT scanning and magnetic resonance imaging are techniques available to further explore the diagnosis. A right-heart catheterization including assessment of PVR and right atrial and ventricular pressures, together with LV pressures, is required to confirm the diagnosis and to define the hemodynamic profile with greater precision. Figure 24-24 outlines an algorithm for the evaluation of PAH. The number of patients with PAH related to pulmonary venous hypertension (systolic and diastolic heart failure with PAH), chronic lung disease with hypoxemia, and thromboembolic pulmonary disease is far greater than the number of patients with IPAH. The term *secondary PAH* is being used less because of the many therapies for PAH regardless of cause, and the underlying disease often overshadows the clinical manifestations of PAH. Once the cause of PAH is identified, treatment should begin immediately because it is most effective if instituted before the onset of right-heart failure.

Unfortunately, PAH often has progressed to the point that the value of any treatment is limited to palliation of incapacitating symptoms. Decisions about whether specific therapy should be undertaken and how to take care of such patients should be made on a case-by-case basis by experienced PAH centers. RV function plays a major role in prognosis of PAH. A combination of echocardiography and catheterization is needed to effectively diagnose RV failure.

The Right Ventricle and Pathophysiology of Right Ventricular Failure

The right ventricle is a unique, asymmetric, crescent-shaped structure that is designed to accommodate the entire venous return while maintaining a low RA pressure and to provide sustained low-pressure perfusion through the lungs. The right ventricle receives coronary blood supply throughout the cardiac cycle, that is, during systole and diastole, because of the continuous coronary perfusion pressure gradient between the aorta and the right ventricle. Any attempts to treat PAH or increase RV pressure can compromise RV perfusion pressure because RV perfusion pressure is directly proportional to systemic pressure and inversely proportional to RV pressure. The right ventricle ejects blood from the right atrium to the lungs because of the low-pressure, low-resistance, and high-compliance circuit of the pulmonary vascular bed. In contrast, the LV generates high pressure

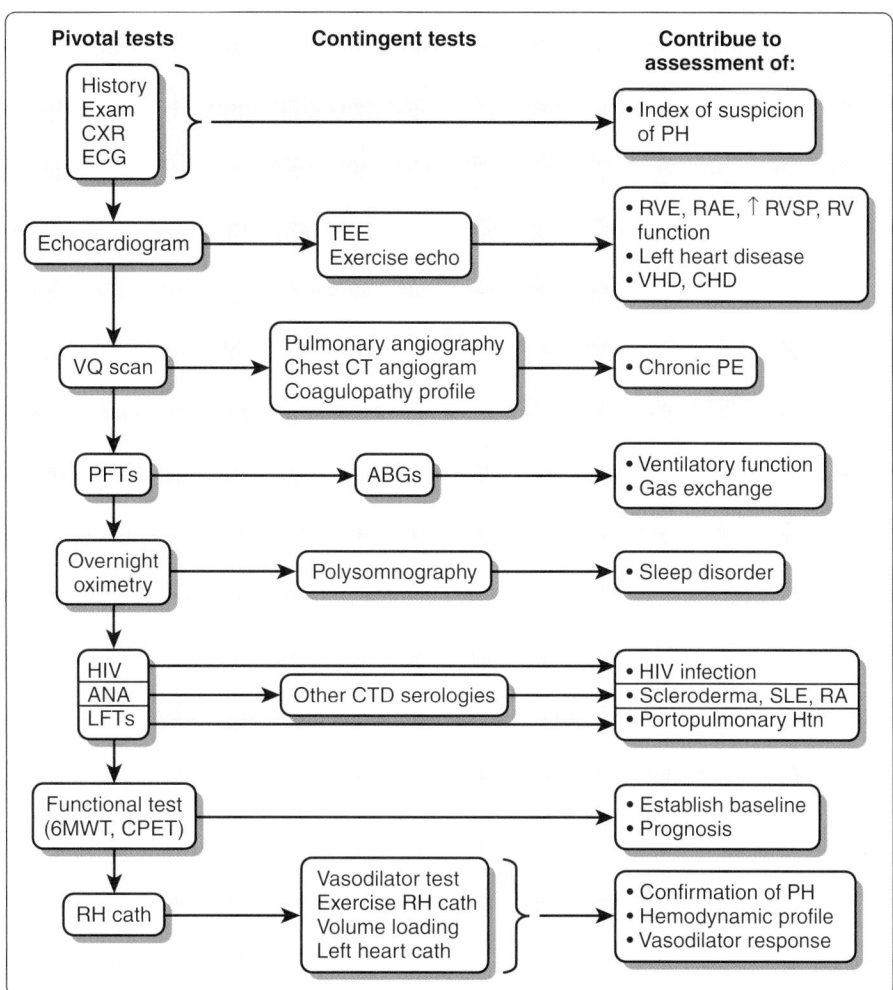

Figure 24-24   Diagnostic approach to pulmonary arterial hypertension (PAH). The diagnosis of idiopathic pulmonary arterial hypertension (IPAH) is one excluding all other reasonable possibilities. Pivotal tests are those that are essential to establishing a diagnosis of any type of PAH either by identification of criteria of associated disease or exclusion of diagnoses other than IPAH. All pivotal tests are required for a definitive diagnosis and baseline characterization. An abnormality of one assessment (such as obstructive pulmonary disease on pulmonary function test [PFTs]) does not preclude that another abnormality (chronic thromboembolic disease on ventilation-perfusion scintigram [V/Q scan] and pulmonary angiogram) is contributing or predominant. Contingent tests are recommended to elucidate or confirm results of the pivotal tests and need only be performed in the appropriate clinical context. The combination of pivotal and appropriate contingent tests contributes to assessment of the differential diagnoses in the right-hand column. It should be recognized that definitive diagnosis may require additional specific evaluations not necessarily included in this general guideline. 6MWT, 6-minute walk test; ABGs, arterial blood gases; ANA, antinuclear antibody serology; CHD, congenital heart disease; CPET, cardiopulmonary exercise test; CT, computerized tomography; CTD, connective tissue disease; CXR, chest X-ray; ECG, electrocardiogram; HIV, human immunodeficiency virus screening; Htn, hypertension; LFT, liver function test; PE, pulmonary embolism; PH, pulmonary hypertension; RA, rheumatoid arthritis; RAE, right atrial enlargement; RH Cath, right-heart catheterization; RVE, right ventricular enlargement; RVSP, right ventricular systolic pressure; SLE, systemic lupus erythematosus; TEE, transesophageal echocardiography; VHD, valvular heart disease. *(Reprinted from McLaughlin VV Archer SL, Badesch DB, et al: ACCF/AHA 2009 expert consensus document on pulmonary hypertension: A report of the American College of Cardiology Foundation Task Force on Expert Consensus Documents. J Am Coll Cardiol 53:1573, 2009 by permission of the American College of Cardiology Foundation and American Heart Association.)*

with low compliance to optimize organ perfusion. Functionally and anatomically, the right ventricle is adapted for generation of sustained low-pressure perfusion.

The right ventricle is divided by a circular muscular band that separates the inflow portion, the sinus, which generates pressure during systole and the outflow portion, and the conus, which regulates this pressure.[214] RV contraction occurs in three phases: contraction of the papillary muscles; then a bellows-like peristaltic movement of the RV free wall toward the IVS; and, finally, contraction of the LV that causes a "wringing"-type motion of the IVS, which further empties the right ventricle. The net effect is that the sinus generates pressure starting from the apex moving toward the compliant conus, which is able to decrease the peak RV pressure and PAP, thereby prolonging

ejection. The right ventricle tolerates small changes in venous return well without changing end-diastolic pressure or volume; however, this is not true with larger amounts of venous return. The RV pressure-volume loop has a triangular shape, in contrast with the rectangular shape of the LV pressure-volume loop. This means that the right ventricle has longer periods of ejection and shorter periods of isovolumic contraction and relaxation.[215] This implies that the prolonged low-pressure ejection of the right ventricle is very sensitive to any changes in PAPs seen with PAH. Therefore, in PAH, the RV pressure-volume loop adapts to the same rectangular shape, resembling the LV pressure-volume loop,[216] leading to prolonged isovolumic contraction and ejection time, causing increase in myocardial oxygen consumption. When acute or chronic RV dysfunction ensues, the normally thin-walled, crescent shape allows the right ventricle to be highly compliant, accommodating a large increase in preload with minimal changes in RV end-diastolic pressure. Consequently, the initial primary compensatory mechanism of RV dysfunction often is dilatation that is usually well tolerated.[217] Normally, the right ventricle is two-thirds the area of the LV with a wall thickness around 5 mm, compared with the LV, which is double the thickness and performs one-quarter the stroke work. The IVS is responsible for approximately one-third the RV stroke work under normal conditions. Actually, during RV infarction and loss of the RV free wall, it is the septum that continues to generate RV systolic pressure. It is important to note that the afterload effect on RV systolic function typically is more significant than the afterload effect on LV performance. Essentially, the right ventricle is a thin-walled, volume-pumping chamber that is exquisitely sensitive to acute increases in PAP, whereas the thick-walled LV is a pressure-pumping chamber that often can preserve its ejection function with increases in systemic arterial pressure. RV ejection fraction decreases in a linear fashion in response to an increase in PAP. Increase in RV afterload leads to increase in RV wall tension and RV oxygen demand, thereby reducing the oxygen supply, leading to ischemia. In the presence of PAH, the right coronary artery perfusion pressure occurs during diastole if RV systolic pressure is greater than aortic systolic pressure, rather than throughout systole and diastole, further decreasing oxygen supply. Once RV afterload increases and ventricular dilation ensues, decreased RV oxygen supply compromises RV contractility. The decrease in RV CO, as well as septal shift toward the LV, result in decrease LV filling, decreased CO, and systemic hypotension (Box 24-6). Normally, the IVS is shifted toward the RV free wall, contributing to RV ejection. However, when the RV pressure increases, the IVS paradoxically shifts toward the LV, no longer contributing to the RV ejection. Increasing the SVR, that is, aortic constriction, therefore, can restore the contribution of the IVS to RV ejection.[218–220] Therefore, systemic vasoconstrictors can be used in this fashion to restore RV ejection and blood supply. There are several ways to diagnose right ventricular failure (RVF): clinical signs and symptoms that are very nonspecific or diagnostic modalities such as cardiac biomarkers, cardiac magnetic resonance imaging, echocardiography, and right-heart catheterization, which yield better results. Cardiac magnetic resonance imaging accurately assessed RV size and function as predictors of mortality in 64 patients with IPAH. A low RV stroke output, RV dilatation, and impaired LV filling independently predicted mortality.[221]

Predictors of survival after the first year of therapy with epoprostenol included functional class and improvements in exercise tolerance, cardiac index, and mPAP. A 6MW test was found to be an independent predictor of survival in several studies, leading to use of this test as the primary end point for many prospective trials.[222,223] N-terminal

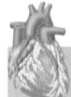

BOX 24-7. ASSESSMENT OF RIGHT VENTRICULAR DYSFUNCTION

A. ECG
- T inversion in leads V1-4 or lead III and aVF
- Sinus tachycardia
- New RBBB
- S1Q3T3 pattern

B. ECHO (+TEE)
- RV dilation (without mitral valve lesion and LV disease)
- RV free wall motion hypokinesia with sparing of apex (McConnell sign)
- Increased RV afterload
- Change to a more concentric RV morphology
- Pulmonary hypertension as tricuspid regurgitation with jet velocity > 2.8 m/sec
- Paradoxical septal motion
- 60/60 sign
- Lack of inspiratory collapse of the IVC
- Pulmonary artery dilation and right atrial enlargement

C. Right-Heart Catheterization
- Evidence of pulmonary arterial obstruction (precapillary pressure > 20 mm Hg with pulmonary capillary wedge pressure < 19 mm Hg)
- Impaired LV diastolic filling

D. Increased Levels of Biomarkers
- cTnT > 0.07 µg/L
- ProBNP ≥ 600 ng/L

The McConnell sign is defined as right ventricular (RV) free wall hypokinesis in the presence of normal RV apical contractility.[226] 60/60 sign is acceleration time of RV ejection < 60 milliseconds in the presence of tricuspid insufficiency pressure gradient < 60 mm Hg.[226] Cardiac troponin T (cTnT) and I (cTnI) are sensitive indicators for cell damage and are present in up to 50% of patients with pulmonary embolism (PE). cTnI, in particular, can be used to triage patients with PE and distinguish between low-, intermediate-, and high-risk patients.[227]
IVC, inferior vena cava; LV, left ventricular; proBNP, pro–brain natriuretic peptide; RBBB, right bundle branch block; TEE, transesophageal echocardiography.

pro–brain natriuretic peptide levels are independent predictors of survival, and they correlate well with RV enlargement and dysfunction.[224] Presence of cardiac troponin T potentially suggests RV ischemia and, therefore, confers poor prognosis[225] (Box 24-7).

Echocardiography is an easy, accessible bedside technique for diagnosing and following patients suspected of having PAH. TTE easily assesses RA and RV enlargement, reduced RV function, displacement of the IVS, and TR. The presence of a pericardial effusion has proved a consistent predictor of mortality.[228] There are two simple visual methods to assess RV chamber size: (1) RV chamber area relative to LV chamber area in the midesophageal four-chamber view; and (2) RV extension relative to the apex of the heart. RV dilation is severe when the RV area is more than the LV area and the RV apex extends beyond the LV apex. Echocardiographic evaluation of RV wall thickness also may serve to evaluate global RV performance in conditions of RV pressure overload causing compensatory RVH. RVH may be diagnosed when the RV free wall thickness is more than 5 mm at end-diastole.[229] Common causes of RV pressure overload causing secondary RVH include pulmonary stenosis, PAH from mitral stenosis, PE, and CTEPH, among other causes. When RV dysfunction ensues, the compensatory RV dilation causes the normal complex RV geometry to change from a triangular, crescent shape to a more ellipsoid, circular, D-shape.[227] Although such changes point to RV dysfunction, they do not distinguish whether the RV dysfunction is related to RV volume overload, RV pressure overload, or both. Echocardiographic evaluation of the shape and motion of the IVS may be useful to differentiate between RV volume overload and RV pressure overload pathology.[230]

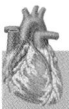

BOX 24-6. CAUSES OF RIGHT VENTRICULAR FAILURE

RV Pressure Overload
- Pulmonary embolism
- Pulmonary hypertension
- Pulmonary stenosis
- Pericardial disease
- Left-sided valvular disease
- Left-sided cardiomyopathy
- RV outflow obstruction
- Postcardiac and lung transplantation

RV Volume Overload
- Tricuspid regurgitation
- Pulmonary regurgitation
- Intracardiac shunt

RV, right ventricular.

Right Ventricular Volume Overload

Normally, the IVS is curved in a convex fashion toward the right ventricle during the entire cardiac cycle as a result of its motion being controlled by the more abundant and centrally located LV muscle mass. As the right ventricle progressively dilates and hypertrophies such that the RV mass increases to equal that of the LV, the convex shape of the IVS toward the LV begins to flatten. Moreover, when RV volume and mass exceed LV volume and mass, paradoxical septal motion appears in that the IVS abnormally bows toward the LV.

The RV volume is largest at end-diastole, which corresponds to the time of peak diastolic filling. With RV volume overload, instead of the normal IVS convex curvature toward the right ventricle, the IVS appears flattened and curves toward the LV at end-diastole, corresponding to peak RV overfilling (Figure 24-25). Additional signs of RV volume overload include RA enlargement, dilatation of the tricuspid annulus, hepatic, or great veins, and/or leftward deviation of the atrial septum. Such findings of RV volume overload suggest severe TR, atrial septal defect, or PAH (because of left-sided heart disease or intrinsic lung disease).[229,230]

Right Ventricular Pressure Overload

Although RV pressure overload alone may occur because of pulmonary stenosis or PAH, pure RV pressure overload is uncommon in the adult heart because RV hypertension usually is associated with TR and RV dilatation. Initially, RV pressure overload reduces the normal motion and curvature of the IVS toward the right ventricle and causes the appearance of abnormal IVS flattening throughout the cardiac cycle. As RV pressure overload progresses to more severe RVH, the center of mass of the heart shifts toward the right ventricle. This causes a characteristic paradoxical septal motion of the IVS bowing toward the LV that is most pronounced at end-systole when RV systolic afterload is at its peak (i.e., the time when RV pressure is the highest) (Figure 24-26). When comparing the paradoxical septal motion of RV pressure overload versus RV volume overload, the key point to remember is that the most pronounced IVS bowing toward the LV occurs at end-systole with RV pressure overload and at end-diastole with RV volume overload.

Tricuspid annular plane systolic excursion (TAPSE) is another method to assess global RV systolic function. TAPSE refers to the long-axis, apex-to-base tricuspid annulus systolic excursion. TAPSE appears more as a hingelike motion secondary to the relatively fixed septal attachment of the tricuspid annulus with the predominant tricuspid annular displacement being asymmetric and more lateral. Normal TAPSE is 20 to 25 mm toward the cardiac apex, and reductions in normal TAPSE values are suggestive of RV systolic dysfunction.[231-233]

Right-heart catheterization remains the gold standard in assessment of hemodynamics in patients with PAH, as well as a confirmatory method for diagnosis. Right-heart catheterization is performed

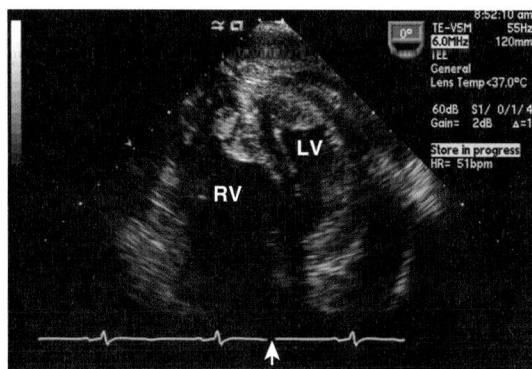

Figure 24-26 Transgastric midpapillary short-axis view demonstrating right ventricular *pressure overload*. Note the interventricular septal flattening yielding a D-shaped left ventricle in systole. *Arrow* points to the associated electrocardiogram denoting end-systole. LV, left ventricle; RV, right ventricle.

in patients who, after the initial screening, have suspected PAH. This procedure focuses on measuring PAPs, PVR, and the effects of vasodilator therapy on the pulmonary circulation. The underlying principle for vasodilator testing as a diagnostic step is identifying patients who are responders to vasodilator therapy because these patients are more likely to benefit from treatments with vasodilators, such as oral calcium channel blockers, than nonresponders.[234] Inhaled NO most commonly is used in acute vasodilator testing, but intravenous epoprostenol and adenosine are acceptable alternatives. Vasodilator testing that is positive with an acute response is defined as a decrease in mPAP of at least 10 mm Hg to an absolute mPAP less than 40 mm Hg, without a decrease in the CO (Figure 24-27).

Treatment Options for Pulmonary Arterial Hypertension

The goal for treatments in patients with PAH is geared toward improving symptoms and quality of life. Another important objective is to reduce PAP and normalize CO as early in the disease process as possible before RVF ensues. Anticoagulation therapy with warfarin has been recommended in patients with IPAH as prospective and retrospective studies proved increased survival.[235] Diuretics are indicated in patients with RVF as manifested with increased jugular venous pressure, lower extremity edema, and ascites. It is not infrequent to maintain these patients on oxygen to keep oxygen saturation above 90% to prevent further vasoconstriction from hypoxemia. Patients whose vasodilator test was positive with an acute response and who meet the criteria may be treated with calcium channel blockers.

Alternative or additional therapy should be instituted if patients do not improve to functional Class I or II on their current treatment. Continuous epoprostenol infusion therapy (Flolan) was found to improve hemodynamics and exercise tolerance and to prolong survival. Several open-label randomized trials demonstrated significant improvements of the primary end point 6MW test. Intravenous epoprostenol is titrated based on relief of symptoms or side effects. Most experts would not exceed a dosage between 25 and 40 ng/kg/min for most adult patients when used as monotherapy.[236] Common adverse effects include headache, jaw pain, flushing, nausea, diarrhea, skin rash, and musculoskeletal pain. Infections and infusion interruptions can lead to severe hypotension and cardiovascular collapse. Epoprostenol use should be limited to centers experienced with its administration and with systematic follow-up of patients.

Because prostaglandin therapy requires continuous intravenous administration to be efficacious, alternate forms have been created: oral (beraprost), subcutaneous (treprostinil), and inhaled (iloprost).

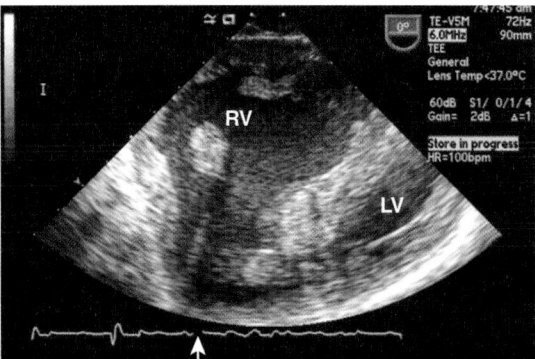

Figure 24-25 Transgastric midpapillary short-axis view demonstrating right ventricular *volume overload*. Note the interventricular septal flattening during end-diastole. *Arrow* points to the associated electrocardiogram denoting end-diastole. LV, left ventricle; RV, right ventricle.

Acute right ventricular failure

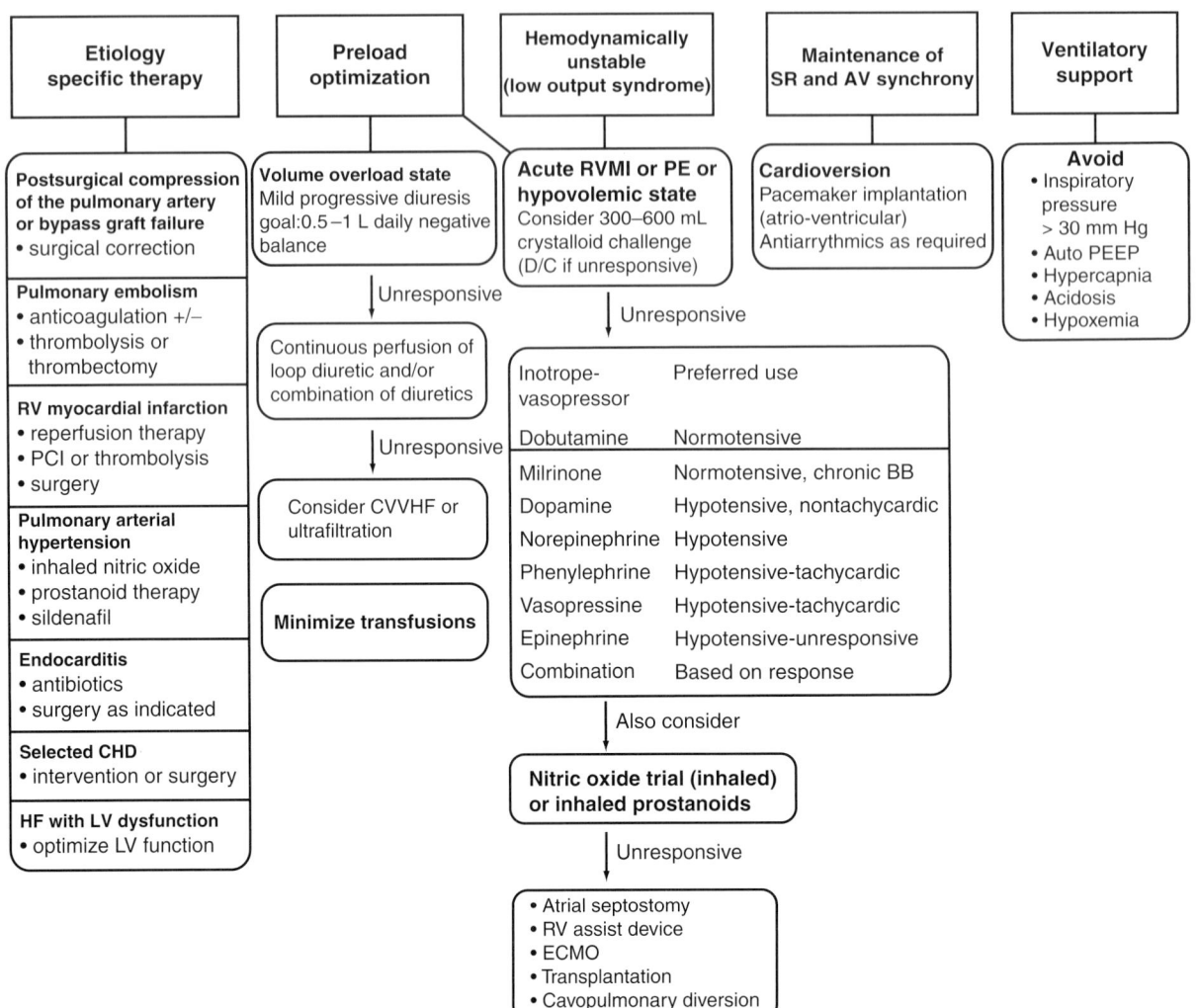

Figure 24-27   **Proposed approach to acute right ventricular failure.** AV, antrioventricular; BB, β-blockade; CHD, congenital heart disease; CVVHF, continuous veno-venous hemofiltration; D/C, discontinue; ECMO, extracorporeal membrane oxygenation; HF, heart failure; L, liter; LV, left ventricular; PCI, percutaneous coronary intervention; PE, pulmonary embolism; PEEP, positive end-expiratory pressure; RV, right ventricular; RVMI, right ventricular myocardial infarction; SR, sinus rhythm. *(Used with permission from Haddad F. Couture P, Tousignant C, Denault AY: The right ventricle in cardiac surgery, a perioperative perspective: II. Pathophysiology, clinical importance, and management, Anesth Anal 108(2):422–433.)*

Prostaglandin therapy contains valuable anti-inflammatory properties and is directed at the various pathologic mechanisms considered responsible for PAH besides pulmonary vasodilatation. Newer agents targeting thromboxane inhibition (terbogrel, riociguat), and endothelin-receptor antagonism (bosentan, and ambrisentan) have been developed. Treprostinil is a stable prostanoid with an elimination half-life of about 4.5 hours that resulted in a modest but statistically significant improvement of 16 minutes on the 6MW test compared with the placebo group.[237] In 2004, intravenous treprostinil was approved by the U.S. Food and Drug Administration (FDA) for use in patients with functional Classes II, III, and IV. Iloprost is another prostanoid that is delivered by inhalation method. Iloprost was used for 12 weeks in a randomized trial comparing its 6MW test with placebo in 207 patients with functional Class III and IV with either IPAH, PAH caused by connective tissue disease, or inoperable patients with CTEPH disease. This study utilized an end point of improvement in functional class by at least one level and improvement in 6MW test by at least 10% in the absence of clinical deterioration. Iloprost had an increase of 36 m on the 6MW test compared with the placebo group ($P = 0.004$).[238] Common adverse effects include cough, headache, flushing, and jaw

pain. Iloprost was approved by the FDA in 2004 for functional Classes III and IV PAH.

Bosentan, a promising endothelin-receptor antagonist, works by blocking the ET-1 vasoconstriction effect on the pulmonary circulation. Patients with PAH were found to have high levels of circulating ET-1, which correlated with the severity and prognosis of IPAH.[239] Bosentan was used in a randomized, double-blind, placebo-controlled, multicenter study in 32 functional Class III or IV IPAH or scleroderma spectrum of diseases with PAH. The median improvements from baseline was 51 m with bosentan versus 6 m with placebo. Bosentan had a great impact on the functional status of these patients with improvements in cardiac index and noticeable decrease in PVR.[240] Bosentan is widely used in patients with PAH. The FDA requires that liver function tests be checked monthly and hematocrit every 3 months to ensure safety in these patients.

PDE inhibitors play a big role in the treatments of PAH. NO exerts its vasodilatory effect by its ability to augment and sustain guanosine 3′, 5′-cyclic monophosphate (cGMP) content in vascular smooth muscle. The brief vasorelaxation effect of cGMP is due to PDEs. That is, decreased endothelial NO levels[241] and increased PDE-5 expression and activity in lung tissue[242,243] and RV myocardium[244] will lead to PAH.

Therefore, PDE-5 inhibitors, such as sildenafil and tadalafil, act by inactivating the phosphodiesterase enzymes that inactivate the second messengers for the vasodilating signals, cyclic adenosine monophosphate (cAMP) and cGMP in lung tissues.[245] The SUPER-1 (Sildenafil Use in Pulmonary Arterial Hypertension) was a double-blinded, placebo-controlled study that randomly assigned 278 symptomatic PAH patients with sildenafil orally three times daily for 12 weeks versus placebo. The primary end point was symptomatic improvement from baseline after 12 weeks in the 6MW test. Sildenafil monotherapy significantly reduced PAP and improved exercise capacity and World Health Organization functional class.[246]

Tadalafil, a longer-acting PDE inhibitor, was evaluated in a randomized, placebo-controlled (PHIRST) study in 405 patients with PAH either treated with bosentan or not for 16 weeks. The primary end point was symptomatic improvement from baseline after 16 weeks. Tadalafil, 40 mg, was well tolerated and improved quality of life and time to clinical deterioration. Patients who were not receiving bosentan fared better.[247]

Sildenafil and tadalafil are both indicated for use in patients with mild to moderately severe symptoms (World Health Organization Class II or III); in patients with severe (Class IV) symptoms, intravenous epoprostenol or treprostinil is preferred. Combination therapy is an attractive option considering the availability of medications with different mechanisms of action. The goal of combination therapy should be to maximize efficacy, whereas reducing side effects. Despite all the advances in the medical treatment for PAH, invasive therapies are still a valid option for patients who are refractory to medical treatments with worsening right-heart failure leading to poor quality of life. It is in these patients, as well as in CTEPH patients, that interventional and surgical therapeutic options should be considered, including atrial septostomy and lung or combined heart and lung transplantation, or PTE as the treatment of choice. With the latest advances in cardiac surgery in patients with severe refractory right-heart failure, left and biventricular assist devices have proved effective and are other viable options for these patients.

A prothrombotic state, with increased levels of tissue plasminogen activator inhibitor-1 and decreased tissue factor pathway inhibitor, has been well documented in those with primary PAH.[248] Consequently, anticoagulation is recommended to prolong survival.[249]

Anesthetic management of individuals with PAH undergoing cardiac or general surgery is challenging because perioperative increases in PVR readily occur and may provoke right-sided heart failure, resulting in death. The tolerance of the right ventricle is a major concern. Anesthetic consideration in PAH patients is discussed in detail in the PTE section of this chapter. In general, intravenous anesthetics have less effect on hypoxic pulmonary vasoconstriction, PVR, and oxygenation than do volatile agents.[250] Nitrous oxide has been reported to increase PVR, but it is not contraindicated in these patients.[250] Isoflurane may be beneficial by decreasing PAP and has been frequently used during noncardiac procedures. Fentanyl may be given as an adjunct or a primary anesthetic agent in these patients because it causes little myocardial depression and excellent circulatory stability.

Successful management of RV failure is an important aspect of PAH and requires a great deal of attention. Treatment of RV failure has focused on optimizing ventricular preload, vasodilators, vasoconstrictors, inotropic support, balance between oxygen supply and demand, maintenance of normal AV conduction, and mechanical assist devices. However, the selection of the most appropriate treatment option depends largely on RV afterload and contractility of the right ventricle. In cases where PVR and RV function are normal, volume expansion is appropriate, though there are conflicting results from several clinical studies that report variable responses to volume challenge.[251–254] Moreover, volume expansion is limited by the pericardium to a ventricular filling pressure of approximately 12 mm Hg, and any further expansion has been shown to distort the IVS, leading to a reduction in both LV compliance and output.[251] In these circumstances, inotropic support is more favorable and required to maintain compliance of both ventricles. Dobutamine is the preferred inotropic agent that has the least deleterious effects on afterload, arrhythmias, and oxygen consumption. Dell'Italia[253] et al demonstrated that volume loading by itself did not improve CO; however, dobutamine administration following appropriate volume loading considerably improved CO and RV ejection fraction even more than nitroprusside. In patients with severe hypotension, agents with pressor effects (such as dopamine) are a better choice to maintain adequate coronary perfusion pressure. Laver[255] demonstrated the ability of vasopressor therapy with phenylephrine to maintain RV perfusion pressure by increasing aortic diastolic pressure while treating RV failure. The "inodilator" agents such as milrinone and isoproterenol both have positive inotropy and pulmonary vasodilatation effects, which are ideal for treatment of patients with increased RV afterload. One potential problem with the use of intravenous vasodilator agents is that their effects are not limited to the pulmonary circulation, and because of the undesirable effect of systemic hypotension, can have a deleterious effect on the RV perfusion pressure[256] (see Chapters 10, 27, 32, and 34).

Inhaled NO, a selective pulmonary vasodilator, has been shown to significantly increase CO and stroke volume by decreasing PVR without exerting any systemic effects.[257] Palmer et al[258] proved that the endothelium relaxing factor that Furchgott and Zawadzki[259] proposed was, in fact, NO, which is produced by the vascular endothelium and acts on vascular smooth muscle, causing vasodilatation. NO is synthesized from the terminal guanidine nitrogen of L-arginine by NO synthetase in endothelial cells. NO exists in gaseous form and is rapidly inactivated by the heme component of hemoglobin. Once it is inhaled through the lungs, NO rapidly diffuses across the alveolar-capillary membrane to exert its relaxing effect by stimulating the production of cGMP. Once in the blood vessel lumen, it immediately binds to hemoglobin and is inactivated. Once bound to hemoglobin, it is converted to nitrosyl hemoglobin, then methemoglobin, which is then converted to nitrates and nitrites by methemoglobin reductase in the erythrocytes.[260] Therefore, NO has a relatively short half-life of less than 1 minute and regional vasodilatory effects. Inhaled NO in humans was first reported in adult patients with primary PAH.[261] Pepke-Zaba et al showed that 40 parts per million (ppm) NO in air given to eight patients with primary PAH decreased PVR significantly with no effect on SVR. Because NO selectively decreases RV afterload and improves RV function, with no effect in the systemic circulation, it offers particular advantage in cardiac surgical patients with PAH. Fullerton et al[262] demonstrated that inhalation of NO (20 and 40 ppm) in patients undergoing CABG produced a significant reduction in PAP and PVR; moreover, there was no difference in the vasodilatory effect achieved between 40 and 20 ppm.

Case 1*

Pulmonary Thromboendarterectomy: Transesophageal Echocardiography, Right Atrial Thrombus

Framing

Patients with CTEPH often suffer from hypercoagulability and chronic thromboembolism with resultant PAH secondary to PE. Evidence of thrombosis may be found throughout the venous system, right heart, and pulmonary vasculature. Although the finding of right-heart thrombi perioperatively is uncommon, the implications may become evident during anesthetic induction, invasive catheter placement, and the surgical procedure.

Where is the thrombus located? What are the nature and mobility of the thrombus? Is dislodgement likely during induction of anesthesia, central catheter placement, or right-heart catheterization? Are there implications with CPB cannulation?

Data Collection

Preoperative data including TTE and cardiac catheterization may reveal imaging evidence of thrombus formation or indirect evidence such as difficulty with internal jugular vein cannulation. In patients with preoperative evidence of vena cava or right-heart thrombus formation,

---

*See Videos on the website.

special consideration must be given to central catheter location and right-heart catheterization. Preprocedural TEE will assist with identification of thrombus location, mobility, and likelihood of dislodgement. Typical fresh thrombus formation will appear as homogenous, round masses that may be adherent to native cardiac structures or intracardiac devices such as pacemaker leads (Figure 24-28A, B). Chronic thrombus may be flatter and laminated in nature. Indirect clues to thrombus formation include dilated right atrium and right ventricle, intracardiac devices, or the presence of spontaneous echo contrast. CTEPH patients may exhibit thrombus throughout the venous circulation, therefore demanding a full examination of the right heart inclusive of vena cava, right atrium, RA appendage, right ventricle, and PAs (see Figure 24-28C). Therefore, the midesophageal four-chamber, midesophageal ascending aortic short-axis, RV inflow-outflow, and bicaval views are essential in such patients.

Discussion

A feared complication of venous or intracardiac thrombus formation is dislodgement and embolization resulting in tricuspid valve obstruction (RV inflow) and/or main PA obstruction (saddle embolism) with resultant cardiovascular collapse. Consideration must be given to paradoxical emboli through a PFO because of the increased RA pressures in CTEPH and resultant opening of a probe PFO.

Identification and knowledge of thrombus formation before surgery assist with anesthetic and surgical planning. Routine intraoperative right-heart catheterization is utilized during PTE to monitor RV function, PAPs, and surgical results. Precentral venous catheter TEE probe placement may aid in detection of thrombus, resulting in TEE-guided

catheterization or simply deferred placement until thrombectomy occurs. Often, CTEPH patients have Jamieson type I disease with large PA thrombus formation in the right or left PAs, which do not necessarily preclude central venous and PA catheterization. Care must be taken when advancing the PA catheter after the PA tracing is identified. Again, preprocedural TEE may provide guidance. More proximal thrombus formation may lead to dislodgement and right-heart obstruction; therefore, careful consideration of risks and benefits of right-heart catheterization is necessary.

Typical CPB venous cannulation for PTE includes bicaval cannulation for blood evacuation of the right heart. Identification of SVC or inferior vena cava thrombus may alter the surgical approach to cannulation; therefore, a thorough discussion of findings with the surgical and perfusion teams is essential. Right atrial and ventricular thrombus formation dictates minimal cardiac manipulation before commencing CPB.

▧ Case 2

Pulmonary Thromboendarterectomy: Transesophageal Echocardiography, Patent Foramen Ovale

Framing

An estimated 25% of the adult population exhibits a probe patient PFO. Secondary to increased RA pressures, a PFO present in CTEPH patients may be complicated by hypoxia from right-to-left shunting, as well as paradoxical emboli. Identification perioperatively is imperative in surgical planning to reduce the risk for hypoxia and systemic embolization.

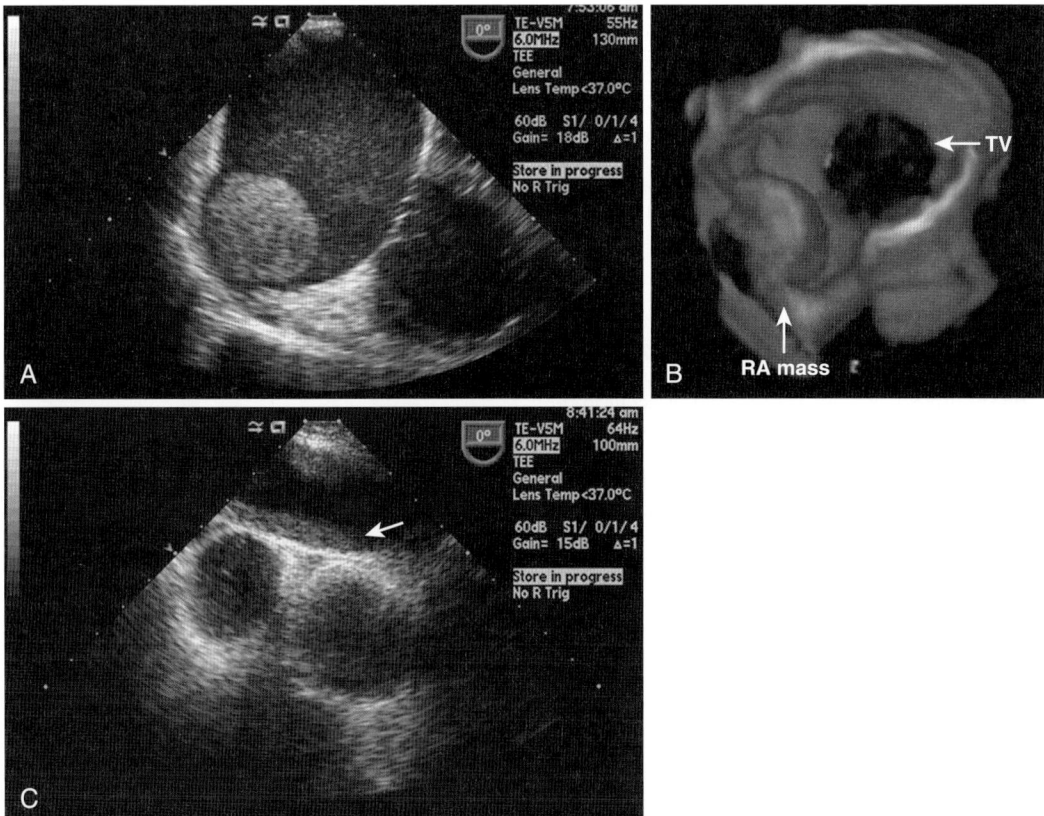

Figure 24-28   **Thrombus formation in a patient with chronic thromboembolic pulmonary hypertension (CTEPH).** A 57-year-old man with CTEPH, hypertension, and poor exercise tolerance was scheduled for pulmonary thromboendarterectomy (PTE). Preoperative transthoracic echocardiography (TTE) demonstrated right atrial and pulmonary artery thrombi. After induction of anesthesia, the TEE probe was placed to further define the location and mobility of various thrombi. *A,* A slightly right-rotated midesophageal four-chamber view demonstrated a severely enlarged right atrium (RA), spontaneous echo contrast, and a 3 × 4 cm homogenous-appearing, round, mobile mass. *B,* Three-dimensional reconstruction demonstrated its relation to the tricuspid valve (TV). *C,* The midesophageal ascending aortic short-axis view demonstrated flat, laminated-appearing thrombus in the right pulmonary artery (PA). A central line sheath was placed using continuous TEE monitoring of the guidewire. The PA catheter was placed after a successful PTE and thrombectomy through a right atriotomy. The application of TEE was critical in identifying thrombus location, guiding invasive line placement, and altering management strategies.

Does the patient have a history suggestive of systemic embolization (i.e., stroke or transient ischemic attack)? Does the patient have a PFO? What is the size of the PFO? What is the degree of intracardiac shunting of blood flow? What is the degree of RV dysfunction and PAH?

Data Collection
A careful history for transient ischemic attacks, strokes, or unexplained hypoxia raises suspicion for the existence of a PFO. The basis of PFO detection consists of 2D echo, color-flow Doppler, and contrast echocardiography in midesophageal views (Figure 24-29A, B). CTEPH patients often have greater RA than LA pressures; however, Valsalva maneuvers to increase RA pressures relative to LA pressure during contrast injection may increase the sensitivity of detection.

Discussion
Patients with CTEPH often exhibit multiple risk factors for paradoxical embolism such as recurrent thromboembolism despite anticoagulation, RV dysfunction, residual PAH after surgery, or previous paradoxical embolism. In fact, a PFO is detected in 25% to 35% of patients undergoing PTE. The surgical procedure typically involves CPB with bicaval cannulation and DHCA. Therefore, the addition of surgical PFO closure via right atriotomy does not change the circulatory management or significantly alter the length of CPB.

Case 3

Pulmonary Thromboendarterectomy: Transesophageal Echocardiography, Right Ventricular Dysfunction

Framing
Patients with CTEPH often present with New York Heart Association Class III or IV cardiac impairment and evidence of RV failure (i.e., jugular venous distention, hepatomegaly, peripheral edema). Induction

of anesthesia and maintenance of anesthesia in the prebypass period may be complicated by profound hemodynamic instability, requiring pharmacologic therapy, and rapid institution of CPB. Identification of the cause of hemodynamic instability, with attention to RV function, is imperative in the proper treatment of such patients. CTEPH patients extend across a large age range, and coexisting diseases such as coronary insufficiency or valvular disease also may be present.

What is the severity of the RV dysfunction? Is there evidence of paradoxical septal motion? RV pressure or volume overload? Is there evidence of increased RA pressure? Does the patient have TR? What is the severity of the right ventricle? What is the estimated PAP? Is there coexisting LV or valvular disease? What is the response to pharmacologic therapy?

Data Collection
Preoperative workup including symptomatology, vital signs, cardiac catheterization, and TTE may provide an impression of baseline RV function before anesthetic induction. TEE has a category I indication in the setting of hemodynamic instability and, therefore, plays a key role in identifying the cause of instability. In addition to an abbreviated, focused examination on all cardiac structures, particular attention to the right heart in CTEPH patients is imperative. Transgastric midpapillary short-axis view allows a view of LV size, as well as the presence of paradoxical septal motion (RV pressure vs. volume overload). The midesophageal four-chamber view allows assessments of RV dilation and RVH, RA size, and tricuspid valve function. Particular to this view, TAPSE allows a quantifiable assessment of RV function. Lastly, the RV inflow-outflow view allows assessments of RV free wall function and right-sided valvular function, as well as parallel alignment with TR jets for PAP estimation (Figure 24-30).

Discussion
Patients with CTEPH have fixed PVR because of the proximal nature of the disease in the pulmonary vascular tree. However, they may still

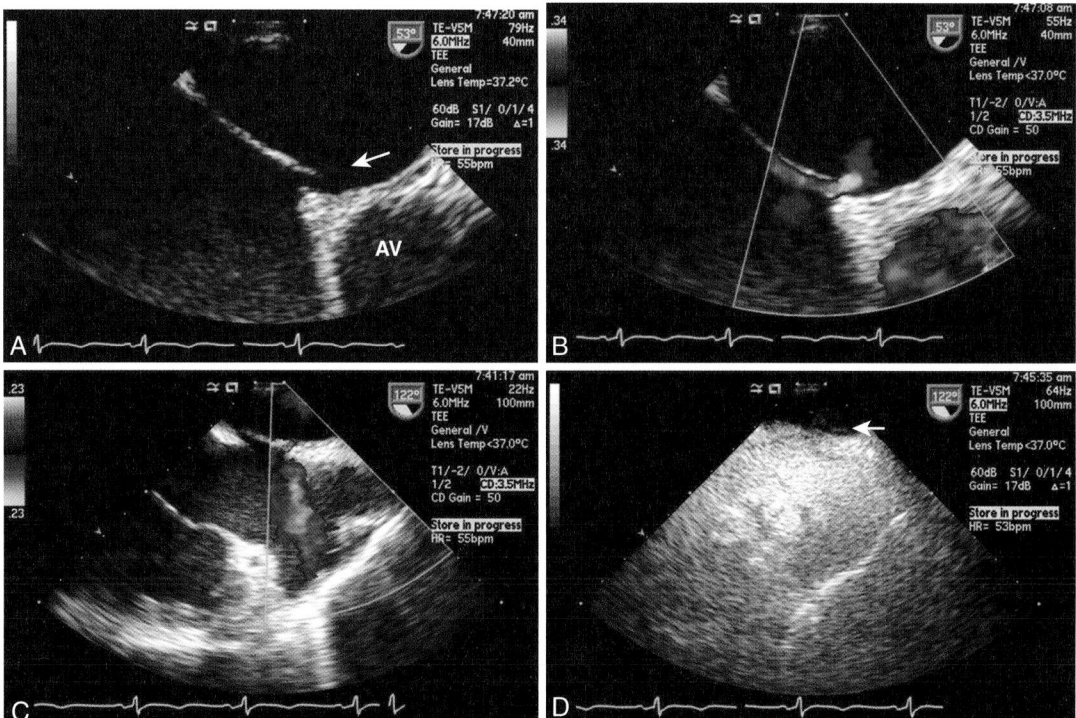

Figure 24-29   Patent foramen ovale (PFO) in a patient with chronic thromboembolic pulmonary hypertension (CTEPH). A 39-year-old woman with history of CTEPH scheduled for pulmonary thromboendarterectomy (PTE). The patient denied history of transient ischemic attacks or stroke; preoperative TTE did not demonstrate a PFO. After induction of anesthesia, the TEE probe was inserted for routine monitoring, which includes evaluation for PFO in CTEPH patients. *A*, A zoomed perspective of the midesophageal RV inflow-outflow view demonstrated the appearance of a PFO. *B* and *C*, Application of color-flow Doppler confirmed transseptal flow, also demonstrated in a modified bicaval view. *D*, Lastly, an agitated saline study confirmed transseptal flow. The patient underwent successful PTE and PFO closure via right atriotomy. TEE played a critical role in the identification of a PFO, altering surgical management and potentially reducing future paradoxical embolic risk. AV, aortic valve.

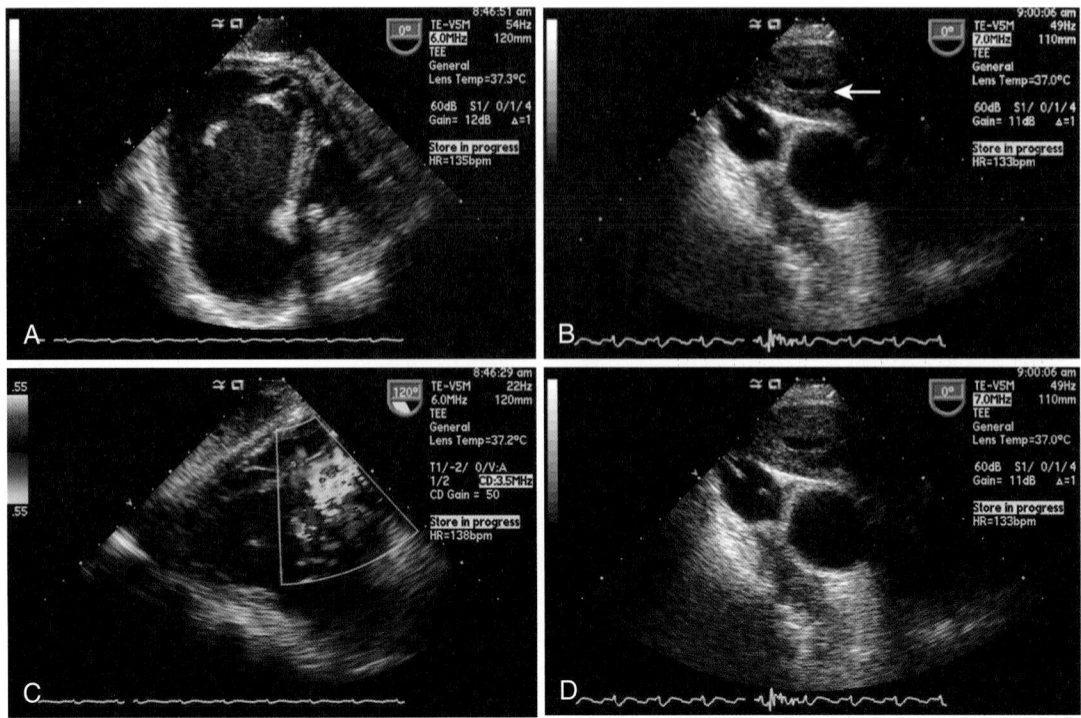

Figure 24-30 **Right ventricular dysfunction in a patient with chronic thromboembolic pulmonary hypertension (CTEPH).** A 49-year-old woman with a medical history of CTEPH and stroke was admitted to the intensive care unit (ICU) for worsening cardiac function and hypoxia (89% on 10 L oxygen by face mask), and scheduled for pulmonary thromboendarterectomy (PTE). During induction of anesthesia, the patient exhibited marked hemodynamic instability prompting rapid median sternotomy and initiation of cardiopulmonary bypass (CPB). *A,* An abbreviated transesophageal echocardiography (TEE) examination revealed a transgastric midpapillary short-axis view with significant right ventricular dilation, paradoxical septal motion, and an underfilled left ventricle. *B,* Midesophageal views were difficult to obtain secondary to significant RA and RV enlargement. *C,* Transgastric RV inflow view demonstrated significant tricuspid regurgitation because of annular dilatation. *D,* Lastly, the midesophageal ascending aortic short-axis view confirmed near-complete occlusion of the right pulmonary artery. After a successful bilateral PTE and PFO closure, the patient had improved RV function after discontinuing CPB. The application of TEE was critical in identifying the cause of hemodynamic instability, directing inotropic therapy, and prompting the rapid institution of CPB.

demonstrate increases in PVR in response to hypoxia, hypercarbia, acidosis, pain, or anxiety. PVRs in excess of 1000 dynes·sec·cm^{-5} are associated with impending decompensation. Therefore, such exacerbating factors should be avoided during induction of anesthesia and prebypass maintenance of anesthesia. In response to chronically increased PVR, the right ventricle both dilates and hypertrophies, taking on a coronary perfusion pattern similar to the LV (primarily during diastole). With an increased RV end-diastolic pressure in the failing right heart, declines in systemic blood pressure result in decreased coronary perfusion pressure and are poorly tolerated. Phenylephrine often is used to maintain systemic blood pressure and, therefore, coronary perfusion pressure.

A decreased CO often is evidenced on preoperative TTE and right-heart catheterization. Identification of increased RV end-diastolic pressure (> 14 mm) and severe TR (typically from annular dilation) also are indicative of impending decompensation. The intraoperative TEE often corroborates this information, in which a decreased TAPSE (< 2.5 cm), paradoxical septal motion, an underfilled LV, and shifted interatrial septum (indicative of RA pressure greater than LA pressure) are observed in patients with poor RV function and decreased CO. Inotropic support, such as dopamine or epinephrine, commonly is used before the induction of anesthesia.

REFERENCES

1. Fedullo PF, Auger WR, Kerr KM, et al: Chronic thromboembolic pulmonary hypertension, *N Engl J Med* 345:1465, 2001.
2. Yi ES, Kim H, Ahn H, et al: Distribution of obstructive intimal lesions and their cellular phenotypes in chronic pulmonary hypertension, *Am J Respir Crit Care Med* 162:1577, 2000.
3. Auger WR, Kim NH, Kerr KM, et al: Chronic thromboembolic pulmonary hypertension, *Clin Chest Med* 28:255, 2007.
4. Dibble JH: Organization and canalization in arterial thrombosis, *J Pathol Bacteriol* 75:1, 1958.
5. Auger WR, Fedullo PF, Moser KM, et al: Chronic major-vessel thromboembolic pulmonary artery obstruction: Appearance at angiography, *Radiograph* 182:393, 1992.
6. Korn D, Gore I, Blenke A: Pulmonary arterial bands and webs an unrecognized manifestation of organized pulmonary emboli, *Am J Pathol* 5:129, 1962.
7. Rosenhek R, Korschineck I, Gharehbaghi-Schnell E, et al: Fibrinolytic balance of the arterial wall: Pulmonary artery displays increased fibrinolytic potential compared with the aorta, *Lab Invest* 83:871, 2003.
8. Olman MA, Marsh JJ, Lang IM, et al: Endogenous fibrinolytic system in chronic large-vessel thromboembolic pulmonary hypertension, *Circulation* 86:1241, 1992.
9. Lang IM, Marsh JJ, Olman MA, et al: Parallel analysis of tissue-type plasminogen derived from patients with chronic pulmonary thromboemboli, *Circulation* 90:706, 1994.
10. Pengo V, Lensing AW, Prins MH, et al: Incidence of chronic Thromboembolic pulmonary hypertension after pulmonary embolism, *N Engl J Med* 350:2257, 2004.
11. Ribeiro A, Lindmarker P, Johnsson H, et al: Pulmonary embolism: One year follow-up with echocardiography Doppler and five-year survival analysis, *Circulation* 99:1325, 1999.
12. Dentali F, Donadini M, Gianni M, et al: Incidence of chronic pulmonary hypertension in patients with previous pulmonary embolism, *Thromb Res* 124:256, 2009.
13. Ryu JH, Olson EJ, Pellikka PA: Clinical recognition of pulmonary embolism: Problem of unrecognized and asymptomatic cases, *Mayo Clin Proc* 73:873, 1998.
14. Bonderman D, Wilkens H, Wakounig S, et al: Risk factors for chronic thromboembolic pulmonary hypertension, *Eur Respir J* 33:325, 2009.
15. Wolf M, Boyer-Neumann C, Parent F, et al: Thrombotic risk factors in pulmonary hypertension, *Eur Respir J* 116:503, 2000.
16. Bonderman D, Turecek PL, Jakowitsch J, et al: High prevalence of elevated clotting factor VIII in chronic thromboembolic pulmonary hypertension, *Thromb Haemost* 90:372, 2003.
17. Morris TA, Marsh JJ, Chiles PG, et al: Fibrin derived from patients with chronic thromboembolic pulmonary hypertension is resistant to lysis, *Am J Respir Crit Care Med* 173:1270, 2006.
18. Morris TA, Marsh JJ, Chiles PG, et al: High prevalence of dysfibrinogenemia among patients with chronic thromboembolic pulmonary hypertension, *Blood* 114:1929, 2009.
19. Jamieson SW, Kapelanski DP, Sakakibara N, et al: Pulmonary endarterectomy: experience and lessons learned in 1,500 cases, *Ann Thorac Surg* 76:1457, 2003.
20. Lang IM: Chronic thromboembolic pulmonary hypertension—not so rare after all, *N Engl J Med* 350:2236, 2004.

21. Auger WR, Moser KM: Pulmonary flow murmurs: A distinctive physical sign found in chronic pulmonary thromboembolic disease, *Clin Res* 37:145A, 1989.

22. Kapitan KS, Buchbinder M, Wagner PD, et al: Mechanisms of hypoxemia in chronic pulmonary hypertension, *Am Rev Respir Dis* 139:1149, 1989.

23. Moser KM, Daily PO, Peterson K: Thromboendarterectomy for chronic, major-vessel thromboembolic pulmonary hypertension. Immediate and long-term results in 42 patients, *Ann Intern Med* 107:560, 1987.

24. Woodruff WW III, Hoeck BE, Chitwood WR, et al: Radiographic finding in pulmonary hypertension from unresolved embolism, *Am J Roentgenol* 144:681, 1985.

25. Morris TA, Auger WR, Ysreal MZ, et al: Parenchymal scarring is associated with restrictive spirometric defects in patients with chronic thromboembolic pulmonary hypertension, *Chest* 110:399, 1996.

26. Steenhuis LH, Groen HJM, Keoter GH, et al: Diffusing capacity and hemodynamics in primary and chronic thromboembolic pulmonary hypertension, *Eur Respir J* 16:276, 2000.

27. Menzel T, Wagner S, Kramm T, et al: Pathophysiology of impaired right and left ventricular function in chronic embolic pulmonary hypertension: Changes after pulmonary thromboendarterectomy, *Chest* 118:897, 2000.

28. Lisbona R, Kreisman H, Novales-Diaz J, et al: Perfusion lung scanning differentiation of primary from thromboembolic pulmonary hypertension, *AJR Am J Roentgenol* 144:27, 1985.

29. Fishmann AJ, Moser KM, Fedullo PF: Perfusion lung scans vs. pulmonary angiography in evaluation of suspected primary pulmonary hypertension, *Chest* 84:679, 1983.

30. Ryan KL, Fedullo PF, Davis GB, et al: Perfusion scan finding understate the severity of angiographic and hemodynamic compromise in chronic thromboembolic pulmonary hypertension, *Chest* 93:1180, 1988.

31. Bailey CL, Channick RN, Auger WR, et al: "High probability" perfusion lung scans in pulmonary veno-occlusive disease, *Am J Respir Crit Care Med* 162:1974, 2000.

32. Kerr KM, Auger WR, Fedullo PF, et al: Large vessel pulmonary arteritis mimicking chronic thromboembolic disease, *Am J Respir Crit Care Med* 152:367, 1995.

33. King MA, Ysreal M, Bergin CJ: Chronic thromboembolic pulmonary hypertension: CT findings, *Am J Roentgenol* 170:955, 1998.

34. Hoeper MM, Barbera JA, Channick RN, et al: Diagnosis, assessment and treatment of non-pulmonary arterial hypertension pulmonary hypertension, *J Am Coll Cardiol* 54:S85, 2009.

35. Moser KM, Fedullo PF, Finkbeiner WE, et al: Do patients with primary pulmonary hypertension develop extensive central thrombi? *Circulation* 91:741, 1995.

36. Russo A, De Luca M, Vigna C, et al: Central pulmonary artery lesions in chronic obstructive pulmonary disease. A transesophageal echocardiography study, *Circulation* 100:1808, 1999.

37. Reichelt A, Hoeper MM, Laganski M, et al: Chronic thromboembolic pulmonary hypertension: Evaluation with 64-detector row CT versus digital subtraction angiography, *Eur J Radiol* 71:49, 2009.

38. Suga K, Kawakami Y, Hayashi N, et al: Comprehensive assessment of lung CT attenuation alteration at perfusion defects of acute pulmonary thromboembolism with breath-hold SPECT-CT fusion images, *J Comput Assist Tomogr* 30:83, 2006.

39. Nikolaou K, Schoenberg SO, Attenberger U, et al: Pulmonary arterial hypertension: Diagnosis with fast perfusion MR imaging and high-spatial-resolution MR angiography—preliminary experience, *Radiology* 236:694, 2005.

40. Kreitner KF, Kunz RP, Ley S, et al: Chronic thromboembolic pulmonary hypertension—assessment by magnetic resonance imaging, *Eur Radiol* 17:11, 2007.

41. Hoeper MM, Lee SH, Voswinckel R, et al: Complications of right heart catheterization procedures in patients with pulmonary hypertension in experienced centers, *J Am Coll Cardiol* 48:2546, 2006.

42. Thistlethwaite PA, Kaneko K, Madani MM, et al: Technique and outcomes of pulmonary endarterectomy surgery, *Ann Thorac Cardiovasc Surg* 14:274, 2008.

43. Archibald CJ, Auger WR, Fedullo PF, et al: Long-term outcome after pulmonary thromboendarterectomy, *Am J Respir Crit Care Med* 160:523, 1999.

44. Condliffe R, Kiely DG, Gibbs JSR: Improved outcomes in medically and surgically treated chronic thromboembolic pulmonary hypertension, *Am J Respir Crit Care Med* 177:1122, 2008.

45. Corsico AG, D'Armini AM, Cerveri I, et al: Long-term outcome after pulmonary endarterectomy, *Am J Respir Crit Care Med* 178:419, 2008.

46. Kim NH, Fesler P, Channick RN, et al: Preoperative partitioning of pulmonary vascular resistance correlates with early outcome after thromboendarterectomy for chronic thromboembolic pulmonary hypertension, *Circulation* 109:18, 2004.

47. Hardziyenka M, Reesink HJ, Bouma BJ, et al: A novel echocardiographic predictor of in-hospital morality and mid-term hemodynamic improvement after pulmonary endarterectomy for chronic thrombo-embolic pulmonary hypertension, *Am J Respir Crit Care Med* 28:842, 2007.

48. Riedel M, Stanek V, Widimsky J, et al: Longterm follow-up of patients with pulmonary thromboembolism. Late prognosis and evolution of hemodynamic and respiratory data, *Chest* 81:151–158, 1982.

49. Ono F, Nagaya N, Okumura H, et al: Effect of orally active prostacyclin analogue on survival in patients with chronic thromboembolic pulmonary hypertension without major vessel obstruction, *Chest* 123:1583, 2003.

50. Bonderman D, Nowotny R, Skoro-Sajer N, et al: Bosentan therapy for inoperable chronic thromboembolic pulmonary hypertension, *Chest* 128:2599, 2005.

51. Archer SL, Michelakis ED: Phosphodiesterase type 5 inhibitors for pulmonary arterial hypertension, *N Engl J Med* 361:1864, 2009.

52. McLaughlin VV, Archer SL, Badesch DB: Expert Consensus Document on Pulmonary Hypertension, *J Am Coll Cardiol* 53:1573, 2009.

53. Nagaya N, Sasaki N, Ando M, et al: Prostacyclin therapy before pulmonary thromboendarterectomy in patients with chronic thromboembolic pulmonary hypertension, *Chest* 123:338, 2003.

54. Augoustides JG, Culp K, Smith S: Rebound pulmonary hypertension and cardiogenic shock after withdrawal of inhaled prostacyclin, *Anesthesiology* 100:1023, 2004.

55. Hurwitt ES, Schein CJ, Rifkin H, et al: A surgical approach to the problem of chronic pulmonary artery obstruction due to thrombosis or stenosis, *Ann Surg* 147:157, 1958.

56. Chitwood WR, Sabiston DC Jr, Wechsler AS: Surgical treatment of chronic unresolved pulmonary embolism, *Clin Chest Med* 5:507, 1984.

57. Winkler MH, Rohrer CH, Ratty SC, et al: Perfusion techniques of profound hypothermia and circulatory arrest for pulmonary thromboendarterectomy, *J Extra Corpor Technol* 22:57, 1990.

58. Madani MM, Jamieson SW: Pulmonary embolism and thromboendarterectomy. In Cohn LH, editor: *Cardiac surgery in the adult*, ed 3, New York, 2007, McGraw Hill, pp 1309–1331.

59. Jamieson SW: Pulmonary thromboendarterectomy. In Franco KL, Putnam JB, editors: *Advanced Therapy in Thoracic Surgery*, Hamilton, Ontario, Canada, 1998, BC Decker, pp 310–318.

60. Hartz RS, Byme JG, Levitsky S, et al: Predictors of mortality in pulmonary thromboendarterectomy, *Ann Thorac Surg* 62:12559, 1996.

61. Mohr R, Lavee J, Goor DA: Inaccuracy of radial artery pressure measurement after cardiac operations, *J Thorac Cardiovasc Surg* 94:286, 1987.

62. Baba T, Goto T, Yoshitake A, et al: Radial artery diameter decreases with increased femoral to radial arterial pressure gradient during cardiopulmonary bypass, *Anesth Analg* 85:252–258, 1997.

63. Goldman S, Sutter F, Ferdinand F, et al: Optimizing intraoperative cerebral oxygen delivery using noninvasive cerebral oximetry decreases the incidence of stroke for cardiac surgical patients, *Heart Surg Forum* 7:E376, 2004.

64. Yao FSF, Tseng C-C, Ho CYA, et al: Cerebral oxygen desaturation is associated with early postoperative neuropsychological dysfunction in patients undergoing cardiac surgery, *J Cardiothoracic Vasc Anesth* 18:552, 2004.

65. Schuhmann MU, Suhr DF, Gosseln HH, et al: Local brain surface temperature compared to temperatures measured at standard extracranial monitoring sites during posterior fossa surgery, *J Neurosurg Anesthesiol* 11:90–95, 1999.

66. Dittrich HC, McCann HA, Wilson WC: Identification of interatrial communication in patients with elevated right atrial pressure using surface and transesophageal contrast echocardiography, *J Am Coll Cardiol* 21(Suppl):135A, 1993.

67. Amsel BJ, Rodrigus I, De Paep R, et al: Right-to-left flow through a patent foramen ovale in acute right ventricular infarction. Two case reports and a proposal for management, *Chest* 108:1468, 1995.

68. Langley SM, Chai PJ, Jaggers JJ, et al: Preoperative high dose methylprednisolone attenuates the cerebral response to deep hypothermic circulatory arrest, *Eur J Cardiothorac Surg* 17:279, 2000.

69. Carlsson C, Harp JR, Siesjo BK: Metabolic changes in the cerebral cortex of the rat induced by intravenous pentothal sodium, *Acta Anaesthesiol Scand Suppl* 57:1, 1975.

70. Astrup J, Sorensen PM, Sorensen HR: Inhibition of cerebral oxygen and glucose consumption in the dog by hypothermia, pentobarbital and lidocaine, *Anesthesiology* 55:263, 1981.

71. Nussmeier NA, Arlund C, Slogoff S: Neuropsychiatric complications after cardiopulmonary bypass: Cerebral protection by a barbiturate, *Anesthesiology* 64:165, 1986.

72. Manecke GR, Wilson WC, Auger WR, Jamieson SW: Chronic thromboembolic pulmonary hypertension and pulmonary thromboendarterectomy, *Semin Cardiothorac Vasc Anesh* 9:189–204, 2005.

73. Harris B, Manecke GR Jr, Niemann J, et al: Deep hypothermia and the vascular response to thiopental, *J Cardiothorac Vasc Anesth* 20:678, 2006.

74. Dittrich HC, Nicod PH, Chow LC, et al: Early changes of right heart geometry after pulmonary thromboendarterectomy, *J Am Coll Cardiol* 11:937, 1988.

75. Blanchard DG, Malouf PJ, Gurudevan SV, et al: Utility of right ventricular Tei index in noninvasive evaluation of chronic thromboembolic pulmonary hypertension before and after pulmonary thromboendarterectomy, *JACC Cardiovasc Imaging* 2:143, 2009.

76. Mahmud E, Raisinghani A, Hassankhani A, et al: Correlation of left ventricular diastolic filling characteristics with right ventricular overload and pulmonary artery pressure in chronic thromboembolic pulmonary hypertension, *J Am Coll Cardiol* 40:318, 2002.

77. Manecke GR Jr, Kotzur A, Atkins G, et al: Massive pulmonary hemorrhage after pulmonary thromboendarterectomy, *Anesth Analg* 99:672, 2004.

78. Adams A, Fedullo PF: Postoperative management of the patient undergoing pulmonary endarterectomy, *Semin Cardiothorac Vasc Anesth* 18:250–256, 2006.

79. Thistlethwaite PA, Madani MM, Kemp AD, et al: Venovenous extracorporeal life support after pulmonary endarterectomy: Indications, techniques, and outcomes, *Ann Thorac Surg* 82:2139, 2006.

80. Berman M, Tsui S, Vuylsteke A, et al: Successful extracorporeal membrane oxygenation support after pulmonary thromboendarterectomy, *Ann Thorac Surg* 86:1261, 2008.

81. Olman MA, Auger WR, Fedullo PF, et al: Pulmonary vascular steal in chronic thromboembolic pulmonary hypertension, *Chest* 98:1430, 1990.

82. Moser KM, Metersky ML, Auger WR, et al: Resolution of vascular steal after pulmonary thromboendarterectomy, *Chest* 104:1441, 1993.

83. Wragg RE, Dimsdale JE, Moser KM, et al: Operative predictors of delirium after pulmonary thromboendarterectomy. A model for postcardiotomy delirium? *J Thorac Cardiovasc Surg* 96:524, 1988.

84. Yung GL, Channick RN, Fedullo PF, et al: Successful pulmonary thromboendarterectomy in two patients with sickle cell disease, *Am J Respir Crit Care Med* 157:1690, 1998.

85. Moser KM, Shea JG: The relationship between pulmonary infarction, cor pulmonale, and the sickle cell states, *Am J Med* 27:561, 1957.

86. Collins FS, Orringer E: Pulmonary hypertension and cor pulmonale in the sickle hemoglobinopathies, *Am J Med* 73:814, 1982.

87. Sutton LL, Castro O, Cross DJ, et al: Pulmonary hypertension in sickle cell disease, *Am J Cardiol* 74:626, 1994.

88. Simmons BE, Santhanam V, Castaner A, et al: Sickle cell disease: Two-dimensional echo and Doppler ultrasonographic findings in hearts of adult patients with sickle anemia, *Arch Intern Med* 148:1526, 1988.

89. Métras D, Coulibaly AO, Ouattara K, et al: Open-heart surgery in sickle-cell hemoglobinopathies: Report of 15 cases, *Thorax* 37:486, 1982.

90. Balasundaram S, Duran CG, al-Halees Z, et al: Cardiopulmonary bypass in sickle cell anaemia. Report of five cases, *J Cardiovasc Surg* 32:271, 1991.

91. Hockmuth D, Mills N: Management of unusual problems encountered in initiating and maintaining cardiopulmonary bypass. In *Cardiopulmonary bypass: principles and practice*, Baltimore, 1993, Williams & Wilkins, pp 750–751.

92. Deleval M, Taswell HF, Bowie EJW, et al: Open heart surgery in patients with inherited hemoglobinopathies, red cell dyscrasias and coagulopathies, *Arch Surg* 109:618, 1974.

93. Aldrich TK, Dhuper SK, Patwa NS, et al: Pulmonary entrapment of sickle cells: The role of regional alveolar hypoxia, *J Appl Physiol* 80:531, 1996.

94. Vichinsky EP, Haberkern CM, Neumayr L: A comparison of conservative and aggressive transfusion regimens in the perioperative management of sickle cell disease: The perioperative transfusion in sickle cell disease study group, *N Engl J Med* 333:206, 1995.

95. Rubens FD, Sabloff M, Wells PS: Use of recombinant-hirudin in pulmonary thromboendarterectomy, *Ann Thorac Surg* 69:1942, 2000.

96. Warkentin TE, Greinacher A: Heparin-induced thrombocytopenia and cardiac surgery, *Ann Thorac Surg* 76:2121, 2003.

97. Potzsch B, Madlener K, Seelig C, et al: Monitoring of r-hirudin anticoagulation during cardiopulmonary bypass—assessment of the whole blood ecarin clotting time, *Thromb Haemost* 77:920, 1997.

98. Riess FC, Lower C, Seelig C, et al: Recombinant hirudin as a new anticoagulant during cardiac operations instead of heparin: Successful for aortic valve replacement in man, *J Thorac Cardiovasc Surg* 110:265, 1995.

99. von Segesser LK, Mueller X, Marty B, et al: Alternatives to unfractionated heparin for anticoagulation in cardiopulmonary bypass, *Perfusion* 16:411, 2001.

100. Mertzlufft F, Kuppe H, Koster A: Management of urgent high-risk cardiopulmonary bypass in patients with heparin-induced thrombocytopenia type II and coexisting disorders of renal function: Use of heparin and epoprostenol combined with on-line monitoring of platelet function, *J Cardiothorac Vasc Anesth* 14:304, 2000.

101. Koster A, Meyer O, Fischer T, et al: One-year experience with the platelet glycoprotein IIb/IIIa antagonist tirofiban and heparin during cardiopulmonary bypass in patients with heparin-induced thrombocytopenia type II, *J Thorac Cardiovasc Surg* 122:1254, 2001.

102. Warkentin TE, Greinacher A: Heparin-induced thrombocytopenia and cardiac surgery, *Ann Thorac Surg* 76:2121, 2003.

103. Warkentin TE, Greinacher A, Koster A: Treatment and prevention of heparin-induced thrombocytopenia: American College of Chest Physicians evidence-based clinical practice guidelines (8th) edition, *Chest* 133:340S, 2008.

104. Corsico AG, D'Armini AM, Cerveri I, et al: Long-term outcome after pulmonary endarterectomy, *Am J Respir Crit Care Med* 178:419, 2008.

105. Task Force Report of the European Society of Cardiology: Guidelines on diagnosis and management of acute pulmonary embolism, *Eur Heart J* 21:1301, 2000.
106. Heit JA, Melton LJ III, Lohse CM, et al: Incidence of venous thromboembolism in hospitalized patients versus community residents, *Mayo Clin Proc* 76:1102, 2001.
107. Silverstein MD, Heit JA, Mohr DN, et al: Trends in the incidence of deep vein thrombosis and pulmonary embolism: A 25-year population-based, cohort study, *Arch Intern Med* 158:585, 1998.
108. Heit JA, Cohen AT, Anderson FA Jr: Estimated annual number of incident and recurrent, non-fatal and fatal venous thromboembolism (VTE) events in the US, *Blood* 106:267a, 2005.
109. Cushman M, Tsai AW, White RH, et al: Deep vein thrombosis and pulmonary embolism in two cohorts: The longitudinal investigation of thromboembolism etiology, *Am J Med* 117:19, 2004.
110. White RH, Zhou H, Romano PS: Incidence of idiopathic deep venous thrombosis and secondary thromboembolism among ethnic groups in California, *Ann Intern Med* 128:737, 1998.
111. White RH, Zhou H, Murin S, et al: Effect of ethnicity and gender on the incidence of venous thromboembolism in a diverse population in California in 1996, *Thromb Haemost* 93:298, 2005.
112. Heit JA, Mohr DN, Silverstein MD, et al: Predictors of recurrence after deep vein thrombosis and pulmonary embolism: a population-based cohort study, *Arch Intern Med* 160:761, 2000.
113. Prandoni P, Lensing AW, Cogo A, et al: The long-term clinical course of acute deep venous thrombosis, *Ann Intern Med* 125:1, 1996.
114. Goldhaber SZ, Visani L, De Rosa M: Acute pulmonary embolism: Clinical outcomes in the International Cooperative Pulmonary Embolism Registry (ICOPER), *Lancet* 353:1386, 1999.
115. Kasper W, Konstantinides S, Geibel A, et al: Management strategies and determinants of outcome in acute major pulmonary embolism: Results of a multicenter registry, *J Am Coll Cardiol* 30:1165, 1997.
116. Heit JA, Rooke TW, Silverstein MD, et al: Trends in the incidence of venous stasis syndrome and venous ulcer: A 25-year population-based study, *J Vasc Surg* 33:1022, 2001.
117. Mohr DN, Silverstein MD, Heit JA, et al: The venous stasis syndrome after deep venous thromboembolism or pulmonary embolism: A population-based study, *Mayo Clin Proc* 75:1249, 2000.
118. Kahn SR, Kearon C, Julian JA, et al: Predictors of post-thrombotic syndrome during long-term treatment of proximal deep vein thrombosis, *J Thromb Haemost* 3:718, 2005.
119. Dalen JE: Pulmonary embolism: What have we learned since Virchow? Natural history, pathophysiology, and diagnosis, *Chest* 122:1440–1456, 2002.
120. Elliott CG: Pulmonary physiology during pulmonary embolism, *Chest* 101:163S, 1992.
121. Wood KE: Major pulmonary embolism: Review of a pathophysiological approach to the golden hour of hemodynamically significant pulmonary embolism, *Chest* 121:877, 2002.
122. Seligsohn U, Lubetsky A: Genetic susceptibility to venous thrombosis, *N Engl J Med* 344:1222–1231, 2001.
123. Larsen T, Sorensen H, Skytthe A, et al: Major genetic susceptibility for venous thromboembolism in men: A study of Danish twins, *Epidemiology* 14:328, 2003.
124. Heit JA, Phelps M, Ward S, et al: Familial segregation of venous thromboembolism, *J Thromb Haemost* 2:731, 2004.
125. Heit JA, Silverstein MD, Mohr DN, et al: Risk factors for deep vein thrombosis and pulmonary embolism: A population-based case-control study, *Arch Intern Med* 160:809, 2000.
126. Samama MM: An epidemiologic study of risk factors for deep vein thrombosis in medical outpatients: The Sirius study, *Arch Intern Med* 160:3415, 2000.
127. Kobbervig C, Heit J, Petterson T, et al: The effect of patient age on the incidence of idiopathic vs. secondary venous thromboembolism: A population-based cohort study, *Blood* 104:957a, 2004.
128. Gomes MPV, Deitcher SR: Risk of venous thromboembolic disease associated with hormonal contraceptives and hormone replacement therapy, *Arch Intern Med* 164:1965, 2004.
129. Heit JA, Kobbervig CE, James AH, et al: Trends in the incidence of deep vein thrombosis and pulmonary embolism during pregnancy or the puerperium: A 30-year population-based study, *Ann Intern Med* 143:697, 2005.
130. Stein PD: Acute pulmonary embolism, *Dis Mon* 40:467, 1994.
131. Elliott CG, Coldhaber SZ, Jensen RL: Delays in diagnosis of deep vein thrombosis and pulmonary embolism, *Chest* 128:3372, 2005.
132. Hamspon NB: Pulmonary embolism: Difficulties in the clinical diagnosis, *Semin Respir Infect* 10:123, 1995.
133. The PIOPED Investigators: Value of the ventilation/perfusion scan in acute pulmonary embolism. Results of the Prospective Investigation of Pulmonary Embolism Diagnosis (PIOPED), *JAMA* 263:2753, 1990.
134. Kearon C, Hirsh J: The diagnosis of pulmonary embolism, *Haemostasis* 25:72, 1995.
135. Goldhaber SZ, Elliott CG: Acute pulmonary embolism: Part I: epidemiology, pathophysiology, and diagnosis, *Circulation* 108:2726, 2003.
136. Powell T, Muller NL: Imaging of acute pulmonary thromboembolism: Should spiral computed tomography replace the ventilation-perfusion scan? *Clin Chest Med* 24:29, 2003.
137. Hampson NB: Pulmonary embolism: Difficulties in the clinical diagnosis, *Semin Respir Infect* 10:123, 1995.
138. Stein PD, Terrin ML, Hales CA, et al: Clinical, laboratory, roentgenographic and electrocardiographic findings in patients with acute pulmonary embolism and no pre-existing cardiac or pulmonary disease, *Chest* 100:598, 1991.
139. Sreeram N, Cheriex EC, Smeets JL, et al: Value of the 12-lead electrocardiogram at hospital admission in the diagnosis of pulmonary embolism, *Am J Cardiol* 73:298, 1994.
140. Stein PD, Hull RD, Patel KC, et al: D-dimer for the exclusion of acute venous thrombosis and pulmonary embolism: A systematic review, *Ann Intern Med* 140:589, 2004.
141. Di Nisio M, Squizzato A, Rutjes AW, et al: Diagnostic accuracy of D-dimer test for exclusion of venous thromboembolism: A systematic review, *J Thromb Haemost* 5:296, 2007.
142. Dunn KL, Wolf JP, Dorfman DM, et al: Normal D-dimer levels in emergency department patients suspected of acute pulmonary embolism, *J Am Coll Cardiol* 40:1475, 2002.
143. Wells PS, Anderson DR, Rodger M, et al: Excluding pulmonary embolism at the bedside without diagnostic imaging: Management of patients with suspected pulmonary embolism presenting to the emergency department by using a simple clinical model and D-dimer, *Ann Intern Med* 135:98, 2001.
144. Wells PS, Ginsberg JS, Anderson DR, et al: Use of a clinical model for safe management of patients with suspected pulmonary embolism, *Ann Intern Med* 129:997, 1998.
145. Wicki J, Perneger TV, Junod AF, et al: Assessing clinical probability of pulmonary embolism in the emergency ward: A simple score, *Arch Intern Med* 161:92, 2001.
146. Le Gal G, Righini M, Roy PM, et al: Prediction of pulmonary embolism in the emergency department: The revised Geneva score, *Ann Intern Med* 144:165, 2006.
147. Miniati M, Prediletto R, Forcichi B, et al: Accuracy of clinical assessment in the diagnosis of pulmonary embolism, *Am J Respir Crit Care Med* 159:864, 1999.
148. Miniati M, Monti S, Bottai M: A structured clinical model for predicting the probability of pulmonary embolism, *Am J Med* 114:173, 2003.
149. Kearon C, Ginsberg JS, Douketis J, et al: An evaluation of D-dimer in the diagnosis of pulmonary embolism: A randomized trial, *Ann Intern Med* 144:812, 2006.
150. Righini M, Aujesky D, Roy PM, et al: Clinical usefulness of D-dimer depending on clinical probability and cutoff value in outpatients with suspected pulmonary embolism, *Arch Intern Med* 164:2483, 2004.
151. Kruip MJ, Söhne M, Nijkeuter M, et al: A simple diagnostic strategy in hospitalized patients with clinically suspected pulmonary embolism, *J Intern Med* 260:459, 2006.
152. van Strijen MJ, de Monye W, Schiereck J, et al: Single-detector helical computed tomography as the primary diagnostic test in suspected pulmonary embolism: A multicenter clinical management study of 510 patients, *Ann Intern Med* 138:307, 2003.
153. Perrier A, Howarth N, Didier D, et al: Performance of helical computed tomography in unselected outpatients with suspected pulmonary embolism, *Ann Intern Med* 135:88, 2001.
154. DeMonaco NA, Dang Q, Kapoor WN, et al: Pulmonary embolism incidence is increasing with use of spiral computed tomography, *Am J Med* 121:611, 2008.
155. Swenson SJ, Sheedy PFII, Ryu JH, et al: Outcomes after withholding anticoagulation from patients with suspected acute pulmonary embolism and negative computed tomographic findings: A cohort study, *Mayo Clin Proc* 77:130, 2002.
156. Task Force on Pulmonary Embolism, European Society of Cardiology: Guidelines on diagnosis and management of acute pulmonary embolism, *Eur Heart J* 21:1301, 2000.
157. Goldhaber SZ: Recent advances in the diagnosis and lytic therapy of pulmonary embolism, *Chest* 99:173S, 1991.
158. Loud PA, Katz DS, Bruce DA, et al: Deep venous thrombosis with suspected pulmonary embolism: Detection with combined CT venography and pulmonary angiography, *Radiology* 219:498, 2001.
159. Stein PD, Fowler SE, Goodman LR, et al: Multidetector computed tomography for acute pulmonary embolism, *N Engl J Med* 354:2317, 2006.
160. Goldhaber SZ: Echocardiography in the management of pulmonary embolism, *Ann Intern Med* 136:691, 2002.
161. Kucher N, Goldhaber SZ: Cardiac biomarkers for risk stratification of patients with acute pulmonary embolism, *Circulation* 108:2191, 2003.
162. Goldhaber SZ: Unsolved issues in the treatment of pulmonary embolism, *Thromb Res* 103:V245, 2001.
163. Dehring DJ, Arens JF: Pulmonary thromboembolism: Disease recognition and patient management, *Anesthesiology* 73:146, 1990.
164. Mangano DT: Immediate hemodynamic and pulmonary changes following pulmonary thromboembolism, *Anesthesiology* 52:173, 1980.
165. Levine MN: Thrombolytic therapy for venous thromboembolism. Complications and contraindications, *Clin Chest Med* 16:321, 1995.
166. Lualdi JC, Goldhaber SZ: Right ventricular dysfunction after acute pulmonary embolism: Pathophysiologic factors, detection, and therapeutic implications, *Am Heart J* 130:1276, 1995.
167. Gossage JR: Early intervention in massive pulmonary embolism. A guide to diagnosis and triage for the critical first hour, *Postgrad Med* 111:27, 33, 39–40, 2002.
168. Hirsh J: Treatment of pulmonary embolism, *Annu Rev Med* 38:91, 1987.
169. Hull RD, Pineo GF: Current concepts of anticoagulation therapy, *Clin Chest Med* 16:269, 1995.
170. Simonneau G, Sors H, Charbonnier B, et al: A comparison of low-molecular weight heparin with unfractionated heparin for acute pulmonary embolism, *N Engl J Med* 337:663, 1997.
171. Hull RD, Raskob GE, Brant RF, et al: Low-molecular-weight heparin vs. heparin in the treatment of patients with pulmonary embolism, *Arch Intern Med* 160:229, 2000.
172. The Matisse Investigators: Subcutaneous fondaparinux versus intravenous unfractionated heparin in the initial treatment of pulmonary embolism, *N Engl J Med* 349:1695, 2003.
173. The Columbus Investigators: Low-molecular-weight heparin in the treatment of patients with venous thromboembolism, *N Engl J Med* 337:657, 1997.
174. McCowan TC, Eidt JF, Ferris EJ: Interventions in pulmonary embolism, *J Thorac Imaging* 4:67, 1989.
175. Kearon C, Kahn SR, Agnelli G, et al: Antithrombotic therapy for venous thromboembolic disease: American College of Chest Physicians Evidence-Based Clinical Practice Guidelines, 8th ed. *Chest* 133:454–545, 2008.
176. Wan S, Quinlan DJ, Agnelli G, et al: Thrombolysis compared with heparin for the initial treatment of pulmonary embolism: A meta-analysis of the randomized controlled trials, *Circulation* 110:744, 2004.
177. Gray HH, Miller GA, Paneth M: Pulmonary embolectomy: Its place in the management of pulmonary embolism, *Lancet* 1:1441, 1988.
178. Goldhaber SZ: A contemporary approach to thrombolytic therapy for pulmonary embolism, *Vasc Med* 5:115, 2000.
179. Goldhaber SZ, Kessler CM, Heit JA, et al: Recombinant tissue type plasminogen activator versus a novel dosing regimen of urokinase in acute pulmonary embolism: A randomized controlled multicenter trial, *J Am Coll Cardiol* 20:24, 1992.
180. Tsai SK, Wang MJ, Ko WJ, et al: Emergent bedside transesophageal echocardiography in the resuscitation of sudden cardiac arrest after tricuspid inflow obstruction and pulmonary embolism, *Anesth Analg* 89:1406, 1999.
181. Kucher N: Catheter embolectomy for acute pulmonary embolism, *Chest* 132:657, 2007.
182. Fava M, Loyola S: Applications of percutaneous mechanical thrombectomy in pulmonary embolism, *Tech Vasc Interv Radiol* 6:53, 2003.
183. Steenberg RW, Warren R, Wilson RE, et al: New look at pulmonary embolectomy, *Surg Gynecol Obstet* 107:214, 1958.
184. Cooley DA, Beall AC, Alexander JK: Acute massive pulmonary embolism: Successful surgical treatment using temporary cardiopulmonary bypass, *JAMA* 177:79, 1961.
185. Sharp EH: Pulmonary embolectomy: Successful removal of a massive pulmonary embolus with the support of cardiopulmonary bypass: A case report, *Ann Surg* 156:1, 1962.
186. Dauphine C, Omari B: Pulmonary embolectomy for acute massive pulmonary embolism, *Ann Thorac Surg* 79:1240, 2005.
187. Aklog L, Williams CS, Byrne JG, et al: Acute pulmonary embolectomy: A contemporary approach, *Circulation* 105:1416, 2002.
188. Meyer G, Tamisier D, Sors H, et al: Pulmonary embolectomy: A 20-year experience at one center, *Ann Thorac Surg* 51:232, 1991.
189. Shimokawa S, Uehara K, Toyohira H, et al: Massive endobronchial hemorrhage after pulmonary embolectomy, *Ann Thorac Surg* 61:1241, 1996.
190. Layish DT, Tapson VF: Pharmacologic hemodynamic support in massive pulmonary embolism, *Chest* 111:218, 1997.
191. Molloy DW, Lee KY, Jones D, et al: Effects of noradrenaline and isoproterenol on cardiopulmonary function in a canine model of acute pulmonary hypertension, *Chest* 88:432, 1985.
192. Leacche M, Unic D, Goldhaber SZ, et al: Modern surgical treatment of massive pulmonary embolism: Results in 47 consecutive patients after rapid diagnosis and aggressive surgical approach, *J Thorac Cardiovasc Surg* 129:1018, 2005.
193. McLaughlin VV, Archer SL, Badesch DB, et al; American College of Cardiology Foundation Task Force on Expert Consensus Documents; American Heart Association; American College of Chest Physicians; American Thoracic Society, Inc; Pulmonary Hypertension Association: ACCF/AHA 2009 expert consensus document on pulmonary hypertension a report of the American College of Cardiology Foundation Task Force on Expert Consensus Documents and the American Heart Association developed in collaboration with the American College of Chest Physicians; American Thoracic Society, Inc.; and the Pulmonary Hypertension Association, *J Am Coll Cardiol* 53:1573–1619, 2009.
194. Dresdale DT, Schultz M, Mitchom RJ: Primary pulmonary hypertension: Clinical and hemodynamic study, *Am J Med* 11:686, 1951.

195. Rich S, Kaufmann E, Levy PS: The effect of high doses of calcium-channel blockers on survival in primary pulmonary hypertension, *N Engl J Med* 327:76, 1992.
196. Sitbon O, Humbert M, Jais X, et al: Long-term response to calcium channel blockers in idiopathic pulmonary arterial hypertension, *Circulation* 111:3105, 2005.
197. Cool CD, Kennedy D, Voelkel NF, et al: Pathogenesis and evolution of plexiform lesions in pulmonary hypertension with scleroderma and human immunodeficiency virus, *Hum Pathol* 28:434, 1997.
198. Voelkel NF, Cool C, Lee SD, et al: Primary pulmonary hypertension between inflammation and cancer, *Chest* 114:225S, 1998.
199. Lee SD, Shroyer KR, Markham NE, et al: Monoclonal endothelial cell proliferation is present in primary but not secondary pulmonary hypertension, *J Clin Invest* 101:927, 1998.
200. Nichols WC, Koller DL, Slovis B, et al: Localization of the gene for familial primary pulmonary hypertension to chromosome 2q31-31, *Nat Genet* 15:277, 1997.
201. Loyd JE, Butler MG, Foroud TM, et al: Genetic anticipation and abnormal gender ratio at birth in familial primary pulmonary hypertension, *Am J Respir Crit Care Med* 152:93, 1995.
202. Thenappan T, Shah SJ, Rich S, et al: A USA-based registry for pulmonary arterial hypertension: 1982–2006, *Eur Respir J* 30:1103, 2007.
203. Rich S, Dantzker DR, Ayres S, et al: Primary pulmonary hypertension: A national prospective study, *Ann Intern Med* 107:216, 1987.
204. D'Alonzo G, Barst R, Ayres S, et al: Survival in patients with primary pulmonary hypertension: Results from a national prospective registry, *Ann Intern Med* 115:343, 1991.
205. Thomson Jr, Machado RD, Pauciulo MW, et al: Sporadic primary pulmonary hypertension is associated with germline mutations of the gene encoding BMPR-II, a receptor member of the TGF-beta family, *J Med Genet* 37:741, 2000.
206. Budhiraja R, Tuder RM, Hassoun PM: Endothelial dysfunction in pulmonary hypertension, *Circulation* 109:159, 2004.
207. Galie N, Manes A, Branzi A: The new clinical trials on pharmacological treatment in pulmonary arterial hypertension, *Eur Respir J* 20:1037, 2002.
208. Welsh CH, Hassell KL, Badesch DB, et al: Coagulation and fibrinolytic profiles in patients with severe pulmonary hypertension, *Chest* 110:710, 1996.
209. Cacoub P, Dorent R, Nataf P, et al: Endothelin-1 in the lungs of patients with pulmonary hypertension, *Cardiovasc Res* 33:196, 1997.
210. Ishikawa S, Miyauchi T, Sakai S, et al: Elevated levels of plasma endothelin-1 in young patients with pulmonary hypertension caused by congenital heart disease are decreased after successful surgical repair, *J Thorac Cardiovasc Surg* 110:271, 1995.
211. Stewart DJ, Levy RD, Cernacek P, et al: Increased plasma endothelin-1 in pulmonary hypertension: Marker or mediator of disease? *Ann Intern Med* 114:464, 1991.
212. Giaid A, Yanagisawa M, Langleben D, et al: Expression of endothelin-1 in the lungs of patients with pulmonary hypertension, *N Engl J Med* 328:1732, 1993.
213. Weir EK, Archer SL: The mechanism of acute hypoxic pulmonary vasoconstriction: The tale of two channels, *FASEB J* 9:183, 1995.
214. Stephanazzi J, Guidon-Attali C, Escarment J: Right ventricular function: Physiological and pathophysiological features, *Ann Fr Anesth Reanim* 16:165, 1997.
215. Redington AN, Gray JJ, Hodson ME, et al: Characterization of the normal right ventricular pressure-volume relation by biplane angiography and simultaneous micro manometer pressure measurements, *Br Heart J* 59:23, 1988.
216. Redington AN, Rigby ML, Shinebourne EA, et al: Changes in the pressure-volume relation of the right ventricle when its loading conditions are modified, *Br Heart J* 63:45, 1990.
217. Brooks H, Kirk ES, Vokonas PS, et al: Performance of the right ventricle under stress: Relation to right coronary flow, *J Clin Invest* 50:2176, 1971.
218. Goldstein JA: Pathophysiology and management of right heart ischemia, *J Am Coll Cardiol* 40:841, 2002.
219. Piazza G, Goldhaber SZ: The acutely decompensated right ventricle: Pathways for diagnosis and management, *Chest* 128:1836, 2005.
220. Woods J, Monteiro P, Rhodes A: Right ventricular dysfunction, *Curr Opin Crit Care* 13:532, 2007.
221. van Wolferen SA, Marcus JT, Boonstra A, et al: Prognostic value of right ventricular mass, volume, and function in idiopathic pulmonary arterial hypertension, *Eur Heart J* 28:1250, 2007.
222. Barst RJ, Rubin LJ, Long WA, et al: A comparison of continuous intravenous epoprostenol (prostacyclin) with conventional therapy for primary pulmonary hypertension. The primary pulmonary hypertension study group, *N Engl J Med* 334:296, 1996.
223. McLaughlin VV, Shillington A, Rich S: Survival in primary pulmonary hypertension: The impact of epoprostenol therapy, *Circulation* 106:1477, 2002.
224. Nagaya N, Uematsu M, Satoh T, et al: Serum uric acid levels correlate with the severity and the mortality of primary pulmonary hypertension, *Am J Respir Crit Care Med* 160:487, 1999.
225. Torbicki A, Kurzyna M, Kuca P, et al: Detectable serum cardiac troponin T as a marker of poor prognosis among patients with chronic precapillary pulmonary hypertension, *Circulation* 108:844, 2003.
226. McConnell MV, Solomon SD, Rayan ME, et al: Regional right ventricular dysfunction detected by echocardiography in acute pulmonary embolism, *Am J Cardiol* 78:469, 1996.
227. Konstantinides S, Geibel A, Olschewski M, et al: Importance of cardiac troponins I and T in risk stratification of patients with acute pulmonary embolism, *Circulation* 106:1263, 2002.
228. Eysmann SB, Palevsky HI, Reichek N, et al: Two-dimensional and Doppler-echocardiographic and cardiac catheterization correlates of survival in primary pulmonary hypertension, *Circulation* 80:353, 1989.
229. Haddad F, Couture P, Tousignant C, et al: The right ventricle in cardiac surgery, a perioperative perspective: I. Anatomy, physiology, and assessment, *Anesth Analg* 108:407, 2009.
230. Raymond RJ, Hinderliter AL, Willis PW, et al: Echocardiographic predictors of adverse outcomes in primary pulmonary hypertension, *J Am Coll Cardiol* 39:1214, 2002.
231. Tamborini G, Pepi M, Galli CA, et al: Feasibility and accuracy of a routine echocardiographic assessment of right ventricular function, *Int J Cardiol* 115:86, 2007.
232. Zeineh NS, Champion HC: Utility of tricuspid annular plane systolic excursion in the assessment of right ventricular function, *PVRI Review* 2:17, 2010.
233. van Wolferen SA, Marcus JT, Boonstra A, et al: Prognostic value of right ventricular mass, volume, and function in the idiopathic pulmonary arterial hypertension, *Eur Heart J* 28:1250, 2007.
234. Sitbon O, Humbert M, Jais X, et al: Long-term response to calcium channel blockers in idiopathic pulmonary arterial hypertension, *Circulation* 111:3105, 2005.
235. Frank H, Mlczoch J, Huber K, et al: The effect of anticoagulant therapy in primary and anorectic drug-induced pulmonary hypertension, *Chest* 112:714, 1997.
236. Rich S, McLaughlin VV: The effects of chronic prostacyclin therapy on cardiac output and symptoms in primary pulmonary hypertension, *J Am Coll Cardiol* 34:1184, 1999.
237. Simonneau G, Barst RJ, Galie N, et al: Continuous subcutaneous infusion of treprostinil, a prostacyclin analogue, in patients with pulmonary arterial hypertension: A double-blind, randomized, placebo-controlled trial, *Am J Respir Crit Care Med* 165:800, 2002.
238. Olschewski H, Simonneau G, Gaile N, et al: Inhaled iloprost for severe pulmonary hypertension, *N Engl J Med* 347:322, 2002.
239. Rubens C, Ewert R, Halank M, et al: big endothelin-1 and endothelin-1 plasma levels are correlated with the severity of primary pulmonary hypertension, *Chest* 120:1562, 2001.
240. Channick RN, Simonneau G, Sitbon O, et al: Effects of the dual endothelin-receptor antagonist bosentan in patients with pulmonary hypertension: A randomized placebo-controlled study, *Lancet* 358:1119, 2001.
241. Giaid A, Saleh D: Reduced expression of endothelial nitric oxide synthase in the lungs of patients with pulmonary hypertension, *N Engl J Med* 333:214, 1995.
242. Murray F, MacLean MR, Pyne NJ: Increased expression of the cGMP-inhibited cAMP-specific (PDE3) and cGMP binding cGMP-specific (PDE5) phosphodiesterases in models of pulmonary hypertension, *Br J Pharmacol* 137:1187, 2002.
243. Wharton J, Strange JW, Møller GM, et al: Antiproliferative effects of phosphodiesterase type 5 inhibition in human pulmonary artery cells, *Am J Respir Crit Care Med* 172:105, 2005.
244. Nagendran J, Archer SL, Soliman D, et al: Phosphodiesterase type 5 is highly expressed in the hypertrophied human right ventricle, and acute inhibition of phosphodiesterase type 5 improves contractility, *Circulation* 116:238, 2007.
245. Humbert M, Sitbord O, Simonneau G: Treatment of pulmonary arterial hypertension, *N Engl J Med* 351:1425, 2004.
246. Galie N, Ghofrani HA, Torbicki A, et al: Sildenafil citrate therapy for pulmonary arterial hypertension, *N Engl J Med* 353:2148, 2005.
247. Gaile N, Brundage BH, Ghofrani HA, et al: Tadalafil therapy for pulmonary arterial hypertension, *Circulation* 119:2894–2903, 2009.
248. Altman R, Scazziota A, Rouvier J, et al: Coagulation and fibrinolytic parameters in patients with pulmonary hypertension, *Clin Cardiol* 19:549, 1996.
249. Gaine SP, Rubin LJ: Primary pulmonary hypertension, *Lancet* 352:719, 1998.
250. Fischer LG, Van Aken H, Burkle H: Management of pulmonary hypertension: Physiological and pharmacological considerations for anesthesiologists, *Anesth Analg* 96:1603, 2003.
251. Dell'Italia LJ, Starling MR, Crawford MH, et al: Right ventricular infarction: Identification by hemodynamic measurements before and after volume loading and correlation with noninvasive techniques, *J Am Coll Cardiol* 4:931–939, 1984.
252. Goldstein JA, Barzilai B, Rosamond TL, et al: Determinants of hemodynamic compromise with severe right ventricular infarction, *Circulation* 82:359–368, 1990.
253. Dell'Italia LJ, Starling MR, Blumhardt R, et al: Comparative effects of volume loading, dobutamine, and nitroprusside in patients with predominant right ventricular infarction, *Circulation* 72:1327–1335, 1985.
254. Ferrario M, Poli A, Previtali M, et al: Hemodynamics of volume loading compared with dobutamine in severe right ventricular infarction, *Am J Cardiol* 74:329–333, 1994.
255. Laver MB: Myocardial ischaemia: Dilemma between information available and information demand, *Br Heart J* 50:222–230, 1983.
256. Radermacher P, Santak B, Wust HJ, et al: Prostacyclin and right ventricular function in patients with pulmonary hypertension associated with ARDS, *Intensive Care Med* 16:227–232, 1990.
257. Bhorade S, Christenson J, O'Connor M, et al: Response to inhaled nitric oxide in patients with acute right heart syndrome, *Am J Respir Crit Care Med* 159:571–579, 1999.
258. Palmer RM, Ferrige AG, Moncada S: Nitric oxide release accounts for the biological activity of endothelium-derived relaxing factor, *Nature* 327:524–526, 1987.
259. Furchgott RF, Zawadzki JV: The obligatory role of endothelial cells in the relaxation of arterial smooth muscle by acetaylcholine, *Nature* 288:373–376, 1980.
260. Roberts JD, Chen TY, Kawai N, et al: Inhaled nitric oxide reverses pulmonary vasoconstriction in the hypoxic and acidotic newborn lamb, *Circ Res* 72:246–254, 1993.
261. Pepke-Zaba J, Higenbottam TW, Dinh-Xuan AT, et al: Inhaled nitric oxide as a cause of selective pulmonary vasodilatation in pulmonary hypertension, *Lancet* 338:1173–1174, 1991.
262. Fullerton DA, Jones SD, Jaggers J, et al: Effective control of pulmonary vascular resistance with inhaled nitric oxide following cardiac operation, *J Thorac Cardiovasc Surg* 111:753–763, 1996.

25 Cardiac Pacing and Defibrillation

MARC A. ROZNER, PHD, MD

KEY POINTS

Preoperative Key Points

1. Identify the manufacturer and model of the generator.
2. Have the pacemaker or defibrillator interrogated by a competent authority shortly before the procedure.
3. Obtain a copy of this interrogation. Ensure that the device will appropriately pace the heart.
4. Consider replacing any device near its elective replacement period in a patient scheduled to undergo either a major operation or surgery within 25 cm of the generator.
5. Determine the patient's underlying rate, rhythm, and pacing dependency to determine the need for backup pacing support.
6. If magnet use is planned, ensure that a magnet mode exists; for pacemakers, verify the magnet rate and pacing mode.
7. Consider programming minute ventilation and other rate responsiveness features off, if present.
8. Consider programming rate enhancements off, if present.
9. Consider increasing the pacing rate to optimize oxygen delivery to tissues for major operations.
10. Disable antitachycardia therapy, if present, if electromagnetic interference is likely, or if a central venous catheter guidewire will be placed into the chest. Although a magnet might work, magnet therapy has been associated with inappropriate implantable cardioverter-defibrillator (ICD) discharge.

Intraoperative Key Points

1. Monitor cardiac rhythm/peripheral pulse with pulse oximeter (plethysmography) or arterial waveform.
2. Disable the "artifact filter" on the electrocardiograph monitor.
3. Avoid use of the monopolar electrosurgical unit (ESU), or limit ESU bursts to less than 5 seconds.
4. Use bipolar ESU if possible; if not possible, then pure cut (monopolar ESU) is better than "blend" or "coag."
5. Place the ESU current return pad in such a way to prevent electricity from crossing the generator-heart circuit, even if the pad must be placed on the distal forearm and the wire covered with sterile drape.

6. If the ESU causes ventricular oversensing and pacer quiescence, limit the period(s) of asystole.
7. Temporary pacing might be necessary, and consideration should be given to the possibility of pacemaker or defibrillator failure.
8. Consider avoiding sevoflurane, isoflurane, or desflurane in the patient with long QT syndrome.

Postoperative Key Points

1. Have the device interrogated by a competent authority after surgery. Some rate enhancements can be reinitiated, and optimum heart rate and pacing parameters should be determined. The ICD patient must be monitored until the antitachycardia therapy is restored.

Battery-operated, implantable pacing devices were first introduced in 1958, just 4 years after the invention of the transistor. The complexity, calculation, and data storage abilities of these devices have grown in a manner similar to that seen within the computer industry. The natural progression of pacemaker developments led to the invention of the implantable cardioverter-defibrillator (ICD) around 1980. As this technology has advanced, the lines between these devices have become less clear. For example, every ICD currently implanted has antibradycardia pacing capability; and patients, news media, and even physicians often misidentify an implanted defibrillator as a pacemaker. The consequence of mistaking an ICD for a conventional pacemaker can lead to patient harm, either because of electromagnetic interference (EMI) issues resulting in inappropriate ICD therapy, or the unintentional disabling of ICD therapies in some ICDs that can be permanently disabled by magnet placement.[1] Figure 25-1 shows a three-lead defibrillation system and identifies the right ventricular (RV) shock coil, which differentiates an ICD system from a conventional pacemaking system. The complexity of cardiac pulse generators and the multitude of programmable parameters limit the number of sweeping generalizations that can be made about the perioperative care of the patient with an implanted pulse generator. Population aging, continued enhancements in implantable technology, and new indications for implantation will lead to growing numbers of patients with these devices in the new millennium. Both the American College of Cardiology and the North American Society for Pacing and Electrophysiology/The Heart Rhythm Society (HRS-NASPE)* have taken note of these issues, and guidelines have been published regarding the care of the perioperative patient with a device.[2,3] Pinski and Trohman[4,5] also have reviewed this subject,

---

*The North American Society of Pacing and Electrophysiology changed their name in 2004 to the Heart Rhythm Society. The abbreviation HRS-NASPE is used in this chapter to avoid confusion.

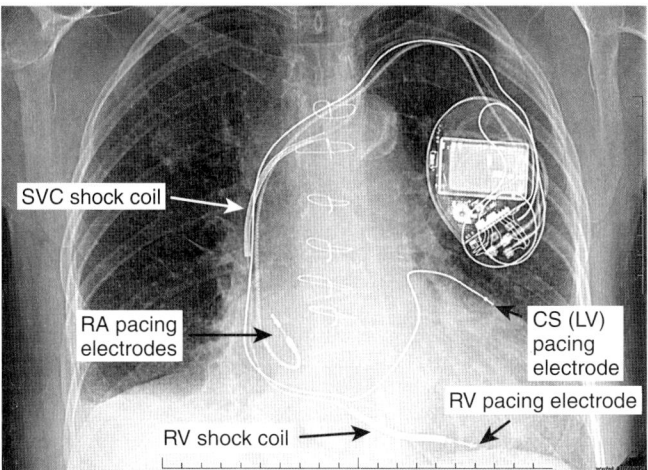

Figure 25-1   A defibrillator system with biventricular (BiV) antibradycardia pacemaker capability. Note that three leads are placed: a conventional bipolar lead to the right atrium (RA), a tripolar lead to the right ventricle (RV), and a unipolar lead to the coronary sinus (CS). This system is designed to provide "resynchronization (antibradycardia) therapy" in the setting of a dilated cardiomyopathy with a prolonged QRS (and frequently with a prolonged P-R interval as well). The bipolar lead in the right atrium will perform both sensing and pacing function. In the RV, the tip electrode functions as the cathode for pacing and sensing functions. The presence of a "shock" conductor (termed *shock coil*) on the RV lead in the RV distinguishes a defibrillation system from a conventional pacemaking system. In this particular patient, the RV shock coil also functions as the pacing and sensing anode (this is called an *integrated bipolar defibrillator lead;* true bipolar leads have a ring electrode between the tip electrode and the shock coil). The lead in the CS depolarizes the left ventricle, and the typical current pathway includes the anode in the RV. Because of the typically wide QRS complex in a left bundle branch pattern, failure to capture the left ventricle can lead to ventricular oversensing (and inappropriate antitachycardia therapy) in an implanted cardioverter-defibrillator (ICD) system. Many defibrillation systems also have a shock coil in the superior vena cava (SVC), which is electrically identical to the defibrillator case (called the *can*). When the defibrillation circuit includes the ICD case, it is called *active can configuration*. Incidental findings on this chest radiograph include the presence of sternal wires from prior sternotomy, as well as the lung cancer seen in the right upper lobe.

and they have published similar recommendations. Additional reviews have been published, and the American Society of Anesthesiologists has issued a practice advisory.[6–8]

PACEMAKERS

Since 1958, more than 26 companies have produced more than 2000 pacemaker models. Determining the actual number of implants and prevalence of devices is difficult. A variety of economic and market reports suggest that more than 300,000 adults and children in the United States underwent pacemaker placement (new or revision) in 2009. It is likely that more than 3 million patients have pacemakers today. Many factors lead to confusion regarding the behavior of a

device and the perioperative care of a patient with a device, especially because case reports, textbooks, and literature reviews have not kept pace with technologic developments, and many of these reviews contain incorrect statements.[9,10] In addition, sometimes the preoperative consultation process leads to improper advice as well.[11] Most patients with a pacemaker have significant comorbid disease. The care of these patients requires attention to both their medical and psychological problems. In addition, an understanding of pulse generators and their likely idiosyncrasies in the operating or procedure room is needed. Whether the patient with a pacemaker is at increased perioperative risk remains unknown, but two reports suggest that these patients deserve extra perioperative attention. In 1995, Badrinath et al[12] retrospectively reviewed ophthalmic surgery cases in one hospital in Madras, India, from 1979 through 1988 (14,787 cases), and wrote that the presence of a pacemaker significantly increased the probability of a mortal event within 6 weeks after surgery, regardless of the anesthetic technique. In 2007, Pili-Floury et al[13] reported a prospective study of 65 consecutive patients undergoing any anesthetic for any invasive noncardiac procedure unrelated to their device; they found seven (11%) postoperative myocardial infarctions, two (3%) patients experienced development of left ventricular failure, and two (3%) patients died of cardiac causes during their hospitalization.

No discussion of pacemakers can take place without an understanding of the generic pacemaker code (NBG; Table 25-1), which has been published by the North American Society of Pacing and Electrophysiology (HRS-NASPE) and British Pacing and Electrophysiology Group. This code, initially published in 1983, was revised in 2002.[14] The code describes the basic behavior of the pacing device. Pacemakers also come with a variety of terms generally unfamiliar to the anesthesiologist, many of which are shown in the Glossary at the end of this chapter.

Pacemaker Indications

Indications for permanent pacing are shown in Box 25-1 and are reviewed in detail elsewhere.[15] Devices have also been approved by the U.S. Food and Drug Administration (FDA) for three-chamber pacing (right atrium, both ventricles) to treat dilated cardiomyopathy (DCM[16,17]; also called *biventricular pacing* [BiV] or *cardiac resynchronization therapy* [CRT]). Also, specially programmed devices are used to treat hypertrophic obstructive cardiomyopathy in both adults and children.[18,19] BiV and hypertrophic obstructive cardiomyopathy indications require careful attention to pacemaker programming because effective pacing in these patients often requires a pacing rate greater than native sinus or junctional escape rate (often accomplished with drugs) and an atrioventricular delay shorter than the native P-R interval so that

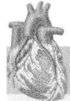

BOX 25-1. PACEMAKER INDICATIONS

Symptomatic sinus node disease
Symptomatic atrioventricular node disease
Long QT syndrome
Hypertrophic obstructive cardiomyopathy*
Dilated cardiomyopathy*

*See text and Pacemaker Programming for special precautions.

TABLE 25-1	North American Society of Pacing and Electrophysiology/British Pacing and Electrophysiology Group Revised (2002) Generic Pacemaker Code (NBG)				
Position I	*Position II*	*Position III*	*Position IV*	*Position V*
Pacing Chamber(s)	**Sensing Chamber(s)**	**Response(s) to Sensing**	**Programmability**	**Multisite Pacing**
O = None	O = None	O = None	O = None	O = None
A = Atrium	A = Atrium	I = Inhibited	R = Rate Modulation	A = Atrium
V = Ventricle	V = Ventricle	T = Triggered		V = Ventricle
D = Dual (A+V)	D = Dual (A+V)	D = Dual (T+I)		D = Dual (A+V)

the ventricle is paced 100% of the time.[20] Inhibition or loss of pacing (i.e., from native conduction, atrial irregularity, ventricular irregularity, development of junctional rhythm, or EMI) can lead to deteriorating hemodynamics in these patients. BiV can lengthen the Q-T interval in some patients, producing torsade de pointes.[21] Multisite atrial pacing to prevent or treat atrial arrhythmias remains in clinical trial.[22,23]

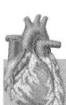 Pacemaker Magnets

Despite oft-repeated folklore, most pacemaker manufacturers warn that magnets were never intended to treat pacemaker emergencies or prevent EMI effects. Rather, magnet-activated switches, both electronic (Hall-effect sensor) and mechanical (reed switch), were incorporated to produce pacing behavior that demonstrates remaining battery life and, sometimes, pacing threshold safety factors. Newer pacemakers provide telephonic data "uplinks" that are routed directly to the patient's pacemaker physician.

Placement of a magnet over a generator might produce no change in pacing because *not all pacemakers switch to a continuous asynchronous mode when a magnet is placed.* Also, not all models from a given company behave the same way. Although more than 90% of pacemakers have "high-rate (80 to 100 beats/min)" asynchronous pacing with magnet application, some switch to asynchronous pacing at program rate, and some respond with only a brief (60 to 100 beats) asynchronous pacing event. Possible effect(s) of magnet placement are shown in Box 25-2.[24–26] In many devices, magnet behavior can be altered via programming. Also, any pacemaker from Boston Scientific (Natick, MA)* will ignore magnet placement after any electrical reset, which is a possibility in the presence of strong EMI. Appendix 25-1 lists pacemakers by manufacturers and has a complete listing of all magnet behaviors.

For all generators, calling the manufacturer remains the most reliable method for determining magnet response and using this response to predict remaining battery life. A list of telephone numbers is shown in Appendix 25-2 at the end of this chapter.

BOX 25-2. PACEMAKER MAGNET BEHAVIOR

Asynchronous pacing without rate responsiveness using parameters possibly not in patient's best interest—this is the most common behavior, although pacemakers manufactured by Biotronik, Boston Scientific, and St. Jude Medical have programmable magnet behavior
Unexpected behavior (e.g., VOO in Medtronic or VDD in Biotronik dual-chamber pacemaker) suggests elective replacement has been reached and the pacemaker should be interrogated promptly
No apparent rhythm or rate change
Magnet mode disabled permanently by programming (possible with Biotronik, Boston Scientific, St. Jude Medical) or temporarily suspended (see Medtronic)
Program rate pacing in already paced patient (many older pacemakers)
Improper monitor settings with pacing near the current heart rate (pace filter on)
No magnet sensor (some pre-1985 Cordis, Telectronics models)
Brief (10–100 beats) asynchronous pacing, then return to program values (most Biotronik and Intermedics pacemakers)
Continuous or transient loss of pacing
Discharged battery (some pre-1990 devices)
Pacer enters diagnostic "Threshold Test Mode" (some Intermedics, Medtronic, St. Jude Medical devices, depending on model and programming)

Also see Appendix 25-1.

---

*Boston Scientific purchased the Guidant Medical Corporation in 2005, thus becoming the owner of the Guidant and CPI trademarks.

For generators with programmable magnet behavior (Biotronik [Berlin, Germany; US Headquarters: Lake Oswego, OR], Boston Scientific, and St. Jude Medical [Syl Mar, CA]), only an interrogation with a programmer can reveal current settings. Most manufacturers publish a reference guide, although not all of these guides list all magnet idiosyncrasies.

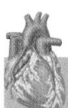 Preanesthetic Evaluation and Pacemaker Reprogramming

Preoperative management of the patient with a pacemaker includes evaluation and optimization of coexisting disease(s). No special laboratory tests or radiographs (chest films are remarkably insensitive for determination of lead problems) are needed for the patient with a pacemaker. Such testing should be dictated by the patient's underlying disease(s), medication(s), and planned intervention. For programmable devices, interrogation with a programmer remains the only reliable method for evaluating lead performance and obtaining current program information. A chest film might be useful to document the position of the coronary sinus lead in a patient with a BiV pacemaker or defibrillator, especially if central venous catheter placement is planned, because spontaneous coronary sinus lead dislodgement was found in more than 11% of patients in early studies.[27,28] A chest radiograph is certainly indicated for the patient with a device problem discovered during his or her pacemaker evaluation.

The prudent anesthesiologist will review the patient's pacemaker history and follow-up schedule. Under the name NASPE, the HRS has published a consensus statement suggesting that pacemakers should be evaluated routinely with telephone checks for battery condition at least every 3 months. NASPE also recommends a comprehensive evaluation (interrogation) at least once per year. There are additional checks for devices implanted fewer than 6 or greater than 48 (dual chamber) or 72 (single chamber) months.[29] In abstract form, Rozner et al[30] reported a two-year retrospective review of follow-up intervals in patients who presented for an anesthetic, finding that more than 32% of 172 patients presenting for an anesthetic at their hospital did not meet the HRS-NASPE guideline for comprehensive evaluation. They also reported that 5% of the patients presented for their anesthetic with a pacemaker in need of replacement for battery depletion, and nearly 10% of patients had less than optimal pacing settings.[30] Note that a recent preoperative interrogation remains a part of the American College of Cardiology guidelines.[2]

Important features of the preanesthetic device evaluation are shown in Box 25-3. Determining pacing dependency might require temporary reprogramming to a VVI mode with a low rate. In patients from countries where pacemakers might be reused,[31,32] battery performance might not be related to length of implantation in the current patient. Clinicians also should note that in a registry of 345 pacemaker generator failures, 7% of failures were not related to battery depletion.[33]

BOX 25-3. PREANESTHETIC PULSE GENERATOR (PACEMAKER, IMPLANTED CARDIOVERTER-DEFIBRILLATOR) EVALUATION

Determining the indication for and date of initial device placement
Identifying the number and types of leads
Determining the last generator test date and battery status
Obtaining a history of generator events (if any)
Obtaining the current program information (device interrogation)
Ensuring that generator discharges become mechanical systoles with adequate safety margins
Ensuring that magnet detection is enabled
Determining whether the pacing mode should be reprogrammed

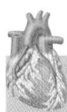

BOX 25-4. PACEMAKER REPROGRAMMING PROBABLY NEEDED

Any rate-responsive device (problems are well-known,[151,152] problems have been misinterpreted with potential for patient injury,[24,42,44,153] and the FDA has issued an alert regarding devices with minute ventilation sensors; see Box 25-5 for pacemakers with minute ventilation sensors[49])
Special pacing indication (hypertrophic obstructive cardiomyopathy, dilated cardiomyopathy, pediatric patient)
Pacing-dependent patient
Major procedure in the chest or abdomen
Special procedures (see Box 25-6)

Appropriate reprogramming (Box 25-4) might be the safest way to avoid intraoperative problems, especially if monopolar "Bovie" electrocautery will be used. For lithotripsy, consideration should be given to programming the pacing function from an atrial-paced mode, as some lithotriptors are designed to fire on the R wave, and the atrial pacing stimulus could be misinterpreted as the contraction of the ventricle.[34]

Most cardiac rhythm management device manufacturers stand ready to assist with this task (see Appendix 25-2 for company telephone numbers). Reprogramming a pacemaker to asynchronous pacing at a rate greater than the patient's underlying rate usually ensures that no oversensing or undersensing during EMI will take place, thus protecting the patient. Reprogramming a device *will not* protect it from internal damage or reset caused by EMI.

Experts do not agree on the appropriate reprogramming for the pacing-dependent patient. Setting a device to asynchronous mode to prevent inappropriate oversensing and ventricular output suppression can cause the pacemaker to ignore premature atrial or ventricular systoles, which could have the potential to create a malignant rhythm in the patient with significant structural compromise of the myocardium.[35] Reviews by Stone and McPherson,[7] as well as Rozner,[36] and several case reports[37,38] demonstrate inappropriate R-on-T pacing with the development of a malignant ventricular rhythm. Hayes and Strathmore[39] suggest the VVT mode for the pacing-dependent patient because EMI will generally increase the pacing rate rather than inhibit the pacing output. However, they do not consider the upper pacing rate for this mode. Although some pacemakers limit VVT pacing rates to the maximum tracking rate (i.e., Boston Scientific), others will pace to the lower of the runaway pacing rate (typically around 200 beats/min) or the minimum V-V interval defined by the ventricular refractory period (i.e., Medtronic Corporation, Minneapolis, MN), which is typically 200 milliseconds (representing 300 beats/min). There are two other caveats for this mode: for the patient with a dual-chamber device and in need of atrioventricular synchrony to sustain cardiac output, hemodynamics might be compromised during VVT operation because ventricular pacing will take place without regard to atrial activity. In addition, in the VVT mode without rate-smoothing enabled, considerable increases and decreases in paced rate could result during EMI. If VVT reprogramming is to be considered, the manufacturer should be contacted regarding programming for the upper rate.

In general, rate responsiveness and other "enhancements" (hysteresis, sleep rate, atrioventricular search, etc.) should be disabled by programming because many of these can mimic pacing system malfunction (see Figure 25-2).[40-42] Note that for many CPI Boston Scientific devices,

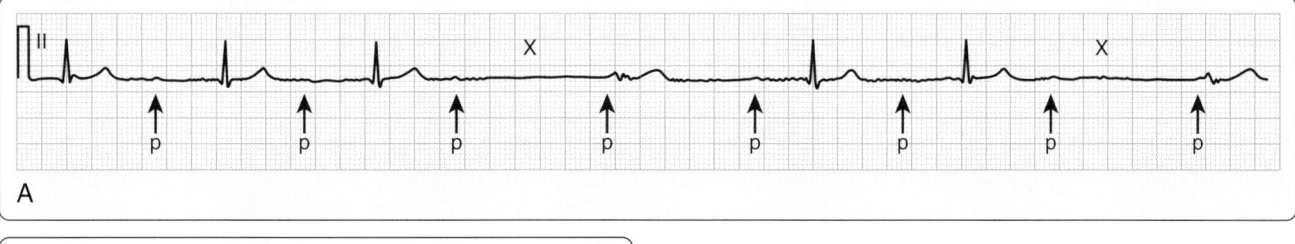

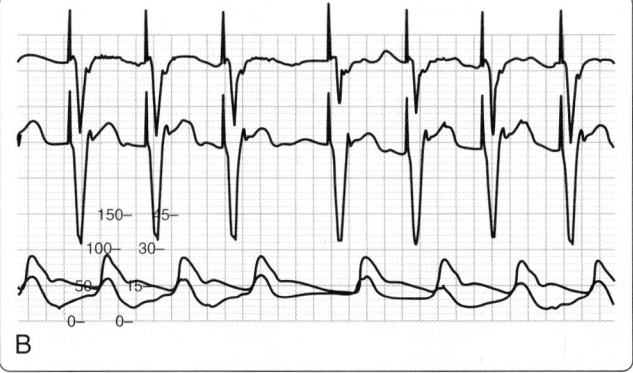

Figure 25-2 *A,* The search feature "managed ventricular pacing" mimics pacing system malfunction. This is a patient with a sinus rate of 50 and a native PR interval of nearly 500 milliseconds. Her Medtronic pacing device was set to AAIR-DDDR (called *managed ventricular pacing* [MVP]), which does not pace the ventricle in response to an atrial event until a native QRS is not conducted (dropped). The next atrial event will be followed by an immediate (60-millisecond) paced QRS. Two such events (marked *X*) are shown after the third and seventh P waves. The subsequent paced QRS morphology axis is nearly orthogonal to the sensing axis, which is labeled (but might not actually be) lead 2, depending on the placement of the actual leads. MVP does not permit two consecutive dropped QRS events, and if two of any four QRS events are dropped, the pacing device paces in DDD mode for at least 1 minute before resuming MVP. However, because oversensing from monopolar electrosurgery can convince a pacing device that ventricular systoles are present, a patient with atrioventricular nodal disease undergoing surgery with monopolar electrosurgery could demonstrate many dropped QRS events. *B,* The feature "search hysteresis" mimics pacemaker malfunction. This patient has a single-chamber VVI pacemaker set to a lower rate of 70/min. It was placed for complete atrioventricular block. This programmable feature causes the pacemaker to delay pacing every 256th event for 1400 milliseconds (equal to a rate of 50/min). This delay in pacing is shown between the third and fourth QRS complexes. From top to bottom, the tracings are lead II, lead V5, the invasive arterial pressure, and the central venous pressure. Hysteresis (where the pacemaker delays pacing after an intrinsic event) and search hysteresis often confuse caregivers regarding pacemaker malfunction (called *pseudomalfunction*). This electrocardiographic tracing could also result from ventricular oversensing, usually related to the T wave.

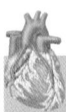

BOX 25-5. PACEMAKERS WITH MINUTE VENTILATION (BIOIMPEDANCE) SENSORS

Boston Scientific/Guidant/CPI—Pulsar, Pulsar Max I and II (1170, 1171, 1172, 1180, 1181, 1270, 1272, 1280); Insignia Plus or Ultra (1190, 1194, 1290, 1291, 1297, 1298); Altrua 40 or 60 (S401, S402, S403, S404, S601, S602, S603, S606)
ELA Medical—Brio (212, 220, 222); Chorus RM (7034, 7134); Opus RM (4534); Reply DR (no number); Rhapsody (D2410 [outside United States only], DR2530); Symphony (DR2550); Talent (113, 133, 213, 223, 233)
Medtronic—Kappa 400 series (KDR401, KDR403, KSR401, KSR403)
Telectronics/St. Jude—Meta (1202, 1204, 1206, 1230, 1250, 1254, 1256); Tempo (1102, 1902, 2102, 2902)

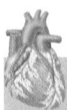

BOX 25-6. SPECIAL PROCEDURES IN PATIENTS WITH IMPLANTABLE GENERATORS

Lithotripsy—acceptable with precautions to protect the generator and, possibly, programming out of an atrial pacing mode[34]
TUR and uterine hysteroscopy—procedures using monopolar electrocautery that can be easily accomplished after device reprogramming
Magnetic resonance imaging (MRI)—**absolutely contraindicated** by most generator manufacturers, and deaths have been reported[62]; however, a recent report suggests that appropriate patients can safely undergo MRI,[64] but not without appropriate precautions[65]
Electroconvulsive therapy—requires asynchronous (nonsensing) mode[154]
Nerve stimulator testing/therapy—inappropriate detection of transcutaneous electrical nerve stimulation (TENS), neuromuscular, and chiropractic electrical muscle stimulation as ventricular tachycardia or ventricular fibrillation has been reported[155,156]

the physician's manual recommends increasing the pacing voltage to "5 volts or higher" in any case in which the monopolar electrosurgical unit (ESU) will be used. In 1986, Levine et al[43] noted an increase in the amount of energy required to pace the ventricle (i.e., a pacing threshold increase) in the setting of intrathoracic surgery and monopolar ESU use. Both Pili-Floury et al[13] and Rozner et al[30] have reported increases in atrial (Rozner only) and ventricular (both reports) pacing thresholds after operations involving pacemaker (but not ICD) cases in which the monopolar ESU was used, large volume and blood shifts were observed, or both. Although many of the operations were thoracic explorations, no pacing threshold changes were noted for these cases. No cardiopulmonary bypass cases were in these cohorts.

Special attention must be given to any device with a minute ventilation (bioimpedance) sensor (Box 25-5), because inappropriate tachycardia has been observed secondary to mechanical ventilation,[44,45] monopolar "Bovie" ESU,[44,46,47] and connection to an electrocardiographic (ECG) monitor with respiratory rate monitoring.[48,49]

Intraoperative (or Procedure) Management

No special monitoring or anesthetic technique is required for the patient with a pacemaker. However, ECG monitoring of the patient must include the ability to detect pacemaker discharges. Often, noise filtering on the ECG monitor must be changed to permit demonstration of the pacemaker pulse, and devices such as a nerve stimulator can interfere with detection and display of the pacemaker pulses.[50]

In addition, patient monitoring must include the ability to ensure that myocardial electrical activity is converted to mechanical systoles. Mechanical systoles are best evaluated by pulse oximetry plethysmography or arterial waveform display. Some patients might need an increased pacing rate during the perioperative period to meet an increased oxygen demand. A pulmonary artery catheter (PAC), an esophageal Doppler monitor, or a transesophageal echocardiogram can be used to evaluate pacing frequency and its relation to cardiac output. In addition to blood pressure and systemic vascular resistance, the monitoring of acid-base status might be needed to determine adequacy of cardiac output.

With respect to anesthetic technique, no studies have championed one over another. Nevertheless, a number of reports of prolongation of the QT interval with the use of isoflurane or sevoflurane have been published. Halothane appears to reduce this interval.[51-55] No interactions have been reported for enflurane or desflurane.

Monopolar "Bovie" electrocautery (ESU) use remains the principal intraoperative issue for the patient with a pacemaker. Between 1984 and 1997, the FDA was notified of 456 adverse events with pulse generators, 255 from electrocautery, and a "significant number" of device failures.[56] Monopolar ESU is more likely to cause problems than bipolar ESU, and patients with unipolar electrode configuration are more sensitive to EMI than those with bipolar configurations. Coagulation ESU will likely cause more problems than nonblended "cutting" ESU.[57] Magnet placement during electrocautery might allow reprogramming of an

older (pre-1990) generator; however, newer generators are relatively immune to such effects. In fact, most devices from Boston Scientific, as well as St. Jude, cannot be reprogrammed in the presence of a magnet. Note, however, that strong EMI can produce an electrical reset or a detection of battery depletion, which might change the programming mode or rate, or both. If monopolar electrocautery is to be used, then the current return pad should be placed to ensure that the electrocautery current path does not cross the pacemaking system. For cases such as head and neck surgery, the pad might be best placed on the shoulder contralateral to the implanted device. For breast and axillary cases, the pad might need to be placed on the ipsilateral arm with the wire prepped into the field by sterile plastic cover. Procedures with special pacing ramifications are shown in Box 25-6.

The use of an ultrasonic cutting device, commonly called a *harmonic scalpel*, has been championed to prevent EMI while providing the surgeon with the ability to both cut and coagulate tissue. A number of case reports demonstrate successful surgery without EMI issues in these patients.[58-61]

At this time, MRI deserves special mention. In general, MRI has been contraindicated in pacemaker and ICD patients.[62,63] However, a landmark article showing that MRI could be conducted safely in some patients has led to performance of MRI evaluations in these patients.[64] Nevertheless, not all MRI sequences and energy levels have been studied, and judicious monitoring and caution are advised.[65,66] Medtronic Corporation is testing a pacing generator and lead system called Enrhythm MRI SureScan (current model is EMDR01), which has special programming modes and leads for MRI scanning.[67] It is already approved in several European countries.

Pacemaker Failure

Pacemaker failure has three causes: (1) failure of capture, (2) lead failure, or (3) generator failure. Failure of capture because of a defect at the level of the myocardium (i.e., the generator continues to fire but no myocardial depolarization takes place) remains the most difficult problem to treat. Myocardial changes that result in noncapture include myocardial ischemia/infarction, acid-base disturbance, electrolyte abnormalities, or abnormal levels of antiarrhythmic drug(s). Note that temporary pacing (transvenous, transcutaneous, transthoracic, or transesophageal) might inhibit pacemaker output at voltages that will not produce myocardial capture.[68] Sympathomimetic drugs generally lower pacing threshold. Outright generator or lead failure is rare.

Temporary Pacemakers

Several techniques are available to the anesthesiologist to establish reliable temporary pacing during the perioperative period or in the intensive care unit.[69] Cardiovascular anesthesiologists are more likely than the generalists to routinely use temporary transvenous or epicardial pacing in their practices. Temporary cardiac pacing can serve as definitive therapy for transient bradyarrhythmias or as a bridge to permanent generator placement.

The various forms of temporary pacing include many transvenous catheter systems, transcutaneous pads, transthoracic wires, and esophageal pacing techniques. This section reviews the indications for temporary cardiac pacing and discusses the techniques available to the anesthesiologist. Many of the references in this section are older because temporary pacing is a well-established technique and not many advances have taken place since the early 1990s. Table 25-2 summarizes these techniques.

Regardless of temporary modality, most implanted pacemakers or ICDs need to be reprogrammed when placing any temporary pacing device. Electrical energy entering the body from a temporary pacing device can be sensed by the permanent device on the atrial lead, the ventricular lead, or both. Energy sensed on a ventricular lead can result in an inappropriate shock from an ICD or pacing inhibition from a pacemaker or ICD. Pacing inhibition in a pacing-dependent patient will produce asystole. If energy enters the cardiac rhythm management device on the atrial lead in a dual-chamber device, then rapid ventricular pacing might result (intrinsic atrial rate plus temporary atrial rate). The cardiac rhythm management device might "detect" an atrial arrhythmia condition, resulting in ventricular pacing only, which might produce untoward hemodynamics.

Indications for Temporary Pacing

Temporary pacemakers are commonly used after cardiac surgery,[70] in the treatment of drug toxicity resulting in arrhythmias, with certain arrhythmias complicating myocardial infarction, and for intraoperative bradycardia caused by β-blocker use. On occasion, the placement of a temporary pacing system can assist in the hemodynamic management in the perioperative period. Abnormal electrolytes, preoperative β-blocker use, and many intraoperative drugs have the potential to aggravate bradycardia and bradycardia-dependent arrhythmias.[71] Because drugs used to treat bradyarrhythmias have a number of important disadvantages compared with temporary pacing, hemodynamically unstable perioperative bradyarrhythmias should be considered an indication for temporary pacing (Table 25-3). If the patient already has epicardial wires or a pacing catheter or wires, or transesophageal pacing is feasible, pacing is preferred to pharmacologic therapy. However, transcutaneous and ventricular-only transvenous pacing, even if feasible, may exacerbate hemodynamic problems in patients with heart disease because these pacing modalities do not preserve atrioventricular synchrony (i.e., produce ventricular or global activation).

TABLE 25-3	Temporary Pacing Indications
Patient Condition	*Event Requiring Temporary Pacing*
Acute myocardial infarction	Symptomatic bradycardia, medically refractory
	New bundle branch block with transient complete heart block
	Complete heart block
	Postoperative complete heart block
	Symptomatic congenital heart block
	Mobitz II with anterior myocardial infarction
	New bifascicular block
	Bilateral bundle branch block and first-degree atrioventricular block
	Symptomatic alternating Wenckebach block
	Symptomatic alternating bundle branch block
Tachycardia treatment or prevention	Bradycardia-dependent VT
	Torsade de pointes
	Long QT syndrome
	Treatment of recurrent SVT or VT
Prophylactic	Pulmonary artery catheter placement with left bundle branch block (controversial)
	New atrioventricular block or bundle branch block in acute endocarditis
	Cardioversion with sick sinus syndrome
	Postdefibrillation bradycardia
	Counteract perioperative pharmacologic treatment causing hemodynamically significant bradycardia
	AF prophylaxis postcardiac surgery
	Postorthotopic heart transplantation

AF, atrial fibrillation; SVT, supraventricular tachycardias, VT, ventricular tachycardia.

Nearly every indication for a permanent pacemaker is an indication for temporary pacing in patients without a pacemaker who, because of circumstances (emergency surgery, critically ill), cannot have elective permanent pacemaker implantation. Temporary pacing also may be needed before implantation of a permanent pacemaker to stabilize patients with hemodynamically significant bradycardia.

Temporary pacing is also indicated if a patient with a myocardial infarction complicated by second- or third-degree heart block is scheduled for emergency surgery. Bifascicular block in an asymptomatic patient is not reason enough for temporary pacing before surgery.[72] Bellocci et al[73] reported no occurrence of complete heart block in 98 patients with preoperative bifascicular block undergoing general anesthesia, despite 14% having prolonged conduction through their His-Purkinje system. The development of new bifascicular block immediately after surgery, though, suggests perioperative myocardial ischemia or infarction, and temporary pacing might be required.

TABLE 25-2	Comparison of Temporary Pacing Techniques					
Temporary Pacing Method	*Time to Initiate*	*Chambers Paced*	*Advantages*	*Disadvantages*	*Uses*
Transcutaneous	1–2 minutes	Right ventricle	Simple, rapid, safe	Variable capture, chest wall movement, patient discomfort	Arrest, intraoperative, prophylactic
Transesophageal	Minutes	Left atrium	Reliable atrial capture, safe, simple	Requires special generator	Prophylactic atrial pacing, overdrive pacing for supraventricular tachyarrhythmia, monitoring atrial electrogram
Transvenous semirigid	3–20 minutes	Atrium and/or ventricle	Most reliable, well tolerated	Invasive, time, consuming, potential complications	Arrest, prophylactic, maintenance
Transvenous flow-directed	3–20 minutes	Right ventricle	Simple, does not require fluoroscopy	Invasive, stability questions, less readily available	Arrest, intraoperative, prophylactic, maintenance
Pacing pulmonary artery catheter (PAC)	Minutes (if PAC in place)	Atrium and/or ventricle	Reliable ventricular capture, well tolerated	Requires specific PAC, which must be placed first	Arrest, intraoperative, prophylactic, maintenance
Epicardial pacing wires	< 1 minute	Atrium and/or ventricle	Reliable short-term	Postoperative only, early lead failure	Arrest, prophylactic, maintenance
Transthoracic	10–60 seconds	Ventricle	Rapid and simple	Many potential complications	Arrest only

Surgical resection of neck and carotid sinus tumors may cause bradyarrhythmias requiring temporary cardiac pacing during surgical manipulation. Neurosurgical procedures involving the brainstem also may be associated with significant bradycardia.

Temporary antitachycardia pacing is most commonly used after cardiac surgery.[74] With increased availability of effective noninvasive pacing technology, antitachycardia pacing might be offered to other perioperative patients as well. Even when used properly, these techniques can induce more dangerous arrhythmias, and proper resuscitation equipment should be available.

Atrioventricular junctional tachycardia can occur after cardiopulmonary bypass, when it could be a manifestation of reperfusion injury or, possibly, inadequate myocardial protection during perfusion. Atrioventricular junctional tachycardia does not respond well to most drug therapy, although its rate (≤ 120 beats/min in adults) may be slowed by β-adrenergic blockers or edrophonium. Atrioventricular junctional tachycardia is best managed by atrial or atrioventricular sequential overdrive pacing because both of these modalities will preserve atrioventricular synchrony. Frequently, there is resumption of sinus rhythm on withdrawal of temporary pacing.

Most sudden-onset paroxysmal supraventricular tachycardia (PSVT) is initiated by a premature beat, which could be of atrial, atrioventricular junctional, or ventricular origin. PSVT may be terminated by competitive, atrial underdrive pacing (paced rate < PSVT rate) if, by chance, an atrial capture beat interferes with the circulating wavefront perpetuating the tachycardia. In contrast, with overdrive pacing, PSVT is paced at a rate 10% to 15% in excess of the tachycardia rate until there is evidence of 1:1 capture with paced beats. Pacing is continued at this rate for 20 to 30 seconds, then gradually slowed to some predetermined rate, and finally terminated. As with all pacing modalities, a gradual reduction in pacing rate is recommended in patients known to have sinus node dysfunction to reduce the risk for prolonged asystole when pacing is terminated. If pacing fails to terminate PSVT, or PSVT produces circulatory collapse, immediate DC cardioversion is recommended.

Type I atrial flutter (flutter rate < 320 to 340 beats/min) is pace terminable, but type II flutter (> 340 beats/min) is not. Type I flutter is treated by atrial overdrive pacing at a rate 15 to 20 beats/min more than the flutter rate and is increased by 10 to 20 beats/min if the first attempt is not successful. Once atrial capture is evident, pacing is continued for 20 to 30 seconds and then slowed as for PSVT. Usually, type I atrial flutter can be terminated by overdrive pacing, with prompt restoration of normal sinus rhythm.

Relative contraindications to transvenous ventricular pacing include digitalis toxicity with ventricular tachycardia (VT), tricuspid valve prostheses, or the presence of a coagulopathy. Pacing in the setting of severe hypothermia might induce ventricular fibrillation (VF) or alter the normal compensatory physiologic mechanisms to the hypothermia, although one prospective study in dogs using transcutaneous pacing suggests that pacing decreases rewarming time.[75] Atrial fibrillation, multifocal atrial tachycardia, and significant atrioventricular conduction system disease are contraindications to transvenous *atrial* pacing.

Transvenous Temporary Pacing

Transvenous cardiac pacing provides the most reliable means of temporary pacing. Temporary transvenous pacing is dependable and well tolerated by patients. With a device that can provide both atrial and ventricular pacing, transvenous pacing can maintain atrioventricular synchrony and improve cardiac output. Disadvantages include the need for practitioner experience, time to appropriately place the wire(s) to provide capture, the potential complications of line placement and manipulation, and the need for fluoroscopy in many cases. Three different types of typical transvenous leads are shown in Figure 25-3. (See Videos on the website.)

Rapid catheter positioning is most easily obtained by using the right internal jugular vein, even without fluoroscopy,[76] although a prudent practitioner might want to clearly document the final position(s) of the catheters. The left subclavian vein is also easily utilized in emergent situations. Other sites are often impassable without fluoroscopy. In addition, brachial and femoral venous routes can increase the frequency of lead dislodgments during motion of the extremities, especially during patient transport.

Once central access is obtained, the lead is guided into position using hemodynamic data (not possible with the simple bipolar lead catheter) or by fluoroscopic guidance. Electrocardiographic guidance is less desirable. The right atrial appendage and RV apex provide the most stable catheter positions. Techniques for placement into these positions are part of cardiology training and likely are foreign to most anesthesiologists. When fluoroscopy is unavailable or in emergency situations, a flow-directed catheter can be attempted using pressure or ECG guidance. Once the right ventricle is entered, the balloon is deflated, if used, and the catheter gently advanced until electrical capture is noted. Flow-directed catheters and a right internal jugular approach afford the shortest insertion times.[77] The reported incidence of successful capture in urgent situations without fluoroscopy ranges from 30% to 90%.[76,78,79]

Once catheters are positioned, pacing is initiated using the distal electrode as the cathode and the proximal electrode as the anode. Ideally, the capture thresholds should be less than 1 mA and generator output should be maintained at three times threshold as a safety margin. In dual-chamber pacing, atrioventricular delays of between 100 and 200 milliseconds are used. Many patients are sensitive to this parameter. Cardiac output optimization with echocardiography and/or mixed venous oxygen saturation can be used to maximize hemodynamics when adjusting atrioventricular delay.[80] Atrioventricular sequential pacing is clearly beneficial in many patients,[80–84] but it should be remembered that emergency pacing starts with *ventricular* capture alone. There is a potential risk of interference of external pacemaker generators by walkie-talkies and digital cellular phones.[85,86] Clinicians should also be aware of all complications related to transvenous lead placement.[87]

Pacing Pulmonary Artery Catheters

The pulmonary artery atrioventricular pacing TD catheter (see Figure 25-3C) was described by Zaidan in 1983.[88] It allows for atrioventricular sequential pacing via electrodes attached to the outside of the catheter, as well as routine PAC functions. Combination of the two functions into one catheter eliminates the need for separate insertion of temporary transvenous pacing electrodes. However, several potential disadvantages exist with this catheter including: (1) varying success in initiating and maintaining capture,[88] (2) external electrode displacement from the catheter,[89] and (3) relatively high cost as compared with standard PACs. The Paceport PAC (see Figure 25-3B) provides ventricular pacing with a separate bipolar pacing lead (Chandler probe), which allows for more stable ventricular pacing, as well as hemodynamic measurements.[90] This catheter has been used for successful resuscitation after cardiac arrest during closed-chest cardiac massage when attempts to capture with transcutaneous and transvenous flow-directed bipolar pacing catheters had failed. However, this unit does not provide the potential advantages associated with atrial pacing capability. The newer pulmonary artery A-V Paceport adds a sixth lumen to the older Paceport to allow placement of an atrial J-wire, flexible tip bipolar pacing lead. Both of these Paceport catheters are placed by transducing the RV port to assure correct positioning of the port 1 to 2 cm distal to the tricuspid valve. This position usually guides the ventricular wire (Chandler probe) to the apex where adequate capture should occur with minimal current requirements. Although ventricular capture is easily obtained, atrial capture can be more difficult and less reliable.[80] This catheter has been used successfully after cardiac surgery.[80,91] The atrial wire can be used to diagnose supraventricular tachyarrhythmias (SVTs) by atrial electrograms and to overdrive atrial flutter and reentrant SVTs.[92]

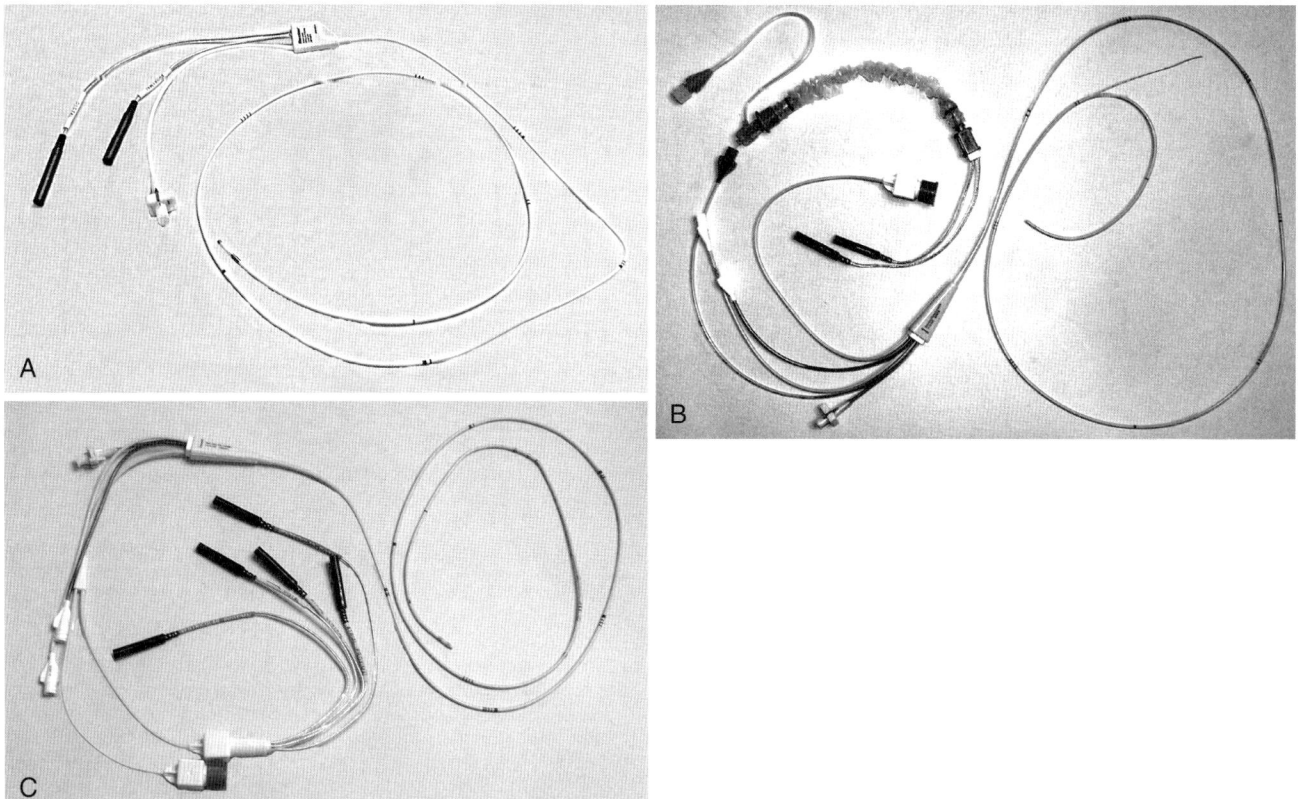

Figure 25-3 **A variety of transvenous pacing leads is shown.** *A*, A simple, flow-directed, bipolar pacing wire. This lead is placed through a 6F introducer sheath, and it is advanced (usually under fluoroscopy) into the atrium or ventricle until mechanical systoles result from the electrical pacing event (called *pacing capture*). The principal disadvantage of this lead is the lack of hemodynamic measurements to guide placement. *B*, A specially adapted pulmonary artery catheter with a channel for a bipolar, ventricular pacing wire. The bipolar pacing wire, side-port adapter, and condom are packaged separately from the pulmonary artery catheter. Note that the electrode is shown protruding from its orifice just distal to the 20-cm mark on the pulmonary artery catheter. *C*, An atrioventricular-capable, pacing pulmonary artery catheter. Five electrodes are present: two for ventricular pacing and three for atrial pacing. This catheter is positioned to provide adequate ventricular capture, after which atrial pacing is attempted using two of the three atrial electrodes. Sometimes the entire PA catheter must be repositioned to obtain atrial capture. In the setting of a functioning atrioventricular node, atrial capture can be determined by the presence of a narrow complex QRS following the atrial pace. In the setting of a significant atrioventricular block, atrial capture can be difficult to assess.

Transcutaneous Pacing

Transcutaneous pacing, first described by Zoll,[93] is readily available and can be implemented rapidly in emergency situations. Capture rate is variable and the technique may cause pain in awake patients, but usually it is tolerated until temporary transvenous pacing can be instituted. It may be effective even when endocardial pacing fails.[94] It is now considered by many to be the method of choice for prophylactic and emergent applications.[95]

The large patches typically are placed anteriorly (negative electrode or cathode) over the palpable cardiac apex (or V$_3$ lead location) and posteriorly (positive electrode or anode) at the inferior aspect of the scapula. The anode also has been placed on the anterior right chest with success in healthy volunteers.[96] The skin should be cleaned with alcohol (but not abraded) to reduce capture threshold and improve patient comfort. Abraded skin can cause more discomfort. Typical thresholds are 20 to 120 mA, but pacing may require up to 200 mA at long pulse durations of 20 to 40 milliseconds.[97] Transcutaneous pacing appears to capture the right ventricle, followed by near-simultaneous activation of the entire left ventricle. The hemodynamic response is similar to that of RV endocardial pacing. Both methods can cause reductions in left ventricular systolic pressure, a decrease in stroke volume, and an increase in right-sided pressures because of atrioventricular dyssynchrony. Capture should be confirmed by palpation or display of a peripheral pulse. Maintenance current is set 5 to 10 mA above threshold as tolerated by the patient. Success rates appear to be greatest when the system is used

prophylactically or early after arrest, upward of 90%.[98,99] When used in emergent situations, successful capture rates are usually lower but range from 10% to 93%.[100-102] A 3-year study of out-of-hospital asystolic arrest showed no difference in survival for the group that received early transcutaneous pacing compared with the group that received basic CPR without pacing.[103] Similarly, early use during in-hospital arrests may not alter long-term survival.[104] This technique also has been used to terminate VT, atrioventricular nodal reentrant tachycardia, and atrioventricular reciprocating tachycardia.[102,105]

Coughing and discomfort from cutaneous stimulation are the most frequent problems. The technique poses no electrical threat to medical personnel, and complications are rare. There have been no reports of significant damage to myocardium, skeletal muscle, skin, or lungs in humans despite continuous pacing for up to 108 hours and intermittent pacing for up to 17 days.[93,98,106] Several commercially available defibrillators include transcutaneous pacing generators as standard equipment.

Esophageal Pacing

The newest technique available to anesthesiologists is esophageal pacing, and it has been shown to be quite reliable,[107-109] even in children.[110] Significant bradycardia, secondary to underlying sinus node pathology or pharmacologic effects, can occur during anesthesia. The response to pharmacologic therapy for significant bradycardia with vagolytic drugs can be unpredictable and difficult to sustain accurately.[111] Chronotropic drugs may have little effect, or they can produce tachyarrhythmias or myocardial ischemia, or both. Esophageal pacing is relatively noninvasive and well tolerated, even in the majority of awake patients, and it appears to be devoid of serious complications. This modality is useful for heart rate support of cardiac output, overdrive suppression of reentrant SVT, and for diagnostic atrial electrograms. Ventricular capture must be excluded before attempts at rapid atrial pacing for overdrive suppression to prevent potential VT or VF. Some surgical positions (e.g., three-quarter prone) can increase the chance of unintentional ventricular capture.[112]

Problems with esophageal pacing include (1) the necessity for special generators that must provide 20 to 30 mA of current with wide pulse widths of 10 to 20 milliseconds and (2) the ability to pace only the left atrium reliably and not the left ventricle, which can be a significant problem in emergency situations.[107] In comparison, typical temporary generators designed for endocardial pacing have a maximum output of 20 mA with pulse width durations of only 1 to 2 milliseconds.

A typical transesophageal pacing generator and lead are shown in Figure 25-4. As noted in Figure 25-4, the pacing stimulus is delivered

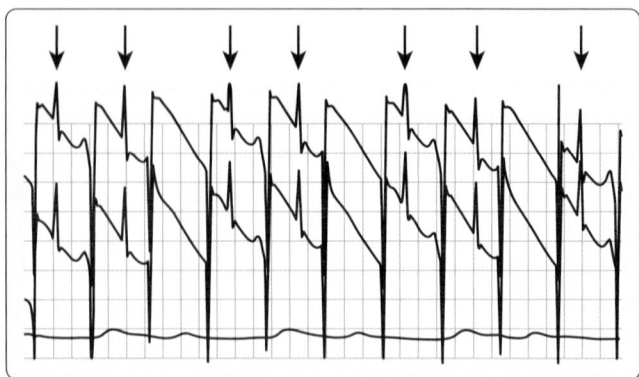

Figure 25-5 An electrocardiographic strip from a patient with a transesophageal pacemaker demonstrating atrial capture and Wenckebach second-degree A-V nodal block. An 84-year-old man with coronary artery disease and taking atenolol developed a sinus bradycardia (rate, 37/min) with hypotension during a general anesthetic for transurethral bladder resection. An esophageal pacemaker was placed and the rate was set to 85 beats/min (this is AOO pacing mode). The top two tracings are electrocardiographic leads II and V5. The downward depolarization artifacts are the pacing stimuli from the esophageal pacemaker (15-mA output). The upward depolarization events are the QRS inscriptions, which are highlighted by the *downward arrows*. Atrial P waves can be found shortly after the esophageal pulse. Note the lengthening PR interval with the dropped ventricular depolarizations. Also note how distorted the electrocardiographic signal becomes in the setting of an esophageal pacemaker. The third tracing is the pulse oximeter plethysmographic waveform. The small graticules (representing the 40-millisecond time points) and the monitor text were digitally removed from this strip to increase the contrast.

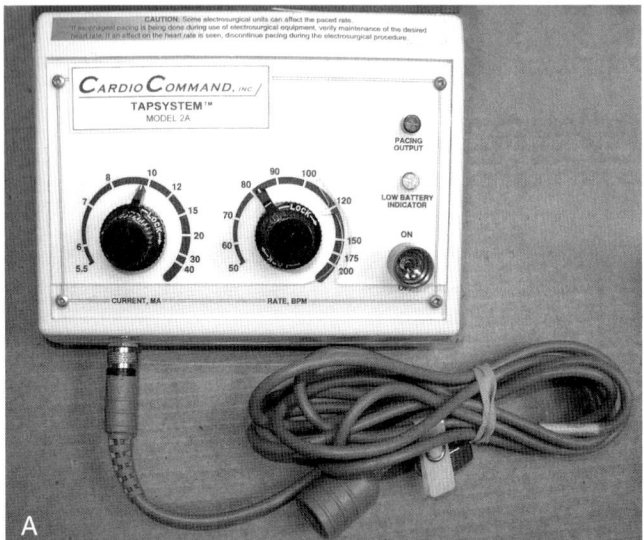

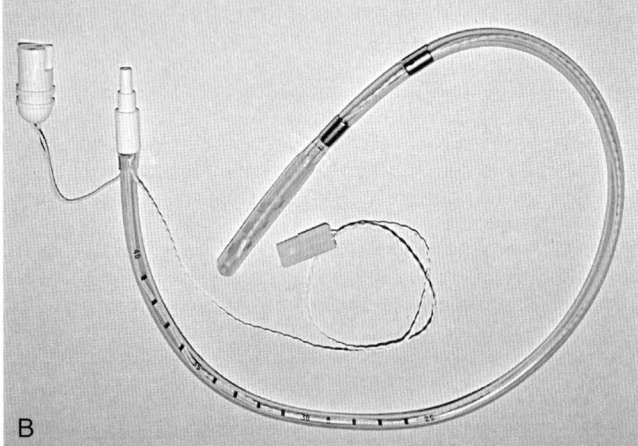

Figure 25-4 A typical transesophageal pacing generator *(A)* and esophageal stethoscope with bipolar electrodes *(B)*. The esophageal stethoscope is placed to between 30 and 40 cm from the teeth, and pacing is initiated at a rate greater than the patient's native heart rate using an output setting of at least 20 mA. Atrial capture is determined by an increase in peripheral pulse rate. Detection of capture using only electrocardiographic monitoring can be difficult to discern because the pacing impulse from these generators produces a large artifact and often distorts the surface electrocardiogram.

in asynchronous atrial-only mode through a modified esophageal stethoscope. Pacing is initiated by connecting the system and placing the esophageal stethoscope to a depth of 30 to 40 cm from the teeth. Capture should be confirmed using the peripheral pulse (i.e., from the pulse oximeter plethysmogram or an invasive hemodynamic monitor) because the pacing stimulus often is large relative to the QRS and frequently fools the ECG counting algorithm on the monitor (Figure 25-5). Atrial capture is obtained in virtually all patients using outputs of 8 to 20 mA, and the output should be set to two to three times the threshold for capture. Thresholds are not influenced by weight, age, atrial size, or previous cardiac surgery.[109] Because there is no sensing element involved, esophageal pacing is AOO mode pacing.

Transesophageal *ventricular* pacing is generally unreliable, yet the optimal site appears to be 2 to 4 cm distal to the atrial site.[113] The esophageal stethoscope also can be used (with a special adapter) to record the intra-atrial electrogram.

No long-term complications with this modality have been described. Induction of ventricular tachyarrhythmias during rapid atrial pacing has been noted. No significant esophageal trauma has been reported despite long-term use of up to 60 hours.[114] Phrenic nerve stimulation has been described.[108]

▆ Transthoracic Pacing

Transthoracic pacing involves the direct introduction of a pacing wire or needle through the thorax into the ventricular cavity. Several commercial kits are available, and even the use of a spinal needle has been described. The technique is rapid, is simple, and does not require venous access or fluoroscopy. In contrast with other temporary pacing modalities, there is a large potential for misadventure, and no study demonstrates any benefit in survival. Transcutaneous techniques have supplanted this procedure in essentially all situations.

Postanesthesia Pacemaker Evaluation

Any pacemaker that was reprogrammed for the perioperative period should be re-evaluated and programmed appropriately. For nonreprogrammed devices, most manufacturers recommend interrogation to ensure proper functioning and remaining battery life if any monopolar electrosurgery was used. In their retrospective review, Trankina et al[115] reported 6% of 169 patients showed a problem during postoperative checks of pacemakers. Senthuran et al[116] suggested that failure to perform a postoperative pacemaker check led to an unexpected postoperative death in Great Britain, and both Pili-Floury et al[13] and Rozner et al[30] reported perioperative pacing issues that could be found and mitigated at the postoperative check. American College of Cardiology guidelines recommend a postprocedure interrogation.[2]

IMPLANTABLE CARDIOVERTER-DEFIBRILLATORS

The development of an implantable, battery-powered device able to deliver sufficient energy to terminate VT or VF has represented a major medical breakthrough for patients with a history of ventricular tachyarrhythmias. These devices prevent death in the setting of malignant ventricular tachyarrhythmias,[117–119] and they clearly remain superior to antiarrhythmic drug therapy.[120,121] Initially approved by the FDA in 1985, the implantation rate currently exceeds 10,000 ICDs per month in the United States.[122] Industry sources report that more than 300,000 patients have these devices today.

A significant number of technologic advances have been applied since the first ICD was placed, including considerable miniaturization (pectoral pocket placement with transvenous leads is the norm), as well as battery improvements that now permit permanent pacing with these devices. Thus, clinicians could easily confuse a pectoral ICD with a pacemaker. Like pacemakers, ICDs have a generic code to indicate lead placement and function (see Table 25-4).[123] The most robust form of identification, called the *label form*, expands the fourth character into its component generic pacemaker code (NBG; see Table 25-1).

ICDs have many programmable features, but essentially they measure each cardiac R-R interval and categorize the rate as normal, too fast (short R-R interval), or too slow (long R-R interval). When the device detects a sufficient number of short R-R intervals within a period of time (all programmable), it will begin an antitachycardia event. The internal computer will decide to choose antitachycardia pacing (less energy use, better tolerated by patient) or shock, depending on the presentation and device programming. If shock is chosen, an internal capacitor is charged. Most newer devices are programmed to reconfirm VT or VF after charging to prevent inappropriate shock therapy (IST). Some ICDs will deliver immediate antitachycardia pacing while charging the capacitor in preparation for a shock. Typically, ICDs have six to eight therapies available for each type of event (VT, fast VT, VF), and some of these therapies can be repeated before moving to the next higher energy sequence. Thus, ICDs can deliver many shocks per event. In an ICD with antitachycardia pacing, once a shock is delivered, no further antitachycardia pacing will take place.

IST occurs in 20% to 40% of ICD patients, with shocks for rhythm other than VT or VF.[124–126] Atrial fibrillation with rapid ventricular response and supraventricular tachycardia remain the most common cause of IST.[127] Whether inappropriate shocks injure patients remains a subject of considerable debate, but a significant number of patients who receive an inappropriate shock will demonstrate increased troponin levels in the absence of an ischemic event,[128] and a death has been reported.[129] Also, IST predicts increased mortality,[130] and statin therapy might reduce the incidence of IST through a reduction in atrial fibrillation.[131] Dual-chamber ICD technology might reduce IST from atrial fibrillation as well. Programmable features in current ICDs to differentiate VT from a tachycardia of supraventricular origin (SVT) include[132]:

1. Onset criteria—in general, onset of VT is abrupt, whereas onset of SVT has sequentially shortening R-R intervals
2. Stability criteria—in general, the R-R interval of VT is relatively constant, whereas the R-R interval of atrial fibrillation with rapid ventricular response is quite variable
3. QRS width criteria—some ICDs measure the QRS width using the RV lead tip to ICD case-sensing pathway; in general, the QRS width in SVT is narrow (<110 milliseconds), whereas the QRS width in VT is wide (>120 milliseconds)
4. "Intelligence" in dual-chamber devices attempting to associate atrial activity with ventricular activity
5. Morphology waveform analysis with comparison with stored historic templates

Note that once the R-R interval becomes sufficiently short for VF detection, the ICD will begin a shock sequence. As noted earlier, once the device delivers any shock therapy, no further antitachycardia pacing will take place. An ICD with antibradycardia pacing capability will begin pacing when the R-R interval is too long. In July 1997, the FDA approved devices with sophisticated dual-chamber pacing modes and rate-responsive behavior for ICD patients who need permanent pacing (about 20% of ICD patients).

Implantable Cardioverter-Defibrillator Indications

Initially, ICDs were placed for hemodynamically significant VT or VF. Newer indications associated with sudden death include long QT syndrome, Brugada syndrome (right bundle branch block, ST-segment elevation in leads V_1-V_3), and arrhythmogenic RV dysplasia.[133] Recent studies suggest that ICDs can be used for primary prevention of sudden death (i.e., before the first episode of VT or VF) in young patients with hypertrophic cardiomyopathy,[134] and data from the second Multicenter Automatic Defibrillator Intervention Trial (MADIT II) suggest that any post-MI patient with ejection fraction (EF) less than 30% should undergo prophylactic implantation of an ICD.[135] Currently, however, the Centers for Medicare and Medicaid (CMS) requires a prolonged QRS interval (to > 120 milliseconds) to qualify for ICD placement in this group.

Several newer trials have included patients with nonischemic cardiomyopathy as well. Data from the Sudden Cardiac Death–Heart Failure Trial (SCD-HeFT),[121] as well as the Defibrillators In Non-Ischemic Cardiomyopathy Treatment Evaluation (DEFINITE)[136] study, now suggest that ICD placement will lower mortality in any patient with EF less than 35% regardless of the cause of the cardiomyopathy. The DEFINITE results are important because these patients were randomized only after initiation of β-blockade and angiotensin-converting enzyme inhibitor therapy, which form the backbone of medical therapy for cardiomyopathy.

Three-chamber (leads placed in atrium, right ventricle, and coronary sinus) ICDs (see Figure 25-1) for CRT (also called *biventricular pacing* [BiV]) have been FDA approved for patients with DCM and prolonged QRS intervals. Two-chamber (leads placed in atrium and right ventricle) ICDs are in clinical trial for patients with hypertrophic obstructive cardiomyopathy who have experienced VT or VF. Box 25-7 reviews ICD indications.

Dilated Cardiomyopathy

With the advent of CRT pacing (CRT-P) for the patient with DCM and prolonged QRS interval,[137] and the approval of ICDs with CRT capability (CRT-D), the presence of a defibrillator with BiV pacing will become

TABLE 25-4	North American Society of Pacing and Electrophysiology/British Pacing and Electrophysiology Group Generic Defibrillator Code (NBD)		
Position I	*Position II*	*Position III*	*Position IV*
Shock Chambers(s)	Antitachycardia Pacing Chamber(s)	Tachycardia Detection	Antibradycardia Pacing Chamber(s)
O = None	O = None	E = Electrogram	O = None
A = Atrium	A = Atrium	H = Hemodynamic	A = Atrium
V = Ventricle	V = Ventricle		V = Ventricle
D = Dual (A+V)	D = Dual (A+V)		D = Dual (A+V)

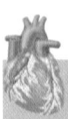

> ### BOX 25-7. IMPLANTED CARDIOVERTER-DEFIBRILLATOR INDICATIONS
>
> Ventricular tachycardia
> Ventricular fibrillation
> Brugada syndrome (right bundle branch block, S-T elevation V_1-V_3)
> Arrhythmogenic right ventricular dysplasia
> Long QT syndrome
> Hypertrophic cardiomyopathy
> Prophylactic use after myocardial infarction, ejection fraction < 30%

more common. Currently, about 550,000 new diagnoses of congestive heart failure are made annually in the United States,[138] and the prevalence of this disease includes 5.7 million patients.[139] Significant risk factors for the development of congestive heart failure include both ischemic heart disease and hypertension.[140] These data, combined with the recent results from SCD-HeFT[121] and MADIT II trials (ICD is indicated in any patient with cardiomyopathy and EF < 30–35%),[135] suggest that the number of patients eligible to receive a defibrillator to include CRT-P will increase dramatically. Whether any country's economy can absorb this economic burden remains to be seen. Currently, CRT-P improves functional status and quality of life[141] and reduces congestive heart failure events,[142] primarily by decreasing the dyssynchrony between the two ventricles in the dilated heart (see Videos on the website.) whether the CRT device includes ICD capability (CRT-D) or not (CRT-P). In addition, CRT-D has been shown to reduce mortality in some but not all studies.[17] However, about 30% of patients who undergo CRT implantation achieve no additional benefit from the multichamber pacing.[143]

Implantable Cardioverter-Defibrillator Magnets

Like pacemakers, magnet behavior in some ICDs can be altered by programming. Most devices will suspend tachyarrhythmia detection (and therefore therapy) when a magnet is appropriately placed to activate the magnet sensor. Some devices from Angeion, Boston Scientific, Pacesetter, and St. Jude Medical can be programmed to ignore magnet placement. *Antitachycardia therapy in some CPI devices can be permanently disabled by magnet placement for 30 seconds,1* although recent upgrades to the Boston Scientific programmer have eliminated this setting after a programming session in most of their Guidant ICDs. In general, magnet application will not affect antibradycardia pacing rate (except ELA* [Milano, Italy; U.S. Headquarters: Arvado, CO]) or pacing mode (except pacing is disabled in Telectronics Guardian 4202/4203*). Interrogating the device and calling the manufacturer remain the most reliable methods for determining magnet response. Magnet effects on ICDs are shown in Appendix 25-3.

Note that reliable confirmation of appropriate magnet placement, and therefore, suspension of antitachyarrhythmic therapy, is present only in Boston Scientific ICDs (tone) and ELA ICDs (pacing rate changes to 90 beats/min if the battery is good; 80 if the battery is at elective replacement). Medtronic marketed a Smart-Magnet device that houses a magnet and electronics to show appropriate disablement of the ICD functions in their device, but this device is not generally available. When using a Smart-Magnet, the "FOUND" light is often extinguished during EMI from the electrosurgical cautery, even though the magnet remains in place. Despite these features in Medtronic and Boston Scientific ICDs, numerous anecdotal reports exist of IST during electrocautery, most often a result of movement of the magnet during patient repositioning.

---

*These two device families were implanted during clinical trials only. Thus, the likelihood of encountering these devices is low; they are included for completeness.

Preanesthetic Evaluation and Implantable Cardioverter-Defibrillator Reprogramming

In general, ALL ICDs should have their antitachycardia therapy disabled before the commencement of any procedure (see American College of Cardiology guidelines[2]), although such action might be unnecessary in a setting without EMI or placement of a metal guidewire into the chest.[144] The comments in the pacing section apply here for any ICD with anti-bradycardia pacing. Guidelines from HRS-NASPE suggest that every patient with an ICD have an in-office comprehensive evaluation every 1 to 4 months.[145] Devices with CRT-P must have a sufficiently short atrioventricular delay for sensed events to ensure that all ventricular activity is paced. Failure of ventricular pacing (either right or left) because of native atrioventricular conduction or threshold issues has been associated with inappropriate antitachycardia therapy (i.e., shock).[146]

Intraoperative (or Procedure) Management

Currently, no special monitoring (because of the ICD) is required for the patient with an ICD. Electrocardiographic monitoring and the ability to deliver external cardioversion or defibrillation must be present during the time of ICD disablement. Although many recommendations exist for defibrillator pad placement to protect the ICD, it should be remembered that the patient, not the ICD, is being treated.

In addition, no special anesthetic techniques have been championed for the patient with an ICD. Most of these patients will have severely depressed systolic function, dilated ventricular cavities, and significant valvular regurgitation, and the choice of anesthetic technique should be dictated by the underlying physiologic derangements that are present. Conflicting data have been published regarding the choice of anesthetic agent(s) and changes to defibrillation threshold (DFT). In 1992, Gill et al[147] examined DFT in dogs and concluded that neither halothane nor isoflurane changed DFT in open-chest defibrillation compared with a pentobarbital infusion. However, Weinbroum et al[148] evaluated DFTs in humans during ICD implant and found that halothane, isoflurane, and fentanyl increased DFT. Even with these increases, though, the increased DFTs found were still substantially lower than the maximum energy generally available in ICDs, and these increases would not have been noted under usual ICD testing conditions. As noted earlier, both isoflurane and sevoflurane have been reported to lengthen the QT interval, which could increase the risk for torsades de pointe in certain patients.

Caution should be observed when placing a central venous catheter in any patient with an ICD. In the patient with an integrated bipolar ventricular sensing configuration, an inappropriate 30-joule shock was delivered because of noise artifact created by the guidewire hitting the ventricular shock coil (which was serving as the heart rate sensor). The output of the ICD was short-circuited because of the presence of a shock coil in the superior vena cava, and the ICD was unknowingly rendered ineffective. Only after failure to deliver subsequent therapy was this problem noted, and the patient subsequently expired.[149] It is important to note that some ICDs are configured to the "integrated bipolar sensing configuration" even in the presence of a true bipolar RV lead.

Postanesthesia Implantable Cardioverter-Defibrillator Evaluation

The ICD must be reinterrogated and re-enabled. All events should be reviewed, and counters should be cleared because the next device evaluator might not receive information about the EMI experience of the patient and make erroneous conclusions regarding the patient's arrhythmia events. One patient death has been reported to the FDA because of failure to reactivate tachyarrhythmia therapy in an ICD patient after a cardiac ablation procedure.[150]

SUMMARY

Electronic miniaturization has permitted the design and use of sophisticated electronics in patients who have need for artificial pacing and/or automated cardioversion/defibrillation of their heart. Both the aging of the population and the ability to care for patients with increasingly complex disease suggest that many more patients with these devices will require subsequent surgery. Safe and efficient clinical management of these patients depends on an understanding of implantable systems, indications for their use, and the perioperative needs that they create.

Glossary

Atrioventricular Delay The time that a dual-chamber system waits after detecting (or initiating) an atrial event before pacing the ventricle. Some generators shorten this time as heart rate increases (termed *rate-adaptive atrioventricular delay* or *dynamic atrioventricular delay*). Some generators can be programmed to extend the atrioventricular delay to search for intrinsic conduction ("search atrioventricular delay"). Some generators will prolong an atrioventricular delay after any atrial event in which the last ventricular event was intrinsic ("atrioventricular delay hysteresis"). In a patient with a conducting atrioventricular node, the sensed A-V delay will be slightly longer than the "P-R" interval on the surface electrocardiogram (see "Fusion Beat" and "Pseudofusion Beat") because the ventricular sensing element is attached to the apex of the right ventricle and detects the depolarization only after right ventricular activation.

Bipolar Lead An electrode with two conductors. Bipolar sensing is more resistant to oversensing from muscle artifact or stray electromagnetic fields. Some pacing generators can be programmed to unipolar mode even in the presence of bipolar electrodes.

Dynamic Atrioventricular Delay see Atrioventricular Delay

EGM Mode Passive acquisition and internal storage of electrocardiographic data for diagnostic purposes while pacing (or monitoring) with programmed parameters.

Fusion Beat (PFB) A pacemaker spike delivered shortly before a native depolarization of the ventricle that alters the morphology of the QRS, often misdiagnosed as undersensing. It is caused by the position of the sensing electrode relative to the depolarizing wavefront. Confirmation of appropriate sensing behavior can be made by lengthening the sensing interval (i.e., lengthening the atrioventricular delay). Fusion beats suggest ventricular capture.

Generator The device with a power source and circuitry to produce an electrical impulse designed to be conducted to the heart. Typically, pacing generators are placed in a pectoral pocket and leads are inserted into the right atrium, right ventricle, or both. Since 1995, though, implantable cardioverter-defibrillators (ICDs) also have been approved for pectoral pocket placement.

Hysteresis If present, the amount by which the patient's intrinsic rate must decline below the programmed rate before the generator begins pacing. Some pacers periodically decrease the pacing rate to search for resumption of intrinsic activity (called *search hysteresis*). These functions, when present, can mimic pacemaker malfunction.

ICD Mode The designation of chamber(s) shocked, chamber(s) paced for antitachycardia pacing, method of tachycardia detection, and chambers paced for antitachycardia therapy. Table 25-4 shows the North American Society for Pacing and Electrophysiology/British Pacing and Electrophysiology Group (NASPE/BPEG) generic implantable cardioverter-defibrillator (ICD) code.

Managed Ventricular Pacing Some evidence exists that right ventricular (RV) pacing increases mortality in patients with intact atrioventricular nodal conduction. As a result, several companies have algorithms to reduce the incidence of RV pacing. Pacing modes called Managed Ventricular Pacing (Medtronic) or AAI Safe-R (ELA Medical) can permit an occasional dropped QRS (more likely with MVP than AAI Safe-R). However, no pacing device should allow two consecutive dropped QRS events. After several beats with a dropped QRS, however, these devices begin pacing in a true DDD mode for several cardiac cycles. These dropped QRS events can mimic pacing system malfunction (pseudomalfunction).

Oversensing Detection of undesired signals that are interpreted as cardiac activity. Oversensing can lead to pacemaker-driven tachycardia (pacing device, DDD mode with atrial oversensing and ventricular tracking); ventricular pause (pacing device with electrosurgically induced ventricular oversensing, leading the pacer to "detect" ventricular activity); or inappropriate shock (defibrillator, event oversensing).

Pacing Mode The designation of chamber(s) paced, chamber(s) sensed, sensing response, rate responsiveness, and antitachyarrhythmia function for a pacemaker system. Table 25-1 shows the North American Society for Pacing and Electrophysiology/British Pacing and Electrophysiology Group (NASPE/BPEG) generic pacemaker code.

Postventricular Atrial Blanking Period (PVAB) Present only in a dual-chamber pacemaker, the PVAB is the period immediately after any ventricular event during which atrial events will not be detected by the atrial sensing circuitry. In general, PVAB is used to determine where, in the postventricular period, atrial event counting should resume for mode switch determination. PVAB is the early part of postventricular atrial refractory period.

Postventricular Atrial Refractory Period (PVARP) Present only in a dual-chamber pacemaker, the PVARP is the period immediately after any ventricular event during which atrial events are ignored (for the purpose of pacing the ventricle). In some devices, atrial events during PVARP (but after the expiration of the postventricular atrial blanking period timer) will be counted for atrial rate determinations leading to possible mode switch. The duration of PVARP added to the atrioventricular delay (called *total atrial refractory period* [TARP]) determines the 2:1 block rate of pacing. Some devices allow the PVARP to vary based on the heart rate.

Programmed Rate (also Automatic Rate) The lowest sustained regular rate at which the generator will pace. Typically, the device begins pacing when the patient's intrinsic rate declines below this value.

Pseudofusion Beat (PFB) A pacemaker spike delivered shortly after a native depolarization without alteration of the QRS morphology. PFBs are often misdiagnosed as undersensing, and they result from the position of the sensing electrode relative to the depolarizing wavefront (see "Fusion Beat"). Confirmation of appropriate sensing behavior can be made by lengthening the sensing interval (i.e., decreasing the program rate [atrial FB] or lengthening the atrioventricular delay [ventricular PFB]). PFB cannot be used to confirm electronic capture.

Rate Enhancements The features such as rate adaptive atrioventricular delay (shortens the atrioventricular delay with increasing heart rate); atrioventricular search hysteresis (lengthens/shortens the atrioventricular delay to produce intrinsic atrioventricular conduction); AF suppression (also called *dynamic atrial overdrive;* increases the lower rate on appearance of native atrial depolarization to create nearly constant atrial pacing but at a rate only slightly higher than the patient's intrinsic rate); rate smoothing (limits changes in ventricular paced rates because of changes in atrial rates; increasing and decreasing rate limits can be programmed); sleep rate (see later); ventricular rate regulation (similar to rate smoothing but used to prevent atrial fibrillation); and hysteresis (see earlier). Each of these enhancements can produce pacing/nonpacing that can mimic pacemaker dysfunction, and these enhancements should be programmed "OFF" before any anesthetic.

Rate Modulation The ability of the generator to sense the need to increase heart rate. Mechanisms include (1) a mechanical sensor in the generator to detect motion or vibration; (2) electronic detection of Q-T interval (shortens during exercise) or transthoracic impedance to measure changes in respiration; or (3) sensor(s) for central venous blood temperature or oxygen saturation. Some generators now incorporate multiple sensors.

Runaway Pacing Rate   The highest pacing rate (typically around 200 beats/min) that could occur in the setting of multiple internal component failures in a cardiac generator.

Sleep Rate (also Circadian Rate)   The rate (lower than the programmed rate) at which the pacing generator will pace during programmed "nighttime" hours.

Total Atrial Refractory Period (TARP)   Present only in dual-chamber pacing devices, the TARP refers to the sum of the postventricular atrial refractory period (PVARP) and the atrioventricular delay, and it determines the point at which the pacing device will pace the ventricle every other atrial event. This 2:1 block rate can be calculated by dividing 60,000 (msec/min) by the TARP (measured in milliseconds). This 2:1 block results from the ignoring of the atrial event during the PVARP, so these 2:1 blocks appear only when ventricular pacing is needed in a patient and the 2:1 block rate is lower than the maximum tracking rate. In some pacing devices, the dynamic atrioventricular delay will make the calculation of TARP dependent on atrial rate, and many of the programmers will report the final 2:1 block rate for any given combination of programmed parameters.

Undersensing   Failure to detect a desired event.

Unipolar Lead   An electrode with only one conductor. Some devices with bipolar leads are programmed to the unipolar lead mode. Systems with unipolar leads produce larger spikes on the electrocardiogram than bipolar leads. Systems with unipolar leads utilize the generator case as the second conductor.

Upper Sensor Rate (USR; also Upper Activity Rate [UAR])   The maximum rate to which a rate-modulated pacemaker can drive the heart. USR is not affected by UTR because when USR becomes active, the pacemaker is pacing the atrium.

Upper Tracking Rate (UTR; also called Upper Rate Limit [URL])   Pacemakers programmed to VDDxx or DDDxx mode cause the ventricles to track atrial activity. Should a patient develop an atrial tachyarrhythmia, such as a supraventricular tachycardia, atrial fibrillation, or atrial flutter, the generator acts to limit ventricular pacing. When the atrial rate exceeds the UTR, the generator can change mode (i.e., switch to DDI) or introduce second-degree A-V block. Second-degree blocks can be Mobitz type I (Wenckebach) or Mobitz type II, depending on a variety of programmed settings within the pacemaker.

Ventricular Refractory Period (VRP)   The period immediately after any ventricular event during which the pacing device will not respond to a sensed event on the ventricular channel. Depending on the manufacturer and programming, though, events sensed during VRP might be counted for determining a high-rate ventricular condition.

APPENDIX 25-1	Pacemaker Response to Magnet Placement

Pacemaker Company		Magnet Mode Designation	Explanation
Biotronik	INOS	ASYNCH	Asynchronous VOO (even if dual-chamber device) pacing at 70 or 90 beats/min, depending on programming, if battery okay. 80 at ERI.* There is no way to tell what the magnet rate will be without the programmer.
		SYNCH	VVI (even if dual-chamber device) pacing at 70 or 90 beats/min, depending on programming, if battery okay. 80 at ERI.* There is no way to tell what the magnet rate will be without the programmer. Also, if the patient's intrinsic ventricular rate is greater than 80 beats/min, there will be no way to identify ERI.*
	DROMOS	ASYNCH	See "AUTO."
		SYNCH	See "SYNCH."
	All Others	AUTO	If battery is okay, 10 asynchronous events at 90 beats/min, then returns to original programmed mode, without rate responsiveness. Pacing is at lowest available rate (LRL, sleep rate, or hysteresis rate). If battery at ERI,* 10 asynchronous events at 80 beats/min in VOO mode, then either VDD (dual chamber) or VVI (single-chamber) pacing at 11% lower than lowest available rate. For any dual-chamber mode (DDD, DDI, or VDD), the atrioventricular delay shortens to 100 milliseconds while the magnet is in place.
		ASYNCH	Asynchronous pacing at 90 beats/min if battery okay. At ERI,* 80 beats/min (single-step change) in VOO mode regardless of original programming. For any dual-chamber mode (DDD, DDI, or VDD), the atrioventricular delay shortens to 100 milliseconds while the magnet is in place.
		SYNCH	If battery is okay, pacing in original programmed mode, without rate responsiveness. Pacing is at lowest available rate (LRL, sleep rate, or hysteresis rate). If battery at ERI,* then either VDD (dual-chamber) or VVI (single-chamber) pacing at 11% lower than lowest available rate. For any dual-chamber mode (DDD, DDI, or VDD), the atrioventricular delay shortens to 100 milliseconds while the magnet is in place.
Boston Scientific includes Guidant Medical CPI		ASYNCH	Asynchronous pacing with 100-millisecond atrioventricular delay at 100 beats/min if okay, 85 beats/min at ERT (single-step change). The Insignia and Altrua models have an intermediate step (90 beats/min) at IFI. Most models shorten the pulse width to 50% on the third paced ventricular event (TMT). For Triumph and Prelude models, see Medtronic pacemakers.
		OFF	No change, magnet is ignored. OFF is the magnet mode after a "power on reset," which can occur secondary to EMI.
		EGM mode	No change in pacing. Magnet application initiates data collection.
ELA Medical			Asynchronous pacing at 96 beats/min gradually declining to 80 beats/min at ERI.* ELA pacemakers take eight additional asynchronous pacing cycles (the final two cycles are at LRL with long atrioventricular delay) on magnet removal.
Intermedics (purchased by Guidant, 1998, now Boston Scientific; requires special programmer)			Five asynchronous events at 90 beats/min (regardless of battery voltage), then 60 additional asynchronous events at LRL if battery is okay, 90 beats/min if ERI,* and 80 beats/min if EOL. The fifth paced event is emitted at 50% of the originally programmed pulse width (TMT). After the 65th asynchronous event, the magnet is ignored.

	APPENDIX 25-1	Pacemaker Response to Magnet Placement—Cont'd	

Pacemaker Company	Magnet Mode Designation		Explanation
Medtronic[†]			Asynchronous pacing at 85 beats/min if okay, 65 SSI regardless of original programming if ERI* (single-step change). Most Medtronic pacemakers pace the first three events at 600-millisecond intervals (rate = 100 beats/min) with a short atrioventricular delay. During the first 3–7 asynchronous events, most Medtronic pacemakers emit one or more ventricular pulses at a reduced pulse width or voltage (TMT). Also, all Medtronic pacemakers default to SSI pacing at 65 beats/min, without rate responsiveness, on detection of ERI,* regardless of whether a magnet is present. Note that a dual-chamber pacemaker in AAI mode will revert to VVI on ERI* or reset, which might be a problem for some patients.
St. Jude Medical	"SJM" X-ray logo	Battery Test	Asynchronous pacing at 98.6 beats/min gradually decreasing to 86.3 beats/min at ERI.*
		OFF	No magnet response.
		Event snapshots	No change in pacing. Magnet application causes pacemaker to collect data. Identity and Entity models lack this feature.
		Event snapshots + Battery Test	For a magnet placed 2 seconds, pacing mode and rate are unchanged and the device stores an electrogram. If the magnet is placed ≥5 seconds, the Battery Test mode (see earlier) is activated. Identity and Entity models lack this feature.
	Pacesetter X-ray logo (ψ)	Battery Test	Asynchronous pacing, and the rate depends on specific model. In general, a pacing rate < 90 beats/min should prompt further evaluation.
		OFF	No magnet response.
		VARIO mode (present in some models)	VARIO results in a series of 32 asynchronous pacing events. The rate of the first 16 paces reflects battery voltage, gradually declining from 100 beats/min to 85 beats/min at ERI.* The next 15 paces are used to document ventricular pacing capture safety margin. The rate will be 119 beats/min with gradually declining pacing voltage. The 16th pace of this group is at no output. The next pace restarts the 32-event sequence. The 32-event sequence repeats while the magnet remains in place.
Telectronics	Meta 1202		Asynchronous pacing at 99 beats/min gradually declining to < 93 at ERI.*
	Meta 1204 1206 1256		Asynchronous pacing at 100 beats/min gradually declining to < 82.5 beats/min at ERI.*
	Meta 1230 1250 1254		Asynchronous VOO pacing (regardless of original programming) at > 85 beats/min gradually declining to < 78 beats/min at ERI.*
	Tempo		Asynchronous pacing at 100 beats/min gradually declining to 80 beats/min at ERI.*
	All Others		Contact St. Jude Medical.

The effect(s) of appropriately placing a magnet over a pacemaker are shown. Column 1 shows the pacemaker manufacturer. Some manufacturers have multiple responses, which can be determined by the X-ray identifier. If the magnet response is programmable, then Column 2 shows the various magnet modes available. The first mode shown is the default mode, and it will be active at device startup or after a device reset. Column 3 shows the effect on pacing therapy for the magnet mode shown in Column 2. Unless otherwise specified, asynchronous pacing takes place, without rate responsiveness, in the chambers originally programmed. Thus, a dual-chamber program would result in DOO pacing, and a single-chamber program would result in VOO (unless an atrial device, which would be AOO) pacing, and a biventricular, dual-chamber device would be DOOOV.

EOL, end of life (the device should be replaced immediately); ERI, elective replacement indicator (the device should be replaced promptly); ERT, elective replacement time (the device should be replaced promptly); IFI, intensified follow-up interval (the device should undergo monthly battery checks); LRL, lower rate limit (the programmed lower rate, or set point, of the pacemaker); SSI, single chamber, inhibited mode (if implanted for ventricular pacing, then SSI = VVI; for an atrial pacemaker, SSI = AAI).

*ERI notes: Biotronik dual-chamber pacemakers switch to VDD pacing at 90% of the programmed lower rate on reaching elective replacement. St. Jude pacemakers add 100 milliseconds to the basic pacing interval (LRL) on ERI. For example, an LRL of 60 beats/min should be an interval of rate responsiveness and other features (if programmed) are suspended. Medtronic dual-chamber pacemakers switch to VVI pacing at 65 beats/min on reaching elective replacement.

†Caution for Medtronic pacemakers: All Medtronic pacemakers except Enrhythm (P1501, EMDR series) suspend magnet detection for 60 minutes after removal of the programming head after an interrogation session, unless specific programming action (which requires multiple "button" depressions) is taken before removing the programming head.

	APPENDIX 25-2	Company Phone Numbers

AM Pacemaker Corp. (Guidant Medical)	800-227-3422	Edwards Pacemaker Systems (Medtronic)	800-325-2518
Angeion*	800-264-2466	ELA Medical*	800-352-6466
Arco Medical (Guidant Medical)	800-227-3422	Guidant Medical*	800-227-3422
Biotronik*	800-547-0394	Intermedics (Guidant Medical)*	800-227-3422
Cardiac Control Systems[†]	unavailable	Medtronic*	800-505-4636
Cardio Pace Medical, Inc (Novacon)[†]	unavailable	Pacesetter (St. Jude Medical)*	800-722-3774
Cardiac Pacemakers, Inc–CPI (Guidant Medical)*	800-227-3422	Siemens–Elema (St. Jude Medical)	800-722-3774
Cook Pacemaker Corp.	800-245-4715	Telectronics Pacing (St. Jude Medical)*	800-722-3774
Coratomic (Biocontrol Technology)[†]	unavailable	Ventritex (St. Jude Medical)*	800-722-3774
Cordis Corporation (St. Jude Medical)	800-722-3774	Vitatron (Medtronic)	800-328-2518
Diag/Medcor (St. Jude Medical)	800-722-3774		

*Market defibrillators.
†Companies are no longer available.

APPENDIX 25-3	Implantable Cardioverter-Defibrillator Response to Magnet Placement				
ICD Manufacturer	**Magnet Mode Designation**	**Effect on Tachy Therapy**	**Effect on Bradytherapy (regular pacing)**	**Magnet Mode Confirmation**	
Angeion	ENABLE	Disables	No effect	None	
	DISABLE	No effect	No effect		
Biotronik		Disables	No effect	None	
Boston Scientific (Guidant Medical, CPI)	"GDT," "CPI," "BOS 119," "BOS 203" X-ray label	ON	Disables	No effect	Short beep with each detected heartbeat or constant tone*
		OFF	No effect	No effect	None
	All other "BOS" X-ray label	ON	Disables	No effect	Short beep every second or constant tone*
		OFF	No effect	No effect	None
ELA Medical (Sorin)		Disables	The pacing rate, but not mode, changes to 80–90 beats/min; 80 beats/min indicates elective replacement time	None	
Medtronic	AT-500†	Disables	No effect	None‡	
	All others	Disables	No effect		
Pacesetter and St. Jude Medical	NORMAL	Disables	No effect	None	
	IGNORE	No effect	No effect		

The effect(s) of appropriately placing a magnet over an implantable cardioverter-defibrillator (ICD) are shown. Column 1 shows the manufacturer. Some manufacturers have multiple responses that can be determined by the X-ray identifier. If the magnet response is programmable, then Column 2 shows the various magnet modes available. The first mode shown is the default mode, and it will be active at device startup or after a device reset. Column 3 shows the effect on antitachycardia therapy (defibrillation, cardioversion, and antitachycardia pacing) for the magnet mode shown in Column 2. Only ICDs from ELA Medical alter their antibradycardia pacing rate on magnet placement (Column 4), and this pacing rate can be used to predict remaining battery life provided that the patient's native heart rate is less than the magnet rate. Only ICDs from Boston Scientific/Guidant/CPI produce reliable audio feedback for confirmation of magnet placement (Column 5). For devices from Angeion, Pacesetter, and St. Jude Medical, a device interrogation is required to determine the magnet mode.

*For Boston Scientific/Guidant/CPI ICDs, if magnet mode is programmed to "ON," appropriate magnet placement immediately disables tachy detection and therapy, and tachy therapies remain disabled for as long as the magnet remains appropriately applied. When magnet mode is enabled in these devices, the ICD will emit either a constant tone or "beep" to identify appropriate magnet placement. If the device emits a constant tone, then tachy therapy is disabled regardless of whether a magnet is present, and tachy therapy will not be present even after the magnet is removed. If any of these ICDs emit a "beep" (ICDs with "GDT," "CPI, " "BOS 119," or "BOS 203" X-ray codes emit each beep with either paced or sensed R waves; all newer Boston Scientific ICDs [all will have "BOS" X-ray code] emit a beep every second), then a properly working ICD will be enabled for tachy therapy on magnet removal. If the "Change Tachy Mode with Magnet" feature also is programmed "ON," after 30 seconds of continuous magnet application, the tachy mode changes; that is, it will switch from enabled when the magnet is removed (beeping with magnet correctly applied) to permanently disabled (constant tone when magnet is correctly applied) or vice versa. This mode has been phased out, and properly updated Boston Scientific programmers contain software designed to disable and eliminate this feature. Any Boston Scientific/CPI/Guidant ICD that does not emit sound when a magnet is applied should undergo an immediate device interrogation.

†The Medtronic AT-500 series defibrillators provide antitachycardia pacing in the atrium *only*, and usually after a delay often exceeding 1 minute from onset of atrial tachyarrhythmia. They have no shock coil on any lead, and they are difficult to distinguish from a conventional two-chamber pacemaker on X-ray. They have *no* apparent magnet response. The X-ray identifier on these devices includes the Medtronic "M," but the first character is "I." All other Medtronic cardiac generators have the Medtronic "M" with the first letter identifier "P."

‡Some Medtronic ICDs will emit a tone for 15–20 seconds when a magnet is placed on the device. However, this tone will not be interrupted with immediate magnet removal, and as a result, the tone cannot be used for confirmation of appropriate magnet placement.

REFERENCES

1. Rasmussen MJ, Friedman PA, Hammill SC, et al: Unintentional deactivation of implantable cardioverter-defibrillators in health care settings, *Mayo Clin Proc* 77:855–859, 2002.
2. Fleisher LA, Beckman JA, Brown KA, et al: ACC/AHA 2007 guidelines on perioperative cardiovascular evaluation and care for noncardiac surgery: A report of the American College of Cardiology/American Heart Association Task Force on practice guidelines (writing committee to revise the 2002 guidelines on perioperative cardiovascular evaluation for noncardiac surgery), *Circulation* 116:e418–e500, 2007.
3. Goldschlager N, Epstein A, Friedman P, et al: Environmental and drug effects on patients with pacemakers and implantable cardioverter/defibrillators: A practical guide to patient treatment, *Arch Intern Med* 161:649–655, 2001.
4. Pinski SL, Trohman RG: Interference in implanted cardiac devices, part I, *Pacing Clin Electrophysiol* 25:1367–1381, 2002.
5. Pinski SL, Trohman RG: Interference in implanted cardiac devices, part II, *Pacing Clin Electrophysiol* 25:1496–1509, 2002.
6. Practice advisory for the perioperative management of patients with cardiac rhythm management devices: Pacemakers and implantable cardioverter-defibrillators: A report by the American Society of Anesthesiologists Task Force on Perioperative Management of Patients with Cardiac Rhythm Management Devices, *Anesthesiology* 103:186–198, 2005.
7. Stone KR, McPherson CA: Assessment and management of patients with pacemakers and implantable cardioverter defibrillators, *Crit Care Med* 32:S155–S165, 2004.
8. Salukhe TV, Dob D, Sutton R: Pacemakers and defibrillators: Anaesthetic implications, *Br J Anaesth* 93:95–104, 2004.
9. Rozner MA: Corrections to electrosurgery in patients with cardiac pacemakers or implanted cardioverter defibrillators, *Ann Plast Surg* 58:226–227, 2007.
10. Rozner MA: Pacemakers and implantable cardioverter defibrillators, *Crit Care Med* 32:1809–1812, 2004.
11. Rozner MA: Pacemaker misinformation in the perioperative period: Programming around the problem, *Anesth Analg* 99:1582–1584, 2004.
12. Badrinath SS, Bhaskaran S, Sundararaj I, et al: Mortality and morbidity associated with ophthalmic surgery, *Ophthalmic Surg Lasers* 26:535–541, 1995.
13. Pili-Floury S, Farah E, Samain E, et al: Perioperative outcome of pacemaker patients undergoing non-cardiac surgery, *Eur J Anaesthesiol* 25:514–516, 2008.
14. Bernstein AD, Daubert JC, Fletcher RD, et al: The revised NASPE/BPEG generic code for antibradycardia, adaptive-rate, and multisite pacing. North American Society of Pacing and Electrophysiology/British Pacing and Electrophysiology Group, *Pacing Clin Electrophysiol* 25: 260–264, 2002.
15. Atlee J, Bernstein A: Cardiac rhythm management devices part I, *Anesthesiology* 95:1265–1280, 2001.
16. Auricchio A, Stellbrink C, Sack S, et al: The pacing therapies for congestive heart failure (PATH-CHF) study: Rationale, design, and endpoints of a prospective randomized multicenter study, *Am J Cardiol* 83:130D–135D, 1999.
17. Bristow MR, Saxon LA, Boehmer J, et al: Cardiac-resynchronization therapy with or without an implantable defibrillator in advanced chronic heart failure, *N Engl J Med* 350:2140–2150, 2004.
18. Hayes DL: Evolving indications for permanent pacing, *Am J Cardiol* 83:161D–165D, 1999.
19. Bevilacqua L, Hordof A: Cardiac pacing in children, *Curr Opin Cardiol* 13:48–55, 1998.
20. Gras D, Mabo P, Tang T, et al: Multisite pacing as a supplemental treatment of congestive heart failure: Preliminary results of the Medtronic Inc. InSync Study, *Pacing Clin Electrophysiol* 21:2249–2255, 1998.
21. Medina-Ravell VA, Lankipalli RS, Yan GX, et al: Effect of epicardial or biventricular pacing to prolong QT interval and increase transmural dispersion of repolarization: Does resynchronization therapy pose a risk for patients predisposed to long QT or torsade de pointes? *Circulation* 107:740–746, 2003.
22. Delfaut P, Saksena S: Electrophysiologic assessment in selecting patients for multisite atrial pacing, *J Interv Card Electrophysiol* 4(Suppl 1):81–85, 2000.
23. Prakash A, Saksena S, Ziegler PD, et al: Dual site right atrial pacing can improve the impact of standard dual chamber pacing on atrial and ventricular mechanical function in patients with symptomatic atrial fibrillation: Further observations from the dual site atrial pacing for prevention of atrial fibrillation trial, *J Interv Card Electrophysiol* 12:177–187, 2005.
24. Rozner MA, Nishman RJ: Pacemaker-driven tachycardia revisited, *Anesth Analg* 88:965, 1999.
25. Purday JP, Towey RM: Apparent pacemaker failure caused by activation of ventricular threshold test by a magnetic instrument mat during general anaesthesia, *Br J Anaesth* 69:645–646, 1992.
26. Bourke ME: The patient with a pacemaker or related device, *Can J Anaesth* 43:24–41, 1996.
27. Valls-Bertault V, Mansourati J, Gilard M, et al: Adverse events with transvenous left ventricular pacing in patients with severe heart failure: Early experience from a single centre, *Europace* 3:60–63, 2001.
28. Alonso C, Leclercq C, d'Allonnes FR, et al: Six year experience of transvenous left ventricular lead implantation for permanent biventricular pacing in patients with advanced heart failure: Technical aspects, *Heart* 86:405–410, 2001.
29. Bernstein AD, Irwin ME, Parsonnet V, et al: Report of the NASPE Policy Conference on antibradycardia pacemaker follow-up: Effectiveness, needs, and resources. North American Society of Pacing and Electrophysiology, *Pacing Clin Electrophysiol* 17:1714–1729, 1994.
30. Rozner MA, Roberson JC, Nguyen AD: Unexpected high incidence of serious pacemaker problems detected by pre-and postoperative interrogations: A two-year experience, *J Am Coll Cardiol* 43:113A, 2004.

31. Sethi KK, Bhargava M, Pandit N, et al: Experience with recycled cardiac pacemakers, *Indian Heart J* 44:91–93, 1992.
32. Panja M, Sarkar CN, Kumar S, et al: Reuse of pacemaker, *Indian Heart J* 48:677–680, 1996.
33. Hauser R, Hayes D, Parsonnet V, et al: Feasibility and initial results of an Internet-based pacemaker and ICD pulse generator and lead registry, *Pacing Clin Electrophysiol* 24:82–87, 2001.
34. Kato Y, Hou K, Hori J, et al: Extracorporeal shock wave lithotripsy for ureteral stone in patient with implanted cardiac pacemaker: A case report, *Nippon Hinyokika Gakkai Zasshi* 94:626–629, 2003.
35. Preisman S, Cheng DC: Life-threatening ventricular dysrhythmias with inadvertent asynchronous temporary pacing after cardiac surgery, *Anesthesiology* 91:880–883, 1999.
36. Rozner MA: Implantable cardiac pulse generators: Pacemakers and cardioverter-defibrillators. In Miller RD, Fleisher L, Johns R, Savarese J, editors: *Anesthesia*, ed 6, New York, 2004, Churchill Livingstone.
37. Ren X, Hongo RH: Polymorphic ventricular tachycardia from R-on-T pacing, *J Am Coll Cardiol* 53:218, 2009.
38. Vogelgesang D, Vogelgesang S: Pacemaker-induced ventricular tachycardia, *Europace* 10:46–47, 2008.
39. Hayes DL, Strathmore NF: Electromagnetic interference with implantable devices. In Ellenbogen KA, Kay GN, Wilkoff BL, editors: *Clinical cardiac pacing and defibrillation*, ed 2, Philadelphia, 2000, WB Saunders Company, pp 939–952.
40. Augoustides JG, Fleisher LA: The future for B-type natriuretic peptide in preoperative assessment, *Anesthesiology* 108:332–333, 2008.
41. Andersen C, Madsen GM: Rate-responsive pacemakers and anaesthesia. A consideration of possible implications, *Anaesthesia* 45:472–476, 1990.
42. Levine PA: Response to "rate-adaptive cardiac pacing: implications of environmental noise during craniotomy", *Anesthesiology* 87:1261, 1997.
43. Levine PA, Balady GJ, Lazar HL, et al: Electrocautery and pacemakers: Management of the paced patient subject to electrocautery, *Ann Thorac Surg* 41:313–317, 1986.
44. Madsen GM, Andersen C: Pacemaker-induced tachycardia during general anaesthesia: A case report, *Br J Anaesth* 63:360–361, 1989.
45. von Knobelsdorff G, Goerig M, Nagele H, et al: Interaction of frequency-adaptive pacemakers and anesthetic management. Discussion of current literature and two case reports, *Anaesthesist* 45:856–860, 1996.
46. Van Hemel NM, Hamerlijnck RP, Pronk KJ, et al: Upper limit ventricular stimulation in respiratory rate responsive pacing due to electrocautery, *Pacing Clin Electrophysiol* 12:1720–1723, 1989.
47. Wong DT, Middleton W: Electrocautery-induced tachycardia in a rate-responsive pacemaker, *Anesthesiology* 94:710–711, 2001.
48. Wallden J, Gupta A, Carlsen HO: Supraventricular tachycardia induced by Datex patient monitoring system, *Anesth Analg* 86:1339, 1998.
49. Center for Devices and Radiologic Health: *Interaction between minute ventilation rate-adaptive pacemakers and cardiac monitoring and diagnostic equipment*, Published October 14, 1998. Available at: http://www.fda.gov/cdrh/safety/minutevent.html. Accessed April 8, 2009.
50. Rozner MA: Peripheral nerve stimulators can inhibit monitor display of pacemaker pulses, *J Clin Anesth* 16:117–120, 2004.
51. Michaloudis D, Fraidakis O, Lefaki T, et al: Anaesthesia and the QT interval in humans. The effects of isoflurane and halothane, *Anaesthesia* 51:219–224, 1996.
52. Michaloudis D, Fraidakis O, Petrou A, et al: Anaesthesia and the QT interval. Effects of isoflurane and halothane in unpremedicated children, *Anaesthesia* 53:435–439, 1998.
53. Paventi S, Santevecchi A, Ranieri R: Effects of sevoflurane versus propofol on QT interval, *Minerva Anestesiol* 67:637–640, 2001.
54. Gallagher JD, Weindling SN, Anderson G, et al: Effects of sevoflurane on QT interval in a patient with congenital long QT syndrome, *Anesthesiology* 89:1569–1573, 1998.
55. Michaloudis D, Fraidakis O, Lefaki T, et al: Anaesthesia and the QT interval in humans: Effects of halothane and isoflurane in premedicated children, *Eur J Anaesthesiol* 15:623–628, 1998.
56. Pressly N: *Review of MDR Reports reinforces concern about EMI*, 1997. FDA User Facility Reporting #20 Published 1997. Available at: http://www.fda.gov/cdrh/fuse20.pdf Accessed April 8, 2009.
57. Rozner MA: Review of electrical interference in implanted cardiac devices, *Pacing Clin Electrophysiol* 26:923–925, 2003.
58. Nandalan SP, Vanner RG: Use of the harmonic scalpel in a patient with a permanent pacemaker, *Anaesthesia* 59:621, 2004.
59. Epstein MR, Mayer JE Jr, Duncan BW: Use of an ultrasonic scalpel as an alternative to electrocautery in patients with pacemakers, *Ann Thorac Surg* 65:1802–1804, 1998.
60. Ozeren M, Dogan OV, Duzgun C, et al: Use of an ultrasonic scalpel in the open-heart reoperation of a patient with pacemaker, *Eur J Cardiothorac Surg* 21:761–762, 2002.
61. Erdman S, Levinsky L, Strasberg B, et al: Use of the Shaw Scalpel in pacemaker operations, *J Thorac Cardiovasc Surg* 89:304–307, 1985.
62. Gimbel JR, Johnson D, Levine PA, et al: Safe performance of magnetic resonance imaging on five patients with permanent cardiac pacemakers, *Pacing Clin Electrophysiol* 19:913–919, 1996.
63. Gimbel JR, Kanal E: Can patients with implantable pacemakers safely undergo magnetic resonance imaging? *J Am Coll Cardiol* 43:1325–1327, 2004.
64. Martin ET, Coman JA, Shellock FG, et al: Magnetic resonance imaging and cardiac pacemaker safety at 1.5-Tesla, *J Am Coll Cardiol* 43:1315–1324, 2004.
65. Rozner MA, Burton AW, Kumar AJ: Pacemaker complication during MRI, *J Am Coll Cardiol* 45:161–162, 2005.
66. Gimbel JR, Wilkoff BL, Kanal E, et al: Safe, sensible, sagacious: Responsible scanning of pacemaker patients, *Eur Heart J* 26:1683–1684, 2005.
67. Mitka M: Researchers seek MRI-safe pacemakers, *JAMA* 301:476, 2009.
68. Mychaskiw G, Eichhorn JH: Interaction of an implanted pacemaker with a transesophageal atrial pacemaker: Report of a case, *J Clin Anesth* 11:669–671, 1999.
69. Kaushik V, Leon AR, Forrester JS Jr, et al: Bradyarrhythmias, temporary and permanent pacing, *Crit Care Med* 28:N121–N128, 2000.
70. Kashima I, Shin H, Yozu R, et al: Optimal positioning of temporary epicardial atrial pacing leads after cardiac surgery, *Jpn J Thorac Cardiovasc Surg* 49:307–310, 2001.
71. Atlee JL III, Pattison CZ, Mathews EL, et al: Evaluation of transesophageal atrial pacing stethoscope in adult surgical patients under general anesthesia, *Pacing Clin Electrophysiol* 15:1515–1525, 1992.
72. Zaidan JR: Pacemakers, *Anesthesiology* 60:319–334, 1984.
73. Bellocci F, Santarelli P, Di Gennaro M, et al: The risk of cardiac complications in surgical patients with bifascicular block. A clinical and electrophysiologic study in 98 patients, *Chest* 77:343–348, 1980.
74. Del Nido P, Goldman BS: Temporary epicardial pacing after open heart surgery: Complications and prevention, *J Card Surg* 4:99–103, 1989.
75. Dixon RG, Dougherty JM, White LJ, et al: Transcutaneous pacing in a hypothermic-dog model, *Ann Emerg Med* 29:602–606, 1997.
76. Syverud SA, Dalsey WC, Hedges JR, et al: Radiologic assessment of transvenous pacemaker placement during CPR, *Ann Emerg Med* 15:131–137, 1986.
77. Lang R, David D, Klein HO, et al: The use of the balloon-tipped floating catheter in temporary transvenous cardiac pacing, *Pacing Clin Electrophysiol* 4:491–496, 1981.
78. Hazard PB, Benton C, Milnor JP: Transvenous cardiac pacing in cardiopulmonary resuscitation, *Crit Care Med* 9:666–668, 1981.
79. Phillips SJ, Butner AN: Percutaneous transvenous cardiac pacing initiated at beside: Results in 40 cases, *J Thorac Cardiovasc Surg* 59:855–858, 1970.
80. Trankina MF, White RD: Perioperative cardiac pacing using an atrioventricular pacing pulmonary artery catheter, *J Cardiothorac Anesth* 3:154–162, 1989.
81. Befeler B, Hildner FJ, Javier RP, et al: Cardiovascular dynamics during coronary sinus, right atrial, and right ventricular pacing, *Am Heart J* 81:372–380, 1971.
82. Benchimol A, Ellis JG, Dimond EG: Hemodynamic consequences of atrial and ventricular pacing in patients with normal and abnormal hearts. Effect of exercise at a fixed atrial and ventricular rate, *Am J Med* 39:911–922, 1965.
83. Hartzler GO, Maloney JD, Curtis JJ, et al: Hemodynamic benefits of atrioventricular sequential pacing after cardiac surgery, *Am J Cardiol* 40:232–236, 1977.
84. Curtis J, Walls J, Boley T, et al: Influence of atrioventricular synchrony on hemodynamics in patients with normal and low ejection fractions following open heart surgery, *Am Surg* 52:93–96, 1986.
85. Trigano AJ, Azoulay A, Rochdi M, et al: Electromagnetic interference of external pacemakers by walkie-talkies and digital cellular phones: Experimental study, *Pacing Clin Electrophysiol* 22:588–593, 1999.
86. Betts TR, Simpson IA: Inhibition of temporary pacing by a mobile phone, *Heart* 87:130, 2002.
87. Cooper JP, Swanton RH: Complications of transvenous temporary pacemaker insertion, *Br J Hosp Med* 53:155–161, 1995.
88. Zaidan JR, Freniere S: Use of a pacing pulmonary artery catheter during cardiac surgery, *Ann Thorac Surg* 35:633–636, 1983.
89. Heiselman DE, Maxwell JS, Petno V: Electrode displacement from a multipurpose Swan-Ganz catheter, *Pacing Clin Electrophysiol* 9:134–136, 1986.
90. Colardyn F, Vandenbogaerde J, De Niel C, et al: Ventricular pacing via a Swan Ganz catheter: A new mode of pacemaker therapy, *Acta Cardiol* 41:23–29, 1986.
91. Lumb PD: Atrioventricular sequential pacing with transluminal atrial and ventricular pacing probes inserted via a pulmonary artery catheter: A preliminary comparison with epicardial wires, *J Clin Anesth* 1:292–296, 1989.
92. Trankina MF: Pacemakers and automatic implantable cardiac defibrillators, *Semin Anesth* 12:165–167, 1993.
93. ZOLL PM: Resuscitation of the heart in ventricular standstill by external electric stimulation, *N Engl J Med* 247:768–771, 1952.
94. Estes NA III, Deering TF, Manolis AS, et al: External cardiac programmed stimulation for noninvasive termination of sustained supraventricular and ventricular tachycardia, *Am J Cardiol* 63:177–183, 1989.
95. Zoll PM: Noninvasive cardiac stimulation revisited, *Pacing Clin Electrophysiol* 13:2014–2016, 1990.
96. Falk RH, Ngai ST: External cardiac pacing: Influence of electrode placement on pacing threshold, *Crit Care Med* 14:931–932, 1986.
97. Gauss A, Hubner C, Meierhenrich R, et al: Perioperative transcutaneous pacemaker in patients with chronic bifascicular block or left bundle branch block and additional first-degree atrioventricular block, *Acta Anaesthesiol Scand* 43:731–736, 1999.
98. Zoll PM, Zoll RH, Falk RH, et al: External noninvasive temporary cardiac pacing: Clinical trials, *Circulation* 71:937–944, 1985.
99. Madsen JK, Meibom J, Videbak R, et al: Transcutaneous pacing: Experience with the Zoll noninvasive temporary pacemaker, *Am Heart J* 116:7–10, 1988.
100. Falk RH, Ngai ST, Kumaki DJ, et al: Cardiac activation during external cardiac pacing, *Pacing Clin Electrophysiol* 10:503–506, 1987.
101. Kelly JS, Royster RL: Noninvasive transcutaneous cardiac pacing, *Anesth Analg* 69:229–238, 1989.
102. Altamura G, Bianconi L, Boccadamo R, et al: Treatment of ventricular and supraventricular tachyarrhythmias by transcutaneous cardiac pacing, *Pacing Clin Electrophysiol* 12:331–338, 1989.
103. Cummins RO, Graves JR, Larsen MP, et al: Out-of-hospital transcutaneous pacing by emergency medical technicians in patients with asystolic cardiac arrest, *N Engl J Med* 328:1377–1382, 1993.
104. Knowlton AA, Falk RH: External cardiac pacing during in-hospital cardiac arrest, *Am J Cardiol* 57:1295–1298, 1986.
105. Altamura G, Bianconi L, Toscano S, et al: Transcutaneous cardiac pacing for termination of tachyarrhythmias, *Pacing Clin Electrophysiol* 13:2026–2030, 1990.
106. Luck JC, Markel ML: Clinical applications of external pacing: A renaissance? *Pacing Clin Electrophysiol* 14:1299–1316, 1991.
107. Pattison CZ, Atlee JL III, Mathews EL, et al: Atrial pacing thresholds measured in anesthetized patients with the use of an esophageal stethoscope modified for pacing, *Anesthesiology* 74:854–859, 1991.
108. Backofen JE, Schauble JF, Rogers MC: Transesophageal pacing for bradycardia, *Anesthesiology* 61:777–779, 1984.
109. Atlee JL III, Pattison CZ, Mathews EL, et al: Transesophageal atrial pacing for intraoperative sinus bradycardia or AV junctional rhythm: Feasibility as prophylaxis in 200 anesthetized adults and hemodynamic effects of treatment, *J Cardiothorac Vasc Anesth* 7:436–441, 1993.
110. Yamanaka A, Kitahata H, Tanaka K, et al: Intraoperative transesophageal ventricular pacing in pediatric patients, *J Cardiothorac Vasc Anesth* 22:92–94, 2008.
111. Smith I, Monk TG, White PF: Comparison of transesophageal atrial pacing with anticholinergic drugs for the treatment of intraoperative bradycardia, *Anesth Analg* 78:245–252, 1994.
112. Trankina MF, Black S, Mahla ME: Cardiac pacing using a pacing esophageal stethoscope in patients undergoing posterior fossa craniotomy in the three quarter prone position, *J Neurosurg Anesth* 6:340, 1994.
113. Roth JV, Brody JD, Denham EJ: Positioning the pacing esophageal stethoscope for transesophageal atrial pacing without P-wave recording: Implications for transesophageal ventricular pacing, *Anesth Analg* 83:48–54, 1996.
114. Burack B, Furman S: Transesophageal cardiac pacing, *Am J Cardiol* 23:469–472, 1969.
115. Trankina MF, Black S, Gibby G: Pacemakers: Perioperative evaluation, management and complications, *Anesthesiology* 93:A1193, 2000.
116. Senthuran S, Toff WD, Vuylsteke A, et al: Editorial III—Implanted cardiac pacemakers and defibrillators in anaesthetic practice, *Br J Anaesth* 88:627–631, 2002.
117. Hernandez AF, Fonarow GC, Hammill BG, et al: Clinical effectiveness of implantable cardioverter-defibrillators among medicare beneficiaries with heart failure, *Circ Heart Fail* 3:7–13, 2010.
118. Moss AJ, Hall WJ, Cannom DS, et al: Improved survival with an implanted defibrillator in patients with coronary disease at high risk for ventricular arrhythmia. Multicenter Automatic Defibrillator Implantation Trial Investigators, *N Engl J Med* 335:1933–1940, 1996.
119. A.V.I.D. Investigators: A comparison of antiarrhythmic-drug therapy with implantable defibrillators in patients resuscitated from near-fatal ventricular arrhythmias. The Antiarrhythmics versus Implantable Defibrillators (AVID) Investigators, *N Engl J Med* 337:1576–1583, 1997.
120. Buxton AE, Lee KL, Fisher JD, et al: A randomized study of the prevention of sudden death in patients with coronary artery disease. Multicenter Unsustained Tachycardia Trial Investigators, *N Engl J Med* 341:1882–1890, 1999.
121. Bardy GH, Lee KL, Mark DB, et al: Amiodarone or an implantable cardioverter-defibrillator for congestive heart failure, *N Engl J Med* 352:225–237, 2005.
122. Hammill SC, Kremers MS, Kadish AH, et al: Review of the ICD Registry's third year, expansion to include lead data and pediatric ICD procedures, and role for measuring performance, *Heart Rhythm* 6:1397–1401, 2009.

123. Bernstein AD, Camm AJ, Fisher JD, et al: North American Society of Pacing and Electrophysiology policy statement. The NASPE/BPEG defibrillator code, *Pacing Clin Electrophysiol* 16:1776–1780, 1993.

124. Poole JE, Johnson GW, Hellkamp AS, et al: Prognostic importance of defibrillator shocks in patients with heart failure, *N Engl J Med* 359:1009–1017, 2008.

125. Mishkin JD, Saxonhouse SJ, Woo GW, et al: Appropriate evaluation and treatment of heart failure patients after implantable cardioverter-defibrillator discharge: Time to go beyond the initial shock, *J Am Coll Cardiol* 54:1993–2000, 2009.

126. Begley DA, Mohiddin SA, Tripodi D, et al: Efficacy of implantable cardioverter defibrillator therapy for primary and secondary prevention of sudden cardiac death in hypertrophic cardiomyopathy, *Pacing Clin Electrophysiol* 26:1887–1896, 2003.

127. Rinaldi CA, Simon RD, Baszko A, et al: A 17 year experience of inappropriate shock therapy in patients with implantable cardioverter-defibrillators: Are we getting any better? *Heart* 90:330–331, 2004.

128. Hasdemir C, Shah N, Rao AP, et al: Analysis of troponin I levels after spontaneous implantable cardioverter defibrillator shocks, *J Cardiovasc Electrophysiol* 13:144–150, 2002.

129. Veltmann C, Borggrefe M, Schimpf R, et al: Fatal inappropriate ICD shock, *J Cardiovasc Electrophysiol* 18:326–328, 2007.

130. Daubert JP, Zareba W, Cannom DS, et al: Inappropriate implantable cardioverter-defibrillator shocks in MADIT II: Frequency, mechanisms, predictors, and survival impact, *J Am Coll Cardiol* 51:1357–1365, 2008.

131. Bhavnani SP, Coleman CI, White CM, et al: Association between statin therapy and reductions in atrial fibrillation or flutter and inappropriate shock therapy, *Europace* 10:854–859, 2008.

132. Swerdlow CD: Supraventricular tachycardia-ventricular tachycardia discrimination algorithms in implantable cardioverter defibrillators: State-of-the-art review, *J Cardiovasc Electrophysiol* 12:606–612, 2001.

133. Brugada P, Geelen P: Some electrocardiographic patterns predicting sudden cardiac death that every doctor should recognize, *Acta Cardiol* 52:473–484, 1997.

134. Maron BJ, Shen WK, Link MS, et al: Efficacy of implantable cardioverter-defibrillators for the prevention of sudden death in patients with hypertrophic cardiomyopathy, *N Engl J Med* 342:365–373, 2000.

135. Moss A, Zareba W, Hall W, et al: Prophylactic implantation of a defibrillator in patients with myocardial infarction and reduced ejection fraction, *N Engl J Med* 346:877–883, 2002.

136. Kadish A, Dyer A, Daubert JP, et al: Prophylactic defibrillator implantation in patients with nonischemic dilated cardiomyopathy, *N Engl J Med* 350:2151–2158, 2004.

137. Peters RW, Gold MR: Pacing for patients with congestive heart failure and dilated cardiomyopathy, *Cardiol Clin* 18:55–66, 2000.

138. Hunt SA, Abraham WT, Chin MH, et al: 2009 focused update incorporated into the ACC/AHA 2005 Guidelines for the Diagnosis and Management of Heart Failure in Adults: A Report of the American College of Cardiology Foundation/American Heart Association Task Force on Practice Guidelines Developed in Collaboration with the International Society for Heart and Lung Transplantation, *J Am Coll Cardiol* 53:e1–e90, 2009.

139. Adams KF, Lindenfeld J, Arnold JMO, et al: HFSA 2006 Comprehensive heart failure practice guideline, *J Card Fail* 12:e1–e119, 2006.

140. Lloyd-Jones DM, Larson MG, Leip EP, et al: Lifetime risk for developing congestive heart failure: The Framingham Heart Study, *Circulation* 106:3068–3072, 2002.

141. Gras D, Leclercq C, Tang AS, et al: Cardiac resynchronization therapy in advanced heart failure the multicenter InSync clinical study, *Eur J Heart Fail* 4:311–320, 2002.

142. Moss AJ, Hall WJ, Cannom DS, et al: Cardiac-resynchronization therapy for the prevention of heart-failure events, *N Engl J Med* 361:1329–1338, 2009.

143. Mullens W, Grimm RA, Verga T, et al: Insights from a cardiac resynchronization optimization clinic as part of a heart failure disease management program, *J Am Coll Cardiol* 53:765–773, 2009.

144. Rozner MA: Management of implanted cardiac defibrillators during eye surgery, *Anesth Analg* 106:671–672, 2008.

145. Winters SL, Packer DL, Marchlinski FE, et al: Consensus statement on indications, guidelines for use, and recommendations for follow-up of implantable cardioverter defibrillators. North American Society of Electrophysiology and Pacing, *Pacing Clin Electrophysiol* 24:262–269, 2001.

146. Garcia-Moran E, Mont L, Brugada J: Inappropriate tachycardia detection by a biventricular implantable cardioverter defibrillator, *Pacing Clin Electrophysiol* 25:123–124, 2002.

147. Gill RM, Sweeney RJ, Reid PR: The defibrillation threshold: A comparison of anesthetics and measurement methods, *Pacing Clin Electrophysiol* 16:708–714, 1993.

148. Weinbroum AA, Glick A, Copperman Y, et al: Halothane, isoflurane, and fentanyl increase the minimally effective defibrillation threshold of an implantable cardioverter defibrillator: First report in humans, *Anesth Analg* 95:1147–1153, 2002.

149. Varma N, Cunningham D, Falk R: Central venous access resulting in selective failure of ICD defibrillation capacity, *Pacing Clin Electrophysiol* 24:394–395, 2001.

150. U.S. Food and Drug Administration: *MAUDE adverse event report—ICD not re-enabled*, Published 2008. Available at: http://www.accessdata.fda.gov/scripts/cdrh/cfdocs/cfMAUDE/Detail.cfm?MDRFOI__ ID=868724 Accessed January 22, 2010.

151. Schwartzenburg CF, Wass CT, Strickland RA, et al: Rate-adaptive cardiac pacing: Implications of environmental noise during craniotomy, *Anesthesiology* 87:1252–1254, 1997.

152. Aldrete JA, Brown C, Daily J, et al: Pacemaker malfunction due to microcurrent injection from a bioimpedance noninvasive cardiac output monitor, *J Clin Monit* 11:131–133, 1995.

153. Rozner MA, Nishman RJ: Electrocautery-induced pacemaker tachycardia: Why does this error continue? *Anesthesiology* 96:773–774, 2002.

154. Alexopoulos GS, Frances RJ: ECT and cardiac patients with pacemakers, *Am J Psychiatry* 137:1111–1112, 1980.

155. Philbin DM, Marieb MA, Aithal KH, et al: Inappropriate shocks delivered by an ICD as a result of sensed potentials from a transcutaneous electronic nerve stimulation unit, *Pacing Clin Electrophysiol* 21:2010–2011, 1998.

156. Vlay SC: Electromagnetic interference and ICD discharge related to chiropractic treatment, *Pacing Clin Electrophysiol* 21:2009, 1998.

26

Procedures in the Hybrid Operating Room

JOANNA CHIKWE, MD | JACK F. KERR, AIA | BARRY A. LOVE, MD

KEY POINTS

1. Hybrid cardiovascular suites are likely to become a key feature of more institutions as the number of patients undergoing hybrid procedures increase, and the technologic and procedural demands outstrip what can be supported by conventional cardiac operating rooms, endovascular suites, and catheterization laboratories.
2. Surgical and imaging equipment should meet the specifications for cardiac surgery and intervention, respectively, and investment in an integrated audiovisual system with linked conferencing capability can facilitate live case discussion.
3. Myocardial revascularization, transcatheter aortic valve implantation, thoracic aortic repair, and congenital cardiac surgery offer clinical outcomes that increasingly are comparable with those of conventional surgical approaches in selected patients and currently represent the bulk of hybrid cardiovascular procedures.

Transcatheter techniques are being used increasingly as an adjunct to, rather than a replacement for, cardiac surgery; the primary aim is to improve clinical outcomes by reducing the size and number of incisions and cardiopulmonary bypass (CPB) time, without compromising the long-term results offered by conventional cardiac surgery.[1] Increasingly, it is only possible to perform these hybrid procedures in suites combining conventional cardiac operating room capability with standard cardiovascular imaging equipment, particularly because most existing cardiac operating rooms and catheterization laboratories do not meet the requirements for performing both surgery and interventional imaging.[2] Hybrid operating rooms first emerged in vascular surgery, driven by lack of access to interventional radiology facilities at a time of expansion in endovascular techniques; more recently, an increase in the number of hybrid procedures has emphasized the need for suites specifically designed for this purpose. This chapter provides an overview of the rationale for building a hybrid cardiovascular suite and the planning, logistics, and design challenges that must be met to create and run it successfully. There is relatively little available on the design and logistics of hybrid operating rooms in the medical literature; the reference articles,[3–5] including an excellent case study by Hirsch[4] and detailed review by Nollert and Wich,[5] were the primary source materials for this chapter and cover most of the aspects outlined here in more depth.

RATIONALE

Key aspects of building design depend on the intended use of the room. Given total costs of between \$2 and \$4 million, there may be a desire to ensure that the room is suitable for the full gamut of cardiovascular hybrid procedures (Table 26-1) to maximize use; and key stakeholders from adult and pediatric cardiac surgery, interventional cardiology, electrophysiology, vascular surgery, and anesthesiology should, therefore, be involved in planning at the earliest stages. It is vital to decide early in the process whether the aim is to build a cardiac catheterization laboratory that can be used for surgical procedures, a cardiac operating room that may be used for cardiovascular imaging, or a true hybrid suite meeting the specifications for cardiac surgery and catheterization and designed to allow state-of-the-art imaging, intervention, and surgery to take place at the same time.

HYBRID CARDIOVASCULAR PROCEDURES

Coronary Revascularization

Coronary artery surgery, which represents more than 90% of adult cardiac procedures nationally, offers some scope for a hybrid approach. The impact of graft failure after coronary artery bypass grafting (CABG) is well documented. In a recent prospective, multicenter study, the 1-year failure rate of saphenous vein grafts was reported to be more than 30%, that of the left internal mammary artery 8%, and the common end point of death or new myocardial infarction was 14% in these patients compared with 1% in patients with patent grafts.[6] More recent data suggested saphenous vein failure rates of more than 40% at 12 to 18 months.[7] Early graft failure, present in 5% to 20% of patients at discharge from the hospital, commonly is attributed to technical error and is the rationale for completion angiography with the option for percutaneous coronary intervention before leaving the operating room. In a recent series of 366 consecutive patients undergoing CABG surgery with completion angiography, 6% of all grafts required percutaneous coronary intervention to address technical problems compromising patency (including vein valves impeding flow [$n = 9$], left internal mammary artery dissection [$n = 6$], vein graft kinks [$n = 7$], and incorrect location or vessel [$n = 8$]). In an additional 49 cases (6.2% of grafts), angiography revealed problems that could be corrected either by minor adjustments such as removing a clip or adjustment of conduit lie or by traditional surgical revision[8] (see Chapter 18).

The relatively high rate of early saphenous graft failure and the lack of clear prognostic benefit conferred by surgical revascularization of non–left anterior descending coronary artery territories has led some groups to explore the option of hybrid revascularization. In the earlier series, 60% ($n = 67$) of patients underwent planned percutaneous coronary intervention either immediately before or after CABG surgery. The majority of patients were selected for hybrid revascularization in an attempt to decrease the perceived risk for conventional surgical revascularization or because lesion anatomy favored stenting over surgery. There was one death in this group because of stent thrombosis in a patient who underwent left internal mammary artery grafting to

Procedures That Can Be Included in the Business Plan for a Hybrid Cardiovascular Suite

Interventional Cardiology

Diagnostic and therapeutic cardiac catheterization, including percutaneous coronary intervention

Diagnostic and therapeutic electrophysiology procedures, including endocardial ablation, pacemaker and defibrillator device insertion and changes

Conventional Cardiac Surgery

All adult and pediatric cardiac surgery

Transplant, ventricular assist device, and extracorporeal membrane oxygenation

Trauma surgery

Fetal interventions

Endovascular Surgery

Abdominal aortic aneurysm stenting

Thoracic aortic aneurysm stenting

Carotid stenting

Hybrid Procedures

Pediatric

Hybrid stage I procedure for hypoplastic left-heart syndrome (modified Norwood)

Patent ductus arteriosus stenting with surgical Blalock-Taussig shunt

Pulmonary artery stenting

Percutaneous atrial septal defect with option to convert to on-bypass open procedure

Preventricular ventricular septal defect closure for muscular apical septal defects

Pulmonary valve replacement

Adult

Coronary artery bypass grafting in multivessel disease with either endoscopic, minithoracotomy or robotic mammary harvest, with direct or robotic left anterior descending coronary artery anastomosis, percutaneous intervention on other lesions, and operative angiography of bypass grafts

Transcatheter aortic valve implantation

Thoracoabdominal aneurysm stenting with surgical debranching or bypass

the left anterior descending artery, and a hybrid stent to the left main stem coronary artery. There are no robust data on long-term outcomes in what are typically small, single-center studies.

The authors emphasized the importance of a collaborative working environment. Although they concluded that routine completion graft imaging should become the standard of care in coronary artery surgery, the authors identified several key considerations. Performing percutaneous revascularization immediately before chest closure, as opposed to 1 or 2 days after surgery, means that the patient is submitted to one, rather than two, procedures, and graft patency may be evaluated and addressed as described earlier. The disadvantages of this approach include the requirement for nephrotoxic contrast at the time of surgery, the additional procedural time and cost, the risk for acute stent thrombosis on reversing heparin with protamine, cardiac catheterization-related complications such as stroke or arterial injury, infection risk, and the need to give patients clopidogrel before surgery, with potential impact on bleeding complications.

Transcatheter Valve Replacement

An emerging modality that will likely become a mainstay of hybrid operating rooms is transcatheter valve replacements.[9] Aortic valve replacement is the treatment of choice for symptomatic severe aortic stenosis; medical management is associated with high mortality, and balloon valvuloplasty offers temporary symptomatic relief without any associated survival benefit. Despite the low operative mortality of isolated primary aortic valve replacement, up to 40% of patients with American Heart Association/American College of Cardiology Class I indications for aortic valve replacement are denied surgery. Reasons most commonly cited by clinicians include advanced patient age and morbidity, and this is a driving force behind the development of transcatheter aortic valve implantation. Transcatheter aortic valve replacement has been performed via either the transfemoral or transapical approach in several thousand patients in Europe, and as of 2010, the U.S. Food and Drug Administration approved the procedure in the United States (see Chapter 19).

These techniques allow aortic valves to be replaced without CPB, large incisions, and in some cases, under sedation rather than general anesthesia. The device consists of a delivery catheter system (now as small as 18F in some devices), a disposable compression and loading system for the prosthesis, and the valve prosthesis. Several such prostheses are available and consist of pericardial valves mounted on compressible metal stents, which can be re-expanded once in position, allowing the valve to be delivered in a retrograde fashion without recourse to CPB, via a catheter placed in the femoral or axillary artery, or antegradely via the apex of the left ventricle, once the native aortic valve has been fractured and displaced by balloon inflation into the coronary sinuses. One key difference between the devices is how the valve is re-expanded once in position. The Cribier–Edwards valve (Edwards Labs, Irvine, CA) is expanded by inflating a balloon inside the valve once in position; cardiac output is zero for the few seconds required to expand the stent. In comparison, the CoreValve prosthesis (Core Valve, Inc., Irvine, CA) is mounted on a large, self-expanding nitinol stent, which allows left ventricular ejection to continue during stent expansion.

The device is guided into position with a combination of real-time transesophageal echocardiography (TEE) and fluoroscopy. Transcatheter valve replacement requires state-of-the-art imaging capability, as well as the ability to secure surgical access, potentially institute CPB, and convert emergently to general anesthesia and conventional aortic valve replacement. If the risk for conversion to open chest surgery declines as experience with the technique increases, the main obstacle preventing standard cardiac catheterization laboratories from being the optimal place to perform transcatheter valve replacement may become one of sterility because current building specifications between catheter laboratories and operating rooms in many countries differ in this regard.

The likelihood is that transfemoral aortic valve replacement will become the dominant treatment modality in high-risk patients requiring aortic valve replacement, greatly expanding the growing pool of eligible patients. Results have improved as both experience with the procedures and technology have developed, and currently mortality, associated stroke, major morbidity, and echocardiographic outcomes appear to offer very-high-risk and nonoperable patients a safe alternative to conventional surgery. Indications for transcatheter aortic valve implantation eventually may be expanded to lower-risk groups, based on outcomes of the large prospective clinical trials currently under way. Interventions for mitral and tricuspid valve repair are at a much earlier stage of development and are less likely to contribute significantly to the volume of hybrid procedures in the next decade.[10]

Hybrid Thoracic Aortic Surgery

Thoracoabdominal aortic disease increasingly is treated with hybrid procedures in which open repair, debranching, or bypasses are performed in conjunction with endovascular stenting. These procedures are particularly suited to hybrid suites capable of providing high-quality imaging, CPB capability, and optimal surgical conditions (see Chapter 21).

Hybrid Congenital Cardiac Surgery

Combined open and interventional approaches have been used successfully to treat multiple muscular ventricular septal defects, pulmonic stenosis, and hypoplastic left-heart syndrome. Hybrid techniques address the barriers to transcatheter approaches such as poor vascular access and hemodynamic compromise, as well as reduce the need for high-risk resternotomy and long CPB times (see Chapter 20).

Cardiac Electrophysiology

A hybrid suite would be the optimal location for totally endoscopic approaches to epicardial ablation combined with a modified transcatheter endocardial strategy, which may provide better long-term freedom from atrial fibrillation and stroke than patients treated using these methods in isolation, although data are currently limited to small, single-center series (see Chapter 4).

PLANNING

The process of building a hybrid operating room, from initial proposal to official opening, takes around 21 months (Table 26-2). All involved parties should establish a clear, early understanding of the primary role of the hybrid room, the statutory requirements, and site limitations that must be met.

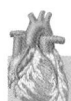 Construction

An operating room and an interventional catheterization laboratory are basically the same. In design and construction, many states enforce the *2006 Guidelines for Design and Construction of Health Care Facilities*. This document has been revised and was published in 2010 (Box 26-1). In the guidelines, both rooms have virtually the same requirements for ventilation, cleanliness, and room finishes. These are 15 room-air changes per hour, relative humidity should be maintained between 30% and 60%, and temperature should be maintained at 68° C to 73° C in operating rooms and 70° C to 75° C in interventional catheterization laboratories. The major differences are in the suite support infrastructure; a surgical suite has requirements for support services that are not required in an interventional catheterization suite. These include:

- The surgical suite should be divided into three designated areas—unrestricted, semirestricted, and restricted—defined by the physical activities performed in each area
- Anesthesia workroom
- Substerile room contiguous to the operating room
- Direct access to Central Sterile Processing with separate paths for clean and soiled.

TABLE 26-2	Design and Construction Timeline	
Time Required	*Activity*	
Months 1–6	Agree on planning group	
	Initial architectural plans and quotes produced	
	Obtain vendor quotes and costs	
	Produce business plan	
	Administration approve business plan	
Month 7	Formal presentation to institutional planning committee	
Month 8	Architectural plans finalized	
	Engineering plans finalized	
	Information technology (IT) and audiovisual plans finalized	
	Vendors selected	
Month 8	Budget completed	
Month 10	Presentation to institutional capital expenditure committee	
Month 11–18	Construction of hybrid room	
Month 18–20	Hybrid room outfitted	
Month 20	Testing hybrid room equipment and setup	
Month 21	Hybrid room official opening	

Historically, catheterization suites have been located within or adjacent to the facility's imaging department. Occasionally, the catheterization suite is standalone within the cardiology service area. Like surgical suites, interventional cardiology suites are required to have support areas including adjacent scrub facilities; patient preparation, holding and recover areas; control room, viewing suite, and electrical

---

BOX 26-1. EXCERPTS FROM 2010 GUIDELINES FOR DESIGN AND CONSTRUCTION OF HEALTH CARE FACILITIES

Surgical Suites
Layout
(1) The surgical suite shall be located and arranged to prevent nonrelated traffic through the suite.
(2) The clinical practice setting shall be designed to facilitate movement of patients and personnel into, through, and out of defined areas within the surgical suite. Signs shall clearly indicate the surgical attire required.
(3) An operating room suite design with a sterile core shall provide for no cross-traffic of staff and supplies from the soiled/decontaminated areas to the sterile/clean areas. The use of facilities outside the operating room for soiled/decontaminated processing and clean assembly and sterile processing shall be designed to move the flow of goods and personnel from dirty to clean/sterile without compromising universal precautions or aseptic techniques in both departments.

Operating and Procedure Rooms
General operating room(s)
(1) New construction
  (a) Space requirements
    (i) Each room shall have a minimum clear area of 400 square feet (37.16 square meters) exclusive of fixed or wall-mounted cabinets and built-in shelves, with a minimum of 20 feet (6.10 meters) clear dimension between fixed cabinets and built-in shelves.
  (b) Communication system. Each room shall have a system for emergency communication with the surgical suite control station.
  (c) X-ray viewers. X-ray film viewers for handling at least four films simultaneously or digital image viewers shall be provided.
  (d) Construction requirements. Operating room perimeter walls, ceiling, and floors, including penetrations, shall be sealed.

Room(s) for cardiovascular, orthopedic, neurological, and other special procedures that require additional personnel and/or large equipment
(1) Space requirements. When included, these room(s) shall have, in addition to the above requirements for general operating rooms, a minimum clear area of 600 square feet (55.74 square meters), with a minimum of 20 feet (6.10 meters) clear dimension exclusive of fixed or wall-mounted cabinets and built-in shelves.
(2) Pump room. Where open-heart surgery is performed, an additional room in the restricted area of the surgical suite, preferably adjoining this operating room, shall be designated as a pump room where extracorporeal pump(s), supplies, and accessories are stored and serviced.
(3) Plumbing and electrical connections. Appropriate plumbing and electrical connections shall be provided in the cardiovascular, orthopedic, neurosurgical, pump, and storage rooms.

Cardiac Catheterization Laboratory (Cardiology)
Location
The cardiac catheterization laboratory is normally a separate suite, but location in the imaging suite shall be permitted provided the appropriate sterile environment is provided.

Space requirements
(1) Procedure rooms
  (a) The number of procedure rooms shall be based on expected utilization.
  (b) The procedure room shall be a minimum of 400 square feet (37.16 square meters) exclusive of fixed cabinets and shelves.

Electrophysiology labs
(1) If electrophysiology labs are also provided in accordance with the functional program, these labs may be located within and integral to the catheterization suite or located in a separate functional area proximate to the cardiac care unit.
(2) These procedure rooms shall comply with all the requirements of Section 2.1-5.4, Cardiac Catheterization Lab.

Excerpted from *2010 Guidelines for Design and Construction of Health Care Facilities.* Dallas, TX: The Facility Guidelines Institute, 2010.

equipment rooms; clean and soiled workrooms; housekeeping closet; and staff clothing change areas. A key consideration to determine early in the planning process is who holds primary responsibility for the hybrid suite—radiology, interventional radiology, interventional cardiology, or cardiac surgery. Once this is established, the physical construction is easier to develop.

Personnel

To address the key needs of the interdisciplinary teams that will be using the hybrid suite, clinicians and technicians from adult and congenital cardiac surgery, interventional cardiology, anesthesiology, perfusion, vascular surgery, and interventional radiology should be involved from the earliest planning stages (Table 26-3). A multidisciplinary planning team should produce a list of requirements, as well as identify key constraints, such as the existing location of services. These include intensive care, cardiac operating room, and cardiac catheterization laboratories. Initial plans then are produced and refined in conjunction with specialist architects, working closely with equipment vendors. Visiting established hybrid rooms, reviewing plans with teams already familiar with the process and outcomes, and three-dimensional reconstructions are all essential parts of the design process because few hybrid rooms are identical, and it is usually difficult to visualize how a setup will function based purely on architectural drawings.

Location

Frequently, the greatest challenge in establishing a hybrid room is identifying a suitable space. If the existing cardiac operating rooms are located separately from the cardiac catheterization laboratories, the hybrid operating room should probably be constructed in proximity to the cardiac operating rooms so that access to cardiac instruments and equipment, CPB machines, perfusionists, cardiac anesthesiologists, extracorporeal membrane oxygenators, and the intensive care unit is optimized. It usually is not possible to convert a single existing cardiac operating room to a hybrid room; a maximally efficient hybrid room requires 900 to 1200 square feet, compared with most operating rooms and catheterization laboratories, which are no more than 400 to 700 square foot. Biplane imaging has a rigid vertical room height requirement of 9'6" to 9'9", and this may be difficult to achieve within an existing operating room complex. The existing space between the ceiling and the floor above is usually full of heating, ventilation, and air conditioning (HVAC) ducts, power and data conduits and cabling,

TABLE 26-3	Key Members of Planning Group for Hybrid Cardiovascular Suite
Clinical Staff	
Adult and pediatric cardiothoracic surgeons	
Interventional cardiologist	
Cardiac anesthesiologist	
Vascular surgeon	
Perfusionist	
Microbiologist	
Operating room nurse manager	
Cardiac catheterization nurse manager	
Business Administrators	
Financial officer	
Construction and Design	
Specialist architect	
Specialist interior designer	
Hospital estates and facilities manager	
Specialist construction manager	
Electronic engineer	
Information technology manager	
Audiovisual specialist	
Internal applications specialist	

and medical gas pipes. The presence of an interstitial floor above or below the site is a great advantage but is the exception rather than the rule in medical center construction. In the absence of constructing additional space, which often is not feasible in urban locations, potential solutions include combining two existing operating rooms or an operating room and a support area for renovation/expansion into an adjacent space. These also cause a domino effect because of the loss of a functioning space.

Infrastructure

Regulatory guidance covering operating rooms and catheterization laboratories varies from state to state, and by country, and the more stringent of the two standards should be met in each case. This usually includes floor area excluding fixed-storage space, nonpaneled ceiling design, air circulation and filtration, and full-scale temperature and humidity control. With rooms 900 to 1200 square feet in size, infrastructural design must incorporate one or more booms housing all perfusion and anesthetic gases, power outlets, data ports, suction, and waste gas scavenging requirements. The booms may additionally house fiberoptic light sources, electrocautery machines, radiofrequency ablation devices, near-infrared spectroscopy, and blood chemistry and hematology analyzers. The booms usually consist of a perfusion boom at one side of the operating table and an anesthetic boom at the head of the table. It may be useful to install a third boom so that the CPB machine may be set up on the opposite side of the table according to surgeon preference. The aim is to ensure that all cabling and conduits are kept off the floor to facilitate cleaning, maintenance, and safety. The brakes on the booms may be powered by compressed nitrogen.

Ergonomics

Several problems commonly are seen in hybrid rooms adapted from catheterization laboratories or operating rooms. The anesthesia area around the head of the bed is typically crowded; positioning of imaging and hemodynamic recording devices may significantly impede flow or movement in the room; sight lines to vital monitoring and imaging may be poor; and moving overhead operating lights and monitors results in collisions with other equipment. One successful solution, described in an excellent case study on setting up a hybrid pediatric cardiac surgery operating room, was to convert the future hybrid suite from a rectangle into a T shape, with the top of the "T" extending from the head of the bed on either side. This provided ample space for the anesthesia boom, anesthetic machine, echocardiography machine, defibrillators, storage cart, and personnel while facilitating access to the patient. Moving bulky hemodynamic and imaging recorders out of the main operating room to a glass-paneled control room linked by a voice-activated microphone system further enhances flow in the main operating room. Creating mobile storage carts dedicated to specific procedures that can be removed from the room when not required frees up additional floor space and further improves flow, particularly if they are located in the horizontal bar of a T-shaped room, so nursing staff no longer have to move around the patient to access equipment. Touch-panel automated doors wide enough to accommodate a bed together with a CPB or extracorporeal membrane oxygenator circuit should be included in the design.

EQUIPMENT

Lights, Monitors

Surgical lights and banks of four to six imaging monitors (or, preferably, large flat-panel screens that can support multiple video inputs) are housed on overhead gantries. Optimally, monitors that display continuous invasive and noninvasive monitoring of vital signs should be placed in four quadrants of the room, in addition to the imaging monitors, which should be located opposite the surgeon, as well as in the control room. A specific plan should be created, including all ceiling-mounted

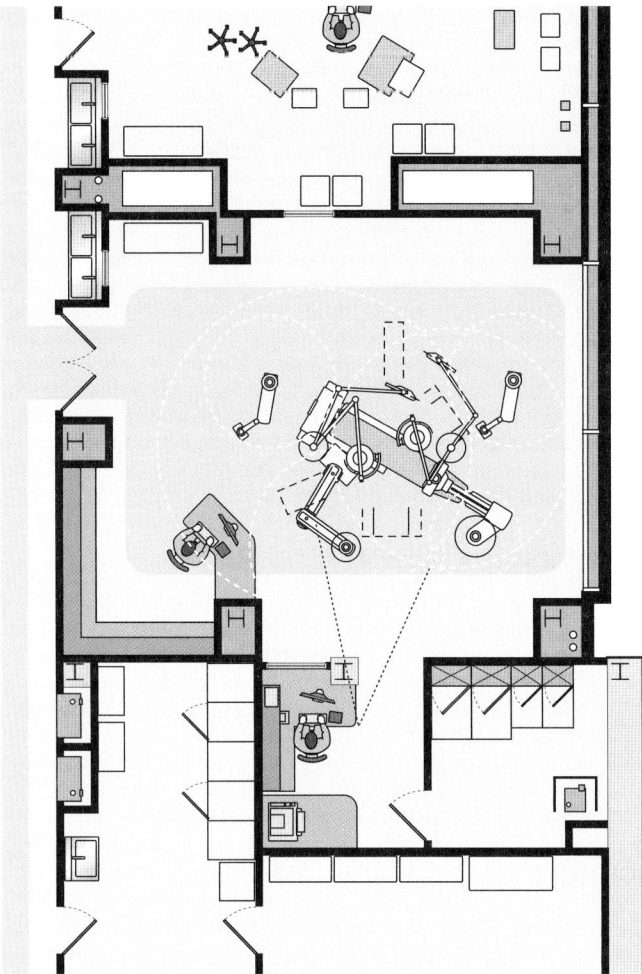

Figure 26-1 Floor plan showing the layout of a hybrid cardiovascular suite, including the working arcs of three booms, C-arm, operating lights, and monitoring gantries; location for bypass circuit; and ancillary rooms. *(Courtesy of Alfred I. Dupont Hospital for Children.)*

components (lights, monitors, booms, air-conditioning, C-arms, etc.) to minimize collisions between devices (Figure 26-1). Conventional surgical lights are often mounted on very long gantries. It can be difficult to position the lights adequately and maintain sterility without assistance, without interfering with sight lines or other equipment, particularly the overhead monitors. A video camera integrated in the main overhead light enables nonsurgical personnel to obtain a view of the surgical field.

Infection Control

The two main focuses of infection control are preventing contamination of the hybrid site and adjacent operating rooms during construction and maintaining hygiene once the room is in use. It frequently is necessary to change or limit access to existing facilities and utilities during building work, and eliminating low-level contamination of nearby rooms is challenging. Rigorous infection control risk assessments are mandatory before and during construction. Requirements for infection control once construction is completed differ between surgical disciplines and between countries. Standard provision by many centers now includes laminar air flow with specified volume changes. Ceiling skirts, which are often used in conjunction with laminar flow systems, preclude ceiling-mounted imaging gantries. Furthermore, ceiling-mounted systems are more difficult to clean than floor-mounted systems, interfere with air flow, and may increase the risk for dust contaminating the

surgical field if running parts cross the ceiling above the operating table. Their main advantage is that they can move up and down the entire operating field without putting tension onto lines and catheters. Touch panel–operated doors and daily terminal cleaning contribute to optimal infection control once the hybrid room is running.

Both a surgical suite, in which the operating room is located, and a cardiac catheterization suite are required to have staff locker facilities that encourage one-way changing from street clothes to scrubs. A catheterization suite should maintain the same semirestricted and restricted areas that are required in a surgical suite. In terms of dress codes, the standard two-step policy for surgical attire is applied to the hybrid operating room. Education of nonsurgical personnel, who are less familiar with the strict antisepsis requirements required in a cardiac operating room, is mandatory.

Imaging Equipment

Fluoroscopy is the basic imaging mode provided by all angiography systems, and is the predominantly used modality during surgery because it exposes the patient to less radiation and provides high-resolution, real-time images. Biplanar rather than monoplanar imaging is essential for interventional cardiology-based procedures. Two kinds of C-arms are available: mobile and fixed. Mobile C-arms, which surgeons currently use routinely for screening for missing instruments and catheter placement, are not adequate for visualizing thin guidewires or fine stents or quantifying stenosis of small vessels. The technical specifications for power, frame rate, and heat storage capacity of mobile C-arms are well below those set by the regulatory bodies, and for a room to work as a true hybrid cardiovascular suite, a fixed C-arm should be installed (Figure 26-2). Where available space is lacking, a semimobile system with a fixed generator may be a reasonable compromise. Flat-panel detectors are preferable to image intensifiers because contrast resolution is higher; there is no edge distortion effect, and flat-panel detectors offer three-dimensional (3D) imaging capabilities (see Chapter 3).

Postprocessing of fluoroscopic images allows 3D images to be generated, as well as fusion of fluoroscopic images with any previously acquired 3D images including computerized tomography, magnetic resonance imaging, positron emission tomography, and single-photon emission tomography. The C-arm must be integrated with the operating table if 3D imaging is planned. Fixed C-arms may be ceiling or floor mounted. Although floor-mounted systems are preferred for hygiene reasons outlined earlier, ceiling-mounted systems can image the whole

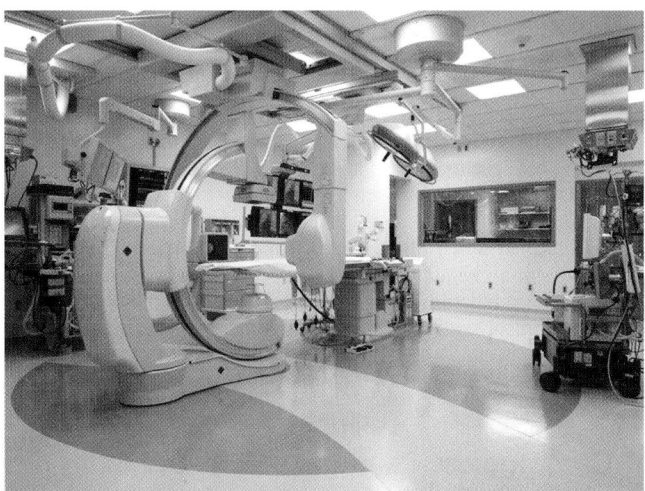

Figure 26-2 View of a hybrid cardiovascular operating room. The cardiopulmonary bypass circuit is on the far right with its own boom. The operating table is in the middle of the picture, with a floor-mounted, fixed biplanar C-arm to the left. *(Courtesy of Alfred I. Dupont Hospital for Children.)*

patient without the need to move the operating table, associated lines, catheters, and monitoring and easily can be moved in and out of the operative field as required. Careful attention needs to be paid to idle and working positions. It often is difficult to mobilize a ceiling-mounted C-arm left at the head of the patient during a procedure without interfering with anesthesia and monitoring equipment. Designing a hybrid suite where large imaging equipment must routinely be stored outside defeats the purpose of a true hybrid operating room.

Operating Equipment

Deciding on a table that meets the needs of both surgeon and interventionalist is challenging. If fixed imaging equipment is installed, then the table also must be fixed. The table must be radiolucent, with a floating tabletop controlled by a touch panel in the surgeon's field providing fast, fine movements during angiography, allowing the whole patient to be imaged. Carbon-fiber tables meet this requirement but do not meet the surgeon's need for a breakable table, although some models do permit lateral and Trendelenburg tilt, and these should be selected for cardiovascular hybrid suites. Most additional positioning can be accomplished with inflatable cushions, which should be checked to establish they do not interfere with any imaging modalities. If robotic procedures are planned, then particularly careful attention needs to be paid to both working space and storage, as well as access between the two because the robot console and arms are particularly bulky pieces of equipment that are preferably stored outside the immediate area of the operating table. As the robot arms surround the operating table, it is not possible to leave the C-arm in space, and options for parking this during robotic procedures should be planned carefully in advance of installation. A fixed C-arm may not be feasible in a room in which the dominant procedure is robotic surgery.

Anesthetic Equipment

Anesthesia for hybrid procedures presents particular challenges, and careful attention must be paid to the design and ergonomics of the anesthesia area. Patients undergoing hybrid procedures may be selected because of substantial frailty or morbidity, contraindicating conventional surgery. Procedures starting out without endotracheal intubation may need urgent conversion. In addition to providing anesthesia for procedures that, in the case of transcatheter aortic valve replacement, for example, may require rapid pacing with periods of complete loss of cardiac output, the anesthetic team is simultaneously required to provide accurate transesophageal echocardiographic guidance to interventionalists. Providing real-time image guidance during time-critical parts of the procedure when the patient is often maximally unstable is a different dynamic from providing routine prebypass and postbypass imaging. Primary consideration, therefore, in designing the anesthesia area is ensuring adequate space to accommodate the anesthetic adjuncts to hybrid procedures such as transesophageal echocardiographic machines, somatosensory-evoked potential and cerebral perfusion monitoring, pacing and defibrillator devices, standard invasive monitoring, and drugs and equipment required for cardiac surgery, while ensuring the anesthesia team has optimal access to the patient at all times. The T-shaped design described earlier offers a particularly effective layout, facilitating flow to patient and equipment. Additional improvements in work flow can be obtained by creating an anesthetic room for induction; these are widely used in conventional cardiac operating rooms in Europe because they increase the efficiency with which the rooms can be used by almost eliminating anesthetic turnaround time.

Communication and Audiovisual Equipment

Imaging routing is helpful, so that all prior patient imaging can be brought up on monitoring screens, which also can display any combination of the real-time imaging or monitoring as required. Integration of multiple video inputs, such as echocardiography, angiography, film

of the operative field, physiologic monitoring, electrophysiologic mapping, and live processing to produce 3D imaging, can greatly facilitate hybrid procedures but requires careful planning. Cameras may be usefully mounted high on the wall of the hybrid suite and within the central light handle, and if high-definition equipment is used with sufficient zooming and remote control capability, it can provide high-quality video footage for monitoring and education purposes. Fixed cameras can be combined with handheld thoracoscopic cameras for minimally invasive procedures. Voice-activated microphones (both fixed to the wall and mounted on headsets) are most useful for communicating with a separate control room during cardiac catheterization but also can allow the surgical team to communicate outside the operating room without breaking sterility if telephone routers are integrated. Well-planned audiovisual systems also facilitate live teaching, case discussions, and conferencing if video footage is linked to remote monitoring screens and projection centers. Dedicated Ethernet and data ports for each imaging modality, as well as standard Internet access, are necessary for uploading large image files onto hospital mainframes. Hybrid rooms should have DVD recording capability.

Opening a New Hybrid Room

Despite painstaking planning and exhaustive testing, initial wrinkles in the smooth functioning of a hybrid room are inevitable; staff need time to familiarize themselves with new layouts, equipment, and ways of working, and unforeseen challenges are inevitable. It, therefore, makes sense to ensure that, for the first week or so of operation, procedures scheduled for the hybrid operating room are routine operations with which all staff are familiar. Building complex and novel approaches in an incremental fashion should minimize adverse events and build institutional confidence in what is, by any measure, a huge investment for all concerned.

HYBRID TRAINING

The growth in hybrid procedures may require a cadre of clinicians trained in both cardiovascular interventional and surgical skills, rather than relying on teams composed of traditionally trained interventionalists and surgeons. The training requirements of the American Board of Thoracic Surgeons have evolved to reflect this perception, already prevalent in vascular surgery, and several residency and fellowship training programs have been developed to provide training in catheter-based skills, diagnostic cardiology, and cardiac surgery, with a view to producing cardiovascular specialists rather than cardiothoracic surgeons. Barriers preventing wholesale adoption of this hybrid approach to training include established conventional referral and working practices; the difficulties inherent in acquiring and maintaining skills in highly technical procedures that are not performed routinely in most centers; the challenge of designing a robust curriculum providing high-quality education and training in a new field that is evolving rapidly; and problems associated with workforce planning. Simulation and wet-labs address some of the training and educational challenges, as well as provide a useful platform for building professional working relationships within hybrid cardiovascular teams. Changing established working practice may prove more challenging; in the hybrid procedures described earlier, the roles of the surgeon and interventionalist still fit traditional patterns even if they are working together in the same room. The likelihood is that, as technology continues to favor percutaneous rather than surgical approaches, hybrid procedures will fall predominantly within the realm of traditionally trained interventionalists who not only already possess the necessary technical and clinical skill set but also are the gatekeepers to the patients.

SUMMARY

Hybrid cardiovascular suites are likely to become a key feature of more institutions as the number of patients undergoing hybrid procedures increase, and the technologic and procedural demands outstrip what can be supported by conventional cardiac operating rooms, endovascular suites, and catheterization laboratories. Surgical and imaging equipment should meet the specifications for cardiac surgery and intervention, respectively, and investment in an integrated audiovisual system with linked conferencing capability can facilitate live case discussion, which is likely to be of particular value in complex, innovative hybrid procedures. Complex coronary artery procedures, transcatheter aortic valve implantation, thoracic aortic repair, and congenital cardiac surgery offer clinical outcomes that increasingly are comparable with those of conventional surgical approaches in selected patients and currently represent the bulk of hybrid cardiovascular procedures. Hybrid training programs providing diagnostic, interventional, and surgical skills may provide cardiovascular specialists with the necessary skill set, but in the longer term, hybrid cardiovascular care is most likely to be dominated by interventionalists. Anesthesiologists have a pivotal role to play in the safe delivery of technology-driven patient care, in the high-stakes environment of the hybrid cardiovascular suite.

REFERENCES

1. King SB 3rd: Who are interventionalists? What about surgeons? *JACC Cardiovasc Interv* 1:109–110, 2008.
2. Byrne JG, Leacche M, Vaughan DE, et al: Hybrid cardiovascular procedures, *JACC Cardiovasc Interv* 1:459–468, 2008.
3. Kpodonu J, Raney A: The cardiovascular hybrid room a key component for hybrid interventions and image guided surgery in the emerging specialty of cardiovascular hybrid surgery, *Interact Cardiovasc Thorac Surg* 9:688–692, 2009.
4. Hirsch R: The hybrid cardiac catheterization laboratory for congenital heart disease: From conception to completion, *Catheter Cardiovasc Interv* 71:418–428, 2008.
5. Nollert G, Wich S: Planning a cardiovascular hybrid operating room: The technical point of view, *Heart Surg Forum* 12:E125–E130, 2009.
6. Alexander JH, Hafley G, Harrington RA, et al: Efficacy and safety of edifoligide, an E2F transcription factor decoy, for prevention of vein graft failure following coronary artery bypass graft surgery: PREVENT IV: A randomized controlled trial, *JAMA* 294:2446–2454, 2005.
7. Lopes RD, Hafley GE, Allen KB, et al: Endoscopic versus open vein-graft harvesting in coronary-artery bypass surgery, *N Engl J Med* 361:235–244, 2009.
8. Zhao DX, Leacche M, Balaguer JM, et al: Routine intraoperative completion angiography after coronary artery bypass grafting and 1-stop hybrid revascularization results from a fully integrated hybrid catheterization laboratory/operating room, *J Am Coll Cardiol* 53:232–241, 2009.
9. Chiam PT, Ruiz CE: Percutaneous transcatheter aortic valve implantation: Assessing results, judging outcomes, and planning trials: The interventionalist perspective, *JACC Cardiovasc Interv* 1:341–350, 2008.
10. Feldman T, Kar S, Rinaldi M, et al: Percutaneous mitral repair with the MitraClip system: Safety and midterm durability in the initial EVEREST (Endovascular Valve Edge-to-Edge REpair Study) cohort, *J Am Coll Cardiol* 54:686–694, 2009.

27

New Approaches to the Surgical Treatment of End-Stage Heart Failure

MARC E. STONE, MD | KORAY ARICA, MD | MASAO HAYASHI, MD | GREGORY W. FISCHER, MD

KEY POINTS

1. Congestive heart failure (CHF) is a chronic progressive disease of epidemic proportion that costs billions of dollars annually.
2. Current medical management alone is incapable of preventing the progression of CHF to the advanced stages of the disease.
3. Surgical options for the management of CHF exist and are being increasingly used at an earlier stage in the course of the disease.
4. Electrophysiologic maneuvers (e.g., biventricular pacing) often can improve cardiac output and decrease mortality in patients with advanced CHF.
5. Surgical procedures (e.g., revascularization, mitral valve repair/replacement, ventricular restoration) can alleviate symptoms and prolong survival in appropriately selected patients.
6. Implantation of a mechanical circulatory assist device remains an attractive management option for advanced cardiac failure because the underlying problem is mechanical pump failure. The new generation of continuous-flow devices is performing admirably, with demonstrably fewer complications, and is rapidly supplanting the first generation of pulsatile devices worldwide for long-term support of the failing heart.
7. New therapies (e.g., transplantation of skeletal myoblasts, stem cells, gene therapies) that potentially can reverse the adverse ventricular remodeling accompanying CHF and improve ventricular function are under development and in various stages of human clinical trials, but they are years away from routine clinical applicability.
8. The anesthetic management of patients presenting for "heart-failure surgery" can be challenging, but diligent preoperative identification of comorbidities, preoperative optimization, appropriate intraoperative monitoring, careful titration of anesthetic agents, and continuous optimization of hemodynamics throughout the perioperative period are necessary for a good outcome.
9. Attention to postoperative pain management is critical in this population if exacerbations of hemodynamic instability are to be avoided.

EPIDEMIOLOGY, PATHOPHYSIOLOGY, AND LIMITATIONS OF CURRENT MANAGEMENT

Scope of the Problem

According to the American Heart Association, approximately 6 million people in the United States have congestive heart failure (CHF). Available statistics indicate that the incidence of CHF in the population approaches 15.2 per 1000 after age 65, 31.7 per 1000 after age 75, and 65.2 per 1000 after age 85, with 1,106,000 hospital discharges for heart failure (HF) in 2006 alone.[1] HF is the leading cause of hospitalization in patients older than 65,[2] with a reported associated cost of $24 to $50 billion annually.[1-4] On a global scale, HF reportedly affects 0.4% to 2.0% of the adult population.[5]

Despite great advances in the understanding of the pathophysiology of HF and the development of medications that can potentially attenuate the progression of that pathophysiology, morbidity and mortality from this disease remain high. The incidence rate of hospitalization for HF increased by 70% during the 1990s,[2] and patients with New York Heart Association (NYHA) Class IV symptoms currently have a reported 1-year mortality rate of 30% to 50%.[6] By comparison, the corresponding rates for NYHA Class I-II patients and Class II-III patients are 5% and 10% to 15%, respectively. (Table 27-1 defines the NYHA symptomatic classes.[7]) Thus, one of the major goals in the management of HF is the prevention of progression to advanced stages.

Although many patients successfully achieve temporary relief of HF *symptoms* with medical management, the underlying pathophysiology inevitably progresses, and pharmacologic interventions alone eventually will become inadequate in most patients. A variety of surgical procedures can be performed to improve cardiac function and potentially arrest (or even reverse) the progression to severe dysfunction; but until very recently, surgical intervention (short of transplantation or placement of a ventricular assist device [VAD]) was considered contraindicated in patients with advanced HF. Surprisingly, good outcomes with "corrective" interventions, however, now have resulted in patients presenting for surgical treatment of their HF on a regular basis. This chapter describes the procedures typically performed in this population and the anesthetic considerations for patients with advanced HF.

Brief Review of the Pathophysiology

The current understanding of the pathophysiology of chronic HF maintains that initial increases in end-diastolic ventricular volume and pressure trigger the release of endogenous natriuretic peptides that promote diuresis.[8-10] Concurrent activation of the sympathetic nervous system causes peripheral vasoconstriction and increases the inotropic state of the myocardium. Initially, these mechanisms act to decrease excessive preload (which restores wall tension to normal) and maintain cardiac output (CO) and arterial blood pressure (BP) in the face of mildly depressed ventricular function. Eventually, however, the carotid, ventricular, and aortic arch baroreceptors are activated by the relative hypovolemia, which leads to further activation of the sympathetic nervous system (via the medullary vasomotor regulatory center), as well as

TABLE 27-1	New York Heart Association (NYHA) Functional Capacity	
Functional Capacity	**Objective Assessment**	
Class I. Patients with cardiac disease but without resulting limitation of physical activity. Ordinary physical activity does not cause undue fatigue, palpitation, dyspnea, or anginal pain.	A. No objective evidence of cardiovascular disease	
Class II. Patients with cardiac disease resulting in slight limitation of physical activity. They are comfortable at rest. Ordinary physical activity results in fatigue, palpitation, dyspnea, or anginal pain.	B. Objective evidence of minimal cardiovascular disease	
Class III. Patients with cardiac disease resulting in marked limitation of physical activity. They are comfortable at rest. Less than ordinary activity causes fatigue, palpitation, dyspnea, or anginal pain.	C. Objective evidence of moderately severe cardiovascular disease	
Class IV. Patients with cardiac disease resulting in inability to carry on any physical activity without discomfort. Symptoms of heart failure or the anginal syndrome may be present even at rest. If any physical activity is undertaken, discomfort is increased.	D. Objective evidence of severe cardiovascular disease.	

From The Criteria Committee of the New York Heart Association: *Nomenclature and Criteria for Diagnosis of Diseases of the Heart and Great Vessels*, 9th edition. Boston: Little, Brown & Co, 1994, pp 253–256.

the renin-angiotensin-aldosterone axis, and the release of vasopressin. The resultant peripheral vasoconstriction, mild fluid retention, and further increases in heart rate and inotropy will again compensate for the failing heart. Ultimately, however, chronic sympathetic stimulation causes myocardial β_1-adrenergic receptors to downregulate, and as ventricular function deteriorates, left ventricular (LV) end-diastolic volumes and pressures again increase, resulting in increased ventricular wall tension. During this time, increased levels of angiotensin II result in adverse myocardial remodeling. Remodeling is a key event in the progression of HF and refers to changes in not only ventricular geometry (e.g., dilation) but also myocardial composition (e.g., myocyte hypertrophy, lengthening, hyperplasia, fibrosis). In addition, increased circulating levels of angiotensin II may enhance myocyte apoptosis (programmed cell death) via a protein kinase C–mediated increase in cytosolic calcium levels.[11]

Alterations in chamber geometry (dilation) and myocardial remodeling lead to progressively decreased forward CO, perpetuating the vicious cycle of adverse neurohumoral activation and transient, tenuous compensation. Myocardial oxygen demand increases, whereas oxygen supply potentially decreases because of shortened diastolic periods and increased diastolic wall tension. This developing diastolic dysfunction (ventricular "stiffness") leads to increased left atrial and pulmonary pressures, pulmonary congestion, and increased right ventricular (RV) afterload. This eventually may progress to signs and symptoms of right-sided HF.

Modern medical management of chronic CHF, therefore, uses agents that have been shown to decelerate the progression to severe failure, reduce adverse myocardial remodeling, and enhance survival (e.g., angiotensin-converting enzyme inhibitors,[12–14] β-blockers,[15–18] and aldosterone antagonists[19,20]), in combination with other agents that improve the symptoms but have not been shown to improve long-term survival alone (e.g., diuretics, digoxin). (See Chapter 10.)

▓ Limitations of Current Medical Management

Given that there are currently between 300,000 and 800,000 patients in the United States who have progressed to NYHA Class III and IV status despite modern medical management,[21] it appears that current treatment strategies have significant limitations. Part of the failure of medical management alone to control the progression of the disease may be that treatment has traditionally focused on systolic dysfunction.

Four classic stages of HF have been described: (1) an initial cardiac injury or insult, (2) activation of specific neurohormonal axes with resultant cardiac remodeling, (3) compensatory fluid retention and peripheral vasoconstriction, and (4) ultimate contractile failure.[22] In contrast with this traditional conception, it is now known that diastolic dysfunction (decreased lusitropic function) is the primary problem in an estimated 30% to 50% of patients with HF. Pharmacologic interventions aimed at improving diastolic dysfunction and attenuating (if not reversing) remodeling currently are the subject of randomized trials worldwide.

SURGICAL OPTIONS FOR HEART FAILURE

A growing number of surgical procedures exist (or have been developed) to relieve CHF symptoms and arrest the progression of the disease through correction of abnormal myocardial depolarization, enhancement of myocardial blood supply, improvement in ventricular loading conditions, and restoration of more normal ventricular geometry. Box 27-1 provides a list of current surgical interventions for CHF.

Cumulative worldwide experience with the interventions listed in Box 27-1 suggests that these procedures not only relieve symptoms but may attenuate or possibly arrest the progressive myocardial remodeling that accompanies chronic HF.[23–27] In some cases, partial reversal of the adverse myocardial remodeling has been demonstrated, and combination therapy (surgical intervention with targeted pharmacologic treatment) intended to enhance reverse remodeling is actively being investigated.[28]

Thus, interventions previously considered contraindicated by low ejection fraction (EF) are now being used precisely for that indication. It remains to be determined, however, which procedures ultimately will benefit which subpopulations of patients with HF. Despite the common final pathway that leads to dilated pathophysiology seen in the majority of these patients, an individual's initial underlying causative factor may again become an important consideration because these procedures are used earlier and earlier in the course of deterioration as a treatment intended to halt the progression of the disease.

▓ Revascularization

Coronary artery disease has become the most common cause of HF.[29] Of those patients currently listed for heart transplantation, 36% carry a primary diagnosis of ischemic heart disease, and 31% of those transplanted in 2007 had ischemia as their primary indication. Commonly used terms describing the extent of myocardial injury are defined in Table 27-2.

Where viable myocardium and feasible targets exist, revascularization of chronically ischemic, hibernating myocardium can improve ventricular function, downgrade NYHA functional class, and improve prognosis.[30,31] Although the primary benefit of revascularization appears to

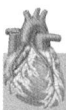

BOX 27-1. SURGICAL OPTIONS FOR THE MANAGEMENT OF CONGESTIVE HEART FAILURE

- Cardiac resynchronization therapy with biventricular pacing
- Revascularization (coronary artery bypass grafting or percutaneous coronary artery stenting)
- Mitral valve repair or replacement
- Surgical ventricular restoration
- Implantation of a left ventricular assist device
- Cardiac transplantation
- New therapies for congestive heart failure in various stages of development include transplantation of skeletal myoblasts and stem cells, "gene" therapy, and xenotransplantation

TABLE 27-2	Commonly Used Terms Describing the Extent of Myocardial Injury and the Potential for Recovery
Term	*Definition*
Ischemic	Insufficient oxygen supply to meet myocardial oxygen demand
Stunned	Acute myocardial dysfunction after an ischemic event with potential for full recovery
Hibernating	Chronically ischemic, dysfunctional myocardium with potential for full recovery
Maimed	Dysfunctional myocardium on the basis of ischemia that does not fully recover
Infarcted	Myocardial necrosis caused by ischemia with no potential for recovery

be functional improvement of the left ventricle, reducing ischemic substrate for arrhythmias and retarding adverse myocardial remodeling are important secondary benefits.[24]

Despite an increased perioperative risk for morbidity and mortality in this population, the world's literature reports current survival rates between 57% and 75% at 5 years, with in-hospital mortality rates between 1.7% and 11%.[31] A review reported an 83.5% survival rate at 2 years after revascularization compared with only 57.2% survival in patients with CHF who were not revascularized.[30] In general, morbidity and mortality tend to correlate inversely with EF and directly with NYHA functional class. Additional factors predisposing patients to greater morbidity and mortality include advanced age, female sex, hypertension, diabetes, and emergent operations[32] (see Chapter 18). The decreases in morbidity and mortality after revascularization in this high-risk population in recent years are at least partially attributable to improvements in surgical technique and myocardial protection, but the concurrent performance of mitral valve repair and ventricular reshaping address the adverse ventricular loading conditions present and also may contribute to improved outcomes. The results of ongoing clinical trials evaluating combinations of surgical procedures (e.g., revascularization plus ventricular reshaping vs. revascularization alone) are discussed in detail later.

The importance of determining the viability of myocardium in the area to be revascularized cannot be overstated because the potential for recovery of function depends on residual contractile reserve, integrity of the sarcolemma, and metabolically preserved cellular function.[31] Methods to detect viable myocardium include dobutamine stress echocardiography, single-photon emission computed tomography, positron emission tomography, and cardiac magnetic resonance imaging (see Chapters 1 and 2). Although dobutamine stress echocardiography often has been shown to have the greatest predictive accuracy,[33] important limitations need to be taken into account. Dobutamine stress echocardiography does not demonstrate viability directly, but improvement in mechanical contraction under pharmacologic stimulation. An example for a false-negative result can be seen if there is loss of contractile proteins in the presence of preserved function of the muscle fiber membrane.[31] Some centers report using only the intraoperative assessment of myocardial wall thickness and contractility to determine potential viability with revascularization of the target region.[34] Regardless of the specific method used, the important point is that there needs to be viable tissue to revascularize, and the best results will be obtained in properly selected individuals. Overwhelmingly, encouraging results worldwide suggest that, when feasible, revascularization is of benefit and provides survival advantage to patients with significant ventricular dysfunction.

Correction of Mitral Regurgitation

The mitral valve is a complex apparatus consisting of the anterior and posterior leaflets, the mitral annulus, the chordae tendineae, the papillary muscles, and the wall of the left ventricle. The posterior portion of the annulus is only rudimentarily developed and flexible. This explains why this portion of the annulus is prone to dilation during pathologic

volume-overloaded states and mandates some form of mechanical stabilization when surgical valve repair is undertaken. The normal annulus has a three-dimensional (3D) saddle shape that is exacerbated during systole because of apical displacement of the commissures.[35] In addition, the aortic root bulges posteriorly during systole. These dynamic phenomena lead to the ability of the annulus to change its shape during the cardiac cycle. During systole, an elliptical shape is assumed that facilitates coaptation of the leaflets. During diastole, a more circular form increases orifice dimensions, decreasing resistance to LV inflow.[36] Consequently, the LV free wall, papillary muscles, and chordae play an important role in the competence of the valve, as well as in LV function during systole.

The mechanism responsible for mitral regurgitation can best be understood by utilizing the Carpentier classification (Table 27-3). This classification describes the motion of the mitral leaflets and position of the coaptation zone relative to the annular plane. The mitral regurgitation seen in patients with CHF is most often functional, primarily because of apical displacement of the papillary muscles resulting in tethering of the leaflets leading to systolic restriction of leaflet motion (type IIIb).

Historically, many physicians considered mitral regurgitation advantageous for the failing left ventricle. It was believed that a low-pressure atrial "pop off" allowed the failing ventricle to protect itself from the high afterload of the systemic circulation and gave the illusion that the heart had a better overall contractile state than really existed. This misconception was "supported" by the fact that surgical replacement of the mitral valve was associated with a very high mortality rate in patients with depressed LV function.[37]

Romano and Bolling's[38] work disproved this misconception, showing that despite increased operative risk, mitral valve repair or replacement was beneficial to patients with severely depressed LV function, CHF, and mitral regurgitation. Operative mortality rates of 5% were reported, with 1- and 2-year survival rates of 80% and 70%, respectively.[38] Not only was long-term mortality reduced, but the increase in LV systolic function (on average by 10%) enabled a downgrading of NYHA class and resulted in an improved quality of life (see Chapter 19).

Although the majority of patients with end-stage HF will exhibit functional mitral regurgitation (as discussed earlier), there may be additional concurrent valvular pathology present in a given patient. An intraoperative transesophageal echocardiography (TEE) evaluation of the valvular anatomy, the mechanism of the mitral regurgitation, and direct surgical inspection will determine the feasibility of repair. Data obtained from patients suffering from organic mitral valve regurgitation have been extrapolated to the functional mitral regurgitation group in the belief that valve repair is preferable to valve replacement, because there are demonstrated hemodynamic advantages associated with preservation of the subvalvular apparatus,[39] and long-term anticoagulation is not required. However, review of the literature cannot unequivocally support this assumption. Magne et al[40] were unable to show a survival advantage between MV repair and

TABLE 27-3	Carpentier Classification of Mitral Regurgitation	
Carpentier Class	*Leaflet Motion*	*Typical Pathology*
Type I	Normal leaflet motion	Annular dilation, leaflet perforation
Type II	Excessive leaflet motion	Leaflet prolapse or flail, chordal rupture or elongation
Type IIIa	Restricted leaflet motion	Rheumatic leaflet(s), thickened or fused leaflets or chordae
Type IIIb	Restricted leaflet motion	Papillary muscle displacement/dysfunction (dilated cardiomyopathy or ischemic)

From Carpentier A, Chauvaud S, Fabiani JN, et al: Reconstructive surgery of mitral valve incompetence: Ten-year appraisal. *J Thorac Cardiovasc Surg* 79:338, 1980.

replacement in patients with ischemic mitral regurgitation. Gillinov et al[41] showed that a survival benefit could be obtained by repairing the mitral valve as opposed to replacing it, especially in lower-risk patients. However, in high-risk patients, defined as patients with extremely low EF and dilated ventricles, this survival benefit was lost, prompting them to recommend MV replacement.[41] Braun et al[42] showed that end-diastolic diameter larger than 65 mm was associated with poorer survival in 108 patients undergoing restrictive mitral annuloplasty and CABG. Reverse remodeling was seen in all patients with end-diastolic diameter smaller than 65 mm; however, it was seen in only 25% with end-diastolic diameter larger than 65 mm, making them question whether MV repair/CABG is justified in grossly dilated ventricles. Most likely a ventricular solution will need to be considered in this subset of patients.

A common dilemma that is encountered by the perioperative team is what to do with a patient with ischemic cardiomyopathy and moderate mitral regurgitation. In the setting of severe mitral regurgitation, most would agree to perform concurrent mitral regurgitation repair, and in the setting of mild mitral regurgitation, to leave the mitral valve dysfunction unaddressed. Penicka et al's[43] study potentially could help shed light on this topic. They found improvement in moderate ischemic mitral regurgitation only in patients in whom viable myocardium in the region of the papillary muscles could be identified by preoperative single-photon emission computed tomographic testing. Patients with nonviable myocardium and dyssynchrony between the papillary muscles showed postoperative worsening of ischemic mitral regurgitation. Consequently, the authors argued to perform annuloplasty in all patients with nonviable myocardium and perform isolated CABG in patients with viable myocardium.[43]

The primary repair technique in the setting of type IIIb dysfunction consists of downsized annuloplasty. Although much debate exists regarding whether the annuloplasty should be performed with the aid of a complete semirigid ring or band, most experts agree that the annulus needs to be remodeled and stabilized. Although this technique results in excellent short-term results, most surgeons realize that addressing a ventricular problem at the annular level cannot represent the ideal solution. Magne et al[44] showed that the use of annuloplasty rings eliminated severe mitral regurgitation; however, this was at the cost of leaving patients with functional mitral stenosis. One valvular disorder could be exchanged for another by undersizing the annulus (see Chapter 19).

After the procedure, TEE is used to assess the adequacy of the repair and potential improvement of overall cardiac function. Often, hemodynamic improvement is not immediately apparent, and TEE is used to optimize preload and guide pharmacologic interventions (see Chapters 12 to 14, 32, and 34).

Left Ventricular Restoration

In 1985, building on work by Cooley, Jatene, and others,[45–47] Dor et al introduced a ventricular reshaping procedure intended to improve systolic performance by excluding akinetic/dyskinetic and aneurysmal portions of the left ventricle with a circular stitch at the transitional zone between contractile and noncontractile myocardium. A small patch was used within the ventricular cavity as needed to reestablish ventricular wall continuity at the level of the purse-string suture.[48]

This procedure generally was performed in conjunction with revascularization (and included mitral repair/replacement as needed) and thus helped establish important principles for a surgical ventricular restoration: revascularization of ischemic myocardium, decreasing of ventricular volume, and the restoration of ventricular shape. A subsequent publication by the same group described the results of this procedure in 130 patients (35% of whom had "heart failure" as the indication for the operation) and reported a 6% in-hospital mortality rate and a 3% late mortality rate because of recurrence of cardiac failure.[49]

In 1996, Batista et al[50] introduced a procedure for the reshaping of the nonischemic, dilated, and failing left ventricle of NYHA Class IV patients through resection of a wedge of normal myocardium from the LV apex to the base (laterally, between the papillary muscles). This "partial left ventriculectomy" restored more normal ventricular geometry and decreased wall tension. Functional mitral regurgitation also was addressed during the Batista procedure by a mitral valve replacement or repair. Although many patients did benefit initially from this procedure (reduction of NYHA functional class to NYHA Class I in 57% and NYHA Class II in 33.3%),[51] perioperative mortality was high (20% in both Batista's own series and in the large Cleveland Clinic experience).[51,52] In addition, the experience of several centers was that many patients required rescue mechanical circulatory assistance after the procedure, and many patients experienced a redilatation of their left ventricle resulting in a return to NYHA Class IV status.[53–55] Thus, despite the short-lived period of initial enthusiasm in the mid- to late-1990s, the Batista procedure essentially has been abandoned. The concept of ventricular reshaping, however, remains of interest.

The modified Dor procedure (endoventricular circular patch plasty) has been used successfully to reshape large, dilated, spherical left ventricles of patients who have had an anterior wall myocardial infarction (MI) with resulting aneurysm and akinesis/dyskinesis. Essentially, a Dacron patch is placed within the LV cavity to exclude the large akinetic/dyskinetic area of the anterior wall. This restores LV geometry to a more normal elliptical shape and improves systolic function. When performed concurrently with CABG, significant early and late improvements in both NYHA functional class and EF have been demonstrated, with an in-hospital mortality rate of 12%.[56,57] A trial of 439 patients undergoing this procedure found an improved in-hospital mortality rate of 6.6% and an 18-month survival rate of 89.2%. In this series, CABG was performed concurrently in 89%, mitral valve repair in 22%, and mitral valve replacement in 4%.[58]

Surgical ventricular restoration is the modern name for a modified Dor procedure, in which, in addition to exclusion of the akinetic aneurysmal segment of the anterior and/or septal wall and revascularization, a sizing balloon (or other sizer) is used to create an elliptical left ventricle of 30% to 40% smaller volume than baseline. Despite a worldwide surgical ventricular restoration database already in place including more than 5000 surgical ventricular restoration patients, a randomized, controlled trial was designed named "The Surgical Treatment for Heart failure (STICH)," with the intention to scientifically prove the efficacy of this procedure as an adjunct to revascularization. The results of this important trial have been eagerly awaited for years. Unfortunately, STICH did *not* demonstrate that the addition of surgical ventricular restoration to revascularization was associated with a greater improvement in symptoms or exercise tolerance, or with a reduction in the rate of death or hospitalization for cardiac causes when compared with revascularization alone.[59] The negative results from this trial have caused much controversy and the validity questioned.[60] Noted areas of concern revolve around participant eligibility for anatomic reasons, lack of standardized volumetric assessments in large numbers of participants, and alteration of the primary objective after trial commencement. In essence, the expert opinion is that the STICH trial was "well conceived, but poorly executed." At the time of this writing, surgical ventricular restoration continues to be performed for true LV aneurysms but has fallen out of favor as a routine adjunct for the dilated end-stage left ventricle.

Cirillo's[61] recent publication described a further modification of the Dor concept wherein the shape and orientation of the patch, as well as the manner of suturing, ostensibly maintained more physiologic orientation of the myocardial fibers. Named the "KISS" procedure (**K**eep fibers orientation with **S**trip patch re**S**haping), this methodology reportedly allowed for a return of normal apical rotation and ventricular torsion to optimize systolic performance. Long-term results of this new approach await further study.

Cardiac Resynchronization Therapy and Implantable Cardioverter-Defibrillators

The progression of disease resulting in advanced cardiac failure is typically accompanied by conduction defects and arrhythmias, and pacemakers and implantable cardioverter-defibrillators (ICDs) are common in this population. In addition to the well-known defects in sinus or atrioventricular node function, intraventricular conduction defects delay the onset of RV or LV systole in 30% to 50% of patients with advanced HF.[62,63] This lack of coordination of LV and RV contractions further impairs CO[64–67] and has been reported to increase the risk for death in this population[68,69] (see Chapters 4 and 25).

Cardiac resynchronization therapy (CRT) entails biventricular pacing (not to be confused with dual-chamber atrioventricular sequential pacing) to optimize the timing of RV and LV contractions. The right atrium is paced by a lead in the right atrium, the right ventricle by a lead in the right ventricle, and the left ventricle by a lead in a coronary vein (accessed via the coronary sinus). Although CRT is more an interventional cardiology procedure than a surgical procedure per se, anesthesiologists frequently are asked to provide sedation (if not general anesthesia) for these sometimes lengthy implantation procedures.

Studies have shown that atrial-synchronized biventricular pacing (pacing the left and right ventricles in a carefully timed manner) can resynchronize RV and LV contraction, improving CO and overall hemodynamics. This enhances these patients' ability to exercise, which improves their NYHA functional class, and decreases the length and frequency of their hospitalizations, which improves their quality of life.[70–74]

Sudden death from ventricular fibrillation accounts for approximately 350,000 deaths annually in the United States.[1] Patients with advanced HF experience ventricular fibrillation with a frequency six to nine times that of the general population,[1] and ventricular fibrillation causes 40% of all deaths in this population even in the absence of apparent disease progression based on symptoms.[75] Thus, ICDs commonly are indicated for patients with advanced cardiac failure. An ICD is a device capable of arrhythmia detection and automatic defibrillation. ICDs successfully terminate ventricular fibrillation in greater than 98% of episodes, and studies have demonstrated that an ICD increases survival and decreases the risk for sudden death in patients with ischemic cardiomyopathy and decreased LV function.[76–78]

The COMPANION trial (Comparison of Medical Therapy, Pacing, and Defibrillation in Heart Failure) studied 1500 patients with NYHA Class III/IV HF, a QRS interval of greater than 120 milliseconds, PR interval greater than 150 milliseconds, and an LVEF less than or equal to 35%. Compared with optimal pharmacologic therapy alone, CRT decreased the risk of the combined end point of death from or hospitalization for HF by 34%. The combination of CRT and ICD implantation reduced these risks by 40%.[79]

The CARE-HF (Cardiac Resynchronization in Heart Failure) trial enrolled 800 patients with NYHA Class III/IV HF, a QRS interval of more than 150 milliseconds, a QRS interval of more than 120 milliseconds with echocardiographic evidence of dyssynchrony, and an LVEF of 35% or less. Compared with optimal medical therapy alone, CRT (without ICD functionality) reduced all-cause mortality by 36%. In addition, CRT showed significant improvement of cardiac dyssynchrony, ventricular function, and mitral regurgitation based on echocardiographic criteria.[68]

Most recent guidelines give a Class I recommendation for placement of a CRT device with or without ICD in patients with LVEF ≤ 35%, QRS ≥ 120 milliseconds, presence of sinus rhythm, and NYHA Class III/IV symptoms on optimal medical therapy.[80] However, two recent trials have investigated the effects of CRT on patients with NYHA Class I/II HF. The REVERSE trial (Resynchronization Reverses Remodeling in Systolic Left Ventricular Dysfunction) randomized 610 NYHA Class I/II patients with QRS ≥ 120 milliseconds and LVEF ≤ 40% to receive a CRT device (±ICD) that was either active (CRT-ON) or disabled (CRT-OFF). This study showed a significant delay in time to first hospitalization and improvement in measures of LV remodeling in the CRT-ON group.[81] The MADIT-CRT trial (Multicenter Automatic Defibrillator Implantation Trial–Cardiac Resynchronization Therapy) randomized 1820 NYHA Class I/II patients with QRS ≥ 130 milliseconds and LVEF ≤ 30% to receive CRT and ICD or ICD alone. The CRT-ICD group had a significant 41% decrease in risk for first HF event, significant reduction in LV volumes, and increase in LVEF as compared with the ICD only group.[82] Thus, although CRT previously has been about reduction in symptoms, it is anticipated that results such as those reported from MADIT-CRT will lead to an increased utilization of CRT in relatively asymptomatic patients with developing HF to prevent the progression of the disease.

MECHANICAL CIRCULATORY SUPPORT

Mechanical support of the failing heart has become a mainstay of the modern management of patients with both acute and chronic HF refractory to pharmacologic and other usual interventions. Recent advances in device technology, new understandings of risk factors that may result in complications, increased patient management experience, favorable published data from clinical trials with the new continuous-flow devices, and the experience of high-volume centers not only have resulted in more widespread acceptance of VADs as a management strategy but also an earlier utilization of VADs in the course of a patient's cardiac deterioration. This section discusses the current theory and practice of mechanical circulatory support (MCS), highlighting new and innovative devices that rapidly are becoming the new standard.

Ventricular Assist Devices: Implementation of Support

VADs can be used to take over the pumping function of the failing ventricle and provide effective CO to the arterial circulation downstream from the failing ventricle. In the case of the failing right ventricle, a right ventricular assist device (RVAD) can divert the deoxygenated venous return to the heart and pump it directly to the pulmonary arterial circulation. In the case of the failing left ventricle, a left ventricular assist device (LVAD) can divert the oxygenated blood returning to the left side of the heart and pump it directly into the aorta. Figure 27-1 demonstrates common cannulation strategies in the heart and great vessels by which MCS is implemented. Although there are a few notable exceptions (discussed later), these basic cannulation strategies are common to all manufacturers' devices currently in use, regardless of the type of output they produce.

In addition to maintaining the circulation, decompression (or emptying) of the failing ventricle provides additional benefit because decompression will decrease the wall tension (and, therefore, myocardial oxygen demand) in the volume- and pressure-overloaded failing ventricle, potentially allowing for recovery of ventricular function. This is particularly relevant to short-term support of the acutely failing ventricle, but recovery of function (to varying degrees) also can be seen with chronically failing ventricles.

Mechanical Circulatory Support: Modern Practice

In prior years, VADs were regarded as either a last-ditch hope for recovery after an acute cardiac event that resulted in refractory cardiogenic shock ("bridge-to-recovery"), or as a "bridge-to-transplantation" for patients with chronic HF who were doing poorly. This has all changed now. More widespread acceptance of MCS, the recognition that outcomes are better when the support is instituted earlier rather than later, the development and use of risk scores to appropriately select patients and support strategies,[83–94] the demonstration that there is often significant improvement in multiorgan function during the time spent on VAD support,[95–97] the advent of new and improved devices, and a

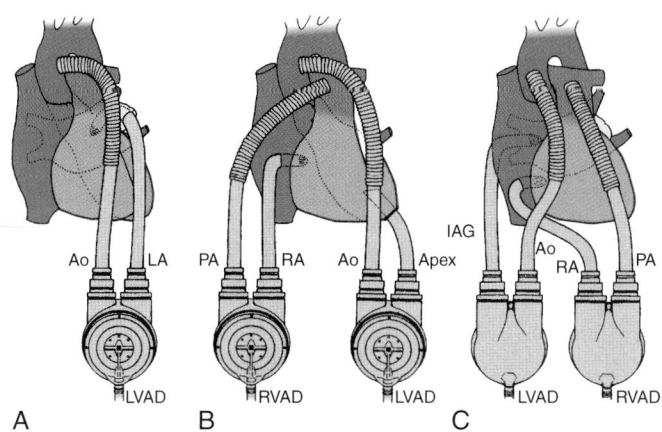

Figure 27-1 The Thoratec ventricular assist device (VAD) and three cannulation approaches for univentricular left-heart support *(A)* and biventricular support *(B, C)*. Potential cannulation strategies for VADs are shown. *B,* The most commonly used cannulation approaches for most currently available VADs. Cannulas are placed in the heart and great vessels to divert blood returning to the failing side of the heart to the pump. The blood collected in the VAD blood chamber is then ejected into the arterial circulation immediately downstream of the failing ventricle. AO, aorta; Apex, left ventricular apex; IAG, cannula inserted via the interatrial groove and directed toward the LA roof; LA, left atrial appendage; PA, pulmonary artery; RA, right atrium. *(Reproduced from Thoratec Corporation, Pleasanton, CA.)*

TABLE 27-4	Conditions or Comorbidities That Make Ventricular Assist Device Placement or Use Difficult, Make the Patient More Likely to Have Major Complications, or Make Meaningful Recovery Unlikely

- Prosthetic valves
- Aortic regurgitation
- Congenital heart disease
- Intracardiac shunts
- Prior cardiac surgery
- Small BSA
- Advanced systemic disease (severe chronic obstructive pulmonary disease, malignancy, ESLD, ESRD, sepsis, progressive neurologic disorder, etc.)

BSA, body surface area; ESLD, end stage liver disease; ESRD, end stage renal disease.

The traditional concept of the temporary or short-term use of a VAD as a "bridge-to-recovery" has thus been expanded to include concepts such as "bridge-to-immediate survival," "bridge-to-next decision," and "bridge-to-a-bridge."

- "Bridge-to-immediate survival" refers to the urgent institution of MCS at the first diagnosis of refractory cardiac failure, often with a rapidly deployable, short-term device to ensure the immediate survival of the patient from the acute cardiac event. Current devices used as a "bridge-to-immediate-survival" include an intra-aortic balloon pump (IABP; see Chapter 32), the TandemHeart (CardiacAssist, Pittsburgh, PA; Figure 27-2), and the Impella (Abiomed, Danvers, MA; Figure 27-3).

substantially decreased rate of VAD-associated complications[98–101] have allowed for an increased and an improved clinical utilization of this life-saving technology in the management of both acute and chronic HF.

Short-Term Ventricular Assist Device Use

The main indication for the short-term use of VADs always has revolved around the concept that the acutely failed myocardium could potentially recover after a short period of support. Depending on the cause of the acute failure (e.g., ischemic stunning, viral myocarditis), early experience revealed that myocardial recovery typically took a week or two in the majority of well-managed patients, who were then theoretically able to be weaned from support. Most short-term VAD use in prior decades was with extracorporeal, pulsatile devices, although standard centrifugal pumps producing continuous flow were also occasionally used, especially for the pediatric population and for extracorporeal membrane oxygenation (ECMO). In reality, however, regardless of the device used as a bridge-to-recovery, support often was initiated too late, complications (e.g., bleeding, thromboembolism, infection, multisystem organ failure) were frequent, and the percentage of patients who were able to be weaned from support (much less discharged from the hospital) was often disappointing.

Early experience also demonstrated that specific patient conditions or comorbidities (Table 27-4) potentially increased the risk for complications during VAD support or made support difficult to implement. It also was proposed that patients who were not potential transplant candidates should probably not be considered for VAD support. Finally, it commonly was believed for many years that patients unlikely to survive regardless of the reestablishment of effective systemic perfusion should probably not even be considered for temporary VAD support. However, society currently demands that everyone (no matter how critically ill) be given an opportunity to recover, and the new and improved MCS technology is often now used with the understanding that improvement in clinical status will allow for a continuation of support, whereas a worsening of the clinical picture will prompt a discontinuation of support. Nevertheless, it is the advancements of the technology and an increased patient management experience that have brought a new flexibility to the arena of short-term MCS.

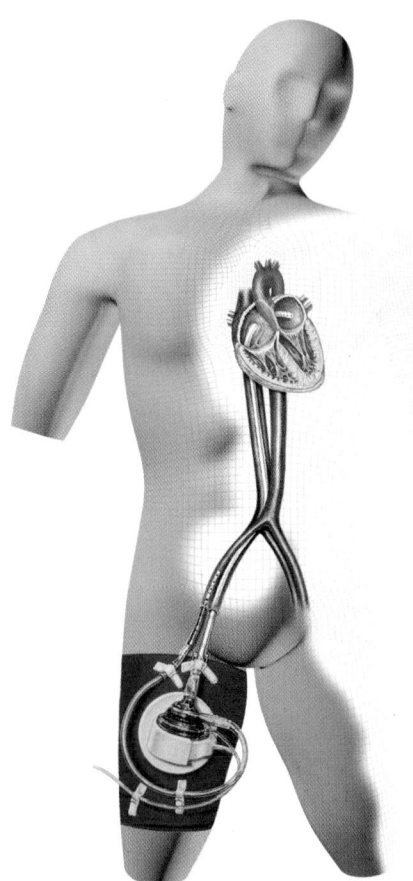

Figure 27-2 The Tandem Heart percutaneous Ventricular Assist Device (pVAD). This recently introduced device provides circulatory support with a centrifugal pump head and the potential advantages of percutaneous cannula insertion. Partial left-heart bypass is accomplished via an interatrial septal cannulation into the left atrium across the area of the fossa ovalis, and oxygenated blood is returned to the femoral artery. *(Courtesy of CardiacAssist Inc., Pittsburgh, PA.)*

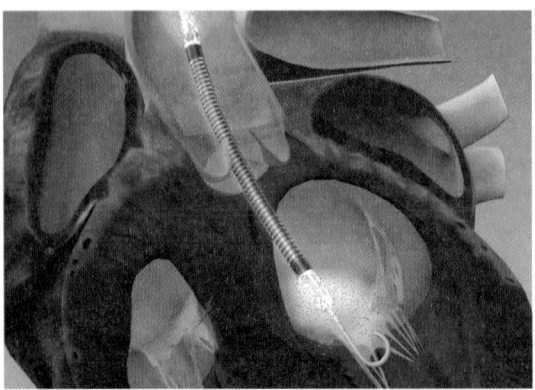

Figure 27-3   The Impella. The Impella 2.5 is a minimally invasive, catheter-based cardiac assist device designed to unload the left ventricle (thereby reducing myocardial oxygen consumption), while increasing overall cardiac output to maintain systemic perfusion. The Impella 2.5 can be percutaneously inserted into the left ventricle from the femoral artery. The tip of the catheter rests in the left ventricle during support, generating flows up to 2.5 L/min in the ascending aorta. *(Reproduced from Abiomed, Inc., Danvers, MA.)*

- "Bridge-to-next-decision" refers to the temporary use of ECMO or a short-term MCS device to assure continued systemic perfusion while assessments are made regarding improvement or worsening of major organ function, neurologic intactness, recoverability of myocardial function, and overall patient survivability. Evidence of deterioration often prompts discussion of a timely withdrawal of support, but evidence of overall stabilization, neu-

rologic intactness, and improvement of major organ function lead to a continuation of support to allow the myocardium an opportunity to recover ("Bridge-to-recovery"). In some cases, this requires the subsequent deployment of a different device, capable of providing a longer term of support. Current U.S. Food and Drug Administration (FDA)–approved devices used as a "Bridge-to-next-decision" and potential "Bridge-to-recovery" include the Abiomed BVS5000 (Abiomed; Figure 27-4), the Thoratec pVAD (Thoratec Laboratories, Pleasanton, CA; Figure 27-5), the AB5000 ventricle (Abiomed; Figure 27-6), and the CentriMag (Thoratec Laboratories; Figure 27-7). ECMO is also commonly used when respiratory failure is part of the clinical picture.

- "Bridge-to-a-bridge" refers (often retrospectively) to the use of a short-term MCS device as a bridge to the placement of another MCS device capable of providing a longer term of support in a patient who has survived but whose myocardium has not recovered despite short-term support.

Though useful conceptually, the apparent distinctions between these indications can sometimes appear somewhat artificial in the clinical arena, and the current practice of short-term MCS is really more of a continuous spectrum beginning with the immediate survival of the patient.

Bridge-to-Immediate Survival

Since the late 1960s, the IABP has been the most commonly used "bridge-to-immediate survival" because it simultaneously increases myocardial O_2 supply and decreases O_2 demand, interrupting the otherwise inexorable cycle leading to ventricular failure. It is estimated that 5% to 10% of patients will experience development of cardiogenic

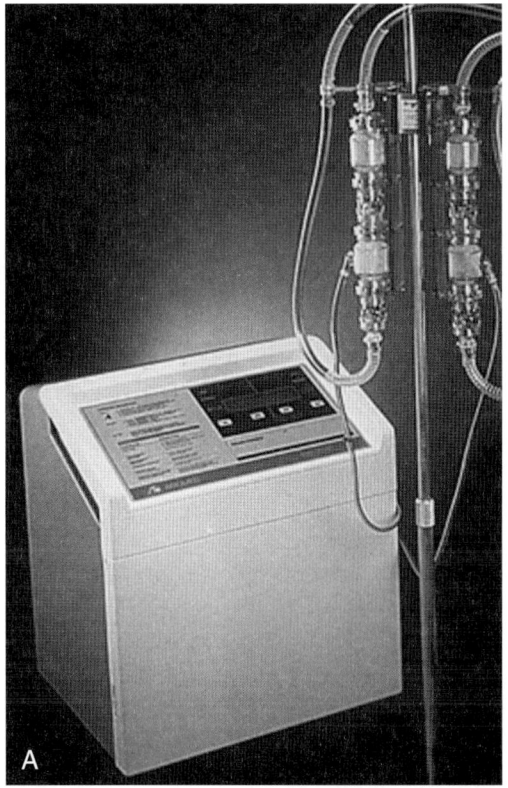

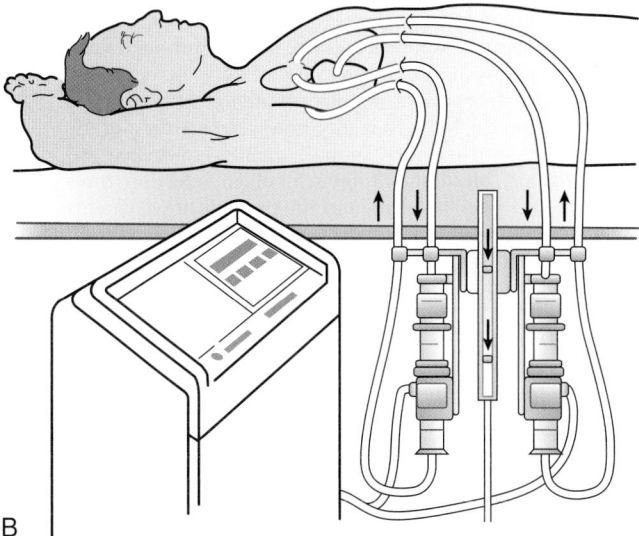

Figure 27-4   *A,* The Abiomed BVS5000. *B,* Biventricular support with the Abiomed BVS5000. Cannulas are placed in the heart and great vessels to divert blood to the extracorporeal BVS5000 pumps. Blood collected in the pumps is ejected into the ascending aorta (left ventricular assist device [LVAD]) and main pulmonary artery (right ventricular assist device [RVAD]). Note that the pumps fill by gravity drainage and are, therefore, generally mounted below the level of the heart. Adjustments can be made to pump height to optimize filling and pump ejection. For example, lowering a pump can augment device filling but will increase the afterload against which the device must eject. Conversely, raising a pump can facilitate pump emptying but will decrease filling of the device. *(Reproduced from Abiomed Corporation, Danvers, MA.)*

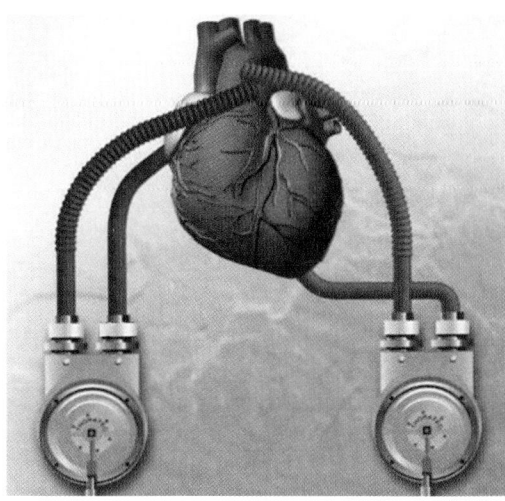

Figure 27-5 **The Thoratec pVAD (percutaneous ventricular assist device).** *(Reproduced from Thoratec Corporation, Pleasanton, CA.)*

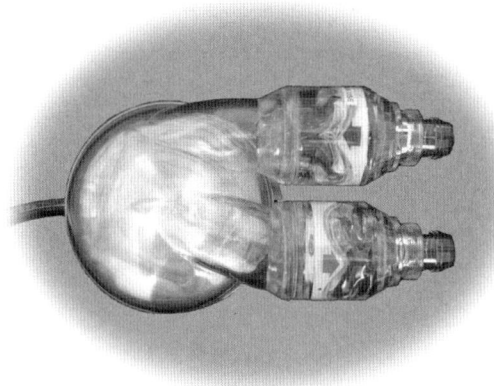

Figure 27-6 **The Abiomed AB5000 ventricle.** Hookups for the inflow and outflow cannulas are at the right. Although *arrows* indicate the direction of flow, they also serendipitously point at the artificial unidirectional valves that mandate anticoagulation during support with this device. The driveline, which alternately provides vacuum to assist filling and compressed air to accomplish ejection, is at the left. *(Reproduced from Abiomed Corporation, Danvers, MA.)*

shock after an acute MI, and early survival rates for these patients are on the order of 5% to 21%.[102] However, 75% of such patients who are unresponsive to pharmacologic interventions will exhibit hemodynamic improvement with IABP therapy alone,[103] and early survival rates in these patients are reported to approach 93% when treated with IABP counterpulsation.[104]

Although a balloon pump can improve the output from an acutely stunned ventricle, it only can augment forward CO by about 25% to 30% at maximum depending on the afterload,[105,106] and it is clear that there will be no augmentation of forward CO if there is a complete absence of LV function; thus, by itself, an IABP cannot be expected to rescue a patient from catastrophic myocardial failure (see Chapter 32).

ECMO has heretofore been the mainstay of emergent temporary MCS when there is intractable cardiorespiratory failure, and ECMO is making a comeback as an integral part of resuscitative protocols in many institutions, but the development of effective devices that can be deployed rapidly, at the first recognition of refractory ventricular insufficiency, has made "bridge-to-immediate survival" more of a reality than ever.

A key determinant of the overall survivability of acute cardiac failure is the rapidity with which the failing ventricle can be decompressed and resumption of adequate systemic perfusion assured. Although immediate implementation of support with conventional short-term VADs could potentially achieve these goals, sternotomy and CPB typically are utilized for the implantation of the requisite cannulae in the heart and great vessels. Furthermore, delays may be experienced while awaiting the availability of the operating room and necessary perioperative staff, prolonging the period of time during which the failing ventricle is pressure and volume overloaded, and the splanchnic beds and peripheral tissues are underperfused. It was considerations such as these that drove the development of several new and innovative short-term assist devices. Once immediate survival is assured, such a device conceivably can be changed later to another capable of providing longer term support.

The TandemHeart pVAD

Centrifugal pumps long have been used as MCS via both intrathoracic and percutaneous femoral cannulation strategies.[107] Although standard intrathoracic cannulations require sternotomy, percutaneous femoral arterial and venous cannulations can be performed outside of an operating room setting. A disadvantage of femoral venous cannulation, however, is that ventricular decompression is often inadequate to substantially reduce myocardial oxygen demand.

The TandemHeart pVAD (percutaneous VAD; Cardiac Assist) uses a percutaneous Seldinger-type cannula deployment system that enables rapid cannula placement to assure rapid resumption of systemic perfusion without the requisite need for patient transfer to an operating room.

With this device, a 21-French venous inflow cannula is percutaneously advanced retrograde from the femoral vein through the right atrium and across the interatrial septum into the left atrium (see Figure 27-2); 2.5 to 5 L/min of continuous, nonpulsatile outflow from the centrifugal device is returned to the femoral artery to support the circulation. Heparinization to an ACT of 180 to 200 seconds is used during support. Although a theoretical downside to cannulation of the femoral artery for device outflow is retrograde arterial perfusion through the potentially diseased aorta of a patient with atherosclerosis, cerebral embolism has not been reported as a significant problem.

The primary use of this innovative device has thus far been as a margin of safety in high-risk patients undergoing a variety of high-risk percutaneous coronary interventions.[108–110] Recent publications document the utility of the TandemHeart as a "bridge-to-immediate survival" from cardiogenic shock after acute MI,[111] after postcardiotomy failure to wean from CPB,[112] and in cases of acute myocarditis.[113] With respect to outcomes, a prospective comparison of the TandemHeart and the IABP in 41 patients with cardiogenic shock after acute MI found that, although hemodynamic and metabolic indices were significantly improved by the TandemHeart (with respect to the IABP), complications (including bleeding and limb ischemia) were more frequent with the VAD. There was no significant difference in 30-day mortality between the two groups.[114]

The utility of the TandemHeart as active hemodynamic support during off-pump coronary artery bypass surgery has also been reported.[115] Thus, the TandemHeart can serve as a "bridge-to-next decision," a "bridge-to-recovery," a "bridge-to-a-bridge," and even as a "bridge-to-transplantation"[116] (if the wait time is very short for a donor organ). Currently, the TandemHeart holds a CE mark (Conformité Européene) in Europe and is FDA-cleared in the United States for up to 6 hours of use.

Impella

The Impella Pump System (Abiomed) is a recently introduced family of axial flow devices that can be used to support the left, right, or both ventricles. Although the directly implantable Impella LD and RD remain the subject of clinical trials in the United States at the time of this writing, the Impella LP 2.5 has been FDA-cleared since June 2008 to provide partial circulatory support for periods up to 6 hours. The LP 2.5 is a catheter-based miniaturized axial flow pump that can provide

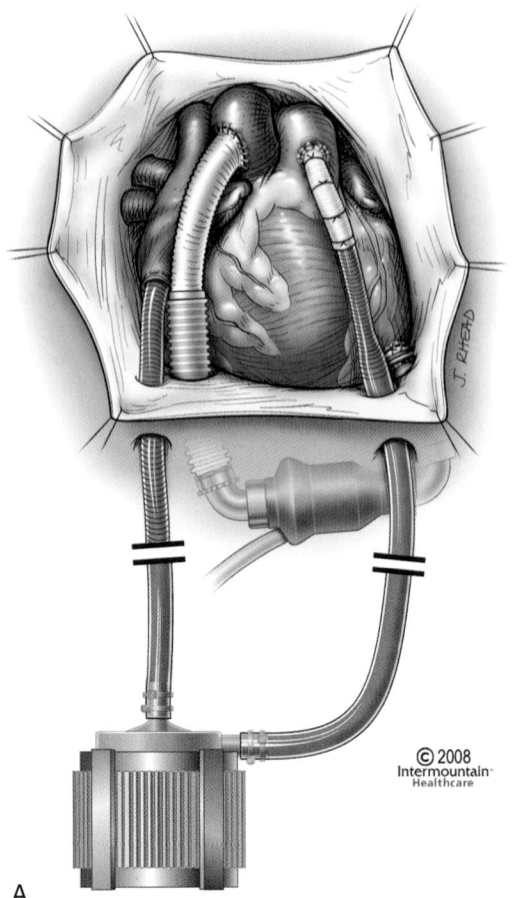

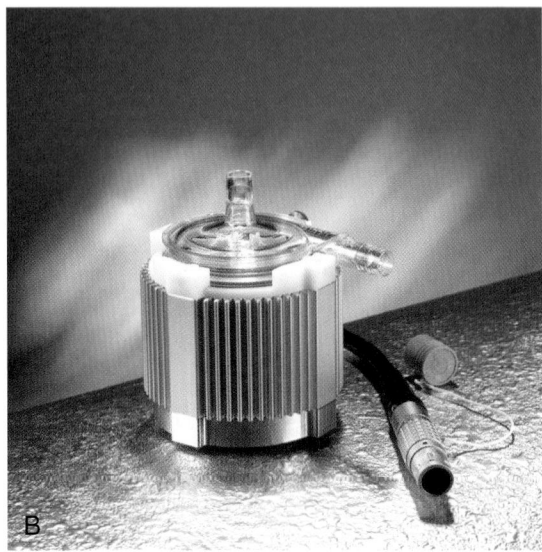

Figure 27-7 **The Thoratec CentriMag.** *(From Thoratec Corporation, Pleasanton, CA.)*

up to 2.5 L/min of flow. Like the Hemopump available in the late 1980s and early 1990s, the LP 2.5 is inserted percutaneously into the femoral artery and then passed retrograde up the aorta and across the aortic valve into the left ventricle. Oxygenated blood is then impelled from the left ventricle to the ascending aorta (see Figure 27-3).

Early clinical experience with the Impella LP 2.5 in patients with cardiogenic shock reported significantly increased CO, decreased pulmonary capillary wedge pressure, and decreased lactate levels by 6 hours of support[117]; 68% of the patients studied were successfully weaned from support, although only 38% survived. Among the observed complications were clinically significant hemolysis in 38% of the patients and one instance of pump displacement.

When compared with an IABP, a prospective study of 26 patients with cardiogenic shock caused by AMI reported that the use of a percutaneously placed LVAD (Impella LP 2.5) is feasible and safe and provides superior hemodynamic support compared with standard treatment using an IABP.[118]

Though potentially useful as a bridge-to-immediate-survival, the main use of the Impella thus far has been as an extra margin of safety in patients undergoing high-risk percutaneous coronary intervention. The safety and feasibility of the Impella LP 2.5 for hemodynamic support for this indication were demonstrated in the recently published PROTECT I trial.[119] The LP 2.5 also may be of use in high-risk patients undergoing off-pump coronary artery bypass surgery or as a margin of safety in high-risk patients undergoing noncardiac surgery.[120]

A mechanical or severely calcified aortic valve contraindicates the use of the Impella for LV support. Significant aortic insufficiency also may represent a relative contraindication.

Lifebridge (Lifebridge AG, Munich, Germany)

The Lifebridge represents one of the new generation of devices specifically designed for "bridge-to-immediate survival." This compact device essentially provides a maximum of 3.5 L/min of ECMO in a "plug-and-play" manner via percutaneous femoral arterial and venous cannulations. The 18-kg unit consists of a disposable patient module (which contains a CPB circuit, including an oxygenator), a centrifugal pump, a control module containing a driving motor, and an automated gas detection and bubble removing system. In situations of cardiac arrest, a heat exchanger can be configured in line with the bypass circuit to provide protective cooling of the patient. The safety and efficacy of this device were recently discussed in a publication from Germany, where this novel device was successfully used in the resuscitation and management of a patient with post-MI cardiogenic shock.[121]

Bridge-to-Recovery, Bridge-to-Next Decision

It is now well-known that the success of "bridge-to-recovery" with a VAD hinges on appropriate patient selection and prompt intervention. If the myocardium is going to recover after an acute insult, it generally tends to do so within a week or two (although the process may take longer than a month in some patients), and the patient may then be weaned from MCS. Although dismal in the past, rates of successful weaning from short-term support have improved. In the postcardiotomy cardiogenic shock population, survival rates approaching 50% have been reported with the Abiomed BVS5000 and AB5000 ventricle in "experienced centers with well-defined protocols for patient selection and timing of intervention."[122,123] Survival from acute MI cardiogenic shock has been reported at 42% with the AB5000 ventricle (mean number of days supported, 25.4) and 27% with the BVS 5000 (mean number of days supported, 5.2).[124] Limited information is available at the time of this writing regarding current rates of recovery from short-term support with the new devices (discussed later), but the strategies of support have changed dramatically in recent years and current data may no longer be directly comparable with the pure "bridge-to-recovery" strategy used in prior decades.

Regardless, prompt intervention to restore adequate systemic perfusion and careful patient selection are the key considerations if a patient is to be successfully bridged to recovery with any VAD. Despite the new technology currently available and the new strategies surrounding mechanical circulatory assistance, any patient who is unlikely to survive regardless of the reestablishment of effective systemic perfusion should not even be considered for VAD support. In contrast, if the myocardial injury is deemed likely to recover and the clinical assessment is otherwise favorable, VAD support may be considered. Although time is of the essence, a balance must be struck in the decision-making process and clinicians cannot wait until cardiogenic shock has resulted in multisystem organ failure before initiating mechanical circulatory assistance because experience has shown that the patient is unlikely to survive.

Early information[125] based on the experience with the Abiomed BVS5000 indicated that the best outcomes tended to occur in the following situations:

- Support is commenced to correct marginal hemodynamics within 30 to 45 minutes of attempted pharmacologic treatment (with or without an IABP).
- The time between the first attempt to wean from CPB and BVS implant is less than 6 hours.
- The BVS implant occurs as part of the initial operation.
- Due consideration is given to whether the patient requires univentricular or biventricular support.
- Hemostasis is ensured before leaving the operating room.

Poor outcomes occur in the following situations:

- Signs of other end-organ failure are present.
- The patient is older than 75 years.
- The patient is brought back to the operating room for implantation after a period of time.

Although the use of the BVS5000 device has decreased in recent years, the experience with this pioneering "bridge-to-recovery" device formed the basis of the current understanding that careful patient selection and prompt intervention to restore adequate systemic perfusion are critical if a patient is to be successfully bridged to recovery with MCS.

Additional considerations revolve around whether univentricular or biventricular support is required, but often this is a decision now made in retrospect in the arena of short-term support, once LVAD support has been engaged and the clinical situation is reassessed. Severe RV dysfunction has been reported to occur in up to 30% of LVAD-supported patients[126,127] because of unfavorable alterations in RV geometry (e.g., leftward shift of the interventricular septum) resulting in increased RV compliance and decreased RV contractility in the presence of increased RV preload[128] and potentially increased RV afterload. Although the overall incidence of RV failure in the setting of LVAD support appears to be decreased with continuous flow not intended to completely decompress the left ventricle during support, the perioperative management of RV preload and afterload continues to play an enormous role in the potential for RV dysfunction after implementation of LVAD support. The issue of RV failure during LVAD support is more of an issue during long-term support and is discussed in more detail later.

When severe cardiopulmonary failure is present, and there is uncertainty about the recoverability of the situation (or the neurologic status of the patient), ECMO again has become a popular circulatory support strategy.[129] ECMO has significant disadvantages, however, including a somewhat limited potential duration of support, the need for dedicated personnel to manage the flows and the anticoagulation, and a high incidence of complications as the duration of support increases.

Until recently, pulsatile, extracorporeal devices such as the Abiomed BVS5000 (FDA-approved in 1992), the Thoratec pVAD (FDA-approved in 1998), and the more recently approved AB5000 ventricle (FDA-approved in 2003) were the standard short-term bridge-to-recovery devices for patients with refractory cardiac failure. However, advances in technology and device engineering have supplanted the time-honored, pulsatile devices, and the CentriMag rapidly is becoming the short-term support device of choice.

The CentriMag

The CentriMag (Thoratec Laboratories; see Figure 27-7) is a small centrifugal pump with a magnetically levitated impeller. As with other short-term devices, the pump head itself remains paracorporeal during support, connected to cannulae in the heart and great vessels.

The impeller of the CentriMag is magnetically levitated and hydrodynamically suspended in the patient's blood; there is no central bearing (which has advantages), and without a bearing, there is less heat produced and potentially less thrombus formation.[130] There is also less hemolysis associated with the design of the CentriMag,[131] and, therefore, potentially less inflammatory response and less peripheral vasoconstriction from the plasma-free hemoglobin. The derangement of liver function tests generally seen after a few days with a standard biohead are reportedly not seen with the CentriMag (Monique Boshell, Thoratec Corporation, personal communication).

Despite its small size, the pump itself can provide flow rates of up to 9.9 L/min and can pump through a membrane oxygenator if ECMO is desired, so it is versatile. Overall, the CentriMag has now become the device of choice for short-term support in many institutions worldwide.

Published clinical experiences with the CentriMag have reported the safety and efficacy of this device as a bridge-to-immediate survival, a bridge-to-next decision, a bridge-to-a-bridge, a bridge-to-recovery, and a bridge-to-transplantation for patients with acute cardiogenic shock of causative factors ranging from acute MI cardiogenic shock to postcardiotomy cardiogenic shock (including failed heart transplantation) to RV failure while on LVAD support.[132-134]

At the time of this writing, the CentriMag has been FDA approved to provide circulatory support as a bridge to recovery for up to 30 days as an RVAD, but only for up to 6 hours as a bridge-to-next decision as an LVAD. A nonrandomized pivotal trial in adults is in progress in the United States evaluating the CentriMag as a longer-term bridge-to-recovery, bridge-to-transplantation, or bridge-to-a-bridge. A smaller version called the *pediVAS* is approved for 6 hours of use as either an LVAD or an RVAD for pediatric patients.

Table 27-5 describes the basic characteristics of the devices currently used for short-term support, and Box 27-2 provides common clinical scenarios in which short-term VAD use may be indicated.

Long-Term Ventricular Assist Device Use

Permanent replacement of the failing heart was the original intent of the research and development in the field of mechanical circulatory assistance, and this dream is alive and well in the latest version of the total artificial heart, the AbioCor Implantable Replacement Heart (Abiomed; Figure 27-8), but most long-term VAD use has been as a bridge-to-transplantation.

The traditional concept of the intermediate or long-term use of a VAD as a "bridge-to-transplantation" has now been expanded to include the concept of "destination therapy" (DT), a final management strategy for end-stage HF in patients who are not transplant eligible. However, as mentioned earlier, time spent on VAD support often improves multisystem organ function and can potentially convert high-risk transplant-ineligible patients into transplant-eligible patients. Thus, another intermediate or perhaps long-term use for VADs might be termed "bridge-to-improved candidacy."

Current FDA-approved devices used as a bridge-to-transplantation in the United States include the Thoratec pVAD (Thoratec Laboratories;

TABLE 27-5	Basic Characteristics of the Devices Currently Used for Short-Term Support (e.g., Bridge-to-Recovery)			
Device	*Type of Support*	*Fill Mechanism*	*Drive Mechanism*	*System Control and Output*
Abiomed BVS5000	Pulsatile	Gravity drainage	Pneumatic compression of blood chamber	Automatically adjusts rate of pumping to provide up to 5 L/min of outflow (output depends on intravascular volume status and downstream vascular resistances)
Thoratec	Pulsatile	Vacuum assisted	Pneumatic compression of blood chamber	Depending on the mode of operation, user-defined settings determine the output (intravascular volume status is important)
Abiomed AB5000 ventricle	Pulsatile	Vacuum assisted	Pneumatic compression of blood chamber	Automatically adjusts rate of pumping to provide up to 6 L/min of outflow (output depends on intravascular volume status and downstream vascular resistances)
Centrifugal pumps	Nonpulsatile	Gravity drainage assisted by vortex	Centrifugal force drives blood	Output is dependent on user-defined speed of impeller rotation and afterload
CentriMag	Nonpulsatile	Gravity drainage assisted by vortex	Centrifugal force drives blood	Output is dependent on user-defined speed of impeller rotation and afterload

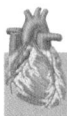

BOX 27-2. COMMON CLINICAL SCENARIOS IN WHICH SHORT-TERM VENTRICULAR ASSIST DEVICE USE (E.G., AS A BRIDGE-TO-RECOVERY) MAY BE INDICATED

- Postcardiotomy ventricular failure
- Cardiogenic shock after myocardial infarction
- Myocardial failure after heart transplantation
- Failed catheterization laboratory intervention
- Acute myocarditis
- Right ventricular failure while on a left ventricular assist device

see Figure 27-5), the HeartMate XVE (Thoratec Corporation, Woburn, MA; Figure 27-9), the IVAD (implanted vascular assist device; Thoratec Laboratories; Figure 27-10), the HeartMate II (Thoratec Laboratories; Figure 27-11), and the CardioWest TAH (total artificial heart; SynCardia Systems, Tucson, AZ; Figure 27-12). Currently,

the HeartMate XVE and the HeartMate II are the only devices FDA approved in the United States for DT. The Novacor LVAS (World Heart, Ottawa, Canada) was approved as a bridge-to-transplantation in 1998 but is no longer being implanted. Despite arguably superior engineering regarding device longevity in comparison with other devices available at the time, as well as comparable rates of successful bridging to transplantation, the Novacor was associated with a high incidence of thromboembolic complications. Table 27-6 summarizes the basic characteristics of devices used for long-term support.

Intermediate- or long-term VAD support potentially is indicated as a bridge-to-transplantation in situations in which no myocardial recovery is expected (e.g., end-stage cardiomyopathy) or when an acutely stunned or infarcted left ventricle fails to recover despite support with a short-term VAD. By providing effective CO in place of the failed native heart, this technology can stave off the end-organ damage resulting from a rapidly deteriorating CO and allows severely decompensated transplant-eligible patients to potentially survive long enough to receive a donor heart. An additional benefit of this application of VADs is an improved quality of life, often as an outpatient, while awaiting a new heart. Further, significant improvements in multiorgan function

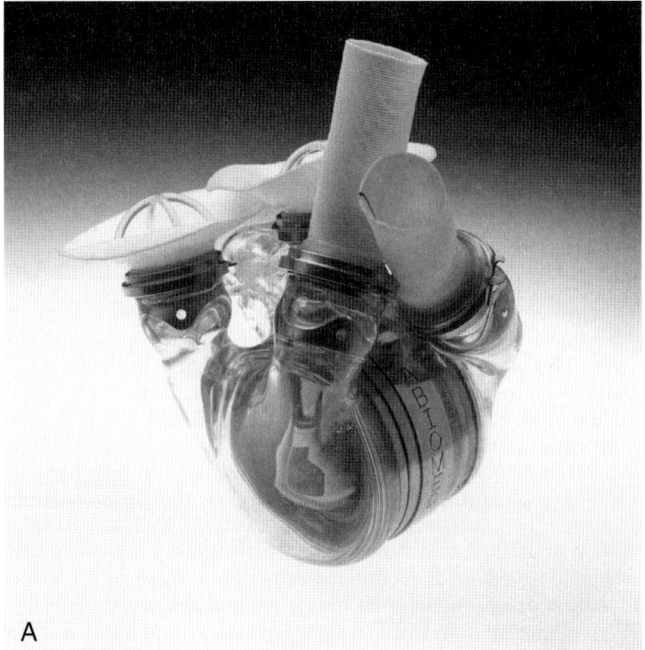

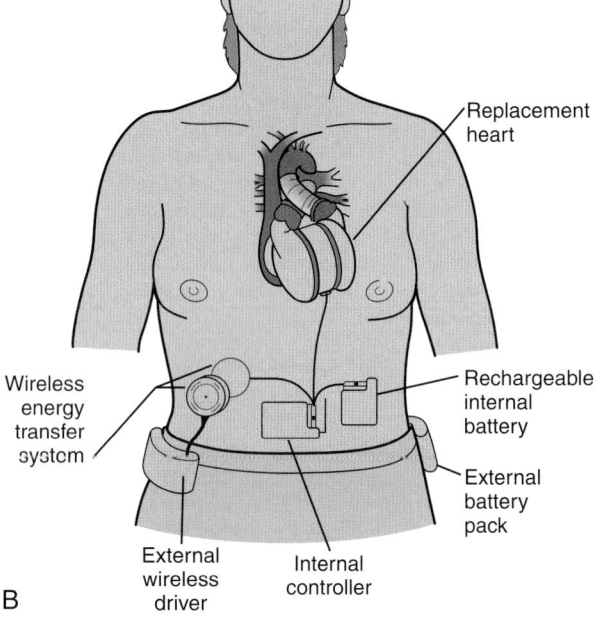

Figure 27-8 *A*, The AbioCor Implantable Replacement Heart. *B*, Orthotopic implantation of the AbioCor Implantable Replacement Heart. The native failed heart is removed, and the AbioCor is implanted orthotopically, anastomosed to cuffs of native atria and the great vessels. Transcutaneous energy transfer technology eliminates the need for percutaneous wires. *(From Abiomed, Inc., Danvers, MA.)*

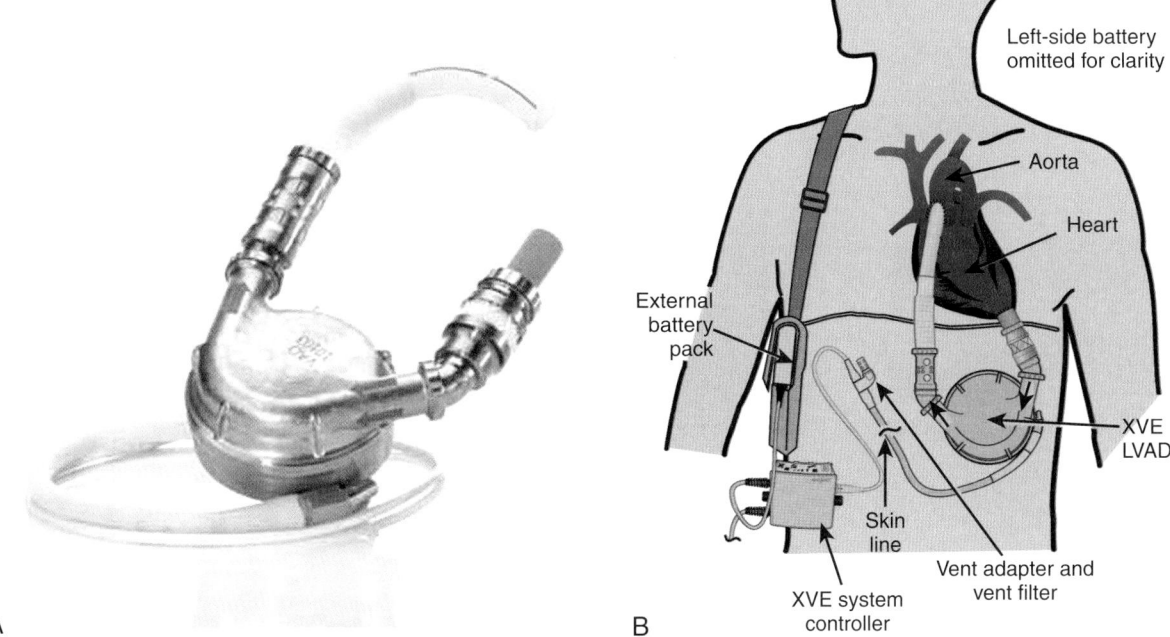

A **B**

Left-side battery omitted for clarity

Aorta

Heart

External battery pack

XVE LVAD

Skin line

Vent adapter and vent filter

XVE system controller

Figure 27-9   **The HeartMate XVE.** *(From Thoratec Corporation, Pleasanton, CA.)*

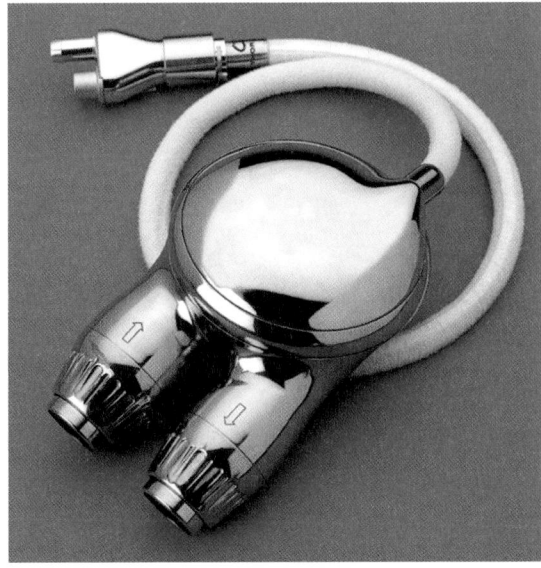

Figure 27-10   **The IVAD (implanted vascular assist device).** *(From Thoratec Corporation, Pleasanton, CA.)*

have been demonstrated during the time spent on VAD support,[95-97] and it is unusual nowadays for a patient to present for heart transplantation without an LVAD in situ.

The HeartMate I (World Heart, Oakland, CA; see Figure 27-9) has heretofore been the most commonly used bridge-to-transplantation device for patients with advanced LV failure. The original pneumatically powered HeartMate IP was FDA-approved for this indication in 1994, and the electrically powered version (the VE, vented electric) was approved in 1998. Data from prior years indicated a 67% success rate of bridging-to-transplantation with the HeartMate VE.[135] The major advantage of the pulsatile HeartMate LVAS always has been the "antithrombogenic" lining of its blood chamber that obviated the need for formal anticoagulation with warfarin once a neointima was established. The major disadvantages of the HeartMate included infections of the large percutaneous lead and in the preperitoneal

pocket where the device was implanted, as well as a limited durability beyond 18 months.

The current incarnation (the XVE) is the result of improvements to the device, and it has been in use since approximately 2002. According to the manufacturer, more than 4500 patients have been implanted with the HeartMate XVE in 186 centers worldwide. The average age has been 51 years old, with a range from 8 to 74, and the longest duration of support (ongoing patient on one device) has been 1854 days.[136]

Patients with biventricular failure generally have been bridged to transplantation with the Thoratec pVAD (FDA-approved for this indication in 1995) or, potentially, the IVAD (the implantable, titanium-coated version of the Thoratec device). According to the manufacturer, more than 4000 patients have been supported by the Thoratec pVAD at more than 240 medical centers in 26 countries. The longest duration of support is reportedly 1204 days, with 858 of those patients discharged to home, and the rate of successful bridge-to-transplantation is reported at 69%.[136] For the IVAD, more than 500 patients reportedly have been implanted at 95 medical centers in 9 countries, with the longest duration of support being 979 days,[136] and a reported rate of successful bridge-to-transplantation of 69%.[137]

The CardioWest total artificial heart (SynCardia Systems; see Figure 27-12) is available in select centers internationally as a bridge-to-transplantation for patients with biventricular failure, and a resurgence of interest in this device has been seen recently. A successful bridge-to-transplantation rate of 79% was observed in prior years.[138]

Complications such as infection of percutaneous drivelines, perioperative bleeding, RV failure, sepsis, and multisystem organ failure were always an enormous issue with the first-generation, pulsatile VADs. Thromboembolism was less prevalent with the HeartMate because of the antithrombogenic lining of its blood chamber, but it did occur. A review of 228 patients on long-term support with the Thoratec, Novacor, and HeartMate as a bridge to transplantation reported cerebral embolism in 24%, 39%, and 16%, respectively, despite adherence to recommended anticoagulation protocols.[139]

Updated information from recent clinical experiences is not available for these first-generation devices at the time of this writing, but it may be moot because the nonpulsatile HeartMate II was approved as a bridge-to-transplantation in April 2008, and it rapidly has become an intermediate and long-term support device of choice.

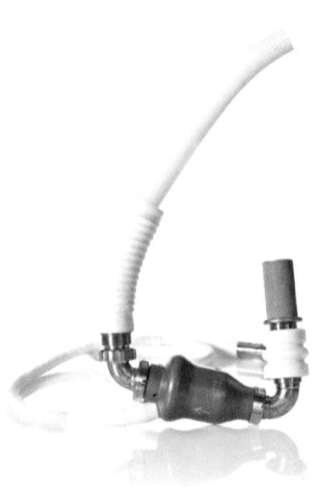

A

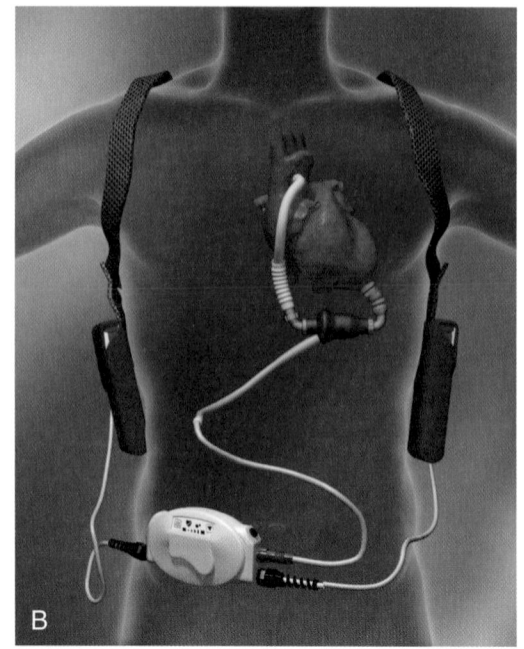

B

Figure 27-11 **The HeartMate II.** *(From Thoratec Corporation, Pleasanton, CA.)*

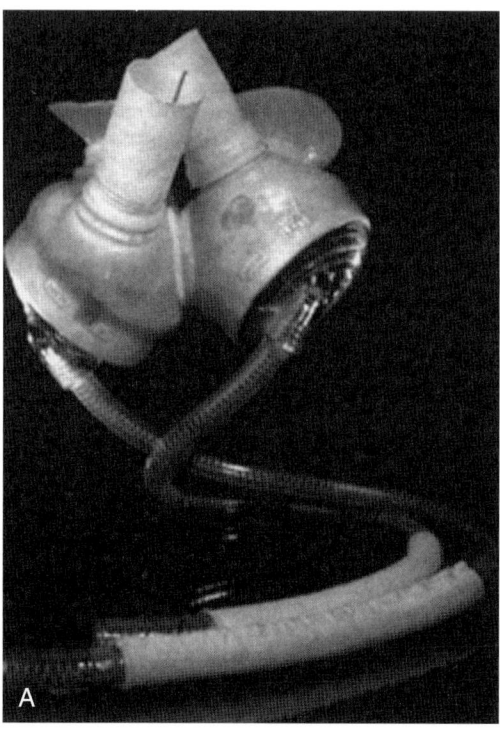

A

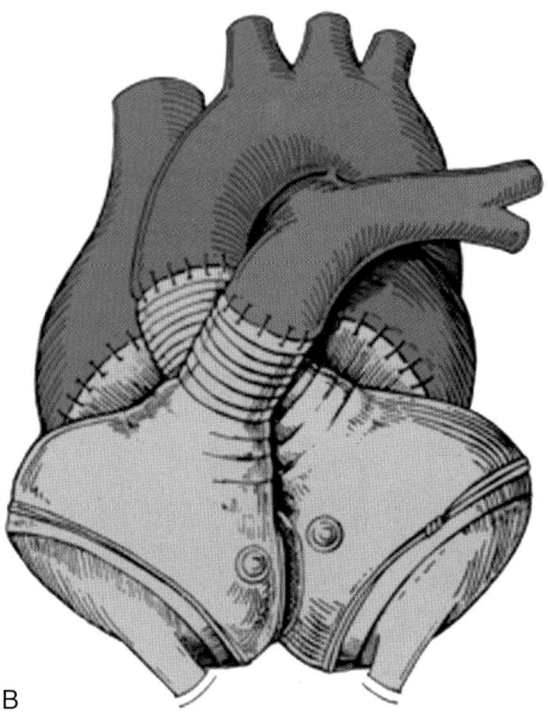

B

Figure 27-12 *A,* The CardioWest Total Artificial Heart. *B,* Orthotopic implantation of the CardioWest Total Artificial Heart. The failed native heart is removed, and the CardioWest TAH is implanted orthotopically, anastomosed to cuffs of native atria and the great vessels. *(Reproduced from SynCardia Systems, Tucson, AZ.)*

TABLE 27-6	Basic Characteristics of Devices Used for Long-Term Support			
Device	*Type of Support*	*Fill Mechanism*	*Drive Mechanism*	*System Control and Output*
HeartMate XVE	Pulsatile; LVAD only	Gravity drainage	Electrically powered compression of blood chamber	Fixed rate and automatic modes available; 85-mL blood chamber; maximum flow
Thoratec	Pulsatile; BiVAD possible	Vacuum assisted	Pneumatic compression of blood chamber	Depending on the mode of operation, user-defined settings determine the output (intravascular volume status is important)
IVAD	Pulsatile; BiVAD possible	Vacuum assisted	Pneumatic compression of blood chamber	Depending on the mode of operation, user-defined settings determine the output (intravascular volume status is important)
HeartMate II	Nonpulsatile flow; axial device; LVAD only	Gravity drainage assisted by vortex	Continuous rotation of axial pump impels blood forward	Output is dependent on user-defined speed of impeller rotation, available volume in ventricle, and afterload
CardioWest TAH	Pulsatile; replaces natural heart	All venous and pulmonary arterial blood returns to device	Pneumatic compression of blood chambers	Maximum stroke volume 70 mL, can deliver more than 9 L/min of output

BiVAD, biventricular assist device; IVAD, implanted vascular assist device; LVAD, left ventricular assist device; TAH, total artificial heart.

The HeartMate II

The HeartMate II (see Figure 27-11) is a small, nonpulsatile axial flow pump that has demonstrated a significantly decreased incidence of complications and a significantly improved durability compared with its predecessor. According to the manufacturer, more than 5000 patients worldwide have been implanted with the HeartMate II, with the longest duration of support (ongoing patient on one device) greater than 5 years, and 79% of patients successfully transplanted, recovered, or supported to 18 months.[136]

The smaller size of the HeartMate II has simplified implantation, and the rates of common complications have been shown to be significantly decreased by comparison with the pulsatile HeartMate I. Published series using identical definitions of certain complications have reported a 64% decrease in reoperation for bleeding, a 10-fold decrease in percutaneous lead infections, a 55% decrease in stroke, and a 70% decrease in RV failure after implementation of HeartMate II LVAD support.[140-142] The reason for the decreased incidence of these specific complications is likely multifactorial (e.g., improved surgical techniques and lack of a need for a large preperitoneal pocket, the routine use of antifibrinolytics during device implantation in the modern era, a smaller percutaneous lead, improved perioperative care protocols and patient management, improved anticoagulation protocols).

The decreased incidence of severe RV failure requiring RVAD seen with the HeartMate II[143] may be because of the nature of the type of flow it produces. The first generation of LVADs (e.g., the HeartMate VE and the XVE) produced pulsatile flow and, therefore, had to capture the entire potential output from the left ventricle to eject a physiologic stroke volume with each pump cycle. Consequently, the left ventricle frequently was emptied to the point where the interventricular septum was displaced significantly to the left during support, resulting in decreased function of the interventricular septum[144] and overall RV dysfunction from the change in its overall geometry. The nonpulsatile next generation of LVADs (whether axial or centrifugal) produce continuous flow and do not fully decompress the left ventricle during support, theoretically preserving RV function, at least in part, because the interventricular septum is not significantly displaced to the left. In contrast with the reported 25% to 30% rates of RV failure in the past with first-generation pulsatile devices, the rate of RV failure with HeartMate II recently was reported at 5%.[145]

Despite the improved durability and the decreased incidence of observed complications, one potential disadvantage of the HeartMate II compared with the HeartMate XVE is the requisite need for anticoagulation with warfarin.

The HeartMate II is the only next-generation continuous-flow device approved for use as a bridge-to-transplantation in the United States at the time of this writing. Other axial and centrifugal continuous-flow devices (e.g., the Heart Assist 5 [formerly the DeBakey VAD; MicroMed Technologies, Houston, TX], the Flowmaker [formerly the Jarvik 2000; Jarvik Heart, New York, NY], the Berlin Heart INCOR [Berlin Heart, Berlin, Germany], the VentrAssist [Ventracor Ltd., Sydney, Australia], the DuraHeart [Terumo Heart, Ann Arbor, MI], the HeartWare LVAS [HeartWare International, Framingham, MA]) have demonstrated safety and efficacy, and many are already CE marked in Europe, but none is yet approved and clinically available in the United States.

Permanent Ventricular Assist Device Use: Destination Therapy

A relatively new indication for long-term VAD use is called *destination therapy* (DT), which refers to the intentionally permanent use of an LVAD as a permanent management solution for end-stage cardiac failure. From a certain perspective, the field of MCS has come full circle because the original concept of ventricular support devices was for the permanent replacement of the failing heart. From a certain perspective, this dream is alive and well in the latest version of the total artificial heart, the AbioCor Implantable Replacement Heart discussed later.

The REMATCH trial (Randomized Evaluation of Mechanical Assistance for the Treatment of Congestive Heart Failure) established that the use of a left-sided VAD was not only an effective tool to treat patients with advanced HF but resulted in more than twice the survival rate and an improved quality of life in comparison with optimal medical management.[146] Based on the results of REMATCH, the FDA approved the HeartMate VE in November 2002 for transplant-ineligible patients as DT, but improvements to the HeartMate device resulted in the HeartMate XVE by the time FDA approval was granted, and it is the XVE that has been implanted for DT patients in the United States. Although use of the XVE quickly was associated with fewer adverse events and a better survival rate than in the REMATCH trial,[147] increased experience with patient management likely also played a role in the observed improved outcomes.

To date, DT has been indicated only for transplant-ineligible patients, but it may be anticipated that this indication may be broadened going forward because although cardiac transplantation remains the gold standard therapy for end-stage disease, the number of donor organs is severely limited in comparison with the number of patients who would benefit, and most patients with end-stage cardiac disease cannot realistically expect to be transplanted. Another factor that may lead to a potential broadening of the indication is the FDA approval of the HeartMate II for DT in January 2010, after the completion of the HeartMate II DT pivotal clinical trial.[148] In this prospective, randomized trial, the HeartMate II was pitted against the HeartMate XVE on a 2:1 basis. Not only was the incidence of adverse events, including infection, sepsis, right-heart failure, and mechanical problems, significantly lower in HeartMate II patients compared with patients implanted with the XVE, but HeartMate II patients experienced shorter hospital stays. After approval of the HeartMate II for DT, the number of patients implanted with the XVE as DT has dropped off significantly, though the VXE may remain useful for patients who cannot be anticoagulated.

New Risk Scores: Optimizing Survival while Minimizing Risk during Long-Term Ventricular Assist Device Support

Just as with the short-term devices used as a short-term bridge-to-recovery, it has been demonstrated that the best outcomes with long-term devices used as DT are obtained through careful patient selection and earlier implantation. Large retrospective analyses have allowed for a new understanding of how specific clinical derangements play out in terms of perioperative morbidity and mortality and have provided insight into how intensive medical therapy can optimize patients before VAD use.

Lietz–Miller Risk Score

Lietz et al[149] described the outcomes of nearly the entire U.S. DT population in the post-REMATCH era from the fall of 2002 through December 2006 and identified the most important determinants of in-hospital mortality. In this landmark study,[149] the main preoperative determinants of mortality in this population were shown to be poor nutrition (resulting in subsequent sepsis), hematologic abnormalities (resulting in subsequent stroke), RV dysfunction (resulting in postimplantation RV dysfunction), lack of inotropic support, and preexisting end-organ dysfunction (resulting in ultimate multisystem organ failure), though it should be noted that people did die of other things, including technical problems with their LVAD. Approximately 25% either required LVAD replacement or died as a result of pump failure or complications, but the death of only 6% was directly attributable to device failure. Of concern was the reported probability of device exchange or fatal device failure, which was approximately 18% at 1 year and 73% at 2 years with the HeartMate XVE.

Furthermore, Lietz et al[149] were able to stratify patients into risk categories based on a risk score calculated from these predictors that correlates well with survival. According to their analysis, the highest-risk patients have severe deterioration in their medical condition (as evidenced by poor nutritional status with low serum albumin), impaired renal function, and markers of significant right-heart failure such as low PA pressures or congestive levels of hepatic enzymes. Probable infection, as evidenced by increased white blood cell counts and anemia and coagulation abnormalities such as declining platelet counts and increased international normalized ratio, worsen the chance of operative survival. Thus, if operative risk derives from comorbidities, then initially high risk because of correctable factors should not dissuade physicians from considering LVAD therapy in certain cases because intensive medical treatment can convert high-risk patients to acceptable candidates.

INTERMACS Profile

INTERMACS (Interagency Registry for Mechanically Assisted Circulatory Support) is a relatively new registry of patients supported by FDA-approved "durable" MCS devices for DT, bridge-to-transplantation, and/or recovery. Analysis of the growing registry has allowed for the development of a classification scheme (INTERMACS "profile") that helps guide medical and surgical decision making regarding the timing of interventions and therapies (e.g., VAD insertion), provides a conventional frame of reference that facilitates communication between practitioners, and allows for an understanding of risks associated with various interventions.[150]

The INTERMACS profile describes the status of the HF patient who might benefit from MCS. INTERMACS stratifies HF patients into seven levels of clinical acuity, defined as 1 ("critical cardiogenic shock"), 2 ("progressive decline despite inotropes"), 3 ("stable but inotrope-dependent"), 4 ("recurrent advanced HF"), 5 ("exertion-intolerant"), 6 ("exertion-limited"), and 7 ("advanced NYHA III"). The assigned profile is modifiable by the coexistence of arrhythmias, the need for temporary circulatory support, and the frequency of requisite hospitalization.[151]

Given the increased risk for complications known to be associated with late intervention in this population, current thinking holds that interventions such as the implementation of MCS are likely best performed for patients with an INTERMACS status 3 or 4.

It also is anticipated that the INTERMACS registry will allow for the collection of outcomes data, as well as assess the efficacy of specific therapeutic interventions. A recent analysis of the INTERMACS registry data reported that cardiogenic shock, advanced age, and severe right-heart failure manifested as ascites or increased bilirubin are predictors of death in patients supported by MCS devices. Furthermore, although biventricular HF patients who require biVAD support have a transplant rate similar to that of LVAD-only patients, an increased mortality is seen at 6 and 12 months.[152]

Seattle Heart Failure Model

The Seattle Heart Failure Model[153] was developed to predict survival in patients with HF. This multivariate risk score uses 21 parameters (age, sex, NYHA class, weight, EF, systolic BP, presence of ischemic cardiomyopathy, daily furosemide-equivalent dose, inotrope use, statin use, allopurinol use, angiotensin-converting enzyme use, β-blocker use, angiotensin-receptor blocker use, potassium-sparing diuretic use, ICD use, hemoglobin, lymphocyte percent on complete blood count differential, serum uric acid, serum cholesterol, and serum sodium). The model subsequently was modified for LVAD patients by adding two variables: IABP-implanted or ventilated, or both, and inotrope therapy.[154] Overall, the Seattle Heart Failure Model reportedly provides an accurate estimate of mean, 1-, 2-, and 3-year survival, and allows estimation of effects of adding medications or devices to a patient's regimen. A recent comparison of available risk indices (including the Lietz–Miller risk score, the Columbia risk score, APACHE II, and INTERMACS) found the Seattle score to best predict mortality in continuous-flow LVAD patients.[155]

Ventricular Assist Device Use and the Potential for Myocardial Recovery

In cases of acute ventricular failure, removal of the sudden volume and pressure overload and improvement in the balance of myocardial oxygen supply and demand may allow for myocardial recovery

and weaning from mechanical support. Clinical experience has shown that if recovery from an acute insult is going to occur, it generally does so over the course of 1 to 2 weeks. In cases of long-standing, progressive failure, decompression of the dilated and chronically failing left ventricle by an LVAD also may allow for some degree of recovery over time.

Although echocardiographic and histologic support for this general premise has been available since the mid 1990s,[156] the underlying biochemical mechanisms of remodeling (and its reversal) are only now being elucidated. Patten et al showed that therapy with a VAD normalizes inducible nitric oxide synthase expression in association with decreased cardiomyocyte apoptosis.[156] Decompression of the left ventricle by an LVAD has been reported to allow for normalization of LV geometry, regression of myocyte hypertrophy,[157] favorable changes in LV collagen content,[158] and normalized expression of genes controlling excitation-contraction coupling and the calcium content of the sarcoplasmic reticulum.[159] It has been reported that maximum structural reverse remodeling is complete after around 40 days of LV decompression, with reversal of some of the molecular aspects of remodeling by 20 days.[160]

It should be appreciated, however, that although a great deal of knowledge regarding myocardial remodeling (and its reversal) has been elucidated, long-lasting ventricular recovery after chronic HF is a relatively infrequent event, reportedly occurring primarily in patients with dilated cardiomyopathy, and the actual number of patients who recover sufficiently to have their long-term VAD explanted is small. Worldwide efforts to understand the nature of adverse ventricular remodeling and its reversal are ongoing, and the relevant literature is rapidly burgeoning.

Abiocor Implantable Replacement Heart

From the original pneumatically driven devices with their massive external control consoles to the totally implantable computer-controlled AbioCor Implantable Replacement Heart (Abiomed) now in clinical trials, the mechanical TAH has been the subject of intensive research and development for decades.

The first TAH was a pneumatically driven biventricular pump developed by Dr. Domingo Liotta and colleagues in the 1960s. This device (the Liotta TAH) was implanted in a 47-year-old patient with severe HF by Dr. Denton Cooley on April 4, 1969, and was used for 64 hours as a bridge-to-heart transplantation.[160] The patient died of *Pseudomonas* pneumonia 32 hours after his transplantation, but the Liotta heart proved that a mechanical device could be successfully used clinically to sustain a patient.

The second human implantation of a TAH also was performed by Dr. Cooley. In July 1981, the Akutsu III TAH was used successfully for 55 hours as bridge-to-transplantation in a 36-year-old patient with end-stage HF.[161] The Jarvik-7 TAH was first implanted as a permanent replacement heart in August 1985 in a 61-year-old man with primary cardiomyopathy and chronic obstructive pulmonary disease.[162] Although the patient survived only 112 days, the duration of his survival was encouraging. Since 1991, the Jarvik-7 has been known as the CardioWest TAH. As discussed earlier, this device is still in use today as a bridge-to-human heart transplantation in selected centers in the United States, France, and Canada.

The AbioCor Implantable Replacement Heart (see Figure 27-8) represents a major advance in artificial heart technology because it is truly totally implantable; there are no percutaneous cables, conduits, or wires. The device is motor driven, so a source of compressed air to drive the pumping action is not required, allowing patients complete mobility. The device itself weighs approximately 2 pounds and is orthotopically implanted. Transcutaneous energy transfer is used (in lieu of a percutaneous cable) to supply the motor-driven hydraulic pumping of the artificial ventricles with power and system control. Artificial unidirectional valves within the device mandate anticoagulation during support.

Initial implantations of the AbioCor were performed in 14 patients between 2001 and 2003. Although the device performed well, with one patient supported longer than 1 year, there were a lot of strokes and only one patient actually was discharged to home. Results from the initial implants were submitted to the FDA in September 2004 for marketing approval, but the FDA ultimately denied the application, citing concerns about patient inclusion criteria and device labeling, potential benefit versus risk of the device, anticoagulation protocols, and quality-of-life versus quantity-of-life issues.

However, because of its limited market, in September 2006, the AbioCor was FDA approved as a Humanitarian Use Device. Currently, the AbioCor Implantable Replacement Heart is FDA approved for patients younger than 75 years with end-stage biventricular failure who are not transplant eligible and who cannot be treated with an LVAD alone as DT. No new information is available at the time of this writing regarding recent implantations of the AbioCor Implantable Replacement Heart.

CARDIAC TRANSPLANTATION

Cardiac transplantation remains the ultimate surgical intervention for advanced HF and greatly impacts the lives of those patients who receive a new heart, but considering the massive scope of this public health issue, this management strategy is epidemiologically and biostatistically small because of the extremely limited number of donor organs available each year. Although it is estimated that at least 100,000 patients could meet the transplant criteria at any given time,[21] only 3153 are currently listed to potentially receive one.[163] Furthermore, it is apparent that the number of available donor hearts is limited to approximately 2200 each year in the United States. Thus, transplantation simply is not a realistic expectation for the majority of patients with advanced end-stage HF. Although survival varies slightly by blood type (AB > B > A > O), patients fortunate enough to get a donor organ can currently expect a 1-year survival rate of approximately 87%, a 3-year survival rate of approximately 78%, and a 5-year survival rate of approximately 73%[163] (see Chapter 23).

NEW THERAPIES

Cellular Transplantation into the Myocardium

A novel approach to treating severe systolic dysfunction is the injection of harvested autologous skeletal muscle cells into the failing myocardium. This procedure can be performed either surgically at the end of a revascularization procedure or percutaneously in the catheterization laboratory.

The use of cell transplantation is not a novel approach to treating disease. Skin and bone-marrow transplantations were the first replacement therapies described. These were followed by embryologic neuron transplantation in patients with Parkinson's disease and islet cell transplantation for the treatment of diabetes mellitus.[164]

The basic understanding of the remodeling process is that viable and contractile cardiomyocytes undergo apoptosis and become replaced by noncontractile tissue; this, in turn, leads to systolic and diastolic dysfunction. In an attempt to restore functionality, contractile cells are injected into this region. In clinical practice, myoblasts from the patient's quadriceps muscle have been used. Using the patient's own tissue has several advantages. First, the complications of pharmacologic immunosuppression are avoided. Second, there are no ethical problems in contrast with those frequently observed when fetal cells are used. Finally, the ease of harvest and processing make this tissue ideal for this purpose.

Skeletal muscle cells, however, are histologically different from native cardiomyocytes. Adhesion molecules, which are found in native cardiomyocytes, are not found in skeletal myocytes (N-cadherin and connexin-43).[104] These adhesion molecules are important for adhesion to the extracellular matrix and for intercellular communication.

Clinically, a Phase I study from Poland, the POZNAN trial,[165] showed that myoblasts can be implanted safely via a percutaneous route into a scarred region of the left ventricle. Only 10 patients were enrolled into this study. Nine were transplanted. One could not be transplanted because of technical reasons. Six patients of the nine were followed up. Improvement of NYHA class and EF were observed in all of them. Similar results were seen by Menasche et al.[164] A frequently encountered occurrence in the phase I studies was the fact that many patients had episodes of ventricular tachycardia after the procedure. They were successfully treated with amiodarone or electric cardioversion. Phase II studies are now in progress in the United States and Europe. Many other cell types are now being experimentally injected into the myocardium or given intravenously in an attempt to regrow cardiac myocytes.[166–168] These cells include adult bone marrow stem cells, embryonic stem cells, and cardiac progenitor cells found mainly in the atrium. They have been injected alone or with multiple growth factors such as granulocyte-macrophage colony-stimulating factor, vasoactive endothelial growth factor, and angiopoietan-1, which mobilize progenitor cells and induce new cell growth. The transplanted cells may morph into new cardiac muscle cells, or they may improve cardiac function by boosting the growth of new blood vessels, or releasing other growth factors that encourage cell proliferation and survival. Any of these effects could explain some of the early positive results seen to date.

Gene Transfer in Cardiac Myocytes

Gene therapy has received much interest by the media. Multiple research groups are trying to cure or at least alleviate symptoms brought on by CHF through gene therapy. It is necessary to inoculate the cell with DNA to change the genetic programming of a cell. Vectors are being used to achieve this goal. Vectors commonly used range from plasmid DNA to different virus types (e.g., adenovirus, herpes virus). The two cellular pathways that are being targeted are the sarcoplasmic reticulum and the β-adrenergic pathway.[169] The targets of gene therapy are to increase β-adrenergic function, adenylyl cyclase, the V_2 vasopressin receptor, and sarcoplasmic reticulum Ca^{2+} ATPase *(SERCA2a)*, while also decreasing phospholamban and β-adrenoreceptor kinase *(BARK 1)*. All of these new therapies hold great promise, and many trials are under way.[170]

ANESTHETIC CONSIDERATIONS IN THE PATIENT WITH SEVERELY IMPAIRED CARDIAC FUNCTION

Essential Considerations

Cardiac failure can be the common outcome of a variety of underlying causative factors, and patients may, therefore, present with widely varying clinical status. Some may appear quite compromised, whereas others may appear surprisingly well-compensated despite significant underlying pathophysiology. Regardless of what is planned surgically, achieving hemodynamic stability during the induction and maintenance of anesthesia requires a preoperative knowledge of the status of the coronary arteries (including prior bypass grafts or stents), the extent of any valvular regurgitation and/or stenosis that may be present, and whether there is significant pulmonary hypertension. In addition, all patients with significant ventricular dysfunction require a thorough preoperative evaluation of the major organ systems (particularly the renal, hepatic, and central nervous systems) for impairment. The anesthetic plan can then take any existing organ dysfunction into consideration.

Preoperative Optimization

Patients with cardiac failure are medically optimized by pharmacologic manipulations of afterload, β-blockade, and diuresis. Most medications should be continued throughout the perioperative period, but the decision whether to withhold angiotensin-converting enzyme inhibitors and diuretics should be made on an individual basis. Patients with HF often require preinduction optimization of intravascular volume status, pharmacologic manipulations of inotropy and afterload, adjustments to pacemaker settings (where present), and, on occasion, elective placement of an IABP. It is prudent to provide supplemental oxygen and monitor vital signs during the preoperative period. This is especially important if anxiolytic medications are given because this population will not tolerate sudden decreases in sympathetic tone, hypoxemia, or the potentially increased pulmonary vascular resistance that may accompany a respiratory acidosis if hypoventilation results from anxiolysis.

Intraoperative Considerations

Most procedures intended to improve cardiac function will require CPB, but the potential availability of bypass cannot be taken for granted because the function of even a severely depressed ventricle can still get worse, and it is well-known that having to emergently institute CPB significantly increases morbidity and mortality. In the prebypass period, further depression of cardiac function and significant increases in ventricular afterload must be avoided because these will increase myocardial oxygen demand and may cause ischemia. Preload, afterload, heart rate, and contractility must be continuously optimized for each patient at all times.

Where CPB will be used, it is generally prudent to consider using an antifibrinolytic agent (e.g., ε-aminocaproic acid or tranexamic acid) in an attempt to decrease bleeding in the postbypass period. In some patients, CPB may not be necessary to insert an LVAD.

Anesthetic Agents and Technique

Although the usual sedative and hypnotic agents may be tolerated in patients with mild cardiac failure, the failing heart is chronically compensated by a heightened adrenergic state, and removal of that sympathetic tone may lead to rapid decompensation with cardiovascular collapse during anesthetic induction. Patients with severely decreased ventricular function tend to decompensate quickly from physiologic and hemodynamic aberrations (e.g., hypercarbia, hypoxemia, hypotension, bradycardia/tachycardia, sudden alterations in volume status, and loss of sinus rhythm); agents should be chosen and used in a manner likely to maintain hemodynamic stability. In addition, agent selection should take into account any coexisting renal or hepatic insufficiency. Intravascular volume status needs to be carefully considered and continuously optimized for each individual patient. Inotropic and vasoactive agents including ephedrine, phenylephrine, dopamine, epinephrine, milrinone, vasopressin, nitroglycerin, and nitroprusside should be available and judiciously used at the first sign of refractory hemodynamic instability.

There can be no cookbook approach to these patients. Despite the perceived similarity of one patient with cardiac failure to another, each individual's underlying pathophysiology must be carefully considered and then anesthetic agents chosen that will best maintain the hemodynamic goals for that patient.

Traditionally, a technique based on high-dose opioid (e.g., total fentanyl dose, 50 to 100 µg/kg, or total sufentanil dose, 5 to 10 µg/kg), together with a neuromuscular blocking agent, has been used for patients with severely depressed cardiac function. Although such a technique likely will result in many hours of hemodynamic stability, potential disadvantages of this technique are that amnesia may not be adequate and the bradycardia and initial chest wall rigidity that typically accompany such an induction must be pharmacologically countered (see Chapter 9).

Etomidate (0.2 to 0.3 mg/kg intravenously) is usually the induction agent of choice in these patients because it causes neither a significant reduction in surgical ventricular restoration nor a significant decrease in myocardial contractility. The decreases in vascular tone and myocardial contractility that accompany induction with propofol make this drug unsuitable for those with severely depressed cardiac function.

Similarly, thiopental, with its propensity to cause myocardial depression and venodilation, with consequent decreases in CO, is not often used for these patients.

As a general rule, high doses of the potent inhalation agents are poorly tolerated in this population. Although all of the inhalation agents (including nitrous oxide) are myocardial depressants to varying extents, enflurane and halothane are particularly potent in this regard and generally are avoided in patients with depressed ventricular function. Isoflurane, sevoflurane, and desflurane are more likely to be compatible with hemodynamic stability in the well-optimized patient, although isoflurane and desflurane must be used with caution because of their particular tendency to decrease systemic vascular resistance. In comparison with the other currently available agents, sevoflurane appears to cause less myocardial depression and decrease in surgical ventricular restoration. In addition to direct myocardial depression and vasodilation, the inhaled anesthetic agents also may affect myocardial automaticity, impulse conduction, and refractoriness, potentially resulting in reentry phenomena and arrhythmias.

Although its use in adults has decreased dramatically in recent years, ketamine remains an extremely useful agent in patients with severely decreased ventricular function. A ketamine induction (1 to 2.5 mg/kg intravenously or 2.5 to 5 mg/kg intramuscularly), followed by a maintenance infusion (50 to 100 µg/kg/min), usually will provide excellent hemodynamic stability while assuring adequate analgesia and amnesia. Where feasible, midazolam generally is provided before giving ketamine in an attempt to lessen the potential postemergence psychiatric side effects that may occur in some patients. Additional small doses (1 to 2 mg every 2 to 3 hours) or an infusion of midazolam (0.5 µg/kg/min) often are provided when a ketamine infusion is in use. For adults and older pediatric patients, a small dose of glycopyrrolate (e.g., 0.2 mg IV) generally is provided to act as an antisialagogue. Atropine (10 µg/kg) is used for this purpose in neonates and infants. Once on CPB, the ketamine infusion can be stopped, and moderate-to-high doses of narcotics administered.

Central venous access and pulmonary artery catheterization (PAC) are extremely useful (if not mandatory) in this patient population for several reasons. First, pharmacologic interventions are frequently necessary, and potent inotropic and vasoactive agents are preferably administered to the circulation through a central route. Second, despite recent controversy regarding the usefulness and potentially increased morbidity and mortality with a PAC in critically ill patients, the ability to follow and optimize trends of CO and other hemodynamic indices, as well as the ability to assess the efficacy of pharmacologic interventions to manipulate pulmonary vascular resistance, cannot be overlooked.[171] The studies critical of routine PAC use do not directly address the cardiac surgical population and thus cannot reasonably be used to exclude this patient population from their use. Third, an extraordinarily useful monitor for evaluating the adequacy of oxygen delivery is measurement of mixed venous oxygen saturation (see Chapter 14). It might be argued that a central venous catheter alone can be used to estimate central filling pressures, and Mangano et al[172] demonstrated the ability to assess LV filling pressures using a central venous catheter, but only if the EF was greater than 40%. The population in question, however, will (by definition) present to the operating room with severely depressed LV function, justifying the use of a PAC in the majority of cases.

TEE is now considered one of the main monitoring devices used by a cardiac anesthesiologist. In addition to all the other 2D and Doppler information obtainable, the main advantage of TEE over a PAC lies in the ability to directly visualize and optimize filling volumes. When using a PAC, the clinician assumes a certain filling volume by measuring filling pressures. However, this assumed correlation is accurate only when the pressure-volume curve is known, and this is rarely the case in clinical practice. This patient population with severe CHF, usually presenting with concurrent diastolic dysfunction, will have pathologic compliance curves, requiring higher than normal filling pressures to obtain normal filling volumes. In addition, the Doppler capabilities of modern TEE systems can give the clinician a wealth of knowledge to help fine-tune pharmacologic interventions. There are, however, certain limitations to using TEE. In addition to the fact that initial acquisition cost and maintenance of equipment are considerable, TEE *is* an invasive monitoring technique, and injuries to the pharynx and esophagus are well known (though uncommon) complications. Perhaps the biggest limiting factor in using TEE as a routine monitoring device, however, is the fact that interpretation of ultrasound images can be complex and requires an experienced echocardiographer.

Nowhere is TEE a more invaluable intraoperative tool than during surgical procedures intended to improve cardiac function, because the success of many of these procedures depends on specific information provided by the echocardiographer. For example, TEE visualization of the precise mechanism and location of mitral regurgitation often determine the feasibility of valve repair. TEE is used to assess the anatomy of the valve overall, as well as to specifically evaluate the leaflets for abnormal thickening, calcification, mobility, and points of coaptation with respect to the annular plane. Doppler analyses and color-flow mapping complement the 2D evaluation and may provide additional information. The use of a mechanistic classification of mitral regurgitation greatly facilitates communication with the surgeon. The Carpentier classification of mitral regurgitation (see Table 27-3) is often used because it mechanistically distinguishes valves with normal leaflet motion (type I), excessive leaflet motion (type II), and restricted leaflet motion (type III).[173]

◾ Transesophageal Echocardiography and Ventricular Assist Devices

The role of TEE where mechanical VADs are concerned really begins before placement of the device, with a TEE evaluation focused on detecting or ruling out specific anatomic pathologies that may prevent the device from functioning as intended or lead to preventable complications, and often must be surgically addressed before starting support by the device.

To know what to look for, it is important to understand the basics of the device, including where the device or its components reside during support, how they are placed there, and the principles by which the device functions to assist the ventricle and support the circulation. As described earlier, the goal of such assist devices is twofold: (1) to decompress, or to empty, the failing ventricle by diverting blood from the failed side of the heart into the pump; and (2) once the pump is full, the stroke volume in the pump must be ejected into the arterial circulation immediately downstream of the failing ventricle to provide effective forward CO.

Regardless of the specific manufacturer's device attached to the inflow and outflow cannulae, TEE is an invaluable tool before, during, and after the placement of VADs (Table 27-7).

TABLE 27-7	Common Perioperative Echocardiographic Assessment of Patients Undergoing Left Ventricular Assist Device Insertion	
Preoperative LVAD Assessment (Patient Screening)	**Intraoperative and Postoperative LVAD Assessment**
Intracardiac shunts	Intracardiac shunts
Intracavitary thrombus	Deairing (left ventricle and device)
Atherosclerosis or severe calcifications of the aortic arch	Aortic dissection
Aortic regurgitation/mitral stenosis	Aortic regurgitation (valve opening)
Right ventricular function (tricuspid regurgitation)	Positioning and flow dynamics of both cannulae
Ventricular (apical) scars or aneurysms	Left ventricular unloading
	Right ventricular function (tricuspid regurgitation)
	Assessment of cardiac tamponade

LVAD, left ventricular assist device.
From Castillo JG, Anyanwu AC, Adams DH, et al: Real-time 3-dimensional echocardiographic assessment of current continuous-flow rotary left ventricular assist devices. *J Cardiothorac Vasc Anesth* 23:702–710, 2009, Table 3.

Before LVAD placement, TEE is used to detect specific anatomic pathologies that will:
- Impair LVAD filling (e.g., mitral stenosis, severe tricuspid regurgitation, severe RV dysfunction)
- Decrease efficacy of LVAD ejection and LV decompression (e.g., aortic regurgitation)
- Cause complications once the LVAD is functioning (e.g., patent foramen ovale, atrial septal defect, intracardiac thrombus, ascending aortic atherosclerosis, mobile plaques)

During LVAD placement, TEE is used to:
- Ensure proper inflow cannula position in the center of the left ventricle (pointing toward the mitral valve)
- Ensure adequate deairing of the device before startup

After LVAD placement, TEE is used to:
- Ensure adequate LV decompression (but not complete obliteration of the LV cavity)
- Ensure RV function does not deteriorate
- Ensure tricuspid regurgitation does not worsen (or assess the need for a tricuspid valve annuloplasty)
- Reevaluate for patent foramen ovale (must be closed if detected)

For a more detailed description of the utility of TEE before and during VAD placement and in the perioperative period, the interested reader is referred to the many published reviews available in the literature and major textbooks of echocardiography.[174–178] (See Chapters 12 and 13.)

◾ Three-dimensional Transesophageal Echocardiography and Ventricular Assist Devices

Given the increasing number of VADs being implanted worldwide, it is progressively expected of cardiac anesthesiologists to become comfortable providing anesthetic care to this extremely challenging subset of patients. This includes the echocardiographic assessment of VAD placement, as well as the timely detection of potential catastrophic events that are unique to VAD surgery. Three-dimensional echocardiography (3DE) is now a well-established imaging modality. It should never be viewed in isolation, but complementary and supplementary to 2D imaging. Strengths of 3D imaging lie in the interrogation of the positioning and alignment of cannulae, as well as an improved accuracy and reproducibility of ventricular volumes and function leading to a better understanding of ventricular spatial relations.

Volume assessment by 3DE has been shown to be rapid, accurate, and superior to conventional standardized 2D methods. Ventricular volume and mass obtained by 3DE have even compared favorably with those obtained from studies with magnetic resonance imaging, further demonstrating advantages in efficacy and accuracy in assessing volumes in remodeled ventricles after MI.[179–181]

Left and Right Ventricles

Once the LVAD is properly inserted and activated, LV decompression should occur. The reduction in size and distortion of normal LV dimensions make conventional 2D assessment of LV function, based on geometric assumptions, impractical. The ability to quantitate true cavitary volumes and thus calculate an EF, especially in light of possible explantation secondary to myocardial recovery, is appealing to the clinician. With 3DE, it is now possible to acquire full-volume images of the left ventricle and reconstruct a virtual model. This is especially useful in the setting of ventricular aneurysms or when regional wall motion abnormalities are present, which are frequently encountered in this patient population.

RV function is a major concern after LVAD implantation, and it has been the world's experience that up to 30% of patients will develop RV dysfunction after LVAD implantation. A subset of these will require the implantation of an RVAD.[182–184]

Unfortunately, the right ventricle, because of its complex anatomy, does not lend itself to geometric modeling in the same fashion as its left-sided counterpart. 3DE, with its ability to generate true volumetric measurements based on endocardial border detection and recognition, could elegantly sidestep the geometric restraints limiting the usefulness of 2D echocardiography in the functional assessment of this ventricle. Three-dimensional software, which enables the imager to create a model of the right ventricle, is currently available (TomTec Imaging Systems GmbH, Unterschleissheim, Germany).

Inflow Cannula

3DE has made it substantially easier to inspect and visualize the orientation of the inflow cannula, commonly entering the left ventricle from the apex. The echocardiographic examination of the inflow cannula position and orientation using 2DE required at least two orthogonal views (four-chamber and two-chamber long axis). A dataset can be acquired and spatially oriented when using 3DE so that the imager views the mitral valve en face from the left atrial perspective. The cropping tool can now be used to edit away the mitral valve and basal regions of the left ventricle, enabling the echocardiographer to obtain an en face view of the outflow cannula as it enters the LV apex. The cannula orifice should be centrally located entering the apex of the ventricle, aligned to the LV inflow tract (mitral valve orifice), not abutting any ventricular structures (Figure 27-13). Often the cannula ends up being slightly angled toward the anteroseptal ventricular wall. As long as the deviation is less than 30 degrees, no hindrance of ventricular drainage should be encountered. Figure 27-14 depicts the proper positioning of the inflow cannula of the Impella VAD entering the left ventricle in a retrograde fashion through the aortic valve.

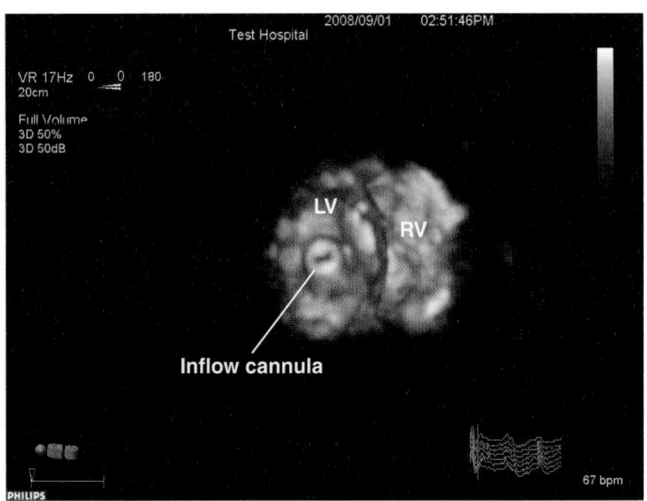

Figure 27-13 The cannula orifice should be centrally located entering the apex of the ventricle, aligned to the left ventricular inflow tract (mitral valve orifice), not abutting any ventricular structures. LV, left ventricle; RV, right ventricle.

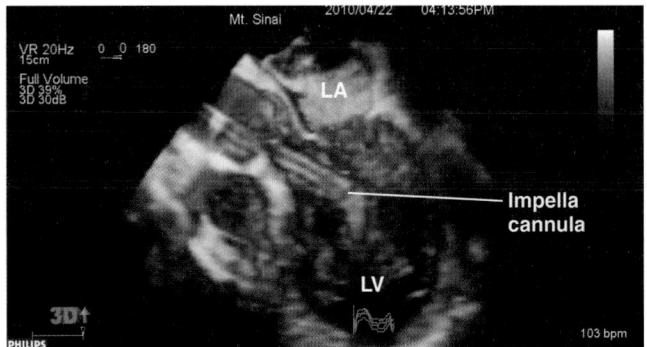

Figure 27-14 The proper positioning of the inflow cannula of the Impella VAD (ventricular assist device) entering the left ventricle (LV) in a retrograde fashion through the aortic valve. LA, left atrium.

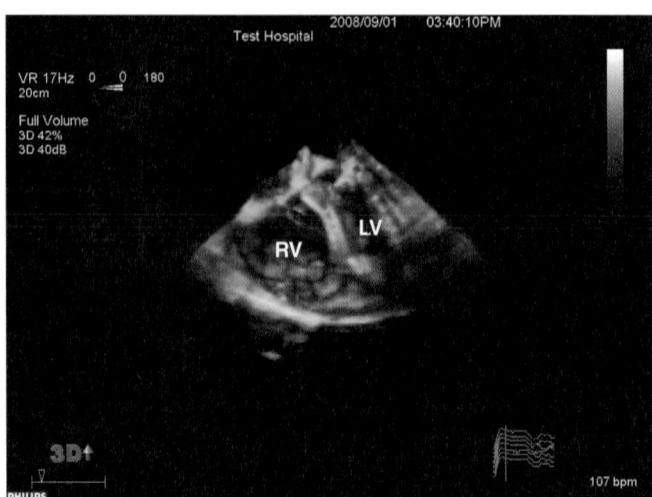

Figure 27-15 Compression of the interventricular septum. LV, left ventricle; RV, right ventricle.

Inflow cannula patency is obviously critical in achieving adequate CO. In general, patients undergoing LVAD insertion who present with severely dilated ventricles are less prone to cannula malalignment-induced hindrance of ventricular drainage. In contrast, patients with ventricles of normal dimension (e.g., acute myocarditis, acute MI) are more dependent on proper cannula alignment. In general, deviations of less than 30 degrees from the LV inflow axis are well tolerated.

In conjunction with color-flow Doppler, the echocardiographer can check for unidirectional laminar flows through the ventricle to the device. The presence of abnormal high-velocity turbulent flows or an aliasing flow at the cannula orifice suggests cannular obstruction. The differential diagnosis can include hypovolemia, a thrombotic episode, malalignment with partial obstruction by ventricular walls, or compression of the interventricular septum ("suck-down" effect; Figure 27-15). Because the treatment for these disorders is different, it is important to have excellent echocardiographic imaging capabilities. In the scenario of malalignment, the surgeon may be able to reposition the cannula by moving the flexible conduit and reassessing the LVAD hemodynamics, routinely done at the time of chest closure. A "suck-down" effect is treated by primarily reducing device flows and volume loading of the patient, as well as potentially providing RV support.

Outflow Cannula

The outflow cannula is anastomosed to the anterolateral aspect of the ascending aorta (alternatively, to the descending aorta in case of the Jarvik 2000) and should be visualized with the ascending aorta long-axis view. Here, too, color-flow Doppler represents the method of choice to evaluate flow patterns and hemodynamics. Several studies have reported the impact that the angulation of the outflow cannula to the ascending aorta has on flow patterns. The incidence of thrombus formation is reduced by decreasing the angle (<90 degrees) between both structures. Outflow graft kinking is seen echocardiographically by visualizing proximal flow acceleration when compared with those flows seen distally to the graft, and color-flow Doppler is characterized by nonlaminar high-velocity flow.

■ Postoperative Considerations

By and large, improvements in ventricular function will not be immediately apparent in this population after the majority of surgical procedures described in this chapter. In fact, ventricular function is often worse after a major cardiotomy because there often has been some degree of myocardial stunning during CPB despite the best of myocardial protective techniques with modern cardioplegia. Generally, it will be necessary to optimize intravascular volume status and use pharmacologic manipulations of afterload and contractility. Temporary pacing with epicardial wires placed during surgery often is used to optimize heart rate. In addition, meticulous management of electrolytes, coagulation status, and red blood cell mass is necessary.

One area that is often neglected in this population with sometimes tenuous hemodynamics is postoperative pain management. Patients with severely decreased ventricular function will not tolerate the stress response and tachycardia that accompany postoperative pain because of the increased myocardial oxygen demand (potentially leading to ischemia) and decreased diastolic filling time (potentially leading to decreased stroke volume). This combination is especially deleterious in patients with poor ventricular function and will exacerbate hemodynamic instability.

Most often, postoperative pain management in this population is with intermittent boluses of opioids delivered by a nurse or via patient-controlled analgesia pumps. Regional techniques (e.g., continuous epidural infusions and single-shot intrathecal opioids) are becoming popular, although concern for central neuraxial hematomas in light of intraoperative heparinization and the coagulopathy that results from CPB still limit their use in the adult population in many centers.

Placement of preservative-free morphine in the subarachnoid space (7.5 to 10 µg/kg) or the epidural space (75 to 100 µg/kg) generally will be well tolerated and can provide adequate analgesia for approximately 16 to 24 hours after cardiac surgical procedures. The main side effects of this technique are itching (usually controllable by a low-dosage infusion of naloxone, 0.5 to 1 µg/kg/hr, titrated to effect) and sedation with potential late respiratory depression (see Chapter 38).

CONCLUSIONS

The preceding sections have summarized the advances made in surgical therapy of CHF. As one of the fastest growing segments of the population of patients with heart disease, CHF patients will be the subject of many ongoing investigations. As the biotechnology industry and practitioners make further advances, the interested reader must pay close attention to the medical literature to remain current on this subject.[185–187]

REFERENCES

1. American Heart Association: *Heart disease and stroke statistics—2010 update*, Dallas, TX, 2010, American Heart Association.
2. Lloyd-Jones DM: The risk of congestive heart failure: Sobering lessons from the Framingham Heart Study, *Curr Cardiol Rep* 3:184, 2001.
3. O'Connell JB, Bristow MR: Economic impact of heart failure in the United States: Time for a different approach, *J Heart Lung Transplant* 13(Suppl):S107, 1994.
4. Zeltsman D, Acker MA: Surgical management of heart failure: An overview, *Annu Rev Med* 53:383, 2002.
5. Vitali E, Colombo T, Fratto P, et al: Surgical therapy in advanced heart failure, *Am J Cardiol* 91(Suppl):88F, 2003.
6. Dec GW: Management of heart failure: Crossing boundary over to the surgical country, *Surg Clin N Am* 84:1, 2004.
7. The Criteria Committee of the New York Heart Association: In *Nomenclature and criteria for diagnosis of diseases of the heart and great vessels*, ed 9 Boston, 1994, Little, Brown & Co, pp 253–256.
8. Francis GS, Tang WH, Sonnenblick EH: Pathophysiology of heart failure. In Furster V, Alexander RW, O'Rourke RA, et al: *Hurst's the heart*, ed 11 New York, 2004, McGraw-Hill, pp 697–722.
9. Massie BM: Pathophysiology of heart failure. In Goldman L, Ausiello D, editors: *Cecil textbook of medicine*, ed 22 Philadelphia, 2005, WB Saunders, pp 291–299.
10. Colucci WS, Braunwald E: Pathophysiology of heart failure. In Braunwald E, editor: *Heart disease: a textbook of cardiovascular medicine*, ed 7 Philadelphia, 2005, WB Saunders, pp 509–538.
11. Kajstura J, Cigola E, Malhotra A, et al: Angiotensin II induces apoptosis of adult ventricular myocytes in-vitro, *J Mol Cell Cardiol* 29:859, 1997.
12. The CONSENSUS Trial Study Group: Effects of enalapril on mortality in severe congestive heart failure. Results of the Cooperative North Scandinavian Enalapril Survival Study (CONSENSUS), *N Engl J Med* 316:1429, 1987.
13. The SOLVD Investigators: Effect of enalapril on survival in patients with reduced left ventricular ejection fractions and congestive heart failure, *N Engl J Med* 325:293, 1991.
14. Pfeffer MA, Braunwald E, Moye LA, et alon behalf of the SAVE Investigators: Effect of captopril on mortality and morbidity in patients with left ventricular dysfunction after myocardial infarction. Results of the Survival and Ventricular Enlargement Trial, *N Engl J Med* 327:669, 1992.
15. Packer M, Bristow MR, Cohn JN, et alfor the US Carvedilol Heart Failure Study Group: The effect of carvedilol on mortality and morbidity in patients with chronic heart failure, *N Engl J Med* 334:1349, 1996.
16. Leizorovicz A, Lechat P, Cucherat M, et al: Bisoprolol for the treatment of chronic heart failure: A meta-analysis on individual data of two placebo-controlled studies. CIBIS and CIBIS II, *Am Heart J* 143:301, 2002.
17. McGavin JK, Keating GM: Bisoprolol: A review of its use in chronic heart failure, *Drugs* 62:2677, 2002.
18. Wikstrand J, Hjalmarson A, Waagstein F, et al: Dose of metoprolol CR/XL and clinical outcome in patients with heart failure. Analysis of the experience in metoprolol CR/XL randomized intervention trial in chronic heart failure, *J Am Coll Cardiol* 40:491, 2002.
19. Pitt B, Zannad F, Remme WJ, et alfor the Randomized Aldactone Evaluation Study Investigators: The effect of spironolactone on morbidity and mortality in patients with severe heart failure, *N Engl J Med* 341:709, 1999.
20. Farquharson CAJ, Struthers AD: Spironolactone increases nitric oxide bioactivity, improves endothelial vasodilator dysfunction, and suppresses angiotensin I/angiotensin II conversion in patients with chronic heart failure, *Circulation* 101:594, 2000.
21. Westaby S, Narula J: Preface: Surgical options in heart failure, *Surg Clin N Am* 84:15, 2004.
22. Packer M: Management of heart failure. In Goldman L, Ausiello D, editors: *Cecil textbook of medicine*, ed 22 Philadelphia, 2005, WB Saunders, pp 300–310.
23. Mickleborough L, Merchant N, Ivanov J, et al: Left ventricular reconstruction: Early and late results, *J Thorac Cardiovasc Surg* 128:27, 2004.
24. Kumpati GS, McCarthy PM, Hoercher KJ: Surgical treatments for heart failure, *Cardiol Clin* 19:669, 2001.
25. Elefteriades J, Edwards R: Coronary bypass in left heart failure, *Semin Thorac Cardiovasc Surg* 14:125, 2002.
26. Bolling SF: Mitral reconstruction in cardiomyopathy, *J Heart Valve Dis* 11(Suppl 1):S26, 2002.
27. Tolis GA Jr, Korkolis DP, Kopf GS, et al: Revascularization alone (without mitral valve repair) suffices in patients with advanced ischemic cardiomyopathy and mild-moderate mitral regurgitation, *Ann Thorac Surg* 74:1476, 2002.
28. Hon JKF, Yacoub MH: Bridge to recovery with the use of left ventricular assist device and clenbuterol, *Ann Thorac Surg* 75:S36, 2003.
29. Miller WL, Tointon SK, Hodge DO, et al: Long-term outcome and the use of revascularization in patients with heart failure, suspected ischemic heart disease, and large reversible myocardial perfusion defects, *Am Heart J* 143:904, 2002.
30. Liao L, Cabell CH, Jollis JG, et al: Usefulness of myocardial viability or ischemia in predicting long-term survival for patients with severe left ventricular dysfunction undergoing revascularization, *Am J Cardiol* 93:1275, 2004.
31. Vitali E, Colombo T, Fratto P, et al: Surgical therapy in advanced heart failure, *Am J Cardiol* 91(Suppl):88F, 2003.
32. Trachiotis GD, Weintraub WS, Johnston T, et al: Coronary artery bypass grafting in patients with advanced left ventricular dysfunction, *Ann Thorac Surg* 66:1632, 1998.
33. Carstensen S: Dobutamine-atropine stress echocardiography, *Heart Drug* 5:101, 2005.
34. Mickleborough LL, Carson S, Tamariz M, et al: Results of revascularization in patients with severe left ventricular dysfunction, *J Thorac Cardiovasc Surg* 119:550, 2000.
35. Salgo IS, Gorman JH 3rd, Gorman RC, et al: Effect of annular shape on leaflet curvature in reducing mitral leaflet stress, *Circulation* 106:711–717, 2002.
36. Geha AS, El-Zein C, Massad MG: Mitral valve surgery in patients with ischemic and nonischemic dilated cardiomyopathy, *Cardiology* 101:15, 2004.
37. Phillips HR, Levine FH, Carter JE, et al: Mitral valve replacement for isolated mitral regurgitation: Analysis of clinical course and late postoperative left ventricular ejection fraction, *Am J Cardiol* 48:647, 1981.
38. Romano MA, Bolling SF: Mitral valve repair as an alternative treatment for heart failure patients, *Heart Fail Monit* 4:7, 2003.
39. Reese TB, Tribble CG, Ellman PI, et al: Mitral repair is superior to replacement when associated with coronary artery disease, *Ann Surg* 239:671–675, 2004.
40. Magne J, Girerd N, Sénéchal M, et al: Mitral repair versus replacement for ischemic mitral regurgitation: Comparison of short-term and long-term survival, *Circulation* 120(11 Suppl):S104–S111, 2009.
41. Gillinov AM, Wierup PN, Blackstone EH, et al: Is repair preferable to replacement for ischemic mitral regurgitation? *J Thorac Cardiovasc Surg* 122:1125–1141, 2001.
42. Braun J, van de Veire NR, Klautz RJ, et al: Restrictive mitral annuloplasty cures ischemic mitral regurgitation and heart failure, *Ann Thorac Surg* 85:430–436, 2008 discussion 436–437.
43. Penicka M, Linkova H, Lang O, et al: Predictors of improvement of unrepaired moderate ischemic mitral regurgitation in patients undergoing elective isolated coronary artery bypass graft surgery, *Circulation* 120:1474–1481, 2009.
44. Magne J, Sénéchal M, Mathieu P, et al: Restrictive annuloplasty for ischemic mitral regurgitation may induce functional mitral stenosis, *J Am Coll Cardiol* 51:1692–1701, 2008.
45. Cooley D: Ventricular endoaneurysmorrhaphy: A simplified repair for extensive postinfarction aneurysm, *J Cardiac Surg* 4:200–205, 1989.
46. Loop FD, Effler DB: Left ventricular aneurysm. In *Gibbon's surgery of the chest*, ed 3 Philadelphia, 1976, WB Saunders, pp 1384.
47. Jatene AD: Left ventricular aneurysmectomy: Resection or reconstruction, *J Thorac Cardiovasc Surg* 89:321–331, 1985.
48. Dor V, Kreitmann P, Jourdan J, et al: Interest of physiological closure (circumferential plasty on contractile areas) of left ventricle after resection and endocardiectomy for aneurysm of akinetic zone: Comparison with classical technique about a series of 209 left ventricular resections [abstract], *J Cardiovasc Surg* 26:73, 1985.
49. Dor V, Saab M, Coste P, et al: Left ventricular aneurysm: a new surgical approach, *Thorac Cardiovasc Surg* 37:11–19, 1989.
50. Batista RJ, Santos JL, Takeshita N, et al: Partial left ventriculectomy to improve left ventricular function in end-stage heart disease, *J Cardiac Surg* 11:96, 1996.
51. Batista RJV, Verde J, Nery P, et al: Partial left ventriculectomy to treat end-stage heart disease, *Ann Thorac Surg* 64:634, 1997.
52. Franco-Cereceda A, McCarthy PM, Blackstone EH, et al: Partial left ventriculectomy for dilated cardiomyopathy: Is this an alternative to transplantation? *J Thorac Cardiovasc Surg* 121:879, 2001.
53. McCarthy JF, McCarthy PM, Starling RC, et al: Partial left ventriculectomy and mitral valve repair for end-stage congestive heart failure, *Eur J Cardiothorac Surg* 13:337, 1998.
54. Etoch SW, Koenig SC, Laureano MA, et al: Results after partial left ventriculectomy versus heart transplantation for idiopathic cardiomyopathy, *J Thorac Cardiovasc Surg* 117:952, 1999.
55. Suma HRESTORE Group: Left ventriculoplasty for nonischemic dilated cardiomyopathy, *Semin Thorac Cardiovasc Surg* 13:514, 2001.
56. Dor V, Sabatier M, DiDonato M, et al: Efficacy of endoventricular patch plasty in large postinfarction akinetic scar and severe left ventricular dysfunction: Comparison with a series of large dyskinetic scars, *J Thorac Cardiovasc Surg* 116:47, 1998.
57. DiDonato M, Sabatier M, Dor V, et al: Effects of the Dor procedure on left ventricular dimension and shape and geometric correlates of mitral regurgitation one year after surgery, *J Thorac Cardiovasc Surg* 121:91, 2001.
58. Athanasuleas CL, Stanley AW Jr, Buckberg GD, et al: Surgical anterior ventricular endocardial restoration (SAVER) in the dilated remodeled ventricle after anterior myocardial infarction. RESTORE Group. Reconstructive Endoventricular Surgery, Returning Torsion Original Radius Elliptical Shape to the LV, *J Am Coll Cardiol* 37:1199, 2001.
59. Jones RH, Velazquez EJ, Michler RM, et al: Coronary bypass surgery with or without surgical ventricular reconstruction, *N Engl J Med* 360:1705–1717, 2009.
60. Buckberg GD, Athanasuleas CL: The STICH trial: Misguided conclusions, *J Thorac Cardiovasc Surg* 138:1060–1064, 2009.

61. Cirillo M: A new surgical ventricular restoration technique to reset residual myocardium's fiber orientation: The "KISS" procedure, *Ann Surg Innov Res* 3:6–14, 2009.
62. Kerwin WF, Botvinick EH, O'Connell JW, et al: Ventricular contraction abnormalities in dilated cardiomyopathy: Effect of biventricular pacing to correct interventricular dyssynchrony, *J Am Coll Cardiol* 35:1221, 2000.
63. Jarcho J: Resynchronizing ventricular contraction in heart failure, *N Engl J Med* 352:1594, 2005.
64. Shamin W, Francis DP, Yousufuddin M, et al: Intraventricular conduction delay: A prognostic marker in chronic heart failure, *Int J Cardiol* 70:171, 1999.
65. Auricchio A, Stellbrink C, et al: The pacing therapies for congestive heart failure study: Rationale, design, and endpoint of a prospective randomized multicenter study, *Am J Cardiol* 83:130D, 1999.
66. Cazeau S, Leclereq C, Lavergne T, et al: The Multisite Stimulation in Cardiomyopathies Study Investigators. Effects of multisite biventricular pacing in patients with heart failure and intraventricular conduction delay, *N Engl J Med* 334:873, 2001.
67. Abraham WT, Fisher WG, et al for the multicenter Insync Randomized Clinical Evaluation Investigators and Coordinators: Double-blind, randomized, controlled trial of cardiac resynchronization in chronic heart failure, *N Engl J Med* 346:1845, 2002.
68. Cleland J, Daubert J, Erdman E, et al: The effect of cardiac resynchronization on morbidity and mortality in heart failure, *N Engl J Med* 352:1539, 2005.
69. Kass DA, Chen CH, Curry C, et al: Improved left ventricular mechanics from acute VDD pacing in patients with dilated cardiomyopathy and ventricular conduction delay, *Circulation* 99:1567, 1999.
70. Auricchio A, Stellbrink C, Block M, et al: Effect of pacing chamber and atrioventricular delay on acute systolic function of paced patients with congestive heart failure, *Circulation* 99:2993, 1999.
71. Gras D, Mabo P, Tang T, et al: Multisite pacing as a supplemental treatment of congestive heart failure: Preliminary results of the Medtronic Inc. InSync Study, *Pacing Clin Electrophysiol* 21:2249, 1998.
72. Cazeau S, Leclercq C, Lavergne T, et al: Effects of multisite biventricular pacing in patients with heart failure and intraventricular conduction delay, *N Engl J Med* 344:873, 2001.
73. Goldman S, Johnson Gfor the V-HeFT VA Cooperative Studies Group: Mechanism of death in heart failure. The Vasodilator-Heart Failure Trials, *Circulation* 87(Suppl VI):VI–V24, 1993.
74. Abraham WT, Fisher WG, Smith ALfor the MIRACLE Investigators and Coordinators: Multicenter InSync Randomized Clinical Evaluation (MIRACLE): Results of a randomized, double-blind, controlled trial to assess cardiac resynchronization therapy in heart failure patients [abstract], *Circulation* 104:II, 2001.
75. Hohnloser S, Kuck K, Dorlan P, et al: Prophylactic use of an implantable cardioverter-defibrillator after acute myocardial infarction, *N Engl J Med* 351:2481, 2004.
76. Bardy E, Lee K, Mark D, et al: Amiodarone or an implanted cardioverter-defibrillator for congestive heart failure, *N Engl J Med* 352:225, 2005.
77. Buxton AE, Lee KL, et al: A randomized study of the prevention of sudden death in patients with coronary artery disease, *N Engl J Med* 341:1882, 1999.
78. Moss AJ, Zareba W, et al: Prophylactic implantation of a defibrillator in patients with myocardial infarction and reduced ejection fraction, *N Engl J Med* 346:877, 2002.
79. Bristow MR, Saxon LA, Boehmer J, et al: Cardiac-resynchronization therapy with or without an implantable defibrillator in advanced chronic heart failure, *N Engl J Med* 350:2140, 2004.
80. Epstein AE, DiMarco JP, et al: ACC/AHA/HRS 2008 guidelines for device-based therapy of cardiac rhythm abnormalities, *Circulation* 117:e350, 2008.
81. Linde C, Abraham WT, et al: Randomized trial of cardiac resynchronization in mildly symptomatic heart failure patients and in asymptomatic patients with left ventricular dysfunction and previous heart failure symptoms, *J Am Coll Cardiol* 52:1834–1843, 2008.
82. Moss AJ, Hall WJ, et al: Cardiac-resynchronization therapy for the prevention of heart failure events, *N Engl J Med* 361:1329, 2009.
83. el-Banayosy A, Arusoglu L, Kizner L, et al: Predictors of survival in patients bridged to transplantation with the Thoratec VAD device: A single-center retrospective study on more than 100 patients, *J Heart Lung Transplant* 19:964–968, 2000.
84. Fukamachi K, McCarthy PM, Smedira NG, et al: Preoperative risk factors for right ventricular failure after implantable left ventricular assist device insertion, *Ann Thorac Surg* 68:2181–2184, 1999.
85. Ochiai Y, McCarthy PM, Smedira NG, et al: Predictors of severe right ventricular failure after implantable left ventricular assist device insertion: Analysis of 245 patients, *Circulation* 106(Suppl 1): I–198–I-202, 2002.
86. Rao V, Oz MC, Flannery MA, et al: Revised screening scale to predict survival after insertion of a left ventricular assist device, *J Thorac Cardiovasc Surg* 125:855–862, 2003.
87. Schenk S, McCarthy PM, Blackstone EH, et al: Duration of inotropic support after left ventricular assist device implantation: Risk factors and impact on outcome, *J Thorac Cardiovasc Surg* 131:447–454, 2006.
88. Farrar DJ: Preoperative predictors of survival in patients with Thoratec ventricular assist devices as a bridge to heart transplantation, *J Heart Lung Transplant* 13:93–100, 1994.
89. Deng MC, Loebe M, el-Banayosy A, et al: Mechanical circulatory support for advanced heart failure: Effect of patient selection on outcome, *Circulation* 103:231–237, 2001.
90. Frazier OH, Rose EA, Oz MC, et al: Multicenter clinical evaluation of the HeartMate vented electric left ventricular assist system in patients awaiting heart transplantation, *J Thorac Cardiovasc Surg* 122:1186–1195, 2001.
91. Miller LW, Pagani FD, Russell RD, et al: Use of a continuous-flow device in patients awaiting heart transplantation, *N Engl J Med* 357:885–896, 2007.
92. Miller LW, Lietz K: Candidate selection for long-term left ventricular assist device therapy for refractory heart failure, *J Heart Lung Transplant* 25:756–764, 2006.
93. Fitzpatrick JR, Frederick JR, Hsu V: Risk score derived from pre-operative data analysis predicts the need for biventricular mechanical circulatory support, *J Heart Lung Transplant* 27:1286–1292, 2008.
94. Holman WL, Kormos RL, Naftel DC, et al: Predictors of death and transplant in patients with a mechanical circulatory support device: A multi-institutional study, *J Heart Lung Transplant* 28:44–50, 2009.
95. Zimpfer D, Zrunek P, Roethy W, et al: Left ventricular assist devices decrease fixed pulmonary hypertension in cardiac transplant candidates, *J Thorac Cardiovasc Surg* 133:689–695, 2007.
96. Radovancevic B, Vrtovec B, de Kort E, et al: End-organ function in patients on long-term circulatory support with continuous- or pulsatile-flow assist devices, *J Heart Lung Transplant* 26:815–818, 2007.
97. Kamdar F, Boyle A, Liao K, et al: Effects of centrifugal, axial, and pulsatile left ventricular assist device support on end-organ function in heart failure patients, *J Heart Lung Transplant* 28:352–359, 2009.
98. Miller LW, Pagani FD, Russell SD, et al: Use of a continuous flow device in patients awaiting heart transplantation, *N Engl J Med* 357:885–896, 2007.
99. Feller ED, Sorensen EN, Haddad M, et al: Clinical outcomes are similar in pulsatile and nonpulsatile left ventricular assist device recipients, *Ann Thorac Surg* 83:1082–1088, 2007.
100. Frazier OH, Gemmato C, Myers TJ, et al: Initial clinical experience with the HeartMate II axial-flow left ventricular assist device, *Tex Heart Inst J* 34:275–281, 2007.
101. John R, Kamdar F, Liao K, et al: Improved survival and decreasing incidence of adverse events with the HeartMate II left ventricular assist device as bridge-to-transplant therapy, *Ann Thorac Surg* 86:1227–1235, 2008.
102. Mueller HS: Role of intra-aortic counterpulsation in cardiogenic shock and acute myocardial infarction, *Cardiology* 84:168, 1994.
103. Braunwald E: Treatment of heart failure-assisted circulation. In *Heart disease: A textbook of cardiovascular medicine*, ed 6 Philadelphia, 2001, WB Saunders Company.
104. Allen BS, Rosenkrantz F, Buckberg GD, et al: Studies on prolonged acute regional ischemia: VI. Myocardial infarction with LV power failure: A medical/surgical emergency requiring urgent revascularization with maximal protection of remote muscle, *J Thorac Cardiovasc Surg* 98:691, 1989.
105. Maccioli G, Lucas W, Norfleet E: The intra-aortic balloon pump: A review, *J Cardiothorac Anesth* 2:365–373, 1988.
106. Dietl CA, Berkheimer MD, Woods EL, et al: Efficacy and cost effectiveness of pre-operative IABP in patients with ejection fraction of 0.25 or less, *Ann Thorac Surg* 62:401–408, 1996.
107. Noon GP, Ball JW, Short HD: Bio-medicus centrifugal ventricular support for postcardiotomy cardiac failure: A review of 129 cases, *Ann Thorac Surg* 61:291–295, 1996.
108. Aragon J, Lee MS, Kar B, et al: Percutaneous left ventricular assist device: "TandemHeart" for high-risk coronary intervention, *Catheter Cardiovasc Interv* 65:346–352, 2005.
109. Vranckx P, Foley DP, de Feijter PJ, et al: Clinical introduction of the TandemHeart as a percutaneous left ventricular assist device for circulatory support during high-risk percutaneous coronary intervention, *Int J Cardiovasc Intervent* 5:35–39, 2003.
110. Kar B, Butkevich A, Civitello AB, et al: Hemodynamic support with a percutaneous left ventricular assist device during stenting of an unprotected left main coronary artery, *Tex Heart Inst J* 31:84–86, 2004.
111. Neuzil P, Kmonicek P, Skoda J, et al: Temporary (short-term) percutaneous left ventricular assist device (Tandem Heart™) in a patient with STEMI, multivessel coronary artery disease, cardiogenic shock and severe peripheral artery disease, *Acute Card Care* 11:146–150, 2009.
112. Pitsis AA, Visouli AN, Burkhoff D, et al: Feasibility study of a temporary percutaneous left ventricular assist device in cardiac surgery, *Ann Thor Surg* 84:1993–1999, 2007.
113. Khalife WI, Kar B: The TandemHeart® pVAD™ in the treatment of acute fulminant myocarditis, *Tex Heart Inst J* 34:209–213, 2007.
114. Thiele H, Sick P, Boudriot E, et al: Randomized comparison of intra-aortic balloon support with a percutaneous left ventricular assist device in patients with revascularized acute myocardial infarction complicated by cardiogenic shock, *Eur Heart J* 26:1276–1283, 2005.
115. Gregoric ID, Poglajen G, Span M, et al: Percutaneous ventricular assist device support during off-pump surgical coronary revascularization, *Ann Thorac Surg* 86:637–639, 2008.
116. Bruckner BA, Jacob JP, Gregoric ID: Clinical experience with the TandemHeart percutaneous ventricular assist device as a bridge to cardiac transplantation, *Tex Heart Inst J* 35:447–450, 2008.
117. Meyns B, Dens J, Sergeant P, et al: Initial experiences with the Impella device in patients with cardiogenic shock, *Thorac Cardiovasc Surg* 51:312–317, 2003.
118. Seyfarth M, Sibbing D, Bauer I: A randomized clinical trial to evaluate the safety and efficacy of a percutaneous left ventricular assist device versus intra-aortic balloon pumping for treatment of cardiogenic shock caused by myocardial infarction, *J Am Coll Cardiol* 52:1584–1588, 2008.
119. Dixon SR, Henriques JPS, Mauri L: A prospective feasibility trial investigating the use of the Impella 2.5 system in patients undergoing high-risk percutaneous coronary intervention (The PROTECT I Trial): Initial U.S. experience, *JACC: Cardiovasc Interv* 2:91–96, 2009.
120. Atoui R, Samoukovic G, Al-Tuwaijri F: The use of the Impella LP 2.5 percutaneous microaxial ventricular assist device as hemodynamic support during high-risk abdominal surgery, *J Card Surg* 25:238–240, 2010.
121. Ferrari M, Poerner TC, Brehm BR: First use of a novel plug-and-play percutaneous circulatory assist device for high-risk coronary angioplasty, *Acute Card Care* 10:111–115, 2008.
122. Abiomed: BVS 5000 clinical update, Available at: www.abiomed.com/clinical_information/BVS5000_Update.cfm Accessed December 27, 2009.
123. Abiomed: AB5000 clinical update, Available at: www.abiomed.com/clinical_information/AB5000_Update.cfm Accessed December 27, 2009.
124. Abiomed: Data presented in video lecture from Dr. Ralph de la Torre: AMI Patients and Mechanical Support, Available at: www.abiomed.com/clinical_information/physician_videos.cfm Accessed December 27, 2009.
125. *BVS5000 Bi-ventricular Support Training Manual*, Danvers, MA, July 1997, Abiomed.
126. Fukumachi K, McCarthy PM, Smedira NG, et al: Preoperative risk factors for right ventricular failure after implantable left ventricular assist device insertion, *Ann Thorac Surg* 68:2181–2184, 1999.
127. Elbeery JR, Owen CH, Savitt MA, et al: Effects of the left ventricular assist device on right ventricular function, *J Thorac Cardiovasc Surg* 99:809–816, 1990.
128. Santamore WP, Gray LA Jr: Left ventricular contributions to right ventricular systolic function during LVAD support, *Ann Thorac Surg* 61:350–356, 1996.
129. Marasco SF, Lukas G, McDonald M, et al: Review of ECMO (Extra Corporeal Membrane Oxygenation) support in critically ill adult patients, *Heart Lung Circ* 17(Suppl 4):S41–S47, 2008.
130. Hoshi H, Shinshi T, Takatani S: Third-generation blood pumps with mechanical noncontact magnetic bearings, *Artif Organs* 30:324–333, 2006.
131. Asama J, Shinshi T, Hoshi H, et al: A compact highly efficient and low hemolytic centrifugal blood pump with a magnetically levitated impeller, *Artif Organs* 30:160–167, 2006.
132. Santise G, Petrou M, Pepper JR, et al: Levitronix CentriMag as a short-term salvage treatment for primary graft failure after heart transplantation, *J Heart Lung Transplant* 25:495–498, 2006.
133. John R, Liao K, Lietz K, et al: Experience with the Levitronix CentriMag circulatory support system as a bridge to decision in patients with refractory acute cardiogenic shock and multisystem organ failure, *J Thorac Cardiovasc Surg* 134:351–358, 2007.
134. Shuhaiber JH, Jenkins D, Berman M, et al: The Papworth experience with the Levitronix CentriMag ventricular assist device, *J Heart Lung Transplant* 27:158–164, 2008.
135. Frazier OH, Rose EA, Oz MC, et al: Multicenter clinical evaluation of the HeartMate vented electric left ventricular assist system in patients awaiting heart transplantation, *J Thorac Cardiovasc Surg* 122:1186–1195, 2001.
136. www.thoratec.com Accessed December 27, 2009.
137. Slaughter M, Tsui SEl-Banayosy A, et al: Results of a multicenter clinical trial with the Thoratec implantable ventricular assist device, *J Thorac Cardiovasc Surg* 133:1573–1580, 2007.
138. Copeland JG, Smith RG, Arabia FA, et al: Cardiac replacement with a total artificial heart as a bridge to transplantation, *N Engl J Med* 351:859–867, 2004.
139. Minami K, El-Banayosy A, Sezai A, et al: Morbidity and outcome after mechanical support using Thoratec, Novacor, and HeartMate for bridging to heart transplantation, *Artif Organs* 24:421–426, 2000.
140. Miller LW, Pagani FD, Russel SD, et al: Use of a continuous-flow device in patients awaiting heart transplantation, *N Engl J Med* 357:885–896, 2007.
141. Frazier OH, Rose EA, Oz MC, et al: Multicenter clinical evaluation of the HeartMate vented electric left ventricular assist system in patients awaiting heart transplantation, *J Thorac Cardiovasc Surg* 122:1186–1195, 2001.
142. Lee S, Kamdar F, Madlon-Kay R, et al: Effects of the HeartMate II continuous-flow left ventricular assist device on right ventricular function, *J Heart Lung Transplant* 29:209–215, 2010.
143. Patel ND, Weiss ES, Schaffer J, et al: Right heart dysfunction after left ventricular assist device implantation: A comparison of the pulsatile HeartMate I and axial-flow HeartMate II devices, *Ann Thorac Surg* 86:832–840, 2008.
144. Saleh S, Liakopoulos OJ, Buckberg GD: The septal motor of biventricular function, *Eur J Cardiothorac Surg* 29S:S126–S138, 2006.
145. Lee S, Kamdar F, Madlon-Kay R, et al: Effects of the HeartMate II continuous-flow left ventricular assist device on right ventricular function, *J Heart Lung Transplant* 29:209–215, 2010.

146. Rose EA, Gelijns AC, Moskowitz AJ, et al: Long-term mechanical left ventricular assistance for end-stage heart failure, *N Engl J Med* 345:1435–1443, 2001.

147. Long JW, Kfoury AG, Slaughter MS, et al: Long term destination therapy with the HeartMate XVE left ventricular assist device: Improved outcomes since the REMATCH study, *Congest Heart Fail* 11:133–138, 2005.

148. Slaughter MS, Rogers JG, Milano CA, et al: Advanced heart failure treated with continuous-flow left ventricular assist device, *N Engl J Med* 361:2282–2285, 2009.

149. Lietz K, Long JW, Kfoury AG, et al: Outcomes of left ventricular assist device implantation as destination therapy in the post-REMATCH era: Implications for patient selection, *Circulation* 116:497–505, 2007.

150. Kirklin JK, Naftel DC, Stevenson LW, et al: INTERMACS database for durable devices for circulatory support: First annual report, *J Heart Lung Transplant* 27:1065–1072, 2008.

151. Stevenson LW, Pagani FD, Young JB, et al: INTERMACS profiles of advanced heart failure: The current picture, *J Heart Lung Transplant* 28:535–541, 2009.

152. Holman WL, Kormos RL, Naftel DC, et al: Predictors of death and transplant in patients with a mechanical circulatory support device: A multi-institutional study, *J Heart Lung Transplant* 28:44–50, 2009.

153. Levy WC, Mozaffarian D, Linker DT, et al: The Seattle Heart Failure Model: Prediction of survival in heart failure, *Circulation* 113:1424–1433, 2006.

154. Levy WC, Mozaffarian D, Linker DT, et al: Can the Seattle Heart Failure Model be used to risk-stratify heart failure patients for potential left ventricular assist device therapy? *J Heart Lung Transplant* 28:231–236, 2009.

155. Schaffer JM, Allen JG, Weiss ES, et al: Evaluation of risk indices in continuous-flow left ventricular assist device patients, *Ann Thorac Surg* 88:1889–1896, 2009.

156. Patten RD, Denofrio D, El-Zaru M, et al: Ventricular assist device therapy normalizes inducible nitric oxide synthate expression and reduces cardiomyocyte apoptosis in the failing human heart, *J Am Coll Cardiol* 45(9):1425–1427, 2005.

157. Zafeirides A, Jeevanandam V, Houser SR, et al: Regression of cellular hypertrophy after left ventricular assist device support, *Circulation* 98:656–662, 1998.

158. Madigan JD, Barbone A, Choudhri AF, et al: Time course of reverse remodeling of the left ventricle during support with a left ventricular assist device, *J Thorac Cardiovasc Surg* 121:902–908, 2001.

159. Terracciano CMN, Hardy J, Birks EJ, et al: Clinical recovery from end-stage heart failure using left ventricular assist device and pharmacological therapy correlates with increased sarcoplasmic reticulum calcium content but not with regression of cellular hypertrophy, *Circulation* 109:2263–2265, 2004.

160. Cooley DA, Liotta D, Hallman GL, et al: Orthotopic cardiac prosthesis for two staged cardiac replacement, *Am J Cardiol* 24:723, 1969.

161. Cooley DA, Akutsu T, Norman JC, et al: Total artificial heart in two-stage cardiac transplantation, *Cardiovasc Dis* 8:305, 1981.

162. DeVries WL, Anderson JL, Joyce LD, et al: Clinical use of the total artificial heart, *N Engl J Med* 310:273, 1984.

163. Organ Procurement and Transplant Network (OPTN) Web site: www.OPTN.org/data Accessed March 8, 2010.

164. Menasche P: Cell transplantation in myocardium, *Ann Thorac Surg* 75:20, 2003.

165. Siminiak T, Fiszer D, Jerzykowska O, et al: *Percutaneous transvenous transplantation of autologous myoblasts in the treatment of postinfarction heart failure: The POZNAN trial*, March 7, 2004 Presented at the American College of Cardiology, 53rd Annual Scientific Session, New Orleans.

166. Len N: Mobilizing cells to the injured myocardium, *J Am Coll Cardiol* 44:1521, 2004.

167. Rosenstrauch D, Poglajen G, Zidar N, et al: Stem cell therapy for ischemic heart failure, *Tex Heart Inst J* 32:339, 2005.

168. Snakumar B, Harry L, Paleolog E: Modulating angiogenesis, *JAMA* 292:972, 2004.

169. Chaudhri BB, del Monte F, Harding SE, et al: Gene transfer in cardiac myocytes, *Surg Clin N Am* 84:141, 2004.

170. Askuri A, Penn M: Targeted gene therapy for the treatment of cardiac dysfunction, *Semin Thorac Cardiovasc Surg* 14:167, 2002.

171. Sandham JD, Hull RD, Brant RF, et al: A randomized, controlled trial of the use of pulmonary-artery catheters in high-risk surgical patients, *N Engl J Med* 348:5, 2003.

172. Mangano DT: Monitoring pulmonary artery pressures in coronary artery disease, *Anesthesiology* 53:364, 1980.

173. Carpentier A, Chauvaud S, Fabiani JN, et al: Reconstructive surgery of mitral valve incompetence: Ten-year appraisal, *J Thorac Cardiovasc Surg* 79:338, 1980.

174. Horton S, Khodaverdian R, Chatelain P, et al: Left ventricular assist device malfunction: An approach to diagnosis by echocardiography, *J Am Coll Cardiol* 45:1435, 2005.

175. Scalia GM, McCarthy PM, Savage RM, et al: Clinical utility of echocardiography in the management of implantable ventricular assist devices, *J Am Soc Echocardiogr* 13:754, 2000.

176. Stone M: Transesophageal echocardiography and surgical devices: Cannulas, catheters, intraaortic balloon pumps, ventricular assist devices, and occluders. In Konstadt S, Shernan S, Oka Y, editors: *Clinical Transesophageal Echocardiography: A Problem Oriented Approach*, ed 2 Philadelphia, 2003, Lippincott Williams & Wilkins.

177. Mets B: Anesthesia for left ventricular assist device placement, *J Cardiothorac Vasc Anesth* 14:316, 2000.

178. Castillo JG, Anyanwu AC, Adams DH, et al: Real-time 3-D echocardiographic assessment of current continuous flow rotary left ventricular assist devices, *J Cardiothorac Vasc Anesth* 23:702–710, 2009.

179. Kuhl HP, Schreckenberg M, Rulands D, et al: High-resolution transthoracic real-time three-dimensional echocardiography: Quantitation of cardiac volumes and function using semi-automatic border detection and comparison with cardiac magnetic resonance imaging, *J Am Coll Cardiol* 43:2083–2090, 2004.

180. Gopal AS, Schnellbaecher MJ, Shen Z, et al: Freehand three-dimensional echocardiography for determination of left ventricular volume and mass in patients with abnormal ventricles: Comparison with magnetic resonance imaging, *J Am Soc Echocardiogr* 10:853–861, 1997.

181. Arai K, Hozumi T, Matsumura Y, et al: Accuracy of measurement of left ventricular volume and ejection fraction by new real-time three-dimensional echocardiography in patients with wall motion abnormalities secondary to myocardial infarction, *Am J Cardiol* 94:552–558, 2004.

182. Ochiai Y, McCarthy PM, Smedira NG, et al: Predictors of severe right ventricular failure after implantable left ventricular assist device insertion: Analysis of 245 patients, *Circulation* 106:I198–I202, 2002.

183. Maeder MT, Leet A, Ross A, et al: Changes in right ventricular function during continuous-low left ventricular assist device support, *J Heart Lung Transplant* 28:360–366, 2009.

184. Farrar DJ, Hill JD, Pennington DG, et al: Preoperative and postoperative comparison of patients with univentricular and biventricular support with the Thoratec ventricular assist device as a bridge to cardiac transplantation, *J Thorac Cardiovasc Surg* 113:202–209, 1997.

185. Adams DH, Anyanwu AC, Chikwe J, et al: The year in cardiovascular surgery, *J Am Coll Cardiol* 53:239–240, 2009.

186. Ramakrishna H, Fassl J, Sinha A, et al: The Year in cardiothoracic and vascular anesthesia: selected highlights from 2009, *J Cardiothorac Vasc Anesth* 24:7–17, 2010.

187. Thunberg C, Gaitan B, Arable F, et al: Ventricular assist devices today and tomorrow, *J Cardiothorac Vasc Anesth* 24:656–680, 2010.

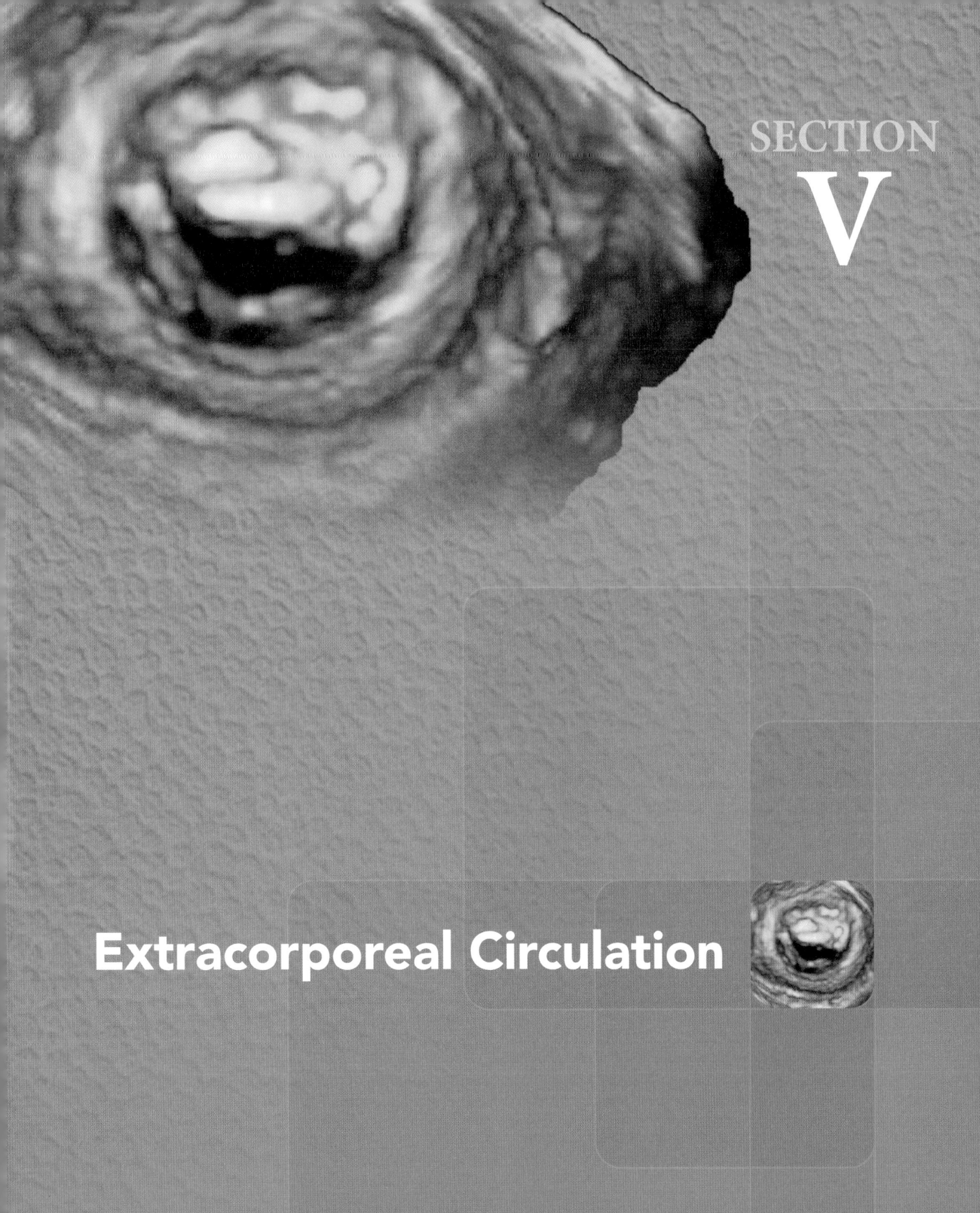

Extracorporeal Circulation

28

Cardiopulmonary Bypass Management and Organ Protection

HILARY P. GROCOTT, MD, FRCPC, FASE | MARK STAFFORD-SMITH, MD, CM, FRCPC | CHRISTINA T. MORA MANGANO, MD, FAHA

KEY POINTS

1. Cardiopulmonary bypass (CPB) provides the extracorporeal maintenance of respiration and circulation at hypothermic and normothermic temperatures. CPB permits the surgeon to operate on a quiet—or nonbeating—heart at hypothermic temperatures, thus facilitating surgery in an ischemic environment.
2. CPB is associated with a number of profound physiologic perturbations. The central nervous system, kidneys, gut, lungs, and heart are especially vulnerable to ischemic events associated with extracorporeal circulation.
3. Advanced age is one of the most important risk factors for stroke and neurocognitive dysfunction after CPB.
4. Acute renal injury from CPB can contribute directly to poor outcomes.
5. Drugs such as dopamine and diuretics do not prevent renal failure after CPB.
6. Myocardial stunning represents injury caused by short periods of myocardial ischemia that can occur with CPB.
7. Blood cardioplegia has the potential advantage of delivering oxygen to ischemic myocardium, whereas crystalloid cardioplegia does not carry much oxygen.
8. Gastrointestinal complications after CPB include pancreatitis, gastrointestinal bleeding, bowel infarction, and cholecystitis.
9. Pulmonary complications such as atelectasis and pleural effusions are common after cardiac surgery with CPB.
10. Embolization, hypoperfusion, and inflammatory processes are central common pathophysiologic mechanisms responsible for organ dysfunction after CPB.
11. Controversy regarding the optimal management of blood flow, pressure, and temperature during CPB remains. Perfusion should be adequate to support ongoing oxygen requirements; mean arterial pressures of more than 70 mm Hg may benefit patients with cerebral or other diffuse arthrosclerosis. Arterial blood temperatures should not exceed 37.0° C.
12. The initiation and termination of CPB are key phases of a cardiac surgery procedure, but the anesthesiologist must remain vigilant throughout the entire bypass period.
13. Total CPB can be tailored to produce deep hypothermic circulatory arrest or partial bypass. These special techniques require sophisticated monitoring and care.
14. Organ dysfunction cannot definitely be prevented during cardiac surgery with off-pump techniques.

An anesthesiologist-in-training posed the question, "Why is my presence necessary during cardiopulmonary bypass [CPB]? The perfusionist has direct control of the patient's blood pressure and respiration. The inhalation anesthetic is attached to the bypass circuit. Drugs are administered into the venous reservoir. What is my role?"[1] The resident's own answer was incomplete but more robust than that argued by many clinicians, who suggest that the presence of a member of the anesthesia care team (e.g., anesthesiologist, nurse anesthetist, credentialed anesthesia assistant) during CPB is not essential. The American Society of Anesthesiologists (ASA) states that the absence of anesthesia personnel during the conduct of a general anesthetic violates the first of the ASA Standards for Basic Anesthesia Monitoring.[2] The absence of a member of the anesthesia care team during CPB is below the accepted standard of care. Moreover, to bill for anesthesia care when an anesthesia provider is not physically present in the patient's operating room constitutes fraud.[3] At a minimum, the anesthesiologist's role during CPB is to maintain the anesthetic state—a more challenging task than the usual case when the patient's blood pressure, heart rate, and movement provide information regarding the depth of anesthesia. The complexities of CPB and the necessary integration of risk factors with the nuances of cardiac surgery warrant the constant thinking and rethinking of how the conduct of CPB and surgery modulates the risk and what protective strategies need implementation. This chapter outlines the tasks, challenges, and responsibilities of the cardiovascular anesthesiologist that extend beyond the maintenance of the anesthetic state, focusing on overall organ protection.

HISTORIC PERSPECTIVE ON CARDIOPULMONARY BYPASS

On May 6, 1953, John Gibbon, Jr., surgically treated a young woman using CPB, and the long-elusive goal of extracorporeal circulation (ECC) was achieved (Figure 28-1). This accomplishment was preceded by 15 years of work by Gibbon and colleagues to develop a device that would provide ECC and support respiration. The 50th anniversary of the first successful use of CPB was celebrated in 2003. A number of insightful perspectives on this important medical landmark accompanied the anniversary of this achievement.[4-7]

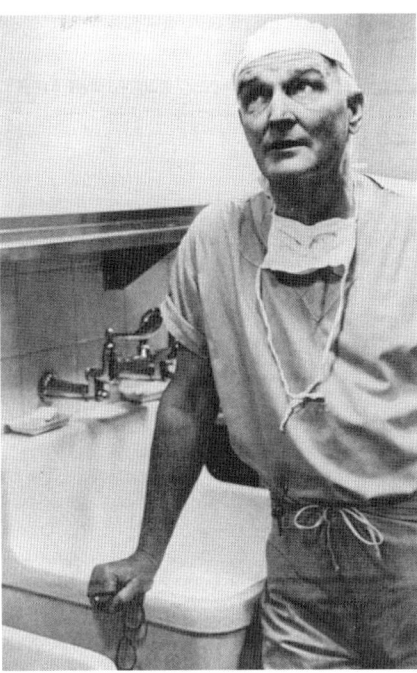

Figure 28-1 Dr. John Gibbon, Jr., before the first successful application of total extracorporeal circulation for cardiac surgery in humans. (Courtesy of Mütter Museum of the College of Physicians of Philadelphia.)

Reviewing the history of CPB and cardiac surgery shows that the development of this lifesaving technology occurred in three distinct phases. In the 1950s, cardiac surgeons adopted ECC to care for patients suffering from previously untreatable congenital heart disease. At the conclusion of the decade, the backlog of patients with surgically correctable congenital heart disease had diminished, and a new frontier emerged: valvular heart disease. Through the early 1960s, Starr and others described their success with prosthetic valves. Previously untreatable anatomic maladies of the heart could be corrected. As the population aged more, the importance of coronary artery bypass grafting (CABG) with extracorporeal support increased. This third

phase includes more than 1 million CABG patients annually. As Pierre Galletti observed, during none of these phases was the next step in perfusion quantitatively anticipated. It is difficult to predict how CPB will be used in this millennium.

This chapter briefly describes modern bypass circuits and highlights the many current controversies regarding the management of patients during CPB. It also deals with perfusion accidents that can be life-threatening events. It is critical that all members of the cardiac surgery team anticipate and respond appropriately to mishaps during CPB (see Chapter 29). More common than the rare catastrophe that can occur are the injurious end-organ effects that can result from the inherently physiologic nature of CPB. The multiple pathophysiologic perturbations precipitated by the process of ECC and the putative effects of these phenomena on end-organ function are discussed in detail.

GOALS AND MECHANICS OF CARDIOPULMONARY BYPASS

The CPB circuit is designed to perform four major functions: oxygenation and carbon dioxide elimination, circulation of blood, systemic cooling and rewarming, and diversion of blood from the heart to provide a bloodless surgical field. Typically, venous blood is drained by gravity from the right side of the heart into a reservoir that serves as a large mixing chamber for all blood return, additional fluids, and drugs. Because (in most instances) negative pressure is not used, the amount of venous drainage is determined by the central venous pressure (CVP), the column height between the patient and reservoir, and resistance to flow in the venous circuitry. Negative pressure will enhance venous drainage and is used in some bypass approaches.

Venous return may be decreased deliberately (as is done when restoring the patient's blood volume before coming off bypass) by application of a venous clamp. From the reservoir, blood is pumped to an oxygenator and heat exchanger unit before passing through an arterial filter and returning to the patient. Additional components of the circuit generally include pumps and tubing for cardiotomy suction, venting, and cardioplegia delivery and recirculation, as well as in-line blood gas monitors, bubble detectors, pressure monitors, and blood sampling ports. A schematic representation of a typical bypass circuit is depicted in Figure 28-2 (see Chapter 29).

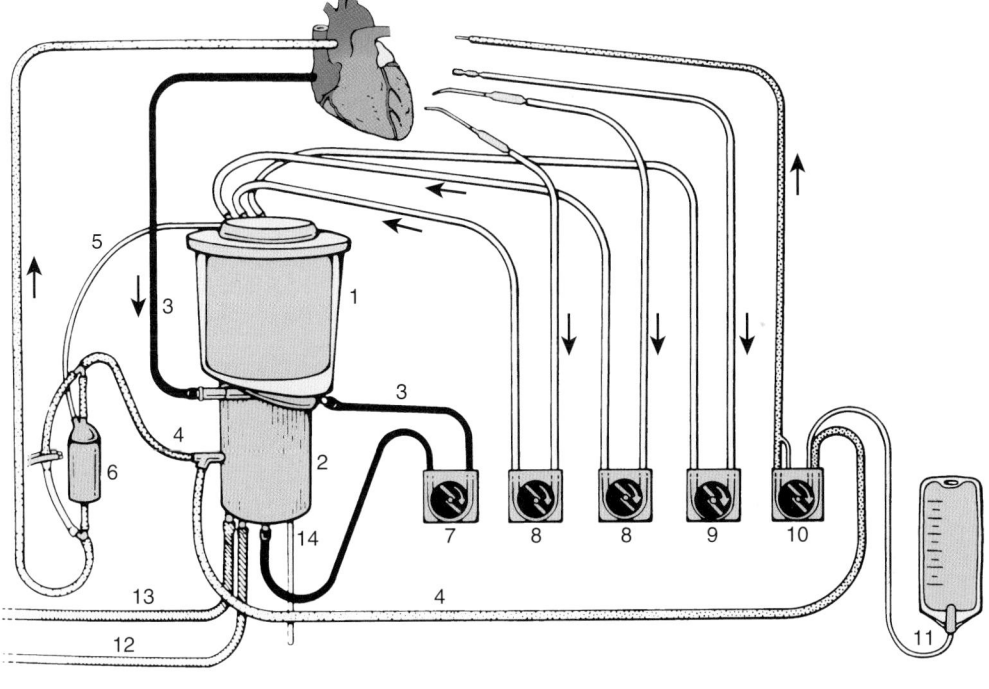

Figure 28-2 Components of the extracorporeal circuit: (*1*) integral cardiotomy reservoir; (*2*) membrane oxygenator bundle; (*3*) venous blood line; (*4*) arterial blood line; (*5*) arterial filter purge line; (*6*) arterial line filter; (*7*) venous blood pump (also called the *arterial pump head*; this pump forces venous blood through the membrane oxygenator and arterialized blood to the patient's aortic root); (*8*) cardiotomy suction pump; (*9*) ventricular vent pump; (*10*) cardioplegia pump; (*11*) crystalloid cardioplegia; (*12*) water inlet line; (*13*) water outlet line; and (*14*) gas inlet line. (*From Davis RB, Kauffman JN, Cobbs TL, Mick SL: Cardiopulmonary Bypass. New York, Springer-Verlag, 1995, p 239.*)

The cannulation sites and type of CPB circuit used are dependent on the type of operation planned.[8] Most cardiac procedures use full CPB, in which the blood is drained from the right side of the heart and returned to the systemic circulation through the aorta. The CPB circuit performs the function of the heart and lungs. Aorto-atriocaval cannulation is the preferred method of cannulation for CPB, although femoral arteriovenous cannulation may be the technique of choice for emergency access, "redo" sternotomy, and other clinical settings in which aortic or atrial cannulation is not feasible. Procedures involving the thoracic aorta often are performed using partial bypass in which a portion of oxygenated blood is removed from the left side of the heart and returned to the femoral artery. Perfusion of the head and upper extremity vessels is performed by the beating heart, and distal perfusion is provided below the level of the cross-clamp by retrograde flow by the femoral artery. All blood passes through the pulmonary circulation, eliminating the need for an oxygenator.

PHYSIOLOGIC PARAMETERS OF CARDIOPULMONARY BYPASS

The primary objective of CPB is maintenance of systemic perfusion and respiration. Controversy arises whether systemic oxygenation and perfusion should be "optimal or maximal" or "adequate or sufficient." Remarkably, after more than a half century of CPB, there is continued disagreement regarding the fundamental management of ECC. Clinicians and investigators disagree on what are the best strategies for arterial blood pressure goals, pump flow, hematocrit, temperature, blood gas management, or mode of perfusion (pulsatile vs. nonpulsatile). Whereas each of these physiologic parameters has to be taken into account individually, the application of each has organ-specific effects. As a result, the ensuing discussion deals with these parameters on an organ-specific basis.

END-ORGAN EFFECTS OF CARDIOPULMONARY BYPASS

Modern cardiac surgery continues to be challenged by the risk for organ dysfunction and the morbidity and mortality that accompany it. Catastrophic organ system failure was common in the early days of CPB, but advances in perfusion, surgical techniques, and anesthesia have allowed most patients to undergo surgery without major morbidity or mortality. However, organ dysfunction, ranging in severity from the most subtle to the most severe, still occurs, manifesting most frequently in patients with decreased functional reserves or extensive comorbidities. With more than 1,000,000 patients worldwide undergoing various cardiac operations annually, understanding organ dysfunction and developing perioperative organ protection strategies are of paramount importance.

A number of injurious common pathways may account for the organ dysfunction typically associated with cardiac surgery. CPB itself initiates a whole-body inflammatory response with the release of various injurious inflammatory mediators. Add to this the various preexisting patient comorbidities and the potential for organ ischemic injury because of embolization and hypoperfusion, and it becomes clear why organ injury can occur. Most cardiac surgery, because of its very nature, causes some degree of myocardial injury. Other body systems can be affected by the perioperative insults associated with cardiac surgery (particularly CPB), including the kidneys, lungs, gastrointestinal (GI) tract, and central nervous system (CNS).

Understanding the fundamentals of organ dysfunction, including the incidence, significance, associated risk factors, etiology, and pathophysiology, provides a framework for discussing various organ-specific protective strategies. The following section describes the various organ dysfunction syndromes that can occur in the cardiac surgical patient, with particular emphasis directed at strategies for reducing these injuries.

CENTRAL NERVOUS SYSTEM INJURY

Incidence and Significance of Injury

CNS dysfunction after CPB represents deficits ranging from neurocognitive deficits, occurring in approximately 25% to 80% of patients, to overt stroke, occurring in 1% to 5% of patients.[9-12] The significant disparity between studies in the incidence of these adverse cerebral outcomes relates, in part, to their definition and to numerous methodologic differences in the determination of neurologic and neurocognitive outcome. Retrospective versus prospective assessments of neurologic deficits account for a significant portion of this inconsistency, as do the experience and expertise of the examiner. The timing of postoperative testing also affects determinations of outcome. For example, the rate of cognitive deficits can be as high as 80% for patients at discharge, between 10% and 35% at approximately 6 weeks after CABG, and 10% to 15% more than a year after surgery. Greater rates of cognitive deficits have been reported 5 years after surgery, when up to 43% of patients have documented deficits.[10] The issue of whether cardiac surgery causes cognitive loss has been greatly debated. Although some have questioned whether long-term deficits result as a consequence of surgery,[13] even if only present in the short term, they are meaningful to patients and families[14] (see Chapter 36).

Although the incidence of these deficits varies greatly, the significance of these injuries cannot be overemphasized. Cerebral injury is a most disturbing outcome of cardiac surgery. To have a patient's heart successfully treated by the planned operation but discover that the patient no longer functions as well cognitively or is immobilized from a stroke can be devastating. There are enormous personal, family, and financial consequences of extending a patient's life with surgery, only to have the quality of the life significantly diminished.[12,15] Mortality after CABG, although having reached relatively low levels in recent years (generally < 1% overall), increasingly is attributable to cerebral injury.[12]

Risk Factors for Central Nervous System Injury

Successful strategies for perioperative cerebral and other organ protection begin with a thorough understanding of the risk factors, causative factors, and pathophysiology involved. Risk factors for CNS injury can be considered from several different perspectives. Most studies outlining risk factors take into account only stroke. Few describe risk factors for neurocognitive dysfunction. Although it often is assumed that their respective risk factors are similar, few studies consistently have reported the preoperative risks for cognitive loss after cardiac surgery. Factors such as a poor baseline (preoperative) cognitive state, years of education (i.e., more advanced education is protective), age, diabetes, and CPB time frequently are described.[16,17]

Stroke is better characterized with respect to risk factors. Although studies differ somewhat as to all the risk factors, certain patient characteristics consistently correlate with an increased risk for cardiac surgery–associated neurologic injury. In a study of 2108 patients from 24 centers conducted by the Multicenter Study of Perioperative Ischemia, incidence of adverse cerebral outcome after CABG surgery was determined and the risk factors analyzed. Two types of adverse cerebral outcomes were defined. Type I included nonfatal stroke, transient ischemic attack, stupor or coma at time of discharge, and death caused by stroke or hypoxic encephalopathy. Type II included new deterioration in intellectual function, confusion, agitation, disorientation, and memory deficit without evidence of focal injury. A total of 129 (6.1%) of the 2108 patients had an adverse cerebral outcome in the perioperative period. Type I outcomes occurred in 66 (3.1%) of 2108 patients, with type II outcomes occurring in 63 (3.0%) of 2108 patients. Stepwise logistic regression analysis identified eight independent predictors of type I outcomes and seven independent predictors of type II outcomes (Table 28-1).

TABLE 28-1	Risk Factors for Adverse Cerebral Outcomes after Cardiac Surgery	
Risk Factor	*Type I Outcomes**	*Type II Outcomes**
Proximal aortic atherosclerosis	4.52 (2.52–8.09)	
History of neurologic disease	3.19 (1.65–6.15)	
Use of IABP	2.60 (1.21–5.58)	
Diabetes mellitus	2.59 (1.46–4.60)	
History of hypertension	2.31 (1.20–4.47)	
History of pulmonary disease	2.09 (1.14–3.85)	2.37 (1.34–4.18)
History of unstable angina	1.83 (1.03–3.27)	
Age (per additional decade)	1.75 (1.27–2.43)	2.20 (1.60–3.02)
Admission systolic BP > 180 mm Hg		3.47 (1.41–8.55)
History of excessive alcohol intake		2.64 (1.27–5.47)
History of CABG		2.18 (1.14–4.17)
Arrhythmia on day of surgery		1.97 (1.12–3.46)
Antihypertensive therapy		1.78 (1.02–3.10)

*Adjusted odds ratio (95% confidence intervals) for type I and II cerebral outcomes
associated with selected risk factors from the Multicenter Study of Perioperative Ischemia.
BP, blood pressure; CABG, coronary artery bypass graft surgery; IABP, intra-aortic balloon
pump.
From Arrowsmith JE, Grocott HP, Reves JG, et al: Central nervous system complications
of cardiac surgery. *Br J Anaesth* 84:378, 2000.

In a subsequent analysis of the same study database, a stroke risk index using preoperative factors was developed (Figure 28-3). This risk index allowed for the preoperative calculation of the stroke risk based on the weighted combination of the preoperative factors, including age, unstable angina, diabetes mellitus, neurologic disease, prior coronary artery or other cardiac surgery, vascular disease, and pulmonary disease.[18] Of all the factors in the Multicenter Study of Perioperative

Ischemia analysis and in multiple other analyses,[12,19-22] age appeared to be the most overwhelmingly robust predictor of stroke and of neurocognitive dysfunction after cardiac surgery.[9,10] Tuman et al[22] demonstrated that age has a greater impact on neurologic outcome than it does on perioperative myocardial infarction or low cardiac output states after cardiac surgery (Figure 28-4).

The influence of sex on adverse perioperative cerebral outcomes after cardiac surgery has been evaluated. Women appear to be at greater risk for stroke after cardiac surgery than men.[23] Hogue et al[24] found that women appear more likely to suffer deficits in the visuospatial cognitive domain after cardiac surgery, although the frequency of cognitive dysfunction after cardiac surgery is similar for women and men.

Other consistent risk factors for stroke after cardiac surgery are the presence of cerebrovascular disease and atheromatous disease of the aorta. With respect to cerebrovascular disease, patients who have had a prior stroke or transient ischemic attack are more likely to suffer a perioperative stroke.[23,25-27] Even in the absence of symptomatic cerebrovascular disease, such as the presence of a carotid bruit, the risk for stroke increases with the severity of the carotid artery disease. Breslau et al[28] reported that Doppler-detected carotid disease increased the risk for stroke after cardiac surgery by threefold. Similarly, Brener et al[29] found that a carotid stenosis greater than 50% increased the risk for stroke from 1.9% to 6.3%.

Although the presence of cerebrovascular disease is a risk factor for perioperative stroke, it does not always correlate well with the presence of significant aortic atherosclerosis.[30] Atheromatous disease of the ascending, arch, and descending thoracic aorta has been consistently implicated as a risk factor for stroke in cardiac surgical patients.[31-34] The increased use of transesophageal echocardiography (TEE) and epiaortic ultrasonography has added new dimensions to the detection of aortic atheromatous disease and the understanding of its relation to stroke risk. These imaging modalities have allowed the diagnosis of atheromatous disease to be made in a more sensitive and detailed manner, contributing greatly to the information regarding potential stroke risk. The risk for cerebral embolism from aortic atheroma was described early in the history of cardiac surgery,[35] and has been described repeatedly in detail since then.[12,36-38] For example, Katz et al[39] found that the incidence rate of stroke was 25% in patients with a mobile atheromatous plaque in the aortic arch, compared with a stroke rate of 2% in those with limited atheromatous disease. Studies consistently have reported greater stroke rates for patients with increasing atheromatous aortic involvement (particularly the ascending and arch segments).[40] This relation is outlined in Figure 28-5.

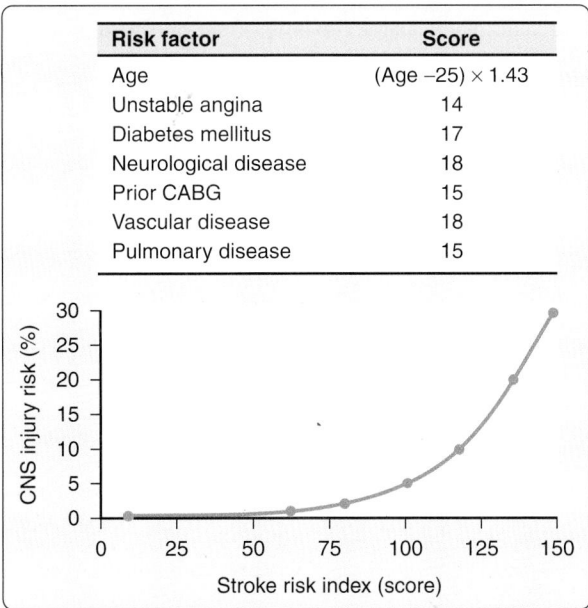

Risk factor	Score
Age	(Age −25) × 1.43
Unstable angina	14
Diabetes mellitus	17
Neurological disease	18
Prior CABG	15
Vascular disease	18
Pulmonary disease	15

Figure 28-3 Preoperative stroke risk for patients undergoing coronary artery bypass graft surgery. The individual patient's stroke risk can be determined from the corresponding cumulative risk index score in the nomogram. CNS, central nervous system. (*From Arrowsmith JE, Grocott HP, Reves JG, et al: Central nervous system complications of cardiac surgery. Br J Anaesth 84:378, 2000.*)

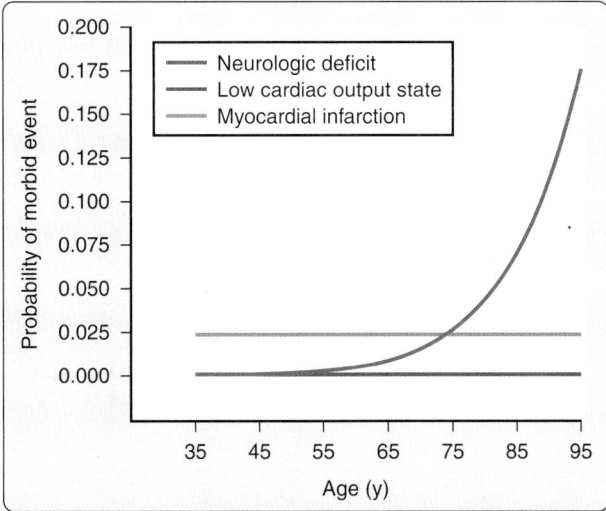

Figure 28-4 Relative effect of age on the predicted probability of neurologic and cardiac morbidity after cardiac surgery. (*From Tuman KJ, McCarthy RJ, Najafi H, et al: Differential effects of advanced age on neurologic and cardiac risks of coronary artery operations. J Thorac Cardiovasc Surg 104:1510, 1992.*)

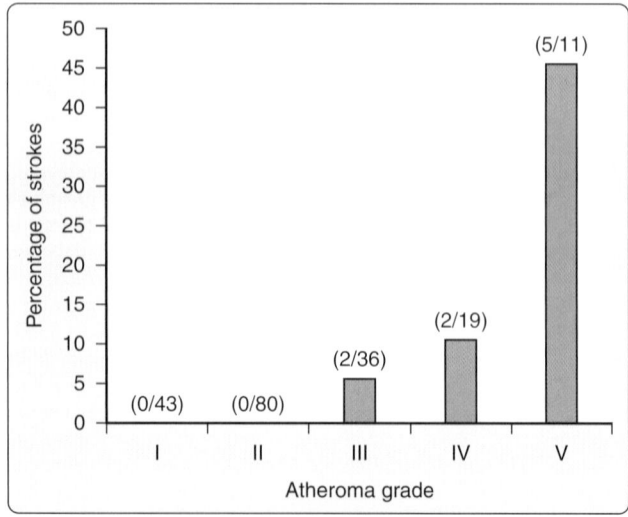

Figure 28-5 **Stroke rate 1 week after cardiac surgery as a function of atheroma severity.** Atheroma was graded by transesophageal echocardiography as follows: I, normal; II, intimal thickening; III, plaque < 5 mm thick; IV, plaque > 5 mm thick; V, any plaque with a mobile segment. *(From Hartman GS, Yao FS, Bruefach M 3rd, et al: Severity of aortic atheromatous disease diagnosed by transesophageal echocardiography predicts stroke and other outcomes associated with coronary artery surgery: A prospective study. Anesth Analg 83:701, 1996.)*

Cause of Perioperative Central Nervous System Injury

Because CNS dysfunction represents a wide range of injuries, differentiating the individual causes of these various types of injuries becomes somewhat difficult (Box 28-1). They frequently are grouped together and superficially discussed as representing different severities on a continuum of brain injury. This likely misrepresents the different causes of these injuries. The following section addresses stroke and cognitive injury (Table 28-2), and their respective causes are differentiated where appropriate.

Cerebral Embolization

Macroemboli (e.g., atheromatous plaque) and microemboli (e.g., gaseous and particulate) are generated during CPB, and many emboli find their way to the cerebral vasculature.[41] Macroemboli are responsible for stroke, with microemboli being implicated in the development of less severe encephalopathies. Sources for the microemboli are numerous and include those generated de novo from the interactions of blood within the CPB apparatus (e.g., platelet-fibrin aggregates) and those generated within the body by the production and mobilization of atheromatous material or entrainment of air from the operative field. Other sources for emboli include lipid-laden debris that can be added by cardiotomy suction.[42] Other gaseous emboli may be generated through injections into the venous reservoir of the CPB apparatus itself.[43,44]

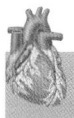

BOX 28-1. CAUSES OF CENTRAL NERVOUS SYSTEM COMPLICATIONS AFTER CARDIOPULMONARY BYPASS

- Cerebral emboli
- Global hypoperfusion
- Inflammation
- Cerebral hyperthermia
- Cerebral edema
- Blood-brain barrier dysfunction
- Genetics

TABLE 28-2	Causes of Cognitive Dysfunction after Cardiac Surgery
Cause	*Possible Settings*
Cerebral microemboli	Generated during cardiopulmonary bypass (CPB); mobilization of atheromatous material or entrainment of air from the operative field; gas injections into the venous reservoir of the CPB apparatus
Global cerebral hypoperfusion	Hypotension, occlusion by an atheromatous embolus leading to stroke
Inflammation (systemic and cerebral)	Injurious effects of CPB, such as blood interacting with the foreign surfaces of pump-oxygenator; upregulation of proinflammatory mediators
Cerebral hyperthermia	Hyperthermia during and after cardiac surgery, such as aggressive rewarming, from hypothermic CPB
Cerebral edema	Edema from global cerebral hypoperfusion or from hyponatremia; increased cerebral venous pressure from cannula misplacement
Blood-brain barrier dysfunction	Diffuse cerebral inflammation; ischemia from cerebral microembolization or increased intracranial pressure
Pharmacologic influences	Anesthetic-related cognitive damage; apoptosis of neonatal brains; proteomic changes
Genetic influences	Effects of single nucleotide polymorphisms on risk for Alzheimer disease or for acute coronary syndromes and other inflammatory disorders

Numerous studies outline the relation between emboli and cognitive decline after cardiac surgery.[45–47] However, one of the major limitations in understanding this relation has been the relative inability to discern between gaseous and particulate microemboli.[48] Typically, Doppler ultrasonography has been used to measure cerebral embolic signals, but Doppler cannot reliably distinguish between gaseous and particulate emboli.[49] In addition to using Doppler evidence, Moody et al[41] performed histologic analyses on brains from cardiac surgical patients and described the presence of millions of cerebral emboli represented as small capillary arteriolar dilations.

The impact of aortic atheroma on cognitive decline is incompletely understood. It is widely known from nonsurgical and cardiac surgical studies that there is a clear relation between aortic atheroma and stroke,[31,50–52] but the relation between cognitive outcome and cerebral atheroma is uncertain. Several studies describe different results.[53,54] Whereas some data suggest that cerebral emboli are more likely with a greater degree of atheroma in the ascending aorta,[55] there is a relative failure to demonstrate that these atheroma correspond to cognitive decline.[53] Part of the discordance between these two findings may reflect the limitation of Doppler technology to discriminate between gaseous and particulate emboli, thereby possibly misrepresenting the true cerebral embolic load.[56]

Global Cerebral Hypoperfusion

The concept that global cerebral hypoperfusion during CPB may lead to neurologic and neurocognitive complications originates from the earliest days of cardiac surgery, when significant (in degree and duration) systemic hypotension was a relatively common event. Although making intuitive sense (i.e., that hypotension would lead to global cerebral hypoperfusion), studies that have examined the relation between mean arterial pressure (MAP) and cognitive decline after cardiac surgery generally have failed to show any significant relation.[17,57,58]

This is not the case for stroke, for which Hartman et al[38] and Gold et al[59] demonstrated a link between hypotension and the presence of a significantly atheromatous aorta with an increased risk for stroke (see Figure 28-5). This is not a clear relation, however, and likely represents an interaction between macroembolism and global cerebral hypoperfusion. It is likely, for example, that if an area of the brain that is being perfused by a cerebral vessel becomes occluded by an atheromatous embolus, it may be more susceptible to hypoperfusion if collateral perfusion is compromised by concomitant systemic hypotension.[60] Other evidence for global cerebral hypoperfusion comes from Mutch et al,[61] who examined magnetic resonance imaging assessments of cerebral blood flow (CBF) showing progressive decreases in CBF during the course of experimental CPB in pigs. However, clinical demonstrations of a reduction in CBF during lengthy CPB have not been seen.[62]

Temperature-Related Factors

The impact of CPB temperature (i.e., hypothermia) on outcome is addressed further in this section. However, with the various trials of hypothermia during CPB and with detailed temperature monitoring, the observation has been made that *hyperthermia* can occur during certain periods during and after cardiac surgery. During rewarming from hypothermic CPB, there can be an overshoot in cerebral temperature because of aggressive rewarming generally aimed at decreasing time on CPB and overall operating room time. This cerebral hyperthermia may well be responsible for some of the injury that occurs in the brain.[63]

The postoperative period is also a critical time in which hyperthermia can contribute to brain injury.[64,65] Grocott et al[64] demonstrated that the peak temperature in the postoperative period (24 hours after surgery) was related to cognitive decline 6 weeks after cardiac surgery. It is not clear whether this hyperthermia causes de novo injury or whether it exacerbates injury that already has occurred (e.g., injury that might be induced by cerebral microembolization or global cerebral hypoperfusion). It is necessary to be cautious in concluding whether these relations are temporal or causal. However, it is assumed that the brain is injured during CPB, and because experimental brain injury is known to cause hyperthermia (resulting from hypothalamic injury[66]), the hyperthermia that is demonstrated in the postoperative period may be caused by the occurrence or extent of brain injury. However, if hyperthermia results from the inflammatory response to CPB, the hyperthermia itself may induce or exacerbate cerebral injury.

Inflammation

Although it is well-known that blood interacts with the foreign surfaces of the pump-oxygenator to stimulate a profound inflammatory response,[67] the systemic end-organ effects of this inflammatory response are less clearly defined. Much of the data relating organ dysfunction in the CNS to the inflammatory response in the cardiac surgical patient have focused on indirect experimental and clinical evidence. It is not clear whether a cerebral inflammatory response occurs as a result of CPB in humans. Hindman et al[68] reported that cyclooxygenase mRNA was upregulated after CPB, suggesting that on the molecular biologic level, CPB induces overexpression of this proinflammatory gene in the brain. What is not clear was whether this was a primary event (i.e., as a direct result of the proinflammatory effects of CPB) or a secondary event as a result of other injurious effects of CPB (e.g., microembolization). In settings other than cardiac surgery, inflammation has been demonstrated to directly injure the brain (e.g., sepsis-mediated encephalopathy),[69] but it also is known to result as a response to various cerebral injuries (e.g., ischemic stroke).[70]

There is no direct evidence that inflammation causes cardiac surgery–associated adverse cerebral outcome; however, there is some supportive indirect evidence. For example, Mathew et al[71] demonstrated a relation between poor cognitive outcome and an impaired immune response to circulating endotoxin, which inevitably translocates from the gut into the bloodstream because of alterations in splanchnic blood flow during CPB. Having a low antibody response to circulating endotoxin is paradoxically associated with an overstimulated inflammatory response,[72] thus demonstrating that the relation between low endotoxin antibodies and poor cognitive outcome may be mediated by an augmented inflammatory response. Increasingly, there is genetic evidence linking inflammation to adverse cerebral outcomes, both stroke and cognitive loss (see Genetic Influences section later in this chapter).

Cerebral Edema

Cerebral edema after CPB has been reported in several studies.[73,74] The explanation for why cerebral edema may occur early in the postbypass period is not clear. It may be caused by cytotoxic edema resulting from global cerebral hypoperfusion or possibly by hyponatremia-induced cerebral edema. Generalized cerebral edema caused by increases in cerebral venous pressure caused by cannula misplacement, which frequently occurs during CPB, is another reason.[75] Specifically, use of a dual-stage venous cannula often can lead to cerebral venous congestion during the vertical displacement of the heart during access to the lateral and posterior epicardial coronary arteries. It is not clear from these studies whether the edema results because of injury that occurs during CPB, leading to cognitive decline, or whether the edema itself directly causes the injury by consequent increases in intracranial pressure with global or regional decreases in CBF and resulting ischemia.

Blood-Brain Barrier Dysfunction

The function of the blood-brain barrier (BBB) is to aid in maintaining the homeostasis of the extracellular cerebral milieu protecting the brain against fluctuations in various ion concentrations, neurotransmitters, and growth factors that are present in the serum.[76] The impact of CPB on the function and integrity of the BBB is not clearly known. Gillinov et al[77] were unable to show any changes in BBB dysfunction 2 hours after CPB in piglets as assessed using carbon 14-aminoisobutyric acid tracer techniques in postbypass brain homogenates. However, Cavaglia et al,[78] measuring the leakage of fluorescent albumin from blood vessels in brain slices after CPB, were able to demonstrate significant breaches in the BBB. Both studies looked at a single time point (i.e., immediately after CPB), and it is not known whether there are temporal changes in the BBB integrity.

It is difficult to determine whether the changes in BBB integrity, if present at all, are a primary cause of brain dysfunction or simply a result of other initiating events such as ischemia (i.e., from cerebral microembolization) or a diffuse cerebral inflammatory event. Changes in the BBB could cause some of the cerebral edema that has been demonstrated, or it could result from cerebral edema if the edema resulted in ischemic injury (from increases in intracranial pressure).[74]

Possible Pharmacologic Influences

Anesthetics have been demonstrated to affect cognitive loss after surgery. Experimental studies of cognitive outcome in young rats exposed to anesthetics have demonstrated that relatively brief (several hours) exposure to isoflurane can lead to long-term cognitive changes in the animals.[79,80] Coupled with the demonstration in other experimental models of apoptosis in neonatal brains exposed to certain anesthetic agents (e.g., isoflurane, midazolam, nitrous oxide),[81] this added to the data suggesting that corresponding proteomic changes can occur in the brain after exposure to anesthetics[82] and highlighted this as a potential area for further research.

Genetic Influences

Genetics may play a role in modifying the degree of CNS injury or in the ability of the brain to recover after an injury has occurred. Several investigations have assessed the genetic influences on cerebral outcome after CPB. The most commonly explored gene variant, or single nucleotide polymorphism (SNP), has been the ε4 allele of the apolipoprotein gene. This gene has been reported to be responsible for increasing the risk for sporadic and late-onset Alzheimer disease (as well as complicating outcome after a variety of other head injuries).[83] Although early reports suggest that this may be an important influence,[84] later reports shed some doubt on how robust this effect is.[85] A second SNP examined relates to the platelet surface receptor glycoprotein IIb/IIIa P1^{A2} (P1^{A2}) receptor polymorphism. This platelet integrin receptor polymorphism is important in the cause of acute coronary syndromes and other thrombotic disorders.[86,87] A small study in cardiac surgery patients demonstrated worse impairments in the Mini-Mental Status Examination in the P1^{A2}-positive patients compared with P1^{A2}-negative patients.[88]

With the multitude of genes that may play a role in injury, it is important to go beyond examining the impact of single SNPs and explore the impact of multiple SNPs, alone or in combination. In a study of 2140 patients examining 26 different SNPs, the presence of the minor alleles of C-reactive protein (CRP), interleukin-6 (IL-6) had a threefold increase in the risk for stroke after cardiac surgery.[89] Of note, no single (or combination of) prothrombotic genes were associated with stroke, suggesting that inflammatory, as opposed to thrombotic, mechanisms may be more important to the risk for a stroke.

With respect to cognitive dysfunction after cardiac surgery, a recent study outlined the impact of genetics on outcome after cardiac surgery. In a study of 513 patients who were extensively genotyped (30 SNPs) and had cognitive testing after cardiac surgery, a link between SNPs of CRP and P-selectin (CRP1059G4/C and SELP1087G/A), and a reduction in cognitive deficit were found.[90] The incidence rate of cognitive deficit was 16.7% in carriers of the minor alleles of both these genes compared with 42.9% of the patients possessing these major alleles. Unique in this study was the mechanism-based genetic effect in which these polymorphisms also were associated with reductions in both CRP and platelet activation, suggesting that an attenuation of perioperative inflammatory and prothrombotic states may be beneficial with respect to reducing the cognitive deficits after cardiac surgery.[91]

Neuroprotective Strategies

Emboli Reduction

There are multiple sources of particulate and gaseous emboli during cardiac surgery. Within the CPB circuit itself, particulate emboli in the form of platelet-fibrin aggregates and other debris are generated. Gaseous emboli can be created in the circuit or augmented, if already present, by factors such as turbulence-related cavitation and, potentially, even by vacuum-assisted venous drainage.[92] Air in the venous return tubing is variably handled by the bypass circuit (i.e., reservoir, oxygenator, and arterial filters). The ability of the circuit to prevent the transit of gaseous emboli through the oxygenator varies considerably between manufacturers and remains a significant source of emboli. The impact of perfusionist interventions on cerebral embolic load also has been studied. Borger et al[44] found that after drug injections into the venous reservoir, gaseous emboli can make a rapid passage through to the arterial outflow. Reducing these perfusionist interventions reduced emboli generation and neurocognitive impairment.

Significant quantities of air can be entrained from the surgical field into the heart itself; flooding the field with carbon dioxide has been proposed as being effective in reducing this embolic source.[93] Its ability to specifically reduce cerebral injury has not been rigorously evaluated, although it has been demonstrated to significantly reduce the number of TEE-detectable bubbles in the heart after cardiac surgery.[94] Even with the use of carbon dioxide in the surgical field, significant amounts of entrained air can be present. Although the oxygenator-venous reservoir design attempts to purge this air before reaching the inflow cannula, the arterial line filter handles a great deal of what is left. The capacity of the arterial filter to remove all sources of emboli (gaseous or particulate) has significant limitations, and despite its use, emboli can pass easily through and on into the aortic root.

The aortic cannula may be very important to reduce cerebral emboli production. Placement of the cannula into an area of the aorta with a large atheroma burden may cause the direct generation of emboli from the "sandblasting" of atherosclerotic material in the aorta.[95] The use of a long aortic cannula, where the tip of the cannula lies beyond the origin of the cerebral vessels, also has been found to reduce emboli load.[96] The type of cannula itself may be an important factor.

Various designs have allowed the reduction of sandblasting-type jets emanating from the aortic cannula. Baffled cannulae and cannulae that allow the incorporation of regional brain hypothermia and diversion of emboli away from the cerebral vessels have been investigated.[97] A cannula that has a basket-like extension that can be inserted just before cross-clamp removal also has been studied.[98] In a large ($N = 1289$) study, this Embol-X cannula was unable to reduce the incidence of CNS dysfunction.[99] A smaller ($N = 24$) study paradoxically showed an increase in embolic signals with its deployment in the aorta.[100] This has been because of air bubbles trapped within the basket or abrasion of the atheromatous aortic wall. Few other emboli-reducing strategies, besides arterial line filtration and reducing perfusion interventions itself,[44,47] have been studied sufficiently to determine their impact on cognitive loss after cardiac surgery. The safety of introducing new techniques also has not been thoroughly studied; the additional risk assumed when significantly altering a standard of practice to use a new device must be considered (see Chapters 3, 29, and 39).

Blood that is returned from the surgical field through the use of the cardiotomy suction may significantly contribute to the particulate load in the CPB circuit and, subsequently, in the brain. The use of cell-salvage devices to process shed blood before returning it to the venous reservoir may minimize the amount of particulate- or lipid-laden material that contributes to embolization.[42,43] Most of this material is small enough or so significantly deformable (due to its high lipid content) that it can pass through standard 40-μm arterial filters. There are several issues with the cell saver, however. One is the cost that is incurred with its use, and the other is its side effects of reducing platelet and coagulation factors through its intrinsic washing processes. Modest use of cell salvage up to a certain, although as yet undefined, volume of blood likely is prudent. Despite this rationale, the results from studies examining neurologic outcome have shown variable effects of cell-saver use on cognitive outcome. A study by Djaiani et al[102] demonstrated a benefit, whereas one by Rubens et al[101] did not. This may have been caused by differences in cell savers used that likely varied in their ability to remove lipid emboli (see Chapter 29).

Management of Aortic Atherosclerosis

Although the previous section dealt with issues related to reduction of emboli, many of which likely are spawned from atheromatous plaque in the aorta, further specific management of the atheromatous aorta, particularly as it relates to stroke risk, requires special attention. The widespread use of TEE and complementary (and preferably routine) epiaortic scanning has had a tremendous impact on the understanding of the risks involved in the patient with a severely atheromatous aorta. There is indisputable evidence linking stroke to atheroma.[31,50–52] However, the strength of association between atheroma and cognitive decline seen after cardiac surgery is less clear.

A small study used a combination of epiaortic scanning and atheroma avoidance techniques (with respect to cannulation, clamping, and vein graft anastomosis placement) to attempt to reduce neurocognitive deficits.[54] In that study, the incidence of cognitive decline was lower in patients who had an avoidance technique guided by epiaortic scanning compared with no epiaortic scanning. It was limited by its small size, but it identified an area that requires more investigation. Others have examined this issue and found the relation between cognitive decline and atheroma to be doubtful.[103] Regardless of whether atheroma cause cognitive dysfunction, their contribution to cardiac surgery–associated stroke is enough to warrant specific strategies for their management.

One of the difficulties in interpreting studies that have evaluated atheroma avoidance strategies is the absence of any form of blinding of the investigators. For the most part, a strategy is chosen based on the presence of known atheroma, and the results of these patients are compared with historic controls. What constitutes the best strategy is unclear. Multiple techniques can be used to minimize atheromatous material liberated from the aortic wall from getting into the cerebral circulation. These range from optimizing placement of the aortic cannula in the aorta up to an area relatively devoid of plaque to the use of specialized cannulae that reduce the sandblasting of the aortic wall. Alternative aortic cannulae and using different locations possess the ability to decrease embolization of atheromatous plaque. The avoidance of partial occlusion clamping for proximal vein graft placement by performing all of the anastomoses made in a single application of an aortic cross-clamp has been demonstrated to have benefit.[104] Specialized cannulae that contain filtering technologies[98] and other means to deflect emboli to more distal sites have been developed and are being studied.[105] Technology is advancing rapidly, and proximal (and distal) coronary artery anastomotic devices are becoming increasingly available and focus on minimizing manipulation of the ascending aorta. None of these aortic manipulations has yet yielded significant neuroprotective results in large, prospective, randomized trials, but the potential holds promise.

Pulsatile Perfusion

A large volume of literature has accumulated comparing the physiology of pulsatile with nonpulsatile perfusion.[106,107] Nevertheless, it remains uncertain whether pulsatile CPB has shown substantive clinical improvement in any outcome measure compared with standard, nonpulsatile CPB. Table 28-3, although by no means complete, represents this highly contradictory body of literature.[108–137] Claims of advantages to pulsatile flow are effectively offset by conflicting studies of similar design (see Chapter 29).

Nonpulsatile CPB is the most commonly practiced form of artificial perfusion. As intuitive as it may seem that this type of nonphysiologic, nonpulsatile pump flow could be injurious, there is an overall lack of data to suggest that using pulsatile flow during clinical CPB has a neurologic benefit. In a large ($N = 316$), double-blind, randomized investigation by Murkin et al,[138] examining the effect of pulsatile versus nonpulsatile CPB on neurologic and neuropsychologic outcome, no significant benefit was demonstrated. One study of balloon pump–induced pulsatile perfusion during CPB failed to show any improvements in jugular venous oxygen saturation of regional brain oxygenation.[139] A significant limitation to most pulsatility studies is that, because of technical limitations, true "physiologic" pulsatility is almost never accomplished. Instead, variations of sinusoidal pulse waveforms are produced that do not replicate the kinetics and hydrodynamics of normal physiologic pulsation. A review by Hickey et al,[107] published in 1983, offered important criticism and insight into this controversy and remains germane to recent reports. A fundamental difference between pulsatile and nonpulsatile flow is that additional hydraulic energy is required and applied to move blood when pulsatile flow is used. This extra kinetic energy is known to improve red blood cell (RBC) transit, increase capillary perfusion, and aid lymphatic function.[133] The hydraulic power of pulsatile flow is the sum over time of the product of instantaneous pressure and instantaneous flow. CPB may influence many of the properties of the blood (viscosity) and the vasculature itself (arterial tone, size, and geometry) as a result of hemodilution, hypothermia, alteration of RBC deformability, and redistribution of flow. As a result of these changes, generation of what appears to be a normal pulsatile *pressure* waveform may not result in a normal pulsatile *flow* waveform. Simply reproducing pulsatile pressure is not sufficient to assure reproduction of pulsatile flow, nor does it allow quantification of energetics.

Virtually no study has quantified the energetics of the pulsatile or nonpulsatile perfusion used. Few studies report representative pressure waveforms.[108–113] Even fewer give *flow* waveforms.[134,135] When pulsatile flow is not quantified, critical features such as vascular impedance and the hydraulic power delivered cannot be evaluated (i.e., whether the pulsatile perfusion used in a particular study was really delivering more hydraulic power than the nonpulsatile perfusion with which it was compared). Grossi et al[135] developed two indices of pulsatility: the pulsatility index, which quantitates the relative sharpness of a given waveform with respect to its mean flow; and the pulse power index, which quantifies the power of a pulsatile waveform compared with nonpulsatile equal flow. They found that despite use of a computer-controlled pulsatile pump, in every case, pulsatility index or pulse power index was considerably less than control (nonbypass pulsatility). Only with specific combinations of pulse rate and pulsatile flow contours, which had high pulsatility index or pulse power index, was lactate production lower than the nonpulsatile perfusion at the same minute flow during pulsatile CPB. This study indicates that not all pulsatile perfusion is the same and that pulsatile modes are not necessarily capable of improved perfusion relative to nonpulsatile systems.

It is, therefore, not surprising that such a wide disparity of results should occur. The authors are unaware of any human study in which pulsatility has been quantitated in terms other than pulse pressures. Consequently, whether the generated pressure waveform is a sine wave or some other pattern cannot be ascertained.[113,114,117,119–123,126–128] The comparatively small size of the arterial inflow cannula effectively can filter out a large component of the pulsatile kinetic energy. Consequently, as achieved clinically, pulsatile flow may actually be quite similar energetically to nonpulsatile flow.

Newer pulsatile technologies may better reproduce the normal biologic state of cardiac pulsatility. Computer technologies that allow creating a more physiologic pulsatile perfusion pattern have, at least experimentally, demonstrated preservation of cerebral oxygenation. This approach showed some promise in a pig model of CPB in which pulsatile flow controlled by a computer to replicate the normal biologic variability in pulsatility was associated with significantly lower jugular venous oxygen desaturation during rewarming after hypothermic CPB.[140] However, most studies do not present convincing evidence to suggest that routine pulsatile flow during CPB, as can be achieved by widely available technology, is warranted.

Acid-Base Management: Alpha-Stat versus pH-Stat

Optimal acid-base management during CPB has long been debated. Theoretically, alpha-stat management maintains normal CBF autoregulation with the coupling of cerebral metabolism ($CMRO_2$) to CBF, allowing adequate oxygen delivery while minimizing the potential for emboli. Although early studies[138] were unable to document a difference in neurologic or neuropsychologic outcome between the two techniques, later studies showed reductions in cognitive performance when pH-stat management was used, particularly in cases with prolonged CPB times.[141] pH-stat management (i.e., CO_2 is added to the fresh oxygenator gas flow) results in a greater CBF than is necessary for the brain's metabolic requirements. This luxury perfusion risks excessive delivery of emboli to the brain. Except for congenital

TABLE 28-3	Comparison of Studies Investigating Pulsatile Flow during Cardiopulmonary Bypass	
	References	
Proposed Beneficial Effect of Pulsatile Flow	*Yes*	*No*
Reduced systemic vascular resistance	108–114	115–123
Changes in systemic blood flow distribution	108, 124	110, 115, 116, 121
Improved microcirculatory flow/aerobic metabolism	108, 109, 111, 123, 125, 126	110, 115, 116, 121–123
Attenuation of hormonal responses		
Catecholamines	127	109, 119
Renin/angiotensin	114, 119, 122	115, 116, 127, 128
Antidiuretic hormone	113, 127	117
Cortisol		117, 128
Thromboxane/prostacyclin	120	
Improved renal blood flow or urine output	111, 113, 115, 124, 126	110, 116–118, 123, 129, 136
Improved pancreatic blood flow	124, 129	
Improved cerebral blood flow, metabolism, or outcome	112, 125, 130–132, 140	137–139

heart surgery, for which most outcome data support the use of pH-stat management[142,143] because of its improvement in homogenous brain cooling before circulatory arrest, adult outcome data support the use of alpha-stat management.

Temperature and Rewarming Strategies

The use of hypothermia remains a mainstay of perioperative management in the cardiac surgical patient. Its widespread use relates to its putative, although not definitively proved, global organ-protective effects. Although hypothermia has a measurable effect on suppressing cerebral metabolism (approximately 6% to 7% decline per 1° C),[144] it is likely that its other neuroprotective effects may be mediated by nonmetabolic actions. In the ischemic brain, for example, moderate hypothermia has multimodal effects, including blocking the release of glutamate,[145] reducing calcium influx,[146] hastening recovery of protein synthesis,[147] diminishing membrane-bound protein kinase C activity,[148] slowing of the time to onset of depolarization,[149] reducing formation of reactive oxygen species,[150] and suppressing nitric oxide (NO) synthase activity.[151] Some or all of these effects in combination may convey some of the neuroprotective effects of hypothermia. Although experimental demonstrations of this are abundant, clinical examples of hypothermia neuroprotection have been elusive until recently.[152-155]

Some of the most meaningful data on CPB temperature and cerebral outcome came from work that had its origins in the late 1980s and early 1990s. It was at that time that warm CPB was used because of its putative myocardial salvaging effects when used with continuous warm cardioplegia.[156-159] However, because CPB was being conducted at higher temperatures than what were considered conventional, the implications for the brain were also studied. Several large studies have been undertaken to elucidate the effects of temperature management on cerebral outcome after cardiac surgery. The Warm Heart Investigators trial,[156] a trial performed at Emory University,[160] and a later trial at Duke University,[161] although having several methodologic differences, had similar results with respect to neurocognitive outcome,[162,163] but some divergent results with respect to stroke. None of the studies, or ones performed since, demonstrated any neuroprotective effect of hypothermia on neurocognitive outcome after cardiac surgery. However, the Emory trial did demonstrate an apparent injurious effect (as manifest by a worse stroke outcome) of what were most likely mild degrees of hyperthermia during CPB. Neither the Warm Heart Investigators trial nor the Duke trial showed any effect of temperature on stroke per se. These data suggest that active warming to maintain temperatures at (or greater) than 37° C may pose an unnecessary risk for stroke.

Just as hypothermia has some likely protective effects on the brain, hyperthermia, in an opposite and disproportionate fashion, has some injurious effects. Although the studies referred to previously[156,160,161] demonstrated no neuroprotective effect, there is emerging evidence that if some degree of neuroprotection is afforded by hypothermia, it may be negated by the obligatory rewarming period that must ensue.[63] Grigore et al[63] demonstrated in a prospective trial that compared with conventional "fast" rewarming, slower rewarming resulted in a lower incidence of neurocognitive dysfunction 6 weeks after cardiac surgery. These lower rewarming rates led to lower peak cerebral temperatures during rewarming, consistent with past observations that rapid rewarming can lead to an overshoot in cerebral temperature resulting in inadvertent cerebral hyperthermia.[164] By reducing this rewarming rate, it reduces the overshoot in temperature and prevents the negative effects of cerebral hyperthermia. Consistent with the concept that preventing some of the rewarming may be protective was a study by Nathan et al[165] that demonstrated an intermediate-term (3 months) neurocognitive benefit for patients who were maintained between 34° C and 36° C for a prolonged (12 hours) period after surgery. That trial may have had its beneficial effect by the avoidance of cerebral hyperthermia during rewarming rather than the prolonged hypothermia.[165] However, the 5-year follow-up rate did not show a sustained benefit.[166]

Although there are numerous sites for monitoring temperature during cardiac surgery, several warrant special consideration. One of the lessons learned from the three warm versus cold trials, as well as from other information regarding temperature gradients between the CPB circuit, nasopharynx, and brain,[164] is that it is important to monitor (and use as a target) a temperature site relevant to the organ of interest. If it is the body, a core temperature measured in the bladder, rectum, pulmonary artery, or esophagus is appropriate. However, if the temperature of the brain is desired, barring implantation of a thermistor directly into the brain (which actually has been done),[167] it is important to look at surrogates of brain temperature. These include nasopharyngeal temperature and tympanic membrane temperature. More invasive surrogates of brain temperature have been obtained using a jugular bulb thermistor.[164,168] Testing these different temperature sites has demonstrated that vast temperature gradients appear across the body and across the brain. It is likely that during periods of rapid flux (e.g., during rewarming), these temperature gradients are maximal.

Mean Arterial Pressure Management during Cardiopulmonary Bypass

The relation between blood pressure during CPB and CBF is pertinent to understanding whether MAP can be optimized to reduce neurologic injury. Tables 28-4 and 28-5 outline some of the pertinent studies regarding the relation (or lack thereof) between blood pressure and neurologic outcome. Plochl et al[169] examined the lower threshold of the autoregulatory curve in dogs whereby further decreasing blood pressure would result in inadequate CBF and oxygen delivery during CPB. In that study, the brain became perfusion pressure dependent below 50 mm Hg. The investigators also demonstrated that hypothermia did not shift this threshold leftward. Clinically, the available data suggest that in an otherwise normal patient, CBF during nonpulsatile hypothermic CPB using alpha-stat blood gas management is largely independent of MAP as long as that MAP is within or near the autoregulatory range for the patient (i.e., 50 to 100 mm Hg).[170]

TABLE 28-4	Studies Supporting Relation between Intraoperative Hypotension and Postoperative Neurologic Dysfunction	
First Author	*Year*	*Patients*
Gilman[746]	1965	35
Javid[747]	1969	100
Tufo[748]	1970	100
Lee[749]	1971	71
Stockard[750]	1973	25
Stockard[751]	1974	75
Branthwaite[752]	1975	538
Savageau[753]	1982	227
Gardner[754]	1985	168
Gold[59]	1995	248

TABLE 28-5	Studies Not Supporting Relation between Intraoperative Hypotension and Postoperative Neurologic Dysfunction	
First Author	*Year*	*Patients*
Kolkka[755]	1980	204
Ellis[756]	1980	30
Sotaniemi[757]	1981	49
Slogoff[758]	1982	204
Govier[170]	1984	67
Nussmeier[57]	1986	182
Fish[759]	1987	100
Townes[760]	1989	90
Slogoff[844]	1990	504
Bashein[761]	1990	86
Stanley[762]	1990	19
Kramer[763]	1994	230
McKhann[764]	1997	456

Although the autoregulatory curve traditionally is considered a horizontal plateau, this plateau has a slightly positive slope, but this slight upward slope is unlikely to have a significant clinically meaningful effect. For example, Newman et al[17] demonstrated that under hypothermic conditions, CBF changed only 0.86 mL/100 g/min for every 10-mm Hg change in MAP. Although this change (1.78 mL/100 g/min) was greater with normothermia,[171] these changes represented a relatively small fraction of the normal CBF of approximately 50 mL/100 g/min. Underlying essential hypertension as a comorbidity, however, likely is the effect of a rightward shift in the autoregulatory curve. The degree to which this rightward shift occurs is not clear, but it would be reasonable to expect that it is at least 10 mm Hg, suggesting that the lower range of autoregulatory blood flow is more likely to be 60 than 50 mm Hg.[172] In addition, diabetes may lead to autoregulatory disturbances that make CBF more pressure passive than in individuals without diabetes.[173,174]

Although the data relating MAP to neurologic and neurocognitive outcome after CABG surgery are inconclusive, most data suggest that MAP during CPB is not the primary predictor of cognitive decline or stroke after cardiac surgery. However, with increasing age, MAP during CPB may play a role in improving cerebral collateral perfusion to regions embolized, improving neurologic and cognitive outcome.[17]

Gold et al[59] added significantly to the understanding of the influence of perfusion pressure on outcome after cardiac surgery in a study of 248 patients randomized to low (50 to 60 mm Hg) or high (80 to 100 mm Hg) MAP during CPB. Although a difference was demonstrated in their composite end point of combined adverse cardiac and neurologic outcome (4.8% high vs. 12.9% low; $P = 0.026$), when the individual outcomes were compared, there were similar trends but no statistical differences. A secondary analysis of the same data performed by Hartman et al[38] found interesting interactions among pressure, aortic atheroma, and stroke; patients who were at risk for cerebral embolic stroke (from having severely atheromatous aortas) were more likely to manifest a stroke if MAP was maintained in the lower range than in the higher range. Intuitively, this is logical. Some experimental data in the noncardiac surgical setting suggest that collateral perfusion to penumbral areas of brain suffering from ischemic injury are relatively protected by higher perfusion pressure.[60] Overall, it appears that MAP (in the normal range) has little effect on cognitive outcome; but in those with significant aortic atheroma, it may be prudent to modestly increase blood pressure.

Glucose Management

Hyperglycemia is a common occurrence during the course of cardiac surgery. Administration of cardioplegia containing glucose and stress response–induced alterations in insulin secretion and resistance increase the potential for significant hyperglycemia.[175] Hyperglycemia has been repeatedly demonstrated to impair neurologic outcome after experimental focal and global cerebral ischemia.[176–178] The explanation for this adverse effect likely relates to the effects that hyperglycemia have on anaerobic conversion of glucose to lactate, which ultimately cause intracellular acidosis and impair intracellular homeostasis and metabolism.[179] A second injurious mechanism relates to an increase in the release of excitotoxic amino acids in response to hyperglycemia in the setting of cerebral ischemia.[177] If hyperglycemia is injurious to the brain, the threshold for making injuries worse appears to be 180 to 200 mg/dL.[180,181]

Despite much experimental data, the role of glucose management on cerebral outcome after clinical CPB is not clear. Although Hindman et al[182] cautioned about the use of glucose-containing prime for CPB, Metz and Keats[183] did not find a difference in neurologic outcome in patients undergoing CPB with a glucose prime (blood glucose during CPB of 600 to 800 mg/dL) versus no glucose prime (blood glucose level of 200 to 300 mg/dL). This finding was supported by Nussmeier et al,[184] who reported that use of a glucose-containing prime was not a risk factor for cerebral injury in nondiabetic or diabetic patients having CABG procedures. In the largest retrospective review, outcome data from 2862 CABG patients showed no association between the intraoperative maximum glucose concentration and major adverse neurologic outcome or in hospital mortality.[185,186]

The appropriate type of perioperative serum glucose management and whether it adversely affects neurologic outcome in patients undergoing CPB remain unclear. The major difficulty in hyperglycemia treatment is the relative ineffectiveness of insulin therapy. Using excessive amounts of insulin during hypothermic periods may lead to rebound hypoglycemia after CPB. Chaney et al[187] attempted to maintain normoglycemia during cardiac surgery with the use of an insulin protocol and came to the conclusion that even with aggressive insulin treatment, hyperglycemia often is resistant and may actually predispose to postoperative hypoglycemia. This concern over potentially increasing adverse effects by exerting tight glycemic controls reportedly has been demonstrated.[188,189] Attempting to mediate injury may actually predispose to additional injury.

Off-Pump Cardiac Surgery

Off-pump coronary artery bypass (OPCAB) surgery frequently is used for the operative treatment of coronary artery disease (CAD). Although its ability to optimally treat CAD (through the demonstration of long-term graft patency) has not yet been shown in a long-term, prospective, randomized, controlled fashion, it is clear that OPCAB and similar operations will continue to be mainstays of cardiac surgery, although in an evolving fashion. Their impact on adverse cerebral outcomes after cardiac surgery has been variably reported.[190]

Although early data suggested less cognitive decline after OPCAB procedures, most studies have not seen it eliminated altogether. The reasons for this are unclear but likely reflect the complex pathophysiology involved. For example, if inflammatory processes play a role in initiating or propagating cerebral injury, OPCAB, with its continued use of sternotomy, heparin administration, and wide hemodynamic swings, all of which may contribute to a stress and inflammatory response, may be a significant reason why cognitive dysfunction is still seen. Ascending aortic manipulation, with its ensuing particulate embolization, is also still commonly used (see Chapter 18).

The results of the largest OPCAB study by Van Dijk et al[191] to examine cognitive dysfunction showed that, although there was a reduction in cognitive decline in the early months after surgery, at 1 year,[192] and even at 5 years,[166] there were no differences between groups. In a subset of patients from this study, jugular bulb saturation was examined. More desaturation (indicative of ischemia risk to the brain) was seen in the OPCAB group. This may have been caused by the low cardiac output that can be seen during manipulation of the heart, as well as jugular venous hypertension.[193] The effects of OPCAB on stroke risk have not been sufficiently analyzed, but one meta-analysis showed no beneficial effect on the incidence of stroke.[194]

Pharmacologic Neuroprotection

In addition to the improvements in CPB technology, knowledge of the molecular workings of the brain has improved significantly, revealing potential pharmacologic neuroprotective targets. The oversimplified concept that depletion of high-energy phosphates and destruction of brain tissue rapidly follow ischemia has been replaced by a considerably more complex temporal, topographic, and biochemical picture. Advanced imaging techniques have discovered spatial gradations of residual CBF in the downstream territory of an occluded cerebral vessel, producing an ischemic penumbra, in which CBF is critically reduced but still sufficient to prevent immediate cell death. There is a marked difference in the temporal association between the ischemic insult and eventual cell death, resulting in a therapeutic window in which intervention (particularly pharmacologic) may attenuate infarct size. This window differs between the profoundly ischemic core and the penumbra. In the ischemic core, restoration of oxygen and glucose supplies is essential where high-energy phosphates have been severely depleted. In contrast, in the penumbra, the decreases in oxygen and glucose delivery are insufficient to kill cells directly.

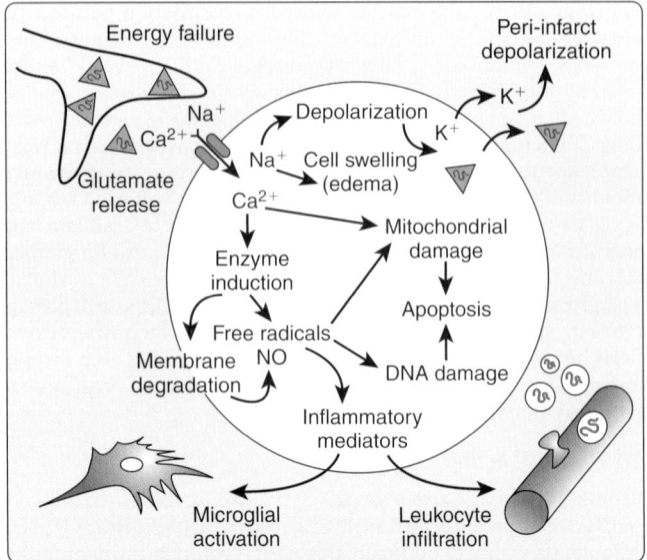

Figure 28-6 Cerebral ischemic cascade. A simplified overview of central nervous system events that occur after energy failure in the ischemic brain. NO, nitric oxide. *(From Dirnagl U, Iadecola C, Moskowitz M: Pathobiology of ischemic stroke: An integrated review.* Trends Neurosci 22:391, 1999.)

TABLE 28-6	Agents Studied as Pharmacologic Neuroprotectants during Cardiac Surgery
Agent	*Study Reference*
Thiopental	57
Propofol	200
Acadesine	205
Aprotinin	209, 210
Nimodipine	220–222
GM$_1$ ganglioside	223
Dextromethorphan	225
Remacemide	225
Lidocaine	230
β-Blockers	232
Pegorgotein	235
C5 complement inhibitor (pexelizumab)	237
Lexiphant (platelet-activating factor antagonist)	239
Clomethiazole	244
Ketamine	251

In these regions, pharmacologic agents with little or no ability to modify CBF have been shown experimentally to effectively reduce cerebral infarct volume, even if administered after the onset of permanent focal ischemia.

The CNS ischemic cascade (Figure 28-6) is triggered by reductions in CBF, globally or regionally, to the point at which the demands of cerebral metabolism can no longer be met.[195] This depletion in cerebral energy stores leads to membrane ionic pump failure, resulting in a number of injurious events mediated by the influx of sodium, the opening of voltage-dependent calcium gates, a release of stored intracellular calcium, and overall membrane depolarization. Membrane depolarization results in the release of excitatory amino acids (e.g., glutamate, aspartate), with subsequent dramatic increases in intracellular calcium. This increase in cytoplasmic calcium propagates the cascade through the activation of a number of calcium-dependent enzymes, including endonucleases, NO synthase, various proteases, protein kinases, and phospholipases. If left unabated, these enzymes will result in neuronal death.

Although some of these events are potentially reversible if reperfusion is quickly reestablished, reperfusion itself initiates a number of other destructive pathways. The reestablishment of oxygen delivery provides substrate for the production of reactive oxygen species, so-called free radicals. Reperfusion initiates a number of other damaging extracellular events, including BBB breakdown, endothelial swelling, and localized thrombosis that together may culminate in microvascular occlusion and further ischemia. Each of these pathways in the ischemic cascade represents discrete groups of potential targets for neuroprotection. The ischemic cascade has formed the basis for the initiation of pharmacologic neuroprotective strategies in the setting of overt stroke and of cardiac surgery-related cerebral injury.

No pharmacologic therapies have been approved by the U.S. Food and Drug Administration or foreign regulatory agencies for the prevention or treatment of cardiac surgery–associated cerebral injury, despite numerous previous investigations of specific pharmacologic agents in this setting (Table 28-6). This has not stopped progress, however, with multiple clinical trials ongoing. The most relevant cardiac surgery pharmacologic neuroprotection strategies, past and present, are reviewed here.

Thiopental

Thiopental was one of the first agents investigated as a potential neuroprotective agent for cardiac surgery. In a study by Nussmeier et al,[57] thiopental was administered until electroencephalographic (EEG) isoelectricity was obtained before cannulation and continued until separation from CPB. In this study, neurologic complications on postoperative day 10 were significantly reduced in the thiopental group versus control subjects. Based on the encouraging results of this trial, high-dose thiopental frequently was used for valvular and other open ventricular procedures. The proposed mechanism of this effect related to the suppressive effects of barbiturates on cerebral metabolism. This mechanism, together with experimental data reporting the beneficial effects of the barbiturates,[196] made it a logical choice for cardiac surgery. However, results of additional investigations of the use of thiopental were not as positive. Studies by Pascoe et al[197] and Zaidan et al[198] failed to support a beneficial effect of thiopental on neurologic outcome after cardiac surgery. These negative trials and the side effects of prolonged sedation with barbiturates served to quell the optimism for barbiturates. Retrospectively examining the initial Nussmeier et al[57] study, the beneficial effects of the thiopental might not have been related to a direct neuroprotective effect, but to an indirect effect on reducing emboli-containing CBF. The well-known cerebral vasoconstricting effects of thiopental (matching CBF with a barbiturate-induced reduction in CMRO$_2$) may have resulted in a reduction in embolic load to the brain during CPB and, as a result, a beneficial effect on neurologic outcome. It subsequently has been shown that isoelectricity itself is not necessary to incur a neuroprotective benefit from barbiturates.[199] Evaluations of subisoelectric doses of thiopental have not been performed.

Propofol

Propofol has effects similar to those of thiopental on CMRO$_2$ and CBF and has some antioxidant and calcium channel antagonist properties.[200] Together with supportive data from experimental cerebral ischemia studies,[201–203] propofol has been evaluated as a neuroprotectant in the setting of cardiac surgery. A prospective, randomized, clinical trial was conducted to determine whether propofol-induced EEG burst suppression would reduce the incidence or severity of cerebral injury during valvular surgery.[204] In a randomized trial ($n = 215$) of burst-suppression doses of propofol, there was no beneficial effect on cognitive outcome at 2 months. The investigators concluded that EEG burst-suppression doses of propofol provided no neuroprotection during valvular cardiac surgery. No other studies in nonvalve cardiac surgery have assessed the effects of propofol on the brain.

Acadesine

The adenosine-regulating agent, acadesine, was studied in the early 1990s with the aim of improving myocardial outcome; stroke was examined as a secondary outcome.[205] Compared with placebo, high- and low-dose infusions of acadesine resulted in a lower stroke rate ($P = 0.016$). Other adenosine-like agents have provided neuroprotection in preclinical experimental settings.[206,207] Despite this positive, albeit indirect, clinical data and supportive experimental data, no further clinical neuroprotection indication for acadesine has been pursued.[208] However, studies of this drug recently have been renewed. Whether this will have any effect on neurologic outcome is not known.

Aprotinin

Aprotinin is a nonspecific serine protease inhibitor that was first used in the 1950s for the treatment of pancreatitis. Its indication in cardiac surgery was for the prevention of blood loss and transfusion. In a large, multicenter trial of aprotinin for primary or redo CABG and valvular surgery evaluating its blood loss–reducing effects, the high-dose aprotinin group also had a lower stroke rate compared with placebo ($P = 0.032$).[209,210] Similarly, Frumento et al[211] retrospectively examined patients at high risk for stroke (because of the presence of significant aortic atheroma), and those who received aprotinin had a significantly lower stroke rate. In a small ($N = 36$) study examining the effect of aprotinin on cognitive deficit after CABG surgery, the incidence of cognitive deficit was reduced in the aprotinin group (58% aprotinin vs. 94% placebo; $P = 0.01$).[212] However, the high rate in the placebo group, the small size of the study, and methodologic concerns limit the applicability of these results to broader populations.[213] Animal investigations in the setting of cerebral ischemia failed to show any direct benefit on functional or neurohistologic outcome after cerebral ischemia.[214]

There has been considerable investigation of the potential mechanism for aprotinin-derived neuroprotection. Initial enthusiasm focused on its anti-inflammatory effects potentially preventing some of the adverse inflammatory sequelae of cerebral ischemia. However, aprotinin may have beneficial effects independent of any direct neuroprotective effect through an indirect effect of modulating cerebral emboli. Brooker et al[42] identified the cardiotomy suction as a major source of cerebral emboli during CPB. By extrapolation, if a drug reduces the amount of particulate-containing blood returning from the operative field to the cardiotomy reservoir (by decreasing overall blood loss), cerebral emboli and the resulting neurologic consequences also may be decreased.

The potential adverse effects of aprotinin were reported by Mangano et al[215] in their observational study of 4,374 patients. In that study, patients having received aprotinin had a significantly greater rate of cerebrovascular complications ($P < 0.001$). The Blood Conservation using Antifibrinolytics: A Randomized Trial (BART) reported a significant reduction in bleeding but an overall mortality risk with aprotinin compared with other antifibrinolytics.[216] However, there were no differences in the stroke rate with aprotinin compared with tranexamic acid (2.5% aprotinin vs. 3.7% tranexamic acid [0.78 odds ratio, 95% confidence interval, 0.45 to 1.35]). Although the Mangano et al[215] study and the BART trial contributed to the market withdrawal of aprotinin, the relevance of the potential neurologic effects of kallikrein inhibition remains. At least two other highly potent kallikrein inhibitors (CU-2010 and ecallantide) are being considered for clinical development, the neurologic effects of which are unknown.[217–219]

Nimodipine

Calcium plays a central role in propagating cerebral ischemic injury. For this reason, as well as a demonstrated beneficial effect of the calcium channel blocker nimodipine in subarachnoid hemorrhage and experimental cerebral ischemia, a randomized, double-blind, placebo-controlled, single-center trial was undertaken to assess the effect of nimodipine on neurologic, neuro-ophthalmologic, and neuropsychologic outcomes after valvular surgery.[220–222] The trial was not completed after safety concerns regarding increased bleeding and death rates in the nimodipine group prompted an external review board to suspend the study after enrolling 150 of 400 patients planned to be studied.

There also was no neuropsychologic deficit difference between the placebo or nimodipine groups at this interim review. As a result, the true effect of this drug or similar calcium blockers may never be fully known in this setting.

GM₁ Ganglioside

The monosialoganglioside GM_1 ganglioside has been investigated as a potential neuroprotectant during cardiac surgery.[223] In addition to the potential beneficial effects of this type of compound on preserving neuronal membranes, some data suggest that it has a potential beneficial effect on reducing excitatory amino acid transmission.[224] In a preliminary (but underpowered) cardiac surgery study, no beneficial effect was demonstrated. However, the study authors used this pilot trial to describe useful statistical methodology needed to measure differences in neurocognitive outcome, thereby constituting a template for later trials. This trial highlights one of the biggest difficulties in this investigative field: the interpretation of negative but underpowered studies.

Dextromethorphan

The N-methyl-D-aspartate (NMDA) receptor plays a major role in cerebral ischemic injury.[195] Although human stroke trials have been limited by distressing psychomimetic side effects, a wealth of experimental data point to NMDA-receptor antagonists as being robust neuroprotective agents with a potential role in CPB-associated cerebral injury.[225] Dextromethorphan, known for its antitussive activity, has some nonspecific NMDA antagonistic properties. A small ($N = 12$) pilot study examined dextromethorphan in the setting of pediatric cardiac surgery using EEG and magnetic resonance imaging end points to determine a difference between treatment groups but saw no difference, probably because of the small size of the study.[226] No other studies have examined NMDA-receptor antagonism in the setting of pediatric cardiac surgery.

Remacemide

A second NMDA-receptor antagonist that has been evaluated for neuroprotection during CABG surgery is remacemide. In a well-designed and well-executed study by Arrowsmith et al,[225] remacemide was given orally for 4 days before CABG. A neurocognitive battery was performed 1 week before and 8 weeks after CABG. A deficit was defined as a decrease in one standard deviation in 2 or more of the 12 tests within the neurocognitive battery. The patients were evaluated for their learning ability by subtracting the postoperative neurocognitive score from the preoperative score (formulating a Z-score). Although there was no difference between groups with respect to the dichotomous outcome of cognitive deficit ($P = 0.6$), examination of a continuous measure of learning ability showed there was a beneficial cognitive effect in the patients who received remacemide ($P = 0.028$). Despite these apparently beneficial results, because of the length of time that it took to perform this single-center trial, initial nonbeneficial preliminary results, and a prolonged period of data analysis and review for publication, this drug was not further pursued for this indication. It has, however, highlighted the potential utility of this class of drugs for this indication, and ongoing investigations examining other NMDA-receptor antagonists continue.[227–229]

Lidocaine

Intravenous lidocaine, because of its properties as a sodium channel blocking agent and potential anti-inflammatory effects, has been investigated as a neuroprotectant in cardiac surgery. In a study of 55 patients undergoing valvular surgery, a lidocaine infusion (in an antiarrhythmic dose of 1 mg/min) was begun preinduction and maintained for 48 hours after surgery.[230] Neurocognitive testing was performed before surgery and 8 days, 2 months, and 6 months after surgery. Compared with placebo, neurocognitive outcome 8 days after surgery was significantly better in the lidocaine group ($P = 0.025$). However, a much larger double-blind, randomized trial in cardiac surgery failed to replicate the finding.[231] Mathew et al,[231] in a study of 241 patients, found no difference in the incidence of cognitive loss with the perioperative administration of lidocaine. Interestingly, they found that in patients with diabetes, and in those receiving high doses of lidocaine, that outcome was worse and may have confounded any potential benefit in the overall cohort receiving it. Lidocaine cannot be recommended at this time as a clinical neuroprotective agent in cardiac surgery, but it continues to be investigated.

β-Blockers

Although the use of β-blockers in patients with cardiac disease has been predominantly directed toward the prevention of adverse myocardial events, in a study of neurologic outcomes after cardiac surgery, β-blockers have been demonstrated to have mixed effects on neurologic outcomes. In a retrospective study of almost 3000 patients, stroke and encephalopathy were studied.[232] Patients receiving β-blocker therapy had a significantly lower incidence of neurologic deficit versus those not receiving β-blockers. Although the reasons for this potential benefit are not clear, there are several potential reasons why β-blockers may be efficacious, including the modulation of cerebrovascular tone and CPB-related inflammatory events. Support for a potential neuroprotective effect from β-blockers has come from a study of carvedilol, which is known to have mixed adrenergic antagonist effects, as well as acting as an antioxidant and inhibitor of apoptosis[233] (see Chapter 10). Any potential benefit to β-blocker therapy needs to be tempered by recent data in the noncardiac surgery population that demonstrated neurologic harm. The perioperative ischemic evaluation (POISE) trial, although demonstrating a reduction in myocardial infarction, demonstrated an increase in stroke rate in patients randomized to receive metoprolol perioperatively.[234] It is unclear how this information pertains to the cardiac surgical population.

Pegorgotein

The generation of reactive oxygen species is a well-described pathophysiologic mechanism of ischemic/reperfusion injury. Combined with the whole-body inflammatory response associated with CPB and its own generation of reactive oxygen species, this mechanism has opened the field of neuroprotection and cardiac surgery to antioxidant therapies. Superoxide dismutase is involved in the catabolism of free radicals, and its mimetics have had beneficial results in the setting of experimental ischemia. Pegorgotein, a monomethyoxy-polyethyleneglycol covalently linked to superoxide dismutase, is protective against reperfusion-mediated cardiac and neuronal injury in animal studies.[235] One study was initiated to examine whether pegorgotein would be associated with a reduced number of neurocognitive deficits after cardiac surgery.[236] In this study of 67 patients undergoing primary elective CABG surgery (n = 22 to 23 in each of three groups: placebo, 200 IU/kg pegorgotein, or 5000 IU/kg pegorgotein), no difference in neurocognitive outcome was found.

C5 Complement Inhibitor: Pexelizumab

The activation of complement is central to the inflammatory response seen as a response to CPB.[237] In a small (n = 18) study using a simple assessment of cognitive function, patients receiving an inhibitor to C5 (h5G1.1-scFv, pexelizumab), demonstrated fewer visuospatial deficits at hospital discharge.[238] Additional large-scale (phase III) investigations of this compound to more adequately delineate any potential longer term neuroprotective effects from this drug in this setting have been performed. Mathew et al[238] assessed pexelizumab in a 914-patient study aimed at evaluating its effect on myocardial outcome and mortality. A secondary end point of neurocognitive outcome demonstrated that pexelizumab, although having no effect on global measures of cognition, appeared to have a benefit with respect to the visuospatial domain.

Platelet-Activating Factor Antagonist: Lexiphant

Platelet-activating factor antagonists have demonstrated neuroprotective effects in experimental models of cerebral ischemia.[239] Platelet-activating factor is thought to modulate postischemic injury by the release of cerebral cellular lipids and free fatty acids that may result in cellular injury and cerebral edema.[240] In an investigation of 150 cardiac surgery patients receiving placebo or one of two different doses of lexiphant, no protective effects were found in neurocognitive outcome 3 months after cardiac surgery. This study was significantly underpowered, which is a recurring and troublesome feature of many studies in this field.[241]

Clomethiazole

Clomethiazole, which enhances γ-aminobutyric acid (GABA)-receptor activity, has been evaluated in CABG surgery. GABA repeatedly has been shown to be an important neuroprotective target in focal and global experimental ischemia.[242,243] However, in a relatively large, well-designed, and well-conducted study, it failed to decrease neurocognitive dysfunction after cardiac surgery.[244]

Steroids

Corticosteroids have long been considered as potential cerebroprotective agents, in part, because of their ability to reduce the inflammatory response. Inflammation is considered an important factor in propagating ischemia-mediated brain injury.[245,246] However, with the exception of spinal cord injury,[247] steroids have never been demonstrated to possess any significant clinical neuroprotective properties. Furthermore, the administration of steroids actually has worsened cerebral outcome in a large trial (N = 10,000). The Corticosteroid Randomization after Significant Head Injury (CRASH) trial demonstrated an increased relative risk for death (1.18 [95% confidence interval, 1.09 to 1.27]; P = 0.0001) in those receiving high-dose steroids within 8 hours of injury.[248,249] Part of their lack of effect may result from the hyperglycemia that generally follows their administration. Hyperglycemia in animal models and several human studies of cerebral injury has been associated with worsened neurologic outcome.[180,250] The administration of steroids with the intent of conferring some degree of neuroprotection during cardiac surgery cannot be recommended. This therapeutic modality remains one that is being actively studied.

Ketamine

The neuroprotective effects of S(+)-ketamine, a frequently used anesthetic that is also an NMDA-receptor antagonist, were evaluated in a small (N = 106) study enrolling cardiac surgery patients.[251] The incidence of neurocognitive dysfunction 10 weeks after surgery trended toward being lower in the ketamine group (20% for ketamine vs. 25% for controls; P = 0.54), but because the study was underpowered, it was not a significant change. Although some experimental evidence supports its role as a neuroprotectant, there is insufficient clinical evidence to support its use for this indication.[252]

Future Neuroprotective Drugs

Despite the failure thus far to discover a robust pharmacologic neuroprotectant, efforts continue in this investigative field. Most of these drug trials are using cognitive dysfunction, or mild cognitive impairment, as primary end points, although stroke is assumed (albeit with little evidence) to be on the same brain injury continuum. Dexanabinol is one such potential neuroprotective compound that is a synthetic noncompetitive NMDA-receptor antagonist. It also possesses some tumor necrosis factor-α antagonist properties. Its neuroprotective potential has been evaluated extensively experimentally in the setting of various models of cerebral ischemia.[253,254] It currently is being evaluated in early-phase clinical trials in CABG for the prevention of neurocognitive dysfunction.

In addition to the dexanabinol trial, other peptides are also under investigation. One of these, AL-208, is an eight–amino acid activity-dependent neurotrophic factor that is secreted by allele cells in response to stimulation by vasoactive intestinal protein. In addition to antiapoptotic activity, it also has been shown to promote neurite outgrowth and stabilize microtubules. It is currently in a phase II trial in CABG surgery. Another growth factor–related peptide, Glypromate (glycine-proline-glutamate), is an insulin-like growth factor 1 that has completed a small phase II trial (N = 30) and has advanced to larger clinical trials. Furthermore, a small phase I CABG trial (N = 20) was undertaken of the energy substrate providing ketone body drug, KTX-0101 (sodium β-hydroxybutyrate), but the results have not been reported. Several other proprietary compounds also are undergoing evaluation and have yet to be reported.

ACUTE RENAL INJURY

Despite concern for almost half a century over the seriousness of renal dysfunction as a complication,[255][258] acute kidney injury (AKI) persists as a prevalent and important postcardiac surgery predictor of early mortality.[259] Even during procedures in which there is no evidence of AKI by serum creatinine, more subtle markers often demonstrate renal tubular injury.[260] Increasing degrees of AKI after cardiac surgery are associated with poorer outcome, greater costs, and more short- and long-term resource utilization.[256,261–263] The degree of AKI also predicts poorer long-term survival in patients returning home.[264–266] Notably, long-term outcome is just as strongly linked to the success of renal recovery as the magnitude of the injury; incomplete return of renal function occurs in up to one third of the patients.[264–266] Although some of the harm associated with AKI simply reflects its accompaniment of other serious complications as an "epiphenomenon" (e.g., sepsis), there is also compelling evidence that AKI itself contributes to adverse outcome.[267–272] Accumulation of "uremic toxins" beyond creatinine has widespread adverse effects on most organ systems,[267,268,273] and where it is best studied in chronic renal disease, inadequate clearance of uremic toxins adversely affects survival.[274] (See Chapter 37.)

Even when postoperative dialysis is avoided, the strong relation of AKI with adverse outcome continues to fuel the search for therapies to protect the kidney. Although practicing avoidance of the numerous recognized renal insults is a well-established approach to reducing AKI rates, the search for renoprotective strategies has otherwise been extremely disappointing. More recently, lack of progress has fueled a strategic reexamination of AKI with agreement that, compared with other conditions such as acute myocardial infarction (AMI) in which advances have been made, progress in AKI therapy has been hampered by its obligate delay in diagnosis (serum creatinine accumulation takes 48 to 72 hours) and poor agreement on its definition.[275,276] Thus, strategic policies have reframed AKI along the lines of AMI, viewing it as a condition with threshold criteria, whose treatment demands prompt diagnosis and acute intervention.[275] On a positive note, consensus serum creatinine thresholds are already available to diagnose AKI and are becoming widely embraced, whereas tools for the kidney allowing earlier diagnosis equivalent to the ST segment, creatine kinase-MB (CK-MB), and troponin for the heart may soon be available clinically.[275–279]

Clinical Course, Incidence, and Significance

Surgical procedure is important when considering postoperative AKI. The incidence varies widely by operation (Figure 28-7), each cardiac surgery having its own characteristic renal insult and pattern of serum creatinine change. For example, creatinine often declines immediately after CABG surgery (presumably because of hemodilution) but then increases, typically peaking on postoperative day 2, then returning toward or even below baseline values in subsequent days. Up to 30% of CABG patients sustain sufficient insult to meet threshold AKI criteria (e.g., RIFLE–injury[275]/AKIN criteria[280]: a creatinine increase > 0.3 mg/dL or 50% within the first 48 hours).[256,261,281,282] The reported incidence varies according to the definition of kidney injury, as well as by the institution reporting their results (Figure 28-8). Even among patients with similar risk factors undergoing the same procedure, however, current models poorly predict the likelihood of AKI. AKI also has been linked to accelerated long-term renal decline that may lead to end-stage disease requiring chronic dialysis.[283–288]

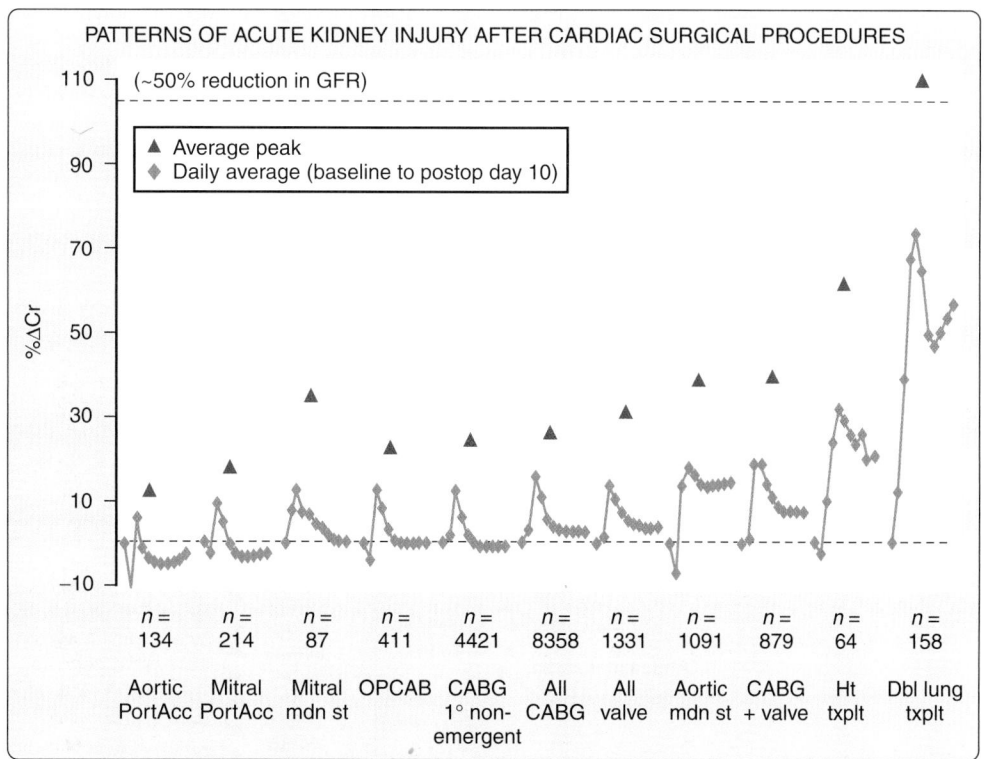

Figure 28-7 Different cardiac surgical procedures are associated with characteristic patterns of acute kidney injury; average daily *(diamonds)* and unadjusted average peak *(triangles)* serum creatinine values are presented. 1°, nonemergent; %ΔCr, peak fractional serum creatinine increase; aortic mdn st, median sternotomy aortic valve replacement; aortic PortAcc, minimally invasive parasternotomy aortic valve replacement; CABG, coronary artery bypass graft surgery; dbl lung txplt, double lung transplant; GFR, glomerular filtration rate; ht txplt, heart transplant; mdn st, median sternotomy mitral valve surgery; OPCAB, off-pump coronary artery bypass surgery; PortAcc, port access mitral valve surgery; postop, postoperative. *(From Stafford-Smith M, Patel UD, Phillips-Bute BG, et al: Acute kidney injury and chronic kidney disease after cardiac surgery. Adv Chronic Kidney Dis 15:257–277, 2008, by permission.)*

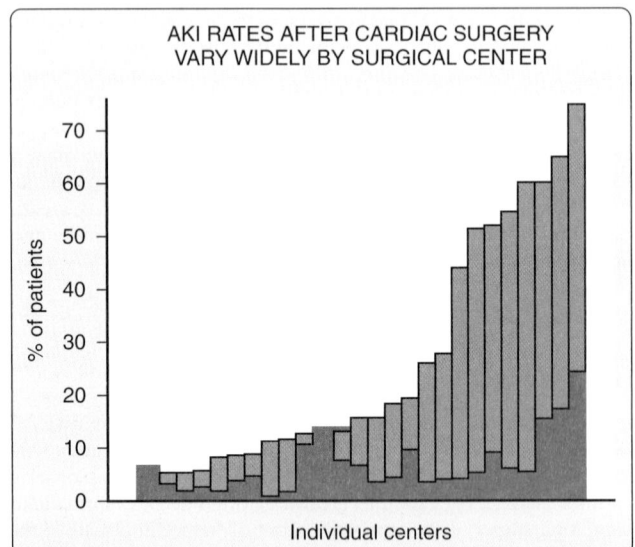

Figure 28-8 Even after adjusting for case complexity, among institutions there is wide variation in acute kidney injury (*shaded bar* represents risk, injury, or failure by ADQI-RIFLE-system)[275] and dialysis (*dark bar*) rates, as exemplified by Heringlake and colleagues[353] in a study of 2003 data from 26 German heart centers. (*Modified from Heringlake M, Knappe M, Vargas Hein O, et al: Renal dysfunction according to the ADQI-RIFLE system and clinical practice patterns after cardiac surgery in Germany. Minerva Anesthesiol 72:645–654, 2006, by permission.*)

Of the 1% to 3% of patients sustaining AKI severe enough to require dialysis after CABG, up to 60% will die before hospital discharge, and many of the survivors will require continuing dialysis or be left with chronic kidney disease.[289] Up to 20% of individuals presenting for nonemergent CABG surgery have chronic kidney disease.[290,291] Although dialysis after cardiac surgery is always important, when this is associated with poor preoperative renal function, postoperative mortality rates more closely resemble similar patients who avoid dialysis.[292] The rate of "renal recovery" after AKI is also difficult to predict, but emerging evidence suggests it is highly associated with outcome and apparently independent of AKI itself.[265,293]

Risk Factors and Surgery-Related Acute Kidney Injury Pathophysiology

Numerous studies have characterized risk factors for nephropathy after cardiac surgery (Figure 28-9).[294] Despite an increasing understanding of perioperative renal dysfunction, known risk factors account for only one third of the observed variability in creatinine increase after cardiac surgery. Procedure-related risk factors include emergent and redo operations,[295,296] valvular procedures,[295,297,298] and operations requiring a period of circulatory arrest[296] or extended durations of CPB.[256,261,299–301] Infection and sepsis,[296,299,302] atrial fibrillation,[303] and indicators of low cardiac output states, including need for inotropic agents and insertion of an intra-aortic balloon pump during surgery, also have been associated with renal impairment.[261,295,296,299,304]

Preoperative demographic risk factors identified include advanced age,[256,261,296,298,304,305] increased body weight,[256] African American ethnicity,[256,306] hypertension and wide pulse pressure,[295,307,308] baseline anemia,[309] peripheral or carotid atherosclerotic disease,[256,295] diabetes, preoperative hyperglycemia and/or increased hemoglobin A1c in individuals without diabetes,[256,261,307,310,311] reduced left ventricular (LV) function, and obstructive pulmonary disease.[256,295,296,299,300] Interestingly, baseline chronic kidney disease is not a risk factor for AKI, but because even small amounts of additional renal impairment may lead to dialysis when severe renal disease is present at baseline, these individuals are at greatest risk for dialysis.

A genetic predisposition to AKI exists and explains more variation in postcardiac surgery AKI than conventional clinical risk factors alone.[312,313] A handful of candidate polymorphisms known to affect inflammation and vasoconstriction have been studied, and several, alone or in combination, demonstrate strong associations with postcardiac surgery AKI.[312,313] For example, CO possession of the IL-6 -572C and angiotensinogen (AGT) 842C polymorphisms in whites (6% of patients) predicts an approximately fourfold greater than average creatinine increase (121%) after CABG surgery.[313] These data add credence to the idea that much of the variability in postoperative AKI may result from genetic influences[313] and suggest that wider genetic profiling and future whole-genome studies may lead to useful preoperative risk prediction tools and may even provide a roadmap in the search for useful renoprotective strategies.

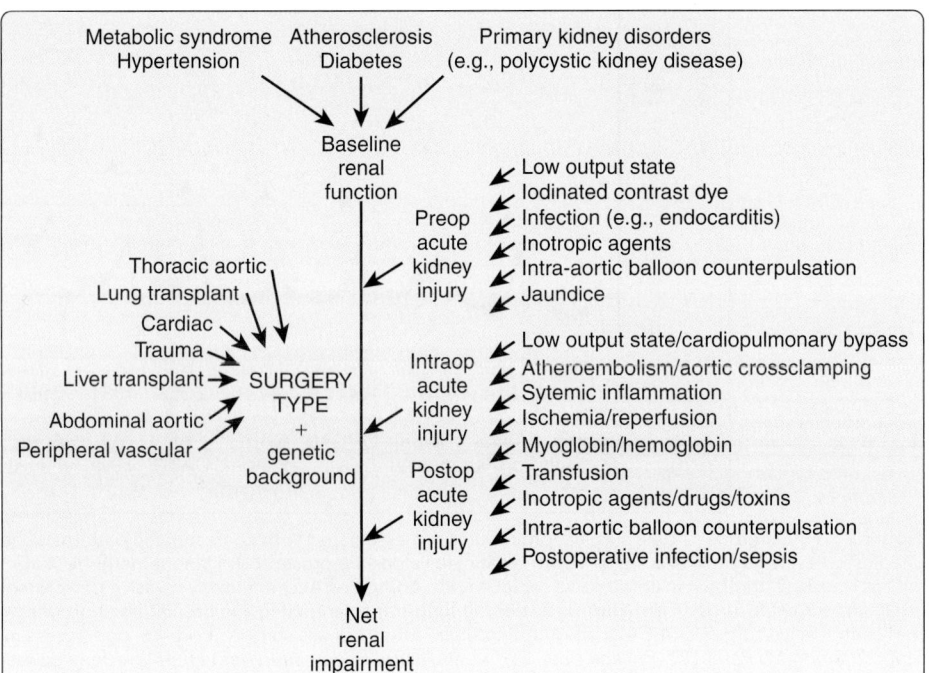

Figure 28-9 Numerous sources of kidney insult are known that play a variably important role for each patient during the perioperative period. (*Modified from Stafford-Smith M, Patel UD, Phillips-Bute BG, et al: Acute kidney injury and chronic kidney disease after cardiac surgery. Adv Chronic Kidney Dis 15:257–277, 2008, by permission.*)

Postcardiac surgery AKI for an individual patient reflects the actual net injury from numerous potential perioperative sources known capable of inflicting insult (see Figure 28-9). Many markers of renal risk hint at causes of perioperative AKI in individuals. Thus, perioperative AKI contrasts with single insult renal injuries such as contrast nephropathy. Nonetheless, a common pathway mediates the consequences of AKI including tubular and vascular cell dysfunction, necrosis, and apoptosis.[314] Although details of the trigger mechanisms for this reflexive component of AKI remain elusive, there is better understanding of the direct renal consequences of some insults specific to cardiac surgery. Although the physiology of perioperative renal recovery is as yet less studied, emerging data suggest this is also likely to be important. A brief overview of AKI pathophysiology focused toward cardiac surgery is pertinent.

Using intraoperative epiaortic scanning, Davila-Roman et al[315] found that ascending aortic atheroma burden correlates with AKI. Sreeram et al[316] noted that postoperative AKI correlates with arterial emboli counts. Conlon et al,[317] however, did not see a relation between renal artery stenosis and AKI. Renal atheroembolism is sometimes a dominant source of cardiac surgical AKI[318] and often observed at autopsy.[319] Filter devices deployed before cross-clamp removal often capture macroscopic atheroemboli.[98] Plaque disruption caused by balloon pump counterpulsation also is a contributor to AKI.[296,320] Antiembolism strategies have been adopted into the conduct of cardiac surgery,[321–324] but evidence that this is decreasing AKI is lacking. One randomized filter device trial in a post hoc analysis found less AKI in higher-risk patients.[99]

Other emboli sources may be relevant to AKI in some circumstances. Fat droplets, particulates, and bubbles are common during cardiac surgery. Renal embolic infarcts from any source are wedge shaped and involve adjacent cortex and medulla, highlighting the vascular arrangement and lack of redundancy of kidney perfusion. Incriminated particulates other than atheroma include thrombus, platelet fibrin debris, septic vegetations, and even normal vessel wall.[98,325] One third of surgery patients with bacterial endocarditis suffer significant AKI.[326] Although sternal marrow lipid droplet reinfusion with red cell salvage is common[327] and may have effects on renal cortical blood flow,[328] its importance is unknown. Air bubbles rarely have been associated with AKI.[329] Surgical field insufflation of CO_2 reduces intravascular emboli,[330] but whether this reduces AKI rates has not been assessed.

Many cardiac surgery patients meet the criteria for systemic inflammatory response syndrome in the early postoperative period. AKI is a major consequence of systemic inflammatory response syndrome.[331] Sepsis is a strong predictor of postoperative AKI, likely mediated through the effects of renal inflammation.[275,296,299,332] A surge of circulating proinflammatory cytokines is typical after trauma, major surgery, and CPB.[333] Local cytokine release also occurs in response to ischemia/reperfusion-mediated renal nuclear factor-kappa B (NF-κB) activation.[334] Finally, impaired renal filtration affects the course of any inflammatory response by influencing the primary clearance mechanism for many cytokines (e.g., IL-6, IL-1β, tumor necrosis factor-α).[335]

Many elements of cardiac surgery contribute to the risk for hypoperfusion and ischemia/reperfusion-mediated AKI. Embolism, low-output syndrome, and exogenous catecholamines can all contribute,[296,316,336] leading to cellular high-energy phosphate depletion, calcium accumulation, oxygen free radical generation, local leukocyte activation, and NF-κB activation.[337] These changes can cause apoptotic cell death through caspase activation (executioner enzymes) or tissue necrosis, or both.[338] Apoptosis instigates more local inflammation and injury,[339,340] and, experimentally, inhibition of caspase or NF-κB attenuates ischemia/reperfusion AKI.

Femoral artery cannulation can be complicated by leg ischemia and has been blamed for myoglobinuric AKI.[341] Although statins can cause myopathy, these agents have not been associated with increased renal risk in vascular and major noncardiac surgery patients.[342] Myoglobin and hemoglobin avidly bind NO and are believed to cause AKI through vasoconstrictor effects, but also through direct cytotoxicity and frank tubular obstruction.[343]

Withdrawal of the antifibrinolytic agent aprotinin from the market eliminates one concern of perioperative renal toxicity for cardiac surgery patients.[344] In contrast, the lysine analog antifibrinolytics ε aminocaproic acid and tranexamic acid can raise concern because of their renal effects of small protein spillage into the urine (tubular proteinuria).[345,346] A single retrospective analysis of 1502 patients involving the introduction of ε aminocaproic acid therapy did not find an increase in AKI.[290] Although tubular proteinuria often heralds tubular injury, with lysine analog antifibrinolytics, this is completely resolved within 15 minutes after the agent is discontinued.[345,346]

Other perioperative nephrotoxins include some antibiotics,[347] α-adrenergic agonist agents,[348] cyclosporine,[349] and nonsteroidal anti-inflammatory agents.[350] However, the net effect on postcardiac surgery AKI of α_1-mediated vasoconstriction and dopaminergic and α_2-mediated renal vasodilation with hemodynamic compromise is unknown. Although experimentally, even short periods of high-dose norepinephrine cause long-lasting AKI,[351] and catecholamines during cardiac surgery also predict AKI,[296,352] disentangling cause and association for these agents is problematic because they are rarely used in the absence of other major risk factors (e.g., low output state). Interestingly, in a survey of German intensive care units (ICUs) involving more than 29,000 cardiac surgery patients, centers with worse AKI rates were more likely to prefer dopamine over other inotropes and avoid norepinephrine as a vasopressor.[353]

Intravenous contrast is known to have nephrotoxic effects. Contrast-associated nephropathy usually is heralded by a significant increase in serum creatinine within 5 days after intravascular contrast injection and occurs in approximately 2% to 7% of patients.[354,355] The pathophysiology primarily results from vasoconstriction and direct renal tubular cell injury. Those at greatest risk typically have preprocedure renal impairment.[356] In a study of 27 CABG patients, Garwood et al[357] found indicators of tubular injury to be increased in those presenting for surgery within 5 days of cardiac catheterization relative to those further separated from an intravenous contrast injection. Use of low-osmolar contrast media and aggressive prestudy hydration have significantly reduced the risk for contrast-associated nephropathy for patients with diabetic nephropathy and other causes of chronic renal disease (Box 28-2).

Strategies for Renal Protection

The sluggish serum creatinine increase consequent to sudden declines in glomerular filtration is now considered inadequate to be the signal for acute renoprotection, much as Q waves are too late to be useful for cardioprotection. When serum creatinine is used, the obligatory delay in AKI recognition has even been suggested to explain some of the disappointing results from past renoprotection studies. Developing and validating tools for more prompt AKI diagnosis has become a priority. The hope is that early AKI biomarkers that can play a role in renal protection, much like CK-MB and troponin currently serve for myocardial protection, can be identified.

Nonetheless, despite its limitations as an early biomarker, serum creatinine remains an important clinical tool because of its many other uses. Indisputably, creatinine accumulation serves as a prognostic "gold standard," heralding AKI that is highly predictive of other major adverse

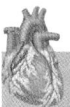

BOX 28-2. CAUSES OF RENAL INJURY DURING CARDIOPULMONARY BYPASS

- Emboli
- Renal ischemia
- Reperfusion injury
- Pigments
- Contrast agents

outcomes including mortality.[256] Validation for even the most promising of newer early AKI biomarkers is limited or lacking in comparison. In addition to injury, serum creatinine characterizes renal recovery unlike most AKI biomarkers. Renal recovery as reflected by declining creatinine levels is highly predictive of short- and long-term outcomes beyond the magnitude of kidney insult.[265] Finally, the generalizability across studies and settings of creatinine-based consensus definitions for AKI, such as RIFLE and AKIN,[280] are gaining popularity.

Unfortunately, the lack of success in developing effective renoprotective responses and the renal monitoring challenges outlined earlier dictate that any review of renal protection still remains limited primarily to strategies to minimize or avoid AKI risk factors. Few to no interventions have consistently proved effective once AKI is established. However, there is hope that the new paradigm, viewing AKI as a threshold diagnosis much like AMI, whose recognition must be swift and intervention immediate if tissue salvage is to occur, will lead to progress in this field.

Early Acute Kidney Injury Biomarkers

Beyond serum creatinine, the race is on to identify one or more "early biomarkers" for AKI. As a condition whose treatment paradigm demands prompt intervention, AKI currently has no equivalents to CK-MB, troponin, and the ST segment for the heart.

The search for better early AKI biomarkers currently involves several contenders involving numerous physiologic mechanisms (Table 28-7). Markers such as creatinine and cystatin C that accumulate to diagnostic

TABLE 28-7	Early Acute Kidney Injury Biomarkers

- **Serum accumulation markers:** reflect AKI much like creatinine, serum accumulation and decreased clearance with decline in glomerular filtration (Note: It is also useful to monitor renal recovery.)
  - Cystatin C
  - Proatrial natriuretic peptide (1–98)
  - Tryptophan glycoconjugate
- **Tubular enzymuria markers:** reflect AKI through leakage of cell contents into urine after tubular cell damage
  - α-Glutathione S-transferase
  - π-Glutathione S-transferase
  - β-N-acetyl-β-D-glucosaminidase
  - γ-Glutamyl transpeptidase
  - Alkaline phosphatase
  - Lactate dehydrogenase
  - Ala-(leu-gly)-aminopeptidase
  - Proximal renal tubular epithelial antigen
  - Urinary sodium hydrogen exchanger isoform 3
- **Tubular proteinuria markers:** reflect AKI through appearance of small proteins in urine that would normally be taken up by tubule cells, reflecting tubular cell dysfunction (Note: These are not useful if using lysine analog antifibrinolytic agents.)
  - α_1-Microglobulin
  - β_2-Microglobulin
  - Albumin
  - Adenosine deaminase binding protein
  - Renal tubular epithelial antigen 1
  - Retinol binding protein
  - Lysozyme
  - Ribonuclease
  - IgG
  - Transferrin
  - Ceruloplasmin
  - λ and κ light chains
  - Urinary total protein
- **Renal stress markers:** reflect AKI through various pathphysiologies reflecting or triggered by acute stress
  - Neutrophil gelatinase-associated lipocalin
  - Urinary interleukin-18
  - Platelet activating factor
  - Kidney injury molecule-1
  - Cysteine rich protein 61
  - Urinary pO2

Early acute kidney injury (AKI) biomarkers reflect renal insult through diverse mechanisms. Understanding of the physiology underpinning each marker can aid in understanding their potential value to improve the diagnosis of AKI.

levels because of decreased clearance are further challenged during the perioperative period because of "signal-to-noise" confounders, such as hemodilution, which complicate early AKI recognition by disrupting steady-state assumptions. Although only a few new early biomarker candidates involve a substitute "ideal" creatinine, most involve one of three other early consequences of AKI: tubular cell damage, tubular cell dysfunction, and the adaptive stress response of the kidney. For example, damaged renal cells leak contents directly into urine; this strategy underpins "tubular enzymuria" AKI biomarkers including β-N-acetyl-β-D-glucosaminidase and at least eight other candidates. Monitoring markers of the kidney's "stress" response provides another strategy for AKI recognition, including some frontrunners; these include neutrophil gelatinase-associated lipocalin, urinary IL-18, and at least three other candidates. Simple urinary P_{O_2} monitoring correlates with changes in renal medullary oxygen levels and predicts subsequent AKI in cardiac surgery patients.

Some early biomarker candidates are poorly suited specifically to perioperative AKI. So-called tubular proteinuria biomarkers, including urine α_1- and α_2-microglobulin and at least 12 other markers, manifest AKI through spillage into the urine of small filtered proteins because of impaired reuptake by the kidney. As outlined earlier, commonly used lysine analog antifibrinolytics (epsilon aminocaproic acid and tranexamic acid) mimic this abnormality by selectively blocking kidney tubule receptors, causing a reversible form of this same proteinuria with apparently benign consequences; these biomarkers are considered of little value in most cardiac surgery settings.

Several large, prospective observational studies are currently under way that may help identify the winner(s) of the early AKI biomarker race. It will be important for surgical and anesthesia advocates to highlight AKI biomarker issues unique to cardiac surgery lest these be overlooked in the broader pursuit of consensus AKI definitions.

Cardiopulmonary Bypass Management and the Kidney

Basic issues in the management of CPB that relate to the kidney involve the balance between oxygen supply and oxygen demand, particularly to the renal medulla. Perfusion pressure (i.e., MAP during CPB) and oxygen-carrying capacity (as related to hemodilution and transfusion) address the supply issues, with the use of hypothermia being directed at modulating renal oxygen demand.

Profound hypothermia is a highly effective component of the protective strategy used during renal transplantation. Mild hypothermia during CPB would, therefore, seem to be a logical component of a perioperative renal protective strategy.[358] However, three separate studies have not found any protective benefit of mild hypothermia during CPB.[359-361] In the largest study, including 298 elective CABG patients who were randomly assigned to normothermic (35.5° C to 36.5° C) or hypothermic (28° C to 30° C) CPB, there was no association between normothermic (as compared with hypothermic) bypass and increased renal dysfunction after cardiac surgery.[361]

Low CPB blood pressure typically is not associated with the hypoperfusion characteristic of hypovolemic shock and low output states, conditions that are highly associated with AKI. Studies addressing the role of CPB perfusion pressure have not shown an association with AKI.[305,310,362,363] A retrospective, multivariable analysis of minute-to-minute CPB blood pressure data from 1404 CABG surgery procedures, including an assessment of a degree-duration integral index of MAP less than 50 mm Hg, found no links between acute or extended episodes of hypotension during CPB and AKI.[310]

Moderate hemodilution is thought to reduce the risk for kidney injury during cardiac surgery through blood viscosity-related improvement in regional blood flow.[364,365] However, the practice of extreme hemodilution (hematocrit < 20%) during CPB has been linked to adverse renal outcome after cardiac surgery.[366,367] Accounting for perfusion pressure, in the study of 1404 CABG patients cited earlier,[310] independent associations were noted for both lowest hematocrit during CPB and transfusion with postoperative AKI. Other studies have reported similar patterns and suggest that profound hematocrit change (e.g., > 50% decline) may be even less well tolerated, highlighting the importance of a clinical strategy including transfusion only after all measures of hemodilution avoidance have been taken.[368–371]

Glycemic control during CPB has been identified as a potential opportunity to attenuate AKI. However, recent evidence has called into question the influential findings of Van den Berghe et al,[372] who reported reduced AKI and dialysis rates with postoperative therapy targeting tight serum glucose control (63% of study patients were postcardiac surgery). Despite widespread adoption of these intensive insulin protocols, numerous subsequent studies have failed to reproduce Van den Berghe et al's findings of benefit. Wiener et al[373] performed a meta-analysis of the available randomized ICU studies involving more than 3500 patients and found no reductions in AKI, dialysis rates, or mortality. In a study combining "Van den Berghe-like" postoperative management of 400 cardiac surgery patients randomized to intensive intraoperative insulin therapy (target, 80 to 100 mg/dL) versus usual management, Gandhi et al[188] found no benefit and similar dialysis rates (6/199 vs. 4/201; $P = 0.54$), even noting an unexpected increase in 30-day mortality and stroke with tight control.

Pharmacologic Intervention

As evidenced by a recent Cochrane database review, few interventions are available to the clinician to pharmacologically prevent or treat established perioperative AKI.[374] Proposed changes to improve the likelihood of success in finding renoprotective strategies have included increasing the size of studies designed to see benefit should it be present and, as outlined earlier, improving timely AKI detection to allow earlier intervention. Researchers have performed meta-analyses for many prevalent therapies by combining data from their randomized clinical trials. In some cases, these reports indicate that study size concerns may have been warranted. Potential optimism comes from a finding of reduced AKI in a meta-analysis of trials involving 934 cardiac surgery patients comparing various natriuretic peptides with placebo (urodilatin: 2 studies; brain natriuretic peptide [BNP]: 3 studies; atrial natriuretic peptide [ANP]: 9 studies)[375]; however, combined evaluation of the most studied single agent, ANP, still remained inconclusive.[376] Another meta-analysis involving 20 studies assessing various methods to guide fluid and inotrope therapy to achieve hemodynamic optimization targets, involving 4220 patients, found reduced AKI and a trend toward reduced mortality.[377] Notably, although hopeful, neither of these meta-analyses has sufficient evidence to make practical recommendations for changes in clinical practice.

Other systematic reviews and meta-analyses of collected AKI cardiac surgery studies recently have been reported. For example, several meta-analyses found N-acetylcysteine not to have renal benefit even in large cardiac surgery populations.[378–381] A meta-analysis limited to randomized cardiac surgery trials of fenoldopam (20 studies, more than 1400 patients) concluded that a larger trial (1700 to 2300 patients) was needed to reconcile promising but conflicting evidence.[382] Another less rigorous fenoldopam analysis of trials and observational studies (1059 patients, 13 studies) by Landoni et al[383] suggested reduced dialysis and death after cardiac surgery. A meta-analysis of statin therapy before cardiac surgery including 3 randomized and 16 observational studies (more than 30,000 patients) found reduced incidence of renal failure with this therapy.[384] A meta-analysis of 61 studies comparing "renal" dose dopamine with placebo (3359 patients) found extremely modest benefit on day 1—increased urine output, slight serum creatinine decline (4%), and GFR increase (6%).[385] However, by day 2, these gains were lost, and there was no effect on mortality, need for dialysis, or adverse events. Meta-analyses of loop diuretics trials and controlled studies in critically ill patients described improvements in markers of renal function (urine output, oliguric period) and reduced need for dialysis, but also concerning trends toward increased mortality, and poorer renal recovery.[386–388] Unfortunately, because of the limitations of current research tools, most potential renoprotective therapies have not been subjected to the rigor of a large randomized trial, or even

meta-analysis, and none has been given the opportunity to be used soon after the onset of AKI. Additional data, including rationale and existing studies for a number of these therapies, are outlined later.

Dopamine

Mesenteric dopamine$_1$ (D$_1$)-receptor agonists increase renal blood flow, decrease renal vascular resistance, and enhance natriuresis and diuresis. Despite the absence of clinical evidence of renoprotection, this rationale has been used to justify the use of low-dose ("renal-dose") dopamine (< 5 µg/kg/min) for decades. However, numerous double-blind, randomized studies in several surgical and nonsurgical settings have failed to demonstrate any renal benefits.[389–391] Concerns have been raised that dopamine in cardiac surgery is not benign, including evidence suggesting impairment of hepatosplanchnic metabolism, despite an increase in regional perfusion,[392] and increased postoperative arrhythmias.[393] Despite the lack of benefit and accumulating concerns regarding the use of low-dose dopamine, many centers continue to use this agent for renoprotection.

Fenoldopam

Fenoldopam mesylate, a derivative of benzazepine, is a selective D$_1$-receptor agonist. Although first approved as an antihypertensive agent, fenoldopam has shown promise in the prevention of contrast-induced nephropathy.[394–396] There are, however, few randomized, controlled studies to evaluate the agent as a therapy for postoperative renal dysfunction. In one prospective, randomized study involving 160 patients with preoperative renal dysfunction, improved renal function with fenoldopam versus placebo was reported after cardiac surgery; however, no long-term benefit was evaluated.[397] Other prospective, randomized, double-blind studies enrolling patients with established postoperative renal injury have proved inconclusive or even indicated possible adverse outcomes in patients with diabetes.[398] More systematic study is necessary before this agent can be recommended for renoprotection in cardiac surgery.

Diuretic Agents

Diuretics increase urine generation by reducing reuptake of tubular contents. This can be achieved by numerous mechanisms, including inhibiting active mechanisms that lead to solute reuptake (e.g., loop diuretics), altering the osmotic gradient in the tubular contents to favor solute remaining in the tubule (e.g., mannitol), or hormonal influences that affect the balance of activities of the tubule to increase urine generation (e.g., ANP). The general renoprotective principle of diuretic agents is that increasing tubular solute flow through injured renal tubules will maintain tubular patency, avoiding some of the adverse consequences of tubular obstruction, including oliguria or anuria and, possibly, the need for dialysis. Other agent-specific properties (e.g., antioxidant effects, reduced active transport) also have been proposed to have beneficial effects in the setting of ischemic renal injury.

Loop diuretics, such as furosemide, produce renal cortical vasodilation and inhibit reabsorptive transport in the medullary thick ascending limb, causing more solute to remain in the renal tubule and increasing urine generation. In animal models, administration of furosemide and other loop diuretics has been shown to increase oxygen levels in the renal medulla,[399] presumably by reducing oxygen consumption by tubular active transport; but it also results in distal tubular hypertrophy.[400] In experimental models, loop diuretics have provided protection from renal tubular damage after ischemia/reperfusion and nephrotoxic injuries.[401–403] In contrast with evidence from animal experiments, several clinical studies have shown no benefit and, possibly, even harm from perioperative diuretic therapy in cardiac surgery patients.[404–406] In a double-blind, randomized, controlled trial comparing infusions of furosemide, low-dose dopamine, or placebo administered during and for 48 hours after surgery in 126 cardiac surgery patients, Lassnigg et al[407] found no benefit of dopamine and a greater postoperative increase in serum creatinine in the group receiving furosemide. Although they may facilitate avoidance of dialysis in responsive patients by maintaining fluid balance in selected patients, there is insufficient evidence to support the routine use of loop diuretics as specific renoprotective agents. However, in situations of severe hemoglobinuria, they may facilitate urine production and tubular clearance of this nephrotoxin.

Mannitol, an osmotic diuretic, has been evaluated in several studies of cardiac surgical patients.[359,408,409] Although an increased diuresis has been documented, few studies have carefully assessed postoperative renal dysfunction in these patients. In an animal model of thoracic aortic clamping, mannitol did not provide evidence of improved renal function after unclamping.[410] In addition to the lack of beneficial effect on the kidney, several studies have identified a nephrotoxic potential of high-dose mannitol, especially in patients with preexisting renal insufficiency.[411]

Several studies have addressed the potential for renoprotection with natriuretic peptides. Three natriuretic peptides have received most of the attention in human trials: ANP (anaritide), urodilatin (ularitide), and BNP (nesiritide).[412] Natriuretic peptides have primary effects, including receptor-mediated natriuresis and vasodilation, and normally are secreted in response to volume expansion. ANP increases glomerular filtration and urinary output by constricting efferent and dilating afferent renal arterioles.[413] In a secondary analysis of randomized data from an ICU study of 504 patients with established AKI, Allgren et al[414] noted a 24-hour intravenous infusion of ANP ($0.2\,\mu g/kg/min$) was associated with improved dialysis-free survival in oliguric patients (8% vs. 27%; $P = 0.008$) but not in nonoliguric patients (59% vs. 48%; $P = 0.03$). Unfortunately, a repeat study designed to reproduce these favorable findings did not see any benefit.[415] Few studies have evaluated urodilatin, and these have all provided inconclusive results.[416] BNP has potent vasodilating properties and is generated in response to ventricular dilatation. Recent evidence from cardiology studies suggests that BNP treatment may worsen renal function in patients with heart failure.[417,418] However, two randomized studies in cardiac surgery patients suggest renoprotective benefit from this agent.[419,420]

N-acetylcysteine

N-acetylcysteine is an antioxidant that enhances the endogenous glutathione scavenging system and has shown promise as a renoprotective agent by attenuating intravenous contrast-induced nephropathy. The weight of evidence, including four meta-analyses, suggests that potential benefits that may exist with contrast nephropathy are not pertinent to the perioperative patient.[378–381,421,422]

Adrenergic Agonists

The α_1- and α_2-adrenergic receptors in the kidney modulate vasoconstrictor and vasodilatory effects, respectively. Agents that attenuate renal vasoconstriction may have potential as renoprotective drugs because vasoconstriction most likely contributes to the pathophysiology of AKI. Clonidine, an α_2-agonist, has been shown experimentally to inhibit renin release and cause a diuresis, and it has been evaluated in an experimental AKI model, confirming its potential as a renoprotective agent.[423–427] Similarly, two clinical trials have demonstrated some promise. A prospective, double-blind, randomized, placebo-controlled clinical trial evaluating preoperative clonidine in 48 CABG patients found that creatinine clearance decreased over the first postoperative night from 98 ± 18 (before surgery) to $68 \pm 19\,mL/min$ ($P < 0.05$) in the placebo-treated group, but it remained unchanged in clonidine-treated patients (90 ± 1 to $92 \pm 17\,mL/min$; $P < 0.05$).[428] The effect was transient, however, with creatinine clearance in both groups being no different at postoperative day 3. Despite being positively supported in a second trial,[429] clonidine has not gained popular acceptance as a renoprotective agent. Notably, decreased afferent α_1-adrenergic receptor–mediated vasoconstriction has been suggested as an explanation for the renoprotective benefit of thoracic epidural blockade in cardiac surgery patients.[430]

Calcium Channel Blockers

Diltiazem is the calcium channel blocker that has been the most evaluated as a renoprotective agent in cardiac surgery, with its ability to antagonize vasoconstricting signals and reports of beneficial effects in experimental models of toxic and ischemic acute renal failure.[431,432] However, in humans, numerous small, randomized trials and a retrospective study combined to provide a confusing picture, including evidence suggesting diltiazem therapy in cardiac surgery patients may have minor renal benefits, no benefit, or even potential harm.[433–438]

Sodium Bicarbonate

The perioperative infusion of sodium bicarbonate recently has attracted attention because of reduced AKI compared with a placebo saline infusion in 100 postcardiac surgery patients.[439] Despite evidence that sodium bicarbonate-based hydration appears to be of benefit in other settings such as contrast-induced nephropathy, the considerable additional fluid and sodium loads required with this therapy have raised concern for some clinicians.[440]

Angiotensin-Converting Enzyme Inhibitor and Angiotensin-1–Receptor Blockers

The renin-angiotensin system mediates vasoconstriction and is important in the paracrine regulation of the renal microcirculation. Angiotensin-converting enzyme inhibitor and angiotensin-1–receptor blocker agents act by inhibiting steps in activation of the renin-angiotensin system. Although angiotensin-converting enzyme inhibitor and angiotensin-1 receptor–blocker agents have demonstrated effects at slowing the progression of most chronic renal diseases,[441] their role in AKI has not been well studied.[442,443] In a study of 249 aortic surgery patients, Cittanova et al[444] reported an increased risk for postoperative renal dysfunction in patients receiving preoperative angiotensin-converting enzyme inhibitor therapy. Animal studies suggest that both groups of drugs have protective properties in experimental AKI.[445] In a small ($N = 18$), double-blind, placebo-controlled clinical trial enrolling CABG patients, preservation of renal plasma flow intraoperatively in patients receiving the angiotensin-converting enzyme inhibitor captopril relative to placebo was demonstrated.[446] A similar study assessing perioperative enalaprilat (an angiotensin-1–receptor blocker) therapy in 14 CABG patients demonstrated greater renal plasma flow in the enalaprilat group before CPB and on postoperative day 7, as well as greater creatinine clearance after CPB.[447,448]

Insulin-Like Growth Factor

The concept of combining AKI prevention with enhanced renal recovery is appealing given the emerging evidence; insulin-like growth factor offers the potential for the importance of the latter, evidenced by promising findings from animal AKI studies and reports in humans with chronic kidney disease of improved renal function and delayed need for dialysis.[449–451] However, unfortunately, the only randomized controlled trial in 72 patients with acute renal failure found no renal benefit and a significant side effect profile.[452]

Alternate Perioperative Renoprotective Strategies

In a survey involving more than 29,000 cardiac surgery patients from 26 German heart programs, Heringlake et al[353] reported extremely wide variation in AKI rates by center, ranging from 3.1% to 75% (mean, 15.4%; see Figure 28-9). Although programs were unaware of their AKI ranking when responding to a questionnaire, centers were asked to provide case mix data and answer questions on their standard practice in patients with increased renal risk. Interestingly, groups of centers with higher and lower AKI rates had similar case mix and urgency/emergency rates, but several differences existed in their responses to standard management questions. High and low AKI centers used loop diuretics at about the same rates but selected norepinephrine in preference to epinephrine or dopamine as a vasopressor, and they were less likely to prefer dopamine for either inotropy or renal prophylaxis. Using monitoring of AKI rates among centers as a tool to identify outliers and alter practice patterns was a useful strategy to improve outcomes in one study.[262]

MYOCARDIAL INJURY

From the earliest days of modern cardiac surgery, perioperative myocardial dysfunction, with its associated morbidity and mortality, has been reported.[453] Evidence, including substantial subendocardial cellular necrosis, led to the conclusion that this injury resulted from an inadequate substrate supply to the metabolically active myocardium.[454] Optimizing myocardial protection during cardiac surgery involves several compromises inherent in allowing surgery to be performed in a relatively immobile, bloodless field while preserving postoperative myocardial function. The fundamental tenets of this protection center on the judicious use of hypothermia together with the induction and maintenance of chemically induced electromechanical diastolic cardiac arrest. Bigelow et al[455] were the first to describe the use of hypothermia for this purpose, and this was complemented by subsequent work by Melrose et al,[456] who first reported the electromechanical arrest of the heart by the administration of potassium-containing cardioplegia. Despite continued efforts directed at myocardial protection, it is clear that myocardial injury, although reduced, still remains a problem, and with it, the representative phenotype of postoperative myocardial dysfunction (see Chapters 29, 32, and 34).

Incidence and Significance of Myocardial Dysfunction after Cardiopulmonary Bypass

Unlike other organs at risk for damage during cardiac surgery, it is assumed, because of the very nature of the target of the operation being performed, that all patients having cardiac surgery will suffer some degree of myocardial injury. Although the injury can be subclinical, represented only by otherwise asymptomatic increases in cardiac enzymes (e.g., myocardial creatine kinase isoenzyme [CK-MB]), frequently it manifests more overtly. The degree to which these enzymes are released by injured myocardium, frequently to levels sufficiently high to satisfy criteria for myocardial infarction, have been related to perioperative outcome after cardiac surgery.[457–459] Chaitman et al[458] reported CK-MB results from the Guard During Ischemia Against Necrosis (GUARDIAN) trial in 11,950 patients with acute coronary syndromes or undergoing high-risk percutaneous intervention or CABG surgery. CK-MB values more than 10 times the upper limit of normal during the initial 48 hours after CABG were significantly associated with 6-month mortality ($P < 0.001$).[458]

Risk Factors for Myocardial Injury

With an increasingly sicker cohort of patients presenting for cardiac surgery,[460] many with acute ischemic syndromes (e.g., often with evolving AMI) or significant LV dysfunction, the need has never been greater for optimizing myocardial protection to minimize the myocardial dysfunction consequent to aortic cross-clamping and cardioplegia.[461] The continued increase in cardiac transplantation and other complex surgeries in the heart failure patient has served to fuel the search for better myocardial protection strategies.

Pathophysiology of Myocardial Injury

Myocardial stunning represents the myocardial dysfunction that follows a brief ischemic event. It is differentiated from the reversible dysfunction associated with chronic ischemia, which is termed *hibernation*.[462] Myocardial stunning typically resolves over the 48 to 72 hours after the ischemic event and frequently is observed after aortic cross-clamping with cardioplegic arrest.[463,464] Important factors that contribute to stunning include not only the metabolic consequences of oxygen deprivation but also the premorbid condition of the myocardium, reperfusion injury, acute alterations in signal transduction systems, and the effects of circulating inflammatory mediators.

The metabolic consequences of oxygen deprivation become apparent within seconds of coronary artery occlusion. With the rapid depletion of high-energy phosphates, accumulation of lactate and intracellular acidosis in the myocytes soon follows, with the subsequent development of contractile dysfunction. When myocyte adenosine triphosphate (ATP) levels decline to a critical level, the subsequent inability to maintain electrolyte gradients requiring active transport (e.g., Na^+, K^+, Ca^{2+}) leads to cellular edema, intracellular Ca^{2+} overload, and loss of membrane integrity.

Predictably, with the release of the aortic cross-clamp and the restoration of blood flow, myocardial reperfusion occurs. With reperfusion, the paradox represented by the balance of substrate delivery restoration needed for normal metabolism that also can serve as the substrate for injurious free radical production, becomes a significant issue for consideration. Reperfusion causes a rapid increase in free radical production within minutes, and it plays a major role initiating myocardial stunning. Bolli et al[465] identified the importance of this effect by demonstrating that antioxidants administered just before reperfusion significantly diminished myocardial stunning, an effect not observed if the same substances were introduced after reperfusion. Sun et al[466,467] subsequently showed the significance of the free radical effect by demonstrating that up to 80% of myocardial stunning could be avoided with an appropriately timed regimen of free radical scavengers.

Free radical insults during myocardial reperfusion result in the near-immediate dysfunction of proteins involved in ion transport and excitation-contraction coupling, as well as injury to membranes through damage mediated through lipid peroxidation.[468] Free radical–mediated myocardial dysfunction is related to a myofilament defect manifested by an impairment in Ca-activated excitation-contraction coupling.[468] Although free radicals can directly injure these myofilament components, injury to other proteins related to ion transport and membrane integrity serve to increase intracellular calcium. Several mechanisms have been proposed to explain this impairment of myofilament function, although the most likely explanation includes physiologic down-regulation of excitation-contraction coupling in response to cellular Ca^{2+} overload. The mechanisms underlying Ca^{2+} overload are not well understood, but they are thought to involve free radical–related and free radical–independent abnormalities in Ca^{2+} homeostasis. Whatever the cause, the rapid calcium influx during myocardial reperfusion quickly can overload the myocyte with Ca^{2+}.[469] The importance of Ca^{2+} overload is demonstrated by the substantial protection from reperfusion injury obtained by pretreatment with traditional Ca^{2+} blocking agents.[470]

A free radical–independent mechanism for Ca^{2+} overload involves activation of the Na^+/H exchanger during reperfusion in an attempt by the cell to correct intracellular pH.[471] The resultant increase in intracellular Na^+ from activation of the Na^+/H^+ exchanger further activates the Na^+/Ca^{2+} exchanger, increasing Ca^{2+} influx.[472] Evidence for the activation of Na^+/H^+ exchangers being responsible for some of the harmful effects of reperfusion is shown by the benefits that Na^+/H^+ exchanger inhibitors have had on myocardial stunning with reductions in arrhythmias, improvements in systolic and diastolic function, and reductions in myocyte injury.[473] In addition to its role in Ca^{2+} overload, activation of the Na^+/H^+ exchanger has been linked to increased phospholipase activity, generation of prostaglandins and other eicosanoids, and activation of platelets and neutrophils—all potentially injurious processes.[471,473]

In addition to free radical upregulation, myocardial reperfusion associated with acute myocardial ischemic injury induces inflammation mediated by neutrophils and an array of humoral inflammatory components.[471,474,475] Several studies using novel neutrophil inhibitors have demonstrated a cardioprotective effect in models of myocardial stunning.[475,476] Prostaglandins also are generated during reperfusion. The adverse effects of prostaglandins appear to be synergistic with increases in intracellular calcium. The relation of leukotriene and cytokine release to reperfusion injury is less clear.[471,474] Consistent with a role for prostaglandins in this injury is the demonstration that inhibition of prostaglandins by nonsteroidal anti-inflammatory agents can significantly diminish myocardial stunning.[477]

A potential additional mechanism for myocardial dysfunction specific to the setting of CPB relates to proposed acute alterations in β-adrenergic signal transduction.[478] Acute desensitization and downregulation of myocardial β-adrenergic receptors during CPB have been demonstrated after cardiac surgery.[478,479] Although the role of the large increases in circulating catecholamines seen with CPB on β-adrenergic malfunction is unclear, it has been proposed that an increased incidence of post-CPB low cardiac output states and reduced responsiveness to inotropic agents may, in part, be attributed to this effect.[480,481]

Myocardial Protection during Cardiac Surgery: Cardioplegia

Optimizing the metabolic state of the myocardium is fundamental to preserving its integrity. The major effects of temperature and functional activity (i.e., contractile and electrical work) on the metabolic rate of myocardium have been extensively described.[454,472,482] With the institution of CPB, the emptying of the heart significantly reduces contractile work and myocardial oxygen consumption (Mvo_2). Nullifying this cardiac work reduces the Mvo_2 by 30% to 60%. With subsequent reductions in temperature, the Mvo_2 further decreases, and with induction of cardiac arrest and hypothermia, 90% of the metabolic requirements of the heart can be reduced (Figure 28-10). Temperature reductions diminish metabolic rate for all electromechanical states (i.e., beating or fibrillating) of the myocardium (Table 28-8).

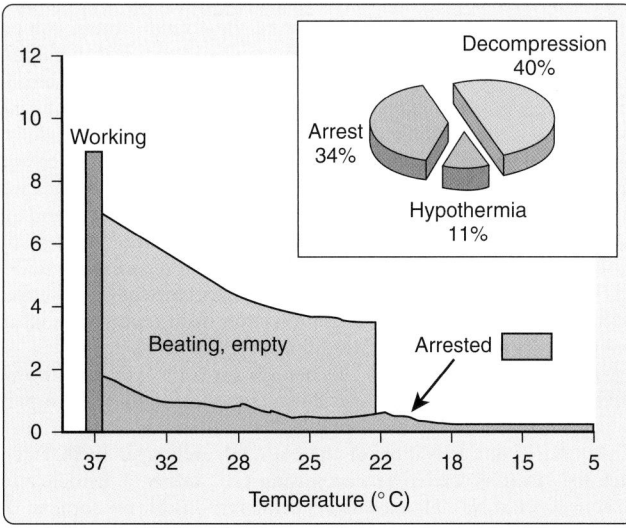

Figure 28-10 **Myocardial oxygen uptake (reflecting oxygen demand) versus temperature.** Compared with the oxygen uptake of a normally beating heart, eliminating cardiac work by venting the beating heart during bypass reduces oxygen demand by 30% to 60%. Arresting the heart reduces demands by another 50%, producing a total reduction of approximately 90%. Hypothermia extends the reductions in oxygen demand. (*From Vinten-Johansen J, Thourani VH: Myocardial protection: An overview.* J Extra Corpor Technol 32:38, 2000.)

TABLE 28-8	Influence of Temperature on Myocardial Oxygen Consumption for Different Work and Electrical Conditions			
	Myocardial Oxygen Consumption (mL/100 mg/min)			
Cardiac Conditions	*37° C*	*32° C*	*28° C*	*22° C*
Beating, empty	5.5	5.0	4.0	2.9
Fibrillating, empty	6.5	3.8	3.0	2.0
K+ cardioplegia	1.8	0.8	0.6	0.3
Beating, full	9.0	—	—	—

Data from Karkouti et al[368] and Stone et al.[396]

Although cardiac surgery on the empty beating heart or under conditions of hypothermic fibrillation (both with the support of CPB) is sometimes performed, aortic cross-clamping with cardioplegic arrest remains the most prevalent method of myocardial preservation. Based on the principle of reducing metabolic requirements, the introduction of selective myocardial hypothermia and cardioplegia (i.e., diastolic arrest) marked a major clinical advance in myocardial protection.[483,484] With the various additives in cardioplegia solutions (designed to optimize the myocardium during arrest and attenuate reperfusion injury) and the use of warm cardioplegia, the idea of delivering metabolic substrates (as opposed to solely reducing metabolic requirements) also is commonplace. Several effective approaches to chemical cardioplegia are used. The clinical success of a cardioplegia strategy may be judged by its ability to achieve and maintain prompt continuous arrest in all regions of the myocardium, early return of function after cross-clamp removal, and minimal inotropic requirements for successful separation from CPB. Composition, temperature, and route of delivery constitute the fundamentals of cardioplegia-derived myocardial protection (see Chapter 29).

Composition of Cardioplegia Solutions

The composition of the various cardioplegia solutions used during cardiac surgery varies as much between institutions as it does between individual surgeons. In general terms, cardioplegia can be classified into blood-containing and nonblood-containing (i.e., crystalloid) solutions. Crystalloid cardioplegia has fallen out of favor, with blood cardioplegia in various combinations of temperatures and routes of delivery being the most used solution. However, even within the category of blood cardioplegia, the individual chemical constituents of the solution vary considerably with respect to the addition of numerous additives. Table 28-9 outlines the various additives to cardioplegia solutions together with their corresponding rationale for use. Although all cardioplegia solutions contain greater than physiologic levels of potassium, solutions used for the induction of diastolic arrest contain the greatest concentrations of potassium as opposed to solutions used for the maintenance of cardioplegia. In addition to adjustment of electrolytes, manipulation of buffers (e.g., bicarbonate, tromethamine), osmotic agents (e.g., glucose, mannitol, potassium), and metabolic

TABLE 28-9	Strategies for the Reduction of Ischemic Injury with Cardioplegia	
Principle	*Mechanism*	*Component*
Reduce O₂ demand	Hypothermia	Blood, crystalloid, ice slush, lavage
	Perfusion	
	Topical/lavage	
	Asystole	KCl, adenosine (?), hyperpolarizing agents
Substrate supply and use	Oxygen	Blood, perfluorocarbons, crystalloid (?)
	Glucose	Blood, glucose, citrate-phosphate-dextrose
	Amino acids	Glutamate, aspartate
	Buffer acidosis	Hypothermia (Rosenthal factor), intermittent infusions
	Buffers	Blood, tromethamine, histidine, bicarbonate, phosphate
	Optimize metabolism	Warm induction (37° C), warm reperfusion
Reduce Ca²⁺ overload	Hypocalcemia	Citrate, Ca²⁺ channel blockers, K channel openers (?)
Reduce edema	Hyperosmolarity	Glucose, KCl, mannitol
	Moderate infusion pressure	50 mm Hg

From Vinten-Johansen J, Thourani VH: Myocardial protection: An overview. *J Extra Corpor Technol* 32:38, 2000.

substrates (e.g., glucose, glutamate, and aspartate) constitute the most common variations in cardioplegia content. Oxygenation of crystalloid cardioplegia before infusion is aimed at increasing aerobic metabolism, but the limited oxygen-carrying capacity of crystalloid makes a rapid decline in metabolic rate through immediate and sustained diastolic arrest critical to effective cardioprotection with this technique.

Blood cardioplegia has the potential advantage of delivering sufficient oxygen to ischemic myocardium to sustain basal metabolism or even augment high-energy phosphate stores, as well as possessing free radical scavenging properties.[485] The introduction of blood cardioplegia in the late 1970s followed recognition of the clinical utility of this technique.[486] Although low-risk cardiac surgical patients appear to do equally well with crystalloid or blood cardioplegic protection, evidence is compelling that more critically ill patients, including those with "energy-depleted" hearts (e.g., cardiogenic shock, AMI before CPB), have improved outcomes using blood cardioplegia.[487,488] Patients at high risk also appear to have better recovery using a combination of antegrade and retrograde blood cardioplegia delivery, when compared with antegrade administration alone.[488]

Because an infusion of oxygenated blood cardioplegia is in many ways similar to myocardial reperfusion, it is not surprising that the composition of blood cardioplegia is based on reperfusate parameters known to minimize myocardial stunning.[489,490] These parameters include maintenance of Ca^{2+} at 1.0 mEq/L (by chelating Ca^{2+} from perfusate blood) to diminish myocyte Ca^{2+} uptake; pH between 7.6 and 7.8 (the pH of water in the hypothermic temperature range used); osmolality between 340 and 360 mOsm to minimize edema-related myocardial dysfunction after reperfusion; and hyperkalemia between 10 and 25 mEq/L to safely sustain electromechanical arrest. Blood is mixed in a ratio of 4:1 with a prepared crystalloid solution to create blood cardioplegia with these characteristics.

Infusion of a single, warm (37° C) reperfusion dose of cardioplegia (so-called hot shot) containing metabolic substrates (i.e., glucose, glutamate, and aspartate) just before aortic cross-clamp removal is preferred by some clinicians. The rationale for this is evidence that normothermia maximally enhances myocardial aerobic metabolism and recovery after an ischemic period. Although some have advocated continuous infusion of hyperkalemic warm cardioplegia throughout the period of aortic cross-clamping,[491] this technique has not gained wide popularity for CABG because of the technical challenges of grafting vessels perfused in this way and the threat of ischemia to nonperfused (warm) myocardium during grafting.

Numerous other cardioplegia additives continue to be assessed involving various buffers, osmotic agents, metabolites, ATP and precursors, enzymes controlling ATP synthesis and catabolism, oxygen radical scavengers and antioxidants. Protection of myocardial β-adrenergic receptor function using intracoronary administration of esmolol appears to hold promise as an alternate cardioprotective method.[492] Alternative cardioplegia strategies potentially extending safe ischemic periods for heart transplantation to up to 24 hours also are being evaluated.[493-495]

Cardioplegia Temperature

The composition of cardioplegia solutions varies considerably; in contrast, myocardial temperature during cardioplegia is almost uniformly reduced to between 8° C and 10° C or less by the infusion of refrigerated cardioplegia and external topical cooling with ice slush. However, the introduction of warm cardioplegia has challenged the once universally accepted necessity of hypothermia for successful myocardial protection.[156] Although hypothermic cardioplegia is the most commonly used, numerous investigations have examined tepid (27° C to 30° C) and warm (37° C to 38° C) temperature ranges for the administration of cardioplegia. Much of the work aimed at determining the optimum temperature of the cardioplegia solution centered on the fact that, although hypothermia clearly offered some advantages to the myocardium in suppressing metabolism (particularly when intermittent cardioplegia was delivered), it may have some detrimental effects.

The deleterious effects of hypothermia include the increased risk for myocardial edema (through ion pump activity inhibition) and the impaired function of various membrane receptors on which some pharmacologic therapy depends (such as the various additives to the cardioplegia solutions). The other disadvantages of hypothermic cardioplegia, in addition to the production of the metabolic inhibition in the myocardium, are an increase in plasma viscosity and a decrease in RBC deformability.[157,482,496] As a result, investigations aimed at using warmer cardioplegia temperatures have been conducted.[156,497] During the initial phase of cardioplegia delivery, hypothermic temperatures, in addition to inhibiting some of the needed drug-receptor interactions, fail to optimize the metabolic rate in the myocardium. Hypothermia results in a leftward shift in the oxygen hemoglobin dissociation curve, inhibiting the release of oxygen into tissues. The myocardium is relatively ischemic during this initial induction phase of cardioplegia, with the uptake of the oxygen to this tissue being low and, as a result, significant oxygen debt occurs.

The adverse effects of hypothermia spawned interest in using warm cardioplegia. With the warm induction of cardiac arrest, metabolic activity is maintained, ion exchanges through cellular membranes are maintained, intracellular acidosis occurring with hypothermia is eliminated, oxygen delivery is optimized by maintaining a near-normal hemoglobin-oxygen dissociation curve, hypothermia-induced changes in viscosity and blood rheology are avoided, and RBC deformability and resulting flow through the myocardial microvasculature are maintained. The principal differences in cold versus warm cardioplegia result from the timing and route of delivery. If the myocardium is maintained at normothermic temperature, continuous cardioplegia must be delivered to adequately supply substrate to the metabolically active myocardium. In most cases, this is done using continuous retrograde cardioplegia (discussed later).

A compromise temperature (tepid, 27° C to 30° C) also has been proposed.[497] Ikonomidis et al[497] compared outcomes for patients receiving warm, tepid, or cold cardioplegia. Although numerous differences were found among the various groups, the recovery of LV stroke work at 1 and 4 hours after surgery was optimal in the tepid group. The researchers concluded that tepid cardioplegia provided better overall protection with superior functional recovery.[498] Hayashida et al[498] conducted a randomized trial comparing the effects of cold (9° C), tepid (29° C), and warm (37° C) cardioplegia in 42 patients undergoing CABG surgery. Overall, the investigators found that Mvo_2 and lactate production were greatest in the warm group, intermediate in the tepid group, and least in the cold cardioplegia group. However, early postoperative LV function was optimized in the tepid cardioplegia group.[498]

Cardioplegia Delivery Routes

If using tepid or warm cardioplegia administration, the continuous administration of this cardioplegia needs to be ensured. Retrograde cardioplegia, in which a cardioplegia catheter is introduced into the coronary sinus, allows for almost continuous cardioplegia administration. Retrograde delivery is also useful in settings in which antegrade cardioplegia is problematic, such as with severe aortic insufficiency or during aortic root or aortic valve (and, frequently, mitral) surgery. It also allows the distribution of cardioplegia to areas of myocardium supplied by significantly stenosed coronary vessels. Retrograde cardioplegia has proved safe and effective for cardioplegia in patients with CAD and in those undergoing valve surgery.[499,500] With the administration of retrograde cardioplegia, certain provisos should be considered. The acceptable perfusion pressure to limit perivascular edema and hemorrhage needs to be limited to less than 40 mm Hg.[501]

Two trials added information about cardioplegia routes of delivery. The CABG patch trial[502] enrolled high-risk CAD patients with impaired LV function and demonstrated the superiority of the combined antegrade and retrograde delivery of blood cardioplegia compared with antegrade cardioplegia alone. The limitation of this trial was that the antegrade group received crystalloid cardioplegia (as opposed to blood cardioplegia in the antegrade-retrograde group), raising questions

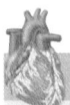

about whether the differences in the groups were seen because of the route of administration or the constituents of the cardioplegia itself. A second trial failed to demonstrate any differences when the administration of intermittent antegrade cold blood cardioplegia was compared with a group receiving antegrade cold blood cardioplegia induction followed by retrograde cold blood maintenance for valve surgery.[503] They did find that the antegrade-retrograde approach was technically more convenient, allowing for shorter aortic cross-clamp times.

Retrograde cardioplegia does have some limitations. Although the retrograde approach has been shown to effectively deliver cardioplegia adequately to the left ventricle, because of shunting and blood flowing into the atrium and ventricles by the thebesian veins and various arteriosinusoidal connections, the right ventricle and septum frequently receive inadequate delivery of cardioplegia. Difficulties with retrograde delivery also can occur if the coronary sinus catheter is placed beyond the great cardiac vein, or if anatomic variants occur that communicate with systemic veins, such as a persistent left superior vena cava (SVC).[501,504,505] Because retrograde cardioplegia is inefficient in producing arrest of the beating heart, induction of arrest with this technique must be achieved by a single antegrade infusion of cardioplegia before its institution (Box 28-3; see Chapter 29).

Ischemic Preconditioning

Myocardial stunning during cardiac surgery is affected by several parameters. The preischemic state of the myocardium can influence the degree of stunning that follows an ischemic event. Ischemic preconditioning (IPC) is endogenous myocardial protection triggered by exposure to brief (5 to 15 minutes) periods of ischemia. IPC is a natural defense mechanism that permits the heart to better tolerate myocardial ischemia. Although brief ischemic episodes in themselves result in stunning, they also build up a temporary resistance to the adverse effects of subsequent more prolonged ischemia.[506,507] IPC has been well described experimentally.[508-510] Several proposed mechanisms are responsible for IPC, including the activation of several myocardial G protein-coupled receptors, most notably A_1 adenosine and α_1-adrenergic receptors.[511] Protein kinase C appears to be a key cellular mediator of IPC, in part through activation of ATP-sensitive potassium channels.[512]

Myocardial protection strategies continue to be an active area of investigation, including assessment of IPC. Attempts to induce IPC by brief ischemia or pharmacologic means before CPB have been assessed in human cardiac surgical patients. Sevoflurane, a frequently used volatile anesthetic, has been demonstrated to pharmacologically replicate IPC.[513] Administration of adenosine, before bypass or in cardioplegic solutions, has been studied as a pharmacologic means to induce IPC. It has been associated with reduced postoperative myocardial injury, reduced inotropic requirements, and improved myocardial recovery.[514,515] The potential for myocardial stunning after beating heart OPCAB has not been fully assessed. Intermittent coronary occlusion before OPCAB to induce IPC, although unclear as to its effect, has also undergone clinical assessment.[516] (See Chapter 9.)

GASTROINTESTINAL COMPLICATIONS

Incidence and Significance

Gastrointestinal (GI) complications after cardiac surgery, although occurring relatively infrequently (0.5% to 5.5%), portend a significantly increased risk for overall adverse patient outcome. The variability in the reported incidence of GI complications is partly a reflection of how they are defined, as well as the variable patient and operative risk factors in the studied cohorts.[517-528] As devastating as they are, because of the relative low incidence, studies of GI complications are few. Although the most commonly considered GI complications include pancreatitis, GI bleeding, cholecystitis, and bowel perforation or infarction, hyperbilirubinemia (total bilirubinemia > 3.0 mg/dL) also has been described as an important complication after cardiac surgery. In one of the largest prospective studies examining these complications after CPB, McSweeney et al[525] studied 2417 patients undergoing CABG (with or without concurrent intracardiac procedures) in a multicenter study in the United States. The overall incidence rate of GI complications in this study was 5.5%, ranging from 3.7% for hyperbilirubinemia to 0.1% for major bowel perforation or infarction (Table 28-10).

In addition to their association with other morbid events, adverse GI complications are significantly associated with increased mortality after cardiac surgery.[525,529-531] The average mortality among subtypes of GI complications in the study by McSweeney et al[525] was 19.6%, and in other reports, the mortality rate ranges from 13% to 87%, with an overall average mortality rate of 33%. Even the seemingly insignificant complication of having an increased laboratory measurement of total bilirubin was associated with a 6.6 odds ratio of death in McSweeney et al's study, compared with a death odds ratio of 8.4 for all adverse GI outcomes combined. Apart from the significant effect on mortality, the occurrence of an adverse GI outcome also significantly increases the incidence of perioperative myocardial infarction, renal failure, and stroke, as well as significantly prolonging ICU and hospital length of stay.[525]

Risk Factors

Many preoperative, intraoperative, and postoperative risk factors for GI complications have been identified in a number of studies.[523,525,532-537] Because many factors are associated with one another, it is only when these risk factors are examined in multivariable analyses that a more accurate understanding of what the most significant risk factors for visceral complications after cardiac surgery are. Table 28-11 represents the most consistently reported risk factors for GI complications after cardiac surgery: Before surgery, age (> 75 years), history of congestive heart failure, presence of hyperbilirubinemia (> 1.2 mg/dL), combined cardiac procedures (e.g., CABG plus valve), repeat cardiac operation, preoperative ejection fraction less than 40%, preoperative increases in partial thromboplastin time, and emergency operations; intraoperatively, prolonged CPB, use of TEE, and blood transfusion; and postoperatively, requirements for prolonged inotropic vasopressor support, IABP use for the treatment of low cardiac output; and prolonged

TABLE 28-10	Adverse Gastrointestinal Outcomes		
	No. of Patients	Percentage of Patients with a Gastrointestinal Event (n = 133)	Percentage of Total Patients (N = 2417)
Hyperbilirubinemia, total*	90	67.7	3.7
3.1–5.0 mg/dL	54	40.6	2.2
5.1–9.0 mg/dL	19	14.2	0.8
>9.0 mg/dL	17	12.8	0.7
Gastrointestinal bleeding	28	21.0	1.2
Pancreatitis	19	14.3	0.8
Cholecystitis	7	5.3	0.3
Bowel perforation	2	1.5	0.1
Bowel infarction	2	1.5	0.1

*Hyperbilirubinemia was defined as maximum total bilirubin after surgery of 3.0 mg/dL.
From McSweeney ME, Garwood S, Levin J, et al: Adverse gastrointestinal complications after cardiopulmonary bypass: Can outcome be predicted from preoperative risk factors? *Anesth Analg* 98:1610, 2004.

TABLE 28-11	Commonly Identified Risk Factors for Visceral Complications after Cardiac Surgery			
Preoperative Risk Factors	*Type of Cardiac Surgery*	*Cardiopulmonary Bypass Factors*	*Postoperative Risk Factors*
Age	Emergency surgery	Duration of CPB	Low cardiac output, use of inotropes, vasopressors, or IABP
History of CHF or low EF	Reoperations	Cross-clamp duration	Reoperation for bleeding
Renal insufficiency	Valve or combined procedures		Loss of normal sinus rhythm
Peptic ulcer disease, chronic lung disease, recent acute myocardial infarction, diabetes mellitus, peripheral vascular disease, use of IABP*	Cardiac transplantation		Renal failure
			Ventilation > 24 hours
			ICU stay > 1 day
			Increased bilirubin or lactate level, mediastinitis*

*Less commonly mentioned risk factors.
CHF, congestive heart failure; CPB, cardiopulmonary bypass; EF, ejection fraction; IABP, intra-aortic balloon bump; ICU, intensive care unit.
From Hessel EA 2nd: Abdominal organ injury after cardiac surgery. *Semin Cardiothorac Vasc Anesth* 8:243, 2004.

ventilatory support are all risk factors. These factors identify patients at high risk, and they lend some credence to the overall pathophysiology and suspected causes of these adverse events. If there is a common link among all these risks, it is that many of these factors would be associated with impairment in oxygen delivery to the splanchnic bed.

Pathophysiology and Causative Factors

Impairments in splanchnic perfusion commonly occur during even the normal conduct of cardiac surgery. When these are superimposed on an already depressed preoperative cardiac output or associated with prolonged postoperative low cardiac output, the impairment in splanchnic blood flow is further perpetuated. The systemic inflammatory response to CPB itself can be initiated by splanchnic hypoperfusion by means of translocation of endotoxin from the gut into the circulation. De novo splanchnic hypoperfusion can be a result of the humoral vasoactive substances that are released by inflammation remote from the gut.[538–540] Another causative factor for GI complications directly related to splanchnic hypoperfusion is atheroembolism. Several studies have directly attributed atheroembolism to splanchnic hypoperfusion and gut infarction.[532,536,541] Prolonged ventilator support is another causative factor for GI complications. Several lines of investigation have described a relation between prolonged ventilation and GI adverse events; this likely results from a direct effect of positive-pressure ventilation impairing cardiac output and, subsequently, splanchnic perfusion.[521,523,535,542] Lung volume reduction surgery and lung transplantation also produce (approximately 9%) GI complications.[543,544]

Protecting the Gastrointestinal Tract during Cardiac Surgery

As with other aspects of organ protection, critical causative factors need to be addressed with specific targeted therapies (Box 28-4). Unfortunately, as with most other organ-protective strategies, the major limitation in making definitive recommendations is an overall lack of large, well-controlled, prospectively randomized studies to

BOX 28-4. PROTECTING THE GASTROINTESTINAL TRACT DURING CARDIOPULMONARY BYPASS

- Avoiding high doses of vasopressors
- Maintaining a high perfusion flow
- Reducing emboli-producing maneuvers
- Decontaminating the gastrointestinal tract (?)

provide supportive data for any one particular technique. However, some recommendations can be made, and attention can be focused on a number of other less well-studied but potentially valid strategies.

Cardiopulmonary Bypass Management

Because CPB itself has been shown to impair splanchnic blood flow, modifications in how it is conducted may have some salutary effects on GI tract integrity. Several studies have focused on the issue of the relative importance of pressure versus flow during CPB, demonstrating that it is likely more beneficial to maintain an adequate bypass flow rate than only maintaining pressure during bypass.[545–547] The addition of significant vasoconstrictors to artificially maintain an adequate MAP in the presence of inadequate flow on CPB may lead to further compromise of splanchnic blood flow. Few definitive data offer guidance about pulsatility. Some studies have shown improvements with pulsatility by indirect measurements (i.e., gastric mucosal intracellular pH), but no studies have found definitive differences in clinical outcomes. Similarly, the optimal bypass temperature to protect the gut also is unknown. Just as aggressive rewarming can be injurious to the brain,[63] there is some evidence that rewarming can cause increases in visceral metabolism, making any overshoot in temperature suspect by adversely altering the balance of gut oxygen consumption and delivery.[548]

Emboli Reduction

Whereas microembolization and macroembolization to the splanchnic bed clearly occur during CPB and possibly even during the postbypass period, there are few data to determine whether emboli reduction strategies can alter GI outcome. Mythen et al[549] found a relation between transcranial Doppler–detected emboli (used as a surrogate for overall microembolic load within the body) and adverse changes in gastric mucosal intracellular pH. However, with respect to microembolization, a trial that used an intra-aortic filter to reduce atheroemboli failed to have any influence on the rate of GI complications.[99] It remains prudent to avoid maneuvers (i.e., aortic cannulation and cross-clamping) in areas of high atheroma burden, which is an overall tenet of cardiac surgery for the prevention of all other complications.

Drugs

A range of vasoactive drugs has been used to enhance splanchnic blood flow during CPB. It is likely that most of these drugs, such as the phosphodiesterase III inhibitors, dobutamine, and other inotropic agents, maintain or enhance splanchnic blood flow not because of a direct effect on the vasculature but by the inherent enhancement in cardiac output. Dobutamine and dopamine have had a paradoxic detrimental effect on the splanchnic vasculature, with some evidence that they cause further mucosal ischemia.[550,551] Dopexamine also has been studied in a small group that did show an improvement in mucosal blood flow (using laser–Doppler flowmetry), but there was no beneficial effect on gastric mucosal intracellular pH.[552] An increasingly common drug in the setting of cardiac surgery is vasopressin. Although vasopressin clearly can augment systemic MAP, it does so at the cost of severe impairments to splanchnic blood flow.[553] Although there are always trade-offs when choosing which vasoactive agent to use, if having a very low MAP is going to be detrimental to other organ systems, the choice to use vasopressin should at least be made with the knowledge that it can have an adverse effect on splanchnic blood flow.

Selective Gastrointestinal Decontamination

Addressing the concept that gut translocation of endotoxin plays a role in inflammation and other organ injuries, one interesting therapy that has been tried in the setting of cardiac surgery involves the administration of oral antibiotics to selectively decontaminate the GI tract before surgery.[554] Although examined in a small (N = 100) study, a combination of oral polymyxin, tobramycin, and amphotericin before surgery for 3 days reduced the degree of endotoxemia, it was not associated with a beneficial effect on patient outcomes. One possible explanation is that there is such an overwhelmingly large depot of gram-negative organisms in the GI tract that the elimination of even a large population of these by oral antibiotics still leaves significant repositories of endotoxin in the gut. Killing these bacteria may in itself cause the release of the endotoxin, which can then be absorbed into the systemic circulation by impairment of mucosal blood flow inherent in the unphysiologic flow during CPB.

Off-Pump Cardiac Surgery

There is little evidence that the use of off-pump cardiac surgery is in any way beneficial to the GI tract. Three retrospective studies[525,533,555] have shown no differences in GI complications. One reason for this lack of apparent difference between on-pump and off-pump cardiac surgery may again be related to the common denominator of splanchnic perfusion. OPCAB surgery is fraught with hemodynamic compromise that may lead to prolonged periods of splanchnic hypoperfusion by itself or as a result of the concurrent administration of vasopressors to maintain normal hemodynamics during the frequent manipulations of the heart.

Anti-inflammatory Therapies

Although the inflammatory response to CPB has been implicated as a causative factor in GI complications after cardiac surgery, few data are available to assess the ability of various anti-inflammatory therapies (e.g., corticosteroids, aprotinin, complement inhibitors) to reduce these types of complications.

LUNG INJURY DURING CARDIAC SURGERY

Incidence and Significance

Pulmonary dysfunction was one of the earliest recognized complications of cardiac surgery using CPB.[556] However, as improvements in operative technique and CPB perfusion technologies occurred, the overall frequency and severity of this complication decreased. Juxtaposed to the improvements in cardiac surgery, which led to an overall reduction in complications, is an evolving patient population that now comprises a higher risk group with a greater degree of pulmonary comorbidities, increasing their risks for postoperative pulmonary dysfunction. With the advent of fast-track techniques,[557] even minor degrees of pulmonary dysfunction have reemerged as significant contributors to patient morbidity and the potential need for extended postoperative ventilation. As with most postoperative organ dysfunction, there is a range of dysfunction severity. Arguably, some degree of pulmonary dysfunction occurs in most patients after cardiac surgery; however, it manifests clinically only when the degree of dysfunction is particularly severe

or the pulmonary reserve is significantly impaired.[558,559] As a result, even minor CPB-related pulmonary dysfunction can cause significant problems in some patients.

The full range of reported pulmonary complications includes simple atelectasis, pleural effusions, pneumonia, cardiogenic pulmonary edema, pulmonary embolism, and various degrees of acute lung injury ranging from the mild to the most severe (i.e., acute respiratory distress syndrome [ARDS]). Although the final common pathway in all these forms of pulmonary dysfunction complications is the occurrence of hypoxemia, these complications vary widely in their incidence, cause, and clinical significance. Understanding that the changes that occur after CPB represent a continuum, it becomes necessary to define what constitutes pulmonary dysfunction and injury.

Definitions have varied. One commonly accepted definition that was used in a large study (N = 1461 patients) performed in the setting of cardiac surgery defined acute pulmonary dysfunction as a patient requiring mechanical ventilation with a Pao_2/Fio_2 ratio of less than 150, irrespective of positive end-expiratory pressure, coupled with a chest radiograph that indicated the development of bilateral pulmonary infiltrates, assuming that other causes of hypoxia such as pneumothorax could be excluded. Using this definition, approximately 12% of patients on admission to the cardiovascular ICU after cardiac surgery met the criteria of early acute pulmonary dysfunction.[560,561] Early acute pulmonary dysfunction should be differentiated from the more severe but less common ARDS that occurs in 1% to 2% of patients.[560,562] Although these two forms likely represent similar processes with different degrees of severity, ARDS differs particularly in its timing. The definition of ARDS in the setting of cardiac surgery generally requires the presence of refractory hypoxemia, diffuse bilateral pulmonary infiltrates on chest radiograph, the requirement for mechanical ventilation with an Fio_2 of more than 0.40, and most importantly, duration of at least 3 days (as opposed to on admission to the ICU). This must be in the presence of a low pulmonary capillary wedge pressure (< 18 mm Hg). In Welsby et al's[563] study of 2609 consecutive adult cardiac surgery patients, 7.5% of whom had pulmonary complications, the overall mortality rate was 21%, with 64% of these patients remaining in the hospital more than 10 days. In another study, the most significantly affected patients (i.e., those with ARDS) had a mortality rate upward of 80%.[564] These significant morbidity and mortality rates lend credence to pulmonary complications remaining as significant and relevant today as in the early days of cardiac surgery.

Atelectasis and pleural effusions are the most common pulmonary abnormalities seen after cardiac surgery, presenting in more than 60% of patients.[565,566] Atelectasis commonly is attributed to a number of intraoperative and postoperative events. With the induction of general anesthesia, physical compression of the left lower lobe to aid exposure of the heart and facilitate in the dissection of the internal mammary artery and the apnea occurring during the conduct of CPB itself have been implicated.[567,568] Postoperative causes include the poor respiratory efforts by patients with impaired coughing, lack of deep inspirations, and pleural effusions.[569] Despite a high incidence of these radiographically recognized complications, the clinical significance is relatively low.[570,571]

Similar to atelectasis, pleural effusions, despite occurring commonly after cardiac surgery (40% to 50%), rarely cause significant perioperative morbidity. More common in the left thorax, likely as a consequence of the bleeding from the dissection of the internal mammary artery, other causes of pleural effusions relate to continued postoperative bleeding, pulmonary edema from cardiogenic and noncardiogenic causes, and pneumonia. Surgical trauma also can disrupt the normal pleural lymphatic flow through the thorax and, rarely, direct damage to the thoracic duct can lead to the development of a chylothorax. Small effusions tend to resolve over time (a few months after surgery) and rarely require any specific treatment. However, large pleural effusions that compromise the underlying lung respond well to thoracentesis and temporary chest tube placement, but if persistent, they may require decortication.

Pneumonia after cardiac surgery also has a variable incidence but a much greater significance to overall patient outcome. Reported rates of pneumonia range widely from 2% to 22%.[572–575] Pneumonia occurring early after cardiac surgery portends a poor outcome, illustrated in one study by a mortality rate of 27%.[576] A number of factors increase the risk for postoperative pneumonia, including smoking, the presence of chronic obstructive pulmonary disease, other pulmonary complications requiring prolonged intubation, significant cardiac failure itself, and the transfusion of large volumes of blood products.

Risk Factors for Pulmonary Dysfunction

Rady et al[560] defined preoperative, operative, and postoperative variables that represent risk factors for early pulmonary dysfunction after cardiac surgery. Although it is not entirely clear whether any of these risk factors can be modified, identifying their presence increases the level of vigilance for the subsequent development of pulmonary dysfunction. The risk factors for the most severe ARDS syndrome as defined by Christenson et al[562] include hypertension, current smoking, emergency surgery, congestive heart failure (New York Heart Association Class III and IV), low postoperative cardiac output, and a LV ejection fraction of less than 40%. More recently, Filsoufi et al reported the risk factors for respiratory failure, focusing on valve surgery patients.[577] They studied 2808 patients having risk factors of preoperative renal failure, female sex, ejection fraction less than 30%, double-valve procedures, active endocarditis, advanced age (> 70 years), congestive heart failure, reoperation, emergent procedures, previous myocardial infarction, and prolonged (> 180 minutes) CPB time.

Pathophysiology and Causative Factors

Studies have demonstrated CPB-induced changes in the mechanical properties (i.e., elastance or compliance and resistance) of the pulmonary apparatus (particularly the lung as opposed to the chest wall) and changes in pulmonary capillary permeability. Impairment in gas exchange has been demonstrated to be a result of atelectasis with concomitant overall loss of lung volume.[556,578–582] Most research has focused on the development of increases in pulmonary vascular permeability (leading to various degrees of pulmonary edema) as the principal cause of the impaired gas exchange that occurs during cardiac surgery and results in a high alveolar-arteriolar gradient (A-a Do_2).

The cause of pulmonary dysfunction and ARDS after cardiac surgery is complex but largely revolves around the CPB-induced systemic inflammatory response with its associated increase in pulmonary endothelial permeability.[583,584] A central causative theme is a significant upregulation in the inflammation induced because of the interaction between the blood and foreign surfaces of the heart-lung machine or the inflammation related to the consequences of splanchnic hypoperfusion with the subsequent translocation of significant amounts of endotoxin into the circulation. Endotoxin is proinflammatory, and it has direct effects on the pulmonary vasculature.[585] Clinical studies have demonstrated an increase in circulating intracellular adhesion molecules after CPB in patients with development of acute lung injury.[586] Pathologic examination of the lungs of patients manifesting ARDS has shown extensive injury to the tissue, including swelling and necrosis of endothelial cells and type I and II pneumocytes.[587] In addition to CPB-mediated inflammation, inflammation mediated by endotoxemia has been reported. Several studies have identified transfusion of packed RBCs (> 4 units) as a risk factor for ARDS in the cardiac surgical patient.[588,589] Transfusion-related ARDS has been repeatedly recorded in noncardiac surgical settings.

Pulmonary Thromboembolism

Although not an injury to the lungs occurring as a direct result of CPB itself, deep vein thrombosis (DVT) and pulmonary embolism occur with regular frequency in the cardiac surgical population. The incidence rate of pulmonary embolism after cardiac surgery ranges from 0.3% to 9.5%, with a mortality rate approaching 20%.[326,590,591] The incidence of pulmonary embolism appears to be lower after valve surgery compared with CABG, which may be because of the anticoagulation that is started soon after valve surgery.[591,592]

The incidence rate of DVT is 17% to 46%, with most cases being asymptomatic.[326,591] The greater incidences were reported from series that used lower extremity ultrasound to more comprehensively examine populations.[326] DVT has been reported for the leg from which the saphenous vein grafts were harvested and for the contralateral leg.[591,593] In a study of post-CABG patients (n = 270) admitted to a rehabilitation unit who underwent lower extremity ultrasound examinations, DVT was detected in 17%, with two patients subsequently experiencing development of pulmonary emboli.[594] In a postmortem study in 147 patients after cardiac surgery, pulmonary embolism was the cause of death for 4% (see Chapter 24).

The recommendations for DVT prophylaxis in cardiac surgery are aspirin and elastic gradient compression stockings in patients who ambulate within 2 to 3 days after surgery, and low-molecular-weight heparin and sequential compression stockings in nonambulatory patients.[326] These recommendations are based on a randomized trial in which prophylaxis with sequential pneumatic compression stockings provided no added protection against DVT in ambulating CABG patients treated with aspirin and elastic gradient-compression stockings.[595]

Pulmonary Protection

Ventilatory Strategies

Several studies have examined the use of continuous positive airway pressure during CPB as a means to minimize the decrement in the A-a Do_2 gradient that can occur after surgery. In a small study by Gilbert et al,[596] the effect of continuous positive airway pressure was examined in a randomized trial of 18 patients undergoing CABG surgery with CPB. Continuous positive airway pressure did not appear to make any difference with respect to changes in measured lung resistance and elastance. In a larger (N = 61) study by Berry et al,[597] continuous positive airway pressure did appear to have some transient beneficial effects on A-a Do_2; however, these minor differences dissipated 4 hours after bypass. Overall, it is unlikely that continuous positive airway pressure plays any major role in preventing or treating the pulmonary dysfunction that occurs in the setting of cardiac surgery.

The inspired oxygen content of the gases that the lungs see during the period of apnea during CPB may have an effect on the A-a Do_2 gradient, probably because of the enhanced effect of greater Fio_2 on the atelectasis (so-called absorption atelectasis). With these findings in mind, it would be prudent to reduce the Fio_2 to room air levels during CPB. Several simple therapies can be introduced before separation from CPB, including adequate tracheobronchial toilet and the delivery of several vital capacity breaths that may reduce the amount of atelectasis that has occurred during CPB[568] (Box 28-5; see Chapter 35).

Ventilatory support of patients with acute lung injury (including ARDS) has undergone changes.[598,599] Although not studied specifically in the setting of cardiac surgery, a study authored by the Acute Respiratory Distress Syndrome network highlighted the avoidance of ventilator-associated pulmonary mechanotrauma.[599] Delivery of

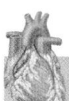

BOX 28-5. STRATEGIES TO PROTECT THE LUNGS

- Reduced Fio_2 during bypass
- Low postoperative tidal volume
- Vital capacity breath before bypass separation
- High-dose steroid avoidance

repeated large tidal volumes may damage the alveoli and other small lung structures, and these mechanical stresses may activate a pulmonary inflammatory response with a local release of cytokines, further enhancing injury to the lungs. As a result, these groups of investigators randomized patients to small (approximately 6 mL/kg) or traditional tidal volumes (12 mL/kg). They demonstrated that the low tidal volume ventilation strategy could reduce mortality in patients with ARDS by up to 25%. It would be prudent to use this beneficial ventilator strategy in the cardiac surgical patient presenting with significant acute lung injury.

Pharmacologic Pulmonary Protection

Steroids

Anti-inflammatory therapies may play a role in moderating the effects of the more significant forms of pulmonary dysfunction that occur after cardiac surgery and that have inflammation as a central causative factor. However, with the exception of corticosteroids, few anti-inflammatory therapies are available for routine use. Corticosteroid use can reduce the amount of systemic inflammation as measured by circulating cytokines.[600-602] However, this has not been coupled with a reduction in pulmonary dysfunction. Chaney et al, in two separate studies,[187,603] demonstrated that relatively high doses of methylprednisolone actually had a detrimental effect on post-CPB pulmonary function. Both studies demonstrated no improvement or worsening in lung compliance, shunt, A-a Do$_2$, and delays in extubation. It was speculated that the A-a Do$_2$ deterioration and delayed pulmonary extubation associated with steroid administration were attributable to steroid-induced sodium retention and vasodilation resulting in increased shunt and increased lung water content with pulmonary edema. Steroid administration led to significant hyperglycemia, which is difficult to treat during CPB.[603] In a similar study by Oliver et al[602] comparing placebo with steroids or hemofiltration, the steroid-treated patients had larger increases in postoperative A-a Do$_2$ gradients. Using a preset mechanical ventilation protocol to guide ventilation weaning, steroids again failed to reduce the time to tracheal extubation (519 ± 293 vs. 618 ± 405 minutes; $P = 0.21$), confirming Chaney et al's[603] findings.

Aprotinin

The nonspecific serum protease inhibitor aprotinin was used to reduce blood loss and transfusion after cardiac surgery, and there is some evidence that it reduced CPB-related systemic inflammation.[604-606] Aprotinin was first investigated for use in the setting of cardiac surgery as a means to protect the lungs from the whole-body inflammatory response initiated as a result of the contact activation of blood with the foreign surfaces of the CPB apparatus.[607,608] These studies serendipitously discovered aprotinin's salutary effect on preventing blood loss and transfusion in cardiac surgery.[609] After these studies, aprotinin was extensively evaluated for its blood loss and transfusion-sparing effects, with little further work focused on the pulmonary effects. Despite being a robust inhibitor of CPB-related inflammatory response, any ability to prevent the pulmonary complications of CPB has not yet been demonstrated.

Nitric Oxide

Consistent sequelae of pulmonary dysfunction include the development of variable degrees of increased pulmonary vascular resistance and pulmonary hypertension. As a result, several pulmonary vasodilators have been used, most notably inhaled NO, in an attempt to reduce the pulmonary artery pressures and with it the workload of the right ventricle.[610-612]

NO has been used in cardiac surgery and in heart and lung transplantation as a selective pulmonary vasodilator.[613] However, no trials have demonstrated any beneficial use for its prophylactic administration in the setting of cardiac surgery. Although it has statistically significantly reduced pulmonary artery pressures in cardiac surgery, it is unclear whether these reductions are reflected in improvements in overall outcome.

MANAGEMENT OF BYPASS: AN OVERVIEW

The Prebypass Period

An important objective is to prepare the patient properly for CPB (Box 28-6). This phase invariably involves two key steps: anticoagulation and vascular cannulation. With rare exception,[614] heparin is still the anticoagulant clinically used for CPB. Dose, method of administration, and opinions as to what constitutes adequate anticoagulation vary. Heparin must be administered before cannulation for CPB, even if cannulation must be done emergently. Failure to do so is to risk thrombosis in both the patient and extracorporeal circuit. Chapters 30 and 31 offer a complete discussion of hemostasis management for the cardiac surgery patient. After heparin has been administered, a period of at least 3 minutes is customarily allowed for systemic circulation and onset of effect. An activated coagulation time or heparin concentration measurement demonstrating actual achievement of adequate anticoagulation is then performed.

Vascular Cannulation

The next major step in the prebypass phase is vascular cannulation. The goal of vascular cannulation is to provide access whereby the CPB pump may divert all systemic venous blood to the pump oxygenator at the lowest possible venous pressures and deliver oxygenated blood to the arterial circulation at pressure and flow sufficient to maintain systemic homeostasis (see Chapter 29).

Arterial Cannulation

Arterial cannulation generally is established before venous cannulation to allow volume resuscitation of the patient, should it be necessary. The ascending aorta is the preferred site for aortic cannulation because it is easily accessible, does not require an additional incision, accommodates a larger cannula to provide greater flow at a reduced pressure, and carries a lower risk for aortic dissection compared with other arterial cannulation sites (femoral or iliac arteries). Because hypertension increases the risk for aortic dissection during cannulation, the aortic pressure may be temporarily reduced (MAP < 70 mm Hg) during aortotomy and cannula insertion. Several potential complications are associated with aortic cannulation including embolization of air or atheromatous debris, inadvertent cannulation of aortic arch vessels, aortic dissection, and other vessel wall injury.[615-620]

Reviews and clinical reports emphasize the importance of embolization as the major mechanism of focal cerebral injury in cardiac surgery patients. Barzilai et al[621] and Wareing et al[616] reported intraoperative use of two-dimensional epiaortic ultrasound imaging as a guide to selection of cross-clamping and cannulation sites. In 24% and 33% of the patients in these studies, respectively, ultrasonic findings led to selection of alternate cannulation sites. A femoral or axillary artery, rather than the ascending aorta, can be cannulated for systemic perfusion. These alternate sites can be used when ascending aortic cannulation is considered relatively contraindicated, as in severe aortic atherosclerosis, aortic aneurysm or dissection, or known cystic medial necrosis.[8,118,622,623] The anesthesiologist can look for evidence of cannula malposition by checking for unilateral blanching of the face, gently palpating carotid artery pulses for new unilateral diminution,

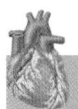

BOX 28-6. MANAGEMENT BEFORE CARDIOPULMONARY BYPASS

- Anticoagulation
- Cannulation of the heart
- Careful monitoring to minimize organ dysfunction

and by measuring blood pressure in both arms to check for new asymmetries. However, robust assessments of CBFs can be made more reliably with the use of near-infrared spectroscopy cerebral oximetry (see Chapter 16).

Venous Cannulation

Venous cannulation can be achieved using a single atrial cannula that is inserted into the right atrium and directed inferiorly (Figure 28-11). Drainage holes in this multistage cannula are located in the inferior vena cava (IVC) and right atrium to drain blood returning from the lower extremities and the SVC and coronary sinus, respectively. This technique has the advantage of being simpler, faster, and requiring only one incision; however, the quality of drainage can be compromised easily when the heart is lifted for surgical exposure.[624] The bicaval cannulation technique, required in cases in which right atrial access is necessary, involves cannulating the SVC and IVC (Figure 28-12). Loops placed around the vessels can be tightened to divert all caval blood flow away from the heart. Blood returning to the right atrium from the coronary sinus will not be drained using this technique, so an additional vent or atriotomy is necessary.

During CPB, blood will continue to return to the left ventricle from a variety of sources, including the bronchial and thebesian veins, as well as blood that traverses the pulmonary circulation. Abnormal sources of venous blood include a persistent left SVC, systemic-to-pulmonary shunts, and aortic regurgitation. It is important to avoid LV filling and distention during CPB to prevent myocardial rewarming, minimize LV wall tension, and limit myocardial oxygen demand.[625] This can be accomplished with the use of a vent placed in the left ventricle via the left superior pulmonary vein. Alternate sites include

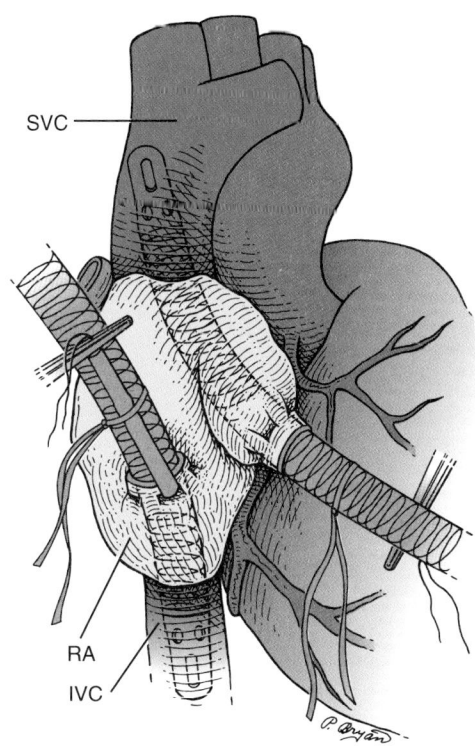

Figure 28-12 Position of two-vessel cannulation of right atrium (RA) with placement of drainage holes into superior vena cava (SVC) and inferior vena cava (IVC). The aortic cannula is not shown. *(From Connolly MW: Cardiopulmonary Bypass. New York, Springer-Verlag, 1995, p 59.)*

the pulmonary artery, the aortic root, or directly into the left ventricle via the ventricular apex.

Venous cannulae, using a multistage or bicaval cannula, are large and can impair venous return from the IVC or SVC. Superior vena caval obstruction is detected by venous engorgement of the head and neck, conjunctival edema, and increased SVC pressure. IVC obstruction is far more insidious, presenting only as decreased filling pressures and lowered venous return to the bypass circuit.

Femoral venous cannulation is sometimes used for CPB without, or before, sternotomy or right atrial cannulation (e.g., redos, ascending aortic aneurysms). Because of their comparatively small size and long length, venous return can be impaired but is optimized when the tip of the cannula is advanced (under TEE guidance) until it is placed at the level of the vena cava–right atrium junction. Kinetic or vacuum-assisted negative pressure can be applied to further enhance drainage.

Other Preparations

Once anticoagulation and cannulation are complete, CPB can be instituted. Because there is redundant pulmonary artery catheter (PAC) length in the right ventricle, and the heart is manipulated during CPB, there is a tendency for distal migration of the catheter into pulmonary artery branches.[626] This distal migration of the catheter increases the risks for "overwedging" and pulmonary artery damage. During the prebypass phase, it is advisable to withdraw the PAC 3 to 5 cm to decrease the likelihood of these untoward events. It also is advisable to check the integrity of all vascular access and monitoring devices. A PAC placed through an external jugular[627,628] or subclavian vein[629] can become kinked or occluded on full opening of the sternal retractor. If TEE is being used, the probe should be placed in the "freeze" mode and the tip of the scope placed in the neutral and unlocked position. Leaving the electronic scanning emitter turned on during hypothermic CPB adds heat (in older TEE equipment models) to the esophagus and posterior wall of the ventricle.

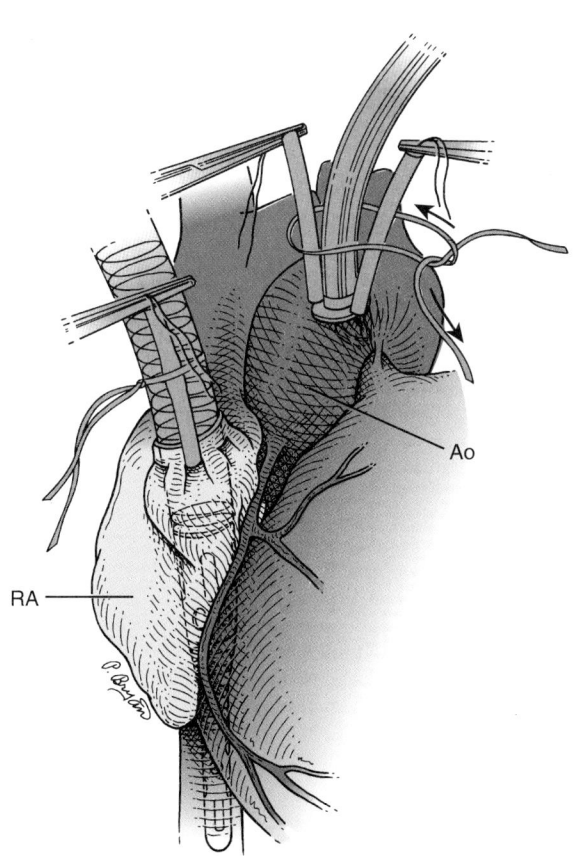

Figure 28-11 Aortic (Ao) and single, double-staged, right atrial (RA) cannulation. Notice the drainage holes of venous cannula in right atrium and inferior vena cava. *(From Connolly MW: Cardiopulmonary Bypass. New York, Springer-Verlag, 1995, p 59.)*

TABLE 28-12	Preparation for Bypass: Prebypass Checklist

1. Anticoagulation
   a. Heparin administered
   b. Desired level of anticoagulation achieved
2. Arterial cannulation
   a. Absence of bubbles in arterial line
   b. Evidence of dissection or malposition?
3. Venous cannulation
   a. Evidence of superior vena cava obstruction?
   b. Evidence of inferior vena cava obstruction?
4. Pulmonary artery catheter (if used) pulled back
5. Are all monitoring/access catheters functional?
6. Transesophageal echocardiograph (if used)
   a. In "freeze" mode
   b. Scope in neutral/unlocked position
7. Supplemental medications
   a. Neuromuscular blockers
   b. Anesthetics, analgesics, amnestics
8. Inspection of head and neck
   a. Color
   b. Symmetry
   c. Venous drainage
   d. Pupils

TABLE 28-13	Checklist for Bypass Procedure

1. Assess arterial inflow
   Is arterial perfusate oxygenated?
   Is direction of arterial inflow appropriate?
   Evidence of arterial dissection?
   Patient's arterial pressure persistently low?
   Inflow line pressure high?
   Pump/oxygenator reservoir level declining?
   Evidence of atrial cannula malposition?
   Patient's arterial pressure persistently high or low?
   Unilateral facial swelling, discoloration?
   Symmetrical cerebral oximetry?
2. Assess venous outflow
   Is blood draining to the pump/oxygenator's venous reservoir?
   Evidence of SVC obstruction?
   Facial venous engorgement or congestion, CVP increased?
3. Is bypass complete?
   High-CVP/low-PA pressure?
   Impaired venous drainage?
   Low-CVP/high-PA pressure?
   Large bronchial venous blood flow?
   Aortic insufficiency?
   Arterial and PA pressure nonpulsatile?
   Desired pump flow established?
4. Discontinue drug and fluid administration
5. Discontinue ventilation and inhalation drugs to patient's lungs

CVP, central venous pressure; PA, pulmonary artery; SVC, superior vena cava.

Before initiating CPB, the anesthesiologist should assess the depth of anesthesia and adequacy of muscle relaxation. It is important to maintain paralysis to prevent patient movement that could result in dislodgment of bypass circuit cannulae and prevent shivering as hypothermia is induced (with the attendant increases in oxygen consumption).[630] It often is difficult to determine the depth of anesthesia during the various stages of CPB. Because blood pressure, heart rate, pupil diameter, and the autonomic nervous system are profoundly affected by ECC (e.g., the heart is asystolic; blood pressure is greatly influenced by circuit blood flow; sweating occurs with rewarming), these variables do not reliably reflect the anesthetic state. Although hypothermia decreases anesthetic requirements, it is necessary to provide analgesia, hypnosis, and muscle relaxation during CPB. Useful adjuncts to assessing depth of anesthesia are available in the form of processed EEG devices. For example, the bispectral index has proved useful in preventing awareness during cardiac surgery.[631] With the initiation of CPB and hemodilution, blood levels of anesthetics and muscle relaxants will acutely decrease. However, plasma protein concentrations also decrease, which increases the free-fraction and active drug concentrations. Every drug has a specific kinetic profile during CPB, and kinetics and pharmacodynamics during CPB will vary greatly among patients. Many clinicians administer additional muscle relaxants and opioids at the initiation of CPB. A vaporizer for potent inhalation drugs may be included in the bypass circuit. Hall et al[632] presented an extended discussion of pharmacokinetics and bypass. A final inspection of the head and neck for color, symmetry, adequacy of venous drainage (neck vein and conjunctiva engorgement), and pupil equality is reasonable to serve as a baseline for the anesthetic state. A summary of preparatory steps to be accomplished during the prebypass phase is given in Table 28-12.

INITIATION AND DISCONTINUATION OF BYPASS SUPPORT

Initiation of Cardiopulmonary Bypass

Uncomplicated Initiation

Once all preparatory steps have been taken, the perfusionist progressively increases delivery of oxygenated blood to the patient's arterial system, as systemic venous blood is diverted from the patient's right side of the heart, maintaining the pump's venous reservoir volume. After full flow is achieved, all systemic venous blood is (ideally) drained from the patient to the pump reservoir. An on-CPB checklist of issues to address shortly after initiation of bypass can serve as a valuable safety tool (Table 28-13). The central venous pressure (CVP) and pulmonary arterial pressure should decrease to near zero (2 to 5 mm Hg), whereas systemic flow, arterial pressure, and oxygenation are maintained at desired values.

Hypotension with Onset of Bypass

Systemic arterial hypotension (MAP = 30 to 40 mm Hg) is relatively common on initiation of CPB. Gordon et al[633] proposed that much of this could be explained by the acute reduction of blood viscosity that results from hemodilution with nonblood priming solutions. These investigators proposed systemic vascular resistance (SVR = MAP − CVP/CO) to be the product of blood viscosity (η) and inherent systemic vascular hindrance: SVR = $\eta \bullet$SVH. MAP increases with initiation of hypothermia-induced vasoconstriction, together with levels of endogenous catecholamines and angiotensin. The hemodilution also results in the loss of NO binding by hemoglobin[634]; the excess free NO can lead to further vasodilation. Treatment with α-agonists *usually* is not necessary if the hypotension is brief (< 60 seconds). Of concern is the potential for myocardial and cerebral ischemia because hypothermia has not yet been achieved.

Until the aortic cross-clamp is applied, the coronary arteries are perfused with hemodiluted, nonpulsatile blood. Schaff et al[635] showed that subendocardial ischemia occurred in the distribution of critical coronary stenosis when MAP was less than 80 mm Hg in the normothermic empty beating heart. If placement of the aortic cross-clamp is delayed, MAP should be maintained in the range of 60 to 80 mm Hg to support myocardial perfusion, especially in the presence of known coronary stenosis or ventricular hypertrophy. This arterial pressure is likely adequate to maintain CBF until hypothermia is induced.

Unless pulsatile perfusion is used, once at full flow, the arterial pressure waveform should be nonpulsatile except for small (5- to 10-mm Hg) sinusoidal deflections created by the roller pump heads. Continued pulsatile arterial pressure indicates that the left ventricle is receiving blood from some source.

Pump Flow and Pressure during Bypass

Pump flow during CPB represents a careful balance between the conflicting demands of surgical visualization and adequate oxygen delivery. Two different approaches exist. The first is to maintain oxygen delivery during ECC at normal levels for a given core temperature. Although this may limit hypoperfusion, it does increase the delivered embolic load. The second approach is to use the lowest flows that do not result in end-organ injury. This approach offers the potential advantage of less embolic delivery, as well as potentially improved myocardial protection and surgical visualization.[636,637] However, some of these advantages are not seen when the left ventricle is vented during CPB.[638]

During CPB, pump flow and pressure are related through overall arterial impedance, a product of hemodilution, temperature, and arterial cross-sectional area. This is important because the first two factors, hemodilution and temperature, are critical determinants of pump flow requirements. Pump flows of $1.2\,L/min/m^2$ perfuse most of the microcirculation when the hematocrit is near 22% and hypothermic CPB is being used.[639] However, at lower hematocrits or periods of higher oxygen consumption, these flows become inadequate.[640–642] Because of changes in oxygen demand with temperature and the plateauing of oxygen consumption with increasing flow, a series of nomograms have been developed for pump flow selection (Figure 28-13).

In addition to use of these nomograms, most perfusion teams also monitor mixed venous saturation, targeting levels of 70% or greater. Unfortunately, this level does not guarantee adequate perfusion of all tissue beds because some (muscle, subcutaneous fat) may be functionally removed from circulation during CPB.[642] Hypothermic venous saturation may overestimate end-organ reserves.[643] Slater et al[547] characterized the hierarchy of regional blood flows during CPB at 27° C. Animals were perfused at pump blood flows of 1.9, 1.6, 1.3, and $1.0\,L/min/m^2$. Regional perfusion of various end organs (brain, kidney, small intestine, pancreas, and muscle) was quantified with a fluorescent microsphere technique. CBF was unchanged at the three highest pump flows. Renal perfusion was maintained at flows of 1.9 and $1.6\,L/min/m^2$. Perfusion to the pancreas was constant at all flows studied, and small-bowel perfusion varied linearly with pump flow. Muscle bed flows were decreased at all flows. This study confirmed previous work regarding end-organ perfusion during CPB and highlighted the vulnerability of the kidneys to reduced flows at moderate hypothermia (see Chapter 29).

During CPB, most of the outcomes studied in relation to pump flow are those related to the organs at high risk for ischemic injury (i.e., kidney and brain). Much work has been devoted to examining the relation between renal dysfunction and pump flow.[300,305,644,645] Preexisting renal disease is a consistent predictor of postoperative renal dysfunction, the incidence of which ranges between 3% and 5%. Renal function appears unaltered when pump flows greater than $1.6\,L/min/m^2$ are used,[644] but whether this management will affect outcomes

in patients with preexisting renal dysfunction is less clear.[645] Because of autoregulation, most studies,[170,646] but not all,[647] suggest that CBF is unaltered by variation in pump flow. At low-flow states, CBF probably is more dependent on perfusion pressure.[648–650]

Preparation for Separation

Before discontinuation of CPB, conditions that optimize cardiac and pulmonary function must be restored. To a great extent, this is achieved by reversing the processes and techniques used to initiate and maintain CPB (Table 28-14).

Potential for Patient Awareness

It is not uncommon for patients to sweat during rewarming. This almost certainly is caused by perfusion of the hypothalamus (i.e., the thermoregulatory site) with blood that is warmer than the latter organ's set point (37° C). The brain is a high-flow organ and can be assumed to equilibrate fairly quickly (10 to 15 minutes) with cerebral perfusate temperature (i.e., nasopharyngeal temperature). A less likely but more disturbing possibility is that restoration of brain normothermia with decreased anesthetic concentration may result in inadequate depth of anesthesia and the potential for awareness. It is estimated that awareness occurs during cardiac surgery in approximately 0.1% of patients.[631]

The following suggestions are made to attempt to limit the possibility and sequelae of awareness during cardiac surgery with CPB. During the preoperative evaluation, the possibility of awareness and why it could occur should be discussed with the patient. Use of volatile agents for their amnestic properties should be considered. During the postoperative visit, a mechanism whereby the patient can freely communicate perioperative experiences should be provided. Necessary support, including counseling, to minimize potential long-term psychologic problems should be provided if awareness is reported.

Patient movement before discontinuation of CPB is, at the least, extremely disruptive and may be genuinely life-threatening if it results in cannula dislodgment or disruption of the procedure. Additional muscle relaxant should be administered. If awareness is suspected, supplemental amnestics or anesthetics should be administered during rewarming. Because sweating stops almost immediately on discontinuation of CPB, continued sweating after emergence from CPB may be a sign of awareness. Neurologic monitors such as the bispectral index can be used to help judge the depth of anesthesia during and after weaning from CPB.[651]

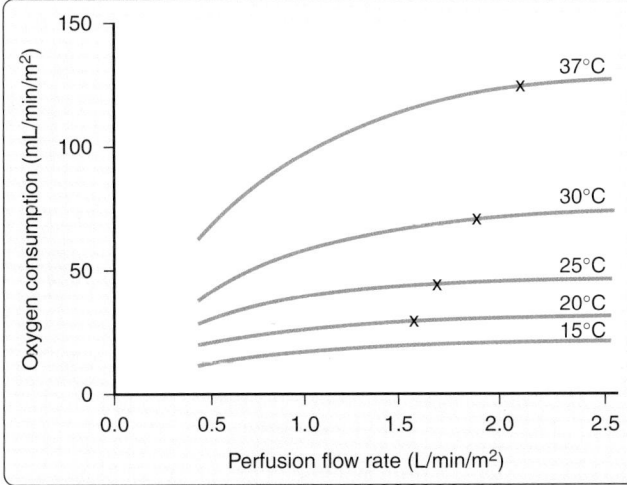

Figure 28-13 Nomogram depicting the relation of oxygen consumption (Vo₂) to perfusion flow rate and temperature. The X on the curves represents common clinically used flow rates at the various temperatures. (From Kirklin JW, Barratt-Boyes BG: Cardiac Surgery. New York, Wiley, 1986, p 35.)

TABLE 28-14 Preparation for Separation-from-Bypass Checklist

1. Air clearance maneuvers completed
2. Rewarming completed
   a. Nasopharyngeal temperature 36–37° C
   b. Rectal/bladder temperature ≥ 35° C, but ≤ 37° C
3. Address issue of adequacy of anesthesia and muscle relaxation
4. Obtain stable cardiac rate and rhythm (use pacing if necessary)
5. Pump flow and systemic arterial pressure
   a. Pump flow to maintain mixed venous saturation ≥ 70%
   b. Systemic pressure restored to normothermic levels
6. Metabolic parameters
   a. Arterial pH, Po₂, Pco₂ within normal limits
   b. Hct: 20–25%
   c. K⁺: 4.0–5.0 mEq/L
   d. Ionized calcium
7. Are all monitoring/access catheters functional?
   a. Transducers rezeroed
   b. TEE (if used) out of freeze mode
8. Respiratory management
   a. Atelectasis cleared/lungs re-expanded
   b. Evidence of pneumothorax?
   c. Residual fluid in thoracic cavities drained
   d. Ventilation reinstituted
9. Intravenous fluids restarted
10. Inotropes/vasopressors/vasodilators prepared

Hct, hematocrit; TEE, transesophageal echocardiography.

Rewarming

When systemic hypothermia is used, body temperature is restored to normothermia by gradually increasing perfusate temperature with the heat exchanger. Time required for rewarming (i.e., heat transfer) varies with arterial perfusate temperature, patient temperature, and systemic flow. Excessive perfusate heating is not advisable for at least three key reasons: possible denaturation of plasma proteins, possible cerebral hyperthermia, and the fact that dissolved gas can come out of solution and coalesce into bubbles if the temperature gradient is too great. Because small increases (0.5° C) in cerebral temperature exacerbate ischemic injury in the brain, it is critical to perfuse the patient with blood temperatures at or below 37° C. Although this will increase the duration of rewarming, the risk for hyperthermic brain injury is increased greatly with hyperthermic blood temperatures. Most centers now use mild hypothermia (i.e., systemic temperature = 31° C to 34° C) instead of moderate hypothermia (26° C to 28° C), reducing the amount of heat transfer required to achieve normothermia during rewarming.

Rewarming may be enhanced by increasing pump flow, which thereby increases heat input. At levels of hypothermia routinely used (25° C to 30° C), the patient behaves as if vasoconstricted (calculated SVR is relatively high). Increasing pump flow in this setting may result in unacceptable hypertension. There are two approaches to this problem: wait out the vasoconstriction or pharmacologically induce patient vasodilation. When rectal or bladder temperature approaches 30° C to 32° C, patients appear to rapidly vasodilate. This is probably the result of decreasing blood viscosity or relaxation of cold-induced vasoconstriction with warming. Increasing pump flow at this point serves several purposes: increased heat transfer, support of systemic arterial pressure, and increased oxygen delivery in the face of increasing oxygen consumption. Often, waiting for the patient to spontaneously "vasodilate" is sufficient, and with subsequent increased pump flows, rewarming will be adequate at separation from ECC support. Circumstances in which more aggressive rewarming may be necessary include profound hypothermia with a large hypoperfused "heat sink" and late initiation of warming by accident or design.

Skeletal muscle and subcutaneous fat are relatively hypoperfused during CPB. These tissues cool slowly and are also slow to warm. Temperatures at high-flow regions (e.g., esophagus, nasopharynx) do not reflect the temperature of these tissues. Davis et al[652] reported that restoration of normothermia (as monitored at high-flow sites) led to a net heat deficit after CPB, with subsequent recooling after emergence (i.e., after-drop). Pharmacologic vasodilation allows an earlier increase in pump flow and delivery of warmed arterial blood to low-flow beds, making the rewarming process more uniform. Noback and Tinker[653] used sodium nitroprusside ($3.5 \pm 0.8 \mu g/kg/min$) to permit increased pump flows during warming, from 4.0 to 4.5 L/min, keeping MAP at approximately 70 mm Hg. Compared with a group who were warmed without sodium nitroprusside for an equivalent period, the sodium nitroprusside group had much greater peripheral warming and a much smaller decline in postbypass temperature. Arteriolar vasodilators (e.g., nicardipine, sodium nitroprusside) are much more likely to be effective in this process than venodilators (e.g., nitroglycerin). Other aids to warming during or after CPB are sterile forced-air rewarming devices and servoregulated systems,[654] as well as heating blankets, warmed fluids,[655] heated humidified gases,[656] and increased room temperature. The issue of after-drop is less of a concern during routine cardiac surgery but manifests frequently in patients after deep hypothermic circulatory arrest (DHCA).

Unfortunately, there is a narrow range for acceptable systemic temperatures at the end of CPB. Just as temperatures that are "too hot" increase the risk for cerebral injury, those that are "too cool" may lead to inadequate rewarming and the problem of shivering, increased oxygen consumption and carbon dioxide production, and coagulopathies. It is imperative to prevent cerebral hyperthermia in patients undergoing CPB. Additional heat may be added to the patient with the use of external heating devices *after* discontinuation of CPB support. This approach can prevent the complications of hypothermia without the use of hyperthermic blood.

Targets for rectal or bladder temperature before separation from CPB vary among institutions. Nathan and Polis[657] surveyed 28 Canadian centers regarding temperature monitoring practices during cardiac surgery and found the use of a variety of monitoring sites (Figure 28-14). Many centers failed to use monitors likely to reflect cerebral temperatures routinely—not one center studied routinely monitored tympanic membrane temperature, and only slightly more than half monitored nasopharyngeal temperatures. The investigators were unable to discern any uniformity of practice regarding monitors or rewarming temperature end points. In general, temperatures measured at highly perfused tissues exceeded 37° C at the end of CPB in most centers.

Cook et al[658] reported that cerebral hyperthermia occurs with rewarming. They studied 10 cardiac surgery patients requiring hypothermic CPB, and measured nasopharyngeal and cerebral venous temperatures (monitored at the jugular bulb). Ten minutes after the onset of rewarming from 27° C, cerebral venous temperature was 37° C, but nasopharyngeal temperature was only 34° C ± 2.9° C. After 18 minutes of rewarming, nasopharyngeal temperature reached 37° C and cerebral venous temperature was 38.2° C ± 1.1° C. Peak central venous temperature exceeded 39° C for an average of 15 minutes in all 10 patients before the termination of CPB.

Nathan and Polis[657] found a substantial difference between tympanic membrane and urinary bladder temperature in 11 patients rewarmed after hypothermic CPB (Figure 28-15). The peak temperature for each patient was aligned at minute zero; temperatures were displayed for 30 minutes before (−30 to 0 minutes) and after (0 to 30 minutes) the peak temperature. There was a smooth increase in bladder temperature from 31.4° C to 36° C, but an "overshoot" in peak tympanic membrane temperature to a mean of 38.6° C (range, 37.7° C to 39.7° C). Because tympanic membrane temperature better reflects cerebral temperature than bladder temperature, it is likely that all 11 patients were exposed to hyperthermic cerebral temperatures.

Restoration of Systemic Arterial Pressure to Normothermic Value

After aortic cross-clamp release, the heart again is perfused through the native coronary arteries. Until the proximal anastomoses are made, myocardial perfusion may be compromised in the presence of a low

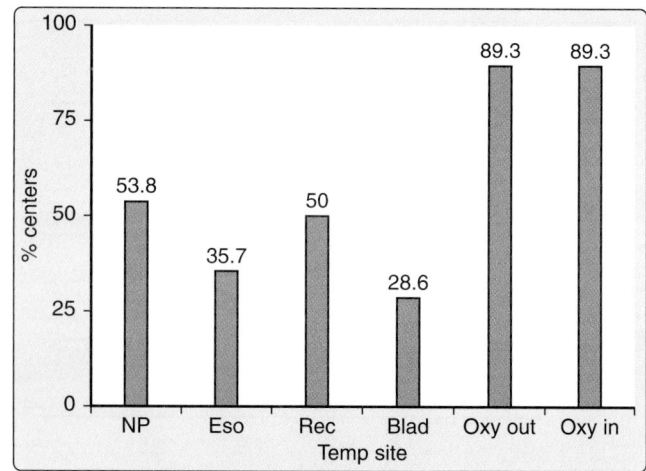

Figure 28-14 **Temperature monitoring sites in 30 adult cardiac surgery centers in Canada.** Blad, bladder; Eso, esophageal; NP, nasopharyngeal; Oxy In, oxygenator inlet; Oxy Out, oxygenator outlet; Rec, rectal. (*From Nathan HJ, Polis T: The management of temperature during hypothermic cardiopulmonary bypass. I. Canadian Survey. Can J Anaesth 42:672, 1995.*)

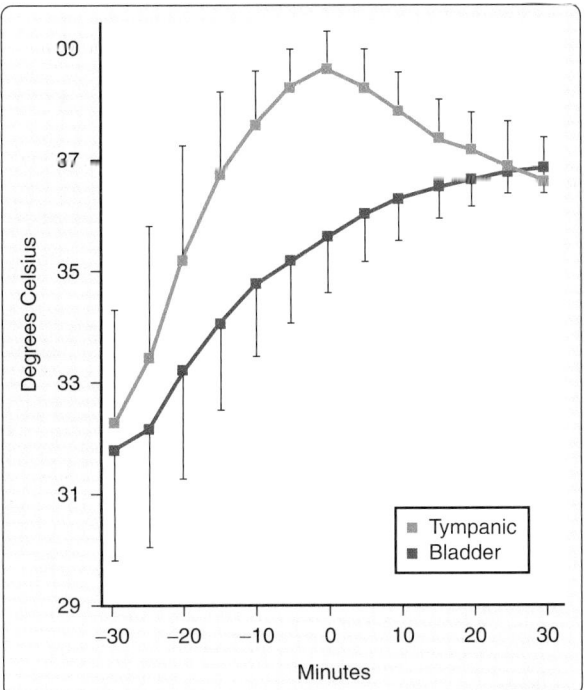

Figure 28-15   Tympanic and bladder temperatures during rewarming. Time 0 = maximum temperature achieved. Means ± standard deviation are shown. *(From Nathan JH, Polis T: The management of temperature during hypothermic cardiopulmonary bypass. I. Canadian Survey. Can J Anaesth 42:672, 1995.)*

MAP. Consequently, it is advisable to gradually increase MAP during rewarming to levels approximately 70 to 80 mm Hg.

With discontinuation of CPB, a marked discrepancy often exists between blood pressure readings measured from the radial artery and the central aorta. Radial arterial catheters may underestimate central aortic systolic pressures by 10 to 40 mm Hg. Discrepancies in MAP tend to be of a lesser magnitude (5 to 15 mm Hg). Such a discrepancy is not present before CPB, nor is it present after CPB in all patients. Mechanisms are undefined, but evidence supports vasodilatory and arteriovenous shunting phenomena in the forearm and hand.[659] Gravlee et al[660] found that systolic pressure differences after CPB were not significantly influenced by duration of CPB, use of sodium nitroprusside or phenylephrine during the final 15 minutes of CPB, SVR, minimum CPB temperature, CPB separation temperature, or duration of rewarming. Blood pressure readings from brachial or femoral arterial catheters tend to more accurately reflect central aortic pressure. It is unknown at what point during CPB radial artery-central aortic blood pressure discrepancies develop, but most investigators report their resolution 20 to 90 minutes after discontinuation of CPB (see Chapter 14).

If measured radial arterial pressure is suspected to be low in relation to central aortic pressure, several actions can be taken. The surgeon can estimate central aortic pressure by palpation of the ascending aorta; the surgeon can place a small needle in the aortic lumen or use an aortic cannula to allow temporary monitoring of aortic pressure, or place a femoral arterial catheter.

Removal of Intracardiac Air

At the end of the procedure, intracardiac air is present in virtually all cases that require opening the heart (i.e., valve repair or replacement, aneurysmectomy, septal defect repair, repair of other congenital lesions).[661] In such cases, it is important to remove as much air as possible before resumption of ejection. Surgical techniques differ. With the aortic cross-clamp still applied, the surgeon or perfusionist can partially limit venous return and LV vent flow, causing the left atrium and left

ventricle to fill with blood. Through a transventricular approach, the left ventricle then can be aspirated. The left atrium and left ventricle are balloted to dislodge bubbles, and the cycle is repeated. The operating table can be rotated from side to side and the lungs ventilated to promote clearance of air from the pulmonary veins. Rather than transventricular aspiration, some surgeons vent air through the cardioplegia cannula or a needle vent in the ascending aorta. Before removal of the aortic cross-clamp, the patient is placed head down so that bubbles will float away from the dependent carotid arteries. Some surgeons favor temporary manual carotid occlusion before cross-clamp removal, but safety and efficacy of this potentially dangerous maneuver are undocumented. A venting cannula often is left in the aorta at a location that should allow air pickup after resumption of ejection.

Oka et al,[661] using TEE, have shown that routine air clearance techniques are not completely effective. Transcranial Doppler studies document a high incidence of intracranial gas emboli on release of the aortic cross-clamp or resumption of ejection. Oka et al[661] described three essential elements of air removal: mobilization of air by positive chamber filling, stretching of the atrial wall, and repeated chamber ballottement; removal of mobilized air by continuous ascending aortic venting; and proof of elimination by TEE. The investigators contended that using these techniques could completely eliminate intracardiac air. Carbon dioxide gas insufflated by gravity into open cardiac chambers during CPB helps replace nitrogen in the bubbles with a more soluble gas. Accordingly, the persistence of gas bubbles observed by TEE after release of the aortic cross-clamp was lower in patients exposed to CO_2 in the chest wound than in the controls. However, CO_2 insufflation should be used in addition to, rather than instead of, other deairing maneuvers.[662]

Intracardiac air may be present in 10% to 30% of closed cardiac cases as well (e.g., CABG).[661] Robicsek and Duncan[663] demonstrated that during aortic cross-clamping, air may enter the aorta and left ventricle retrograde through native coronary arteries opened in the course of CABG surgery, particularly when suction is applied to vent the left side of the heart or aortic root. They suggested that efforts to expel air from the LV and aortic root should be routine before unclamping the aorta. It is unclear to what extent gas emboli originating from the heart and aorta contribute to neurologic injury. Oka et al[661] found most patients in whom LV microbubbles were detected to be free of major neurologic injury. This result is in agreement with the findings of several investigators who detected LV and cerebral microbubbles for various periods after CPB without apparent neurologic sequelae. However, microembolic load correlates with magnitude of cognitive dysfunction.[664] Other studies reported that air ejected from the left ventricle also can travel to the coronary arteries, resulting in sudden and sometimes extreme myocardial ischemia and failure after separation from CPB.

Defibrillation

Before discontinuation of CPB, the heart must have an organized rhythm that is spontaneous or pacer induced. Ventricular fibrillation (VF), common after cross-clamp release and warming, often will spontaneously convert to some other rhythm. Prolonged VF is undesirable during rewarming for at least three reasons: Subendocardial perfusion is compromised in the presence of normothermic VF; myocardial oxygen consumption is greater with VF compared with a beating heart at normothermia; and if the left ventricle receives a large amount of blood (aortic insufficiency or bronchial return) in the absence of mechanical contraction, the left ventricle may distend. LV distention increases wall tension and further compromises subendocardial perfusion. However, early resumption of mechanical contraction may make some surgical procedures difficult (e.g., modification of distal anastomoses).

Defibrillation, when necessary, is accomplished with internal paddles at much lower energies than would be used for external cardioversion. In the adult, starting energies of 5 to 10 J are routine. Defibrillation is less effective when the heart has not fully rewarmed, and it rarely is successful if myocardial (perfusate) temperature is less than 30° C.[665]

Repeated attempts at defibrillation, particularly with escalating energy levels, can lead to myocardial injury. If defibrillation is not successful after two to four attempts, options include further warming, correction of blood gas and electrolyte abnormalities if present (high Po_2 and high normal serum potassium [K^+] seem favorable), increased MAP, and antiarrhythmic therapy. Bolus administration of 100 mg lidocaine before the release of the cross-clamp significantly reduces the incidence of reperfusion VF.[666] Increasing coronary perfusion by increasing MAP is believed to result in myocardial reperfusion and recovery of the energy state. Larger loading doses of antiarrhythmics will be necessary to achieve therapeutic concentrations because of the larger CPB volume of distribution.

Restoration of Ventilation

With discontinuation of CPB, the venous outflow line gradually is occluded and pulmonary arterial blood flow restored. Studies disagree as to the nature and magnitude of pulmonary dysfunction after CPB, and various aspects of this problem were discussed earlier. Some studies have found evidence of increased deadspace/tidal volume ratio (Vd/Vt) after CPB, whereas others have not.[667] Increased Vd/Vt would result in less effective alveolar ventilation than prebypass, which would result in increased $Paco_2$. Other studies reported modest increases in pulmonary shunt fraction after CPB, which leads to less effective oxygenation and decreased Pao_2. Catastrophic bypass-induced pulmonary injury with severe hypoxemia immediately on discontinuation of CPB is exceedingly uncommon in adults.

Before discontinuation of CPB, the lungs must be reinflated. Positive pressure (20 to 40 cm H_2O) is applied repeatedly until all areas of atelectasis are visually reinflated. Attention is specifically directed at the left lower lobe, which seems more difficult to re-expand. Fluid that has collected in the thoracic cavities during CPB is removed by the surgeon, and if the pleural cavity has not been opened, evidence of pneumothorax is also sought. The ventilatory rate can be increased 10% to 20% above prebypass values to compensate for increased Vd/Vt if present. Ventilation is resumed with 100% oxygen, and subsequent adjustments in Fio_2 are made based on arterial blood gas analysis and pulse oximetry.

Correction of Metabolic Abnormalities and Arterial Oxygen Saturation

When rewarming is nearly complete and separation from CPB is anticipated to occur in 10 to 15 minutes, an arterial blood sample is taken and analyzed for acid-base status, Po_2, Pco_2, hemoglobin or hematocrit, potassium, glucose, and ionized calcium.

Oxygen-Carrying Capacity

Generally, a hematocrit of at least 20% to 25% is sought before discontinuation of bypass. The primary compensatory mechanism to ensure adequate systemic oxygen delivery in the presence of normovolemic anemia is increased CO. Increased CO results in an increased myocardial oxygen need, which is met by increased coronary oxygen delivery by coronary vasodilation. The lower limit of the hematocrit, below which increased CO can no longer support systemic oxygen needs, is reported to be 17% to 20% in dogs with *completely healthy hearts.*[668] With increases in systemic Vo_2, such as occur with exercise, fever, or shivering, greater values of the hematocrit are required. Patients with good ventricular function and good coronary reserve (or good revascularization) might be expected to tolerate hematocrit values in the 20s. When ventricular function is impaired or revascularization is incomplete, hematocrit greater than 25% may aid in support of the systemic circulation and concomitantly lower myocardial oxygen requirements on discontinuation of CPB.

When pump or oxygenator reservoir volume is in excess, the hematocrit can be increased by use of hemofiltration. As Klineberg et al[669] described, application of a hydrostatic pressure gradient across a porous membrane results in transport of water and low-molecular-weight solutes (molecular weight, 500 to 50,000). Ultrafiltrate composition is similar to glomerular filtrate with solute concentrations identical to that of plasma water (see Chapter 29).

Arterial pH

Considerable debate has centered on the extent to which acidemia affects myocardial performance and whether correction of arterial pH with sodium bicarbonate is advantageous or deleterious to the heart.[670] Studies have challenged long-held beliefs that acidemia impairs myocardial performance. Nevertheless, most in vivo and clinical studies have found that metabolic acidosis impairs contractility and alters responses to exogenous catecholamines.[671] Hemodynamic deterioration usually is mild above pH 7.2 because of compensatory increases in sympathetic nervous system activity.[671] Attenuation of sympathetic nervous system responses by β-blockade or ganglionic blockade increases the detrimental effect of acidosis. The ischemic myocardium has been found to be particularly vulnerable to detrimental effects of acidosis. Patients with poor contractile function or reduction of myocardial sympathetic responsiveness (e.g., chronic LV failure), those treated with β-blockers, or those with myocardial ischemia are especially susceptible to the adverse effects of acidosis. For these reasons, arterial pH is corrected to near-normal levels before discontinuation of CPB, using sodium bicarbonate. Concerns regarding carbon dioxide generation and acidification of the intracellular space can be obviated by slow administration and appropriate adjustment of ventilation, both of which easily are achieved during CPB.

Electrolytes

Electrolytes most commonly of concern before discontinuation of CPB are potassium and calcium. Serum potassium concentration may be acutely low because of hemodilution with nonpotassium priming solutions, large-volume diuresis during CPB, or the use of insulin to treat hyperglycemia. More commonly, potassium concentration is increased as a result of systemic uptake of potassium-containing cardioplegic solution; values exceeding 6 mEq/L are not uncommon. Other potential causes of hyperkalemia that must be considered are hemolysis, tissue ischemia or necrosis, and acidemia. Hypokalemia can be rapidly corrected during CPB with *relative* safety because the heart and systemic circulation are supported. Increments of 5 to 10 mEq KCl over 1- to 2-minute intervals can be given directly into the pump or oxygenator by the perfusionist, and potassium subsequently is rechecked. Depending on severity and urgency of correction, increased potassium level can be treated or reduced by any of several standard means: alkali therapy, diuresis, calcium administration, or insulin and glucose. Alternatively, hemofiltration can be used to decrease serum potassium. While still on CPB, potassium-containing extracellular fluid is removed from the patient and replaced with fluid not containing potassium.

Ionized calcium is involved in the maintenance of normal excitation-contraction coupling and, therefore, in maintaining cardiac contractility and peripheral vascular tone. Low concentrations of ionized calcium lead to impaired cardiac contractility and reduced vascular tone. Concerns have been raised about the contribution of calcium administration to myocardial reperfusion injury and to the action of various inotropes.[672] Some investigators argue in favor of measuring ionized calcium before discontinuation of CPB and administering calcium in patients with low concentrations to optimize cardiac performance.[673] When confronted with poor myocardial or peripheral vascular responsiveness to inotropes or vasopressors after CPB *in the presence of a low level of ionized calcium,* calcium salts should be administered to restore ionized calcium to normal (not increased) levels in the hope of restoring responsiveness. The same strategy can be used for measuring and administering magnesium.

Other Final Preparations

Before separating from CPB, all monitoring and access catheters should be checked and calibrated. The zero-pressure calibration points of the pressure transducers are checked routinely. Not uncommonly, finger pulse oximeter probes do not have a good signal after CPB. In those cases, a nasal or ear probe is placed to obtain reliable oximetry.

Intravenous infusions are restarted before separation from CPB, and their flow characteristics are assessed for evidence of obstruction or disconnection.

During warming and preparation for separation, an assessment should be made of the functional status of the heart and peripheral vasculature based on visual inspection, hemodynamic indices, and metabolic parameters. Based on this assessment, inotropes, vasodilators, and vasopressors thought likely to be necessary for successful separation from CPB should be prepared and readied for administration.

Separation from Bypass

After all preparatory steps are taken (see Table 28-14), CPB can be discontinued. Venous outflow to the pump or oxygenator is impeded by slowly clamping the venous line, and the patient's intravascular volume and ventricular loading conditions are restored by transfusion of perfusate through the aortic inflow line. When loading conditions are optimal, the aortic inflow line is clamped and the patient is separated from CPB.

At this juncture, it must be determined whether oxygenation, ventilation, and, more commonly, myocardial performance (systemic perfusion) are adequate. A discussion of these issues no longer involves CPB per se, but rather applied cardiopulmonary physiology. Consequently, a discussion of this extremely important topic is detailed in Chapter 32. Should separation fail for any reason, CPB simply can be reinstituted by unclamping the venous outflow and arterial inflow lines and restoring pump flow. This allows for support of systemic oxygenation and perfusion while steps are taken to diagnose and treat those problems that precluded successful separation.

PERFUSION EMERGENCIES

Accidents or mishaps occurring during CPB quickly can evolve into life-threatening emergencies (Box 28-7). Many of the necessary conditions of CPB (cardiac arrest, hypothermia, volume depletion) preclude the ability to resume normal cardiorespiratory function if an accident threatens the integrity of the extracorporeal cir-

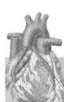

BOX 28-7. PERFUSION EMERGENCIES

- Arterial cannula malposition
- Aortic dissection
- Massive air embolism
- Venous air lock
- Reversed cannulation

cuit. Fortunately, major perfusion accidents occur infrequently and rarely are associated with permanent injury or death (Table 28-15). However, all members of the cardiac surgery team must be able to respond to perfusion emergencies to limit the likelihood of perfusion-related disasters. Some of the most common emergencies are discussed in the subsequent sections.

Arterial Cannula Malposition

Ascending aortic cannulae can be malpositioned such that the outflow jet is directed primarily into the innominate artery,[674-676] the left common carotid artery (rare),[677,678] or the left subclavian artery (rare).[679] The latter two can occur with the use of long arch-type cannulae. In the first two circumstances, unilateral cerebral *hyperperfusion*, usually with systemic hypoperfusion, occurs, whereas flow directed to the subclavian artery results in global cerebral *hypoperfusion*. Despite the fact that not all combinations of arterial pressure monitoring site and cannula malposition produce systemic hypotension, it commonly is regarded as a cardinal sign of cannula malposition. For example, right arm blood pressure monitoring and innominate artery cannulation,[674] or left arm monitoring and left subclavian artery cannulation,[679] may result in *high* arterial pressure on initiation of bypass. With other positioning and monitoring combinations, investigators report persistently low systemic arterial pressure (MAP = 25 to 35 mm Hg), which is poorly responsive to increasing pump flow or vasoconstrictors. Over time (minutes), signs of systemic hypoperfusion (e.g., acidemia, oliguria) develop.[677] Because a variable period of systemic hypotension with CPB initiation nearly always is seen with hemodilution, hypotension alone is not significant evidence to establish a diagnosis of arterial cannula malposition. Ross et al[677] described a case of accidental left common carotid cannulation with unilateral facial and conjunctival edema accompanied by rhinorrhea, otorrhea, and signs of systemic hypoperfusion. In a similar case, Sudhaman[678] found left facial congestion, whereas the right side was pale. Watson[674] described a case of innominate artery cannulation. On initiation of CPB, the skin over the carotid vessels on the right was colder than on the left. Three cases of innominate cannulation produced dramatic unilateral facial blanching with onset of CPB caused by perfusion with nonblood-containing priming solution.[675,676] On initiation of CPB and periodically thereafter, it is advisable to inspect the face for color change and edema, rhinorrhea, or otorrhea and to palpate the neck with onset of cooling for temperature asymmetry. EEG monitoring first was advocated as a method of detecting cannula malposition. In one study, cannula malposition, detected by EEG asymmetry, occurred in 3 (3.5%) of 84 patients.[680] However, transcranial Doppler, and more commonly available cerebral oximetry, is the monitor of choice to detect malperfusion secondary to cannula complications (see Chapter 16).

TABLE 28-15	Comparison of the Five Most Common Accidents from Three Perfusion Surveys					
	Stoney (1972–1977)[686]		Wheeldon (1974–1979)[765]		Kurusz (1982–1985)[766]	
*Complication**	*Incidents*	*PI/D*	*Incidents*	*PI/D*	*Incidents*	*PI/D*
Air embolism	(2) 1.14	0.41	(2) 0.79	0.18	(6) 0.80	0.12
Coagulopathy	(1) 1.26	0.51	(6) 0.26	0.09	(8) 0.21	0.05
Electrical failure	(3) 0.67	0.01	(1) 1.00	0.06	(4) 0.84	0.003
Mechanical failure	(4) 0.38	0.02	(5) 0.27	0	(7) 0.30	0.007
Inadequate oxygenation	(5) 0.33	0.02	(3) 0.59	0	(3) 0.88	0.07
Hypoperfusion	—	—	(4) 0.30	0.18	(2) 0.96	0.15
Protamine reaction	—	—	—	—	(1) 2.80	0.22
Drug error	—	—	—	—	(5) 0.82	0.08

*The five most common complications for each study are listed as incidence per 1000 perfusions, and the number of permanent injuries and mortalities as incidence per 1000 perfusions. The numbers in parentheses are the rank of each complication from most to least.

PI/D, permanent injury or death.

Data from Stoney WS, Alford WC Jr, Burrus GR, et al: Air embolism and other accidents using pump oxygenators. *Ann Thorac Surg* 29:336, 1980; Wheeldon DR: Can cardiopulmonary bypass be a safe procedure? In Longmore DB (ed): *Towards Safer Cardiac Surgery.* London, 1981, MTP, pp 427–446; Kurusz M, Conti VR, Arens JF, et al: Perfusion accident survey. *Proc Am Acad Cardiovasc Perf* 7:57, 1986.

Two other arterial cannula malpositions are possible: abutment of the cannula tip against the aortic intima, which results in high line pressure, poor perfusion, or even acute dissection when CPB is initiated, and the cannula tip directed caudally toward the aortic valve. This may result in acute aortic insufficiency, with sudden left ventricular distention and systemic hypoperfusion on bypass. If the aortic inflow cannula is soft, aortic cross-clamping will occlude the arterial perfusion line, which can rupture the aortic inflow line. Suspicion of any cannula malposition must be brought to the attention of the surgeon immediately.

Aortic or Arterial Dissection

Signs of arterial dissection, often similar to those of cannula malposition, also must be sought continuously, especially on initiation of CPB. Dissection may originate at the cannulation site, aortic cross-clamp site, proximal vein graft anastomotic site, or partial occlusion (side-biting) clamp site. Dissections are due to intimal disruption or, more distally, to fracture of atherosclerotic plaque. In either case, some systemic arterial blood flow becomes extraluminal, being forced into the arterial wall. The dissection propagates mostly in the direction of the systemic flow, but not exclusively. Extraluminal blood compresses the luminal origins (take-offs) of major arterial branches such that vital organs (heart, brain, kidney, intestinal tract, spinal cord) may become ischemic. Because systemic perfusion may be low, and origins of the innominate and subclavian arteries may be compressed, probably the best sign of arterial dissection is persistently low systemic arterial pressure.[681] Venous drainage to the pump decreases (blood is sequestered), and arterial inflow "line pressure" is usually inappropriately high. The surgeon may see the dissection if it involves the anterior or lateral ascending aorta (bluish discoloration), or both.[681,682] It is possible the surgeon may *not* see any sign of dissection because the dissection is out of view (e.g., posterior ascending aorta, aortic arch, descending aorta). Dissection can occur at any time before, during, or after CPB. As with cannula malposition, a suspicion of arterial dissection must be brought to the attention of the surgeon. The anesthesiologist must not assume that something is suddenly wrong with the arterial pressure transducer but should "think dissection."

After a dissection of the ascending aorta is diagnosed, immediate steps to minimize propagation must be taken. If it has occurred before CPB, the anesthesiologist should take steps to reduce MAP and the rate of increase of aortic pressure (dP/dt). If it occurs during CPB, pump flow and MAP are reduced to the lowest acceptable levels. Arterial perfusate frequently is cooled to profound levels (14° C to 19° C) as rapidly as possible to decrease metabolic demand and protect vital organs.[682] A different arterial cannulation site is prepared (e.g., the femoral artery is cannulated or the true aortic lumen is cannulated at a site more distal on the aortic arch). Arterial inflow is shifted to that new site with the intent that perfusing the true aortic lumen will reperfuse vital organs.[682] The ascending aorta is cross-clamped just below the innominate artery, and cardioplegia is administered (into the coronary ostia or coronary sinus). The aorta is opened to expose the site of disruption, which is then resected and replaced. Reimplantation of the coronary arteries or aortic valve replacement, or both, may be necessary. The false lumina at both ends of the aorta are obliterated with Teflon buttresses, and the graft is inserted by end-to-end suture.[622] With small dissections it is sometimes possible to avoid open repair by application of a partial occlusion clamp with plication of the dissection and exclusion of the intimal disruption.[682] Troianos et al[683] described three cases of arterial dissection during CPB in which TEE was found useful. Although provisional diagnoses were made on the basis of traditional signs, TEE allowed assessment of the origin and extent of dissection. Diagnosis of arterial dissection also has been assisted by presence of EEG[684] and cerebral oximetry asymmetry.[685]

Arterial dissections originating from femoral cannulation also necessitate reductions in arterial pressure, systemic flow, and temperature. If the operation is near completion, the heart may be transfused

and CPB discontinued; otherwise, the aortic arch must be cannulated and adequate systemic perfusion restored to allow completion of the operation.[681]

Massive Arterial Gas Embolus

Macroscopic gas embolus is a rare but disastrous CPB complication. Two independent studies in 1980 reported incidence rates of recognized massive arterial gas embolism of 0.1% to 0.2%.[686,687] The current incidence probably is lower because of the widespread use of reservoir level alarms and other bubble detection devices. Between 20% and 30% of affected patients died immediately, with another 30% having transient or nondebilitating neurologic deficits, or both. Circumstances that most commonly contributed to these events were inattention to oxygenator blood level, reversal of LV vent flow, or unexpected resumption of cardiac ejection in a previously opened heart. Rupture of a pulsatile assist device[688] or intra-aortic balloon pump[689] also may introduce large volumes of gas into the arterial circulation.

The pathophysiology of cerebral gas embolism (macroscopic and microscopic) is not well understood. Tissue damage after gas embolization is initiated from simple mechanical blockage of blood vessels by bubbles.[690,691] Although gas emboli may be absorbed or pass through the circulation within 1 to 5 minutes,[690–693] the local reaction of platelets and proteins to the blood/gas interface or endothelial damage is thought to potentiate microvascular stasis,[693–698] prolonging cerebral ischemia to the point of infarction. Areas of marginal perfusion, such as arterial boundary zones, do not clear gas emboli as rapidly as well-perfused zones,[690] producing patterns of ischemia or infarction difficult to distinguish from those caused by hypotension or particulate emboli.

Recommended treatment for massive arterial gas embolism includes immediate cessation of CPB with aspiration of as much gas as possible from the aorta and heart, assumption of steep Trendelenburg position, and clearance of air from the arterial perfusion line. After resumption of CPB, treatment continues with implementation or deepening of hypothermia (18° C to 27° C) during completion of the operation and clearance of gas from the coronary circulation before emergence from CPB.[687,688,699,700] In many reports of patients suffering massive arterial gas embolus, seizures occurred after surgery and were treated with anticonvulsants.[126,700–702] Because seizures after ischemic insults are associated with poor outcomes, perhaps because of hypermetabolic effects, prophylactic phenytoin seems reasonable. Hypotension has been shown to lengthen the residence time of cerebral air emboli and worsen the severity of resulting ischemia.[703] Maintenance of moderate hypertension is reasonable and clinically attainable to hasten clearance of emboli from the circulation and, hopefully, improve neurologic outcome.

Many clinicians have reported dramatic neurologic recovery when hyperbaric therapy is used for arterial gas embolism, even if delayed up to 26 hours after the event.[688,698,699,704] Spontaneous recovery from air emboli also has been reported,[695,700,702,704] and no prospective study of hyperbaric therapy in the cardiac surgery setting has been performed.[705] Few institutions that do cardiac surgery have an appropriately equipped and staffed hyperbaric chamber to allow expeditious and safe initiation of hyperbaric therapy. Nonetheless, immediate transfer by air is often possible and should seriously be considered. It seems reasonable to expect that institutions that do cardiac surgery should have policies regarding catastrophic air embolism.

In 1980, Mills and Ochsner[687] suggested venoarterial perfusion as an alternative to hyperbaric therapy. Retrograde perfusion through the SVC cannula at 1.2 L/min at 20° C for 1 to 2 minutes was used in five of their eight patients with massive gas embolism. The goal was to flush air from the cerebral arterial circulation. None of the patients so treated had evidence of neurologic injury. Other reports using this technique have followed.[706,707] Hendriks et al,[708] in a porcine model of venoarterial perfusion, found that only 50% of injected gas (nitrogen) could be recovered from the aorta. Ninety-eight percent of the removable gas was collected from the aorta in the first 7 to 10 minutes of retrograde perfusion. Although no animal (clinically or pathologically) appeared to sustain neurologic injury, the investigators concluded that venoarterial perfusion did not adequately remove embolized gas, and hyperbaric therapy remained the treatment of choice. The timing of the embolism is also a major consideration. For example, if massive air embolism occurs during connection, serious consideration should be given to abandoning the procedure to allow immediate therapy and awakening the patient to assess the neurologic status. Air embolism and its subsequent cerebral ischemia are likely worsened by the nonphysiologic nature of CPB, as well as its inherent inflammatory processes.

Venous Air Lock

Air entering the venous outflow line can result in complete cessation of flow to the venous reservoir, and this is termed *air lock*. Loss of venous outflow necessitates immediate slowing, even cessation of pump flow, to prevent emptying the reservoir and subsequent delivery of air to the patient's arterial circulation. After an air lock is recognized, a search for the source of venous outflow line air must be undertaken (e.g., loose atrial purse string, atrial tear, open intravenous access) and repaired before reestablishing full bypass.

Reversed Cannulation

In this case, the venous outflow limb of the CPB circuit is incorrectly connected to the arterial inflow cannula and the arterial perfusion limb of the circuit is attached to the venous cannula. On initiation of CPB, blood is removed from the arterial circulation and returned to the venous circulation at high pressure. Arterial pressure is found to be extremely low by palpation and arterial pressure monitoring. Very low arterial pressures also can (more commonly) be caused by dissection in the arterial tree. In the latter case, the perfusionist will rapidly lose volume, whereas with reversed cannulation, the perfusionist will have an immediate gross excess of volume. If high pump flow is established, venous or atrial rupture may occur. The CVP will be dramatically increased, with evidence of facial venous engorgement.

Line pressure is the pressure in the arterial limb of the CPB circuit. Because arterial cannulae are much smaller than the aorta, there is always a pressure decline across the aortic cannula. Arterial inflow line pressure will always be considerably greater than systemic (patient) arterial pressure. The magnitude of the pressure decline depends on cannula size and systemic flow; small cannulae and higher flows result in greater gradients. The CPB pump must generate a pressure that overcomes this gradient to provide adequate systemic arterial pressure. For a typical adult (i.e., MAP of about 60 mm Hg, systemic flow of about 2.4 L/min/m², and a 24 Fr aortic cannula), line pressure in an uncomplicated case usually ranges from 150 to 250 mm Hg. The fittings on the arterial inflow line are plastic; the fittings and the line itself can rupture. Perfusionists typically do not want a line pressure in excess of 300 mm Hg.

CPB must be discontinued and the cannula disconnected and inspected for air. If air is found in the arterial circulation, an air embolus protocol is initiated. Once arterial air is cleared, the circuit is correctly reconnected and CPB restarted. In adults, the venous outflow limb of the CPB circuit is a larger diameter tubing than the arterial inflow tubing, precisely to eliminate reversed cannulation. This is why reversed cannulation is rare in adults, but it has happened. In pediatric cases, the arterial inflow and venous outflow limbs of the CPB circuit are close or equal in size (see Chapter 29).

SPECIAL PATIENT POPULATIONS

Care of the Gravid Patient during Bypass

Studies assessing the effects of cardiac surgery and CPB on obstetric physiology and fetal well-being are lacking. However, several reviews and many case reports describe individual experience in caring for the gravid patient and fetus during cardiac surgery and ECC.[709–714] These surveys and anecdotal reports, together with an understanding of

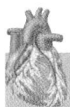

BOX 28-8. SPECIAL PATIENTS WHO MAY NEED CARDIOPULMONARY BYPASS

- Pregnant women
- Accidental hypothermia victims
- Neurosurgical patients with an intracranial aneurysm

the well-documented physiology of pregnancy and the effects of cardiac therapeutics on fetal physiology, can serve as a basis for a rational approach to care for the pregnant patient and fetus during cardiac surgery (Box 28-8).

Several groups have published reports detailing their individual experiences or survey data on maternal and fetal outcomes after cardiac surgery and CPB.[709–714] Jacobs et al[710] reported their experience with three first-trimester gravid patients. All recovered from their operative procedures and delivered normal-term infants. The first survey data on pregnancy and cardiac surgery were reported in 1969 by Zitnik et al[711] from the Mayo Clinic. Among the 20 patients, there was only one maternal death, but seven fetuses died before term. The study authors concluded that cardiac surgery does not increase the likelihood of death in the pregnant patient with heart disease but is associated with substantial fetal mortality. Lapiedra et al[713] and Becker[712] individually published reports in the 1980s on gravid patients undergoing cardiac surgery. Lapiedra et al[713] reviewed their own experiences and found only one fetal death and no instance of maternal death in their review of 23 cases. Becker[712] surveyed members of the Society of Thoracic Surgeons on their experiences with pregnant patients requiring cardiac surgery. Of the 600 surgeons responding, 119 reported on a total of 169 gravid patients undergoing cardiac surgery, 68 of whom were managed with CPB. Pomini et al[714] reviewed 69 case reports of gravid patients undergoing cardiac procedures and CPB. Overall, the embryo-fetal mortality rate was 20.2%, but fetal loss was reduced to 12.5% in the last 40 cases. The reported experience on maternal and fetal outcomes after cardiac procedures with CPB suggests that cardiac surgery is well tolerated by the mother but poses a significant risk to the fetus.

Although most physicians advocate providing perioperative care that can ensure maternal well-being, appropriate investigation would enable clinicians to care optimally for mother and fetus. This section outlines recommendations for perioperative management of the gravid patient requiring cardiac surgery and CPB. The basic principles for the perioperative management of the gravid patient requiring any type of surgery are outlined by Levinson and Shnider[715]: maternal safety, avoidance of teratogenic drugs, avoidance of intrauterine asphyxia, and prevention of preterm labor.

Considerations before Bypass

Premedication and Patient Positioning
Premedication should be appropriate for the specific cardiac lesion and physical status of the patient. Teratogenic drugs should be avoided, especially in the first trimester of pregnancy. After the 34th week of gestation, stomach emptying is delayed and patients are at increased risk for pulmonary aspiration. Although it is not possible to ensure gastric emptying before anesthesia induction, sodium citrate and an H₂-receptor antagonist may provide some protection against aspiration pneumonia. The gravid uterus obstructs aortic flow and IVC blood return to the heart. Gravid patients should never be supine; they must be positioned with left uterine displacement throughout the perioperative period.

Maternal and Fetal Monitor Information
The pregnant patient undergoing cardiac surgery requires the usual monitors used during cardiac surgery, as well as monitors that can assess fetal well-being. Monitors that help assess the adequacy of maternal cardiovascular performance and oxygen delivery to the fetus are of

paramount importance. Little is known about the effects of cardiovascular drugs and other therapeutic measures on the pregnant cardiac patient undergoing CPB. Appropriate monitors permit the assessment of an individual therapy on maternal and fetal oxygen delivery.

Monitors for cardiac surgery and CPB are discussed in detail in chapters in Section III of this textbook. A two-lead (II, V_5) ECG, peripheral pulse oximeter, and blood pressure cuff should be placed first. These monitors provide information concerning cardiorespiratory function as other, more invasive monitors are placed. Before the induction of anesthesia, radial artery and PAC should be placed. An oximetry PAC provides continuous information on venous oxygen saturation—an indirect, approximate measure of the adequacy of maternal tissue oxygen delivery.

Uterine activity should be monitored with a tocodynamometer applied to the maternal abdomen. This monitor transduces the tightening of the abdomen during uterine contractions. As is the case with other types of major surgery, the tocodynamometer should not interfere with the conduct of cardiac surgery; if necessary, the monitor may be intermittently displaced by the operating surgeon. The use of an intra-amniotic catheter to monitor uterine activity and pressure may be inadvisable in a patient who will be fully heparinized. Intraoperative uterine contractions may have a deleterious effect on fetal oxygen delivery (by causing an increase in uterine venous pressure and decrease in uterine blood flow) and signal the onset of preterm labor. Use of the tocodynamometer is imperative because it will provide important information about the state of the uterus and allow intervention if necessary. Various case reports have documented the common occurrence of uterine contractions during cardiac surgery and CPB. Uterine contractions may appear at any time during the perioperative period but occur most frequently immediately after the discontinuation of CPB and in the early ICU period.[716] It is, therefore, important to leave the tocodynamometer in place after the completion of surgery. Although uterine contractions occur frequently in the perioperative course, they usually are effectively treated with magnesium sulfate, ritodrine, or ethanol infusions, and they do not result in preterm labor and fetal demise.[717]

Fetal heart rate (FHR) monitors should be used in all gravid patients after 16 weeks gestation because one of the primary perioperative goals is to avoid fetal loss. Use of an FHR monitor permits recognition of fetal distress and allows the clinician to institute measures to improve fetal oxygen delivery. The FHR monitor recognizes and records the FHR, FHR variability, and uterine contractions. An electrode placed in the fetal scalp gives the most reliable fetal ECG and, therefore, the best FHR information. However, this method may be undesirable in the presence of maternal anticoagulation. External FHR monitoring—using ultrasound, phonocardiography, or external abdominal ECG—is less exact but preferable in this clinical setting.

The cardiac surgeon, perfusionist, and cardiac anesthesiologist may not be familiar with uterine and FHR monitors. As a result, having a perinatologist or an obstetrician present during cardiac surgery is desirable to assess for preoperative fetal distress and the anticipated need for emergency caesarean section during cardiac surgery.

FHR usually is normal in the prebypass period but decreases precipitously with the initiation of CPB and remains below normal for the entire bypass period. There are many potential causes of this observed decrease in FHR. Persistent fetal bradycardia is a classic sign of acute fetal hypoxia. However, in the CPB setting, especially when hypothermia is used, it is difficult to ascribe fetal bradycardia to hypoxia or to decreased fetal oxygen demand. Fetal tachycardia typically occurs after the discontinuation of ECC support. This tachycardia may represent a compensatory mechanism for the oxygen debt incurred during CPB. The FHR usually returns to normal by the end of the operative period.

Interventions optimizing maternal blood oxygen content, correcting any acid-base imbalance, and replenishing fetal glycogen stores may alleviate signs of fetal hypoxia. Some clinicians recommend an increase in CPB pump flow to improve fetal oxygen delivery.[712,714]

After anesthesia induction, a urinary bladder catheter with a temperature probe and TEE probe should be placed. The former provides information on fluid balance and core temperature. TEE is always helpful but is especially important in the patient undergoing valvular or congenital heart surgery because it can document pathologic changes and help assess the adequacy of repair. One of the authors (C.T.M.M.) reported a case of a gravid patient requiring replacement of aortic and mitral porcine prosthetic valves.[717] The patient was thought to have cardiac disease limited to her aortic valve; however, after an unsuccessful attempt to wean from CPB, mitral valve dysfunction was diagnosed and a second period of CPB was required to replace the mitral valve. Prebypass TEE would have identified mitral valve dysfunction before ECC and obviated the need for two separate periods of CPB.

Conducting the Bypass Procedure

The conditions of ECC—nonpulsatile blood flow, hypothermia, anemia, and requisite anticoagulation—will likely have a negative impact on fetal well-being during CPB. No studies recommend a particular CPB management strategy in gravid patients. Recommendations are summarized (Table 28-16) for the management of bypass in pregnant patients, based on the survey and anecdotal reports in the literature (Table 28-17).

Blood Flow

The optimal extracorporeal circuit blood flow in the *nongravid* patient is controversial. Some clinicians recommend that blood flow be maintained

TABLE 28-16	Recommendations for the Conduct of Extracorporeal Circulation in the Gravid Patient	
Variable	*Value/Characteristic*	*Recommended Rationale*
Blood flow	3.0 L/min/m²	Cardiac index normally is increased during pregnancy
Blood pressure (MAP)	60–70 mm Hg	Uterine blood flow depends on maternal MAP
Temperature	32–34° C	Mild hypothermia decreases fetal oxygen requirements and is less likely to cause fetal arrhythmia
Oxygenator type	Membrane	Membrane oxygenators are associated with fewer embolic phenomena than bubblers
Hematocrit	25–27%	The quantity of oxygen carried in maternal blood (and therefore the oxygen available to the fetus) greatly depends on hemoglobin concentration
Duration of perfusion	Minimized	The duration of bypass is dictated by the complexity of the operative procedure
Cardioplegia	?	No data
Pulsatile perfusion	?	No data

MAP, mean arterial pressure.

TABLE 28-17	Prevalence of Maternal and Fetal Mortality after Cardiac Surgery and Cardiopulmonary Bypass in Gravid Patients	
Study	*Maternal Death*	*Fetal Death*
Jacobs/Cooley (1965)[710]	0/3 (0%)	0/3 (0%)
Zitnik (1969)[711]	1/20 (5%)	7/20 (35%)
Becker (1983)[712]	1/68 (1.5%)	11/68 (16%)
Lapiedra (1986)[713]	0/23 (0%)	1/23 (4.3%)
Pomini (1996)[714]*	2/69 (2.9%)	8/69 (20.2%)
Pomini (1996)[714]†	0/40 (0%)	5/40 (12.5%)
Arnoni (2003)[709]	5/58 (8.6%)	11/58 (18.6%)

*All patients from 1958 to 1992.
†Last 40 patients in series only.

at relatively normal values (i.e., cardiac index ≥ 2.3 L/min/m²), but others believe that lower blood flows, especially with hypothermia, are desirable and may decrease the morbidity associated with CPB and embolization of particulate matter.

Optimal CPB blood flow in the gravid patient is unknown. However, the increase in CO associated with pregnancy is well defined, and it might be argued that high blood flows during CPB are more physiologic in the gravid patient. Becker[712] suggested that flow during CPB in the pregnant patient be maintained at a minimum of 3.0 L/min/m². A few reports demonstrate that increasing CPB circuit blood flow improves FHR, suggesting improvement in fetal oxygen delivery. In Koh et al's[718] report, FHR improved when pump flow was increased from 3100 to 3600 mL/min. Similarly, Werch et al[719] reported an improvement in FHR when blood flow was increased from 2800 to 4600 mL/min. However, another report, describing two separate cases of perfusion in which fetal monitors were used, suggested that increasing pump flow did not consistently improve FHR. In one case, flow was increased from 2.3 to 2.9 L/min/m², with a brief, unsustained apparent improvement in fetal oxygen delivery.[719]

Blood Pressure

Under normal conditions, uterine blood flow is determined solely by maternal blood pressure, as the placental vasculature is maximally dilated. However, it is not known what factors determine uterine blood flow during the very abnormal condition of CPB. For example, catecholamine levels increase by several times during CPB; therefore, uterine vascular resistance may increase during ECC in response to increased levels of norepinephrine and epinephrine. However, regardless of the state of uterine vascular resistance during CPB, maternal blood pressure will be an important determinant of uterine blood flow and fetal oxygen delivery. Moderately high pressure (MAP ≥ 65 mm Hg) should be used during perfusion in the gravid patient.[712]

No reports demonstrate that increasing blood pressure during CPB improves FHR or fetal oxygen delivery. Most case reports on CPB in the gravid patient do not include information on blood pressure during CPB. The few blood pressure values reported in gravid perfusion cases ranged from 55 to 95 mm Hg.[717,720]

In theory, the use of short-acting vasodilators, such as nitroglycerin or sodium nitroprusside, may counteract the effects of CPB and norepinephrine- or epinephrine-induced increases in uterine vasculature resistance. If maternal blood pressure is maintained by increasing extracorporeal circuit pump flow, uterine blood flow and fetal oxygen delivery may be increased with vasodilators. Monitoring should be conducted to assess the effect of a given therapy on fetal oxygen delivery during CPB.

Temperature

Although varying degrees of hypothermic CPB have been considered the standard of care, several groups have advocated the use of normothermic CPB and warm blood cardioplegia to improve myocardial protection. However, the effects of warm versus cold cardioplegia on myocardial protection are controversial, and one group has reported an increase in adverse neurologic sequelae in patients treated with normothermic perfusion.[162] Controversy exists regarding temperature management during CPB in the nongravid patient, although most perfusions are conducted under hypothermic conditions. Similarly, there are few data and no consensus regarding temperature management in the gravid patient undergoing CPB.

There are theoretical advantages and disadvantages for normothermic and hypothermic CPB in the gravid patient. Hypothermia can cause fetal bradycardia and may lead to fetal ventricular arrhythmias, resulting in fetal wastage. Rewarming after hypothermic CPB may precipitate uterine contractions and preterm labor.[712] However, others reported the onset of uterine contractions at the time of discontinuation of CPB in spite of normothermic perfusion. Uterine contractions also occur at various times in the postbypass and postoperative periods. The association of uterine contractions with rewarming after hypothermic CPB is unclear.

Hypothermia may be protective to the fetus during ECC by decreasing fetal oxygen requirements. Assali et al[721] demonstrated that hypothermia to 28° C in gravid dogs caused an increase in uterine vascular resistance but did not result in a decrease in uterine blood flow. Hypothermia did not affect fetal survival. Pardi et al,[722] using a fetal lamb model, reported that temperatures above 18° C were well tolerated. More profound hypothermia caused irreversible fetal acidosis and hypoxia. Several reports discussed the effects of deliberately induced and septicemia-associated hypothermia in gravid patients. The investigators observed that the FHR decreased with maternal hypothermia but improved with maternal rewarming.[723]

Perfusion temperatures of 25° C to 37° C have been used in gravid patients undergoing CPB.[712,717,720,724] Because Pomini et al[714] found an apparent decrease in fetal loss when CPB temperatures were maintained at or above 36° C, they recommended normothermic temperatures during CPB. However, they acknowledged the lack of follow-up in many of the case reports they reviewed. The authors reported a case in which hypothermic CPB at 25° C was required for 2 hours 40 minutes, and in which the patient underwent two periods of rewarming. Uterine contractions occurring in the early postoperative period were successfully treated with magnesium sulfate. Despite the magnitude and duration of hypothermia and two periods of rewarming, a healthy infant was delivered 10 days after surgery.[717]

In conclusion, the optimal gravida temperature during CPB has not been established. No data suggest hypothermia is harmful to the mother or fetus undergoing bypass. Normothermic CPB may increase the likelihood of untoward neurologic sequelae in the mother, an event that would be catastrophic in a woman with young children.

Accidental Hypothermia

In the early 1950s, Bigelow et al[455] demonstrated a direct relation between metabolic rate and temperature and postulated that DHCA could facilitate cardiac surgery. Although ECC was not used in these early cardiac cases (a tub of ice and warming coils were used to induce hypothermia and rewarm the patient), the notion that a patient could survive hypothermic arrest was established. With the introduction of CPB in the mid-1950s,[725] the induction of DHCA, followed by resuscitation, was greatly facilitated by the extracorporeal circuit. It was a short leap to consider the use of CPB to resuscitate the victim suffering accidental hypothermia.

This section outlines the care of a subgroup of accidental hypothermia patients. Patients with core temperatures less than 32° C, and without a perfusing cardiac rhythm, are best managed with some type of extracorporeal support.[726] This section discusses the management of hypothermic patients who are optimally managed with CPB for rewarming. Danzl and Pozos[727] outlined treatment algorithms for hypothermic patients who do not require ECC for resuscitation (e.g., patients with preserved circulation and suffering only moderate hypothermia [temperature ≥ 32° C]).

Patient Selection

Clinicians lack consensus regarding the absolute indications or contraindications for the use of CPB in the treatment of accidental deep hypothermia.[728] However, there are theoretical considerations and some data to help guide the decision-making process regarding the rewarming of accidental hypothermia patients. Phenomena that greatly limit the likelihood of successful resuscitation (that leads to an acceptable patient outcome) include the presence of asphyxia before the initiation of hypothermia. (This occurs commonly in avalanche and drowning victims.) Similarly, patients with severe traumatic injury, or extremely increased potassium levels (≥10 mmol/L), are unlikely to benefit from resuscitative efforts.

One report suggested that several factors may increase the likelihood of a desirable patient outcome after accidental hypothermia managed with CPB.[729] Victims suffering profound hypothermia (without prior asphyxia), as opposed to moderate hypothermia, benefit from the substantial slowing of metabolic processes and are less likely to have severe end-organ (brain, heart) damage. Young patients in good health are more likely to survive resuscitative efforts than older, debilitated victims. Patients who have multiple preexisting medical problems are less likely to have a desirable outcome. Initial rescue treatment algorithms may influence the likelihood of surviving profound hypothermia. The maintenance of profound hypothermia in the rescued patient before the initiation of extracorporeal warming may greatly enhance the likelihood of successful recovery. Rewarming with CPB is the most efficient method to resuscitate the hypothermic patient. Tissue perfusion is enhanced by hemodilution, and metabolic perturbations can be easily corrected.

Caring for the Accidental Hypothermia Victim

After the decision is made to resuscitate an accidental hypothermia victim, the patient should be maintained at the hypothermic temperature and rapidly transferred to a facility that can provide extracorporeal rewarming. In the operating room, various vascular sites may be cannulated to initiate rewarming. Femoral vessels or mediastinal vasculature may serve as conduits for rewarming. Because the ventricle is noncompliant at temperatures less than 32° C, sternotomy or thoracotomy may be preferable to facilitate direct cardiac massage and defibrillation. Although hypothermia reduces anesthetic requirements, the prudent use of anesthetics, analgesics, sedative-hypnotics, and volatile drugs is recommended. These agents should be administered through the extracorporeal circuit.

The extracorporeal circuit must include a pump, oxygenator, and heat exchange waterbath to treat an asystolic patient. At flow rates of 2 to 3 L/min, with the waterbath at 37° C, the patient's core temperature can increase by as much as 1° C to 2° C every 3 to 5 minutes. Slowly, the flow rate can be increased as determined by venous return. Given the data regarding the adverse effects of mildly hyperthermic blood on ischemic cerebral damage, the accidental hypothermia patient should not be perfused with blood warmed to temperatures in excess of 37° C. If the victim has a perfusing cardiac rhythm, venovenous rewarming may be used. Indeed, strong arguments can be made for limiting the rewarming to only 32° C to 33° C and then utilizing cardiac arrest protocols that utilize prolonged mild hypothermia to optimize cerebral outcomes.

One study suggests that, under certain circumstances (e.g., profound hypothermia before asphyxia; young, healthy patients; maintenance of hypothermia before CPB-supported rewarming), accidental hypothermia patients have an almost even chance of surviving and not suffering significant end-organ (including cerebral) deficits. Walpoth et al[729] reviewed the hospital records of 234 patients suffering accidental hypothermia. Forty-six of these patients had core temperatures less than 28° C and had circulatory arrest. Of the 32 patients rewarmed with CPB support, 15 were long-term survivors. These 15 patients were re-examined and studied an average of 7 years after their resuscitation from accidental hypothermia. The survivors were uniformly young (25.2 ± 9.9 years) and were resuscitated with CPB 141 ± 15 minutes after discovery. Although neurologic and neuropsychologic deficits were observed in all the victims in the early postresuscitation period, all patients had fully or almost completely recovered at the long-term follow-up. The investigators concluded that otherwise healthy individuals can survive accidental deep hypothermia with a preserved good quality of life.

Intracranial Aneurysm Surgery

Surgery for intracranial aneurysm represents a major challenge for the surgeon and anesthesiologist.[730] For a small number of these cases, DHCA has been applied to improve surgical access and cerebral protection. Like many areas, significant evolution in technique and application has occurred over time. Initial enthusiasm for DHCA in intracranial aneurysm surgery was tempered by the unfortunate occurrence of coagulopathies. Its use was further restricted by advances in neurosurgical microscopic technique (aneurysm wrapping, parent vessel ligation, and use of temporary clips). Improvements in perioperative monitoring and

neuroanesthesia have reserved a use for DHCA in the approach to giant aneurysms that might otherwise be inoperable.

DHCA for intracranial aneurysm requires precise integration of a remarkably large and diverse team, which includes anesthesiologists, nurses, perfusionists, cardiac surgeons, and neurosurgeons. All components and demands of the operation should be thoroughly familiar to all participants. The anesthesiologist primarily is occupied by five areas. The first area is patient selection and consent, which need to include a careful assessment for preexisting coagulation problems or contraindication to TEE. The second area entails careful premedication and induction. This is undertaken to blunt hemodynamic response to invasive monitor placement and intubation, and avoid respiratory depression in that subgroup of patients with increased intracranial pressure. The third area of focus is maintenance and monitoring. This often includes TEE, EEG, and placement of defibrillator pads in addition to the routine anesthetic monitors. Next, the anesthesiologist prepares for initiation of CPB and arrest. Lastly, the anesthesiologist manages rewarming, resumption of native circulation, and correction of coagulation abnormalities. Depending on the length of arrest and adequacy of cardiac protection, these steps may proceed smoothly or be complicated by significant hemodynamic embarrassment.

DHCA has been used for intracranial aneurysm surgery with good success at a number of centers.[731–736] The high percentage of patients surviving is probably the best indicator of the value of this technique, although the relatively small number of cases performed on an annual basis make controlled outcome trials difficult to complete. Silverberg et al[731] reported nine operative cases with no operative deaths, although six modest perioperative complications occurred (i.e., small stroke, transient cranial nerve palsy, frontal lobe hematoma, and pulmonary embolus). Baumgartner et al[732] also had no reported deaths in their series, and all patients went on to live independently. Like Silverberg's series, a fair number of patients experienced modest perioperative complications (i.e., four thromboembolic episodes, three strokes, three transient neurologic palsies). The other reported series[733–736] were similar in the respect that most patients went on to live independently and modest perioperative complications were in the range of 50%. Most recently, Stone et al[167] have studied the use of DHCA for neurosurgery and similarly reported good results. Given that the overall numbers involved are small, it is difficult to develop precise estimates for morbidity and mortality rates. However, given that DHCA in intracranial aneurysm surgery has been reserved for only the most difficult cases, the results seen are encouraging. As in most areas of cardiac surgery, continued developments have led to an evolution in neurosurgery as well and in how these intracranial aneurysms are being addressed. For example, many more are now being addressed with neurovascular radiologic coiling than are being treated open under DHCA. It is likely that this will be a continuing trend in the declining use of DHCA for intracranial aneurysm treatment.

MINIMALLY INVASIVE SURGERY AND CARDIOPULMONARY BYPASS

In the mid-1990s, interest in minimally invasive techniques for cardiac surgery emerged. Today, coronary revascularization and mitral and aortic valvular surgery are being performed in some centers with minimally invasive approaches. The proponents of port-access cardiac surgery (PACS) suggest that this technique permits minimally invasive cardiac surgery while providing the support of ECC. This section describes the current technology and expertise with port-access CPB. Minimally invasive procedures and off-pump cardiac surgery are discussed further in Chapters 18, 19, and 29.

Port-Access Bypass Circuit

The port-access system consists of a series of catheters that are introduced through various puncture sites, including the femoral artery and vein, and threaded through the aorta and venous system to the heart. The perfusion is usually set up from the femoral vein to the oxygenator and then returned via the femoral artery. An inflatable balloon on the end of an endoaortic clamp (EAC) catheter can be used to arrest the blood flow in the aorta, and other catheters help drain and reroute the blood flow to the heart-lung machine. Through two of the catheters, cardioplegia solution can be administered to the heart (Figure 28-16).[737,738]

The EAC is an occlusion balloon that functions as an aortic cross-clamp and permits antegrade cardioplegia infusion into the aortic root and coronary arteries. The lumen used to administer cardioplegia can also function as an aortic root-venting catheter. Some surgeons prefer to use a direct modified aortic cross-clamp inserted through a port in the right chest instead of using the EAC; they depend on administration of cardioplegia in a retrograde fashion via the coronary sinus. Retrograde cardioplegia can be delivered through an endocoronary sinus catheter (ECSC) that is placed with a percutaneous approach (Figure 28-17).

Blood returns to the ECC through the femoral venous catheter that is advanced to the level of the IVC-right atrium junction. Because extrathoracic gravity drainage is usually insufficient in providing adequate blood flow for complete CPB support, kinetic-assisted venous drainage, with controlled suction, is used to augment the drainage of blood to the heart-lung machine (see Chapter 29). Removing all air from the system at the end of surgery is challenging and must be done carefully.

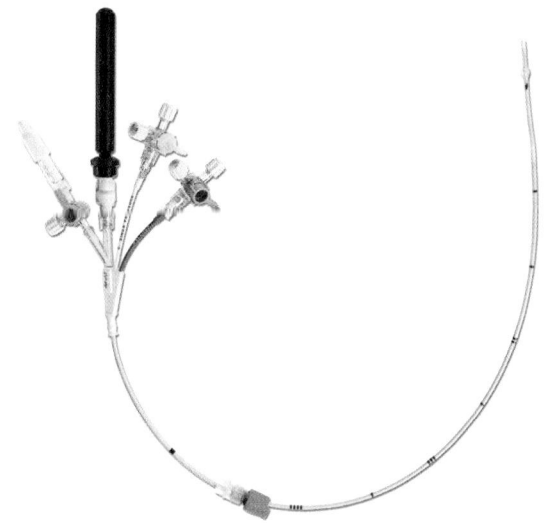

Figure 28-17 **Steerable coronary catheter for port-access surgery.** *(Courtesy Edwards Lifesciences, Irvine, CA.)*

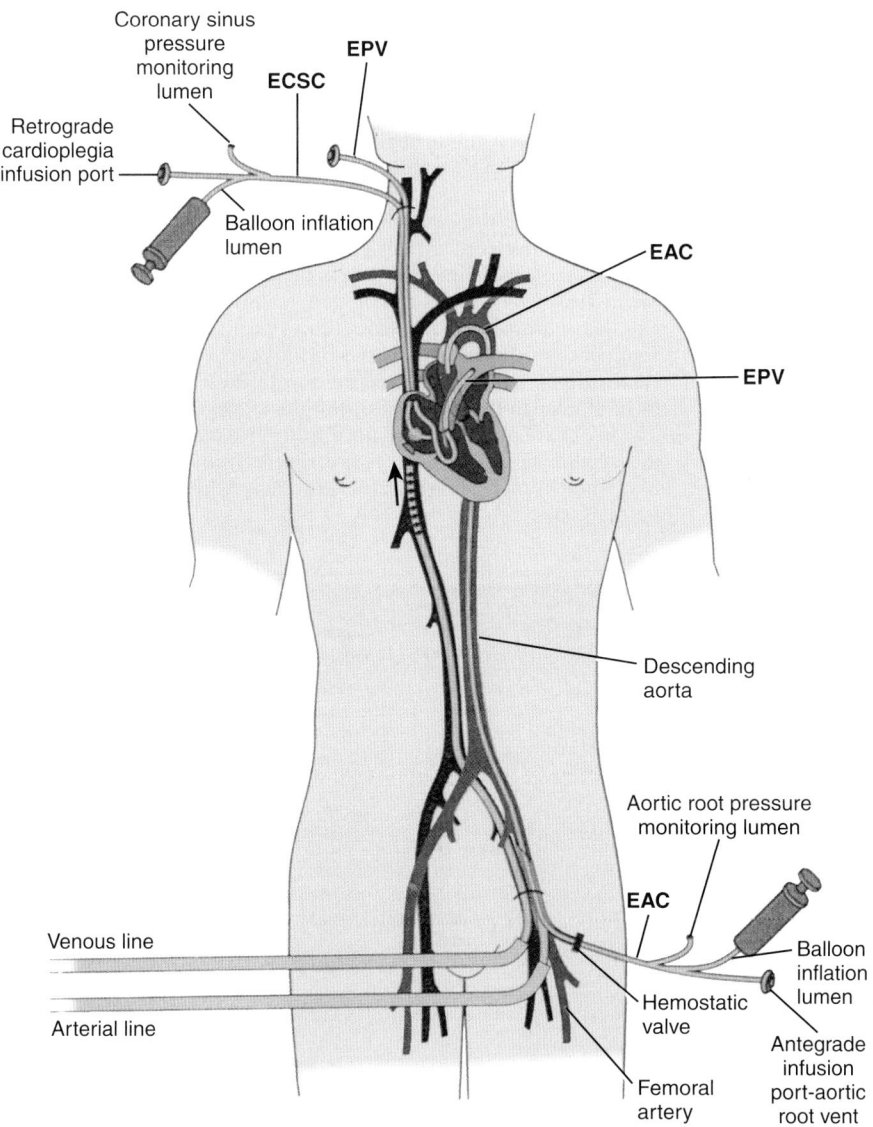

Figure 28-16 **Positioning of endovascular catheters.** The femoral venous drainage catheter tip is positioned at the right atrium-superior vena cava junction by fluoroscopy and transesophageal echocardiography. EAC, endoaortic clamp; ECSC, endocoronary sinus catheter; EPV, cardiopulmonary vent. *(From Toomasian JM, Peters SP, Siegel LC, Stevens JH: Extracorporeal circulation for port-access cardiac surgery. Perfusion 12:83, 1997.)*

Port-access CPB demands an expanded role of the anesthesiologist during CPB. The anesthesiologist is responsible for inserting the ECSC and the endopulmonary vent (EPV) through introducer sheaths placed in the right internal jugular vein. The ECSC should be placed first with the assistance of both fluoroscopy and two-dimensional TEE. The technique was recently described in detail by Lebon et al[739] and Miller et al,[740] who have a combined experience with more than 600 insertions. TEE guidance is used for engaging the coronary sinus and fluoroscopy for advancing the catheter in the coronary sinus. Proper placement is judged by attaining a pressure in the coronary sinus greater than 30 mm Hg during cardioplegia administration at a rate of 150 to 200 mL/min. The mean total procedure time in the series by Lebon et al was 16 ± 14 minutes. Failure can occur for a number of reasons, but the most common reason is displacement of the catheter from the coronary sinus during surgical manipulations. Complications including perforation and dissections have been reported in a small percentage of patients.

The EPV catheter is evolving in design and use. A balloon at the tip of the flow-directed catheter is inflated so that it floats into the pulmonary artery, to assist EPV catheter placement. The EPV is subsequently advanced over the flow-directed catheter until the tip is seated within the pulmonary artery. The balloon-tipped catheter is then withdrawn. In addition to fluoroscopy and TEE, distal catheter pressures facilitate positioning of the catheter.

As with any new procedure or technology, the anesthesiologist should expect a learning curve regarding the skill of placing an ECSC and EPV. A side benefit of port-access bypass is the necessity of increased communication among members of the health care team. It is hoped that this phenomenon will spill over to all CPB cases and decrease the likelihood of perfusion mishaps.

Monitoring for Endovascular Clamp Bypass

Measures of venous drainage, the arterial blood flow, ventricular venting, cardioplegic delivery, regional perfusion, and aortic occlusion must be carefully monitored to ensure safe and adequate CPB and myocardial protection. Although the surgical staff is positioned to assess cardioplegia delivery and LV venting, and the perfusionist monitors arterial flow and venous drainage to and from the CPB circuit, the anesthesiologist is responsible for determining the proper placement of the EAC and adequacy of CBF.[741]

The aorta catheter with the EAC should be positioned in the ascending aorta 2 to 4 cm distal to the aortic valve. Because cephalad migration of the endovascular aortic root clamp may compromise CBF, it is imperative to monitor endovascular clamp position continuously. There are several proposed methods to achieve this essential goal (Table 28-18). TEE and color-flow Doppler aid in visualizing the placement of the EAC balloon in the ascending aorta and in detecting any leakage of blood around the balloon. Right radial artery pressure will decrease acutely if the EAC migrates and obstructs the brachiocephalic artery. Some clinicians choose to measure blood pressure in the left and right radial arteries. The occurrence of acute difference in radial artery pressures may indicate cephalad migration of the EAC. Pulse-wave Doppler of the right carotid artery can verify cerebral perfusion but is frequently difficult to assess under the conditions of nonpulsatile blood flow. The ability of transcranial Doppler monitoring of the middle cerebral artery and cerebral oximetry techniques to determine the adequacy of CBF requires further evaluation. The TEE probe may be useful in visualizing the ascending aorta and location of the balloon; however, many clinicians report the inadequacy of this technique.

Port-Access Cardiac Surgery Outcome Data

Early advocates of PACS hoped that this new approach provided the benefits of minimally invasive surgery with the advantage of extracorporeal support and myocardial preservation during procedures on the heart. A relatively steep learning curve exists, and multiple, unexpected complications have been reported (e.g., inadequate deairing of the ventricle before discontinuation of CPB support, aortic or femoral artery dissection, malposition of the endovascular clamp).

Coronary artery surgery can be done using PACS, but it has not become a popular technique compared with OPCABs and other minimally invasive revascularization procedures. Mohr et al[742] reported a 9.8% mortality rate in their series of 51 patients undergoing elective mitral valve replacement or repair with PACS. Two patients suffered femoral artery dissections (requiring conversion to conventional techniques), and three patients required second operations for repair of postoperative perivalvular leaks. Patients in the port-access group reported the same amount of pain as those undergoing sternal splitting (as measured by a visual analog pain scale), challenging the hypothesis that minimally invasive procedures result in less pain than conventional approaches (see Chapter 38). Two other large series of mitral valve surgery via right thoracotomies with PACS found the outcomes to be similar to the standard operations done via a sternotomy.[743,744] The use of robotic assistance for mitral valve repairs performed via a thoracotomy using PACS has gained popularity in some centers; results have shown good success rates, less transfusion need, and shorter hospital stays.[745]

TABLE 28-18	Potential Strategies to Monitor Cerebral Blood Flow during Port-Access Bypass	
Monitor	Limitations	Observation with Cephalad Migration of Endoaortic Clamp*
Fluoroscopy	1. Must interrupt surgery to use monitor	EAC occluding great vessels
Transesophageal echocardiography	1. May be difficult to visualize EAC position during cardiopulmonary bypass	EAC in area of great vessels
Carotid ultrasound	1. Difficult to monitor signal continuously—depends on index of suspicion 2. Difficult to obtain signal with nonpulsatile blood flow	Sudden loss of blood flow signal
Transcranial Doppler	1. Difficult to monitor MCA blood flow continuously—depends on index of suspicion 2. Difficult to insonate MCA during nonpulsatile blood flow 3. Poor sensitivity/specificity	1. Loss of MCA blood flow velocity signal 2. Change in ratio of RMCA vs. LMCA blood flow velocity 3. Change in RMCA or LMCA blood flow direction
Cerebral venous blood oximetry (R vs. L signal)	1. Sensitivity/specificity?	Decrease in cerebral venous blood oxygen saturation; change in R vs. L signal†
Electroencephalography	1. Hypothermia, anesthetics, and roller pump artifacts limit interpretation of EEG signals	EEG slowing/change in right vs. left EEG signal
Right and left radial arterial pressures	1. Requires cannulation of both radial arteries; increased risk for hand ischemia 2. Left radial arterial free graft conduit not possible	Change in the ratio of right and left radial arteries measured MAP

*Hypothetical observation; the sensitivity and specificity of these monitors in this clinical setting have not been evaluated.
†The rate and magnitude of change depend on many factors, including the patient's cerebral temperature, magnitude of obstruction, and collateral blood flow.
EAC, endoaortic clamp; L, left; MAP, mean arterial pressure; MCA, middle cerebral artery; R, right.

REFERENCES

1. Mora Mangano CT, Chow JL, Kanevsky M: Cardiopulmonary bypass and the anesthesiologist. In Kaplan JA, Reich DL, Lake CL, et al, editors. *Kaplan's Cardiac Anesthesia*, ed 5, Philadelphia, 2006, Saunders Elsevier, pp 893–935.
2. American Society of Anesthesiologists: *Standards for basic anesthetic monitoring*. Available at: www.asahq.org/For-Members/Practice-Management/Practice-Parameters.aspx, accessed December 14, 2010.
3. American Society of Anesthesiologists (ASA): *Compliance with Medicare and Other Payor Billing Requirements*, Park Ridge, IL, 1997, ASA.
4. Braunwald E: The Simon Dack lecture. Cardiology: The past, the present, and the future, *J Am Coll Cardiol* 42:2031–2041, 2003.
5. Edmunds LH: Cardiopulmonary bypass after 50 years, *N Engl J Med* 351:1603–1606, 2004.
6. Cohn LH: Fifty years of open-heart surgery, *Circulation* 107:2168–2170, 2003.
7. Mora CT: *Cardiopulmonary BYPASS*, New York, 1995, Springer-Verlag.
8. Taylor PC, Effler DB: Management of cannulation for cardiopulmonary bypass in patients with adult-acquired heart disease, *Surg Clin North Am* 55:1205–1215, 1975.
9. Wolman RL, Nussmeier NA, Aggarwal A, et al: Cerebral injury after cardiac surgery: Identification of a group at extraordinary risk, *Stroke* 30:514–522, 1999.
10. Newman MF, Kirchner JL, Phillips-Bute B, et al: Longitudinal assessment of neurocognitive function after coronary-artery bypass surgery, *N Engl J Med* 344:395–402, 2001.
11. Nussmeier N: Adverse neurologic events: Risks of intracardiac versus extracardiac surgery, *J Cardiothorac Vasc Anesth* 10:31–37, 1996.
12. Roach GW, Kanchuger M, Mangano CM, et al: Adverse cerebral outcomes after coronary bypass surgery. Multicenter Study of Perioperative Ischemia Research Group and the Ischemia Research and Education Foundation Investigators, *N Engl J Med* 335:1857–1863, 1996.
13. Selnes OA, Grega MA, Bailey MM, et al: Cognition 6 years after surgical or medical therapy for coronary artery disease, *Ann Neurol* 63:581–590, 2008.
14. Leung JM, Sands LP: Long-term cognitive decline: Is there a link to surgery and anesthesia? *Anesthesiology* 111:931–932, 2009.
15. Newman MF, Grocott HP, Mathew JP, et al: Report of the substudy assessing the impact of neurocognitive function on quality of life 5 years after cardiac surgery, *Stroke* 32:2874–2881, 2001.
16. Arrowsmith JE, Grocott HP, Reves JG, et al: Central nervous system complications of cardiac surgery, *Br J Anaesth* 84:378–393, 2000.
17. Newman MF, Croughwell ND, Blumenthal JA, et al: Effect of aging on cerebral autoregulation during cardiopulmonary bypass. Association with postoperative cognitive dysfunction, *Circulation* 90: II243–II249, 1994.
18. Aoki M, Nomura F, Stromski ME, et al: Effects of pH on brain energetics after hypothermic circulatory arrest, *Ann Thorac Surg* 55:1093–1103, 1993.
19. Cosgrove D, Loop F, Lytle B, et al: Primary myocardial revascularizations, *J Thorac Cardiovasc Surg* 88:673–684, 1984.
20. Gardner TJ, Horneffer PJ, Gott VL, et al: Coronary artery bypass grafting in women. A ten-year perspective, *Ann Surg* 201:780–784, 1985.
21. Newman M, Kramer D, Croughwell N, et al: Differential age effects of mean arterial pressure and rewarming on cognitive dysfunction after cardiac surgery, *Anesth Analg* 81:236–242, 1995.
22. Tuman KJ, McCarthy RJ, Najafi H, et al: Differential effects of advanced age on neurologic and cardiac risks of coronary artery operations, *J Thorac Cardiovasc Surg* 104:1510–1517, 1992.
23. Hogue CW Jr, De Wet CJ, Schechtman KB, et al: The importance of prior stroke for the adjusted risk of neurologic injury after cardiac surgery for women and men, *Anesthesiology* 98:823–829, 2003.
24. Hogue CW, Lillie R, Hershey T, et al: Gender influence on cognitive function after cardiac operation, *Ann Thorac Surg* 76:1119–1125, 2003.
25. Martin WR, Hashimoto SA: Stroke in coronary bypass surgery, *Can J Neurol Sci* 9:21–26, 1982.
26. Sotaniemi K: Brain damage and neurological outcome after open-heart surgery, *J Neurol Neurosurg Psychiatry* 43:127–135, 1980.
27. Turnipseed WD, Berkoff HA, Belzer FO: Postoperative stroke in cardiac and peripheral vascular disease, *Ann Surg* 192:365–368, 1980.
28. Breslau PJ, Fell G, Ivey TD, et al: Carotid arterial disease in patients undergoing coronary artery bypass operations, *J Thorac Cardiovasc Surg* 82:765–767, 1981.
29. Brener BJ, Brief DK, Alpert J, et al: The risk of stroke in patients with asymptomatic carotid stenosis undergoing cardiac surgery: A follow-up study, *J Vasc Surg* 5:269–279, 1987.
30. Amarenco P, Duyckaerts C, Tzourio C, et al: The prevalence of ulcerated plaques in the aortic arch in patients with stroke, *N Engl J Med* 1992:221–225, 1992.
31. Blauth CI, Cosgrove DM, Webb BW, et al: Atheroembolism from the ascending aorta. An emerging problem in cardiac surgery, *J Thorac Cardiovasc Surg* 103:1104–1111, 1992 discussion 11–12.
32. Blumenthal J, Mahanna E, Madden D, et al: Methodological issues in the assessment of neuropsychologic function after cardiac surgery, *Ann Thorac Surg* 59:1345–1350, 1995.
33. Borowicz L, Goldsborough M, Selenes O, et al: Neuropsychological changes after cardiac surgery: A critical review, *J Cardiothorac Vasc Anesth* 10:105–112, 1996.
34. Branthwaite MA: Neurological damage related to open-heart surgery. A clinical survey, *Thorax* 27:748–753, 1972.
35. Harris LS, Kennedy JH: Atheromatous cerebral embolism. A complication of surgery of the thoracic aorta, *Ann Thorac Surg* 4:319–326, 1967.
36. Barbut D, Lo YW, Hartman GS, et al: Aortic atheroma is related to outcome but not numbers of emboli during coronary bypass, *Ann Thorac Surg* 64:454–459, 1997.
37. Davila-Roman VG, Barzilai B, Wareing TH, et al: Intraoperative ultrasonographic evaluation of the ascending aorta in 100 consecutive patients undergoing cardiac surgery, *Circulation* 84:III47–III53, 1991.
38. Hartman GS, Yao FS, Bruefach M 3rd, et al: Severity of aortic atheromatous disease diagnosed by transesophageal echocardiography predicts stroke and other outcomes associated with coronary artery surgery: A prospective study, *Anesth Analg* 83:701–708, 1996.
39. Katz ES, Tunick PA, Rusinek H, et al: Protruding aortic atheromas predict stroke in elderly patients undergoing cardiopulmonary bypass: Experience with intraoperative transesophageal echocardiography, *J Am Coll Cardiol* 20:70–77, 1992.
40. Cheng MA, Theard MA, Tempelhoff R: Intravenous agents and intraoperative neuroprotection. Beyond barbiturates, *Crit Care Clin* 13:185–199, 1997.
41. Moody DM, Brown WR, Challa VR, et al: Brain microemboli associated with cardiopulmonary bypass: A histologic and magnetic resonance imaging study, *Ann Thorac Surg* 59:1304–1307, 1995.
42. Brooker RF, Brown WR, Moody DM, et al: Cardiotomy suction: A major source of brain lipid emboli during cardiopulmonary bypass, *Ann Thorac Surg* 65:1651–1655, 1998.
43. Aldea GS, Soltow LO, Chandler WL, et al: Limitation of thrombin generation, platelet activation, and inflammation by elimination of cardiotomy suction in patients undergoing coronary artery bypass grafting treated with heparin-bonded circuits, *J Thorac Cardiovasc Surg* 123:742–755, 2002.
44. Borger MA, Peniston CM, Weisel RD, et al: Neuropsychologic impairment after coronary bypass surgery: Effect of gaseous microemboli during perfusionist interventions, *J Thorac Cardiovasc Surg* 121:743–749, 2001.
45. Stump DA, Rogers AT, Hammon JW, et al: Cerebral emboli and cognitive outcome after cardiac surgery, *J Cardiothorac Vasc Anesth* 10:113–118, 1996, quiz 8–9.
46. Stump DA, Kon NA, Rogers AT, et al: Emboli and neuropsychological outcome following cardiopulmonary bypass, *Echocardiography* 13:555–558, 1996.
47. Pugsley W, Klinger L, Paschalis C, et al: Microemboli and cerebral impairmant during cardiac surgery, *Vasc Surg* 24:34–43, 1990.
48. van Dijk D, Kalkman CJ: Why are cerebral microemboli not associated with cognitive decline? *Anesth Analg* 109:1006–1008, 2009.
49. Tegeler CH, Babikian VL, Gomez CR: *Neurosonology*, St. Louis, 1996, Mosby.
50. Djaiani G, Fedorko L, Borger M, et al: Mild to moderate atheromatous disease of the thoracic aorta and new ischemic brain lesions after conventional coronary artery bypass graft surgery, *Stroke* 35:e356–e358, 2004.
51. Davila-Roman VG, Murphy SF, Nickerson NJ, et al: Atherosclerosis of the ascending aorta is an independent predictor of long-term neurologic events and mortality, *J Am Coll Cardiol* 33:1308–1316, 1999.
52. Amarenco P, Cohen A, Tzourio C, et al: Atherosclerotic disease of the aortic arch and the risk of ischemic stroke, *N Engl J Med* 331:1474–1479, 1994.
53. Bar-Yosef S, Mathew JP, Newman MF, et al: Prevention of cerebral hyperthermia during cardiac surgery by limiting on-bypass rewarming in combination with post-bypass body surface warming: A feasibility study, *Ann Thorac Surg* 99:641–646, 2004.
54. Royse AG, Royse CF, Ajani AE, et al: Reduced neuropsychological dysfunction using epiaortic echocardiography and the exclusive Y graft, *Ann Thorac Surg* 69:1431–1438, 2000.
55. Mackensen GB, Ti LK, Phillips-Bute BG, et al: Cerebral embolization during cardiac surgery: Impact of aortic atheroma burden, *Br J Anaesth* 91:656–661, 2003.
56. Grocott HP, Homi HM, Puskas F: Cognitive dysfunction after cardiac surgery: Revisiting etiology, *Semin Cardiothorac Vasc Anesth* 9:123–129, 2005.
57. Nussmeier N, Arlund A, Slogoff S: Neuropsychiatric complications after cardiopulmonary bypass: Cerebral protection by a barbiturate, *Anesthesiology* 64:165–170, 1986.
58. Newman M, Murkin J, Roach G, et al: Cerebral physiologic effects of burst suppression doses of propofol during nonpulsatile cardiopulmonary bypass, *Anesth Analg* 81:452–457, 1995.
59. Gold JP, Charlson ME, Williams-Russo P, et al: Improvement of outcomes after coronary artery bypass, *J Thorac Cardiovasc Surg* 110:1302–1314, 1995.
60. Sillesen H, Nedergaard M, Schroeder T, et al: Middle cerebral artery occlusion in presence of low perfusion pressure increases infarct size in rats, *Neurol Res* 10:61–63, 1988.
61. Mutch WA, Ryner LN, Kozlowski P, et al: Cerebral hypoxia during cardiopulmonary bypass: A magnetic resonance imaging study, *Ann Thorac Surg* 64:695–701, 1997.
62. Croughwell ND, Reves JG, White WD, et al: Cardiopulmonary bypass time does not affect cerebral blood flow, *Ann Thorac Surg* 65:1226–1230, 1998.
63. Grigore AM, Grocott HP, Mathew JP, et al: The rewarming rate and increased peak temperature alter neurocognitive outcome after cardiac surgery, *Anesth Analg* 94:4–10, 2002.
64. Grocott HP, Mackensen GB, Grigore AM, et al: Postoperative hyperthermia is associated with cognitive dysfunction after coronary artery bypass graft surgery, *Stroke* 33:537–541, 2002.
65. Thong WY, Strickler AG, Li S, et al: Hyperthermia in the forty-eight hours after cardiopulmonary bypass, *Anesth Analg* 95:1489–1495, 2002, table of contents.
66. Gerriets T, Stolz E, Walberer M, et al: Neuroprotective effects of MK-801 in different rat stroke models for permanent middle cerebral artery occlusion: Adverse effects of hypothalamic damage and strategies for its avoidance, *Stroke* 34:2234–2239, 2003.
67. Pintar T, Collard CD: The systemic inflammatory response to cardiopulmonary bypass, *Anesthesiol Clin North Am* 21:453–464, 2003.
68. Hindman BJ, Moore SA, Cutkomp J, et al: Brain expression of inducible cyclooxygenase 2 messenger RNA in rats undergoing cardiopulmonary bypass, *Anesthesiology* 95:1380–1388, 2001.
69. Bogdanski R, Blobner M, Becker I, et al: Cerebral histopathology following portal venous infusion of bacteria in a chronic porcine model, *Anesthesiology* 93:793–804, 2000.
70. Chamorro A: Role of inflammation in stroke and atherothrombosis, *Cerebrovasc Dis* 17(Suppl 3):1–5, 2004.
71. Mathew JP, Grocott HP, Phillips-Bute B, et al: Lower endotoxin immunity predicts increased cognitive dysfunction in elderly patients after cardiac surgery, *Stroke* 34:508–513, 2003.
72. Hamilton-Davies C, Barclay GR, Cardigan RA, et al: Relationship between preoperative endotoxin immune status, gut perfusion, and outcome from cardiac valve replacement surgery, *Chest* 112:1189–1196, 1997.
73. Harris D, Oatridge A, Dob D, et al: Cerebral swelling after normothermic cardiopulmonary bypass, *Anesthesiology* 88:340–345, 1998.
74. Harris D, Bailey S, Smith P, et al: Brain swelling in first hour after coronary artery bypass surgery, *Lancet* 342:586–587, 1993.
75. Murkin JM, Stump DA: Conference on cardiac and vascular surgery: Neurobehavioral assessment, physiological monitoring and cerebral protective strategies. Introduction, *Ann Thorac Surg* 70: 1767–1769, 2000.
76. Kandel ER, Schwartz JH, Jessell TM: *Principles of Neural Science*, ed 3, Norwalk, VA, 1991, Appleton and Lange.
77. Gillinov A, Davis E, Curtis W, et al: Cardiopulmonary bypass and the blood brain barrier. An experimental study, *J Thorac Cardiovasc Surg* 104:1110–1115, 1992.
78. Cavaglia M, Seshadri SG, Marchand JE, et al: Increased transcription factor expression and permeability of the blood brain barrier associated with cardiopulmonary bypass in lambs, *Ann Thorac Surg* 78:1418–1425, 2004.
79. Culley DJ, Baxter M, Yukhananov R, et al: The memory effects of general anesthesia persist for weeks in young and aged rats, *Anesth Analg* 96:1004–1009, 2003, table of contents.
80. Homi HM, Calvi CL, Lynch J, et al: Longitudinal assessment of neurocognitive function in rats after cardiopulmonary bypass: Evidence for long-term deficits, *J Cardiothorac Vasc Anesth* 24:293–299, 2010.
81. Jevtovic-Todorovic V, Beals J, Benshoff N, et al: Prolonged exposure to inhalational anesthetic nitrous oxide kills neurons in adult rat brain, *Neuroscience* 122:609–616, 2003.
82. Futterer CD, Maurer MH, Schmitt A, et al: Alterations in rat brain proteins after desflurane anesthesia, *Anesthesiology* 100:302–308, 2004.
83. Saunders A, Strittmatter W, Schmechel D, et al: Association of apolipoprotein E allele epsilon 4 with late-onset familial and sporadic Alzheimer's disease, *Neurology* 43:1467–1472, 1993.
84. Tardiff BE, Newman MF, Saunders AM, et al: Preliminary report of a genetic basis for cognitive decline after cardiac operations. The Neurologic Outcome Research Group of the Duke Heart Center, *Ann Thorac Surg* 64:715–720, 1997.
85. Gaynor JW, Gerdes M, Zackai EH, et al: Apolipoprotein E genotype and neurodevelopmental sequelae of infant cardiac surgery, *J Thorac Cardiovasc Surg* 126:1736–1745, 2003.
86. Barakat K, Kennon S, Hitman GA, et al: Interaction between smoking and the glycoprotein IIIa P1(A2) polymorphism in non-ST-elevation acute coronary syndromes, *J Am Coll Cardiol* 38: 1639–1643, 2001.
87. Kenny D, Muckian C, Fitzgerald DJ, et al: Platelet glycoprotein Ib alpha receptor polymorphisms and recurrent ischaemic events in acute coronary syndrome patients, *J Thromb Thrombolysis* 13:13–19, 2002.
88. Mathew JP, Rinder CS, Howe JG, et al: Platelet PlA2 polymorphism enhances risk of neurocognitive decline after cardiopulmonary bypass. Multicenter Study of Perioperative Ischemia (McSPI) Research Group, *Ann Thorac Surg* 71:663–666, 2001.

89. Grocott HP, White WD, Morris RW, et al: Genetic polymorphisms and the risk of stroke after cardiac surgery, *Stroke* 36:1854–1858, 2005.
90. Mathew JP, Podgoreanu MV, Grocott HP, et al: Genetic variants in P-selectin and C-reactive protein influence susceptibility to cognitive decline after cardiac surgery, *J Am Coll Cardiol* 49:1934–1942, 2007.
91. Mathew JP, Grocott HP, Podgoreanu MV, et al: Inflammatory and prothrombotic genetic polymorphisms are associated with cognitive decline after CABG surgery, *Anesthesiology* 101:A274, 2004.
92. Lapietra A, Grossi EA, Pua BB, et al: Assisted venous drainage presents the risk of undetected air microembolism, *J Thorac Cardiovasc Surg* 120:856–862, 2000.
93. Webb WR, Harrison LH Jr, Helmcke FR, et al: Carbon dioxide field flooding minimizes residual intracardiac air after open heart operations, *Ann Thorac Surg* 64:1489–1491, 1997.
94. Svenarud P, Persson M, van der Linden J: Effect of CO2 insufflation on the number and behavior of air microemboli in open-heart surgery: A randomized clinical trial, *Circulation* 109:1127–1132, 2004.
95. Swaminathan M, Grocott HP, Mackensen GB, et al: The "sandblasting" effect of aortic cannula on arch atheroma during cardiopulmonary bypass, *Anesth Analg* 104:1350–1351, 2007.
96. Borger MA, Taylor RL, Weisel RD, et al: Decreased cerebral emboli during distal aortic arch cannulation: A randomized clinical trial, *J Thorac Cardiovasc Surg* 118:740–745, 1999.
97. Cook DJ, Zehr KJ, Orszulak TA, et al: Profound reduction in brain embolization using an endoaortic baffle during bypass in swine, *Ann Thorac Surg* 73:198–202, 2002.
98. Reichenspurner H, Navia JA, Berry G, et al: Particulate emboli capture by an intra-aortic filter device during cardiac surgery, *J Thorac Cardiovasc Surg* 119:233–241, 2000.
99. Banbury MK, Kouchoukos NT, Allen KB, et al: Emboli capture using the Embol-X intraaortic filter in cardiac surgery: A multicentered randomized trial of 1,289 patients, *Ann Thorac Surg* 76:508–515, 2003.
100. Eifert S, Reichenspurner H, Pfefferkorn T, et al: Neurological and neuropsychological examination and outcome after use of an intra-aortic filter device during cardiac surgery, *Perfusion* 18(Suppl 1): 55–60, 2003.
101. Rubens FD, Boodhwani M, Mesana T, et al: The cardiotomy trial: A randomized, double-blind study to assess the effect of processing of shed blood during cardiopulmonary bypass on transfusion and neurocognitive function, *Circulation* 116:I89–I97, 2007.
102. Djaiani G, Fedorko L, Borger MA, et al: Continuous-flow cell saver reduces cognitive decline in elderly patients after coronary bypass surgery, *Circulation* 116:1888–1895, 2007.
103. Bar-Yosef S, Anders M, Mackensen GB, et al: Aortic atheroma burden and cognitive dysfunction after coronary artery bypass graft surgery, *Ann Thorac Surg* 78:1556–1563, 2004.
104. Hammon JW, Stump DA, Butterworth JF, et al: Single crossclamp improves 6-month cognitive outcome in high-risk coronary bypass patients: The effect of reduced aortic manipulation, *J Thorac Cardiovasc Surg* 131:114–121, 2006.
105. Cook DJ, Orszulak TA, Zehr KJ, et al: Effectiveness of the Cobra aortic catheter for dual-temperature management during adult cardiac surgery, *J Thorac Cardiovasc Surg* 125:378–384, 2003.
106. Edmunds LH Jr: Pulseless cardiopulmonary bypass, *J Thorac Cardiovasc Surg* 84:800–804, 1982.
107. Hickey PR, Buckley MJ, Philbin DM: Pulsatile and nonpulsatile cardiopulmonary bypass: Review of a counterproductive controversy, *Ann Thorac Surg* 36:720–737, 1983.
108. Nakayama K, Tamiya T, Yamamoto K, et al: High-amplitude pulsatile pump in extracorporeal circulation with particular reference to hemodynamics, *Surgery* 54:798–809, 1963.
109. Shepard RB, Kirklin JW: Relation of pulsatile flow to oxygen consumption and other variables during cardiopulmonary bypass, *J Thorac Cardiovasc Surg* 58:694–702 passim, 1969.
110. Dunn J, Kirsh MM, Harness J, et al: Hemodynamic, metabolic, and hematologic effects of pulsatile cardiopulmonary bypass, *J Thorac Cardiovasc Surg* 68:138–147, 1974.
111. Jacobs LA, Klopp EH, Seamone W, et al: Improved organ function during cardiac bypass with a roller pump modified to deliver pulsatile flow, *J Thorac Cardiovasc Surg* 58:703–712 passim, 1969.
112. Dernevik L, Arvidsson S, William-Olsson G: Cerebral perfusion in dogs during pulsatile and non-pulsatile extracorporeal circulation, *J Cardiovasc Surg (Torino)* 26:32–35, 1985.
113. Philbin DM, Levine FH, Emerson CW, et al: Plasma vasopressin levels and urinary flow during cardiopulmonary bypass in patients with valvular heart disease: Effect of pulsatile flow, *J Thorac Cardiovasc Surg* 78:779–783, 1979.
114. Taylor KM, Bain WH, Russell M, et al: Peripheral vascular resistance and angiotensin II levels during pulsatile and no-pulsatile cardiopulmonary bypass, *Thorax* 34:594–598, 1979.
115. Boucher JK, Rudy LW Jr, Edmunds LH Jr: Organ blood flow during pulsatile cardiopulmonary bypass, *J Appl Physiol* 36:86–90, 1974.
116. Singh RK, Barratt-Boyes BG, Harris EA: Does pulsatile flow improve perfusion during hypothermic cardiopulmonary bypass? *J Thorac Cardiovasc Surg* 79:827–832, 1980.
117. Frater RW, Wakayama S, Oka Y, et al: Pulsatile cardiopulmonary bypass: Failure to influence hemodynamics or hormones, *Circulation* 62:I19–I25, 1980.
118. Salerno TA, Henderson M, Keith FM, et al: Hypertension after coronary operation. Can it be prevented by pulsatile perfusion? *J Thorac Cardiovasc Surg* 81:396–399, 1981.
119. Landymore RW, Murphy DA, Kinley CE, et al: Does pulsatile flow influence the incidence of postoperative hypertension? *Ann Thorac Surg* 28:261–268, 1979.
120. Watkins WD, Peterson MB, Kong DL, et al: Thromboxane and prostacyclin changes during cardiopulmonary bypass with and without pulsatile flow, *J Thorac Cardiovasc Surg* 84:250–256, 1982.
121. Nieminen MT, Philbin DM, Rosow CE, et al: Temperature gradients and rewarming time during hypothermic cardiopulmonary bypass with and without pulsatile flow, *Ann Thorac Surg* 35:488–492, 1983.
122. Nagaoka H, Innami R, Arai H: Effects of pulsatile cardiopulmonary bypass on the renin-angiotensin-aldosterone system following open heart surgery, *Jpn J Surg* 18:390–396, 1988.
123. Lindberg H, Svennevig JL, Lilleaasen P, et al: Pulsatile vs. non-pulsatile flow during cardiopulmonary bypass. A comparison of early postoperative changes, *Scand J Thorac Cardiovasc Surg* 18:195–201, 1984.
124. Mori A, Watanabe K, Onoe M, et al: Regional blood flow in the liver, pancreas and kidney during pulsatile and nonpulsatile perfusion under profound hypothermia, *Jpn Circ J* 52:219–227, 1988.
125. Matsumoto T, Wolferth CC Jr, Perlman MH: Effects of pulsatile and non-pulsatile perfusion upon cerebral and conjunctival microcirculation in dogs, *Am Surg* 37:61–64, 1971.
126. Williams GD, Seifen AB, Lawson NW, et al: Pulsatile perfusion versus conventional high-flow nonpulsatile perfusion for rapid core cooling and rewarming of infants for circulatory arrest in cardiac operation, *J Thorac Cardiovasc Surg* 78:667–677, 1979.
127. Philbin DM, Levine FH, Kono K, et al: Attenuation of the stress response to cardiopulmonary bypass by the addition of pulsatile flow, *Circulation* 64:808–812, 1981.
128. Kono K, Philbin DM, Coggins CH, et al: Adrenocortical hormone levels during cardiopulmonary bypass with and without pulsatile flow, *J Thorac Cardiovasc Surg* 85:129–133, 1983.
129. Murray WR, Mittra S, Mittra D, et al: The amylase-creatinine clearance ratio following cardiopulmonary bypass, *J Thorac Cardiovasc Surg* 82:248–253, 1981.
130. Andersen K, Waaben J, Husum B, et al: Nonpulsatile cardiopulmonary bypass disrupts the flow-metabolism couple in the brain, *J Thorac Cardiovasc Surg* 90:570–579, 1985.
131. Sanderson JM, Wright G, Sims FW: Brain damage in dogs immediately following pulsatile and non-pulsatile blood flows in extracorporeal circulation, *Thorax* 27:275–286, 1972.
132. Tranmer BI, Gross CE, Kindt GW, et al: Pulsatile versus nonpulsatile blood flow in the treatment of acute cerebral ischemia, *Neurosurgery* 19:724–731, 1986.
133. Mavroudis C: To pulse or not to pulse, *Ann Thorac Surg* 25:259–271, 1978.
134. Evans PJ, Ruygrok P, Seelye ER, et al: Does sodium nitroprusside improve tissue oxygenation during cardiopulmonary bypass? *Br J Anaesth* 49:799–803, 1977.
135. Grossi EA, Connolly MW, Krieger KH, et al: Quantification of pulsatile flow during cardiopulmonary bypass to permit direct comparison of the effectiveness of various types of "pulsatile" and "nonpulsatile" flow, *Surgery* 98:547–554, 1985.
136. Badner NH, Murkin JM, Lok P: Differences in pH management and pulsatile/nonpulsatile perfusion during cardiopulmonary bypass do not influence renal function, *Anesth Analg* 75:696–701, 1992.
137. Shaw PJ, Bates D, Cartlidge NE, et al: An analysis of factors predisposing to neurological injury in patients undergoing coronary bypass operations, *Q J Med* 72:633–646, 1989.
138. Murkin J, Martzke J, Buchan A, et al: A randomized study of the influence of perfusion technique and pH management strategy in 316 patients undergoing coronary artery bypass surgery, *J Thorac Cardiovasc Surg* 110:349–362, 1995.
139. Kawahara F, Kadoi Y, Saito S, et al: Balloon pump-induced pulsatile perfusion during cardiopulmonary bypass does not improve brain oxygenation, *J Thorac Cardiovasc Surg* 118:361–366, 1999.
140. Mutch W, Lefevre G, Thiessen D, et al: Computer-controlled cardiopulmonary bypass increases jugular venous oxygen saturation during rewarming, *Ann Thorac Surg* 65:59–65, 1998.
141. Patel RL, Turtle MR, Chambers DJ, et al: Alpha-stat acid-base regulation during cardiopulmonary bypass improves neuropsychologic outcome in patients undergoing coronary artery bypass grafting, *J Thorac Cardiovasc Surg* 111:1267–1279, 1996.
142. Duebener LF, Hagino I, Sakamoto T, et al: Effects of pH management during deep hypothermic bypass on cerebral microcirculation: alpha-Stat versus pH-stat, *Circulation* 106:I103–I108, 2002.
143. Laussen PC: Optimal blood gas management during deep hypothermic paediatric cardiac surgery: alpha-Stat is easy, but pH-stat may be preferable, *Paediatr Anaesth* 12:199–204, 2002.
144. Michenfelder J, Milde J: The relationship among canine brain temperature, metabolism, and function during hypothermia, *Anesthesiology* 75:130–136, 1991.
145. Busto R, Globus M, Dietrich W, et al: Effect of mild hypothermia on ischemia-induced release of neurotransmitters and free fatty acids in rat brain, *Stroke* 20:904–910, 1989.
146. Bickler PE, Buck LT, Hansen BM: Effects of isoflurane and hypothermia on glutamate receptor-mediated calcium influx in brain slices, *Anesthesiology* 81:1461–1469, 1994.
147. Widmann R, Miyazawa T, Hossmann K: Protective effect of hypothermia on hippocampal injury after 30 minutes of forebrain ischemia in rats is mediated by postischemic recovery of protein synthesis, *J Neurochem* 61:200–209, 1993.
148. Busto R, Globus M, Neary J, et al: Regional alterations of protein kinase C activity following transient cerebral ischemia: Effects of intraischemic brain temperature modulation, *J Neurochem* 63:1095–1103, 1994.
149. Nakashima K, Todd MM, Warner DS: The relation between cerebral metabolic rate and ischemic depolarization. A comparison of the effects of hypothermia, pentobarbital, and isoflurane, *Anesthesiology* 82:1199–1208, 1995.
150. Globus M, Busto R, Lin B, et al: Detection of free radical activity during transient global ischemia and recirculation: Effects of intraischemic brain temperature modulation, *J Neurochem* 65:1250–1256, 1995.
151. Kader A, Frazzini V, Baker C, et al: Effect of mild hypothermia on nitric oxide synthesis during focal cerebral ischemia, *Neurosurgery* 35:272–277, 1994.
152. Bernard SA, Gray TW, Buist MD, et al: Treatment of comatose survivors of out-of-hospital cardiac arrest with induced hypothermia, *N Engl J Med* 346:557–563, 2002.
153. Mild therapeutic hypothermia to improve the neurologic outcome after cardiac arrest, *N Engl J Med* 346:549–556, 2002.
154. Clifton GL, Miller ER, Choi SC, et al: Lack of effect of induction of hypothermia after acute brain injury, *N Engl J Med* 344:556–563, 2001.
155. Todd MM, Hindman BJ, Clarke WR, et al: Mild intraoperative hypothermia during surgery for intracranial aneurysm, *N Engl J Med* 352:135–145, 2005.
156. The Warm Heart Investigators: Randomized trial of normothermic versus hypothermic coronary bypass surgery, *Lancet* 343:559–563, 1994.
157. Gaillard D, Bical O, Paumier D, et al: A review of myocardial normothermia: Its theoretical basis and the potential clinical benefits in cardiac surgery, *Cardiovasc Surg* 8:198–203, 2000.
158. Nicolini F, Beghi C, Muscari C, et al: Myocardial protection in adult cardiac surgery: Current options and future challenges, *Eur J Cardiothorac Surg* 24:986–993, 2003.
159. Panos AL, Deslauriers R, Birnbaum PL, et al: Perspectives on myocardial protection: Warm heart surgery, *Perfusion* 8:287–291, 1993.
160. Martin T, Craver J, Gott J, et al: Prospective, randomized trial of retrograde warm blood cardioplegia: Myocardial benefit and neurologic threat, *Ann Thorac Surg* 57:298–302, 1994.
161. Grigore AM, Mathew J, Grocott HP, et al: Prospective randomized trial of normothermic versus hypothermic cardiopulmonary bypass on cognitive function after coronary artery bypass graft surgery, *Anesthesiology* 95:1110–1119, 2001.
162. Mora C, Henson M, Weintraub W, et al: The effect of temperature management during cardiopulmonary bypass on neurologic and neuropsychologic outcomes in patients undergoing coronary revascularization, *J Thorac Cardiovasc Surg* 112:514–522, 1996.
163. McLean RF, Wong BI, Naylor CD, et al: Cardiopulmonary bypass, temperature, and central nervous system dysfunction, *Circulation* 90:II250–II255, 1994.
164. Grocott HP, Newman MF, Croughwell ND, et al: Continuous jugular venous versus nasopharyngeal temperature monitoring during hypothermic cardiopulmonary bypass for cardiac surgery, *J Clin Anesth* 9:312–316, 1997.
165. Nathan HJ, Wells GA, Munson JL, et al: Neuroprotective effect of mild hypothermia in patients undergoing coronary artery surgery with cardiopulmonary bypass: A randomized trial, *Circulation* 104:I85–I91, 2001.
166. van Dijk D, Spoor M, Hijman R, et al: Cognitive and cardiac outcomes 5 years after off-pump vs on-pump coronary artery bypass graft surgery, *JAMA* 297:701–708, 2007.
167. Stone JG, Young WL, Smith CR, et al: Do standard monitoring sites reflect true brain temperature when profound hypothermia is rapidly induced and reversed? *Anesthesiology* 82:344–351, 1995.
168. Cook DJ, Oliver WC Jr, Orszulak TA, et al: A prospective, randomized comparison of cerebral venous oxygen saturation during normothermic and hypothermic cardiopulmonary bypass, *J Thorac Cardiovasc Surg* 107:1020–1028, 1994; discussion 8–9.
169. Plochl W, Liam BL, Cook DJ, et al: Cerebral response to haemodilution during cardiopulmonary bypass in dogs: The role of nitric oxide synthase, *Br J Anaesth* 82:237–243, 1999.
170. Govier AV, Reves JG, McKay RD, et al: Factors and their influence on regional cerebral blood flow during nonpulsatile cardiopulmonary bypass, *Ann Thorac Surg* 38:592–600, 1984.
171. Newman MF, Croughwell ND, White WD, et al: Effect of perfusion pressure on cerebral blood flow during normothermic cardiopulmonary bypass, *Circulation* 94:II353–II357, 1996.
172. Barry DI, Strandgaard S, Graham DI, et al: Cerebral blood flow in rats with renal and spontaneous hypertension: Resetting of the lower limit of autoregulation, *J Cereb Blood Flow Metab* 2:347–353, 1982.
173. Schell RM, Kern FH, Greeley WJ, et al: Cerebral blood flow and metabolism during cardiopulmonary bypass, *Anesth Analg* 76:849–865, 1993.

174. Croughwell N, Lyth M, Quill TJ, et al: Diabetic patients have abnormal cerebral autoregulation during cardiopulmonary bypass, *Circulation* 82:IV407–IV412, 1990.
175. Lanier WL: Glucose management during cardiopulmonary bypass: Cardiovascular and neurologic implications, *Anesth Analg* 72:423–427, 1991.
176. Dietrich WD, Alonso O, Busto R: Moderate hyperglycemia worsens acute blood-brain barrier injury after forebrain ischemia in rats, *Stroke* 24:111–116, 1993.
177. Siesjö B: Acidosis and ischemic brain damage, *Neurochem Pathol* 9:31–88, 1988.
178. Warner DS, Gionet TX, Todd MM, et al: Insulin-induced normoglycemia improves ischemic outcome in hyperglycemic rats, *Stroke* 22:1775–1781, 1992.
179. Feerick AE, Johnston WE, Jenkins LW, et al: Hyperglycemia during hypothermic canine cardiopulmonary bypass increases cerebral lactate, *Anesthesiology* 82:512–520, 1995.
180. Lam AM, Winn HR, Cullen BF, et al: Hyperglycemia and neurological outcome in patients with head injury, *J Neurosurg* 75:545–551, 1991.
181. Li PA, Shuaib A, Miyashita H, et al: Hyperglycemia enhances extracellular glutamate accumulation in rats subjected to forebrain ischemia, *Stroke* 31:183–192, 2000.
182. Hindman B: Con: Glucose priming solutions should not be used for cardiopulmonary bypass, *J Cardiothorac Vasc Anesth* 9:605–607, 1995.
183. Metz S, Keats AS: Benefits of a glucose-containing priming solution for cardiopulmonary bypass, *Anesth Analg* 72:428–434, 1991.
184. Nussmeier N, Marino M, Cooper J, et al: Use of glucose-containing prime is not a risk factor for cerebral injury or infection in nondiabetic or diabetic patients having CABG procedures, *Anesthesiology* 91:A122, 1999.
185. Hill SE, van Wermeskerken GK, Lardenoye JW, et al: Intraoperative physiologic variables and outcome in cardiac surgery: Part I. In-hospital mortality, *Ann Thorac Surg* 69:1070–1075, 2000, discussion 5–6.
186. van Wermeskerken GK, Lardenoye JW, Hill SE, et al: Intraoperative physiologic variables and outcome in cardiac surgery: Part II. Neurologic outcome, *Ann Thorac Surg* 69:1077–1083, 2000.
187. Chaney MA, Nikolov MP, Blakeman BP, et al: Attempting to maintain normoglycemia during cardiopulmonary bypass with insulin may initiate postoperative hypoglycemia, *Anesth Analg* 89:1091–1095, 1999.
188. Gandhi GY, Nuttall GA, Abel MD, et al: Intensive intraoperative insulin therapy versus conventional glucose management during cardiac surgery: A randomized trial, *Ann Intern Med* 146:233–243, 2007.
189. Duncan AE, Abd-Elsayed A, Maheshwari A, et al: Role of intraoperative and postoperative blood glucose concentrations in predicting outcomes after cardiac surgery, *Anesthesiology* 112:860–871, 2010.
190. Bainbridge D, Martin J, Cheng D: Off pump coronary artery bypass graft surgery versus conventional coronary artery bypass graft surgery: A systematic review of the literature, *Semin Cardiothorac Vasc Anesth* 9:105–111, 2005.
191. Van Dijk D, Jansen EW, Hijman R, et al: Cognitive outcome after off-pump and on-pump coronary artery bypass graft surgery: A randomized trial, *JAMA* 287:1405–1412, 2002.
192. Mark DB, Newman MF: Protecting the brain in coronary artery bypass graft surgery, *JAMA* 287: 1448–1450, 2002.
193. Diephuis JC, Moons KG, Nierich AN, et al: Jugular bulb desaturation during coronary artery surgery: A comparison of off-pump and on-pump procedures, *Br J Anaesth* 94:715–720, 2005.
194. Bainbridge D, Cheng DCH, Martin JE: Off-pump versus on-pump coronary artery bypass surgery: A meta-analysis of clinical outcomes from randomized controlled trials, *Anesth Analg* 96:SCA100, 2003.
195. Dirnagl U, Iadecola C, Moskowitz MA: Pathobiology of ischaemic stroke: An integrated view, *Trends Neurosci* 22:391–397, 1999.
196. Michenfelder JD, Theye RA: Cerebral protection by thiopental during hypoxia, *Anesthesiology* 39:510–517, 1973.
197. Pascoe EA, Hudson RJ, Anderson BA, et al: High-dose thiopentone for open-chamber cardiac surgery: A retrospective review, *Can J Anaesth* 43:575–579, 1996.
198. Zaidan J, Klochany A, Martin W: Effect of thiopental on neurologic outcome following coronary artery bypass grafting, *Anesthesiology* 74:406–411, 1991.
199. Warner D, Takaoka S, Wu B, et al: Electroencephalographic burst suppression is not required to elicit maximal neuroprotection from pentobarbital in a rat model of focal cerebral ischemia, *Anesthesiology* 84:1475–1484, 1996.
200. Zhou W, Fontenot HJ, Liu S, et al: Modulation of cardiac calcium channels by propofol, *Anesthesiology* 86:670–675, 1997.
201. Pittman JE, Sheng HX, Pearlstein R, et al: Comparison of the effects of propofol and pentobarbital on neurologic outcome and cerebral infarct size after temporary focal ischemia in the rat, *Anesthesiology* 87:1139–1144, 1997.
202. Young Y, Menon DK, Tisavipat N, et al: Propofol neuroprotection in a rat model of ischaemia reperfusion injury, *Eur J Anaesthesiol* 14:320–326, 1997.
203. Wang J, Yang X, Camporesi CV, et al: Propofol reduces infarct size and striatal dopamine accumulation following transient middle cerebral artery occlusion: A microdialysis study, *Eur J Pharmacol* 452:303–308, 2002.
204. Roach GW, Newman MF, Murkin JM, et al: Ineffectiveness of burst suppression therapy in mitigating perioperative cerebrovascular dysfunction. Multicenter Study of Perioperative Ischemia (McSPI) Research Group, *Anesthesiology* 90:1255–1264, 1999.
205. Mangano D: Effects of acadesine on the incidence of myocardial infarction and adverse cardiac outcomes after coronary artery bypass graft surgery, *Anesthesiology* 83:658–673, 1995.
206. MacGregor DG, Miller WJ, Stone TW: Mediation of the neuroprotective action of R-phenylisopropyl-adenosine through a centrally located adenosine A1 receptor, *Br J Pharmacol* 110:470–476, 1993.
207. Perez-Pinzon MA, Mumford PL, Rosenthal M, et al: Anoxic preconditioning in hippocampal slices: Role of adenosine, *Neuroscience* 75:687–694, 1996.
208. Grocott HP, Nussmeier NA: Neuroprotection in cardiac surgery, *Anesthesiol Clin North Am* 21:487–509, 2003.
209. Levy J, Ramsay J, Murkin J: Aprotinin reduces the incidence of strokes following cardiac surgery, *Circulation* 94:I–535, 1996.
210. Levy JH, Pifarre R, Schaff HV, et al: A multicenter, double-blind, placebo-controlled trial of aprotinin for reducing blood loss and the requirement for donor-blood transfusion in patients undergoing repeat coronary artery bypass grafting, *Circulation* 92:2236–2244, 1995.
211. Frumento RJ, O'Malley CM, Bennett-Guerrero E: Stroke after cardiac surgery: A retrospective analysis of the effect of aprotinin dosing regimens, *Ann Thorac Surg* 75:479–484, 2003.
212. Harmon DC, Ghori KG, Eustace NP, et al: Aprotinin decreases the incidence of cognitive deficit following CABG and cardiopulmonary bypass: A pilot randomized controlled study: [L'aprotinine reduit l'incidence de deficit cognitif a la suite d'un PAC et de la circulation extracorporelle: une etude pilote randomisee et controlee], *Can J Anaesth* 51:1002–1009, 2004.
213. Murkin JM: Postoperative cognitive dysfunction: Aprotinin, bleeding and cognitive testing/ Dysfonction cognitive postoperatoire: Aprotinine, hemorragie et epreuves cognitives, *Can J Anaesth* 51:957–962, 2004.
214. Grocott HP, Sheng H, Miura Y, et al: The effects of aprotinin on outcome from cerebral ischemia in the rat, *Anesth Analg* 88:1–7, 1999.
215. Mangano DT, Tudor IC, Dietzel C: The risk associated with aprotinin in cardiac surgery, *N Engl J Med* 354:353–365, 2006.
216. Fergusson DA, Hebert PC, Mazer CD, et al: A comparison of aprotinin and lysine analogues in high-risk cardiac surgery, *N Engl J Med* 358:2319–2331, 2008.
217. Davis AE 3rd: The pathogenesis of hereditary angioedema, *Transfus Apher Sci* 29:195–203, 2003.
218. Dietrich W, Nicklisch S, Koster A, et al: CU-2010—a novel small molecule protease inhibitor with antifibrinolytic and anticoagulant properties, *Anesthesiology* 110:123–130, 2009.
219. Homi HM, Arepally G, Sheng H, et al: The effect of kallikrein inhibition in a rat model of stroke during cardiopulmonary bypass [Abstract], *Anesthesiology* 107:A2136, 2007.
220. Forsman M, Tubylewicz Olsnes B, Semb G, et al: Effects of nimodipine on cerebral blood flow and neuropsychological outcome after cardiac surgery, *Br J Anesth* 65:514–520, 1990.
221. Gelmers H, Gorter K, de Weerdt C, et al: A controlled trial of nimodipine in acute ischemic stroke, *N Engl J Med* 318:203–207, 1988.
222. Legault C, Furberg C, Wagenknecht L, et al: Nimodipine neuroprotection in cardiac valve replacement. Report of an early terminated trial, *Stroke* 27:593–598, 1996.
223. Grieco G, d'Hollosy M, Culliford A, et al: Evaluating neuroprotective agents for clinical anti-ischemic benefit using neurological changes after cardiac surgery under cardiopulmonary bypass, *Stroke* 27:858–874, 1996.
224. Leon A, Lipartiti M, Seren MS, et al: Hypoxic-ischemic damage and the neuroprotective effects of GM1 ganglioside, *Stroke* 21:III95–III97, 1990.
225. Arrowsmith J, Harrison M, Newman S, et al: Neuroprotection of the brain during cardioulmonary bypass. A randomized trial of remacemide during coronary artery bypass in 171 patients, *Stroke* 29:2357–2362, 1998.
226. Schmitt B, Bauersfeld U, Fanconi S, et al: The effect of the N-methyl-D-aspartate receptor antagonist dextromethorphan on perioperative brain injury in children undergoing cardiac surgery with cardiopulmonary bypass: Results of a pilot study, *Neuropediatrics* 28:191–197, 1997.
227. Ma D, Yang H, Lynch J, et al: Xenon attenuates cardiopulmonary bypass-induced neurologic and neurocognitive dysfunction in the rat, *Anesthesiology* 98:690–698, 2003.
228. Homi HM, Yokoo N, Ma D, et al: The neuroprotective effect of xenon administration during transient middle cerebral artery occlusion in mice, *Anesthesiology* 99:876–881, 2003.
229. Homi HM, Yokoo N, Venkatakrishnan K, et al: Neuroprotection by antagonism of the N-methyl-D-aspartate receptor NR2B subtype in a rat model of cardiopulmonary bypass, *Anesthesiology* A878, 2004.
230. Mitchell SJ, Pellett O, Gorman DF: Cerebral protection by lidocaine during cardiac operations, *Ann Thorac Surg* 67:1117–1124, 1999.
231. Mathew JP, Mackensen GB, Phillips-Bute B, et al: Randomized, double-blinded, placebo controlled study of neuroprotection with lidocaine in cardiac surgery, *Stroke* 40:880–887, 2009.
232. Amory DW, Grigore A, Amory JK, et al: Neuroprotection is associated with beta-adrenergic receptor antagonists during cardiac surgery: Evidence from 2,575 patients, *J Cardiothorac Vasc Anesth* 16: 270–277, 2002.
233. Savitz SI, Erhardt JA, Anthony JV, et al: The novel beta-blocker, carvedilol, provides neuroprotection in transient focal stroke, *J Cereb Blood Flow Metab* 20:1197–1204, 2000.
234. Devereaux PJ, Yang H, Yusuf S, et al: Effects of extended-release metoprolol succinate in patients undergoing non-cardiac surgery (POISE trial): A randomised controlled trial, *Lancet* 371:1839–1847, 2008.
235. Liu TH, Beckman JS, Freeman BA, et al: Polyethylene glycol-conjugated superoxide dismutase and catalase reduce ischemic brain injury, *Am J Physiol* 256:H589–H593, 1989.
236. Butterworth J, Legault C, Stump DA, et al: A randomized, blinded trial of the antioxidant pegorgotein: No reduction in neuropsychological deficits, inotropic drug support, or myocardial ischemia after coronary artery bypass surgery, *J Cardiothorac Vasc Anesth* 13:690–694, 1999.
237. Levy JH, Tanaka KA: Inflammatory response to cardiopulmonary bypass, *Ann Thorac Surg* 75:S715–S720, 2003.
238. Mathew JP, Shernan SK, White WD, et al: Preliminary report of the effects of complement suppression with pexelizumab on neurocognitive decline after coronary artery bypass graft surgery, *Stroke* 35:2335–2339, 2004.
239. Hofer RE, Christopherson TJ, Scheithauer BW, et al: The effect of a platelet activating factor antagonist (BN 52021) on neurologic outcome and histopathology in a canine model of complete cerebral ischemia, *Anesthesiology* 79:347–353, 1993.
240. Panetta T, Marcheselli VL, Braquet P, et al: Effects of a platelet activating factor antagonist (BN 52021) on free fatty acids, diacylglycerols, polyphosphoinositides and blood flow in the gerbil brain: Inhibition of ischemia-reperfusion induced cerebral injury, *Biochem Biophys Res Commun* 149:580–587, 1987.
241. Taggart D, et al: *Neuroprotection during cardiac surgery: A randomized trial of a platelet activating factor antagonist.* Presented at the Fifth International Brain and Cardiac Surgery Conference, London, 2000.
242. Sethy VH, Wu H, Oostveen JA, et al: Neuroprotective effects of the GABA(A) receptor partial agonist U-101017 in 3-acetylpyridine-treated rats, *Neurosci Lett* 228:45–49, 1997.
243. Yang Y, Shuaib A, Li Q, et al: Neuroprotection by delayed administration of topiramate in a rat model of middle cerebral artery embolization, *Brain Res* 804:169–176, 1998.
244. Kong R, Butterworth J, Aveling W, et al: Clinical trial of the neuroportectant clomethiazole in coronary artery bypass graft surgery, *Anesthesiology* 97:585–591, 2002.
245. Clark RK, Lee EV, White RF, et al: Reperfusion following focal stroke hastens inflammation and resolution of ischemic injured tissue, *Brain Res Bull* 35:387–392, 1994.
246. Chopp M, Zhang RL, Chen H, et al: Postischemic administration of an anti-Mac-1 antibody reduces ischemic cell damage after transient middle cerebral artery occlusion in rats, *Stroke* 25:869–875, 1994, discussion 75–76.
247. Bracken MB, Shepard MJ, Collins WF, et al: A randomized, controlled trial of methylprednisolone or naloxone in the treatment of acute spinal-cord injury. Results of the Second National Acute Spinal Cord Injury Study, *N Engl J Med* 322:1405–1411, 1990.
248. Roberts I, Yates D, Sandercock P, et al: Effect of intravenous corticosteroids on death within 14 days in 10008 adults with clinically significant head injury (MRC CRASH trial): Randomised placebo-controlled trial, *Lancet* 364:1321–1328, 2004.
249. Wass CT, Lanier WL: Glucose modulation of ischemic brain injury: Review and clinical recommendations, *Mayo Clin Proc* 71:801–812, 1996.
250. Li P, Kristian T, Shamloo M, et al: Effects of preischemic hyperglycemia on brain damage incurred by rats subjected to 2.5 or 5 minutes of forebrain ischemia, *Stroke* 27:1592–1602, 1996.
251. Nagels W, Demeyere R, Van Hemelrijck J, et al: Evaluation of the neuroprotective effects of s(+)-ketamine during open-heart surgery, *Anesth Analg* 98:1595–1603, 2004.
252. Hudetz JA, Pagel PS: Neuroprotection by ketamine: A review of the experimental and clinical evidence, *J Cardiothorac Vasc Anesth* 24:131–142, 2010.
253. Lavie G, Teichner A, Shohami E, et al: Long term cerebroprotective effects of dexanabinol in a model of focal cerebral ischemia, *Brain Res* 901:195–201, 2001.
254. Leker RR, Shohami E, Abramsky O, et al: Dexanabinol; a novel neuroprotective drug in experimental focal cerebral ischemia, *J Neurol Sci* 162:114–119, 1999.
255. Doberneck RC, Reiser MP, Lillehei CW: Acute renal failure after open-heart surgery utilizing extracorporeal circulation and total body perfusion. Analysis of 1000 patients, *J Urol Nephrol (Paris)* 43:441–452, 1962.
256. Conlon PJ, Stafford-Smith M, White WD, et al: Acute renal failure following cardiac surgery, *Nephrol Dial Transplant* 14:1158–1162, 1999.

257. Abel RM, Wick J, Beck CH Jr, et al: Renal dysfunction following open-heart operations, *Arch Surg* 108:175–177, 1974.

258. Yeh T, Brackney E, Hall D, et al: Renal complications of open-heart surgery: Predisposing factors, prevention and management, *J Thorac Cardiovasc Surg* 47:79–95, 1964.

259. Nicoara A, Patel UD, Phillips-Bute BG, et al: Mortality trends associated with acute renal failure requiring dialysis after CABG surgery in the United States, *Blood Purif* 28:359–363, 2009.

260. Mazzarella V, Gallucci MT, Tozzo C, et al: Renal function in patients undergoing cardiopulmonary bypass operations, *J Thorac Cardiovasc Surg* 104:1625–1627, 1992.

261. Mora-Mangano C, Diamondstone LS, Ramsay JG, et al: Renal dysfunction after myocardial revascularization: Risk factors, adverse outcomes, and hospital resource utilization. The Multicenter Study of Perioperative Ischemia Research Group, *Ann Intern Med* 128:194–203, 1998.

262. Page US, Washburn T: Using tracking data to find complications that physicians miss: The case of renal failure in cardiac surgery, *Jt Comm J Qual Improv* 23:511–520, 1997.

263. Mora-Mangano C, Boisvert D, Zhou S, et al: Small reductions in renal function following CABG independently predict hospitalization, *Anesth Analg* 90:SCA 35, 2000.

264. Coca SG, Yusuf B, Shlipak MG, et al: Long-term risk of mortality and other adverse outcomes after acute kidney injury: A systematic review and meta-analysis, *Am J Kidney Dis* 53:961–973, 2009.

265. Swaminathan M, Hudson CCC, Phillips-Bute BG, et al: Impact of early renal recovery on survival after cardiac surgery-associated acute kidney injury, *Ann Thor Surg* 89:1098–1104, 2010.

266. Bihorac A, Yavas S, Subbiah S, et al: Long-term risk of mortality and acute kidney injury during hospitalization after major surgery, *Ann Surg* 249:851–858, 2009.

267. Kelly KJ: Distant effects of experimental renal ischemia/reperfusion injury, *J Am Soc Nephrol* 14:1549–1558, 2003.

268. Rabb H, Wang Z, Nemoto T, et al: Acute renal failure leads to dysregulation of lung salt and water channels, *Kidney Int* 63:600–606, 2003.

269. Deng J, Hu X, Yuen PS, et al: Alpha-melanocyte-stimulating hormone inhibits lung injury after renal ischemia/reperfusion, *Am J Respir Crit Care Med* 169:749–756, 2004.

270. Kramer AA, Postler G, Salhab KF, et al: Renal ischemia/reperfusion leads to macrophage-mediated increase in pulmonary vascular permeability, *Kidney Int* 55:2362–2367, 1999.

271. Meldrum KK, Meldrum DR, Meng X, et al: TNF-alpha-dependent bilateral renal injury is induced by unilateral renal ischemia-reperfusion, *Am J Physiol Heart Circ Physiol* 282:H540–H546, 2002.

272. Serteser M, Koken T, Kahraman A, et al: Changes in hepatic TNF-alpha levels, antioxidant status, and oxidation products after renal ischemia/reperfusion injury in mice, *J Surg Res* 107:234–240, 2002.

273. Cohen G, Horl WH: Retinol binding protein isolated from acute renal failure patients inhibits polymorphonuclear leucocyte functions, *Eur J Clin Invest* 34:774–781, 2004.

274. Vanholder R, Smet RD, Glorieux G, et al: Survival of hemodialysis patients and uremic toxin removal, *Artif Organs* 27:218–223, 2003.

275. Bellomo R, Ronco C, Kellum JA, et al: Acute renal failure—definition, outcome measures, animal models, fluid therapy and information technology needs: The Second International Consensus Conference of the Acute Dialysis Quality Initiative (ADQI) Group, *Crit Care* 8:R204–R212, 2004.

276. Cuhaci B: More data on epidemiology and outcome of acute kidney injury with AKIN criteria: Benefits of standardized definitions, AKIN and RIFLE classifications, *Crit Care Med* 37:2659–2661, 2009.

277. Haase M, Bellomo R, Devarajan P, et al: Novel biomarkers early predict the severity of acute kidney injury after cardiac surgery in adults, *Ann Thorac Surg* 88:124–130, 2009.

278. Haase-Fielitz A, Bellomo R, Devarajan P, et al: Novel and conventional serum biomarkers predicting acute kidney injury in adult cardiac surgery—a prospective cohort study, *Crit Care Med* 37:553–560, 2009.

279. Han WK, Wagener G, Zhu Y, et al: Urinary biomarkers in the early detection of acute kidney injury after cardiac surgery, *Clin J Am Soc Nephrol* 4:873–882, 2009.

280. Mehta RL, Kellum JA, Shah SV, et al: Acute Kidney Injury Network: Report of an initiative to improve outcomes in acute kidney injury, *Crit Care* 11:R31, 2007.

281. Karkouti K, Wijeysundera DN, Yau TM, et al: Acute kidney injury after cardiac surgery: Focus on modifiable risk factors, *Circulation* 119:495–502, 2009.

282. Massoudy P, Wagner S, Thielmann M, et al: Coronary artery bypass surgery and acute kidney injury—impact of the off-pump technique, *Nephrol Dial Transplant* 23:2853–2860, 2008.

283. Schrier RW, Harris DC, Chan L, et al: Tubular hypermetabolism as a factor in the progression of chronic renal failure, *Am J Kidney Dis* 12:243–249, 1988.

284. Whitworth JA, Ihle BU, Becker GJ, et al: Preservation of renal function in chronic renal failure, *Tohoku J Exp Med* 166:165–183, 1992.

285. Small G, Watson AR, Evans JH, et al: Hemolytic uremic syndrome: Defining the need for long-term follow-up, *Clin Nephrol* 52:352–356, 1999.

286. Kikuchi Y, Koga H, Yasutomo Y, et al: Patients with renal hypouricemia with exercise-induced acute renal failure and chronic renal dysfunction, *Clin Nephrol* 53:467–472, 2000.

287. Schweda F, Blumberg FC, Schweda A, et al: Effects of chronic hypoxia on renal renin gene expression in rats, *Nephrol Dial Transplant* 15:11–15, 2000.

288. Bach PH: Detection of chemically induced renal injury: The cascade of degenerative morphological and functional changes that follow the primary nephrotoxic insult and evaluation of these changes by in-vitro methods, *Toxicol Lett* 46:237–249, 1989.

289. Schiffl H: Renal recovery from acute tubular necrosis requiring renal replacement therapy: A prospective study in critically ill patients, *Nephrol Dial Transplant* 21:1248–1252, 2006.

290. Stafford-Smith M, Phillips-Bute B, Reddan DN, et al: The association of epsilon-aminocaproic acid with postoperative decrease in creatinine clearance in 1502 coronary bypass patients, *Anesth Analg* 91:1085–1090, 2000.

291. Anderson RJ, O'Brien M, MaWhinney S, et al: Renal failure predisposes patients to adverse outcome after coronary artery bypass surgery. VA Cooperative Study #5, *Kidney Int* 55:1057–1062, 1999.

292. Gaudino M, Luciani N, Giungi S, et al: Different profiles of patients who require dialysis after cardiac surgery, *Ann Thorac Surg* 79:825–829, 2005.

293. Pham PT, Slavov C, Pham PC: Acute kidney injury after liver, heart, and lung transplants: Dialysis modality, predictors of renal function recovery, and impact on survival, *Adv Chronic Kidney Dis* 16:256–267, 2009.

294. Stafford-Smith M, Patel UD, Phillips-Bute BG, et al: Acute kidney injury and chronic kidney disease after cardiac surgery, *Adv Chronic Kidney Dis* 15:257–277, 2008.

295. Chertow GM, Lazarus JM, Christiansen CL, et al: Preoperative renal risk stratification, *Circulation* 95:878–884, 1997.

296. Zanardo G, Michielon P, Paccagnella A, et al: Acute renal failure in the patient undergoing cardiac operation. Prevalence, mortality rate, and main risk factors, *J Thorac Cardiovasc Surg* 107:1489–1495, 1994.

297. Mangos GJ, Brown MA, Chan WY, et al: Acute renal failure following cardiac surgery: Incidence, outcomes and risk factors, *Aust N Z J Med* 25:284–289, 1995.

298. Corwin HL, Sprague SM, DeLaria GA, et al: Acute renal failure associated with cardiac operations. A case-control study, *J Thorac Cardiovasc Surg* 98:1107–1112, 1989.

299. Llopart T, Lombardi R, Forselledo M, et al: Acute renal failure in open heart surgery, *Ren Fail* 19:319–323, 1997.

300. Hilberman M, Myers BD, Carrie BJ, et al: Acute renal failure following cardiac surgery, *J Thorac Cardiovasc Surg* 77:880–888, 1979.

301. Fischer UM, Weissenberger WK, Warters RD, et al: Impact of cardiopulmonary bypass management on postcardiac surgery renal function, *Perfusion* 17:401–406, 2002.

302. Domart Y, Trouillet JL, Fagon JY, et al: Incidence and morbidity of cytomegaloviral infection in patients with mediastinitis following cardiac surgery, *Chest* 97:18–22, 1990.

303. Albahrani MJ, Swaminathan M, Phillips-Bute B, et al: Postcardiac surgery complications: Association of acute renal dysfunction and atrial fibrillation, *Anesth Analg* 96:637–643, 2003.

304. Andersson LG, Ekroth R, Bratteby LE, et al: Acute renal failure after coronary surgery—a study of incidence and risk factors in 2009 consecutive patients, *Thorac Cardiovasc Surg* 41:237–241, 1993.

305. Abel RM, Buckley MJ, Austen WG, et al: Etiology, incidence, and prognosis of renal failure following cardiac operations. Results of a prospective analysis of 500 consecutive patients, *J Thorac Cardiovasc Surg* 71:323–333, 1976.

306. Stafford-Smith M, Conlon PJ, White WD, et al: Low hematocrit but not perfusion pressure during CPB is predictive for renal failure following CABG surgery, *Anesth Analg* 86:SCA102, 1998.

307. Ostermann ME, Taube D, Morgan CJ, et al: Acute renal failure following cardiopulmonary bypass: A changing picture, *Intensive Care Med* 26:565–571, 2000.

308. Aronson S, Fontes M, Miao Y, et al: Risk index for perioperative renal dysfunction/failure: Critical dependence on pulse pressure hypertension, *Circulation* 115:733–742, 2007.

309. De Santo L, Romano G, Della Corte A, et al: Preoperative anemia in patients undergoing coronary artery bypass grafting predicts acute kidney injury, *J Thorac Cardiovasc Surg* 138:965–970, 2009.

310. Swaminathan M, Phillips-Bute BG, Conlon PJ, et al: The association of lowest hematocrit during cardiopulmonary bypass with acute renal injury after coronary bypass surgery, *Ann Thorac Surg* 76:784–791, 2003.

311. Hudson C, Welsby I, Phillips-Bute B, et al: Glycosylated hemoglobin levels and outcome in non-diabetic cardiac surgery patients, *Can J Anesth* 57:565–572, 2010.

312. Lu JC, Coca SG, Patel UD, et al: Searching for genes that matter in acute kidney injury: A systematic review, *Clin J Am Soc Nephrol* 4:1020–1031, 2009.

313. Stafford-Smith M, Podgoreanu M, Swaminathan M, et al: Association of genetic polymorphisms with risk of renal injury after coronary artery bypass graft surgery, *Am J Kidney Dis* 45:519–530, 2005.

314. Lieberthal W, Koh JS, Levine JS: Necrosis and apoptosis in acute renal failure, *Semin Nephrol* 18:505–518, 1998.

315. Davila-Roman VG, Kouchoukos NT, Schechtman KB, et al: Atherosclerosis of the ascending aorta is a predictor of renal dysfunction after cardiac operations, *J Thorac Cardiovasc Surg* 117:111–116, 1999.

316. Sreeram GM, Grocott HP, White WD, et al: Transcranial Doppler emboli count predicts rise in creatinine after coronary artery bypass graft surgery, *J Cardiothorac Vasc Anesth* 18:548–551, 2004.

317. Conlon PJ, Crowley J, Stack R, et al: Renal artery stenosis is not associated with the development of acute renal failure following coronary artery bypass grafting, *Ren Fail* 27:81–86, 2005.

318. Barbut D, Hinton RB, Szatrowski TP, et al: Cerebral emboli detected during bypass surgery are associated with clamp removal, *Stroke* 25:2398–2402, 1994.

319. Blauth CI, Cosgrove DM, Webb BW, et al: Atheroembolism from the ascending aorta. An emerging problem in cardiac surgery, *J Thorac Cardiovasc Surg* 103:1104–1111, 1992, discussion 11–12.

320. Tierney G, Parissis H, Baker M, et al: An experimental study of intra aortic balloon pumping within the intact human aorta, *Eur J Cardiothorac Surg* 12:486–493, 1997.

321. Hosaka S, Suzuki S, Kato J, et al: [Modification of the surgical strategy based on intraoperative echographic findings of atherosclerotic ascending aorta], *Nippon Kyobu Geka Gakkai Zasshi* 45:1916–1921, 1997.

322. Muehrcke DD, Cornhill JF, Thomas JD, et al: Flow characteristics of aortic cannulae, *J Card Surg* 10:514–519, 1995.

323. Dietl CA, Madigan NP, Laubach CA, et al: Myocardial revascularization using the "no-touch" technique, with mild systemic hypothermia, in patients with a calcified ascending aorta, *J Cardiovasc Surg (Torino)* 36:39–44, 1995.

324. St Amand M, Murkin J, Menkis A, et al: Aortic atherosclerotic plaque identified by epiaortic scanning predicts cerebral embolic load in cardiac surgery, *Can J Anaesth* 44(Suppl):A7, 1997.

325. Conlon PJ, Jefferies F, Krigman HR, et al: Predictors of prognosis and risk of acute renal failure in bacterial endocarditis, *Clin Nephrol* 49:96–101, 1998.

326. Shammas NW: Pulmonary embolus after coronary artery bypass surgery: A review of the literature, *Clin Cardiol* 23:637–644, 2000.

327. Shann KG, Likosky DS, Murkin JM, et al: An evidence-based review of the practice of cardiopulmonary bypass in adults: A focus on neurologic injury, glycemic control, hemodilution, and the inflammatory response, *J Thorac Cardiovasc Surg* 132:283–290, 2006.

328. Deal DD, Jones TJ, Vernon JC, et al: Real time OPS imaging of embolic injury of the renal micro-circulation during cardiopulmonary bypass, *Anesth Analg* 92:S23, 2001.

329. Murray KD, Binkley PF, Dumond DA, et al: The significance and prevention of air emboli with the total artificial heart, *Artif Organs* 17:734–740, 1993.

330. Al-Rashidi F, Blomquist S, Hoglund P, et al: A new de-airing technique that reduces systemic microemboli during open surgery: A prospective controlled study, *J Thorac Cardiovasc Surg* 138:157–162, 2009.

331. Rangel-Frausto MS, Pittet D, Costigan M, et al: The natural history of the systemic inflammatory response syndrome (SIRS). A prospective study, *JAMA* 273:117–123, 1995.

332. Wan L, Bagshaw SM, Langenberg C, et al: Pathophysiology of septic acute kidney injury: What do we really know? *Crit Care Med* 36:S198–S203, 2008.

333. Hall R, Stafford-Smith M, Rocker G: The systemic inflammatory response to cardiopulmonary bypass: Pathophysiological, therapeutic, and pharmacological considerations, *Anesth Analg* 85:766–782, 1997.

334. Donnahoo KK, Meldrum DR, Shenkar R, et al: Early renal ischemia, with or without reperfusion, activates NFkappaB and increases TNF-alpha bioactivity in the kidney, *J Urol* 163:1328–1332, 2000.

335. Vanholder R, Argiles A, Baurmeister U, et al: Uremic toxicity: Present state of the art, *Int J Artif Organs* 24:695–725, 2001.

336. Sinsteden TD, O'Neil TJ, Hill S, et al: The role of high-energy phosphate in norepinephrine-induced acute renal failure in the dog, *Circ Res* 59:93–104, 1986.

337. Ozden A, Sarioglu A, Demirkan NC, et al: Antithrombin III reduces renal ischemia-reperfusion injury in rats, *Res Exp Med (Berl)* 200:195–203, 2001.

338. Padanilam BJ: Cell death induced by acute renal injury: A perspective on the contributions of apoptosis and necrosis, *Am J Physiol Renal Physiol* 284:F608–F627, 2003.

339. Daemen MA, van 't Veer C, Denecker G, et al: Inhibition of apoptosis induced by ischemia-reperfusion prevents inflammation, *J Clin Invest* 104:541–549, 1999.

340. Daemen MA, de Vries B, Buurman WA: Apoptosis and inflammation in renal reperfusion injury, *Transplantation* 73:1693–1700, 2002.

341. Maccario M, Fumagalli C, Dottori V, et al: The association between rhabdomyolysis and acute renal failure in patients undergoing cardiopulmonary bypass, *J Cardiovasc Surg (Torino)* 37:153–159, 1996.

342. Schouten O, Bax JJ, Dunkelgrun M, et al: Statins for the prevention of perioperative cardiovascular complications in vascular surgery, *J Vasc Surg* 44:419–424, 2006.

343. Haase M, Haase-Fielitz A, Bagshaw SM, et al: Cardiopulmonary bypass-associated acute kidney injury: A pigment nephropathy? *Contrib Nephrol* 156:340–353, 2007.

344. Ferraris VA, Bridges CR, Anderson RP: Aprotinin in cardiac surgery, *N Engl J Med* 354:1953–1957, 2006.

345. Thelle K, Christensen EI, Vorum H, et al: Characterization of proteinuria and tubular protein uptake in a new model of oral L-lysine administration in rats, *Kidney Int* 69:1333–1340, 2006.

346. Stafford-Smith M: Antifibrinolytic agents make alpha1- and beta2-microglobulinuria poor markers of post cardiac surgery renal dysfunction, *Anesthesiology* 90:928–929, 1999.
347. Tune B: Renal tubular transport and nephrotoxicity of beta lactam antibiotics: Structure activity relationships, *Miner Electrolyte Metab* 20:221–231, 1994.
348. Bennett WM, Luft F, Porter GA: Pathogenesis of renal failure due to aminoglycosides and contrast media used in roentgenography, *Am J Med* 69:767–774, 1980.
349. Olyaei AJ, de Mattos AM, Bennett WM: Immunosuppressant-induced nephropathy: Pathophysiology, incidence and management, *Drug Saf* 21:471–488, 1999.
350. Baisac J, Henrich W: Nephrotoxicity of nonsteroidal anti inflammatory drugs, *Miner Electrolyte Metab* 20:187–192, 1994.
351. Baehler RW, Williams RH, Work J, et al: Studies on the natural history of the norepinephrine model of acute renal failure in the dog, *Nephron* 26:266–273, 1980.
352. Santos FO, Silveira MA, Maia RB, et al: Acute renal failure after coronary artery bypass surgery with extracorporeal circulation—incidence, risk factors, and mortality, *Arq Bras Cardiol* 83:150–154, 145–149, 2004.
353. Heringlake M, Knappe M, Vargas Hein O, et al: Renal dysfunction according to the ADQI-RIFLE system and clinical practice patterns after cardiac surgery in Germany, *Minerva Anestesiol* 72:645–654, 2006.
354. Porter GA: Contrast-associated nephropathy: Presentation, pathophysiology and management, *Miner Electrolyte Metab* 20:232–243, 1994.
355. Kahn JK, Rutherford BD, McConahay DR, et al: High-dose contrast agent administration during complex coronary angioplasty, *Am Heart J* 120:533–536, 1990.
356. Gussenhoven MJ, Ravensbergen J, van Bockel JH, et al: Renal dysfunction after angiography; a risk factor analysis in patients with peripheral vascular disease, *J Cardiovasc Surg (Torino)* 32:81–86, 1991.
357. Garwood S, Mathew J, Hines R: Renal function and cardiopulmonary bypass: Does time since catheterization impact renal performance? *Anesthesiology* 87:A90, 1997.
358. Lieberthal W, Rennke H, Sandock K, et al: Ischemia in the isolated erythrocyte-perfused rat kidney. Protective effect of hypothermia, *Ren Physiol Biochem* 11:60–69, 1988.
359. Ip-Yam PC, Murphy S, Baines M, et al: Renal function and proteinuria after cardiopulmonary bypass: The effects of temperature and mannitol, *Anesth Analg* 78:842–847, 1994.
360. Regragui IA, Izzat MB, Birdi I, et al: Cardiopulmonary bypass perfusion temperature does not influence perioperative renal function, *Ann Thorac Surg* 60:160–164, 1995.
361. Swaminathan M, East C, Phillips-Bute B, et al: Report of a substudy on warm versus cold cardiopulmonary bypass: Changes in creatinine clearance, *Ann Thorac Surg* 72:1603–1609, 2001.
362. Urzua J, Troncoso S, Bugedo G, et al: Renal function and cardiopulmonary bypass: Effect of perfusion pressure, *J Cardiothorac Vasc Anesth* 6:299–303, 1992.
363. Bhat JG, Gluck MC, Lowenstein J, et al: Renal failure after open heart surgery, *Ann Intern Med* 84: 677–682, 1976.
364. Shah D, Corson J, Karmody A, et al: Effects of isovolemic hemodilution on abdominal aortic aneurysmectomy in high risk patients, *Ann Vasc Surg* 1:50–54, 1986.
365. Messmer K: Hemodilution, *Surg Clin North Am* 55:659–678, 1975.
366. DeFoe GR, Ross CS, Olmstead EM, et al: Lowest hematocrit on bypass and adverse outcomes associated with coronary artery bypass grafting. Northern New England Cardiovascular Disease Study Group, *Ann Thorac Surg* 71:769–776, 2001.
367. Fang WC, Helm RE, Krieger KH, et al: Impact of minimum hematocrit during cardiopulmonary bypass on mortality in patients undergoing coronary artery surgery, *Circulation* 96:II-194–II-199, 1997.
368. Karkouti K, Beattie WS, Wijeysundera DN, et al: Hemodilution during cardiopulmonary bypass is an independent risk factor for acute renal failure in adult cardiac surgery, *J Thorac Cardiovasc Surg* 129:391–400, 2005.
369. Habib RH, Zacharias A, Schwann TA, et al: Role of hemodilutional anemia and transfusion during cardiopulmonary bypass in renal injury after coronary revascularization: Implications on operative outcome, *Crit Care Med* 33:1749–1756, 2005.
370. Karkouti K, Wijeysundera DN, Beattie WS: Risk associated with preoperative anemia in cardiac surgery: A multicenter cohort study, *Circulation* 117:478–484, 2008.
371. Stafford-Smith M, Newman MF: What effects do hemodilution and blood transfusion during cardiopulmonary bypass have on renal outcomes? *Nat Clin Pract Nephrol* 2:188–189, 2006.
372. Van den Berghe G, Wouters P, Weekers F, et al: Intensive insulin therapy in the critically ill patients, *N Engl J Med* 345:1359–1367, 2001.
373. Wiener RS, Wiener DC, Larson RJ: Benefits and risks of tight glucose control in critically ill adults: A meta-analysis, *JAMA* 300:933–944, 2008.
374. Zacharias M, Conlon NP, Herbison GP, et al: Interventions for protecting renal function in the perioperative period, *Cochrane Database Syst Rev* CD003590, 2008.
375. Nigwekar SU, Hix JK: The role of natriuretic peptide administration in cardiovascular surgery-associated renal dysfunction: A systematic review and meta-analysis of randomized controlled trials, *J Cardiothorac Vasc Anesth* 23:151–160, 2009.
376. Nigwekar SU, Navaneethan SD, Parikh CR, et al: Atrial natriuretic peptide for management of acute kidney injury: A systematic review and meta-analysis, *Clin J Am Soc Nephrol* 4:261–272, 2009.
377. Brienza N, Giglio MT, Marucci M, et al: Does perioperative hemodynamic optimization protect renal function in surgical patients? A meta-analytic study, *Crit Care Med* 37:2079–2090, 2009.
378. Nigwekar SU, Kandula P: N-acetylcysteine in cardiovascular-surgery-associated renal failure: A meta-analysis, *Ann Thorac Surg* 87:139–147, 2009.
379. Baker WL, Anglade MW, Baker EL, et al: Use of N-acetylcysteine to reduce post-cardiothoracic surgery complications: A meta-analysis, *Eur J Cardiothorac Surg* 35:521–527, 2009.
380. Ho KM, Morgan DJ: Meta-analysis of N-acetylcysteine to prevent acute renal failure after major surgery, *Am J Kidney Dis* 53:33–40, 2009.
381. Naughton F, Wijeysundera D, Karkouti K, et al: N-acetylcysteine to reduce renal failure after cardiac surgery: A systematic review and meta-analysis, *Can J Anaesth* 55:827–835, 2008.
382. Landoni G, Poli D, Bove T: Fenoldopamin in cardiac surgery, *Clin Res Cardiol* 2:591–595, 2007.
383. Landoni G, Biondi-Zoccai GG, Marino G, et al: Fenoldopam reduces the need for renal replacement therapy and in-hospital death in cardiovascular surgery: A meta-analysis, *J Cardiothorac Vasc Anesth* 22:27–33, 2008.
384. Liakopoulos OJ, Choi YH, Haldenwang PL, et al: Impact of preoperative statin therapy on adverse postoperative outcomes in patients undergoing cardiac surgery: A meta-analysis of over 30,000 patients, *Eur Heart J* 29:1548–1559, 2008.
385. Friedrich JO, Adhikari N, Herridge MS, et al: Meta-analysis: Low-dose dopamine increases urine output but does not prevent renal dysfunction or death, *Ann Intern Med* 142:510–524, 2005.
386. Karajala V, Mansour W, Kellum JA: Diuretics in acute kidney injury, *Minerva Anestesiol* 75:251–257, 2009.
387. Bagshaw SM, Delaney A, Haase M, et al: Loop diuretics in the management of acute renal failure: A systematic review and meta-analysis, *Crit Care Resusc* 9:60–68, 2007.
388. Sampath S, Moran JL, Graham PL, et al: The efficacy of loop diuretics in acute renal failure: Assessment using Bayesian evidence synthesis techniques, *Crit Care Med* 35:2516–2524, 2007.
389. Marik PE: Low-dose dopamine: A systematic review, *Intensive Care Med* 28:877–883, 2002.
390. Kellum JA, Decker JM: Use of dopamine in acute renal failure: A meta-analysis, *Crit Care Med* 29:1526–1531, 2001.
391. Prins I, Plotz FB, Uiterwaal CS, et al: Low-dose dopamine in neonatal and pediatric intensive care: A systematic review, *Intensive Care Med* 27:206–210, 2001.
392. Jakob SM, Ruokonen E, Takala J: Effects of dopamine on systemic and regional blood flow and metabolism in septic and cardiac surgery patients, *Shock* 18:8–13, 2002.
393. Hoffman TM, Bush DM, Wernovsky G, et al: Postoperative junctional ectopic tachycardia in children: Incidence, risk factors, and treatment, *Ann Thorac Surg* 74:1607–1611, 2002.
394. Stone GW, McCullough PA, Tumlin JA, et al: Fenoldopam mesylate for the prevention of contrast-induced nephropathy: A randomized controlled trial, *JAMA* 290:2284–2291, 2003.
395. Kini AS, Mitre CA, Kim M, et al: A protocol for prevention of radiographic contrast nephropathy during percutaneous coronary intervention: Effect of selective dopamine receptor agonist fenoldopam, *Catheter Cardiovasc Interv* 55:169–173, 2002.
396. Stone GW, Tumlin JA, Madyoon H, et al: Design and rationale of CONTRAST—a prospective, randomized, placebo-controlled trial of fenoldopam mesylate for the prevention of radiocontrast nephropathy, *Rev Cardiovasc Med* 2(Suppl 1):S31–S36, 2001.
397. Caimmi PP, Pagani L, Micalizzi E, et al: Fenoldopam for renal protection in patients undergoing cardiopulmonary bypass, *J Cardiothorac Vasc Anesth* 17:491–494, 2003.
398. Tumlin JA, Finckle K, Murray P, et al: Dopamine receptor 1 agonists in early acute tubular necrosis: A prospective, randomized, double blind, placebo-controlled trial of fenoldopam mesylate [Abstract], *J Am Soc Nephrol* 14:PUB001, 2003.
399. Brezis M, Agmon Y, Epstein FH: Determinants of intrarenal oxygenation. I. Effects of diuretics, *Am J Physiol* 267:F1059–F1062, 1994.
400. Ellison DH, Velazquez H, Wright FS: Adaptation of the distal convoluted tubule of the rat. Structural and functional effects of dietary salt intake and chronic diuretic infusion, *J Clin Invest* 83:113–126, 1989.
401. Liss P: Effects of contrast media on renal microcirculation and oxygen tension. An experimental study in the rat, *Acta Radiol Suppl* 409:1–29, 1997.
402. Lindner A, Cutler R, Goodman W: Synergism of dopamine plus furosemide in preventing acute renal failure in the dog, *Kidney Int* 16:158–166, 1979.
403. Heyman SN, Rosen S, Epstein FH, et al: Loop diuretics reduce hypoxic damage to proximal tubules of the isolated perfused rat kidney, *Kidney Int* 45:981–985, 1994.
404. Hager B, Betschart M, Krapf R: Effect of postoperative intravenous loop diuretic on renal function after major surgery, *Schweiz Med Wochenschr* 126:666–673, 1996.
405. Shilliday IR, Quinn KJ, Allison ME: Loop diuretics in the management of acute renal failure: A prospective, double-blind, placebo-controlled, randomized study, *Nephrol Dial Transplant* 12: 2592–2596, 1997.
406. Nuutinen L, Hollmen A: The effect of prophylactic use of furosemide on renal function during open heart surgery, *Ann Chir Gynaecol* 65:258–266, 1976.
407. Lassnigg A, Donner E, Grubhofer G, et al: Lack of renoprotective effects of dopamine and furosemide during cardiac surgery, *J Am Soc Nephrol* 11:97–104, 2000.
408. Fisher AR, Jones P, Barlow P, et al: The influence of mannitol on renal function during and after open-heart surgery, *Perfusion* 13:181–186, 1998.
409. Nishimura O, Tokutsu S, Sakurai T, et al: Effects of hypertonic mannitol on renal function in open heart surgery, *Jpn Heart J* 24:245–257, 1983.
410. Pass LJ, Eberhart RC, Brown JC, et al: The effect of mannitol and dopamine on the renal response to thoracic aortic cross-clamping, *J Thorac Cardiovasc Surg* 95:608–612, 1988.
411. Visweswaran P, Massin EK, Dubose TD Jr: Mannitol-induced acute renal failure, *J Am Soc Nephrol* 8:1028–1033, 1997.
412. Joffy S, Rosner MH: Natriuretic peptides in ESRD, *Am J Kidney Dis* 46:1–10, 2005.
413. Deegan PM, Ryan MP, Basinger MA, et al: Protection from cisplatin nephrotoxicity by A68828, an atrial natriuretic peptide, *Ren Fail* 17:117–123, 1995.
414. Allgren RL, Marbury TC, Rahman SN, et al: Anaritide in acute tubular necrosis. Auriculin Anaritide Acute Renal Failure Study Group, *N Engl J Med* 336:828–834, 1997.
415. Lewis J, Salem MM, Chertow GM, et al: Atrial natriuretic factor in oliguric acute renal failure. Anaritide Acute Renal Failure Study Group, *Am J Kidney Dis* 36:767–774, 2000.
416. Meyer M, Pfarr E, Schirmer G, et al: Therapeutic use of the natriuretic peptide ularitide in acute renal failure, *Ren Fail* 21:85–100, 1999.
417. Sackner-Bernstein JD, Skopicki HA, Aaronson KD: Risk of worsening renal function with nesiritide in patients with acutely decompensated heart failure, *Circulation* 111:1487–1491, 2005.
418. Teerlink JR, Massie BM: Nesiritide and worsening of renal function: The emperor's new clothes? *Circulation* 111:1459–1461, 2005.
419. Mentzer RM Jr, Oz MC, Sladen RN, et al: Effects of perioperative nesiritide in patients with left ventricular dysfunction undergoing cardiac surgery: The NAPA Trial, *J Am Coll Cardiol* 49:716–726, 2007.
420. Chen HH, Sundt TM, Cook DJ, et al: Low dose nesiritide and the preservation of renal function in patients with renal dysfunction undergoing cardiopulmonary-bypass surgery: A double-blind placebo-controlled pilot study, *Circulation* 116:I–134–I-138, 2007.
421. Kshirsagar AV, Poole C, Mottl A, et al: N-acetylcysteine for the prevention of radiocontrast induced nephropathy: A meta-analysis of prospective controlled trials, *J Am Soc Nephrol* 15:761–769, 2004.
422. Pannu N, Manns B, Lee HH, et al: Systematic review of the impact of N-acetylcysteine in contrast nephropathy, *Kidney Int* 65:1366–1374, 2004.
423. Solez K, Ideura T, Silvia CB, et al: Clonidine after renal ischemia to lessen acute renal failure and microvascular damage, *Kidney Int* 18:309–322, 1980.
424. Ideura T, Solez K, Heptinstall RH: The effect of clonidine on tubular obstruction in postischemic acute renal failure in the rabbit demonstrated by microradiography and microdissection, *Am J Pathol* 98:123–150, 1980.
425. Eknoyan G, Dobyan DC, Senekjian HO, et al: Protective effect of oral clonidine in the prophylaxis and therapy of mercuric chloride–induced acute renal failure in the rat, *J Lab Clin Med* 102:699–713, 1983.
426. Eknoyan G, Bulger RE, Dobyan DC: Mercuric chloride-induced acute renal failure in the rat. I. Correlation of functional and morphologic changes and their modification by clonidine, *Lab Invest* 46:613–620, 1982.
427. Zou AP, Cowley AW Jr: alpha(2)-adrenergic receptor-mediated increase in NO production buffers renal medullary vasoconstriction, *Am J Physiol Regul Integr Comp Physiol* 279:R769–R777, 2000.
428. Kulka PJ, Tryba M, Zenz M: Preoperative alpha2-adrenergic receptor agonists prevent the deterioration of renal function after cardiac surgery: Results of a randomized, controlled trial, *Crit Care Med* 24:947–952, 1996.
429. Myles PS, Hunt JO, Holdgaard HO, et al: Clonidine and cardiac surgery: Haemodynamic and metabolic effects, myocardial ischaemia and recovery, *Anaesth Intensive Care* 27:137–147, 1999.
430. Scott NB, Turfrey DJ, Ray DA, et al: A prospective randomized study of the potential benefits of thoracic epidural anesthesia and analgesia in patients undergoing coronary artery bypass grafting, *Anesth Analg* 93:528–535, 2001.
431. Schramm L, Heidbreder E, Kartenbender K, et al: Effects of urodilatin and diltiazem on renal function in ischemic acute renal failure in the rat, *Am J Nephrol* 15:418–426, 1995.
432. Schramm L, Heidbreder E, Lukes M, et al: Endotoxin-induced acute renal failure in the rat: Effects of urodilatin and diltiazem on renal function, *Clin Nephrol* 46:117–124, 1996.

433. Yavuz S, Ayabakan N, Goncu MT, et al: Effect of combined dopamine and diltiazem on renal function after cardiac surgery, *Med Sci Monit* 8:PI45–PI50, 2002.
434. Piper SN, Kumle B, Maleck WH, et al: Diltiazem may preserve renal tubular integrity after cardiac surgery, *Can J Anaesth* 50:285–292, 2003.
435. Manabe S, Tanaka H, Yoshizaki T, et al: Effects of the postoperative administration of diltiazem on renal function after coronary artery bypass grafting, *Ann Thorac Surg* 79:831–835, 2005, discussion 5–6.
436. Young EW, Diab A, Kirsh MM: Intravenous diltiazem and acute renal failure after cardiac operations, *Ann Thorac Surg* 65:1316–1319, 1998.
437. Bergman AS, Odar-Cederlof I, Westman L, et al: Diltiazem infusion for renal protection in cardiac surgical patients with preexisting renal dysfunction, *J Cardiothorac Vasc Anesth* 16:294–299, 2002.
438. Zanardo G, Michielon P, Rosi P, et al: Effects of a continuous diltiazem infusion on renal function during cardiac surgery, *J Cardiothorac Vasc Anesth* 7:711–716, 1993.
439. Haase M, Haase-Fielitz A, Bellomo R, et al: Sodium bicarbonate to prevent increases in serum creatinine after cardiac surgery: A pilot double-blind, randomized controlled trial, *Crit Care Med* 37:39–47, 2009.
440. Meier P, Ko DT, Tamura A, et al: Sodium bicarbonate-based hydration prevents contrast-induced nephropathy: A meta-analysis, *BMC Med* 7:23, 2009.
441. Kitagawa S, Komatsu Y, Futatsuyama M, et al: Renoprotection of ace inhibitor and angiotensin II receptor blocker for the patients with severe renal insufficiency, *Nephrology* 8(Suppl):A26–A27, 2003.
442. Rady MY, Ryan T: The effects of preoperative therapy with angiotensin-converting enzyme inhibitors on clinical outcome after cardiovascular surgery, *Chest* 114:487–494, 1998.
443. Gamoso MG, Phillips-Bute B, Landolfo KP, et al: Off-pump versus on-pump coronary artery bypass surgery and postoperative renal dysfunction, *Anesth Analg* 91:1080–1084, 2000.
444. Cittanova ML, Zubicki A, Savu C, et al: The chronic inhibition of angiotensin-converting enzyme impairs postoperative renal function, *Anesth Analg* 93:1111–1115, 2001.
445. Welch WJ, Wilcox CS: AT1 receptor antagonist combats oxidative stress and restores nitric oxide signaling in the SHR, *Kidney Int* 59:1257–1263, 2001.
446. Colson P, Ribstein J, Mimran A, et al: Effect of angiotensin converting enzyme inhibition on blood pressure and renal function during open heart surgery, *Anesthesiology* 72:23–27, 1990.
447. Ryckwaert F, Colson P, Ribstein J, et al: Haemodynamic and renal effects of intravenous enalaprilat during coronary artery bypass graft surgery in patients with ischaemic heart dysfunction, *Br J Anaesth* 86:169–175, 2001.
448. Wagner F, Yeter R, Bisson S, et al: Beneficial hemodynamic and renal effects of intravenous enalaprilat following coronary artery bypass surgery complicated by left ventricular dysfunction, *Crit Care Med* 31:1421–1428, 2003.
449. Vijayan A, Franklin S, Behrend T, et al: Insulin-like growth factor I improves renal function in patients with end-stage chronic renal failure, *Am J Physiol* 276:R929–R934, 1999.
450. Miller SB, Martin DR, Kissane J, et al: Rat models for clinical use of insulin-like growth factor I in acute renal failure, *Am J Physiol* 266:F949–F956, 1994.
451. Miller SB, Moulton M, O'Shea M, et al: Effects of IGF-I on renal function in end-stage chronic renal failure, *Kidney Int* 46:201–207, 1994.
452. Hirschberg R, Kopple J, Lipsett P, et al: Multicenter clinical trial of recombinant human insulin-like growth factor I in patients with acute renal failure, *Kidney Int* 55:2423–2432, 1999.
453. Najafi H, Henson D, Dye WS, et al: Left ventricular hemorrhagic necrosis, *Ann Thorac Surg* 7:550–561, 1969.
454. Buckberg GD: Left ventricular subendocardial necrosis, *Ann Thorac Surg* 24:379–393, 1977.
455. Bigelow WG, Lindsay WK, Greenwood WF: Hypothermia; its possible role in cardiac surgery: An investigation of factors governing survival in dogs at low body temperatures, *Ann Surg* 132:849–866, 1950.
456. Melrose DG, Dreyer B, Bentall HH, et al: Elective cardiac arrest, *Lancet* 269:21–22, 1955.
457. Erhardt LR: GUARD During Ischemia Against Necrosis (GUARDIAN) trial in acute coronary syndromes, *Am J Cardiol* 83:23G–25G, 1999.
458. Chaitman BR: A review of the GUARDIAN trial results: Clinical implications and the significance of elevated perioperative CK-MB on 6-month survival, *J Card Surg* 18(Suppl 1):13–20, 2003.
459. Theroux P, Chaitman BR, Danchin N, et al: Inhibition of the sodium-hydrogen exchanger with cariporide to prevent myocardial infarction in high-risk ischemic situations. Main results of the GUARDIAN trial. Guard during ischemia against necrosis (GUARDIAN) Investigators, *Circulation* 102:3032–3038, 2000.
460. Ferguson TB Jr, Hammill BG, Peterson ED, et al: A decade of change—risk profiles and outcomes for isolated coronary artery bypass grafting procedures, 1990-1999: A report from the STS National Database Committee and the Duke Clinical Research Institute. Society of Thoracic Surgeons, *Ann Thorac Surg* 73:480–489, 2002.
461. Ovize M: Still looking for the ultimate mechanism of myocardial stunning, *Basic Res Cardiol* 92 (Suppl 2):16–17, 1997.
462. Braunwald E, Kloner RA: The stunned myocardium: Prolonged, postischemic ventricular dysfunction, *Circulation* 66:1146–1149, 1982.
463. Gray R, Maddahi J, Berman D, et al: Scintigraphic and hemodynamic demonstration of transient left ventricular dysfunction immediately after uncomplicated coronary artery bypass grafting, *J Thorac Cardiovasc Surg* 77:504–510, 1979.
464. Kloner RA, Przyklenk K, Kay GL: Clinical evidence for stunned myocardium after coronary artery bypass surgery, *J Card Surg* 9:397–402, 1994.
465. Bolli R: Mechanism of myocardial "stunning". *Circulation* 82:723–738, 1990.
466. Sun JZ, Kaur H, Halliwell B, et al: Use of aromatic hydroxylation of phenylalanine to measure production of hydroxyl radicals after myocardial ischemia in vivo. Direct evidence for a pathogenetic role of the hydroxyl radical in myocardial stunning, *Circ Res* 73:534–549, 1993.
467. Sekili S, McCay PB, Li XY, et al: Direct evidence that the hydroxyl radical plays a pathogenetic role in myocardial "stunning" in the conscious dog and demonstration that stunning can be markedly attenuated without subsequent adverse effects, *Circ Res* 73:705–723, 1993.
468. Shattock MJ: Myocardial stunning: Do we know the mechanism? *Basic Res Cardiol* 92(Suppl 2):18–22, 1997.
469. Shen AC, Jennings RB: Kinetics of calcium accumulation in acute myocardial ischemic injury, *Am J Pathol* 67:441–452, 1972.
470. Clark RE, Magovern GJ, Christlieb IY, et al: Nifedipine cardioplegia experience: Results of a 3-year cooperative clinical study, *Ann Thorac Surg* 36:654–663, 1983.
471. Karmazyn M: The 1990 Merck Frosst Award. Ischemic and reperfusion injury in the heart. Cellular mechanisms and pharmacological interventions, *Can J Physiol Pharmacol* 69:719–730, 1991.
472. Sarnoff SJ, Braunwald E, Welch GH Jr, et al: Hemodynamic determinants of oxygen consumption of the heart with special reference to the tension-time index, *Am J Physiol* 192:148–156, 1958.
473. Karmazyn M: The sodium-hydrogen exchange system in the heart: Its role in ischemic and reperfusion injury and therapeutic implications, *Can J Cardiol* 12:1074–1082, 1996.
474. Kawamura T, Wakusawa R, Okada K, et al: Elevation of cytokines during open heart surgery with cardiopulmonary bypass: Participation of interleukin 8 and 6 in reperfusion injury, *Can J Anaesth* 40:1016–1021, 1993.
475. Hansen PR: Myocardial reperfusion injury: Experimental evidence and clinical relevance, *Eur Heart J* 16:734–740, 1995.
476. Kofsky ER, Julia PL, Buckberg GD, et al: Studies of controlled reperfusion after ischemia. XXII. Reperfusate composition: Effects of leukocyte depletion of blood and blood cardioplegic reperfusates after acute coronary occlusion, *J Thorac Cardiovasc Surg* 101:350–359, 1991.
477. Karmazyn M: Synthesis and relevance of cardiac eicosanoids with particular emphasis on ischemia and reperfusion, *Can J Physiol Pharmacol* 67:912–921, 1989.
478. Schwinn D, Liggett S, McRae R, et al: Desensitization of myocardial beta-adrenergic receptors during cardiopulmonary bypass. Evidence for early uncoupling and late downregulation, *Circulation* 84:2559–2567, 1991.
479. Smiley RM, Kwatra MM, Schwinn DA: New developments in cardiovascular adrenergic receptor pharmacology: Molecular mechanisms and clinical relevance, *J Cardiothorac Vasc Anesth* 12:80–95, 1998.
480. Reves JG, Buttner E, Karp RB, et al: Elevated catecholamines during cardiac surgery: Consequences of reperfusion of the postarrested heart, *Am J Cardiol* 53:722–728, 1984.
481. Reves JG, Karp RB, Buttner EE, et al: Neuronal and adrenomedullary catecholamine release in response to cardiopulmonary bypass in man, *Circulation* 66:49–55, 1982.
482. Vinten-Johansen J, Thourani VH: Myocardial protection: An overview, *J Extra Corpor Technol* 32: 38–48, 2000.
483. Gay WA Jr: Potassium-induced cardioplegia, *Ann Thorac Surg* 20:95–100, 1975.
484. Gay WA Jr, Ebert PA: Functional, metabolic, and morphologic effects of potassium-induced cardioplegia, *Surgery* 74:284–290, 1973.
485. Julia PL, Buckberg GD, Acar C, et al: Studies of controlled reperfusion after ischemia. XXI. Reperfusate composition: Superiority of blood cardioplegia over crystalloid cardioplegia in limiting reperfusion damage—importance of endogenous oxygen free radical scavengers in red blood cells, *J Thorac Cardiovasc Surg* 101:303–313, 1991.
486. Follette DM, Mulder DG, Maloney JV, et al: Advantages of blood cardioplegia over continuous coronary perfusion or intermittent ischemia. Experimental and clinical study, *J Thorac Cardiovasc Surg* 76:604–619, 1978.
487. Fremes SE, Christakis GT, Weisel RD, et al: A clinical trial of blood and crystalloid cardioplegia, *J Thorac Cardiovasc Surg* 88:726–741, 1984.
488. Loop FD, Higgins TL, Panda R, et al: Myocardial protection during cardiac operations. Decreased morbidity and lower cost with blood cardioplegia and coronary sinus perfusion, *J Thorac Cardiovasc Surg* 104:608–618, 1992.
489. Follette DM, Fey K, Buckberg GD, et al: Reducing postischemic damage by temporary modification of reperfusate calcium, potassium, pH, and osmolarity, *J Thorac Cardiovasc Surg* 82:221–238, 1981.
490. Follette D, Fey K, Mulder D, et al: Prolonged safe aortic clamping by combining membrane stabilization, multidose cardioplegia, and appropriate pH reperfusion, *J Thorac Cardiovasc Surg* 74:682–694, 1977.
491. Salerno TA, Houck JP, Barrozo CA, et al: Retrograde continuous warm blood cardioplegia: A new concept in myocardial protection, *Ann Thorac Surg* 51:245–247, 1991.
492. Mehlhorn U: Improved myocardial protection using continuous coronary perfusion with normothermic blood and beta-blockade with esmolol, *Thorac Cardiovasc Surg* 45:224–231, 1997.
493. Segel LD, Follette DM: Cardiac function and glycogen content after twenty-four-hour preservation with various metabolic substrates, *J Heart Lung Transplant* 17:299–305, 1998.
494. Segel LD, Follette DM, Baker JM, et al: Recovery of sheep hearts after perfusion preservation or static storage with crystalloid media, *J Heart Lung Transplant* 17:211–221, 1998.
495. Smolens IA, Follette DM, Berkoff HA, et al: Incomplete recovery of working heart function after twenty-four-hour preservation with a modified University of Wisconsin solution, *J Heart Lung Transplant* 14:906–915, 1995.
496. Mauney MC, Kron IL: The physiologic basis of warm cardioplegia, *Ann Thorac Surg* 60:819–823, 1995.
497. Ikonomidis JS, Rao V, Weisel RD, et al: Myocardial protection for coronary bypass grafting: The Toronto Hospital perspective, *Ann Thorac Surg* 60:824–832, 1995.
498. Hayashida N, Weisel RD, Shirai T, et al: Tepid antegrade and retrograde cardioplegia, *Ann Thorac Surg* 59:723–729, 1995.
499. Menasche P, Subayi JB, Veyssie L, et al: Efficacy of coronary sinus cardioplegia in patients with complete coronary artery occlusions, *Ann Thorac Surg* 51:418–423, 1991.
500. Menasche P, Subayi JB, Piwnica A: Retrograde coronary sinus cardioplegia for aortic valve operations: A clinical report on 500 patients, *Ann Thorac Surg* 49:556–563, 1990, discussion 63–64.
501. Hammond GL, Davies AL, Austen WG: Retrograde coronary sinus perfusion: A method of myocardial protection in the dog during left coronary artery occlusion, *Ann Surg* 166:39–47, 1967.
502. Flack JE 3rd, Cook JR, May SJ, et al: Does cardioplegia type affect outcome and survival in patients with advanced left ventricular dysfunction? Results from the CABG Patch Trial, *Circulation* 102:III84–III89, 2000.
503. Dagenais F, Pelletier LC, Carrier M: Antegrade/retrograde cardioplegia for valve replacement: A prospective study, *Ann Thorac Surg* 68:1681–1685, 1999.
504. Shahian DM: Retrograde coronary sinus cardioplegia in the presence of persistent left superior vena cava, *Ann Thorac Surg* 54:1214–1215, 1992.
505. Roberts WA, Risher WH, Schwarz KQ: Transesophageal echocardiographic identification of persistent left superior vena cava: Retrograde administration of cardioplegia during cardiac surgery, *Anesthesiology* 81:760–762, 1994.
506. Murry CE, Jennings RB, Reimer KA: Preconditioning with ischemia: A delay of lethal cell injury in ischemic myocardium, *Circulation* 74:1124–1136, 1986.
507. Ikonomidis JS, Weisel RD, Mickle DA: Ischemic preconditioning: Cardioprotection for cardiac surgery, *J Card Surg* 9:526–531, 1994.
508. Finegan BA, Lopaschuk GD, Gandhi M, et al: Ischemic preconditioning inhibits glycolysis and proton production in isolated working rat hearts, *Am J Physiol* 269:H1767–H1775, 1995.
509. Hagar JM, Hale SL, Kloner RA: Effect of preconditioning ischemia on reperfusion arrhythmias after coronary artery occlusion and reperfusion in the rat, *Circ Res* 68:61–68, 1991.
510. Liu GS, Thornton J, Van Winkle DM, et al: Protection against infarction afforded by preconditioning is mediated by A1 adenosine receptors in rabbit heart, *Circulation* 84:350–356, 1991.
511. Perrault LP, Menasche P: Role of preconditioning in cardiac surgery, *Basic Res Cardiol* 92 (Suppl 2):54–56, 1997.
512. Speechly-Dick ME, Grover GJ, Yellon DM: Does ischemic preconditioning in the human involve protein kinase C and the ATP-dependent K+ channel? Studies of contractile function after simulated ischemia in an atrial in vitro model, *Circ Res* 77:1030–1035, 1995.
513. De Hert S, Vermeyen K, Adriensen H: Influence of thiopental, etomidate and propofol on regional myocardial function in the normal and acute ischemic heart segments, *Anesth Analg* 70:600, 1990.
514. Mentzer RM Jr, Rahko PS, Molina-Viamonte V, et al: Safety, tolerance, and efficacy of adenosine as an additive to blood cardioplegia in humans during coronary artery bypass surgery, *Am J Cardiol* 79:38–43, 1997.
515. Lee HT, LaFaro RJ, Reed GE: Pretreatment of human myocardium with adenosine during open heart surgery, *J Card Surg* 10:665–676, 1995.
516. Finegan BA, Cohen M: Myocardial protection: Is there anything better than ice? *Can J Anaesth* 45:R32–R39, 1998.
517. Lawhorne TWJ, Davis JL, Smith GW: General surgical complications after cardiac surgery, *Am J Surg* 136:254–256, 1976.
518. Lucas A, Max MH: Emergency laparotomy immediately after coronary bypass, *JAMA* 244:1829–1830, 1980.
519. Reath DB, Maull KI, Wolfgang TC: General surgical complications following cardiac surgery, *Am Surg* 49:11–14, 1983.

520. Aranha GV, Pickleman J, Pifarre R, et al: The reasons for gastrointestinal consultation after cardiac surgery, *Am Surg* 50:301–304, 1984.
521. Ohri SK, Desai JB, Gaer JA, et al: Intraabdominal complications after cardiopulmonary bypass, *Ann Thorac Surg* 52:826–831, 1991.
522. Rosemurgy AS, McAllister E, Karl RC: The acute surgical abdomen after cardiac surgery involving extracorporeal circulation, *Ann Surg* 207:323–326, 1988.
523. D'Ancona G, Baillot R, Poirier B, et al: Determinants of gastrointestinal complications in cardiac surgery, *Tex Heart Inst J* 30:280–285, 2003.
524. Fitzgerald T, Kim D, Karakozis S, et al: Visceral ischemia after cardiopulmonary bypass, *Am Surg* 66:623–626, 2000.
525. McSweeney ME, Garwood S, Levin J, et al: Adverse gastrointestinal complications after cardiopulmonary bypass: Can outcome be predicted from preoperative risk factors? *Anesth Analg* 98:1610–1617, 2004, table of contents.
526. Filsoufi F, Rahmanian PB, Castillo JG, et al: Predictors and outcome of gastrointestinal complications in patients undergoing cardiac surgery, *Ann Surg* 246:323–329, 2007.
527. Andersson B, Andersson R, Brandt J, et al: Gastrointestinal complications after cardiac surgery—improved risk stratification using a new scoring model, *Interact Cardiovasc Thorac Surg* 10:366–370.
528. Croome KP, Kiaii B, Fox S, et al: Comparison of gastrointestinal complications in on-pump versus off-pump coronary artery bypass grafting, *Can J Surg* 52:125–128, 2009.
529. Halm MA: Acute gastrointestinal complications after cardiac surgery, *Am J Crit Care* 5:109–118, 1996, quiz 19–20.
530. Sakorafas GH, Tsiotos GG: Intra-abdominal complications after cardiac surgery, *Eur J Surg* 165:820–827, 1999.
531. Hessel EA 2nd: Abdominal organ injury after cardiac surgery, *Semin Cardiothorac Vasc Anesth* 8:243–263, 2004.
532. Christenson JT, Schmuziger M, Maurice J, et al: Gastrointestinal complications after coronary artery bypass grafting, *J Thorac Cardiovasc Surg* 108:899–906, 1994.
533. Musleh GS, Patel NC, Grayson AD, et al: Off-pump coronary artery bypass surgery does not reduce gastrointestinal complications, *Eur J Cardiothorac Surg* 23:170–174, 2003.
534. Perugini RA, Orr RK, Porter D, et al: Gastrointestinal complications following cardiac surgery. An analysis of 1477 cardiac surgery patients, *Arch Surg* 132:352–357, 1997.
535. Spotnitz WD, Sanders RP, Hanks JB, et al: General surgical complications can be predicted after cardiopulmonary bypass, *Ann Surg* 221:489–496, 1995, discussion 96–97.
536. Zacharias A, Schwann TA, Parenteau GL, et al: Predictors of gastrointestinal complications in cardiac surgery, *Tex Heart Inst J* 27:93–99, 2000.
537. Sanisoglu I, Guden M, Bayramoglu Z, et al: Does off-pump CABG reduce gastrointestinal complications? *Ann Thorac Surg* 77:619–625, 2004.
538. Lennon MJ, Gibbs NM, Weightman WM, et al: Transesophageal echocardiography-related gastrointestinal complications in cardiac surgical patients, *J Cardiothorac Vasc Anesth* 19:141–145, 2005.
539. Bolke E, Jehle PM, Orth K, et al: Changes of gut barrier function during anesthesia and cardiac surgery, *Angiology* 52:477–482, 2001.
540. Sack FU, Hagl S: Extracorporeal circulation and intestinal microcirculation: Pathophysiology and therapeutical options. An intravital microscopic study in a large animal model, *Eur Surg Res* 34:129–137, 2002.
541. Doty JR, Wilentz RE, Salazar JD, et al: Atheroembolism in cardiac surgery, *Ann Thorac Surg* 75:1221–1226, 2003.
542. Simic O, Strathausen S, Hess W, et al: Incidence and prognosis of abdominal complications after cardiopulmonary bypass, *Cardiovasc Surg* 7:419–424, 1999.
543. Cetindag IB, Boley TM, Magee MJ, et al: Postoperative gastrointestinal complications after lung volume reduction operations, *Ann Thorac Surg* 68:1029–1033, 1999.
544. Smith PC, Slaughter MS, Petty MG, et al: Abdominal complications after lung transplantation, *J Heart Lung Transplant* 14:44–51, 1995.
545. Bastien O, Piriou V, Aouifi A, et al: Relative importance of flow versus pressure in splanchnic perfusion during cardiopulmonary bypass in rabbits, *Anesthesiology* 92:457–464, 2000.
546. Boston US, Slater JM, Orszulak TA, et al: Hierarchy of regional oxygen delivery during cardiopulmonary bypass, *Ann Thorac Surg* 71:260–264, 2001.
547. Slater JM, Orszulak TA, Cook DJ: Distribution and hierarchy of regional blood flow during hypothermic cardiopulmonary bypass, *Ann Thorac Surg* 72:542–547, 2001.
548. Landow L: Splanchnic lactate production in cardiac surgery patients, *Crit Care Med* 21:S84–S91, 1993.
549. Mythen MG, Webb AR: Perioperative plasma volume expansion reduces the incidence of gut mucosal hypoperfusion during cardiac surgery, *Arch Surg* 130:423–429, 1995.
550. Debaveye YA, Van den Berghe GH: Is there still a place for dopamine in the modern intensive care unit? *Anesth Analg* 98:461–468, 2004.
551. Parviainen I, Ruokonen E, Takala J: Dobutamine-induced dissociation between changes in splanchnic blood flow and gastric intramucosal pH after cardiac surgery, *Br J Anaesth* 74:277–282, 1995.
552. Gardeback M, Settergren G: Dopexamine and dopamine in the prevention of low gastric mucosal pH following cardiopulmonary by-pass, *Acta Anaesthesiol Scand* 39:1066–1070, 1995.
553. Westphal M, Freise H, Kehrel BE, et al: Arginine vasopressin compromises gut mucosal microcirculation in septic rats, *Crit Care Med* 32:194–200, 2004.
554. Martinez-Pellus AE, Merino P, Bru M, et al: Endogenous endotoxemia of intestinal origin during cardiopulmonary bypass. Role of type of flow and protective effect of selective digestive decontamination, *Intensive Care Med* 23:1251–1257, 1997.
555. Matheson PJ, Wilson MA, Garrison RN: Regulation of intestinal blood flow, *J Surg Res* 93:182–196, 2000.
556. Rea HH, Harris EA, Seelye ER, et al: The effects of cardiopulmonary bypass upon pulmonary gas exchange, *J Thorac Cardiovasc Surg* 75:104–120, 1978.
557. Cheng DC: Fast track cardiac surgery pathways: Early extubation, process of care, and cost containment, *Anesthesiology* 88:1429–1433, 1998.
558. Branca P, McGaw P, Light R: Factors associated with prolonged mechanical ventilation following coronary artery bypass surgery, *Chest* 119:537–546, 2001.
559. Rankin JS, Hammill BG, Ferguson TB Jr, et al: Determinants of operative mortality in valvular heart surgery, *J Thorac Cardiovasc Surg* 131:547–557, 2006.
560. Rady MY, Ryan T, Starr NJ: Early onset of acute pulmonary dysfunction after cardiovascular surgery. Risk factors and clinical outcome, *Crit Care Med* 25:1831–1839, 1997.
561. Bernard GR, Artigas A, Brigham KL, et al: Report of the American-European consensus conference on ARDS: Definitions, mechanisms, relevant outcomes and clinical trial coordination. The Consensus Committee, *Intensive Care Med* 20:225–232, 1994.
562. Christenson JT, Aeberhard JM, Badel P, et al: Adult respiratory distress syndrome after cardiac surgery, *Cardiovasc Surg* 4:15–21, 1996.
563. Welsby IJ, Bennett-Guerrero E, Atwell D, et al: The association of complication type with mortality and prolonged stay after cardiac surgery with cardiopulmonary bypass, *Anesth Analg* 94:1072–1078, 2002.
564. Ng CS, Wan S, Yim AP, et al: Pulmonary dysfunction after cardiac surgery, *Chest* 121:1269–1277, 2002.
565. Jindani A, Aps C, Neville E, et al: Postoperative cardiac surgical care: An alternative approach, *Br Heart J* 69:59–63, 1993.
566. Jain U, Rao TL, Kumar P, et al: Radiographic pulmonary abnormalities after different types of cardiac surgery, *J Cardiothorac Vasc Anesth* 5:592–595, 1991.
567. Magnusson L, Zemgulis V, Wicky S, et al: Atelectasis is a major cause of hypoxemia and shunt after cardiopulmonary bypass: An experimental study, *Anesthesiology* 87:1153–1163, 1997.
568. Magnusson L, Zemgulis V, Tenling A, et al: Use of a vital capacity maneuver to prevent atelectasis after cardiopulmonary bypass: An experimental study, *Anesthesiology* 88:134–142, 1998.
569. Daganou M, Dimopoulou I, Michalopoulos N, et al: Respiratory complications after coronary artery bypass surgery with unilateral or bilateral internal mammary artery grafting, *Chest* 113:1285–1289, 1998.
570. Johnson D, Kelm C, Thomson D, et al: The effect of physical therapy on respiratory complications following cardiac valve surgery, *Chest* 109:638–644, 1996.
571. Lim E, Callaghan C, Motalleb-Zadeh R, et al: A prospective study on clinical outcome following pleurotomy during cardiac surgery, *Thorac Cardiovasc Surg* 50:287–291, 2002.
572. Lainez RM, Losada M, Nieto E, et al: [Pneumonia in patients undergoing heart surgery], *Enferm Infecc Microbiol Clin* 12:4–8, 1994.
573. Bouza E, Perez A, Munoz P, et al: Ventilator-associated pneumonia after heart surgery: A prospective analysis and the value of surveillance, *Crit Care Med* 31:1964–1970, 2003.
574. Kollef MH, Sharpless L, Vlasnik J, et al: The impact of nosocomial infections on patient outcomes following cardiac surgery, *Chest* 112:666–675, 1997.
575. Leal-Noval SR, Marquez-Vacaro JA, Garcia-Curiel A, et al: Nosocomial pneumonia in patients undergoing heart surgery, *Crit Care Med* 28:935–940, 2000.
576. Gaynes R, Bizek B, Mowry-Hanley J, et al: Risk factors for nosocomial pneumonia after coronary artery bypass graft operations, *Ann Thorac Surg* 51:215–218, 1991.
577. Filsoufi F, Rahmanian PB, Castillo JG, et al: Logistic risk model predicting postoperative respiratory failure in patients undergoing valve surgery, *Eur J Cardiothorac Surg* 34:953–959, 2008.
578. Auler JO Jr, Zin WA, Caldeira MP, et al: Pre- and postoperative inspiratory mechanics in ischemic and valvular heart disease, *Chest* 92:984–990, 1987.
579. Barnas GM, Watson RJ, Green MD, et al: Lung and chest wall mechanical properties before and after cardiac surgery with cardiopulmonary bypass, *J Appl Physiol* 76:166–175, 1994.
580. Hachenberg T, Brussel T, Roos N, et al: Gas exchange impairment and pulmonary densities after cardiac surgery, *Acta Anaesthesiol Scand* 36:800–805, 1992.
581. Raijmakers PG, Groeneveld AB, Schneider AJ, et al: Transvascular transport of 67Ga in the lungs after cardiopulmonary bypass surgery, *Chest* 104:1825–1832, 1993.
582. Messent M, Sinclair DG, Quinlan GJ, et al: Pulmonary vascular permeability after cardiopulmonary bypass and its relationship to oxidative stress, *Crit Care Med* 25:425–429, 1997.
583. Laffey JG, Boylan JF, Cheng DC: The systemic inflammatory response to cardiac surgery: Implications for the anesthesiologist, *Anesthesiology* 97:215–252, 2002.
584. Sinclair DG, Haslam PL, Quinlan GJ, et al: The effect of cardiopulmonary bypass on intestinal and pulmonary endothelial permeability, *Chest* 108:718–724, 1995.
585. Baue AE: The role of the gut in the development of multiple organ dysfunction in cardiothoracic patients, *Ann Thorac Surg* 55:822–829, 1993.
586. Gorlach G, Sroka J, Heidt M, et al: Intracellular adhesion molecule-1 in patients developing pulmonary insufficiency after cardiopulmonary bypass, *Thorac Cardiovasc Surg* 51:138–141, 2003.
587. Wasowicz M, Sobczynski P, Biczysko W, et al: Ultrastructural changes in the lung alveoli after cardiac surgical operations with the use of cardiopulmonary bypass (CPB), *Pol J Pathol* 50:189–196, 1999.
588. Milot J, Perron J, Lacasse Y, et al: Incidence and predictors of ARDS after cardiac surgery, *Chest* 119:884–888, 2001.
589. Asimakopoulos G, Taylor KM, Smith PL, et al: Prevalence of acute respiratory distress syndrome after cardiac surgery, *J Thorac Cardiovasc Surg* 117:620–621, 1999.
590. Gillinov AM, Davis EA, Alberg AJ, et al: Pulmonary embolism in the cardiac surgical patient, *Ann Thorac Surg* 53:988–991, 1992.
591. Josa M, Siouffi SY, Silverman AB, et al: Pulmonary embolism after cardiac surgery, *J Am Coll Cardiol* 21:990–996, 1993.
592. Weissman C: Pulmonary complications after cardiac surgery, *Semin Cardiothorac Vasc Anesth* 8:185–211, 2004.
593. DeLaria GA, Hunter JA: Deep venous thrombosis. Implications after open heart surgery, *Chest* 99:284–288, 1991.
594. Ambrosetti M, Salerno M, Zambelli M, et al: Deep vein thrombosis among patients entering cardiac rehabilitation after coronary artery bypass surgery, *Chest* 125:191–196, 2004.
595. Goldhaber SZ, Hirsch DR, MacDougall RC, et al: Prevention of venous thrombosis after coronary artery bypass surgery (a randomized trial comparing two mechanical prophylaxis strategies), *Am J Cardiol* 76:993–996, 1995.
596. Gilbert TB, Barnas GM, Sequeira AJ: Impact of pleurotomy, continuous positive airway pressure, and fluid balance during cardiopulmonary bypass on lung mechanics and oxygenation, *J Cardiothorac Vasc Anesth* 10:844–849, 1996.
597. Berry CB, Butler PJ, Myles PS: Lung management during cardiopulmonary bypass: Is continuous positive airways pressure beneficial? *Br J Anaesth* 71:864–868, 1993.
598. Lee AH, Gallagher PJ: Post-mortem examination after cardiac surgery, *Histopathology* 33:399–405, 1998.
599. Ventilation with lower tidal volumes as compared with traditional tidal volumes for acute lung injury and the acute respiratory distress syndrome. The Acute Respiratory Distress Syndrome Network, *N Engl J Med* 342:1301–1308, 2000.
600. Hill G, Alonso A, Thiele G, et al: Glucocorticoids blunt neutrophil CD11b surface glycoprotein upregulation during cardiopulmonary bypass in humans, *Anesth Analg* 79:23–27, 1994.
601. Kilger E, Weis F, Briegel J, et al: Stress doses of hydrocortisone reduce severe systemic inflammatory response syndrome and improve early outcome in a risk group of patients after cardiac surgery, *Crit Care Med* 31:1068–1074, 2003.
602. Oliver WC Jr, Nuttall GA, Orszulak TA, et al: Hemofiltration but not steroids results in earlier tracheal extubation following cardiopulmonary bypass: A prospective, randomized double-blind trial, *Anesthesiology* 101:327–339, 2004.
603. Chaney MA, Nikolov MP, Blakeman B, et al: Pulmonary effects of methylprednisolone in patients undergoing coronary artery bypass grafting and early tracheal extubation, *Anesth Analg* 87:27–33, 1998.
604. Bidstrup B, Royston D, Sapsford R, et al: Reduction in blood loss and blood use afer cardiopulmonary bypass with high dose aprotinin (Trasylol), *J Thorac Cardiovasc Surg* 97:364–372, 1989.
605. Hill GE, Alonso A, Spurzem JR, et al: Aprotinin and methylprednislone equally blunt cardiopulmonary bypass-induced inflammation in humans, *J Thorac Cardiovasc Surg* 110:1658–1662, 1995.
606. Royston D, Bidstrup BP, Taylor KM, et al: Effect of aprotinin on need for blood transfusion after repeat open-heart surgery, *Lancet* 2:1289–1291, 1987.
607. Royston D: High dose aprotinin therapy: A review of the first five years' experience, *J Cardiothorac Vasc Anesth* 6:76–100, 1992.
608. Royston D: Aprotinin therapy, *Br J Anaesth* 73:734–737, 1994.
609. van Oeveren W, Jansen N, Bidstrup B, et al: Effects of aprotinin on hemostatic mechanisms during cardiopulmonary bypass, *Ann Thorac Surg* 44:640–645, 1987.

610. Wessel DL, Adatia I, Giglia TM, et al: Use of inhaled nitric oxide and acetylcholine in the evaluation of pulmonary hypertension and endothelial function after cardiopulmonary bypass, *Circulation* 88:2128–2138, 1993.
611. Rich GF, Murphy GD Jr, Roos CM, et al: Inhaled nitric oxide. Selective pulmonary vasodilation in cardiac surgical patients, *Anesthesiology* 78:1028–1035, 1993.
612. Fullerton DA, Jones SD, Jaggers J, et al: Effective control of pulmonary vascular resistance with inhaled nitric oxide after cardiac operation, *J Thorac Cardiovasc Surg* 111:753–762, 1996, discussion 62–63.
613. Bacha EA, Head CA: Use of inhaled nitric oxide for lung transplantation and cardiac surgery, *Respir Care Clin N Am* 3:521–536, 1997.
614. Wasowicz M, Vegas A, Borger MA, et al: Bivalirudin anticoagulation for cardiopulmonary bypass in a patient with heparin-induced thrombocytopenia, *Can J Anaesth* 52:1093–1098, 2005.
615. Mills NL, Everson CT: Atherosclerosis of the ascending aorta and coronary artery bypass. Pathology, clinical correlates, and operative management, *J Thorac Cardiovasc Surg* 102:546–553, 1991.
616. Wareing TH, Davila-Roman VG, Barzilai B, et al: Management of the severely atherosclerotic ascending aorta during cardiac operations. A strategy for detection and treatment, *J Thorac Cardiovasc Surg* 103:453–462, 1992.
617. Ohteki H, Itoh T, Natsuaki M, et al: Intraoperative ultrasound imaging of the ascending aorta in ischemic heart disease, *Ann Thorac Surg* 50:539–542, 1990.
618. Magilligan DJ Jr, Eastland MW, Lell WA, et al: Decreased carotid flow with ascending aortic cannulation, *Circulation* 45:I130–I133, 1972.
619. Benedict JS, Buhl TL, Henney RP: Acute aortic dissection during cardiopulmonary bypass. Successful treatment of three patients, *Arch Surg* 108:810–813, 1974.
620. Still RJ, Hilgenberg AD, Akins CW, et al: Intraoperative aortic dissection, *Ann Thorac Surg* 53:374–379, 1992, discussion 380.
621. Barzilai B, Marshall W, Saffitz J, et al: Avoidance of embolic complications by ultrasonic characterization of the ascending aorta, *Circulation* 80:I275–I279, 1989.
622. Coselli JS, Crawford ES: Aortic valve replacement in the patient with extensive calcification of the ascending aorta (the porcelain aorta), *J Thorac Cardiovasc Surg* 91:184–187, 1986.
623. Pillai R, Venn G, Lennox S, et al: Elective femoro-femoral bypass for operations on the heart and great vessels, *J Thorac Cardiovasc Surg* 88:635–637, 1984.
624. Bennett EV Jr, Fewel JG, Ybarra J, et al: Comparison of flow differences among venous cannulas, *Ann Thorac Surg* 36:59–65, 1983.
625. Rosenfeldt FL, Watson DA II: Interference with local myocardial cooling by heat gain during aortic cross-clamping, *Ann Thorac Surg* 27:13–16, 1979.
626. Johnston WE, Royster RL, Choplin RH, et al: Pulmonary artery catheter migration during cardiac surgery, *Anesthesiology* 64:258–262, 1986.
627. Bromley JJ, Moorthy SS: Acute angulation of a pulmonary artery catheter, *Anesthesiology* 59:367–368, 1983.
628. Campbell FW, Schwartz AJ: Pulmonary artery catheter malfunction? *Anesthesiology* 60:513–514, 1984.
629. Mantia AM, Robinson JN, Lolley DM, et al: Sternal retraction and pulmonary artery catheter compromise, *J Cardiothorac Anesth* 2:430–439, 1988.
630. Baraka A, Darwish R, Mora Mangano CM: Marked mixed venous hemoglobin desaturation in a patient during hypothermic cardiopulmonary bypass, *J Cardiothorac Vasc Anesth* 9:764–767, 1995.
631. Myles PS, Leslie K, McNeil J, et al: Bispectral index monitoring to prevent awareness during anaesthesia: The B-Aware randomised controlled trial, *Lancet* 363:1757–1763, 2004.
632. Hall RI, Thomas BL, Hug CC Jr: Pharmacokinetics and pharmacodynamics during cardiac surgery and cardiopulmonary bypass. In Mora C, editor: *Cardiopulmonary Bypass: Principles and Techniques of Extracorporeal Circulation*, New York, 1995, Springer-Verlag, pp 55.
633. Gordon RJ, Ravin M, Rawitscher RE, et al: Changes in arterial pressure, viscosity and resistance during cardiopulmonary bypass, *J Thorac Cardiovasc Surg* 69:552–561, 1975.
634. Doss DN, Estafanous FG, Ferrario CM, et al: Mechanism of systemic vasodilation during normovolemic hemodilution, *Anesth Analg* 81:30–34, 1995.
635. Schaff HV, Ciardullo RC, Flaherty JT, et al: Development of regional myocardial ischemia distal to a critical coronary stenosis during cardiopulmonary bypass: Comparison of the fibrillating vs. the beating nonworking states, *Surgery* 83:57–66, 1978.
636. Brazier J, Hottenrott C, Buckberg G: Noncoronary collateral myocardial blood flow, *Ann Thorac Surg* 19:426–435, 1975.
637. Lajos TZ, Glicken D: Metabolic measurements in the human heart-lung preparation during hypothermic cardioplegia, *Thorac Cardiovasc Surg* 28:34–41, 1980.
638. Olinger GN, Bonchek LI, Geiss DM: Noncoronary collateral distribution in coronary artery disease, *Ann Thorac Surg* 32:554–557, 1981.
639. Fox LS, Blackstone EH, Kirklin JW, et al: Relationship of whole body oxygen consumption to perfusion flow rate during hypothermic cardiopulmonary bypass, *J Thorac Cardiovasc Surg* 83:239–248, 1982.
640. Hirsch DM Jr, Hadidian C, Neville WE: Oxygen consumption during cardiopulmonary bypass with large volume hemodilution, *J Thorac Cardiovasc Surg* 56:197–202, 1968.
641. Kawamura M, Minamikawa O, Yokochi H, et al: Safe limit of hemodilution in cardiopulmonary bypass—comparative analysis between cyanotic and acyanotic congenital heart disease, *Jpn J Surg* 10:206–211, 1980.
642. Niinikoski J, Laaksonen V, Meretoja O, et al: Oxygen transport to tissue under normovolemic moderate and extreme hemodilution during coronary bypass operation, *Ann Thorac Surg* 31:134–143, 1981.
643. Dexter F, Hindman B: Theoretical analysis of cerebral venous blood hemoglobin oxygen saturation as an index of cerebral oxygenation during hypothermic cardiopulmonary bypass, *Anesthesiology* 83:405–412, 1995.
644. Slogoff S, Reul GJ, Keats AS, et al: Role of perfusion pressure and flow in major organ dysfunction after cardiopulmonary bypass, *Ann Thorac Surg* 50:911–918, 1990.
645. Koning HM, Koning AJ, Defauw JJ: Optimal perfusion during extra-corporeal circulation, *Scand J Thorac Cardiovasc Surg* 21:207–213, 1987.
646. Rogers AT, Prough DS, Roy RC, et al: Cerebrovascular and cerebral metabolic effects of alterations in perfusion flow rate during hypothermic cardiopulmonary bypass in man, *J Thorac Cardiovasc Surg* 103:363–368, 1992.
647. Soma Y, Hirotani T, Yozu R, et al: A clinical study of cerebral circulation during extracorporeal circulation, *J Thorac Cardiovasc Surg* 97:187–193, 1989.
648. Michler RE, Sandhu AA, Young WL, et al: Low-flow cardiopulmonary bypass: Importance of blood pressure in maintaining cerebral blood flow, *Ann Thorac Surg* 60:S525–S528, 1995.
649. Schwartz AE, Sandhu AA, Kaplon RJ, et al: Cerebral blood flow is determined by arterial pressure and not cardiopulmonary bypass flow rate, *Ann Thorac Surg* 60:165–169, 1995, discussion 169–170.
650. Schwartz AE, Kaplon RJ, Young WL, et al: Cerebral blood flow during low-flow hypothermic cardiopulmonary bypass in baboons, *Anesthesiology* 81:959–964, 1994.
651. Liu EH, Dhara SS: Monitoring oxygenator expiratory isoflurane concentrations and the bispectral index to guide isoflurane requirements during cardiopulmonary bypass, *J Cardiothorac Vasc Anesth* 19:485–487, 2005.
652. Davis FM, Parimelazhagan KN, Harris EA: Thermal balance during cardiopulmonary bypass with moderate hypothermia in man, *Br J Anaesth* 49:1127–1132, 1977.
653. Noback C, Tinker J: Hypothermia after cardiopulmonary bypass in man: Amelioration by nitroprusside-induced vasodilation during rewarming, *Anesthesiology* 53:277–280, 1980.
654. Clark JA, Bar-Yosef S, Anderson A, et al: Postoperative hyperthermia following off-pump versus on-pump coronary artery bypass surgery, *J Cardiothorac Vasc Anesth* 19:426–429, 2005.
655. Jani K, Carli F, Bidstrup BP, et al: Changes in body temperature following cardiopulmonary bypass procedures; the effects of active rewarming, *Life Support Syst* 4:269–272, 1986.
656. Ralley FE, Ramsay JG, Wynands JE, et al: Effect of heated humidified gases on temperature drop after cardiopulmonary bypass, *Anesth Analg* 63:1106–1110, 1984.
657. Nathan HJ, Polis T: The management of temperature during hypothermic cardiopulmonary bypass: II—Effect of prolonged hypothermia, *Can J Anaesth* 42:672–676, 1995.
658. Cook D, Orszulak T, Daly R, et al: Cerebral hyperthermia during cardiopulmonary bypass in adults, *J Thorac Cardiovasc Surg* 111:268–269, 1996.
659. Mohr R, Lavee J, Goor DA: Inaccuracy of radial artery pressure measurement after cardiac operations, *J Thorac Cardiovasc Surg* 94:286–290, 1987.
660. Gravlee GP, Wong AB, Adkins TG, et al: A comparison of radial, brachial, and aortic pressures after cardiopulmonary bypass, *J Cardiothorac Anesth* 3:20–26, 1989.
661. Oka Y, Inoue T, Hong Y, et al: Retained intracardiac air. Transesophageal echocardiography for definition of incidence and monitoring removal by improved techniques, *J Thorac Cardiovasc Surg* 91:329–338, 1986.
662. Persson M, Svenarud P, van der Linden J: What is the optimal device for carbon dioxide deairing of the cardiothoracic wound and how should it be positioned? *J Cardiothorac Vasc Anesth* 18:180–184, 2004.
663. Robicsek F, Duncan GD: Retrograde air embolization in coronary operations, *J Thorac Cardiovasc Surg* 94:110–114, 1987.
664. Clark R, Brillman J, Davis D, et al: Microemboli during coronary artery bypass grafting, *J Thorac Cardiovasc Surg* 109:249–258, 1995.
665. Lake CL, Sellers TD, Nolan SP, et al: Energy dose and other variables possibly affecting ventricular defibrillation during cardiac surgery, *Anesth Analg* 63:743–751, 1984.
666. Baraka A, Kawkabani N, Dabbous A, et al: Lidocaine for prevention of reperfusion ventricular fibrillation after release of aortic cross-clamping, *J Cardiothorac Vasc Anesth* 14:531–533, 2000.
667. Fletcher R, Veintemilla F: Changes in the arterial to end-tidal PCO2 differences during coronary artery bypass grafting, *Acta Anaesthesiol Scand* 33:656–659, 1989.
668. Crystal GJ, Ruiz JR, Rooney MW, et al: Regional hemodynamics and oxygen supply during isovolemic hemodilution in the absence and presence of high-grade beta-adrenergic blockade, *J Cardiothorac Anesth* 2:772–779, 1988.
669. Klineberg PL, Kam CA, Johnson DC, et al: Hematocrit and blood volume control during cardiopulmonary bypass with the use of hemofiltration, *Anesthesiology* 60:478–480, 1984.
670. Hindman BJ: Sodium bicarbonate in the treatment of subtypes of acute lactic acidosis: Physiologic considerations, *Anesthesiology* 72:1064–1076, 1990.
671. Kaplan JA, Guffin AV, Yin A: The effects of metabolic acidosis and alkalosis on the response to sympathomimetic drugs in dogs, *J Cardiothorac Anesth* 2:481–487, 1988.
672. Robertie PG, Butterworth JFt, Royster RL, et al: Normal parathyroid hormone responses to hypocalcemia during cardiopulmonary bypass, *Anesthesiology* 75:43–48, 1991.
673. Hosking MP: Should calcium be administered prior to separation from cardiopulmonary bypass? *Anesthesiology* 75:1121–1122, 1991.
674. Watson BG: Unilateral cold neck. A new sign of misplacement of the aortic cannula during cardiopulmonary bypass, *Anaesthesia* 38:659–661, 1983.
675. Dalal FY, Patel KD: Another sign of inadvertent carotid cannulation, *Anesthesiology* 55:487, 1981.
676. Chapin JW, Nance P, Yarbrough JW: Facial paleness, *Anesth Analg* 61:475, 1982.
677. Ross WT Jr, Lake CL, Wellons HA: Cardiopulmonary bypass complicated by inadvertent carotid cannulation, *Anesthesiology* 54:85–86, 1981.
678. Sudhaman DA: Accidental hyperperfusion of the left carotid artery during CPB, *J Cardiothorac Vasc Anesth* 5:100–101, 1991.
679. McLeskey CH, Cheney FW: A correctable complication of cardiopulmonary bypass, *Anesthesiology* 56:214–216, 1982.
680. Salerno TA, Lince DP, White DN, et al: Arch versus femoral artery perfusion during cardiopulmonary bypass, *J Thorac Cardiovasc Surg* 76:681–684, 1978.
681. Carey JS, Skow JR, Scott C: Retrograde aortic dissection during cardiopulmonary bypass: "Nonoperative" management, *Ann Thorac Surg* 24:44–48, 1977.
682. Murphy DA, Craver JM, Jones EL, et al: Recognition and management of ascending aortic dissection complicating cardiac surgical operations, *J Thorac Cardiovasc Surg* 85:247–256, 1983.
683. Troianos CA, Savino JS, Weiss RL: Transesophageal echocardiographic diagnosis of aortic dissection during cardiac surgery, *Anesthesiology* 75:149–153, 1991.
684. Michaels I, Sheehan J: EEG changes due to unsuspected aortic dissection during cardiopulmonary bypass, *Anesth Analg* 63:946–948, 1984.
685. Janelle GM, Mnookin S, Gravenstein N, et al: Unilateral cerebral oxygen desaturation during emergent repair of a DeBakey type 1 aortic dissection: Potential aversion of a major catastrophe, *Anesthesiology* 96:1263–1265, 2002.
686. Stoney WS, Alford WC Jr, Burrus GR, et al: Air embolism and other accidents using pump oxygenators, *Ann Thorac Surg* 29:336–340, 1980.
687. Mills NL, Ochsner JL: Massive air embolism during cardiopulmonary bypass. Causes, prevention, and management, *J Thorac Cardiovasc Surg* 80:708–717, 1980.
688. Tomatis L, Nemiroff M, Riahi M, et al: Massive arterial air embolism due to rupture of pulsatile assist device: Successful treatment in the hyperbaric chamber, *Ann Thorac Surg* 32:604–608, 1981.
689. Haykal HA, Wang AM: CT diagnosis of delayed cerebral air embolism following intraaortic balloon pump catheter insertion, *Comput Radiol* 10:307–309, 1986.
690. Fritz H, Hossmann KA: Arterial air embolism in the cat brain, *Stroke* 10:581–589, 1979.
691. Kort A, Kronzon I: Microbubble formation: In vitro and in vivo observation, *J Clin Ultrasound* 10:117–120, 1982.
692. Feinstein SB, Shah PM, Bing RJ, et al: Microbubble dynamics visualized in the intact capillary circulation, *J Am Coll Cardiol* 4:595–600, 1984.
693. Helps SC, Meyer-Witting M, Reilly PL, et al: Increasing doses of intracarotid air and cerebral blood flow in rabbits, *Stroke* 21:1340–1345, 1990.
694. Hekmatpanah J: Cerebral microvascular alterations in arterial air embolism, *Adv Neurol* 20:245–253, 1978.
695. Menkin M, Schwartzman RJ: Cerebral air embolism. Report of five cases and review of the literature, *Arch Neurol* 34:168–170, 1977.
696. Warren BA, Philp RB, Inwood MJ: The ultrastructural morphology of air embolism: Platelet adhesion to the interface and endothelial damage, *Br J Exp Pathol* 54:163–172, 1973.
697. Butler BD, Kurusz M: Gaseous microemboli: A review, *Perfusion* 5:81–99, 1990.
698. Armon C, Deschamps C, Adkinson C, et al: Hyperbaric treatment of cerebral air embolism sustained during an open-heart surgical procedure, *Mayo Clin Proc* 66:565–571, 1991.
699. Steward D, Williams WG, Freedom R: Hypothermia in conjunction with hyperbaric oxygenation in the treatment of massive air embolism during cardiopulmonary bypass, *Ann Thorac Surg* 24:591–593, 1977.
700. Bayindir O, Paker T, Akpinar B, et al: Case 6—1991. A 58-year-old man had a massive air embolism during cardiopulmonary bypass, *J Cardiothorac Vasc Anesth* 5:627–634, 1991.
701. Bojar RM, Najafi H, DeLaria GA, et al: Neurological complications of coronary revascularization, *Ann Thorac Surg* 36:427–432, 1983.

702. Voorhies RM, Fraser RA: Cerebral air embolism occurring at angiography and diagnosed by computerized tomography. Case report, *J Neurosurg* 60:177–178, 1984.
703. Furlow TW Jr: Experimental air embolism of the brain: An analysis of the technique in the rat, *Stroke* 13:847–852, 1982.
704. Peirce EC 2nd: Specific therapy for arterial air embolism, *Ann Thorac Surg* 29:300–303, 1980.
705. Layon AJ: Hyperbaric oxygen treatment for cerebral air embolism—where are the data? *Mayo Clin Proc* 66:641–646, 1991.
706. Stark J, Hough J: Air in the aorta: Treatment by reversed perfusion, *Ann Thorac Surg* 41:337–338, 1986.
707. Brown JW, Dierdorf SF, Moorthy SS, et al: Venoarterial cerebral perfusion for treatment of massive arterial air embolism, *Anesth Analg* 66:673–674, 1987.
708. Hendriks FF, Bogers AJ, Brutel de la Riviere A, et al: The effectiveness of venoarterial perfusion in treatment of arterial air embolism during cardiopulmonary bypass, *Ann Thorac Surg* 36:433–436, 1983.
709. Arnoni RT, Arnoni AS, Bonini RC, et al: Risk factors associated with cardiac surgery during pregnancy, *Ann Thorac Surg* 76:1605–1608, 2003.
710. Jacobs WM, Cooley D, Goen GP: Cardiac surgery with extracorporeal circulation during pregnancy; report of 3 cases, *Obstet Gynecol* 25:167–169, 1965.
711. Zitnik RS, Brandenburg RO, Sheldon R, et al: Pregnancy and open-heart surgery, *Circulation* 39:I257–I262, 1969.
712. Becker RM: Intracardiac surgery in pregnant women, *Ann Thorac Surg* 36:453–458, 1983.
713. Lapiedra OJ, Bernal JM, Ninot S, et al: Open heart surgery for thrombosis of a prosthetic mitral valve during pregnancy. Fetal hydrocephalus, *J Cardiovasc Surg (Torino)* 27:217–220, 1986.
714. Pomini F, Mercogliano D, Cavalletti C, et al: Cardiopulmonary bypass in pregnancy, *Ann Thorac Surg* 61:259–268, 1996.
715. Levinson G, Shnider SM: Anesthesia for surgery during pregnancy. In Shnider S, Levinson G, editors: *Anesthesia for Obstetrics*, Baltimore, 1987, Williams & Wilkins, p 188.
716. Bahary CM, Ninio A, Gorodesky IG, et al: Tococardiography in pregnancy during extracorporeal bypass for mitral valve replacement, *Isr J Med Sci* 16:395–397, 1980.
717. Mora CT, Grunewald KE: Reoperative aortic and mitral prosthetic valve replacement in the third trimester of pregnancy, *J Cardiothorac Anesth* 1:313–317, 1987.
718. Koh KS, Friesen RM, Livingstone RA, et al: Fetal monitoring during maternal cardiac surgery with cardiopulmonary bypass, *Can Med Assoc J* 112:1102–1104, 1975.
719. Werch A, Lambert HM, Cooley D, et al: Fetal monitoring and maternal open heart surgery, *South Med J* 70:1024, 1977.
720. Trimakas AP, Maxwell KD, Berkay S, et al: Fetal monitoring during cardiopulmonary bypass for removal of a left atrial myxoma during pregnancy, *Johns Hopkins Med J* 144:156–160, 1979.
721. Assali NS, Westin B: Effects of hypothermia on uterine circulation and on the fetus, *Proc Soc Exp Biol Med* 109:485–488, 1962.
722. Pardi G, Ferrari MM, Iorio F, et al: The effect of maternal hypothermic cardiopulmonary bypass on fetal lamb temperature, hemodynamics, oxygenation, and acid-base balance, *J Thorac Cardiovasc Surg* 127:1728–1734, 2004.
723. Jadhon ME, Main EK: Fetal bradycardia associated with maternal hypothermia, *Obstet Gynecol* 72:496–497, 1988.
724. Lamb MP, Ross K, Johnstone AM, et al: Fetal heart monitoring during open heart surgery. Two case reports, *Br J Obstet Gynaecol* 88:669–674, 1981.
725. Gibbon JH Jr, Miller BJ, Dobell AR, et al: The closure of interventricular septal defects in dogs during open cardiotomy with the maintenance of the cardiorespiratory functions by a pump-oxygenator, *J Thorac Surg* 28:235–240, 1954.
726. Splittgerber FH, Talbert JG, Sweezer WP, et al: Partial cardiopulmonary bypass for core rewarming in profound accidental hypothermia, *Am Surg* 52:407–412, 1986.
727. Danzl DF, Pozos RS: Accidental hypothermia, *N Engl J Med* 331:1756–1760, 1994.
728. Walpoth BH, Locher T, Leupi F, et al: Accidental deep hypothermia with cardiopulmonary arrest: Extracorporeal blood rewarming in 11 patients, *Eur J Cardiothorac Surg* 4:390–393, 1990.
729. Walpoth BH, Walpoth-Aslan BN, Mattle HP, et al: Outcome of survivors of accidental deep hypothermia and circulatory arrest treated with extracorporeal blood warming, *N Engl J Med* 337:1500–1505, 1997.
730. Weiss L, Grocott HP, Rosania RA, et al: Case 4—1998. Cardiopulmonary bypass and hypothermic circulatory arrest for basilar artery aneurysm clipping, *J Cardiothorac Vasc Anesth* 12:473–479, 1998.
731. Silverberg GD, Reitz BA, Ream AK: Hypothermia and cardiac arrest in the treatment of giant aneurysms of the cerebral circulation and hemangioblastoma of the medulla, *J Neurosurg* 55:337–346, 1981.
732. Baumgartner WA, Silverberg GD, Ream AK: Reappraisal of cardiopulmonary bypass with deep hypothermia and circulatory arrest for complex neurosurgical operations, *Surgery* 94:242–249, 1983.
733. Richards PG, Marath A, Edwards JM, et al: Management of difficult intracranial aneurysms by deep hypothermia and elective cardiac arrest using cardiopulmonary bypass, *Br J Neurosurg* 1:261–269, 1987.
734. Spetzler R, Hadley M, Rigamonti D, et al: Aneurysms of the basilar artery treated with circulatory arrest, hypothermia, and barbiturate cerebral protection, *J Neurosurg* 68:868–879, 1988.
735. Williams M, Rainer W: Cardiopulmonary bypass, profound hypothermia, and circulatory arrest for neurosurgery, *Ann Thorac Surg* 52:1069–1075, 1991.
736. Solomon R, Smith C, Raps E: Deep hypothermic circulatory arrest for the management of complex anterior and posterior circulation aneurysms, *Neurosurgery* 29:732–738, 1991.
737. Stevens JH, Burdon TA, Peters WS, et al: Port-access coronary artery bypass grafting: A proposed surgical method, *J Thorac Cardiovasc Surg* 111:567, 1996.
738. Schwartz DS, Ribakove GH, Grossi EA, et al: Single and multivessel port-access coronary artery bypass grafting with cardioplegic arrest: Technique and reproducibility, *J Thorac Cardiovasc Surg* 114:46, 1997.
739. Lebon JS, Couture P, Rochon G, et al: The endovascular coronary sinus catheter in minimally invasive mitral and tricuspid valve surgery, *J Cardiothorac Vasc Anesth* 24:746–751, 2010.
740. Miller G, Siwek L, Mokadam N, Bowdle A: Percutaneous coronary sinus catheterization for minimally invasive cardiac surgery, *J Cardiothorac Vasc Anesth* 24:743–745, 2010.
741. Siegel LC, St. Goar FG, Stevens JH, et al: Monitoring considerations for port-access cardiac surgery, *Circulation*, 96:562, 1997.
742. Mohr FW, Falk V, Diegeler A, et al: Minimally invasive port-access mitral valve surgery. *J Thorac Cardiovasc Surg*, 115:567, 1998.
743. Grossi E, Galloway A, LaPietra A, et al: Minimally invasive mitral valve surgery, *Ann Thorac Surg* 74:660–663, 2002.
744. Mishra Y, Khanna S, Wasir H, et al: Port access approach for cardiac surgical procudures, *Indian Heart J* 57:688–693, 2005.
745. Nifong L, Chitwood W, Pappas P, et al: Robotic mitral valve surgery: A USA multicenter trial, *J Thorac Cardiovasc Surg* 129:1395–1404, 2005.
746. Gilman S: Cerebral disorders after open-heart operations, *N Engl J Med* 272:489–498, 1965.
747. Javid H, Tufo HM, Najafi H, et al: Neurological abnormalities following open-heart surgery, *J Thorac Cardiovasc Surg* 58:502–509, 1969.
748. Tufo HM, Ostfeld AM, Shekelle R: Central nervous system dysfunction following open-heart surgery, *JAMA* 212:1333–1340, 1970.
749. Lee WII Jr, Brady MP, Rowe JM, et al: Effects of extracorporeal circulation upon behavior, personality, and brain function. II. Hemodynamic, metabolic, and psychometric correlations, *Ann Surg* 173:1013–1023, 1971.
750. Stockard JJ, Bickford RG, Schauble JF: Pressure-dependent cerebral ischemia during cardiopulmonary bypass, *Neurology* 23:521–529, 1973.
751. Stockard JJ, Bickford RG, Myers RR, et al: Hypotension-induced changes in cerebral function during cardiac surgery, *Stroke* 5:730–746, 1974.
752. Branthwaite MA: Prevention of neurological damage during open-heart surgery, *Thorax* 30:258–261, 1975.
753. Savageau JA, Stanton BA, Jenkins CD, et al: Neuropsychological dysfunction following elective cardiac operation. I. Early assessment, *J Thorac Cardiovasc Surg* 84:585–594, 1982.
754. Gardner TJ, Horneffer PJ, Manolio TA, et al: Stroke following coronary bypass grafting: A ten year study, *Ann Thorac Surg* 40:574–581, 1985.
755. Kolkka R, Hilberman M: Neurologic dysfunction following cardiac operation with low-flow, low-pressure cardiopulmonary bypass, *J Thorac Cardiovasc Surg* 79:432–437, 1980.
756. Ellis RJ, Wisniewski A, Potts R, et al: Reduction of flow rate and arterial pressure at moderate hypothermia does not result in cerebral dysfunction, *J Thorac Cardiovasc Surg* 79:173–180, 1980.
757. Sotaniemi KA, Juolasmaa A, Hokkanen ET: Neuropsychologic outcome after open-heart surgery, *Arch Neurol* 38:2–8, 1981.
758. Slogoff S, Girgis K, Keats A: Etiologic factors in neuropsychiatric complications associated with cardiopulmonary bypass, *Anesth Analg* 61:903–911, 1982.
759. Fish KJ, Helms KN, Sarnquist FH, et al: A prospective, randomized study of the effects of prostacyclin on neuropsychologic dysfunction after coronary artery operation, *J Thorac Cardiovasc Surg* 93:609–615, 1987.
760. Townes BD, Bashein G, Hornbein TF, et al: Neurobehavioral outcomes in cardiac operations. A prospective controlled study, *J Thorac Cardiovasc Surg* 98:774–782, 1989.
761. Bashein G, Townes BD, Nessly ML, et al: A randomized study of carbon dioxide management during hypothermic cardiopulmonary bypass, *Anesthesiology* 72:7–15, 1990.
762. Stanley TE, Smith LR, White WD: Effect of cerebral perfusion pressure during cardiopulmonary bypass on neuropsychiatric outcome following coronary artery bypass grafting, *Anesthesiology* 73:A93, 1990.
763. Kramer DC, Stanley TE, Sanderson I: *Failure to demonstrate relationship between mean arterial pressure during cardiopulmonary bypass and postoperative cognitive dysfunction*. Presented at the Society of Cardiovascular Anesthesiologists, Montreal, Quebec, Canada, 1994, p 211.
764. McKhann GM, Goldsborough MA, Borowicz LM Jr, et al: Predictors of stroke risk in coronary artery bypass patients, *Ann Thorac Surg* 63:516–521, 1997.
765. Wheeldon DR: Can cardiopulmonary bypass be a safe procedure? In Longmore DB, editor: *Towards Safer Cardiac Surgery*, Lancaster, London, 1981, MTP, pp 427–446.
766. Kurusz M, Conti VR, Arens JF, et al: Perfusion accident survey, *Proc Am Acad Cardiovasc Perfusion* 7:57–65, 1986.

29

Extracorporeal Devices and Related Technologies

ROBERT C. GROOM, MS, CCP | ALFRED H. STAMMERS, MSA, CCP, PBMT

KEY POINTS

1. Cardiopulmonary bypass (CPB) has been described as one of the boldest and most successful feats of the human mind.
2. CPB has progressed from experimental to a commonly practiced invasive high-risk procedure as evidenced by a recent randomized trial of off-pump versus on-pump surgery that showed significantly better composite outcomes with on-pump surgery.
3. Two predominant methods of blood propulsion are used: positive displacement roller pumps and constrained vortex or centrifugal-type pumps.
4. Modern heart-lung machines incorporate a number of microprocessor controls that serve to enhance safety and improve the pump-operator interface.
5. Modern heart-lung machines are equipped with a number of alarm systems and redundant backup systems to overcome primary system failures.
6. Blood gas exchange devices have improved over time in terms of reduced blood-surface interface, improved efficiency, and improved blood device-related inflammatory response.
7. Gaseous and particulate microemboli enter the CPB circuit from entrainment in the venous inflow to the circuit and also through the cardiotomy suction system. None of the currently available CPB systems removes all of the emboli.
8. Gaseous emboli may be reduced by correcting air entrainment around venous cannulation sites, avoiding the use of excessive vacuum-assisted venous drainage ($\geq$20 mm Hg), use of an arterial line filter, minimizing use of vent and cardiotomy suction flow, and use of a venous reservoir with a screen filter of 40 μm or less pore size.
9. Coating technology for CPB tubing and circuit components reduces inflammation and thrombus formation.
10. There is growing concern about plasticizers such as di(2-ethylhexyl) phthalate (DEHP) in polyvinyl chloride tubing. New plasticizers such as dioctyl adipate (DOA) that have less leaching are under investigation.
11. Cardioplegia delivery must be delivered accurately to prevent myocardial damage, and new pump delivery systems provide a better operator-interface for effective delivery.
12. Blood conservation is paramount, and an effective system involves proper equipment selection for the size of the patient, careful coagulation management, and the use of advanced techniques such as acute normovolemic hemodilution, retrograde and antegrade priming, ultrafiltration, and autotransfusion.
13. Despite more than 150 studies to evaluate the effectiveness of pulsatile flow during CPB, there is little evidence of the efficacy of pulsatile flow.
14. Numerous techniques to continuously perfuse the cerebral circulation have been developed, reducing the use of deep hypothermia circulatory arrest.
15. Communication and teamwork are of paramount importance during cardiac surgery.
16. The use of simulation and the study of human factor science are emerging areas of research that will help teams to become effective in responding to routine and nonroutine events that may occur during CPB.

The development of surgical interventions for the treatment of cardiovascular disease has resulted in enhancements in the quality of life for an indeterminate number of patients. One of the most influential areas that has aided in the evolution of this discipline has been the development of devices and techniques for extracorporeal circulation (ECC). Indeed, the sheer complexity of how blood behaves in an extravascular environment and the influence of synthetic materials on biologic processes have provided rich areas for research.

On May 6, 1953, Gibbon closed an atrial septal defect with the use of a heart-lung machine, the culmination of more than 20 years of his own research.[1,2] By the early 1950s, Gibbon had completed an extensive series of animal experiments with the heart-lung machine with survival rates of greater than 90%. However, his first attempt in human patients was not successful. On his second attempt, the patient's circulation was supported for less than 20 minutes while the atrial septal defect was repaired. According to Dr. Bernard J. Miller, "Near the termination of the operation, the machine suddenly shut down—reason being, clotting of the blood on the oxygenator took place, and the automatic arterial control sensed the sudden fall in the pool at the bottom and shut the entire machine down."[3,4] However, the patient survived and was discharged from the hospital in 9 days. Gibbon's five subsequent procedures at Jefferson Hospital were not successful and he abandoned the use of ECC. However, his one successful case served to inspire others, including John Kirklin at The Mayo Clinic, C. Walton Lillihei at the University of Minnesota, and Denis Melrose at Hammersmith Hospital in London, to continue the further development of ECC and cardiopulmonary bypass (CPB) in the laboratory and ultimately in the clinical arena. The accomplishments of these early pioneers in cardiac surgery have been described as being "the boldest and most successful feats of man's mind."[4]

Since the 1950s, CPB has undergone a dramatic metamorphosis from a lifesaving, yet life-threatening, technique to an event practiced nearly 1,000,000 times a year throughout the world. It is uncommon in today's medical environment to encounter such an invasive procedure, with such significant risk and inherent morbidity, being practiced as routine. The goal of all techniques of CPB always has been to design an integrated system that could provide nutritive solutions with appropriate hemodynamic driving force to maintain whole-body homeostasis, without causing inherent injury. A recent randomized clinical trial, the Randomized Off-pump or On BYpass (ROOBY) trial, involving 2203 elective or urgent coronary artery bypass grafting (CABG) patients randomized to either off- or on-pump surgery is a testament to the efficacy and safety of CPB as currently practiced. At 1 year, the on-pump group had significantly better composite outcomes (death, myocardial infarction, or repeat revascularization) than the off-pump group (9.9% vs. 7.4%; $P = 0.04$). The overall rate of graft patency was lower in the off-pump group than in the on-pump group as well (82.6% vs. 87.8%; $P < 0.01$).[5]

This chapter is a compilation of information on extracorporeal devices and techniques used in the conduct of cardiovascular perfusion. No attempt is made to chronicle or list the multitude of components and perfusion devices currently manufactured. Rather, examples have been chosen to best represent current technology. Similarly, the techniques described under perfusion practices were chosen because of the current clinical interest, with specific protocols taken from referenced sources.

MECHANICAL DEVICES

Blood Pumps

All extracorporeal flow occurs through processes that incorporate a transfer of energy from mechanical forces to a perfusate, and, ultimately, to the tissue. Methods of achieving this transfer of energy include gravitational and mechanical forces, or a combination of both. It is through the transfer of energy from an electrical power source to the motor of a pumping mechanism and on to the fluid (blood) that causes tissue perfusion.[4,6] Most extracorporeal pumps fall into one of the following categories: positive displacement (PD), centrifugal or constrained vortex (CP), passive filling, pneumatic and electrical pulsation, and axial flow (the latter pumps are used primarily as cardiac assist or replacement devices),[7-9] and are described in Chapter 27.

Positive Displacement Pumps

The PD pump operates by occluding tubing between a stationary raceway and rotating roller(s) or occluder(s) (Figure 29-1). The pumping mechanism is also referred to as the *pump head,* and the tubing that traverses the raceway is referred to as the *pump header.* PD pumps were first proposed for use in cardiovascular medicine in the 1930s by Gibbon.[2] In 1935, an adaptation to the PD pump was described that included tube bushings at the head of the raceway on both inlet and outlet locations to prevent tubing creepage around the roller head.[9] Melrose[10] later modified the pump to include a grooved raceway, which further reduced tubing shimmy. Both of these adaptations were important in reducing the mobility of tubing during the operation of the

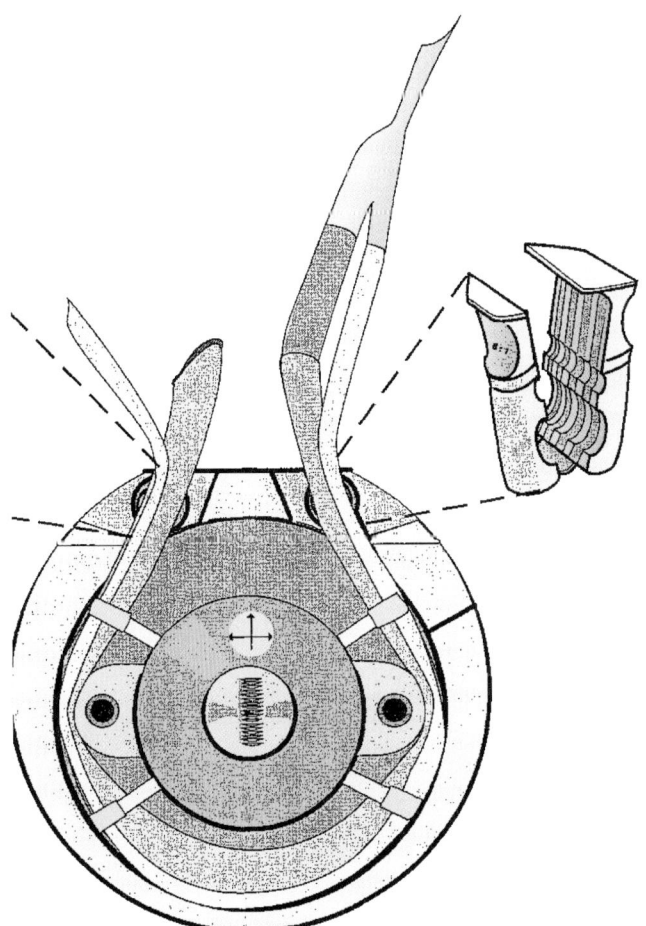

Figure 29-1 Stockert S-3 Twin Roller Pump diagram. A positive displacement pump with a stationary raceway and rotating twin roller pumps. *(Courtesy of The Sorin Group, Arvada CO.)*

pump, which decreased the potential for tubing rupture in the pump head. In a PD pump, fluid is displaced in a progressive fashion from suction to discharge, with the capacity of the displacement dependent both on the volume of the tubing occluded by the rollers and on the number of revolutions per minute (rpm) of the roller. All PD roller pumps (RPs) use the volume in the pump header, which is referred to as a *flow constant,* and is specific to each size of tubing referred to by the internal diameter of tubing, for calculating the flow of the pump. This is displayed on a digital readout and is referred to as the *output* (flow) of the pump. It is measured in liters per minute. Although many types of RPs have been used for CPB, the most common PD pump in use today is the twin-RP.

There are currently at least five manufacturers of PD pumps used in ECC, with each device consisting of minor variations of the twin-RP design (Box 29-1). A modern heart-lung machine consists of between four and five of these RPs positioned on a base console (Figures 29-2 and 29-3). Most machines are modular in design, permitting the rapid change-out of a defective unit in the case of single-pump failure. It is standard practice of perfusionists to rotate the pumps along the base console in different positions so that mechanical wear is distributed evenly while maintaining equitable time utilization. Each pump is independently controlled by a rheostat that functions to regulate the rpm of the rollers. Each pump is calibrated according to specific flow constants that are calculated from the internal diameter of tubing, as well as the tubing length, placed in the pump raceway. Periodically, PD pumps are calibrated by performing a timed collection of pumped fluid to verify that after proper calibration the pump delivers the volume indicated on

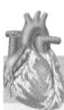

BOX 29-1. ROLLER PUMPS

Composed of twin rollers.
Deliver flow using positive displacement of the fluid in the tubing.
Blood flow is calculated using tubing stroke volume and pump revolutions per minute.
An underocclusive roller pump may result in retrograde flow in the patient and in the cardiopulmonary bypass circuit.
An overocclusive roller pump may increase hemolysis and produce spallation of the perfusion tubing.

the pump flow display. The internal diameters for ECC tubing ranges between 1/8 and 5/8 inch/min. For this reason, a single console can be used to perfuse a wide range of patients whose size may vary from a few kilograms to several hundred. This is accomplished simply by changing the raceway tubing and the shims that hold the tubing in place. It is important to note that the larger the internal diameter of the tubing, the lower the rpm necessary to achieve a desired pump flow. This is especially important because there is a positive correlation between

red blood cell (RBC) hemolysis and the rpm of the pump rotation. The magnitude of hemolysis is related to both the time and exposure of the blood to shear forces generated by the pump. A region of high pressure and shear force is created at the leading edge of the roller where the tubing is compressed, which is followed by a period of negative pressure as the tubing expands behind the roller. This momentary negative pressure under certain conditions may induce the cavitation of air dissolved in the solution. A further related concern is particulate emboli that may be generated by microfragmentation, so-called spallation, of the inner surface of the tubing where the roller contacts the tubing and where the fold at the edges of the tubing occurs.[11] Studies of tubing wear over time have shown that polyvinylchloride fragments generated from RPs are numerous, frequently less than 20 μm in diameter, and begin to occur during the first hour of use.[12] However, the majority of the hemolysis generated during a routine CPB procedure is not related to the occlusiveness of the arterial pump head but rather by the air-surface interface interaction occurring with the use of suction and "vent" lines components of the circuit.[13] An underocclusive arterial pump head will result in retrograde flow. This, in turn, will require increased rpm to ensure adequate forward flow, which increases hemolysis.[14] Overocclusive adjustment of the RP results in both hemolysis of RBCs and spallation (particulate fragmentation from the inner walls of

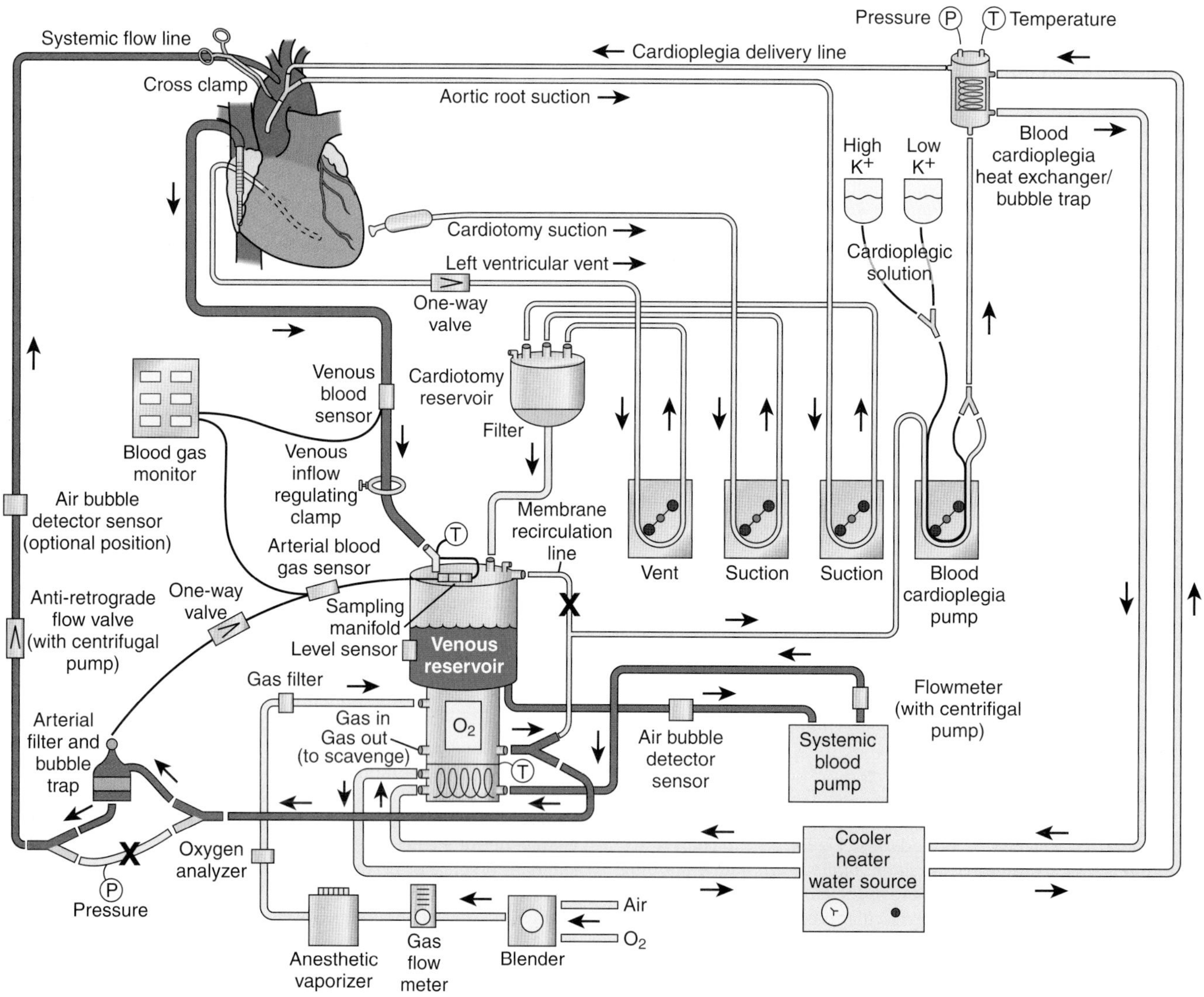

Figure 29-2 Schematic diagram of cardiopulmonary bypass circuit including four roller pumps (one vent pump, two suction pumps, and a cardioplegia deliver pump). A centrifugal blood pump for systemic blood propulsion is shown on the lower right. (From Hensley FA, Martin DE, Gravlee GP: A Practical Approach to Cardiac Anesthesia, 4th ed. Philadelphia, Lippincott Williams & Wilkins, 2008, Figure 18.1.)

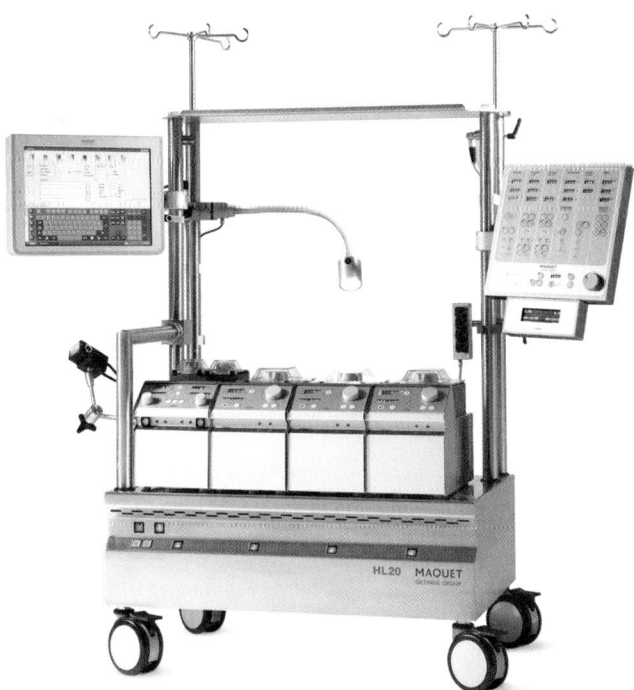

Figure 29-3 **HL20 Heart Lung Machine Console.** *(Courtesy of Maquet Cardiovascular, Wayne, NJ.)*

tubing) that continues with PD pumps.[15] Kurusz[11] identified the erosive and fatiguing action of the RP as a major source for generating tubing particles in CPB circuits.

The setting of occlusion in the pump head is extremely important and varies among the pumps used on the heart-lung machine console. The arterial pump head occlusion should be set by a water-drop method that incorporates a "30-and-1" rule for setting occlusion. In this method, the occlusion of the arterial pump is set by displacing a column of water (perfusate) 30 cm above the highest water level in the venous or cardiotomy reservoir (whichever is highest) and allowing the perfusate to drop 1 cm/min. The same drop rate can be obtained by setting the fluid height difference at 30 inches and the drop rate at 1 inch/min. Of note, if cardioplegic solution is to be delivered through a separate RP, and/or a left ventricular drainage line (left ventricular vent) placed in a roller head, occlusion for these pumps should be set at 100% (full occlusion) with no drop in fluid movement. This ensures that during the time when cardioplegic solution is not delivered, or the left ventricular vent is turned off, the risk for negative pressure in the ascending aorta or coronary sinus, created by a slowly falling column of fluid, does not create a siphon that causes cavitation or the entrainment of air into the infusion lines. Such aspirated air could be infused directly into the patient by restarting the pump. The heart is vented during CPB to facilitate the removal of ventricular blood that accumulates from noncoronary mediastinal collateral vessels, arteriovenous sinusoids, and thebesian veins, all of which drain directly into the left atrium (LA) or left ventricle. Other anatomic locations of venting the heart include the pulmonary artery and the ascending aorta, with the latter usually drained through an antegrade cardioplegia cannula. The remaining pumps usually are denoted as "suckers" and aspirate shed blood from the operative field. Although debated, it generally is thought that a slightly nonocclusive pump sucker leads to reductions in the amounts of RBC trauma and hemolysis. Additional uses for the peripheral PD pumps include ultrafiltration (UF) or dialysis, for topical myocardial cooling devices, or for removing air from collapsible venous reservoirs.

Centrifugal Pumps

The second type of extracorporeal pump is a resistance-dependent pump termed a *centrifugal* (CP), or *constrained vortex* pump.[16-18] The CP conducts fluid movement by the addition of kinetic energy to a fluid through the forced centrifugal rotation of an impeller or cone in a constrained housing (Box 29-2). The greatest force, highest energy, is found at a point most distal to the center axis of rotation (Figures. 29-4 to 29-6). CPs operate as pressure-sensitive pumps, with blood flow directly related to downstream resistance. Blood flow is, therefore, related to both the rpm of the cones or impellers and the total resistance. This represents an important safety feature in coupling blood flow with resistance. During unexpected increases in resistance, the total energy transfer from the CP to blood will not generate forces sufficient to cause arterial line separation. However, when downstream occlusion occurs, either through increases in afterload or through the placement of line clamps, the fluid in the pump head will be heated because of hydrodynamic processes in the magnetic coupling. This increase in temperature could result in increased blood trauma and coagulation defects.[18]

The acceptance of these devices in routine CPB has increased tremendously since first being introduced into clinical practice in 1969,[19] and it is the pump of choice during emergency bypass procedures. The CP also has been used as a ventricular assist device (VAD)

BOX 29-2. CENTRIFUGAL PUMPS

Operate on the constrained vortex principle.
Blood flow is inversely related to downstream resistance.
Flow rate is determined using an ultrasonic flow meter.
Increase in centrifugal pump revolutions per minute may result in heat generation and hemolysis.
If the centrifugal pump is stopped, the line must be clamped to prevent retrograde flow.

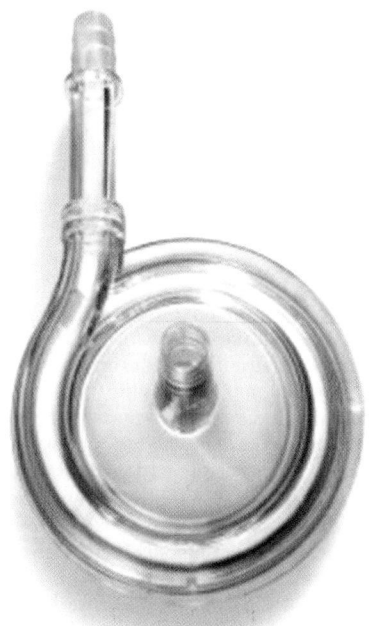

Figure 29-4 Rotaflow Centrifugal Pump disposable with low-friction one-point bearing (sapphire ball and PE calotte). *(Courtesy of Maquet Cardiovascular, Wayne, NJ.)*

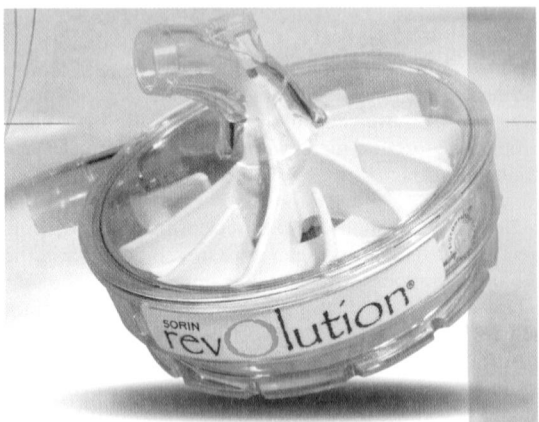

Figure 29-5   Revolution Centrifugal Pump Disposable. *(Courtesy of The Sorin Group Arvada, CO.)*

Laminar flow improves
blood and air handling capabilities

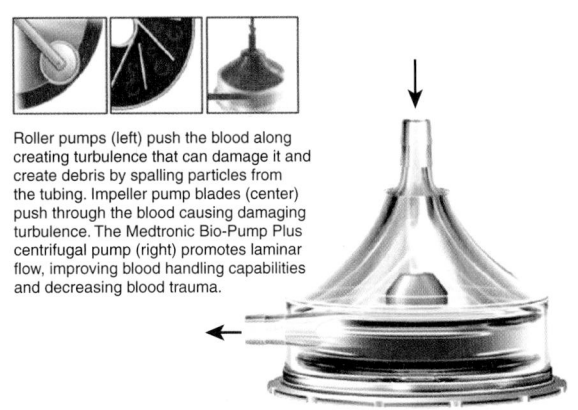

Roller pumps (left) push the blood along creating turbulence that can damage it and create debris by spalling particles from the tubing. Impeller pump blades (center) push through the blood causing damaging turbulence. The Medtronic Bio-Pump Plus centrifugal pump (right) promotes laminar flow, improving blood handling capabilities and decreasing blood trauma.

Figure 29-6   Medtronic Bio-Pump Plus Centrifugal Pump. The manufacturer states that the Bio-Pump laminar flow design is superior to roller pump and impeller pump designs with inherently more turbulent flow characteristics. *(Courtesy of Medtronic Cardiovascular, Eden Prarie, MN.)*

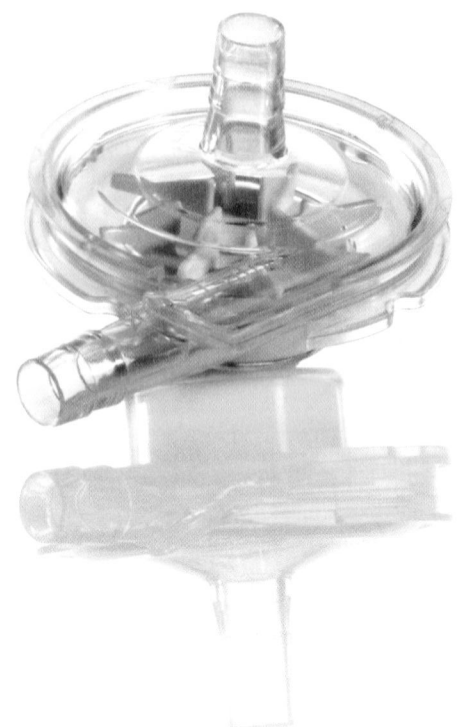

Figure 29-7   CentriMag Blood Pump. Thoratec CentriMag magnetically levitated bearingless blood pump. *(Reprinted with permission from Thoratec Corporation.)*

because of its inherent safety features and pressure sensitivity, as well as relatively low cost. Although these pumps have been used extensively off-label for VADs, none of the CPs has received U.S. Food and Drug Administration clearance for use for systemic circulatory support for more than 6 hours. CP pumps have been used extensively off-label as VADs or in extracorporeal membrane oxygenation (ECMO) circuits. The afterload and preload sensitivity of these pumps make them particularly amenable for use for ECMO in the treatment of reversible respiratory dysfunction and postcardiotomy dysfunction.[20] The Levitronix CentriMag Blood Pumping System (Levitronix, Waltham, MA) recently developed a pump with a novel magnetically levitated *bearingless motor* technology designed to minimize friction and heat generation in the blood path (Figure 29-7), which reduces stasis and minimizes blood trauma. The Centrimag is approved for use for up to 6 hours of support and is undergoing further investigation for prolonged use for patients with heart failure (HF). The Centrimag also recently received approval by the FDA for use as a right ventricular support device, for use up to 14 days to treat patients with right-heart failure—the first approval of this class of pump for use beyond 6 hours. In a recent in vitro study, Guan et al[21] compared mechanical performance characteristics of the Centrimag pump with a conventional CP, the Rotaflow Centrifugal Pump (Maquet, Wayne, NJ) and reported

better mechanical performance characteristics with the rotaflow pump in terms of higher shutoff flow rate, maximal flow, and propensity for retrograde flow.[21] These findings deserve further study given the magnitude of cost for the Centrimag pump system disposable components (Centrimag costs 20 to 30 times more than other CP disposable components).

When gross air is introduced into the CP, as in emptying of the venous reservoir, the pump head will deprime, stopping forward flow, which reduces the risk for gas embolization. However, when small quantities of air are aspirated into the pump head, these bubbles will coalesce and be passed into the outlet stream of fluid movement, and potentially into the patient. Although the CP has been described as exerting less trauma to the cellular elements of blood,[22] variability in individual pump hemolytic potential has been reported.[23,24] Tamari et al[25] have reported that the degree of hemolysis in CP is related to the hemodynamic conditions under which the pump is operated, with lower flows and higher pressure resulting in more hemolysis than similarly operated RPs. There have been reports of thrombus formation when these pumps are used with low anticoagulation or for prolonged periods.[26] Later designs possess fins and channels that prevent these areas of stasis. Improved designs have addressed issues of stasis, heat generation, and bearing wear. One contemporary design has minimal contact area for the cone and the outer housing and incorporates a series of magnets to suspend the moving rotor within the pump housing.[27] Additional advantages of CP over PD RPs include reduced mechanical trauma to extracorporeal tubing and the generation of high-volume output with moderate pressure development. A potential complication associated with nonocclusive-type pumps involves retrograde flow through the aortic cannula when the pressure in the central aorta exceeds that generated by the pump.[28] This may occur during times of power disruption or pump failure when there is an increased risk for drawing air into the arterial line via purse-string sutures placed to secure the arterial cannula (see Safety Mechanisms for Extracorporeal Flow section later in this chapter). Other uses of CPs include supported CPB in high-risk angioplasty patients, left-heart bypass (LHB) during repair of descending thoracic aortic aneurysms or dissections, and veno-venous bypass during hepatic transplantation. Use of CPs to assist venous return for minimally invasive cardiac surgery is described as kinetic-assisted venous return.[29,30]

Currently, six manufacturers produce CPs for extracorporeal use: Biomedicus (Biomedicus-Medtronics, Minneapolis, MN), Delphin (3M Health Care, Ann Arbor, MI), Revolution Pump (The Sorin Group, Arvanda, CO), Capiox-SP (Terumo Medical Corporation, Somerset, NJ), Rotoflow Maquet (Wayne, NJ), and the Centrimag Pump. The operational characteristics are similar among the various systems in which the internal smooth cones or vaned impellers are connected to a central magnet (isolated from contact with blood by encasement in a polycarbonate housing), which couples with the console, where electromagnetic forces are produced. The centrifugal console usually is placed in the arterial pump head position on the heart-lung machine, replacing the main drive. All of the consoles currently available include their own battery backup systems in the event of power failure and a manually operated motor in case of drive motor or console failure. The Revolution pump is equipped with an electronic tubing clamp that may be programmed to deploy automatically if low, zero, or retrograde flow is sensed; if the level sensor in the venous reservoir senses a low level; if a high arterial line pressure is sensed; or if the air detector on the arterial line senses air in the circuit (Figure 29-8). This is an especially important feature when using these machines to transfer patients on ventricular assistance or during the conduct of emergency bypass. Each manufacturer markets disposable software that must be purchased in conjunction with the pump.

A number of investigators have conducted in vitro studies comparing CPs and RPs in terms of blood handling during short-term and long-term use. Oku et al,[31] Jakob et al,[32] Englehardt et al,[33] and Hoerr et al[34] reported less hemolysis with the CP when tested in vitro. Kress et al[35] showed no difference between the two pump types in a rabbit ECMO model. Tamari et al[36] examined hemolysis under various flow and pressure conditions in an in vitro model using porcine blood and concluded that the hemolysis index was related to the duration of blood exposure to shear, the ratio of pump pressure difference between the inflow and outflow, and the flow rate of the pump. From this work they provided guidelines related to pump selection based on the pressure/flow ratio likely to occur in a given application. Rawn et al[37] compared an underocclusive RP with a CP and found a significantly higher index of hemolysis in the CP (3.38 to 14.65 vs. 29.58 g/100 L pumped). In a randomized trial, Salo et al[38] examined inflammatory response mediators in 16 CABG patients with CPB times of less than 2 hours. These mediators included interleukin-1 beta (IL-1β), IL-2, IL-6, phospholipase A_2, endotoxin, fibronectin, and serum C Group II phospholipase A_2. These researchers found no differences in the levels of these inflammatory markers immediately

post-CPB and at 24 hours after surgery. Other randomized clinical trials have been conducted to compare emboli generation, neurocognitive outcome, blood trauma, and patient charges. Wheeldon et al[39] conducted a randomized, controlled trial in 16 patients, in which the only difference in equipment and technique was the type of pump used, and found significantly fewer microemboli, less complement activation, and better preservation of platelet count. Parault and Conrad[40] reported a similar significant improvement in platelet preservation in a retrospective review of 785 cases and further reported that the differences were more profound in patients older than 70 years with CPB times of longer than 2 hours. Klein et al[41] conducted a randomized, prospective clinical study in 1000 adult cardiac patients comparing RPs with the Biomedicus CP (Medtronic, Eden Prairie, MN), using risk stratification methodology, and reported clinical benefits to the CP including blood loss, renal function, and neurologic outcomes, but no significant difference in mortality. Ashraf et al[42] examined S100 beta levels relative to pump type in a randomized, controlled trial that included 32 patients who had CABG and found no significant difference in S100 beta levels between the groups at 2 and 24 hours after bypass. Dickinson et al[43] did a retrospective review of 102 patients examining length of stay, total patient charges, reimbursement, mortality, and major complications but could not identify a single difference. A more recent randomized control trial by Scott et al[44] subjected 103 patients to a battery of 6 standardized tests and found a trend toward fewer abnormal tests in the CP group; however, it failed to reach statistical significance. DeBois et al[45] conducted a trial in 200 elective CABG surgery patients who were randomized to either an RP or CP and found similar patient characteristics including platelet counts, hematocrit, transfusion rate, and mortality; however, they observed differences favoring the CP with regard to weight gain, length of stay, and net hospital financial balance. Alamanni et al[46] evaluated the prevalence of major neurologic complications in 3,438 consecutive patients and found the occurrence of injury to be associated with age and a history of a previous neurologic event. The authors further reported that use of the CP provided a risk reduction for the considered events ranging from 23% to 84%. Babin-Ebell[47] et al conducted a randomized trial of CABG patients and found a significant reduction in tissue factor in the group supported with a CP; however, this did not translate into a measurable reduction in thrombin formation or other apparent clinical benefit. Baufreton et al[48] examined cytokine production (tumor necrosis factor-α, IL-6, IL-8) and circulating adhesion molecules (soluble endothelial-leukocyte adhesion molecule-1 and intercellular adhesion molecule-1) in a randomized, controlled trial of 29 CABG patients. They reported greater SC5b-9 and elastase levels in the CP group, suggesting more favorable performance from the RP with regard to complement and neutrophil activation.

Although nearly all of the randomized trials show significant benefit to systems designed with CPs, it is difficult to separate the improved performance conferred from other characteristics, such as lower prime volume, surface coating, more limited surface area, and reduced air-to-blood contact. Current research would suggest that CPs produce less blood damage; however, this improvement may be masked by blood trauma and inflammation related to contact activation of the blood related to cardiotomy suction, the introduction of gaseous and particulate emboli, and related factors. According to the recently published *Guidelines on Perioperative Blood Transfusion and Blood Conservation in Cardiac Surgery,* jointly endorsed by the Society of Thoracic Surgeons and the Society of Cardiovascular Anesthesiologists, "It is not unreasonable to select a CP rather than a RP but more so for safety reasons rather than blood conservation" (American Heart Association/American College of Cardiology Class IIb level of evidence B).[49] In 2000, approximately 50% of the cardiac centers in the United States routinely used CPs.[50]

Electromagnetic transducers and Doppler ultrasonic flowmeters are the two methods of measuring CP flow, as compared with the digital display of the PD pumps, which is the product of a flow constant and rpm. Electromagnetic flowmeters operate under Faraday's principle, that an electric current can be produced in a wire moved through

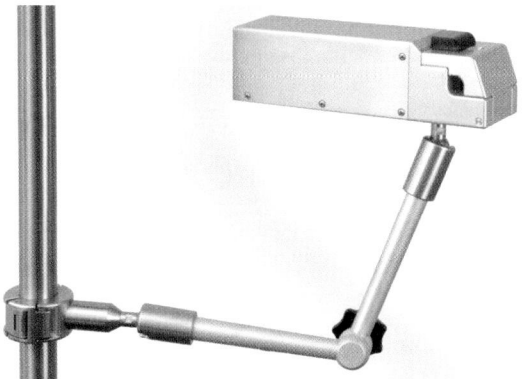

Figure 29-8 E-Clamp electronic line clamp works in conjunction with the Revolution centrifugal pump. The clamp is automatically deployed to clamp the line when retrograde flow is detected or if the air detector or level detector is triggered. *(Courtesy of The Sorin Group, Arvada, CO.)*

a magnetic field. Voltage is generated when an electrical conductor moves through a magnetic field if the movement is perpendicular to the magnetic lines between the poles of the magnet. Because blood is an electrical conductor, voltage is generated when it passes through a magnetic field and the voltage is directly proportional to the velocity of blood movement. The Doppler technology uses digital signal processing to transform the Doppler analog signal received from the flowmeter into digital format. Fast Fourier transformation then matches the incoming signal to recognizable patterns, which are displayed as flow rates.

Safety Mechanisms for Extracorporeal Flow

Some of the most recent advances in pump design have been a result of a heightened awareness of increasing safety associated with complex operating systems. The PD pumps are pressure independent, which means they will continue to pump regardless of downstream resistance. In a CPB circuit, the summation of resistances against which a pump must function includes the total tubing length, the oxygenator, the heat exchanger, the arterial line filter, the cannula, and the patient's systemic vascular resistance (SVR). Additional factors that influence SVR include the viscosity of the perfusate, related to the total formed element concentration, which primarily is dependent on the formed elements of blood and the temperature of the solution. According to Poiseuille's law, the greatest resistance to flow is created at the arterial cannula, where the change in the caliber of the tubing lumen declines the most. Perfusionists routinely monitor the summation of all resistances and record this value as the arterial line, or system, pressure. This always will be greater than the pressure measured at the distal end of the circuit terminating at the cannula tip because the pressure drop across each component in the series circuit will be subtracted from the summation of resistance (resistors) in the entire circuit. Bypass circuitry and components have been designed to incorporate minimal pressure drops; therefore, in routine adult perfusion, the resistance becomes a function of the patient's SVR and the pump flow rate. Establishing a normal value for arterial line resistance is difficult, although normal limits range between 100 and 350 mm Hg. Any acute change in resistance, such as unexpected clamping or kinking of the arterial line, results in an abrupt increase in arterial line pressure, which can lead to catastrophic line separation or circuit fracture anywhere on the high-pressure side of the circuit. A life-threatening event could occur on the initiation of CPB if the tip of the arterial cannula lodges against the wall of the aorta, undermining the intima of the vessel. Under these conditions, aortic dissection can occur as the vessel intima separates from the media, directing blood flow into a newly created false lumen. This dissection can extend throughout the entire length of the aorta. For this reason, perfusionists routinely check the line pressure after cannulation before the onset of CPB to ensure the presence of a pulsatile waveform, indicating proper cannula placement in the central lumen of the aorta. Either the absence of pulsatility or an extremely high line pressure (> 400 mm Hg when CPB is initiated) should immediately be investigated (see Chapter 28).

All heart-lung machines include a microprocessor-controlled safety interface with their pump consoles. These systems monitor and control pump function and serve as the primary mechanical safety control system for regulating extracorporeal flow. Pressure limits are set by the perfusionist and are determined by patient characteristics and the type of intervention performed. These units consist of early-warning alarms that alert the user to abrupt changes in pressure and will automatically turn off a pump when preset limits are exceeded. These safety devices have been used in both the main arterial pump and the cardioplegia pump; the latter become more important with the utilization of retrograde cardioplegia administration into the coronary sinus.[51,52] Currently, the incorporation of a safety monitor for negative pressure sensing, located on the inflow side of the arterial pump head and during pulsatile perfusion when intermittent occlusion is created, still is lacking.

Electrical failure in the operating room can be especially catastrophic in the conduct of ECC when the native heart and lungs are unable to

function. When such an event occurs during CPB, it is imperative that instantaneous actions be instituted to minimize the risk for whole-body hypoperfusion. The perfusionist should be mindful of the power limitations of the electrical outlet used in the cardiac operating room and also be aware of the location of the circuit breaker panel for the room and the specific number of the breaker in the panel for the outlet used for the heart-lung machine and other support equipment. Methods to ensure the safe conduct of CPB involve the incorporation of an emergency power source in the extracorporeal circuit that provides a secondary power source in the event of electrical interruption. Electrical failure during CPB was reported by 42.3% of respondents in a survey on perfusion accidents.[53] Although hospitals are equipped with emergency generators for such events, their availability may be limited to certain electrical circuits within the operating suite. Furthermore, these emergency power systems require a brief interruption in power before a generator or backup source of power is initiated. Most heart-lung machines are equipped with uninterrupted backup power, sometimes referred to as the "Uninterrupted Power Source" (UPS), whereby there is a seamless transfer from the wall power source to an internal battery within the pump should the wall power fail. Thus, with this system, there is no loss of flow from the pumps that could result in retrograde flow and entrainment of air or disruption of settings and timers. Cases of primary power failure with concurrent emergency backup failure also have been reported.[54] As a tertiary fallback measure, emergency hand cranks for CPB pumps are standard features in extracorporeal circuitry, which enable pump operation in the event of total power failure and when emergency systems fail to operate. However, care should be taken to ensure that the direction of blood flow is ascertained because hand cranking in the reverse direction of fluid flow could result in serious patient injury related to exsanguination and the entrainment of air around purse-string sutures at cannulation sites. The Retroguard valve (Quest Medical Incorporated, Allen, TX), a mechanical circuit component to prevent retrograde flow in the arterial outflow of the circuit, is available to prevent retrograde flow in the arterial line and possible entrainment of air into the circuit and into the patient's arterial circulation. It is composed of a simple duck-bill valve that adds minimal resistance to forward flow in the circuit and will close when downstream pressure is greater (Figure 29-9).

Although the chance of infusing massive air boluses to patients has been reduced dramatically since the early days of CPB,[53] this remains a serious potential event during surgery (Box 29-3). Cannulation of the heart with aortic and venting catheters has been identified as the primary cause for air embolization during ECC.[55] Methods of air-bubble detection have improved tremendously, and the sensitivity for detecting small amounts of air has increased in modern heart-lung machines.[56] Ultrasonic and capacitance air-detection systems, used for both level sensing and air detection in arterial and cardioplegia circuit lines, represent dramatic improvements over less sensitive (photoelectric) methods.[57] However, lacking in clinical practice are effective, reliable level-sensing devices that alert the perfusionist to rapid changes in venous reservoir levels, especially during utilization of collapsible venous reservoir systems. Both air-bubble detection and level-sensing devices should be safety techniques used as standards of care in all extracorporeal circuits.

EXTRACORPOREAL CIRCUITRY

Blood Gas Exchange Devices

The ECC of blood incorporating total heart-lung bypass could not be accomplished were it not for the development of devices that could replace the function of the lungs in pulmonary gas exchange. The technology of pumps to replace the mechanical action of the heart was developed well before their incorporation in ECC. Therefore, the limiting factor hindering the progression of CPB was the development of an artificial lung, or blood gas exchange device (BGED), commonly referred to as a *membrane oxygenator* (Box 29-4). The term *membrane* denotes the separation of blood and gas phases by a semipermeable of the most pressing were the design of high-capacity units for gas exchange with low rates of bioreactivity. The latter requirement, also termed *biocompatibility*, was imperative to reduce both RBC trauma and activation of the formed elements of blood.

In the 1940s, the first dialyzer membranes were made of cellulose acetate, and although intended for use in dialysis, they also had gas exchange characteristics.[1] In the 1950s, several membrane materials (including polyethylene and ethyl cellulose) were used in a flat sheet or plate configuration. At the same time, rotating disk oxygenators were introduced whereby gas exchange was accomplished by spreading venous blood in a thin film over a rotating disk, which was exposed to an oxygen-rich environment. In the 1960s, the first disposable membrane oxygenators were introduced and were made primarily of silicone rubber in either a plate or spiral wound design. Silicone offered the distinct advantage of separating both the blood and gas phases, facilitating gas exchange through a semipermeable barrier by diffusion. Teflon was introduced in the 1970s as a membrane material, together with microporous polypropylene, which first appeared in Travenol membrane devices. Today, the majority of commercially available oxygenators are made of polypropylene in either a pleated or folded configuration, or as capillary hollow fibers (Figure 29-10). In the United States, manufacturers develop oxygenators that meet federal regulatory guidelines for performance and biocompatibility. Those devices meeting these requirements are "cleared," approved for use for up to 6 hours of CPB, and represent the majority of oxygenators. Currently, there is only one oxygenator that utilizes silicone membranes that is approved for long-term support such as that occurring for ECMO. However, the "off-label" use of more durable, lower prime, hollow-fiber technology membrane oxygenators and newer polymethylpentane fiber oxygenators is widely reported in the literature.

Historically, oxygenators were divided into two broad classes based on the method of gas exchange: bubble and membrane systems. Bubble-type devices have been shown to denature plasma proteins, increase RBC fragility,[58] activate platelets,[59] and generate substantial gaseous microemboli (GME).[60-62] For these reasons, they are no longer used in most countries and are infrequently encountered in all but a few

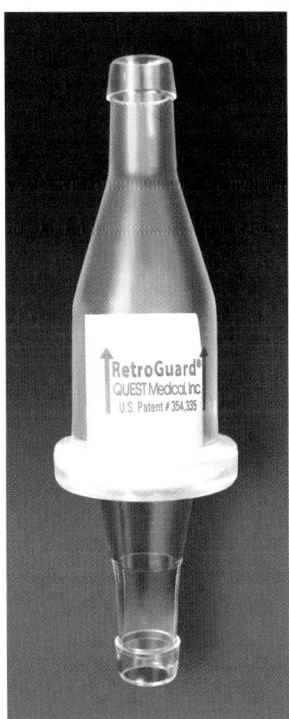

Figure 29-9 Quest Medical RetroGard Valve. Blood enters from the 3/8-inch inlet, passes through a duck-billed valve, and exits through a 3/8-inch outlet. This valve prevents retrograde flow. This valve may also be placed on an inlet port of the venous reservoir to prevent pressurization of the hard shell venous reservoir. *(Courtesy of Quest Medical, Allen, TX.)*

BOX 29-3. SAFETY MASSIVE AIR EMBOLISM

Cannulation of the heart with aortic and venting catheters is a primary source of massive air embolism (MAE).

Air detection and level-sensing safety devices should be used in the cardiopulmonary bypass circuit.

One-way vent valves, positive pressure release valves, and filter purge line valves may prevent MAE related to reversed vent tubing or a pressurized venous reservoir.

BOX 29-4. MEMBRANE OXYGENATORS

Hollow-fiber membrane oxygenators are commonly used for cardiopulmonary bypass.

An oxygen gas mixture flows through microporous polypropylene hollow fibers.

Blood flow is directed over the microporous hollow fibers.

Recently nonporous polymethyl pentene (PMP) hollow fibers have been developed.

PMP fibers provided a more durable surface for prolonged oxygenation such as extracorporeal membrane oxygenation.

PMP fibers do not permit the passage of volatile anesthetics such as isoflurane.

barrier, whereas *oxygenator* refers to the change in oxygen partial pressure that occurs by the arterialization of venous blood. However, "oxygenator" is a misrepresentation of the functional ability of these systems to perform ventilatory control of carbon dioxide. Numerous engineering challenges hindered the development of BGEDs, but two

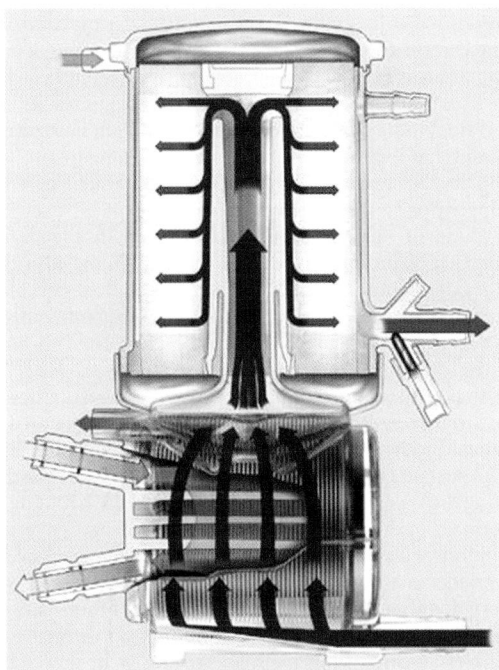

Figure 29-10 Diagram of blood flow path through the Medtronic Affinity Oxygenator. Heat exchange water path shown in blue. Gas flow path shown in green. Blood flow path shown in red. *(Courtesy of Medtronic Cardiovascular, Eden Prarie, MN.)*

remaining places throughout the world. Bubbler systems use a direct gas-blood interface, with gas exchange occurring by the dispersion of gas, either 100% oxygen or a mixture of oxygen and carbon dioxide (carbogen), through a column of desaturated blood. Bubble devices are made of two separate compartments: an oxygenating column and a defoaming chamber. The dispersion of gas in a bubbler occurs through a sparger plate, where a thin film of blood comes in direct contact with gas. This direct blood-gas interface results in the production of foam, where gas exchange occurs. Coalescence of the foam is achieved in the defoaming chamber both through the presence of surface tension–reducing substances and by filtration. Gas exchange is affected by several factors, including the quantity of gas and the size of bubbles produced in the gas sparger.[63] Small bubbles are extremely efficient at oxygen exchange but poor at carbon dioxide exchange, whereas large bubbles are poor in oxygen but good in carbon dioxide exchange.

Membrane oxygenators are made of three distinct compartments: gas, blood, and water (see Figure 29-10). The latter phase is also termed the *heat exchange compartment* and is used for temperature control. Gas and blood are partitioned into separate compartments with either a limited or absent gas-blood interface. Microporous membrane oxygenators initially have a blood-gas interface that becomes diminished only after the inner blood contact surface has been exposed to plasma; and a protein layer is deposited, acting as a diffusible barrier to gas exchange. The most common material in use today in membrane oxygenators is microporous polypropylene, which has excellent capacity for gas exchange and good biocompatibility. Membrane devices made of silicone materials transfer gas directly by diffusion across the semipermeable membrane and effectively never have a blood–gas interface.[64] Despite the improvements made to extracorporeal devices over the past several decades, once blood is exposed to synthetic surfaces, hematologic changes result. Initially, complement is activated mainly through alternative pathways, resulting in the liberation of toxic mediators such as C3a and C5a.[65,66] Both platelets and leukocytes that elicit a complex series of inflammatory and hemostatic reactions that ultimately increase the risk for postoperative complications are activated.[63]

Gas transfer in membrane oxygenators is a function of several factors that include surface area, the partial pressures of venous oxygen and carbon dioxide, blood flow, ventilation flow (called *sweep rate*), and gas flow composition. Membrane devices independently control arterial oxygen and carbon dioxide tensions (Pao_2 and $Paco_2$). Pao_2 is a function of the Fio_2, whereas $Paco_2$ is determined by the sweep rate of the ventilating gas. This independent control of ventilating gas results in arterial blood gas values more closely resembling normal physiologic blood gas status. However, it is common for perfusionists to maintain Pao_2 levels in the 150- to 250-mm Hg range during CPB because of the limited reserve capacity of membrane oxygenators.

A multitude of factors must be considered in the design of a membrane BGED, including total surface area, blood film thickness, diffusion residence time, gas diffusion rate, blood flow rate, blood flow geometrics, and gas flow characteristics. The most influential factors that affect blood trauma in an oxygenator are related to how blood traverses the device and are termed *shear stress* and *stasis*.[67] Design characteristics that minimize these effects by optimizing flow pattern geometry through extracorporeal devices have been generated through mathematical models termed *computational fluid dynamics*.[68] Two of the most important considerations in designing a membrane device are determining the type of membrane material and the handling of water vapor produced in the gas phase of the device. This water vapor would be synonymous with pulmonary exudate and, when excessive, mimics pulmonary edema associated with permeability changes of the alveolar capillary membrane. Another important membrane feature is how blood flows through the membrane. As fluid moves through a conduit, laminae are established, with the highest velocity of flow achieved in the center of the tube. At the same time, the outermost layers, nearest the walls of the conduit, effectively have no velocity because of the drag coefficient of the inside surface. This occurs in both the gas phase and the blood phase of membrane oxygenators. The laminar effect can be

disrupted by several techniques that produce a "secondary flow," facilitating increased gas exchange.[69] In hollow-fiber membrane oxygenators, incorporating blood flow outside of the fibers, mixing is achieved by winding of the fibers, creating a crossing pattern, increasing blood exposure to the membrane surface. Laminar flow is reduced in hollow-fiber oxygenators with blood flow through the fibers by the expansion and contraction of the capillaries via the movement of blood through them, gently disrupting the boundary layers.

Estimating the total surface area of material necessary for gas exchange is a function of the predicted oxygen demands of the patient and is used as a primary determinant for selecting membrane size. As the surface area of an oxygenator increases, the volume of solution necessary to prime the system increases. Microporous polypropylene hollow-fiber membrane devices come in two classifications: those with blood flow through the fiber and those with blood flow around the fiber. Systems that use the latter design require a lower membrane surface area for gas exchange and hence result in lower prime volumes. Microporous polypropylene membranes have the distinct advantage of a greater gas transfer rate per surface area of membrane than that of silicone membranes.

The oxygenator represents the largest source of nonendothelialized surface area in the extracorporeal circuit, ranging in size between 0.5 and $2.5 M^2$. As a consequence, it is imperative that the device is meticulously primed to remove all residual air before establishing CPB. Oxygenators have been shown to possess different abilities to remove gaseous emboli that vary according to the physical CPB conditions including temperature and pressure decline.[70–73] In an effort to reduce surface exposure and prime volume, several membrane oxygenators are now manufactured that either possess integrated arterial line filters (FX Oxygenator Line; Terumo Cardiovascular, Ann Arbor, MI; Figure 29-11) or systems in which the arterial line filter is sequenced in the oxygenator (Synthesis; Sorin Biomedical, Arvada, CO). Some studies suggest that these devices may result in a reduction in gaseous microemboli.[74,75]

Numerous studies have identified the occurrence of GME during cardiac surgery with CPB.[76] Weitkemper et al[77] have shown that currently used microporous membrane oxygenators have widely variable characteristics related to how they handle gas. Furthermore, the design characteristics in some cases cause partial removal of GME,

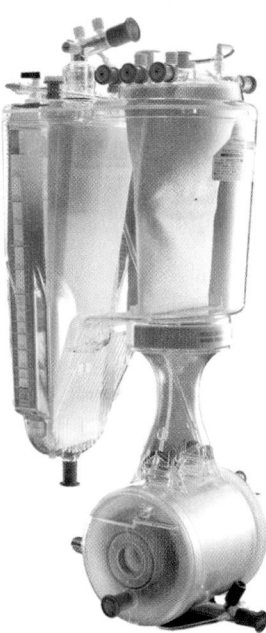

Figure 29-11 Hard-shell venous reservoir with integral cardiotomy and membrane oxygenator (Terumo RX15). *(Courtesy of Terumo Cardiovascular, Ann Arbor, MI)*

as well as a change in size and numbers of microbubbles. Dickinson et al[78] conducted an in vitro analysis that showed significant air-handling differences between the oxygenators from four different manufacturers. They demonstrated how a sonar-based system, the embolus Detection and Classification System (EDAC; Lunar Technology, Blacksburg, VA), could be used to evaluate perfusion systems with regard to their ability to handle gas entrained in the circuit.

A new nonporous membrane surface composed of poly-(4-methyl-1-pentene) (PMP) fibers has shown improved diffusion compared with the conventional polypropylene (PPL) hollow fibers. PPL affords improved durability and biocompatibility when used for long-term support[79,80] and for routine CPB.[81] Although oxygen and carbon dioxide gas exchange are comparable between polypropylene hollow fibers and the PMP nonporous fibers, it is important to note that the transfer of volatile anesthetic agents is not the same. Wiesenack et al[82] demonstrated that the PMP fibers allow only minimal transfer of isoflurane compared with the currently used PPL microporous hollow-fiber oxygenators. During long-term support, it is not uncommon for PMP oxygenators to develop breaches in the surface that lead to plasma leaks after 40 to 90 hours of use, whereas the PPL fibers tend to be more robust and are not prone to plasma leaks, and continue to transfer oxygen and carbon dioxide for many days.

Venous and Cardiotomy Reservoirs

There are two general categories for venous reservoirs: open and closed systems (Box 29-5). Open systems have a hard polycarbonate venous reservoir and usually incorporate a cardiotomy reservoir and defoaming compartment (see Figure 29-11). Closed systems are collapsible polyvinylchloride bags that have a minimal surface area and often a thin single-layer screen filter, and they require a separate external cardiotomy reservoir for cardiotomy suction (Figure 29-12). Filters and defoaming compartments in the venous reservoir and air-trapping ports located at the highest level of the blood flow path within the oxygenator are areas designed to allow passive removal of air. Studies that have examined the air-handling capabilities of oxygenators have shown that all of the currently available oxygenators do not sufficiently remove GME when challenged with air in the inflow.[77,78] The use of an open system offers several distinct advantages. Unlike collapsible reservoirs, it is not necessary to actively aspirate air, which may be entrained in the venous line during CPB. The large buoyant air migrates to the top of the reservoir and escapes through strategically placed vents on the reservoir cover. An additional benefit of the use of "open" hard-shell reservoir systems incorporates the capability of vacuum-assisted venous drainage, although alternative methods have been imple-

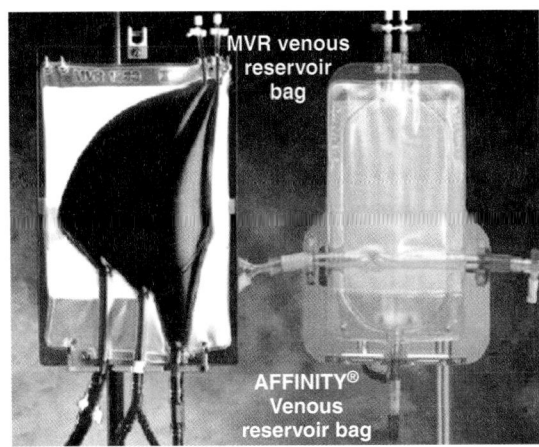

Figure 29-12 **Example of a closed system.** Oxygenator with a collapsable polyvinyl chloride venous reservoir. (*Courtesy of Medtronic Cardiovascular, Minneapolis, MN.*)

mented augmenting venous drainage to closed "bag" systems using CPs or creative vacuum applications applied to the venous line to enhance natural gravity drainage. Furthermore, a number of studies have reported a greater incidence of GME caused by air entrained in the venous line and furthermore that vacuum-assisted venous drainage further increases GME counts.[81,83-87] Wilcox has raised concern that vacuum-assisted venous drainage has been used clinically without any significant redesign of the components of the CPB circuit to improve the gas handling performance in negative pressure conditions.[86] The prime volume may be reduced slightly because the integration of the venous reservoir with the cardiotomy eliminates connecting circuitry and may permit a smaller bore venous line with use of vacuum-assisted venous drainage. With open systems, the circulating blood is exposed to a larger and more complex surface that contains defoaming sponges and antifoam agents.

Air can traverse the oxygenator into the arterial outflow of the CPB circuit and into the patient's arterial circulation, including the cerebral circulation, producing contact activation of the vascular endothelium or obstruction at the microcapillary level. Thousands of GMEs can be introduced into the patient's arterial circulation with these circuits if air becomes continuously entrained into the venous inflow, a condition that could not be tolerated with a collapsible reservoir. Recently, several randomized clinical trials have found superior clinical outcomes with a system equipped with a closed reservoir and a centrifugal arterial pump.[88,89] Schonberger et al[90] prospectively studied differences in inflammatory and coagulation activation of blood in CABG patients treated with open and closed reservoir systems. Levels of complement 3a, thromboxane B_2, fibrin degradation products, and elastase were significantly greater in open reservoir patients. Furthermore, the largest ($P < 0.001$) amount of shed blood loss, greatest ($P < 0.05$) need for colloid-crystalloid infusion, and largest (not significant) need for donor blood (0.8 ± 0.4 vs. 0.2 ± 0.2 units of packed cells) were observed in the patient supported with open reservoir systems.

Aldea et al[91] conducted a randomized, controlled trial to evaluate the effects of cardiotomy suction in CABG patients. Use of cardiotomy suction resulted in significant increases in thrombin, neutrophil, and platelet activation, as well as the release of neuron-specific enolase, after CPB. The authors suggested that limiting increases in these markers would be best accomplished by eliminating cardiotomy suction and routinely using heparin-bonded circuits whenever possible.

Miniaturized Cardiopulmonary Bypass

The principal drawbacks to the conventional CPB circuit include activation of the systemic inflammatory response, aberration in coagulation function, CPB-related gaseous embolism, and excessive hemodilution

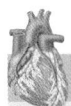

BOX 29-5. VENOUS RESERVOIRS

Open Systems
Open systems have polycarbonate hard-shell reservoirs and are usually equipped with an integral cardiotomy reservoir.
With open systems, venous return may be improved by applying regulated suction to the reservoir (vacuum-assisted venous drainage).
With open systems, buoyant air bubbles escape to the atmosphere at the top of the reservoir.

Closed Systems
Closed systems consist of have collapsable polyvinylchloride bags.
Closed systems require a separate cardiotomy reservoir.
Buoyant air from the venous line accumulates in the bag and must be actively aspirated.
Closed systems have a reduced contact surface of the blood with air or plastic.
A separate centrifugal pump may be used to increase venous return (kinetic-assisted venous drainage).

requiring blood transfusions. A principal design approach to overcome some of these problems has been the introduction of "miniaturized CPB circuits" that reduce the blood–foreign surface contact, blood-air interface, and hemodilution (Figures 29-13 to 29-15). The currently available "mini" systems consist of either an adaptation of standard CPB components or the introduction of new devices by manufacturers that have a striking resemblance to existing devices.[92–126] The manufacturers' "mini" systems all use a single CP to provide kinetic venous drainage and arterial blood propulsion. All have eliminated or isolated the venous reservoir to reduce blood foreign surface contact, and all eliminated the introduction of activated blood from a cardiotomy suction system. Field shed blood is recaptured and washed by an autotransfuser before reintroduction to the "mini" systems. Many of the systems have incorporated multisite bubble detection and innovative air removal systems to automatically remove and isolate micro and macro air entrained in the CPB circuit.

These systems lack several of the characteristics of the old standard CPB systems that made CPB simple. For example, the entrainment of air into the old systems was of little operational consequence because air could escape to the top of open reservoir systems or be aspirated by a vacuum or an RP from closed reservoir systems. Furthermore, shed blood at the surgical field could be readily collected and reintroduced into the circulation with conventional systems using the cardiotomy suction system without the use of an autotransfuser. In other words, variable venous return or excessive suction return can be easily accommodated with regular CPB systems, with minimal or no addition to the basic circuit as opposed to the "mini" systems currently on the market.

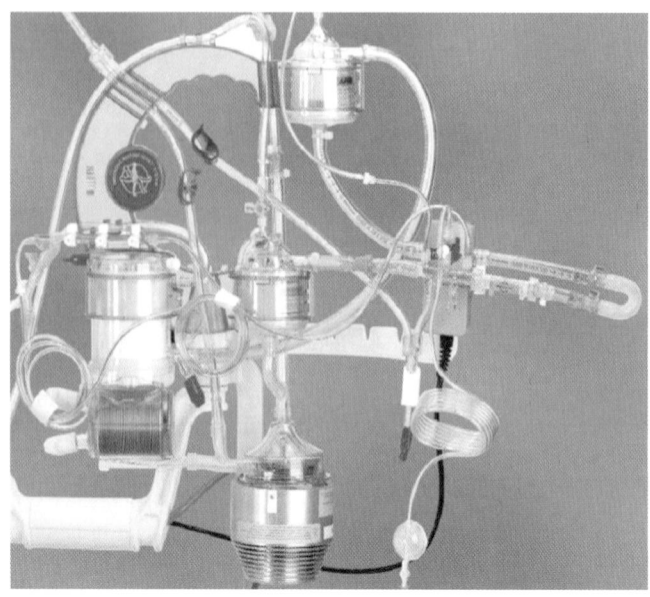

Figure 29-13 **Medtronic resting heart closed "mini-bypass" system.** Includes a centrifugal pump (that provides both kinetic-assisted drainage and propulsion of blood to the patient), venous air detection and evacuation system, a membrane oxygenator, and arterial line filter. *(Courtesy of Medtronic Cardiopulmonary, Minneapolis, MN.)*

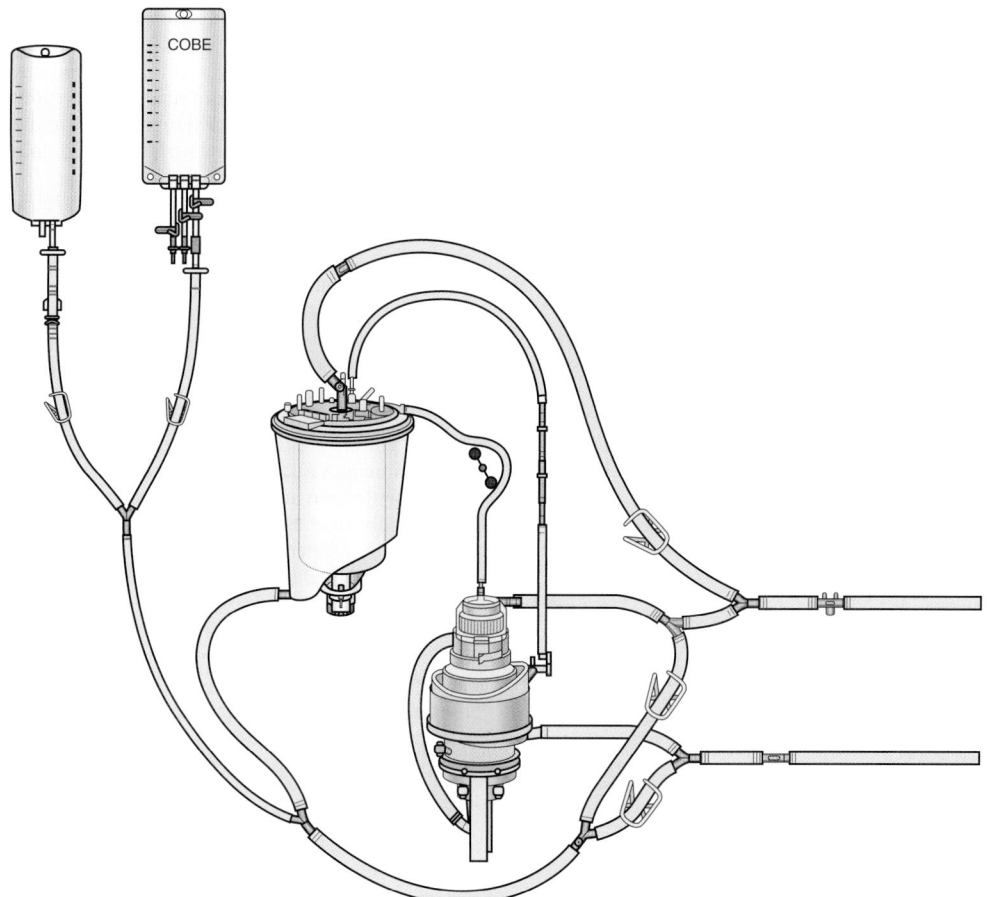

Figure 29-14 **Sorin Group Synthesis mini-bypass system.** The oxygenator has an integral air detection and evacuation system and a single integral revolution centrifugal pump (providing both kinetic-assisted venous drainage and arterial blood propulsion). An integrated arterial line filter surrounds the oxygenator fiber bundle. A separate cardiotomy reservoir is incorporated into the circuit. The system may be converted to an open system by repositioning clamps and redirecting blood flow to the reservoir. *(Courtesy of The Sorin Group, Arvada, CO.)*

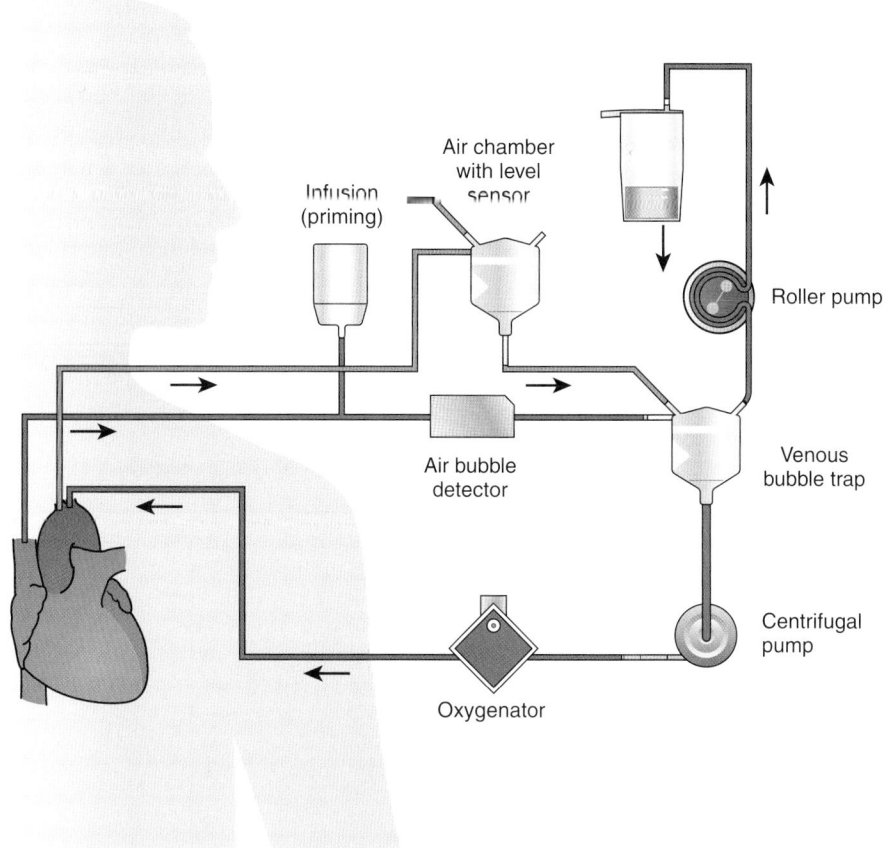

Figure 29-15 Maquet Minimal ExtraCorporeal Circulation (MECC). The system includes venous air bubble detection and venous bubble trap, a single integral pump (providing both kinetic-assisted venous drainage and arterial blood propulsion), and quadrox oxygenator. *(Courtesy of Maquet Cardiovascular, Wayne, NJ.)*

With most of the "mini" systems, minor changes in the circuit or complete major reconfiguration of the "mini" systems may be necessary if excessive bleeding occurs at the surgical field (addition of a venous reservoir, addition of a cardiotomy reservoir, and transfer of a massive amount of blood from the autotransfuser collection reservoir back to the mini system). "Mini" systems do not facilitate emptying of the cardiac chambers, as well as conventional systems. With conventional CPB systems, the cardiac chambers can be passively emptied into a capacitance reservoir where, in the usual configuration, the capacity of the venous system, in the presence of a mini system, is quite fixed. In mini systems, the capacitance reservoir is the patient's venous bed. To empty the heart, blood must be actively diverted to a separate reservoir or to the patient's capacitance reservoir with manipulation of the venous capacitance. For example, if volume is required to maintain safe flows, the venous bed must be increased using vasoactive drugs or elevation of the inferior limbs. If too much volume obscures the surgical field, a venous vasodilation drug may be used to decrease the venous volume traveling through the heart, while attempting to increase the systemic flows. Safe use of these systems requires good communication among the surgeon, anesthesiologist, and the perfusion team, together with careful monitoring. These major differences have caused a reluctance to change to these new systems by some centers.

A recent meta-analysis of randomized, controlled trials conducted by Zangrillo[127] et al sought to determine whether the use of miniaturized CPB translates into decreased morbidity including blood transfusion, neurologic events, and blood loss in patients having cardiac surgery. Sixteen trials met inclusion criteria, 1619 patients (803 to miniaturized CPB and 816 undergoing standard cardiac surgery). Miniaturized CPB proved to be beneficial in terms of decreased transfusion rate and decreased cardiac and neurologic injury. These finding are summarized in Figure 29-16. Current use of such systems is limited. Further studies are necessary to substantiate the benefit of such systems and will likely increase the adoption of this new technology.

Heat Exchangers

Patients who are exposed to ECC will become hypothermic in the absence of an external source of heat to regulate body temperature. Most CPB systems use some form of heat exchanger in the circuit to warm and/or cool the patient's blood. The majority of oxygenators contain integral heat exchangers that blood passes through before undergoing gas exchange (see Figure 29-10). Heat exchangers may be absent from circuits used for ventricular assist or certain types of LHB. However, in either of these scenarios, external warming blankets and ambient room temperature are controlled to restrict declines in patient temperature. Heat exchangers can be made from a variety of materials, although the most often used are aluminum (anodized or silicone-coated anodized), stainless steel, and polypropylene. Stainless steel is the most durable and chemically inert of all commercially used heat exchangers.

Some of the basic performance features that all heat exchangers for extracorporeal blood should possess include a high degree of chemical inertness, high resistance to corrosion, smooth surfaces, and a low-energy surface where RBC and plasmatic residues do not adhere. The ideal heat exchanger must possess the following characteristics: low resistance to blood flow, freedom from defects in material that could facilitate the mixture of blood and water, low priming volume, and disposability. The effectiveness of a heat exchanger is dependent on several factors including total surface area, thickness of the conductor walls, thermal conductivity, and the residence time of blood through the device. As fluid flow through a heat exchanger is increased, the performance characteristics decline, primarily as a function of decreased residence time in the device.

Heat exchanger basic design consists of two separate phases, with water passing on one side and blood, or perfusate, on the other. The direction of blood flow is routinely countercurrent to the flow of water, optimizing heat transfer. The temperature of the water entering the heat exchanger is controlled by either an external cooler/heater device or a wall source, with a temperature range from 4° C to 42° C.

The majority of heat transfer occurs by the process of conduction, in which thermal energy is passed from water to blood.

Heat exchangers can be placed in the circuit in a variety of locations, although the most common location is on the proximal side of the oxygenator, often termed an *integral heat exchanger*. During ECMO a separate heat exchanger is placed distal to the oxygenator for better control of the patient's temperature at normothermia. An alternative to either location uses simultaneous heat and gas exchange. It is hypothesized that with proximal, or venous-side, heat exchange, there is less chance of "outgassing of solution" caused by rapid rewarming of blood after hypothermic CPB, which could generate GME. Of similar concern is

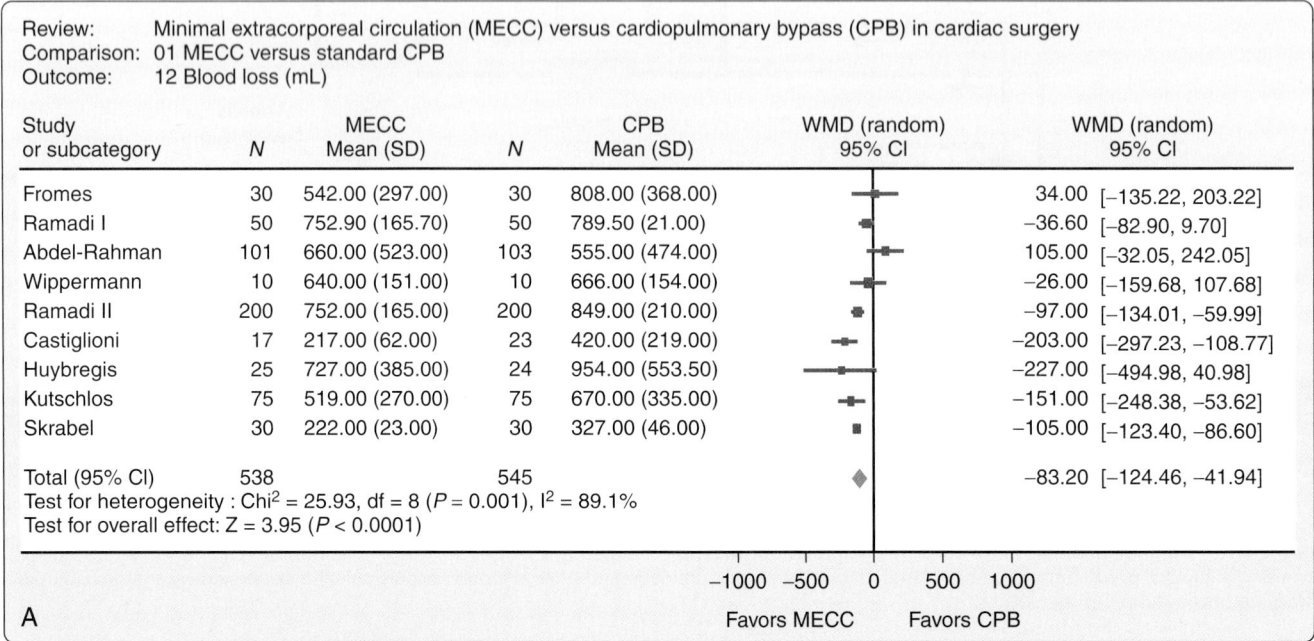

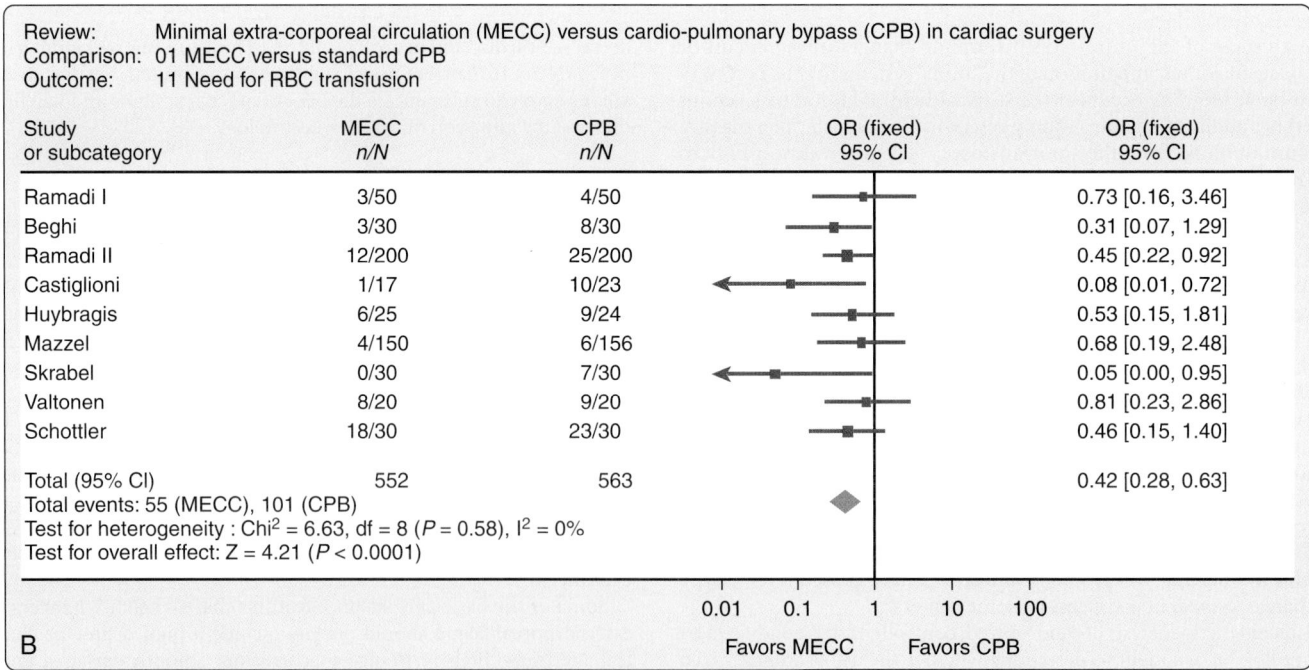

Figure 29-16 A–C, Forest plot for the risk for neurologic events comparing miniaturized cardiopulmonary bypass versus control from nine randomized, controlled trials. CI, confidence interval; df degrees of freedom; OR, odds ratio pooled estimates of neurologic events. (*From Zangrillo A, Garozzo AF, Biondi-Zoccai G, et al: Miniaturized cardiopulmonary bypass improves short-term outcome in cardiac surgery: A meta-analysis of randomized controlled studies. J Thorac Cardiovasc Surg 139:1162–1169, 2010.*)

(Continued)

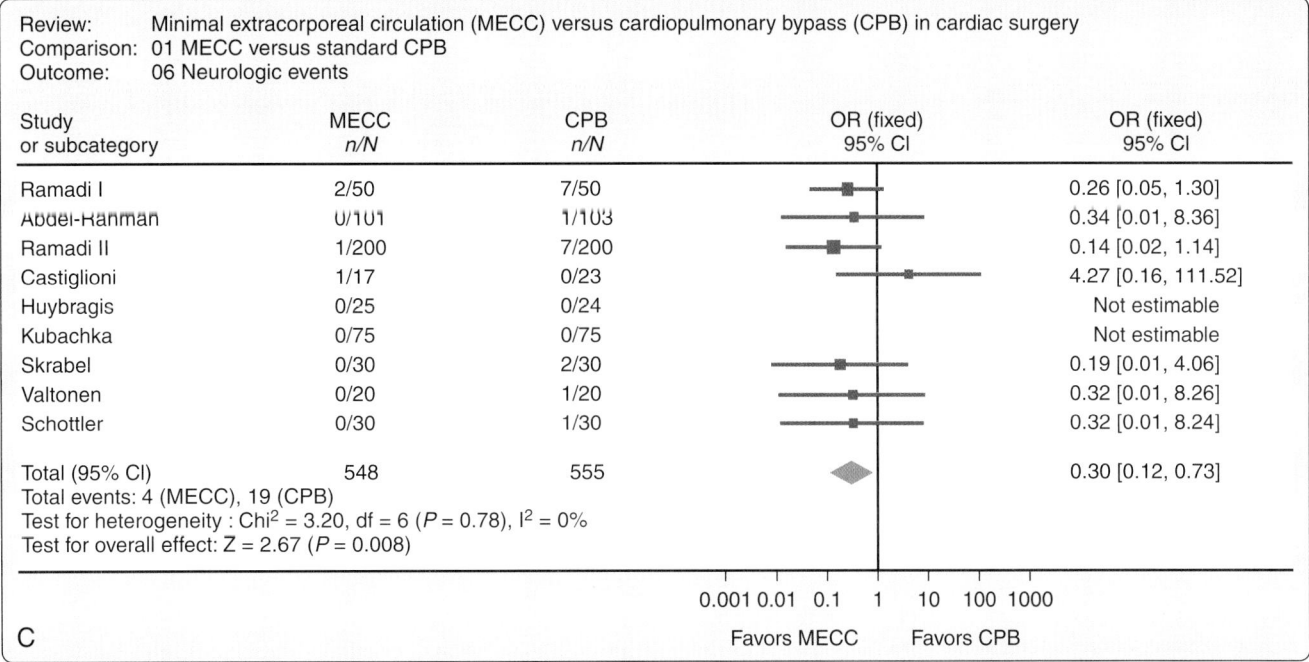

Review: Minimal extracorporeal circulation (MECC) versus cardiopulmonary bypass (CPB) in cardiac surgery
Comparison: 01 MECC versus standard CPB
Outcome: 06 Neurologic events

Study or subcategory	MECC n/N	CPB n/N	OR (fixed) 95% CI	OR (fixed) 95% CI
Ramadi I	2/50	7/50		0.26 [0.05, 1.30]
Abdel-Rahman	0/101	1/103		0.34 [0.01, 8.36]
Ramadi II	1/200	7/200		0.14 [0.02, 1.14]
Castiglioni	1/17	0/23		4.27 [0.16, 111.52]
Huybragis	0/25	0/24		Not estimable
Kubachka	0/75	0/75		Not estimable
Skrabel	0/30	2/30		0.19 [0.01, 4.06]
Valtonen	0/20	1/20		0.32 [0.01, 8.26]
Schottler	0/30	1/30		0.32 [0.01, 8.24]
Total (95% CI)	548	555		0.30 [0.12, 0.73]

Total events: 4 (MECC), 19 (CPB)
Test for heterogeneity : Chi^2 = 3.20, df = 6 (P = 0.78), I^2 = 0%
Test for overall effect: Z = 2.67 (P = 0.008)

0.001 0.01 0.1   1   10   100 1000

Favors MECC   Favors CPB

C

Figure 29-16—Cont'd

the effect of rapid cooling and warming of an organ or tissue, during which temperature fluctuations would create an environment in which the solubility of gas in blood would abruptly decline, increasing the partial pressure so that GME could be generated. Increased risk would be directly proportional to the oxygen tension of blood, which would enhance the rate solubility shifts.

Other potential risks of heat exchangers are associated with the type of material used for construction. Because stainless steel is relatively expensive, aluminum has been used most often as the material for heat exchangers. Aluminum, however, has a high toxicity in humans; when blood levels exceed 100 mg/L, careful patient monitoring is imperative and levels greater than 200 mg/L are toxic.[128] Aluminum oxide concretions were found recently in organs of neonatal patients having undergone ECMO; these concretions most likely formed from aluminum leached from the anodized aluminum heat exchangers used in the circuit.[129]

Heat exchanger performance standards were established in the American Association of Medical Instruments draft report in 1982.[130] Performance testing is conducted by the simultaneous measurement of three temperatures: blood inlet temperature, blood outlet temperature, and water inlet temperature. Heat exchanger performance is reflected through a coefficient for heat transfer calculated by the following equation (where a coefficient of 1 is equal to 100% efficiency):

$$HEC = (TBI - TBO)/(TWI - TBO)$$

where HEC = heat exchanger coefficient; TBI = temperature of blood inlet; TBO = temperature of blood outlet; and TWI = temperature of water inlet. The heat exchange coefficient can be calculated for various devices over steady-state conditions, which would provide comparative analysis data on heat exchanger efficiency.

Arterial Line Filters

Arterial line filters significantly reduce the load of gaseous and particulate emboli and should be used in CPB circuits[131,132] (Figure 29-17). Some studies suggest that 20-µm screen filtration is superior to 40-µm filtration in the reduction of cerebral embolic counts.[132] A dose-response

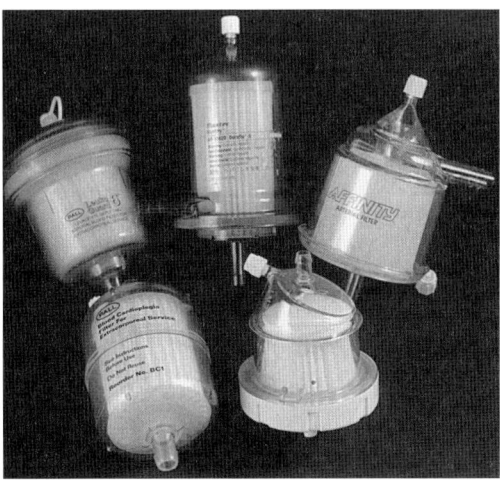

Figure 29-17 Arterial line blood filters for use during extracorporeal circulation.

relation between GME and subtle neurologic injury has been reported, and some studies have demonstrated a protective effect of arterial line filtration on neurologic outcomes[133-135] Whitaker et al's[136] clinical trial showed that the use of a leukocyte-depleting arterial line filter reduced cerebral embolic count and demonstrated a trend (not statistically significant) toward improved postoperative psychometric test scores. The GME separation performance of 10 different arterial line filters in clinical use was recently evaluated.[137] All were found to be moderately effective, and rated pore size did not predict performance. A systematic review of the data related to arterial line filtration reported that the level of evidence supporting this practice was high (Class I level of evidence A).[138] Filter design has been of two principal types: microporous screen filters and depth filters composed of dense fiber material packed in a polycarbonate housing patented by Swank. Screen filters are the predominant type in current use. Screen filters trap particulate and gaseous emboli that are of larger diameter than their effective

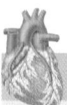

pore size. The filter material is accordion pleated to provide a larger surface area within a lower prime housing. Two contemporary filter designs consist of a larger flat screen surface that is located concentrically around the oxygenator fiber bundle. The Terumo F series filter incorporates the screen material concentrically surrounding the fiber bundle. This design reduces CPB circuit prime volume because the filter media is incorporated into the oxygenator housing, eliminating the prime volume of the separate arterial filter housing.[139] Preston et al[140] found that the F05 series oxygenator released more emboli than a similar model oxygenator used in combination with a separate 32-μm arterial filter, although the difference was not statistically significant. Sorin Group has incorporated a concentric filter design that surrounds the fiber bundle. The screen forms an envelope around the fiber bundle. This design does not effectively reduce prime; however, the larger housing provides an effective bubble trap (Box 29-6).

Cannulae and Tubing

The major devices of CPB are those that replace the systems from which the heart-lung machine has derived its name. However, as with most technologic advances, it is the combination of all component parts that function in toto to ensure success. Besides the pump and oxygenator, a seamless array of tubing is required to connect the patient to the heart-lung machine. Monitoring lines are necessary not only to ensure patient hemodynamic management but also to assess the proper function of the pump. Manufacturers of tubing and circuit packs can attest to the large number of variations in combinations and configurations of circuit assemblies requested by different institutions, as well as by individual clinicians within the same institution. The following discussion of an "ideal" tubing circuit has been generated from the experiences of the authors and may differ somewhat among cardiac centers (Figure 29-18).

The majority of cardiac procedures using CPB are performed with venous cannulation through the right atrium (RA) and arterial return into the ascending aorta. A multitude of cannulae are available for all types of cardiac surgery, which may reflect the developmental philosophy that if a vessel could conceivably be perfused or drained, then a cannula could be made to facilitate entry. The key principles of cannulae design include minimizing turbulence, reducing cannulae exit

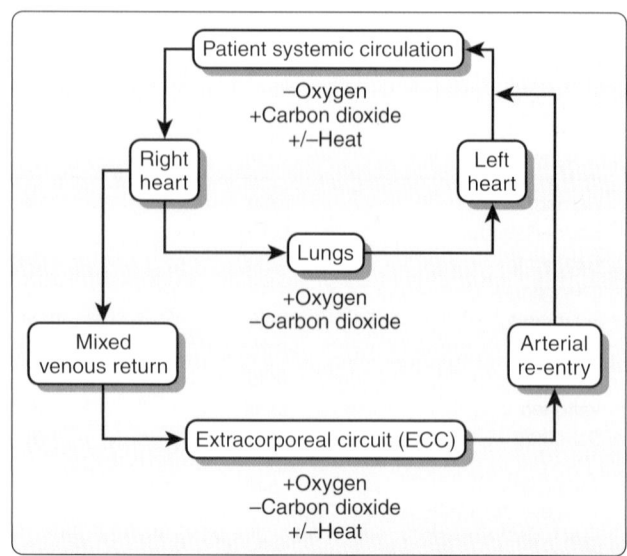

Figure 29-18 Schematic of an "ideal" tubing circuit used during extracorporeal circulation.

velocity, and avoiding areas of stagnant flow so that blood trauma and thrombus formation are minimal (Figure 29-19). In the past, cannulae were constructed of stainless steel or tapered polyvinylchloride. Subsequently, thin-walled stainless steel was used to increase effective orifice diameter and reduce cannulae pressure drop across the cannulae. Currently, most cannulae are fabricated from polyvinylchloride with composite polycarbonate thin wall tips. The ends of the cannulae are formed to permit easy vascular entry while maintaining maximum lumen (caliber) size. According to Poiseuille mechanics, the greatest resistance, measured as pressure drop in a circuit, is going to be found at the smallest opening for fluid flow and has an inverse exponential relation to the fourth power of the radius of the lumen. Therefore, to reduce pressure drops across the circuit, cannulae are selected to facilitate the greatest flow with the least injury to the vessel because of mechanical abrasion. Several arterial cannulae designs have incorporated multiple openings and dispersion tips to reduce velocity at the tip of the cannulae and reduce the likelihood of disruption of atheromatous debris from the intimal surface of the aorta.[141,142] Most cannulae have a wire reinforcement body to prevent kinking when the cannula is curved to accommodate placement in the surgical field and to maintain cannula rigidity. Although cannulation of the ascending aorta is preferred for most procedures, femoral arterial cannulation often is selected for reoperations or minimally invasive surgical procedures (Figure 29-20). The axillary or subclavian artery often is selected for arterial return

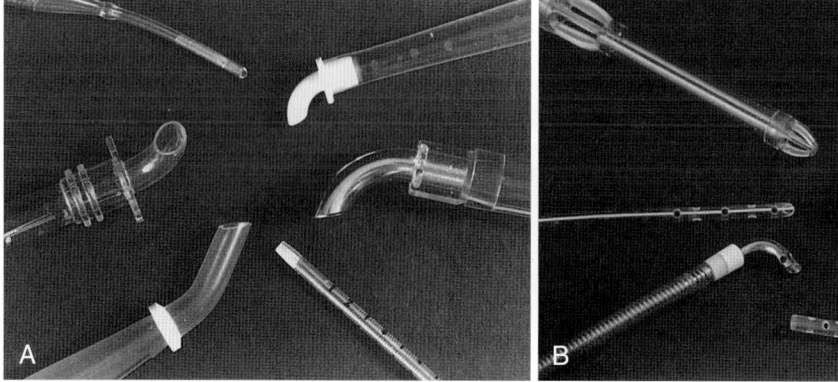

Figure 29-19 **Various commercially available cannulae for extracorporeal circulation.** *A,* Arterial cannulae. *B,* Venous cannulae.

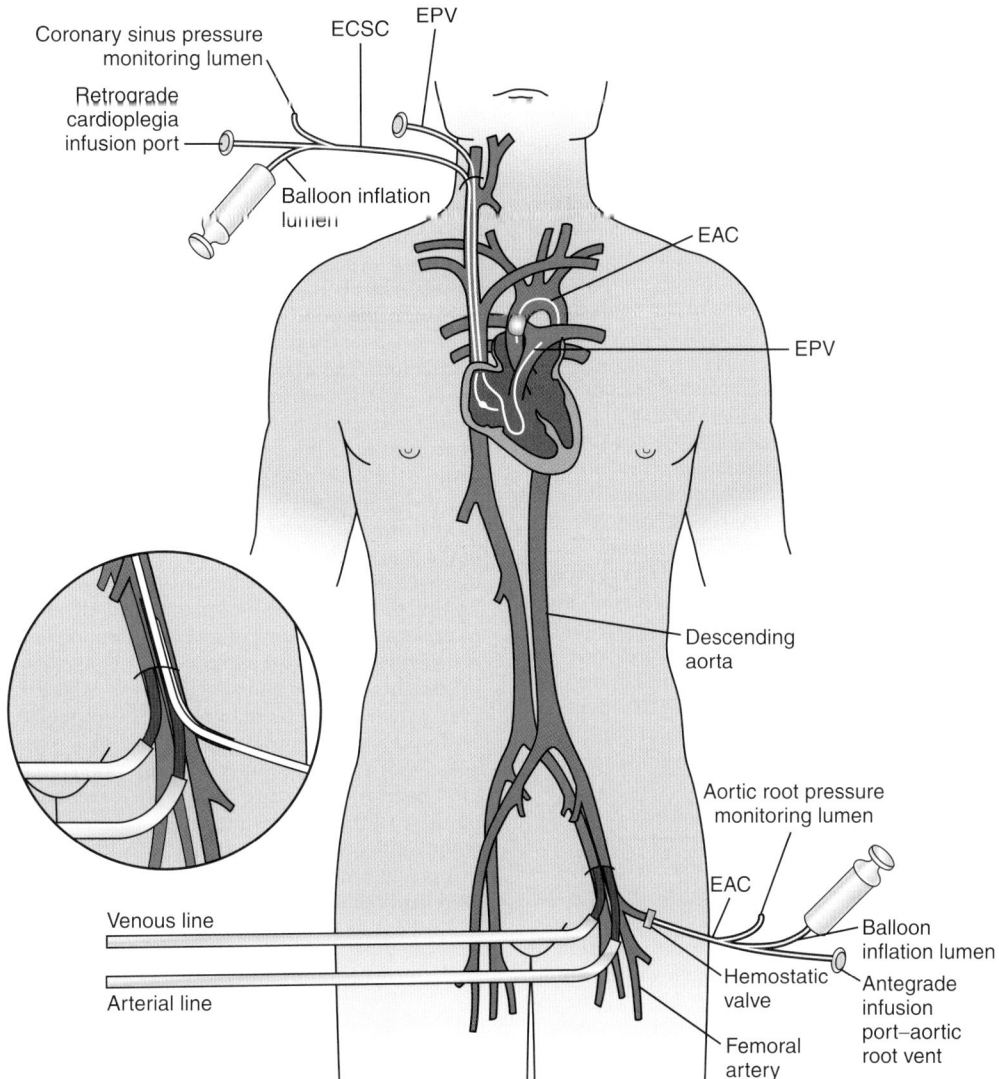

Figure 29-20 Diagram of cannulation used for minimally invasive surgery. EAC, endoaortic occlusion balloon; ECSC, endocoronary sinus catheter; EPV, endopulmonary vent. *(From Toomasian JM, Williams DL, Colvin SB, et al: Perfusion during coronary and mitral valve surgery utilizing minimally invasive port-access technology. J Extra Corpor Technol 29:66–72, 1997.)*

for patients with severe atherosclerosis of the ascending aorta. This site offers the advantage of providing antegrade flow to the arch vessels, protection of the arm and hand, and avoidance of inadvertent cannulation of the false lumen in cases in which type A aortic dissection has occurred. The axillary artery is accessed through a subclavicular incision.[143] Although the vessel may be cannulated directly with a long thin-walled 7- or 8-mm cannula, the preferred technique is to sew a 10- or 12-mm Dacron graft to the right axillary artery and insert a 20- to 24-Fr cannula into the graft. This technique provides uninterrupted flow to the right arm and hand. Transapical aortic cannulation through a 1-cm incision on the anterior wall of the left ventricle also has been described for patients with type A dissection. A 7.0-mm aortic cannula may be placed into the left ventricle and advanced across the aortic valve (Box 29-7).

Venous cannulae come in two broad classifications: single or dual stage. Single-stage cannulae are used during most open heart situations, in which either bicaval cannulation or femoral cannulation will be performed, whereas dual-stage cannulae are used for most closed heart procedures, in which a single cannula is placed into the RA.

Although both silicone (Silastic) and polyurethane tubing have been used in extracorporeal circuits, plasticized polyvinylchloride is exclusively used in CPB circuits. Plasticizers impart flexibility into tubing

BOX 29-7. ARTERIAL CANNULAE

The arterial cannulae tip is the point of highest blood flow velocity in the cardiopulmonary bypass circuit.
Some arterial cannulae have flow-dispersing tips to reduce exit velocity and reduce the risk for atheroma dislodgement from the wall of the aorta.
Cannula placement should be assessed by a test infusion from the pump and observation of a pulsatile pressure excursion.

and comprise as much as 40% of the polymer. The most commonly used plasticizer for medical-grade tubing is di(2-ethylhexyl) phthalate (DEHP). There is growing concern about the migration (leaching) of DEHP from tubing into the blood because DEHP has been shown to cause inflammation and is potentially a carcinogen and a toxic agent.[144,145] Numerous studies since the 1970s have shown that DEHP and its metabolites are present in blood products[146-149] and tissues,[150,151] as well as intravenous solutions[152] and pharmaceuticals.[153] Recently, the release properties of various plasticized polyvinylchloride tubing exposed to electrolyte solutions for up to 28 days were evaluated. Tubing formulations with one dioctyl adipate (DOA) stored in 0.9% sodium chloride solution had significantly less leaching than either DEHP plasticizer or tri(2-ethylhexyl) trimellitate (TOTM).

Blood flows out of the RA cannula and into the venous reservoir when CPB is initiated. The venous line connects the cannula to the venous reservoir. Mixed venous oxygen saturation is measured by optical or chemical fluorescence by flow through cells placed in the venous line. A stopcock is placed in the venous line to facilitate the delivery of medications and for venous sampling. Blood then enters the venous reservoir, which serves as a volume chamber for mixing and acts as a safety feature, providing additional response time to the perfusionist. Venous reservoirs come in two broad categories: hard shell (see Figure 29-11) and soft shell (see Figure 29-12), which refers to the rigidity of the device and its ability to collapse on itself. Hard-shell reservoirs are open to the atmosphere (open systems) through a ventilation port on top of the reservoir and are superior in handling gross quantities of air that may return through the venous or cardiotomy line. Soft-shell reservoirs are called *closed systems* and will collapse on themselves with the inadvertent emptying of the reservoir. The venous reservoir also has an inlet line that drains blood from a cardiotomy reservoir.

A cardiotomy reservoir is simply a second chamber used for collecting and filtering blood aspirated from the surgical field via suction lines. Vented blood from the left ventricle, pulmonary artery, or aortic root also is returned to the venous reservoir through the cardiotomy device. These are hard-shell devices made of polycarbonate housing material with polyurethane and polyester filters and defoamers to reduce the risk for gas embolism into the venous reservoir. Some venous reservoirs also serve as integral cardiotomy reservoirs, obviating the need for a separate unit.

From the venous reservoir, blood is pumped into the heat exchanger of a membrane oxygenator by the actions of the arterial pump. The heat exchanger is connected to an external water source that maintains the perfusate temperature according to the temperature of the water pumped from the cooler/heater. Blood passes directly to the oxygenator, where gas exchange occurs in accordance with the operation of a gas blender that controls the Fio_2 by mixing oxygen with medical-grade air, and a flowmeter that regulates the ventilation rate. The gas blender is attached to the inlet gas port of the oxygenator via a section of 1/4-inch tubing and a bacteriostatic (0.2-µm) filter. Many circuits have a vaporizer for the delivery of volatile anesthetic gases placed in line between the gas blender and the oxygenator.

The oxygenator has two ports on the outflow side by which arterialized blood is accessed: a recirculation port and an arterial outlet port. The recirculation port is used both to provide a safety line for relieving overpressurization and to facilitate easy replacement in the event of device failure. It also is used as an exit port of arterialized blood for sanguineous cardioplegia or in the separate perfusion of a second arterial cannula. The arterial outlet port is where the arterial blood leaves the oxygenator and flows to the arterial line filter. The arterial line filter is a screen device constructed of synthetic material, with a specific pore size effectively blocking particles greater in size than the rating of the filter (20 and 40 µm). Microembolic particles originate from many sources in the extracorporeal circuit, including the BGED, tubing, and heat exchanger, and include various substances including polycarbonate, filter material fibers, silicone, and polyvinylchloride particles.[154,155] Arterial line pressure also is measured between the arterial port and the arterial line filter. An arterial monitoring device can be placed "in line" to reflect arterial oxygen saturations and as a trending device for pH, Pao_2, and $Paco_2$. Just distal to the arterial line filter is a bubble detector that is an essential feature for the conduct of safe perfusion. This device is controlled by a microprocessor and is used to detect microgaseous and macrogaseous emboli. This is the last safety feature in the line before blood returns to the patient through the arterial cannula. When the ascending aorta is the site for arterial perfusion, an aortic cannula is placed through a purse-string suture with positioning of the cannula tip so that flow is directed cephalad toward the brachiocephalic vessels. The location of the aortic cannula and the direction of arterial blood

flow emphasize the importance of assuring safe, continuous flow of filtered perfusate devoid of embolic particles.

CARDIOPLEGIA DELIVERY SYSTEMS

In the previous section, the main tubing circuit for CPB was described and the devices for bypassing the pulmonary and systemic circulation identified. Methods of decoupling electromechanical function of the heart have been developed to achieve a safe surgical field during cardiac surgery. During aortic cross clamping, the heart is rendered globally ischemic by the cessation of coronary blood flow. Some myocardial perfusion undoubtedly occurs through the involvement of noncoronary collateral circulation from mediastinal sources and the bronchial circulation. There are numerous methods of achieving mechanical arrest, and the combination of these techniques is referred to as *myocardial preservation*. Myocardial preservation encompasses both the pharmacologic manipulation of the solutions (cardioplegia) used to protect the heart and methods of mechanical delivery. This section is devoted to methods of mechanical myocardial protection.

Melrose and colleagues[156] were the first to describe chemical arrest of the heart with potassium citrate solution. The arresting solution was delivered with a syringe directly into the aortic root after the application of the aortic cross clamp.[156] Similarly, others described delivery of various formulations of arresting solutions contained in collapsible intravenous bags using a sterile intravenous tubing set that was passed off the surgical field and attached to an inflatable infusion pump bag. This system was replaced by the use of recirculating circuits where the cardioplegia solution was recirculated in a system that consisted of a polycarbonate-filtered reservoir, and cooling of tubing that was placed in a bucket of ice (Figure 29-21). These recirculating systems provided filtration of the solution and improved control of delivery pressure and temperature. A single-pass system for delivery of blood cardioplegia in a predetermined ratio, which subsequently became the most widely used cardioplegia delivery system, was described in 1978 by Buckberg and colleagues[157,158] (Figure 29-22). The ratio of blood to cardioplegia

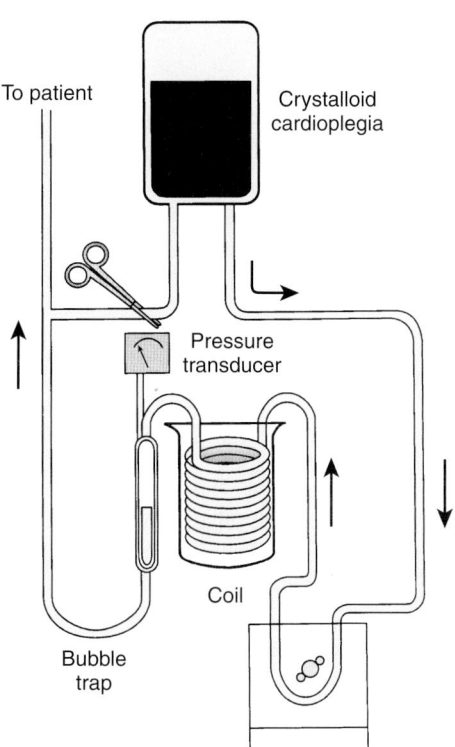

Figure 29-21   Coil-type cardioplegia delivery system. This can be used for sanguineous or asanguineous cardioplegia solution.

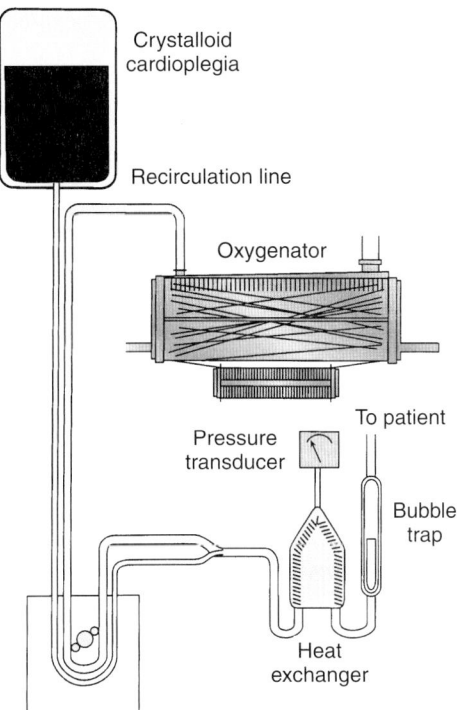

Figure 29-22 Nonrecirculating cardioplegia delivery system for use in blood to crystalloid mixed solutions of various ratios (1:1, 4:1, or 8:1 crystalloid to blood).

could be adjusted by changing the internal diameter of the tubing in the custom delivery set. The blood and crystalloid components are delivered to a miniaturized heat exchanger bubble trap before delivery at the surgical field. With this system, the temperature of the cardioplegia may be regulated from 4° C to 37° C with the use of a cooler/heater device. More recently, Menasché and colleagues[159] described a microplegia system in which arresting additives are added directly to tepid blood from the CPB circuit with a standard infusion pump to arrest the heart. This greatly decreased the volume of crystalloid solutions delivered in a typical CPB procedure and avoided the detrimental consequences of volume overload and subsequent hemodilution. The authors also cited a few particular advantages of minicardioplegia, including improved oxygenation and improved control of blood volume, not to mention reduced cost.

Adjunct means of cooling and protecting the myocardium during aortic cross clamping include the use of topical application of cold solutions to prevent early transmural myocardial rewarming. A common method for cooling the myocardium is achieved by the surgeon creating a "pericardial cradle" in the chest by suspending the pericardium with stay sutures to the chest retractor. Cold (4° C) topical saline solution is then applied to the pericardium, bathing the heart in cold solution while a sucker line is placed in the well to evacuate the saline solution. Topical saline has been shown to cool the epicardium and diminish transmural gradients,[160,161] but it also has resulted in phrenic nerve paresis and myocardial damage.[162,163] An alternate technique involves a topical cooling device, which consists of a coolant flow pad in which cold (4° C) saline flows, separated from the body by a metal skeleton and polyurethane insulator, which protects the posterior mediastinum and phrenic nerve from hypothermic injury.[164] The benefits of a topical cooling device over topical cold saline include a reduction in total hemodilution, procurement of a drier operative field, reduced blood loss in waste suction, and more uniform distribution of cooling.[164–166] However, these devices are costly, require a separate RP for delivery, and may not be applicable for all procedures in which the heart will be lifted and elevated away from the posterior pericardium.

Disposable Cardioplegia Circuits

All cardioplegia delivery systems consist of two distinct components classified as either disposable or nondisposable devices.[167] Effective myocardial protection is ensured only through the precise interface of both disposable and nondisposable components of the cardioplegia delivery system, which function to ensure safe, precise, and accurate administration of cardioplegic solutions. The disposable items that make up a standard cardioplegic circuit consist of three basic parts: a heat exchanger, a bubble trap with an incorporated filter, and various delivery cannulae. The disposable devices are utilized on a single-use basis and, because of their consumptive nature, represent the most significant cost associated with mechanical myocardial protection.

Early methods of cardioplegia delivery consisted of infusions of pharmacologic agents directly into the aortic root, or left ventricle, via handheld syringes. Unfortunately, such methods caused a heterogenous distribution of solution and led to the need for more precise delivery techniques. Many clinicians turned to a pressurized bag method in which a bag of crystalloid solution was placed in a pressure bag and cardioplegia infused at a semicontrolled rate dependent on the degree of pressure and the bore of the cardioplegic needle.[168,169] Although the results were better than those previously obtained, there was a profound lack of safety features that included pressure monitoring and control systems, as well as air-handling capacity, and a lack of temperature control. Vertrees and colleagues[170] described a simple circuit that utilized a coronary perfusion reservoir, a coil submerged in iced water, and an RP. This system was a significant improvement over previous techniques insomuch as it included a means to trap air and to measure pressure within the circuit.

There are two major disposable circuit configurations for cardioplegia delivery: a recirculating system with a coil (polyvinylchloride or stainless steel heat exchanger) for asanguineous delivery, and a sanguineous cardioplegia system for nonrecirculating delivery. In asanguineous systems, crystalloid cardioplegic solution is kept constantly recirculating throughout the cardioplegia circuit and is delivered to the patient by the movement of a clamp, directing flow away from the recirculation line and into the infusion line. These systems generally are the most economic in that they incorporate a coil of polyvinylchloride tubing as the heat-exchanging element, obviating the need for both a metal transfer unit and a separate heater/cooler device to regulate the temperature of the cardioplegic solution. Instead, the coil sits in a Styrofoam container filled with ice. The heat-exchange efficiency of coil systems has been shown to be superior to that of metal units in single-pass trials. These systems also can be used for sanguineous cardioplegia with minor adaptations to the circuit. However, with the increased use of warm sanguineous cardioplegia and the administration of warm reperfusate at the end of aortic cross-clamping, these units are not ideally suitable because of their inability to accurately control delivery temperatures.

The second classification of disposable cardioplegia systems is termed a *sanguineous system*, which involves the shunting of arterialized blood from the oxygenator into the cardioplegia circuit, where it is mixed with a crystalloid base solution, usually of high potassium concentration, before it is delivered into the coronary circulation. The most frequently used port for obtaining saturated blood from the oxygenator is the recirculation port, although some institutions directly shunt blood from the arterial line filter. The majority of sanguineous cardioplegia systems are nonrecirculating and only make a single pass through a heat exchanger before passing to the heart. For this reason, these systems must have a high efficiency rating for caloric exchange between the cardioplegic solution and the cooling, or warming, source. These devices can deliver varying ratios of blood-to-crystalloid base, ranging from a 1:1 to a 1:20 ratio of crystalloid to blood. Most are equipped with temperature monitoring ports and pressure-measuring sites to monitor delivery pressures. An important consideration of sanguineous cardioplegia delivery systems is that the main arterial pump can never be turned lower than the flow rate of the cardioplegic solution pump (i.e., delivering a higher volume of cardioplegic solution to the circuit than is flowing to the patient). If this were to occur, excessive negative pressures would be created in the recirculation line from the oxygenator, increasing the risk for cavitation (outgassing of solution).

Cardioplegic Delivery Catheters

Antegrade Aortic Root Cardioplegia

The delivery of cardioplegia is made possible through special cannulae that are placed within the ascending aorta or directly into the coronary ostia. These have been specifically designed to minimize pressure drop across the tip of the cannula, which has a relatively small bore (12 to 18 gauge). When cardioplegia is administered into the aorta, it is termed *antegrade cardioplegia*. The most common flow rates achieved in adult cardiac surgery are between 200 and 300 mL/min, with corresponding aortic root pressures usually between 60 and 100 mm Hg. In addition, the cardioplegic needle can be used as a "vent" by which residual air in the aortic root is removed by connecting the needle either to an RP or siphon drain. The final point of attachment is the cardiotomy reservoir.

The distribution of cardioplegia to the myocardium with antegrade cardioplegia techniques is hindered in patients with atherosclerotic lesions, where distal perfusion is lost because of vascular obstruction. Furthermore, impaired delivery of cardioplegia may occur because of the retrograde escape of cardioplegia across the aortic valve. This commonly occurs if the patient has aortic insufficiency. However, it may occur in patients with a competent aortic valve that becomes distorted by the placement of the aortic cross clamp.[171] Some antegrade cardioplegia cannulae have an integrated pressure monitoring lumen that allows measurement and display of the antegrade cardioplegia infusion pressure. It also is common to measure the cardioplegia delivery system pressure from a site distal to the cardioplegia delivery pump. A high system pressure alerts the team to an obstruction or malplacement of the cardioplegia delivery cannula. A low system pressure would occur from aortic insufficiency or from some breach of the delivery system. Conditions such as aneurysmal deformation of the ascending aorta and aortic valvular lesions both compromise the delivery of cardioplegia when administered via the antegrade direction. This concern has led to the search for alternative administration techniques for cardioplegic delivery.

Retrograde Coronary Sinus Cardioplegia

Retrograde delivery of blood to the heart via the coronary sinus and venous circulation was first proposed by C. Walton Lillehei. In 1982, Menasche and colleagues[172] revisited the application of retrograde coronary sinus cardioplegia (RCSC), and with this technique they found superior maintenance of left ventricular function when compared with direct coronary artery perfusion in patients with coronary artery disease. Initially, this technique was proposed as a means of delivering cardioplegia as a replacement for direct coronary artery cannulation in procedures involving the aortic valve or root. However, the utility of RCSC quickly expanded as a means of delivering nutritive flow to the distal myocardium in patients with severe coronary artery disease.[173,174] The delivery of RCSC, provided catheter position in the sinus and seal of the sinus by the balloon are optimal, results in a more uniform distribution of cardioplegia than antegrade and causes minimal disturbance of the operative field during administration.

Coronary sinus cardioplegia cannulae come in numerous configurations varying in catheter size, balloon configuration, stylet characteristics, and inflation mode (Figure 29-23). Various cannula designs are available incorporating geometric design to promote better fit into the sinus. The terminal end of the cannula is fitted with a balloon, which serves the function of seating the cannula in the coronary sinus so that cardioplegia is delivered into the coronary venous system, minimizing the amount of cardioplegia leakage into the right atrium. Some have textured balloon surfaces to minimize dislodgement of the catheter from the coronary sinus but result in leakage of the cardioplegia solution into the right atrium. Some designs have balloons that automatically inflate

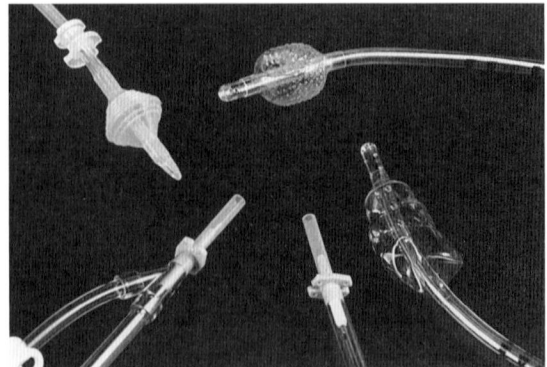

Figure 29-23 Antegrade and retrograde cardioplegia cannulae.

when flow is initiated through the catheter. Others require manual filling of the balloon with a syringe. In an animal model, Menasche and colleagues[175] have shown that autoinflated retrograde catheters leak as much as 22% of cardioplegic flow, whereas manually inflated catheters had a leakage rate less than 1%. Several authors have described the efficacy of combining both antegrade and retrograde cardioplegic delivery methods in a single integrated system.[176,177] These authors believe that the delivery of both antegrade and retrograde cardioplegia concomitantly supplies better perfusion to all regions of the myocardium despite the degree of coronary occlusive disease. Drainage is ensured through both thebesian and arteriosinusoidal vessels. Ihnken et al[178] found in a large series of high-risk patients (New York Heart Association Class III and IV) that simultaneous delivery of warm cardioplegia directly into the bypass grafts and the coronary sinus was both safe and efficacious in assuring myocardial protection. A major disadvantage of this multisite simultaneous delivery method is that most of the flow will be directed down the path of least resistance and not necessarily uniformly to all segments of the heart muscle.

Despite the excellent results achieved with RCSC, complications resulting from cannulation and excessive pressurization of the coronary sinus occasionally are reported. These include rupture of the coronary sinus, poor perfusion of the right ventricle and posterior septum, and nonhomogenous flow patterns.[179,180] In addition, controversy exists concerning the optimal delivery flow rate of RCSC. In one study of 62 patients, retrograde flow rates less than 100 mL/min resulted in reduced coronary venous effluent pH, with the authors recommending that maintenance of a minimum flow rate of 200 mL/min be considered whenever RCSC is used.[181] The optimal delivery pressure also is controversial. Most centers use a guideline of 20 to 40 mm Hg pressure measured in the delivery catheter at a point distal to the balloon. It has been suggested by one researcher that pressures as high as 50 mm Hg are safe.[182]

Nondisposable Cardioplegia Pumping Mechanisms

The currently used nondisposable devices consist of two major components: the mechanical pump and the temperature control unit. The PD twin RP is the most commonly used mechanical pump for cardioplegia. The temperature control module also is termed a *heater/cooler* and serves the function of the caloric transfer of heat by convective means between the circulating water of the heater/cooler and the cardioplegic perfusate.

Historically, commercial delivery systems for blood cardioplegia used a fixed-ratio delivery system of blood-to-crystalloid components. Cardioplegia solution mixing was achieved via a two-line RP system that combined arterialized blood and a crystalloid base solution on the distal side of the occlusive pump in a dual-lumen outlet. The ratio of blood to crystalloid was determined by the lumen size of the tubing within the raceway of the pump. Although these systems are considered as industry standards, they offered little flexibility in altering the ratio of blood or crystalloid components, and the only means of changing ionic or substrate concentration was to make up several base crystalloid bags that contained varying concentrations of solute. Several devices that address these shortcomings recently have been marketed: the Jostra HL20 Hl30 systems, the Sorin Group S-3 and S-5 Console (Sorin Biomedical, Irvine, CA), Terumo System 1 (Terumo Cardiovascular, Tustin, CA), and the Myocardial Protection System (MPS; Quest Medical, Allen, TX).

The Sorin Group S-3 and S-5 heart-lung machines have an integrated cardioplegia delivery system that consists of twin RPs, monitoring and control systems, and an internal heater/cooler for temperature regulation. Two 3-inch RPs are used, containing hybrid direct-drive systems with optical encoders, which permit accurate solution delivery at low-flow delivery rates. The two-roller-pump system was designed to allow the user to select variable ratios of blood-to-crystalloid solutions. Available ratios include 1:1 through 16:1, all blood, and all crystalloid. The system may be stop-linked to a pressure monitor, bubble detector, or to the arterial pump. The system has temperature monitors, automatic dose and ischemic time interval timers, and displays of infused blood, crystalloid, and cardioplegic solution volumes.

The Quest MPS consists of a microprocessor-controlled electromechanical instrument and disposable delivery set that is integral to the device (Figure 29-24). There is a main pumping mechanism and a pumping subsystem that operates by a set of four pistons, each driven by a stepper motor, that align with several pouches in the disposable cartridge to mechanically displace the pouch contents. The subsystem pouches contain an arresting agent and one additional additive if required. The main pumping mechanism consists of two motor-driven piston pumps and valved pouches that alternately fill and pump extracorporealized blood and crystalloid solutions, providing constant cardioplegia flow. A number of sensors become activated when the cartridge is placed into the console, and the system software completes a series of self-checks before operation. The cardioplegic solution passes through a stainless-steel heat exchanger, which controls the

caloric transfer of heat in congruence with the integral heater/cooler. There are four temperature sensors to provide temperature-controlled cardioplegia delivery, and the inlet water and cardioplegia temperatures are continuously displayed.

The MPS provides the selection of variable blood-to-crystalloid ratios that range from 1:1 to 20:1, as well as the capability to deliver all blood or all crystalloid solutions. However, the MPS allows variable ratio control, which is accomplished without changing the arresting agent concentration. This independent control of cardioplegic additive and total blood delivery is an attractive feature when optimizing oxygen-carrying capacity and enhancing aerobiosis, while assuring chemical arrest. Likewise, the MPS allows the user to change the arresting agent concentration without altering the ratio of blood to crystalloid solution. The MPS has an auto-flow mode that will vary infusion flow to maintain a set delivery pressure. The MPS is capable of pulsatile cardioplegia delivery, although few studies have demonstrated the efficacy of this delivery feature.

PRIMING SOLUTIONS AND CONTROVERSIES

Before ECC can be attempted, the patient must be connected to the CPB machine, necessitating the creation of a fluid-filled circuit to ensure continuity with the patient. Not only is it important that the circuit be "primed," but it also must be completely devoid of any gaseous bubbles or particulate matter that potentially could embolize. For this reason, perfusionists often perform painstaking maneuvers to rid the circuit of bubbles before bypass. Historically, early priming solutions were formulated to closely match the patient's own rheologic characteristics, which necessitated the use of fresh whole blood.[183] Priming the early oxygenating circuits required vast quantities of blood and balanced electrolyte solutions, and cardiac operations often were scheduled around the availability of blood donors. Eight to 10 units of heparinized blood was required to prime the average CPB circuit,[184] and the risk for contracting viral hepatitis was substantial. The addition of blood to priming solutions also induced the capillary leak syndrome,[185] which may implicate histamine as a contributing factor in leading to postpump pulmonary dysfunction. As a result of the excellent work on hemodilution by Messmer and colleagues[186,187] and others,[188] it is now the rare adult patient who receives any blood in the circuit before the initiation of CPB. Instead, balanced electrolyte solutions are the first choice in priming bypass circuits. In pediatric circuits, however, where the circuit volume often exceeds the patient's circulating blood volume, allogeneic blood products often are added to the prime to reduce the risk for anemia and hypoproteinemia (see Chapters 28, 30, and 31).

When nonhemic primes are used during CPB, there is a concomitant reduction in SVR at the onset of ECC as a result of the reduced viscosity of the blood.[189] Although the oxygen-carrying capacity of the pump perfusate is reduced by hemodilution, overall oxygen delivery may not be significantly affected because the reduced viscosity enhances perfusion. Safe levels of hemodilution are dependent on multiple factors that include the patient's metabolic rate, cardiovascular function and reserve, degree of atherosclerotic disease and resultant tissue perfusion, and core temperature. Although an absolute value for the degree of hemodilution tolerated will vary among individual patients, the studies of Kessler and Messmer support a minimal hematocrit value of 20% to ensure oxygen delivery and tissue extraction.[190,191] Much progress has been made in understanding absolute tolerances of hemodilution through treating patients of certain religious groups who refuse the transfusion of allogeneic blood products.[192]

For years controversy has raged over the inclusion of colloids in pump primes, with specific emphasis placed on the value of albumin as a routine prime constituent.[193,194] The nonphysiologic effects of CPB, with both nonpulsatile and pulsatile perfusion, are known to alter various hemodynamic and physiologic forces affecting the extravascularization of plasma water, especially in the lungs, which leads to respiratory dysfunction.[195] Total body water is increased after CPB,

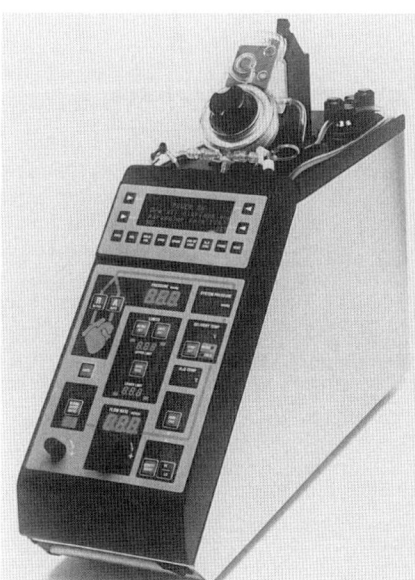

Figure 29-24 **Quest Myocardial Protection System (MPS).** Cardioplegia is pumped by a system actuated by a stepper motor. Arrest solution and additive solutions are contained in 50-mL pouches and may be precisely added to the delivery solution. The disposable heat exchanger component is attached to the top of the console. The MPS has system and delivery pressure sensors, as well as an air detection and elimination system. Blood-to-crystalloid ratio, temperature, and additive drug concentrations may be adjusted in real time during delivery. (Courtesy of Quest Medical, Allen, TX.)

leading to tissue edema and altered organ function.[196] Total body fluid shifts may take several days after CPB to correct because of the degree of hypotonicity created during bypass.[197] Although the pathophysiology related to tissue edema is appreciated, the influence of factors such as total bypass time and pressure gradients during CPB remains to be elucidated. Priming of the CPB circuit with crystalloid solutions alone reduces colloid oncotic pressure, and this reduction is directly related to the total volume of prime solution and the overall level of hemodilution. Hypo-oncotic primes promote tissue edema through interstitial expansion with plasma water.[193] A significant decline in plasma albumin occurs after CPB in patients who have been exposed to crystalloid-only primes.[198] Albumin[199] and various high-molecular-weight colloid solutions are added by some groups to the prime to offset these changes, although the benefits associated with each practice remain controversial.

Both high- and low-molecular-weight hydroxyethyl starch (HES), synthetic colloids that are derived from amylopectin, have been used as volume-expanding adjuncts to crystalloid primes.[200,201] HES is an effective colloid oncotic increasing agent that has colloidal properties similar to that of 5% albumin and is relatively inexpensive.[202] In postoperative pulmonary function studies of extravascular lung water accumulation and alveolar-arterial differences in oxygen tension, there was no significant difference seen when either 6% HES or 25% albumin was used in the pump prime.[203] Platelet counts tend to be lower when hetastarch (the high-molecular-weight form of HES) is used in CPB primes, but this reduction has questionable clinical significance.[92] When HES is infused in cardiac patients in the immediate post-CPB period, significant derangements in hemostasis have been reported, despite not being present when the solution was given to patients on entry to the intensive care unit.[204] The authors hypothesized that the infusion of HES in the immediate post-CPB period, when fibrinolytic stimulation is at a maximum and platelet count is at a nadir, could be responsible. The low-molecular-weight HES compound pentastarch may offer future promise as a more potent volume expander than hetastarch by causing fewer alterations in hemostasis.[99] One study failed to show a positive correlation between extravascular lung water and plasma colloid oncotic pressure/pulmonary capillary wedge pressure gradient after CPB when bubble oxygenators were used.[205] The use of hypertonic saline solutions (7.2% NaCl) in combination with hetastarch was recently shown to result in better patient hemodynamics with lower fluid requirements during CPB.[206] There also was evidence that this combination technique may result in better postoperative pulmonary function compared with hetastarch alone.

The addition of glucose to prime solutions remains an area of controversy because of the relation between high glucose concentrations on CPB and neurologic dysfunction.[207,208] Metz and Keats[209] reported that when glucose was included in prime solutions of 107 patients undergoing CPB, there was a lower fluid balance as evidenced by significant reductions in crystalloid administration and there was no increased neurologic dysfunction. Although there is a paucity of prospective studies on the neurologic outcome of cardiac patients after perioperative glucose administration, there is evidence that glucose administration is associated with greater morbidity after cerebral ischemia.[210,211] The hypothesis for this pathophysiologic phenomenon is related to a shift in glycolysis from aerobic to anaerobic pathways during ischemia, which results in a metabolic end-product accumulation of lactate and decline in intracellular pH.[212] Until further work is done in which tightly controlled preoperative and postoperative neurologic examinations are performed, it may be advantageous to manage glucose conservatively, restricting glucose-containing solutions in cardiac patients.[213]

Marelli and colleagues studied perioperative fluid balance in 100 adult patients divided into two groups who either did or did not receive albumin (50 g) in the bypass prime.[214] They were unable to show any improvement in more than 40 clinical parameters affecting patient outcome when albumin was included in the prime. It is known that, within the first few seconds of CPB, a proteinaceous film is deposited on the surface of all extracorporeal circuit surfaces.[215] Priming the pump

circuitry with albumin is thought to decrease the initial adsorption of protein components, which would increase biocompatibility. Bonser et al[216] examined complement activation in 36 patients who received priming solutions of either crystalloid, crystalloid plus albumin, or crystalloid plus the plasma expander polygeline. They measured products of both the alternate and common complement pathways and found a significantly greater level of activation in both the crystalloid and crystalloid plus albumin groups when compared with the polygeline patients. A similar study examined both plasma and dextran 70 in priming solutions and their effects on complement activation.[217] When plasma was added to the prime, a significant increase in the plasma concentration of C3 activation products (C3c and C3dg) was observed, which was not present in the dextran 70 group. A study of the effects of postbypass hypoalbuminemia demonstrated that this reduction was well tolerated except in patients with poor left ventricular function.[97]

Further important considerations in choosing a priming solution for CPB circuits include alterations induced by changes in electrolyte activity. Balanced electrolyte solutions are the first-choice base solutions of most prime solution "cocktails" used by perfusionists. Lactated Ringer's solution, Normosol-A, and Plasmalyte are used frequently because of their electrolyte compositions and isotonicity. One potential concern with the latter solutions focuses on the absence of calcium and potential for hypocalcemia. Calcium concentration varies depending on the type of prime constituents, as well as the presence of citrate in allogeneic blood products. Hysing et al[218] reported substantial differences in the calcium concentrations among five different prime solutions throughout the bypass period. They reported an initial decline in ionized calcium with the initiation of CPB followed by a normalization over the first 30 minutes of ECC and emphasized the importance of frequent monitoring of this cation. In pediatric ECC and in certain adult patients who have preoperative deficiencies in either hemoglobin or coagulation proteins, it may be necessary to prime the heart-lung machine with allogeneic blood products. When calcium-containing prime solutions, such as lactated Ringer's, are used, additional anticoagulation is necessary to prevent circuit thrombus from forming before the initiation of CPB. The most frequently used ratio of heparinization for CPB is 2500 IU heparin for each liter of prime solution, which would ensure adequate anticoagulation for both sanguineous and asanguineous prime solutions.

COMPUTERS IN PERFUSION

Microprocessors are ubiquitous, and their incorporation into the CPB circuit is profound and encompassing.[219] The acceptance of computers in clinical practice has been a gradual process among perfusionists,[220] which may reflect an overall tendency to resist the unknown coupled with reluctance to confront the anticipated complexity of advancing technologies. Microprocessors can be manipulated easily by user requirements to mimic logic and related functions. They are able to function without interruption through all processes involved in cardiac surgery, with minimal downtime ensured with proper utilization and maintenance. Microprocessors have proved to effectively decrease communication delays by processing vast quantities of information quickly, satisfying the demand of immediate output to facilitate decision processes. Their utility in organizing and analyzing large datasets aids in producing trending information, as well as identifying aberrant situations.

The practice of ECC is represented by a multitude of physiologic and mechanical events, which are closely interrelated and constantly changing. The continuous generation of information during these events provides a perfect situation for data capture and processing, optimizing the conduct of perfusion.[221–223] Most heart-lung machine manufacturers market data processing systems that, through a microprocessor, interface with various operating room equipment including bedside monitors and anesthesia machines. Peripheral components of the ECC, such as online blood gas analyzers, coagulation monitoring devices, heater/cooler units, and autotransfusion devices are all microprocessor controlled and easily can be integrated into a single operating system.

This organized feedback acts as an information source that centralizes data handling. The information obtained during ECC is formidable and is best manipulated by a database management system. The database management system controls how the computer stores and retrieves data and is nothing more than a tool enabling multiple complex calculations to be performed quickly.

Some of the data types obtained and analyzed during ECC include patient anthropomorphic information and perfusion and/or oxygen requirements calculated from body surface area and anticipated metabolic demands. The determinations of prime constituents and medication dosing are routinely performed via simple computer programs, together with predicting postdilutional hematocrits.[224] The conduct of CPB is reflected by terminals that display information on pump dynamics, perfusion flow, SVR, ventilatory needs, and cardiac index. In-line arterial blood gas monitors can process changes in both gas exchange and pH as often as every second. Arterial and venous samples can be measured continuously, and arterial-venous oxygen differences, oxygen delivery and consumption, and oxygen extraction ratios calculated. Input and output ratios can be determined quickly by loading values for volume input (crystalloid, colloid, blood products) and volume output (urine, aspirated waste, ultrafiltration [UF], and autotransfusion). Graphic interpretation of data is facilitated by trending summaries over the CPB period, which could incorporate "flags" as markers of events that deviated from standard treatment. This information could then be tabulated as norms and indices that could alter patient management strategies and be used in quality management assessment. A case summary then can be generated that could be used for review and interpretation, or as an official record of the case.[225]

Some of the additional benefits of computers in perfusion include their utilization as educational and training aids,[226] for assessment of the patient's physiologic status[227] and optimization of metabolite delivery.[228] Perhaps no area is more critical in the application of microprocessors in perfusion than that of safety. No matter how integrated a circuit becomes, or how technologically enhanced are the CPB components that evolve, without the conduct of safe, uneventful bypass, the advances are meaningless. Advances in bubble detection devices that incorporate ultrasonic systems have greatly reduced the risk for gross air embolism. One shortcoming in safety devices remains the absence of reliable level-detection systems that monitor venous reservoir volumes. Arterial pressure monitoring with feedback loops that will interrupt pump operation in the event of high pressure, or gas emboli detection, has greatly enhanced the quality of CPB.

The future of computers in ECC is probably as much a function of education as technologic advance. The most advanced systems, with the highest price tags, are of absolutely no value without the fundamental knowledge of how to operate them. Nevertheless, some of the future goals of microprocessor-enhanced perfusion include inexpensive, menu-driven software programs that would reduce the time spent learning terminology and functions. A reduction in system complexity with succinct troubleshooting guides may decrease technical support required for system maintenance. Finally, computers will serve as valuable training tools to assess skills and competencies before actual clinical situations.[229–231] Indeed, several perfusion education programs incorporate clinical computer simulation as a means of assessing student proficiency in didactic areas before operating the pump in the operating room.

PERIOPERATIVE METHODS OF RED BLOOD CELL CONSERVATION

Homologous blood is a precious resource, the transfusion of which confers both benefits and risks. The practice of transfusion began in the 1930s with the Nobel Prize–winning work of Landsteiner.[232] Transfusion medicine expanded through experience gained in battlefield medicine and the development of cardiac surgery, vascular surgery, and oncology. Of the 29 million transfusions administered each year, it is estimated that one third to half are not administered in accordance with evidence-based indications.[233] Cardiac surgery programs are one of the leading consumers of blood and blood products. More than 80% of the blood used in cardiac surgery is transfused in 15% to 20% of the patients undergoing surgery.[234] In the late 1970s and early 1980s, there was concern about transfusion-related hepatitis B and C, HIV, and bacterial infections. With modern blood bank processes and screening, these risks have become extremely low; however, other associated risks including transfusion-related lung injury, leukocyte-related target organ injury, transfusion errors, and bacterial infections are comparatively common. Furthermore, there is a growing confirmation of the relation between transfusion and reduced short-term survival, long-term survival, and HF in cardiac surgery patients.[235–241] Transfusion of stored blood and blood products is related to a host of adverse effects including release of bioactive compounds that cause inflammation, reduced oxygen availability to tissues, and other immunomodulatory effects, all of which contribute to increased morbidity and mortality[242] (see Chapters 30 and 31).

Transfusion practice varies widely, and this variation is based largely on individual physician practice.[243] The administration of allogeneic blood products during cardiac surgery continues to be a major concern for both patients and clinicians. The changing population of patients undergoing cardiac surgery has presented new transfusion-related challenges that are being addressed through both pharmacologic and mechanical means. A combination of increasing age of patients undergoing cardiac surgery and a greater percentage of patients undergoing resternotomy procedures has increased the challenge of bloodless cardiac surgery. Although the safety of receiving allogeneic blood has increased dramatically, risks remain and need to be understood when considering patient transfusion. These risks include both hemolytic and nonhemolytic reactions, disease transmission, graft-versus-host disease, recipient alloimmunization, and hypervolemia.[244] Results generated when meticulous attention and adherence to conventional blood conservation techniques have been followed are promising.[245,246] However, the diversity in surgical practices, anesthesia management, and postoperative care all represent a multifactorial process rendering reproducibility difficult from center to center.

Isovolumic hemodilution combined with hypotensive anesthesia is an effective strategy for limiting allogeneic transfusions. Intraoperative phlebotomy before ECC is performed easily with volume replacement consisting of either colloid or crystalloid solutions ranging, respectively, from 1 to 3 mL for every milliliter of phlebotomized blood. Relative contraindications to performing intraoperative donation may be left main stenosis, unstable angina, critical aortic stenosis, hemodynamic instability, and a history of cerebrovascular disease.[132] The increased risks associated with allogeneic blood are well-known. Although the dangers of receiving contaminated blood vary among geographic regions, it is accepted that the incidence of post-transfusion hepatitis C has decreased markedly,[247] whereas the risk for HIV transmission has been reported to be as high as 1 in 100,000 transfusions. The emphasis on reducing the risks associated with blood exposure has long been evident within hospitals. Standing blood utilization committees are charged with the responsibility of reviewing transfusion practices within hospitals. Some states have enacted laws that protect the rights of patients undergoing elective surgical procedures in regard to blood transfusions. Legislative actions in California have established specific mandates for physician involvement in ensuring that patients at risk for transfusion are informed of the availability of alternate techniques for reducing the risk for allogeneic blood exposure. Clearly, the impetus directing specific blood replacement practices associated with cardiovascular surgery will come under intense scrutiny from both internal and external sources of review.

The term *autotransfusion* has been used generically to represent the process of reinfusing blood collected from a patient at some time before infusion. Autotransfusion can be broken down into three distinct categories delineated by both the time of collection and the methods used to collect the blood. Preoperative donation, intraoperative salvage, and postoperative collection are techniques used in varying degrees at most cardiac centers. Each category is further subdivided according to the techniques used; however, the underlying goal that firmly links all processes together is the reduction in exposure of patients to allogeneic blood.

Preoperative Donation

Predonation before surgery would seem to be a plausible means of obtaining blood and avoiding homologous transfusion, particularly in this era of heightened awareness of the dangers associated with receiving allogeneic blood products. The use of autologous blood not only is nonimmunogenic but reduces the hospital's dependence on blood banks. However, this technique has had limited success in treating the cardiac surgery patient.[248] From a blood bank perspective, predonation of blood is a logistic nightmare. Furthermore, there are many contraindications to autologous blood collection in cardiac patients, including aortic stenosis, left main coronary artery disease, idiopathic hypertrophic subaortic stenosis, unstable angina, cardiac failure, recent myocardial infarction, ventricular arrhythmia, symptoms on the day of donation, and the emergency need for surgery. Only 10% of transfusion recipients may be eligible for self-donation[249]; therefore, the majority of surgical candidates require alternative measures to reduce exposure to the general blood supply.

Plasmapheresis

Plasmapheresis is the separation of whole blood into plasma (which may be platelet poor or platelet rich), platelets, and RBCs. The first clinical utilization of plasmapheresis in thoracic surgery was reported by Ferrari and colleagues[250] in 1987. The benefits of plasmapheresis in the cardiac surgical patient are derived from the production of autologous blood products that, because of their separation into isolated components, can be administered to treat specific deficiencies related to the patient's hemostatic needs. One of the most critical advantages involves the treatment of patients who would otherwise not be candidates for predonation of blood. The logistic difficulties are easily overcome when this method is used in the operating room with the patient under the direct care of the anesthesiologist.

As with any new treatment, potential disadvantages do exist and are related to exsanguination phenomena. Plasmapheresis reduces circulating albumin and total protein levels before surgery, which, when combined with noncolloidal fluid replacement, may lead to extravascularization of plasma water. In addition, there may exist select patients who cannot tolerate the anemia associated with use of this technique before CPB. The expenses associated with plasmapheresis are minimal because most cardiac centers have purchased cell-washing autotransfusion devices for alternate reasons, and these machines easily can perform intraoperative plasmapheresis.

The technique of plasmapheresis uses similar technology to that of cell-washing autotransfusion devices. Both systems use centrifuges, peristaltic pumps, and collection reservoirs. The process for plasmapheresis is unique in several ways, including its processing of whole blood collected using protocols for isovolumic hemodilution, before heparinization. During plasmapheresis the clinician has the ability to alter the collection process to obtain either platelet-poor or platelet-rich plasma (PRP). The platelet-poor plasma is collected at greater centrifuge speeds (5200 to 5600 rpm), resulting in tighter packing of the RBC layer, restricting the separation of platelets into a buffy coat layer. At slower centrifuge speeds (2400 to 3600 rpm), the platelet fraction is sequestered in the buffy coat layer that is then collected, together with a small volume of RBCs, as PRP.

In the operating room, removal of whole blood should begin as soon as central venous access is established. The most common site is the internal jugular vein, although external jugular, saphenous, and antecubital veins all have been used. The anticoagulant used is sodium citrate, which should be delivered at a rate of 1 mL/12 mL whole blood. The blood is drawn into a collection bag and then transferred to a processing bowl in the autotransfusion device via a peristaltic pump. The calculated plasma volume to be removed has generally been set as 20%

of the patient's circulating plasma volume,[251] which ranges from 10 to 12 mL/kg.[252] Approximately 200 mL whole blood can be processed in 12 to 14 minutes.[251,252] The number of cycles necessary to complete the calculated draw volume is dependent on the patient's RBC mass and plasma volume. Volume replacement should be carried out both before and during the sequestration process. Replacement therapy varies among institutions, but the solutions most often reported include high-molecular-weight HES (6% HES),[252] crystalloid solutions, and 5% albumin.[253] After the plasma has been removed, the RBCs can either be reinfused to the patient via the return mode of the machine or saved and returned after CPB. The product yield is dependent on the patient's predraw platelet level and plasma volume but generally is between 1.0 and 2.5×10^{11} platelets/600 mL product.[251–253]

Storage of collected products should follow established practices of the blood bank at the individual institution. Platelet clumping has been reduced by placing the removed plasma in a rocker or agitation device. The temperature at which to store the sequestered plasma is controversial, although room temperature has been used. In some operating rooms where the ambient temperature is kept quite low, wrapping the reinfusion bag in a warm blanket has been advocated. The product should be returned to the patient after reversal of heparin by protamine, as ascertained by monitoring activated coagulation times.

The results of plasmapheresis in thoracic surgery have been encouraging, although questions have been raised concerning efficacy.[254,255] When the use of autotransfusion alone has been compared with plasmapheresis, the patients treated with PRP have had lower positive fluid balances than patients who had cell washing used as a method of hemoconcentration.[252] Several clinical trials have shown a decreased usage of allogeneic blood products, including plasma and platelets, during the hospitalization of patients treated with PRP.[252,256–258] After the reinfusion of autologous PRP, patients have had greater operative platelet counts,[139] decreased postoperative bleeding,[250,259] and greater fibrinogen and antithrombin III (AT III) concentrations.[260] Giordano et al reported that the concomitant use of autotransfusion and PRP reduced transfusions from 13.67 to 6.32 allogeneic blood exposures per patient.[253]

Stammers et al[261] have described additional benefits of plasmapheresis in the immediate postinfusion period and can be related to an overall reduction in fibrinolytic tendency. It also has been shown that, through reductions in blood transfusion, PRP administration to patients in a hyperfibrinolytic state ameliorates the effect of fibrinolytic substances. Although specific factors in the plasma product have not been identified, the rapid reduction in fibrinolysis suggests the presence of endogenous antifibrinolytic substances.

The effects of platelet-affecting drugs on both platelet-poor plasma and PRP are germane because a substantial number of cardiac patients are exposed to these medications before surgery. Giordano and colleagues[256] studied patients who received warfarin (Coumadin), heparin, or nonsteroidal anti-inflammatory agents up to the day before surgery. When these patients were treated with PRP, there was no effect on postoperative bleeding after reinfusion of PRP. The contraindications to plasmapheresis are based mainly on the patient's inability to withstand low hemoglobin concentrations before the initiation of CPB. Patients with hemoglobin concentrations of less than 10 g/dL generally have their RBCs returned in between cycles.

Autologous Priming Techniques

The process of displacing crystalloid prime solution with the patient's own blood to reduce hemodilution during the onset of CPB, known as autologous priming (AP), has become a widely adopted method of reducing the burden of hemodilution that occurs at the initiation of CPB. The process involves slowly removing the clear prime from the pump with the patient's own blood through both the arterial and venous limbs of the perfusion circuit, once the patient has been given heparin and the activated coagulation time is adequately prolonged. It is necessary to position the patient in Trendelenburg position to improve right atrial filling pressure and maintain arterial blood pressure during this process. It often is necessary to also infuse phenylephrine to maintain an acceptable arterial blood pressure during this process.

Rosengart et al's[262] prospective trial led the way for other investigators. Their study, conducted on 60 first-time CABG patients, established that AP limits hemodilution and reduces the number of patients needing RBC transfusions. Since their report, other randomized and observational trials have reported similar benefits.[263–267] However, Murphy et al[268] concluded that AP does not offer a clinical benefit as a blood conservation technique. Their trial was limited by design (retrospective cohort, single surgeon), and the limited reporting of AP techniques and volume management strategies prevents replication. More recently, Trowbridge et al[269] designed a prospective study aimed at identifying optimal characteristics of the AP process and found that when used effectively, defined as removal of at least 1300 mL or when less than 10% of AP volume was returned to the patient, greater hematocrit values were obtained and fewer patients received transfusions. Furthermore, they reported that the amount of removed prime returned to the patient was related to the patient's urinary output and the amount of blood loss during the procedure.[269]

Perioperative Salvage and Autotransfusion

Cardiotomy Suction

Shed blood from the surgical field and blood vented from the LA, left ventricle, pulmonary artery, or the aorta is collected and reinfused into the CPB circuit through the cardiotomy suction system. This system is composed of tubing usually 1/4-inch internal diameter directed through an RP into a filtered reservoir. Cardiotomy suction blood contains fat, bone, lipids, and other debris from the surgical field. This blood is also exposed to air, shear forces, and artificial surfaces that cause exacerbation of the systemic inflammatory response and result in microcirculatory dysfunction. These substances may traverse the CPB circuit, enter into the arterial line, and ultimately obstruct the microcapillary circulation of the patient. Brown et al[270] identified thousands of embolic lesions in the brains of patients who died within 3 weeks of cardiac surgery and reported an association between embolic lesions and duration of CPB. For each 1-hour increase in the duration of CPB, the embolic load increased by 90.5%. Cardiotomy suction blood has been identified as a major source of lipid emboli in several studies.[271–273] For this reason, some have advocated eliminating the use of cardiotomy suction, which is returned directly to the ECC. Several clinical studies have examined the effects of eliminating cardiotomy suction. In a randomized trial enrolling CABG patients, use of cardiotomy suction resulted in significant increases in thrombin generation, neutrophil and platelet activation, as well as the release of neuron-specific enolase.[274] Nuttall et al,[275] in a study of patients in whom an open venous reservoir was used, compared the return of cardiotomy suction directly to the ECC, versus sequestration and processing of cardiotomy blood to a cell saver. A battery of blood tests were performed to evaluate platelet function, and no significant difference in any of the tests or in blood transfusion requirements was observed.

Cell Salvaging through Centrifugation and Washing Techniques

One of the simplest forms of autotransfusion is the use of a cell-salvaging system that uses aspiration and anticoagulation to collect shed blood and return it to the patient. The simplest products to perform this function include collection sets consisting of double-lumen tubes through which an anticoagulant (usually heparin or citrate-phosphate-dextrose) is mixed with shed operative blood, aspirated by negative pressure through a vacuum source, collected in a reservoir, and directly reinfused to the patient through a filter. Inherent problems with this technique include questionable quality of reinfused blood because of contamination with particulate matter aspirated from the field that includes bone fragments, fat particles, and suture

materials. In addition, the anticoagulant remains present in the reinfusate. However, this technique is a relatively easy and quick means of returning lost blood in the event of unexpected acute blood loss.

Another form of autotransfusion uses specific machines that salvage and process shed blood and include a cell washing step. The term *cell saving* has come to denote the process of autotransfusion that involves centrifugation of collected operative blood and processing with a wash solution, 0.9% NaCl, and reinfusing the product back to the patient. The basic operating principles found in autotransfusion include aspiration, anticoagulation, centrifugation, washing, and reinfusion. The ensuing discussion focuses specifically on the processes of cell washing and separation by centrifugation as autotransfusion methods.

The major components of any automated or manual device used for cell processing in autotransfusion are listed in Table 29-1. The process begins with the aspiration of blood from the surgical site together with an anticoagulant via a double-lumen line. The blood, together with other operative contaminants including bone chips and adipose tissue, is then collected in a cardiotomy reservoir, functioning as the first filtration, with depth and screen filters ranging in size from 40 to 120 μm. A peristaltic pump then transfers the contents from the cardiotomy reservoir into a centrifuge bowl that has been specifically designed to separate blood according to specific particulate density. Centrifugation necessary for this separation process generally is between 4800 and 5600 rpm (Figure 29-25). The volume of the bowl is an important characteristic of these devices because the volume of the bowl has a role in the minimum amount of shed blood required to obtain an acceptable

TABLE 29-1	Basic Components of a Typical Autotransfusion Device	
Centrifuge		
Centrifugal bowl		
Aspiration set		
Anticoagulant		Cardiotomy reservoir
Wash fluid		
Waste bag		
Reinfusion bag		

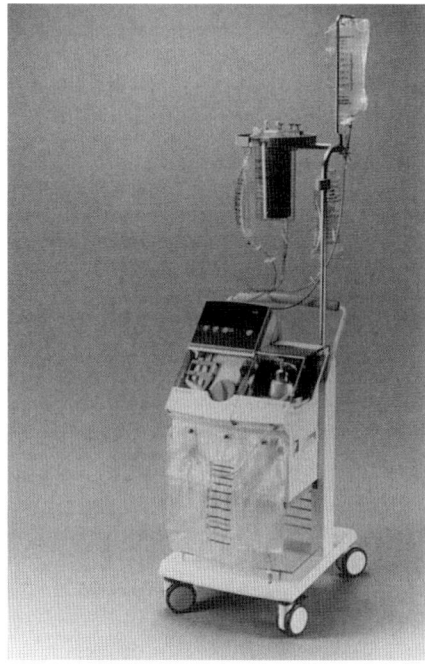

Figure 29-25 Autotransfusion cell processing device using a peristaltic pump and centrifuge for processing of shed blood. *(Courtesy of Haemonetics Corporation, Braintree, MA.)*

hematocrit in the returned product. Some of the systems come with 125-mL bowls for use with small patients or when smaller amounts of shed blood are anticipated. The heavier RBCs are packed farthest from the axis of rotation, whereas the lighter plasma and crystalloid fractions remain closest to the center of the bowl. A wash mode is initiated when the centrifuge bowl has reached its optimal packed RBC level, with sterile physiologic saline pumped through the RBC layer, removing plasma-free hemoglobin, clotting factors, anticoagulant, and nonautogenous particles.

After the wash cycle, the washed product is pumped out of the centrifuge bowl into a collection reservoir and then transferred to a reinfusion bag for administration to the patient. The quality of the finished product is affected by several operating parameters, including the absolute aspiration pressure, the fill speed of the bowl, the wash rate, and the quantity of wash volume used. The percent hematocrit of the processed blood also is dependent on filling rate and wash rate, and when these are kept within the manufacturer's recommendations, the final product should have a hematocrit between 45% and 60%.

One new cell-saver design, the Continuous Autotransfusion System (CATS; Terumo Cardiovascular, Tustin, CA), does not have a Latham bowl and functions in a continuous manner such that the packed RBC product is harvested during centrifugation (Figures 29-26 and 29-27). This approach has several advantages: a lower minimum amount of shed blood is required before packed RBCs may be harvested, a greater RBC concentration of resultant product is obtained, and, most importantly, the separated lipid layer remains suspended during the process. With the traditional Latham bowl systems in which the centrifugation is stopped between cycles, lipids may remix with the final RBC product and be returned to the patient. Several recent studies have shown that the use of a continuous processing system is superior to the Latham bowl-type systems in terms of lipid removal and neurocognitive outcomes.[276,277] Kincaid et al[278] studied effects of blood processing technique on production of lipid emboli in the brain (Small Capillary Arterial Dilations) in a canine model. Two recent randomized trials were designed to determine whether use of a cell saver reduced neurocognitive dysfunction after CPB. In Rubens et al's study,[279] 266 patients undergoing CABG surgery were randomized to two groups: an unprocessed cardiotomy suction blood group (control) and that processed by centrifugal cell washing (treatment group). Greater blood

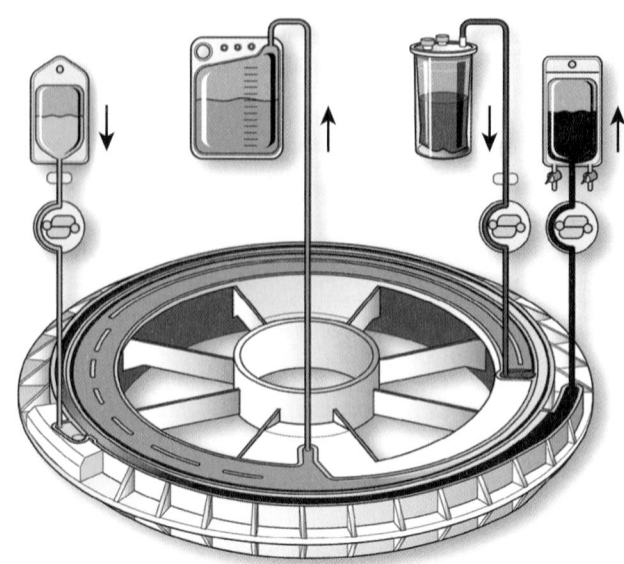

Figure 29-27 **Continuous Autotransfusion System Cell processing cassette.** *(Courtesy of Terumo Cardiovascular Systems, Ann Arbor, MI.)*

product administration and blood loss were observed in the treatment group. No differences in microemboli generation, neurocognitive dysfunction, or other adverse events were demonstrated between groups. In another study by Djaiani et al,[276] patients randomized to cell processing with a continuous autotransfusion system had reduced transfusion requirements and improved neurocognitive function. The latter study used a continuous cell processing system that has been shown to reduce blood lipid content. The former study used a Latham bowl intermittent system, which previously has been shown to be ineffective at lipid removal. Further studies are necessary to define the impact of cardiotomy suction on clinical outcomes.

All of the currently manufactured machines contain microprocessors and operate in either manual or automated modes. In the manual mode, the operator has control over the processing cycle and must be present during each stage of the process. The machines that contain automatic mode capabilities also provide the user with the option of completing several cycles of blood processing without operator dedication. Some models also permit online programming at the user site, which enables the perfusionist to modify the processing program according to the level of aspirated blood contamination, producing an optimal quality product.

The safety features available on autotransfusion machines vary according to the manufacturer. Some of the more prominent features include air-sensing capabilities, level detectors, air and foam detectors, hand-cranking capabilities, two-bag reinfusion systems, and waste bag overfill automatic shutoff. The reinfusion bag from an autotransfusion device should never be directly connected to a patient through an infusion line. The peristaltic pump of the autotransfusion device is connected to the cardiotomy reservoir, which is often emptied during the filling process. The potential, therefore, is that air could be pumped into the reinfusion bag, which could then be passed on to the patient, especially in the situation in which the reinfusion bag is placed under pressure. A second transfer collection bag should be filled from the reinfusion bag and separated from the autotransfusion machine, to reduce the risks for air embolization.

Autotransfusion as a routine practice in cardiac surgery has received mixed acceptance. Cost-effectiveness always has been a concern, with the prevailing belief that the utilization of autotransfusion should be considered only when anticipated blood loss would result in a reinfusion of 1 to 2 units of processed RBCs.[280] However, the active interest in minimizing patient exposure, combined with the use of

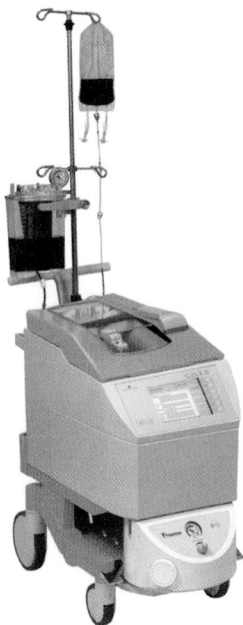

Figure 29-26 **Continuous Autotransfusion System (CATS).** *(Courtesy of Terumo Cardiovascular Systems, Ann Arbor, MI.)*

smaller-volume centrifuge bowls, have prompted increased use of autotransfusion during cardiac surgery. Young et al[281] reported a reduction in allogeneic RBC transfusion from 4.2 to 1.5 units/patient when autotransfusion was used in cardiac patients. The quality of RBCs processed via autotransfusion during cardiac surgery also has been compared with fresh autologous blood, with RBCs collected from the operative field having an in vivo survival comparable with that of phlebotomized blood.[282] Schwieger et al's[283] study examined autotransfusion collected blood for risk for infection and found that patients who had blood salvaged and processed by cell-washing equipment had no higher rate of infection than patients who had no autotransfusion but received banked blood.

In addition to aspirating shed blood from cardiac patients, the autotransfusion device can be used to concentrate the pump perfusate at the termination of CPB. Although this process is known to reduce the protein concentration of the perfusate when compared with reinfusion of the unprocessed pump contents, this method significantly reduced allogeneic banked blood exposure.[284] Many centers will infuse the blood contained in the CPB circuit at the termination of bypass. The blood in the CPB circuit is displaced with a balanced electrolyte solution so that the pump remains primed should it be necessary to return to bypass. Sometimes vasodilators are administered to the patient to increase capacitance and allow this blood to be reinfused. It is common practice in neonate and pediatric cardiac surgery to use a technique referred to as "modified ultrafiltration" (MUF). With this technique, UF is conducted to remove plasma water, while at the same time the blood remaining in the CPB circuit is slowly infused into the patient. Similarly, this technique may be performed using a device called a *hemobag,* where the contents of the CPB circuit are infused into a collection bag and the contents of the bag are then ultrafiltered and returned to the patient.[285,286] The product returned to the patient has a lower water content and greater concentration of RBCs, platelets, white blood cells, and plasma proteins.

Dilutional coagulopathy is a potential problem with overuse of autotransfusion. When large quantities of blood are processed, the washout of clotting factors may induce bleeding purely from a dilutional effect. However, the use of waste or wall suction would result in a similar reduction in clotting factors, as well as the loss of RBCs. Autotransfusion also is used to treat patients with rare blood types or who are sensitized to donor blood and respond poorly to transfusion. In addition, certain religious beliefs will not allow the acceptance of allogeneic blood but will consider the use of autotransfusion on an individual basis.

The contraindications to the use of autotransfusion are relative and are evaluated on a per-case basis. Therefore, the relative contraindications include contaminated wound sites and/or septic procedures, malignancy, aspiration during caesarean sections, and concurrent use when microfibular collagen agents are present. The risks assumed with using cell salvaging and reinfusion techniques in these patients must be weighed against the inherent benefits of autologous versus allogeneic transfusion. Hemoglobinemia resulting from RBC destruction caused by exposure of blood to disposable autotransfusion circuitry and trauma caused by aspiration and mechanical treatment has been reported.[287] The reinfusion of packed RBCs may also lead to pulmonary insufficiency if inadequate filtering of the product results in microaggregate embolization in the pulmonary vasculature. The risk for air embolism also is increased whenever extracorporeal devices are used; therefore, proper precautions with operator vigilance are paramount in assuring patient safety.

Postoperative Shed Mediastinal Blood Collection

The collection and reinfusion of postoperative mediastinal blood after cardiac surgery have been described as postoperative autotransfusion (PAT)[288,289] and have been used in cardiac surgery since 1978.[290] This process consists of connecting either a dedicated collection device or a cardiotomy reservoir from the extracorporeal circuit directly to mediastinal chest tubes and a negative pressure source. Blood flows from the mediastinal tubes into the collection reservoir, where it undergoes gross filtration (40 to 120 μm). The collected product then is reinfused back to the patient via an infusion pump and through an additional 20-μm filter. The volume collected after the operation varies from center to center and according to procedure but may range from 400 to 1200 mL over the first 24 hours. Shed mediastinal blood is defibrinogenated; therefore, levels of fibrin(ogen) split products are increased after reinfusion.[291]

Morris and Tan[292] commented on the use of PAT in 155 consecutive cardiac patients. These authors found a substantial and significant reduction of approximately 30% in the use of allogeneic blood products in patients undergoing cardiac surgery with PAT. Other authors have found that when the postoperative blood loss was less than 500 mL, PAT conferred no benefit in reducing banked blood requirements.[293,294] In a prospective, randomized study of cardiac patients undergoing CABG surgery, Bouboulis et al[295] found no benefit to the use of PAT, and patients receiving autotransfusion had greater incidences of febrile reactions. These authors and others have advocated the concurrent use of a cell-washing device to process the PAT product before reinfusion.[296] A portable cell-washing device, the CardioPAT, is now available for processing shed blood from thoracic and pleural drainage. This device functions similarly to the centrifugal cell-washing systems. The major differences are a smaller footprint and a slower rate of processing than the traditional cell-saver systems. The processing of this blood removes activated white blood cells and fibrinolytic mediators, which may be associated with hemolytic reactions found when unwashed blood is reinfused. Schmidt et al[297] have shown that the reinfusion of PAT blood in CABG patients caused an increase in levels of cardiac enzymes including creatine kinase-MB activity. These increases may result in a compromised assessment of myocardial injury in patients undergoing cardiac surgery with PAT.

Ultrafiltration

UF is a process in which plasma water is filtered from whole blood via a semipermeable membrane (see Figure. 29-34). Although primarily a method of removing plasma water, it is also an effective means of blood conservation in that it indirectly increases the volume of RBCs, platelets, and coagulation factors. The technology used in UF was initially developed as a treatment for dialysis patients who became volume overloaded.[298] UF is used synonymously with hemofiltration and diafiltration and uses similar devices and principles to those seen in continuous arteriovenous hemofiltration and slow continuous UF. Continuous arteriovenous hemodiafiltration uses a dialysate that flows countercurrent to the direction of blood flow around the fibers, removing plasma solutes and electrolytes by diffusion. When UF is used exclusively to remove excessive fluid from CPB circuits, it has been referred to as *hemoconcentration.*

Cardiac patients are particularly susceptible to volume overloading via crystalloid administration for hemodynamic maintenance and prime solution of the heart-lung machine. Priming of the extracorporeal circuit with nonhemic solutions results in hemodilution that ranges from 33% to 200% of the patient's volume. After cardiac surgery, the amount of extravascular fluid load may increase by greater than one third of the adult patient's prebypass blood volume,[299] whereas in pediatric perfusion, the total volume of hemodilution may far exceed the patient's preoperative blood volume.[300] It is well-known that the body responds to hemodilution by increasing cardiac index as a result of reduced SVR.[301] In sick or compromised hearts, however, there is less myocardial reserve, which may result in inadequate oxygen delivery and hypoperfusion because of decreased output. UF not only reduces the risk for volume overload in these patients, but it can be used to correct electrolyte and acid-base imbalances.

UF is a hemoconcentration technique by which plasma water and certain low-molecular-weight plasma solutes are separated from circulating whole blood by free convective transport. A semipermeable

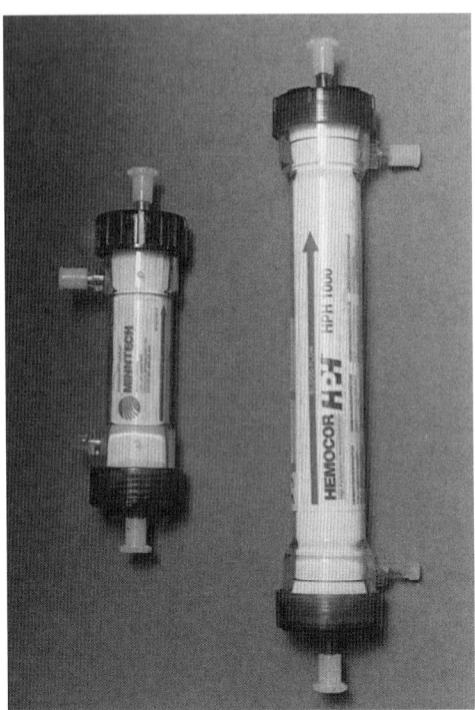

Figure 29-28   Ultrafiltration device. (*Courtesy of Minntech Corp., Minneapolis.*)

hollow-fiber membrane operates on the principle of a hydrostatic pressure differential generated across the membrane to separate an ultrafiltrate from blood (Figure 29-28).[302] The composition of the ultrafiltrate is similar to that of glomerular filtrate.[303] Uremic toxins also are selectively removed from the circulating perfusate,[304] which may decrease the incidence of acute tubular necrosis as a result of CPB. Sieving coefficients that are based on the molecular weight of plasma solutes and the porosity of the UF device have been established by the various manufacturers. These are determined by dividing the concentration of the solute in the filtrate by the concentration in the plasma. Generally, solutes greater than 50,000 Daltons do not pass through the membrane pores (albumin has a molecular mass of 65,000 Daltons).

The advantages of UF in the cardiac patient are:
1. Hemoconcentration without removing the protein segment of whole blood, thus maintaining plasma constituents including albumin and clotting factors
2. The concentration of the albumin fraction increases colloid oncotic pressure and reduces edema by drawing fluid out of the extravascular area
3. The reduction of pulmonary dysfunction after CPB by decreasing the amount of extravascular lung fluid[305]
4. In patients with renal impairment, its concomitant use with dialysis before surgery may prepare the patient for anesthetic induction by optimizing the electrolyte and blood urea nitrogen levels[306]

UF differs from dialysis in that dialysis is the diffusion of solutes through a semipermeable membrane via a concentration gradient into a dialysate solution. UF uses the hydrostatic pressure gradient in removing plasma water without an osmotic gradient. The principle of operation involves a transmembrane pressure gradient (TMP), which is the force by which solutes are separated from the solution. The calculation of TMP uses the arterial inlet pressure (P_a), venous outlet pressure (P_v), ultrafiltrate pressure of outlet (P_n), and oncotic pressure at the inlet (P_i) and the outlet (P_o):

$$TMP = P_a/2 + P_v + P_n - P_i/2 + P_o$$

The UF rate is the rate at which plasma volume is removed from the blood passing through the ultrafiltrator and is dependent on TMP and the surface area of the hemoconcentrator.[307]

Ultrafiltrators traditionally have been designed in either parallel-plate or hollow-fiber configuration. The hollow-fiber types are used in hemoconcentration and are manufactured out of cellulose, polyacrylonitrile, or polysulfone materials. Blood passes along the inside of the hollow fiber, with the outside of the hollow fiber open to siphon drainage or negative pressure created by a vacuum suction. The TMP forces created by the movement of blood through the fibers and UF pressure force plasma water and dissolved solutes through the pores in the synthetic material. The pore size of hollow-fiber ultrafiltrators varies among manufacturers but is generally between 30 and 40 angstroms. The wall thickness of the hollow fiber is around 40 μm, and the diameter of the fiber reaches 200 μm. Other factors that influence UF rates include the rate of blood flow through the device, the RBC and protein concentrations, and the temperature of the perfusate passing through the device.

There are few contraindications to hemoconcentration with an ultrafiltrator. As with any nonendothelialized material, biocompatibility becomes an important issue. Leukopenia and complement activation have both been reported when blood is exposed to cellulosic membrane material.[308,309] Excessive TMP may lead to increased RBC trauma and release of plasma-free hemoglobin. When concentrating the pump contents, care must be taken during reinfusion because of the retention of heparin in the hemoconcentrated product. The heterogenous molecular size of heparin varies the amount of heparin retained in the hemoconcentrate. Strict cost analysis during routine cardiac surgery is difficult to quantify because patients are known to tolerate positive fluid balances of up to 4 L without adverse pathologic effects.[173] Therefore, the benefits of UF in these patients have yet to be established.

Modified Ultrafiltration

In 1991, Naik et al[310] described a modification to the technique of UF that has since been extensively applied to pediatric patients undergoing cardiac surgery. Nearly 75% of all pediatric centers in North America routinely use MUF for neonate, infant, and pediatric cardiac surgery.[311] Pediatric patients are thought to be more susceptible to the injurious effects of fluid overloading and may benefit from this technique because of the greater reoperation rate and use of profound and deep hypothermia seen in pediatric cardiac surgery. The technique is applied after CPB and allows the UF of both the circuit contents and the patient. The timing of MUF is critical and permits a rapid increase in patient hematocrit by the removal of plasma water.[312] The results associated with MUF have been very encouraging and have included reductions in postoperative morbidity,[313] reduced blood loss and blood utilization,[310,314] reduced inflammatory mediators,[315,316] and improvements in myocardial function[317] and cerebral oxygenation.[314]

MUF generally is performed shortly after termination of CPB and is completed with a typical ultrafiltrator. In pediatric operations, these devices are routinely set up and primed together with the entire ECC. The ultrafiltrator is placed in-line at a point distal to the membrane oxygenator with the inlet of the device connected to the arterial line and the outlet connected to the venous return line (Figure 29-29). An RP controls the flow rate through the MUF circuit and is located in a parallel circuit between the arterial and venous cannulae. Such a configuration allows conventional UF to take place during the CPB procedure. On separation from CPB, the patient becomes the source for blood for MUF by clamping both the arterial and venous lines proximal to the MUF circuit, draining from the arterial cannula, and reinfusing directly into the venous cannula. The remaining pump contents also are concentrated during MUF and serve as a volume replacement for the removed plasma water. Blood flows during MUF vary with patient size and hemodynamic stability.

During MUF, there is an increase in mean arterial pressure (MAP) that may be related to changes in SVR associated with increasing

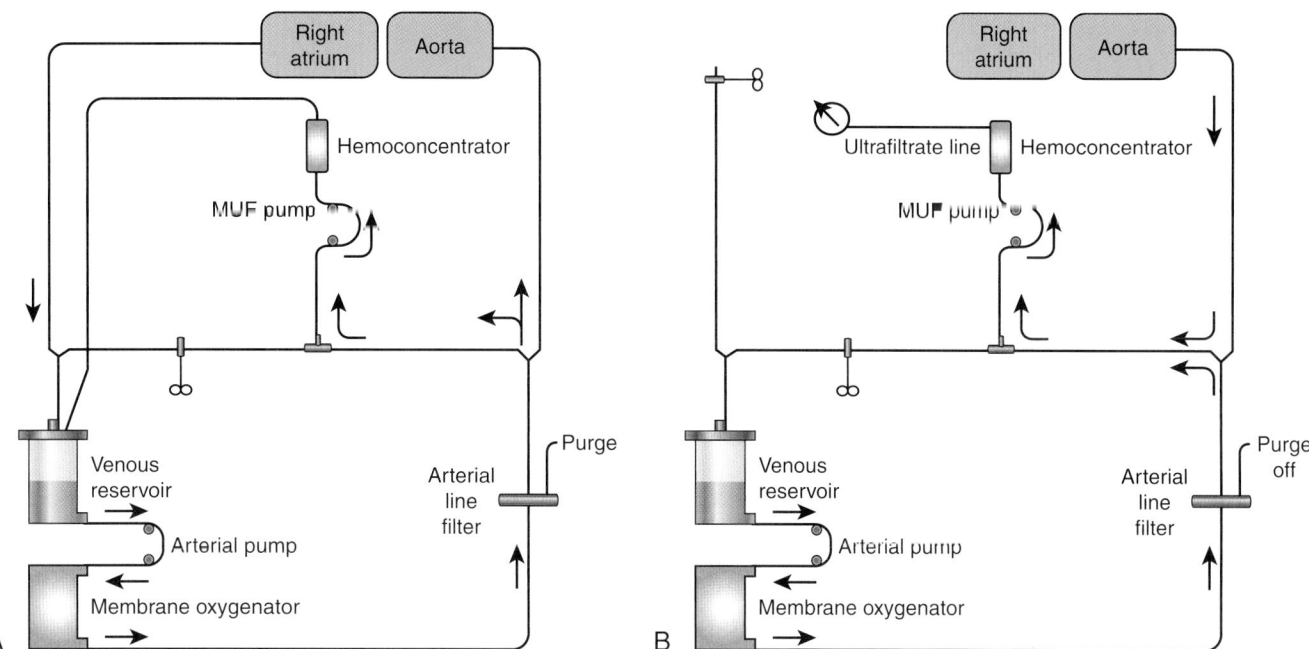

Figure 29-29 Modified ultrafiltration (MUF) circuit used for pediatric cardiac surgery. *A*, Conventional ultrafiltration. *B*, MUF. *(From Darling EM, Shearer IR, Nanry C, et al: Modified ultrafiltration in pediatric cardiopulmonary bypass. J Extra Corpor Technol 26:205, 1994.)*

blood viscosity and via the removal of vasoactive substances.[314,318] The obvious benefit of MUF is the removal of plasma water and the concentration of cellular and acellular elements of blood. However, a number of investigators have shown that UF reduces the production of other potential harmful substances including cytokines and endogenous pyrogens.[316,319] This reduction in number is independent of the effects of hemoconcentration and is instead related to a reduction in the whole-body inflammatory response associated with CPB.[316] The benefits of MUF are accentuated when aggressive UF is utilized during the rewarming period of CPB. This is more than likely a result of the removal of the activated complement fragment C3a, which is easily sieved in the ultrafiltrate.[316] Patients treated with MUF have been shown to have a significantly faster rate of pulmonary function recovery than nonultrafiltrated patients, which may be because of a leukocyte stability and a reduced degranulation of polymorphonuclear neutrophils in the pulmonary capillaries.[316,319]

COATED CIRCUITS

Bypass-induced coagulopathy represents one of the most prevalent pathophysiologic events associated with the exposure of blood to foreign surfaces.[320] Identifying patients at risk for development of postoperative coagulopathies has long challenged clinicians involved with cardiac surgery. Abnormal postoperative bleeding usually is classified as resulting from a preexisting coagulopathy, acquired hemostatic deficiencies, or inadequate surgical hemostasis (although a single patient can suffer from all of the above maladies). The activation of various humoral and cellular systems is associated with the exposure of blood to negatively charged foreign surfaces, with arguably the primary causative factor related to platelet dysfunction.[321–324] It has long been thought that, during ECC, thrombin formation is initiated through contact activation with factor XII (Hageman factor), with subsequent activation of the intrinsic pathway of coagulation.[325] However, recent research has shown that activation of tissue factor pathway and the extrinsic limb play an important role in the stimulation of thrombin during CPB.[326] The bypass circuit is composed of various synthetic materials, including polypropylene, polyvinylchloride, stainless steel and/or anodized aluminum, Dacron, and various plasticizers, all of which evoke contact activation of platelets, granulocytes, and proteins

associated with the intrinsic pathway. The pathologic events associated with ECC-induced complement activation are poorly understood,[327] although potent mediators such as C3a, C4a, and C5a are thought to play a major role in postbypass whole-body inflammation[328,329] (see Chapter 31).

Surface coatings play a role in the interface between the blood and the circuit components. Attenuation of the inflammatory and coagulation pathways should translate into decreased postoperative morbidity directly related to platelet dysfunction, bleeding complications, and end-organ damage. The desire to avoid anticoagulation of patients undergoing extensive thoracic aortic surgery led to the first reported use of a shunt with a graphite-benzalkonium-heparin coating by Gott et al.[330] Heparin-coating of the CPB circuit was originally intended to supplant systemic anticoagulation with heparin. Subsequently, this concept of eliminating systemic heparin was dismissed, and a strategy combining the use of low-dose systemic heparin with a heparin-coated CPB circuit was introduced.[331–335] In vitro and in vivo studies of these surfaces demonstrated reductions in coagulation and systemic inflammatory processes. Numerous studies have been conducted to evaluate the effectiveness of heparin-treated surfaces compared with circuits without heparin coatings.[336–361] Most studies have shown evidence of reduced platelet activation,[340–343] reductions in inflammation characterized by complement activation,[344–351] and improvements in clinical outcomes including bleeding and transfusions,[352–354] pulmonary function,[355,356] and cognitive function.[357–359] One randomized trial in patients undergoing redo CABG surgery showed no differences in biomarkers of inflammation or differences in blood loss and transfusion.[360] A larger randomized trial from the same center, which included redo valve patients, suggested that heparin-coated circuits imparted benefits including a trend of fewer reoperations for bleeding (0% vs. 4.0%; $P = 0.058$) in CABG patients, significantly fewer major bleeding episodes (1.2% vs. 5.4%; $P = 0.035$), and significantly lower blood transfusion requirements in the intensive care unit ($P = 0.013$).[361] The authors further commented that the material-independent blood activation (e.g., blood-air interface and cardiotomy suction) may have blunted the total effect of the heparin-coated surface (HCS).

Unfortunately, most of the studies were small and substantially different in anticoagulation management with heparin, the use of a partially or completely coated circuits, the method by which cardiotomy blood was managed, different heparin coatings, and variations in measuring different end points across studies. The heterogeneity of the randomized trials related to heparin coatings precludes the use of meta-analysis as a method of summarizing the effectiveness of these circuits.[49,336] Stammers et al[336] used weighted means in an effort to summarize the effects of 27 randomized controlled trials of heparin-coated circuits that included 1515 patients. The authors concluded that heparin-coated circuits have shown statistically better results than similar noncoated circuits by decreasing hospital costs attributable to shorter intensive care unit length of stay and bleeding-related complications; and further, that immunologic factors were maintained better with the use of the Carmeda-coated circuits, whereas hematologic factors, excluding platelet count, favored the Duraflo II heparin coating. Two new heparin coatings have been developed: Hyaluronan-coated heparin coating (GBSTM Coating; Gish Biomedical, Rancho Santa Margarita, CA) and Bioline (Maquet); however, comparative studies of these surfaces are promising but limited.[362]

Numerous surface modifications rendering the CPB surfaces more thromboresistant and biologically inert including X-Coating PMEA (poly-(2-methoxyethyl acrylate); Terumo Cardiovascular), SMARxT (Sorin Biomedical), P.H.I.S. I.O. phosphorylcholine inert surface (Sorin Group), Softline heparin-free synthetic polymer (Maquet), and Safeline synthetic-immobilized albumin (Maquet) are commercially available. Preliminary findings indicate that these surfaces provide some improvements, including reduction of platelet activation, leukocyte activation, bradykinin release, and, to some extent, reduction in the release of cytokines compared with noncoated surfaces.[363-367] Gu et al[368] compared circuits with the SMA coating with noncoated circuits and reported improved platelet preservation and function, but no difference in complement activation. Ereth et al[369] compared hematocrit, leukocyte count, platelet count, terminal complement complex, complement activation, myeloperoxidase, β-thromboglobulin, prothrombin fragment 1.2, plasmin-antiplasmin, heparin concentration, activated coagulation time, fibrinogen, blood loss, and blood-product usage in 36 cardiac surgery patients randomized to a trillium-coated circuit or an uncoated circuit. No significant differences were observed between the trillium-coated and uncoated group. Ferraris et al[49] concluded that "heparin-coated bypass circuits (oxygenator alone or the entire circuit) are not unreasonable for blood conservation (Class IIb, Level of evidence B)." Similarly, Shann et al[370] have stated, "Reduction of circuit surface and the use of biocompatible surface-modified circuits might be useful; effective in reducing the systemic inflammatory response (Class IIA, Level of Evidence B)."

Heparin-coating, or bonding, of extracorporeal circuit surfaces (HCSs) increases the hemocompatibility of nonendothelialized substances.[322,371,372] The specific benefits of HCS center on a reduction in the activation of humoral protein systems involved in hemostasis and complement systems, together with a benign deposition of platelets and protein on the extracorporeal surface.[373] Bound heparin inhibits the binding of factors Xa, IIa, and XII, inhibiting thrombus formation by restricting the initiation of coagulation.[374,375] Several authors have shown a reduction in granulocyte activation by reduced liberation of primary granule proteins (myeloperoxidase, lactoferrin) during in vitro whole-blood circulation in HCS circuits.[322,376] The amelioration of blood-surface interactions through the use of HCS may reflect similar responses seen in vivo at the endothelial lining of the vasculature.[372] Palatianos et al[377] examined the effect of HCS on platelet preservation in a pig model of ECC, finding no reduction in platelet consumption or platelet count when HCS were used during CPB periods of 3 hours. However, their model did not include functional studies of the residual platelets, nor did they report results of hemostatic differences after ECC. In a similar animal model using calves during CPB with HCS, Tong et al[378] were able to show superior platelet preservation and function compared with noncoated bypass circuits. Fibrinopeptide levels were reduced in the HCS group, and there was no evidence of thrombus formation in any of the coated circuits.

Once blood comes in contact with HCS, AT III attaches to the bound heparin in an accelerated fashion. Thrombin then combines with AT III,

forming an inactivated complex that leaves the HCS, enabling the process to be repeated.[379] HCSs have been evaluated in various clinical settings that have included ECMO,[379] hepatic transplantation,[380] aortic aneurysm repair,[381] pulmonary artery catheters,[382] and during routine cardiac surgery. The efficacy of heparinless bypass may be especially evident when used to treat patients suffering from hypothermic exposure or in trauma patients suffering from head or severe soft-tissue injuries.

The use of HCS may result in the reevaluation of heparin therapy necessary for systemic anticoagulation during certain ECC procedures.[383-385] Reducing heparin levels has the desired effect of limiting the potential for postoperative coagulopathy that is due to heparin-related platelet defects and heparin reappearance after protamine administration (heparin-rebound effect). This may be especially attractive in patients at increased risk for adverse sequelae of heparin exposure (i.e., heparin-induced thrombocytopenia, neurosurgical procedures, protamine intolerances). In some studies, the reduced level of heparinization resulted in lower postoperative blood loss.[383,385] Aldea et al[386] have shown in patients undergoing CABG surgery that when HCSs were used in conjunction with lower heparinization protocols, there was a marked improvement in hemostasis, as well as reduced blood loss and transfusion rates. These benefits were accentuated in patients who were at a greater risk because of the urgent need for care.

Because heparin is the primary means of anticoagulation during CPB, any method that suggests reducing circulating levels must be critically evaluated.[387] Kuitunen et al[388] prospectively evaluated HCS in patients undergoing CPB who received either a reduced heparinization protocol (100 IU/kg) or a full heparinization dose (300 IU/kg). These authors found that thrombin was formed during CPB, and that there was an increased risk for microembolic, intravascular, and circuit clotting with low heparin levels. This was also confirmed in an in vitro model in which whole blood exposed to an extracorporeal heparin-coated circuit with low heparin concentrations demonstrated evidence of contact activation after 120 minutes of simulated bypass.[389] In a retrospective analysis of patients undergoing first-time valve surgery, Shapira et al[390] compared patients with HCS who had received low (100 IU/kg) heparinization with patients with normal (300 IU/kg) heparinization and non-HCS circuits. The heparin-coated group had significantly better clinical outcomes and lower allogeneic blood transfusions than the conventional group but also had an increased risk for early valve thrombosis. For this reason, the authors recommended using full-dose heparinization protocols in patients undergoing valve surgery with HCS.

One of the major difficulties in developing HCS was the bonding technique used to attach heparin to the various components used during bypass. An early technique for heparin bonding was described by Gott[391] and involved the substance tridodecylmethylammonium chloride (TDMAC). This method of ionic bonding is currently used in the production of shunts for aneurysm surgery and hepatic transplantation (Gott shunts; Sherwood Medical, St. Louis, MO).[380]

The difficulty in bonding heparin to extracorporeal circuits is compounded by both the diversity of synthetic compounds used during bypass and the geometric variations of cardiovascular devices that may produce areas of stagnation and flow stasis. In addition, the benefits associated with HCS are dependent on heparin being minimally eluted from the surface after contact with blood. The quantity of surface-bound heparin necessary to inhibit clot formation generally is greater than $1.0 \, mg/cm^2$ of circuit surface area but is dependent on the distribution of heparin on the surface. It is well-known that heparin is not a single unique compound, but rather is a heterogenous class of mucopolysaccharides, which also may influence binding characteristics.

Quaternary ammonium salts have been used to bond heparin ionically to synthetic surfaces, because heparin forms a highly nondissociable complex with quaternary ammonium salt. One manufacturer of HCS (Bentley Duraflow II; Baxter Health Care Corporation, Irvine, CA) uses a water-insoluble complex between heparin (porcine intestinal mucosa) and alkylbenzyldimethylammonium chloride. When ionically bound heparin surfaces are exposed to blood, there is an initial early

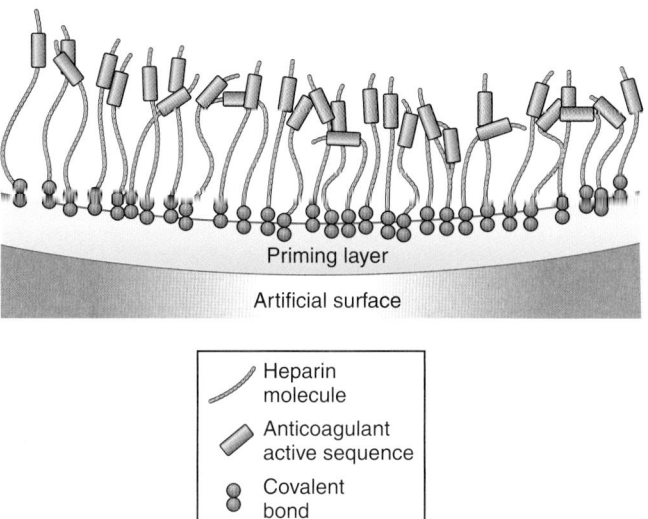

Figure 29-30 **Carmeda Bio-Active Surface.** Covalent bonded heparin coating. *(Courtesy of Carmeda, Stockholm, Sweden)*

5% elution of bound heparin when blood first contacts the surface, but the remaining concentration stays stable for many hours. Synthetic materials that have been used successfully in covalent bonding include silicone and natural rubber, polypropylene, and polyethylene.

Heparin contains a hydroxyl group, carboxylic acid, and an amino group, which are all suited for covalent attachment to artificial surfaces. Covalent bonding of heparin has also been termed *end-point attachment of heparin,* in which an intermediate layer of substrate is first deposited onto the surface to which heparin is affixed by binding to a primary amine.[379] Partially degraded heparin is covalently end-point attached to extracorporeal circuits by a process developed by engineers from the Carmeda Corporation (Carmeda Bio-Active Surface; Carmeda, Stockholm, Sweden; Figure 29-30).[379,381]

The effectiveness of HCSs is dependent on blood flow dynamics within the circuit, with thrombus inhibition related to the ratio of circuit surface area to blood volume.[392,393] HCSs are effective only when exposed to blood; therefore, blood must be kept in constant circulation. Systemic heparinization still would be necessary to decrease clot formation in stagnant or low-flow capillary beds within the body, such as occurs in the pulmonary circulation. Therefore, it is not likely that HCS will totally supplant the use of systemic heparinization. However, the use of heparin bonding to these circuits may necessitate the reevaluation of the total concentration of heparin necessary for systemic heparinization and may result in the identification of a more controlled protocol for the administration of heparin.[394]

PERFUSION PRACTICES

Minimally Invasive Cardiac Surgery

The changing economics of health care have forced the reevaluation of how techniques and technologies are utilized in the delivery of care. Despite the proven benefits of the heart-lung machine as a resource that enabled cardiac surgery to evolve, the morbidity associated with its use continues to plague clinicians. In a recent survey of cardiac surgeons, the question of which procedure would be preferable to eliminate, median sternotomy or CPB, more than 80% responded with the latter.[395] The development of endoscopic instruments and high-resolution video equipment has shaped the conduct of minimally invasive surgery and changed the conventional wisdom by which surgical practice is directed. The most promising results in applying these techniques in cardiac surgery have been seen in patients requiring CABG surgery. When the procedure is performed through a left anterior minithoracotomy, it is designated as minimally invasive

direct coronary artery bypass grafting. The major benefit to patients who undergo this procedure has been described as being cosmetic, at least when comparing single-vessel disease patients with those undergoing conventional therapy.[396] Although one of the primary goals of minimal invasion is the avoidance of the heart-lung machine, there are situations in which ECC is used to support the patient. This is true in patients with decreased ventricular function or in whom it is necessary to manipulate the heart for posterior access. The degree of involvement will vary from institution to institution, but in general these processes involve specialized cannulae that are most often placed transfemorally, with venous drainage accomplished with a CP (KVAD).[29,30]

When cardiac surgery is performed in patients without the use of a conventional midline sternotomy, it is referred to as *keyhole surgery.* When this technique is combined with CPB, it is referred to as port-access cardiac surgery and has been used for both CABG and valve surgery.[397,398] The success of this operative technique is dependent on a number of factors including surgical expertise and the correct utilization of specialty instruments and cannulae (Heartport EndoCPB; Heartport, Redwood City, CA) (Figures 29-20 and 29-31). The primary cannula is termed an *endoaortic clamp* that has been specifically designed to occlude the aorta, deliver cardioplegia, and vent the ascending aorta. In this way, myocardial protection can be achieved while enabling the surgeon to work in a quiescent, flaccid heart. The endoaortic clamp is positioned under fluoroscopic and echocardiographic guidance. Improper positioning can result in inadequate myocardial protection, left ventricular distention, or occlusion of the arch vessels.[398] A pulmonary artery venting catheter is placed through the jugular vein and used to assist ventricular unloading. The final cannula is a coronary sinus cardioplegia cannula that is used for retrograde cardioplegia administration (see Chapter 28).

The venous return is augmented by the use of KVAD and a CP. Negative pressure is measured at the inlet port to the CP and is regulated by controlling pump inertia.[29] The KVAD pressure is maintained between −50 and −80 mm Hg, which ensures adequate flow rates. The outlet of the CP is connected directly to an integrated cardiotomy/venous reservoir, which, in turn, is connected to an arterial pump and the oxygenator (see Figure 29-31). Patient management during port-access cardiac surgery is performed using similar protocols to those of conventional bypass. Additional monitoring is necessary for the CP and various cannulae that are used to vent the heart and to administer cardioplegia. Once the endoaortic clamp is correctly positioned, the balloon is inflated with a mixture of contrast media and saline, and cardioplegia solution infused. During antegrade cardioplegia administration, the aortic root pressure will increase to between 60 and 90 mm Hg, and a pressure gradient of 20 to 40 mm Hg will be seen with the MAP. After cardioplegia administration, the aortic root vent is started and a −80 mm Hg pressure relief valve ensures that excessive negative pressure does not occur.

Weaning from CPB is accomplished in a normal fashion with the KVAD siphon gradually reduced, which diverts blood from the heart-lung machine into the patient. The aortic root and endopulmonary vents are removed, the femoral vessels repaired, and the thoracic incision sites are closed in a standard fashion. Although limited data have thus far been collected to assess this technology, it offers the surgeon a unique ability to perform minimally invasive surgery in a controlled environment with high-resolution stereoscopic visualization.

Monitoring during Cardiopulmonary Bypass

Technologic advancements in physiologic monitoring have made the process of CPB safe, comprehensive, and reliable. Monitoring devices measure both physiologic and mechanical functions of the patient–device interface. From a historic perspective, perfusionists had few devices that functioned as monitors relaying information other than hemodynamic data. Technologic advancement has generated new classes of devices for monitoring that at one time either were cost-prohibitive or viewed by perfusionists as superfluous. However, two

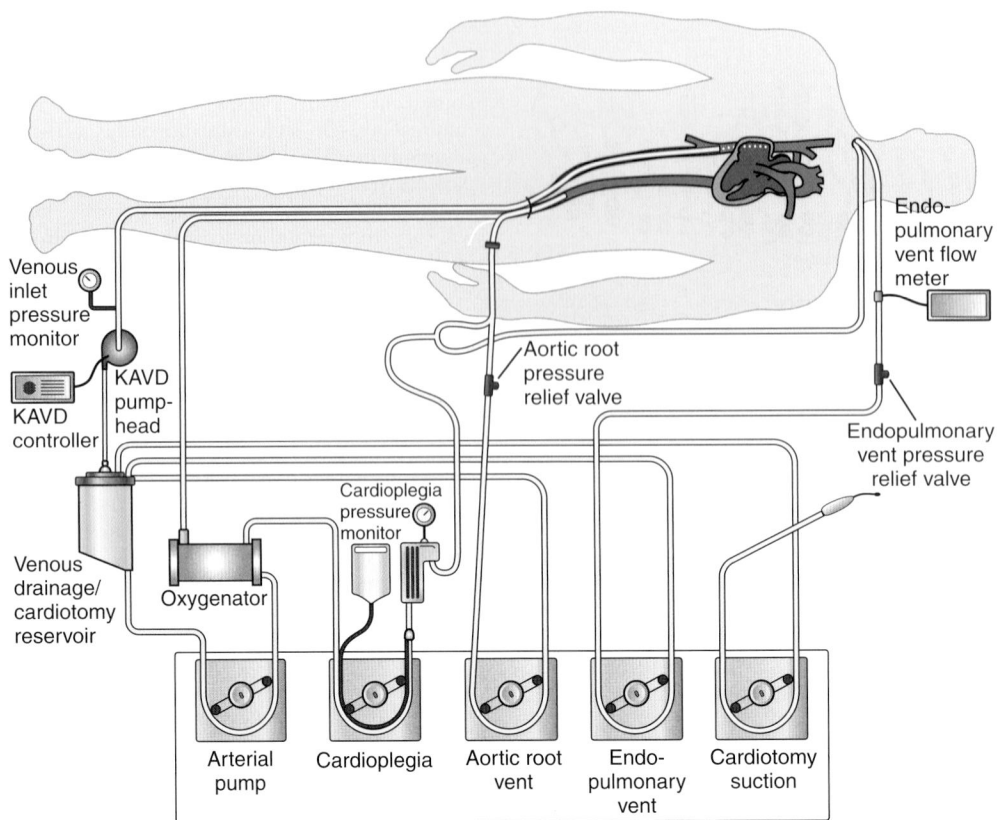

Figure 29-31 Circuit diagram for the endovascular port-access cardiopulmonary bypass system. (*From Toomasian JM, Williams DL, Colvin SB, et al: Perfusion during coronary and mitral valve surgery utilizing minimally invasive port-access technology.* J Extra Corpor Technol 29:66, 1997.)

developments occurred in the field that have greatly increased the safe conduct of CPB. First, the quantity and quality of information produced during a typical procedure increased and became more specific and sensitive in reflecting patient status. Second, the tremendous resurgence in research on the pathophysiologic events associated with CPB shifted the performance of perfusionists from relying primarily on instinctive reasoning to relying on deduction. This could only be accomplished through stricter methods of monitoring and analyzing both the patient's and machine's response to CPB. This section highlights the major variables monitored in the operation of the heart-lung machine.

After ensuring that an appropriate level of anticoagulation has been achieved, the perfusionist initiates CPB. Undoubtedly, the most important assessment of CPB after initiation of perfusion is the function of the oxygenator. This can be compared with establishing an airway in a patient before initiating basic life support. Without the proper delivery of oxygen to the venous blood and the removal of carbon dioxide, the arterial pump serves no purpose. Traditionally, isolated blood analysis was performed at a distant site from the operating room and provided the clinician with a historic marker of oxygenator and patient performance. Unfortunately, this event is only a "snapshot" of one point during CPB and will not reflect ongoing changes or trends in the operation. Routine sampling of blood gases normally occurs every 15 to 30 minutes on bypass, and in the event of oxygenator failure, periods of hypoxemia and/or hypercapnia could result during those intervals. For this reason, the use of inline blood gas monitoring is imperative and should not be considered as a "luxury" because of its added cost.[399] Indeed, in this litigious society, it is questionable not to use readily available technologies that may reduce unnecessary patient risk.

Optical fluorescence technology has made reliable in-line blood gas and electrolyte monitoring a reality, providing minute-to-minute accurate surveillance of these parameters during CPB.[400,401] In-line

blood gas monitoring allows for real-time monitoring of the "adequacy of perfusion," and one device currently available for use in CPB is the CDI500 (Terumo Cardiovascular Systems, Ann Arbor, MI; Figures 29-32 and 29-33). The CDI500 provides continuous real-time blood gas and electrolyte measurements for Po_2, Pco_2, pH, HCO_3^-, and K^+. The enhanced safety conferred by the use of this technology has been documented in the literature.[402] A survey of anesthesiologists in the United Kingdom and Ireland in 1994 concerning monitoring device utilization revealed that 98% of the 42 hospitals surveyed intermittently monitored blood-gas tensions during cardiac surgery, and 33% utilized continuous blood-gas monitoring.[403] In the United States, it has been estimated that approximately 40% of institutions utilize continuous blood-gas monitoring during CPB.[399,404,405] Practice surveys indicate that the use of in-line monitoring is increasingly widespread.[406-408]

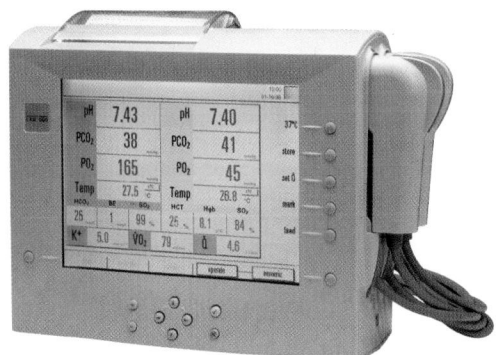

Figure 29-32 **CDI500 continuous blood gas and saturation monitor.** Measures arterial and venous pH, Pco_2, Po_2, potassium, hemoglobin saturation, hematocrit, and hemoglobin. (*Courtesy of Terumo Cardiovascular Systems, Ann Arbor, MI.*)

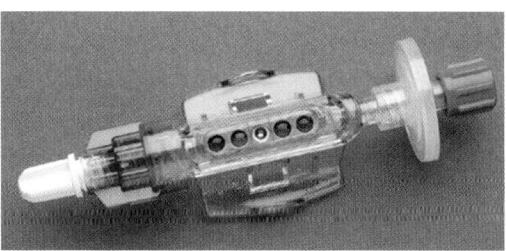

Figure 29-33 CDI500 sensor. Blood flows through the sensor so that continuous monitoring may be accomplished. *(Courtesy of Terumo Cardiovascular Systems, Ann Arbor, MI)*

TABLE 29-3	Reasons for Monitoring during Cardiopulmonary Bypass
Assessment of oxygenator and/or device performance	
Calculation of patient conditions	
Oxygen delivery	
Oxygen extraction	
Oxygen consumption	
Carbon dioxide production	
Analysis of therapeutic interventions	
Quality assurance	

However, approximately two thirds of the cardiac surgical centers worldwide do not use this technology. Ottens et al[409] suggested that this may be attributed to the lack of scientific evidence and cost associated with the use of this technology.

Arterial blood oxygen saturation always should be maintained at greater than 99%, with Po_2 tensions between 150 and 250 mm Hg. Arterial Pco_2 levels will vary depending on whether alpha-stat or pH-stat blood-gas management is used (see Chapter 28). Currently, there are several devices for measuring oxygenator gas exchange performance, including in-line continuous monitors. These monitors must meet basic criteria before they can be viewed as safe and accurate (Table 29-2). They must possess a rapid response time, be as accurate as standard blood-gas analysis methods, be unaffected by hemodilution and temperature, and be easy to use. Alpha-stat blood gas management is achieved by maintaining electrochemical neutrality of blood as temperature declines, by keeping the pH alkalotic during hypothermic perfusion. During alpha-stat management, the rule of thumb for controlling carbon dioxide is to maintain Pco_2 levels equal to the temperature of arterial blood. For pH-stat management, the Pco_2 is kept constant at 40 mm Hg, and the pH at 7.4 at all temperatures. Therefore, when blood gases are temperature-uncorrected, a respiratory acidosis is seen. The venous oxygen saturation (Svo_2) will vary during the operative procedure depending on the metabolic state of the patient but is generally maintained at around 80%.

Clinical decisions for using in-line blood gas monitors ultimately must be determined by the ability of these devices to improve patient outcomes with a value that exceeds that of the total costs associated with use. Complications arising from the cardiac surgical procedure remain significant in terms of the expense associated with their management.[410,411] The improvement in patient outcomes by the incorporation of a technology assumes that the intended problem is significant enough to warrant an intervention, a fact not always clear in the manufacturing and marketing of medical devices. For a practice to qualify as a standard of care, there must be some evidence that failure to incorporate the technique potentially could result in patient harm. Some of the reasons for monitoring during CPB are listed in Table 29-3.

Although overall mortality associated with CPB has declined over the past several decades, an increase in death (7.2% to 19.6%) resulting from neurologic injury has been shown.[412] Gill and Murkin[413] reported

TABLE 29-2	Characteristics of an Ideal Point-of-Care Monitoring System for Cardiopulmonary Bypass
High degree of accuracy, precision, and reliability	
Rapid response time	
Minimally affected by hemodynamic conditions	
Wide parameter measurement range	
Easy calibration and alignment processes	
Stable measurement ranges (low drift) over 6 hours	
Self-contained instrumentation with minimal disposable use	
High degree of biocompatibility	
Cost-effective	
Input and output data-handling capabilities	

on post-CPB neuropsychologic dysfunction and have implicated cerebral microemboli generated from the bypass circuit as a major source of morbidity. These authors emphasized that microembolic phenomena are generated secondarily to alterations in bypass temperature, oxygenator type, pH management, and the use of arterial line filtration, and that modifications of these parameters reduce the overall incidence of neurologic dysfunction.

Acid-base alterations during CPB have been studied intensely both in animal and in human models, and the results are equivocal. Neurologic dysfunction has been reported in patients maintained using the pH-stat blood gas regimen, which more than likely resulted from the ensuing cerebral hyperemia consistent with the respiratory acidosis created during this condition.[414] This was confirmed by a clinical study in which 70 CABG patients were randomized either to an alpha-stat or pH-stat protocol and evaluated via neuropsychologic assessment at a mean of 42 days after the procedure.[415] The authors found that patients maintained by the pH-stat strategy had significantly impaired cerebral autoregulation and neuropsychologic impairment, when compared with their alpha-stat counterparts. Nevin et al[416] have shown that hypocapnia during CPB also results in neurologic injury, whereas others have been unable to confirm that either acid-base strategy for hypothermic perfusion resulted in significant differences.[417] Fullerton et al[418] have shown that respiratory acidemia in patients with pulmonary hypertension from mitral stenosis results in exacerbation of pulmonary hypertension, and that a hypocarbic state may benefit these patients.

The effects of CPB-induced hyperoxia have been thought to exacerbate the pathophysiologic events associated with free oxygen radical formation and GME. In vivo animal studies have further confirmed that hyperoxia induces a reduction in functional capillary density caused by perturbations in leukocyte adherence to the vascular endothelium.[419] In a prospective, randomized study of 48 patients, half of whom had oxygen tensions maintained during CPB between 190 and 300 mm Hg, and half between 75 and 112 mm Hg, patient outcomes were significantly affected by the hyperoxic condition.[420] The patients in the hyperoxic group had decreased RBC rheology, increased bleeding diathesis that required greater transfusion rates, longer ventilator times, and a greater post-CPB complication rate when compared with the normoxic group. Hyperoxemia also has been shown to alter microcirculatory response during both normothermic and hypothermic CPB but was most pronounced during normothermia with increased vascular resistance and a decline in oxygen consumption.[421] A recent randomized, controlled trial involving 67 cyanotic infants found that low-to-normal oxygen tension at the onset of CPB is associated with reduced myocardial damage, reduced oxidative stress, and reduced cerebral and hepatic injury compared with hyperoxic CPB.[422]

The benefits of venous blood-gas monitoring have been well accepted in cardiovascular medicine, and the information gained from such assessment has been used to guide therapeutic interventions in numerous clinical situations including critical and intensive care, internal medicine, and surgical services. Changes in both venous Pco_2 and Po_2 levels have been shown to correlate well with changes in global tissue perfusion.[423] During CPB, the importance of mixed venous oxygen saturation monitoring cannot be overemphasized. This parameter has global utility and is the one parameter universally monitored during most extracorporeal procedures. The mixed venous oxygen saturation

TABLE 29-4	Point-of-Care Monitoring Devices

Online monitors or analyzers
Inline monitors
Intra-arterial monitors
Exhaust gas monitoring (capnography)
Transcutaneous monitors (pulse oximetry)

is used to calculate whole-body oxygen consumption when, according to the Fick equation, perfusion flow and the oxygen content of arterial blood are also known. As a cautionary note, the interpretation of the mixed venous oxygen saturation must be made with a sound knowledge of any patient conditions that could overestimate or underestimate oxygen delivery and uptake, such as in the presence of anatomic or physiologic shunts, or concentrations of abnormal hemoglobin types. It is beyond the scope of this chapter to review all the currently available in-line blood gas monitors. Readers are referred elsewhere for this information (Table 29-4).[424]

The simplest device for measuring oxygen saturation of blood is an optically coupled dual-wavelength (660 and 900 nm) oximeter that reflects oxygen saturation in flowing blood (Bentley Oxysat Meter; Baxter Health Care Corporation, Irvine, CA).[425,426] The device consists of an optical transmission cell that can be placed in both the arterial and venous lines and uses light-emitting diodes and a photosensitive transistor to measure saturations. Limitations of on-line saturation monitoring are seen when blood flow is less than 100 mL/min, at which the accuracy greatly declines and the oximeter reads falsely high. Also, simultaneous display of arterial and venous values cannot be performed with this device.

A second type of blood-gas monitor uses a microprocessor coupled via two fiberoptic cables with disposable flow-through cells and sensors that have both arterial and venous monitoring capabilities (CDI; Cardiovascular Devices Inc., 3M Health Care, Irvine, CA; see Figures 29-32 and 29-33).[425,427] The sensors contain pads of fluorescent chemicals, which emit light in response to gas and hydrogen ion changes, with intensity of the light correlated to concentration. The microprocessor then uses predetermined algorithms to calculate bicarbonate levels and base deficit on the arterial side and Svo_2. Calibration of the microsensor is achieved before each operation using tonometered gases. This process takes approximately 20 minutes but can be bypassed and a single-point calibration performed in the event of an emergency.

An alternate technology is the use of on-line systems for blood-gas analysis (Gem Systems; Instrumentation Laboratories, Ann Arbor, MI).[428,429] These machines differ from in-line monitors in a number of ways. First, they provide discrete sampling of blood from either an arterial or a venous line. Therefore, they can be used independently of the heart-lung machine and do not require blood flow through cells and sensors for operation. They also function by continuously correcting for sensor drifts through automatic washings and calibrations. In addition to measuring Po_2, Pco_2, and pH, they also measure ionized calcium, potassium, sodium, and hematocrit.

As with the use of any device, standards must be set to ensure that performance is accurate and reproducible, incorporating sensitivity and specificity. In the operating room, these standards are usually set by blood-gas analyzer machines calibrated and maintained by medical technologists or pathologists according to national regulations and guidelines. The accuracy of in-line monitors compared with standard blood-gas analyzers recently has come under question.[429-431] Nevertheless, they provide important information on blood gas and acid-base trends, which are subject to rapid change during CPB.

If inadequate oxygenator gas exchange is suspected, several immediate actions should be performed in troubleshooting the problem. The first step is to check that the gas line is properly connected to the gas inlet port of the oxygenator, and to ensure that there are no obstructions, kinks, or leaks in the line impeding the delivery of ventilating gas. An important preoperative check would be to ensure that the disposable 0.2-mm gas line filter is set in the proper direction, and that gas passes freely through the filter. Second, the air-oxygen mixer (blender) and flowmeter should be examined to ensure that they are functioning properly. A breach in the gas delivery system may be exacerbated by the use of excessive vacuum on the anesthetic gas scavenging system.[432] The integrity of the gas delivery system may be tested by temporarily occluding the gas supply line near the oxygenator and observing the increase in the gas system pressure on a manometer or by observing a decline in the level of the gas flow meter's indicator ball. Use of a suction bulb to test the gas supply system is an alternative method.[433] Algorithms for solving poor gas exchange have been described.[434] The placement of an in-line oxygen monitor in the gas delivery line will reflect the Fio_2 of the ventilating gas. If a blender malfunction or gas supply leak is suspected, the problem may be mitigated by attaching a separate supply of 100% oxygen (i.e., a regulated E cylinder of oxygen) directly to the oxygenator gas inlet port. This maneuver will exclude any breach in the gas delivery system, including the oxygen and air sources, the gas blender and flowmeter, and anesthetic vaporizer. If inadequate gas exchange continues, additional checks should include the following: the oxygen consumptive rate of the patient (reflecting metabolic activity), whether the oxygenator was correctly sized to the patient, and oxygenator failure (or any combination of the three). An oxygenator may fail because of deposition of clotted blood or platelets on the membrane surface that interfere with gas exchange. This disruption of the gas exchange surface is characterized by increased pressure excursion across the oxygenator. Measurement of the transmembrane pressure (preoxygenator minus postoxygenator) may be used to confirm this type of malfunction. Separation from CPB and change out of the oxygenator are indicated should poor gas exchange and an increase transmembrane pressure occur. Groom et al[435] described a technique for rapid change-out of an oxygenator during CPB that may be conducted in less than 90 seconds without necessarily discontinuing CPB. Early recognition of an oxygenation problem is paramount because prolonged exposure to hypoxic conditions can cause patient injury. Practice drills aimed at detection and correction of an oxygenator failure should be periodically performed to improve detection and correction of a device failure.

Arguably, the most important parameter measured during CPB is either Svo_2 or venous Po_2.[436-438] In the absence of anatomic or synthetic shunts, the relation between oxygen delivery and uptake is reflected in Svo_2. A further indicator of the adequacy of perfusion is the development of acidosis caused by either a loss of blood buffers or an excess of carbon dioxide. Low Svo_2 values are treated by either increasing the delivery of oxygen to the tissues or decreasing oxygen demand. This is accomplished by decreasing the metabolic rate (through hypothermia or anesthesia), increasing pump flow, or increasing the hemoglobin level of the pump perfusate. Each patient must be assessed individually for the condition causing the decline in SvO_2, with specific treatment administered that best corrects the deficit.[439]

In addition to monitoring oxygenator function and maintaining blood gas homeostasis, the perfusionist is charged with controlling hemodynamic indices of adequate perfusion. What value of MAP provides optimal perfusion remains controversial. The majority of research on target MAP during CPB has centered on cerebral blood flow. However, distant organ and tissue function may be altered by setting standards based on single organ characteristics. Many factors influence cerebral blood flow, including autoregulation,[440] pump flow rate, and acid-base balance.[441,442] It generally is accepted that autoregulation is maintained during CPB when MAP is kept between 30 and 110 mm Hg[440,442] (see Chapter 28). This is true in patients who are neither hypertensive nor suffering from cerebrovascular disease. In both these conditions, standards have yet to be established for MAP control that would ensure adequate perfusion, although most would agree that maintenance of greater perfusion pressures is justified. In the presence of atherosclerosis, the changes in viscosity induced through hemodilution will increase flow to the microcirculation by reducing SVR. Pulsatile CPB will result in increased capillary patency when compared with nonpulsatile perfusion, even at the same MAP; this is discussed in the next section.

Pulsatile versus Nonpulsatile Flow

When designing early extracorporeal systems, engineers and clinicians attempted to mimic the body's normal hemodynamic state. The earliest pumps, therefore, were designed to deliver a pulse waveform and were complicated devices that required specific engineering skills to operate. In the late 1950s and early 1960s, several events led to the decline of pulsatile flow as a preferred method in the conduct of perfusion. These included the complexity of pumping systems and the realization that patients tolerated periods of nonpulsatile flow without significant morbidity. The physiologic benefits of pulsatile flow are a direct function of the transmission of energy into the blood, from which it is transduced to tissue.[443] It is now realized that earlier comparisons between the two methods of CPB were fraught with methodologic insufficiencies that may have artificially negated the beneficial effects of pulsatile perfusion. The elegant studies of Taylor[444] and others[445–449] have resurrected interest in pulsatile perfusion and resulted in a heightened awareness of its potential benefits. Wright[450] summarized the relationship of the human heart and pulsatile flow in transmitting power to the microcirculatory bed to facilitate fluid movement into the tissues.

The two major operational methods used to generate a pulse wave are roller heads and alternating occlusion systems. Pulsatility is produced in a roller head by the pump accelerating during the systolic phase and decelerating in diastole. Alternating occlusion systems, such as those used in VADs and artificial hearts, use intermittent occlusive-phase generators to produce a pulse wave. The physiologic benefits of pulsatile perfusion are related to the geometry of the pulse waveform. These include the rate of rise of flow and/or pressure in the central aorta, as well as the total amplitude of the pulsation.[444,445]

Pulsatile perfusion has been classified by three general theories that attempt to establish quantitative methods of comparison.[444] The theory of *energy-equivalent pressure* (EEP) states that the benefits of a pulse wave are related to the energy content within the pulsation.[445] The pulsatile arterial wave dissipates energy, used to produce the pulse wave, to the tissues:

$$EEP = \int P\,f dT / \int f dT$$

where P = pressure (mm Hg), f = flow (mL/sec), dT = change in time. The increase in energy developed by a pulse waveform is made available to the tissue, which results in maintaining capillary patency, increasing tissue lymph flow, and stimulating cellular metabolism.[467,448] The second theory is that of *capillary critical closing pressure*, which states that peaks of pulsatile systolic pressure will ensure greater flow through the microcirculation by maintaining capillary caliber for greater periods, when compared with nonpulsatile flow. The critical closing pressure at precapillary arterioles, which obliterates tissue perfusion, occurs at higher levels with pulsatile perfusion. Finally, the theory of *neuroendocrine reflex mechanism* is based on the fact that baroreceptors respond to both static and pulsatile aspects of an arterial pressure wave. The baroreceptor mechanism of nonpulsatile perfusion causes a marked increase in discharge frequency of the carotid sinus baroreceptors, inducing reflex vasoconstriction in the systemic circulation.

The benefits of pulsatile perfusion during CPB include increased blood flow in the microcirculation,[447] reduced fluid overloading and "third spacing,"[448] and decreased release of baroreceptor reflex hormones, which limit reflex vasoconstriction.[448] Pulsatile perfusion has been shown to increase renal, cerebral,[447] and pancreatic[446] flow. In a prospective, double-blind study, Murkin et al[451] recently identified nonpulsatile perfusion as a significant risk factor for postoperative morbidity. In a review of pulsatile perfusion, Hornick and Taylor[452] have identified certain high-risk patients as being particularly susceptible to postoperative morbidity when nonpulsatile perfusion techniques are used. They identified patients as being at risk if they presented with any of the following conditions: occult coronary artery disease, significant preexisting atherosclerosis, chronic arterial hypertension, and chronic organ insufficiency. The authors advocated pulsatile perfusion as a treatment of choice.

More than 150 basic science and clinical investigations that directly compared pulsatile and nonpulsatile perfusion have been published. Although there is an extensive body of literature, there remains uncertainty about the effects of pulsatile perfusion on clinical outcomes.[453] Henze et al[454] compared patients undergoing CABG surgery and found no difference in neurologic outcome in patients treated with either pulsatile or nonpulsatile CPB. In a similar study, Azariades et al[455] questioned the benefits of pulsatile flow on the stress-related release of cortisol and were unable to show any differences between patients treated with either pulsatile or nonpulsatile flow. Taggart et al[456] studied pulsatile perfusion and its effects on limiting post-CPB endotoxemia in a prospective randomized study of 60 patients. There were no differences in endotoxin levels, complement fragments, or granulocyte elastase between nonpulsatile or pulsatile perfusion groups at any time. Ohri et al[457] evaluated pulsatile and nonpulsatile perfusion on gastric mucosal perfusion and found that pulsatility showed clinical benefit only during normothermic periods and was lost when moderate (28°C) hypothermia was used (see Chapter 28).

METHODS OF EXTRACORPOREAL CIRCULATION

The techniques involved in the practice of ECC have evolved largely from the conduct of CPB during CABG surgery, valvular surgery, congenital cardiac surgery, or a combination of the three. Applications involving alternate means of ECC transcend the conduct of routine CPB and have included various specialties such as neurosurgery, vascular surgery, and general thoracic surgery. The limitations of incorporating ECC in the treatment of disorders once thought not to be amenable to this process now are being reevaluated because of advances in enhancing the biocompatibility of extracorporeal circuits and components.[458,459] This section focuses on the evaluation of new techniques, as well as the reexamination and elucidation of previously accepted practices.

Left-Heart Bypass

Total CPB is attempted in most situations in which the heart will be rendered quiescent to facilitate surgical manipulation and repair, usually involving the administration of cardioplegia. In certain situations, however, the need to arrest the heart is obviated when the surgical repair can be performed without interfering with normal circulatory flow patterns. An alternate situation also arises when the surgery is performed at some point distant from the heart, through incisions not suitable for normal cannulation sites for CPB. *Left-heart bypass* (LHB) and *right-heart bypass* are terms used to denote the process whereby univentricular diversion of flow is performed by the creation of a parallel circuit to blood flow. Although this definition also serves as a description for a VAD, in the operating room, each term has a specific distinctive meaning, and they are not used interchangeably. LHB is a technique often used in repair of descending thoracic aortic aneurysms (see Chapter 21). Without the use of LHB, cross clamping of the descending aorta results in a tremendous increase in afterload and a decrease in CO, most likely the result of increased ventricular end-diastolic volumes and reduced ejection fractions.[460] The major purpose of LHB is to ensure adequate perfusion to the distal body, which should reduce the potential for paraplegia caused by hypotension and tissue hypoxia.[461,462] The ensuing discussion primarily focuses on LHB because of its predominant use, although right-heart bypass is performed during certain procedures in pediatric cardiac surgery, such as reoperation for right ventricle-to-pulmonary artery conduit replacement.

The term *left-heart bypass (LHB)* is somewhat of a misnomer because it denotes the bypassing of *all* flow through an ECC around the left ventricle. This rarely occurs. Instead, the technique is a form of partial LHB that enables the perfusionist to vary the preload of the left ventricle, thereby controlling the volume of blood ejected into the aorta. This alteration in preload, therefore, directly affects the patient's hemodynamic status and is influenced by the rate at which volume is shifted from the left heart. It has been reported that during LHB with seemingly adequate reduction of preload, ventricular dysfunction, as evidenced by TEE, can occur.[463] The most frequently used applications of LHB include repair of thoracic aneurysms or dissections involving the descending aorta, thoracoabdominal aneurysms,[464] and coarctation of the aorta. The bypass circuit used in LHB is an extremely different variation from that used during total CPB, and these differences must be understood by the anesthesiologist to facilitate patient management.

The most prominent difference in the conduct of partial LHB compared with total CPB is the absence of an oxygenator from the circuit. Therefore, it is impossible to augment the ventilatory capacity of the patient during LHB. Figure 29-34 shows the typical LHB circuitry with the use of a CP as the main drive unit.[461] The entire circuit usually consists of two 6- to 8-foot sections of 3/8-inch polyvinylchloride tubing, which have been attached to the inflow and outflow ports of the centrifugal head. Besides not having an oxygenator, the circuit contains neither a cardiotomy reservoir nor a venous reservoir, so that fluids cannot be added to the circuit. The cannulation sites vary, with the most frequent techniques involving drainage from the LA and return to the femoral artery. Purse-string sutures are placed in either the left atrial appendage or superior pulmonary veins for draining blood from the LA. Left atrial cannula size varies, but in most adult patients, the typical single cannula ranges from 32 Fr to 40 Fr. Alternate cannula locations for draining blood from the heart involve the ascending aorta or the left ventricular apex. Blood is returned to the patient via isolation of the femoral artery by cutdown technique, with retrograde flow into the abdominal aorta. The typical cannula sizes used for femoral artery cannulation range from 16 Fr to 22 Fr. Alternate cannulation sites for the return of blood include the descending thoracic aorta.

Management of the patient during LHB can be accomplished only by a combined effort between the anesthesiologist and perfusionist. The risk for perioperative bleeding is high because of the combined use of prosthetic graft materials and large anastomotic sites.[464] For this reason, minimal anticoagulation is used, with a low dose of systemic heparin to increase the activated coagulation time to approximately two times baseline. The use of heparin-bonded circuits in these patients may offer distinct benefits in reducing bleeding associated with systemic heparinization.[458] The regulation of volume is primarily controlled by the rate of blood removal from the LA, which

is a function of pump flow. As the pump flow is increased, the rate of emptying of the LA concomitantly increases, reducing the flow into the ascending aorta, which reduced MAP. At the same time, the return of flow to the femoral artery is increased. Likewise, as the pump flow is decreased, the amount of blood ejected into the ascending aorta is increased, with a resultant increase in proximal aortic MAP. With the initiation of LHB, MAPs remain identical in the absence of significant restrictions in the descending aorta. When the upper body circulation is isolated from the lower body circulation by the placement of vascular clamps, the two circulations are separated and pulsatile flow is lost in the lower body. At the time of aortic clamping, the proximal aortic pressure increases precipitously as a result of the dramatic change in afterload. The next several minutes of LHB are usually the most difficult to control, with frequent shifts in pressure and flow most likely a function of baroreceptor response. Radial artery pulsatile pressure is maintained at around 120/80 mm Hg, whereas the femoral artery MAP is maintained between 50 and 70 mm Hg, with a flow rate of 50 mL/kg. Filling pressures, measured with a pulmonary artery catheter or left atrial catheter, usually decline by approximately 50%. Once these flow parameters have stabilized, any alteration in hemodynamics should be adjusted either by pharmacologic control or by fluid replacement. Drugs used most often to treat the initial hypertension are nitroprusside, nitroglycerin, and inhalation agents. Other commonly used drugs are phenylephrine, epinephrine, dobutamine, and dopamine.

Methods of volume replacement during repair of thoracic aortic aneurysms must be considered carefully before the start of the case because the potential for rapid blood loss is high. Rapid-infuser devices capable of large volume transfusions over short periods often are used because the LHB circuit has no capability for replacing volume. The success of LHB is directly dependent on the establishment of excellent communication among the surgeon, anesthesiologist, and perfusionist.

Cerebral Protection during Circulatory Arrest

As mentioned in the previous section, aneurysms of the descending thoracic and abdominal aorta represent a major challenge to the anesthesiologist, surgeon, and perfusionist in developing plans for patient management. Aneurysms involving the ascending and/or transverse aortic arch represent a distinctly different challenge for which the plan of ECC differs greatly. The current options for managing patients with these lesions include deep hypothermic circulatory arrest (DHCA),[465–468] retrograde cerebral perfusion (RCP),[469–471] and selective cerebral perfusion of one or more brachiocephalic vessels[472–474] (see Chapters 21, 24, and 28). The next three sections review some of the specific practices involved in managing a patient with these challenging lesions.

Deep Hypothermic Circulatory Arrest

Use of various methods of DHCA has long been standard practice in treating pediatric patients with congenital heart disease. This technique also has been efficacious in treating various other critical disease processes, including neurologic lesions and renal cell carcinoma.[475–477] More recent adaptations in ECC practices have questioned the need for DHCA in select patients[286,478] and have stressed the benefits of low-flow hypothermic perfusion in preserving neurologic function.[479]

The primary determinant in selecting an extracorporeal technique for treating various lesions is assuring cerebral protection through the maintenance of either adequate perfusion or sustained protection. Although the morbidity associated with CPB has declined significantly over time, perturbations of the central nervous system remain a significant factor in assessing postoperative neuropsychologic dysfunction[480] (see Chapter 36). Many factors have been shown to affect cerebral blood flow during CPB, including MAP, viscosity of the perfusate, cannula placement, and/or the presence of carotid stenoses. However, in the absence of mechanical limitations, one of the most influential factors affecting cerebral blood flow is acid-base management,[481] specifically, the control of

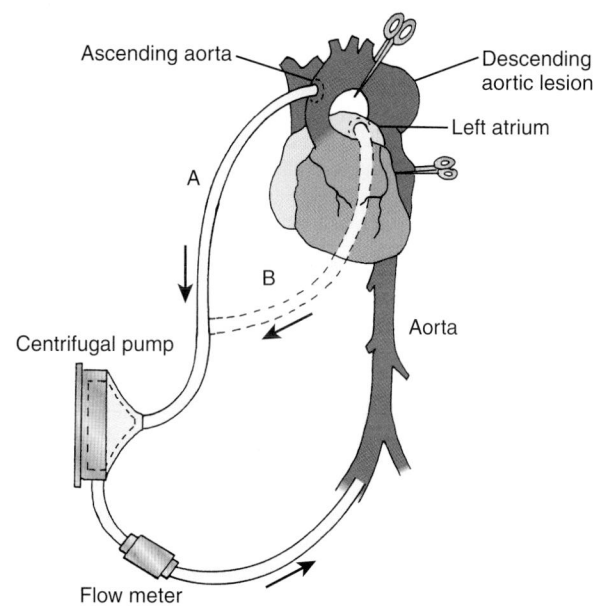

Figure 29-34 Left-heart bypass with use of a centrifugal pump.

Ascending aorta
Descending aortic lesion
Left atrium
A
B
Aorta
Centrifugal pump
Flow meter

Paco$_2$.[482,483] Concurrent use of hypothermia with CPB has been shown to be an effective treatment in reducing organ and tissue oxygen demands. However, the use of DHCA results in metabolic deregulation and changes in membrane integrity, altering cellular maintenance.[484] Hemorrhagic complications induced by DHCA frequently are encountered, necessitating the use of prophylactic transfusion replacement therapy to correct bleeding diathesis.[485,486] Fox et al[487] have shown that, when cerebral temperatures of monkeys were cooled to 20° C, the whole-brain blood flow was decreased concomitantly with the reduction in systemic flow, but the proportion of total flow to the brain was increased. Furthermore, brain oxygen extraction increased as perfusion flow declined, which was unlike other tissue beds in the body. It has been shown that even when nasopharyngeal temperatures are reduced to 15° C, severe cerebral hypoxia quickly develops once DHCA is achieved.[488]

The extracorporeal techniques of DHCA are centered around the regulation and control of circuit and patient temperatures. Core cooling of the patient is achieved through high-flow CPB with cooling temperatures never exceeding 10° C differences between the perfusate temperature (circuit) and the patient core (rectal, bladder) temperature. The perfusate temperature is maintained between 10° C and 15° C during cooling. Other temperatures that can be measured include esophageal, nasopharyngeal, tympanic, and skin temperature. Both tympanic and nasopharyngeal temperatures are remeasured to reflect brain temperatures. The depth of cooling remains controversial, with most clinicians choosing to monitor electroencephalographic activity. Once the electroencephalogram is isoelectric, usually between 15° C and 20° C nasopharyngeal temperature, the patient is cooled for another 5 to 10 minutes before initiating DHCA. Such a technique promotes further global cooling. Some authors advocate monitoring jugular venous bulb oxygen saturation and terminating perfusion only after the saturation is greater than 95%.[489] The period of safe circulatory arrest will vary from patient to patient and depends on a large number of variables including the degree of preexisting neuropathy, the transmural cooling profile of the brain, and reperfusion-related phenomena. In general, the limit of safe circulatory arrest time in adult patients undergoing profound hypothermia is between 40 and 50 minutes.[489,490] Other authors have successfully monitored brainstem activity with somatosensory-evoked potentials for determining the optimal temperature for circulatory arrest.[491] Surface cooling of the cranium is performed by packing the head with ice at the onset of cooling and throughout the DHCA period.

Warming should be accomplished following the same principle of no greater than a 10° C temperature differential between the core and perfusate temperatures. Patients tend to warm at the same rate at which they were cooled. However, the warming rate should never exceed 1° C core temperature increase per 3 minutes of bypass time. Use of vasodilators to facilitate distal perfusion is warranted and treatment of metabolic acidosis should proceed vigorously. Termination of warming should occur when the nasopharyngeal temperature is between 35° C and 36° C. This mild hypothermia provides additional cerebral protection in the early postoperative period.

The use of barbiturates in providing added cerebral protection has not been clearly defined, and their benefits in cardiac surgery may be related to their early use at the onset of surgery.[492] Barbiturates may possibly provide protection by reducing intracranial blood volume, pressure, and edema, as well as acting as oxygen free radical scavengers.[493–495] The level at which barbiturates provided effective protection was seen at doses that abolished synaptic transmission and electrical activity,[193] which in one study was achieved with a mean thiopental dose of 39.5 mg/kg.[492] However, these patients had depressed myocardial contractility and required longer pulmonary recovery periods. It is not known whether barbiturates and hypothermia have an additive effect on cephaloplegia, but profound cerebral depressant effects are seen during CPB with thiopental doses of 8 to 24 mg/kg at 25° C to 30° C.[495]

The term *cerebroplegia* has appeared in the literature, and it reflects isolated pharmacologic manipulation of the perfusate delivered to the brain.[474,496] The authors in both studies advocated the use of either sanguineous[474] or asanguineous[496] oxygen-rich solutions to protect the brain via carotid perfusion during low-flow hypothermic CPB.

Retrograde Cerebral Perfusion

Despite the relative safety of DHCA, there is a finite time limit for nutrient decoupling before irreversible central nervous system damage occurs. In 1990, Ueda et al[469] described a technique of RCP and circulatory arrest that provided perfusion of arterialized blood to the cerebral vasculature during the period of circulatory arrest. The use of RCP had been described previously as a treatment for catastrophic air embolism arising during CPB.[497] This technique provides an alternative to selective cerebral perfusion that requires cannulation of one or more of the brachiocephalic vessels and is considered technologically challenging. Although there are similarities in patient management between DHCA and RCP, the major difference has to do with the placement of a cannula into the superior vena cava (SVC) (Figure 29-35). This can be accomplished with either bicaval cannulation or with an isolated SVC cannula and a dual-stage right atrial cannula.[498] The use of a retrograde cardioplegia cannula placed in the SVC may be desirable because it also contains an end lumen pressure port for monitoring infusion pressure. During the period of circulatory arrest, blood flow is directed away from the systemic circulation and into the SVC retrograde into the cerebral venous system. The perfusion pressure of RCP as measured in the SVC or jugular vein should be maintained between 20 and 40 mm Hg. Flow rates for RCP range between 250 and 500 mL/min. The temperature of the cerebral perfusate usually ranges between 15° C and 18° C, and despite these cold temperatures, desaturated blood is seen returning from the arch vessels.[489]

Some of the benefits of RCP include the maintenance of cerebral temperature via the delivery of a hypothermic perfusate, a decreased risk for air and atheromatous debris from open brachiocephalic vessels, and a continuous delivery of nutrients to the cerebral tissue. Stroke rates also have been shown to be significantly reduced with the use of RCP.[470] Potential problems with RCP include increased cerebral venous resistance caused by cortical vein collapse, the presence of competent jugular valves, which restrict perfusate delivery, and questionable delivery of nutritive flow to the target tissue.[471]

Selective Cerebral Perfusion

Initial efforts to protect the brain during repair of lesions requiring circulatory arrest included the isolated cannulation of brachiocephalic vessels.[499,500] The primary mandate for ECC is the protection of the central nervous system, and selective cerebral perfusion remains attractive because it supplies a continuous source of nutritive perfusate to metabolically active brain tissue during circulatory arrest. Similar to RCP, by continuously perfusing the brain, the extracorporeal management of the patient can be modified with the lower levels of hypothermia and an extension of the period for surgical repair.[472,473]

The technique of selective cerebral perfusion involves the cannulation of one or more of the brachiocephalic vessels or axillary arteries with small (8 Fr to 14 Fr) cannulae that are connected to a separate circuit with a dedicated heat exchanger (Figure 29-36). During this technique, the systemic ECC continues to perfuse the patient via femoral cannulation with cold (20° C to 28° C) perfusate at a rate of 60 to 70 mL/kg/min. Arterialized blood is drawn from the oxygenator through a separate pump, either roller or centrifugal, and passed through a cardioplegia heat exchanger (Figure 29-37) that decreases the temperature to approximately 15° C. The perfusate then passes through a 40-μm filter before perfusing the brachiocephalic vessels. Flow rates to the brain are controlled between 5 and 10 mL/kg/min, with a perfusion pressure at the circuit kept under 150 mm Hg. As with RCP, acid-base homeostasis is maintained according to alpha-stat principles. Oxygen extraction is assessed through measurement of the venous oxygen saturation returning to the SVC cannula. Because autoregulatory mechanisms in the brain have been shown to be maintained at low blood temperatures (20° C), cerebral blood flow should be adequate under these conditions.[501]

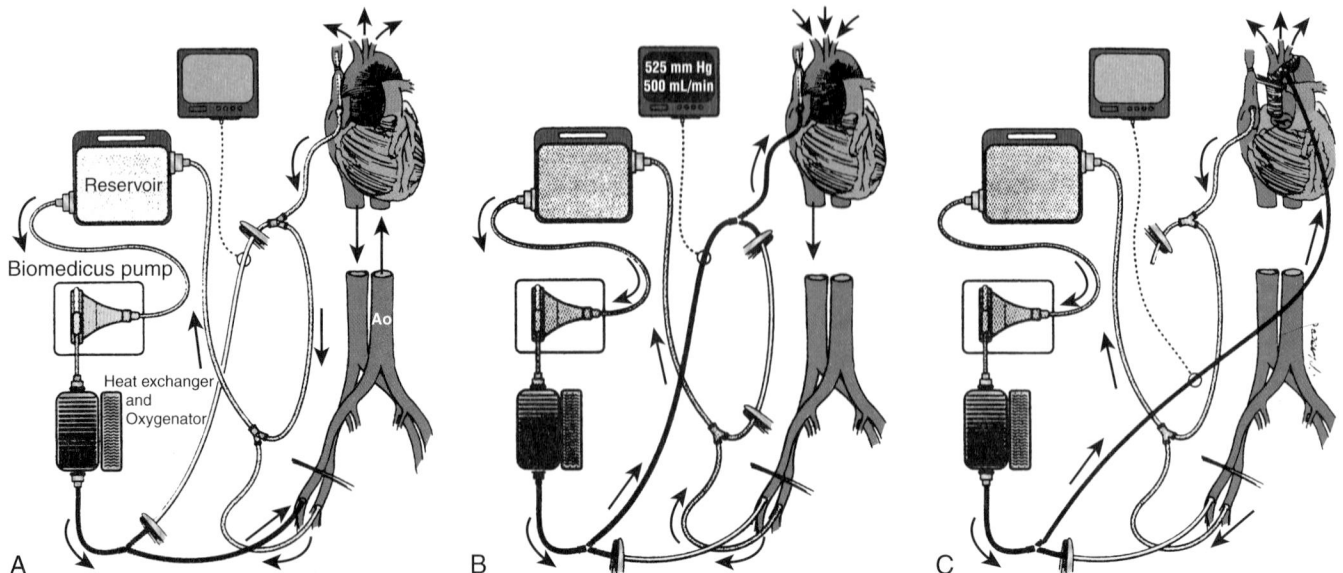

Figure 29-35 **Extracorporeal circuit design for retrograde cerebral perfusion.** *A,* Cooling period. Venous drainage occurs from superior vena cava and femoral vein cannulae with arterial return to the femoral artery. *B,* Retrograde cerebral perfusion with circulatory arrest. Oxygenated blood flows from the arterial line into the superior vena cava, and pressure and flow are monitored. *C,* Warming period. A side arm arterial cannula is placed into the transverse arch graft. *(From Safi HJ, Letsou GV, Iliopoulos DC, et al: Impact of retrograde cerebral perfusion on ascending aortic arch and arch aneurysm repair. Ann Thorac Surg 63:1601, 1997.)*

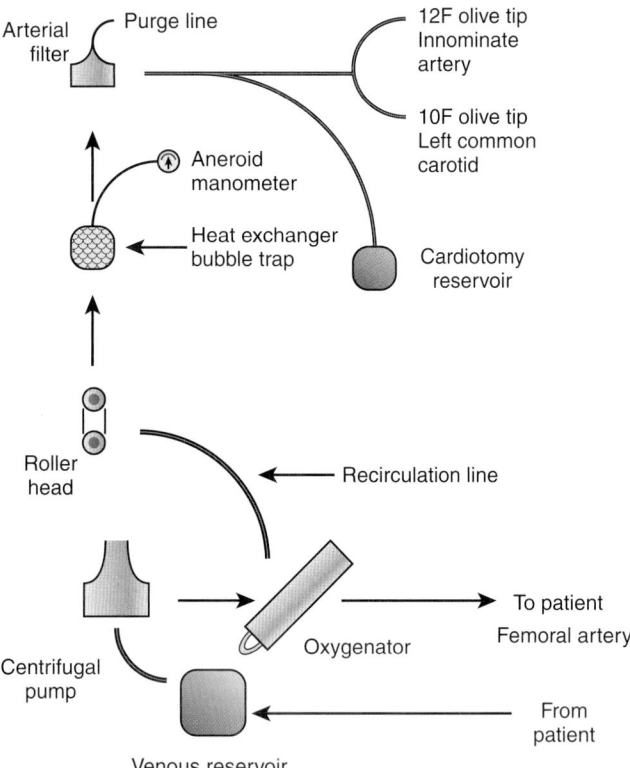

Figure 29-36 **Extracorporeal circuit design for selective cerebral perfusion.** *(From Stammers AH, Butler RR, Kirsh MM: Extracorporeal circulation during treatment of aneurysms of the ascending aorta. Proc Am Soc Extra-Corp Tech 28:72, 1990.)*

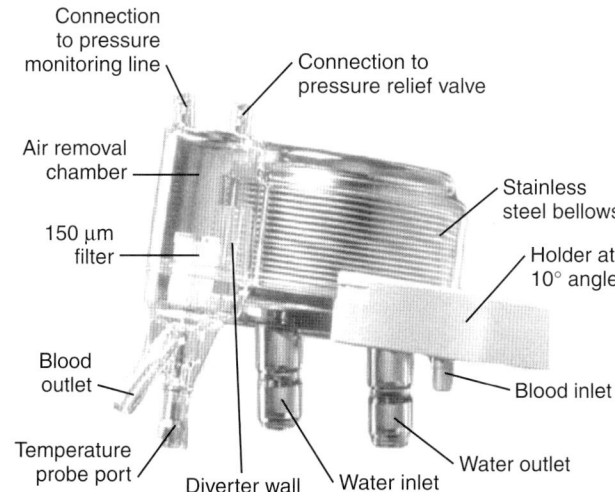

Figure 29-37 **Cardioplegia heat exchanger.** *(Courtesy of Medtronic Cardiovascular Inc.)*

cannulae are utilized connected to a single RP, the downstream flow cannot be independently determined without individual monitoring devices for each line. This is not of major concern because of the anatomic nature of the circle of Willis and distribution of cerebral blood flow. The improved safety resulting from technologic enhancements to pressure control modules and air detection systems of heart-lung machines makes these arguments moot. Monitoring of jugular bulb oxygen saturations or cerebral oxygenation with near-infrared spectroscopy provides feedback information that is used to adjust flow rates and delivery pressures so that adequate delivery of oxygen is matched with extraction rates.[472,502]

Communication and Teamwork

Most human errors emanate from three specific failures: a failure of perception (things are not as they appear), a failure of assumption (the 10-mL vial in the middle drawer with a blue label is always heparin),

The problems associated with selective cerebral perfusion arise from the use of a secondary circuit and additional cannulation sites. The risk for embolization of atheromatous matter may be of concern because of the additional manipulation of the arch vessels, and the presence of additional cannulae also clutters the field.[489] When multiple and failed communication. It is possible for an individual to fail; however, through teamwork and communication, a system can be designed that is highly reliable in which potential errors are mitigated through situational awareness and communication. Although one team member's perception may be distorted at times, another team member may detect a problem. Clinicians are prone to assume that aspects of the working environment are reliable. In highly functional teams, the members have an expectation that there will be failure and are constantly observing and questioning. In highly functional teams, there is a shared mental model of expectations and trust when everyone in the operating room is comfortable speaking up if they observe something that is of concern. Communication failures are the leading cause of inadvertent patient harm. Analysis of 2455 recent sentinel events reported to the Joint Commission for Hospital Accreditation showed that the primary root cause in more than 70% was communication failure, and approximately 75% of these patients died of their injuries.[503,504] An estimated 234 million patients undergo surgical procedures and more than 1 million succumb from complications related to the surgery, many of which are related to how the surgical team interacts and communicates. Use of a simple checklist could have prevented half of these deaths each year.[505] The World Health Organization has designed a checklist that serves as a tool to enhance communication within a team. The checklist has been tested in eight cities around the world and resulted in a reduction of mortality from 1.5% to 0.8% ($P = 0.003$) and a reduction of inpatient complications from 11.0% to 7.0% ($P > 0.001$). Checklists also should be used to improve reliability of infrequent tasks or unexpected occurrences. For example, a checklist may be used to improve the reliability of completing all of the required interventions before the initiation of DHCA (head packed in ice, cooling blanket on, steroids given, acid-base balance corrected, and timer started). Checklists help clinicians to perform the simple tasks reliably and allow more cognitive engagement for the things that are complicated and complex.

Communication and safety training transformed aviation into a highly reliable industry. Gladwell[506] described a pathologic type of communication that he referred to as "mitigated speech." Mitigated speech is a tendency to downplay or sugarcoat the meaning of what is being said. This occurs when an individual experiences a problem but there is a reluctance to speak up about it, when trying to be polite, when ashamed or embarrassed, or when being deferential to authority. The key to breaking this pattern of flawed communication is for leaders to understand that their number one job is to get the best performance possible out of their team, acknowledge their own humanity, and let those who work on the team know that they are expected to speak up about anything unusual or anything that is of concern.

More commonly, communication may be difficult because of an abrasive or difficult team member whose behavior exasperates staff. Recipients of this type of behavior can be at a loss for words to respond to this type of abuse. The danger is that communication may be avoided with difficult individuals because it is too painful and frightening to engage such an individual. Frankel[507] has described the "Five Cs," a pattern for responding to individuals who exhibit this type of abusive behavior. The scripted responses to this abuse are designed in a way that one learns to escalate until the pattern is broken. A respondent begins with 1: "I'm Curious about why you…" If this is not effective, then escalate to 2, "I'm Concerned that…" or 3, "I'm feeling Challenged by this problem we are having…" then 4, "We need to Collaborate with ____ to get another point of view…" If all else fails, then the fifth "C" is to activate the "Chain of Command" and involve leadership in resolving the issue.

Often leaders are not aware of how disruptive their behavior is to the team. They perceive themselves as good communicators and collaborators. Makary et al[508] used a survey to examine the perceptions of collaboration among 3000 team members in the operating room. The survey revealed drastic differences in how professional groups in the operating room perceived the quality of collaboration of other professionals. For example, 84% of surgeons reported good collaboration with anesthesiologists; however, only 70% of anesthesiologists reported good collaboration with surgeons. Furthermore, 88% of surgeons

thought there was good collaboration between surgeons and nurses, whereas only 48% of nurses considered surgeons good collaborators with nurses. Until recently, relationship issues have been unexplored. There is a growing interest in studying the culture in the operating room. The Agency for Healthcare Research and Quality (AHRQ) has responded to requests from hospitals interested in comparing their safety culture survey results to other hospitals. AHRQ funded the development of a comparative database on the survey in 2006.[509] The database is composed of voluntarily submitted data from U.S. hospitals that administered the survey. Comparative database reports were produced in 2007 and 2008 and will be produced yearly through at least 2012. Survey elements for the AHRQ survey are shown in Table 29-5.

Overall, survey respondents to the AHRQ survey reported that the level of teamwork is generally quite good. The areas surveyed that appeared to be opportunities for improvement include development of a nonpunitive response to error, handoffs and transitions, and the number of events reported. These surveys are valuable in that they identify areas where there is an opportunity to improve. The survey results can be used as a tool to help leaders to become knowledgeable about the culture within units and professional groups and lead to the development of training and exercises to improve the safety culture.

Perfusion Simulation

Catastrophic perfusion incidents require the delivery of a complex, coordinated response by the perfusionist within a very short timeframe.[510] Human factors research has shown that simulation of clinical events prepares the clinician for an unexpected event by attenuating a clinician's emotional arousal to a level that allows optimal performance.[511] Pioneering work in CPB simulation was reported by Riley et al in 1977[512] and 1984,[513] who built their system on an IBM personal computer platform and predicted that these systems would mature as processing power, storage, and display technology improved. The aim of their work was to develop systems that would simulate important processes that occur during CPB and would reinforce thought processes that would be dangerous and impractical to conduct in the clinical setting. Later, Austin et al[514] emulated the Air Force's flight simulation model by designing a simulation training model for cardiovascular perfusion education. Orpheus, the first commercially available system, is a computer-controlled hydraulic model of human circulation, intended for use in the training of personnel involved in the procedure of CPμ[10] (Figure 29-38). The system can be used in a number of educational settings (Table 29-6). It may be easily configured to simulate a number of routine and nonroutine scenarios (Table 29-7). In the educational setting, a simulator provides a standardized experience and evaluation process for students. The simulation setting allows the student to experience the cognitive challenge, stress, and physical demands in a setting far removed from an operating room. Students or experienced perfusionists may be subjected to a particularly challenging clinical problem over and over again, and their response to the clinical problem can be accurately evaluated.[515] Ninomiya et al have developed a simulator for adult and infant perfusion crisis management.[516] The system reports

TABLE 29-5	Agency for Healthcare Research and Quality Survey Elements

Communication openness
Feedback and communication about error
Frequency of events reported
Handoffs and transitions
Management support for patient safety
Nonpunitive response to error
Organizational learning–continuous improvement
Overall perceptions of patient safety
Staffing
Supervisor/manager expectations and actions promoting safety
Teamwork across units and within units

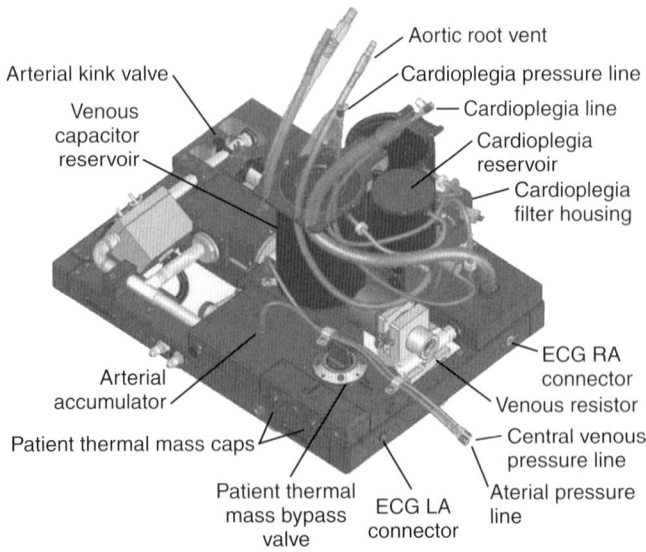

Figure 29-38 Orpheus, the first commercially available system, is a computer-controlled hydraulic model of human circulation. ECG, electrocardiograph; LA, left atrium; RA, right atrium. *(From Morris RW, Pybus DA: "Orpheus" cardiopulmonary bypass simulation system. J Extra Corpor Technol 39:228–233, 2007.)*

TABLE 29-6	Proposed Uses of the Orpheus Simulator

Training in perfusion crisis resource management

Training in the use of other forms of cardiorespiratory support devices

Proficiency checking of experienced perfusionists

Continuing education of experienced perfusionists

Recertification of perfusionists

Demonstration of bypass techniques to surgeons, anesthesiologists, and intensivists

Evaluation of new circuits and/or equipment

TABLE 29-7	Routine and Nonroutine Perfusion Simulation Scenarios

Routine bypass

Initiation of bypass

Weaning from bypass

Cooling and rewarming

Use of centrifugal pumps

Variations in patient resistance

Variations in patient coagulability

Patient emergencies

Blood loss

Left ventricular dysfunction

Cardiac arrhythmias

Failure of anticoagulation

Air embolism

Anaphylaxis

Use of vasodilators

Use of vasoconstrictors

Oxygen consumption changes

Protamine reaction

Transfusion reaction

Blood gas abnormalities

Drug errors

Equipment malfunctions

Aortic cannula obstruction

Aortic cannula displacement

Venous line kinking/venous cannula obstruction

Oxygen supply failure

Pump power supply failure

Heat exchanger failure

Monitor failure

Oxygenator failure

Venous air entrainment

Circuit leaks

the relative percent of the time the adult's or infant's hemodynamic parameters are maintained within range. The authors believe that these systems will supplant recertification requirements based on completing an actual number of clinical cases with periodic required simulation examinations (see Chapters 40 and 41).

Periodic performances of drills that simulate various CPB crises may be conducted in any operating room setting using a mock setup and scripted scenarios. A survey of 314 perfusionists from centers in the Northeastern region of the United States in 2002 revealed that 97% of the perfusionists surveyed believed that such practice drills would be beneficial; however, only 17% reported that such drills are conducted at their centers.[517] Reasons for not doing so ranged from: left up to the individuals to maintain proficiency (19 [39%]), not motivated (11 [22%]), confident of proficiency (9 [19%]), no time (8 [17%]), dubious value (1 [2%]), and cost prohibitive (1 [2%]).

SUMMARY

There have been substantial innovations and improvements in CPB devices and techniques over the past six decades, and the use of CPB has increased from a few hundred procedures per year at a handful of centers around the world in 1955 to the current rate of more than a million procedures performed per year at a few thousand centers worldwide. Great strides have been made in conserving blood and reducing transfusions, attenuation of the systemic inflammatory response, and organ protection. Despite the many advances and widespread use of CPB, there remain substantial opportunities to improve devices, techniques, and safety. Perfusion devices will continue to improve with the introduction of improved device design and the introduction of improved gas exchange surfaces and biocompatible surface coatings. The use of computer technology, human factors science, and simulation training will improve the operator-machine interface, further enhancing safety and improving patient outcomes.

REFERENCES

1. Stammers AH: Historical aspects of cardiopulmonary bypass: From antiquity to acceptance, *J Cardiothorac Vasc Anesth* 11:266, 1997.
2. Gibbon JH: Artificial maintenance of circulation during experimental occlusion of pulmonary artery, *Arch Surg* 34:1105, 1937.
3. Miller BJ: Laboratory work preceding the first clinical application of cardiopulmonary bypass, *Proc Am Acad Cardiovasc Perfusion* 24:19, 2003.
4. Eloesser L: Milestones in chest surgery, *J Thorac Cardiovasc Surg* :157, 1970.
5. Shroyer AL, Grover FL, Hattler B, et al: Veterans Affairs Randomized On/Off Bypass (ROOBY) Study Group: On-pump versus off-pump coronary-artery bypass surgery, *N Engl J Med* 361:1827–1837, 2009.
6. Munoz HR, Sacco CM: Cardiac mechanical energy and effects on the arterial tree, *J Cardiothorac Vasc Anesth* 11:289, 1997.
7. Wright G: Mechanical simulation of cardiac function by means of pulsatile blood pumps, *J Cardiothorac Vasc Anesth* 11:298, 1997.
8. Quaal S: *Cardiac mechanical assistance: Beyond Balloon Pumping*, St. Louis, MO, 1993, Mosby-Year Book.

9. Cooley DA: Development of the roller pump for use in the cardiopulmonary bypass circuit, *Tex Heart Inst J* 14:113, 1987.
10. Melrose DG: Pumping and oxygenating systems, *Br J Anaesth* 31:393, 1959.
11. Kurusz M: Roller pump induced tubing wear: Another argument in favor of arterial line filtration, *J Extra Corpor Technol* 12:49–59, 1980.
12. Peek GJ, Thompson A, Killer HM, et al: Spallation performance of extracorporeal membrane oxygenation tubing, *Perfusion* 15:457–466, 2000.
13. de Jong JCF, ten Duis HJ, Smit Sibinga CT, et al: Hematologic aspects of cardiotomy suction in cardiac operations, *J Thorac Cardiovasc Surg* 79:227, 1980.
14. Noon GP, Kane LE, Feldman L, et al: Reduction of blood trauma in roller pumps for long-term perfusion, *World J Surg* 9:65, 1985.
15. Hubbard LC, Kletschka HD, Olson DA, et al: Spallation using roller pumps and its clinical implications, *Proc Am Soc Extra-Corp Tech* 3:27, 1975.
16. Noon GP, Sekela E, Glueck J, et al: Comparison of Delphin and Biomedicus pumps, *Trans Am Soc Artif Intern Organs* 36:M616, 1990.

17. Leschinsky BM, Itkin GP, Zimin NK: Centrifugal blood pumps—A brief analysis: Development of new designs, *Perfusion* 6:115, 1991.
18. Kijima T, Oshiyama H, Horiuchi K, et al: A straight path centrifugal blood pump concept in the Capiox centrifugal pump, *Artif Organs* 17:593, 1993.
19. Dorman F, Bernstein EF, Blackshear PL Jr, et al: Progress in the design of a centrifugal cardiac assist pump with transcutaneous energy transmission by magnetic coupling, *Trans ASAIO* 15:441, 1969.
20. Pedersen TH, Videm V, Svennevig JL, et al: Extracorporeal membrane oxygenation using a centrifugal pump and a Servo regulator to prevent negative pressure, *Ann Thorac Surg* 63:1333, 1997.
21. Guan Y, Su X, McCoach R, et al: Mechanical performance comparison between RotaFlow and CentriMag centrifugal blood pumps in an adult ECLS model, *Perfusion* 25:71–76, 2010.
22. Lynch MF: Centrifugal blood pumping for open heart surgery, *Minn Med* 61:536, 1988.
23. Rawn DJ, Harris HK, Riley JB, et al: An underoccluded roller pump is less hemolytic than a centrifugal pump, *J Extra Corpor Technol* 29:1518, 1997.
24. Kawahito K, Nose Y: Hemolysis in different centrifugal pumps, *Artif Organs* 21:323, 1997.
25. Tamari Y, Lee-Sensiba K, Leonard EF, et al: The effects of pressure and hemolysis caused by Biomedicus centrifugal pumps and roller pumps, *J Thorac Cardiovasc Surg* 106:997–1007, 1993.
26. Morin BJ, Riley JB: Thrombus formation in centrifugal pumps, *J Extra Corpor Technol* 24:20–25, 1992.
27. Horton S, Thuys C, Bennett M, et al: Perfusion. Experience with the Jostra Rotaflow and QuadroxD oxygenator for ECMO, *Perfusion* 19:17–23, 2004.
28. Kolff J, McClurken JB, Alpern JB: Beware centrifugal pumps: Not a one-way street, but a potentially dangerous "siphon" [Letter], *Ann Thorac Surg* 50:512, 1991.
29. Toomasian JM, Williams DL, Colvin SB, et al: Perfusion during coronary and mitral valve surgery utilizing minimally invasive port-access technology, *J Extra Corpor Technol* 29:66, 1997.
30. Toomasian JM, Peters WS, Siegel LC, et al: Extracorporeal circulation for port-access cardiac surgery, *Perfusion* 12:83, 1997.
31. Oku T, Haraski H, Smith W, et al: Hemolysis. A comparative study of four nonpulsatile pumps, *ASAIO Trans* 34:500–504, 1988.
32. Jakob H, Kutschera Y, Palzer B, et al: In-vitro assessment of centrifugal pumps for ventricular assist, *Artif Organs* 14:278–283, 1990.
33. Englehardt H, Vogelsang B, Reul H, et al: Hydrodynamical aand hemodynamical evaluation of rotary blood pumps. In Thoma H, Schima H, editors: *Proceeding of the International Workshop on Rotary Blood Pumps*, Vienna, Austria, 1988.
34. Hoerr HR, Kraemer MF, Williams JL, et al: In vitro comparison of the blood handling by the constrained vortex and twin roller pumps, *J Extra Corpor Technol* 19:316–321, 1987.
35. Kress DC, Cohen DJ, Swanson DK, et al: Pump-induced hemolysis in rabbit model of neonatal ECMO, *Trans Am Soc Artif Intern Organs* 33:446–452, 1987.
36. Tamari Y, Kerri L-S, Leonard EF, et al: The effects of pressure and flow on hemolysis caused by biomedicus centrifugal pumps and roller pumps, *J Thorac Cardiovasc Surg* 106:997–1007, 1993.
37. Rawn D, Harris H, Riley J, et al: An under-occluded roller pump is less hemolytic than a centrifugal pump, *J Extra Corpor Technol* 29:15–18, 1997.
38. Salo M, Perttila J, Pulkki K, et al: Proinflammatory mediator response to coronary bypass surgery using a centrifugal or a roller pump, *J Extra Corpor Technol* 27:146–151, 1995.
39. Wheeldon DR, Bethune DW, Gill RD: Vortex pumping for routine cardiac surgery: A comparative study, *Perfusion* 5:135–143, 1990.
40. Parault BG, Conrad SA: The effect of extracorporeal circulation time and patient age on platelet retention during cardiopulmonary bypass: A comparison of roller and centrifugal pumps, *J Extra Corpor Technol* 23:34–38, 1991.
41. Klein M, Dauben HP, Schulte HD, et al: Centrifugal pumping during routine open heart surgery improves clinical outcome, *Artif Organs* 22:326–336, 1998.
42. Ashraf S, Bhattacharya K, Zacharias S, et al: Serum S100beta release after coronary artery bypass grafting: Roller versus centrifugal pump, *Ann Thorac Surg* 66:1958–1962, 1998.
43. Dickinson TA, Prichard J, Rieckens F: A comparison of the benefits of roller pump versus constrained vortex pump in adult open-heart operations utilizing outcomes research, *J Extra Corpor Technol* 26:108–113, 1994.
44. Scott DA, Silbert BS, Doyle TJ, et al: Centrifugal versus roller head pumps for cardiopulmonary bypass: Effect on early neuropsychologic outcomes after coronary artery surgery, *J Cardiothorac Vasc Anesth* 16:715–722, 2002.
45. DeBois W, Brennan R, Wein E, et al: Centrifugal pumping: The patient outcome benefits following coronary artery bypass surgery, *J Extra Corpor Technol* 27:77–80, 1995.
46. Alamanni F, Parolari A, Zanobini M, et al: Centrifugal pump and reduction of neurological risk in adult cardiac surgery, *J Extra Corpor Technol* 33:4–9, 2001.
47. Babin-Ebell J, Misoph M, Müllges W, et al: Reduced release of tissue factor by application of a centrifugal pump during cardiopulmonary bypass, *Heart Vessels* 13:147–151, 1998.
48. Baufreton C, Intrator L, Jansen PG, et al: Inflammatory response to cardiopulmonary bypass using roller or centrifugal pumps, *Ann Thorac Surg* 67:972–977, 1999.
49. Society of Thoracic Surgeons Blood Conservation Guideline Task Force, Ferraris VA, Ferraris SP, et al, Society of Cardiovascular Anesthesiologists Special Task Force on Blood Transfusion et al. Perioperative blood transfusion and blood conservation in cardiac surgery: The Society of Thoracic Surgeons and The Society of Cardiovascular Anesthesiologists clinical practice guideline, *Ann Thorac Surg* 83(Suppl 5):S27–S86, 2007.
50. Mejak B, Stammers A, Rauch E, et al: A retrospective study on perfusion incidents and safety devices, *Perfusion* 15:51–61, 2000.
51. Kshettry VR, Salerno CT, Lakhanpal S, et al: Coronary sinus injury during retrograde cardioplegia: A report of three cases, *J Card Surg* 11:359, 1996.
52. Guarracino F, Benussi S, Triggiani M, et al: Delayed presentation of coronary sinus rupture after retrograde cardioplegia, *J Cardiothorac Vasc Anesth* 11:89, 1997.
53. Kurusz M, Conti VR, Arens JF, et al: Perfusion accident survey, *Proc Am Acad Cardiovasc Perf* 7:57, 1986.
54. Greenhalgh D, Thomas W: Blackout during cardiopulmonary bypass, *Anesthesia* 45:175, 1990.
55. Reed CC, Kurusz M, Lawrence AE: Air embolism. In Reed CC, editor: *Safety and Techniques in Perfusion*, Stafford, TX, 1988, Quali-Med Inc., p 239.
56. Myers GJ: Sorin low level detector II: A new concept on an old design, *Canad Perf* 7:11, 1995.
57. Kriewall TJ: Safety systems in perfusion, *Perfusion Life* 11:18, 1994.
58. van Oeveren W, Kazatchkine MD, Descamps-Latscha B, et al: Deleterious effects of cardiopulmonary bypass: A prospective study of bubble versus membrane oxygenation, *J Thorac Cardiovasc Surg* 89:888, 1985.
59. de Jong JC, Smit Sibinga CTH, Wildevuur CRH: Platelet behavior in extracorporeal circulation, *Transfusion* 19:72, 1979.
60. Bastianen GW: The use of air with bubble oxygenators and its influence on the formation of microgas emboli, *J NeSECC* 9:25, 1984.
61. Pearson DT, Holden MP, Waterhouse PS, et al: Gaseous microemboli during open heart surgery: Detection and prevention, *Proc Am Acad Cardiovasc Perf* 4:103, 1983.
62. Yost G: The bubble oxygenator as a source of gaseous microemboli, *Med Instrum* 19:67, 1985.
63. Pearson DT: Gas exchange: Bubble and membrane oxygenators, *Semin Thorac Cardiovasc Surg* 2:313, 1990.
64. Shimono T, Shomura Y, Hioki I, et al: Silicone-coated polypropylene hollow-fiber oxygenator: Experimental evaluation and preliminary evaluation and preliminary clinical use, *Ann Thorac Surg* 63:1730, 1997.
65. Hammerschmidt DE, Stroneck DF, Bowers TM, et al: Complement activation and neutropenia occurring during cardiopulmonary bypass, *J Thorac Cardiovasc Surg* 81:370, 1981.
66. Chenoweth DE, Cooper SW, Hugli TE, et al: Complement activation during cardiopulmonary bypass, *N Engl J Med* 304:497, 1981.
67. Wegner J: Oxygenator anatomy and function, *J Cardiothorac Vasc Anesth* 11:275, 1997.
68. Goodin MS, Thor EJ, Haworth WS: Use of computational fluid dynamics in the design of the Avecor Affinity oxygenator, *Perfusion* 9:217, 1994.
69. Galletti PM: Cardiopulmonary bypass: A historical perspective, *Artif Organs* 17:675, 1993.
70. Beckley PD, Shinko PD, Sites JP: A comparison of gaseous emboli release in five membrane oxygenators, *Perfusion* 12:133–141, 1997.
71. De Somer F: Impact of oxygenator characteristics on its capability to remove gaseous microemboli, *J Extra Corpor Technol* 39:271–273, 2007.
72. Weitkemper HH, Oppermann B, Spilker A, et al: Gaseous microemboli and the influence of microporous membrane oxygenators, *J Extra Corpor Technol* 37:256–264, 2005.
73. Guan Y, Palanzo D, Kunselman A, et al: Evaluation of membrane oxygenators and reservoirs in terms of capturing gaseous microemboli and pressure drops, *Artif Organs* 33:1037–1043, 2009.
74. Preston TJ, Gomez D, Olshove VF Jr, et al: Clinical gaseous microemboli assessment of an oxygenator with integral arterial filter in the pediatric population, *J Extra Corpor Technol* 41:226–230, 2009.
75. Gomez D, Preston TJ, Olshove VF, et al: Evaluation of air handling in a new generation neonatal oxygenator with integral arterial filter, *Perfusion* 24:107–112, 2009.
76. Taylor RL, Borger MA, Weisel RD, et al: Cerebral microemboli during cardiopulmonary bypass: Increased emboli during perfusionist interventions, *Ann Thorac Surg* 68:89–93, 1999.
77. Weitkemper HH, Oppermann B, Spilker A, et al: Gaseous microemboli and the influence of microporous membrane oxygenators, *J Extra Corpor Technol* 37:256–264, 2005.
78. Dickinson T, Riley JB, Crowley JC, et al: In vitro evaluation of the air separation ability of four cardiovascular manufacturer extracorporeal circuit designs, *J Extra Corpor Technol* 38:206–213, 2006.
79. Horton S, Thuys C, Bennett M, et al: Experience with the Jostra Rotaflow and QuadroxD oxygenator for ECMO, *Perfusion* 19:17–23, 2004.
80. Khoshbin E, Roberts N, Harvey C, et al: Poly-methyl pentene oxygenators have improved gas exchange capability and reduced transfusion requirements in adult extracorporeal membrane oxygenation, *ASAIO J* 51:281–287, 2005.
81. Peek GJ, Killer HM, Reeves R, et al: Early experience with a polymethyl pentene oxygenator for adult extracorporeal life support, *ASAIO J* 48:480–482, 2002.
82. Wiesenack C, Wiesner G, Keyl C, et al: In vivo uptake and elimination of isoflurane by different membrane oxygenators during cardiopulmonary bypass, *Anesthesiology* 97:133–138, 2002.
83. Rider SP, Simon LV, Rice BJ, et al: Assisted venous drainage, venous air, and gaseous microemboli transmission into the arterial line: An in-vitro study, *J Extra Corpor Technol* 30:160–165, 1998.
84. Willcox TW, Mitchell SJ, Gorman DF: Venous air in the bypass circuit: A source of arterial line emboli exacerbated by vacuum-assisted drainage, *Ann Thorac Surg* 68:1285–1289, 1999.
85. Jones TJ, Deal DD, Vernon JC, et al: Does vacuum-assisted venous drainage increase gaseous microemboli during cardiopulmonary bypass? *Ann Thorac Surg* 74:2132–2137, 2002.
86. Willcox TW: Vacuum-assisted venous drainage: To air or not to air, that is the question. Has the bubble burst? *J Extra Corpor Technol* 34:24–28, 2002.
87. Groom RC, Likosky DS, Forest RJ, et al: A model for cardiopulmonary bypass redesign, *Perfusion* 19:257–261, 2004.
88. Jensen E, Andreasson S, Bengtsson A, et al: Influence of two different perfusion systems on inflammatory response in pediatric heart surgery, *Ann Thorac Surg* 75:919–925, 2003.
89. Morgan IS, Codispoti M, Sanger K, et al: Superiority of centrifugal pump over roller pump in paediatric cardiac surgery: Prospective randomised trial, *Eur J Cardiothorac Surg* 13:526–532, 1998.
90. Schonberger JP, Everts PA, Hoffmann JJ: Systemic blood activation with open and closed venous reservoirs, *Ann Thorac Surg* 59:1549–1555, 1995.
91. Aldea GS, Soltow LO, Chandler WL, et al: Limitation of thrombin generation, platelet activation, and inflammation by elimination of cardiotomy suction in patients undergoing coronary artery bypass grafting treated with heparin-bonded circuits, *J Thorac Cardiovasc Surg* 123:742–755, 2002.
92. Vaislic C, Bical O, Farge C, et al: Totally minimized extracorporeal circulation: An important benefit for coronary artery bypass grafting in Jehovah's witnesses, *Heart Surg Forum* 6:307–310, 2003.
93. Remadi JP, Rakotoarivelo Z, Marticho P, et al: Prospective randomized study comparing coronary artery bypass grafting with the new mini-extracorporeal circulation Jostra System or with a standard cardiopulmonary bypass, *Am Heart J* 151:198, 2006.
94. Fromes Y, Gaillard D, Ponzio O, et al: Reduction of the inflammatory response following coronary bypass grafting with total minimal extracorporeal circulation, *Eur J Cardiothorac Surg* 22:527–533, 2002.
95. Wippermann J, Albes JM, Hartrumpf M, et al: Comparison of minimally invasive closed circuit extracorporeal circulation with conventional cardiopulmonary bypass and with off-pump technique in CABG patients: Selected parameters of coagulation and inflammatory system, *Eur J Cardiothorac Surg* 28:127–132, 2005.
96. Immer FF, Pirovino C, Gygax E, et al: Minimal versus conventional cardiopulmonary bypass: Assessment of intraoperative myocardial damage in coronary bypass surgery, *Eur J Cardiothorac Surg* 28:701–704, 2005.
97. Skrabal CA, Steinhoff G, Liebold A: Minimizing cardiopulmonary bypass attenuates myocardial damage after cardiac surgery, *ASAIO J* 53:32–35, 2007.
98. Folliguet TA, Philippe F, Larrazet F, et al: Beating heart revascularization with minimal extracorporeal circulation in patients with a poor ejection fraction, *Heart Surg Forum* 6:19–23, 2002.
99. Brest van Kempen AB, Gasiorek JM, Bloemendaal K, et al: Low-prime perfusion circuit and autologous priming in CABG surgery on a Jehovah's Witness: A case report, *Perfusion* 1769–1772, 2002.
100. Folliguet TA, Villa E, Vandeneyden F, et al: Coronary artery bypass graft with minimal extracorporeal circulation, *Heart Surg Forum* 6:297–301, 2003.
101. Gerritsen WB, van Boven WJ, Wesselink RM, et al: Significant reduction in blood loss in patients undergoing minimal extracorporeal circulation, *Transfus Med* 16:329–334, 2006.
102. Rex S, Brose S, Metzelder S, et al: Normothermic beating heart surgery with assistance of miniaturized bypass systems: The effects on intraoperative hemodynamics and inflammatory response, *Anesth Analg* 102:352–362, 2006.
103. Wiesenack C, Liebold A, Philipp A, et al: Four years' experience with a miniaturized extracorporeal circulation system and its influence on clinical outcome, *Artif Organs* 28:1082–1088, 2004.
104. van Boven WJ, Gerritsen WB, Waanders FG, et al: Mini extracorporeal circuit for coronary artery bypass grafting: Initial clinical and biochemical results: A comparison with conventional and off-pump coronary artery bypass grafts concerning global oxidative stress and alveolar function, *Perfusion* 19:239–246, 2004.
105. Abdel-Rahman U, Martens S, Risteski P, et al: The use of minimized extracorporeal circulation system has a beneficial effect on hemostasis—a randomized clinical study, *Heart Surg Forum* 9:E543–E548, 2006.

106. Beghi C, Nicolini F, Agostinelli A, et al: Mini-cardiopulmonary bypass system: Results of a prospective randomized study, *Ann Thorac Surg* 81:1396–1400, 2006.
107. Loubser PG, Morell RI, Loubser IA: Impact of extracorporeal circuit prime volume reduction on whole blood sequestration during acute normovolemic hemodilution for adult cardiac surgery patients, *J Extra Corpor Technol* 36:329–335, 2004.
108. Beholz S, Zheng L, Kessler M, et al: A new PRECiSe (priming reduced extracorporeal circulation setup) minimizes the need for blood transfusions: First clinical results in coronary artery bypass grafting, *Heart Surg Forum* 8:E132–E135, 2005.
109. Perthel M, Kseibi S, Sagebiel F, et al: Comparison of conventional extracorporeal circulation and minimal extracorporeal circulation with respect to microbubbles and microembolic signals, *Perfusion* 20:329–333, 2005.
110. Abdel-Rahman U, Ozaslan F, Risteski PS, et al: Initial experience with a minimized extracorporeal bypass system: Is there a clinical benefit? *Ann Thorac Surg* 80:238–243, 2005.
111. Beholz S, Kessler M, Konertz WF: PRECiSe (priming reduced extracorporeal circulation setup): Results of a safety study, *Heart Surg Forum* 6:311–315, 2003.
112. Remadi JP, Marticho P, Butoi I, et al: Clinical experience with the mini-extracorporeal circulation system: An evolution or a revolution? *Ann Thorac Surg* 77:2172–2175, 2004 discussion 2176.
113. Remadi JP, Rakotoarivello Z, Marticho P, et al: Aortic valve replacement with the minimal extracorporeal circulation (Jostra MECC System) versus standard cardiopulmonary bypass: A randomized prospective trial, *J Thorac Cardiovasc Surg* 128:436–441, 2004.
114. Takai H, Eishi K, Yamachika S, et al: The efficacy of low prime volume completely closed cardiopulmonary bypass coronary artery revascularization, *Ann Thorac Cardiovasc Surg* 10:178–182, 2004.
115. Liebold A, Khosravi A, Westphal B, et al: Effect of closed minimized cardiopulmonary bypass on cerebral tissue oxygenation and microembolization, *J Thorac Cardiovasc Surg* 131:268–276, 2006.
116. Vang SN, Brady CP, Christensen KA, et al: Clinical evaluation of poly(2-methoxyethylacrylate) in primary coronary artery bypass grafting, *J Extra Corpor Technol* 37:23–31, 2005.
117. Koster A, Bottcher W, Merkel F, et al: The more closed the bypass system the better: A pilot study on the effects on reduction of cardiotomy suction and passive venting on hemostatic activation during on-pump coronary artery bypass grafting, *Perfusion* 20:285–288, 2005.
118. Nollert G, Schwabenland I, Maktav D, et al: Miniaturized cardiopulmonary bypass in coronary artery bypass surgery: Marginal impact on inflammation and coagulation but loss of safety margins, *Ann Thorac Surg* 80:2326–2332, 2005.
119. Fransen EJ, Ganushchak YM, Vijay V, et al: Evaluation of a new condensed extra-corporeal circuit for cardiac surgery: A prospective randomized clinical pilot study, *Perfusion* 20:91–99, 2005.
120. Montiglio F, Dor V, Lecompte J, et al: Cardiac surgery in adults and children without use of blood, *Ann Thorac Cardiovasc Surg* 4:3–11, 1998.
121. Castiglioni A, Verzini A, Pappalardo F, et al: Minimally invasive closed circuit versus standard extracorporeal circulation for aortic valve replacement, *Ann Thorac Surg* 83:586–591, 2007.
122. Beholz S, Kessler M, Tholke R, et al: Priming Reduced Extracorporeal Circulation Setup (PRECiSe) with the DeltaStream diagonal pump, *Artif Organs* 27:1110–1115, 2003.
123. Rousou JA, Engelman RM, Flack JE 3rd, et al: The 'primeless pump': A novel technique for intraoperative blood conservation, *Cardiovasc Surg* 7:228–235, 1999.
124. Wasowicz M, Sobczynski P, Drwila R, et al: Air-blood barrier injury during cardiac operations with the use of cardiopulmonary bypass (CPB). An old story? A morphological study, *Scand Cardiovasc J* 37:216–221, 2003.
125. De Somer F, Foubert L, Poelaert J, et al: Low extracorporeal priming volumes for infants: A benefit? *Perfusion* 11:455–460, 1996.
126. Honek H, Horvath P, Kucera V, et al: Miniaturized extracorporeal circulation for infants, *Rozhl Chir* 69:515–518, 1990.
127. Zangrillo A, Garozzo AF, Biondi-Zoccai G, et al: Miniaturized cardiopulmonary bypass improves short-term outcome in cardiac surgery: A meta-analysis of randomized controlled studies, *J Thorac Cardiovasc Surg* 139:1162–1169, 2010.
128. Savory J, Berlin A, Courtoux C, et al: Summary report of an international workshop on the "Role of biological monitoring in the prevention of aluminum toxicity in man: Aluminum analysis in biological fluids" *Ann Clin Lab Sci* 13:444, 1983.
129. Vogler C, Sotelo-Avila C, Lagunoff D, et al: Aluminum containing emboli in infants treated with extracorporeal membrane oxygenation, *N Engl J Med* 319:75, 1988.
130. *Standard for Blood/Gas Exchange Devices (draft)*, Washington, DC, February 1982, revision. Association for the Advancement of Medical Instruments.
131. Loop F, Szabo J: Events related to microembolism in man during CPB, *Ann Thorac Surg* 21:412–420, 1976.
132. Paddyachee TS: The effect of arterial line filtration on GME in the middle cerebral arteries, *Ann Thorac Surg* 45:647–649, 1988.
133. Pugsley W, Klinger C, Paschalis, et al: : The impact of microemboli on neuropsychological functioning, *Stroke* 25:1393–1399, 1994.
134. Clark RE, Brillman J, Davis DA, et al: Microemboli during coronary artery bypass grafting. Genesis and effect on outcome, *J Thorac Cardiovasc Surg* 109:249–257, 1995.
135. Stump DA, Rogers AT, Hammon JW, et al: Cerebral emboli and cognitive outcome after cardiac surgery, *J Cardiothorac Vasc Anesth* 10:113–118, 1996.
136. Whitaker DC, Stanton P: The effect of leucocyte-depleting arterial line filters on cerebral microemboli and neuropsychological outcome following CPB, *Eur J Cardiothorac Surg* 25:267–274, 2004.
137. Riley JB: Arterial line filters ranked for gaseous micro-emboli separation performance: An in vitro study, *J Extra Corpor Technol* 40:21–26, 2008.
138. Shann KG, Likosky DS, Murkin JA, et al: An evidence-based review of the practice of cardiopulmonary bypass in adults: A focus on neurologic injury, glycemic control, hemodilution, and the inflammatory response, *J Thorac Cardiovasc Surg* 132:283–290, 2006.
139. Deptula J, Valleley M, Glogowski K, et al: Clinical evaluation of the Terumo Capiox® FX05 Hollow Fiber Oxygenator with integrated arterial line filter, *J Extra Corpor Technol* 41:220–225, 2009.
140. Preston TJ, Gomez D, Olshove VF, et al: Clinical gaseous microemboli assessment of an oxygenator with integral arterial filter in the pediatric population, *J Extra Corpor Technol* 41:226–230, 2009.
141. Groom RC, Hill AG, Kuban B, et al: Aortic cannula velocimetry, *Perfusion* 10:183–188, 1995.
142. Muehrcke DD, Cornhill JF, Thomas JD, et al: Flow characteristics of aortic cannulae, *J Card Surg* 10(Suppl 4):514–519, 1995.
143. Wada S, Yamamoto S, Honda J, et al: Transapical aortic cannulation for cardiopulmonary bypass in type A aortic dissection operations, *J Thorac Cardiovasc* 132:369–372, 2006.
144. Gourlay T, Samartzis I, Stefanou DC, et al: Inflammatory response of rat and human neutrophils exposed to di-(2-ethylhexyl)-phthalate and di-(2-ethyl-hexyl)-phthalate plasticized polyvinyl chloride, *Artif Organs* 27:256–260, 2003.
145. Kavlock R, Boeckelheide K, Chapin R, et al: NTP: Phthalates expert panel report on the reproductive and developmental toxicity of di(2-ethylhexyl) phthalate, *Reprod Toxicol* 16:529–553, 2002.
146. Baker RWR: Diethylhexyl phthalate as a factor in blood transfusion and haemodialysis, *Toxicology* 9:319–329, 1978.
147. Rock G, Labow RD, Tocchi M: Distribution of di(2-ethylhexyl) phthalate and products in blood and blood components, *Environ Health Perspect* 65:309–316, 1986.
148. Dine T, Luyckx M, Cazin M, et al: Rapid determination by high-performance liquid chromatography of di-2-ethylhexyl phthalate in plasma stored in plastic bags, *Biomed Chromatogr* 5:94–97, 1991.
149. Jaeger RJ, Rubin RJ: Plasticizers from plastic devices: Extraction, metabolism, and accumulation by biological systems, *Science* 170:460–462, 1970.
150. Jaeger RJ, Rubin RJ: Leakage of a phthalate ester plasticizer from polyvinyl chloride blood bags into stored human blood and its localization in human tissues, *N Engl J Med* 287:1114–1118, 1972.
151. Kambia K, Dine T, Azar R, et al: Comparative study of the leachability of di(2-ethylhexyl) phthalate and tri(2-ethylhexyl) trimellitate from haemodialysis tubing, *Int J Pharm* 229:139–146, 905–912, 2001.
152. Hanawa T, Muramatsu E, Asakawa K, et al: Investigation of the release behaviour of diethylhexyl phthalate from polyvinyl-chloride tubing for intravenous administration, *Int J Pharm* 210:109–115, 2000.
153. Gotardo MA, Monteiro M: Migration of diethylhexyl phthalate from PVC bags into intravenous cyclosporine solutions, *J Pharm Biomed Anal* 38:709–713, 2005.
154. Uretzky G, Landsburg G, Cohn D, et al: Analysis of microembolic particles originating in extracorporeal circuits, *Perfusion* 2:9, 1987.
155. Taylor KM: Microemboli: Gaseous and particulate. In Taylor KM, editor: *Cardiopulmonary Bypass*, Baltimore, 1986, Williams & Wilkins, pp 313.
156. Baker JB, Bentall HH, Dreyer B, et al: Arrest of isolated heart with potassium citrate, *Lancet* 273:555–559, 1957.
157. Dyson CW, Follette D, Buckberg G, et al: Intraoperative myocardial protection III. Blood cardioplegia. 1978, *J Extra Corpor Technol* 142–144, 1978.
158. Dyson C, Emerson R, Buckberg G: A hemodilution cardioplegia and a proposed delivery system, *J Extra Corpor Technol* 12:86–88, 1980.
159. Menasché P: Blood cardioplegia: Do we still need to dilute? *Ann Thorac Surg* 62:957–960, 1996.
160. Stiles QR, Hughes RK, Lindensmith GG: The effectiveness of topical cardiac hypothermia, *J Thorac Cardiovasc Surg* 73:176, 1977.
161. Rosenfeldt FL, Watson DA: Local cardiac hypothermia: Experimental comparison of Shumway's technique and perfusion cooling, *Ann Thorac Surg* 27:17, 1979.
162. Rousou JA, Parker T, Engleman RM, et al: Phrenic nerve paresis associated with the use of ice slush and the cooling jacket for topical hypothermia, *J Thorac Cardiovasc Surg* 89:921, 1985.
163. Speicher CE, Ferrigan L, Wolfson SK, et al: Cold injury of myocardium and pericardium in cardiac hypothermia, *Surg Gynecol Obstet* 114:659, 1962.
164. Daily PO, Kinney TB: Optimizing myocardial hypothermia: II. Cooling jacket modifications and clinical results, *Ann Thorac Surg* 51:284, 1991.
165. Boncheck LI, Olinger GN: An improved method of topical hypothermia, *J Thorac Cardiovasc Surg* 82:878, 1981.
166. Daily PO, Pfeffer TA, Wisniewski JB, et al: Clinical comparison of methods of myocardial protection, *J Thorac Cardiovasc Surg* 93:324, 1987.
167. Stammers AH: Advances in myocardial protection: The role of mechanical devices in providing cardioprotective strategies, *Int Anesthesiol Clin* 34:61, 1996.
168. Molina JE, Gani KS, Voss DM: Pressurized rapid cardioplegia versus administration of exogenous substrate and topical hypothermia, *Ann Thorac Surg* 33:434, 1982.
169. Mitchell BA, Litwak RS: Myocardial protection with cold, ischemic potassium-induced cardioplegia: An overview, *Proc Am Soc Extra-Corp Tech* 6:127, 1978.
170. Vertrees RA, Auvil J, Rousou JH, et al: A technique of myocardial preservation perfusion, *Ann Thorac Surg* 78:601, 1979.
171. Voci P, Bilotta F, Caretta F, et al: Mechanisms of incomplete cardioplegia distribution during coronary artery bypass grafting, *Anesthesiology* 79:904, 1993.
172. Menasche P, Koral S, Fauchest M, et al: Retrograde coronary sinus perfusion: A safe alternative for ensuring cardioplegic delivery in aortic valve surgery, *Ann Thorac Surg* 34:647, 1982.
173. Quintilio C, Voci P, Bilotta F, et al: Risk factors of incomplete distribution of cardioplegic solution during coronary artery grafting, *J Thorac Cardiovasc Surg* 109:439, 1995.
174. Gundry SR, Kirsh MM: A comparison of retrograde cardioplegia versus antegrade cardioplegia in the presence of coronary artery obstruction, *Ann Thorac Surg* 38:124, 1984.
175. Menasche P, Piwnica A: Cardioplegia by the way of the coronary sinus for valvular and coronary surgery, *J Am Coll Cardiol* 18:628, 1991.
176. Buckberg GD, Beyersdorf F, Allen BS, et al: Integrated myocardial management: Background and application, *J Card Surg* 10:68, 1995.
177. Lee J, Gates RN, Laks H, et al: A comparison of distribution between simultaneously or sequentially delivered antegrade/retrograde blood cardioplegia, *J Card Surg* 11:111, 1996.
178. Ihnken K, Morita K, Buckberg GD, et al: The safety of simultaneous antegrade and coronary sinus perfusion: Experimental background and initial clinical results, *J Card Surg* 9:15, 1994.
179. Fleisher AG, Sarabu MR, Reed GE: Repair of coronary sinus rupture secondary to retrograde cardioplegia, *Ann Thorac Surg* 57:476, 1994.
180. Kshettry VR, Salerno CT, Lakhanpal S, et al: Coronary sinus injury during retrograde cardioplegia: A report of three cases, *J Card Surg* 11:359, 1996.
181. Ikonomidis JS, Yau IM, Weisel RD, et al: Optimal flow rates for retrograde warm cardioplegia, *J Thorac Cardiovasc Surg* 107:510, 1994.
182. Eke CC, Gundry SR, Fukushima N, et al: Is there a safe limit to coronary sinus pressure during retrograde cardioplegia? *Am Surg* 63:417–420, 1997.
183. Dow JW, Dickson JF, Hamer NA, et al: Anaphylactoid shock due to homologous blood exchange in the dog, *J Cardiovasc Surg* 39:449, 1960.
184. Austin JW, Harner DL: In *The Heart-Lung Machine and Related Technologies of Open Heart Surgery*, Phoenix, AZ, 1990, Phoenix Medical Communication, pp 136.
185. Marath A, Man W, Taylor KM: Histamine release in pediatric cardiopulmonary bypass—a possible role in the capillary leak syndrome, *Agents Action* 20:299, 1987.
186. Messmer K, Lewis DH, Sunder-Plassman WP, et al: Acute normovolemic hemodilution, *Eur Surg Res* 4:55, 1972.
187. Messmer K, Sunder-Plassman WP, Klovekorn WP, et al: Circulatory significance of hemodilution: Rheological changes and limitations, *Adv Microsc* 4:1, 1972s.
188. Chapler CK, Cain SM: The physiologic reserve in oxygen-carrying capacity: Studies in experimental hemodilution, *Can J Physiol Pharmacol* 64:7, 1986.
189. Gordon RJ, Ravin M, Rawitscher RE, et al: Changes in arterial pressure, viscosity and resistance during cardiopulmonary bypass, *J Thorac Cardiovasc Surg* 69:552, 1975.
190. Kessler M, Messmer K: Tissue oxygenation during hemodilution. In Messmer K, Schmid-Schonbein H, editors: *International Hemodilution, Bibliotheca Hematologica. Basel*, Switzerland, 1975, S. Karger, pp 16.
191. Messmer K: Acute preoperative hemodilution: An alternative to transfusion of donor blood, *Acta Univ Uppsala* 3:93, 1977.
192. Henderson AM, Maryniak JK, Simpson JC: Cardiac surgery in Jehovah's Witness, *Anaesthesia* 41:748, 1986.
193. London MJ: Colloids versus crystalloids in cardiopulmonary bypass. Pro: Colloids should be added to the pump prime, *J Cardiothorac Anesth* 4:401, 1990.
194. D'Ambra MN, Philbin DM: Colloids versus crystalloids in cardiopulmonary bypass. Con: Colloids should not be added to the pump prime, *J Cardiothorac Vasc Anesth* 4:406, 1990.
195. Hachenberg T, Tenling A, Rothen HU, et al: Thoracic intravascular and extravascular fluid volumes in cardiac surgical patients, *Anesthesiology* 79:976, 1993.

196. Hindman BJ, Funatsu N, Cheng DCH, et al: Differential effect of oncotic pressure on cerebral and extracerebral water content during cardiopulmonary bypass in rabbits, *Anesthesiology* 73:951, 1990.
197. Beattie HW, Evans G, Garnett ES, et al: Sustained hypovolemia and extracellular fluid volume expansion following cardiopulmonary bypass, *Surgery* 71:891, 1972.
198. Kaul TK, Bhatnagar NK, Mercer JL: Plasma albumin and calcium levels following cardiopulmonary bypass, *Int J Artif Organs* 12:461, 1989.
199. Hoeft A, Korb H, Mehlhorn U, et al: Priming of cardiopulmonary bypass with human albumin or Ringer's lactate: Effect on colloid osmotic pressure and extravascular lung water, *Br J Anaesth* 66:73, 1991.
200. Strauss RG, Stansfield C, Henriksen RA, et al: Pentastarch may exert fewer effects on coagulation than hetastarch, *Transfusion* 28:257, 1988.
201. Boldt J, Kling D, Weidler B, et al: Acute preoperative hemodilution in cardiac surgery: Volume replacement with a hypertonic saline-hydroxyethyl starch solution, *J Cardiothorac Vasc Anesth* 5:23, 1991.
202. Lazrove S, Waxman K, Shippy C, et al: Hemodynamic, blood volume, and oxygen transport responses to albumin and hydroxyethyl starch infusions in critically ill postoperative patients, *Crit Care Med* 8:302, 1980.
203. Lumb PD: A comparison between 25% albumin and 6% hydroxyethyl starch solutions on lung water accumulation during and immediately after cardiopulmonary bypass, *Ann Surg* 206:210, 1987.
204. Cope JT, Banks D, Mauney MC, et al: Intraoperative hetastarch infusion impairs hemostasis after cardiac operations, *Ann Thorac Surg* 63:78, 1997.
205. Auler-Junior JO, Saldiva PH: Pulmonary structure and extravascular lung water after cardiopulmonary bypass, *Braz J Med Biol Res* 19:707, 1987.
206. Boldt J, Zickman B, Ballestros M, et al: Cardiorespiratory responses to hypertonic saline solution in cardiac operations, *Ann Thorac Surg* 51:610, 1991.
207. Slogoff S, Girgis KZ, Keats AS: Etiologic factors in neuropsychiatric complications associated with cardiopulmonary bypass, *Anesth Analg* 61:903, 1982.
208. Steward DL, Da Silva CA, Flegel T: Elevated blood glucose levels may increase the danger of neurological deficit following profoundly hypothermic cardiac arrest [Letter], *Anesthesiology* 68:653, 1988.
209. Metz S, Keats AS: Benefit of glucose-containing priming solution for cardiopulmonary bypass, *Anesth Analg* 72:428, 1991.
210. Lanier WL, Stangland KJ, Scheithauer BW, et al: The effects of dextrose infusion and head position on neurologic outcome after complete cerebral ischemia in primates: Examination of a model, *Anesthesiology* 66:39, 1987.
211. Nakakimura K, Fleischer JE, Drummond JC, et al: Glucose administration before cardiac arrest worsens neurologic outcome in cats, *Anesthesiology* 72:1005, 1990.
212. Nicolson SC: Glucose: Enough versus too much, *J Cardiothorac Vasc Anesth* 11:409, 1997.
213. Lanier WL: Glucose management during cardiopulmonary bypass: Cardiovascular and neurologic implications, *Anesth Analg* 72:423, 1991.
214. Marelli D, Paul A, Samson R, et al: Does the addition of albumin to the prime solution in cardiopulmonary bypass affect clinical outcome? A prospective randomized study, *J Thorac Cardiovasc Surg* 98:751, 1989.
215. Baier RE, Dutton RC: Initial events in interactions of blood with a foreign surface, *J Biomed Mater Res* 3:196, 1969.
216. Bonser RS, Dave JR, Davies ET, et al: Reduction of complement activation during bypass by prime manipulation, *Ann Thorac Surg* 49:278, 1990.
217. Mellbye DJ, Froland SS, Lilleaasen P, et al: Complement activation during cardiopulmonary bypass: Comparison between the use of large volumes of plasma and Dextran 70, *Eur Surg Res* 20:101, 1988.
218. Hysing ES, Kofstad J, Lilleaasen P, et al: Ionized calcium in plasma during cardiopulmonary bypass, *Scand J Clin Lab Invest* 184:119, 1986.
219. Wells ES, Griewski R, Jasperson K, et al: Microprocessors and perfusion equipment, *Int Anesthesiol Clin* 34:15, 1996.
220. Gorlay T: Computers in perfusion practice, *Perfusion* 2:79, 1987.
221. Jerabek CF, Walton HG, Sugden EH: An inexpensive real-time computer system for cardiac surgery, *Proc Am Soc Extra-Corp Tech* 26:23, 1988.
222. Wilt SL, Silvershein JL: Applications of a laptop microcomputer during cardiopulmonary bypass, *Proc Am Soc Extra-Corp Tech* 26:32, 1988.
223. Clark RE, Ferguson TB, Hagen RW, et al: Experimental and clinical use of an automated perfusion system and a membrane oxygenator, *Circulation* 50(Suppl II):II–213, 1974.
224. Fletcher RW: A model for estimating post-dilution hematocrit with minimal blood loss, *J Extra Corpor Technol* 20:89, 1988.
225. Dilworth RL, Lawrence AE: A microcomputer-generated perfusionist's record, *Proc Am Acad Cardiovasc Perf* 5:43, 1984.
226. Riley JB, O'Kane KC: A computer simulation of maintaining total heart-lung bypass for basic education, *Proc Am Soc Extra-Corp Tech* 5:42, 1977.
227. Hankins T, Roberts AJ: Perfusion technology. In Roberts AJ, Conti CR, editors: *Current Surgery of the Heart*, Philadelphia, 1987, JB Lippincott, pp 75.
228. Hankins T: Computer-assisted bypass management, *Proc Am Soc Extra-Corp Tech* 12:95, 1980.
229. Riley JB, Winn BA, Hurdle MB: A computer simulation of cardiopulmonary bypass: Version two, *J Extra Corpor Technol* 16:130, 1984.
230. Leonard RJ: A total heart/lung bypass simulator, *Trans Am Soc Artif Intern Organs* 34:739, 1988.
231. Davis RB: The heart-lung pump/human interface: A real-time microcomputer-based simulation, *Proc Am Soc Extra-Corp Tech* 28:96, 1990.
232. Landsteiner K: Individual differences in human blood, *Science* 73:403–409, 1931.
233. Paxton A: Soon, all eyes on better blood management, *CAP Today* January 2009 Accessed January 21, 2009. Available at: www.cap.org/apps/cap.portal?_nfpb-true&cntvwrPtlt_actionOverride-%2Fportlets%2FcontentViewer%2Fshow&_windowLabel-cntvwrPtlt&cntvwrPtlt%7BactionForm.contentReference%7D-cap_today%2F1208%2F1208_soon_all_eyes_03.html&_state-maximized&_pageLabel-cntwr. Accessed December 17, 2010.
234. Society of Thoracic Surgeons Blood Conservation Guideline Task Force, Ferraris VA, Ferraris SP, et al: Society of Cardiovascular Anesthesiologists Special Task Force on Blood Transfusion, et al: Perioperative blood transfusion and blood conservation in cardiac surgery: The Society of Thoracic Surgeons and The Society of Cardiovascular Anesthesiologists clinical practice guideline, *Ann Thorac Surg* 83(Suppl 5):S27–S86, 2007.
235. Surgenor SD, DeFoe GR, Fillinger MP, et al: Intraoperative red blood cell transfusion during coronary artery bypass graft surgery increases the risk of postoperative low-output heart failure, *Circulation* 114(Suppl 1):I43–I48, 2006.
236. Habib RH, Zacharias A, Schwann TA, et al: Role of hemodilutional anemia and transfusion during cardiopulmonary bypass in renal injury after coronary revascularization: Implications on operative outcome, *Crit Care Med* 33:1749–1756, 2005.
237. Habib RH, Zacharias A, Schwann TA, et al: Role of hemodilutional anemia and transfusion during cardiopulmonary bypass in renal injury after coronary revascularization: Implications on operative outcome, *Crit Care Med* 33:1749–1756, 2005.
238. Engoren MC, Habib RH, Zacharias A, et al: Effect of blood transfusion on long-term survival after cardiac operation, *Ann Thorac Surg* 74:1180–1186, 2002.
239. Engoren MC, Habib RH, Zacharias A, et al: Effect of blood transfusion on long-term survival after cardiac operation, *Ann Thorac Surg* 74:1180–1186, 2002.
240. Koch CG, Li L, Duncan AI, et al: Transfusion in coronary artery bypass grafting is associated with reduced long term survival, *Ann Thorac Surg* 81:1650, 2006.
241. Kamper-Jørgensen M, Ahlgren M, Rostgaard K, et al: Survival after blood transfusion, *Transfusion* 48:2577–2584, 2008.
242. Ho J, Sibbald WJ, Chin-Yee IH: Effects of storage on efficacy of red cell transfusion: When is it not safe? *Crit Care Med* 31(Suppl 12):S687–S697, 2003.
243. Stover EP, Siegel LC, Parks R, et al: Variability in transfusion practice for coronary artery bypass surgery persists despite national consensus guidelines: A 24-institution study. Institutions of the Multicenter Study of Perioperative Ischemia Research Group, *Anesthesiology* 88:327–333, 1998.
244. Testa LD, Tobias JD: Techniques of blood conservation, *Am J Anesthesiol* 23:20, 1996.
245. Parolari A, Antona C, Rona P, et al: The effect of multiple blood conservation techniques on donor blood exposure in adult coronary and valve surgery performed with a membrane oxygenator, *J Card Surg* 10:227, 1995.
246. Ovrum E, Am Holen E, Abdelnoor M, et al: Conventional blood conservation techniques in 500 consecutive coronary artery bypass operations, *Ann Thorac Surg* 52:500, 1991.
247. Donahue JG, Munoz A, Ness PM, et al: The declining risk of post-transfusion hepatitis C virus infection, *N Engl J Med* 327:369, 1992.
248. Sayers MH: Autologous blood donation by cardiac surgery patients: Wisdom or folly? In Massei LM, Thurer RL, editors: *Autologous Blood Transfusion: Current Issues*, Arlington, VA, 1989, American Association of Blood Banks, pp 111.
249. The American Red Cross: *Blood Services Annual Report 1986–1987*, Washington, DC, 1988, ARC, p 4.
250. Ferrari M, Zia S, Henriquet F, et al: A new technique for hemodilution, preparation of autologous platelet-rich plasma and intraoperative blood salvage in cardiac surgery, *Int J Artif Organs* 10:47, 1987.
251. Tawes RL, Sydorak GR, Duvall TB, et al: The plasma collection system: A new concept in autotransfusion, *Ann Vasc Surg* 64:304, 1988.
252. Boldt J, Kling D, Zickman B, et al: Acute preoperative plasmapheresis and established blood conservation techniques, *Ann Thorac Surg* 50:62, 1990.
253. Giordano GF, Rivers SL, Chung GKT, et al: Autologous platelet-rich plasma in cardiac surgery: Effect of intraoperative and postoperative transfusion requirements, *Ann Thorac Surg* 46:416, 1988.
254. Tobe CE, Vocelka C, Sepulvada R, et al: Infusion of autologous platelet-rich-plasma does not reduce blood loss and product use after coronary artery bypass, *J Thorac Cardiovasc Surg* 105:1007, 1993.
255. Wong CA, Franklin ML, Wade LD: Coagulation tests, blood loss, and transfusion requirements in platelet-rich plasmapheresed versus nonpheresed cardiac surgery patients, *Anesth Analg* 78:29, 1994.
256. Giordano GF Sr, Giordano GF Jr, Rivers SL, et al: Determinants of homologous blood usage utilizing autologous platelet-rich plasma in cardiac operations, *Ann Thorac Surg* 47:897, 1989.
257. Giordano GF Sr, Giordano GF Jr, Rivers SL, et al: Determinants of homologous blood usage utilizing autologous platelet-rich plasma in cardiac operations, *Ann Thorac Surg* 47:897, 1989.
258. Jones JW, McCoy TA, Rawitscher RE, et al: Effects of intraoperative plasmapheresis on blood loss in cardiac surgery, *Ann Thorac Surg* 49:585, 1990.
259. Stammers AH, Kratz J, Johnson T, et al: Hematological assessment of patients undergoing plasmapheresis during cardiac surgery, *J Extra Corpor Technol* 25:6, 1993.
260. Boldt J, von Borman B, Kling D, et al: Preoperative plasmapheresis in patients undergoing cardiac surgery, *Anesthesiology* 72:282, 1990.
261. Stammers AH, Rasmussen CR, Kratz JM: The effects of platelet-rich-plasma on postcardiopulmonary bypass fibrinolysis, *J Extra Corpor Technol* 25:122, 1993.
262. Rosengart TK, DeBois W, O'Hara M, et al: Retrograde autologous priming for cardiopulmonary bypass: A safe and effective means of decreasing hemodilution and transfusion requirements, *J Thorac Cardiovasc Surg* 115:426438, 1998.
263. Zelinka ES, Ryan P, McDonald J, et al: Retrograde autologous prime with shortened bypass circuits decreases blood transfusion in high-risk coronary artery surgery patients, *J Extra Corp Technol* 36:343–347, 2004.
264. Eising GP, Pfauder M, Niemeyer M, et al: Retrograde autologous priming: Is it useful in elective on-pump coronary artery bypass surgery? *Ann Thorac Surg* 75:23–27, 2003.
265. Balachandran S, Cross MH, Karthikeyan S, et al: Retrograde autologous priming of the cardiopulmonary bypass circuit reduces blood transfusion after coronary artery surgery, *Ann Thorac Surg* 73:1912–1918, 2002.
266. Rousou JA, Engelman RM, Flack JE 3rd, et al: The 'primeless pump': A novel technique for intraoperative blood conservation, *Cardiovasc Surg* 7:228–235, 1999.
267. Sobieski M.A.I.I., Slaughter MS, Hart DE, et al: Prospective study on cardiopulmonary bypass prime reduction and its effect on intraoperative blood product and hemoconcentrator use, *Perfusion* 20:31–37, 2005.
268. Murphy GS, Szokol JW, Nitsun M, et al: The failure of retrograde autologous priming of the cardiopulmonary bypass circuit to reduce blood use after cardiac surgical procedures, *Anesth Analg* 98:1201–1207, 2004.
269. Trowbridge C, Stammers AH, Klayman M, et al: Factors that influence the ability to perform autologous priming, *J Extra Corpor Technol* 40:43–51, 2008.
270. Brown WR, Moody DM, Challa VR, et al: Longer duration of cardiopulmonary bypass is associated with greater numbers of cerebral microemboli, *Stroke* 31:707–713, 2000.
271. Ajzan A, Modine T, Punjabi P, et al: Quantification of fat mobilization in patients undergoing coronary artery revascularization using off-pump and on-pump techniques, *J Extra Corpor Technol* 38:122–129, 2006.
272. Jewell AE, Akowuah EF, Suvarna SK, et al: A prospective randomized comparison of cardiotomy suction and cell saver for recycling shed blood during cardiac surgery, *Eur J Cardiothorac Surg* 23:633–636, 2003.
273. Brooker RF, Brown WR, Moody DM, et al: Cardiotomy suction: A major source of brain lipid emboli during cardiopulmonary bypass, *Ann Thorac Surg* 65:1651–1655, 1998.
274. Aldea GS, Soltow LO, Chandler WL, et al: Limitation of thrombin generation, platelet activation, and inflammation by elimination of cardiotomy suction in patients undergoing coronary artery bypass grafting treated with heparin-bonded circuits, *J Thorac Cardiovasc Surg* 123:742–755, 2002.
275. Nuttall GA, Oliver WC, Fass DN, et al: A prospective, randomized platelet-function study of heparinized oxygenators and cardiotomy suction, *J Cardiothorac Vasc Anesth* 20:554–561, 2006.
276. Djaiani G, Fedoroko L, Borger M, et al: Continuous-flow cellsaver reduces cognitive decline in elderly coronary artery bypass patients, *Circulation* 116:1888–1895, 2007.
277. Booke M, Fobker M, Fingerhut D, et al: Fat elimination during intraoperative autotransfusion: An in vitro investigation, *Anesth Analg* 85:959–962, 1997.
278. Kincaid EH, Jones TJ, Stump DA, et al: Processing scavenged blood with a cell saver reduces cerebral lipid microembolization, *Ann Thorac Surg* 70:1296–1300, 2000.
279. Rubens FD, Boodhwani M, Mesana T, et al: Cardiotomy Investigators: The cardiotomy trial: A randomized, double-blind study to assess the effect of processing of shed blood during cardiopulmonary bypass on transfusion and neurocognitive function, *Circulation* 116(Suppl 11):I89–I97, 2007.
280. Vertrees RA, Jackson A, Roher C, et al: Intraoperative blood conservation during cardiac surgery, *J Extra Corpor Technol* 12:60, 1980.

281. Young JN, Ecker RR, Moretti RL, et al: Autologous blood retrieval in thoracic, cardiovascular, and orthopedic surgery, *Am J Surg* 144:48, 1982.
282. Young JN, Ecker RR, Moretti RL, et al: Autologous blood retrieval in thoracic, cardiovascular, and orthopedic surgery, *Am J Surg* 144:48, 1982.
283. Schwieger IM, Gallagher CJ, Finlayson DC, et al: Incidence of cell-saver contamination during cardiopulmonary bypass, *Ann Thorac Surg* 48:51, 1989.
284. Moran JM, Babka R, Silberman S, et al: Immediate centrifugation of oxygenator contents after cardiopulmonary bypass, *J Thorac Cardiovasc Surg* 76:510, 1978.
285. Beckmann SR, Carlile D, Bissinger RC, et al: Improved coagulation and blood conservation in the golden hours after cardiopulmonary bypass, *J Extra Corpor Technol* 39:103–108, 2007.
286. Moskowitz DM, Klein JJ, Shander A, et al: Use of the Hemobag® for modified ultrafiltration in a Jehovah's Witness patient undergoing cardiac surgery, *J Extra Corpor Technol* 38:265–270, 2006.
287. Autotransfusion machines, *Health Devices* 17:219–242, 1988.
288. Dietrich W, Barankay A, Dilthey G, et al: Reduction of blood utilization during myocardial revascularization, *J Thorac Cardiovasc Surg* 97:213, 1989.
289. Bryer RH, Engleman RM, Rousou JA, et al: Blood conservation for myocardial revascularization; is it cost-effective? *J Thorac Cardiovasc Surg* 93:512, 1987.
290. Schaff HV, Hauer J, Gardner TJ, et al: Routine use of autotransfusion following cardiac surgery: Experience in 700 patients, *Ann Thorac Surg* 27:49, 1978.
291. Hartz RS, Smith JA, Green D: Autotransfusion after cardiac operation, *J Thorac Cardiovasc Surg* 96:178, 1988.
292. Morris JJ, Tan YS: Autotransfusion: Is there a benefit in a current practice of aggressive blood conservation, *Ann Thorac Surg* 58:502, 1994.
293. Thurer RL, Lytle BW, Cosgrove DM, et al: Autotransfusion following cardiac operations: A randomized, prospective study, *Ann Thorac Surg* 27:500, 1978.
294. Page R, Russell GN, Fox MA, et al: Hard-shell cardiotomy reservoir for reinfusion of shed mediastinal blood, *Ann Thorac Surg* 48:514, 1989.
295. Bouboulis N, Kardara M, Kesteven PJ, et al: Autotransfusion after coronary artery bypass surgery: Is there any benefit? *J Card Surg* 9:314, 1994.
296. Griffith LD, Billman GF, Daily PO, et al: Apparent coagulopathy caused by infusion of shed mediastinal blood and its prevention by washing of the infusate, *Ann Thorac Surg* 47:400, 1989.
297. Schmidt H, Mortensen PE, Folsgaard SL, et al: Cardiac enzymes and autotransfusion of shed mediastinal blood after myocardial revascularization, *Ann Thorac Surg* 63:1288, 1997.
298. Kolff WJ, Watschinger B: Further development of a coil kidney: Disposable artificial kidney, *J Lab Clin Med* 47:969, 1956.
299. Breckinridge DM, Digerness SB, Kirklin JW: Increased extracellular fluid after open intracardiac operation, *Surg Gynecol Obstet* 131:53, 1970.
300. Naik AK, Knight A, Elliot MJ: A successful modification of ultrafiltration for cardiopulmonary bypass in children, *Perfusion* 6:41, 1991.
301. Naik AK, Knight A, Elliot MJ: A successful modification of ultrafiltration for cardiopulmonary bypass in children, *Perfusion* 6:41, 1991.
302. Boldt J, Zickmann B, Fedderson B, et al: Six different hemofiltration devices for blood conservation in cardiac surgery, *Ann Thorac Surg* 51:747, 1991.
303. Silverstein ME, Ford CA, Lysaght MJ, et al: Treatment of severe fluid overload by ultrafiltration, *N Engl J Med* 291:747, 1974.
304. Henderson LW, Livoti LG, Ford CA, et al: Clinical experience with intermittent hemodiafiltration, *Trans Am Soc Artif Int Organs* 19:119, 1973.
305. Magilligan DJ, Oyama C: Ultrafiltration during cardiopulmonary bypass: Laboratory evaluation and initial clinical experience, *Ann Thorac Surg* 37:33, 1984.
306. Magilligan DJ: Indications for ultrafiltration in the cardiac surgical patient, *J Thorac Cardiovasc Surg* 83:183, 1985.
307. Holt DW, Landis GH, Dumond DA, et al: Hemofiltration as an adjunct to cardiopulmonary bypass for total oxygenator volume control, *J Extra Corpor Technol* 14:373, 1982.
308. Chenoweth DE, Cooper SW, Hugh TE, et al: Complement activation during cardiopulmonary bypass: Evidence of generation of C3a and C5a anaphylatoxins, *N Engl J Med* 304:497, 1981.
309. Craddick PR, Fehr J, Brigham KL: Complement and leucocyte-mediated pulmonary dysfunction in hemodialysis, *N Engl J Med* 296:769, 1977.
310. Naik SK, Knight A, Elliot MJ: A prospective randomized study of a modified technique of ultrafiltration during pediatric open-heart surgery, *Circulation* 84(Suppl 3):422, 1991.
311. Groom RC, Froebe S, Martin J, et al: Update on pediatric perfusion practice in North America: 2005 survey, *J Extra Corpor Technol* 37:343–350, 2005.
312. Darling EM, Shearer IR, Nanry C, et al: Modified ultrafiltration in pediatric cardiopulmonary bypass, *J Extra Corpor Technol* 26:205, 1994.
313. Koutlas TC, Gaynor JW, Nicolson SC, et al: Modified ultrafiltration reduces postoperative morbidity after cavopulmonary connection, *Ann Thorac Surg* 64:37, 1997.
314. Skaryak LA, Kirshbom PM, DiBernardo LR, et al: Modified ultrafiltration improves cerebral metabolic recovery after circulatory arrest, *J Thorac Cardiovasc Surg* 109:744, 1995.
315. Wang MJ, Chiu IS, Hsu CM, et al: Efficacy of ultrafiltration in removing inflammatory mediators during pediatric cardiac operations, *Ann Thorac Surg* 61:651, 1996.
316. Journois D, Israel-Biet D, Pouard P, et al: High-volume, zero-balanced hemofiltration to reduce delayed inflammatory response to cardiopulmonary bypass in children, *Anesthesiology* 85:965, 1996.
317. Elliot MJ: Ultrafiltration and modified ultrafiltration in pediatric open heart operations, *Ann Thorac Surg* 56:1518, 1993.
318. Draaisma AM, Hazekamp MG, Frank M, et al: Modified ultrafiltration after cardiopulmonary bypass in pediatric cardiac surgery, *Ann Thorac Surg* 64:521, 1997.
319. Journois D, Pouard P, Greeley WJ, et al: Hemofiltration during cardiopulmonary bypass in pediatric cardiac surgery: Effects of hemostasis, cytokines and complement components, *Anesthesiology* 81:1181, 1994.
320. Woodman RC, Harker LA: Bleeding complications associated with cardiopulmonary bypass, *Blood* 76:1680, 1990.
321. Harker LA, Malpass TW, Branson HE, et al: Mechanism of abnormal bleeding in patients undergoing cardiopulmonary bypass: Acquired transient platelet dysfunction associated with selective alpha-granule release, *Blood* 56:824, 1980.
322. Videm V, Nilsson L, Venge P, et al: Reduced granulocyte activation with a heparin-coated device in an in vitro model of cardiopulmonary bypass, *Artif Organs* 15:90, 1991.
323. Addonizio VP: Platelet function in cardiopulmonary bypass and artificial organs, *Hematol Oncol Clin North Am* 4:145, 1990.
324. Wenger RK, Lukasiewicz H, Mikuta BS, et al: Loss of platelet fibrinogen receptors during clinical cardiopulmonary bypass, *J Thorac Cardiovasc Surg* 97:235, 1989.
325. Velthuis HT, Baufreton C, Jansen PGM, et al: Heparin coating of extracorporeal circuits inhibits contact activation during cardiac operations, *J Thorac Cardiovasc Surg* 114:117, 1997.
326. Gorman RC, Ziats NP, Koneti A, et al: Surface-bound heparin fails to reduce thrombin formation during clinical cardiopulmonary bypass, *J Thorac Cardiovasc Surg* 111:1, 1996.
327. Videm V, Mollnes TE, Garred P, et al: Biocompatibility of extracorporeal circulation, *J Thorac Cardiovasc Surg* 101:654, 1991.
328. Mollnes TE, Lachmann P: Regulation of complement, *Scand J Immunol* 27:127, 1988.
329. Tennenberg SD, Clardy CW, Bailey WW, et al: Complement activation and lung permeability during cardiopulmonary bypass, *Ann Thorac Surg* 50:597, 1990.
330. Gott VL, Whiffen JD, Koepke DE, et al: Techniques of applying a graphite-benzalkonium-heparin coating to various plastics and metals, *Trans Am Soc Artif Intern Organs* 10:213–217, 1964.
331. Aldea GS, Doursounian M, O'Gara P, et al: Heparinbonded circuits with a reduced anticoagulation protocol in primary CABG: A prospective, randomized study, *Ann Thorac Surg* 62:410–418, 1996.
332. von Segesser LK, Weiss BM, Garcia E, et al: Reduction and elimination of systemic heparinization during cardiopulmonary bypass, *J Thorac Cardiovasc Surg* 103:790–799, 1992.
333. Sinci V, Kalaycioglu S, Gunaydin S, et al: Evaluation of heparin-coated circuits with full heparin dose strategy, *Ann Thorac Cardiovasc Surg* 5:156–163, 1999.
334. von Segesser LK, Weiss BM, Pasic M, et al: Risk and benefit of low systemic heparinization during open heart operations, *Ann Thorac Surg* 58:391–398, 1994.
335. Kuitunen AH, Heikkila LJ, Salmenpera MT: Cardiopulmonary bypass with heparin-coated circuits and reduced systemic anticoagulation, *Ann Thorac Surg* 63:438–444, 1997.
336. Stammers AH, Christensen KA, Lynch J, et al: Quantitative evaluation of heparin-coated versus non-heparin-coated bypass circuits during cardiopulmonary bypass, *J Extra Corpor Technol* 31:135–141, 1999.
337. Grossi EA, Kallenbach K, Chau S, et al: Impact of heparin bonding on pediatric cardiopulmonary bypass: A prospective randomized study, *Ann Thorac Surg* 70:191–196, 2000.
338. Ozawa T, Yoshihara K, Koyama N, et al: Superior biocompatibility of heparin-bonded circuits in pediatric cardiopulmonary bypass, *Jpn J Thorac Cardiovasc Surg* 47:592–599, 1999.
339. Jensen E, Andreasson S, Bengtsson A, et al: Changes in hemostasis during pediatric heart surgery: Impact of a biocompatible heparin-coated perfusion system, *Ann Thorac Surg* 77:962–967, 2004.
340. Boonstra PW, Gu YJ, Akkerman C, et al: Heparin coating of an extracorporeal circuit partly improves hemostasis after cardiopulmonary bypass, *J Thorac Cardiovasc Surg* 107:289–292, 1994.
341. Thelin S, Bagge L, Hultman J, et al: Heparin-coated cardiopulmonary bypass circuits reduce blood cell trauma. Experiments in the pig, *Eur J Cardiothorac Surg* 5:486–491, 1991.
342. van der Kamp KW, van Oeveren W: Contact, coagulation and platelet interaction with heparin treated equipment during heart surgery, *Int J Artif Organs* 16:836–842, 1993.
343. Palatianos GM, Dewanjee MK, Smith W, et al: Platelet preservation during cardiopulmonary bypass with iloprost and Duraflo-II heparin-coated surfaces, *ASAIO Trans* 37:620–622, 1991.
344. Svennevig JL, Geiran OR, Karlsen H, et al: Complementactivation during extracorporeal circulation. In vitro comparison of Duraflo II heparin-coated and uncoated oxygenator circuits, *J Thorac Cardiovasc Surg* 106:466–472, 1993.
345. Fosse E, Thelin S, Svennevig JL, et al: Duraflo II coating of cardiopulmonary bypass circuits reduces complement activation, but does not affect the release of granulocyte, *Eur J Cardiothorac Surg* 11:320–327, 1997.
346. Videm V, Svennevig JL, Fosse E, et al: Reduced complement activation with heparincoated oxygenator and tubings in coronary bypass operations, *J Thorac Cardiovasc Surg* 103:806–813, 1992.
347. Mollnes TE, Videm V, Gotze O, et al: Formation of C5a during cardiopulmonary bypass: Inhibition by precoating with heparin, *Ann Thorac Surg* 52:92–97, 1991.
348. Gu YJ, van Oeveren W, Akkerman C, et al: Heparin-coated circuits reduce the inflammatory response to cardiopulmonary bypass, *Ann Thorac Surg* 55:917–922, 1993.
349. Belboul A, Akbar O, Lofgren C, et al: Improved blood cellular biocompatibility with heparin coated circuits during cardiopulmonary bypass, *J Cardiovasc Surg (Torino)* 41:357–362, 2000.
350. Moen O, Fosse E, Brockmeier V, et al: Disparity in blood activation by two different heparin-coated cardiopulmonary bypass systems, *Ann Thorac Surg* 60:1317–1323, 1995.
351. Moen O, Hogasen K, Fosse E, et al: Attenuation of changes in leukocyte surface markers and complement activation with heparin-coated cardiopulmonary bypass, *Ann Thorac Surg* 63:105–111, 1997.
352. Ranucci M, Mazzucco A, Pessotto R, et al: Heparin-coated circuits for high-risk patients: A multicenter, prospective, randomized trial, *Ann Thorac Surg* 67:994–1000, 1999.
353. Mahoney CB: Heparin-bonded circuits: Clinical outcomes andcosts, *Perfusion* 13:192–204, 1998.
354. Mahoney CB, Lemole GM: Transfusion after coronary artery bypass surgery: The impact of heparin-bonded circuits, *Eur J Cardiothorac Surg* 16:206–210, 1999.
355. Ranucci M, Cirri S, Conti D, et al: Beneficial effects of Duraflo II heparin-coated circuits on postperfusion lung dysfunction, *Ann Thorac Surg* 61:76–81, 1996.
356. Redmond JM, Gillinov AM, Stuart RS, et al: Heparin-coated bypass circuits reduce pulmonary injury, *Ann Thorac Surg* 56:474–478, 1993.
357. Heyer EJ, Lee KS, Manspeizer HE, et al: Heparin-bonded cardiopulmonary bypass circuits reduce cognitive dysfunction, *J Cardiothorac Vasc Anesth* 16:37–42, 2002.
358. Svenmarker S, Haggmark S, Jansson E, et al: Use of heparin-bonded circuits in cardiopulmonary bypass improves clinical outcome, *Scand Cardiovasc J* 36:241–246, 2002.
359. Mongero LB, Beck JR, Manspeizer HE, et al: Cardiac surgical patients exposed to heparin-bonded circuits develop less postoperative cerebral dysfunction than patients exposed to non-heparin-bonded circuits, *Perfusion* 16:107–111, 2001.
360. Muehrcke DD, McCarthy PM, Kottke-Marchant K, et al: Biocompatibility of heparin-coated extracorporeal bypass circuits: A randomized, masked clinical trial, *J Thorac Cardiovasc Surg* 112: 472–483, 1996.
361. McCarthy PM, Yared JP, Foster RC, et al: A prospective randomized trial of Duraflo II heparin-coated circuits in cardiac reoperations, *Ann Thorac Surg* 67:1268–1273, 1999.
362. Gunaydin S, McCusker V: Clinical performance and biocompatibility of novel hyaluronan-based heparin-bonded extracorporeal circuits, *J Extra Corpor Technol* 37:290–295, 2005.
363. Noguchi M, Eishi K, Tada S, et al: Biocompatibility of poly2methoxyethylacrylate coating for cardiopulmonary bypass, *Ann Thorac Cardiovasc Surg* 9:22–28, 2003.
364. Gunaydin S, Farsak B, Kocakulak M, et al: Clinical performance and biocompatibility of poly (2-methoxyethylacrylate)–coated extracorporeal circuits, *Ann Thorac Surg* 74:819–824, 2002.
365. Rubens FD, Labow RS, Lavallee GR, et al: Hematologic evaluation of cardiopulmonary bypass circuits prepared with a novel block copolymer, *Ann Thorac Surg* 67:689–696, 1999.
366. Dickinson T, Mahoney CB, Simmons M, et al: Trillium-coated oxygenators in adult open-heart surgery: A prospective randomized trial, *J Extra Corpor Technol* 34:248–253, 2002.
367. Defraigne JO, Pincemail J, Dekoster G, et al: SMA circuits reduce platelet consumption and platelet factor release during cardiac surgery, *Ann Thorac Surg* 70:2075–2081, 2000.
368. Gu YJ, Boonstra PW, Rijnsburger AA, et al: Cardiopulmonary bypass circuit treated with surface-modifying additives: A clinical evaluation of blood compatibility, *Ann Thorac Surg* 65:1342–1347, 1998.
369. Ereth MH, Nuttall GA, Clarke SH, et al: Biocompatibility of trillium biopassive surface-coated oxygenator versus uncoated oxygenator during cardiopulmonary bypass, *J Cardiothorac Vasc Anesth* 15:545–550, 2001 discussion 539–541.
370. Shann KG, Likosky DS, Murkin JM, et al: An evidence-based review of the practice of cardiopulmonary bypass in adults: A focus on neurologic injury, glycemic control, hemodilution, and the inflammatory response, *J Thorac Cardiovasc Surg* 132:283–290, 2006.
371. Fosse E, Moen O, Johnson E, et al: Reduced complement and granulocyte activation with heparin-coated cardiopulmonary bypass, *Ann Thorac Surg* 58:472, 1994.
372. Ovrum E, Fosse E, Mollnes TE, et al: Complete heparin-coated cardiopulmonary bypass and low heparin dose reduce complement and granulocyte activation, *Eur J Cardiothorac Surg* 10:54, 1996.

373. Videm V, Svennevig JL, Fosse E, et al: Reduced complement activation with heparin-coated oxygenator and tubing in coronary bypass operations, *J Thorac Cardiovasc Surg* 103:806, 1992.
374. Boonstra PWAikkerman C, Van Oeveren W, et al: Cardiopulmonary bypass with a heparin-coated extracorporeal circuit. Clinical evaluation in 30 patients. In *Abstracts of the European Association for Cardio-Thoracic Surgery, Perfusion* 6:235–242, 1991.
375. Merrill EW, Salzman EW, Wong PSL, et al: Polyvinyl alcohol-heparin hydrogel "G", *J Appl Physiol* 29:723, 1970.
376. Lundblad R, Moen O, Fosse E: Endothelin-1 and neutrophil activation during heparin-coated cardiopulmonary bypass, *Ann Thorac Surg* 63:1361, 1997.
377. Palatianos GM, Dewanjee MK, Kapadvanjwala M, et al: Cardiopulmonary bypass with a surface heparinized extracorporeal perfusion system, *Trans Am Soc Artif Intern Organs* 36:M476, 1990.
378. Tong SD, Rolfs MR, Hsu LC: Evaluation of Duraflo II heparin-immobilized cardiopulmonary bypass circuits, *Trans Am Soc Artif Intern Organs* 36:M654, 1990.
379. Bindslev L: Adult ECMO performed with surface-heparinized equipment, *Trans Am Soc Artif Intern Organs* 34:1009, 1988.
380. Garavet SP, Crowley JC: Extracorporeal circulation in liver transplantation, *J Extra Corpor Technol* 18:81, 1986.
381. von Segesser LK, Lachat M, Gallino A, et al: Performance characteristics of centrifugal pumps with heparin surface coating, *J Thorac Cardiovasc Surg* 38:224, 1990.
382. Hoar PF, Wilson RM, Mangano DT, et al: Heparin bonding reduces thrombogenicity of pulmonary artery catheters, *N Engl J Med* 305:993, 1981.
383. von Segesser LK, Weiss BM, Garcia E, et al: Reduction and elimination of systemic heparinization during cardiopulmonary bypass, *J Thorac Cardiovasc Surg* 103:790, 1992.
384. Sellevold OFM, Berg TM, Rein KA, et al: Heparin-coated circuit during cardiopulmonary bypass. A clinical study using closed circuit, centrifugal pump and reduced heparinization, *Acta Anaesthesiol Scand* 38:372, 1994.
385. Ovrum E, Brosstad FA, Holen E, et al: Completely heparinized cardiopulmonary bypass and reduced systemic heparin: Clinical and hemostatic effects, *Ann Thorac Surg* 60:365, 1995.
386. Aldea GS, Zhang X, Memmolo CA, et al: Enhanced blood conservation in primary coronary artery bypass surgery using heparin-bonded circuits with lower anticoagulation, *J Card Surg* 11:85, 1996.
387. Edmunds LH: Surface-bound heparin—panacea or peril? *Ann Thorac Surg* 58:285, 1994.
388. Kuitunen AH, Heikkila LJ, Salmenpera MT: Cardiopulmonary bypass with heparin-coated circuits and reduced systemic anticoagulation, *Ann Thorac Surg* 63:438, 1997.
389. Bannan S, Danby A, Cowan D, et al: Low heparinization with heparin-bonded bypass circuits: Is it a safe strategy? *Ann Thorac Surg* 63:663, 1997.
390. Shapira OM, Aldea GS, Zelingher J, et al: Enhanced blood conservation and improved clinical outcome after valve surgery using heparin-bonded cardiopulmonary bypass circuits, *J Card Surg* 11:307, 1996.
391. Gott VL: Heparinized shunts for thoracic vascular operations, *Ann Thorac Surg* 14:219, 1972.
392. von Segesser LK, Turina M: Heparin-coated hollow-fiber oxygenator without systemic heparinization in comparison to classic bubble and membrane oxygenators, *J Extra Corpor Technol* 20:76, 1988.
393. Bindslev L, Eklund J, Norlander D, et al: Treatment of acute respiratory failure by extracorporeal carbon dioxide elimination performed with a surface-heparinized artificial lung, *Anesthesiology* 67:117, 1987.
394. von Segesser LK, Weiss BM, Garcia E, et al: Reduction and elimination of systemic heparinization during cardiopulmonary bypass, *J Thorac Cardiovasc Surg* 103:790, 1992.
395. Shennib H, Mack MJ, Lee AGL: A survey of minimally invasive coronary artery bypass grafting, *Ann Thorac Surg* 64:110, 1997.
396. Izzat MB, Yim APC: Didn't they do well? *Ann Thorac Surg* 64:1, 1997.
397. Stevens JH, Burdon TA, Siegel LC, et al: Port-access coronary artery bypass with cardioplegic arrest: Acute and chronic canine studies, *Ann Thorac Surg* 62:435, 1996.
398. Fann JI, Pompili MF, Stevens JH, et al: Port-access cardiac operations with cardioplegic arrest, *Ann Thorac Surg* 63:s35, 1997.
399. Rubsamen DS: Continuous blood gas monitoring during cardiopulmonary bypass—How soon will it be the standard of care, *J Cardiothorac Anesth* 4:1, 1990.
400. Trowbridge C, Vasquez M, Stammers AH, et al: The effects of continuous blood gas monitoring during cardiopulmonary bypass: A prospective, randomized study. Part 1, *J Extra Corpor Technol* 32:121–128, 2000.
401. Southworth R, Sutton R, Mize S, et al: Clinical evaluation of a new In-line Continuous blood gas monitor, *J Extra Corpor Technol* 30:166–170, 1998.
402. Hiong YT: Failure of a membrane oxygenation module during cardiopulmonary bypass and its implications for the cardiac anesthesiologist, *J Cardiothorac Vasc Anesth* 9:620–621, 1995.
403. Cockroft A: Use of monitoring devices during anesthesia for cardiac surgery: A survey of practices at public hospitals within the UK and Ireland, *J Cardiothorac Vasc Anesth* 8:382, 1994.
404. McDonald J, Cleland A, et al: The use of in-line oxygen analysers during cardiopulmonary bypass, *Proc Am Acad Card Perf* 13:81–85, 1992.
405. Rubsamen DS: Continuous blood gas monitoring during cardiopulmonary bypass: How soon will it be the standard of care? *J Cardiothorac Anesth* 4:1–4, 1990.
406. Charriere JM, Pelissie J, Verd C, et al: Survey: Retrospective survey of monitoring/safety devices and incidents of cardiopulmonary bypass for cardiac surgery in France, *J Extra Corpor Technol* 39: 142–157, 2007.
407. Baker RA, Wilcox T: Australian and New Zealand Perfusion Survey: Equipment and monitoring, *J Extra Corpor Technol* 38:220–229, 2006.
408. Stammers AH, Mejak BS, Rauch BS, et al: Factors affecting perfusionists' decisions on equipment utilization: Results of a United States Survey, *J Extra Corpor Technol* 32:5–10, 2000.
409. Ottens J, Tuble SC, Sanderson AJ, et al: Improving cardiac surgery: Does continuous blood gas monitoring have a role to play? *J Extra Corpor Technol* 42:199–202, 2010.
410. Mauldin PD, Wentraub WS, Becker ER: Predicting hospital costs for first-time coronary artery bypass grafting from preoperative and postoperative variables, *Am J Cardiol* 74:772, 1994.
411. Mangano DT: Multicenter outcome research, *J Cardiovasc Thorac Anesth* 8:10, 1994.
412. The Warm Heart Investigators: Randomized trial of normothermic versus hypothermic coronary bypass surgery, *Lancet* 343:559, 1994.
413. Gill R, Murkin JM: Neuropsychologic dysfunction after cardiac surgery: What is the problem? *J Cardiovasc Thorac Anesth* 10:91, 1996.
414. Stephan H, Weyland A, Kazmaier S, et al: Acid-base management during hypothermic CPB does not affect cerebral metabolism but does affect blood flow and neurologic outcome, *Br J Anesth* 69:51, 1992.
415. Patel RL, Turtle MR, Chambers DJ, et al: Alpha-stat regulation during cardiopulmonary bypass improves neuropsychological outcome in patients undergoing coronary artery bypass grafting, *J Thorac Cardiovasc Surg* 111:1267, 1996.
416. Nevin M, Colchester ACF, Adams S, et al: Evidence for the involvement of hypocarbia and hypoperfusion in the etiology of neurological deficits, *Lancet* 11:1493, 1987.
417. Bashien G, Townes BD, Nessly BS, et al: A randomized study of carbon dioxide management during hypothermic cardiopulmonary bypass, *Anesthesiology* 72:7, 1990.
418. Fullerton DA, McIntyrre RC, Kirson LE, et al: Impact of respiratory acid-base status in patients with pulmonary hypertension, *Ann Thorac Surg* 61:696, 1996.
419. Kamler M, Wendt D, Pizanis N, et al: Deleterious effects of oxygen during extracorporeal circulation to the microcirculation in Vivo, *Eur J Cardiothorac Surg* 26:564–570, 2004.
420. Belboul A, Al-Khaja N, Ericson C, et al: The effect of hyperoxia during cardiopulmonary bypass on blood cell rheology and postoperative morbidity associated with cardiac surgery, *J Extra Corpor Technol* 23:43, 1991.
421. Joachimsson PO, Sjoberg F, Forsman M, et al: Adverse effects of hyperoxemia during cardiopulmonary bypass, *J Thorac Cardiovasc Surg* 112:812, 1996.
422. Caputo M, Mokhtari A, Rogers CA, et al: The effects of normoxic versus hyperoxic cardiopulmonary bypass on oxidative steee and inflammatory response in cyanotic pediatric patients underging open cardiac surgery: A randomized controlled trial, *J Thorac Cardiovasc Surg* 138:206–214, 2009.
423. Oropello JM, Manasia A, Hannon E, et al: Continuous fiberoptic arterial and venous blood gas monitoring in hemorrhagic shock, *Chest* 109:1049, 1996.
424. Stammers AH: Monitoring controversies during cardiopulmonary bypass: How far have we come? *Perfusion* 13:35, 1998.
425. Brown ME, Rawleigh JD, Gallagher JM: In vitro evaluation of continuous mixed venous oxygen saturation and hematocrit monitors, *J Extra Corpor Technol* 26:189, 1994.
426. Appleblad M, Svenmarker S, Haggmark S, et al: Continuous venous oximetry: A comparative study between the CDI 100 and the Bentley Oxy-Sat II, *J Extra Corpor Technol* 26:185, 1994.
427. Appleblad M, Svenmarker S, Haggmark S, et al: Continuous venous oximetry: A comparative study between the CDI 100 and the Bentley Oxy-Sat II, *J Extra Corpor Technol* 26:185, 1994.
428. Bennett JB: A comparison of three blood gas analyzers: Ciba-Corning 288, Gem Premier and Stat Pal II, *Proc Am Acad Card Perf* 16:61, 1995.
429. Parault B: Technique for improved patient care: Initial experience with the GEM-6, *J Extra Corpor Technol* 20:47, 1988.
430. Alston P: A clinical evaluation of a monitor for in-line measurement of PO2, PCO2, and pH during cardiopulmonary bypass, *Perfusion* 3:225, 1988.
431. Riley JB, Fletcher RW, Jenusaitis M, et al: Comparison of the response time of various sensors for continuous monitoring of blood gases, pH and O2 saturation during cardiopulmonary bypass, *Proc Am Soc Extra-Corp Tech* 26:1, 1988.
432. Kurusz M, Andrews JJ, Arens JF, et al: Monitoring oxygen concentration prevents potential adverse patient outcome caused by a scavenging malfunction: Case report, *Proc Am Acad Cardiovasc Perfus* 12:162–165, 1991.
433. Gautam NK, Schmitz ML, Zabala LM, et al: Anesthetic vaporizer mount malfunction resulting in oxygenation failure after initiating cardiopulmonary bypass: Specific recommendations for the pre-bypass checklist, *J Extra Corpor Technol* 41:183–186, 2009.
434. Webb DP, Deegan RJ, Greelish JP, et al: Oxygenation failure during cardiopulmonary bypass prompts new safety algorithm and training initiative, *J Extra Corpor Technol* 39:188–191, 2007.
435. Groom RC, Forest RJ, Cormack JE, et al: Parallel replacement of the oxygenator that is not transferring oxygen: The PRONTO procedure, *Perfusion* 17:447–450, 2002.
436. Swan H, Tyndal M, et al: Quality control of cardiopulmonary bypass: Monitoring mixed venous saturation, *J Thorac Cardiovasc Surg* 99:868, 1990.
437. Justison GA, Pelley W: Hemodynamic management during closed circuit percutaneous cardiopulmonary bypass, *Proc Am Soc Extra-Corp Tech* 27:88, 1989.
438. Sutton RG, Salisbury MM III, Barrett RK, et al: Comparison of venous oxygen partial pressure (PvO2) and oxygen saturation (SvO2) in hypothermic blood flow control, *Proc Am Soc Extra-Corp Tech* 26:7, 1988.
439. Baraka A: Continuous venous oximetry should be used routinely during cardiopulmonary bypass, *J Cardiothorac Anesth* 6:105, 1992.
440. Govier AV, Reves JG, McKay RD, et al: Factors and their influence on regional cerebral blood flow during nonpulsatile cardiopulmonary bypass, *Ann Thorac Surg* 38:592, 1984.
441. Murkin JM, Farrar JK, Tweed WA, et al: Cerebral autoregulation and flow/metabolism coupling during cardiopulmonary bypass: The influence of PaCO2, *Anesth Analg* 66:825, 1987.
442. Johnsson P, Messeter K, Ryding E, et al: Cerebral blood flow and autoregulation during hypothermic cardiopulmonary bypass, *Ann Thorac Surg* 43:386, 1987.
443. McMaster PD, Parsons RJ: The effect of the pulse on the spread of substances through the tissues, *J Exp Med* 68:377, 1938.
444. Taylor KM: Pulsatile perfusion. In Taylor KM, editor: *Cardiopulmonary Bypass*, Baltimore, 1986, Williams & Wilkins, pp 85.
445. Shepard RB, Simpson MS, Sharp JF: Energy-equivalent pressure, *Arch Surg* 93:730, 1966.
446. Nagoka H, Innami R, Watanabe M: Preservation of pancreatic beta-cell function with pulsatile cardiopulmonary bypass, *Ann Thorac Surg* 48:798, 1990.
447. Watanabe T, Miura M, Orita H, et al: Brain tissue pH, oxygen tension, and carbon dioxide tension in profoundly hypothermic cardiopulmonary bypass. Pulsatile assistance for circulatory arrest, low-flow perfusion, and moderate-flow perfusion, *J Thorac Cardiovasc Surg* 100:274, 1990.
448. Minami K, Korner MM, Vyska K, et al: Effects of pulsatile perfusion on plasma catecholamine levels and hemodynamics during and after cardiac operations with cardiopulmonary bypass, *J Thorac Cardiovasc Surg* 99:82, 1990.
449. Alston RP, Singh M, McLaren AD: Systemic oxygen uptake during hypothermic cardiopulmonary bypass, *J Thorac Cardiovasc Surg* 98:757, 1989.
450. Wright G: Mechanical simulation of cardiac function by means of pulsatile blood pumps, *J Cardiothorac Vasc Anesth* 11:299, 1997.
451. Murkin J, Martzke J, Buchan A, et al: A randomized study of the influence of perfusion technique and pH management strategy in 316 patients undergoing coronary artery bypass surgery, *J Thorac Cardiovasc Surg* 110:340, 1995.
452. Hornick P, Taylor K: Pulsatile and nonpulsatile perfusion: The continuing controversy, *J Cardiothorac Vasc Anesth* 11:310, 1997.
453. Murphy G, Hessel E, Groom RC: Optimal cardiopulmonary bypass; an evidence based review, *Anesth Analg* 108:1394–1417, 2009.
454. Henze T, Stephan H, Sonntag H: Cerebral dysfunction following extracorporeal circulation for aortocoronary bypass surgery: No differences in neuropsychological outcome after pulsatile versus nonpulsatile flow, *J Thorac Cardiovasc Surg* 38:65, 1990.
455. Azariades M, Wood AJ, Awnag Y, et al: A qualitative analysis of pulsatile perfusion: Effects on cortisol response to cardiopulmonary bypass surgery, *J Thorac Cardiovasc Surg* 34:163, 1986.
456. Taggart DP, Sundaram S, McCartney C, et al: Endotoxemia, complement, and white blood cell activation in cardiac surgery: A randomized trial of laxatives and pulsatile perfusion, *Ann Thorac Surg* 57:376, 1994.
457. Ohri SK, Bowles CW, Mathie RT, et al: Effect of cardiopulmonary bypass perfusion protocols on gut tissue oxygenation and blood flow, *Ann Thorac Surg* 64:163, 1997.
458. Von Segesser LK, Weiss BM, Gallino A, et al: Superior hemodynamics in left-heart bypass without systemic heparinization, *Eur J Cardiothorac Surg* 4:384, 1990.
459. Mollnes TE, Videm V, Gotze O, et al: Formation of C5a during cardiopulmonary bypass: Inhibition by precoating with heparin, *Ann Thorac Surg* 52:92, 1991.
460. Gregoretti S, Gelman S, Henderson T, et al: Hemodynamics and oxygen uptake below and above aortic occlusion during cross-clamping of the thoracic aorta and sodium nitroprusside infusion, *J Thorac Cardiovasc Surg* 100:830, 1990.
461. Vasilakis A, Rozar GE, Hill RC, et al: Left atrial to femoral arterial bypass using the Biomedicus pump for operations of the thoracic aorta, *Am Surg* 56:802, 1990.

462. Vasilakis A, Rozar GE, Hill RC, et al: Left atrial to femoral arterial bypass using the Biomedicus pump for operations of the thoracic aorta, *Am Surg* 56:802, 1990.

463. Gordon G, Panza W, Bojar R: Failure of left heart bypass to prevent acute left ventricular failure associated with proximal thoracic aortic cross-clamping, *J Cardiothorac Vasc Anesth* 11:80, 1997.

464. Kazui T, Komatsu S, Yokoyama H: Surgical treatment of aneurysms of the thoracic aorta with the aid of partial bypass: An analysis of 95 patients, *Ann Thorac Surg* 43:622, 1987.

465. Griepp RB, Stinson EB, Hollingsworth JF, et al: Prosthetic replacement of the aortic arch, *J Thorac Cardiovasc Surg* 70:1051, 1975.

466. Sweeney MS, Cooley DA, Reul GJ, et al: Hypothermic circulatory arrest for cardiovascular lesions: Technical considerations and results, *Ann Thorac Surg* 40:498, 1985.

467. Graham JM, Stinnett DM: Operative management of acute aortic dissection using profound hypothermia and circulatory arrest, *Ann Thorac Surg* 44:192, 1987.

468. Crawford ES, Snyder DM: Treatment of aneurysms of the aortic arch, *J Thorac Cardiovasc Surg* 85:237, 1983.

469. Ueda Y, Miki S, Kusuhara K, et al: Surgical treatment of aneurysm or dissection involving the ascending aorta and aortic arch, utilizing circulatory arrest and retrograde cerebral perfusion, *J Cardiovasc Surg* 31:553, 1990.

470. Safi HJ, Letsou GV, Iliopoulos DC, et al: Impact of retrograde cerebral perfusion on ascending aortic arch and arch aneurysm repair, *Ann Thorac Surg* 63:1601, 1997.

471. Ganzel BL, Edmonds HL, Pank JR, et al: Neurophysiologic monitoring to assure delivery of retrograde cerebral perfusion, *J Thorac Cardiovasc Surg* 113:748, 1997.

472. Matsuda H, Nakano S, Shirakura R, et al: Surgery for aortic arch aneurysm with selective cerebral perfusion and hypothermic cardiopulmonary bypass, *Circulation* 80(Suppl I):I–243, 1989.

473. Stammers AH, Butler RR, Kirsh MM: Extracorporeal circulation during treatment of aneurysms of the ascending aorta, *Proc Am Soc Extra-Corp Tech* 28:72, 1990.

474. Bachet J, Guilmet D, Goudot B, et al: Cold cerebroplegia, *J Thorac Cardiovasc Surg* 102:85, 1991.

475. Kouchoukos NT, Wareing TH, Izumoto H, et al: Elective hypothermic cardiopulmonary bypass and circulatory arrest for spinal cord protection during operations on the thoracoabdominal aorta, *J Thorac Cardiovasc Surg* 99:659, 1990.

476. Thelin S, Almgren B, Hasson HE, et al: Surgery of extracranial carotid artery aneurysm using cardiopulmonary bypass, hypothermia and circulatory arrest, *J Cardiovasc Surg* 29:332, 1988.

477. Janosko EO, Powell CS, Spence PA, et al: Surgical management of renal cell carcinoma with extensive intracaval involvement using a venous bypass system suitable for rapid conversion to total cardiopulmonary bypass, *J Urol* 145:555, 1991.

478. Stewart JR, Carey JA, McDougal WS, et al: Cavoatrial tumor thrombectomy using cardiopulmonary bypass without circulatory arrest, *Ann Thorac Surg* 51:717, 1991.

479. Swain JA, McDonald TJ, Griffith PK, et al: Low-flow hypothermic cardiopulmonary bypass protects the brain, *J Thorac Cardiovasc Surg* 102:76, 1991.

480. Roach GW, Kanchuger M, Mangano CM, et al: Adverse cerebral outcomes after coronary artery bypass surgery, *N Eng J Med* 335:1857, 1996.

481. Swan H: The importance of acid-base management for cardiac and cerebral preservation during open heart operations, *Surg Gynecol Obstet* 158:391, 1984.

482. Johnston WE, Vinten-Johansen J, DeWitt DS, et al: Cerebral perfusion during canine hypothermic cardiopulmonary bypass: Effect of arterial carbon dioxide tension, *Ann Thorac Surg* 52:479, 1991.

483. van der Linden J, Wesslen O, Ekroth R, et al: Transcranial Doppler-estimated versus thermodilution-estimated cerebral blood flow during cardiac operations, *J Thorac Cardiovasc Surg* 102:95, 1991.

484. Hochachka PW: Defense strategies against hypoxia and hypothermia, *Science* 231:234, 1986.

485. Drakley SK, Fisher AR, O'Riordan JB, et al: The use of cardiopulmonary bypass with profound hypothermia and circulatory arrest during the surgical treatment of giant intracranial aneurysms, *Perfusion* 5:203, 1990.

486. Spetzler FR, Hadley MN, Rigamonti D, et al: Aneurysms of the basilar artery treated with circulatory arrest, hypothermia, and barbiturate cerebral protection, *J Neurosurg* 68:868, 1988.

487. Fox LS, Blackstone EH, Kirklin JW, et al: Relationship of brain blood flow and oxygen consumption to perfusion flow rate during profoundly hypothermic cardiopulmonary bypass, *J Thorac Cardiovasc Surg* 87:658, 1984.

488. Hilberman M, Barlow CH, Haselgrove JC, et al: Cerebral mitochondrial oxygenation during CPB in dogs, *Anesthesiology* 53:693, 1980.

489. Ergin MA, Griepp EB, Lansman SL, et al: Hypothermic circulatory arrest and other methods of cerebral protection during operations on the thoracic aorta, *J Card Surg* 9:525, 1994.

490. Raskin SA, Fuselier VW, Reeves-Viets JL, et al: Deep hypothermic circulatory arrest with and without retrograde cerebral perfusion, *Int Anesthesiol Clin* 34:177, 1996.

491. Guerit JM, Verhelst R, Rubay J, et al: The use of somatosensory evoked potentials to determine the optimal degree of hypothermia during circulatory arrest, *J Card Surg* 9:596, 1994.

492. Nussmeier NA, Arlund C, Slogoff S: Neuropsychiatric complications after cardiopulmonary bypass: Cerebral protection by a barbiturate, *Anesthesiology* 64:165, 1986.

493. Tan PSK: The anaesthetic management of circulatory arrest, *Br J Hosp Med* 43:38, 1990.

494. Thomas AN, Anderton JM, Harper NJN: Anesthesia for the treatment of a giant cerebral aneurysm under hypothermic circulatory arrest, *Anesthesia* 45:383, 1990.

495. Quasha AL, Tinker JH, Sharbrough FW: Hypothermia plus thiopental: Prolonged electroencephalographic suppression, *Anesthesiology* 55:636, 1981.

496. Robbins RC, Balaban RS, Swain JA: Intermittent hypothermic asanguineous cerebral perfusion (cerebroplegia) protects the brain during prolonged circulatory arrest: A phosphorus 31 nuclear magnetic resonance study, *J Thorac Cardiovasc Surg* 99:878, 1990.

497. Mills NL, Ochsner JL: Massive air embolism during cardiopulmonary bypass: Causes, prevention, and management, *J Thorac Cardiovasc Surg* 102:85, 1980.

498. Cope JT, Tribble RW, Komorowski B, et al: A simple technique for retrograde cerebral perfusion during circulatory arrest, *J Card Surg* 11:65, 1996.

499. Philips PA, Miyamoto AM: Use of hypothermia and cardiopulmonary bypass in resection of aortic arch aneurysms, *Ann Thorac Surg* 17:398, 1974.

500. Crawford ES, Saleh SA, Schuessler JS: Treatment of aneurysms of the transverse aortic arch, *J Thorac Cardiovasc Surg* 78:383, 1979.

501. Fox LS, Blackstone EH, Kirklin JW, et al: Relationship of whole body oxygen consumption to perfusion flow rate during hypothermic cardiopulmonary bypass, *J Thorac Cardiovasc Surg* 83:239, 1982.

502. Katoh T, Esato K, Gohra H, et al: Evaluation of brain oxygenation during selective cerebral perfusion by near-infrared spectroscopy, *Ann Thorac Surg* 64:432, 1997.

503. Leonard M, Grahm S, Bonocum D: The human factor: The critical importance of effective teamwork and communication in providing safe care, *Qual Saf Health Care* 13(Suppl 1):i85–i90, 2004.

504. Joint Commission on Accreditation of Healthcare Organizations: June 29 *Sentinel event statistics,* 2004. Available at: www.jcaho.org/accredited+organizations/ambulatory+care/sentinel+events/sentinel+event+statistics.html. Accessed July 5, 2010.

505. World Health Organization: *Endorsement of the "WHO Surgical Safety Checklist".* Available at: www.who.int/patientsafety/safesurgery/endorsements/en/index.html. Accessed July 5, 2010.

506. Gladwell Malcolm: *Outliers: The Story of Success,* Penguin, 2008, p 194.

507. Available at: https://www.bluecrossma.com/staticcontent/frankel_presentation.pdf. Accessed December 17, 2010.

508. Makary MA, Sexton JB, Freischlag JA, et al: Operating room teamwork among physicians and nurses: Teamwork in the eye of the beholder, *J Am Coll Surg* 202:746–752, 2006.

509. Agency for Healthcare Research and Quality: *Surveys on patient safety culture,* 2010. Available at: http://www.ahrq.gov/qual/patientsafetyculture Accessed February 3,.

510. Morris RW, Pybus DA: "Orpheus" cardiopulmonary bypass simulation system, *J Extra Corpor Technol* 39:234–233, 2007.

511. Yerkes RM, Dodson JD: The relation of strength of stimulus to rapidity of habit-formation, *J Comp Neurol Psychol* 18:459–482, 1908.

512. Riley JB, O'Kane KC: A computer simulation of maintaining total heart lung bypass for basic education. In 15th International Conference of the American Society for Extra-Corporeal Technology, Chicago, 1977pp 4249.

513. Riley JB, Winn BA, Hurdle MB: A computer simulation of cardiopulmonary bypass: Version two, *J Extra Corpor Technol* 16:130–136, 1984.

514. Austin J, Cassidy B, Olson T, et al: Transferring air force flight simulation training effectiveness to university-based cardiopulmonary bypass simulation training: "A model for success" [Abstract], *J Extra Corp Technol* 34:45, 2002.

515. Bruce Searles, Assistant Professor of Surgery, Syracuse NY, Upstate University Medical Center: Personal Communication

516. Ninomiya S, Tokaji M, Tokumine A, et al: Virtual patient simulator for the perfusion resource management drill, *J Extra Corpor Technol* 41:206–212, 2009.

517. Ginther R, Darling E, Fillingham R, et al: Departmental use of perfusion crisis management drills: 2002 survey results, *Perfusion* 18:299–302, 2003.

30

Blood and Fluid Management during Cardiac Surgery

COLLEEN KOCH, MD, MS, MBA | SIMON C. BODY, MBCHB, MPH

KEY POINTS

1. Practice guidelines are useful tools to guide patient management in the setting of wide practice variation or costly therapies.
2. Practice guidelines often are not effective in changing clinical practice for a variety of reasons.
3. Effective guidelines require effective implementation and the tools to follow the guidelines.
4. ABO and Rh blood groups are defined by the presence or absence of surface antigens on the red blood cell membrane.
5. The purpose of cross-matching is to reduce the mixing of patient and donor antigens and antibodies that elicit immune consequences.
6. Complications related to transfusion can be immune-mediated such as graft-versus-host disease, or transfusion-related acute lung injury (TRALI), as well as nonimmune-mediated complications such as infectious transmission and transfusion-associated circulatory overload (TACO).
7. Genetic variations affect circulating levels of coagulation factors and platelet numbers.
8. It is likely that genetic variation influences risk for perioperative hemorrhage.
9. Reoperation for bleeding is associated with increased postoperative morbidity and mortality.
10. Implementation of a massive transfusion protocol and consideration for higher fresh frozen plasma-to-red blood cell ratio may improve hemorrhage and patient outcomes.
11. Factor replacement with recombinant factor VIIa is effective for treatment of refractory bleeding in the perioperative setting; however, it may be associated with an increased risk for thrombotic complications.
12. Human fibrinogen concentrates are approved for use in patients with dysfibrinogenemias. Use in patients with low-normal levels of fibrinogen undergoing surgery is uncertain and may place the patient at risk for thrombotic complications.
13. Prothrombin complex concentrates are prepared from pooled plasma and contain four vitamin K–dependent clotting factors: II, VII, IX, and X.
14. Appropriate volume replacement to avoid tissue hypoperfusion is more important than specific choice of colloid or crystalloid.
15. Despite decades of research, currently, there are no approved blood substitutes for clinical use in the United States.
16. Anemia on cardiopulmonary bypass has been associated with increased perioperative renal injury and patient morbidity. However, results of the observational studies are not entirely consistent, and a specific cutoff value for "safe" hematocrit on cardiopulmonary bypass has not been determined.

Appropriate perioperative blood and fluid management are critical to the care of patients undergoing cardiac surgical procedures. A conservative strategy to minimize use of red blood cells (RBCs) and component therapy is strongly recommended. Transfusion guidelines have been developed to assist clinicians with transfusion decisions, as have clinical studies examining the use of component therapy and choice of fluid therapy for maintaining adequate intravascular volume. This chapter reviews transfusion guidelines as they apply to cardiothoracic surgical patients, examines genetic background of blood type groupings, explains immunologic and nonimmunologic-related complications associated with RBC transfusion, and explores risk factors and treatment strategies for perioperative bleeding.

TRANSFUSION GUIDELINES

Rationale for Guidelines

Clinical guidelines are a ubiquitous part of medicine that are "systematically developed statements to assist practitioner and patient decisions about appropriate healthcare for specific clinical circumstances."[1] The U.S. National Guideline Clearinghouse (http://www.guideline.gov) includes more than 2480 recently generated guidelines. Guidelines are valuable methods for reducing practice variation, errors, and to ensure efficient use of healthcare resources.[2] Despite the availability of well-constructed guidelines, clinicians often are reluctant to implement guidelines in daily practice. Several studies have shown that guidelines may do little to change practice behavior.[3]

Formulation of Guidelines

Groups developing guidelines require support from a national or international society that can endorse and disseminate guidelines. Members

TABLE 30-1	Requirements for Successful Guideline Development and Implementation

Guideline Writing Group Formation
Support at a societal level
Perception of need to define practice standards
Senior leadership for guideline preparation
Statistical support for examination of evidence
Guideline Preparation
Sufficient evidence base for guideline preparation
Sufficient expertise for guideline preparation
Dedicated time and effort for guideline generation
Dissemination to content and structure experts for commentary
Guideline Dissemination
Wide dissemination using an authoritative journal within the field
Wide dissemination using traditional and nontraditional mechanisms such as Web sites, conferences, and special interest groups
Guideline Conformity at the local institutional level
Senior leadership within the institution
Incorporation of guidelines into the local context of clinical practice
Providing practitioners with the resources to conform to the guidelines
Providing practitioners with timely, accurate, and pertinent feedback on measured conformity with guidelines

of the guideline committee should be recognized experts in the field and be assisted by people with expertise in guideline preparation. American Heart Association guidelines are the model for well-crafted guidelines, developed using well-conducted peer-reviewed studies as their evidence base (Table 30-1).

Guidelines can be based on a spectrum of evidence from case reports, series without control groups, or randomized, controlled trials. The Society of Thoracic Surgeons/Society of Cardiovascular Anesthesiologists Transfusion Guidelines published in 2007[4] are a good example of generally well-crafted guidelines, but based on limited available evidence. There were 57 recommendations in the guidelines. For level of evidence, only 13 were level A (best level of evidence), 27 were level B (limited evidence), and 17 were level C (very limited evidence). For class of recommendation, only 7 were class I (benefit strongly outweighs risk), 18 were Class IIa (benefit outweighs risk), 23 were Class IIb (benefit may outweigh risk), and 10 were class III (risk outweighs benefit).[5] The relatively low level of evidence for the guidelines likely is reflected by a lack of wide implementation by clinicians.

Implementation of Guidelines

To be effective, guidelines should be widely disseminated using commercial marketing tools. Anesthesia and surgical societies have been comparatively slow in adopting guidelines. Although the recently announced Society of Thoracic Surgeons/Society of Cardiovascular Anesthesiologists Transfusion Guidelines were widely distributed throughout both societies and to the perfusion community, many practitioners were not aware of the content of the guidelines. Several other studies have found similar lack of awareness of other guidelines.[6,7]

A number of other factors may hinder effective implementation of guidelines by practitioners such as guidelines that are too complicated and difficult to implement or lack rigorous scientific evidence as

a basis. In other fields, such as general medicine practices, several studies have demonstrated low rates of change in response to guidelines.[8-10] Furthermore, in the surgical environment that relies on multispecialty teams, there is a need for the entire team to understand the rationale for practice guideline implementation. However, it is equally important to realize that "guidelines need to remain flexible enough to permit a degree of patient-specific departures from specified prevention, diagnostic, and treatment protocols."[11]

Other key components for successful implementation of guidelines lie in senior institution leadership and endorsement,[12] as well as practice-specific feedback of performance. Implementation of guidelines in cardiac surgery previously has been reported to be poor,[13,14] but focused implementation of guidelines at single institutions has been reported to be successful.[15,16] Quality improvement initiatives used in industry such as Total Quality Management and Six Sigma, which appear applicable to surgical processes, are dependent on collection of verifiable data concerning processes.[17,18] The notion that clinicians can improve cardiac surgical care and the performance of individual members of the team without proper timely feedback is not reasonable. In fact, real-time feedback has been demonstrated to be particularly effective.[19] In summary, individuals involved in the management of cardiac surgical patients are obligated to provide the best possible clinical care, often guided by guidelines. Societies have a key role in endorsement, dissemination, and use of guidelines to improve care.

BLOOD GROUPS AND TRANSFUSION
ABO Blood Groups

ABO and Rh blood groups are the most well-known of more than 30 antigen-based classifications of human blood types. The ABO blood group system is based on identification of A and B antigens present on RBCs and was originally described by Janský and Landsteiner.[20] Wide variation exists in the frequency of the ABO groups across different populations, with group B being the most common in Asians but comparatively rare in whites.[21]

ABO blood grouping is defined by presence or absence of surface antigens on the RBC membrane. The *ABO* gene is located on chromosome 9q34 and has three principal isoforms (A, B, and O) that are determined by single nucleotide polymorphisms (SNPs) and single-base deletions within the ABO gene (Table 30-2). Four missense SNPs determine the structural and functional differences between the A and B transferases. The different transferases result from four amino acid substitutions at amino acid positions (codons) 176, 235, 266, and 268 and nearly always occur together as a group. Two of these SNPs (L266M and G268A) change the substrate specificity of the ABO enzyme for galactose. The protein produced by the *ABO* gene is not the antigen. Rather, O, A, and B antigens are formed by the action of three different glycosyltransferases (isoforms) encoded by the *ABO* gene that modifies a cell membrane glycoprotein (H antigen).[22]

The O blood group is caused by a single base deletion (261delG) in exon 6 of the *ABO* gene that results in a frameshift mutation and translation of a truncated ABO protein, the O isoform, with no enzymatic activity; therefore, the A and B antigens are not present (the H antigen is unmodified).[23]

TABLE 30-2	Genetic Causes of the ABO Blood Groups					
ABO gene exon		6			7	
Nucleotide position		261	526	703	796	803
Common allele		G	C	G	C	G
Rare allele		del	G	A	A	C
Amino acid position		118	176	235	266	268
Blood group	O	Deleted	Deleted	Deleted	Deleted	Deleted
	A	Leucine	Arginine	Glycine	Leucine	Glycine
	B	Leucine	Glycine	Serine	Methionine	Alanine

In the A transferase, the amino acids are leucine (L) and glycine (G) at codons 266 and 268, respectively. The A isoform (L266 and G268) encodes a glycosyltransferase (A transferase) that bonds α-N-acetylgalactosamine to the H antigen, producing the A antigen of the ABO blood group system. Individuals who exclusively synthesize A isoforms are blood group A and have the genotype AA (homozygotes; same A allele on both chromosomes) or AO (heterozygotes; A allele only present on one chromosome).[23]

In the B transferase, the amino acids are methionine (M) and alanine (A) at the same codons 266 and 268, respectively. The B isoform (M266 and A268) encodes a glycosyltransferase (B transferase) that joins α-D-galactose to the H antigen, creating the B antigen. Blood group B individuals have the genotype BB (homozygotes) or BO (heterozygotes). Individuals who express both A and B isoforms of the ABO gene (an A allele on one chromosome 9 and a B allele on the other chromosome 9) are blood group AB.[23]

Other variations in the ABO gene that create functionally similar antigens also exist. For example, the A(2) isoform, comprising only 20% of group A individuals, is caused by deletion of a protein coding termination point, thus extending the enzyme by 21 extra amino acids and altering its specificity. These structural differences reflect the different catalytic activities of the enzymes encoded by the A(1) and A(2) alleles and result in different antigenic properties of A(1) and A(2) antigens.[24] Different molecular mechanisms may be responsible for seemingly identical ABO blood groups. For example, the B3 phenotype may be caused by either a missense mutation (D291N), a splicing mutation (B303), or the combination of a missense mutation and a single nucleotide deletion (V277M and 1060delC).

ABO blood groups also could be measured by genotyping the variants in the ABO gene instead of measuring the presence or absence of the A and B antigens. The ABO antigens are also expressed on the surface of many other cells types, indicating the importance of ABO cross-matching of organ transplants. Several other rare variants of the ABO gene that change activity and/or specificity of the enzyme have been identified and generate several rare blood groups.[25]

Anti-A and anti-B antibodies (isohemagglutinins) are IgM antibodies that appear in the first years of life. Early in the postnatal period, the immune system generates IgM antibodies against ABO antigen(s) even when they are absent from the individual's RBCs. The IgM antibodies, if present in the fetus, are too large to cross the placenta, and thus are not a relevant cause of hemolytic disease of the newborn. The antibodies are thought to be produced in response to infantile exposure to influenza virus and gram-negative bacteria. Antibodies usually are not generated against the H antigen. Therefore, an individual with blood group A will make IgM antibodies against the B antigen. An individual with blood group B will make IgM antibodies against the A antigen. An individual with blood group AB will not make IgM antibodies to the A and B antigens. Finally, an individual with blood group O will make IgM antibodies against both the A and B antigens.[23]

If an individual of blood group A receives group B RBCs, anti-B IgM isohemagglutinins in the recipient plasma bind to the B antigen on donor RBCs, generating a locus for complement-mediated lysis of transfused donor RBCs and generation of a hemolytic transfusion reaction. Similar events occur in group O and B individuals receiving RBCs containing non–self-antigens. However, blood group AB individuals do not generate anti-A and anti-B antibodies. Therefore, they can receive RBCs from all groups and are universal RBC recipients.[23]

Rhesus Blood Groups

The rhesus (Rh) blood group system consists of ~50 blood group antigens among which five antigens—D, C, c, E, and e—are the most important. The proteins that carry the Rh antigens form a transmembrane transporter complex that resembles NH_3 and CO_2 transporters of evolutionary origin.[26] The proteins are encoded by two adjacent genes on chromosome 1p36.13-p34.3: the *RHD* gene that encodes the RhD protein with the frequent D antigen and the *RHCE* gene that encodes the RhCE protein with the C, E, c, and e antigens.[27] The term *Rh factor* refers

only to the D antigen that is normally present. Unlike the ABO system, the absence of the normally present D antigen is called the *d antigen*, but there is no protein corresponding to the d antigen. Lowercase "d" indicates the absence of the D antigen, often as a result of the deletion of the gene or other variants that prevent expression of the antigenic protein on RBCs.[27] To be Rh negative, the individual must have the gene absent on both chromosomes.

The frequency of Rh-negative individuals ranges from ~16% in white populations to less than 1% in Asian populations.[28] Rh incompatibility of an RhD-negative mother and RhD-positive fetus is the predominant cause of hemolytic disease of the newborn, which occurs when maternal IgG anti-RhD antibodies pass through the placenta into the fetal circulation and cause hemolysis of RhD antigen-positive fetal RBCs.[29]

Other Blood Groups

At least 30 other antigens are expressed on the RBC surface including the Kell–Cellano, MNS, and Lewis blood groups. These blood groups are capable of causing transfusion reactions, though most are less common and produce less severe transfusion reactions than ABO incompatibility. Several are capable of producing hemolytic disease of the newborn.[29]

The Kell–Cellano antigens are variants of a transmembrane glycoprotein (*ET3*) encoded on chromosome 7q33. In contrast with many other blood groups, the function of the enzyme is known and is responsible for producing endothelin-3, a potent bioactive peptide with multiple biologic roles. There are several variants of the gene, of which K_1 (Kell) and K_2 (Cellano) are the most common and result from an SNP generating a $Thr193(K_2)$ from the more frequent $Met193(K_1)$ isoform. Kell incompatibility is second to Rh incompatibility for generation of hemolytic disease of the newborn.[29]

The MNS antigens are variants of two genes, glycophorin A (containing the M and N alleles) and glycophorin B (containing the S and s alleles), adjacent to each other on chromosome 4q28-q31. The glycophorins are the most common sialoglycoproteins present on the RBC membrane, but their function is not clear. Unlike most other blood group systems in which individual SNPs or deletions create the antigens, the MNS antigens are created by complex rearrangements of the protein structure that generate antigens.[30]

The Lewis blood group antigens are structurally similar to the ABO and the H blood group systems. The antigens are generated by variants in the fucosyl transferase gene (FUT3), residing on chromosome 19p13.3, that acts on the Lewis antigens in a similar fashion to the galactose transferase function of the ABO gene acting on the H antigen. The Lewis antigens are not synthesized in erythrocyte progenitor cells like the ABO antigens, more likely in the gut. The Le-a or Le-b antigens circulate in plasma bound to serum lipoproteins and are adsorbed to circulating erythrocytes, usually only after birth.[31]

Cross-matching

The use of citrate, refrigeration, and a nascent understanding of blood incompatibility during the First World War enabled the development of blood banking.[32] The first U.S. hospital blood bank was created at Cook County Hospital in 1937.[32] About 16 million units of blood was transfused in the United States in 2008.[33] Cross-matching of donor blood products to an individual recipient is a sequence of procedures performed to prevent transfusion reactions. American Association of Blood Banks' Standards for Blood Banks and Transfusion Services has defined the procedures performed before blood is transfused to a recipient. The first laboratory component for the recipient blood specimen is a "type and screen," which consists of two separate tests.[34] First, the recipient's ABO and RhD blood groups are determined (typed) by using commercially produced anti-A and anti-B antibodies that will react with the A or B antigens, if present, on the recipient's RBCs, causing the RBCs to agglutinate. The RhD antigen is tested in the same manner, with commercially available anti-D antibodies mixed with the recipient's RBCs.[34]

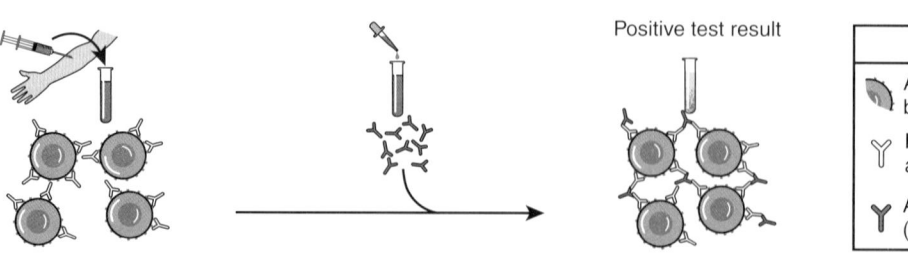

DIRECT COOMBS TEST/DIRECT ANTIGLOBULIN TEST

	Positive test result

Legend

- Antigens on the red blood cell's surface
- Human anti-RBC antibody
- Antihuman antibody (*Coombs reagent*)

Blood sample from a patient with immune-mediated hemolytic anaemia: antibodies are shown attached to antigens on the RBC surface.

The patient's washed RBCs are incubated with antihuman antibodies (*Coombs reagent*).

RBCs agglutinate: antihuman antibodies form links between RBCs by binding to the human antibodies on the RBCs.

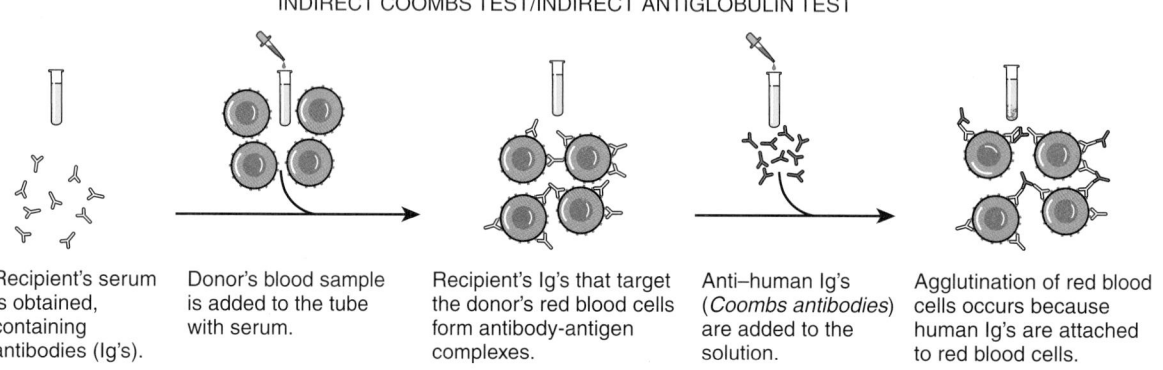

INDIRECT COOMBS TEST/INDIRECT ANTIGLOBULIN TEST

Recipient's serum is obtained, containing antibodies (Ig's).

Donor's blood sample is added to the tube with serum.

Recipient's Ig's that target the donor's red blood cells form antibody-antigen complexes.

Anti–human Ig's (*Coombs antibodies*) are added to the solution.

Agglutination of red blood cells occurs because human Ig's are attached to red blood cells.

Figure 30-1   The indirect and direct Coombs (antiglobulin) tests. The recipient's serum or plasma is separately mixed with three or more commercially available type O washed red blood cells that are known to express ~20 of the most "clinically significant" red cell antigens, to detect unexpected red cell antibodies. The recipient's serum and reagent red cells are incubated at 37° C for 30 minutes and examined. Spun cells are then washed and tested with anti–human immunoglobulin and then reexamined for hemolysis or agglutination. If antibodies have bound to red cell surface antigens, red cells will agglutinate when incubated with an anti–human globulin (also known Coombs reagent), and the indirect Coombs test will be positive. (*Modified from Wikipedia: Coombs test schematic. Available at: http://en.wikipedia.org/wiki/File:Coombs_test_schematic.png.*)

Second, antibody screening is to identify whether the recipient has formed antibodies to nonself blood groups, such as Duffy, MNS, Kell, Kidd, and P system antigens, using an updated version of the classic Coombs test, also called the *indirect antiglobulin test* (Figure 30-1). The recipient's serum or plasma is mixed separately with three or more commercially available type O washed RBCs that are known to express ~20 of the most "clinically significant" RBC antigens, to detect unexpected RBC antibodies. If transfusion is required, the recipient sample that is already typed and screened is cross-matched with donor units. Provided recipient antibodies were not identified on the type and screen, it is possible to perform a cross-match either serologically, using an immediate spin cross-match, or by an electronic match. If clinically significant antibodies have been found on the type and screen, electronic cross-matching is not sufficient and antiglobulin cross-match must be performed.[34] An electronic or computerized cross-match is performed by identifying donor units on hand that have appropriate ABO and RhD blood groups for the recipient.[35] Electronic cross-matching only can be used if a patient has a negative antibody screen, which means that they do not have any active RBC atypical antibodies. It is assumed that the proper testing (type and screen) on the recipient and donor blood are sufficient to identify clinically important incompatibility and to identify matching donor blood.[36]

When serologic cross-matching (immediate-spin cross-match) is performed, RBCs from an ABO and RhD-compatible RBC unit are mixed with the recipient's plasma. The mixture is centrifuged and examined for hemolysis or agglutination. Agglutination is considered a positive reaction, indicating that the donor unit is incompatible for that specific patient. If both are absent, ABO compatibility is verified and the RBC unit issued. This procedure is repeated for each donor RBC

unit. If agglutination or hemolysis occurs, additional screening of the recipient's plasma is performed to identify the unexpected antibodies.[36] Performing a serologic cross-match, over electronic cross-matching, before transfusing RBCs is preferred by some laboratories because it detects rare ABO errors and also detects most recipient IgM antibodies to antigens on donor RBCs.[37] In an emergency, "uncross-matched blood" can be transfused and risk for a serious transfusion reaction minimized by administration of type O and RhD-negative RBCs.[38]

Components

Because plasma contains the anti-ABO, RhD, and other antibodies of the donor, only ABO and RhD-compatible units are transfused. Thus, the recipient and donor unit must undergo a type and screen; however, cross-matching is not performed. Platelets have ABO antigens on their surface. However, ABO compatibility for platelet transfusion is desirable but not required because of the relatively small volume of plasma present in a bag of platelets. If ABO-incompatible platelets are administered for operational reasons, the recipient subsequently may have a positive direct antiglobulin test result, but significant hemolysis is rare. Furthermore, a donor–recipient ABO mismatch may result in poor function of donor platelets after transfusion.[39–41]

■ Immediate Immune-Mediated Complications of Transfusion

Hemolytic transfusion reaction is the result of complement-mediated destruction of transfused RBCs, nearly always because of incompatibility of antigen on the transfused RBCs with antibody in the recipient's circulation. The most common cause of acute hemolytic reactions is transfusion of ABO-incompatible blood; rarely, undetected serologic incompatibility is a cause of acute hemolysis.[18]

Transfusion has been associated with greater pulmonary morbidity after cardiac surgery.[43] Transfusion-related acute lung injury (TRALI) occurs when increased permeability of the pulmonary endothelium causes pulmonary edema, usually within a few hours of transfusion. Hypotension and fever also may occur.[44,45] TRALI constitutes the majority of transfusion-associated mortality in the United States.[45,46] The specific cause of TRALI is unknown; however, in many cases, the occurrence of TRALI is associated with the presence of antibodies in donor plasma directed toward the recipient's leukocyte or neutrophil antigens.[45,46] These antibodies are seen more frequently in multiparous women and individuals with prior transfusion.[47] Transfusion of blood components, especially products containing high volumes of plasma such as fresh-frozen plasma (FFP), have the greatest risk for TRALI.[47] Thus, plasma from women is usually, but not exclusively, used for processed protein fractions rather than transfusion. No routinely available pretransfusion testing is available.

Immune-mediated platelet destruction is the result of recipient antibodies being present to human leukocyte or platelet-specific antigens present on transfused platelets. Most cases of immune-mediated platelet destruction occur in individuals who have had several prior platelet transfusions. In some patients, platelet matching may be required.[41]

Anaphylactoid reactions rarely occur in transfusion of IgA-containing plasma present in any blood product given to IgA-deficient patients who have anti-IgA antibodies. The reaction is characterized by hypotension, bronchospasm, and laryngeal edema.[48]

Febrile nonhemolytic reactions are relatively frequent and typically manifested by a temperature increase of 1° C or more occurring during or shortly after transfusion. They may result from antibodies to white blood cells or from the presence of high levels of cytokines in transfused blood products.[49]

Delayed Immune-Mediated Complications of Transfusion

Delayed hemolytic reactions occur in patients who have had previous exposure to incompatible blood but who do not have circulating antibodies. Re-exposure to the antigen provokes delayed production of antibody that reaches a significant circulating level while the transfused RBCs are still present in the circulation, usually 2 to 14 days after transfusion.[50]

Graft-versus-host disease (GVHD) is a rare condition that occurs when viable donor T lymphocytes in the transfused blood product successfully engraft in the recipient. Normally, donor T cells are recognized as foreign by the recipient's immune system. However, in immunocompromised patients, and rarely when the donor is homozygous and the recipient is heterozygous for an HLA haplotype (as can occur in directed donations from first-degree relatives), the recipient's immune system is not able to destroy the donor T cells. This can result in graft-versus-host disease. Irradiation of the donor unit prevents T-cell proliferation and graft-versus-host disease.[51,52]

Nonimmune Complications of Transfusion

Transmission of infectious disease may occur with transfusion despite standard blood-banking operational procedures. Routine testing of donor blood is performed for Chagas disease, hepatitis B and C, human immunodeficiency viruses types 1 and 2, human T-lymphotropic virus, syphilis, West Nile virus, and, in some situations, cytomegalovirus.[33] Bacterial contamination occurs rarely and is manifested by fever and hemodynamic instability surrounding transfusion of the blood product.[53] Circulatory overload, hypothermia, and metabolic and electrolyte derangements are other complications that may occur in high-volume transfusion.[54]

Transfusion and Morbidity Outcomes

Although transfusion of RBCs is necessary for some patients, its use has been associated with a dose-dependent greater prevalence of morbidity after cardiac surgery.[55] Greater rates of postoperative infectious complications, prolonged postoperative ventilatory support, renal injury, and reductions in short and long term survival are more common in patients transfused with RBCs.[43,55–57] Greater rates of bacteremia, septicemia, and deep and superficial sternal wound infections are thought to be secondary to a downregulation of the immune system.[38,58] Transfusion has been related to an increased development of postoperative atrial fibrillation thought to be secondary to the influence of RBC transfusion on inflammation. RBC transfusion results in a direct infusion of inflammatory mediators, as well as augmenting the inflammatory response to cardiopulmonary bypass (CPB) and cardiac surgery.[59,60]

Storage duration of the RBC product also may be a contributing factor for observed adverse outcomes. The storage lesion consists of a series of structural and functional changes occurring with increasing RBC storage. Some of these changes are reversible, others are not, and together may result in decreased microvascular tissue flow.[61–63] A recent investigation reported transfusion of RBCs stored longer than 14 days was associated with a greater risk for death and complications after cardiac surgery.[64] A recent laboratory investigation from Sweeney et al[65] reported increased thrombin generation for RBC units of increasing storage duration, suggesting a cause for increased complications observed with transfusion of RBCs of increased storage duration.

GENETIC CAUSES OF HEMORRHAGE

In general, the coagulation system can be thought of as being highly optimized toward rapid cessation of hemorrhage. There likely has been a strong evolutionary pressure toward rapid coagulation and wound healing. Of course, there must be an equally highly developed system that prevents overwhelming coagulation of the entire blood volume in response to a trivial intravascular insult. In contrast, there was likely little or no pressure to avoid a deep venous thrombosis in older age because most individuals did not live beyond 40 years until a few centuries ago. Similarly, there has been no evolutionary pressure to successfully undergo blood exposure to foreign surfaces such as the CPB circuit. Because severe bleeding abnormalities are strongly selected against, in evolutionary terms, they are rare. A sentinel example is the hemophilias, in which a rare variant causes production of a nonfunctional protein with severe consequences. In contrast, trivial abnormalities have not undergone marked evolutionary pressures and are likely to be more common. A good example of this is the wide, but seemingly unimportant, heritable variation seen in the circulating level of many coagulation proteins.[66–69]

In some individuals, the coagulation system is not optimized to achieve rapid coagulation. Most abnormalities are either a quantitative deficiency of a normal protein or a qualitatively defective (hypofunctional) protein present in normal concentration. The measurement of protein concentration and activity are importantly different. Protein concentrations usually are measured by the amount of binding of a manufactured antibody against a portion of the protein (antigen). Antibody-based assays will detect quantitative deficiencies of the protein but will not be able to detect qualitative defects unless the antibody is specifically directed toward the structural abnormality of the protein. The function of a protein usually is measured by the enzyme or other functional activity of the protein, often by measuring the amount of enzyme product formed. Activity-based assays may be reduced because the amount of the protein is reduced or its activity is reduced, so the cause of reduced function likely will also include the measurement of the amount of protein using a quantitative assay.

Genetic causes of impaired coagulation can be somewhat simplistically thought of as either a qualitative defect arising from abnormal protein structure because of a coding genetic variant or a quantitative defect arising from abnormal, usually reduced, production of a normal protein because of a noncoding (promoter) genetic variant. This approach is rudimentary but gives the best basic understanding of the genetic mechanisms of coagulation disorders. Like all genetic disorders, the overall effect of a genetic variant on the whole human or surgical population is a product of the frequency of the genetic variant and the biologic effect of the variant.[70] If the variant is rare, such as the hemophilias, although the disease is problematic for a single individual, the overall effect on day-to-day practice is low because of its rarity. By contrast, a more common variant may have greater effect. Similarly, for two variants of equal frequency, the one with low biologic effect will have less overall influence than one with a higher biologic effect. To date, no frequent variants with high biologic effect on coagulation have been identified.[69]

Variation in Coagulation Protein Levels

Several studies have demonstrated the strong heritability of levels of plasma proteins and platelet levels in normal populations.[68,71-74] This type of research is undertaken by examining the plasma level of coagulation proteins in multigenerational families and estimating the within-family variation compared with the whole-population variation.[75] In accordance with the believed strong evolutionary importance of coagulation function, there is similar strong inheritance within families, with up to 70% of the variation in plasma protein levels determined by genetic heritability. Similar heritability of platelet count and platelet volume has been observed.[76,77]

Genetic variation associated with the circulating level of a coagulation protein is usually in or around the gene for that coagulation protein. For example, the circulating level of plasminogen activator inhibitor 1 (PAI-1) principally is determined by a common promoter variant that alters the binding of the transcription factor inhibitor.[66,67] Similarly, the circulating level of thrombin-activated fibrinolysis inhibitor is determined by two variants,[78] and circulating prothrombin levels are determined by a single variant.[79] However, some coagulation protein levels are regulated by genetic variation that is not in or around the protein's gene. Similarly, platelet count and platelet volume are regulated by genes that would not be intuitive choices.[76,77]

Hemophilias

Hemophilias are the most well-known example of a rare severe genetic disorder of coagulation. Hemophilia A (factor VIII deficiency) is the most common hemophilia, occurring in about 1 in 5000 male births.[80] Hemophilia B (factor IX deficiency) occurs in about 1 in 34,000 male births. Both genes lie on the X chromosome, meaning that in male individuals, only one copy of the chromosome is present and a single variant may result in hemophilia (often called a *sex-linked* or *X-linked disease*). Accordingly, female hemophiliacs must have two copies of the rare variant—an event that usually occurs only in consanguineous births in which the father has hemophilia. Although most hemophilias are maternally inherited, about 30% are spontaneous mutations not present in the mother. An obvious question is why female individuals do not have twice the factor VIII and IX levels as male individuals. The reason is that in female individuals, one of the X chromosomes is usually "turned off" and does not generate messenger RNA for translation of proteins. However, it is possible for female carriers to have mild hemophilia because of lyonization (inactivation) of the X chromosome that carries the normal gene, leaving the abnormal gene to be the most active. Adult women may experience menorrhagia because of the bleeding tendency. Hemophilia C is an autosomal genetic disorder (not X-linked) involving a lack of functional clotting factor XI. Hemophilia C is not completely recessive because heterozygous individuals also show increased bleeding.[81]

The gene *F8* encodes factor VIII of the intrinsic pathway. Factor VIII is a cofactor for factor IXa, which converts factor X to the activated form Xa. There are almost 700 known coding variations of the *F8* gene, many of which have been seen in only one individual or family. More than 170 give severe forms of hemophilia A, and more than 180 produce milder forms.[82,83] Some of these mutations change one amino acid; many of these have little effect on protein function because only one amino acid is changed, often to a similar type of amino acid.[84] Others cause a frameshift mutation that usually truncates the protein

and markedly reduces its function. Another severe mutation is an inversion of a portion of the genome and, therefore, the sequence of a portion of the protein is "back-to-front" with marked reduction in function. Rarely, the entire gene is deleted so that both quantitative and qualitative assays show the absence of factor VIII. The diagnosis of hemophilia A is made by reduced factor VIII activity, prolonged activated partial thromboplastin time except in mild disease, and a normal PT and platelet count.[84]

The gene *F9* encodes the vitamin K–dependent factor IX of the intrinsic pathway. Factor IX is activated by factor XI to factor IXa. Because hemophilia B is rarer than hemophilia A, fewer mutations have been described, but the mechanisms of protein dysfunction from genetic variation are similar. The diagnosis of hemophilia B is made by reduced factor IX activity, prolonged activated partial thromboplastin time except in mild disease, and a normal PT and platelet count.[84]

Hemophilia is not a contraindication for cardiac surgery, but it is an absolute indication for involvement of a hematologist and blood banker. Most experience has been small case series or single case reports, but all emphasize the need for prolonged factor therapy and subsequent excellent outcomes. For hemophilia A, the factor VIII activity level should be corrected to 100% of normal for cardiac surgery, although some hematologists use 50% to 70% of normal as a goal. One unit of factor VIII is the normal amount of factor VIII in 1 mL plasma, by definition. Because the volume of distribution of factor VIII is that of plasma, the amount of factor VIII in an individual is ~50 mL/kg. The factor VIII dose needed to correct the level is calculated as follows[85,86]:

$$\text{Units factor VIII} = (\text{weight in kg}) * (50 \text{ mL plasma}/\text{kg}) * (\text{desired } \% \text{ factor VIII level} - \text{the current } \% \text{ factor VIII level})/100$$

Approximately 30% of people with severe hemophilia A develop antibodies to transfused factor VIII. These antibodies (also called *inhibitors*) bind to transfused factor VIII and reduce its activity so increased doses of factor VIII are required.[87] The next dose should be administered 6 to 12 hours after the initial dose, together with repeated factor VIII activity monitoring with the goal of keeping the trough activity greater than 50%. During hemorrhage, cryoprecipitate and FFP can be given to restore levels of factor VIII and other coagulation factors, as well as blood volume. 1-Deamino-8-D-arginine vasopressin (DDAVP) at a dose of 0.3 µg/kg can be used in mild or moderate hemophilia A, and works by increasing circulating factor VIII and von Willebrand factor (vWF) levels. DDAVP works only when some normal factor VIII activity is present and usually with only modest success.[88]

For hemophilia B, the factor IX activity level should be corrected to 100% of normal for cardiac surgery, although some hematologists use 50% to 70% of normal as a goal. One unit of factor IX is the normal amount of factor IX in 1 mL plasma, by definition. Unlike factor VIII, the volume of distribution of factor IX in an individual is 100 mL/kg. The factor IX dose needed to correct the level is calculated as follows[89]:

$$\text{Units factor IX} = (\text{weight in kg}) * (100 \text{ mL plasma}/\text{kg}) * (\text{desired } \% \text{ factor IX level} - \text{the current } \% \text{ factor IX level})/100$$

The next dose should be administered 12 to 24 hours after the initial dose, together with repeated factor IX activity monitoring with the goal of keeping the trough activity greater than 50%. During hemorrhage, FFP can be given to restore levels of factor IX and other coagulation factors, as well as blood volume. DDAVP is not effective.[88]

Von Willebrand Disease

Von Willebrand disease (vWD) is the most common inherited coagulation abnormality in humans, occurring in about 1% of individuals.[90] vWD also can be an acquired disease. It arises from quantitative (reduced amounts of usually normal protein) or qualitative (normal amounts of a defective protein) deficits of vWF, which is a multimeric plasma glycoprotein produced by endothelium and platelets. The protein binds factor VIII, the platelet GPIb receptor, the activated form of the GPIIb/IIIa receptor, and collagen.[71]

Unlike the serine proteases of the intrinsic and extrinsic pathways of the coagulation system, vWF is not an enzyme and serves its functions by binding to other proteins.[91] It has an important role in platelet adhesion to exposed subendothelial collagen by binding to exposed collagen and also to the GPIb receptor of circulating platelets, especially in high shear environments such as arterial bleeding. vWF decelerates platelets from rapid flow by uncoiling; thus, it appears to be the critical initiator of platelet adhesion in high-flow environments. Platelet adhesion initiates rapid platelet activation, with switching of the most common platelet receptor, GPIIb/IIIa, from a quiescent protein that poorly binds to fibrinogen and fibrin, to an activated protein that strongly binds fibrinogen and fibrin. Subsequently, vWF also can bind to activated GPIIb/IIIa receptors expressed on activated platelets.

There are four types of hereditary vWD caused by mutations in the gene *vWF* (Figure 30-2).[92,93] Other factors, including having an O blood group, increase the clinical severity of vWD. Type 1 vWD (60% to 80% of all vWD) is a mild quantitative defect of normal vWF, with individuals having about 10% to 50% of normal vWF levels and often having low levels of factor VIII. The disease is inherited in an autosomal dominant fashion, and most individuals are heterozygous (possess one copy) of the abnormal gene with variants principally found between exons 18 and 28 of the gene.[94] Rarely, homozygotes (two copies of the abnormal gene) have extremely low levels of vWF. Most heterozygotes have normal or near-normal coagulation and are identified by having abnormal bleeding after tooth extraction or surgery, or having menorrhagia.[95]

Type 2 vWD (20% to 30%) is a qualitative defect with four subtypes: 2A, 2B, 2M, and 2N.[90] Type 2A vWD is caused by decreased activity, but normal levels, of vWF. The vWF multimers are structurally abnormal and usually small. In contrast with hemophilia, type 2A vWD is inherited in an autosomal dominant fashion and is caused by variants in exons 12 to 16, 28, and 52 of the gene. Type 2B vWF is a rare "gain-of-function" defect leading to spontaneous binding to platelets and subsequent rapid clearance of the platelets and large vWF multimers. Patients with this subtype should not receive desmopressin because it can induce platelet aggregation. Type 2M vWD is characterized by a platelet function defect caused by a decrease in high-molecular-weight multimers. Type 2N vWD is caused by the inability of vWF to bind factor VIII but has an autosomal recessive inheritance and is most often associated with variants in exons 18 to 20. This type gives a normal vWF antigen level and normal functional test results, but has a low factor VIII. This probably has led to some 2N patients being misdiagnosed in the past as having hemophilia A, and should be suspected if the patient has the clinical findings of hemophilia A but a pedigree suggesting autosomal, rather than X-linked, inheritance.[90]

Type 3 vWD is caused by a quantitative lack of vWF and premature proteolysis of factor VIII, similar to type 2A vWD, but in an autosomal recessive fashion. Type 3 is the most severe form of vWD because individuals are homozygous for the defective gene and protein. They have no detectable vWF antigen and may have sufficiently low factor VIII that they have hemarthroses, similar to hemophilia.[95]

Acquired vWD can occur in patients with autoantibodies. In this case, the function of vWF is not inhibited, but the vWF-antibody complex is rapidly cleared from the circulation by antibody binding. A form of vWD occurs in patients with aortic valve stenosis, leading to gastrointestinal bleeding (Heyde syndrome).[96] This form of acquired vWD may be more prevalent than is currently thought. Acquired vWD also has been described in Wilms tumor and hypothyroidism.

Laboratory diagnosis is made by usually normal hemoglobin, activated partial thromboplastin time, and partial thromboplastin time, but reduced quantity of vWF measured by an antigenic assay, reduced vWF:ristocetin cofactor assay (vWF:RCo), or reduced functional factor VIII assay.[92] If abnormalities in these three tests are identified, specialized coagulation studies also may be performed to determine the subtype of vWD. Bleeding can be treated with plasma-derived clotting factor concentrates containing both vWF and FVIII; depending on the vWD type, mild bleeding episodes usually respond to DDAVP.[97]

Platelet-type or pseudo-vWD is an autosomal dominant type of vWD caused by gain-of-function coding mutations of the vWF receptor (GPIb) on platelets, not of the vWF gene.[93] GPIb is a dimeric protein that is part of the larger complex (GPIb/V/IX), which forms the full vWF receptor on platelets. The loss of large vWF multimers is similar to that seen in type 2B vWD, but genetic testing of the vWF gene does not find mutations. The hyper-responsiveness of the platelet receptor results in increased interaction with vWF in response to minimal or no stimulation in vivo. This leads to a decline in plasma vWF and typically to a decreased or low normal platelet count.[91] Replacement therapy in the form of VIII/vWF preparations or drugs aimed at increasing the release of endogenous vWF will exacerbate the condition and lead to further reduction of the platelet count. Platelet transfusions are therapeutic.

Factor V

Normal factor Va and its cofactor, factor Xa, are the first members of the *final common pathway* or *thrombin pathway* and combine to form the prothrombinase complex.[98,99] The prothrombinase complex catalyzes the conversion of prothrombin (factor II) to thrombin (factor IIa).

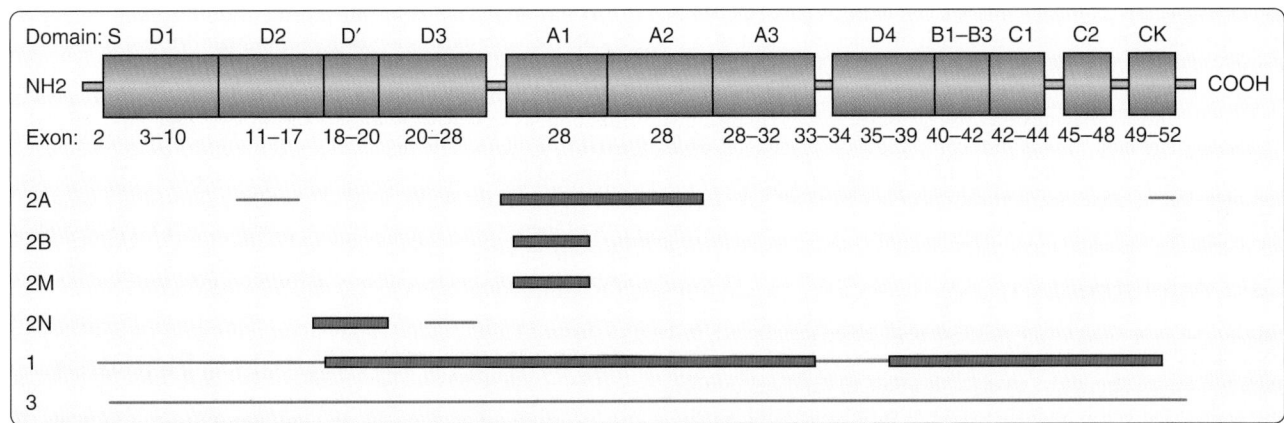

Figure 30-2 **Location of von Willebrand factor *(vWF)* mutations by von Willebrand disease (vWD) type.** *Green horizontal lines* indicate the approximate position of exons where mutations are most prevalent; *thinner lines* indicate exons with mutations of lower frequency. Mutations that result in type 2 vWD affect vWF function and cluster in domains primarily disrupted by missense mutations. *(From http://www.ncbi.nlm.nih .gov/bookshelf/br.fcgi?book=gene&part=von-willebrand&rendertype=figure&id=von-willebrand.F1 and http://www.ncbi.nlm.nih.gov/bookshelf/br .fcgi?book=gene&part=von-willebrand. Source: www.genetests.org. Copyright University of Washington, Seattle, WA.)*

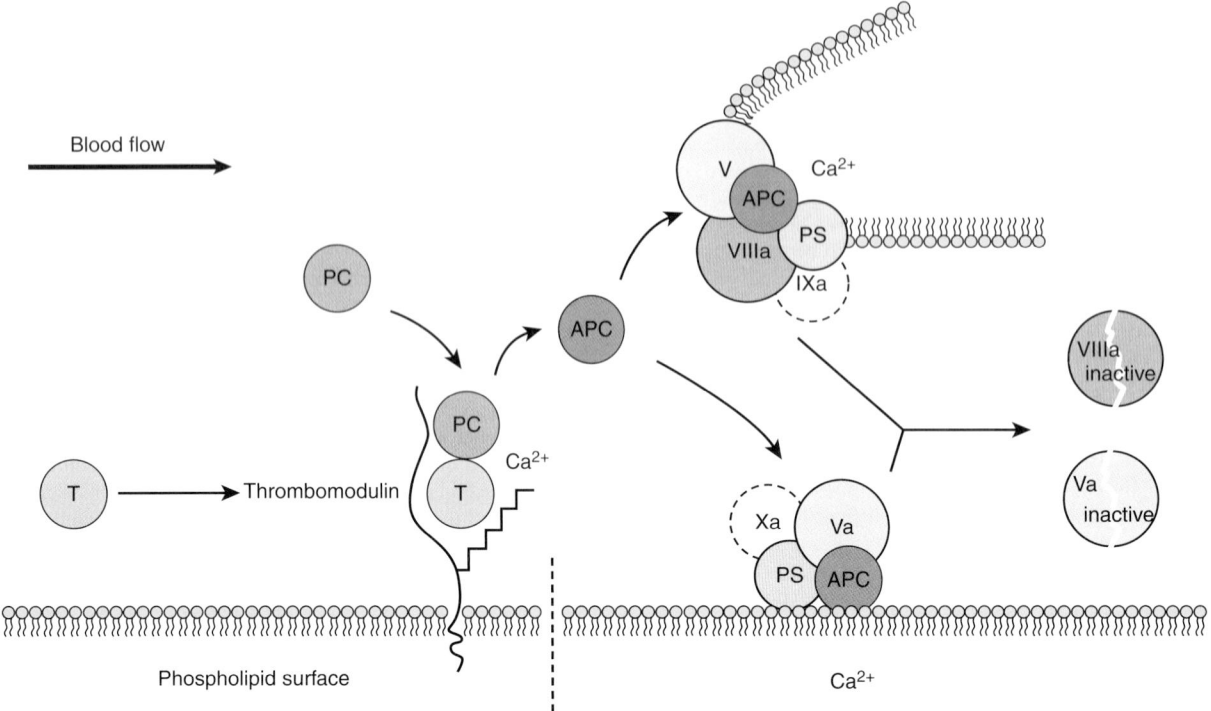

Figure 30-3 Protein C anticoagulant pathway: Activated protein C (aPC) functions as a circulating anticoagulant, which specifically degrades factors Va and VIIIa. This effectively downregulates the coagulation cascade and limits clot formation to sites of vascular injury. APC, activated protein C, PC, protein C; PS, protein S; T, thrombin. *(From Wikipedia: Protein C anticoagulant. Available at: http://en.wikipedia.org/wiki/File:Protein_C_anticoagulant.jpg)*

To produce thrombin, the prothrombinase complex cleaves two peptide bonds in prothrombin. The action of factor Va is terminated by cleavage by activated protein C (aPC) (Figure 30-3).

Factor V Leiden is a common SNP that results in a factor V variant that cannot be as easily degraded by aPC.[100] The nucleotide variant (G1691A) results in conversion of an arginine to a glycine (Arg506Gln). This amino acid is normally the cleavage site for aPC, and the protein change markedly reduces the activity of aPC on factor Va.[99] When factor Va remains active, it facilitates overproduction of thrombin, leading to excess fibrin generation and excess clotting. In essence, it is creating a gain of function by inhibiting the termination of factor Va. The clotting is almost always venous, resulting in deep vein thrombosis or pulmonary embolus.[99]

About 5% of whites in North America have factor V Leiden.[100] The SNP is less common in Hispanics and African Americans, and is rare in Asians. About 30% of people who have a deep vein thrombosis or pulmonary embolism, especially in younger patients, carry the SNP. Having the SNP and also having other risk factors for deep vein thrombosis including smoking, taking oral contraceptives, pregnancy, and recent surgery, markedly increase risk. Efforts to show that the prothrombotic factor V Leiden variant results in *less* bleeding have been mixed.[101,102]

Cold Agglutinins

Cold agglutinin disease is rare (~2/100,000). Causes include a lymphoma-induced monoclonal gammopathy, renal cell carcinoma, or infection; but most commonly, no cause is found.[103] Cold agglutinins are usually IgM autoantibodies that react at cold temperatures with RBC polysaccharide antigens. Low titers (1:16) of cold agglutinins often are found in the sera of healthy individuals, but the presence of high titers of cold agglutinins (titers over 1:1000 at 4°C) can lead to hemagglutination and thrombosis at low temperatures, followed by complement activation and subsequent hemolysis on rewarming.[104,105]

It generally is agreed that screening for cold agglutinins before cardiac surgery is not warranted because of their rarity.[104]

In contrast with the warm agglutinins, patients with cold agglutinins do not respond to steroids or splenectomy but sometimes respond to rituximab.[103] Rituximab destroys both normal and malignant B lymphocytes and is used to treat B-cell lymphomas and rheumatoid arthritis. It specifically targets the CD20 antigen, but the function of CD20 is unknown.[103]

Variation in Platelet Count and Volume

There are wide variabilities in platelet counts and volumes in normal individuals coming for surgery. In addition, platelet function is often markedly depressed from purposeful administration of antiplatelet agents such as aspirin, clopidogrel, and other drugs.

Mean platelet volume is a measurement of the average size of platelets found in blood and is positively correlated with platelet count and function, as well as with adverse thrombotic outcomes. Genetic variants associated with mean platelet volume and platelet count have been identified in or near the genes *WDR66, ARGHEF3, TAOK1, TMCC2, TPM1, PIK3CG, EHD3, ATXN2, PTPN11,* and *AK3,* among others.[77] Few of these associations are intuitive or supported by well-understood biologic mechanisms; nevertheless, they indicate the complexity and importance of genetic causes of normal coagulation function.

BLEEDING AFTER CARDIAC SURGERY

Do genetics affect bleeding after cardiac surgery? For many of the well-identified bleeding diatheses mentioned earlier, the answer is yes. However, clinicians rarely encounter these patients in their practice. More commonly, they see a patient who is bleeding for no apparent reason—without a surgical bleeding site, without a drug cause, and with normal or near-normal coagulation tests. The reason for this occurring in an individual patient is almost never known, and the patient is treated symptomatically until the bleeding stops. It is possible, but unproved, that these patients have a genetically inherited bleeding diathesis. Few studies have examined this question, and their limited findings are unreplicated.[102,106–108] (See Chapter 31.)

Reoperation for Bleeding

Re-exploration for bleeding is a serious complication, which significantly impacts a patient's subsequent postoperative course by increasing both morbidity and mortality. Approximately 2% to 4% of patients undergoing cardiac surgery require reoperation for bleeding with greater reported rates for more complex procedures. A recent investigation evaluating incidence, risk factors, and outcomes for patients requiring reoperation for bleeding in 528,686 CABG patients from the Society of Thoracic Surgeons National Cardiac Database (2004–2007) reported a 2.4% rate of reoperation. Risk factors for reoperation were older age, male sex, comorbidity such as peripheral vascular and cerebrovascular disease, chronic lung disease, renal insufficiency, heart failure, previous interventions, urgent or emergent surgery, preoperative intra-aortic balloon pump, PCI less than 6 hours before CABG, and thienopyridine use less than 24 hours before surgical intervention. Patients requiring reoperation had greater risk for morbidity such as septicemia, stroke, and prolonged ventilatory support after surgery. Risk-adjusted mortality was significantly greater for patients requiring reoperation: 5.9% vs. 1.97%. Of note, risk was not increased in patients receiving aspirin therapy less than 24 hours before surgery.[109]

Additional studies have characterized risk factors for reoperation and its relation to patient outcome. Moulton et al[110] identified a 4.2% reoperation rate and identified increasing age, renal insufficiency, reoperative procedures, and prolonged CPB time as risk factors for this complication. Interestingly, antiplatelet drugs, such as preoperative aspirin, and preoperative use of heparin or thrombolytic agents were not significant predictors. In addition, the authors reported that incidence of death, renal failure, sepsis, and need for prolonged ventilatory support were significantly greater in patients who underwent reoperation for bleeding.[110] Choong et al[111] reported demographic and comorbidity risk factors previously described, as well as cessation of aspirin within 4 days of surgery, preoperative use of clopidogrel, lack of antifibrinolytic agents during surgery, type of operation, and CPB duration as risk factors for postoperative bleeding necessitating re-exploration.

In a contemporary cohort of patients, Karthik et al[112] examined risk factors for reoperation and effect of time delay on morbidity after surgery. The rate of reoperation in their investigation was 3.1%. Factors associated with the need for reoperation included demographics such as increasing age, smaller body mass index, and surgery that was non-elective. They similarly reported that reoperation was associated with increased morbidity, hemodynamic instability, and transfusion of RBC and component therapy. Among the 89 patients requiring reoperation, 31 had greater than 12 hours time delay to re-exploration (4 deaths in delayed reoperation group). The authors concluded that mortality outcomes were worse if the time delay was greater than 12 hours after surgery and recommended an early re-exploration policy for bleeding.[112] Ranucci et al[113] reported an increased risk for reoperation and noted that much of the morbidity risk was attributable to the amount of RBCs transfused; delay for reoperation was related to risk only if the delay involved excess use of blood products.

Hall et al[114] sought to differentiate coagulopathy versus hemorrhage from surgical causes in patients undergoing reoperation for bleeding. Both groups had increased morbidity and mortality compared with those not requiring reoperation. Excess risk was attributed to more hemodynamic instability, transfusions, and inotropic support, which were more common in patients undergoing reoperation. The authors recommended normalization of coagulation profiles within 4 hours of intensive care unit admission, and if significant bleeding persisted with a normal coagulation profile, re-exploration.[114]

Ratios in Resuscitation: Implications for Massive Transfusion in Cardiac Surgery

Patients requiring massive transfusion in the perioperative period may become coagulopathic secondary to loss, hemodilution, consumption of coagulation factors, and insufficient component replacement. Furthermore, hypothermia is common in the perioperative period and can lead to platelet dysfunction via its effect on platelet activation and adhesion.[115] Hypothermia also may contribute to reductions in clotting factor functional activity.[116–119] Development of acidosis may act synergistically with hypothermia to further worsen coagulopathy through its impact on pH-sensitive enzyme complexes involved in the clotting cascade.[120–122] Furthermore, choice of volume administration (i.e., hetastarch) may further worsen coagulopathy in patients with massive blood loss.[120]

A number of investigations propose a modification of more traditional component replacement therapy in massively transfused patients to one that considers a greater FFP:RBC ratio. The optimal ratio has not been well clarified, and the impact on patient morbid outcomes is variable; however, a number of publications report improved outcomes after traumatic injury for patients receiving a greater ratio of FFP to RBC. These recommendations have considerable implications in terms of product supply and associated morbidity risk to patients.

Borgman et al[123] recommended implementation of massive transfusion protocols consisting of greater FFP:RBC (1:1) ratio, noting evidence of improved survival and possibly less use of RBCs primarily in the trauma literature. Holcomb et al[124] recommended a massive transfusion protocol that included a 1:1:1 ratio of FFP/platelets/RBC to favorably impact patient outcomes. They analyzed four groups based on high and low plasma and platelet/RBC ratios. The combination of high plasma/RBC and high platelet/RBC ratios was associated with decreased truncal hemorrhage and increased 6-hour, 24-hour, and 30-day survival. Gunter et al[125] reported a significant reduction in 30-day mortality for patients who received FFP/RBC of 2:3 or greater compared with those who received less than 2:3. Patients receiving platelets to RBC at a greater ratio (≥ 1:5) also had lower 30-day mortality when compared with patients with less than 1:5 ratio. Similarly, Zink et al[126] reported improved survival and decreased overall RBC transfusion in trauma patients receiving early high FFP and platelet-to-RBC transfusion ratios within the first 6 hours of hemorrhage. The authors appropriately addressed the difficulty of basing component therapy on laboratory testing because of time delay for test results.

Others have suggested a U-shaped curve depicting higher mortality at low and higher FFP/RBC ratios, and better outcomes when the ratio was 1:2 or 1:3. A 1:1 ratio of FFP/RBC reduced coagulopathy but failed to improve survival, prompting authors to caution against adopting the 1:1 ratio without further testing.[120,127] Interestingly, some have criticized proponents of the greater FFP-to-RBC transfusion protocols, noting that these studies may have a "survival bias" present; that is, the most severely injured patients simply did not survive long enough to receive FFP, which often is not immediately available.[120]

In a computer simulation model of dilutional coagulopathy, Hirshberg et al[128] reported that current massive transfusion protocols in bleeding patients underestimate dilution of clotting factors to correct dilutional coagulopathy. The authors provided a sensitivity analysis of a wide range of replacement protocols by programming their model to administer FFP and platelets after transfusion of a predefined number of RBC units. (Model was calibrated to data from 44 patients.) They determined that the optimal replacement ratios are 2:3 for plasma and 8:10 for platelets with RBC[128] (Figures 30-4 and 30-5).

Massive transfusion protocols improve survival in patients with exsanguinating hemorrhage. Early activation of a massive transfusion protocol and achieving predefined ratios have been associated with improved survival.[129] Others have reported on benefits of predefined massive transfusion protocols in terms of improved patient outcome in severely injured patients.[129] Riskin et al[130] reported that it was the implementation of a protocol for massive transfusion that included

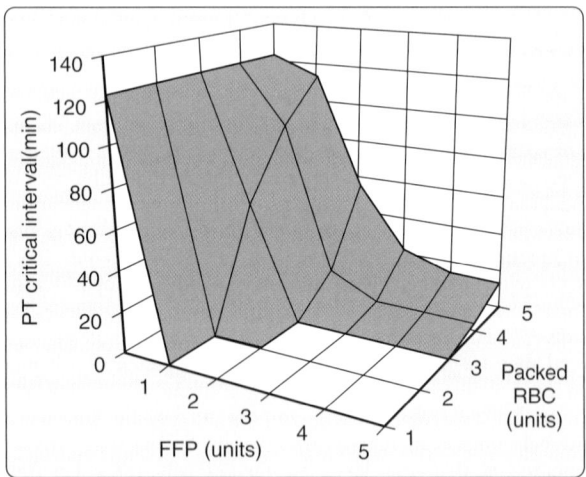

Figure 30-4   A response surface of the effect of a matrix of fresh frozen plasma/red blood cell (RBC) replacement ratios on the prothrombin time (PT) critical interval. The optimal ratio (2:3) is the point at the edge of the surface where the highest value for red blood cells intersects with the lowest value for fresh frozen plasma (FFP) to maintain a critical interval of zero. *(From Hirshberg A, Dugas M, Banez EI, et al: Minimizing dilutional coagulopathy in exsanguinating hemorrhage: A computer simulation. J Trauma 54:454–463, 2003, by permission.)*

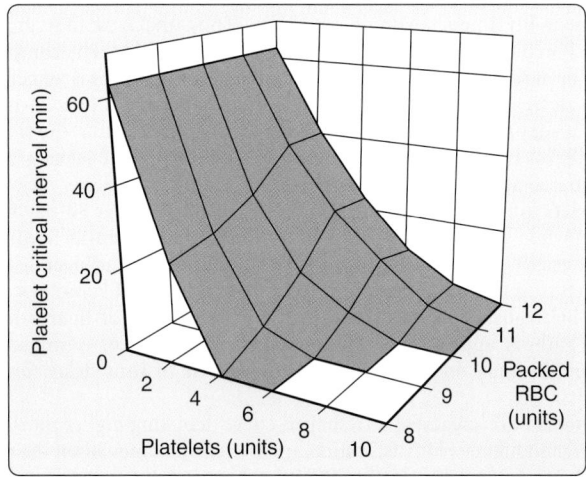

Figure 30-5   A response surface of the effect of a matrix of platelets/red blood cell (RBC) replacement ratios on the platelet critical interval. The optimal ratio is 8:10. *(From Hirshberg A, Dugas M, Banez EI, et al: Minimizing dilutional coagulopathy in exsanguinating hemorrhage: A computer simulation. J Trauma 54:454–463, 2003, by permission.)*

improved access and availability of blood products that reduced mortality in their patient population rather than use of a greater FFP/RBC ratio. They emphasized the importance of expeditious product availability because survival benefit did not appear to have been related to any alteration in the volume or ratio of blood components used.

REPLACEMENT THERAPY

Factor VIIa

Recombinant factor VIIa (rFVIIa, NovoSeven trademark; Novo Nordisk, Bagsvaerd, Denmark) is approved for the treatment of bleeding in patients with hemophilia A or B with inhibitors against factors VIII and IX. Factor VII acts locally at the site of vessel injury by binding to tissue factor on subendothelial cells and facilitates transformation of factors IX and X to active forms, ultimately resulting in thrombin

generation and clot formation.[131,132] A laboratory investigation examined the effect of rFVIIa-mediated thrombin generation on platelet adhesion and aggregation at normal and reduced platelet counts. Their results suggested that administration of rFVIIa in patients with and without thrombocytopenia enhanced platelet deposition and aggregation at the site of vascular injury, which may explain, in part, the efficacy of rFVIIa in thrombocytopenic patients.[133]

Off-label use of rFVIIa has been reported as a rescue therapy for patients with hemorrhage refractory to conventional therapy. However, the safety of rFVIIa in the cardiac surgical setting has not been well clarified. Safety concerns relate to the risk for thrombosis, and case reports of thrombotic events have tempered consideration for use in patients beyond rescue therapy, that is, prophylactically in patients at high risk for bleeding to avoid blood transfusion.

In a comprehensive evaluation of off-label use of rFVIIa in Canada, Karkouti et al[134] noted rFVIIa was associated with significant reductions in transfusion after administration without increases in mortality or major morbid events. Filsoufi et al[131] reported improvement in coagulation variables, blood loss, and reduced need for blood products in patients receiving rFVIIa for management of refractory bleeding after surgery. Similarly, a retrospective investigation from Von Heymann et al[135] reported significant reductions in blood loss and transfusion requirements after rFVIIa administration for perioperative bleeding refractory to conventional treatment. Mortality was similar between groups, and no thromboembolic complications were observed in the rFVIIa group. A number of other investigations have reported on use of rFVIIa for treatment of refractory bleeding. Most report that rFVIIa is effective in reducing bleeding and decreasing RBC and component therapy requirements. Clinical use beyond rescue therapy is unclear because of the safety profile of the medication.[136–138]

A large case series of rFVIIa use from the Australian and New Zealand Hemostasis Registry reported rFVIIa was associated with fewer blood products; however, it was associated with a 7% adverse event rate, 4% of which was related to thromboembolic events.[139] In a review of rFVIIa, DiDomenico et al[140] noted that 10% of patients had what was believed to be thromboembolic complications after the administration of rFVIIa and addressed the primary concerns with the use of rFVIIa, that is, promoting a hypercoagulable state. Gill et al[141] reported that patients who received rFVIIa had fewer transfusions after randomization and fewer reoperations for bleeding; however, they also reported an increase in serious adverse events in patients randomized to rFVIIa compared with placebo; this increase was not significantly different. Similarly, Bowman et al[142] reported benefits in controlling hemorrhage and reductions in blood product requirements with rFVIIa; however, patients who received rFVIIa had a greater prevalence of postoperative renal failure, pneumonia, and an 11% incidence rate of thrombosis. Review of the U.S. Food and Drug Administration Adverse Event Reporting System found a total of 431 adverse events related to the use of factor VIIa, among which 185 were thromboembolic events.[143]

Fibrinogen Concentrates

Human fibrinogen concentrates have been used for substitution therapy in cases of hypofibrinogenemia, dysfibrinogenemia, and afibrinogenemia. Accumulating data suggest that fibrinogen plays a critical role in hemostasis, especially in bleeding patients with an acquired fibrinogen deficiency.[144] Clinical use of fibrinogen concentrates is based on the supposition that plasma fibrinogen concentrations may become critically reduced somewhat early in a bleeding patient, and that this may contribute to the coagulopathy associated with hemorrhage. Furthermore, a functional fibrinogen deficiency may develop with excessive hemodilution with colloid plasma expanders. Correction of fibrinogen deficits has included administration of FFP, cryoprecipitate, and plasma-derived fibrinogen concentrates.[145]

Riastap USA is a commercially available virally inactivated fibrinogen concentrate derived from human plasma. Benefits over FFP and cryoprecipitate include viral inactivation and rapid reconstitution in addition to lower volume of administration. In a pilot study,

Rahe-Meyer et al[146] reported a reduction in transfusion with administration of fibrinogen concentrate, targeting a greater plasma fibrinogen concentration compared with conventional therapy. Fenger-Eriksen et al[145] reported significant reductions in blood loss and RBC, FFP, and platelet transfusion with fibrinogen concentrate without serious adverse events. Others have described benefits of fibrinogen concentrate with outcome measures of fewer transfusions and improved clot firmness.[147]

Karlsson et al[148] hypothesized that preoperative fibrinogen plasma concentrations within the reference range may be a limiting factor for hemostasis. The authors randomized CABG patients with preoperative plasma fibrinogen levels less than 3.8 g/L to an infusion of 2 g fibrinogen concentrate or placebo. End points were vessel occlusion assessed by multislice computed tomography (CT), blood loss, transfusion, and hemoglobin levels 24 hours after surgery. One subclinical vein graft occlusion was reported in the fibrinogen group, with similar global measures of hemostasis assessed by thromboelastography. The fibrinogen group had lower postoperative blood loss and greater hemoglobin concentrations. The authors appropriately addressed the concern of creating a prothrombotic state with increased incidence of graft occlusion. Interesting, they were not able to clarify the mechanism behind the reduced bleeding. Fibrinogen plasma levels were increased in the fibrinogen group immediately after infusion, but there were no differences between the groups 2 hours after surgery, and measures of hemostasis also were similar.[148]

Prothrombin Complex Concentrates

Prothrombin complex concentrates (PCCs) are prepared from pooled plasma and contain four vitamin K–dependent clotting factors II, VII, IX, and X. PCC can be used for rapid reversal of oral anticoagulants (vitamin K antagonists) in patients with life-threatening bleeding and less commonly for patients with congenital or acquired deficiencies of factor II or X. The U.S. Food and Drug Administration has not approved PCCs for reversal of bleeding associated with warfarin. Although FFP commonly has been used for emergent reversal of vitamin K antagonists, it has a greater volume of administration, it must be patient matched and thawed, and has risks associated with exposure. PCC is virally inactivated and more efficacious in normalizing international normalized ratio in patients treated with vitamin K antagonists. Some have suggested PCC may have a role in the management of massive bleeding; however, side effects include potential for thromboembolic complications.[149–152]

Volume Replacement: Colloids and Crystalloids

Maintenance of intravascular volume is a common goal for perioperative management in cardiovascular surgery. Merits of specific choices for fluid therapy to replace ongoing fluid loss continue to be debated. Although there may be theoretical advantages of colloid or crystalloid as a choice for volume replacement, clinical trial data do not definitively support one over the other in terms of mortality outcomes. Both have distinct advantages and disadvantages.[153] In general, more important than choice of volume replacement is appropriate volume replacement to avoid tissue hypoperfusion.

Volume of distribution for a particular fluid administered will depend on fluid composition. Generally, saline-based crystalloids will result in expansion of plasma volume by approximately 200 to 250 mL for each 1 L administered; glucose-based solutions will expand plasma volume less (approximately 60 to 70 mL/1 L infused); and colloid solutions will result in expansion of plasma volume generally similar to volume infused. Of note, within the semisynthetic colloid solutions there is variability in degree of plasma volume expansion, as well as a differential influence on hemostasis and inflammatory processes.[154,155]

Broadly, those favoring crystalloids for volume replacement note problems with hemostasis, adverse reactions, and greater risk for volume overload with colloidal fluids. Those favoring colloids highlight larger volumes of crystalloid required to achieve volume resuscitation,

tissue edema, and potential for reduction in tissue oxygen delivery.[156] It is unclear whether the type of fluid therapy for hypovolemia impacts development of pulmonary edema. Verheij et al[157] reported that type of fluid given to patients with pulmonary vascular injury without fluid overloading did not influence pulmonary vascular permeability or pulmonary edema.

A key characteristic of colloid solutions is their persistence within the intravascular space, which is determined by rate of loss from the circulation.[155] Albumin is monodisperse (uniformity of particle size molecular weight), whereas semisynthetic colloids are polydisperse (wide distribution of particle molecular weight). The molecular weight of a colloid has pharmacokinetic implications in terms of degree of oncotic effect, viscosity, intravascular persistence, and initial degree of volume expansion. In addition to molecular weight, other properties of colloids such as surface charge impact the degree of loss through capillary endothelium, as well as rate of glomerular filtration.[154,155,158]

Albumin is derived from pooled human plasma and has minimal side effects or contraindications. Results from the Saline versus Albumin Evaluation (SAFE) trial, which randomized 7000 critically ill medical and surgical patients to 4% albumin or normal saline, provided evidence on the safety of albumin in critically ill patients. The groups had similar mortality outcomes at 28-day follow-up, as well as similar secondary outcomes of length of stay, ventilatory requirements, and renal replacement therapy.[159–161]

Semisynthetic colloids are dissolved in a crystalloid carrier solvent consisting of either isotonic or hypertonic saline or glucose, or isotonic balanced electrolyte solution. Clinical data provide supportive evidence in terms of patient outcomes for colloids with a balanced solvent solution mirroring composition of plasma.[154,155] Semisynthetic colloids have been reported to increase the risk for bleeding largely attributed to hemodilution of clotting factors, reductions in factor VIII/vWF also caused by hemodilution, and/or functional platelet abnormalities.[154,155,160,162,163] A retrospective chart review concluded that intraoperative use of hetastarch in cardiac surgery requiring CPB increased bleeding and transfusion requirements.[164]

A laboratory investigation in a rabbit model examined the effect of fluid resuscitation with three colloids (Hextend, Dextran 70, 5% albumin) on coagulation and uncontrolled bleeding in rabbits subjected to a splenic injury. Although the prothrombin and partial thromboplastin times were prolonged in all rabbits, thromboelastography and thrombin generation assays identified more severe coagulopathy with Hextend and Dextran than with albumin. Their results suggested resuscitation with albumin maintained coagulation function, decreased blood loss, and improved survival time compared with synthetic colloids.[165]

Lang et al[166] examined the impact of volume replacement with 6% hydroxyethyl starch or lactated Ringer solutions on tissue oxygen tension during and after major surgical procedures. Patients who received 6% hydroxyethyl starch had improved tissue oxygenation compared with a crystalloid-based volume replacement strategy. Improvements in tissue oxygen tension in the hydroxyethyl starch–treated group were thought to be due to improved microperfusion and less endothelial swelling.

Jacob et al[155] examined the impact of albumin, hydroxyethyl starch, and saline as resuscitation fluids on vascular integrity in an isolated guinea pig perfused heart model. The authors hypothesized that fluid extravasation might lead to myocardial edema and consequent reduction in ventricular function. Albumin more effectively prevented fluid extravasation in the heart than crystalloid or artificial colloid, and this effect was partly independent of colloid osmotic pressure. Others have noted that using albumin for the CPB prime better preserved platelet counts than crystalloid prime and more favorably influenced colloid oncotic pressure, positive fluid balance, and postoperative weight gain.[167]

Blood Substitutes

Risks associated with RBC transfusion in terms of morbidity, mortality, survival, and availability of supply have been issues that have spurred development of alternatives to blood transfusion for decades. Ideal characteristics of a blood substitute include long shelf-life, no need to cross-match, immediate availability, and lack of toxic side effects.[168] Hemoglobin-based oxygen carriers (HBOCs) are engineered human, animal, or recombinant hemoglobin products in a cell-free hemoglobin preparation. There are currently no approved products in the United States.[169,170] Perfluorocarbon-based oxygen carriers are aqueous emulsions of perfluorocarbon derivative that dissolve relatively large amounts of oxygen and generally require patients to breathe oxygen-enriched air.[169]

Failure to bring a product to the clinical arena has been primarily because of toxicity-related issues. First-generation HBOC had issues with the way oxygen was carried and released from RBCs. A number of adverse events have been reported in clinical trials of oxygen carriers that include death, stroke, hypertension, anemia, and abdominal pain.[171] Others have reported on adverse effects that included skin rash, diarrhea, hemoglobinuria, elevated lipase, vasoconstrictive effects, and increased hemostatic effect because of reversal of inhibition effect of nitric oxide on platelet aggregation. Free plasma hemoglobin in addition to generating reactive oxygen species is also a potent scavenger of nitric oxide[170] (Figure 30-6 and Table 30-3).

In a review of the current state of oxygen carriers, Winslow[171] noted these solutions exhibit side effects of vasoconstriction, which has been one of the limiting factors for clinical use. Vasoconstriction is thought to be due to either scavenging nitric oxide by hemoglobin or an oversupply of oxygen from free hemoglobin via facilitated diffusion. An understanding of the proposed mechanisms of vasoconstriction (i.e., the oversupply theory) led to new product development involving modification of hemoglobin with lower P50 and increased molecule size, thereby reducing release of oxygen in resistance vessels and resultant vasoconstriction.[172]

Similarly, Yu et al[173] noted profound vasoconstrictor side effects limiting clinical utility of HBOC and attributed this side effect to nitric oxide scavenging. The authors noted that by inhaling nitric oxide, changes occur in body stores of nitric oxide metabolites without producing hypotension and may prevent hypertensive side effects of HBOC infusion. Others have reported on nitric oxide scavenging properties of HBOC as a likely mechanism of vasoconstriction associated with infusion and proposed modifications that could potentially ameliorate this side effect.[174,175]

A basic science working group from the National Heart, Lung and Blood Institute Division of Blood Diseases and Resources summarized and provided recommendations for basic science focus in the area of blood substitutes. The working group highlighted impediments to further HBOC product development secondary to significant side effects of excessive cardiovascular and cerebrovascular events and mortality.[176]

LOWEST HEMATOCRIT ON CARDIOPULMONARY BYPASS

Both anemia on CPB and transfusion of RBCs have been associated with adverse perioperative outcomes. Hemodilution secondary to fixed priming volume and pre-CPB fluid administration contribute to anemia and transfusion need.[177,178] Minimum hematocrit values less than or equal to 14% on CPB have been associated with postoperative mortality in CABG; and in high-risk patients, values less than 17% increase mortality risk.[179] Morbidity risk associated with hemodilutional anemia is thought to be due to inadequate oxygen delivery leading to organ dysfunction.[180] Lowest hematocrit on CPB also has been a risk factor for postoperative low-output syndrome and renal failure. Ranucci et al[181] reported a cutoff hematocrit value of 23% for renal failure and 24% for development of the low-output syndrome. Transfusion of RBCs also was associated with both renal failure and the low-output syndrome in their investigation. Risk for renal injury further increased when RBC transfusions were associated with a nadir hematocrit on CPB of less than 23%.

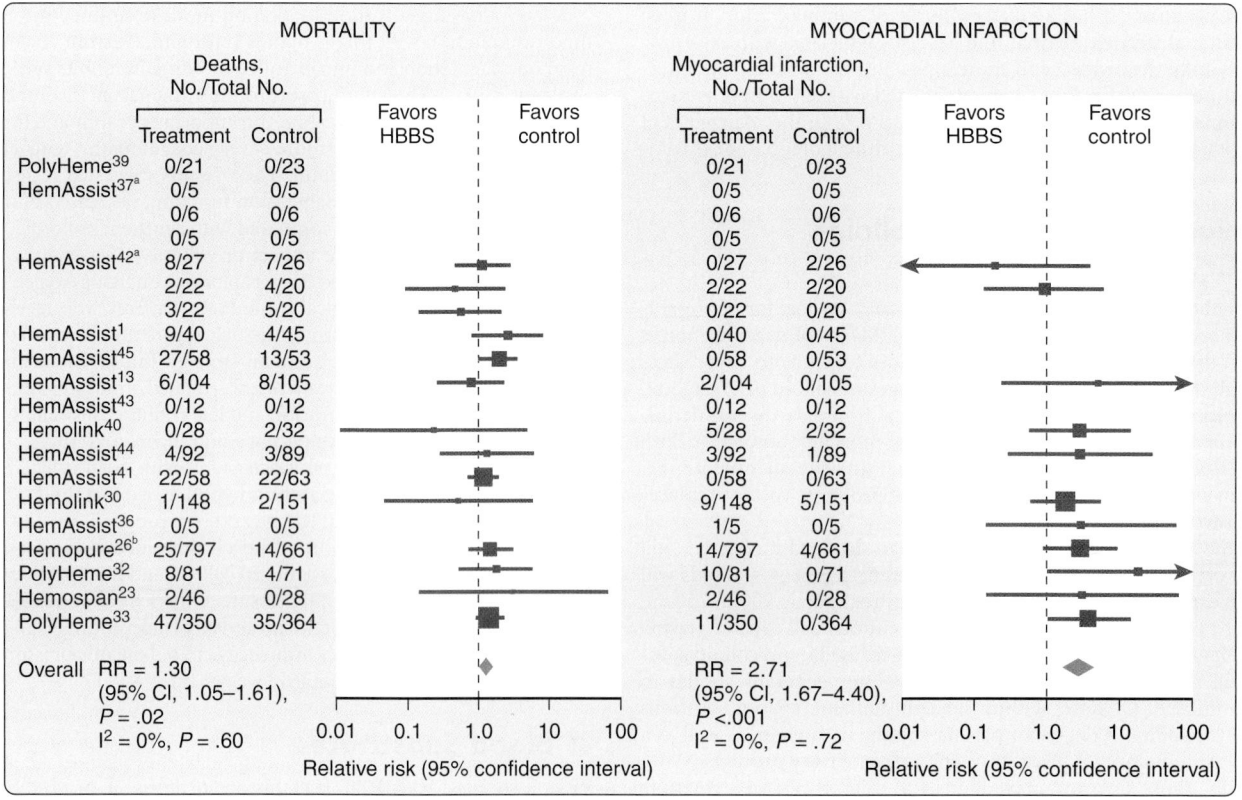

Figure 30-6 **Mortality and myocardial infarction associated with hemoglobin-based blood substitutes (HBBS). CI, confidence interval; RR, relative risk.** *(From Natanson C, Kern SJ, Lurie P, et al: Cell-free hemoglobin-based blood substitutes and risk of myocardial infarction and death: A meta-analysis. JAMA 299:2304–2312, 2008, by permission.)*

TABLE 30-3 Summary of Adverse Events Reported in the Literature or Publicly Available

Cohort	Apex Test	Apex Ctl	Baxter[24-26,37,65-73] Test	Baxter Ctl	Biopure[71,74-81]* Test	Biopure Ctl	Enzon Test	Enzon Ctl	Hemosol[82-84] Test	Hemosol Ctl	Northfield Laboratories[19,85-87]† Test	Northfield Ctl	Sangart[17,18] Test	Sangart Ctl	Somatogen[30,88,89] Test	Somatogen Ctl
No. of Subjects	Not reported		504	505	708	618	Not reported		209	192	623	457	85	45	64	26
1. Death	‡	‡	78	61	25	14	‡	‡	1	4	73	39	2	0	2	‡
2. Hypertension	‡	‡	76	38	166	59	‡	‡	113	75	‡	‡	7	1	8	0
3. Pulmonary hypertension	‡	‡	1	0	3	0	‡	‡	‡	‡	‡	‡	‡	‡	‡	‡
4. Chest pain/chest tightness	‡	‡	‡	‡	21	16	‡	‡	‡	‡	‡	‡	‡	‡	12	0
5. Congestive heart failure	‡	‡	0	1	54	22	‡	‡	0	2	17	20	‡	‡	‡	‡
6. Cardiac arrest	‡	17	6	‡	‡	1	‡	14	9	‡	‡	‡	‡	‡	‡	‡
7. Myocardial infarction	‡	‡	6	1	14	4	1	1	14	7	29	2	2	0	‡	‡
8. Cardiac arrhythmias/conduction abnormalities	‡	‡	23	17	153	100	‡	‡	1	1	‡	‡	15	5	1	1
9. Cerebrovascular accident, cerebrovascular ischemia, TIA	‡	‡	‡	‡	16	3	‡	‡	2	1	3	1	‡	‡	‡	‡
10. Pneumonia	‡	‡	‡	‡	35	22	‡	‡	‡	‡	27	21	‡	‡	‡	‡
11. Respiratory distress/failure	‡	‡	‡	‡	22	12	‡	‡	‡	‡	21	17	‡	‡	‡	‡
12. Acute renal failure	‡	‡	1	3	10	4	‡	‡	2	2	‡	‡	‡	‡	‡	‡
13. Hypoxia, cyanosis, decreased oxygen saturation	‡	‡	‡	‡	76	35	‡	‡	1	1	‡	‡	2	1	2	1
14. Hypovolemia	‡	‡	‡	‡	19	4	‡	‡	‡	‡	‡	‡	‡	‡	‡	‡
15. Gastrointestinal	‡	‡	51	31	345	195	‡	‡	23	1	‡	‡	57	20	36	6
16. Liver, LFTs abnormal	‡	‡	27	8	20	5	‡	‡	8	0	‡	‡	‡	‡	6	3
17. Pancreatitis	‡	‡	11	0	5	3	‡	‡	1	0	‡	‡	‡	‡	‡	‡
18. Coagulation defect, thrombocytopenia, thrombosis	‡	‡	‡	‡	45	17	‡	‡	1	0	13	4	‡	‡	‡	‡
19. Hemorrhage/bleeding/anemia	‡	‡	33	22	108	55	‡	‡	1	1	20	17	‡	‡	‡	‡
20. Sepsis, septic shock, MOF	‡	‡	2	2	15	6	‡	‡	0	1	26	20	‡	‡	‡	‡
21. Pancreatic enzyme inc	‡	‡	13	4	3	0	‡	‡	‡	‡	‡	‡	‡	‡	‡	‡
22. Lipase increase	‡	‡	29	9	48	12	‡	‡	19	2	‡	‡	8	4	7	1
23. Amylase increase	‡	‡	48	45	‡	‡	‡	‡	35	20	‡	‡	7	2	4	1

Not all clinical trials conducted by commercial sponsors have been published, and the published results are not synonymous with line listings that would be found in a comprehensive final study report. For each paper, editorial decisions were made about what information should be included or excluded and data presentation (numbers vs. percentages), making derivation of number of subjects experiencing an event and aggregation of information to derive a comprehensive list of adverse events difficult and potentially incomplete. Not all studies were controlled. Not all enzyme elevations were captured as adverse events, and in some instances, the number of subjects experiencing enzyme elevations was not captured. Differences in reporting methods may have resulted in counting subjects more than once in each category of events (row).

*See also http://www.fda.gov/ohrms/dockets/ac/cber06.html#BloodProducts.
†See also http://northfieldlabs.com.
‡No information available.

Ctl, control; LFT, liver function tests; MOF, multisystem organ failure; TIA, transient ischemic attack.
Reproduced from Silverman TA, Weiskopf RB: Hemoglobin-based oxygen carriers: Current status and future directions. Transfusion 49:2495–2515, 2009.

Swaminathan et al[182] reported more perioperative renal injury with hemodilution, targeting CPB hematocrit levels of 22% to 24%. The authors highlighted renal benefits of hemodilution relating to reductions in blood viscosity and improved regional blood flow; however, they noted that a well-defined cutoff for hemodilution has not been well clarified. They were unable to find an "elbow" for a cutoff between hematocrit and change in creatinine values. The significant association between lowest CPB hematocrit and change in creatinine values was highly influenced by body weight in their investigation.[182] Others have reported that hemodilution on CPB to hematocrit values less than 24% and associated renal injury were further exacerbated by longer CPB times and with RBC transfusion.[180]

Karkouti et al[183] suggested a U-shaped relation between nadir hematocrit on CPB and renal failure requiring dialysis. Moderate hemodilution (hematocrit values between 21% and 25%) were associated with lowest risk for acute renal failure; risk increased as nadir hematocrit concentrations decreased to less than 21% or were greater than 25%. In congenital heart surgery, Jonas et al[184] reported that lower hematocrit strategies (21% ± 2.9%) versus higher hematocrit strategies (28% ± 3.2%) were associated with higher serum lactate levels 60 minutes after CPB, greater percentage of increase in total body water on postoperative day 1, and at age 1 year, worse scores on the Psychomotor Development Index. The authors concluded that a lower hematocrit strategy was associated with increased risk for developmental impairment.

DeFoe et al[185] reported a risk-adjusted increased risk for mortality, need for intra-aortic balloon pump, and return to CPB after initial separation with nadir hematocrit on CPB. Smaller patients and those with lower preoperative hematocrit values were at greater risk for development of lower CPB values. They reported trends toward increasing risk for death in patients with hematocrit values less than 23%; and for those with hematocrit values less than 19%, mortality was almost twice as high as in patients with hematocrit values of 25% or more.[185] Others

have reported on the association between hemodilution to hematocrit values of 24%, RBC transfusion, and increased risk for renal and splanchnic injury.[186]

Notably, not all investigations reported adverse consequences with lower nadir hematocrit values on CPB. von Heymann et al[187] examined oxygen delivery, oxygen consumption, and outcomes in low-risk CABG patients assigned CPB hematocrit values of 20% or 25%. They reported similar oxygen delivery, oxygen consumption, and blood lactate levels between the two groups, as well as clinical outcome measures. The authors concluded that CPB hematocrit values of 20% were adequate to maintain calculated whole-body oxygen delivery above critical levels. Similarly, Berger et al randomized patients to profound hemodilution with CPB hematocrit values between 19% and 21% versus standard values of 24% to 26%. They reported similar changes in intestinal permeability and cytokine release between the two groups and concluded that CPB hematocrit values between 19% and 21% did not adversely impact outcomes.[188]

Orlov et al[189] reported on the clinical utility of using oxygen extraction ratio as an adjunct to hemoglobin concentration for guiding cardiac surgical RBC transfusion decisions. The authors suggested that a normal oxygen extraction ratio in patients with anemia with no evidence of organ dysfunction indicated adequate tissue oxygen delivery, and by incorporating this into the transfusion decisions, RBC transfusions could be reduced.

CONCLUSION

Proper blood and fluid management in the perioperative period are critical to the care of cardiac surgical patients and can significantly influence patient outcomes. A better understanding of the role of genetics in perioperative bleeding may enable a more proactive approach to managing these patients before surgical intervention. Technologic advances in measurement of tissue oxygenation will allow for better evidenced-based transfusion decisions in the future.

REFERENCES

1. Field M, Lohr K, editors: *Clinical Practice Guidelines: Directions for a New Program*, Committee to Advise the Public Health Service on Clinical Practice Guidelines. Washington, DC, 1990, National Academy Press, Institute of Medicine.
2. DioDato CP, Likosky DS, DeFoe GR, et al: Cardiopulmonary bypass recommendations in adults: The northern New England experience, *J Extra Corpor Technol* 40:16–20, 2008.
3. Woolf SH, Grol R, Hutchinson A, et al: Clinical guidelines: Potential benefits, limitations, and harms of clinical guidelines, *BMJ* 318:527–530, 1999.
4. Ferraris VA, Ferraris SP, Saha SP, et al: Perioperative blood transfusion and blood conservation in cardiac surgery: The Society of Thoracic Surgeons and the Society of Cardiovascular Anesthesiologists clinical practice guideline, *Ann Thorac Surg* 83(Suppl 5):S27–S86, 2007.
5. Guidelines MaPftAATFoP: *Methodology Manual for ACCF/AHA Guideline Writing Committees*, January 1, 2010. Available at: http://www.americanheart.org/downloadable/heart/126047705973012 09Methodology_Manual_for_ACC_AHA_Writing_Committees.pdf Accessed February 2, 2010.
6. Arroll B, Jenkins S, North D, et al: Management of hypertension and the core services guidelines: Results from interviews with 100 Auckland general practitioners, *N Z Med J* 108:55–57, 1995.
7. Christakis DA, Rivara FP: Pediatricians' awareness of and attitudes about four clinical practice guidelines, *Pediatrics* 101:825–830, 1998.
8. Grilli R, Lomas J: Evaluating the message: The relationship between compliance rate and the subject of a practice guideline, *Med Care* 32:202–213, 1994.
9. Rhew DC, Riedinger MS, Sandhu M, et al: A prospective, multicenter study of a pneumonia practice guideline, *Chest* 114:115–119, 1998.
10. Grol R, Dalhuijsen J, Thomas S, et al: Attributes of clinical guidelines that influence use of guidelines in general practice: Observational study, *BMJ* 317:858–861, 1998.
11. Merritt TA, Palmer D, Bergman DA, et al: Clinical practice guidelines in pediatric and newborn medicine: Implications for their use in practice, *Pediatrics* 99:100–114, 1997.
12. Fleming M, Wentzell N: Patient safety culture improvement tool: Development and guidelines for use, *Healthc Q* 11(3 spec no.):10–15, 2008.
13. Hıratzka LF, Eagle KA, Liang L, et al: Atherosclerosis secondary prevention performance measures after coronary bypass graft surgery compared with percutaneous catheter intervention and nonintervention patients in the Get With the Guidelines database, *Circulation* 116(Suppl 11):I207–I212, 2007.
14. Steinberg BA, Steg PG, Bhatt DL, et al: Comparisons of guideline-recommended therapies in patients with documented coronary artery disease having percutaneous coronary intervention versus coronary artery bypass grafting versus medical therapy only (from the REACH International Registry), *Am J Cardiol* 99:1212–1215, 2007.
15. Yam FK, Akers WS, Ferraris VA, et al: Interventions to improve guideline compliance following coronary artery bypass grafting, *Surgery* 140:541–547, 2006; discussion 547–552.
16. Berry SA, Doll MC, McKinley KE, et al: ProvenCare: Quality improvement model for designing highly reliable care in cardiac surgery, *Qual Saf Health Care* 18:360–368, 2009.
17. Grimshaw JM, Thomson MA: What have new efforts to change professional practice achieved? Cochrane Effective Practice and Organization of Care Group, *J R Soc Med* 91(Suppl 35):20–25, 1998.
18. Mowatt G, Grimshaw JM, Davis DA, et al: Getting evidence into practice: The work of the Cochrane Effective Practice and Organization of Care Group (EPOC), *J Contin Educ Health Prof* 21:55–60, 2001.
19. Vasaiwala S, Nolan E, Ramanath VS, et al: A quality guarantee in acute coronary syndromes: The American College of Cardiology's Guidelines Applied in Practice program taken real-time, *Am Heart J* 153:16–21, 2007.
20. Bayne-Jones S: Dr. Karl Landsteiner Nobel Prize Laureate in Medicine, 1930, *Science* 73:599–604, 1931.
21. *Racial and Ethnic Distribution of ABO blood types*, July 13, 2008. Available at: http://www.bloodbook.com/world-abo.html. Accessed February 2, 2010.
22. Yamamoto F, Clausen H, White T, et al: Molecular genetic basis of the histo-blood group ABO system, *Nature* 345:229–233, 1990.
23. Reid M, Lomas-Francis C: *The Blood Group Antigen Facts Book*, ed 2, New York, 2004, Elsevier Academic Press.
24. Yamamoto F, McNeill PD, Hakomori S: Human histo-blood group A2 transferase coded by A2 allele, one of the A subtypes, is characterized by a single base deletion in the coding sequence, which results in an additional domain at the carboxyl terminal, *Biochem Biophys Res Commun* 187:366–374, 1992.
25. Yamamoto F: *Molecular Genetic Basis of the Blood Group ABO System*, 2008. Available at: http://sites.google.com/site/abobloodgroup/17.aboalleles2008. Accessed February 2, 2010.
26. Kustu S, Inwood W: Biological gas channels for NH3 and CO2: Evidence that Rh (rhesus) proteins are CO2 channels, *Transfus Clin Biol* 13:103–110, 2006.
27. Avent N, Reid M: The Rh blood group system: A review, *Blood* 95:375–387, 2002.
28. Mwangi J: Blood group distribution in an urban population of patient targeted blood donors, *East Afr Med J* 76:615–618, 1999.
29. Urbaniak S, Greiss M: RhD haemolytic disease of the fetus and the newborn, *Blood Rev* 14:44–61, 2000.
30. National Center for Biotechnology Information: *MNS (MNS) Blood Group System*, December 11, 2009. Available at: http://www.ncbi.nlm.nih.gov/gv/mhc/xslcgi.cgi?cmd=bgmut/systems_info&system=mns. Accessed February 2, 2010.
31. National Center for Biotechnology Information: *Lewis (LE) Blood Group System*, January 29 2009. Available at: http://www.ncbi.nlm.nih.gov/projects/gv/mhc/xslcgi.cgi?cmd=bgmut/systems_info&system=lewis Accessed February 2, 2010.
32. Blood Bank: January 28, 2010. Available at: http://en.wikipedia.org/wiki/Blood_bank. Accessed February 2, 2010.
33. U.S. Food and Drug Administration: *Fatalities Reported to FDA Following Blood Collection and Transfusion: Annual Summary for Fiscal Year 2008*. February 19, 2010. Available at: http://www.fda.gov/BiologicsBloodVaccines/SafetyAvailability/ReportaProblem/TransfusionDonationFatalities/ucm113649.htm. Accessed February 2, 2010.
34. Napier JA: The crossmatch, *Br J Haematol* 78:1–4, 1991.
35. Chapman JF, Milkins C, Voak D: The computer crossmatch: A safe alternative to the serological crossmatch, *Transfus Med* 10:251–256, 2000.
36. Roback J, Combs M, Grossman B, et al: *AABB Technical Manual*, ed 16, Bethesda, MD, 2008, American Association of Blood Banks.
37. Judd WJ: Requirements for the electronic crossmatch, *Vox Sang* 74(Suppl 2):409–417, 1998.
38. Inaba K, Teixeira PG, Shulman I, et al: The impact of uncross-matched blood transfusion on the need for massive transfusion and mortality: Analysis of 5,166 uncross-matched units, *J Trauma* 65:1222–1226, 2008.

39. Lee EJ, Schiffer CA: ABO compatibility can influence the results of platelet transfusion. Results of a randomized trial, *Transfusion* 29:384–389, 1989.
40. Julmy F, Ammann RA, Taleghani BM, et al: Transfusion efficacy of ABO major-mismatched platelets (PLTs) in children is inferior to that of ABO-identical PLTs, *Transfusion* 49:21–33, 2009.
41. Kanda J, Ichinohe T, Matsuo K, et al: Impact of ABO mismatching on the outcomes of allogeneic related and unrelated blood and marrow stem cell transplantations for hematologic malignancies: IPD-based meta-analysis of cohort studies, *Transfusion* 49:624–635, 2009.
42. [illegible] Pedal I: Diagnostic approaches to acute transfusion reactions, *Forens Sci Med Pathol* 6: 135–145, 2010.
43. Koch C, Li L, Figueroa P, et al: Transfusion and pulmonary morbidity after cardiac surgery, *Ann Thorac Surg* 88:1410–1418, 2009.
44. Cherry T, Steciuk M, Reddy VV, et al: Transfusion-related acute lung injury: Past, present, and future, *Am J Clin Pathol* 129:287–297, 2008.
45. Curtis BR, McFarland JG: Mechanisms of transfusion-related acute lung injury (TRALI): Anti-leukocyte antibodies, *Crit Care Med* 34(Suppl 5):S118–123, 2006.
46. Popovsky MA: Transfusion and lung injury, *Transfus Clin Biol* 8:272–277, 2001.
47. Holness L, Knippen MA, Simmons L, et al: Fatalities caused by TRALI, *Transfus Med Rev* 18:184–188, 2004.
48. Sandler SG: How I manage patients suspected of having had an IgA anaphylactic transfusion reaction, *Transfusion* 46:10–13, 2006.
49. Hirayama F: Recent advances in laboratory assays for nonhemolytic transfusion reactions, *Transfusion* 50:252–263, 2010.
50. Davenport RD: Pathophysiology of hemolytic transfusion reactions, *Semin Hematol* 42:165–168, 2005.
51. Hendrickson JE, Hillyer CD: Noninfectious serious hazards of transfusion, *Anesth Analg* 108: 759–769, 2009.
52. Ruhl H, Bein G, Sachs UJ: Transfusion-associated graft-versus-host disease, *Transfus Med Rev* 23: 62–71, 2009.
53. Hsueh JC, Ho CF, Chang SH, et al: Blood surveillance and detection on platelet bacterial contamination associated with septic events, *Transfus Med* 19:350–356, 2009.
54. Dzik WH, Kirkley SA: Citrate toxicity during massive blood transfusion, *Transfus Med Rev* 2:76–94, 1988.
55. Koch CG, Li L, Duncan AI, et al: Transfusion in coronary artery bypass grafting is associated with reduced long-term survival, *Ann Thorac Surg* 81:1650–1657, 2006.
56. Banbury MK, Brizzio ME, Rajeswaran J, et al: Transfusion increases the risk of postoperative infection after cardiovascular surgery, *J Am Coll Surg* 202:131–138, 2006.
57. Koch CG, Li L, Duncan AI, et al: Morbidity and mortality risk associated with red blood cell and blood-component transfusion in isolated coronary artery bypass grafting, *Crit Care Med* 34: 1608–1616, 2006.
58. Blajchman MA: Immunomodulation and blood transfusion, *Am J Ther* 9:389–395, 2002.
59. Koch CG, Li L, Van Wagoner DR, et al: Red cell transfusion is associated with an increased risk for postoperative atrial fibrillation, *Ann Thorac Surg* 82:1747–1756, 2006.
60. Fransen E, Maessen J, Dentener M, et al: Systemic inflammation present in patients undergoing CABG without extracorporeal circulation, *Chest* 113:1290–1295, 1998.
61. Bennett-Guerrero E, Veldman TH, Doctor A, et al: Evolution of adverse changes in stored RBCs, *Proc Natl Acad Sci U S A* 104:17063–17068, 2007.
62. Relevy H, Koshkaryev A, Manny N, et al: Blood banking-induced alteration of red blood cell flow properties, *Transfusion* 48:136–146, 2008.
63. Rigamonti A, McLaren AT, Mazer CD, et al: Storage of strain-specific rat blood limits cerebral tissue oxygen delivery during acute fluid resuscitation, *Br J Anaesth* 100:357–364, 2008.
64. Koch CG, Li L, Sessler DI, et al: Duration of red-cell storage and complications after cardiac surgery, *N Engl J Med* 358:1229–1239, 2008.
65. Sweeney J, Kouttab N, Kurtis J: Stored red blood cell supernatant facilitates thrombin generation. *Transfusion* 49: 1569–1579, 2009.
66. Burzotta F, Iacoviello L, Di Castelnuovo A, et al: 4G/5G PAI-1 promoter polymorphism and acute-phase levels of PAI-1 following coronary bypass surgery: A prospective study, *J Thromb Thrombolysis* 16:149–154, 2003.
67. de Lange M, Snieder H, Ariens RA, et al: The genetics of haemostasis: A twin study, *Lancet* 357:101–105, 2001.
68. Freeman MS, Mansfield MW, Barrett JH, et al: Genetic contribution to circulating levels of hemostatic factors in healthy families with effects of known genetic polymorphisms on heritability, *Arterioscler Thromb Vasc Biol* 22:506–510, 2002.
69. Muehlschlegel JD, Body SC: Impact of genetic variation on perioperative bleeding, *Am J Hematol* 83:732–737, 2008.
70. Souto JC, Almasy L, Borrell M, et al: Genetic susceptibility to thrombosis and its relationship to physiological risk factors: The GAIT study. Genetic Analysis of Idiopathic Thrombophilia, *Am J Hum Genet* 67:1452–1459, 2000.
71. de Lange M, de Geus EJ, Kluft C, et al: Genetic influences on fibrinogen, tissue plasminogen activator-antigen and von Willebrand factor in males and females, *Thromb Haemost* 95(3):414–419, 2006.
72. Dunn EJ, Ariens RA, de Lange M, et al: Genetics of fibrin clot structure: A twin study, *Blood* 103: 1735–1740, 2004.
73. Miller CH, Haff E, Platt SJ, et al: Measurement of von Willebrand factor activity: Relative effects of ABO blood type and race, *J Thromb Haemost* 1:2191–2197, 2003.
74. Eriksson-Berg M, Deguchi H, Hawe E, et al: Influence of factor VII gene polymorphisms and environmental factors on plasma coagulation factor VII concentrations in middle-aged women with and without manifest coronary heart disease, *Thromb Haemost* 93:351–358, 2005.
75. Eyre-Walker A: Evolution in health and medicine Sackler colloquium: Genetic architecture of a complex trait and its implications for fitness and genome-wide association studies, *Proc Natl Acad Sci U S A* 107(Suppl 1):1752–1756, 2010.
76. Ganesh SK, Zakai NA, van Rooij FJ, et al: Multiple loci influence erythrocyte phenotypes in the CHARGE Consortium, *Nat Genet* 41:1191–1198, 2009.
77. Soranzo N, Spector TD, Mangino M, et al: A genome-wide meta-analysis identifies 22 loci associated with eight hematological parameters in the HaemGen consortium, *Nat Genet* 41:1182–1190, 2009.
78. Miah MF, Boffa MB: Functional analysis of mutant variants of thrombin-activatable fibrinolysis inhibitor resistant to activation by thrombin or plasmin, *J Thromb Haemost* 7:665–672, 2009.
79. Peyvandi F, Jayandharan G, Chandy M, et al: Genetic diagnosis of haemophilia and other inherited bleeding disorders, *Haemophilia* 12(Suppl 3):82–89, 2006.
80. Coppola A, Franchini M, Tagliaferri A: Prophylaxis in people with haemophilia, *Thromb Haemost* 101:674–681, 2009.
81. Seligsohn U: Factor XI deficiency in humans, *J Thromb Haemost* 7(Suppl 1):84–87, 2009.
82. National Institutes of Health: *Genetic Home Reference*, February 21, 2010. Available at: http://ghr.nlm.nih.gov/condition=hemophilia#genes. Accessed February 25, 2010.
83. James P, Lillicrap D: The role of molecular genetics in diagnosing von Willebrand disease, *Semin Thromb Hemost* 34:502–508, 2008.
84. Wagenman BL, Townsend KT, Mathew P, et al: The laboratory approach to inherited and acquired coagulation factor deficiencies, *Clin Lab Med* 29:229–252, 2009.
85. Brettler DLevine P: Clinical manifestations and therapy of inherited coagulation factor deficiencies. In Colman R, Hirsh J, Marder V, Salzman E, editors: *Hemostasis and Thrombosis: Basic Principles and Clinical Practice*, ed 3 1993, pp 169–183.
86. ClinLab Navigator: *Factor VIII concentrate*, 2010. Available at: http://www.clinlabnavigator.com/transfusion/factorviiiconcentrate.html Accessed February 2, 2010.
87. ClinLab Navigator: Factor VIII inhibitors, Available at: http://www.clinlabnavigator.com/transfusion/factorviiiinhibitors.html. Accessed February 2, 2010.
88. Levy JH: Pharmacologic methods to reduce perioperative bleeding, *Transfusion* 48(Suppl 1): [illegible]
89. ClinLab Navigator: Factor IX complex & concentrates. Available at: http://www.clinlabnavigator.com/transfusion/factorixcomplex.html. Accessed February 2, 2010.
90. Michiels JJ, Berneman Z, Gadisseur A, et al: Classification and characterization of hereditary types 2A, 2B, 2C, 2D, 2E, 2M, 2N, and 2U (unclassifiable) von Willebrand disease, *Clin Appl Thromb Hemost* 12:397–420, 2006.
91. Federici AB: Classification of inherited von Willebrand disease and implications in clinical practice, *Thromb Res* 124(Suppl 1):S2–S6, 2009.
92. Favaloro EJ: Laboratory identification of von Willebrand disease: Technical and scientific perspectives, *Semin Thromb Hemost* 32:456–471, 2006.
93. Lillicrap D: Von Willebrand disease—phenotype versus genotype: Deficiency versus disease, *Thromb Res* 120(Suppl 1):S11–16, 2007.
94. Lillicrap D: Genotype/phenotype association in von Willebrand disease: Is the glass half full or empty? *J Thromb Haemost* 7(Suppl 1):65–70, 2009.
95. Budde U: Diagnosis of von Willebrand disease subtypes: Implications for treatment, *Haemophilia* 14(Suppl 5):27–38, 2008.
96. Pate GE, Chandavimol M, Naiman SC, et al: Heyde's syndrome: A review, *J Heart Valve Dis* 13: 701–712, 2004.
97. Cattaneo M. The use of desmopressin in open-heart surgery, *Haemophilia* 14(Suppl 1):40–47, 2008.
98. Nicolaes GA, Dahlback B: Factor V and thrombotic disease: Description of a janus-faced protein, *Arterioscler Thromb Vasc Biol* 22:530–538, 2002.
99. Segers K, Dahlback B, Nicolaes GA: Coagulation factor V and thrombophilia: Background and mechanisms, *Thromb Haemost* 98:530–542, 2007.
100. Andreassi MG, Botto N, Maffei S: Factor V Leiden, prothrombin G20210A substitution and hormone therapy: Indications for molecular screening, *Clin Chem Lab Med* 44:514–521, 2006.
101. Boehm J, Grammer JB, Lehnert F, et al: Factor V Leiden does not affect bleeding in aprotinin recipients after cardiopulmonary bypass, *Anesthesiology* 106:681–686, 2007.
102. Donahue BS, Gailani D, Higgins MS, et al: Factor V Leiden protects against blood loss and transfusion after cardiac surgery, *Circulation* 107:1003–1008, 2003.
103. Berentsen S, Beiske K, Tjonnfjord GE: Primary chronic cold agglutinin disease: An update on pathogenesis, clinical features and therapy, *Hematology* 12:361–370, 2007.
104. Agarwal SK, Ghosh PK, Gupta D: Cardiac surgery and cold-reactive proteins, *Ann Thorac Surg* 60:1143–1150, 1995.
105. Fischer GD, Claypoole V, Collard CD: Increased pressures in the retrograde blood cardioplegia line: An unusual presentation of cold agglutinins during cardiopulmonary bypass, *Anesth Analg* 84:454–456, 1997.
106. Welsby IJ, Jones R, Pylman J, et al: ABO blood group and bleeding after coronary artery bypass graft surgery, *Blood Coagul Fibrinolysis* 18:781–785, 2007.
107. Welsby IJ, Podgoreanu MV, Phillips-Bute B, et al: Association of the 98G/T ELAM-1 polymorphism with increased bleeding and transfusion after cardiac surgery, *Anesth Analg* 104:SCA39, 2007.
108. Welsby IJ, Podgoreanu MV, Phillips-Bute B, et al: Genetic factors contribute to bleeding after cardiac surgery, *J Thromb Haemost* 3:1206–1212, 2005.
109. Mehta RH, Sheng S, O'Brien SM, et al: Reoperation for bleeding in patients undergoing coronary artery bypass surgery: Incidence, risk factors, time trends, and outcomes, *Circulation* 2:583–590, 2009.
110. Moulton MJ, Creswell LL, Mackey ME, et al: Reexploration for bleeding is a risk factor for adverse outcomes after cardiac operations, *J Thorac Cardiovasc Surg* 111:1037–1046, 1996.
111. Choong CK, Gerrard C, Goldsmith KA, et al: Delayed re-exploration for bleeding after coronary artery bypass surgery results in adverse outcomes, *Eur J Cardiothorac Surg* 31:834–838, 2007.
112. Karthik S, Grayson AD, McCarron EE, et al: Reexploration for bleeding after coronary artery bypass surgery: Risk factors, outcomes, and the effect of time delay, *Ann Thorac Surg* 78:527–534, 2004.
113. Ranucci M, Bozzetti G, Ditta A, et al: Surgical reexploration after cardiac operations: Why a worse outcome? *Ann Thorac Surg* 86:1557–1562, 2008.
114. Hall TS, Brevetti GR, Skoultchi AJ, et al: Re-exploration for hemorrhage following open heart surgery differentiation on the causes of bleeding and the impact on patient outcomes, *Ann Thorac Cardiovasc Surg* 7:352–357, 2001.
115. Kermode JC, Zheng Q, Milner EP: Marked temperature dependence of the platelet calcium signal induced by human von Willebrand factor, *Blood* 94:199–207, 1999.
116. Johnston TD, Chen Y, Reed RL 2nd: Functional equivalence of hypothermia to specific clotting factor deficiencies, *J Trauma* 37:413–417, 1994.
117. Wolberg AS, Meng ZH, Monroe DM 3rd, et al: A systematic evaluation of the effect of temperature on coagulation enzyme activity and platelet function, *J Trauma* 56:1221–1228, 2004.
118. Meng ZH, Wolberg AS, Monroe DM 3rd, et al: The effect of temperature and pH on the activity of factor VIIa: Implications for the efficacy of high-dose factor VIIa in hypothermic and acidotic patients, *J Trauma* 55:886–891, 2003.
119. Martini WZ, Pusateri AE, Uscilowicz JM, et al: Independent contributions of hypothermia and acidosis to coagulopathy in swine, *J Trauma* 58:1002–1009, 2005 discussion 1009–1010.
120. Alam HB, Bice LM, Butt MU, et al: Testing of blood products in a polytrauma model: Results of a multi-institutional randomized preclinical trial, *J Trauma* 67:856–864, 2009.
121. Dirkmann D, Hanke AA, Gorlinger K, et al: Hypothermia and acidosis synergistically impair coagulation in human whole blood, *Anesth Analg* 106:1627–1632, 2008.
122. Maani CV, DeSocio PA, Holcomb JB: Coagulopathy in trauma patients: What are the main influence factors? *Curr Opin Anaesthesiol* 22:255–260, 2009.
123. Borgman MA, Spinella PC, Perkins JG, et al: The ratio of blood products transfused affects mortality in patients receiving massive transfusions at a combat support hospital, *J Trauma* 63:805–813, 2007.
124. Holcomb JB, Wade CE, Michalek JE, et al: Increased plasma and platelet to red blood cell ratios improves outcome in 466 massively transfused civilian trauma patients, *Ann Surg* 248:447–458, 2008.
125. Gunter OL Jr, Au BK, Isbell JM, et al: Optimizing outcomes in damage control resuscitation: Identifying blood product ratios associated with improved survival, *J Trauma* 65:527–534, 2008.
126. Zink KA, Sambasivan CN, Holcomb JB, et al: A high ratio of plasma and platelets to packed red blood cells in the first 6 hours of massive transfusion improves outcomes in a large multicenter study, *Am J Surg* 197:565–570, 2009.
127. Kashuk JL, Moore EE, Johnson JL, et al: Postinjury life threatening coagulopathy: Is 1:1 fresh frozen plasma:packed red blood cells the answer? *J Trauma* 65:261–270, 2008; discussion 270–271.
128. Hirshberg A, Dugas M, Banez EI, et al: Minimizing dilutional coagulopathy in exsanguinating hemorrhage: A computer simulation, *J Trauma* 54:454–463, 2003.

129. Cotton BA, Au BK, Nunez TC, et al: Predefined massive transfusion protocols are associated with a reduction in organ failure and postinjury complications, *J Trauma* 66:41–48, 2009 discussion 48–49.

130. Riskin DJ, Tsai TC, Riskin L, et al: Massive transfusion protocols: The role of aggressive resuscitation versus product ratio in mortality reduction, *J Am Coll Surg* 209:198–205, 2009.

131. Filsoufi F, Castillo JG, Rahmanian PB, et al: Effective management of refractory postcardiotomy bleeding with the use of recombinant activated factor VII, *Ann Thorac Surg* 82:1779–1783, 2006.

132. Hoffman M, Monroe DM 3rd: A cell-based model of hemostasis, *Thromb Haemost* 85:958–965, 2001.

133. Lisman T, Adelmeijer J, Cauwenberghs S, et al: Recombinant factor VIIa enhances platelet adhesion and activation under flow conditions at normal and reduced platelet count, *J Thromb Haemost* 3:742–751, 2005.

134. Karkouti K, Beattie WS, Arellano R, et al: Comprehensive Canadian review of the off-label use of recombinant activated factor VII in cardiac surgery, *Circulation* 118:331–338, 2008.

135. von Heymann C, Redlich U, Jain U, et al: Recombinant activated factor VII for refractory bleeding after cardiac surgery—a retrospective analysis of safety and efficacy, *Crit Care Med* 33:2241–2246, 2005.

136. McCall P, Story DA, Karalapillai D: Audit of factor VIIa for bleeding resistant to conventional therapy following complex cardiac surgery, *Can J Anaesth* 53:926–933, 2006.

137. Tatoulis J, Theodore S, Meswani M, et al: Safe use of recombinant activated factor VIIa for recalcitrant postoperative haemorrhage in cardiac surgery, *Interact Cardiovasc Thorac Surg* 9:459–462, 2009.

138. Bishop CV, Renwick WE, Hogan C, et al: Recombinant activated factor VII: Treating postoperative hemorrhage in cardiac surgery, *Ann Thorac Surg* 81:875–879, 2006.

139. Dunkley S, Phillips L, McCall P, et al: Recombinant activated factor VII in cardiac surgery: Experience from the Australian and New Zealand Haemostasis Registry, *Ann Thorac Surg* 85:836–844, 2008.

140. DiDomenico RJ, Massad MG, Kpodonu J, et al: Use of recombinant activated factor VII for bleeding following operations requiring cardiopulmonary bypass, *Chest* 127:1828–1835, 2005.

141. Gill R, Herbertson M, Vuylsteke A, et al: Safety and efficacy of recombinant activated factor VII: A randomized placebo-controlled trial in the setting of bleeding after cardiac surgery, *Circulation* 120:21–27, 2009.

142. Bowman LJ, Uber WE, Stroud MR, et al: Use of recombinant activated factor VII concentrate to control postoperative hemorrhage in complex cardiovascular surgery, *Ann Thorac Surg* 85:1669–1676, 2008; discussion 1676–1667.

143. O'Connell KA, Wood JJ, Wise RP, et al: Thromboembolic adverse events after use of recombinant human coagulation factor VIIa, *JAMA* 295:293–298, 2006.

144. Fenger-Eriksen C, Ingerslev J, Sorensen B: Fibrinogen concentrate—a potential universal hemostatic agent, *Expert Opin Biol Ther* 9:1325–1333, 2009.

145. Fenger-Eriksen C, Lindberg-Larsen M, Christensen AQ, et al: Fibrinogen concentrate substitution therapy in patients with massive haemorrhage and low plasma fibrinogen concentrations, *Br J Anaesth* 101:769–773, 2008.

146. Rahe-Meyer N, Pichlmaier M, Haverich A, et al: Bleeding management with fibrinogen concentrate targeting a high-normal plasma fibrinogen level: A pilot study, *Br J Anaesth* 102:785–792, 2009.

147. Fenger-Eriksen C, Jensen TM, Kristensen BS, et al: Fibrinogen substitution improves whole blood clot firmness after dilution with hydroxyethyl starch in bleeding patients undergoing radical cystectomy: A randomized, placebo-controlled clinical trial, *J Thromb Haemost* 7:795–802, 2009.

148. Karlsson M, Ternstrom L, Hyllner M, et al: Prophylactic fibrinogen infusion reduces bleeding after coronary artery bypass surgery. A prospective randomised pilot study, *Thromb Haemost* 102:137–144, 2009.

149. Samama CM: Prothrombin complex concentrates: A brief review, *Eur J Anaesthesiol* 25:784–789, 2008.

150. Riess HB, Meier-Hellmann A, Motsch J, et al: Prothrombin complex concentrate (Octaplex) in patients requiring immediate reversal of oral anticoagulation, *Thromb Res* 121:9–16, 2007.

151. Leissinger CA, Blatt PM, Hoots WK, et al: Role of prothrombin complex concentrates in reversing warfarin anticoagulation: A review of the literature, *Am J Hematol* 83:137–143, 2008.

152. Warren O, Simon B: Massive, fatal, intracardiac thrombosis associated with prothrombin complex concentrate, *Ann Emerg Med* 53:758–761, 2009.

153. Vincent JL: Fluid resuscitation: Colloids vs crystalloids, *Acta Clin Belg Suppl* 408–411, 2007.

154. Sakka SG: Resuscitation of hemorrhagic shock with normal saline versus lactated Ringer's: Effects on oxygenation, extravascular lung water, and hemodynamics, *Crit Care* 13:128, 2009.

155. Jacob M, Bruegger D, Rehm M, et al: Contrasting effects of colloid and crystalloid resuscitation fluids on cardiac vascular permeability, *Anesthesiology* 104:1223–1231, 2006.

156. Grocott MP, Hamilton MA: Resuscitation fluids, *Vox Sang* 82:1–8, 2002.

157. Verheij J, van Lingen A, Raijmakers PG, et al: Effect of fluid loading with saline or colloids on pulmonary permeability, oedema and lung injury score after cardiac and major vascular surgery, *Br J Anaesth* 96:21–30, 2006.

158. Dieterich HJ: Recent developments in European colloid solutions, *J Trauma* 54(Suppl 5):S26–S30, 2003.

159. Finfer S, Bellomo R, Boyce N, et al: A comparison of albumin and saline for fluid resuscitation in the intensive care unit, *N Engl J Med* 350:2247–2256, 2004.

160. Boldt J, Suttner S: Plasma substitutes, *Minerva Anestesiol* 71:741–758, 2005.

161. Fan E, Stewart TE: Albumin in critical care: SAFE, but worth its salt? *Crit Care* 8:297–299, 2004.

162. Vercueil A, Grocott MP, Mythen MG: Physiology, pharmacology, and rationale for colloid administration for the maintenance of effective hemodynamic stability in critically ill patients, *Transfus Med Rev* 19:93–109, 2005.

163. Roberts JS, Bratton SL: Colloid volume expanders. Problems, pitfalls and possibilities, *Drugs* 55:621–630, 1998.

164. Knutson JE, Deering JA, Hall FW, et al: Does intraoperative hetastarch administration increase blood loss and transfusion requirements after cardiac surgery? *Anesth Analg* 90:801–807, 2000.

165. Kheirabadi BS, Crissey JM, Deguzman R, et al: Effects of synthetic versus natural colloid resuscitation on inducing dilutional coagulopathy and increasing hemorrhage in rabbits, *J Trauma* 64:1218–1228, 2008; discussion 1228–1229.

166. Lang K, Boldt J, Suttner S, et al: Colloids versus crystalloids and tissue oxygen tension in patients undergoing major abdominal surgery, *Anesth Analg* 93:405–409, 403rd contents page, 2001.

167. Russell JA, Navickis RJ, Wilkes MM: Albumin versus crystalloid for pump priming in cardiac surgery: Meta-analysis of controlled trials, *J Cardiothorac Vasc Anesth* 18:429–437, 2004.

168. Jahr JS, Walker V, Manoochehri K: Blood substitutes as pharmacotherapies in clinical practice, *Curr Opin Anaesthesiol* 20:325–330, 2007.

169. Kim HW, Greenburg AG: Artificial oxygen carriers as red blood cell substitutes: A selected review and current status, *Artif Organs* 28:813–828, 2004.

170. Napolitano LM: Hemoglobin-based oxygen carriers: First, second or third generation? Human or bovine? Where are we now? *Crit Care Clin* 25:279–301, Table of Contents 2009.

171. Winslow RM: Current status of oxygen carriers ('blood substitutes'): 2006, *Vox Sang* 91:102–110, 2006.

172. Winslow RM: Cell-free oxygen carriers: Scientific foundations, clinical development, and new directions, *Biochim Biophys Acta* 1784:1382–1386, 2008.

173. Yu B, Bloch KD, Zapol WM: Hemoglobin-based red blood cell substitutes and nitric oxide, *Trends Cardiovasc Med* 19:103–107, 2009.

174. Raat NJ, Liu JF, Doyle MP, et al: Effects of recombinant-hemoglobin solutions rHb2.0 and rHb1.1 on blood pressure, intestinal blood flow, and gut oxygenation in a rat model of hemorrhagic shock, *J Lab Clin Med* 145:21–32, 2005.

175. Hermann J, Corso C, Messmer KF: Resuscitation with recombinant hemoglobin rHb2.0 in a rodent model of hemorrhagic shock, *Anesthesiology* 107:273–280, 2007.

176. Estep T, Bucci E, Farmer M, et al: Basic science focus on blood substitutes: A summary of the NHLBI Division of Blood Diseases and Resources Working Group Workshop, March 1, 2006, *Transfusion* 48:776–782, 2008.

177. Campbell JA, Holt DW, Shostrom VK, et al: Influence of intraoperative fluid volume on cardiopulmonary bypass hematocrit and blood transfusions in coronary artery bypass surgery, *J Extra Corpor Technol* 40:99–108, 2008.

178. Pappalardo F, Corno C, Franco A, et al: Reduction of hemodilution in small adults undergoing open heart surgery: A prospective, randomized trial, *Perfusion* 22:317–322, 2007.

179. Fang WC, Helm RE, Krieger KH, et al: Impact of minimum hematocrit during cardiopulmonary bypass on mortality in patients undergoing coronary artery surgery, *Circulation* 96(Suppl 9):II-194–II-199, 1997.

180. Habib RH, Zacharias A, Schwann TA, et al: Role of hemodilutional anemia and transfusion during cardiopulmonary bypass in renal injury after coronary revascularization: Implications on operative outcome, *Crit Care Med* 33:1749–1756, 2005.

181. Ranucci M, Biagioli B, Scolletta S, et al: Lowest hematocrit on cardiopulmonary bypass impairs the outcome in coronary surgery: An Italian Multicenter Study from the National Cardioanesthesia Database, *Tex Heart Inst J* 33:300–305, 2006.

182. Swaminathan M, Phillips-Bute BG, Conlon PJ, et al: The association of lowest hematocrit during cardiopulmonary bypass with acute renal injury after coronary artery bypass surgery, *Ann Thorac Surg* 76:784–791, 2003; discussion 792.

183. Karkouti K, Beattie WS, Wijeysundera DN, et al: Hemodilution during cardiopulmonary bypass is an independent risk factor for acute renal failure in adult cardiac surgery, *J Thorac Cardiovasc Surg* 129:391–400, 2005.

184. Jonas RA, Wypij D, Roth SJ, et al: The influence of hemodilution on outcome after hypothermic cardiopulmonary bypass: Results of a randomized trial in infants, *J Thorac Cardiovasc Surg* 126:1765–1774, 2003.

185. DeFoe GR, Ross CS, Olmstead EM, et al: Lowest hematocrit on bypass and adverse outcomes associated with coronary artery bypass grafting. Northern New England Cardiovascular Disease Study Group, *Ann Thorac Surg* 71:769–776, 2001.

186. Huybregts RA, de Vroege R, Jansen EK, et al: The association of hemodilution and transfusion of red blood cells with biochemical markers of splanchnic and renal injury during cardiopulmonary bypass, *Anesth Analg* 109:331–339, 2009.

187. von Heymann C, Sander M, Foer A, et al: The impact of an hematocrit of 20% during normothermic cardiopulmonary bypass for elective low risk coronary artery bypass graft surgery on oxygen delivery and clinical outcome—a randomized controlled study [ISRCTN35655335], *Crit Care* 10:R58, 2006.

188. Berger K, Sander M, Spies CD, et al: Profound haemodilution during normothermic cardiopulmonary bypass influences neither gastrointestinal permeability nor cytokine release in coronary artery bypass graft surgery, *Br J Anaesth* 103:511–517, 2009.

189. Orlov D, O'Farrell R, McCluskey SA, et al: The clinical utility of an index of global oxygenation for guiding red blood cell transfusion in cardiac surgery, *Transfusion* 49:682–688, 2009.

31

Transfusion Medicine and Coagulation Disorders

BRUCE D. SPIESS, MD, FAHA | JAY HORROW, MD, MS, FAHA | JOEL A. KAPLAN, MD, CPE, FACC

KEY POINTS

1. It is easiest to think of coagulation as a wave of biologic activity occurring at the site of tissue injury consisting of initiation, acceleration, control, and lysis.
2. Hemostasis is part of a larger body system: inflammation. The protein reactions in coagulation have important roles in signaling inflammation.
3. Thrombin is the most important coagulation modulator, interacting with multiple coagulation factors, platelets, tissue plasminogen activator, prostacyclin, nitric oxide, and various white blood cells.
4. The serine proteases that compose the coagulation pathway are balanced by serine protease inhibitors, termed *serpins*. Antithrombin is the most important inhibitor of blood coagulation.
5. Platelets are the most complex part of the coagulation process, and antiplatelet drugs are important therapeutic agents.
6. Heparin requires antithrombin to anticoagulate blood and is not an ideal anticoagulant for cardiopulmonary bypass. Newer anticoagulants are actively being sought to replace heparin.
7. Protamine can have many adverse effects. Ideally, a new anticoagulant will not require reversal with a toxic substance such as protamine.
8. Antifibrinolytic drugs are often given during cardiac surgery; these drugs include ε-aminocaproic acid and tranexamic acid.
9. Recombinant factor VIIa is the latest drug to be studied as a "rescue agent" to stop bleeding during cardiac surgery.
10. Every effort should be made to avoid transfusion of banked blood products during routine cardiac surgery. In fact, bloodless surgery is a reality in many cases.

Coagulation and bleeding assume particular importance when surgery is performed on the heart and great vessels using extracorporeal circulation. This chapter provides an understanding of the depth and breadth of hemostasis relating to cardiac procedures, beginning with coagulation pathophysiology. The pharmacology of heparin and protamine follows. This background is then applied to treatment of the bleeding patient. Coagulation monitoring is covered in Chapter 17, and fluid and blood management is further discussed in Chapter 30.

OVERVIEW OF HEMOSTASIS

Blood cannot coagulate to stop hemorrhage unless there is closure of large vessels. Any vascular structure larger than 50 μm cannot contract enough to allow platelets and proteins to perform their actions. Superb, meticulous surgical technique is the single most important variable in decreasing postoperative bleeding/blood transfusion requirements. Those centers with not only fast surgeons but ones willing to spend a few extra minutes conserving blood by detailed hemostasis will exhibit better outcomes.

Proper hemostasis requires the participation of innumerable biologic elements (Box 31-1). This section groups them into four topics to facilitate understanding: coagulation factors, platelet function, the endothelium, and fibrinolysis. The reader must realize this is for simplicity of learning, and that in biology, the activation creates many reactions and control mechanisms, all interacting simultaneously. The interaction of the platelets, endothelial cells, and proteins to either activate or deactivate coagulation is a highly buffered and controlled process. It is perhaps easiest to think of coagulation as a wave of biologic activity occurring at the site of tissue injury (Figure 31-1).[1] Although there are subcomponents to coagulation itself, the injury/control leading to hemostasis is a four-part event: initiation, acceleration, control, and lysis (recanalization/fibrinolysis). The initiation phase begins with tissue damage, which really is begun with endothelial cell destruction or dysfunction. This initiation phase leads to binding of platelets, as well as protein activations; both happen nearly simultaneously, and each has feedbacks into the other. Platelets adhere, creating an activation or acceleration phase that gathers many cells to the site of injury. From that adhesion a large number of events of cellular/protein messaging cascade. As the activation phase ramps up into an explosive set of reactions, counter-reactions are spun off, leading to control proteins damping the reactions. It is easiest, conceptually, to think of these control mechanisms as analogous to a nuclear reactor. The activation phase would continue to grow and overcome the whole organism unless control rods were inserted (e.g., thrombomodulin, proteins C and S, and tissue plasminogen activator [t-PA]) to stop the spread of the reaction. The surrounding normal endothelium acts quite differently from the disturbed (ischemic) endothelium. Eventually, the control reactions overpower the acceleration reactions and lysis comes into play.

BOX 31-1. COMPONENTS OF HEMOSTASIS

- Coagulation factor activation
- Platelet function
- Vascular endothelium
- Fibrinolysis and modulators of coagulation

949

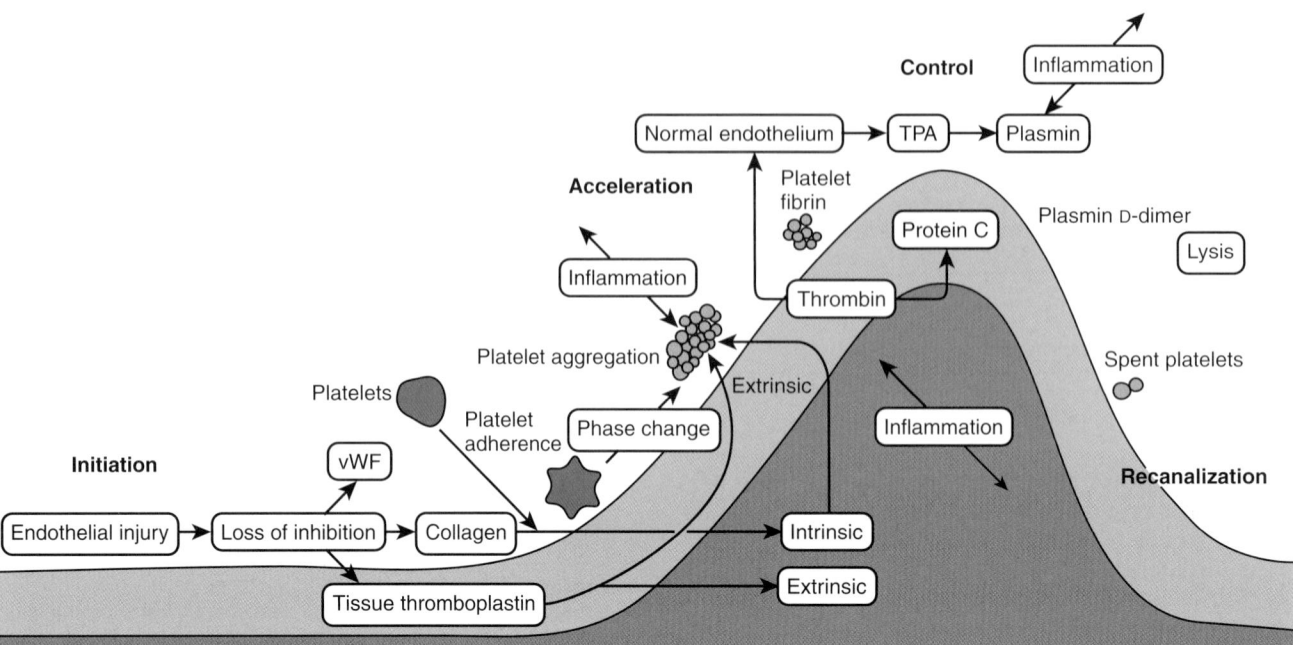

Figure 31-1 Coagulation is a sine wave of activity at the site of tissue injury. It goes through four stages: initiation, acceleration, control, and lysis/recanalization. TPA, tissue plasminogen activator; vWF, von Willebrand factor. *(Redrawn from Spiess BD: Coagulation function and monitoring. In Lichtor JL [ed]: Atlas of Clinical Anesthesia. Philadelphia, 1996, Current Medicine.)*

The diagram in Figure 31-1 shows lysis as relatively quick, but it can take 24 hours to days to have its full effects. A key concept is that hemostasis is part of a larger body system: inflammation. Most, if not all, of the protein reactions of coagulation control have importance in signaling inflammation leading to other healing mechanisms. Entire books have been written merely to examine these fascinating interactions. It is no wonder that cardiopulmonary bypass (CPB) has such profound inflammatory effects when it is considered that each of the activated coagulation proteins and cell lines then feeds into upregulation of inflammation.

During cardiac surgery, the endothelium (locally and systemically) is disturbed.[2] The coronary arteries are made either partially or fully ischemic for periods with cardioplegia (perfused CPB being relatively rare today). Little known is that high concentrations of potassium are particularly insulting to endothelial cells. Ischemia/reperfusion injury is, therefore, the norm for every cardiac surgical case using CPB.[3] Systemic ischemia and reperfusion occur throughout every capillary bed because microair, thrombus, and fat emboli are by-products of CPB[4] (see Chapters 28 to 30 and 36). It is quite possible that transfusion of red blood cell (RBC) products, through blocking of the microcirculation, actually may contribute to ischemia/reperfusion injury. Transfusion has been shown to evoke endothelial cell hyper-reactivity mediated through cell membrane microparticles.[4]

The coagulation proteins and platelets are both hemodiluted and consumed during CPB. Platelets are activated/inhibited by various means. Coagulation dysfunction in cardiac surgery has been studied for more than 50 years. The complexity of the myriad number of dysfunctions should impress the student of this area. Unfortunately, when a patient is bleeding in the operating room or ICU, there is no universal way to quickly sort out the causative events. Furthermore, the interventions are limited, yet an educated and planned approach (algorithm-driven transfusion/coagulation intervention) does decrease transfusion and influences subsequent bleeding.

▪ Protein Coagulation Activations

Coagulation Pathways

The coagulation factors participate in a series of activating and feedback inhibition reactions, ending with the formation of an insoluble clot.[5] A *clot* is the sum total of platelet-to-platelet interactions, leading to the formation of a platelet plug (initial stoppage of bleeding). The cross-linking of platelets to each other by way of the final insoluble fibrin leads to a stable clot. Clot is not simply the activation of proteins leading to more protein deposition. Clinicians have been shaped in their thinking about coagulation by the historic way that coagulation proteins were discovered and the resulting coagulation tests. It is that teaching of the coagulation cascade, with resultant monitoring technology, that has led to some transfusion behaviors. The way coagulation has been classically taught (protein cascades) is not the way coagulation proceeds biologically.

With few exceptions, the coagulation factors are glycoproteins (GPs) synthesized in the liver, which circulate as inactive molecules termed *zymogens*. Factor activation proceeds sequentially, each factor serving as substrate in an enzymatic reaction catalyzed by the previous factor in the sequence. Hence this classically has been termed a *cascade* or *waterfall* sequence. Cleavage of a polypeptide fragment changes an inactive zymogen to an active enzyme. The active form is termed a *serine protease* because the active site for its protein-splitting activity is a serine amino acid residue. Many reactions require the presence of calcium ion (Ca^{2+}) and a phospholipid surface (platelet phosphatidylserine). The phospholipids occur most often either on the surface of an activated platelet or endothelial cell and occasionally on the surface of white cells. So anchored, their proximity to one another permits reaction rates profoundly accelerated (up to 300,000-fold) from those measured when the enzymes remain in solution. The factors form four interrelated *arbitrary* groups (Figure 31-2): the contact activation, intrinsic, extrinsic, and common pathways. They were so labeled historically by the human need for order. In biology, they are all highly interactive, occur simultaneously on the surface of cells, and have feedback loops with cross-reactions.

Contact Activation

Factor XII, high-molecular-weight kininogen (HMWK), prekallikrein (PK), and factor XI form the contact or surface activation group. The in vivo events that activate factor XII remain unconfirmed. Clinicians do know that ex vivo contact with ionically charged surfaces will activate factor XII. Because factor XII autoactivates by undergoing a shape change in the presence of a negative charge, in vitro coagulation tests use glass, silica, kaolin, and other compounds with negative surface charge (see Chapter 17). The glycocalyx of endothelial cells has a repelling charge for coagulation proteins. One potential in vivo mechanism

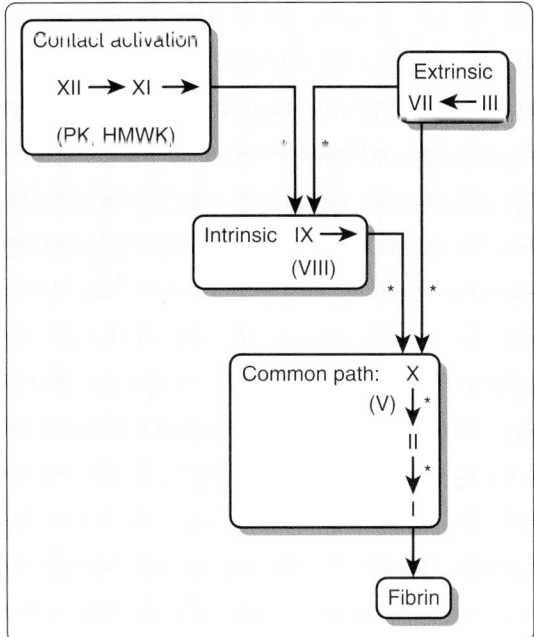

Figure 31-2 **Depiction of coagulation protein activation sequence.** *Asterisks* denote participation of calcium ion. HMWK, high-molecular-weight kininogen; PK, prekallikrein.

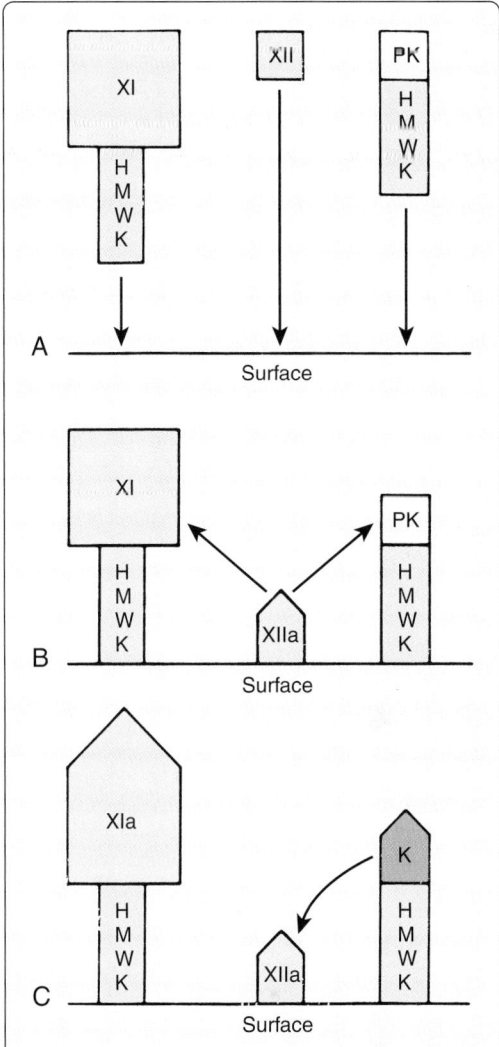

Figure 31-3 *A–C,* Activation of the contact factors XII, XI, and prekallikrein (PK). The cofactor, high-molecular-weight kininogen (HMWK), binds factor XI and PK to the endothelial surface. Kallikrein (K) amplifies factor XII activation. *(From Colman RW, Marder VJ, Salzman EW, Hirsh J: Overview of hemostasis. In Colman RW, Hirsh J, Marder VJ, Salzman EW [eds]: Hemostasis and Thrombosis, 3rd ed. Philadelphia: JB Lippincott, 1994, p 3.)*

for factor XII activation is disruption of the endothelial cell layer, which exposes the underlying negatively charged collagen matrix. Activated platelets also provide negative charges on their membrane surfaces. HMWK anchors the other surface activation molecules, PK and factor XI, to damaged endothelium or activated platelets. Factor XIIa cleaves both factor XI, to form factor XIa, and PK, to form kallikrein. Figure 31-3 depicts the events of surface activation.

This system also interlinks to the complement cascade and fibrinolytic process as follows. Kallikrein converts HMWK to bradykinin, which activates the complement proteins. Kallikrein also may convert plasminogen to plasmin (see later). This latter function is quite weak, however, and of unknown significance in vivo.

It was rather tempting historically to attribute all coagulation abnormalities to activation of the contact system. This seemed an obvious explanation for the coagulopathy of CPB. The circuits are most often made of polyvinylchloride with a negatively charged surface. Today, it is known that the effects of contact activation in the entire scheme of CPB coagulation dysfunction are actually quite small. Of note, patients with completely absent factor XII do just fine and do not exhibit excess bleeding, nor are they particularly dry after CPB. Therefore, the presence or absence of factor XII in the evolution of humankind seems to not be critical for survival. It also should reveal that the surface activation mechanism is not the driving force behind the bleeding/consumptive coagulopathy of CPB.

Intrinsic System

Intrinsic activation forms factor XIa from the products of surface activation. Factor XIa splits factor IX to form factor IXa, with Ca^{2+} required for this process. Then factor IXa activates factor X with help from Ca^{2+}, a phospholipid surface (platelet-phosphatidylserine), and a GP cofactor, factor VIIIa. Figure 31-4 displays a stylized version of factor X activation. The phospholipids and GP cofactors are on the surface of platelets.

Extrinsic System

Activation of factor X can proceed independently of factor XII by substances classically thought to be extrinsic to the vasculature. This is of historic interest because today it is known that the expression of tissue factor is actually a highly regulated event in endothelial cells. Any number of endothelial cell insults can lead to the production of

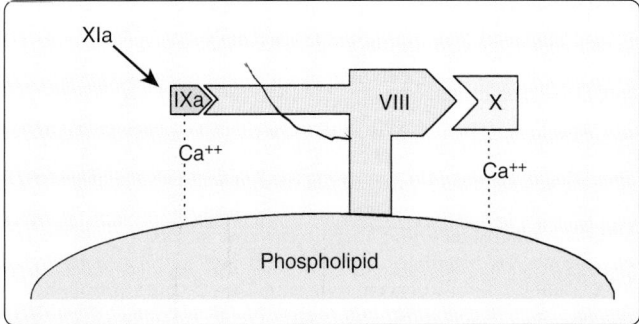

Figure 31-4 Factor VIII facilitates the activation of factor X by factor IXa. Calcium tethers the molecules to the phospholipid surface. *(From Horrow JC: Desmopressin and antifibrinolytics. Int Anesthesiol Clin 28:230, 1990.)*

tissue factor by the endothelial cell.[3-10] At rest, the endothelial cell is quite antithrombotic. However, with ischemia, reperfusion, sepsis, or cytokines (particularly interleukin-6), the endothelial cell will stimulate its production of intracellular nuclear factor-κB and send messages for the production of messenger RNA for tissue factor production.[6] This can happen quickly and the resting endothelial cell can turn out large amounts of tissue factor. It is widely held today that the activation of tissue factor is what drives many of the abnormalities of coagulation after cardiac surgery, rather than contact activation.[7,8] In some tissues, cells outside the vasculature contain large amounts of tissue factor. They are released when cells are damaged/ruptured. Thromboplastin, also known as tissue factor, released from tissues into the vasculature, acts as a cofactor for initial activation of factor X by factor VII. Factors VII and X then activate one another with the help of platelet phospholipid and Ca^{2+}, thus rapidly generating factor Xa. (Factor VIIa also activates factor IX, thus linking the extrinsic and intrinsic paths.)

Thromboplastin straddles the extravascular cell membrane, with its extracellular portion available to bind factor VIIa. Cytokines (particularly tumor necrosis factor-α and interleukin-6) and endotoxins can stimulate its expression on endothelium.[9,10] It anchors factor VIIa to the cell surface, thus facilitating activation of factor X. The amount of available factor Va also seems to be quite important for the adequate functioning of the normal coagulation cascades.

Common Pathway

Using membrane phospholipids (phosphatidylserine) as a catalyst site, Ca^{2+} as a ligand, and factor Va as cofactor, factor Xa splits prothrombin (factor II) to thrombin (factor IIa). The combination of factors Xa, Va, and Ca^{2+} is termed the *prothrombinase complex*. Factor Xa anchors to the membrane surface (of platelets) via Ca^{2+}. Factor Va, assembling next to it, initiates a rearrangement of the complex, vastly accelerating binding of the substrate, prothrombin. Most likely, the factor Xa formed from the previous reaction is channeled along the membrane to this next reaction step without detaching from the membrane.

Figure 31-5 depicts the steps involved in formation of thrombin from its precursor, prothrombin. The by-product, fragment F1.2, serves as a plasma marker of prothrombin activation. An alternative scheme generates a different species, meizothrombin, involved more specifically in activation of coagulation inhibitors.[11]

Thrombin cleaves the fibrinogen molecule to form soluble fibrin monomer and polypeptide fragments termed *fibrinopeptides A and B*. Fibrin monomers associate to form a soluble fibrin matrix. Factor XIII, activated by thrombin, cross-links these fibrin strands to form an insoluble clot. Patients with lower levels of factor XIII have been found to have more bleeding after cardiac surgery.[11,12]

Vitamin K

Those factors that require calcium (II, VII, IX, X) depend on vitamin K to add between 9 and 12 γ-carboxyl groups to glutamic acid residues near their amino termini. Calcium tethers the negatively charged carboxyl groups to the phospholipid surface (platelets), thus facilitating molecular interactions. Some inhibitory proteins also depend on vitamin K (proteins C and S).

Modulators of the Coagulation Pathway

Thrombin, the most important coagulation modulator, exerts a pervasive influence throughout the coagulation factor pathways. It activates factors V, VIII, and XIII; cleaves fibrinogen to fibrin; stimulates platelet recruitment, chemotaxis of leukocytes and monocytes; releases t-PA, prostacyclin, and nitric oxide from endothelial cells; releases interleukin-1 from macrophages; and with thrombomodulin, activates protein C, a substance that then inactivates factors Va and VIIIa.[12] Note the negative feedback aspect of this last action (Figure 31-6). Coagulation function truly centers around the effects of thrombin. The platelets, tissue factor, and contact activation all are interactive and are activated by a rent in the surface of the endothelium or through the loss of endothelial coagulation control. Platelets adhere to a site of injury and, in turn, are activated, leading to sequestration of other platelets.

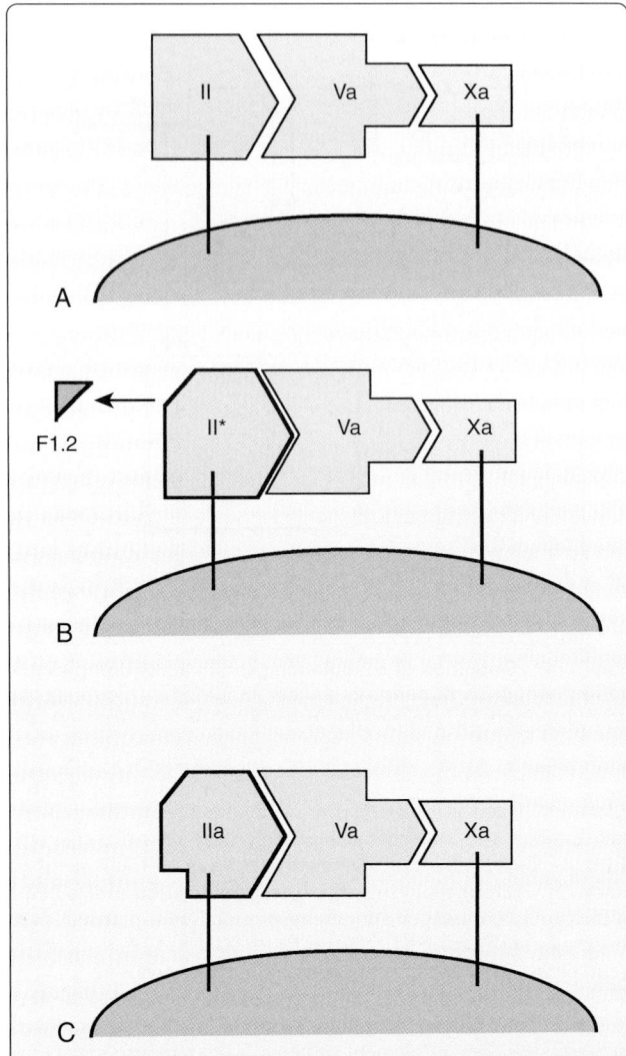

Figure 31-5 **Activation of prothrombin by factor Xa proceeds in a multistep fashion.** *A,* On the phospholipid surface, the prothrombinase complex consists of prothrombin (factor II), factor Xa, and factor Va. *B,* The first activation step in which the prothrombin fragment F1.2 is split from prothrombin to form prethrombin (II*). *C,* Molecular rearrangement of prethrombin yields thrombin.

It is the interaction of all of those factors together that eventually creates a critical mass. Once enough platelets are interacting together, with their attached surface concomitant serine protease reactions, then a thrombin burst is created. Only when enough thrombin activation has been encountered in a critical time point is a threshold exceeded, and the reactions become massive and much larger than the sum of the whole. It is thought that the concentration and ability of platelets to react fully affect the ability to have a critical thrombin burst. CPB may affect the ability to get that full thrombin burst because of its effects on platelet number, platelet-to-platelet interactions, and the decreased amounts of protein substrates.

The many serine proteases that compose the coagulation pathways are balanced by serine protease inhibitors, termed *serpins*.[13] This biologic yin and yang leads to an excellent buffering capacity. It is only when the platelet-driven thrombin burst so overwhelms the body's localized anticoagulation or inhibitors that clot proceeds forward. Serpins include α_1-antitrypsin, α_2-macroglobulin, heparin cofactor II, α_2-antiplasmin, antithrombin (AT; also termed *antithrombin III* [AT III]), and others.

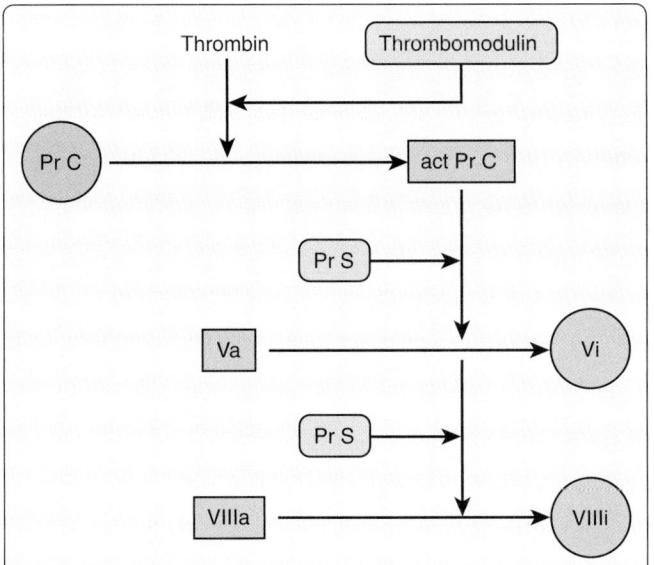

Figure 31-6 Modulating effects of protein C on coagulation. Thrombomodulin from endothelial cells accelerates thrombin activation of protein C (Pr C). In the presence of protein S (Pr S), activated protein C [(act Pr C)a] inactivates factors V and VIII. Protein C and protein S are vitamin K dependent.

AT III constitutes the most potent and widely distributed inhibitor of blood coagulation. It binds to the active site (serine) of thrombin, thus inhibiting action of thrombin. It also inhibits, to a much lesser extent, the activity of factors XIIa, XIa, IXa, and Xa; kallikrein; and the fibrinolytic molecule, plasmin. Thrombin bound to fibrin is protected from the action of AT, thus explaining the poor efficacy of heparin in treating established thrombosis. AT III is a relatively inactive zymogen. To be most effective, AT must bind to a unique pentasaccharide sequence contained on the wall of endothelial cells in the glycosaminoglycan surface known as heparan; the same active sequence is present in the drug heparin.

An important note is that activated AT III is active only against free thrombin (fibrin-bound thrombin cannot be seen by AT III).[14] Prothrombin circulates in the plasma but is not affected by heparin-AT III complexes; it is only thrombin, and thrombin does not circulate freely. Most thrombin in its active form is either bound to GP binding sites of platelets or in fibrin matrices. When blood is put into a test tube and clot begins to form (such as in an activated coagulation time [ACT]), 96% of thrombin production is yet to come. Most thrombin generation is on the surface of platelets and on clot-held fibrinogen. Platelets, through their GP binding sites and phospholipid folds, protect activated thrombin from attack by AT III. Therefore, the biologic role of AT III is to create an anticoagulant surface on endothelial cells. It is not present biologically to sit and wait for a dose of heparin before CPB.

CPB dilutes AT III substantially, and the further consumption of AT III during CPB (thrombin generation) leads, in some patients, to profoundly low levels of this important inhibitor.[15] Research work adding AT III back to the CPB circuit has shown promise in that by doing so there is better preservation of serine protease proteins and platelets. Unfortunately, no pharmaceutical company has decided to pursue this line of research to the point that it would be either commonplace or economically feasible to add large amounts of AT III to CPB and, therefore, avoid consumptive coagulopathies. Congenital AT III deficiency can lead to in utero fetal destruction if the fetus is homozygous for the abnormal AT III. However, patients who are heterozygous for AT III abnormalities have about 40% to 60% of normal AT III activity. They have a particularly high risk for deep vein thrombosis. Low AT III levels have been described during extracorporeal membrane oxygenation,

and the addition of AT III to the extracorporeal membrane oxygenation circuit has been effective in improving outcome and decreasing bleeding in some circumstances.[16] It is not known how useful it would be in all patients on CPB because only small trials have been performed, but these have been encouraging.[17,18] Both human AT III concentrate (harvested from multiple plasma donors and pasteurized) and a pharmaceutically engineered, goat milk–produced AT III (slightly different structure than human AT III) are commercially available.

Heparin cofactor II also inhibits thrombin, once it is activated. Although large doses of heparin activate heparin cofactor II, dermatans on endothelial cell surfaces activate it far more effectively, suggesting dermatans as alternative drugs to heparin.[19] Dermatan sulfates are not available for use today in the United States.

Another serpin, *protein C*, degrades factors Va and VIIIa. Like other vitamin K–dependent factors, it requires Ca^{2+} to bind to phospholipid. Its cofactor, termed *protein S*, also exhibits vitamin K dependence. Genetic variants of protein C are less active and lead to increased risk for deep vein thrombosis and pulmonary embolism. When endothelial cells release thrombomodulin, thrombin then accelerates by 20,000-fold its activation of protein C[20] (see Figure 31-6). Activated protein C also promotes fibrinolysis through a feedback loop to the endothelial cells to release t-PA.[21]

Regulation of the extrinsic limb of the coagulation pathway occurs via tissue factor pathway inhibitor (TFPI), a glycosylated protein that associates with lipoproteins in plasma.[22] TFPI is not a serpin. It impairs the catalytic properties of the factor VIIa-tissue factor complex on factor X activation. Both vascular endothelium and platelets appear to produce TFPI.[23,24] Heparin releases TFPI from endothelium, increasing TFPI plasma concentrations by as much as sixfold, which should be viewed as a biologic indicator of how poor heparin is as an anticoagulant. TFPI is not tested for in routine coagulation testing. It may be that some individuals with certain types of TFPI or who have very large amounts of circulating TFPI could be at risk for severe adverse bleeding after cardiac surgery.[25–30] This area is just beginning to be examined today both in terms of whether TFPI is responsible for abnormal bleeding and whether its genetic variants have abnormal bleeding or thrombosis.

von Willebrand factor (vWF), a massive molecule composed of disulfide-linked glycosylated peptides, associates with factor VIII in plasma, protecting it from proteolytic enzymes. It circulates in the plasma in its coiled inactive form.[31] Disruption of the endothelium either allows for binding of vWF from the plasma or allows for expression of vWF from tissue and from endothelial cells. Once bound, vWF uncoils to its full length and exposes a hitherto cryptic domain in the molecule. This A-1 domain has a very high affinity for platelet GPs. Initially, vWF attaches to the glycoprotein Iα (GPIα) platelet receptor, which slows the platelet forward movements against the shear forces of blood flow. Shear forces are activators of platelets. As the platelet's forward movement along the endothelial brush border is slowed (because of vWF attachment), shear forces actually increase; thus, the binding of vWF to GP1 acts to provide a feedback loop for individual platelets, further activating them. The activation of vWF and its attachment to the platelet are not enough to bind the platelet to the endothelium, but it creates a membrane signal that allows for early shape change and expression of other GPs, GPIb and GPIIb/IIIa. Then, secondary GPIb binding connects to other vWF nearby, binding the platelet and beginning the activation sequence. It bridges normal platelets to damaged subendothelium by attaching to the GPIb platelet receptor. An ensuing platelet shape change then releases thromboxane, β-thromboglobulin, and serotonin, and exposes GPIIb/IIIa, which binds fibrinogen.

Deficiency States

Decreased amounts of coagulation proteins may be inherited or acquired. Deficiencies of each part of the coagulation pathway are considered in turn. Table 31-1 summarizes the coagulation factors, their activation sequences, and vehicles for factor replacement when deficient.

TABLE 31-1	The Coagulation Pathway Proteins, Minimal Amounts Needed for Surgery, and Replacement Sources				
Factor	Activated By	Acts On	Minimal Amount Needed	Replacement Source	Alternate Name and Comments
XIII	IIa	Fibrin	< 5%	FFP, CRYO	Fibrin-stabilizing factor; not a serine protease, but an enzyme
XII	Endothelium	XI	None	Not needed	Hageman factor; activation enhanced by XIIa
XI	XIIa	IX	15–25%	FFP	Plasma thromboplastin antecedent
X	VIIa or IXa	II	10–20%	FFP, 9C	Stuart–Prower factor; vitamin K dependent
IX	VIIa or XIa	X	25–30%	FFP, 9C, PCC	Christmas factor; vitamin K dependent
VIII	IIa	X	> 30%	CRYO, 8C, FFP	Antihemophilic factor; a cofactor; RES synthesis
VII	Xa	X	10–20%	FFP, PCC	Serum prothrombin conversion accelerator; vitamin K dependent
V	IIa	II	< 25%	FFP	Proaccelerin; a cofactor; RES and liver synthesis
IV	—	—	—	—	Calcium ion; binds II, VII, IX, X to phospholipid
III	—	X	—	—	Thromboplastin/tissue factor; a cofactor
II	Xa	I	20–40%	FFP, PCC	Prothrombin; vitamin K dependent
I	IIa	—	1 g/L	CRYO, FFP	Fibrinogen; activated product is soluble fibrin
vWF	—	VIII	See VIII	CRYO, FFP	von Willebrand factor; endothelial cell synthesis

Unless otherwise specified, all coagulation proteins are synthesized in the liver. Note that there is no factor VI. For von Willebrand factor, cryoprecipitate or fresh frozen plasma (FFP) is administered to obtain a factor VIII coagulant activity > 30%.

8C, factor VIII concentrate; 9C, purified factor IX complex concentrate; CRYO, cryoprecipitate; PCC, prothrombin complex concentrate; RES, reticuloendothelial system.

Contact Activation

Although decreased amounts of factor XII, PK, and HMWK can occur, these defects do not have clinical sequelae. The autosomal dominant deficiency of factor XI is very rare. However, its incidence among Ashkenazi Jews is as high as 0.1% to 0.3%.[32] Most of these patients require factor replacement with fresh-frozen plasma (FFP) for surgery. Spontaneous bleeding does not occur, but increased bleeding after a surgical event or trauma is possible. Factor XI concentrations do not directly correlate with bleeding after trauma or surgery, suggesting that factor XI deficiency can be easily overcome by activation of platelets, factor IX, and other signaling mechanisms. An FFP dose of 10 mL/kg will yield target concentrations of 20% activity, and it is often given for this rare deficiency.

Intrinsic

Hemophilia occurs worldwide, with a prevalence of 1 in 10,000. Hemophilia A, which constitutes about 80% to 85% of cases, originates from decreased activity of factor VIII. Because platelet function remains normal, minor cuts and abrasions do not bleed excessively. Joint and muscle hemorrhages ensue from minor trauma or, seemingly, spontaneously. Airway issues include epistaxis and obstruction from bleeding into the tongue. The bleeding time and prothrombin time (PT) remain normal, whereas the activated partial thromboplastin time (aPTT) is prolonged.[33] Desmopressin, a synthetic analog of vasopressin, will increase factor VIII activity by releasing vWF from endothelial cells, except in patients with severe hemophilia A who have too little functional factor VIII available for vWF.[34] Major surgery requires replenishment of factor VIII functional activity to greater than 80% of normal with FFP, cryoprecipitate, or factor VIII concentrate.[35] Factor VIII concentrate is the preferred method today. After surgery, factor VIII concentrations should be maintained greater than 30% for 2 weeks with repeat doses. Current plasma-derived concentrates are solvent detergent and heat-treated to remove lipid-coated viruses (human immunodeficiency virus [HIV], hepatitis B, human T-lymphotropic virus [HTLV]. However, this was not historically the case, and in Europe during the early parts of the HIV/acquired immune deficiency syndrome (AIDS) crisis, most individuals with hemophilia contracted HIV/AIDS from contaminated products. A recombinant product also is available but costs about three times that of the plasma-derived one.

Factor IX deficiency manifests as hemophilia B, constituting 15% to 20% of all hemophilia cases. Patients present with symptoms identical to those with hemophilia A. No study has demonstrated a salutary effect of desmopressin here. Prothrombin complex (factor IX) concentrates will replenish levels, but consumptive coagulopathy remains a possible complication, stemming from the presence of activated coagulation factors, principally factor VIIa, in the preparation.[36]

Purified factor IX concentrate, a plasma-derived, solvent detergent and heat-treated product, currently constitutes the replacement vehicle of choice for patients with hemophilia B.[37] Recombinant pure factor IX concentrate will be available, but at considerable expense (factor VIIa is now available as well). Consultation with an experienced hematologist aids in the care of patients with hemophilia undergoing surgery.

Extrinsic

Inheritance of factor VII deficiency follows an autosomal recessive pattern, with a prevalence of 1 in 500,000. Although factor VII deficiency may mimic hemophilia in presentation, most often, clinical bleeding is absent and surgery is well tolerated without replacement. The PT is elevated, whereas the PTT is normal. When necessary, replacement of factor VII levels to 10% to 20% of normal with FFP suffices.

Common Pathway

Deficiency of either factor V or factor X, both extremely rare autosomal recessive disorders, increases both the PT and PTT. The bleeding time is normal in factor X deficiency but prolonged in one third of patients with factor V deficiency. The bleeding time prolongation arises from the role of factor V in platelet function.[38] Prothrombin complex concentrate or FFP supplies prothrombin, factor V, and factor X. Numerous inherited abnormalities (polymorphisms) of prothrombin and fibrinogen occur, with varying characteristics. Cryoprecipitate, which contains 250 mg fibrinogen and 100 units factor VIII per 10-mL bag, as well as vWF and factor XIII, treats inherited or acquired disorders of fibrinogen. Many of these polymorphisms are associated with hypercoagulability and, perhaps, accelerated atherosclerosis rather than bleeding.

Liver Disease

Hepatic compromise decreases the circulating amounts of factors II, VII, and X, but the level of factor IX is often normal. Decreases in factor V are variable. Factor VIII levels, in contrast, can reach as much as five times normal in acute hepatitis. Factors XIII, XII, and XI, HMWK, and PK suffer mild decreases. Administration of FFP restores these factors to normal levels. Liver disease also leads to decreases in the production of AT III and protein S. Therefore, the buffering capacity of coagulation is thrown off. A small change in activation could, therefore, lead to a large and diffuse whole-body event such as consumptive coagulopathy.

Warfarin

Administration of this vitamin K antagonist affects plasma levels of factors II, VII, IX, and X, as well as proteins C and S.[39] Protein C has the shortest half-life, followed by factors VII (6 hours), IX (24 hours), X (2 days), and II (3 days).[36] Substantial PT prolongation and some PTT prolongation accompany warfarin therapy. For immediate restoration of clotting function, FFP is given. Otherwise, parenteral vitamin K or cessation of warfarin (Coumadin) suffices. Clinicians should be extremely careful in administering these compounds if a patient is suspected of having heparin-induced thrombocytopenia (HIT). Treatment with commercially available factor VIIa restores PT to normal and appears to stop bleeding when warfarin therapy has not had time to be reversed. The use of factor VIIa for this intervention before surgery is both effective and, perhaps, worthwhile as it avoids the use of FFP. The time scale of factor VIIa effectiveness may not be as long as if one normalized circulating levels through FFP administration. It makes sense, therefore, that if the PT is prolonged again approximately 8 to 12 hours after a dose of factor VIIa, then redosage of the drug be given.

Inherited Thrombotic Disorders

A number of genetic abnormalities lead to thrombosis. The most prevalent (2% to 5%) in European-derived populations is factor V Leiden, in which a point mutation at residue 1691 on factor V renders it resistant to inactivation by activated protein C.[40] Venous thromboembolism risk increases 7-fold in heterozygotes and 80-fold in homozygotes, but episodes are less severe than in other thrombotic disorders. Pregnancy and oral contraceptives greatly exacerbate the thrombotic tendency.[41]

Congenital AT III deficiency (1:1000 patients) causes venous thromboembolism and heparin resistance. This autosomal dominant disorder involves three types: absence of AT (type I), dysfunctional AT (type II), and AT with dysfunction limited to a reduced response to heparin (type III). Clinical presentation begins at age 15 or later, with venous thrombosis occurring with surgery, pregnancy, or bed rest. Replacement AT III is now available for use in the United States.

Protein C or S deficiencies, if homozygous, present at birth as neonatal purpura fulminans. Protein C deficiency heterozygotes demonstrate 40% to 60% protein C activity and present with venous thrombosis beginning in adolescence. The role of reduced concentrations of protein S in causing thrombosis has come into question.[41] Together, deficiencies of AT, protein C, and protein S account for 10% to 15% of inherited thrombosis.[42]

Deficiency of heparin cofactor II is rare. Its role in thrombosis is uncertain. Other conditions that cause thrombosis are dysfibrinogenemia with lysis-resistant fibrinogen, plasminogen deficiency, t-PA deficiency, excess plasminogen activator inhibitor 1 activity (plasminogen activator inhibitor 1 inhibits t-PA), and homocysteinemia.

Homocysteinemia is the mild heterozygous state of cystathione β-synthetase deficiency, known as homocystinuria in its more serious homozygous form. Increased plasma concentrations of homocysteine induce endothelial cell tissue factor activity, stimulate factor V activation, and impair protein C activation, all of which contribute to thrombosis. Folic acid and vitamins B_6 and B_{12} reduce homocysteine plasma concentrations.[43]

Platelet Function

Most clinicians think first of the coagulation proteins when considering hemostasis. Although no one element of the many that participate in hemostasis assumes dominance, platelets may be the most complex.[44] Without platelets, there is no coagulation and no hemostasis, so it could be argued that they are most important. Without the proteins, there is hemostasis, but it lasts only about 10 to 15 minutes as the platelet plug is inherently unstable and breaks apart under the shear stress of the vasculature. Platelets provide phospholipid for coagulation factor reactions; contain their own microskeletal system and release coagulation factors; secrete active substances affecting themselves, other platelets, the endothelium, and other coagulation factors; and alter shape (through active actin-myosin contraction) to expose membrane GPs essential to hemostasis. Their cell signaling is highly regulated, is present in other cell lines (RBCs, leukocytes, and endothelial cells), and has been intensively studied. Platelets have perhaps as many as 30 to 50 different types of cell receptors, with many ways of these being activated and inhibited.

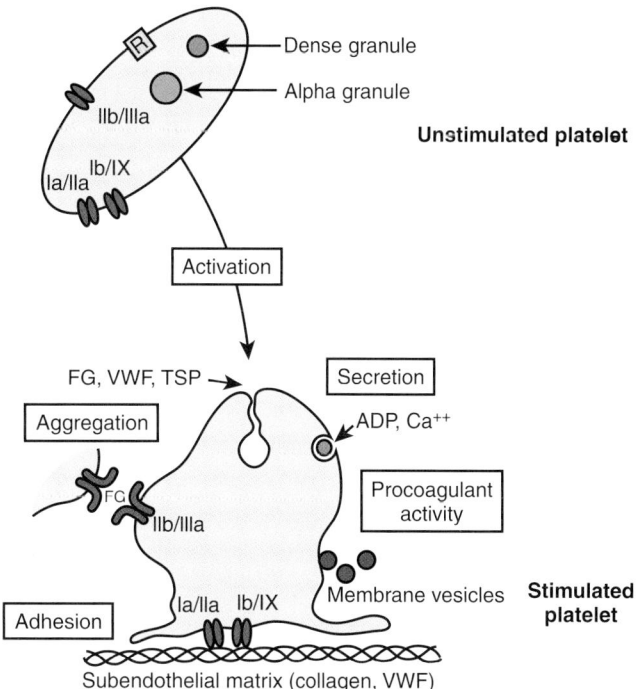

Figure 31-7 **Platelet function in hemostasis.** Glycoproteins Ib and IX and von Willebrand factor (VWF) mediate adhesion to the vessel wall. Glycoproteins IIb and IIIa and integrin molecules (FG [fibrinogen], TSP [thrombospondin]) mediate platelet aggregation. ADP, adenosine diphosphate. *(From George J, Shattil SJ: The clinical importance of acquired abnormalities of platelet function. N Engl J Med 324:27, 1991.)*

The initial response to vascular injury is formation of a platelet plug. Good hemostatic response depends on proper functioning of platelet adhesion, activation, and aggregation (Figure 31-7). This section first discusses these aspects and then follows with the effects of platelet disorders and platelet-inhibiting pharmaceuticals. Clinicians talk about platelet dysfunction, which is largely overarching and grossly too general a term. The complexity that is platelet function really needs careful study.

Platelet Adhesion

Capillary blood exhibits laminar flow, which maximizes the likelihood of interaction of platelets with the vessel wall. Red cells and white cells stream near the center of the vessels and marginate platelets. However, turbulence causes reactions in endothelium that lead to the secretion of vWF, adhesive molecules, and tissue factor. Shear stress is high as fast-moving platelets interact with the endothelium. When the vascular endothelium becomes denuded or injured, the platelet has the opportunity to contact vWF, which is bound to the exposed collagen of the subendothelium. A platelet membrane component, GPIb, attaches to vWF, thus anchoring the platelet to the vessel wall. Independently, platelet membrane GPIa and GPIIa and IX may attach directly to exposed collagen, furthering the adhesion stage.[44-46]

After activation (see later), additional adhesive mechanisms come into play. Release of selectin GPs from α-granules allows their membrane expression, thus promoting platelet-leukocyte adhesion. This interaction ultimately may allow expression of tissue factor on monocytes, thus amplifying coagulation.[47]

The integrin GPs form diverse types of membrane receptors from combinations of 20 α and 8 β subunits.[48] One such combination is GPIIb/IIIa, a platelet membrane component that initially participates in platelet adhesion. Platelet activation causes a conformational change in GPIIb/IIIa, which results in its aggregator activity.

Platelet adhesion begins rapidly—within 1 minute of endothelial injury—and completely covers exposed subendothelium within 20 minutes.[45] It begins with decreased platelet velocity when GPIb/IX and vWF mediate adhesion, followed by platelet activation, GPIIb/IIIa conformational change, then vWF binding and platelet arrest on the endothelium at these vWF ligand sites.[44,46]

Adhesion requires margination of platelets; high hematocrits concentrate RBCs in the central regions of a vessel, promoting marginal placement of platelets. Dilute hematocrit (e.g., post-CPB) impairs this effect, thus adversely affecting platelet adhesion. Low hematocrit also may affect platelet prostaglandin levels as RBCs are required for preprocessing of arachidonic acid before platelets make thromboxane. Because of rheology, RBC transfusions have been thought by some to improve hemostasis. However, transfusion should not be used primarily to achieve this goal because RBC concentrates carry a high concentration of cytokines and platelet-activating factor, which may contribute to platelet dysfunction or consumptive coagulopathy. Some of the most recent data-based studies looking at only several units of blood transfusion have noted that when transfusion is used, the postoperative chest tube output is greater. That observation is, however, fundamentally different from one in which if a patient is bleeding and has a particularly low hematocrit, the use of RBCs may well increase margination of platelets.

Platelet Activation and Aggregation

Platelet activation results after contact with collagen, when adenosine diphosphate (ADP), thrombin, or thromboxane A_2 binds to membrane receptors, or from certain platelet-to-platelet interactions. Platelets then release the contents of their dense (δ) granules and α granules. Dense granules contain serotonin, ADP, and Ca^{2+}; α granules contain platelet factor V (previously termed platelet factor 1), β-thromboglobulin, platelet factor 4 (PF4), P-selectin, and various integrin proteins (vWF, fibrinogen, vitronectin, and fibronectin). Simultaneously, platelets use their microskeletal system to change shape from a disk to a sphere, which changes platelet membrane GPIIb/IIIa exposure. Released ADP recruits additional platelets to the site of injury and stimulates platelet G protein, which, in turn, activates membrane phospholipase. This results in the formation of arachidonate, which platelet cyclooxygenase converts to thromboxane A_2. Other platelet agonists besides ADP and collagen include serotonin, a weak agonist, and thrombin and thromboxane A_2, both potent agonists. Thrombin is by far the most potent platelet agonist, and it can overcome all other platelet antagonists, as well as inhibitors. In total, more than 70 agonists can produce platelet activation and aggregation.

Agonists induce a graded platelet shape change (the amount based on the relative amount of stimulation), increase platelet intracellular Ca^{2+} concentration, and stimulate platelet G protein. In addition, serotonin and thromboxane A_2 are potent vasoconstrictors (particularly in the pulmonary vasculature).[49] The presence of sufficient agonist material results in platelet aggregation. Aggregation occurs when the integrin proteins (mostly fibrinogen) released from α granules form molecular bridges between the GPIIb/IIIa receptors of adjacent platelets (the final common platelet pathway).

Platelet Disorders

Dysfunctional vWF produces von Willebrand disease (vWD), an autosomal dominant disorder of variable expressivity.[34] With an incidence of 1.4 to 5 cases per 1000 population, vWD is the most common inherited coagulopathy. Patients present with mucocutaneous hemorrhages rather than hemarthroses. Common symptoms include epistaxis, ecchymoses, and excessive bleeding after trauma, with surgery, or during menses. Because vWF concentrations vary greatly with time, symptoms have variable expressivity. Desmopressin reverses the prolonged bleeding time in patients with mild vWD.[50] As with hemophilia A, severe cases of vWD do not benefit from desmopressin therapy. In one rare class of vWD (type IIB, 3% to 5% of vWD), desmopressin aggregates platelets, inducing thrombocytopenia and worsening rather than helping hemostasis. Table 31-2 summarizes features of the more common types of vWD. When blood products are needed, cryoprecipitate constitutes the replacement vehicle of choice in vWD, although recent factor VIII concentrates retain vWF activity and have been used successfully during cardiac surgery.[51]

The addition of agonist (ADP or collagen) to platelets allows measurement of platelet aggregation in vitro. In Glanzmann thrombasthenia, the GPIIb/IIIa receptor is absent, preventing aggregation. However, ristocetin, a cationic antibiotic similar to vancomycin, can agglutinate platelets directly via GPIb receptors and vWF. Absence of the GPIb receptor, Bernard–Soulier syndrome, prevents adhesion and agglutination with ristocetin, but aggregation to ADP is normal, because the GPIIb/IIIa receptor is intact. Patients with vWD also exhibit impaired platelet adhesion and normal aggregation. Decreased amounts of vWF antigen distinguish it from the Bernard–Soulier syndrome. In platelet storage pool deficiency, impairment of dense granule secretion yields no ADP on adhesion. In vitro addition of collagen will not aggregate platelets because of absence of ADP release, whereas added ADP will initiate some aggregation. Table 31-3 summarizes these diagnostic findings. Uremia impairs the secretory and aggregating functions of platelets, resulting in an increased bleeding time.

TABLE 31-2	**Major Types of von Willebrand Disease**				
Classification	*Prevalence Rate*	*vWf:Ag*	*R:Co*	*Molecular Pathology*	
I (Classic)	70–80%	Decreased	Decreased	Normal multimers; decreased quantity	
IIA	10–12%	Decreased	Decreased	Intermediate and large multimers decreased	
IIB	3–5%	Decreased	Near normal	Abnormal, large multimers that bind platelets	
III	1–3%	None	None	No vWF present	
Platelet-type	0–1%	Decreased	Decreased	Normal vWF; platelet glycoprotein Ib receptors bind large multimers	

R:Co, ristocetin cofactor activity measurement; vWF:Ag, von Willebrand factor antigen measurement.
Data from Montgomery RR, Colier BS: von Willebrand disease. In Colman RW, Hirsh J, Marder VJ, Salzman EW (eds): *Hemostasis and Thrombosis*, 3rd ed. Philadelphia, 1994, JB Lippincott, pp 134–168.

TABLE 31-3	**Diagnosis of Some Inherited Platelet Disorders**				
Disorder	*Deficiency*	*Platelet Adhesion*	*Platelet Aggregation*	*Ristocetin Agglutination*	*vWF:Ag Level*
Glanzmann thrombasthenia	GPIIb/IIIa	Normal	Absent	Occurs	Normal
Bernard–Soulier syndrome	GPIb	Absent	Normal	Absent	Normal
Storage pool deficiency	Dense granule secretion	Normal	Impaired	Occurs	Normal
von Willebrand disease	vWF	Absent	Normal	Absent or decreased	Low

GP, glycoprotein receptor; vWF, von Willebrand factor; vWF:Ag, von Willebrand factor antigen.

However, the most common effect of renal dysfunction is hypercoagulability. It is only with severe uremia that the platelets are poisoned. It is, therefore, a common misconception in the operating room that a patient with mild-to-moderate renal failure will be at increased risk for bleeding. The utilization of thromboelastography (TEG) can help in deciding whether the extent of renal failure is causing hypocoagulability. The cause and clinical significance remain poorly defined (see Chapter 17).

Prostaglandins and Aspirin

Endothelial cell cyclooxygenase synthesizes prostacyclin, which inhibits aggregation and dilates vessels. Platelet cyclooxygenase forms thromboxane A_2, a potent aggregating agent and vasoconstrictor. Aspirin irreversibly acetylates cyclooxygenase, rendering it inactive. Low doses of aspirin, 80 to 100 mg, easily overcome the finite amount of cyclooxygenase available in the nucleus-free platelets. However, endothelial cells can synthesize new cyclooxygenase. Thus, with low doses of aspirin, prostacyclin synthesis continues whereas thromboxane synthesis ceases, decreasing platelet activation and aggregation. High doses of aspirin inhibit the enzyme at both cyclooxygenase sites.[49]

Reversible platelet aggregation is blocked by aspirin, as the platelet cyclooxygenase is inhibited. However, the more powerful agonists that yield the calcium release response can still aggregate and activate platelets, because cyclooxygenase is not required for those pathways (Figure 31-8).

In many centers, a majority of the patients presenting for coronary artery bypass grafting (CABG) will have received aspirin within 7 days of surgery in hopes of preventing coronary thrombosis.[52] Aspirin is a drug for which an increased risk for bleeding often has been demonstrated.[53] Although most early research studies stated that aspirin leads to increased bleeding, since the mid-1990s, that early impression has

not been confirmed. Today, it probably is more likely that, in some patients, a mild-to-moderate increased risk for bleeding is possible.

Unfortunately, most of the early studies of aspirin were not blinded, and it may be that the pervading belief that aspirin caused increased bleeding was actually self-fulfilling. Since the early 1990s, there have been a number of therapeutic changes including use of lower doses and greater use of antifibrinolytics. These changes alone may have decreased the overall risk for bleeding from aspirin. Follow-up prospective studies have, thus, yielded varied results. In the largest cohort of 772 men, aspirin increased bleeding after CABG by 33%,[54] and a group of 101 aspirin-taking patients bled 25% to 56% more than a control group.[55] In another study, the need to explore the mediastinum for excessive bleeding nearly doubled (factor of 1.82) in patients taking aspirin.[56] However, many other studies have not shown increased bleeding with aspirin.[57–62] Although a single aspirin can irreversibly inhibit platelet cyclooxygenase for the life of the platelet, aspirin-related bleeding after surgery usually requires more extensive exposure to the drug.

Drug-Induced Platelet Abnormalities

Many other agents inhibit platelet function. β-Lactam antibiotics coat the platelet membrane, whereas the cephalosporins are rather profound but short-term platelet inhibitors.[63] Many cardiac surgeons may not realize that their standard drug regimen for antibiotics may be far more of a bleeding risk than aspirin. Hundreds of drugs can inhibit platelet function. Calcium channel blockers, nitrates, and β-blockers are ones commonly used in cardiac surgery. Nitrates are effective antiplatelet agents, and that may be part of why they are of such benefit in angina, not just for their vasorelaxing effect on large blood vessels. Nonsteroidal anti-inflammatory drugs reversibly inhibit both endothelial cell and platelet cyclooxygenase. In addition, anecdotal reports of platelet inhibition, without clear confirmatory studies, exist for many pharmaceuticals including dextran, and for innumerable foods (e.g., onion, garlic, alcohol) and spices (e.g., ginger, tumeric, cloves).[24]

Rofecoxib (Vioxx), a cyclooxygenase 2 (COX-2) inhibitor, was withdrawn from the U.S. market because of its cardiovascular risk profile (a small increase in associated acute myocardial infarctions).[64] This COX-2 inhibitor has the highest selectivity for COX-2 versus COX-1 and thus leads to an imbalance between thromboxane A_2 and prostacyclin production. The other COX-2 inhibitors are currently also undergoing cardiovascular investigation.

In addition to the partial inhibitory effects of aspirin and the other drugs mentioned earlier, new therapies that inhibit platelet function in a more specific manner have been developed. These drugs include platelet adhesion inhibitor agents, platelet-ADP-receptor antagonists, and GPIIb/IIIa receptor inhibitors (Table 31-4).[65]

Adhesion Inhibitors

Dipyridamole (Persantine) and cilostazol (Pletal) alter platelet adhesion by various mechanisms including cyclic adenosine monophosphate, phosphodiesterase III, and thromboxane A_2 inhibition. Dipyridamole has been used with warfarin in some patients with artificial valves and with aspirin in patients with peripheral vascular disease.

Adenosine Diphosphate (ADP) Receptor Antagonists

Clopidogrel (Plavix), prasugrel (Effient), and ticlopidine (Ticlid) are thienopyridine derivatives that inhibit the ADP receptor pathway to platelet activation. They have a slow onset of action because they must be converted to active drugs, and their potent effects last the lifetime of the platelets affected (5 to 10 days). Clopidogrel and prasugrel are the preferred drugs. They are administered orally once daily to inhibit platelet function and are quite effective in decreasing myocardial infarctions after percutaneous coronary interventions (see Chapter 3). The combination of aspirin and clopidogrel has led to increased bleeding but is sometimes used in an effort to keep vessels and stents open. The TEG and now the RoTEM (a modified TEG) with ADP or other additives can be used to determine the degree of inhibition caused by these drugs (see Chapter 17). Other new tests are coming onto the market to

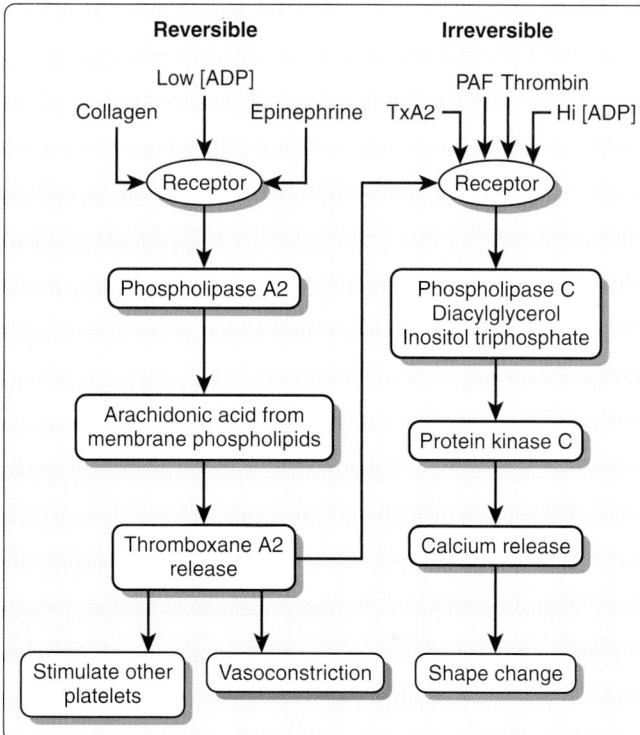

Figure 31-8 Pathways for reversible (left column) and irreversible (right column) platelet aggregation. Note the different agents that activate distinct receptors. Aspirin inhibits reversible platelet aggregation via the phospholipase A_2 pathway by affecting the arachidonic acid enzyme cyclooxygenase, but it does not prevent more powerful agonists from aggregating platelets by directly stimulating phospholipase C pathway receptors. (*Adapted from Kroll MH, Schafer A: Biochemical mechanisms of platelet activation. Blood 74:1181, 1989.*)

TABLE 31-4	Antiplatelet Therapy						
Drug Type	*Composition*	*Mechanism*	*Indications*	*Route*	*Half-life*	*Metabolism*
Aspirin	Acetylsalicylic acid	Irreversible COX inhibition	CAD, AMI, PVD, PCI, ACS	Oral	10 days	Liver, kidney
NSAIDs	Multiple	Reversible COX inhibition	Pain	Oral	2 days	Liver, kidney
Adhesion inhibitors (e.g., dipyridamole)	Multiple	Block adhesion to vessels	VHD, PVD	Oral	12 hours	Liver
ADP receptor antagonists (e.g., clopidogrel)	Thienopyridines	Irreversible inhibition of ADP binding	AMI, CVA, PVD, ACS, PCI	Oral	5 days	Liver
GPIIb/IIIa receptor inhibitors						
Abciximab (ReoPro)	Monoclonal antibody	Nonspecific—binds to other receptors	PCI, ACS	IV	12–18 hours	Plasma proteinase
Eptifibatide (Integrilin)	Peptide	Reversible—specific to GPIIb/IIIa	PCI, ACS	IV	2–4 hours	Kidney
Tirofiban (Aggrastat)	Nonpeptide-tyrosine derivative	Reversible—specific to GPIIb/IIIa	PCI, ACS	IV	2–4 hours	Kidney

ACS, acute coronary syndrome; AMI, acute myocardial infarction; CAD, coronary artery disease; COX, cyclooxygenase; CVA, cerebrovascular disease; IV, intravenous; NSAID, nonsteroidal anti-inflammatory drug; PCI, percutaneous coronary intervention; PVD, peripheral vascular disease; VHD, valvular heart disease.

allow testing for relative platelet inhibition caused by thienopyridines. Some of these are modifications of platelet flow cytometry or automated platelet aggregometers. Verify Now (Accumetrics, San Diego, CA) and the PFA-100 (Siemens USA, Deerfield, IL) have been used in dosing clopidogrel for cardiology procedures. These new platelet function tests are now finding their way into hospitals, and some are starting to use them before or after surgery.[66–72] In the past, aprotinin was able to partially reverse the effects of these drug; however, it is currently not available. Today, treatment for bleeding caused by platelet dysfunction after cardiac surgery involves using factor VIIa, as well as repeated platelet transfusions. Although one report notes that in addition to factor VIIa, the investigators found it useful to infuse fibrinogen (available in Europe as a purified product) and factor XIII.[73]

Glycoprotein IIb/IIIa Receptor Inhibitors
GPIIb/IIIa receptor inhibitors are the most potent (> 90% platelet inhibition) and important platelet inhibitors because they act at the final common pathway of platelet aggregation with fibrinogen, no matter which agonist began the process. All of the drugs mentioned earlier work at earlier phases of activation of platelet function. These drugs are all administered by intravenous infusion, and they do not work orally. The GPIIb/IIIa inhibitors often are used in patients taking aspirin because they do not block thromboxane A_2 production. The dose of heparin usually is reduced when used with these drugs (i.e., percutaneous coronary intervention to avoid bleeding at the vascular puncture sites). Platelet activity can be monitored to determine the extent of blockade. Excessive bleeding requires allowing the short-acting drugs to wear off, while possibly administering platelets to patients receiving the long-acting drug abciximab (see Table 31-4). Most studies have found increased bleeding in patients receiving these drugs who required emergency CABG.

New ultra-short-acting agents of the above two classes are undergoing testing. These drugs could prove to be of great utility to cardiac anesthesiologists. If they were able to block surface membrane activation of the platelet during CPB ("platelet anesthesia"), then a number of deleterious secondary events might be reduced in severity.

Vascular Endothelium

The cells that form the intima of vessels provide an excellent nonthrombogenic surface. Characteristics of this surface, which may account for its nonthrombogenicity, include negative charge; incorporation of heparan sulfate in the grid substance; the release of prostacyclin, nitric oxide, adenosine, and protease inhibitors by endothelial cells; binding and clearance of activated coagulation factors both directly, as occurs with thrombin, and indirectly, as evidenced by the action of thrombomodulin to inactivate factors Va and VIIIa via protein C; and stimulation of fibrinolysis.

Nitric oxide vasodilates blood vessels and inhibits platelets. Its mechanism involves activation of guanylate cyclase with eventual uptake of calcium into intracellular storage sites. Prostacyclin (prostaglandin I_2) possesses powerful vasodilator and antiplatelet properties. Endothelium-derived prostacyclin opposes the vasoconstrictor effects of platelet-produced thromboxane A_2. Prostacyclin also inhibits platelet aggregation, disaggregates clumped platelets, and at high concentrations, inhibits platelet adhesion. Prostacyclin increases intracellular concentrations of cyclic adenosine monophosphate, which inhibits aggregation. Thromboxane acts in an opposite manner. The mechanism of prostacyclin action is stimulation of adenylyl cyclase, leading to reduced intracellular calcium concentrations. Some vascular beds (e.g., lung) and atherosclerotic vessels secrete thromboxane, endothelins, and angiotensin, all vasoconstrictors, as well as prostacyclin. Activation of platelets releases endoperoxides and arachidonate. These substances, used by nearby damaged endothelial cells, provide substrate for prostacyclin production.[5]

The endothelial cell also participates in coagulation factor activation. Playing a role similar to that of platelet phospholipid, the endothelial surface facilitates activation of factor IX. Thrombospondin, a substance formed in endothelial cells and platelets, helps complete platelet aggregation and binds plasminogen. The latter effect decreases the amount of locally available plasmin, thus inhibiting fibrin breakdown.

Fibrinolysis

Fibrin breakdown, a normal hematologic activity, is localized to the vicinity of a clot. It remodels formed clot and removes thrombus when endothelium heals. Like clot formation, clot breakdown may occur by intrinsic and extrinsic pathways. As with clot formation, the extrinsic pathway plays the dominant role in clot breakdown. Each pathway activates plasminogen, a serine protease synthesized by the liver, which circulates in zymogen form. Cleavage of plasminogen by the proper serine protease forms plasmin. Plasmin splits fibrinogen or fibrin at specific sites. Plasmin is the principal enzyme of fibrinolysis, just as thrombin is principal to clot formation. Plasma normally contains no circulating plasmin because a scavenging protein, α_2-antiplasmin, quickly consumes any plasmin formed from localized fibrinolysis. Thus, localized fibrinolysis, not systemic fibrinogenolysis, accompanies normal hemostasis.

Extrinsic Fibrinolysis

Endothelial cells synthesize and release t-PA. Both t-PA and a related substance, urokinase plasminogen activator, are serine proteases that split plasminogen to form plasmin. The activity of t-PA magnifies on binding to fibrin. In this manner, also, plasmin formation remains localized to sites of clot formation. Epinephrine, bradykinin, thrombin, and factor Xa cause endothelium to release t-PA, as do venous occlusion and CPB.[74] Fibrinolysis during and after CPB is discussed later.

Intrinsic Fibrinolysis

Factor XIIa, formed during the contact phase of coagulation, cleaves plasminogen to plasmin. The plasmin so formed then facilitates additional cleavage of plasminogen by factor XIIa, forming a positive feedback loop. Kallikrein also can activate plasminogen; the physiologic importance of this pathway for fibrin breakdown has not been established.

Exogenous Activators

Streptokinase (made by bacteria) and urokinase (found in human urine) both cleave plasminogen to plasmin, but do so with low fibrin affinity. Thus, systemic plasminemia and fibrinogenolysis, as well as fibrinolysis, ensue. Acetylated streptokinase plasminogen activator complex provides an active site, which is not available until deacetylation occurs in blood. Its systemic lytic activity lies intermediate to those of t-PA and streptokinase. Recombinant t-PA (Alteplase) is a second-generation agent that is made by recombinant DNA technology and is relatively fibrin specific.

Clinical Applications

Figure 31-9 illustrates the fibrinolytic pathway, with activators and inhibitors. Streptokinase, acetylated streptokinase plasminogen activator complex, and t-PA find application in the lysis of thrombi associated with myocardial infarction. These intravenous agents "dissolve" clots that form on atheromatous plaque. Clinically significant bleeding may result from administration of any of these exogenous activators or streptokinase.[75]

Fibrinolysis also accompanies CPB. This undesirable breakdown of clot after surgery may contribute to postoperative hemorrhage and the need to administer allogeneic blood products. Regardless of how they are formed, the breakdown products of fibrin intercalate into sheets of normally forming fibrin monomers, thus preventing cross-linking. In this way, extensive fibrinolysis exerts an antihemostatic action. Factor XIII is an underappreciated coagulation protein. It circulates and, when activated, cross-links fibrin strands and protects fibrin from the lytic actions of plasmin. It has been known for some time that low levels of factor XIII are associated with increased hemorrhage after CPB. Factor XIII levels are reduced by hemodilution, but it also appears that there is active destruction in some patients with CPB. Several new studies have begun testing adding factor XIII to patients and assessing bleeding.[76–78] The problem, however, is that currently there is no good way to assess factor XIII levels. Clearly, factor XIII will be quite expensive, and using it for most patients may well be ill advised.

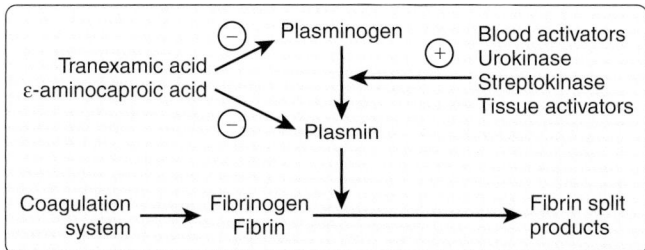

Figure 31-9   The fibrinolytic pathway. Antifibrinolytic drugs inhibit fibrinolysis by binding to both plasminogen and plasmin. Intrinsic blood activators (factor XIIa), extrinsic tissue activators (tissue plasminogen activator, urokinase plasminogen activator), and exogenous activators (streptokinase, acetylated streptokinase plasminogen activator complex) split plasminogen to form plasmin. *(From Horrow JC, Hlavacek J, Strong MD, et al: Prophylactic tranexamic acid decreases bleeding after cardiac operations. J Thorac Cardiovasc Surg 99:70, 1990.)*

HEPARIN

In 1916, in the course of experiments to determine whether the phospholipid component of cephalin caused clotting, a second-year medical student, Jay McLean, instead discovered a substance derived from liver that prolonged coagulation.[79] His mentor, William Howell, named this substance *heparin*. Heparin has been used almost exclusively as the anticoagulant for CPB for more than 50 years.

Pharmacology

Chemical Structure

In the 1920s, Howell's group isolated heparin and identified it as a carbohydrate containing glucuronic acid residues. In the 1930s, Jorpes demonstrated a hexosamine component to heparin (glucosamine, in particular) that is present in a ratio of 1:1 with glucuronic acid. Of greater importance, he discovered that heparin contains many sulfate groups—two per uronic acid residue—making it one of the strongest acids found in living things. In the 1950s, Jorpes' group identified the sulfate groups at the N-position on glucosamine, where solely acetyl groups previously were thought to reside. In the 1960s, they corrected identification of the uronic acid as L-iduronic acid, an epimer of D-glucuronic acid, and refined its structural detail.[80]

The *N*-sulfated-D-glucosamine and L-iduronic acid residues of heparin alternate in copolymer fashion to form chains of varying length (Figure 31-10). As a linear anionic polyelectrolyte, the negative charges being supplied by sulfate groups, heparin demonstrates a wide spectrum of activity with enzymes, hormones, biogenic amines, and plasma proteins. A pentasaccharide segment binds to AT.[81] Heparin is a heterogenous compound; the carbohydrates vary in both length and side-chain composition, yielding a range of molecular weights from 5000 to 30,000, with most chains between 12,000 and 19,000.[82] Today, the standard heparin is called *unfractionated heparin* (UFH).

Heparin versus Heparan

Heparan, a glycosaminoglycan found in the connective tissue and the coating of the endothelial surfaces of nearly all species, can be distinguished from heparin by the following characteristics: (1) a predominance of glucuronic acid over iduronic acid; and (2) N-acetylation, rather than N-sulfation, of more than 20% of glucosamine residues. Bound to cellular proteins, heparan resides inside cells, on cell surfaces, and in the extracellular matrix.[80–84]

Source and Biologic Role

Heparin is found mostly in the lungs, intestines, and liver of mammals, with skin, lymph nodes, and thymus providing less plentiful sources.[84] Abundance of heparin in tissues rich in mast cells suggests these as the source of the compound. Its presence in tissues with environmental contact suggests a biologic role relating to immune function. Heparin may assist white blood cell movements in the interstitium after an immunologic response has been triggered. Mollusks have no coagulation system yet possess heparin, arguing against a biologic role in hemostasis. It is clear that heparin, per se, was never intended biologically to be circulating in large dosages throughout the vascular tree.

Most commercial preparations of heparin now use pig intestine, 40,000 pounds of which yield 5 kg heparin.[80] Prevention of postoperative thrombosis constituted the initial clinical use of heparin in 1935 by Best, Jaques, and colleagues in Toronto, and by Crafoord in Stockholm.[80]

Potency

Heparin potency is determined by comparing the test specimen against a known standard's ability to prolong coagulation.[85] Current United States Pharmacopeia (USP) and British Pharmacopoeia (BP) assays use a PT-like method on pooled sheep's plasma obtained from slaughterhouses. The plasma commonly is contaminated with tissue extracts or other hemostatically active substances. The European Pharmacopoeia's

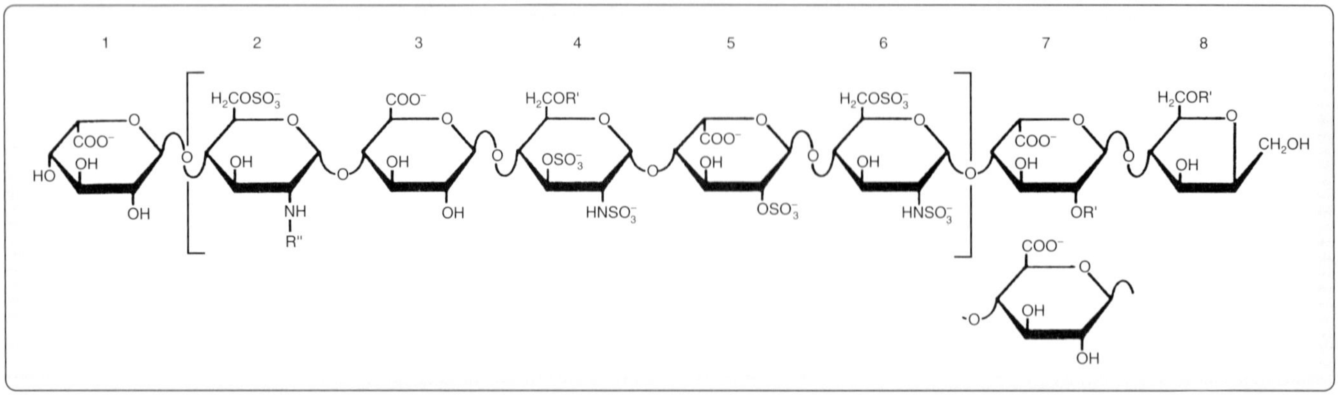

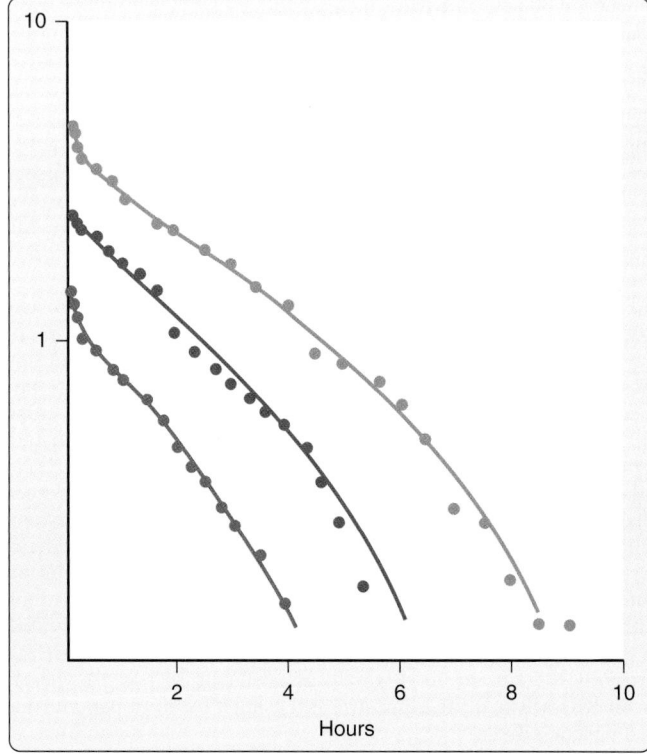

Figure 31-10   An octasaccharide fragment of heparin, a substituted alternating copolymer of iduronic acid and glucosamine. The leftmost sugar is iduronic acid. Note the numerous sulfate groups and the acetyl substitution on the second sugar. Variations in sugar substitutions and in chain length produce molecular heterogeneity. Brackets indicate the pentasaccharide sequence that binds to antithrombin. *(From Rodén L: Highlights in the history of heparin. In Lane DA, Lindahl U [eds]: Heparin. Boca Raton, FL: CRC Press, 1989, p 1.)*

method, an aPTT on fresh sheep's plasma, is superior to that of the USP.[86] Modern research assays use human FFP, an aPTT-like method, and require linear log versus log plots of standard and test samples.[85]

UFH dose should not be specified by weight (milligrams) because of the diversity of anticoagulant activity expected from so heterogenous a compound. Unfortunately, because of the flawed USP assay, even units of activity often do not reflect clinical effects. As originally defined, 1 unit heparin prolongs the clotting of cat's blood for only 24 hours at 0°C.[87] Milligram usage, introduced in 1937 as a Swedish standard, was superseded by the first international standard, in which 130 units of activity corresponded to 1 mg. The fourth international standard uses a porcine mucosal preparation.[85]

One USP unit of heparin activity is the quantity that prevents 1.0 mL of citrated sheep's plasma from clotting for 1 hour after addition of calcium.[88] Units cannot be cross-compared among heparins of different sources, such as mucosal versus lung, or low-molecular-weight heparin (LMWH) versus UFH, or even lot to lot, because the assay used may or may not reflect actual differences in biologic activity. None of these measures has anything to do with the effect of a unit on anticoagulation effect for human cardiac surgery.

Pharmacokinetics and Pharmacodynamics

The heterogeneity of UFH molecules produces variability in the relation of dose administered to plasma level of drug. In addition, the relation of plasma level to biologic effect varies with the test system. A three-compartment model describes heparin kinetics in healthy humans: rapid initial disappearance, saturable clearance observed in the lower dose range, and exponential first-order decay at greater doses[89,90] (Figure 31-11). The rapid initial disappearance may arise from endothelial cell uptake.[91,92] The reticuloendothelial system, with its endoglycosidases and endosulfatases, and uptake into monocytes, may represent the saturable phase of heparin kinetics. Finally, renal clearance via active tubular secretion of heparin, much of it desulfated, explains heparin's exponential clearance.

Male sex and cigarette smoking are associated with more rapid heparin clearance.[93] The resistance of patients with deep vein thrombosis or pulmonary embolism to heparin therapy may be caused by the release from thrombi of PF4, a known heparin antagonist.[94,95] Chronic renal failure prolongs elimination of high, but not low, heparin doses.[93] Chronic liver disease does not change elimination.[96]

Loading doses for CPB (200 to 400 U/kg) are substantially greater than those used to treat venous thrombosis (70 to 150 U/kg). Plasma heparin levels, determined fluorometrically, vary widely (2 to 4 units/mL) after doses of heparin administered to patients about to undergo CPB.[97] The ACT response to these doses of heparin displays even greater dispersion. Gravlee et al[98] identified thrombocytosis and advanced age

Figure 31-11   Decay of heparin anticoagulant activity (U/mL on a logarithmic scale) after injections of 75, 150, and 250 U/kg to a single healthy volunteer. Note the rapid initial decline in all curves and nonlinearity at greater doses. *(From deSwart CAM, Nijmeyer B, Roelofs JMM, Sixma JJ: Kinetics of intravenously administered heparin in normal humans. Blood 60:1251, 1982.)*

as causing a decreased ACT response to administered heparin. This effect may arise from alterations in pharmacokinetics, pharmacodynamics, or both. Interpatient variability in heparin response (pharmacodynamics) does affect the clotting time[99,100]; however, the clinical response to heparin administered to various patients is more consistent than suggested by in vitro measurements.

Although not substantiated formally, most clinicians would agree that hypothermia prolongs the effect of heparin. Precise documentation remains impeded by inability to warm the patient's blood immediately to 37° C for standardized measurement of its ACT. Delayed metabolism or excretion, or both, most likely account for the prolongation of heparin presence during systemic hypothermia, whereas prolongation of the ACT more likely relates to decreased activity of coagulation enzymatic processes (see later).

Actions and Interactions

Heparin exerts its anticoagulant activity via AT III, one of the many circulating serine protein inhibitors (serpins), which counter the effects of circulating proteases.[101] The major inhibitor of thrombin and factors IXa and Xa is AT III; that of the contact activation factors XIIa and XIa is α_1-proteinase inhibitor; kallikrein inhibition arises mostly from C1 inhibitor. AT activity is greatly decreased at a site of vascular damage, underscoring its primary role as a scavenger for clotting enzymes that escape into the general circulation.

AT inhibits serine proteases even without heparin. The extent to which heparin accelerates AT inhibition depends on the substrate enzyme; UFH accelerates the formation of the thrombin-AT complex by 2000-fold, but accelerates formation of the factor Xa-AT complex by only 1200-fold[102] (Table 31-5). In contrast, LMWH fragments preferentially inhibit factor Xa. Enzyme inhibition proceeds by formation of a ternary complex consisting of heparin, AT, and the proteinase to be inhibited (e.g., thrombin, factor Xa). For UFH, inhibition of thrombin occurs only on simultaneous binding to both AT and thrombin. This condition requires a heparin fragment of at least 18 residues.[101,103] A pentasaccharide sequence binds to AT (see Figure 31-10). LMWHs, consisting of chains 8 to 16 units long, preferentially inhibit factor Xa. In this case, the heparin fragment activates AT, which then sequentially inactivates factor Xa; heparin and factor Xa do not directly interact (Figure 31-12).[104,105]

Several investigators have demonstrated continued formation of fibrinopeptides A[106,107] and B[108] (Figure 31-13), as well as prothrombin fragment F1.2 and thrombin-AT complexes,[109] despite clearly acceptable anticoagulation for CPB by many criteria. These substances indicate thrombin activity. The clinical significance of this ongoing thrombin activity has had limited study. The ACT must be more prolonged to prevent fibrin formation during cardiac surgery compared with during extracorporeal circulation without surgery because surgery itself incites coagulation. UFH in conjunction with AT appears to work in plasma only on free thrombin. When considering what is known today about thrombin burst and thrombin activity, heparin appears to be relatively inefficient because there is not much free thrombin. Thrombin is held on the surface of activated platelets at various GP binding sites including the GPIIb/IIIa site. Most thrombin is fibrin bound, and heparin-AT complexes do not bind at all to this thrombin unless the level of heparin is pushed far above what is used routinely for CPB. The idea behind using heparin for CPB is that by creating a large circulating concentration of activated AT, whenever a thrombin molecule is produced, an available AT molecule will be there to immediately bind to it before it can have any further activating effect. Clearly, that is unrealistic with the knowledge that thrombin exerts its main activity by binding to the surface of platelets.

Bovine versus Porcine Preparations

Bovine lung heparin contains greater amounts of iduronic acid and sulfoamino groups than pork mucosal heparin. Because endothelial endoglycosidases degrade heparin at sulfoamino groups, elimination

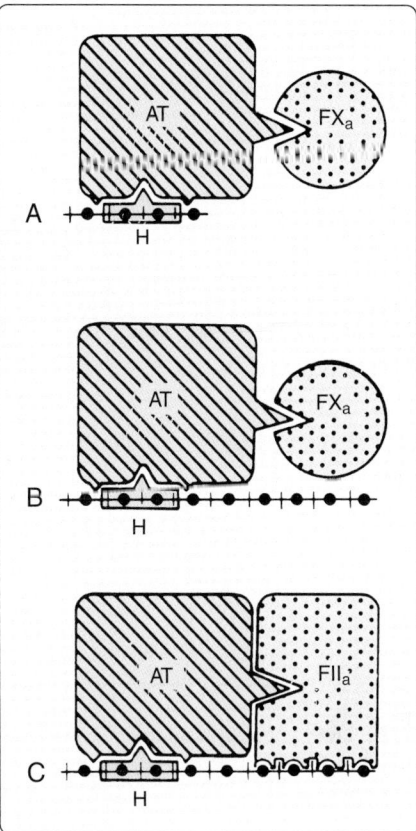

Figure 31-12 Antithrombin interaction with factor Xa may occur with either low-molecular-weight heparin (A) or standard unfractionated heparin (B). Inhibition of thrombin (factor IIa), however, requires simultaneous binding of the heparin molecule to both antithrombin and thrombin (C). (From Holmer E, Soderberg K, Bergqvist D, Lindahl U: Heparin and its low-molecular-weight derivatives. Anticoagulant and antithrombotic properties. Haemostasis 16[Suppl 2]:1, 1986.)

of beef lung heparin proceeds more quickly than that of pork mucosal heparin. Its AT III affinity and anticoagulant activity are less than those of porcine heparin. Either preparation can establish suitable anticoagulation for CPB. Beef lung heparin may be more amenable to protamine neutralization than the pork mucosal preparation because it exerts less anti–factor Xa activity.[110] HIT is less common with pork heparin (see later). This information may be of historic value only because bovine heparin is no longer available in the United States.

Heparin Resistance

In the course of continuous infusions of UFH to treat venous thrombosis, some patients experience development of tachyphylaxis, requiring increasing amounts of heparin to maintain the laboratory measurement of anticoagulation, the aPTT, at its designated therapeutic level. In some reports, up to 22% of patients do not adequately respond to heparin and are termed *heparin resistant*.[111–114] To most practitioners, that number seems high, but the definition of what constitutes heparin resistance is highly variable from institution to institution. Likewise, patients receiving UFH infusions exhibit a much diminished ACT response to full anticoagulating doses of UFH for CPB (200 to 400 U/kg). With widespread use of heparin infusions to treat myocardial ischemia and infarction, heparin resistance or, more appropriately, "altered heparin responsiveness" has become more problematic during cardiac surgery (Box 31-2).[115,116]

TABLE 31-5	Some Coagulation Factor Inhibitors and the Effects of Heparin	
Factor	*Major Inhibitor*	*Acceleration of Antithrombin Activity by Heparin*
Kallikrein	C1 inhibitor	—
XIIa	α_1-Proteinase inhibitor	—
XIa	α_1-Proteinase inhibitor	40-fold
Xa	Antithrombin	1,200-fold
IXa	Antithrombin	10,000-fold
IIa	Antithrombin	2,000-fold

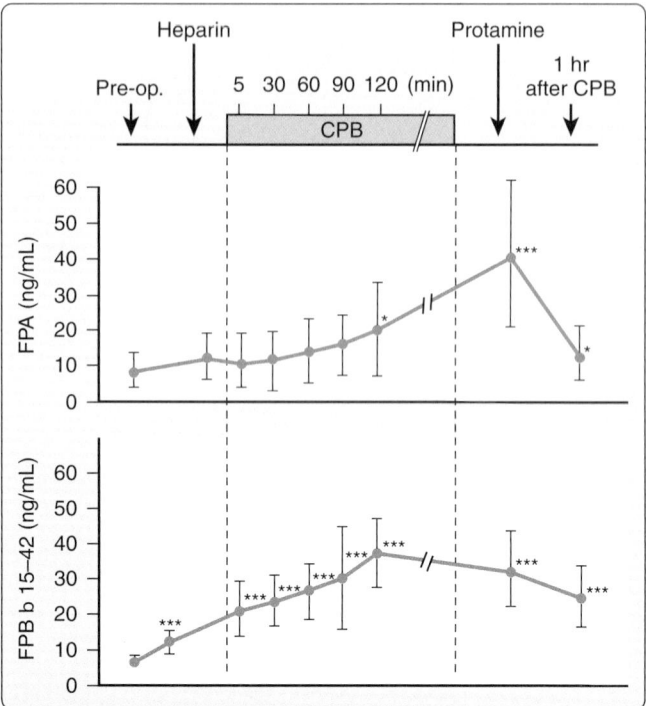

Figure 31-13 Serial measurements of fibrinopeptides A (top) and B (bottom) during cardiopulmonary bypass (CPB) in 20 patients. *Asterisks* denote statistically significant changes compared with the preoperative measurement. Note continued presence of these markers of thrombin activity despite heparin administration. *(From Tanaka K, Takao M, Yada I, et al: Alterations in coagulation and fibrinolysis associated with cardiopulmonary bypass during open heart surgery. J Cardiothorac Anesth 3:181, 1989.)*

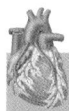

BOX 31-2. PROBLEMS WITH HEPARIN AS AN ANTICOAGULANT FOR CARDIOPULMONARY BYPASS

- Heparin resistance
- Heparin-induced thrombocytopenia
- Heparin rebound
- Heparin's heterogeneity and variable potency
- AT-III decrease

AT-III, antithrombin.

Mechanism

Although several observations suggest that decreased levels of AT III mediate heparin resistance, these observations lack sufficient evidence to establish this relation.[116] In one study of 500 CABG patients, 21% demonstrated heparin resistance, and 65% of these responded to added AT III; this translates into 35% being nonresponders.[112] First, a patient with congenital AT III deficiency displayed heparin resistance[117]; this hardly proves that all heparin resistance stems from AT III deficiency. Second, of six patients with venous thrombosis, three receiving heparin infusions displayed a 25% shorter half-life for AT III compared with the three untreated patients.[118] Accelerated AT III consumption could have resulted from the thrombotic process rather than the heparin infusion. Third, plasma levels of AT III decreased by 17% to 33% during heparin administration by intravenous or subcutaneous routes.[119–124] It is possible that this measurement resulted merely from formation of heparin-AT complexes. Perhaps accelerated elimination of AT III arises from some modification of the protein during or after its interaction with heparin.[123] Also, it has been postulated that

excesses of platelet activity, releases of PF4, could neutralize heparin in these patients. That has yet to be studied, as has a great deal to do with hypercoagulable states in cardiac surgery.[125]

Hemodilution accompanying CPB decreases AT levels to about half of normal levels.[97] There are, however, outlier patients who have profoundly low AT levels. It is possible to see AT III levels as low as 20% of normal, and these levels correspond to levels seen in septic shock and diffuse intravascular coagulation.[15] However, supplemental AT may not prolong the ACT, which means that the heparin available has been bound to sufficient or available AT. The only way that the ACT would be prolonged is if there is excess heparin beyond available AT. Reports of heparin resistance for CPB ascribe its occurrence variously to the use of autotransfusion,[124] previous heparin therapy,[126–129] infection,[130,131] and ventricular aneurysm with thrombus.[128,130] The differential diagnosis also includes hypereosinophilia, oral contraceptive therapy, consumptive coagulopathy, thrombocytosis, and congenital AT deficiency.[128] Heparin resistance also might occur in patients with subclinical thrombotic processes releasing PF4.

The individual anticoagulant response to heparin varies tremendously.[132] Some presumed cases of heparin resistance may represent nothing more than this normal variation. Regardless of cause, measurement of each individual's anticoagulant response to heparin therapy for CPB is warranted.[133] Heparin resistance helps focus the debate regarding whether anticoagulation monitoring should measure heparin concentrations or heparin effect; the goal of anticoagulation is not to achieve heparin presence in plasma but to inhibit the action of thrombin on fibrinogen, platelets, and endothelial cells (see Chapter 17). Therefore, the effect of heparin usually is measured.

Treatment

Most commonly, additional heparin prolongs the ACT sufficiently for the conduct of CPB. Amounts up to 800 U/kg may be necessary to obtain an ACT of 400 to 480 seconds or longer. Although administration of FFP, which contains AT,[134] should correct AT depletion (Figure 31-14) and suitably prolong the ACT,[135] such exposure to transfusion-borne infectious diseases should be avoided whenever possible. Today, the risks of blood transfusion have shifted away from blood-borne viral transmission, with transfusion-related acute lung injury being noted as the greatest mortality-associated event with transfusion. FFP and platelet transfusions carry the greatest risk for transfusion-related acute lung injury.[136,137] Although transfusion-related acute lung injury has not been studied in relation to use of FFP for heparin resistance, it makes great sense to use one of the AT products. This modality is reserved for

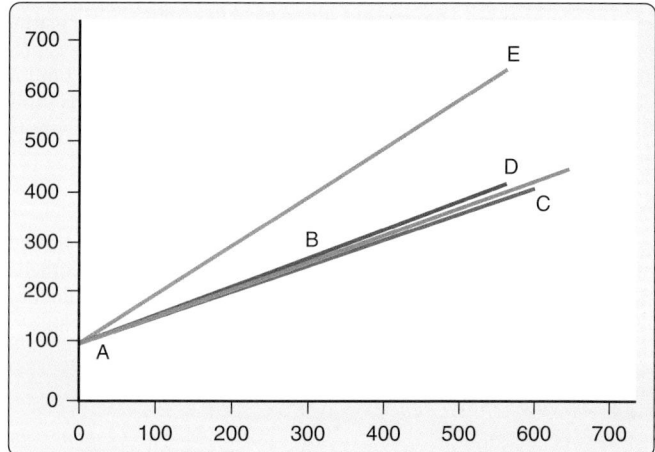

Figure 31-14 Activated coagulation time response in seconds (vertical axis) to heparin administered in units per kilogram (horizontal axis) to a single patient. A, Baseline measurement; (B) after 300 U/kg; (C) after an additional 300 U/kg; (D) soon after C; (E) after 2 units of fresh frozen plasma. *(From Sabbagh AH, Chung GKT, Shuttleworth P, et al: Fresh frozen plasma: A solution to heparin resistance during cardiopulmonary bypass. Ann Thorac Surg 37:466, 1984.)*

the rare refractory case. Rather than administer FFP, centers normally accepting only ACTs of 480 seconds or longer for CPB might consider accepting 400 seconds or less, or administering AT III concentrate.[135,138]

AT concentrate specifically addresses AT deficiency.[15-18,134] Two products are available for utilization. One is a recombinant DNA engineered product made from goat's milk and the other is a purified human plasma harvest derivative. There are currently no head-to-head studies to recommend one over the other at this time. The literature supports success in treating heparin resistance during cardiac surgery.[116,139] A multicenter study on the efficacy of using a recombinant human antithrombin in heparin-resistant patients undergoing CPB was published.[140] The patients received 75 U/kg recombinant human AT, which was effective in restoring heparin responsiveness in most patients. However, some patients still required FFP, and the patients bled more than did a control group after surgery.

Heparin Rebound

Several hours after protamine neutralization for cardiac surgery, some patients experience development of clinical bleeding associated with prolongation of coagulation times. This phenomenon is often attributed to reappearance of circulating heparin. Theories accounting for "heparin rebound" include late release of heparin sequestered in tissues, delayed return of heparin to the circulation from the extracellular space via lymphatics, clearance of an unrecognized endogenous heparin antagonist, and more rapid clearance of protamine in relation to heparin.[141,142] Studies demonstrating uptake of heparin into endothelial cells suggest that these cells may slowly release the drug into the circulation once plasma levels decline with protamine neutralization.[92] It is questionable how much heparin rebound contributes to actual bleeding. This phenomenon may be caused by TFPI release from the surface of endothelial cells or other causes of bleeding.

Incidence and Timing

Although initial reports placed the incidence of heparin rebound after cardiac surgery at about 50%, modifications in the timing and amount of protamine administration decreased the incidence.[143,144] Heparin rebound can occur as soon as 1 hour after protamine neutralization.[127] When present, prolonged coagulation times or more direct evidence of circulating heparin may persist for 6 hours or longer.[97,144-147]

Treatment and Prevention

Although still debated by a few, most clinicians accept heparin rebound as a real phenomenon. However, clinical bleeding does not always accompany heparin rebound. When it does, administration

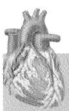
of supplemental protamine will neutralize the remaining heparin (Box 31-3). Can the initial protamine dose be adjusted to prevent heparin rebound? Available studies yield conflicting results. All six patients who received protamine based on the estimated amount of *remaining* heparin developed heparin rebound, compared with none of six who received protamine based on the total administered dose of heparin.[144] However, 42% of patients receiving large, fixed doses of both drugs experienced heparin rebound and increased bleeding compared with patients whose doses were titrated to clotting assays[145] (Figure 31-15). Likewise, patients receiving smaller doses of protamine bled less than those receiving protamine doses based on the total amount of heparin administered.[147] In contrast, a fourth study recommended that the ratio of protamine given to heparin remaining be as much as 1.6 mg/100 units.[97]

It should be noted that in vitro work shows that as little as one-third the heparin dose is all the protamine that is actually required to reverse the heparin in a test tube. It is still difficult to know exactly what the best heparin reversal dose is by protamine. Some effort at titration with a heparin dose–response curve seems worthwhile.

Although larger initial doses of protamine may decrease the likelihood of heparin rebound, two potential complications of protamine overdosage must be considered: adverse cardiovascular sequelae of protamine administration and the anticoagulant effects of protamine itself. Although protamine is an in vitro anticoagulant, doses up to 6 mg/kg in volunteers, in the absence of heparin, do not prolong the clotting time.[148] However, doses four times in excess of a neutralizing dose doubled the ACT in dogs.[149] The dose after CPB that causes anticoagulation in patients remains unknown. Clinical studies comparing fixed-ratio protamine doses with protocols that gauge protamine dose to remaining heparin activity and protamine drug lot potency demonstrated decreased doses of protamine, decreased chest tube drainage after surgery, and fewer transfusions.[150,151]

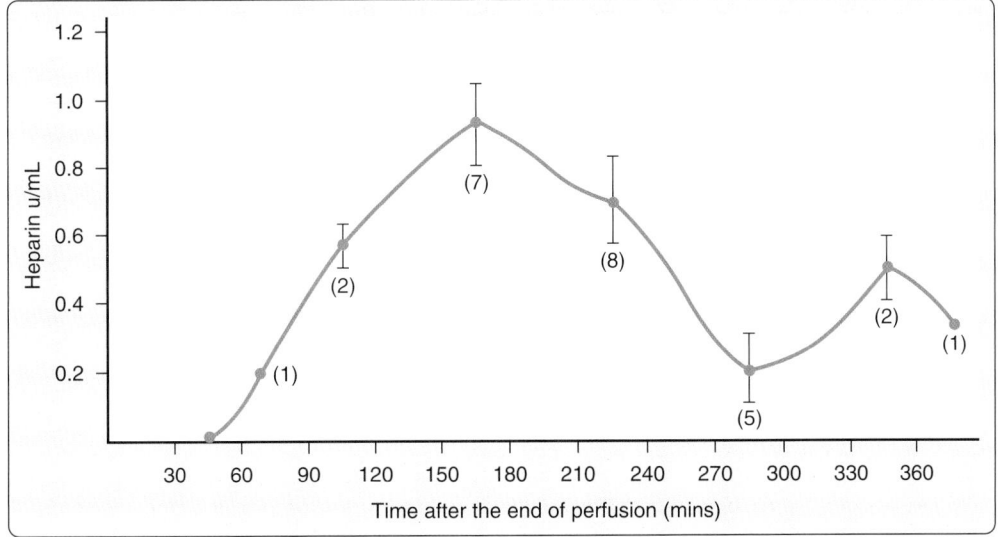

Figure 31-15 Heparin rebound measured by protamine titration in 10 of 24 patients given heparin by a fixed-time protocol. Parentheses denote number of patients. (*From Kaul TK, Crow MJ, Rajah SM, et al: Heparin administration during extracorporeal circulation. J Thorac Cardiovasc Surg 78:95, 1979.*)

Heparin Effects Other Than Anticoagulation

UFH was never biologically intended to circulate freely in plasma.[152,153] As such, it has a number of underappreciated and untoward effects. All too often the effects of CPB have been asserted as causing a coagulopathy; however, the effect of heparin contributing to this has not been widely studied. This is because there has not been an alternative anticoagulant to compare with heparin until now. In the future, there may be better anticoagulants to use during cardiac surgery (see later).

Heparin exerts its anticoagulant activity by activating a binding site on AT III, and without AT, heparin has no intrinsic anticoagulation effect. AT does have anticoagulant effects of its own, but its ability to bind to thrombin is increased 100- to 2000-fold by the presence of the pentasaccharide sequence of heparin. Less than one third of all mucopolysaccharides present in a dose of heparin contain the active pentasaccharide sequence. The other molecules may have a number of adverse properties.

Heparin binds AT III during CPB, and through ongoing thrombin generation, the AT III levels are decreased over time, as well as via hemodilution. Thus, the AT III levels may become quite low, in the range seen during disseminated intravascular coagulopathy, septic shock, and eclampsia.[15,154–156] AT III is not able to be constitutively increased by production. Therefore, the level at the beginning of a CPB case is all that is available. The liver will manufacture more AT III, but it may take 1 to 3 days to return to normal after cessation of CPB. In at least one study in which AT III was repleted to normal, the levels of coagulation proteins were much improved after CPB in patients who received exogenous AT III.[15,134]

UFH chelates calcium.[157] When a large bolus dose of heparin is given, there is a slow and steady decline in blood pressure, probably because of decreased vascular resistance and decreased preload. Both arterial and venous vessels are dilated by the decrease in the calcium level. The heparin is given while patients are being prepared for CPB, and there are numerous mechanical events (i.e., catheters being inserted into the right atrium and vena cava and arrhythmias) that can be blamed for the hypotension, rather than the heparin itself.

Heparin, even in very small doses, partially and reversibly activates platelets and forces them to express many, if not all, of their GP binding sites.[158–160] This fact alone makes clinicians wonder if there is not a better anticoagulant that might not do this. Heparan, the endothelial analog of heparin, does not break off freely into the circulation; and if it does, it is immediately neutralized by platelets through expression of PF4 and adsorption. Thus, it makes sense that platelets seeing loose heparin would suspect a site of tissue injury nearby and, therefore, an evolutionary advantage would be created by making these cells react and get ready to create a thrombus. Every coagulation activation is also an inflammatory signal. The fact that platelets take this reactive step means that they are now primed to either become highly reactive or contribute to the inflammatory events, or have their receptors targeted by other subsequent events. After CPB, platelets have many of their membrane GPs either destroyed or competitively occupied by a number of products of inflammation produced during CPB. The expression of binding sites in response to heparin, therefore, is important and probably has profound implications.

Heparin causes the competitive release of some heparan from endothelial cells and the release of TFPI.[25,26] Endothelial cells all over the body change from being anticoagulant producing to rapidly producing tissue factor. What role large doses of heparin have in this whole-body event is hard to define, but it is known that heparin also causes the release of single-chain urokinase from endothelial cells.[161] The amount of fibrinolysis caused by heparin infusion is not as great as the release of t-PA, which probably is mediated by cytokines as a result of the inflammatory reactions. When released from mast cells, heparin promotes leukocyte chemotaxis and movement through the interstitium.[152,153] However, it is unclear whether heparin upregulates or decreases white cell activations.[153]

Heparin is important for a number of angiogenesis and repair activities of tissue,[153] and these effects may have something to do with its antineoplastic effect.[153] Heparin also affects lipid, sodium and potassium, and acid-base metabolism. These effects are not usually seen acutely but come into play when patients have been on heparin infusions for days in the ICU.

The immunologic effects of heparin are profound. The next section discusses HIT, but recent work shows that 30% to 50% of cardiac surgery patients have heparin antibodies present in their blood by the time of hospital discharge.[162] The clinical implications of these prevalent antibodies remain unknown and are the subject of investigation.

Heparin-Induced Thrombocytopenia

Heparin normally binds to platelet membranes at GPIb and other sites, and aggregates normal platelets by releasing ADP.[162,163] A moderate, reversible HIT, now termed type I, has been known for half a century.[164] The fact that heparin actually triggers an acute decline in platelet count should be considered a biologic event, because heparin, even in trace amounts, triggers the expression of many different platelet GPs. This has been termed "activation of platelets," but it is not total activation. Heparin's prolongation of the bleeding time probably is related to activation of the platelets, as well as heparin binding to the GPIb surface. It may be that a number of platelets adhere to endothelial cells simply because of their expression of these GP binding sites. Margination, particularly within the pulmonary vasculature, may be an event of HIT type I.

In contrast with these predictable effects of heparin, occasional patients experience development of progressive and severe thrombocytopenia (< 100,000/mm³), sometimes accompanied by a debilitating or fatal thrombosis. This syndrome is termed type II heparin-induced thrombocytopenia (HIT II). A platelet count in excess of 100,000/mm³ does not mean that HIT II is not present. A decline in platelet count in excess of 30% to 50% over several days in a patient who is receiving or who has just finished receiving heparin is probably caused by HIT II.

Mechanism

These patients with HITT demonstrate a heparin-dependent antibody, usually IgG, although others are described, which aggregates platelets in the presence of heparin.[161,162] During heparin therapy, measured antibody titers remain low because of antibody binding to platelets. Titers rise after heparin therapy ceases; but paradoxically, antibody may be undetectable a few months later.[165] Two other features are unexpected: First, the antibody does not aggregate platelets in the presence of excess heparin; and second, not all re-exposed patients experience development of thrombocytopenia.[166–168]

The platelet surface contains complexes of heparin and PF4. Affected patients have an antibody to this complex. Antibody binding activates platelets via their FcγII receptors and activates endothelium[169–171] (Figure 31-16). The activation of the platelet surface triggers a secondary thrombin release. Platelets can attach to each other creating what is known as a white-clot syndrome; but if secondary thrombin generation is created through antibody activation of the platelets, then a fibrin clot can be the result. In the absence of heparin, the heparin-PF4 antigen cannot form. However, there seems to be some sort of continuum between idiopathic thrombocytopenia and HIT.

In the absence of an endothelial defect, the only responses to the antibody-antigen interaction are platelet consumption and thrombocytopenia. Atheroma rupture, endovascular interventions such as balloon angioplasty, vascular surgery, and other procedures that disrupt endothelium can provide a nidus for platelet adhesion and subsequent activation. PF4, released with platelet activation, binds to heparin locally, thus not only removing the inhibition of coagulation but also generating additional antigenic material (Figure 31-17). Clumps of

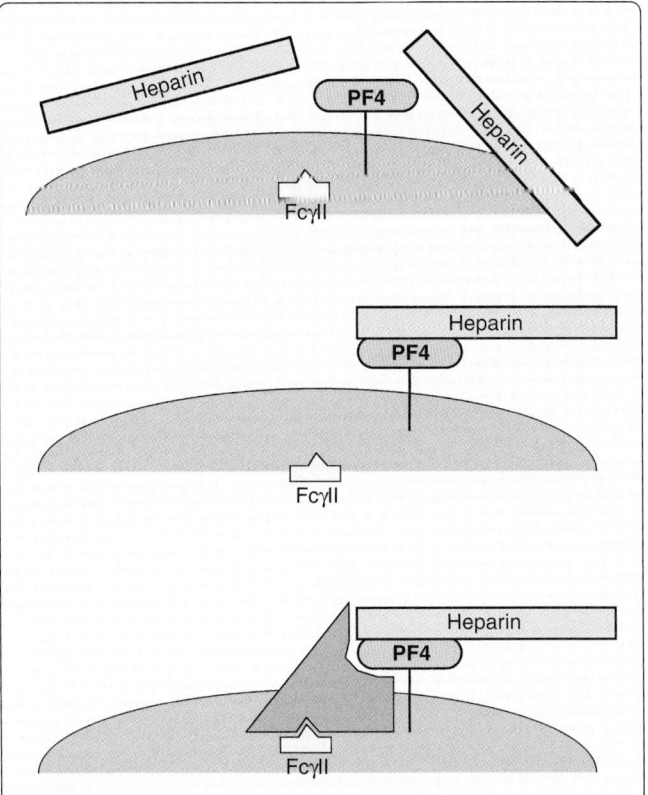

Figure 31-16 **Presumed mechanism of the interaction among heparin, platelets, and antibody in heparin-induced thrombocytopenia.** *Top,* Platelet factor 4 (PF4) released from platelet granules is bound to the platelet surface. *Middle,* Heparin and PF4 complexes form. *Bottom,* The antibody binds to the PF4-heparin complex and activates platelet FcγII receptors.

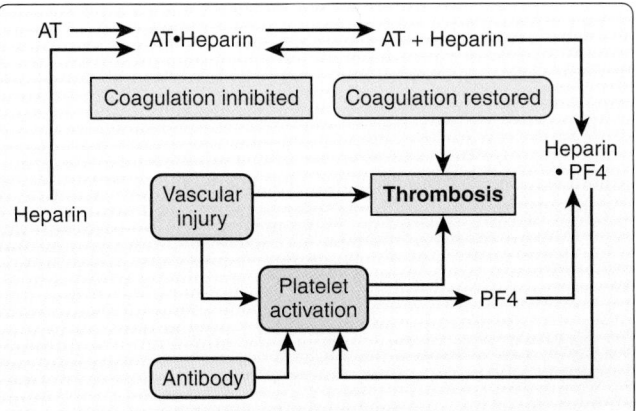

Figure 31-17 **Mechanism of thrombosis accompanying heparin-induced thrombocytopenia.** Normally, heparin and antithrombin (AT) form a complex that inhibits coagulation. Platelet factor 4 (PF4), released from platelets on activation, binds heparin and drives the dissociation reaction of the AT-heparin complex to the right, restoring coagulation locally. Restored coagulation mechanisms and activated platelets form thrombus in the presence of vascular injury. *(Adapted from Parmet JL, Horrow JC: Hematologic diseases. In Benumof J [ed]: Anesthesia and Uncommon Diseases, 3rd ed. Philadelphia: WB Saunders Company, 1997.)*

aggregated platelets thrombose vessels, resulting in organ and limb infarction. Amputation, death, or both often occur with established HIT with thrombosis (HITT). The presence of heparin-PF4 antibodies recently has been associated with other adverse effects. It appears that if a patient undergoes cardiac surgery with positive antibodies, the risk for mortality or myocardial infarction, or both, may at least double.

Incidence and Diagnosis

Estimates of the true incidence of HIT are confounded by different diagnostic thresholds for platelet count, varying efforts to detect other causes, and incomplete reports.[172,173] After 7 days of therapy with UFH, probably 1% of patients experience development of HIT; after 14 days of therapy, the prevalence rate is 3%.[171] Using a platelet count of 100,000/mm³, multiple reports comprising more than 1200 patients revealed an overall incidence rate of HIT of 5.5% with bovine heparin and 1.0% with porcine heparin.[161] Other recent research has found the preoperative incidence rate of enzyme-linked immunosorbent assay (ELISA)–positive patients to be between 6.5% to 10%. This means that antibodies are present, and that may not mean that thrombocytopenia is occurring. Of great interest is that many more patients develop positive tests for ELISA antibodies by days 7 to 30 after cardiac surgery. Somewhere between 25% and 50% of patients develop these antibodies.[162] In a study of patients after cardiac surgery wherein all patients were screened for HIT antibodies, the group also looked for platelet counts well less than the patient's baseline[174]; 21 of 153 patients (14%) tested positive for antibodies by heparin induced platelet activation (HIPA) testing. Those patients with a low platelet count and a high HIT antibody titer after surgery were at very high risk for mortality (59%). Therefore, a decline in platelet count or persistence of a low platelet count after cardiac surgery should be considered HIT until proved otherwise and taken very seriously. Anticoagulation with alternative nontriggering anticoagulants is imperative.[174] Warfarin should be avoided until such time as the platelet count is recovered and vitamin K therapy can be instituted; this is because the use of warfarin compounds will decrease protein C, which has been known to trigger an HITT crisis.

In the bivalirudin trials, wherein patients thought to have HIT were given an alternative anticoagulant, the presence of antibodies after surgery was associated with adverse events. Particularly worrisome were the presence of a low platelet count or a blunted return toward a normal platelet count after surgery.[175–177]

Some particular lots of heparin may be more likely to cause HIT than others.[178] HIT can occur not only during therapeutic heparin administration but with low prophylactic doses, although the incidence is dose related. Even heparin flush solution or heparin-bonded intravascular catheters can incite HIT.[179–182] Cases of platelet-to-platelet adhesion creating a "white clot" in otherwise normal patients have been observed in the oxygenator and the reservoir of CPB machines. The fact that such events have been reported even when all other tests appeared normal signals the unpredictable nature of the heparin-PF4 antibody, as well as the biologic activity of UFH.

Although HIT usually begins 3 to 15 days (median, 10 days) after heparin infusions commence, it can occur within hours in a patient previously exposed to heparin. Platelet count steadily decreases to a nadir between 20,000 and 150,000/mm³. Absolute thrombocytopenia is not necessary; only a significant decrease in platelet count matters, as witnessed by patients with thrombocytosis who experience development of thrombosis with normal platelet counts after prolonged exposure to heparin. Occasionally, thrombocytopenia resolves spontaneously despite continuation of heparin infusion.[183]

Clinical diagnosis of HIT requires a new decrease in platelet count during heparin infusion. Laboratory confirmation is obtained from several available tests. In the serotonin release assay, patient plasma, donor platelets, and heparin are combined. The donor platelets contain radiolabeled serotonin, which is released when donor platelets are activated by the antigen-antibody complex. Measurement of serotonin release during platelet aggregation at both low and high heparin concentrations provides excellent sensitivity and specificity.[166]

A second assay measures more traditional markers of platelet degranulation in a mixture of heparin, patient plasma, and donor platelets.[184] The most specific test is an ELISA for antibodies to the heparin-PF4 complex.[160,161,185,186]

The type, source, and lot of heparin used affect the outcome of these tests. The heterogenous nature of heparin demands that a lot-specific drug be used in serotonin release assays, especially when used to determine suitability of future administration. For example, if LMWH administration is planned for a patient who experienced development of HIT II with UFH, testing of patient plasma with the lot of LMWH to be given should precede its administration.

Measurement of platelet-associated IgG is poorly specific for HIT because of numerous other causes of antiplatelet IgG. This test should not be used in the diagnosis of HIT.

Heparin-Induced Thrombocytopenia with Thrombosis

The incidence rate of HITT is 1.7% with bovine heparin and 0.3% with porcine heparin; thus, thrombosis accompanies more than one in five cases of HIT.[161,162] It is clear that the longer patients are on heparin, the more likely it is that they will develop antibody; and with the knowledge that today close to 50% of cardiac patients develop antibodies, it is possible that a significant number of long-term or early mortalities might be because of undiagnosed HITT.[162] In several studies in the catheterization laboratory, it has been shown that if HITT antibodies are present before the performance of angioplasty, the mortality and combined morbidity are greatly increased, perhaps double or more.[187,188] One study has been conducted in almost 500 patients undergoing CABG surgery looking for the presence of antibodies and outcome. The incidence rate of antibody-positive patients was approximately 15%, and their length of stay in the hospital and mortality were more than doubled. Occasional rare situations in which the CPB circuit suddenly clots or when there is early graft thrombosis or whole-body clotting may all be variants of HITT, but none of these cases can be readily studied because they are so rare.[187] If such an occurrence does happen, HITT should be in the differential diagnosis. The occurrence of thrombosis at first seems paradoxic. However, HITT has as its hallmark a huge thrombin burst that can occur all over the body. With such massive thrombin generation, the triggering of thrombosis is natural. Thrombosis may then activate the fibrinolytic system to produce a picture of consumptive coagulopathy.[179]

From 15% to 30% of patients who experience development of HITT will have severe neurologic complications, require amputation of a limb, or die. Lower limb ischemia constitutes the most frequent presentation. Venous clots occur probably as frequently as arterial ones but are not detected as often. Unfortunately, no test predicts the thrombosis component of HIT; thrombosis should be anticipated in the presence of vascular injury, such as puncture sites for catheterization.

Warkentin and others[189] have stressed the use of the 4Ts system (Thrombocytopenia, Timing, Thrombosis, and oTher [lack of other reasons]) to increase the index of suspicion with regard to HIT. The use of this scoring system is quite effective, but after cardiac surgery, the decline in platelet count is expected for at least 24 hours. If platelet count stays down after that time, then a high index of suspicion should be for HIT. A study of critically ill patients (noncardiac) using the 4Ts showed an incidence rate of 4.1% for HIT. Low scoring appears to be reliable, whereas high and intermediate scoring showed patients with antibody-positive tests.

Treatment and Prevention

In the absence of surgery, bleeding from thrombocytopenia with HIT is rare. In contrast with other drug-induced thrombocytopenia, in which severe thrombocytopenia commonly occurs, more moderate platelet count nadirs characterize HIT. Platelet transfusions are not indicated and may incite or worsen thrombosis. Heparin infusions must be discontinued, and an alternative anticoagulant should be instituted. LMWHs can be tested in the laboratory using serotonin release before patient administration. Although thrombosis may be treated with fibrinolytic therapy,[190] surgery often is indicated. No heparin should be given for vascular surgery. Monitoring catheters should be purged of heparin flush, and heparin-bonded catheters should not be placed. Antiplatelet agents, such as aspirin, ticlopidine, or dipyridamole, which block adhesion and activation and, thus, PF4 release, provide ancillary help (see Table 31-4).

The patient presenting for cardiac surgery who has sustained HIT in the past presents a therapeutic dilemma. Antibodies may have regressed; if so, a negative serotonin release assay using the heparin planned for surgery will predict that transient exposure during surgery will be harmless. However, no heparin should be given at catheterization or in flush solutions after surgery.[162,163]

Patients with HIT who require urgent surgery may receive heparin once platelet activation has been blocked with aspirin and dipyridamole[156–193] or, in the past, the prostacyclin analog iloprost.[194–197] Unfortunately, iloprost is no longer available. The problem with this strategy is obtaining sufficient blockade of platelet activity. In the future, there may be ultra-short-acting platelet surface blocking agents available, and these would then seem perfect to create "platelet anesthesia."

Another alternative, delaying surgery to wait for antibodies to regress, may fail because of the variable offset of antibody presence and the unpredictable nature of platelet response to heparin rechallenge. Plasmapheresis may successfully eliminate antibodies and allow benign heparin administration.[198] Finally, methods of instituting anticoagulation without heparin may be chosen (see later). Of these, the alternative thrombin antagonists pose the greatest risk for uncontrolled bleeding, whereas LMWHs and heparinoids afford the greatest chance of success.[199,200]

LMWH heparin, as an alternative to UFH, has been used for urgent surgery.[201–203] Although LMWHs also can induce thrombocytopenia,[204–206] by displaying different antigenic determinants, they may prove acceptable alternatives for patients who experience development of HIT from UFH. Table 31-6 summarizes the therapeutic options available for urgent cardiac surgery in patients with HIT. For additional information on HIT, see reviews by Warkentin and Greinacher,[162] Godal,[163] and Chong.[207]

New Modes of Anticoagulation

The hemostatic goal during CPB is complete inhibition of the coagulation system. Unfortunately, even large doses of heparin do not provide this, as evidenced by formation of fibrinopeptides during surgery.[107–109] Despite being far from the ideal anticoagulant, heparin still performs better than its alternatives. Heparans, dermatans, and other glycosaminoglycans with minimal antihemostatic properties may replace heparin in the future. Current substitutes for heparin include ancrod, a proteinase obtained from snake venom that destroys fibrinogen; heparin

TABLE 31-6	Therapeutic Options for Anticoagulation for Bypass in Patients with Heparin-Induced Thrombocytopenia

1. Ancrod
2. Low-molecular-weight heparin or heparinoid (test first!)
3. Alternative thrombin inhibitor (hirudin, bivalirudin, argatroban)
4. Use a single dose of heparin, promptly neutralize with protamine, *and*
   a. Delay surgery so antibodies can regress; *or*
   b. Use plasmapheresis to decrease antibody levels; *or*
   c. Inhibit platelets with iloprost, aspirin and Persantine, abciximab, or RGD blockers

In all cases:
1. No heparin in flush solutions
2. No heparin-bonded catheters
3. No heparin lock intravenous ports

No agent is currently indicated for anticoagulation in cardiopulmonary bypass.
RGD, receptor glycoprotein derived.

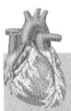

BOX 31-4. POTENTIAL REPLACEMENTS AS AN ANTICOAGULANT FOR CARDIOPULMONARY BYPASS

- Ancrod
- Low-molecular-weight heparins
- Factor Xa inhibitors
- Bivalirudin or other direct thrombin inhibitors (hirudin, argatroban)
- Platelet receptor inhibitors

fragments, which provide less thrombin inhibition than the parent, unfractionated molecule; direct factor Xa inhibitors; and direct thrombin inhibitors (Box 31-4).

Ancrod

Ancrod abnormally cleaves fibrinogen, resulting in its rapid clearance by the reticuloendothelial system. Thrombin, thus, has no substrate on which to act. Proper patient preparation for CPB (plasma fibrinogen, 0.4 to 0.8 g/L) requires more than 12 hours. Figure 31-18 demonstrates the extent of fibrinogen depletion (from normal value of 1.5 to 4.5 g/L) and repletion for cardiac surgery using ancrod.[208] Replenishment of fibrinogen via hepatic synthesis is slow; cryoprecipitate or FFP administration, or both, will speed restoration of coagulation. Patients anticoagulated in this fashion bleed more and require more cryoprecipitate and FFP compared with heparin-anticoagulated patients.[208] One case was done with ancrod in which the coagulation activation was carefully studied.[209] Unbridled thrombin production led to massive platelet activation with a secondary precipitous decline in platelet count. No clot formed, but a gray slime of platelets adhered to the wall of the oxygenator and the reservoir. The platelet count declined to less

than 1000/mm³. However, transfusion with platelet concentrates and cryoprecipitate reestablished normal coagulation, and the patient had less than 500 mL of blood loss for the first 24 hours. No neurologic deficits occurred. However, ancrod is not commercially available in the United States.[209]

Low-Molecular-Weight Heparins

Figure 31-19 displays the effect of polysaccharide chain length on the inhibition of thrombin and factor Xa. Note that thrombin inhibition requires chains longer than 18 saccharide units and aPTT activity follows anti–factor IIa activity more closely than it does anti–factor Xa activity.[103] Thrombin must bind to a portion of the heparin chain for AT to inhibit it. In contrast, factor Xa inhibition by AT does not require interaction of factor Xa with the heparin molecule. Only about 1% to 2% of standard heparin consists of low-molecular-weight (molecular weight, 6000 to 7000) fragments.[93] Short polysaccharide chains of heparin can be synthesized, or extracted from standard heparin, but both processes cost much more than depolymerization of standard heparin utilizing nitric acid, peroxides, or the enzyme heparinase. Preparations of LMWH formed by these methods include Fraxiparine, dalteparin, and enoxaparin.

Standard heparin can inhibit thrombus formation in vivo (antithrombotic activity) and prolong in vitro clotting tests (anticoagulant activity). It also leads to clinical bleeding (antihemostatic activity). Table 31-7 highlights these definitions. LMWHs may dissociate these activities, displaying greater antithrombotic activity and less antihemostatic activity.[93] Unfortunately, coagulation tests sensitive to thrombin inhibition and insensitive to inhibition of factor Xa, namely, the aPTT and ACT (see Figure 31-19), do not adequately monitor the antithrombotic effects of LMWHs. For additional information regarding LMWHs, there are several good reviews.[210–212]

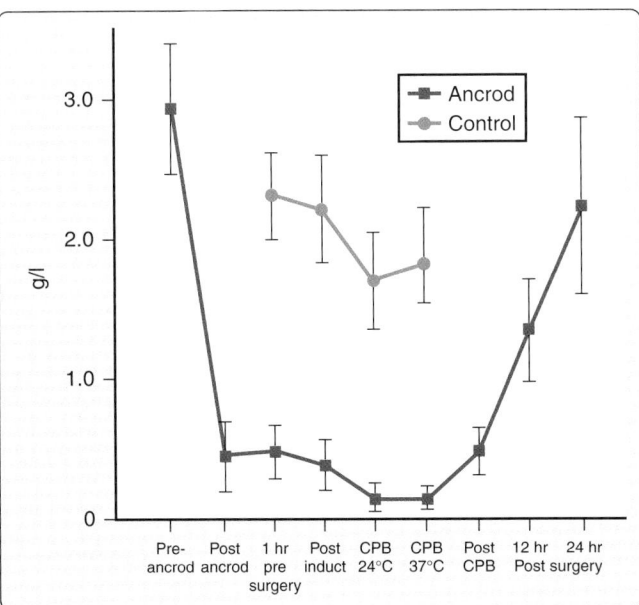

Figure 31-18 Plasma fibrinogen concentrations (normal, 1.5 to 4.5 g/L) in 20 patients who received snake venom (Ancrod; *squares*) and 20 patients who received heparin (control; *circles*) for anticoagulation during cardiopulmonary bypass (CPB). Note the slow return of plasma fibrinogen, despite administration of 9.3 ± 16.3 SD units of cryoprecipitate and 5.6 ± 3.1 units of fresh frozen plasma to the Ancrod group. (*From Zulys VJ, Teasdale SJ, Michel ER, et al: Ancrod [Arvin] as an alternative to heparin anticoagulation for cardiopulmonary bypass. Anesthesiology 71:870, 1989.*)

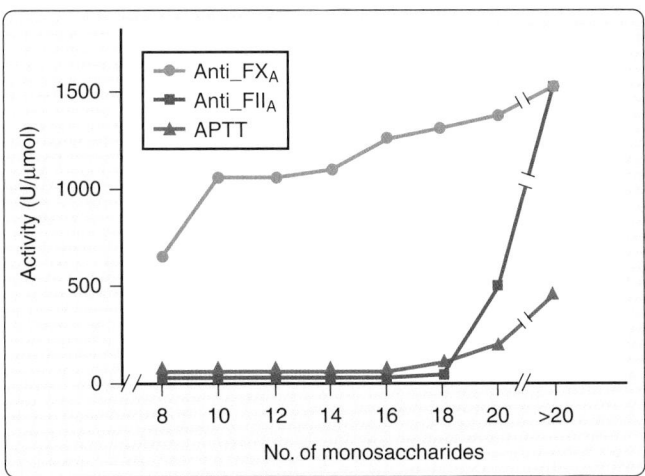

Figure 31-19 Heparin activity as a function of chain length. Oligosaccharides containing 8 to 16 units exhibit strong anti–factor Xa (FX_A) activity, whereas anti–factor IIa (FII_A) activity requires 20 or more units. Note that prolongation of the activated partial thromboplastin time (APTT) tracks anti–factor IIa activity. (*From Holmer E, Soderberg K, Bergqvist D, Lindahl U: Heparin and its low-molecular-weight derivatives. Anticoagulant and antithrombotic properties. Haemostasis 16[Suppl 2]:1, 1986.*)

TABLE 31-7	Properties of Unfractionated Heparin
1. Anti*thrombotic**—prevents thrombus formation in vivo	
2. Anti*coagulant**—prolongs clotting time in vitro	
3. Anti*hemostatic*—promotes bleeding	
4. Anti*platelet*—activates platelets	

*Properties of an ideal agent.

LMWHs have undergone clinical trials for antithrombosis after orthopedic procedures and for prevention of deep vein thrombosis.[213-215] The traditional LMWHs, such as enoxaparin, have not been used for CPB cases because of a limited ability of protamine to neutralize them.[216,217]

Heparinoids

Danaparoid (Orgaran), a mixture of LMWHs and dermatans, can provide anticoagulation for CPB, but lack of readily available monitoring and sure neutralization limit its application to cases in which UFH clearly is contraindicated.[217,218] Dermatans alone might prove suitable, but much more investigative work must first occur.[7,218] Case reports of these agents have shown severe bleeding and, in some cases, death from hemorrhage after cardiac surgery. It appears at this point that dermatan sulfate will not be used for cardiac surgery, and danaparoid was removed from the U.S. market.

Fondaparinux (Arixtra) is a synthetic pentasaccharide identical to that in heparin. It is a primary factor Xa inhibitor that requires AT III, which does not affect thrombin, platelets, or fibrinolytic activity. It is being used for prophylaxis of deep vein thrombosis after surgery, but it does not alter routine coagulation tests (requires a factor Xa assay).[219] Since 2008, there have been some reports of patients with HIT not responding successfully to therapy with fondaparinux.[220,221] Supratherapeutic dosages for fondaparinux were required to inhibit binding of antibodies to platelets. Danaparoid in very low concentrations increased PF4 antibodies; however, in therapeutic concentrations, it decreased production of antibodies.[221] There is no direct antidote for either of these agents, but patients may respond to factor VIIa (see later).

Direct Thrombin Inhibitors

Hirudin, a single-chain polypeptide containing 65 amino acids with a molecular weight of 7000 and produced by the medicinal leech *Hirudo medicinalis*, binds directly to thrombin without need of a cofactor or enzyme, inhibiting all the proteolytic functions of thrombin. This inhibition includes actions on fibrinogen; factors V, VIII, and XIII; and platelets.

Modifications of hirudin include hirugen, a synthetic peptide containing residues 53 to 64 of the native hirudin, and Hirulog, formed by attaching the amino acid sequence d-phe-pro-arg-pro-(gly) to the amino-terminal end of hirugen. Hirugen inhibits the action of thrombin on fibrinogen, but not on factor V. Hirulog has full inhibitory properties but is slowly cleaved by thrombin itself to a hirugen-like molecule.

Hirudin depends on renal excretion; renal failure prolongs its elimination half-life of 0.6 to 2.0 hours. Although there are no known direct neutralizing agents for these drugs, administration of prothrombin complex may partially restore coagulation by enhancing thrombin generation. Clinical trials of hirudin compounds have yielded mixed results. It has been used for patients with HITT, but the longer half-life of approximately 90 minutes means that many of these patients bleed after cardiac surgery.[222] Hirudin is highly antigenic and will lead to immune complexes being created to itself in about 40% of patients. If it is used a second time, the overall incidence rate of anaphylaxis may be as high as 10% of all patients who have received it before.[222] Currently, it is not recommended to turn to hirudin as a primary agent to perform CPB even if a patient has HIT antibodies.

New direct thrombin inhibitors are now available (Figure 31-20). These include argatroban and bivalirudin. Argatroban is a derivative of L-arginine, is a relatively small molecule, and functions as a univalent direct thrombin inhibitor.[223,224] It binds at the active cleavage site of thrombin and stops thrombin's action on serine proteases. It is completely hepatically cleared and has a reported half-life of 45 to 55 minutes with prolongation when liver function is depressed or liver blood flow is decreased. One case report examined argatroban's half-life after CPB. It was found to be prolonged to 514 minutes in a patient undergoing heart transplantation.[225] This led to the use of massive transfusion

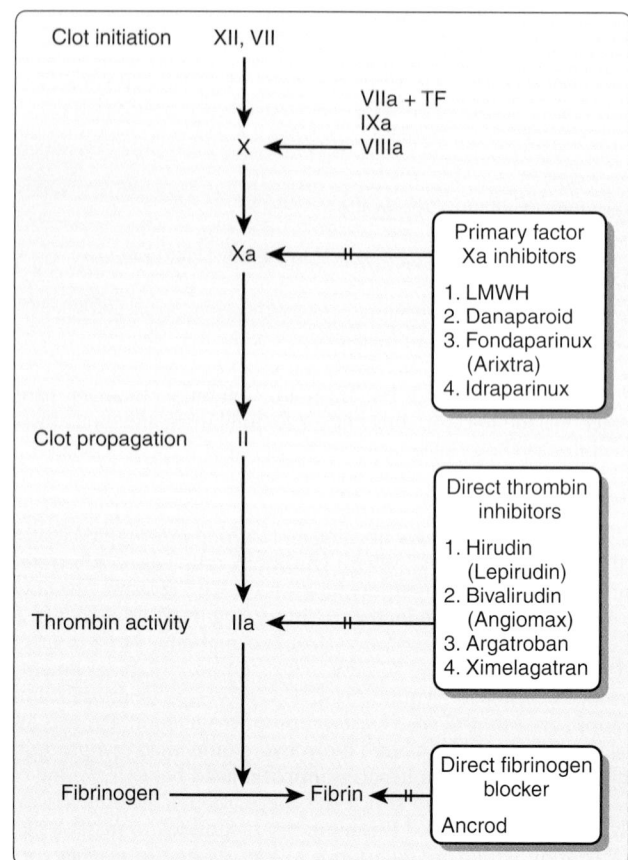

Figure 31-20   Alternatives to heparin. New modes of anticoagulation are shown in the boxes on the right side of the figure where they inhibit either factor Xa, thrombin, or fibrinogen. LMWH, low-molecular-weight heparin.

(55 units of RBCs, 42 units of FFP, 40 units of cryoprecipitate, 40 units of platelets, as well as 3 doses of factor VIIa).

There is no reversal agent for argatroban, although factor VIIa has been given to increase thrombin generation. It has been U.S. Food and Drug Administration (FDA)–approved for anticoagulation in the face of HITT, but there has not been, to date, a large-scale, prospective, randomized trial for cardiac surgery or any type of comparison with heparin/protamine. Some case reports do exist of successful usage of argatroban in patients with HITT both on- and off-pump with acceptable amounts of postoperative bleeding.[226-230] The dosing for off-pump cases has been reported to be about 2 to 3 μg/kg/min, with a goal of an ACT longer than 200 seconds. For on-pump cases, the dose is at least doubled (5 to 10 μg/kg/min), with an effort to achieve an ACT of 300 to 400 seconds.[229] There is no safe and effective dose that has been clinically studied, so any use of this drug for cardiac surgery is off-label and based on experience, as well as case reports. Successful case completions have been noted without undue excess bleeding. However, as noted earlier in the transplant case, some very large bleeds have been encountered. Some cases of thrombosis also have occurred.[231-236] It has been more commonly used in the ICU for patients with hypercoagulable syndromes and HITT.[237,238] Argatroban is a viable direct thrombin inhibitor for use in the cardiac catheterization laboratory. It is far more likely that anesthesiologists will encounter the drug either in the ICU being used for patients with HIT or in patients who have come from the catheterization laboratory directly to the operating rooms.

Bivalirudin is a bivalent synthetic 20-amino acid peptide based on the structure of hirudin (previously called *Hirulog*).[239-248] Pharmacologists have taken the active amino acids at either end of the hirudin molecule and biosynthesized them. One active site competitively binds to the fibrinogen-binding site of thrombin; and the other end of the molecule, the amino-terminal sequence, binds to the active serine cleavage site of thrombin. The two sequences of amino acids are connected together by a tetraglycine spacer. This fully manufactured molecule is highly specific for thrombin and has the unique property that it binds to both clot-bound and free thrombin. Heparin binds only to free plasma thrombin. Bivalirudin has a shorter half-life than argatroban and hirudin; the $t_{1/2}$ is approximately 20 to 25 minutes (with normal renal function and not on CPB). One of the most unique features of bivalirudin is that its binding to thrombin is reversible and the molecule itself is cleaved by thrombin.

Like the other direct thrombin inhibitors, it also has no reversal agent analogous to protamine; so when it is used, it must wear off. Bivalirudin undergoes destruction by the molecule to which it binds and deactivates, thrombin; it is destroyed by thrombin (proteolytic cleavage). The more thrombin activation that is present (i.e., the less bivalirudin that is present), the shorter is the half-life. Only about 20% of the molecular activity is eliminated by renal clearance.[240] In mild-to-moderate renal failure, the effect on bivalirudin clearance is thought to be small, but bleeding in patients with renal failure has been noted.

Several clinical trials of bivalirudin for cardiology procedures or cardiac surgery have been completed and published.[240–248] Two pivotal trials aiming for FDA approval of bivalirudin for cardiac surgery with known/suspected HIT were conducted several years ago.[175,176] In trials comparing bivalirudin with either heparin/protamine alone or heparin plus the use of a GP IIb/IIIa inhibitor for percutaneous interventions, bivalirudin was found to have at least equal or better safety and less bleeding than either of the other therapies. When compared with heparin/protamine alone in percutaneous coronary intervention, bivalirudin was found to be superior, not just in bleeding, but also in terms of morbidity and mortality (as a combined end point).[247] In a trial of 100 off-pump routine CABG patients without suspected HIT, patients were randomized to receive either bivalirudin or heparin/protamine, and bleeding and outcome were equal between the groups.[240] These patients underwent recatheterization at 3 months, and it was found that the bivalirudin patients had overall better flow down their grafts than did the patients who had received heparin/protamine. That finding is consistent with the work noted in the HIT section earlier wherein the presence of antibodies bodes poorly for postoperative complications. It also suggests that heparin-protamine in the face of ischemia and reperfusion may lead to adverse thrombotic outcomes with or without heparin-PF4 antibodies. This trial, in conjunction with subsequent trials, raises questions with regard to heparin-protamine and suggests that for off-pump CABG, a more routine usage of bivalirudin might produce improved outcomes.

A phase I/II safety trial of bivalirudin in 30 on-pump CABG patients has also shown good safety, but no comparison was conducted to look at advantages against heparin/protamine. When used, the doses for CPB have been a 0.50- to 0.75-mg/kg bolus followed by an infusion at 1.75 to 2.5 mg/kg/hr titrated to the ACT (target, 2.5 times baseline). The CPB system also was primed with 50 mg, and no stasis can be allowed in the CPB circuit because of metabolism of bivalirudin during CPB. The infusion is stopped about 15 to 30 minutes before CPB is discontinued, and patients bleed for up to 4 to 6 hours. OPCAB cases have used similar doses to ACT targets of 350 to 450 seconds.[240] There certainly are some tricks to using bivalirudin for cardiac cases. The drug itself is broken down by thrombin, and thrombin is produced by CPB, as well as through tissue destruction. Any blood left alone without a continuous infusion of bivalirudin will, because of its generation of thrombin, overcome the anticoagulation of bivalirudin in time. Therefore, it is expected that stagnant blood in the mediastinal or the chest cavities, or both, will clot. This is alarming to the first-time user of bivalirudin and completely different from what is seen in cases with heparin anticoagulation. Also, the use of mediastinal suction during bypass is not recommended because the mediastinum is a source of a great deal of thrombin activity. Suctioning that back into the CPB reservoir has led to clots being present in a hard-shell reservoir wherein there is stasis or incomplete mixing of bivalirudin. Once the patient is separated from CPB, it is important to make a decision regarding whether the patient is likely to need to return to bypass. The bypass

system, if left stagnant, will have ongoing production of thrombin. Over time, that thrombin will overcome the bivalirudin present in the plasma. Therefore, within 10 minutes of separation from CPB, it is wise to decide to either drain the blood from the pump, process it through a cell-saver machine, or reestablish flow and have a slow infusion of bivalirudin into the pump. The reestablishment of flow can be easily accomplished by reattaching the ends of the venous and arterial cannulae. If it is necessary to reestablish CPB, the system should be maintained warm and either a bolus (25 to 50 mg) of bivalirudin should be put into the pump or the infusion that had been running to the patient should be switched to the pump.[241] Furthermore, some surgeons have suggested that in areas of stasis, such as in an internal mammary artery, it is important to flush the artery every 10 to 15 minutes to allow for new bivalirudin to be perfused, or clot could build up in the "dead end" if it is clamped. The other option is to not completely clamp off the internal mammary artery until just before it is to be anastomosed.

There has been some confusion regarding how best to monitor anticoagulation with bivalirudin for cardiac surgery. Originally, Koster et al [222] utilized the ecarin clotting time (ECT) to follow circulating levels of bivalirudin. The ECT has a straight-line dose-response relation in the critical range between 300 and 550 seconds. The ACT has a less specific and more variable relation. With circulating bivalirudin concentrations of 10 to 15 μg/mL, the ECT will be 400 to 450 seconds. It is known that clot will not be able to be generated with a bivalirudin concentration greater than 3 to 5 μg/mL, so a level of 10 to 12 will be well greater than a therapeutic threshold to ensure that fibrin formation does not occur on bypass. The dose-responsiveness of bivalirudin is highly predictable. There is no secondary reaction necessary such as with AT III and UFH. Therefore, when bivalirudin is given, there is an absolute amount of AT available. Debates among researchers have gone forward as to whether ACT or ECT monitoring is even necessary at all. The consensus is that ACT will work (the ECT is no longer commercially available). The other reason for using an ACT is that during CPB, if a drug pump malfunctions or the infusion is somehow disconnected, it is important to know that earlier rather than later. If the ACT begins to elevate to more than 500 seconds, then the team really does not know whether to back off on the bivalirudin infusion, stop it altogether, or attribute the effect to some other ACT-prolonging situation such as hemodilution or hypothermia. It is known that hypothermia retards the production of thrombin, but no studies have been done of bivalirudin half-lives in the face of mild-to-moderate hypothermia.

The two trials of bivalirudin in the face of known or suspected HIT antibodies did show effectiveness and safety.[176,177] The CABG Hit On and Off-pump Safety and Efficacy (CHOOSE) and Evaluation of patients during coronary artery bypass Operation: Linking UTilization of bivalirudin to Improved Outcomes and New anticoagulant strategies (EVOLUTION) trials were performed as parts of a program to get bivalirudin approved for patients undergoing cardiac surgery with known or suspected HIT. EVOLUTION (ON and OFF) trials randomized patients to receive either heparin-protamine or bivalirudin as the primary anticoagulant regimen for either on- or off-pump CABG surgery. In EVOLUTION-OFF, 157 patients were scheduled for OPCAB at 21 centers. The dosing of bivalirudin was 0.75 mg/kg as a bolus and 1.75 mg/kg/hr while the grafts were being prepared and anastomosed. Heparin was dosed to reach an ACT target of 300 seconds and reversed with protamine. There were no differences in death, myocardial infarction, or need for repeat revascularization. However, there was a significant reduction in strokes seen with the use of bivalirudin. Bleeding was about the same with both groups. In the EVOLUTION-On trial, 150 patients underwent a number of cardiac procedures at the 21 sites. There were, again, no major differences in procedural success (death, MI, need for redo) in the heparin versus bivalirudin groups. There was a statistically, but clinically insignificant, difference (78 mL) in blood loss at 2 hours and not at 24 hours with bivalirudin.

The CHOOSE trials undertook to use bivalirudin in patients with known or suspected HIT. In the CHOOSE-On trial, 50 patients were enrolled. Immediate success of surgery was achieved in 94% of patients (treated with bivalirudin); at 30 days, success was 86%, and at 12 weeks that had decreased to 82%. Unfortunately, only historic controls could be examined to compare, and conjecture comes into play as to what might happen in such a high-risk group with known/suspected HIT. Bleeding and transfusion were greater in patients who received bivalirudin. In a single German center with a large experience using bivalirudin, 40 patients had heparin antibodies.[242] These investigators noted that their procedural success rate was 99.4%; however, they did have an increased use of transfusion in those patients who received bivalirudin.

In the face of HITT syndrome, case reports continue to show effectiveness and utility of bivalirudin.[244,245,248] This is an off-label use of the drug because it has not been FDA approved. In animal studies, bivalirudin does not activate platelets, and those animals that have received the drug for CPB have a better platelet count at the end of surgery. Other inflammatory mediators such as cytokines also may be decreased with bivalirudin administration as compared with heparin/protamine administration. Heparin, even in small doses, activates platelets to express their binding sites, whereas bivalirudin seems to leave the platelets quiescent. It also has no cross-reactivity with any immunoglobulin that is present to heparin/PF4 and does not produce an immune response of its own, which can be seen with hirudin.

The latest direct thrombin inhibitors being developed are for long-term oral use. Ximelagatran was in active phase III clinical trials, but they have been stopped. This is a prodrug that is rapidly biotransformed into the active drug Melagatran. The drug produces a predictable anticoagulant response, and no laboratory monitoring is required. This drug may be able to replace warfarin, which is a difficult drug to manage. Unfortunately, the FDA turned down ximelagatran in 2004 because of increased ALT levels in 6% of patients. It is approved in Europe for short-term use, and the FDA will reevaluate it after further clinical trials.[249–252]

Nonthrombogenic Surface

Considered the "Holy Grail" of extracorporeal circulation, an artificial surface that does not incite thrombus formation remains undiscovered. The endothelial surface, which the artificial one should mimic, performs a host of biochemical functions related to antithrombosis. Two that appear crucial are (1) secretion of substances that inhibit both platelet activation and aggregation and (2) surface and matrix adsorption of heparin and heparan, which may locally potentiate AT.[253]

Heparin may be immobilized onto surfaces by ionic bonding onto cationic surfactants. Unfortunately, both heparin and surfactant leach off the coated surface on exposure to blood. Covalent binding or surface grafting of heparin provides a more stable preparation. A properly heparin-bonded surface should bind AT sufficiently to prevent fibrinogen-induced platelet adhesion. Heparin-coated CPB tubing reduces the need for systemic heparin but has not been sufficiently effective to replace systemic anticoagulation.[254–256] Other approaches include increasing surface hydrophilicity with polyethylene oxide and sequestration of the thrombogenic surface by endothelialization, albumin activation, or phospholipid mimicking.[257] New materials might permit cardiac surgery with minimal doses of heparin or even without it (see Chapter 29).

PROTAMINE

Pharmacology

Protamine neutralizes heparin-induced anticoagulation. This section considers the history, pharmacology, and clinical use of protamine during cardiovascular surgery, including toxic and idiosyncratic adverse effects. Alternatives to protamine complete the discussion.

History

Miescher, investigating cell nuclei in 1868, discovered and named protamine, a nitrogenous alkaline substance in sperm heads of salmon.[258] Composed of nearly two-thirds arginine, protamines contain many

HOOC – Gln – **Arg** – Thr – Cys – **Arg**
                                    |
                                   Ile
                                    |
Gly – **Arg** – **Arg** – **Arg** – **Arg** – **Arg** – **Arg** – Val – Cys – Tyr – Thr – Val
|
Phe
|
Arg   Ala – **Arg** – Tyr – **Arg** – Cys – Cys – Leu – Thr – His – Ser – Gly
|
Arg   H₂N   Ser
| |
Arg   **Arg**
| |
Arg – **Arg** – **Arg** – Cys – **Arg** – **Arg** – **Arg** – **Arg** – **Arg** – **Arg** – Cys

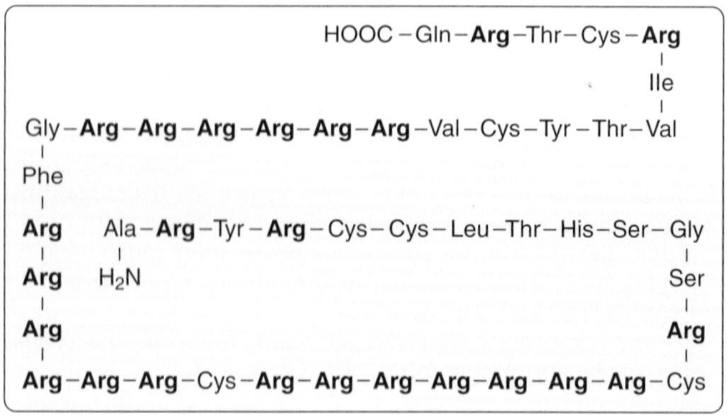

Figure 31-21 The complete amino acid sequence of protamine from steer. Note the abundance of arginine residues (50% for this species). *(Modified from Coelingh JP, Monfoort CH, Rozijn TH, et al: The complete amino acid sequence of the basic nuclear protein of bull spermatozoa. Biochim Biophys Acta 285:1, 1972.)*

positive charges (Figure 31-21). Their biologic role is to associate with the negatively charged phosphate groups of nucleic acids[259] (Figure 31-22).

In 1936, Hagedorn and colleagues used protamine to delay the absorption of insulin administered subcutaneously. They (correctly) chose protamine, hoping that its alkaline pH would maintain insulin in an ionized, slowly absorbed state. When others attempted to mix

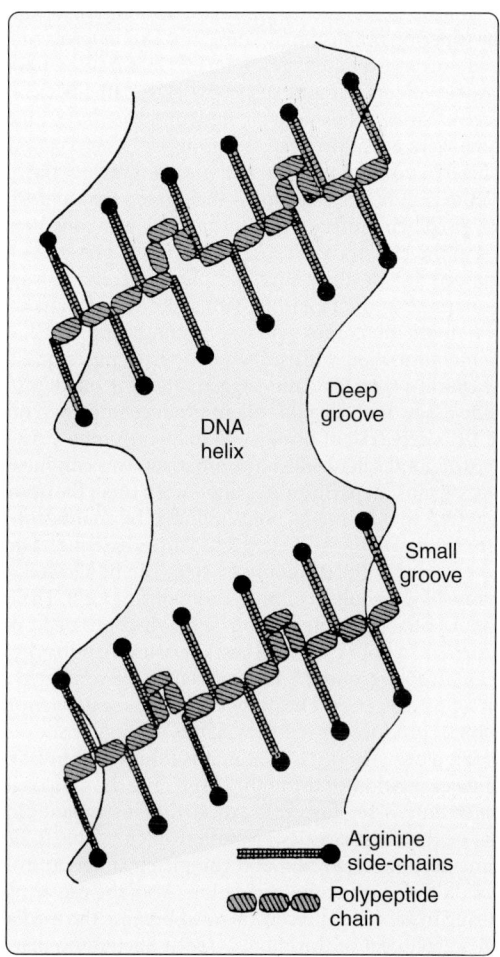

Figure 31-22 The polypeptide chain of protamine with its arginine residues seen residing in the small groove of the DNA helix. *(From Wilkins MHF: Physical studies of the molecular structure of deoxyribonucleic acid and nucleoprotein. Cold Spring Harbor Symp Quant Biol 21:83, 1956.)*

protamine with heparin to make a long-acting subcutaneous preparation for thrombosis prophylaxis, they obtained a white precipitate instead of a useful mixture.[260] Chargaff and Olson[261] recognized that this precipitate represented the salt of polycationic protamine and polyanionic heparin. They established protamine as the neutralizing drug for heparin's anticoagulant effect. Jacques[262,263] developed the in vitro protamine titration test for blood heparin levels and documented ~~inhibition of blood coagulation by excess protamine.~~

Source and Preparation

Most vertebrate species synthesize a protamine residing in the heads of sperm. Human protamine closely resembles that of other species.[264] Salmon milt provides the pharmaceutical source of protamine. The crushed gonads of male salmon undergo a crude extraction and filtration process using salt and alcohol. The final product, a dried powder, commonly is reconstituted as a 10-mg/mL solution. Like insulin and some other protein products, it is stable without refrigeration for several weeks. Protamine is available as sulfate and chloride salts. Protamine chloride may have a more rapid onset compared with protamine sulfate.[265] Nevertheless, clinical study reveals no superiority of one preparation over the other.[266]

Uses and Actions

Two long-acting insulin preparations contain protamine. Protamine-zinc insulin contains 10 to 15 μg protamine per unit of insulin, whereas NPH (neutral protamine Hagedorn) insulin contains 3 to 6 μg/unit. The former compound, with more protamine, exhibits a 36-hour duration, compared with 24 hours for the NPH insulin. Both heparin and protamine alter cell division and influence angiogenesis and tumor size.[267,268] However, these effects have not yet developed into therapeutic modalities. In addition, both protamine and its substitute polycation, hexadimethrine, possess broad antimicrobial activity, suggesting application as a topical antibiotic.[269]

Neutralization of heparin-induced anticoagulation remains the primary use of protamine. Formation of complexes with the sulfate groups of heparin forms the basis for this "antidote" effect. Protamine neutralizes the AT effect of heparin far better than its anti–factor Xa effect.[110] This distinction may arise from the need for thrombin, but not factor Xa, to remain complexed to heparin for AT to exert its inhibitory effect. Because porcine mucosal heparin has more potent anti–factor Xa activity than bovine lung heparin,[270] today's available heparin may prove to be more difficult to neutralize with protamine. Protamine's poor efficacy in neutralizing anti–factor Xa activity limits the utility of LMWH compounds as anticoagulants for CPB.

Protamine exhibits antihemostatic properties by affecting platelets and by releasing t-PA from endothelial cells.[110] Thrombocytopenia follows protamine administration in dogs[263,271] and in humans.[271,272] Heparin-protamine complexes inhibit thrombin-induced platelet aggregation.[273–275] In addition, protamine appears to bind to thrombin, inhibiting its ability to convert fibrinogen to fibrin.[276] Initial attempts to document an in vivo antihemostatic effect of protamine proved unsuccessful.[148] Rapid degradation of protamine by circulating proteases may account for this discrepancy.

Administration, Distribution, and Fate

Neutralization of heparin occurs by intravenous injection of protamine. Subcutaneous administration is limited to prolongation of insulin absorption. Presumably, these highly charged polycations distribute only to the extracellular space.

In the presence of circulating heparin, protamine forms large complexes with heparin.[277] Excess protamine creates larger complexes. The reticuloendothelial system may then dispose of these particles by endocytosis. Although this action has not been proved, macrophages in the lung may constitute the site for elimination of these complexes because intravenous administration of protamine permits formation of heparin-protamine complexes in the pulmonary circulation first. Protamine also may bind to circulating plasma proteins, the

significance of which remains unclear.[278] Proteolytic degradation of the protamine complexed to heparin conceivably results in free heparin. Protamine degradation in vivo proceeds by the action of circulating proteases, among them carboxypeptidase N, an enzyme that also clears anaphylatoxins and kinin pathway products.[279] The time course of protamine disappearance from plasma in patients remains poorly investigated.

Dosage

The recommended dose of protamine to neutralize heparin varies widely. Table 31-8 lists factors accounting for this variability. The first factor is the proper ratio of protamine to heparin. Reports of the optimal ratio of milligrams of protamine to units of heparin cite values as low as zero (i.e., they do not neutralize heparin)[280] to as much as 4 mg/100 units.[158] This variability has been accounted for by differences in timing, temperature, and other environmental factors; choices for coagulation tests and outcome variables; and speculation and unproven assumptions. Second, the basis for calculating protamine dose, the total amount of heparin given or the amount remaining in the patient, must be determined. Protamine titration tests at the conclusion of CPB can determine the amount of heparin remaining in the patient. With automated versions of this test and simple assumptions regarding the volume of distribution of heparin, the amount needed to neutralize the heparin detected in the patient's vasculature can be calculated. However, this technique may invite heparin rebound, the third concern (see Chapter 17).

An alternative regimen splits a 1 mg/100 units calculated dose of protamine into two separate doses: an initial dose (75% of the total) after CPB, with the remainder after reinfusion of blood from the bypass circuit. This regimen prevented increased plasma heparin levels and prolongation of the aPTT, compared with a control group.[281] The ACT remained unchanged, perhaps a reflection of its insensitivity to small amounts of circulating heparin. Protamine chloride did not prove superior to protamine sulfate in preventing the occurrence of heparin rebound.[266]

A system using coagulation test tubes that contain lyophilized heparin and protamine matched by lot to that administered to the patient permits calculation of dosages to account for variations arising from patient and pharmaceutical factors. It results in increased doses of heparin and decreased doses of protamine compared with those calculated by weight alone. Nevertheless, decreased bleeding and less use of allogeneic blood products result.[150]

Finally, lest fear of heparin rebound prompt the clinician to administer protamine in excess, gross overdosage may likely anticoagulate patients. Dogs given excess protamine exhibited a dose-dependent prolongation of the ACT, with the ACT nearly doubling after a protamine dose four times that needed to neutralize heparin. At a 10-fold dose, the aPTT prolonged and thrombocytopenia developed[149] (Figure 31-23). Without prior heparin, the coagulation test abnormalities occurred at lower protamine doses. The cautious clinician realizes that the protease enzyme system that degrades protamine can be saturated. Prolongation of coagulation times may conceivably result from protamine overdose, as well as from unneutralized heparin. Fortunately, the safe range of protamine dose regarding neutralization of anticoagulation is large; therefore, the prudent clinician will not hesitate to administer a small additional dose of protamine should incomplete neutralization or heparin rebound be suspected, while limiting administration so as not to overwhelm the proteases that degrade protamine.

TABLE 31-8	Basis for Variability in Protamine Dose
Ratio of protamine to heparin	
Amount of heparin to neutralize	
Heparin rebound	
Protamine overdose	

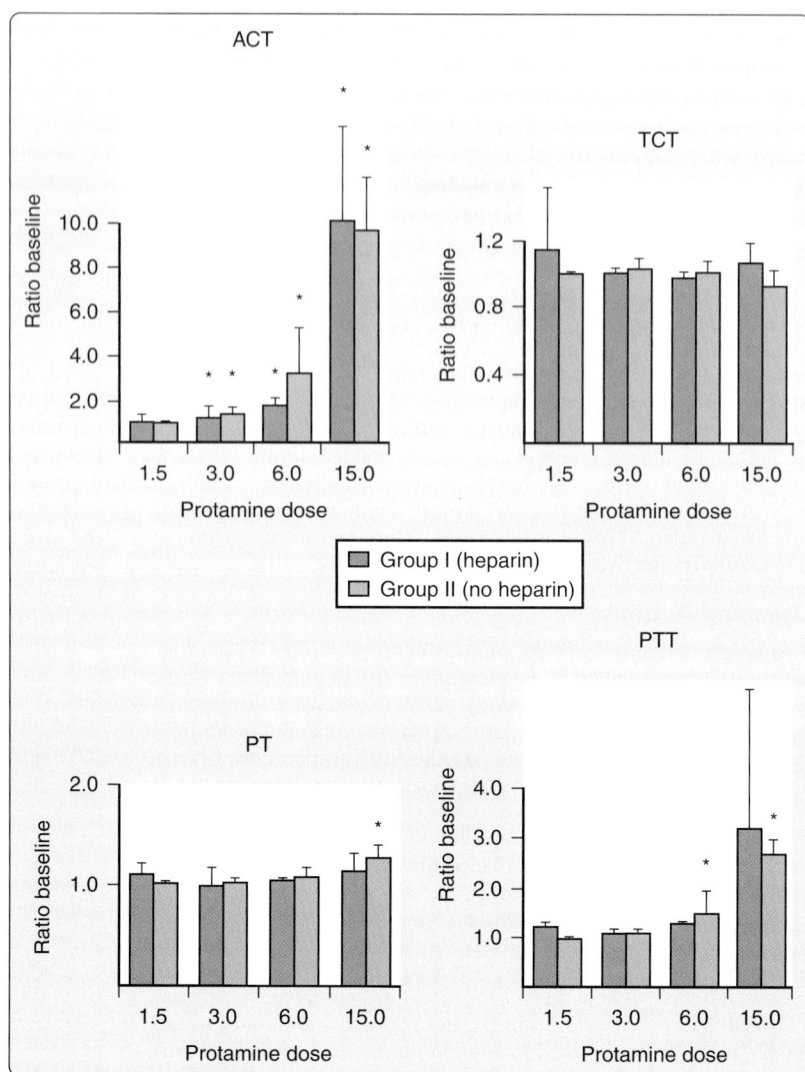

Figure 31-23 Effect on the activated coagulation time (ACT), thrombin clotting time (TCT), prothrombin time (PT), and activated partial thromboplastin time (aPTT) of protamine dose (in mg/kg) given to dogs 10 minutes after 150 U/kg heparin *(dark bars)* or without prior heparin *(light bars)*. Error bars represent standard deviation (SD). *Asterisks* denote statistical significance compared with baseline values. *(From Kresowik TF, Wakefield TW, Fessler RD, Stanley JC: Anticoagulant effects of protamine sulfate in a canine model. J Surg Res 45:8, 1988.)*

Adverse Reactions

The potential for a deleterious response to protamine administration raises serious questions and difficult choices in clinical care before, during, and after cardiac operations. This section presents the spectrum of adverse reactions, the presumed mechanism for each, and treatment options. These adverse events can be reduced with proper clinical technique. Thus, a clinical perspective at the end of this section discusses preventive measures to guard against untoward responses. The causes of hypotension after protamine (rapid administration, anaphylactic reaction, and pulmonary vasoconstriction) are considered in turn.

Rapid Administration

Peripheral Cardiovascular Changes
Jaques determined initially that systemic hypotension from protamine administered to dogs required a rapid (15-second) injection. Subsequent studies confirmed that hypotension accompanies intravenous protamine.[263,282–289] However, repeat doses are benign when given slowly or rapidly within 4 to 6 hours of an initial reaction unless heparin is given before the second dose.[283,290] Pulmonary arterial pressures also increase.[283,291] Although increased pulmonary arterial pressure and pulmonary vascular resistance follow protamine predictably in dogs, pigs, and sheep, humans respond in a more idiosyncratic fashion. Decreased systemic vascular resistance accompanies the

systemic hypotension,[271,286,287] whereas venous return and cardiac filling pressures decrease.[286,287] Rapid volume administration may avert systemic hypotension in both dogs and humans.[286,292]

Slow administration of a neutralizing dose over 5 minutes or longer rarely will engender cardiovascular changes.[293] Systemic hypotension from rapid injection in humans has been ascribed to pharmacologic displacement of histamine from mast cells by the highly alkaline protamine, similar to the mechanism by which curare, morphine, and alkaline antibiotics (e.g., vancomycin and clindamycin) cause hypotension. However, protamine alone, in concentrations similar to those expected in vivo, fails to release histamine from minced animal lung tissue,[294] or from dispersed human mast cells.[295] More recent investigations linked hypotension to the release of nitric oxide from endothelium.[296]

Effects on Cardiac Inotropy
Cardiac output (CO) predictably decreases after rapid administration to animals when preload is allowed to decrease.[271,282,284,285,289,291] Most human studies document no change in CO with rapid[297–299] or slow administration.[300–304] When volume infusion accompanies protamine, CO increases[292]; however, the effects of protamine on CO do not assess its impact on inotropy, which constitutes only one of many determinants of CO.

Initial reports indicated a myocardial depressant effect.[282,284,285,287] Studies using strips of myocardium bathed in concentrated protamine solutions produced similar results[305–308]; clinically relevant bath concentrations yielded conflicting results regarding depressed myocardial mechanics.[309,310] One study suggested that only concentrated noncomplex protamine would compromise patients clinically.[308] Another suggested that patients with established ventricular compromise might suffer further degradation of contractile performance on exposure to unbound protamine.[311] The mechanism may relate to altered membrane ion conductances that increase intracellular calcium.[311] Well-conducted studies in intact organisms revealed no effect of protamine on contractility in animals[288,313] or humans[283,313–319] (Figure 31-24).

Left-Sided Injection

Based on early reports claiming protection from adverse responses, injection of protamine directly into the left side of the circulation (left atrium or aortic root) became popular.[316,317] Some subsequent animal investigations confirmed a left-sided advantage[318,319]; others demonstrated no advantage[313,320] or more compromised hemodynamics[313] compared with a control right-sided group. Left-sided injection provides no protection from pulmonary hypertension.[321] In humans, the published evidence weighs against left-sided injection; three separate investigations in a total of 130 patients demonstrated more hypotension from left-sided than right-sided injection.[299,322,323] The clinician must consider that left-sided injection also increases the risk for systemic particulate and air embolization.

Platelet Reactions

The most underappreciated reaction to protamine is thrombocytopenia. The heparin-protamine complex activates the microcirculation. For a quick graphic example, the reader should merely mix heparin and protamine in a well or syringe. A milky precipitate is observed that grows into larger beads of precipitate. It is clear that when protamine is administered, it binds heparin wherever it comes into contact with it. It may find heparin attached to the surface of platelets and then coat the surface of the platelets with heparin–protamine complexes. It also is possible that heparin and protamine could form cross-links between platelets because the protamine is polycationic and can bind a number of heparin molecules. The end result is a decrease in platelet count within 10 to 15 minutes of administration of protamine. The usual is roughly a 10% decline in platelet count, but it can be larger, when normalization of coagulation is expected. It appears that the platelets are sequestered by the reticuloendothelial and pulmonary vasculature. It is unclear whether those patients with the largest drop in platelets develop the worst bleeding or whether they are at the greatest risk for

pulmonary vasoconstriction and pulmonary hypertension secondary to thromboxane release. The sequestered platelets come back into the circulation over the next few hours, and by 1 to 4 hours, the platelet count returns toward normal.

Anaphylactoid Reaction

Allergy, Anaphylaxis, and Adverse Responses

Not all adverse responses to protamine are allergic reactions. Rapid protamine injection decreases blood pressure just as morphine induces nausea; neither side effect is allergic. Immediate hypersensitivity allergic reactions involve release of vasoactive mediators resulting from antigen-antibody interaction. The broader term *anaphylactoid reactions* includes not only severe immediate hypersensitivity allergy, termed *anaphylaxis,* but also other life-threatening idiosyncratic responses of nonimmunologic origin[324,325] (Figure 31-25). The initial classification of protamine reactions split the anaphylactoid category (type II) into three subsets: anaphylaxis (IIA), nonimmunologic anaphylactoid reaction (IIB), and delayed noncardiogenic pulmonary edema (IIC).[326] The last two are poorly defined phenomena. Complement-mediated nonimmunologic effects do occur but are not discussed here.[327] This section deals mainly with allergic responses and polycation lung injury.[326–328]

Diabetes Mellitus

Patients receiving protamine-containing insulin develop antibodies to protamine. Between 38% and 91% of these patients demonstrate an antiprotamine IgG[329–331]; far fewer patients develop an antiprotamine IgE. Do these antibodies cause adverse responses to protamine administration? Few patients with diabetes actually experience development of hemodynamic compromise from protamine.[331] The numerous case

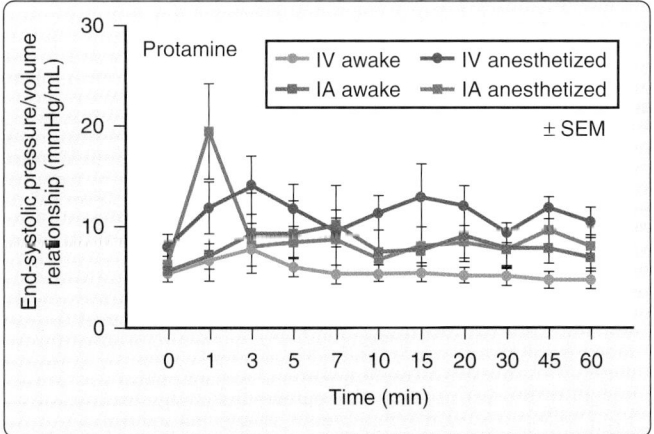

Figure 31-24 Effect of protamine infusion to dogs on a measure of inotropic state, the end-systolic pressure-volume relation. Neither route of administration (intra-aortic [IA], intravenous [IV]) nor the presence of anesthesia modified the absence of an effect of protamine on inotropic state. (*From Taylor RL, Little WC, Freeman GL, et al: Comparison of the cardiovascular effects of intravenous and intraaortic protamine in the conscious and anesthetized dog. Ann Thorac Surg 42:22, 1986.*)

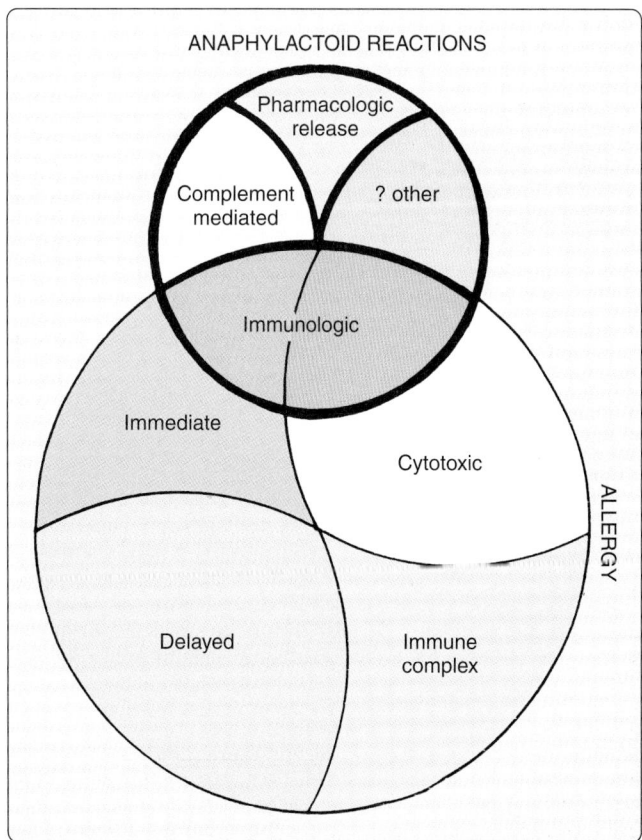

Figure 31-25 Venn diagram depicting the spectrum of allergy and of anaphylactoid reactions. Anaphylaxis to protamine is an immunologic-type anaphylactoid reaction classified as an immediate allergic reaction. (*From Horrow JC: Protamine allergy. J Cardiothorac Vasc Anesth 2:225, 1988.*)

TABLE 31-9	Studies on the Incidence of Protamine Reactions (Type Unspecified)						
Authors	Type	Size	Situation	Nondiabetics	Diabetics, No Insulin	Diabetics-NPH
Stewart et al[344]	Retrospective	651	Catheterization	0.50%	0.0%	27.0% (4/15)
Gottschlich et al[345]	Retrospective	2996	Catheterization	0.07%	—	2.9% (2/68)
Levy et al[294]	Prospective	3245	Surgery	0.06%	—	0.6% (1/160)
Weiss et al[346]	Case control	27	Various	25 × (IgG)*	—	95 × (IgE)†

*Nondiabetics who sustained an adverse response to protamine were 25 times more likely to demonstrate an antiprotamine IgG than nondiabetics who did not suffer an adverse protamine response.

†Diabetics taking NPH insulin who sustained an adverse response to protamine were 95 times more likely to demonstrate an antiprotamine IgE than NPH-taking diabetics who did not suffer an adverse protamine response.

reports of diabetic patients who had adverse responses to protamine reflected either a truly increased incidence of adverse response in this population or merely a reporting bias, because cases in nondiabetics are not published.[332–343] Retrospective attempts to determine the risk for protamine reaction in diabetic patients yield diverse results.[344,345] A case-control study found a 95-fold increase in risk relative to patients taking NPH insulin,[346] whereas prospective studies[331,347] demonstrated no increased risk. Table 31-9 displays these data. If risk is increased, it remains quite small (0.6%).[331]

Prior Exposure to Protamine

Previous protamine exposure may occur at catheterization,[334,348] at prior vascular surgery,[332,335] at dialysis,[349] or during blood component donation,[350] although modern techniques for the latter two procedures no longer use heparin and protamine. Multiple exposures at intervals of about 2 weeks maximize the chance of an allergic response.[351]

A single intravenous exposure to protamine will engender an IgG or IgE antibody response in 28% of patients.[352] Nevertheless, many thousands of patients each year receive protamine at both catheterization and then later at surgery without sequelae. They offer evidence of the safety of this sequence and the rarity of intravenous exposure to protamine generating clinically significant antibodies.

Fish Allergy

Salmon is a vertebrate or true fish (also known as "fin" fish), as opposed to shellfish, which are invertebrates. Patients allergic to fin fish can respond to protamine with anaphylaxis. Several case reports support this statement.[353,354] As with patients with diabetes, patients with fish allergy followed prospectively do not exhibit an adverse response to protamine challenge.[331] One of the authors (J.H.) has documented negative skin tests in several patients with fish allergy in whom subsequent protamine administration was benign, as well as a positive skin test in one patient who did not receive protamine (unpublished data). Because skin tests have high sensitivity and poor specificity, negative results suggest lack of allergy. No data link shellfish and protamine allergies.

Vasectomy

Within 1 year of vasectomy, 22% of men develop cytotoxic (IgG) antibody to human protamine, which may cross-react with salmon protamine because of similarity among protamines.[355] These autoantibodies exist in weak titers, however. Prospective studies demonstrate that patients with prior vasectomy receive protamine during cardiac surgery without adverse response.[355,356] Case reports of vasectomy-related protamine allergy[357] display insufficient evidence to demonstrate a causal relation[326,358]; thus, vasectomy remains only a theoretic risk for protamine allergy.

Noncardiogenic Pulmonary Edema

Systemic hypotension accompanied by massive pulmonary capillary leak, accumulation of alveolar fluid, decreased pulmonary compliance, wheezing, and pulmonary edema can occur after CPB. Originally attributed to protamine, these rare responses occur sporadically at least 20 minutes after protamine administration.[338,359–362] Others have attributed the problem to administration of banked blood products[363,364] or other substances.[365] CPB itself activates complement via the alternate pathway, which can (but usually does not) result in leukocyte aggregation, free radical formation, and lung injury.[324,366]

Many polycations, including protamine, hexadimethrine, and polylysine, can directly induce delayed pulmonary vascular damage.[366] Verapamil may attenuate polycation injury via its inhibitory effects on calcium channels.[367] The delayed noncardiogenic pulmonary edema seen clinically might arise from protamine, from administration of leukocytes that accompany banked blood products,[364] or from CPB.[368,369] Perhaps the marked decrease in occurrence of this phenomenon since 2000 arises from less frequent use of FFP, more widespread administration of calcium channel blockers perioperatively, or both.

Pulmonary Vasoconstriction

Clinical Features

Several years after PACs achieved common usage and case reports sensitized clinicians to adverse responses to protamine, Lowenstein et al[370] reported a series of patients in whom protamine caused systemic hypotension, decreased left atrial pressure, increased rather than decreased pulmonary arterial pressure, and RV distention and failure. This syndrome resembles the predictable response seen in certain laboratory animals.[370–374] Unlike in anaphylaxis, plasma histamine levels do not change during this idiosyncratic, catastrophic pulmonary vasoconstriction,[372] thus justifying a separate classification for this unusual response.[373]

The duration of pulmonary hypertension may vary substantially from brief episodes[374] (Figure 31-26) to those requiring reinstitution of CPB.[370,374,375] Rechallenge with protamine immediately after recovery from this type III reaction can be benign,[374] similar to the results in laboratory animals.[225] However, because rechallenge could induce repeat pulmonary vasoconstriction, it is best avoided whenever possible.

Proposed Mechanism

Animal models of type III protamine responses demonstrate that heparin must precede the protamine,[252,376] that heparin–protamine complexes activate the complement pathway,[377] and that blockade of complement activation attenuates pulmonary damage.[378] Furthermore, leukocytes respond to complement activation by forming free radicals, which stimulate the arachidonate pathway.[367,379] Blockade of this pathway mitigates the pulmonary response,[380,381] whereas antihistamines do not.[321,372]

Unlike the immediate pulmonary damage induced by heparin–protamine complexes, polycations alone (e.g., poly-L-lysine) induce pulmonary damage in a more delayed fashion. Polycation-induced injury probably involves pulmonary macrophages and arachidonate metabolites.[367,377,382–385] Heparin-protamine complex size varies with the molar ratios of heparin and protamine present[338]; an excess of protamine forms larger complexes.[277] Rapid protamine administration in humans may not predictably cause pulmonary hypertension because, unlike those of the pig and sheep, human lungs do not contain large numbers of macrophages.[338,367] Polycations can block nitric oxide synthetase, leading to speculation that this pathway also participates in the development of pulmonary vasoconstriction. Figure 31-27 summarizes the speculative mechanisms of various adverse responses to protamine.

Treatment and Prevention

Theoretically, slow administration should limit type III reactions because large heparin–protamine complexes would less likely form. Slow dilute infusion (see later) has decreased this adverse response to protamine.

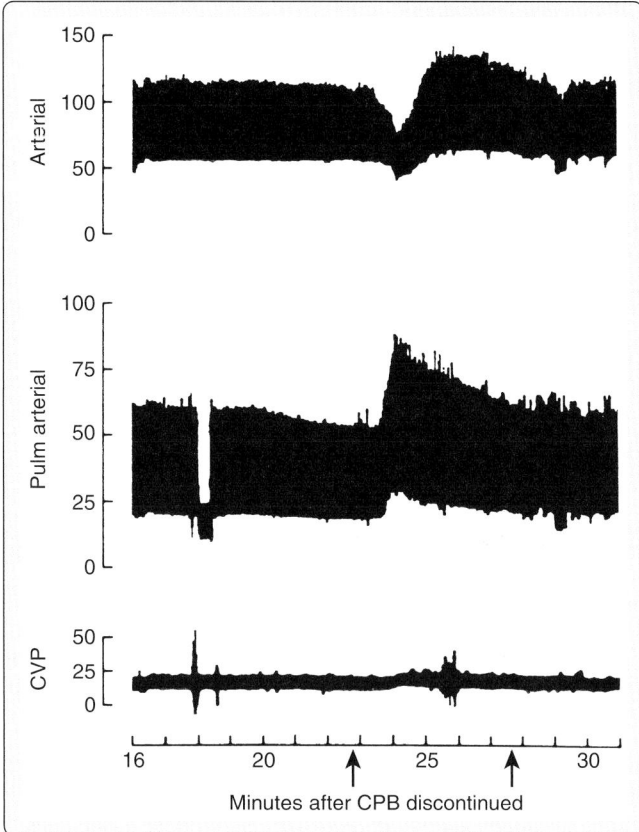

Figure 31-26 Example of a type III protamine reaction of brief duration. Compressed waveforms of radial arterial, pulmonary arterial, and central venous pressures (CVP; all in mm Hg) demonstrate sudden systemic hypotension and pulmonary hypertension soon after administration of 10 mg protamine sulfate (arrow at 23 minutes after bypass). Note lack of adverse response to an additional 10 mg protamine sulfate 5 minutes later. *(From Horrow JC: Thrombocytopenia accompanying a reaction to protamine sulfate. Can Anesth Soc J 32:49, 1985.)*

Some have suggested routine administration of antihistamines to prevent protamine-induced circulatory changes. For type III reactions, in which histamine has no mechanistic role, such a plan should fail. Indeed, antihistamines confer no advantage in general.[386] Hydrocortisone or aminophylline prophylaxis may lessen any circulatory changes with protamine administration, but for nonspecific reasons.[387,388]

On detection of sudden pulmonary hypertension and systemic hypotension, protamine infusion should cease, as should administration of any cardiovascular depressant. Administration of a heparin bolus should be considered in an attempt to reduce heparin–protamine complex size.[375] Excess heparin would theoretically attract protamine away from large complexes to yield a larger number of smaller size particles. If hemodynamics have not deteriorated sufficiently to warrant immediate reinstitution of CPB, 70 U/kg heparin should be tried first, then 300 U/kg if that fails. Inotropic support should be selected so as not to worsen the pulmonary hypertension; isoproterenol (0.1 to 0.2 μg/kg bolus followed by 0.1 to 0.3 μg/kg/min) or milrinone appear best suited for this purpose. Milder cases may revert without intervention,[374] merely by halting protamine administration,[389] a highly desirable outcome insofar as the treatments outlined earlier all extract a price, whether it be arrhythmias from inotropes or bleeding from heparin. Rechallenge with protamine should be avoided.

Guidelines for Clinical Use

The most important principle in avoiding adverse responses to protamine is to administer the drug slowly. Dilution aids this goal by limiting the impact of an undetected rapid administration. A neutralizing dose (3 mg/kg, or 21 mL on average of 10 mg/mL solution) can be added to 50 mL clear fluid; then the diluted drug can be administered into a central vein by a small-drop infusion (60 drops/mL) over 10 to 15 minutes. It is important to provide a carrier flow when administering by peripheral vein so that the long tubing does not slowly fill with drug rather than the drug entering the patient. Additional doses of undiluted protamine are given from small syringes (5 mL) at a maximum rate of 20 mg/min to adults. Proper choice of materials (small syringes, small-drop administration sets, and use of diluent) helps protect against too-rapid drug delivery.

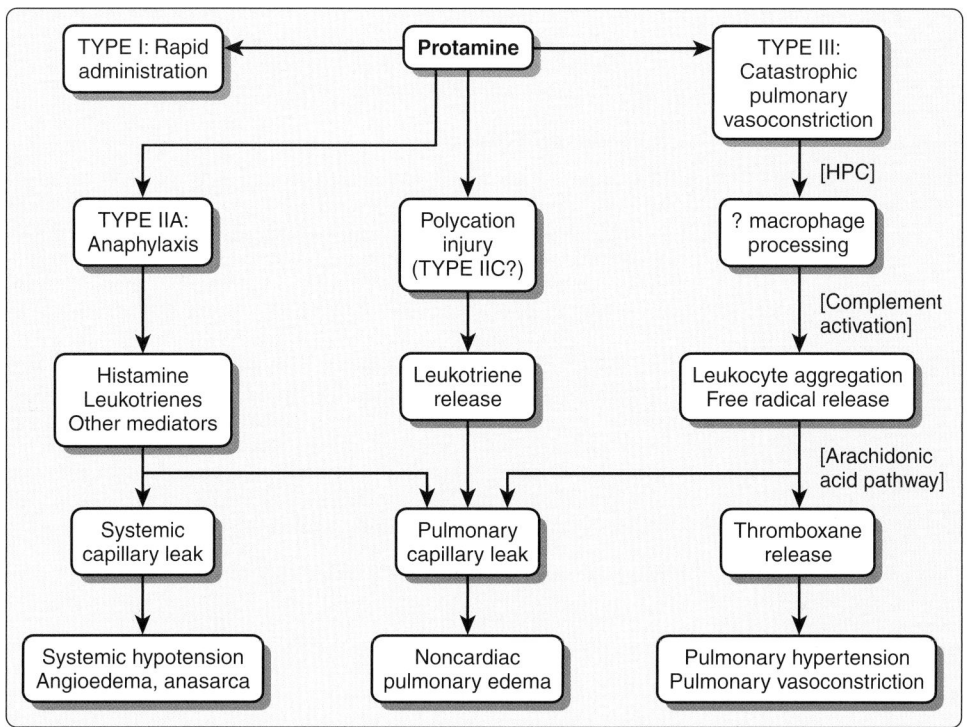

Figure 31-27 Speculative mechanisms of some protamine reactions to heparin-protamine complex (HPC). *(From Horrow JC: Heparin reversal of protamine toxicity: Have we come full circle? J Cardiothorac Vasc Anesth 4:539, 1990.)*

Slow administration should decrease the likelihood of a type I and III adverse response. However, anaphylactic response (type IIA) may occur at any delivery rate. Preparation for groups at risk to receive protamine is discussed in the following sections.

Patients with Diabetes

No screening test predicts an adverse response to protamine; serum IgE levels are nonspecific; and skin tests do not correlate with antiprotamine antibody measurements.[390,391] Using too concentrated a protamine solution in performing skin tests may produce false-positive results.[392,393] Antiprotamine antibody determinations, available by radio allergosorbent test or ELISA, appear equally nonspecific and are expensive.[390,391] Although most patients with diabetes have antiprotamine immunoglobulin (38% to 91%), most receive protamine without adverse sequelae (> 99.4%).

Vasectomy and Patients with Fish Allergy

Like patients with diabetes, vasectomy patients demonstrate antibodies but show a benign response to protamine. All skin tests on vasectomy patients by these authors have displayed negative results and benign responses to protamine after CPB, including one who demonstrated an anaphylactoid reaction at catheterization, probably arising from radio-contrast administration.

Patients with strong evidence by history or laboratory tests of allergy to fin fish are uncommon. After CPB, these patients receive 1 mg protamine diluted in 50 mL intravenous fluid over 10 minutes. If hemodynamics do not deteriorate, the neutralizing dose is administered as previously outlined. Otherwise, protamine is withheld. Skin testing may predict this allergy but would not change the approach, because false-positive skin tests are common, and too few reported cases of protamine–fin fish cross-allergy exist to warrant more aggressive drug administration to those demonstrating negative skin tests. Heparin has been successfully neutralized in a patient with a history of fin fish anaphylaxis and positive skin tests to protamine by using the enzyme heparinase I (Neutralase). This case is unpublished.

Prior Reaction to Protamine

For patients with prior reaction to protamine, skin testing, radio allergosorbent test, and ELISA are appropriate, because negative responses provide greater comfort in attempting a rechallenge. If the historic or laboratory evidence for protamine sensitivity is poor, then a challenge as described for patients with fish allergy may be attempted. Otherwise, an alternative to protamine should be chosen. Availability of a safe alternative would save the cost of these tests and any prolonged hospitalization that accompanies them.

■ Alternatives to Protamine

This section discusses techniques for neutralizing heparin other than with administration of protamine. Substitutes for protamine in long-acting insulin preparations are not considered.

Hexadimethrine

This synthetic polycation (Figure 31-28) is 1.1 to 2.0 times more potent than protamine.[394,395] Hexadimethrine (Polybrene) engenders the same biologic responses as protamine when administered rapidly:

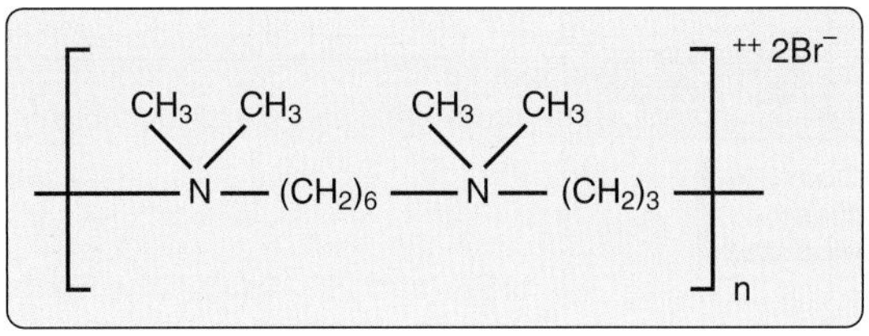

Figure 31-28 Hexadimethrine, a synthetic polycationic polymer. (From Horrow JC: Protamine. A necessary evil. In Ellison N, Jobes DR [eds]: Effective Hemostasis in Cardiac Surgery. Philadelphia: WB Saunders Company 1988, p 15.)

systemic hypotension, decreased systemic vascular resistance, and rapid disappearance from plasma.[395,396] Pulmonary hypertension occurs after hexadimethrine neutralization of UFH.[397] Patients allergic to protamine have received hexadimethrine without adverse effects.[334] The small group of patients with true anaphylaxis, as demonstrated by clinical history and antiprotamine IgE, may benefit from hexadimethrine insofar as this protamine substitute may not cross-react with the antibodies present.

After reports of renal toxicity, hexadimethrine was withdrawn from clinical use in the United States.[398,399] Animal studies confirmed glomerular injury from hexadimethrine. Urinary excretion of lactic dehydrogenase, aspartase aminotransferase, and other enzymes occurs.[400] Binding of the polycation to the carboxyl groups of proteoglycans in the glomerular basement membrane probably mediates this injury.[401] Although protamine also causes renal toxicity, larger doses are required.[402,403] Hexadimethrine appears unlikely to replace protamine for routine clinical use.[404]

Platelet Factor 4

Platelets contain the potent antiheparin compound PF4. An early attempt to neutralize heparin by platelet concentrate transfusion in two patients produced poor results, however. Despite 18 units of platelets and 400 mL FFP, 1 patient bled 4 L, whereas 12 units platelets and 1100 mL FFP accompanied more than 2 L of blood loss in another.[340]

Rather than bind to heparin electrostatically, like protamine, PF4 utilizes lysine residues at its C termini to neutralize heparin. Both native and recombinant PF4 effectively neutralize heparin in rats without adverse effects at one-fifth the potency of protamine, that is, 5 mg/100 U heparin.[94] In heparinized human blood, recombinant PF4 was half as potent as protamine in restoring the ACT and whole-blood clotting time.[405] Doses of 2.5 and 5.0 mg/kg recombinant PF4 neutralized the 5000 units heparin given for cardiac catheterization.[406] Doses of 5 mg/kg recombinant PF4 to a small number of patients successfully neutralized the 300 U/kg heparin given for CPB.[407]

Does PF4 avoid the adverse effects of protamine? Kurrek et al[408] demonstrated pulmonary hypertension in lambs when neutralizing heparin with PF4. The lamb, like the dog, responds predictably to protamine with increased pulmonary pressures, and thus serves as a model for predicting the idiosyncratic effects of protamine in humans. Those patients likely to respond to protamine with pulmonary hypertension might respond likewise to PF4.[408] Another less likely explanation is that PF4 constitutes a foreign protein to the lamb, thus engendering the adverse pulmonary hemodynamic response.[409] Further clinical work on PF4 as a protamine substitute appears to have slowed.

Interposed Filters

The enzyme, heparinase, bonded to an exit filter of an experimental bypass circuit and interposed at the conclusion of CPB, decreased blood heparin levels within two passes[410]; current filters achieve 90% heparin removal with a single pass.

A modification of this concept uses a hollow-fiber filter to which protamine has been immobilized. Although not a true alternative to protamine, the protamine filter traps heparin extracorporeally, limiting tissue interaction with heparin-protamine complexes.[411,412] This "protamine filter" attenuates both thrombocytopenia and leucopenia. The clinical efficacy and safety of this technique have not yet been clearly demonstrated. Heparin removal proceeds much too slowly, requiring 10 minutes to remove half of circulating heparin; the potential for clot formation in the circuit from return of unheparinized blood for successive passes through the filter remains an unresolved problem.

Methylene Blue

This positively charged chemical dye binds to heparin in an electrostatic fashion similar to that of protamine. Sloan et al[413] administered 2 mg/kg to a patient who had sustained a severe reaction to protamine, successfully restoring the ACT and aPTT, and decreasing chest tube output. Follow-up work ex vivo confirmed a potential benefit.[414]

However, more rigorous laboratory testing[415] and a clinical trial of ascending doses of methylene blue to neutralize heparin administered for elective CPB demonstrated no efficacy whatsoever in restoring the ACT to normal.[416] Furthermore, doses greater than 6 mg/kg resulted in moderate-to-severe pulmonary hypertension, necessitating administration of inotropic support.[417] Methylene blue, an inhibitor of nitric oxide synthetase, predictably increases pulmonary and systemic vascular resistances at greater doses. Methylene blue should not be used to neutralize heparin.

Omit Neutralization

Heparin activity will decay spontaneously with time because of drug elimination. Castaneda omitted heparin neutralization in 92 patients[280]; despite lower doses of heparin and meticulous hemostasis, most of those patients bled excessively. Another patient in whom heparin was not neutralized bled 5 L over 13 hours and required more than 15 units of blood products.[417] Although this option avoids exposure to protamine, hemodynamic instability and consumptive coagulopathy may result from massive hemorrhage. Substantial exposure to transfusion-related viral disease also creates serious concern for the clinician.

Heparinase

Systemic administration of the enzyme heparinase I, produced by *Flavobacterium,* resulted in a return of the ACT to normal in an ex vivo model,[418] animal models of CPB,[418] and healthy volunteers.[419] Initial investigation in patients undergoing elective CABG operations confirmed the utility of heparinase in neutralizing heparin-induced anticoagulation.[420]

Because the enzyme remains in the vasculature for some time after administration (the half-life is 12 minutes in healthy subjects), should an immediate need arise to reinstitute CPB, patients would require not only repeat doses of heparin, but an infusion of heparin to counter the lingering effects of the enzyme. All work on the development of heparinase has stopped after failure of initial clinical trials.

Designer Polycations

If the action of protamine is derived from its polycationic structure, could artificial polycations be developed to retain the heparin-neutralizing property while minimizing or eliminating adverse effects? Wakefield et al[421,422] have generated a series of designed molecules with this purpose in mind.

Unfortunately, adverse effects appear to correlate with the ability to neutralize UFH. However, some of the polycations developed can neutralize LMWH species without adverse sequelae, suggesting replacement of both UFH and protamine with a doubly superior regimen for achieving anticoagulation for CPB.[384] Much more investigation must precede clinical trials. The future may be in using the new direct thrombin inhibitors and completely avoiding the need for protamine.

BLEEDING PATIENT

After cardiac surgery, some patients bleed excessively. Prompt diagnostic and therapeutic action will avoid impaired hemodynamics from hemorrhage, decreased oxygen-carrying capacity from anemia, and impaired hemostasis from depletion of endogenous hemostatic resources. The surgical act creates the potential for hemorrhage, sometimes aided by preoperative attempts to lyse intracoronary thromboses. Beyond that, however, many factors govern whether a particular patient will experience excessive bleeding after cardiac surgery. This section details the causes, prevention, and management of the bleeding patient (see Chapters 17, 28 to 30, and 34).

Although many different criteria can define excessive bleeding, chest tube drainage of more than 10 mL/kg in the first hour after operation or a total of more than 20 mL/kg over the first 3 hours after operation for patients weighing more than 10 kg is considered significant.

Also, any sudden increase of 300 mL/hr or greater after minimal initial drainage in an adult usually indicates anatomic disruption warranting surgical intervention.[421]

Patient Factors

The medical history can reveal information relevant to hemostasis. Any patient with a personal or family history of abnormal bleeding after surgery deserves specific coagulation testing for an inherited disorder. Routine PT, aPTT, and bleeding times probably offer little as screening tests.[423–425] The bleeding time has been investigated in a meta-analysis of more than 800 published articles, and it was concluded that it has no correlation with postoperative coagulopathic bleeding.[426] The other routine tests have less than a 50% accuracy for predicting who will bleed and who will have normal chest tube outputs.

The thromboelastograph has been tested extensively both alone and in conjunction with a number of other tests including PT, platelet count, and fibrinogen. The TEG has been shown to have the best predictive accuracy for postoperative bleeding.[427–435] In work using an algorithm based on the TEG and other tests, blood product utilization was cut considerably.[434] Chest tube bleeding was not different, but the TEG did predict which patients might bleed abnormally. Work with TEG monitoring has shown that it can detect both hypocoagulable and hypercoagulable states. New additives to the testing make it sensitive to the ADP-receptor platelet antagonists, as well as the IIb/IIIa inhibitors (see Chapter 17).

Concurrent systemic disease affects hemostasis during surgery as well. Uremia from renal failure results in platelet dysfunction. Severe hepatic compromise impairs every aspect of hemostasis: PK and most coagulation factors circulate in decreased concentration; additional sialic acid residues on fibrinogen and other coagulation factors impair clotting function; splenomegaly induces thrombocytopenia; maldistribution of vWF multimers impairs platelet adhesiveness and aggregation; impaired clearance of endogenous plasminogen activators accentuates fibrinolysis; and decreased levels of coagulation inhibitors induce a consumptive coagulopathy.[436]

Medications significantly affect surgical bleeding. Many patients taking aspirin or other platelet-inhibiting drugs regularly cannot halt that therapy within 7 days of surgery. No antidote can correct the platelet defect. Fortunately, most patients taking aspirin within 7 days of surgery do not exhibit excessive bleeding. The new antiplatelet drugs can all lead to postoperative bleeding (see Table 31-4).

Patients taking warfarin require 2 to 5 days without therapy for correction of the international normalized ratio. Patients for urgent surgery may receive parenteral vitamin K or FFP, which corrects the warfarin defect more quickly. Some patients may receive thrombolytic therapy for acute ischemic events just before surgery. Systemic fibrinogenolysis resulting from use of nonspecific thrombolytic agents such as streptokinase should respond to antifibrinolytic therapy with ε-aminocaproic acid (EACA) or tranexamic acid (TA).

Insult of Cardiopulmonary Bypass

More so than patient factors, CPB itself acts to impair hemostasis. Bypass activates fibrinolysis, impairs platelets, and affects coagulation factors. Hypothermia, used in most centers during CPB, adversely affects hemostasis as well.

Fibrinolysis

Numerous investigations support the notion that CPB activates the fibrinolytic pathway.[437–439] Despite clinically adequate doses and blood concentrations of heparin, coagulation pathway activity persists. Formation of prothrombin and fibrinopeptide fragments and thrombin-AT complexes document continued thrombin activity in this setting (see Figure 31-13). The site of thrombin activity probably resides in the extracorporeal circuit, which contains a large surface of thrombogenic material. Thrombin activation results in fibrinolytic activity; activation of fibrinolysis may be localized to those external sites of fibrin formation. Plasminogen activator concentrations increase during CPB, whereas levels of its inhibitor plasminogen activator inhibitor 1 remain unchanged. This scenario is consistent with activation of fibrinolysis during CPB. Neither of the labels "primary" or "secondary" applies to the fibrinolysis peculiar to CPB.

Does fibrin formation during CPB constitute a consumptive coagulopathy? It is not a systemic event. Presuming that plasminogen activation occurs only where fibrin is formed (extracorporeally), a systemic fibrinogenolytic state should not ensue. Should α_2-antiplasmin become overwhelmed by plasmin formation, however, systemic manifestations may result. Previous generations of oxygenators may have engendered systemic fibrinogenolysis more easily because of their more thrombogenic designs. In these (now more uncommon) instances of fibrinolysis, the TEG may demonstrate clot lysis. Even when fibrinolysis remains limited to the sites of extravascular fibrin formation, the fibrin degradation products so formed might impair hemostasis. In many cases, the mild fibrinolytic state engendered during CPB resolves spontaneously with little clinical impact.

Platelet Dysfunction

Thrombocytopenia occurs during CPB as a result of hemodilution, heparin, hypothermia-induced splenic sequestration of platelets, and platelet destruction from the blood-gas and blood-tissue interfaces created by cardiotomy suction, filters, and bubble oxygenators.[440–442] Platelet count rarely declines to less than 50,000/mm³, however.

Not only does the number of platelets decrease during CPB, but remaining platelets become impaired by partial activation. Fibrinogen and fibrin, which adhere to artificial surfaces of the extracorporeal circuit, form a nidus for platelet adhesion and aggregation. A reduced content of platelet α-granules constitutes the evidence for partial activation[443]; nearly one third of circulating platelets undergo α-granule release during CPB.[444] Bypass also depletes platelet GP receptors Ib and IIb/IIIa.[444,445] These platelets cannot respond fully when subsequent hemostatic stimuli call for release of granule contents. Use of frequent cardiotomy suction and bubble oxygenators aggravates the extent of platelet activation.

Activation of the fibrinolytic system may contribute to platelet dysfunction. Local formation of plasmin affects platelet membrane receptors.[445] Antifibrinolytic medications preserve platelet function and prevent some platelet abnormalities that occur during CPB[446–449] (Figure 31-29).

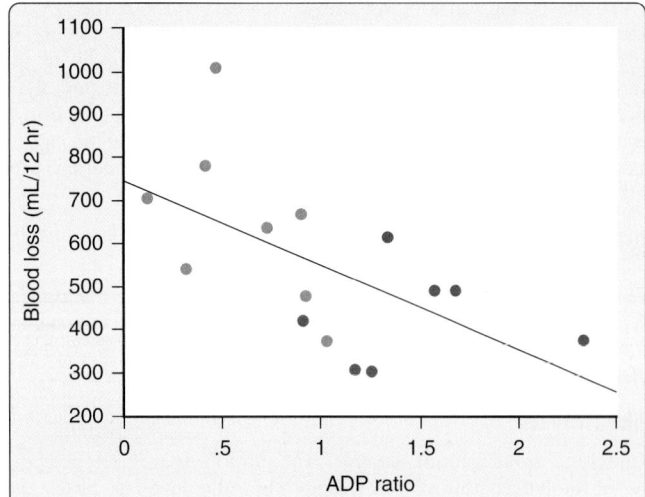

Figure 31-29 Antifibrinolytics may aid hemostasis by platelet preservation. Here, blood loss appears as a function of platelet adenosine diphosphate (ADP), expressed as a ratio (after bypass/before bypass). *Purple circles* represent patients who received prophylactic tranexamic acid. Placebo-treated patients appear as *green circles.* Note that the antifibrinolytic afforded less bleeding after operation and greater platelet ADP. *(From Soslau G, Horrow JC, Brodsky I: The effect of tranexamic acid on platelet ADP during extracorporeal circulation. Am J Hematol 38:113, 1991.)*

Clotting Factors

Denaturation of plasma proteins, including the coagulation factors, occurs at blood-air interfaces. Liberal use of cardiotomy suction and prolonged use of bubble oxygenators potentially impair coagulation by decreasing coagulation factor availability. Hemodilution also decreases factor concentrations. However, rarely do coagulation factor levels decline to less than the thresholds for adequate formation of fibrin in adult surgery. In infants, however, the smallest achievable pump priming volumes can dilute factors to less than 30% of normal levels.

Hypothermia

Hypothermia potentially affects hemostasis in many ways. First, the splanchnic circulation responds to hypothermia with sequestration of platelets.[450–452] After warming, the accompanying thrombocytopenia reverses over 1 hour. Second, transient platelet dysfunction occurs, evidenced by a platelet shape change, increased adhesiveness, inhibition of ADP-induced aggregation, and decreased synthesis of both thromboxane and prostacyclin.[450,451] Third, a specific heparin-like inhibitor of factor Xa becomes more active[452]; protamine cannot neutralize this factor, which might be heparan. Fourth, hypothermia slows the enzymatic cleavage on which activation of coagulation factors depends. Many biologic phenomena display a 7% attenuation of activity for each decrease of 1° C in temperature.[453] Although coagulation factor structure remains unaltered, formation of fibrin may be sluggish when the patient is cold. Fifth, hypothermia accentuates fibrinolysis[454]; the fibrin degradation products so formed then impair subsequent fibrin polymerization. Cold-induced injury of vascular endothelium can release thromboplastin, which then incites fibrin formation and activates fibrinolysis. Table 31-10 summarizes these effects.

▣ Prevention of Bleeding

The possible transmission of serious viral illness and impairment of immune function during transfusion of blood products may generate great concern among clinicians and patients. Many techniques attempt to limit viral exposure, including donation of autologous blood or directed blood, blood scavenging during and after surgery, and efforts to limit perioperative hemorrhage (Table 31-11). Advances in blood banking have decreased infectious disease transmission.[455] Blood sterilization techniques may render such concerns moot.[456]

Preoperative Factors

What can be done before surgery to minimize the extent of bleeding during and after surgery? Existing disorders of hemostasis must be identified and treated. The bleeding diathesis of uremia responds to hemodialysis, RBC transfusion, and administration of desmopressin.[457,458] Because impaired hemostasis from hepatic failure may respond to intravenous desmopressin, preoperative verification of an appropriate response will permit proper administration of this drug after protamine neutralization of heparin after CPB.[459] Likewise, patients with hematologic disorders potentially amenable to desmopressin therapy, such as hemophilia and vWD, should receive desmopressin before surgery to determine the extent of response, if any.[460] When specific factor replacement is indicated, withholding it until after neutralization of heparin will provide less extensive exposure to allogeneic blood products.

TABLE 31-10	Antihemostatic Effects of Hypothermia	
Hemostatic Component	*Effect of Hypothermia*
Factors	Increased anti–factor Xa activity; heparan?
	Slows enzymes of the coagulation cascade
Platelets	Splanchnic sequestration
	Partial activation
Fibrinolysis	Enhanced
Endothelium	Tissue factor release

TABLE 31-11	Ways to Prevent* Excessive Bleeding in Decreasing Order of Importance
Intervention†	Purpose
Ligatures	Repair all vascular trespass
Neutralize	Heparin fully neutralized
Blood pressure	Avoid hypertension after aortotomy
Suction	Limit cardiotomy suction
Drugs	Cease platelet-inhibiting drugs in advance
Preoperative	Diagnose and treat first
Oxygenator	Membrane oxygenators for long cases
ε-Aminocaproic acid (EACA)	Antifibrinolytic prophylaxis
Temperature	Rewarm sufficiently
Go	Act with deliberate speed (tardiness begets bleeding)
Intravenous	Limit fluids, hemoconcentrate, and diurese
Extracorporeal circuit	Minimize volume

*These maneuvers do not all apply to the treatment of excessive bleeding after operation.
†The entries in this column form a mnemonic device: the initial letters of each entry, when rearranged, form the words STOP BLEEDING.

Administration of platelet-inhibiting drugs should cease before surgery. Two to 3 days should elapse for nonsteroidal anti-inflammatory medications, which cause reversible inhibition of cyclooxygenase. Seven to 10 days are required for regeneration of platelets after administration of aspirin, which irreversibly acetylates cyclooxygenase and some other platelet inhibitors (see Table 31-4).

Physical Factors

Hypothermia still forms an essential component of organ protection during CPB in many centers. Sufficient rewarming with adequate distribution of heat from central to intermediate and peripheral zones should help prevent hypothermia-induced impairment of hemostasis.

Incomplete surgical hemostasis may occur from a slipped ligature, unclipped vessel branch, loose anastomosis, unattended open vessel at the wound edge, or sternal wire placed through the internal mammary artery. Because few fresh aortic suture lines fail to leak at high systemic pressures (systolic pressure > 180 mm Hg or mean arterial pressure > 120 mm Hg), control of hypertension after CPB promotes hemostasis (see Chapter 34).

Limiting the intensity and frequency of use of the cardiotomy suction fosters platelet preservation during CPB and improves hemostasis after surgery.[461] Selection of a membrane rather than a bubble-type oxygenator for cases involving prolonged CPB limits platelet destruction and fibrinolysis, thus aiding hemostasis.[462]

A small priming volume of the extracorporeal circuit restricts the extent of hemodilution. Hemodilution engenders bleeding not only by providing decreased concentrations of clotting factors and platelets, it also decreases margination of platelets, making them less available for adhesion and aggregation. Other measures that help include regulating cardioplegia volumes, restricting intravenous fluids, administering mannitol or loop diuretics, and providing hemoconcentration with filtration devices during CPB.

Removal of platelet-rich plasma at the induction of anesthesia for return to the patient after CPB by plasmapheresis supplies autologous, functional thrombocytes when they are most needed.[463–468] Previously, some centers collected autologous whole blood from patients at the beginning of surgery, reinfusing it after CPB, with controversial benefit.

Speed of surgery receives less attention now than in the past, when the therapeutic index of available anesthetics was less favorable. However, patients undergoing short surgery enjoy several advantages. Shorter CPB duration preserves platelet function and limits the coagulant stimulus for subsequent fibrinolysis; more rapid closure after CPB limits tissue exposure to the hypothermic operating room environment.

Pharmacologic Factors

Heparin and Protamine

The prudent clinician's admonition to administer no drug to excess applies well to this pair of essential drugs. Too little heparin invites active fibrin formation during CPB with consumption of clotting factors and platelets, and excessive activation of the fibrinolytic system; too much heparin risks postoperative heparin rebound. With too little protamine, the remaining unneutralized heparin impairs hemostasis by its anticoagulant action. Doses of protamine excessive enough to overwhelm the endogenous proteases may exert an anticoagulant effect, as well as invite polycation-induced lung injury and pulmonary vasoconstriction. The optimal approach utilizes coagulation testing to estimate the appropriate heparin and protamine doses, and confirm both adequate anticoagulation and its neutralization.

Desmopressin

Desmopressin, an analog of vasopressin (Figure 31-30), provides more potent and longer-lasting antidiuretic activity than vasopressin, with little vasoconstriction (Box 31-5). Like the parent compound and like epinephrine and insulin, desmopressin releases coagulation system

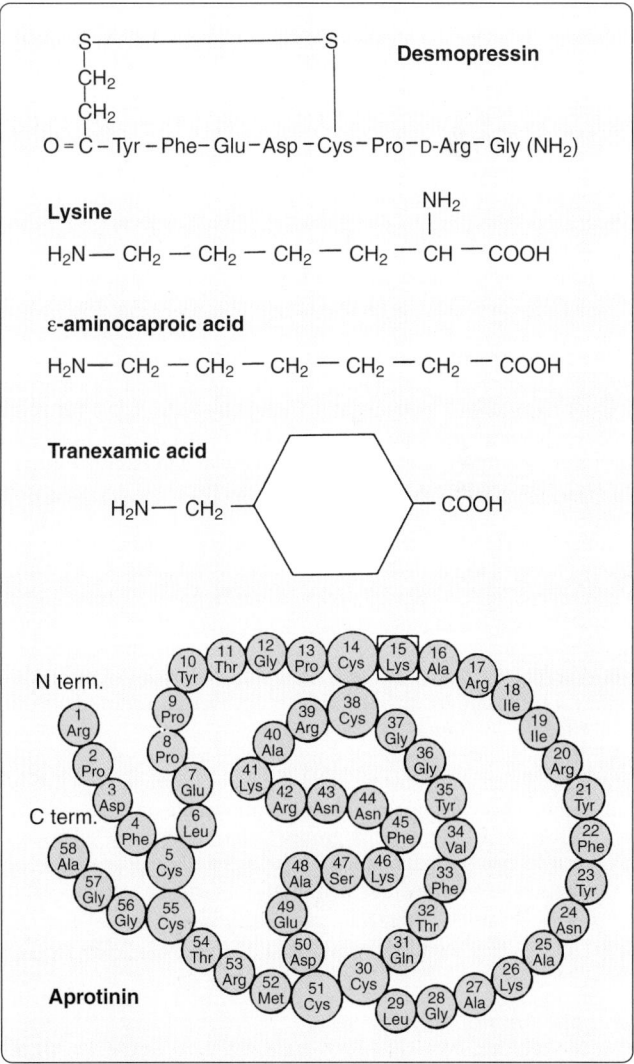

Figure 31-30 Molecular configurations of drugs used to decrease surgical bleeding. For comparison, the amino acid lysine is also depicted. (Modified from Horrow JC: Desmopressin and antifibrinolytics. Int Anesthesiol Clin 28:230, 1990; and Fritz H, Wunderer G: Biochemistry and applications of aprotinin, the kallikrein inhibitor from bovine organs. Drug Res 33:479, 1983.)

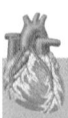

mediators from vascular endothelium. Factor VIII coagulant activity increases 2- to 20-fold and is maximal about 30 to 90 minutes after injection.[458,469–489] Factor XII levels also increase.[469] In response to desmopressin, endothelium releases the larger multimers of vWF, as well as t-PA and prostacyclin.[470] The latter two compounds potentially thwart clot formation and stability. Nevertheless, the overall effect of desmopressin is procoagulant, perhaps because of the impact of factor VIII and vWF.

The optimal dose of desmopressin is 0.3 µg/kg. Intravenous, subcutaneous, and intranasal routes are all acceptable. After plasma redistribution with an 8-minute half-life, metabolism in liver and kidney and urinary excretion yield a plasma half-life of 2.5 to 4 hours.[458] Levels of factor VIII persist in plasma long after desmopressin excretion because of the release of vWF. Depletion of vWF stores in endothelial cells accounts for the drug's tachyphylaxis. Rapid intravenous administration decreases systemic blood pressure and systemic vascular resistance, possibly by prostacyclin release or stimulation of extrarenal vasopressin V_2 receptors.[472–476] The antidiuretic action of the drug poses no problem in the absence of excessive free water administration.[477]

Specific applications of desmopressin's hemostatic benefit include uremia, cirrhosis, aspirin therapy, and surgery of various types. Correction of prolonged bleeding times in patients with uremia follows desmopressin administration, making desmopressin the treatment of choice for bleeding emergencies in uremia.[458] Administration of desmopressin to patients with cirrhosis also shortens prolonged bleeding times.[460] Desmopressin corrected the aspirin-induced prolongation in bleeding time in 2 patients and 10 healthy volunteers.[478] It is also effective in some rare platelet disorders.[469] Evidence of a hemostatic effect during surgery is varied. Early success in adolescents undergoing Harrington rod placement was not confirmed with subsequent studies.[479]

Initial reports of a hemostatic effect during cardiac surgery were largely unsubstantiated by subsequent investigations.[480–489] vWF activity increased in both control and desmopressin-treated patient groups, thus explaining the absence of a salutary effect of desmopressin on blood loss[485] (Figure 31-31). Desmopressin-induced release of t-PA does not overcome its hemostatic action during cardiac surgery because antifibrinolytic therapy fails to uncover an additional hemostatic effect of desmopressin.[487]

Which subgroups of patients undergoing cardiac surgery might benefit from desmopressin? Certainly, those with uremia or cirrhosis. Those who display decreased maximum amplitude on TEG for whatever reason constitute a third group.[489] The heparinase-augmented TEG permits timely identification of patients in this subgroup.

Desmopressin afforded no hemostatic benefit to patients taking aspirin before cardiac surgery,[486,487] and the bulk of evidence currently points away from desmopressin as a prophylactic hemostatic agent for patients undergoing elective cardiac surgery.[430]

Synthetic Antifibrinolytics

Synthetic antifibrinolytics, simple molecules (see Figure 31-30) and analogs of the amino acid lysine, bind to plasminogen and plasmin, thus inhibiting binding of plasminogen at the lysine residues of fibrinogen. Antifibrinolytics may be administered intravenously or orally and undergo renal concentration and excretion with a plasma half-life of about 80 minutes. Effective fibrinolysis inhibition requires an intravenous loading dose of 10 mg/kg for TA followed by 1 mg/kg/hr or

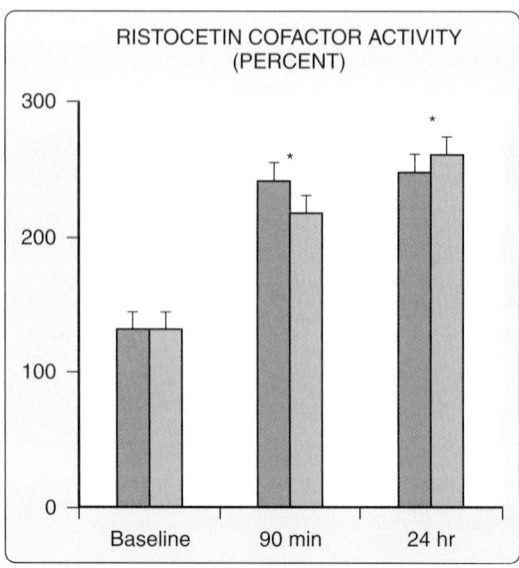

Figure 31-31 At 90 minutes and 24 hours after receiving desmopressin (*green bars*), ristocetin cofactor (von Willebrand factor) activity was not different from a placebo-treated group (*purple bars*). However, in each group, ristocetin cofactor activity increased (*asterisks*) from baseline values, possibly from surgical stress. Blood loss did not differ in the two groups. Error bars denote standard error of the mean. (*Modified from Hackmann T, Gascoyne RD, Naiman SC, et al: A trial of desmopressin [1-desamino, 8-D-arginine vasopressin] to reduce blood loss in uncomplicated cardiac surgery. N Engl J Med 321:1437, 1989.*)

50 mg/kg of EACA followed by infusion of 25 mg/kg/hr.[490,491] Infusion rates require downward adjustment when serum creatinine concentration is increased. Plasma concentrations of TA achieve greater values with decreasing glomerular function. The author's practice is to administer only a loading dose of TA to patients with serum creatinine concentrations in excess of 2.0 mg/dL. Antifibrinolytics are not given to patients with significant upper urinary tract bleeding or consumptive coagulopathy because they prevent the clot lysis needed for continued patency of the ureters or circulatory system, respectively. However, they can also halt ongoing consumption.[492]

Pharmacokinetic studies demonstrated a need to readminister a bolus of EACA on institution of CPB.[491,493] This may not apply to TA,[494] perhaps because of a larger volume of distribution of this drug, although definitive data are still lacking.

Antifibrinolytics aid clotting in patients with hemophilia and patients with vWD by blocking lysis of whatever clot can form.[495,496] Spontaneous bleeding after chemotherapy is decreased with oral TA.[497] Prostate surgery, well known for excessive bleeding from release of t-PA, responds beneficially to antifibrinolytic therapy.[498] Fibrinolysis contributes to bleeding during the anhepatic phase of liver transplantation; antifibrinolytic therapy proves useful in this setting.

Ongoing thrombin activity with varied activation of fibrinolysis plagues cardiac surgery. Figure 31-13 demonstrates thrombin activity as reflected in continuing formation of fibrinopeptides despite adequate heparin anticoagulation. For decades, antifibrinolytics have been proposed as potential hemostatic agents during cardiac surgery. Initial investigations of the efficacy of synthetic antifibrinolytics as hemostatic agents during or after cardiac surgery lacked blinding, randomization, and control groups.[499–507] Most subsequent studies administered EACA after CPB. One study demonstrated a salutary effect in cyanotic children, but not in acyanotic children.[502]

Several investigations, using prophylactic antifibrinolytics, documented savings in blood loss, as well as in blood transfused in a general population of cardiac surgery patients[487,505–507] (Figure 31-32). By commencing administration of TA before CPB, chest tube drainage in the first 12 hours after surgery decreased by 30%, and the likelihood

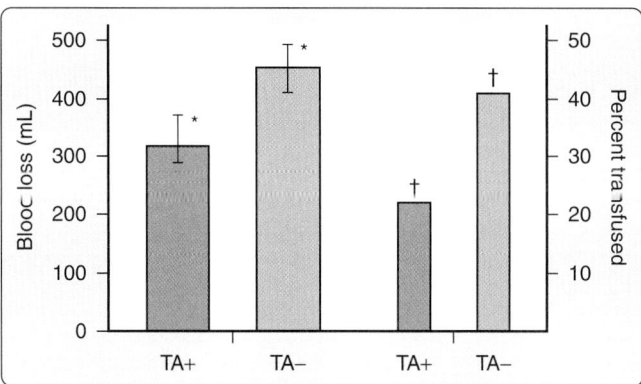

Figure 31-32 Effect of prophylactic tranexamic acid on blood loss (left vertical axis) and on the percentage of patients receiving homologous red blood cell transfusion within 5 days of surgery (right vertical axis). *Purple bars* denote patients who received tranexamic acid; *green bars* denote those not receiving tranexamic acid. *$P < 0.0001$; †$P = 0.011$. *(From Horrow JC, Van Riper DF, Strong MD, et al: The hemostatic effects of tranexamic acid and desmopressin during cardiac surgery. Circulation 84:2063, 1991.)*

of receiving banked blood within 5 days of operation decreased from 41% to 22%.[486] Prophylactic antifibrinolytics may spare platelet function by inhibiting the deleterious effects of plasmin,[508] but administration of very large doses of antifibrinolytics appears to offer no greater savings.[509] Cardiac surgery patients undergoing repeat operation may benefit particularly from prophylactic antifibrinolytic administration.[510]

Some recent reports noted that TA is associated with increased risks for seizure. This has been known for some time in the neurosurgical literature wherein it is considered unwise to place TA directly on the surface of the brain. The mechanism for this potential neurologic toxicity is unknown.[511–515]

Aprotinin

Bovine lung provides the source of the 58-residue polypeptide serine protease inhibitor aprotinin.[516] Aprotinin inhibits a host of proteases, including trypsin, plasmin, kallikrein, and factor XIIa activation of complement[517] (Figure 31-33). The adult intravenous dose for surgical hemostasis is 2 million kallikrein inhibitor units (KIU) for both

patient and CPB circuit, followed by 600,000 KIU/hr.[518,519] The elimination half-life of aprotinin, 7 hours, is considerably longer than that of the synthetic antifibrinolytics; after 6 days, aprotinin continues to be excreted in the urine. Volume-loaded rats respond to aprotinin with decreases in glomerular filtration rate, renal plasma flow, and sodium and potassium excretion; however, no significant renal impairment follows routine clinical use.[520]

Decades ago, several investigations failed to show decreased bleeding after cardiac operations with moderate doses of aprotinin.[521,522] After the serendipitous discovery of unusually dry surgical fields while investigating high-dose aprotinin for respiratory distress syndrome, Royston et al[523] documented more than a fourfold reduction in blood loss during repeat cardiac surgery. Subsequent studies using high-dose aprotinin confirmed conservation of blood products and a reduction in bleeding, ranging from 29% to 50%.[524–530] Figure 31-34 demonstrates the efficacy of aprotinin in this regard. Although studies clearly demonstrated decreased fibrinolysis in aprotinin-treated patient groups, preservation of platelet GPIb or blockade of a plasmin-mediated platelet defect may better explain the hemostatic mechanism of aprotinin.[439,446,447,528]

High-dose aprotinin alone prolonged the celite ACT, leading some investigators to limit use of heparin during CPB.[530] Reports of clot formation during CPB, however, mandated continued use of heparin despite administration of aprotinin. Most investigators simply avoided the celite ACT and used kaolin ACT. The kaolin ACT adsorbs about 98% of aprotinin and any intrinsic AT effect that aprotinin had was mitigated. It was recommended to use the kaolin ACT and keep the length of ACT time the same as if aprotinin was not being used.[531–534] An animal protein, aprotinin caused anaphylaxis, although uncommon (< 1 in 1000).[528–535] Aprotinin cost significantly more than equivalent doses of synthetic antifibrinolytic drugs.[536,537] The group at Duke University analyzed overall cost-effectiveness of aprotinin therapy and found it highly cost-effective.[538] That is in light of its effects on stroke and blood transfusion utilization alone.[539]

Aprotinin has been reviewed in great detail and its usage scrutinized since the last writing of this chapter for the fifth edition of this

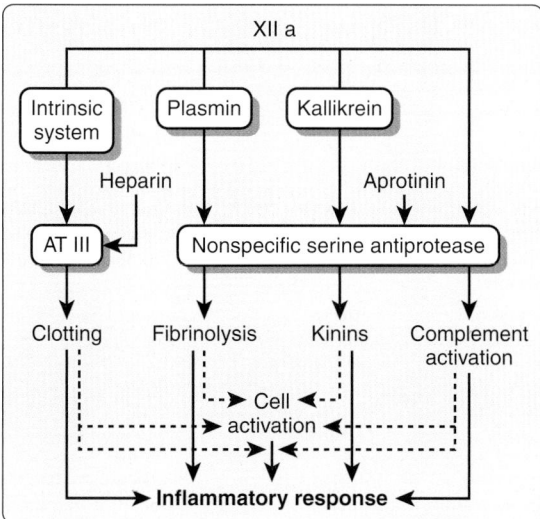

Figure 31-33 Actions of aprotinin on the contact coagulation system, fibrinolytic pathway, and complement activation. ATIII, antithrombin III. *(From Royston D: The serine antiprotease aprotinin [Trasylol]: A novel approach to reducing postoperative bleeding. Blood Coag Fibrin 1:55, 1990.)*

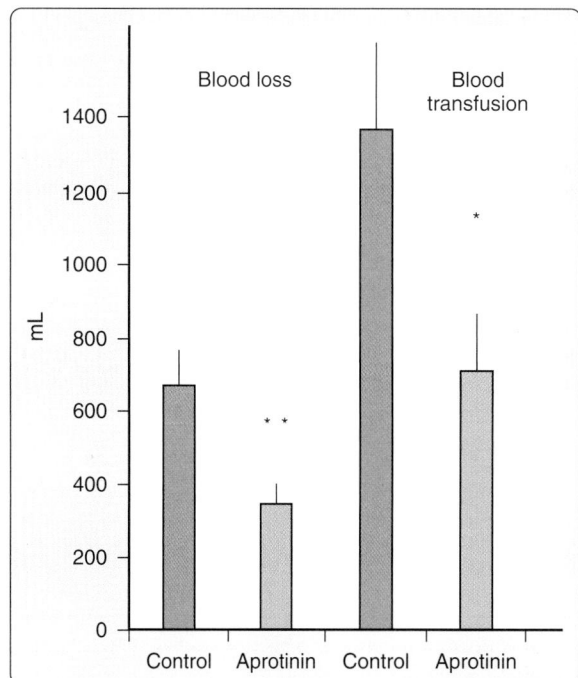

Figure 31-34 Savings in blood loss and blood transfused with aprotinin in a representative study of 22 patients. *Asterisks* denote statistical significance. *(From van Oeveren W, Jansen NJG, Bidstrup BP, et al: Effects of aprotinin on hemostatic mechanisms during cardiopulmonary bypass. Ann Thorac Surg 44:640, 1987.)*

textbook. It was voluntarily withdrawn from the market after two reviews of adverse outcomes by the FDA. Published reports of an association between high-dose aprotinin utilization and renal dysfunction/failure occurred in 2005 and 2006. These publications arose from the Multicentered Study of Perioperative Ischemia EPI-II database.[540] The study was complex, involving more than 4300 cases, and used sophisticated statistical analysis. Unfortunately, the patients who received aprotinin had been selected to get that drug, as opposed to two other antifibrinolytics, by physician choice. This channeling of therapy meant that those patients who were more ill would get aprotinin. To separate out cause and effect from such data becomes impossible; yet, with elegant propensity analysis methods, weighting of certain covariates can be accounted for. The study, although landmark, was widely criticized for all the potential covariates not examined, such as sites (European countries had different practice patterns) and the use of FFP and platelet transfusions. At the same time, a separate report from the University of Toronto examined cases within their own institution.[541] Their study used aprotinin in only the sickest patients (approximately 400 of a total of 10,000 patients). From their large series, they carefully propensity-matched the 400 plus patients to ones of similar age and risk in the overall group of 10,000. There was a propensity for those patients to have more renal dysfunction once the statistics controlled for the other confounders. A third study performed using the Medicare billing database also found that patients who received aprotinin had worse overall outcomes.[542] The use of billing databases has always been fraught with problems in that they are incomplete. Billing data are only summary data and give little of the medical history necessary when trying to balance risk in terms of covariates. Finally, Fergusson et al's[543] study in Canada (BART study) confirmed a greater mortality rate with use of aprotinin compared with either EACA or TA and led to the immediate withdrawal of the drug by the manufacturer and the FDA.[544] Many questions remain about aprotinin and whether it should be available for high-risk cardiac surgical patients in the future. Some clinicians believe that its withdrawal has led to more bleeding and use of blood products and drugs to improve coagulation, all of which have their own complications.

▣ Management of the Bleeding Patient

The initial approach to perioperative bleeding violates the medical paradigm of treatment based on diagnosis. The clinician must simultaneously initiate diagnostic tests, begin treating a presumed cause, and replace lost hemostatic resources. The latter two actions influence all three. The all-encompassing ("shotgun") approach to bleeding after operation should be shunned. Avoiding it will simplify patient management and yield superior results.

Determine the Cause

The complexity of human hemostasis, augmented by unexpected behavior of coagulation tests, can lead to confusion in the diagnosis of bleeding after cardiac surgery. For example, warfarin (Coumadin) inhibits the vitamin K–dependent factors II, VII, IX, and X; yet the aPTT, which involves factors II, IX, and X, typically is not markedly prolonged with warfarin therapy. Likewise, heparin inhibits factors II, IX, X, and XI, yet the PT, which tests factors II and X, remains normal with heparin plasma concentrations less than 1.5 U/mL. As a third example, the thrombin time tests only the ability of activated factor II to convert fibrinogen to fibrin; why should it be much more sensitive to heparin than the ACT or aPTT, which also depend on other heparin-inhibited factors? These examples emphasize to the clinician the importance of seeking expert consultation in hemostasis instead of using inference and theory to diagnose postoperative hemorrhage.

Anatomic sources of bleeding frequently present once systemic blood pressure achieves sufficient magnitude. Some clinicians prefer to identify these sources before chest closure with a provocative test, that is, allowing brief periods of hypertension. Generous chest tube drainage early after surgery suggests an anatomic source. Retained mediastinal clot may engender a consumptive coagulopathy. A widened mediastinum on chest radiograph suggests the need for surgical drainage.

Nonsurgical causes of bleeding (platelets, coagulation factors, and fibrinolysis) usually manifest as a generalized ooze. Inspection of vascular access puncture sites aids in this diagnosis. Bleeding from other areas not manipulated during surgery (stomach, bladder) also may occur.

Coagulation tests aid diagnosis. Because the PT and aPTT usually are prolonged by several seconds after CPB, only values more than 1.5 times control suggest factor deficiency. Increase of the ACT should first suggest unneutralized heparin, then factor deficiency.

A decreased platelet count, usually denoting hemodilution or consumption, requires correction with exogenous platelets in any bleeding patient. However, bleeding patients with insufficient functional platelets may demonstrate normal platelet counts early after operation. For this reason, clinicians have sought rapid diagnostic tests of platelet function and attempted correlation with bleeding after CPB[537,545] (see Chapter 17).

Low plasma fibrinogen occurs from excessive hemodilution or factor consumption and is corrected with cryoprecipitate or FFP. The thrombin time is useful here. Most clinical laboratories can perform this test with rapid turnaround. A prolonged thrombin time denotes unneutralized heparin, insufficient fibrinogen, or high concentrations of fibrin degradation products. Finally, direct measurement of fibrin degradation products denotes fibrinolytic activity. In the absence of a cause for a consumptive coagulopathy, antifibrinolytic therapy may be useful.

Table 31-12 lists a treatment plan for excessive bleeding after cardiac surgery. Interventions appear not in order of likelihood, but rather by priority of consideration. Thus, surgical causes should be ruled out before seizing on the diagnosis of a consumptive coagulopathy. The priority will also vary among institutions, depending on the availability and cost of resources. This table provides a simple algorithm for treating postoperative bleeding. More complete schemes present a daunting level of complexity that deters implementation (Figure 31-35). The material presented in this chapter is intended to assist the clinician in developing, refining, and implementing a personal approach to this problem.

Adjunctive Therapy

Warming

Bleeding patients with core or intermediate zone temperatures less than 35° C will benefit from warming efforts, both passive (warm

TABLE 31-12	Treatment Plan for Excessive Bleeding after Cardiac Surgery	
Action	**Amount**	**Indication**
Rule out surgical cause	—	No oozing at puncture sites; chest radiograph
More protamine	0.5–1 mg/kg	ACT > 150 seconds or aPTT > 1.5 times control
Warm the patient	—	"Core" temperature < 35° C
Apply PEEP*	5–10 cm H_2O	—
Desmopressin	0.3 µg/kg IV	Prolonged bleeding time
Aminocaproic acid	50 mg/kg, then 25 mg/kg/hr	Increased D-dimer or teardrop-shaped TEG tracing
Tranexamic acid	10 mg/kg, then 1 mg/kg/hr	Increased D-dimer or teardrop-shaped TEG tracing
Platelet transfusion	1 U/10 kg	Platelet count < 100,000/mm^3
Fresh frozen plasma	15 mL/kg	PT or aPTT > 1.5 times control
Cryoprecipitate	1 U/4 kg	Fibrinogen < 1 g/L or 100 mg/dL

*Positive end-expiratory pressure (PEEP) is contraindicated in hypovolemia.
ACT, activated coagulation time; aPTT, activated partial thromboplastin time; TEG, thromboelastograph.

Management of the Bleeding Cardiac Surgical Patient

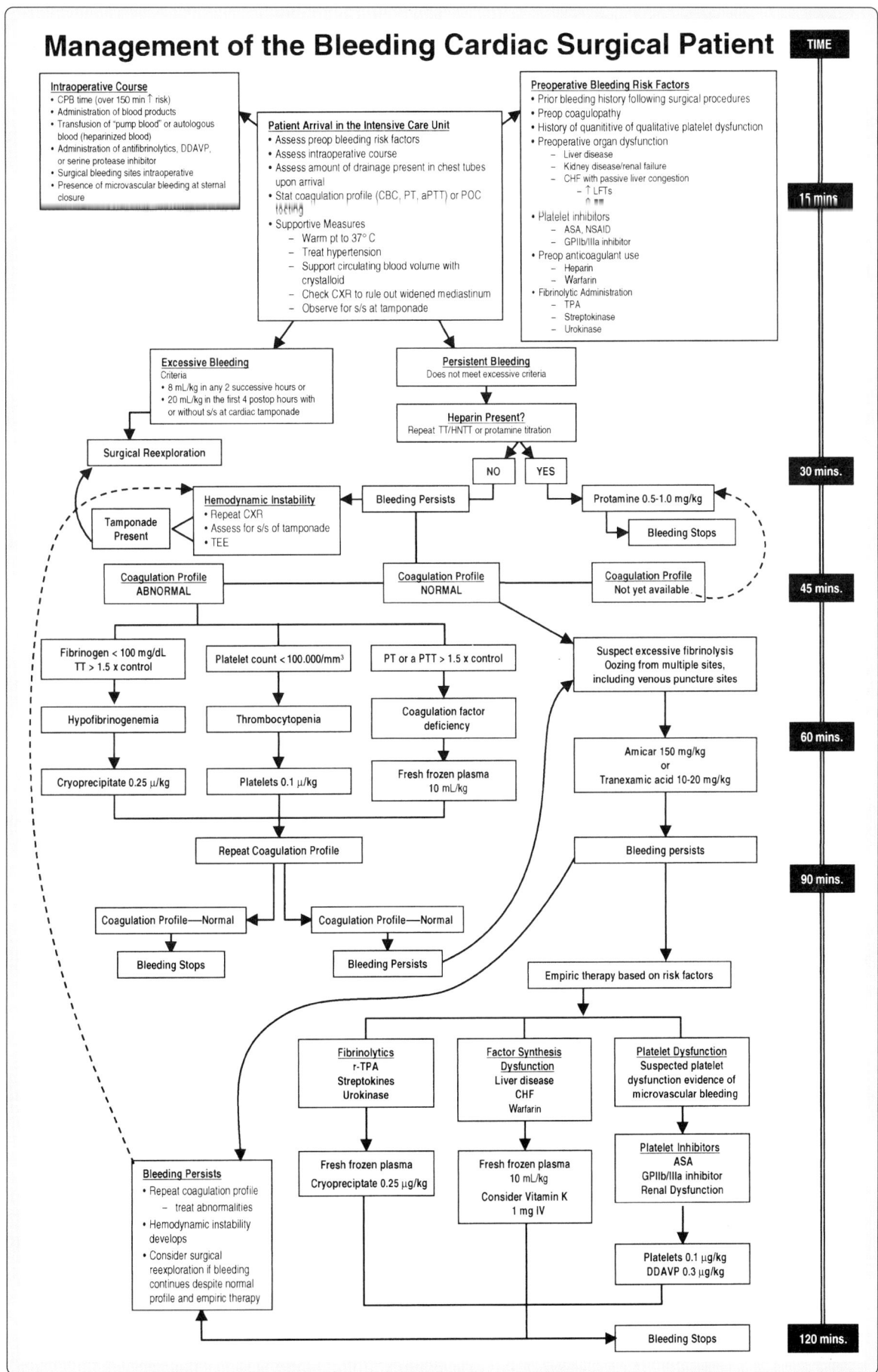

Figure 31-35 **Example of a scheme for treating excessive bleeding.** aPTT, activated partial thromboplastin time; ASA, acetylsalicylic acid; CBC, complete blood cell count; CHF, congestive heart failure; CPB, cardiopulmonary bypass; CXR, chest radiograph; GP, glycoprotein; NSAID, nonsteroidal anti-inflammatory drug; POC, point of care; PT, prothrombin time; r-TPA, recombinant tissue plasminogen activator; TEE, transesophageal echocardiography; TPA, tissue plasminogen activator. (*From Milas B, Johes D, Gorman R: Management of bleeding and coagulopathy after heart surgery. Semin Thorac Cardiovasc Surg 12:326, 2000.*)

ambient temperature, adequate body coverings, low ventilator fresh gas flows, airway heat and humidity exchangers) and active (heated humidifiers, warmed intravenous fluids, forced air convective warming blankets). All too often, in the effort to maintain intravascular volume, intensive care unit personnel administer liters of room-temperature ($\leq 20°$ C) or refrigerated ($0°$ C to $4°$ C) fluids, which render patients hypothermic. Ready availability of fluid warmers reduces the possibility of the treatment of hemorrhage becoming its continuing cause.

Positive End-Expiratory Pressure

One popular method to limit bleeding after cardiac surgery is application of positive end-expiratory pressure (5 to 10 cm H_2O).[546,547] A tamponade effect in the mediastinum may explain this salutary effect. Unfortunately, controlled studies have not confirmed this benefit.[548,549] In addition, excessive pressure impedes venous return, worsening hemodynamics in the patient with hypovolemia.

Blood Pressure

Maintenance of systemic blood pressure in the low-normal range promotes tissue perfusion while limiting leakage around suture lines. Adequate depth of anesthesia during surgery and sufficient postoperative analgesia and sedation should be verified before initiating vasodilator therapy.

Blood Products

The bleeding patient becomes subject to additional hemostatic derangements. The need to maintain intravascular blood volume arises in nearly all cases before identification of the cause of bleeding. Protracted hypovolemia can lead to shock. Consumptive coagulopathy accompanies prolonged shock,[550] and failure to treat hypovolemia from bleeding may induce this second hemostatic abnormality. Clear fluid or colloid will replenish intravascular volume; however, RBCs, platelets, and coagulation factors become diluted when continued bleeding is treated with such replacement. Also, packed RBCs and banked whole blood do not provide platelets or sufficient factor V or factor VIII to maintain hemostasis. Although routine prophylactic administration of FFP or platelets plays no role in modern cardiac surgical care,[551] demonstration of a platelet count less than 100,000/mm³ or prolongation of the PT or aPTT despite adequate heparin neutralization *in a patient actively bleeding* is an indication for platelet or plasma replacement.[551]

Banked blood should be infused to maintain a hemoglobin concentration that allows appropriate oxygen delivery to tissues. In the absence of coagulation tests to guide therapy, when reconstituted RBCs adequately replace blood lost, platelets should be given after 15 units of RBCs to patients undergoing noncardiac surgery.[551,552] Because patients undergoing cardiac surgery also experience the hemodiluting and antihemostatic effects of CPB, the prudent clinician will commence platelet and factor replenishment earlier in the course of hemorrhage while awaiting laboratory confirmation. Each unit of platelet concentrate supplies about 10¹¹ platelets, which increases platelet count by about 20,000/mm³ in the adult. Enough plasma accompanies platelet concentrates to supply the equivalent of 1.0 to 1.5 units plasma for each 6 units platelets.[551]

Shed mediastinal blood can be collected and given back to patients using a closed drainage system. The drainage fluid, often collected in citrate, contains little fibrinogen. Presence of tissue and other debris in this fluid suggests the need for filtration before reinfusion. Shed mediastinal fluid supplies RBCs without risk for viral transmission via allogeneic blood products (see Chapter 29).[552]

Drugs

Desmopressin often fails in the treatment of established bleeding,[553] despite initial uncontrolled studies to the contrary.[482,554] The efficacy of desmopressin in treating surgical hemorrhage associated with aspirin therapy also remains anecdotal.[555] Of course, desmopressin

administration carries no risk for viral disease transmission; therefore, its substitution for otherwise unneeded, prophylactic FFP or platelets prevents potential patient harm.

Although antifibrinolytic therapy initiated before CPB decreases bleeding after surgery, its efficacy after CPB or once bleeding is established remains controversial. Two studies of adult patients undergoing CABG yielded opposite conclusions regarding a savings of blood.[503,504] Lack of sufficient antifibrinolytic dose (only 4 or 5g EACA loading) confounds both investigations. In the control of postoperative hemorrhage, antifibrinolytic therapy is suggested by any of the following: a TEG demonstrating clot lysis, fibrin degradation products of 40 µg/mL or more, or increased thrombin time coexisting with normal fibrinogen and known absence of heparin.

Recombinant factor VIIa (rFVIIa; NovoSeven) has been approved for use in patients with hemophilia who are resistant to factor VIII concentrates. When rFVIIa is administered, it binds to tissue factor and activates factor X, leading to thrombin and fibrin formation, which then activate platelets. Thrombin generation and clotting take place on the surface of platelets and at sites of injury.[556–559] Numerous reports have been published of the off-label use of this "rescue agent" to stop bleeding in surgical patients, including cardiac surgical patients after CPB.

In patients with hemophilia, the recommended dose is 90 µg/kg. However, reports in cardiac surgical patients have suggested doses of 30 µg/kg, while continuing ongoing component therapy and monitoring the PT/international normalized ratio. The half-life is about 2 hours, and the dose may have to be repeated if bleeding continues. Most of the anecdotal reports have been positive with a marked decrease in bleeding taking place.[560–562] This treatment should not be used in the presence of disseminated intravascular coagulation or sepsis. Other potential indications for it include warfarin reversal, thrombocytopenia, factor XI deficiency, hepatic failure, vWD, reversal of fondaparinux, and in cardiac surgery after DHCA or after use of direct thrombin inhibitors. Further studies are necessary to determine dosing, safety, and efficacy for these potential uses.

Perspective on Bleeding after Cardiac Surgery

The differential diagnosis of bleeding after cardiac surgery derives from the elements of hemostasis outlined in the first section of this chapter. After initiating action to determine the cause, the prudent clinician ensures continued adequacy of circulating volume and, when indicated, of platelets and coagulation factors. Above all, it is important to avoid embracing one possibility, no matter how obvious, as the cause of bleeding until confirmatory evidence becomes available. In this way, the actual cause will not go undisclosed.[563]

CONCLUSIONS

The basic science and clinical knowledge of coagulation, hemostasis, and thrombosis have evolved dramatically since 1980. Continued insights and advances in understanding pathophysiology and in developing pharmaceutical preparations will continue to have significant impact on clinical practice in the future. Perhaps the future will hold great strides in genetics and other realms. Of particular interest is a new focus on short-and long-term outcomes after CABG surgery. Genetics is just now beginning to be studied in the coagulation field, and although a number of genetic polymorphisms have been discovered, it is not known which ones are the most important. It is also not known yet what the implications are if a particular patient has one or more of these genetic polymorphisms. Some genetic abnormalities make patients more likely to thrombose or have early graft atherosclerosis, whereas others may affect drug metabolism or the way in which patients react with inflammation. The future may also involve genetic engineering and correction of defects (see Chapter 30).[564–566]

REFERENCES

1. Spiess BD: Coagulation function and monitoring. In Lichtor JL, editor: *Atlas of Clinical Anesthesia*, Philadelphia, 1996, Current Medicine.
2. Spiess BD: *The Relationships Between Coagulation, Inflammation and Endothelium—A Pyramid Towards Outcome [SCA monograph]*, Baltimore, 2002, Lippincott Williams & Wilkins.
3. Boyle EM Jr, Morgan EN, Verrier ED: The endothelium disturbed: The procoagulant response. In Spiess BD, editor: *The Relationship Between Coagulation, Inflammation and Endothelium—A Pyramid Towards Outcome [SCA monograph]*, Baltimore, 2002, Lippincott Williams & Wilkins, p 79.
4. [illegible] response, *Ann Thorac Surg* 62:1549, 1996.
5. Colman RW, Marder VJ, Salzman EW, et al: Overview of hemostasis. In Colman RW, Hirsh J, Marder VJ, Salzman EW, editors: *Hemostasis and Thrombosis*, ed 3, Philadelphia, 1994, JB Lippincott, p 3.
6. Mackman N: Regulation of tissue factor gene expression in human monocytic and endothelial cells, *Haemostasis* 26(Suppl 1):17, 1996.
7. Edmunds LH Jr: Blood-surface interactions during cardiopulmonary bypass, *J Card Surg* 8:404, 1993.
8. Boisclair MD, Lane DA, Philippau H, et al: Mechanisms of thrombin generation during surgery and cardiopulmonary bypass, *Blood* 82:3350, 1993.
9. Almus FE, Rao LV, Rapaport SI: Decreased inducibility of tissue factor activity on human umbilical vein endothelial cells cultured with endothelial cell growth factor and heparin, *Thromb Res* 50:339, 1988.
10. Rao LV, Rapaport SI, Lorenzi M: Enhancement by human umbilical vein endothelial cells of factor Xa-catalyzed activation of factor VII, *Blood* 71:791, 1988.
11. Krishnaswamy S, Mann KG, Nesheim ME: The prothrombinase-catalyzed activation of prothrombin proceeds through the intermediate meizathrombin in an ordered, sequential reaction, *J Biol Chem* 261:8977, 1986.
12. Jones A, Geczy CL: Thrombin and factor Xa enhance the production of interleukin, *Immunology* 71:236, 1990.
13. Salvesen G, Pizzo SV: Proteinase inhibitors: Alpha-macroglobulins, serpins, and kinins. In Colman RW, Hirsh J, Marder VJ, Salzman EW, editors: *Hemostasis and Thrombosis*, ed 3, Philadelphia, 1994, JB Lippincott, p 241.
14. Spiess BD: Heparin: Beyond an anticoagulant. In Spiess BD, editor: *The Relationship Between Coagulation, Inflammation and Endothelium—A Pyramid Towards Outcome*, Baltimore, 2002, Lippincott Williams & Wilkins, pp 169.
15. Van Norman GA, Gernsheimer T, Chandler WL, et al: Indicators of fibrinolysis during cardiopulmonary bypass after exogenous antithrombin III administration for antithrombin deficiency, *J Cardiothorac Vasc Anesth* 11:760, 1997.
16. Hashimoto Y, Yamgishi M, Sasaki T, et al: Heparin and antithrombin III levels during cardiopulmonary bypass: Correlation with subclinical plasma coagulation, *Ann Thorac Surg* 58:799, 1994.
17. Despotis GJ, Levine V, Joist JH, et al: Antithrombin III during cardiac surgery: Effect on response of activated clotting time to heparin and relationship to markers of hemostatic activation, *Anesth Analg* 85:498, 1997.
18. Levy JH, Despotis GJ, Szlam F, et al: Recombinant human transgenic antithrombin in cardiac surgery: A dose finding study, *Anesthesiology* 96:1095, 2002.
19. Brister SJ, Buchanan MR: Heparinless cardiopulmonary bypass revisited: A newer strategy to avoid heparin-related bleeding using dermatan sulfate, *J Thorac Cardiovasc Anesth* 9:317, 1995.
20. Esmon CT, Owen WG: Identification of an endothelial cell cofactor for thrombin-catalyzed activation of protein C, *Proc Natl Acad Sci U S A* 78:2249, 1981.
21. DeFouw NJ, van Hinsbergh VW, deJong YF, et al: The interaction of activated protein C and thrombin with the plasminogen activator inhibitor released from human endothelial cells, *Thromb Haemost* 57:176, 1987.
22. Novotny WF, Girard TJ, Miletich JP, et al: Purification and characterization of the lipoprotein-associated coagulation inhibitor from human plasma, *J Biol Chem* 264:18832, 1989.
23. Bajaj MS, Kuppuswamy MN, Saito H, et al: Cultured normal human hepatocytes do not synthesize lipoprotein-associated coagulation inhibitor: Evidence that endothelium is the principal site of its synthesis, *Proc Natl Acad Sci USA* 87:8869, 1990.
24. Novotny WF, Girard TJ, Miletich JP, et al: Platelets secrete a coagulation inhibitor functionally and antigenically similar to the lipoprotein-associated coagulation inhibitor, *Blood* 72:2020, 1988.
25. Hansen JB, Sarset PM: Differential effects of low molecular weight heparin and unfractionated heparin on circulating levels of antithrombin and tissue factor pathway inhibitor (TFPI): A possible mechanism for difference in therapeutic efficacy, *Thromb Res* 91:177, 1998.
26. Soejima H, Ogawa H, Yasue H, et al: Plasma tissue factor pathway inhibitor and tissue factor antigen levels after administration of heparin in patients with angina pectoris, *Thromb Res* 93:17, 1999.
27. Jeske W, Hoppensteadt D, Callas D, et al: Pharmacologic profiling of recombinant tissue factor pathway inhibitor, *Semin Thromb Hemost* 22:213, 1996.
28. Kojima T, Gando S, Kemmotsu O, et al: Another point of view on the mechanism of thrombin generation during cardiopulmonary bypass: Role of tissue factor inhibitor, *J Cardiothorac Vasc Anesth* 15:60, 2001.
29. Adams MJ, Cardigan RA, Marchant WA, et al: Tissue factor pathway inhibitor antigen and activity in 96 patients receiving heparin for cardiopulmonary bypass, *J Cardiothoracic Vasc Anesth* 16:59, 2002.
30. Fischer R, Kuppe H, Koster A: Impact of heparin management on release of tissue factor pathway inhibitor during cardiopulmonary bypass, *Anesthesiology* 100:1040, 2004.
31. Tsai H, Sussman I, Nagel R: Shear stress enhances the proteolysis of von Willebrand factor in normal plasma, *Blood* 83:2171, 1994.
32. Asakai R, Chung DW, Davie EW, et al: Factor XI deficiency in Ashkenazi Jews in Israel, *N Engl J Med* 325:153, 1991.
33. Brettler DB, Levine PH: Clinical manifestations and therapy of inherited coagulation factor deficiencies. In Colman RW, Hirsh J, Marder VJ, et al: *Hemostasis and Thrombosis*, ed 3, Philadelphia, 1994, JB Lippincott, p 169.
34. Mannucci PM: Desmopressin: A nontransfusional form of treatment for congenital and acquired bleeding disorders, *Blood* 72:1449, 1988.
35. Blajchman MA, Hirst R, Perrault RA: Blood component therapy in anaesthetic practice, *Can Anaesth Soc J* 30:382, 1983.
36. Van Aken WG: Preparation of plasma derivatives. In Rossi EC, Simon TL, Moss GS, et al: *Principles of Transfusion Medicine*, ed 2, Baltimore, 1996, Williams & Wilkins, p 403.
37. Palenzo DA, Sadr FS: Coronary artery bypass grafting in a patient with haemophilia B, *Perfusion* 10:265, 1995.
38. Flier JS, Underhill LH: Molecular and cellular biology of blood coagulation, *N Engl J Med* 326:800, 1992.
39. Bertina RM, Koeleman BPC, Koster T, et al: Mutation in blood coagulation factor V associated with resistance to activated protein C, *Nature* 369:64, 1994.
40. Florell SR, Rodgers GM: Inherited thrombotic disorders. An update, *Am J Hematol* 54:53, 1997.
41. Koster T, Rosendaal FR, Briet E, et al: Protein C deficiency in a controlled series of unselected outpatients: An infrequent but clear risk for venous thrombosis, *Blood* 85:2756, 1995.
42. Rodgers GM, Chandler WL: Laboratory and clinical aspects of inherited thrombotic disorders, *Am J Hematol* 41:113, 1992.
43. Mayer O, Filipovsky J, Hromadka M, et al: Treatment of hyperhomocysteinemia with folic acid, *J Cardiovasc Pharmacol* 39:851, 2002.
44. Rinder CS: Platelet and their interactions. In Spiess BD, editor: *The Relationship Between Coagulation,* [illegible], Baltimore, [illegible], Lippincott [illegible] Wilkins, p 107.
45. Kroll MH, Schafer A: Biochemical mechanisms of platelet activation, *Blood* 74:1181, 1989.
46. Savage B, Saldivar E, Ruggeri ZM: Initiation of platelet adhesion by arrest onto fibrinogen or translocation on von Willebrand factor, *Cell* 84:289, 1996.
47. Celi A, Pellegrini G, Lorenzet R, et al: P-selectin induces the expression of tissue factor on monocytes, *Proc Natl Acad Sci U S A* 91:8767, 1994.
48. Hynes RO: Integrins: Versatility, modulation, and signaling in cell adhesion, *Cell* 69:11, 1992.
49. Kessler CM: The pharmacology of aspirin, heparin, coumarin, and thrombolytic agents, *Chest* 99:97S, 1991.
50. Montgomery RR: Coller BS: von Willebrand disease. In Colman RW, Hirsh J, Marder VJ, et al: *Hemostasis and Thrombosis*, ed 3, Philadelphia, 1994, JB Lippincott, p 134.
51. Slaughter TF, Mody EA, Oldham HN Jr, et al: Management of a patient with type IIC von Willebrand's disease during coronary artery bypass graft surgery, *Anesthesiology* 78:195, 1993.
52. Steering Committee of the Physicians' Health Study Research Group: Final report on the aspirin component of the ongoing Physicians' Health Study, *N Engl J Med* 321:129, 1989.
53. George J, Shattil SJ: The clinical importance of acquired abnormalities of platelet function, *N Engl J Med* 324:27, 1991.
54. Goldman S, Copeland J, Moritz T, et al: Improvement in early saphenous vein graft patency after coronary artery bypass surgery with antiplatelet therapy: Results of a Veterans Administration cooperative study, *Circulation* 77:1324, 1988.
55. Taggart DP, Siddiqui A, Wheatley DJ: Low-dose preoperative aspirin therapy, postoperative blood loss and transfusion requirements, *Ann Thorac Surg* 50:425, 1990.
56. Bashein G, Nessly ML, Rice AL, et al: Preoperative aspirin therapy and reoperation for bleeding after coronary artery bypass surgery, *Arch Intern Med* 151:89, 1991.
57. Weksler BB, Pett SB, Aloso D, et al: Differential inhibition by aspirin of vascular and platelet prostaglandin synthesis in atherosclerotic patients, *N Engl J Med* 308:800, 1983.
58. Rajah SM, Salter MCP, Donaldson DR: Acetylsalicylic acid and dipyridamole improve the early patency of aorta-coronary bypass grafts, *J Thorac Cardiovasc Surg* 90:373, 1985.
59. Karwande S, Weksler BB, Gay WA, et al: Effect of preoperative antiplatelet drugs on vascular prostacyclin synthesis, *Ann Thorac Surg* 43:318, 1987.
60. Rawitscher RE, Jones JW, McCoy TA, et al: A prospective study of aspirin effect on red blood cell loss in cardiac surgery, *J Cardiovasc Surg* 32:1, 1991.
61. Tuman KJ, McCarthy RJ, O'Connor CJ, et al: Aspirin does not increase allogeneic blood transfusion in reoperative coronary artery surgery, *Anesth Analg* 83:1178, 1996.
62. Reich DL, Patel GC, Vela-Cantos F, et al: Aspirin does not increase homologous blood requirements in elective coronary bypass surgery, *Anesth Analg* 79:4, 1994.
63. Baeuerle JJ, Mongan PD, Hosking MP: An assessment of the duration of cephapirin-induced coagulation abnormalities as measured by thromboelastography, *J Cardiothorac Vasc Anesth* 7:422, 1993.
64. Juni P, Nartey L, Reichenbach S, et al: Risk of cardiovascular events and rofecoxib: Cumulative meta-analysis, *Lancet* 364:2021, 2004.
65. Lange RA, Hillis LD: Antiplatelet therapy for ischemic heart disease, *N Engl J Med* 350:277, 2004.
66. Kobasr AL, Koessler J, Rajkovic MS, et al: Prostacyclin receptor stimulation facilitates detection of human platelet P2Y (12) inhibition by the PFA-100 system, *Platelets* 21:112–116, 2010.
67. Linnemann B, Schwonberg J, Rechner AR, et al: Assessment of clopidogrel non-response by the PFA-100 system using the new test cartridge INNOVANCE PFA P2Y, *Ann Hematol* 89:597–605, 2010.
68. Bouman H, Parlak E, van Werkum J, et al: Which platelet function test is suitable to monitor clopidogrel responsiveness? A pharmokinetic analysis on the active metabolite of clopidogrel, *J Thromb Haemost* 8:482–488, 2010.
69. Eriksson AC, Jonasson L, Lindahl TL, et al: Static platelet adhesion, flow cytometry and serum TXB2 levels for monitoring platelet inhibiting treatment with ASA and clopidogrel in coronary artery disease: A randomized cross-over study, *J Transl Med* 9:42, 2009.
70. Gibbs NM: Point-of-care assessement of antiplatelet agenst in the perioperative period: A review, *Anaesth Intensive Care* 37:354–369, 2009.
71. Varenhorst C, James S, Erlinge D, et al: Assessment of P2Y(12) inhibition with the point-of-care device VerifyNow P2Y12 in patients treated with prasugrelor clopidogrel coadministered with aspirin, *Am Heart J* 157:562 e1–562 e9, 2009.
72. Scharbert G, Auer A, Kozek-Langenecker S: Evaluation of the platelet mapping assay on rotational thromboelastometry ROTEM, *Platelets* 20:125–130, 2009.
73. von Heyman C, Schoenfeld H, Sander M, et al: Clopidogrel-related refractory bleeding after coronary artery bypass graft surgery: A rationale fo r the use of coagulation factor concentrates? *Heart Surg Forum* 8:E–39–E-41, 2005.
74. Teufelsbauer H, Proidl S, Havel M, et al: Early activation of hemostasis during cardiopulmonary bypass. Evidence for thrombin-mediated hyperfibrinolysis, *Thromb Haemost* 68:250, 1992.
75. Goldberg M, Colonna-Romano P, Babins N: Emergency coronary artery bypass surgery following intracoronary streptokinase, *Anesthesiology* 61:601, 1984.
76. Levy JH, Gill R, Nussmeier NA, et al: Repletion of factor XIII following cardiopulmonary bypass using a recombinant A-subunit homodimer. A preliminary report, *Thromb Haemost* 102:765–771, 2009.
77. Shigemura N, Kawamura T, Minami M, et al: Successful factor XIII administration for persistent chylothorax after lung transplantation for lymphangioleiomyomatosis, *Ann Thorac Surg* 88:1003–1006, 2009.
78. Gödje O, Gallmeier U, Schelian M, et al: Coagulation factor XIII reduces postoperative bleeding after coronary surgery with extracorporeal circulation, *Thorac Cardiovasc Surg* 54:26–33, 2006.
79. McLean J: The discovery of heparin, *Circulation* 19:75, 1959.
80. Rodén L: Highlights in the history of heparin. In Lane DA, Lindahl U, editors: *Heparin*, Boca Raton, FL, 1989, CRC Press, p 1.
81. Casu B: Structure of heparin and heparin fragments. In Ofosu FA, Danishefsky I, Hirsh J, editors: *Heparin and Related Polysaccharides*, New York, 1989, New York Academy of Sciences, p 1.
82. Holmer E: Low-molecular-weight heparin. In Lane DA, Lindahl U, editors: *Heparin*, Boca Raton, FL, 1989, CRC Press, p 575.
83. Freedman JE, Loscalzo J: New antithrombitic strategies. In Loscalzo J, Schafer AI, editors: *Thrombosis and Hemorrhage*, ed 3, Philadelphia, 2003, Lippincott Williams & Wilkins, p 978–995.
84. Nader HB, Dietrich CP: Natural occurrence and possible biological role of heparin. In Lane DA, Lindahl U, editors: *Heparin*, Boca Raton, FL, 1989, CRC Press, p 81.

85. Barrowcliffe TW: Heparin assays and standardization. In Lane DA, Lindahl U, editors: *Heparin*, Boca Raton, FL, 1989, CRC Press, p 393.
86. Coyne E, Outschoorn AS: Some thoughts on a new USP heparin assay—Aren't we ready for an upgrade? *Pharmacopeial Forum* 1492:1991.
87. Howell WH: Heparin, an anticoagulant, *Am J Physiol* 631:434, 1922.
88. Majerus PW, Broze GJ, Miletich JP, et al: Anticoagulant, thrombolytic, and antiplatelet drugs. In Hardman JG, Limbird LE, Molinoff PB, et al: *Goodman & Gilman's The Pharmacological Basis of Therapeutics*, ed 9, New York, 1996, McGraw-Hill, p 1341.
89. Albada H, Nieuwenhuis HK, Sixma JJ: Pharmacokinetics of standard and low-molecular-weight heparin. In Lane DA, Lindahl U, editors: *Heparin*, Boca Raton, FL, 1989, CRC Press, p 417.
90. deSwart CAM, Nijmeyer B, Roelofs JMM, et al: Kinetics of intravenously administered heparin in normal humans, *Blood* 60:1251, 1982.
91. Mahadoo J, Heibert L, Jaques LB: Vascular sequestration of heparin, *Thromb Res* 12:79, 1978.
92. Glimelius B, Busch C: Binding of heparin on the surface of cultured human endothelial cells, *Thromb Res* 12:773, 1978.
93. Cipolle RJ, Seifert RD, Neilan BA, et al: Heparin kinetics: Variables related to disposition and dosage, *Clin Pharmacol Ther* 29:387, 1981.
94. Cook JJ, Niewiarowski S, Yan Z, et al: Platelet factor 4 efficiently reverses heparin anticoagulation in the rat without adverse effects of the heparin-protamine complexes, *Circulation* 85:1102, 1992.
95. Okuno T, Crockatt D: Platelet factor, activity and thromboembolic episodes, *Am J Clin Pathol* 67:351, 1977.
96. Sette H, Hughes RD, Langley PG, et al: Heparin response and clearance in acute and chronic liver disease, *Thromb Haemost* 54:591, 1985.
97. Kesteven PJ, Ahred A, Aps C, et al: Protamine sulphate and rebound following open heart surgery, *J Cardiovasc Surg* 27:600, 1986.
98. Gravlee GP, Brauer SD, Roy RC, et al: Predicting the pharmacodynamics of heparin: A clinical evaluation of the Hepcon System 4, *J Cardiothorac Anesth* 1:379, 1987.
99. Estes JW: Kinetics of the anticoagulant effect of heparin, *JAMA* 212:1492, 1970.
100. Seifert R, Borchert W, Letendre P, et al: Heparin kinetics during hemodialysis: Variation in sensitivity, distribution volume, and dosage, *Ther Drug Monit* 8:32, 1986.
101. Ofosu FA: Antithrombotic mechanisms of heparin and related compounds. In Lane DA, Lindahl U, editors: *Heparin*, Boca Raton, FL, 1989, CRC Press, p 433.
102. Jordan RE, Oosta GM, Gardner WT, et al: The kinetics of hemostatic enzyme-antithrombin interactions in the presence of low-molecular-weight heparin, *J Biol Chem* 225:10,081, 1980.
103. Barrowcliffe TW, Thomas DP: Anticoagulant activities of heparin and fragments. In Ofosu FA, Danishefsky I, Hirsh J, editors: *Heparin and Related Polysaccharides*, New York, 1989, New York Academy of Sciences, p 132.
104. Bjork I, Olson ST, Shore JD: Molecular mechanisms of the accelerating effect of heparin on the reactions between antithrombin and clotting proteinases. In Lane DA, Lindahl U, editors: *Heparin*, Boca Raton, FL, 1989, CRC Press, p 229.
105. Holmer E, Soderberg K, Berggvist D, et al: Heparin and its low-molecular-weight derivatives: Anticoagulant and antithrombotic properties, *Haemostasis* 16(Suppl 2):1, 1986.
106. Gravlee GP, Haddon WS, Rothberger HK, et al: Heparin dosing and monitoring for cardiopulmonary bypass, *J Thorac Cardiovasc Surg* 99:518, 1990.
107. Tanaka K, Takao M, Yada I, et al: Alterations in coagulation and fibrinolysis associated with cardiopulmonary bypass during open heart surgery, *J Cardiothorac Anesth* 3:181, 1989.
108. Davies GC, Sobel M, Salzman EW: Elevated plasma fibrinopeptide A and thromboxane B2 levels during cardiopulmonary bypass, *Circulation* 61:808, 1980.
109. Slaughter TF, LeBleu TH, Douglas JM Jr, et al: Characterization of prothrombin activation during cardiac surgery by hemostatic molecular markers, *Anesthesiology* 80:520, 1994.
110. Racanelli A, Fareed J, Walenga JM, et al: Biochemical and pharmacologic studies on the protamine interactions with heparin, its fractions and fragments, *Semin Thromb Hemost* 11:176, 1985.
111. Avidan MS, Levy JH, Scholz J, et al: A phase II double-blind placebo controlled, multicenter study on the efficacy of recombinant human anti-thrombin in heparin-resistant patients scheduled to undergo cardiopulmonary bypass, *Anesthesiology* 102:276–284, 2005.
112. Rannucci M, Isgrò G, Cazzaniga A, et al: Different patterns of heparin resistance: Therapeutic implications, *Perfusion* 17:199–204, 2002.
113. Staples MH, Dunton RF, Karlson KJ, et al: Heparin resistance after preoperative heparin therapy or intraaortic balloon pumping, *Ann Thorac Surg* 57:1211–1216, 1994.
114. Williams MR, D'Ambra AB, Beck JR, et al: A randomized trial of antithrombin concentrate for treatment of heparin resistance, *Ann Thorac Surg* 70:873–877, 2000.
115. Levy JH: Heparin resistance and antithrombin: Should it still be called heparin resistance? *J Cardiothorac Vasc Anesth* 18:129, 2004.
116. Koster A, Fischer T, Grunendel M, et al: Management of heparin: Resistance and cardiopulmonary bypass: The effect of 5 different anticoagulation strategies on hemostatic activation, *J Cardiothorac Vasc Anesth* 18:131, 2004.
117. Soloway HB, Christansen TW: Heparin anticoagulation during cardiopulmonary bypass in an antithrombin III-deficient patient. Implications relative to the etiology of heparin, *Am J Clin Pathol* 73:723, 1980.
118. Collen D, Schetz J, deCock F, et al: Metabolism of antithrombin III (heparin cofactor) in man: Effects of venous thrombosis and of heparin administration, *Eur J Clin Invest* 7:27, 1977.
119. Linden MD, Schneider M, Baker S, et al: Decreased concentration of antithrombin after preoperative therapeutic heparin does not cause heparin resistance during cardiopulmonary bypass, *J Cardiothorac Vasc Anesth* 18:131–135, 2004.
120. Andersson G, Fagrell B, Holngren K, et al: Antithrombin III in patients with acute deep vein thrombosis during heparin treatment (subcutaneous and intravenous) and during and after treatment with oral coumarins, *Thromb Res* 34:333, 1984.
121. Holm HA, Kalvenes S, Abidgaard U: Changes in plasma antithrombin (heparin cofactor activity) during intravenous heparin therapy: Observations in 198 patients with deep venous thrombosis, *Scand J Haematol* 35:564, 1985.
122. Marciniak E, Gockerman JP: Heparin-induced decrease in circulating antithrombin III, *Lancet* 1:581, 1977.
123. deSwart CA, Nijmeyer B, Andersson LO, et al: Elimination of intravenously administered radiolabeled antithrombin III and heparin in humans, *Thromb Haemost* 52:66, 1984.
124. Mummaneni N, Istanbouli M, Pifarri R, et al: Increased heparin requirements with autotransfusion, *J Thorac Cardiovasc Surg* 86:446, 1983.
125. Spiess BD: Treating heparin resistance with antithrombin or fresh frozen plasma, *Ann Thorac Surg* 85:2153–2160, 2008.
126. Hicks GL: Heparin resistance during cardiopulmonary bypass [Letter], *J Thorac Cardiovasc Surg* 86:633, 1983.
127. Esposito RA, Culliford AT, Colvin SB, et al: Heparin resistance during cardiopulmonary bypass, *J Thorac Cardiovasc Surg* 85:346, 1983.
128. Anderson EF: Heparin resistance prior to cardiopulmonary bypass, *Anesthesiology* 64:504, 1986.
129. Rivard DC, Thompson SJ, Cameron D: The role of antithrombin III in heparin resistance. In *Proceedings of the 28th International Conference of the American Society of Extracorporeal Technology*, Dallas, TX, 1990, p 66.
130. Chung F, David TE, Watt J: Excessive requirement for heparin during cardiac surgery, *Can Anaesth Soc J* 28:280, 1981.
131. Mabry CD, Read RC, Thompson BW, et al: Identification of heparin resistance during cardiac and vascular surgery, *Arch Surg* 114:129, 1979.
132. Young JA, Kisker T, Doty DB: Adequate anticoagulation during cardiopulmonary bypass determined by activated clotting time and the appearance of fibrin monomer, *Ann Thorac Surg* 26:231, 1978.
133. Jobes DR: Tight control of anticoagulation, not empiric management, improves outcome from cardiopulmonary bypass, *J Cardiothorac Anesth* 3:655, 1989.
134. Jackson MR, Olsen SB, Gomez ER, et al: Use of antithrombin III concentrates to correct antithrombin III deficiency during vascular surgery, *J Vasc Surg* 22:804, 1995.
135. Sabbagh AH, Chung GKT, Shuttleworth P, et al: Fresh frozen plasma: A solution to heparin resistance during cardiopulmonary bypass, *Ann Thorac Surg* 37:466, 1984.
136. Rana R, Fernández-Pérez ER, Khan SA, et al: Transfusion-related acute lung injury and pulmonary edema in critically ill patients: A retrospective study, *Transfusion* 46:1478–1483, 2006.
137. Gajic R, Rana, Winters JL, et al: Transfusion-related acture lung injury in the critically ill: Prospective nested case-control study, *Am J Respir Crit Care Med* 176:839–840, 2007.
138. Metz S, Keats AS: Low activated coagulation time during cardiopulmonary bypass does not increase postoperative bleeding, *Ann Thorac Surg* 49:440, 1990.
139. Lemmer JH, Despotis GJ: Antithrombin III concentrate to treat heparin resistance in patients undergoing cardiac surgery, *J Thorac Cardiovasc Surg* 123:213, 2002.
140. Avidan M, Levy J, Scholz J, et al: A phase III, double blind, placebo-controlled, multicenter study on the efficacy of recombinant human antithrombin in heparin-resistant patients scheduled to undergo cardiac surgery necessitating cardiopulmonary bypass, *Anesthesiology* 102:276, 2005.
141. Milas B, Jobes D, Gorman R: Management of bleeding and coagulopathy after heart surgery, *Semin Thorac Cardiovasc Surg* 12:326, 2000.
142. Frick PG, Brogli H: The mechanism of heparin rebound after extracorporeal circulation for open cardiac surgery, *Surgery* 59:721, 1966.
143. Gollub S: Heparin rebound in open heart surgery, *Surg Gynecol Obstet* 124:337, 1967.
144. Ellison N, Beatty P, Blake DR, et al: Heparin rebound, *J Thorac Cardiovasc Surg* 67:723, 1974.
145. Kaul TK, Crow MJ, Rajah SM, et al: Heparin administration during extracorporeal circulation, *J Thorac Cardiovasc Surg* 78:95, 1979.
146. Fiser WP, Read RC, Wright FE, et al: A randomized study of beef lung and pork mucosal heparin in cardiac surgery, *Ann Thorac Surg* 35:615, 1983.
147. Guffin AV, Dunbar RW, Kaplan JA, et al: Successful use of a reduced dose of protamine after cardiopulmonary bypass, *Anesth Analg* 55:110, 1976.
148. Ellison N, Ominsky AJ, Wollman H: Is protamine a clinically important anticoagulant? *Anesthesiology* 35:621, 1971.
149. Kresowik TF, Wakefield TW, Fessler RD, et al: Anticoagulant effects of protamine sulfate in a canine model, *J Surg Res* 45:8, 1988.
150. Jobes DR, Aitken GL, Shaffer GW: Increased accuracy and precision of heparin and protamine dosing reduces blood loss and transfusion in patients undergoing primary cardiac operations, *J Thorac Cardiovasc Surg* 110:36, 1995.
151. DeLaria GA, Tyner JJ, Hayes CL, et al: Heparin-protamine mismatch. A controllable factor in bleeding after open heart surgery, *Arch Surg* 129:944, 1994.
152. Spiess BD: Heparin: Beyond an anticoagulant. In Spiess BD, editor: *The Relationship Between Coagulation, Inflammation and Endothelium—A Pyramid Towards Outcome*, Baltimore, 2002, Lippincott Williams & Wilkins, p 169.
153. Day JRS, Landis RC, Taylor KM: Heparin is more than just an anticoagulant, *J Cardiothorac Vasc Anesth* 18:93, 2004.
154. Chang CH, Chang FM, Chen CP, et al: Antithrombin III activity in normal and toxemic preganancies, *J Formosa Med Assoc* 91:680, 1992.
155. Saveliega GM, Efinov VS, Grislin VL, et al: Blood coagulation changes in pregnant women at risk of developing preeclampsia, *Int J Gynaecol Obstet* 48:3, 1995.
156. Fourrier F, Chopin C, Hwart JJ, et al: Double blind placebo-controlled trial of antithrombin III concentrate in septic shock with disseminated intravascular coagulation, *Chest* 104:882, 1993.
157. Urban P, Scheidegger D, Buchmann B, et al: The hemodynamic effects of heparin and their relation to ionized calcium levels, *J Thorac Cardiovasc Surg* 91:303, 1986.
158. Thomson C, Forkes CD, Prentice CR: Potentiation of platelet aggregation and adhesion by heparin both in vitro and in vivo, *Clin Sci Mol Med* 33:63, 1973.
159. Schneider DJ, Tracy PB, Mann KG, et al: Differential effects of anticoagulants on the activation of platelets ex vivo, *Circulation* 96:2877, 1997.
160. Warkentin TE, Kelton JG: Heparin and platelets, *Hematol Oncol Clin North Am* 4:243, 1990.
161. Fareed J, Walenga JM, Hoppensteadt DA, et al: Studies on the profibrinolytic actions of heparin and its factors, *Semin Thromb Hemost* 11:199, 1985.
162. Warkentin TE, Greinacher A: Heparin induced thrombocytopenia and cardiac surgery, *Ann Thorac Surg* 18:2121, 2003.
163. Godal HC: Heparin-induced thrombocytopenia. In Lane DA, Lindahl U, editors: *Heparin*, Boca Raton, FL, 1989, CRC Press, p 533.
164. Fidlar E, Jaques LB: The effects of commercial heparin on the platelet count, *J Lab Clin Med* 33:1410, 1948.
165. Sandler RM, Seifer DB, Morgan K, et al: Heparin-induced thrombocytopenia and thrombosis. Detection and specificity of a platelet-aggregating IgG, *Am J Clin Pathol* 83:760, 1985.
166. Sheridan D, Carter C, Kelton JC: A diagnostic test for heparin-induced thrombocytopenia, *Blood* 67:27, 1986.
167. Rhodes GR, Dixon RH, Silver D: Heparin-induced thrombocytopenia with thrombotic and hemorrhagic manifestations, *Surg Gynecol Obstet* 136:409, 1973.
168. Eika C, Godal AC, Laake K, et al: Low incidence of thrombocytopenia during treatment with hog mucosa and beef lung heparin, *Scand J Haematol* 25:19, 1980.
169. Kelton JG, Smith JW, Warkentin TE, et al: Immunoglobulin G from patients with heparin-induced thrombocytopenia binds to a complex of heparin and platelet factor 4, *Blood* 83:3232, 1994.
170. Amiral J, Bridey F, Dreyfus M: Platelet factor 4 complexed to heparin is the target for antibodies generated in heparin-induced thrombocytopenia [Letter], *Thromb Haemost* 68:95, 1992.
171. Hirsh J, Raschke R, Warkentin TE, et al: Heparin: Mechanism of action, pharmacokinetics, dosing considerations, monitoring, efficacy, and safety, *Chest* 108:258S, 1995.
172. Chong BH, Castaldi PA: Heparin-induced thrombocytopenia: Further studies of the effects of heparin-dependent antibodies on platelets, *Br J Haematol* 64:347, 1986.
173. Schwartz KA, Roger G, Kaufman DB, et al: Complications of heparin administration in normal individuals, *Am J Hematol* 19:355, 1985.
174. Thielmann M, Bunschkowski M, Tossios P, et al: Perioperative thrombocytopenia in cardiac surgical patients-incidence of heparin-induced thrombocytopenia, morbidies and mortality, *Eur J Cardiothroac Surg* 37:1391–1395, 2010.
175. Ortel TL: Heparin-induced thrombocytopenia: When a low platelet count is a mandate for anticoagulation, *Hematl Am Soc Hematol Educ Program* 225–232, 2009.
176. Dyke CM, Aldea G, Koster A, et al: Off-pump coronary artery bypass with bivalirudin for patients with heparin-induced thrombocytopenia or antiplatelet factor four/heparin antibodies, *Ann Thorac Surg* 84:836–839, 2007.

177. Koster A, Dyke CM, Aldea G, et al: Bivalidruidn during cardiopulmonary bypassin patients with previous or acute heparin-induced thrombocytopenia and heparin antibodies: Results of the CHOOSE-ON trial, *Ann Thorac Surg* 83:572–577, 2007.
178. Stead RB, Schafer AI, Rosenberg RD, et al: Heterogeneity of heparin lots associated with thrombocytopenia and thromboembolism, *Am J Med* 77:185, 1984.
179. Godal HC: Thrombocytopenia and heparin, *Thromb Haemost* 43:222, 1980.
180. Rizzoni WE, Miller K, Rick M, et al: Heparin-induced thrombocytopenia and thromboembolism in the postoperative period, *Surgery* 103:470, 1988.
181. Moberg PQ, Geary VM, Sheich FM: Heparin-induced thrombocytopenia: A possible complication of heparin coated pulmonary artery catheters, *J Cardiothorac Anesth* [illegible]
182. Laster J, Silver D: Heparin-coated catheters and heparin-induced thrombocytopenia, *J Vasc Surg* 7:667, 1988.
183. Ansell J, Slepchuk N Jr, Kumar R, et al: Heparin-induced thrombocytopenia: A prospective study, *Thromb Haemost* 43:61, 1980.
184. Kelton JG, Sheridan D, Brain M: Clinical usefulness of testing for a heparin-dependent platelet-aggregating factor in patients with suspected heparin-induced thrombocytopenia, *J Lab Clin Med* 103:6062, 1984.
185. Arepally G, Reynolds C, Tomaski A, et al: Comparison of PF4/heparin ELISA with the 14C-serotonin release assay in the diagnosis of heparin-induced thrombocytopenia, *Am J Clin Pathol* 104:648, 1995.
186. Nelson JC, Lerner RG, Goldstein R, et al: Heparin-induced thrombocytopenia, *Arch Intern Med* 138:548, 1978.
187. Taylor-Williams R, Damaraju LV, Mascelli MA, et al: Antiplatelet factor 4/heparin antibodies, *Circulation* 107:2307, 2003.
188. Mattioli AV, Bonetti L, Sternieri S, et al: Heparin-induced thrombocytopenia in patients treated with unfractionated heparin: Prevalence of thrombosis in a 1 year follow-up, *Ital Heart J* 1:39, 2000.
189. Crowther MA, Cook DJ, Albert M, et al: The 4Ts scoring system for heparin-induced thrombocytopenia in medical-surgical intensive care unit patients, *J Crit Care* 25:287–293, 2010.
190. Mehta DP, Yoder EL, Appel J, et al: Heparin-induced thrombocytopenia and thrombosis, *Am J Hematol* 36:275, 1991.
191. Kappa JR, Cottrell ED, Berkowitz HD, et al: Carotid endarterectomy in patients with heparin-induced platelet activation: Comparative efficacy of aspirin and Iloprost (ZK36374), *J Vasc Surg* 5:693, 1987.
192. Makhoul RG, McCann RL, Austin EH, et al: Management of patients with heparin-associated thrombocytopenia and thrombosis requiring cardiac surgery, *Ann Thorac Surg* 43:617, 1987.
193. Smith JP, Walls JT, Muscato MS, et al: Extracorporeal circulation in a patient with heparin-induced thrombocytopenia, *Anesthesiology* 62:363, 1985.
194. Addonizio VP, Fisher CA, Kappa JR, et al: Prevention of heparin-induced thrombocytopenia during open heart surgery with iloprost (ZK36374), *Surgery* 102:796, 1987.
195. Kappa JR, Horn D, McIntosh CL, et al: Iloprost (ZK36374): A new prostacyclin analogue permits open cardiac operation in patients with heparin-induced thrombocytopenia, *Surg Forum* 36:285, 1985.
196. Kraezler EJ, Starr NJ: Heparin-associated thrombocytopenia: Management of patients for open heart surgery, *Anesthesiology* 69:964, 1988.
197. Ellison N, Kappa JR, Fisher CA, et al: Extracorporeal circulation in a patient with heparin-induced thrombocytopenia, *Anesthesiology* 63:336, 1985.
198. Vender JS, Matthew EB, Silverman IM, et al: Heparin-associated thrombocytopenia: Alternative managements, *Anesth Analg* 65:520, 1986.
199. Magnani HN: Heparin-induced thrombocytopenia (HIT). An overview of 230 patients treated with Orgaran (ORG 10172), *Thromb Haemost* 70:554, 1993.
200. Bretelle C, Leude E, Quilici J, et al: Utilisation de l'Orgaran pour une circulation extra-corporelle chez une patiente allergique à l'héparine, *Presse Méd* 25:1846, 1996.
201. Gouault-Heilmann M, Huet Y, Contant G, et al: Cardiopulmonary bypass with a low-molecular-weight heparin fraction, *Lancet* 2:1374, 1983.
202. Roussi JH, Houbouyan LL, Goguel AF: Use of low-molecular-weight heparin in heparin-induced thrombocytopenia with thrombotic complications, *Lancet* 1:1183, 1984.
203. Rowlings PA, Mansberg R, Rozenberg MC, et al: The use of a low-molecular-weight heparinoid (Org 10172) for extracorporeal procedures in patients with heparin-dependent thrombocytopenia and thrombosis, *Aust NZ J Med* 21:52, 1991.
204. Roynard JL, Pourriat JL, LeRoux G, et al: Hyperaggrabilité plaquettaire induit par une héparine de bas poids molculaire au cours d'un syndrome de détresse respiratoire de l'adulte, *Ann Fr Anesth Reanim* 10:70, 1991.
205. Lecompte T, Luo S, Stieltjes N, et al: Thrombocytopenia associated with low-molecular-weight heparin, *Lancet* 338:1217, 1991.
206. Leroy J, Leclerc MH, Delahousse B, et al: Treatment of heparin-associated thrombocytopenia and thrombosis with low-molecular-weight heparin (CY 216), *Semin Thromb Hemost* 11:326, 1985.
207. Chong BH: Heparin-induced thrombocytopenia, *Br J Haematol* 89:431, 1995.
208. Zulys VJ, Teasdale SJ, Michel ER, et al: Ancrod (Arvin) as an alternative to heparin anticoagulation for cardiopulmonary bypass, *Anesthesiology* 71:870, 1989.
209. Spiess BD, Gernsheimer T, Vocelka C, et al: Hematologic changes with ancrod anticoagulated cardiopulmonary bypass: A case report, *J Cardiothorac Vasc Anesth* 10:918, 1996.
210. Samama MM, Bara L, Gouin-Thibault I: New data on the pharmacology of heparin and low-molecular-weight heparins, *Drugs* 52(Suppl 7):8, 1996.
211. Bergqvist D: Low-molecular-weight heparins, *J Intern Med* 240:63, 1996.
212. Weitz JI: Low-molecular-weight heparin(s), *N Engl J Med* 337:688, 1997.
213. Planes A, Vochelle N, Fagola M, et al: Efficacy and safety of a perioperative enoxaparin regimen in total hip replacement under various anesthesia, *Am J Surg* 161:525, 1991.
214. Turpie AG: Efficacy of a postoperative regimen of enoxaparin in deep vein thrombosis prophylaxis, *Am J Surg* 161:532, 1991.
215. Hirsh J: Rationale for development of low-molecular-weight heparin and their clinical potential in the prevention of postoperative venous thrombosis, *Am J Surg* 161:512, 1991.
216. Van Ryn-McKenna J, Cai L, Ofosu FA, et al: Neutralization of enoxaparin-induced bleeding by protamine sulfate, *Thromb Haemost* 63:271, 1990.
217. Massonnet-Castel S, Pelissier E, Bara L, et al: Partial reversal of low-molecular-weight heparin (PK10169) anti-Xa activity by protamine sulfate: In vitro and in vivo study during cardiac surgery with extracorporeal circulation, *Haemostasis* 16:139, 1986.
218. Gravlee GP: Dermatan sulfate anticoagulation: Future replacement for heparin [Editorial]? *J Cardiothorac Vasc Anesth* 9:237, 1995.
219. Bauer KA, Ericksson BI, Lassen MR, et al: Fondaparinux compared with enoxaparin for the prevention of venous thromboembolism after elective major knee surgery, *N Engl J Med* 345:1305, 2001.
220. Maurer SH, Wilimas JA, Wang WC, et al: Heparin induced thrombocytopenia and re-thromboisis associated with warfarin and fondaparinux in a child, *Pediatr blood Cancer* 53:468–471, 2009.
221. Krauel K, Fürli B, Warkentin TE, et al: Heparin-induced thrombocytopenia-therapeutic concentrations of danaproid, unlike fondaparinux and direct thrombin inhibitors, inhibit formation of platelet factor 4-heparin complexes, *J Thromb Haemost* 6:2160–2167, 2008.
222. Koster A, Hansen R, Kuppe H, et al: Recombinant hirudin as an alternative for anticoagulation during cardiopulmonary bypass with HIT II, *J Cardiothorac Vasc Anesth* 14:243, 2000.
223. Dinisio M, Middeldorp S, Buller H: Direct thrombin inhibitors, *N Engl J Med* 353:1028, 2005.
224. Lewis BE, Wallis DE, Berkowitz SD, et al: Argatroban anticoagulant therapy in patients with heparin-induced thrombocytopenia, *Circulation* 103:1838, 2002.
225. Genzen JR, Fareed J, Hoppensteadt D, et al: Prolonged elevation of plasma argatroban in a cardiac transplant patient with a suspected history of heparin-induced thrombocytopenia with thrombosis, *Transfusion* 50:801–807, 2010.
226. Furukawa K, Ohteki H, Hirahara K, et al: The use of Argatroban as an anticoagulant for cardiopulmonary bypass in cardiac operations, *J Thorac Cardiovasc Surg* 122:1255–1256, 2001.
227. Edwards JT, Hambly JK, Worrall NK: Successful use of argatroban as a heparin substitute dduring cardiopulmonary bypass: Heparin-induced thrombocytopenia in a high-risk cardiac surgical patient, [illegible]
228. Cannon MA, Butterworth J, Riley RD, et al: Failure of argatroban anticoagulation during off-pump coronary artery bypass surgery, *Ann Thorac Surg* 77:711–713, 2004.
229. Kieta DR, McCammon AT, Holman WL, et al: Hemostatic analysis of a patient undergoing off-pump coronary artery bypass surgery with Argatroban anticoagulation, *Anesth Analg* 96:956–958, 2003.
230. Murphy GS, Marymont JH: Alternative anticoagulation management strategies for the patient with heparin-induced thrombocytopenia undergoin cardiac surgery, *J Cardiothorac Vasc Anesth* 21:113–126, 2007.
231. Follis F, Filippone G, Montalbanl G, et al: Argatroban as a substitute of a heparin alternative during cardiopulmonary bypass: A safe alternative? *Interact Cardiovasc Thorac Surg* 10:592–596, 2010.
232. Smith AI, Stroud R, Damiani P, et al: Use of argatroban for anticoagulation during cardiopulmonary bypass in a patient with heparin allergy, *Eur J Cardiothorac Surg* 34:1113–1114, 2008.
233. Samuels LE, Kohout J, Casanova-Ghosh E, et al: Argatroban as a primary or secondary postoperative anticoagulant in patients implanted with ventricular assist devices, *Ann Thorac Surg* 85:1651–1655, 2008.
234. Martin ME, Kloeker GH, Laber DA: Argatroban for anticoagulation during cardiac surgery, *Eur J Haematol* 78:161–166, 2007.
235. Kurup V, Transue S, Wu Y, et al: Cardiac surgery in a patient with heparin-induced thrombocytopenia-cautions with use of the direct thrombin inhibitor, Argatroban, *Conn Med* 70:245–250, 2006.
236. Azuma K, Koichi M, Hirokazu I, et al: Difficult management of anticoagulation with argatroban in a patient undergoing on-pump cardiac surgery, *J Cardiothoracvasc Anesth* 24:831–833, 2010.
237. Lewis BE, Walenga JM, Wallis DE: Anticoagulation with Novastatin (argatroban) in patients with heparin induced thrombocytopenia and heparin-induced thrombocytopenia and thrombosis syndrome, *Semin Thromb Haemost* 23:197, 1997.
238. McKeage K, Plosker GL: Argatroban, *Drugs* 61:515, 2001.
239. Koster A, Chew D, Grundel M, et al: An assessment of different filter systems for extracorporeal elimination of bivalirudin: An in vitro study, *Anesth Analg* 96:1316, 2003.
240. Merry AF, Raudkivi P, White HD, et al: Anticoagulation with bivalirudin (a direct thrombin inhibitor) vs heparin. A randomized trial in OPCAB graft surgery, *Ann Thorac Surg* 77:925, 2004.
241. Veale JJ, McCarthy HM, Palmer G, et al: Use of bivalirudin as an anticoagulant during cardiopulmonary bypass, *J Extracorpor Technol* 37:296–302, 2005.
242. Koster A, Buz S, Krbatsch T, et al: Bivalirduin anticoagulation during cardiac surgery: A single center experience in 141 patients, *Perfusion* 24:7–11, 2009.
243. Koster A, Spiess BD, Chew DP, et al: Effectiveness of bivalirudin as a replacement for heparin during cardiopulmonary bypass in patients undergoing coronary artery bypass grafting, *Am J Cardiol* 93:356, 2004.
244. Koster A, Chew D, Grundel M, et al: Bivalirudin monitored with the ecarin clotting time for anticoagulation during cardiopulmonary bypass, *Anesth Analg* 96:383, 2003.
245. Vasquez JC, Vichiendilokkul A, Mahmood S, et al: Anticoagulation with bivalirudin during cardiopulmonary bypass in cardiac surgery, *Ann Thorac Surg* 74:2177, 2002.
246. Gurm H, Sarembock I, Kereiakes D, et al: Use of bivalirudin during percutaneous coronary intervention in patients with diabetes mellitus, *J Am Coll Cardiol* 45:1932, 2005.
247. Lincoff M, Bittle J, Harrington R, et al: Bivalirudin and provisional gycoprotein IIb/IIIa blockade compared to heparin and GIIb/IIIa inhibition during PCI: Replace-2, *JAMA* 289:853, 2003.
248. Spiess B, Deanda A, McCarthy H, et al: Off pump CABG surgery anticoagocation with bivalirudin, *J Cardiothorac Vasc Anesth* 20:106–111, 2006.
249. Francis CW, Davidson BL, Berkowitz SD, et al: Ximalagatran versus warfarin for the prevention of venous thromboembolism after total knee arthroplasty, *Ann Intern Med* 137:548, 2002.
250. Eriksson H, Wahlander K, Gustafsson D, et al: Randomized, controlled, dose-guiding study of the oral direct thrombin ximelagatran compared with standard therapy for treatment of acute deep venous thrombosis, *J Thromb Haemost* 1:41, 2002.
251. Heit JA, Colwell CW, Francis CA, et al: Comparison of ximelagatran with enoxaparin as prophylaxis against venous thromboembolism, *Arch Intern Med* 161:2215, 2001.
252. Schulman S, Wahlander K, Lundstrom T, et al: Secondary prevention of venous thromboembolism with the oral direct thrombin inhibitor ximelagatran, *N Engl J Med* 349:1713, 2003.
253. Larm O, Larsson R, Olsson P: Surface-immobilized heparin. In Lane DA, Lindahl U, editors: *Heparin*, Boca Raton, FL, 1989, CRC Press, p 597.
254. Von Segesser LK, Weiss BM, Garcia E, et al: Reduction and elimination of systemic heparinization during cardiopulmonary bypass, *J Thorac Cardiovasc Surg* 103:790, 1992.
255. Videm V, Svennevig JL, Fosse E, et al: Reduced complement activation with heparin-coated oxygenator and tubings in coronary bypass operations, *J Thorac Cardiovasc Surg* 103:806, 1992.
256. Gravlee GP: Heparin-coated cardiopulmonary bypass circuits [Review], *J Cardiothoracic Vasc Anesth* 8:213, 1994.
257. Engbers GH, Feijen J: Current techniques to improve the blood compatibility of biomaterial surfaces [Editorial], *Int J Artif Organs* 14:199, 1991.
258. Ando T, Yamasaki M, Suzuki K: Protamines. In Kleinzeller A, Springer GF, Wittmann HG, editors: *Molecular Biology, Biochemistry and Biophysics*, 12, Berlin, 1973, Springer-Verlag, p 1.
259. Wilkins MHF: Physical studies of the molecular structure of deoxyribonucleic acid and nucleoprotein, *Cold Spring Harbor Symp Quant Biol* 21:83, 1956.
260. Jaques LB: Personal communication, February 14, 1986.
261. Chargaff E, Olson KB: Studies on the chemistry of blood coagulation, part VI, *J Biol Chem* 122:153, 1937.
262. Jaques LB: Protamine-antagonist to heparin, *J Can Med Assoc* 108:1291, 1973.
263. Jaques LB: A study of the toxicity of the protamine, salmine, *Br J Pharmacol* 4:135, 1949.
264. Samuel T, Kolk A: Auto-antigenicity of human protamines. In Lepow IH, Crozier R, editors: *Vasectomy. Immunologic and Pathophysiologic Effects in Animals and Man*, New York, 1979, Academic Press, p 203.
265. Moriou M, Masure R, Hurlet A, et al: Haemostasis disorders in open heart surgery with extracorporeal circulation, *Vox Sang* 32:41, 1977.
266. Kuitunen AH, Salmenpera MT, Heinonen J, et al: Heparin rebound: A comparative study of protamine chloride and protamine sulfate in patients undergoing coronary artery bypass surgery, *J Cardiothorac Vasc Anesth* 5:221, 1991.
267. Folkman J, Langer R, Linhardt RJ, et al: Angiogenesis inhibition and tumor regression caused by heparin or a heparin fragment in the presence of cortisone, *Science* 221:719, 1983.
268. Taylor S, Folkman J: Protamine is an inhibitor of angiogenesis, *Nature* 297:307, 1982.
269. Mulholland B, Mellersh AR: The antimicrobial activity of protamine and polybrene, *J Hosp Infect* 10:305, 1987.

270. O'Reilly RA: Anticoagulant, antithrombotic and thrombolytic drugs. In Gilman AG, Goodman LS, Rall TW, Murad F, editors: *The Pharmacological Basis of Therapeutics*, ed 7, New York, 1985, Macmillan, p 1340.
271. Radegran K, McAshlan C: Circulatory and ventilatory effects of induced platelet aggregation and their inhibition by acetylsalicylic acid, *Acta Anaesthesiol Scand* 16:76, 1972.
272. Bjoraker DG, Ketcham TR: In vivo platelet response to clinical protamine sulfate infusion, *Anesthesiology* 57:A7, 1982.
273. Ellison N, Edmunds LH, Colman RW: Platelet aggregation following heparin and protamine administration, *Anesthesiology* 48:65, 1978.
274. Lindblad B, Wakefield TW, Whitehouse WM, et al: The effect of protamine sulfate on platelet function, *Scand J Thorac Cardiovasc Surg* 22:55, 1988.
275. Eika C: On the mechanism of platelet aggregation induced by heparin, protamine and polybrene, *Scand J Haematol* 9:248, 1972.
276. Cobel-Geard RJ, Hassouna HI: Interaction of protamine sulfate with thrombin, *Am J Hematol* 14:227, 1983.
277. Shanberge JN, Murato M, Quattrociocchi-Longe T, et al: Heparin-protamine complexes in the production of heparin rebound and other complications of extracorporeal bypass procedures, *Am J Clin Pathol* 87:210, 1987.
278. DePaulis R, Mohammed SF, Chiariello L, et al: The role of plasma proteins in formation of obstructive protamine complexes, *J Cardiothorac Vasc Anesth* 5:227, 1991.
279. Tan F, Jackman H, Skidgel RA, et al: Protamine inhibits plasma carboxypeptidase N, the inactivator of anaphylatoxins and kinins, *Anesthesiology* 70:267, 1989.
280. Castaneda AR: Must heparin be neutralized following open-heart operations? *J Thorac Cardiovasc Surg* 52:716, 1966.
281. Arn C, Feddersen K, Radegran K: Comparison of two protocols for heparin neutralization by protamine after cardiopulmonary bypass, *J Thorac Cardiovasc Surg* 94:539, 1987.
282. Welsby I, Newman M, Phillips-Bute B, et al: Hemodynamic changes after protamine administration, *Anesthesiology* 102:308, 2005.
283. Radegran K, Taylor GA, Olsson P: Mode of action of protamine in regard to its circulatory and respiratory side effects, *Eur Surg Res* 3:139, 1971.
284. Fadali MA, Ledbetter M, Papacostas CA, et al: Mechanism responsible for the cardiovascular depressant effect of protamine sulfate, *Ann Surg* 180:232, 1974.
285. Marin-Neto JA, Sykes MK, Marin JLB, et al: Effect of heparin and protamine on left ventricular performance in the dog, *Cardiovasc Res* 13:254, 1979.
286. Gourin A, Streisand RL, Greineder JK, et al: Protamine sulfate administration and the cardiovascular system, *J Thorac Cardiovasc Surg* 62:193, 1971.
287. Gourin A, Streisand RL, Stuckey JH: Total cardiopulmonary bypass, myocardial contractility, and the administration of protamine sulfate, *J Thorac Cardiovasc Surg* 61:160, 1971.
288. Greene CE, Higgins CB, Kelley MI, et al: Cardiovascular effects of protamine sulfate, *Invest Radiol* 16:324, 1981.
289. Jones MM, Hill AB, Nahrwold ML, et al: Effect of protamine on plasma ionized calcium in the dog, *Can Anaesth Soc J* 29:65, 1982.
290. Komatsu H, Enzan K: Repeated administration of protamine attenuates protamine-induced systemic hypotension [in Japanese], *Masui Jpn J Anesth* 45:1319, 1996.
291. Stefaniszyn HJ, Novick RJ, Salerno TA: Toward a better understanding of the hemodynamic effects of protamine and heparin interaction, *J Thorac Cardiovasc Surg* 87:678, 1984.
292. Pauca AL, Graham JE, Hudspeth AS: Hemodynamic effects of intraaortic administration of protamine, *Ann Thorac Surg* 35:637, 1983.
293. Wakefield TW, Hantler CB, Wrobleski SK, et al: Effects of differing rates of protamine reversal of heparin anticoagulation, *Surgery* 119:123, 1996.
294. Levy JH, Faraj BA, Zaidan JR, et al: Effects of protamine on histamine release from human lung, *Agents Actions* 28:70, 1989.
295. Sauder RA, Hirshman CA: Protamine-induced histamine release in human skin mast cells, *Anesthesiology* 73:165, 1990.
296. Raikar GV, Hisamochi K, Raikar BL, et al: Nitric oxide inhibition attenuates systemic hypotension produced by protamine, *J Thorac Cardiovasc Surg* 111:1240, 1996.
297. Frater RWM, Oka Y, Hong Y, et al: Protamine-induced circulatory changes, *J Thorac Cardiovasc Surg* 87:687, 1984.
298. Masone R, Hong YOka, YW, et al: Cardiovascular effects of right atrial injection of protamine sulfate as compared to left atrial injection, *Anesthesiology* 57:A6, 1982.
299. Milne B, Rogers K, Cervenko F, et al: The haemodynamic effects of intraaortic versus intravenous administration of protamine for reversal of heparin in man, *Can Anaesth Soc J* 30:347, 1983.
300. Jastrzebski J, Sykes MK, Woods DG: Cardiorespiratory effects of protamine after cardiopulmonary bypass in man, *Thorax* 29:534, 1974.
301. Conahan TJ, Andrews RW, MacVaugh H: Cardiovascular effects of protamine sulfate in man, *Anesth Analg* 60:33, 1981.
302. Sethna DH, Moffitt E, Gray RJ, et al: Effects of protamine sulfate on myocardial oxygen supply and demand in patients following cardiopulmonary bypass, *Anesth Analg* 61:247, 1982.
303. Michaels IA, Barash PG: Hemodynamic changes during protamine administration, *Anesth Analg* 62:831, 1983.
304. Hanowell ST, Jones M, Pierce E, et al: Protamine titration: What degree of precision is necessary? *Anesthesiology* 59:A91, 1983.
305. Iwatsuki N, Matsukawa S, Iwatsuki K: A weak negative inotropic effect of protamine sulfate upon the isolated canine heart muscle, *Anesth Analg* 59:100, 1980.
306. Caplan RA, Su JY: Differences in threshold for protamine toxicity in isolated atrial and ventricular tissue, *Anesth Analg* 63:1111, 1984.
307. Hendry PJ, Taichman GC, Keon WJ: The myocardial contractile responses to protamine sulfate and heparin, *Ann Thorac Surg* 44:263, 1987.
308. Wakefield TW, Bies LE, Wrobleski SK, et al: Impaired myocardial function and oxygen utilization due to protamine sulfate in an isolated rabbit heart preparation, *Ann Surg* 212:387, 1990.
309. Housmans PR, Ferguson DM: Inotropic effects of protamine sulfate on isolated mammalian cardiac muscles: Mechanisms of action, *Anesthesiology* 67:A24, 1987.
310. Hird RB, Wakefield TW, Mukherjee R, et al: Direct effects of protamine sulfate on myocyte contractile processes. Cellular and molecular mechanisms, *Circulation* 92(Suppl II):II–433, 1995.
311. Hird RB, Crawford FA, Spinale FG: Differential effects of protamine sulfate on myocyte contractile function with left ventricular failure, *J Am Coll Cardiol* 25:773, 1995.
312. Park WK, Pancrazio JJ, Lynch C 3rd: Mechanical and electrophysiological effects of protamine on isolated ventricular myocardium. Evidence for calcium overload, *Cardiovasc Res* 28:505, 1994.
313. Taylor RL, Little WC, Freeman GL, et al: Comparison of the cardiovascular effects of intravenous and intraaortic protamine in the conscious and anesthetized dog, *Ann Thorac Surg* 42:22, 1986.
314. Humphrey LS, Topol EJ, Casella ES, et al: Absence of direct myocardial depression by protamine, *Anesthesiology* 61:A50, 1984.
315. Oe M, Asou T, Morita S, et al: Protamine-induced hypotension in heart operations. Application of the concept of ventricular-arterial coupling, *J Thorac Cardiovasc Surg* 112:462, 1996.
316. Aris A, Solanes H, Bonnin JO, et al: Intraaortic administration of protamine: Method for heparin neutralization after cardiopulmonary bypass, *Cardiovasc Dis Bull Texas Heart Inst* 8:23, 1981.
317. Iida Y, Tsuchiya K, Sakakibara N, et al: Intraaortic administration of protamine, *Kyobu Geka* 35:704, 1982.
318. Wakefield TW, Whitehouse WM, Stanley JC: Depressed cardiovascular function and altered platelet kinetics following protamine sulfate reversal of heparin activity, *J Vasc Surg* 1:346, 1984.
319. Casthely PA, Goodman K, Fyman PN, et al: Hemodynamic changes after the administration of protamine, *Anesth Analg* 65:78, 1986.
320. Rogers K, Milne B, Salerno TA: The hemodynamic effects of intraaortic versus intravenous administration of protamine for reversal of heparin in pigs, *J Thorac Cardiovasc Surg* 85:851, 1983.
321. Habezettl H, Conzen PF, Vollmar B: Pulmonary hypertension after heparin-protamine: Roles of left-sided infusion, histamine, and platelet-activating factor, *Anesth Analg* 71:637, 1990.
322. Cherry DA, Chiu RCJ, Wynands JE, et al: Intraaortic vs intravenous administration of protamine: A prospective randomized clinical study, *Surg Forum* 36:238, 1985.
323. Procaccini B, Clementi G, Bersanetti L, et al: Cardiopulmonary effects of protamine sulfate in man: Intraaortic vs intra-right atrial rapid administration after cardiopulmonary bypass, *J Cardiovasc Surg* 28:112, 1987.
324. Levy JH: *Anaphylactic Reactions in Anesthesia and Intensive Care*, Boston, 1986, Butterworth's, p 39.
325. Dockhorn RJ: Diagnostic tests for allergic disease. In Korenblat PE, Wedner HJ, editors: *Allergy: Theory and Practice*, Philadelphia, 1984, Grune & Stratton, p 57.
326. Horrow JC: Protamine allergy, *J Cardiothorac Vasc Anesth* 2:225, 1988.
327. Kirklin JK, Chenoweth DE, Naftel DC: Effects of protamine administration after cardiopulmonary bypass on complement, blood elements, and the hemodynamic state, *Ann Thorac Surg* 41:193, 1986.
328. Horrow JC: Heparin reversal of protamine toxicity: Have we come full circle? *J Cardiothorac Vasc Anesth* 4:539, 1990.
329. Kurtz AB, Gray RS, Markanday S, et al: Circulating IgG antibodies to protamine in patients treated with protamine-insulins, *Diabetologia* 25:322, 1983.
330. Nell LJ, Thomas JW: Frequency and specificity of protamine antibodies in diabetic and control subjects, *Diabetes* 37:172, 1988.
331. Levy JH, Schwieger IA, Zaidan JR, et al: Evaluation of patients at risk for protamine reactions, *J Thorac Cardiovasc Surg* 98:200, 1989.
332. Jackson DR: Sustained hypotension secondary to protamine sulfate, *Angiology* 21:295, 1970.
333. Moorthy SS, Pond W, Rowland RG: Severe circulatory shock following protamine (an anaphylactic reaction), *Anesth Analg* 59:77, 1980.
334. Doolan L, McKenzie I, Kratchek J, et al: Protamine sulfate hypersensitivity, *Anaesth Intensive Care* 9:147, 1981.
335. Cobb CA, Fung DL: Shock due to protamine hypersensitivity, *Surg Neurol* 17:245, 1981.
336. Vontz FK, Puestow EC, Cahill DJ: Anaphylactic shock following protamine administration, *Ann Surg* 48:549, 1982.
337. Vierthaler LD, Becker KE Jr: Protamine anaphylaxis. Protocols for therapy in acute reactions, *J Kans Med Soc* 84:454, 1983.
338. Holland CL, Singh AK, McMaster PRB, et al: Adverse reactions to protamine sulfate following cardiac surgery, *Clin Cardiol* 7:157, 1984.
339. Chung F, Miles J: Cardiac arrest following protamine administration, *Can Anaesth SocJ* 31:314, 1984.
340. Walker WS, Reid KG, Hider CF, et al: Successful cardiopulmonary bypass in diabetics with anaphylactoid reactions to protamine, *Br Heart J* 52:112, 1984.
341. Grant JA, Cooper JR, Albyn KC, et al: Anaphylactic reactions to protamine in insulin-dependent diabetics during cardiovascular procedures [Abstract], *J Allergy Clin Immunol* 73:180, 1984.
342. Sharath MD, Metzger WJ, Richerson HB, et al: Protamine-induced fatal anaphylaxis: Prevalence of antiprotamine immunoglobulin E antibody, *J Thorac Cardiovasc Surg* 90:86, 1985.
343. Menk EJ: Cardiac arrest following protamine sulfate infusion during regional anesthesia, *Milit Med* 151:318, 1986.
344. Stewart WJ, McSweeney SM, Kellett MA, et al: Increased risk of severe protamine reactions in NPH insulin-dependent diabetics undergoing cardiac catheterization, *Circulation* 70:788, 1984.
345. Gottschlich G, Gravlee GP, Georgitis JW: Adverse reactions to protamine sulfate during cardiac surgery in diabetic and non-diabetic patients, *Ann Allergy* 61:277, 1988.
346. Weiss ME, Nyhan D, Peng Z, et al: Association of protamine IgE and IgG antibodies with life-threatening reactions to intravenous protamine, *N Engl J Med* 320:886, 1989.
347. Reed DC, Gascho JA: The safety of protamine sulfate in diabetics undergoing cardiac catheterization, *Cathet Cardiovasc Diagn* 144:19, 1988.
348. Best N, Teisner B, Grudzinskas JG, et al: Classical pathway activation during an adverse response to protamine sulfate, *Br J Anaesth* 55:1149, 1983.
349. Andersen JM, Johnson TA: Hypertension associated with protamine sulfate administration, *Am J Hosp Pharm* 38:701, 1981.
350. Lakin JD, Blocker TJ, Strong DM, et al: Anaphylaxis to protamine sulfate by a complement-dependent IgG antibody, *J Allergy Clin Immunol* 61:102, 1978.
351. Stoelting RK: Allergic reactions during anesthesia, *Anesth Analg* 63:341, 1983.
352. Nyhan DP, Shampaine EL, Hirshman CA, et al: Single doses of intravenous protamine result in the formation of protamine-specific IgE and IgG antibodies, *J Allergy Clin Immunol* 97:991, 1996.
353. Knape JTA, Schuller JL, de Haan P, et al: An anaphylactic reaction to protamine in a patient allergic to fish, *Anesthesiology* 55:324, 1981.
354. Caplan SN, Berkman EM: Protamine sulfate and fish allergy [Letter], *N Engl J Med* 295:172, 1976.
355. Samuel T, Kolk AHJ, Rumke P, et al: Autoimmunity to sperm antigens in vasectomized men, *Clin Exp Immunol* 21:65, 1975.
356. Sheridan P, Blain R, Vezina D, Bleau G: Prospective evaluation of the safety of heparin reversal with protamine in vasectomized patients after cardiopulmonary bypass. In *Proceedings of the 10th Annual Meeting of the Society of Cardiovascular Anesthesiologists*, New Orleans, 1988, p 140.
357. Watson RA, Ansbacher R, Barry M, et al: Allergic reaction to protamine: A late complication of elective vasectomy? *Urology* 22:493, 1983.
358. Metz S: Prior vasectomy and anaphylaxis following protamine. No cause and effect [Letter], *Anesthesiology* 79:617, 1993.
359. Olinger GN, Becker RM, Bonchek LI: Noncardiac pulmonary edema and peripheral vascular collapse following cardiopulmonary bypass: Rare protamine reaction? *Ann Thorac Surg* 29:20, 1980.
360. Baimbridge MV: Fulminating noncardiogenic pulmonary edema (discussion), *J Thorac Cardiovasc Surg* 80:868, 1980.
361. Just-Viera JO, Fischer CR, Gago O, et al: Acute reaction to protamine its importance to surgeons, *Am Surg* 50:52, 1984.
362. Pajuelo A, Otero C, Jiminez D, et al: Edema pulmonary no cardiogenico tras circulacion extracorporea: Implicaciones del sulfato de protamina, *Rev Espanola Anest Rean* 33:187, 1986.
363. Culliford AT, Thomas S, Spencer FC: Fulminating noncardiogenic pulmonary edema, *J Thorac Cardiovasc Surg* 80:868, 1980.
364. Hashim SW, Kay HR, Hammond GL, et al: Noncardiogenic pulmonary edema after cardiopulmonary bypass: An anaphylactic reaction to fresh frozen plasma, *Am J Surg* 147:560, 1984.
365. Frater RWM: Fulminating noncardiogenic pulmonary edema (discussion), *J Thorac Cardiovasc Surg* 80:868, 1980.
366. Chang S-W, Voelkel NF: Charge-related lung microvascular injury, *Am Rev Resp Dis* 139:534, 1989.

367. Toyofuku T, Koyama S, Kobayashi T, et al: Effects of polycations on pulmonary vascular permeability in conscious sheep, *J Clin Invest* 83:2063, 1989.
368. Iglesias A, Nuez L: Pulmonary edema [Letter], *Ann Thorac Surg* 33:304, 1982.
369. Kirklin JK: Prospects for understanding and eliminating deleterious effects of cardiopulmonary bypass, *Ann Thorac Surg* 51:529, 1991.
370. Lowenstein E, Johnston WE, Lappas DG, et al: Catastrophic pulmonary vasoconstriction associated with protamine reversal of heparin, *Anesthesiology* 59:470, 1983.
371. Jastrzebski J, Hilgard P, Sykes MK: Pulmonary vasoconstriction produced by protamine and protamine-heparin complex in the isolated cat lung perfused with blood or dextran, *Cardiovasc Res* 9:691, 1975.
372. Morel DR, Zapol WM, Thomas SJ, et al: C5a and thromboxane generation associated with pulmonary vaso- and bronchoconstriction during protamine reversal of heparin, *Anesthesiology* 66:597, 1987.
373. Horrow JC: Protamine—a review of its toxicity, *Anesth Analg* 64:348, 1985.
374. Horrow JC: Thrombocytopenia accompanying a reaction to protamine sulfate, *Can Anaesth Soc J* 32:49, 1985.
375. Lock R, Hessel EA: Probable reversal of protamine reactions by heparin administration, *J Cardiothorac Vasc Anesth* 4:604, 1990.
376. Fiser WP, Fewell JE, Hill DE, et al: Cardiovascular effects of protamine sulfate are dependent on the presence and type of circulation heparin, *J Thorac Cardiovasc Surg* 89:63, 1985.
377. Rent R, Ertel N, Eisenstein R, et al: Complement activation by interaction of polyanions and polycations: I. Heparin-protamine-induced consumption of complement, *J Immunol* 114:120, 1975.
378. Kreil E, Montalescot G, Greene E, et al: Nafamstat mesilate attenuates pulmonary hypertension in heparin-protamine reactions, *J Appl Physiol* 67:1463, 1989.
379. Colman RW: Humoral mediators of catastrophic reactions associated with protamine neutralization, *Anesthesiology* 66:595, 1987.
380. Hobbhahn J, Conzen PF, Zenker B, et al: Beneficial effect of cyclooxygenase inhibition on adverse hemodynamic responses after protamine, *Anesth Analg* 67:253, 1988.
381. Conzen PF, Habazettl H, Gutman R, et al: Thromboxane mediation of pulmonary hemodynamic responses after neutralization of heparin by protamine in pigs, *Anesth Analg* 68:25, 1989.
382. Nuttall GA, Murray MJ, Bowie EJW: Protamine-heparin-induced pulmonary hypertension in pigs: Effects of treatment with a thromboxane receptor antagonist on hemodynamics and coagulation, *Anesthesiology* 74:138, 1991.
383. Schumacher WA, Heran CL, Ogletree ML: Protamine-induced pulmonary hypertension in heparinized monkeys and pigs is inhibited by the thromboxane receptor antagonist SQ 30,741, *Eicosanoids* 3:87, 1990.
384. Wakefield TW, Wrobleski SK, Stanley JC: Reversal of depressed oxygen consumption accompanying in vivo protamine sulphate-heparin interactions by the prostacyclin analogue, iloprost, *Eur J Vasc Surg* 4:25, 1990.
385. Degges RD, Foster ME, Dang AQ, et al: Pulmonary hypertensive effect of heparin and protamine interaction: Evidence for thromboxane B2 release from the lung, *Am J Surg* 154:696, 1987.
386. Kanbak M, Kahraman S, Celebioglu B, et al: Prophylactic administration of histamine, and/or histamine-receptor blockers in the prevention of heparin- and protamine-related haemodynamic effects, *Anaesth Intensive Care* 24:559, 1996.
387. Baraka A, Choueiry P, Taha S, et al: Hydrocortisone pretreatment for attenuation of protamine-induced adverse hemodynamic reactions [Letter], *J Cardiothorac Vasc Anesth* 9:481, 1995.
388. Katircioglu SF, Kucukaksu DS, Buzdayi M, et al: The beneficial effects of aminophylline administration on heparin reversal with protamine, *Surg Today* 24:99, 1994.
389. Van der Starre PJA, Solinas C: Ketanserin in the treatment of protamine-induced pulmonary hypertension, *Texas Heart Inst J* 23:301, 1996.
390. Horrow JC, Pharo G, Levit LS, et al: Neither skin tests nor serum enzyme-linked immunosorbent assay tests provide specificity for protamine allergy, *Anesth Analg* 82:386, 1996.
391. Weiler JM, Gellhaus MA, Carter JG, et al: A prospective study of the risk of an immediate adverse reaction to protamine sulfate during cardiopulmonary bypass surgery, *J Allerg Clin Immunol* 85:713, 1990.
392. Kindler CH, Bircher AJ: Anaphylactoid reactions to protamine [Letter], *Anesthesiology* 85:1209, 1996.
393. Fisher M: Intradermal testing after anaphylactoid reaction to anaesthetic drugs: Practical aspects of performance and interpretation, *Anaesth Intensive Care* 12:115, 1984.
394. Wright JS, Osborn JJ, Perkins HA, et al: Heparin levels during and after hypothermic perfusion, *J Cardiovasc Surg* 5:244, 1964.
395. Godal HC: A comparison of two heparin-neutralizing agents: Protamine and polybrene, *Scand J Clin Lab Invest* 12:446, 1960.
396. Egerton WS, Robinson CLN: The anti-heparin, anticoagulant and hypotensive properties of hexadimethrine and protamine, *Lancet* 2:635, 1961.
397. Montalescot G, Zapol WM, Carvalho A, et al: Neutralization of low-molecular-weight heparin by polybrene prevents thromboxane release and severe pulmonary hypertension in awake sheep, *Circulation* 82:1754, 1990.
398. Haller JA, Ransdell HT, Stowens D, et al: Renal toxicity of polybrene in open heart surgery, *J Thorac Cardiovasc Surg* 44:486, 1962.
399. Ransdell HT, Haller JA, Stowens D, et al: Renal toxicity of polybrene (hexadimethrine bromide), *J Surg Res* 5:195, 1965.
400. Ohata H, Momose K, Takahashi A, et al: Urinalysis for detection of chemically induced renal damage-changes in urinary excretions of enzymes and various components caused by p-aminophenol, puromycin aminonucleoside and hexadimethrine, *J Toxicol Sci* 12:357, 1987.
401. Bertolatus JA, Hunsicker LG: Polycation binding to glomerular basement membrane, *Lab Invest* 56:170, 1987.
402. Messina A, Davies DJ, Ryan GB: Protamine sulfate-induced proteinuria: The roles of glomerular injury and depletion of polyanion, *J Pathol* 158:147, 1989.
403. Saito T, Sumithran E, Glasgow EF, et al: The enhancement of aminonucleoside nephrosis by the co-administration of protamine, *Kidney Int* 32:691, 1987.
404. Schapira M, Christman BW: Neutralization of heparin by protamine, *Circulation* 82:1877, 1990.
405. Levy JH, Cormack JG, Morales A: Heparin neutralization by recombinant platelet factor 4 and protamine, *Anesth Analg* 81:35, 1995.
406. Dehmer GJ, Fisher M, Tate DA, et al: Reversal of heparin anticoagulation by recombinant platelet factor 4 in humans, *Circulation* 91:2188, 1995.
407. Giesecke M, Cooper J, Keats A, et al: Recombinant platelet factor r (rPF4) neutralizes heparin in patients undergoing coronary artery bypass, *Anesth Analg* 80:SCA131, 1995.
408. Kurrek MM, Winkler M, Robinson DR, et al: Platelet factor 4 injection produces acute pulmonary hypertension in the awake lamb, *Anesthesiology* 82:183, 1995.
409. Giesecke M, Alexander A: rPF4 does not cause pulmonary hypertension in humans [Letter], *Anesthesiology* 83:644, 1995.
410. Bernstein H, Yang BC, Cooney CL, et al: Immobilized heparin lysis system for blood deheparinization, *Methods Enzymol* 137:515, 1988.
411. Kim J-S, Vincent C, Teng C-LC, et al: A novel approach to anticoagulation control, *ASAIO Trans* 35:644, 1989.
412. Yang VC, Port FK, Kim J-S, et al: The use of immobilized protamine in removing heparin and preventing protamine-induced complications during extracorporeal blood circulation, *Anesthesiology* 75:288, 1991.
413. Sloand EM, Kessler CM, McIntosh CL, et al: Methylene blue for neutralization of heparin, *Thromb Res* 54:677, 1989.
414. Kikura M, Lee MK, Levy JH: What is the concentration of hexadimethrine and methylene blue required for neutralization of heparin following cardiopulmonary bypass [Abstract]? *Anesthesiology* 81:A177, 1994.
415. Kikura M, Lee MK, Levy JH: Heparin neutralization with methylene blue, hexadimethrine, or vancomycin after cardiopulmonary bypass, *Anesth Analg* 83:223, 1996.
416. Metz S, Horrow JC, Goel IP, et al: Methylene blue does not neutralize heparin after cardiopulmonary bypass, *J Cardiothorac Vasc Anesth* 10:474, 1996.
417. Campbell FW, Goldstein MF, Atkins PC: Management of the patient with protamine hypersensitivity for cardiac surgery, *Anesthesiology* 61:761, 1984.
418. Michelsen LG, Kikura M, Levy JH, et al: Heparinase I (Neutralase) reversal of systemic anticoagulation, *Anesthesiology* 85:339, 1996.
419. Zimmerman J, McIntosh C, Clementi W, et al: Heparin reversal with Neutralase (heparinase I) in adult male volunteers, *Anesth Analg* 82:SCA93, 1996.
420. Van Riper DF, Heres E, Bennett JA, et al: Neutralase 7 mcg/kg reverses heparin-induced prolongation of ACT better than 5 mcg/kg in patients undergoing CABG [Abstract], *Anesthesiology* 87:A95, 1997.
421. DeLucia A 3rd, Wakefield TW, Andrews PC, et al: Efficacy and toxicity of differently charged polycationic protamine-like peptides for heparin anticoagulation reversal, *J Vasc Surg* 18:49, 1993.
422. Wakefield TW, Andrews PC, Wrobleski SK, et al: Effective and less toxic reversal of low-molecular-weight heparin anticoagulation by a designer variant of protamine, *J Vasc Surg* 21:839, 1995.
423. Kirklin JWBarratt-Boyes BG: Postoperative care. In *Cardiac Surgery*, New York, 1986, Churchill Livingstone, p 139.
424. Erban SB, Kinman JL, Schwartz S: Routine use of the prothrombin and partial thromboplastin times, *JAMA* 262:2428, 1989.
425. Ratnatunga CP, Rees GM, Kovacs IB: Preoperative hemostatic activity and excessive bleeding after cardiopulmonary bypass, *Ann Thorac Surg* 52:250, 1991.
426. Rodgers RP, Levin J: Bleeding time revisited, *Blood* 79:2495, 1992.
427. Horrow JC: Desmopressin and antifibrinolytics, *Int Anesthesiol Clin* 28:230, 1990.
428. Spiess BD, Wall MH, Gillies BS, et al: A comparison of thromboelastography with heparinase or protamine sulfate added in-vitro during heparinized cardiopulmonary bypass, *Thromb Haemost* 78:820, 1997.
429. Spiess BD: Thromboelastogram and postoperative hemorrhage, *Ann Thorac Surg* 54:810, 1992.
430. Ostrowsky J, Foes J, Warchol M, et al: Plateletworks platelet function test compared to the Thrombelastograph for prediction of postoperative outcomes, *J Extra Corpor Technol* 36:149, 2004.
431. Cammerer U, Dietrich W, Rampf T, et al: The predictive value of modified computerized thromboelastography and platelet function analysis for postoperative blood loss in routine cardiac surgery, *Anesth Analg* 96:51, 2003.
432. Royston D, von Kier S: Reduced haemostatic factor transfusion using heparinase-modified thromboelastography during cardiopulmonary bypass, *Br J Anaesth* 86:575, 2001.
433. Shore-Lesserson L, Manspeizer HE, DePerio M, et al: Thromboelastography-guided transfusion algorithm reduces transfusions in complex cardiac surgery, *Anesth Analg* 88:312, 1999.
434. Tuman KJ, McCarthy RJ, Djuric M, et al: Evaluation of coagulation during cardiopulmonary bypass with a heparinase modified thromboelstographic assay, *J Cardiothorac Vasc Anesth* 8:144, 1994.
435. Essell JH, Martin TJ, Salinas J, et al: Comparison of thromboelastography to bleeding time and standard coagulation tests in patients after cardiopulmonary bypass, *J Cardiothoracic Vasc Anesth* 7:410, 1993.
436. Marengo-Rowe AJ, Leveson JE: Fibrinolysis: A frequent cause of bleeding. In Ellison N, Jobes DR, editors: *Effective Hemostasis in Cardiac Surgery*, Philadelphia, 1988, WB Saunders, p 41.
437. Umlas J: Fibrinolysis and disseminated intravascular coagulation in open heart surgery, *Transfusion* 16:460, 1976.
438. Stibbe J, Kluft C, Brommer EJ, et al: Enhanced fibrinolytic activity during cardiopulmonary bypass in open-heart surgery in man is caused by extrinsic (tissue-type) plasminogen activator, *Eur J Invest* 14:375, 1984.
439. Havel M, Teufelsbauer H, Knöbl P, et al: Effect of intraoperative aprotinin administration on postoperative bleeding in patients undergoing cardiopulmonary bypass operation, *J Thorac Cardiovasc Surg* 101:968, 1991.
440. Villalobos TJ, Aderson E, Barila TG: Hematologic changes in hypothermic dogs, *Proc Soc Exp Biol Med* 89:192, 1985.
441. Hessell EA, Schmer G, Dillard DH: Platelet kinetics during deep hypothermia, *J Surg Res* 28:23, 1980.
442. Harker LA, Malpass TW, Branson HE: Mechanism of abnormal bleeding in patients undergoing cardiopulmonary bypass: Acquired transient platelet dysfunction associated with selective α-granule release, *Blood* 56:824, 1980.
443. Rinder CS, Bohnert J, Rinder H, et al: Platelet activation and aggregation during cardiopulmonary bypass, *Anesthesiology* 75:388, 1991.
444. Rinder CS, Mathew JP, Rinder HM, et al: Modulation of platelet surface adhesion receptors during cardiopulmonary bypass, *Anesthesiology* 75:563, 1991.
445. Adelman B, Rizk A, Hanners E: Plasminogen interactions with platelets in plasma, *Blood* 72:1530, 1988.
446. van Oeveren W, Eijsman L, Roozendaal KJ, et al: Platelet preservation by aprotinin during cardiopulmonary bypass, *Lancet* 1:644, 1988.
447. van Oeveren W, Harder MP, Roozendaal KJ, et al: Aprotinin protects platelets against the initial effect of cardiopulmonary bypass, *J Thorac Cardiovasc Surg* 99:788, 1990.
448. Soslau G, Horrow J, Brodsky I: The effect of tranexamic acid on platelet ADP during extracorporeal circulation, *Am J Hematol* 38:113, 1991.
449. Khuri SF, Wolfe JA, Josa M, et al: Hematologic changes during and after bypass, *J Thorac Cardiovasc Surg* 104:94, 1992.
450. Valeri CR, Khabbaz K, Khuri SF, et al: Effect of skin temperature on platelet function in patients undergoing bypass, *J Thorac Cardiovasc Surg* 104:108, 1992.
451. Paul J, Cornillon B, Baguet J, et al: In vivo release of a heparin-like factor in dogs during profound hypothermia, *J Thorac Cardiovasc Surg* 82:45, 1981.
452. Cornillon B, Mazzorana M, Dureau G, et al: Characterization of a heparin-like activity released in dogs during deep hypothermia, *Eur J Clin Invest* 18:160, 1988.
453. Michenfelder JD, Theye RA: Hypothermia: Effects on canine brain and whole-body metabolism, *Anesthesiology* 29:1107, 1968.
454. Yoshihara H, Yamamoto T, Mihara H: Changes in coagulation and fibrinolysis occurring in dogs during hypothermia, *Thromb Res* 37:503, 1985.
455. Lackritz EM, Satten GA, Aberle-Grasse J, et al: Estimated risk of the transmission of the human immunodeficiency virus by screened blood in the United States, *N Engl J Med* 333:1721, 1995.
456. Corash L: Photochemical decontamination of cellular blood components. In Horrow JC: Pharmacology of Blood and Haemostasis, *Anaesth Pharmacol Rev* 3:138, 1995.

457. Castaldi PA, Gorman DJ: Disordered platelet function in renal disease. In Colman R, Hirsh J, Marder VJ, et al: *Hemostasis and Thrombosis*, ed 2 Philadelphia, 1987, JB Lippincott, p 960.
458. Mannucci PM, Remuzzi G, Pusineri F, et al: Deamino, 8-D-arginine vasopressin shortens the bleeding time in uremia, *N Engl J Med* 308:8, 1983.
459. Mannucci PM, Vicente V, Vianello L, et al: Controlled trial of desmopressin in liver cirrhosis and other conditions associated with a prolonged bleeding time, *Blood* 67:1148, 1986.
460. Mannucci PM: Desmopressin: A nontransfusional form of treatment for congenital and acquired bleeding disorders, *Blood* 72:1449, 1988.
461. Boonstra PW, van Imhoff GW, Eysman L, et al: Reduced platelet activation and improved hemostasis after controlled cardiotomy suction during clinical membrane oxygenator perfusions, *J Thorac Cardiovasc Surg* 89:900, 1985.
462. van den Dungen JJ, Karliczek GF, Brenken U, et al: Clinical study of blood trauma during perfusion with membrane and bubble oxygenators, *J Thorac Cardiovasc Surg* 83:108, 1982.
463. Giordano GF, Rivers SL, Chung GK, et al: Autologous platelet-rich plasma in cardiac surgery: Effect on intraoperative and postoperative transfusion requirements, *Ann Thorac Surg* 46:416, 1988.
464. Giordano GF Sr, Giordano GF Jr, Rivers SL, et al: Determinants of homologous blood usage utilizing autologous platelet-rich plasma in cardiac operations, *Ann Thorac Surg* 47:897, 1989.
465. Boldt J, Von Bormann B, Kling D, et al: Preoperative plasmapheresis in patients undergoing cardiac surgery procedures, *Anesthesiology* 72:282, 1990.
466. Pliam MB, McGoon DC, Tarhan S: Failure of transfusion of autologous whole blood to reduce banked-blood requirements in open heart surgical patients, *J Thorac Cardiovasc Surg* 70:338, 1975.
467. Silver H: Banked and fresh autologous blood in cardiopulmonary bypass surgery, *Transfusion* 15:600, 1975.
468. Ereth MH, Oliver WC Jr, Beynen FM, et al: Autologous platelet-rich plasma does not reduce transfusion of homologous blood products in patients undergoing repeat valvular surgery, *Anesthesiology* 79:540, 1993.
469. DiMichele DM, Hathaway WE: Use of DDAVP in inherited and acquired platelet dysfunction, *Am J Hematol* 33:39, 1990.
470. MacGregor IR, Roberts EN, Provose CV, et al: Fibrinolytic and haemostatic responses to desamino-D-arginine vasopressin (DDAVP) administered by intravenous and subcutaneous routes in healthy subjects, *Thromb Haemost* 59:34, 1988.
471. Williams TD, Dunger DB, Lyon CC, et al: Antidiuretic effect and pharmacokinetics of oral 1-desamino, 8-D-arginine vasopressin. 1. Studies in adults and children, *J Clin Endocrinol Metab* 63:129, 1986.
472. D'Alauro FS, Johns RA: Hypotension related to desmopressin administration following cardiopulmonary bypass, *Anesthesiology* 69:962, 1988.
473. Salmenpera M, Kuitunen A, Hynynen M, et al: Hemodynamic responses to desmopressin acetate after CABG: A double-blind trial, *J Cardiothorac Vasc Anesth* 5:146, 1991.
474. Jahr JS, Marquez J, Cottington E, et al: Hemodynamic performance and histamine levels after desmopressin acetate administration following cardiopulmonary bypass in adult patients, *J Cardiothorac Vasc Anesth* 5:139, 1991.
475. Reich DL, Hammerschlag BC, Rand JH, et al: Desmopressin acetate is a mild vasodilator that does not reduce blood loss in uncomplicated cardiac surgical procedures, *J Cardiothorac Vasc Anesth* 5:142, 1991.
476. Bichet DG, Razi M, Lonergan M, et al: Hemodynamic and coagulation responses to 1-desamino (8-D-arginine) vasopressin in patients with congenital nephrogenic diabetes insipidus, *N Engl J Med* 318:881, 1988.
477. Weinstein RE, Bona RD, Althman AJ, et al: Severe hyponatremia after repeated intravenous administration of desmopressin, *Am J Hematol* 32:258, 1989.
478. Kobrinsky NL, Gerrard JM, Watson CM, et al: Shortening of bleeding time by 1-desamino, 8-D-arginine vasopressin in various bleeding disorders, *Lancet* 1:1145, 1984.
479. Guay J, Reinberg C, Poitras B, et al: A trial of desmopressin to reduce blood loss in patients undergoing spinal fusion for idiopathic scoliosis, *Anesth Analg* 75:405, 1992.
480. Salzman EW, Weinstein MJ, Weintraub RM, et al: Treatment with desmopressin acetate to reduce blood loss after cardiac surgery, *N Engl J Med* 314:1402, 1986.
481. Czer LSC, Bateman TM, Gray RJ, et al: Treatment of severe platelet dysfunction and hemorrhage after cardiopulmonary bypass: Reduction in blood product usage with desmopressin, *J Am Coll Cardiol* 9:1139, 1987.
482. Seear MD, Wadsworth LD, Rogers PC, et al: The effect of desmopressin acetate (DDAVP) on postoperative blood loss after cardiac operations in children, *J Thorac Cardiovasc Surg* 98:217, 1989.
483. Rocha E, Llorens R, Paramo JA, et al: Does desmopressin acetate reduce blood loss after surgery in patients on cardiopulmonary bypass? *Circulation* 77:1319, 1988.
484. Andersson TLG, Solem JO, Tengborn L, et al: Effects of desmopressin acetate on platelet aggregation, von Willebrand factor, and blood loss after cardiac surgery with extracorporeal circulation, *Circulation* 81:872, 1990.
485. Hackmann T, Gascoyne RD, Naiman SC, et al: A trial of desmopressin (1-desamino, 8-D-arginine vasopressin) to reduce blood loss in uncomplicated cardiac surgery, *N Engl J Med* 321:1437, 1989.
486. Lazenby WD, Russo I, et al: Treatment with desmopressin acetate in routine coronary artery bypass surgery to improve postoperative hemostasis, *Circulation* 82(Suppl IV):IV–413, 1990.
487. Horrow JC, Van Riper DF, Strong MD, et al: The hemostatic effects of tranexamic acid and desmopressin during cardiac surgery, *Circulation* 84:2063, 1991.
488. Reynolds LM, Nicolson SC, Jobes DR, et al: Desmopressin does not decrease bleeding after cardiac operation in young children, *J Thorac Cardiovasc Surg* 106:954, 1993.
489. Mongan PD, Hosking MP: The role of desmopressin acetate in patients undergoing coronary artery bypass surgery, *Anesthesiology* 77:38, 1992.
490. Verstraete M: Clinical application of inhibitors of fibrinolysis, *Drugs* 29:236, 1985.
491. Butterworth J, James R, Lin Y, et al: Pharmacokinetics of episilon aminocaproic acid in patients undergoing coronary artery bypass surgery, *Anesthesiology* 90:1624, 1999.
492. Takada A, Takada Y, Mori T, et al: Prevention of severe bleeding by tranexamic acid in a patient with disseminated intravascular coagulation, *Thromb Res* 58:101, 1990.
493. Butterworth JF, James RL, Kennedy DJ, et al: Pharmacokinetics of ε-aminocaproic acid in adult patients undergoing coronary artery surgery, *Anesthesiology* 85:A151, 1996.
494. Horrow JC, DiGregorio GJ, Ruch E: The dose-plasma concentration relationship of tranexamic acid during surgery, *Am J Ther* 1:206, 1994.
495. Williamson R, Eggleston DJ: DDAVP and EACA used for minor oral surgery in von Willebrand disease, *Aust Dent J* 33:32, 1988.
496. Blomback M, Johansson G, Johnsson H, et al: Surgery in patients with von Willebrand disease, *Br J Surg* 76:398, 1989.
497. Avvisati G, Büller HR, ten Cate JW, et al: Tranexamic acid for control of haemorrhage in acute promyelocytic leukaemia, *Lancet* 2:122, 1989.
498. Sharifi R, Lee M, Ray P, et al: Safety and efficacy of intravesical aminocaproic acid for bleeding after transurethral resection of prostate, *Urology* 27:214, 1986.
499. Sterns LP, Lillehei CW: Effect of epsilon aminocaproic acid upon blood loss following open heart surgery: An analysis of 340 patients, *Can J Surg* 10:304, 1967.
500. Gomes MMR, McGoon DC: Bleeding patterns after open heart surgery, *J Thorac Cardiovasc Surg* 60:87, 1970.
501. Midell AI, Hallman GL, Bloodwell RD, et al: Epsilon-aminocaproic acid for bleeding after cardiopulmonary bypass, *Ann Thorac Surg* 11:577, 1971.
502. McClure PD, Izsak J: The use of epsilon-aminocaproic acid to reduce bleeding during cardiac bypass in children with congenital heart disease, *Anesthesiology* 40:604, 1974.
503. Saussine M, Delpech S, Allien M, et al: Saignement apres circulation extracorporelle et acide epsilon amino-caproque, *Ann Fr Anesth Reanim* 4:403, 1985.
504. Vander Salm T, Ansell JE, Okike ON, et al: The role of epsilon-aminocaproic acid in reducing bleeding after cardiac operation: A double-blind randomized study, *J Thorac Cardiovasc Surg* 95:538, 1988.
505. Del Rossi AJ, Cernaianu AC, Botros S, et al: Prophylactic treatment of postperfusion bleeding using EACA, *Chest* 96:27, 1989.
506. Horrow JC, Hlavacek J, Strong MD, et al: Prophylactic tranexamic acid decreases bleeding after cardiac operations, *J Thorac Cardiovasc Surg* 99:70, 1990.
507. Isetta C, Samat C, Kotaiche M, et al: Low-dose aprotinin or tranexamic acid treatment in cardiac surgery [Abstract], *Anesthesiology* 75:A80, 1991.
508. Karski JM, Teasdale SJ, Norman P, et al: Prevention of bleeding after cardiopulmonary bypass with high-dose tranexamic acid, *J Thorac Cardiovasc Surg* 110:835, 1995.
509. Horrow JC, Van Riper DF, Strong MD, et al: The dose-response relationship of tranexamic acid, *Anesthesiology* 82:383, 1995.
510. Shore-Lesserson L, Reich DL, Vela-Cantos F, et al: Tranexamic acid reduces transfusions and mediastinal drainage in repeat cardiac surgery, *Anesth Analg* 83:18, 1996.
511. Ngaage DL, Bland JM: Lessons from aprotinin: Is the routine use and inconsistent dosing of tranexamic acid prudent? Meta-analysis of randomized and large matched observational studies, *Eur J Cardiothorac Surg* 37:1375–1383, 2010.
512. Murkin JM, Falter F, Granton J, et al: High dose tranexamic acid is associated with nonischemic clinical seizures in cardiac surgical patients, *Anesth Analg* 110:350–353, 2010.
513. Breuer T, Martin K, Wilhelm M, et al: The blood sparing effect and the safety of aprotinin compared to tranexamic acid in paediatric surgery, *Eur J Cardiothroac Surg* 35:167–171, 2009.
514. Mohseni K, Jafari A, Nobahar MR, et al: Polymyoclonus seizure resulting from accidental injection of tranexamic acid in spinal anesthesia, *Anesthanalg* 108:1984–1986, 2009.
515. Furtmüller R, Schlag MG, Berger M, et al: Tranexamic acid, a widely used antifibrinolytic agent, causes convulsions by a gamma-aminobutyric acid receptor antagonist effect, *J Pharmacol Exp Ther* 301:168–173, 2002.
516. Fritz H, Wunderer G: Biochemistry and applications of aprotinin, the kallikrein inhibitor from bovine organs, *Drug Res* 33:479, 1983.
517. Royston D: The serine antiprotease aprotinin (Trasylol): A novel approach to reducing postoperative bleeding, *Blood Coag Fibrin* 1:55, 1990.
518. Royston D: High-dose aprotinin therapy: A review of the first five years experience, *J Cardiothorac Vasc Anesth* 6:76, 1992.
519. D'Ambra MN, Risk SC: Aprotinin, erythropoietin, and blood substitutes, *Int Anesthesiol Clin* 28:237, 1990.
520. Lemmer JH, Stanford W, Bonney SL, et al: Aprotinin for coronary artery bypass grafting: Effect on postoperative renal function, *Ann Thorac Surg* 59:132, 1995.
521. Tice DA, Woeth MH, Clauss RH, et al: The inhibition of Trasylol of fibrinolytic activity associated with cardiovascular operations, *Surg Gynecol Obstet* 119:71, 1964.
522. Mammen EF: Natural proteinase inhibitors in extracorporeal circulation, *Ann NY Acad Sci* 146:754, 1968.
523. Royston D, Taylor KM, Bidstrup BP, et al: Effect of aprotinin on need for blood transfusion after repeat open heart surgery, *Lancet* 2:1289, 1987.
524. van Oeveren W, Jansen NJG, Bidstrup BP, et al: Effects of aprotinin on hemostatic mechanisms during cardiopulmonary bypass, *Ann Thorac Surg* 44:640, 1987.
525. Bidstrup BP, Royston D, Sapsford RN, et al: Reduction in blood loss and use after cardiopulmonary bypass with high-dose aprotinin (Trasylol), *J Thorac Cardiovasc Surg* 97:364, 1989.
526. Dietrich W, Barankay A, Dilthey G, et al: Reduction of homologous blood requirements in cardiac surgery by intraoperative aprotinin application-clinical experience in 152 cardiac surgical patients, *Thorac Cardiovasc Surg* 37:92, 1989.
527. Royston D: Aprotinin versus lysine analogues: The debate continues, *Ann Thorac Surg* 65:59, 1998.
528. Blauhut B, Gross C, Necek S, et al: Effects of high-dose aprotinin on blood loss, platelet function, fibrinolysis, complement, and renal function after cardiopulmonary bypass, *J Thorac Cardiovasc Surg* 101:958, 1991.
529. Edmunds LH, Niewiarowski S, Colman RW: Aprotinin [Letter], *J Thorac Cardiovasc Surg* 101:1103, 1991.
530. deSmet AAEA, Joen MCN, van Oeveren W, et al: Increased anticoagulation during cardiopulmonary bypass by aprotinin, *J Thorac Cardiovasc Surg* 100:520, 1990.
531. Dietrich W, Dilthey G, Spannagl M, et al: Influence of high-dose aprotinin on anticoagulation, heparin requirement, and celite- and kaolin-activated clotting time in heparin-pretreated patients undergoing open heart surgery. A double-blind, placebo-controlled study, *Anesthesiology* 83:679, 1995.
532. Wang J, Lin C, Hung W, et al: Monitoring of heparin-induced anticoagulation with kaolin-activated clotting time in cardiac surgical patients treated with aprotinin, *Anesthesiology* 77:1080, 1992.
533. Dietrich W, Jochum M: Effect of celite and kaolin on activated clotting time in the presence of aprotinin: Activated clotting time is reduced by binding of aprotinin to kaolin, *J Thorac Cardiovasc Surg* 109:177, 1995.
534. Huyzen RJ, Harder MP, Huet RC, et al: Alternative perioperative anticoagulation monitoring during cardiopulmonary bypass in aprotinin-treated patients, *J Cardiothorac Vasc Anesth* 8:153, 1994.
535. Bohrer H, Bach A, Fleischer F, et al: Adverse haemodynamic effects of high-dose aprotinin in a paediatric cardiac surgical patient, *Anaesthesia* 45:853, 1990.
536. Harmon DE: Cost/benefit analysis of pharmacologic hemostasis, *Ann Thorac Surg* 61(Suppl 2):S21, 1996.
537. Greilich PE, Carr ME Jr, Carr SL, et al: Reductions in platelet force development by cardiopulmonary bypass are associated with hemorrhage, *Anesth Analg* 80:459, 1995.
538. Smith PK, Datta SK, Muhlbaier LH, et al: Cost analysis of aprotinin for coronary artery bypass patients: Analysis of the randomized trials, *Ann Thorac Surg* 77:635, 2004.
539. Smith PK, Shah AS: The role of aprotinin in a blood-conservation program, *J Cardiothoracic Vasc Anesth* 18(Suppl):S24, 2004.
540. Mangano DT, Tudor JC, Dietzel C, et al: Multicenter Study of Perioperative Research Group of the Ischemic Research Foundation. The Risk Associated with Aprotinin in Cardiac Surgery, *N Engl J Med* 254:353–365, 2006.
541. Karkouti K, Beattie WS, Dattilo KM, et al: Propensity score case-controlled comparison of aprotinin and tranexamic acid in high transfusion-risk cardiac surgery, *Transfusion* 46:327–338, 2006.
542. Mangano DT, Miao Y, Vuylsteke A, et al: Mortality associated with aprotinin during 5 year followup after CABG surgery, *JAMA* 297:471–479, 2007.
543. Fergusson D, Hebert P, Mazar CD, et al: A comparison of aprotinin and lysine analogues in high-risk cardiac surgery, *N Engl J Med* 358:2319–2331, 2008.
544. Spiess B: Pro: Withdrawal of aprotinin has led to changes in our practice, *J Cardiothorac Vasc Anesth* 24:875–878, 2010.
545. Despotis GJ, Levine V, Filos KS, et al: Evaluation of a new point-of-care test that measures PAF-mediated acceleration of coagulation in cardiac surgical patients, *Anesthesiology* 85:1311, 1996.
546. Thomson DS: Effect of positive end-expiratory pressure on postoperative bleeding [Letter], *J Thorac Cardiovasc Surg* 88:457, 1984.

547. Ilabaca PA, Ochsner JL, Mills NL: Positive end-expiratory pressure in the management of the patient with a postoperative bleeding heart, *Ann Thorac Surg* 30:281, 1980.

548. Murphy DA, Finlayson DC, Craver JM, et al: Effect of positive end-expiratory pressure on excessive mediastinal bleeding after cardiac operations, *J Thorac Cardiovasc Surg* 85:864, 1983.

549. Zurick AM, Urzua J, Ghattas M, et al: Failure of positive end-expiratory pressure to decrease postoperative bleeding after cardiac surgery, *Ann Thorac Surg* 34:608, 1982.

550. Marder VJ, Feinstein DI, Francis CW, et al: Consumptive thrombohemorrhagic disorders. In Colman RW, Hirsh J, Marder VJ, et al, editors: *Hemostasis and Thrombosis*, ed 3 Philadelphia, 1994, JB Lippincott, p 1023.

551. Gravlee GP: Optimal use of blood components, *Int Anesthiol Clin* 28:216, 1990.

552. Murray DJ, Olson J, Strauss R, et al: Coagulation changes during packed red cell replacement of major blood loss, *Anesthesiology* 69:839, 1988.

553. de Prost D, Barbier-Boehm G, Hazebroucq J, et al: Desmopressin has no beneficial effect on excessive postoperative bleeding or blood product requirements associated with cardiopulmonary bypass, *Thromb Haemost* 68:106, 1992.

554. Shiffrin JS, Glass DD: Desmopressin is of value in the treatment of post-cardiopulmonary bypass bleeding, *J Cardiothorac Vasc Anesth* 5:285, 1991.

555. Chard RB, Kam CA, Nunn GR, et al: Use of desmopressin in the management of aspirin-related and intractable hemorrhage after cardiopulmonary bypass, *Aust N Z J Surg* 60:125, 1990.

556. Erhardtsen E: Pharmacokinetics of recombinant activated factor VII, *Semin Thromb Hemost* 26:385, 2000.

557. Roberts H, Monroe D, Hoffman M: Safety profile of recombinant factor VIIa, *Semin Hematol* 41(Suppl 1):101, 2004.

558. O'Connell N, Perry D, Hudgson A, et al: Recombinant FVIIa in the management of uncontrolled hemorrhage, *Transfusion* 43:1711, 2003.

559. Key N: Recombinant FVIIa for intractable hemorrhage: More questions than answers, *Transfusion* 43:1649, 2003.

560. Tanaka K, Waly A, Cooper W, et al: Treatment of excessive bleeding in Jehovah's Witness patients after cardiac surgery with recombinant factor VIIa, *Anesthesiology* 98:1513, 2003.

561. Zietkiewicz M, Garlicki M, Domagala J, et al: Successful use of activated recombinant factor VII to control bleeding abnormalities in a patient with left ventricular assist device, *J Thorac Cardiovasc Surg* 123:384, 2002.

562. Hendriks H, van der Maaten J, de Wolf J, et al: An effective treatment of severe intractable bleeding after valve repair by one single dose of activated recombinant factor VII, *Anesth Analg* 93:287, 2001.

563. Milas B, Jobes D, Gorman, R: Management of bleeding and coagulopathy after heart surgery, *Semin Thorac Cardiovasc Surg* 12:326, 2000.

564. Body SC, Shernan SK: Genetic basis of cardiovascular disease and perioperative pain. In Van Aken H, editor: *Clinical Anesthiology*, London, 2001, Baillière Tindall.

565. Ginsburg G, Donahue M, Newby L: Prospects for personalized cardiovascular medicine, *J Am Coll Cardiol* 46:1615, 2005.

566. Podgoreanu M, Schwinn D: New paradigms in cardiovascular medicine, *J Am Coll Cardiol* 46:1965, 2005.

32

Discontinuing Cardiopulmonary Bypass

JACK S. SHANEWISE, MD, FASE | JOEL A. KAPLAN, MD, CPE, FACC

KEY POINTS

1. The key to success in weaning from cardiopulmonary bypass (CPB) is proper preparation.
2. After rewarming the patient, correcting any abnormal blood gases, and inflating the lungs, make sure to turn on the ventilator.
3. To prepare the heart for discontinuing CPB, optimize the cardiac rhythm, heart rate, myocardial contractility, preload, and afterload.
4. The worse the heart's condition, the more gradually CPB should be weaned. If hemodynamic values are not adequate, immediately return to CPB. Assess the problem, and choose an appropriate pharmacologic, surgical, or mechanical intervention before trying to terminate CPB again.
5. Perioperative ventricular dysfunction usually is caused by myocardial stunning and is a temporary state of contractile dysfunction that should respond to positive inotropic drugs.
6. In addition to left ventricular dysfunction, right ventricular failure is a possible source of morbidity and mortality after cardiac surgery.
7. Epinephrine is frequently the inotropic drug of choice when terminating CPB because of its mixed α- and β-adrenergic stimulation.
8. Milrinone is an excellent inodilator drug that can be used alone or combined with other drugs such as epinephrine for discontinuing CPB in patients with poor ventricular function.
9. In patients with high preloads, vasodilators such as nitroglycerin or nitroprusside may markedly improve ventricular function.
10. Intra-aortic balloon pump counterpulsation increases coronary blood flow during diastole and unloads the left ventricle during systole. These effects can help in weaning patients with poor left ventricular function and severe myocardial ischemia.

Cardiopulmonary bypass (CPB) has been used since the 1950s to facilitate surgery on the heart and great vessels, and even with the increased interest in off-pump coronary artery bypass grafting, CPB remains a critical part of most cardiac operations. Managing patients with CPB remains one of the defining characteristics of cardiac surgery and cardiac anesthesiology (see Chapters 28 to 31). Discontinuing CPB is a necessary part of every operation involving extracorporeal

circulation. Through this process, the support of the circulation by the bypass pump and oxygenator is transferred back to the patient's heart and lungs. This chapter reviews important considerations involved with discontinuing CPB and presents an approach to managing this critical component of a cardiac operation, which may be routine and easy or extremely complex and difficult. The key to success in discontinuing CPB is proper preparation. The period during and immediately after weaning from CPB usually is busy for the anesthesiologist, and having to do things that could have been accomplished earlier in the operation is not helpful. The preparations for bringing a patient off CPB may be organized into several parts: general preparations, preparing the lungs, preparing the heart, and final preparations.

GENERAL PREPARATIONS

Temperature

Because at least moderate hypothermia is used during CPB in most cardiac surgery cases, it is important that the patient is sufficiently rewarmed before attempting to wean from CPB (Table 32-1).[1] Initiation of rewarming is a good time to consider whether additional drugs need to be given to keep the patient anesthetized. Anesthetic vaporizers need to be off for 20 to 30 minutes before coming off CPB to clear the agent from the patient if so desired.[2] However, currently, the patient is frequently removed from CPB with low doses of the inhalation agent still on to continue the anesthetic preconditioning of the heart (see Chapter 9). Monitoring the temperature of a highly perfused tissue such as the nasopharynx is useful to help prevent overheating the brain during rewarming, but these temperatures may increase more rapidly than others, such as bladder, rectum, or axilla temperatures, leading to inadequate rewarming and temperature drop-off after CPB as the heat continues to distribute throughout the body.[3] Different institutions have various protocols for rewarming, but the important point is to warm gradually, avoiding hyperthermia of the central nervous system while getting enough heat into the patient to prevent significant drop-off after CPB[4] (see Chapters 28 and 29). After CPB, there is a tendency for the patient to lose heat, and measures to keep the patient warm such as fluid warmers, a circuit heater-humidifier, and forced-air warmers should be set up and turned on before weaning from CPB. The temperature of the operating room may need to be increased as well; this is probably an effective measure to keep a patient warm after CPB, but it may make the scrubbed and gowned personnel uncomfortable.

Laboratory Results

An arterial blood gas should be measured before weaning from CPB and any abnormalities corrected. Severe metabolic acidosis depresses the myocardium and should be treated with $NaHCO_3$ or THAM.[5–8] The optimal hematocrit for weaning from CPB is controversial and probably varies from patient to patient.[9,10] It makes sense that sicker patients with lower cardiovascular reserve may benefit from a higher hematocrit (optimal is considered to be 30%), but the risks and adverse consequences of transfusion need to be considered as well. Suffice it to say that the hematocrit should be measured and optimized before weaning from CPB (see Chapters 30 and 31). Serum potassium level should be measured before weaning from CPB and may be high because of dysfunction after CPB may require positive end-expiratory pressure, an intensive care unit–type ventilator, or nitric oxide (see Chapters 33, 35, and 37). If needed, this equipment should be obtained before attempting to wean the patient from CPB.

TABLE 32-1	General Preparations for Discontinuing Cardiopulmonary Bypass
Temperature	*Laboratory Results*
Adequately rewarm before weaning from CPB	Correct metabolic acidosis
Avoid overheating the brain	Optimize hematocrit
Start measures to keep patient warm after CPB	Normalize K^+
Use fluid warmer, forced air warmer	Consider giving Mg^{2+} or checking Mg^{2+} level
Warm operating room	Check Ca^{2+} level and correct deficiencies

CPB, cardiopulmonary bypass.

cardioplegia or low, especially in patients receiving loop diuretics. Hyperkalemia may make establishing an effective cardiac rhythm difficult and can be treated with $NaHCO_3$, $CaCl_2$, or insulin, but the levels usually decrease quickly after cardioplegia has been stopped. Low serum potassium levels probably should be corrected before coming off CPB, especially if arrhythmias are present. Administration of magnesium (Mg^{2+}) to patients on CPB decreases postoperative arrhythmias and may improve cardiac function, and many centers routinely give all CPB patients magnesium sulfate.[11] Theoretic disadvantages include aggravation of vasodilation and inhibition of platelet function.[12] If Mg^{2+} is not given routinely, the level should be checked before weaning from CPB and deficiencies corrected. The ionized calcium level should be measured and significant deficiencies corrected before discontinuing CPB. Many centers give all patients a bolus of calcium chloride just before coming off CPB because it transiently increases contractility and systemic vascular resistance (SVR).[13] However, it has been argued that this practice is to be avoided because Ca^{2+} may interfere with catecholamine action and aggravate reperfusion injury.[14]

PREPARING THE LUNGS

As the patient is weaned from CPB and the patient's heart starts to support the circulation, the lungs again become the site of gas exchange, delivering oxygen and eliminating carbon dioxide. Before weaning from CPB, the lung function must be restored (Table 32-2). The trachea should be suctioned and, if necessary, lavaged with saline to clear secretions. If the abdomen appears to be distended, the stomach should be suctioned so that gastric distention does not impair ventilation after CPB. The lungs are reinflated by hand gently and gradually, with sighs using up to 30 cm H_2O pressure, and then mechanically ventilated with 100% oxygen. Care should be taken not to allow the left lung to injure an in situ internal mammary artery graft as the lung is reinflated. The compliance of the lungs can be judged by their feel with hand ventilation, with stiff lungs suggesting more difficulty with oxygenation or ventilation after CPB. If visible, both lungs should be inspected for residual atelectasis, and they should be rising and falling with each breath. Ventilation alarms and monitors should be activated. If prolonged expiration or wheezing is detected, bronchodilators should be given. The surgeon should inspect both pleural spaces for pneumothorax, which should be treated with opening the pleural space. Any fluid present in the pleural spaces should be removed before attempting to wean the patient from CPB. In its most severe form, pulmonary

TABLE 32-2	Preparing the Lungs for Discontinuing Cardiopulmonary Bypass

Suction trachea and endotracheal tube.

Inflate lungs gently by hand.

Ventilate with 100% oxygen.

Treat bronchospasm with bronchodilators.

Check for pneumothorax and pleural fluid.

Consider need for positive end-expiratory pressure, intensive care unit ventilator, and nitric oxide.

PREPARING THE HEART

Preparing the heart to resume its function of pumping blood involves optimizing the five hemodynamic parameters that can be controlled: rhythm, rate, contractility, afterload, and preload (Table 32-3).

Rhythm

There must be an organized, effective, and stable cardiac rhythm before attempting to wean from CPB. This can occur spontaneously after removal of the aortic cross clamp, but the heart may resume electrical activity with ventricular fibrillation. If the blood temperature is greater than 30° C, the heart may be defibrillated with internal paddles applied directly to the heart using 10 to 20 J. Defibrillation at lower temperatures may be unsuccessful because extreme hypothermia can cause ventricular fibrillation.[15-17] If ventricular fibrillation persists or recurs repeatedly, antiarrhythmic drugs such as lidocaine or amiodarone may be administered to help achieve a stable rhythm. It is

TABLE 32-3	Preparing the Heart for Discontinuing Cardiopulmonary Bypass
Hemodynamic Parameters	*Preparation*
Rhythm	Normal sinus rhythm is ideal.
	Defibrillate if necessary when temperature > 30° C.
	Consider antiarrhythmic drugs if ventricular fibrillation persists more than a few minutes.
	Try synchronized cardioversion for atrial fibrillation or flutter.
	Look at the heart to diagnose atrial rhythm.
	Try atrial pacing if AV conduction exists.
	Try AV pacing for heart block.
Heart rate	Rate should be between 75 and 95 beats/min in most cases.
	Treat slow rates with electrical pacing.
	Treat underlying causes of fast heart rates.
	Heart rate may decrease as the heart fills.
	Control fast supraventricular rates with drugs and then pace as needed.
	Always have pacing immediately available during heart surgery.
Contractility	Inotropic support is more likely needed with depressed cardiac function before CPB, advanced age, long bypass or clamp time, poor preservation, or incomplete revascularization.
	Look for the vigorous "snap" of a heartbeat with good contractility.
	If depressed contractility is likely, begin inotropic drugs before weaning from CPB.
	Severely impaired function may require mechanical support.
Afterload	Systemic vascular resistance is a major component of afterload.
	Keep MAP between 60 and 80 mm Hg at full CPB flow.
	Consider a vasoconstrictor if the MAP is low and a vasodilator if the MAP is high.
Preload	End-diastolic volume is the best measure of preload and can be seen with TEE.
	Filling pressures provide a less direct measure of preload.
	Consider baseline filling pressures.
	Assess RV volume and function with direct inspection.
	Assess LV volume and function with TEE.
	Cardiac distention may cause MR and TR.

AV, atrioventricular; CPB, cardiopulmonary bypass; LV, left ventricular; MAP, mean arterial pressure; MR, mitral regurgitation; RV, right ventricular; TEE, transesophageal echocardiography; TR, tricuspid regurgitation.

not unusual for the rhythm to remain unstable for several minutes immediately after cross clamp removal, but persistent or recurrent ventricular fibrillation should prompt concern about impaired coronary blood flow. Because it provides an atrial contribution to ventricular filling and a normal, synchronized contraction of the ventricles, normal sinus rhythm is the ideal cardiac rhythm for weaning from CPB.[18,19] Atrial flutter or fibrillation, even if present before CPB, often can be converted to normal sinus rhythm with synchronized cardioversion, especially if antiarrhythmic drugs are administered. It often is helpful to look directly at the heart when there is any question about the cardiac rhythm. Atrial contraction, flutter, and fibrillation are easily seen on CPB when the heart is visible. Ventricular arrhythmias should be treated by correcting underlying causes such as potassium or magnesium deficits and, if necessary, with antiarrhythmic drugs such as amiodarone.[20] If asystole or complete heart block occurs after cross clamp removal, electrical pacing with temporary epicardial pacing wires may be needed to achieve an effective rhythm before weaning from CPB. If atrioventricular conduction is present, atrial pacing should be attempted because, as with normal sinus rhythm, it provides atrial augmentation to filling and synchronized ventricular contraction. Atrioventricular sequential pacing is used when there is heart block, which frequently is present for 30 to 60 minutes as the myocardium recovers after cross clamp removal. Ventricular pacing remains the only option if no organized atrial rhythm is present, but this sacrifices the atrial "kick" to ventricular filling and the more efficient synchronized ventricular contraction of the normal conduction system[21,22] (see Table 32-3).

Rate

In most situations for adult patients, the heart rate (HR) should be between 75 and 95 beats/min for weaning from CPB. Lower rates theoretically may be desirable for hearts with residual ischemia or incomplete revascularization. Higher HRs may be needed for hearts with limited stroke volume such as after ventricular aneurysmectomy. Slow HRs are best treated with electrical pacing, but β-agonist or vagolytic drugs also may be used to increase the HR. Tachycardia before weaning from CPB is more worrisome and difficult to deal with, and treatable causes such as inadequate anesthesia, hypercarbia, and ischemia should be identified and corrected. The HR often decreases as the heart is filled in the weaning process, and electrical pacing always should be immediately available during cardiac surgery. Supraventricular tachycardias should be electrically cardioverted if possible, but drugs such as β-antagonists or calcium channel antagonists may be needed to control the ventricular rate if they persist, most typically occurring in patients with chronic atrial fibrillation. If drug therapy decreases the rate too much, pacing may be used.

Contractility

The contractile state of the myocardium should be considered before attempting to wean from CPB. The likelihood of decreased contractility requiring inotropic support after CPB is greater with preexisting ventricular impairment (e.g., low ejection fraction, high left ventricular end-diastolic pressure before surgery or before CPB), advanced age, long CPB time, long aortic cross clamp time, inadequate myocardial preservation, and incomplete revascularization.[23] A heart with good contractility often has a vigorous snap with contraction that can be seen while on CPB, in contrast with the weak contractions of a heart with impaired contractility, but it may be difficult to assess global ventricular function while the heart is empty and on CPB. If significant depression of contractility is likely, inotropic support can be started before attempting to wean the patient from CPB. If depressed myocardial contractility becomes evident during weaning, the safest approach is to prevent cardiac distention by resuming CPB and resting the heart for 10 to 20 minutes while inotropic therapy with a catecholamine or phosphodiesterase (PDE) inhibitor drug is started. Extreme depression of contractile function of the myocardium may require mechanical

support with an intra-aortic balloon pump (IABP) or ventricular assist device (see Pharmacologic Management of Ventricular Dysfunction section later in this chapter; see also Chapters 27 and 34).

Afterload

Afterload is the tension developed within the ventricular muscle during contraction. An important component of afterload in patients is the SVR (see Chapters 5, 14, and 34).[24] While on CPB at full flow, usually about 2.2 L/min/m², mean arterial pressure (MAP) is directly related to SVR and indicates whether the SVR is appropriate, too high, or too low. Low SVR after CPB can cause inadequate systemic arterial perfusion pressure, and high SVR can significantly impair cardiac performance, especially in patients with poor ventricular function. SVR usually is within a reasonable range when the arterial pressure is between 60 and 80 mm Hg at full pump flow. If below that range, infusion of a vasopressor may be needed to increase SVR before attempting to wean from CPB. If the MAP is high while on CPB, vasodilator therapy may be needed.

Preload

Preload is the amount of stretch on the myocardial muscle fibers just before contraction. In the intact heart, the best measure of preload is end-diastolic volume. Less direct clinical measures of preload include left atrial pressure (LAP), pulmonary artery occlusion pressure, and pulmonary artery diastolic pressure, but there may be a poor relation between end-diastolic pressure and volume during cardiac surgery[25,26] (see Chapters 5, 14, and 34). Transesophageal echocardiography (TEE) is a useful tool for weaning from CPB because it provides direct visualization of the end-diastolic volume and contractility of the left ventricle[27–29] (see Chapters 11 to 13). The process of weaning a patient from CPB involves increasing the preload (i.e., filling the heart from its empty state on CPB) until an appropriate end-diastolic volume is achieved. When preparing to discontinue CPB, some thought should be given to the appropriate range of preload for the particular patient at hand. The filling pressures before CPB may indicate what they need to be after CPB; a heart with high filling pressures before CPB may require high filling pressures after CPB to achieve an adequate preload.

FINAL PREPARATIONS

The final preparations before discontinuing CPB include leveling the operating table, rezeroing the pressure transducers, ensuring the proper function of all monitoring devices, confirming that the patient is receiving only intended drug infusions, ensuring the immediate availability of resuscitation drugs and appropriate fluid volume, and verifying that the lungs are being ventilated with 100% oxygen (Table 32-4).

The surgeon must confirm that he or she has completed the necessary preparations in the surgical field before discontinuing CPB. Macroscopic collections of air in the heart should be evacuated before starting to wean from CPB. These are detected most easily with TEE,

TABLE 32-4	Final Preparations for Discontinuing Cardiopulmonary Bypass	
Anesthesiologist's Preparations	*Surgeon's Preparations*	
Level operating table.	Remove macroscopic collections of air from the heart.	
Rezero transducers.	Control major sites of bleeding.	
Activate monitors.	Ensure CABG is lying nicely without kinks.	
Check drug infusions.	Turn off or remove cardiac vents.	
Have resuscitation drugs and fluid volume at hand.	Take clamps off the heart and great vessels.	
Reestablish TEE/PAC monitoring.	Loosen tourniquets around caval cannulas.	

CABG, coronary artery bypass graft; PAC, pulmonary artery catheter; TEE, transesophageal echocardiography.

which also can be helpful in monitoring and directing the deairing process.[30] Major sites of bleeding should be controlled, cardiac vent suction should be off, all clamps on the heart and great vessels should be removed, coronary artery bypass grafts should be checked for kinks and bleeding, and tourniquets around the caval cannulas should be loosened or removed before starting to wean a patient from CPB.

ROUTINE WEANING FROM CARDIOPULMONARY BYPASS

There should be close and clear communication among the perfusionist, the surgeon, and the anesthesiologist while weaning a patient from CPB, and the surgeon or the anesthesiologist should be in charge of the process. The anesthesiologist should be positioned at the head of the table, able to readily see the CPB pump and perfusionist, the heart, and the surgeon, and the anesthesia monitor display. The TEE display also should be easily in view. Weaning a patient from CPB is accomplished by diverting blood back into the patient's heart by occluding the venous drainage to the CPB pump. The arterial pump flow is decreased simultaneously as the pump reservoir volume empties into the patient and the heart's contribution to systemic flow increases. This can be accomplished most abruptly by simply clamping the venous return cannula and transfusing blood from the pump until the heart fills and the preload appears to be adequate. Some patients will tolerate this method of discontinuing CPB, but many will not, and a more gradual transfer from the pump to the heart usually is desirable. The worse the function of the heart, the slower the transition from full CPB to off CPB needs to be.

Before beginning to wean the patient from CPB, the perfusionist should communicate to the physicians involved three important parameters: the current flow rate of the pump, the volume in the pump reservoir, and the oxygen saturation of venous blood returning to the pump from the patient. The current flow rate of the pump indicates the stage of weaning as it is decreased. Weaning is just beginning at full flow, is well under way when down to 2 or 3 L/min in adults, and is almost finished at less than 2 L/min. The reservoir volume indicates how much blood is available for transfusion to fill the heart and lungs as CPB is discontinued. If the volume is low, less than 400 to 500 mL in adults, more fluid may need to be added to the reservoir before weaning from CPB. The oxygen saturation of the venous return (Svo_2) gives an indication of the adequacy of peripheral perfusion during CPB. If the Svo_2 is greater than 60%, oxygen delivery during CPB is adequate; if less than 50%, oxygen delivery is inadequate, and measures to improve delivery (e.g., increase pump flow or hematocrit) or decrease consumption (e.g., give more anesthetic agents or neuromuscular blocking drugs) need to be taken before coming off CPB. An Svo_2 between 50% and 60% is marginal and must be followed closely. As the patient is weaned from CPB, an increasing Svo_2 suggests that the net flow to the body is increasing and that the heart and lungs will support the circulation; a declining Svo_2 indicates that tissue perfusion is decreasing and that further intervention to improve cardiac performance will be needed before coming off CPB.

The actual process of weaning from CPB begins with partially occluding the venous return cannula with a clamp (Figure 32-1). This may be done in the field by the surgeon or at the pump by the perfusionist. This causes blood to flow into the right ventricle. As the right ventricle fills and begins to pump blood through the lungs, the left heart will begin to fill. When this occurs, the left ventricle will begin to eject and the arterial waveform will become pulsatile. Next, the perfusionist will gradually decrease the pump flow rate. As more of the venous return goes through the heart and less to the pump reservoir, it becomes necessary to gradually decrease the pump flow to avoid emptying the pump reservoir. One approach to weaning from CPB is to bring the filling pressure being monitored (e.g., central venous pressure, pulmonary artery occlusion pressure, LAP) to a specific, predetermined level somewhat lower than may be necessary and then assess the hemodynamics. Volume (preload) of the heart also may be judged

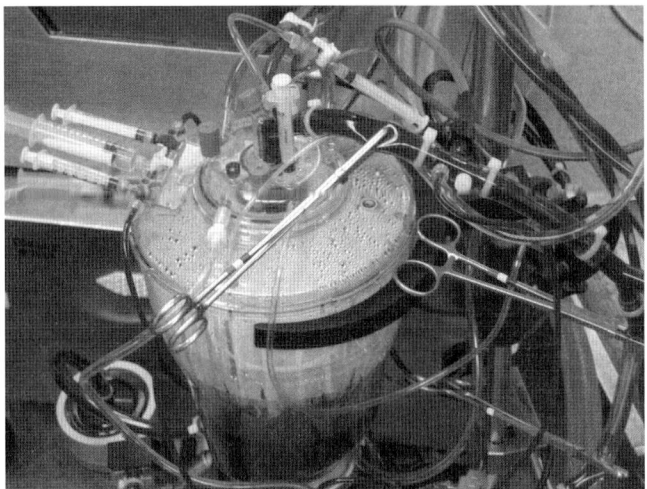

Figure 32-1 The process of weaning from cardiopulmonary bypass is started by partially occluding the venous return cannula with a clamp.

by direct observation of its size or with TEE. Further filling is done in small increments (50 to 100 mL) while closely monitoring the preload until the hemodynamics appear satisfactory as judged by the arterial pressure, the appearance of the heart, and the trend of the Svo_2. It typically is easy to see the right-heart volume and function directly in the surgical field and the left heart with TEE, and combining the two observations is a useful approach for weaning from CPB. Overfilling and distention of the heart should be avoided because it may stretch the myofibrils beyond the most efficient length and dilate the annuli of the mitral and tricuspid valves, rendering them incompetent, which easily is detected with TEE. If the patient has two venous cannulas, the smaller of the two may be removed when the pump flow is half of the full flow rate to improve movement of blood from the great veins into the right atrium. When the pump flow has been decreased to 1 L/min or less in an adult and the hemodynamics are satisfactory, the venous cannula may be completely clamped and the pump flow turned off. At this point, the patient is "off bypass" (Figure 32-2).

This is a critical juncture in the operation. The anesthesiologist should pause a moment to make a brief scan of the patient and monitors to confirm that the lungs are being ventilated with oxygen, the hemodynamic status is acceptable and stable, the electrocardiogram shows no new signs of ischemia, the heart does not appear to be

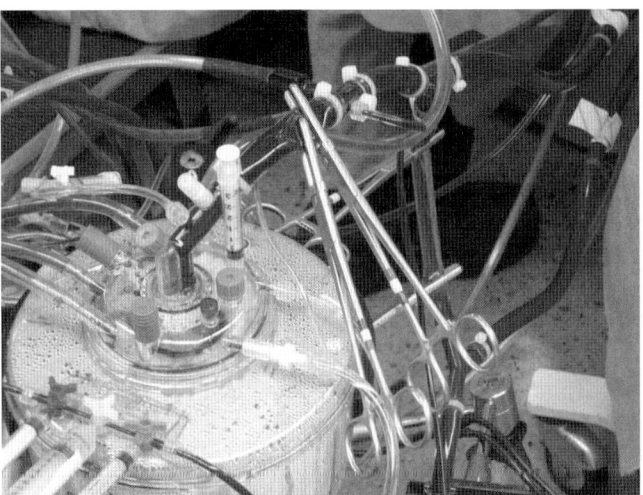

Figure 32-2 When the venous return cannula is completely clamped, the patient is "off bypass."

distending, and the drug infusions are functioning as desired. Further fine-tuning of the preload is accomplished by transfusing 50- to 100-mL boluses from the pump reservoir through the arterial cannula and observing the effect on hemodynamics. If there is acute failure of the circulation as evidenced by an unstable rhythm, falling arterial and rising filling pressures, or visible distention of the heart, the patient is put back on CPB by unclamping the venous return cannula and turning on the arterial pump flow. Once back on CPB, an assessment of the cause of failure to wean is made and appropriate interventions undertaken before attempting to wean again. When the hemodynamics appear to be stable and adequate, the surgeon may remove the venous cannula from the heart.

The next step in discontinuing CPB is to transfuse as much as possible of the blood remaining in the pump reservoir into the patient before removal of the arterial cannula. This is usually easier and quicker than transfusing through the intravenous infusions after decannulation. The blood in the venous cannula and tubing (usually about 500 mL) may be drained into the reservoir for transfusion. The patient's venous capacitance can be increased by raising the head of the bed (i.e., reverse Trendelenburg position) or giving nitroglycerin, being more cautious with these maneuvers in patients with impaired cardiac function. Filling the vascular space with the head up and while infusing nitroglycerin increases the ability to cope with volume loss after decannulation by allowing rapid augmentation of the central vascular volume by leveling the bed and decreasing the nitroglycerin infusion rate.

After discontinuing CPB, the anticoagulation by heparin is reversed with protamine. Depending on institutional preference, protamine may be administered before or after removal of the arterial cannula. Giving it before removal allows for continued transfusion from the pump and easier return to CPB if there is a severe protamine reaction (see Chapter 31). Giving protamine after removal of the arterial cannula may decrease the risk for thrombus formation and systemic embolization. After the infusion of protamine is started, pump suction return to the reservoir should be stopped to keep protamine out of the pump circuit in case subsequent return to CPB becomes necessary. Protamine should be given slowly through a peripheral intravenous catheter over 5 to 15 minutes while watching for systemic hypotension and pulmonary hypertension, which may indicate that an untoward (allergic) reaction to protamine is occurring.[31-33] Technically flawed coronary artery bypass grafts may thrombose after protamine administration, causing acute ischemia mimicking a protamine reaction.

When transfusion of the pump reservoir blood is completed, a thorough assessment of the patient's condition should be made before removing the arterial cannula, because after this is done, returning to CPB becomes much more difficult. The cardiac rhythm should be stable. Cardiac function is assessed by evaluating pressures, cardiac output, and TEE. Hemodynamics should be satisfactory and stable. Adequate oxygenation and ventilation should be confirmed by arterial blood gas or pulse oximetry and capnography. Bleeding from the heart should be at a manageable level before removal of the arterial cannula. The perfusionist should not have to transfuse significant amounts of blood through the arterial cannula before removing it, because it may be difficult to keep up with the blood loss through intravenous infusions alone. Bleeding sites behind the heart may have to be repaired on CPB if the patient cannot tolerate lifting the heart to expose the problem area. At the time of arterial decannulation, the systolic pressure should be between 85 and 100 mm Hg to minimize the risk for dissection or tearing of the aorta.[34] The head of the bed may be raised, or small boluses of a short-acting vasodilator (e.g., nitroglycerin, nitroprusside) may be given to lower the systemic blood pressure as necessary. Tight control of the arterial blood pressure may be needed for a few minutes until the cannulation site is secure.

When the arterial cannula has been removed, the heparin effects are reversed with protamine, and the hemodynamic status remains stable, the routine process of discontinuing CPB is complete. However, in patients with poor ventricular function after CPB, multiple drugs or even mechanical assist devices may be required throughout the rest of the operation and continued in the intensive care unit.

PHARMACOLOGIC MANAGEMENT OF VENTRICULAR DYSFUNCTION

Perioperative ventricular dysfunction usually is a transient state of contractile impairment that may require temporary support with positive inotropic agents. In a subset of patients, contractility may be significantly depressed such that combination therapy with positive inotropes and vasodilator agents is needed to effectively improve cardiac output and tissue perfusion. The use of mechanical assist devices is reserved for conditions of overt or evolving cardiogenic shock.

Severe ventricular dysfunction, specifically the low cardiac output syndrome (LCOS), occurring after CPB and cardiac surgery differs from chronic congestive heart failure (CHF) (Box 32-1). Patients emerging from CPB have hemodilution, moderate hypocalcemia, hypomagnesemia, and altered potassium levels. Depending on temperature and depth of anesthesia, these individuals may demonstrate low, normal, or high SVR. Increasing age, female sex, decreased LVEF, and increased duration of CPB are associated with a greater likelihood that inotropic support will be needed after CABG surgery[23] (Table 32-5).

Contractile dysfunction during or after cardiac surgery can result from preexisting impairment in contractility or be a new-onset condition. Abnormal contraction, especially in the setting of coronary artery disease (CAD), usually is caused by myocardial injury resulting in ischemia or infarction. The magnitude of contractile dysfunction

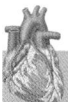

BOX 32-1. RISK FACTORS FOR THE LOW CARDIAC OUTPUT SYNDROME AFTER CARDIOPULMONARY BYPASS

- Preoperative ventricular dysfunction
- Myocardial ischemia
- Poor myocardial preservation
- Reperfusion injury
- Inadequate cardiac surgical repair or revascularization

TABLE 32-5	Patient Characteristics Associated with the Use of Inotropic Drug Support		
Variable	*No Inotropic Drug Support** (n = 58)	*Inotropic Drug Support** (n = 70)	*P*
Age (yr)	57 ± 8	62 ± 8	0.005
Sex			
Female (%)	10	26	0.027
Male (%)	90	74	
Collateral circulation (%)	64	73	0.271
WMA (%)	78	84	0.334
Patients demonstrating cardiac enlargement (%)	7	21	0.021
Baseline LVEDP (mm Hg)	14 ± 7	16 ± 6	0.044
Postcontrast LVEDP (mm Hg)	21 ± 8	24 ± 7	0.054
Change in LVEDP (mm Hg)	7 ± 6	7 ± 7	0.534
EF (%)	61 ± 11	54 ± 13	0.002
PT (min)	106 ± 30	125 ± 37	0.004
IT (min)	42 ± 15	50 ± 19	0.009

*All values except for sex, collateral circulation, WMA, and patients demonstrating cardiac enlargement are expressed as mean ± SD.

EF, preoperative ejection fraction calculated from end-diastolic and end-systolic measurements from radiograph-contrast ventriculography; IT, duration of aortic cross-clamping (ischemic time); LVEDP, left ventricular end-diastolic pressure; PT, total duration of cardiopulmonary bypass (pump time); WMA, wall motion abnormalities identified during preoperative radiographic-contrast ventriculography.

From Royster RL, Butterworth JF, Prough DS, et al: Preoperative and intraoperative predictors of inotropic support and long-term outcome in patients having coronary bypass grafting. *Anesth Analg* 72:729, 1991.

corresponds to the extent and duration of injury. Brief periods of myocardial oxygen deprivation (< 10 minutes) produce regional contractile dysfunction, which can be rapidly reversed by reperfusion. Extension of the ischemia to 15 to 20 minutes also is associated with restoration of cardiac function with reperfusion; however, this process is very slow and can take hours to days. This condition of postischemic reversible myocardial dysfunction in the presence of normal flow is referred to as *myocardial stunning.*[35-37] Irreversible cell injury will occur with longer periods of ischemia, producing a myocardial infarction characterized by release of intracellular enzymes, disruption of cell membranes, influx of calcium, persistent contractile dysfunction, and eventual cellular swelling and necrosis.[38]

In addition to the previously described factors, right ventricular (RV) dysfunction and failure are potential sources of morbidity and mortality after cardiac surgery. Numerous factors may predispose patients to the development of perioperative RV dysfunction, including CAD, RV hypertrophy, previous cardiac surgery, and operative considerations such as inadequate revascularization or hypothermic protection. Technical and operative difficulties are associated with various cardiac surgical procedures (e.g., right ventriculotomy), RV trauma, rhythm and conduction abnormalities, injury to the right ventricle during cessation of CPB, or protamine reaction (see Chapter 31).

The following discussion provides an overview of the pharmacologic approach to management of perioperative ventricular dysfunction in the setting of cardiac surgery. Management goals are described in Table 32-6.[39] These are extensions of the routine preparations made for discontinuing CPB shown in Table 32-3.

Sympathomimetic Amines

Sympathomimetic drugs (i.e., catecholamines) are pharmacologic agents capable of providing inotropic and vasoactive effects (Box 32-2). Catecholamines exert positive inotropic action by stimulation of the β_1 receptor. The predominant hemodynamic effect of a specific catecholamine depends on the degree to which the various α, β, and dopaminergic receptors are stimulated (Tables 32-7 and 32-8).

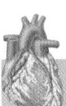

BOX 32-2. PHARMACOLOGIC APPROACHES TO VENTRICULAR DYSFUNCTION

- Inotropic drugs
- Phosphodiesterase inhibitors
- Vasodilators
- Vasopressors
- Metabolic supplements

The physiologic effect of an adrenergic agent is determined by the sum of its actions on α, β, and dopaminergic receptors. The effectiveness of any adrenergic agent will be influenced by the availability and responsiveness of adrenergic receptors. Chronically increased levels of plasma catecholamines (e.g., chronic CHF and long CPB time) cause downregulation of the number and sensitivity of β receptors.[40] Maintenance of normal acid-base status, normothermia, and electrolytes also improve the responsiveness to adrenergic-receptor stimulation.

The selection of a drug to treat ventricular dysfunction is influenced by pathophysiologic abnormalities, as well as by the physician's experience and preference. If LV performance is decreased primarily as a result of diminished contractility, the drug chosen should increase contractility. Although β-agonists improve contractility and tissue perfusion, their effects may increase myocardial oxygen consumption (Mvo_2) and reduce coronary perfusion pressure (CPP). However, if the factor most responsible for decreased cardiac function is hypotension with concomitantly reduced CPP, use of an α-adrenergic agonist can increase blood pressure and improve diastolic coronary perfusion.

Catecholamines also are effective for treating primary RV contractile dysfunction, with all of the β_1-adrenergic agonists augmenting RV contractility. Studies have documented the efficacy of epinephrine, norepinephrine, dobutamine, isoproterenol, dopamine, and PDE-III inhibitors in managing RV contractile dysfunction. When decreased RV contractility is combined with increased afterload, agents that exert vasodilator and positive inotropic effects should be used, including epinephrine, isoproterenol, dobutamine, and the PDE-III inhibitors (see Chapters 10, 24, and 34).[41-44]

Epinephrine

Epinephrine stimulates α- and β-adrenergic receptors in a dose-dependent fashion. It frequently is the inotrope of choice after CPB (Box 32-3). Dosages of 10, 20, and 40 ng/kg/min increased stroke volume by 2%, 12%, and 22%, respectively, and increased cardiac index by 0.1, 0.7, and 1.2 L/min/m². The HR also increased, but by no more than 10 beats/min at any dose.[45] Epinephrine frequently is used after cardiac surgery to support the function of the "stunned" reperfused heart. During emergence from CPB, Butterworth et al[46] showed epinephrine (30 ng/kg/min) increased cardiac index and stroke volume by 14% without increasing HR. In cardiac surgical patients, epinephrine infusion (0.01 to 0.4 µg/kg/min) effectively increases cardiac output, minimally increases HR, and has acceptable side effects (see Table 32-8; see Chapters 10 and 34).

Dobutamine

Dobutamine is a synthetic catecholamine that generally produces dose-dependent increases in cardiac output and reductions in diastolic filling pressures. The effects of epinephrine (30 ng/kg/min) were compared with dobutamine (5 µg/kg/min) in 52 patients recovering from CABG surgery.[46] Both drugs significantly and similarly increased stroke volume index, but epinephrine increased the HR by only 2 beats/min, whereas dobutamine increased the HR by 16 beats/min.

In addition to increasing contractility, dobutamine may have favorable metabolic effects on ischemic myocardium. Intravenous and

TABLE 32-6	Management of Cardiac Dysfunction
Variable	*Physiologic Management*
Heart rate and rhythm	Maintain normal sinus rhythm, avoid tachycardia; for tachycardia or bradycardia, consider pacing or chronotropic agents (atropine, isoproterenol, epinephrine), correct acid-base, electrolytes, and review of current medications
Preload	Reduce increased preload with diuretics or venodilators (nitroglycerin or sodium nitroprusside); monitor CVP, PCWP, and SV; obtain echocardiogram to rule out ischemia, valvular lesions, tamponade, and intracardiac shunts; consider using inotropes, IABP, or both
Afterload	Avoid increased afterload (increased wall tension), use vasodilators (sodium nitroprusside); avoid hypotension; maintain coronary perfusion pressure; consider IABP, inotropes devoid of α_1-adrenergic effects (dobutamine or milrinone), or both IABP and inotropes
Contractility	Assess hemodynamics, rule out ischemia/infarction, assess rate/rhythm, preload, and afterload, use inotropes; if uncertain, obtain echocardiogram to assess cardiac function; consider combination therapy with inotropes and vasodilators and/or assist devices (IABP/LVAD/RVAD)
Oxygen delivery	Increase Fio_2 and CO; check ABGs and chest radiograph; mechanical ventilation if indicated; correct acid-base disturbances

ABG, arterial blood gas; CO, cardiac output; CVP, central venous pressure; Fio_2, inspired oxygen concentration; IABP, intraaortic balloon pump; LVAD, left ventricular assist device; PCWP, pulmonary capillary wedge pressure; RVAD, right ventricular assist device; SV, stroke volume.

TABLE 32-7	**Sympathomimetics**					
	Dosage		**Site of Action**			
Drug	*Intravenous*	*Infusion*	*α*	*β*	*Mechanism of Action*	
Methoxamine	2–10 mg	—	++++		Direct	
Phenylephrine	50–500 μg	10 mg/500 mL 20 μg/mL 10–50 μg/min	++++	±	Direct	
Norepinephrine	—	8 mg/500 mL 16 μg/mL 2–16 μg/min	++++	+++	Direct	
Metaraminol	100 μg	20–200 mg/500 mL 40–400 μg/mL 40–500 μg/min	++++	+	Direct and indirect	
Epinephrine	2–16 μg	4 mg/500 mL 8 μg/mL 2–10 μg/min	+++	+++	Direct	
Ephedrine	5–25 mg	—	+	++	Direct and indirect	
Dopamine	—	400 mg/500 mL 800 μg/mL 2–30 μg/kg/min	++	+++	Direct and indirect	
Dobutamine	—	250 mg/500 mL 500 μg/mL 2–20 μg/kg/min	+	++++	Direct	
Dopexamine	—	0.5–4 μg/kg/min		++	Direct	
Isoproterenol	1–4 μg	2 mg/500 mL 4 μg/mL 1–5 μg/min		++++	Direct	

TABLE 32-8	**Hemodynamic Effects of Catecholamines and Phosphodiesterase Inhibitors**						
Drug	*CO*	*dP/dt*	*HR*	*SVR*	*PVR*	*PCWP*	*Mvo₂*
Dobutamine							
2–12 μg/kg/min*	↑↑↑	↑	↑↑	↓	↓	↓ or ⇌	↑
Dopamine							
0–3 μg/kg/min	↑	↑	↑	↓	↓	↑	↑
3–8 μg/kg/min	↑↑	↑	↑	↓	↓	↑	↑
>8 μg/kg/min	↑↑	↑	↑↑	↑	⇌ (↑)	↑ or ⇌	↑↑
Isoproterenol							
0.5–10 μg/min	↑↑	↑↑	↑↑	↓↓	↓	↓	↑↑
Epinephrine							
0.01–0.4 μg/kg/min	↑↑	↑	↑	↑ (↓)	(↑)	↑ or ⇌	↑↑
Norepinephrine							
0.01–0.3 μg/kg/min	↑	↑	⇌ (↑↓)	↑↑	⇌	⇌	↑
PDE inhibitors†	↑↑	↑	↑	↓↓	↓↓	↓↓	↓

*The indicated dosages represent the most common dosage ranges. For the individual patient, a deviation from these recommended doses might be indicated.

†Phosphodiesterase (PDE) inhibitors are usually given as a loading dose followed by a continuous infusion: amrinone: 0.5–1.5 mg/kg loading dose, 10–30 μg/kg/min continuous infusion; milrinone: 50 μg/kg loading dose, 0.375–0.75 μg/kg/min continuous infusion.

CO, cardiac output; dP/dt, myocardial contractility; HR, heart rate; Mvo₂, myocardial oxygen consumption; PCWP, pulmonary capillary wedge pressure; PVR, pulmonary vascular resistance; SVR, systemic vascular resistance.

Modified from Lehmann A, Boldt J: New pharmacologic approaches for the perioperative treatment of ischemic cardiogenic shock. *J Cardiothorac Vasc Anesth* 19:97–108, 2005.

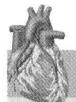

BOX 32-3. INOTROPIC DRUGS

- Epinephrine
- Norepinephrine
- Dopamine
- Dobutamine
- Isoproterenol

intracoronary injections of dobutamine increase coronary blood flow in animal studies.[47] In paced cardiac surgical patients, dopamine increased oxygen demand without increasing oxygen supply, whereas dobutamine increased myocardial oxygen uptake and coronary blood flow. However, because increases in HR are a major determinant of Mvo₂, these favorable effects of dobutamine could be lost if dobutamine induces tachycardia. During dobutamine stress echocardiography, segmental wall motion abnormalities suggestive of myocardial ischemia can occur as a result of tachycardia and increases in Mvo₂[48] (see Chapters 2 and 12).

Dopamine

Dopamine is an endogenous catecholamine and an immediate precursor of norepinephrine and epinephrine. Its actions are mediated by stimulation of adrenergic receptors and specific postjunctional dopaminergic receptors (D_1 receptors) in the renal, mesenteric, and coronary arterial beds.[49] In low doses (0.5 to 3.0 μg/kg/min), dopamine predominantly stimulates the dopaminergic receptors; at doses ranging from 3 to 7 μg/kg/min, it activates most adrenergic receptors in a nonselective fashion; and at higher doses (> 10 μg/kg/min), dopamine behaves as a vasoconstrictor. The dose-dependent effects of dopamine are not very specific and can be influenced by multiple factors such as receptor regulation, concomitant drug use, and interindividual and intraindividual variability.

Dopamine is unique in comparison with other endogenous catecholamines because of its effects on the kidneys. It has been shown to increase renal artery blood flow by 20% to 40% by causing direct vasodilation of the afferent arteries and indirect vasoconstriction of the efferent arteries.[50] This results in increases in glomerular filtration rate and in oxygen delivery to the juxtamedullary nephrons.

Despite favorable effects, dopamine has several undesirable features that may limit its use. Its propensity to increase HR and cause tachyarrhythmias can result in demand-related myocardial ischemia. After cardiac surgery, dopamine causes more frequent and less predictable degrees of tachycardia than dobutamine or epinephrine at doses that produce comparable improvement in contractile function.[51]

Norepinephrine

Norepinephrine is used primarily to treat vasodilated patients after CPB. Meadows et al[52] treated 10 patients with severe sepsis and hypotension unresponsive to volume expansion, dopamine, and dobutamine. Norepinephrine infusion (0.03 to 0.89 μg/kg/min) alone improved arterial blood pressure, left ventricular stroke work index, urine output, and, in most cases, cardiac index. Desjars et al[53] studied the renal effects of prolonged norepinephrine infusion in hypotensive patients with sepsis. Norepinephrine (0.5 to 1.0 μg/kg/min) plus low-dose dopamine improved urine flow and renal function compared with dopamine alone.[53] The α-adrenergic agonists benefit certain patients with circulatory failure refractory to inotropic and fluid therapy. Phenylephrine, norepinephrine, or vasopressin may be used to restore MAP in patients with a low SVR after CPB (i.e., vasoplegia syndrome).[54] When RV dysfunction is primarily a result of decreased CPP, vasoconstrictors can be used to optimize RV performance.[55]

Isoproterenol

Isoproterenol is a potent, nonselective β-adrenergic agonist, devoid of α-adrenergic agonist activity. Isoproterenol dilates skeletal, renal, and mesenteric vascular beds and decreases diastolic blood pressure. The potent chronotropic action of isoproterenol, combined with its propensity to decrease CPP, limit its usefulness in patients with CAD. Applications include treatment of bradycardia (especially after orthotopic heart transplantation), pulmonary hypertension, and heart failure after congenital cardiac surgery.[55] Isoproterenol remains the inotrope of choice for stimulation of cardiac pacemaker cells in the management of acute bradyarrhythmias or atrioventricular heart block. Its use for this purpose during cardiac surgery is limited because artificial pacing is usually easily accomplished in this setting. It reduces refractoriness to conduction and increases automaticity in myocardial tissues. The tachycardia seen with isoproterenol is a result of direct effects of the drug on the sinoatrial and atrioventricular nodes and reflex effects caused by peripheral vasodilation. It is routinely used in the setting of cardiac transplantation for increasing automaticity and inotropy, as well as for its vasodilatory effect on the pulmonary arteries (see Chapter 23).

Phosphodiesterase Inhibitors

The PDE-III inhibitors amrinone (inamrinone) and milrinone increase cyclic adenosine monophosphate, calcium flux, and calcium sensitivity of contractile proteins. These drugs have a similar mode of

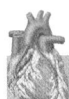

BOX 32-4. INODILATOR DRUGS

- Inamrinone
- Milrinone
- Dobutamine
- Epinephrine plus nitroprusside ("epipride")

action because they are noncatecholamine and nonadrenergic agents. They do not rely on β-receptor stimulation for their positive inotropic activity. As a result, the effectiveness of the PDE-III inhibitors is not altered by previous β-blockade, nor is it reduced in patients who may experience β-receptor downregulation.[40] In addition to their positive inotropic effects, these agents produce systemic and pulmonary vasodilation. As a result of this combination of hemodynamic effects (i.e., positive inotropic support and vasodilation), the term *inodilator* has been used to describe these drugs (Box 32-4).

Amrinone is more effective than dobutamine for weaning from CPB, with increases in stroke volume and cardiac output, and decreases in SVR and pulmonary vascular resistance (PVR).[56,57] Because these agents exert their hemodynamic effects by a nonadrenergic mechanism of action, when used in combination with β-agonists, they have an additive effect on myocardial performance. Gage et al[58] reported that when amrinone was used in combination with dobutamine, cardiac output was significantly increased compared with therapy with dobutamine alone. Since this initial report, other investigators have demonstrated the clinical application of combination therapy using PDE-III inhibitors and dopamine, phenylephrine, epinephrine, and nitroglycerin.[59]

A second-generation PDE-III inhibitor milrinone has a similar hemodynamic profile to amrinone; however, its positive inotropic action is approximately 15 to 30 times that of amrinone. Thrombocytopenia has been a potential clinical concern with the administration of PDE-III inhibitors, particularly amrinone. However, George et al[60] were unable to demonstrate any significant reduction in platelet count after 48 hours of milrinone infusion in cardiac surgical patients. Intravenous milrinone has been studied extensively and demonstrates a favorable short-term effect in CHF and ventricular dysfunction after CPB[61] (see Chapters 10 and 34).

Milrinone, like other PDE-III inhibitors, appears to increase cardiac output without increasing overall Mvo₂. Monrad et al[62] administered milrinone to patients with CHF, increasing cardiac index by 45%, but overall Mvo₂ did not change. Data also suggest that milrinone may improve myocardial diastolic relaxation (i.e., positive "lusitropic" effect) and augment coronary perfusion. The proposed mechanism for this effect on diastolic performance is that by decreasing LV wall tension, ventricular filling is enhanced, and myocardial blood flow and oxygen delivery are optimized (see Table 32-8).

The ability of short-term administration of milrinone to augment ventricular performance in patients undergoing cardiac surgery was shown in the results from the European Milrinone Multicentre Trial Group.[63] In this prospective study, intravenous milrinone was studied in patients after CPB. All patients received a bolus infusion of milrinone at 50 μg/kg over 10 minutes, followed by a maintenance infusion of 0.375, 0.5, or 0.75 μg/kg/min for 12 hours. Significant increases in stroke volume and cardiac index were observed. In addition, significant decreases in pulmonary capillary wedge pressure, central venous pressure, pulmonary artery pressure, MAP, and SVR were seen. Eighteen patients (14%) had arrhythmias; most occurred in the group receiving 0.75 μg/kg/min. Two arrhythmic events were deemed serious; both were bouts of rapid atrial fibrillation occurring with the greater dose.

Bailey et al[64] showed that after CPB, a loading dose of milrinone at 50 μg/kg, followed by a continuous infusion of 0.5 μg/kg/min, resulted in a significant increase in cardiac output. Butterworth et al[65] also studied the pharmacokinetics and pharmacodynamics of milrinone in adult patients undergoing cardiac surgery; milrinone (25, 50, or 75 μg/kg) was given if the cardiac index was less than 3.0 L/min/m² after separation from CPB. All three doses of milrinone significantly increased cardiac index. The 50- and 75-μg/kg doses produced significantly greater increases in cardiac index than the 25-μg/kg dose. The 75-μg/kg dose produced increases in cardiac index comparable with the 50-μg/kg dose, but it was associated with more hypotension, despite administration of intravenous fluid, blood, and a phenylephrine infusion. The initial redistribution half-lives were 4.6, 4.3, and 6.9 minutes, and the terminal elimination half-lives were 63, 82, and 99 minutes for the 25-, 50-, and 75-μg/kg doses, respectively. The results of these investigations suggest that for optimizing hemodynamic performance (while minimizing any potential for arrhythmias), the middle dose range (i.e., loading dose of 50 μg/kg) of milrinone may be most efficacious with a continuous infusion of 0.5 μg/kg/min, leading to a plasma concentration of more than 100 ng/mL. In patients with poor LV function, the loading dose should be given during CPB to avoid a decrease in MAP and to minimize the need for other inotropes on discontinuing CPB.[66]

Vasodilators

The indications for using vasodilators such as nitroglycerin or nitroprusside in cardiac surgery include management of perioperative systemic or pulmonary hypertension, myocardial ischemia, and ventricular dysfunction complicated by excessive pressure or volume overload[67] (Box 32-5). In most conditions, nitroglycerin or nitroprusside may be used. Both share common features such as rapid onset, ultra-short half-lives (several minutes), and easy titratability. Nevertheless, there are important pharmacologic differences between nitroglycerin and nitroprusside. In the setting of ischemia, nitroglycerin is preferred because it selectively vasodilates coronary arteries without producing a coronary "steal" (see Chapters 6, 10, and 18). Likewise, in the management of ventricular volume overload or RV pressure overload, nitroglycerin may offer some advantage over nitroprusside. It has a predominant influence on the venous bed such that preload can be reduced without significantly compromising systemic arterial pressure. The benefits of nitroglycerin are improvement in stroke volume, reduction in wall tension and Mvo₂, increased perfusion to the subendocardium as a result of a lower left ventricular end-diastolic pressure, and maintenance of CPP. Nitroprusside is a more potent arterial vasodilator and may potentiate myocardial ischemia because of a coronary steal phenomenon or a reduction in CPP. Its greater potency, however, makes nitroprusside the vasodilator of choice for management of perioperative hypertensive disorders and for afterload reduction during or after surgery for regurgitant valvular lesions (see Chapter 19).

Additional uses of vasodilators include management of RV dysfunction. Sodium nitroprusside can augment cardiac output by decreasing RV afterload and PVR.[68] Similarly, nitroglycerin has been shown to decrease PVR, transpulmonary pressure, and mean pulmonary artery pressure and to increase cardiac output in patients with increased PVR resulting from mitral valve disease.[69] Although nitroglycerin and nitroprusside decrease the impedance to RV ejection and increase the RV ejection fraction by reducing afterload, they are nonspecific pulmonary vasodilators. As a result, newer studies have focused on the ability

of agents such as prostaglandins (particularly prostaglandin E₁), nitric oxide, and the PDE-III inhibitors to more specifically decrease PVR (see Chapters 10, 24, and 34).

Despite proven benefits of vasodilator therapy in the management of CHF, they can be difficult drugs to use in treatment of perioperative ventricular dysfunction. This is most evident in cases of the LCOS when impaired pump function is complicated by inadequate perfusion pressure. In these situations, multidrug therapy with vasoactive and cardioactive agents is warranted (i.e., nitroglycerin or nitroprusside plus epinephrine or milrinone and norepinephrine). Combination therapy enables greater selectivity of effect. The unwanted side effects of one drug can be avoided while supplementing the desired effects with another agent.[70,71] To maximize the desired effects of any particular combination of agents, frequent assessment of cardiac performance with a PAC and TEE is needed. This allows the Starling curve and the pressure-volume loops to be visualized as they are shifted up and to the left with therapy (see Chapters 5, 14, and 34).

Vasoplegic Syndrome and Cardiopulmonary Bypass

The concept of the vasoplegic syndrome, hypotension associated with profound vasodilation unresponsive to conventional catecholamines or vasopressors, was introduced in association with CPB in the late 1990s.[72] It has been linked with preoperative use of vasodilators and shown to be a risk factor for increased morbidity and mortality after cardiac surgery.[73] Two pharmacologic agents have been reported to be used to treat vasoplegic syndrome after CPB: vasopressin and methylene blue.

Vasopressin

Arginine vasopressin (antidiuretic hormone) is a peptide hormone normally produced in the posterior pituitary that plays a crucial role in water homeostasis by controlling water resorption in the renal collecting ducts.[74] Administered as an intravenous infusion, vasopressin was initially used as a potent vasoconstrictor for vasodilatory shock associated with sepsis[75] and ventricular assist device implantation.[76] Because its vasopressor effect is mediated through a different mechanism (VP1 receptors) from the catecholamines, vasopressin can be infused at a constant rate as a strategy to decrease high doses of catecholamines such as norepinephrine and has been used in this way to treat vasodilation occurring after CPB.[77] The vasoconstricting effects of vasopressin may spare the pulmonary vasculature, making it an attractive choice to treat hypotension associated with right-heart dysfunction, but this effect has not been clearly demonstrated in intact humans.[78] Reported infusion doses vary widely from 0.01 to 0.6 IU/min.[79] Use of vasopressin has been associated with necrotic lesions of the skin and should be used with caution and in the lowest possible effective dose.[80]

Methylene Blue

Methylene blue, a substance commonly used intravenously during surgery for its ability to dye certain tissues, inhibits guanylate cyclase and hence the production of cyclic guanosine monophosphate, a substance known to increase vascular smooth muscle relaxation.[81] It has been used as a rescue treatment for profound vasodilatory shock in a number of settings, including cardiac surgery.[82,83] Methylene blue in a dose of 3 mg/kg given while on CPB was shown to increase SVR and MAP without adverse effects in a randomized trial of patients taking angiotensin-converting enzyme inhibitors, as well as decrease pressor requirements and serum lactate levels after CPB.[84] In another randomized trial, methylene blue, 2 mg/kg, was given 1 hour before surgery to patients at risk for CPB-associated vasoplegic syndrome. None of the treatment group developed vasoplegic syndrome, while 26% of the control group did.[85] Methylene blue causes transient discoloration of the urine and the skin and interferes with pulse oximetry measurements of arterial oxygen saturation. Although a number of

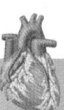

BOX 32-5. VASODILATOR MECHANISMS HELPFUL IN DISCONTINUING CARDIOPULMONARY BYPASS

- Decreased right and left ventricular wall stress (afterload)
- Decreased venous return (preload)
- Improved lusitropy
- Improved coronary blood flow

transient adverse side effects of methylene blue have been reported in other contexts, no serious side effects have been reported in its use for vasoplegia associated with CPB.[86]

Additional Pharmacologic Therapy

Following the steps outlined in Tables 32-3 and 32-6, most patients can be weaned off of CPB. However, a small percentage will be difficult to remove safely from CPB because of their chronic end-stage CHF or an acute insult during cardiac surgery producing cardiogenic shock. These patients probably will require mechanical circulatory support (e.g., IABP), as discussed subsequently or in Chapter 27 (e.g., ventricular assist device). However, while instituting these further steps, some clinicians try additional pharmacologic therapy.

Controversial Older Treatments

Some studies suggest that a reduction in plasma thyroid hormone concentration may be the cause of decreased myocardial function after CPB.[87,88] Some patients exhibit signs of hypothyroidism, including decreases in HR, cardiac index, and myocardial and systemic oxygen consumption, and increases in arteriovenous oxygen difference and SVR. Multiple investigators have documented declines in the circulating triiodothyronine (T_3) concentration during and after CPB, and the most dramatic decreases in T_3 are seen at the end of CPB and during the first few hours after CPB.[87,88] The reduced thyroid hormone concentrations after CPB may exacerbate myocardial stunning and the LCOS encountered in the post-CPB period. Thyroid hormone in the form of an intravenous T_3 infusion (2 μg/hr to a total dose of 0.5 μg/kg) has been used during cardiac surgery. This therapy has resulted in increases in the MAP and HR, as well as reductions in LAP and central venous pressure in patients who initially could not be weaned from CPB. Some of these patients have been successfully weaned from CPB and have required lower doses of dobutamine and other cardiac drug support after the treatment with thyroid hormone.[89-91]

The administration of glucose-insulin-potassium (GIK) or just glucose and insulin has been found to be useful for metabolic support of the heart after CPB. The trauma of cardiac surgery produces insulin resistance, which restricts the availability of carbohydrates to the heart. The increased level of catecholamines during CPB also may put further strain on the energy metabolism of the heart, whereas insulin may improve this situation.[92-94] The administration of high-dose insulin has been compared with dopamine in patients undergoing CABG surgery. The infusion of dopamine (7 μg/kg/min) alone induced metabolic changes unfavorable to the myocardium, whereas dopamine plus insulin increased carbohydrate use with cessation of cardiac uptake of free fatty acids.[95] Gradinac et al[96] studied GIK in patients with refractory CHF after CPB. All of the patients started with a low cardiac index and were receiving cardiac support with an inotropic drug and an IABP. There was a significant increase in cardiac index in the GIK patients at 12 and 24 hours, the need for inotropic and IABP support was decreased, and the 30-day survival rate was increased.[81] A recent study using high-dose insulin therapy during CABG surgery found

significant hypolipidemia with a large lowering of the plasma free fatty acid concentration in the treatment group.[97] The importance of this finding requires further investigation before high-dose insulin therapy becomes part of the everyday armamentarium in dealing with poor ventricular function.

New Treatments for Heart Failure and Cardiogenic Shock

Levosimendan is a new positive inotropic drug belonging to the class of calcium sensitizers. The drug stabilizes the calcium-induced conformational change in cardiac troponin C and prolongs the effective cross-bridging time. In contrast with other positive inotropic drugs, levosimendan does not increase intracellular calcium. The drug has vasodilating and anti-ischemic properties produced by opening K^+-ATP channels[98-100] (Table 32-9; see Chapters 10 and 34).

Levosimendan is recommended by the European Society of Cardiology for treatment of acute worsening of heart failure and for acute heart failure after myocardial infarction.[101] It also has been found to enhance contractile function of stunned myocardium in patients with acute coronary syndromes.[102] It is available clinically in Europe and is undergoing evaluation in the United States. The use of levosimendan has been reported in cardiac surgical patients with high perioperative risk, compromised LV function, difficulties in weaning from CPB, and severe RV failure after mitral valve replacement.[103,104] The doses used were 12 μg/kg as a 10-minute loading dose, followed by an infusion of 0.1 μg/kg/min. It has been used before surgery, during emergence from CPB, and in the postoperative period for up to 28 days. The potential for levosimendan to produce increased contractility, decreased resistance, minimal metabolic cost, and no arrhythmias makes it a potentially useful addition to the treatments for patients with the LCOS or RV failure. Randomized trials have demonstrated that levosimendan can facilitate weaning from CPB and decrease the need for additional inotropic support during CABG surgery.[105,106]

Nesiritide is a recombinant human brain-type natriuretic peptide with vasodilatory and diuretic effects. In patients with heart failure, intravenous nesiritide acts as a vasodilator and reduces preload; SVR is decreased, and cardiac index subsequently increases.[107-109] The drug has no positive inotropic effects (see Chapter 10). Compared with nitroglycerin and dobutamine, nesiritide had a greater effect on decreasing preload than nitroglycerin, and it did not cause as many arrhythmias as dobutamine.[110,111] Its ultimate role in the treatment of acute heart failure is uncertain, but it may augment the vasodilators or diuretics. There also is some evidence suggesting nesiritide may have a role in preserving renal function during cardiac surgery.[112,113]

Numerous other drugs are being studied for their uses in patients with acute decompensated heart failure and cardiogenic shock. These drugs include positive inotropic agents such as toborinone (a PDE-III inhibitor), vasodilators such as tezosentan (a specific and potent dual endothelin-receptor antagonist), and vasopressors such as L-NAME (a nitric oxide inhibitor; see Table 32-9).[98] These various drugs may prove useful for certain types of cardiovascular problems in the future.

TABLE 32-9	Emerging Drugs for Heart Failure and Cardiogenic Shock								
Drug*	CO	PCWP	AP	HR	Arrhyth.	Onset	Offset	Diur.	Shock
Toborinone	↑↑↑	↓↓	↑ or ↓	⇌	↑↑↑	Short	Moderate	⇌	No
L-Simendan	↑↑	↓	↓	↑	⇌	Short	Very long	⇌	Yes
Tezosentan	↑↑	↓	↓	⇌	⇌	Short	Short	⇌	No
Nesiritide	↑	↓↓	↓	⇌	⇌	Short	Long	↑↑	No
L-NAME	↓	↑↑	↑↑↑	(↓)	?	Short	Moderate	↑	Yes

*Positive inotropic drugs: toborinone; phosphodiesterase inhibitor. L-Simendan: levosimendan, calcium sensitizer. Vasodilating drugs: tezosentan: endothelin antagonist. Nesiritide: natriuretic peptide. Vasoconstricting drug: L-NAME: N^G-nitro-L-arginine-methyl ester, inhibitor of nitric oxide synthase.
AP, arterial pressure; Arrhyth., arrhythmogenic potential; CO, cardiac output; Diur., diuresis; HR, heart rate; No, not yet used in patients with cardiogenic shock; PCWP, pulmonary capillary wedge pressure; Shock, cardiogenic shock; Yes, already used in patients with cardiogenic shock.
Modified from Lehman A, Boldt J: New pharmacologic approaches for the perioperative treatment of ischemic cardiogenic shock. *J Cardiothorac Vasc Anesth* 19:97, 2005.

INTRA-AORTIC BALLOON PUMP COUNTERPULSATION

The IABP is a device that is designed to augment myocardial perfusion by increasing coronary blood flow during diastole and unloading the left ventricle during systole. This is accomplished by mass displacement of a volume of blood (usually 30 to 50 mL) by alternately inflating and deflating a balloon positioned in the proximal segment of the descending aorta. The gas used for this purpose is carbon dioxide (because of its great solubility in blood) or helium (because of its inertial properties and rapid diffusion coefficients). Inflation and deflation are synchronized to the cardiac cycle by the electronics of the balloon console producing counterpulsations. The results of effective use of the IABP are often quite dramatic. Improvements in cardiac output, ejection fraction, coronary blood flow, and MAP frequently are seen, as well as decreases in aortic and ventricular systolic pressures, left ventricular end-diastolic pressure, pulmonary capillary wedge pressure, LAP, HR, frequency of premature ventricular contractions, and suppression of atrial arrhythmias.

Indications and Contraindications

Since its introduction, the indications for the IABP have grown (Table 32-10). The most common use of the IABP is for treatment of cardiogenic shock. This may occur after CPB or after cardiac surgery in patients with preoperative shock, with acute postinfarction ventricular septal defects or mitral regurgitation, those who require stabilization before surgery, or patients who decompensate hemodynamically during cardiac catheterization. Patients with myocardial ischemia refractory to coronary vasodilation and afterload reduction are stabilized with an IABP before cardiac catheterization, and some patients with severe CAD will prophylactically have an IABP inserted before undergoing CABG or off-pump CABG surgery.[114–118]

Contraindications to IABP use are relatively few (see Table 32-10). The presence of severe aortic regurgitation (AR) or aortic dissection is listed as an absolute contraindication for the IABP, although successful reports of its use in patients with aortic insufficiency or acute trauma to the descending thoracic aorta have appeared. Other relative contraindications are listed; use of the IABP in these instances is at the discretion of the physician. Because the hemodynamic changes caused by an IABP theoretically would tend to worsen dynamic outflow tract

TABLE 32-10	Intra-aortic Balloon Pump Counterpulsation Indications and Contraindications	
Indications	*Contraindications*

1. Cardiogenic shock
  a. Myocardial infarction
  b. Myocarditis
  c. Cardiomyopathy
2. Failure to separate from CPB
3. Stabilization of preoperative patient
  a. Ventricular septal defect
  b. Mitral regurgitation
4. Stabilization of noncardiac surgical patient
5. Procedural support during coronary angiography
6. Bridge to transplantation
	1. Aortic valvular insufficiency
	2. Aortic disease
	  a. Aortic dissection
	  b. Aortic aneurysm
	3. Severe peripheral vascular disease
	4. Severe noncardiac systemic disease
	5. Massive trauma
	6. Patients with "do not resuscitate" instructions
	7. Mitral SAM with dynamic outflow tract obstruction

obstruction caused by systolic anterior motion (SAM) of the mitral valve, it should be used with caution, if at all, in these patients.

Insertion Techniques

In the initial development of the IABP, insertion was by surgical access to the femoral vessels. In the late 1970s, refinements in IABP design allowed the development of percutaneous insertion techniques. Now the technique most commonly used, percutaneous IABP insertion is performed rapidly with commercially available kits.

The femoral artery with the greater pulse is sought by careful palpation. The length of the balloon to be inserted is estimated by laying the balloon tip on the patient's chest at Louis' angle and appropriately marking the distal point corresponding to the femoral artery. Care must be taken when removing the balloon from its package to follow the manufacturer's procedures exactly so as not to cause perforation of the balloon before insertion. Available balloons come wrapped and need only be appropriately deflated before removal from the package. The femoral artery is entered with the supplied needle, a J-tipped guidewire is inserted to the level of the aortic arch, and the needle is removed. The arterial puncture site is enlarged with the successive placement of an 8-Fr dilator and then a 10.5- or 12-Fr dilator and sheath combination (Figure 32-3). In the adult-sized (30- to 50-mL) balloons, only the dilator needs to be removed, leaving the sheath and guidewire in the artery. The balloon is threaded over the guidewire into the central aorta and into the

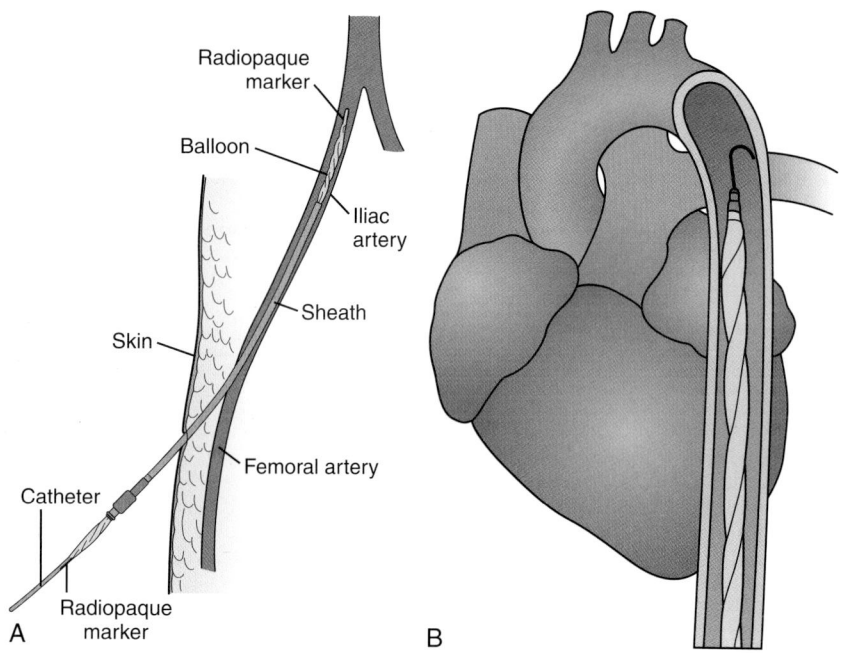

Radiopaque marker

Balloon

Iliac artery

Skin

Sheath

Catheter

Femoral artery

Radiopaque marker

A

B

Figure 32-3 **Diagram of intra-aortic balloon pump (IABP) insertion.** *A,* Cannulation and insertion of the balloon through the femoral artery. Notice the tightly wrapped balloon as it traverses the sheath. A guidewire is not visible in this drawing. *B,* Correct positioning of balloon in proximal descending aorta. The J-tipped guidewire is seen exiting from the balloon's central lumen. (A, *Courtesy of Datascope Corporation;* B, *Courtesy of Kontron, Inc.*)

previously estimated correct position in the proximal segment of the descending aorta. The sheath is gently pulled back to connect with the leak-proof cuff on the balloon hub, ideally so that the entire sheath is out of the arterial lumen to minimize risk for ischemic complications to the distal extremity. Alternatively, the sheath may be stripped off the balloon shaft much like a peel-away pacemaker lead introducer, thereby entirely removing the sheath from the insertion site. At least one manufacturer offers a "sheathless" balloon for insertion.

If fluoroscopy is available during the procedure, correct placement is verified before fixing the balloon securely to the skin. Position also may be checked by radiography or echocardiography after insertion. If an indwelling left radial arterial catheter is functioning at the time of insertion, a reasonable estimate of position may be made by watching balloon-mediated alteration of the arterial pulse waveform (Figure 32-4). After appropriate positioning and timing of the balloon, 1:1 counterpulsation may be initiated. The entire external balloon assembly should be covered in sterile dressings.

Removal of a percutaneously inserted IABP may be by the open (surgical removal) or closed technique. If a closed technique is chosen, the artery should be allowed to bleed for several seconds while pressure is maintained on the distal artery after balloon removal to flush any accumulated clot from the central lumen. This maneuver helps prevent distal embolization of clot. Pressure is then applied for 20 to 30 minutes on the puncture site for hemostasis. If surgical removal is chosen, embolectomy catheters may be passed antegrade and retrograde before suture closure of the artery.

Alternate routes of IABP insertion exist. The balloon may be placed surgically through the femoral artery. This is now performed without the use of an end-to-side vascular conduit, although this placement still requires a second surgical procedure for removal. In patients in whom extreme peripheral vascular disease exists or in pediatric patients in whom the peripheral vasculature is too small, the ascending aorta or aortic arch may be entered for balloon insertion. These approaches necessitate median sternotomy for insertion and usually require reexploration for removal. Other routes of access include the abdominal aorta and the subclavian, axillary, and iliac arteries. The iliac approach may be especially useful for pediatric cases.

▦ Timing and Weaning

A number of different manufacturers of IABP systems are commercially available. The basic console design includes electrocardiographic and arterial blood pressure waveform monitoring and printing, balloon volume monitoring, triggering selection switches, adjustments for inflation and deflation timing, battery backup power sources, and gas reservoir. Some of these systems have become quite sophisticated, with advanced computer microprocessor circuits allowing triggering based on pacemaker signals or detection of and compensation for aberrant rhythms such as atrial fibrillation. Portable models exist for transportation of patients by ground, helicopter, or air ambulances.

For optimal effect of the IABP, inflation and deflation need to be correctly timed to the cardiac cycle. Although a number of variables, including positioning of the balloon within the aorta, balloon volume (Figure 32-5), and the patient's cardiac rhythm, can affect the performance of the IABP, basic principles regarding the function of the balloon must be followed. Balloon inflation should be timed to coincide with aortic valve (AV) closure, or aortic insufficiency and LV strain will result. Similarly, late inflation will result in a diminished perfusion pressure to the coronary arteries. Early deflation will cause inappropriate loss of afterload reduction, and late deflation will increase LV work by causing increased afterload, if only transiently. These errors and correct timing diagrams are shown in Figures 32-4 and 32-6.

As the patient's cardiac performance improves, the IABP support must be removed in stages rather than abruptly. Judicious application and dosing of vasodilator and inotropic medications can assist this procedure. The balloon augmentation may be reduced in steps from 1:1 counterpulsation to 1:2 and then to 1:4, with appropriate intervals at each stage to assess hemodynamic and neurologic stability, cardiac output, and mixed venous oxygen saturation changes. After appropriate observation at 1:4 or 1:8 counterpulsation, balloon assistance can be safely discontinued, and the device can be removed by one of the methods discussed. If percutaneous removal is chosen, an appropriate interval for reversal of anticoagulation (if employed) before removal of the balloon should be allowed.

▦ Complications

Several complications have been associated with IABP use (Table 32-11). The most frequently seen complications are vascular injuries, balloon malfunction, and infection.[114-118] Treatment for these respective problems is straightforward. Flaps, dissections, perforations, embolic events, and pseudoaneurysms should be dealt with directly by surgical intervention and repair. Steal syndromes or ischemia, if not severe, may be dealt with expectantly, but if severe extremity compromise is observed, the balloon should be moved to another site. An alternative means of treatment is a femoral-to-femoral crossover graft placed surgically to help alleviate the affected extremity.

Problems associated with the balloon are managed directly by removal or replacement or, if necessary, repositioning. Gas embolization, although rare, has been successfully treated with hyperbaric oxygen.

Infections usually require removal or replacement of the balloon in an alternate site. Appropriate antibiotic coverage should be instituted and adjusted as culture results become available. Prosthetic materials should be removed if present, and debridement of the insertion site conducted as necessary. Septicemia can occur and have detrimental effects if not aggressively treated.

Because of multiple improvements in medical and anesthetic management, myocardial preservation (see Chapters 28 and 29), and surgical techniques, most patients can be safely weaned off CPB after successful surgery. However, perioperative heart failure and the LCOS still occur in high-risk patients who require complex pharmacologic support to discontinue CPB. Other patients may require treatment of arrhythmias with drugs or pacemakers. Patients with the most severe ventricular dysfunction will require mechanical support (e.g., IABP, left ventricular assist device, RV assist device) and possibly an artificial heart (e.g., AbioCor; Abiomed, Danvers, MA) or heart transplantation (see Chapters 23 and 27).

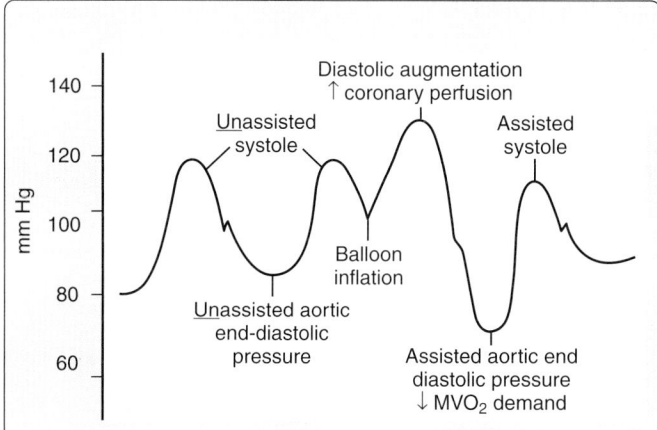

Figure 32-4 Arterial waveforms seen during intra-aortic balloon pump (IABP) assist. The first two waveforms are unassisted, and the last is assisted. Notice the decreased end-systolic and end-diastolic pressures and augmented diastolic pressures caused by IABP augmentation and the (correct) point at which balloon inflation occurs. These are waveforms generated by a correctly positioned and timed balloon. *(Courtesy of Datascope Corporation.)*

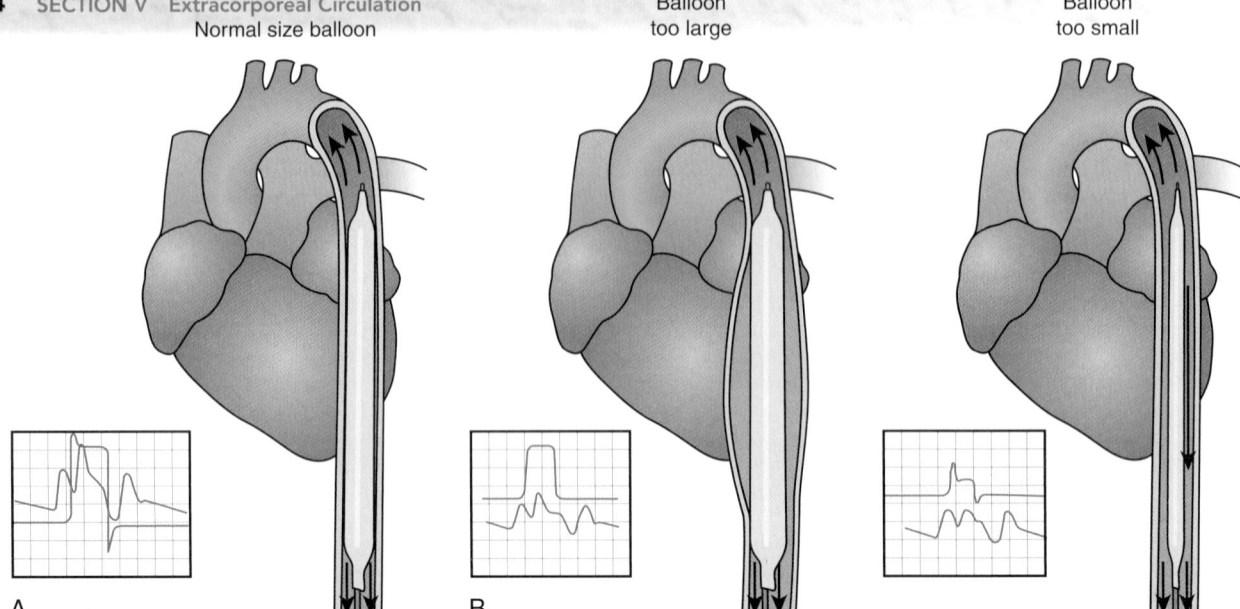

Balloon
Normal size balloon

Balloon
too large

Balloon
too small

A

B

Figure 32-5   Variations in waveform caused by incorrect balloon size. *A,* The balloon is correctly positioned and appropriately sized for the aorta. Notice the arterial waveform diagram in lower left corner. *B,* Examples of too large *(left)* or too small *(right)* balloon sizes with their correspondingly altered arterial waveforms. A similar effect can result from overinflation and underinflation of balloon. Compare waveforms in *B* with the ideal waveform in *A.* *(Courtesy of Kontron, Inc.)*

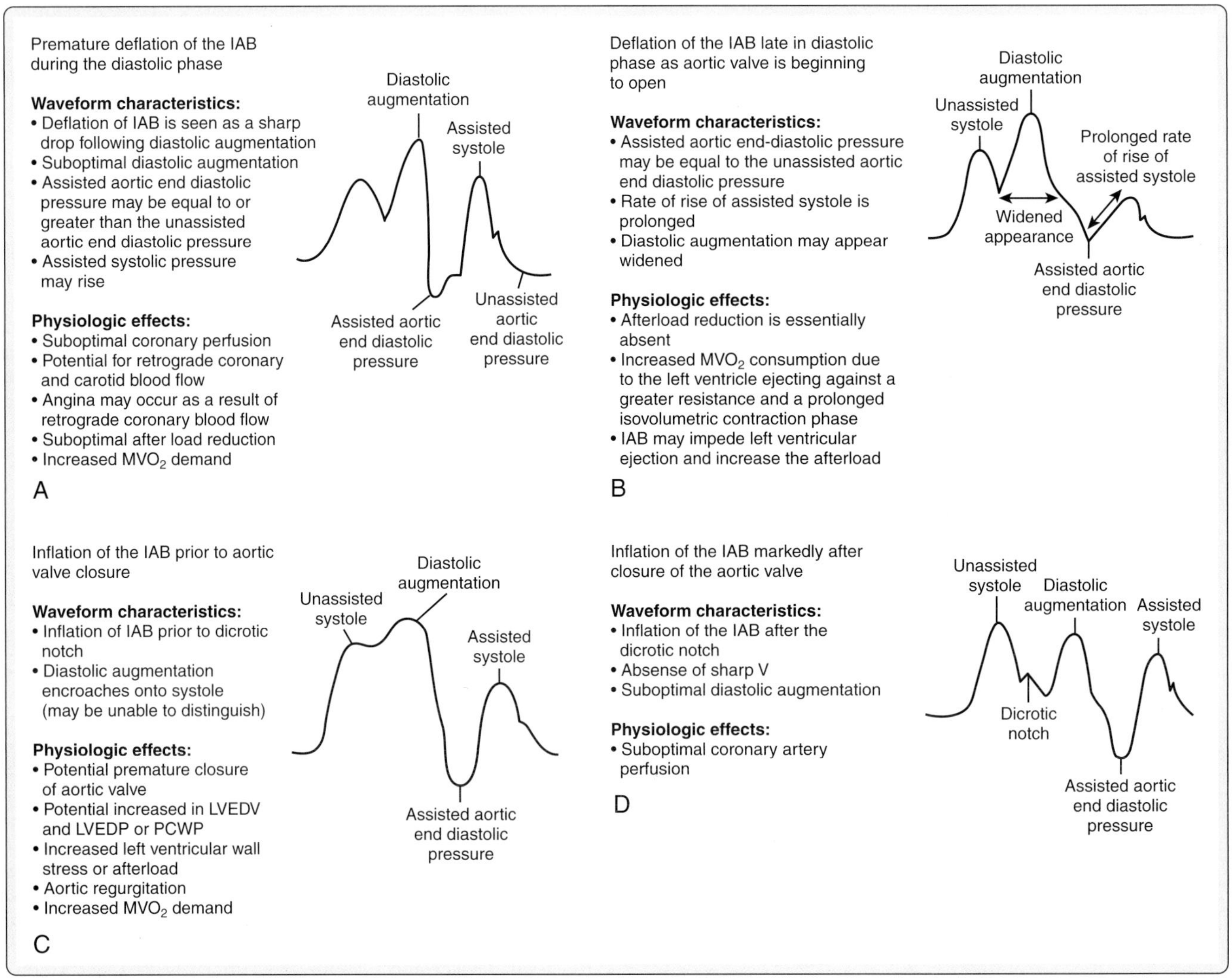

Premature deflation of the IAB
during the diastolic phase

Waveform characteristics:
• Deflation of IAB is seen as a sharp
  drop following diastolic augmentation
• Suboptimal diastolic augmentation
• Assisted aortic end diastolic
  pressure may be equal to or
  greater than the unassisted
  aortic end diastolic pressure
• Assisted systolic pressure
  may rise

Physiologic effects:
• Suboptimal coronary perfusion
• Potential for retrograde coronary
  and carotid blood flow
• Angina may occur as a result of
  retrograde coronary blood flow
• Suboptimal after load reduction
• Increased MVO_2 demand

Diastolic
augmentation

Assisted
systole

Assisted aortic
end diastolic
pressure

Unassisted
aortic
end diastolic
pressure

A

Deflation of the IAB late in diastolic
phase as aortic valve is beginning
to open

Waveform characteristics:
• Assisted aortic end-diastolic pressure
  may be equal to the unassisted aortic
  end diastolic pressure
• Rate of rise of assisted systole is
  prolonged
• Diastolic augmentation may appear
  widened

Physiologic effects:
• Afterload reduction is essentially
  absent
• Increased MVO_2 consumption due
  to the left ventricle ejecting against a
  greater resistance and a prolonged
  isovolumetric contraction phase
• IAB may impede left ventricular
  ejection and increase the afterload

Diastolic
augmentation

Unassisted
systole

Prolonged rate
of rise of
assisted systole

Widened
appearance

Assisted aortic
end diastolic
pressure

B

Inflation of the IAB prior to aortic
valve closure

Waveform characteristics:
• Inflation of IAB prior to dicrotic
  notch
• Diastolic augmentation
  encroaches onto systole
  (may be unable to distinguish)

Physiologic effects:
• Potential premature closure
  of aortic valve
• Potential increased in LVEDV
  and LVEDP or PCWP
• Increased left ventricular wall
  stress or afterload
• Aortic regurgitation
• Increased MVO_2 demand

Diastolic
augmentation

Unassisted
systole

Assisted
systole

Assisted aortic
end diastolic
pressure

C

Inflation of the IAB markedly after
closure of the aortic valve

Waveform characteristics:
• Inflation of the IAB after the
  dicrotic notch
• Absense of sharp V
• Suboptimal diastolic augmentation

Physiologic effects:
• Suboptimal coronary artery
  perfusion

Unassisted
systole

Diastolic
augmentation

Assisted
systole

Dicrotic
notch

Assisted aortic
end diastolic
pressure

D

Figure 32-6   Alterations in arterial waveform tracings caused by errors in timing of intra-aortic balloon pump (IABP). *A,* The balloon was deflated too early. *B,* The balloon was deflated too late. *C,* The balloon was inflated too early. *D,* The balloon was inflated too late. LVEDP, left ventricular end-diastolic pressure; LVEDV, left ventricular end-diastolic volume; PCWP, pulmonary capillary wedge pressure. *(Courtesy of Datascope Corporation.)*

TABLE 32-11	Intra-aortic Balloon Pump Counterpulsation Complications	
Vascular	*Miscellaneous*	*Balloon*
Arterial injury (perforation, dissection)	Hemolysis	Perforation (preinsertion)
Aortic perforation	Thrombocytopenia	Tear (during insertion)
Aortic dissection	Infection	Incorrect positioning
Femoral artery thrombosis	Claudication (postremoval)	Gas embolization
Peripheral embolization	Hemorrhage	Inadvertent removal
Femoral vein cannulation	Paraplegia	
Pseudoaneurysm of femoral vessels	Entrapment	
Lower extremity ischemia	Spinal cord necrosis	
Compartment syndrome	Left internal mammary artery occlusion	
Visceral ischemia	Aggravation of dynamic outflow tract obstruction	

DECISION MAKING WITH TRANSESOPHAGEAL ECHOCARDIOGRAPHY WHILE DISCONTINUING CARDIOPULMONARY BYPASS

Case Study 1

Evacuation of Intracardiac Air

Framing

Air enters the heart in any procedure in which a chamber or the ascending aorta is opened while on CPB. Maneuvers to evacuate any air in the LA or LV need to be performed in these cases in preparation for discontinuing CPB to avoid the adverse consequences of systemic air embolism. Also, air in the right side of the heart may pass through an intracardiac communication such as a patent foramen ovale and result in systemic air embolization if not properly evacuated. TEE can be helpful in identifying and locating air in the heart and assisting in de-airing before coming off CPB.

Data Collection

The time to begin looking with TEE for intracardiac air on CPB is usually after all the chambers and the aorta are closed and the aortic cross-clamp is removed. Microscopic air bubbles are highly echogenic and can be seen with TEE as tiny white spots within the blood and are probably not of great concern (see Air Video 1, which is part of the online materials). It is most important to identify macroscopic accumulations of air within the left heart. These float to the highest point within the chamber and appear in TEE images as a mobile line perpendicular to the direction of gravity that is caused by the air-fluid level as it wobbles with the motion of the heart (see Air Video 2, available online). With a supine patient, air in the LA floats to the superior aspect of the atrial septum, often adjacent to the entrance of the right upper pulmonary vein (see Air Video 3, available online). In the LV, macroscopic accumulations of air float up against the apical septum (see Air Video 4, available online). Air also may be trapped in the left atrial appendage and cause an air-fluid level seen with TEE at its base. The air usually can be identified with TEE at zero degrees multiplane angle with a midesophageal four-chamber view scanning proximal and distal in the esophagus through the entire three-dimensional extents of the left-heart chambers. The midesophageal long-axis view at about 130-degree multiplane angle also may be used to examine the apical septum for air-fluid levels.

Discussion

Although a correlation with the amount of intracardiac air seen with TEE and neurologic outcome has not been shown, one of the major concerns with systemic air embolization after CPB is the potential for cerebral injury. It is reasonable to proceed with the assumption that the less air pumped into the systemic circulation during and after CPB the better. Another adverse consequence of intracardiac air that is well-known and frequently seen is coronary artery embolization leading to myocardial ischemia. Because in a supine patient the right coronary artery takes off from the high point of the aortic root, coronary air embolization is most commonly manifested by dramatic inferior ST-segment elevation and acute right-heart dysfunction. Saphenous vein grafts typically are anastomosed to the anterior aspect of the ascending aorta and susceptible to air emboli as well. If this occurs while still on CPB or before decannulation, it is a simple matter to go back on pump and wait a few minutes until the air clears from the coronary circulation, the ST segments normalize, and ventricular function improves before trying to wean from CPB again. If, however, coronary air embolization occurs after decannulation, the hemodynamics can quickly deteriorate to cardiac arrest. Smaller air emboli can be moved through the coronary vessel by acutely increasing the BP with a vasopressor while dilating the coronary artery with NTG. Perhaps the worst-case scenario is when a macroscopic air bubble in the left heart is shaken loose moving the patient off of the operating table at the end of the case; acute right-heart failure and circulatory collapse may then occur, or may occur while the patient is being transported to the intensive care unit.

Deairing maneuvers may include shaking the vented heart on partial CPB to jar loose any pockets of air, elevating and aspirating LV air directly from the apex, applying positive pressure to the lungs to squeeze air out of the pulmonary veins, and tipping the table from side to side to help the passage of bubbles through the heart to the ascending aorta where they are released through a vent. Additional air may appear in the left heart while weaning from CPB as increasing flow through the pulmonary veins flushes it out from the lungs to the left atrium. Passage of air from the LA to the LV may be facilitated with the head and right-side-down position, as well as from the LV to the ascending aorta with the head and right-side up. It may be impossible to evacuate every last trace of air from the left heart before discontinuing CPB, especially tiny bubbles trapped in the trabeculae of the LV, so it becomes a matter of judgment and experience to know when enough is enough. But the persistence of a macroscopic air-fluid level in the left heart visible with TEE suggests that more deairing probably is needed before closing the vent in the ascending aorta and weaning from CPB.

Case Study 2

Aortic Regurgitation on Cardiopulmonary Bypass

Framing

AR has a special significance for patients on CPB. The primary concern is the potential for distention of the LV once effective contractions of the heart have ceased. Undetected, this can damage the myocardium, causing impaired ventricular function when trying to discontinue CPB. TEE is useful to detect the presence of AR before and while on CPB, and to identify distention of the LV when it occurs.

Data Collection

Before CPB, the AV is examined using the midesophageal AV short-axis and long-axis TEE views with 2-D imaging and color-flow Doppler to detect abnormalities of the valve structure and the presence and severity of AR. Transgastric long-axis and deep transgastric long-axis TEE views are used to display with continuous-wave Doppler the velocity profile of any AR present, and the AR pressure half-time is measured to provide a rough index of severity (see Chapters 12 and 13). Pulsed-wave Doppler is used to detect pan-diastolic flow reversal in the distal descending thoracic aorta, a somewhat insensitive but specific sign of severe AR. The same TEE views are used to check for AR while on CPB, which may occur with a normal AV that is distorted by manipulation of the heart or partial clamping of the aorta. Midesophageal and transgastric views of the LV are used to monitor its size before and after aortic cross-clamp removal while on CPB. The presence of arterial pulsatility on CPB may be an indication of AR. Distention of the LV may cause increased pressure to back up across the mitral valve, through the pulmonary veins and lungs to the pulmonary artery, causing an increasing pressure that can be detected with a pulmonary artery catheter. On CPB, excessive left-heart vent return may be an indication of AR when the aorta is not cross-clamped.

Discussion

The anesthesiologist and the surgeon both need to be aware when patients have AR on CPB to avoid harmful distention of the left ventricle. With AR, as soon as the ventricle is unable to keep itself empty with effective contractions, it becomes progressively fuller. Unchecked, this leads to equalization of the pressures between the LV and the aorta, which on CPB is typically at a systemic level. This high pressure can impair myocardial perfusion and stretch the myofibrils, resulting in subsequent poor contractility. As the ventricle distends, the mitral valve becomes incompetent and the increased pressure can back up into the pulmonary vessels, causing injury at the level of the pulmonary capillaries. This dangerous sequence of events may occur even if the AR is trivial before CPB because, given enough time, it will persist until the aortic and ventricular pressures are equal (see AR Video 1, available online). Normal AVs without AR before CPB may be rendered incompetent if distorted by surgical manipulation of the heart or partial clamping of the aorta, leading to ventricular distention in a few minutes. When AR is present on CPB, the LV must eject the regurgitant volume or it will distend. This ejection provides a clue to the presence of AR by causing persistent arterial pulsatility despite adequate venous drainage to the pump (Figure 32-7).

There are three approaches to preventing left ventricular distention on CPB from AR: maintaining effective contractions of the heart, venting, and cross clamping the aorta. Ventricular fibrillation may be treated with defibrillation, bradycardia with positive chronotropic drugs, or artificial pacing. The surgeon may be able to keep the ventricle from distending until more definitive measures can be taken

by gently squeezing it, ejecting blood through the AV. Left ventricular distention on CPB from AR may be prevented and treated by placing a vent cannula into the heart, typically into the left atrium or ventricle through the right upper pulmonary vein or into the main pulmonary artery, allowing the regurgitant volume to be removed from the heart and returned to the bypass circuit. In urgent situations, the left atrial appendage may be cut open quickly to decompress the left heart and then repaired later. Venting through the atrium is not effective until the mitral valve becomes incompetent, allowing blood to pass from the ventricle to the vent. With severe AR, the vent return may be so large as to compromise flow to the rest of the body and may not provide complete resolution of an urgent situation. Cross clamping the aorta resolves the issue of distention from AR by isolating the AV from the systemic pump flow. An important time to monitor for AR and distention is immediately after removal of the cross clamp, before effective cardiac contractions begin. Awareness of the issue of distention from AR is especially critical in patients having minimally invasive or reoperative procedures in which the surgeon may not have complete access to the heart for palpating to detect distention, defibrillating, pacing, venting, or cross clamping. In such cases, TEE may be the only way to detect ventricular distention from AR before the damage is done.

Case Study 3

Mitral Systolic Anterior Motion after Cardiopulmonary Bypass

Framing

Systolic anterior motion (SAM) of the mitral valve is an abnormal physiology that has two adverse consequences: dynamic left ventricular outflow tract (LVOT) obstruction and mitral regurgitation. It is most commonly associated with hypertrophic obstructive cardiomyopathy but also arises in susceptible individuals in hyperdynamic, hypovolemic states, as often occurs while weaning from CPB. Although SAM may be difficult to differentiate from ventricular dysfunction using conventional hemodynamic monitoring, it is easy to diagnose with TEE. The distinction is critical because the treatments are diametrically opposed.

Data Collection

Mitral SAM should be suspected when encountering unexpected hemodynamic instability while weaning from CPB, especially in situations known to be associated with this physiology: hypertrophic obstructive cardiomyopathy, mitral valve repair for myxomatous disease, and AV replacement for aortic stenosis. Standard TEE views of the mitral valve are used to detect the characteristic, abnormal motion of the mitral leaflets during systole (see SAM Video 1, available online). Color-flow Doppler will demonstrate high-velocity, turbulent flow in the LVOT from the level of the abnormally anterior mitral leaflets through the AV and the mitral regurgitation (see SAM Video 2, available online). Continuous-wave Doppler is directed through the LVOT from the transgastric long-axis or deep transgastric long-axis TEE view to reveal the typical dagger-shaped, late-peaking systolic velocity profile caused by SAM (Figure 32-8). The severity of the dynamic LVOT obstruction is calculated from the continuous-wave Doppler peak velocity by the Bernoulli equation (peak LVOT gradient in mm Hg = $4 V^2$, where V = peak velocity in m/sec) and is considered severe if more than 50 mm Hg. Pulsed-wave Doppler is used to localize the level of the outflow obstruction by moving the sample volume from the midventricular level into the LVOT toward the AV until the high velocity of the obstruction is detected. Mitral SAM causes increase of the left heart filling pressures and decline of the cardiac output that may be detected with a pulmonary artery catheter, but these findings also are consistent with ventricular dysfunction. Because the outflow tract obstruction is dynamic, the arterial blood pressure may be extremely labile, depending mainly on the volume status of the left heart (see SAM Videos 3 through 6 on the website).

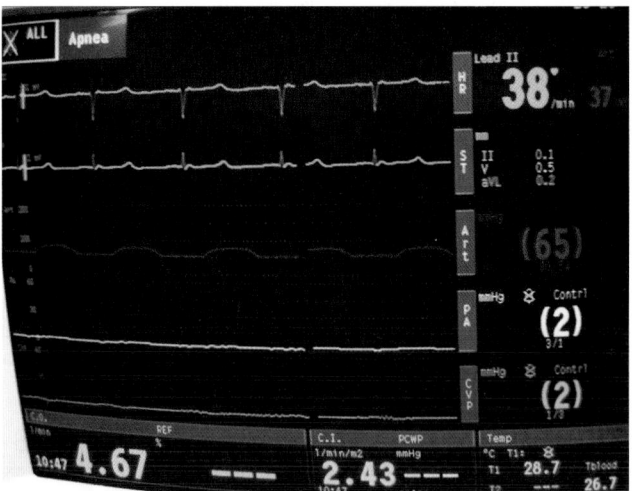

Figure 32-7 A screen shot of a monitor in a patient with aortic regurgitation (AR) on cardiopulmonary bypass (CPB) before aortic cross clamping. The heart is still beating, and the arterial trace is pulsatile, suggesting the presence of AR. Both the pulmonary artery and central venous traces are nonpulsatile, indicating that all the venous blood is being drained to the CPB circuit and that the source for persistent filling of the left ventricle is AR. Transesophageal echocardiography may be used to confirm the presence of AR and to monitor the size of the ventricle for distention. Such pulsatility of the arterial trace should raise the suspicion of AR before and after aortic cross clamping while on CPB.

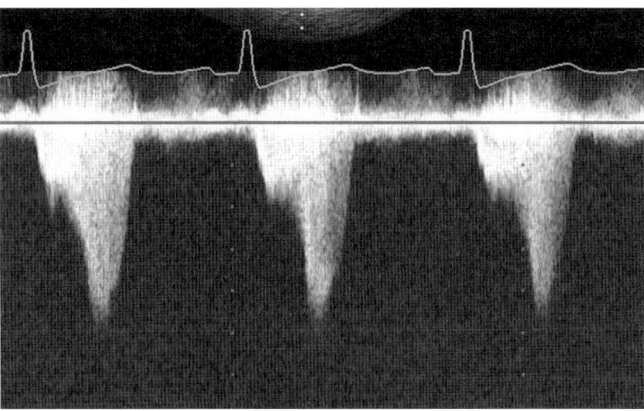

Figure 32-8 A continuous-wave Doppler spectral display of the left ventricular outflow tract (LVOT) velocity profile of a patient with mitral SAM made by directing the Doppler cursor through the LVOT and the aortic valve from a deep transgastric long-axis transesophageal echocardiographic view. The profile has the late peaking "dagger" shape typical of dynamic outflow tract obstruction. Each dot on the vertical scale represents 1 m/sec, indicating a peak instantaneous outflow tract gradient of almost 100 mm Hg.

Discussion

Although classically associated with hypertrophic obstructive cardiomyopathy, mitral SAM has been reported in a number of other situations involving patients having cardiac surgery. SAM after mitral valve repair for myxomatous degeneration is due to excessively redundant residual leaflet tissue and is a well-recognized complication of this surgery. It also has been reported after AV replacement for aortic stenosis in which the relief of an extremely high afterload unmasks the physiology when trying to come off CPB.[119] There seems to be a small number of cardiac surgery patients who are prone to development of SAM when they are hypovolemic and hyperdynamic, even though they appear to have otherwise normal ventricles and mitral valves, especially when coming off CPB.[120]

Hemodynamic changes that decrease the end-systolic volume of the left ventricle increase mitral SAM and its adverse effects. These include hypovolemia, increased myocardial contractility, and decreased afterload. Measures that enlarge the left ventricle will decrease SAM and include volume administration, decreasing myocardial contractility (β-antagonist drugs, e.g., esmolol), and increasing afterload (α-agonist drugs, e.g., phenylephrine). Atrioventricular pacing also has been used effectively in patients with hypertrophic obstructive cardiomyopathy and theoretically could be used to treat SAM in other clinical settings, such as cardiac surgery, in which artificial pacing easily is accomplished. Most patients who experience development of mitral SAM when attempting to discontinue CPB can be successfully managed if the correct diagnosis is made and appropriate interventions are administered (giving volume is probably the most important and helpful maneuver; see SAM Videos 3 through 6 on the website) and inappropriate treatments avoided (milrinone and IABP counterpulsation are especially harmful). Although mitral SAM after mitral valve repair does not cause severe LVOT obstruction and responds to conservative treatment in most patients,[121] if severe and persistent despite optimization of hemodynamics, consideration should be given to revision of the repair or valve replacement.

It is important to realize that the hemodynamic picture caused by mitral SAM, (i.e., high pulmonary artery pressure, and low cardiac output), may be confused with impaired myocardial contractility, leading the clinician to begin afterload reduction or inotropic therapy, both of which will aggravate SAM and its hemodynamic consequences. This may lead to a downward spiral wherein as the patient's hemodynamics worsen, treatment is increased, further worsening SAM and its adverse effects, prompting even further increase of inappropriate treatment. The possibility of mitral SAM in patients with apparent impairment of myocardial contractility as assessed by hemodynamic data, especially if unexpected or not responding appropriately to therapy, should be considered. Mitral SAM easily is diagnosed by echocardiography, which can also be used to monitor the response to therapy.

REFERENCES

1. Cook DJ: Changing temperature management for cardiopulmonary bypass, *Anesth Analg* 88:1254, 1999.
2. Nussmeier NA, Moskowitz GJ, Weiskopf RB, et al: In vitro anesthetic washin and washout via bubble oxygenators, *Anesth Analg* 67:982, 1988.
3. Stone JG, Young WL, Smith CR, et al: Do standard monitoring sites reflect true brain temperature when profound hypothermia is rapidly induced and reversed? *Anesthesiology* 82:344, 1995.
4. Grigore AM, Grocott HP, Mathew JP, et al: Neurologic Outcome Research Group of the Duke Heart Center. The rewarming rate and increased peak temperature alter neurocognitive outcome after cardiac surgery, *Anesth Analg* 94:4, 2002.
5. Gerst PH, Fleming WH, Malm JR: Increased susceptibility of the heart to ventricular fibrillation during metabolic acidosis, *Circ Res* 19:63, 1966.
6. Cingolani HE, Mattiazzi AR, Blesa ES, et al: Contractility in isolated mammalian heart muscle after acid-base changes, *Circ Res* 26:269, 1970.
7. Kassirer JP: Serious acid-base disorders, *N Engl J Med* 291:773, 1974.
8. Bleich HL, Schwartz WB: TRIS buffer (THAM), *N Engl J Med* 274:782, 1966.
9. Jonas RA: Optimal hematocrit for adult cardiopulmonary bypass, *J Cardiothorac Vasc Anesth* 15:672, 2001.
10. Spiess BD: Blood transfusion for cardiopulmonary bypass: The need to answer a basic question, *J Cardiothorac Vasc Anesth* 16:535, 2002.
11. Boyd WC, Thomas SJ: Pro: Magnesium should be administered to all coronary artery bypass graft surgery patients undergoing cardiopulmonary bypass, *J Cardiothorac Vasc Anesth* 14:339, 2000.
12. Grigore AM, Mathew JP: Con: Magnesium should not be administered to all coronary artery bypass graft surgery patients undergoing cardiopulmonary bypass, *J Cardiothorac Vasc Anesth* 14:344, 2000.
13. DiNardo JA: Pro: Calcium is routinely indicated during separation from cardiopulmonary bypass, *J Cardiothorac Vasc Anesth* 11:905, 1997.
14. Prielipp R, Butterworth J: Con: Calcium is not routinely indicated during separation from cardiopulmonary bypass, *J Cardiothorac Vasc Anesth* 11:908, 1997.
15. Tofler OB: Electrocardiographic changes during profound hypothermia, *Br Heart J* 24:265, 1962.
16. Schwab RH, Lewis DW, Killough JH, et al: Electrocardiographic changes occurring in rapidly induced deep hypothermia, *Am J Med Sci* 248:290, 1964.
17. Trevino A, Razi B, Beller BM: The characteristic electrocardiogram of accidental hypothermia, *Arch Intern Med* 127:470, 1971.
18. Braunwald E: The hemodynamic significance of atrial systole, *Am J Med* 37:665, 1964.
19. Konstadt SN, Reich DL, Thys DM, et al: Importance of atrial systole to ventricular filling predicted by transesophageal echocardiography, *Anesthesiology* 72:971, 1990.
20. England MR, Gordon G, Salem M, et al: Magnesium administration and dysrhythmias after cardiac surgery, *JAMA* 268:2395, 1992.
21. Abraham WT, Hayes DL: Cardiac resynchronization therapy for heart failure, *Circulation* 108:2596, 2003.
22. Dubin AM, Feinstein JA, Reddy VM, et al: Electrical resynchronization: A novel therapy for the failing right ventricle, *Circulation* 107:2287, 2003.
23. Royster RL, Butterworth JF, Prough DS, et al: Preoperative and intraoperative predictors of inotropic support and long-term outcome in patients having coronary artery bypass grafting, *Anesth Analg* 72:729, 1991.
24. Evans GL, Smulyan H, Eich RH: Role of peripheral resistance in the control of cardiac output, *Am J Cardiol* 20:216, 1967.
25. Hansen RM, Viquerat CE, Matthay MA, et al: Poor correlation between pulmonary arterial wedge pressure and left ventricular end-diastolic volume after coronary artery bypass graft surgery, *Anesthesiology* 64:764, 1986.
26. Entress JJ, Dhamee S, Olund T, et al: Pulmonary artery occlusion pressure is not accurate immediately after cardiopulmonary bypass, *J Cardiothorac Anesth* 4:558, 1990.
27. Cheung AT, Savino JS, Weiss SJ, et al: Echocardiographic and hemodynamic indexes of left ventricular preload in patients with normal and abnormal ventricular function, *Anesthesiology* 81:376, 1994.
28. Konstadt SN, Thys D, Mindich BP, et al: Validation of quantitative intraoperative transesophageal echocardiography, *Anesthesiology* 65:418, 1986.
29. Abel MD, Nishimura RA, Callahan MJ, et al: Evaluation of Intraoperative transesophageal echocardiography, *Anesthesiology* 66:64, 1987.
30. Hoka S, Okamoto H, Yamaura K, et al: Removal of retained air during cardiac surgery with transesophageal echocardiography and capnography, *J Clin Anesth* 9:457, 1997.
31. Park KW: Protamine and protamine reactions, *Int Anesthesiol Clin* 42:135, 2004.
32. Horrow JC: Protamine: A review of its toxicity, *Anesth Analg* 64:348, 1985.
33. Kimmel SE, Sekeres M, Berlin JA, et al: Mortality and adverse events after protamine administration in patients undergoing cardiopulmonary bypass, *Anesth Analg* 94:1402, 2002.
34. Murphy DA, Craver JM, Jones EL, et al: Recognition and management of ascending aortic dissection complicating cardiac surgical operations, *J Thorac Cardiovasc Surg* 85:247, 1983.
35. Branwald E, Kloner RA: The stunned myocardium: Prolonged postischemic ventricular dysfunction, *Circulation* 66:1146, 1982.
36. Bolli R: Mechanism of myocardial "stunning", *Circulation* 82:723, 1990.
37. Bolli R: Myocardial 'stunning' in man, *Circulation* 86:1671, 1976.
38. Ferrari R, Ceconi C, Cerullo S, et al: Myocardial damage during ischaemia and reperfusion, *Eur Heart J* 14:25, 1993.
39. Fontes ML, Hines RL: Pharmacologic management of perioperative left and right ventricular dysfunction. In Kaplan JA, editor: *Cardiac anesthesia*, Philadelphia, 1999, WB Saunders, pp 1155–1191.
40. Bristow MR, Ginsburg R, Minobe W, et al: Decreased catecholamine sensitivity and beta-adrenergic-receptor density in failing human hearts, *N Engl J Med* 307:205, 1982.
41. Givertz M, Hare J, Loh E, et al: Effect of milrinone on hemodynamics and pulmonary vascular resistance, *J Am Coll Cardiol* 28:1775, 1986.
42. Mentzer RM, Alegre C, Nolan SP: The effects of dopamine and isoproterenol on the pulmonary circulation, *J Thorac Cardiovasc Surg* 71:807, 1976.
43. Cuffe MS, Califf RM, Adams KF Jr, et al: Short-term intravenous milrinone for acute exacerbation of chronic heart failure: A randomized controlled trial, *JAMA* 287:1541, 2002.
44. Stevenson LW: Inotropic therapy for heart failure, *N Engl J Med* 339:1848, 1998.

45. Leenen FH, Chan YK, Smith DL, et al: Epinephrine and left ventricular function in humans: Effects of beta-1 vs nonselective beta-blockade, *Clin Pharmacol Ther* 43:519, 1988.
46. Butterworth JF 4th, Prielipp RC, Royster RL, et al: Dobutamine increases heart rate more than epinephrine in patients recovering from aortocoronary bypass surgery, *J Cardiothorac Vasc Anesth* 6:535, 1992.
47. Miura T, Yoshida S, Iimura O, et al: Dobutamine modifies myocardial infarct size through supply-demand balance, *Am J Physiol* 254(Pt 2):H855, 1988.
48. Kertai MD, Poldermans D: The utility of dobutamine stress echocardiography for perioperative and long-term cardiac risk assessment, *J Cardiothorac Vasc Anesth* 19:520, 2005.
49. Frishman WH, Hotchkiss H: Selective and nonselective dopamine receptor agonists: An innovative approach to cardiovascular disease treatment, *Am Heart J* 132:861, 1996.
50. Richer M, Robert S, Lebel M: Renal hemodynamics during norepinephrine and low-dose dopamine infusions in man, *Crit Care Med* 24:1150, 1996.
51. Steen PA, Tinker JH, Pluth JR, et al: Efficacy of dopamine, dobutamine, and epinephrine during emergence from cardiopulmonary bypass in man, *Circulation* 57:378, 1978.
52. Meadows D, Edwards JD, Wilkins RG, et al: Reversal of intractable septic shock with norepinephrine therapy, *Crit Care Med* 16:663, 1988.
53. Desjars P, Pinaud M, Potel G, et al: A reappraisal of norepinephrine therapy in human septic shock, *Crit Care Med* 15:134, 1987.
54. Kristof AS, Magder S: Low vascular resistance state in patients undergoing cardiopulmonary bypass, *Crit Care Med* 27:1121, 1999.
55. Molloy DW, Lee KY, Jones D, et al: Effects of noradrenaline and isoproterenol on cardiopulmonary function in a canine model of acute pulmonary hypertension, *Chest* 88:432, 1985.
56. Dupuis JY, Bondy R, Cattran C, et al: Amrinone and dobutamine as primary treatment of low-cardiac-output syndrome following coronary artery surgery: A comparison of their effects on hemodynamics and outcome, *J Cardiothorac Vasc Anesth* 6:542, 1992.
57. Butterworth JF, Royster RL, Prielipp RC, et al: Amrinone in cardiac surgical patients with left ventricular dysfunction. A prospective, randomized placebo-controlled trial, *Chest* 104:1660, 1993.
58. Gage J, Rutman H, Lucido E, et al: Additive effects of dobutamine and amrinone on myocardial contractility and ventricular performance in patients with severe heart failure, *Circulation* 74:367, 1986.
59. Royster RL, Butterworth JF 4th, Prielipp RC, et al: Combined inotropic effects of amrinone and epinephrine after cardiopulmonary bypass in humans, *Anesth Analg* 77:662, 1993.
60. George M, Lehot JJ, Estanove S: Haemodynamic and biological effects of intravenous milrinone in patients with a low-cardiac-output syndrome following cardiac surgery: Multicentre study, *Eur J Anaesthesiol Suppl* 5:31, 1992.
61. Levy JH, Bailey JM, Deeb JM: Intravenous milrinone in cardiac surgery, *Ann Thorac Surg* 73:325, 2002.
62. Monrad ES, Baim DS, Smith HS, et al: Effects of milrinone on coronary hemodynamics and myocardial energetics in patients with congestive heart failure, *Circulation* 71:972, 1985.
63. Feneck RO: Intravenous milrinone following cardiac surgery. I. Effects of bolus infusion followed by variable dose maintenance infusion. The European Milrinone Multicentre Trial Group, *J Cardiothorac Vasc Anesth* 6:554, 1992.
64. Bailey JM, Levy JH, Kikura M, et al: Pharmacokinetics of intravenous milrinone in patients undergoing cardiac surgery, *Anesthesiology* 81:616, 1994.
65. Butterworth JF 4th, Hines RL, Royster RL, et al: A pharmacokinetic and pharmacodynamic evaluation of milrinone in adults undergoing cardiac surgery, *Anesth Analg* 81:783, 1995.
66. Kikura M, Sato S: The efficacy of preemptive milrinone or amrinone therapy in patients undergoing coronary artery bypass grafting, *Anesth Analg* 94:22, 2002.
67. Leien CV, Banbach D, Thompson MJ, et al: Central and regional hemodynamic effects of intravenous isosorbide dinitrate, nitroglycerin, and nitroprusside in patients with congestive heart failure, *Am J Cardiol* 48:115, 1981.
68. Lee KY: Effects of hydralazine and nitroprusside on cardiopulmonary function when cardiac output is acutely reduced by pulmonary vascular resistance, *Circulation* 69:1299, 1983.
69. Ziskind Z, Pohoryles L, Mohr R, et al: The effect of low-dose intravenous nitroglycerin on pulmonary hypertension immediately after replacement of a stenotic mitral valve, *Circulation* 72:164, 1985.
70. Felker JM: Inotropic therapy for heart failure: An evidence-based approach, *Am Heart J* 142:393, 2001.
71. Stevenson LW, Massie BM, Francis GS, et al: Optimizing therapy for complex or refractory heart failure, *Am Heart J* 135:S293, 1998.
72. Gomes WJ, Carvalho AC, Palma JH, et al: Vasoplegic syndrome after open heart surgery, *J Cardiovasc Surg* 39:619–623, 1998.
73. Levin MA, Lin HM, Castillo JG, et al: Early on-cardiopulmonary bypass hypotension and other factors associated with vasoplegic syndrome, *Circulation* 120:1664–1671, 2009.
74. Treschan TA, Peters J: The vasopressin system: Physiology and clinical strategies, *Anesthesiology* 105:599–612, 2006.
75. Landry DW, Levin HR, Gallant EM, et al: Vasopressin pressor hypersensitivity in vasodilatory septic shock, *Crit Care Med* 25:1279–1282, 1997.
76. Argenziano M, Chen JM, Choudhri AF, et al: Management of vasodilatory shock after cardiac surgery: Identification of predisposing factors and use of a novel pressor agent, *J Thorac Cardiovasc Surg* 116:973–980, 1998.
77. Masetti P, Murphy SF, Kouchoukos NT: Vasopressin therapy for vasoplegic syndrome following cardiopulmonary bypass, *J Card Surg* 17:485–489, 2002.
78. Garcia-Villalon AL, Garcia JL, Fernandez N, et al: Regional differences in the arterial response to vasopressin: Role of endothelial nitric oxide, *Br J Pharmacol* 118:1848–1854, 1996.
79. Russell JA: Vasopressin in vasodilatory and septic shock, *Curr Opin Crit Care* 13:383–391, 2007.
80. Dunser MW, Mayr AJ, Tur A, et al: Ischemic skin lesions as a complication of continuous vasopressin infusion in catecholamine-resistant vasodilatory shock: Incidence and risk factors, *Crit Care Med* 31:1394–1398, 2003.
81. Leone RJ Jr, Weiss HR, Scholz PM: Positive functional effects of milrinone and methylene blue are not additive in control and hypertrophic canine hearts, *J Surg Res* 77:23–28, 1998.
82. Evora PR, Ribeiro PJ, de Andrade JC: Methylene blue administration in SIRS after cardiac operations, *Ann Thorac Surg* 63:1212–1213, 1997.
83. Shanmugam G: Vasoplegic syndrome—the role of methylene blue, *Eur J Cardiothorac Surg* 28:705–710, 2005.
84. Maslow AD, Stearns G, Butala P, et al: The hemodynamic effects of methylene blue when administered at the onset of cardiopulmonary bypass, *Anesth Analg* 103:2–8, 2006.
85. Ozal E, Kuralay E, Yildirim V, et al: Preoperative methylene blue administration in patients at high risk for vasoplegic syndrome during cardiac surgery, *Ann Thorac Surg* 79:1615–1619, 2005.
86. Shanmugam G: Vasoplegic syndrome—the role of methylene blue, *Eur J Cardiothorac Surg* 28:705–710, 2005.
87. Holland FW 2nd, Brown PS, Weintraub BD, Clark RE: Cardiopulmonary bypass and thyroid function: A "euthyroid sick syndrome," *Ann Thorac Surg* 52:46, 1991.
88. Chu SH, Huang TS, Hsu RB, et al: Thyroid hormone changes after cardiovascular surgery and clinical implications, *Ann Thorac Surg* 52:791, 1991.
89. Salter DR, Dyke CM, Wechsler CS: Triiodothyronine (T₃) and cardiovascular therapeutics: A review, *J Card Surg* 7:363, 1991.
90. Gomberg-Maitland M, Frishman W: Thyroid hormone and cardiovascular disease, *Am Heart J* 135:187, 1998.
91. Novitzky D, Cooper DK, Swanepoel A: Ionotropic effect of triiodothyronine (T₃) in low cardiac output following cardioplegic arrest and cardiopulmonary bypass: An initial experience in patients undergoing open heart surgery, *Eur J Cardiothorac Surg* 3:140, 1989.
92. Smith A, Grattan A, Harper M, et al: Coronary revascularization: A procedure in transition from on-pump to off-pump? The role of glucose-insulin-potassium revisited in a randomized, placebo-controlled study, *J Cardiothorac Vasc Anesth* 16:413, 2002.
93. Van den Berghe G, Wouters P, Weekers F, et al: Intensive insulin therapy and critically ill patients, *N Engl J Med* 245:1359, 2001.
94. Wallin M, Barr G, Owall A, et al: The influence of glucose-insulin-potassium on GH/IGF-1/IGFBP-1 axis during elective coronary artery bypass surgery, *J Cardiothorac Vasc Anesth* 17:470, 2003.
95. Svedjeholm R, Hallhagen S, Ekroth R, et al: Dopamine and high-dose glucose-insulin-potassium after a cardiac operation: Effects on myocardial metabolism, *Ann Thorac Surg* 51:262, 1991.
96. Gradinac S, Coleman G, Taegtmeyer H, et al: Improved cardiac function with glucose-insulin-potassium after aortocoronary artery bypass grafting, *Ann Thorac Surg* 48:484, 1989.
97. Zuurbier CJ, Hoek FJ, van Dijk J, et al: Perioperative hyperinsulinaemic normoglycaemic clamp causes hypolipidaemia after coronary artery surgery, *Br J Anaesth* 100:442–450, 2008.
98. Lehmann A, Boldt J: New pharmacologic approaches for the perioperative treatment of ischemic cardiogenic shock, *J Cardiothorac Vasc Anesth* 19:97, 2005.
99. Haikala H, Pollesello P: Calcium sensitivity enhancers, *Drugs* 3:1199, 2000.
100. Lehmann A, Boldt J, Kirchner J: The role of calcium sensitizers for the treatment of heart failure, *Curr Opin Crit Care* 9:337, 2003.
101. Remme W, Swedberg K: Task Force for the Diagnosis and Treatment of Heart Failure, European Society of Cardiology: Guidelines for the diagnosis and treatment of chronic heart failure, *Eur Heart J* 22:1527, 2001.
102. Sonntag S, Sundberg S, Lehtonen L, et al: The calcium sensitizer levosimendan improves the function of stunned myocardium after percutaneous transluminal coronary angioplasty and acute myocardial ischemia, *J Am Coll Cardiol* 43:2177, 2004.
103. Morais R: Levosimendan in severe right ventricular failure following mitral valve replacement, *J Cardiothorac Vasc Anesth* 20:82–84, 2006.
104. Siirila-Waris K, Suojaranta-Ylinen R, Harjola VP: Levosimendan in cardiac surgery, *J Cardiothorac Vasc Anesth* 19:345, 2005.
105. Eriksson HI, Jalonen JR, Heikkinen LO, et al: Levosimendan facilitates weaning from cardiopulmonary bypass in patients undergoing coronary artery bypass grafting with impaired left ventricular function, *Ann Thorac Surg* 87:448–454, 2009.
106. Tritapepe L, De Santis V, Vitale D, et al: Levosimendan pre-treatment improves outcomes in patients undergoing coronary artery bypass graft surgery, *Br J Anaesth* 102:198–204, 2009.
107. Mills R, Hobbs R: Nesiritide in perspective: Evolving approaches to the management of acute decompensated heart failure, *Drugs Today* 39:767, 2003.
108. Keating G, Goa K: Nesiritide: A review of its use in acute decompensated heart failure, *Drugs* 63:47, 2003.
109. Zineh I, Schofield R, Johnson J: The evolving role of nesiritide in advanced decompensated heart failure, *Pharmacotherapy* 23:1266, 2003.
110. Publications Committee for the VMAC Investigators: Intravenous nesiritide versus nitroglycerin for treatment of decompensated congestive heart failure: A randomized, controlled trial, *JAMA* 287:1531, 2002.
111. Burger A, Horten D, LeJemel T, et al: The effect of nesiritide and dobutamine on ventricular arrhythmias in the treatment of patients with acutely decompensated heart failure, *Am Heart J* 144:1102, 2002.
112. Mentzer RM Jr, Oz MC, Sladen RN, et al: Effects of perioperative nesiritide in patients with left ventricular dysfunction undergoing cardiac surgery: The NAPA Trial, *J Am Coll Cardiol* 49:716–726, 2007.
113. Chen HH, Sundt TM, Cook DJ, et al: Low dose nesiritide and the preservation of renal function in patients with renal dysfunction undergoing cardiopulmonary-bypass surgery: A double-blind placebo-controlled pilot study, *Circulation* 116(11 Suppl):I134–I138, 2007.
114. Goldstein D, Oz M: Mechanical support for postcardiotomy cardiogenic shock, *Semin Thorac Cardiovasc Surg* 12:220, 2000.
115. Stone G, Ohman E, Miller M, et al: Contemporary utilization and outcomes of intra-aortic balloon counterpulsation in acute myocardial infarction: The Benchmark Registry, *J Am Coll Cardiol* 41:1940, 2003.
116. Craver J, Murrah C: Elective intra-aortic balloon counterpulsation for high-risk off-pump coronary artery bypass operations, *Ann Thorac Surg* 71:1220, 2001.
117. Babatasi G, Massetti M, Bruno P, et al: Preoperative balloon counterpulsation and off-pump coronary artery surgery for high-risk patients, *Cardiovasc Surg* 11:145, 2003.
118. Ferguson J, Cohen M, Freedan R, et al: The current practice of intra-aortic balloon counterpulsation: Results from the Benchmark Registry, *J Am Coll Cardiol* 38:1456, 2001.
119. Cutrone F, Coyle JP, Novoa R, et al: Severe dynamic left ventricular outflow tract obstruction following aortic valve replacement diagnosed by intraoperative echocardiography, *Anesthesiology* 72:563–566, 1990.
120. Krenz HK, Mindich BP, Guarino T, et al: Sudden development of intraoperative left ventricular outflow obstruction: Differential and mechanism. An Intraoperative two-dimensional echocardiographic study, *J Card Surg* 5:93–101, 1990.
121. Brown ML, Abel MD, Click RL, et al: Systolic anterior motion after mitral valve repair: Is surgical intervention necessary? *J Thorac Cardiovasc Surg* 133:136–143, 2007.

SECTION VI

Postoperative Care

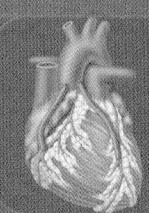

33

Postoperative Cardiac Recovery and Outcomes

DANIEL BAINBRIDGE, MD, FRCPC | DAVY C.H. CHENG, MD, MSC, FRCPC, FCAHS

KEY POINTS

1. Cardiac anesthesia has fundamentally shifted from a high-dose narcotic technique to a more balanced approach using moderate-dose narcotics, shorter-acting muscle relaxants, and volatile anesthetics.
2. This new paradigm has also led to renewed interest in perioperative pain management involving multimodal techniques that facilitate rapid tracheal extubation such as regional blocks, intrathecal morphine, and supplementary nonsteroidal anti-inflammatory drugs.
3. This has prompted a shift from the classic model of recovering patients in the traditional intensive care unit manner, with weaning protocols and intensive observation, to management more in keeping with the recovery room practice of early extubation and rapid discharge, which has shifted the care of cardiac patients to more specialized postcardiac surgical recovery units.
4. Fast-track cardiac anesthesia appears to be safe in comparison with conventional high-dose narcotic anesthesia, but if complications occur that would prevent early tracheal extubation, then the management strategy should be modified accordingly.
5. The goal of a postcardiac surgery recovery model is a postoperative unit that allows variable levels of monitoring and care based on patient needs.
6. The initial management in the postoperative care of fast-track cardiac surgical patients consists of ensuring an efficient transfer of care from the operating room staff to cardiac recovery area staff, while at the same time maintaining stable patient vital signs.
7. It is important to know the risk factors associated with cardiac surgery and to review treatment options for patients with specific reference to outcomes, all placed within the context of cost and resource utilization, especially as medicine increasingly involves economic realities.

Cardiac anesthesia itself has fundamentally shifted from a high-dose narcotic technique to a more balanced approach using moderate-dose narcotics, shorter-acting muscle relaxants, and volatile anesthetics. This primarily has been driven by a realization that high-dose narcotics delay extubation and recovery after surgery. This new paradigm

also has led to renewed interest in perioperative pain management involving multimodal techniques that facilitate rapid tracheal extubation such as regional blocks, intrathecal morphine (ITM), and supplementary nonsteroidal anti-inflammatory drugs (NSAIDs). In addition to changes in anesthetic practice, the type of patients presenting for cardiac surgery is changing. Patients are now older and have more associated comorbidities (stroke, myocardial infarction [MI], renal failure). Treatment options for coronary artery disease have expanded, ranging from medical therapy only to percutaneous interventions and surgery. Surgical options, however, also have expanded and include conventional coronary artery bypass graft surgery (CABG), off-pump coronary artery bypass surgery (OPCAB), minimally invasive direct coronary artery bypass, and robotically assisted coronary artery bypass techniques. Change also has taken place in the recovery of cardiac patients. Although cardiac surgical procedures often were associated with a high mortality and long intensive care unit (ICU) stays, the use of moderate doses of narcotics has allowed for rapid ventilator weaning and discharge from the ICU within 24 hours. This has prompted a shift from the classic model of recovering patients in the traditional ICU manner, with weaning protocols and intensive observation, to management more in keeping with the recovery room practice of early extubation and rapid discharge. This, in turn, has shifted the care of cardiac patients to more specialized postcardiac surgical recovery units.

Finally, hard clinical outcomes have driven change in the ongoing management of cardiac patients and are increasingly the focus of research. Intraoperative management now exists within the continuum of preoperative assessment and postoperative care. The outcomes of a patient within the hospital setting are only one small aspect of success. Long-term mortality, morbidity, and quality-of-life indicators are becoming the gold standard in determining benefit or harm for interventions.

This chapter reviews fast-track cardiac anesthesia (FTCA) and its impact on cardiac recovery. The initial perioperative care of routine cardiac surgical cases, including postoperative pain management techniques such as regional blockade and ITM, are discussed, followed by specific management issues of commonly occurring problems in the cardiac ICU. Finally, important cardiac outcomes are reviewed, focusing on the different treatment options available to patients with coronary artery disease and discussing available evidence for their implementation.

FAST-TRACK CARDIAC SURGERY CARE

Anesthetic Techniques

Few trials have compared inhalation agents for FTCA. A single trial comparing sevoflurane and isoflurane in patients undergoing valve surgery was unable to demonstrate reductions in tracheal extubation times.[1] Several studies have examined the effectiveness of propofol versus inhalation agent, which demonstrated reductions in myocardial enzyme release (creatine kinase-MB, troponin I) and preservation of myocardial function in patients receiving inhalation agents.[2-5] Although this end point is a surrogate for myocardial damage and does not show improved outcome per se, creatine kinase-MB release post-CABG may be associated with poor outcome[6] (Box 33-1).

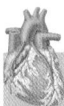

BOX 33-1. BENEFITS OF FAST-TRACK CARDIAC ANESTHESIA

- Decreased duration of intubation
- Decreased length of intensive care unit stay
- Decreased cost

The choice of muscle relaxant in FTCA is important to reduce the incidence of muscle weakness in the cardiac recovery area (CRA), which may delay tracheal extubation.[7] Several randomized trials have compared rocuronium (0.5 to 1 mg/kg) versus pancuronium (0.1 mg/kg) and found significant differences in residual paralysis in the ICU.[8-11] Two studies found statistically significant delays in the time to extubation in the pancuronium group.[9,10] None of the trials used reversal agents, so the use of pancuronium appears acceptable as long as neostigmine or edrophonium is administered to patients with residual neuromuscular weakness.

Several trials have examined the use of different short-acting narcotic agents during FTCA. In these trials, fentanyl, remifentanil, and sufentanil all were found to be efficacious for early tracheal extubation.[12-14] The anesthetic drugs and their suggested dosages are listed in Table 33-1.

Evidence Supporting Fast-Track Cardiac Recovery

Several randomized trials and one meta-analysis of randomized trials have addressed the question of safety of FTCA.[15-21] None of the trials was able to demonstrate differences in outcomes between the fast-track

TABLE 33-1	Suggested Dosages for Fast-Track Cardiac Anesthesia
Induction	
Narcotic	
Fentanyl, 5–10 µg/kg	
Sufentanil, 1–3 µg/kg	
Remifentanil infusions of 0.5–1.0 µg/kg/min	
Muscle relaxant	
Rocuronium, 0.5–1 mg/kg	
Vecuronium, 1–1.5 mg/kg	
Hypnotic	
Midazolam, 0.05–0.1 mg/kg	
Propofol, 0.5–1.5 mg/kg	
Maintenance	
Narcotic	
Fentanyl, 1–5 µg/kg	
Sufentanil, 1–1.5 µg/kg	
Remifentanil infusions of 0.5–1.0 µg/kg/min	
Hypnotic	
Inhalational 0.5–1 MAC	
Propofol, 50–100 µg/kg/min	
Transfer to CRA	
Narcotic	
Morphine, 0.1–0.2 mg/kg	
Hypnotic	
Propofol, 25–75 µg/kg/min	

CRA, cardiac recovery area; MAC, minimum alveolar concentration.
From Mollhoff T, Herregods L, Moerman A, et al: Comparative efficacy and safety of remifentanil and fentanyl in 'fast track' coronary artery bypass graft surgery: A randomized, double-blind study. Br J Anaesth 87:718, 2001; Engoren M, Luther G, Fenn-Buderer N: A comparison of fentanyl, sufentanil, and remifentanil for fast-track cardiac anesthesia. Anesth Analg 93:859, 2001; and Cheng DC, Newman MF, Duke P, et al: The efficacy and resource utilization of remifentanil and fentanyl in fast-track coronary artery bypass graft surgery: A prospective randomized, double-blinded controlled, multi-center trial. Anesth Analg 92:1094, 2001.

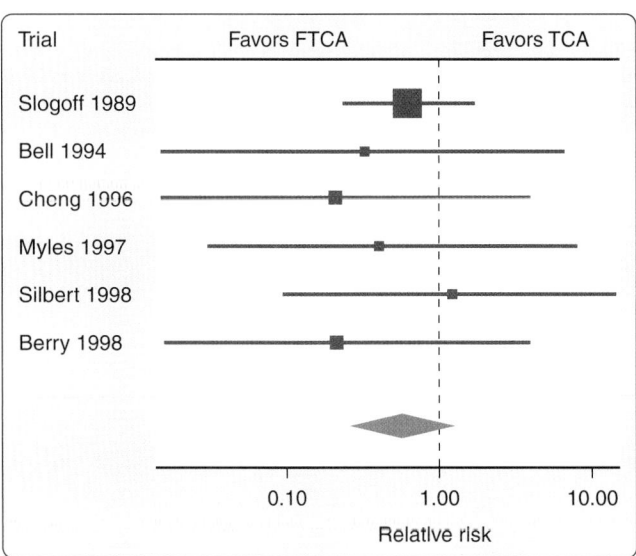

Figure 33-1 Forrest plot of mortality indicating no difference when fast-track cardiac anesthesia (FTCA) was compared with conventional high-dose narcotic anesthesia. TCA, traditional cardiac anesthesia.

group and the conventional anesthesia group (Figure 33-1). The meta-analysis of randomized trials demonstrated a reduction in the duration of intubation by 8 hours (Figure 33-2) and the ICU length of stay (LOS) by 5 hours in favor of the fast-track group. However, the length of hospital stay was not statistically different.

One concern with FTCA is the potential for an increase in the incidence of adverse events, notably awareness. Awareness in patients undergoing FTCA was systematically investigated in a single trial, a prospective observational study of 617 FTCA patients. The reported incidence rate of explicit intraoperative awareness was 0.3% (2/608).[22] This is comparable with the reported incidence during conventional cardiac surgery.[23] This suggests that FTCA does not increase the incidence of awareness compared with conventional cardiac surgery.

FTCA appears safe in comparison with conventional high-dose narcotic anesthesia. It reduces the duration of ventilation and ICU LOS considerably without increasing the incidence of awareness or other

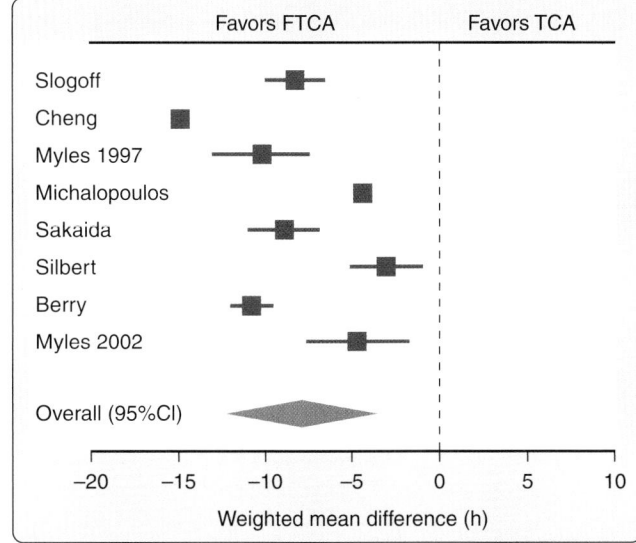

Figure 33-2 Forrest plot showing the weighted mean difference in extubation times. The overall effect was an 8.1-hour reduction in extubation times. CI, confidence interval; FTCA, fast-track cardiac anesthesia; TCA, traditional cardiac anesthesia.

adverse events.[20,21] It appears effective at reducing costs and resource utilization.[24] As such, it is becoming the standard of care in many cardiac centers. The usual practice at many institutions is to treat all patients as fast-track candidates with the goal of allowing early tracheal extubation for every patient. However, if complications occur that would prevent early tracheal extubation, then the management strategy is modified accordingly. It has been demonstrated that the risk factors for delayed tracheal extubation (> 10 hours) are increased by age, female sex, postoperative use of intra-aortic balloon pump (IABP), inotropes, bleeding, and atrial arrhythmia. The risk factors for prolonged ICU LOS (> 48 hours) are those of delayed tracheal extubation plus preoperative MI and postoperative renal insufficiency.[25] Care should be taken to avoid excess bleeding (antifibrinolytics) and to treat arrhythmias either prophylactically or on occurrence (β-blockers, amiodarone).

Postcardiac Surgical Recovery Models

The failure of many randomized FTCA trials to show reductions in resource utilization likely stems from the traditional ICU models used by these centers during the study period. Even when trials were combined in a meta-analysis, the ICU LOS was reduced only by 5 hours despite patients being extubated a mean of 8 hours earlier.[21] Typically, patients who are extubated within the first 24 hours of ICU admission are transferred to the ward on postoperative day 1 in the morning or early afternoon. This allows the following daytime cardiac cases to have available ICU beds but prevents patient transfers during nighttime hours. Two models have been proposed to deal with this issue: the parallel model and the integrated model (Figure 33-3). In the parallel model, patients are admitted directly to a CRA, where they are monitored with 1:1 nursing care until tracheal extubation. After this, the level of care is reduced to reflect reduced nursing requirements with ratios of 1:2 or 1:3. Any patients requiring overnight ventilation are transferred to the ICU for continuation of care. The primary drawback with the parallel model is the physical separation of the CRA and ICU, which leads to two separate units and, thus, does not eliminate the requirement to transfer patients. The integrated model overcomes

these limitations because all patients are admitted to the same physical area, but postoperative management such as nursing-to-patient ratio is variable based on patient requirements.[26–28] Because nursing care accounts for 45% to 50% of ICU costs, reducing the nursing requirements where possible creates the greatest saving. Other cost savings from reductions in arterial blood gases (ABGs) measurement, use of sedative drugs, and ventilator maintenance are small. The goal is a postoperative unit that allows variable levels of monitoring and care based on patient need.[28] Furthermore, FTCA has been demonstrated to be a safe and cost-effective practice that decreases resource utilization after patient discharge from the index hospitalization up to 1-year follow-up.[29]

INITIAL MANAGEMENT OF FAST-TRACK CARDIAC ANESTHESIA PATIENTS: THE FIRST 24 HOURS

On arrival in the CRA, initial management of cardiac patients consists of ensuring an efficient transfer of care from operating room (OR) staff to CRA staff, while at the same time maintaining stable patient vital signs. The anesthesiologist should relay important clinical parameters to the CRA team. To accomplish this, many centers have devised hand-off sheets to aid in the transfer of care. Initial laboratory work should be sent (Table 33-2). An electrocardiogram should be ordered, but a chest radiograph is required only in certain circumstances (Table 33-3). The patient's temperature should be recorded, and if low, active rewarming measures should be initiated with the goal of rewarming the patient to 36.5°C. Shivering may be treated with low doses of meperidine (12.5 to 25 mg intravenously). Hyperthermia, however, is common within the first 24 hours after cardiac surgery and may be associated with an increase in neurocognitive dysfunction, possibly a result of hyperthermia exacerbating cardiopulmonary bypass (CPB)–induced neurologic injury[30,31] (Box 33-2).

TABLE 33-2	Suggested Initial Laboratory Work in Routine Cases, with Additional Laboratory Work to Be Ordered Where Indicated
Routine	
CBC	
Electrolytes	
BUN/creatinine	
aPTT/INR	
ABGs	
As indicated	
Fibrinogen	
LFTs (AST/ALT)	
Calcium	
Magnesium	
Cardiac enzymes (CK-MB, CK, troponin I)	

ABG, arterial blood gas; ALT, alanine aminotransferase; aPTT, activated partial thromboplastin time; AST, aspartate aminotransferase; BUN, blood urea nitrogen; CBC, complete blood count; CK, creatine kinase; CK-MB, creatine kinase myocardium band; INR, international normalized ratio; LFT, liver function test.

TABLE 33-3	Suggested Indications for Ordering a Chest Radiograph
Respiratory	
Pao_2/Fio_2 ratio > 200	
Peak pressure > 30 cm H_2O	
Asymmetric air entry	
Circulatory	
Uncertainty of pulmonary artery catheter position (poor trace, unable to wedge)	
Hypotension resistant to treatment	
Excessive bleeding	
Gastrointestinal	
Nasogastric/orogastric tube feeding	

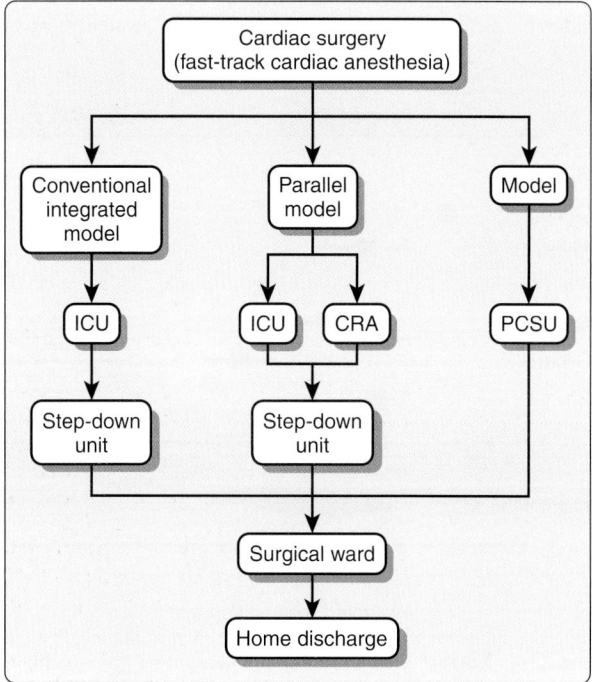

Figure 33-3 Postcardiac surgical recovery models. CRA, cardiac recovery area; ICU, intensive care unit; PCSU, postcardial surgical unit.

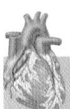

BOX 33-2. INITIAL MANAGEMENT OF THE FAST-TRACK CARDIAC ANESTHESIA PATIENT

- Normothermia
- Hemoglobin > 7 g/dL
- $Paco_2$ 35 to 45 mm Hg
- Sao_2 > 95%
- Mean blood pressure > 50 to 70 mm Hg
- Potassium 3.5 to 5.0 mEq/L
- Blood sugar < 10.0 mmol/L (< 200 mg/dL)

Ventilation Management: Admission to Tracheal Extubation

Ventilatory requirements should be managed with the goal of early tracheal extubation in patients (Table 33-4). ABGs are initially drawn within 1/2 hour after admission and then repeated as needed. Patients should be awake and cooperative, be hemodynamically stable, and have no active bleeding with coagulopathy. Respiratory strength should be assessed by hand grip or head lift to ensure complete reversal of neuromuscular blockade. The patient's temperature should be more than 36° C, preferably normothermic. When these conditions are met and ABG results are within the reference range, tracheal extubation may take place. ABGs should be drawn about 30 minutes after tracheal extubation to ensure adequate ventilation with maintenance of Pao_2 and $Paco_2$. Inability to extubate patients as a result of respiratory failure, hemodynamic instability, or large amounts of mediastinal drainage will necessitate more complex weaning strategies (see Chapter 35). Some patients may arrive after extubation in the OR. Careful attention should be paid to these patients because they may subsequently develop respiratory failure. The patient's respiratory rate should be monitored every 5 minutes during the first several hours. An ABG should be drawn on admission and 30 minutes later to ensure the patient is not retaining carbon dioxide. If the patient's respirations become compromised, ventilatory support should be provided. Simple measures such as reminders to breathe may be effective in the narcotized/anesthetized patient. Low doses of naloxone (0.04 mg intravenously) also may be beneficial. Trials of continuous positive airway pressure or bilevel positive airway pressure may provide enough support to allow adequate ventilation. Reintubation should be avoided because it may delay recovery; however, it may become necessary if the earlier mentioned measures fail, resulting in hypoxemia, hypercarbia, and a declining level of consciousness.

TABLE 33-4	Ventilation Management Goals during the Initial Trial of Weaning from Extubation
Initial ventilation parameters	
A/C at 10–12 beats/min	
TV 8 –10 mL/kg	
PEEP 5 cm H_2O	
Maintain ABGs	
pH 7.35–7.45	
$Paco_2$ 35–45	
Pao_2 > 90	
Saturations > 95%	
Extubation criteria	
ABGs as above	
Awake and alert	
Hemodynamically stable	
No active bleeding (< 400 mL/2 hr)	
Temperature > 36°C	
Return of muscle strength (> 5 seconds, head lift/strong hand grip)	

ABG, arterial blood gas; A/C, assist-controlled ventilation; PEEP, positive end-expiratory pressure; TV, tidal volume.

Regulation of Hemoglobin Level

Anemia is common during and after cardiac surgery as a result of both dilutional changes and bleeding. Although a hemoglobin transfusion threshold of 10 g% was once common, increasing evidence suggests that a threshold of 7 g% is reasonably safe.[32] However, in the post-CPB period, patients with incomplete revascularization or with poor target vessels may require a higher transfusion threshold.[32] As a result, blood transfusions should be individualized for each patient but certainly should be used to maintain a minimal hemoglobin level of 7 g%.

Management of Bleeding

Chest tube drainage should be checked every 15 minutes after ICU admission to assess a patient's coagulation status. Although blood loss is commonly divided into two types, surgical or medical, determining the cause of bleeding is often difficult. When bleeding exceeds 400 mL/hr during the first hour, 200 mL/hr for each of the first 2 hours, or 100 mL/hr over the first 4 hours, returning to the OR for chest reexploration should be considered. The clinical situation must be individualized for each patient, however, and in the face of a known coagulopathy, more liberal blood loss before chest re-exploration may be acceptable. There are numerous medical causes for bleeding after cardiac surgery. Platelet dysfunction after cardiac surgery is common. The CPB circuit itself leads to contact activation and degranulation of platelets, resulting in their dysfunction. Residual heparinization is common postcardiac surgery and frequently occurs when either heparinized pump blood is transfused after CPB or insufficient protamine is administered. Fibrinolysis is also common after CPB, predominantly caused by a host of activated inflammatory and coagulation pathways. Coagulation factors may decrease from activation at air–blood interfaces or from dilution with the CPB pump-priming solution. Hypothermia also may aggravate the coagulation cascade and lead to further bleeding. Conventional coagulation tests are helpful to identify the coagulation abnormality contributing to the bleeding. Common laboratory testing includes activated partial thromboplastin time, international normalized ratio (INR), platelet count, fibrinogen level, and D-dimers. Unfortunately, most conventional measures take 20 to 40 minutes before results are available. This has led to the development of new methods to help guide treatment. These bedside point-of-care tests are providing more rapid, clinically relevant results compared with laboratory testing. The use of point-of-care testing such as thromboelastography has been demonstrated to reduce transfusion requirements without increasing blood loss and is commonly used, especially following difficult cardiac cases[33,34] (see Chapters 17 and 28 to 31).

Initial medical treatment of excessive blood loss consists of 50 to 100 mg intravenous protamine to ensure complete heparin reversal. This may need to be repeated if heparinized CPB pump blood has been administered after protamine reversal. Although the reinfusion of chest tube blood was common to avoid exposure to donor packed red blood cells, it is no longer used routinely in practice because this blood is known to contain activated coagulation and inflammatory mediators that may predispose to an increased risk for infection.[35]

Fresh-frozen plasma usually is given in the setting of an increased INR (> 1.5). Platelet levels of less than 100,000/mm³ may warrant platelet transfusion, but caution must be exercised when considering this course. Platelet transfusions carry the greatest risk for transfusion-related complications of any blood component, typically sepsis from bacterial contamination. Platelets should be used only when platelet counts are low or the patient has a known platelet dysfunction, secondary to the use of acetylsalicylic acid, glycoprotein IIb/IIIa inhibitors, or clopidogrel.[36] Certain physical measures should be instituted, including warming of the hypothermic patient. The benefit of positive end-expiratory pressure on postoperative bleeding is equivocal and likely has little benefit in the face of surgical bleeding or in patients who are coagulopathic.[37,38] The use of antifibrinolytics after cardiac surgery is likely of little benefit because several randomized

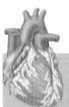

BOX 33-3. MANAGEMENT OF THE BLEEDING PATIENT

- Review activated coagulation time, prothrombin time, international normalized ratio, platelet count
- Protamine if due to excess heparin (reinfusion of pump blood)
- Treat medical cause: platelets, fresh-frozen plasma, cryoprecipitate if secondary to decreased fibrinogen
- Factor VIIa should be considered if bleeding continues despite normal coagulation profile
- Treat surgical cause: re-exploration

trials were unable to demonstrate the efficacy of antifibrinolytics used after surgery[39,40] (Box 33-3).

Factor VIIa recently has become available and initially was introduced for treatment of hemophiliacs who present with bleeding. It was introduced in cardiac surgery as rescue therapy in patients with uncontrolled bleeding, usually in the presence of normal coagulation results and no surgical evidence of bleeding.[41] Although frequently used in the OR before returning to the ICU, it is still given frequently in the ICU setting. Doses initially were in the range of 75 to 100 μg/kg, but concern over thrombotic complications has led to dosage reductions ranging down to as little as 17 μg/kg.[41–43]

Electrolyte Management

Hypokalemia is common after cardiac surgery, especially if diuretics were given intraoperatively. Hypokalemia contributes to increased automaticity and may lead to ventricular arrhythmias, ventricular tachycardia, or ventricular fibrillation. Treatment consists of potassium infusions (20 mEq potassium in 50 mL D_5W infused over 1 hour) until the potassium exceeds 3.5 mEq/mL. In patients with frequent premature ventricular contractions caused by increased automaticity, 5.0 mEq/mL potassium may be desirable. Hypomagnesemia contributes to ventricular pre-excitation and may contribute to atrial fibrillation (AF). It is common in malnourished and sick patients, a frequent occurrence in the cardiac surgical setting. Management consists of intermittent boluses of magnesium—1 to 2 g over 15 minutes. Hypocalcemia also is frequent during cardiac surgery and may reduce cardiac contractility. Intermittent boluses of calcium chloride or calcium gluconate (1 g) may be required (Table 33-5).

TABLE 33-5	Common Electrolyte Abnormalities and Possible Treatment Options
Hypokalemia (K⁺ < 3.5 mmol/L)	
SSx: muscle weakness, ST-segment depression, "u" wave, T-wave flat, ventricular pre-excitation	
Rx: IV KCl at 10–20 mEq/hr via central catheter	
Hyperkalemia (K⁺ > 5.2 mmol/L)	
SSx: muscle weakness, peaked T wave, loss of P wave, prolonged PR/QRS	
Rx: $CaCl_2$ 1 g, insulin/glucose, HCO_3^-, diuretics, hyperventilation, dialysis	
Hypocalcemia (ionized Ca²⁺ < 1.1 mmol/L)	
SSx: hypotension, heart failure, prolonged QT interval	
Rx: $CaCl_2$ or Ca gluconate	
Hypercalcemia (Ionized Ca²⁺ > 1.3 mmol/L)	
SSx: altered mental state, coma, ileus	
Rx: dialysis, diuretics, mithramycin, calcitonin	
Hypermagnesemia (Mg²⁺ > 0.7 mmol/L)	
SSx: weakness, absent reflexes	
Rx: stop Mg infusion, diuresis	
Hypomagnesemia (Mg²⁺ < 0.5 mmol/L)	
SSx: arrhythmia, prolonged PR and QT intervals	
Rx: Mg infusion 1 to 2 g	

IV, intravenous; Rx, treatment; SSx, signs and symptoms.

Glucose Management

Diabetes is a common comorbidity (up to 30%) and is a known risk factor for adverse outcome in patients presenting for cardiac surgery.[44–46] Hyperglycemia itself is common during CPB. The risk factors for hyperglycemia include diabetes, administration of steroids before CPB, volume of glucose-containing solutions administered, and use of epinephrine infusions.[47] Poor perioperative glucose control is associated with increases in mortality and morbidity, including an increased risk for infection and a prolonged duration of ventilation.[48–52] In a large prospective, randomized, controlled trial of tight glucose control (blood glucose levels of 4.1 to 6.5 mmol/L) during postoperative ICU stay, reductions in mortality were shown by the authors compared with more liberal glucose control (blood glucose levels of 12 mmol/L).[52] This trial enrolled both diabetic and nondiabetic hyperglycemic patients who underwent cardiothoracic surgery and demonstrated that tight management of glucose is beneficial in the CRA. However, another recent multicenter trial, as well as a meta-analysis of tight glucose control in the ICU, suggest an increase in harm, likely related to an increase in episodic hypoglycemia.[53,54] Therefore, it may be prudent to accept a more liberal blood sugar level (< 10.0 mmol/L) to reduce hypoglycemic episodes.

Pain Control

Pain control after cardiac surgery has become a concern as narcotic doses have been reduced to facilitate fast-track protocols. Intravenous morphine is still the mainstay of treatment for postcardiac surgery patients. The most common approach is patient-demanded, nurse-delivered intravenous morphine, and this treatment remains popular because of 1:1 to 1:2 nursing typically provided during cardiac recovery. However, with a change to more flexible nurse coverage and, therefore, higher nurse-to-patient ratios, patient-controlled analgesia morphine is becoming increasingly popular. Several studies have examined patient-controlled analgesia morphine use in patients after cardiac surgery.[55–61] A meta-analysis looking at patient-controlled analgesia morphine for postoperative pain showed small incremental benefits. However, young patients, those who use narcotics before surgery or are transferred to a regular ward within 24 hours, may benefit from patient-controlled analgesia for pain management[62] (Table 33-6; see Chapter 38).

Regional Analgesia Techniques

Intrathecal Morphine
ITM has been investigated in randomized trials as an adjuvant for pain control in cardiac surgical patients, with doses ranging from 500 μg to 4 mg.[63–72] A meta-analysis of 17 randomized, controlled trials compared ITM with standard treatment. There was no difference in mortality, MI, or time to extubation. There were modest reductions in morphine use and pain scores, whereas the incidence of pruritus was increased.

Thoracic Epidural Analgesia
Thoracic epidural analgesia has gained some popularity as a method of providing intraoperative and postoperative pain control in cardiac surgery (see Table 33-6). The best evidence for benefit comes from a meta-analysis of 15 randomized, controlled trials.[73] Thoracic epidural analgesia did not significantly affect the incidence of mortality or MI. It did significantly reduce arrhythmias, pulmonary complications, and time to tracheal extubation. All the randomized trials were performed in CABG patients. There were no reported complications as a result of epidural insertion, specifically epidural hematoma; however, all trials were inadequately powered to detect this complication. Attempts have been made to calculate the risk for epidural hematoma using available published series, with estimates of maximum risk ranging from 1:1000 to 1:3500 depending on the confidence limits chosen (99% vs. 95%).[74] A large retrospective review reported no epidural hematomas in 727 patients undergoing cardiac surgery with CPB receiving thoracic epidural analgesia the day of surgery (on entrance into the OR).[75]

TABLE 33-6	Pain Management Options after Cardiac Surgery

Patient-Controlled Analgesia

May be of benefit in a stepdown unit

Reduced 24-hour morphine consumption demonstrated in 2 of 7 randomized trials

Intrathecal Morphine

Doses studied: 500 µg to 4 mg

May be of benefit to reduce IV morphine use

May be of benefit in reducing VAS pain scores

*Potential for respiratory depression

Ideal dosing not ascertained; range, 250–400 µg

Thoracic Epidurals

Common dosages from literature

Ropivacaine 1% with 5 µg/mL fentanil at 3–5 mL/hr

Bupivacaine 0.5% with 25 µg/mL morphine at 3–10 mL/hr

Bupivacaine 0.5% to 0.75% at 2–5 mL/hr

Reduced pain scores

Shorter duration of intubation

*Risk for epidural hematoma difficult to quantify

Nonsteroidal Anti-inflammatory Drugs

Common dosages from literature

Indomethacin 50–100 mg PR BID

Diclofenac 50–75 mg PO/PR q8h

Ketorolac 10–30 mg IM/IV q8h

Reduces narcotic utilization

Many different drugs studied; difficult to determine superiority of a given agent

*May increase serious adverse events (one trial using cyclooxygenase-2–specific inhibitors)

BID, twice daily; IM, intramuscular; IV, intravenous; PO, orally; PR, rectally; VAS, visual analogue scale.

At least 1 hour elapsed between the insertion of the epidural catheter and heparin administration. There were 9 failed catheter insertions and 4 failed analgesia blocks with 11 bloody taps in this study.[75] Unfortunately, the population of cardiac surgical patients is increasingly on antiplatelet medication, such as clopidogrel or prasugrel, which increase the risk for epidural hematoma.[76] The risk for epidural hematoma and the potential delay of surgery from a bloody tap have limited the widespread adoption of thoracic epidural analgesia for cardiac surgery, especially in the United States (see Chapter 38).

Nonsteroidal Anti-inflammatory Drugs

The use of NSAIDs has gained popularity in a multimodal approach, allowing reductions in both pain levels and narcotic side effects (see Table 33-6). The conventional NSAIDs, which nonselectively block the cyclooxygenase-2 (COX-2) isoenzyme, reduce inflammation, fever, and pain, and also block the COX-1 isoenzyme resulting in the side effects of gastrointestinal toxicity and platelet dysfunction.[77] Numerous randomized trials have examined the benefit of NSAID use for postoperative pain control.[61,78–88] In addition, a meta-analysis looking at the benefit of NSAIDs in the setting of cardiac and thoracic surgery demonstrated reductions in narcotic consumption in patients given NSAIDs.[89] Most patients were younger than 70 years and had no coexisting renal dysfunction. The NSAIDs used in this meta-analysis were nonselective COX inhibitors. Several trials have suggested increased adverse events, especially in patients with coronary artery disease, who receive the COX-2 selective NSAIDs both in the perioperative cardiac setting and in ambulatory patients. For this reason, COX-2 selective NSAIDs are no longer used in most cardiac centers.[90] Therefore, although NSAIDs have theoretic side effects, the benefit in reduced narcotic consumption and improved visual analogue scale pain scores is well demonstrated; many centers continue to use nonselective NSAIDs as analgesia adjuvants in cardiac surgery.[91] However, NSAIDs should be avoided in patients with renal insufficiency, a history of gastritis, or peptic ulcer disease. Adjuvant ranitidine treatment should be considered to prevent gastric irritation.

Medications for Risk Reduction after Coronary Artery Bypass Graft Surgery

CABG surgery itself reduces the risk for mortality and angina recurrence, but several medical management issues may help maintain the long-term benefit after CABG surgery. Specifically, the use of aspirin, β blockers, and lipid lowering agents has been demonstrated to prolong survival or reduce graft restenosis, or both (Box 33-4).

Aspirin

Several studies have demonstrated the efficacy of aspirin (acetylsalicylic acid) use on graft patency and reductions in MI and mortality after CABG surgery.[92–96] A large observational study showed a reduction in mortality of nearly 3% and a reduction in MI rate of 48% with the early use of aspirin after surgery (within 48 hours).[96] Acetylsalicylic acid dosages have ranged from 100 mg once daily to 325 mg three times daily orally or by suppository up to 48 hours after ICU admission. There was no additional benefit from the use of aspirin before surgery.[97] The beneficial effect on saphenous vein graft patency appears to be lost after 1 year, with prolonged use of aspirin having no further benefit.[98] However, because aspirin, in dosages of 75 to 325 mg/day, reduces mortality and morbidity in patients at risk for cardiovascular disease, its continued long-term use is clearly warranted.[99] Ticlopidine, clopidogrel, or prasugrel may be suitable alternatives in patients who are allergic to aspirin. Clopidogrel, through reductions in all-cause mortality, stroke, and MI, may be superior to acetylsalicylic acid in patients who return with recurrent ischemic events after cardiac surgery.[100] Ticlopidine, however, should be used with caution because it may cause neutropenia (necessitating white blood cell counts to be monitored during initial use). Clopidogrel has a lower incidence of adverse reactions compared with ticlopidine and is, therefore, preferred as a second-line agent when aspirin is contraindicated.

β-Blockers

The use of β-blockers in patients after CABG surgery has not been shown to improve mortality.[101] They also have failed to reduce myocardial ischemia rate, unlike the angiotensin-converting enzyme inhibitors, which have, in a single study, demonstrated efficacy at reducing ischemic events after CABG.[102] However, patients who received β-blockers after perioperative MI had reductions in mortality at 1 year.[103] Patients with a previous history of MI should be continued on β-blocker therapy.

Statins

Statin use in the cardiac surgical population has focused on its ability to prolong the patency of SVG grafts and, more recently, its possible role in reducing the incidence of AF. Statin use has been shown to reduce the amount and speed of atherosclerotic plaque formation within saphenous vein grafts. This resulted in reductions in the need for subsequent revascularization in one trial.[104,105] It was recently suggested that statin use before surgery may reduce the incidence of AF in the postoperative period.[105–107]

Anticoagulation for Valve Surgery

Anticoagulation should be started in the early postoperative period for patients who have undergone valve replacement, with either a

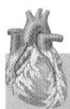

BOX 33-4. MEDICATIONS FOR CARDIAC RISK REDUCTION AFTER CORONARY ARTERY BYPASS GRAFTING SURGERY

- Aspirin: all patients after bypass grafting
- Clopidogrel: patients who have contraindication to aspirin (may have superior efficacy compared with aspirin)
- β-Blockers: especially with perioperative myocardial infarction
- Lipid-lowering agents: especially statin drugs

TABLE 33-7	Suggested Antithrombotic Therapy for Heart Valve Prophylaxis			
	Aspirin (75–100 mg)	Warfarin (INR 2.0–3.0)	Warfarin (2.5–3.5)	No Warfarin
Mechanical Prosthetic Valves				
AVR—low risk				
Less than 3 months	Class I	Class I	Class IIa	
Greater than 3 months	Class I	Class I		
AVR—high risk	Class I		Class I	
MVR	Class I		Class I	
Biological Prosthetic Valves				
AVR—low risk				
Less than 3 months	Class I	Class IIa		Class IIb
Greater than 3 months	Class I			Class IIa
AVR—high risk	Class I	Class I		
MVR—low risk				
Less than 3 months	Class I	Class IIa		
Greater than 3 months	Class I			Class IIa
MVR—high risk	Class I	Class I		

Depending on patients' clinical status, antithrombotic therapy must be individualized. In patients receiving warfarin, aspirin is recommended in virtually all situations. Risk factors: atrial fibrillation, left ventricular dysfunction, previous thromboembolism, and hypercoagulable condition. International normalized ratio (INR) should be maintained between 2.5 and 3.5 for aortic disc valves and Starr-Edwards valves.

AVR, aortic valve replacement; MVR, mitral valve replacement.

From Bonow RO, Carabello BA, Chatterjee K, et al: 2008 focused update incorporated into the ACC/AHA 2006 guidelines for the management of patients with valvular heart disease: A report of the American College of Cardiology/American Heart Association Task Force on Practice Guidelines (Writing Committee to revise the 1998 guidelines for the management of patients with valvular heart disease). Endorsed by the Society of Cardiovascular Anesthesiologists, Society for Cardiovascular Angiography and Interventions, and Society of Thoracic Surgeons. *J Am Coll Cardiol* 52:e1–142, 2008.

mechanical or bioprosthesis and also should be considered when AF complicates the postoperative course.[108] The recommended prophylactic regimens for patients with both mechanical and bioprosthetic heart valves are shown in Table 33-7. AF management is discussed later.

MANAGEMENT OF COMPLICATIONS

Complications are frequent after cardiac surgery. Although many are short-lived, some complications, like stroke, are long-term catastrophic events that seriously affect a patient's functional status (see Chapters 36 and 37). The incidence and predisposing risk factors are well studied for many of the complications (Table 33-8). Many of these complications have specific management issues, which may improve recovery after surgery (Box 33-5).

Stroke

Stroke after cardiac surgery occurs in 2% to 4% of patients and carries a very high 1-year mortality rate of 15% to 30%.[45,109–111] Known risk factors for stroke include age, diabetes, previous history of stroke or transient ischemic attack, peripheral vascular disease, and unstable angina.[45,110] The most common cause is emboli sheared off the aorta during aortic manipulation (proximal anastomosis of the vein grafts, clamping and unclamping of the aorta). However, hemorrhagic and watershed infarcts do occur secondary to the use of large doses of heparin and the frequent occurrence of hypotension during surgery, respectively. AF in the postoperative period also appears to be an important cause of strokes in cardiac patients.[112] Resource utilization is increased in patients who sustained a stroke, with prolonged ICU and hospital

TABLE 33-8	Common Complications after Heart Surgery	
Complication	Incidence Rate	Risk Factors
Stroke	2–4%	Age
		Previous stroke/TIA
		PVD
		Diabetes
		Unstable angina
Delirium	8–15%	Age
		Previous stroke
		Duration of surgery
		Duration of aortic cross-clamp
		AF
		Blood transfusion
Atrial fibrillation	Up to 35%	Age
		Male sex
		Previous AF
		Mitral valve surgery
		Previous CHF
Renal failure	1%	Low postoperative CO
		Repeat cardiac surgery
		Valve surgery
		Age
		Diabetes

AF, atrial fibrillation; CHF, congestive heart failure; CO, cardiac output; PVD, peripheral vascular disease; TIA, transient ischemic attack.

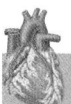

BOX 33-5. TREATMENT FOR COMPLICATIONS AFTER CARDIAC SURGERY

Stroke
- Supportive treatment
- Avoid potential aggravating factors such as hyperglycemia, hyperthermia, and severe anemia

Delirium
- Usually self-limited
- Requires close observation
- May require sedatives (midazolam, lorazepam)

Atrial Fibrillation
- Rate control: calcium channel blockers, β-blockers, digoxin
- Rhythm control: amiodarone, sotalol, procainamide
- Thromboembolic prophylaxis: for atrial fibrillation > 48 hours

Left Ventricular Dysfunction
- Volume
- Inotropes: epinephrine, milrinone, norepinephrine
- Mechanical support: intra-aortic balloon pump

Renal Failure
- Remove the causative agent (nonsteroidal anti-inflammatory drugs, antibiotics)
- Hemodynamic support if necessary
- Supportive care

stays.[110] There are numerous proposed methods of preventing neurologic injury during the intraoperative period including epiaortic scanning, alpha-stat pH management during CABG with CPB, and OPCAB surgery with no-touch surgical techniques.[113–117] Prevention of postoperative neurologic injury may be possible with the aggressive treatment of AF (antiarrhythmics, anticoagulants, early cardioversion) to prevent thromboembolism (see Atrial Fibrillation section later in this chapter). Patients who sustain an intraoperative stroke should be managed with the goal of preventing further brain injury. Hyperglycemia should be avoided because it is associated with poor outcome in brain injury patients.[118–120] Hyperthermia also is known to exacerbate brain injury and should be avoided.[121] Hemoglobin concentrations certainly should be maintained above 7 g%. Whether there is benefit to maintaining hemoglobin levels greater than 10 g% is uncertain, but this may be prudent in patients with perioperative stroke.

Delirium

Delirium is defined generally as an acute transient neurologic condition with impairment of cognitive function, attention abnormalities, and altered psychomotor activity. It often includes a disorder with the sleep/wake cycle. It is fairly common after cardiac surgery, with a prevalence rate of 8% to 15%.[122,123] Risk factors associated with delirium include age, previous history of stroke, duration of surgery, duration of aortic cross-clamp, AF, and blood transfusion.[122–125] Interestingly, delirium is self-limited and does not adversely affect patient outcome or hospital LOS.[124,125] Treatment is supportive, involving close observation of patients and sedatives (midazolam, diazepam) or antipsychotics (haloperidol) as required.

Atrial Fibrillation

AF after cardiac surgery is common and occurs in up to 35% of patients.[126] Although the cause of AF is not completely understood, it is associated with increases in mortality, stroke, and prolonged hospital stay.[110,112,127] Known risk factors include age, male sex, previous AF, mitral valve surgery, and a history of congestive heart failure.[110,128] Prevention and treatment of AF can be achieved effectively with amiodarone, sotalol, magnesium, or β-blockers.[129] Biatrial pacing also may be effective prophylaxis.[129,130] Management of AF consists of rate control with conversion to sinus rhythm or anticoagulation. Several studies conducted to determine which strategy was superior were unable to find a difference between treatment strategies (AFFIRM [Atrial Fibrillation Follow-up Investigation of Rhythm Management] and RACE [Rate Control Versus Electrical Cardioversion] trials).[131–133]

Rate control may be achieved with a β-blocker or a calcium channel blocker. Digoxin also may be effective, but it is difficult to achieve therapeutic levels quickly. An observational review of the AFFIRM trial suggests that β-blockers are superior to either calcium channel blockers or digoxin for rate control in AF.[134] Conversion to sinus rhythm in the stable patient may be achieved with amiodarone, sotalol, or procainamide. Amiodarone is more commonly used in acute management of postoperative AF (150 to 300 mg intravenously) than other antiarrhythmics, particularly in patients with compromised ventricular function, because it causes little cardiac depression. Finally, persistent AF over 48 to 72 hours requires thromboembolic prophylaxis. Warfarin is recommended for patients at high risk of thromboembolic complications. Patients at high risk include those with previous stroke or TIA or thromboembolism. Moderate risk factors include congestive heart failure, ejection fraction less than 35%, diabetes mellitus, or age 75 or older. Patients with one high-risk factor or two or more moderate-risk factors should be treated with warfarin with an INR between 2 and 3 considered therapeutic.[135] In a meta-analysis of randomized trials, warfarin reduced the risk for stroke by 67% and 32% compared with placebo or acetylsalicylic acid, respectively. However, the incidence of hemorrhagic complications also was greater with warfarin (0.3% absolute risk rate increase per year).[136] Aspirin, 325 mg once daily, may be sufficient for patients with a low thromboembolic risk[135,137,138] (Table 33-9).

Left Ventricular Dysfunction

Patients with poor left ventricular (LV) function commonly require inotropes or mechanical support after cardiac surgery. Preoperative factors that predict inotrope use in patients undergoing cardiac surgery include age, underlying LV dysfunction, and female sex.[139,140] The significance of inotrope use on postoperative outcome is uncertain because some centers routinely use these drugs after CPB.[139]

TABLE 33-9 Suggested Atrial Fibrillation Thromboembolic Prophylaxis

Risk Category	Recommended Therapy
No risk factors	Aspirin, 81–325 mg daily
One moderate-risk factor	Aspirin, 81–325 mg daily or warfarin (INR 2.0–3.0, target 2.5)
Any high-risk factor or more than one moderate-risk factor	Warfarin (INR 2.0–3.0, target 2.5)

INR, international normalized ratio.
From Estes NA 3rd, Halperin JL, Calkins H, et al: ACC/AHA/Physician Consortium 2008 clinical performance measures for adults with nonvalvular atrial fibrillation or atrial flutter: A report of the American College of Cardiology/American Heart Association Task Force on Performance Measures and the Physician Consortium for Performance Improvement (Writing Committee to Develop Clinical Performance Measures for Atrial Fibrillation): Developed in collaboration with the Heart Rhythm Society. *Circulation* 117:1101–1120, 2008.

Although pulmonary artery (PA) catheters are useful for monitoring trends in cardiac function, transesophageal echocardiography (TEE) provides more detailed information for diagnosing the cause of acute hypotensive episodes and cardiac function. TEE is used commonly in the ICU to assess patients after cardiac surgery and has demonstrated efficacy for diagnosing cardiac tamponade, cardiac ischemia, and valve dysfunction, resulting in improvements in the postoperative course for these patients.[141–144] TEE also provides information on the filling volumes after CPB.[145–147]

Patients who have an unstable intraoperative course should have PA filling pressures correlated to TEE findings and the results then passed to the recovery unit to allow for optimal initial management in the recovery unit. If the patient remains unstable in the ICU, then TEE is used and cardiac function is reassessed. When hypovolemia is thought to be the underlying cause of hypotension/low cardiac output, then colloids (Pentaspan, Voluven) initially may be used to optimize filling, because third spacing of fluids is common after CPB. The intravascular hypovolemia is best treated with the use of small intermittent boluses of colloid with continuous reassessment of central venous pressure (CVP), PA pressures, systemic pressures, or LV end-diastolic area.[145]

If ventricular dysfunction is the main cause of hypotension/low cardiac output state, then inotropes and vasopressors should be added (see Chapter 34). Unfortunately, few articles have been published examining the superiority of one inotrope over another. Epinephrine (0.02 to 0.04 μg/kg/min) or dopamine (3 to 5 μg/kg/min) is commonly used to support patients coming off CPB and is usually continued into the ICU. If systolic pressure remains low, then the epinephrine infusion is usually increased to allow for greater α-receptor action (vasoconstriction). For patients with a low cardiac output or poor myocardial function on TEE, milrinone commonly is used (with or without a full loading dose). Milrinone has the advantage of bypassing β-adrenergic receptors, which are downregulated after cardiac surgery.[148] Phosphodiesterase inhibitors appear to improve myocardial performance even with the concomitant use of epinephrine.[149] If despite this blood pressure remains low, then a vasopressin infusion may be started with doses ranging from 1 to 10 U/hr. When volume and medical strategies are insufficient, especially in the presence of ischemic heart disease, mechanical support is added (see Chapters 27 and 32). IABPs are used in approximately 3% of cardiac surgical patients. The IABP can be placed before surgery in patients with unstable angina unresponsive to medical treatment, intraoperatively in high-risk patients (redosternotomy with poor LV function), in patients who fail to wean from CPB, or in patients on maximal inotropic support after CPB.

For patients who do not successfully wean from CPB, one retrospective study found 85% success in weaning with the institution of an IABP; however, the overall mortality rate was 35%.[150] Several studies have looked at the timing of IABP insertion and found reductions in mortality in patients who received the IABP before initiation of CPB.[151–154] Complications from the use of IABP are numerous and include wound site infections, leg ischemia, and renal dysfunction. Several retrospective reviews have examined the outcomes after IABP insertion; again, mortality rates were high in patients who received an IABP in the OR or recovery unit (35%).[155,156] Finally, in patients who require long-term inotropic support and use of an IABP, angiotensin-converting enzyme inhibitors may help to reduce mortality. One small trial investigated the use of captopril in patients who required more than two inotropes and/or IABP placement and showed reductions in mortality in patients randomized to receive captopril.[157]

Right Ventricular Dysfunction

Right ventricular (RV) dysfunction may present in patients before cardiac surgery, immediately after surgery, or many days after the operation. It is seen commonly in heart transplant recipients, usually secondary to LV failure. It is also seen in patients with pulmonary hypertension or may be caused by an RV MI.

RV dysfunction presents with features of peripheral edema, hypotension, confusion, and abdominal pain or cramping. Liver function tests may be elevated, including the INR, aspartate aminotransferase, and alanine aminotransferase. Thus, the differential diagnosis frequently includes renal failure, sepsis, bowel ischemia, and liver failure.[158,159]

In patients with invasive monitoring, assessment of RV function may be done indirectly through measurement of CVP, cardiac output, and PA pressures. Unless there is direct myocardial dysfunction, PA pressures are almost always increased. Echocardiography also is useful in assessing patients with suspected RV failure. RV volume overload presents with an enlarged RV and an associated small and underfilled LV (because of both poor RV output and ventricular interdependence). Tricuspid regurgitation is also frequently present. If the RV also is pressure overloaded, the interventricular septum shifts to the left and the LV is said to have a D shape. Tricuspid annular plane systolic excursion (TAPSE) may be helpful in measuring the degree of RV failure.[158–162]

Management of RV failure consists of reducing afterload, increasing systemic pressures to prevent RV ischemia, and ensuring adequate RV filling. Volume, although often useful in LV failure and in cases of RV failure associated with normal PA pressures, often is detrimental in high-pressure RV failure; caution must be exercised to prevent overloading patients. Inotropes, often in combination with afterload reduction, will increase both blood pressure and cardiac output. Norepinephrine, phenylephrine, and vasopressin may all help to increase systemic pressures and, thus, reduce RV ischemia. Afterload reduction with agents specific to the pulmonary vascular tree also may be beneficial. Nitric oxide and inhaled prostaglandin may be selective for pulmonary vasodilation. Milrinone (0.125 to 0.5 µg/kg/hr) or sildenafil (up to 25 mg orally three times a day) also may be of benefit to reduce pulmonary vascular resistance and improve cardiac output (see Chapters 24, 27, 32, and 34).

In the ICU setting, supportive measures should be instituted including providing adequate oxygenation, preventing acidosis and atelectasis, and ensuring minimal amounts of ventilatory support to prevent alveolar collapse.

Renal Insufficiency

Renal failure in the postoperative period is rare, occurring in approximately 1% of patients after cardiac surgery. Not surprisingly, when it does occur, it prolongs CRA LOS and hospital LOS and increases mortality.[46,163] Unfortunately, no clear definition exists as to what constitutes renal impairment or failure after CPB. Although the need for dialysis is a straightforward and easily measured outcome, unfortunately, it ignores patients who have reductions in creatinine clearance but do not require dialysis.[46,163] Change in calculated creatinine clearance, which is predictive of need for dialysis, prolonged hospitalization, and mortality may be a more suitable outcome measurement of renal failure.[164] There are several risk factors for postoperative renal failure, including postoperative low cardiac output, repeat cardiac surgery, valve surgery, age older than 65, and diabetes.[46,163,165] Management of these patients consists of supportive treatment, determining the primary cause, and then directing specific treatment as needed. Supportive treatment consists of ensuring adequate cardiac output, perfusion pressure, and intravascular volume. The cause of renal failure is broadly defined as prerenal, renal, or postrenal failure. Prerenal causes commonly are related to poor cardiac output or low systemic pressure and may be associated with the use of angiotensin-converting enzyme inhibitors and NSAIDs. Renal causes include acute tubular necrosis from an ischemic insult or interstitial nephritis caused by a host of medications including NSAIDs and antibiotics.

Although uncommon in the face of bladder catheterization, the potential for postrenal obstruction is possible. Management of renal failure usually requires correction of the underlying problem, which may include improving renal blood flow (volume, inotropes) or discontinuing the offending agent (NSAIDs, antibiotic). To date, there is no specific treatment to prevent acute tubular necrosis. Although dopamine and diuretics were once both thought to be renoprotective, neither has demonstrated efficacy to prevent renal failure.[166] Fenoldopam, a D1-receptor agonist, may improve renal function in cardiac surgical patients.[167] There is a suggestion that diuretics may be potentially harmful in patients experiencing development of renal failure.[168] If patients do require dialysis, continuous dialysis may be better than intermittent dialysis.[169] N-acetylcysteine has demonstrated efficacy in preventing further renal failure from radiocontrast agent in patients with chronic renal insufficiency.[170] This, however, does not appear to translate to cardiac surgery because several meta-analyses of randomized trials have shown little benefit to N-acetylcysteine.[170–172]

Postoperative Outcomes

Treatment Options for Coronary Artery Disease

Until the advent of CABG surgery, medical management was the only treatment option for patients with coronary artery disease. Today, treatment can be broadly categorized as medical or invasive management, with invasive management divided geographically into interventions performed in the cardiac catheterization laboratory or in the OR. Catheterization procedures commonly performed include balloon angioplasty, cardiac stenting, and drug-eluting stents, which release drugs capable of preventing restenosis (see Chapter 3). OR procedures include conventional CABG (with the use of the CPB machine) and OPCAB (without the use of the CPB machine). OPCAB surgery may include full sternotomy, thoracotomy (minimally invasive direct coronary artery bypass), or robotically assisted thoracotomy surgery. With the ever-increasing number of available options, it becomes crucial to establish which option is superior with regard to angina recurrence, graft patency, and long-term survival with the least morbidity (MI, stroke, AF) at the lowest costs (hospital LOS, ICU LOS, blood transfusions).

Medical Treatment versus Surgical Management

Several large randomized trials have examined the efficacy of medical versus surgical management in patients with symptomatic coronary artery disease (Table 33-10). Most trials were conducted between 1974 and 1984. A meta-analysis was published in 1994 that incorporated seven trials addressing medical versus surgical management with a 10-year follow-up.[173] Although surgical and medical management have advanced since then (i.e., only 9% of patients received IMA grafts), the findings clearly support the benefits of surgery in high-risk patients. This study reviewed 2600 patients and observed an absolute risk reduction in mortality for patients undergoing CABG of 5.6% at 5 years, 5.9% at 7 years, and 4.1% at 10 years. This improvement was most marked in patients with left main disease, proximal left anterior descending coronary artery disease, or triple-vessel disease. The results tended to underestimate the benefits of surgical treatment because 37.4% of medically treated patients eventually underwent surgery.

CABG surgery reduces mortality significantly compared with medical management alone. This benefit is significantly improved beyond 10 years. In addition, many patients initially treated medically eventually require surgical revascularization.

TABLE 33-10	Treatment Options and Outcomes for Coronary Artery Disease	
Comparison	**Outcome**	**Revascularization**
Medical vs. surgical management	Absolute risk reduction in mortality	37% of medically treated patients converted to surgery
	5.6% at 5 years	
	5.9% at 7 years	
	4.1% at 10 years	
	Benefit of surgery greatest in LM, three-vessel disease	
Angioplasty vs. surgical management	Absolute risk reduction in mortality	50% rate of revascularization at 5 years in angioplasty group
	1.9% at 5 years	
	Rates of in-hospital MI and stroke significantly lower in angioplasty group	
	Benefit of surgery greatest in diabetics, multivessel revascularization	
Stent vs. surgical management	Mortality mixed results, relative reduction ranged from a 50% reduction in favor of CABG to a 75% reduction in favor of stenting	15–25% rate of revascularization in stent group
	MI rates at 1-year equivalent	
OPCAB vs. conventional surgical management	No difference in mortality	Most OPCAB patients received fewer grafts than CCAB group (0.2 fewer grafts per patient)
	No difference for in-hospital stroke	
	No difference for in-hospital MI	

CABG, coronary artery bypass grafting; CCAB, conventional coronary artery bypass; LM, left main disease; MI, myocardial infarction; OPCAB, off-pump coronary artery bypass.

Balloon Angioplasty versus Conventional Coronary Artery Bypass Graft Surgery

A number of randomized trials comparing percutaneous transluminal coronary angioplasty (PTCA) with CABG have been performed (see Chapters 3 and 18). One of the largest trials was the Bypass Angioplasty Revascularization Investigation (BARI), which enrolled 1829 patients who were randomized to undergo either PTCA or CABG.[174] It found no significant differences in survival at both 1 and 5 years, with the 5-year survival rates of 89.3% in the CABG group and 86.3% in PTCA group. The rates of in-hospital MI and stroke were greater in the CABG patients compared with the PTCA group (4.6% and 2.1% for Q-wave MI, $P < 0.01$; 0.8% and 0.2% for stroke). For patients with diabetes, 5-year survival rate was 80.6% in the CABG group compared with 65.5% in the PTCA group ($P = 0.003$). The need for repeated revascularization after initial intervention was greater in the PTCA group; at 5 years, only 8% of the patients assigned to CABG had undergone additional revascularization procedures, compared with 54% of those assigned to PTCA (31% of PTCA patients eventually underwent CABG). Several smaller randomized trials found similar results.[175,176]

A meta-analysis of randomized trials was recently published comparing PTCA with CABG for the management of symptomatic coronary artery disease. A total of 13 trials involving 7964 patients were included.[177] They reported a 1.9% absolute survival advantage favoring CABG over PTCA at 5 years ($P < 0.02$). There was no significant difference at 1, 3, or 8 years. In subgroup analysis of patients with multivessel disease, CABG provided a significant survival advantage at both 5 and 8 years. Patients randomized to PTCA had more repeat revascularizations

at all time points. This meta-analysis included some coronary stent trials, in which angina recurrence was reduced by 50% at 1 and 3 years, and the stent cohort had a significant decrease in nonfatal MI at 3 years compared with CABG.

These trials focused primarily on patients with multivessel disease. In patients with single-vessel left anterior descending coronary artery disease, few randomized trials have been conducted. One trial enrolled 134 patients randomized to PTCA or CABG. After 5 years, six patients (9%) had died in the PTCA group versus two (3%) in the CABG group (not significant). MI was more frequent after PTCA (15% vs. 4%, $P = 0.0001$), but there were no differences in the rates of Q-wave infarction (6% in the PTCA group vs. 3% in the CABG group, not significant). Repeat revascularization was required in significantly more patients assigned to the PTCA group (38% vs. 9%, $P = 0.0001$).[178]

When compared with coronary angioplasty, CABG surgery reduces mortality at 5 years. It also reduces the need for additional revascularization procedures. This benefit is greatest in patients with multivessel disease.

Stenting versus Conventional Coronary Artery Bypass Graft Surgery

Surprisingly similar results have been seen when stent implantation (bare metal stents) was compared with CABG surgery[179-181] (see Chapters 3 and 18). Two trials found no difference in the mortality rate at 1 year.[180,181] One trial found a greater mortality rate in the percutaneous coronary intervention (PCI) patients (5% PCI vs. 2% CABG, $P = 0.01$), whereas another trial found reduced mortality in the PCI group (0.9% vs. 5.7%, $P < 0.013$).[179,182] For Q-wave MI, the studies demonstrated equivalent or slightly greater rates with CABG at 1 year. The requirement for repeat revascularizations was still high in all the stent trials, ranging from approximately 15% to 25% (over 1 to 2 years). The costs associated with both PTCA and PCI stents are lower than the cost of CABG. The greatest cost difference is seen at 1 year and decreases after this, because of the high rate of repeat revascularization in the PCI and PTCA groups. Although drug-eluting stents offer the promise of reductions in restenosis, too few trials are published to make a meaningful comment on the effect of this new technology.

A meta-analysis comparing off-pump CABG with PTCA for predominantly single-vessel left internal mammary artery to left anterior descending coronary artery also supported the superiority of surgery. Disease-free survival and need for reintervention were reduced in the surgical group at a cost of longer hospital stay. Most studies used bare metal stents, and thus the impact of drug eluting stents remains to be investigated.[183]

Coronary stenting with bare metal stents demonstrates a similar rate of mortality compared with CABG. The benefit of stenting is a reduction in morbidity outcomes in the short term (MI). However, patients are less likely to be symptom free after stenting, and the need for further revascularization procedures is greater.

Off-Pump Coronary Artery Bypass Surgery versus Coronary Artery Bypass Graft Surgery

The use of OPCAB techniques has increased in popularity, and its greatest benefit will likely be in patients at greatest risk for stroke (e.g., elderly patients, patients with high-grade aortic atheromatous disease).[184-186] A number of randomized trials have investigated the benefits of OPCAB surgery.[187-190] A comprehensive meta-analysis of randomized trials was published demonstrating that OPCAB reduces the rate of blood transfusion, AF, infections, and resource utilization (hospital LOS, ICU LOS, and ventilation time). OPCAB surgery may minimize midterm cognitive dysfunction compared with CABG.[191] OPCAB should be considered a safe alternative to CABG with respect to risk for mortality. However, most trials to date have focused on relatively healthy patients and have been underpowered to determine benefits in the high-risk cohort group purported to benefit the most by OPCAB surgery.[184-186] A large randomized trial, involving more than

2200 patients, drew similar conclusions. It found no difference in stroke, mortality, or MI outcomes, while suggesting that blood transfusions were reduced. Again, however, this was not a high-risk cohort.[192]

The number of coronary vessels bypassed was usually lower in the OPCAB group for all randomized trials. Whether this will translate into worsened outcomes at 1 or 5 years is unknown. Finally, concern has been raised over graft patency.[190] Reports on graft patency after OPCAB are conflicting, with some studies suggesting reduced patency and others suggesting no difference.[192,193] Ultimately, long-term outcomes are needed to assess whether important direct outcomes like mortality, angina recurrence, MI, and reoperation differ in patients undergoing OPCAB versus CABG. In healthy patients, OPCAB has similar rates of mortality and major morbidity compared with CABG, while reducing the rate of AF and blood transfusions.

ECHOCARDIOGRAPHY CASES

In general, in the ICU, TEE is performed for three main indications: (1) hemodynamic deterioration of unknown cause; (2) hemodynamic deterioration of known cause, but not responding to therapy; or (3) hemodynamic deterioration requiring return to OR if the suspected cause is confirmed. It may be performed rarely for detection of aortic dissection and detection of right-to-left shunt in patients with refractory hypoxemia, but these cases are unusual.

Case Study 1

A 57-year-old woman returned to the ICU from the floor 7 days after CABG with a 3-day history of upper abdominal pain and fatigue. Over the past 12 hours, the patient had become more disoriented and obtunded, describing shortness of breath. Her blood pressure had progressively fallen to 100/55 mm Hg from 156/75 mm Hg on discharge from the ICU. Her liver function tests and INR were increased (INR 2.4). The patient was brought back down to the ICU and required urgent intubation; inotropes were started, and an arterial catheter and CVP were inserted (CVP was 14 mm Hg). An ultrasound examination of her abdomen was normal. A transthoracic echocardiogram revealed normal LV function, moderate TR, with an estimated PA pressure of 60 mm Hg.

Framing

The differential diagnosis in this case was broad. Intra-abdominal pathology, including infarcted bowel/bowel perforation, abscess, or cholecystitis, was considered based on symptoms. Infection should always be considered and antibiotics initiated early because this is common in the postoperative period (wound infection, pneumonia) and may present as a series of vague complaints. Any patient with an increased INR, either from warfarin or liver dysfunction, may have pericardial tamponade, even if the presentation is remote from surgery. Presentation within several days of initiation of anticoagulation is not uncommon. Finally, acute deterioration of LV or RV function may present as vague complaints of abdominal pain (RV) or shortness of breath (LV).

Data Collection

For all cases of hemodynamic deterioration in the ICU, data from the arterial catheter, electrocardiogram, CVP (or PA catheter), ABGs (lactate, pH, Po_2), and indicators of organ perfusion (urine output, central nervous system function) need to be assessed to determine whether the patient is in failure and whether this failure is biventricular, left-sided, or right-sided predominantly. In the case presented, there was a suggestion of biventricular failure; because the cause of the problem was unclear, it was decided to proceed with TEE. Assessment consisted of LV assessment (wall motion, ejection fraction estimation, mitral valve function) and RV assessment (RV TAPSE, wall motion, and tricuspid valve function). After this, a comprehensive examination was completed. In this case, the TEE showed an empty LV with a normal

ejection fraction of 50% to 60%, and no regional wall motion abnormalities were noted. The RV TAPSE was depressed at 0.9 cm. Tricuspid regurgitation (TR) was severe and the RV was dilated. This was in keeping with a previous transthoracic echocardiogram from 3 days prior that suggested pulmonary hypertension (Figures 33-4 through 33-8; also see Videos 1 through 3, available online).

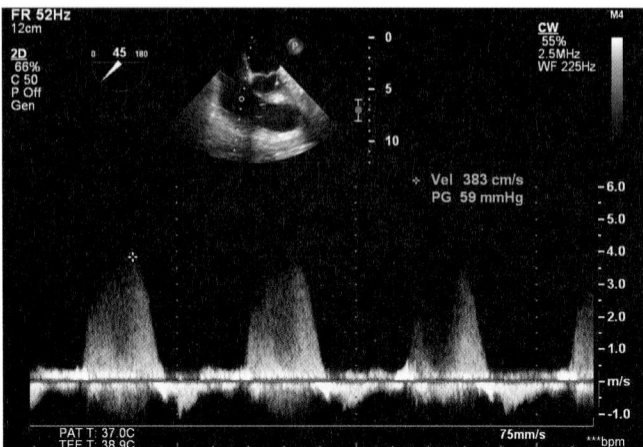

Figure 33-4   Continuous-wave Doppler through the tricuspid valve.

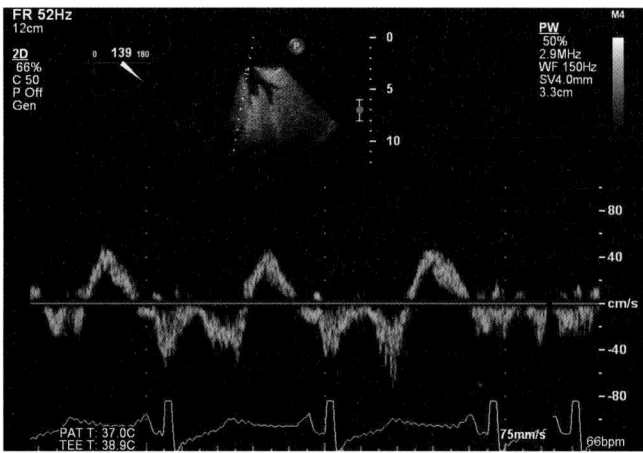

Figure 33-5   Hepatic veins showing flow reversal from atrial contraction to the beginning of diastole.

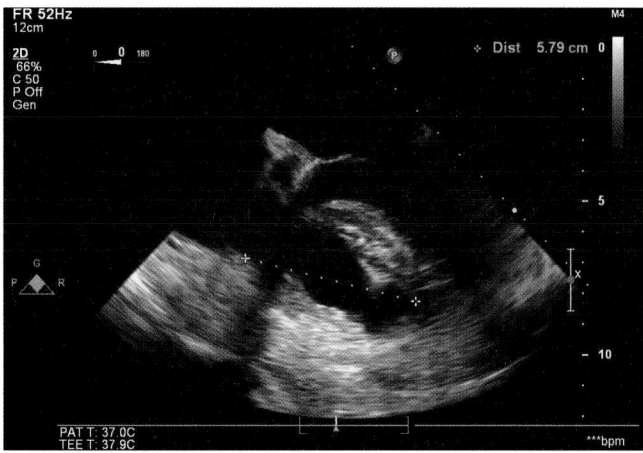

Figure 33-6   After treatment, systolic tricuspid annular plane systolic excursion measurement.

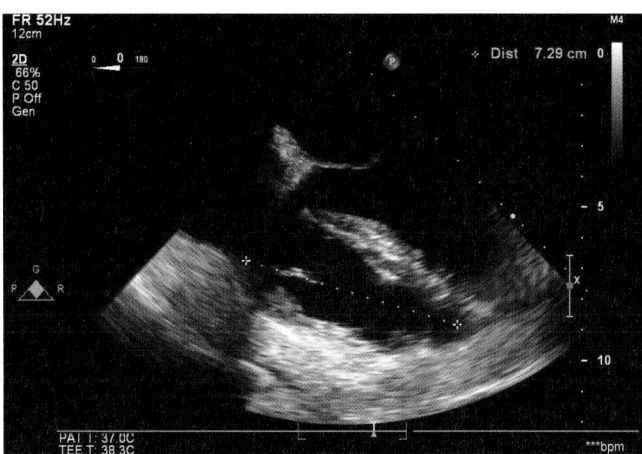

Figure 33-7 After treatment, diastolic tricuspid annular plane systolic excursion measurement.

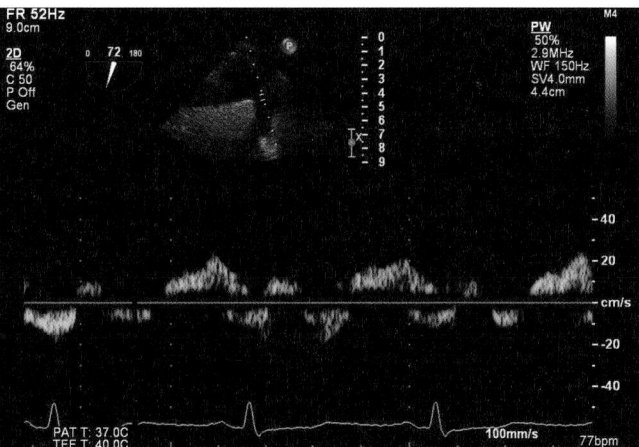

Figure 33-8 After treatment, a normal hepatic flow pattern.

Decision Making and Reassessment

The diagnosis of RV failure was entertained. The cause was either secondary to long-standing pulmonary hypertension (exacerbated by surgery) or secondary to a new cause (pneumonia, pleural effusions, pulmonary embolism). It was decided to initiate treatment for RV failure with milrinone and nitric oxide. The chest radiograph was significant for an effusion, which was drained; no evidence of pneumonia was seen; and spiral CT showed no pulmonary emboli. TEE was planned for the following day. TAPSE and degree of TR were used as repeat measures of treatment efficacy (with TAPSE being more objective and TR being more subjective). Follow-up TEE 24 hours later showed mild TR and improved TAPSE (1.5 cm). This was associated with a decline in liver function tests (LFTs) and INR. Blood cultures the following day were negative and antibiotics were stopped.

Case Study 2

A 47-year-old man underwent urgent three-vessel CABG surgery for left mainstem coronary artery disease. He was previously healthy with comorbidities of hypertension and hypercholesterolemia. He quit smoking 5 years ago. He had been admitted to the hospital for chest pain and ST-segment elevation. An angiogram showed left main stenosis of 90% with preserved LV function. He was taken to the OR for urgent bypass surgery.

After surgery in the ICU, the main concern was intermittent hypotension treated with an epinephrine infusion at 5 μg/min. Lactic acidosis, with serum lactate of 4 mmol/L, and a large chest tube

drainage of 100 to 150 mL/hr over the last 6 hours were treated with 4 units of fresh-frozen plasma and 6 units of packed red blood cells. Over the previous hour, his blood pressure and cardiac index had trended down and lactate had trended up. Chest tube drainage had decreased to 40 to 60 mL/hr. Urine output started to decrease, and vasopressin and norepinephrine were added to maintain blood pressure.

Framing the Problem

This case was considered hemodynamic deterioration of unknown cause. The goals were to assess the function of the LV and RV and, if one or both sides were found to be failing, to determine the cause. Assessment included vital signs (including PA pressure and cardiac index); measures of systemic perfusion (lactate, urine output); and other important indicators (chest tube drainage). The differential in this case was broad, with divergent treatment options; thus, a TEE was extremely important to assess the underlying pathology. Included in the differential diagnosis was hypovolemia, ventricular dysfunction (LV or RV), valvular incompetence (most likely mitral valve), or pericardial tamponade (either fluid or blood clot).

Data Collection

Interpretation of the TEE showed an underfilled LV with normal ejection fraction. The RV was normal to slightly underfilled, with evidence of compression of the RA. The likely diagnosis of cardiac tamponade was entertained and the patient taken to the OR for drainage of the tamponade. Tamponade in the perioperative setting presents a unique set of diagnostic dilemmas on TEE. Free fluid often is not present, and the use of positive pressure ventilation makes RV and RA collapse unusual, especially in the early phases. The presence of clot may result in isolated effects on the RA or RV and, occasionally, the IVC or SVC. If tamponade is suspected, careful examination of all these areas is essential. Edema of the myocardium or tissue surrounding the pericardium may be mistaken for clot, thus producing a false-positive assessment (see Videos 4 through 8, available online). It must be remembered that tamponade is a clinical diagnosis (increased filling pressure in the presence of underfilled ventricles and reduced cardiac output) and TEE should be used to confirm this suspicion. It is also possible, in spite of chest tubes within the pericardium, to develop tamponade either because the chest tubes become obstructed or because clot forms within the pericardium itself. After diagnosis, follow-up should occur with the surgeon to correlate findings on re-exploration with those seen on TEE.

Case Study 3

A 65-year-old woman underwent three-vessel CABG. Her medical history was significant for a 70-pack-year smoking history, hypertension, and colon cancer, treated 4 years previously. Her preoperative investigations revealed three-vessel disease and a normal LV. Preoperative blood work including ABG was unremarkable, as was the chest radiograph. Pulmonary function testing showed moderate obstructive airways disease. The surgical procedure was uneventful, but there was difficulty oxygenating the patient in the post-CPB period.

The patient arrived in the ICU on 100% oxygen with oxygen saturations of 92%. During the first 4 hours after surgery, the patient continued to experience intermittent desaturation on 100% Fio$_2$. Hemodynamically, the patient was stable and was weaned off all inotropes but continued to have intermittent and persistent oxygen desaturation.

Framing the Problem

Desaturation after CABG surgery is not uncommon and is usually successfully treated by increasing inspired oxygen, adding positive end-expiratory pressure, and waiting for the lungs to re-expand. The differential diagnosis is broad and includes preexisting lung disease, anesthesia, supine position, atelectasis, pulmonary edema, and transfusion or CPB-induced acute lung injury. One potential cause often overlooked is a right-to-left shunt. An atrial septal defect (ASD), ventricular septal defect, or large patent foramen ovale may cause shunting, which is usually left-to-right, but in conditions in which PA pressure is increased, systemic pressure is decreased, or TR is increased, the shunting can reverse and become right-to-left, resulting in desaturation not responsive to oxygen. These conditions are more likely in the postoperative period, especially in intubated patients.

Data Collection and Interpretation

Although TEE examination is not the first diagnostic test to be performed in patients in the ICU on high Fio_2, it may be used when other causes have been ruled out or when there is a known ASD or suspicion of one. Although intraoperative echocardiography should detect a patent foramen ovale or ASD, it may sometimes be missed or identified and ignored in closed-chamber procedures (see Video 9, available online). If no TEE was performed, then a TEE should be done in the postoperative period looking for an ASD with right-to-left shunting (which may be intermittent). Color flow will help determine the direction of blood flow. A bubble study can be performed to confirm the potential of right-to-left shunting (especially if shunting occurs without provocative maneuvers like a Valsalva maneuver). Treatment focuses on reducing the right-sided pressures and increasing the left-sided pressures. However, in severe cases unresponsive to medical management, a return to the OR for repair of the ASD may be warranted. If medical management was successful, then the patient should be made aware of the condition and followed by a cardiologist. If the patient returns to the OR, then the findings on reopening should be correlated with the TEE images. If an intraoperative echocardiogram was performed with the initial surgery, this should be reviewed for indications that an ASD was present.

REFERENCES

1. Bennett SR, Griffin SC: Sevoflurane versus isoflurane in patients undergoing valvular cardiac surgery, *J Cardiothorac Vasc Anesth* 15:175–178, 2001.
2. De Hert SG, Cromheecke S, ten Broecke PW, et al: Effects of propofol, desflurane, and sevoflurane on recovery of myocardial function after coronary surgery in elderly high-risk patients, *Anesthesiology* 99:314–323, 2003.
3. De Hert SG, ten Broecke PW, Mertens E, et al: Sevoflurane but not propofol preserves myocardial function in coronary surgery patients, *Anesthesiology* 97:42–49, 2002.
4. Julier K, Da Silva R, Garcia C, et al: Preconditioning by sevoflurane decreases biochemical markers for myocardial and renal dysfunction in coronary artery bypass graft surgery: A double-blinded, placebo-controlled, multicenter study, *Anesthesiology* 98:1315–1327, 2003.
5. Belhomme D, Peynet J, Louzy M, et al: Evidence for preconditioning by isoflurane in coronary artery bypass graft surgery, *Circulation* 100:II340–II344, 1999.
6. Boyce SW, Bartels C, Bolli R, et al: Impact of sodium-hydrogen exchange inhibition by cariporide on death or myocardial infarction in high-risk CABG surgery patients: Results of the CABG surgery cohort of the GUARDIAN study, *J Thorac Cardiovasc Surg* 126:420–427, 2003.
7. Van Oldenbeek C, Knowles P, Harper NJ: Residual neuromuscular block caused by pancuronium after cardiac surgery, *Br J Anaesth* 83:338–339, 1999.
8. McEwin L, Merrick PM, Bevan DR: Residual neuromuscular blockade after cardiac surgery: Pancuronium vs rocuronium, *Can J Anaesth* 44:891–895, 1997.
9. Murphy GS, Szokol JW, Marymont JH, et al: Impact of shorter-acting neuromuscular blocking agents on fast-track recovery of the cardiac surgical patient, *Anesthesiology* 96:600–606, 2002.
10. Thomas R, Smith D, Strike P: Prospective randomised double-blind comparative study of rocuronium and pancuronium in adult patients scheduled for elective 'fast-track' cardiac surgery involving hypothermic cardiopulmonary bypass, *Anaesthesia* 58:265–271, 2003.
11. Murphy GS, Szokol JW, Marymont JH, et al: Recovery of neuromuscular function after cardiac surgery: Pancuronium versus rocuronium, *Anesth Analg* 96:1301–1307, 2003, table of contents.
12. Mollhoff T, Herregods L, Moerman A, et al: Comparative efficacy and safety of remifentanil and fentanyl in 'fast track' coronary artery bypass graft surgery: A randomized, double-blind study, *Br J Anaesth* 87:718–726, 2001.
13. Engoren M, Luther G, Fenn-Buderer N: A comparison of fentanyl, sufentanil, and remifentanil for fast-track cardiac anesthesia, *Anesth Analg* 93:859–864, 2001.
14. Cheng DC, Newman MF, Duke P, et al: The efficacy and resource utilization of remifentanil and fentanyl in fast-track coronary artery bypass graft surgery: A prospective randomized, double-blinded controlled, multi-center trial, *Anesth Analg* 92:1094–1102, 2001.
15. Quasha AL, Loeber N, Feeley TW, et al: Postoperative respiratory care: A controlled trial of early and late extubation following coronary-artery bypass grafting, *Anesthesiology* 52:135–141, 1980.
16. Cheng DC, Karski J, Peniston C, et al: Morbidity outcome in early versus conventional tracheal extubation after coronary artery bypass grafting: A prospective randomized controlled trial, *J Thorac Cardiovasc Surg* 112:755–764, 1996.
17. Berry PD, Thomas SD, Mahon SP, et al: Myocardial ischaemia after coronary artery bypass grafting: Early vs late extubation, *Br J Anaesth* 80:20–25, 1998.
18. Silbert BS, Santamaria JD, O'Brien JL, et al: Early extubation following coronary artery bypass surgery: A prospective randomized controlled trial. The Fast Track Cardiac Care Team, *Chest* 113:1481–1488, 1998.
19. Ovrum E, Tangen G, Schiott C, et al: Rapid recovery protocol applied to 5,658 consecutive "on-pump" coronary bypass patients, *Ann Thorac Surg* 70:2008–2012, 2000.
20. Meade MO, Guyatt G, Butler R, et al: Trials comparing early vs late extubation following cardiovascular surgery, *Chest* 120:445S–453S, 2001.
21. Myles PS, Daly DJ, Djaiani G, et al: A systematic review of the safety and effectiveness of fast-track cardiac anesthesia, *Anesthesiology* 99:982–987, 2003.
22. Dowd NP, Cheng DC, Karski JM, et al: Intraoperative awareness in fast-track cardiac anesthesia, *Anesthesiology* 89:1068–1073, 1998, discussion 9A.
23. Liu WH, Thorp TA, Graham SG, et al: Incidence of awareness with recall during general anaesthesia, *Anaesthesia* 46:435–437, 1991.
24. Cheng DC, Karski J, Peniston C, et al: Early tracheal extubation after coronary artery bypass graft surgery reduces costs and improves resource use. A prospective, randomized, controlled trial, *Anesthesiology* 85:1300–1310, 1996.
25. Wong DT, Cheng DC, Kustra R, et al: Risk factors of delayed extubation, prolonged length of stay in the intensive care unit, and mortality in patients undergoing coronary artery bypass graft with fast-track cardiac anesthesia: A new cardiac risk score, *Anesthesiology* 91:936–944, 1999.
26. Brown MM: Implementation strategy: One-stop recovery for cardiac surgical patients, *AACN Clin Issues* 11:412–423, 2000.
27. Joyce L, Pandolph P: One Stop Post Op cardiac surgery recovery—a proven success, *J Cardiovasc Manag* 12:16–18, 2001.
28. Cheng DC, Byrick RJ, Knobel E: Structural models for intermediate care areas, *Crit Care Med* 27:2266–2271, 1999.
29. Cheng DC, Wall C, Djaiani G, et al: Randomized assessment of resource use in fast-track cardiac surgery 1-year after hospital discharge, *Anesthesiology* 98:651–657, 2003.
30. Grocott HP, Mackensen GB, Grigore AM, et al: Postoperative hyperthermia is associated with cognitive dysfunction after coronary artery bypass graft surgery, *Stroke* 33:537–541, 2002.
31. Nathan HJ, Wells GA, Munson JL, et al: Neuroprotective effect of mild hypothermia in patients undergoing coronary artery surgery with cardiopulmonary bypass: A randomized trial, *Circulation* 104:I85–I91, 2001.
32. Hebert PC: Transfusion requirements in critical care (TRICC): A multicentre, randomized, controlled clinical study. Transfusion Requirements in Critical Care Investigators and the Canadian Critical Care Trials Group, *Br J Anaesth* 81(Suppl 1):25–33, 1998.
33. Shore-Lesserson L, Manspeizer HE, DePerio M, et al: Thromboelastography-guided transfusion algorithm reduces transfusions in complex cardiac surgery, *Anesth Analg* 88:312–319, 1999.
34. Spiess BD, Gillies BS, Chandler W, et al: Changes in transfusion therapy and reexploration rate after institution of a blood management program in cardiac surgical patients, *J Cardiothorac Vasc Anesth* 9:168–173, 1995.
35. Body SC, Birmingham J, Parks R, et al: Safety and efficacy of shed mediastinal blood transfusion after cardiac surgery: A multicenter observational study. Multicenter Study of Perioperative Ischemia Research Group, *J Cardiothorac Vasc Anesth* 13:410–416, 1999.
36. Hillyer CD, Josephson CD, Blajchman MA, et al: Bacterial contamination of blood components: Risks, strategies, and regulation: Joint ASH and AABB educational session in transfusion medicine, *Hematology Am Soc Hematol Educ Program* 575–589, 2003.
37. Zurick AM, Urzua J, Ghattas M, et al: Failure of positive end-expiratory pressure to decrease postoperative bleeding after cardiac surgery, *Ann Thorac Surg* 34:608–611, 1982.
38. Collier B, Kolff J, Devineni R, et al: Prophylactic positive end-expiratory pressure and reduction of postoperative blood loss in open-heart surgery, *Ann Thorac Surg* 74:1191–1194, 2002.
39. Forestier F, Belisle S, Robitaille D, et al: Low-dose aprotinin is ineffective to treat excessive bleeding after cardiopulmonary bypass, *Ann Thorac Surg* 69:452–456, 2000.
40. Ray MJ, Hales MM, Brown L, et al: Postoperatively administered aprotinin or epsilon aminocaproic acid after cardiopulmonary bypass has limited benefit, *Ann Thorac Surg* 72:521–526, 2001.
41. Hardy JF, Belisle S, Van der Linden P: Efficacy and safety of activated recombinant factor VII in cardiac surgical patients, *Curr Opin Anaesthesiol* 22:95–99, 2009.
42. Gill R, Herbertson M, Vuylsteke A, et al: Safety and efficacy of recombinant activated factor VII: A randomized placebo-controlled trial in the setting of bleeding after cardiac surgery, *Circulation* 120:21–27, 2009.
43. Diprose P, Herbertson MJ, O'Shaughnessy D, et al: Activated recombinant factor VII after cardiopulmonary bypass reduces allogeneic transfusion in complex non-coronary cardiac surgery: Randomized double-blind placebo-controlled pilot study, *Br J Anaesth* 95:596–602, 2005.
44. BARI: Seven-year outcome in the Bypass Angioplasty Revascularization Investigation (BARI) by treatment and diabetic status, *J Am Coll Cardiol* 35:1122–1129, 2000.
45. Newman MF, Wolman R, Kanchuger M, et al: Multicenter preoperative stroke risk index for patients undergoing coronary artery bypass graft surgery. Multicenter Study of Perioperative Ischemia (McSPI) Research Group, *Circulation* 94:II74–II80, 1996.
46. Conlon PJ, Stafford-Smith M, White WD, et al: Acute renal failure following cardiac surgery, *Nephrol Dial Transplant* 14:1158–1162, 1999.
47. London MJ, Grunwald GK, Shroyer AL, et al: Association of fast-track cardiac management and low-dose to moderate-dose glucocorticoid administration with perioperative hyperglycemia, *J Cardiothorac Vasc Anesth* 14:631–638, 2000.
48. Golden SH, Peart-Vigilance C, Kao WH, et al: Perioperative glycemic control and the risk of infectious complications in a cohort of adults with diabetes, *Diabetes Care* 22:1408–1414, 1999.
49. Guvener M, Pasaoglu I, Demircin M, et al: Perioperative hyperglycemia is a strong correlate of postoperative infection in type II diabetic patients after coronary artery bypass grafting, *Endocr J* 49:531–537, 2002.
50. McAlister FA, Man J, Bistritz L, et al: Diabetes and coronary artery bypass surgery: An examination of perioperative glycemic control and outcomes, *Diabetes Care* 26:1518–1524, 2003.
51. Latham R, Lancaster AD, Covington JF, et al: The association of diabetes and glucose control with surgical-site infections among cardiothoracic surgery patients, *Infect Control Hosp Epidemiol* 22:607–612, 2001.
52. van den Berghe G, Wouters P, Weekers F, et al: Intensive insulin therapy in the critically ill patients, *N Engl J Med* 345:1359–1367, 2001.
53. Griesdale DE, de Souza RJ, van Dam RM, et al: Intensive insulin therapy and mortality among critically ill patients: A meta-analysis including NICE-SUGAR study data, *CMAJ* 180:821–827, 2009.
54. Finfer S, Chittock DR, Su SY, et al: Intensive versus conventional glucose control in critically ill patients, *N Engl J Med* 360:1283–1297, 2009.
55. Munro AJ, Long GT, Sleigh JW: Nurse-administered subcutaneous morphine is a satisfactory alternative to intravenous patient-controlled analgesia morphine after cardiac surgery, *Anesth Analg* 87:11–15, 1998.
56. Tsang J, Brush B: Patient-controlled analgesia in postoperative cardiac surgery, *Anaesth Intensive Care* 27:464–470, 1999.
57. O'Halloran P, Brown R: Patient-controlled analgesia compared with nurse-controlled infusion analgesia after heart surgery, *Intensive Crit Care Nurs* 13:126–129, 1997.
58. Myles PS, Buckland MR, Cannon GB, et al: Comparison of patient-controlled analgesia and nurse-controlled infusion analgesia after cardiac surgery, *Anaesth Intensive Care* 22:672–678, 1994.
59. Searle NR, Roy M, Bergeron G, et al: Hydromorphone patient-controlled analgesia (PCA) after coronary artery bypass surgery, *Can J Anaesth* 41:198–205, 1994.
60. Boldt J, Thaler E, Lehmann A, et al: Pain management in cardiac surgery patients: Comparison between standard therapy and patient-controlled analgesia regimen, *J Cardiothorac Vasc Anesth* 12:654–658, 1998.
61. Gust R, Pecher S, Gust A, et al: Effect of patient-controlled analgesia on pulmonary complications after coronary artery bypass grafting, *Crit Care Med* 27:2218–2223, 1999.

62. Bainbridge D, Martin JE, Cheng DC: Patient-controlled versus nurse-controlled analgesia after cardiac surgery—a meta-analysis, *Can J Anaesth* 53:492–499, 2006.
63. Chaney MA, Smith KR, Barclay JC, et al: Large-dose intrathecal morphine for coronary artery bypass grafting, *Anesth Analg* 83:215–222, 1996.
64. Bettex DA, Schmidlin D, Chassot PG, et al: Intrathecal sufentanil-morphine shortens the duration of intubation and improves analgesia in fast-track cardiac surgery, *Can J Anaesth* 49:711–717, 2002.
65. Boulanger A, Perreault S, Choiniere M, et al: Intrathecal morphine after cardiac surgery, *Ann Pharmacother* 36:1337–1343, 2002.
66. Zarate E, Latham P, White PF, et al: Fast-track cardiac anesthesia: Use of remifentanil combined with intrathecal morphine as an alternative to sufentanil during desflurane anesthesia, *Anesth Analg* 91:283–287, 2000.
67. Fitzpatrick GJ, Moriarty DC: Intrathecal morphine in the management of pain following cardiac surgery. A comparison with morphine i.v, *Br J Anaesth* 60:639–644, 1988.
68. Aun C, Thomas D, St John-Jones L, et al: Intrathecal morphine in cardiac surgery, *Eur J Anaesthesiol* 2:419–426, 1985.
69. Shroff A, Rooke GA, Bishop MJ: Effects of intrathecal opioid on extubation time, analgesia, and intensive care unit stay following coronary artery bypass grafting, *J Clin Anesth* 9:415–419, 1997.
70. Lena P, Balarac N, Arnulf JJ, et al: Intrathecal morphine and clonidine for coronary artery bypass grafting, *Br J Anaesth* 90:300–303, 2003.
71. Chaney MA, Nikolov MP, Blakeman BP, et al: Intrathecal morphine for coronary artery bypass graft procedure and early extubation revisited, *J Cardiothorac Vasc Anesth* 13:574–578, 1999.
72. Chaney MA, Furry PA, Fluder EM, et al: Intrathecal morphine for coronary artery bypass grafting and early extubation, *Anesth Analg* 84:241–248, 1997.
73. Liu SS, Block BM, Wu CL: Effects of perioperative central neuraxial analgesia on outcome after coronary artery bypass surgery: A meta-analysis, *Anesthesiology* 101:153–161, 2004.
74. Ho AM, Chung DC, Joynt GM: Neuraxial blockade and hematoma in cardiac surgery: Estimating the risk of a rare adverse event that has not (yet) occurred, *Chest* 117:551–555, 2000.
75. Pastor MC, Sanchez MJ, Casas MA, et al: Thoracic epidural analgesia in coronary artery bypass graft surgery: Seven years' experience, *J Cardiothorac Vasc Anesth* 17:154–159, 2003.
76. Horlocker TT, Wedel DJ, Benzon H, et al: Regional anesthesia in the anticoagulated patient: Defining the risks, *Reg Anesth Pain Med* 29:1–12, 2004.
77. Lipsky PE: Defining COX-2 inhibitors, *J Rheumatol Suppl* 60:13–16, 2000.
78. Bigler D, Moller J, Kamp-Jensen M, et al: Effect of piroxicam in addition to continuous thoracic epidural bupivacaine and morphine on postoperative pain and lung function after thoracotomy, *Acta Anaesthesiol Scand* 36:647–650, 1992.
79. Carretta A, Zannini P, Chiesa G, et al: Efficacy of ketorolac tromethamine and extrapleural intercostal nerve block on post-thoracotomy pain. A prospective, randomized study, *Int Surg* 81:224–228, 1996.
80. Fayaz K, Abel R, Pugh S, et al: Opioid sparing and side effect profile of three different analgesic techniques for cardiac surgery, *Eur J Anesth* 20:A6, 2003.
81. Hynninen MS, Cheng DC, Hossain I, et al: Non-steroidal anti-inflammatory drugs in treatment of postoperative pain after cardiac surgery, *Can J Anaesth* 47:1182–1187, 2000.
82. Immer FF, Immer-Bansi AS, Trachsel N, et al: Pain treatment with a COX-2 inhibitor after coronary artery bypass operation: A randomized trial, *Ann Thorac Surg* 75:490–495, 2003.
83. Jones RM, Cashman JN, Foster JM, et al: Comparison of infusions of morphine and lysine acetyl salicylate for the relief of pain following thoracic surgery, *Br J Anaesth* 57:259–263, 1985.
84. Kavanagh BP, Katz J, Sandler AN, et al: Multimodal analgesia before thoracic surgery does not reduce postoperative pain, *Br J Anaesth* 73:184–189, 1994.
85. Keenan DJ, Cave K, Langdon L, et al: Comparative trial of rectal indomethacin and cryoanalgesia for control of early postthoracotomy pain, *Br Med J (Clin Res Ed)* 287:1335–1337, 1983.
86. McCrory C, Diviney D, Moriarty J, et al: Comparison between repeat bolus intrathecal morphine and an epidurally delivered bupivacaine and fentanyl combination in the management of post-thoracotomy pain with or without cyclooxygenase inhibition, *J Cardiothorac Vasc Anesth* 16:607–611, 2002.
87. Merry AF, Wardall GJ, Cameron RJ, et al: Prospective, controlled, double-blind study of i.v. tenoxicam for analgesia after thoracotomy, *Br J Anaesth* 69:92–94, 1992.
88. Ott E, Nussmeier NA, Duke PC, et al: Efficacy and safety of the cyclooxygenase 2 inhibitors parecoxib and valdecoxib in patients undergoing coronary artery bypass surgery, *J Thorac Cardiovasc Surg* 125:1481–1492, 2003.
89. Bainbridge D, Cheng DC, Martin JE, et al: NSAID-analgesia, pain control and morbidity in cardiothoracic surgery: [L'analgesie avec des AINS, le controle de la douleur et la morbidite en chirurgie cardiothoracique], *Can J Anaesth* 53:46–59, 2006.
90. Nussmeier NA, Whelton AA, Brown MT, et al: Complications of the COX-2 inhibitors parecoxib and valdecoxib after cardiac surgery, *N Engl J Med* 352:1081–1091, 2005.
91. Camu F, Beecher T, Recker DP, et al: Valdecoxib, a COX-2-specific inhibitor, is an efficacious, opioid-sparing analgesic in patients undergoing hip arthroplasty, *Am J Ther* 9:43–51, 2002.
92. Collaborative overview of randomised trials of antiplatelet therapy—II: Maintenance of vascular graft or arterial patency by antiplatelet therapy. Antiplatelet Trialists' Collaboration, *BMJ* 308:159–168, 1994.
93. Weber M, von Schacky C, Lorenz R, et al: [Low-dose acetylsalicylic acid (100 mg/day) following aortocoronary bypass operation], *Klin Wochenschr* 62:458–464, 1984.
94. Goldman S, Copeland J, Moritz T, et al: Starting aspirin therapy after operation. Effects on early graft patency. Department of Veterans Affairs Cooperative Study Group, *Circulation* 84:520–526, 1991.
95. Goldman S, Copeland J, Moritz T, et al: Saphenous vein graft patency 1 year after coronary artery bypass surgery and effects of antiplatelet therapy. Results of a Veterans Administration Cooperative Study, *Circulation* 80:1190–1197, 1989.
96. Mangano DT: Aspirin and mortality from coronary bypass surgery, *N Engl J Med* 347:1309–1317, 2002.
97. Sethi GK, Copeland JG, Goldman S, et al: Implications of preoperative administration of aspirin in patients undergoing coronary artery bypass grafting. Department of Veterans Affairs Cooperative Study on Antiplatelet Therapy, *J Am Coll Cardiol* 15:15–20, 1990.
98. Goldman S, Zadina K, Krasnicka B, et al: Predictors of graft patency 3 years after coronary artery bypass graft surgery. Department of Veterans Affairs Cooperative Study Group No. 297, *J Am Coll Cardiol* 29:1563–1568, 1997.
99. Antiplatelet Trialists' Collaboration: Collaborative overview of randomised trials of antiplatelet therapy—I: Prevention of death, myocardial infarction, and stroke by prolonged antiplatelet therapy in various categories of patients, *BMJ* 308:81–106, 1994.
100. Bhatt DL, Chew DP, Hirsch AT, et al: Superiority of clopidogrel versus aspirin in patients with prior cardiac surgery, *Circulation* 103:363–368, 2001.
101. Effect of metoprolol on death and cardiac events during a 2-year period after coronary artery bypass grafting. The MACB Study Group, *Eur Heart J* 16:1825–1832, 1995.
102. Oosterga M, Voors AA, Pinto YM, et al: Effects of quinapril on clinical outcome after coronary artery bypass grafting (The QUO VADIS Study). QUinapril on Vascular Ace and Determinants of Ischemia, *Am J Cardiol* 87:542–546, 2001.
103. Chen J, Radford MJ, Wang Y, et al: Are beta-blockers effective in elderly patients who undergo coronary revascularization after acute myocardial infarction? *Arch Intern Med* 160:947–952, 2000.
104. The effect of aggressive lowering of low-density lipoprotein cholesterol levels and low-dose anticoagulation on obstructive changes in saphenous-vein coronary-artery bypass grafts. The Post Coronary Artery Bypass Graft Trial Investigators, *N Engl J Med* 336:153–162, 1997.
105. Ouattara A, Benhaoua H, Le Manach Y, et al: Perioperative statin therapy is associated with a significant and dose-dependent reduction of adverse cardiovascular outcomes after coronary artery bypass graft surgery, *J Cardiothorac Vasc Anesth* 23:633–638, 2009.
106. Miceli A, Fino C, Fiorani B, et al: Effects of preoperative statin treatment on the incidence of postoperative atrial fibrillation in patients undergoing coronary artery bypass grafting, *Ann Thorac Surg* 87:1853–1858, 2009.
107. Liakopoulos OJ, Choi YH, Kuhn EW, et al: Statins for prevention of atrial fibrillation after cardiac surgery: A systematic literature review, *J Thorac Cardiovasc Surg* 138:678–686e1, 2009.
108. Bonow RO, Carabello BA, Chatterjee K, et al: 2008 focused update incorporated into the ACC/AHA 2006 guidelines for the management of patients with valvular heart disease: A report of the American College of Cardiology/American Heart Association Task Force on Practice Guidelines (Writing Committee to revise the 1998 guidelines for the management of patients with valvular heart disease). Endorsed by the Society of Cardiovascular Anesthesiologists, Society for Cardiovascular Angiography and Interventions, and Society of Thoracic Surgeons, *J Am Coll Cardiol* 52:e1–e142, 2008.
109. Naylor AR, Mehta Z, Rothwell PM, et al: Carotid artery disease and stroke during coronary artery bypass: A critical review of the literature, *Eur J Vasc Endovasc Surg* 23:283–294, 2002.
110. Stamou SC, Hill PC, Dangas G, et al: Stroke after coronary artery bypass: Incidence, predictors, and clinical outcome, *Stroke* 32:1508–1513, 2001.
111. Salazar JD, Wityk RJ, Grega MA, et al: Stroke after cardiac surgery: Short- and long-term outcomes, *Ann Thorac Surg* 72:1195–1201, 2001 discussion 201–202.
112. Lahtinen J, Biancari F, Salmela E, et al: Postoperative atrial fibrillation is a major cause of stroke after on-pump coronary artery bypass surgery, *Ann Thorac Surg* 77:1241–1244, 2004.
113. Murkin JM, Martzke JS, Buchan AM, et al: A randomized study of the influence of perfusion technique and pH management strategy in 316 patients undergoing coronary artery bypass surgery. II. Neurologic and cognitive outcomes, *J Thorac Cardiovasc Surg* 110:349–362, 1995.
114. Murkin JM: Attenuation of neurologic injury during cardiac surgery, *Ann Thorac Surg* 72:S1838–S1844, 2001.
115. Royse AG, Royse CF, Ajani AE, et al: Reduced neuropsychological dysfunction using epiaortic echocardiography and the exclusive Y graft, *Ann Thorac Surg* 69:1431–1438, 2000.
116. Sharony R, Bizekis CS, Kanchuger M, et al: Off-pump coronary artery bypass grafting reduces mortality and stroke in patients with atheromatous aortas: A case control study, *Circulation* 108(Suppl 1):II15–II20, 2003.
117. Leacche M, Carrier M, Bouchard D, et al: Improving neurologic outcome in off-pump surgery: The "no touch" technique, *Heart Surg Forum* 6:169–175, 2003.
118. Bruno A, Levine SR, Frankel MR, et al: Admission glucose level and clinical outcomes in the NINDS rt-PA Stroke Trial, *Neurology* 59:669–674, 2002.
119. Williams LS, Rotich J, Qi R, et al: Effects of admission hyperglycemia on mortality and costs in acute ischemic stroke, *Neurology* 59:67–71, 2002.
120. Quast MJ, Wei J, Huang NC, et al: Perfusion deficit parallels exacerbation of cerebral ischemia/reperfusion injury in hyperglycemic rats, *J Cereb Blood Flow Metab* 17:553–559, 1997.
121. Dietrich WD, Busto R, Valdes I, et al: Effects of normothermic versus mild hyperthermic forebrain ischemia in rats, *Stroke* 21:1318–1325, 1990.
122. Bucerius J, Gummert JF, Borger MA, et al: Predictors of delirium after cardiac surgery delirium: Effect of beating-heart (off-pump) surgery, *J Thorac Cardiovasc Surg* 127:57–64, 2004.
123. van der Mast RC, van den Broek WW, Fekkes D, et al: Incidence of and preoperative predictors for delirium after cardiac surgery, *J Psychosom Res* 46:479–483, 1999.
124. Gokgoz L, Gunaydin S, Sinci V, et al: Psychiatric complications of cardiac surgery postoperative delirium syndrome, *Scand Cardiovasc J* 31:217–222, 1997.
125. Rolfson DB, McElhaney JE, Rockwood K, et al: Incidence and risk factors for delirium and other adverse outcomes in older adults after coronary artery bypass graft surgery, *Can J Cardiol* 15:771–776, 1999.
126. Ommen SR, Odell JA, Stanton MS: Atrial arrhythmias after cardiothoracic surgery, *N Engl J Med* 336:1429–1434, 1997.
127. Zimmer J, Pezzullo J, Choucair W, et al: Meta-analysis of antiarrhythmic therapy in the prevention of postoperative atrial fibrillation and the effect on hospital length of stay, costs, cerebrovascular accidents, and mortality in patients undergoing cardiac surgery, *Am J Cardiol* 91:1137–1140, 2003.
128. Mathew JP, Fontes ML, Tudor IC, et al: A multicenter risk index for atrial fibrillation after cardiac surgery, *JAMA* 291:1720–1729, 2004.
129. Crystal E, Connolly SJ, Sleik K, et al: Interventions on prevention of postoperative atrial fibrillation in patients undergoing heart surgery: A meta-analysis, *Circulation* 106:75–80, 2002.
130. Toraman F, Karabulut EH, Alhan HC, et al: Magnesium infusion dramatically decreases the incidence of atrial fibrillation after coronary artery bypass grafting, *Ann Thorac Surg* 72:1256–1261, 2001 discussion 1261–1262.
131. Blackshear JL, Safford RE: AFFIRM and RACE trials: Implications for the management of atrial fibrillation, *Card Electrophysiol Rev* 7:366–369, 2003.
132. Wyse DG, Waldo AL, DiMarco JP, et al: A comparison of rate control and rhythm control in patients with atrial fibrillation, *N Engl J Med* 347:1825–1833, 2002.
133. Hagens VE, Ranchor AV, Van Sonderen E, et al: Effect of rate or rhythm control on quality of life in persistent atrial fibrillation. Results from the Rate Control Versus Electrical Cardioversion (RACE) Study, *J Am Coll Cardiol* 43:241–247, 2004.
134. Olshansky B, Rosenfeld LE, Warner AL, et al: The Atrial Fibrillation Follow-up Investigation of Rhythm Management (AFFIRM) study: Approaches to control rate in atrial fibrillation, *J Am Coll Cardiol* 43:1201–1208, 2004.
135. Estes NA 3rd, Halperin JL, Calkins H, et al: ACC/AHA/Physician Consortium 2008 clinical performance measures for adults with nonvalvular atrial fibrillation or atrial flutter: A report of the American College of Cardiology/American Heart Association Task Force on Performance Measures and the Physician Consortium for Performance Improvement (Writing Committee to Develop Clinical Performance Measures for Atrial Fibrillation): Developed in collaboration with the Heart Rhythm Society, *Circulation* 117:1101–1120, 2008.
136. Hart RG, Benavente O, McBride R, et al: Antithrombotic therapy to prevent stroke in patients with atrial fibrillation: A meta-analysis, *Ann Intern Med* 131:492–501, 1999.
137. Prystowsky EN, Benson DW Jr, Fuster V, et al: Management of patients with atrial fibrillation. A Statement for Healthcare Professionals. From the Subcommittee on Electrocardiography and Electrophysiology, American Heart Association, *Circulation* 93:1262–1277, 1996.
138. Fuster V, Ryden LE, Asinger RW, et al: ACC/AHA/ESC guidelines for the management of patients with atrial fibrillation: Executive summary. A Report of the American College of Cardiology/American Heart Association Task Force on Practice Guidelines and the European Society of Cardiology Committee for Practice Guidelines and Policy Conferences (Committee to Develop Guidelines for the Management of Patients With Atrial Fibrillation): Developed in Collaboration With the North American Society of Pacing and Electrophysiology, *J Am Coll Cardiol* 38:1231–1266, 2001.
139. Butterworth JFt, Legault C, Royster RL, et al: Factors that predict the use of positive inotropic drug support after cardiac valve surgery, *Anesth Analg* 86:461–467, 1998.
140. Royster RL, Butterworth JFt, Prough DS, et al: Preoperative and intraoperative predictors of inotropic support and long-term outcome in patients having coronary artery bypass grafting, *Anesth Analg* 72:729–736, 1991.
141. Krivec B, Voga G, Zuran I, et al: Diagnosis and treatment of shock due to massive pulmonary embolism: Approach with transesophageal echocardiography and intrapulmonary thrombolysis, *Chest* 112:1310–1316, 1997.

142. van der Wouw PA, Koster RW, Delemarre BJ, et al: Diagnostic accuracy of transesophageal echocardiography during cardiopulmonary resuscitation, *J Am Coll Cardiol* 30:780–783, 1997.

143. Cicek S, Demirilic U, Kuralay E, et al: Transesophageal echocardiography in cardiac surgical emergencies, *J Card Surg* 10:236–244, 1995.

144. Wake PJ, Ali M, Carroll J, et al: Clinical and echocardiographic diagnoses disagree in patients with unexplained hemodynamic instability after cardiac surgery, *Can J Anaesth* 48:778–783, 2001.

145. Tousignant CP, Walsh F, Mazer CD: The use of transesophageal echocardiography for preload assessment in critically ill patients, *Anesth Analg* 90:351–355, 2000.

146. Swenson JD, Bull D, Stringham J: Subjective assessment of left ventricular preload using transesophageal echocardiography: Corresponding pulmonary artery occlusion pressures, *J Cardiothorac Vasc Anesth* 15:580–583, 2001.

147. Fontes ML, Bellows W, Ngo L, et al: Assessment of ventricular function in critically ill patients: Limitations of pulmonary artery catheterization. Institutions of the McSPI Research Group, *J Cardiothorac Vasc Anesth* 13:521–527, 1999.

148. Schwinn DA, Leone BJ, Spahn DR, et al: Desensitization of myocardial beta-adrenergic receptors during cardiopulmonary bypass. Evidence for early uncoupling and late downregulation, *Circulation* 84:2559–2567, 1991.

149. Royster RL, Butterworth JFt, Prielipp RC, et al: Combined inotropic effects of amrinone and epinephrine after cardiopulmonary bypass in humans, *Anesth Analg* 77:662–672, 1993.

150. Tokmakoglu H, Farsak B, Gunaydin S, et al: Effectiveness of intraaortic balloon pumping in patients who were not able to be weaned from cardiopulmonary bypass after coronary artery bypass surgery and mortality predictors in the perioperative and early postoperative period, *Anadolu Kardiyol Derg* 3:124–128, 2003.

151. Marra C, De Santo LS, Amarelli C, et al: Coronary artery bypass grafting in patients with severe left ventricular dysfunction: A prospective randomized study on the timing of perioperative intraaortic balloon pump support, *Int J Artif Organs* 25:141–146, 2002.

152. Christenson JT, Badel P, Simonet F, et al: Preoperative intraaortic balloon pump enhances cardiac performance and improves the outcome of redo CABG, *Ann Thorac Surg* 64:1237–1244, 1997.

153. Christenson JT, Simonet F, Badel P, et al: Optimal timing of preoperative intraaortic balloon pump support in high-risk coronary patients, *Ann Thorac Surg* 68:934–939, 1999.

154. Christenson JT, Schmuziger M, Simonet F: Effective surgical management of high-risk coronary patients using preoperative intra-aortic balloon counterpulsation therapy, *Cardiovasc Surg* 9:383–390, 2001.

155. Torchiana DF, Hirsch G, Buckley MJ, et al: Intraaortic balloon pumping for cardiac support: Trends in practice and outcome, 1968 to 1995, *J Thorac Cardiovasc Surg* 113:758–764, 1997 discussion 764–769.

156. Castelli P, Condemi A, Munari M, et al: Intra-aortic balloon counterpulsation: Outcome in cardiac surgical patients, *J Cardiothorac Vasc Anesth* 15:700–703, 2001.

157. Sirivella S, Gielchinsky I, Parsonnet V: Angiotensin converting enzyme inhibitor therapy in severe postcardiotomy dysfunction: A prospective randomized study, *J Card Surg* 13:11–17, 1998.

158. Haddad F, Couture P, Tousignant C, et al: The right ventricle in cardiac surgery, a perioperative perspective: II. Pathophysiology, clinical importance, and management, *Anesth Analg* 108:422–433, 2009.

159. Haddad F, Couture P, Tousignant C, et al: The right ventricle in cardiac surgery, a perioperative perspective: I. Anatomy, physiology, and assessment, *Anesth Analg* 108:407–421, 2009.

160. Haddad F, Doyle R, Murphy DJ, et al: Right ventricular function in cardiovascular disease, part II: Pathophysiology, clinical importance, and management of right ventricular failure, *Circulation* 117:1717–1731, 2008.

161. Haddad F, Hunt SA, Rosenthal DN, et al: Right ventricular function in cardiovascular disease, part I: Anatomy, physiology, aging, and functional assessment of the right ventricle, *Circulation* 117:1436–1448, 2008.

162. Cecconi M, Johnston E, Rhodes A: What role does the right side of the heart play in circulation? *Crit Care* 10(Suppl 3):S5, 2006.

163. Abrahamov D, Tamariz M, Fremes S, et al: Renal dysfunction after cardiac surgery, *Can J Cardiol* 17:565–570, 2001.

164. Wijeysundera DN, Rao V, Beattie WS, et al: Evaluating surrogate measures of renal dysfunction after cardiac surgery, *Anesth Analg* 96:1265–1273, 2003 table of contents.

165. Wang F, Dupuis JY, Nathan H, et al: An analysis of the association between preoperative renal dysfunction and outcome in cardiac surgery: Estimated creatinine clearance or plasma creatinine level as measures of renal function, *Chest* 124:1852–1862, 2003.

166. Kellum JA: The use of diuretics and dopamine in acute renal failure: A systematic review of the evidence, *Crit Care* 1:53–59, 1997.

167. Landoni G, Biondi-Zoccai GG, Tumlin JA, et al: Beneficial impact of fenoldopam in critically ill patients with or at risk for acute renal failure: A meta-analysis of randomized clinical trials, *Am J Kidney Dis* 49:56–68, 2007.

168. Mehta RL, Pascual MT, Soroko S, et al: Diuretics, mortality, and nonrecovery of renal function in acute renal failure, *JAMA* 288:2547–2553, 2002.

169. Kellum JA, Angus DC, Johnson JP, et al: Continuous versus intermittent renal replacement therapy: A meta-analysis, *Intensive Care Med* 28:29–37, 2002.

170. Adabag AS, Ishani A, Bloomfield HE, et al: Efficacy of N-acetylcysteine in preventing renal injury after heart surgery: A systematic review of randomized trials, *Eur Heart J* 30:1910–1917, 2009.

171. Naughton F, Wijeysundera D, Karkouti K, et al: N-acetylcysteine to reduce renal failure after cardiac surgery: A systematic review and meta-analysis, *Can J Anaesth* 55:827–835, 2008.

172. Misra D, Leibowitz K, Gowda RM, et al: Role of N-acetylcysteine in prevention of contrast-induced nephropathy after cardiovascular procedures: A meta-analysis, *Clin Cardiol* 27:607–610, 2004.

173. Yusuf S, Zucker D, Peduzzi P, et al: Effect of coronary artery bypass graft surgery on survival: Overview of 10-year results from randomised trials by the Coronary Artery Bypass Graft Surgery Trialists Collaboration, *Lancet* 344:563–570, 1994.

174. BARI: Comparison of coronary bypass surgery with angioplasty in patients with multivessel disease. The Bypass Angioplasty Revascularization Investigation (BARI) Investigators, *N Engl J Med* 335:217–225, 1996.

175. Carrie D, Elbaz M, Puel J, et al: Five-year outcome after coronary angioplasty versus bypass surgery in multivessel coronary artery disease: Results from the French Monocentric Study, *Circulation* 96:II-1–II-6, 1997.

176. Hamm CW, Reimers J, Ischinger T, et al: A randomized study of coronary angioplasty compared with bypass surgery in patients with symptomatic multivessel coronary disease. German Angioplasty Bypass Surgery Investigation (GABI), *N Engl J Med* 331:1037–1043, 1994.

177. Hoffman SN, TenBrook JA, Wolf MP, et al: A meta-analysis of randomized controlled trials comparing coronary artery bypass graft with percutaneous transluminal coronary angioplasty: One- to eight-year outcomes, *J Am Coll Cardiol* 41:1293–1304, 2003.

178. Goy JJ, Eeckhout E, Moret C, et al: Five-year outcome in patients with isolated proximal left anterior descending coronary artery stenosis treated by angioplasty or left internal mammary artery grafting. A prospective trial, *Circulation* 99:3255–3259, 1999.

179. Rodriguez A, Bernardi V, Navia J, et al: Argentine Randomized Study: Coronary Angioplasty with Stenting versus Coronary Bypass Surgery in patients with Multiple-Vessel Disease (ERACI II): 30-day and one-year follow-up results. ERACI II Investigators, *J Am Coll Cardiol* 37:51–58, 2001.

180. Serruys PW, Unger F, Sousa JE, et al: Comparison of coronary-artery bypass surgery and stenting for the treatment of multivessel disease, *N Engl J Med* 344:1117–1124, 2001.

181. Legrand VM, Serruys PW, Unger F, et al: Three-year outcome after coronary stenting versus bypass surgery for the treatment of multivessel disease, *Circulation* 109:1114–1120, 2004.

182. SOS: Coronary artery bypass surgery versus percutaneous coronary intervention with stent implantation in patients with multivessel coronary artery disease (the Stent or Surgery trial): A randomised controlled trial, *Lancet* 360:965–970, 2002.

183. Bainbridge D, Cheng D, Martin J, et al: Does off-pump or minimally invasive coronary artery bypass reduce mortality, morbidity, and resource utilization when compared with percutaneous coronary intervention? A meta-analysis of randomized trials, *J Thorac Cardiovasc Surg* 133:623–631, 2007.

184. D'Ancona G, Karamanoukian H, Kawaguchi AT, et al: Myocardial revascularization of the beating heart in high-risk patients, *J Card Surg* 16:132–139, 2001.

185. Hoff SJ, Ball SK, Coltharp WH, et al: Coronary artery bypass in patients 80 years and over: Is off-pump the operation of choice? *Ann Thorac Surg* 74:S1340–S1343, 2002.

186. Yokoyama T, Baumgartner FJ, Gheissari A, et al: Off-pump versus on-pump coronary bypass in high-risk subgroups, *Ann Thorac Surg* 70:1546–1550, 2000.

187. Lee JD, Lee SJ, Tsushima WT, et al: Benefits of off-pump bypass on neurologic and clinical morbidity: A prospective randomized trial, *Ann Thorac Surg* 76:18–26, 2003.

188. Puskas J, Sharoni E, Williams W, et al: Is routine use of temporary epicardial pacing wires necessary after either OPCAB or conventional CABG/CPB? *Heart Surg Forum* 6(Suppl 1):s47, 2003.

189. Angelini GD, Taylor FC, Reeves BC, et al: Early and midterm outcome after off-pump and on-pump surgery in Beating Heart Against Cardioplegic Arrest Studies (BHACAS 1 and 2): A pooled analysis of two randomised controlled trials, *Lancet* 359:1194–1199, 2002.

190. Khan NE, De Souza A, Mister R, et al: A randomized comparison of off-pump and on-pump multivessel coronary-artery bypass surgery, *N Engl J Med* 350:21–28, 2004.

191. Cheng DC, Bainbridge D, Martin JE, et al: Does off-pump coronary artery bypass reduce mortality, morbidity, and resource utilization when compared with conventional coronary artery bypass? A meta-analysis of randomized trials, *Anesthesiology* 102:188–203, 2005.

192. Shroyer AL, Grover FL, Hattler B, et al: On-pump versus off-pump coronary-artery bypass surgery, *N Engl J Med* 361:1827–1837, 2009.

193. Puskas JD, Williams WH, Mahoney EM, et al: Off-pump vs conventional coronary artery bypass grafting: Early and 1-year graft patency, cost, and quality-of-life outcomes: A randomized trial, *JAMA* 291:1841–1849, 2004.

34

Postoperative Cardiovascular Management

JERROLD H. LEVY, MD, FAHA | JAMES G. RAMSAY, MD | KENICHI TANAKA, MD, MSC |
JAMES M. BAILEY, MD, PHD

KEY POINTS

1. Maintaining oxygen transport and oxygen delivery appropriately to meet the tissue metabolic needs is the goal of postoperative circulatory control.
2. Multiple parameters of cardiac function worsen after cardiac surgery. Therapeutic approaches to reversing this dysfunction are important.
3. Myocardial ischemia often occurs after surgery, and it is associated with adverse cardiac outcomes. Multiple strategies have been studied to reduce this complication.
4. Postoperative biventricular dysfunction is common, requiring interventions to optimize the heart rate and rhythm, provide an acceptable preload, and adjust afterload and contractility. In most patients, pharmacologic interventions can be weaned rapidly or stopped within the first 24 hours after surgery.
5. Supraventricular tachyarrhythmias are common in the first postoperative days, with atrial fibrillation predominating. Preoperative and immediate postoperative pharmacotherapy can reduce the incidence and slow the ventricular response.
6. Postoperative hypertension has been a common complication of cardiac surgery; newer vasodilator drugs are more arterial selective and allow greater circulatory stability than older nonselective drugs.
7. Catecholamines, phosphodiesterase inhibitors, and the calcium sensitizer levosimendan have been studied for treating biventricular dysfunction.
8. Phosphodiesterase inhibitors and levosimendan are clinically effective inodilators. Natriuretic peptides such as nesiritide also may have a role as a vasodilator to improve cardiac output in this setting.
9. A prolonged bypass run may cause a refractory vasodilated state ("vasoplegia") requiring combinations of pressors such as norepinephrine and vasopressin.
10. Positive-pressure ventilation has multiple effects on the cardiovascular system, with complex interactions that should be considered in patients after cardiac surgery.

Postoperative cardiovascular dysfunction is increasingly common as older and potentially more critically ill patients undergo cardiac surgery. Biventricular dysfunction and circulatory changes occur after cardiopulmonary bypass (CPB) but also can occur in patients undergoing off-pump surgery. Pharmacologic therapy with suitable monitoring and mechanical support may be necessary for patients in the postoperative period until ventricular or circulatory dysfunction improves. This chapter reviews management considerations of postoperative circulatory failure.

OXYGEN TRANSPORT

Maintaining oxygen transport (i.e., oxygen delivery [Do_2]) satisfactory to meet the tissue metabolic needs is the goal of postoperative circulatory control. Oxygen transport is the product of cardiac output (CO) times arterial content of oxygen (Cao_2; i.e., hemoglobin concentration $\times$ 1.34 mL oxygen per 1 g hemoglobin $\times$ oxygen saturation), and it can be affected in many ways by the cardiovascular and respiratory systems, as shown in Figure 34-1. Low CO, anemia from blood loss, and pulmonary disease can decrease Do_2. Before altering the determinants of CO, including the inotropic state of the ventricles, an acceptable hemoglobin concentration and adequate oxygen saturation (Sao_2) should be provided, enabling increases in CO to provide the maximum available Do_2. As hemoglobin concentration increases, so does blood viscosity and, therefore, the work of the heart to eject the blood. In normal hearts (e.g., athletes), increasing hemoglobin levels to supranormal will increase performance, suggesting that in this setting the increased viscosity is less important than the increase in oxygen-carrying capacity.[1] This has not been examined in patients with cardiac disease. Model analysis of data from animal investigations suggests that maintenance of the hematocrit between 30% and 33% provides the best balance between oxygen-carrying capacity and viscosity.[2] This analysis also suggests that, in ischemic states, a hematocrit in this range may be desirable. Patients needing continued inotropic or mechanical support of ventricular function beyond the first few postoperative hours, especially those in need of intravascular volume expansion, should probably be transfused to a hematocrit in this

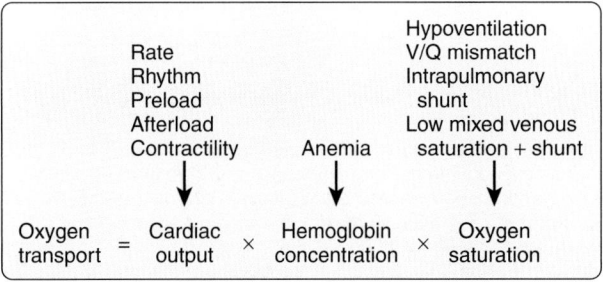

Figure 34-1 Important factors that contribute to abnormal oxygen transport.

range, bearing in mind that blood transfusion has been associated with decreased organ function and increased mortality in critically ill patients. A randomized trial suggested a transfusion threshold of 7 g, rather than 9 g, was associated with at least equivalent outcomes in critically ill patients who did not have acute myocardial infarction (MI) or unstable angina.[3-5] Neither of these studies identified cohorts of patients who had undergone cardiac surgery. Wu et al[5] found transfusion for a hematocrit of 30% or lower in elderly patients with acute MI was associated with better outcome. This study supports the concept that this is the desirable hematocrit, especially in elderly cardiac surgery patients or those experiencing a complicated course.

Hypoxemia from any cause reduces Do_2, and acceptable arterial oxygenation (Pao_2) may be achieved with the use of an increased inspired oxygen concentration (Fio_2) or positive end-expiratory pressure (PEEP) in the ventilated patient. Use of PEEP or continuous positive airway pressure in the spontaneously breathing patient may improve Pao_2 by reducing intrapulmonary shunt; however, venous return may be reduced, causing a decrease in CO, with DO_2 decreased despite an increased Pao_2 (Figure 34-2).[6] It is important to measure CO as PEEP is applied. Intravascular volume expansion may be used to offset this damaging effect of PEEP[7] (see Chapter 35).

In patients with marginal arterial oxygenation, pulmonary function must be monitored closely to allow prompt therapy to be undertaken for abnormalities. Measurements of airway resistance and respiratory system compliance should be made. When resistance is increased, treatment of bronchospasm may improve the Pao_2 and CO, because decreases in intrathoracic pressure improve venous return. Treatment of lung overinflation may decrease pulmonary vascular resistance (PVR), benefiting right ventricular (RV) function.[8] If compliance is decreased, application of PEEP or continuous positive airway pressure may help promote re-expansion of atelectatic areas and move the tidal volume to a more compliant section of the pressure-volume relation of the respiratory system[9] (Figure 34-3). This will reduce the work expended by the patient during spontaneous efforts and may reduce PVR[10] (see Chapter 35).

Unexplained hypoxemia may be caused by right-to-left intracardiac shunting, most commonly by a patent foramen ovale. This is most likely to occur when right-sided pressures are abnormally increased; an example is the use of high levels of PEEP.[11] If suspected, echocardiography should be performed, and therapy to reduce right-sided pressures should be initiated.

Patients with pulmonary disease may experience dramatic worsening of oxygenation when vasodilator therapy is started because of release of hypoxic pulmonary vasoconstriction in areas of diseased lung.[12] Although CO may be increased, the worsening in Cao_2 will result in a decrease in Do_2. Reduced dosage of direct-acting vasodilators or trials of different agents may be indicated.

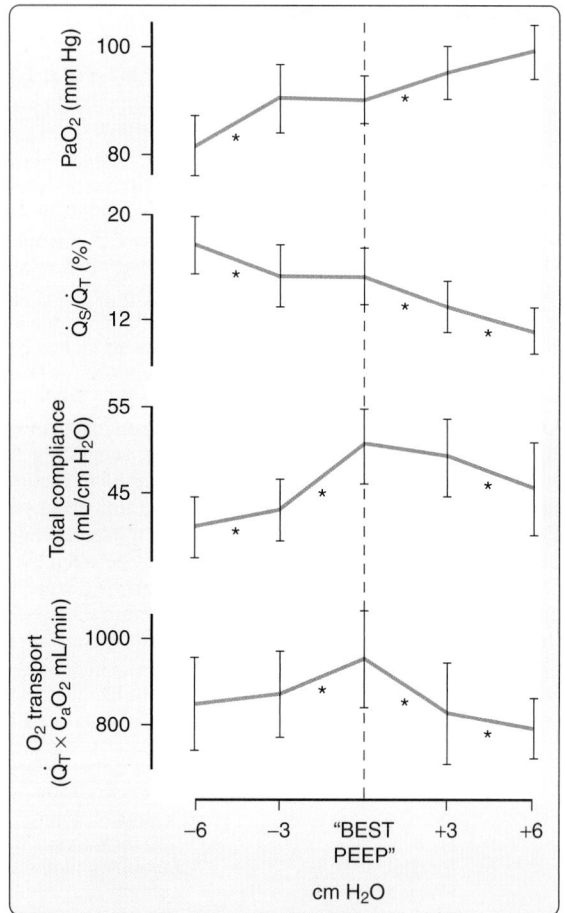

Figure 34-2 Mean values ± standard error of the mean of arterial oxygen tension (Pao_2), intrapulmonary shunt (Q_S/Q_T), total static compliance, and oxygen transport, measured at the level of positive end-expiratory pressure (PEEP), resulting in maximum oxygen transport ("best PEEP") compared with values obtained at 3 and 6 cm H_2O of PEEP above and below that level in 15 patients with acute respiratory failure. *$P < 5.005$ versus the value at best PEEP. (*From Suter PM, Fairley HB, Isenberg MD: Optimum end-expiratory pressure in patients with acute pulmonary failure. N Engl J Med 292:284, 1975.*)

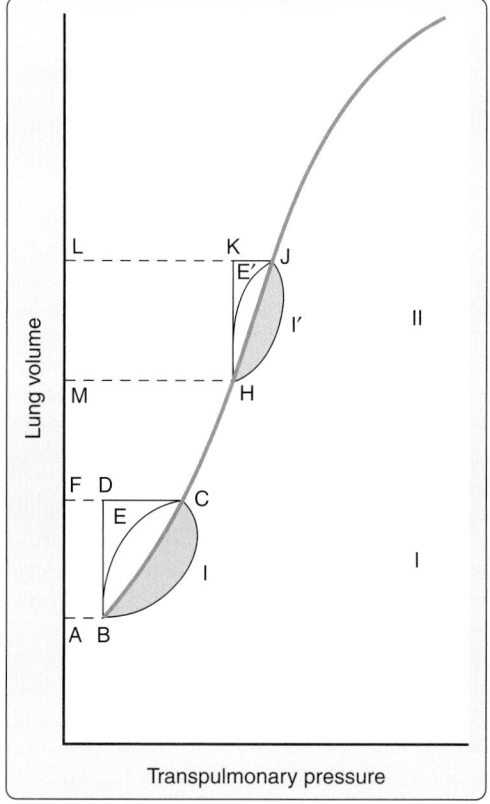

Figure 34-3 Pressure-volume diagram of elastic and resistive (nonelastic) work done on noncompliant lungs. Breathing at ambient airway pressure and low lung volume (by T tube) (I) versus breathing with continuous positive airway pressure (CPAP) at increased lung volume (II). *Solid line* BCHJ is the elastic pressure-volume curve for the lung, determined by measuring transpulmonary pressures at the instant of zero flow. *Hatched areas* represent nonelastic work (BIC and HI'J), whereas elastic work is represented by BCD and HJK. With CPAP, both types of work are reduced. Without CPAP, the area ABDF is additional elastic work partly done by the patient and partly by elastic recoil of the chest wall, whereas with CPAP, the additional work represented by MHKL is mostly done by the CPAP system. (*From Katz JA, Marks JD: Inspiratory work with and without continuous positive airway pressure in patients with acute respiratory failure. Anesthesiology 63:598, 1985.*)

When Do_2 cannot be increased to an acceptable level as judged by decreased organ function or development of lactic acidemia, measures to decrease oxygen consumption ($\dot{V}o_2$) may be taken while awaiting improvement in cardiac or pulmonary function. For example, sedation and paralysis may buy time to allow reversible postoperative myocardial dysfunction to improve.

TEMPERATURE

Patients often *are* admitted to the intensive care unit (ICU) after cardiac surgery with core temperatures less than 35° C, especially after off-pump cardiac surgery. The typical pattern of temperature change during and after cardiac surgery and the hemodynamic outcomes are illustrated in Figure 34-4. Decreases in temperature after CPB occur, in part, because of redistribution of heat within the body and because of heat loss. Noback and Tinker[13] found that administration of nitroprusside and the use of high flows (> 2.2 L/min/m²) during rewarming on CPB could improve the uniformity of rewarming and reduce this afterdrop from 4° C to about 2° C. Monitoring of body sites other than the blood and brain (e.g., urinary bladder, tympanic membrane temperatures) can help provide more complete rewarming, but the body temperature usually declines after bypass, especially when difficulties are encountered and the chest remains open for an extended period, and some degree of hypothermia is an almost unavoidable result.[14,15] Intraoperative use of newer forced air warming blankets or cutaneous gel pads[16] can help reduce the temperature loss during and after surgery.

The normal thermoregulatory and metabolic responses to hypothermia remain intact after cardiac surgery, resulting in peripheral vasoconstriction that contributes to the hypertension commonly seen early in the ICU.[17] As temperature decreases, CO is decreased because of bradycardia, whereas oxygen consumed per beat is actually increased.[18] Coagulation, platelet, and immune functions are impaired by hypothermia to potentiate postoperative bleeding and infection.[19–21] Other adverse consequences of postoperative hypothermia

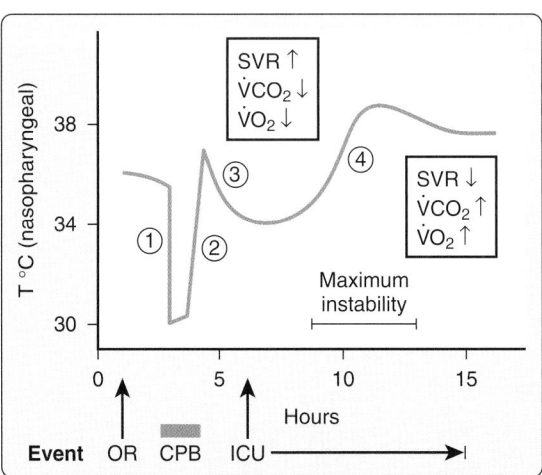

Figure 34-4 **Nasopharyngeal temperature during and after cardiac surgery.** *(1)* Core (i.e., blood) cooling on cardiopulmonary bypass (CPB). *(2)* Core warming on CPB. *(3)* Afterdrop in temperature (T) after separation from CPB. *(4)* Rewarming after admission to the intensive care unit (ICU). Systemic vascular resistance (SVR) is increased, and carbon dioxide production ($\dot{V}co_2$) and oxygen consumption ($\dot{V}o_2$) are decreased on admission to the ICU because of residual hypothermia. During rapid rewarming, SVR decreases and $\dot{V}co_2$ and $\dot{V}o_2$ increase, which can cause marked cardiac and ventilatory instability. OR, operating room. *(From Sladen RN: Management of the adult cardiac patient in the intensive care unit. In Ream AK, Fogdall RP [eds]: Acute Cardiovascular Management: Anesthesia and Intensive Care. Philadelphia, JB Lippincott, 1982, p 495.)*

are large increases in $\dot{V}o_2$ and CO_2 production during rewarming.[22] When patients cannot increase CO (i.e., O_2 delivery), the effects of this large increase in $\dot{V}o_2$ include mixed venous desaturation and metabolic acidosis. Unless end-tidal carbon dioxide is monitored or arterial blood gases are analyzed often to show the increased CO_2 production and guide increases in ventilation, hypercarbia will occur, causing catecholamine release, tachycardia, and pulmonary hypertension.[23] These effects of rewarming are most intense when patients shiver.[24] Shivering may be treated effectively with meperidine, which lowers the threshold for shivering. Muscle relaxation may provide more stable hemodynamics than meperidine but needs accompanying sedation to avoid having an awake and paralyzed patient.[25,26]

As the temperature increases, usually to about 36° C, the vasoconstriction and hypertension are replaced by vasodilation, tachycardia, and hypotension, even without hypercarbia. Often, over minutes, a patient who needs vasodilators for hypertension transforms into one requiring vasopressors or large volumes of fluid for hypotension. Volume loading during the rewarming period can help to reduce the rapid swings in blood pressure (BP) that may occur. It is important to recognize when these changes result from changes in body temperature to avoid attributing them to other processes that may call for different therapy.

ASSESSMENT OF THE CIRCULATION
Physical Examination

Surgical dressings, chest tubes attached to suction, fluid in the mediastinum and pleural spaces, peripheral edema, and temperature gradients can distort or mask information obtained by the classic techniques of inspection, palpation, and auscultation in the postoperative period. However, the physician should not be deterred from applying these basic techniques in view of the potential benefit. Physical examination may be of great value in diagnosing gross or acute pathology, such as pneumothorax, hemothorax, or acute valvular insufficiency, but it is of limited value in diagnosing and managing ventricular failure. For example, in the critical care setting, experienced clinicians (e.g., internists) using only physical findings often misjudge cardiac filling pressures by a large margin.[27] Low CO, in particular, is not consistently recognized by clinical signs, and systemic BP does not correlate with CO after cardiac surgery. Oliguria and metabolic acidosis, classic indicators of a low CO, are not always reliable because of the polyuria induced by hypothermia, oxygen debts induced during CPB causing acidosis, and medications or fluids given during or immediately after bypass.[28]

Although clinicians are taught that the adequacy of CO can be assessed by the quality of the pulses, capillary refill, and peripheral temperature, there is no relationship between these indicators of peripheral perfusion and CO or calculated systemic vascular resistance (SVR) in the postoperative period.[29] By the first postoperative day, there is a crude correlation between peripheral temperature and cardiac index (CI; $r = -0.60$). Many patients arrive in the ICU in a hypothermic state, and residual anesthetic agents can decrease the threshold for peripheral vasoconstriction in response to this condition.[30] A patient's extremities may therefore remain warm despite a hypothermic core or a decreasing CO. Even after temperature stabilization on the first postoperative day, the relation between peripheral perfusion and CO is too crude to be used for hemodynamic management.

Invasive Monitoring

Concepts regarding invasive monitoring with a pulmonary artery catheter (PAC) have been revolutionized in the past decade because of several studies in a variety of settings that fail to show a benefit from its use. In addition, there is a poor relation between filling pressures and end-diastolic volume, stroke volume (SV), or volume responsiveness. A recent review of patients admitted to medical ICUs in the United States demonstrated a reduction of more than 40% in PAC use in the 10 years before 2004.[31] The same trend was evident in surgical patients, including those undergoing cardiac surgery. The PAC rarely is used in cardiac surgery patients in many other countries. Greater availability of high-quality bedside echocardiography, often performed by intensivists, has made this modality a technique of choice in the postoperative period. Measures of volume responsiveness in mechanically ventilated patients, such as pulse pressure or SV variability (from arterial waveform analysis devices), are widely recognized as more sensitive and specific indicators of the need for intravascular volume expansion than filling pressures.[32]

Despite the lack of a proven benefit with PAC use, many patients in North America continue to have this monitor placed for cardiac surgery. Cardiac anesthesiologists believe the lack of evidence about the PAC may reflect the lack of a well-designed randomized trial. There are no such trials in cardiac surgery patients, probably attesting to the reluctance of cardiac surgeons and anesthesiologists to manage their patients without what they consider to be important information. After surgery, many cardiac surgical centers do not have in-house physicians, and surgeons believe the "objective" PAC data obtained over telephone are valuable. As less invasive tools such as echocardiography or arterial waveform analysis devices become better known and available, it seems likely that PAC use will diminish in cardiac surgery patients.

Specialized PACs have been developed that permit continuous mixed venous oxygen saturation ($S\dot{V}o_2$) monitoring, continuous CO measurement, calculation of RV volumes and ejection fraction, or have either imbedded electrodes or channels to pass atrial or ventricular pacing wires. The ability to pace through a PAC is particularly valuable in patients undergoing "minimally invasive" procedures in which the surgeon does not have adequate access to the heart to place epicardial leads. The Svo_2 catheter helps evaluate the adequacy of Do_2 and allows continuous assessment of the response to therapy, which may affect Do_2 or $\dot{V}o_2$ (e.g., PEEP therapy). The trend in the Svo_2 may function as an early warning signal of worsening in the oxygen supply/demand relation as Do_2 declines or VO_2 increases. In the postoperative period, the Svo_2 does not correlate with CO because the latter is only one of the factors in the oxygen supply/demand relation.[33] On the continuous CO catheter, a wire coil warms the blood, passing by it at time intervals determined by an algorithm, and the measured changes in temperature at the tip of the catheter are used to provide a continuous display of the CO. Although the CO displayed needs gathering of information over several minutes and is therefore not as quick as conventional thermodilution, and it does not provide beat-to-beat SV, it avoids having to give injected volumes to the patient (which can add up to a significant amount every 24 hours) and provides trends that may give earlier warning than intermittent injections. The "volumetric" PAC-computer system (REF-1; Edwards Lifesciences, Irvine, CA) uses a high-sensitivity thermistor to permit calculation of accurate right-sided volumes[34] (see Chapter 14).

Echocardiography

Echocardiography is the technique of choice for acute assessment of cardiac function. Just as transesophageal echocardiography (TEE) has become essential for intraoperative management in various conditions, several studies document its utility in the postoperative period in the presence and absence of the PAC.[35–38] It provides information that may lead to urgent surgery or prevent unnecessary surgery, gives important information about cardiac preload, and can detect acute structural and functional abnormalities. Although transthoracic echocardiography can be performed more rapidly in this setting, satisfactory images can be obtained only in about 50% of patients in the ICU[39] (see Chapters 11 to 14).

POSTOPERATIVE MYOCARDIAL DYSFUNCTION

Studies using hemodynamic, nuclear scanning, and metabolic techniques have documented worsening in cardiac function after coronary artery bypass grafting (CABG) surgery.[40–53] Although improvements in myocardial protection, surgical techniques, and operative care

have been reported, similar incidences of early biventricular dysfunction (90%) were reported between 1979 and 1990. All of these studies showed significant declines in left ventricular (LV) or biventricular (when measured) function in the first postoperative hours, with gradual return to preoperative values by 8 to 24 hours. In one study, this decline was evident in only half the patients[44]; but in the other studies, more than 90% of patients showed at least a transient decrease in function. Decreased ventricular performance at normal or increased filling pressures occurs, suggesting decreased contractility. Similarly, "flattening" of the ventricular function curves is usually obvious, suggesting that preload expansion much greater than 10 mm Hg for CVP or 12 mm Hg for pulmonary capillary wedge pressure is of little benefit. In the classic study by Mangano,[45] patients with an LV ejection fraction of less than 0.45 or ventricular dyssynergy showed more marked and prolonged dysfunction than did those patients with normal ventricles.

Satisfactory myocardial protection is important to prevent postoperative dysfunction. In off-pump surgery, the idea is to preserve coronary perfusion; but during mechanical manipulation, changes in CO and BP can occur. For CABG with CPB, most surgeons use some combination of hypothermia and crystalloid or blood cardioplegia to arrest the heart and reduce its metabolism. Although there is little consensus that any one technique is preferable in all circumstances, cold intermittent crystalloid cardioplegia with systemic hypothermia is the most widely used technique clinically and in the reported studies. Salerno et al[54] recommended continuous, warm, retrograde blood cardioplegia without systemic hypothermia. Mullen et al[50] suggested that blood cardioplegia had at least short-term benefit with less myocardial damage and better function; however, other studies of blood cardioplegia have showed mixed results[47–52] (see Chapters 28 and 29).

Other proposed factors that contribute to postoperative ventricular dysfunction include myocardial ischemia,[55] residual hypothermia,[46,47] preoperative medications such as β-adrenergic antagonists,[53] and ischemia/reperfusion injury (Box 34-1). Inflammatory cell activation from cytokine generation, upregulation of neutrophil adhesion molecules with neutrophil activation, oxygen free radical formation, and lipoperoxidation after ischemia/reperfusion injury may be important pathways accounting for the dysfunction. Multiple studies have showed the importance of limiting myocardial ischemia/reperfusion injury.[56,57] Breisblatt et al[40] observed the timing of ventricular dysfunction, and recovery after CPB for CABG was similar to what had been suggested in animal models of reperfusion injury.[58–60] This nadir at 4 hours corresponds to the peak in cytokine levels. Cytokines can release nitric oxide from endothelium, which produces myocardial depression. Data evaluating complement inhibition with pexelizumab in improving outcomes represent a novel strategy[61] (see Chapter 8).

POSTOPERATIVE MYOCARDIAL ISCHEMIA

Although intraoperative myocardial ischemia has been a focus, studies have shown that ischemia often occurs after surgery and is associated with adverse cardiac outcomes. Leung et al[55] found the electrocardiographic

BOX 34-1. RISK FACTORS FOR LOW CARDIAC OUTPUT SYNDROME AFTER CARDIOPULMONARY BYPASS

- Preoperative left ventricular dysfunction
- Valvular heart disease requiring repair or replacement
- Long aortic cross-clamp time and total cardiopulmonary bypass time
- Inadequate cardiac surgical repair
- Myocardial ischemia and reperfusion
- Residual effects of cardioplegia solution
- Poor myocardial preservation
- Reperfusion injury and inflammatory changes

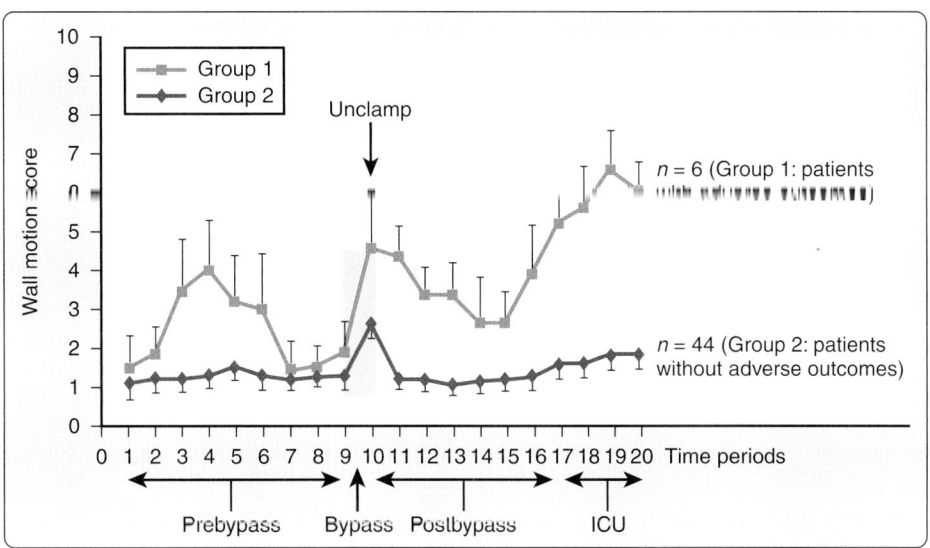

Figure 34-5 Sequential changes in wall motion score, as measured by transesophageal echocardiography, in patients undergoing elective coronary artery bypass grafting. Score is defined as follows: 0 = normal; 1 = mild hypokinesis; 2 = severe hypokinesis with myocardial thickening; 3 = akinesis; and 4 = dyskinesis. Adverse outcomes were myocardial infarction, death, or congestive heart failure. The time periods were as follows: 1 = after tracheal intubation; 2 = before incision; 3 = after incision; 4 = before sternotomy; 5 = after sternotomy; 6 and 7 = internal mammary dissection; 8 = after pericardiotomy; 9 = immediately before bypass; 10 = unclamping of aortic side-clamp; 11 to 14 = off bypass; 15 = after chest closure; 16 = skin closure; 17 to 20 = intensive care unit (ICU) for the first 4 hours. *Shaded area* indicates the bypass period. *(From Leung JM, O'Kelly B, Browner WS, et al: Prognostic importance of postbypass regional wall motion abnormalities in patients undergoing coronary artery bypass graft surgery. Anesthesiology 71:16, 1989.)*

(ECG) and segmental wall motion abnormality evidence of ischemia early after surgery in up to 40% of patients undergoing CABG surgery. Postbypass segmental wall motion abnormalities were significantly associated with adverse outcomes (e.g., MI, death; Figure 34-5). Surprisingly, these abnormalities most often appeared in the regions of the heart that had been revascularized. Hemodynamic changes rarely preceded ischemia; however, postoperative heart rates (HRs) were, as reported in other studies, significantly greater than intraoperative or preoperative values. Jain et al[62] found major ECG changes in the 8 hours after cross-clamp release in 58% of CABG patients, and these changes were independent predictors of perioperative MI. Whether such changes occur because of surgery-reperfusion or events after CPB is not known. These findings do suggest that monitoring for ischemia must continue after revascularization. It may be that early recognition and treatment of ischemia or prophylactic medication can help prevent or reduce myocardial ischemia and dysfunction occurring after CABG surgery (see Chapters 6, 10, 12, 15, and 18).

Early recovery, or fast-tracking, of the cardiac surgical patient has led to some concern that ischemia will occur as patients awaken early after surgery in pain, especially because Mangano et al[63] showed that sedation with a sufentanil infusion could reduce ischemia in this period. A randomized study by Cheng et al[64] dispelled this concern because awakening and extubation within 6 hours of CABG were not associated with more CK-MB (isoenzyme of creatine kinase with muscle and brain subunits) release or ECG changes than overnight ventilation. Wahr et al[65] showed that even with the use of propofol sedation, hemodynamic episodes (significant changes in HR and BP) were common in the 12 hours after surgery, and ST-segment changes occurred in 12% to 13% of patients.

THERAPEUTIC INTERVENTIONS

Therapeutic interventions for postoperative biventricular dysfunction include the standard concerns of managing low CO states by controlling the HR and rhythm, providing an acceptable preload, and adjusting afterload and contractility. In most patients, pharmacologic interventions can be rapidly weaned or stopped within the first 24 hours after surgery.

Postoperative Arrhythmias

Patients with preoperative or newly acquired noncompliant ventricles need a correctly timed atrial contraction to provide satisfactory ventricular filling, especially when they are in sinus rhythm before surgery (see Chapters 4, 5, 10, 19, and 25). Although atrial contraction provides around 15% to 20% of ventricular filling, this may be more important in postoperative patients, when ventricular dysfunction and reduced compliance may be present. For example, in medical patients with acute MI, atrial systole contributed 35% of the SV.[66] The SV is relatively fixed in patients with ventricular dysfunction, and the HR is an important determinant of CO. Rate and rhythm disorders need to be corrected when possible, using epicardial pacing wires. Approaches to postoperative rate and rhythm disturbances are listed in Table 34-1. The use of a PAC with atrial or ventricular pacing electrodes or use of lumens for pacing wires can facilitate temporary pacing if epicardial wires are not functioning. Failing that, temporary transvenous pacing wires can be placed (see Chapter 25).

Later in the postoperative period (days 1 through 3), supraventricular tachyarrhythmias become a major problem, with atrial fibrillation (AF) predominating. The overall incidence rate is between 30% and 40%, but with increasing age and valvular surgery, the incidence rate may be in excess of 60%.[67] There are many reasons for this, including genetic factors, inadequate atrial protection during surgery, electrolyte abnormalities, change in atrial size with fluid shifts, epicardial inflammation, stress, and irritation.[68] Randomized trials of off-pump coronary artery bypass have found a similar incidence of postoperative AF compared with on-pump CABG.[69,70]

Advanced age, a history of AF, and valvular heart surgery are the most consistently identified risk factors for AF.[68] Because AF is difficult to treat and potentially increases duration and cost of hospitalization, there is a great interest in effective therapy and prophylaxis.[67] Many studies have showed that β-blockade significantly reduces the incidence of postoperative AF and that withdrawal of β-blockers in patients receiving them before surgery is an important risk factor. Guidelines published by the American Heart Association, American College of Cardiology, and North American Society of Pacing and Electrophysiology recommend administration of β-blockers to prevent postoperative AF if there are no contraindications.[71] Sotalol, which also

TABLE 34-1	Postoperative Rate and Rhythm Disturbances	
Disturbance	**Usual Causes**	**Treatments**
Sinus bradycardia	Preoperative/ intraoperative β-blockade	Atrial pacing β-Agonist Anticholinergic
Heart block (first, second, and third degree)	Ischemia Surgical trauma	Atrioventricular sequential pacing Catecholamines
Sinus tachycardia	Agitation/pain Hypovolemia Catecholamines	Sedation/analgesia Volume administration Change or stop drug
Atrial tachyarrhythmias	Catecholamines Chamber distention Electrolyte disorder (hypokalemia, hypomagnesemia)	Change or stop drug Treat underlying cause (e.g., vasodilator, give K^+/Mg^{2+}) May require synchronized cardioversion or pharmacotherapy
Ventricular tachycardia or fibrillation	Ischemia Catecholamines	Cardioversion Treat ischemia, may require pharmacotherapy Change or stop drug

has some class III actions, is also effective[72] and is currently available in the intravenous form in North America (see Chapters 4 and 10).

Several studies have examined the use of amiodarone for prophylaxis or treatment and report both oral and intravenous amiodarone. Intravenous amiodarone is most often used in clinical practice because "acute" loading with oral therapy often is not feasible. Two pivotal studies of amiodarone deserve mention.

In the PAPABEAR study, oral amiodarone (10 mg/kg daily) or placebo was given 6 days before surgery through 6 days after surgery (13 days).[73] Atrial tachyarrhythmias occurred in fewer amiodarone patients (48/299; 16.1%) than in placebo patients (89/302; 29.5%) overall, in patients younger than 65 years (19 [11.2%] vs. 36 [21.1%], in patients older than 65 years (28 [21.7%] vs. 54 [41.2%]), in patients who had CABG surgery only (22 [11.3%] vs. 46 [23.6%]), in patients who had valve replacement/repair surgery (25 [23.8%] vs. 44 [44.1%]), in patients who received preoperative β-blocker therapy (27 [15.3%] vs. 42 [25.0%]), and in patients who did not receive preoperative β-blocker therapy (20 [16.3%] vs. 48 [35.8%]), respectively. Postoperative sustained ventricular tachyarrhythmias occurred less frequently in amiodarone patients (1/299; 0.3%) than in placebo patients (8/302; 2.6%) ($P = 0.04$).[73]

In another study, Guarnieri et al[74] evaluated 300 patients randomized in a double-blind fashion to intravenous amiodarone (1 g/day for 2 days) or to placebo immediately after cardiac surgery. The primary end points of the trial were incidence of AF and length of hospital stay. AF occurred in 67 (47%) of 142 patients on placebo versus 56 (35%) of 158 on amiodarone ($P = 0.01$). Length of hospital stay for the placebo group was 8.2 ± 6.2 days, and 7.6 ± 5.9 days for the amiodarone group.

After AF or other supraventricular arrhythmias develop, treatment often is urgently needed for symptomatic relief or hemodynamic benefit. The longer a patient remains in AF, the more difficult it may be to convert, and the greater the risk for thrombus formation and embolization.[68,72] Treatable underlying conditions such as electrolyte disturbances or pain should be corrected while specific pharmacologic therapy is being instituted. Paroxysmal supraventricular tachycardia (uncommon in this setting) can be abolished or converted by intravenous adenosine, and atrial flutter can sometimes be converted by overdrive atrial pacing by temporary wires placed at the time of surgery. Electrical cardioversion may be necessary if hypotension is caused by the rapid rate; however, atrial arrhythmias recur in this setting.[67] Rate control for AF or flutter can be achieved with various atrioventricular

nodal blocking drugs, and conversion is facilitated by many of these drugs as well. Table 34-2 summarizes the various treatment modalities for supraventricular arrhythmias. If conversion to sinus rhythm does not occur, electrical cardioversion in the presence of antiarrhythmic drug therapy should be attempted or anticoagulation with warfarin started (see Chapters 4, 10, and 25).

In summary, AF is a frequent complication of cardiac surgery, but the incidence can be significantly reduced with suitable prophylactic therapy. β-Adrenergic blockers should be administered to patients without contraindication, and prophylactic amiodarone can be considered for patients at high risk for postoperative AF. Patients who are poor candidates for β-blockade may not tolerate sotalol, whereas amiodarone does not have this limitation. More studies need to be performed to better assess the role of prophylactic therapy in off-pump cardiac surgery. After AF occurs, there is a high incidence of recurrence, so treatment with specific continuing pharmacologic therapy is usually necessary.

Preload

The Frank-Starling law states that myocardial work increases as the resting length of the myocardial fiber increases.[75] In vivo, this implies that SV will increase with increasing end-diastolic volume, although there is a limit at which SV reaches a plateau (and possibly decreases), with further increases in end-diastolic volume caused by excessive muscle stretch. In the normal myocardium, the Frank-Starling mechanism is the most important mechanism for increasing CO, and hypovolemia is a common cause of decreased CO and hypotension in the perioperative period. Assessment of preload is probably the single most important clinical skill for managing hemodynamic instability. Preload rapidly changes in the postoperative period because of bleeding, spontaneous diuresis, vasodilation during warming, the effects of positive-pressure ventilation and PEEP on venous return, capillary leak, and other causes.

Direct assessment of preload is clinically feasible using echocardiography. Several studies have demonstrated a fair-to-good correlation between echocardiographic and radionuclide measures of end-diastolic volume, and there is a good correlation between end-diastolic area by TEE and SV.[76-79] Although the use of echocardiography to assess preload must always be tempered by the realization the clinician is viewing a two-dimensional image of a three-dimensional object, this is the most direct technique clinically available. Increased awareness of the value of TEE in the ICU and increased availability of echocardiography in general have made this modality a first choice in acute assessment of preload in the setting of unexplained or refractory hypotension. Without echocardiography, pressure measurements are used as surrogates for volume measurements. For example, in the absence of mitral valve disease, left atrial pressure is almost equal to LV end-diastolic pressure, and pulmonary artery occlusion pressure (PAOP) is almost equivalent to these two pressures. In patients without left atrial pressure catheters, the PAOP or, when shown to be equivalent to this latter number, the pulmonary artery diastolic (PA_d) pressure is used (see Chapters 5 and 14).

The use of PAOP as a measure of preload may be misleading in various settings, including after cardiac surgery, when changes in pressure may not accurately reflect changes in ventricular end-diastolic volume. Studies by Ellis et al[80] and Calvin et al[81] suggest that fluid therapy in postoperative patients could cause a large increase in LV end-diastolic volume, with minimal or no change in PAOP. Mangano et al[45,82] reported that fluid loading after CPB can uncover LV dysfunction and have also shown there is little benefit to be derived from exceeding a PAOP of about 12 mm Hg. Whether this is secondary to an open pericardium, which allows overdistention of the left ventricle, the use of PEEP causing RV distention, or other factors is unclear. Breisblatt et al[83] evaluated changes in ventricular pressure-volume relations after CABG surgery while keeping a low-to-normal PAOP (10 to 15 mm Hg). The increase seen in LV end-diastolic volume was not

TABLE 34-2	Treatment Modalities for Supraventricular Arrhythmias	
Treatment	**Specifics***	**Indications**
Overdrive pacing by atrial wires[†]	Requires rapid pacer (up to 800/min); start above arrhythmia rate and slowly decrease	PAT, atrial flutter
Adenosine	Bolus dose of 6–12 mg; may cause 10 seconds of complete heart block	AV nodal tachycardia Bypass-tract arrhythmia Atrial arrhythmia diagnosis
Amiodarone	150 mg IV over 10 minutes, followed by infusion	Rate control/conversion to NSR in atrial fibrillation/flutter
β-Blockade	Esmolol, up to 0.5 mg/kg load over 1 minute, followed by infusion if tolerated	Rate control/conversion to NSR in atrial fibrillation/flutter
	Metoprolol, 0.5–5 mg, repeat effective dose q4-6h	Rate control/conversion to NSR in atrial fibrillation/flutter
	Propranolol, 0.25–1 mg; repeat effective dose q4h[‡]	
	Labetalol, 2.5–10 mg; repeat effective dose q4hr[‡]	Conversion of atrial fibrillation/flutter to NSR
	Sotalol, 40–80 mg PO q12h	Conversion of PAT to NSR
Ibutilide	1 mg over 10 minutes; may repeat after 10 minutes	Rate control/conversion to NSR in atrial fibrillation/flutter
Verapamil	2.5–5 mg IV, repeated PRN[‡]	
Diltiazem	0.2 mg/kg over 2 minutes, followed by 10–15 mg/hr[§]	Rate control/conversion to NSR in atrial fibrillation/flutter
Procainamide	50 mg/min up to 1 g, followed by 1–4 mg/min	Rate control/conversion to NSR in atrial fibrillation/flutter Prevention of recurrence of arrhythmias Treatment of wide-complex tachycardias[¶¶]
Digoxin[¶]	Load of 1 mg in divided doses over 4–24 hours**; may give additional 0.125-mg doses 2 hours apart (3–4 doses)	Rate control/conversion to NSR in atrial fibrillation/flutter
Synchronized cardioversion	50–300 J (external); most effective with anteroposterior patches	Acute tachyarrhythmia with hemodynamic compromise (usually atrial fibrillation or flutter)

*See specific drug monographs for full description of indications, contraindications, and dosage. Doses are for intravenous administration; use lowest dose and administer slowly in patients with hemodynamic compromise.
[†]Verify pacer is not capturing ventricle.
[‡]Infusion may provide better control. This drug is less useful than diltiazem because of myocardial depression.
[§]Limited experience; may cause less hypotension than verapamil.
[¶¶]When diagnosis is unclear (ventricular vs. supraventricular) and there is no acute hemodynamic compromise (i.e., cardioversion not indicated).
[¶]Rate of administration depending on urgency of rate control.
**Less useful than other drugs because of slow onset and modest effect.
AV, atrioventricular; IV, intravenously; NSR, normal sinus rhythm; PAT, paroxysmal atrial tachycardia; PO, orally; PRN, as needed; SVT, supraventricular tachycardia.

significant enough to explain the degree of ventricular dysfunction they noted. Bouchard et al[84] compared ventricular performance assessments from the PAC (i.e., LV stroke work index) with fractional area change and regional wall motion score index from TEE in 60 patients during and after cardiac surgery. They found no correlation between LV stroke work index and fractional area change and postulated that changes in ventricular compliance, loading conditions, and ventricular function alter the pressure-volume relation of the left ventricle in a manner that leads to discordant interpretations between the two techniques.

When ventricular compliance is normal and the ventricle is not distended, small changes in end-diastolic volume are usually accompanied by small changes in end-diastolic pressure. In patients with noncompliant ventricles from preexisting congestive heart failure (HF), chronic hypertrophy resulting from hypertension or valvular disease, postoperative MI, or ventricular dysfunction, small increases in ventricular volume may produce rapid increases in end-diastolic pressure, requiring therapeutic intervention.[83–89] Increased intraventricular pressure will increase myocardial oxygen demand ($M\dot{V}o_2$) and decrease subendocardial coronary blood flow.[90] Myocardial ischemia may be the result. Increases in LV end-diastolic pressure are transmitted to the pulmonary circulation, causing congestion and, possibly, hydrostatic pulmonary edema. Although PAOP or left atrial pressure may not always show true preload, there are still good reasons to monitor them. The periods when patients are at particular risk for increases in end-diastolic pressure include awakening, endotracheal suctioning, and rapid-volume resuscitation. If myocardial ischemia or acute HF occurs, sudden increases in the end-diastolic pressure may result.

Many drugs may be used to reduce cardiac preload. Direct-acting vasodilators, especially nitroglycerin, increase venous capacitance, decreasing end-diastolic volume and pressure.[89–91] Intravenous furosemide, besides its diuretic effect, increases venous capacitance.[92]

Diuretics are important to help remove the fluid that is mobilized in the days after surgery. In patients who may not tolerate the acute volume loss that is induced by the loop diuretics, a furosemide infusion allows a more gradual diuresis. Such infusions have been shown to be effective in patients with renal dysfunction.[93,94] In a patient who appears refractory to diuresis, it is important to evaluate the circulatory state. Such refractoriness may suggest that a renal insult has been suffered, but it may also suggest underperfusion of the kidneys. In the latter case, the preload must be kept at the upper range of normal and CO augmented.

A new agent used in treatment of acute decompensated left-heart failure is recombinant B-type natriuretic peptide (nesiritide). The mechanism of action occurs by specific cell-surface receptors, stimulation of which increases levels of intracellular cyclic guanosine monophosphate (cGMP). The physiologic effects are mainly vasodilation, natriuresis, and renin inhibition. The result is balanced vasodilation, reducing preload and afterload, while simultaneously increasing SV and CO and promoting diuresis.[95] Nesiritide has not been studied widely in the cardiac surgery population, but it has been used anecdotally in patients with poor right ventricular function and high filling pressures, pulmonary hypertension, or RV failure.[96] A related drug, human atrial natriuretic peptide, was shown in a small, randomized trial to reduce the need for dialysis and to improve dialysis-free survival after complicated cardiac surgery.[97]

Angiotensin-converting enzyme (ACE) inhibitors also can cause venodilation and reduce preload. Alternatively, opioids or benzodiazepines, or both, used to reduce endogenous catecholamine release, should be considered in the patient who needs mechanical ventilation. Morphine causes histamine release, which directly induces venodilation. In the patient with oliguria and renal failure who is fluid overloaded, peritoneal dialysis, hemodialysis, or continuous hemofiltration or dialysis may be needed.[98,99]

Contractility

Contractility is a well-defined concept in vitro, where it can be measured by the velocity of shortening of isolated muscle strips. However, it has been more complex to quantify the contractility of the intact heart because it has been difficult to find a variable to measure contractility that is also independent of preload and afterload. The pioneering work of Suga and Sagawa[100,101] has shown that contractility can be measured by the end-systolic elastance of the ventricle, defined as

$$E_{ES} = P_{ES} / (V_{ES} - V_0)$$

in which P_{ES} is the end-systolic pressure, V_{ES} is the end-systolic volume, and V_0 is a dead-space term. E_{ES} is strictly determined by evaluating ventricular pressure-volume loops for different preloads or afterloads and by defining end-systole as the point in time at which the time-varying elastance is maximal.[102] The slope of the line connecting the points at end-systole is E_{ES}. This parameter varies with changes in inotropic state but is *nearly* independent of preload and afterload. Routine measurement of end-systolic elastance is not clinically feasible. However, consideration of the above definition underscores the utility of TEE for the qualitative evaluation of contractility in the clinical setting. A decrease in contractility is manifested as some combination of a decrease in pressure or an increase in V_{ES} (i.e., a decrease in SV). End-systolic volume can be estimated using TEE. A large V_{ES} (implying a low ejection fraction) with a low or normal BP suggests a low value for E_{ES} and poor contractility. If BP is high, a large value of V_{ES} may be seen even if contractility is normal. By interpreting end-diastolic volume, end-systolic volume, and ejection fraction in the context of BP, an assessment of contractility is possible with TEE (see Chapters 5 and 12 to 14).

An alternative measure of contractility is the preload-recruitable stroke work, which is the slope of the line relating stroke work to preload.[103] In the operating room or ICU, it often is estimated by the extent of the increase in CO that accompanies an increase in preload and is not dependent on the availability of TEE. If preload is increased by a change in patient position, BP can be a surrogate for CO because it is unlikely that SVR will change in the short time needed for the position change. A change in BP, therefore, is proportional to the change in CO.

Therapy for decreased contractility should be directed toward correcting any reversible causes, such as myocardial depressants, metabolic abnormalities, or myocardial ischemia. If the cause of depressed myocardial contractility is irreversible, positive inotropic agents may be necessary to keep a CO satisfactory to support organ function (see Chapters 5, 10, 28, and 32).

Afterload

Afterload is a concept that is well defined in vitro, where it refers to the added tension imposed on isolated muscle strips with contraction, but it is harder to define in vivo. In analogy with in vitro studies, afterload can be equated with ventricular wall stress, expressed as the product of cavity radius times transmural pressure divided by wall thickness, as described by the law of Laplace. However, many investigators find this definition unsatisfactory because it implies the heart generates its own afterload and because afterload would be viewed as changing during the cardiac cycle.[104] If afterload is viewed as the external forces opposing ejection, possibly the best definition is the aortic input impedance, the complex ratio of pressure to flow, expressed in terms of magnitude, and the phase angle between flow and pressure for any given frequency. However, it has been difficult to quantitatively analyze the impact of impedance on overall cardiac performance (see Chapter 5). Sunagawa et al[105] proposed a simplified theory of ventricular-vascular coupling within the framework of the end-systolic pressure-volume relation. Using the definition of end-systolic elastance produces the following:

$$E_{ES} = P_{ES} / (V_{ES} - V_0)$$

Equating SV with $V_E - V_{ES}$ (ignoring the difference between end-ejection and end-systole), it is a matter of algebra to show that

$$P_{ES} = E_{ES}(V_{ED} - V_0) - E_{ES} \bullet SV$$

This means that an increase in SV implies a decrease in P_{ES}. The interpretation of this from the perspective of the heart is that the work that can be done is finite, and that a greater SV can only be achieved by decreasing the end-systolic pressure, if contractility (E_{ES}) is fixed. At the same time, it is known that from the perspective of the vasculature, if the SV increases, BP increases when vascular tone does not change.

The application of an electrical law describing constant voltages and flows to the circulation, in which pulsatile flow is generated by a pump, has resulted in estimates of afterload that are questionable.[104] Although SVR is a component of impedance, it cannot be equated with it. The correct downstream pressure is probably not the CVP.[106] There is instead a critical opening pressure that should be used in calculating SVR that is not measurable in routine clinical care.[106] Clinical use of such calculated resistances is made complex by the relation of CO to body size; the normal resistance of a small patient is much higher than that of a large one. The use of a resistance index (i.e., using CI instead of CO) partly overcomes this problem, but it is not widely used.

Calculated SVR continues to be widely used in guiding therapy or drawing conclusions about the state of the circulation. This should only be done with caution, if at all. SVR is not a complete indicator of afterload. Even if SVR were an accurate measure of impedance, the response to vasoactive agents depends on the coupling of ventricular-vascular function, not on impedance alone. Hemodynamic therapy should be guided based on the primary variables, BP and CO. If preload is appropriate, low BP and low CO are treated with an inotropic drug. If BP is acceptable (and preload appropriate) but CO is low, a vasodilator alone or in combination with an inotropic drug is used. If the patient is hypertensive (with low CO), vasodilators are indicated; if the patient is vasodilated (low BP and high CO), vasoconstrictors are used (Box 34-2).

POSTOPERATIVE HYPERTENSION

Hypertension has been a common complication of cardiac surgery, reported to occur in 30% to 80% of patients from studies in the 1970s when CABG was common in patients with normal ventricular function.[107–109] The current population of older, sicker patients appears to have fewer problems with hypertension than with low-output syndromes or vasodilation. Although hypertension most commonly occurs in patients with normal preoperative ventricular function, after aortic valve replacement, or a prior history, any patient may experience development of hypertension. Multiple reasons contribute to postoperative hypertension, including preoperative hypertension, preexisting atherosclerotic vascular disease, awakening from general anesthesia, increases in endogenous catecholamines, activation of the plasma renin-angiotensin system, neural reflexes (e.g., heart, coronary arteries, great vessels), and hypothermia.[110] Arterial vasoconstriction with various degrees of intravascular hypovolemia is the hallmark of perioperative hypertension.

The hazards of untreated postoperative hypertension include depressed LV performance, increased MVo_2, cerebrovascular accidents,

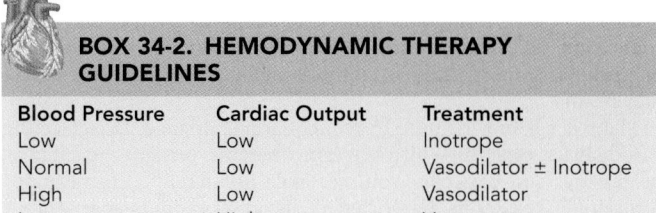

BOX 34-2. HEMODYNAMIC THERAPY GUIDELINES

Blood Pressure	Cardiac Output	Treatment
Low	Low	Inotrope
Normal	Low	Vasodilator ± Inotrope
High	Low	Vasodilator
Low	High	Vasopressor

suture line disruption, MI, rhythm disturbances, and increased bleeding.[108,111,112] Historically, therapy for hypertension in cardiac surgery was sodium nitroprusside because of its rapid onset and short duration of action.[113] With multiple vasodilators available in the current era, sodium nitroprusside is no longer the drug of choice for many reasons. Nitroprusside is a potent venodilator, increasing venous capacitance (decreasing preload) and can produce arterial vasodilation, often leading to precipitous decreases in BP and a hyperdynamic cardiac state. Sodium nitroprusside can cause coronary arteriolar dilation with the potential for a steal phenomenon, resulting in myocardial ischemia.[114] In patients with renal failure, the elimination of sodium nitroprusside is reduced, potentially leading to toxic effects of its metabolites cyanide or thiocyanate. This can occur if large doses are given to patients with normal renal function.

There are many alternative drugs to sodium nitroprusside for treating hypertension after cardiac surgery, including nitroglycerin,[115] adrenergic-blocking agents such as β-adrenergic blockers,[116] and the mixed α- and β-adrenergic blocker labetalol.[117] Direct-acting vasodilators, dihydropyridine calcium channel blockers (e.g., nicardipine,[118] isradipine,[119] clevidipine,[120-123]) ACE inhibitors,[119] and fenoldopam (a dopamine$_1$ [D$_1$] receptor agonist)[124,125] also have been used. Novel therapeutic approaches are listed in Table 34-3.

Dihydropyridine calcium channel blockers are particularly effective in cardiac surgical patients because they relax arterial resistance vessels without negative inotropic actions or effects on atrioventricular nodal conduction and are important therapeutic options. Dihydropyridines are arterial-specific vasodilators of peripheral resistance arteries, resulting in a generalized vasodilation, including the renal, cerebral, intestinal, and coronary vascular beds. In doses that effectively reduce BP, the dihydropyridines have little or no direct negative effect on cardiac contractility or conduction. Although the dihydropyridines are more vasoselective than verapamil and diltiazem, there are also differences between dihydropyridines in this respect. Nifedipine is the least vasoselective of the dihydropyridines, isradipine and clevidipine are the most selective, and nicardipine and nimodipine are intermediately selective.[120] Nicardipine is available for intravenous administration and is an important therapeutic agent to consider because of its lack of effects on vascular capacitance vessels and preload in patients after cardiac surgery.[126] The pharmacokinetic profile of nicardipine suggests that effective administration requires variable rate infusions when trying to treat hypertension because of the half-life of 40 minutes. If even more rapid control is essential, a dosing strategy consisting of a loading bolus or rapid infusion dose with a constant-rate infusion may be more efficient. The effect of nicardipine may persist even though the infusion is stopped. Clevidipine, a new ultra-short-acting dihydropyridine approved in 2008 in the United States for clinical use, has a half-life of only minutes, represents a potential alternative to sodium nitroprusside, and has been studied extensively in cardiac surgical patients.[121-123]

Fenoldopam is a short-acting dopamine agonist approved for short-term intravenous therapy that causes arterial-specific vasodilation by stimulation of D$_1$ receptors. Unlike sodium nitroprusside, D$_1$-receptor stimulation also increases renal blood flow to produce diuresis and natriuresis. Fenoldopam and sodium nitroprusside were similarly effective in reducing BP in patients who experienced development of hypertension after CABG surgery.[124] Fenoldopam often needs greater doses for severe hypertension that may be associated with increases in HR.

TABLE 34-3	Novel Vasodilators	
Drug	*Mechanism of Action*	*Half-Life*
Nicardipine	Calcium channel blocker	Intermediate
Clevidipine	Calcium channel blocker	Ultra-short
Fenoldopam	Dopamine$_1$-receptor agonist	Ultra-short
Nesiritide	Brain natriuretic agonist	Short
Levosimendan	K$^+$-ATP channel modulator	Intermediate

The ACE inhibitors are used in treating chronic hypertension and ventricular dysfunction. Enalaprilat is the intravenous preparation used for administration in the postoperative setting.[127] These drugs are indirect vasodilators that function by inhibiting angiotensin II formation and breakdown of bradykinin. Intravenous enalaprilat has an unpredictable effect and may be long acting. A suitable role is for replacing intravenous ACE inhibitors in a patient being weaned from short-acting agents or with HF.

POSTOPERATIVE VASODILATION

Vasodilation and a need for vasoconstrictor support are relatively frequent complications of cardiac surgery with and without CPB. The reported incidence rate is 4% to 44%, but this wide range largely results from lack of a common definition.[128-130] Vasodilation alone should be associated with a hyperdynamic circulatory state presenting as systemic hypotension, in association with an increased CO (and a low calculated SVR). More commonly, after cardiac surgery, a combination of vasodilation and myocardial dysfunction occurs, requiring vasoconstrictor and inotropic therapy. Gomez et al[131-133] coined the term *vasoplegia syndrome* for the condition that requires high doses of vasoconstrictors, and they reported its occurrence after off-pump and on-pump surgery.

Multiple humoral and inflammatory cascades are activated by surgery alone and by CPB, aortic cross-clamping, and reperfusion, generating complement anaphylatoxins, kinins, and cytokines, many of which cause vasodilation by direct and indirect vascular mechanisms.[134-136] Another potential cause of systemic vasodilation is splanchnic circulatory insufficiency resulting in endotoxemia, and this, too, has been noted after off-pump surgery[137,138] (see Chapter 8). The cellular mechanisms and pathogenesis of vasodilatory shock were summarized by Landry and Oliver.[135] Although the most common clinical context of vasodilatory shock is sepsis, the similarity in the cytokine response and clinical syndrome seen in sepsis with the vasodilated state seen after cardiac surgery is striking. As Landry and Oliver[135] described, the stimuli of cytokines and increased tissue lactate lead to increased nitric oxide synthase and the generation of vasodilating GMP. Nitric oxide and metabolic acidosis activate potassium channels, which hyperpolarize the cell membrane, making it refractory to calcium entry and thereby refractory to norepinephrine and angiotensin II action. At this time, plasma vasopressin levels are low because of central depletion. Reports of marked vasodilatory shock after CPB responsive to vasopressin appeared when this pathophysiology was investigated.[139] The ability of vasopressin to block the potassium channels and interfere with nitric oxide signaling makes it an important therapy for this syndrome. Provided there is an acceptable CO, vasopressin is a valuable agent for treating vasodilation after cardiac surgery, significantly reducing the dose requirement for norepinephrine. Systemic vasodilation also can result from hyperthermia caused by excessive warming during CPB (see Chapters 8, 28, and 29) and during warming in the ICU.

When patients experience development of acute systemic vasodilation after administration of drugs or blood products, an anaphylactic reaction should be considered. Acute anaphylaxis caused by immunoglobulin E (IgE)–mediated responses can present with systemic vasodilation and increased CO.[140] Alternatively, complement-mediated transfusion reactions to any blood product can present with hypotension produced by systemic vasodilation or by thromboxane-mediated acute pulmonary vasoconstriction and RV dysfunction. Antibodies in the donor blood called *leukoagglutinins,* when directed against recipient white cell antigens, can actively produce white cell aggregation and thromboxane generation. These reactions have been called *transfusion-related acute lung injury,* which can manifest with hypotension, RV failure, and noncardiogenic pulmonary edema.[140] Monitoring of RV function may, therefore, help to identify these transfusion reactions.

While underlying causes are being sought and treated, the therapeutic approach to systemic vasodilation includes intravascular volume expansion, α-adrenergic agents, and vasopressin. Administration of vasoconstrictors for more than a brief period must be guided by measures of cardiac performance because restoration of BP may camouflage a low-output state. There are no established guidelines for beginning vasoconstrictor therapy; autoregulation in vital organs is lost at mean arterial pressures (MAPs) less than 60 mm Hg, and it is reasonable to try to achieve this pressure in normotensive patients (possibly higher in hypertensive patients). A study in septic shock patients was unable to show a benefit from MAPs greater than 65 mm Hg.[141]

Clinicians often are concerned about the potential for constricting supply vessels or the microcirculation to vital beds (e.g., brain, kidney); although not fully evaluated in the postoperative setting, giving vasoconstrictors in septic states does not appear to have such harmful effects.[142] Use of relatively low doses of vasopressin to restore responsiveness to catecholamines is physiologically sensible, but there is no clear evidence to suggest that use of vasopressin besides or instead of norepinephrine is associated with better outcome. However, dopamine was recently demonstrated to increase mortality in cardiogenic shock.[143]

CORONARY ARTERY SPASM

Coronary artery or internal mammary artery vasospasm can occur after surgery. Mechanical manipulation and underlying atherosclerosis of the native coronary circulation and the internal mammary artery have the potential to produce transient endothelial dysfunction. The endothelium is responsible for releasing endothelium-derived relaxing factor, which is nitric oxide, a potent endogenous vasodilator substance that preserves normal endogenous vasodilation (see Chapters 6 and 8). Thromboxane can be liberated because of heparin-protamine interactions, CPB, platelet activation, or anaphylactic reactions to produce coronary vasoconstriction.[144,145] Calcium administration, increased α-adrenergic tone from vasoconstrictor administration (especially in bolus doses), platelet thromboxane liberation, and calcium channel blocker withdrawal represent added reasons that may put the cardiac surgical patient at risk for spasm of native coronary vessels and arterial grafts. Engelman et al[145] reported four patients who experienced development of coronary artery spasm after discontinuation of their calcium channel blockers 8 to 18 hours before surgery. In three of these patients, spasm was identified by the ECG pattern and documented as the cause of ischemia in the distribution of a nondiseased right coronary artery, with the fourth patient developing spasm in a bypassed native vessel. In two of the patients, the problem was recognized retrospectively; MIs developed, and one patient died. In the other two patients, spasm was recognized, and intravenous nitroglycerin was given (1 to 3 μg/kg/min) in combination with nifedipine, 10 mg sublingually every 5 to 6 hours, to reverse the ischemic process. The therapy of choice remains empirical. Nitroglycerin is a first-line drug, but nitrate tolerance can occur. Phosphodiesterase (PDE) inhibitors represent novel approaches to this problem and have been reported to be effective in vascular models of spasm.[146] Intravenous dihydropyridine calcium channel blockers are also important therapeutic considerations.[147]

Reports of successful use of the radial artery as a bypass conduit have rekindled interest in this vessel.[148–150] In the early days of CABG surgery, this conduit was abandoned because of its propensity to spasm. In later reports, techniques developed in the use of the internal mammary artery have been applied to the radial artery, as well as prophylactic use of diltiazem infusions.[148,150] Which components of this approach are responsible for the reported success are not known, but use of a calcium channel blocking drug is recommended by many surgeons. The arterial selectivity of the dihydropyridine drugs (e.g., nicardipine) should be an advantage in this setting. However, addition of a vasodilator drug to prevent spasm of the radial artery in a patient needing a vasopressor for systemic vasodilation makes no pharmacologic sense.

DECREASED CONTRACTILITY

Drugs that increase contractility all result in increased calcium mobilization from intracellular sites to and from the contractile proteins or sensitize these proteins to calcium. Although calcium chloride has been used to increase inotropy, evidence suggests that after CPB, its

principal action is peripheral vasoconstriction.[151] The same group of investigators has shown that exogenously administered calcium chloride attenuates the response to catecholamines in this setting.[152] The administration of calcium salts will improve myocardial performance if there is severe hypocalcemia or hyperkalemia and may be indicated during rapid transfusion of citrated blood.[153]

Catecholamines, through β_1-receptor stimulation in the myocardium, increase intracellular cyclic adenosine monophosphate (cAMP). This second messenger increases intracellular calcium, causing an improvement in myocardial contraction.[154] Inhibition of the breakdown of cAMP by PDE inhibitors increases intracellular cAMP independent of the β receptor.[155] Intracellular calcium availability can be increased by inhibiting Na^+/K^+-ATPase with digitalis glycosides, promoting transmembranous Na^+/Ca^{++} exchange. However, the use of digoxin to increase myocardial contractility for postoperative ventricular dysfunction is limited by its slow onset, low potency, and narrow therapeutic safety margin. The "calcium sensitizers" constitute a new class of inotropic agents. One drug in this class, levosimendan, is being evaluated in clinical trials (Box 34-3).

Catecholamines

The catecholamines used after surgery include dopamine, dobutamine, epinephrine, norepinephrine, and isoproterenol (Box 34-4). These drugs have various effects on α and β receptors and, therefore, various effects on HR, rhythm, and myocardial metabolism (see Chapters 10 and 32). Dosing recommendations for the catecholamines are provided in Table 34-4.

Isoproterenol

Isoproterenol is the most potent β-agonist in the heart (β_1) and in the periphery (β_2). Its positive inotropic effect is accompanied by an increase in HR and a propensity for arrhythmias. In patients with coronary artery disease, tachycardia and associated peripheral vasodilation increase $M\dot{V}O_2$ and decrease coronary perfusion pressure. In patients with bradycardias in whom pacing is not an immediate or practical option, or in those in whom an increased HR is desirable (e.g., cardiac transplant recipients, patients with regurgitant valvular lesions), isoproterenol may be used with caution bearing in mind its rather narrow therapeutic window. Although used for its β_2 effects in the pulmonary vasculature, it is a weak pulmonary vasodilator.

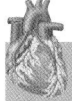

BOX 34-3. PHARMACOLOGIC APPROACHES FOR PERIOPERATIVE VENTRICULAR DYSFUNCTION

Inotropic agents
Catecholamines
Phosphodiesterase inhibitors
Levosimendan
Vasodilator therapy
Pulmonary vasodilators
Phosphodiesterase inhibitors (milrinone, sildenafil)
Inhaled nitric oxide
Prostaglandins (PGI_2, PGE_1, iloprost, and derivatives)

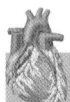

BOX 34-4. DISADVANTAGES OF CATECHOLAMINES

- Increased myocardial oxygen consumption
- Tachycardia
- Arrhythmias
- Excessive peripheral vasoconstriction
- Coronary vasoconstriction
- β-Receptor downregulation and decreased drug efficacy

TABLE 34-4	Catecholamines Used after Surgery
Drug	*Infusion Dose (μg/kg/min)*
Dopamine*†	2–10
Dobutamine‡	2–10
Epinephrine‡	0.03–0.20
Norepinephrine†	0.03–0.20
Isoproterenol‡	0.02–0.10

*Less than 2 μg/kg/min predominantly "dopaminergic" (renal and mesenteric artery dilatation).
†If 10 μg/kg/min is ineffective, change to epinephrine or norepinephrine.
‡Dose to effect; may require greater dose than indicated.

Epinephrine

Epinephrine is a potent adrenergic agonist with the desirable feature that, in low doses (< 3 μg/min), β_1- and β_2-receptor effects predominate. As the dose is increased, α effects (e.g., vasoconstriction) and tachycardia occur. However, in the acutely failing heart after surgery, only drugs such as epinephrine or norepinephrine provide adequate positive inotropy and perfusion pressure. These features and its low cost make it a common first-line drug in the postoperative setting. Despite what is often stated in older literature, epinephrine causes less tachycardia than dopamine[156] or dobutamine[157] at equivalent inotropic doses.[158] Epinephrine is a first-line therapy for anaphylaxis and, when titrated, does not produce ventricular arrhythmias. Because of the metabolic actions of β_2-receptor stimulation, epinephrine infusion can cause hyperglycemia and increased serum lactate levels.[159]

Norepinephrine

Norepinephrine, which has potent β_1- and α-receptor effects, preserves coronary perfusion pressure while not increasing HR, actions that are favorable to the ischemic, reperfused heart. When norepinephrine is used alone without a vasodilator or PDE inhibitor, the potent α_1-receptor effects may have variable effects on CO. Ventricular filling pressures usually increase when this drug is given because of constriction of the capacitance vessels. Administration of a vasodilator, including the PDE inhibitors, with norepinephrine may partially oppose the vasoconstriction. Clinicians may express concern for the renal blood flow when norepinephrine is given for hypotension; however, norepinephrine has long been used as a first-line agent for hypotension and shock in ICU settings and after cardiac surgery. Despite perceived concerns, when norepinephrine is infused to increase MAP to more than 70 mm Hg in sepsis, increased urine flow and increased creatinine clearance rate occurred after 24 hours.[160] Furthermore, its use in circulatory shock did not increase mortality.[161] End-organ ischemia would appear to be unlikely if CO can be preserved at normal levels when norepinephrine is given. PDE inhibitors in combination with norepinephrine attenuate the arterial vasoconstrictive effects.[146]

Dopamine

A precursor of norepinephrine, dopamine probably achieves its therapeutic effects by releasing myocardial norepinephrine or preventing its reuptake, especially when administered in high doses.[162] This indirect action may result in reduced effectiveness when given to patients with chronic HF or shock states because the myocardium becomes depleted of norepinephrine stores.[163] In contrast with dobutamine, the α-agonist properties of dopamine cause increases in pulmonary artery pressure (PAP), PVR, and LV filling pressure.[164-166] At low doses (< 2 μg/kg/min), dopamine stimulates renal dopaminergic receptors to increase renal perfusion more than can be explained by an increase in CO.[167] Despite this action, a multicenter study demonstrated that use of low-dose dopamine in critically ill patients confers no protection from renal dysfunction.[168] One review suggests there is no justification

for low-dose dopamine in the ICU and that it is "bad medicine."[169] At doses greater than 10 μg/kg/min, tachycardia and vasoconstriction become the predominant actions of this drug. Tachycardia is a consistent side effect, and in patients with cardiogenic shock, dopamine was recently shown to increase mortality.[142,161]

Dobutamine

In contrast with dopamine, dobutamine shows mainly β_1-agonist properties, with decreases in diastolic BP, and sometimes, decreased systemic BP being observed.[170,171] Dobutamine is functionally similar to isoproterenol, with less tendency to induce tachycardia in the postoperative setting.[172] However, Romson et al[173] demonstrated that after CPB, the principal effect of dobutamine is a dose-related increase in HR. A modest effect on SV was observed in patients with poor ventricular function. Salomon et al[174] showed that dobutamine increased Mvo_2, which was matched by an increase in coronary blood flow, whereas dopamine increased Mvo_2 but failed to increase coronary blood flow. However, the favorable actions of dobutamine may be limited if a tachycardia develops, and like dopamine, its inotropic potency is modest in comparison with that of epinephrine or norepinephrine.[174]

Phosphodiesterase Inhibitors

The PDE inhibitors are nonglycosidic, nonsympathomimetic drugs that have positive inotropic effects independent of the β_1-adrenergic receptor and unique vasodilatory actions independent of endothelial function or nitrovasodilators.[154,155] Patients with HF have downregulation of the β_1-receptor, with a decrease in receptor density and altered responses to catecholamine administration.[154,175] Milrinone, amrinone, and enoximone bypass the β_1 receptor, causing increases in intracellular cAMP by selective inhibition of PDE fraction III, a cAMP-specific PDE enzyme.[155,176] In vascular smooth muscle, these agents cause vasodilation in the arterial and capacitance beds.[177] PDE inhibitors increase CO, decrease pulmonary capillary wedge pressure, and decrease SVR and PVR in patients with biventricular dysfunction, and they are important therapeutic approaches in postoperative cardiac surgical patients. Sildenafil and other PDE5 inhibitors also are being used increasingly for pulmonary hypertension.[178] The PDE5 inhibitor sildenafil, marketed with a different name from Viagra, called Revatio, was approved for the treatment of pulmonary arterial hypertension by the U.S. Food and Drug Administration and by the European Medicines Agency in 2005[178] (see Chapters 10 and 24).

Effects on Vascular Responses

Any drug that increases cyclic nucleotides (e.g., cAMP, cGMP) in vascular smooth muscle will produce vasodilation.[176-178] The concentration of cGMP can be increased by the release of nitric oxide produced by nitroglycerin, sodium nitroprusside, and inhaled nitric oxide, and cAMP can be increased by prostaglandin E_1 (PGE_1) or PGI_2, or by inhibiting its breakdown by PDE inhibition. Increasing cAMP in vascular smooth muscle promotes calcium uptake by the sarcoplasmic reticulum, decreasing calcium available for contraction. The net effect of increasing calcium uptake is smooth muscle relaxation. This effect can also occur through stimulation by drugs that inhibit the breakdown of cGMP (e.g., nonspecific PDE inhibitor). Sildenafil and its congeners are PDE5 inhibitors that were originally developed for nitrate tolerance but are marketed for erectile dysfunction and pulmonary hypertension.[178]

PDE III inhibitors have a clinical effect as inodilators; they produce dilation of arterial and venous beds, decreasing the MAP and central filling pressures. Increases in CO are induced by multiple mechanisms, including afterload reduction and positive inotropy, but not by increasing HR.[179-189] The net effect is a decrease in myocardial wall tension, representing an important contrast with most sympathomimetic agents.[181] Catecholamine administration often needs the simultaneous administration of vasodilators to reduce ventricular wall tension.

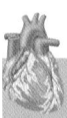

BOX 34-5. ADVANTAGES OF PREEMPTIVE PHOSPHODIESTERASE INHIBITOR ADMINISTRATION

- Increased myocardial contractility (left and right ventricles)
- Pulmonary vasodilation
- Resolution and prevention of ischemia
- Minimal drug side effects while on cardiopulmonary bypass
- Dilation of internal mammary artery
- Avoidance of mechanical intervention
- Prevention of a "failed wean"

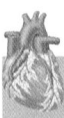

BOX 34-6. ACUTE HEART FAILURE: THERAPEUTIC GOALS AND TREATMENT SUMMARY

Goals	Treatment
Reduce impedance to ventricular ejection	Vasodilator
Reduce wall stress	Vasodilator
Reduce filling pressures	Diuretics, venodilators
Increase contractility	Inotropic agents, phosphodiesterase inhibitors

TABLE 34-5	Dosing for Phosphodiesterase Inhibitors (Cyclic Adenosine Monophosphate–Specific) Used after Surgery	
Drug	*Loading Dose**	*Infusion Rate*
Amrinone	1.5–2.0 mg/kg	5–20 µg/kg/min
Milrinone	50 µg/kg	0.375–0.75 µg/kg/min
Enoximone	0.5–1.0 mg/kg	5–10 µg/kg/min

*Loading doses should be administered over 5 to 10 minutes to avoid excessive vasodilation.

Milrinone and other PDE inhibitors also have unique mechanisms of vasodilation that may be favorable for coronary artery and internal mammary artery flow[146] (Box 34-5).

Sildenafil inhibits PDE5, an enzyme that metabolizes cGMP, thereby increasing the cGMP-mediated relaxation.[178] The current treatment modalities for pulmonary hypertension include conventional supportive therapies and more specific pharmacologic therapies that are targeted at abnormalities of endothelial function. NO and PDE5 inhibitors induce pulmonary vasodilation by increasing intracellular cGMP concentrations. Sildenafil citrate is a selective inhibitor of PDE5. Investigations in animal models and recent clinical case reports with some studies in the pediatric population suggest that sildenafil may be a promising agent in treating pulmonary hypertension. The effect of sildenafil on pulmonary vasculature appears to be independent of the underlying cause, thereby providing a role in idiopathic pulmonary arterial hypertension, pulmonary arterial hypertension associated with congenital heart disease, pulmonary hypertension secondary to lung disease, or persistent pulmonary hypertension of the newborn. It also may be beneficial in postoperative pulmonary hypertension and in patients who are difficult to wean from inhaled NO. It is administered easily and effectively and has minimal adverse systemic effects[182] (see Chapter 24).

Combination Therapy: Catecholamines and Phosphodiesterase Inhibitors

Catecholamine therapy depends on the capacity of the myocardial cell to respond to β_1-agonist activity. In patients with preoperative HF, the number of effective β_1 receptors decreases because of downregulation, which refers to reduced density or uncoupling, such that fewer receptors are available for binding with the β_1-agonist.[154,175] When postoperative ventricular dysfunction is treated, a pharmacologic ceiling effect may occur with increasing doses of a single β_1-agonist or even when other catecholamines are added.[176] Combining PDE inhibitors with a catecholamine may significantly increase cAMP levels in patients with β_1-receptor downregulation, such as patients after cardiac surgery.[190] The two forms of therapy may attenuate each other's adverse effects. Catecholamine stimulation of vascular α_1 receptors induces vasoconstriction, which is attenuated by PDE inhibitors.[146] Catecholamines with potent α_1-agonist effects may be necessary to prevent hypotension when PDE inhibitors are given after surgery; or, alternatively, when an α agent is necessary to obtain an acceptable perfusion pressure, PDE inhibitors may be administered to augment CO. The additive improvement in hemodynamic effects of catecholamines plus amrinone, milrinone, or enoximone has been also described.[187,191–195] Combined therapy may theoretically avoid dose-related adverse effects of high doses of each individual agent and is useful in RV failure[196] (Box 34-6; see Chapter 10).

Dosage and Administration

Suggested dosing is provided in Table 34-5. Available drugs are reviewed in the following sections.

Amrinone

Amrinone, the first bipyridine evaluated for HF during and after cardiac surgery, has a half-life of ~3.5 hours.[197–201] In HF patients, an intravenous loading dose of 1.5 mg/kg and an infusion of 10 µg/kg/min resulted in a plasma concentration of 1.7 µg/mL and produced a 30% increase in CI.[197] The original recommended dosing included a bolus dose of 0.75 mg/kg given intravenously over 2 to 3 minutes, followed by a maintenance infusion of 5 to 10 µg/kg/min. This dose regimen produced subtherapeutic concentrations after 5 to 10 minutes, and it failed to show any hemodynamic effect after it was given 10 minutes before termination of CPB.[201,202] A loading dose of 1.5 to 2.0 mg/kg of this drug during CPB will produce therapeutic concentrations for 30 to 60 minutes, after which an infusion is required to keep therapeutic blood levels. With prolonged administration, amrinone will produce thrombocytopenia. Amrinone has been replaced with milrinone for the most part.

Milrinone

Milrinone, an analog of amrinone, is a bipyridine derivative with an inotropic activity that is almost 20 times more potent than that of amrinone, and it has a shorter half-life.[183] Milrinone is an effective inodilator for patients with decompensated HF and low CO after cardiac surgery. Suggested dosing for milrinone is a loading dose of 50 µg/kg over 10 minutes, followed by an infusion of 0.5 µg/kg/min (0.375 to 0.75 µg/kg/min). By using slower loading doses, high peak concentrations can be prevented, and the vasodilation that is observed with rapid loading can be attenuated.[183] A milrinone loading dose of 50 µg/kg, in combination with an infusion of 0.5 µg/kg/min, consistently maintained plasma concentrations more than 100 ng/mL. Clearance was 3.8 ± 1.7 mL/kg/min, volume of distribution was 465 ± 159 mL/kg, and terminal elimination half-time was 107 ± 77 minutes (values expressed as mean ± SD).[183] Pharmacokinetic parameters were independent of dose. The relation between plasma concentration and pharmacodynamic effects produced about a 30% improvement in CI with plasma levels of 100 ng/mL, and there was a curvilinear relation between plasma levels and improvement in CI. Bailey et al[183] observed that a dose of 50 µg/kg with an infusion rate of 0.5 µg/kg/min can keep plasma concentrations near the threshold of its therapeutic effects. Compared with amrinone, milrinone has a shorter context-sensitive half-time after administration is stopped, without adverse effects on platelet function.[189]

Kikura et al[194] reported the effects of milrinone on hemodynamics and LV function in cardiac surgical patients who were already treated with catecholamines. After emergence from CPB, patients were randomly assigned to a control group ($n = 10$) or to one of the milrinone dosing groups: intravenous milrinone at $50\,\mu g/kg$ ($n = 8$), $50\,\mu g/kg + 0.5\,\mu g/kg/min$ ($n = 10$), or $75\,\mu g/kg + 0.75\,\mu g/kg/min$ ($n = 9$). Hemodynamics and TEE were recorded while constant filling pressures were maintained by volume reinfusion. In all three milrinone groups, CI and velocity of circumferential fiber shortening significantly increased from the baseline, and both were significantly greater at 5 and 10 minutes than those in the control group. The plasma concentration of milrinone with half of the maximal increase in velocity of circumferential fiber shortening was 139 ng/mL on the dose-response curve. Milrinone improves hemodynamics and LV function when constant loading conditions are maintained.[194]

Feneck et al[203] studied 99 adult patients with a low CO after elective cardiac surgery. Milrinone was administered as a loading dose of $50\,\mu g/kg$ over a 10-minute period, followed by a continuous infusion of 0.375, 0.5, or $0.75\,\mu g/kg/min$ (low-, middle-, and high-dose groups, respectively) for a minimum of 12 hours. They observed that milrinone therapy was associated with a rapid and well-sustained increase in CO and a decrease in PAOP in all groups. They found the increase in CI was associated with increases in SV and HR (Table 34-6).

Enoximone

Enoximone, an imidazolone derivative, is eliminated mostly by sulfoxidation, is solubilized in propylene glycol, and cannot be diluted when administered intravenously. The loading dose is 0.5 to 1.0 mg/kg, followed by an infusion of 5 to $10\,\mu g/kg/min$. Gonzalez et al[187] reported using enoximone in managing a CI less than $2.2\,L/min/m^2$ despite a pulmonary capillary wedge pressure of 15 mm Hg, catecholamine administration (e.g., dobutamine, dopamine), or IABP counterpulsation after cardiac surgery. Enoximone was administered as a 1-mg/kg loading dose over 10 minutes after a minimum of 4 hours of unsuccessful conventional therapy. An extra dose (0.5 mg/kg) was given if the increase in CO was less than 20%. A continuous infusion of the drug was administered at 3 to $10\,\mu g/kg/min$ and continued for at least 8 hours. In all patients, significant increases in CI and a significant decrease in pulmonary capillary wedge pressure occurred. Naeije et al[204] also reported variable effects on BP, HR, and CO of enoximone in a dose of 0.5 mg/kg after cardiac surgery. Boldt et al[193] demonstrated potentiating effects of enoximone, 0.5 mg/kg, with epinephrine in a dose of $0.1\,\mu g/kg/min$.

Levosimendan

Levosimendan is a calcium-sensitizing drug that exerts positive inotropic effects through sensitization of myofilaments to calcium and vasodilation through opening of ATP-dependent potassium channels on vascular smooth muscle. These effects occur without increasing intracellular cAMP or calcium and without an increase in $M\dot{V}o_2$

at therapeutic doses. As would be expected with an inodilator, the hemodynamic effects include a decrease in PAOP in association with an increase in CO. β-Blockade does not block the hemodynamic effects of this drug. Levosimendan itself has a short elimination half-life, but it has active metabolites with elimination half-lives up to 80 hours. A study in patients with decompensated HF found hemodynamic improvements at 48 hours were similar whether patients received the drug for 24 or 48 hours. Increasing plasma levels of the active metabolite were found for 24 hours after the drug infusion was stopped.[205] Currently, levosimendan is not approved for use in the United States.

A randomized study enrolling 203 low-output HF patients found that levosimendan improved hemodynamics more effectively than dobutamine and was associated with a lower 6-month mortality rate.[206] However, the latter finding may be caused more by adverse effects related to dobutamine than by a positive effect of levosimendan. Another study in 504 patients with LV dysfunction after acute MI demonstrated better 6-month survival with levosimendan, this time compared with placebo.[207] In a small study after cardiac surgery, patients were given levosimendan; of 11 patients with severely impaired CO and hemodynamic compromise, 8 patients (73%) showed evidence of hemodynamic improvement within 3 hours after the start of levosimendan infusion. Specifically, CI and SV were increased significantly, whereas MAP, indexed SVR, mean PAP, right atrial pressure (RAP), and PAOP were decreased significantly.[208] Clinical studies continue to evaluate the potential role for this new positive inotropic agent in patients with HF.

RIGHT-HEART FAILURE

HF after cardiac surgery usually results from LV impairment. Although an isolated right-sided MI can occur perioperatively, most perioperative inferior MIs show variable involvement of the right ventricle.[209] The myocardial preservation techniques that are best for the left ventricle may not offer ideal RV protection because the right ventricle is thin walled and more exposed to body and atmospheric temperature. Cardioplegic solution given through the coronary sinus (retrograde) may not reach parts of the right ventricle because of positioning of the cardioplegia cannula in relation to the venous outflow from this chamber and because the thebesian veins do not drain into the coronary sinus.[210] Impairment of RV function after surgery is more severe and persistent when preoperative right coronary artery stenosis is present.[211] Although depression of the ejection fraction is compensated by preload augmentation, right ventricular ejection fraction (RVEF) cannot be preserved if coronary perfusion pressure is reduced or impedance to ejection is increased.

Certain aspects of the physiology of the right ventricle make it different from the left. Normally, the RV free wall receives its blood flow during systole and diastole; however, systemic hypotension or increased RV systolic and diastolic pressures may cause supply-dependent depression of contractility when $M\dot{V}o_2$ is increased, whereas coronary perfusion pressure is decreased.[212] The normal thin-walled right ventricle is at least twice as sensitive to increases in afterload as is the left ventricle[213] (Figure 34-6). Relatively modest increases in outflow impedance from multiple causes in the postoperative period can exhaust preload reserve, causing a decrease in RVEF with ventricular dilation. RV pressure overload may be complicated by volume overload caused by functional tricuspid regurgitation.[214] Decreases in RV SV will decrease LV filling, and dilation of the right ventricle can cause a leftward shift of the interventricular septum, interfering with diastolic filling of the left ventricle (i.e., ventricular interaction; Figure 34-7). A distended right ventricle limited by the pericardial cavity further decreases LV filling. RV failure has the potential to affect LV performance by decreasing pulmonary venous blood flow, decreasing diastolic distending pressure, and decreasing LV diastolic compliance. The resulting decrease in LV output will further impair RV pump function. The mechanical outcomes of RV failure in postoperative cardiac surgical patients are depicted in Figure 34-8. It can, therefore, be appreciated how, once established, RV failure is self-propagating, and aggressive treatment interventions may be needed to interrupt the vicious cycle (see Chapter 24).

TABLE 34-6	Hemodynamic Effect of Milrinone after Cardiac Surgery			
	% Change (Mean ± SEM)			
Parameter	*15 Minutes*	*60 Minutes*	*12 Hours*	*Post*
CI (L/min/m²)				
Low	+40* (4.2)	+42* (4.9)	+58* (8.8)	+44* (6.3)
Mid	+30* (4.5)	+34* (4.5)	+49* (5.1)	+27* (3.8)
High	+36* (4.9)	+44* (4.7)	+66* (6.5)	+47* (6.6)
PCWP (mm Hg)				
Low	−30* (4.7)	−20* (4.7)	−15† (7.2)	+22‡ (6.3)
Mid	−34* (4.5)	−25* (4.1)	−20* (4.3)	−3 (6.7)
High	−35* (4.0)	−22* (4.3)	−15† (6.0)	−6‡ (6.3)

Loading dose of $50\,\mu g/kg$ over 10 minutes, then 0.375 (low, $n = 34$), 0.5 (mid, $n = 34$), and 0.75 (high, $n = 31$) $\mu g/kg/min$.
*$p < 0.001$ vs. control.
†$p < 0.05$ vs. control.
‡$p < 0.01$ vs. control.
CI, cardiac index; PCWP, pulmonary capillary wedge pressure.
From Feneck RO: Effects of variable dose milrinone in patients with low cardiac output after cardiac surgery. *Am Heart J* 121(Suppl 2):1995, 1991.

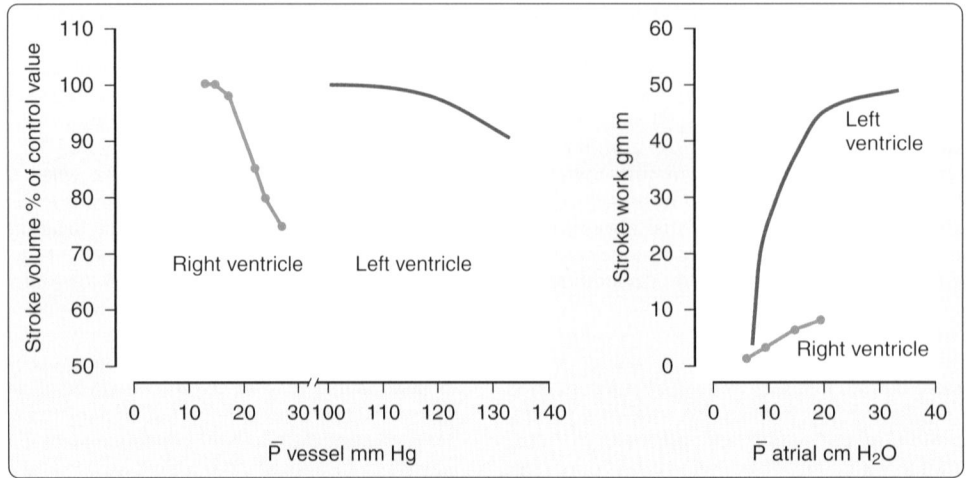

Figure 34-6 Various effects of afterload and preload seen in ventricular function curves from the right and left ventricle. The right ventricular output is more afterload dependent and less preload dependent than the left ventricular output. *(From McFadden ER, Braunwald E: Cor pulmonale and pulmonary thromboembolism. In Braunwald E [ed]:* Textbook of Cardiovascular Medicine. *Philadelphia, WB Saunders Company, 1980, pp 1643–1680.)*

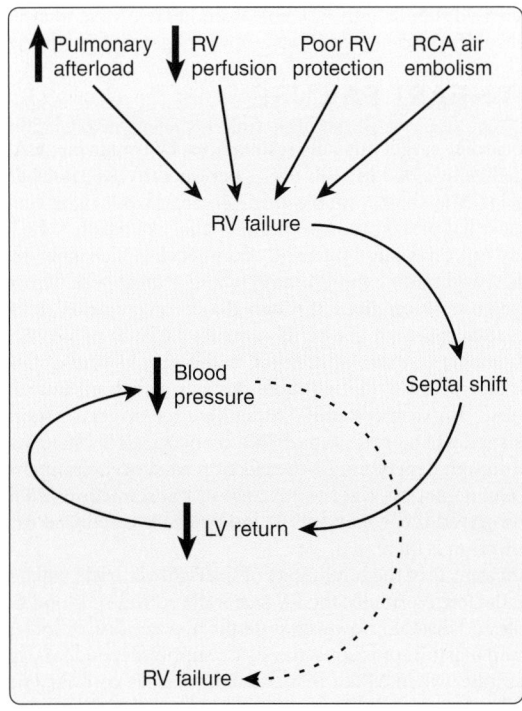

Figure 34-7 **Sequence inducing right ventricular (RV) failure and causing a downward spiral of events.** LV, left ventricular; RCA, right coronary artery.

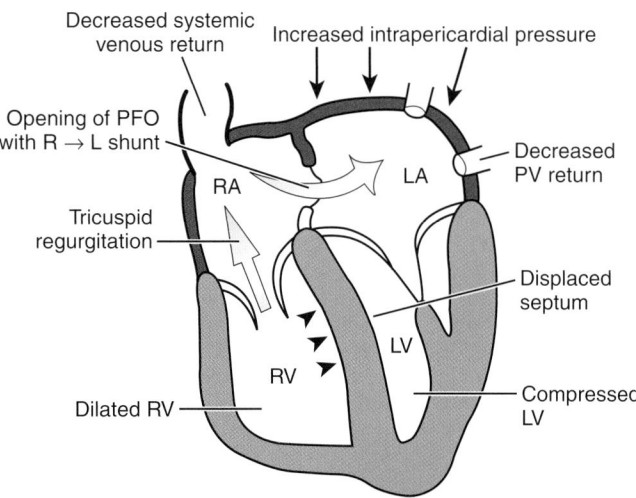

Figure 34-8 **Mechanical changes produced by acute right ventricular failure.** LA, left atrium; LV, left ventricle; PFO, patent foramen ovale; PV, pulmonary veins; RA, right atrium; R→L, right to left; RV, right ventricle.

depression of the RVEF and increased RV end-diastolic volume, and these changes were immediately reversed when normocarbia was reinstituted.[223]

▓ Diagnosis

In the postoperative cardiac surgical patient, a low CI with RAP increased disproportionately compared with changes in left-sided filling pressures is highly suggestive of RV failure. The PAOP also may increase because of ventricular interaction, but the relation of RAP to PAOP stays close to or greater than 1.0. The absence of a step-up in pressure in going from the right atrium (RA) to the pulmonary artery (mean), provided PVR is low, suggests that RV failure is severe and the right side of the heart is acting only as a conduit. This hemodynamic presentation is typical of cardiogenic shock associated with RV infarction. The venous waveforms are accentuated with a prominent Y descent similar to constrictive pericarditis, suggesting reduced RV compliance.[224] Large V waves also may be discernible and may relate to tricuspid regurgitation.

The use of a volumetric PAC to calculate right-sided volumes and ejection fraction could potentially guide management in the setting

Although not consistently proved, PVR has been shown to be reversibly increased immediately after CPB and for several hours into the postoperative period.[215,216] The possible mechanisms include extravascular compression by increased lung water,[216] endocrine-mediated or autonomic nervous system–mediated increases in pulmonary vascular tone,[217] vasoactive substances released from activated platelets and leukocytes,[218] and leukocytes or platelet aggregates obstructing pulmonary vascular beds.[219] Hypoxic pulmonary vasoconstriction may result in increased PVR; more commonly, hypercarbia causes an important increase in PAP.[220,221] The pulmonary vascular bed has been shown to be more sensitive to the vasoconstrictor influences of respiratory acidosis after CPB as compared with the preoperative situation.[222] Moderate respiratory acidosis was shown to cause of RV failure, because increased end-diastolic volume in association with a decreased RVEF indicates decompensation. This catheter-computer system has been validated in comparison with radionuclear and ventriculographic measures, but it may not be accurate when there is tricuspid regurgitation[34,225,226] (see Chapter 14). Unfortunately, tricuspid regurgitation is a common finding with RV dilation.

Echocardiography allows a qualitative interpretation of RV size, contractility, and configuration of the interventricular septum and can provide a definitive diagnosis of RV dysfunction or failure. Because of the crescent shape of the right ventricle, volume determination is not easy, but the qualitative examination and assessment for tricuspid regurgitation are valuable. TEE is also useful to determine whether the increased RAP opens a patent foramen ovale, producing a right-to-left shunt (see Chapters 12, 13, and 22). This is important because traditional methods to treat hypoxemia such as PEEP and larger tidal volumes in this setting will only increase the afterload of the right ventricle and potentially increase the shunt and hypoxemia.

Treatment

Treatment approaches in postoperative RV failure may differ from those used in LV failure, and they are affected by the presence of pulmonary hypertension (Table 34-7). In all cases, preload should be increased to the upper range of normal; however, the Frank–Starling relation is flat in RV failure, and to avoid ventricular dilation, the CO response to an increasing CVP should be determined. Volume loading should be stopped when the CVP exceeds 10 mm Hg and CO does not increase despite increases in this pressure.[227,228] If a volumetric PAC is in use, an increase in the end-diastolic volume with unchanged or declining RVEF suggests there will be no advantage to further volume loading. The CVP should not be permitted to exceed the PAOP because if these pressures equalize, any increase obtained in pulmonary blood flow will be offset by decreased diastolic filling of the left ventricle by ventricular interdependence.[229] The atrial contribution to RV filling is important when the ventricle is dilated and noncompliant. Maintenance of sinus rhythm and use of atrial pacing are important components of treating postoperative RV failure (see Chapters 4, 5, 10, 13, 14, 19, 23–25 and 32).

TABLE 34-7	Treatment Approaches in Postoperative Right-Heart Failure

Preload Augmentation

Volume, vasopressors, or leg elevation (CVP/PCWP < 1)

Decrease juxtacardiac pressures (pericardium and/or chest open)

Establish atrial kick and treat atrial arrhythmias (sinus rhythm, atrial pacing)

Afterload Reduction (pulmonary vasodilation)

Nitroglycerin, isosorbide dinitrate, nesiritide

cAMP-specific phosphodiesterase inhibitors, B$_2$-adrenergic agonists

Inhaled nitric oxide

Nebulized PGI$_2$

Intravenous PGE$_1$ (+left atrial norepinephrine)

Inotropic Support

cAMP-specific phosphodiesterase inhibitors, isoproterenol, dobutamine

Norepinephrine

Levosimendan

Ventilatory Management

Lower intrathoracic pressures (tidal volume < 7 mL/kg, low PEEP)

Attenuation of hypoxic vasoconstriction (high F$_I$O$_2$)

Avoidance of respiratory acidosis (Paco$_2$ 30–35 mm Hg, metabolic control with meperidine or relaxants)

Mechanical Support

Intra-aortic counterpulsation

Pulmonary artery counterpulsation

Right ventricular assist devices

cAMP, cyclic adenosine monophosphate; CVP/PCWP, central venous pressure/pulmonary capillary wedge pressure; PEEP, positive end-expiratory pressure; PGE$_1$, prostaglandin E$_1$; PGI$_2$, prostaglandin I$_2$.

Although vasodilators may lead to cardiovascular collapse in RV infarction (as a result of decreases in RV filling and coronary perfusion), postoperative RV failure is often associated with increased PVR and pulmonary hypertension. In this context, attempts to decrease RV outflow impedance may be worthwhile. Intravenous vasodilators invariably reduce systemic BP, mandating the simultaneous administration of a vasoconstrictor. One way to reduce the pulmonary effects of the needed vasoconstrictor is to administer the vasoconstrictor through a left atrial catheter, treating RV dysfunction with intravenous PGs and left atrial norepinephrine.[230] The PDE inhibitors commonly are used for their effect on the pulmonary vasculature and RV function. In recent years, there have been an increased interest in and availability of aerosolized pulmonary vasodilators. This route of administration reduces or even abolishes the undesirable systemic vasodilation. Delivery of the drug directly to the alveoli improves pulmonary blood flow to these alveoli, potentially improving oxygenation by better matching blood flow to ventilation. Three drugs have been used: nitric oxide, PGI$_2$ (i.e., epoprostenol or prostacyclin), and milrinone.[231,232]

Nitric oxide is an important signaling molecule throughout the body. In the lung, it rapidly diffuses across the alveolar-capillary membrane and activates soluble guanylate cyclase, leading to smooth muscle relaxation by several mechanisms.[231] Inhaled nitric oxide is given through a specialized delivery system in a concentration of 5 to 80 parts per million. It is available commercially in the United States, but it is costly. It has been used successfully to treat RV dysfunction associated with pulmonary hypertension after cardiac surgery,[231] mitral valve replacement,[233] cardiac transplantation,[234] and placement of LV assist devices.[235] Although it is used widely to treat the same problem in lung transplantation, a randomized trial of prophylactic inhaled nitric oxide in this population failed to show a benefit.[236] This finding should not prevent its use should RV dysfunction occur in the lung transplant recipient. Potential adverse effects of inhaled nitric oxide include toxicity from forming nitrogen dioxide (NO$_2$) and methemoglobin, rebound pulmonary hypertension from abrupt disconnection or withdrawal, and pulmonary vascular congestion because of increased pulmonary blood flow in patients with poor LV function. If administered at the recommended dosage, toxicity should not be observed; patients should have the drug gradually withdrawn, and those with poor ventricular function should be monitored closely for increases in left-sided filling pressures.

A less expensive alternative to inhaled nitric oxide is aerosolized epoprostenol (i.e., prostacyclin or PGI$_2$). This compound binds to cell-surface PG receptors, activating adenylate cyclase, which activates protein kinase A to cause a decrease in cytosolic free calcium. It also stimulates endothelial release of nitric oxide. It is a profound vasodilator and inhibitor of platelet aggregation. Similar to inhaled nitric oxide, its delivery to ventilated alveoli can improve oxygenation by augmenting blood flow to these alveoli. Aerosolized PGI$_2$ has been used successfully to treat pulmonary hypertension after cardiac surgery,[232,237] pulmonary embolism,[238] and to treat hypoxemia in patients with lung injury.[239,240] Its use needs collaboration with pharmacy and respiratory therapy, as well as suitable care and monitoring of the nebulizer device. Adverse effects include the possibility of vagus-mediated bradycardia at low doses and risks similar to those of inhaled nitric oxide for abrupt withdrawal or left-sided HF.

Haraldsson et al[241] studied the use of inhaled (i.e., aerosolized) milrinone in patients with mild pulmonary hypertension after CPB. They found that when delivered by this route, milrinone was an effective pulmonary vasodilator without causing systemic hypotension, and the pulmonary vasodilation was additive to that caused by inhaled PGI$_2$.

Even a moderate increase in arterial carbon dioxide tension (Paco$_2$) should be avoided in patients with RV failure. Although induced hypocarbia is of proven benefit in controlling PVR in neonates, the evidence in adults does not warrant this as a standard therapy because mechanical ventilation-induced changes in intrathoracic pressure have important therapeutic implications[242,243] (see Chapter 35). An IABP may be of great benefit, even in patients in whom the right ventricle is mainly responsible for circulatory decompensation. This beneficial effect is mediated by increased coronary perfusion. Right-heart assist devices have a place as temporizing measures in severe intractable failure. Pulmonary artery counterpulsation is experimental, and its clinical role is uncertain.[244] In cases of severe RV failure, it may be necessary to leave the sternum open or to reopen the chest if it has been closed. This decreases the tamponade-like compression of the left ventricle by the distended right ventricle, RA, and edematous mediastinal tissues.

Effects of Mechanical Ventilation in Heart Failure

HF at the time of surgery has been identified as a significant predictor of postoperative respiratory complications.[245] Maintenance of gas exchange in these situations usually mandates prolonged ventilatory support. Besides improving Pao_2, mechanical ventilation can influence Do_2 through its effects on CO. Suppression of spontaneous respiratory efforts may substantially decrease the work of breathing and improve the oxygen supply/demand relation (see Chapter 35). Traditionally, the influence of mechanical ventilation on hemodynamics has been viewed as negative. The unavoidable increase in intrathoracic pressure caused by positive-pressure ventilation or PEEP is associated with a decreased CO.[246] However, in the presence of HF or myocardial ischemia, increased intrathoracic pressure has the potential to favorably affect the determinants of global cardiac performance. Understanding these heart-lung interactions is essential for the integrated management of the ventilated patient with HF after cardiac surgery. The effects of ventilation on RV and LV failure need to receive independent consideration.

Systemic venous return is proportional to the pressure gradient between the systemic veins and the RA. Changes in intrathoracic pressure imposed by positive-pressure ventilation or PEEP are transmitted to the compliant RA, causing an increase in RAP. This decreases the driving pressure for venous return, with a decrease in RV preload as the clinically most important mechanism of the decrease in RV SV caused by ventilatory support.[247] The effects of mechanical ventilation on RV preload may be accentuated by hypovolemia or by an increase in venous capacitance caused by vasodilator administration.[248] The effects of increased intrathoracic pressure can be overcome by fluid administration, leg elevation, or even vasopressors to increase the systemic venous pressure. Preload augmentation must be done with caution with RV failure.

Two other factors related to increased intrathoracic pressure potentially impede the diastolic filling of the left ventricle. If positive-pressure ventilation or PEEP causes an increase in PVR, RV systolic emptying may be impaired and the right ventricle will dilate. This may cause leftward displacement of the interventricular septum and decrease LV compliance.[229] Independent of ventricular interaction, increased lung volume also increases juxtacardiac pressures, decreasing the transmural distending pressure.[249]

The end-diastolic volume and systolic BP are directly proportional to systolic wall stress or ventricular afterload. Because ventricles and the outflow vessels are surrounded by intrathoracic pressure, increases in this pressure by positive-pressure ventilation decrease the transmural pressure load (aortic or PAP relative to intrathoracic pressure) of each ventricle.[250] On the right side of the heart, the hemodynamic effects of ventilatory support usually result from changes in PVR. To the extent that PEEP increases lung volume above functional residual capacity, PVR may decrease from reduced compression of extraalveolar vessels.[251] Beyond that, large tidal volumes and high levels of PEEP increase PVR.[252] The increase in PVR may be obvious even with normal tidal volumes in airflow-limited diseases. The effects of increased PVR in RV failure are decreased CO and further dilation.

Increased intrathoracic pressure may significantly improve LV performance as a result of the reduced transmural pressure needed to achieve an acceptable systemic BP.[253] This can be viewed as afterload reduction, a favorable effect separate from the resistance to venous return that also may help such patients. Clinically significant improvements in cardiac function have been documented in patients ventilated

for cardiogenic respiratory failure produced by myocardial ischemia and after CABG surgery.[254,255] High LV filling pressures may help identify a subgroup benefiting from reduced afterload with increased intrathoracic pressure.[256]

Increased intrathoracic pressure and PEEP also have been suggested to affect the inotropic state of the ventricles. Dilation of the right ventricle in response to an increase in afterload increases the RV distending pressure, which can reduce the pressure gradient for subendocardial coronary blood flow. Decreased RV contractility related to a decreased coronary blood flow has been described with high levels of PEEP in an animal model with critical right coronary artery obstruction[212] and in patients with significant right coronary artery disease.[256] Left ventricular contractility does not seem to be affected by this mechanism.[257] Increased intrathoracic pressure and lung distention also may modulate contractility by stimulating vagal afferents[258] and releasing PGs.[259] The impairment of contractility by these mechanisms appears to be minimal.

The circulatory responses to changes in ventilation always should be assessed in patients with cardiac disease; the goal of improving or maintaining Do_2 must be kept in mind. This usually requires measurement of arterial oxygenation and CO. In right and biventricular failure, the increase in the airway pressure caused by ventilatory support should be kept, at a minimum, compatible with acceptable gas exchange. This means avoidance of high levels of PEEP and trials of decreased inspiratory times, flow rates, and tidal volumes. Breathing modes that emphasize spontaneous efforts such as intermittent mandatory ventilation, pressure support, or continuous positive airway pressure should be considered. Alternatively, if isolated LV failure is the reason for ventilatory therapy, improvements in cardiac performance may be achieved by positive-pressure ventilation with PEEP. In particular, patients with increased LV filling pressures, mitral regurgitation, and reversible ischemic dysfunction may improve from afterload reduction related to increased airway and intrathoracic pressures. Newer modes of ventilatory support that decrease mean airway pressure, such as cardiac cycle–specific, high-frequency jet ventilation[260] and airway pressure release ventilation,[261] and their roles in supporting heart function are discussed in Chapter 35.

Effects of Ventilatory Weaning on Heart Failure

Traditional criteria for weaning of ventilatory support assess the adequacy of gas exchange and peak respiratory muscle strength.[262] In the patient with HF, the response of global hemodynamics to spontaneous respirations must also be considered. The changes of the loading conditions of the heart brought about by resuming spontaneous ventilation can induce a vicious cycle resulting in hypoxemia and pulmonary edema.

Pulmonary congestion, often present in patients with LV dysfunction, decreases pulmonary compliance. Thus, large decreases in inspiratory intrathoracic pressure are necessary to cause satisfactory lung inflation. These negative swings of intrathoracic pressure increase venous return.[263] Increased diaphragmatic movements may increase intra-abdominal pressure, further increasing the pressure gradient for venous return.[264] Decreased intrathoracic pressure also increases the ventricular transmural pressures, increasing the impedance to ventricular emptying. The increased afterload causes further increases in preload, with these changes jeopardizing the myocardial oxygen balance. Accordingly, worsening of myocardial ischemia as shown by ST-segment deviations was demonstrated when ventilatory support was removed in patients ventilated after MI.[265] Spontaneous ventilation episodes also precipitated ischemic dysfunction, causing LV dilation and altered thallium-201 uptake, in ventilator-dependent patients after lung injury caused by infection or complications of surgery.[266]

In the patient with severe ventricular dysfunction, one of the main methods of improving cardiac performance to allow separation from CPB and to maintain function in the postoperative period is to augment preload with fluid therapy. The unavoidable consequence is a positive fluid balance and a weight gain of several kilograms, even after uncomplicated surgery. Diuretic therapy to reduce this hypervolemia, as well as vasodilator therapy to reduce ventricular wall stress, should be considered before these patients are exposed to the afterload stress of ventilatory weaning.[263,267]

CARDIAC TAMPONADE

Cardiac tamponade is an important cause of the low CO state after cardiac surgery and occurs when the heart is compressed by an external agent, most commonly blood accumulated in the mediastinum. Hemodynamic compromise, to some degree attributable to the constraining effect of blood accumulating within the chest, is often observed in the 3% to 6% of patients needing multiple blood transfusions for hemorrhage after cardiac surgery.[268] Postoperative cardiac tamponade usually manifests acutely during the first 24 hours after surgery, but delayed tamponade may develop 10 to 14 days after surgery, and it has been associated with postpericardiotomy syndrome or postoperative anticoagulation.[269-271]

The mechanism of hemodynamic deterioration during tamponade is discussed in Chapter 22 and mainly is the result of impaired filling of one or more of the cardiac chambers. As the external pressure on the heart increases, the distending or transmural pressure (external intracavitary pressure) is decreased. The intracavitary pressure increases in compensation lead to impaired venous return and elevation of the venous pressure. If the external pressure is high enough to exceed the ventricular pressure during diastole, diastolic ventricular collapse occurs. These changes have been documented in the right and the left hearts after cardiac surgery.[272] As the end-diastolic volume and end-systolic volume decrease, there is a concomitant decrease in SV. In the most severe form of cardiac tamponade, ventricular filling occurs only during atrial systole. Adrenergic and endocrine mechanisms are activated in an effort to maintain venous return and perfusion pressure.[273,274] Intense sympathoadrenergic activation increases venous return by constricting venous capacitance vessels. Tachycardia helps to maintain CO in the face of a reduced SV. Adrenergic mechanisms may also explain decreased urinary output and sodium excretion, but these phenomena also may be caused by reduced CO or a reduction in atrial natriuretic factor from decreased distending pressure of the atria.[273]

The diagnosis of cardiac tamponade depends on a high degree of suspicion. Tamponade after heart surgery is a clinical entity distinct from the tamponade typically seen in medical patients in whom the pericardium is intact and the heart is surrounded by a compressing fluid. In the setting of cardiac surgery, the pericardial space is often left open and in communication with one or both of the pleural spaces, and the compressing blood is, at least in part, in a clotted, nonfluid state and able to cause localized compression of the heart. Serious consideration should be given to the possibility of tamponade after cardiac surgery in any patient with inadequate or worsening hemodynamics, as evidenced by hypotension, tachycardia, increased filling pressures, or low CO, especially when there has been excessive chest tube drainage. A more subtle presentation of postoperative tamponade is gradually increasing needs for inotropic and pressor support. Many of the classic signs of tamponade may not be present in these patients, partly because they are usually sedated and ventilated, but also because the pericardium is usually left open, resulting in a more gradual increase in the restraining effects of blood accumulation. There may be localized accumulations that affect one chamber more than another.[275] The classic findings of increased CVP or equalization of CVP, PA_d, and PAOP may not occur.[276,277] It may, therefore, be difficult in the face of a declining CO and increased filling pressures to distinguish tamponade from biventricular failure. A useful clue may be pronounced respiratory variation in BP with mechanical ventilation in association with high filling pressures and low CO because the additional external pressure applied to the heart by positive-pressure ventilation may further impair the already compromised ventricular filling in the presence of tamponade.

Echocardiography may provide strong evidence for the diagnosis of tamponade.[277-280] Echolucent crescents between the RV wall and the pericardium or the posterior LV wall and the pericardium are visible with transthoracic imaging or TEE. Echogenicity of grossly bloody pericardial effusions, especially when clots have been formed, may sometimes make delineation of the borders of the pericardium and the ventricular wall difficult, compromising the sensitivity of this technique. A classic echocardiographic sign of tamponade is diastolic collapse of the RA or right ventricle, with the duration of collapse bearing a relation to the severity of the hemodynamic alteration, but such findings are often absent in the postcardiac surgery patient.[277,281,282] Often, transthoracic imaging is difficult because of mechanical ventilation, and TEE is required for satisfactory imagining (see Chapters 12 and 13).

The definitive treatment of tamponade is surgical exploration with evacuation of hematoma. The chest may have to be opened in the ICU if tamponade proceeds to hemodynamic collapse. For delayed tamponade, pericardiocentesis may be acceptable. Medical palliation in anticipation of re-exploration consists of reinforcing the physiologic responses that are already occurring while preparing for definitive treatment. Venous return can be increased by volume administration and leg elevation. The lowest tidal volume and PEEP compatible with adequate gas exchange should be used.[283] Epinephrine in high doses gives the needed chronotropic and inotropic boost to the ventricle and increases systemic venous pressures. Sedatives and opioids should be given with caution because they may interfere with adrenergic discharge and precipitate abrupt hemodynamic collapse. Occasionally, patients experience development of significant cardiac tamponade without accumulation of blood in the chest. Edema of the heart, lungs, and other tissues in the chest after CPB may not allow chest closure at the first operation and need staged chest closure after the edema has subsided.[284] Similarly, it was found that some patients with inadequate hemodynamics after cardiac surgery despite maximum support in the ICU improved with opening of the chest because of relief of this tamponade effect. Reclosure of the chest in the operating room often is possible after a few days of continued cardiovascular support and diuresis.

TRANSPLANTED HEART

Postoperative circulatory control in the heart transplant recipient differs from that of the nontransplant population in three major respects: The transplanted heart is noncompliant with a relatively fixed SV, acute rejection must be considered when cardiac performance is poor or suddenly deteriorates, and these patients are at risk for acute RV failure if pulmonary hypertension develops.[285]

The fixed SV combined with denervation of the donor heart means that maintenance of CO often is dependent on therapy to maintain an increased HR (110 to 120 beats/min). The drug most commonly used is isoproterenol because it is a potent inotropic agent and because it causes a dose-related increase in HR. Its vasodilating β_2-receptor effect on the pulmonary vasculature may be of benefit if PVR is above normal. Alternatively, atrial pacing may be used to maintain HR if contractility appears normal. Pacing is often used to allow the withdrawal of isoproterenol in the first postoperative days. Parasympatholytic drugs, such as atropine, do not have any effect on the transplanted heart (see Chapter 23).

Major concerns in monitoring and therapy for the transplant recipient are the potential for infection and rejection. Immunosuppressive therapy regimens include cyclosporine and usually steroids or azathioprine, or both. These drugs also suppress the patient's response to infection, and steroid therapy may induce increases in the white blood cell count, further confusing the issue. Protocols for postoperative care stress strict aseptic technique and frequent careful clinical evaluations for infection.

The adequacy of immunosuppression is monitored by percutaneous myocardial biopsy, usually performed at weekly intervals in the first month. Less invasive techniques, such as echocardiographic evaluation of diastolic function and sophisticated ECG analysis, are being evaluated.[286] Although acute rejection is diagnosed histologically, if suspected clinically (i.e., acute deterioration in cardiac function), it must be treated with intense immunosuppressive therapy. The agents and doses used vary from institution to institution, but they usually include high-dose steroids and monoclonal antibody to T_3 lymphocytes (OKT3).[287] Pharmacologic management and sometimes mechanical support of biventricular function are required because severe impairment of contractility, ventricular dilation, and even cardiovascular collapse may occur.

Preoperative evaluation helps screen patients with fixed pulmonary hypertension because the normal donor right ventricle may fail acutely if presented with an increased PAP in the recipient.[285] However, patients may have progression of disease between the time of evaluation and surgery, or the right ventricle may be inadequately protected during harvest or transport. When separation from CPB is attempted, acute RV dilation and failure occur, and such patients may emerge from the operating room on multiple drug therapy, including the inhaled agents nitric oxide and prostacyclin, as described earlier. Gradual withdrawal of these drugs occurs in the first postoperative days, with close monitoring of PAPs and oxygenation.

There is a heightened concern for fluid balance in the perioperative period because transplant recipients are often fluid overloaded due to chronic biventricular failure and the potential for edema in the donor heart. It is not unusual for vigorous diuretic therapy to be initiated within 24 hours of surgery, with the goals of negative fluid balance and a PAOP less than 12 mm Hg. Inotropic agents rather than preload augmentation are used to keep CO at an acceptable level while this is being done. Electrolyte abnormalities induced by this therapy and the use of cyclosporine (which causes potassium and magnesium wasting) are common in this period.

REFERENCES

1. Jones M, Tunstall-Pedow DS: Blood doping—a literature review, *Br J Sports Med* 23:84, 1989.
2. Mirhashemi S, Ertefai S, Merrmer K, Intaglietta M: Model analysis of the enhancement of tissue oxygenation by hemodilution due to increased microvascular flow velocity, *Microvasc Res* 34:290, 1987.
3. Vincent JL, Baron JF, Reinhart K, et al: Anemia and blood transfusion in critically ill patients, *JAMA* 288:1499, 2002.
4. Hebert PC, Wells G, Blajchman MA, et al: A multicenter, randomized, controlled clinical trial of transfusion requirements in critical care, *N Engl J Med* 340:409, 1999.
5. Wu WC, Rathore SS, Wang Y, et al: Blood transfusions in elderly patients with acute myocardial infarction, *N Engl J Med* 345:1230, 2001.
6. Suter PM, Fairley HB, Isenbery MD: Optimum end-expiratory pressure in patients with acute pulmonary failure, *N Engl J Med* 292:284, 1975.
7. Dhainaut JF, Devaux JY, Monsallier JE, et al: Mechanisms of decreased left ventricular preload during continuous positive-pressure ventilation in ARDS, *Chest* 90:74, 1986.
8. Robotham JL, Scharf SM: Effects of positive and negative pressure ventilation on cardiac performance, *Clin Chest Med* 4:161, 1983.
9. Katz JA, Marks JD: Inspiratory work with and without continuous positive airway pressure in patients with acute respiratory failure, *Anesthesiology* 63:598, 1985.
10. Rasanen J, Vaisanen IT, Heikkil J, et al: Acute myocardial infarction complicated by left ventricular dysfunction and respiratory failure. The effects of continuous airway pressure, *Chest* 87:158, 1987.
11. Sukernik MR, Mets B, Bennett-Guerrero E: Patent foramen ovale and its significance in the perioperative period, *Anesth Analg* 93:137, 2001.
12. Radermacher P, Santak B, Becker H, et al: Prostaglandin E_1 and nitroglycerin reduce pulmonary capillary pressure but worsen Va/Q distribution in patients with ARDS, *Anesthesiology* 70:601, 1989.
13. Noback CR, Tinker JH: Hypothermia after cardiopulmonary bypass in man; amelioration by nitroprusside-induced vasodilation during rewarming, *Anesthesiology* 53:277, 1980.
14. Ramsay JG, Ralley FE, Whalley DG, et al: Site of temperature monitoring and prediction of afterdrop after open heart surgery, *Can Anaesth Soc J* 32:607, 1985.
15. Pujol A, Fusciardi J, Ingrand P, et al: Afterdrop after hypothermic cardiopulmonary bypass: The value of tympanic membrane temperature monitoring, *J Cardiothorac Vasc Anesth* 10:336, 1996.
16. Grocott HP, Mathew JP, Carver EH, et al: A randomized controlled trial of the Arctic Sun temperature management system versus conventional methods for preventing hypothermia during off-pump cardiac surgery, *Anesth Analg* 98:298, 2004.
17. Licker M, Schweizer A, Ralley FE: Thermoregulatory and metabolic responses following cardiac surgery, *Eur J Anaesthesiol* 13:502, 1996.
18. Buckberg GD, Brazier JR, Nelson RL, et al: Studies of the effects of hypothermia on regional myocardial blood flow and metabolism during cardiopulmonary bypass. 1. The adequately perfused beating, fibrillating, and arrested heart, *J Thorac Cardiovasc Surg* 73:87, 1977.
19. Reed LR II, Bracey AW Jr, Hudson JD, et al: Hypothermia and blood coagulation: Dissociation between enzyme activity and clotting factor levels, *Circ Shock* 32:141, 1990.
20. Valeri CR, Khabbaz K, Khuri SF, et al: Effect of skin temperature on platelet function in patients undergoing extracorporeal bypass, *J Thorac Cardiovasc Surg* 104:108, 1992.
21. Valeri CR, Feingold H, Cassidy G, et al: Hypothermia-induced reversible platelet dysfunction, *Ann Surg* 205:175, 1987.
22. Donati F, Maille JG, Blain R, et al: End-tidal carbon dioxide tension and temperature changes after coronary artery bypass surgery, *Can Anaesth Soc J* 32:272, 1985.
23. Sladen RN: Temperature and ventilation after hypothermic cardiopulmonary bypass, *Anesth Analg* 64:816, 1985.
24. Ralley FE, Wynands JE, Ramsay JG, et al: The effects of shivering on oxygen consumption and carbon dioxide production in patients re-warming from hypothermic cardiopulmonary bypass, *Can J Anaesth* 35:332, 1988.
25. Kurz A, Ikeda T, Sessler DI, et al: Meperidine decreases the shivering threshold twice as much as the vasoconstriction threshold, *Anesthesiology* 86:1046, 1997.
26. Sladen RN, Berend JZ, Fassero JS, Zehnder EB: Comparison of vecuronium and meperidine on the clinical and metabolic effects of shivering after hypothermic cardiopulmonary bypass, *J Cardiothorac Vasc Anesth* 9:147, 1995.
27. Connors AF, McCaffree DR, Gray BA: Evaluation of right heart catheterization in the critically ill patient with acute myocardial infarction, *N Engl J Med* 308:263, 1983.
28. Ariza M, Gothard JW, Macnaughton P, et al: Blood lactate and mixed venous-arterial Pco_2 gradient as indices of poor peripheral perfusion following cardiopulmonary bypass surgery, *Intensive Care Med* 17:320, 1991.
29. Bailey JM, Levy JH, Kopel MA, et al: Relationship between clinical evaluation of peripheral perfusion and global hemodynamics in adults after cardiac surgery, *Crit Care Med* 18:1353, 1990.
30. Sessler D: Mild perioperative hypothermia, *N Engl J Med* 336:1730, 1997.
31. Wiener RS, Welch HG: Trends in the use of pulmonary artery catheters in the US, 1993-2004, *JAMA* 298:423, 2007.
32. Mayer J, Boldt J, Poland R, et al: Continuous arterial pressure waveform-based cardiac outputs using the FloTrac/Vigeleo: Review & meta-analysis, *J Cardiothorac Vasc Anesth* 23:401, 2009.
33. Magilligan DJ, Teasdall R, Eisinminger R, Peterson E: Mixed venous oxygen saturation as a predictor of cardiac output in the postoperative cardiac surgical patient, *Ann Thorac Surg* 44:260, 1987.
34. Spinale FG, Smith AC, Crawford FA: Right ventricular function using thermodilution, *Surg Forum* 39:242, 1988.
35. Reichert CLA, Visser CA, Doolen JJ, et al: Transesophageal echocardiography in hypotensive patients after cardiac operations. Comparison with hemodynamic parameters, *J Thorac Cardiovasc Surg* 104:321, 1992.
36. Kochar GS, Jacobs LE, Kotler MN: Right atrial compression in post-operative cardiac patients: Detection by transesophageal echocardiography, *J Am Coll Cardiol* 16:511, 1990.
37. Chan K-L: Transesophageal echocardiography for assessing cause of hypotension after cardiac surgery, *Am J Cardiol* 62:1142, 1988.
38. Costachescu T, Denault A, Guimond JG, et al: The hemodynamically unstable patient in the intensive care unit: Hemodynamic vs TEE monitoring, *Crit Care Med* 30:1214, 2002.
39. Hwang JJ, Shyu KG, Chen JJ, et al: Usefulness of transesophageal echocardiography in the treatment of critically ill patients, *Chest* 104:861, 1993.
40. Breisblatt WM, Stein KL, Wolfe CJ, et al: Acute myocardial dysfunction and recovery: A common occurrence after cardiopulmonary bypass surgery, *J Am Coll Cardiol* 15:1261, 1990.
41. Roberts AJ, Spies M, Meyers SN, et al: Early and long-term improvement in left ventricular performance following coronary bypass surgery, *Surgery* 88:467, 1980.
42. Roberts AJ, Spies M, Sanders JH, et al: Serial assessment of left ventricular performance following coronary artery bypass grafting, *J Thorac Cardiovasc Surg* 81:69, 1981.
43. Gray R, Maddahi J, Berman D, et al: Scintigraphic and hemodynamic demonstration of transient left ventricular dysfunction immediately after uncomplicated coronary artery bypass grafting, *J Thorac Cardiovasc Surg* 77:504, 1979.
44. Reduto LA, Lawrie GM, Reid JW, et al: Sequential postoperative assessment of left ventricular performance with gated cardiac blood pool imaging following aortocoronary bypass surgery, *Am Heart J* 101:59, 1981.
45. Mangano DT: Biventricular function after myocardial revascularization in humans: Deterioration and recovery patterns during the first 24 hours, *Anesthesiology* 62:571, 1985.
46. Czer L, Hamer A, Murthey F, et al: Transient hemodynamic dysfunction after myocardial revascularization, *J Thorac Cardiovasc Surg* 86:226, 1983.
47. Fremes SE, Weisel RD, Mickle DG, et al: Myocardial metabolism and ventricular function following cold potassium cardioplegia, *J Thorac Cardiovasc Surg* 89:531, 1985.
48. Codd JE, Barner HB, Pennington DG, et al: Intraoperative myocardial protection: Comparison of blood and asanguineous cardioplegia, *Ann Thorac Surg* 39:125, 1985.
49. Roberts AJ, Woodhall DD, Knauf DG, Alexander JA: Coronary artery bypass graft surgery: Clinical comparison of cold blood potassium cardioplegia, warm cardioplegic induction, and secondary cardioplegia, *Ann Thorac Surg* 40:483, 1985.
50. Mullen JC, Christakis GT, Weisel RD, et al: Late postoperative ventricular function after blood and crystalloid cardioplegia, *Circulation* 74(Suppl III):89, 1986.
51. Rousou JA, Engleman RM, Breyer RH, et al: The effect of temperature and hematocrit level of oxygenated cardioplegic solutions of myocardial preservation, *J Thorac Cardiovasc Surg* 95:625, 1988.
52. Khuri SF, Warner KG, Josa M, et al: The superiority of continuous cold blood cardioplegia in the metabolic protection of the hypertrophied human heart, *J Thorac Cardiovasc Surg* 95:442, 1988.
53. Phillips HR, Carter JE, Okada RD, et al: Serial changes in left ventricular ejection in the early hours after aortocoronary bypass grafting, *Chest* 83:28, 1983.
54. Salerno TA, Houck JP, Barrozo CAM, et al: Retrograde continuous warm blood cardioplegia: A new concept in myocardial protection, *Ann Thorac Surg* 51:245, 1991.
55. Leung JM, O'Kelly B, Browner WS, et al: Prognostic importance of postbypass regional wall-motion abnormalities in patients undergoing coronary artery bypass graft surgery, *Anesthesiology* 71:16, 1989.
56. Shernan SK: Perioperative myocardial ischemia reperfusion injury, *Anesthesiol Clin North America* 21:465, 2003.
57. Verrier ED, Shernan SK, Taylor KM: Terminal complement blockade with pexelizumab during coronary artery bypass graft surgery requiring cardiopulmonary bypass: A randomized trial, *JAMA* 291:2319, 2004.
58. Bolli R: Oxygen-derived free radicals and postischemic myocardial dysfunction, *J Am Coll Cardiol* 12:239, 1988.
59. Entman M, Michael M, Rossen R, et al: Inflammation in the course of early myocardial ischemia, *FASEB J* 5:2529, 1991.
60. Maxwell S, Lip G: Reperfusion injury: A review of the pathophysiology, clinical manifestations and therapeutic options, *Int J Cardiol* 58:95, 1997.
61. Shernan SK, Fitch JC, Nussmeier NA, et al: Impact of pexelizumab, an anti-C5 complement antibody, on total mortality and adverse cardiovascular outcomes in cardiac surgical patients undergoing cardiopulmonary bypass, *Ann Thorac Surg* 77:942, 2004.
62. Jain U, Laflamme CJA, Aggarwal A, et al: Electrocardiographic and hemodynamic changes and their association with myocardial infarction during coronary artery bypass surgery, *Anesthesiology* 86:576, 1997.
63. Mangano DT, Siciliano D, Hollenberg M, et al: Postoperative myocardial ischemia. Therapeutic trials using intensive analgesia following surgery, *Anesthesiology* 76:342, 1992.
64. Cheng DCH, Karski J, Peniston C, et al: Morbidity outcome in early versus conventional tracheal extubation after coronary artery bypass grafting: A prospective randomized controlled trial, *J Thorac Cardiovasc Surg* 112:755, 1996.
65. Wahr JA, Plunkett JJ, Ramsay JG, et al: Cardiovascular responses during sedation after coronary revascularization, *Anesthesiology* 84:1350, 1996.

66. Rahimtoola SH, Ehsani A, Sinno MZ, et al: Left atrial transport function in myocardial infarction: Importance of its booster function, *Am J Med* 59:686, 1975.
67. Mathew JP, Fontes ML, Tudor IC, et al: A multicenter risk index for atrial fibrillation after cardiac surgery, *JAMA* 291:1720, 2004.
68. Hill LL, Kattapuram M, Hogue CW: Management of atrial fibrillation after cardiac surgery. Part 1. Pathophysiology and risks, *J Cardiothorac Vasc Anesth* 16:483, 2002.
69. Van Dijk D, Nierich AP, Jansen EWL, et al: Early outcome after off-pump versus on-pump coronary bypass surgery, *Circulation* 104:1761, 2001.
70. Puskas JD, Williams WH, Mahoney EM, et al: Off-pump versus conventional coronary artery bypass grafting: Early and 1-year graft patency, cost, and quality of life outcomes, *JAMA* 291:1841, 2004.
71. Fuster V, Ryden LE, Asinger RW, et al: ACC/AHA/ECC guidelines for the management of patients with atrial fibrillation (executive summary), *J Am Coll Cardiol* 38:1231, 2001.
72. Hill LL, De Wet C, Hogue CW: Management of atrial fibrillation after cardiac surgery. Part II. Prevention and treatment, *J Cardiothorac Vasc Anesth* 16:626, 2002.
73. Mitchell LB, Exner DV, Wyse DG, et al: Prophylactic Oral Amiodarone for the Prevention of Arrhythmias that Begin Early After Revascularization, Valve Replacement, or Repair: PAPABEAR: A randomized controlled trial, *JAMA* 294:3093, 2005.
74. Guarnieri T, Nolan S, Gottlieb SO, et al: Intravenous amiodarone for the prevention of atrial fibrillation after open heart surgery: The Amiodarone Reduction in Coronary Heart (ARCH) trial, *J Am Coll Cardiol* 34:343, 1999.
75. Sarnoff ST, Berglund E: Ventricular function. I. Starling's law of the heart studied by means of simultaneous right and left ventricular function curves in the dog, *Circulation* 9:706, 1954.
76. Urbanowicz JH, Shaaban MJ, Cohen NH, et al: Comparison of transesophageal echocardiographic and scintigraphic estimates of left ventricular end-diastolic volume index and ejection fraction in patients following coronary artery bypass grafting, *Anesthesiology* 72:607, 1990.
77. Harpole DH, Clements FM, Quill T, et al: Right and left ventricular performance during and after abdominal aortic aneurysm repair, *Ann Surg* 209:356, 1989.
78. Thys DM, Hillel Z, Goldman ME, et al: A comparison of hemodynamic indices derived by invasive monitoring and two-dimensional echocardiography, *Anesthesiology* 67:630, 1987.
79. Smith MD, MacPhail B, Harrison MR, et al: Value and limitations of transesophageal echocardiography in determination of left ventricular volumes and ejection fraction, *J Am Coll Cardiol* 19:1213, 1992.
80. Ellis RJ, Mangano DT, Van Dyke DC: Relationship of wedge pressure to end-diastolic volume in patients undergoing myocardial revascularization, *J Thorac Cardiovasc Surg* 78:605, 1974.
81. Calvin JE, Driedger AA, Sibbald WJ: Does the pulmonary capillary wedge pressure predict left ventricular preload in critically ill patients? *Crit Care Med* 9:437, 1981.
82. Mangano DT, Van Dyke DC, Ellis RJ: The effect of increasing preload on ventricular output and ejection in man, *Circulation* 62:535, 1980.
83. Breisblatt WM, Vita N, Armuchastegui M, et al: Usefulness of serial radionuclide monitoring during graded nitroglycerin infusion for unstable angina pectoris for determining left ventricular function and individualized therapeutic dose, *Am J Cardiol* 61:685, 1988.
84. Bouchard MJ, Denault A, Couture P, et al: Poor correlation between hemodynamic and echocardiographic indexes of left ventricular performance in the operating room and intensive care unit, *Crit Care Med* 32:644, 2004.
85. Breisblatt WM, Navratil DL, Burns MJ, Spaccavento LJ: Comparable effects of intravenous nitroglycerin and intravenous nitroprusside in acute ischemia, *Am Heart J* 116:465, 1988.
86. Ghani MF, Parker BM, Smith JR: Recognition of myocardial infarction after cardiac surgery and its relation to cardiopulmonary bypass, *Am Heart J* 88:18, 1974.
87. Chiarello M, Gold WK, Leinbach RC, et al: Comparison between the effects of nitroprusside and nitroglycerin on ischemic injury during acute myocardial infarction, *Circulation* 54:766, 1976.
88. Marchionni N, Schneeweiss A, Di Bari M, et al: Age-related hemodynamic effects of intravenous nitroglycerin for acute myocardial infarction and left ventricular failure, *Am J Cardiol* 61:81E, 1988.
89. Natarajan D, Khurana TR, Karnade V, et al: Sustained hemodynamic effects with therapeutic doses of intravenous nitroglycerin in congestive heart failure, *Am J Cardiol* 62:319, 1988.
90. Katz AM: Cardiomyopathy of overload: A major determinant of prognosis in congestive heart failure, *N Engl J Med* 322:100, 1990.
91. Muir AL, Nolan J: Modulation of venous tone in heart failure, *Am Heart J* 6:1948, 1991.
92. Dikshit K, Vyden JK, Forrester JS, et al: Renal and extrarenal hemodynamic effects of furosemide in congestive heart failure after acute myocardial infarction, *N Engl J Med* 288:1087, 1973.
93. Copeland JG, Campbell DW, Plachetka JR, et al: Diuresis with continuous infusion of furosemide after cardiac surgery, *Am J Surg* 146:796, 1983.
94. Krasna MJ, Scott GE, Scholz PM, et al: Postoperative enhancement of urinary output in patients with acute renal failure using continuous furosemide therapy, *Chest* 89:294, 1986.
95. Adams KF, Mathur VS, Gheorghiade M: B-type natriuretic peptide: From bench to bedside, *Am Heart J* 145:S34, 2003.
96. Moazami N, Damiano DJ, Bailey MS, et al: Nesiritide (BNP) in the management of postoperative cardiac patients, *Ann Thorac Surg* 75:1974, 2003.
97. Sward K, Valsson F, Odencrants P, et al: Recombinant human atrial natriuretic peptide in ischemic acute renal failure: A randomized placebo-controlled trial, *Crit Care Med* 32:1310, 2004.
98. Caver A, Saccaggi A, Ronco C, et al: Continuous arteriovenous hemofiltration in the critically ill patient. Clinical use and operational characteristics, *Ann Intern Med* 99:455, 1983.
99. Lamer C, Valleaux T, Plaisance P, et al: Continuous arteriovenous hemodialysis for acute renal failure after cardiac operations [Letter], *J Thorac Cardiovasc Surg* 99:175, 1990.
100. Sagawa K: The end-systolic pressure-volume relation of the ventricle: Definition, modifications, and clinical use, *Circulation* 63:1223, 1981.
101. Suga H, Sagawa K, Shoukas AA: Load independence of the instantaneous pressure-volume ratio of the canine left ventricle and effects of epinephrine and heart rate on the ratio, *Circ Res* 32:314, 1973.
102. Kass DA, Maughan WL: From "Emax" to pressure-volume relations: A broader view, *Circulation* 77:1203, 1988.
103. Glower DD, Spratt JA, Snow ND, et al: Linearity of the Frank-Starling relationship in the intact heart: The concept of preload recruitable stroke work, *Circulation* 71:994, 1985.
104. Hettrick DA, Warltier DC: Ventriculoarterial coupling. In Warltier DC, editor: *Ventricular Function*, Baltimore, 1995, Williams & Wilkins, pp 153–179.
105. Sunagawa K, Maughan WL, Sagawa K: Optimal arterial resistance for the maximal stroke work studied in isolated canine left ventricle, *Circ Res* 56:586, 1985.
106. Urzua J, Meneses G, Fajardo C, et al: Arterial pressure-flow relationships in patients undergoing cardiopulmonary bypass, *Anesth Analg* 84:958, 1997.
107. Estafanous FG, Tarazi RC: Systemic arterial hypertension associated with cardiac surgery, *Am J Cardiol* 46:685, 1980.
108. Roberts AJ, Niarchos AP, Subramanian VA, et al: Systemic hypertension associated with coronary artery bypass surgery. Predisposing factors, hemodynamic characteristics, humoral profile, and treatment, *J Thorac Cardiovasc Surg* 74:846, 1977.
109. Vuylsteke A, Feneck RO, Jolin-Mellgard A, et al: Perioperative blood pressure control: A prospective survey of patient management in cardiac surgery, *J Cardiothorac Vasc Anesth* 14:269, 2000.
110. Wallach R, Karp RB, Reves JG, et al: Pathogenesis of paroxysmal hypertension developing during and after coronary bypass surgery: A study of hemodynamic and humoral factors, *Am J Cardiol* 46:559, 1980.
111. Stinson EB, Holloway EL, Derby GC, et al: Control of myocardial performance early after open-heart operations by vasodilator treatment, *J Thorac Cardiovasc Surg* 73:523, 1977.
112. Aronson S, Boisvert D, Lapp W: Isolated systolic hypertension is associated with adverse outcomes from coronary artery bypass grafting surgery, *Anesth Analg* 94:1079, 2002.
113. Roberts AJ, Niarchos AP, Subramanian VA, et al: Hypertension following coronary artery bypass surgery. Comparison of hemodynamic responses to nitroprusside, phentolamine and converting enzyme inhibitor, *Circulation* 58(Suppl I):49, 1978.
114. Becker LC: Conditions of vasodilator-induced coronary steal in experimental myocardial ischemia, *Circulation* 57:1103, 1978.
115. Flaherty JT, MaGee PA, Gardner TL, et al: Comparison of intravenous nitroglycerin and sodium nitroprusside for treatment of acute hypertension developing after coronary artery bypass surgery, *Circulation* 65:1072, 1982.
116. Gray RJ, Bateman JM, Czer LSC, et al: Comparison of esmolol and nitroprusside for acute postcardiac surgical hypertension, *Am J Cardiol* 59:887, 1987.
117. Morel DR, Forster A, Suter PM: IV labetalol in the treatment of hypertension following coronary artery surgery, *Br J Anaesth* 54:1191, 1982.
118. David D, Dubois C, Loria Y: Comparison of nicardipine and sodium nitroprusside in the treatment of paroxysmal hypertension following aortocoronary bypass surgery, *J Cardiothorac Vasc Anesth* 5:357, 1991.
119. Leslie J, Brister NW, Levy JH, et al: Treatment of postoperative hypertension following coronary artery bypass surgery: Double-blind comparison of intravenous isradipine and sodium nitroprusside, *Circulation* 90(Suppl II):256, 1994.
120. Bailey JM, Lu W, Levy JH, et al: Clevidipine in adult cardiac surgical patients: A dose-finding study, *Anesthesiology* 96:1086, 2002.
121. Levy JH, Mancao MY, Gitter R: Clevidipine effectively and rapidly controls blood pressure preoperatively in cardiac surgery patients: Results of the efficacy study of clevidipine assessing its preoperative antihypertensive effect in cardiac surgery-1 (ESCAPE-1) Trial, *Anesth Analg* 105:918–925, 2007.
122. Aronson S, Dyke CM, Stierer KA, et al: The ECLIPSE Trials: Comparative studies of clevidipine to nitroglycerin, sodium nitroprusside, and nicardipine for acute hypertension treatment in cardiac surgery patients, *Anesth Analg* 107:1110–1121, 2008.
123. Singla H, Wartier DC, Gandhi SD, et al: Treatment of Acute Postoperative Hypertension in Cardiac Surgical Patients (ESCAPE 2), *Anesth Analg* 107:59, 2008.
124. Hill AJ, Feneck RO, Walesby RK: A comparison of fenoldopam and nitroprusside in the control of hypertension following coronary artery surgery, *J Cardiothorac Vasc Anesth* 7:279, 1993.
125. Goldberg ME, Cantillo J, Nemiroff MS, et al: Fenoldopam infusion for the treatment of postoperative hypertension, *J Clin Anesth* 5:386, 1993.
126. Levy JH, Huraux C, Nordlander M: Treatment of perioperative hypertension. In Epstein M, editor: *Calcium Antagonists in Clinical Medicine*, Philadelphia, 1997, Hanley & Belfus.
127. Demarco T, Daly PA, Liv N, et al: Enalaprilat, a new parenteral angiotensin-converting enzyme inhibitor: Rapid changes in systemic and coronary hemodynamics and humoral profile in chronic heart failure, *J Am Coll Cardiol* 9:1131, 1987.
128. Mekontso-Dessap A, Houel R, Soustelle C, et al: Risk factors for post-cardiopulmonary bypass vasoplegia in patients with preserved left ventricular function, *Ann Thorac Surg* 71:1428, 2001.
129. Tuman KJ, McCarthy RJ, O'Connor CJ, et al: Angiotensin-converting enzyme inhibitors increase vasoconstrictor requirements after cardiopulmonary bypass, *Anesth Analg* 80:473, 1995.
130. Kristoff AS, Magder S: Low systemic vascular resistance state in patients undergoing cardiopulmonary bypass, *Crit Care Med* 27:1121, 1999.
131. Gomez WJ, Erlichman MR, Batista-Filho ML, et al: Vasoplegic syndrome after off-pump coronary artery bypass surgery, *Eur J Cardiothorac Surg* 23:165, 2003.
132. Biglioli P, Cannata A, Alamanni F, et al: Biological effects of off pump vs on pump coronary artery surgery: Focus on inflammation, hemostasis and oxidative stress, *Eur J Cardiothorac Surg* 24:260, 2003.
133. Gomez WJ, Carvalho AC, Palma JH, et al: Vasoplegic syndrome: A new dilemma, *J Thorac Cardiovasc Surg* 107:942, 1994.
134. Chenoweth DE, Cooper SW, Hugli TE, et al: Complement activation during cardiopulmonary bypass: Evidence of generation of C3a and C5a anaphylatoxins, *N Engl J Med* 304:497, 1981.
135. Landry DW, Oliver JA: The pathogenesis of vasodilatory shock, *N Engl J Med* 345:588, 2001.
136. Haeffner-Cavaillon N, Roussellier N, Ponzio O, et al: Induction of interleukin-1 production in patients undergoing cardiopulmonary bypass, *J Thorac Cardiovasc Surg* 98:1100, 1989.
137. Bennett-Guerrero E, Barclay GR, Weng PL, et al: Endotoxin-neutralizing capacity of serum from cardiac surgical patients, *J Cardiothorac Vasc Anesth* 15:451, 2001.
138. Aydin NB, Gercekoglu H, Aksu B, et al: Endotoxemia in coronary artery bypass surgery: A comparison of the off-pump technique and conventional cardiopulmonary bypass, *J Thorac Cardiovasc Surg* 125:843, 2003.
139. Argenziano M, Chen JM, Choudhri AF, et al: Management of vasodilatory shock after cardiac surgery: Identification of predisposing factors and use of a novel pressor agent, *J Thorac Cardiovasc Surg* 116:973, 1998.
140. Levy JH, Adkinson NF: Anaphylaxis during cardiac surgery: Implications for clinicians, *Anesth Analg* 106:392, 2008.
141. LeDoux D, Astiz ME, Carpati CM, et al: Effects of perfusion pressure on tissue perfusion in septic shock, *Crit Care Med* 28:2729, 2000.
142. Desjars P, Pinaud M, Potel G, et al: A reappraisal of norepinephrine therapy in human septic shock, *Crit Care Med* 15:134, 1987.
143. Levy JH: Treating shock—old drugs, new ideas, *N Engl J Med* 362:841–843, 2010.
144. Addonizio VP, Smith JB, Strauss JF, et al: Thromboxane synthesis and platelet secretion during cardiopulmonary bypass with bubble oxygenator, *J Thorac Cardiovasc Surg* 79:91, 1980.
145. Engelman RM, Harji-Rovsov I, Breyer RH, et al: Rebound vasospasm after coronary revascularization, *Ann Thorac Surg* 37:469, 1984.
146. Salmenpera MT, Levy JH: Effects of phosphodiesterase inhibitors on the human internal mammary artery, *Anesth Analg* 82:954, 1996.
147. Huraux C, Makita T, Szlam F, et al: Vasodilator effects of clevidipine on human internal mammary artery, *Anesth Analg* 85:1000, 1997.
148. Acar C, Jebara VA, Portoghese M, et al: Revival of the radial artery for coronary artery bypass grafting, *Ann Thorac Surg* 54:652, 1992.
149. da Costa FDA, da Costa IA, Poffo R, et al: Myocardial revascularization with the radial artery: A clinical and angiographic study, *Ann Thorac Surg* 62:475, 1996.
150. Dietl CA, Benoit CH: Radial artery graft for coronary revascularization: Technical considerations, *Ann Thorac Surg* 60:102, 1995.
151. Royster RL, Butterworth J.F.I.V., Prielipp RC, et al: A randomized, blinded, placebo-controlled evaluation of calcium chloride and epinephrine for inotropic support after emergence from cardiopulmonary bypass, *Anesth Analg* 74:3, 1992.
152. Zaloga GP, Strickland RA, Butterworth J.F.I.V., et al: Calcium attenuated epinephrine's beta-adrenergic effects in postoperative heart surgery patients, *Circulation* 81:196, 1991.
153. Drop LJ: Ionized calcium, the heart, and hemodynamic function, *Anesth Analg* 64:432, 1985.
154. Bristow MR, Ginsburg R, Umans V, et al: β_1- and β_2-adrenergic receptor subpopulations in normal and failing human ventricular myocardium. Coupling of both receptor subtypes to muscle contraction and selective β_1-receptor down-regulation in heart failure, *Circ Res* 59:297, 1986.
155. Levy JH, Bailey JM, Deeb M: Intravenous milrinone in cardiac surgery, *Ann Thorac Surg* 73:325, 2002.

156. Stephenson LW, Blackstone EH, Kouchoukos NT: Dopamine vs. epinephrine in patients following cardiac surgery: Randomized study, *Surg Forum* 27:272, 1976.
157. Butterworth JF, Prielipp RC, Zaloga GP, et al: Is dobutamine less chronotropic than epinephrine after coronary bypass surgery? *Anesthesiology* 73(Suppl 3A):A61, 1990.
158. Sung BH, Robinson C, Thadani U, et al: Effects of L-epinephrine on hemodynamics and cardiac function in coronary disease: Dose-response studies, *Clin Pharmacol Ther* 43:308, 1988.
159. Totaro RJ, Raper RF: Epinephrine-induced lactic acidosis following cardiopulmonary bypass, *Crit Care Med* 25:1693, 1997.
160. Albanese J, Leone M, Garnier F, et al: Renal effects of norepinephrine in septic and nonseptic patients, *Chest* 126:534, 2004.
161. De Backer D, Biston P, Devriendt J, et al: Comparison of dopamine and norepinephrine in the treatment of shock, *N Engl J Med* 362:779–789, 2010.
162. Leier CV, Heran PT, Huss P, et al: Comparative systemic and regional hemodynamic effects of dopamine and dobutamine in patients with cardiomyopathic heart failure, *Circulation* 58:466, 1978.
163. Port JD, Gilbert EM, Larrabee P, et al: Neurotransmitter depletion compromises the ability of indirect acting amines to provide inotropic support in the failing human heart, *Circulation* 81:929, 1990.
164. Lehmann A, Boldt J: New pharmacologic approaches for the perioperative treatment of ischemic cardiogenic shock, *J Cardiothorac Vasc Anesth* 19:97, 2005.
165. DiSesa V, Gold J, Shemin R, et al: Comparison of dopamine and dobutamine in patients requiring postoperative circulatory support, *Clin Cardiol* 9:253, 1986.
166. Royster RL: Intraoperative administration of inotropes in cardiac surgery patients, *J Cardiothorac Anesth* 4:17, 1990.
167. Davis RF, Cappas DG, Kirklin JK, et al: Acute oliguria after cardiopulmonary bypass: Renal functional improvement with low-dose dopamine infusion, *Crit Care Med* 10:852, 1982.
168. Bellomo R, Chapman M, Finfer S, et al: Low-dose dopamine in patients with early renal dysfunction: A placebo-controlled randomized trial: Australian and New Zealand Intensive Care Society (ANZICS) Clinical Trials Group, *Lancet* 356:2139, 2000.
169. Holmes C, Walley KR: Bad medicine: Low-dose dopamine in the ICU, *Crit Care Med* 123:1266, 2003.
170. Ward HB, Einzig S, Wang T, et al: Enhanced cardiac efficiency with dobutamine after global ischemia, *J Surg Res* 33:32, 1982.
171. Stephens J, Ead H, Spurrell R: Haemodynamic effects of dobutamine with special reference to myocardial blood flow: A comparison with dopamine and isoprenaline, *Br Heart J* 42:269, 1981.
172. Fowler MB, Alderman EL, Oesterle SN, et al: Dobutamine and dopamine after cardiac surgery: Greater augmentation of myocardial blood flow with dobutamine, *Circulation* 70(Suppl I):103, 1984.
173. Romson JL, Leung JM, Bellows WH, et al: Effects of dobutamine on hemodynamics and left ventricular performance after cardiopulmonary bypass in cardiac surgical patients, *Anesthesiology* 91:1318, 1999.
174. Salomon NW, Plachetka JR, Copeland JG: Comparison of dopamine and dobutamine following coronary artery bypass grafting, *Ann Thorac Surg* 33:48, 1982.
175. Bristow MR, Ginsburg R, Minobe W, et al: Decreased catecholamine sensitivity and beta-adrenergic receptor density in failing human hearts, *N Engl J Med* 307:205, 1982.
176. Gain KR, Appleman MM: Distribution and regulation of the phosphodiesterases of muscle tissues, *Adv Cyclic Nucleotide Res* 10:221, 1978.
177. Weishaar RE, Burrows SD, Kobylarz DC, et al: Multiple molecular forms of cyclic nucleotide phosphodiesterase in cardiac and smooth muscle and in platelets. Isolation, characterization, and effects of various reference phosphodiesterase inhibitors and cardiotonic agents, *Biochem Pharmacol* 35:787, 1986.
178. Archer SL, Michelakis ED: Phosphodiesterase type 5 inhibitors for pulmonary arterial hypertension, *N Engl J Med* 361:1864, 2009.
179. Benotti JR, Grossman W, Braunwald E, et al: Hemodynamic assessment of amrinone, *N Engl J Med* 299:1373, 1987.
180. Levy JL, Bailey JM: Amrinone: Its effects on vascular resistance and capacitance in human subjects, *Chest* 105:62, 1994.
181. Benotti JR, Grossman W, Braunwald E, et al: Effects of amrinone on myocardial energy metabolism and hemodynamics in patients with severe congestive heart failure due to coronary artery disease, *Circulation* 62:28, 1980.
182. Galie N, Ghofrani HA, Torbicki A, et al: Sildenafil citrate therapy for pulmonary arterial hypertension, *N Engl J Med* 353:2148, 2005.
183. Bailey JM, Levy JH, Kikura M, et al: Pharmacokinetics of milrinone during cardiac surgery, *Anesthesiology* 81:616, 1994.
184. Konstam MA, Cohen SR, Weiland DS, et al: Relative contribution of inotropic and vasodilator effects to amrinone-induced hemodynamic improvement in congestive heart failure, *Am J Cardiol* 57:242, 1986.
185. Firth BG, Ratner AV, Grassman ED, et al: Assessment of the inotropic and vasodilator effects of amrinone versus isoproterenol, *Am J Cardiol* 54:1331, 1984.
186. Baim DS, McDowell AV, Cherniles J, et al: Evaluation of a new bipyridine inotropic agent—Milrinone—in patients with severe congestive heart failure, *N Engl J Med* 309:748, 1983.
187. Gonzalez M, Desager J-P, Jacquemart J-L, et al: Efficacy of enoximone in the management of refractory low-output states following cardiac surgery, *J Cardiothorac Anesth* 2:409, 1988.
188. Boldt J, Kling D, Zickmann B, et al: Efficacy of the phosphodiesterase inhibitor enoximone in complicated cardiac surgery, *Chest* 98:53, 1990.
189. Kikura M, Lee MK, Safon R, et al: Effect of milrinone on platelets in patients undergoing cardiac surgery, *Anesth Analg* 81:44, 1995.
190. Gilbert EM, Mealey P, Volkman K, et al: Combination therapy with enoximone and dobutamine is superior to nitroprusside and dobutamine in heart failure, *Circulation* 78:109, 1988.
191. Gage J, Rutman H, Lucido D, et al: Additive effects of dobutamine and amrinone on myocardial contractility and ventricular performance in patients with severe heart failure, *Circulation* 74:367, 1986.
192. Prielipp RC, MacGregor DA, Butterworth JF, et al: Pharmacodynamics and pharmacokinetics of milrinone administration to increase oxygen delivery in critically ill patients, *Chest* 109:1291, 1996.
193. Boldt J, Kling D, Moosdorf R, Hempelmann G: Enoximone treatment of impaired myocardial function during cardiac surgery: Combined effects with epinephrine, *J Cardiothorac Anesth* 4:462, 1990.
194. Kikura M, Levy JH, Bailey JM, et al: Effects of milrinone on ventricular function after emergence from cardiopulmonary bypass, *Anesth Analg* 85:16, 1997.
195. Kikura M, Levy JH, Bailey JM, et al: A bolus dose of 1.5mg/kg amrinone effectively improves low cardiac output state following separation from cardiopulmonary bypass in cardiac surgical patients, *Acta Anaesthesiol Scand* 42:825, 1998.
196. Bondy R, Ramsay JG: Reversal of refractory right ventricular failure with amrinone, *J Cardiothorac Anesth* 5:255, 1991.
197. Edelson J, LeJemtel TH, Alousi AA, et al: Relationship between amrinone plasma concentration and cardiac index, *Clin Pharmacol Ther* 29:723, 1981.
198. Park GB, Kershner RP, Angelotti J, et al: Oral bioavailability and intravenous pharmacokinetics of amrinone in humans, *J Pharm Sci* 72:817, 1983.
199. Kikura M, Levy JH: New cardiac drugs, *Int Anesthesiol Clin* 33:21, 1995.
200. Rocci ML, Wilson H, Likoff M, et al: Amrinone pharmacokinetics after single and steady-state doses in patients with chronic cardiac failure, *Clin Pharmacol Ther* 33:260, 1983.
201. Bailey JM, Levy JH, Rogers G, et al: Pharmacokinetics of amrinone during cardiac surgery, *Anesthesiology* 75:961, 1991.
202. Ramsay JG, DeJesus JM, Wynands JE, et al: Amrinone before termination of cardiopulmonary bypass: Hemodynamic variables and oxygen utilization in the postbypass period, *Can J Anaesth* 39:342, 1992.
203. Feneck RO: Effects of variable dose milrinone in patients with low cardiac output after cardiac surgery, *Am Heart J* 121(Suppl 2):1995, 1991.
204. Naeije R, Carlier E, DeSmet JM, et al: Enoximone in low-output states following cardiac surgery, *J Crit Care* 4:112, 1989.
205. Kivikko M, Lehtonen L, Colucci WS, et al: Sustained hemodynamic effects of intravenous levosimendan, *Circulation* 107:81, 2003.
206. Follath F, Cleland JG, Just H, et al: Efficacy and safety of intravenous levosimendan compared with dobutamine in severe low-output heart failure (the LIDO study): A randomized double-blind trial, *Lancet* 360:196, 2002.
207. Moiseyev VS, Poder P, Anderjevs N, et al: Safety and efficacy of a novel calcium sensitizer, levosimendan, in patients with left ventricular failure due to an acute myocardial infarction. A randomized, placebo-controlled, double-blind study (RUSSLAN), *Eur Heart J* 23:1422, 2002.
208. Labriola C, Siro-Brigiani M, Carrata F, et al: Hemodynamic effects of levosimendan in patients with low-output heart failure after cardiac surgery, *Int J Clin Pharmacol Ther* 42:204, 2004.
209. Jacobs A, Leopold J, Bates E, et al: Cardiogenic shock caused by right ventricular infarction: A report from the SHOCK registry, *J Am Coll Cardiol* 41:1273, 2003.
210. Hayashida N, Ikonomidis JS, Weisel RD, et al: Adequate distribution of warm cardioplegic solution, *J Thorac Cardiovasc Surg* 110:800, 1995.
211. Boldt J, Kling D, Thiel A, et al: Revascularization of the right coronary artery: Influence on thermodilution right ventricular ejection fraction, *J Cardiothorac Anesth* 2:140, 1988.
212. Schulman DS, Biondi JW, Zohgbi S, et al: Coronary flow and right ventricular performance during positive end-expiratory pressure, *Am Rev Respir Dis* 141:1531, 1990.
213. Matthay RA, Ellis JH, Steele PP: Methoxamine-induced increase in afterload. Effect on left ventricular performance in chronic obstructive pulmonary disease, *Am Rev Respir Dis* 117:871, 1978.
214. Mikami T, Kudo T, Sakurai N, et al: Mechanisms for development of functional tricuspid regurgitation determined by pulsed Doppler and two-dimensional echocardiography, *Am J Cardiol* 53:160, 1984.
215. Heinonen J, Salmenpera M, Takkunen O: Increased pulmonary artery diastolic-pulmonary wedge pressure gradient after cardiopulmonary bypass, *Can Anaesth Soc J* 32:165, 1985.
216. Byrick RJ, Kay JC, Noble WH: Extravascular lung water accumulation in patients following coronary artery surgery, *Can Anaesth Soc J* 24:332, 1977.
217. Chernow B, Rainey TG, Lake CR: Endogenous and exogenous catecholamines in critical care medicine, *Crit Care Med* 10:407, 1982.
218. Colman RW: Platelet and neutrophil activation in cardiopulmonary bypass, *Ann Thorac Surg* 49:32, 1990.
219. Chenoweth DE, Cooper SW, Hugli TE, et al: Complement activation during cardiopulmonary bypass. Evidence for generation of C3a and C5a anaphylatoxins, *N Engl J Med* 304:497, 1991.
220. Anjoyu-Lindskog E, Broman L, Broman M, Holmgren A: Effects of oxygen on central hemodynamics and VA/Q distribution after coronary bypass surgery, *Acta Anaesthesiol Scand* 27:378, 1983.
221. Salmenpera M, Heinonen J: Pulmonary vascular responses to moderate changes in $Paco_2$ after cardiopulmonary bypass, *Anesthesiology* 64:311, 1986.
222. Viitanen A, Salmenpera M, Hynynen M, Heinonen J: Pulmonary vascular resistance before and after cardiopulmonary bypass. The effect of $Paco_2$, *Chest* 95:773, 1989.
223. Viitanen A, Salmenpera M, Heinonen J: Right ventricular response to hypercarbia after cardiac surgery, *Anesthesiology* 73:393, 1990.
224. Lloyd EA, Gersh BJ, Kennelly BM: Hemodynamic spectrum of "dominant" right ventricular infarction in 19 patients, *Am J Cardiol* 48:1016, 1981.
225. Kay H, Afshari M, Barash P, et al: Measurement of ejection fraction by thermal dilution techniques, *J Surg Res* 34:337, 1983.
226. Spinale FG, Smith AC, Carabello BA, Crawford FA: Right ventricular function computed by thermodilution and ventriculography; a comparison of methods, *J Thorac Cardiovasc Surg* 99:141, 1990.
227. Dell'Italia LJ, Starling MR, Blumhardt R, et al: Comparative effects of volume loading, dobutamine, and nitroprusside in patients with predominant right ventricular infarction, *Circulation* 72:1327, 1985.
228. Berisha S, Kastrati A, Goda A, Popa Y: Optimal value of filling pressure in the right side of the heart in acute myocardial infarction, *Br Heart J* 63:98, 1990.
229. Brinker JA, Weiss JL, Lapp DL, et al: Leftward septal displacement during right ventricular loading in man, *Circulation* 61:626, 1980.
230. D'Ambra MN, LaRaia PJ, Philbin DM, et al: Prostaglandin E_1—a new therapy for refractory right heart failure and pulmonary hypertension after mitral valve replacement, *J Thorac Cardiovasc Surg* 89:567, 1985.
231. Ichinose F, Roberts JD, Zapol WM: Inhaled nitric oxide: A selective pulmonary vasodilator; current uses and therapeutic potential, *Circulation* 109:3106, 2004.
232. De Wet CJ, Affleck DG, Jacobsohn E, et al: Inhaled prostacyclin is safe, effective, and affordable in patients with pulmonary hypertension, right heart dysfunction, and refractory hypoxemia after cardiothoracic surgery, *J Thorac Cardiovasc Surg* 127:1058, 2004.
233. Girard C, Lehot J-J, Pannetier J-C, et al: Inhaled nitric oxide after mitral valve replacement in patients with chronic pulmonary artery hypertension, *Anesthesiology* 77:880, 1992.
234. Ardehali A, Hughes K, Sadeghi A, et al: Inhaled nitric oxide for pulmonary hypertension after cardiac transplantation, *Transplantation* 72:638, 2001.
235. Argenziano M, Choudhri AF, Moazami N, et al: Randomized, double-blind trial of inhaled nitric oxide in LVAD recipients with pulmonary hypertension, *Ann Thorac Surg* 65:340, 1998.
236. Meade MO, Granton JT, Matte-Martyn A, et al: A randomized trial of inhaled nitric oxide to prevent ischemia-reperfusion injury after lung transplantation, *Am J Respir Crit Care Med* 167:1483, 2003.
237. Haraldsson A, Kieler-Jensen N, Ricksten S-E: Inhaled prostacyclin for treatment of pulmonary hypertension after cardiac surgery or heart transplantation: A pharmacodynamic study, *J Cardiothorac Vasc Anesth* 10:864, 1996.
238. Webb SA, Scott S, van Heerden PV: The use of inhaled aerosolized prostacyclin (IAP) in the treatment of pulmonary hypertension secondary to pulmonary embolism, *Intensive Care Med* 22:353, 1996.
239. Heerden PV, Barden A, Michalopoulos N, et al: Dose-response to inhaled aerosolized prostacyclin for hypoxemia due to ARDS, *Chest* 117:819, 2000.
240. Domenighetti G, Stricker H, Waldispuehl B: Nebulized prostacyclin (PGI_2) in acute respiratory distress syndrome: Impact of primary (pulmonary injury) and secondary (extrapulmonary injury) on gas exchange response, *Crit Care Med* 29:57, 2001.
241. Haraldsson A, Kieler-Jensen N, Ricksten SE: The additive pulmonary vasodilatory effects of inhaled prostacyclin and inhaled milrinone in postcardiac surgical patients with pulmonary hypertension, *Anesth Analg* 93:1439, 2001.
242. Drummond WH, Gregory GA, Heyman MA, Phibbs RA: The independent effects of hyperventilation, tolazoline, and dopamine on infants with persistent pulmonary hypertension, *J Pediatr* 98:603, 1981.

243. Mahdi M, Salem MR, Joseph NJ, et al: Influence of moderate hypocapnia on pulmonary vascular tone following mitral valve replacement, *Anesthesiology* 75:A166, 1991.
244. Miller DC, Moreno-Cabral RJ, Stinson EB, et al: Pulmonary artery balloon counterpulsation for acute right ventricular infarction, *J Thorac Cardiovasc Surg* 80:760, 1980.
245. Higgins TL, Yared JP, Paranandi L, et al: Risk factors for respiratory complications after cardiac surgery, *Anesthesiology* 75:A258, 1991.
246. Vuori A, Jalonen J, Laaksonen V: Continuous positive airway pressure during mechanical ventilation and spontaneous ventilation: Effects on central hemodynamics and oxygen transport, *Acta Anaesthesiol Scand* 23:453, 1979.
247. Morgan BC, Abel FL, Mullins GL, Guntheroth WG: Flow patterns in cavae, pulmonary artery, pulmonary vein and aorta in intact dogs, *Am J Physiol* 210:903, 1966.
248. Harken HA, Brennan MF, Smith B, Barsamian EM: The hemodynamic response to positive end-expiratory pressure ventilation in hypovolemic patients, *Surgery* 76:786, 1974.
249. Wallis TW, Robotham JL, Compean R, Kindred MK: Mechanical heart-lung interaction with positive end-expiratory pressure, *J Appl Physiol* 54:1039, 1983.
250. Pinsky MR, Matuschak GM, Klain M: Determinants of cardiac augmentation by elevations in intrathoracic pressure, *J Appl Physiol* 58:1189, 1985.
251. Canada E, Benumof JL, Tousdale FR: Pulmonary vascular resistance correlates in intact normal and abnormal canine lungs, *Crit Care Med* 10:719, 1982.
252. Permutt S, Howell JBL, Proctor DF, Riley RL: Effect of lung inflation on static pressure-volume characteristics of pulmonary vessels, *J Appl Physiol* 16:64, 1961.
253. McGregor M: Pulsus paradoxus, *N Engl J Med* 301:480, 1979.
254. Grace MP, Greenbaum DM: Cardiac performance in response to PEEP in patients with cardiac dysfunction, *Crit Care Med* 10:358, 1982.
255. Mathru M, Rao TLK, El-Etr AA, Pifarre R: Hemodynamic response to changes in ventilatory patterns in patients with normal and poor left ventricular reserve, *Crit Care Med* 10:423, 1982.
256. Schulman DS, Biondi JW, Matthay RA, et al: Effect of positive end-expiratory pressure on right ventricular performance-importance of baseline right ventricular function, *Am J Med* 84:57, 1988.
257. Calvin JE, Driedger AA, Sibbald WJ: Positive end-expiratory pressure (PEEP) does not depress left ventricular function in patients with pulmonary edema, *Am Rev Respir Dis* 124:121, 1981.
258. Glick G, Wechsler AS, Epstein SE: Reflex cardiovascular depression produced by stimulation of pulmonary stretch receptors in the dog, *J Clin Invest* 48:467, 1979.
259. Dunham BM, Grindlinger GA, Utsunomiya T, et al: Role of prostaglandins in positive end-expiratory pressure-induced negative inotropism, *Am J Physiol* 241:783, 1981.
260. Pinsky MR, Marquez J, Martin D, Klain M: Ventricular assist by cardiac cycle–specific increases in intrathoracic pressure, *Chest* 91:709, 1987.
261. Garner W, Downs JB, Stock MC, Rasanen J: Airway pressure release ventilation (APRV)—a human trial, *Chest* 94:779, 1988.
262. Cane RD, Shapiro BA: Ventilator discontinuance and weaning, *Anesthesiol Clin North America* 5:749, 1987.
263. Lemaire F, Teboul J-L, Cinotti L, et al: Acute left ventricular dysfunction during unsuccessful weaning from mechanical ventilation, *Anesthesiology* 69:171, 1988.
264. Permutt S: Circulatory effects of weaning from mechanical ventilation: The importance of transdiaphragmatic pressure, *Anesthesiology* 69:157, 1988.
265. Rasanen J, Nikki P, Heikkila J: Acute myocardial infarction complicated by respiratory failure. The effects of mechanical ventilation, *Chest* 85:21, 1984.
266. Hurford WE, Lynch KE, Strauss W, et al: Myocardial perfusion as assessed by thallium 201 scintigraphy during the discontinuance of mechanical ventilation in ventilator-dependent patients, *Anesthesiology* 74:1007, 1991.
267. Tahvanainen J, Salmenpera M, Nikki P: Extubation criteria after weaning from intermittent mandatory ventilation and continuous positive airway pressure, *Crit Care Med* 11:702, 1983.
268. Russo A, O'Connor W, Waxman H: Atypical presentations and echocardiographic findings in patients with cardiac tamponade occurring early and late after cardiac surgery, *Chest* 104:71, 1993.
269. Yilmaz AT, Arslan M, Demirklic U, et al: Late posterior cardiac tamponade after open heart surgery, *J Cardiovasc Surg* 37:615, 1996.
270. Borkon AM, Schaff HV, Gardner TI, et al: Diagnosis and management of postoperative pericardial effusions and late cardiac tamponade following open heart surgery, *Ann Thorac Surg* 31:512, 1981.
271. King TE, Stelzner TJ, Steven A, Sahn SA: Cardiac tamponade complicating the postpericardiotomy syndrome, *Chest* 83:500, 1983.
272. Chuttani K, Pandian NG, Mohanty PK, et al: Left ventricular diastolic collapse. An echocardiographic sign of regional cardiac tamponade, *Circulation* 83:1999, 1991.
273. Fowler NO: Physiology of cardiac tamponade and pulsus paradoxus. Physiological, circulatory, and pharmacologic responses in cardiac tamponade, *Mod Concepts Cardiovasc Dis* 47:115, 1978.
274. Hynynen M, Salmenpera M, Harjula ALJ, et al: Atrial pressure and hormonal and renal responses to acute cardiac tamponade, *Ann Thorac Surg* 49:632, 1990.
275. Kochar GS, Jacobs LE, Kotler MN: Right atrial compression in postoperative cardiac patients: Detection by transesophageal echocardiography, *J Am Coll Cardiol* 16:511, 1990.
276. Bommer WJ, Follette D, Pollock M, et al: Tamponade in patients undergoing cardiac surgery: A clinical-echocardiographic diagnosis, *Am Heart J* 130:1216, 1995.
277. Chuttani K, Tischler MD, Pandian NG, et al: Diagnosis of cardiac tamponade after cardiac surgery: Relative value of clinical, echocardiographic, and hemodynamic signs, *Am Heart J* 127:913, 1994.
278. D'Cruz IA, Kensey K, Campbell C, et al: Two-dimensional echocardiography in cardiac tamponade occurring after cardiac surgery, *J Am Coll Cardiol* 5:1250, 1985.
279. Reichert CL, Visser CA, Koolen JJ, et al: Transesophageal echocardiography in hypotensive patients after cardiac operations. Comparison with hemodynamic parameters, *J Thorac Cardiovasc Surg* 104:321, 1992.
280. Settle HP, Adolph RJ, Fowler NO, et al: Echocardiographic study of cardiac tamponade, *Circulation* 56:951, 1977.
281. Singh SM, Wann LS, Schuchard GH, et al: Right ventricular and right atrial collapse in patients with cardiac tamponade—a combined echocardiographic and hemodynamic study, *Circulation* 70:966, 1984.
282. Russo AM, O'Connor WH, Waxman HL: Atypical presentations and echocardiographic findings in patients with cardiac tamponade occurring early and late after cardiac surgery, *Chest* 104:71, 1993.
283. Mattila I, Takkunen O, Mattila P, et al: Cardiac tamponade and different modes of artificial ventilation, *Acta Anaesthesiol Scand* 23:236, 1984.
284. Ziemer G, Karck M, Muller H, Luhmer I: Staged chest closure in pediatric cardiac surgery preventing typical and atypical cardiac tamponade, *Eur J Cardiothorac Surg* 6:91, 1992.
285. Addonizio LJ, Gersony WM, Robbins RC, et al: Elevated pulmonary vascular resistance and cardiac transplantation, *Circulation* 76(Suppl V):52, 1987.
286. Valantine HA, Schroeder JS: Cardiac transplantation, *Intensive Care Med* 15:283, 1989.
287. O'Connell JB, Renlund DG, Bristow MR: Murine monoclonal CD3 antibody (OKT3) in cardiac transplantation: Three-year experience, *Transplant Proc* 21(Suppl 2):31, 1989.

35

Postoperative Respiratory Care

THOMAS L. HIGGINS, MD, MBA, FACP, FCCM | JEAN-PIERRE YARED, MD | AHMAD ADI, MD

KEY POINTS

1. Pulmonary complications after cardiopulmonary bypass are relatively common, with up to 12% of patients experiencing acute lung injury and about 1.5% tracheostomy for long-term ventilation.
2. Risk factors for respiratory insufficiency include advanced age, presence of diabetes or renal failure, smoking, chronic obstructive lung disease, peripheral vascular disease, prior cardiac operations, and emergency or unstable status.
3. Patients with preexisting chronic obstructive pulmonary disease have greater rates of pulmonary complications, atrial fibrillation, and death.
4. Operating room events that increase risk include reoperation, blood transfusion, prolonged cardiopulmonary bypass time, and low cardiac output states, particularly if a mechanical support device is required.
5. Transesophageal color-Doppler echocardiography is an important tool for real-time bedside monitoring in the postoperative period and has additional applications in assessing ability to wean from chronic ventilatory support.
6. Hospital-acquired infections are an important cause of postoperative morbidity and nosocomial pneumonia. Strategies to reduce the incidence of ventilator-associated pneumonia include early removal of gastric and tracheal tubes, formal infection control programs, hand washing, semirecumbent positioning of the patient, use of disposable heat and moisture exchangers, and scheduled drainage of condensate from ventilator circuits.
7. Patients at risk for acute lung injury and those experiencing development of acute respiratory distress syndrome should be switched to a lung-protective ventilation strategy, which involves maintaining peak inspiratory pulmonary pressure less than 35 cm H_2O and restricting tidal volumes to less than 6 mL/kg of ideal body weight.
8. Permissive hypercapnia may be necessary to accomplish lung-protective ventilatory strategy. It should be used judiciously in patients with pulmonary hypertension because acidosis can exacerbate pulmonary vasoconstriction and further impair right ventricular function and cardiac output.
9. Impediments to weaning and extubation include delirium, unstable hemodynamics, respiratory muscle dysfunction, renal failure with fluid overload, and sepsis.
10. Short-term weaning success can be achieved with any variety of ventilation modes. The long-term patient requires an individualized approach, which may encompass pressure-support ventilation, synchronized intermittent mandatory ventilation weaning, or T-piece trials.
11. Although a number of parameters exist to assess respiratory strength and endurance, the single best parameter is the frequency-to-tidal volume ratio (f/V_T).
12. Long-term administration of neuromuscular blocking agents is associated with persistent muscle weakness. Possible causes include accumulation of drug metabolites, critical illness polyneuropathy, or neurogenic atrophy.
13. A very small percentage of patients will not be able to wean from ventilation support. Characteristics of these patients include persistent low-output state with multisystem organ failure. Echocardiography can be helpful in establishing ventricular filling, contractility, and cardiac output at baseline and during weaning trials. Long-term weaning may be best accomplished in a specialized unit rather than an acute cardiovascular recovery area.

Patients undergoing cardiac surgery experience physiologic stresses from anesthesia, thoracotomy, surgical manipulation, and cardiopulmonary bypass (CPB). Each of these interventions can create transient deleterious effects on pulmonary function even with normal lungs; the effects may be exaggerated in the presence of preexisting pulmonary pathology. Important pulmonary changes after cardiac surgery include diminished functional residual capacity after general anesthesia and muscle relaxants,[1] transient reduction in vital capacity (VC) after median sternotomy and intrathoracic manipulation, atelectasis, and increased intravascular lung water.[2] Acute functional residual capacity reduction creates arterial hypoxemia because of a mismatch between ventilation and perfusion, and diminishes lung compliance with increased work of breathing. This additional work of breathing, which increases oxygen consumption by up to 20% in spontaneously breathing patients,[3] also increases myocardial work at a time when

TABLE 35-1	Pulmonary Complications					
Reference	No. of Patients	Median Time to Extubation (days)	Mechanical Ventilation	Reintubation	Tracheostomy	In-hospital Mortality Rate
Rady et al (1993–1996)[18]	11,330	2.2	NR	6.6%	NR	3.5%
Branca et al (1996–1997)[17]	4,863	2 (1–105)	5.9% (> 72 hours)	3.2%	0.8%	1.95%
Cleveland Clinic Experience (1998–2001, unpublished data)	13,191	0.32	4.11%	7%	1.4%	NR

NR, not reported.

myocardial reserves may be limited. Changes in spirometric measurements and respiratory muscle strength can last up to 8 weeks after surgery.[4]

Thus, a sizeable proportion of cardiac surgical patients can be expected to have respiratory complications. In our experience, about a fourth of cardiac surgical patients were extubated in the operating room or within 4 hours of intensive care unit (ICU) arrival, and about half within 8 hours of ICU arrival. Median postprocedure intubation time was 7.6 hours. About 8% of patients experienced prolonged mechanical ventilation (defined as ≥ 72 hours after ICU arrival), and about 7% required reintubation of the trachea either shortly after initial extubation or because of delayed respiratory failure. Acute lung injury (ALI), sometimes progressing to acute respiratory distress syndrome (ARDS), can occur in up to 12% of postoperative cardiac patients.[5] Tracheostomy was performed in 1.4% of post-CPB patients to facilitate recovery and weaning from ventilatory support. Although these figures represent the experience of one referral center, others have reported similar results (Table 35-1). A more recent study at this same institution showed a trend toward less ventilator dependency but little change in the rate of tracheostomy.[6] In this study, 5.5% experienced ventilator dependency, whereas 1.45% required tracheostomy.

RISK FACTORS FOR RESPIRATORY INSUFFICIENCY

The lung is especially vulnerable because disturbances may affect it directly (atelectasis, effusions, pneumonia) or indirectly (via fluid overload in heart failure, as the result of mediator release from CPB, shock states, or infection, or via changes in respiratory pump function as with phrenic nerve injury). Postoperative status will be determined, in part, by the patient's preoperative pulmonary reserve, as well as by the level of stress imposed by the procedure. Thus, a patient with reduced VC caused by restrictive lung disease undergoing minimally invasive surgery may have fewer postoperative pulmonary issues than a relatively healthy patient undergoing simultaneous CABG and valve replacement with its longer accompanying operative/anesthetic and CPB times. Respiratory muscle weakness contributes to postoperative pulmonary dysfunction, and prophylactic inspiratory muscle training has been shown to improve respiratory muscle function, pulmonary function tests, and gas exchange. Training reduces the percentage of patients requiring more than 24 hours of postoperative ventilation support from 26% to 5%.[7]

Assessing Risk Based on Preoperative Status

A number of robust models are available to stratify mortality outcome by preoperative risk factors in patients undergoing cardiac surgery.[8] The independent (predictive) variables and their weighting vary somewhat from model to model and vary between models predicting mortality versus those predicting morbidity or length-of-stay outcomes,[9] but the commonalities are greater than the differences. The Society of Thoracic Surgeons National Adult Cardiac Surgery Database is widely used in the United States and offers, in addition to a mortality prediction, a model customized to predict prolonged ventilation.[10,11] The EuroSCORE is

commonly used in Europe.[12] Factors common to outcome risk adjustment models include age, sex, body surface area, presence of diabetes or renal failure, chronic lung disease, peripheral vascular disease, cerebrovascular disease, prior cardiac surgery, and emergency or unstable status.[9–11] Chronic obstructive pulmonary disease (COPD) might be expected to be a major risk for postoperative respiratory morbidity and mortality and appears as a factor in many models. However, hospital mortality with mild to moderate COPD is not especially high; it is the minority of patients with severe COPD, especially those older than 75 years and receiving steroids, who are at greatest risk.[13] Patients with preexisting COPD have greater rates of pulmonary complications (12%), atrial fibrillation (27%), and death (7%).[13] Obesity, defined by increased body mass index, does not appear to increase the risk for postoperative respiratory failure.[14] In contrast, even modest increases of serum creatinine concentration (> 1.5 mg/dL) are independently associated with greater morbidity and mortality.[9,15]

At least four studies have used multivariate regression techniques to elucidate factors specifically associated with postoperative respiratory failure (Table 35-2). The studies differ in their end points for outcome and in their choice of preoperative versus operative versus postoperative variables. Spivack et al[16] examined 513 consecutive patients undergoing CABG and identified reduced left ventricular ejection fraction, preexisting congestive heart failure, angina, current smoking, and diabetes mellitus as predictors of mechanical ventilation support beyond 48 hours. In this study, pulmonary diagnosis, lung mechanics, and blood gas parameters were not independently useful in predicting outcome. Branca et al[17] found that the mortality rate predicted by the Society of Thoracic Surgeons model[10] was the single best predictor of mechanical ventilation support for longer than 72 hours, but also identified mitral valvular disease, age, vasopressor and inotrope use, renal failure, operative urgency, type of operation, preoperative ventilation, prior cardiac surgery, female sex, myocardial infarction within 30 days, and previous stroke as contributors.[17] Rady et al[18] examined both preoperative and intraoperative factors and noted that transfusion of more than 10 units of blood products or total CPB time in excess of 120 minutes were important operative events in addition to the usual preoperative predictors of extubation failure. Canver and Chandra[19] looked only at operative and postoperative predictors versus the end point of mechanical ventilation for more than 72 hours; they found that prolonged CPB time, sepsis and endocarditis, gastrointestinal bleeding, renal failure, deep sternal wound infection, new stroke, and bleeding requiring reoperation were important predictors of prolonged ventilatory support. None of these models, general or specific for respiratory complications, is sufficiently sensitive or specific to prohibit consideration of surgery for an individual patient, but they do provide the clinician with early warning for patients at high risk.

Operating Room Events

Identification of the patient who is difficult to intubate is important for planning extubation for a time when sufficient personnel and equipment are available to deal with a potentially difficult reintubation. Opioids and neuromuscular blocking agents with long half-lives might be expected to influence extubation time. It is not the specific duration of action of these drugs but rather the skill of the anesthesiologist in knowing how to use them well that influences extubation time.

TABLE 35-2	Factors Predicting Postoperative Respiratory Outcome			
	Spivack et al[16]	*Branca et al[17]*	*Rady et al[18]*	*Canver and Chandra[19]*
End point	Mechanical ventilation > 48 hours	Mechanical ventilation > 72 hours	Extubation failure (reintubation after initial extubation)	Mechanical Ventilation > 72 hours
Risk factors	• Reduced LVEF • Preexisting CHF • Angina • Current smoking • Diabetes	• STS-predicted mortality estimate • Mitral valve disease • Advanced age • Pressors/Inotropes • Renal failure • Operative urgency • Type of operation • Preoperative ventilation • Prior CABG • Female sex • MI within 30 days • Previous stroke	• Age ≥ 65 years • Inpatient • Vascular disease • COPD/asthma • Pulmonary hypertension • Reduced LVEF • Cardiac shock • Hct ≤ 34% • BUN ≥ 24 mg/dL • Serum albumin ≤ 4.0 mg/dL • $DO_2 ≤ 320mL/mm/L^2$ • 1 prior CABG • Thoracic aortic surgery • 10 units of blood products • Total CPB time ≥ 120 minutes	• CPB time • Sepsis and endocarditis • GI bleeding • Renal failure • Deep sternal wound infection • New CVA • Bleeding requiring reoperation

BUN, blood urea nitrogen; CABG, coronary artery bypass grafting; CHF, congestive heart failure; CPB, cardiopulmonary bypass; COPD, chronic obstructive pulmonary disease, DO_2, systemic oxygen delivery; GI, gastrointestinal, Hct, hematocrit; LVEF, left ventricular ejection fraction; MI, myocardial infarction; STS, Society of Thoracic Surgeons.

Reoperative patients are at risk[18-20] partly because of longer CPB time, increased blood transfusion, and the additional likelihood of bleeding in this population. CPB time is repeatedly identified as a risk,[18-20] and a correlation between CPB time and inflammatory cytokine release has been demonstrated.[21] However, levels of C-reactive protein, an inflammatory marker, do not correlate with outcomes such as time on mechanical ventilation.[22] Genetic polymorphisms are associated with respiratory complications,[23] suggesting that risk prediction may require more sophisticated understanding of individual patient variables. Recent observations of dose-dependent reductions in adverse events after CABG in patients receiving statins are also intriguing.[24,25]

Low cardiac output states may be important predictors of prolonged ventilation because prolonged periods of inadequate perfusion result in additional mediator release. Patients maintained on an intra-aortic balloon pump (IABP) or a ventricular assist device may have borderline or insufficient cardiac output; it makes little sense to impose the additional work of breathing[3] until their cardiac issues have resolved. Cardiovascular collapse occasionally occurs at the time of chest closure secondary to severe distension or edema of the lungs. Physiologically, this acts much like cardiac tamponade, and the solution is to leave the chest open for 24 to 48 hours. An open chest delays early extubation

and also has a potential to produce long-term ventilator dependency should infection or sternal osteomyelitis develop.

The prognostic and therapeutic implications of an IABP depend on the reasons for which the device was inserted (Figure 35-1). Not surprisingly, mortality and ventilation-dependency rates are lowest in those not requiring any mechanical support. In patients in whom the IABP was placed before surgery for unstable angina, definitive surgery should correct the problem and removal of the IABP and extubation need not be delayed. In all other scenarios, intubation and ventilatory support may be required beyond the time of removal of the IABP because of residual cardiac dysfunction, fluid overload, or associated organ injury. Patients whose IABP was placed for preoperative cardiogenic shock, as an assist to separating from CPB, or for low output states in the postoperative period have a high mortality risk and frequently need prolonged ventilatory support.

Positive end-expiratory pressure (PEEP) while on CPB has been advocated as one method to prevent atelectasis. This turns out to be impractical in patients with COPD because air trapping interferes with surgical exposure. Recruitment maneuvers after CPB have variable impact on intubation time; most studies show it to be ineffective in reducing the need for long-term ventilatory support. Alveolar

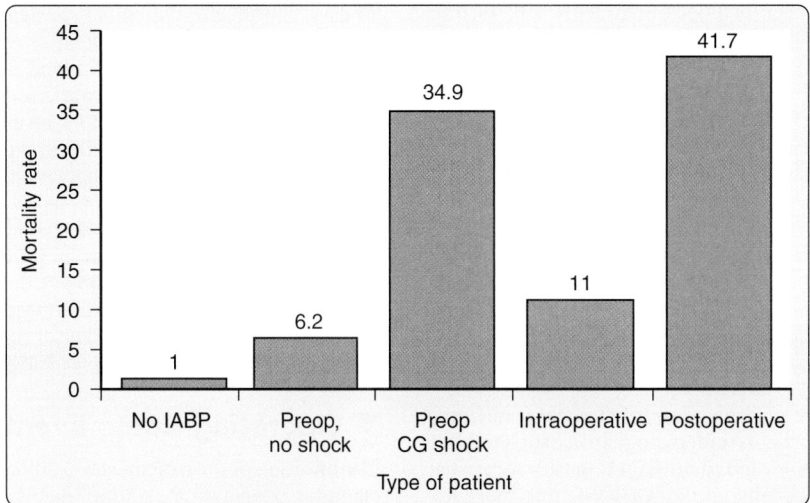

Figure 35-1 The prognostic implications of an intra-aortic balloon pump (IABP) depend on the timing and reason for insertion. In patients undergoing isolated coronary artery bypass grafting, the basal mortality rate is less than 1%. Patients who received a preoperative IABP for unstable angina have a 6.2% mortality rate. Preoperative insertion for cardiogenic (CG) shock has the worst prognosis, with nearly 35% mortality. Intraoperative insertion of a balloon pump, generally to facilitate separation from cardiopulmonary bypass, carries an 11% mortality rate. The worst prognosis is if a balloon pump is required after surgery for any reason. Patients in the highest-risk category are likely to require prolonged ventilatory support.

recruitment maneuvers can be performed without deleterious effects, even in morbidity obese patients, as long as intravascular volume is adequate.[26] There are no compelling data that fluid management choices or the use of steroids before CPB have substantial effects on intubation time or respiratory failure. A number of studies[27,28] suggest that infusion of small volumes of hypertonic saline prepared in a hydroxyethyl starch solution may reduce total fluid needs, improve cardiac index, and lessen the pulmonary gas exchange compromise, but studies have not examined whether these differences in the operating room translate to improved outcome or shorter length of stay.

Postoperative Events

The expected postoperative course is a short period of ventilatory support while the patient is warmed, allowed to awaken, and observed for bleeding or hemodynamic instability. Preoperative risks, issues with difficult intubation, and operating room events should be communicated from the operating room team to the ICU team at the time of ICU admission. Box 35-1 outlines criteria to be met before routine extubation. Reduced cuff leak volume reliably identifies patients at risk for laryngeal edema. Intravenous methylprednisolone can reduce the incidence of postextubation stridor.[29] Prophylactic nasal continuous positive airway pressure (CPAP) at 10 cm H_2O for a minimum of 6 hours has been shown to reduce hypoxemia, pneumonia, and reintubation rates after elective cardiac surgery.[30]

Aspiration of mouth flora or gastric contents is a major risk factor for later pulmonary compromise. Oral rather than nasal routes should be used for the endotracheal and gastric sump tubes, and these devices removed at the earliest possible opportunity. Before extubation, a quick neurologic examination should be performed to rule out new cerebrovascular events, presence of excess opioids, or residual neuromuscular blocking agents. Knowing that the work of breathing can consume up to 20% of cardiac output should preclude immediate extubation in the hemodynamically unstable patient. Although patients may be successfully extubated while on IABP, the need to lie flat after balloon and sheath removal may interfere with their ability to resolve atelectasis and clear secretions. This limitation often dictates continued temporary ventilator support until the patient is able to sit up.

Although postoperative care of low-risk cardiac surgical patients has come to resemble a recovery room model, high-risk patients benefit from postoperative involvement of anesthesiologists, cardiologists, and critical care specialists.[31] Numerous individual studies and systematic reviews[32] have confirmed the value of full-time intensive care specialists in a variety of settings, although there is at least one dissenting

opinion.[33] Wide variation continues in adherence to the Leapfrog group physician staffing standard,[34] despite demonstrated financial return on investment.[35] It is likely that a robust organizational environment, rather than the mere presence of intensivists, is necessary to achieve the best results.[36]

Hospital-acquired infections are an important cause of postoperative morbidity and nosocomial pneumonia is common in patients receiving continuous mechanical ventilation. The historic risk for ventilator-associated pneumonia (VAP) appears to be around 1% per day when diagnosed using protected specimen brush and quantitative culture techniques.[37] More recent data suggest that VAP rates can be decreased by an order of magnitude with careful attention to patient management.[38,39] Strategies believed to be effective at reducing the incidence of VAP include early removal of nasogastric or endotracheal tubes, formal infection control programs, hand washing, semirecumbent positioning of the patient,[40] daily sedation "vacation,"[41] avoiding unnecessary reintubation, providing adequate nutritional support, avoiding gastric overdistention, use of the oral rather than the nasal route for intubation, scheduled drainage of condensate from ventilator circuits,[42] and maintenance of adequate endotracheal tube cuff pressure.[43] Strategies that are *not* considered effective include routine changes of the ventilator circuit, dedicated use of disposable suction catheters, routine changes of in-line suction catheters, daily replacement of heat and moisture exchangers, and chest physiotherapy.[44] The literature supports both continuous aspiration of subglottic secretions and use of silver-coated endotracheal tubes to reduce the incidence of VAP.[45-47]

DIAGNOSIS OF ACUTE LUNG INJURY AND ACUTE RESPIRATORY DISTRESS SYNDROME

ARDS may develop as a sequela of CPB or, more commonly, in the postoperative patient with cardiogenic shock, sepsis, or multisystem organ failure. Components of ARDS include diffuse alveolar damage resulting from endothelial and type I epithelial cell necrosis, as well as noncardiogenic pulmonary edema caused by breakdown of the endothelial barrier with subsequent vascular permeability. The exudative phase of ARDS occurs in the first 3 days after the precipitating event and is thought to be mediated by neutrophil activation and sequestration. Neutrophils release mediators causing endothelial damage. Ultimately, the alveolar spaces fill up with fluid as a result of increased endothelial permeability.

Intravascular and intra-alveolar fibrin deposition are common. Procoagulant activity becomes enhanced in ARDS, and bronchoalveolar lavage will reveal increased tissue factor levels.[48] The clinical presentation is typically an acute onset of severe arterial hypoxemia refractory to oxygen therapy, with a PaO_2 to F_IO_2 (P/F ratio) of less than 200 mm Hg. ARDS is classically diagnosed only in the absence of left ventricular failure, which complicates the diagnosis in the postoperative cardiac patient who may also be in heart failure. Other findings in ARDS include decreased lung compliance (< 80 mL/cm H_2O) and bilateral infiltrates on chest radiograph.[49] Murray et al[50] created a Lung Injury Score that awards points for affected quadrants on chest radiograph, P/F ratio, amount of PEEP applied, and the static compliance of the lung. Scores above zero, but less than 2.5, are considered ALI, and scores greater than 2.5 meet the threshold for ARDS.

The proliferative phase of ARDS occurs on days 3 to 7 as inflammatory cells accumulate as a result of chemoattractants released by the neutrophils. At this stage, the normal repair process would remove debris and begin repair, but a disordered repair process may result in exuberant fibrosis, stiff lungs, and inefficient gas exchange. Evidence suggests that careful fluid and ventilator management may affect this process.[51,52] Conventional ventilator support after cardiac surgery is to maintain large tidal volumes (V_T; typically 10 mL/kg) to reopen atelectatic but potentially functional alveolae. The problem is that the compromised lung is no longer homogenous, and high pressures can further damage the remaining normal lung. Direct mechanical injury

---

BOX 35-1. CRITERIA TO BE MET BEFORE EARLY POSTOPERATIVE EXTUBATION

- *Neurological:* Awake, neuromuscular blockade fully dissipated (head lift ≥ 5 seconds); following instructions, able to cough and protect airway
- *Cardiac:* Stable without mechanical support; cardiac index ≥ 2.2 L/min/m²; MAP ≥ 70 mm Hg, no serious arrhythmias
- *Respiratory:* Acceptable CXR and ABGs (pH ≥ 7.35); minimal secretions, comfortable on CPAP or T-piece with spontaneous respiratory rate ≤ 20 breaths/min, MIP at least 25 cm H_2O; Alternatively, a successful SBT defined as RSBI < 100 and a PaO_2/FiO_2 ≥ 200
- *Renal:* Diuresing well; urine output > 0.8 mL/kg/hr; not markedly fluid overloaded from operative/CPB fluid administration or SIRS
- *Hematologic:* Chest tube drainage minimal
- *Temperature:* Fully rewarmed; not actively shivering

ABG, arterial blood gas; CPAP, continuous positive airway pressure; CPB, cardiopulmonary bypass; CXR, chest radiograph; MAP, mean arterial pressure; MIP, maximal inspiratory pressure; RSBI, rapid shallow breathing index; SBT, spontaneous breathing trial; SIRS, systemic immune response syndrome.

may occur as a result of overdistention (volutrauma), high pressures (barotrauma), or shear injury from repetitive opening and closing. "Biotrauma" also may occur as a result of inflammatory mediator release and impaired antibacterial barriers. Nahum et al[53] showed that dissemination of *Escherichia coli* via bacterial translocation from the lung was highest in dogs ventilated with a high-V_T strategy. Thus, current clinical practice with known or suspected lung injury is to limit inflation pressures. The maximal "safe" inflation pressure is not known, but evidence favors keeping peak inspiratory pressures less than 35 cm H_2O and restricting V_T to ≤ 6 mL/kg of ideal body weight in patients at risk for ALI.[54] The landmark ARDSNet trial randomized patients to 6 versus 12 mL/kg of ideal body weight and demonstrated a significant difference in 28-day survival with the low-V_T group.[55] The same study showed significant decreases in interleukin-6 (IL-6) release when the low-V_T strategy was used. Most recently, ventilation with lower V_T has been shown to be beneficial in critically ill patients even without ALI, as measured by plasma IL-6 levels and progression to lung injury,[56] but this issue has not yet been studied in the cardiac surgical population. A conservative strategy of fluid administration has been shown to improve oxygenation and shorten the duration of mechanical ventilation.[51]

THERAPY WITH ACUTE LUNG INJURY/ ACUTE RESPIRATORY DISTRESS SYNDROME

Maintaining a lung protective ventilatory strategy can involve permissive hypercapnia,[57] if normal PCO_2 levels cannot be achieved with low V_T. The acid-base changes must be monitored carefully, especially in patients with reactive pulmonary vasculature. Prone positioning can be useful in achieving oxygenation.[58] A short daily turn to the prone position does not appear to improve outcome in ARDS, although one post hoc analysis found lower mortality in the sickest patients.[59] Lower V_T with increasing amounts of PEEP may increase alveolar recruitment and thus improve oxygenation.[60] Taken to an extreme, patients with ALI may be ventilated with high-frequency oscillation, which is essentially high PEEP with tiny (smaller than dead space), frequently delivered V_T. Other techniques for patients who did not respond successfully to conventional therapy include extracorporeal CO_2 removal,[61] extracorporeal membrane oxygenation,[62] partial liquid ventilation,[63] inhaled nitric oxide,[64,65] and inhaled prostacyclin.[66] Although clearly beneficial to some individuals in extreme circumstances, prospective controlled trials are lacking. High-dose corticosteroids have been in and then out of fashion for treatment of ARDS. More recently, Miduri et al gave prolonged lower dose methylprednisolone therapy for unresolving ARDS and were able to document improvements in P/F ratio, better ICU survival, and shortened duration of mechanical ventilation.[67]

In the healthy cardiac surgical population, the use of PEEP usually is not necessary.[68,69] Increased levels of PEEP may decrease cardiac output, unless volume loading is used to stabilize preload by maintaining transmural filling pressures.[70] The effects of PEEP are most marked in the presence of abnormal right ventricular function, particularly if the right coronary artery is compromised.[71] PEEP neither protects against the development of ARDS[72] nor reduces the amount of mediastinal bleeding after cardiac surgical procedures involving CPB.[73] Most clinicians will routinely use 5 cmH_2O of PEEP in ventilated patients. However, greater levels of PEEP (often 8 to 15+ cmH_2O) are usually necessary to maintain adequate oxygenation with ALI or developing ARDS; application of PEEP in the postoperative patient usually involves a trade-off between cardiac and pulmonary goals.

Lung Recruitment

In laboratory and clinical models, an important component of a lung protective ventilatory strategy is recruitment of the lung. This is the closed-chest analogy to the open-chest recruitment maneuver typically done at the end of CPB to re-expand the collapsed lung. The goal of opening the lung is to allow ventilation to occur at a point on the pressure-volume curve that avoids repetitive atelectasis (by staying above a critical closing pressure) and at the same time avoids overinflation.[74] ARDSNet data suggest that the short-term effects of recruitment maneuvers are highly variable and that further study is necessary to determine the role of recruitment maneuvers in the management of ALI/ARDS.[75] With anesthetic techniques geared to early extubation, suboptimal oxygenation in the early postoperative period appears to be more common today. In most instances, impaired oxygenation is due to atelectasis and responds quickly to brief recruitment maneuvers. These should be performed with caution because of the adverse impact of increased airway pressure on venous return and cardiac output if the patient is intravascularly "empty." Although the benefits of early application of the lung protective ventilatory strategy in the high-risk cardiac surgical patient have not been studied formally, the benefits of lung protective ventilatory strategy in other populations suggest that this strategy should be considered as soon as ALI is identified, and perhaps even prophylactically in high-risk patients.[56]

Permissive Hypercapnia

Conventional management is to maintain $PaCO_2$ within a "normal" or eucapnic range, classically between 35 and 45 mm Hg. A patient who chronically retains CO_2 would be considered eucapnic at his or her higher baseline $PaCO_2$. The traditional reason for maintaining eucapnia is primarily that acute deviation from a normal or acclimatized $PaCO_2$ will result in alkalemia or acidemia to which the kidneys will respond by retaining or excreting bicarbonate ion. Normal kidneys can compensate for a PCO_2-induced pH change in 12 to 36 hours.[76] If high airway pressures would be required to maintain a "normal" $PaCO_2$, then $PaCO_2$ values up to 60 mm Hg are acceptable as long as cardiovascular stability is present and the pH remains greater than 7.30. It has been hypothesized that increased PCO_2 levels might even be protective and that low levels of PCO_2 could play a role in organ injury.[77] Permissive hypercapnia should be used judiciously in patients with pulmonary hypertension because acidosis can exacerbate pulmonary vasoconstriction and further impair right ventricular function and cardiac output.[78] (See Chapter 24.)

Cardiopulmonary Interactions

An understanding of cardiopulmonary interactions associated with mechanical ventilation is critical to the cardiothoracic intensivist. Hemodynamic changes may occur secondary to changes in lung volume and intrathoracic pressure even when V_T remains constant.[79] Pulmonary vascular resistance and mechanical heart-lung interactions play prominent roles in determining the hemodynamic response to mechanical ventilation. Because lung inflation alters pulmonary vascular resistance and right ventricular wall tension, there are limits to intrathoracic pressure that a damaged heart will tolerate. High lung volumes also may mechanically limit cardiac volumes. In patients with airflow obstruction, occult PEEP (auto-PEEP) may also contribute to hypotension and low cardiac output.[80] Auto-PEEP can be detected by respiratory waveform monitoring or by pressure monitoring with the ventilator's expiratory port held closed at end-exhalation. Auto-PEEP may respond to bronchodilators and/or increased expiratory time to permit more complete exhalation.

General Support Issues

Patients requiring long-term ventilatory support are prone to a number of complications including venous thromboembolism, central venous catheter–related bloodstream infections, surgical site infections, VAP, pressure ulcers, nutritional depletion, delirium, and gastrointestinal bleeding. The Agency for Healthcare Research and Quality has identified a number of patient safety practices applicable to the ICU patient; high on the list are appropriate venothromboembolism prophylaxis, use of perioperative β-blockers, use of maximum sterile barriers

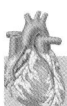

during catheter insertion, and appropriate use of antibiotic prophylaxis.[81] Standard practice in long-term ventilator patients includes prophylaxis against gastrointestinal bleeding with histamine blockers or proton pump inhibitors (unless the patient is receiving continuous gastric feedings), head of bed elevation to 30 degrees or more in hemodynamically stable patients,[40] a brief daily wake up from sedation,[82] use of in-line suction catheters, glucose control,[83] and appropriate venothromboembolism prophylaxis. Box 35-2 summarizes these risk-reduction efforts. Ensuring that each of these goals is met on each patient every day requires extra work but can be accomplished with a daily goals form[84] or with information technology.[85]

IMPEDIMENTS TO WEANING AND EXTUBATION

Factors that limit the removal of mechanical ventilatory support include delirium, neurologic dysfunction, unstable hemodynamics, respiratory muscle dysfunction, renal failure with fluid overload, and sepsis. Figure 35-2 outlines one approach to identifying readiness to wean and possible alternative approaches to weaning.

Neurological Complications

Delirium is common in long-stay ICU patients and is associated with greater costs in the ICU and for the entire hospital stay.[86] Delirium after cardiac surgery is a common complication in cardiovascular ICUs; estimated incidence rates are approximately 30% in the general cardiac surgical population to 83% in mechanically ventilated patients.[87,88] Delirium resolves spontaneously or with pharmacologic intervention in almost all patients by postoperative day 6. Evidence from a large trial of mostly medical critical care patients suggests dexmedetomidine is associated with less delirium than midazolam.[89] Dexmedetomidine has been shown to be safe and effective in the post-CABG population.[90] Alcohol or benzodiazepine withdrawal should be considered in the differential diagnosis of delirium. Recent evidence suggests that ketamine may attenuate delirium in CPB patients, possibly because of anti-inflammatory effects.[91] Initial postoperative management of agitation consists of reassurance and orientation of the patient, as well as control of pain with opioids. Agitation accompanied by disorientation may be worsened by benzodiazepines, which should be restricted to treatment of oriented but anxious patients or for prophylaxis of alcohol and

benzodiazepine withdrawal. If the patient remains agitated and disoriented, haloperidol is useful.[92] Newer agents such as risperidone, olanzapine, and quetiapine also may be useful, but they have not been well studied in the cardiothoracic ICU setting.

Diaphragmatic paralysis may complicate any procedure, but it is more common in patients undergoing reoperation, because of the difficulty in identifying the phrenic nerve in fibrotic pericardial tissue. In our experience, permanent bilateral diaphragmatic paralysis occurs in less than 0.1% of patients after CPB, but temporary diaphragmatic weakness may occur in 4% or more. The diagnosis of diaphragmatic paralysis should be suspected whenever a patient does not successfully wean from mechanical ventilation; it should be documented by observing paradoxic movement of the diaphragm during inspiration, and by comparing VC and V_T in the supine and seated positions. Differences in supine and seated VC of more than 10% to 15% should prompt fluoroscopic examination of the diaphragm ("sniff" test). Bilateral paralysis may be missed by this test, because comparison of left and right diaphragmatic excursion has lower specificity when both diaphragms are involved. Transient diaphragmatic paralysis can occur secondary to cold injury to the phrenic nerve.[93] Less often, the phrenic nerve is injured or transected during dissection of the internal mammary arteries or during mobilization of the heart in patients undergoing reoperation.

Patients with respiratory failure and systemic inflammatory response syndrome frequently develop critical illness polyneuropathy, the first sign of which may be failure to wean from the ventilator.[94] Disuse atrophy[95] and steroid administration[96] also contribute to muscle weakness. Patients with severe COPD who are dependent on diaphragmatic breathing before surgery are most likely to manifest diaphragmatic weakness as postoperative ventilator dependency. Full recovery of diaphragmatic function may take from 4 months to more than 2 years, and partial recovery is apparent when the patient can lie flat without dyspnea.[97] Adjuncts to improving diaphragmatic strength include inspiratory muscle training,[7] normalizing calcium and phosphate levels, and possibly the use of aminophylline.[98]

Cardiac Complications

Acute myocardial dysfunction occurs in almost all post-CPB patients, reaching a nadir about 4 hours (range, 2 to 6) after CPB. Patients with persistent low-output syndrome have an increased risk for cardiac death, as well as complications such as renal failure, respiratory failure, disseminated intravascular coagulation, gastrointestinal bleeding, and neurologic sequelae. Regional differences in blood flow also can occur even in the presence of an adequate overall cardiac output, so a normal whole-body cardiac index does not guarantee adequate perfusion of individual organs. Multiorgan failure may be precipitated by a period of gut ischemia or hyperpermeability followed by translocation of gut bacteria and release of endotoxin and other vasoactive substances, leading to generalized inflammation and organ injury.[99]

Patients maintained on chronic amiodarone therapy are prone to postoperative respiratory failure, longer intubation times, and longer ICU stays, even with only subclinical evidence of pulmonary amiodarone toxicity.[100] Rarely, patients taking amiodarone experience development of life-threatening pulmonary complications, including ARDS. Histologic lung examination of these patients demonstrates marked interstitial fibrosis with enlarged air spaces ("honeycomb" appearance) and hyperplasia of type II pneumocytes.[101]

Acute left ventricular dysfunction may occur in patients with COPD during the shift from mechanical to spontaneous ventilation.[102] Attention to fluid balance and aggressive diuresis or use of ultrafiltration help with weaning. Although it is useful to compare the patient's current and preoperative body weights, catabolic states arising after surgery, and especially during sepsis, reduce lean body weight. Patients may be "unweanable" until fluid removal reduces body weight to several kilograms less than the preoperative value.

Patients with valvular disease have significantly higher respiratory system and lung elastances and resistances than those undergoing

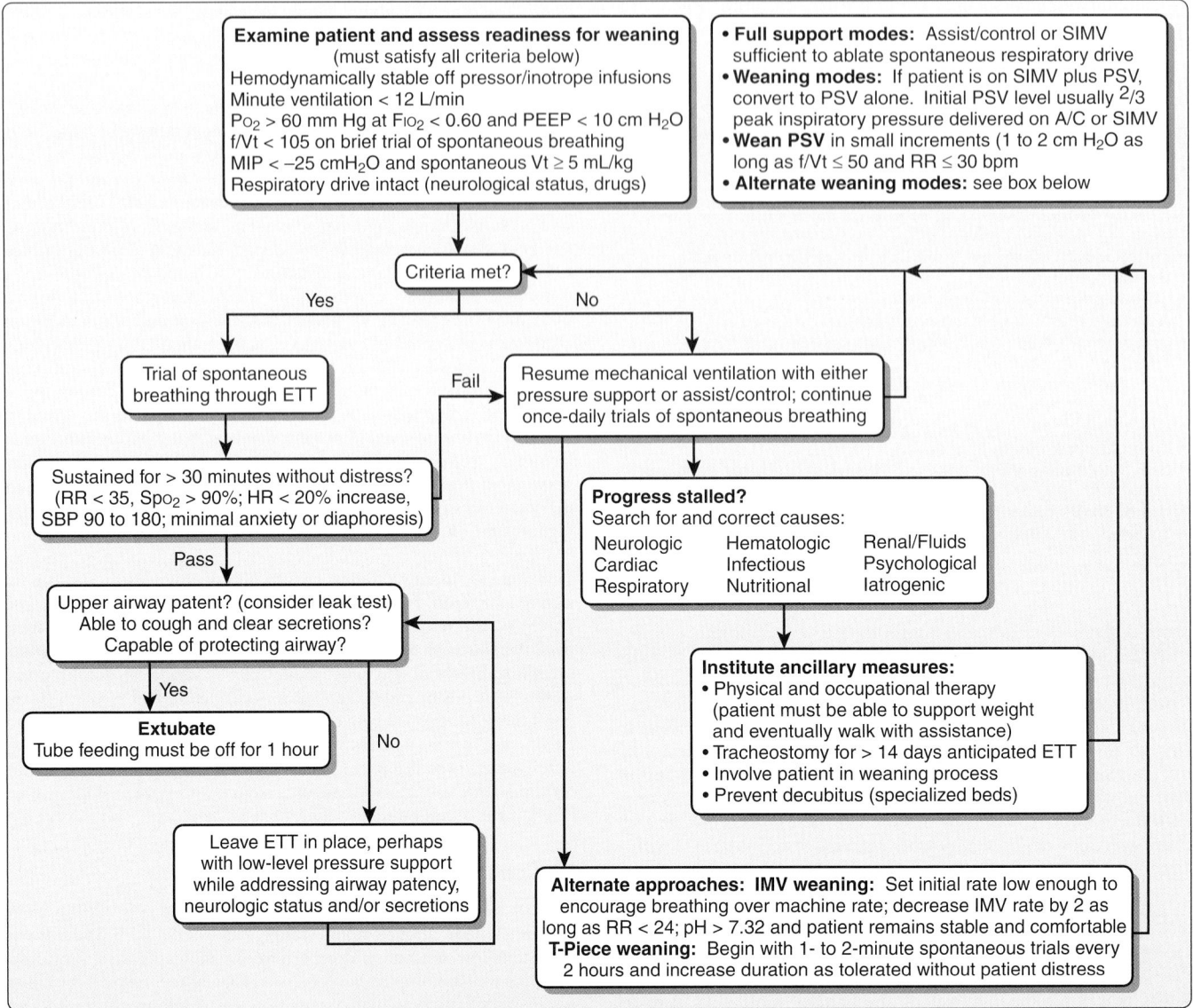

Examine patient and assess readiness for weaning
(must satisfy all criteria below)
Hemodynamically stable off pressor/inotrope infusions
Minute ventilation < 12 L/min
Po_2 > 60 mm Hg at Fio_2 < 0.60 and PEEP < 10 cm H_2O
f/Vt < 105 on brief trial of spontaneous breathing
MIP < −25 cmH_2O and spontaneous Vt ≥ 5 mL/kg
Respiratory drive intact (neurological status, drugs)

• **Full support modes:** Assist/control or SIMV sufficient to ablate spontaneous respiratory drive
• **Weaning modes:** If patient is on SIMV plus PSV, convert to PSV alone. Initial PSV level usually 2/3 peak inspiratory pressure delivered on A/C or SIMV
• **Wean PSV** in small increments (1 to 2 cm H_2O as long as f/Vt ≤ 50 and RR ≤ 30 bpm
• **Alternate weaning modes:** see box below

Criteria met?

Yes — No

Trial of spontaneous breathing through ETT

Fail

Resume mechanical ventilation with either pressure support or assist/control; continue once-daily trials of spontaneous breathing

Sustained for > 30 minutes without distress?
(RR < 35, Spo_2 > 90%; HR < 20% increase, SBP 90 to 180; minimal anxiety or diaphoresis)

Progress stalled?
Search for and correct causes:

Neurologic	Hematologic	Renal/Fluids
Cardiac	Infectious	Psychological
Respiratory	Nutritional	Iatrogenic

Pass

Upper airway patent? (consider leak test)
Able to cough and clear secretions?
Capable of protecting airway?

Institute ancillary measures:
• Physical and occupational therapy (patient must be able to support weight and eventually walk with assistance)
• Tracheostomy for > 14 days anticipated ETT
• Involve patient in weaning process
• Prevent decubitus (specialized beds)

Yes

Extubate
Tube feeding must be off for 1 hour

No

Leave ETT in place, perhaps with low-level pressure support while addressing airway patency, neurologic status and/or secretions

Alternate approaches: IMV weaning: Set initial rate low enough to encourage breathing over machine rate; decrease IMV rate by 2 as long as RR < 24; pH > 7.32 and patient remains stable and comfortable
T-Piece weaning: Begin with 1- to 2-minute spontaneous trials every 2 hours and increase duration as tolerated without patient distress

Figure 35-2 This flow chart addresses the broad categorization of patients, both short and long term, in the cardiothoracic intensive care unit. All patients require periodic assessment for readiness for weaning, and if they meet criteria are eligible for spontaneous trials leading to extubation. Patients who do not meet the criteria should have mechanical ventilation maintained until criteria are met. Pressure-support weaning may be possible; if not, alternative approaches include intermittent mandatory ventilation weaning and TP weaning. Patients who stall in their weaning progress should have a comprehensive examination and an assessment of organ systems to search for correctable causes. A/C, assist control; ETT, endotracheal tube; f/V$_T$, frequency-to-tidal volume ratio; HR, heart rate; IMV, intermittent mandatory ventilation; MIP, maximal inspiratory pressure; PEEP, positive end-expiratory pressure; PSV, pressure-support ventilation; RR, respiratory rate; SBP, systolic blood pressure; SIMV, synchronized intermittent mandatory ventilation; TP, T-piece.

surgery for ischemic heart disease, but these may correct with successful surgery.[103] Thus, valve surgery patients have less work of breathing and improved respiratory function after correction of the valvular pathology, but CABG patients are less likely to show dramatic improvement after surgery.

Utility of Echocardiography in the Intensive Care Unit Setting

For many years, echocardiography has been practiced routinely in the operating room to assess ventricular function and valvular pathology. In recent years, transesophageal color-Doppler echocardiography (TEE) or transthoracic echocardiography (TTE) has moved to the bedside.[104–106] High-quality images from TEE/TTE can be a valuable diagnostic tool in the management of critically ill patients, as well as in the diagnosis and treatment of respiratory disease related

to cardiopulmonary dysfunction.[107] Use of a focused cardiovascular examination frequently alters perioperative management.[108]

Pleural Effusion

Accumulation of fluid in the pleural space from bleeding or collection of fluid can compress the lung parenchyma and cause basal atelectasis, resulting in impaired gas exchange. An undetected pleural effusion also may act as a potential source of postoperative infection. As with the ultrasound probe used by radiologists, the TTE probe can be used to assess the size of a pleural effusion, mark the skin at the site that is optimal for needle insertion to drain the effusion, and verify that there is no lung tissue in the area where the physician plans to insert the needle (Figure 35-3). Orihashi et al[109] have described the TEE appearance of pleural fluid. When the patient is supine, fluid pools in the dorsal and caudal portions of the pleural space. From the four-chamber view, the TEE probe is rotated counterclockwise to obtain the short-axis view

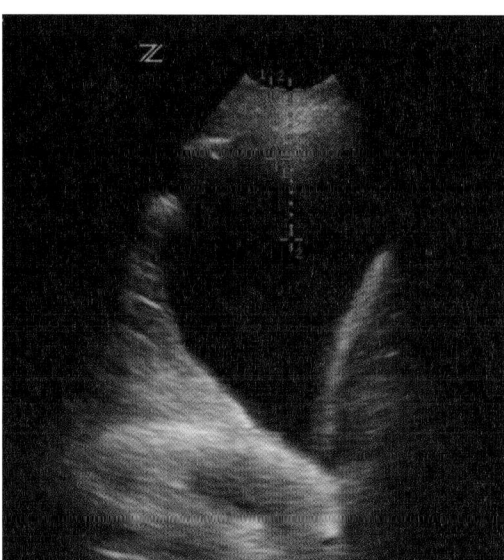

Figure 35-3 Pleural effusion, left hemithorax. With the patient seated erect, the transducer is oriented perpendicular to the left chest wall at the skin mark, and the following measurements are obtained: depth to enter the fluid collection: 1.7 cm; depth to midfluid collection: 3.7 cm.

of the descending aorta. In the presence of left-side pleural effusion, a crescent shape linked to a tiger's claw could be noted. The probe is rotated clockwise from the four-chamber view position to examine for a right pleural effusion. A crescent-shaped, echo-free space adjacent to the transducer is noted.

Treatment of pleural effusion is thoracentesis or placement of tube thoracostomy. Talmor et al[110] showed that drainage of pleural fluid resulted in a significant improvement in oxygenation in patients with acute respiratory failure with pleural effusions who were refractory to treatment with mechanical ventilation and PEEP.

Patent Foramen Ovale

When a mechanically ventilated patient becomes more hypoxemic despite efforts to improve ventilation, shunt-induced hypoxemia caused by a patent foramen ovale should be suspected, among other causes such as pulmonary embolism. Only echocardiography can identify such specific abnormalities in mechanically ventilated patients, when weaning is difficult or refractory hypoxemia is not explained by pulmonary disease alone.[111]

Septic Shock

The treatment of critically ill patients frequently requires a comprehensive evaluation of the hemodynamic status. Pulmonary artery catheters are widely used but have not been shown to improve survival[112] and have substantial limitations.[113] Echocardiography appears to be an alternative modality for assessment of patients with circulatory failure in the ICU,[114] allowing rapid assessment and differentiation of the cause of shock.

The diagnostic accuracy of TEE has been superior to that of TTE in identifying the cardiac source of shock, especially in ventilated patients.[115] Inotropic support may be necessary to facilitate weaning from mechanical ventilation.[116] In the presence of tricuspid regurgitation, the measurement of cardiac output by thermodilutional techniques will underestimate its value. Balik et al[117] confirmed that the severity of tricuspid regurgitation, an abnormality frequently observed in mechanically ventilated ICU patients,[118] reduces the agreement between thermodilution and TEE for the cardiac output determination.

Inadequate fluid administration can be detrimental, but avoiding inefficient and potentially deleterious volume expansion is equally

important. Bedside echocardiography is one option for goal-directed therapy.[119] Pulse-pressure variation under volume-controlled ventilation has been used successfully to predict the response to a fluid challenge in patients with sepsis because this variation is mainly based on the respiratory change in the left ventricular stroke volume. Feissel et al[120] were able to measure the variation of aortic blood flow velocity by echo Doppler and predict preload responsiveness in septic ventilated patients. Variation of aortic Doppler velocities was calculated as the ratio of the difference between maximal (inspiratory) and minimal (expiratory) velocities to the mean of these two velocities, and responders were defined as patients who increased their cardiac index by at least 15% after fluid challenge. Passive leg raising has been shown, using esophageal Doppler and respiratory variation in pulse pressure, to predict fluid responsiveness.[121] Vieillard-Baron et al[122] showed that the collapsibility index (maximal diameter on expiration - minimal diameter on inspiration/maximal diameter on expiration expressed as a percentage) of the superior vena cava greater than 36% using TEE accurately distinguished responders from nonresponders to a fluid challenge. The pathophysiology and treatment of ARDS often impose additional strain on the right ventricle. Echocardiography can be useful in helping in the assessment of the management of fluids, mechanical ventilation, and inotropic support on right ventricular function.[123] A recent review summarized the advantages and disadvantages of minimally invasive cardiac output monitoring in the perioperative setting (see Chapter 14).[124]

Pericardial Effusion

The Beck triad of jugular venous distention, muffled heart sounds, and hypotension are present in less than 40% of patients with tamponade. When these signs are present, it is not until late in the clinical scenario. TEE is an essential tool in making the accurate diagnosis of pericardial effusion, especially in a hypotensive patient who does not respond to volume expansion or inotropic support. Findings of a pericardial effusion include systolic collapse of the right atrium, diastolic collapse of the right ventricle, and mitral valve inflow decrease by 25% during inspiration (in spontaneously breathing patients) or tricuspid valve inflow decrease in ventilated patients are all consistent with tamponade.

Renal Failure and Fluid Overload

Significant oliguria or anuric renal failure occurs after 1% to 4% of cardiac surgical procedures, and lesser degrees of renal dysfunction, marked by increased serum creatinine concentration, occur in up to 30%. Univariate predictors of serious acute renal failure include low cardiac output at the end of CPB, advanced age, preoperative heart failure, need for postoperative circulatory support or blood transfusions, and prolonged time on CPB.[125]

When renal failure occurs, it often follows one of three well-defined patterns.[126] Abbreviated acute renal failure occurs after an isolated insult, results in a peak in serum creatinine around the fourth postevent day and generally resolves if no other events occur. The second pattern initially resembles the first, except that the acute insult is accompanied by prolonged circulatory failure. This pattern runs a longer course, with recovery typically occurring in the second or third week after injury, in tandem with improvements in cardiac output. In the third pattern, recovery is complicated by a second insult such as sepsis, massive gastrointestinal bleeding, or myocardial infarction, and permanent renal failure may result. Because fluid overload with renal failure may precipitate respiratory and cardiac failure, early application of hemodialysis and related techniques to remove excess fluid can facilitate separation from ventilator support.[127]

Infectious Complications

Mediastinitis, sternal dehiscence, or both, are complications of CABG, with an incidence rate of about 1%, a mortality rate of about 13%, and a tendency to prolong ventilator dependency. Predisposing factors for wound complications after cardiac surgery include diabetes, low cardiac output, use of bilateral internal mammary grafts, and reoperation for control of bleeding.[128] Keeping the blood glucose less than 200 mg/dL in the perioperative period reduces the sternal wound infection rate from 2.4% to 1.5%.[129] Mediastinal infection manifests as unexplained fever, an unstable sternum, and sometimes, failure to wean. In addition to selective antibiotic therapy, surgical debridement and drainage of the wound are usually necessary. Polymicrobial isolates are associated with poor outcome. Additional management of mediastinitis may include primary or delayed sternal closure using pectoralis or omental flaps.

Pneumonia, tracheobronchitis, catheter sepsis, and urinary tract infections are frequent in the ventilator-dependent patient. Continuous lateral rotational therapy reduces the prevalence of pneumonia but may not affect mortality or length of mechanical support.[130] The diagnosis of VAP[131-157] can be difficult to confirm because upper airway organism can contaminate the sputum specimen. Special suction catheters with a protected tip may be used for a "mini"-bronchoalveolar lavage to improve the yield of sputum cultures. Because typical perioperative antibiotic prophylaxis consists of an antistaphylococcal penicillin or cephalosporin, nosocomial pneumonia is likely to occur with organisms such as *Pseudomonas, Klebsiella, Serratia, Acinetobacter,* or methicillin-resistant *Staphylococcus aureus.* Treatment of the secondary infection may be followed by a tertiary infection with more difficult organisms, such as *Candida, Torulopsis,* or other fungal species.

Gastrointestinal Complications

Gastrointestinal complications requiring intervention occur in 1% to 3% of patients. Postoperative ileus can affect diaphragmatic excursion and increase work of breathing. Upper gastrointestinal bleeding is common. Pancreatitis, mesenteric ischemia, perforation, and bleeding elsewhere in the gastrointestinal tract are problems of any critically ill patient with multisystem failure. Mesenteric ischemia can be the result of low perfusion or embolic atheroma from large-vessel manipulation. Gut ischemia is a potential source of bacteremia, especially problematic for patients with artificial valves. The risk for gastrointestinal bleeding can be minimized with antacid therapy, histamine blockers, or barrier protection agents. Enteral nutritional support also appears to protect the gastric mucosa.

Diarrhea can occur as the result of mesenteric ischemia, but is also frequently caused by *Clostridium difficile* overgrowth in patients treated with antibiotics, especially later-generation cephalosporins. Patients on prolonged mechanical ventilation have a significantly greater risk for concurrent *C. difficile*–associated diarrhea, with attendant increases in hospital length of stay and costs. The rapid assay for *C. difficile* can miss certain strains; culture of stool is not as rapid but is more reliable. Treatment of *C. difficile* colitis can be accomplished with oral or intravenous metronidazole or enteral (*not* intravenous) vancomycin. Toxic megacolon is a surgical emergency requiring immediate attention. Nutrition depletion is common in long-term ventilated patients, and early enteral feeding should be implemented in high-risk patients unless there are specific contraindications such as ongoing bowel ischemia.

Nutritional Support and Weaning

Respiratory failure can be precipitated by high carbohydrate loads delivered during attempts to provide nutritional support, so the goals should be to institute support early before serious depletion occurs, and to use an appropriate mix of fat and carbohydrate to maintain a respiratory quotient less than 1.0. Weekly monitoring of transferrin or prealbumin levels screens for changes in nutritional status; more sophisticated analysis including metabolic monitoring and nitrogen balance can identify reasons for poor response to therapy.

The adequacy of nutritional support has a strong influence on the ability to wean from ventilation. Successful weaning occurs in about 93% of those with adequate nutritional support but only 50% of those

with inadequate nutrition. Increases in albumin and transferrin level with parenteral nutrition predict eventual ability to wean.

MODES OF VENTILATOR SUPPORT

Positive-pressure ventilators used outside the operating room have a nonrebreathing circuit, may be volume or pressure limited, and may be triggered by changes in flow or changes in pressure. All modern ventilators contain multiple modes of ventilatory support that accommodate both mandatory and patient-triggered breaths. The most common modes of positive-pressure ventilation are assist control, synchronized intermittent mandatory ventilation (SIMV), and pressure-support ventilation (PSV). With volume modes, the inspiratory flow rate, targeted volume, and inspiratory time are set by the clinician, and inspiratory peak pressure will vary depending on the patient's lung compliance and synchrony with the ventilator. Volume cycling ensures consistent delivery of a set V_T as long as the pressure limit is not exceeded. With non-homogenous lung pathology, however, delivered volume tends to flow to areas of low resistance, which may result in overdistension of healthy segments of lung and underinflation of atelectatic segments and consequent ventilation/perfusion (V/Q) mismatching. Figure 35-4 demonstrates pressure and flow tracings with volume ventilation. Volume breaths may be triggered by a timer (control mode ventilation) or by patient effort between the control mode breaths (assist control ventilation). In either case, the V_T delivered will be determined by the ventilator settings. This can present a problem in a patient with tachypnea as a response to neurologic injury. If the patient breathes inappropriately in response to normal arterial levels of carbon dioxide, significant respiratory alkalosis will result. Assist-control mode is most appropriate for the patient whose respiratory drive is normal but muscles are weak, or when neuromuscular blockade is used, in which case assist control essentially becomes control-mode ventilation.

Intermittent mandatory ventilation (IMV) and SIMV were developed to facilitate weaning from mechanical ventilatory support. With

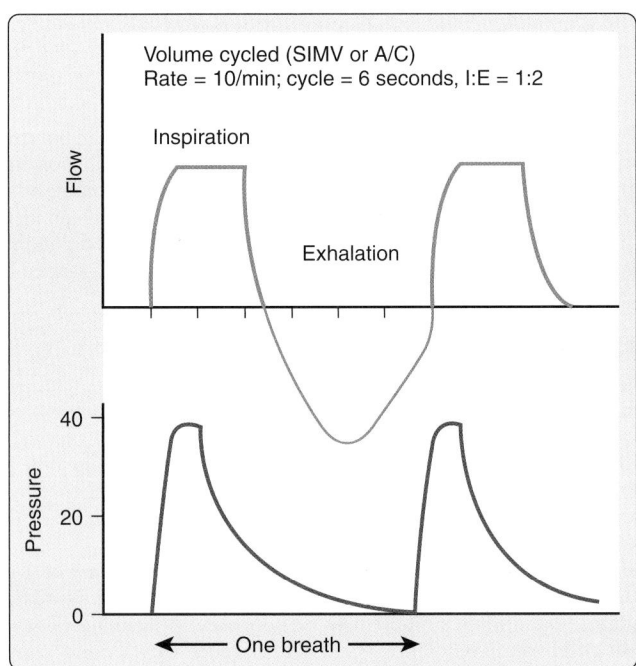

Figure 35-4 Top tracing shows the inspiratory flow, which is close to a square wave. Originally this flow pattern was dictated by the function of mechanical valves but may now be duplicated electronically. Note that the flow waveform becomes negative during the exhalation phase. The typical volume cycle breath with a square waveform results in a rapid increase to peak inspiratory pressure followed by a gradual decline. If the safety pressure limit is exceeded, the peak of the pressure waveform may be truncated.

either IMV modality, a basal respiratory rate is set by the clinician, which may be supplemented by patient-initiated breaths. In contrast with assist-control ventilation, however, the V_T of the patient's spontaneous breaths will be determined by their own respiratory strength and lung compliance rather than delivered as a preset volume. SIMV mode is appropriate for patients with normal lungs recovering from opioid anesthesia. Weaning is accomplished by reducing the mandatory IMV rate and allowing the patient to assume more and more of the respiratory effort over time. SIMV mode has been used for weaning complex patients, but the weaning effort may stall at very low IMV rates if the patient cannot achieve spontaneous volumes sufficient to activate their pulmonary stretch receptors. Under these circumstances, the patient is likely to become tachypneic and not respond to weaning attempts. Thus, other methods of weaning from ventilatory support may need to be used.

Pressure-Controlled Ventilation

Pressure-controlled ventilation is available on most newer ventilators and allows the clinician to specify a target inspiratory pressure; the ventilator then calculates and delivers the optimal flow rate to achieve the desired V_T and inspiratory-to-expiratory ratio. Figure 35-5 demonstrates the difference between pressure- and volume-controlled ventilation with regard to inspiratory flow. Pressure-controlled inverse ratio ventilation (PC-IRV) is pressure-controlled ventilation with an inspiratory time that exceeds expiratory time (I:E ratio > 1.0). Opening alveoli with damaged lungs sometimes requires exceeding a critical opening pressure for an adequate amount of time (Figure 35-6). With standard ventilation, this time above the critical pressure only

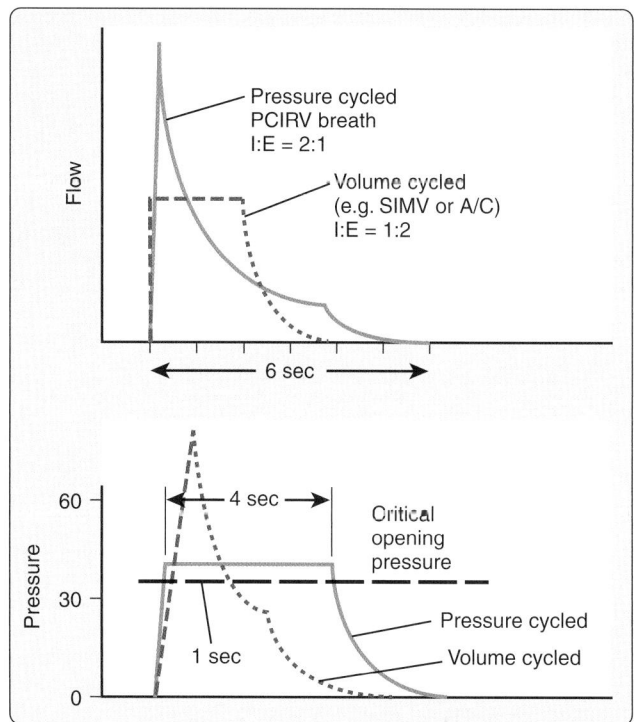

Figure 35-6 Volume- and pressure-cycle modes are compared as in Figure 35-5. If there is a critical opening pressure to recruit atelectatic lung segments, a pressure-controlled ventilation mode, particularly if the inspiration-to-expiration (I:E) ratio is inverted, is far more successful at maintaining an inspiratory pressure above the critical opening pressure for a greater length of time. Attempting to increase the volume-cycled flow would result in unacceptably high peak inspiratory pressures in an attempt to achieve more time above the critical opening pressure. But even in volume control, inspiratory pauses or changes to the flow rate in I:E ratio may be able to achieve longer sustained inspiratory pressures. PCIRV, pressure-controlled inverse ratio ventilation; SIMV, synchronized intermittent mandatory ventilation.

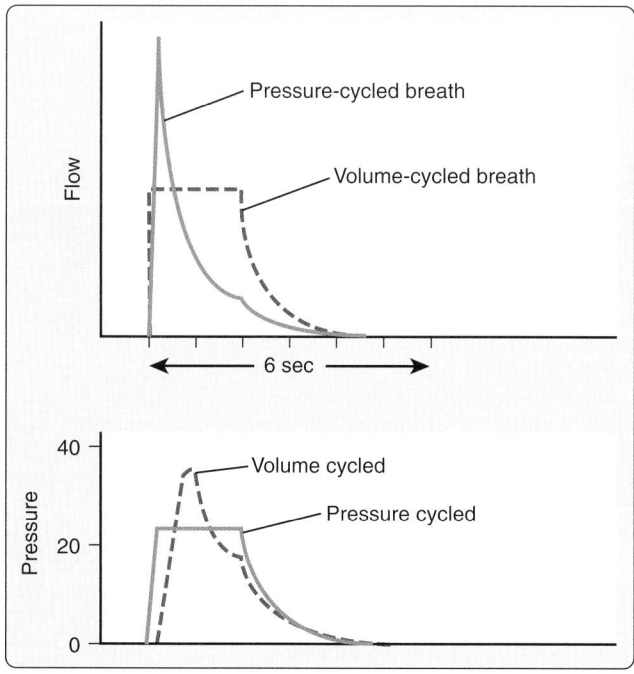

Figure 35-5 The difference between pressure-cycled breaths and volume-cycled breaths is demonstrated. With a pressure-cycle breath, the flow is titrated by a feedback mechanism to maintain a set inspiratory pressure. Thus, flow is very rapid at the beginning of the inspiratory cycle and rapidly tapers, in contrast with a volume-cycled breath in which the waveform is more or less consistent throughout the inspiratory cycle. Bottom graph shows the difference in pressure tracings. As noted earlier, volume-cycled ventilation reaches a peak and then falls back. In contrast, pressure-cycled ventilation reaches a lower, but sustained, pressure limit and holds at that level for the inspiratory time. In the absence of significant pulmonary disease, either mode of ventilation results in a rapid decrease of pressure once exhalation occurs.

can be lengthened by increasing the peak inspiratory pressure, which is generally undesirable with a damaged lung. With PC-IRV, the pressure waveform is optimized to allow a long inspiratory time above the critical opening pressure while avoiding high peak pressures. The disadvantage of PC-IRV is that the increased inspiratory time necessarily reduces exhalation time, which may lead to stacking of breaths or auto-PEEP in patients with abnormal lungs. Tharat et al[137] demonstrated that PC-IRV allowed a reduction in minute ventilation and reduced peak pressures while increasing mean airway pressures in patients with ARDS. At a given plateau pressure (similar end-inspiratory distention), lower V_T and increased PEEP are associated with better recruitment and oxygenation.

Changing a patient from conventional volume ventilation to pressure-control or PC-IRV can be accomplished by noting the existing V_T, inspiratory pressures, and inspiration-to-expiration (I:E) ratio, and switching to pressure-controlled ventilation mode with similar inspiratory peak pressure, rate, and inspiratory time. The level of inspiratory pressure is then titrated to deliver a V_T similar to what the patient was receiving with volume-control ventilation. Then, the inspiratory time can be lengthened to achieve better oxygenation or decreased to allow sufficient exhalation time if auto-PEEP is evident. In any patient with abnormal lungs, but particularly if an IRV mode is used, the patient must be monitored for the development of auto-PEEP, identified either by monitoring failure of the pressure waveform to return to baseline between breaths or instituting an expiratory hold and noting the difference in pressure between the ventilator's pressure gauge and the level of PEEP that was specified. Sedation and neuromuscular blockade are often necessary if the I:E ratio is inverted. Adjusting the ventilator settings in pressure-control mode is not always intuitive. Increased rates may paradoxically decrease CO_2 elimination if V_T decreases. Improvements in oxygenation may not occur until the patient is stabilized and given time to recruit atelectatic segments. Recruitment maneuvers when initiating pressure-controlled ventilation may help to open up atelectatic segments, and the hope is that these segments will remain open once recruited. Airway pressure release ventilation is functionally similar to PC-IRV in terms of recruitment but often can be accomplished in spontaneously breathing patients. Adaptive support ventilation, a microprocessor-controlled mode that maintains preset minute ventilation, also has been used in the cardiothoracic surgical population.

Pressure-Support Ventilation

PSV, which is primarily a weaning technique, must be distinguished from pressure-control ventilation, which is generally utilized during the maintenance phase of ALI. PSV may be used in conjunction with CPAP or SIMV modes. Pressure support augments the patient's spontaneous inspiratory effort with a clinician-selected level of pressure. Putative advantages include improved patient comfort, reduced ventilatory work, and more rapid weaning. The volume delivered with each PSV breath depends on the pressure set for inspiratory assist, as well as the patient's lung compliance. The utility of PSV in weaning from chronic ventilatory support is that it allows the patient's ventilatory muscles to assume part of the workload while augmenting V_T, thus preventing atelectasis, sufficiently stretching lung receptors, and keeping the patient's spontaneous respiratory rate within a reasonable physiologic range. With some older (and now mostly obsolete) ventilators, the inspiratory phase of PSV is terminated when flow falls to less than 25% of the initial value. In the presence of a cuff leak around the endotracheal tube, the flow rate may not decline to sufficiently low levels to terminate the breath, and the patient will struggle trying to exhale against the inspiratory flow. This problem is rare or nonexistent with the newer ventilators. V_T will vary markedly with the patient's lung compliance, so close clinical observation is necessary with the initiation of PSV. Monitoring end-tidal CO_2, as well as pulse oximetry readings, during the PSV weaning phase helps limit the need for arterial blood gases.

LIBERATION FROM MECHANICAL SUPPORT (WEANING)

An important concept to consider is that weaning from ventilatory support is not synonymous with extubation. There are conditions in which weaning is possible, but extubation is not—for example, upper airway edema or compression, glottic dysfunction with aspiration, neurologic dysfunction, or any other inability to protect the airway. A second important concept is that a formal weaning process is not essential in a normal postoperative patient, although SIMV or PSV weaning may be convenient. In the absence of significant cardiopulmonary dysfunction, extubation depends more on a stable clinical condition, adequate warming, elimination and metabolism of anesthetics, and reversal of neuromuscular blockade. Weaning strategies, however, are almost always required after more than 3 days of ventilatory support.

When terminating mechanical ventilation, two phases of decision making are involved. First, there should be resolution of the initial process for which mechanical ventilation was begun. The patient cannot be septic, hemodynamically unstable, or burdened with excessive respiratory secretions. If these general criteria are met, then specific weaning criteria can be examined. These include oxygenation (typically a Pao_2 > 60 mm Hg on 35% inspired oxygen and low levels of PEEP), adequate oxygen transport (measurable by O_2 extraction ratio or assumed if the cardiac index is adequate and lactic acidosis is not present), adequate respiratory mechanics (V_T, maximal inspiratory pressure), adequate respiratory reserve (minute ventilation at rest of < 10 L/min), and a low frequency-to-tidal volume ratio (f/V_T < 100), indicating adequate volume at a sustainable respiratory rate.

Objective Measures of Patient Strength and Endurance

Although clinicians may use a variety of parameters to determine readiness for extubation, few have been examined carefully. VC, defined as the volume of gas exhaled after maximal inspiration, is normally greater than 70 mL/kg. A clinical readiness threshold of 10 to 15 mL/kg has been proposed but is neither sensitive nor specific. For short-term ventilated patients, VC is less reliable than the ability to maintain a pH value greater than 7.35 while the IMV rate is decreased to CPAP. Maximal inspiratory pressure is often referred to as inspiratory force, negative inspiratory force, or peak negative pressure, and quantifies inspiratory effort as a marker of respiratory muscle strength. The proper technique involves airway occlusion for up to 20 seconds starting at full exhalation using a one-way valve that allows the patient to exhale after attempted inspiration. Normal values of maximal inspiratory pressure should exceed 100 cm H_2O in male patients and 80 cm H_2O in female patients. Values are usually expressed as an absolute to avoid confusion with "less than" or "greater than" when referring to a negative number. The classic cutoff value of 20 to 30 cm H_2O is associated with a 26% false-positive and 100% false-negative rate. Maximal inspiratory pressure is best used for serial evaluation of patients and is more a measure of strength than endurance.

Attempts have been made to predict endurance using the resting minute ventilation rate, but using the common value of 10 L/min as the cutoff results in a false-positive rate of 11% and a false-negative rate of 75% in predicting successful extubation. Similarly, the ability to sustain maximum voluntary ventilation twice the minute ventilation correctly predicts in only about 75% of the patients. More sophisticated measurement of endurance can be accomplished using a diaphragmatic or intercostal electromyogram power spectrum, but these are not practical for routine clinical use. Yang and Tobin[142] attempted to develop a scoring system for weaning that integrated lung compliance, respiratory rate, oxygenation levels, and maximum inspiratory pressure to predict weaning success. Although all of these elements and the total score have some predictive value, the best index turned out to be the f/V_T. An f/V_T greater than 105 has a predictive value of 89% for weaning failure. The tension-time index of the diaphragm (TT_{di}) integrates the inspiratory pressure with time and is a reliable measurement of endurance, but it is difficult to perform in the clinical setting. If the percentage of inspiratory time over total time in a spontaneously breathing patient is more than 15%, respiratory failure will eventually ensue, probably because of limitations of diaphragmatic blood flow, which occurs only during the expiratory phase. The tension time of the human diaphragm (TT_{DI}) is calculated by plotting the inspiratory time on the y-axis against the ratio of transdiaphragmatic pressure with normal and maximal effort on the x-axis. Fatigue is unlikely with values of TT_{DI} less than 0.15; values greater than 0.18 define the fatigue zone. Commercially available equipment such as the BiCor CP-100 pulmonary monitor can provide Ti/T total, f/V_T, and P 0.1, a marker of respiratory drive. Some newer ventilators also incorporate this technology. A problem with all measured respiratory parameters or scoring systems relying on pulmonary function is that they do not include the nonrespiratory parameters affecting weaning (Box 35-3).

Weaning: The Process

The actual process of weaning from mechanical ventilatory support must be individualized. There is no "one size fits all" method. Although gradually decreasing the SIMV rate in increments of 2 breaths/min generally works for short-term ventilatory support, long-term patients often have difficulty making the transition from SIMV rates of 2 to CPAP. The time-honored method of weaning by maintaining a patient on full ventilatory support alternating with increasingly longer periods of spontaneous ventilation on a T-piece is effective but time-consuming, because it requires setting up additional equipment and requires a nurse or respiratory therapist to be immediately available at bedside during each weaning attempt. Diaphragmatic effort

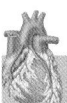

BOX 35-3. NONRESPIRATORY FACTORS THAT AFFECT WEANING

- Nutrition status
- Renal function
- Fluid balance
- Sepsis/Infection
- Hematologic status/anemia
- Metabolic disturbance
- Cardiac function
- Pharmacologic therapy
- Neurologic compromise
- Neuropsychiatric issues/delirium
- Sleep deprivation
- Endotracheal tube size
- Perception of breathing

is significantly lower during a T-piece trial with a deflated tracheostomy tube cuff than with the cuff inflated. Weaning trials with the cuff deflated may thus be more physiologic when attempting to wean the difficult patient. Breath-to-breath monitoring, display of V_T, and ventilator alarms will not be available during a T-piece trial. More commonly, pressure support is used as an adjunct to weaning either with IMV or CPAP, while still connected to the ventilator and its alarm system. Our preference is to conduct CPAP weaning with pressure support alone (i.e., no additional IMV rate) because mechanical ventilation introduces one more variable into the evaluation of a patient's progress. Sufficient CPAP is applied to maintain open alveoli (generally 5 to 8 cm H_2O, but often higher, when recovering from ALI/ARDS) and then the pressure-support level is titrated to provide the patient with sufficient volume and a respiratory rate less than 24. As the patient's exercise tolerance improves, the pressure-support level can be decreased in increments of 2 to 3 cm H_2O. It is usually necessary to address fluid overload, nutritional support, and other nonpulmonary factors to achieve the pressure-support reduction.

Regardless of which weaning method is chosen, it is important to end each weaning trial with success rather than to stress the patient to the point of fatigue. Cohen et al[146] identified the clinical sequence of inspiratory muscle fatigue. The earliest sign of inspiratory muscle fatigue was a spectrum shift in the electromyogram power spectrum, which is impractical in the clinical setting. However, the next most sensitive sign was an increase in respiratory rate, which occurred before respiratory alternans, abdominal paradox, and increase in the $Paco_2$ level, or acidemia. Thus, respiratory rate can serve as a sensitive marker of weaning progress.

Specific Impediments to Weaning

Weaning from ventilator support affects cardiac output because of changes in pulmonary vascular resistance. Increased pulmonary vascular resistance can lead to septal shifts and consequent changes in the efficiency of right and left ventricular function. Thus, it makes little sense to attempt weaning in the hemodynamically unstable patient. Our approach has been to keep these patients on full ventilator support with sedation and neuromuscular blockade, if necessary, until the acute cardiac problem is resolved.

Older ventilators with demand-valve systems impose an additional work of breathing, although it would be rare to see such ventilators (Bear I & II, Puritan Bennett MA-II) in clinical use today. Most newer ventilators use computer-assisted demands valve technology to supply a variable flow rate, unlike older ventilators in which a fixed low gas flow rate occasionally resulted in the inability to supply peak flow on demand. Nonetheless, if the patient is demonstrating apparent air hunger during the weaning process, a quick check of the inspiratory flow rates often can solve the problem. Pulmonary effusions

and pneumothorax can develop in otherwise stable patients and also may present as stalled weaning. Stacking of breaths or auto-PEEP can occur if the expiratory time is too short for patients, particularly those with obstructive disease, to exhale fully before the next breath is delivered. Brown and Pierson[147] demonstrated that the magnitude of auto-PEEP varied between 0 and 16 cm H_2O during routine ventilator checks.

Ventilator Dyssynchrony

Increases in intercostal muscle tone and increases in abdominal muscle tone, pressure, or contents will decrease chest cage compliance. During volume-cycled ventilation, a decrease in chest cage compliance results in increased intrathoracic pressure that may reduce venous return to the right heart. A patient also may actively attempt to impede flow during the inspiratory cycle, a process referred to as "fighting," being "out of phase," or "breathing against" the ventilator. This should not be confused with a patient making ventilatory efforts during the ventilator's expiratory cycle, which has little, if any, detrimental effect.

The most common reasons for fighting the ventilator are (1) inadequate ventilation (hypercarbia), (2) acidemia, (3) inadequate oxygenation, (4) central nervous system dysfunction, and (5) pain or anxiety. Assisting the patient with manual ventilation or switching to assist modes for a short time will allow the patient to settle down and return to synchrony with the ventilator. These maneuvers are temporizing during evaluation and treatment of the underlying cause for the patient/ventilator dyssynchrony. Endotracheal cuff leak, misplaced endotracheal tube, inadequate inspiratory flow rates, pneumothorax, abdominal distention, pain, and anxiety should all be considered in the differential diagnosis.

Muscle Weakness and Critical Illness Polyneuropathy

Long-term administration of neuromuscular blocking agents, particularly those such as vecuronium with a steroid structure, has been associated with persistent paralysis. One explanation may be the accumulation of the metabolite 3-desacetylvecuronium, which rarely is seen in patients with normal renal function but is quite common in patients with delayed recovery.[148] However, prolonged paralysis also can be seen after treatment with other drugs such as pancuronium, metocurine, and cisatracurium, which do not necessarily share the same structure or have persistent metabolism. The suspicion is that neurogenic atrophy occurs with prolonged paralysis resulting in a flaccid quadriplegia or more localized weakness of respiratory muscles.

Prolonged ICU stay also may precipitate psychiatric problems even in normal patients, although in our experience, these difficulties are more common in patients with an underlying psychiatric history. Light, noise, and lack of sleep can change a patient's perception of reality. Psychological dependency on the ventilator also may develop, although this is rare. Although this issue has not been examined with controlled trials, it is believed that careful attention to maintaining a normal day/night sleep cycle, assuring adequate sleep, creating a quiet ICU environment, judicious use of pharmacologic agents such as haloperidol or quetiapine, and involving the patient and family as participants in the weaning process are all helpful when there are psychological impediments to weaning.

Tracheostomy

Prolonged endotracheal intubation results in damage to the respiratory epithelium and cilia and may lead to vocal cord damage and airway stenosis.[150,151] If mechanical ventilation is anticipated for longer than 14 days, consideration should be given to early tracheostomy.[152,153] Other indications for tracheostomy include copious or tenacious secretions in debilitated patients who are unable to clear secretions spontaneously. Tracheostomy is relatively contraindicated with ongoing mediastinitis or local infection at the tracheostomy site because of the potential for mediastinal contamination with respiratory secretions. Tracheostomy is not a risk-free procedure, and complications include pneumothorax, pneumomediastinum, subcutaneous emphysema, incisional hemorrhage, late tracheal stenosis or tracheomalacia, stomal infections, and rarely, tracheoinnominate fistula. Early tracheostomy can be accomplished at the bedside with commercially available kits such as the Cook-Ciaglia or the "Rhino" device.[154,155] Swallowing dysfunction may occur after tracheostomy or after prolonged endotracheal intubation, introducing the risk for aspiration pneumonia or respiratory failure. A swallowing evaluation is indicated before allowing a tracheostomy patient to attempt oral feeding. This is usually accomplished with a formal speech pathology consult, but swallowing difficulty also may be noted by the nurses during attempted feedings. The predictors and outcome of cardiac surgical patients requiring tracheotomy were recently studied.[6] Hemodynamic status on ICU admission (low cardiac output, vasopressor use, pulmonary hypertension) and early postoperative events (stroke, bacteremia) were more important than preoperative and intraoperative variables in predicting ventilatory dependency. Survival at 30 days, 1 year, and 5 years thereafter was 76%, 49%, and 33%, respectively, and was strongly associated with favorable hemodynamic status.

Inability to Wean

A small percentage of patients will not be able to wean from ventilator support despite all efforts. Predictive models, however, are rarely useful for deciding which individuals will not benefit from further intensive care.[5,9,16,20,156]

Our experience has been that it is rarely a single problem, but the interaction among multiple morbidities that creates a situation in which the patient may never be able to separate from the ventilator. At this point, a frank discussion with the patient (if he/she has decisional capacity) or the health care proxy can be helpful in defining the benefits and burdens of further therapy and the patient's desires. Consultation from the hospital's ethics team may be helpful.[157] Patients who remain in a low cardiac output state and who have sustained multiple organ failure rarely, if ever, end their dependence on high-technology support including ventilation and hemodialysis. In contrast, malnutrition and deconditioning in the absence of ongoing sepsis and organ system failure sometimes respond to prolonged rehabilitation, which may be better handled by a long-term ventilation facility than an acute-care hospital. The critical issue is patient reserve, for without adequate cardiac and pulmonary reserve to tolerate stress once all remediable problems have been addressed, a patient is unlikely to remain technology independent.

CONCLUSIONS

Success in weaning from mechanical ventilation requires an individualized and holistic approach to the patient. Weaning should be the first priority for the day, and all other demands minimized if possible. If trips to the computed tomography scanner or therapeutic intervention such as wound debridement are anticipated, weaning may not be possible for part of the day. Thus, it is wise to try to minimize interruptions and to group them so as not to interrupt the weaning process. With that goal in mind, it is also essential to avoid disrupting the patient's nighttime sleep so that the patient can be well rested and ready to participate in the weaning process. Detailed and full instructions need to be given to the patient, and it frequently is helpful to include family members in the discussion so that they can serve as adjunct respiratory coaches. We try to avoid pushing the patient to the point of exhaustion or panic and use a planned, conservative approach such that weaning always ends in a sense of accomplishment for the patient rather than failure. Windows of opportunity for weaning from mechanical support are few and often must be created. Box 35-4 summarizes the recommendations for the difficult-to-wean cardiac surgical patient.

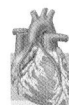

BOX 35-4. THE DIFFICULT TO WEAN PATIENT

1. Recognize patients at risk based on preoperative and operating room events (see Table 35-2).
2. Where possible, minimize risk (see Box 35-2).
3. Prioritize organ system support: without adequate perfusion, all other systems will fail.
4. Maintain full ventilator support during acute phase of respiratory insufficiency or circulatory failure.
5. Adopt a lung-protective ventilation strategy for acute lung injury/acute respiratory distress syndrome patients.
6. Expect and defend against common problems (see Box 35-3).
7. Pay attention to general support measures and safety issues including sedation holidays and infection control.
8. Prepare patient and family for involvement in rehabilitation phase.
9. Have a clear weaning plan or protocol and follow it.
10. Recognize when the burdens of treatment are disproportionate and initiate appropriate discussions with the patient or health care proxy.

REFERENCES

1. Westbrook RR, Stuvs SE, Sessler AD, et al: Effects of anesthesia and muscle paralysis on respiratory mechanisms in normal man, *J Appl Physiol* 34:81, 1973.
2. Sivak ED, Wiedemann HP: Clinical measurement of extravascular lung water, *Crit Care Clin* 2:511–526, 1986.
3. Wilson RS, Sullivan SF, Malm JR, et al: The oxygen cost of breathing following anesthesia and cardiac surgery, *Anesthesiology* 99:387, 1973.
4. Johnson D, Hurst T, Thompson D, et al: Respiratory function after cardiac surgery, *J Cardiothorac Vasc Anesth* 10:571, 1996.
5. Rady MY, Ryan T, Starr NJ: Early onset of acute pulmonary dysfunction after cardiovascular surgery: Risk factors and clinical outcome, *Crit Care Med* 25(11):1831, 1997.
6. Murthy SC, Arroliga AC, Walts PA, et al: Ventilatory dependency after cardiovascular surgery, *J Thorac Cardiovasc Surg* 134:484–490, 2007.
7. Weiner P, Zeidan F, Zamir D, et al: Prophylactic inspiratory muscle training in patients undergoing coronary artery bypass graft, *World J Surg* 22:427–431, 1998.
8. Higgins TL: Quantifying risk in assessing outcome in cardiac surgery, *J Cardiothor Vasc Anesth* 12:330–340, 1998.
9. Higgins TL, Estafanous EG, Loop FD, et al: Stratification of morbidity and mortality outcome by preoperative risk factors in coronary artery bypass patients. A clinical severity score, *JAMA* 267:2344–2348, 1992.
10. Hatler BG, Armitage JM, Haristy RL, et al: Risk stratification using the Society of Thoracic Surgeons Program, *Ann Thorac Surg* 58:1348–1352, 1994.
11. The Society of Thoracic Surgeons: 30-Day operative mortality and morbidity risk models, *Ann Thorac Surg* 75:1856–1865, 2003.
12. Nashef SAM, Roques F, Michel P, et al: EuroSCORE Study Group: European system for cardiac operative risk evalauation (EuroSCORE), *Eur J Cardiothorac Surg* 16:9–13, 1999.
13. Samuels LE, Kaufman MS, Rohinton BA, et al: Coronary artery bypass grafting in patients with COPD, *Chest* 113:878–882, 1998.
14. Rockx MA, Fox SA, Stitt LW, et al: Is obesity a predictor of mortality, morbidity and readmission after cardiac surgery? *Can J Surg* 47:34–38, 2004.

15. O'Brien MM, Gonzales R, Shroyer AL, et al: Modest serum creatinine elevation affects adverse outcome after general surgery, *Kidney Int* 62:585, 2002.
16. Spivack SD, Shinozaki T, Albertini JJ, et al: Preoperative prediction of postoperative respiratory outcome. Coronary artery bypass grafting, *Chest* 109:1222–1230, 1996.
17. Branca P, McGaw P, Light RW, et al: Factors associated with prolonged mechanical ventilation following coronary artery bypass surgery, *Chest* 119:537–546, 2001.
18. Rady MY, Ryan T: Perioperative predictors of extubation failure and the effect on clinical outcomes after cardiac surgery, *Crit Care Med* 27:340–347, 1999.
19. Canver CC, Chanda J: Intraoperative and postoperative risk factors for respiratory failure after coronary bypass, *Ann Thorac Surg* 75:853–857, 2003.
20. Higgins TL, Estafanous FG, Loop FD, et al: ICU admission score for predicting morbidity and mortality risk after coronary artery bypass grafting, *Ann Thorac Surg* 64:1050–1058, 1997.
21. Hall RI, Smith MS, Rocker G: The systemic inflammatory response to cardiopulmonary bypass—pathophysiological, therapeutic and pharmacological considerations, *Anesth Analg* 85:766, 1997.
22. Corral L, Carrio ML, Ventura JL, et al: Is C-reactive protein a biomarker for immediate clinical outcome after cardiac surgery? *J Cardiothorac Vasc Anesth* 23:166–169, 2009.
23. Yende S, Quasney MW, Tolley EA, et al: Clinical relevance of angiotensin-converting enzyme gene polymorphisms to predict risk of mechanical ventilation after coronary artery bypass graft surgery, *Crit Care Med* 32:922–927, 2004.
24. Huffmyer JL, Mauermann WJ, Thiele RH, et al: Preoperative statin administration is associated with lower mortality and decreased need for postoperative hemodialysis in patients undergoing coronary artery bypass graft surgery, *J Cardiothorac Vasc Anesth* 23:468–473, 2009.
25. Ouattara A, Benhaoua H, Le Manach Y, et al: Perioperative statin therapy is associated with a significant and dose-dependent reduction of adverse cardiovascular outcomes after coronary artery bypass graft surgery, *J Cardiothorac Vasc Anesth* 23:633–638, 2009.
26. Bohm SH, Thamm OC, von Sandersleben A, et al: Alveolar recruitment strategy and high positive end-expiratory pressure levels do not affect hemodynamics in morbidly obese intravascular volume-loaded patients, *Anesth Analg* 109:160–163, 2009.

27. Boldt J, Kling D, Weidler B, et al: Acute preoperative hemodilution in cardiac surgery: Volume replacement with a hypertonic saline-hydroxyethyl starch solution, *J Cardiothorac Vasc Anesth* 5:23–28, 1991.
28. Boldt J, Zickman B, Ballesteros M, et al: Cardiorespiratory responses to hypertonic saline solution in cardiac operations, *Ann Thorac Surg* 51:610–615, 1991.
29. Cheng KC, Hou CC, Huang HC, et al: Intravenous injection of methylprednisolone reduces the incidence of postextubation stridor in intensive care unit patients, *Crit Care Med* 34:1345–1350, 2006.
30. Zarbock A, Mueller E, Netzer S, et al: Prophylactic nasal continuous positive airway pressure following cardiac surgery protects from postoperative pulmonary complications, *Chest* 135:1252–1259, 2009.
31. Jacobs MC, Hussain E, Hall MH, et al: Stranger in a strange land: Internists in cardiothoracic intensive care, *New Horizons* 7:562–568, 1999.
32. Pronovost PJ, Angus DC, Dorman T, et al: Physician staffing patterns and clinical outcomes in critically ill patients. A systematic review, *JAMA* 288:2151–2162, 2002.
33. Levy MM, Rapoport J, Lemeshow S, et al: Association between critical care physician management and patient mortality in the intensive care unit, *Ann Intern Med* 148:801–809, 2008.
34. Pronovost PJ, Thompson DA, Holzmueller CG, et al: The organization of intensive care unit physician services, *Crit Care Med* 25:2256–2261, 2007.
35. Pronovost PJ, Needham DM, Waters H, et al: Intensive care unit physician staffing: Financial modeling of the Leapfrog standard, *Crit Care Med* 32:1247–1253, 2004.
36. Gajic O, Afessa B: Physician staffing models and patient safety in the ICU, *Chest* 135:1038–1044, 2009.
37. Fagon J-Y, Chastre J, Domart Y, et al: Nosocomial pneumonia in patients receiving continuous mechanical ventilation. Prospective analysis of 52 episodes with use of a protected specimen brush and quantitative culture techniques, *Am Rev Respir Dis* 139:877–884, 1989.
38. Weireter LJ, Collins JN, Britt RC, et al: Impact of a monitored program of care on incidence of ventilator-associated pneumonia: Results of a longterm performance-improvement project, *J Am Coll Surg* 208:700–705, 2009.
39. Guidelines for the management of adults with hospital-acquired, ventilator-associated, and healthcare-associated pneumonia, *Am J Respir Crit Care Med* 171:388–416, 2005.
40. Drakulovic MB, Torres A, Bauer TT, et al: Supine body position as a risk factor for nosocomial pneumonia in mechanically ventilated patients: A randomized trial, *Lancet* 354:1851–1858, 1999.
41. Schweickert WD, Gehlbach BK, Pohlman AS, et al: Daily interruption of sedative infusions and complications of critical illness in mechanically ventilated patients, *Crit Care Med* 32:1272–1276, 2004.
42. Craven DE, Goularte TA, Make BJ: Contaminated condensate in mechanical ventilator circuits: A risk factor for nosocomial pneumonia? *Am Rev Respir Dis* 129:625–628, 1984.
43. Sonora R, Jubert P, Artigas A, et al: Pneumonia in intubated patients: Role of respiratory airway care, *Am J Respir Crit Care Med* 154:111–115, 1996.
44. Kollef MH: The prevention of ventilator-associated pneumonia, *N Engl J Med* 340:627–634, 1999.
45. Dezfulian C, Shojania K, Collard HR, et al: Subglottic secretion drainage for preventing ventilator-associated pneumonia: A meta-analysis, *Am J Med* 118:11–18, 2005.
46. Kollef MH, Afessa B, Anzueto A, et al: Silver-coated endotracheal tubes and incidence of ventilator-associated pneumonia. The NASCENT randomized trial, *JAMA* 300:805–813, 2008.
47. Collard HR, Sanjay S, Matthay MA: Prevention of ventilator-associated pneumonia: An evidence-based systemic review, *Ann Intern Med* 138:494–501, 2003.
48. Ware LB, Matthay MA: Protein C and thrombomodulin in human acute lung injury, *Am J Physiol Lung Cell Mol Physiol* 285:L514–L521, 2003.
49. Bernard GR, Artigas A, Brigham KL, et al: The American-European Consensus Conference on ARDS. Definitions, mechanisms, relevant outcomes, and clinical trial coordination, *Am J Respir Crit Care Med* 149:818–824, 1994.
50. Murray JF, Matthay MA, Luce JM, et al: An expanded definition of the adult respiratory distress syndrome, *Am Rev Respir Dis* 138:720–723, 1988.
51. The National Heart, Lung, and Blood Institute Acute Respiratory Distress Syndrome (ARDS) Clinical Trials Network: Comparison of two fluid-management strategies in acute lung injury, *N Engl J Med* 354:2564–2575, 2006.
52. Kallet RH, Jasmer RM, Pittet J-F, et al: Clinical implementation of the ARDS network protocol is associated with reduced hospital mortality compared with historical controls, *Crit Care Med* 33: 925–929, 2005.
53. Nahum A, Hoyt J, Schmitz L, et al: Effect of mechanical ventilation strategy on dissemination of intratracheally instilled Escherichia coli in dogs, *Crit Care Med* 25:1733–1743, 1997.
54. Amato MB, Barbas CS, Medeiros DM, et al: Beneficial effects of the "open lung approach" with low distending pressures in acute respiratory distress syndrome: A prospective randomized study on mechanical ventilation, *Am J Respir Crit Care Med* 152:1835–1846, 1995.
55. The Acute Respiratory Distress Syndrome Network: Ventilation with lower tidal volumes as compared with traditional tidal volumes for acute lung injury and the acute respiratory distress syndrome, *N Engl J Med* 342:1301–1308, 2000.
56. Determan RM, Royakkers A, Wolthuis EK, et al: Ventilation with lower tidal volumes as compared to conventional tidal volumes for patients without acute lung injury—a preventive randomized controlled trial, *Crit Care* 14:R1, 2010.
57. Bidani A, Tzouanakis AE, Cardenas VJ, et al: Permissive hypercapnea in acute respiratory failure, *JAMA* 272:957–962, 1994.
58. Tidswell M: Prone ventilation, *Clin Intensive Care* 12:193–201, 2001.
59. Gattinoni L, Tognoni G, Pesenti A, et al: Effect of prone positioning on the survival of patients with acute respiratory failure, *N Engl J Med* 345:568–573, 2001.
60. Richard J-C, Brochard L, Vandelet P, et al: Respective effects of end-expiratory and end-inspiratory pressures on alveolar recruitment in acute lung injury, *Crit Care Med* 31:89–92, 2003.
61. Morris AH, Wallace CJ, Menlove Rl, et al: Randomized clinical trial of pressure-controlled inverse ratio ventilation and extracorporeal CO2 removal for adult respiratory distress syndrome, *Am J Respir Crit Care Med* 149:295–305, 1994.
62. Pranikoff T, Hirschl RB, Steimle CN, et al: Mortality is directly related to the duration of mechanical ventilation before the initiation of extracorporeal life support for severe respiratory failure, *Crit Care Med* 25:28–32, 1997.
63. Hirschl RB, Pranikoff T, Wise C, et al: Initial experience with partial liquid ventilation in adult patients with the acute respiratory distress syndrome, *JAMA* 275:383–389, 1996.
64. Body SC, Shernan SK: The utility of nitric oxide in the postoperative period, *Semin Cardiothorac Vasc Anesth* 2:4–30, 1998.
65. Ullrich R, Lorber C, Röder G, et al: Controlled airway pressure therapy, nitric oxide inhalation, prone position, and extracorporeal membrane oxygenation (ECMO) as components of an integrated approach to ARDS, *Anesthesiology* 91:1577–1586, 1999.
66. Walmrath D, Schneider T, Schermuly R, et al: Direct comparison of inhaled nitric oxide and aerosolized prostacyclin in acute respiratory distress syndrome, *Am J Respir Crit Care Med* 153: 991–996, 1996.
67. Miduri GU, Headley AS, Golden E, et al: Effect of prolonged methylprednisolone therapy in unresolving acute respiratory distress syndrome, *JAMA* 280:159–165, 1998.
68. Michalopoulos A, Anthi A, Rellos K, et al: Effects of positive end-expiratory pressure (PEEP) in cardiac surgery patients, *Respir Med* 92:858–862, 1998.
69. Calzia E, Lindner KH, Radermacher P, et al: Effects of continuous positive airway pressure on respiratory mechanics and work of breathing after cardiac surgery, *Clin Intensive Care* 9:105–110, 1998.
70. Guyton RA, Chiavarelli M, Padgett CA, et al: The influence of positive-end expiratory pressure on intrapericardial pressure and cardiac function after coronary artery bypass surgery, *J Cardiothorac Vasc Anesth* 1:98, 1987.
71. Boldt J, Kling D, Bormann BV, et al: Influence of PEEP ventilation immediately after cardiopulmonary bypass on right ventricular function, *Chest* 94:566, 1988.
72. Pepe PE, Hudson LD, Carrico CJ: Early application of positive end-expiratory pressure in patients at risk for the adult respiratory distress syndrome, *N Engl J Med* 311:281, 1984.
73. Zurick AM, Urzua J, Ghattas M, et al: Failure of positive end-expiratory pressure to decrease postoperative bleeding after cardiac surgery, *Ann Thorac Surg* 34:608, 1982.
74. Rimensberger PC, Pristine G, Mullen BM, et al: Lung recruitment during small tidal volume ventilation allows minimal positive end-expiratory pressure without augmenting lung injury, *Crit Care Med* 27:1940–1944, 1999.
75. The ARDS Clinical Trials Network, National Heart, Lung and Blood Institute, National Institutes of Health: Effects of recruitment maneuvers in patients with acute lung injury and acute respiratory distress syndrome ventilated with high positive end-expiratory pressure, *Crit Care Med* 31:2592–2597, 2003.
76. Hood VL, Tannen RL: Protection of acid-base balance by pH regulation of acid production, *N Engl J Med* 339:819–826, 1998.
77. Laffrey JG, Kavanagh BP: Carbon dioxide and the critically ill—too little of a good thing? *Lancet* 354:1283–1286, 1999.
78. Mekontso DA, Charron C, Devaquet J, et al: Impact of acute hypercapnia and augmented positive end-expiratory pressure on right ventricle function in severe acute respiratory distress syndrome, *Intensive Care Med* 11:1850–1858, 2009.
79. Steingrub JS, Tidswell MA, Higgins TL: Hemodynamic consequences of heart-lung interactions, *J Intensive Care Med* 18:92–99, 2003.
80. Pepe PE, Marini JJ: Occult positive end-expiratory pressure in mechanically ventilated patients with airflow obstruction, *Am Rev Respir Dis* 126:166, 1982.
81. Agency for Healthcare Research and Quality: Available at: http://www.AHRQ.gov/clinic/ptsafety/addend.htm Accessed May 20, 2004.
82. Kress JP, Pohlman AS, O'Connor MF, et al: Daily interruption of sedative infusions in critically ill patients undergoing mechanical ventilation, *N Engl J Med* 342:1471–1477, 2000.
83. Van den Berghe G, Wouters P, Welkes F, et al: Intensive insulin therapy in the critically ill patient, *N Engl J Med* 345:1359–1367, 2001.
84. Pronovost P, Berenholtz S, Dorman T, et al: Improving communication in the ICU using daily goals, *J Crit Care* 18:71–75, 2003.
85. Bates DW, Gawande AA: Improving safety with information technology, *N Engl J Med* 348:2526–2534, 2003.
86. Milbrandt EB, Deppen S, Harrison PL, et al: Costs associated with delirium in mechanically ventilated patients, *Crit Care Med* 31:955–962, 2004.
87. Smith LW, Dimsdale JE: Postcardiotomy delirium: Conclusions after 25 years, *Am J Psychiatry* 146:452–458, 1989.
88. Eli EW, Inouye SK, Bernard GR, et al: Delirium in mechanically ventilated patients. Validity and reliability of the Confusion Assessment Method for the Intensive Care Unit (CAM-ICU), *JAMA* 286:2703–2710, 2001.
89. Riker RR, Shehabi Y, Bokesch PM, et al: Dexmedetomidine vs. midazolam for sedation of critically ill patients, *JAMA* 301:489–499, 2009.
90. Herr DL, Sum-Ping St, England M: ICU sedation after coronary artery bypass graft surgery: Dexmedetomidine-based versus propofol-based sedation regimens, *J Cardiothorac Vasc Anesth* 17:576–584, 2003.
91. Hudetz JA, Patterson KM, Iqbal Z, et al: Ketamine attenuates delirium after cardiac surgery with cardiopulmonary bypass, *J Cardiothorac Vasc Anesth* 23:651–657, 2009.
92. Tesar GE, Murray GB, Cassem NH: Use of high-dose intravenous haloperidol in the treatment of agitated cardiac patients, *J Clin Psychopharmacol* 5:344, 1985.
93. Wilcox P, Baile EM, Hards J, et al: Phrenic nerve function and its relationship to atelectasis after coronary artery bypass surgery, *Chest* 93:693, 1988.
94. Lorin S, Sivak M, Nierman DM: Critical illness polyneuropathy: What to look for in at-risk patients. Diagnosis requires a high index of suspicion, *J Crit Illness* 13:608, 1998.
95. Ibebunjo C, Martyn JAJA: Fiber atrophy, but not changes in acetylcholine receptor expression, contributes to the muscle dysfunction after immobilization, *Crit Care Med* 27:275, 1999.
96. Van Balkom RHH, Dekhuijzen R, Folgering HTM, et al: Effects of long-term low-dose methylprednisone on rat diaphragm function and structure, *Muscle Nerve* 20:983, 1997.
97. Abd AG, Braun NMT, Baskin MI, et al: Diaphragmatic dysfunction after open heart surgery; treatment with a rocking bed, *Ann Intern Med* 111:881, 1989.
98. Aubier M, Detroyer A, Sampson M, et al: Aminophylline improves diaphragmatic contractility, *N Engl J Med* 305:249, 1981.
99. Riddington DW, Venkatesh B, Boivin CM, et al: Intestinal permeability, gastric intramucosal pH and systemic endotoxemia in patients undergoing cardiopulmonary bypass, *JAMA* 275:1007, 1996.
100. Tuzcu EM, Maloney JD, Sangani BH, et al: Cardiopulmonary effects of chronic amiodarone therapy in the early postoperative course of cardiac surgery patients, *Cleve Clin J Med* 54:491, 1987.
101. Nalos PC, Kass RM, Gang ES, et al: Life-threatening postoperative pulmonary complications in patients with previous amiodarone pulmonary toxicity undergoing cardiothoracic operations, *J Thorac Cardiovasc Surg* 93:904, 1987.
102. Manthous CA, Zarich S: Myocardial ischemia during weaning from mechanical ventilation, *Semin Cardiothorac Vasc Anesth* 2:78, 1998.
103. Zin WA, Caldeira MPR, Cardoso WV, et al: Expiratory mechanics before and after uncomplicated heart surgery, *Chest* 1:21, 1989.
104. Guillory RK, Gunter OL: Ultrasound in the surgical intensive care unit, *Curr Opin Crit Care* 14:415–422, 2008.
105. Melamed R, Sprenkle MD, Ulstad VK, et al: Assessment of left ventricular function by intensivists using hand-held echocardiography, *Chest* 135:1416–1420, 2009.
106. Beaulieu Y, Marik PE: Bedside ultrasonography in the ICU: Part 2, *Chest* 128:1766–1781, 2005.
107. Omoto R, Kyo S, Matsumara M, et al: Evaluation of biplane color Doppler Transesophageal echocardiography in 200 consecutive patients, *Circulation* 85:1237–1247, 1992.
108. Cowie B: Focused cardiovascular ultrasound performed by anesthesiologists in the perioperative period: Feasible and alters patient management, *J Cardiothorac Vasc Anesth* 23:450–456, 2009.
109. Orihashi K, Hong YW, Chung G, et al: New application of two-dimensional echocardiography in cardiac surgery, *J Cardiothorac Vasc Anesth* 5:33–39, 1991.
110. Talmor M, Hydo L, Gershenwald JG, et al: Beneficial effects of chest tube drainage of pleural effusion in acute respiratory failure refractory to positive end-expiratory pressure ventilation, *Surgery* 123:137–143, 1998.
111. Seward JB, Khanderia BK, Edwards WD, et al: Biplanar transesophageal echocardiography: Anatomic correlation, image orientation and clinical application, *Mayo Clin Proc* 65:1193–1213, 1990.
112. American Society of Anesthesiologists Task Force on Pulmonary artery Catheterization: Practice guidelines for pulmonary artery catheterization, *Anesthesiology* 99:988–1014, 2003.

113. Jardin F, Bourdarias JP: Right heart catheterization at bedside: A critical view, *Intensive Care Med* 21:291–295, 1995.
114. Joseph MX, Disney PJS, Da Costa R, et al: Transthoracic echocardiography to identify or exclude cardiac cause of shock, *Chest* 126:1592–1597, 2004.
115. Subramaniam B, Talmor D: Echocardiography for management of hypotension in the intensive care unit, *Crit Care Med* 35(8 Suppl):S401–S407, 2007.
116. Sterba M, Banerjee A, Mudaliar Y: Prospective observational study of levosimendan and weaning of difficult-to-wean ventilator dependent intensive care patients, *Crit Care Resusc* 10:182–186, 2008.
117. Balik M, Pachl J, Hendl J: Effect of the degree of tricuspid regurgitation on cardiac output measurements by thermodilution, *Intensive Care Med* 28:1117–1121, 2002.
118. Jullien T, Valtier B, Hongnat JM, et al: Incidence of tricuspid regurgitation and vena cava backward flow in mechanically ventilated patients. A color Doppler and contrast echocardiography study, *Chest* 107:488–493, 1995.
119. Beaulieu Y: Bedside echocardiography in the assessment of the critically ill, *Crit Care Med* 35:S235–S249, 2007.
120. Feissel M, Teboul JL, Merlani P, et al: Plethysmographic dynamic indices predict fluid responsiveness in septic ventilated patients, *Intensive Care Med* 33:993–999, 2007.
121. Monnet X, Rienzo M, Osman D, et al: Passive leg raising predicts fluid responsiveness in the critically ill, *Crit Care Med* 34:1402–1407, 2006.
122. Vieillard-Baron A, Charron C: Preload responsiveness or right ventricular dysfunction? *Crit Care Med* 37:2662–2663, 2009.
123. Vieillard-Baron AI: Is right ventricular function the one that matters in ARDS patients? Definitely yes, *Intensive Care Med* 35:4–6, 2009.
124. Funk DJ, Moretti EW, Gan TJ: Minimally invasive cardiac output monitoring in the perioperative setting, *Anesth Analg* 108:887–897, 2009.
125. Koning HM, Koning AJ, Leusink JA: Serious acute renal failure following open heart surgery, *J Thorac Cardiovasc Surg* 33:283, 1985.
126. Myers BD, Moran SM: Hemodynamically mediated acute renal failure, *N Engl J Med* 314:97, 1987.
127. Joy MS, Matske GR, Armstrong DK, et al: A primer on continuous renal replacement therapy for critically ill patients, *Ann Pharmacother* 32:362, 1998.
128. Loop FD, Lytle BW, Cosgrove DM, et al: Sternal wound complications after isolated coronary artery bypass grafting: Early and late mortality, morbidity, and cost of care, *Ann Thorac Surg* 49:179, 1990.
129. Zerr KJ, Furnary AP, Grunkemeier GL, et al: Glucose control lowers the risk of wound infection in diabetics after open heart operations, *Ann Thorac Surg* 63:356, 1997.
130. Kirschenbaum L, Azzi E, Sfeir T, et al: Effect of continuous lateral rotational therapy on the prevalence of ventilator-associated pneumonia in patients requiring long-term ventilatory care, *Crit Care Med* 30:1983–1986, 2002.
131. Chastre J, Fagon J-Y: Ventilator-associated pneumonia, *Am J Respir Crit Care Med* 165:867–903, 2002.
132. Krasna MJ, Flanchbaum L, Trooskin ZS, et al: Gastrointestinal complications after cardiac surgery, *Surgery* 104:733, 1988.
133. Ephgrave KS, Kleinman-Wexler RL, Adar CG: Enteral nutrients prevent stress ulceration and increase intragastric volume, *Crit Care Med* 18:621, 1990.
134. Zilberberg MD, Nathanson B, Higgins TL, et al: Epidemiology and outcomes of *Clostridium difficile*-associated disease among patients on prolonged acute mechanical ventilation, *Chest* 136:752–758, 2009.
135. Bassilli HR, Deitel M: Effect of nutritional support on weaning patients off mechanical ventilators, *J Parenter Enteral Nutr* 5:161, 1981.
136. Larca L, Greenbaum DM: Effectiveness of intensive nutritional regimes in patients who fail to wean from mechanical ventilation, *Crit Care Med* 10:297–300, 1982.
137. Tharratt RS, Allen RP, Albertson TE: Pressure controlled inverse ratio ventilation in severe adult respiratory failure, *Chest* 94:755–762, 1988.
138. Richard J-C, Brochard L, Vandelet P, et al: Respective effects of end-expiratory and end-inspiratory pressures on alveolar recruitment in acute lung injury, *Crit Care Med* 31:89–92, 2003.
139. Stock AC, Downs JB, Frolicher DA: Airway pressure release ventilation, *Crit Care Med* 15:462–466, 1987.
140. Dongelmans DA, Veelo DP, Bindels A, et al: Determinants of tidal volumes with adaptive support ventilation: A multicenter observational study, *Anesth Analg* 107:932–937, 2008.
141. Millbern SM, Downs JB, Jumper LC, et al: Evaluation of criteria for discontinuing mechanical ventilator, *Arch Surg* 113:1441–1443, 1978.
142. Yang KL, Tobin MJ: A prospective study of indexes predicting the outcome of trials of weaning from mechanical ventilation, *N Engl J Med* 324:1445–1450, 1991.
143. Bellemare F, Grassino A: Effect of pressure and timing of contraction on human diaphragm fatigue, *J Appl Physiol* 53:1190–1195, 1982.
144. Grassino A, Bellemare F, Laporta D: Diaphragm fatigue and the strategy of breathing in COPD, *Chest* 85:515–535, 1984.
145. Ceriana P, Carlucci A, Navalesi P, et al: Physiological responses during a T-piece weaning trial with a deflated tube, *Intensive Care Med* 32:1399–1403, 2006.
146. Cohen CA, Zagelbaum G, Cross D, et al: Clinical manifestations of inspiratory muscle fatigue, *Am J Med* 73:308–316, 1982.
147. Brown DG, Pierson DJ: Auto-PEEP is common in mechanically ventilated patients: A study of incidence, severity, and detection, *Respir Care* 31:1069–1074, 1986.
148. Segredo V, Caldwell JE, Matthay MA, et al: Persistent paralysis in critically ill patients after long-term administration of Vecuronium, *N Engl J Med* 327:524–528, 1992.
149. Rosenthal LJ, Kim V, Kim D: Weaning from prolonged mechanical ventilation using an antipsychotic agent in a patient with acute stress disorder, *Crit Care Med* 35:2417–2419, 2007.
150. Kastanos N, Estopa R, Peez AM, et al: Laryngotracheal injury due to endotracheal intubation: Incidence, evolution, and predisposing factors. A prospective long-term study, *Crit Care Med* 11:362–367, 1983.
151. Norwood S, Vallina VL, Short K, et al: Incidence of tracheal stenosis and other late complications after percutaneous tracheostomy, *Ann Surg* 232:233–241, 2000.
152. Gibbons KJ: Tracheostomy: Timing is everything, *Crit Care Med* 28:1663–1664, 2000.
153. Brook AD, Sherman G, Malen J, et al: Early versus late tracheostomy in patients who require prolonged mechanical ventilation, *Am J Crit Care* 9:352–359, 2000.
154. Westphal K, Byhahn C, Rinne T, et al: Tracheostomy in cardiosurgical patients: Surgical tracheostomy versus Ciaglia and Fantoni methods, *Ann Thorac Surg* 68:486–492, 1999.
155. Freeman BD, Isabella K, Cobb P, et al: A prospective, randomized study comparing percutaneous with surgical tracheostomy in critically ill patients, *Crit Care Med* 29:926–930, 2001.
156. Holmes L, Loughead K, Treasure T, et al: Which patients will not benefit from further intensive care after cardiac surgery, *Lancet* 344:1200–1202, 1994.
157. Baldyga AP: Ethical issues in the postoperative intensive care unit, *Semin Cardiothorac Vasc Anesth* 2:90, 1998.

36

Central Nervous System Dysfunction after Cardiopulmonary Bypass

JOHN M. MURKIN, MD, FRCPC

KEY POINTS

1. Despite a progressive decrease in cardiac surgical mortality since the 1980s, the incidence of postoperative neurologic complications has remained relatively unchanged. The age, acuity, and extent of comorbidities in cardiac surgical patients have also increased during this same interval.
2. There is a progressive increase in risk for stroke for coronary artery surgery with increasing age ranging from 0.5% for patients younger than 55 years to 2.3% for those older than 75 years.
3. Neurologic events in cardiac surgical patients are associated with increased postoperative mortality, prolonged intensive care unit, hospital stay, decreased quality of life, and decreased long-term survival.
4. Neurologic complications range from coma, stroke, and visual field deficits to impairments of cognitive processes (e.g., delirium, impaired memory and attention, mood alterations).
5. Mechanisms for neurologic injury in cardiac surgery include some combination of cerebral embolism, hypoperfusion, and inflammation; associated vascular disease; and altered cerebral autoregulation, rendering the brain more susceptible to injury. Progression of underlying disease is a confounder in assessing late postoperative complications.
6. Perioperative risk factors for neurologic complications include renal dysfunction, diabetes mellitus, hypertension, prior cerebrovascular disease, aortic atheromatosis, manipulation of ascending aorta, complex surgical procedures, bypass time longer than 2 hours, hypothermic circulatory arrest, hemodynamic instability during and after bypass, new-onset atrial fibrillation, hyperglycemia, hyperthermia, and hypoxemia.
7. Routine epiaortic scanning before instrumentation of the ascending aorta is a sensitive and specific technique to detect nonpalpable aortic atheromatosis.
8. In patients with significant ascending aorta atheromatosis, avoidance of aortic manipulation ("no-touch technique") can decrease perioperative stroke.
9. Strategies to decrease the impact of cardiopulmonary bypass on embolization, inflammation, and coagulation will decrease neurologic complications.
10. Cerebral near-infrared spectroscopy can detect cerebral ischemia and has been associated with improved outcomes after cardiac surgery.
11. There is a greater incidence of early postoperative cognitive dysfunction in patients exposed to cardiopulmonary bypass compared with off-pump and noncardiac surgery patients.
12. The incidence of late cognitive dysfunction appears to be similar between groups whether exposed to cardiopulmonary bypass, percutaneous coronary intervention, or medical management, implying progression of underlying disease as a primary mechanism.

Overt and subclinical perioperative cerebral injury remains a complex problem. As Ferguson et al[1] reported, although overall mortality for patients undergoing coronary artery bypass grafting (CABG) has decreased by 23% during the 1990s, despite a projected risk-adjusted mortality predicting a 33% increase in mortality, the incidence of stroke has remained relatively unchanged.

AGE-ASSOCIATED RISK FOR CENTRAL NERVOUS SYSTEM INJURY

In 1985, Gardner et al[2] reported a retrospective review of 3279 patients who underwent CABG between 1974 and 1983. They noted that despite an overall decrease in mortality, there was a corresponding increase in the incidence of stroke over that same decade.[2] They also observed a progressive increase in the average age of the patients and noted an increased stroke rate of 7.1% in patients older than 75 years compared with an incidence rate of 0.42% in patients younger than 50 years. Notably, at that time, septuagenarians accounted for only 14.7% of their operative population. Approximately a decade later, Tuman et al[3] undertook a prospective study of 2000 patients undergoing CABG and also demonstrated a disproportionately increased risk for neurologic complications as compared with cardiac complications in elderly patients (Figure 36-1). Neurologic events, defined as new sensory, motor, or reflex abnormalities, occurred with an overall frequency rate of 2.8%, having an incidence rate of 0.9% in those patients younger than 65 years, 3.6% in those aged 65 to 74 years, and 8.9% in those patients older than 75 years. Notably, they observed that patients with a neurologic event had a ninefold increase in mortality: 35.7% versus 4.0%.

Current data confirm a persistent association between increased age and cerebral injury after cardiac surgery.[4-14] In a review of 67,764 cardiac surgical patients, of whom 4743 were octogenarians, and who

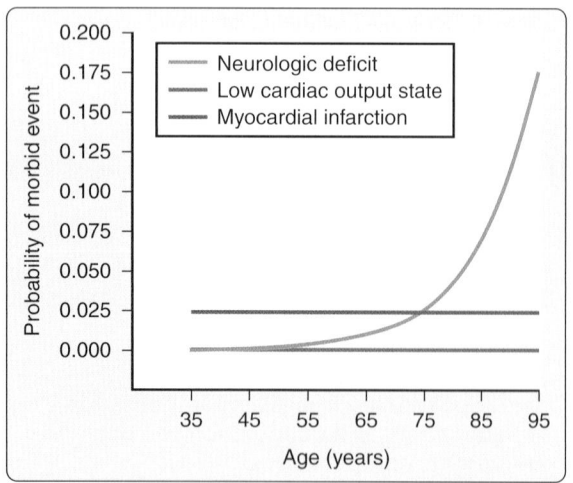

Figure 36-1 **Effect of advanced age on the predicted probability of neurologic and cardiac morbidity.** *(From Tuman KJ, McCarthy RJ, Najafi H, et al: Differential effects of advanced age on neurologic and cardiac risks of coronary artery operations. J Thorac Cardiovasc Surg 104:1510, 1992.)*

underwent cardiac surgery at 22 centers in the National Cardiovascular Network, Alexander et al[12] reported that the incidence of type I cerebral injury, defined by Roach et al[14] as stroke, transient ischemic attack (TIA), or coma,[13] was 10.2% in patients older than 80, versus 4.2% in patients younger than 80. Importantly, although global mortality for cardiac surgery in octogenarians was greater than in younger patients, the authors reported that *when octogenarians without significant comorbidities were considered, their mortality rates were similar to those of younger patients.*[12] In a more recent review from the Society of Thoracic Surgeons National Adult Cardiac Surgery Database of 774,881 patients undergoing isolated CABG between January 2002 and December 2006, the overall incidence rate of stroke was 1.4%, increasing to 2.3% in patients aged 75 years and older.[13] Interestingly, stroke rate was inversely related to body surface area and directly proportional to serum creatinine concentration, as well as presence of valvular heart disease and other comorbidities.[13]

In this respect, in addition to the age-related factor, reports from Europe and North America consistently describe previous cerebrovascular disease, diabetes mellitus, hypertension, peripheral vascular disease, aortic atherosclerosis, and intraoperative and postoperative complications as all being additional factors increasing the incidence of cerebral injury in cardiac surgical patients (Box 36-1). The presence of preoperative comorbidities further increases the age-associated risk for central nervous system (CNS) complications. For example, in a population of 149 patients older than 70 years who also had significant

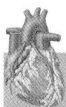

BOX 36-1. FACTORS RELATED TO CEREBRAL INJURY IN CARDIAC SURGERY

- Hemodynamic instability[4,5,27,132]
- Diabetes mellitus[4,8,26,226]
- Age[5,13,19,87,133]
- Combined/complex procedures[4,5]
- Prolonged cardiopulmonary bypass time[4,27,40]
- Prior stroke[5,7,26,87]
- Renal dysfunction[301]
- Aorta atheromatosis[6,8,85–89]
- Peripheral vascular disease[6,40]

Risk factors consistently reported for perioperative cerebral injury in cardiac surgery patients; see reference numbers and discussion in the text.

comorbidities including aortic atheroma, diabetes mellitus, and history of previous CNS event, and who underwent cardiac surgery with cardiopulmonary bypass (CPB), Frumento et al[8] reported a stroke incidence rate of 16%.

The impact of age-associated cerebral injury in cardiac surgery is becoming more relevant because of the progressive increase in the average age of the general population and, in particular, of the cardiac surgical population.[10,11,13–16] As overall survival and quality of life after cardiac surgery continue to improve in elderly patients, advanced age alone is no longer considered a deterrent when evaluating a patient for cardiac surgery.[10–12,17] *The presence and extent of comorbidities should be considered as being of equal or greater importance than age itself as a risk factor for cerebral injury in cardiac surgical patients.*

CENTRAL NERVOUS SYSTEM INJURY

Roach et al[14] classified cerebral injury in two broad categories: type I (focal injury, stupor, or coma at discharge) and type II (deterioration in intellectual function, memory deficit, or seizures).[14] A similar classification was adopted by the American College of Cardiology/American Heart Association (ACC/AHA) guidelines for CABG.[18] Cerebral injury can also be broadly classified as stroke, TIA, delirium (encephalopathy), or cognitive dysfunction. Perioperative cognitive performance is assessed through the administration of a series of standardized psychometric tests, ideally administered before and after surgery.

Stroke is defined clinically as any new focalized sensorimotor deficit persisting longer than 24 hours, identified either on clinical grounds only or, ideally, as confirmed by magnetic resonance imaging (MRI), computed tomography, or other form of brain imaging.

TIA is defined as brief neurologic dysfunction persisting for less than 24 hours. Neurologic dysfunction lasting longer than 24 hours but less than 72 hours is termed a *reversible ischemic neurologic deficit.*

Delirium is described as a transient global impairment of cognitive function, reduced level of consciousness, profound changes in sleep pattern, and attention abnormalities.

Cognitive dysfunction is defined as a decrease in score falling below some predetermined threshold, such as a decrease in postoperative score of magnitude 1 standard deviation or more derived from the preoperative performance of the study group as a whole.

The incidence of stroke or type I injury after closed-chamber cardiac procedures is generally considered to be approximately 1% to 4%, increasing to about 8% to 9% in open-chamber (e.g., valvular surgery) or combined/complex procedures. The incidence of cognitive dysfunction (type II) is reported as ranging in incidence rate from 30% to 80% in the early postoperative period.[4,18–25] To some extent, there is a difference in the incidence of cerebral injury after cardiac surgery related to the type and complexity of the procedure, such as open chamber, combined valvular, and CABG.[4,10,26,27]

Overall, the increased length of stay and increased mortality rates associated with any form of cerebral complication in cardiac surgical patients are especially striking findings.[15,18,20,21] Despite the relatively greater impact on mortality of stroke as opposed to cognitive dysfunction, type II injury is still associated with a fivefold increase in mortality. In their study, Roach et al[14] evaluated 2108 patients undergoing CABG at 24 U.S. institutions and recorded adverse cerebral outcomes in 6.1% of patients overall. Of these, 3.1% experienced type I focal injury, stupor, or coma and had an associated in-hospital mortality rate of 21%, whereas 3.0% of patients experienced deterioration of intellectual function or seizures and had a mortality rate of 10%. In contrast, a significantly lower overall mortality rate of 2% was seen in those patients without adverse cerebral outcomes. In addition, patients with neurologic complications had, on average, a twofold increase in hospital length of stay and a sixfold likelihood of discharge to a nursing home. Independent risk factors were identified for both type I and II cerebral injury. Predictors of both types of cerebral complications included advanced age of older than 70 years and a history or the presence of significant hypertension. *Predictors of type I deficits include the presence of proximal aortic atherosclerosis as defined by the surgeon at the time of surgery, a history of prior neurologic disease, use of the intra-aortic balloon pump, diabetes, a history of hypertension, a history of unstable angina, and increasing age.* Perioperative hypotension and the use of ventricular venting were also weakly associated with this type of outcome.[14]

An important caveat that must be borne in mind when interpreting Roach et al's[14] results is that type II injury as identified in their study is not necessarily equivalent to perioperative cognitive dysfunction as demonstrated in other studies. Type II injury was detected on clinical grounds alone rather than on the basis of a deterioration in performance on a predefined series of specific cognitive tests. The latter are a much more sensitive measure of performance and thus detect cognitive dysfunction with a considerably greater frequency, and as such potentially have a much different, although not necessarily benign, implication from the increased mortality associated with type II injury demonstrated by Roach et al.[14,28]

Using a risk-stratification analysis of this same database, Newman et al[29] developed a preoperative index predicting major perioperative neurologic events of which key predictors were age, history of neurologic disease, diabetes, previous CABG, unstable angina, and history of pulmonary disease (Figure 36-2).[14,29] The Stroke Risk Index allows neurologic risk to be estimated for each patient, thus enabling the most appropriate perioperative therapy to be used, whether surgical modification, change in perfusion management, applied neuromonitoring, or administration of putative pharmacologic cerebroprotectants. It is also useful as a scale to compare risk indices, and thus the efficacy of different interventions across clinical outcome studies.[8,21]

Retrospective versus Prospective Neurologic Assessment

The detection of CNS injury depends critically on the methodology used, and retrospective studies have been deemed insensitive by different authors.[23,24,30,31] As Sotaniemi[31] demonstrated, a retrospective chart review is inadequate as an assessment of the overall incidence of postoperative neurologic dysfunction. In a study of 100 patients in whom a 37% incidence rate of neurologic dysfunction had been diagnosed by careful neurologic examination, the prevalence rate of cerebral abnormalities detected by retrospective analysis of the same patient pool was only 4%. The reasons for the inability of retrospective chart audit to detect the majority of patients with neurologic dysfunction are readily apparent and include incompleteness of records, a reluctance to document apparently minor complications, and most important, an insensitivity to subtle neurologic dysfunction. Many of the types of neurologic impairment now being documented are subclinical and not readily detectable by a standard "foot-of-the-bed" assessment. The timing, thoroughness, and reproducibility (single examiner) of the neurologic examinations, as well as the incorporation of a preoperative assessment for comparison, all determine the sensitivity and accuracy with which postoperative CNS injury can be detected.[23,24,30,32]

Valvular versus Coronary Artery Bypass Graft Surgery

It appears that increasing the complexity or undertaking open chamber–type procedures increases the risk for CNS injury. Ebert et al[33] prospectively studied 42 patients who underwent valve replacement surgery and 42 patients for CABG, with both groups matched post hoc for age, sex, and preoperative cognitive status.

Patients were investigated before surgery, as well as 2 and 7 days after surgery, with a comprehensive neuropsychological and neuropsychiatric assessment. Valve replacement surgery patients exhibited more severe neuropsychological deficits and showed a slower recovery than patients who underwent CABG.[33] In Alexander et al's[12] study of 64,467 patients who underwent CABG alone and 3297 patients who underwent CABG in conjunction with aortic valve replacement or CABG in conjunction with mitral valve repair or replacement, the incidence rate

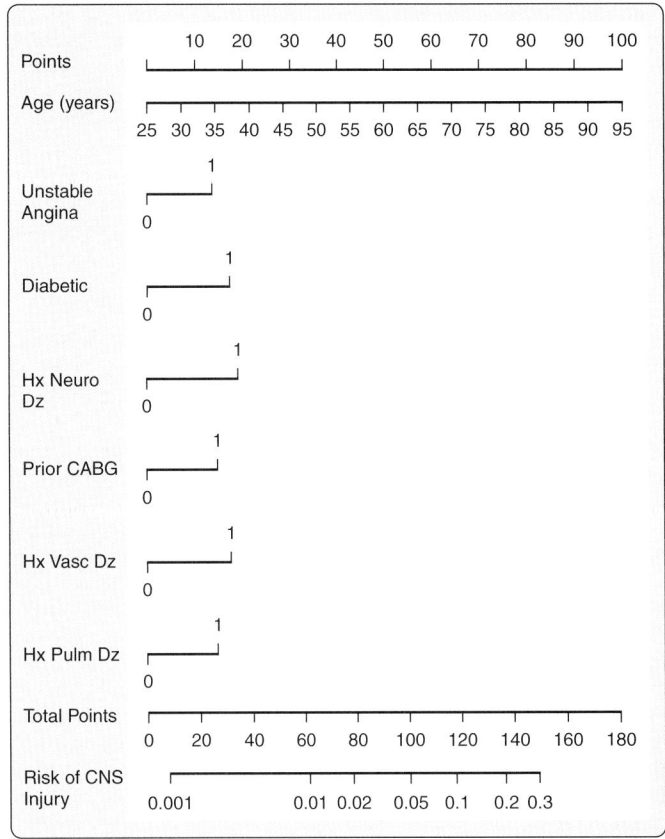

Figure 36-2. Nomogram for computing risk of central nervous system (CNS) injury. Neurologic risk is determined by assigning points for age and positive history of the predictors listed. Total points for each variable are read from the points line at the top of the nomogram. After the total points for an individual patient are computed, the risk for CNS injury can be determined by plotting the total points received against the risk score at the bottom of the nomogram. For example, 100 total points predict a risk for CNS injury of 5%. CABG, coronary artery bypass graft; Hx Neuro Dz, history of symptomatic neurologic disease; Hx Pulm Dz, history of emphysema, chronic bronchitis, asthma, or restrictive lung disease; Hx Vasc Dz, history of atherosclerotic vascular disease or previous vascular surgery. *(From Newman MF, Wolman R, Kanchuger M, et al: Multicenter preoperative stroke risk index for patients undergoing coronary artery bypass graft surgery. Multicenter Study of Perioperative Ischemia [McSPI] Research Group. Circulation 49[suppl II]:II-74, 1996.)*

of type I cerebral injury in patients younger than 80 years was 4.2% for CABG, 9.1% for CABG with aortic valve replacement, and 11.2% for CABG with mitral valve repair or replacement.[12] Notably, the total CPB time was 96 minutes for CABG, 148 minutes for CABG in conjunction with aortic valve replacement, and 161 minutes for CABG with mitral valve repair or replacement. It thus remains unclear whether it is the procedure itself or the prolonged duration of CPB, either acting directly or as a marker of a greater surgical difficulty and thus perioperative hemodynamic instability, that is fundamentally causative.[34]

Wolman et al[20] prospectively studied 273 patients from 24 U.S. medical centers who underwent combined intracardiac surgery and CABG. Included were clinical, historic, specialized testing, neurologic outcome, and autopsy data, and measures of resource utilization. Adverse cerebral outcomes occurred in 16% of patients (43/273), being nearly equally divided between type I cerebral injury (8.4%; 5 cerebral deaths, 16 nonfatal strokes, and 2 new TIAs) and type II cerebral injury (7.3%; 17 new intellectual deteriorations persisting at hospital discharge and 3 newly diagnosed seizures), rates of injury 2- to 3-fold greater than demonstrated after CABG alone by this same group of investigators.[20] Associated resource utilization was significantly increased according to type of CNS injury: prolonging median intensive care unit (ICU) stay from 3 days (no adverse cerebral outcome) to 8 days associated with type I injury and from 3 to 6 days in those patients with type II injury. Significant risk factors for type I cerebral injury related primarily to embolic phenomena, including proximal aortic atherosclerosis, intracardiac thrombus, and intermittent clamping of the aorta during surgery. Risk factors for type II cerebral injury included proximal aortic atherosclerosis, as well as a preoperative history of endocarditis, alcohol abuse, perioperative arrhythmia, or poorly controlled hypertension, and the development of a low-output state after CPB.[20]

CO₂ Insufflation during Open-Chamber Procedures

A primary determinant of the number and duration of microgaseous emboli during open-chamber procedures relates to methodologies for removal of intracavitary air. Although needle aspiration and/or aortic root venting are standard techniques for air removal, use of CO_2 insufflation, either continuously or immediately before closure of ventriculotomy, has been shown to significantly increase the efficacy of deairing resulting in decreased systemic gaseous emboli.[35,36] However, although there has been a general expectation of improvements in neurologic and cognitive outcomes resulting from such CO_2 insufflation, it has been surprisingly difficult to demonstrate. In a recent prospective study of 80 patients undergoing valve surgery and randomized to CO_2 insufflation versus conventional deairing, although postoperative auditory-evoked potential monitoring did demonstrate shorter P-300 latency in the CO_2-insufflated group, there was no detectable difference in clinical outcomes or in the incidence of cognitive dysfunction between groups.[37] In a recent review of the role of CO_2 insufflation, the authors concluded that although the use of CO_2 field flooding has been observed to be associated with a significantly lower count of intracardiac air bubbles and improved survival in two small studies, so far there is no evidence of a sustained reduction of cerebrovascular complications.[38]

Fewer systemic and cerebral emboli were demonstrated in patients undergoing open-chamber surgery in whom bilateral pleurotomy and passive lung deflation associated with staged perfusion and ventilation of lungs during deairing was used in comparison with those in whom pleural cavities were unopened and dead space ventilation was continued during CPB.[39] In this study, CO_2 insufflation was not used, and the authors reported that deairing time was significantly shorter in the treatment group.

Neurocognitive Dysfunction Unrelated to Cerebral Microgaseous Emboli

Interestingly, there is some evidence that the incidence of subtle neurologic dysfunction and cognitive abnormalities is similar in all adult patients undergoing surgical coronary artery revascularization, which some studies have related to the duration of CPB.[4,12,24,40–43] Increasing age has been repeatedly shown to be one of the major risk factors for stroke after CABG, likely related to the greater prevalence of severe aortic atherosclerosis in the elderly. This suggests that *there may be different factors operative in the production of gross neurologic damage than in the genesis of cognitive dysfunction.* Whereas calcific or atheromatous macroembolic debris from the ascending aorta or aortic arch appears to be a prime factor in the production of clinical stroke syndromes and it was formerly thought that microembolic elements, either gaseous or particulate, produced cognitive dysfunction, studies from beating-heart surgery in which CPB is avoided, despite a much lower incidence of embolic events, appear to have a relatively similar incidence of cognitive dysfunction to CABG using conventional CPB.[44–46]

A series of longitudinal studies by Selnes[47] and others in patients undergoing off-pump cardiac surgery, as well as those treated medically, have suggested that *long-term changes in cognitive function* are not specific to CABG or use of CPB and may rather reflect progression of underlying disease.[47–50] Other longitudinal studies have, however, demonstrated a greater incidence of cognitive dysfunction in CABG patients in comparison with various nonsurgical control groups,[51,52] though the comparability of underlying disease processes between groups remains a significant confound in many such studies.

However, as there is general agreement that the incidence of *early postoperative cognitive dysfunction* is greater in CABG patients compared with other noncardiac surgical groups, and because correlations have been made between such early postoperative cognitive dysfunction and new ischemic lesions on MRI studies in valve surgery patients,[53] and between cerebral oxygen desaturation and early postoperative cognitive dysfunction in CABG patients,[54] it does appear as though *early postoperative cognitive dysfunction is, in part, reflective of subclinical brain injury; as such, efforts to mitigate against early postoperative cognitive dysfunction are warranted.*

▣ Circulatory Arrest

Retrograde and Selective Anterograde Cerebral Perfusion

During complex aortic arch repair, surgical access may require interruption of systemic perfusion for relatively protracted periods. Although moderate (25° C to 30° C) and deep (< 25° C) hypothermia remain a mainstay for cerebral and systemic protection, the duration of safe cerebral ischemia time and the nature and techniques for provision of cerebral perfusion during times of hypothermic circulatory arrest (HCA) have been an area of active interest.

In a nonrandomized study, Reich et al[55] performed preoperative and postoperative cognitive testing on 56 patients undergoing HCA, of whom 12 patients underwent retrograde cerebral perfusion (RCP). Memory dysfunction and the overall incidence of cognitive dysfunction had strong associations with RCP even when controlling separately for age and cerebral ischemia time, suggesting worsened outcome with RCP. Okita and colleagues[56] separately evaluated 60 patients who were nonrandomized but were sequentially stratified to receive either RCP or selective antegrade cerebral perfusion (ACP) using serial brain imaging, brain isoenzyme measurement, and limited cognitive testing. They also demonstrated that the prevalence of clinically defined transient brain dysfunction was significantly greater in patients with RCP. Svensson and colleagues[57] used cognitive testing in a subset of 30 of 139 patients undergoing HCA and prospectively randomized 3 three groups to receive either HCA alone, HCA and RCP, or HCA and selective ACP. Comparison of postoperative mean cognitive test scores showed that the HCA alone group did significantly better than either the RCP or ACP group patients.

Despite its conceptual attractiveness and relative ease of application, RCP has not been demonstrated to result in clinically significant cerebral blood flow (CBF) even under conditions of hypothermia-induced decreased cerebral metabolism. In a primate study comparing HCA alone with HCA combined with RCP, Boeckxstaens and Flameng[58] demonstrated that less than 1% of the RCP inflow returned to the aortic arch, and that on histologic analysis, slightly more glial edema was found in the RCP group. Similarly, during HCA in 14 pigs, use of RCP or RCP with inferior vena cava occlusion also resulted in negligible CBFs, and it was similarly observed that less than 13% of retrograde superior vena caval inflow blood returned to the aortic arch with either technique.[59]

It does appear as though modified RCP may be effective in flushing emboli from the cerebral circulation, though at the cost of some mild cerebral ischemic damage. Juvonen et al[60] studied the impact on histologic and behavioral outcome of an interval of RCP with and without inferior vena cava occlusion, versus ACP control, after cerebral arterial embolization in a chronic porcine model. Microsphere recovery from the brain revealed significantly fewer emboli after RCP with inferior vena cava occlusion but demonstrated that significant mild ischemic damage occurred after RCP even in nonembolized animals, but not in the other groups. Behavioral scores by day 7 were considerably lower in all groups after embolization, with no significant differences between groups.

pH Management

The milieu in which HCA is conducted may well also have an important impact on CNS outcomes but has not yet been systematically investigated in adult patients. Although clinical studies and experimental evidence point to a benefit of pH-stat management in infants and children undergoing HCA, it should be noted that neither the clinical studies in pediatric patients[61] nor the experimental models using nonatheromatous animals are necessarily relevant to the adult patient who invariably has substantial atheromatous disease within the ascending aorta, often with concomitant extracranial and intracranial involvement. For adults undergoing moderate hypothermic CPB at least, the weight of evidence from CNS outcomes of at least three separate, prospective, randomized, clinical trials supports alpha-stat pH management over pH-stat.[62-64] In this context, alpha-stat has also been associated with decreased cerebral embolization[65] and preservation of cerebral autoregulation,[63,66] factors likely of paramount importance in perioperative CNS injury in adult patients undergoing HCA.

In none of these studies were stroke rate, mortality, or other measures of morbidity influenced by treatment mode, though all were underpowered to detect such outcomes. However, Hagl et al[67] retrospectively analyzed outcomes in 717 survivors of ascending aortic and aortic arch surgery. They determined that the method of cerebral protection did not influence the occurrence of stroke, but that ACP did result in a significant reduction in the incidence of temporary neurologic dysfunction, a result not seen after RCP. Directionally similar results demonstrating that antegrade perfusion was associated with significantly lower incidences of temporary neurological complications, earlier extubation, shorter ICU stay, and shorter hospitalization in comparison with patients managed with RCP has been shown by Apostolakis and colleagues.[68] Halkos et al[69] demonstrated that during proximal aortic surgery, selective ACP was associated with lower mortality, as well as improved resource utilization and fewer pulmonary and renal complications.

It is unlikely that pH management will substantially change the results of RCP versus ACP discussed earlier; however, Harrington et al's[70] study used alpha-stat management, whereas Reich et al's[55] study used pH-stat management, both with similar directional results relatively unfavorable to RCP. Whether pH management will influence the overall incidence of CNS dysfunction after HCA is unknown. A recent meta-analysis has concluded that in the absence of randomized trials, pH-stat management for infants and alpha-stat for adults would appear to be most appropriate strategies for patients undergoing HCA.[71] Based on the impact of pH management on CBF, *a strong argument could be made to use pH-stat during the cooling phase before circulatory arrest followed by alpha-stat during rewarming,* as practiced in some institutions.[72]

During HCA, meticulous clinical management with systemic hypothermia combined with topical cooling of the head, avoidance of cerebral hyperthermia during rewarming and in the immediate postoperative interval, maintenance of normal perioperative blood glucose concentrations, careful deairing of graft and arteries, ideally with carbon dioxide flushing before reperfusion, all coupled with an expeditious surgical repair designed to minimize the duration of HCA, should be the goal.

Aortic Atherosclerosis

Atheroembolism from an atheromatous ascending aorta and aortic arch is recognized as a major risk factor in the patient undergoing cardiac surgery and is a widespread problem.[73-79] In a study of 298 asymptomatic members from the Framingham cohort aged 60 ± 9 years and of whom 51% were women, subjects underwent thoracoabdominal aortic cardiovascular MRI and demonstrated aortic plaque of 1-mm radial thickness in 38% of the women and 41% of the men.[73] The Stroke Prevention: Assessment of Risk in the Community (SPARC) study used transesophageal echocardiography (TEE) in 581 people older than 44.[76] Atheroma was identified in 51.3% of patients, of whom 7.6% had severe atheroma (> 4 mm thick, ulcerated or mobile). The prevalence rate of aortic arch atheroma increased with age, such that severe atheroma was seen in more than 20% of patients older than 74.[79]

Atheroembolism in cardiac surgery has a broad spectrum of clinical presentations, including devastating injuries and death, yet its true incidence is probably underestimated.[80-83] Thoracic aorta atheromatosis is associated with coronary artery disease and stroke in the general population.[74,75,77-79] In Macleod et al's[74] review, the evidence shows that the risk for stroke is four times greater in patients with severe arch atheroma. Yahia et al[77] prospectively studied patients with diagnoses of TIA or stroke using TEE for assessment of aortic atheromatosis. Thoracic aortic atheromas were present in 141 of 237 patients (59%); mild plaque (< 2 mm) was present in 5%, moderate plaque (2 to 4 mm) in 21%, severe plaque (≥ 4 mm) in 33%, and complex plaque in 27%. Plaques were more frequently present in the descending aorta and the arch of the aorta than in the ascending aorta.[77] Watanabe et al[78] investigated whether thoracic aorta calcification on computed tomography and coronary risk factors had any correlation with obstructive coronary artery disease on angiography. Two hundred twenty-five consecutive patients underwent both thoracic conventional helical computed tomography and coronary angiography. Thoracic aorta calcification was detected in 185 patients; 141 of 225 patients had significant obstructive coronary artery disease. All of the 13 patients without thoracic aorta calcification and no coronary risk factors had no coronary artery disease.[78] *Overall, it can be seen that atherosclerosis of the ascending aorta is present in 20% to 40% of cardiac surgical patients, the percentage increasing with age* (Figure 36-3), *and it is an independent risk factor for type I cerebral injury.*[6-8,84-90]

Transesophageal Echocardiography versus Epiaortic Scanning

The detection of ascending aorta atheromatosis is a cornerstone of strategies to decrease cerebral injury in cardiac surgery. Despite its widespread utilization, manual palpation of the aorta has a very low sensitivity for this purpose.[91,92] The association of severe thoracic aortic plaques (defined as 5-mm-thick focal hyperechogenic zones of the aortic intima and/or lumen irregularities with mobile structures or ulcerations) and coronary artery disease is well established.[89] Identifying severe aortic disease has important clinical implications because surgical technique, including surgical procedure and siting of cannulation and anastomotic sites for proximal grafts, may be altered to avoid producing emboli and stroke. *Intraoperative epiaortic ultrasound scanning (EAS) has emerged as a most helpful tool for the diagnosis of ascending*

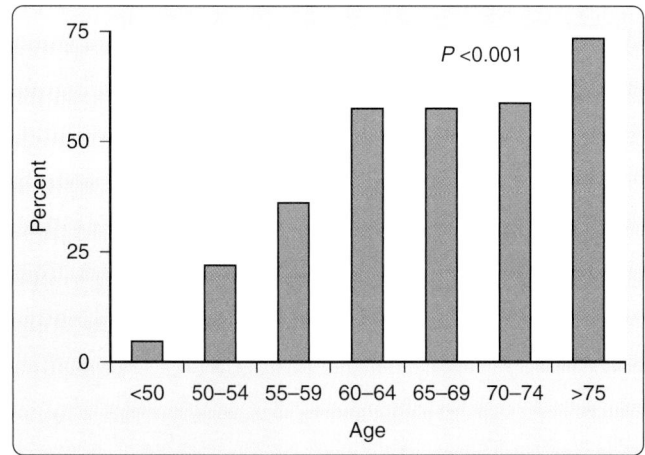

Figure 36-3. Prevalence of severe atherosclerosis of the ascending aorta at autopsy after operations for coronary and valvular heart disease, 1982 through 1989. (*From Blauth CI, Cosgrove DM, Webb BW, et al: Atheroembolism from the ascending aorta. An emerging problem in cardiac surgery.* J Thorac Cardiovasc Surg *103:1104, 1992.*)

aortic atherosclerosis and has revealed major insights into the nature and distribution of this disease.

Djaiani et al[90] performed TEE and EAS to assess the severity of aortic atherosclerosis in the ascending aorta and the aortic arch. Patients were allocated to either low- or high-risk groups according to aorta intimal thickness. Transcranial Doppler (TCD) was used to monitor the middle cerebral artery. Diffusion-weighted MRI was performed 3 to 7 days after surgery. The NEECHAM Confusion Scale was used for assessment and monitoring patient consciousness level. In the high-risk group (intimal thickness > 2 mm), confusion was present in six (16%) patients versus five (7%) patients in the low-risk group, and there was a threefold increase in median embolic count, 223.5 versus 70.0. Diffusion-weighted MRI-detected brain lesions were present only in patients from the high-risk group, 61.5% versus 0%. There was significant correlation between the NEECHAM scores and embolic count in the high-risk group.[87] Multiple studies have documented that most of the significant atherosclerotic lesions in the ascending aorta are missed by intraoperative palpation by the surgeon, and intraoperative echocardiographic studies of the aorta have been recommended[22,86,88,90–96] (Figure 36-4). However, the ability of TEE to reliably detect all ascending aorta and aortic arch lesions is limited.

The high acoustic reflectance attributable to the air-tissue interface resulting from overlying right main bronchus and trachea limits TEE assessment of the upper ascending aorta where cannulation is generally undertaken.[91,92,96,97] Intraoperative EAS has emerged as a most helpful tool for the diagnosis of ascending aortic atherosclerosis and has revealed major insights into the nature and distribution of this disease. Konstadt et al[93,97] investigated 81 patients (57 male and 24 female; aged 32 to 88 years, mean age, 64 years) scheduled for elective cardiac surgery. A comprehensive examination of the entire thoracic aorta in both the longitudinal and transverse planes was performed by biplane TEE. In both echocardiographic examinations, the presence and location of protruding plaques and intimal thickening greater than 3 mm were recorded. Fourteen (17%) of the 81 patients had significant atherosclerotic disease of the ascending aorta as diagnosed by EAS echocardiography. The sensitivity of TEE was 100%, the specificity was 60%, the positive predictive value was 34%, and the negative predictive value was 100%. According to the authors, if the complete biplane TEE examination is negative for plaque, it is highly unlikely that there is significant plaque in the ascending aorta. *If the TEE examination is positive for plaque, there is a 34% chance that there is significant disease of the ascending aorta, and EAS should be considered. TEE is a sensitive but only mildly specific method of determining whether ascending aortic atherosclerosis is present.*[93–97]

The standard for aortic assessment before instrumentation continues to be visual inspection and palpation by the surgeon, despite the fact that this has been shown to identify atheromatous disease in only 25% to 50% of patients, and even then to significantly underestimate its severity.[91,92,98–100] Identification of ascending aorta atheromatous disease would prompt the surgical team for strategies to either modify, decrease, or avoid aortic manipulation. Management strategies for the diseased ascending aorta range from minimally invasive aortic "no-touch" techniques (NTTs) to maximally invasive procedures, including ascending aorta replacement or extensive aortic debridement under deep HCA.[101] A recent review has outlined specific techniques for EAS, as well as steps to be used by the surgical team to mitigate aortic athero-emboli.[102] *Operative modifications in CABG include avoidance of aortic cross-clamping, alternative sites of aortic cross-clamping, and avoidance of proximal anastomoses by usage of all arterial conduit or Y-grafts.* A decreased incidence of stroke and CNS dysfunction has been associated with this approach (Figure 36-5).[103]

"No-Touch" Technique

Avoidance of instrumentation of the ascending aorta in patients with severe aortic atheromatosis has been advocated. Leacche et al[85] retrospectively reviewed data from 640 off-pump CABG (OPCAB) patients and identified 84 patients in whom they adopted an NTT. In these patients, revascularization was performed with single or bilateral internal thoracic arteries and by connecting additional coronary grafts (saphenous vein, radial artery) in a T or Y configuration. The right gastroepiploic artery was used as a conduit in two patients, whereas the brachiocephalic artery was used as an alternative inflow site for arterial cannulation in three reoperations. Age, sex, risk factors, functional class, and history of congestive heart failure were comparable in the two groups. In the NTT group, the frequencies were greater for severe atherosclerosis of the aorta (13% vs. 0%), carotid disease (25% vs. 16%), and history of previous cerebrovascular accidents (17% vs. 8%). In the NTT group, weak trends toward a lower incidence of postoperative delirium

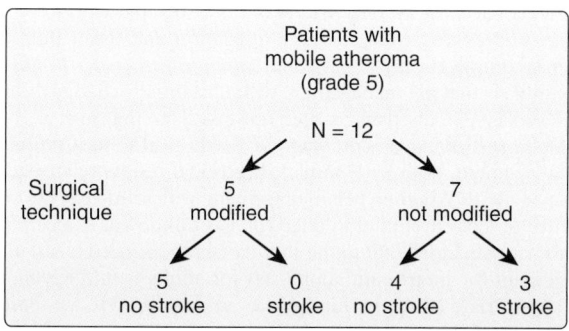

Figure 36-5 **Influence on neurologic outcome of altering operative technique on the basis of the finding of mobile aortic atheromas on transesophageal echocardiography.** *(Reprinted from Katz ES, Tunick PA, Rusinek H, et al: Protruding aortic atheromas predict stroke in elderly patients undergoing cardiopulmonary bypass: Experience with intraoperative transesophageal echocardiography. J Am Coll Cardiol 20:70–77, 1992.)*

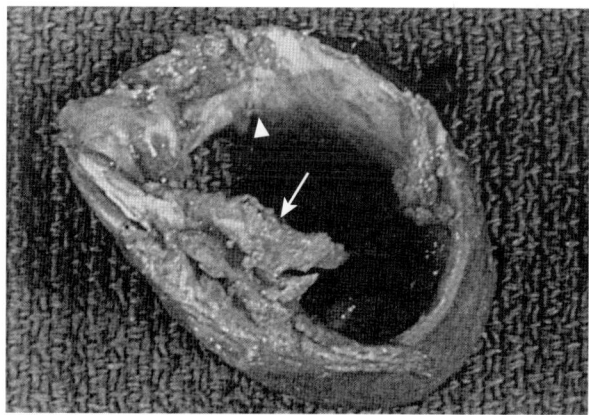
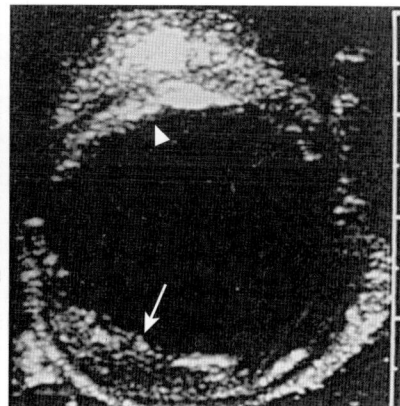

Figure 36-4 Transverse ultrasonic image of the ascending aorta and the corresponding segment of aorta in a patient with severe atherosclerosis. Note the calcification *(arrowhead)* and the projection of atheroma *(arrow)* into the lumen. *(From Wareing TH, Davila-Roman VG, Barzilai B, et al: Management of the severely atherosclerotic ascending aorta during cardiac operations. A strategy for detection and treatment. J Thorac Cardiovasc Surg 103:453, 1992.)*

(8% vs. 15%; $P = 0.12$), a lower incidence rate of stroke (0% vs. 1%; $P = 0.85$), and a shorter ICU stay ($P = 0.07$) were observed.[85] In a review of 1993 beating-heart surgery patients, Calafiore et al[104] observed that in patients with evidence of peripheral vascular disease, use of aortic partial occlusion clamp was associated with a similar stroke rate as in patients in whom conventional CPB was used. They concluded that in patients with extracoronary vasculopathy, aortic manipulation must be avoided to reduce the incidence of stroke. Gaspar et al[96] used EAS and TEE in 22 patients considered to be at high risk for stroke in whom severe aortic atheroma (maximum aortic wall thickness > 5 mm or mobile plaque) was detected, and with the use of aortic NTT and beating-heart surgery, no strokes occurred.

Royse et al[91] performed screening of the aorta for atheroma before aortic manipulation and used an exclusive Y-graft revascularization technique, which has no aortic coronary anastomoses. Aortic atheroma was detected using EAS and TEE. In the control group, aortic atheroma was assessed by manual palpation, whereas TCD of the right middle cerebral artery was used to detect cerebral microemboli. Neuropsychological dysfunction was assessed using a battery of 10 psychometric tests, and they demonstrated that at 60 days after surgery, dysfunction in the control group was 38.1%, whereas in the TEE/Y-graft group, it was reduced to 3.8%. Microemboli detected by TCD during periods of aortic manipulation were greater for those with late dysfunction (5.2 ± 3.0 compared with 0.5 ± 0.2), consistent with an embolic cause for cognitive dysfunction.[91]

NEUROPSYCHOLOGICAL DYSFUNCTION

Compared with stroke, cognitive dysfunction (neurocognitive dysfunction [NCD]) is a considerably more frequent sequela of cardiac surgery and has been demonstrated in up to 80% of patients early after surgery.[24,105–107] The pathogenesis of cognitive dysfunction after cardiac surgery is still uncertain. Variables that have been postulated to explain the development of postoperative neurocognitive decline include advanced age, concomitant cerebrovascular disease, and severity of cardiovascular disease, as well as progression of underlying disease. Various intraoperative factors such as embolization, cerebral hypoperfusion or hypoxia, activation of inflammatory processes, aortic cross-clamp or CPB time, and low mean arterial pressure (MAP) and cerebral venous hypertension have all been implicated. In many instances, subtle signs of neuropsychological dysfunction are detectable only with sophisticated cognitive testing strategies, although depression and personality changes may be noted by family members. It should be recognized that formalized cognitive testing is reproducible and quantifiable and represents an objective outcome measure; as such, it can act as a benchmark to assess various therapeutic interventions (e.g., the efficacy of putative cerebroprotectants, equipment modifications, pH management strategies). In addition, a number of studies have made correlations between early postoperative cognitive dysfunction and intraoperative cerebral oxygen desaturation, as well as new ischemic lesions on MRI.[53,54] *Assessment of early cognitive dysfunction can be used to discriminate between various intraoperative treatment modalities (e.g., pH management, use of cell saver, epiaortic scanning).*

However, whether early postoperative cognitive dysfunction represents permanent neurologic damage remains controversial.[48] In a long-term follow-up study of 97 patients having undergone CABG an average of 39 months earlier, Murkin et al[106] demonstrated an incidence rate of neuropsychological dysfunction of 22%, and 18% of patients exhibited abnormal neurologic findings. The overall incidence rate of combined neurobehavioral dysfunction was 35%, similar to the incidence at 2 to 3 months after surgery in this same group.[62] Knipp et al[105] prospectively investigated cerebral injury early and 3 months after CABG. Patients were studied at three points in time: before operation, early before discharge, and 3 months after operation using a well-validated battery of 13 standardized psychometric tests. Neurocognitive assessment early after surgery disclosed a significant decline in performance in 4 of the 11 psychometric tests compared with the preoperative status, whereas at the 3-month follow-up examination, 3 of the 4 tests disclosed early

cognitive decline, and both depression and mood scores had returned to their baseline values. However, the test score for verbal learning ability remained significantly lower at 3 months.[105] Newman et al[52] sought to determine the course of cognitive change 5 years after CABG and the effect of perioperative decline on long-term cognitive function. They performed neurocognitive tests in 261 patients who underwent CABG; tests were administered before surgery (at baseline), before discharge, and 6 weeks, 6 months, and 5 years after CABG. Among the patients studied, the incidence rate of cognitive decline was 53% at discharge, 36% at 6 weeks, 24% at 6 months, and 42% at 5 years. Cognitive function at discharge was a significant predictor of long-term function. Their results confirmed the relatively high prevalence and persistence of cognitive decline after CABG and suggested a pattern of early improvement followed by a later decline that is predicted by the presence of early postoperative cognitive decline.[52] What is interesting is the apparent lack of association between cognitive dysfunction and aortic atherosclerosis, at least in one study. Of 162 CABG patients who had a perioperative neurocognitive evaluation and evaluable intraoperative TEE images, *no significant relation was found between cognitive dysfunction and atheroma burden in the ascending arch or descending aorta, suggesting that aortic atherosclerosis may not be the primary factor in the pathogenesis of post-CABG cognitive changes.*[108]

In the systematic review and meta-analysis by van Dijk et al,[24] data from six highly comparable studies were pooled and demonstrated an incidence of cognitive deficit, defined as a decrease of at least 1 standard deviation in at least 2 of 9 or 10 neuropsychological tests, of 22.5% (95% confidence interval, 18.7 to 26.4) in CABG patients at 2 months after surgery. In a prospective study of 316 CABG patients, Murkin et al[62] reported a perioperative stroke rate of 2.8% and demonstrated that 33% of 239 patients assessed 2 months after surgery evidenced cognitive dysfunction, and that 45% experienced either neurologic or cognitive dysfunction, in comparison with their preoperative performance.

One important confounder in many of the earlier studies is the absence of a nonsurgical control cohort with similar comorbidities also followed longitudinally with cognitive testing. Several more recent studies have demonstrated similar incidences of later cognitive dysfunction whether patients underwent CABG, off-pump surgery, percutaneous coronary interventions (PCIs), or were managed medically.[47,48] *These results strongly imply that underlying comorbidities and progression of atherosclerotic disease are the most relevant factors in late postoperative cognitive dysfunction rather than cardiac surgery per se.*

The mid- and long-term impact of cognitive dysfunction on quality of life after cardiac surgery has been addressed by different studies.[28,109,110] Ahlgren et al[109] prospectively evaluated neurocognitive function and driving performance after CABG in 27 patients who underwent neuropsychological examination involving 12 cognitive tests, including a standardized on-road driving test and a test in an advanced driving simulator before and 4 to 6 weeks after surgery. Twenty patients who underwent PCIs under local anesthesia served as a control group. After surgery, 48% of patients in the CABG group showed cognitive decline, whereas significantly fewer patients in the PCI group, only 10%, showed cognitive decline after intervention. Of particular relevance to functional quality of life, patients demonstrating cognitive decline also tended to drop in the on-road driving scores to a larger extent than did patients without a cognitive decline.[109] Di Carlo et al[110] administered a series of cognitive tests before and 6 months after the operation to 110 patients (mean age, 64.1 years; 70.9% male sex) undergoing cardiac surgery. The degree of the impairment was determined by two independent neuropsychologists in relation to its impact on everyday life activities. At 6-month assessment, 10 patients (9.1%) were ranked as having severe deterioration, 22 (20%) as having mild or moderate deterioration, and 78 (70.9%) as unchanged or improved.[110] At 5-year follow-up, Newman et al[28] also found a significant correlation between cognitive function and quality of life in patients after cardiac surgery. Lower overall cognitive function scores at 5 years were associated with lower general health and a less productive working status.

Overall, it appears that underlying patient comorbidities rather than use of CPB or even surgery or PCI or medical management are most important in the genesis of long-term cognitive outcome. Although cognitive testing can be used to discriminate and optimize among various perioperative treatment modalities, because of the high variability in methodologies among studies (i.e., differing definitions of NCD, choice of tests, employment of relevant comparator groups), the incidence of NCD between studies is potentially unreliable as an index of the absolute incidence of NCD associated with a given procedure (e.g., CAB surgery). *Cognitive testing is best used as a comparator tool to discriminate between treatment modalities.*

Neuropsychological Testing

As noted in the studies discussed, neuropsychological testing has been increasingly used in an attempt to discriminate the efficacy of various treatment modalities or as an index of cognitive functioning after CPB. In large measure, the sensitivity of this type of testing is such that very small decrements in performance can be assessed and quantified. It appears that a patient may have a consistent decrease in cognitive performance, with or without evidence of subtle neurologic abnormalities, yet may be apparently oblivious to it, whether because of denial or an absence of awareness. Commonly, such a patient's family may have noted some nonspecific alteration in mood or behavior, likely a manifestation of the same dysfunction as detected on cognitive testing.

Preoperative Cognitive Function

One of the earliest prospective reports of neurobehavioral sequelae of cardiac surgery appeared in 1954, and it focused on the acute and chronic stress responses manifested as psychobehavioral syndromes in patients undergoing valvular surgery.[111] As Tufo and others[112,113] noted, this led to a tendency for some investigators to focus on postoperative emotional reactions, regarding them as primarily psychiatric syndromes, rather than systematically investigating cardiac patients for neurologic deficits. Millar et al[114] examined the effect of preexisting cognitive impairment on cognitive outcome in 81 patients undergoing CABG. Patients performed the Stroop Neuropsychological Screening Test and other psychometric assessments before and at 6 days and 6 months after CABG. Those with preexisting cognitive deficits were significantly more likely to display impairment at 6-day and 6-month follow-ups than were those without preexisting deficits, possibly reflecting underlying intrinsic pathology rather than specific intraoperative events. Rankin et al[115] used a 1-hour neuropsychological battery administered before surgery to 43 patients before prospective randomization to either CABG or OPCAB and again to 34 of those patients 2 to 3 months after surgery by an examiner blind to surgical condition. Neuropsychological status did not change 2.5 months after surgery between OPCAB or CABG groups. However, both groups showed dramatic presurgical cognitive deficits in multiple domains, particularly verbal memory and psychomotor speed. This corroborates previous research suggesting that patients requiring CABG may evidence significant presurgical cognitive deficits as a result of existing vascular disease. In Di Carlo et al's[110] study of 110 patients undergoing cardiac surgery, the previous level of education was protective against cognitive decline (odds ratio per year of increment, 0.53; 95% confidence interval, 0.31 to 0.90). It is speculative whether this suggests that greater education reflects greater intellectual capacity, and thus a better ability to compensate for perioperative stresses.

Neuropsychological Test Selection

Research examining cognitive functioning in patients undergoing CPB has frequently focused on the assessment of cognitive functioning within the domains of attention/concentration, psychomotor speed, motor dexterity, and verbal learning. Under the "best-case scenario," it might be desirable to use a complete battery of neuropsychological tests assessing the entire spectrum of cognitive functions. However, the cost of such a procedure and the time demands make such an approach unrealistic. This is especially the case if patients are to be assessed in the

perioperative period, when practical time limitations or patient fatigue levels are likely to be prohibitive. A more practical approach is to use tests that can be administered relatively quickly and easily, and that assess functions particularly dependent, for successful execution, on brain areas most vulnerable to insult (i.e., "watershed" areas).

An additional criterion in test selection is that tests chosen be sensitive to brain dysfunction, broadly defined. In perioperative cardiac surgical patients, the evaluation is necessarily limited by constraints of time and fatigue; thus, tests used should have good sensitivity to dysfunction, even if at the expense of specificity. Tests that can be administered quickly and reliably and are highly sensitive, particularly to dysfunction within cognitive domains localized to brain regions vulnerable to effects of microemboli or transient hypoxia, should be selected.

Research suggests that among the tests most appropriate under these circumstances are tests of attention/concentration, psychomotor speed, motor dexterity, and verbal learning. Research as to the behavioral consequences of hypoxia (and other conditions associated with more diffuse brain damage) suggests these domains are likely to be compromised.[116,117] This presumption has also been supported by research to date examining behavioral consequences of CPB. Frequently, the Grooved Pegboard Test (motor dexterity), various subtests of the Wechsler Adult Intelligence Scale-Revised (Digit Symbol [psychomotor speed]), some of the seven subtests of the Wechsler Memory Scale (Mental Control [Attention], Digit Span [concentration], Paired Associates Verbal Learning [verbal learning]), as well as the Halstead Reitan Trail Making Test (Trails A and B), have been used in whole or in part for the assessment of cognitive impairment after CPB.[28,33,40,52,62,91,105,109,110,114,118–123]

Methodologic Issues in Neurobehavioral Assessment

The Statement of Consensus on Assessment of Neurobehavioral Outcomes after Cardiac Surgery encouraged a more standardized and comparable methodology in assessment of cognitive injury, identifying several key issues of concern in perioperative cognitive testing.[32]

1. A spectrum of postoperative CNS dysfunction both acute and persistent occurs in a proportion of patients after cardiac surgery, including brain death, stroke, subtle neurologic signs, and neuropsychological impairment.
2. A number of patients presenting for cardiac surgery have preexisting CNS abnormalities. Patients' neurologic and neuropsychological states need to be assessed at a time before surgery to provide accurate baseline information.
3. The individual change in performance from baseline to a time after surgery is essential to any evaluation of the impact of surgery or any intervention associated with it.
4. When indicated, designs should incorporate the use of a control or comparison group. This is arguably one of the most important recommendations that was made, but as noted earlier, until recently it has not been consistently applied, resulting in discordant results in the literature.
5. Because of the time constraints and physical limitations of the patient in performing a neuropsychological assessment in the context of cardiac surgery, care must be taken to select appropriate tests. Selection of tests should take the following issues into consideration:
   - Cognitive domain of the test
   - Sensitivity and reliability of the test
   - Time taken to perform the test
   - Degree to which learning may occur in the test
   - Availability of parallel forms of the test
   - Physical effort required to perform the test
   - Overall balance of the cognitive domains assessed in the battery
6. Tests should be free from sex, race, and ethnic bias, and be structured to avoid floor and ceiling effects.

7. Because of the multifocal nature of the potential lesion locations, no single test will always detect postoperative neurobehavioral dysfunction.

8. Care must be taken in performing the assessments because neurobehavioral performance can be influenced by environmental, psychiatric, physiologic, and pharmacologic factors.

9. Because the performance of neuropsychological tests may be influenced by mood state and mood state variations, it is important that mood state assessments be performed concurrently with the neuropsychological assessments.

10. To ensure objectivity and reliability of the assessment, for each patient, the testing should be performed by the same suitably qualified and trained individual, and tests should minimize subjectivity and be performed in a standardized manner. The examiner should be blinded to any treatment.

11. A comprehensive and concise neurologic examination should be performed by a suitably qualified and trained individual.

12. Because the incidence of postoperative neurobehavioral dysfunction is greatest in the immediate postoperative period and then declines, care must be taken to perform at least one assessment when performance is more stable. Ideally, this should be at least 3 months after surgery.

13. Investigators should be aware that new events may occur in the days after surgery.

14. Cognitive testing may be associated with improvement in performance on repeated testing, recognized as "practice effect." This improvement needs to be taken into consideration in any analyses of the data. In addition, study design incorporating procedures to minimize practice effects (i.e., providing sufficient practice trials on each test at each assessment period) is encouraged.[26]

Based on the proceedings of these consensus conferences, the following cognitive tests were recommended as necessary but not sufficient components of any neuropsychological test battery *based on their availability in multiple languages, and availability of paper and pencil versions* for use in cardiac surgical patients:

Rey Auditory Verbal Learning Test
Trail Making A
Trail Making B
Grooved Pegboard

MECHANISMS OF BRAIN INJURY

Determining which factor or, more likely, which combination of factors is responsible for postoperative neurologic or behavioral dysfunction in patients undergoing cardiac surgery using CPB is problematic (Box 36-2). From the few studies in which a surgical control group has been used, it appears that elements inherent to CPB are causative, particularly in dysfunction occurring in the immediate postoperative period.[62,123] How much of this dysfunction is as a direct result of exposure to CABG and CPB or occurs as a result of underlying comorbid disease, such as aortic and cerebrovascular atherosclerosis, hypertension, and diabetes, which predispose such patients to CNS dysfunction as a result of nonspecific "stress" associated with major surgery independent of CABG,

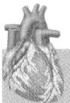

BOX 36-2. RISK FACTORS FOR NEUROLOGIC COMPLICATIONS IN CARDIAC SURGERY

- Hemodynamic instability
- Diabetes mellitus
- Advanced age
- Combined/complex procedures
- Prolonged cardiopulmonary bypass time
- Prior stroke/cerebrovascular disease
- Aortic atheromatosis
- Renal dysfunction
- Peripheral vascular disease

is an area of active ongoing investigation. Based on postmortem studies, as well as correlative analyses of intraoperative events with neurologic outcomes, two primary mechanisms appear to be responsible for brain injury in otherwise uncomplicated cardiac operations: cerebral hypoperfusion and cerebral emboli.

Intraoperative cerebral embolization of particulate and microgaseous elements has been demonstrated to have a significant role in the genesis of cerebral events in postoperative cardiac surgical patients.[42,81,107,124–131] Increasing attention is also being paid to the role of perioperative hypoperfusion, particularly in patients with intracranial and extracranial atherosclerosis, and to the effect of inflammatory processes triggered during exposure to surgery and CPB.[27,36,100]

In a prospective study of 151 consecutive Japanese patients (115 men and 36 women ranging in age from 41 to 82 years) scheduled for CABG, carotid and intracranial arteries were examined for occlusive lesions with magnetic resonance angiography.[137] Cervical carotid artery stenoses of more than 50% narrowing were detected in 16.6% of the subjects, and intracranial artery stenoses of more than 50% narrowing were detected in 21.2% of the subjects.[137] In a similar study of 201 Korean patients presenting for CABG, *more than 50% had evidence of either extracranial or intracranial atherosclerotic disease*, whereas 13% of patients had evidence of both.[135] In this series, 25.4% of patients had single or multiple postoperative CNS complications, and intracranial atherosclerotic disease was found to have a strong independent association with the development of CNS complications. The presence of both extracranial and intracranial atherosclerotic disease was even more strongly associated with adverse perioperative CNS outcomes than was intracranial atherosclerotic disease alone.[138]

In those studies in which a control group (subjected to a noncardiac procedure) was used, the incidence of both new neurologic signs and cognitive dysfunction was significantly greater in the patients undergoing CABG in the first several postoperative days compared with the surgical cohort.[62,79]

Cognitive dysfunction after noncardiac surgery can also be persistent on long-term follow-up, although to a variable extent compared with the incidence reported for cardiac surgery (see earlier). Abildstrom et al[139] reported that 1% of patients showed persistent cognitive dysfunction 2 years after major noncardiac surgery. Several studies have also demonstrated the release of markers of cerebral injury and demonstrated a lesser but significant incidence of cognitive dysfunction after noncardiac surgery.[140,141] The occurrence of cerebral emboli during noncardiac surgery has also been demonstrated.[141–144] Accordingly, it appears as though some of the same mechanisms operative in CABG may also be culpable. Edmonds et al[142] recorded TCD signals from the middle cerebral artery in 23 patients undergoing total hip arthroplasty and demonstrated that, in 8 of 20 patients, there were embolic signals ranging in number from 1 to 200. In all eight of these patients, signals were recorded during impaction of a cemented component or after relocation of the hip. In 2 patients, there were 150 and 200 embolic signals; mild respiratory symptoms developed in both of these patients, and one patient also became overtly agitated during a flurry of emboli.

There is also evidence of a greater stroke rate in cardiac surgery from the recently published SYNTAX trial in which 1800 patients with three-vessel or left mainstem coronary artery disease were randomized to PCI or conventional CABG surgery.[145] This study demonstrated no difference in mortality at 1 year but a significantly ($P = 0.002$) lower incidence of primary composite end point of major adverse cardiac or cerebrovascular event in CABG (12.4%) versus PCI (17.8%) patients. However, although the overall outcome should argue strongly in favor of CAB surgery, the stroke rate was significantly greater in CAB (2.2%) than PCI (0.6%) patients.

Neuropathologic Studies

In an early series from 1962 to 1970 that examined 206 patients dying after cardiac surgery or CABG and a group of 110 patients dying after non-CPB vascular surgery, Aguilar et al[146] reported that there was a

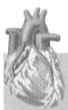

high correlation between the use of CPB and the incidence of brain lesions. They reported that the most significant abnormalities found, in both severity and frequency of occurrence, were emboli in small cerebral vessels; acute petechial, perivascular, and focal subarachnoid hemorrhages; and acute ischemic neuronal damage (Box 36-3). They noted the virtual disappearance from the brain of nonfat emboli such as fibrin, platelet aggregates, polarizable crystalline material, xanthomatous debris, striated muscle, and calcium in cases examined after the introduction of arterial line filtration, whereas they reported that cerebral embolization of such debris was commonly observed in patients dying after CPB before the introduction of arterial line filtration.[146] Other early studies showed that measures taken to decrease the duration of CPB, as well as the introduction of arterial line filtration and filtration of the cardiotomy suction return, decreased overt neurologic dysfunction.[124,125,147]

A review of autopsy findings from 221 patients dying after CABG or valve surgery between 1982 and 1989 reported a direct correlation among age, severe atherosclerosis of the ascending aorta, and presence of atheroemboli. Atheroemboli were significantly more common in patients who underwent CABG versus valvular surgery, and there was a high correlation of atheroemboli with severe atherosclerosis of the ascending aorta, being present in 37.4% of patients with severe disease of the aorta versus only 2% of those without. Of all patients who had evidence of atheroemboli, 95.8% had severe atherosclerosis of the ascending aorta.[80] Doty et al[81] reviewed the records of 49,377 autopsy cases and surgical specimens from the Johns Hopkins Hospital between 1973 and 1995. Three hundred twenty-seven patients (0.7%) had an identifiable atheroembolism on histologic examination. Of these patients, 29 (0.2%) had undergone a cardiac surgical procedure within 30 days of autopsy or surgical resection. Six of the 29 patients (21%) had atheroembolism to the heart, 7 patients (24%) had embolism to the CNS, 19 patients (66%) had embolism to the gastrointestinal tract, 14 patients (48%) had embolism to one or both kidneys, and 5 patients (17%) had embolism to a lower extremity. Sixteen patients (55%) had atheroembolism in two or more areas. In six patients (21%), death was directly attributable to atheroembolism, including intraoperative cardiac failure from coronary embolism (three), massive stroke (two), and extensive gastrointestinal embolization (one).[81]

In a neuropathologic study of brains from 262 patients dying after having undergone CABG, valve replacement, or heart transplantation surgery, 49% of cases demonstrated evidence of circulatory disturbances identified as macrohemorrhages and microhemorrhages, infarcts, subarachnoid hemorrhages, or hypoxemic brain damage.[148] The infarcts were caused by local arteriosclerosis of cerebral arteries, fat emboli, arterial emboli from operative sites, or foreign body emboli. These authors concluded that histologically overt microemboli did not play a major role in their findings, and that nonfatal white matter

microhemorrhages were found with varying frequency, especially after valve operations. These observations are not inconsistent with the apparent lack of correlation seen in several beating-heart surgery studies between differing incidences of TCD-detected cerebral emboli and cognitive dysfunction.[44,45]

Watershed Infarctions

Watershed, or boundary zone, infarcts are ischemic lesions that are situated along borderzones between the territories of two major cerebral arteries (e.g., the middle and posterior, or the anterior and middle cerebral arteries) where terminal arteriolar anastomoses exist[149-152] (Figure 36-6). In a series reported by Malone et al,[152] a correlation was made between the presence of intraoperative electroencephalographic (EEG) abnormalities (virtual or complete electrical silence) usually seen in conjunction with sustained hypotensive episodes and neuropathologic lesions found at necropsy. In all nine patients with clinical evidence of brain damage, cortical boundary zone (watershed) lesions were observed in the parieto-occipital areas. They suggest that this location is the most sensitive area for placement of recording EEG electrodes because it is where minimal boundary zone ischemic lesions occurred in the absence of other lesions, and it is also where ischemic lesions were found in their maximal severity and extent.

A profound reduction in systemic blood pressure is the most frequent cause of watershed infarcts. These areas are thought to be more susceptible to ischemia resulting from hypotension because of their critical dependence on a single blood supply. Wityk et al[153] studied the pattern of ischemic changes on diffusion- and perfusion-weighted MRI in 14 patients with neurologic complications after cardiac surgery, of whom 8 patients presented with encephalopathy, which was associated with focal neurologic deficits in 4, 4 with focal deficits alone, and 2 with either fluctuating symptoms or TIAs. Acute ischemic lesions were classified as having a territorial, watershed, or lacunar pattern of infarction. Patients with multiple territorial infarcts in differing vascular distributions that were not explained by occlusive vascular lesions were classified as having multiple emboli. Acute infarcts were found in 10 of 14 patients by diffusion-weighted imaging. Among patients with encephalopathy, seven of eight had patterns of infarction suggestive of multiple emboli, including three of four patients with no focal neurologic deficits. Several patients had combined watershed and multiple embolic patterns of ischemia. Diffusion-weighted MRI findings were abnormal in two of four patients, showing diffusion–perfusion mismatch; both patients had either fluctuating deficits or TIAs, and their conditions improved with blood pressure increase.[153]

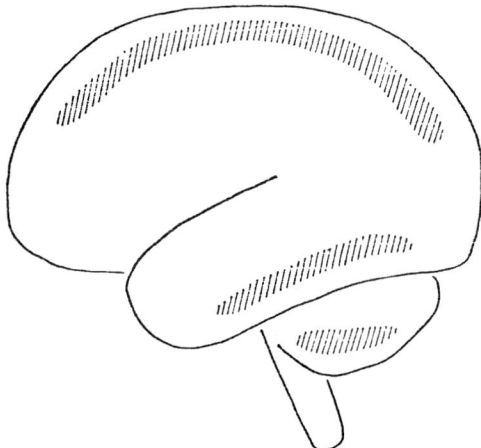

Figure 36-6 Hatched areas showing the most frequent locations of boundary area, or watershed zone infarcts in the brain, situated between the territories of major cerebral or cerebellar arteries. *(From Torvik A: The pathogenesis of watershed infarcts in the brain. Stroke 2:221, 1984.)*

By the same rationale, however, these areas are also highly suscep-tible to ischemia because of end-artery embolization, and it is also rec-ognized that although severe hypotension is the most common cause, showers of microemboli may lodge preferentially in these areas and cause infarcts in the underlying brain.[153–156] As such, although they are commonly due to profoundly hypotensive episodes, watershed lesions are not pathognomonic of a hypotensive episode and may be the result of cerebral emboli. Embolization and hypoperfusion acting together play a synergistic role and either cause or magnify the brain damage of cardiac surgical patients. The negative influence of hemodynamic instability and hypoxia has been demonstrated by several authors, showing improved outcomes by an early and aggressive recognition and correction of hypoperfusion.[5,27,40,157–159]

Cerebral Perfusion Pressure

Intraoperative hypotension during cardiac surgery has been related to postoperative neurologic dysfunction.[4,5,21,27,42,160] Ridderstolpe et al[27] published a retrospective study of 3282 patients of mean age of 65.6 years who underwent cardiac surgery in the period from July 1996 through June 2000. Cerebral complications occurred in 107 patients (3.3%). Of these, 60 (1.8%) were early, 33 (1.0%) were delayed, and in 14 (0.4%) patients the onset was unknown. Predictors of early cere-bral complications were older age, preoperative hypertension, aortic aneurysm surgery, prolonged CPB time, hypotension at CPB comple-tion and soon after CPB, and postoperative arrhythmia and supraven-tricular tachyarrhythmia. Predictors of delayed cerebral complications were female sex, diabetes, previous cerebrovascular disease, combined valve and CABG, postoperative supraventricular tachyarrhythmia, and prolonged ventilator support. Early cerebral complications seemed to be more serious, with more permanent deficits and a greater over-all mortality (35.0% vs. 18.2%). The results of this study suggest that aggressive antiarrhythmic treatment and blood pressure control may improve the cerebral outcome after cardiac surgery.[27]

EEG patterns consistent with ischemia—increased slow wave activ-ity, diffuse slowing of EEG activity—have been reported to occur during CPB episodes thought to be associated with cerebral hypoperfusion.[161–163] Episodes of flow reduction during normothermia frequently produced ischemic changes, whereas similar decreases during stable hypothermia were not associated with EEG changes.[162] Ischemic EEG changes are also frequently seen in association with reductions in perfusion flow rate during the initiation of CPB[161,162] (see Chapters 16, 28, and 29). Using computerized EEG to quantitate episodes of low-frequency power as an index of cerebrocortical ischemia in 96 patients undergo-ing CABG, a correlation was made among episodes of hypotension, focal increases in low-frequency EEG power, and the occurrence of postoperative disorientation.[164]

During the transition to CPB, the brain is particularly vulnerable to ischemia, inasmuch as cerebral metabolic rate for oxygen ($CMRO_2$) is apparently unchanged, yet the brain is initially perfused with an asan-guineous prime, and even after equilibration during established CPB, hematocrit is generally maintained at a range between 20% and 30%. As a result, any further decreases in cerebral perfusion, in the absence of concomitant decreases in $CMRO_2$, are poorly tolerated. During hypo-thermic conditions, there is a profound decrease in $CMRO_2$, exceeding 50% for a 10° C reduction in temperature.[66] Without need to postulate an extension of the lower limit of cerebral autoregulation, it is clear that under anesthesia, and particularly during hypothermic CPB, CBF is maintained at very low levels of cerebral perfusion pressure. As dis-cussed later, this was initially reported by Govier et al[165] and further explored by Murkin et al[66] and Prough et al.[166] As the average age and extent of disease in patients presenting for CABG continue to increase, however, the number of patients with concomitant cerebrovascular disease, and thus potentially deranged cerebral autoregulation, pres-ents an increasingly important group.

Using radioisotope techniques for measurement of CBF, and incorporating a jugular venous catheter for calculation of $CMRO_2$, it was determined that there is a profound reduction in $CMRO_2$ during hypothermic CPB, and that CBF is decreased proportionately and will autoregulate down to a cerebral perfusion pressure of 20 mm Hg, in the presence of alpha-stat pH management.[66] Low arterial pressure dur-ing the hypothermic phase of CPB is thus unlikely to result in cerebral ischemia *in the absence of cerebrovascular disease*. In a study of high versus low arterial pressure management during CPB in 248 patients undergoing CABG, however, an apparently lower rate of postopera-tive complications was reported by Gold et al[167] for those patients in the high-pressure group. Although specific CNS morbidity, cognitive and functional status outcomes, and mortality did not differ signifi-cantly between groups, the overall complication rate for combined cardiac and neurologic complications was significantly lower in the high-pressure group. This is not inconsistent with data demonstrating a high incidence of cerebrovascular disease in coronary revasculariza-tion patients.[108,109]

Cerebral Venous Obstruction

It should also be appreciated that during CPB, cerebral venous hyper-tension can result from partial obstruction of the superior vena cava (Figure 36-7), particularly in the presence of a single two-stage venous cannula, and may cause cerebral edema, as well as produce a dispropor-tionate decline in cerebral perfusion pressure relative to arterial pres-sure.[168] In a study by Avraamides,[169] surgical dislocation of the heart during CPB produced increases in proximal superior vena cava pres-sure and resulted in significant decreases in CBF velocity as measured with TCD, despite stable arterial pressure and pump flow rates. This strongly suggests that cerebral venous hypertension, as can occur dur-ing CPB with myocardial dislocation and impaired drainage of supe-rior vena cava, may result in cerebral ischemia if unrecognized and untreated. It is feasible that such unrecognized cerebral venous hyper-tension has resulted in some of the postoperative neurologic syndromes that have been reported.[170]

Although the association between hypotension during CPB and cerebral dysfunction remains contentious, there is some evidence that certain subsets of patients may be at particular risk. Newman et al[171] used preoperative and postoperative cognitive testing to assess the effects of MAP and rate of rewarming on cognitive decline in 237 patients. They demonstrated significant interactions between cogni-tive decline and MAP less than 50 mm Hg on one measure of cogni-tive performance and between rate of rewarming and age on another. They concluded that although MAP and rewarming were not primary determinants of cognitive decline, hypotension and rapid rewarming contributed significantly to cognitive dysfunction in the elderly. Again, because elderly patients comprise an increasing segment of the cardiac surgical population, these aspects are becoming increasingly important clinical management issues.

Hemodynamic Instability

The interaction of emboli, perfusion pressure, and the particular con-ditions of the regional cerebral circulation (e.g., preexisting cerebral intravascular lesions) will determine the final expression of brain dam-age in the cardiac surgical patient. In a retrospective study, Ganushchak et al[172] tested the hypothesis that combinations of hemodynamic events from apparently normal CPB procedures are related to the develop-ment of postoperative neurologic complications and affect the impact of common clinical risk factors. A multivariate statistical procedure (cluster analysis) was applied to a data set of automatically recorded perfusions from 1395 patients who underwent CABG. The following five parameters emerged for cluster analysis: MAP, dispersion of MAP, dispersion of systemic vascular resistance, dispersion of arterial pulse pressure, and the maximum value of mixed venous saturation. Using these parameters, they found four clusters that were significantly dif-ferent by CPB performance (first cluster, 389 patients; second clus-ter, 431 patients; third cluster and fourth cluster, 229 patients each). Patients in the fourth cluster had the greatest dispersion of MAP, that is, greatest instability on CPB. The frequency of postoperative neurologic

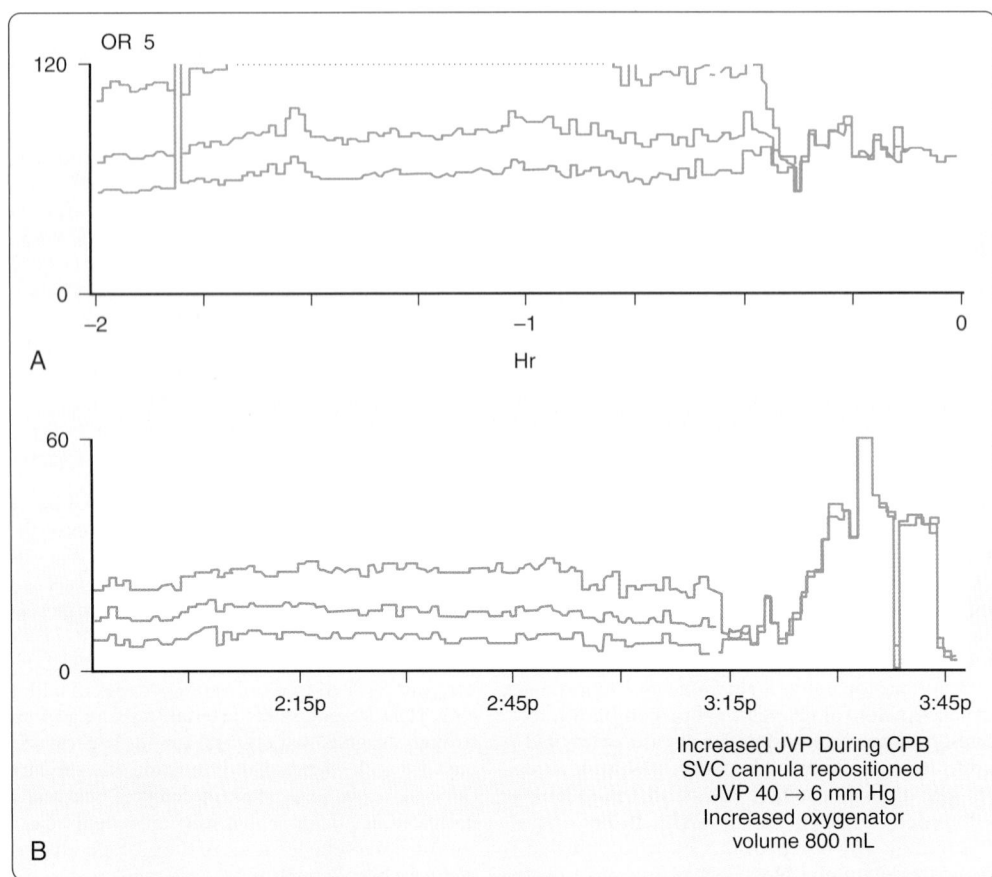

Figure 36-7. *A,* Systolic, mean, and diastolic arterial blood pressures, with commencement of cardiopulmonary bypass (CPB) indicated at 3:15 PM, after which mean arterial pressure (MAP) is shown. *B,* Pulmonary artery systolic, mean, and diastolic pressures with proximal jugular venous pressure (JVP) recorded at 3:15 PM, with commencement of CPB. A single two-stage venous cannula was used for CPB and, with rotation of the heart, venous return to the oxygenator decreased and JVP approached MAP values. SVC, superior vena cava. *(Modified from Murkin JM: Intraoperative management. In Estaphanous FG, Barash PG, Reves JG [eds]: Cardiac Anesthesia Principles and Clinical Practice. Philadelphia, Lippincott, 1994, p 326.)*

complications was 0.3% in the first cluster and increased to 3.9% in the fourth cluster. Importantly, the impact of common clinical risk factors for postoperative neurologic complications was affected by the performance of the CPB procedure. For example, the frequency of neurologic complications among patients with cerebrovascular disease in their medical history was 22% in the fourth cluster, whereas it was zero in the second cluster. *Patients who underwent CPB procedures with large fluctuations in hemodynamic parameters showed a particularly increased risk for the development of postoperative neurologic complications.*[172]

Cerebral Emboli and Outcome

Two different types of cerebral emboli appear to occur during CPB composed of solid or gaseous matter, such as macroemboli (e.g., atherosclerotic debris) and microemboli (e.g., microgaseous bubbles, microparticulate matter). Overt and focal neurologic damage likely reflects the occurrence of cerebral macroemboli (e.g., calcific and atheromatous debris generated during valve tissue removal or instrumentation of an atheromatous aorta), whereas less focal neurologic dysfunction has been ascribed to cerebral microemboli.[14] Microemboli appear to have some role in diffuse, subtle neurologic and cognitive disturbances, whereas macroemboli likely produce clinically apparent catastrophic strokes. Whatever the nature of the cerebral insult, however, it seems that coexistent inflammatory processes can exacerbate the magnitude of injury.

In a study to assess the impact of surgical manipulation of the aorta and correlations with postoperative stroke, Ura et al[173] performed EAS before aortic cannulation and after decannulation in 472 patients

undergoing cardiac surgery with CPB. *A new lesion in the ascending aortal intima was identified in 16 patients (3.4%) after aortic decannulation, of whom 10 patients sustained neurologic complications.* New lesions were severe, with mobile lesions or disruption of the intima in 10 patients. Six of the severe lesions were related to aortic clamping and the other four to aortic cannulation. Three patients in this group had postoperative stroke. *The incidence rate of new lesions was directly related to extent of aortic atheroma, being 11.8% if the atheroma was approximately 3 to 4 mm thick and as high as 33.3% if the atheroma was greater than 4 mm, but only 0.8% when it was less than 3 mm.*[173] Again, this underscores the need to reliably detect and ultimately avoid disruption of aortic atherosclerotic plaque.

Sylivris et al[174] studied 41 consecutive patients undergoing CABG with TCD monitoring and preoperative and postoperative MRI brain scans. A subgroup of 32 patients underwent neuropsychological testing the day before and 5 to 6 days after the operation, of whom 27 had TCD data. Among the subgroup of patients with reliable TCD data and neuropsychological studies, early neuropsychological deficit after CABG was found in 17 (63%) of the 27 patients. On univariate analysis, the time duration on CPB, total microembolic load during bypass, and microembolic rates during bypass were all significantly greater in the group with neuropsychological decline. Actual rates of emboli detected per minute were greatest during release of the aortic cross-clamp. Five patients had strokes, of which four had a significant decline in neuropsychological functioning. Unlike the association between microembolic signals (MESs) during bypass and neuropsychological deficits, there was no relation between these factors and radiologic evidence of cerebral infarction. Not inconsistent with the findings of Ura et al[173] described earlier, there was a significantly greater microembolic load at cannulation in patients with cerebral infarction, temporally suggestive of particulate emboli, which was not apparent in comparison with patients with neuropsychological deficits alone.[174]

A study with a newer generation of TCD, which uses two different frequencies for insonation and purportedly discriminates between gaseous and particulate emboli, compared the number and nature of intraoperative microemboli in patients undergoing on-pump and off-pump cardiac surgery procedures in 45 patients (15 OPCAB, 15 on-pump CABG, and 15 open cardiac procedures).[128] They demonstrated significantly fewer emboli in the OPCAB versus on-pump CABG and open procedure groups, averaging 40 (28 to 80), 275 (199 to 472), and 860 (393 to 1321) emboli, respectively ($P < 0.01$). Twelve percent of microemboli in the OPCAB group were defined as solid compared with 28% and 22% in the on-pump CABG and open procedure groups, respectively. In the on-pump groups, 24% of microemboli occurred during CPB, and 56% occurred during aortic manipulation for cannulation, decannulation, application, and removal of cross clamp or side clamp, again underscoring the importance of minimizing aortic instrumentation.[11]

Gaseous emboli are not innocuous, however. It has been demonstrated that the effects of air emboli on the cerebral vasculature not only are due to bubble entrapment with direct blockage of cerebral vessels but represent the effects that such bubbles have on vascular endothelial cells.[175] Ultrastructural examinations of pial vessels in rats exposed to cerebral air emboli demonstrated severe injury to endothelial plasmalemma, leading to loss of cellular integrity and endothelial cell swelling.[176] Such endothelial damage produces disruptions of vasoreactivity, as has been observed in cat pial vessels exposed to air emboli. In these capillary beds, the endothelial layer demonstrated ultrastructural abnormalities that included degradation of intercellular junctions, flattening of nuclei, and crenation of the plasmalemma. Air embolism also produces changes in blood elements leading to formation of a proteinaceous capsule around the bubbles, marked dilation of pial vessels, platelet sequestration, and damage to endothelial cells.[177–179] Air-induced mechanical trauma to the endothelium causes basement membrane disruption, thrombin production, release of P-selectin from intracellular vesicles, synthesis of platelet-activating factor, and a reperfusion-like injury with perturbations in inflammation and thrombotic processes. These phenomena likely impair nitric oxide production, causing alterations in cerebral microvascular regulation.[180–182]

In Moody et al's[126] study, four of five patients dying after CPB, two patients dying after proximal aortography, and six dogs placed on CPB were all found to have small cerebral capillary and arteriolar dilations (SCADs), consistent with sites of gas bubbles or fat emboli (Figure 36-8). These microvascular anomalies were only found in conjunction with utilization of CPB or proximal aortic instrumentation. In a subsequent series of elegant studies by this same group, use of colored microspheres was able to "time-lock" the development of SCADs to the period associated with CPB[183] (Figure 36-9). In further studies from this group, Challa et al[184] identified SCADs in thick colloidin sections of the brains of eight patients who died after cardiac surgery supported with a membrane oxygenator and in two dogs that underwent CPB with a bubble oxygenator. In SCADs of the eight patients who had cardiac surgery, both aluminum and silicone values were higher, and silicone values were also high in the two dogs in which a bubble oxygenator was used. Their results indicated that contamination with aluminum and silicone occurred during cardiac surgery assisted by CPB, and that switching to membrane oxygenators from bubble oxygenators for CPB may have reduced silicone contamination of blood.[184] Kincaid et al[185] used a cell saver to process the cardiotomy blood in dogs that underwent hypothermic CPB. The brain tissue from two groups of dogs (group I, cardiotomy suction blood reinfused through arterial line filter; group II, cardiotomy suction blood collected and processed in a cell saver) was examined for the presence of SCADs. Mean SCAD density in the cell-saver group was less than the arterial filter group (11 ± 3 vs. 24 ± 5; $P = 0.02$). The authors concluded that using a cell saver to scavenge shed blood during CPB decreases cerebral lipid microembolization.[185]

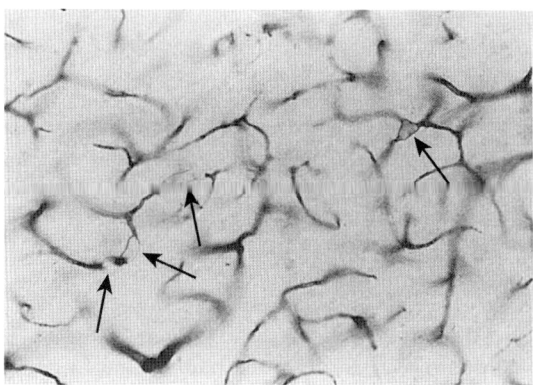

Figure 36-8 Microemboli or small capillary and arteriolar dilations (SCADs) in arterioles of human brain 1 day after cardiopulmonary bypass. The afferent microvessels are black. The SCADs are dilated clear areas (*arrows*); the largest one here measures 25 μm in diameter. It is believed these represent the "footprints" of emboli that were almost completely removed by the reagents used in this histochemical staining method (alkaline phosphatase–stained 100-μm-thick celloidin section; magnification ×300 before 50% reduction). (*Reprinted from Moody DM, Brown WR, Challa VR, et al: Brain microemboli associated with cardiopulmonary bypass: A histologic and magnetic resonance imaging study. Ann Thorac Surg 59:1304, 1995.*)

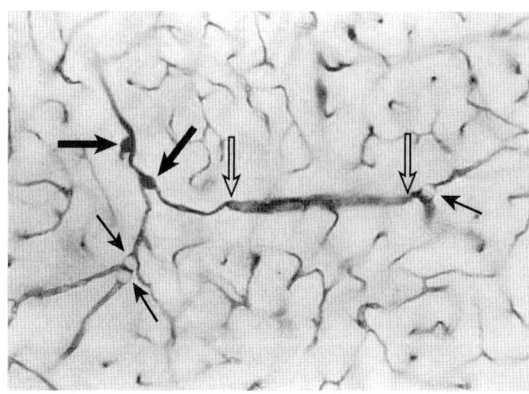

Figure 36-9. Microemboli (*white arrows*) "bracketed in time" by sequentially injected microspheres of different colors. Clear microspheres (*small black arrows*) and black microspheres (*large black arrows*) can be seen distal to proximal order in a single arteriolar complex. In this experiment, clear spheres were injected into the carotid artery of a dog, followed in succession by injection of corn oil and then black spheres. Direction of blood flow in the arteriole is from top to bottom (alkaline phosphatase–stained 100-μm-thick celloidin section; microspheres = 15 μm). (*Reprinted from Moody DM, Brown WR, Challa VR, et al: Brain microemboli associated with cardiopulmonary bypass: A histologic and magnetic resonance imaging study. Ann Thorac Surg 59:1304, 1995.*)

More recently, two separate randomized, prospective studies in cardiac surgical patients have assessed the impact of cell-saver usage on cognitive dysfunction after cardiac surgery.[186,187] A series of 226 patients older than 60 years undergoing CABG surgery were randomly allocated to either cell-saver or control groups.[186] Anesthesia and surgical management were standardized. Epiaortic scanning of the proximal thoracic aorta was performed in all patients, and TCD was used to measure cerebral embolic rates. Standardized neuropsychological testing was conducted 1 week before and 6 weeks after surgery. Cognitive dysfunction was present in 6% of patients in the cell-saver group and 15% of patients in the control group 6 weeks after surgery ($P = 0.038$). However, significantly ($P = 0.018$) more patients in the cell-saver group required transfusion of fresh frozen plasma (25%) versus the control group (12%). In a remarkably similar study from Rubens et al,[187] patients undergoing coronary and/or aortic valve surgery using CPB were randomized to receive unprocessed blood (control, $n = 134$) or cardiotomy blood that had been processed by centrifugal washing and lipid filtration (treatment, $n = 132$). The treatment group received more intraoperative red blood cell transfusions (0.23 ± 0.69 vs. 0.08 ± 0.34 units; $P = 0.004$), and both red blood cell and non–red blood cell blood product use was greater in the treatment group. Postoperative bleeding was greater in the treatment group. Patients also underwent neuropsychometric testing before surgery and at 5 days and 3 months after surgery. There was no difference in the incidence of postoperative cognitive dysfunction in the two groups (relative risk: 1.16, 95% CI: 0.86 to 1.57 at 5 days after surgery; relative risk: 1.05, 95% CI: 0.58 to 1.90 at 3 months). Similarly, there was no difference in the quality of life, nor was there a difference in the number of emboli detected in the two groups. These authors concluded that processing of cardiotomy blood before reinfusion results in greater blood product use with greater postoperative bleeding in patients undergoing cardiac surgery, and that there was no clinical evidence of any neurologic benefit with this approach in terms of postoperative cognitive function. In summary, both these studies showed an increase in utilization of allogeneic blood products and perioperative blood loss as a consequence of routine cell-saver usage, with either no or minor improvements in incidence of postoperative cognitive decline. *In view of the variable impact on NCD demonstrated in these studies and the detrimental impact of perioperative allogeneic transfusion,*[188] *routine usage of cell saver for processing of cardiotomy suction blood is probably unwarranted.*

CEREBRAL BLOOD FLOW

In the mid-1960s, Wollman et al[189] used changes in the arterial and jugular venous oxygen content differences (A-Vdo$_2$) to estimate changes in CBF during alterations of MAP and arterial carbon dioxide tensions (Paco$_2$) in patients undergoing CPB. They observed a direct correlation between Paco$_2$ and A-Vdo$_2$ (CBF), but no relation between A-Vdo$_2$ and MAP. Although the concepts of alpha-stat and pH-stat pH management had not been formulated at that time, these authors recommended maintaining temperature-corrected Paco$_2$ between 30 and 40 mm Hg during hypothermic CPB (see Chapter 28).

In 1968, a Japanese investigator, using the recently developed technique of radioisotope clearance, measured CBF and CMRO$_2$ during CPB.[190] In a series of 40 patients, krypton-85 clearance, with concomitant cannulation of the superior jugular bulb, was used to measure CBF and calculate CMRO$_2$ during CPB. The influence of nonpulsatile CPB on the cerebral vasculature was also directly observed using retinal photomicrography. Although critical data such as esophageal temperatures and hematocrits were not reported, the observed 35% decrease in CBF with institution of CPB, 63% decrease in CMRO$_2$ during hypothermia, 23% decrease in CMRO$_2$ during rewarming and retinal venous engorgement during rewarming are consistent with subsequent research findings. This report apparently also marked the first observations in humans of retinal microembolism occurring during CPB, consistent with but markedly preceding the reports of Blauth and colleagues.[127]

Few subsequent radioisotope CBF studies during CPB in humans were reported for the next 15 years. Other investigators used indirect estimates of CBF (e.g., A-Vdo$_2$, TCD CBF velocities, or thermodilution techniques) to estimate CBF.[191]

pH Management and Cerebral Blood Flow

Relatively little new information regarding the cerebral circulation in human beings during CPB appeared until 1983, when Henriksen et al[192] reported evidence of cerebral hyperemia occurring during CPB. This report was followed in 1984 by a seminal paper from Govier et al,[165] who not only incited controversy with their observations of ischemic threshold levels of CBF during CPB, in direct contrast with

the hyperperfusion reported by Henriksen, but also made preliminary observations on many of the other critical variables thought to influence CBF during CPB.

Without the measurement of concomitant cerebral metabolism, these apparently discordant observations of CBF could not be reconciled. Murkin et al[66] subsequently reported their observations of both CBF and CMRO$_2$ during hypothermic CPB in humans, using a xenon-133 clearance technique for measurement of CBF, similar to techniques used by Kubota, Govier et al, and Henriksen et al, but with the addition of a jugular bulb catheter for sampling effluent cerebral venous blood for measurement of cerebral metabolic activity. It was hypothesized that differences in pH management accounted for the divergent values previously reported for CBF during hypothermic CPB. Accordingly, patients were managed with either alpha-stat or pH-stat pH management during hypothermic CPB. A similar and pronounced reduction in CMRO$_2$ was observed in both groups during hypothermia (Figure 36-10), and in the alpha-stat group, global cerebral flow/metabolism coupling was preserved in comparison with the group managed with pH-stat (Figure 36-11). Decreases in CBF and CMRO$_2$, significantly lower than similar measures before and after CPB, were still evident after rewarming during normothermic nonpulsatile CPB. These low values for CBF and CMRO$_2$ were restored to control levels shortly after separation from CPB. Alpha-stat management preserved autoregulation and the relation between CBF and metabolism.[66]

Temperature and Coronary Artery Bypass Grafting

How much does cerebral hyperthermia superimposed on a brain suffused with focal ischemic lesions contribute to postoperative CNS dysfunction? It is known that the vulnerability of the normothermic brain to focal ischemic insult demonstrates a surprising variability in the presence of small gradations in temperature. Busto et al[194] demonstrated that at 33° C, expression of cerebral ischemia was virtually

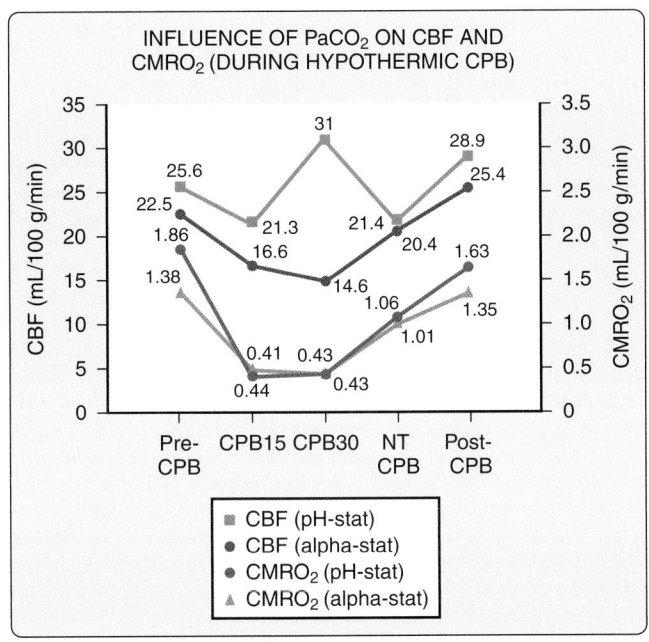

Figure 36-10 Cerebral blood flow (CBF) and cerebral metabolic rate for oxygen (CMRO$_2$) in the alpha-stat (non–temperature-corrected) and pH-stat (temperature-corrected) groups. Note the convergence of CMRO$_2$ and divergence of CBF between groups during the hypothermic phase of cardiopulmonary bypass (CPB). *(From Murkin JM: Cerebral hyperperfusion during cardiopulmonary bypass: The influence of PaCO$_2$. In Mark Hilberman [ed]: Brain Injury and Protection During Heart Surgery. Boston, Martinus Nijhoff, 1988, p 57.)*

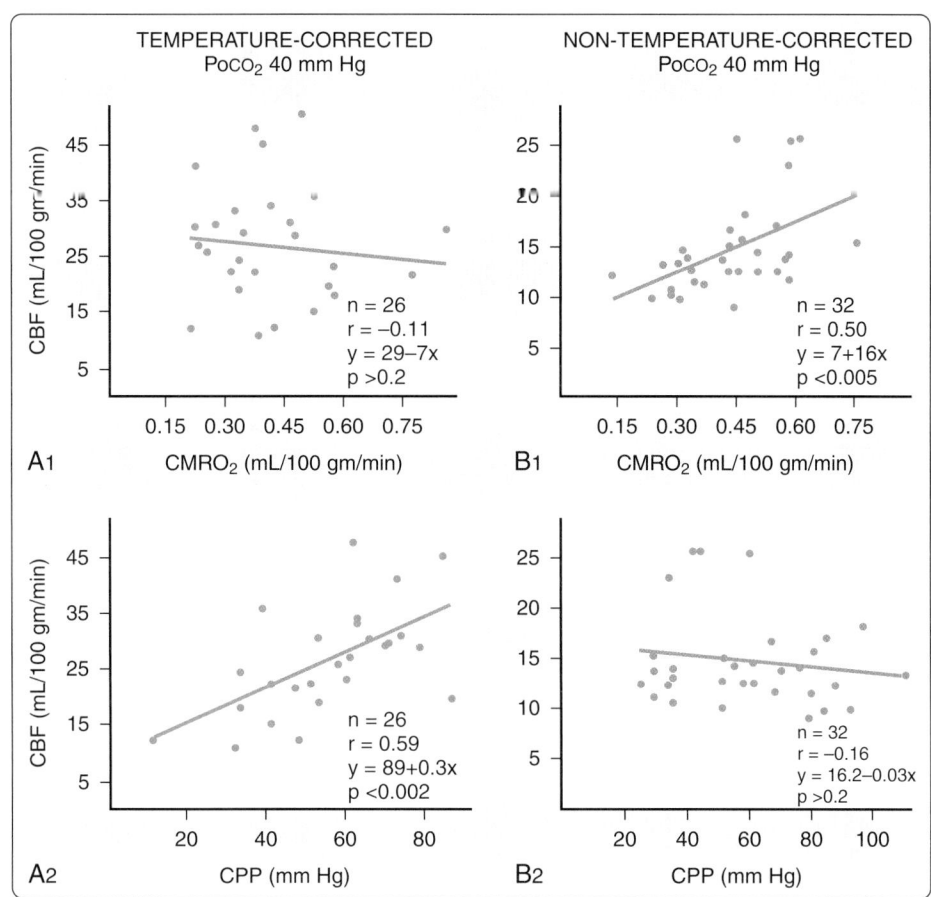

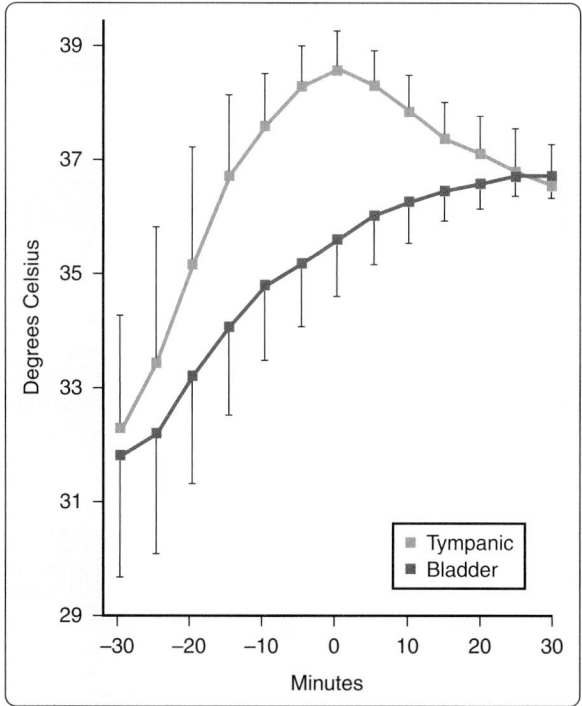

Figure 36-11 Simple linear regression of cerebral blood flow (CBF) versus cerebral perfusion pressure or cerebral oxygen consumption for temperature-corrected and non–temperature-corrected groups. There is no significant correlation between CBF and cerebral metabolic rate for oxygen ($CMRO_2$) in the temperature-corrected group (A1), whereas CBF significantly correlates with $CMRO_2$ in the non–temperature-corrected group (B1). CBF is significantly correlated with cerebral perfusion pressure (CPP) in the temperature-corrected group (A2), whereas CBF is independent of CPP in the non–temperature-corrected group (B2). (From Murkin JM, Farrar JK, Tweed A, et al: Cerebral autoregulation and flow/metabolism coupling during cardiopulmonary bypass: The influence of PaCO_2. Anesth Analg 66:825, 1987.)

eliminated compared with controls maintained at 36° C. In fact, a large measure of the apparent cerebroprotective efficacy of the glutamate-receptor antagonist MK-801 in global ischemia was demonstrated by Buchan and Pulsinelli[195] to be mediated by just such a small secondary decrease in brain temperature. Conversely, small increases in brain temperature, such as to 39° C increments as may occur during CABG (Figure 36-12), have been shown to profoundly enhance the susceptibility of the brain to focal ischemic insult and result in ischemic lesions of much greater extent in comparison with controls at 37° C.[196]

Normothermic Cardiopulmonary Bypass

The demonstration of apparently improved myocardial performance and shorter CPB and operating room times after normothermic CPB has prompted several outcome studies to assess the efficacy of this therapy, with particular focus now centered on CNS outcomes. Hypothermia reduces cerebral metabolic rate; thus, mild hypothermia might protect the brain by preferentially suppressing energy utilization to maintain cellular integrity.[197] In support of this are results from a subset of 138 patients randomized to normothermic or hypothermic CPB, in whom a detailed prospective neurologic examination and a series of cognitive tests were performed before surgery, at postoperative days 1 to 3 and 7 to 10, and again at 1 month after surgery.[198] Seven of 68 patients in the normothermic group were found to have a central neurologic deficit compared with none of the patients in the hypothermic group, a significantly greater incidence. In a separate study of 96 patients undergoing CABG and randomized to CPB at either 28° C, 32° C, or 37° C, patients managed at 37° C had a significantly greater incidence of deterioration on cognitive test scores than did those managed at either 28° C or 32° C. No additional benefit in terms of cognitive function was conferred by cooling to 28° C versus 32° C.[199] Nathan et al[200] reported on CABG patients operated under hypothermic (32° C) CPB and then randomly

Figure 36-12 Tympanic and bladder temperatures during rewarming. Time 0 = maximal temperature achieved. Mean ± standard deviation values are shown. (From Nathan JH, Lavallee G: The management of temperature during hypothermic cardiopulmonary bypass: I. Canadian survey. Can J Anaesth 42:669, 1995.)

assigned to rewarming to 37° C (control) or 34° C (hypothermic), with no further intraoperative warming. Neurocognitive testing was performed 1 week and 3 months after surgery. Eleven tests were combined into three cognitive domains: memory, attention, and psychomotor speed and dexterity. The incidence of cognitive deficits 1 week after surgery was 62% in the control group and 48% in the hypothermic group (relative risk, 0.77; $P = 0.048$). In the hypothermic group, the magnitude of deterioration in attention and in speed and dexterity was reduced by 55.6% ($P = 0.038$) and 41.3% ($P = 0.042$), respectively. At 3 months, the hypothermic group still performed better on one test of speed and dexterity.[201]

Other studies have demonstrated apparently different results, however. Engelman et al[201] randomized a series of 291 patients undergoing coronary revascularization to either hypothermic or tepid/normothermic perfusion. Twelve intraoperative ischemic strokes occurred; six of these were in the group receiving hypothermic perfusion, and six were in the group receiving the tepid/normothermic perfusion. Measuring the infarct volume documented that three of the strokes in each group resulted in minor or small infarcts, and that three in each group were significant, major strokes. The volume of infarction, whether including all six patients in each group or only those with major strokes, was no different between the hypothermic and the tepid/normothermic groups. The authors observed no relation between the size of a cerebral ischemic infarct and the perfusate temperature during coronary revascularization.[201] Similarly, Dworschak et al[202] found no difference in brain isoenzyme S-100β release pattern or in clinical neurologic complications between two groups of CABG patients randomly assigned to normothermic or hypothermic (32° C) CPB. In a large, prospective study, Grigore et al[118] randomly assigned 300 patients undergoing elective CABG to tepid/normothermic (35.5° C to 36.5° C) or hypothermic (28° C to 30° C) CPB and used a battery of neurocognitive tests evaluating four distinct cognitive domains administered before surgery and at 6 weeks after surgery. Again, there were no differences in neurologic or neurocognitive outcomes between normothermic and hypothermic groups in multivariable models. In a separate study, Grimm et al[203] actually found subclinical impairment of cognitive brain function to be more pronounced in CABG patients undergoing mildly hypothermic CPB compared with normothermic CPB. Accordingly, *a protective effect of hypothermia on neurologic outcome in CABG has not been verified in most clinical trials,* possibly because of too fast and/or excessive rewarming of patients or, more likely, because the impact of only transient cooling during CPB does not extend into the postoperative interval when cerebral hyperthermia has also been demonstrated and correlated with impaired cognitive performance at 6 weeks after surgery.[21,204–208]

Cerebral Hyperthermia

Cerebral hyperthermia during the rewarming phase of CPB can exacerbate a preexisting injury before rewarming and may be detrimental in itself. Hyperthermia can have a strong impact on cerebral oxygen transfer and neurologic outcome. Glutamate levels can increase during cerebral hyperthermia, leading to eventual cell death. Rapid rewarming decreases jugular venous hemoglobin saturation, creating a mismatch between cerebral oxygen consumption and delivery.[209,210] Okano et al[211] assessed the effects of normothermia and mild hypothermia (32° C) during CPB on jugular oxygen saturation ($Sjvo_2$) in 20 patients scheduled for elective CABG. The $Sjvo_2$ in the normothermic group was decreased significantly at 20 and 40 minutes after the onset of CPB compared with pre-CPB, whereas there was no change in $Sjvo_2$ in the mild hypothermic group during the study. The authors concluded that cerebral oxygenation, as assessed by $Sjvo_2$, was increased during mild hypothermic CPB compared with normothermic CPB. Kawahara et al[210] examined the effect of rewarming rates on $Sjvo_2$ in 100 patients scheduled for elective CABG and randomly divided into two groups: a control group and a slow rewarming group. Cerebral desaturation (defined as an $Sjvo_2$ value < 50%) during rewarming was more frequent in the control group than in the slow group. Cerebral

desaturation time was defined as duration when $Sjvo_2$ was less than 50% and the ratio of the cerebral desaturation time to the total CPB time in the control group differed significantly from those in the slow group (control group: 17 ± 11 minutes, 12% ± 4%; slow group: 10 ± 8 minutes, 7% ± 4%, respectively; $P < 0.05$).[210] Consistent with this, in a study of the impact of rate of rewarming on cognitive outcomes in 165 CABG patients randomized to two differing rewarming strategies, Grigore et al[118] demonstrated a significant association between change in cognitive function and rate of rewarming.

Grocott et al[208] recorded hourly postoperative temperatures in 300 patients undergoing CABG on CPB and determined the degree of postoperative hyperthermia using the maximum temperature within the first 24 hours, as well as by calculating the area under the curve for temperatures greater than 37° C. Patients underwent a battery of cognitive testing both before surgery and 6 weeks after surgery. The maximum temperature within the first 24 hours after CABG ranged from 37.2° C to 39.3° C, and these investigators demonstrated that the maximum postoperative temperature was independently associated with cognitive dysfunction at 6 weeks.[176] Accordingly, slower rewarming rate with lower peak temperatures during CPB may be an important factor in the prevention of neurocognitive decline after hypothermic CPB, and interventions to avoid postoperative hyperthermia may be warranted to improve cerebral outcome after cardiac surgery.

Cerebrovascular Disease

Relatively few studies have examined the cerebrovascular responses to CPB in patients with known cerebrovascular disease. Because of the vasodilatory effects of increased carbon dioxide in patients with cerebrovascular disease, pH-stat management could theoretically induce redistribution of regional CBF from marginally perfused to well-perfused regions (i.e., an intracerebral steal). Gravlee et al[212] investigated patients with cerebrovascular disease undergoing CABG and assessed the CBF responses to varying pH management, between alpha-stat and pH-stat. They confirmed the responsiveness of the cerebral vasculature to changes in $Paco_2$ during hypothermic CPB but did not demonstrate evidence of intracerebral steal at greater $Paco_2$ levels in any of these patients. In all patients, however, arterial perfusion pressure was greater than 65 mm Hg during CBF measurements, which may have offset any tendency for regional CBF inhomogeneities.

Using TCD monitoring of CBF velocity, 18 patients with severe carotid stenosis and 37 with no or mild stenosis were monitored during CPB.[213] Although not specified, it appears as though pH-stat management was used, because flow velocities correlated with $Paco_2$ and arterial pressure. There were no significant differences detectable in flow velocity between patients with or without significant carotid stenosis. In a case report of a single patient with bilateral carotid stenoses, alpha-stat pH management was used and arterial pressure was varied from 35 to 85 mm Hg, whereas CBF was measured during hypothermic CPB.[214] The CBF values obtained from contralateral hemispheres were essentially equal and remained so throughout the range of different perfusion pressures used. These studies suggest that the cerebrovascular responses to CPB in patients with cerebrovascular disease do not differ significantly from those of normal patients with respect to gross measures of cerebrovascular responsiveness. This suggests that other factors, including associated aortic atherosclerosis, may be a more important factor.

Hogue et al[7] examined demographic and perioperative data prospectively collected from 2972 patients undergoing cardiac surgery. Carotid artery ultrasound examination was performed before surgery for patients aged 65 years or older or when there was a history of TIAs or prior stroke. Epiaortic ultrasound was performed at the time of surgery in all patients to assess for atherosclerosis of the ascending aorta. Strokes occurred after surgery in 30 women and 18 men ($P < 0.0001$). A history of a stroke was the strongest predictor of new stroke for both women and men. A prior cerebrovascular event was a more important predictor of stroke for men than women.[7]

Delirium

In Bucerius et al's study[5] assessing CNS outcomes from 16,184 patients undergoing cardiac operations, the overall prevalence rate of postoperative delirium was 8.4%. Stepwise logistic regression revealed history of cerebrovascular disease, peripheral vascular disease, atrial fibrillation, diabetes mellitus, left ventricular ejection fraction of 30% or less, preoperative cardiogenic shock, urgent operation, intraoperative hemofiltration, operation time of 3 hours or more, and a high perioperative transfusion requirement as being independent predictors of delirium. In a prospective follow-up study of 112 cardiac surgical patients, the incidence rate of postoperative delirium was 21% and was associated with significantly increased mortality and readmission to hospital, as well as significantly greater incidences of cognitive and sleep disturbances.[215]

Carotid Endarterectomy

In the current cardiac surgical population, 17% to 22% of patients have a moderate carotid artery stenosis of 50% or more, and 6% to 12% have a severe stenosis of 80% or more.[21] The risk for postoperative stroke is 10% in patients with moderate and 11% to 19% in patients with severe stenosis, whereas it remains 2% or less in patients with a stenosis of less than 50%. Although in patients presenting for cardiac surgery severe bilateral carotid artery disease is rare, the risk for perioperative stroke is as high as 20%.[21,216–218] It is not clear that carotid endarterectomy decreases this rate, however, because in a meta-analysis, pooled data for stroke or death did not support carotid endarterectomy for risk reduction from asymptomatic carotid stenosis during CABG (relative risk, 0.9; $P = 0.5$).[219] In a review, it was estimated that only about 40% of perioperative strokes (at most) could be directly attributable to ipsilateral carotid artery disease.[220] Accordingly, in a patient with asymptomatic carotid stenosis, combined surgery should not be undertaken unless the surgical team is very experienced in combined carotid endarterectomy/CABG procedures. *Concomitant carotid endarterectomy is unlikely to decrease a patient's stroke risk. Rather, carotid stenosis should be regarded as indicating a high likelihood of aortic and/or concomitant intracerebral disease, and there is increasing evidence that use of EAS with appropriate modification of surgical approach and, potentially, applied neuromonitoring can be of particular benefit in this high-risk group.*

Diabetes Mellitus and Hyperglycemia

The presence of diabetes is recognized as a factor related to increased morbidity and mortality in cardiac surgical patients.[221–225] The incidence of diabetes mellitus increases with age, and its presence is known to accelerate the damage caused by atherosclerosis; thus, an increasingly greater percentage of patients coming for CABG have concomitant diabetes, currently estimated as a comorbidity in approximately 30% to 40% of CABG patients. Bucerius et al[226] found diabetes to be associated with increased incidence of stroke and delirium, and prolonged ICU and hospital stay. Mortasawi et al[227] and Nussmeier[26] describe diabetes mellitus as associated with increased incidences of stroke and mortality. In a large study, McKhann et al[19] prospectively collected data on 2711 CABG patients and identified diabetes mellitus as an independent risk factor for both stroke and encephalopathy. Part of the risk may involve cerebral hypoperfusion because cerebral oxygen desaturation during CPB has been documented in diabetic patients, with patients with insulin-dependent diabetes demonstrating the lowest values as measured via jugular oximetry and the poorest response to increases in MAP.[228]

Studies identify normoglycemia as a desirable perioperative goal in cardiac surgical patients regardless of whether they are diabetic.[223,225] There is both experimental and clinical evidence that hyperglycemia is associated with exacerbation of neurologic injury.[229] Approaches to maintain serum glucose values less than 150 mg/dL have shown favorable results. Furnary et al[221] reported on 3554 patients who underwent

CABG from 1987 through 2001, demonstrating that the observed mortality in the group managed with tighter glucose values was lower and concluded that continuous intravenous insulin infusion added a protective effect against death. Carvalho et al[224] used an aggressive approach to maintain serum glucose values between 80 and 110 mg/dL and reported that this is a safely attainable goal. One study positively correlated average blood glucose on the first postoperative day with a variety of adverse outcomes (stroke, myocardial infarction, septic complication, or death). For each 1-mmol/L increase greater than 6.1 mmol/L (1 mmol = 18 mg/dL), risk increased by 17%.[230] The ideal value of serum glucose in cardiac surgical patients remains unknown, but the evidence available suggests that maintenance of euglycemia is related to a better prognosis.

In accordance with these data, recent Society of Thoracic Surgeons guidelines have been published outlining recommendations for glucose control in diabetic and nondiabetic patients undergoing cardiac surgery with an overall recommendation that in both diabetic and nondiabetic patients, blood glucose levels should be maintained at less than or equal to 180 mg/dL with intravenous insulin as required.[231] However, because of concerns regarding potential adverse effects associated with hypoglycemia, including both increased risk for mortality associated with even a single episode of severe hypoglycemia as seen in medical/surgical intensive care patients,[232] and because in a randomized, prospective study of 400 cardiac surgical patients managed either with tight glucose control (intravenous insulin to maintain intraoperative glucose between 80 and 100 mg/dL) or conventional management (glucose level < 200 mg/dL) a significantly greater incidence of stroke was found in the treatment group,[233] avoidance of hypoglycemia should be paramount. Accordingly, an important caveat recommending preservation of lower limit of glucose level greater than 100 mg/dL should be appended to the guidelines.[234] Overall, it would appear that *maintenance of perioperative serum glucose between 100 and 180 mg/dL in both diabetic and nondiabetic patients is desirable.*

Hemodynamic Instability

Hemodynamic complications, either before, during, or after surgery, have been found to increase cerebral injury in cardiac surgical patients. In Bucerius et al's[5] report, ejection fraction less than 30%, urgent operations, and preoperative cardiogenic shock were related to increased postoperative delirium. Ridderstolpe et al[27] found that hypotension and postoperative arrhythmias were related to cerebral complications, whereas Stanley et al[132] reported that postoperative atrial fibrillation was related to increased cognitive decline. Ganushchak et al[172] reported in a retrospective analysis of 1395 patients that the frequency of neurologic complications was 3.9% in the group of patients who experienced large fluctuations in hemodynamic parameters while on CPB, whereas in the group of patients with more stable values on CPB, the incidence rate of neurologic complications was 0.3%. These studies indicate an increased susceptibility of the brain in cardiac surgical patients to apparently "benign" hemodynamic alterations that either produce or enhance cerebral injury, probably through hypoperfusion of the brain tissue, particularly because it has been estimated that more than 50% of CABG patients have coexisting cerebrovascular disease.[137,138]

CEREBROPROTECTIVE STRATEGIES

Cardiopulmonary Bypass Equipment

Early studies demonstrated increased microemboli in patients undergoing CPB using bubble oxygenators, with a reduction in cerebral embolization with the use of membrane oxygenators and arterial line filtration[124,127,235–237] (Box 36-4). Using intraoperative fluorescein retinal angiography, Blauth et al[124] reported retinal microembolizations occurring during CPB with much greater frequency in patients in whom bubble versus membrane oxygenators were used. Using TCD for detection of cerebral emboli, Padayachee et al[236] demonstrated continuous generation of cerebral emboli in all patients managed using bubble

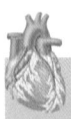

BOX 36-4 CLINICAL STRATEGIES THAT MAY DECREASE NEUROLOGIC COMPLICATIONS IN CARDIAC SURGERY

- Early and aggressive control of hemodynamic instability
- Perioperative euglycemia between 100 and 180 mg/dL
- Routine epiaortic scanning before manipulation of ascending aorta
- Avoidance of manipulation of ascending aorta in severe atheromatosis
- Maintenance of adequate cerebral perfusion pressure (neuromonitoring/cerebral oximetry)
- Monitoring of cerebral venous pressure via a proximal central venous pressure catheter or the introducer port of a pulmonary artery catheter
- Alpha-stat pH management during moderate hypothermic cardiopulmonary bypass (CPB)
- Avoidance of arterial inflow temperature greater than 37°C
- Use of CPB circuitry incorporating membrane oxygenator and 40-μm arterial line filter
- Use of surface-modified and reduced-area CPB circuitry
- Use of cerebral oximetry

oxygenators and none in patients in whom a membrane oxygenator was used. They also demonstrated the efficacy of arterial line filtration to significantly decrease cerebral embolic load.[237] It is apparent that emboli may be generated continuously during CPB and that equipment modification (e.g., arterial line microfiltration and preferential usage of membrane oxygenators) can decrease the generation of such emboli.[238] Membrane oxygenators are currently recommended for CPB.[131] (See Chapters 28 and 29.)

It is equally evident that equipment modifications, although decreasing the embolic load, cannot completely eliminate it.[94,236] Georgiadis et al[239] used Doppler ultrasound and evaluated the percentage of MES reduction caused by the arterial filter and the proportion of MES actually reaching the brain by comparing the MES counts detected before the arterial filter, after the arterial filter, and in both middle cerebral arteries. Eleven patients underwent surgery using normothermic CPB, alpha-stat, a membrane oxygenator, and a 40-μm arterial filter. Evaluation of MES was only performed during extracorporeal circulation, was initiated after cannulation and clamping of the ascending aorta, and was terminated shortly before the aortic clamp was removed. The arterial filter resulted in a 58.9% reduction of MES, with only 4.4% (2624/59,132) of the MES detected after the arterial filter. The proportion of MES detected in the middle cerebral artery corresponded to the total cerebral perfusion under CPB, estimated as 5% to 10% of the total perfusion volume.[239]

Schoenburg et al[240] used a dynamic bubble trap, incorporated in the arterial line after a 40-μm filter, to reduce the number of gaseous microemboli in 50 patients undergoing CABG. In 26 patients, a dynamic bubble trap was placed between the arterial filter and the aortic cannula (group 1), and in 24 patients, a placebo dynamic bubble trap was used (group 2) with TCD continuously measured on both sides during bypass, which was separated into four periods: phase 1, start of bypass until aortic clamping; phase 2, aortic clamping until rewarming; phase 3, rewarming until clamp removal; and phase 4, clamp removal until end of bypass. The bubble elimination rate during bypass was 77% in group 1 and 28% in group 2. The number of high-intensity signals was lower in group 1 during phase 1 (5.8 ± 7.3 vs. 16 ± 15.4; $P < 0.05$ vs. group 2) and phase 2 (6.9 ± 7.3 vs. 24.2 ± 27.3; $P < 0.05$ vs. group 2) but not during phases 3 and 4.[240] The authors found that the dynamic bubble trap can remove gaseous microemboli. Unfortunately, no psychometric studies were performed on either group of patients, but future research in this area might yield positive influence on neurologic outcome by decreasing gas microemboli. Other investigators have demonstrated that air within the venous line

of the CPB circuit, resulting from air entrainment at the venous cannulation site, injection of drugs into the venous line, or use of cardiotomy suction can pass through the oxygenator and appear as microemboli within the arterial line, even in the presence of a venous line defoamer and with use of a membrane oxygenator.[239,240] Georgiadis et al[239] used tubing systems that included an arterial line 40-μm filter and demonstrated that the arterial filter resulted in a 58.9% reduction of microemboli signals with only 4.4% of the MESs detected after the arterial filter being actually detected in the middle cerebral artery.

Modification of the inflammatory response to the CPB using modified surface CPB circuits and leukocyte-depleting filters has been explored. Hamada et al[134] examined the combined use of heparin coating of the CPB circuit and a leukocyte-depleting arterial line filter in 30 patients allocated randomly to equal groups with a conventional circuit and arterial line filter, a heparin-coated circuit with a conventional filter, or a heparin-coated circuit with a leukocyte-depleting arterial line filter. Plasma interleukin-6 and -8 concentrations in the heparin bonded with leukocyte-depleting filter group were lower than in the conventional circuit group. Although a decrease in inflammatory mediator release has been observed by using leukocyte-depleting filters, the impact of these types of filters on neurologic outcome is less clear. In a meta-analysis of 28 relevant clinical studies, Whitaker et al[243] concluded that conventional arterial line filtration had a definite effect in reducing neuropsychological deficit post-CPB. The results of studies using the leucocyte-depleting filter were less clear-cut.

In an attempt to decrease emboli originating from the surgical field, cell savers have been used for processing cardiotomy suction blood before returning it to the CPB circuit. Jewell et al[244] reported on 20 patients prospectively randomized to either cell saver or cardiotomy suction and demonstrated that compared with cardiotomy suction, cell saver removed significantly more fat from shed blood, such that the percentage reduction in fat weight achieved by cell saver or cardiotomy suction was 87% compared with 45%. de Vries et al[245] published a study on patients randomly assigned to have a fat removal filter for the cardiotomy suction. The fat filter removed 40% fat, leukocytes, and platelets from cardiotomy suction blood during cardiac surgery compared with the control group without the filter.

In addition, various intraoperative manipulations, particularly instrumentation of the atherosclerotic aorta, are independent risks for the generation of cerebral emboli and likely produce particulate or macrogaseous emboli, rather than oxygenator-generated microgaseous and microaggregate emboli.[80,84,246,247] Avoidance of manipulation of a diseased aorta seems to decrease embolization and cerebral injury.[91,97,248] An alternative approach, emboli reduction by capture using an intra-aortic filter inserted through a side chamber of a modified aortic cannula, has also been assessed (Figure 36-13).

In a nonrandomized study, Schmitz et al[133] examined the impact of intra-aortic filtration during CPB.[134,249] Three hundred four cardiac surgical patients had intra-aortic filtration using a 150-μm net deployed through the aortic cannula, whereas a further 278 patients formed the control group. Patients in the filter group experienced a lower incidence of adverse neurologic outcomes than patients in the control group (4.3% vs. 11.9%), with significantly fewer TIAs (0% vs. 1.4%), delirium (3.0% vs. 6.5%), and memory deficit (1.3% vs. 6.2%). There were also fewer strokes in the filter group compared with the control group (0.7% vs. 2.2%). Although the sample size was relatively small and the patients were not randomly assigned, the study findings suggest a protective effect of intra-aortic filters on CNS injury.[133] In a large, multi-institutional, prospective, randomized trial of 1289 patients in whom intra-aortic filtration or conventional CPB cannula was used, emboli were identified in 598 (96.8%) of 618 filters successfully deployed, and their post hoc analysis indicated a reduction in postoperative renal complications.[249] In other studies, intra-aortic emboli trapping devices have been used with varied results.[97,239] In a small study by Eifert et al[94] in 24 patients, the use of the intra-aortic filter device did not show any difference in neurologic, neuroradiographic, or neuropsychological outcomes, yet the intra-aortic filter was effective in capturing particulate material. Similar efficacy in

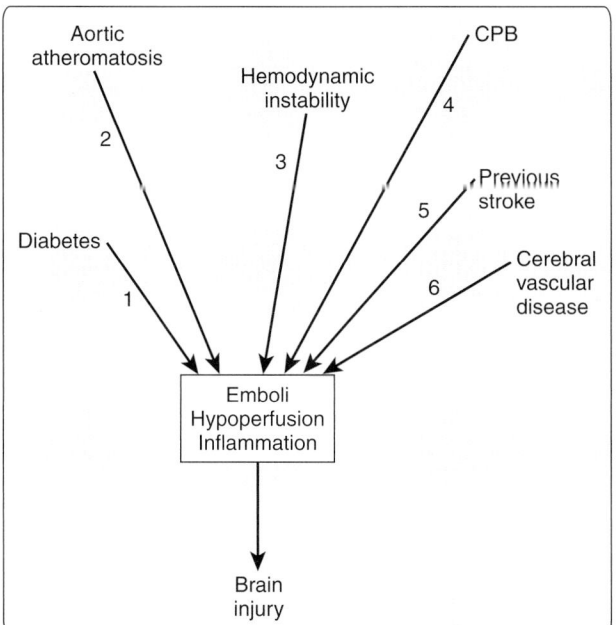

Figure 36-13 The "Brain Milieu" concept. Cerebral injury in cardiac surgery is the product of concurrent risk factors related to the surgical procedure and the patient's previous condition. This unique combination of embolic, perfusion, inflammatory, coagulation, and metabolic events yields a broad spectrum of neurologic manifestations. The graphic shows factors and potential interventions to decrease neurologic morbidity in cardiac surgery. These are numbered clockwise: 1, tight perioperative control of glycemia; 2, epiaortic scanning to detect severe atheromatosis of ascending aorta; modified surgical technique to decrease or avoid aortic manipulation; 3, early pharmacologic and/or mechanical support to attain stable circulatory conditions; 4, cardiopulmonary bypass (CPB) circuitry of reduced and modified surface, use of arterial line 40-μm filters, alpha-stat CO_2 management, mild/moderate hypothermia, use of cell savers to process shed blood before reinfusing to CPB circuitry, arterial inflow temperature less than 37°C; and 5 and 6, intraoperative neurophysiologic monitoring (central venous pressure on CPB, brain oximetry [near-infrared spectrophotometry], retinal and transcranial Doppler, evoked potentials), and maintenance of cerebral perfusion pressure greater than 60 mm Hg.

capturing intraoperative material using intraaortic filters during CPB was reported by Reichenspurner et al.[250] It does appear as though intraaortic filters can be safely deployed, and that they do capture particulate emboli, the predominant origin of which is atheromatous.

In a recent study of 150 CABG patients randomized to either intraaortic filtration, dynamic bubble trap or conventional management, no difference was found in the overall incidence of postoperative MRI-detected small ischemic brain lesions (17/143) between groups, whereas dynamic bubble trap was associated with significantly fewer TCD-detected cerebral emboli and improved cognitive performance at 3 months after surgery in comparison with control and intra-aortic filtration groups.[251]

Applied Neuromonitoring

Intraoperative neurophysiologic monitoring may be of benefit to decrease CNS injury.[252] Intraoperative TCD has been demonstrated to detect embolic events in real time and allows modification of perfusion and surgical techniques. It has been shown that the numbers of emboli generated by perfusionist interventions (e.g., drug injection, blood return), as well as episodes of entrainment of air from the surgical field, are rapidly identified and corrected by TCD detection of intraoperative emboli.[253] (See Chapter16.)

Brain oximetry studies using noninvasive near-infrared spectrophotometry (NIRS) have shown promising results.[254-260] In Goldman's[259] large, nonrandomized cohort study, NIRS was used to monitor cerebral oxygen saturation in 1034 cardiac surgical patients and was compared with outcomes in 1245 patients who underwent cardiac surgery immediately before cerebral oximetry was incorporated. The study group had significantly more patients in New York Heart Association (NYHA) Classes III and IV than the control group, but the study group overall had fewer permanent strokes (10 [0.97%] vs. 25 [2.5%]; $P < 0.044$) and the proportion of patients requiring prolonged ventilation was significantly smaller in the study group, as was the length of hospital stay.[259] Murkin et al[260] reported a prospective, blinded, randomized study of NIRS cerebral oximetry in 200 cardiac surgical patients and demonstrated significantly fewer adverse clinical outcomes in NIRS versus control groups ($P = 0.027$).

Even during beating-heart procedures, compromised cerebral perfusion can occur relatively frequently, and if unrecognized, may account for the relative lack of difference in CNS outcomes between CABG and OPCAB surgery.[261] Combined EEG and cerebral oximetry identified episodes of cerebral ischemia in 15% of a series of 550 beating-heart patients; all were treated successfully by a combination of pharmacologically improved cardiac output, increased perfusion pressure, and cardiac repositioning.[261]

In a study utilizing cerebral oximetry in 265 patients undergoing primary CAB surgery and randomized to active monitoring and a series of interventions designed to improve rSo_2 or to a control group in which blinded monitoring was used, a significant association was found between prolonged cerebral desaturation and early cognitive decline, as well as a threefold increased risk for prolonged hospital stay.[54] However, cerebral desaturation rates were similar between groups and ascribed to poor compliance with the treatment protocol, resulting in no difference in the incidence of cognitive dysfunction between groups. In a study of 103 patients undergoing valvular heart surgery in whom blinded cerebral NIRS monitoring was used, cerebral oxygen desaturation was again found to be associated with significantly longer duration of postoperative hospitalization.[262] In a prospective, randomized, blinded study in 200 patients undergoing coronary artery grafting, Murkin et al[260] demonstrated that active treatment of declining cerebral rSo_2 values prevented prolonged cerebral desaturations and was associated with a shorter ICU length of stay and a significantly reduced incidence of major organ morbidity or mortality in comparison with a similar control group. In this study, the intervention protocol undertaken to return rSo_2 to baseline resulted in a rapid improvement in rSo_2 in 84% of cases and did not add undue risk to the patient, including no increase in allogeneic blood transfusions.[260,263] There were also numerically fewer clinical cerebrovascular accidents in the monitored patients directionally consistent with previous studies.[259] As such, a physiologically derived treatment algorithm for management of perioperative cerebral oxygen desaturation has been proposed and is shown in Figure 36-14.[264] *An important confounder in evaluating the role of cerebral NIRS devices is the efficacy of treatment for cerebral desaturation.*

Neuromonitoring during Deep Hypothermic Circulatory Arrest

Moderate (25° C to 30° C) and deep (< 25° C) hypothermia remain a mainstay for cerebral and systemic protection during complex aortic arch repair because surgical access may require interruption of systemic perfusion for relatively protracted periods. As there is relatively little ability to monitor cerebral well-bring during such times because EEG becomes progressively attenuated at less than 25° C, cerebral NIRS has been advocated as a means of monitoring and detecting onset of cerebral ischaemia during deep HCA.[265,266] Although some groups monitor jugular venous oxygen saturation (Sjo_2) using retrograde cannulation of the internal jugular vein as an index of cerebral metabolic suppression during cooling, correlation has not been demonstrated between Sjo_2 and cerebral NIRS during deep HCA,[267] likely indicative of the fact that NIRS is a highly regional measure of cerebral cortical oxygen tissue saturation, whereas Sjo_2 is a measure of cerebral mixed venous

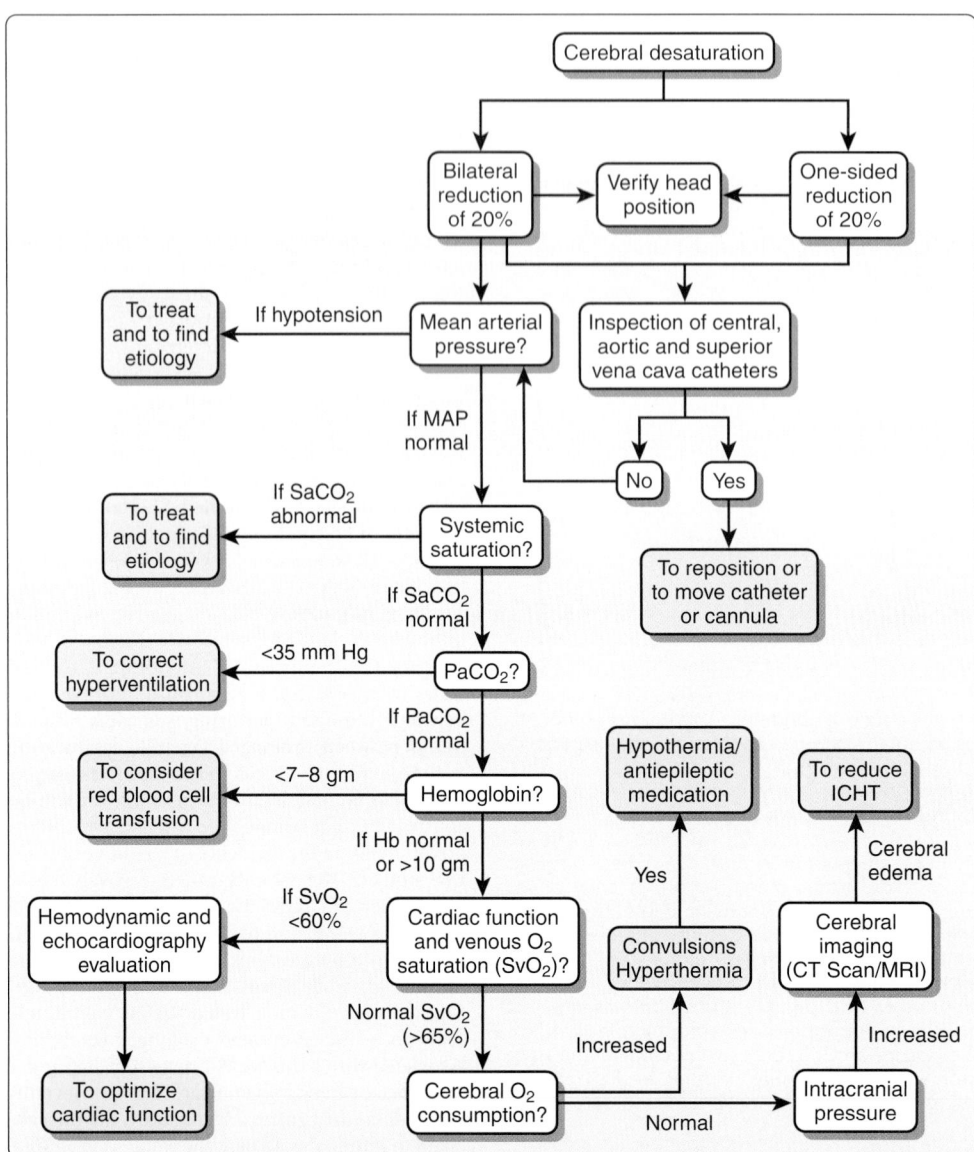

Figure 36-14 Algorithm for the use of brain oximetry. CT, computed tomography; ICHT, intracranial hypertension; MAP, mean arterial pressure; MRI, magnetic resonance imaging. *(Reprinted from Denault A, Deschamps A, Murkin JM: A proposed algorithm for the intraoperative use of cerebral near-infrared spectroscopy. Semin Cardiothorac Vasc Anesth 11:274–281, 2007.)*

oxygen saturation, and thus reflective of global changes in venous oxygenation, and as such, potentially less sensitive to regional perfusion inhomogeneities.

In addition to deep HCA, some centers use RCP via the superior vena cava or, increasingly, selective anterograde cerebral perfusion (SACP) via the innominate or subclavian artery. There have been a variety of case reports of the ability of cerebral NIRS to detect onset of cerebral ischemia during aortic arch surgeries, and there is growing interest in the role of cerebral NIRS as a measure of adequacy of perfusion in this setting.[268–272] There is increasing recognition that RCP does not provide sufficient nutritive flow to sustain cerebral integrity for an extended interval,[273] as has been reflected in lower rSo₂ values seen during NIRS monitoring in RCP versus SACP.[271–273]

In a review of the role of NIRS monitoring during SACP, a study was undertaken in 46 consecutive patients in whom SACP was established by separate concomitant perfusion of the innominate and the left carotid arteries or by perfusion of the right subclavian artery (with or without left carotid artery perfusion), and during which bilateral regional cerebral tissue oxygen saturation index was monitored by

INVOS 4100 NIRS (Somanetics Corporation, Troy, MI) and that used stroke as the primary clinical end point, together with indices of diagnostic performance of the NIRS device.[274] In this series, six patients died in the hospital and six patients (13%) in whom regional cerebral tissue oxygen saturation values were significantly lower during SACP experienced a perioperative stroke. Regional cerebral tissue oxygen saturation decreasing to between 76% and 86% of baseline during SACP had a sensitivity of up to 83% and a specificity of up to 94% in identifying individuals with stroke. It was concluded that using NIRS monitoring of regional cerebral tissue oxygen saturation during SACP allows detection of clinically important cerebral desaturations and can help predict perioperative neurologic sequelae, supporting its use as a noninvasive trend monitor of cerebral oxygenation.[274]

In adult patients, cerebral malperfusion can occur either as a consequence of ascending aortic dissection with occlusion of carotid lumen,[275] kinking or obstruction of perfusion cannula during selective cerebral perfusion for circulatory arrest procedures, or due to migration of aortic endoclamp cannula during minimal-access cardiac surgery with potential compromise of cerebral perfusion.[276,277] There are increasing reports that bilateral rSo$_2$ monitoring can detect contralateral desaturation during unilateral selective cerebral perfusion. This can result from an incomplete circle of Willis, which in some series has a prevalence rate of up to 50% and has been estimated to be a factor in cerebral malperfusion in approximately 15% of patients.[278,279] In a more recent case report, cerebral rSo$_2$ monitoring was used during selective cerebral perfusion in the absence of systemic CPB during repair of traumatic aortic arch rupture and detected both episodes of cerebral malperfusion and, most critically, acute thrombosis of carotid artery graft leading to thrombectomy and restoration of flow.[280]

There have also been a number of case reports of aortic arch surgery in which cerebral oximetry has been shown to detect cerebral hypoperfusion from a variety of factors including diminished Blalock–Taussig shunt flow after pediatric cardiac surgery.[281]

Pharmacologic Cerebral Protection

In general, pharmacologic protection from cerebral ischemia remains an elusive goal. Although there had been one clinical study in which a significant reduction in persistent neurologic defects after open-chamber cardiac surgery was reported after administration of high-dose thiopental, this was not confirmed in closed-chamber CABG procedures.[282,283] Other data have suggested that if there is any such thiopental-derived cerebroprotective effect, the mechanism may be caused by a metabolically driven decrease in CBF, with a concomitant reduction in the delivery of emboli into the brain, rather than occurring primarily as a result of a decrease in CMRO$_2$.[284] However, a three-center study in 225 patients undergoing mitral or aortic valve surgery and randomized to high-dose propofol with induction of burst-suppression on EEG or a sufentanil control group was unable to detect any significant differences in neurologic or neuropsychological outcomes between groups.[285] These authors concluded that neither cerebral metabolic suppression nor reduction in CBF reliably provides neuroprotection in open-chamber cardiac surgery. A large trial of perioperative nimodipine in valve replacement surgery had to be terminated prematurely after enrollment of only 150 of 400 patients because of a significant increase in major bleeding and an increased mortality in the 6-month follow-up period.[286]

There are some interesting associations between certain drug therapies having anti-inflammatory properties and lowered incidences of stroke and adverse CNS events. In a retrospective review of 2575 CABG patients, Amory et al[287] reported that patients who received perioperative β-blockers had a significantly lower incidence of severe neurologic outcomes versus those who did not receive these drugs, demonstrating a 1.9% incidence rate of stroke and coma versus 4.3%.

However, concerns regarding perioperative β-blocker therapy has been raised by the results of the PeriOperative ISchemic Evaluation (POISE) trial in which 8351 patients with, or at risk for, atherosclerotic disease who were undergoing noncardiac surgery were randomized to receive extended-release metoprolol ($n = 4174$) or placebo ($n = 4177$).[288] Although significantly fewer patients in the metoprolol group than in the placebo group had a myocardial infarction, there were more deaths in the metoprolol group than in the placebo group (3.1% vs. 2.3%), and more patients in the metoprolol group than in the placebo group had a stroke (1.0% vs. 0.5%).[285] The implications of this study for cardiac surgical patients remains unclear, but there does not appear to be any increased risk for perioperative stroke in noncardiac surgery patients chronically maintained on β-blocker therapy.[289]

The serine protease inhibitor aprotinin has been shown to positively impact coagulation and inflammatory alterations triggered by CPB and has also been associated with decreased incidences of stroke and major

CNS injury in cardiac surgical patients.[135,136] Aprotinin has also been demonstrated to have anti-inflammatory and antithrombotic effects.[290] Frumento et al[8] retrospectively analyzed stroke outcomes in 1524 patients undergoing cardiac surgery and identified a subset of 149 patients older than 70, with history of hypertension, diabetes mellitus, stroke or TIA, and presence of aortic atheroma who were deemed to be at similarly high risk for stroke. The authors reported that in this high-risk subset of patients, intraoperative administration of full-dose aprotinin, but not half dose, was associated with a lower incidence of stroke. However, because the clinical usage of aprotinin has been suspended indefinitely because of several reports of increased mortality and adverse events associated with aprotinin therapy in cardiac surgical patients,[291-293] the future of this drug remains controversial.[294,295]

In a prospective study of 5065 patients undergoing CABG conducted at 70 centers in 17 countries, the relation between early aspirin use and fatal and nonfatal outcomes was investigated.[296] Among patients who received aspirin within 48 hours after revascularization, subsequent mortality rate was 1.3% compared with 4% among those who did not receive aspirin during this period. Aspirin therapy was associated with a 48% reduction in the incidence of myocardial infarction (2.8% vs. 5.4%; $P < 0.001$), a 50% reduction in the incidence of stroke (1.3% vs. 2.6%; $P = 0.01$), a 74% reduction in the incidence of renal failure (0.9% vs. 3.4%; $P < 0.001$), and a 62% reduction in the incidence of bowel infarction (0.3% vs. 0.8%; $P = 0.01$). Taken together, these studies seem to indicate that therapies associated with decreased inflammatory and sympathetic responses appear to be associated with decreased incidence of stroke and adverse CNS events.

Several preliminary studies had suggested that intraoperative administration of lidocaine infusion during cardiac surgery was associated with a decreased incidence of postoperative cognitive dysfunction.[297,298] However, in larger, randomized, prospective trials, this was not demonstrated.[299] In view of these divergent results, whether lidocaine infusion will have any further role as a cerebroprotectant remains uncertain.[300] An increasingly promising line of investigation for cerebral protection is the role of perioperative statin therapy, with evidence accruing that increased statin dosages and combination with other antiinflammatory agents such as angiotensin converting enzyme inhibitors can significantly decrease inflammatory markers and associated stroke risk.[301,302]

Although these results suggest that there is as yet no pharmacologic "magic bullet" that can be used to reduce neurologic injury in patients undergoing cardiac surgery, a combination of technical and pharmacologic measures is currently available that might positively affect the CNS outcomes of these patients.[160] In patients identified as being at risk for perioperative cerebral injury, preventive measures as outlined in Box 36-4 should be instituted with organ-targeted management to guide the whole intraoperative and postoperative period. The Best Practice Cardiopulmonary Bypass Group summarized these measures as the avoidance of embolic injury by means of intraoperative EAS before aortic instrumentation, the employment of arterial line filters, modified-surface and reduced-area CPB circuits and membrane oxygenators, minimization of transfusion of unprocessed cardiotomy suction blood, the use of alpha-stat pH management during moderate hypothermic CPB, monitoring cerebral venous outflow pressure via proximal jugular venous pressure, avoidance of hypotension, the avoidance of cerebral hyperthermia during rewarming, maintenance of euglycemia, and the use of "tepid" rather than normothermic perfusion during CPB. As the age and incidence of comorbid disease in the cardiac surgical population continue to increase, the importance of these issues becomes ever more acute. In summary, primary prevention continues to be the only effective measure to decrease cerebral injury in cardiac surgical patients.

REFERENCES

1. Ferguson TB Jr, Hammill BG, Peterson ED, et al: A decade of change—risk profiles and outcomes for isolated coronary artery bypass grafting procedures, 1990-1999: A report from the STS National Database Committee and the Duke Clinical Research Institute. Society of Thoracic Surgeons, Ann Thorac Surg 73:480, 2002.
2. Gardner TJ, Horneffer PJ, Manolio TA, et al: Stroke following coronary artery bypass grafting: A ten year study, Ann Thorac Surg 40:574, 1985.
3. Tuman KJ, McCarthy RJ, Najafi H, et al: Differential effects of advanced age on neurologic and cardiac risks of coronary artery operations, J Thorac Cardiovasc Surg 104:1510, 1992.
4. Bucerius J, Gummert JF, Borger MA, et al: Stroke after cardiac surgery: A risk factor analysis of 16,184 consecutive adult patients, Ann Thorac Surg 75:472, 2003.
5. Bucerius J, Gummert JF, Borger MA, et al: Predictors of delirium after cardiac surgery: Effect of beating-heart (off-pump) surgery, J Thorac Cardiovasc Surg 127:57, 2004.
6. Ricotta JJ, Char DJ, Cuadra SA, et al: Modeling stroke risk after coronary artery bypass and combined coronary artery bypass and carotid endarterectomy, Stroke 34:1212, 2003.
7. Hogue CW Jr, De Wet CJ, Schechtman KB, et al: The importance of prior stroke for the adjusted risk of neurologic injury after cardiac surgery for women and men, Anesthesiology 98:823, 2003.
8. Frumento RJ, O'Malley CM, Bennett-Guerrero E: Stroke after cardiac surgery: A retrospective analysis of the effect of aprotinin dosing regimens, Ann Thorac Surg 75:479, 2003.
9. Ridderstolpe L, Ahlgren E, Gill H, et al: Risk factor analysis of early and delayed cerebral complications after cardiac surgery, J Cardiothorac Vasc Anesth 16:278, 2002.

10. D'Alfonso A, Mariani MA, Amerini A, et al: Off-pump coronary surgery improves in-hospital and early outcomes in octogenarians, *Ital Heart J* 5:197, 2004.
11. Gerrah R, Izhar U, Elami A, et al: Cardiac surgery in octogenarians—a better prognosis in coronary artery disease, *Isr Med Assoc J* 510:713, 2003.
12. Alexander KP, Anstrom KJ, Muhlbaier LH, et al: Outcomes of cardiac surgery in patients ≥80 years: Results from the National Cardiovascular Network, *J Am Coll Cardiol* 135:731, 2000.
13. Shahian DM, O'Brien SM, Filardo G, et al: Society of Thoracic Surgeons Quality Measurement Task Force. The Society of Thoracic Surgeons 2008 cardiac surgery risk models: Part 1—coronary artery bypass grafting surgery, *Ann Thorac Surg* 88(Suppl 1):S2–S22, 2009.
14. Roach GW, Kanchuger M, Mangano CM, et al: Adverse cerebral outcomes after coronary bypass surgery. Multicenter Study of Perioperative Ischemia Research Group and the Ischemia Research and Education Foundation Investigators, *N Engl J Med* 525:1857, 1996.
15. Blacker DJ, Flemming KD, Link MJ, et al: The preoperative cerebrovascular consultation: Common cerebrovascular questions before general or cardiac surgery, *Mayo Clin Proc* 79:223, 2004.
16. Naylor AR, Mehta Z, Rothwell PM, et al: Carotid artery disease and stroke during coronary artery bypass: A critical review of the literature, *Eur J Vasc Endovasc Surg* 23:283, 2002.
17. Hewitt TD, Santa Maria PL, Alvarez JM: Cardiac surgery in Australian octogenarians: 1996-2001, *Aust N Z J Surg* 73:749, 2003.
18. Eagle KA, Guyton RA, Davidoff R, et al: ACC/AHA guidelines for coronary artery bypass graft surgery: A report of the American College of Cardiology/American Heart Association Task Force on Practice Guidelines Committee to Revise the 1991 Guidelines for Coronary Artery Bypass Graft Surgery. American College of Cardiology/American Heart Association, *J Am Coll Cardiol* 34:1262, 1999.
19. McKhann GM, Grega MA, Borowicz LM Jr, et al: Encephalopathy and stroke after coronary artery bypass grafting: Incidence, consequences, and prediction, *Arch Neurol* 59:1422, 2002.
20. Wolman RL, Nussmeier NA, Aggarwal A, et al: Cerebral injury after cardiac surgery: Identification of a group at extraordinary risk. Multicenter Study of Perioperative Ischemia Research Group (McSPI) and the Ischemia Research Education Foundation (IREF) Investigators, *Stroke* 30:514, 1999.
21. Ahonen J, Salmenpera M: Brain injury after adult cardiac surgery, *Acta Anaesthesiol Scand* 48:4, 2004.
22. Arrowsmith JE, Grocott HP, Reves JG, et al: Central nervous system complications of cardiac surgery, *Br J Anaesth* 84:378, 2000.
23. Baker RA, Andrew MJ, Knight JL: Evaluation of neurologic assessment and outcomes in cardiac surgical patients, *Semin Thorac Cardiovasc Surg* 13:149, 2001.
24. van Dijk D, Keizer AM, Diephuis JC, et al: Neurocognitive dysfunction after coronary artery bypass surgery: A systematic review, *J Thorac Cardiovasc Surg* 120:632, 2000.
25. Hogue CW Jr, Barzilai B, Pieper KS, et al: Sex differences in neurological outcomes and mortality after cardiac surgery: A Society of Thoracic Surgery National Database report, *Circulation* 12:133, 2001.
26. Nussmeier NA: A review of risk factors for adverse neurologic outcome after cardiac surgery, *J Extra Corpor Technol* 34:4, 2002.
27. Ridderstolpe L, Ahlgren E, Gill H, et al: Risk factor analysis of early and delayed cerebral complications after cardiac surgery, *J Cardiothorac Vasc Anesth* 16:278, 2002.
28. Newman MF, Grocott HP, Mathew JP, et al: Report of the substudy assessing the impact of neurocognitive function on quality of life 5 years after cardiac surgery, *Stroke* 1:2874, 2001.
29. Newman MF, Wolman R, Kanchuger M, et al: Multicenter preoperative stroke risk index for patients undergoing coronary artery bypass graft surgery. Multicenter Study of Perioperative Ischemia (McSPI) Research Group, *Circulation* 1949(Suppl II):II–174, 1996.
30. Maruff P, Silbert B, Evered L: Cognitive decline following cardiac surgery, *Br J Anaesth* 87:518, 2001.
31. Sotaniemi KA: Cerebral outcome after extracorporeal circulation. Comparison between prospective and retrospective evaluations, *Arch Neurol* 40:75, 1983.
32. Murkin JM, Newman SP, Stump DA, et al: Statement of consensus on assessment of neurobehavioral outcomes after cardiac surgery, *Ann Thorac Surg* 59:1289, 1995.
33. Ebert AD, Walzer TA, Huth C, et al: Early neurobehavioral disorders after cardiac surgery: A comparative analysis of coronary artery bypass graft surgery and valve replacement, *J Cardiothorac Vasc Anesth* 15:15, 2001.
34. Murkin JM: Neurologic dysfunction after CAB or valvular surgery: Is the medium the miscreant? *Anesth Analg* 76:213, 1993.
35. Kalpokas MV, Nixon IK, Kluger R, et al: Carbon dioxide field flooding versus mechanical de-airing during open-heart surgery: A prospective randomized controlled trial, *Perfusion* 18:291–294, 2003.
36. Svenarud P, Persson M, van der Linden J: Effect of CO2 insufflation on the number and behavior of air microemboli in open-heart surgery: A randomized clinical trial, *Circulation* 109:1127–1132, 2004.
37. Martens S, Neumann K, Sodemann C, et al: Carbon dioxide field flooding reduces neurologic impairment after open heart surgery, *Ann Thorac Surg* 85:543–547, 2008.
38. Giordano S, Biancari F: Does the use of carbon dioxide field flooding during heart valve surgery prevent postoperative cerebrovascular complications? *Interact Cardiovasc Thorac Surg* 9:323–326, 2009.
39. Al-Rashidi F, Blomquist S, Höglund P, et al: A new de-airing technique that reduces systemic microemboli during open surgery: A prospective controlled study, *J Thorac Cardiovasc Surg* 138: 157–162, 2009.
40. Ho PM, Arciniegas DB, Grigsby J, et al: Predictors of cognitive decline following coronary artery bypass graft surgery, *Ann Thorac Surg* 77:597, 2004.
41. Arrowsmith JE, Grocott HP, Newman MF: Neurologic risk assessment, monitoring and outcome in cardiac surgery, *J Cardiothorac Vasc Anesth* 13:736, 1999.
42. Fearn SJ, Pole R, Wesnes K, et al: Cerebral injury during cardiopulmonary bypass: Emboli impair memory, *J Thorac Cardiovasc Surg* 121:1150, 2001.
43. Almassi GH, Sommers T, Moritz TE, et al: Stroke in cardiac surgical patients: Determinants and outcome, *Ann Thorac Surg* 68:391, 1999.
44. Omar Y, Balacumaraswami L, Pigott DW, et al: Solid and gaseous cerebral microembolization during off-pump, on-pump, and open cardiac surgery procedures, *J Thorac Cardiovasc Surg* 127:1759, 2004.
45. Watters MP, Cohen AM, Monk CR, et al: Reduced cerebral embolic signals in beating heart coronary surgery detected by transcranial Doppler ultrasound, *Br J Anaesth* 84:629, 2000.
46. van DD, Jansen EW, Hijman R, et al: Cognitive outcome after off-pump and on-pump coronary artery bypass graft surgery: A randomized trial, *JAMA* 287:1405, 2002.
47. Selnes OA, Gottesman RF: Neuropsychological outcomes after coronary artery bypass grafting, *J Int Neuropsychol Soc* 16:221–226, 2010.
48. Selnes OA, Grega MA, Bailey MM, et al: Do management strategies for coronary artery disease influence 6-year cognitive outcomes? *Ann Thorac Surg* 88:445–454, 2009.
49. Shroyer AL, Grover FL, Hattler B, et al: Veterans Affairs Randomized On/Off Bypass (ROOBY) Study Group: On-pump versus off-pump coronary-artery bypass surgery, *N Engl J Med* 361:1827–1837, 2009.
50. Sweet JJ, Finnin E, Wolfe PL, et al: Absence of cognitive decline one year after coronary bypass surgery: Comparison to nonsurgical and healthy controls, *Ann Thorac Surg* 85:1571–1578, 2008.
51. Tully PJ, Baker RA, Knight JL, et al: Neuropsychological function 5 years after cardiac surgery and the effect of psychological distress, *Arch Clin Neuropsychol* 24:741–751, 2009.
52. Newman MF, Kirchner JL, Phillips-Bute B, et al: Longitudinal assessment of neurocognitive function after coronary-artery bypass surgery, *N Engl J Med* 8344:395, 2001.
53. Barber PA, Hach S, Tippett LJ, et al: Cerebral ischemic lesions on diffusion-weighted imaging are associated with neurocognitive decline after cardiac surgery, *Stroke* 39:1427–1433, 2008.
54. Slater JP, Guarino T, Stack J, et al: Cerebral oxygen desaturation predicts cognitive decline and longer hospital stay after cardiac surgery, *Ann Thorac Surg* 87:36–44, 2009.
55. Reich DL, Uysal S, Ergin MA, et al: Retrograde cerebral perfusion during thoracic aortic surgery and late neuropsychological dysfunction, *Eur J Cardiothorac Surg* 19:594–600, 2001.
56. Okita Y, Minatoya K, Tagusari O, et al: Prospective comparative study of brain protection in total aortic arch replacement: Deep hypothermic circulatory arrest with retrograde cerebral perfusion or selective antegrade cerebral perfusion, *Ann Thorac Surg* 72:72–79, 2001.
57. Svensson LG, Nadolny EM, Penney DL, et al: Prospective randomized neurocognitive and S-100 study of hypothermic circulatory arrest, retrograde brain perfusion, and antegrade brain perfusion for aortic arch operations, *Ann Thorac Surg* 71:1905–1912, 2001.
58. Boeckxstaens CJ, Flameng WJ: Retrograde cerebral perfusion does not perfuse the brain in nonhuman primates, *Ann Thorac Surg* 60:319–327, 1995.
59. Ehrlich MP, Hagl C, McCullough JN, et al: Retrograde cerebral perfusion provides negligible flow through brain capillaries in the pig, *J Thorac Cardiovasc Surg* 122:331–338, 2001.
60. Juvonen T, Weisz DJ, Wolfe D, et al: Can retrograde perfusion mitigate cerebral injury after particulate embolization? A study in a chronic porcine model, *J Thorac Cardiovasc Surg* 115:1142–1159, 1998.
61. du Plessis AJ, Jonas RA, Wypij D, et al: Perioperative effects of alpha-stat versus pH-stat strategies for deep hypothermic cardiopulmonary bypass in infants, *J Thorac Cardiovasc Surg* 114:991–1000, 1997.
62. Murkin JM, Martzke JS, Buchan AM, et al: A randomized study of the influence of perfusion technique and pH management strategy in 316 patients undergoing coronary artery bypass surgery. II. Neurologic and cognitive outcomes, *J Thorac Cardiovasc Surg* 110:349–362, 1995.
63. Patel RL, Turtle MR, Chambers DJ, et al: Alpha-stat acid-base regulation during cardiopulmonary bypass improves neuropsychologic outcome in patients undergoing coronary artery bypass grafting, *J Thorac Cardiovasc Surg* 111:1267–1279, 1996.
64. Stephan H, Weyland A, Kazmaier S, et al: Acid-base management during hypothermic cardiopulmonary bypass does not affect cerebral metabolism but does affect blood flow and neurological outcome, *Br J Anaesth* 69:51–57, 1992.
65. Cook DJ, Plochl W, Orszulak TA: Effect of temperature and PaCO2 on cerebral embolization during cardiopulmonary bypass in swine, *Ann Thorac Surg* 69:415–420, 2000.
66. Murkin JM, Farrar JK, Tweed WA, et al: Cerebral autoregulation and flow/metabolism coupling during cardiopulmonary bypass: The influence of PaCO2, *Anesth Analg* 66:825–832, 1987.
67. Hagl C, Ergin MA, Galla JD, et al: Neurologic outcome after ascending aorta-aortic arch operations: Effect of brain protection technique in high-risk patients, *J Thorac Cardiovasc Surg* 121:1107–1121, 2001.
68. Apostolakis E, Koletsis EN, Dedeilias P, et al: Antegrade versus retrograde cerebral perfusion in relation to postoperative complications following aortic arch surgery for acute aortic dissection type A, *J Card Surg* 23:480–487, 2008.
69. Halkos ME, Kerendi F, Myung R, et al: Selective antegrade cerebral perfusion via right axillary artery cannulation reduces morbidity and mortality after proximal aortic surgery, *J Thorac Cardiovasc Surg* 138:1081–1089, 2009.
70. Harrington DK, Bonser M, Moss A, et al: Neuropsychometric outcome following aortic arch surgery: A prospective randomized trial of retrograde cerebral perfusion, *J Thorac Cardiovasc Surg* 126: 638–644, 2003.
71. Abdul, Aziz KA, Meduoye A: Is pH-stat or alpha-stat the best technique to follow in patients undergoing deep hypothermic circulatory arrest? *Interact Cardiovasc Thorac Surg* 10:271–282, 2010.
72. Sundt TM 3rd, Orszulak TA, Cook DJ, et al: Improving results of open arch replacement, *Ann Thorac Surg* 86:787–796, 2008.
73. Jaffer FA, O'Donnell CJ, Larson MG, et al: Age and sex distribution of subclinical aortic atherosclerosis: A magnetic resonance imaging examination of the Framingham Heart Study, *Arterioscler Thromb Vasc Biol* 122:849, 2002.
74. Macleod MR, Amarenco P, Davis SM, et al: Atheroma of the aortic arch: An important and poorly recognised factor in the aetiology of stroke, *Lancet Neurol* 3:408, 2004.
75. Macleod MR, Donnan GA: Atheroma of the aortic arch: The missing link in the secondary prevention of stroke? *Expert Rev Cardiovasc Ther* 1:487, 2003.
76. Li AE, Kamel I, Rando F, et al: Using MRI to assess aortic wall thickness in the multiethnic study of atherosclerosis: Distribution by race, sex, and age, *AJR Am J Roentgenol* 182:593, 2004.
77. Yahia AM, Kirmani JF, Xavier AR, et al: Characteristics and predictors of aortic plaques in patients with transient ischemic attacks and strokes, *J Neuroimaging* 14:16, 2004.
78. Watanabe K, Hiroki T, Koga N: Relation of thoracic aorta calcification on computed tomography and coronary risk factors to obstructive coronary artery disease on angiography, *Angiology* 54:433, 2003.
79. Agmon Y, Khandheria BK, Meissner I, et al: Relation of coronary artery disease and cerebrovascular disease with atherosclerosis of the thoracic aorta in the general population, *Am J Cardiol* 189:262, 2002.
80. Blauth CI, Cosgrove DM, Webb BW, et al: Atheroembolism from the ascending aorta. An emerging problem in cardiac surgery, *J Thorac Cardiovasc Surg* 103:1104, 1992.
81. Doty JR, Wilentz RE, Salazar JD, et al: Atheroembolism in cardiac surgery, *Ann Thorac Surg* 75:1221, 2003.
82. Goodwin AT, Goddard M, Taylor GJ, et al: Clinical versus actual outcome in cardiac surgery: A postmortem study, *Eur J Cardiothorac Surg* 17:747, 2000.
83. Mackensen GB, Swaminathan M, Ti LK, et al: Preliminary report on the interaction of apolipoprotein E polymorphism with aortic atherosclerosis and acute nephropathy after CABG, *Ann Thorac Surg* 78:520, 2004.
84. Davila-Roman VG, Barzilai B, Wareing TH, et al: Atherosclerosis of the ascending aorta. Prevalence and role as an independent predictor of cerebrovascular events in cardiac patients, *Stroke* 25: 2010–2016, 1994.
85. Leacche M, Carrier M, Bouchard D, et al: Improving neurologic outcome in off-pump surgery: The "no touch" technique, *Heart Surg Forum* 6:169, 2003.
86. Mackensen GB, Ti LK, Phillips-Bute BG, et al: Cerebral embolization during cardiac surgery: Impact of aortic atheroma burden, *Br J Anaesth* 91:656, 2003.
87. Sharony R, Bizekis CS, Kanchuger M, et al: Off-pump coronary artery bypass grafting reduces mortality and stroke in patients with atheromatous aortas: A case control study, *Circulation* 9(Suppl I):II–115, 2003.
88. Wareing TH, Davila-Roman VG, Daily BB, et al: Strategy for the reduction of stroke incidence in cardiac surgical patients, *Ann Thorac Surg* 55:1400, 1993.
89. Sekoranja L, Vuille C, Bianchi-Demicheli F, et al: Thoracic aortic plaques, transoesophageal echocardiography and coronary artery disease, *Swiss Med Wkly* 134:75–78, 2004.
90. Djaiani G, Fedorko L, Borger M, et al: Mild to moderate atheromatous disease of the thoracic aorta and new ischemic brain lesions after conventional coronary artery bypass graft surgery, *Stroke* 35:e356–e358, 2004.
91. Royse AG, Royse CF, Ajani AE, et al: Reduced neuropsychological dysfunction using epiaortic echocardiography and the exclusive Y graft, *Ann Thorac Surg* 69:1431, 2000.
92. St Amand MA, Murkin JM, Menkis AH, et al: Aortic atherosclerotic plaque identified by epiaortic scanning predicts cerebral embolic load in cardiac surgery, *Can J Anaesth* 44:A7, 1997.
93. Konstadt SN, Reich DL, Kahn R, et al: Transesophageal echocardiography can be used to screen for ascending aortic atherosclerosis, *Anesth Analg* 81:225, 1995.
94. Eifert S, Reichenspurner H, Pfefferkorn T, et al: Neurological and neuropsychological examination and outcome after use of an intra-aortic filter device during cardiac surgery, *Perfusion* 18(Suppl 1):55, 2003.
95. Bonatti J: Ascending aortic atherosclerosis—a complex and challenging problem for the cardiac surgeon, *Heart Surg Forum* 2:125, 1999.

96. Gaspar M, Laufer G, Bonatti J, et al: Epiaortic ultrasound and intraoperative transesophageal echocardiography for the thoracic aorta atherosclerosis assessment in patient undergoing CABG. Surgical technique modification to avoid cerebral stroke, *Chirurgia (Bucur)* 97:529, 2002.
97. Konstadt SN, Reich DL, Quintana C, et al: The ascending aorta: How much does transesophageal echocardiography see? *Anesth Analg* 78:240, 1994.
98. Wareing TH, Davila-Roman VG, Barzilai B, et al: Management of the severely atherosclerotic ascending aorta during cardiac operations. A strategy for detection and treatment, *J Thorac Cardiovasc Surg* 103:453, 1992.
99. Ohteki H, Itoh T, Natsuaki M, et al: Intraoperative ultrasonic imaging of the ascending aorta in ischemic heart disease, *Ann Thorac Surg* 50:539, 1990.
100. Murkin JM: Attenuation of neurologic injury during cardiac surgery, *Ann Thorac Surg* 72:S1838, 2001.
101. Takami Y, Tajima K, Terazawa S, et al: Safer aortic crossclamping during short-term moderate hypothermic circulatory arrest for cardiac surgery in patients with a bad ascending aorta, *J Thorac Cardiovasc Surg* 137:875–880, 2009.
102. Royse AG, Royse CF: Epiaortic ultrasound assessment of the aorta in cardiac surgery, *Best Pract Res Clin Anaesthesiol* 23:335–341, 2009.
103. Bergman P, Hadjinikolaou L, Dellgren G, et al: A policy to reduce stroke in patients with extensive atherosclerosis of the ascending aorta undergoing coronary surgery, *Interact Cardiovasc Thorac Surg* 3:28–32, 2004.
104. Calafiore AM, Di MM, Teodori G, et al: Impact of aortic manipulation on incidence of cerebrovascular accidents after surgical myocardial revascularization, *Ann Thorac Surg* 73:1387, 2002.
105. Knipp SC, Matatko N, Wilhelm H, et al: Evaluation of brain injury after coronary artery bypass grafting. A prospective study using neuropsychological assessment and diffusion-weighted magnetic resonance imaging, *Eur J Cardiothorac Surg* 25:791, 2004.
106. Murkin JM: Long-term neurological and neuropsychological outcome 3 years after coronary artery bypass surgery, *Anesth Analg* 82:S328, 1996.
107. Taggart DP, Westaby S: Neurological and cognitive disorders after coronary artery bypass grafting, *Curr Opin Cardiol* 16:271, 2001.
108. Bar-Yosef S, Anders M, Mackensen GB, et al: Aortic atheroma burden and cognitive dysfunction after coronary artery bypass graft surgery, *Ann Thorac Surg* 78:1556, 2005.
109. Ahlgren E, Lundqvist A, Nordlund A, et al: Neurocognitive impairment and driving performance after coronary artery bypass surgery, *Eur J Cardiothorac Surg* 23:334, 2003.
110. Di Carlo CA, Perna AM, Pantoni L, et al: Clinically relevant cognitive impairment after cardiac surgery: A 6-month follow-up study, *J Neurol Sci* 188:85–93, 2001.
111. Fox HM, Rizzo ND, Gifford S: Psychological observations of patients undergoing mitral surgery: A study of stress, *Psychosom Med* 16:186, 1954.
112. Tufo HM, Ostfeld AM, Shekelle R: Central nervous system dysfunction following open-heart surgery, *JAMA* 212:1333, 1970.
113. Kornfeld DS, Heller SS, Frank KA, et al: Delirium after coronary artery bypass surgery, *J Thorac Cardiovasc Surg* 76:93, 1978.
114. Millar K, Asbury AJ, Murray GD: Pre-existing cognitive impairment as a factor influencing outcome after cardiac surgery, *Br J Anaesth* 86:63, 2001.
115. Rankin KP, Kochamba GS, Boone KB, et al: Presurgical cognitive deficits in patients receiving coronary artery bypass graft surgery, *J Int Neuropsychol Soc* 9:913, 2003.
116. Muramoto O, Kuru Y, Sugishita M, et al: Pure memory loss with hippocampal lesions: A pneumoencephalographic study, *Arch Neurol* 36:54, 1979.
117. Grant I: Neuropsychological findings in hypoxemic chronic obstructive pulmonary disease. In *Proceedings of the 10th Annual Meeting of the International Neuropsychology Society*, Pittsburgh PA, 1982.
118. Grigore AM, Grocott HP, Mathew JP, et al: The rewarming rate and increased peak temperature alter neurocognitive outcome after cardiac surgery, *Anesth Analg* 94:4, 2002.
119. Harrington DK, Bonser M, Moss A, et al: Neuropsychometric outcome following aortic arch surgery: A prospective randomized trial of retrograde cerebral perfusion, *J Thorac Cardiovasc Surg* 126:638, 2003.
120. Rasmussen LS, Sperling B, Abildstrom HH, et al: Neuron loss after coronary artery bypass detected by SPECT estimation of benzodiazepine receptors, *Ann Thorac Surg* 74:1576, 2002.
121. Wang D, Wu X, Li J, et al: The effect of lidocaine on early postoperative cognitive dysfunction after coronary artery bypass surgery, *Anesth Analg* 95:1134, 2002.
122. Basile AM, Fusi C, Conti AA, et al: S-100 protein and neuron-specific enolase as markers of subclinical cerebral damage after cardiac surgery: Preliminary observation of a 6-month follow-up study, *Eur Neurol* 45:151, 2001.
123. Shaw PJ, Bates D, Cartlidge NE, et al: Neurologic and neuropsychological morbidity following major surgery: Comparison of coronary artery bypass and peripheral vascular surgery, *Stroke* 18:700, 1987.
124. Blauth CI, Smith PL, Arnold JV, et al: Influence of oxygenator type on the prevalence and extent of microembolic retinal ischemia during cardiopulmonary bypass. Assessment by digital image analysis, *J Thorac Cardiovasc Surg* 99:61, 1990.
125. Harrison MJ, Pugsley W, Newman S, et al: Detection of middle cerebral emboli during coronary artery bypass surgery using transcranial Doppler sonography, *Stroke* 2110:1512, 1990.
126. Moody DM, Bell MA, Challa VR, et al: Brain microemboli during cardiac surgery or aortography, *Ann Neurol* 28:477, 1990.
127. Blauth C, Arnold J, Kohner EM, et al: Retinal microembolism during cardiopulmonary bypass demonstrated by fluorescein angiography, *Lancet* 2:837, 1986.
128. bu-Omar Y, Balacumaraswami L, Pigott DW, et al: Solid and gaseous cerebral microembolization during off-pump, on-pump, and open cardiac surgery procedures, *J Thorac Cardiovasc Surg* 127:1759, 2004.
129. Motallebzadeh R, Kanagasabay R, Bland M, et al: S100 protein and its relation to cerebral microemboli in on-pump and off-pump coronary artery bypass surgery, *Eur J Cardiothorac Surg* 25:409, 2004.
130. Wimmer-Greinecker G: Reduction of neurologic complications by intra-aortic filtration in patients undergoing combined intracardiac and CABG procedures, *Eur J Cardiothorac Surg* 23:159, 2003.
131. Hindman BJ: Emboli, inflammation, and CNS impairment: An overview, *Heart Surg Forum* 5:249, 2002.
132. Stanley TO, Mackensen GB, Grocott HP, et al: The impact of postoperative atrial fibrillation on neurocognitive outcome after coronary artery bypass graft surgery, *Anesth Analg* 94:290, 2002.
133. Schmitz C, Weinreich S, White J, et al: Can particulate extraction from the ascending aorta reduce neurologic injury in cardiac surgery? *J Thorac Cardiovasc Surg* 126:1829, 2003.
134. Hamada Y, Kawachi K, Nakata T, et al: Antiinflammatory effect of heparin-coated circuits with leukocyte-depleting filters in coronary bypass surgery, *Artif Organs* 25:1004, 2001.
135. Greilich PE, Brouse CF, Whitten CW, et al: Antifibrinolytic therapy during cardiopulmonary bypass reduces proinflammatory cytokine levels: A randomized, double-blind, placebo-controlled study of epsilon-aminocaproic acid and aprotinin, *J Thorac Cardiovasc Surg* 126:1498, 2003.
136. Murkin JM: Inflammatory responses and CNS injury: Implications, prophylaxis, and treatment, *Heart Surg Forum* 6:193, 2003.
137. Uehara T, Tabuchi M, Kozawa S, et al: MR angiographic evaluation of carotid and intracranial arteries in Japanese patients scheduled for coronary artery bypass grafting, *Cerebrovasc Dis* 11:341, 2001.
138. Yoon BW, Bae HJ, Kang DW, et al: Intracranial cerebral artery disease as a risk factor for central nervous system complications of coronary artery bypass graft surgery, *Stroke* 32:94, 2001.
139. Abildstrom H, Rasmussen LS, Rentowl P, et al: Cognitive dysfunction 1-2 years after noncardiac surgery in the elderly. ISPOCD group. International Study of Post-Operative Cognitive Dysfunction, *Acta Anaesthesiol Scand* 44:1246, 2000.
140. Linstedt U, Meyer O, Kropp P, et al: Serum concentration of S-100 protein in assessment of cognitive dysfunction after general anesthesia in different types of surgery, *Acta Anaesthesiol Scand* 46:384, 2002.
141. Connolly ES Jr, Winfree CJ, Rampersad A, et al: Serum S100B protein levels are correlated with subclinical neurocognitive declines after carotid endarterectomy, *Neurosurgery* 49:1076, 2001.
142. Edmonds CR, Barbut D, Hager D, et al: Intraoperative cerebral arterial embolization during total hip arthroplasty, *Anesthesiology* [illegible]
143. Colonna DM, Kilgus D, Brown W, et al: Acute brain fat embolization occurring after total hip arthroplasty in the absence of a patent foramen ovale, *Anesthesiology* 96:1027, 2002.
144. Kinoshita H, Iranami H, Fujii K, et al: The use of bone cement induces an increase in serum astroglial S-100B protein in patients undergoing total knee arthroplasty, *Anesth Analg* 97:1657, 2003.
145. Serruys PW, Morice MC, Kappetein AP, et al, SYNTAX Investigators: Percutaneous coronary intervention versus coronary-artery bypass grafting for severe coronary artery disease, *N Engl J Med* 360:961–972, 2009.
146. Aguilar MJ, Gerbode F, Hill JD: Neuropathologic complications of cardiac surgery, *J Thorac Cardiovasc Surg* 61:676, 1971.
147. Aberg T, Kihlgren M: Cerebral protection during open-heart surgery, *Thorax* 32:525, 1977.
148. Emmrich P, Hahn J, Ogunlade V, et al: [Neuropathological findings after cardiac surgery—retrospective study over 6 years], *Z Kardiol* 92:925, 2003.
149. Torvik A: The pathogenesis of watershed infarcts in the brain, *Stroke* 15:221, 1984.
150. Salazar JD, Wityk RJ, Grega MA, et al: Stroke after cardiac surgery: Short- and long-term outcomes, *Ann Thorac Surg* 72:1195, 2001.
151. Koga M, Shimokawa S, Moriyama Y, et al: Watershed infarction after combined coronary and axillobifemoral bypass surgery, *Jpn J Thorac Cardiovasc Surg* 48:258, 2000.
152. Malone M: Brain damage after cardiopulmonary bypass: Correlations between neurophysiological and neuropathological findings, *J Neurol Neurosurg Psychiatry* 44:924, 1981.
153. Wityk RJ, Goldsborough MA, Hillis A, et al: Diffusion- and perfusion-weighted brain magnetic resonance imaging in patients with neurologic complications after cardiac surgery, *Arch Neurol* 58:571, 2001.
154. Torvik A, Skullerud K: Watershed infarcts in the brain caused by microemboli, *Clin Neuropathol* 1:99, 1982.
155. Boyajian RA, Otis SM: Embolic stroke syndrome underlies encephalopathy and coma following cardiac surgery, *Arch Neurol* 60:291, 2003.
156. Boyajian RA, Otis SM, Tyner JJ, et al: Study design validation for consolidating global with focal neurological events in cardiac surgery stroke risk factor analyses, *Eur J Neurol* 10:71, 2003.
157. Browne SM, Halligan PW, Wade DT, et al: Postoperative hypoxia is a contributory factor to cognitive impairment after cardiac surgery, *J Thorac Cardiovasc Surg* 126:1061, 2003.
158. Koga M, Shimokawa S, Moriyama Y, et al: Watershed infarction after combined coronary and axillobifemoral bypass surgery, *Jpn J Thorac Cardiovasc Surg* 48:258, 2000.
159. Caplan LR, Hennerici M: Impaired clearance of emboli (washout) is an important link between hypoperfusion, embolism, and ischemic stroke, *Arch Neurol* 5511:1475, 1998.
160. Shann KG, Likosky DS, Murkin JM, et al: An evidenced-based review of the practice of cardiopulmonary bypass in adults, *J Thorac Cardiovasc Surg* 132:283–290, 2006.
161. Bolsin SN: Detection of neurological damage during cardiopulmonary bypass, *Anaesthesia* 41:61, 1986.
162. Levy WJ: Electroencephalographic evidence of cerebral ischemia during acute extracorporeal hypoperfusion, *J Cardiothorac Anesth* 1:300, 1987.
163. Russ W, Kling D, Sauerwein G, et al: Spectral analysis of the EEG during hypothermic cardiopulmonary bypass, *Acta Anaesthesiol Scand* 31:111, 1987.
164. Edmonds HL Jr, Griffiths LK, Slater AD, et al: Quantitative electroencephalographic monitoring during myocardial revascularization predicts postoperative disorientation and improves outcome, *J Thorac Cardiovasc Surg* 103:555, 1992.
165. Govier AV, Reves JG, McKay RD, et al: Factors and their influence on regional cerebral blood flow during nonpulsatile cardiopulmonary bypass, *Ann Thorac Surg* 38:592, 1984.
166. Prough DS, Stump DA, Roy RC, et al: Response of cerebral blood flow to changes in carbon dioxide tension during hypothermic cardiopulmonary bypass, *Anesthesiology* 64:576, 1986.
167. Gold JP, Charlson ME, Williams-Russo P, et al: Improvement of outcomes after coronary artery bypass. A randomized trial comparing intraoperative high versus low mean arterial pressure, *J Thorac Cardiovasc Surg* 110:1302, 1995.
168. Lundar T, Froysaker T, Lindegaard KF, et al: Some observations on cerebral perfusion during cardiopulmonary bypass, *Ann Thorac Surg* 39:318, 1985.
169. Avraamides EJ: The effect of surgical dislocation of the heart on cerebral blood flow in the presence of a single, two-stage venous cannula during cardiopulmonary bypass, *Can J Anaesth* 43:A36, 1996.
170. Russell RW, Bharucha N: The recognition and prevention of border zone cerebral ischaemia during cardiac surgery, *Q J Med* 47187:303, 1978.
171. Newman MF, Kramer D, Croughwell ND, et al: Differential age effects of mean arterial pressure and rewarming on cognitive dysfunction after cardiac surgery, *Anesth Analg* 81:236, 1995.
172. Ganushchak YM, Fransen EJ, Visser C, et al: Neurological complications after coronary artery bypass grafting related to the performance of cardiopulmonary bypass, *Chest* 125:2196, 2004.
173. Ura M, Sakata R, Nakayama Y, et al: Ultrasonographic demonstration of manipulation-related aortic injuries after cardiac surgery, *J Am Coll Cardiol* 35:1303, 2000.
174. Sylivris S, Levi C, Matalanis G, et al: Pattern and significance of cerebral microemboli during coronary artery bypass grafting, *Ann Thorac Surg* 66:1674, 1998.
175. Eckmann DM, Armstead SC, Mardini F: Surfactants reduce platelet-bubble and platelet-platelet binding induced by in vitro air embolism, *Anesthesiology* 103:1204, 2005.
176. Persson LI, Johansson BB, Hansson HA: Ultrastructural studies on blood-brain barrier dysfunction after cerebral air embolism in the rat, *Acta Neuropathol (Berl)* 1344:53, 1978.
177. Philp RB, Inwood MJ, Warren BA: Interactions between gas bubbles and components of the blood: Implications in decompression sickness, *Aerosp Med* 43:946, 1972.
178. Warren BA, Philp RB, Inwood MJ: The ultrastructural morphology of air embolism: Platelet adhesion to the interface and endothelial damage, *Br J Exp Pathol* 54:163, 1973.
179. Helps SC, Parsons DW, Reilly PL, et al: The effect of gas emboli on rabbit cerebral blood flow, *Stroke* 21:94, 1990.
180. Haller C, Sercombe R, Verrecchia C, et al: Effect of the muscarinic agonist carbachol on pial arteries in vivo after endothelial damage by air embolism, *J Cereb Blood Flow Metab* 7:605, 1987.
181. Mangano CM: Scuds, scads, and other air-borne hazards, *Anesthesiology* 87:476, 1997.
182. Mitchell S, Gorman D: The pathophysiology of cerebral arterial gas embolism, *J Extra Corpor Technol* 34:18, 2002.
183. Moody DM, Brown WR, Challa VR, et al: Brain microemboli associated with cardiopulmonary bypass: A histologic and magnetic resonance imaging study, *Ann Thorac Surg* 59:1304, 1995.
184. Challa VR, Lovell MA, Moody DM, et al: Laser microprobe mass spectrometric study of aluminum and silicon in brain emboli related to cardiac surgery, *J Neuropathol Exp Neurol* 57:140, 1998.
185. Kincaid EH, Jones TJ, Stump DA, et al: Processing scavenged blood with a cell saver reduces cerebral lipid microembolization, *Ann Thorac Surg* 70:1296, 2000.

186. Djaiani G, Fedorko L, Borger MA, et al: Continuous-flow cell saver reduces cognitive decline in elderly patients after coronary bypass surgery, *Circulation* 116:1888–1895, 2007.
187. Rubens FD, Boodhwani M, Mesana T, et al: Cardiotomy Investigators: The cardiotomy trial: A randomized, double-blind study to assess the effect of processing of shed blood during cardiopulmonary bypass on transfusion and neurocognitive function, *Circulation* 116(Suppl 11):I89–I97, 2007.
188. Koch CG, Li L, Duncan AI, et al: Morbidity and mortality risk associated with red blood cell and blood-component transfusion in isolated coronary artery bypass grafting, *Crit Care Med* 34: 1608–1616, 2006.
189. Wollman H, Stephen GW, Clement AJ, et al: Cerebral blood flow in man during extracorporeal circulation, *J Thorac Cardiovasc Surg* 52:558, 1966.
190. Kubota Y: Clinical study of the cerebral hemodynamics during extracorporeal circulation, *Nagoya J Med Sci* 31:117, 1968.
191. Branthwaite MA: Cerebral blood flow and metabolism during open-heart surgery, *Thorax* 29:633, 1974.
192. Henriksen L, Hjelms E, Lindeburgh T: Brain hyperperfusion during cardiac operations. Cerebral blood flow measured in man by intra-arterial injection of xenon 133: Evidence suggestive of intraoperative microembolism, *J Thorac Cardiovasc Surg* 86:202, 1983.
193. Taylor KM: Brain damage during cardiopulmonary bypass, *Ann Thorac Surg* 654(Suppl):S20, 1998.
194. Busto R, Dietrich WD, Globus MY, et al: The importance of brain temperature in cerebral ischemic injury, *Stroke* 20:1113, 1989.
195. Buchan A, Pulsinelli W: Hypothermia but not the N-methyl-D-aspartate antagonist, MK801, attenuates neuronal damage in gerbils subjected to transient global ischemia, *J Neurosci* 10:311, 1990.
196. Chopp M, Knight R, Tidwell CD, et al: The metabolic effects of mild hypothermia on global cerebral ischemia and recirculation in the cat: Comparison to normothermia and hyperthermia, *J Cereb Blood Flow Metab* 9:141, 1989.
197. Nemoto EM, Klementavicius R, Melick JA, et al: Suppression of cerebral metabolic rate for oxygen CMRO(2) by mild hypothermia compared with thiopental, *J Neurosurg Anesthesiol* 8:52, 1996.
198. Mora CT, Henson MB, Weintraub WS, et al: The effect of temperature management during cardiopulmonary bypass on neurologic and neuropsychological outcomes in patients undergoing coronary revascularization, *J Thorac Cardiovasc Surg* 112:514, 1996.
199. Murkin JM: Hypothermic cardiopulmonary bypass—time for a more temperate approach, *Can J Anaesth* 42:663, 1995.
200. Nathan HJ, Wells GA, Munson JL, et al: Neuroprotective effect of mild hypothermia in patients undergoing coronary artery surgery with cardiopulmonary bypass: A randomized trial, *Circulation* 18(Suppl I):I–85, 2001.
201. Engelman RM, Pleet AB, Hicks R, et al: Is there a relationship between systemic perfusion temperature during coronary artery bypass grafting and extent of intraoperative ischemic central nervous system injury? *J Thorac Cardiovasc Surg* 119:230, 2000.
202. Dworschak M, Lassnigg A, Tenze G, et al: Perfusion temperature during cardiopulmonary bypass does not affect serum S-100beta release, *Thorac Cardiovasc Surg* 52:29, 2004.
203. Grimm M, Czerny M, Baumer H, et al: Normothermic cardiopulmonary bypass is beneficial for cognitive brain function after coronary artery bypass grafting—a prospective randomized trial, *Eur J Cardiothorac Surg* 18:270, 2000.
204. Arrowsmith JE, Dunning JL: Normothermic cardiopulmonary bypass is beneficial for cognitive brain function after coronary artery bypass grafting—a prospective randomized trial, *Eur J Cardiothorac Surg* 19:732, 2001.
205. Engelman R, Pleet AB: Cardiopulmonary bypass temperature and extension of intraoperative brain damage: Controversies persist, *J Thorac Cardiovasc Surg* 120:1014, 2000.
206. Gaudino M, Possati G: Cardiopulmonary bypass temperature and extension of intraoperative brain damage: Controversies persist, *J Thorac Cardiovasc Surg* 120:1013, 2000.
207. Murkin JM: Pathophysiological basis of CNS injury in cardiac surgical patients: Detection and prevention, *Perfusion* 21:203–208, 2006.
208. Grocott HP, Mackensen GB, Grigore AM, et al: Postoperative hyperthermia is associated with cognitive dysfunction after coronary artery bypass graft surgery, *Stroke* 33:537, 2002.
209. Scheffer T, Sanders DB: The neurologic sequelae of cardiopulmonary bypass-induced cerebral hyperthermia and cerebroprotective strategies, *J Extra Corpor Technol* 35:317, 2003.
210. Kawahara F, Kadoi Y, Saito S, et al: Slow rewarming improves jugular venous oxygen saturation during rewarming, *Acta Anaesthesiol Scand* 47:419, 2003.
211. Okano N, Owada R, Fujita N, et al: Cerebral oxygenation is better during mild hypothermic than normothermic cardiopulmonary bypass, *Can J Anaesth* 47:131, 2000.
212. Gravlee GP, Roy RC, Stump DA, et al: Regional cerebrovascular reactivity to carbon dioxide during cardiopulmonary bypass in patients with cerebrovascular disease, *J Thorac Cardiovasc Surg* 99:1022, 1990.
213. von Reutern GM, Hetzel A, Birnbaum D, et al: Transcranial Doppler ultrasonography during cardiopulmonary bypass in patients with severe carotid stenosis or occlusion, *Stroke* 19:674, 1988.
214. Brusino FG, Reves JG, Prough DS, et al: Cerebral blood flow during cardiopulmonary bypass in a patient with occlusive cerebrovascular disease, *J Cardiothorac Anesth* 3:87, 1989.
215. Koster S, Hensens AG, van der Palen J: The long-term cognitive and functional outcomes of postoperative delirium after cardiac surgery, *Ann Thorac Surg* 87:1469–1474, 2009.
216. Berens ES, Kouchoukos NT, Murphy SF, et al: Preoperative carotid artery screening in elderly patients undergoing cardiac surgery, *J Vasc Surg* 15:313, 1992.
217. Schwartz LB, Bridgman AH, Kieffer RW, et al: Asymptomatic carotid artery stenosis and stroke in patients undergoing cardiopulmonary bypass, *J Vasc Surg* 21:146, 1995.
218. Salasidis GC, Latter DA, Steinmetz OK, et al: Carotid artery duplex scanning in preoperative assessment for coronary artery revascularization: The association between peripheral vascular disease, carotid artery stenosis, and stroke, *J Vasc Surg* 21:154, 1995.
219. Palerme LP, Hill AB, Obrand D, et al: Is Canadian cardiac surgeons' management of asymptomatic carotid artery stenosis at coronary artery bypass supported by the literature? A survey and a critical appraisal of the literature, *Can J Surg* 43:93, 2000.
220. Naylor AR: A critical review of the role of carotid disease and the outcomes of staged and synchronous carotid surgery, *Semin Cardiothorac Vasc Anesth* 8:37, 2004.
221. Furnary AP, Gao G, Grunkemeier GL, et al: Continuous insulin infusion reduces mortality in patients with diabetes undergoing coronary artery bypass grafting, *J Thorac Cardiovasc Surg* 125:1007, 2003.
222. Latham R, Lancaster AD, Covington JF, et al: The association of diabetes and glucose control with surgical-site infections among cardiothoracic surgery patients, *Infect Control Hosp Epidemiol* 22:607, 2001.
223. Coursin DB, Prielipp RC: The new anesthesia diet plan: Keeping perioperative carbs in check, *Anesth Analg* 99:316, 2004.
224. Carvalho G, Moore A, Qizilbash B, et al: Maintenance of normoglycemia during cardiac surgery, *Anesth Analg* 99:319, 2004.
225. Jessen ME: Glucose control during cardiac surgery: How sweet it is, *J Thorac Cardiovasc Surg* 125:985, 2003.
226. Bucerius J, Gummert JF, Walther T, et al: Impact of diabetes mellitus on cardiac surgery outcome, *Thorac Cardiovasc Surg* 51:11, 2003.
227. Mortasawi A, Arnrich B, Rosendahl U, et al: Is age an independent determinant of mortality in cardiac surgery as suggested by the EuroSCORE? *BMC Surg* 72:8, 2002.
228. Kadoi Y, Saito S, Yoshikawa D, et al: Increasing mean arterial blood pressure has no effect on jugular venous oxygen saturation in insulin-dependent patients during tepid cardiopulmonary bypass, *Anesth Analg* 95:266, 2002.
229. Murkin JM: Pro: Tight intraoperative glucose control improves outcome in cardiovascular surgery, *J Cardiothorac Vasc Anesth* 14:475, 2000.
230. McAlister FA, Man J, Bistritz L, et al: Diabetes and coronary artery bypass surgery: An examination of perioperative glycemic control and outcomes, *Diabetes Care* 26:1518, 2003.
231. Lazar HL, McDonnell M, Chipkin SR, et al: Society of Thoracic Surgeons Blood Glucose Guideline Task Force: The Society of Thoracic Surgeons practice guideline series: Blood glucose management during adult cardiac surgery, *Ann Thorac Surg* 87:663–669, 2009.
232. Krinsley JS, Grover A: Severe hypoglycemia in critically ill patients: Risk factors and outcomes, *Crit Care Med* 35:2262–2267, 2007.
233. Gandhi GY, Nuttall GA, Abel MD, et al: Intensive intraoperative insulin therapy versus conventional glucose management during cardiac surgery: A randomized trial, *Ann Intern Med* 146:233–243, 2007.
234. Sheehy AM, Coursin DB, Keegan MT: Risks of tight glycemic control during adult cardiac surgery, *Ann Thorac Surg* 88:1384–1385, 2009.
235. Blauth CI, Arnold JV, Schulenberg WE, et al: Cerebral microembolism during cardiopulmonary bypass. Retinal microvascular studies in vivo with fluorescein angiography, *J Thorac Cardiovasc Surg* 95:668, 1988.
236. Padayachee TS, Parsons S, Theobold R, et al: The detection of microemboli in the middle cerebral artery during cardiopulmonary bypass: A transcranial Doppler ultrasound investigation using membrane and bubble oxygenators, *Ann Thorac Surg* 44:298, 1987.
237. Padayachee TS, Parsons S, Theobold R, et al: The effect of arterial filtration on reduction of gaseous microemboli in the middle cerebral artery during cardiopulmonary bypass, *Ann Thorac Surg* 45:647, 1988.
238. Williams IM, Stephens JF, Richardson EP Jr, et al: Brain and retinal microemboli during cardiac surgery, *Ann Neurol* 30:736, 1991.
239. Georgiadis D, Hempel A, Baumgartner RW, et al: Doppler microembolic signals during cardiac surgery: Comparison between arterial line and middle cerebral artery, *J Thorac Cardiovasc Surg* 126:1638, 2003.
240. Schoenburg M, Kraus B, Muehling A, et al: The dynamic air bubble trap reduces cerebral microembolism during cardiopulmonary bypass, *J Thorac Cardiovasc Surg* 126:1455, 2003.
241. Edmunds LH Jr: Advances in the heart-lung machine after John and Mary Gibbon, *Ann Thorac Surg* 76:S2220, 2003.
242. Haworth WS: The development of the modern oxygenator, *Ann Thorac Surg* 76:S2216, 2003.
243. Whitaker DC, Stygall JA, Newman SP, et al: The use of leukocyte-depleting and conventional arterial line filters in cardiac surgery: A systematic review of clinical studies, *Perfusion* 16:433, 2001.
244. Jewell AE, Akowuah EF, Suvarna SK, et al: A prospective randomised comparison of cardiotomy suction and cell saver for recycling shed blood during cardiac surgery, *Eur J Cardiothorac Surg* 23:633, 2003.
245. de Vries AJ, Gu YJ, Douglas YL, et al: Clinical evaluation of a new fat removal filter during cardiac surgery, *Eur J Cardiothorac Surg* 25:261, 2004.
246. Marschall K, Kanchuger M, Kessler K, et al: Superiority of transesophageal echocardiography in detecting aortic arch atheromatous disease: Identification of patients at increased risk of stroke during cardiac surgery, *J Cardiothorac Vasc Anesth* 8:5, 1994.
247. Hosoda Y, Watanabe M, Hirooka Y, et al: Significance of atherosclerotic changes of the ascending aorta during coronary bypass surgery with intraoperative detection by echography, *J Cardiovasc Surg (Torino)* 32:301, 1991.
248. Van Boven WJ, Berry G: Intra-aortic filtration captures particulate debris in OPCAB cases using anastomotic devices, *Heart Surg Forum* 5(Suppl 4):S461, 2002.
249. Banbury MK, Kouchoukos NT, Allen KB, et al: Emboli capture using the Embol-X intraaortic filter in cardiac surgery: A multicentered randomized trial of 1,289 patients, *Ann Thorac Surg* 76:508, 2003.
250. Reichenspurner H, Navia JA, Berry G, et al: Particulate emboli capture by an intra-aortic filter device during cardiac surgery, *J Thorac Cardiovasc Surg* 119:233, 2000.
251. Gerriets T, Schwarz N, Sammer G, et al: Protecting the brain from gaseous and solid micro-emboli during coronary artery bypass grafting: A randomized controlled trial, *Eur Heart J* 31:360–368, 2010.
252. Murkin JM: Perioperative multimodality neuromonitoring: An overview, *Semin Cardiothorac Vasc Anesth* 8:167, 2004.
253. Borger MA, Djaiani G: Reduction of cerebral emboli during cardiac surgery: Influence of surgeon and perfusionist feedback, *Heart Surg Forum* 6:204, 2003.
254. Bar-Yosef S, Sanders EG, Grocott HP: Asymmetric cerebral near-infrared oximetric measurements during cardiac surgery, *J Cardiothorac Vasc Anesth* 17:773, 2003.
255. Daubeney PE, Smith DC, Pilkington SN, et al: Cerebral oxygenation during paediatric cardiac surgery: Identification of vulnerable periods using near-infrared spectroscopy, *Eur J Cardiothorac Surg* 13:370, 1998.
256. Austin EH III, Edmonds HL Jr, Auden SM, et al: Benefit of neurophysiologic monitoring for pediatric cardiac surgery, *J Thorac Cardiovasc Surg* 114:707, 1997.
257. Chen CS, Leu BK, Liu K: Detection of cerebral desaturation during cardiopulmonary bypass by cerebral oximetry, *Acta Anaesthesiol Sin* 34:173, 1996.
258. Murkin JM, Arango M: Near-infrared spectroscopy as an index of brain and tissue oxygenation, *Br J Anaesth* 103(Suppl 1):i3–i13, 2009.
259. Goldman S: Optimizing intraoperative cerebral oxygen delivery using noninvasive cerebral oximetry decreases the incidence of stroke for cardiac surgical patients, *Heart Surg Forum* 7:E376–E381, 2004.
260. Murkin JM, Adams SJ, Novick RJ, et al: Monitoring brain oxygen saturation during coronary bypass surgery: A randomized, prospective study, *Anesth Analg* 104:51–58, 2007.
261. Novitzky D, Boswell BB: Total myocardial revascularization without cardiopulmonary bypass utilizing computer-processed monitoring to assess cerebral perfusion, *Heart Surg Forum* 3:198, 2000.
262. Hong SW, Shim JK, Choi YS, et al: Prediction of cognitive dysfunction and patients' outcome following valvular heart surgery and the role of cerebral oximetry, *Eur J Cardiothorac Surg* 33: 560–565, 2008.
263. Murkin JM, Bainbridge D, Novick R: In response. Do the data really support the conclusion [Letter]? *Anesth Analg* 105:536–538, 2007.
264. Denault A, Deschamps A, Murkin JM: A proposed algorithm for the intraoperative use of cerebral near-infrared spectroscopy, *Semin Cardiothorac Vasc Anesth* 11:274–281, 2007.
265. Kurth CD, Steven JM, Nicolson SC: Cerebral oxygenation during pediatric cardiac surgery using deep hypothermic circulatory arrest, *Anesthesiology* 82:74–82, 1995.
266. Kurth CD, Steven JM, Nicolson SC, et al: Kinetics of cerebral deoxygenation during deep hypothermic circulatory arrest in neonates, *Anesthesiology* 77:656–661, 1992.
267. Leyvi G, Bello R, Wasnick JD, et al: Assessment of cerebral oxygen balance during deep hypothermic circulatory arrest by continuous jugular bulb venous saturation and near-infrared spectroscopy, *J Cardiothorac Vasc Anesth* 20:826–833, 2006.

268. Ogino H, Ueda Y, Sugita T, et al: Monitoring of regional cerebral oxygenation by near-infrared spectroscopy during continuous retrograde cerebral perfusion for aortic arch surgery, *Eur J Cardiothorac Surg* 14:415–418, 1998.

269. Orihashi K, Sueda T, Okada K, et al: Near-infrared spectroscopy for monitoring cerebral ischemia during selective cerebral perfusion, *Eur J Cardiothorac Surg* 26:907–911, 2004.

270. Hofer A, Haizinger B, Geiselseder G, et al: Monitoring of selective antegrade cerebral perfusion using near infrared spectroscopy in neonatal aortic arch surgery, *Eur J Anaesthesiol* 22:293–298, 2005.

271. Higami T, Kozawa S, Asada T, et al: A comparison of changes of cerebrovascular oxygen saturation in retrograde and selective cerebral perfusion during aortic arch surgery, *Nippon Kyobu Geka Gakkai Zasshi* 43:1010–1023, 1995.

272. Matalanis G, Hata M, Buxton BF: A retrospective comparative study of deep hypothermic circulatory arrest, retrograde, and antegrade cerebral perfusion in aortic arch surgery, *Ann Thorac Cardiovasc Surg* 9:174–179, 2003.

273. Higami T, Kozawa S, Asada T, et al: Retrograde cerebral perfusion versus selective cerebral perfusion as evaluated by cerebral oxygen saturation during aortic arch reconstruction, *Ann Thorac Surg* 67:1091–1096, 1999.

274. Olsson C, Thelin S: Regional cerebral saturation monitoring with near-infrared spectroscopy during selective antegrade cerebral perfusion: Diagnostic performance and relationship to postoperative stroke, *J Thorac Cardiovasc Surg* 131:371–379, 2006.

275. Janelle GM, Mnookin S, Gravenstein N, et al: Unilateral cerebral oxygen desaturations during emergent repair of DeBakey type 1 aortic dissection: Potential aversion of a major catastrophe, *Anesthesiology* 96:1263–1265, 2002.

276. Sakaguchi G, Komiya T, Tamura N, et al: Cerebral malperfusion in acute type A dissection: Direct innominate artery cannulation, *J Thorac Cardiovasc Surg* 129:1190–1191, 2005.

277. Schneider F, Falk V, Walther T, et al: Control of endoaortic clamp position during port-access mitral valve operations using transcranial Doppler echography, *Ann Thorac Surg* 65:1481, 1998.

278. Hoksbergen AW, Legemate DA, Csiba L, et al: Absent collateral function of the circle of Willis as risk factor for ischemic stroke, *Cerebrovasc Dis* 16:191–198, 2003.

279. Merkkola P, Tulla H, Ronkainen A, et al: Incomplete circle of Willis and right axillary artery perfusion, *Ann Thorac Surg* 82:74–79, 2006.

280. Santo KC, Barrios A, Dandekar U, et al: Near-infrared spectroscopy: An important monitoring tool during hybrid aortic arch replacement, *Anesth Analg* 107:793–796, 2008.

281. Rossi M, Tirotta CF, Laguereula RG, et al: Diminished Blalock-Taussig shunt flow detected by cerebral oximetry, *Paediatr Anaesth* 17:72–74, 2007.

282. Nussmeier NA, Arlund C, Slogoff S: Neuropsychiatric complications after cardiopulmonary bypass: Cerebral protection by a barbiturate, *Anesthesiology* 64:165, 1986.

283. Zaidan JR, Klochany A, Martin WM, et al: Effect of thiopental on neurologic outcome following coronary artery bypass grafting, *Anesthesiology* 74:406, 1991.

284. Woodcock TE, Murkin JM, Farrar JK, et al: Pharmacologic EEG suppression during cardiopulmonary bypass: Cerebral hemodynamic and metabolic effects of thiopental or isoflurane during hypothermia and normothermia, *Anesthesiology* 67:218, 1987.

285. Roach GW, Newman MF, Murkin JM, et al: Ineffectiveness of burst suppression therapy in mitigating perioperative cerebrovascular dysfunction. Multicenter Study of Perioperative Ischemia (McSPI) Research Group, *Anesthesiology* 90:1255–1264, 1999.

286. Legault C, Furberg CD, Wagenknecht LE, et al: Nimodipine neuroprotection in cardiac valve replacement: Report of an early terminated trial, *Stroke* 27:593, 1996.

287. Amory DW, Grigore A, Amory JK, et al: Neuroprotection is associated with beta-adrenergic receptor antagonists during cardiac surgery: Evidence from 2,575 patients, *J Cardiothorac Vasc Anesth* 16:270, 2002.

288. POISE Study Group, Devereaux PJ, Yang H: Effects of extended-release metoprolol succinate in patients undergoing non-cardiac surgery (POISE trial): A randomised controlled trial, *Lancet* 371:1839–1847, 2008.

289. van Lier F, Schouten O, van Domburg RT, et al: Effect of chronic beta-blocker use on stroke after noncardiac surgery, *Am J Cardiol* 104:429–433, 2009.

290. Landis RC, Asimakopoulos G, Poullis M, et al: The antithrombotic and antiinflammatory mechanisms of action of aprotinin, *Ann Thorac Surg* 72:2169, 2001.

291. Mangano DT, Tudor IC, Dietzel C, Multicenter Study of Perioperative Ischemia Research Group. Ischemia Research and Education Foundation: The risk associated with aprotinin in cardiac surgery, *N Engl J Med* 354:353–365, 2006.

292. Fergusson DA, Hébert PC, Mazer CD, et al, BART Investigators: A comparison of aprotinin and lysine analogues in high-risk cardiac surgery, *N Engl J Med* 358:2319–2331, 2008.

293. Mangano DT, Miao Y, Vuylsteke A, et al, Investigators of The Multicenter Study of Perioperative Ischemia Research Group, Ischemia Research and Education Foundation: Mortality associated with aprotinin during 5 years following coronary artery bypass graft surgery, *JAMA* 297:471–479, 2007.

294. Later AF, Maas JJ, Engbers FH, et al: Tranexamic acid and aprotinin in low- and intermediate-risk cardiac surgery: A non-sponsored, double-blind, randomised, placebo-controlled trial, *Eur J Cardiothorac Surg* 36:322–329, 2009.

295. Immer FF, Jent P, Englberger L, et al: Aprotinin in cardiac surgery: A different point of view, *Heart Surg Forum* 11:E9–E12, 2008.

296. Mangano DT: Aspirin and mortality from coronary bypass surgery, *N Engl J Med* 2434:1309, 2002.

297. Wang D, Wu X, Li J, et al: The effect of lidocaine on early postoperative cognitive dysfunction after coronary artery bypass surgery, *Anesth Analg* 95:1134–1141, 2002.

298. Mitchell SJ, Merry AF, Frampton C, et al: Cerebral protection by lidocaine during cardiac operations: A follow-up study, *Ann Thorac Surg* 87:820–825, 2009.

299. Mathew JP, Mackensen GB, Phillips-Bute B, et al: Neurologic Outcome Research Group (NORG) of the Duke Heart Center: Randomized, double-blinded, placebo controlled study of neuroprotection with lidocaine in cardiac surgery, *Stroke* 40:880–887, 2009.

300. Mitchell SJ, Merry AF: Lignocaine: Neuro-protective or wishful thinking? *J Extra Corpor Technol* 41:37–42, 2009.

301. Aboyans V, Labrousse L, Lacroix P, et al: Productive factors of stroke in patients undergoing coronary bypass grafting: Statins are protective, *Eur J Cardiothorac Surg* 30:300–304, 2006.

302. Radaelli A, Loardi C, Cazzaniga M, et al: Inflammatory activation during coronary artery surgery and its dose-dependent modulation by statin/ACE-inhibitor combination, *Arteriosclcer Thromb Vasc Biol* 27(12):2750–2755, 2007.

37

Long-Term Complications and Management

MICHAEL J. MURRAY, MD, PHD | ALYSSA B. CHAPITAL, MD, PHD | DEAN T. GIACOBBE, MD

KEY POINTS

1. After undergoing cardiac surgical procedures, patients usually follow a fairly predictable postoperative course: the hemodynamic sequelae of cardiopulmonary bypass abate; the patient is weaned from mechanical ventilation and extubated; and within 24 hours, most patients are discharged from the intensive care unit (ICU).
2. After undergoing cardiac operations, a small percentage of patients have complicated courses and prolonged stays in the ICU.
3. Patients with extended stays in the ICU have a higher-than-average mortality rate because of noncardiac organ dysfunction.
4. Anesthesiologists and intensivists caring for patients who have prolonged stays in the ICU and who have complex medical issues must take into account all organ systems when determining the correct diagnosis and prescribing appropriate treatment.
5. Meticulous attention to detail and the application of recent evidence-based treatments will result in improved survival in patients who have extended stays in the ICU.

Most patients who have undergone cardiac surgical procedures have brief stays in the intensive care unit (ICU; < 24 hours), and these stays typically follow a predictable pattern. During this time, most instability and morbidity are attributable to the cardiopulmonary organ systems, bleeding, hypothermia, and the emergence from anesthesia.[1] A small minority of patients, however, have prolonged ICU stays, characterized by multisystem complications involving both the cardiac and noncardiac systems. This group of patients consumes a disproportionate number of ICU resources; generates enormous hospital costs; and, ultimately, has a much worse prognosis (both in-hospital and long term).[1-3] For example, Bashour et al[1] described a series of 2618 patients who had undergone cardiac operations, 5.4% of whom had an ICU length of stay (LOS) of longer than 10 days. In the prolonged LOS group, the in-hospital mortality rate was 33.1% (vs. 1.5% in a group with an LOS < 10 days). Of those patients with a prolonged ICU LOS who survived to discharge, 46.8% died within 30 months. Welsby et al[2] analyzed types of complications in a cohort of patients who had undergone cardiac surgical procedures and who had a prolonged LOS in the ICU; they demonstrated that noncardiac complications are more deleterious than are isolated cardiac complications. In another series of 1280 patients, only 3.8% of patients had an ICU LOS longer than 14 days. The hospital mortality rate in the prolonged LOS group was 25.8% (vs. 5.3% in a short LOS group), and only 62% of patients discharged after an extended stay in the ICU were alive at 2 years.[3]

These data underscore the fact that, when caring for the minority of patients who require a prolonged stay in the ICU after undergoing a cardiac procedure, health care providers must distinctly shift their orientation—from a "recovery-room" mode, focusing primarily on the cardiovascular organ system, to a true ICU mode, focusing on preventing and treating dysfunction in multiple organ systems. At the same time, the physicians who continue to prescribe aggressive treatment must temper this decision with a realistic view of the patient's prognosis and an assessment of the "cost" of that treatment to the patient, family, and society. The following sections of this chapter highlight the issues that must be addressed in those patients with an extended LOS in the ICU.

SEDATION IN THE INTENSIVE CARE UNIT

Most patients who have an extended LOS in the ICU will require a different approach to sedation and pain control than do patients who do not have an extended LOS. The major goals of sedation in the ICU are to provide anxiolysis and to improve the patient's perceptual experience during this physiologically and emotionally stressful period (Box 37-1).[4] Secondarily, sedation reduces the physiologic stress response and attendant cardiovascular work, may facilitate the maintenance of circadian rhythms, and lessens delirium and agitation.[5] These goals are distinct from those associated with analgesia, which are the alleviation of pain through nonpharmacologic and pharmacologic means and to facilitate diagnostic and therapeutic procedures.[4] Although sedation and analgesia are separate therapeutic goals usually provided by individual drugs, combining anxiolytic and analgesic drugs often results in a synergistic effect, and some newer agents provide elements of both analgesia and anxiolysis, thus blurring the distinction in clinical practice (see Chapter 38).

In 1995, the Society of Critical Care Medicine (SCCM) published guidelines for sedation in the ICU,[6] revised the guidelines in 2002,[7] and is in the process of again updating the guidelines (Michael J. Murray, MD, PhD, Personal Communication, December 2010). The guidelines emphasize the need for the goal-directed delivery of psychoactive medications. Using goal-directed sedation is supported by an increasing body of literature that shows that daily interruption of sedation, intermittent sedation, and sedation protocols all reduce the duration of mechanical ventilation and, in some instances, decrease ICU LOS.[8]

Sedation Scoring Systems

Several scoring systems are available to assess a patient's degree of sedation in the ICU and to facilitate goal-directed therapy. When using the seven-item Riker Sedation-Agitation Scale,[9] which was

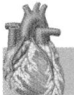

BOX 37-1. SEDATION GOALS

- Use specific agents targeted to therapeutic goals (e.g., sedative agents for the treatment of agitation; opioid agents to provide analgesia).
- Use goal-directed sedation therapy titrated to an objective scoring system.
- Wean sedative agents daily to assess the patient and reevaluate the need for sedation.

TABLE 37-1	Ramsay Sedation Scale

The patient

1. Is anxious and agitated or restless, or both
2. Is cooperative, oriented, and tranquil
3. Responds only to commands
4. Exhibits a brisk response to a light glabellar tap or loud auditory stimulus
5. Exhibits a sluggish response to a light glabellar tap or loud auditory stimulus
6. Is unresponsive

the first scale proved to be reliable and valid for use in critically ill adults, the clinician assigns a score based on the patient's behavior. The Motor Activity Assessment Scale[10] includes seven categories to describe patients' behavior in response to stimulation. Like the Sedation-Agitation Scale, it has been validated in critically ill adults.

Most comparative clinical studies of sedation in critically ill patients have used the Ramsay Scale.[11] Scoring with this six-point scale of motor activity ranges from 1 (patient anxious, agitated or restless, or both) to 6 (no response to light glabellar tap or loud auditory stimulus; Table 37-1).[5] Originally designed as a research tool, the Ramsay Scale has been used for decades in clinical practice.

Other sedation scales that have been validated in critically ill adults include the Vancouver Interaction and Calmness Scale,[12] the COMFORT scale,[13] the Richmond Agitation-Sedation Scale,[14,15] and the Minnesota Sedation Assessment Tool.[16] Increasing recognition of the long-term sequelae of delirium has led to the development and use of other scoring systems. The Confusion Assessment Method for the ICU (CAM-ICU) recently was validated in one ICU study and it is increasingly being used.[17]

More objective parameters to assess sedation are being pursued. The bispectral index is a monitor that measures a simple, three-lead, frontal-montage that, through proprietary software, converts the electroencephalographic activity to a digital scale from 1 to 100. When specific sedative agents are used, the bispectral index reading typically correlates well with the level of sedation in patients in the ICU[18] (see Chapter 16).

Sedative Agents

Benzodiazepines

Many drugs are available for sedating patients in the cardiothoracic ICU. The most frequently used agents for sedation include benzodiazepines (midazolam, lorazepam), propofol, and the α_2-receptor agonist, dexmedetomidine. Although multiple medications can be used to allay anxiety, the traditional approach has been to use benzodiazepines. These drugs act by binding to benzodiazepine receptors (subunits of the $GABA_A$ [γ-aminobutyric acid] receptors, in the limbic area of the brain). This binding enhances the effects of GABA in a dose-dependent fashion. Benzodiazepines can be titrated to effect, with the effect ranging from light sedation to coma. Side effects such as respiratory depression are also dose dependent and are more likely to appear in patients with comorbid conditions such as chronic obstructive pulmonary disease, very young and very old patients, and in patients receiving drugs with synergistic properties, such as opioids.

Midazolam, a short-acting, water-soluble benzodiazepine, can only be given parenterally. Its intravenous administration causes no pain or venous irritation (and, therefore, thrombosis), and its potency is two to four times that of diazepam. Midazolam is readily redistributed in tissues and is rapidly cleared by the liver and kidneys. It is enzymatically degraded in the liver to α-hydroxy-midazolam, which has minimal, if any, clinical sedative or hypnotic

effects. The clinical effects of midazolam are short-lived because of an elimination half-life of 1.5 to 3.5 hours. These properties make midazolam ideal as an anxiolytic benzodiazepine for short-term use in the ICU.[19] Depending on the situation, intermittent boluses of midazolam can be given, or a continuous infusion of 0.5 to 5.0 mg/hr can be used. Greater doses may be required, and infusions of up to 20 mg/hr have been used safely in mechanically ventilated patients.[20]

In patients whose condition deteriorates while they are in the ICU, such as the patient who experiences development of sepsis or multiple organ dysfunction syndrome, midazolam elimination may be decreased, and its clinical effect prolonged. This prolongation of effect may be because of the increased volume of distribution that occurs in patients with multiple organ dysfunction syndrome, whose renal clearance is decreased.

Lorazepam is a long-acting agent with sedative effects that last 6 to 8 hours after a single dose. Lorazepam has minimal effect on cardiovascular and respiratory function and can be given orally or parenterally.[21] Because its potency is two to four times that of midazolam, the dose must be adjusted accordingly. Because of the long half-life of lorazepam and despite the fact that its time of onset of action is considerably longer than that of midazolam, the use of lorazepam is preferred to midazolam for patients requiring long-term sedation.[6] Because of different volumes of distribution, elimination half-lives, and so on, especially in patients with multiple organ dysfunction syndrome and in critically ill patients who require benzodiazepines for longer than 24 hours, lorazepam has a clinical half-life similar to that of midazolam.[22]

Diazepam, the most well-known benzodiazepine, can be given orally or intravenously. It is considered to be a long-acting benzodiazepine because of its prolonged elimination half-life (up to 50 hours, with active metabolites that also have hypnotic effects). After an intravenous bolus is administered, diazepam is rapidly redistributed in body tissues; therefore, its initial sedative effect quickly diminishes. However, drug clearance becomes dependent on hepatic metabolism when tissues are saturated during prolonged use. This saturation causes a prolongation of clinical effect even in patients with normal liver function. Because diazepam is not water soluble and because its diluent is ethyl alcohol, propylene glycol, and sodium benzoate, with a pH of 6.6, it is irritating to veins and frequently causes pain on administration. The usual dose of diazepam is 2 to 5 mg given by slow intravenous injection every 1 to 4 hours and is titrated to achieve the desired effect. Very high doses may be required in some patients, especially those with a history of ethanol abuse.

If a benzodiazepine is used to manage the sedation of patients in the ICU, the benzodiazepine antagonist, flumazenil, should be readily available.[23] Flumazenil is a highly specific benzodiazepine antagonist that reverses all known central nervous system effects of the benzodiazepines. It reaches maximum concentration in the brain within 5 to 10 minutes after intravenous administration. The mean terminal half-life of flumazenil is approximately 1 hour. It is completely metabolized to free carboxylic acid and glucuronide, both of which are inactive metabolites and renally excreted.

Propofol

Propofol, an intravenously administered alkyl-phenol anesthetic agent that is chemically unrelated to other anesthetic agents, has been used to provide sedation for patients in ICUs and is the preferred drug for "fast-tracking" patients. Because it is so hydrophobic, it is formulated in a lipid emulsion (10% Intralipid), which must be taken into account when it is administered to patients. It is short-acting and rapidly redistributed and metabolized, making it suitable for use as a continuous infusion. Because it allows for a rapid recovery and has a favorable side-effect profile, propofol often is used not only to sedate patients but also for use in certain procedures such as cardioversions, chest tube insertions or withdrawal, and pleurodesis (see Chapter 9).

Compared with midazolam, propofol allows for more rapid weaning of patients from mechanical ventilation; because of this property, propofol is used more commonly for fast-tracking patients after cardiac operations.[24] When used for sedation, propofol should be administered as an initial dose of 0.5 to 1.0 mg/kg followed by an infusion of approximately 25 to 100 μg/kg/min. Because case reports have recounted mortality in patients who received excessively high doses of propofol, the maximum dose should probably be less than 100 μg/kg/min.[23,25] Propofol infusion syndrome has been reported to occur in patients who have received propofol for a very short period, indicating that this may be an idiosyncratic reaction.[26]

When given by bolus administration, propofol may cause a decrease in mean arterial pressure because of peripheral vasodilation, not direct myocardial depression. Reports have been published of death with the use of propofol in both adults and children.[27] The U.S. Food and Drug Administration requires the following boxed warning on product labeling for propofol, "While causality has not been established, Diprivan injectable emulsion is not indicated for sedation in pediatric patients until further studies have been performed to document its safety in that population."

Myoclonic activity versus frank seizures has been reported to occur in patients receiving propofol,[28] and individuals have become chemically dependent on propofol. These side effects, however, are rare (with the exception of the hypotension after bolus infusion) and should not limit the use of propofol in patients after cardiac surgical procedures, particularly given the effectiveness of propofol in fast-tracked patients. Studies have specifically addressed the issue of sedation in patients after cardiac operations; most of the studies compared midazolam with propofol and, in general, showed no specific advantage of one agent over another.[29,30]

Dexmedetomidine

Significant interest has been shown in using the α_2-receptor agonist dexmedetomidine for postoperative cardiac sedation. α_2-Receptor agonists bind to noradrenergic receptors in the brain, spinal cord, and elsewhere in the body. The benefit with the use of these agents is that sedation is provided with supplemental analgesic effects without respiratory depression. Dexmedetomidine was compared with benzodiazepines for the sedation of all groups of critically ill patients in four separate randomized, controlled trials.[9,31-33] The findings of the Safety and Efficacy of Dexmedetomidine Compared with Midazolam (SEDCOM) study group[9] revealed that dexmedetomidine-treated patients experienced less time on mechanical ventilation, less tachycardia, and less hypertension, with the most common adverse effect being bradycardia. The Maximizing Efficacy of Targeted Sedation and Reducing Neurological Dysfunction (MENDS) group showed similar findings, with a longer duration of delirium for those treated with lorazepam, as compared with patients treated with dexmedetomidine.[33]

The results of trials specific to patients after cardiac surgery have not been as strong. Dexmedetomidine was used in a fast-track setting without a shorter duration on the ventilator, compared with opioids, at a $50-per-patient greater cost.[31] The dexmedetomidine-treated group did have a lower incidence of postoperative delirium and reduction in opioid requirements.[31] Herr et al[32] conducted a multicenter trial comparing dexmedetomidine and propofol for sedation after coronary artery bypass grafting. They found no significant difference between groups in time to extubation, but the dexmedetomidine-treated patients required significantly fewer supplemental analgesics, antiemetics, epinephrine, and diuretics. In a more recent multicenter study of 356 patients in the ICU, the overall costs associated with the use of dexmedetomidine, compared with midazolam, were lower because the dexmedetomidine-treated patients had a shorter LOS in the ICU.[34] After examining the literature applying to all critical care patients, not only those after cardiac operations, the committee that developed the SCCM sedation guidelines made multiple recommendations (Table 37-2; these recommendations predate the introduction of dexmedetomidine).[7]

TABLE 37-2	Society for Critical Care Medicine Sedation Guidelines

1. Midazolam or diazepam should be used for rapid sedation of acutely agitated patients.
2. Propofol is the preferred sedative agent when rapid awakening is important. Triglyceride concentrations should be monitored after 2 days of propofol infusion, and total caloric intake from lipids should be included in the nutrition assessment.
3. Midazolam is recommended for short-term use only because it produces unpredictable awakening and time to extubation when infusions continue longer than 48 to 72 hours.
4. Lorazepam is recommended for the sedation of most patients via either intermittent intravenous administration or continuous infusion.
5. Dexmedetomidine can be used for chemically dependent patients and for patients who have failed any of the above. If dexmedetomidine is used for longer than 48 hours, the infusion should be discontinued with caution because a withdrawal-hypertensive crisis could occur.

Neuromuscular Blocking Agents

Occasionally, some patients are so critically ill that they cannot be adequately sedated to receive appropriate care. This most commonly happens in an agitated patient requiring mechanical ventilation in whom the level of sedation would mimic a general anesthetic and whose hemodynamic status does not tolerate this degree of deep sedation. In these circumstances, neuromuscular blocking agents (NMBAs) are used.

An NMBA binds the nicotinic acetylcholine receptor on the muscle membrane, thus preventing the receptor from binding two molecules of acetylcholine, which open the sodium channel, allowing the influx of sodium and other electrolytes, with activation of actin and myosin and muscle contraction. NMBAs in current use fall into one of two categories: depolarizing or nondepolarizing agents. Succinylcholine is a classic depolarizing NMBA, which structurally resembles acetylcholine and, when it binds to the nicotinic acetylcholine receptor, results in depolarization of the membrane and a muscle fasciculation. Depolarizing NMBAs rarely are used outside the operating room except for rapid-intubation protocols in the emergency department and ICU, and by emergency response teams.

Nondepolarizing NMBAs are divided into two classes: benzylisoquinolinium compounds and the aminosteroid compounds. Both classes of drugs can be used to chemically paralyze a patient in the ICU, which occasionally is required to intubate the trachea of a patient with acute respiratory failure.[35] Patients in the ICU who are receiving NMBAs must be mechanically ventilated; they typically have acute lung injury or acute respiratory distress syndrome that requires mechanical ventilation but that cannot be appropriately managed without the use of an NMBA.[36]

If NMBAs are used, it cannot be overemphasized that the patient must be adequately sedated before the initiation of the NMBA—it has been several decades since reports first appeared of chemically paralyzed awake patients,[37] but it is a situation that all individuals working in an ICU must strive to avoid. Once an adequate degree of sedation (usually to include an analgesic medication such as an opioid) is achieved, the patient is administered a bolus and then a continuous infusion of an NMBA. Although several NMBAs are available, the drugs most commonly used in the ICU are the aminosteroid compounds (e.g., rocuronium) and the benzylisoquinolinium compounds (e.g., cisatracurium). Because these drugs are infused continuously, the duration of action is not as important as if they were given as a single bolus, but duration of action does become of consequence when the medication is discontinued and the physician is assessing the return of the patient's neuromuscular function. When infusing these medications, a twitch monitor should be used, and the physician should strive to achieve a train-of-4 of one or two twitches.[38] If no twitches are observed, the patient may have received an overdose of medication and may be at risk for development of acute quadriplegic myopathy syndrome (AQMS), a situation that develops in patients receiving NMBAs in which, when the medication is discontinued, the patient remains flaccid for much longer than would be predicted simply based on the pharmacokinetics of the medications that were infused.[39] The cause of this syndrome is unknown but is most likely secondary to the destruction of myosin by the NMBA or one of its metabolites. Differentiating between AQMS and critical illness polyneuropathy often is difficult, but in the latter, profound muscle necrosis—as is seen with AQMS—would not be expected to occur. Bolus administration of NMBAs, when tolerated, is advantageous for monitoring the effects of sedation and analgesia, as well as decreasing the incidence of tachyphylaxis.[38]

Another way to minimize the incidence of AQMS is to institute a daily drug holiday. Not only is this beneficial in decreasing the incidence of AQMS, but in patients receiving opioids and benzodiazepines, the incidence of drug withdrawal also decreases. When using NMBAs in the ICU, following the algorithm listed in Figure 37-1 is recommended.[38]

INFECTIONS IN PATIENTS IN THE INTENSIVE CARE UNIT

Microbiologic infections are some of the most common and frequently serious secondary complications that plague patients in the ICU.[40] The following is a brief review of the most frequent infectious complications occurring in critically ill patients after cardiothoracic operations (Box 37-2). Pneumonia and acute respiratory distress syndrome are reviewed in Chapter 35.

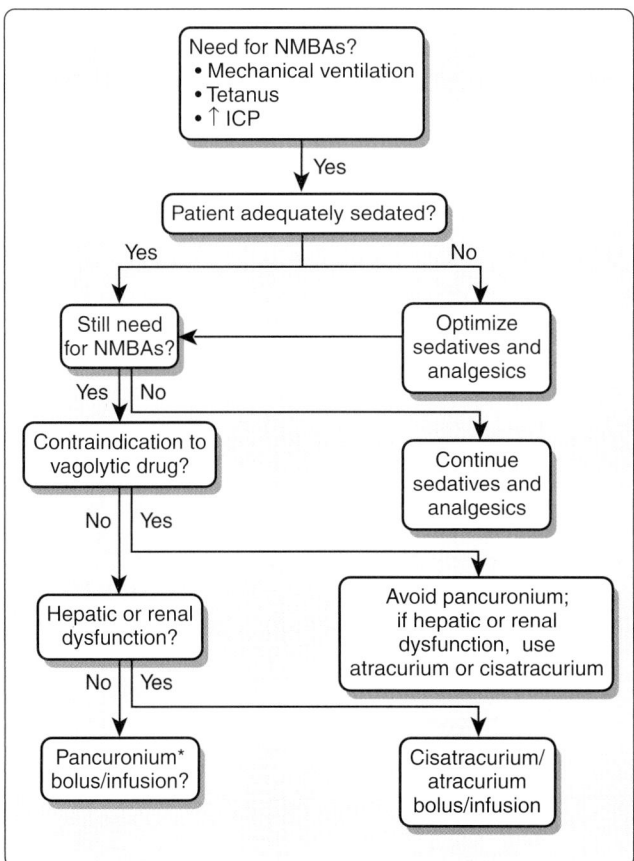

Figure 37-1   Use of neuromuscular blocking agents (NMBAs) in the intensive care unit. Monitor train-of-4 ratio, protect the patient's eyes, position the patient to protect pressure points, and address deep venous thrombosis prophylaxis. Reassess every 12 to 24 hours for continued NMBA indication. ICP, intracranial pressure. *(Redrawn from Murray MJ, Cowen J, DeBlock H, et al: Clinical practice guidelines for sustained neuromuscular blockade in the adult critically ill patient.* **Crit Care Med** *30:142, 2002.)*

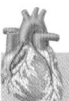

BOX 37-2. LATENT SOURCES OF INFECTION IN THE CARDIOTHORACIC INTENSIVE CARE UNIT

- Intravascular device-related bloodstream infections
- Sternal wound infections
- Prosthetic valve endocarditis
- Sepsis
- Urinary tract infection
- *Clostridium difficile* enterocolitis
- Sinusitis

Intravascular Device–Related Infections

Virtually all adult patients having cardiac operations are monitored with invasive intravascular devices (IVDs), such as arterial, central venous, and pulmonary artery catheters (see Chapter 14). Unfortunately, patients who have IVDs in place frequently acquire bloodstream infections (BSIs). IVD-related BSIs are associated with an attributable mortality rate of 12% to 15%, prolonged hospitalization (mean of 7 days), and an increased hospital cost of approximately $35,000.[41,42]

Approximately 90% of all IVD-related BSIs occur with the short-term use of IVDs.[43] IVDs that are present for a short period are most commonly colonized from the skin surrounding the insertion site.[44,45] Organisms migrate along the external surface of the catheter and then the intercutaneous and subcutaneous segments, leading to colonization of the intravascular segment of the catheter.[46,47] Once the catheter is colonized, it is difficult to eradicate organisms from the intravascular segment without catheter removal because the microbes adhere to and are covered by either a biofilm layer that they produce or the thrombin layer that the host forms on the device.[48] Because the skin is the most common site of colonization, coagulase-negative staphylococci and *Staphylococcus aureus* from the host's skin and the hands of hospital personnel caring for the patient are the most common infecting pathogens.[49] However, with the long-term use of IVDs, contamination of the catheter hub also contributes to intraluminal colonization.[46,47]

Several factors have been associated with an increased risk for patients acquiring IVD-related bacteremia. These factors include site of insertion (femoral > internal jugular > subclavian), number of lumens (multiple > single), duration of catheter in situ, established infection elsewhere in the body, the presence of bacteremia, and the experience of the personnel placing the catheter. Although some practitioners support the use of peripherally inserted IVDs, the risk for patients acquiring BSIs approaches that of patients with short centrally placed catheters.[50] In an effort to reduce the incidence of IVD-related BSIs, a Centers for Disease Control and Prevention advisory committee formulated pertinent evidence-based guidelines[51]:

- IVDs should be placed by designated individuals with documented competence in insertion. Personnel who are learning techniques to obtain central vascular access should be adequately supervised.
- When inserting catheters, maximal sterile barrier precautions (gowns, sterile gloves, mask, maximal draping) should be used.
- Two percent chlorhexidine is the agent of choice to prevent bacterial colonization of catheters and BSI. (The use of alcohol tinctures of iodine, 10% povidone-iodine combination, and alcohol alone are acceptable but should be given secondary consideration).
- Chlorhexidine-impregnated sponge dressings are associated with a 60% reduction in IVD-related BSIs.
- The use of sulfadiazine- and chlorhexidine- or minocycline-rifampin–impregnated catheters is associated with a reduction in BSI in patients with IVDs that are used for a short period. There is no evidence of an increase in bacterial resistance in studies to date. Guidelines recommend using these catheters in high-risk patients if institutional IVD-related BSI rates are unacceptable after other prevention strategies have been instituted.
- CVCs should not be routinely changed to prevent infection.

- Gauze dressings should be changed every 2 days and transparent dressings every 7 days. Dressings should be replaced sooner if they become soiled or contaminated, or a site inspection is required.
- No advice is provided regarding the use of sutureless securement devices.
- Catheters do not need to be replaced in bacteremic or febrile patients if the catheter is not suspected to be the source of infection.
- If there is evidence of an exit-site infection or if the patient is bacteremic with a suspected IVD-related BSI, the catheter should be removed and placed at a new site. Changing catheters over a wire is not recommended.

These guidelines are summarized in Box 37-3.

The diagnosis of IVD-related BSI can be challenging. The diagnosis should be suspected in patients with evidence of infection (e.g., fever, leukocytosis, positive blood cultures) when another source is not evident. Careful inspection of the catheter site is warranted; the presence of exit-site erythema or purulence strongly supports the diagnosis. If the patient has no visible signs of infection, clinical suspicion and supporting data must be used to guide therapy. The most frequently used technique to culture IVDs is the semiquantitative roll-plate technique. With this technique, the most common threshold to define colonization is growth of at least 15 colony-forming units (cfu).[48,52] Siegman-Igra and colleagues[49] and others[53,54] have shown that quantitative culture of sonicated catheters is superior to the roll-plate technique. However, because these techniques require catheter removal, paired concomitant qualitative blood cultures are drawn through the device and percutaneously. IVD-related BSI is diagnosed if both cultures are positive for the presence of microorganisms and the concentration of microorganisms from the device is twofold to fivefold greater than the concentration from the peripherally drawn culture.[55]

The first clinical decision to make when managing a suspected IVD-related BSI is to remove the catheter or leave it in place. This decision is influenced by whether the risk for IVD-related BSI is low, intermediate, or high. Risk, in turn, is determined by the infecting organism and whether the IVD-related BSI is complicated or uncomplicated. Complicated infections are those associated with shock; the persistence of positive blood cultures for longer than 48 hours after appropriate antibiotics are administered; and IVD-related BSIs associated with septic thrombosis, septic emboli, or deep-seated infections (e.g., endocarditis or a tunnel or port-pocket infection[46,47]; Figure 37-2). A low-risk IVD-related BSI is caused by organisms of low virulence (e.g., coagulase-negative staphylococci) in a patient without complications of infection. A moderate-risk IVD-related BSI is characterized by uncomplicated infections with moderate to highly virulent organisms (*S. aureus*, *Candida* species). A high-risk IVD-related BSI is a complicated IVD-related BSI.

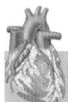

BOX 37-3. CENTRAL VENOUS CATHETER MANAGEMENT

- Central venous catheters should be placed only by practitioners with documented competency.
- Catheters should be placed under maximal sterile-barrier precautions.
  - Preferably, the skin should be prepared with 2% chlorhexidine.
  - Chlorhexidine-impregnated sponge dressings should be used.
  - Antibiotic-impregnated catheters should be used in high-risk patients.
- Catheters should not be "routinely" replaced.
- Catheters should be removed as soon as clinically feasible.

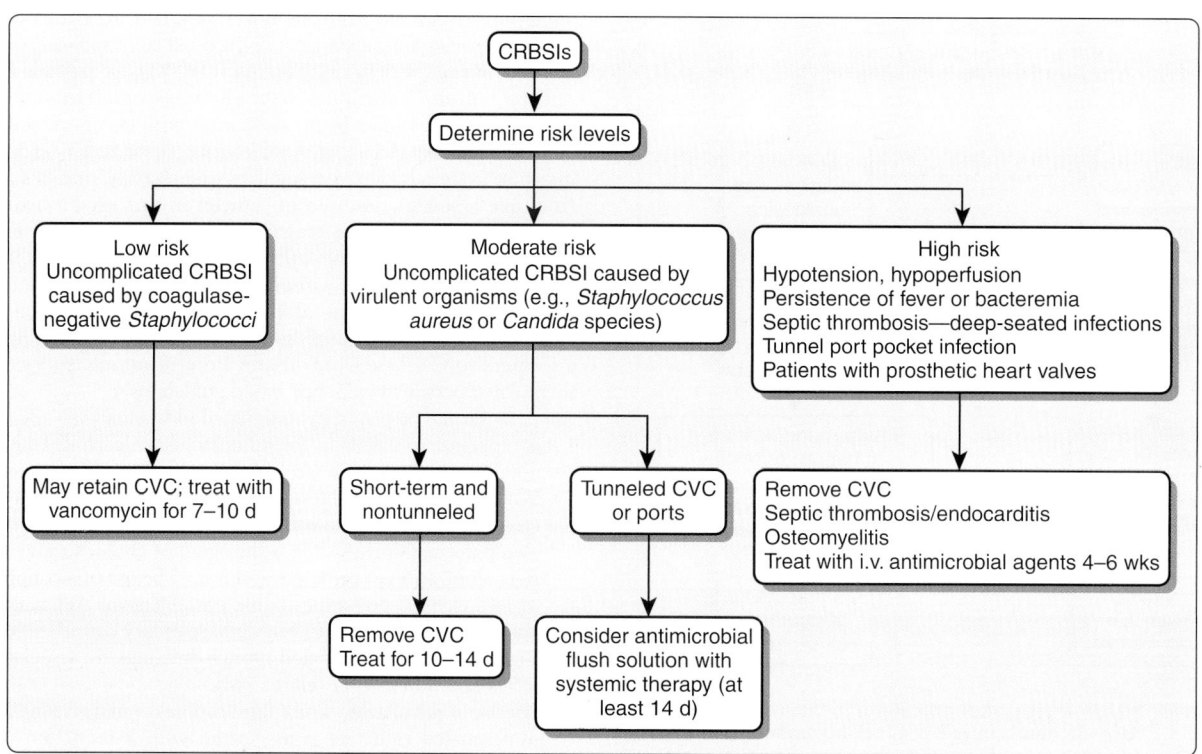

Figure 37-2 **Algorithm for the management of intravascular catheter-related bloodstream infections (CRBSIs).** A prelude to appropriate management involves confirming the diagnosis of a CRBSI through simultaneous blood cultures (5:1 of colony-forming units from blood cultures drawn through the catheter compared with the peripheral vein or differential time to positivity of 2 hours) or colonization of the catheter demonstrated through semiquantitative or quantitative catheter cultures with the same organism isolated from the peripheral blood culture. CVC, central venous catheter; i.v., intravenous. (*Redrawn from Raad II, Hanna HA: Intravascular catheter-related infections. New horizons and recent advances.* Arch Intern Med *162:871, 2002, by permission of the American Medical Association.*)

Low-risk IVD-related BSIs can be treated without catheter removal.[46,47] However, catheters should be removed in low-risk patients with prosthetic heart valves. In intermediate-risk patients, the catheters should be removed and the patients treated with a 10- to 14-day course of antibiotics. In high-risk patients, catheters should be removed and the duration of antibiotic use should be based on the nature of the complication. In deep-seated infections, such as septic thrombosis or endocarditis, antimicrobials should be administered for 4 to 6 weeks.[56]

Sternal Wound Infections

Deep and superficial surgical site infections occur infrequently but are morbid complications after cardiac operations, with an incidence rate of approximately 1% to 4%.[57] Deep sternal infections are defined as those infections involving muscle and fascial layers, any other organ spaces manipulated during the operation, or organ involvement.[58] They are associated with a 250% greater mortality rate, as compared with matched individuals without infection, and postoperative wound infections double the length of hospitalization.[59] A host of preoperative, intraoperative, and postoperative risk factors have been identified for chest wall infections (Table 37-3).[57-63]

The diagnosis of sternal infections is based on the presence of wound tenderness, drainage, cellulitis, fever, leukocytosis, and sternal instability.[60] S. aureus and coagulase-negative staphylococci account for approximately 50% of the organisms causing sternal wound infections after coronary artery bypass graft procedures.[58] Several preventive strategies have been proposed to reduce the rates of surgical-site infection after cardiac operations. Martorell et al[64] reported a reduction in the incidence rate of chest wall infections from greater than 8% to less than 2% after an intensive surveillance and intervention program that included the nasal application of mupirocin and having the patient shower before surgery with chlorhexidine. Other variables that are being investigated to reduce infection rates include perioperative antibiotic timing and redosing, adequacy of glycemic control, perioperative temperature control, and conservative transfusion protocols.[65] The treatment of mediastinitis involves the prompt institution of antibiotics (empirically covering staphylococci species before obtaining culture results), debridement, open packing, and frequent dressing changes. On resolution, the chest is closed by primary closure or flap transposition in patients with large chest wall defects.[60]

Prosthetic Valve Endocarditis

Prosthetic valve endocarditis (PVE)—the infection of a prosthetic heart valve, the surrounding cardiac tissues, or both the valve and surrounding tissue—is a rare but serious source of infection in patients after cardiac surgery.[65] The incidence rate of PVE is between 0.3% and 0.8% after valve-replacement operations.[66-70] S. aureus is the most common organism related to PVE; timing of infection can be helpful to illustrate the pathophysiology and causative pathogen. PVE cases can be clustered into two groups according to the time of infection. In early PVE (within 2 months of valve implantation), the valve and sewing ring have not yet endothelialized; hence microorganisms

frequently invade the surrounding tissue planes, causing perivalvular abscess and perivalvular leak. In early PVE, the responsible microorganisms are nosocomial pathogens, such as staphylococci, gram-negative bacilli, and Candida species, which are introduced at the time of the operation or are hematogenously seeded in the immediate postoperative period. The pathophysiology of late PVE probably resembles that of native valve endocarditis; that is, platelet-fibrin thrombi form on the valve leaflet and are then hematogenously seeded during episodes of transient bacteremia. In late PVE, the infecting organisms are usually streptococci, S. aureus, enterococci, and fastidious gram-negative organisms (the HACEK group).[71-75] Infection appears to occur with equal frequency in both the mitral and aortic valves and is exceedingly rare in tricuspid prostheses (excluding intravenous drug abusers).[67]

In the ICU, cases of early PVE present more dramatically than do either native-valve endocarditis or late PVE. The clinical signs that suggest PVE include new or changing murmurs, congestive heart failure, new electrocardiographic conduction disturbances, and the presence of systemic emboli. In fact, 40% of patients have clinically apparent central nervous system emboli.[76-79] The diagnosis is confirmed by positive results of blood cultures and findings on transesophageal echocardiography (TEE). If blood cultures are obtained before institution of antibiotic therapy, more than 90% of culture results will be positive. Transesophageal echocardiography is the diagnostic imaging modality of choice because it has a sensitivity of 82% to 96%, as compared with 17% to 36% with transthoracic echocardiography.[80,81] Transesophageal echocardiography also allows the detection of abscesses, fistulas, and perivalvular leaks.[82] The treatment of early PVE involves the administration of antibiotics directed at the cultured organism and prompt surgical intervention in cases of complicated PVE (Table 37-4).[83] Mortality is related to older age, S. aureus infection, and patients with persistent bacteremia with the occurrence of septic shock.[84,85] In complicated PVE, survival is improved with the institution of both medical and surgical therapy versus medical therapy alone.[77,86,87]

Systemic Inflammatory Response Syndrome and Sepsis

Systemic inflammatory response syndrome (SIRS) and sepsis are part of a spectrum of disorders that produce dysfunction in a variety of organ systems and arise from a combination of tissue injury and the host's response to that injury. In 1992,[88] 1997,[89] and 2001,[90] the American College of Chest Physicians, the SCCM, the European Society of Intensive Care Medicine, the American Thoracic Society, and the Surgical Infection Society published consensus statements to clarify the definitions used to describe this spectrum. In 1991, the consensus statement introduced the now widely used term SIRS to describe a syndrome with multiple, clinically evident, organ-system effects (e.g., fever, oliguria, mental-status changes) that occurred as the result of the body's inflammatory response activated by a variety of causes.[88] Historically, it had been thought that infection, particularly gram-negative infection, was the sole source of this clinical phenomenon.[91,92] It is now accepted that any major tissue injury (burns, sterile pancreatitis, major trauma) can precipitate such a dramatic inflammatory response with or without the presence of infection.[91,92] However, in the most recent consensus statement, the authors acknowledge that,

TABLE 37-3	Risk Factors for Chest Wall Infections		
Host Factors	**Surgical Factors**	**Postoperative Factors**	
Obesity, diabetes mellitus, hyperglycemia, use of internal mammary artery grafts (especially bilateral), advanced age, male sex, COPD, smoking, prolonged mechanical ventilation, steroids, preoperative hospital stay longer than 5 days	Duration of surgery and bypass, use of IABP balloon pump, postoperative bleeding, reoperation, sternal rewiring, extensive electrocautery, shaving with razors, and use of bone wax	Postoperative bleeding, prolonged ventilation, chest re-exploration, blood transfusion, and use of an IABP	

COPD, chronic obstructive pulmonary disease; IABP, intra-aortic balloon pump.

TABLE 37-4	Indications for Surgical Intervention in Patients with Prosthetic Valve Endocarditis
Valvular regurgitation with or without heart failure	
Uncontrollable infection* caused by:	
Periannular extension	
Difficult-to-treat microorganisms	
Abscess	
Large vegetation with high risk for embolization or recurrent emboli	

*Uncontrollable infection includes persistent fever and positive results of blood culture.

although SIRS exists, it is too broad and lacks the specificity to make it a useful, working "diagnosis" at this time.[90]

Sepsis is defined as the clinical syndrome that occurs as the result of an infection (or suspected infection) and an inflammatory response (Table 37-5).[90,92] Severe sepsis is associated with organ dysfunction, hypoperfusion, or hypotension. Septic shock includes sepsis-induced hypotension and organ-perfusion abnormalities that persist despite fluid resuscitation.[88] A detailed description of the current understanding of the pathophysiology of SIRS and sepsis is beyond the scope of this chapter; see Chapter 8 and reviews of this topic[93–97] for more detailed discussions.

Sepsis is the leading reason for admission to surgical ICUs and, despite recent advances in therapy, remains the leading cause of mortality in ICUs.[88,92,96] The mortality rate increases across the inflammatory spectrum from SIRS to septic shock.[40,98,99] Because of the unacceptably high mortality rate associated with sepsis and the inflammatory disorders, an international group of experts in sepsis convened in 2003 and launched the "surviving sepsis campaign" with the goal of producing treatment recommendations that could be used to reduce the mortality from sepsis.[99–101] These recommendations (summarized in Table 37-6) were formulated from an evidence-based review of the medical literature

TABLE 37-5	Diagnostic Criteria for Sepsis in Adults

Documented or suspected infection plus some of the following:[a]

General variables
 Fever[b]
 Hypothermia[c]
 Tachycardia[d]
 Tachypnea
 Altered mental status
 Significant edema or positive fluid balance[e]
 Hyperglycemia in the absence of diabetes[f]

Inflammatory variables
 Leukocytosis[g]
 Leukopenia[h]
 Normal WBC count with > 10% immature forms
 Increased plasma C-reactive protein concentration[i]
 Increased plasma procalcitonin concentration[i]

Hemodynamic variables
 Arterial hypotension[j]
 Svo_2 > 70%
 Cardiac index > 3.5 L/min/m2

Organ-dysfunction variables
 Arterial hypoxemia[k]
 Acute oliguria[l]
 Creatinine concentration increase > 0.5 mg/dL
 Coagulation abnormalities[m]
 Ileus
 Thrombocytopenia[n]
 Hyperbilirubinemia[o]

Tissue-perfusion variables
 Hyperlactatemia[p]
 Decreased capillary refill or mottling

[a]Defined as a pathologic process induced by a microorganism.
[b]Defined as core temperature > 38.3° C.
[c]Defined as core temperature < 36° C.
[d]Defined as > 90 beats/min or > 2 standard deviations (SDs) above the normal value for age.
[e]Defined as > 20 mL/kg over 24 hours.
[f]Defined as a plasma glucose concentration > 120 mg/dL or 7.7 mmol/L.
[g]Defined as a white blood cell (WBC) count > 12,000/μL.
[h]Defined as a WBC count < 4000/μL.
[i]Defined as > 2 SDs above the normal value.
[j]Defined as a systolic blood pressure (SBP) < 90 mm Hg, mean arterial pressure < 70, or a decrease in SBP > 40 mm Hg in adults or < 2 SDs below normal for age.
[k]Defined as a Pa_{O_2}/Fi_{O_2} < 300.
[l]Defined as urine output < 0.5 mL/kg/hr.
[m]Defined as an international normalized ratio (INR) > 1.5 or activated partial thromboplastin time (aPTT) > 60 seconds.
[n]Defined as platelet count < 100,000/μL.
[o]Defined as plasma total bilirubin concentration > 4 mg/dL or 70 mmol/L.
[p]Defined as > 1 mmol/L.
Modified from Levy MM, Fink MP, Marshall JC, et al: 2001 SCCM/ESICM/ACCP/ATS/SIS International Sepsis Definitions Conference. *Crit Care Med* 31:1250, 2001.

and expert opinion when high-level evidence was absent. They reflect the "state of the art" in the management of critically ill patients with sepsis in 2008 (when the recommendations were last revised). Adoption of the recommendations set forth in these guidelines is associated with improved outcome.[102]

Urinary Tract Infection

Urinary tract infections (UTIs) are the most common hospital-acquired infections[103] and are thought to represent 25% to 50% of ICU-acquired infections.[104] Traditionally, hospital-acquired UTIs have been defined as the presence of more than 10^5 cfu/mL urine in patients during bladder catheterization. In the early 1980s, Platt et al[105] showed that hospitalized patients meeting this definition of nosocomial UTI had a 2.8-fold increase in mortality. However, more data suggest that many of these cases may represent asymptomatic bacteriuria rather than invasive infection and perhaps do not merit treatment.[104] Stark and Maki[106] have demonstrated that, in catheterized patients, colonic bacteria rapidly proliferate in the urinary system and exceed 10^5 cfu/mL. In fact, up to 30% of catheterized hospitalized patients have more than 10^5 cfu/mL urine.[107] In addition, pyuria is not helpful in differentiating between infection and colonization because most catheter-associated bacteriuria has accompanying pyuria.[108] The rate of UTI-associated bacteremia is quite low (Box 37-4). A large Canadian case series demonstrated a UTI rate in an ICU of 9%, with only a 0.4% incidence rate of bacteremic UTI.[103]

Bladder irrigation with antibiotic solutions does not reduce the likelihood of patients acquiring catheter-related UTI,[109] nor does the prophylactic use of systemic antibiotics.[110] The use of antimicrobial agent–impregnated urinary catheters does appear to reduce infection rates.

In light of the clinical uncertainty in the diagnosis of nosocomial, catheter-related UTI, patients with asymptomatic catheter-related bacteriuria should not be treated. However, symptomatic patients or patients with signs of infection and urine cultures demonstrating more than 10^5 cfu/mL and no other obvious source of infection merit 10 to 14 days of antimicrobial treatment.

Clostridium difficile Enterocolitis

The anaerobic, gram-positive rod *Clostridium difficile* was first described in 1935 by Hall and O'Toole.[111] It was not until 1978, however, that its two toxigenic exotoxins (toxins A and B) were identified to be the cause of antibiotic-associated pseudomembranous enterocolitis.[112,113] Although *C. difficile* is part of the normal fecal flora in 50% of newborns, it is not found in adults until the normal microbial barrier is altered by antibiotic therapy.[111,112] *C. difficile* colonization occurs via the fecal-oral route and can follow exposure to any antibiotic. It is unclear why only a small percentage of patients exposed to a given antibiotic become colonized, nor is it clear why only some of those colonized develop symptomatic infection.[112,114] There is some speculation that antibody titers to the toxins may play a role.[115,116]

C. difficile diarrhea is the most common enteric infection in hospitalized patients, infecting approximately 10% of individuals who are hospitalized for longer than 2 days.[117] The organism enters the hospital environment via asymptomatic carriers and is then transmitted from patient to patient primarily via contact from hospital personnel. The risk factors that predispose a patient to development of *C. difficile* colonization include the severity of illness at admission, multiple antibiotic exposures, gastrointestinal operations, enteral feeding, an infected roommate, and the use of proton-pump inhibitors.[117–119] Once the patient's gut is colonized, clinical infection occurs after the secretion and adherence of toxin to receptors on the host's colonocyte brush border. The bound toxins cause necrosis of the epithelial cells, an intense inflammatory response, and exudative secretion into the bowel lumen. This cellular response is visible on endoscopy as "volcano" or "summit" lesions and pseudomembranes.[120] Hospital and unit epidemics of *C. difficile* are common, are often attributable to a single strain (despite multiple strains being present in the environment), and are associated with the use of clindamycin.[121,122]

TABLE 37-6	Recommendations from the Surviving Sepsis Campaign

1. Initial Resuscitation—first 6 hours

   Resuscitation should begin as soon as possible—do not delay for ICU admission.

   The goals of resuscitation include:

   CVP: 8–12 mm Hg (12–15 mm Hg in mechanically ventilated patients or if high abdominal pressure)

   MAP: > 65 mm Hg

   Urine output: > 0.5 mL/kg/hr

   Svo_2 or $Scvo_2$ > 70%

   If unable to increase Svo_2 or $Scvo_2$ > 70% with ventilation, transfuse to hematocrit > 30%, administer dobutamine (to a maximum dose of 20 µg/kg/min), or both transfuse and administer dobutamine.

2. Diagnosis

   Always obtain appropriate cultures before initiating antibiotics.

   Obtain at least two blood cultures—one from peripheral and one from each vascular access device.

   Culture other sites[a] as clinically indicated.

   Promptly perform diagnostic and imaging studies to identify the source of infection.

3. Antibiotic Therapy

   IV antibiotic therapy should be started within the first hour of recognition of severe sepsis.[b]

   Empiric antibiotics should include one with activity against the most likely pathogen and that can penetrate the likely source.

   Empiric antibiotics should be broad spectrum until the causative organism is identified.

   The antibiotic regimen should be reassessed after 48 to 72 hours on the basis of clinical and microbiologic data. The goal is to use a narrow-spectrum antibiotic to limit toxicity, cost, and development of superinfection and microbial resistance.

   Once the causative organism is identified, use monotherapy for 7–10 days.[c]

   Most experts use combination therapy for neutropenic patients and treat for the duration of neutropenia

4. Source Control

   Every patient should be evaluated for the presence of a focus of infection that is amenable to source-control measures.[d]

   Risks vs. benefits of source-control procedures must be weighed; source control with the least physiologic insult generally is best.

   Source-control measures should be instituted as soon as possible after initial resuscitation.

5. Fluid Therapy

   Fluid challenge with crystalloids or colloids in cases of suspected hypovolemia

   Repeat boluses based on response[f] and tolerance[g]

   No evidence to support preference of crystalloid or colloid

6. Inotropic Therapy

   In patients with low CO despite fluid resuscitation, dobutamine is the agent of choice to increase CO.

   A vasopressor can be added to increase BP, once CO is normalized.

7. Steroids

   IV corticosteroids[h] can be used for patients with septic shock who require vasopressor therapy despite adequate fluid resuscitation.

   Some experts recommend using a 250-µg ACTH stimulation test to identify responders[i] and only treat nonresponders.

   Dose should not exceed 300 mg hydrocortisone daily.

   Some experts add 50 µg fludrocortisone orally.[j]

   No evidence to recommend fixed-duration therapy over taper or clinically guided regimen.

8. rhAPCl

   The use of rhAPC is recommended in patients with high risk for death and who do not have any contraindications.

   Contraindications to the use of rhAPC:

   Active internal bleeding

   Recent, within 3 months, hemorrhagic stroke

   Recent, within 2 months, intracranial or intraspinal surgery or severe head trauma

   Trauma with increased risk for life-threatening bleeding

   Presence of epidural catheter

   Intracranial neoplasm, mass lesion, or cerebral herniation

9. Blood Product Administration

   Once tissue hypoperfusion has resolved, pRBC transfusion should only occur when hemoglobin decreases to < 7.0 g/dL and target a hemoglobin of 7.0–9.0 g/dL.

   Erythropoietin is not recommended to treat anemia of sepsis.[m]

   FFP should not be administered to correct laboratory abnormalities in the absence of bleeding or planned invasive procedures.

   Antithrombin administration is not recommended to treat severe sepsis or septic shock.

   Platelet transfusion

   Administer if counts < 5000/mm^3

   Consider when counts 5000–30,000/mm^3 and the patient has a significant risk for bleeding.

   Counts > 50,000/mm^3 are typically required for surgery or invasive procedures.

10. Mechanical Ventilation of SI-ALI/ARDS

    Use low V_T (6 mL/kg) with goal of plateau pressure less than 30 cm H_2O.

    Permissive hypercapnia is tolerated to minimize plateau pressures and V_T.

    A minimum amount of PEEP should be set to minimize lung collapse at end expiration.

    Prone positioning may be considered in patients requiring potentially injurious levels of plateau pressure or Fio_2 who are not at high risk for development of adverse consequences of prone positioning.

    Unless contraindicated, mechanically ventilated patients should be maintained with the head of the bed raised to 30 degrees to prevent the development of ventilator-associated pneumonia.

    A weaning protocol should be in place.

    When stable, patients should undergo daily, spontaneous-breathing trials with a T-piece or 5 cm H_2O CPAP.

    If spontaneous breathing trials are successful, consideration should be given to extubation.

TABLE 37-6	Recommendations from the Surviving Sepsis Campaign—Cont'd

11. Sedation, Analgesia, and Neuromuscular Blockade

    Sedation protocols should be used that include the use of a sedation goal, measured by a standardized subjective sedation scale.

    Use either continuous infusion or intermittent bolus to achieve predetermined end points.

    Sedation should be interrupted or lightened daily to evaluate patients.

    NMBAs should be avoided, if possible; when NMBAs are used, train-of-4 monitoring of depth of blockade should be used.

12. Glucose Control

    Maintain blood glucose levels < 150 mg/dL with the use of insulin infusion.

    Monitor blood glucose every 30 minutes initially and then regularly (every 4 hours) once glucose concentration has stabilized.

    Glycemic control should include the use of a nutrition protocol that favors enteral feeding.

13. Renal Replacement

    In ARF, continuous venovenous hemofiltration and intermittent hemodialysis are equivalent.

    Venovenous hemofiltration may be tolerated better in hemodynamically unstable patients.

    There is no evidence to support hemofiltration in sepsis independent of renal replacement needs.

14. Bicarbonate Therapy

    No evidence supports the use of bicarbonate therapy for the treatment of hypoperfusion-induced lactic acidemia.

15. DVT Prophylaxis

    Patients with severe sepsis should receive DVT prophylaxis with low-dose unfractionated heparin or LMWH.

    Mechanical prophylaxis should be used in patients with contraindications to the use of heparin.

    In extremely high-risk patients—i.e., with a history of DVT—a combination of pharmacologic and mechanical therapy is recommended.

16. Stress Ulcer Prophylaxis

    All patients with sepsis should receive stress-ulcer prophylaxis.

    H_2-receptor antagonists are more efficacious than sucralfate.

    No studies have directly compared the use of proton-pump inhibitors with H_2-receptor antagonists, so their efficacy is unknown.

17. Consideration of Limitation of Support

    Advance-care planning, including the communication of likely outcomes and realistic treatment goals, should be discussed with patients and their families.

    Less aggressive therapy and withdrawal of therapy may be in the patient's best interest.

ACTH, adrenocorticotropic hormone; ARF, acute renal failure; BP, blood pressure; CO cardiac output; CPAP, continuous positive airway pressure; CVP, central venous pressure; DVT, deep vein thrombosis; FFP, fresh frozen plasma; IV, intravenously administered; LMWH, low-molecular-weight heparin; NMBA, neuromuscular blocking agents; PEEP, positive end-expiratory pressure; pRBC, packed red blood cells; rhAPC, recombinant human activated protein C; Scvo2, central venous oxygen saturation; SI-ALI, sepsis-induced acute lung injury; Svo2, mixed venous oxygen saturation; VT, tidal volume.

[a]Cerebrospinal fluid, wounds, urine, respiratory secretions, other body fluids.

[b]After cultures are obtained.

[c]Some experts prefer combination therapy for *Pseudomonas* infections.

[d]For example, drainage of abscess, removal of infected vascular access device.

[e]For example, percutaneous rather than surgical abscess drainage.

[f]Increased blood pressure (BP) and urine output.

[g]Evidence of intravascular volume overload.

[h]Hydrocortisone, 200 to 300 mg/day for 7 days in 3 or 4 divided doses or by continuous infusion.

[i]More than 9-μg/dL increase in cortisol after 30 to 60 minutes.

[j]Controversial because hydrocortisone has mineralocorticoid activity.

[k]APACHE II score > 25, sepsis-induced multiple organ dysfunction syndrome (MODS), septic shock, or sepsis-induced acute respiratory distress syndrome (ARDS).

[l]Because support for this recommendation was based on a single randomized trial, practitioners must truly weigh the risk-to-benefit ratio before initiating therapy until other trials confirm the results.

[m]May use if other coexisting conditions merit treatment with erythropoietin, (e.g., renal failure).

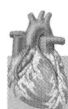

BOX 37-4. NOSOCOMIAL URINARY TRACT INFECTION

- Traditional diagnostic criteria are misleading because they are common in hospitalized patients with bladder catheters.*
- UTIs should be treated only when signs of a UTI are present, and the patient has signs or symptoms of infection and *no other obvious source of infection.*
- UTIs should be treated with 10 to 14 days of culture-directed antimicrobial therapy.

*Traditional diagnostic criteria for urinary tract infection (UTI) include the presence of pyuria and > 10^5 cfu/mL urine.

C. difficile diarrhea produces a spectrum of clinical disease. After the administration of antibiotics, the typical presentation includes low-grade fever, leukocytosis, frequent watery bowel movements (10 to 15 per day), and abdominal pain. However, at its most severe, the disease results in fulminant illness with "toxic megacolon."[122] It is important to note that the majority of antibiotic-associated diarrhea results from an osmotic diarrhea and not from *C. difficile* infection. In osmotic diarrhea, antibiotics inhibit the intestinal flora from metabolizing carbohydrates, which results in increased intraluminal osmotic pressure, the transloca-tion of water into the bowel lumen, and diarrhea.[123] The diagnosis of *C. difficile* infection is suggested by the presence of fecal leukocytes (not present in osmotic diarrhea), systemic toxicity (fever, leukocytosis), and the persistence of diarrhea despite the discontinuation of enteral feeding (which will decrease the carbohydrate source in osmotic diar-rhea). The diagnosis is confirmed by bioassay of *C. difficile* cytotoxins.[124] Endoscopy is reserved for use in suspected cases of *C. difficile* in which diagnosis is not confirmed by toxin assay or when a diagnosis must be made before assay results are available. In these instances, colonoscopy is superior to sigmoidoscopy (lesions are often proximal in the colon), and the presence of pseudomembranes in a patient with antibiotic-associated diarrhea is pathognomonic of *C. difficile* diarrhea.[125,126]

C. difficile diarrhea is treated with oral metronidazole (500 mg, 3 times daily) or oral vancomycin (125 mg, 4 times daily) for 10 to 14 days. Metronidazole is considered to be the first choice because it and vancomycin have a similar efficacy but metronidazole is less expensive.[127] However, oral vancomycin has been shown to be supe-rior to metronidazole for severe *C. difficile* when patients are stratified by severity of illness.[128] In severely ill patients, oral vancomycin (up to 500 mg, 4 times daily) is supplemented with intravenously administered metronidazole.[129] Relapse occurs in 10% to 25% of patients, is not from antibiotic resistance (not described to date), and should be treated by repeating the same therapy for another 10 to 14 days. Increases in the incidence and severity of *C. difficile* prompted investigators across the United States to identify a virulent strain of infection, which appears to be related to the use of cephalosporin and fluoroquinolone antibiotics.[130] The strain is known as BI/NAP1/027, which is restriction endonuclease analysis group BI, pulse-field gel electrophoresis type NAP1, and polymerase chain reaction ribotype 027. Although this strain has not shown resistance to metronidazole, the use of oral vancomycin is recommended because of the hypervirulence of this strain.[130]

When caring for patients with *C. difficile* infection, health care workers always should wear gloves because none of the antiseptic agents is reliably sporicidal against *C. difficile*. After removing the gloves, health care workers should wash with nonantimicrobial or antimicrobial soap.

Sinusitis

Sinusitis is a frequent and clinically silent source of infection in intubated patients.[104] The presence of nasogastric tubes predisposes patients to developing ethmoid and maxillary sinusitis. Sinusitis is also particularly common after nasal intubation, with an incidence rate of up to 85% after 1 week of intubation.[104,131-134] The diagnosis is suggested by the presence of air-fluid levels or total opacification of the sinuses on computed tomography scan.[134] However, opacification of the sinuses is common after intubation. In one series, 96% of nasotracheally intubated and 23% of orotracheally intubated patients with previously clear sinuses had new sinus opacification after 1 week of intubation.[134] The diagnosis can be confirmed by the presence of pus and high quantitative cultures that can be obtained via either transnasal puncture of the maxillary sinus or open ethmoidectomy or sphenoidectomy.[104,133] Case series have reported a resolution of fever and leukocytosis after the treatment of sinusitis.[133,134] Treatment consists of removal of all nasal tubes, drainage of the maxillary sinuses, and the use of broad-spectrum antibiotics.

▨ Hematology

Transfusion

Blood products frequently are transfused into critically ill patients. In a general ICU population, patients receive an average of 0.2 unit blood products per day; this incidence increases to 1.3 units per day in cardiothoracic ICUs.[135,136] Although transfusion of blood products is often necessary to either improve oxygen delivery or restore the coagulation system (Box 37-5), a growing body of literature suggests that transfusion carries substantial risk for patients after cardiac operations.

Several large studies have identified the use of transfusion as increasing patients' risk for development of infection after cardiac operations. A review of 19 retrospective studies found that, in 17 studies, transfusion was found to be a significant factor related to postoperative infection and was frequently the best predictor of postoperative infection.[135,137] Transfusion has been cited as a risk factor for development of mediastinitis,[58] early bacteremia,[138] and pneumonia,[139] as well as for increased mortality rate and increased LOS after cardiac operations.[140]

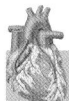

BOX 37-5. TRANSFUSION STRATEGY IN THE CARDIOTHORACIC INTENSIVE CARE UNIT

- For patients who are not actively bleeding (e.g., chest tube drainage < 100 mL/hr), decisions to transfuse pRBCs should be guided by laboratory data: maintain Hgb concentration ≥ 7 g/dL
- For patients who are actively bleeding

Transfuse	If
• Platelets	• Platelet count ≤ 100,000
• FFP	• INR ≥ 1.5
• Cryoprecipitate	• Fibrinogen ≤ 200 mg/dL

ICU, intensive care unit; pRBCs, packed red blood cells; Hgb, hemoglobin; FFP, fresh frozen plasma; INR, international normalized ratio.

In 2001, Leal-Noval et al[135] published a large cohort study that identified transfusion as a risk factor for severe postoperative infections. In their series of 738 cardiac surgical patients at a large Spanish teaching hospital, a transfusion of more than 4 units blood components was associated with a statistically significant increased risk for pneumonia, mediastinitis, mortality, and longer ICU LOS (Figure 37-3).[135]

In 2007, Murphy et al[141] published the results of a review of the cardiac surgical databases in the United Kingdom, finding that those patients who had received transfusions of packed red blood cells (pRBCs) had a greater incidence of infection and increased rates of ischemic postoperative morbidity. Two articles published in *Critical Care Medicine* had similar conclusions. An observational cohort study of 11,963 patients at the Cleveland Clinic found that perioperative transfusion of pRBCs was the single factor most reliably associated with morbidity in patients who had undergone isolated coronary artery bypass grafting.[142] Marik and Corwan,[143] after systematically reviewing the literature, came to a similar conclusion—in patients in the ICU, pRBC transfusions are associated with increased rates of not only morbidity but also mortality. As transfusion practices continue to be evaluated, additional data suggest that allogeneic and not autologous blood is associated with the twofold increased risk for hospital infection, signifying an immunologic relation[144] (see Chapters 30 and 31).

In 1999, Hebert et al[145] published a landmark study that has fundamentally altered the approach to transfusion in critically ill patients. This large, multicenter, randomized, prospective trial of 838 patients admitted to Canadian ICUs found no difference in 30-day mortality between patients assigned to a liberal (hemoglobin, 10–12 g/dL) and conservative pRBC transfusion protocol (hemoglobin, 7–9 g/dL). Mortality was lower in less ill patients (APACHE II [Acute Physiology and Chronic Health Evaluation II] score ≤ 20) and in younger patients (< 55 years of age). Also, the restrictive strategy resulted in a 54% reduction in pRBC transfusions. Before this study, pRBC transfusion

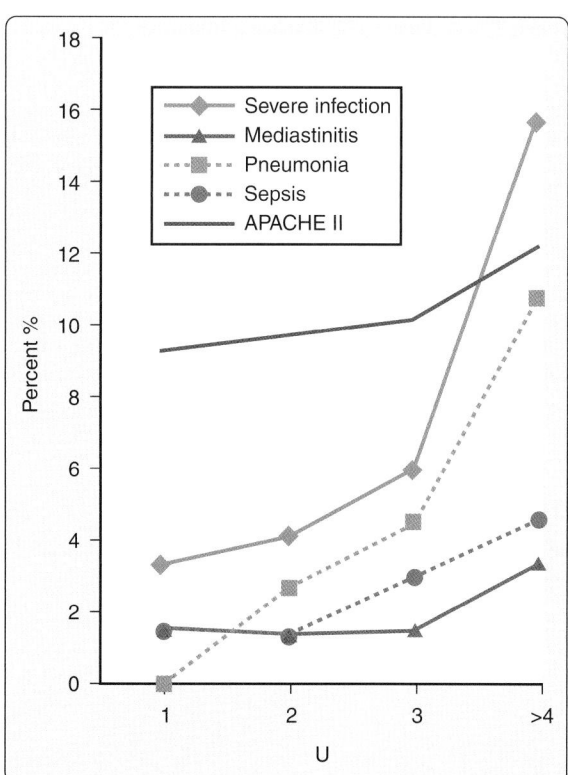

Figure 37-3 **Relation between the units of blood transfused and the percentage of infections.** *(Redrawn from Leal-Noval SR, Rincon-Ferrari MD, Carcia-Curiel A, et al: Transfusion of blood components and postoperative infection in patients undergoing cardiac surgery.* Chest *119:1461, 2001.)*

had been extensively investigated as a component of the now-dated paradigm that supranormal oxygen delivery was associated with increased survival in critically ill patients.[135] Hebert et al's study[145] showed that a conservative strategy was associated with no increase in mortality and halved the number of transfused units, with attendant decreases in infectious risk, immunomodulation, and cost associated with the lower transfusion rate. Two similar small trials in patients after cardiac operations showed no difference in outcome between conservative and liberal transfusion strategies.[146,147]

These data, combined with evidence supporting the use of early "goal-directed" therapy in sepsis, are what led to the transfusion recommendations cited in the Surviving Sepsis Campaign Guidelines.[101,148,149] Although no consensus guidelines exist for transfusion practices after cardiac operations, an extrapolation of these recommendations for patients who have had cardiac surgical procedures seems prudent. That is, in the initial 24 to 48 hours of "resuscitation," a more liberal transfusion strategy targeting oxygen delivery (with objective end points, e.g., lactate levels, mixed venous oxygen saturation) and resolution of coagulopathy or bleeding seems appropriate. Once stabilized, patients in the cardiothoracic ICU long term should probably be subjected to a conservative (hemoglobin, 7–9 g/dL) transfusion strategy. A multi-center retrospective review of patients after myocardial infarction suggested that a more liberal goal of transfusing to achieve a hemoglobin concentration of 10 g/dL is associated with increased mortality rates.[150] Although not directly applicable to a cardiothoracic ICU setting, the results of this study do suggest that improving oxygen delivery in patients with coronary artery disease by transfusing pRBCs to a hemoglobin of 10g/dL is not the panacea clinicians once thought.

ACUTE RENAL FAILURE

Acute renal failure (ARF), like many of the clinical syndromes frequently encountered in the ICU, has been difficult to precisely define.[151] If it is agreed that the principal functions of the kidney are to create urine and excrete water-soluble waste products of metabolism, then ARF is the sudden loss of these functions.[151]

Renal solute excretion is a function of glomerular filtration. The glomerular filtration rate (GFR) is a convenient and time-honored way of quantifying renal function. It must be appreciated, however, that GFR varies considerably under normal circumstances as a function of protein intake.[152] A normal GFR is 120 ± 25 mL/min for men and 95 ± 20 mL/min for women. Serum creatinine concentration is the most frequently used surrogate of GFR and, hence, solute excretion. When measured in the *steady state* and analyzed in the context of age, sex, and race, the GFR loosely reflects renal function. In fact, when baseline serum creatinine is unknown, standardized tables allow the estimation of baseline creatinine that can then be compared with actual serum creatinine levels to estimate decremental changes in renal function (Table 37-7).[152]

The use of creatinine concentration is much less accurate in estimating renal function in non–steady-state conditions (e.g., ARF in the critically ill). Creatinine is formed from nonenzymatic dehydration of creatine (98% muscular in origin) in the liver. Because critical illness affects liver function, muscle mass, tubular excretion of creatinine, and the volume of distribution of creatinine, its limitations as a useful marker of renal function become apparent.[152] Nonetheless, changes in serum creatinine concentration and the rate of change in creatinine concentration remain the most convenient and frequently used surrogates of renal dysfunction.

Urine output is the other frequently measured parameter of renal function in the ICU. Oliguria is defined by a urine output of less than 0.5 mL/kg/hr.[152] Under a wide range of normal physiologic conditions, urine output primarily reflects changes in renal hemodynamics and volume status rather than representing renal parenchymal function and reserve. Hence, it is very nonspecific for renal dysfunction unless urine output is severely reduced or absent.[152] And although oliguric renal failure has a greater mortality rate than does nonoliguric renal failure, no data demonstrate that the pharmacologic creation of urine in patients with renal failure reduces mortality.[153]

The incidence of ARF after cardiovascular operations is high and is associated with a "formidable" mortality rate.[154] A cohort study from Duke University described a 0.7% incidence rate of dialysis-dependent ARF that was associated with an increase in mortality rate from 1.8% to 28%.[155] Another cohort described an incidence rate of dialysis-dependent ARF of 1.1% after cardiac surgery that was associated with a mortality rate of 63.7%.[154] In critically ill patients (noncardiac), the mortality rate for ARF is 50% to 80% and has not declined significantly since the advent of acute dialysis therapy.[153]

The pathogenesis of ARF after cardiac operations is thought to primarily result from hypoperfusion and ischemia.[155] Other contributing factors include exposure to nephrotoxins, nonpulsatile flow during cardiopulmonary bypass, and aortic emboli. The two most important determinants of ARF after cardiopulmonary bypass are preexisting renal insufficiency and postoperative low-cardiac-output states.[156,157]

The Acute Dialysis Quality Initiative Workgroup formulated a classification system for ARF in 2004 to develop consensus-based recommendations.[158] Termed the *RIFLE criteria* (risk, injury, failure, loss, and end-stage renal disease; Table 37-8), stratification from risk for development of acute renal dysfunction to end-stage renal disease is based on GFR and urine output. Since the RIFLE criteria were instituted, three studies[159–161] have been conducted in the cardiac surgical population that confirmed that the development of renal injury is an independent risk factor for 90-day mortality.[152]

TABLE 37-8	RIFLE Criteria for Categorizing Acute Renal Dysfunction	
Category	*P_{cr} and GFR Criteria*	*UO Criteria*
Risk	↑ $P_{cr} \times 1.5$ or GFR ↓ > 25%	< 0.5 mL·kg⁻¹·hr⁻¹ for 6 hours
Injury	↑ $P_{cr} \times 2$ or GFR ↓ > 50%	< 0.5 mL·kg⁻¹·hr⁻¹ for 12 hours
Failure	↑ $P_{cr} \times 3$, or serum creatinine ≥ 4 mg/100 mL with an acute rise > 0.5 mg/dL, or GFR ↓ > 75%	< 0.3 mL·kg⁻¹·hr⁻¹ for 24 hours or anuria for 12 hours
Loss	Persistent ARF = complete loss of kidney function > 4 weeks	
ESRD	ESRD < 3 months	

For conversion of creatinine expressed in conventional units to ST units, multiply by 88.4. Renal function is categorized based on serum creatinine concentration (P_{cr}) or urinary output (UO), or both, and the criteria that led to the worst classification are used. Glomerular filtration rate (GFR) criteria are calculated as an increase of P_{cr} above the baseline P_{cr}. When the baseline P_{cr} is unknown and the patient has no history of chronic renal disease, P_{cr} is calculated using the Modification of Diet in Renal Disease formula (GFR = 170 × [P_{cr} {mg/dL}]⁻⁰·⁹⁹⁹ × [Age]⁻⁰·¹⁷⁶ × [0.762 if patient is female] [1.180 if patient is black] × [serum urea nitrogen concentration {mg/dL}]⁻⁰·¹⁷⁰ × [serum albumin concentration {g/dL}]⁺⁰·³¹⁸). Acute kidney injury should be considered when kidney dysfunction is abrupt (within 1–7 days) and sustained (> 24 hours).
ARF, acute renal failure; ESRD; end-stage renal disease.

TABLE 37-7	Estimated Baseline Creatinine Concentration				
	Men			**Women**	
Age, yr	*African American*	*White*		*African American*	*White*
20–24	1.5 (133)	1.3 (115)		1.2 (106)	1.0 (88)
25–29	1.5 (133)	1.2 (106)		1.1 (97)	1.0 (88)
30–39	1.4 (124)	1.2 (106)		1.1 (97)	0.9 (80)
40–54	1.3 (115)	1.1 (97)		1.0 (88)	0.9 (80)
55–65	1.3 (115)	1.1 (97)		1.0 (88)	0.8 (71)
> 65	1.2 (106)	1.0 (88)		0.9 (80)	0.8 (71)

Data are presented as mg/dL (μmol/L). Estimated glomerular filtration rate: GFR (mL/min/1.73 m²) = 175 × (Scr) − 1.154 × (Age) −0.203 × (0.742 if female) × (1.212 if African American) (conventional units). The equation does not require weight because the results are reported normalized to 1.73 m² body surface area, which is an accepted average adult surface area.

Several strategies for preventing perioperative renal failure have been evaluated in patients who have undergone cardiac operations. "Renal-dose" dopamine has been shown to have no effect on either renal function or mortality after both cardiac and vascular operations.[162–164] Similarly, the use of the diuretics furosemide and mannitol has demonstrated no renal-protective effect. In fact, a small study demonstrated a significantly worse renal outcome in patients prophylactically treated with furosemide infusion versus control subjects.[163] Results with pulsatile perfusion during cardiopulmonary bypass have been similarly disappointing.[151]

The recombinant brain atrial natriuretic peptide nesiritide has demonstrated some initial promise in treating perioperative renal failure in patients after cardiac operations. In a randomized, prospective, double-blinded trial in two cardiothoracic ICUs in Sweden, patients with an increase in serum creatinine concentration more than 50% above baseline had improved renal excretion, a decreased need for hemodialysis, and improved survival after treatment with brain atrial natriuretic peptide, compared with control subjects.[165] Nesiritide works via a cyclic guanosine monophosphate–coupled receptor (NPR-A) in vascular smooth muscle cells. Physiologically, it produces arterial and venous vasodilation and inhibition of aldosterone production and increases urine volume and sodium excretion.[166] Further trials are under way to more clearly define this agent's role in cardiac surgical patients (see Chapters 10 and 34).

Treatment and Renal Replacement Therapies

Just as the diagnosis and prevention of ARF remain enigmatic, so, too, does the treatment of ARF. In the critically ill patient who experiences development of ARF, the initial treatment strategy is to create an optimal "environment" for the kidney to heal; that is, to maximize oxygen delivery to the renal parenchyma via the manipulation of hemodynamics and volume status while simultaneously avoiding exposure to nephrotoxins (e.g., contrast agents, aminoglycosides) and ensuring that no postrenal obstruction exists. The administration of furosemide in this setting, long advocated to maintain urine output, has not been associated with an improvement in outcome but has been associated with an increase in oxygen consumption in the renal cortex,[167] which may be deleterious in patients with decreased renal perfusion pressure.

If optimization is provided and the kidney does not recover, the clinician must provide renal replacement therapy (RRT). Many of the classic indications for RRT are noncontroversial (Table 37-9).[168] In the absence of these indications, the decision to initiate RRT in critically ill patients is a matter of clinical judgment. Typical laboratory parameters that suggest the need for RRT include a blood urea nitrogen concentration greater than 100 mg/dL or a creatinine concentration greater than 4.5 mg/dL.[164]

Once the decision to initiate RRT has been made, the mode of replacement must be chosen. In broad terms, RRT can be divided into

TABLE 37-9	Indications for Renal Replacement Therapy

- Uremic symptoms
  - Anorexia
  - Nausea
  - Vomiting
- Uremic signs
  - Uremic pericarditis
  - Bleeding
  - Encephalopathy
- Hyperkalemia refractory to medical therapy
- Volume overload unresponsive to restriction and diuretics
- Metabolic acidosis
- Dialyzable intoxications
  - Lithium
  - Toxic alcohols
  - Salicylate
- Some cases of hypocalcemia, hypercalcemia, or hyperphosphatemia

TABLE 37-10	Criteria for Weaning of Continuous Renal Replacement Therapy

- Criteria to initiate RRT have resolved
- Urine output averages 1 mL/kg/hr over 24 hours
- Fluid balance can be maintained with present urine output
- Complications of continuous RRT outweigh benefits

RRT, renal replacement therapy.

intermittent hemodialysis or continuous RRT. The latter comes in a wide variety of forms, each associated with its own unique acronym (e.g., slow continuous ultrafiltration [SCUF], slow low-efficiency daily dialysis [SLEDD], continuous venovenous hemofiltration [CVVH], continuous venovenous hemofiltration-dialysis [CVVH-D]). The differences between these different forms of continuous RRT lie in the membrane used, the mechanism of solute transport, the presence or absence of a dialysis solution, and the type of vascular access.[164,168,169] In the United States, most patients with ARF are treated with hemodialysis, but the trend is toward the increased use of continuous RRT, whereas in other countries, continuous RRT predominates.[164,170–172] Currently, no studies support the use of one modality over another, but most intensivists prefer using continuous RRT in hemodynamically unstable patients or in patients in whom the hypotension associated with hemodialysis may lead to adverse effects.[164,168] A trial of weaning of continuous RRT should be considered when established criteria have been met (Table 37-10).[168]

NUTRITION SUPPORT

Patients who are anticipated to have an extended stay in the ICU (longer than 2 to 3 days) will require nutrition assessment, and patients who are malnourished or who will remain non per os (NPO) without parenteral nutrition should be examined and assessment made whether they should receive enteral or parenteral nutrition support. In the 1970s, several articles in the nutrition literature concluded that anywhere from 40% to 70% of patients in the hospital, and by extension in the ICU, were malnourished.[173] Three decades of providing aggressive intervention have not yet changed that assessment. Because of chronic illness and the sequelae of acute illness, many patients remain cachectic and hypermetabolic, and though aggressive nutrition support may not completely reverse the sequelae of malnutrition in these patients, the lack of support will likely make the malnutrition worse.[174,175]

The stress response that many, if not all, critically ill patients have is responsible for this ongoing altered metabolic state. With any form of injury or acute illness, a number of hormones and cytokines that affect metabolism, including catecholamines, glucagons, tumor necrosis factor, and so on are released. These hormones create a state in which metabolic rate is increased, protein synthetic rate is decreased, and glycolysis and lipolysis are increased. Patients who remain NPO and have an ongoing critical illness—such that the stress response does not abate as it normally would after a surgical procedure—require a nutrition assessment; after the assessment, a decision must be made whether the patient should be fed and by what means.

Nutrition Assessment

The nutrition assessment of any patient in the ICU begins by obtaining a history of the patient's eating habits, weight loss or gain, medication use, alcohol use, and symptoms that would be compatible with a nutrient or vitamin deficiency. A history of an unplanned weight loss of 10% in the preceding 6 months places patients at increased risk for development of perioperative complications, and such patients should receive further evaluation, additional tests, and perhaps earlier intervention from a nutrition standpoint. Patients who have increased alcohol intake (i.e., two or more drinks per day for a man and one or more drinks for a woman), alcoholics, and patients with malabsorption are at risk for having a nutrient deficiency and for the sequelae associated with the deficiency. In addition, while making the initial nutrition assessment, the clinician should assess the integrity of the patient's gastrointestinal tract to determine whether the patient might be a candidate for enteral feeding if nutrition support is indicated or, if not, should identify potential intravenous access sites.

A thorough physical examination should include an assessment of the patient's general appearance and overall condition, a brief neurologic examination specifically looking at ability to swallow and protect the airway, muscle stores (in the temporal fossa), fat stores (usually in the triceps area), and evidence of jaundice, glossitis, edema, and cheilosis. A subjective global assessment of the patient's overall nutrition status has been validated and is becoming the gold standard by which patients' nutrition status is assessed.[176]

For the final part of the nutrition assessment, laboratory tests should be conducted. Many nutritionists rely on measurement of serum albumin concentration, but because of the long half-life of serum albumin, others prefer measurement of serum prealbumin concentrations. Concentrations of the plasma proteins often will be decreased, but they do serve as a marker for adequacy of anabolism that can be measured at baseline and weekly thereafter to assess the efficacy of nutrition interventions. Other laboratory tests that should be assessed on a regular basis include acid-base status; electrolyte concentrations, to include phosphorus, magnesium, and calcium; and measures of renal and liver function. Finally, all patients in the ICU who are receiving nutrition support should have a serum glucose concentration measured on a regular basis.

Every attempt should be made to keep the serum glucose concentration less than 150 to 180 mg/dL, with minimum variability in glucose concentrations ensured.[177] One study found that patients with a mean absolute change in glucose concentration of more than 15.8 mg/dL/hr had a greater mortality rate than did a group with a change of less than 7.1 mg/dL/hr.[178] Caloric support should not be decreased merely to meet this goal, but any patient receiving nutrition intervention should have blood glucose monitored.

Measuring resting energy expenditure is a test that is used for the extremely obese patient and the profoundly anorexic patient to help guide support. Otherwise, using a simple measure, such as a Harris-Benedict equation, allows the calculation of an estimation of the number of calories patients require.

$$\text{For men}: RMR = 66.4 + (13.8 \times W) + (5 \times H) + (6.8 \times A)$$

$$\text{For women}: RMR = 655(9.6 \times W) + (1.8 \times H) + (4.7 \times A)$$

where RMR is the resting metabolic rate, W is weight (kg), H is height (cm), and A is age (years). However, in reality, most intensivists use a simple goal of providing 1 kcal/kg/hr.

After the initial nutrition assessment, the patient is classified as having mild, moderate, or severe malnutrition. Patients who are moderately to severely malnourished should have more attention paid to their nutrition support. If the patient is anticipated to remain NPO for several days, many intensivists and nutrition-support personnel would implement nutrition support early in the hospital course, within the first 1 to 3 days. The data for this recommendation are lacking, except in trauma patients in whom there are studies that justify early nutrition support.[179] As long as there are no side effects, there should be no danger to early intervention using a tube placed through the pylorus to aliment the patient.

Depending on the institution, enteral feeding tubes are placed fluoroscopically by a radiologist, endoscopically by a gastroenterologist, or at the bedside by an intensivist using several different techniques and approaches. There are several complications from enteral nutrition, including, among others, placement of the feeding tube past the tracheal tube and into the trachea and the feeding tube remaining in the stomach and not passing through the pylorus. Bloating is one of the more frequent side effects of enteral nutrition; significant ileus with gastric residual volumes increases the risk for aspiration of gastric contents. In addition, distention of the large or small intestine can increase intra-abdominal pressure, displacing the diaphragm in a cephalad direction and interfering with weaning from mechanical ventilation if the patient is mechanically ventilated. Another frequent side effect of enteral nutrition is diarrhea, which can be secondary to bacterial overgrowth, the osmolality of the nutrition formula, or the administration through the enteral feeding tube of medications containing sorbitol or glycerol or be caused by *C. difficile* infection.

Although enteral nutrition is preferred and has been reported to decrease the incidence of infectious complications in some patient populations, occasionally, some patients cannot be fed enterally and must be fed parenterally. If the parenteral route is chosen, placement of the central venous access line using a sterile technique is critical.[51] Furthermore, keeping blood glucose levels at or less than 150 to 180 mg/dL decreases the incidence of IVD-related BSI and pneumonia.[180]

Formulas

Enteral formulas, which can be provided via tube feeding or orally, are listed in Tables 37-11 and 37-12.

TABLE 37-11	Nutrient Analysis of Tube-Feeding Formulas[a]												
Product	Kcal/mL	Volume[b]	H_2O, mL	Osmolality, mOsm	Protein, g (%)	Fat, g (%)	CHO, g (%)	Fiber, g	Na, mEq	K, mEq	Ca, mg	Phos, mg	Mg, mg	Comments
Jevity														
1.0	1.06	1321	829	300	44.3 (16.7)	34.7 (29)	154.7 (54.3)	14.4	40.4	40.2	910	760	305	Isotonic, with fiber
1.5	1.5	1000	760	525	63.8 (17)	49.8 (29.4)	215.7 (53.6)	22	60.9	47.4	1200	1200	400	Calorically dense, with fiber
Nepro	1.8	948	725	600	81 (18)	96 (48)	166.8 (34)	15.6	346.1	27.2	1060	700	210	Low electrolyte for renal failure
NutriHep	1.5	100	760	790	40 (11)	21.2 (12)	290 (77)	0	7	33.8	956	1000	376	High BCAA for hepatic encephalopathy
Osmolite	1.2	1000	820	360	55 (18.5)	39.3 (29)	157.5 (52.5)	0	58.3	46.4	1200	1200	400	Calorically dense
Peptamen	1	1500	850	270	40 (16)	39 (33)	127 (51)	0	24.3	28.5	800	700	300	Elemental
TwoCal HN	2	948	701	725	83.5 (16.7)	90.5 (40.1)	218.5 (43.2)	5	63	62.6	1050	1050	425	Calorically dense, high protein

[a]Nutrients per 1000 mL.
[b]Volume required to achieve 100% minimum recommended dietary intake.
BCAA, branched-chain amino acids; CHO, carbohydrate.

TABLE 37-12	Nutrient Analysis of Oral Supplements[a]										
Product	kcal	Pro, g	Fat, g	CHO, g	Fiber	Na, mEq	K, mEq	Ca, mg	Phos, mg	Mg, mg	Flavors
Boost[c]	240	10	4	0	41	5.7					Strawberry, vanilla, chocolate
CIB[b] (mg)	160	4.5	1	28	0–1	4.3	8.9	300	250	105	Strawberry, vanilla, chocolate
CIB[b], sugar free (mg)	70	4.5	1	12	0–1	4	8.9	300	250	80	Strawberry, vanilla, chocolate
Enlive[c]	250	10	0	65	0	1.96	1.2	50	280	14	Apple, mixed berry
Ensure Plus[c]	355	13	11.4	50.1	0	10.4	11.3	200	200	100	Strawberry, vanilla, chocolate
Glucerna Shake[c]	220	10	8.5	29	3	210	9.5	250	250	100	Strawberry, vanilla, chocolate, butter pecan
Nepro[c]	425	19.1	22.7	39.4	3.7	10.9	6.4	250	165	50	Vanilla, butter pecan, mixed berry
Resource Breeze[c]	250	9	0	54	0	3.5	0.3	10	150	1	Orange, peach, wild berry
TwoCal HN[c]	475	19.9	21.5	51.8	1–2	15	14.8	250	250	100	Vanilla, butter pecan

[a]Nutrients per serving
[b]A serving equals 1 package.
[c]A serving equals 8 oz.
CHO, Carbohydrate; CIB, Carnation Instant Breakfast; Pro, protein.

Protein

Most authorities currently recommend 1.0 to 1.5 g protein/kg/day based on the patient's average weight, including the admission weight, current weight, and ideal body weight. Unless the patient has renal insufficiency and is not on dialysis or unless the patient has hepatic encephalopathy that responds to administration of branched-chain amino acids, there are no unique protein formulas that should be used to feed enterally or parenterally.

Lipids and Carbohydrates

Most of a patient's energy needs should be met with a combination of carbohydrate (glucose) and lipids (lipid emulsion). The amount of glucose that a critically ill patient can oxidize is limited to 6 g glucose/kg/day or 4 mg/kg/min. Patients who receive more glucose than this are at increased risk for development of complications such as hyperglycemia, diuresis, increased carbon-dioxide production (which, in some circumstances, may keep the patient mechanically ventilated), and a fatty liver.

Lipids are the other mainstay for supplying calories to a critically ill patient. They are not adequately oxidized if more than 1.0 to 1.5 g lipid emulsion/kg/day is administered to the patient. When lipids are used as part of a parenteral nutrition regimen, serum triglyceride concentrations should be checked on a regular basis to ensure that the patient does not experience development of hypertriglyceridemia, with its attendant side effects and toxicity.

Electrolytes

Electrolyte abnormalities are common in patients in the ICU. For patients fed parenterally who have renal failure, formulas are available that have low levels of potassium and phosphate, among others. In patients receiving parenteral nutrition, it is relatively easy to manipulate the concentration of deficient or excessive electrolytes in the total parenteral nutrition formula.

Vitamins

Most enteral products contain 100% of the recommended daily dose of nutrients, but some patients may require supplementation of vitamins.

Patients who are alcoholic should receive supplemental thiamin; patients with short-bowel syndrome who are deficient in fat-soluble vitamins may benefit from the administration of these vitamins; and unless patients are on anticoagulants, they need to be supplemented with vitamin K. Fluid balance in patients fed enterally and parenterally also must be monitored, and, occasionally, formulas for both enteral and parenteral nutrition may need to be changed to accommodate fluid excess or dehydration.

Several formulas have been recommended for delivery to critically ill patients, including formulas that contain glutamine, arginine, essential γ-3 fatty acids, nucleotides, and structured lipids. The SCCM-American Society for Parenteral and Enteral Nutrition guidelines for support in critically ill patients gave a Grade A recommendation to administering an enteral formulation with anti-inflammatory properties (fish and borage oils and antioxidants) to patients with acute lung injury and acute respiratory distress syndrome.[181] Yet within a year of this publication, the EDEN-Omega Study (early vs. delayed enteral feeding and omega-3 fatty acid/antioxidant supplementation for treating people with acute lung injury and acute respiratory distress syndrome) was terminated early because of futility.[182]

Electrolyte Abnormalities

Fluid and electrolyte abnormalities occur often after cardiac operations. Diagnosis and treatment algorithms are shown in Figures 37-4 and 37-5 for hypernatremia and hyponatremia, Figure 37-6 and Table 37-13 for hyperkalemia, and Figure 37-7 for hypokalemia. Symptoms of hypercalcemia (serum Ca^{2+} > 13.0 mEq) include anorexia, nausea, vomiting, lethargy, dehydration, coma, and death. The treatment of hypercalcemia is listed in Table 37-14. Hypomagnesemia is common, and the underlying cause should be identified, if possible, and then treated with an intravenous infusion of 0.1 to 0.2 mEq/kg/day or orally at 0.4 mEq/kg/day. Close monitoring is necessary with the treatment of any electrolyte disorder.

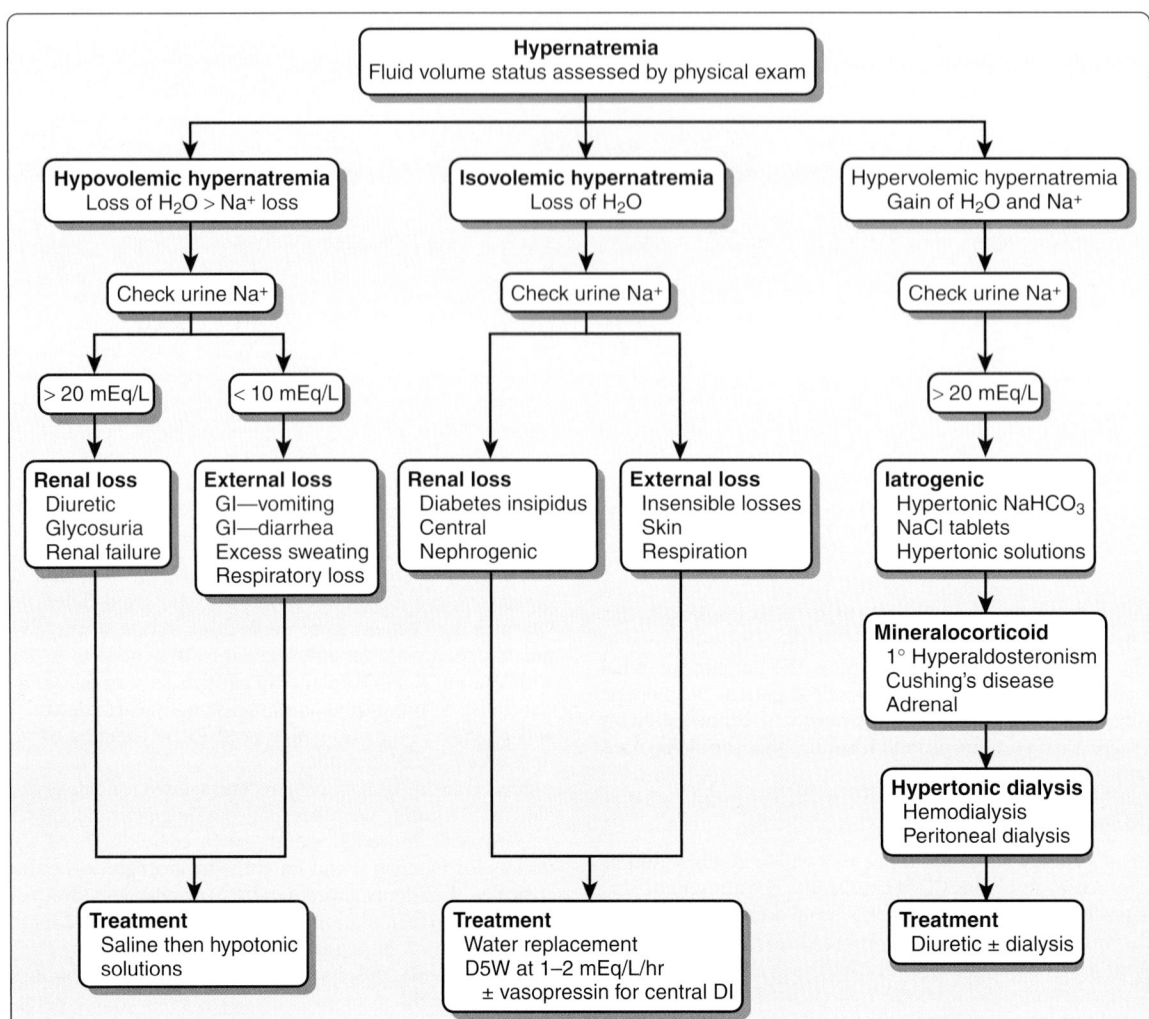

Figure 37-4 **Assessment and treatment of hypernatremia.** D5W, 5% dextrose in water; DI, diabetes insipidus; GI, gastrointestinal. *(Modified from Torres N: Electrolyte abnormalities: Sodium. In Faust RJ [ed]: Anesthesiology Review, 3rd ed. Philadelphia: Churchill Livingstone, 2002, p 28, by permission of Mayo Foundation.)*

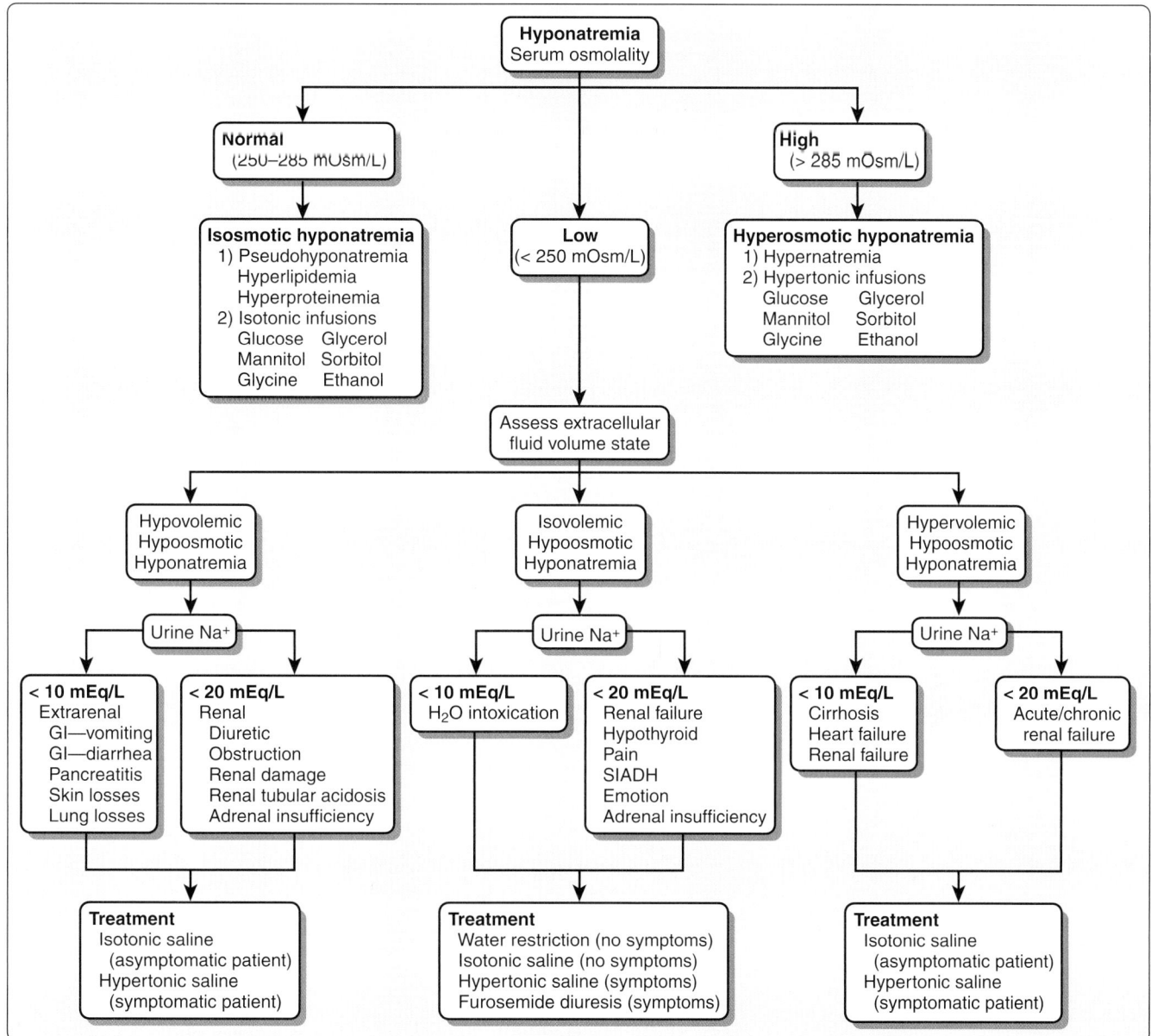

Figure 37-5   **Assessment and treatment of hyponatremia.** GI refers to gastrointestinal; SIADH, syndrome of inappropriate antidiuretic hormone. *(Modified from Torres N: Electrolyte abnormalities: Sodium. In Faust RJ [ed]: Anesthesiology Review, 3rd ed. Philadelphia, 2002, Churchill Livingstone, p 29, by permission of Mayo Foundation.)*

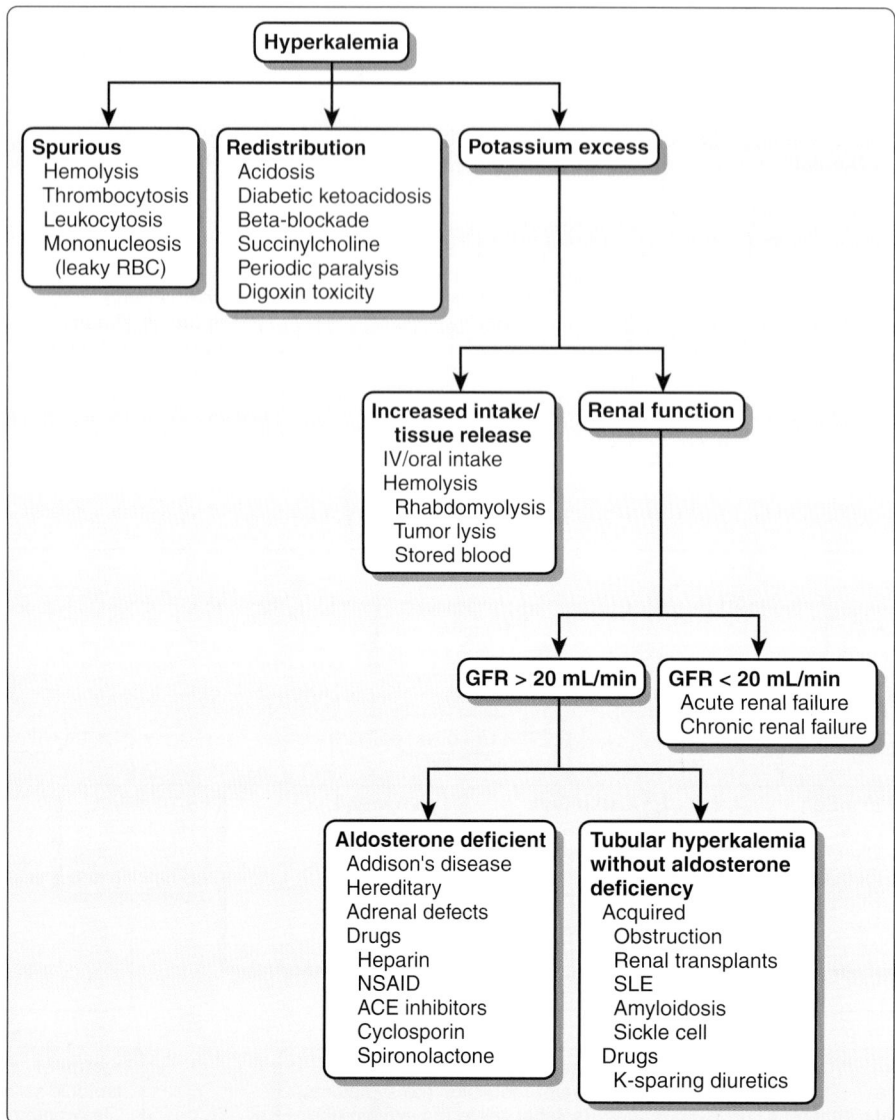

Figure 37-6 **Causes of hyperkalemia.** ACE inhibitor, acetylcholine esterase inhibitor; GFR, glomerular filtration rate; IV, intravenous; NSAID, non-steroidal antiinflammatory drugs; RBC, red blood cells; SLE, systemic lupus erythematosus. *(Modified from Torres N: Electrolyte abnormalities: Potassium. In Faust RJ [ed]: Anesthesiology Review, 3rd ed. Philadelphia, 2002, Churchill Livingstone, p 31, by permission of Mayo Foundation.)*

TABLE 37-13	Treatment of Hyperkalemia			
Treatment	*Dose*	*Mechanism*	*Onset*	*Duration*
Calcium chloride	7–14 mg/kg	Direct antagonism	Instantly	15–30 min
Sodium bicarbonate	0.7–1.4 mEq/kg	Direct antagonism; redistribution	15–30 min	3–6 hr
Glucose + insulin	25 g + 10–15 units	Redistribution	15–30 min	3–6 hr
Kayexalate	30 ga	Elimination of K+	1–3 hr	NA
Peritoneal dialysis	NA	Elimination of K+	1–3 hr	NA
Hemodialysis	NA	Elimination of K+	Rapid	NA

aMay be given orally or rectally.
NA, not applicable.

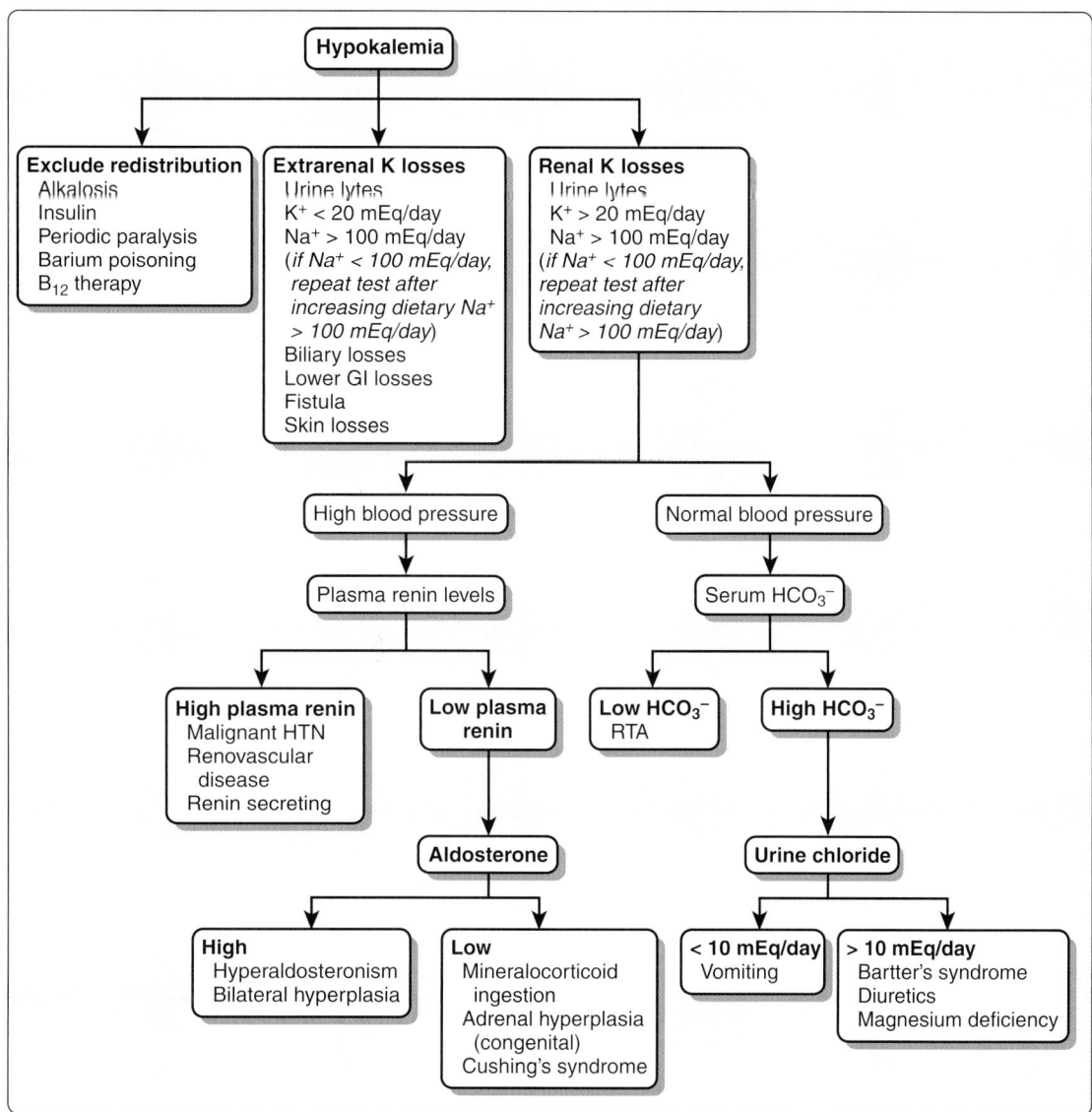

Figure 37-7 Causes of hypokalemia. GI, gastrointestinal; RTA, renal tubular acidosis. *(Modified from Torres N: Electrolyte abnormalities: Potassium. In Faust RJ [ed]: Anesthesiology Review, 3rd ed. Philadelphia, 2002, Churchill Livingstone, p 32, by permission of Mayo Foundation.)*

TABLE 37-14	Treatment of Hypercalcemia				
Treatment, dose	*Onset of Action*	*Duration of Action*	*Normalization, %*	*Advantages*	*Disadvantages*
Saline, 200–500 mL/hr[a]	Hours	During infusion	0–10	Rehydration	May produce cardiac failure, electrolyte changes, hypokalemia, hypomagnesemia; requires intensive monitoring
Saline + furosemide, 40–80 mg q2h	Hours	During treatment[b]	0–10	Enhanced calcium elimination	May produce cardiac failure, electrolyte changes, hypokalemia, hypomagnesemia; requires intensive monitoring
Zoledronate[c], 4 mg IV over 15 minutes	1–2 days	32–39 days	60–80	Potent and effective	Increases serum phosphate concentration; requires 3-day infusion
Calcitonin[d], 4 U/kg SQ or IM q12h	Hours	2–3 days	10–20	Nontoxic, rapid onset of normalization	Only decreases serum calcium level by 2–3 mg/dL, may produce tachyphylaxis
Gallium nitrate, 200 mg/ m²/day	2–3 days	10–14 days	70–80	Potent	Long infusion time, cannot be used in patients with renal failure

IM, intramuscularly; IV, intravenously; SQ, subcutaneously.
[a]Increases urine calcium concentration and excretion.
[b]Saline flow rate equals urine flow rate.
[c]Most potent biphosphonate available.
[d]Inhibits osteoclasts and stimulates calciuresis.

REFERENCES

1. Bashour CA, Yared JP, Ryan TA, et al: Long-term survival and functional capacity in cardiac surgery patients after prolonged intensive care, *Crit Care Med Dec* 28:3847–3853, 2000.
2. Welsby IJ, Bennett-Guerrero E, Atwell D, et al: The association of complication type with mortality and prolonged stay after cardiac surgery with cardiopulmonary bypass, *Anesth Analg* 94:1072–1078, 2002.
3. Williams MR, Wellner RB, Hartnett EA, et al: Long-term survival and quality of life in cardiac surgical patients with prolonged intensive care unit length of stay, *Ann Thorac Surg* 73:1472–1478, 2002.
4. Maze M, Scarfini C, Cavaliere F: New agents for sedation in the intensive care unit, *Crit Care Clin* 17:881–897, 2001.
5. Young C, Knudsen N, Hilton A, et al: Sedation in the intensive care unit, *Crit Care Med* 28:854–866, 2000.
6. Shapiro BA, Warren J, Egol AB, et al: Practice parameters for intravenous analgesia and sedation for adult patients in the intensive care unit: An executive summary. Society of Critical Care Medicine, *Crit Care Med* 23:1596–1600, 1995.
7. Nasraway SA Jr, Jacobi J, Murray MJ, et al: Sedation, analgesia, and neuromuscular blockade of the critically ill adult: Revised clinical practice guidelines for 2002, *Crit Care Med* 30:117–118, 2002.
8. Pun BT, Ely EW: The importance of diagnosing and managing ICU delirium, *Chest* 132:624–636, 2007.
9. Riker RR, Shehabi Y, Bokesch PM, et al: Dexmedetomidine vs midazolam for sedation of critically ill patients: A randomized trial, *JAMA* 301:489–499, 2009.
10. Devlin JW, Boleski G, Mlynarek M, et al: Motor Activity Assessment Scale: A valid and reliable sedation scale for use with mechanically ventilated patients in an adult surgical intensive care unit, *Crit Care Med* 27:1271–1275, 1999.
11. Ramsay MA, Savege TM, Simpson BR, et al: Controlled sedation with alphaxalone-alphadolone, *Br Med J* 2:656–659, 1974.
12. de Lemos J, Tweeddale M, Chittock D: Measuring quality of sedation in adult mechanically ventilated critically ill patients: The Vancouver Interaction and Calmness Scale. Sedation Focus Group, *J Clin Epidemiol* 53:908–919, 2000.
13. Wielenga JM, De Vos R, de Leeuw R, et al: COMFORT scale: A reliable and valid method to measure the amount of stress of ventilated preterm infants, *Neonatal Netw* 23:39–44, 2004.
14. Ely EW, Truman B, Shintani A, et al: Monitoring sedation status over time in ICU patients: Reliability and validity of the Richmond Agitation-Sedation Scale (RASS), *JAMA* 289:2983–2991, 2003.
15. Sessler CN, Gosnell MS, Grap MJ, et al: The Richmond Agitation-Sedation Scale: Validity and reliability in adult intensive care unit patients, *Am J Respir Crit Care Med* 166:1338–1344, 2002.
16. Weinert C, McFarland L: The state of intubated ICU patients: Development of a two-dimensional sedation rating scale for critically ill adults, *Chest* 126:1883–1890, 2004.
17. Luetz A, Heymann A, Radtke FM, et al: Different assessment tools for intensive care unit delirium: Which score to use? *Crit Care Med* 38:409–418, 2010.
18. Adesanya AO, Rosero E, Wyrick C, et al: Assessing the predictive value of the bispectral index vs patient state index on clinical assessment of sedation in postoperative cardiac surgery patients, *J Crit Care* 24:322–328, 2009.
19. Dundee J, Halliday NJ, Fee JP: Midazolam in intensive care, *Br Med J (Clin Res Ed)* 289:1540, 1984.
20. Woo E, Greenblatt DJ: Massive benzodiazepine requirements during acute alcohol withdrawal, *Am J Psychiatry* 136:821–823, 1979.
21. Deppe SA, Sipperly ME, Sargent AI, et al: Intravenous lorazepam as an amnestic and anxiolytic agent in the intensive care unit: A prospective study, *Crit Care Med* 22:1248–1252, 1994.
22. Pohlman AS, Simpson KP, Hall JB: Continuous intravenous infusions of lorazepam versus midazolam for sedation during mechanical ventilatory support: A prospective, randomized study, *Crit Care Med* 22:1241–1247, 1994.
23. Park GR, Navapurkar V, Ferenci P: The role of flumazenil in the critically ill, *Acta Anaesthesiol Scand Suppl* 108:23–34, 1995.
24. Myles PS, Buckland MR, Weeks AM, et al: Hemodynamic effects, myocardial ischemia, and timing of tracheal extubation with propofol-based anesthesia for cardiac surgery, *Anesth Analg* 84:12–19, 1997.
25. Strickland RA, Murray MJ: Fatal metabolic acidosis in a pediatric patient receiving an infusion of propofol in the intensive care unit: Is there a relationship? *Crit Care Med* 23:405–409, 1995.
26. Vasile B, Rasulo F, Candiani A, et al: The pathophysiology of propofol infusion syndrome: A simple name for a complex syndrome, *Intensive Care Med* 29:1417–1425, 2003.
27. Wysowski DK, Pollock ML: Reports of death with use of propofol (Diprivan) for nonprocedural (long-term) sedation and literature review, *Anesthesiology* 105:1047–1051, 2006.
28. Drummond JC, Iragui-Madoz VJ, Alksne JF, et al: Masking of epileptiform activity by propofol during seizure surgery, *Anesthesiology* 76:652–654, 1992.
29. Searle NR, Cote S, Taillefer J, et al: Propofol or midazolam for sedation and early extubation following cardiac surgery, *Can J Anaesth* 44:629–635, 1997.
30. Sherry KM, McNamara J, Brown JS, et al: An economic evaluation of propofol/fentanyl compared with midazolam/fentanyl on recovery in the ICU following cardiac surgery, *Anaesthesia* 51:312–317, 1996.
31. Barletta JF, Miedema SL, Wiseman D, et al: Impact of dexmedetomidine on analgesic requirements in patients after cardiac surgery in a fast-track recovery room setting, *Pharmacotherapy* 29:1427–1432, 2009.
32. Herr DL, Sum-Ping ST, England M: ICU sedation after coronary artery bypass graft surgery: Dexmedetomidine-based versus propofol-based sedation regimens, *J Cardiothorac Vasc Anesth* 17:576–584, 2003.
33. Pandharipande PP, Pun BT, Herr DL, et al: Effect of sedation with dexmedetomidine vs lorazepam on acute brain dysfunction in mechanically ventilated patients: The MENDS randomized controlled trial, *JAMA* 298:2644–2653, 2007.
34. Dasta JF, Kane-Gill SL, Pencina M, et al: A cost-minimization analysis of dexmedetomidine compared with midazolam for long-term sedation in the intensive care unit, *Crit Care Med* 38:497–503, 2010.
35. Murray MJ, Strickland RA, Weiler C: The use of neuromuscular blocking drugs in the intensive care unit: A US perspective, *Intensive Care Med* 19(Suppl 2):S40–S44, 1993.
36. Klessig HT, Geiger HJ, Murray MJ, et al: A national survey on the practice patterns of anesthesiologist intensivists in the use of muscle relaxants, *Crit Care Med* 20:1341–1345, 1992.
37. Shovelton DS: Reflections on an intensive therapy unit, *Br Med J* 1:737–738, 1979.
38. Murray MJ, Cowen J, DeBlock H, et al: Clinical practice guidelines for sustained neuromuscular blockade in the adult critically ill patient, *Crit Care Med* 30:142–156, 2002.
39. Hund E: Myopathy in critically ill patients, *Crit Care Med* 27:2544–2547, 1999.
40. Alberti C, Brun-Buisson C, Burchardi H, et al: Epidemiology of sepsis and infection in ICU patients from an international multicentre cohort study, *Intensive Care Med* 28:108–121, 2002.
41. Garland JS, Henrickson K, Maki DG: The 2002 Hospital Infection Control Practices Advisory Committee Centers for Disease Control and Prevention guideline for prevention of intravascular device-related infection, *Pediatrics* 110:1009–1013, 2002.
42. Maki DG, Weise CE, Sarafin HW: A semiquantitative culture method for identifying intravenous-catheter-related infection, *N Engl J Med* 296:1305–1309, 1977.
43. Maki DG: Yes, Virginia, aseptic technique is very important: maximal barrier precautions during insertion reduce the risk of central venous catheter-related bacteremia, *Infect Control Hosp Epidemiol* 15(4 Pt 1):227–230, 1994.
44. Linares J, Sitges-Serra A, Garau J, et al: Pathogenesis of catheter sepsis: A prospective study with quantitative and semiquantitative cultures of catheter hub and segments, *J Clin Microbiol* 21:357–360, 1985.
45. Mermel LA, McCormick RD, Springman SR, et al: The pathogenesis and epidemiology of catheter-related infection with pulmonary artery Swan-Ganz catheters: A prospective study utilizing molecular subtyping, *Am J Med* 91:197S–205S, 1991.
46. Raad II, Hanna HA: Intravascular catheter-related infections: New horizons and recent advances, *Arch Intern Med* 162:871–878, 2002.
47. Raad I, Hanna H, Maki D: Intravascular catheter-related infections: Advances in diagnosis, prevention, and management, *Lancet Infect Dis* 7:645–657, 2007.
48. Sitges-Serra A, Puig P, Linares J, et al: Hub colonization as the initial step in an outbreak of catheter-related sepsis due to coagulase negative staphylococci during parenteral nutrition, *JPEN J Parenter Enteral Nutr* 8:668–672, 1984.
49. Siegman-Igra Y, Anglim AM, Shapiro DE, et al: Diagnosis of vascular catheter-related bloodstream infection: A meta-analysis, *J Clin Microbiol* 35:928–936, 1997.
50. Safdar N, Maki DG: Risk of catheter-related bloodstream infection with peripherally inserted central venous catheters used in hospitalized patients, *Chest* 128:489–495, 2005.
51. O'Grady NP, Alexander M, Dellinger EP, et al: Guidelines for the prevention of intravascular catheter-related infections. Centers for Disease Control and Prevention, *MMWR Recomm Rep* 51(RR-10): 1–29, 2002.
52. Fidalgo S, Vazquez F, Mendoza MC, et al: Bacteremia due to Staphylococcus epidermidis: Microbiologic, epidemiologic, clinical, and prognostic features, *Rev Infect Dis* 12:520–528, 1990.
53. Sherertz RJ, Heard SO, Raad II: Diagnosis of triple-lumen catheter infection: Comparison of roll plate, sonication, and flushing methodologies, *J Clin Microbiol* 35:641–646, 1997.
54. Slobbe L, El Barzouhi A, Boersma E, et al: Comparison of the roll plate method to the sonication method to diagnose catheter colonization and bacteremia in patients with long-term tunnelled catheters: A randomized prospective study, *J Clin Microbiol* 47:885–888, 2009.
55. Safdar N, Fine JP, Maki DG: Meta-analysis: Methods for diagnosing intravascular device-related bloodstream infection, *Ann Intern Med* 142:451–466, 2005.
56. Baddour LM, Wilson WR, Bayer AS, et al: Infective endocarditis: Diagnosis, antimicrobial therapy, and management of complications: A statement for healthcare professionals from the Committee on Rheumatic Fever, Endocarditis, and Kawasaki Disease, Council on Cardiovascular Disease in the Young, and the Councils on Clinical Cardiology, Stroke, and Cardiovascular Surgery and Anesthesia, American Heart Association: Endorsed by the Infectious Diseases Society of America, *Circulation* 111:e394–e434, 2005.
57. Roy MC: Surgical-site infections after coronary artery bypass graft surgery: Discriminating site-specific risk factors to improve prevention efforts, *Infect Control Hosp Epidemiol* 19:229–233, 1998.
58. Mekontso-Dessap A, Kirsch M, Brun-Buisson C, et al: Poststernotomy mediastinitis due to *Staphylococcus aureus*: Comparison of methicillin-resistant and methicillin-susceptible cases, *Clin Infect Dis* 32:877–883, 2001.
59. Risk factors for deep sternal wound infection after sternotomy: A prospective, multicenter study, *J Thorac Cardiovasc Surg* 111:1200–1207, 1996.
60. Hollenbeak CS, Murphy DM, Koenig S, et al: The clinical and economic impact of deep chest surgical site infections following coronary artery bypass graft surgery, *Chest* 118:397–402, 2000.
61. Hughes JM, Culver DH, White JW, et al: Nosocomial infection surveillance, 1980–1982, *MMWR CDC Surveill Summ* 32:1SS–16SS, 1983.
62. Lazar HL, Fitzgerald C, Gross S, et al: Determinants of length of stay after coronary artery bypass graft surgery, *Circulation* 92(9 Suppl):II20–II24, 1995.
63. Zacharias A, Habib RH: Factors predisposing to median sternotomy complications. Deep vs superficial infection, *Chest* 110:1173–1178, 1996.
64. Martorell C, Engelman R, Corl A, et al: Surgical site infections in cardiac surgery: An 11-year perspective, *Am J Infect Control* 32:63–68, 2004.
65. Edwards MB, Ratnatunga CP, Dore CJ, et al: Thirty-day mortality and long-term survival following surgery for prosthetic endocarditis: A study from the UK heart valve registry, *Eur J Cardiothorac Surg* 14:156–164, 1998.
66. Arvay A, Lengyel M: Incidence and risk factors of prosthetic valve endocarditis, *Eur J Cardiothorac Surg* 2:340–346, 1988.
67. de Gevigney G, Pop C, Delahaye JP: The risk of infective endocarditis after cardiac surgical and interventional procedures, *Eur Heart J* 16(Suppl B):7–14, 1995.
68. Grover FL, Cohen DJ, Oprian C, et al: Determinants of the occurrence of and survival from prosthetic valve endocarditis. Experience of the Veterans Affairs Cooperative Study on Valvular Heart Disease, *J Thorac Cardiovasc Surg* 108:207–214, 1994.
69. Kuyvenhoven JP, van Rijk-Zwikker GL, Hermans J, et al: Prosthetic valve endocarditis: Analysis of risk factors for mortality, *Eur J Cardiothorac Surg* 8:420–424, 1994.
70. Vlessis AA, Khaki A, Grunkemeier GL, et al: Risk, diagnosis and management of prosthetic valve endocarditis: A review, *J Heart Valve Dis* 6:443–465, 1997.
71. Agnihotri AK, McGiffin DC, Galbraith AJ, et al: The prevalence of infective endocarditis after aortic valve replacement, *J Thorac Cardiovasc Surg* 110:1708–1720, 1995, discussion 1720–1704.
72. Calderwood SB, Swinski LA, Waternaux CM, et al: Risk factors for the development of prosthetic valve endocarditis, *Circulation* 72:31–37, 1985.
73. Horstkotte D, Piper C, Niehues R, et al: Late prosthetic valve endocarditis, *Eur Heart J* 16(Suppl B): 39–47, 1995.
74. Ivert TS, Dismukes WE, Cobbs CG, et al: Prosthetic valve endocarditis, *Circulation* 69:223–232, 1984.
75. Piper C, Korfer R, Horstkotte D: Prosthetic valve endocarditis, *Heart* 85:590–593, 2001.
76. Ben Ismail M, Hannachi N, Abid F, et al: Prosthetic valve endocarditis. A survey, *Br Heart J* 58:72–77, 1987.
77. Keyser DL, Biller J, Coffman TT, et al: Neurologic complications of late prosthetic valve endocarditis, *Stroke* 21:472–475, 1990.
78. Masur H, Johnson WD Jr: Prosthetic valve endocarditis, *J Thorac Cardiovasc Surg* 80:31–37, 1980.
79. Tornos P, Sanz E, Permanyer-Miralda G, et al: Late prosthetic valve endocarditis. Immediate and long-term prognosis, *Chest* 101:37–41, 1992.
80. Morguet AJ, Werner GS, Andreas S, et al: Diagnostic value of transesophageal compared with transthoracic echocardiography in suspected prosthetic valve endocarditis, *Herz* 20:390–398, 1995.
81. Vered Z, Mossinson D, Peleg E, et al: Echocardiographic assessment of prosthetic valve endocarditis, *Eur Heart J* 16(Suppl B):63–67, 1995.
82. Daniel WG, Mugge A, Martin RP, et al: Improvement in the diagnosis of abscesses associated with endocarditis by transesophageal echocardiography, *N Engl J Med* 324:795–800, 1991.
83. Karchmur AW: Infections of prosthetic valves and intravascular devices. In Mandell GL, Bennett JE, Dolin R, editors: *Principles and Practice of Infectious Disease*, vol 1, Philadelphia, 1999, Churchill Livingstone, pp. 903–917.
84. Calderwood SB, Swinski LA, Karchmer AW, et al: Prosthetic valve endocarditis. Analysis of factors affecting outcome of therapy, *J Thorac Cardiovasc Surg* 92:776–783, 1986.
85. Yu VL, Fang GD, Keys TF, et al: Prosthetic valve endocarditis: Superiority of surgical valve replacement versus medical therapy only, *Ann Thorac Surg* 58:1073–1077, 1994.
86. Gordon SM, Serkey JM, Longworth DL, et al: Early onset prosthetic valve endocarditis: The Cleveland Clinic experience 1992–1997, *Ann Thorac Surg* 69:1388–1392, 2000.

87. Habib G, Hoen B, Tornos P, et al: Guidelines on the prevention, diagnosis, and treatment of infective endocarditis (new version 2009): The Task Force on the Prevention, Diagnosis, and Treatment of Infective Endocarditis of the European Society of Cardiology (ESC), *Eur Heart J* 30:2369–2413, 2009.

88. Bone RC, Balk RA, Cerra FB, et al: Definitions for sepsis and organ failure and guidelines for the use of innovative therapies in sepsis. The ACCP/SCCM Consensus Conference Committee. American College of Chest Physicians/Society of Critical Care Medicine, *Chest* 101:1644–1655, 1992.

89. Muckart DJ, Bhagwanjee S: American College of Chest Physicians/Society of Critical Care Medicine Consensus Conference definitions of the systemic inflammatory response syndrome and allied disorders in relation to critically injured patients, *Crit Care Med* 25:1789–1795, 1997.

90. Levy MM, Fink MP, Marshall JC, et al: 2001 SCCM/ESICM/ACCP/ATS/SIS International Sepsis Definitions Conference, *Crit Care Med* 31:1250–1256, 2003.

91. Natanson C, Hoffman WD, Suffredini AF, et al: Selected treatment strategies for septic shock based on proposed mechanisms of pathogenesis, *Ann Intern Med* 120:771–783, 1994.

92. Orbach S, Weiss Y, Deutschman CS: The patient with sepsis or the systemic inflammatory response syndrome. In Murray MJ, Coursin DB, Pearl RG, et al: *Critical Care Medicine: Perioperative Management*, ed 2, Philadelphia, 2002, Lippincott Williams & Wilkins, pp. 601–615.

93. Vandijck DM: Severe sepsis in critically ill patients: Early recognition and outcome, *Acta Anaesthesiol Scand* 54:658–659, 2010.

94. Tsalik EL, Woods CW: Sepsis redefined: The search for surrogate markers, *Int J Antimicrob Agents* 34(Suppl 4):S16–S20, 2009.

95. Nduka OO, Parrillo JE: The pathophysiology of septic shock, *Crit Care Clin* 25:677–702, vii, 2009.

96. Hotchkiss RS, Karl IE: The pathophysiology and treatment of sepsis, *N Engl J Med* 348:138–150, 2003.

97. Landry DW, Oliver JA: The pathogenesis of vasodilatory shock, *N Engl J Med* 345:588–595, 2001.

98. Danai P, Martin GS: Epidemiology of sepsis: Recent advances, *Curr Infect Dis Rep* 7:329–334, 2005.

99. Levy MM, Dellinger RP, Townsend SR, et al: The Surviving Sepsis Campaign: Results of an international guideline based performance improvement program targeting severe sepsis, *Crit Care Med* 38:367–374, 2010.

100. Dellinger RP, Carlet JM, Masur H, et al: Surviving Sepsis Campaign guidelines for management of severe sepsis and septic shock, *Intensive Care Med* 30:536–555, 2004.

101. Dellinger RP, Levy MM, Carlet JM, et al: Surviving Sepsis Campaign: International guidelines for management of severe sepsis and septic shock: 2008, *Intensive Care Med* 34:17–60, 2008.

102. Levy MM, Dellinger RP, Townsend SR, et al: The Surviving Sepsis Campaign: Results of an international guideline-based performance improvement program targeting severe sepsis, *Crit Care Med* 38:367–374, 2010.

103. Laupland KB, Zygun DA, Davies HD, et al: Incidence and risk factors for acquiring nosocomial urinary tract infection in the critically ill, *J Crit Care* 17:50–57, 2002.

104. Marik PE: Fever in the ICU, *Chest* 117:855–869, 2000.

105. Platt R, Polk BF, Murdock B, et al: Mortality associated with nosocomial urinary-tract infection, *N Engl J Med* 307:637–642, 1982.

106. Stark RP, Maki DG: Bacteriuria in the catheterized patient. What quantitative level of bacteriuria is relevant? *N Engl J Med* 311:560–564, 1984.

107. Brown DF, Warren RE: Effect of sample volume on yield of positive blood cultures from adult patients with haematological malignancy, *J Clin Pathol* 43:777–779, 1990.

108. Warren JW: Catheter-associated urinary tract infections, *Infect Dis Clin North Am* 11:609–622, 1997.

109. Warren JW, Platt R, Thomas RJ, et al: Antibiotic irrigation and catheter-associated urinary-tract infections, *N Engl J Med* 299:570–573, 1978.

110. Sandock DS, Gothe BG, Bodner DR: Trimethoprim-sulfamethoxazole prophylaxis against urinary tract infection in the chronic spinal cord injury patient, *Paraplegia* 33:156–160, 1995.

111. Hall IC, O'Toole E: Intestinal flora in new-born infants with a description of a new pathogenic anaerobe *Bacillus difficilis*, *Am J Dis Child* 49:390–402, 1935.

112. Bartlett JG, Moon N, Chang TW, et al: Role of *Clostridium difficile* in antibiotic-associated pseudomembranous colitis, *Gastroenterology* 75:778–782, 1978.

113. George RH, Symonds JM, Dimock F, et al: Identification of *Clostridium difficile* as a cause of pseudomembranous colitis, *Br Med J* 1:695, 1978.

114. Thomas C, Stevenson M, Riley TV: Antibiotics and hospital-acquired *Clostridium difficile*-associated diarrhoea: A systematic review, *J Antimicrob Chemother* 51:1339–1350, 2003.

115. Kyne L, Warny M, Qamar A, et al: Asymptomatic carriage of *Clostridium difficile* and serum levels of IgG antibody against toxin A, *N Engl J Med* 342:390–397, 2000.

116. Kyne L, Warny M, Qamar A, et al: Association between antibody response to toxin A and protection against recurrent *Clostridium difficile* diarrhoea, *Lancet* 357:189–193, 2001.

117. McFarland LV, Mulligan ME, Kwok RY, et al: Nosocomial acquisition of *Clostridium difficile* infection, *N Engl J Med* 320:204–210, 1989.

118. Cunningham R, Dale B, Undy B, et al: Proton pump inhibitors as a risk factor for *Clostridium difficile* diarrhoea, *J Hosp Infect* 54:243–245, 2003.

119. Kyne L, Sougioultzis S, McFarland LV, et al: Underlying disease severity as a major risk factor for nosocomial *Clostridium difficile* diarrhea, *Infect Control Hosp Epidemiol* 23:653–659, 2002.

120. Riegler M, Sedivy R, Pothoulakis C, et al: *Clostridium difficile* toxin B is more potent than toxin A in damaging human colonic epithelium in vitro, *J Clin Invest* 95:2004–2011, 1995.

121. Johnson S, Samore MH, Farrow KA, et al: Epidemics of diarrhea caused by a clindamycin-resistant strain of *Clostridium difficile* in four hospitals, *N Engl J Med* 341:1645–1651, 1999.

122. Kelly CP, Pothoulakis C, LaMont JT: *Clostridium difficile* colitis, *N Engl J Med* 330:257–262, 1994.

123. Rao SS, Edwards CA, Austen CJ, et al: Impaired colonic fermentation of carbohydrate after ampicillin, *Gastroenterology* 94:928–932, 1988.

124. Bartlett JG: Clinical practice. Antibiotic-associated diarrhea, *N Engl J Med* 346:334–339, 2002.

125. Tedesco FJ: Antibiotic associated pseudomembranous colitis with negative proctosigmoidoscopy examination, *Gastroenterology* 77:295–297, 1979.

126. Triadafilopoulos G, Hallstone AE: Acute abdomen as the first presentation of pseudomembranous colitis, *Gastroenterology* 101:685–691, 1991.

127. Wenisch C, Parschalk B, Hasenhundl M, et al: Comparison of vancomycin, teicoplanin, metronidazole, and fusidic acid for the treatment of *Clostridium difficile*-associated diarrhea, *Clin Infect Dis* 22:813–818, 1996.

128. Zar FA, Bakkanagari SR, Moorthi KM, et al: A comparison of vancomycin and metronidazole for the treatment of *Clostridium difficile*-associated diarrhea, stratified by disease severity, *Clin Infect Dis* 45:302–307, 2007.

129. Bolton RP, Culshaw MA: Faecal metronidazole concentrations during oral and intravenous therapy for antibiotic associated colitis due to *Clostridium difficile*, *Gut* 27:1169–1172, 1986.

130. O'Connor JR, Johnson S, Gerding DN: *Clostridium difficile* infection caused by the epidemic BI/NAP1/027 strain, *Gastroenterology* 136:1913–1924, 2009.

131. Deutschman CS, Wilton P, Sinow J, et al: Paranasal sinusitis associated with nasotracheal intubation: A frequently unrecognized and treatable source of sepsis, *Crit Care Med* 14:111–114, 1986.

132. Fassoulaki A, Pamouktsoglou P: Prolonged nasotracheal intubation and its association with inflammation of paranasal sinuses, *Anesth Analg* 69:50–52, 1989.

133. Grindlinger GA, Niehoff J, Hughes SL, et al: Acute paranasal sinusitis related to nasotracheal intubation of head-injured patients, *Crit Care Med* 15:214–217, 1987.

134. Rouby JJ, Laurent P, Gosnach M, et al: Risk factors and clinical relevance of nosocomial maxillary sinusitis in the critically ill, *Am J Respir Crit Care Med* 150:776–783, 1994.

135. Leal-Noval SR, Rincon-Ferrari MD, Garcia-Curiel A, et al: Transfusion of blood components and postoperative infection in patients undergoing cardiac surgery, *Chest* 119:1461–1468, 2001.

136. Mezrow CK, Bergstein I, Tartter PI: Postoperative infections following autologous and homologous blood transfusions, *Transfusion* 32:27–30, 1992.

137. Gu YJ, de Vries AJ, Boonstra PW, et al: Leukocyte depletion results in improved lung function and reduced inflammatory response after cardiac surgery, *J Thorac Cardiovasc Surg* 112:494–500, 1996.

138. Goodnough LT, Despotis GJ, Hogue CW Jr, et al: On the need for improved transfusion indicators in cardiac surgery, *Ann Thorac Surg* 60:473–480, 1995.

139. van de Watering LM, Hermans J, Houbiers JG, et al: Beneficial effects of leukocyte depletion of transfused blood on postoperative complications in patients undergoing cardiac surgery: A randomized clinical trial, *Circulation* 97:562–568, 1998.

140. Blumberg N, Heal JM: Transfusion and recipient immune function, *Arch Pathol Lab Med* 113:246–253, 1989.

141. Murphy GJ, Reeves BC, Rogers CA, et al: Increased mortality, postoperative morbidity, and cost after red blood cell transfusion in patients having cardiac surgery, *Circulation* 116:2544–2552, 2007.

142. Koch CG, Li L, Duncan AI, et al: Morbidity and mortality risk associated with red blood cell and blood-component transfusion in isolated coronary artery bypass grafting, *Crit Care Med* 34:1608–1616, 2006.

143. Marik PE, Corwin HL: Efficacy of red blood cell transfusion in the critically ill: A systematic review of the literature, *Crit Care Med* 36:2667–2674, 2008.

144. Rogers MA, Blumberg N, Saint S, et al: Hospital variation in transfusion and infection after cardiac surgery: A cohort study, *BMC Med* 7:37, 2009.

145. Hebert PC, Wells G, Blajchman MA, et al: A multicenter, randomized, controlled clinical trial of transfusion requirements in critical care. Transfusion Requirements in Critical Care Investigators, Canadian Critical Care Trials Group, *N Engl J Med* 340:409–417, 1999.

146. Johnson RG, Thurer RL, Kruskall MS, et al: Comparison of two transfusion strategies after elective operations for myocardial revascularization, *J Thorac Cardiovasc Surg* 104:307–314, 1992.

147. Weisel RD, Charlesworth DC, Mickleborough LL, et al: Limitations of blood conservation, *J Thorac Cardiovasc Surg* 88:26–38, 1984.

148. Dellinger RP, Carlet JM, Masur H, et al: Surviving Sepsis Campaign guidelines for management of severe sepsis and septic shock, *Crit Care Med* 32:858–873, 2004.

149. Dellinger RP, Levy MM, Carlet JM, et al: Surviving Sepsis Campaign: International guidelines for management of severe sepsis and septic shock: 2008, *Crit Care Med* 36:296–327, 2008.

150. Rao SV, Jollis JG, Harrington RA, et al: Relationship of blood transfusion and clinical outcomes in patients with acute coronary syndromes, *JAMA* 292:1555–1562, 2004.

151. Lee HT, Sladen RN: Perioperative renal protection. In Murray MJ, Coursin DB, Pearl RG, et al: *Critical Care Medicine: Perioperative Management*, ed 2, Philadelphia, 2002, Lippincott Williams & Wilkins, pp. 501–520.

152. Bellomo R, Kellum JA, Ronco C: Defining acute renal failure: Physiological principles, *Intensive Care Med* 30:33–37, 2004.

153. Block CA, Manning HL: Prevention of acute renal failure in the critically ill, *Am J Respir Crit Care Med* 165:320–324, 2002.

154. Chertow GM, Levy EM, Hammermeister KE, et al: Independent association between acute renal failure and mortality following cardiac surgery, *Am J Med* 104:343–348, 1998.

155. Conlon PJ, Stafford-Smith M, White WD, et al: Acute renal failure following cardiac surgery, *Nephrol Dial Transplant* 14:1158–1162, 1999.

156. Higgins TL, Estafanous FG, Loop FD, et al: Stratification of morbidity and mortality outcome by preoperative risk factors in coronary artery bypass patients. A clinical severity score, *JAMA* 267:2344–2348, 1992.

157. Hilberman M, Derby GC, Spencer RJ, et al: Sequential pathophysiological changes characterizing the progression from renal dysfunction to acute renal failure following cardiac operation, *J Thorac Cardiovasc Surg* 79:838–844, 1980.

158. Bellomo R, Ronco C, Kellum JA, et al: Acute renal failure—definition, outcome measures, animal models, fluid therapy and information technology needs: The Second International Consensus Conference of the Acute Dialysis Quality Initiative (ADQI) Group, *Crit Care* 8:R204–R212, 2004.

159. Heringlake M, Knappe M, Vargas Hein O, et al: Renal dysfunction according to the ADQI-RIFLE system and clinical practice patterns after cardiac surgery in Germany, *Minerva Anestesiol* 72 (7–8):645–654, 2006.

160. Kuitunen A, Vento A, Suojaranta-Ylinen R, et al: Acute renal failure after cardiac surgery: Evaluation of the RIFLE classification, *Ann Thorac Surg* 81:542–546, 2006.

161. Lin CY, Chen YC, Tsai FC, et al: RIFLE classification is predictive of short-term prognosis in critically ill patients with acute renal failure supported by extracorporeal membrane oxygenation, *Nephrol Dial Transplant* 21:2867–2873, 2006.

162. Baldwin L, Henderson A, Hickman P: Effect of postoperative low-dose dopamine on renal function after elective major vascular surgery, *Ann Intern Med* 120:744–747, 1994.

163. Lassnigg A, Donner E, Grubhofer G, et al: Lack of renoprotective effects of dopamine and furosemide during cardiac surgery, *J Am Soc Nephrol* 11:97–104, 2000.

164. Murray P, Hall J: Renal replacement therapy for acute renal failure, *Am J Respir Crit Care Med* 162(3 Pt 1):777–781, 2000.

165. Sward K, Valsson F, Odencrants P, et al: Recombinant human atrial natriuretic peptide in ischemic acute renal failure: A randomized placebo-controlled trial, *Crit Care Med* 32:1310–1315, 2004.

166. de Denus S, Pharand C, Williamson DR: Brain natriuretic peptide in the management of heart failure: The versatile neurohormone, *Chest* 125:652–668, 2004.

167. Textor SC, Glockner JF, Lerman LO, et al: The use of magnetic resonance to evaluate tissue oxygenation in renal artery stenosis, *J Am Soc Nephrol* 19:780–788, 2008.

168. Bellomo R, Ronco C: Continuous renal replacement therapy in the intensive care unit, *Intensive Care Med* 25:781–789, 1999.

169. Forni LG, Hilton PJ: Continuous hemofiltration in the treatment of acute renal failure, *N Engl J Med* 336:1303–1309, 1997.

170. Lewis J, Chertow GM, Paganini EP, et al: A multicenter survey of patient characteristics, practice patterns, and outcomes in critically ill patients with ARF [Abstract], *J Am Soc Nephrol* 8:A0673, 2000.

171. Mehta RL, Letteri JM: Current status of renal replacement therapy for acute renal failure. A survey of US nephrologists. The National Kidney Foundation Council on Dialysis, *Am J Nephrol* 19:377–382, 1999.

172. Silvester W: Outcome studies of continuous renal replacement therapy in the intensive care unit, *Kidney Int Suppl* 66:S138–S141, 1998.

173. Butterworth CE Jr: Editorial: Malnutrition in the hospital, *JAMA* 230:879, 1974.

174. The skeleton in the hospital closet—20 years later: Malnutrition in patients with GI disease, cancer and AIDS, Proceedings of a conference. Los Angeles, California, October 1–2, 1994, *Nutrition* 11(2 Suppl):192–254, 1995.

175. Blackburn GL, Ahmad A: Skeleton in the hospital closet—then and now, *Nutrition* 11(2 Suppl): 193–195, 1995.

176. Hirsch S, de Obaldia N, Petermann M, et al: Subjective global assessment of nutritional status: further validation, *Nutrition* 7:35–37, 1991, discussion 37–38.

177. Akhtar S, Barash PG, Inzucchi SE: Scientific principles and clinical implications of perioperative glucose regulation and control, *Anesth Analg* 110:478–497, 2010.

178. Hermanides J, Vriesendorp TM, Bosman RJ, et al: Glucose variability is associated with intensive care unit mortality, *Crit Care Med* 38:838–842, 2010.

179. Kompan L, Kremzar B, Gadzijev E, et al: Effects of early enteral nutrition on intestinal permeability and the development of multiple organ failure after multiple injury, *Intensive Care Med* 25:157–161, 1999.

180. Murrary MJ, Brull SJ, Coursin DB: Strict blood glucose control in the ICU: Panacea or Pandora's box? *J Cardiothorac Vasc Anesth* 18:687–689, 2004.

181. Martindale RG, McClave SA, Vanek VW, et al: Guidelines for the provision and assessment of nutrition support therapy in the adult critically ill patient: Society of Critical Care Medicine and American Society for Parenteral and Enteral Nutrition: Executive Summary, *Crit Care Med* 37:1757–1761, 2009.

182. National Heart, Lung, and Blood Institute: *Early Versus Delayed Enteral Feeding and Omega-3 Fatty Acid/Antioxidant Supplementation for Treating People With Acute Lung Injury or Acute Respiratory Distress Syndrome (The EDEN-Omega Study)*, 2008. Available at: http://clinicaltrials.gov/ct2/show/results/NCT00609180. Accessed March 10, 2010.

38

Postoperative Pain Management for the Cardiac Patient

MARK A. CHANEY, MD

KEY POINTS

1. Inadequate postoperative analgesia and/or an uninhibited perioperative surgical stress response has the potential to initiate pathophysiologic changes in all major organ systems, including the cardiovascular, pulmonary, gastrointestinal, renal, endocrine, immunologic, and/or central nervous systems, all of which may lead to substantial postoperative morbidity. Adequate postoperative analgesia prevents unnecessary patient discomfort, may decrease morbidity, may decrease postoperative hospital length of stay, and thus may decrease cost.

2. Pain after cardiac surgery may be intense and originates from many sources, including the incision (sternotomy or thoracotomy), intraoperative tissue retraction and dissection, vascular cannulation sites, vein-harvesting sites, and chest tubes, among others. Achieving optimal pain relief after cardiac surgery is often difficult, yet may be attained via a wide variety of techniques, including local anesthetic infiltration, nerve blocks, intravenous agents, intrathecal techniques, and epidural techniques.

3. Traditionally, analgesia after cardiac surgery has been obtained with intravenous opioids (specifically morphine). However, intravenous opioid use is associated with definite detrimental side effects (nausea/vomiting, pruritus, urinary retention, respiratory depression), and longer-acting opioids such as morphine may delay tracheal extubation during the immediate postoperative period via excessive sedation and/or respiratory depression. Thus, in the current era of early extubation ("fast-tracking"), cardiac anesthesiologists are exploring unique options other than traditional intravenous opioids for control of postoperative pain in patients after cardiac surgery.

4. Although patient-controlled analgesia is a well-established technique (used for more than two decades) and offers potential unique benefits (reliable analgesic effect, improved patient autonomy, flexible adjustment to individual needs, etc.), whether it truly offers significant

clinical advantages (compared with traditional nurse-administered analgesic techniques) to patients immediately after cardiac surgery remains to be determined.

5. Cyclooxygenase-2 (COX-2) inhibitors possess analgesic (opioid-sparing) effects and lack deleterious effects on coagulation (in contrast with nonselective nonsteroidal anti-inflammatory drugs [NSAIDs]). However, current evidence does not suggest that COX-2 inhibitors provide major advantages over traditional NSAIDs. Furthermore, potential links between this class of drugs and cardiovascular complications, sternal wound infections, and thromboembolic complications need to be fully evaluated.

6. Administration of intrathecal morphine to patients initiates reliable postoperative analgesia after cardiac surgery. Intrathecal opioids or local anesthetics cannot reliably attenuate the perioperative stress response associated with cardiac surgery that persists during the immediate postoperative period. Although intrathecal local anesthetics (not opioids) may induce perioperative thoracic cardiac sympathectomy, the hemodynamic changes associated with a "total spinal" make the technique unpalatable in patients with cardiac disease.

7. Administration of thoracic epidural opioids or local anesthetics to patients initiates reliable postoperative analgesia after cardiac surgery. The quality of analgesia obtained with thoracic epidural anesthetic techniques is sufficient to allow cardiac surgery to be performed in "awake" patients (without general endotracheal anesthesia). Administration of thoracic epidural local anesthetics (not opioids) can both reliably attenuate the perioperative stress response associated with cardiac surgery that persists during the immediate postoperative period and induce perioperative thoracic cardiac sympathectomy.

8. Use of intrathecal and epidural techniques in patients undergoing cardiac surgery, although seemingly increasing in popularity, remains extremely controversial. Concerns regarding hematoma risk and the fact that the numerous

clinical investigations regarding this topic are suboptimally designed and use a wide array of disparate techniques have prevented clinically useful conclusions.

9. As a general rule, it is best to avoid intense, single-modality therapy for the treatment of acute postoperative pain. The administration of two analgesic agents that act by different mechanisms ("multimodal" or "balanced" analgesia) provides superior analgesic efficacy with equivalent or reduced adverse effects. Analgesic therapies should be used only after thoughtful consideration of the risks and benefits for each individual patient. The therapy (or therapies) selected should reflect the individual anesthesiologist's expertise, as well as the capacity for safe application of the chosen modality in each practice setting. The choice of medication, dose, route, and duration of therapy always should be individualized.

Adequate postoperative analgesia prevents unnecessary patient discomfort, may decrease morbidity, may decrease postoperative hospital length of stay, and thus may decrease cost. Because postoperative pain management has been deemed important, the American Society of Anesthesiologists has published practice guidelines regarding this topic.[1] Furthermore, in recognition of the need for improved pain management, the Joint Commission on Accreditation of Healthcare Organizations has developed new standards for the assessment and management of pain in accredited hospitals and other health care settings.[2] Patient satisfaction (no doubt linked to adequacy of postoperative analgesia) has become an essential element that influences clinical activity of not only anesthesiologists but all healthcare professionals.

Achieving optimal pain relief after cardiac surgery is often difficult. Pain may be associated with many interventions, including sternotomy, thoracotomy, leg-vein harvesting, pericardiotomy, and/or chest tube insertion, among others. Inadequate analgesia and/or an uninhibited stress response during the postoperative period may increase morbidity by causing adverse hemodynamic, metabolic, immunologic, and hemostatic alterations.[3–5] Aggressive control of postoperative pain, associated with an attenuated stress response, may decrease morbidity and mortality in high-risk patients after noncardiac surgery[6,7] and may also decrease morbidity and mortality in patients after cardiac surgery.[8,9] Adequate postoperative analgesia may be attained via a wide variety of techniques (Table 38-1). Traditionally, analgesia after cardiac surgery has been obtained with intravenous opioids (specifically morphine). However, intravenous opioid use is associated with definite detrimental side effects (nausea/vomiting, pruritus, urinary retention, respiratory depression), and longer-acting opioids such as morphine may delay tracheal extubation during the immediate postoperative period via excessive sedation and/or respiratory depression. Thus,

in the current era of early extubation ("fast-tracking"), cardiac anesthesiologists are exploring unique options other than traditional intravenous opioids for control of postoperative pain in patients after cardiac surgery.[10,11] No single technique is clearly superior; each possesses distinct advantages and disadvantages. It is becoming increasingly clear that a multimodal approach/combined analgesic regimen (utilizing a variety of techniques) is likely the best way to approach postoperative pain (in all patients after surgery) to maximize analgesia and minimize side effects. When addressing postoperative analgesia in cardiac surgical patients, choice of technique (or techniques) is made only after a thorough analysis of the risk/benefit ratio of each technique in the specific patient in whom analgesia is desired.

PAIN AND CARDIAC SURGERY

Surgical or traumatic injury initiates changes in the peripheral and central nervous systems (CNSs) that must be addressed therapeutically to promote postoperative analgesia and, it is hoped, positively influence clinical outcome (Boxes 38-1 and 38-2). The physical processes of incision, traction, and cutting of tissues stimulate free nerve endings and a wide variety of specific nociceptors. Receptor activation and activity are further modified by the local release of chemical mediators of inflammation and sympathetic amines released via the perioperative surgical stress response. The perioperative surgical stress response peaks during the immediate postoperative period and exerts major effects on many physiologic processes. The potential clinical benefits of attenuating the perioperative surgical stress response (above and beyond simply attaining adequate clinical analgesia) have received much attention during the 2000s and remain fairly controversial.[12] However, it is clear that inadequate postoperative analgesia and/or an uninhibited perioperative surgical stress response has the potential to initiate pathophysiologic changes in all major organ systems, including the cardiovascular, pulmonary, gastrointestinal, renal, endocrine, immunologic, and/or CNSs, all of which may lead to substantial postoperative morbidity.

Pain after cardiac surgery may be intense and it originates from many sources, including the incision (sternotomy, thoracotomy, etc.), intraoperative tissue retraction and dissection, vascular cannulation sites, vein-harvesting sites, and chest tubes, among others.[13,14] Patients in whom an internal mammary artery (IMA) is surgically exposed and used as a bypass graft may have substantially more postoperative pain.[15]

A prospective clinical investigation involving 200 consecutive patients undergoing cardiac surgery via median sternotomy assessed the location, distribution, and intensity of postoperative pain.[13] All patients

TABLE 38-1	Techniques Available for Postoperative Analgesia

- Local anesthetic infiltration
- Nerve blocks
- Opioids
- Nonsteroidal anti-inflammatory agents
- α-Adrenergic agents
- Intrathecal techniques
- Epidural techniques
- Multimodal analgesia

BOX 38-1. PAIN AND CARDIAC SURGERY

- Originates from many sources
- Most commonly originates from chest wall
- Preoperative expectations influence postoperative satisfaction
- Quality of postoperative analgesia may influence morbidity/mortality

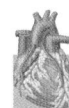

BOX 38-2. POTENTIAL CLINICAL BENEFITS OF ADEQUATE POSTOPERATIVE ANALGESIA

- Hemodynamic stability
- Metabolic stability
- Immunologic stability
- Hemostatic stability
- Stress response attenuation
- Decreased morbidity/mortality

received 25 to 50 μg/kg intraoperative intravenous fentanyl, were subjected to routine cardiopulmonary bypass (CPB), had their arms positioned along their body on the operating table, had their sternum closed with five peristernal wires, and received mediastinal and thoracic drains passed through the rectus abdominis muscle just below the xiphoid. A subgroup (127 patients) also underwent long saphenous vein harvesting either from the calf (men) or thigh (women). All patients were extubated before the first postoperative morning. Postoperative analgesic management was standardized and included intravenous morphine, oral paracetamol, oral tramadol, and subcutaneous morphine. Pain location, distribution, and intensity were documented in the morning on the first, second, third, and seventh postoperative days using a standardized picture dividing the body into 32 anatomic areas. A numerical rating scale of 0 to 10 (with 0 representing no pain and 10 representing worst possible pain) was used to assess maximal pain intensity.

These investigators found that maximal pain intensity was highest on the first postoperative day and lowest on the third postoperative day. However, maximal pain intensity was only graded as "moderate" (mean pain score was approximately 3.8) and did not diminish during the first 2 postoperative days, yet started to decline between postoperative days 2 and 3. Pain distribution did not appear to vary throughout the postoperative period, yet location did (more shoulder pain observed on the seventh postoperative day). As time after surgery increased, pain usually moved from primarily incisional/epigastric to osteoarticular. Another source of postoperative pain in patients after cardiac surgery is thoracic cage rib fractures, which may be common.[16,17] Furthermore, sternal retraction, causing posterior rib fracture, may lead to brachial plexus injury. In these patients, routine chest radiographs may be normal despite the presence of fracture. Thus, bone scans (better at detecting rib fractures than chest radiographs) are recommended whenever there is unexplained postoperative nonincisional pain in a patient who has undergone sternal retraction.[17] Other studies have indicated that the most common source of pain in patients after cardiac surgery is the chest wall. Age also appears to impact pain intensity; patients younger than 60 often have greater pain intensity than patients older than 60. Although maximal pain intensity after cardiac surgery is usually only moderate, there remains ample room for clinical improvement in analgesic control to minimize pain intensity, especially during the first few postoperative days.

Persistent pain after cardiac surgery, although rare, can be problematic.[18-20] The cause of persistent pain after sternotomy is multifactorial, yet tissue destruction, intercostal nerve trauma, scar formation, rib fractures, sternal infection, stainless-steel wire sutures, and/or costochondral separation may all play roles. Such chronic pain is often localized to the arms, shoulders, or legs. Postoperative brachial plexus neuropathies also may occur and have been attributed to rib fracture fragments, IMA dissection, suboptimal positioning of patients during surgery, and/or central venous catheter placement. Postoperative neuralgia of the saphenous nerve has also been reported after harvesting of saphenous veins for coronary artery bypass grafting (CABG). Younger patients appear to be at greater risk for development of chronic, long-lasting pain. The correlation of severity of acute postoperative pain and development of chronic pain syndromes has been suggested (patients requiring more postoperative analgesics may be more likely to develop chronic pain), yet the causative relation is still vague.

Ho and associates[18] assessed via survey 244 patients after cardiac surgery and median sternotomy and found that persistent pain (defined as pain still present 2 or more months after surgery) was reported in almost 30% of patients. The incidence rate of persistent pain at any site was 29% (71 patients) and for sternotomy was 25% (61 patients). Other common locations of persistent pain reported to these investigators were the shoulders (17.4%), back (15.9%), and neck (5.8%). However, such persistent pain was usually reported as mild, with only 7% of patients reporting interference with daily living. The most common words used to describe the persistent pain were "annoying" (57%), "nagging" (33%), "dull" (30%), "sharp" (25%), "tiring" (22%), "tender" (22%), and "tight" (22%). The temporal nature of this pain was mostly reported as being brief/transient and periodic/intermittent.

Twenty patients (8%) also described symptoms of numbness, burning pain, and tenderness over the IMA-harvesting site, symptoms suggestive of IMA syndrome. Thus, it was concluded that mild persistent pain after cardiac surgery and median sternotomy is common yet only infrequently substantially interferes with daily life.

Although the most common source of pain in patients after cardiac surgery remains the chest wall, leg pain from vein-graft harvesting can be problematic as well. Such pain may not become apparent until the late postoperative period, which may be related to the progression of patient mobilization, as well as the decreasing impact of sternotomy pain (unmasking leg incisional pain). The recent utilization of minimally invasive vein-graft harvesting techniques (endoscopic vein-graft harvesting) decreases postoperative leg pain intensity and duration compared with conventional open techniques.[21] Although initial harvest times may be prolonged, harvest times become equivalent between the two techniques (endoscopic vs. conventional) once a short learning curve is overcome. Furthermore, leg morbidity (infection, dehiscence, etc.) may be less in patients undergoing endoscopic vein harvest compared with patients undergoing conventional open techniques because of different incisional lengths.

Patient satisfaction with quality of postoperative analgesia is as much related to the comparison between anticipated and experienced pain as it is to the actual level of pain experienced. Satisfaction is related to a situation that is better than predicted, dissatisfaction to one that is worse than expected. Patients undergoing cardiac surgery remain concerned regarding the adequacy of postoperative pain relief and tend to preoperatively expect a greater amount of postoperative pain than that which is actually experienced.[14] Because of these unique preoperative expectations, patients after cardiac surgery who receive only moderate analgesia postoperatively will likely still be satisfied with their pain control. Thus, patients may experience pain of moderate intensity after cardiac surgery yet still express very high satisfaction levels.[14,15]

Scientific advances have allowed a better understanding of how and why pain occurs, leading to unique and possibly clinically beneficial pain management strategies. Clinicians now know that noxious input from acute injury may trigger a state of CNS sensitization, called *wind-up*. In essence, dorsal horn neurotransmitter release via nociceptive input conditions the CNS such that there is enhanced responsiveness (secondary hyperalgesia). Although experimental evidence exists indicating that enhanced responsiveness outlasts the initial provocative insult (induced sensitivity outlasts stimulus), the exact clinical relevance remains to be determined. Advances regarding spinal cord neuropharmacology have led to research aimed at modifying or blocking N-methyl-d-aspartate (NMDA) receptors to influence pain control and to the concept of preemptive analgesia. The concept of preemptive analgesia is predicated on addressing pain before it initiates peripheral and central sensitization. However, given the redundancy in the neurotransmitter receptor systems in the CNS, it is unlikely that blocking only one component will result in clear clinical benefits. Although the use of NMDA-receptor antagonists and the concept of preemptive analgesia are intriguing and certain clinical investigations appear to support their utility, clear and definite clinical benefits in humans remain to be determined. Debate continues over the potential benefits of NMDA-receptor antagonists and the utility of preemptive analgesic treatment, as well as direction in which research and conceptual development in this exciting field need to proceed.

POTENTIAL CLINICAL BENEFITS OF ADEQUATE POSTOPERATIVE ANALGESIA

Inadequate analgesia (coupled with an uninhibited stress response) during the postoperative period may lead to many adverse hemodynamic (tachycardia, hypertension, vasoconstriction), metabolic (increased catabolism), immunologic (impaired immune response), and hemostatic (platelet activation) alterations. In patients undergoing cardiac surgery, perioperative myocardial ischemia (diagnosed by electrocardiography [ECG] and/or transesophageal echocardiography) is most commonly observed during the immediate postoperative period and appears to be related to outcome.[22,23] Intraoperatively, initiation of CPB causes substantial increases in stress response hormones (norepinephrine, epinephrine, etc.) that persist into the immediate postoperative period and may contribute to myocardial ischemia observed during this time.[24–26] Furthermore, postoperative myocardial ischemia may be aggravated by cardiac sympathetic nerve activation, which disrupts the balance between coronary blood flow and myocardial oxygen demand.[27] Thus, during the pivotal immediate postoperative period after cardiac surgery, adequate analgesia (coupled with stress–response attenuation) may potentially decrease morbidity and enhance health-related quality of life.[27,28]

Evidence exists indicating that aggressive control of postoperative pain in patients after noncardiac surgery may beneficially affect outcome.[6,7] In 1987, Yeager et al,[7] in a small ($n = 53$ patients), randomized, controlled clinical trial involving patients undergoing major thoracic/vascular surgery, revealed that patients who were managed with more intense perioperative anesthesia and analgesia demonstrated decreased postoperative morbidity and improved operative outcome. In 1991, Tuman et al,[6] in another small ($n = 80$ patients), randomized, controlled clinical trial involving patients undergoing lower extremity revascularization, revealed that patients who were managed with more intense perioperative anesthesia and analgesia demonstrated improved outcome compared with patients receiving routine on-demand narcotic analgesia.

Evidence also exists that aggressive control of postoperative pain in patients after cardiac surgery may beneficially affect outcome. Two intriguing clinical investigations published in 1992 hint at such possibilities.[8,9] Mangano et al[8] prospectively randomized 106 adult patients undergoing elective CABG to receive either standard postoperative analgesia or intensive analgesia during the immediate postoperative period. Standard-care patients received low-dose intermittent intravenous morphine for the first 18 postoperative hours, whereas intensive-analgesia patients received a continuous intravenous sufentanil infusion during the same time period. Patients receiving sufentanil demonstrated a lesser severity of myocardial ischemia episodes (detected by continuous ECG monitoring) during the immediate postoperative period. The authors postulated that the administration of intensive analgesia during the immediate postoperative period may have more completely suppressed sympathetic nervous system activation, thereby having numerous beneficial clinical effects, including beneficial alterations in sensitivity of platelets to epinephrine, beneficial alterations in fibrinolysis, enhanced regional left ventricular function, and decreased coronary artery vasoconstriction, all potentially leading to a reduced incidence/severity of myocardial ischemia. Anand and Hickey[9] prospectively randomized 45 neonates undergoing elective cardiac surgery (mixed procedures) to receive either standard perioperative care or deep opioid anesthesia. Standard-care patients received a halothane/ketamine/morphine anesthetic with intermittent intravenous morphine for the first 24 postoperative hours, whereas deep-opioid patients received an intravenous sufentanil anesthetic with a continuous infusion of either intravenous fentanyl or intravenous sufentanil during the same postoperative time period. Neonates receiving continuous postoperative opioid infusions demonstrated a reduced perioperative stress response (assessed via multiple blood mediators), less perioperative morbidity (hyperglycemia, lactic acidemia, sepsis, metabolic acidosis, disseminated intravascular coagulation), and significantly fewer deaths than the control group (0/30 vs. 4/15, respectively; $p < 0.01$).

The accompanying editorial accurately summarizes this clinical investigation: "What Anand and Hickey have shown is that this reluctance to treat pain adequately is not a necessary evil. It markedly contributes to a bad outcome."[29] Unfortunately, aggressive control of postoperative pain in patients after cardiac surgery with relatively large amounts of intravenous opioids in this manner does not allow tracheal extubation in the immediate postoperative period (a goal of current practice).

TECHNIQUES AVAILABLE FOR POSTOPERATIVE ANALGESIA

Although the mechanisms of postoperative pain and the pharmacology of analgesic drugs are relatively well understood, the delivery of effective postoperative analgesia remains far from universal. Many techniques are available (see Table 38-1). In general, the American Society of Anesthesiologists Task Force on Acute Pain Management in the Perioperative Setting reports that the existing literature supports the efficacy and safety of three techniques used by anesthesiologists for perioperative pain control: regional analgesic techniques (including but not limited to intercostal blocks, plexus blocks, and local anesthetic infiltration of incisions), patient-controlled analgesia (PCA) with systemic opioids, and intrathecal/epidural opioid analgesia.[1] Regarding regional analgesic techniques, the existing literature supports the analgesic efficacy of peripheral nerve blocks and postincisional infiltration with local anesthetics for postoperative analgesia, yet is equivocal regarding the analgesic benefits of preincisional infiltration. Regarding PCA with systemic opioids, the existing literature supports its efficacy (compared with intramuscular techniques) for postoperative pain management, yet the existing literature is equivocal regarding the efficacy of PCA techniques compared with nurse- or staff-administered intravenous analgesia. In addition, the existing literature is equivocal regarding the comparative efficacy of epidural PCA versus intravenous PCA techniques.

When background opioid infusions are included with PCA techniques, patients report better analgesia and greater morphine consumption without increased incidence of nausea, vomiting, pruritus, or sedation. Although greater morphine consumption during PCA with continuous background infusion might predispose patients to respiratory depression, the existing literature is insufficient to reveal this potential adverse effect. Finally, regarding intrathecal and epidural opioid analgesia, the existing literature supports the efficacy of epidural morphine and fentanyl for perioperative analgesia but is insufficient to characterize the spectrum of risks and benefits associated with the use of other specific opioids given by these routes. Pruritus and urinary retention occur more frequently when morphine is given intrathecally or epidurally compared with systemic (intravenous or intramuscular) administration. Furthermore, epidural morphine provides more effective pain relief than intramuscular morphine. Similarly, epidural fentanyl provides more effective postoperative analgesia than intravenous fentanyl. The existing literature is insufficient to evaluate the effects of epidural techniques administered at different times (preincisional, postincisional, postoperative).

LOCAL ANESTHETIC INFILTRATION

Pain after cardiac surgery is often related to median sternotomy (peaking during the first 2 postoperative days). Because of problems associated with traditional intravenous opioid analgesia (nausea and vomiting, pruritus, urinary retention, respiratory depression) and the more recently introduced nonsteroidal anti-inflammatory drugs (NSAIDs) and cyclooxygenase (COX) inhibitors (gastrointestinal bleeding, renal dysfunction), alternative methods of achieving postoperative analgesia in cardiac surgical patients have been sought. One such alternative method that may hold promise is continuous infusion of local anesthetic (Box 38-3). In a prospective, randomized, placebo-controlled, double-blind clinical trial, White et al[30] studied 36 patients undergoing cardiac surgery. Intraoperative management was standardized. All patients had

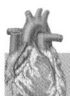

BOX 38-3. LOCAL ANESTHETIC INFILTRATION

- Advantage: Simple, reliable analgesia
- Disadvantage: Tissue necrosis?

two indwelling infusion catheters placed at the median sternotomy incision site at the end of surgery (one in the subfascial plane above the sternum, one above the fascia in the subcutaneous tissue). Patients received 0.25% bupivacaine (*n* = 12), 0.5% bupivacaine (*n* = 12), or normal saline (*n* = 12) via a constant-rate infusion through the catheter (4 mL/hr) for 48 hours after surgery. Average times to tracheal extubation were similar in the three groups (approximately 5 to 6 hours). Compared with the control group (normal saline), there was a statistically significant reduction in verbal rating scale pain scores and intravenous PCA morphine use in the 0.5% bupivacaine group. Patient satisfaction with their pain management was also improved in the 0.5% bupivacaine group (vs. control). However, there were no significant differences in PCA morphine use between the 0.25% bupivacaine and control groups. Although tracheal extubation time and the duration of the intensive care unit (ICU) stay (30 vs. 34 hours, respectively) were not significantly altered, time to ambulation (1 vs. 2 days, respectively) and duration of hospital stay (4.2 vs. 5.7 days, respectively) were lower in the 0.5% bupivacaine group than in the control group.

Serum bupivacaine concentrations in patients were reasonable, yet one complication related to the local anesthetic delivery system was encountered when a catheter tip was inadvertently broken off during its removal from the incision site, which required surgical reexploration of the wound under local anesthesia. The authors concluded that continuous infusion of 0.5% bupivacaine at 4 mL/hr is effective for decreasing postoperative pain and the need for postoperative supplemental opioid analgesic medication, as well as for improving patient satisfaction (earlier ambulation, reduced length of hospital stay) with pain management after cardiac surgery.

Another clinical investigation revealed the potential benefits of using a continuous infusion of local anesthetic in patients after cardiac surgery.[31] In this prospective, randomized, placebo-controlled, double-blind clinical trial, Dowling et al[31] studied 35 healthy patients undergoing cardiac surgery. Patients undergoing elective CABG via median sternotomy were randomized to either "ropivacaine" or "placebo" groups. At the end of the operation, before wound closure, bilateral intercostal nerve injections from T1 to T12 were performed using 20 mL of either 0.2% ropivacaine or normal saline. After sternal reapproximation with wires, two catheters with multiple side openings were placed anterior to the sternum (Figure 38-1). These catheters were connected to a pressurized elastomeric pump containing a flow regulator, which allowed for delivery of 0.2% ropivacaine or normal saline at approximately 4 mL/hr. The intraoperative anesthetic technique was standardized (short-acting anesthetics were used to minimize the presence of residual anesthetic agents in the postoperative period), as was postoperative pain management via intravenous PCA morphine (for 72 hours).

Both groups exhibited similar postoperative extubation times (approximately 8 hours). The sternal catheters were removed in both groups after 48 hours. Total mean PCA morphine consumption during the immediate postoperative period (72 hours) was significantly decreased in the ropivacaine group compared with the placebo group (47.3 vs. 78.7 mg, respectively; *p* = 0.038). Mean overall pain scores (scale ranging from 0 for no pain to 10 for maximum pain imaginable) also were significantly decreased in the ropivacaine group compared with the placebo group (1.6 vs. 2.6, respectively; *p* = 0.005). Most interestingly, patients receiving ropivacaine had a mean hospital length of stay of 5.2 ± 1.3 days compared with 8.2 ± 7.9 days for patients receiving normal saline, a difference that was statistically significant (*P* = 0.001). One patient in the placebo group had an extremely long postoperative hospitalization (39 days). However, the difference between the two groups regarding length of hospital stay remained statistically significant even if this outlier was removed (5.2 ± 1.3 days vs. 6.3 ± 2.8 days, respectively; *p* < 0.01). Despite differences in postoperative analgesia, postoperative pulmonary function (assessed via forced expiratory volume in 1 second and peak expiratory flow) was similar between the two groups. There was no difference in wound infections or wound healing between the two groups during hospitalization or after hospital discharge. No complications related to placement of the sternal wound catheters or performance of the intercostal nerve blocks were encountered.

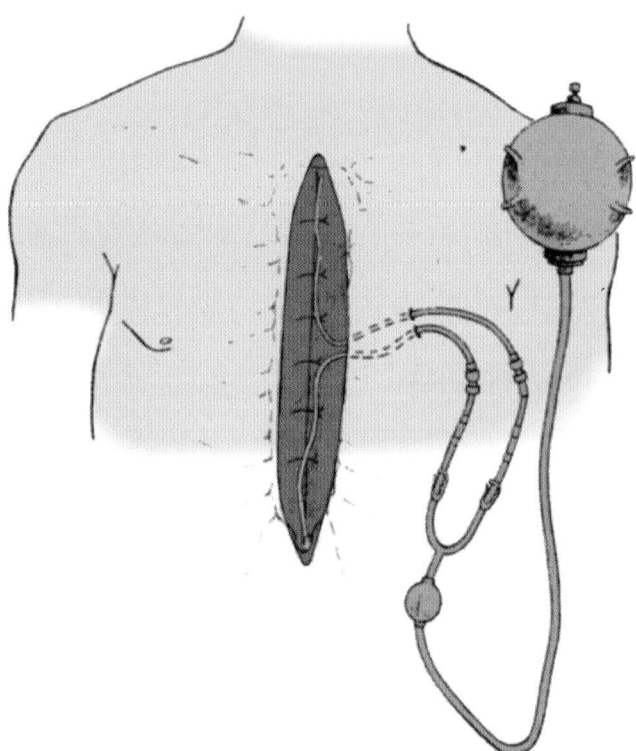

Figure 38-1 Intraoperative placement of the pressurized elastomeric pump and catheters. *(From Dowling R, Thielmeier K, Ghaly A, et al: Improved pain control after cardiac surgery: Results of a randomized, double-blind, clinical trial. J Thorac Cardiovasc Surg 126:1271, 2003.)*

The authors concluded that their analgesic technique significantly improves postoperative pain control while decreasing the amount of opioid analgesia required in patients subjected to standard median sternotomy. The significant decrease in hospital length of stay observed by the investigators is intriguing, may result in substantial cost reductions, and deserves further study.

The management of postoperative pain with continuous direct infusion of local anesthetic into the surgical wound has been described after a wide variety of surgeries other than cardiac (inguinal hernia repair, upper abdominal surgery, laparoscopic nephrectomy, cholecystectomy, knee arthroplasty, shoulder surgery, and gynecologic operative laparoscopy).[32] The infusion pump systems used for anesthetic wound perfusion are regulated by the U.S. Food and Drug Administration as medical devices. Thus, adverse events involving these infusion pump systems during direct local anesthetic infusion into surgical wounds are reported to this organization.

Complications encountered with these infusion pump systems reported to the U.S. Food and Drug Administration include tissue necrosis, surgical wound infection, and cellulitis after orthopedic, gastrointestinal, podiatric, and other surgeries. None of these reported adverse events has involved patients undergoing cardiac surgery. The most commonly reported complication is tissue necrosis, an adverse event almost never seen after normal surgical procedures. Furthermore, consequences of these reported adverse events were typically severe and required intervention and additional medical and/or surgical treatment. Although these initial reports may be isolated incidents, they may also represent an early warning that is representative of a problem that is widespread. Nevertheless, these reports provide a potentially important signal, suggesting the need for further investigation into the relation between use of these infusion pumps for direct continuous infusion of local anesthetics and other drugs into surgical wounds and tissue necrosis, serious infections, or cellulitis. Neither of the two clinical investigations involving local anesthetic infusion in patients after cardiac surgery with median sternotomy reported such wound complications.[30,31] Regardless, these safety issues merit careful consideration because of the importance of sternal wound complications in this setting.

The anterior and posterior branches of the intercostal nerves innervate the sternum. Parasternal infiltration of local anesthetic, therefore, is a possible means of improving postoperative analgesia. Although the use of parasternal blocks has not been extensively investigated, one small, prospective, randomized, placebo-controlled, double-blind clinical study indicated that parasternal block and local anesthetic infiltration of the sternotomy wound and mediastinal tube sites with local anesthetic may be a useful analgesic adjunct for patients who are expected to undergo early tracheal extubation after cardiac surgery.[33]

NERVE BLOCKS

With the increasing popularity of minimally invasive cardiac surgery, which uses nonsternotomy incisions (minithoracotomy), the use of nerve blocks for the management of postoperative pain has increased as well[34–39] (Box 38-4). Thoracotomy incisions (transverse anterolateral minithoracotomy, vertical anterolateral minithoracotomy), because of costal cartilage trauma tissue damage to ribs, muscles, or peripheral nerves, may induce more intense postoperative pain than that resulting from median sternotomy. Adequate analgesia after thoracotomy is important because pain is a key component in alteration of lung function after thoracic surgery. Uncontrolled pain causes a reduction in respiratory mechanics, reduced mobility, and increases in hormonal and metabolic activity. Perioperative deterioration in respiratory mechanics may lead to pulmonary complications and hypoxemia, which may, in turn, lead to myocardial ischemia/infarction, cerebrovascular accidents, thromboembolism, and delayed wound healing, leading to increased morbidity and prolonged hospital stay. Various analgesic techniques have been developed to treat postoperative thoracotomy pain. The most commonly used techniques include intercostal nerve blocks, intrapleural administration of local anesthetics, and thoracic paravertebral blocks. Intrathecal techniques and epidural techniques also are effective in controlling postthoracotomy pain and are covered in detail later in this chapter.

Intercostal nerve blocks have been used extensively for analgesia after thoracic surgery.[34–36] They can be performed either intraoperatively or postoperatively and usually provide sufficient analgesia lasting approximately 6 to 12 hours (depending on amount and type of local anesthetic used) and may need to be repeated if additional analgesia is required. Local anesthetics may be administered as a single treatment under direct vision, before chest closure, as a single preoperative percutaneous injection, as multiple percutaneous serial injections, or via an indwelling intercostal catheter. Blockade of intercostal nerves interrupts C-fiber afferent transmission of impulses to the spinal cord. A single intercostal injection of a long-acting local anesthetic can provide pain relief and improve pulmonary function in patients after thoracic surgery for up to 6 hours. A continuous extrapleural intercostal nerve block technique may be used in which a catheter is placed percutaneously into an extrapleural pocket by the surgeon to achieve longer duration of analgesia. A continuous intercostal catheter allows frequent dosing or infusions of local anesthetic agents and avoids multiple needle injections. Various clinical studies have confirmed the analgesic efficacy of this technique, and the technique compares favorably with thoracic epidural analgesic techniques.[34] A major concern associated with intercostal nerve block is the potentially high amount of local anesthetic systemic absorption, yet multiple clinical studies

involving patients undergoing thoracic surgery have documented safe blood levels with standard techniques. Clinical investigations involving patients undergoing thoracic surgery indicate that intercostal nerve blockade by intermittent or continuous infusion of 0.5% bupivacaine with epinephrine is an effective method, as is continuous infusion of 0.25% bupivacaine through indwelling intercostal catheters for supplementing systemic intravenous opioid analgesia for postthoracotomy pain. The value of single preclosure injections remains doubtful.

Intrapleural administration of local anesthetics initiates analgesia via mechanisms that remain incompletely understood. However, the mechanism of action of extrapleural regional anesthesia seems to depend primarily on diffusion of the local anesthetic into the paravertebral region. Local anesthetic agents then affect not only the ventral nerve root but also afferent fibers of the posterior primary ramus. Posterior ligaments of the posterior primary ramus innervate posterior spinal muscles and skin and are traumatized during posterolateral thoracotomy. Intrapleural administration of local anesthetic agent to this region through a catheter inserted in the extrapleural space thus creates an anesthetic region in the skin. The depth and width of the anesthetic region depend on diffusion of the local anesthetic agent in the extrapleural space. With this technique, local anesthetics may be administered via an indwelling intrapleural catheter placed between the parietal and visceral pleura by intermittent or continuous infusion regimens. Concerns regarding systemic absorption of local anesthetic and toxicity are always a concern with this technique, yet have not been substantiated in clinical studies that assayed plasma levels. A handful of clinical investigations involving patients undergoing thoracic surgery via thoracotomy incision suggests that 0.25% to 0.5% bupivacaine may improve analgesia in patients after thoracic surgery, yet its true efficacy as a postoperative analgesic in this patient population remains somewhat controversial.[37] The analgesic benefits are of short duration and there does not appear to be a significant overall opioid-sparing effect. Furthermore, the optimum concentration and duration regimen remains to be defined. However, a prospective, randomized, clinical study involving 50 patients undergoing minimally invasive direct CABG (via minithoracotomy) indicated that an intrapleural analgesic technique (with 0.25% bupivacaine) is safe, effective, and compares favorably (provided superior postoperative analgesia) with a conventional thoracic epidural technique.[38] These investigators noted, however, that careful catheter positioning, chest tube clamping, and anchoring of the catheter are mandatory for postoperative intrapleural analgesia to be effective. A major factor implicated in lack of efficacy regarding intrapleural techniques is loss of local anesthetic solution through intercostal chest drainage tubes. Although clamping the chest tubes during the postoperative period will increase analgesic efficacy, it may not be safe to clamp chest tubes because they provide important drainage of hemorrhage and air and allow for enhanced lung patency and expansion. Apart from proper catheter positioning (insertion of catheter under direct vision and anchoring catheter to skin are essential), effective analgesia with this technique also appears to depend on whether lung surgery is performed or whether the pleural anatomy and physiology are relatively intact.

Thoracic paravertebral block involves injection of local anesthetic adjacent to the thoracic vertebrae close to where the spinal nerves emerge from the intervertebral foramina (Figure 38-2). Thoracic paravertebral block, compared with thoracic epidural analgesic techniques, appears to provide equivalent analgesia, is technically easier, and may harbor less risk. Several different techniques exist for successful thoracic paravertebral block and recently have been extensively reviewed.[35] The classic technique, most commonly used, involves eliciting loss of resistance. Injection of local anesthetic results in ipsilateral somatic and sympathetic nerve blockade in multiple contiguous thoracic dermatomes above and below the site of injection (together with possible suppression of the neuroendocrine stress response to surgery). These blocks may be effective in alleviating acute and chronic pain of unilateral origin from the chest, abdomen, or both. Bilateral use of thoracic paravertebral block also has been described. Continuous thoracic paravertebral infusion of local anesthetic via a catheter placed under direct

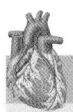

BOX 38-4. NERVE BLOCKS

- Advantage: Simple, long-lasting analgesia
- Disadvantage: Unreliable?

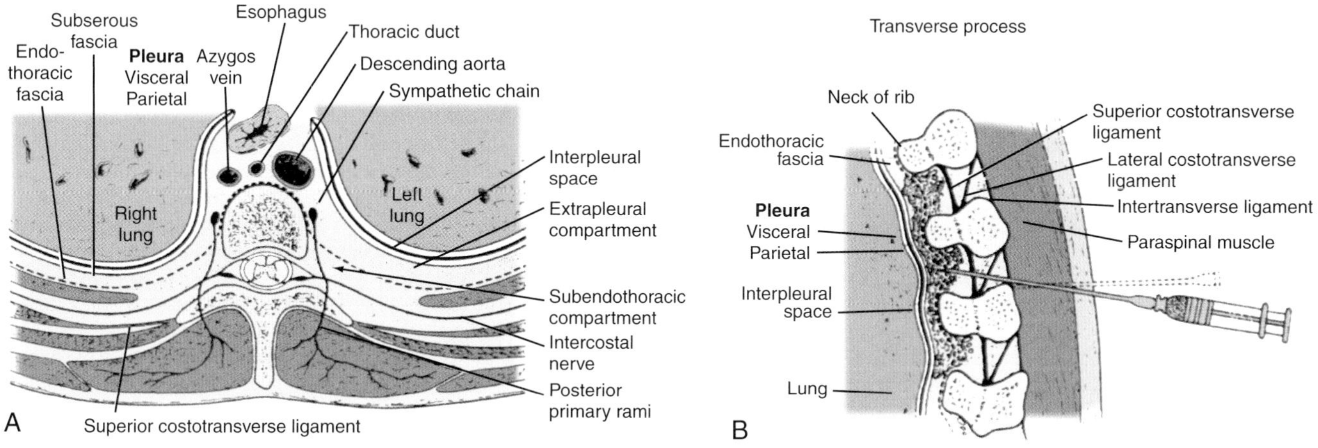

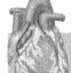

Figure 38-2 Anatomy of the thoracic paravertebral space *(A)* and sagittal section through the thoracic paravertebral space showing a needle that has been advanced above the transverse process *(B)*. *(From Karmakar MK: Thoracic paravertebral block [review article]. Anesthesiology 95:771, 2001.)*

vision at thoracotomy is also a safe, simple, and effective method of providing analgesia after thoracotomy. It is usually used in conjunction with adjunct intravenous medications (opioid or other analgesics) to provide optimum relief after thoracotomy.

Although supplemental intravenous analgesics are usually required, opioid requirements are substantially reduced. Unilateral paravertebral block is useful for attaining post-thoracotomy analgesia because pain after lateral thoracotomy is essentially always unilateral. The role of bilateral thoracic paravertebral block remains to be defined. The benefits of unilateral paravertebral blockade are a lesser incidence of adverse events (hypotension, urinary retention) and a decreased risk for systemic local anesthetic toxicity because less local anesthetic is used. Few clinical investigations involve unilateral paravertebral block in patients undergoing thoracic surgery. Therefore, it is not possible to determine from the available literature whether the technique of paravertebral blockade (single injection) is truly useful in the postoperative analgesic management of patients after thoracotomy. However, continuous thoracic paravertebral block, as part of a balanced analgesic regimen, may provide effective pain relief with few adverse effects after thoracotomy and appears to be comparable with thoracic epidural analgesia.[35]

Intercostal nerve blocks, intrapleural administration of local anesthetics, and thoracic paravertebral blocks offer the advantages of simplicity and efficacy in controlling postoperative pain in patients after thoracic surgery. However, although analgesic efficacy of these techniques sometimes is comparable with intrathecal techniques and epidural techniques, these techniques appear to work best as a part of a multimodal analgesic regimen (supplementing other analgesic techniques). Complications associated with infiltrations of large quantities of local anesthetic (often required) are always a concern when utilizing these analgesic techniques.

For a wide variety of reasons (increased use of small thoracic incisions by cardiac surgeons, etc.), the last decade has seen a resurgence of nerve blocks (usually catheter-based techniques) in patients undergoing cardiac surgery. Specifically, recent clinical studies using intercostal catheters,[40] intrapleural catheters,[41,42] and paravertebral blockade[43,44] indicate that these techniques may have unique advantages, even when compared with traditional intrathecal/epidural techniques.[45–47]

OPIOIDS

Beginning in the 1960s (and continuing for essentially 30 years), large doses of intravenous opioids (starting with morphine) have been administered to patients undergoing cardiac surgery[48,49] (Box 38-5). Because even very large amounts of intravenous opioids do not initiate "complete anesthesia" (unconsciousness, muscle relaxation, suppression of reflex responses to noxious surgical stimuli), other intravenous/

> **BOX 38-5 OPIOIDS**
>
> - Advantage:
>   - Time-tested, reliable analgesia
> - Disadvantages:
>   - Pruritus
>   - Nausea and vomiting
>   - Urinary retention
>   - Respiratory depression

inhalation agents must be administered during the intraoperative period.[50] Analgesia is the best known and most extensively investigated opioid effect, yet opioids also are involved in a diverse array of other physiologic functions, including control of pituitary and adrenal medulla hormone release and activity, control of cardiovascular and gastrointestinal function, and in the regulation of respiration, mood, appetite, thirst, cell growth, and the immune system.[51] A number of well-known and potential side effects of opioids (nausea and vomiting, pruritus, urinary retention, respiratory depression) may limit postoperative recovery when they are used for postoperative analgesia.

Opioids interact with specific receptors that are widely distributed within the CNS to produce a variety of pharmacologic effects. Currently, three distinct opioid-receptor types are recognized: μ, κ, and δ. The μ receptor has two subtypes: a high-affinity μ_1 receptor and a low-affinity μ_2 receptor. The supraspinal mechanisms of analgesia are thought to involve μ_1 receptors, whereas spinal analgesia, respiratory depression, and gastrointestinal effects are associated with the μ_2 receptor. Other subtypes of the μ receptor have been isolated, yet their clinical relevance remains to be elucidated. Likewise, subtypes of the κ and δ receptors also have been isolated. Selective κ-agonists may have therapeutic potential as analgesics, lacking the adverse side effects produced by the current μ-receptor agonists. δ_1-Receptors appear to mediate spinal analgesia, whereas δ_2-receptors appear to mediate supraspinal analgesia. Unfortunately, despite extensive pharmacologic and functional studies of the wide variety of opioid receptors, understanding of the structural basis of their actions remains quite limited.

The classic pharmacologic effect of opioids is analgesia, and these drugs have traditionally been the initial choice when a potent postoperative analgesic is required. Two anatomically distinct sites exist for opioid receptor–mediated analgesia: supraspinal and spinal. Systemically administered opioids produce analgesia at both sites. Supraspinally, the μ_1 receptor is primarily involved in analgesia, whereas the μ_2 receptor is the one predominantly involved in the spinal modulation of nociceptive processing. κ receptors are important in mediating spinal and supraspinal analgesia as well. δ ligands may have a modulatory rather than a primary analgesic role. All three types of opioid receptors (μ,κ, and δ) have been demonstrated in peripheral terminals of sensory nerves. Activation of these receptors seems to require an inflammatory reaction because locally applied opioids do not produce analgesia in healthy tissue. The inflammatory process also may activate previously inactive opioid receptors.

Although nausea and vomiting, pruritus, and urinary retention are more commonly encountered, respiratory depression remains the most feared complication associated with use of opioids. All μ-receptor agonist opioids produce dose-related respiratory depression, which appears to be mediated via $μ_2$ receptors. Pure κ agonists have little effect on respiration, and the role of δ receptors in respiratory control remains to be elucidated. The primary respiratory effect of opioids is a reduction in the sensitivity of the respiratory center to carbon dioxide (together with depression of both medullary and peripheral chemoreceptors). Initially, respiratory rate is affected more than tidal volume, which may even increase. With increasing doses of opioids, respiratory rhythmicity is disturbed, resulting in the irregular gasping breathing characteristic of opioid overdose. In addition to retention of carbon dioxide, respiratory depression also may result in hypoxia (the hypoxic drive to ventilation is depressed by the opioids as well). Elderly patients seem to be more sensitive to the respiratory depressant effects of opioids than younger patients, and the dose used needs to be adjusted accordingly. It also is important to keep in mind that all other CNS depressants, such as benzodiazepines, barbiturates, and/or inhalation anesthetics, will potentiate the respiratory depressant effects of the opioids. Furthermore, in addition to the parent opioid drug, metabolites may, in some circumstances, contribute to respiratory depression. For instance, metabolites of morphine (morphine-6-β-glucuronide) may occur in substantial quantities after intravenous administration and may be responsible for a considerable proportion of the clinical effects of intravenous morphine.

Morphine is the prototype opioid agonist with which all opioids are compared. Morphine is perhaps the most popular analgesic used in patients after cardiac surgery. Many semisynthetic derivatives are made by simple modifications of the morphine molecule. Morphine is poorly lipid soluble and binds approximately 35% to plasma proteins, particularly albumin. Morphine is primarily metabolized in the liver, principally by conjugation to water-soluble glucuronides. The liver is the predominant site for morphine biotransformation, although extrahepatic metabolism also occurs in the kidney, brain, and possibly gut. Extrahepatic clearance accounts for approximately 30% of the total body clearance. The terminal elimination half-life of morphine is on the order of 2 to 3 hours. In patients with liver cirrhosis, morphine pharmacokinetics are variable, probably reflecting the variability of liver disease in patients. Morphine's terminal elimination half-life in patients with renal disease is comparable with that of normal patients. Although morphine is perhaps the most popular intravenous analgesic used in patients after cardiac surgery, other synthetically derived opioids have been developed and may be used as well. These include fentanyl, alfentanil, sufentanil, and remifentanil.

Fentanyl is considerably more potent (60 to 80 times) than morphine. However, at the opioid receptor, the intrinsic affinities of fentanyl and morphine differ by only a factor of 2 to 3. The differences between receptor affinities and clinical potency ratios arise from differing physiochemical and pharmacokinetic properties of the drugs (in particular, the differences in lipid solubility). Fentanyl is highly lipid soluble, which influences rate of entry and exit to and from organs and tissues, especially the CNS, which has a high lipid content.

Fentanyl is rapidly transferred across the blood–brain barrier, resulting in a rapid onset of action after intravenous injection. The relative potential for entering the CNS is approximately 150 times greater for fentanyl than for morphine. However, the large quantities of fentanyl taken up by adipose tissues may act as a reservoir (depending on dosage amounts) that slowly releases fentanyl back into the circulation when plasma concentrations decline to less than that in fat. This slow reentry may serve to maintain the plasma concentration and is one factor in the relatively long plasma terminal elimination half-life of fentanyl. Fentanyl is rapidly and extensively metabolized by the liver to inactive metabolites. After bolus intravenous injection, plasma fentanyl concentrations decrease rapidly because of distribution from the plasma to tissues, so that after moderate (10 μg/kg) doses, fentanyl has a short duration of action (see Chapter 9).

Larger doses convert fentanyl from a short-acting to a long-acting drug. With increased doses, the distribution phase is completed before the fentanyl concentration declines to threshold levels, so duration of action becomes dependent on the decrease in concentration during the much slower elimination phase. Thus, to avoid accumulation of fentanyl, successive doses at regular intervals should be progressively reduced in amount, or the interval between doses of the same size should be progressively lengthened. When fentanyl is given by continuous intravenous infusion, the rate of decline of fentanyl plasma concentration is markedly dependent on the duration of the infusion. Fentanyl undergoes substantial first-pass uptake in the lungs (approximately 80% of the injected dose). Hepatic extraction of fentanyl is also high, making its clearance dependent on liver blood flow. Thus, factors that reduce liver blood flow also will decrease fentanyl clearance. It is likely that fentanyl metabolites accumulate in patients with impaired renal function, yet this is unlikely to have clinical consequences because they are pharmacologically inactive. Because the liver is the principal organ for fentanyl biotransformation, decreases in hepatic function caused by liver disease will be expected to alter fentanyl pharmacokinetics.

The popularity of fentanyl as an intraoperative analgesic agent relates directly to the cardiovascular stability it provides, even in critically ill patients. Also, its analgesic efficacy relative to the intensity of side effects has prompted much interest in its use as an analgesic after surgery and/or in critically ill patients.[52] Fentanyl (as well as any opioid) can be administered intravenously for postoperative analgesia in many ways: using a loading dose with a continuous fixed or variable infusion, a fixed background infusion with PCA, or PCA alone. An intravenous bolus of 1 to 2 μg/kg usually is administered before initiating an infusion. If variable, the infusion rate is usually 1 to 2 μg/kg/hr and may be adjusted upward or downward as required by fluctuations in analgesic requirements or appearance of side effects. Before the infusion rate is increased, small intravenous bolus doses of fentanyl may be administered. Infusion rates of 1.5 to 2.5 μg/kg/hr usually provide good-to-excellent postoperative analgesia. At rest, the quality of analgesia remains stable; however, with movement, analgesia may not be sufficient, even with greater infusion rates.

A background low-dose intravenous infusion of fentanyl may be combined with PCA to provide satisfactory analgesia with potentially fewer adverse effects. PCA bolus doses typically range from 5 to 50 μg, and background infusion rates may be fixed (ranging from 5 to 50 μg/hr) or be variable (adjusted up and down according to clinical criteria). Generally, the larger the background infusion rate, the smaller the PCA bolus dose. Lockout intervals (minimum time period between doses) range from "on demand" (no lockout) to 15 minutes, the most common interval being 1 to 5 minutes. The technique of using a background infusion plus PCA produces excellent postoperative analgesia. Fentanyl is rarely used alone for PCA because of its brief duration of action. The most commonly administered opioid used in this manner (PCA alone) remains morphine. Transdermal delivery of fentanyl also has been investigated extensively. This modality is simple, noninvasive, and allows continuous release of fentanyl into the systemic circulation. However, the steady release of fentanyl in such a manner does not allow flexibility in dose adjustment, which may result in inadequate treatment of postoperative pain during rapidly changing intensity. Thus, intravenous opioids often are necessary to supplement analgesia when transdermal fentanyl is used to manage acute postoperative pain.

Alfentanil is about 5 to 10 times less potent than fentanyl. The drug acts rapidly; peak effect being reached within minutes after intravenous administration. Its duration of action after bolus administration also is shorter than fentanyl. Alfentanil is highly lipid soluble (about 100 times more lipid soluble than morphine) and rapidly crosses the blood–brain barrier. Alfentanil pharmacokinetics are minimally affected by renal disease, and hepatic extraction is more a function of intrinsic hepatic enzyme capacity and protein binding than liver blood flow.

The performance of a patient-demand, target-controlled alfentanil infusion system has compared favorably with traditional morphine PCA in patients after cardiac surgery.[53] Checketts et al[53] prospectively randomized 120 patients undergoing elective cardiac surgery to receive either morphine PCA or alfentanil PCA for postoperative analgesia (nonblinded). All patients received a similar standardized intraoperative anesthetic technique and were extubated during the immediate postoperative period. Overall median visual analog pain scores were significantly lower in patients receiving alfentanil, yet both alfentanil and morphine delivered high-quality postoperative analgesia (Figure 38-3). Although the clinical impression by these investigators was that alfentanil patients were less sedated in the immediate postoperative period, this clinical observation was not substantiated after statistical analysis of sedation scores. The two groups did not differ with respect to overall sedation scores, frequency of nausea and vomiting, hemodynamic instability, myocardial ischemia, or hypoxemia during the immediate postoperative period.

Sufentanil is approximately 10 times more potent than fentanyl. The drug is extremely lipid soluble and highly bound to plasma proteins. Because of its high potency, conventional clinical doses of sufentanil result in plasma concentrations that rapidly decline to less than the sensitivity of most assay methods, making it difficult to determine accurate pharmacokinetic parameters. However, sufentanil pharmacokinetics appear not to be altered in patients with renal disease. Because hepatic sufentanil clearance approaches liver blood flow, it is expected that the drug's pharmacokinetics would change with hepatic disease, yet the clinical relevance remains undetermined. Sufentanil undergoes substantial (approximately 60%) first-pass uptake in the lungs.

Remifentanil has a very fast onset and an ultrashort duration of action, and is unique in that it is readily susceptible to rapid hydrolysis by nonspecific esterases in the blood and tissues. Remifentanil is moderately lipophilic and is half as potent as fentanyl when blood concentrations causing equivalent analgesia are compared. Remifentanil has an elimination half-life of 10 to 20 minutes. The time required for a 50% reduction in blood concentration after discontinuation of an infusion that has attained steady state is about 3 minutes and does not increase with duration of infusion. Available evidence suggests that

neither pharmacokinetics nor pharmacodynamics of remifentanil is significantly altered in patients with severe hepatic or renal disease. These properties should confer ease of titration to changing analgesic conditions. However, the quick offset of action, although desirable, may result in inadequate postoperative analgesia. Because of the rapid offset of effect of remifentanil, the continued requirement for postoperative analgesia needs to be considered before the remifentanil is discontinued. A transition must be made from remifentanil to some other longer-acting analgesic for substantial postoperative pain. Although the transition to postoperative pain management can be made using a remifentanil infusion alone, this appears to be associated with a high incidence of adverse respiratory effects.

In 1996, Bowdle et al[54] evaluated the use of a remifentanil infusion to provide postoperative analgesia during recovery from total intravenous anesthesia with remifentanil and propofol from a wide variety of noncardiac surgeries (abdominal, spine, joint replacement, thoracic surgery). This multi-institutional study involving 157 patients had a detailed protocol that specified doses and method of administration of all anesthetic drugs. In essence, total intraoperative intravenous anesthesia consisted of midazolam (premedication only), remifentanil, propofol, and vecuronium. Propofol was stopped immediately before intraoperative extubation, and the remifentanil infusion was continued for postoperative analgesia. During the immediate postoperative period, intravenous morphine was administered during tapering of remifentanil infusion. Adverse respiratory events (oxygen saturation via pulse oximetry < 90%, respiratory rate less than 12 per minute, apnea) affected 45 patients (29%, 2 required naloxone). Apnea occurred in 11 patients (7% treated with mask ventilation and downward titration of remifentanil infusion; 1 required naloxone). The administration of a bolus of remifentanil preceded the onset of adverse respiratory events in 19 of 45 cases and in 9 of 11 cases of apnea.

These data suggest that remifentanil boluses plus an infusion are particularly likely to produce clinically significant adverse respiratory events. The authors of this open, dose-ranging study concluded that although remifentanil certainly initiates analgesia, its use in the immediate postoperative period may pose dangers. Additional studies are needed to investigate the transition from remifentanil to longer-lasting analgesics and to refine strategies that minimize respiratory depression whereas optimizing pain control. The administration of a potent, rapidly acting opioid such as remifentanil by continuous infusion for postoperative analgesia must be performed with meticulous attention to detail and constant vigilance. Extreme caution should be exercised in the postoperative administration of bolus doses of remifentanil because substantial respiratory depression (including apnea) may develop. Furthermore, the remifentanil infusion should be inserted into the intravenous line as close as possible to the patient to minimize dead space, and the rate of the main intravenous infusion should be controlled at a rate that is high enough to continuously flush remifentanil from the tubing. A more dilute remifentanil solution that would run at greater rates (on a volume per time basis) would help to minimize the effect of variations in flow rate of the main intravenous tubing on delivery of remifentanil to the patient. Remifentanil also may possess detrimental cardiovascular effects via bradycardia and decreases in systemic vascular resistance, leading to decreased cardiac output and hypotension.[55] Such changes may occur during clinically utilized doses for cardiac surgery (0.1 to 1.0 μg/kg/min), inducing significant cardiovascular disturbances that are potentially deleterious to patients with cardiac disease.[55]

PATIENT-CONTROLLED ANALGESIA

When intravenous opioids are used for controlling postoperative pain (most commonly morphine and fentanyl), PCA technology generally is used. Essentials in the successful use of PCA technology include "loading" the patient with intravenous opioids to the point of patient comfort before initiating PCA, ensuring that the patient wants to control analgesic treatment, using an appropriate PCA dose and lockout

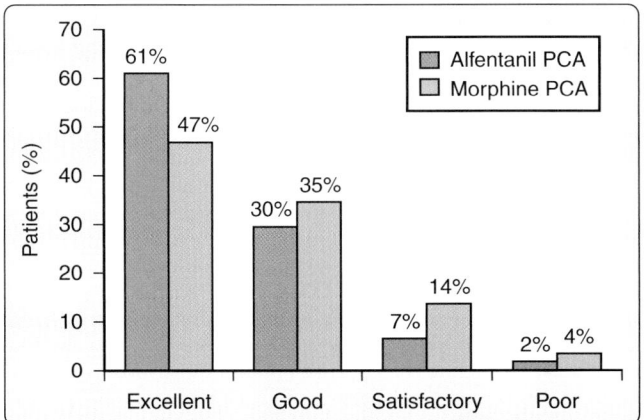

Figure 38-3 **Overall patient satisfaction with postoperative analgesia.** Ninety-one percent of patients using alfentanil rated their postoperative analgesia as excellent or good, whereas 82% of patients using morphine rated their postoperative analgesia similarly (differences not statistically significant). PCA, patient-controlled analgesia. (*From Checketts MR, Gilhooly CJ, Kenny GNC: Patient-maintained analgesia with target-controlled alfentanil infusion after cardiac surgery: A comparison with morphine PCA. Br J Anaesth 80:748, 1998 ©The Board of Management and Trustees of the British Journal of Anaesthesia, by permission of Oxford University Press/British Journal of Anaesthesia.*)

interval, and considering the use of a basal rate infusion. Focused guidance of PCA dosing by a dedicated acute pain service, compared with surgeon-directed PCA, may result in more effective analgesia with fewer adverse effects. Patient-controlled epidural analgesic techniques, with opioids and/or local anesthetics, also have been proved reliable, effective, and safe.[56,57]

Although PCA is a well-established technique (used for more than two decades) and offers potential unique benefits (reliable analgesic effect, improved patient autonomy, flexible adjustment to individual needs, etc.), whether it truly offers significant clinical advantages (compared with traditional nurse-administered analgesic techniques) to patients immediately after cardiac surgery remains to be determined.[58-63] A clinical investigation by Gust et al[59] indicated that PCA techniques provide a higher quality of postoperative analgesia, which may lead to a reduction in postoperative respiratory complications. In this prospective, randomized, clinical investigation involving 120 healthy patients after extubation after elective CABG, patients received either intravenous PCA piritramide, intravenous PCA piritramide plus rectal indomethacin, or conventional nurse-controlled analgesia with intravenous piritramide and/or rectal indomethacin for 3 days. Postoperative assessment included daily visual analog pain scoring and chest radiographs graded for the extent of atelectasis by a radiologist blinded to treatment. Perioperative management (surgical treatment, intraoperative anesthetic management) was standardized. Although chest radiography atelectasis scores and visual analog pain score values were similar among the three groups on the first and second postoperative days, on the third postoperative day, chest radiography atelectasis scores and visual analog pain score values were significantly better in the two PCA groups compared with the control (nurse-controlled analgesia) group.

At the end of the study, all patients retrospectively graded their postoperative pain management on average as good, but significantly more patients in the two PCA groups assessed their pain management as excellent compared with the control group. These investigators concluded that treatment with PCA may reduce respiratory complications in patients after CABG. However, no difference was observed regarding perioperative oxygenation values among the three groups during the entire study period, and not a single patient in any group met prospectively defined criteria for diagnosis of pneumonia. Other clinical investigations also have indicated that PCA techniques, compared with standard nurse-based pain therapy, may provide higher quality analgesia leading to reduced cardiopulmonary morbidity after cardiac surgery.[60,63]

Despite the popularity of PCA techniques and the results of the earlier quoted studies, other clinical investigations demonstrated no major benefits offered.[58,61,62] Tsang and Brush[58] prospectively evaluated 69 patients after cardiac surgery via median sternotomy. Thirty-nine were randomized to receive PCA morphine after surgery, whereas 30 were randomized to receive nurse-administered morphine after surgery. Perioperative care was standardized, visual analog pain scores were used for pain assessment, and pulmonary function tests were performed before surgery and every 6 hours after surgery until discharge from the ICU. These clinical investigators found no difference between the two groups regarding postoperative morphine consumption (Figure 38-4), postoperative visual analog pain scores, postoperative sedation scores, and postoperative pulmonary function (Figure 38-5). These investigators concluded that there are no significant advantages achieved when using PCA routinely in patients after cardiac surgery. Interestingly, in this study, opinions expressed by the nursing staff on the use of PCA were not as positive as expected (repetition of PCA instruction to patients was often required during the study period). Potential reasons for required repeated instructions on PCA include poor retention of preoperative learning because of anxiety after hospital admission, incomplete recovery of higher cognitive function after prolonged general anesthesia and CPB, and/or ICU-induced disorientation.

These results suggest that there may be additional patient limitations to the effective use of PCA immediately after cardiac surgery even

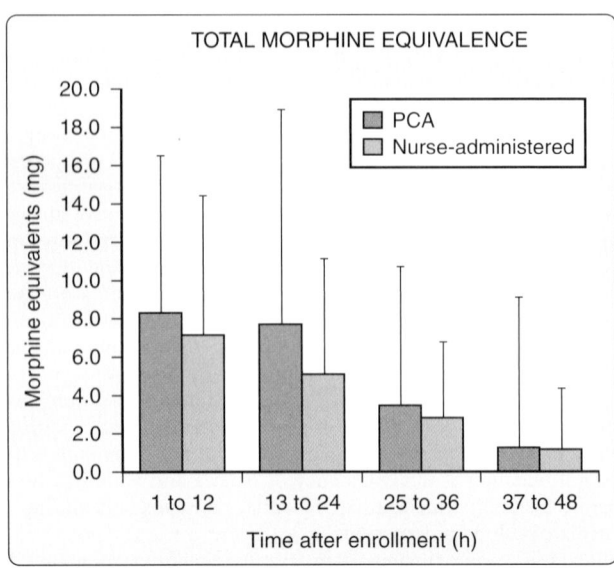

Figure 38-4 **Total morphine equivalents.** Dosages of morphine equivalents in the patient-controlled analgesia (PCA) nurse-administered groups during each observation period. No differences existed between the two groups at any observation period. (*From Tsang J, Brush B: Patient-controlled analgesia in postoperative cardiac surgery.* Anaesth Intensive Care 27:464, 1999.)

though patients can obey simple commands and acknowledge discomfort. Munro and associates,[61] when comparing intravenous PCA morphine and nurse-administered subcutaneous morphine, detailed similar findings. They prospectively randomized 92 patients undergoing elective cardiac surgery to receive either intravenous PCA morphine or nurse-administered subcutaneous morphine during the postoperative period. They found no differences between the two groups regarding many postoperative variables, including total postoperative morphine requirements, postoperative visual analog pain scores at rest and with movement, daily verbal pain relief scores, side effect profiles, and physiotherapist's evaluation of effectiveness of analgesia for chest physiotherapy. Subcutaneous techniques are attractive because they have low equipment and disposable costs, eliminate the need for bulky pumps in ambulating patients, and may be more effective for the elderly or mildly confused postoperative patient.

Myles et al[62] also were unable to find any specific clinical benefits during use of PCA techniques in patients after cardiac surgery. In their prospective clinical investigation, 72 patients undergoing elective cardiac surgery were randomized to receive either intravenous PCA morphine or intravenous nurse-titrated morphine during the immediate postoperative period. They found no differences between the two groups regarding many postoperative variables, including postoperative morphine consumption, postoperative pain scores, postoperative nausea scores, and postoperative serum cortisol levels (Figure 38-6). Much like Munro and associates, they noted that patients also had variable ability and understanding of the requirements of PCA, particularly in the early postoperative period when they were confused or too weak to operate the demand button. These investigators also noted that overall pain management in their patients was optimized by receiving experienced one-to-one nursing care (other studies evaluating PCA also have found that nurse-administered techniques may provide the highest quality analgesia). It could, therefore, be argued that these studies support increased staff education and involvement to optimize postoperative analgesia. The nurses in these clinical investigations all raised concerns regarding the time required for PCA setup and the inability of patients to cope with the demands of PCA in the early stages of their recovery, particularly if elderly, confused, or both. However, PCA was well received later in the recovery process and was found to be less demanding on nursing time.

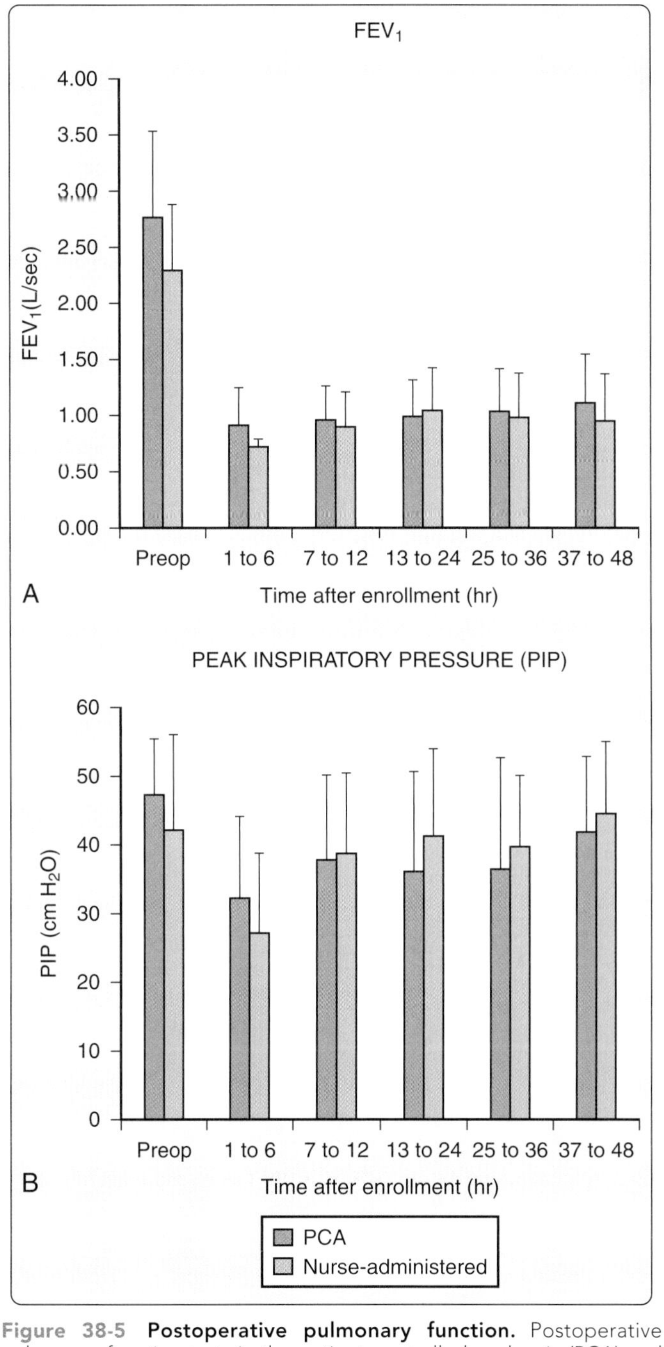

FEV1
4.00
3.50
3.00
2.50
2.00
1.50
1.00
0.50
0.00
FEV1(L/sec)
Preop
1 to 6
7 to 12
13 to 24
25 to 36
37 to 48
A
Time after enrollment (hr)
PEAK INSPIRATORY PRESSURE (PIP)
60
50
40
30
20
10
0
PIP (cm H2O)
Preop
1 to 6
7 to 12
13 to 24
25 to 36
37 to 48
B
Time after enrollment (hr)
PCA
Nurse-administered

Figure 38-5 Postoperative pulmonary function. Postoperative pulmonary function tests in the patient-controlled analgesia (PCA) and nurse-administered groups during each observation period. A significant decrease in forced expiratory volume in 1 second (FEV_1) in both groups was observed immediately after surgery (and lasting 48 hours). No differences existed between the two groups at any observation period. *(From Tsang J, Brush B: Patient-controlled analgesia in postoperative cardiac surgery.* Anaesth Intensive Care *27:464, 1999.)*

1200
1000
800
600
400
200
0
Serum cortisol (nmol/L)
PCA
STD
24 hr
48 hr
Time after CPB

Figure 38-6 Postoperative serum cortisol. Mean serum cortisol level at 24 and 48 hours after cardiopulmonary bypass (CPB) for patients receiving intravenous patient-controlled analgesia (PCA) morphine or intravenous nurse-titrated morphine (STD). *(From Myles PS, Buckland MR, Cannon GB, et al: Comparison of patient-controlled analgesia and nurse-controlled infusion analgesia after cardiac surgery.* Anaesth Intensive Care *22:672, 1994.)*

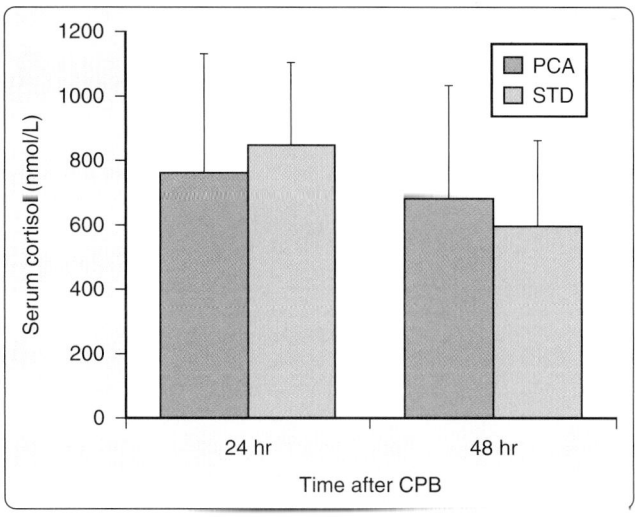

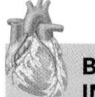

BOX 38-6. NONSTEROIDAL ANTI-INFLAMMATORY AGENTS

- Advantage:
  - Opioid-sparing, reliable analgesia
- Disadvantages:
  - Gastric mucosal dysfunction?
  - Renal tubular dysfunction?
  - Inhibition of platelet aggregation?
  - Sternal wound infection?
  - Thromboembolic complications?

NONSTEROIDAL ANTI-INFLAMMATORY AGENTS

NSAIDs, in contrast with the opioids' CNS mechanism of action, mainly exert their analgesic, antipyretic, and anti-inflammatory effects peripherally by interfering with prostaglandin synthesis after tissue injury[64,65] (Box 38-6). NSAIDs inhibit COX, the enzyme responsible for the conversion of arachidonic acid to prostaglandin (Figure 38-7). Combining NSAIDs with traditional intravenous opioids may allow a patient to achieve an adequate level of analgesia with fewer side effects than if a similar level of analgesia was obtained with intravenous opioids alone. Numerous clinical investigations reveal the potential value (opioid-sparing effects) of NSAIDs when combined with traditional intravenous opioids during the postoperative period after noncardiac surgery. In fact, the administration of NSAIDs is one of the most common nonopioid analgesic techniques currently used for postoperative pain management. The efficacy of NSAIDs for postoperative pain has been demonstrated repeatedly in many analgesic clinical trials. Unlike opioids, which preferentially reduce spontaneous postoperative pain, NSAIDs have comparable efficacy for both spontaneous and movement-evoked pain, the latter of which may be more important in causing postoperative physiologic impairment. Certainly, NSAIDs reduce postoperative opioid consumption, accelerate postoperative recovery, and represent an integral component of balanced postoperative analgesic regimens after noncardiac surgery. However, little is known regarding NSAID use in the management of pain after cardiac surgery. It is likely that concerns regarding NSAID side effects, including alterations in the gastric mucosal barrier, renal tubular function, and inhibition of platelet aggregation, have made clinicians reluctant to use NSAIDs in patients undergoing cardiac surgery. Other rare adverse effects of NSAIDs (from COX inhibition) include hepatocellular injury, asthma exacerbation, anaphylactoid reactions, tinnitus, and urticaria. Despite these fears, a small number of clinical investigations seem to indicate that NSAIDs may provide analgesia in patients after cardiac surgery

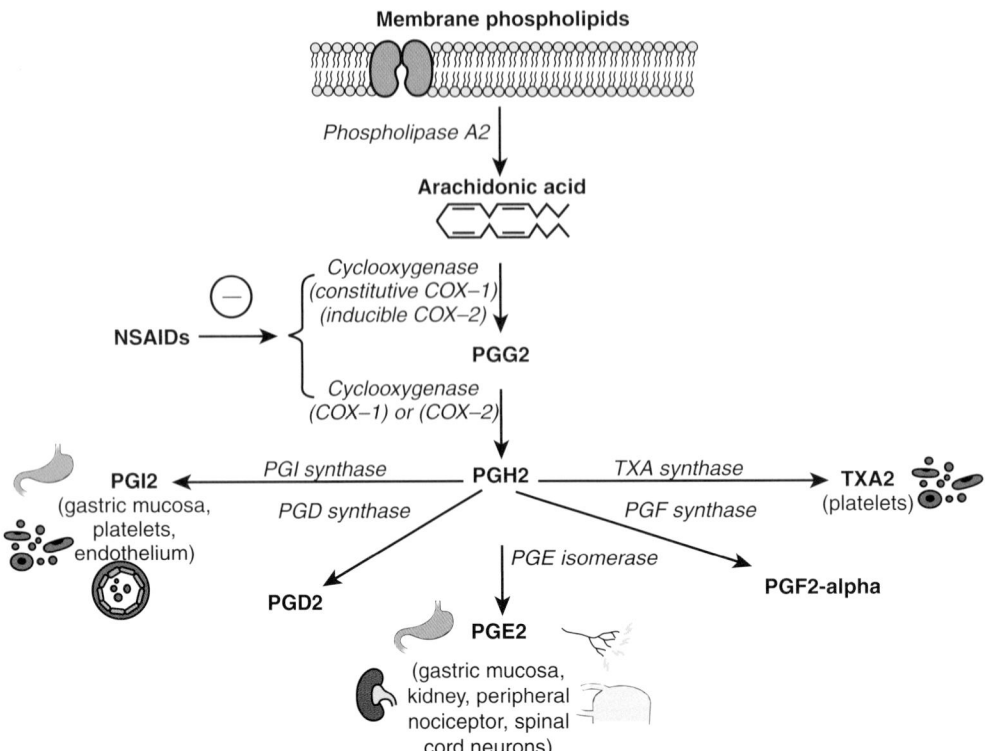

Figure 38-7 **The role of cyclooxygenase in prostaglandin (PG) synthesis.** Prostaglandin and thromboxanes (TX), which are important in inflammation and homeostasis, are products of a biochemical cascade by which membrane phospholipids are converted to arachidonic acid, then to intermediate prostaglandins by cyclooxygenase, and to their final products by a series of synthases. COX, cyclooxygenase; NSAID, nonsteroidal anti-inflammatory drug. *(From Gilron I, Milne B, Hong M: Cyclooxygenase-2 inhibitors in postoperative pain management: Current evidence and future directions [review article].* Anesthesiology 99:1198, 2003.)

without untoward effects (gastrointestinal ulceration, renal dysfunction, excessive bleeding). Although NSAIDs have been associated with reports of increased postoperative blood loss, other studies have failed to corroborate this.

NSAIDs are not a homogenous group and vary considerably in analgesic efficacy as a result of differences in pharmacodynamic and pharmacokinetic parameters. NSAIDs are nonspecific inhibitors of COX, which is the rate-limiting enzyme involved in the synthesis of prostaglandins. A major scientific discovery revealed that COX exists in multiple forms. Most important, a constitutive form is present in normal conditions in healthy cells (COX-1) and an inducible form (COX-2) exists, which is the major isozyme induced by and associated with inflammation. Simplistically, COX-1 is ubiquitously and constitutively expressed, and has a homeostatic role in platelet aggregation, gastrointestinal mucosal integrity, and renal function, whereas COX-2 is inducible and expressed mainly at sites of injury (and kidney and brain) and mediates pain and inflammation. NSAIDs are nonspecific inhibitors of both forms of COX, yet vary in their ratio of COX-1 to COX-2 inhibition. Recent molecular studies distinguishing between constitutive COX-1 and inflammation-inducible COX-2 enzymes have led to the exciting hypothesis that the therapeutic and adverse effects of NSAIDs could be uncoupled[66–71] (Figure 38-8). Subsequently, over the past ten years, clinicians have witnessed an exponential increase in publications and the growing use of COX-2 inhibitors in the perioperative period after noncardiac surgery. A compelling body of evidence now exists that COX-2 inhibitors, like their predecessors the nonselective NSAIDs, in general provide postoperative analgesia, decrease intravenous opioid requirements, and provide greater patient satisfaction compared with placebo. There is also some evidence that opioid sparing by COX-2 inhibitors also spares opioid side effects. The primary advantage of COX-2 inhibitors, compared with NSAIDs, is their lack of effect on platelet function and bleeding, hence the opportunity for perioperative administration.

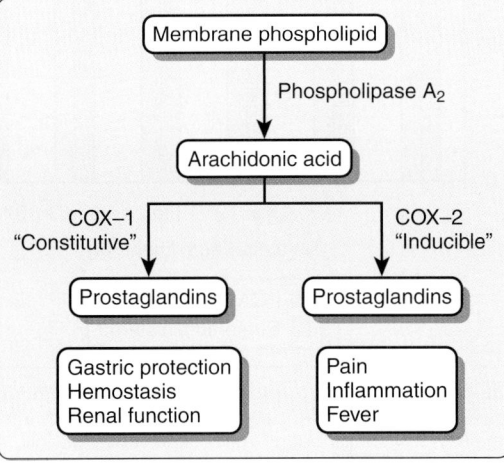

Figure 38-8 **Cyclooxygenase (COX) pathways.** Recent molecular studies distinguishing between COX-1 and COX-2 enzymes have led to the exciting hypothesis that the therapeutic and adverse effects of the nonspecific inhibitors (nonsteroidal anti-inflammatory drugs [NSAIDs]) could be uncoupled. *(From Gajraj NM: Cyclooxygenase-2 inhibitors [review article].* Anesth Analg 96:1720, 2003.)

Only a handful of clinical studies have investigated the potential of NSAIDs in the management of postoperative pain after cardiac surgery.[72–75] One well-designed clinical investigation showed that a combination of NSAID and intravenous opioid may provide superior analgesia after cardiac surgery without untoward effects. Rapanos et al[74] prospectively randomized 57 patients to receive either indomethacin suppositories or placebo suppositories in a double-blinded fashion during the immediate postoperative period after elective

CABG. Patients receiving indomethacin suppositories demonstrated significantly less ($P = 0.019$) morphine consumption (assessed via PCA morphine) and significantly lower ($P = 0.006$) pain scores (assessed via visual analog pain scores) during the immediate postoperative period compared with controls. Postoperative morphine use during the first 24 postoperative hours was 22.40 ± 12.55 mg in the indomethacin group and 35.99 ± 25.84 mg in the placebo group. There were no differences between groups regarding tracheal extubation time or postoperative blood loss (assessed via chest tube output). None of the study subjects (either group) developed postoperative renal dysfunction. In fact, a moderate reduction in serum creatinine concentration was observed in both groups. These investigators concluded that the combination of indomethacin suppositories with morphine after cardiac surgery results in reduced postoperative pain scores and opioid consumption without an increase in side effects.

However, two well-designed clinical investigations demonstrated that the use of NSAIDs or NSAID-like drugs (acetaminophen) in patients after cardiac surgery may not offer any substantial clinical benefits.[72,75] Hynninen et al,[72] in a prospective, double-blind, placebo-controlled study, randomized patients to receive either diclofenac ($n = 28$ patients), ketoprofen ($n = 28$ patients), indomethacin ($n = 27$ patients), or placebo ($n = 31$ patients) for postoperative analgesia after elective CABG via a median sternotomy. All patients received standardized fast-track cardiac anesthesia and standardized postoperative analgesia treatment. Mean morphine consumption in the immediate postoperative period was significantly reduced only in the diclofenac group when compared with placebo (12.4 vs. 19.0 mg, respectively; $P < 0.05$). Total analgesic consumption calculated as morphine equivalents was also significantly lower only in the diclofenac group compared with placebo (18.1 vs. 26.5 mg, respectively; $P \leq 0.05$). No additional important differences were observed when doses of other analgesics were compared. The visual analog pain scores at rest were comparable among the four groups at all times. Also, there were no postoperative differences among the four groups regarding creatinine concentration, percentage of patients with 20% and greater increases in creatinine level after surgery, and 24-hour blood loss. These findings indicate that although some NSAIDs may offer opioid-sparing effects, others may not.

Lahtinen et al,[75] in a prospective, double-blind, placebo-controlled study, randomized patients to receive either propacetamol, a prodrug of acetaminophen ($n = 40$ patients), or placebo ($n = 39$ patients) for postoperative analgesia after elective CABG via a median sternotomy. Acetaminophen (not an NSAID) might be a safer nonopioid analgesic in cardiac surgery because it does not depress platelet function or renal function as much as traditional NSAIDs. The mechanism behind the analgesic action of acetaminophen remains unclear. Acetaminophen has only a weak inhibitory influence on peripheral COXs and has no substantial anti-inflammatory activity. Acetaminophen-induced analgesia may be partially centrally mediated, and the peak cerebrospinal fluid concentrations may reflect analgesic actions. Intravenous propacetamol is quickly hydrolyzed to acetaminophen in the bloodstream. In the clinical investigation by Lahtinen et al,[75] a standardized intraoperative anesthetic technique was used for all patients, and extubation times were identical between the two groups (approximately 5.3 hours). From the time of extubation, all patients had access to PCA oxycodone using a standardized protocol. The variation of oxycodone consumption was large in both groups, and although postoperative cumulative oxycodone consumption (combined amount administered via PCA and given as rescue doses) was less in the propacetamol group compared with the placebo group, the difference was not statistically significant (123.5 ± 51.3 mg vs. 141.8 ± 57.5 mg, respectively; $P = 0.15$). Postoperative visual analog pain scores (obtained at rest and during a deep breath) were similar, as well as patients' satisfaction with analgesia, between the two groups. Furthermore, no differences existed between the two groups regarding postoperative pulmonary function tests (forced expiratory volume in 1 second, peak expiratory volume, forced vital capacity), blood gas analysis, bleeding, renal function tests, and liver function tests. Postoperative nausea and vomiting were the most common adverse events, which occurred with identical frequency

in both groups. These investigators concluded that propacetamol neither enhances postoperative opioid-based analgesia in patients after CABG, nor does it decrease cumulative opioid consumption or reduce adverse effects.

One prospective, randomized clinical study investigated the potential advantages and disadvantages of using COX inhibitors in patients after cardiac surgery.[76] Immer et al[76] prospectively randomized 60 patients scheduled for elective CABG with conventional sternotomy to receive either a COX-2 inhibitor (etodolac), a nonselective COX inhibitor (diclofenac), or a weak opioid (tramadol) for postoperative analgesia. Postoperative pain was assessed via a visual analog scale, perioperative blood samples were obtained for serum creatinine and urea levels, and creatinine clearance was determined on the first postoperative day (before starting study medication) and on the fourth postoperative day (after receiving study medication). In patients with insufficient postoperative analgesia (defined via predetermined visual analog scale score), supplemental subcutaneous morphine was administered. Total morphine consumption and occurrence of nausea were recorded daily. At the doses analyzed by these investigators, etodolac and diclofenac produced slightly better postoperative analgesia (assessed via visual analog scale scores and morphine consumption) with fewer adverse effects (assessed via antiemetic therapy) than tramadol. However, a short-lasting impairment of renal function was found in patients treated with etodolac and diclofenac (assessed via serum creatinine and urea levels; Figures 38-9 and 38-10). However, at hospital discharge, no significant differences existed among the three groups regarding serum creatinine and urea levels (see Figures 38-9 and 38-10). Furthermore, all three groups experienced similar decreases in postoperative creatinine clearance.

Another clinical investigation in CABG patients suggested a proportionately, but not significantly, greater incidence of serious cardiac and cerebrovascular adverse events in patients taking COX-2 inhibitors.[77] In this multicenter (58 institutions), prospective, randomized, double-blind, parallel-group trial performed by Ott et al,[77] 462 patients undergoing CABG were allocated at a ratio of 2:1 to parecoxib/valdecoxib (311 patients) or standard care (151 patients; control) groups, respectively. Patients in the parecoxib/valdecoxib group required significantly less morphine or morphine equivalents than patients in the control group during the postoperative period (up to 6 days). Both patients and physicians evaluated the study medication (parecoxib/valdecoxib) as significantly better than control therapy. Pain questionnaires detected significant improvements in the parecoxib/valdecoxib group beginning on day 4 and continuing for at least 4 days. However, although there were no differences between the groups in overall

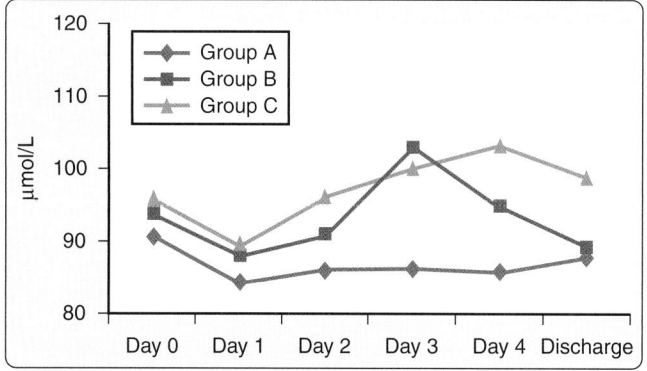

Figure 38-9 Serum creatinine values. Serum creatinine values for groups A (tramadol), B (diclofenac), and C (etodolac) on postoperative days 1 to 4 and at discharge. Results are displayed as mean values. Serum creatinine levels were significantly greater on postoperative days 3 and 4 in groups B and C compared with group A ($p < 0.05$). However, at discharge, no significant differences were found among the three groups. *(From Immer FF, Immer-Bansi AS, Trachsel N, et al: Pain treatment with a COX-2 inhibitor after coronary artery bypass operation: A randomized trial. Ann Thorac Surg 75:490, 2003.)*

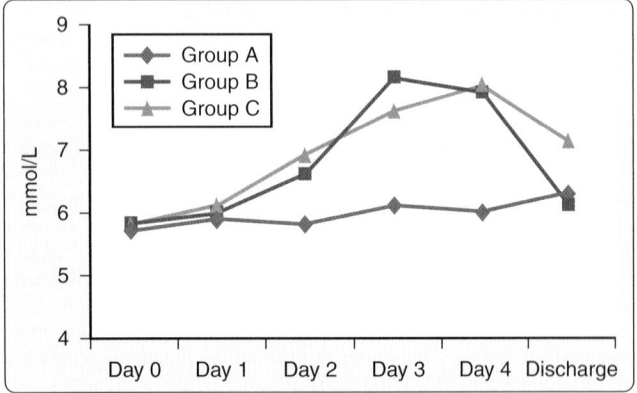

Figure 38-10 **Serum urea values.** Serum urea values for groups A (tramadol), B (diclofenac), and C (etodolac) on postoperative days 1 to 4 and at discharge. Results are displayed as mean values. Serum urea levels were significantly greater on postoperative days 3 and 4 in groups B and C compared with group A ($P < 0.05$). However, at discharge, no significant differences were found among the three groups. (From Immer FF, Immer-Bansi AS, Trachsel N, et al: Pain treatment with a COX-2 inhibitor after coronary artery bypass operation: A randomized trial. Ann Thorac Surg 75:490, 2003.)

adverse events, serious adverse events occurred twice as frequently in parecoxib/valdecoxib-treated patients than in control patients (19.0% vs. 9.9%, respectively; $P = 0.015$).

Regarding individual serious adverse events, a greater incidence rate in sternal wound infection was found in the parecoxib/valdecoxib patients (3.2%) versus control patients (0.0%) ($P = 0.035$). The effects of NSAIDs on sternal wound complications had not been reported previously. The COX-2 enzyme enables prostaglandin release and the inflammatory response; inhibition of this enzyme by nonspecific COX inhibitors (NSAIDs), as well as specific COX-2 inhibitors, might impede reparative inflammatory responses and increase susceptibility to sternal wound infections. An alternative hypothesis is that reduced fever and tachycardia in NSAID/COX-2 inhibitor–treated patients may delay detection of infection, resulting in further progression and greater consequence. Regardless of the mechanism, these safety issues merit careful consideration because of the importance of sternal wound complications in this setting. The incidence of other individual serious adverse events, including cerebrovascular complications, myocardial infarction, and renal dysfunction, were proportionally greater in the parecoxib/valdecoxib patients but not significantly different between the two groups. Specifically, when the groups were compared, more patients in the treatment group (parecoxib/valdecoxib) experienced cerebrovascular disorders (2.9% vs. 0.7%; $P = 0.177$), myocardial infarction (1.6% vs. 0.7%; $P = 0.669$), and renal dysfunction (1.9% vs. 0.0%; $P = 0.184$) compared with control patients.

Such thrombosis-mediated complications also merit careful consideration. In cardiac surgery patients exposed to CPB, the delicate balance among platelets, endothelial cells, and serum clotting factors is disturbed, with consequent thrombosis and clot lysis occurring disparately and unpredictably throughout the vascular system. Given that COX-2 inhibitors are platelet sparing, they might tip the balance toward thrombosis during periods of platelet activation. In addition, because COX-1 is unaffected, consequent release of thromboxane A_2 may further promote platelet activation and thrombosis. Of note, some analyses addressing these issues in chronically treated patients with arthritis indicate a potential association between COX-2 inhibition and thrombogenic events (myocardial infarction, stroke, vascular death).[78] Ott et al[77] concluded that, in patients undergoing CABG, the COX-2 inhibitor combination of parecoxib/valdecoxib is effective in controlling postoperative analgesia. However, the treatment regimen may be associated with an increased incidence of serious adverse events overall and sternal wound infections in particular. Their study,

therefore, raises important concerns requiring a comprehensive evaluation of the potential link between this class of drugs and perioperative complications in a large-scale clinical trial before the COX-2 inhibitors are routinely used in patients undergoing cardiac surgery.

Over the next decade, much more will be learned about COX-2 inhibitors. Their analgesic (opioid-sparing) effects and lack of deleterious effects on coagulation (in contrast with nonselective NSAIDs) certainly are desirable. The evidence to date does not suggest that COX-2 inhibitors provide major advantages over traditional NSAIDs. It is possible that their continued development will lead to specific drugs with a superior therapeutic profile. Many important questions regarding their safety remain to be answered, such as effects on CNS sensitization, perioperative renal function, preemptive analgesia, clinically significant blood loss, the gastrointestinal system, the cardiovascular system, chronic postsurgical pain, bone/wound healing, blood pressure, and peripheral edema, among others. Specifically regarding patients undergoing cardiac surgery, the potential links between this class of drugs and sternal wound infections and thromboembolic complications need to be fully evaluated. Lastly, the recent and unprecedented retraction of more than 20 peer-reviewed articles and abstracts (spanning 15 years) published by a leading investigator in the perioperative use of NSAIDs and COX-2 inhibitors raises important questions as to the potential adverse impact of this investigator's fraudulent work on the practice of acute postoperative pain management.[79] Simply put, such unprecedented retraction forces clinicians to question all that was previously "known" (assumed true) of the advantages/disadvantages of using NSAIDs and COX-2 inhibitors, prompting the need for future clinical analysis studies to address these important issues.

α_2-ADRENERGIC AGONISTS

The α_2-adrenergic agonists provide analgesia, sedation, and sympatholysis (Box 38-7). The initial impetus for the use of α_2-agonists in anesthesia resulted from astute clinical observations made in patients during intraoperative anesthesia who were receiving clonidine therapy. Soon thereafter, investigators revealed that clonidine substantially reduced anesthetic requirements (minimal alveolar concentration). More recently, dexmedetomidine has undergone extensive clinical evaluation for perioperative use. Dexmedetomidine exerts profound effects on cardiovascular parameters and thus appears to affect its own pharmacokinetics. At high doses, there is marked vasoconstriction, which probably reduces the drug's volume of distribution. The elimination half-life of dexmedetomidine is 2 to 3 hours.

α_2-Adrenergic agonists produce clinically sedative effects via stimulation of α_2 receptors in the locus ceruleus and clinically analgesic effects via stimulation of α_2 receptors within the locus ceruleus and the spinal cord.[80] Evidence exists indicating that α_2-agonists enhance the analgesic effects of the opioids via an unknown mechanism of action. Several mechanisms of action have been postulated for the analgesia noted with α_2-adrenergic agonists, including supraspinal, ganglionic, spinal, and peripheral mechanisms. Clinically, systemic administration of these agents produces antinociception and sedation, whereas intrathecal administration usually produces only antinociception. Like other adrenergic receptors, the α_2-adrenergic agonists demonstrate tolerance after prolonged administration.

As with all clinically used analgesics, the α_2-adrenergic agonists possess clinically important side effects that may limit their usefulness.

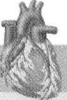

BOX 38-7 α_2-ADRENERGIC AGONISTS

- Advantage:
  - Cardiovascular stability?
- Disadvantages:
  - Sedation
  - Hypotension

The effects of dexmedetomidine on the respiratory system include a decrease in tidal volume, minimal changes in respiratory rate, and a rightward shift and depression of slope of the carbon dioxide response curve (all of which may cause hypercarbia). However, respiratory depression associated with the drug is usually clinically unimportant even during profound levels of sedation. The effects of dexmedetomidine on the cardiovascular system are many, and in contrast with the respiratory effects, may become clinically important. Physiologic changes include decreased heart rate, decreased systemic vascular resistance, and possibly indirectly decreased myocardial contractility, all potentially leading to decreased cardiac output and decreased blood pressure in susceptible patients. By developing more highly selective α_2-adrenergic agonists, it is hoped that these detrimental cardiovascular effects will be minimized while maximizing desired analgesic and sedative properties. Currently, the clinical role of these drugs includes preoperative sedation, an intraoperative adjuvant during anesthesia to reduce sedative and analgesic requirements, and postoperative sedation and analgesia. The potential ability of the α_2-adrenergic agonists to reduce and/or prevent perioperative myocardial ischemia, although intriguing, remains to be determined.[81]

The potential perioperative analgesic benefits of α_2-agonists, when administered to patients undergoing cardiac surgery, were demonstrated almost 20 years ago.[82] In 1987, Flacke et al,[82] in prospective, nonblinded fashion, randomized patients undergoing elective CABG to receive either perioperative oral clonidine supplementation (10 patients) or serve as control patients (10 patients). Outside of oral clonidine supplementation, management of the two study groups was identical. Patients receiving oral clonidine required significantly less preinduction diazepam and significantly less intraoperative sufentanil (Figure 38-11) and isoflurane to maintain intraoperative normotension (clearly establishing clonidine's sedative/analgesic properties). Furthermore, patients receiving oral clonidine were extubated earlier during the postoperative period compared with control patients (approximately 11 vs. 16 hours, respectively; $P < 0.05$). However, 4 of 10 patients receiving oral clonidine required atropine for treatment of intraoperative bradycardia. Unfortunately, postoperative analgesia was not assessed in this clinical investigation.

Although the analgesic properties of α_2-adrenergic agonists are undisputed, most of the clinical investigations regarding perioperative use of this class of drugs remain focused on exploiting the sedative effects and beneficial cardiovascular effects (decreasing hypertension and tachycardia) associated with their use.[83–86] α_2-Adrenergic agonists have been used perioperatively in patients undergoing cardiac surgery, yet the focus of such clinical investigations has been on the intraoperative period and the potential for enhanced postoperative hemodynamic stability, potentially leading to reduced postoperative myocardial ischemia (not specifically to enhanced postoperative analgesia).[87–90] Taken together, these clinical investigations indicated that perioperative administration of α_2-adrenergic agonists to patients undergoing cardiac surgery decreases intraoperative anesthetic requirements, may enhance perioperative hemodynamic stability, and may decrease perioperative myocardial ischemia, yet may cause excessive postoperative sedation and aggravate postoperative hemodynamic instability via bradycardia and/or decreased systemic vascular resistance (leading to hypotension and increased pacing requirements in susceptible patients). The potential ability of this class of drugs to initiate reliable postoperative analgesia awaits definitive investigation.

INTRATHECAL AND EPIDURAL TECHNIQUES

It is clear from numerous clinical investigations that intrathecal or epidural techniques, or both (using opioids and/or local anesthetics), initiate reliable postoperative analgesia in patients after cardiac surgery[91] (Boxes 38-8 and 38-9). Additional potential advantages of using intrathecal or epidural techniques, or both, in patients undergoing cardiac surgery include stress-response attenuation and thoracic cardiac sympathectomy.

An uninhibited stress response during the postoperative period may lead to many adverse hemodynamic (tachycardia, hypertension, vasoconstriction), metabolic (increased catabolism), immunologic (impaired immune response), and hemostatic (platelet activation) alterations. Intrathecal or epidural anesthesia and analgesia (with local anesthetics or opioids) can effectively inhibit the stress response associated with surgical procedures.[27] Local anesthetics appear to possess greater efficacy than opioids in perioperative stress-response attenuation, perhaps because of their unique mechanism of action.

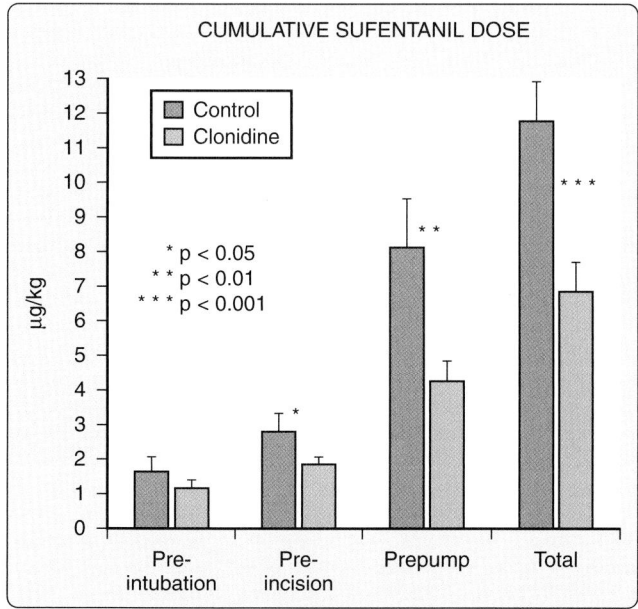

Figure 38-11 **Cumulative sufentanil dose.** Mean cumulative sufentanil doses are shown for the periods before intubation, before incision, before CPB, and for the entire anesthetic period. *(From Flacke JW, Bloor BC, Flacke WE, et al: Reduced narcotic requirement by clonidine with improved hemodynamic and adrenergic stability in patients undergoing coronary bypass surgery. Anesthesiology 67:11, 1987.)*

BOX 38-8. INTRATHECAL TECHNIQUES

- Advantages:
  - Simple, reliable analgesia
  - Stress-response attenuation
  - Less hematoma risk than epidural techniques
- Disadvantages:
  - No cardiac sympathectomy
  - Hematoma risk increased
  - Side effects of intrathecal opioids

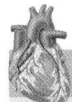

BOX 38-9. EPIDURAL TECHNIQUES

- Advantages:
  - Reliable analgesia
  - Stress-response attenuation
  - Cardiac sympathectomy
- Disadvantages:
  - Labor intensive
  - Hematoma risk increased
  - Side effects of epidural opioids

Although still a matter of some debate, perioperative stress-response attenuation with epidural local anesthetics and/or opioids in high-risk patients after major noncardiac surgery may decrease morbidity and mortality.[6,7,27] In patients undergoing cardiac surgery, initiation of CPB causes significant increases in stress-response hormones that persist into the immediate postoperative period.[24–26] Attenuation of this component of the perioperative stress response with intravenous opioids also may decrease morbidity and mortality in these patients.[8,9] Unfortunately, perioperative stress-response attenuation in patients undergoing cardiac surgery with intravenous opioids in this manner does not allow tracheal extubation to occur in the immediate postoperative period. Intrathecal or epidural anesthesia and analgesia techniques (particularly with local anesthetics) are attractive alternatives to intravenous opioids in this setting for their potential to attenuate the perioperative stress response, yet still allow tracheal extubation to occur in the immediate postoperative period.

The myocardium and coronary vasculature are densely innervated by sympathetic nerve fibers that arise from T1 to T5 and profoundly influence total coronary blood flow and distribution.[92] Cardiac sympathetic nerve activation initiates coronary artery vasoconstriction[93] and paradoxic coronary vasoconstriction in response to intrinsic vasodilators.[94] In patients with CAD, cardiac sympathetic nerve activation disrupts the normal matching of coronary blood flow and myocardial oxygen demand.[95,96] Animal models have revealed an intense poststenotic coronary vasoconstrictive mechanism mediated by cardiac sympathetic nerve activation that attenuates local metabolic coronary vasodilation in response to myocardial ischemia.[97,98] Furthermore, myocardial ischemia initiates a cardiocardiac reflex mediated by sympathetic nerve fibers, which augments the ischemic process.[99] Cardiac sympathetic nerve activation likely plays a central role in initiating postoperative myocardial ischemia by decreasing myocardial oxygen supply via the mechanisms listed earlier.[27,100]

Thoracic epidural anesthesia (TEA) with local anesthetics effectively blocks cardiac sympathetic nerve afferent and efferent fibers.[27] Opioids, administered similarly, are unable to effectively block such cardiac sympathetic nerve activity.[27] Patients with symptomatic CAD benefit clinically from cardiac sympathectomy, and the application of thoracic sympathetic blockade in the management of angina pectoris was described as early as 1965.[101] TEA with local anesthetics increases the diameter of stenotic epicardial coronary artery segments without causing dilation of coronary arterioles,[95] decreases determinants of myocardial oxygen demand,[96] improves left ventricular function,[102] and decreases anginal symptoms.[96,103] Furthermore, cardiac sympathectomy increases the endocardial-to-epicardial blood flow ratio,[104,105] beneficially affects collateral blood flow during myocardial ischemia,[105] decreases poststenotic coronary vasoconstriction,[98] and attenuates the myocardial ischemia-induced cardiocardiac reflex.[98] In an animal model, TEA with local anesthetics actually decreased myocardial infarct size after coronary artery occlusion.[104] Of note, these beneficial effects are not caused by systemic absorption of the local anesthetic.[104] In short, TEA with local anesthetics may benefit patients undergoing cardiac surgery by effectively blocking cardiac sympathetic nerve activity and improving the myocardial oxygen supply/demand balance.

▓ Intrathecal Techniques

Application of intrathecal analgesia to patients undergoing cardiac surgery was initially reported by Mathews and Abrams in 1980.[106] They described the administration of intrathecal morphine (1.5 to 4.0 mg) to 40 adults after the induction of general anesthesia for cardiac surgery. Somewhat remarkably, all 40 patients awakened pain free at the end of surgery (before leaving the operating room), and 36 patients were tracheally extubated before transfer to the ICU. After surgery, all 40 patients were entirely pain free for the first 27.5 postoperative hours, and 17 did not require any supplemental analgesics before discharge from the hospital. Of the 17 patients who received 4.0 mg intrathecal morphine, 11 did not require any postoperative analgesic drugs.

Mathews and Abrams[106] summarized: "The benefits of recovering from surgery free from pain have been impressive. This has been particularly appreciated by patients who have had previous operations with conventional anesthesia and postoperative analgesic drugs. The patients have been remarkably comfortable, able to move more easily in bed, and more cooperative, thus greatly helping their nursing care." After this impressive clinical display, other investigators have subsequently applied intrathecal anesthesia and analgesia techniques to patients undergoing cardiac surgery.[107–132]

Most clinical investigators have used intrathecal morphine in hopes of providing prolonged postoperative analgesia. Some clinical investigators have used intrathecal fentanyl, sufentanil, and/or local anesthetics for intraoperative anesthesia and analgesia (with stress–response attenuation) and/or thoracic cardiac sympathectomy. An anonymous survey of members of the Society of Cardiovascular Anesthesiologists indicated that almost 8% of practicing anesthesiologists incorporate intrathecal techniques into their anesthetic management of adults undergoing cardiac surgery.[133] Of these anesthesiologists, 75% practice in the United States, 72% perform the intrathecal injection before induction of anesthesia, 97% use morphine, 13% use fentanyl, 2% use sufentanil, 10% use lidocaine, and 3% use tetracaine.[133]

Two randomized, blinded, placebo-controlled clinical studies revealed the ability of intrathecal morphine to induce significant postoperative analgesia after cardiac surgery.[119,126] In 1988, Vanstrum et al[126] prospectively randomized 30 patients to receive either intrathecal morphine (0.5 mg) or intrathecal placebo before induction of anesthesia. Intraoperative anesthetic management was standardized, and after surgery all patients received only intravenous morphine administered by a nurse who attempted to keep the linear analog pain score at less than 4 (a score of 1 represented no pain, 10 represented the worst pain imaginable; the scale was 25 cm long). Although pain scores between groups were not significantly different at any postoperative time interval tested, patients who received intrathecal morphine required significantly less intravenous morphine than placebo controls (2.4 vs. 8.3 mg, respectively; $P < 0.02$) during the initial 30 hours after intrathecal injection (Figure 38-12). Associated with this enhanced analgesia in patients receiving intrathecal morphine was a substantially decreased need for antihypertensive medications (sodium nitroprusside, nitroglycerin, hydralazine) during the immediate postoperative period. Time to tracheal extubation (approximately 20 hours) and postoperative arterial blood gas tensions after anesthesia were not significantly affected by the use of intrathecal morphine. In 1996, Chaney and associates[119] prospectively randomized 60 patients to receive either intrathecal morphine (4.0 mg) or intrathecal placebo before induction of anesthesia for elective CABG. Intraoperative anesthetic management was standardized, and after tracheal extubation, all patients received intravenous morphine via PCA exclusively. The mean time from ICU arrival to tracheal extubation was similar in all patients (approximately 20 hours). However, patients who received intrathecal morphine required significantly less intravenous morphine than placebo controls (33.2 vs. 51.1 mg, respectively; $P < 0.05$) during the initial postoperative period (Table 38-2). Despite enhanced analgesia, no clinical differences between groups existed regarding postoperative morbidity (pruritus, nausea, vomiting, urinary retention, prolonged somnolence, atrial fibrillation, ventricular tachycardia, myocardial infarction, cerebral infarction), mortality, or duration of postoperative hospital stay (approximately 9 days in each group).

The mid-1990s saw the emergence of fast-track cardiac surgery, with the goal being tracheal extubation in the immediate postoperative period. Chaney and associates in 1997[118] were the first to study the potential clinical benefits of intrathecal morphine when used in patients undergoing cardiac surgery and early tracheal extubation. They prospectively randomized 40 patients to receive either intrathecal morphine (10 µg/kg) or intrathecal placebo before induction of anesthesia for elective CABG. Intraoperative anesthetic management was standardized (intravenous fentanyl, 20 µg/kg, and intravenous midazolam, 10 mg), and after surgery all patients received intravenous morphine via

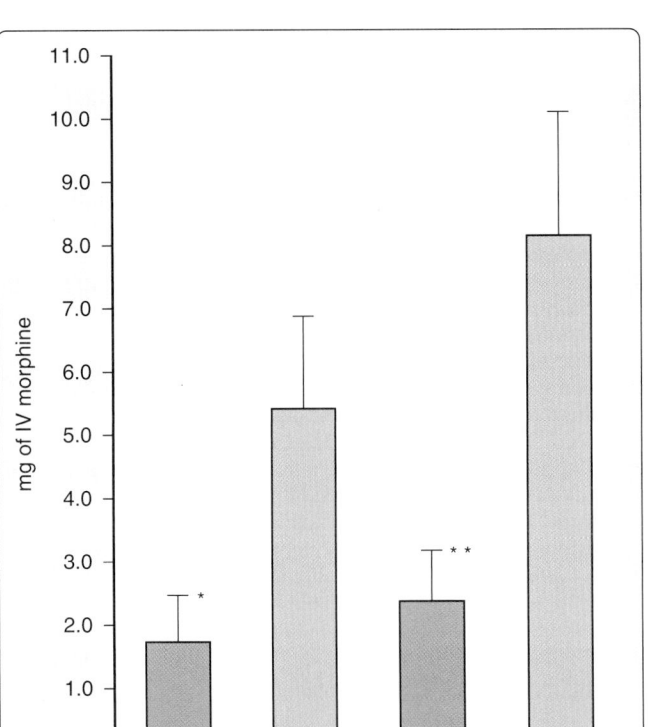

Figure 38-12 Postoperative supplemental intravenous (IV) morphine requirements. Patients receiving intrathecal morphine (Group I) required significantly less supplemental intravenous morphine during the initial 24 postoperative hours (*, $P < 0.048$) and during the initial 30 postoperative hours (**, $P < 0.02$) compared with patients receiving intrathecal placebo (Group II). *(From Vanstrum GS, Bjornson KM, Ilko R: Postoperative effects of intrathecal morphine in coronary artery bypass surgery. Anesth Analg 67:261, 1988.)*

TABLE 38-2	Postoperative Supplemental Intravenous Midazolam and Morphine Requirements	
	Group MS (n = 27)	**Group NS** (n = 29)
Midazolam use from ICU arrival to extubation, mg (range)	8.7 ± 15.8 (0–80)	8.3 ± 15.4 (0–66)
Morphine use from ICU arrival to 8:00 AM POD 2, mg (range)	33.2 ± 15.8 (4–74)	51.1 ± 45.7 (4–254)
Morphine use from 8:00 AM POD 2 to 8:00 AM POD 3, mg (range)	14.2 ± 16.4 (0–68)	12.1 ± 12.6 (0–42)

Patients receiving intrathecal morphine (group MS) required significantly less supplemental intravenous morphine during the immediate postoperative period compared with patients receiving intrathecal placebo (group NS; 33.2 vs. 51.1 mg, respectively; $P < 0.05$).
ICU, intensive care unit; POD, postoperative day.
From Chaney MA, Smith KR, Barclay JC, Slogoff S: Large-dose intrathecal morphine for coronary artery bypass grafting. *Anesth Analg* 83:215, 1996.

PCA exclusively. Of the patients who were tracheally extubated during the immediate postoperative period, the mean time from ICU arrival to tracheal extubation was significantly ($P = 0.02$) prolonged in patients who received intrathecal morphine (10.9 ± 4.4 hours) compared with placebo controls (7.6 ± 2.5 hours). Three patients who received intrathecal morphine had tracheal extubation substantially delayed (12 to 24 hours) because of prolonged ventilatory depression (likely secondary to intrathecal morphine). Although the mean postoperative intravenous morphine use for 48 hours was less in patients who received intrathecal morphine (42.8 mg) compared with patients who received intrathecal placebo (55.0 mg), the difference between groups was not statistically significant. No clinical

differences existed between groups regarding postoperative morbidity, mortality, or duration of postoperative hospital stay (approximately 9 days in each group).

These somewhat discouraging findings (absence of enhanced analgesia, prolongation of tracheal extubation time) stimulated the same group of investigators in 1999 to try again, this time decreasing the amount of intraoperative intravenous fentanyl patients received (hoping to decrease the effect of fentanyl on augmenting postoperative respiratory depression associated with intrathecal morphine).[116] Forty patients were prospectively randomized to receive either intrathecal morphine (10 μg/kg) or intrathecal placebo before induction of anesthesia for elective CABG. Intraoperative anesthetic management was standardized (intravenous fentanyl, 10 μg/kg, and intravenous midazolam, 200 μg/kg), and after surgery all patients received intravenous morphine exclusively via PCA. Of the patients tracheally extubated during the immediate postoperative period, mean time to tracheal extubation was similar in patients who received intrathecal morphine (6.8 ± 2.8 hours) compared with intrathecal placebo patients (6.5 ± 3.2 hours). However, once again, four patients who received intrathecal morphine had tracheal extubation substantially delayed (14, 14, 18, and 19 hours) because of prolonged respiratory depression (likely secondary to intrathecal morphine). The mean postoperative intravenous morphine use during the immediate postoperative period was actually greater in patients receiving intrathecal morphine (49.8 mg) compared with patients receiving intrathecal placebo (36.2 mg), yet the difference between groups was not statistically significant. No clinical differences existed between groups regarding postoperative morbidity, mortality, or duration of postoperative hospital stay (approximately 6 days in each group). Thus, Chaney and associates, from their three prospective, randomized, double-blind, placebo-controlled, clinical investigations in the late 1990s involving 140 healthy adults undergoing elective CABG, concluded that although intrathecal morphine certainly can initiate reliable postoperative analgesia, its use in the setting of fast-track cardiac surgery and early tracheal extubation may be detrimental by potentially delaying tracheal extubation in the immediate postoperative period.[116,118,119]

Since this time, however, other clinical investigators have revealed that certain combinations of intraoperative anesthetic techniques, coupled with appropriate doses of intrathecal morphine, will allow tracheal extubation after cardiac surgery within the immediate postoperative period together with enhanced analgesia. Alhashemi et al[108] prospectively randomized 50 adults undergoing elective CABG to receive either one of two doses of intrathecal morphine (250 μg or 500 μg) or intrathecal placebo. Intraoperative anesthetic management was standardized (fentanyl, midazolam), and all patients received intermittent morphine by a blinded practitioner during the postoperative period. Tracheal extubation times were similar in the placebo group, 250 μg intrathecal morphine group, and 500 μg intrathecal morphine group (7.3, 5.4, and 6.8 hours, respectively; $P = 0.270$). However, postoperative morphine requirements in the placebo group (21.3 ± 6.2 mg), 250 μg intrathecal morphine group (13.6 ± 7.8 mg), and the 500 μg intrathecal morphine group (11.7 ± 7.4 mg) were substantially different. There was at least a 36% reduction in postoperative intravenous morphine requirements among those patients who received intrathecal morphine. Although there were no differences in postoperative intravenous morphine requirements between patients randomized to receive either 250 or 500 μg intrathecal morphine, both groups required significantly less intravenous morphine during the immediate postoperative period compared with control patients ($p = 0.001$). However, despite enhanced analgesia, there were no differences among the study groups in regard to midazolam, nitroglycerin, and sodium nitroprusside requirements in the postoperative period (Table 38-3). Furthermore, postextubation blood gas analysis, use of supplemental inspired oxygen, and ICU length of stay (approximately 22 hours in all groups) were comparable among the three groups.

These investigators, as well as others, revealed that the use of intrathecal morphine in patients undergoing fast-track cardiac surgery and early tracheal extubation may (if used appropriately) provide enhanced

TABLE 38-3	Analysis of Outcome Measures in Patients Receiving Either Placebo, 250 μg Intrathecal Morphine, or 500 μg Intrathecal Morphine			
	Placebo (n = 19)	*250 μg (n = 16)*	*500 μg (n = 15)*	*P*
Ventilatory time (min)	441 ± 207	325 ± 187	409 ± 245	0.270
Morphine (mg)	21.3 ± 6.2	13.6 ± 7.8	11.7 ± 7.4	0.001
Midazolam (mg)	2.3 ± 3.5	0.9 ± 1.8	1.5 ± 2.7	0.346
Nitroglycerin (mg)	52.5 ± 37.6	55.0 ± 38.4	52.8 ± 43.0	0.982
Nitroprusside (mg)	7.9 ± 22.7	0.1 ± 0.4	1.4 ± 4.0	0.230

From Alhashemi JA, Sharpe MD, Harris CL, et al: Effect of subarachnoid morphine administration on extubation time after coronary artery bypass graft surgery. *J Cardiothorac Vasc Anesth* 14:639, 2000.

postoperative analgesia without delaying tracheal extubation. The authors also interestingly postulated that limiting the amounts of intraoperative intravenous opioids and intravenous sedatives, and the application of a postoperative tracheal extubation protocol may be more important in achieving the goal of early tracheal extubation after cardiac surgery than adequate pain control during the immediate postoperative period.

Many other suboptimally designed clinical investigations (retrospective, observational, etc.) attest to the ability of intrathecal morphine to induce substantial postoperative analgesia in patients after cardiac surgery (Table 38-4). Intrathecal doses of 0.5 to 10.0 mg administered before CPB initiate reliable postoperative analgesia, the quality of which depends not only on the intrathecal dose administered but on the type and amount of intravenous analgesics and sedatives used for the intraoperative baseline anesthetic. The optimal dose of intrathecal morphine for achieving the maximum postoperative analgesia with minimum undesirable drug effects is uncertain. Naturally, when larger doses of intrathecal morphine are used, more intense and prolonged postoperative analgesia is obtained at the expense of more undesirable drug effects (nausea and vomiting, pruritus, urinary retention, respiratory depression).

Because of morphine's low lipid solubility, analgesic effects after intrathecal injection are delayed. Thus, even large doses of intrathecal morphine administered to patients before cardiac surgery will not initiate reliable intraoperative analgesia[126–128,131] and, therefore, would not be expected to potentially attenuate the intraoperative stress response associated with CPB. Only an extremely large dose of intrathecal morphine (10.0 mg) may initiate reliable intraoperative analgesia in this

TABLE 38-4	Reports of Intrathecal Anesthesia and Analgesia for Cardiac Surgery					
First Author	*Year*	*Study Design*	*Total Patients*	*Drugs: Dose*	*Intraoperative Management*	*Remarks*
Lee[134]	2003	Prospective, randomized blind, placebo-controlled	38	Bupivacaine: 37.5 mg	Standardized	Potential stress-response attenuation
Bowler[107]	2002	Prospective, randomized	24	Morphine: 2.0 mg	Not standardized	No benefit
Bettex[132]	2002	Prospective, randomized	24	Morphine: 0.5 mg Sufentanil: 50 μg	Not standardized	Reliable postoperative analgesia. Facilitated early extubation
Alhashemi[108]	2000	Prospective, randomized, blind, placebo-controlled	0	Morphine: 250 or 500 μg	Standardized	Significant postoperative analgesia
Latham[109]	2000	Prospective, randomized	40	Morphine: 8 μg/kg	Standardized	No benefit
Zarate[110]	2000	Prospective, randomized	40	Morphine: 8 μg/kg	Standardized	Reliable postoperative analgesia
Peterson[113]	2000	Retrospective	18	Morphine: 5 to 10 μg/kg Tetracaine: 1 to 2 mg/kg	Not standardized	No benefit
Hammer[114]	2000	Retrospective	25	Morphine: 7 to 10 μg/kg Tetracaine: 0.5 to 2 mg/kg	Not standardized	No benefit
Chaney[116]	1999	Prospective, randomized, blind, placebo-controlled	40	Morphine: 10 μg/kg	Standardized	No benefit
Shroff[117]	1997	Prospective, randomized	21	Morphine: 10 μg/kg Fentanyl: 25 μg	Not standardized	Reliable postoperative analgesia, facilitated early extubation
Chaney[118]	1997	Prospective, randomized, blind, placebo-controlled	40	Morphine: 10 μg/kg	Standardized	Hindered early extubation
Chaney[119]	1996	Prospective, randomized, blind, placebo-controlled	60	Morphine: 4.0 mg	Standardized	Significant postoperative analgesia, no stress-response attenuation
Taylor[121]	1996	Retrospective	152	Morphine: 30 μg/kg	Not standardized	Reliable postoperative analgesia
Kowalewski[122]	1994	Retrospective	18	Morphine: 0.5 to 1.0 mg Bupivacaine: 23 to 30 mg Lidocaine: 150 mg	Not standardized	Reliable postoperative analgesia, possible thoracic cardiac sympathectomy
Swenson[123]	1994	Retrospective	10	Morphine: 0.5 mg Sufentanil: 50 μg	Not standardized	Reliable postoperative analgesia, facilitated early extubation
Fitzpatrick[125]	1988	Prospective, randomized	44	Morphine: 1.0 to 2.0 mg	Not standardized	Significant postoperative analgesia
Vanstrum[126]	1988	Prospective, randomized, blind, placebo-controlled	30	Morphine: 0.5 mg	Standardized	Significant postoperative analgesia, possible stress–response attenuation
Casey[127]	1987	Prospective, randomized, blind, placebo-controlled	40	Morphine: 20 μg/kg	Standardized	No benefit
Cheun[128]	1987	Prospective, observational	180	Morphine: 0.1 mg/kg Meperidine: 1.5 mg/kg	Not standardized	Reliable postoperative analgesia
Aun[129]	1985	Prospective, randomized	60	Morphine: 2.0 to 4.0 mg	Not standardized	Significant postoperative analgesia
Jones[131]	1984	Postospective, observational	56	Morphine: 20 to 30 μg/kg	Not standardized	Reliable postoperative analgesia
Mathews[106]	1980	Retrospective	40	Morphine: 1.5 to 4.0 mg	Not standardized	Reliable postoperative analgesia

setting.[130] Only one clinical investigation has examined the ability of intrathecal morphine to potentially attenuate the intraoperative stress response associated with CPB as measured by blood catecholamine levels.[119] In Chaney and associates' clinical investigation,[119] patients were prospectively randomized to receive either intrathecal morphine (4.0 mg) or intrathecal placebo before induction of anesthesia for elective CABG with CPB. Intraoperative anesthetic management was standardized, and multiple arterial blood samples were obtained perioperatively to ascertain norepinephrine and epinephrine levels. Patients who were administered intrathecal morphine experienced similar perioperative increases in blood catecholamine levels when compared with placebo controls. Thus, it appears that intrathecal morphine (even in relatively large doses) is unable to reliably attenuate the perioperative stress response associated with cardiac surgery and CPB.

Although intrathecal morphine cannot reliably prevent the perioperative stress response associated with CPB, it may (by initiating postoperative analgesia) potentially attenuate the stress response during the immediate postoperative period.[126] Vanstrum et al[126] revealed that patients who were administered 0.5 mg intrathecal morphine before the induction of anesthesia not only required significantly less intravenous morphine after surgery compared with placebo control patients, but also required significantly less intravenous nitroprusside (58.1 vs. 89.1 mg, respectively; $p < 0.05$) during the initial 24 postoperative hours to control hypertension, which suggests partial postoperative stress-response attenuation.

Some clinical investigators have used intrathecal fentanyl, sufentanil, and/or local anesthetics for patients undergoing cardiac surgery, hoping to provide intraoperative anesthesia and analgesia (and stress–response attenuation), with mixed results (see Table 38-4). Administration of intrathecal local anesthetics to patients after the induction of anesthesia for cardiac surgery may help promote intraoperative hemodynamic stability,[120,122] whereas intrathecal sufentanil (50 μg) administered before the induction of anesthesia for cardiac surgery can reduce volatile anesthetic requirements during mediastinal dissection but is unable to reliably block intraoperative hemodynamic responses to laryngoscopy and intubation.[123]

Most clinical attempts at inducing thoracic cardiac sympathectomy in patients undergoing cardiac surgery have used TEA with local anesthetics. However, a small number of clinical investigators have attempted cardiac sympathectomy in this setting with an intrathecal injection of local anesthetic. In 1994, as reviewed retrospectively, 18 adult patients were administered lumbar intrathecal hyperbaric bupivacaine (23 to 30 mg) and/or hyperbaric lidocaine (150 mg) mixed with morphine (0.5 to 1.0 mg) after the induction of anesthesia.[122] In an attempt to produce a "total spinal" and, thus, thoracic cardiac sympathectomy, Trendelenburg position was maintained for at least 10 minutes after intrathecal injection. Heart rate decreased significantly (baseline mean 67 beats/min to postinjection mean 52 beats/min) after the intrathecal injection (indicating cardiac sympathectomy was obtained), and not a single patient exhibited ECG evidence of myocardial ischemia before CPB. Although these authors reported that the technique provided stable perioperative hemodynamics, 17 of 18 patients required intravenous phenylephrine at some time intraoperatively to increase blood pressure. In 1996, the same group of investigators reported similar hemodynamic changes in a case report involving a 10-year-old child with Kawasaki disease who underwent CABG and received intrathecal hyperbaric bupivacaine mixed with morphine via a lumbar puncture after induction of anesthesia.[120] Although Kowalewski's group reported that these patients experienced enhanced postoperative analgesia, definite conclusions cannot be reached regarding this technique because of study design formats (retrospective review, case report).

A small ($n = 38$ patients), prospective, randomized, blinded clinical investigation showed that large doses of intrathecal bupivacaine (37.5 mg) administered to patients immediately before induction of general anesthesia (19 patients received intrathecal bupivacaine, 19 patients served as controls) for elective CABG may potentially initiate intraoperative stress–response attenuation (assessed via serum

mediator levels, hemodynamics, and qualitative/quantitative alterations in myocardial β receptors).[134] However, no effect on clinical outcome parameters (tracheal extubation times, respiratory function, perioperative spirometry, etc.) was observed. Mean tracheal extubation times (measured from the time of sternotomy dressing application) were extremely short in both groups (11 to 19 minutes). Specifically regarding postoperative analgesia, postoperative pain scores and morphine use via PCA did not differ between the two groups. Not surprisingly, phenylephrine use was more common in patients who received intrathecal bupivacaine compared with control patients.

The many clinical investigations involving the use of intrathecal analgesic techniques in patients undergoing cardiac surgery indicate that the administration of intrathecal morphine to patients before CPB initiates reliable postoperative analgesia after cardiac surgery. Intrathecal opioids or local anesthetics cannot reliably attenuate the perioperative stress response associated with CPB that persists during the immediate postoperative period. Although intrathecal local anesthetics (not opioids) may induce perioperative thoracic cardiac sympathectomy, the hemodynamic changes associated with a "total spinal" make the technique unpalatable in patients with cardiac disease. Indeed, a recently published meta-analysis of randomized, controlled trials (25 randomized trials, 1106 patients) concluded that spinal analgesia does not improve clinically relevant outcomes in patients undergoing cardiac surgery.[135]

Epidural Techniques

The initial description of TEA and analgesia applied to a cardiac surgical patient occurred in 1954, during the formative years of CPB.[136] Clowes et al[136] described their presurgical anesthetic technique in a 55-year-old man with severe cardiac failure: "An endotracheal tube was passed with topical anesthesia. Under extradural block of the upper thorax, hypotension developed but responded to the administration of a vasopressor drug. At this time the patient became comatose" (Figure 38-13). The patient eventually died. Application of TEA to patients undergoing cardiac surgery during the modern surgical era was initially reported by Hoar et al in 1976.[137] They described the intraoperative insertion of thoracic epidural catheters in 12 patients after CABG (after intravenous protamine, before transfer to ICU). The epidural catheters were injected with lidocaine and bupivacaine during the immediate postoperative period to promote analgesia and effectively control hypertension. Administration of epidural local anesthetics to these patients significantly decreased postoperative blood pressure in hypertensive and normotensive patients, and not a single patient required cardiac or peripheral vascular stimulants during the immediate postoperative study period. The 1987 report by El-Baz and Goldin[138] was the first to describe the insertion of thoracic epidural catheters in patients before performance of cardiac surgery. In prospective, randomized fashion, patients undergoing elective CABG received either routine treatment for postoperative pain ($n = 30$ patients, intravenous morphine) or a continuous infusion of morphine (0.1 mg/hr) via a thoracic epidural catheter ($n = 30$ patients). Thoracic epidural catheters were inserted at T3-4 immediately before induction of anesthesia on the day of surgery. Intraoperative anesthetic technique was standardized and mean postoperative tracheal extubation time was significantly shorter in patients receiving TEA compared with control patients (9 ± 3 hours vs. 18 ± 5 hours, respectively; $P < 0.01$).

Continuous thoracic epidural infusion of morphine also achieved better postoperative pain relief in patients than intravenous morphine (significantly better pain scores, significantly less supplemental intravenous morphine). Furthermore, in a subgroup of 20 patients (10 per group), postoperative "stress" was assessed via serum cortisol and β-endorphin levels. Patients receiving TEA had significantly lower postoperative levels of these mediators compared with control patients, indicating potential postoperative stress-response attenuation. Continuous thoracic epidural infusion of morphine (compared with controls) also was associated with a lower incidence of opioid-related side effects during the immediate postoperative period. The insertion

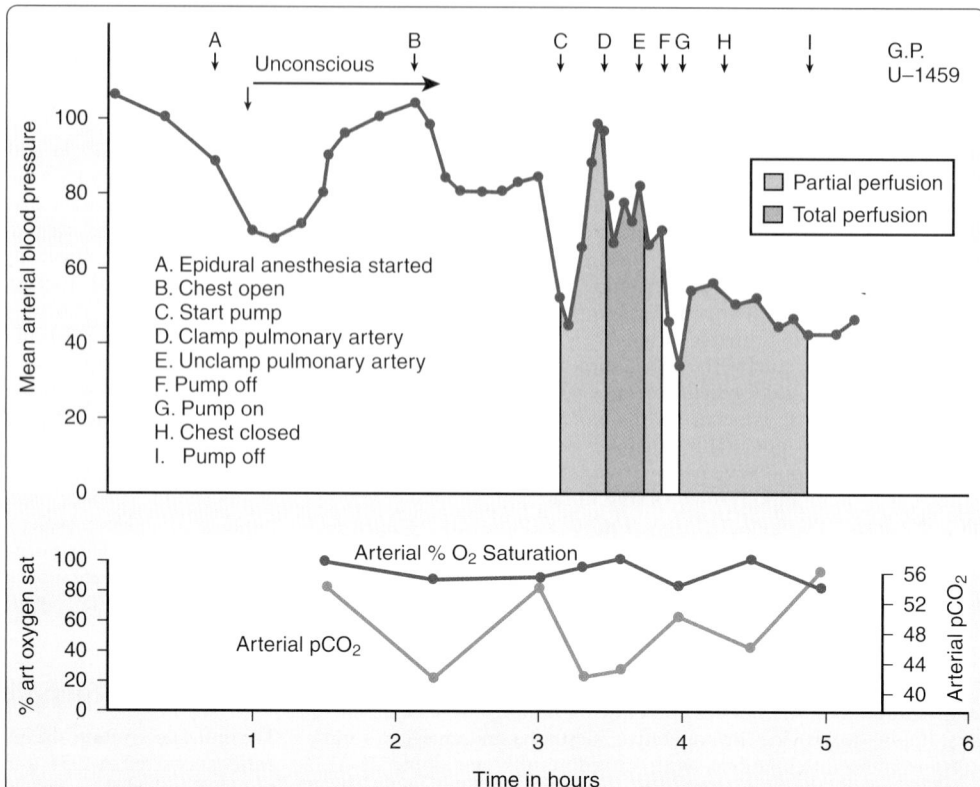

Figure 38-13 **Graph of clinical course of initial cardiac patient receiving pre-surgical epidural anesthesia in 1954.** *(From Clowes GHA, Neville WE, Hopkins A, et al: Factors contributing to success or failure in the use of a pump oxygenator for complete by-pass of the heart and lung: Experimental and clinical. Surgery 36:557, 1954.)*

of the thoracic epidural catheter immediately before systemic heparin administration was not associated with any neurologic problems. Since this initial impressive display of potential benefits (reliable postoperative analgesia, stress-response attenuation, facilitation of early tracheal extubation), other clinical investigators have subsequently applied TEA to patients undergoing cardiac surgery.[139–174] Most clinical investigators have used thoracic epidural local anesthetics in hopes of providing perioperative stress-response attenuation and/or perioperative thoracic cardiac sympathectomy. Some clinical investigators have used thoracic epidural opioids to provide intraoperative and/or postoperative analgesia. An anonymous survey of members of the Society of Cardiovascular Anesthesiologists indicated that 7% of practicing anesthesiologists incorporate thoracic epidural techniques into their anesthetic management of adults undergoing cardiac surgery.[133] Of these anesthesiologists, 58% practice in the United States. Regarding the timing of epidural instrumentation, 40% perform instrumentation before induction of general anesthesia, 12% perform instrumentation after induction of general anesthesia, 33% perform instrumentation at the end of surgery, and 15% perform instrumentation on the first postoperative day.[133]

TEA and analgesia with local anesthetics and/or opioids induce significant postoperative analgesia in patients after cardiac surgery. Patients randomized to receive a continuous thoracic epidural morphine infusion (0.1 mg/hr) after cardiac surgery required significantly less postoperative supplemental intravenous morphine compared with patients without thoracic epidural catheters (5 vs. 18 mg/day per patient, respectively; $p < 0.05$) during the initial 3 postoperative days.[138] Children (aged 2 to 12 years) randomized to receive caudal epidural morphine (75 µg/kg) intraoperatively after cardiac surgery required significantly less postoperative supplemental intravenous morphine compared with patients who did not receive epidural morphine (0.32 vs. 0.71 mg/kg, respectively; $p < 0.01$) during the initial 24 postoperative hours.[158] Numerous additional clinical studies further attest to the ability of TEA with local anesthetics and/or opioids to induce substantial postoperative analgesia in patients after cardiac surgery (Table 38-5).

One unique clinical investigation directly compared TEA and intravenous clonidine in patients undergoing cardiac surgery. Loick et al[142] prospectively randomized 70 patients undergoing elective CABG to receive TEA supplementation (bupivacaine, sufentanil continuous infusion) perioperatively to general anesthesia ($n = 25$ patients), to receive intravenous clonidine supplementation (continuous infusion) perioperatively to general anesthesia ($n = 24$ patients), or to receive only general anesthesia ($n = 21$ patients, controls). Hemodynamics, plasma epinephrine and norepinephrine levels, plasma cortisol levels, the myocardium-specific contractile protein troponin T levels, and other plasma cardiac enzymes were assessed perioperatively. Both the TEA and intravenous clonidine groups experienced postoperative decreases in heart rate compared with the control group (without jeopardizing cardiac output or perfusion pressure). The effects on stress-response mediators were unpredictable and variable. Electrocardiographic evidence of ischemia (ST-segment elevation, ST-segment depression) occurred in 70% of control patients, 50% of TEA patients, and 40% of intravenous clonidine patients. The release of troponin T was attenuated (compared with control patients) in the TEA group only (no effect in the intravenous clonidine group). Interestingly enough, the highest quality of postoperative analgesia was found in the patients receiving intravenous clonidine. In the intravenous clonidine group, visual analog pain scores were nearly halved when compared with the two other groups. Sedation scores were similar among the three groups, with the exception of the 24-hour value in the intravenous clonidine group, which was greater than that in the TEA group. The postoperative comfort scores (rated between excellent and good) did not differ among the three groups.

Many clinical investigations have proved that TEA with local anesthetics also significantly attenuates the perioperative stress response in patients undergoing cardiac surgery. Patients randomized to receive intermittent boluses of thoracic epidural bupivacaine intraoperatively followed by continuous infusion postoperatively exhibited significantly decreased blood levels of norepinephrine and epinephrine perioperatively when compared with patients managed similarly

| | | | | **Total** | | **Intraoperative** | |
TABLE 38-5	**Reports of Epidural Anesthesia and Analgesia for Cardiac Surgery**						
First Author	*Year*	*Study Design*		*Total Patients*	*Drugs: Dosage Method*	*Intraoperative Management*	*Remarks*
Royse[179]	2003	Prospective, randomized		80	Ropivacaine, fentanyl infusion	Not standardized	Reliable postoperative analgesia
Pastor[161]	2003	Prospective, observational		714	Bupivacaine or ropivacaine boluses plus infusion	Not standardized	No hematoma formation
Priestley[180]	2002	Prospective, randomized		100	Ropivacaine, fentanyl infusion	Not standardized	Reliable postoperative analgesia
de Vries[165]	2002	Prospective, randomized		90	Bupivacaine: bolus plus infusion Sufentanil: bolus plus infusion	Standardized	Reliable postoperative analgesia Facilitated early extubation Possible decreased hospital stay
Canto[166]	2002	Prospective, observational		305	Ropivacaine: bolus plus infusion	Not standardized	No hematoma formation
Fillinger[167]	2002	Prospective, randomized		60	Bupivacaine: bolus plus infusion Morphine: bolus plus infusion	Not standardized	No benefit
Jideus[139]	2001	Prospective, randomized		41	Bupivacaine: bolus plus infusion Sufentanil: infusion	Not standardized	Stress-response attenuation Thoracic cardiac sympathectomy
Scott[140]	2001	Prospective, randomized		206	Bupivacaine: bolus plus infusion Clonidine: infusion	Standardized	Decreased postoperative arrhythmias Improved postoperative pulmonary function Decreased postoperative renal failure Decreased postoperative confusion
Dhole[168]	2001	Prospective, randomized		41	Bupivacaine: bolus plus infusion	Not standardized	No benefit
Djaiani[169]	2001	Retrospective		37	Bupivacaine: bolus plus infusion	Not standardized	Facilitated early extubation
Warters[141]	2000	Retrospective		278	Not specified	Not standardized	No hematoma formation
Loick[142]	1999	Prospective, randomized		25	Bupivacaine: bolus plus infusion Sufentanil: bolus plus infusion	Standardized	Stress-response attenuation Thoracic cardiac sympathectomy Facilitated early extubation
Tenling[143]	1999	Prospective, randomized		14	Bupivacaine: bolus plus infusion	Not standardized	Reliable postoperative analgesia Facilitated early extubation
Sanchez[144]	1998	Prospective, observational		571	Bupivacaine: boluses	Not standardized	No hematoma formation
Fawcett[172]	1997	Prospective, randomized		16	Bupivacaine: bolus plus infusion	Standardized	Reliable postoperative analgesia Improved pulmonary function Stress-response attenuation
Turfrey[173]	1997	Retrospective		218	Bupivacaine: bolus plus infusion Clonidine: infusion	Not standardized	Facilitated early extubation Possible thoracic cardiac sympathectomy
Shayevitz[147]	1996	Retrospective		54	Morphine: bolus plus infusion	Not standardized	Reliable postoperative analgesia Facilitated early extubation
Stenseth[174]	1996	Prospective, randomized		54	Bupivacaine: bolus plus infusion	Not standardized	Facilitated early extubation Possible thoracic cardiac sympathectomy
Moore[149]	1995	Prospective, randomized		17	Bupivacaine: bolus plus infusion	Standardized	Stress-response attenuation Possible thoracic cardiac sympathectomy
Stenseth[150]	1995	Prospective, randomized		30	Bupivacaine: bolus plus infusion	Standardized	Thoracic cardiac sympathectomy
Kirno[151]	1994	Prospective, randomized		20	Mepivacaine: bolus	Standardized	Stress-response attenuation Thoracic cardiac sympathectomy
Stenseth[152,153]	1994	Prospective, randomized		30	Bupivacaine: bolus plus infusion	Standardized	Stress-response attenuation Possible thoracic cardiac sympathectomy
Liem[155–157]	1992	Prospective, randomized		54	Bupivacaine: bolus plus infusion Sufentanil: bolus plus infusion	Not standardized	Reliable postoperative analgesia Stress-response attenuation Possible thoracic cardiac sympathectomy
Rosen[158]	1989	Prospective, randomized		32	Morphine: bolus	Not standardized	Reliable postoperative analgesia Facilitated early extubation
Joachimsson[159]	1989	Observational		28	Bupivacaine: boluses	Not standardized	Reliable postoperative analgesia
El-Baz[138]	1987	Prospective, randomized		60	Morphine: infusion	Standardized	Reliable postoperative analgesia Stress-response attenuation Facilitated early extubation
Robinson[160]	1986	Prospective, observational		10	Meperidine: bolus	Standardized	Reliable postoperative analgesia
Hoar[137]	1976	Prospective, observational		12	Lidocaine: boluses	Not standardized	Reliable postoperative analgesia
					Bupivacaine: boluses		Possible stress response attenuation

without thoracic epidural catheters.[152] Furthermore, increased blood catecholamine levels in these patients were associated with increased systemic vascular resistance.[152] Patients randomized to receive continuous thoracic epidural bupivacaine infusion perioperatively exhibited significantly decreased blood levels of norepinephrine and cortisol perioperatively when compared with patients managed similarly without thoracic epidural catheters.[149] Patients randomized to receive a continuous thoracic epidural bupivacaine and sufentanil infusion perioperatively exhibited significantly decreased blood levels of norepinephrine after sternotomy when compared with patients managed similarly without thoracic epidural catheters.[155]

Other clinical studies further attest to the ability of TEA with local anesthetics to promote perioperative hemodynamic stability in patients undergoing cardiac surgery, which suggests perioperative stress-response attenuation.[137,151,152,155] Although most clinical attempts at stress-response attenuation involve thoracic epidural administration of local anesthetics, one investigation indicated that TEA with opioids may significantly attenuate the perioperative stress response in patients undergoing cardiac surgery.[138] In this clinical investigation, patients randomized to receive a continuous thoracic epidural morphine infusion after surgery exhibited significantly decreased blood levels of cortisol and β-endorphin after surgery when compared with patients managed similarly without thoracic epidural catheters.[138]

Two provocative clinical studies demonstrated the ability of TEA to induce significant thoracic cardiac sympathectomy in patients undergoing cardiac surgery.[150,151] In the first study, patients undergoing CABG were evaluated with reverse thermodilution catheters that had been inserted into the midcoronary sinus under fluoroscopic guidance before the induction of anesthesia.[150] Intraoperative anesthetic management was standardized. Coronary sinus blood flow was measured by a constant-infusion technique, and coronary vascular resistance was calculated using coronary perfusion pressure (arterial diastolic pressure minus pulmonary capillary wedge pressure) and coronary sinus blood flow. Patients who had been randomized to receive intermittent boluses of thoracic epidural bupivacaine intraoperatively followed by a continuous infusion after surgery exhibited significant decreases in coronary vascular resistance after CPB when compared with pre-CPB values, whereas patients managed similarly without thoracic epidural catheters exhibited significant increases in coronary vascular resistance after CPB. In the second study, patients undergoing CABG were evaluated with catheters that had been inserted into the coronary sinus under fluoroscopic guidance and continuous pressure monitoring before the induction of anesthesia.[151] Intraoperative anesthetic management was standardized and all patients received a continuous intravenous infusion of tritiated norepinephrine (allowed assessment of cardiac norepinephrine spillover to plasma via isotope dilution technique). Blood samples were obtained from the coronary sinus and radial artery and the rate of norepinephrine spillover from the heart was calculated according to the Fick principle to assess cardiac sympathetic activity.

Patients randomized to receive a single bolus of thoracic epidural mepivacaine immediately after induction of anesthesia exhibited significantly decreased cardiac norepinephrine spillover after sternotomy when compared with patients managed similarly without thoracic epidural catheters. Furthermore, 20% of patients managed without thoracic epidural catheters exhibited ECG evidence of myocardial ischemia after sternotomy, whereas no patient managed with a thoracic epidural catheter exhibited myocardial ischemia during this time.

Perioperative cardiac sympathectomy induced via TEA with local anesthetics may clinically benefit patients undergoing cardiac surgery by increasing myocardial oxygen supply.[95,104,105] However, such a cardiac sympathectomy may offer additional benefits to patients undergoing cardiac surgery. Multiple clinical studies demonstrated that TEA with local anesthetics significantly decreases heart rate before[155] and after[149,155] initiation of CPB, and significantly decreases the need to administer β-blockers after CPB.[152] Multiple clinical studies also demonstrated that TEA with local anesthetics significantly decreases systemic vascular resistance before[151,152] and after[155,159] initiation of CPB. Furthermore, patients undergoing cardiac surgery who receive TEA with

local anesthetics not only exhibit significant decreases in postoperative heart rate and systemic vascular resistance but also significant decreases in postoperative ECG evidence of myocardial ischemia when compared with patients managed similarly without thoracic epidural catheters.[155]

A relatively large clinical investigation highlighted the potential clinical benefits of TEA in cardiac surgical patients.[140] Scott et al[140] prospectively randomized (nonblinded) 420 patients undergoing elective CABG to receive either TEA (bupivacaine/clonidine) and general anesthesia or general anesthesia alone (control group). The two groups received similar intraoperative anesthetic techniques. In TEA patients, the thoracic epidural infusion was continued for 96 hours after surgery (titrated according to need). In control patients, target-controlled infusion alfentanil was used for the first 24 postoperative hours, then followed by PCA morphine for the next 48 hours. After surgery, striking clinical differences were observed between the two groups (Table 38-6). Postoperative incidence of supraventricular arrhythmia, lower respiratory tract infection, renal failure, and acute confusion all were significantly lower in patients receiving TEA compared with control patients. However, data from this clinical investigation must be viewed with caution. The clinical protocol dictated that β-adrenergic blocker therapy could not be used intraoperatively or postoperatively for the 5 days of the study period (except in those patients who developed a new arrhythmia requiring additional therapy). Because approximately 90% of this study's patients were taking β-adrenergic blockers before surgery, this unique perioperative management clouds interpretation of postoperative supraventricular arrhythmia data.

Despite prospective randomization, substantially fewer patients receiving TEA were current active smokers before surgery compared with control patients (5.8% vs. 13.4%, respectively), which clouds interpretation of postoperative lower respiratory tract infection data. These investigators also found that postoperative pre-extubation maximal expiratory lung volumes were increased in TEA patients (compared with control patients), and postoperative tracheal extubation was facilitated via TEA as well (yet TEA patients and control patients were managed somewhat differently during the immediate postoperative period). Although postoperative analgesia was not definitively assessed in this clinical investigation, 11.9% of control patients were converted to TEA during the first 24 postoperative hours because of suboptimal postoperative analgesia, whereas only 2.9% of TEA patients were converted to target-controlled infusion alfentanil or PCA morphine because of suboptimal postoperative analgesia. The results of this clinical investigation are certainly intriguing, but definitive conclusions regarding the use of thoracic epidural techniques in patients undergoing cardiac surgery cannot be drawn because of the study's substantial limitations, highlighted by an accompanying editorial[175] and three subsequent letters to the editor.[176–178]

TABLE 38-6	Various Outcomes of Patients		
Outcome	*TEA (N = 206), n (%)*	*GA (N = 202), n (%)*	
Supraventricular arrhythmia	21 (10.2)	45 (22.3)	
Lower respiratory tract infection	31 (15.3)	59 (29.2)	
Renal failure	4 (2.0)	14 (6.9)	
Cerebrovascular accident	2 (1.0)	6 (3.0)	
Acute confusion	3 (1.5)	11 (5.5)	
Significant bleeding	35	23	
Any complications	84	108	

Significant (unadjusted) differences existed between groups regarding supraventricular arrhythmia (*P* = 0.0012), lower respiratory tract infection (*P* = 0.0007), renal failure (*P* = 0.016), acute confusion (*P* = 0.031), and any complications (*P* = 0.011).
GA, general anesthesia; TEA = thoracic epidural analgesia.
From Scott NB, Turfrey DJ, Ray DAA, et al: A prospective randomized study of the potential benefits of thoracic epidural anesthesia and analgesia in patients undergoing coronary artery bypass grafting. *Anesth Analg* 93:528, 2001.

In contrast with the encouraging findings of Scott et al's[140] clinical investigation, two prospective, randomized, nonblinded clinical investigations revealed that using TEA techniques in patients undergoing cardiac surgery may not offer substantial clinical benefits.[179,180] In 2002, Priestley et al[180] prospectively randomized 100 patients undergoing elective CABG to receive either TEA (ropivacaine/fentanyl) and general anesthesia or general anesthesia alone (control group). The two groups received quite different intraoperative anesthetic techniques. Before surgery, TEA patients received epidural ropivacaine/fentanyl for 48 hours (supplemental analgesics available if needed), whereas control patients received nurse-administered intravenous morphine, followed by PCA morphine. Patients receiving TEA were extubated sooner than control patients (3.2 vs. 6.7 hours, respectively; $P < 0.001$), yet this difference may have been secondary to the different amounts of intraoperative intravenous opioid administered to the two groups (intraoperative intravenous anesthetic technique not standardized).

Postoperative pain scores at rest were significantly lower in patients receiving TEA only on postoperative days 0 and 1 (equivalent on days 2 and 3). Postoperative pain scores during coughing were significantly lower in patients receiving TEA only on postoperative day 0 (equivalent on days 1, 2, and 3; Figure 38-14). There were no significant differences between the two groups in postoperative oxygen saturation on room air, chest radiograph changes, or spirometry (Table 38-7).

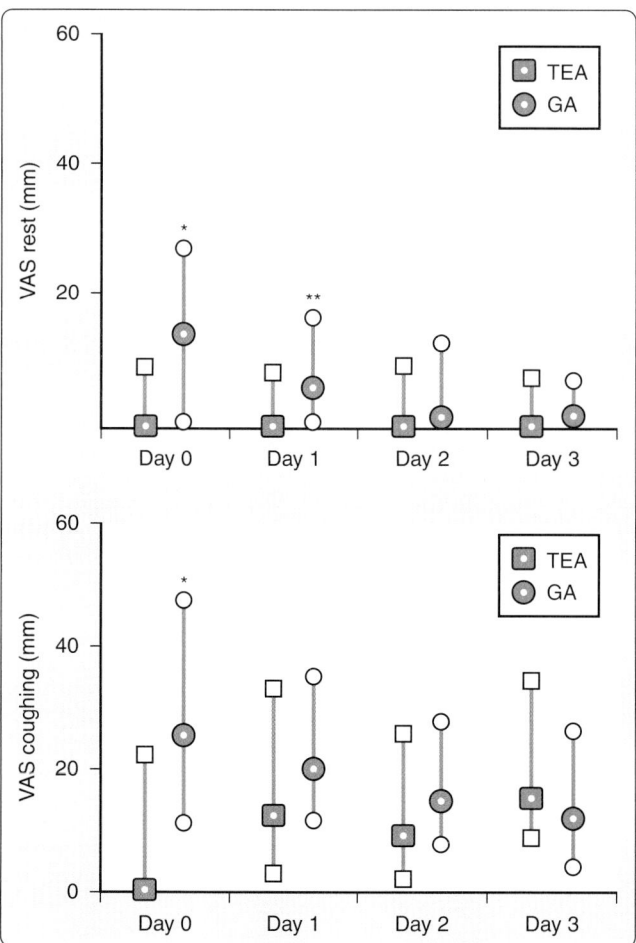

Figure 38-14   **Visual analog scale (VAS) scores.** VAS scores for pain at rest (*top*) and with coughing (*bottom*) on the day of surgery and the first 3 postoperative days. Significant differences ($P < 0.03$) existed between the two groups only on day 0 (rest and coughing) and on day 1 (rest only). GA, general anesthesia; TEA, thoracic epidural analgesia. (*From Priestley MC, Cope L, Halliwell R, et al: Thoracic epidural anesthesia for cardiac surgery: The effects on tracheal intubation time and length of hospital stay. Anesth Analg 94:275, 2002.*)

TABLE 38-7   Spirometry Results

Variable	Mean FEV₁ (SD)		Mean FVC (SD)	
	TEA (L)	GA (L)	TEA (L)	GA (L)
Predicted	2.9 (0.4)	2.9 (0.5)	3.9 (0.5)	3.9 (0.6)
Preoperative	2.5 (0.4)	2.6 (0.8)	3.3 (0.8)	3.4 (0.9)
Postoperative day 1	1.0 (0.3)	1.0 (0.4)	1.2 (0.4)	1.4 (0.5)
Postoperative day 2	1.1 (0.3)	1.1 (0.4)	1.4 (0.4)	1.5 (0.5)
Postoperative day 4	1.4 (0.4)	1.3 (0.5)	1.8 (0.6)	1.7 (0.6)

No significant differences existed between patients receiving thoracic epidural analgesia (TEA) and control (general anesthesia [GA]) patients.

FEV₁, forced expiratory volume in 1 second; FVC, forced vital capacity; SD, standard deviation.

From Priestley MC, Cope L, Halliwell R, et al: Thoracic epidural anesthesia for cardiac surgery: The effects on tracheal intubation time and length of hospital stay. *Anesth Analg* 94:275, 2002.

Furthermore, no clinical differences were detected between the two groups regarding postoperative mobilization goals, atrial fibrillation, postoperative hospital discharge eligibility, or actual postoperative hospital discharge. In short, this clinical investigation revealed that TEA may provide enhanced postoperative analgesia (though brief) and enhance early postoperative tracheal extubation, yet has no effect on important clinical parameters (morbidity, hospital length of stay, etc.). In 2003, Royse and associates[179] prospectively randomized 80 patients undergoing elective CABG to receive either TEA (ropivacaine/fentanyl) and general anesthesia or general anesthesia alone (control group). The two groups received very different intraoperative anesthetic techniques. After surgery, TEA patients received epidural ropivacaine/fentanyl until the third postoperative day, whereas control patients received nurse-administered intravenous morphine followed by PCA morphine. Patients receiving TEA were tracheally extubated sooner during the immediate postoperative period than control subjects (2.6 vs. 5.4 hours, respectively; $P < 0.001$); yet, this difference may have been secondary to the different amounts of intraoperative intravenous anesthetics administered (intraoperative anesthetic technique not standardized). Postoperative pain scores at rest and with cough were significantly lower in patients receiving TEA on postoperative days 1 and 2 only (equivalent on postoperative day 3; Table 38-8). Much like Priestley et al's[180] investigation, there were no substantial differences between the two groups regarding important postoperative clinical parameters (respiratory function, renal function, atrial fibrillation, ICU length of stay, hospital length of stay).

Most recently, in 2006, Hansdottir et al (via the best-designed study to date) provided additional evidence that thoracic epidural techniques offer no real clinical benefits to patients undergoing cardiac surgery.[181] This relatively large (113 patients) prospective trial randomized patients undergoing elective cardiac surgery to receive either patient-controlled TEA (catheter inserted the day before surgery; using bupivacaine, fentanyl, and epinephrine) or patient-controlled intravenous morphine analgesia during the immediate postoperative period.

TABLE 38-8   Visual Analog Scale Scores

Pain Score	High Thoracic Epidural Analgesia (mean ± SD)	Control (mean ± SD)
Rest day 1	0.02 ± 0.2	0.8 ± 1.8
Cough day 1	1.2 ± 1.7	4.4 ± 3.1
Rest day 2	0.1 ± 0.4	1.2 ± 2.7
Cough day 2	1.5 ± 2.0	3.6 ± 3.1
Rest day 3	0.2 ± 1.0	0.3 ± 1.1
Cough day 3	1.7 ± 2.3	2.7 ± 3.0

Mean pain scores at rest and with cough for days 1, 2, and 3. Significant differences ($P < 0.05$) existed between groups on days 1 and 2 (at rest and with cough) yet not on day 3.

From Royse C, Royse A, Soeding P, et al: Prospective randomized trial of high thoracic epidural analgesia for coronary artery bypass surgery. *Ann Thorac Surg* 75:93, 2003.

Perioperative care was standardized (all patients underwent general anesthesia and received a median sternotomy). When the two groups were compared, the only difference was a shorter time to postoperative tracheal extubation in patients receiving TEA (2.3 vs. 7.3 hours). Absolutely no differences were observed regarding postoperative analgesia (at rest and during cough), degree of sedation, lung volumes (forced vital capacity, forced vital capacity at 1 second, peak expiratory flow), degree of ambulation, global quality of recovery score (including all five domains studied), cardiac morbidity (myocardial infarction, atrial fibrillation, etc.), renal morbidity (peak serum creatinine), neurologic outcome (stroke, confusion), ICU stay, or hospital length of stay. Furthermore, this group of experienced investigators reported a very high (17%) "failure" rate for the use of thoracic epidural catheters in these patients.

Despite enhanced postoperative analgesia offered via thoracic epidural techniques, such analgesia does not appear to decrease the incidence of persistent pain after cardiac surgery. Ho and associates[18] assessed via survey 244 patients after cardiac surgery via median sternotomy. One hundred fifty patients received perioperative supplementation of general anesthesia with TEA (ropivacaine/fentanyl infusion initiated before induction of anesthesia and continued after surgery for 2 to 3 days), and 94 patients received general anesthesia and routine postoperative nurse-controlled intravenous morphine infusion for analgesia (together with intraoperative wound infiltration with ropivacaine at chest wall closure). Persistent pain (defined as pain still present 2 or more months after surgery) was similar in the two cohorts (reported in almost 30% of patients). However, persistent pain reported by these patients was mild in most cases, infrequently interfering with daily life.

The quality of analgesia obtained with TEA techniques is sufficient to allow cardiac surgery to be performed in awake patients without general endotracheal anesthesia. The initial report of awake cardiac surgery was published in the *Annals of Thoracic Surgery* in 2000. Karagoz and associates,[182] from Turkey, described the perioperative course of five patients who underwent elective off-pump single-vessel CABG via minithoracotomy with only TEA (spontaneous ventilation throughout). All five patients did well, and none had to be converted to general endotracheal anesthesia. Soon thereafter, a group of investigators from Germany described the perioperative course of 12 patients who underwent elective off-pump multivessel CABG via complete sternotomy with only TEA.[183] All patients did well, yet two patients required conversion to general endotracheal anesthesia (one for incomplete analgesia, one for pneumothorax). Also in 2002, investigators from Brazil revealed that "outpatient" CABG was possible (discharge to home within 24 hours of hospital admission) in a small ($n = 20$) group of patients undergoing cardiac surgery solely via TEA.[184] Since these initial small clinical reports appeared, larger series of patients have been published, demonstrating that "awake" cardiac surgery is feasible and safe.[185–195] In 2003, the first case report of awake cardiac surgery requiring CPB was published.[196] In this astonishing case report from Austria, a 70-year-old man with aortic stenosis underwent aortic valve replacement with assistance of normothermic CPB (total time: 123 minutes; cross-clamp time: 82 minutes) solely via TEA. Verbal communication with the patient was possible on demand throughout CPB. The patient did well and experienced an unremarkable postoperative course.

The many clinical investigations involving the use of epidural analgesic techniques in patients undergoing cardiac surgery indicate that administration of thoracic epidural opioids or local anesthetics before and/or after CPB initiates reliable postoperative analgesia after cardiac surgery. Administration of thoracic epidural local anesthetics (not opioids) can both reliably attenuate the perioperative stress response associated with CPB (that persists during the immediate postoperative period) and induce perioperative thoracic cardiac sympathectomy. Enhanced postoperative analgesia likely facilitates early tracheal extubation after cardiac surgery, yet patients may be extubated after cardiac surgery (with or without CPB) in the operating room without assistance of thoracic epidural techniques.[197]

All clinical reports involving utilization of intrathecal anesthesia and TEA and analgesia techniques for cardiac surgery involve small numbers of patients, and few (if any) are well designed (see Tables 38-4 and 38-5). Only a handful of clinical studies involving intrathecal analgesia are prospective, randomized, blinded, and placebo-controlled (see Table 38-4). There are no blinded, placebo-controlled clinical studies involving epidural techniques (see Table 38-5). Furthermore, none of the existing clinical studies involving intrathecal anesthesia and TEA and analgesia techniques for cardiac surgery uses clinical outcome as a primary end point. Thus, there are clear deficiencies in the literature that prohibit definitive analysis of the risk/benefit ratio of intrathecal anesthesia and TEA and analgesia techniques as applied to patients undergoing cardiac surgery.

A 2004 meta-analysis by Liu et al[198] assessed effects of perioperative central neuraxial analgesia on outcome after CABG. These authors, via MEDLINE and other databases, searched for randomized, controlled trials in patients undergoing CABG with CPB. Fifteen trials enrolling 1178 patients were included for TEA analysis, and 17 trials enrolling 668 patients were included for intrathecal analysis. Thoracic epidural techniques did not affect the incidences of mortality or myocardial infarction, yet reduced risk for arrhythmias (atrial fibrillation and tachycardia), reduced risk for pulmonary complications (pneumonia and atelectasis), reduced time to tracheal extubation, and reduced analog pain scores. Intrathecal techniques did not affect incidences of mortality, myocardial infarction, arrhythmias, or time to tracheal extubation, and only modestly decreased systemic morphine utilization and pain scores (while increasing incidence of pruritus). These authors concluded that central neuraxial analgesia does not affect rates of mortality or myocardial infarction after CABG yet is associated with improvements in faster time to tracheal extubation, decreased pulmonary complications and cardiac arrhythmias, and reduced pain scores. However, the authors also noted that the majority of potential clinical benefits offered by central neuraxial analgesia (earlier extubation, decreased arrhythmias, enhanced analgesia) may be reduced and/or eliminated with changing cardiac anesthesia practice using fast-track techniques, use of β-adrenergic blockers or amiodarone, and/or use of NSAIDs or COX-2 inhibitors. These authors also noted that the risk for spinal hematoma (addressed later in this chapter) because of central neuraxial analgesia in patients undergoing full anticoagulation for CPB remains uncertain.

The use of intrathecal and/or epidural techniques in patients undergoing thoracotomy incisions (rare during cardiac surgery, yet sometimes used in certain circumstances) deserves brief mention.[199] Many factors are involved in the occurrence of pulmonary dysfunction after thoracotomy. Postoperative changes in pulmonary function result from lung resection, atelectasis, and/or volume loss caused by pneumothorax and inspiratory muscle dysfunction. Pain after thoracotomy can be intense, which may produce pulmonary complications after surgery. Somewhat surprisingly, patients undergoing a "clamshell" incision (transverse thoracosternotomy) for bilateral lung transplantation do not experience more postoperative pain than patients undergoing a standard thoracotomy for single-lung transplantation, and lung transplant recipients undergoing thoracotomy have a lower incidence of adequate pain relief than patients undergoing thoracotomy for other indications.[200] These clinical observations emphasize that the condition of the patient may play a major role (together with type of incision) regarding adequacy of postoperative pain control.[200] Clearly, compared with standard thoracotomy incisions, patients receiving minithoracotomy incisions experience less postoperative pain and consume fewer supplemental analgesics during the immediate postoperative period. Furthermore, up to half of all patients undergoing thoracotomy incision will experience chronic pain related to the surgical site.

Evidence exists that indicates adequate postoperative pain control after thoracotomy may help prevent the development of chronic postoperative thoracotomy pain. Therefore, an effective postoperative analgesic plan must be developed for these patients. In contrast with median sternotomy incisions and minithoracotomy incisions, there appears to be some clinical evidence indicating that use of regional anesthetic techniques may decrease postoperative complications after thoracotomy incisions. Specifically, Ballantyne et al[201] and Licker et al[202] provide ample evidence that postoperative pain control with epidural techniques after thoracotomy incision may reduce pulmonary morbidity and overall patient mortality. However, although ample evidence exists suggesting that TEA (superiority of thoracic over lumbar routes has been recently called into question) offers superior postoperative analgesia, not all clinical studies have shown that such techniques truly improve postoperative pulmonary function and reduce postoperative pulmonary complications.

Side Effects of Intrathecal and Epidural Local Anesthetics

The most troubling and undesirable drug effect of intrathecal and epidural local anesthetics is hypotension. Spinal anesthesia to upper thoracic dermatomes produces a decrease in mean arterial blood pressure that is accompanied by a parallel decrease in coronary blood flow.[203,204] Exactly what percentage of blood pressure decrease is acceptable remains speculative, especially in patients with CAD. Disturbances in myocardial oxygenation appear to occur in patients with CAD if coronary perfusion pressure is allowed to decrease by more than 50% during induction of TEA with local anesthetics.[205] Furthermore, if α-adrenergic agonists are used to increase blood pressure during this time, there may be detrimental effects (vasoconstriction) on the native coronary arteries and bypass grafts.[206,207] Of the 19 patients who received intrathecal local anesthetics to produce a "total spinal" for cardiac surgery, 18 required intravenous phenylephrine intraoperatively to increase blood pressure, indicating that hypotension is a substantial problem with this technique.[120,122] Hypotension also appears to be relatively common when thoracic epidural local anesthetics are used in this setting. Volume replacement, β-adrenergic agonists, and/or α-adrenergic agonists are required in a fair proportion of patients, and coronary perfusion pressure may decrease in susceptible patients after CPB.

After epidural administration, local anesthetics can produce blood concentrations of drug that may initiate detrimental cardiac electrophysiologic effects and myocardial depression.[208] In fact, myocardial depression has been detected in patients receiving TEA with bupivacaine, a clinical effect at least partially caused by increased blood concentrations of the drug.[209] Concomitant use of β-adrenergic blockers may further decrease myocardial contractility in this setting.[210,211] Patients undergoing cardiac surgery who were randomized to receive intermittent boluses of thoracic epidural bupivacaine intraoperatively, followed by continuous infusion after surgery, exhibited significantly increased pulmonary capillary wedge pressures after CPB when compared with patients managed similarly without epidural catheters (10.8 vs. 6.4 mm Hg, respectively; $P < 0.001$), which suggests myocardial depression.[152]

Two case reports also indicated that the use of epidural anesthesia and analgesia may either mask myocardial ischemia or initiate myocardial ischemia.[212,213] Oden and Karagianes[213] described the perioperative course of an elderly patient who had a history of exertional angina and underwent uneventful cholecystectomy. After surgery, analgesia was achieved with continuous lumbar epidural fentanyl. On the second postoperative day, with continuous lumbar epidural fentanyl being administered, ST-segment depression was noted on the electrocardiogram. The patient was awake, alert, and did not experience angina. Initiation of intravenous nitroglycerin at this time resulted in normalization of ischemic ECG changes. It was thought by these authors that epidural fentanyl-induced analgesia masked the patient's typical anginal pain. Easley et al[212] described the perioperative course of a middle-aged patient without cardiovascular symptoms ("borderline" hypertension) who was scheduled for exploratory laparotomy. Before surgery, a low thoracic epidural catheter was inserted and local anesthetic was administered (sensory level peaked

by pinprick at T2). The patient at this time began complaining of left-sided jaw pain, and substantial (2.7 mm) ST-segment depression was noted on the electrocardiogram. Surgery was canceled and the patient was treated with aspirin and nitroglycerin. The ECG normalized, yet based on ECG changes, troponin levels, and creatine kinase-MB fractions, the patient was diagnosed with a non–Q-wave myocardial infarction. Coronary angiography on the following day was unremarkable, and a presumptive diagnosis of coronary artery spasm was made. It was thought by these authors that low thoracic epidural-induced sympathectomy led to alterations in the sympathetic–parasympathetic balance (i.e., vasoconstriction above level of block) leading to coronary artery spasm.

Side Effects of Intrathecal and Epidural Opioids

Although many have been described, the four clinically relevant undesirable drug effects of intrathecal and epidural opioids are pruritus, nausea and vomiting, urinary retention, and respiratory depression.[214] After administration of intrathecal or epidural opioids, the most common side effect is pruritus. The incidence rate varies widely (from 0% to 100%) and is often identified only after direct questioning of patients. Severe pruritus is rare, occurring in only approximately 1% of patients. The incidence of nausea and vomiting is approximately 30%. The incidence of urinary retention varies widely (from 0% to 80%) and occurs most frequently in young male patients. When intrathecal or epidural opioids are used in patients undergoing cardiac surgery, the incidences of pruritus, nausea and vomiting, and urinary retention are similar to that described earlier. Of note, if a large dose (4.0 mg) of intrathecal morphine is administered, prolonged postoperative urinary retention may occur.[119]

The most important undesirable drug effect of intrathecal and epidural opioids is respiratory depression. Only 4 months after the initial use of intrathecal[215] and epidural[216] opioids in humans, life-threatening respiratory depression was reported.[217-219] The incidence of respiratory depression that requires intervention after conventional doses of intrathecal and epidural opioids is approximately 1%, the same as that after conventional doses of intramuscular and intravenous opioids. Early respiratory depression occurs within minutes of opioid injection and is associated with administration of intrathecal or epidural fentanyl or sufentanil. Delayed respiratory depression occurs hours after opioid injection and is associated with administration of intrathecal or epidural morphine. Delayed respiratory depression results from cephalad migration of morphine in cerebrospinal fluid and the subsequent stimulation of opioid receptors located in the ventral medulla.[220] Factors that increase the risk for respiratory depression include large and/or repeated doses of opioids, intrathecal utilization, advanced age, and concomitant use of intravenous sedatives.[214] The magnitude of postoperative respiratory depression is profoundly influenced by the dose of intrathecal or epidural morphine administered, and the type and amount of intravenous analgesics and amnestics used for the intraoperative baseline anesthetic. Prolonged postoperative respiratory depression may delay tracheal extubation, and naloxone may be required in some patients.

Children may be more susceptible to developing postoperative respiratory depression when intrathecal morphine is used in this setting. Of 56 children (aged 1 to 17 years) administered either 20 or 30 μg/kg intrathecal morphine before surgical incision for cardiac surgery, 3 of 29 who received 20 μg/kg and 6 of 27 who received 30 μg/kg required naloxone after surgery for respiratory depression.[131]

One clinical study indicated that administration of intrathecal morphine to patients undergoing cardiac surgery may be contraindicated if early extubation is planned.[118] Patients were randomized to receive either intrathecal morphine (10 μg/kg) or intrathecal placebo before the induction of anesthesia. Intraoperative anesthetic management was standardized and consisted of intravenous fentanyl (20 μg/kg) and intravenous midazolam (10 mg total) together with inhaled isoflurane and/or intravenous nitroglycerin, if required. Regarding patients extubated during the immediate postoperative period, the mean time from ICU arrival to extubation was significantly increased in those who received intrathecal morphine compared with those who received intrathecal placebo (10.9 vs. 7.6 hours, respectively; $P = 0.02$). However, other clinical studies indicated that intrathecal or epidural morphine may yet prove to be a useful adjunct for cardiac surgery and early extubation. The optimal dose of intrathecal or epidural morphine in this setting, together with the optimal intraoperative baseline anesthetic that will provide significant postoperative analgesia yet not delay tracheal extubation in the immediate postoperative period, remains to be elucidated. In contrast with intrathecal and epidural opioids, epidural local anesthetics (which initiate no respiratory depression) should not delay tracheal extubation in the immediate postoperative period.

Risk for Hematoma Formation

Intrathecal or epidural instrumentation entails risk, the most feared complication being epidural hematoma formation. The estimated incidence of hematoma formation is approximately 1:220,000 after intrathecal instrumentation.[221] Hematoma formation is more common (approximately 1:150,000) after epidural instrumentation because larger needles are used, catheters are inserted, and the venous plexus in the epidural space is prominent.[221] Furthermore, hematoma formation does not occur exclusively during epidural catheter insertion; almost half of all cases develop after catheter removal.[221]

Although spontaneous hematomas can occur in the absence of intrathecal or epidural instrumentation,[222] most occur when instrumentation is performed in a patient with a coagulopathy (from any cause) or when instrumentation is difficult or traumatic.[221] Paradoxically, intrathecal or epidural instrumentation has been performed safely in patients with known clinical coagulopathy.[223,224] Of 1000 epidural catheterizations performed in 950 patients receiving oral anticoagulants at time of catheter insertion, none experienced signs or symptoms of hematoma formation.[224] Of 336 epidural injections performed in 36 patients with chronic cancer pain either fully anticoagulated (oral anticoagulants or intravenous heparin) or profoundly thrombocytopenic (platelet count < 50,000/mm^3) at the time of instrumentation, none had signs or symptoms of hematoma formation.[223]

Risk is increased when intrathecal or epidural instrumentation is performed before systemic heparinization, and hematoma formation has occurred in patients when diagnostic or therapeutic lumbar puncture has been followed by systemic heparinization.[225–228] When lumbar puncture is followed by systemic heparinization, concurrent use of aspirin, difficult or traumatic instrumentation, and administration of intravenous heparin within 1 hour of instrumentation increase the risk for hematoma formation.[227] However, by observing certain precautions, intrathecal or epidural instrumentation can be performed safely in patients who will subsequently receive intravenous heparin.[229,230] By delaying surgery 24 hours in the event of a traumatic tap, by delaying heparinization 60 minutes after catheter insertion, and by maintaining tight perioperative control of anticoagulation, more than 4000 intrathecal or epidural catheterizations were performed safely in patients undergoing peripheral vascular surgery who received intravenous heparin after catheter insertion.[230] A retrospective review involving 912 patients further indicates that epidural catheterization before systemic heparinization for peripheral vascular surgery is safe.[229] However, the magnitude of anticoagulation in these two studies (activated partial thromboplastin time of approximately 100 seconds[229] and activated coagulation time approximately twice the baseline value[230]) involving patients undergoing peripheral vascular surgery was substantially less than the degree of anticoagulation required in patients subjected to CPB.

Most clinical studies investigating the use of intrathecal or epidural anesthesia and analgesia techniques in patients undergoing cardiac surgery included precautions to decrease risk for hematoma formation. Some used the technique only after the demonstration of laboratory evidence of normal coagulation parameters, delayed surgery 24 hours

in the event of traumatic tap, or required that the time from instrumentation to systemic heparinization exceed 60 minutes. Although most clinicians investigating use of epidural anesthesia and analgesia techniques in patients undergoing cardiac surgery insert catheters the day before scheduled surgery, investigators have performed instrumentation on the same day of surgery. Institutional practice (same-day admit surgery) may eliminate the option of epidural catheter insertion on the day before scheduled surgery. An alternative is to perform epidural instrumentation postoperatively (before or after tracheal extubation), after the demonstration via laboratory evidence of normal coagulation parameters.

Although most investigators agree that risk for hematoma is likely increased when intrathecal or epidural instrumentation is performed in patients before systemic heparinization required for CPB, the absolute degree of increased risk is somewhat controversial; some believe the risk rate may be as high as 0.35%.[225] An extensive mathematical analysis by Ho et al[231] of the approximately 10,840 intrathecal injections in patients subjected to systemic heparinization required for CPB (without a single episode of hematoma formation) reported in the literature as of 2000 estimated that the minimum risk for hematoma formation was 1:220,000, and the maximum risk for hematoma formation was 1:3600 (95% confidence level); however, the maximum risk may be as high as 1:2400 (99% confidence level). Similarly, of the approximately 4583 epidural instrumentations in patients subjected to systemic heparinization required for CPB (without a single episode of hematoma formation) reported in the literature as of 2000, the minimum risk for hematoma formation was 1:150,000 and the maximum risk for hematoma formation was 1:1500 (95% confidence level); however, the maximum risk may be as high as 1:1000 (99% confidence level).[231]

Certain precautions, however, may decrease the risk.[221,225] The technique should not be used in a patient with known coagulopathy from any cause. Surgery should be delayed 24 hours in the event of a traumatic tap, and time from instrumentation to systemic heparinization should exceed 60 minutes. In addition, systemic heparin effect and reversal should be tightly controlled (smallest amount of heparin used for the shortest duration compatible with therapeutic objectives), and patients should be closely monitored after surgery for signs and symptoms of hematoma formation. An obvious economic disadvantage of intrathecal or epidural instrumentation in patients before cardiac surgery is the possible delay in surgery in the event of a traumatic tap. However, one study involving more than 4000 intrathecal or epidural catheterizations via a 17-gauge Tuohy needle indicated that the incidence of traumatic tap (blood freely aspirated) is rare (< 0.10%).[230]

In 2004, the first case report of an epidural hematoma associated with a thoracic epidural catheter inserted in a patient before cardiac surgery was published.[232] This 18-year-old man had a thoracic (T9-10) epidural catheter uneventfully inserted after induction of general anesthesia (the patient had intense fear of needles) immediately before initiation of CPB for aortic valve replacement surgery. Three hours elapsed from instrumentation to systemic heparinization. The entire intraoperative course and immediate postoperative course were uneventful (tracheally extubated soon after surgery, ambulating without difficulty on the first postoperative day). At 49 hours after surgery, intravenous heparin therapy was initiated (prosthetic valve thromboprophylaxis). At 53 hours after surgery, alteplase (thrombolytic drug) was used to flush a dysfunctional intravenous catheter. Within 2 hours of intravenous alteplase administration, the patient reported intense back pain while ambulating. At this point, the epidural catheter was removed. The activated partial thromboplastin time assessed at this time (during catheter removal) was 87.4 seconds (reference range, 24.8 to 37.3 seconds). The patient also was thrombocytopenic at this time. On catheter removal, the patient experienced sudden onset of numbness and weakness distal to T9. Intravenous heparin was discontinued, a computed tomographic scan was inconclusive, requiring a magnetic resonance imaging scan, which revealed an epidural hematoma. Five hours from the onset of neurologic symptoms, the patient underwent surgical evacuation of the hematoma (which extended from the T8 to T11 levels). Intraoperatively, intravenous methylprednisolone (30 mg/kg) was administered, followed by an infusion (5.4mg/kg/hr), which was continued for 72 hours. Twenty-four hours after laminectomy, the patient demonstrated mild residual lower extremity motor and sensory deficits. Six weeks later, his neurologic examination had returned to normal. The authors noted the factors affecting coagulation in this patient (heparin, alteplase, thrombocytopenia) that likely led to hematoma formation and theorized that removing the catheter may have increased bleeding, further compounding the problem.

Since 2004, numerous such reports (with catastrophic consequences, such as permanent paralysis) have appeared in the literature.[233-235] In addition, thromboembolic complications (neurologic, stroke) may occur during the postoperative period when normalization of coagulation parameters (in a patient requiring anticoagulation) is achieved to safely remove the epidural catheter.[236] Thus, bleeding and/or thromboembolic complications associated with these techniques in this setting are very real and potentially catastrophic.

Use of regional anesthetic techniques in patients undergoing cardiac surgery, although seemingly increasing in popularity, remains extremely controversial, prompting numerous editorials by recognized experts in the field of cardiac anesthesia.[237-240] One of the main reasons such controversy exists (and likely will continue for some time) is that the numerous clinical investigations regarding this topic are suboptimally designed and use a wide array of disparate techniques, preventing clinically useful conclusions on which all can agree.[241,242]

MULTIMODAL ANALGESIA

The possibility of synergism between analgesic drugs is a concept that is nearly a century old.[243,244] Although subsequent research has demonstrated the difference between additivity and synergy, the fundamental strategy behind such combinations ("multimodal" or "balanced" analgesia) remains unchanged: enhanced analgesia with minimization of adverse physiologic effects. Use of analgesic combinations during the postoperative period, specifically the combination of traditional intravenous opioids with other analgesics (NSAIDs, COX-2 inhibitors, ketamine, etc.), has been proved clinically effective in noncardiac patients for decades. Early clinical investigations simply reported analgesic efficacy, whereas more recent clinical investigations have additionally evaluated and described specific opioid-sparing effects (which should lead to a reduction in side effects). For example, in the late 1980s, initial clinical studies involving ketorolac (the first parenteral NSAID available in the United States) revealed significant opioid-sparing effects (analgesia) together with a reduction in respiratory depression. Subsequently, substantial clinical research has clearly established the perioperative analgesic efficacy and opioid-sparing effects of NSAIDs (together with reduction of side effects).

The American Society of Anesthesiologists Task Force on Acute Pain Management in the Perioperative Setting reported that the literature supports the administration of two analgesic agents that act by different mechanisms via a single route for providing superior analgesic efficacy with equivalent or reduced adverse effects.[1] Potential examples include epidural opioids administered in combination with epidural local anesthetics or clonidine and intravenous opioids in combination with ketorolac or ketamine. Dose-dependent adverse effects reported with administration of a medication occur whether it is given alone or in combination with other medications (opioids may cause nausea, vomiting, pruritus, or urinary retention, and local anesthetics may produce motor block). The literature is insufficient to evaluate the postoperative analgesic effects of oral opioids combined with NSAIDs, COX-2 inhibitors, or acetaminophen compared with oral opioids alone. The Task Force believed that NSAIDs, COX-2 inhibitors, or acetaminophen administration has a dose-sparing effect for systemically administered opioids. The literature also suggests that two routes of administration, when compared with a single route, may be more effective in providing perioperative analgesia. Examples include intrathecal or epidural opioids combined with intravenous, intramuscular, oral, transdermal, or

subcutaneous analgesics versus intrathecal or epidural opioids alone. Another example is intravenous opioids combined with oral NSAIDs, COX-2 inhibitors, or acetaminophen versus intravenous opioids alone. The literature is insufficient to evaluate the efficacy of pharmacologic pain management combined with nonpharmacologic, alternative, or complementary pain management compared with pharmacologic pain management alone.

HOW IMPORTANT IS POSTOPERATIVE PAIN AFTER CARDIAC SURGERY?

Cardiac surgery is unique, and because of this, it involves unique risks not routinely associated with noncardiac surgery.[245] Furthermore, as all are aware, for a wide variety of reasons, patients presenting for cardiac surgery continue to get older and "sicker" (more comorbidities: neurologic dysfunction, myocardial dysfunction, renal dysfunction, etc.). Multiple factors interact in a complicated manner during the perioperative period that affect outcome and quality of life after cardiac surgery, including type and quality of surgical intervention, extent of postoperative neurologic dysfunction, extent of postoperative myocardial dysfunction, extent of postoperative pulmonary dysfunction, extent of postoperative renal dysfunction, extent of postoperative coagulation abnormalities, extent of systemic inflammatory response, and quality of postoperative analgesia. Obviously, depending on specific clinical situations, certain factors will be more important than others. It is extremely difficult (if not impossible) to determine exactly how important attaining adequate or "high-quality" postoperative analgesia truly is in relation to all these important clinical factors surrounding a patient undergoing cardiac surgery. For example, how important is it to obtain "high-quality" postoperative analgesia in an 80-year-old patient with preoperative myocardial dysfunction, renal dysfunction, and a heavily calcified aorta after double-valve replacement? It could be argued that factors other than quality of postoperative analgesia will determine clinical outcome in this patient. On the other hand, how important is it to obtain "high-quality" postoperative analgesia in an otherwise healthy 50-year-old patient after routine CABG? It is likely that this patient's clinical outcome will be satisfactory even if postoperative analgesia is suboptimal. In essence, for cardiac and noncardiac surgery patients, there is insufficient evidence to confirm or deny the ability of postoperative analgesic techniques to affect postoperative morbidity or mortality.[246,247]

CONCLUSIONS

Multiple factors are important during the perioperative period that potentially affect outcome and quality of life after cardiac surgery, including type and quality of surgical intervention, extent of postoperative neurologic dysfunction, myocardial dysfunction, pulmonary dysfunction, renal dysfunction, coagulation abnormalities, quality of postoperative analgesia and/or extent of systemic inflammatory response, among others[248] (Table 38-9). This list of factors is presented in no particular order; obviously, depending on specific clinical situations (surgical procedure, patient comorbidity, etc.), certain factors will be more important than others. It is extremely difficult (if not impossible) to determine exactly how important attaining adequate postoperative analgesia truly is in relation to all of these clinical factors

TABLE 38-9	Factors Affecting Outcome after Cardiac Surgery

- Type and quality of surgical intervention
- Extent of postoperative neurologic dysfunction
- Extent of postoperative myocardial dysfunction
- Extent of postoperative pulmonary dysfunction
- Extent of postoperative renal dysfunction
- Extent of postoperative coagulation abnormalities
- Quality of postoperative analgesia
- Extent of systemic inflammatory response

surrounding a patient undergoing cardiac surgery. A clear link between "adequate" or "high-quality" postoperative analgesia and outcome in patients after cardiac surgery has yet to be established.[249-251]

However, despite the absence of substantiating scientific evidence, most clinicians intuitively believe that attaining high-quality postoperative analgesia is important because it may prevent adverse hemodynamic, metabolic, immunologic, and hemostatic alterations, all of which may potentially increase postoperative morbidity. Although many analgesic techniques are available, intravenous systemic opioids form the cornerstone of postcardiac surgery analgesia. Opioids have been used for many years in the treatment of postoperative pain in patients after cardiac surgery, with good results. Although NSAIDs (specifically COX-2 inhibitors) have received much recent attention, important clinical issues regarding their safety (gastrointestinal effects, renal effects, hemostatic effects, immunologic effects) need to be resolved. Although PCA techniques are commonly used, their clear superiority over traditional nurse-controlled analgesic techniques remains unproved. As a general rule, it is likely best to avoid intense, single-modality therapy for the treatment of acute postoperative pain. Clinicians should strive for an approach that uses a number of different therapies (multimodal therapy), each counteracting pain via different mechanisms. Preemptive analgesia, although intriguing, needs further study to determine its role in affecting postoperative analgesia and outcome.[252-255]

Finally, the American Society of Anesthesiologists Task Force on Acute Pain Management in the Perioperative Setting offered sound advice.[1] It recommends that anesthesiologists who manage perioperative pain use analgesic therapeutic options only after thoughtfully considering the risks and benefits for the individual patient. The therapy (or therapies) selected should reflect the individual anesthesiologist's expertise, as well as the capacity for safe application of the chosen modality in each practice setting. This includes the ability to recognize and treat adverse effects that emerge after initiation of therapy. Whenever possible, anesthesiologists should use multimodal pain management therapy. Dosing regimens should be administered to optimize efficacy while minimizing the risk for adverse events. The choice of medication, dose, route, and duration of therapy always should be individualized.

REFERENCES

1. American Society of Anesthesiologists Task Force on Acute Pain Management: Practice guidelines for acute pain management in the perioperative setting: An updated report by the American Society of Anesthesiologists Task Force on Acute Pain Management, *Anesthesiology* 100:1573, 2004.
2. Joint Commission on Accreditation of Healthcare Organizations: *Pain assessment and management—an organizational approach*, 2000. Available at: http://www.jcaho.org. Accessed October 15, 2005.
3. Weissman C: The metabolic response to stress: An overview and update, *Anesthesiology* 73:308, 1990.
4. Kehlet H: Surgical stress: The role of pain and analgesia, *Br J Anaesth* 63:189, 1989.
5. Roizen MF: Should we all have a sympathectomy at birth? Or at least preoperatively [Editorial]? *Anesthesiology* 68:482, 1988.
6. Tuman KJ, McCarthy RJ, March RJ, et al: Effects of epidural anesthesia and analgesia on coagulation and outcome after major vascular surgery, *Anesth Analg* 73:696, 1991.
7. Yeager MP, Glass DD, Neff RK, et al: Epidural anesthesia and analgesia in high-risk surgical patients, *Anesthesiology* 66:729, 1987.
8. Mangano DT, Siliciano D, Hollenberg M, et al: Postoperative myocardial ischemia: Therapeutic trials using intensive analgesia following surgery, *Anesthesiology* 76:342, 1992.
9. Anand KJS, Hickey PR: Halothane-morphine compared with high-dose sufentanil for anesthesia and postoperative analgesia in neonatal cardiac surgery, *N Engl J Med* 326:1, 1992.
10. Wallace AW: Is it time to get on the fast track or stay on the slow track [Editorial]? *Anesthesiology* 99:774, 2003.
11. Myles PS, Daly DJ, Djaiani G, et al: A systematic review of the safety and effectiveness of fast-track cardiac anesthesia, *Anesthesiology* 99:982, 2003.
12. Royston D, Kovesi T, Marczin N: The unwanted response to cardiac surgery: Time for a reappraisal [Editorial]? *J Thorac Cardiovasc Surg* 125:32, 2003.
13. Mueller XM, Tinguely F, Tevaearai HT, et al: Pain location, distribution, and intensity after cardiac surgery, *Chest* 118:391, 2000.
14. Nay PG, Elliott SM, Harrop-Griffiths AW: Postoperative pain. Expectation and experience after coronary artery bypass grafting, *Anaesthesia* 51:741, 1996.
15. Meehan DA, McRae ME, Rourke DA, et al: Analgesic administration, pain intensity, and patient satisfaction in cardiac surgical patients, *Am J Crit Care* 4:435, 1995.
16. Moore R, Follette DM, Berkoff HA: Poststernotomy fractures and pain management in open cardiac surgery, *Chest* 106:1339, 1994.
17. Greenwald LV, Baisden CE, Symbas PN: Rib fractures in coronary bypass patients: Radionuclide detection, *Radiology* 148:553, 1983.
18. Ho SC, Royse CF, Royse AG, et al: Persistent pain after cardiac surgery: An audit of high thoracic epidural and primary opioid analgesia therapies, *Anesth Analg* 95:820, 2002.
19. Kalso E, Mennander S, Tasmuth T, et al: Chronic post-sternotomy pain, *Acta Anaesth Scand* 45:935, 2001.
20. Chaney MA, Morales M, Bakhos M: Severe incisional pain and long thoracic nerve injury after port-access minimally invasive mitral valve surgery, *Anesth Analg* 91:288, 2000.
21. Davis Z, Jacobs HK, Zhang M, et al: Endoscopic vein harvest for coronary artery bypass grafting: Technique and outcomes, *J Thorac Cardiovasc Surg* 116:228, 1998.
22. Smith RC, Leung JM, Mangano DT, SPI Research Group: Postoperative myocardial ischemia in patients undergoing coronary artery bypass graft surgery, *Anesthesiology* 74:464, 1991.
23. Leung JM, O'Kelly B, Browner WS, et al: Prognostic importance of postbypass regional wall-motion abnormalities in patients undergoing coronary artery bypass graft surgery, *Anesthesiology* 71:16, 1989.
24. Philbin DM, Rosow CE, Schneider RC, et al: Fentanyl and sufentanil anesthesia revisited: How much is enough? *Anesthesiology* 73:5, 1990.
25. Reves JG, Karp RB, Buttner EE, et al: Neuronal and adrenomedullary catecholamine release in response to CPB in man, *Circulation* 66:49, 1982.
26. Roberts AJ, Niarchos AP, Subramanian VA, et al: Systemic hypertension associated with coronary artery bypass surgery: Predisposing factors, hemodynamic characteristics, humoral profile, and treatment, *J Thorac Cardiovasc Surg* 74:846, 1977.
27. Liu S, Carpenter RL, Neal MJ: Epidural anesthesia and analgesia: their role in postoperative outcome, *Anesthesiology* 82:1474, 1995.
28. Wu CL, Naqibuddin M, Rowlingson AJ, et al: The effect of pain on health-related quality of life in the immediate postoperative period, *Anesth Analg* 97:1078, 2003.
29. Rogers MC: Do the right thing. Pain relief in infants and children [Editorial], *N Engl J Med* 326:55, 1992.
30. White PF, Rawal S, Latham P, et al: Use of a continuous local anesthetic infusion for pain management after median sternotomy, *Anesthesiology* 99:918, 2003.
31. Dowling R, Thielmeier K, Ghaly A, et al: Improved pain control after cardiac surgery: Results of a randomized, double-blind, clinical trial, *J Thorac Cardiovasc Surg* 126:1271, 2003.
32. Brown SL, Morrison AE: Local anesthetic infusion pump systems adverse events reported to the Food and Drug Administration, *Anesthesiology* 100:1305, 2004.
33. McDonald SB, Jacobsohn E, Kopacz DJ, et al: Parastenal block and local anesthetic infiltration with levobupivacaine after cardiac surgery with desflurane: The effect on postoperative pain, pulmonary function, and tracheal extubation times, *Anesth Analg* 100:75, 2005.
34. Soto RG, Fu ES: Acute pain management for patients undergoing thoracotomy, *Ann Thorac Surg* 75:1349, 2003.
35. Karmakar MK: Thoracic paravertebral block, *Anesthesiology* 95:771, 2001.
36. Kavanagh BP, Katz J, Sandler AN: Pain control after thoracic surgery. A review of current techniques, *Anesthesiology* 81:737-759, 1994.
37. Bilgin M, Akcali Y, Oguzkaya F: Extrapleural regional versus systemic analgesia for relieving postthoracotomy pain: A clinical study of bupivacaine compared with metamizol, *J Thorac Cardiovasc Surg* 126:1580, 2003.
38. Mehta Y, Swaminathan M, Mishra Y, et al: A comparative evaluation of intrapleural and thoracic epidural analgesia for postoperative pain relief after minimally invasive direct coronary artery bypass surgery, *J Cardiothorac Vasc Anesth* 12:162, 1998.
39. Riedel BJ: Regional anesthesia for major cardiac and noncardiac surgery: More than just a strategy for effective analgesia [editorial]? *J Cardiothorac Vasc Anesth* 15:279, 2001.
40. Allen MS, Halgren L, Nichols FC, et al: A randomized controlled trial of bupivacaine through intracostal catheters for pain management after thoracotomy, *Ann Thorac Surg* 88:903, 2009.
41. Maurer K, Blumenthal S, Rentsch KM, et al: Continuous extrapleural infusion of ropivacaine 0.2% after cardiovascular surgery via the lateral thoracotomy approach, *J Cardiothorac Vasc Anesth* 22:249, 2008.
42. Wheatley GH, Rosenbaum DH, Paul MC, et al: Improved pain management outcomes with continuous infusion of a local anesthetic after thoracotomy, *J Thorac Cardiovasc Surg* 130:464, 2005.
43. Myles PA, Bain C: Underutilization of paravertibral block in thoracic surgery, *J Cardiothorac Vasc Anesth* 20:635, 2006.
44. Marret E, Bazelly B, Taylor G, et al: Paravertebral block with ropivacaine 0.5% versus systematic analgesia for pain relief after thoracotomy, *Ann Thorac Surg* 79:2109, 2005.
45. Joshi GP, Bonnet F, Shah R, et al: A systematic review of randomized trials evaluating regional techniques for post thoracotomy analgesia, *Anesth Analg* 107:126, 2008.
46. Gottschalk A, Cohen SP, Yang S, et al: Preventing and treating pain after thoracic surgery, *Anesthesiology* 104:594, 2006.
47. Detterbeck FC: Efficacy of methods of intercoastal nerve blockade for pain relief after thoracotomy, *Ann Thorac Surg* 80:1550, 2005.
48. Raja SN, Lowenstein E: The birth of opioid anesthesia (classic papers revisited), *Anesthesiology* 100:1013, 2004.
49. Bovill JG, Sebel PS, Stanley TH: Opioid analgesics in anesthesia: With special reference to their use in cardiovascular anesthesia, *Anesthesiology* 61:731, 1984.
50. Hug CC: Does opioid "anesthesia" exist [editorial]? *Anesthesiology* 73:1, 1990.
51. Kehlet H, Rung GW, Callesen T: Postoperative opioid analgesia: Time for a reconsideration? *J Clin Anesth* 8:441, 1996.
52. Peng PWH, Sandler AN: A review of the use of fentanyl analgesia in the management of acute pain in adults, *Anesthesiology* 90:576, 1999.
53. Checketts MR, Gilhooly CJ, Kenny GNC: Patient-maintained analgesia with target-controlled alfentanil infusion after cardiac surgery: A comparison with morphine PCA, *Br J Anaesth* 80:748, 1998.
54. Bowdle TA, Camporesi EM, Maysick L, et al: A multicenter evaluation of remifentanil for early postoperative analgesia, *Anesth Analg* 83:1292, 1996.
55. Ouattara A, Boccara G, Kockler U, et al: Remifentanil induces systemic arterial vasodilation in humans with a total artificial heart, *Anesthesiology* 100:602, 2004.
56. Liu SS, Allen HW, Olsson GL: Patient-controlled epidural analgesia with bupivacaine and fentanyl on hospital wards: Prospective experience with 1,030 surgical patients, *Anesthesiology* 88:688, 1998.
57. Boylan JF, Katz J, Kavanagh BP, et al: Epidural bupivacaine-morphine analgesia versus patient-controlled analgesia following abdominal aortic surgery: Analgesic, respiratory, and myocardial effects, *Anesthesiology* 89:585, 1998.
58. Tsang J, Brush B: Patient-controlled analgesia in postoperative cardiac surgery, *Anaesth Intensive Care* 27:464, 1999.
59. Gust R, Pecher S, Gust A, et al: Effect of patient-controlled analgesia on pulmonary complications after coronary artery bypass grafting, *Crit Care Med* 27:2218, 1999.

60. Boldt J, Thaler E, Lehmann A, et al: Pain management in cardiac surgery patients: Comparison between standard therapy and patient-controlled analgesia regimen, *J Cardiothorac Vasc Anesth* 12:654, 1998.
61. Munro AJ, Long GT, Sleigh JW: Nurse-administered subcutaneous morphine is a satisfactory alternative to intravenous patient-controlled analgesia morphine after cardiac surgery, *Anesth Analg* 87:11, 1998.
62. Myles PS, Buckland MR, Cannon GB, et al: Comparison of patient-controlled analgesia and nurse-controlled infusion analgesia after cardiac surgery, *Anaesth Intensive Care* 22:672, 1994.
63. Searle NR, Roy M, Bergeron G, et al: Hydromorphone patient-controlled analgesia (PCA) after coronary artery bypass surgery, *Can J Anaesth* 41:198, 1994.
64. Ralley FE, Day FJ, Cheng DCH: Pro: Nonsteroidal anti-inflammatory drugs should be routinely administered for postoperative analgesia after cardiac surgery, *J Cardiothorac Vasc Anesth* 14:731, 2000.
65. Griffin M: Con: Nonsteroidal anti-inflammatory drugs should not be routinely administered for postoperative analgesia after cardiac surgery, *J Cardiothorac Vasc Anesth* 14:735, 2000.
66. Kharasch ED: Perioperative COX-2 inhibitors: Knowledge and challenges [Editorial], *Anesth Analg* 98:1, 2004.
67. Gilron I, Milne B, Hong M: Cyclooxygenase-2 inhibitors in postoperative pain management: Current evidence and future directions, *Anesthesiology* 99:1198, 2003.
68. Gajraj NM: Cyclooxygenase-2 inhibitors, *Anesth Analg* 96:1720, 2003.
69. McCrory CR, Lindahl SGE: Cyclooxygenase inhibition for postoperative analgesia, *Anesth Analg* 95:169, 2002.
70. FitzGerald GA, Patrono C: The coxibs, selective inhibitors of cyclooxygenase-2, *N Engl J Med* 345:433, 2001.
71. Crofford LJ: Rational use of analgesic and antiinflammatory drugs [Editorial], *N Engl J Med* 345:1844, 2001.
72. Hynninen MS, Cheng DCH, Hossain I, et al: Non-steroidal antiinflammatory drugs in treatment of postoperative pain after cardiac surgery, *Can J Anesth* 47:1182, 2000.
73. Lin JC, Szwerc MF, Magovern JA: Nonsteroidal anti-inflammatory drug-based pain control for minimally invasive direct coronary artery bypass surgery, *Heart Surg Forum* 2:169, 1999.
74. Rapanos T, Murphy P, Szalai JP, et al: Rectal indomethacin reduces postoperative pain and morphine use after cardiac surgery, *Can J Anesth* 46:725, 1999.
75. Lahtinen P, Kokki H, Hendolin H, et al: Propacetamol as adjunctive treatment for postoperative pain after cardiac surgery, *Anesth Analg* 95:813, 2002.
76. Immer FF, Immer-Bansi AS, Trachsel N, et al: Pain treatment with a COX-2 inhibitor after coronary artery bypass operation: A randomized trial, *Ann Thorac Surg* 75:490, 2003.
77. Ott E, Nussmeier NA, Duke PC, et al: Efficacy and safety of the cyclooxygenase 2 inhibitors parecoxib and valdecoxib in patients undergoing coronary artery bypass surgery, *J Thorac Cardiovasc Surg* 125:1481, 2003.
78. Mukherjee D, Nissen SE, Topol EJ: Risk of cardiovascular events associated with selective COX-2 inhibitors, *JAMA* 286:954, 2001.
79. White PF, Kehlet H, Liu S: Perioperative analgesia: What do we still know? *Anesth Analg* 108:1364, 2009.
80. Guo TZ, Jiang JY, Buttermann AE, et al: Dexmedetomidine injection into the locus ceruleus produces antinociception, *Anesthesiology* 84:873, 1996.
81. Nishina K, Mikawa K, Uesugi T, et al: Efficacy of clonidine for prevention of perioperative myocardial ischemia: A critical appraisal and meta-analysis of the literature, *Anesthesiology* 96:323, 2002.
82. Flacke JW, Bloor BC, Flacke WE, et al: Reduced narcotic requirement by clonidine with improved hemodynamic and adrenergic stability in patients undergoing coronary bypass surgery, *Anesthesiology* 67:11, 1987.
83. Ebert TJ, Hall JE, Barney JA, et al: The effects of increasing plasma concentrations of dexmedetomidine in humans, *Anesthesiology* 93:382, 2000.
84. Multz AS: Prolonged dexmedetomidine infusion as an adjunct in treating sedation-induced withdrawal, *Anesth Analg* 96:1054, 2003.
85. Arain SR, Ebert TJ: The efficacy, side effects, and recovery characteristics of dexmedetomidine versus propofol when used for intraoperative sedation, *Anesth Analg* 95:461, 2002.
86. Triltsch AE, Welte M, von Homeyer P, et al: Bispectral index-guided sedation with dexmedetomidine in intensive care: A prospective, randomized, double-blind, placebo-controlled phase II study, *Crit Care Med* 30:1007, 2002.
87. Myles PS, Hunt JO, Holdgaard HO, et al: Clonidine and cardiac surgery: Haemodynamic and metabolic effects, myocardial ischaemia and recovery, *Anaesth Intensive Care* 27:137–147, 1999.
88. Boldt J, Rothe G, Schindler E, et al: Can clonidine, enoximone, and enalaprilat help to protect the myocardium against ischaemia in cardiac surgery? *Heart* 76:207, 1996.
89. Abi-Jaoude F, Brusset A, Ceddaha A, et al: Clonidine premedication for coronary artery bypass grafting under high-dose alfentanil anesthesia: Intraoperative and postoperative hemodynamic study, *J Cardiothorac Vasc Anesth* 7:35, 1993.
90. Dorman BH, Zucker JR, Verrier ED, et al: Clonidine improves perioperative myocardial ischemia, reduces anesthetic requirement, and alters hemodynamic parameters in patients undergoing coronary artery bypass surgery, *J Cardiothorac Vasc Anesth* 7:386, 1993.
91. Chaney MA: Intrathecal and epidural anesthesia and analgesia for cardiac surgery, *Anesth Analg* 84:1211, 1997.
92. Feigl E: Coronary physiology, *Physiol Rev* 63:1, 1983.
93. Lee DDP, Kimura S, DeQuattro V: Noradrenergic activity and silent ischaemia in hypertensive patients with stable angina: Effect of metoprolol, *Lancet* 1:403, 1989.
94. Vanhoutte PM, Shimokawa H: Endothelium-derived relaxing factor and coronary vasospasm, *Circulation* 80:1, 1989.
95. Blomberg S, Emanuelsson H, Kvist H, et al: Effects of thoracic epidural anesthesia on coronary arteries and arterioles in patients with coronary artery disease, *Anesthesiology* 73:840, 1990.
96. Blomberg S, Curelaru I, Emanuelsson H, et al: Thoracic epidural anaesthesia in patients with unstable angina pectoris, *Eur Heart J* 10:437–444, 1989.
97. Heusch G, Deussen A, Thamer V: Cardiac sympathetic nerve activity and progressive vasoconstriction distal to coronary stenosis: Feed-back aggravation of myocardial ischemia, *J Auton Nerv Syst* 13:311, 1985.
98. Heusch G, Deussen A: The effects of cardiac sympathetic nerve stimulation on perfusion of stenotic coronary arteries in the dog, *Circ Res* 53:8, 1983.
99. Uchida Y, Murao S: Excitation of afferent cardiac sympathetic nerve fibers during coronary occlusion, *Am J Physiol* 226:1094, 1974.
100. Mangano DT: Perioperative cardiac morbidity, *Anesthesiology* 72:153, 1990.
101. Birkett DA, Apthorp GH, Chamberlain DA, et al: Bilateral upper thoracic sympathectomy in angina pectoris: Results in 52 cases, *Br Med J* 2:187, 1965.
102. Kock M, Blomberg S, Emanuelsson H, et al: Thoracic epidural anesthesia improves global and regional left ventricular function during stress-induced myocardial ischemia in patients with coronary artery disease, *Anesth Analg* 71:625, 1990.
103. Blomberg SG: Long-term home self-treatment with high thoracic epidural anesthesia in patients with severe coronary artery disease, *Anesth Analg* 79:413, 1994.
104. Davis RF, DeBoer LWV, Maroko PR: Thoracic epidural anesthesia reduces myocardial infarct size after coronary artery occlusion in dogs, *Anesth Analg* 65:711, 1986.
105. Klassen GA, Bramwell RS, Bromage PR, et al: Effect of acute sympathectomy by epidural anesthesia on the canine coronary circulation, *Anesthesiology* 52:8, 1980.
106. Mathews ET, Abrams LD: Intrathecal morphine in open heart surgery [Correspondence], *Lancet* 2:543, 1980.
107. Bowler I, Djaiani G, Abel R, et al: A combination of intrathecal morphine and remifentanil anesthesia for fast-track cardiac anesthesia and surgery, *J Cardiothorac Vasc Anesth* 16:709, 2002.
108. Alhashemi JA, Sharpe MD, Harris CL, et al: Effect of subarachnoid morphine administration on extubation time after coronary artery bypass graft surgery, *J Cardiothorac Vasc Anesth* 14:639, 2000.
109. Latham P, Zarate E, White PF, et al: Fast-track cardiac anesthesia: A comparison of remifentanil plus intrathecal morphine with sufentanil in a desflurane-based anesthetic, *J Cardiothorac Vasc Anesth* 14:645, 2000.
110. Zarate E, Latham P, White PF, et al: Fast-track cardiac anesthesia: Use of remifentanil combined with intrathecal morphine as an alternative to sufentanil during desflurane anesthesia, *Anesth Analg* 91:283, 2000.
111. Bowler I, Djaiani G, Hall J, et al: Intravenous remifentanil combined with intrathecal morphine decreases extubation times after elective coronary artery bypass graft (CABG) surgery [Abstract], *Anesth Analg* 90:S33, 2000.
112. Lee TWR, Jacobsohn E, Maniate JM, et al: High spinal anesthesia in cardiac surgery: Effects on hemodynamics, perioperative stress response, and atrial β-receptor function [Abstract], *Anesth Analg* 90:SCA90, 2000.
113. Peterson KL, DeCampli WM, Pike NA, et al: A report of two hundred twenty cases of regional anesthesia in pediatric cardiac surgery, *Anesth Analg* 90:1014, 2000.
114. Hammer GB, Ngo K, Macario A: A retrospective examination of regional plus general anesthesia in children undergoing open heart surgery, *Anesth Analg* 90:1020, 2000.
115. Djaiani G, Bowler I, Hall J, et al: A combination of remifentanil and intrathecal morphine improves pulmonary function following CABG surgery [Abstract], *Anesth Analg* 90:SCA64, 2000.
116. Chaney MA, Nikolov MP, Blakeman BP, et al: Intrathecal morphine for coronary artery bypass graft procedure and early extubation revisited, *J Cardiothorac Vasc Anesth* 13:574, 1999.
117. Shroff A, Rooke GA, Bishop MJ: Effects of intrathecal opioid on extubation time, analgesia, and ICU stay following coronary artery bypass grafting, *J Clin Anesth* 9:415, 1997.
118. Chaney MA, Furry PA, Fluder EM, et al: Intrathecal morphine for coronary artery bypass grafting and early extubation, *Anesth Analg* 84:241, 1997.
119. Chaney MA, Smith KR, Barclay JC, et al: Large-dose intrathecal morphine for coronary artery bypass grafting, *Anesth Analg* 83:215, 1996.
120. Kowalewski R, MacAdams C, Froelich J, et al: Anesthesia supplemented with subarachnoid bupivacaine and morphine for coronary artery bypass surgery in a child with Kawasaki disease, *J Cardiothorac Vasc Anesth* 10:243, 1996.
121. Taylor A, Healy M, McCarroll M, et al: Intrathecal morphine: One year's experience in cardiac surgical patients, *J Cardiothorac Vasc Anesth* 10:225, 1996.
122. Kowalewski RJ, MacAdams CL, Eagle CJ, et al: Anaesthesia for coronary artery bypass surgery supplemented with subarachnoid bupivacaine and morphine: A report of 18 cases, *Can J Anaesth* 41:1189, 1994.
123. Swenson JD, Hullander RM, Wingler K, et al: Early extubation after cardiac surgery using combined intrathecal sufentanil and morphine, *J Cardiothorac Vasc Anesth* 8:509, 1994.
124. Shroff AB, Bishop MJ: Intrathecal morphine analgesia speeds extubation and shortens ICU stay following coronary artery bypass grafting (CABG) [Abstract], *Anesthesiology* 81:A129, 1994.
125. Fitzpatrick GJ, Moriarty DC: Intrathecal morphine in the management of pain following cardiac surgery. A comparison with morphine i.v, *Br J Anaesth* 60:639, 1988.
126. Vanstrum GS, Bjornson KM, Ilko R: Postoperative effects of intrathecal morphine in coronary artery bypass surgery, *Anesth Analg* 67:261, 1988.
127. Casey WF, Wynands JE, Ralley FE, et al: The role of intrathecal morphine in the anesthetic management of patients undergoing coronary artery bypass surgery, *J Cardiothorac Vasc Anesth* 1:510, 1987.
128. Cheun JK: Intraspinal narcotic anesthesia in open heart surgery, *J Kor Med Sci* 2:225, 1987.
129. Aun C, Thomas D, John-Jones L, et al: Intrathecal morphine in cardiac surgery, *Eur J Anaesth* 2:419, 1985.
130. Vincenty C, Malone B, Mathru M, et al: Comparison of intrathecal and intravenous morphine in post coronary bypass surgery [Abstract], *Crit Care Med* 13:308, 1985.
131. Jones SEF, Beasley JM, Macfarlane DWR, et al: Intrathecal morphine for postoperative pain relief in children, *Br J Anaesth* 56:137, 1984.
132. Bettex DA, Schmidlin D, Chassot PG, et al: Intrathecal sufentanil-morphine shortens the duration of intubation and improves analgesia in fast-track cardiac surgery, *Can J Anesth* 49:711, 2002.
133. Goldstein S, Dean D, Kim SJ, et al: A survey of spinal and epidural techniques in adult cardiac surgery, *J Cardiothorac Vasc Anesth* 15:158, 2001.
134. Lee TWR, Grocott HP, Schwinn D, et al: High spinal anesthesia for cardiac surgery: Effects on β-adrenergic receptor function, stress response, and hemodynamics, *Anesthesiology* 98:499, 2003.
135. Zangrillo A, Bignami E, Biondi-Zuccai GGL, et al: Spinal analgesia in cardiac surgery: A meta-analysis of randomized controlled trials, *J Cardiothorac Vasc Anesth* 23:813, 2009.
136. Clowes GHA, Neville WE, Hopkins A, et al: Factors contributing to success or failure in the use of a pump oxygenator for complete by-pass of the heart and lung, experimental and clinical, *Surgery* 36:557, 1954.
137. Hoar PF, Hickey RF, Ullyot DJ: Systemic hypertension following myocardial revascularization. A method of treatment using epidural anesthesia, *J Thorac Cardiovasc Surg* 71:859, 1976.
138. El-Baz N, Goldin M: Continuous epidural infusion of morphine for pain relief after cardiac operations, *J Thorac Cardiovasc Surg* 93:878, 1987.
139. Jideus L, Joachimsson PO, Stridsberg M, et al: Thoracic epidural anesthesia does not influence the occurrence of postoperative sustained atrial fibrillation, *Ann Thorac Surg* 72:65, 2001.
140. Scott NB, Turfrey DJ, Ray DAA, et al: A prospective randomized study of the potential benefits of thoracic epidural anesthesia and analgesia in patients undergoing coronary artery bypass grafting, *Anesth Analg* 93:528, 2001.
141. Warters D, Knight W, Koch SM, et al: Thoracic epidurals in coronary artery bypass surgery, *Anesth Analg* 90:767, 2000.
142. Loick HM, Schmidt C, Van Aken H, et al: High thoracic epidural anesthesia, but not clonidine, attenuates the perioperative stress response via sympatholysis and reduces the release of troponin T in patients undergoing coronary artery bypass grafting, *Anesth Analg* 88:701, 1999.
143. Tenling A, Joachimsson PO, Tyden H, et al: Thoracic epidural anesthesia as an adjunct to general anesthesia for cardiac surgery: Effects on ventilation-perfusion relationships, *J Cardiothorac Vasc Anesth* 13:258, 1999.
144. Sanchez R, Nygard E: Epidural anesthesia in cardiac surgery: Is there an increased risk? *J Cardiothorac Vasc Anesth* 12:170, 1998.
145. Loick HM, Mollhoff T, Erren M, et al: Thoracic epidural anesthesia lowers catecholamine and TNFa release after CABG in humans [Abstract], *Anesth Analg* 86:S81, 1998.
146. Warters RD, Koch SM, Luehr SL, et al: Thoracic epidural anesthesia in CABG surgery [Abstract], *Anesth Analg* 86:S116, 1998.
147. Shayevitz JR, Merkel S, O'Kelly SW, et al: Lumbar epidural morphine infusions for children undergoing cardiac surgery, *J Cardiothorac Vasc Anesth* 10:217, 1996.

148. Frank RS, Boltz MG, Sentivany SK, et al: Combined epidural-general anesthesia for the repair of atrial septal defects in children results in shorter ICU stays [Abstract], *Anesthesiology* 83:A1176, 1995.
149. Moore CM, Cross MH, Desborough JP, et al: Hormonal effects of thoracic extradural analgesia for cardiac surgery, *Br J Anaesth* 75:387, 1995.
150. Stenseth R, Berg EM, Bjella L, et al: Effects of thoracic epidural analgesia on coronary hemodynamics and myocardial metabolism in coronary artery bypass surgery, *J Cardiothorac Vasc Anesth* 9:503, 1995.
151. Kirno K, Friberg P, Grzegorczyk A, et al: Thoracic epidural anesthesia during coronary artery bypass surgery: Effects on cardiac sympathetic activity, myocardial blood flow and metabolism, and central hemodynamics, *Anesth Analg* 79:1075, 1994.
152. Stenseth R, Bjella L, Berg EM, et al: Thoracic epidural analgesia in aortocoronary bypass surgery, I: Haemodynamic effects, *Acta Anaesthesiol Scand* 38:826, 1994.
153. Stenseth R, Bjella L, Berg EM, et al: Thoracic epidural analgesia in aortocoronary bypass surgery, II: Effects on the endocrine metabolic response, *Acta Anaesthesiol Scand* 38:834, 1994.
154. Shapiro JH, Wolman RL, Lofland GK: Epidural morphine as an adjunct for early extubation following congenital cardiac surgery [Abstract], *Anesth Analg* 78:S385, 1994.
155. Liem TH, Booij LHDJ, Hasenbos MAWM, et al: Coronary artery bypass grafting using two different anesthetic techniques: Part I: Hemodynamic results, *J Cardiothorac Vasc Anesth* 6:148, 1992.
156. Liem TH, Hasenbos MAWM, Booij LHDJ, et al: Coronary artery bypass grafting using two different anesthetic techniques: Part 2: Postoperative outcome, *J Cardiothorac Vasc Anesth* 6:156, 1992.
157. Liem TH, Booij LH, Gielen MJ, et al: Coronary artery bypass grafting using two different anesthetic techniques: Part 3: Adrenergic responses, *J Cardiothorac Vasc Anesth* 6:162, 1992.
158. Rosen KR, Rosen DA: Caudal epidural morphine for control of pain following open heart surgery in children, *Anesthesiology* 70:418, 1989.
159. Joachimsson PO, Nystrom SO, Tyden H: Early extubation after coronary artery surgery in efficiently rewarmed patients: A postoperative comparison of opioid anesthesia versus inhalational anesthesia and thoracic epidural analgesia, *J Cardiothorac Anesth* 3:444, 1989.
160. Robinson RJS, Brister S, Jones E, et al: Epidural meperidine analgesia after cardiac surgery, *Can Anaesth Soc J* 33:550, 1986.
161. Pastor MC, Sanchez MJ, Casas MA, et al: Thoracic epidural analgesia in coronary artery bypass graft surgery: Seven years' experience, *J Cardiothorac Vasc Anesth* 17:154, 2003.
162. Vlachtsis H, Vohra A: High thoracic epidural with general anesthesia for combined off-pump coronary artery and aortic aneurysm surgery, *J Cardiothorac Vasc Anesth* 17:226, 2003.
163. Sisillo E, Salvi L, Juliano G, et al: Thoracic epidural anesthesia as a bridge to redo coronary artery bypass graft surgery, *J Cardiothorac Vasc Anesth* 17:629, 2003.
164. Varadarajan B, Whitaker DK, Vohra A, et al: Case 2-2002. Thoracic epidural anesthesia in patients with ankylosing spondylitis undergoing coronary artery surgery, *J Cardiothorac Vasc Anesth* 16:240, 2002.
165. de Vries AJ, Mariani MA, van der Maaten JM, et al: To ventilate or not after minimally invasive direct coronary artery bypass surgery: The role of epidural anesthesia, *J Cardiothorac Vasc Anesth* 16:21, 2002.
166. Canto M, Casas A, Sanchez MJ, et al: Thoracic epidurals in heart valve surgery: Neurologic risk evaluation, *J Cardiothorac Vasc Anesth* 16:723, 2002.
167. Fillinger MP, Yeager MP, Dodds TM, et al: Epidural anesthesia and analgesia: Effects on recovery from cardiac surgery, *J Cardiothorac Vasc Anesth* 16:15, 2002.
168. Dhole S, Mehta Y, Saxena H, et al: Comparison of continuous thoracic epidural and paravertebral blocks for postoperative analgesia after minimally invasive direct coronary artery bypass surgery, *J Cardiothorac Vasc Anesth* 15:288, 2001.
169. Djaiani GN, Ali M, Heinrich L, et al: Ultra-fast-track anesthetic technique facilitates operating room extubation in patients undergoing off-pump coronary revascularization surgery, *J Cardiothorac Vasc Anesth* 15:152, 2001.
170. Visser WA, Liem TH, Brouwer RM: High thoracic epidural anesthesia for coronary artery bypass graft surgery in a patient with severe obstructive lung disease, *J Cardiothorac Vasc Anesth* 15:758, 2001.
171. Liem TH, Williams JP, Hensens AG, et al: Minimally invasive direct coronary artery bypass procedure using a high thoracic epidural plus general anesthetic technique, *J Cardiothorac Vasc Anesth* 12:668, 1998.
172. Fawcett WJ, Edwards RE, Quinn AC, et al: Thoracic epidural analgesia started after CPB. Adrenergic, cardiovascular and respiratory sequelae, *Anaesthesia* 52:294, 1997.
173. Turfrey DJ, Ray DAA, Sutcliffe NP, et al: Thoracic epidural anaesthesia for coronary artery bypass graft surgery. Effects on postoperative complications, *Anaesthesia* 52:1090, 1997.
174. Stenseth R, Bjella L, Berg EM, et al: Effects of thoracic epidural analgesia on pulmonary function after coronary artery bypass surgery, *Eur J Cardiothorac Surg* 10:859–865, 1996.
175. O'Connor CJ, Tuman KJ: Epidural anesthesia and analgesia for coronary artery bypass graft surgery: Still forbidden territory [editorial]? *Anesth Analg* 93:523, 2001.
176. Amar D: Beta-adrenergic blocker withdrawal confounds the benefits of epidural analgesia with sympathectomy on supraventricular arrhythmias after cardiac surgery [Correspondence], *Anesth Analg* 95:1119, 2002.
177. Riedel BJ, Shaw AD: Thoracic epidural anesthesia and analgesia in patients undergoing coronary artery bypass surgery [Correspondence], *Anesth Analg* 94:1365, 2002.
178. Alston RP: Thoracic epidurals and coronary artery bypass grafting surgery [Correspondence], *Anesth Analg* 94:1365, 2002.
179. Royse C, Royse A, Soeding P, et al: Prospective randomized trial of high thoracic epidural analgesia for coronary artery bypass surgery, *Ann Thorac Surg* 75:93, 2003.
180. Priestley MC, Cope L, Halliwell R, et al: Thoracic epidural anesthesia for cardiac surgery: The effects on tracheal intubation time and length of hospital stay, *Anesth Analg* 94:275, 2002.
181. Hansdottir V, Philip J, Olsen MF, et al: Thoracic epidural versus intravenous patient-controlled analgesia after cardiac surgery, *Anesthesiology* 104:142, 2006.
182. Karagoz HY, Sonmez B, Bakkaloglu B, et al: Coronary artery bypass grafting in the conscious patient without endotracheal general anesthesia, *Ann Thorac Surg* 70:91, 2000.
183. Aybek T, Dogan S, Neidhart G, et al: Coronary artery bypass grafting through complete sternotomy in conscious patients, *Heart Surg Forum* 5:17, 2002.
184. Souto GLL, Junior CSC, de Souza JBS, et al: Coronary artery bypass in the ambulatory patient, *J Thorac Cardiovasc Surg* 123:1008, 2002.
185. Aybek T, Kessler P, Dogan S, et al: Awake coronary artery bypass grafting: Utopia or reality? *Ann Thorac Surg* 75:1165, 2003.
186. Aybek T, Kessler P, Khan MF, et al: Operative techniques in awake coronary artery bypass grafting, *J Thorac Cardiovasc Surg* 125:1394, 2003.
187. Karagoz HY, Kurtoglu M, Bakkaloglu B, et al: Coronary artery bypass grafting in the awake patient: Three years' experience in 137 patients, *J Thorac Cardiovasc Surg* 125:1401, 2003.
188. Chakravarthy M, Jawali V, Patil TA, et al: High thoracic epidural anesthesia as the sole anesthetic for redo off-pump coronary artery bypass surgery, *J Cardiothorac Vasc Anesth* 17:84, 2003.
189. Chakravarthy MR, Jawali V, Patil TA, et al: High thoracic epidural anaesthesia as the sole anaesthetic technique for minimally invasive direct coronary artery bypass in a high-risk patient, *Ann Cardiac Anaesth* 6:62, 2003.
190. Kessler P, Neidhart G, Bremerich DH, et al: High thoracic epidural anesthesia for coronary artery bypass grafting using two different surgical approaches in conscious patients, *Anesth Analg* 95:791, 2002.
191. Vanek T, Straka Z, Brucek P, et al: Thoracic epidural anesthesia for off-pump coronary artery bypass without intubation, *Eur J Cardiothorac Surg* 20:858, 2001.
192. Anderson MB, Kwong KF, Furst AJ, et al: Thoracic epidural anesthesia for coronary bypass via left anterior thoracotomy in the conscious patient, *Eur J Cardiothorac Surg* 20:415, 2001.
193. Paiste J, Bjerke RJ, Williams JP, et al: Minimally invasive direct coronary artery bypass surgery under high thoracic epidural, *Anesth Analg* 93:1486, 2001.
194. Zenati MA, Paiste J, Williams JP, et al: Minimally invasive coronary bypass without general endotracheal anesthesia, *Ann Thorac Surg* 72:1380, 2001.
195. Chakravarthy M, Jawali V, Patil TA, et al: High thoracic epidural anesthesia as the sole anesthetic for performing multiple grafts in off-pump coronary artery bypass surgery, *J Cardiothorac Vasc Anesth* 17:160, 2003.
196. Schachner T, Bonatti J, Balogh D, et al: Aortic valve replacement in the conscious patient under regional anesthesia without endotracheal intubation, *J Thorac Cardiovasc Surg* 125:1526, 2003.
197. Straka Z, Brucek P, Vanek T, et al: Routine immediate extubation for off-pump coronary artery bypass grafting without thoracic epidural analgesia, *Ann Thorac Surg* 74:1544, 2002.
198. Liu SS, Block BM, Wu CL: Effects of perioperative central neuraxial analgesia on outcome after coronary artery bypass surgery: A meta-analysis, *Anesthesiology* 101:153, 2004.
199. Ochroch EA, Gottschalk A, Augostides J, et al: Long-term pain and activity during recovery from major thoracotomy using thoracic epidural analgesia, *Anesthesiology* 97:1234, 2002.
200. Richard C, Girard F, Ferraro P, et al: Acute postoperative pain in lung transplant recipients, *Ann Thorac Surg* 77:1951–1955, 2004.
201. Ballantyne JC, Carr DB, deFerranti S, et al: The comparative effects of postoperative analgesic therapies on pulmonary outcome: Cumulative meta-analyses of randomized, controlled trials, *Anesth Analg* 86:598, 1998.
202. Licker M, de Perrot M, Hohn L, et al: Perioperative mortality and major cardiopulmonary complications after lung surgery for non-small-cell carcinoma, *Eur J Cardiothorac Surg* 15:314, 1999.
203. Sivarajan M, Amory DW, Lindbloom LE, et al: Systemic and regional blood-flow changes during spinal anesthesia in the rhesus monkey, *Anesthesiology* 43:78, 1975.
204. Hackel DB, Sancetta SM, Kleinerman J: Effect of hypotension due to spinal anesthesia on coronary blood flow and myocardial metabolism in man, *Circulation* 13:92, 1956.
205. Reiz S, Nath S, Rais O: Effects of thoracic epidural block and prenalterol on coronary vascular resistance and myocardial metabolism in patients with coronary artery disease, *Acta Anaesth Scand* 24:11, 1980.
206. DiNardo JA, Bert A, Schwartz MJ, et al: Effects of vasoactive drugs on flows through left internal mammary artery and saphenous vein grafts in man, *J Thorac Cardiovasc Surg* 102:730, 1991.
207. Heusch G: α-Adrenergic mechanisms in myocardial ischemia, *Circulation* 81:1, 1990.
208. Reiz S, Nath S: Cardiotoxicity of local anaesthetic agents, *Br J Anaesth* 58:736, 1986.
209. Wattwil M, Sundberg A, Arvill A, et al: Circulatory changes during high thoracic epidural anaesthesia—influence of sympathetic block and of systemic effect of the local anaesthetic, *Acta Anaesth Scand* 29:849, 1985.
210. Blomberg S, Ricksten SE: Effects of thoracic epidural anaesthesia on central haemodynamics compared to cardiac beta-adrenoceptor blockade in conscious rats with acute myocardial infarction, *Acta Anaesth Scand* 34:1, 1990.
211. Hotvedt R, Refsum H, Platou ES: Cardiac electrophysiological and hemodynamic effects of β-adrenoceptor blockade and thoracic epidural analgesia in the dog, *Anesth Analg* 63:817, 1984.
212. Easley RB, Rosen RE, Lindeman KS: Coronary artery spasm during initiation of epidural anesthesia, *Anesthesiology* 99:1015, 2003.
213. Oden RV, Karagianes TG: Postoperative myocardial ischemia possibly masked by epidural fentanyl analgesia, *Anesthesiology* 74:941, 1991.
214. Chaney MA: Side effects of intrathecal and epidural opioids, *Can J Anaesth* 42:891, 1995.
215. Wang JK, Nauss LA, Thomas JE: Pain relief by intrathecally applied morphine in man, *Anesthesiology* 50:149, 1979.
216. Behar M, Magora F, Olshwang D, et al: Epidural morphine in treatment of pain, *Lancet* 1:527, 1979.
217. Glynn CJ, Mather LE, Cousins MJ, et al: Spinal narcotics and respiratory depression [Correspondence], *Lancet* 2:356, 1979.
218. Liolios A, Andersen FH: Selective spinal analgesia [Correspondence], *Lancet* 2:357, 1979.
219. Scott DB, McClure J: Selective epidural analgesia [Correspondence], *Lancet* 1:1410, 1979.
220. Shook JE, Watkins WD, Camporesi EM: Differential roles of opioid receptors in respiration, respiratory disease, and opiate-induced respiratory depression, *Am Rev Respir Dis* 142:895, 1990.
221. Vandermeulen EP, Van Aken H, Vermylen J: Anticoagulants and spinal-epidural anesthesia, *Anesth Analg* 79:1165, 1994.
222. Markham JW, Lynge HN, Stahlman EB: The syndrome of spontaneous spinal epidural hematoma. Report of three cases, *J Neurosurg* 26:334, 1967.
223. Waldman SD, Feldstein GS, Waldman HJ, et al: Caudal administration of morphine sulfate in anticoagulated and thrombocytopenic patients, *Anesth Analg* 66:267, 1987.
224. Odoom JA, Sih IL: Epidural analgesia and anticoagulant therapy. Experience with one thousand cases of continuous epidurals, *Anaesthesia* 38:254, 1983.
225. Owens EL, Kasten GW, Hessel EA: Spinal subarachnoid hematoma after lumbar puncture and heparinization: A case report, review of the literature, and discussion of anesthetic implications, *Anesth Analg* 65:1201, 1986.
226. Brem SS, Hafler DA, Van Uitert RL, et al: Spinal subarachnoid hematoma: A hazard of lumbar puncture resulting in reversible paraplegia, *N Engl J Med* 303:1020, 1981.
227. Ruff RL, Dougherty JH: Complications of lumbar puncture followed by anticoagulation, *Stroke* 12:879, 1981.
228. Varkey GP, Brindle GF: Peridural anaesthesia and anticoagulant therapy, *Can Anaesth Soc J* 21:106, 1974.
229. Baron HC, LaRaja RD, Rossi G, et al: Continuous epidural analgesia in the heparinized vascular surgical patient: A retrospective review of 912 patients, *J Vasc Surg* 6:144, 1987.
230. Rao TLK, El-Etr AA: Anticoagulation following placement of epidural and subarachnoid catheters: An evaluation of neurologic sequelae, *Anesthesiology* 55:618, 1981.
231. Ho AMH, Chung DC, Joynt GM: Neuraxial blockade and hematoma in cardiac surgery: Estimating the risk of a rare adverse event that has not (yet) occurred, *Chest* 117:551, 2000.
232. Rosen DA, Hawkinberry DW, Rosen KR, et al: An epidural hematoma in an adolescent patient after cardiac surgery, *Anesth Analg* 98:966, 2004.
233. Chaney MA: Thoracic epidural anaesthesia in cardiac surgery—the current standing, *Ann Cardiac Anaesth* 12:1, 2009.
234. Chaney MA: Intrathecal and epidural anesthesia and analgesia for cardiac surgery, *Anesth Analg* 102:45, 2006.
235. Ho AM, Li PT, Kasmakar MK: Risk of hematoma after epidural anesthesia and analgesia for cardiac surgery, *Anesth Analg* 103:1327, 2006.
236. Chaney MA, Labovsky JK: Case report of surgery: Balancing postoperative risks associated with hematoma formation and thromboembolic phenomenon, *J Cardiothorac Vasc Anesth* 19:798, 2005.
237. Mora Mangano CT: Risky business [Editorial], *J Thorac Cardiovasc Surg* 125:1204, 2003.
238. Castellano JM, Durbin CG: Epidural analgesia and cardiac surgery: Worth the risk [Editorial]? *Chest* 117:305, 2000.

239. Schwann NM, Chaney MA: No pain, much gain [Editorial]? *J Thorac Cardiovasc Surg* 126:1261, 2003.
240. Gravlee GP: Epidural analgesia and coronary artery bypass grafting: The controversy continues [Editorial], *J Cardiothorac Vasc Anesth* 17:151, 2003.
241. de Leon-Casasola OA: When it comes to outcome, we need to define what a perioperative epidural technique is [Editorial], *Anesth Analg* 96:315, 2003.
242. Rosenquist RW, Birnbach DJ: Epidural insertion in anesthetized adults: Will your patients thank you [Editorial]? *Anesth Analg* 96:1545, 2003.
243. White PF: The role of non-opioid analgesic techniques in the management of pain after ambulatory surgery, *Anesth Analg* 94:577, 2002.
244. Kehlet H, Dahl JB: The value of "multimodal" or "balanced analgesia" in postoperative pain treatment, *Anesth Analg* 77:1048, 1993.
245. Chaney MA: How important is postoperative pain after cardiac surgery? *J Cardiothorac Vasc Anesth* 19:705, 2005.
246. Liu SS, Wu CL: Effect of postoperative analgesia on major postoperative complications: A systematic update of the evidence, *Anesth Analg* 104:689, 2007.
247. White PF, Kehlet HK: Postoperative pain management and patient outcome: Time to return to work!, *Anesth Analg* 104:487, 2007.
248. Myles PS, Hunt JO, Fletcher H, et al: Relation between quality of recovery in hospital and quality of life at 3 months after cardiac surgery, *Anesthesiology* 95:862, 2001.
249. Fleron MH, Weiskopf RB, Bertrand M, et al: A comparison of intrathecal opioid and intravenous analgesia for the incidence of cardiovascular, respiratory, and renal complications after abdominal aortic surgery, *Anesth Analg* 97:2, 2003.
250. Beattie WS, Badner NH, Choi P: Epidural analgesia reduces postoperative myocardial infarction: A meta-analysis, *Anesth Analg* 93:853, 2001.
251. Wu CL, Raja SN: Optimizing postoperative analgesia: The use of global outcome measures [Editorial], *Anesthesiology* 97:533, 2002.
252. Gottschalk A, Ochroch EA: Preemptive analgesia: What do we do now [Correspondence]? *Anesthesiology* 98:280, 2003.
253. Hogan QH: No preemptive analgesia: Is that so bad [Editorial]? *Anesthesiology* 96:526, 2002.
254. Moiniche S, Kehlet H, Dahl JB: A qualitative and quantitative systematic review of preemptive analgesia for postoperative pain relief: The role of timing of analgesia, *Anesthesiology* 96:725, 2002.
255. Katz J, Cohen L, Schmid R, et al: Postoperative morphine use and hyperalgesia are reduced by preoperative but not intraoperative epidural analgesia: Implications for preemptive analgesia and the prevention of central sensitization, *Anesthesiology* 98:1449, 2003.

SECTION

VII

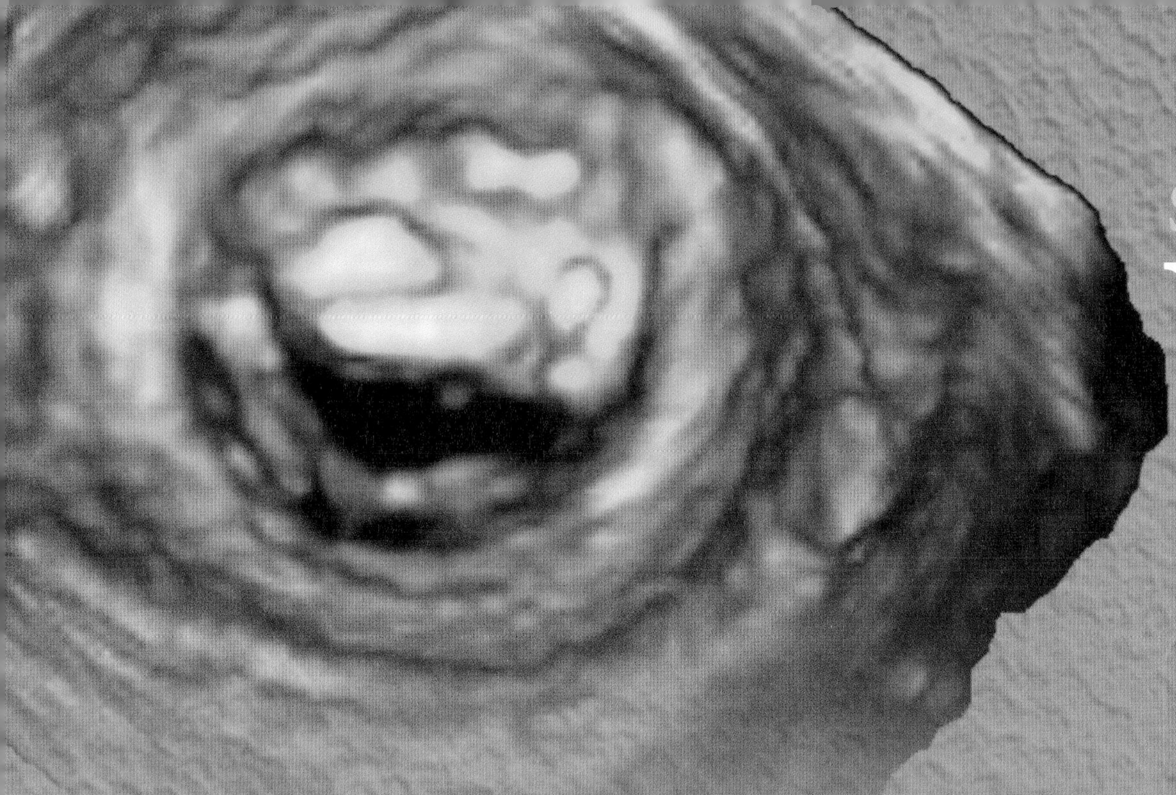

Education in Cardiac Anesthesia

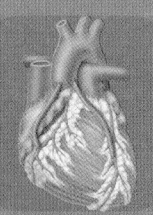

39

Reducing Errors in Cardiac Anesthesiology

T. ANDREW BOWDLE, MD, PHD | **MARK EDWARDS, MBCHB, FANZCA** |
KAREN B. DOMINO, MD, MPH

KEY POINTS

1. Evidence-based recommendations for reducing complications from central catheters include use of maximum sterile barriers, real-time ultrasound guidance during central catheter insertion and selective use of antibiotic-impregnated central venous catheters.
2. Most cases of cardiac tamponade caused by central venous catheters should be preventable by taking a chest x-ray following placement to confirm that the position of the tip of the catheter is outside the pericardial sac and parallel to the walls of the vena cava.
3. Evidence suggests that the most reliable method for avoiding inadvertant cannulation of an artery during central venous catheter insertion is measurement of the intravascular pressure by use of a transducer or manometry.
4. The reported risk of intraoperative awareness during cardiac surgery is around 0.4–1%, a 10-fold increase compared with the overall level of around 0.1–0.2%.
5. Evidence suggests that the use of processed EEG to monitor the depth of anesthesia may significantly reduce the risk of intraoperative awarness.
6. Errors related to drug adminstration are common in anesthesia practice, with self-reporting studies finding a rate of error of approximately 0.75% of anesthetics.
7. Anecdotal evidence suggests that infusion pumps with advisory systems known as "error reduction systems" can significantly reduce drug administration errors resulting from incorrect manual entry of dosing information at the point of care; these pumps utilize predefined dosing limits and warn the practitioner if the dosing parameters that are entered at the point of care will result in an inappropriate dose.
8. Anecdotal evidence suggests that bar coding of patient identifiers, drugs, and infusion pumps at the point of care may significantly reduce the rate of errors related to drug administration.
9. Evidence suggests that fatigue may contribute significantly to errors, although specific studies in cardiac anesthesiology are lacking.
10. The American Society of Anesthesiologists Closed Claims database contains 327 claims related to cardiac anesthesia, with an increased proportion of claims for brain damage, stroke, and awareness during anesthesia and decreased proportion of claims for airway injury compared with 4986 other claims for other surgical procedures under general anesthesia.

Although the safety of anesthesiology has improved over recent years, with an attributable mortality on the order of 1 in 53,500 anesthetics,* errors still occur. Like other medical practitioners, anesthesiologists are prone to human error. The complex arena of cardiac anesthesia provides an opportunity for making just about any of the errors that can possibly be made by an anesthesiologist. It is just because of the complexity and the high stakes encountered in the cardiac anesthesia environment that cardiac anesthesiologists should be most interested in methods for reducing errors. This is particularly relevant now as regulatory agencies and the public in general have become acutely aware of medical errors since the publication of the Institute of Medicine's landmark report on the subject.[1] In response, initiatives have been developed by a wide range of organizations with the intention of reducing errors and improving safety for surgical patients. These have been aimed at the entire surgical patient population (e.g., the World Health Organization's safe surgery saves lives checklist)[2,3] and, more specifically, at cardiac surgical patients. The Society of Cardiovascular Anesthesiologists (SCA) Foundation has undertaken an initiative called Flawless Operative Cardiovascular Unified Systems (FOCUS). They intend to take a multidisciplinary approach to identifying and mitigating hazards. One of the interventions they envision developing is peer-to-peer assessment. An overview of the project and an outline of their plan have been recently published.[4]

The purpose of this chapter is not to catalogue the errors that may be made in cardiac anesthesia, but rather to point to specific areas in which there are data in support of methods for significantly reducing errors. These specific areas are:

1. Errors involving the placement of central catheters
2. Errors in the assessment of anesthetic depth that may result in intraoperative awareness
3. Errors involving the process of administering drugs, such as giving the wrong drug (The principles also apply to errors in administering blood products.)
4. Errors related to diminished vigilance because of fatigue and the use of transesophageal echocardiography (TEE)

In each of these categories of errors, anesthesiologists will see that there are methods that should enable them to reduce error. The reader also may find previous descriptions of mechanisms of error in anesthesia useful.[5–7]

---

*http://www.anzca.edu.au/resources/books-and-publications/reports/mortality/Safety%20of%20Anaesthesia%20in%20Australia.pdf

ERRORS INVOLVING THE PLACEMENT OF CENTRAL CATHETERS

Central catheters have long been regarded as dangerous by practitioners, manufacturers, and the U.S. Food and Drug Administration. (FDA). Complications from central catheters have been reviewed recently.[8–11] Hall and Russell[12] have authored an editorial that provides, in three pages, a concise but complete description of safe practices for placing central catheters; if the reader has time to read only a single article on this topic, it is highly recommended. This section concentrates on errors related to the internal jugular vein (IJV) route of central catheter insertion because this is the most common insertion route used by cardiac anesthesiologists (Box 39-1).

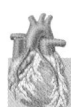 Agency for Healthcare Research and Quality

The Agency for Healthcare Research and Quality (AHRQ) is a part of the Public Health Service of the federal Department of Health and Human Services. The mission of the AHRQ is "to support research designed to improve the quality, safety, efficiency, and effectiveness of healthcare for all Americans." In 2001, AHRQ published a document entitled, "Making Health Care Safer: A Critical Analysis of Patient Safety Practices," an evidence-based review of practices intended to improve patient safety.[13] There were 11 practices that were most highly rated of 79 practices that were reviewed in detail, based on the strength of evidence supporting their widespread implementation. These included three practices related to the management of central venous catheters (CVCs):

1. Use of maximum sterile barriers while placing central intravenous catheters to prevent infections
2. Use of real-time ultrasound guidance during central catheter insertion to prevent complications
3. Use of antibiotic-impregnated CVCs to prevent catheter-related infections

These recommendations clearly have implications for the practice of cardiac anesthesiology. Before examining these recommendations in more detail, the authors will take a broader look at complications from central catheters.

Central Venous Catheter Complications and the American Society of Anesthesiologists Closed Claims Project Database

The American Society of Anesthesiologists (ASA) Closed Claims Project database is a standardized collection of case summaries of adverse anesthesia-related outcomes derived from closed liability claims collected from 35 insurance organizations. Although it is impossible to know the true incidence of the adverse events that appear in the Closed Claims Project database (there is no "denominator" for the database), this relatively large set of cases may reveal patterns of events that contribute to patient injury and subsequent legal action, which would not be possible to discern by looking at individual cases.

> ### BOX 39-1. REDUCING ERRORS FROM USE OF CENTRAL VENOUS CATHETERS
>
> - Sterile barrier precautions during catheter placement
> - Ultrasound guidance for location of the internal jugular vein
> - Pressure waveform monitoring or manometry to avoid cannulation of an artery
> - Tip of a central venous catheter should be outside of the heart
> - Chest radiograph to confirm a safe location of the tip of a central venous catheter
> - Consider use of antibiotic-impregnated central venous catheters

The authors' review of the Closed Claims Project database confirmed the hazards previously associated with central catheters.[14] Among the 6449 claims reported through December 2002, there were 110 claims for injuries related to CVCs (1.7%). Claims related to CVCs had a high severity of patient injury with an increased proportion of death (47%) compared with other claims in the database (29%; $P < 0.01$).

The main results of the review are shown in Table 39-1. Inspection of this table reveals that the most important injuries, both in terms of numbers and death rate, are cardiac tamponade and injuries to major arteries and veins (combining "carotid artery puncture/cannulation," "hemothorax," and "miscellaneous other vessel injury"), representing 16 of 110 and 39 of 110 cases, respectively, not including pulmonary artery (PA) injuries. This impression is reinforced when the injuries reported after 1990 are compared with those reported before 1990 (Figure 39-1). Since 1990, most injuries have been accounted for by vascular injuries.

Although a great deal of attention has been paid to PA injuries caused by pulmonary artery catheters (PACs), it is interesting that they make up only 7 of 110 central catheter-related cases in the Closed Claims Project database.[14] In addition, the anecdotal literature suggests that injuries to pulmonary arteries by PACs are sporadic and probably not related to specific errors or problems with technique. Although highly lethal[15] and certainly to be feared, probably the main thing the

TABLE 39-1	Central Catheter-Related Injuries from the American Society of Anesthesiologists Closed Claims Project Database		
Type of Complication		**n**	**Death, n (%)**
Wire/catheter embolus		20	1 (5)*
Cardiac tamponade		15	12 (80)*
Carotid artery injury		14	5 (36)
Hemothorax		14	12 (92)*
Pneumothorax		12	2 (15)*
Miscellaneous vessel injury		7	2 (29)
Pulmonary artery rupture		6	6 (100)
Hydrothorax		5	2 (40)
Air embolism		4	3 (75)
Fluid extravasation in neck		4	2 (50)
Cardiac arrhythmia		1	0 (0)

*$P < 0.05$ compared with other complications.
Data from Domino KB, Bowdle TA, Posner KL, et al: Injuries and liability related to central vascular catheters. *Anesthesiology* 100:1411–1418, 2004.

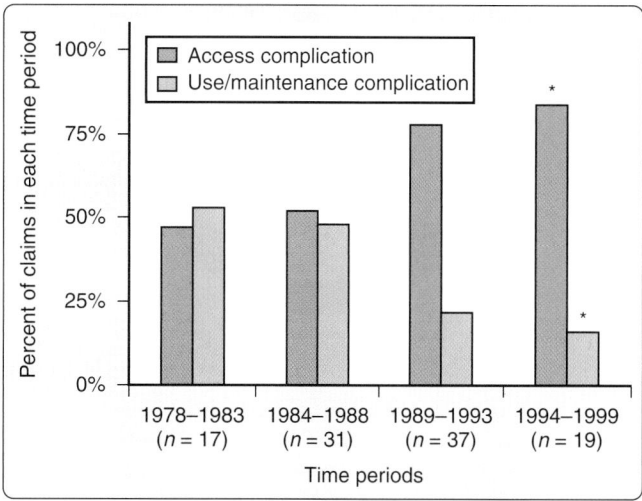

Figure 39-1 Central catheter-related claims or injuries from the American Society of Anesthesiologists (ASA) Closed Claims Project database. A greater proportion of claims from 1989 to 1999 involved complications related to access (i.e., mostly vascular injuries). *$P < 0.05$, 1994–1999 compared with other periods.

practitioner can do to reduce the likelihood of PA injury is to avoid using a PAC in the first place. The appropriate use of PACs has been highly contentious,[16–29] and because the literature is not clear regarding the safety of PACs, they will not be considered further in this chapter (see Chapter 14).

Preventing Cardiac Tamponade

Cardiac tamponade from a central catheter occurs when the tip of a CVC is allowed to remain in the right atrium, or up against the wall of the vena cava at an acute angle, resulting in perforation of the atrium or cava. Perforation can occur immediately after placement or, more commonly, after hours to days. This problem has been documented by numerous case reports[30–36] and accounted for 16 of 110 cases of central catheter-related claims in the ASA Closed Claims Project database; 13 of these 16 cases resulted in death.[14] Perforation can occur immediately after placement, or more commonly after hours to days. Package inserts in CVC kits contain vigorous warnings against placing a CVC into the right atrium or with the CVC tip at an acute angle to the superior vena cava (SVC; Figure 39-2). Despite some controversy, most authors have concluded that the catheter tip should be outside of the pericardial sac and parallel to the walls of the vena cava.[37] It is a widely accepted practice to obtain a chest radiograph after CVC placement, usually in the recovery room or intensive care unit (ICU) after surgery. This allows the position of the catheter tip to be assessed and adjusted if necessary (Figures 39-3 and 39-4).[38,39] The carina is a useful structure for assessing the position of the catheter tip on the chest radiograph because the vena cava is outside the pericardium at the level of the carina.[40,41] Locating the catheter tip at or above the level of the carina should ensure that the catheter tip lies outside of the pericardial sac. The carina may be a better landmark than the radiographic cardiac sillouette because several centimeters of the SVC may lie inside the pericardium but outside of the radiographic cardiac sillouette.[40,41] Kwon et al[42] made measurements of the SVC in vivo in 61 cardiac surgery patients and found that approximately half of the length of the SVC is within the pericardium. Particular caution should be exercised when catheters are placed from the left side (left internal jugular or subclavian veins) that the catheter tip either remains within the innominate vein[37] or makes the turn into the SVC, ending with the tip parallel to the cava and not abutting the wall of the cava at an acute or right angle. Many catheters can be inserted to a depth

sufficient to reach the right atrium (Figure 39-5), and this should be avoided by placing the CVC only to a depth of 10 to 12 cm from the right IJV approach in the typical adult. Because of anatomic variation, the placement should be confirmed by chest radiograph. Alternative approaches to verifying the position of the catheter tip include intravascular electrocardiography[43] and TEE.[44] An interesting editorial regarding tip location of CVCs is available.[37]

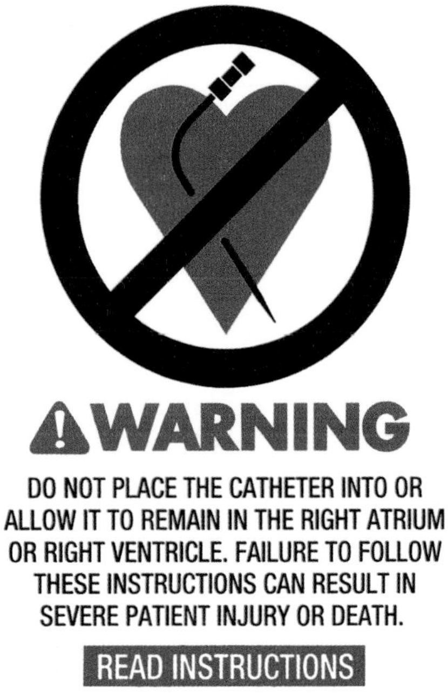

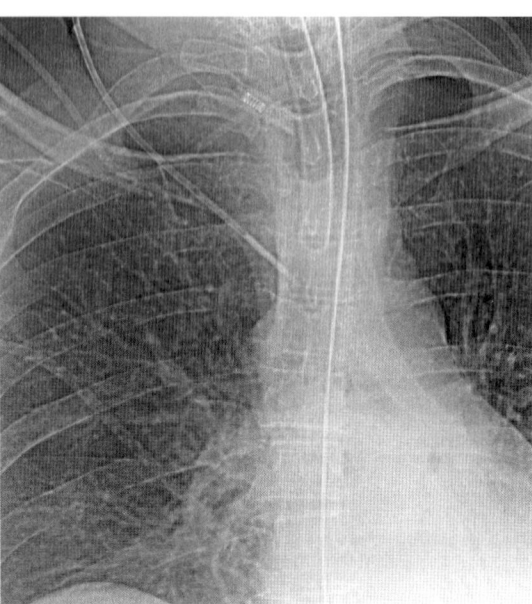

Figure 39-3   Routine chest radiograph taken in the recovery room showed the central venous catheter pointing toward the wall of the superior vena cava at an acute angle. Such positioning may increase the risk for perforation of the vena cava by the tip of the catheter. This catheter was repositioned as shown in Figure 39-4.

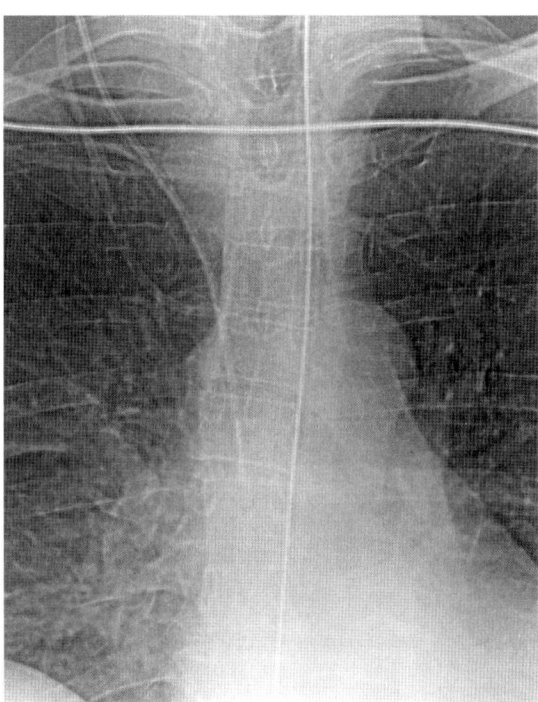

Figure 39-4   The central venous catheter shown in Figure 39-3 was repositioned so that the catheter was parallel to the walls of the superior vena cava. This position is thought to be safer than the original position shown in Figure 39-3 in which the catheter was pointed toward the wall of the vena cava at an acute angle.

⚠️**WARNING**

DO NOT PLACE THE CATHETER INTO OR ALLOW IT TO REMAIN IN THE RIGHT ATRIUM OR RIGHT VENTRICLE. FAILURE TO FOLLOW THESE INSTRUCTIONS CAN RESULT IN SEVERE PATIENT INJURY OR DEATH.

READ INSTRUCTIONS

Figure 39-2   Package insert of a central venous catheter (CVC) kit.

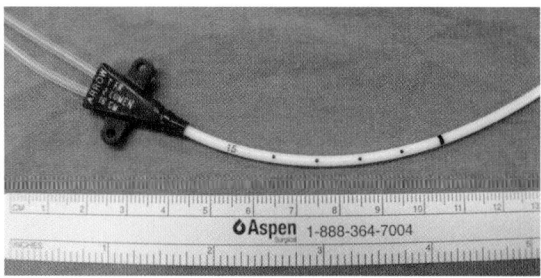

Figure 39-5 A central venous catheter is shown with markings to indicate the distance to the tip of the catheter. The dark band is 10 cm from the tip of the catheter. Inserting this catheter as far as possible will result in the tip being 16 cm from the skin puncture site. If this catheter were inserted 16 cm into the right internal jugular vein from a skin puncture site low in the neck, the tip of the catheter could easily be in the right atrium. Allowing the catheter tip to reside in the right atrium may result in perforation of the atrial wall. Before obtaining a chest radiograph to confirm the location of the catheter tip, limiting the insertion to 10 to 12 cm for the right internal jugular approach in a typical adult patient will usually avoid right atrial placement.

Preventing Vascular Injury

Vascular injury related to central catheters is conveniently divided into injuries to cervical arteries and injuries to intrathoracic veins or arteries. The mechanisms of injury and the methods of prevention are different in each category.

Preventing Injuries to Arteries

The most common injury to arteries is related to puncture or cannulation of the carotid artery. Puncturing the carotid artery with a small needle, although undesirable, does not generally produce any harm. However, if the arterial puncture is not recognized and a guidewire is placed into the artery and followed with a CVC or PAC introducer sheath, there is the possibility of a major problem. Pressure waveform measurement and ultrasound are two methods commonly used to reduce the chances of injury to the carotid artery.

Pressure Waveform Measurement

In 1983, Jobes et al[45] reported on a retrospective study of 1021 attempts at IJV access in which there were 43 arterial punctures; 5 of 43 arterial punctures were unrecognized, resulting in the placement of 8-French introducer sheaths into an artery and resulting in one fatality from hemothorax. Subsequently, these investigators performed a prospective trial of 1284 attempts at IJV access in which they measured a pressure waveform from the vessel before inserting the guidewire. Before measuring the pressure waveform, a clinical assessment was made as to whether the needle was in an artery or vein, based on the usual criteria of color and pulsatility. There were 51 arterial punctures, 10 of which were incorrectly identified as being venous based on color and pulsatility but were determined to be arterial from the pressure waveform. Thus, 10 inadvertant cannulations of the carotid artery were avoided by pressure waveform monitoring.

Ezaru et al[46] recently published a retrospective analysis of 9348 CVC placements requiring mandatory use of manometry to verify venous access. In a single institution, over a 15-year period, there were no cases of arterial injury. During the final year of the study, 511 catheters were placed. Arterial puncture (defined as placement of an 18-gauge finder needle or catheter into an artery) occurred in 28 patients (5%). Arterial puncture was recognized from color and pulsatility in 24 cases, without manometry; but in four cases, the arterial placement was only recognized with manometry. Despite these findings, and the anecdotal experiences of many anesthesiologists who have placed catheters and sheaths into carotid arteries, many anesthesiologists continue to rely

on color and pulsatility of blood in the hub of a needle to differentiate arterial from venous puncture.

The pressure waveform can be most conveniently measured using the setup shown in Figure 39-6.[47] This setup has the advantage of giving the pressure waveform without the need to disconnect the syringe and connect monitoring tubing to the needle, with the risk for dislodging the needle from the vein. An alternative method used by many anesthesiologists uses manometry. The syringe is disconnected from the needle and a length of tubing is connected, allowed to fill with blood, and then held vertically to identify the pressure from the height of the blood column. There are no data comparing these alternative methods of pressure measurement; however, the manometry technique requires an additional step to connect the manometry tubing. A novel approach to measuring a pressure waveform with a miniature, single-use in-line pressure transducer is illustrated in Figure 39-7.

Ultrasound Guidance

The availability of relatively inexpensive, portable ultrasound equipment led to the application of two-dimensional ultrasound imaging to guide CVC placement. Ultrasound imaging allows the presence of the

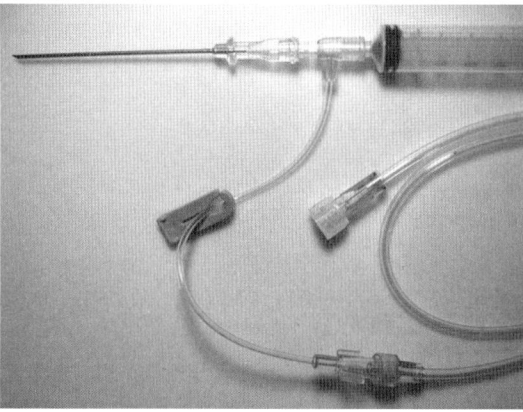

Figure 39-6 This setup is used by the authors for obtaining a pressure waveform during central venous catheter (CVC) placement. The T-shaped adapter and a length of pressure tubing are added to a standard CVC kit, and the device is assembled as shown using the needle and syringe found in the kit. The pressure tubing is handed off to the assistant who connects it to a transducer and flushes the system. When blood is aspirated into the syringe indicating entry into the blood vessel, inspection of the waveform on the monitor immediately allows differentiation between artery and vein. Once the presence of a venous waveform is confirmed, the syringe or T-adapter is removed and the wire is inserted.

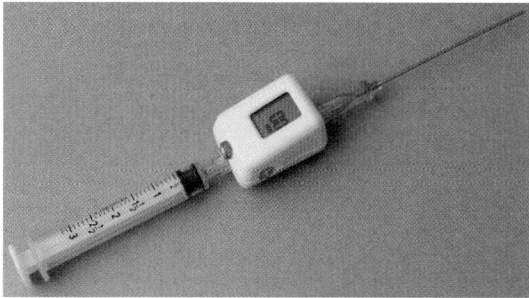

Figure 39-7 **The Compass Vascular Access Device manufactured by Mirador Biomedical, Inc.** This single-use device measures the intravascular pressure, which is displayed digitally and also as an analog representation of the pressure waveform. A wire may be passed either through the syringe connection port after removing the syringe or through a separate valved port. The pressure may be measured continuously during the placement of the wire.

IJV to be confirmed, its patency can be demonstrated, and its anatomic relation to the carotid artery can be defined. Real-time use can guide needle placement into the vein and confirm the presence of a wire in the vein. Troianos et al[48] first reported the use of ultrasound-guided central vascular access in the anesthesia literature in 1991. Their prospective, randomized study of ultrasound guidance versus the traditional landmark method found a greater overall success rate, a greater success rate on the first attempt, and reduced rate of arterial puncture with ultrasound guidance. Numerous studies of ultrasound guidance and two major meta-analyses have appeared subsequently. As noted earlier, a review commissioned by the AHRQ strongly advocated the use of ultrasound guidance.[10] In the United Kingdom, the National Institute of Clinical Excellence (NICE) recommends routine use of ultrasound for central venous catheterization.*

The two major meta-analyses of ultrasound guidance concluded that ultrasound guidance was superior to landmarks for overall success rate, a greater success rate on the first attempt, and reduced complications from arterial puncture for the IJV approach.[49,50] The advantage of ultrasound guidance for the subclavian approach was less clear.

The authors examined CVC complications from the ASA Closed Claims Project database in an attempt to determine whether the use of pressure waveform monitoring or ultrasound guidance would have prevented the complications. This is clearly inferential; nevertheless, it is interesting that nearly half (48/110) of the complications were judged to be possibly preventable by the use of either pressure waveform monitoring or ultrasound guidance, only by ultrasound guidance, only by pressure waveform monitoring, or by chest radiograph (Table 39-2).[14]

Wigmore et al[51] reported their experience in a single tertiary referral center in Britain after implementation of the National Institute of Clinical Excellence guideline. This is a particularly interesting study because it illustrates the effect in a single center of attempting to implement a national guideline. During the study, adoption of ultrasound guidance increased from less than 10% to more than 80%. There were 19 of 152 complications during a preguideline audit, 18 of which

involved the landmark technique without ultrasound guidance. After introduction of the guideline, there were 13 of 286 complications, 10 from cases in which only the landmark technique was used (8.7%) and 3 from cases in which ultrasound guidance was used (1.7%), an absolute risk reduction of 6.9% with ultrasound. Complications consisted of arterial punctures, neck hematomas, and a pneumothorax. There was also a significant reduction in failed insertions with ultrasound guidance (7/115 for the landmark group and 1/169 for the ultrasound group; $P < 0.01$).

Recently, Hosokawa et al[53] have demonstrated the utility of ultrasound guidance in neonates and infants less than 7.5 kg. They compared ultrasound guidance with the traditional anatomic landmark method, and later they compared ultrasound guidance for skin marking (without live ultrasound during needle puncture) with live ultrasound guidance. There was a 97% success rate for ultrasound guidance compared with a 62% success rate for the anatomic landmark method.[52] Live ultrasound compared with ultrasound for skin marking (without live ultrasound during needle puncture) resulted in significantly faster cannulation and fewer needle passes.[53] Fewer than three attempts at puncture were made in 100% of patients in the live ultrasound group compared with 74% of patients in the ultrasound for skin marking group.

An important caveat for the use of ultrasound guidance is that the needle and/or wire may not always be visualized in the vein, depending on the type of ultrasound equipment used and the skill of the operator. Although it may be possible to visualize the tip of the needle with ultrasound,[54] because of the tomographic nature of an ultrasound beam, it may be difficult to distinguish the shaft of the needle from the tip. Needles with a special echogenic surface that may enhance ultrasound visualization are available (see Chapter 14).

Anecdotal experience has shown that despite the use of ultrasound guidance and the appearance that the needle is pointed toward the vein, the needle may hit the artery, particularly when the artery is posterior to the vein. A guidewire can often be visualized more reliably than a needle; however, it is preferable to correctly identify the vessel before placing the guidewire because blindly inserting a guidewire into the carotid or other major artery is undesirable. If the needle and/or wire is not definitely visualized in the vein, measurement of a pressure waveform in conjunction with ultrasound guidance is strongly recommended. In the authors' practice, ultrasound guidance and pressure waveform monitoring are both available, and at least one technique is used routinely after vessel puncture to confirm that the vein has been entered. One important caveat is the possibility that the needle can be inadvertently moved *after* confirmation of venous puncture by ultrasound or pressure waveform and subsequently enter an artery, which may result in cannulation of the artery. This can be avoided by puncturing the vessel with a small (i.e., 18-gauge) angiocatheter instead of a needle before measuring a pressure waveform because the angiocatheter once inserted is less likely to be dislodged. Alternatively, visualizing the wire in the vein with ultrasound can serve as a final check of correct venous placement.

Given the abundance of data in favor of the use of ultrasound guidance, it is reasonable to consider the use of ultrasound guidance to be the "preferred method of insertion."[55] Interestingly, several surveys have found relatively low rates of using ultrasound guidance. A survey of pediatric anesthesiologists in the United Kingdom found that only 39% used ultrasound routinely.[56] A more recent survey of pediatric anesthesiologists in the United Kingdom found that only 26% always used ultrasound.[57] Another recent survey in the United Kingdom of senior members of the Association of Anaesthetists of Great Britain and Ireland found that only 27% used ultrasound guidance as their first choice.[58] A survey of members of the SCA found that only 15% always used ultrasound.[59] A shortage of suitable ultrasound equipment is sometimes a reason for not using ultrasound guidance. A study in the United Kingdom found that 86% of anesthetic departments had ultrasound equipment for CVC placement[60]; however, Bailey et al[59] found that 33% of anesthesiologists in their survey of members of the SCA never or almost never had ultrasound equipment available.

TABLE 39-2	Potential Effect of Ultrasound Guidance or Pressure Waveform Monitoring on Central Venous Catheter–Related Injuries from the American Society of Anesthesiologists Closed Claims Project Database	
Possibly preventable by either ultrasound guidance or pressure waveform monitoring (n = 19)		
Carotid artery puncture/cannulation		16
Hemothorax		1
Wire/catheter embolus		1
Miscellaneous other vessel injury		1
Possible preventable by pressure waveform monitoring only (n = 6)		
Miscellaneous other artery injury		5
Hemothorax		1
Possibly preventable by ultrasound guidance only (n = 9)		
Hemothorax		4
Pneumothorax		4
Miscellaneous other vessel injury		1
Possibly preventable by chest radiograph (n = 14)		
No chest radiograph taken (n = 7)		
Carotid tamponade		2
Wire/catheter embolus		1
Pneumothorax		4
Misread, not read, or inappropriate action taken (n = 7)		
Cardiac tamponade		4
Wire/catheter embolus		3

The cases related to central venous catheters from the ASA Closed Claims database were examined to determine whether the use of ultrasound guidance, pressure waveform monitoring, or chest radiograph (after placement) might have prevented the injuries.
A total of 48 of 110 injuries were thought to be potentially preventable by these means.
Data from Domino KB, Bowdle TA, Posner KL et al: Injuries and liability related to central vascular catheters. *Anesthesiology* 100:1411–1418, 2004.

*http://guidance.nice.org.uk/TA49

Preventing Injuries to Intrathoracic Arteries or Veins

Pressure waveform monitoring and ultrasound guidance are valuable primarily for avoiding injury to arteries, especially to the carotid artery during attempted IJV cannulation. There is another category of vascular injury that is not addressed by pressure waveform monitoring or ultrasound guidance, which is injury to intrathoracic veins or arteries, made clear from anecdotal reports and from the ASA Closed Claims Project database, which contains 15 cases of hemothorax, 14 of which were fatal. A large puncture or tear in a large intrathoracic vein or artery can bleed profusely and may be difficult to repair surgically in time to prevent exsanguination. Although the mechanism of these injuries is not known in every case, certain mechanisms appear to be particularly likely.

Guidewires can take a circuitous route so that when devices are advanced over them, the device may trap the wire up against the wall of the vein, and if the device is stiff enough, perforation of the vein may occur (Figure 39-8).[61] The inner dilators of PAC introducer sheaths are very stiff and may be particularly likely to cause this kind of perforation. The dilator is intended to create a passage through the skin and fascia but has no useful role once the device has entered the vein. Therefore, it is prudent to advance the dilator the minimum distance necessary to reach the vein and no farther. The introducer sheath may then be advanced over the dilator into the vein.

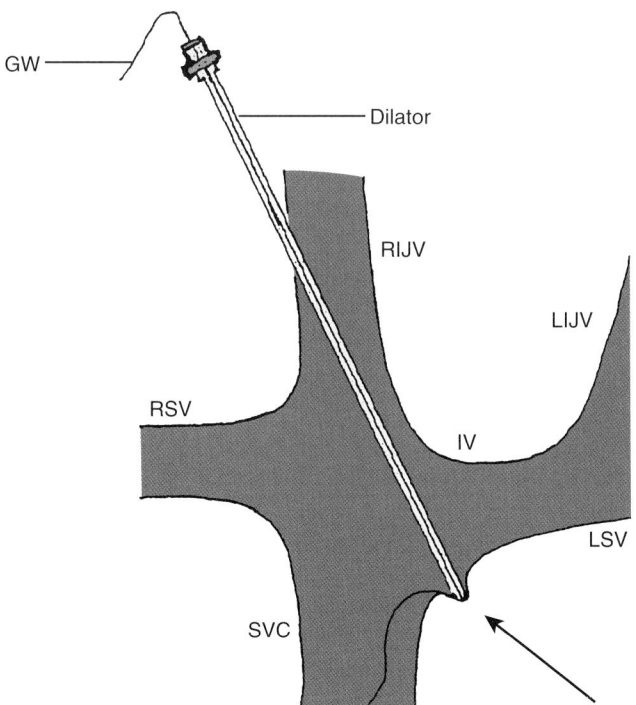

Figure 39-8   A hypothetical mechanism of perforation of a great vein inside the chest (in this case, the innominate vein-vena cava junction) by a dilator (the pulmonary artery catheter introducer sheath, normally loaded onto the dilator, is not shown for simplicity) is shown. The dilator traps the guidewire against the wall of the vein and then perforates the vein as it is advanced. Numerous anecdotal reports of injuries could be explained by this mechanism. Direct observation of the progress of the insertion of the wire and intravascular device under fluoroscopy may be useful for avoiding this potentially fatal complication. GW, guidewire; IV, innominate vein; LIJV, left internal jugular vein; LSV, left subclavian vein; RIJV, right internal jugular vein; RSV, right subclavian vein; SVC, superior vena cava. *(From Oropello JM, Leibowitz AB, Manasia A, et al: Dilator-associated complications of central vein catheter insertion: Possible mechanisms of injury and suggestions for prevention. J Cardiothorac Vasc Anesth 10:634–637, 1996.)*

Kulvatunyou et al[62] reviewed a collection of cases of injury to the right subclavian artery during attempted right IJV cannulation. The right subclavian artery is in close proximity when the right IJV is approached low in the neck. Because of interference from the clavicle, puncture of the subclavian artery may not be seen with ultrasound but will be detected by pressure waveform monitoring. The authors have seen several instances of presumed subclavian artery puncture during attempted IJV cannulation low in the neck, in which ultrasound guidance was used, but the needle tip was not visualized in the vein and arterial puncture was detected with pressure waveform monitoring.

The left IJV approach may be particularly hazardous because the innominate (brachiocephalic) vein crosses the IJV at a right angle. A device inserted into the left IJV could perforate the innominate vein, and anecdotal reports verify that this is indeed the case. The right IJV should be preferred to the left IJV primarily for this reason. If the left IJV is used, special care should be exercised not to advance the dilator of a PAC introducer beyond the IJV. The authors prefer to use a shorter-than-normal introducer sheath in this situation (Figure 39-9). Another potential problem with the left-sided approach is injury to the thoracic duct, which terminates variably in the left IJV, the left subclavian vein, or the left innominate vein. The duct may be perforated in the process of placing a CVC, or rarely, the duct may actually be cannulated. Chylothorax and chylopericardium may result, and infusion of fluids into the thoracic duct may produce cardiac tamponade or constrictive pericarditis by retrograde flow into the pericardial lymphatics.[63]

The use of fluoroscopy is an important consideration in avoiding injuries to intrathoracic veins. Fluoroscopy allows visualization of the guidewire and the intravascular device as it passes over the guidewire in real time. Fluoroscopy is used routinely by interventional radiologists, cardiologists, and surgeons (the latter when placing surgically implanted central catheters). Fluoroscopy is not often used in anesthesia, emergency medicine, or critical care medicine, but perhaps it should be. In the authors' opinion, anesthesiologists wanting to place CVCs in the safest possible manner should strongly consider the use of fluoroscopy, especially when there is difficulty passing wires or catheters into the central circulation. However, availability of fluoroscopy equipment and radiology technical support are significant obstacles to using fluoroscopy for most anesthesiologists. It should be noted that TEE is an alternative method for confirming the presence of a wire in the SVC or right atrium before inserting a catheter.

Treatment of Inadvertent Cannulation of Arteries

Although prevention of inadvertent arterial cannulation with large-bore CVCs is paramount, an approach to treating inadvertent arterial cannulation may be needed in rare circumstances. There have been no

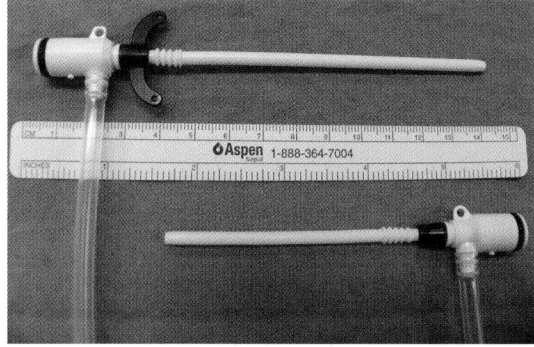

Figure 39-9   A "standard" pulmonary artery catheter introducer sheath (top) is compared with a shorter sheath (bottom). The authors prefer the shorter sheath for the left internal jugular vein (IJV) approach with the intention to avoid having to push the longer sheath past the right angle junction between the left IJV and the innominate (brachiocephalic) vein. Perforation of the innominate vein is a potentially fatal complication of left IJV cannulation.

guidelines in the literature for the treatment of accidental cannulation of arteries with large-bore catheters, but two recently published case series documented better outcomes with surgical or endovascular intervention when compared with removal and compression ("pull/pressure").[64,65] Guilbert et al[65] published a proposed algorithm for dealing with inadvertent arterial cannulation based on cases from their institutions and review of the literature. They found that the "pull/pressure" method was associated with a large incidence of serious complications (47%), including death, whereas the surgical or endovascular approach was not (Figure 39-10). Based on this, they suggested the

algorithm shown in Figure 39-11. Interestingly, a survey of vascular surgeons presented with a hypothetical case of an 8.5-French catheter in a carotid artery found that the respondents saw this complication one to five times per year, and two thirds would simply pull the catheter and apply pressure. However, when vascular surgeons were shown the data from the study by Guilbert et al[65] at a meeting, most of them changed their management to the surgical or endovascular approach as judged by pretest and post-test questions. Several of the specific findings of Guilbert et al's[65] study are worth noting:

1. Arterial cannulation can occur despite the use of ultrasound guidance.
2. The low IJV approach can injure the subclavian or innominate veins, or even the aorta. Arterial injury below the sternoclavicular joint cannot be repaired through a cervical approach. Clinical suspicion of an intrathoracic injury should prompt imaging to locate the site of injury and plan surgical or endovascular treatment.
3. Prolonged arterial cannulation can result in thrombus formation and stroke.
4. A normal carotid duplex examination after removal of a catheter from the carotid artery does not rule out the possibility of a stroke. Because of this, postponing elective surgery has been recommended to avoid unrecognized stroke in an anesthetized patient.
5. False aneurysms or arteriovenous fistulas can occur late after the pull/pressure technique, so close follow-up is needed.

Preventing Infections Related to Central Catheters

Catheter-related bloodstream infections occur 0.5 to 4.8 times per 1000 catheter days, have an attributable mortality rate of 0% to 11%, cause an excess hospital stay of 9 to 12 days per episode, and are expensive for the health care system.[66–68] Infections from central catheters and PACs are related to the time that the catheter is in place and increase significantly after 3 days.[69,70] Because many CVCs placed by anesthesiologists for intraoperative monitoring are removed soon after surgery, the risk for infection is reduced. Nevertheless, anesthesiologists should use the evidence-based methods for preventing

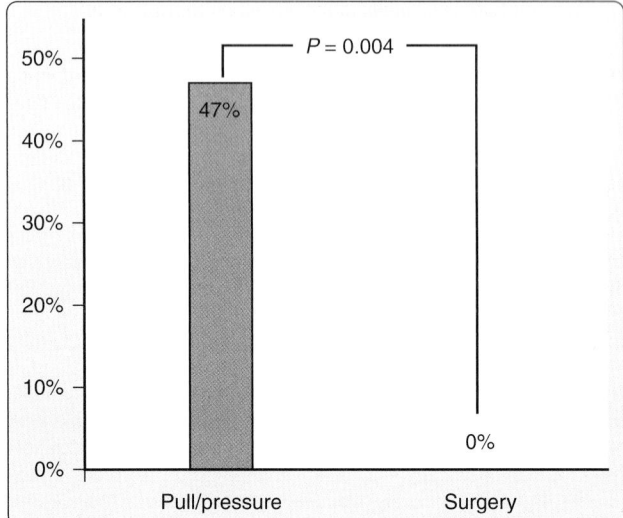

Figure 39-10 Complications from the "pull/pressure" technique of removing a large-bore cannula in an artery were significantly greater than surgical removal with direct repair of the artery or endovascular repair. *(From Guilbert M-C, Elkouri S, Bracco D et al: Arterial trauma during central venous catheter insertion: Case series, review and proposed algorithm. J Vasc Surg 48:918–985, 2008.)*

Figure 39-11 A proposed algorithm for management of inadvertent cannulation of a cervical or thoracic artery with a large-bore catheter during attempted central venous catheter placement. *(From Guilbert M-C, Elkouri S, Bracco D, et al: Arterial trauma during central venous catheter insertion: Case series, review and proposed algorithm. J Vasc Surg 48:918–985, 2008.)*

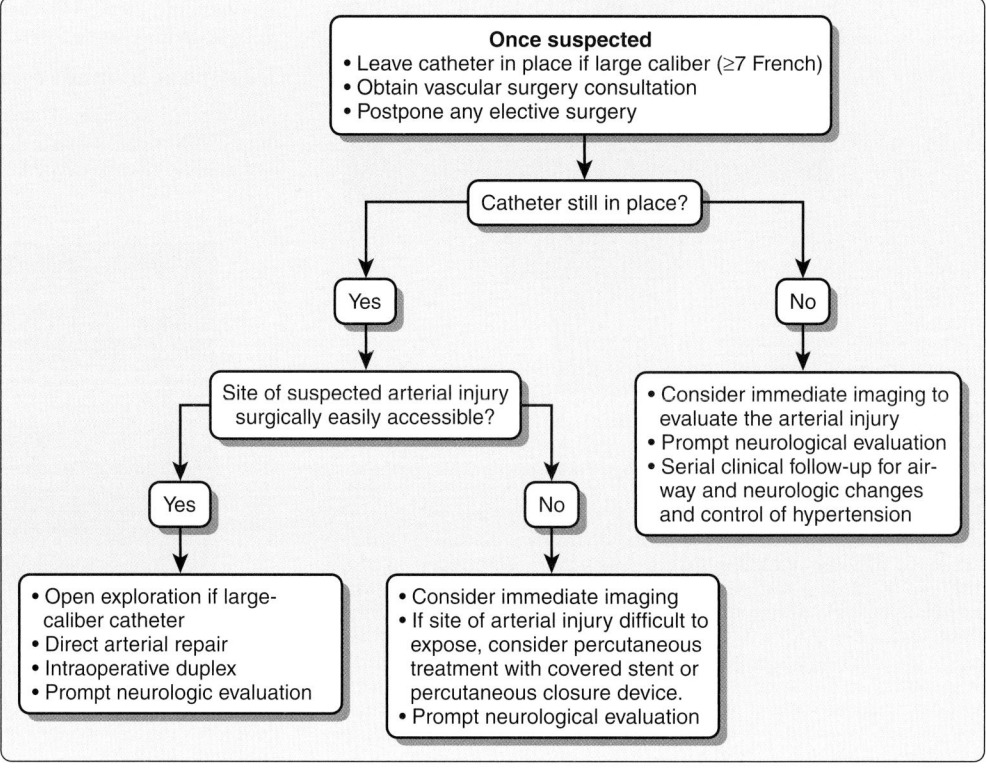

CVC infections.[71] Implementation of a CVC insertion "care bundle" can significantly reduce infection rates. The bundle of interventions used in Pronovost et al's[72] study included appropriate hand hygiene, use of chlorhexidine for skin antisepsis, use of maximal sterile barrier precautions (mask, sterile gown, sterile gloves, and large sterile drapes) during catheter insertion, avoidance of the femoral vein, if possible, and prompt removal of unnecessary catheters. There is substantial evidence that chlorhexidine is a more effective skin cleaning solution than povidone-iodine. Antibiotic ointments applied to the skin puncture site do not affect the risk for bloodstream infection and may actually increase the rate of colonization by fungi and promote antibiotic-resistant bacteria. Recent data suggest that the use of a chlorhexidine-impregnated sponge dressing at the line insertion site may reduce the rate of catheter-related infections.[73] The use of antimicrobial-impregnated catheters reduces the incidence of bloodstream infections related to CVCs, and their use should be considered.[74-76] As noted earlier, antimicrobial-impregnated catheters are recommended in the AHRQ report on evidence-based safety measures. However, these catheters are more expensive and may not be cost-effective when the catheters are going to be removed soon after surgery. For catheters that are intended to remain in place or for high-risk patients (e.g., immunosuppression), antibiotic-impregnated catheters may be worthwhile.[76]

PREVENTING INTRAOPERATIVE AWARENESS

Three large, prospective, multicenter studies of intraoperative awareness have reported similar overall rates of intraoperative awareness of around 0.1% to 0.2% (Box 39-2).[77-79] A recent report from China found a larger incidence rate of about 0.4% in that country.[80] An analysis of cases of awareness during anesthesia from the ASA Closed Claims Project was reported in 1999.[81] Undergoing cardiac surgery increases the risk for intraoperative awareness from the overall level of around 0.1% to 0.2%[78,79] to around 0.4% to 1%,[79,82-86] an increased risk of up to 10-fold. Ghoneim et al[87] recently conducted a review of awareness cases in the literature and confirmed that cardiac surgery is associated with an increased risk. Intraoperative awareness may be a minor or a major complication depending on the severity of the episode of awareness and the response of the individual patient. Intraoperative awareness may result in a significant psychiatric condition such as post-traumatic stress disorder.[88] The explanation for increased risk for intraoperative awareness during cardiac surgery is unknown. Possible causes include deliberately light anesthesia during periods of hemodynamic instability and gaps in anesthetic delivery during separation from cardiopulmonary bypass (CPB) when the volatile anesthetic being administered into the CPB circuit is discontinued. Although vasoactive drugs used during cardiac surgery may mask hemodynamic responses to light anesthesia, it is clear that intraoperative awareness often occurs in the absence of hemodynamic clues, rendering that explanation less likely. Whatever the cause may be, cardiac anesthesiologists should be concerned about the high incidence of intraoperative awareness during cardiac surgery.

Some anesthesiologists are skeptical about an incidence rate of intraoperative awareness of 0.1% to 1%. This skepticism is usually based on personal experience such that individual anesthesiologists believe that the rate of intraoperative awareness in their personal practice is much less than this. However, caution should be used in applying personal experience because of observations in the literature showing that anesthesiologists frequently may miss cases of intraoperative awareness for a variety of reasons, not the least of which is that patients do not always have the opportunity to relate their experience to the anesthesiologist.[89] Several studies have shown that the patient may not report their awareness experience immediately after surgery.[78,79]

Electroencephalography (EEG) has been used extensively by neuropharmacologists since the 1960s to study the effects of anesthetic drugs. As the power of desktop computers increased, it became possible to process raw EEG using fast Fourier transforms and other mathematical methods to make the information contained in the raw EEG immediately accessible in the operating room to those without formal training in its interpretation. The original use of processed EEG in the operating room was for the detection of cerebral ischemia during carotid endarterectomy, and it has been only in recent years that attention has turned once again to the use of EEG to measure the effects of anesthetic drugs. The technologic obstacles to reliably measuring the effects of anesthetic drugs in the operating room with EEG and providing clinically useful information to the anesthesiologist were daunting. Many individuals who were familiar with EEG technology believed that it would never be possible to measure "anesthetic depth" in real time in the typical operating room setting. Nevertheless, the major obstacles have been overcome, and now several commercial products are available for this purpose. The processed EEG monitor known as BIS (bispectral index) is by far the most prevalent, and by far the best documented. Therefore, most of the information here will be concerned with BIS. However, it should be clearly understood that there are other commercial products that purport to provide similar data for clinical monitoring (see Chapter 16). BIS monitoring recently has been reviewed.[90,91]

The result of EEG processing by the BIS monitor is a number ranging from 0 to 100, where 0 is an isoelectric (flat) EEG and 100 is "awake." Assuming that artifacts, interference, signal quality, and other idiosyncrasies of EEG processing have been appropriately evaluated by the user (see later), a BIS value less than 60 should be associated with an extremely low probability of awareness during anesthesia.[92,93] It is possible that if BIS monitoring were used and BIS values kept to less than 60, the incidence of intraoperative awareness could be reduced to a very low level. However, an alternative notion has been proposed[94] that the use of BIS monitoring might actually increase the incidence of intraoperative awareness because of the well-documented tendency of anesthesiologists to administer lower doses of anesthetic drugs when BIS monitoring is used as a guide to anesthetic drug administration.[95,96]

Three studies have been published that support the hypothesis that the use of BIS monitoring can result in a lower incidence of intraoperative awareness. In a retrospective case-comparison study, 5057 consecutive BIS-monitored patients were compared with 7826 non-BIS monitored cases from the same institutions.[97] There were two cases of intraoperative awareness (during intubation; both had BIS values > 60) in the BIS-monitored series compared with 14 in the non-BIS–monitored series ($P < 0.039$). In a prospective, randomized multicenter trial, 2503 "high-risk" (e.g., cardiac anesthesia, trauma, obstetrics) patients were randomized to BIS or non-BIS monitoring.[86] There were 2 cases of intraoperative awareness in the BIS-monitored group (in 1 case, the BIS was <60), compared with 11 in the non-BIS monitoring group (odds ratio, 0.18; 95% adjusted confidence interval, 0.02–0.84; $P = 0.022$). A single-center randomized trial compared BIS monitoring with "targeted end-tidal anesthetic gas analysis" (target range, 0.7–1.3 minimum alveolar concentration) in 2000 patients at "high risk" for intraoperative awareness; 25% of the patients

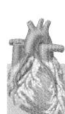

BOX 39-2. AVOIDING INTRAOPERATIVE AWARENESS

- Overall rate of intraoperative awareness is 0.1% to 0.2%.
- Intraoperative awareness during cardiac surgery is greater, 0.4% to 1%.
- Severity of intraoperative awareness experiences varies from mild to profound.
- Some patients experience posttraumatic stress disorder.
- Evidence suggests that the use of computerized electroencephalographic monitoring may help to reduce the incidence of intraoperative awareness.
- Limitation and artifacts encountered with computerized EEG monitoring must be understood by the user.

underwent cardiac surgery.[98] The authors predicted an incidence rate of awareness of 1% but found that either BIS monitoring or "targeted end-tidal gas analysis" reduced the incidence rate to 0.2%. These studies suggest that BIS monitoring may be a useful tool for helping to reduce the incidence of intraoperative awareness.

Although BIS monitoring for the reduction of intraoperative awareness remains controversial, the currently available evidence suggests that cardiac anesthesiologists should seriously consider the use of BIS or other similar processed EEG monitor, especially given the high rate of intraoperative awareness that has been consistently demonstrated in patients undergoing cardiac surgery. BIS is an additional piece of information for use in conducting the anesthetic, but it does not replace the conventional judgments that anesthesiologists make in the absence of BIS.

Although it is not the purpose of this chapter to completely review processed EEG monitoring, there are several important caveats for BIS or other processed EEG monitoring that should be familiar to clinicians.

- Using processed EEG to evaluate anesthetic depth depends on certain fundamental similarities in the effects of anesthetic drugs on the EEG. Ketamine and nitrous oxide[99] have distinct EEG effects that are not taken into account by the BIS algorithm.
- EEG signals are of very low amplitude and, therefore, electrical artifacts are a significant problem. Common sources of electrical artifact include cautery, electromyographic activity, 60-Hz noise from electrical appliances, and high-frequency artifact from temporary external pacing devices (but usually not permanently implanted internal pacemakers). The later is particularly relevant during cardiac surgery. All of these sources of high-frequency electrical noise tend to increase the BIS because their frequency spectrum overlaps the EEG spectrum (2 to 60 Hz), and high-frequency EEG is associated with wakefulness or light anesthesia and greater BIS values. The BIS monitor identifies the presence of high-frequency artifacts and notifies the user by displaying the signal strength of the electromyographic activity. In the presence of high-frequency artifact, the BIS number cannot be interpreted in the usual manner. Small doses of muscle relaxant will usually obliterate high-frequency artifact caused by muscle activity.
- Processing of the raw EEG and data smoothing occur over 15 or 30 seconds (user configurable). This means that the BIS number will lag slightly behind clinical events. This is particularly noticeable during induction, when the patient obviously may be unconscious before the BIS number begins to change.
- BIS numbers reflect the EEG state of the brain but do not reveal how the brain arrived at that state. For example, BIS declines during sleep,[100] yet clearly natural sleep is not the same as anesthesia. Moreover, a BIS number does not reveal what will happen in the future. For example, although BIS may be 45 at one moment, a change in surgical stimulus could result in a BIS of 75 moments later. The propensity of response to a surgical stimulus is more likely with an anesthetic consisting mostly of volatile anesthetic and less likely with an anesthetic that includes a substantial amount of opioid[101]; however, the BIS number does not distinguish between the various possible combinations of opioid and hypnotic drugs.[102]

Kunisawa et al[103] and Kakinohana et al[104] have pointed out that during thoracic aortic surgery with partial left-heart bypass when the descending thoracic aorta is cross-clamped, BIS values can be altered substantially depending on whether the drugs are administered in the circulation above or below the cross-clamp. If the drugs are administered into a vein in the lower body, cross-clamping the aorta may result in a reduction in drug concentrations in the circulation and the brain above the cross-clamp,[103] whereas if the drugs are administered into a vein in the upper body, the concentration in the circulation and the brain above the cross-clamp may increase,[104] presumably because of pharmacokinetic changes relating to the altered circulation with partial left-heart bypass. The change in drug concentrations will be reflected in the BIS, which may increase if the drugs are administered below the cross-clamp, or decrease if the drugs are administered above the cross-clamp.

DRUG ERRORS

Adverse drug events are a major cause of morbidity and mortality in hospitalized patients, affecting more than 770,000 patients per year in the United States. Hospital costs for treating patients who suffer adverse drug events are enormous, estimated at between $1.6 and $5.6 billion annually. Most adverse drug events in hospitalized patients are caused by errors of various kinds,[105] as brought to wide public attention in the Institute of Medicine's report, "To Err Is Human: Building a Safer Health System."[1] This is an international problem, as shown by a recent investigation that used "disguised observation" to discover that one or more errors occurred in the preparation and administration of 58 of 122 intravenous drug doses on the nursing wards of a German hospital. Many of the errors were minor, but there were three cases of wrong dose, one omitted dose, and two "unauthorized" doses.[106] A review of medication errors in the ICU setting is available.[107]

A great deal of attention has been directed at errors that occur in the process of writing and transcribing physician's orders for drugs. There is evidence that computerization of physician ordering (computerized physician order entry [CPOE]), together with computerized advice (clinical decision support), can significantly reduce these types of errors.[108] The AHRQ review "Making Health Care Safer: A Critical Analysis of Patient Safety Practices" rated CPOE and clinical decision support as patient safety practices with medium strength of evidence.[13] The Leapfrog Group ("a coalition of more than 150 public and private organizations...created to help save lives and reduce preventable medical mistakes by mobilizing employer purchasing power to initiate breakthrough improvements in the safety of health care and by giving consumers information to make more informed hospital choices"), founded by the Business Roundtable, a national association of *Fortune 500* CEOs, has made CPOE one of its "safety standards" (http://www.leapfroggroup.org). On balance, CPOE appears to be useful and probably can reduce drug errors[109,110]; however, there is the possibility of harm from unintended consequences,[111,112] as with any technology. In a particularly dramatic example of unintended consequences, introduction of CPOE at the University of Pittsburgh apparently resulted in an increase in mortality rate from 2.8% to 6.3% of children transported to the university for special care, because of unintended delays in delivery of critically important medications.[112] Clearly, the details of implementing technologies intended to reduce drug errors are extremely important, as illustrated for CPOE.[113] This theme is repeated for bar coding and smart pumps later in this chapter.

Because most anesthesiologists seldom write orders for drugs (critical care settings such as the ICU being a notable exception), CPOE is of less interest than the administration of drugs by the anesthesiologist at the "point of care." There is substantial evidence that drug administration errors are common in anesthetic practice (Box 39-3). In 1993, the Australian Incident Monitoring Study identified 144 instances of a wrong drug being given or nearly given to a patient among the first 2000 incidents reported to the study.[114] There was the potential for serious harm in 74% of reports, but no deaths occurred. In 1995, Merry and Peck[115]

BOX 39-3. REDUCING ERRORS RELATED TO DRUG ADMINISTRATION

- Drug administration errors are common in anesthetic practice.
- A multifaceted approach is required to reduce drug administration errors.
- Bar coding patient identifiers, drugs, infusion pumps, and blood products at the point of care may help to reduce errors.
- The FDA requires bar-code labeling of most prescription drugs and blood products.
- "Error-reduction systems" for infusion pumps may reduce errors related to incorrect manual entry of dosing information at the point of care.
- Perfusionists administer drugs during cardiopulmonary bypass and should be included in error reduction strategies.

reported on a survey of 75 anesthesiologists in New Zealand, 89% of whom indicated they had made at least one error of drug administration, with 12.5% indicating that they had harmed a patient by a drug-related error. Subsequently, Merry's group performed a survey of 10,806 anesthetics in two hospitals in New Zealand. Anesthesiologists volunteered information about drug errors using a standardized reporting form.[116] The overall rate of drug error was 0.75%, or 1 in 133 anesthetics. Drug errors resulted in 1 case of intraoperative awareness, 2 cases of prolonged neuromuscular blockade, and 47 cases of transient physiologic effects, 5 of which required intervention. A similar survey of 687 anesthesiologists in Canada found that 85% of the respondents had made at least one drug error or "near miss."[117] Four deaths resulted from a total of 1038 reported errors. A report based on annual surveys conducted by the Japanese Society of Anesthesiologists between 1999 and 2002, reflecting 4,201,925 anesthetics,[118] found an incidence of "critical events" caused by drug administration error rate of 0.02%. The incidence rate of death resulting from drug error was 0.00044%. Additional recent reports from Australia,[119] Japan,[120,121] and South Africa[122] suggest that anesthetic drug error continues to be a significant problem around the world.

The incidence of drug administration errors in an academic practice in the United States appears to be similar to that reported from elsewhere in the world. In a study modeled after the New Zealand study cited earlier, anesthesiologists and nurse anesthetists at the University of Washington completed survey forms; 6066 forms were returned for 6709 anesthetics, a response rate of 90%[123] (Table 39-3). There were 41 reports of errors (0.68%) and 23 reports of pre-errors (near misses; 0.38%). Drug administration errors resulted in transient unintended drug effects (<5 minutes) in 17 cases and prolonged unintended drug effects (>5 minutes) in 12 cases. Of these 29 cases of unintended drug effect, 14 were associated with drug infusions administered by a pump. One patient had possible intraoperative awareness associated with an empty vaporizer, and one patient had a longer than expected hospital stay because of inadvertent administration of neuraxial morphine. There were no cases of drug-related permanent physical injury.

Analysis of the ASA Closed Claims Project database also reveals interesting information about anesthetic drug administration errors in the United States.[124] As of 2003 (a more current update is pending), there were 205 drug errors, 4% of the database of 5803 cases. Drug errors were categorized into the following categories (after Webster et al[116]):

Omission—drug not given
Repetition—extra dose of an intended drug
Substitution—incorrect drug instead of the desired drug; a swap
Insertion—a drug that was not intended to be given at a particular time or at any time

TABLE 39-3	Drug Errors in a University Anesthesia Practice	
Anesthetics		6705
Forms completed		6066
Total errors		41 (0.68%)
Incorrect dose		18
Substitution		7
Insertion		6
Repetition		2
Incorrect route		2
Omission		3
Incorrect label		1
Unintended effects		31
< 5 minutes		18
> 5 minutes		13

A study of self-reported drug-related errors by anesthesiology attendings, residents, and certified registered nurse anesthetists (CRNAs) in a university medical center found the errors shown in the table. The overall rate of drug-related error was 0.68% of anesthetics. There were no permanent injuries; however, in 31 of 41 cases unintended drug effects occurred. One patient had possible intraoperative awareness associated with an empty vaporizer, and one patient had a longer than expected hospital stay because of inadvertent administration of neuraxial morphine.

Data from Bowdle A, Kruger C, Grieve R, et al: Anesthesia drug administration errors in a university hospital. *Anesthesiology* 99:A1358, 2003.

Incorrect dose—wrong dose of an intended drug
Incorrect route—wrong route of an intended drug*
Other—usually a more complex event not fitting the previous categories

The numbers of cases in each category and the types of drugs involved are shown in Figures 39-12 and 39-13. The most common distinct mechanisms of drug administration error were substitution, insertion, and incorrect dose. Drug errors were also a significant factor in claims that involved multiple problems in patient management ("other"). Two drugs in particular were most involved.

Succinylcholine was involved in 35 cases (17%), and epinephrine was involved in 17 cases (8%). Twelve of the 35 cases involving

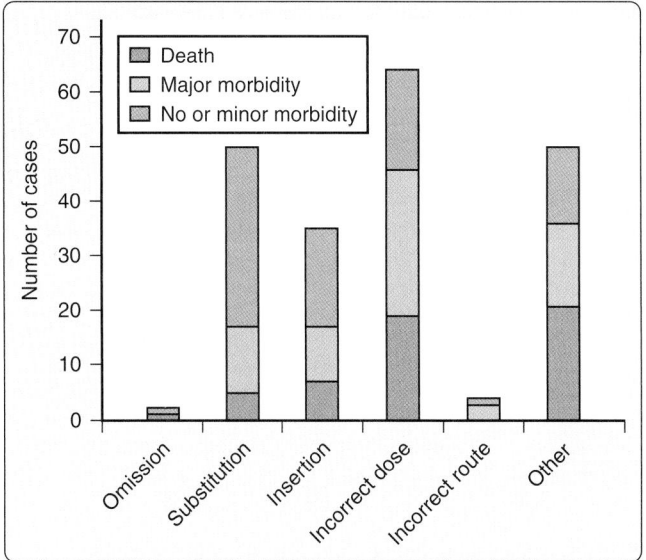

Figure 39-12 A review of claims related to drug errors in the American Society of Anesthesiologists (ASA) Closed Claims database found the mechanisms of error shown in the figure. (*Data from Bowdle TA: Drug administration error from the ASA closed claims project.* American Society of Anesthesiologists Newsletter 67:11–13, 2003.)

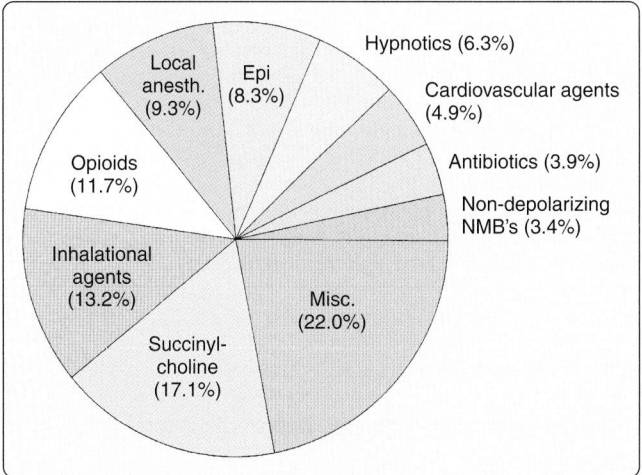

Figure 39-13 A review of claims related to drug errors in the American Society of Anesthesiologists (ASA) Closed Claims database found the drugs shown in the figure. The two individual drugs implicated most frequently were epinephrine and succinylcholine. (*Data from Bowdle TA: Drug administration error from the ASA closed claims project.* American Society of Anesthesiologists Newsletter 67:11–13, 2003.)

*Inadvertent injection of intravenous medications into epidural catheters has prompted efforts to design unique neuraxial injection ports that would prevent such errors.[125]

succinylcholine resulted in patients being awake while paralyzed because of succinylcholine boluses given before induction agents or succinylcholine infusions that were started inadvertently in awake patients. Succinylcholine was administered to five patients with a previous history of definite or probable pseudocholinesterase deficiency, resulting in prolonged neuromuscular blockade. Hyperkalemic cardiac arrest occurred in two paraplegic patients and a patient with Guillain-Barré syndrome who received succinylcholine. Succinylcholine infusions were involved in 14 of the 35 succinylcholine-related cases. Drug administration errors involving epinephrine were particularly dangerous, with death or major morbidity resulting in 11 of the 17 epinephrine-related cases. Six of the 17 cases involving epinephrine were caused by ampoule swaps. Drugs interchanged with epinephrine were ephedrine (two cases), oxytocin (three cases), and hydralazine (one case). An informative case report describing the nearly fatal results of inadvertent epinephrine administration because of an ampoule swap has been published.[126]

There were 19 cases of intraoperative awareness (9%), 14 of which involved inadvertent administration of muscle relaxant to awake patients; a patient who received vecuronium instead of cefazolin experienced development of post-traumatic stress disorder as a result of being paralyzed awake. The remaining five cases of awareness were either unexplained (one case), related to omission of an induction agent (one case), or were apparently related to inadequate doses of general anesthetic agents (three cases).

ASA Closed Claims Project reviewers judged the care to be "less than appropriate" in 84% of the drug error claims, compared with 35% in nondrug error claims. Payments were made to plaintiffs in 72% of the drug error claims compared with 52% of the nondrug error claims.

An analysis of litigation against the National Health Service in England related to anesthetic drug errors found a spectrum of errors that were similar to those found by the ASA Closed Claims Project.[127]

Drug Errors by Perfusionists

Cardiac surgery requiring CPB presents the relatively unusual situation in which the anesthesiologist may not be the only person in the operating room administering drugs intravenously to the patient. Perfusionists frequently administer anesthetic drugs during CPB and may administer a variety of other drugs as well. Rarely, the perfusionist also may be an anesthesiologist (particularly in Australia). Whether the anesthesiologist supervises the perfusionist in the administration of drugs varies depending on the particular practice setting. In some practice settings, the anesthesiologist may leave the operating room during some portion of the time on CPB. Although the suggestion has been made that the anesthesiologist should not leave the operating room during CPB (http://www.asawebapps.org/Newsletters/2004/04_04/gravlee04_04.html), the practice of doing so probably is widespread, particularly outside of academic institutions. Apparently, there are no studies documenting drug errors made by perfusionists, despite several general reports on error and incidents during CPB.[128–131] Any comprehensive effort to reduce drug errors during cardiac surgery should include the perfusionist. Common sense suggests that the perfusionist and anesthesiologist should work together as much as possible to ensure that the patient receives drugs appropriately during CPB.

Prevention of Drug Administration Errors—Bar Coding

Although drug administration errors are clearly important, relatively little is known about preventing these errors. A recent review evaluated the evidence for various measures for reducing drug administration errors in anesthetic practice and made recommendations; however, most of the evidence available for review was anecdotal.[132] Recommendations included carefully reading the label on any ampoule or syringe, optimizing legibility and contents of labels, labeling syringes, formal organization of drugs drawers and workspaces, and double-checking drugs with another person or a device.

A bar-code reader represents just such a device, and bar-coding drugs at the point of care to verify the correctness of the drug and the dose is widely regarded as a technologic solution that might improve the accuracy of drug administration. The Healthcare Information and Management Systems Society has a position statement in support of bar coding in the healthcare environment for a variety of purposes (http://www.himss.org/content/files/BarCoding StatementFINAL20020603_19028.pdf). ECRI, the nonprofit health services research agency, also has published a review concerning the bar coding of medications.[133,134] The proceedings of the Healthcare Information and Management Systems Society from 2000 ("Veterans Affairs: Eliminating Medication Errors Through Point-of-Care Devices"; available online at: http://www.himss.org/content/files/proceedings/2000/sessions/ses073.pdf) contains interesting anecdotal information about the experience of the Department of Veterans Affairs with bar coding. According to this report, wireless, point-of-care bar coding of patient wristbands and medications was used at the Comery-O'Neil Veterans Affairs Medical Center to deliver 5.7 million doses and in the process prevented 378,000 errors. The report claims that "no medication errors occurred when the technology was used as designed," although errors continued to occur when the technology was not properly used. Application of bar-coding technology reduced wrong medication errors by 74%, wrong dose errors by 57%, wrong patient errors by 91%, wrong time errors by 92%, and omission errors by 70%. Clearly, these are promising results that should cause clinicians to look carefully at the prospects for bar coding in the anesthesia environment. Interestingly, the Veterans Affairs medical centers experienced some significant difficulties with point-of-care bar coding, which is described in an article by Mills et al.[135] Some of the most common problems were simple but critically important, such as nonreadable bar codes on patients wrist bands and drug containers. According to Mills et al,[135] "Several anecdotal reports have indicated that bar-coding systems successfully lower medication administrations errors…Nevertheless, within the VA, there have been significant negative effects since introducing the bar-coded medication administration (BCMA) system. More generally, the VA discovered that introducing new technology to complex medical systems, while beneficial, also presents new challenges."

A study of point-of-care bar-code medication administration in a network of six community hospitals examined error logs and determined the likely severity of outcomes associated with errors that were prevented by the bar-code system.[136] Only 1% of prevented errors were judged to be likely to produce severe adverse effects, and 8% moderate adverse effects. However, given that 18 million doses were administered in the hospital network since the bar-code system was implemented, 17,000 errors expected to produce severe or moderate adverse effects may have been prevented.

The FDA issued a rule in February 2004 that requires bar codes on most prescription drugs, certain over-the-counter drugs, and blood products (http://www.accessdata.fda.gov/scripts/cdrh/cfdocs/cfcfr/CFRSearch.cfm?fr=201.25). The FDA believes that bar codes would be used in the following manner:

- A patient is admitted to the hospital. The hospital gives the patient a bar-coded identification bracelet to link the patient to his or her computerized medical record.
- As required by the rule, most prescription drugs and certain over-the-counter drugs would have a bar code on their labels. The bar code would reflect the drug's NDC (National Drug Code) number.
- The hospital would have bar code scanners or readers that are linked to the hospital's computer system of electronic medical records.
- Before a healthcare worker administers a drug to the patient, the healthcare worker scans the patient's bar code. This allows the computer to pull up the patient's computerized medical record.
- The healthcare worker then scans the drug(s) that the hospital pharmacy has provided to be administered to the patient. This scan informs the computer which drug is being administered.
- The computer then compares the patient's medical record with the drug(s) being administered to ensure that they match. If there is a problem, the computer sends an error message and the healthcare worker investigates the problem.

- The problem could be one of many things:
  - Wrong patient
  - Wrong dose of drug
  - Wrong drug
  - Wrong time to administer the drug
  - The patient's chart has been updated and the prescribed medication has changed

The FDA has estimated that this scheme would result in a 50% reduction in medication errors, preventing 500,000 adverse events and transfusion errors, while saving $93 billion over 20 years.

To the best of the authors' knowledge, there are two commercially available systems designed specifically for bar-coding drugs in the anesthesia clinical environment. One was designed by an anesthesiologist and marketed by DocuSys (Hartland, WI); another was designed by an anesthesiologist and marketed by Safer Sleep (Cambridge, United Kingdom).[137] Unfortunately, there are no prospective, randomized data showing that the use of these devices affects outcome, although a recent study of user ratings of the Safer Sleep system gave results in favor of the bar-coding system in comparison with the traditional system of drug administration.[138] The Safer Sleep system was reported to result in a 19% increase in revenue from drug charges in a cardiac anesthesiology practice by improving documentation for billing.[139] Hypothetically, automated anesthesia record-keeping systems provided by other vendors could be adapted to bar coding of drugs because bar-code readers can be operated by most desktop computer systems.

Prevention of Drug Errors—Infusion Pumps

As noted earlier, the study of drug errors at the University of Washington found that among 29 cases of unintended drug effect, 14 were associated with drug infusions administered by a pump.[123] Although there is no comprehensive assessment of the incidence and nature of errors related to infusion pumps, it is clear from anecdotal reports that programming errors are a significant source of error. Obviously, infusion pumps play a major role in drug administration in cardiac surgery patients, so errors related to infusion pumps are of significant concern to cardiac anesthesiologists.

ECRI, the nonprofit health services research agency, recently made recommendations concerning improvements in the safety of infusion pumps. Based on reports of pump-related problems and accident investigations, ECRI has found that pump incidents typically involve either unintentional free-flow of a drug or the delivery of an incorrect dose because of a practitioner error in programming the pump.[140]

Pump sets that prevent free-flow when the set is removed from the pump have been available for many years, but not all pumps in current use require the use of sets that prevent free-flow, and unprotected sets continue to be available. ECRI recommends the use of pumps with tubing sets that prevent free-flow when the set is removed from the pump, and that only pumps that *require* the use of sets with free-flow prevention be purchased. They rate pumps that do not require set-based free-flow protection as "unacceptable."[140]

Some infusion pumps have advisory systems known as "error reduction systems" that use predefined dosing limits and warn the practitioner if the dosing parameters that are entered at the point of care will result in a dose that is out of the predefined dosing limits. Such systems also can keep a computerized log that yields data regarding the incidence of "reprogramming" in response to an alert message; this is essentially the incidence of potential errors because of programming errors. Anecdotal information suggests that error reduction systems may be valuable for helping practitioners to recognize and avoid administering incorrect doses because of programming errors. A recent report of experience with 135 pumps with an error reduction system installed in a community hospital found that 40,644 infusion starts generated 693 alert messages (1.7%), resulting in 158 programming changes.[141] The 1400-bed hospital projected that if all of their pumps had error reduction systems, that in a year more than 1 million infusion starts would result in 18,500 alert messages and 4000 programming changes. All pumps rated "preferred" or "acceptable" by ECRI include dose error reduction systems, whereas pumps without such systems are rated "not recommended" for new purchase.[142] A prospective, randomized trial of "smart" infusion pumps conducted in 2002 in a cardiac surgery ICU found numerous serious medication errors related to pumps (approximately 2 serious errors per 100 patient pump-days).[143] There was no significant improvement with the use of smart pumps, although the investigators observed that the pumps were frequently not used as intended. For example, the drug library that is intended to prevent manual programming errors was bypassed 25% of the time. This study demonstrates that technology alone may not solve a problem, and that close attention to the details of implementing the technology and making it work properly are essential (as noted for bar coding at the point-of-care; see earlier). Nuckols et al[144] also found that the smart pumps they tested were capable of preventing only 4% of the adverse drug events in the ICU, with many of the events having to do with bolus dosing and failure to adequately monitor for and respond to drug-related problems. However, they did not conclude that smart pumps should be abandoned; to the contrary, they advocated smarter and more capable pumps.

An error programming the concentration of morphine in a patient-controlled analgesia pump caused the death of a patient who received a fivefold overdose of morphine because of the programming error. The authors of the case report made an estimate of the likely death rate from similar programming errors of the particular patient-controlled analgesia pump involved in this incident, based on an FDA database and other reports, using a denominator supplied by the pump manufacturer. The estimate was adjusted to take the likely under-reporting of incidents into account. Their estimate was a range of 1 death in 33,000 pump uses to 1 in 338,800, amounting to 65 to 667 deaths for 22,000,000 pump uses in the period 1988 to 2000.[145]

Although error reduction systems help to recognize programming errors that may result in an incorrect dose, they do not recognize that a wrong drug has been placed in the pump or that the drug is being administered to the wrong patient. Bar coding may be a solution to this problem. A bar code on a medication bag can be scanned, together with the patient's bar-coded identification, to electronically prompt the pump with the appropriate drug and drug concentration, preventing misidentification of the drug or the patient, as well as preventing pump programming errors that can occur during manual entry. Furthermore, if the pump is connected to the electronic medical record (or automated anesthesia record in the operating room), all of the dosing information from the pump can be automatically documented in the record. Application of bar coding to infusion pumps is a relatively new and evolving technology.

Transfusion Safety

Although bar coding of drugs has received greater publicity, bar coding of blood units and the use of bar coding to ensure accurate matching of blood component to recipient is another promising avenue for application of bar coding technology to prevent error. ABO mismatched transfusion because of administering the wrong blood is a classic example of a preventable medical error and is a significant cause for concern in the practice of cardiac anesthesia. A study of transfusion errors in New York State estimated the incidence of ABO mismatched transfusion at 1:12,000 to 1:33,000.[146] A recent report from a hospital in Japan specializing in cardiovascular disease described a computer-assisted transfusion management system with bar coding at the bedside; 60,000 blood components were transfused without error, and one human error was prevented. The system also improved the efficiency of blood component management, reducing the outdate rate on red blood cells from 3.9% to 0.32%.[147] Bar coding blood components in the operating room could contribute to both efficiency and accuracy, especially if the data from the bar coding operation were automatically entered in a computerized anesthesia record. As noted earlier, the FDA has mandated bar codes on blood products, as well as drugs.

FATIGUE AND ERROR IN CARDIAC ANESTHESIA

The Institute of Medicine Committee on Optimizing Graduate Medical Trainee Hours and Work Schedules to Improve Patient Safety conducted a comprehensive review of the medical and scientific literature and concluded that working for more than 16 consecutive hours is unsafe for both trainees, because of a marked increase risk for a motor vehicle accident while driving home, and for their patients, because of an increase in attentional failure, serious errors, and diagnostic mistakes.[3] After being awake for 24 hours, impairment of reaction time is comparable with that produced by a blood alcohol concentration of 0.10 g/dL (the equivalent of 4 drinks for a 70-kg individual, and over the legal limit for driving while intoxicated in most countries).[148,149] A survey of resident physicians suggested that fatigue-related errors resulting in death or injury of a patient are not uncommon (Box 39-4).[150]

Interestingly, there is significant variability between individuals in susceptibility to the effects of sleep deprivation. The effect of a single night of acute sleep deprivation on neurobehavioral functions is greater in younger people than in people older than 55 years.[151] This may explain the fact that 55% of sleep-related motor vehicle accidents occur in drivers 25 or younger.[152] However, older people are more vulnerable to the effects of a sequence of night shifts because of greater difficulty obtaining recovery sleep in an adverse portion of the circadian cycle.[153] There also are inter-individual differences in the effects of sleep deprivation on otherwise healthy young people, and these differences may be specific for particular tasks. These differences have been linked to particular genetic polymorphisms.[154,155] Czeisler[156] has speculated that, in the future, it may be possible to identify from a cheek swab the genetic subset of individuals who tolerate sleep deprivation relatively well from those who are very sensitive.

Sleep-deprived individuals develop the subjective experience of sleepiness early, and if sleep deprivation persists, they have a poor capacity to recognize their fatigue, rendering them with a reduced capacity to work safely.[157] Recognition that sleep deprivation adversely affects performance has led to policies that limit work hours. Limitations on work hours for pilots date from the 1950s. In the United States, the Accreditation Council for Graduate Medical Education limits the hours of trainees in approved programs. In other countries, a variety of regulations may apply. For example, in New Zealand, a labor agreement limits consecutive work hours for trainees to 16. There are no work-hour limitations in the United States for nontrainee physicians. In the European Union, all occupations are limited to 13 consecutive work hours and 48-hour work weeks. Whether limiting trainee work hours lessens the effectiveness of training programs has been the subject of much debate, which recently was reviewed.[158] There has been widespread noncompliance with work hour limits in Accreditation Council for Graduate Medical Education–accredited training programs.[159] However, given the available evidence connecting sleep deprivation with impairment in performance, it seems likely that work hour limitations will become more stringent rather than less. Moreover, it seems likely that consideration will be given to extending the limitations applied currently to trainees to physicians in practice.

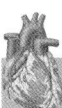

BOX 39-4. REDUCING ERRORS RELATED TO FATIGUE AND DISTRACTION

- Fatigue may contribute to critical incidents and errors.
- Sleep deprivation impairs psychomotor and cognitive performance.
- Anesthesiologists older than 50 may be more vulnerable to the effects of repeated episodes of sleep deprivation and fatigue.
- Operating room logistics and scheduling of personnel should take the demonstrated effects of fatigue and sleep deprivation into account.
- Transesophageal echocardiographic interpretation and monitoring may be a distraction from fundamental patient care.

Effects of Fatigue on Error in Anesthesia

Fatigue has been implicated as a contributor to impaired performance, critical incidents, and errors in anesthesia.[160,161] The work hours and schedules of anesthesiologists expose them to circadian disruption, and both acute and chronic sleep deprivation cause fatigue. The performance of anesthesiologists may be more susceptible to the effects of even mild sleep deprivation compared with other medical specialties because of the vigilance required to provide safe anesthesia care. However, study of the effects of fatigue on the clinical performance of anesthesiologists is difficult, and to date, no clinical studies have shown a definite link between fatigued anesthesiologists and errors.

In a well-designed, realistic, simulation-based trial, Howard et al[162] studied 12 residents who anesthetized a simulated patient for 4 hours in both a sleep-deprived state and a rested state. In the sleep-deprived group, there was a trend to poorer vigilance with slower response to vigilance probes during the simulation. In clinical tasks, the sleep-deprived group took longer to detect and correct abnormal clinical events, but this was not statistically significant. During the simulated anesthetic, nearly one third of the sleep-deprived group fell asleep at some stage.

In an analysis of the first 5700 critical incidents reported to the Australian Incident Monitoring Study database, 2.7% of incidents listed fatigue as a factor contributing to the incident.[161] Drug errors (syringe swaps/wrong drug, underdose and overdose) were more frequent, and anesthesiologists reported that haste, distraction, inattention, failure to check equipment, fault of technique, and pressure to proceed with surgery were all more common in fatigue-related than non–fatigue-related incidents. Experience and training did not render an anesthesiologist any less likely to make a fatigue-related error. A healthy patient and relief anesthesiologist/staff change were factors identified that tended to minimize the critical incident. In a survey of 301 anesthesiologists and trainees in New Zealand, 86% responded that they had at some time made an error in patient care related to fatigue.[163] Fifty percent of trainees and 27% of anesthesiologists believed that their average working week exceeded what they believed they could do on an ongoing basis while maintaining patient safety. In addition, the anesthesiologists who exceeded their self-defined safety limits for continuous anesthesia administration (with breaks) or their weekly safe working hours were more likely to report a fatigue-related error in the 6 months before the survey when compared with those who had not exceeded their limits. The conclusions from these two studies are limited because they are based on retrospective, self-reported data, but the majority of respondents consistently indicate that quality of care is compromised and attribute some errors to working while fatigued.

A Scottish study raised different issues. Flin et al[164] surveyed 222 anesthesiologists. When questioned about stress and fatigue, 83% agreed they were less effective when stressed or tired, but 37% thought they performed effectively during the critical phases of surgery even when tired. Eighty-four percent had made errors during patient care, but they did not attribute any causation to fatigue and did not list being rested or changing work schedules/reducing work hours as methods for reducing errors. The authors conclude, "With regard to attitudes suggesting invulnerability to the effects of stress and fatigue, a significant number of anesthetists were found to show these beliefs" and this "suggests that anesthetists (like pilots) may benefit from additional training in human performance limitations, both in postgraduate education or for consultants through continuing professional development programs."

Gander et al[165] studied work patterns, sleep, and performance on a psychomotor vigilance task of 28 anesthesia trainees and 20 specialists (practicing physicians) during a 2-week work cycle in 2 urban public hospitals in New Zealand. This study is significant because it included specialists and trainees. Reaction times of trainees were slower after night shifts than after day shifts, and after night shifts, poorer performance was associated with longer shift length, longer time since waking, greater acute sleep loss, and more total work over 24 hours. Reaction times of specialists slowed in a progressive, linear fashion over 12 consecutive days of duty (without any days off), and poorer performance was associated with greater acute sleep loss and longer time since waking. Work hours of trainees, but not specialists, are limited in New Zealand by a labor agreement.

Sleep quality and quantity become impaired in those around age 50 and older.[166,167] There have been no formal studies assessing how these changes might affect the performance of older anesthesiologists. However, there is reduced tolerance of late-night and shift work with aging.[167] Thus, many of the fatigue-related performance impairments identified in residents are potentially worse in older anesthesiologists.

Although working at night may contribute to error, the nature of anesthetic work makes it difficult to avoid at least some work during night-time hours. Therefore, work patterns need to be designed to minimize the possibility of fatigue-related error. These designs should not only involve consideration of total individual work hours, but the importance of the effects of shift work on sleep and circadian rhythm. Useful overviews for individual practitioners on the impact of fatigue on learning and good sleep hygiene to mitigate the impact of fatigue and for departments on the impacts of different rostering systems are available.[168–172] Some areas to address to limit fatigue and fatigue-related error in anesthesia providers are listed in Table 39-4.

EFFECTS OF THE USE OF TRANSESOPHAGEAL ECHOCARDIOGRAPHY ON VIGILANCE

The introduction and subsequent widespread use of TEE has been a major advance in cardiac surgery and anesthesia for both diagnosis and monitoring intraoperatively. Anecdotally, the authors have noticed times when all attention in the operating room is focused on the TEE machine rather than the patient. This seems to be more noticeable during the phase of learning TEE than with those who are more experienced. The surgical team also may comment that the anesthesia providers are all looking at the TEE rather than the patient! The authors are aware of only one study that has addressed this issue. During a study on task distribution, workload, and vigilance during cardiac anesthesia, Weinger et al[173] found that there was a significant increase in response time to vigilance probes (a light was illuminated on the monitor screen) when the TEE was being manipulated and analyzed compared with times when it was not. The authors concluded, "The use of the TEE may decrease vigilance to changes in other clinical data." Several factors limit the applicability of this study—it involved anesthesia residents with limited cardiac anesthesia experience and limited TEE experience. The operating room setup had the TEE machine placed opposite to the anesthesia machine and monitor display (where the vigilance light was located) and the study involved only 20 cases. The findings of the study were questioned in a subsequent letter to the editor.[174]

This area needs further investigation before definite conclusions can be reached. However, an important factor may be the operating room setup. In particular, where the TEE machine is placed in relation to the patient and the other monitors may be important. To date, no studies have addressed operating room ergonomics with regard to optimizing TEE machine and anesthesia machine setup for ease of reviewing both patient monitors and the TEE machine. The anesthesiologist working alone may be more vulnerable to this problem given that there is only one place attention can be focused at a time.

AMERICAN SOCIETY OF ANESTHESIOLOGISTS CLOSED CLAIMS PROJECT RESULTS FOR CARDIAC ANESTHESIA

The ASA Closed Claims database contains 327 claims related to cardiac anesthesia. When compared with 4986 other claims for other surgical procedures under general anesthesia, cardiac surgery claims had an increased proportion of claims for brain damage, stroke, and awareness during anesthesia and a decreased proportion of claims for airway injury (Table 39-5). The primary damaging event, for example, the specific incident that led to the injury, was more often related to equipment problems, particularly with central or peripheral catheters (Table 39-6). In addition, a greater proportion of cardiac claims were related to surgical technique or patient condition than other surgical claims in the database (see Table 39-6). Approaches for avoiding problems with intraoperative awareness and central venous access have been reviewed in this chapter. Brain damage and stroke during cardiac anesthesia is a vast topic unto itself that is addressed in Chapter 36.

TABLE 39-4	Some Areas to Address to Limit Fatigue and Fatigue-Related Error in Anesthesia Providers

Individual
Length of time without break
Length of time for shifts
Length of break between shifts
Handover[170,175]
Sleep hygiene education
Education on effects of fatigue on performance and increased likelihood of errors
Naps
Pharmacologic aids (e.g., modafinil[176–179])
Tighten monitor alarm limits after hours
Departmental
Roster design to limit circadian rhythm disruption
Staffing levels
Stop after hours or night work for older anesthesiologists
Sleep hygiene education
Use of written protocols/checklists, especially for complex cases after hours
Hospital
Lighting levels after hours
Nap rooms
Food and drink provision
Limit after-hours work to emergency cases

These topics are intended as a starting point for consideration of possible ways in which errors related to fatigue might be reduced.

TABLE 39-5	Influence of Type of Surgery on Severity of Injury	
Injury	*Cardiac Surgery, n (%)*	*Other Surgery, n (%)*
Major Category		
Death	103 (31%)	1746 (35%)
Brain damage	60 (18%)*	548 (11%)*
Nerve damage	54 (17%)	770 (15%)
Specific Complications		
Stroke	30 (9%)*	156 (3%)*
Airway injury	21 (6%)†	501 (10%)†
Awareness	20 (6%)*	99 (2%)*
Myocardial infarction	5 (2%)	157 (3%)

Cases related to cardiac surgery from the American Society of Anesthesiologists Closed Clams Project database (N = 8954) were compared with noncardiac surgery cases (only cases of general anesthesia were considered).
*P < 0.01 cardiac surgery vs. other surgery by Fisher's exact test.
†P < 0.05 cardiac surgery vs. other surgery by Fisher's exact test.

TABLE 39-6	Influence of Type of Surgery on Primary Damaging Event	
Damaging Event	*Cardiac Surgery, n (%)*	*Other Surgery, n (%)*
Respiratory	33 (10%)*	1507 (30%)*
Cardiovascular	53 (16%)	788 (16%)
Wrong blood administered	4 (1%)	19 (< 1%)
Equipment	104 (32%)*	579 (12%)*
Peripheral catheter	38 (12%)*	99 (2%)*
Central catheter	28 (9%)*	112 (2%)*
Adverse drug reaction/drug error	30 (9%)	336 (7%)
Surgical/patient condition	35 (11%)†	315 (6%)†

Cases related to cardiac surgery from the American Society of Anesthesiologists Closed Clams Project database (N = 8954) were compared with noncardiac surgery cases (only cases of general anesthesia were considered).
*P < 0.01 cardiac surgery vs. other surgery by Z-test.
†P < 0.05 cardiac surgery vs. other surgery by Z-test.

REFERENCES

1. Institute of Medicine: *To Err Is Human. Building a Safer Health Care System*, Washington, DC, 2000, National Academy Press.
2. Haynes AB, Weiser TG, Berry WR, et al: A surgical safety checklist to reduce morbidity and mortality in a global population, *N Engl J Med* 360:491–499, 2009.
3. Resident Duty Hours: *Enhancing Sleep, Supervision and Safety*, Washington, DC, 2008, The National Academies Press.
4. Martinez EA, Marsteller JA, Thompson DA, et al: The Society of Cardiovascular Anesthesiologists' FOCUS initiative: Locating Errors through Networked Surveillance (LENS) project vision, *Anesth Analg* 110:307–311, 2010.
5. Arnstein F: Catalogue of human error, *Br J Anaesth* 79:645–656, 1997.
6. Gaba DM, Fish KJ, Howard SK: *Crisis Management in Anesthesiology*, New York, 1994, Churchill Livingstone, pp 5–53.
7. Reason J: Human error: Models and management, *BMJ* 320:768–770, 2000.
8. McGee DC, Gould MK: Preventing complications of central venous catheterization, *N Engl J Med* 348:1123–1133, 2003.
9. Bowdle T: Complications of invasive monitoring, *Anesthesiol Clin North America* 20:333–350, 2002.
10. Polderman KH, Girbes ARJ: Central venous catheter use. Part 1: Mechanical complications, *Intensive Care Med* 28:1–17, 2002.
11. Polderman KH, Girbes ARJ: Central venous catheter use. Part 2: Infectious complications, *Intensive Care Med* 28:18–28, 2002.
12. Hall AP, Russell WC: Toward safer central venous access: Ultrasound guidance and sound advice, *Anaesthesia* 60:1–4, 2005.
13. Making health care safer: *A critical analysis of patient safety practices*, 2001 Evidence report/technology assessment: Number 43. AHRQ Publication No. 01-E058.
14. Domino KB, Bowdle TA, Posner KL, et al: Injuries and liability related to central vascular catheters, *Anesthesiology* 100:1411–1418, 2004.
15. Urschel JD, Myerowitz D: Catheter-induced pulmonary artery rupture in the setting of cardiopulmonary bypass, *Ann Thorac Surg* 56:585–589, 1993.
16. Harvey S, Harrison DA, Singer M, et al: Assessment of the clinical effectiveness of pulmonary artery catheters in management of patients in intensive care (PAC-Man): A randomised controlled trial, *Lancet* 366:472–477, 2005.
17. Shah MR, Hasselblad V, Stevenson LW, et al: Impact of the pulmonary artery catheter in critically ill patients: Meta-analysis of randomized clinical trials, *JAMA* 294:1664–1670, 2005.
18. Connors AF, Speroff T, Dawson NV, et al: The effectiveness of right heart catheterization in the initial care of critically ill patients, *JAMA* 276:889–897, 1996.
19. Dalen JE, Bone RC: Is it time to pull the pulmonary catheter? *JAMA* 276:916–918, 1996.
20. Isaacson IJ, Lowdon JD, Berry AJ, et al: The value of pulmonary artery and central venous monitoring in patients undergoing abdominal aortic reconstructive surgery: A comparative study of two selected, randomized groups, *J Vasc Surg* 12:754–760, 1990.
21. Mimoz O, Rauss A, Rekik N, et al: Pulmonary artery catheterization in critically ill patients: A prospective analysis of outcome changes associated with catheter-prompted changes in therapy, *Crit Care Med* 22:573–579, 1994.
22. Ramsey SD, Saint S, Sullivan SD, et al: Clinical and economic effects of pulmonary artery catheterization in non-emergent coronary artery bypass graft surgery, *J Cardiothorac Vasc Anesth* 14:113–118, 2000.
23. Tuman KJ, McCarthy RJ, Spiess BD, et al: Effect of pulmonary artery catheterization on outcome in patients undergoing coronary artery surgery, *Anesthesiology* 70:199–206, 1989.
24. Bashein G, Johnson PW, Davis KB, et al: Elective coronary bypass surgery without pulmonary artery catheter monitoring, *Anesthesiology* 63:451–454, 1985.
25. Bender JS, Smith-Meek MA, Jones CE: Routine pulmonary artery catheterization does not reduce morbidity and mortality of elective vascular surgery: Results of a prospective, randomized trial, *Ann Surg* 226:229–236, 1997.
26. Coles NA, Hibberd M, Russell M, et al: Potential impact of pulmonary artery catheter placement on short-term management decisions in the medical intensive care unit, *Am Heart J* 126:815–819, 1993.
27. Mueller HS, Chatterjee K, Davis KB, et al: Present use of bedside right heart catheterization in patients with cardiac disease, *JACC J Am Coll Cardiol* 32:840–864, 1998.
28. Richard C, Warszawski J, Anguel N, et al: Early use of the pulmonary artery catheter and outcomes in patients with shock and acute respiratory distress syndrome: A randomized controlled trial, *Jama* 290:2713–2720, 2003.
29. Sandham JD, Hull RD, Brant RF, et al: A randomized, controlled trial of the use of pulmonary-artery catheters in high-risk surgical patients, *N Engl J Med* 348:5–14, 2003.
30. Bar-Joseph G, Galvis AG: Perforation of the heart by central venous catheters in infants: Guidelines to diagnosis and management, *J Pediatr Surg* 18:284–287, 1983.
31. Brandt RL, Foley WJ, Fink GH, et al: Mechanism of perforation of the heart with production of hydropericardium by a venous catheter and its prevention, *Am J Surg* 119:311–316, 1970.
32. Collier PE, Ryan JJ, Diamond DL: Cardiac tamponade from central venous catheters—a report of a case and review of english literature, *Angiology* 35:595–600, 1984.
33. Jiha JG, Weinberg GL, Laurito CE: Intraoperative cardiac tamponade after central venous cannulation, *Anesth Analg* 82:664–665, 1996.
34. Maschke SP, Rogove HJ: Cardiac tamponade associated with a multilumen central venous catheter, *Crit Care Med* 12:611–612, 1984.
35. Scott WL: Complications associated with central venous catheters, *Chest* 94:1221–1224, 1988.
36. Sheep RE, Guiney WB: Fatal cardiac tamponade: Occurrence with other complications after left internal jugular vein catheterization, *JAMA* 248:1632–1635, 1982.
37. Fletcher SJ, Bodenham AR: Safe placement of central venous catheters: Where should the tip of the catheter lie? *Br J Anaesth* 85:188–191, 2000.
38. Tocino IM, Watanabe A: Impending catheter perforation of superior vena cava: Radiographic recognition, *Am J Roentgenol* 146:487–490, 1986.
39. Trigaux JP, Goncette L, Van Beers B, et al: Radiologic findings of normal and compromised thoracic venous catheters, *J Thorac Imaging* 9:246–254, 1994.
40. Albrecht K, Nave H, Breitmeir D, et al: Applied anatomy of the superior vena cava—the carina as a landmark to guide central venous catheter placement, *Br J Anaesth* 92:75–77, 2004.
41. Schuster M, Nave H, Piepenbrock S, et al: The carina as a landmark in central venous catheter placement, *Br J Anaesth* 85:192–194, 2000.
42. Kwon TD, Kim KH, Ryu HG, et al: Intra- and extra-pericardial lengths of the superior vena cava in vivo: Implication for the positioning of central venous catheters, *Anaesth Intensive Care* 33:384–387, 2005.
43. Gebhard RE, Szmuk P, Pivalizza EG, et al: The accuracy of electrocardiogram-controlled central line placement, *Anesth Analg* 104:65–70, 2007.
44. Jeon Y, Ryu HG, Yoon SZ, et al: Transesophageal echocardiographic evaluation of ECG-guided central venous catheter placement, *Can J Anaesth* 53:978–983, 2006.
45. Jobes DR, Schwartz AJ, Greenhow DE, et al: Safer jugular vein cannulation: Recognition of arterial puncture and preferential use of the external jugular route, *Anesthesiology* 59:353–355, 1983.
46. Ezaru CS, Mangione MP, Oravitz TM, et al: Eliminating arterial injury during central venous catheterization using manometry, *Anesth Analg* 109:130–134, 2009.
47. Bowdle A, Kharasch E, Schwid H: Pressure waveform monitoring during central venous catheterization, *Anesth Analg* 109:2030–2031, 2009 author reply 2031.
48. Troianos CA, Jobes DR, Ellison N: Ultrasound-guided cannulation of the internal jugular vein. A prospective, randomized study, *Anesth Analg* 72:823–826, 1991.
49. Randolph AG, Cook DJ, Gonzales CA, et al: Ultrasound guidance for placement of central venous catheters: A meta-analysis of the literature, *Crit Care Med* 24:2053–2058, 1996.
50. Hind D, Calvert N, McWilliams R, et al: Ultrasonic locating devices for central venous cannulation: Meta-analysis, *BMJ* 327:361–368, 2003.
51. Wigmore TJ, Smythe JF, Hacking MB, et al: Effect of the implementation of NICE guidelines for ultrasound guidance on the complication rates associated with central venous catheter placement in patients presenting for routine surgery in a tertiary referral centre, *Br J Anaesth* 99:662–665, 2007.
52. Shime N, Nomura M, Matsuyama H, et al: Internal jugular vein cannulation in infants and children using a new portable ultrasound designed for vascular access, *J Jpn Soc Intensive Care Med* 12: 407–411, 2005.
53. Hosokawa K, Shime N, Kato Y, et al: A randomized trial of ultrasound image-based skin surface marking versus real-time ultrasound-guided internal jugular vein catheterization in infants, *Anesthesiology* 107:720–724, 2007.
54. Chapman GA, Johnson D, Bodenham AR: Visualisation of needle position using ultrasonography, *Anaesthesia* 61:148–158, 2006.
55. *Guidance on the Use of Ultrasound Locating Devices for Placing Central Venous Catheters*, vol 2005, London, 2002, National Institute for Clinical Excellence.
56. Bosman M, Kavanagh RJ: Two dimensional ultrasound guidance in central venous catheter placement; a postal survey of the practice and opinions of consultant pediatric anesthetists in the United Kingdom, *Paediatr Anaesth* 16:530–537, 2006.
57. Tovey G, Stokes M: A survey of the use of 2D ultrasound guidance for insertion of central venous catheters by UK consultant paediatric anaesthetists, *Eur J Anaesthesiol* 24:71–75, 2007.
58. McGrattan T, Duffty J, Green JS, et al: A survey of the use of ultrasound guidance in internal jugular venous cannulation, *Anaesthesia* 63:1222–1225, 2008.
59. Bailey PL, Glance LG, Eaton MP, et al: A survey of the use of ultrasound during central venous catheterization, *Anesth Analg* 104:491–497, 2007.
60. Harris N, Hodzovic I, Latto P: A national survey of the use of ultrasound during central venous cahteterization, *Anaesthesia* 62:306–307, 2007.
61. Oropello JM, Leibowitz AB, Manasia A, et al: Dilator-associated complications of central vein catheter insertion: Possible mechanisms of injury and suggestions for prevention, *J Cardiothorac Vasc Anesth* 10:634–637, 1996.
62. Kulvatunyou N, Heard SO, Bankey PE: A subclavian artery injury, secondary to internal jugular vein cannulation, is a predictable right-sided phenomenon, *Anesth Analg* 95:564–566, 2002 table of contents.
63. Welliver MD, Masoud PJ: Thoracic duct cannulation during central venous catheterization: A case report, *Am J Anesthesiol* 28:199–202, 2001.
64. Shah PM, Babu SC, Goyal A, et al: Arterial misplacement of large-caliber cannulas during jugular vein catheterization: Case for surgical management, *J Am Coll Surg* 198:939–944, 2004.
65. Guilbert MC, Elkouri S, Bracco D, et al: Arterial trauma during central venous catheter insertion: Case series, review and proposed algorithm, *J Vasc Surg* 48:918–925; discussion 925, 2008.
66. Soufir L, Timsit JF, Mahe C, et al: Attributable morbidity and mortality of catheter-related septicemia in critically ill patients: A matched, risk-adjusted, cohort study, *Infect Control Hosp Epidemiol* 20:396–401, 1999.
67. Renaud B, Brun-Buisson C: Outcomes of primary and catheter-related bacteremia. A cohort and case-control study in critically ill patients, *Am J Respir Crit Care Med* 163:1584–1590, 2001.
68. Maki DG, Kluger DM, Crnich CJ: The risk of bloodstream infection in adults with different intravascular devices: A systematic review of 200 published prospective studies, *Mayo Clin Proc* 81:1159–1171, 2006.
69. Raad II, Bodey GP: Infectious complications of indwelling cascular catheters, *Clin Infect Dis* 15:197–208, 1992.
70. Mermel LA, Maki DG: Infectious complications of Swan-Ganz pulmonary artery catheters. Pathogenesis, epidemiology, prevention and management, *Am J Respir Crit Care Med* 149:1020–1036, 1994.
71. Saint S, Matthay MA: Risk reduction in the intensive care unit, *Am J Med* 105:515–523, 1998.
72. Pronovost P, Needham D, Berenholtz S, et al: An intervention to decrease catheter-related bloodstream infections in the ICU, *N Engl J Med* 355:2725–2732, 2006.
73. Timsit JF, Schwebel C, Bouadma L, et al: Chlorhexidine-impregnated sponges and less frequent dressing changes for prevention of catheter-related infections in critically ill adults: A randomized controlled trial, *JAMA* 301:1231–1241, 2009.
74. Hockenhull JC, Dwan KM, Smith GW, et al: The clinical effectiveness of central venous catheters treated with anti-infective agents in preventing catheter-related bloodstream infections: A systematic review, *Crit Care Med* 37:702–712, 2009.
75. Casey AL, Mermel LA, Nightingale P, et al: Antimicrobial central venous catheters in adults: A systematic review and meta-analysis, *Lancet Infect Dis* 8:763–776, 2008.
76. Gilbert RE, Harden M: Effectiveness of impregnated central venous catheters for catheter related blood stream infection: A systematic review, *Curr Opin Infect Dis* 21:235–245, 2008.
77. Myles PS, Williams DL, Hendrata M, et al: Patient satisfaction after anaesthesia and surgery: Results of a prospective survey of 10,811 patients, *Br J Anaesth* 84:6–10, 2000.
78. Sandin RH, Enlund G, Samuelsson P, et al: Awareness during anaesthesia: A prospective case study, *Lancet* 355:707–711, 2000.
79. Sebel PS, Bowdle TA, Ghoneim MM, et al: The incidence of awareness during anesthesia: A multicenter United States study, *Anesth Analg* 99:833–839, 2004.
80. Xu L, Wu AS, Yue Y: The incidence of intra-operative awareness during general anesthesia in China: A multi-center observational study, *Acta Anaesthesiol Scand* 53:873–882, 2009.
81. Domino KB, Posner KL, Caplan RA, et al: Awareness during anesthesia: A closed claims analysis, *Anesthesiology* 90:1053–1061, 1999.
82. Ranta SO-V, Hernanen P, Hynynen M: Patient's conscious recollections from cardiac anesthesia, *J Cardiothorac Vasc Anesth* 16:426–430, 2002.
83. Ranta S, Jussila J, Hynynen M: Recall of awareness during cardiac anesthesia: Influence of feedback information to the anesthesiologist, *Acta Anaesthesiol Scand* 40:554–560, 1996.
84. Dowd NP, Cheng DCH, Karski JM, et al: Intraoperative awareness in fast-track cardiac anesthesia, *Anesthesiology* 89:1068–1073, 1998.
85. Phillips AA, McLean RF, Devitt JH, et al: Recall of intraoperative events after general anaesthesia and cardiopulmonary bypass, *Can J Anaesth* 40:922–966, 1993.
86. Myles PS, Leslie K, McNeil J, et al: Bispectral index monitoring to prevent awareness during anaesthesia: The B-Aware randomized controlled trial, *Lancet* 363:1757–1763, 2004.
87. Ghoneim MM, Block RI, Haffarnan M, et al: Awareness during anesthesia: Risk factors, causes and sequelae: A review of reported cases in the literature, *Anesth Analg* 108:527–535, 2009.

88. Osterman JE, Hopper J, Heran WJ, et al: Awareness under anesthesia and the development of posttraumatic stress disorder, *Gen Hosp Psychiatry* 23:198–204, 2001.
89. Moerman N, Bonke B, Oosting J: Awareness and recall during general anesthesia. Facts and feelings, *Anesthesiology* 79:454–464, 1993.
90. Bowdle TA: Can we prevent recall during anesthesia? In Fleisher L, editor: *Evidence-Based Practice of Anesthesiology*, ed 2. Philadelphia, 2009, Saunders.
91. Bowdle TA: The Bispectral Index (BIS): An update, *Curr Rev Clin Anesth* 25:17–28, 2004.
92. Glass PS, Bloom M, Kearse L, et al: Bispectral analysis measures sedation and memory effects of propofol, midazolam, isoflurane, and alfentanil in healthy volunteers, *Anesthesiology* 86:836–847, 1997.
93. Islein-Chaves IA, Flaishon R, Sebel PS, et al: The effect of the interaction of propofol and alfentanil on recall, loss of consciousness, and the bispectral index, *Anesth Analg* 87:949–955, 1998.
94. Kalkman CJ, Drummond J: Monitors of depth of anesthesia, quo vadis? *Anesthesiology* 96:784–787, 2002.
95. Gan T, Glass P, Windsor A, et al: Bispectral index monitoring allows faster emergence and improved recovery from propofol, alfentanil and nitrous oxide anesthesia, *Anesthesiology* 87:808–815, 1997.
96. Liu SS: Effects of bispectral index monitoring on ambulatory anesthesia. A meta-analysis of randomized controlled trials and a cost analysis, *Anesthesiology* 101:311–315, 2004.
97. Ekman A, Lindholm M-L, Lennmarken C, et al: Reduction in the incidence of awareness using BIS monitoring, *Acta Anaesthesiol Scand* 48:20–26, 2004.
98. Avidan MS, Zhang L, Burnside BA, et al: Anesthesia awareness and the bispectral index, *N Engl J Med* 358:1097–1108, 2008.
99. Rampil IJ, Kim JS, Lenhardt R, et al: Bispectral EEG index during nitrous oxide administration, *Anesthesiology* 89:671–677, 1998.
100. Nieuwenhuijs D, Coleman EL, Douglas NJ, et al: Bispectral index values and spectral edge frequency at different stages of physiologic sleep, *Anesth Analg* 94:125–129, 2002.
101. Sebel PS, Lang E, Rampil IJ, et al: A multicenter study of bispectral electroencephalogram analysis for monitoring anesthetic effect, *Anesth Analg* 84:891–899, 1997.
102. Bouillon TW, Bruhn J, Radulescu L, et al: Pharmacodynamic interaction between propofol and remifentanil regarding hypnosis, tolerance of laryngoscopy, bispectral index, and electroencephalographic approximate entropy, *Anesthesiology* 100:1353–1372, 2004.
103. Kunisawa T, Ueno M, Suzuki A, et al: Bispectral index monitor prevented intraoperative awareness during partial cardiopulmonary bypass, *J Cardiothorac Vasc Anesth* 24:740, 2010.
104. Kakinohana M, Miyata Y, Kawabata T, et al: Bispectral index decreased to "0" in propofol anesthesia after a cross-clamping of descending thoracic aorta, *Anesthesiology* 99:1223–1225, 2003.
105. Bates DW, Cullen DJ, Laird N, et al: Incidence of adverse drug events and potential adverse drug events: Implications for prevention, *JAMA* 274:29–34, 1995.
106. Taxis K, Barber N: Incidence and severity of intravenous drug errors in a German hospital, *Eur J Clin Pharmacol* 59:815–817, 2004.
107. Camire E, Moyen E, Stelfox HT: Medication errors in critical care: Risk factors, prevention and disclosure, *CMAJ* 180:936–943, 2009.
108. *Reducing and preventing adverse drug events to decrease hospital costs*, [AHRQ Publication No. 01-0020] Research in Action, March 2001.
109. Eslami S, de Keizer NF, Abu-Hanna A: The impact of computerized physician medication order entry in hospitalized patients—a systematic review, *Int J Med Inform* 77:365–376, 2008.
110. Kaushal R, Shojania KG, Bates DW: Effects of computerized physician order entry and clinical decision support systems on medication safety: A systematic review, *Arch Intern Med* 163:1409–1416, 2003.
111. Koppel R, Metlay JP, Cohen A, et al: Role of computerized physician order entry systems in facilitating medication errors, *JAMA* 293:1197–1203, 2005.
112. Han YY, Carcillo JA, Venkataraman ST, et al: Unexpected increased mortality after implementation of a commercially sold computerized physician order entry system, *Pediatrics* 116:1506–1512, 2005.
113. Khajouei R, Jaspers MW: The impact of CPOE medication systems' design aspects on usability, workflow and medication orders: A systematic review, *Methods Inf Med* 49:3–19, 2010.
114. Currie M, Mackay P, Morgan C, et al: The "wrong drug" problem in anaesthesia: An analysis of 2000 incident reports, *Anaesth Intens Care* 21:596–601, 1993.
115. Merry AF, Peck DJ: Anaesthetists, errors in drug administration and the law, *N Z Med J* 108:185–187, 1995.
116. Webster CS, Merry AF, Larsson L, et al: The frequency and nature of drug administration error during anaesthesia, *Anaesth Intensive Care* 29:494–500, 2001.
117. Orser BA, Chen RJB, Yee DA: Medication errors in anesthetic practice: A survey of 687 practitioners, *Can J Anesth* 48:139–146, 2001.
118. Irita K, Kawashima Y, Iwao Y, et al: [Annual mortality and morbidity in operating rooms during 2002 and summary of morbidity and mortality between 1999 and 2002 in Japan: A brief review], *Masui* 53:320–335, 2004.
119. Abeysekera A, Bergman IJ, Kluger MT, et al: Drug error in anaesthetic practice: A review of 896 reports from the Australian Incident Monitoring Study database, *Anaesthesia* 60:220–227, 2005.
120. Yamamoto M, Ishikawa S, Makita K: Medication errors in anesthesia: An 8-year retrospective analysis at an urban university hospital, *J Anesth* 22:248–252, 2008.
121. Sakaguchi Y, Tokuda K, Yamaguchi K, et al: Incidence of anesthesia-related medication errors over a 15-year period in a university hospital, *Fukuoka Igaku Zasshi* 99:58–66, 2008.
122. Gordon PC, Llewellyn RL, James MF: Drug administration errors by South African anaesthetists—a survey, *S Afr Med J* 96:630–632, 2006.
123. Bowdle A, Kruger C, Grieve R, et al: Anesthesia drug administration errors in a university hospital, *Anesthesiology* 99:A1358, 2003.
124. Bowdle TA: Drug administration errors from the ASA closed claims project, *ASA Newsl* 67:11–13, 2003.
125. Bell D: Recurrent wrong-route drug error—a professional shame, *Anaesthesia* 62:541–545, 2007.
126. Orser BA, Oxorn DC: An anaesthetic drug error: Minimizing the risk, *Can J Anaesth* 41:120–124, 1994.
127. Cranshaw J, Gupta KJ, Cook TM: Litigation related to drug errors in anaesthesia: An analysis of claims against the NHS in England 1995-2007, *Anaesthesia* 64:1317–1323, 2009.
128. Svenmarker S, Soren H, Jansson E, et al: Quality assurance in clinical perfusion, *Eur J Cardiothorac Surg* 14:409–414, 1998.
129. Jenkins OF, Morris R, Simpson JM: Australasian perfusion incident survey, *Perfusion* 12:279–288, 1997.
130. Mejak BL, Stammers A, Rauch E, et al: A retrospective study on perfusion incidents and safety devices, *Perfusion* 15:51–61, 2000.
131. Stammers A, Mejak BL: An update on perfusion safety: Does the type of perfusion practice affect the rate of incidents related to cardiopulmonary bypass, *Perfusion* 16:189–198, 2001.
132. Jensen LS, Merry AF, Webster CS, et al: Evidence-based strategies for preventing drug administration errors during anaesthesia, *Anaesthesia* 59:493–504, 2004.
133. ECRI: Bar-coded medication administration systems (BCMA) systems: Future promise, present challenges, *Health Devices* 32:373–381, 2003.
134. Bruhn J, Bouillon TW, Radulescu L, et al: Correlation of approximate entropy, bispectral index, and spectral edge frequency 95 (SEF95) with clinical signs of "anesthetic depth" during coadministration of propofol and remifentanil, *Anesthesiology* 98:621–627, 2003.
135. Mills PD, Neily J, Mims E, et al: Improving the bar-coded medication administration system at the Department of Veterans Affairs, *Am J Health Syst Pharm* 63:1442–1447, 2006.
136. Sakowski J, Newman JM, Dozier K: Severity of medication administration errors detected by a bar-code medication administration system, *Am J Health Syst Pharm* 65:1661–1666, 2008.
137. Merry AF, Webster CS, Mathew DJ: A new, safety-oriented, integrated drug administration and automated anesthesia record system, *Anesth Analg* 93:385–390, 2001.
138. Webster CS, Merry AF, Gander PH, et al: A prospective, randomized clinical evaluation of a new safety-oriented injectable drug administration system in comparison with conventional methods, *Anaesthesia* 59:80–87, 2004.
139. Nolen AL, Rodes WD 2nd: Bar-code medication administration system for anesthetics: Effects on documentation and billing, *Am J Health Syst Pharm* 65:655–659, 2008.
140. New perspectives on general-purpose infusion pumps. Advances in the technology, changes in our ratings, *Health Devices* 31:354–359, 2002.
141. Eskew JA, Jacobi J, Buss WF, et al: Using innovative technologies to set new saety standards for the infusion of intravenous medications, *Hosp Pharm* 1179–1189, 2002.
142. Eye on medical errors: Dose error reduction systems—A valuable tool for reducing iv medication errors, *Health Devices* 31:356–358, 2002.
143. Rothschild JM, Keohane CA, Cook EF, et al: A controlled trial of smart infusion pumps to improve medication safety in critically ill patients, *Crit Care Med* 33:533–540, 2005.
144. Nuckols TK, Bower AG, Paddock SM, et al: Programmable infusion pumps in ICUs: An analysis of corresponding adverse drug events, *J Gen Intern Med* 23(Suppl 1):41–45, 2008.
145. Vicente KJ, Kada-Bekhaled K, Hillel G, et al: Programming errors contribute to death from patient-controlled analgesia: Case report and estimate of probability, *Can J Anesth* 50:328–332, 2003.
146. Linden JV, Paul B, Dressler KP: A report of 104 transfusion errors in New York state, *Transfusion* 32:601–606, 1992.
147. Miyata S, Kawai T, Yamamoto S, et al: Network computer-assisted transfusion-management system for accurate blood component-recipient identification at the bedside, *Transfusion* 44:364–372, 2004.
148. Cajochen C, Khalsa SB, Wyatt JK, et al: EEG and ocular correlates of circadian melatonin phase and human performance decrements during sleep loss, *Am J Physiol* 277:R640–R649, 1999.
149. Dawson D, Reid K: Fatigue, alcohol and performance impairment, *Nature* 388:235, 1997.
150. Barger LK, Ayas NT, Cade BE, et al: Impact of extended-duration shifts on medical errors, adverse events, and attentional failures, *PLoS Med* 3:e487, 2006.
151. Duffy JF, Willson HJ, Wang W, et al: Healthy older adults better tolerate sleep deprivation than young adults, *J Am Geriatr Soc* 57:1245–1251, 2009.
152. Pack AI, Pack AM, Rodgman E, et al: Characteristics of crashes attributed to the driver having fallen asleep, *Accid Anal Prev* 27:769–775, 1995.
153. Folkard S: Shift work, safety, and aging, *Chronobiol Int* 25:183–198, 2008.
154. Viola AU, Archer SN, James LM, et al: PER3 polymorphism predicts sleep structure and waking performance, *Curr Biol* 17:613–618, 2007.
155. Groeger JA, Viola AU, Lo JC, et al: Early morning executive functioning during sleep deprivation is compromised by a PERIOD3 polymorphism, *Sleep* 31:1159–1167, 2008.
156. Czeisler CA: Medical and genetic differences in the adverse impact of sleep loss on performance: Ethical considerations for the medical profession, *Trans Am Clin Climatol Assoc* 120:249–285, 2009.
157. Van Dongen HP, Maislin G, Mullington JM, et al: The cumulative cost of additional wakefulness: Dose-response effects on neurobehavioral functions and sleep physiology from chronic sleep restriction and total sleep deprivation, *Sleep* 26:117–126, 2003.
158. Olson EJ, Drage LA, Auger RR: Sleep deprivation, physician performance, and patient safety, *Chest* 136:1389–1396, 2009.
159. Landrigan CP, Barger LK, Cade BE, et al: Interns' compliance with accreditation council for graduate medical education work-hour limits, *JAMA* 296:1063–1070, 2006.
160. Gravenstein JS, Cooper JB, Orkin FK: Work and rest cycles in anesthesia practice, *Anesthesiology* 72:737–742, 1990.
161. Morris GP, Morris RW: Anaesthesia and fatigue: An analysis of the first 10 years of the Australian Incident Monitoring Study 1987-1997, *Anaesth Intensive Care* 28:300–304, 2000.
162. Howard SK, Gaba DM, Smith BE, et al: Simulation study of rested versus sleep-deprived anesthesiologists, *Anesthesiology* 98:1345–1355, 2003 discussion 1345A.
163. Gander PH, Merry A, Millar MM, et al: Hours of work and fatigue-related error: A survey of New Zealand anaesthetists, *Anaesth Intensive Care* 28:178–183, 2000.
164. Flin R, Fletcher G, McGeorge P, et al: Anaesthetists' attitudes to teamwork and safety, *Anaesthesia* 58:233–242, 2003.
165. Gander P, Millar M, Webster C, et al: Sleep loss and performance of anaesthesia trainees and specialists, *Chronobiol Int* 25:1077–1091, 2008.
166. Kryger M, Monjan A, Bliwise D, et al: Sleep, health, and aging. Bridging the gap between science and clinical practice, *Geriatrics* 59:24–26, 29–30, 2004.
167. Reilly T, Waterhouse J, Atkinson G: Aging, rhythms of physical performance, and adjustment to changes in the sleep-activity cycle, *Occup Environ Med* 54:812–816, 1997.
168. Anonymous: Shift work, the anaesthetist and Santayana's warning, *Anaesthesia* 59:735–737, 2004.
169. Howard SK, Rosekind MR, Katz JD, et al: Fatigue in anesthesia: Implications and strategies for patient and provider safety, *Anesthesiology* 97:1281–1294, 2002.
170. *Fatigue and Anaesthetists*, London, 2004, Association of Anaesthetists of Great Britain and Ireland.
171. *Best Practice Rostering: Training and Resource Kit. Practical Tools for Rostering Doctors*, Kingston, 2003, Australian Capital Territory: Australian Medical Association.
172. Jha A, Duncan B, Bates D: *Fatigue, Sleepiness and Medical Errors. Making Health Care Safer: A Critical Analysis of Patient Safety Practices*, Evidence Report/Technology Assessment: Number 43 [AHRQ Publication No. 01-E058]. Rockville, MD, 2001, Agency for Healthcare Research and Quality.
173. Weinger MB, Herndon OW, Gaba DM: The effect of electronic record keeping and transesophageal echocardiography on task distribution, workload, and vigilance during cardiac anesthesia, *Anesthesiology* 87:144–155, 1997 discussion 129A–130A.
174. Aronson S, Cook R: Vigilance—a main component of clinical quality, *Anesthesiology* 88:1122–1124, 1998.
175. *Guidelines on the Handover of Responsibility during an Anaesthetic*, Melbourne, Australia, 2004, Australian and New Zealand College of Anaesthetists.
176. Batejat DM, Lagarde DP: Naps and modafinil as countermeasures for the effects of sleep deprivation on cognitive performance, *Aviat Space Environ Med* 70:493–498, 1999.
177. Buguet A, Montmayeur A, Pigeau R, et al: Modafinil, d-amphetamine and placebo during 64 hours of sustained mental work. II. Effects on two nights of recovery sleep, *J Sleep Res* 4:229–241, 1995.
178. Caldwell JA, Caldwell JL, Smith JK, et al: Modafinil's effects on simulator performance and mood in pilots during 37 h without sleep, *Aviat Space Environ Med* 75:777–784, 2004.
179. Caldwell JA Jr, Caldwell JL, Smythe NK 3rd, et al: A double-blind, placebo-controlled investigation of the efficacy of modafinil for sustaining the alertness and performance of aviators: A helicopter simulator study, *Psychopharmacology (Berl)* 150:272–282, 2000.

40

Cardiac Anesthesia
Training, Qualifications, Teaching, and Learning

ALAN JAY SCHWARTZ, MD, MSED

KEY POINTS

1. Education is change in behavior based on experience. The fact that 81.1 million Americans present with one or more types of cardiovascular disease (CVD), and that an estimated 7,235,000 inpatient cardiovascular operations and procedures were performed in the United States in 2006, speaks directly to the point that anesthesiologists treating patients with CVD have vast experience that requires and results in considerable education.

2. The complexity of many cardiothoracic diseases requires that there be a cadre of specialty educated cardiothoracic anesthesiologists. Specialty educated cardiothoracic anesthesiologists care for more complex patients, and they are the individuals who educate residents and fellows about these special, high-acuity patients.

3. Essential ingredients of clinical cardiothoracic anesthesiology education are completion of a 3-year core residency in anesthesiology followed by an additional 1-year adult cardiothoracic anesthesiology fellowship during which an exhaustive list of didactic topics for study is coupled with mastery of an inclusive set of psychomotor skills, including basic and advanced perioperative echocardiography.

4. Through concentrated full immersion in a minimum 1-year fellowship devoted exclusively to adult cardiothoracic anesthesiology, an anesthesiologist will be able to gain sufficient and sophisticated knowledge and skill to be a subspecialist able to care for patients with very-high-acuity CVD. In similar fashion, it will only be through accredited fellowship education that subspecialists in cardiac anesthesiology will be on par with the large number of fellowship-educated cardiologists, cardiothoracic surgeons, and all other medical, pediatric, surgical, and diagnostic subspecialists who care for patients with CVD.

5. Being a "qualified" cardiothoracic anesthesiologist implies having met standard criteria and complied with specified requirements defined by the Accreditation Council for Graduate Medical Education. These requirements include: (1) having successfully completed postgraduate medical education in an accredited training program, (2) having successfully completed a certification process (examination) when available, and (3) being credentialed and granted clinical privileges to practice within the scope of the subspecialty within a health care facility.

6. The American Board of Anesthesiology (ABA) oral examination process is designed "to assess the candidate's ability to demonstrate the attributes of an ABA Diplomate [understand and apply complex cognitive functions] when managing patients presented in clinical scenarios. The attributes are appropriate application of scientific principles to clinical problems, sound judgment in decision-making and management of surgical and anesthetic complications, adaptability to unexpected changes in the clinical situations, and logical organization and effective presentation of information. The oral examination emphasizes the scientific rationale underlying clinical management decisions."[21]

7. Simulation is imitation of real-life clinical situations using stand-in devices that assume the patient role, providing learner experience while permitting teaching and learning in repetitive fashion with zero risk to both the provider and recipient of the simulated care.

8. Simulation adds sophisticated aspects to education that are not possible from traditional textbook learning, classroom lectures, or single-learner computer-based programs. These missing ingredients are teamwork and improved processes of care, including, among others, interpersonal communication, situational awareness, appropriate management of available patient care resources, fatigue management, adverse event recognition, team decision making, and performance feedback.

9. Improved patient outcome from simulation education is intuitively obvious, yet scant evidence-based medicine exists to prove this.

10. Student evaluation will be meaningless without the ability to: (1) provide the resident/fellow

constructive feedback, on as frequent a basis as daily (formative evaluation); and (2) have the faculty attest to the resident's/fellow's competence at the completion of the educational process (summative evaluation).

11. Collection of data about an individual faculty member's "teaching abilities, commitment to the educational program, clinical knowledge, and scholarly activities" arms the chair with ammunition for constructive suggestions for change of teaching techniques by the faculty member and provides institutional appointment and promotion committees information on which to base faculty academic recognition.

12. Resident performance on certification examinations and review of patient care data are prime educational assessment techniques for educational program evaluation. A department and its institutional continuous quality improvement programs serve as effective analysis methods for documenting the success of the educational program and clinical care provided to patients by ongoing review of data showing that unacceptable morbidity and mortality are not present and that the educational program does not result in and may, in fact, improve these parameters.

Is cardiovascular disease (CVD) an issue that the anesthesiologist must be aware of, educated about, and qualified to deal with clinically? An obvious and resounding "yes" is the answer to this question. Anesthesiologists are confronted with the patient care dilemmas posed by the presence of CVD as a primary or comorbid diagnosis in an enormous number of patients spanning all age groups. Consider the following CVD statistics for the United States, as compiled and published in the American Heart Association's Heart Disease and Stroke Statistics—2010 Update.[1]

I. PREVALENCE
Some 81.1 million Americans have one or more types of CVD; 38.1 million are estimated to be age 60 and older; one in three has CVD.[1]
A. High blood pressure—74.5 million (defined as systolic pressure 140 mm Hg or greater and/or diastolic pressure 90 mm Hg or greater or taking antihypertensive medication)
B. Coronary heart disease—17.6 million
Myocardial infarction—8.5million
Angina pectoris—10.2 million
C. Congestive heart failure—5.8 million
D. Stroke—6.4 million
E. Congenital cardiovascular defects—1.3 million
II. INCIDENCE
A. The average annual rates of first major cardiovascular events increase from 3 per 1000 men at ages 35 to 44 to 74 per 1000 at ages 85 to 94.
B. The aging of the population will undoubtedly result in an increased incidence of chronic diseases, including coronary artery disease, heart failure, and stroke; the U.S. Census estimates that there will be 55 million Americans aged 65 and older in 2020.
C. There has been an explosive increase in the prevalence of obesity and type 2 diabetes. Their related complications, hypertension, hyperlipidemia, and atherosclerotic vascular disease also have increased.

III. MORTALITY
A. CVD accounted for 34.3% of all deaths, or 1 of every 2.9 deaths in the United States in 2006. CVD mortality rate was about 56% of "total mortality." This means that of more than 2,426,000 deaths from all causes, CVD was listed as a primary or contributing cause on about 1,347,000 death certificates.
B. Since 1900, CVD has been the number one killer in the United States every year except 1918. Nearly 2300 Americans die of CVD each day, an average of 1 death every 38 seconds. CVD claims more lives each year than cancer, chronic lower respiratory diseases, and accidents combined.
IV. HOSPITAL/PHYSICIAN/NURSING HOME VISITS
A. From 1996 to 2006, the number of Americans discharged from short-stay hospitals with CVD as the first listed diagnosis varied from 6,107,000 to 6,161,000. In 2006, CVD ranked highest among all disease categories in hospital discharges.
B. In 2007, there were 4,048,000 visits to emergency departments with a primary diagnosis of CVD.
V. COST
A. In 2010, the estimated direct and indirect cost of CVD is $503.2 billion.[1]
VI. OPERATIONS AND PROCEDURES
A. In 2006, an estimated 7,235,000 inpatient cardiovascular operations and procedures were performed in the United States; 4.1 million were performed on male patients and 3.1 million were performed on female patients.[1]
B. If the focus is on coronary artery disease alone, the statistics highlight the same striking message. In 2006, an estimated 1,313,000 percutaneous coronary intervention procedures, 448,000 inpatient bypass procedures, 1,115,000 inpatient diagnostic cardiac catheterizations, 114,000 inpatient implantable defibrillators, and 418,000 pacemaker procedures were performed in the United States.[1]
C. CVD is not only a geriatric phenomenon. Congenital heart disease (CHD) is a major issue for the pediatric anesthesiologist. In addition, an ever-increasing number of patients with CHD are living longer after surgical palliation or repair, forming an adult CHD population that presents for anesthetic care for surgical and nonsurgical therapeutic and diagnostic procedures.
D. Incidence of CHD is 9.0 defects per 1000 live births, or 36,000 babies per year in the United States.
E. In 2004, hospitalization costs for CHD were $2.6 billion.[1]

With statistics such as those listed, there is quite a compelling argument that being aware of, educated about, and qualified to deal with patients with CVD is essential for all anesthesiologists. *The complexity of cardiothoracic diseases requires that there be a cadre of specialty-educated cardiothoracic anesthesiologists who care for these high-acuity patients and educate residents and fellows about these special patients.* The Anesthesiology Residency Review Committee (RRC) is quite clear about this in its statements defining *faculty* in the program requirements for graduate medical education (GME) in the core residency in anesthesiology and fellowship in adult cardiothoracic anesthesiology[2,3]:

The physician faculty must possess the requisite specialty expertise and competence in clinical care and teaching abilities, as well as documented educational and administrative abilities and experience in their field. There must be evidence of active participation by qualified physicians with training and/or expertise in adult cardiothoracic anesthesiology beyond the requirement for completion of a core anesthesiology residency. The faculty must possess training and experience in the care of adult cardiothoracic patients that would generally meet or exceed that associated with the completion of a one-year adult cardiothoracic anesthesiology program, and must have a continuous and meaningful role in the program...

The faculty may include members from the core anesthesiology program who have subspecialty expertise, including critical care and pediatric anesthesiology...

The responsibility for establishing and maintaining an environment of inquiry and scholarship rests with the faculty, and an active research component must be included in each program...

Complementary to the above scholarship is the regular participation of the teaching staff in clinical discussions, rounds, journal clubs, and research conferences in a manner that promotes a spirit of inquiry and scholarship (e.g., the offering of guidance [mentoring] and technical support for fellows involved in research such as research design and statistical analysis); and the provision of support [mentoring] for fellows' participation, as appropriate, in scholarly activities that pertain specifically to the care of cardiothoracic patients.[2]

It is these same specialists who conduct the basic science and clinical research that advances new knowledge and understanding of CVD and its anesthetic implications. What is the education available and required for cardiothoracic anesthesiologists?

FORMALIZED EDUCATION OF CARDIOTHORACIC ANESTHESIOLOGISTS

The continuum of education in anesthesiology is defined by the Accreditation Council for Graduate Medical Education (ACGME)[2,3] and the American Board of Anesthesiology (ABA).[4] The continuum begins with an initial 4 years of postgraduate (post–medical school) education and constitutes the "core" anesthesiology residency.

Clinical Base Year

The first year is a clinical nonanesthesiology (clinical base) year.
   According to the ACGME:

*The **clinical base year** should provide the resident with 12 months of broad education in medical disciplines relevant to the practice of anesthesiology.[2]*

   According to the ABA:

*The **clinical base year** must include at least six months of clinical rotations during which the resident has responsibility for the diagnosis and treatment of patients with a variety of medical and surgical problems, of which at most one month may involve the administration of anesthesia and one month of pain medicine. Acceptable clinical base experiences include training in internal medicine, pediatrics, surgery or any of their subspecialties, obstetrics and gynecology, neurology, family medicine or any combination of these as approved for residents by the directors of their training programs in anesthesiology. The clinical base year should also include rotations in critical care and emergency medicine, with at least one month, but no more than two months, devoted to each. Other rotations completing the 12 months of broad education should be relevant to the practice of anesthesiology.[4]*

Clinical Anesthesia Years

The next 3 years are clinical anesthesiology years:

*The three-year **clinical anesthesia** curriculum (CA 1-3) consists of experience in basic anesthesia training, subspecialty anesthesia training and advanced anesthesia training. It is a graded curriculum of increasing difficulty and learning that is progressively more challenging of the resident's intellect and technical skills.*

*(1) Experience in **basic anesthesia training** is intended to emphasize basic and fundamental aspects of the management of anesthesia. It is recommended that at least 12 months of the CA-1 and CA-2 years be spent in basic anesthesia training with a majority of this time occurring during the CA-1 year.*

*(2) **Subspecialty anesthesia training** is required to emphasize the theoretical background, subject material and practice of subdisciplines of anesthesiology. These subdisciplines include obstetric anesthesia, pediatric anesthesia, cardiothoracic anesthesia, neuroanesthesia, anesthesia for outpatient surgery, recovery room care, perioperative evaluation, regional anesthesia and pain medicine. It is recommended that these experiences be subspecialty rotations and occur in the CA-1 and CA-2 years. The sequencing of these rotations in the CA-1 and CA-2 years is left to the discretion of the program director.[4]*

The ability to provide extensive specialized education in cardiac anesthesiology during the core residency is restricted primarily because of the time-limited nature of clinical anesthesia training, that is, a total of 36 months. The fundamental cardiac anesthesiology education commonly occurs during the CA-1 or CA-2 year.
   The goals, timing, and minimum required perioperative clinical experiences in cardiothoracic anesthesiology include and are not limited to:

20 patients undergoing cardiac surgery. The majority of these cardiac procedures must involve the use of cardiopulmonary bypass;

20 patients undergoing open or endovascular procedures on major vessels, including carotid surgery, intrathoracic vascular surgery, intraabdominal vascular surgery, or peripheral vascular surgery. Excluded from this category is surgery for vascular access or repair of vascular access;

20 patients undergoing non-cardiac intrathoracic surgery, including pulmonary surgery and surgery of the great vessels, esophagus, and the mediastinum and its structures;

Patients who require specialized techniques for their perioperative care. There must be significant experience with a broad spectrum of airway management techniques (e.g., performance of fiberoptic intubation and lung isolation techniques such as double lumen endotracheal tube placement and endobronchial blockers). Residents also should have significant experience with central vein and pulmonary artery catheter placement and the use of transesophageal echocardiography.[2]

   There is an opportunity for more extensive education about cardiac anesthesiology in the CA-3 year of the core residency:

Experience in advanced anesthesia training constitutes the CA-3 year. The program director, in collaboration with the resident, will design the resident's CA-3 year of training. The CA-3 year is a distinctly different experience from the CA 1-2 years, requiring progressively more complex training experiences and increased independence and responsibility for the resident. Resident assignments in the CA-3 year should include the more difficult or complex anesthetic procedures and care of the most seriously ill patients.[2]

   More extensive education about cardiac anesthesiology in the CA-3 year would be most appropriate for those practitioners electing to subspecialize; however, the CA-3, 6-month subspecialty education option is out of vogue. In 1988–1989, the ABA extended the core anesthesiology residency to a required CA-3 year. In 1989–1990, 56% (606/1084) of CA-3 residents elected more than 6 months of subspecialty training (all anesthesiology subspecialties are represented in this composite number).[5,6] By 1993–1994, only 29%, by 1995–1996, only 21%, and by 2000–2001, a mere 6% (66/1043) elected more than 6 months of subspecialty training in the CA-3 year.[5,6]
   At the same time that CA-3 subspecialty education was becoming rare, the absolute number and percentage of total CA-4 residents who electively enrolled in a 12-month postresidency fellowship program increased (1989–1990: 63/105 [60%]; 1998–1999: 523/605 [86%]; and 2000–2001: 383/525 [73%] CA-4 residents enrolled in a 12-month subspecialty fellowship).[5,6]

It is quite apparent from the residency curriculum outlined earlier that a graduating core resident will most likely be, at best, modestly educated as a specialist cardiac anesthesiologist. More complete subspecialty education is provided through a fellowship (minimum 1-year clinical GME program) that follows the core residency. Over the years, a significant number of individuals have elected CA-4 cardiac anesthesiology subspecialty fellowship education (in 2000–2001, 69 of 383 [18%] CA-4 residents selected cardiac anesthesiology as their fellowship track).[5] This blends well with the fact that many other medical, surgical, and diagnostic disciplines offer accredited fellowship education to develop so-called subspecialists in their respective specialties. Accredited subspecialty graduate education programs of a year or more in duration exist in anesthesiology and medical, pediatric, surgical, and diagnostic disciplines related to cardiac anesthesiology[7] (Table 40-1).

At the same time that the number of CA-3 residents electing cardiac anesthesiology subspecialty education was dwindling and becoming almost nonexistent, and the number of CA-4 residents electing a full 1-year cardiac anesthesiology fellowship was increasing dramatically, standardized cardiothoracic anesthesiology fellowship education did not exist. Standardized and accredited anesthesiology fellowship subspecialty education in critical care, pain management, and pediatric anesthesiology exists. An Anesthesiology RRC–developed standardized curriculum in cardiac anesthesiology had been resisted for many years. Reluctance to accredit specialty education in cardiac anesthesiology related to a desire to avoid creating divisions in clinical practice among anesthesiologists. It had been reasoned that all anesthesiologists care for patients with CVD; therefore, all anesthesiologists need and gain, through core residency education, the requisite knowledge and skills. The data cited earlier negate this supposition.

The Society of Cardiovascular Anesthesiologists (SCA) championed a different viewpoint.[8] The SCA reasoned that, although it is true that all anesthesiologists care for patients with cardiac disease, there has developed, since the 1980s, a highly sophisticated knowledge base (e.g., physiology of deep hypothermic circulatory arrest, clinical management of anticoagulation, anesthetic management of patients undergoing electrophysiologic diagnostic and therapeutic procedures, and physiologic management of mechanical assist devices bridging to heart and lung transplantation) and a technically demanding set of psychomotor skills (e.g., pulmonary artery catheterization, intra-aortic balloon counterpulsation, and transesophageal echocardiography [TEE]) that enable the safe and effective care of patients with very-high-acuity CVD.

Cardiothoracic anesthesiology has blossomed into a subdiscipline that exists adjunctively to the core discipline of anesthesiology. More than 6000 anesthesiologists (approximately 14% of the total American Society of Anesthesiologists [ASA] membership) are SCA members identifying themselves as individuals who recognize that cardiac anesthesiology constitutes more than the basic discipline of anesthesiology. Scientific and educational meetings to disseminate this subspecialty knowledge and develop practice protocols, research programs, and projects devoted specifically to cardiac anesthesiology exist to serve the needs of these subspecialists.[8]

The SCA believes that only through concentrated full immersion in a minimum 1-year clinical fellowship devoted exclusively to cardiothoracic anesthesiology will an anesthesiologist be able to gain sufficient and sophisticated enough knowledge and skill to be a subspecialist able to care for patients with very-high-acuity CVD. In similar fashion, it will only be through accredited fellowship education that subspecialists in cardiac anesthesiology will be on par with the large number of fellowship-educated cardiologists, cardiothoracic surgeons, and all other medical, pediatric, surgical, and diagnostic subspecialists who care for patients with CVD (see Table 40-1).

In 2006, the ACGME, through the sponsorship of the Anesthesiology RRC, established program requirements for standardized adult cardiothoracic anesthesiology fellowship education as had been recommended by the SCA[3] (see Appendix 40-1). *The recommended essential ingredients of clinical cardiothoracic anesthesiology fellowship education are a minimum one-year time frame during which an exhaustive list of didactic topics for study is coupled with mastery of a much more inclusive set of psychomotor skills (including Basic and Advanced Perioperative Echocardiograph (see Chapter 41) than that which is required for core resident education.*[3]

QUALIFICATIONS OF CARDIOTHORACIC ANESTHESIOLOGISTS

Being a "qualified" cardiothoracic anesthesiologist implies having met standard criteria and complied with specified requirements. The standard criteria and specified requirements are "defined and regulated" by agencies vested with the authority to delineate and maintain the "qualified" status. *Qualified,* therefore, implies a minimum achievement that is accomplished and available for public review. Having met the qualifications ensures the public trust because it defines for the public a "common yardstick" by which educational programs, physicians, and medical practices can be measured. For cardiothoracic anesthesiology, qualifications refer to (1) GME programs *(accreditation),* (2) physicians who have completed and subsequently demonstrated mastery of the proscribed GME *(certification),* and (3) physician practice settings where anesthesia patient care takes place *(credentialing and clinical privileging).*

Accreditation

The "ACGME is responsible for the accreditation of post-MD medical training programs within the United States. Accreditation is accomplished through a peer review process and is based upon established standards and guidelines."[9]

The mission of the ACGME is to improve the quality of health in the United States by ensuring and improving the quality of graduate medical education experience for the physicians in training. The

Specialty/Subspecialty	No. of Programs	No. of Fellows
Internal Medicine		
Cardiovascular disease	180	2434
Clinical cardiac electrophysiology	96	155
Critical care medicine	32	136
Pulmonary disease	22	81
Pulmonary disease and critical care medicine	133	1266
Pediatrics		
Pediatric cardiology	48	336
Pediatric critical care medicine	61	357
Pediatric pulmonary	47	125
Radiology-diagnostic		
Cardiothoracic radiology	2	2
Vascular and interventional radiology	93	148
Surgery		
Surgical critical care	94	153
Thoracic surgery	76	230
Congenital cardiac surgery	6	2
Subtotal	**890**	**5425**
Anesthesiology		
Adult cardiothoracic anesthesiology	**44**	**86**
Critical care medicine	47	81
Pediatric anesthesiology	45	129
Total	**8694**	**11,146**

TABLE 40-1 Number of Resident Physicians (Fellows) on Duty December 1, 2008 in Selected Accreditation Council for Graduate Medical Education–Accredited Subspecialty and Combined Specialty Graduate Medical Education Programs Related to Cardiothoracic Anesthesiology (Anesthesiology Subspecialty Programs for Comparison)[7]

ACGME establishes national standards for graduate medical education by which it approves and continually assesses educational programs under its aegis. It uses the most effective methods available to evaluate the quality of graduate medical education programs. It strives to develop evaluation methods and processes that are valid, fair, open and ethical.[10]

GME programs voluntarily apply for accredited status and agree to meet the defined program requirements and undergo periodic scrutiny to document compliance. Accredited status brings with it public recognition and the benefits of being subject to specialty-specific and general institutional ACGME standards. As an example of such a benefit, common program requirements that provide a "level playing field" for all GME programs have been published by the ACGME.[11]

In 2006, the ACGME, through the sponsorship of the Anesthesiology RRC, established program requirements for standardized adult cardiothoracic anesthesiology fellowship education as had been recommended by the SCA (see Appendix 40-1).[3]

Certification

A physician who successfully completes an accredited fellowship program may voluntarily apply to become identified as a board-certified specialist. Board certification is under the auspices of the American Board of Medical Specialties:

The American Board of Medical Specialties (ABMS) is an organization of 24 approved medical specialty boards. The intent of the certification of physicians is to provide assurance to the public that those certified by an ABMS Member Board have successfully completed an approved training program and an evaluation process assessing their ability to provide quality patient care in the specialty.[12]

An increasing amount of scientific evidence exists that attests to the fact that board certification status relates directly to better patient outcome. Silber et al's[13–15] studies, in particular, suggest that quality of patient care improves when anesthesiologists are board certified. Brennan et al[16] provide considerable evidence making the case for viewing certification status as an evidence-based quality measure.

The ABMS serves to coordinate the activities of its Member Boards and to provide information to others concerning issues involving specialization and certification of medical specialists.[12] The ABA is one of the ABMS Member Boards.

A Board certified anesthesiologist is a physician who provides medical management and consultation during the perioperative period, in pain medicine and in critical care medicine. At the time of application and at the time of initial certification, a Diplomate of the Board must possess knowledge, judgment, adaptability, clinical skills, technical facility and personal characteristics sufficient to carry out the entire scope of anesthesiology practice without accommodation or with reasonable accommodation. An ABA Diplomate must logically organize and effectively present rational diagnoses and appropriate treatment protocols to peers, patients, their families and others involved in the medical community. A Diplomate of the Board can serve as an expert in matters related to anesthesiology, deliberate with others, and provide advice and defend opinions in all aspects of the specialty of anesthesiology. A Board certified anesthesiologist is able to function as the leader of the anesthesiology care team.

Because of the nature of anesthesiology, the ABA Diplomate must be able to manage emergent life threatening situations in an independent and timely fashion. The ability to independently acquire and process information in a timely manner is central to assure individual responsibility for all aspects of anesthesiology care. Adequate physical and sensory faculties, such as eyesight, hearing, speech and coordinated function of the extremities, are essential to the independent performance of the Board certified Anesthesiologist. Freedom from the influence of or dependency on chemical substances that impair cognitive, physical, sensory or motor function also is an essential characteristic of the Board certified anesthesiologist.[4]

Board certification in cardiac anesthesiology does not currently exist in the United States.

Credentialing and Clinical Privileges

Anesthesiologists may practice as cardiac subspecialists even though board certification does not exist in the United States. Hospital medical staffs have the privilege and obligation to define what physicians can and cannot do with respect to patient care in their institution. This process is medical credentialing.

To be awarded medical staff privileges in anesthesiology, a physician must fully meet certain required criteria. It is possible to make all the following criteria mandatory or to have a mixture of required and optional criteria. Organizations [Hospital Medical Staffs] should determine which criteria to include and whether to include additional criteria based on the institution's individual requirements and preferences. For example, some facilities may decide that certification by the [ABA] is a requirement for clinical privileges in anesthesiology, while others may deem board certification to be desirable but not essential. Similarly, some institutions may decide that subspecialty fellowship training is needed for certain clinical privileges, while others may not. Some organizations may wish to recognize residency training obtained or certification awarded outside the United States. Institutions granting subspecialty clinical privileges may wish to recognize experience as an alternative to formal training in a subspecialty of anesthesiology. Some institutions may wish to modify certain requirements for physicians who have recently completed their residency or fellowship training.[17]

The ASA has published guidelines for delineating clinical privileges in anesthesiology taking into consideration educational, licensure, performance improvement, personal qualifications, and practice pattern criteria.[17] Many physicians are recognized as credentialed cardiac anesthesiologists and are granted specific clinical privileges defined by their practice group and hospital medical staff while at the same time they are not certified by the ABA. These cardiac anesthesiologists are "experts" in their subspecialty and clearly qualified to care for patients with CVD.

TEACHING AND LEARNING CARDIAC ANESTHESIOLOGY

Teachers and the Teaching/Learning Environment

Teaching and learning cardiac anesthesiology best takes place in an environment conducive to the educational process with a set of goals and objectives to guide the endeavor. This has been defined by the Anesthesiology RRC in their program requirements for GME in adult cardiothoracic anesthesiology (see Appendix 40-1).[3]

The fellowship program must require its fellows to obtain competence in the six areas listed below to the level expected of a new practitioner. Programs must define the specific knowledge, skills, behaviors, and attitudes required, and provide educational experiences as needed in order for their fellows to demonstrate the following:

Patient care that is compassionate, appropriate, and effective for the treatment of health problems and the promotion of health;

Medical Knowledge about established and evolving biomedical, clinical, and cognate sciences, as well as the application of this knowledge to patient care;

Practice-based learning and improvement that involves the investigation and evaluation of care for their patients, the appraisal and assimilation of scientific evidence, and improvements in patient care;

Interpersonal and communication skills that result in the effective exchange of information and collaboration with patients, their families, and other health professionals;

Professionalism, as manifested through a commitment to carrying out professional responsibilities, adherence to ethical principles, and sensitivity to patients of diverse backgrounds;

Systems-based practice, as manifested by actions that demonstrate an awareness of and responsiveness to the larger context and system of health care, as well as the ability to call effectively on other resources in the system to provide optimal health care.[3]

A key factor for successful education is the commitment of effective teachers. A description of the effective clinical teacher has been put forth that, although written about the internal medicine teaching setting, is applicable to all disciplines and certainly cardiothoracic anesthesiology.[18] Effective teachers demonstrate, among other traits, the characteristics outlined in Box 40-1.[18] Effective teachers are also role-models and teach professionalism.[19]

Curriculum

There are three fundamental categories of curricular material for all educational topics that certainly apply to the curriculum for cardiothoracic anesthesiology: cognitive, psychomotor, and affective.

The *cognitive* or knowledge base of cardiothoracic anesthesiology is readily recognized as the basic medical sciences applied clinically. Cardiac embryology, histology, and gross anatomy; cardiorespiratory physiology; and adrenergic, anticoagulation, and antiarrhythmic pharmacology and pathophysiology of cardiac valve disorders are examples of some of the required cognitive base of cardiothoracic anesthesiology. An expansive topical content of cardiothoracic anesthesiology is listed in the ACGME Program Requirements for Graduate Medical Education in Adult Cardiothoracic Anesthesiology (see Appendix 40-1).[3]

The didactic curriculum provided through lectures, conferences, and workshops should supplement clinical experience as necessary for the fellow to acquire the knowledge to care for adult cardiothoracic patients and meet the conditions outlined in the guidelines for the minimum clinical experience for each fellow.[3]

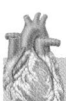

BOX 40-1. CHARACTERISTICS OF AN EFFECTIVE CLINICAL TEACHER[18]

- Allocates dedicated time for teaching
- Creates a trusting learning environment
- Demonstrates clinical credibility
- Provides an initial orientation and final evaluation for the teaching event
- Engages learners by expecting them to present cases, the pertinent details and educational benefit of which are managed by the teacher
- Enhances clinical case material with complementary didactic sessions
- Role-models physician/patient relationships through bedside teaching
- Encourages student consideration of and interactive discussions about the psychosocial aspects of medical care
- Transfers the teaching responsibility to the students who are the future medical educators

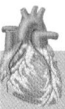

BOX 40-2. BLOOM'S TAXONOMY OF COGNITIVE LEARNING OUTLINING A HIERARCHY FROM SIMPLE (KNOWLEDGE) TO COMPLEX (EVALUATION) PROCESSES[20]

- Knowledge—recall
- Comprehension—understanding
- Application—use of abstractions
- Analysis—break down; seeing the relationship of parts
- Synthesis—put together; creating a new entity
- Evaluation—judgment of value

Complete cognitive learning is a process whereby the facts are considered in a variety of ways that take them beyond simple uninterpreted and unapplied statements. Teaching in the content area requires attention to increasingly complex cognitive functions described by Bloom[20] (Box 40-2).

Bloom's taxonomy fits well with the ABA oral examination process that is designed "to assess the candidate's ability to demonstrate the attributes of an ABA Diplomate [understand and apply complex cognitive functions] when managing patients presented in clinical scenarios. The attributes are (a) appropriate application of scientific principles to clinical problems, (b) sound judgment in decision-making and management of surgical and anesthetic complications, (c) adaptability to unexpected changes in the clinical situations, and (d) logical organization and effective presentation of information. The oral examination emphasizes the scientific rationale underlying clinical management decisions"[21] (Box 40-3).

When confronted with a patient with an ascending aortic arch dissection, for example, the clear expectation for teaching and learning is more than to just know the anatomy; it is to understand the interrelations of the aortic and coronary anatomy, the effect of the aortic dissection on coronary artery blood flow, ventricular function, and total body perfusion, and to be able to develop an anesthetic management plan that considers all of these codependent factors, and selects anesthetic and cardiovascular medications and physiologic monitoring appropriate to the care of the specific patient in question.

Although much of medical knowledge is broadly applicable to a wide variety of specialties, *psychomotor* learning is often quite specific to the specialty in question. Psychomotor skills that must be learned by the cardiac anesthesiologist, for example, do not apply at all to the dermatologist. Bedside cardiac catheterization with the balloon flotation pulmonary artery catheter, administration of carefully titrated vasoactive infusions, manipulation of cardiac output using the intra-aortic balloon pump, and TEE are examples of the required psychomotor skills of cardiothoracic anesthesiology. TEE is a prime example of a psychomotor skill set that, once learned, distinguishes the cardiac anesthesiologist from all other anesthesiologists unskilled in this technique. (See Chapter 41 for educational principles related to mastery of perioperative TEE.)

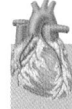

BOX 40-3. ATTRIBUTES OF AN AMERICAN BOARD OF ANESTHESIOLOGY DIPLOMATE TO BE EVALUATED DURING THE ORAL EXAMINATION AND NOT BY THE WRITTEN EXAMINATION[21]

- Appropriate application of scientific principles to clinical problems
- Sound judgment in decision making and management of surgical and anesthetic complications
- Adaptability to unexpected changes in the clinical situations
- Logical organization and effective presentation of information

The psychomotor skill lesson is vital to effective learning in cardiothoracic anesthesiology. Cardiac anesthesiology psychomotor techniques such as internal jugular catheterization and fiberoptic bronchoscopy are most effectively and efficiently taught with less potential harm to patients when using a systematically applied skill lesson plan.

Developing a psychomotor skill lesson is an example of how understanding instructional methodology can lead to effective teaching and learning. The old adage about teaching psychomotor skills in medicine is "see one, do one, teach one." The absurd nature of this approach has been highlighted in the following way: "This is akin to a piano instructor playing 'The Minute Waltz' for a beginner and then saying, 'Now, try it yourself.'"[22,23]

Rather than the repetitive trial-and-error approach to teaching/learning psychomotor skills, a systemic methodology can be used[23] (Box 40-4).

Affective teaching and learning is perhaps the least understood and most underappreciated of the categories of curricular material. Affective teaching/learning deals with feelings or emotions. The taxonomy of affective learning addresses the following[22,24]: Receiving, Responding, Valuing, Organizing, Value Complexing. Although anesthesiologists actively and consciously teach in the cognitive and psychomotor areas, they are much less aware of their affective teaching. Even though clinicians may not be aware of it, they are constantly teaching in the affective arena by the role modeling performed…an example of how affective teaching and learning takes place [is] described.[22]

Picture the educational setting in which an anesthesiology resident [cardiothoracic anesthesiology fellow] is learning how to use epinephrine when weaning a patient from cardiopulmonary bypass. The knowledge and skills that must be learned include application of the pharmacologic principles of catecholamines to the pathophysiology of cardiovascular disease by turning on a mechanical infusion pump to deliver the indicated dose of a medication while technically monitoring for dose response and toxicity. Learning these facts and the skills sufficient to employ them is much different when done from a textbook or a preoperative conference with a staff preceptor than when done during the operating room interaction between the surgeon and anesthesiologist, where varied opinions may consider dopamine a more sound physiologic choice or intermittent boluses a better administration technique. The interposition of the concerned surgeon and real-time patient setting between the student and the knowledge and skills to be learned changes the learning environment and, hence, the educational experience for the resident [fellow]. More is learned than the facts and psychomotor skills. As the attitudes of both the anesthesiologist and the surgeon are displayed during the resolution of the questions about the "best" drug to use and the "right" way to give it, the resident [subspecialty fellow] learns how these two types of practitioners are supposed to relate to one another.

In the real-life setting, the aggressive, passive-aggressive, or passive posture of the anesthesiology teacher interacting with the surgeon

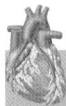

BOX 40-4. SYSTEMATIC METHODOLOGY FOR PSYCHOMOTOR SKILL LESSONS[22,23]

1. Analyze and separate the skills into component parts and determine which aspects of the skill are most difficult to perform.
2. Provide students with a model of the skill they are expected to perform, demonstrated effectively in its entirety.
3. Make provisions for students to practice until the expected behavior is mastered.
4. Provide adequate supervision and an evaluation of the final performance.

provides a lasting lesson in the affective domain for the resident [fellow] anesthesiology learner.[22] Simulation may be the educational solution to issues described in the psychomotor and affective learning scenarios (see later).

TEACHING PROCESS AND CONTENT RESOURCES

The actual teaching process may take the form of one of many time-tested methods available, including formal classroom didactic lectures, interactive teaching conferences, problem-based learning discussions, journal club review of the pertinent and current literature, bedside (e.g., operating room, intensive care unit, and preanesthesia evaluation clinic) patient interactive care/teaching, "surfing the Web," and simulation exercises.

Print materials (textbooks and journals) offering information about cardiothoracic anesthesiology and its related subjects are so numerous and constantly being updated and added to that it is impossible to have a current, complete, and comprehensive library. The Internet solves the problem of constantly being out-of-date with one's print library. The Internet has opened up the teaching environment to an enormous wealth of didactic and interactive teaching materials. Search engines, databases, and Internet links make an encyclopedic amount of up-to-date information available to the learner in cardiothoracic anesthesiology. Utilization of these web resources gives the cardiothoracic anesthesiology fellow access to learning materials and teaching methods that she or he might never have known existed. In addition, using Web-based resources reduces the need for the cardiothoracic anesthesiology fellow to "reinvent the wheel," as she or he can take advantage of what others have already discovered and "published" on the Internet. Appendix 40-2 offers a catalogue of cardiothoracic anesthesiology Web-based resources. Although it would be nice to state that this catalogue is all-inclusive, by its very nature, the Internet is never exhausted and more cardiothoracic anesthesiology Web-based resources exist and will be listed in the future. The cardiothoracic anesthesiology student and practitioner are encouraged to use the Web-based resource listing as a springboard to continually explore this vast educational reservoir as a lifelong learning exercise.

▣ Simulation

Atul Gawande has made a critically important medical education dichotomy and dilemma transparent to the public in his book *Complications: A Surgeon's Notes on an Imperfect Science* in the chapter entitled "Education of a Knife." Gawande[25] writes that there is an "imperative to give patients the best possible care and [at the same time] to provide novices with experience [education is change in behavior based on experience(s)]." To accomplish these two conflicting imperatives in the past, learning clinical care (e.g., cardiac anesthesia) was most often a process of application of knowledge and trial of techniques, both new to the student, on high-acuity/low-physiologic reserve patients in real-time patient care settings. This scenario was characterized by high anxiety for the student and significant risk for complications to the patient cared for by the novice. For the present and future, Gawande[25] makes it clear that the traditional medical education paradigm is no longer acceptable: "By traditional ethics and public insistence (not to mention court rulings), a patient's right to the best care possible must trump the objective of training novices."

The aviation industry long ago recognized this dilemma when teaching pilots. Acknowledging the high-stakes nature of flying, simulation technology was instituted to teach and evaluate a pilot's competence rather than allow her or him to fly a jumbo jet and risk loss of hundreds of lives. Learning to apply the knowledge and perform the techniques before entering the "cockpit" reduces the risk for a "crash disaster." Medical care in general and anesthesia patient care in particular, especially of very-high-risk patients with CVD, is analogous to the jumbo jet situation and logically calls for a similar approach to education, that is, use of simulation.[26] The public is no longer willing to accept teaching on patients. In the cardiothoracic patient care arena, for example, education has moved to virtual reality training for cardiac operating room and catheterization procedures.[27]

Imitation of a real-life clinical situation, using stand-in devices that assume the patient role, provides learner experience while permitting teaching and learning in repetitive fashion with zero risk to both the provider and recipient of the simulated care.[28] An exponential growth of simulation devices has occurred in medicine over the past several decades, many of which are directly applicable to education of cardiothoracic anesthesiologists. Flat-screen computer and mannequin-based simulators have been developed to mimic many patient care settings. Examples of relatively high-fidelity high-technology simulators especially pertinent to learning cardiothoracic anesthesiology include "Harvey," the cardiology patient simulator,[29–31] multimedia computer-assisted cardiology simulation,[32] anesthesia simulators,[33–35] and bronchoscopy simulators.[36] Evidence has been accumulated that simulation results in a better educational outcome for the learner. Schwid and colleagues[37] randomized anesthesiology residents and faculty into two learning groups (textbook reading vs. computerized ACLS [Advanced Cardiac Life Support] simulation education) preparing for performance evaluation at an ACLS mock resuscitation. Computer simulation–prepared learners were judged to perform better than textbook-prepared learners during standardized mega codes that required treatment protocols for clinical simulation of cardiovascular life-threatening scenarios with supraventricular tachycardia, ventricular fibrillation, and second-degree type II atrioventricular block.[37] Pulmonary artery catheterization and cardiovascular physiologic management can be effectively presented through a computer-based critical care training simulation.[38]

Simulation adds other, more sophisticated aspects to education that are not possible from traditional textbook learning, classroom lectures, or single-learner computer-based programs. These missing ingredients are teamwork and improved processes of care. Multidiscipline teams working effectively together must develop if the best medical care is to be provided to patients. Aviation's *crew resource management* (CRM) concepts can be effectively taught through group simulation exercises.[39] The potential for CRM teaching to positively impact care of patients with CVD is enormous when the team of cardiac anesthesiologists is educated with others who care for the same patients, including cardiac surgeons, cardiologists, cardiac operating room nurses, perfusionists, and respiratory therapists. Holzman and colleagues[40] and Grogan and colleagues[39] have demonstrated that CRM (also called *anesthesia crisis resource management* [ACRM]) enhances (1) interpersonal communication, situational awareness, and appropriate management of available patient care resources[40]; and (2) fatigue management, adverse event recognition, team decision making, and performance feedback.[39] CRM is so timely a topic that an entire supplement issue of *Quality & Safety in Health Care* entitled "Simulation and Team Training" described the state of the art.[41]

Although improved patient outcome from simulation education is intuitively obvious, scant evidence-based medicine exists to prove this. Sedlack and colleagues,[42] for example, have demonstrated that patients reported more comfort, a direct benefit to the patient, during gastrointestinal endoscopy provided by computer-based, simulation-trained endoscopists than when the same procedure was performed by patient-based trained endoscopists. Combing the literature for similar studies that document "direct patient benefit" and "improved patient outcome" related to simulation education of anesthesiologists results in virtually nothing of scientific significance. However, studies do document the educational benefit of simulation technology.[43] The clear challenge is to devise methods to scientifically prove that simulation education does benefit patients.

EVALUATION

Completion of the educational loop requires more than what has been described so far. In addition to providing a rationale for learning cardiothoracic anesthesiology, considering who the students and teachers are, describing the teaching/learning environment, defining the concepts of curricular development, and cataloging teaching methodology, evaluation processes must be instituted to complete the educational circle of planning and implementing the teaching process. Evaluation of all aspects of the educational endeavor, including students, teachers, program, and patient outcome, is essential.

Resident/Fellow Evaluation

The Anesthesiology RRC and the ABA outline the process for evaluation of the resident and fellow.[2–4]

The ACGME states[2,3]:

Formative Evaluation [see Appendix 40-1 for complete requirements of formative evaluation]

The faculty must evaluate in a timely manner the fellows whom they supervise. In addition, the fellowship program must demonstrate that it has an effective mechanism for assessing fellow performance throughout the program, and for utilizing the results to improve fellow performance. Faculty responsible for teaching must provide critical evaluations of each fellow's progress and competence to the cardiothoracic anesthesiology Program Director at the end of 6 and 12 months of training.

Final Evaluation

The Program Director must provide a final evaluation for each fellow who completes the program. This evaluation must include a review of the fellow's performance during the final period of education and should verify that the fellow has demonstrated sufficient professional ability to practice competently and independently. The final evaluation must be part of the fellow's permanent record maintained by the institution. Fellows in adult cardiothoracic anesthesiology must obtain overall satisfactory evaluations at the completion of 12 months training to receive credit for training.

The ABA states[4]:

Certification Requirements

At the time of certification by the ABA, the candidate must:

A. Hold an unexpired license to practice medicine or osteopathy in at least one state or jurisdiction of the United States or province of Canada that is permanent, unconditional and unrestricted. Further, every United States and Canadian medical license the applicant holds must be free of restrictions. Candidates for initial certification and ABA diplomates have the affirmative obligation to advise the ABA of any and all restrictions placed on any of their medical licenses and to provide the ABA with complete information concerning such restrictions within 60 days after their imposition or notice, whichever first occurs. Such information shall include, but not be limited to, the identity of the State Medical Board imposing the restriction as well as the restriction's duration, basis, and specific terms and conditions. Candidates and diplomates discovered not to have made disclosure may be subject to sanctions on their candidate or Diplomate status.

B. Have fulfilled all the requirements of the continuum of education in anesthesiology.

C. Have on file with the ABA a Certificate of Clinical Competence with an overall satisfactory rating covering the final six-month period of clinical anesthesia training in each anesthesiology residency program.

D. Have satisfied all examination requirements of the Board.

E. Have a professional standing…satisfactory to the ABA.

F. Be capable of performing independently the entire scope of anesthesiology practice… without accommodation or with reasonable accommodation.

Key components of student evaluation cited earlier include "…regular and timely performance feedback" and "…satisfactory Certificate of Clinical Competence…" Without the ability to (1) provide the resident/fellow constructive feedback, on as frequent a basis as daily, and (2) have the faculty attest to the resident's/fellow's competence at the completion of the educational process, student evaluation will be meaningless.

■ Faculty Evaluation

The ACGME guides department chairs about evaluation of the faculty[2,3]:

The performance of the faculty must be evaluated by the program no less frequently than at the midpoint of the accreditation cycle, and again prior to the next site visit. The evaluations should include a review of their teaching abilities, commitment to the educational program, clinical knowledge, and scholarly activities. This evaluation must include annual written confidential evaluations by fellows.

Collection of these data about an individual faculty member's educational skill, teaching commitment, clinical knowledge, and scholarship arms the chair with ammunition for constructive suggestions for change of teaching techniques by the faculty member and provides institutional appointment and promotion committees information on which to base faculty academic recognition.

■ Program Evaluation

The educational effectiveness of a program must be evaluated at least semiannually in a systematic manner[2,3]:

Representative program personnel (i.e., at least the Program Director, representative faculty, and one fellow) must be organized to review program goals and objectives, and the effectiveness with which they are achieved. This group must conduct a formal documented meeting at least annually for this purpose. In the evaluation process, the group must take into consideration written comments from the faculty, the most recent report of the GMEC of the sponsoring institution, and the fellows' confidential written evaluations. If deficiencies are found, the group should prepare an explicit plan of action, which should be approved by the faculty and documented in the minutes of the meeting.

The program should use fellow performance and outcome assessment in its evaluation of the educational effectiveness of the fellowship program. Performance of program graduates on the certification examination should be used as one measure of evaluating program effectiveness. The program should maintain a process for using assessment results together with other program evaluation results to improve the fellowship program.

Review of patient care data is another prime educational assessment technique for program evaluation. A department and its institutional CQI (continuous quality improvement) programs serve as an effective analysis method for documenting the success of the educational program and clinical care provided to patients by ongoing review of data showing that unacceptable morbidity and mortality are not present, and that the educational program does not result in and, in fact, may improve these parameters. The CQI program

serves as a basis for continuing medication education (CME) of the residents, fellows, and faculty.

LIFELONG LEARNING, CONTINUING MEDICAL EDUCATION, AND MAINTENANCE OF CERTIFICATION

The American Medical Association definition of CME is as follows:

CME consists of educational activities which serve to maintain, develop, or increase the knowledge, skills, and professional performance and relationships that a physician uses to provide services for patients, the public or the profession. The content of CME is the body of knowledge and skills generally recognized and accepted by the profession as within the basic medical sciences, the discipline of clinical medicine, and the provision of health care to the public [AMA House of Delegates policy #300.988].[44]

Continued physician licensure, hospital/medical staff appointment, and maintenance of board certification status require documentation of lifelong learning and participation in accredited CME activities. Since January 1, 2000, the ABA issues 10-year time-limited certificates. Anesthesiologists wishing to renew their board certification status will have to complete the 10-year Maintenance of Certification Process in Anesthesiology (MOCA).[45] The MOCA process serves as the formal mechanism for recertification of board certification status and its principles serve as a lifelong learning process for cardiothoracic anesthesiologists.

SUMMARY

The following practical advice on learning cardiothoracic anesthesia includes pearls to consider.[46]

> ***Education is a change in behavior based upon experiences.*** The first and foremost perspective that the student of cardiothoracic anesthesiology must have is to engage in experiences related to this subspecialty.
>
> *Pearl 1:* To gain experiences, immerse yourself in every conceivable clinical and didactic activity related to cardiothoracic anesthesiology.
>
> Enhance every experience by raising its cognitive level. Full understanding of cardiothoracic anesthesiology can only come from questioning each scenario.[46]
>
> *Pearl 2:* Seek the answer to the most important question related to learning—why?
>
> In order to ensure that the resident [fellow] has had sufficient experiences from which to learn and has asked "why" to fully understand, **insist that the resident [fellow] become a teacher**.[46]
>
> *Pearl 3:* Learn how to teach cardiothoracic anesthesiology to others, and you will ensure that you have learned it![46]
>
> *Pearl 4:* Continue to learn the ever-changing landscape of cardiothoracic anesthesiology. Enroll in and maintain an interest and activity in lifelong learning CME.
>
> Be a lifelong participant in cardiothoracic anesthesiology CME and a MOCA-like program even in the absence of accredited cardiothoracic residency/fellowship educational programs and board certification of the subspecialty of cardiothoracic anesthesiology.
>
> CME consists of educational activities that serve to maintain, develop, or increase the knowledge, skills, and professional performance and relationships a physician uses to provide services for patients, the public, or the profession. CME represents that body of knowledge and skills generally recognized and accepted by the profession as within the basic medical sciences, the discipline of clinical medicine, and the provision of health care to the public.[44]

▣ APPENDIX 40-1

Accreditation Council for Graduate Medical Education Program Requirements for Graduate Medical Education in Adult Cardiothoracic Anesthesiology[3]

Effective: February 14, 2006

In addition to complying with the Program Requirements for Fellowship Education in the Subspecialties of Anesthesiology, programs must comply with the following requirements, which in some cases exceed the Common Requirements.

I. Introduction

I.A. Definition and Scope of the Fellowship

Adult cardiothoracic anesthesiology is the anesthesiology fellowship devoted to the preoperative, intraoperative, and postoperative care of adult patients undergoing cardiothoracic surgery and related invasive procedures.

I.B. Duration and Scope of Education

Fellowship education in adult cardiothoracic anesthesiology shall comprise a minimum of 12 months duration, beginning after satisfactory completion of a residency program in anesthesiology. Because cardiothoracic anesthesiology education requires an intensive continuum of training, it should not be interrupted by frequent and/or prolonged periods of absence. The majority of the training must be spent in caring for patients in the operating room, other anesthetizing locations, and intensive care units. The training shall include experience in providing anesthesia for cardiac, noncardiac thoracic, and intrathoracic vascular surgical procedures. It may also include anesthesia for nonoperative diagnostic and interventional cardiac and thoracic procedures outside of the operating room. Preanesthesia preparation and postanesthesia care, pain management, and Advanced Cardiac Life Support [ACLS] shall also be included. Fellows must be educated in advanced cardiac life support and must be an ACLS provider.

I.C. Goals and Objectives

The program must be structured to ensure optimal patient care while providing fellows the opportunity to develop skills in clinical care and judgment, teaching, and research. The adult cardiothoracic anesthesiology fellow should be proficient in providing anesthesia care for patients undergoing cardiac surgery with and without extracorporeal circulation, and thoracic surgery including operations on the lung, esophagus, and thoracic aorta. The curriculum should also include experience with patients undergoing nonoperative diagnostic and interventional cardiac, thoracic, and electrophysiological procedures. In addition, the cardiothoracic anesthesiology fellow should develop skills in the conduct of preoperative patient evaluation and interpretation of cardiovascular and pulmonary diagnostic test data, hemodynamic and respiratory monitoring, advanced-level perioperative TEE, management of cardiopulmonary bypass (CPB), pharmacological and mechanical hemodynamic support, perioperative critical care, including ventilatory support and perioperative pain management. To meet these goals, the program should expose fellows to the wide variety of clinical problems in cardiothoracic patients as outlined below in Section V.B., which are necessary for the development of these clinical skills. The fellow should also be able to function as a consultant in the anesthetic care of cardiothoracic patients.

II. Institutions

II.A. Sponsoring Institution

One sponsoring institution must assume ultimate responsibility for the program, as described in the Institutional Requirements, and this responsibility extends to fellow assignments at all participating institutions.

II.B. Participating Institutions

II.B.1. Assignment to an institution must be based on a clear educational rationale, integral to the program curriculum, with clearly stated activities and objectives. When multiple participating institutions are used, there should be assurance of the continuity of the educational experience.

II.B.2. Assignment to a participating institution requires a letter of agreement with the sponsoring institution. Such a letter of agreement should:

II.B.2.a) identify the faculty who will assume both educational and supervisory responsibilities for fellows;

II.B.2.b) specify their responsibilities for teaching, supervision, and formal evaluation of fellows, as specified later in this document;

II.B.2.c) specify the duration and content of the educational experience; and

II.B.2.d) state the policies and procedures that will govern fellow education during the assignment.

II.C. Relationship to the Core Residency Program

Accreditation of the fellowship program will be granted only when the program is associated with an ACGME-accredited core residency program by formal agreement. There must be close cooperation between the core program and the fellowship training program. The division of responsibilities between the fellows in the core program and the adult cardiothoracic fellows must be clearly delineated. The presence of an adult cardiothoracic anesthesiology fellowship must not be permitted to compromise the clinical experience and the number of cases available to the residents in a core program in anesthesiology.

II.D. Institutional Policy

There should be an institutional policy governing the educational resources committed to the adult cardiothoracic anesthesiology program.

III. Program Personnel and Resources

III.A. Program Director

III.A.1. There must be a single Program Director responsible for the program. The person designated with this authority is accountable for the operation of the program. In the event of a change of either Program Director or department chair, the Program Director should promptly notify the executive director of the Residency Review Committee (RRC) through the Web Accreditation Data System of the ACGME.

III.A.2. The Program Director, together with the faculty, is responsible for the general administration of the program, and for the establishment and maintenance of a stable educational environment. Adequate lengths of appointment for both the Program Director and faculty are essential to maintaining such an appropriate continuity of leadership.

III.A.3. Qualifications of the Program Director are as follows:

III.A.3.a) The Program Director must possess the requisite specialty expertise, as well as documented educational and administrative abilities. She or he must have training and/or experience in providing anesthesia care for adult cardiothoracic surgical patients beyond the requirements for completion of a core anesthesiology residency. The Program Director should have training and experience that meet or exceed that associated with the completion of a one-year adult cardiothoracic anesthesiology fellowship.

III.A.3.b) The Program Director must be an anesthesiologist who is certified in the specialty by the American Board of Anesthesiology, or possess qualifications judged to be acceptable by the RRC.

III.A.3.c) The Program Director must be appointed in good standing and based at the primary teaching site. The program director must have an appointment to the medical staff of an institution participating in the program. The Clinical Director of the cardiothoracic anesthesiology service may be someone other than the Program Director.

III.A.3.d) The Program Director also must be licensed to practice medicine in the state where the institution that sponsors the program is located. (In certain federal programs unrestricted medical licensure in any state may be accepted.)

III.A.4. Responsibilities of the Program Director are as follows:

III.A.4.a) The Program Director must oversee and organize the activities of the educational program in all institutions that participate in the program. This includes selecting and supervising the faculty and other program personnel at each participating institution, appointing a local site director, and monitoring appropriate fellow supervision at all participating institutions.

III.A.4.b) The Program Director is responsible for preparing an accurate statistical and narrative description of the program as requested by the RRC, as well as updating annually both program and fellow records through the ACGME's Accreditation Data System.

III.A.4.c) The Program Director must ensure the implementation of fair policies, grievance procedures, and due process, as established by the sponsoring institution and in compliance with the Institutional Requirements.

III.A.4.d) The Program Director must seek the prior approval of the RRC for any changes in the program that may significantly alter the educational experience of the fellows. Such changes, for example, include:

III.A.4.d).(1) the addition or deletion of a participating institution;

III.A.4.d).(2) a change in the format of the educational program;

III.A.4.d).(3) a change in the approved fellow complement for those specialties that approve fellow complement. On review of a proposal for any such major change in a program, the RRC may determine that a site visit is necessary.

III.A.4.e) The Program Director must prepare a written outline of the educational goals of the program with respect to the knowledge, skills, and other attributes of fellows for each rotation or other aspect of the program assignment. This statement must be distributed to fellows and members of the teaching staff, and should be readily available for review.

III.A.4.f) She or he must devote sufficient time to provide substantial leadership to the program and supervision for the fellows.

III.A.4.g) The Program Director is responsible for the selection of fellows in accordance with institutional and departmental policies and procedures.

III.A.4.h) The Program Director must provide adequate supervision of the fellows through explicit written descriptions of supervisory lines of responsibility for the care of patients. Such guidelines must be communicated to all members of the program staff. Fellows must be provided with prompt, reliable systems for communication and interaction with supervisory physicians.

III.A.4.i) The Program Director must ensure that all fellows maintain accurate logs, and that this information should be submitted as requested by the RRC.

III.B. Faculty

III.B.1. At each participating institution, there must be a sufficient number of faculty with documented qualifications to instruct and supervise adequately all fellows in the program. Although the number of faculty members involved in teaching will vary, at least 3 faculty members must be involved, and these should be equal to or greater than 2 full-time equivalents, including the Program Director. A ratio of no less than one full-time equivalent faculty member to one fellow shall be maintained. The RRC understands that full-time means that the faculty member devotes essentially all professional time to the program.

III.B.2. The faculty, furthermore, must devote sufficient time to the educational program to fulfill their supervisory and teaching responsibilities. They must demonstrate a strong interest in the education of fellows, and must support the goals and objectives of the educational program of which they are a member.

III.B.3. Qualifications of the physician faculty are as follows:

III.B.3.a) The physician faculty must possess the requisite specialty expertise and competence in clinical care and teaching abilities, as well as documented educational and administrative abilities and experience in their field. There must be evidence of active participation by qualified physicians with training and/or expertise in adult cardiothoracic anesthesiology beyond the requirement for completion of a core anesthesiology residency. The faculty must possess training and experience in the care of adult cardiothoracic patients that would generally meet or exceed that associated with

the completion of a one-year adult cardiothoracic anesthesiology program, and must have a continuous and meaningful role in the program.

III.B.3.b) The physician faculty must be certified in the specialty by the American Board of Anesthesiology, or possess qualifications judged to be acceptable by the RRC.

III.B.3.c) The physician faculty must be appointed in good standing to the staff of an institution participating in the program.

III.B.3.d) The faculty must include at least one individual who has successfully completed advanced perioperative echocardiography education according to echocardiography training objectives of the American Society of Echocardiography and the Society of Cardiovascular Anesthesiologists' "Guidelines for Training in Perioperative Echocardiography"; this individual must also have successfully completed the certification examination of Special Competence in Advanced Perioperative Transesophageal Echocardiography.

III.B.3.e) Faculty in cardiology, cardiothoracic surgery, pediatrics, intensive care, and pulmonary medicine should provide teaching in multidisciplinary conferences.

III.B.3.f) The faculty may include members from the core anesthesiology program who have subspecialty expertise, including critical care and pediatric anesthesiology.

III.B.4. The responsibility for establishing and maintaining an environment of inquiry and scholarship rests with the faculty, and an active research component must be included in each program. Scholarship is defined as the following:

III.B.4.a) the scholarship of discovery, as evidenced by peer-reviewed funding or by publication of original research in a peer-reviewed journal;

III.B.4.b) the scholarship of dissemination, as evidenced by review articles or chapters in textbooks;

III.B.4.c) the scholarship of application, as evidenced by the publication or presentation of, for example, case reports or clinical series at local, regional, or national professional and scientific society meetings.

Complementary to the above scholarship is the regular participation of the teaching staff in clinical discussions, rounds, journal clubs, and research conferences in a manner that promotes a spirit of inquiry and scholarship (e.g., the offering of guidance and technical support for fellows involved in research such as research design and statistical analysis); and the provision of support for fellows' participation, as appropriate, in scholarly activities that pertain specifically to the care of cardiothoracic patients. The Program Director and faculty responsible for teaching fellows must maintain an active role in scholarly pursuits pertaining to cardiothoracic anesthesiology, as evidenced by participation in continuing medical education, as well as by involvement in research that pertains to the care of adult cardiothoracic patients.

III.B.5. Qualifications of the nonphysician faculty are as follows:

III.B.5.a) Nonphysician faculty must be appropriately qualified in their field.

III.B.5.b) Nonphysician faculty must possess appropriate institutional appointments.

III.C. Other Program Personnel

Additional necessary professional, technical, and clerical personnel must be provided to support the program.

III.D. Resources

The program must ensure that adequate resources (e.g., sufficient laboratory space and equipment, computer and statistical consultation services) are available. The following resources and facilities are necessary to the program:

III.D.1. Intensive care units for both surgical and nonsurgical cardiothoracic patients. These units may provide care to patients other than adult cardiothoracic patients, but there must be adequate support and expertise to care for cardiothoracic patients.

III.D.2. An emergency department in which cardiothoracic patients are effectively managed 24 hours a day.

III.D.3. Operating rooms adequately designed and equipped for the management of cardiothoracic patients. A postanesthesia care area adequately designed and equipped for the management of cardiothoracic patients must be located near the operating room suite.

III.D.4. Cardiothoracic patients in sufficient volume and variety to provide a broad educational experience for the program. Physicians with special training and/or experience in cardiovascular disease, clinical cardiac electrophysiology, cardiac and noncardiac thoracic surgery, general vascular surgery, pediatrics, and pulmonary diseases must be available.

III.D.5. Monitoring and advanced life support equipment representative of current levels of technology.

III.D.6. Allied health staff and other support personnel who have experience and expertise in the care of cardiothoracic patients.

III.D.7. Facilities that are readily available at all times to provide prompt laboratory measurement pertinent to the care of cardiothoracic patients. These include, but are not limited to, the measurement of blood chemistries, blood gas and acid base analysis oxygen saturation, hematocrit/hemoglobin and coagulation function.

III.D.8. Facilities that are readily available at all times to provide prompt noninvasive and invasive diagnostic and therapeutic cardiothoracic procedures. These include, but are not limited to, echocardiography, cardiac stress testing, cardiac catheterization, electrophysiological testing and therapeutic intervention, cardiopulmonary scanning procedures and pulmonary function testing.

III.D.9. Conveniently located library facilities and space for research and teaching conferences in cardiothoracic anesthesiology.

IV. Fellow Appointments

IV.A. Eligibility Criteria

The Program Director must comply with the criteria for fellow eligibility as specified in the Institutional Requirements and in departmental policies and procedures.

IV.B. Number of Fellows

The RRC may approve the number of fellows based upon established written criteria that include the adequacy of resources for fellow education (e.g., the quality and volume of patients and related clinical material available for education), faculty-fellow ratio, institutional funding, and the quality of faculty teaching. Clinical resources must be adequate to support the education of fellows and of fellows in the affiliated core residency program in anesthesiology.

IV.C. Fellow Transfers

To determine the appropriate level of education for fellows who are transferring from another fellowship program, the Program Director must receive written verification of previous educational experiences and a statement regarding the performance evaluation of the transferring fellow prior to their acceptance into the program. A Program Director is required to provide verification of fellowship education for fellows who may leave the program prior to completion of their education.

IV.D. Appointment of Fellows and Other Students

The appointment of fellows and other specialty fellows or students must not dilute or detract from the educational opportunities available to regularly appointed fellows.

V. Program Curriculum

V.A. Program Design

V.A.1. Format

The program design and sequencing of educational experiences will be approved by the RRC as part of the review process. All educational components should be related to the program goals.

V.A.2. Goals and Objectives

The program must possess a written statement that outlines its educational goals with respect to the knowledge, skills, and other attributes of fellows for each major assignment and for each level of the program. This statement must be distributed to fellows and faculty, and must be reviewed with fellows prior to their assignments.

V.B. Specialty Curriculum

The program must possess a well-organized and effective curriculum, both didactic and clinical. The curriculum must also provide fellows with direct experience in progressive responsibility for patient management.

V.B.1. Clinical Components

The fellow in cardiothoracic anesthesiology should gain both significant clinical experience that provides direct clinical care of patients and supervisory experience. At a minimum, one-half of the total minimum required case numbers should be obtained with the fellow as the primary anesthesia provider under the supervision of a faculty anesthesiologist. Supervision of fellows and other anesthesia providers by the fellow should be under the direct supervision of a faculty anesthesiologist. The goal of having fellows teach and supervise core fellows and other anesthesia providers is to prepare fellows to become faculty supervisors and teachers. The following represents the guidelines for the minimum clinical experience for each fellow:

V.B.1.a) Six months of clinical anesthesia activity experience with a minimum of 70 surgical procedures involving adult patients and requiring CPB, to include a minimum of 40 anesthetics involving valve repair or replacement, and a minimum of 50 myocardial revascularization procedures with or without CPB. The fellow should provide anesthetic management for patients undergoing minimally invasive cardiac surgery, and for congenital cardiac procedures performed on adult patients. The fellow must gain sufficient experience to independently manage intra-aortic balloon counterpulsation, and should be actively involved in the management of patients with left ventricular assist devices.

V.B.1.b) Additional required clinical experience within the full one-year fellowship should include at least one month or its equivalent of anesthetic management of patients undergoing noncardiac thoracic surgery, and the anesthetic management of 10 adult patients undergoing surgery on the ascending or descending thoracic aorta requiring full CPB, left heart bypass and/or deep hypothermic circulatory arrest. Thoracic aortic stent placements performed under anesthesia may be counted among these cases. The scope of thoracic experience provided, however, should not be limited to stent placement.

V.B.1.c) The fellow is required to have experience in the anesthetic management of adult patients for cardiac pacemaker and automatic implantable cardiac defibrillator placement, surgical treatment of cardiac arrhythmias, cardiac catheterization, and cardiac electrophysiologic diagnostic/therapeutic procedures. The majority of this experience should be obtained in nonoperating room environments to encourage multidisciplinary interaction.

V.B.1.d) Additional clinical experience within the full one-year fellowship must include successful completion of advanced perioperative echocardiography education according to the training objectives from the American Society of Echocardiography and the Society of Cardiovascular Anesthesiologists' "Guidelines for Training in Perioperative Echocardiography." This will include the study of 300 complete perioperative echocardiographic examinations, of which at least 150 are comprehensive intraoperative TEE examinations performed, interpreted, and reported by the fellow.

V.B.1.e) The fellow is required to have a one-month experience managing adult cardiothoracic surgical patients in a critical care (ICU) setting. This experience may include the management of nonsurgical cardiothoracic patients.

V.B.1.f) Two months of elective rotations (none fewer than 2 weeks in duration) from the following categories: inpatient or outpatient cardiology or pulmonary medicine, invasive cardiology, medical or surgical critical care and extracorporeal perfusion technology. Experience with pediatric cardiothoracic anesthesia is encouraged. One to 2 months devoted to a research project in cardiothoracic anesthesiology may be substituted for the 2 months of clinical elective rotations.

V.B.2. Didactic Curriculum

The didactic curriculum provided through lectures, conferences, and workshops should supplement clinical experience as necessary for the fellow to acquire the knowledge to care for adult cardiothoracic patients and meet the conditions outlined in the guidelines for the minimum clinical experience for each fellow. Didactic components should include the following areas, with emphasis on how cardiothoracic diseases affect the administration of anesthesia and life support to adult cardiothoracic patients. These represent guidelines for the minimum didactic experience for each fellow:

V.B.2.a) embryological development of the cardiothoracic structures;

V.B.2.b) pathophysiology, pharmacology, and clinical management of patients with cardiac disease, including cardiomyopathy, heart failure, cardiac tamponade, ischemic heart disease, acquired and congenital valvular heart disease, congenital heart disease, electrophysiologic disturbances and neoplastic and infectious cardiac diseases;

V.B.2.c) pathophysiology, pharmacology, and clinical management of patients with respiratory disease, including pleural, bronchopulmonary, neoplastic, infectious and inflammatory diseases;

V.B.2.d) pathophysiology, pharmacology, and clinical management of patients with thoracic vascular, tracheal, esophageal, and mediastinal diseases, including infectious, neoplastic and inflammatory processes;

V.B.2.e) noninvasive cardiovascular evaluation: electrocardiography, transthoracic echocardiography, TEE, stress testing, cardiovascular imaging. (TEE education must be based upon the training objectives for advanced perioperative echocardiography of the American Society of Echocardiography and the Society of Cardiovascular Anesthesiologists outlined in "Guidelines for Training in Perioperative Echocardiography.")

V.B.2.f) cardiac catheterization procedures and diagnostic interpretation: invasive cardiac catheterization procedures, including angioplasty, stenting, and transcatheter laser and mechanical ablations;

V.B.2.g) noninvasive pulmonary evaluation: pulmonary function tests, blood gas and acid-base analysis, oximetry, capnography, pulmonary imaging;

V.B.2.h) preanesthetic evaluation and preparation of adult cardiothoracic patients;

V.B.2.i) pharmacokinetics and pharmacodynamics of medications prescribed for medical management of adult cardiothoracic patients;

V.B.2.j) perianesthetic monitoring: noninvasive and invasive (intra-arterial, central venous, pulmonary artery, mixed venous saturation, cardiac output);

V.B.2.k) pharmacokinetics and pharmacodynamics of anesthetic medications prescribed for cardiothoracic patients;

V.B.2.l) extracorporeal circulation, including myocardial preservation, effects of CPB on pharmacokinetics and pharmacodynamics, cardiothoracic, respiratory, neurological, metabolic, endocrine, hematological, renal, and thermoregulatory effects of CPB and coagulation/anticoagulation before, during, and after CPB;

V.B.2.m) pharmacokinetics and pharmacodynamics of medications prescribed for management of hemodynamic instability: inotropes, chronotropes, vasoconstrictors, vasodilators;

V.B.2.n) circulatory assist devices: intra-aortic balloon counterpulsation, left and right ventricular assist devices, and biventricular assist devices;

V.B.2.o) pacemaker insertion and modes of action;

V.B.2.p) cardiac surgical procedures: minimally invasive myocardial revascularization, valve repair and replacement, pericardial, neoplastic procedures, and heart and lung transplantation;

V.B.2.q) thoracic aortic surgery: ascending, transverse, and descending aortic surgery with circulatory arrest, CPB employing low flow and or retrograde perfusion;

V.B.2.r) esophageal surgery: varices, neoplastic, colon interposition, foreign body, stricture, tracheoesophageal fistula;

V.B.2.s) pulmonary surgery: thoracoscopic or open, lung reduction, bronchopulmonary lavage, one-lung ventilation, lobectomy, pneumonectomy and bronchoscopy: endoscopic, fiberoptic, rigid, laser resection;

V.B.2.t) postanesthetic critical care of adult cardiothoracic surgical patients;

V.B.2.u) perioperative ventilator management: intraoperative anesthetic, and critical care unit ventilators and techniques;

V.B.2.v) pain management of adult cardiothoracic surgical patients;

V.B.2.w) research methodology/statistical analysis;

V.B.2.x) quality assurance/improvement;

V.B.2.y) ethical and legal issues; and

V.B.2.z) practice management.

Conferences, including lectures, interactive conferences, hands-on workshops, morbidity and mortality conferences, cardiac catheterization and echocardiography conferences, cardiothoracic surgery case review conferences, journal reviews, and research seminars should be regularly attended. Active participation of the fellow in the planning and production of these conferences is essential. The faculty should be the leaders in the majority of the sessions. Attendance at multidisciplinary conferences, especially in cardiovascular medicine, pulmonary medicine, cardiothoracic surgery, vascular surgery, and pediatrics relevant to cardiothoracic anesthesiology, is encouraged.

V.C. Fellows Scholarly Activities

Each program must provide an opportunity for fellows to participate in research or other scholarly activities, and fellows must participate actively in such scholarly activities related to cardiothoracic anesthesiology. The fellow must complete a minimum of one academic assignment. Academic projects may include grand rounds presentations, preparation and publication of review articles, book chapters, and manuals for teaching or clinical practice, clinical, translational, or basic research investigation, or similar scholarly activities. A faculty supervisor must be in charge of each project.

V.D. ACGME Competencies

The fellowship program must require its fellows to obtain competence in the six areas listed below to the level expected of a new practitioner. Programs must define the specific knowledge, skills, behaviors, and attitudes required, and provide educational experiences as needed in order for their fellows to demonstrate the following:

V.D.1. Patient care that is compassionate, appropriate, and effective for the treatment of health problems and the promotion of health;

V.D.2. Medical knowledge about established and evolving biomedical, clinical, and cognate sciences, as well as the application of this knowledge to patient care;

V.D.3. Practice-based learning and improvement that involves the investigation and evaluation of care for their patients, the appraisal and assimilation of scientific evidence, and improvements in patient care;

V.D.4. Interpersonal and communication skills that result in the effective exchange of information and collaboration with patients, their families, and other health professionals;

V.D.5. Professionalism, as manifested through a commitment to carrying out professional responsibilities, adherence to ethical principles, and sensitivity to patients of diverse backgrounds;

V.D.6. Systems-based practice, as manifested by actions that demonstrate an awareness of and responsiveness to the larger context and system of health care, as well as the ability to call effectively on other resources in the system to provide optimal health care.

VI. Fellow Duty Hours and the Working Environment

Providing fellows with a sound didactic and clinical education must be carefully planned and balanced with concerns for patient safety and fellow well-being. Each program must ensure that the learning objectives of the program are not compromised by excessive reliance on fellows to fulfill service obligations. Didactic and clinical education must have priority in the allotment of fellows' time and energy. Duty hour assignments must recognize that faculty and fellows collectively have responsibility for the safety and welfare of patients.

VI.A. Supervision of Fellows

VI.A.1. All patient care must be supervised by qualified faculty. The Program Director must ensure, direct, and document adequate supervision of fellows at all times. Fellows must be provided with rapid, reliable systems for communicating with supervising faculty.

VI.A.2. Faculty schedules must be structured to provide fellows with continuous supervision and consultation.

VI.A.3. Faculty and fellows must be educated to recognize the signs of fatigue, and adopt and apply policies to prevent and counteract its potential negative effects.

VI.B. Duty Hours

VI.B.1. Duty hours are defined as all clinical and academic activities related to the fellowship program; i.e., patient care (both inpatient and outpatient), administrative duties relative to patient care, the provision for transfer of patient care, time spent in-house during call activities, and scheduled activities such as conferences. Duty hours do not include reading and preparation time spent away from the duty site.

VI.B.2. Duty hours must be limited to 80 hours per week, averaged over a four-week period, inclusive of all in-house call activities.

VI.B.3. Fellows must be provided with 1 day in 7 free from all educational and clinical responsibilities, averaged over a 4-week period, inclusive of call. One day is defined as 1 continuous 24-hour period free from all clinical, educational, and administrative duties.

VI.B.4. Adequate time for rest and personal activities must be provided. This should consist of a 10-hour time period provided between all daily duty periods and after in-house call.

VI.C. On-call Activities

The objective of on-call activities is to provide fellows with continuity of patient care experiences throughout a 24-hour period. In-house call is defined as those duty hours beyond the normal work day, when fellows are required to be immediately available in the assigned institution.

VI.C.1. In-house call must occur no more frequently than every third night, averaged over a 4-week period.

VI.C.2. Continuous on-site duty, including in-house call, must not exceed 24 consecutive hours. Fellows may remain on duty for up to 6 additional hours to participate in didactic activities, transfer care of patients, conduct outpatient clinics, and maintain continuity of medical and surgical care.

VI.C.3. No new patients may be accepted after 24 hours of continuous duty.

VI.C.4. At-home call (or pager call) is defined as a call taken from outside the assigned institution.

VI.C.4.a) The frequency of at-home call is not subject to the every third night limitation. At-home call, however, must not be so frequent as to preclude rest and reasonable personal time for each fellow. Fellows taking at-home call must be provided with 1 day in 7 completely free from all educational and clinical responsibilities, averaged over a 4-week period.

VI.C.4.b) When fellows are called into the hospital from home, the hours fellows spend in-house are counted toward the 80-hour limit.

VI.C.4.c) The Program Director and the faculty must monitor the demands of at-home call in their programs, and make scheduling adjustments as necessary to mitigate excessive service demands and/or fatigue.

VI.D. Moonlighting

VI.D.1. Because fellowship education is a full-time endeavor, the Program Director must ensure that moonlighting does not interfere with the ability of the fellow to achieve the goals and objectives of the educational program.

VI.D.2. The Program Director must comply with the sponsoring institution's written policies and procedures regarding moonlighting, in compliance with the ACGME Institutional Requirements.

VI.D.3. Any hours a fellow works for compensation at the sponsoring institution or any of the sponsor's primary clinical sites must be considered part of the 80-hour weekly limit on duty hours. This refers to the practice of internal moonlighting.

VI.E. Oversight

VI.E.1. Each program must have written policies and procedures consistent with the Institutional and Program Requirements for fellow duty hours and the working environment. These policies must be distributed to the fellows and the faculty. Duty hours must be monitored with a frequency sufficient to ensure an appropriate balance between education and service.

VI.E.2. Back-up support systems must be provided when patient care responsibilities are unusually difficult or prolonged, or if unexpected circumstances create fellow fatigue sufficient to jeopardize patient care.

VI.F. Duty Hours Exceptions

An RRC may grant exceptions for up to 10% of the 80-hour limit to individual programs based on a sound educational rationale. Prior permission of the institution's GMEC, however, is required.

VII. Evaluation

VII.A. Fellow

VII.A.1. Formative Evaluation

The faculty must evaluate in a timely manner the fellows whom they supervise. In addition, the fellowship program must demonstrate that it has an effective mechanism for assessing fellow performance throughout the program, and for utilizing the results to improve fellow performance. Faculty responsible for teaching must provide critical evaluations of each fellow's progress and competence to the cardiothoracic anesthesiology Program Director at the end of 6 and 12 months of training.

VII.A.1.a) Assessment should include the use of methods that produce an accurate assessment of fellows' competence in patient care, medical knowledge, practice-based learning and improvement, interpersonal and communication skills, professionalism, and systems-based practice.

VII.A.1.b) Assessment should include the regular and timely performance feedback to fellows that includes at least semiannual written evaluations. Such evaluations are to be communicated to each fellow in a timely manner, and maintained in a record that is accessible to each fellow. The Program Director or designee must inform each fellow of the results of the evaluations at least every 6 months during training, and advise the fellow of areas needing improvement and document the communication.

VII.A.1.c) Assessment should include the use of assessment results, including evaluation by faculty, patients, peers, self, and other professional staff, to achieve progressive improvements in fellows' competence and performance.

VII.A.1.d) Assessment should include essential character attributes, acquired character attributes, fund of knowledge, clinical judgment, and clinical psychomotor skills, as well as specific tasks and skills for patient management and critical analysis of clinical situations.

VII.A.1.e) Periodic evaluation of patient care (quality assurance) is mandatory. Fellows in adult cardiothoracic anesthesiology should be involved in continuing quality improvement and risk management.

VII.A.2. Final Evaluation

The Program Director must provide a final evaluation for each fellow who completes the program. This evaluation must include a review of the fellow's performance during the final period of education, and should verify that the fellow has demonstrated sufficient professional ability to practice competently and independently. The final evaluation must be part of the fellow's permanent record maintained by the institution. Fellows in adult cardiothoracic anesthesiology must obtain overall satisfactory evaluations at the completion of 12 months training to receive credit for training.

VII.B. Faculty

The performance of the faculty must be evaluated by the program no less frequently than at the midpoint of the accreditation cycle, and again prior to the next site visit. The evaluations should include a review of their teaching abilities, commitment to the educational program, clinical knowledge, and scholarly activities. This evaluation must include annual written confidential evaluations by fellows.

VII.C. Program

The educational effectiveness of a program must be evaluated at least annually in a systematic manner.

VII.C.1. Representative program personnel (i.e., at least the Program Director, representative faculty, and one fellow) must be organized to review program goals and objectives, and the effectiveness with which they are achieved. This group must conduct a formal documented meeting at least annually for this purpose. In the evaluation process, the group must take into consideration written comments from the faculty, the most recent report of the GMEC of the sponsoring institution, and the fellows' confidential written evaluations. If deficiencies are found, the group should prepare an explicit plan of action, which should be approved by the faculty and documented in the minutes of the meeting.

VII.C.2. The program should use fellow performance and outcome assessment in its evaluation of the educational effectiveness of the fellowship program. Performance of program graduates on the certification examination should be used as one measure of evaluating program effectiveness. The program should maintain a process for using assessment results together with other program evaluation results to improve the fellowship program.

VIII. Experimentation and Innovation

Since responsible innovation and experimentation are essential to improving professional education, experimental projects along sound educational principles are encouraged. Requests for experimentation or innovative projects that may deviate from the program requirements must be approved in advance by the RRC, and must include the educational rationale and method of evaluation. The sponsoring institution and program are jointly responsible for the quality of education offered to fellows for the duration of such a project.

IX. Certification

Fellows who plan to seek certification by the American Board of Anesthesiology should communicate with the office of the board regarding the full requirements for certification.

ACGME Approved: February 14, 2006
Effective: February 14, 2006
Editorial Revision: July 1, 2009

Appendix 40-2

Department of Anesthesiology and Critical Care Medicine, Children's Hospital of Philadelphia, Cardiac Anesthesiology Web-Based Resources

Organizations

Accreditation Council for Graduate Medical Education: www.acgme.org
Agency for Healthcare Research and Quality: www.ahrq.gov
American Academy of Pediatrics: www.aap.org
American Association of Blood Banks: www.aabb.org
American Association of Health Plans: www.aahp.org
American Board of Anesthesiology: www.theaba.org
American Board of Internal Medicine: www.abim.org
American Board of Medical Specialties: www.abms.org
American Board of Pediatrics: www.abp.org
American Board of Surgery: www.absurgery.org
American Heart Association: www.americanheart.org
American Medical Association: www.ama-assn.org
Anesthesia Patient Safety Foundation: www.apsf.org
American Red Cross: www.redcross.org
Association of University Anesthesiologists: www.auahq.org
British Medical Association: www.bma.org.uk/ap.nsf/content/splashpage
Centers for Disease Control and Prevention: www.cdc.gov
Food and Drug Administration: www.fda.gov
Foundation for Anesthesia Education & Research: www.faer.org

Joint Commission: www.jointcommission.org
National Board of Echocardiography: www.echoboards.org
National Institutes of Health: www.nih.gov
Resuscitation Council (UK): www.resus.org.uk/siteindx.htm

Specialty Societies

American College of Cardiology: www.acc.org
American Society of Anesthesiologists: www.asahq.org
American Society of Critical Care Anesthesiologists: www.ascca.org
American Society of Echocardiography: http://asecho.org/
American Society of Extra-Corporeal Technology: www.amsect.org
American Society of PeriAnesthesia Nurses: www.aspan.org
American Society of Regional Anesthesia and Pain Medicine: www.asra.com
Association of Cardiothoracic Anaesthetists: www.acta.org.uk
Association of Anaesthetists of Great Britain and Ireland: www.aagbi.org
Association of Paediatric Anaesthetists of Great Britain and Ireland: www.apagbi.org.uk
Australian Society of Anaesthetists: www.asa.org.au
British Society of Echocardiography: www.bsecho.org
Canadian Anesthesiologists' Society: www.cas.ca
European Association of Cardiothoracic Anaesthesiologists: www.eacta.org
European Society of Anaesthesiologists: www.euroanesthesia.org
European Society of Intensive Care Medicine: www.esicm.org
International Anesthesia Research Society: www.iars.org
International Society for Minimally Invasive Cardiothoracic Surgery: www.ismics.org
Royal College of Anaesthetists: www.rcoa.ac.uk
Society for Ambulatory Anesthesia: www.sambahq.org
Society of Cardiovascular Anesthesiologists: www.scahq.org
Society of Critical Care Medicine: www.sccm.org
Society for Education in Anesthesia: www.seahq.org
Society of Neurosurgical Anesthesia and Critical Care: www.snacc.org
Society for Obstetric Anesthesia and Perinatology: www.soap.org
Society for Pediatric Anesthesia: www.pedsanesthesia.org
Congenital Cardiac Anesthesia Society: www.pedsanesthesia.org/ccas/
Society for Technology in Anesthesia: www.anestech.org
Society of Thoracic Surgeons: www.sts.org
The Heart Surgery Forum (Official Publication of the International Society for Minimally Invasive Cardiothoracic Surgery): www.hsforum.com
World Federation of Societies of Anaesthesiologists: www.nda.ox.ac.uk/wfsa
World Federation of Societies of Intensive and Critical Care Medicine: www.world-critical-care.org

Journals

Anesthesia and Analgesia: www.anesthesia-analgesia.org
Anesthesiology: www.anesthesiology.org
Annals of Thoracic Surgery: http://ats.ctsnetjournals.org/
American Society of Anesthesiologists Refresher Courses in Anesthesiology: www.asa-refresher.com
British Journal of Anaesthesia: www.bja.oupjournals.org
British Medical Journal: http://bmj.bmjjournals.com/
Canadian Journal of Anesthesia: www.cja-jca.org
Circulation: http://circ.ahajournals.org/
Circulation Research: http://circres.ahajournals.org/
Journal of the American College of Cardiology: www.cardiosource.com/jacc.html
Journal of the American Medical Association: http://jama.ama-assn.org/
Journal of Cardiothoracic and Vascular Anesthesia: www.jcardioanesthesia.com
Journal of Clinical Anesthesia: www.journals.elsevierhealth.com/periodicals/JCA
Journal of Extracorporeal Technology: www.ject.org

Journal of Thoracic and Cardiovascular Surgery: http://jtcs.ctsnetjournals
.org/
New England Journal of Medicine: www.nejm.org
Paediatric Anaesthesia: www.blackwellpublishing.com/journal.asp?ref
=1155-5645
Pediatrics: www.pediatrics.org
Quality & Safety in Health Care: http://qhc.bmjjournals.com/

Literature Search Sites
The Review Group
Cochrane Anaesthesia Review Group: http://carg.cochrane.org
National Center for Biotechnology Information: www.ncbi.nlm.nih.gov
National Library of Medicine: www.nlm.nih.gov
National Library of Medicine: www.pubmed.gov
Medline Plus: http://medlineplus.gov/

Educational Resource Sites
American Society of Anesthesiologists Closed Claims Project: http://
depts.washington.edu/asaccp/
American Society of Anesthesiologists (ASA) Closed Claims Project
Home page: http://depts.washington.edu/asaccp/ASA/index.shtml
Pediatric Perioperative Cardiac Arrest (POCA) Registry: http://depts
.washington.edu/asaccp/POCA/index.shtml
The Postoperative Visual Loss Registry: http://depts.washington.edu/
asaccp/eye/index.shtml
The ASA Committee on Professional Liability: http://depts.washington
.edu/asaccp/prof/index.shtml
Anesthesia, Critical Care Medicine and Emergency Medicine: www
.invivo.net/bg/index2.html
GASNet: http://anestit.unipa.it/HomePage.html
Cardiac Web Links—Martin J. London, MD, University of California
San Francisco: http://mjlworld.tripod.com/page19.htm
Cardiothoracic Surgery Network on the Internet: www.ctsnet.org
Family of educational Web sites for the medical professional: www
.theanswerpage.com
  Anesthesiology, pain management, hospital and CCM, newborn
  medicine and ob-gyn; specialty sites feature Question of the Day
  with a peer-reviewed, referenced answer
Health Information Site: www.healthfinder.gov
Medical information from WebMD: www.medscape.com
National Guideline Clearinghouse (NGC): www.guideline.gov
  A public resource for evidence-based clinical practice guide-
  lines; NGC is sponsored by the Agency for Healthcare Research
  and Quality (formerly the Agency for Health Care Policy and
  Research) in partnership with the American Medical Association
  and the American Association of Health Plans
Online Mendelian Inheritance in Man (database catalog of human
  genes and genetic disorders) (syndrome clinical synopsis): www
  .ncbi.nlm.nih.gov/omim/
Paediatric Anaesthesia Conference—Discussion Group: Hospital for
  Sick Children, Toronto, Canada: www.sickkids.ca/Anaesthesia/pac_
  list.asp
Pediatric Critical Care Education Site: http://pedsccm.org/clinical_
  resources.php
The Perfusion Home Page: www.perfusion.com

Pulmonary Artery Catheter Education Project: www.pacep.org
Society for Simulation in Healthcare: www.ssih.org

Practice Guidelines and Advisories
ASA Practice Parameters: https://ecommerce.asahq.org/c-4-practice-
parameters.aspx
Practice Guidelines for Pulmonary Artery Catheterization: https://
ecommerce.asahq.org/p-179-practice-guidelines-for-pulmonary-
artery-catheterization.aspx
Practice Guidelines for Perioperative Transesophageal Echocardiography: https://ecommerce.asahq.org/p-351-practice-guidelines-for-
perioperative-transesophageal-echocardiography.aspx
Practice Guidelines for Perioperative Blood Transfusion and Adjuvant
Therapies: https://ecommerce.asahq.org/p-116-practice-guidelines-
for-perioperative-blood-transfusion-and-adjuvant-therapies.aspx
Perioperative Management of Patients with Cardiac Rhythm Management
Devices: Pacemakers and Implantable Cardioverter-Defibrillators:
https://ecommerce.asahq.org/p-114-perioperative-mgmt-of-
patients-with-cardiac-rhythm-mgmt-devices-pacemakers-and-
implantable-cardioverter-defibrillators.aspx
Practice Alert for the Perioperative Management of Patients with
Coronary Artery Stents: https://ecommerce.asahq.org/p-323-
practice-alert-for-the-perioperative-management-of-patients-with-
coronary-artery-stents.aspx
Practice Guidelines for Management of the Difficult Airway: https://
ecommerce.asahq.org/p-177-practice-guidelines-for-management-
of-the-difficult-airway.aspx

Research Resource Sites
National Institutes of Health tutorial on the Do's and Don'ts for grant
writing: www.niaid.nih.gov/ncn/grants
Useful information on other sections of an application including
human subjects, training grants, and budgets: www.niaid.nih.gov/
ncn

Pharmacology Resource Sites
Medication information: www.epocrates.com
Physicians Desk Reference: www.pdr.net

General Search Engines
www.altavista.com
www.google.com
www.lycos.com
www.msn.com
www.yahoo.com
www.searchengineguide.com/searchengines.html

Computer-Palm Resource Sites
AetherPalm: www.aether.com
Handheld Med: www.handheldmed.com
Palm: www.palm.com/us
Palm computer resource: http://avantgo.com/frontdoor/index/html
Yahoo Anesthesiology: http://dir.yahoo.com/Health/medicine/
anesthesiology/

REFERENCES
1. American Heart Association: *Heart disease and stroke statistics*. Available at: http://www.americanheart.org/downloadable/heart/1265665152970DS-3241%20HeartStrokeUpdate_2010.pdf. Accessed February 22, 2010.
2. Accreditation Council for Graduate Medical Education: *ACGME Anesthesiology program requirements*. Available at: http://www.acgme.org/acWebsite/downloads/RRC_progReq/040pr703_u804.pdf. Accessed February 22, 2010.
3. Accreditation Council for Graduate Medical Education: *ACGME Adult Cardiothoracic Anesthesiology program requirements*. Available at: http://acgme.org/acWebsite/downloads/RRC_progReq/041pr206.pdf. Accessed February 22, 2010.
4. American Board of Anesthesiology: *Certification and Maintenance of Certification*, February 2001. Available at: http://viewer.zmags.com/publication/8418a33c#/8418a33c/1. Accessed February 23, 2010.
5. Reves JG: *Resident subspecialty training*, Park Ridge, IL, 2000–2001, ASA (Section on Representation).
6. Havidich JE, Haynes GR, Reves JG: The effect of lengthening anesthesiology residency on subspecialty education, *Anesth Analg* 99:844, 2004.
7. Appendix II: Graduate medical education, 2008-2009, *JAMA* 302:1357, 2009.
8. Available at: http://www.scahq.org/sca3/fellowships/Criteria_for_Recognition-2004.pdf. Accessed December 7, 2004.
9. Accreditation Council for Graduate Medical Education: Available at: http://www.acgme.org/acWebsite/home/home.asp. Accessed February 28, 2010.
10. Accreditation Council for Graduate Medical Education: *The purpose of accreditation*. Available at: http://www.acgme.org/acWebsite/about/ab_purposeAccred.asp. Accessed February 28, 2010.
11. Accreditation Council for Graduate Medical Education: Available at: http://www.acgme.org/acWebsite/dutyHours/dh_dutyhoursCommonPR07012007.pdf. Accessed February 28, 2010.
12. American Board of Medical Specialties: Available at: http://www.abms.org/. Accessed February 28, 2010.
13. Silber JH, Williams SV, Krakauer H, et al: Hospital and patient characteristics associated with death after surgery. A study of adverse occurrence and failure to rescue, *Med Care* 30:615, 1992.
14. Silber JH, Kennedy SK, Even-Shoshan O, et al: Anesthesiologist direction and patient outcomes, *Anesthesiology* 93:152, 2000.

15. Silber JH, Kennedy SK, Even-Shoshan O, et al: Anesthesiologist board certification and patient outcomes, *Anesthesiology* 96:1044, 2002.
16. Brennan TA, Horwitz RI, Duffy FD, et al: The role of physician specialty board certification status in the quality movement, *JAMA* 292:1038, 2004.
17. *Guidelines for delineation of clinical privileges in anesthesiology.* Available at: http://www.asahg.org/For_Healthcare_Professionals/Standards_Guidelines_and_Statements.aspx. Accessed December 12, 2010.
18. Mattern WD, Weinholtz D, Friedman CP: The attending physician as teacher, *N Engl J Med* 308:1129, 1983.
19. Gaiser RR: The teaching of professionalism during residency: Why it is failing and a suggestion to improve its success, *Anesth Analg* 108:948, 2009.
20. Bloom BS, editor: *Taxonomy of Educational Objectives. Handbook I: Cognitive Domain*, New York, 1956, David McKay.
21. American Board of Anesthesiology: *An overview of the certification process with emphasis on the oral examination.* Available at: http://www.theaba.org/pdf/oral-overview.pdf. Accessed February 23, 2010.
22. Schwartz AJ: Teaching anesthesiology. In Miller RD, editor: *Miller's Anesthesia*, 7th ed. Philadelphia, 2010, Elsevier Churchill Livingstone Elsevier, pp 193–207.
23. Foley RP, Smilansky: *Teaching Techniques. A Handbook for Health Professionals*, New York, 1980, McGraw-Hill.
24. Krathwohl DR, Bloom BS, Masia BB: *Taxonomy of Educational Objectives. Handbook. II: Affective Domain*, New York, 1964, David McKay.
25. Gawande A: *Complications: A Surgeon's Notes on an Imperfect Science*, New York, 2002, Henry Holt and Company, pp 11–34.
26. Issenberg SB, McGaghie WC, Hart IR, et al: Simulation technology for health care professional skills training and assessment, *JAMA* 282:861, 1999.
27. Gallagher AG, Cates CU: Virtual reality for the operating room and cardiac catheterisation laboratory, *Lancet* 364:1538, 2004.
28. Friedrich MJ: Practice makes perfect: Risk-free medical training with patient simulators, *JAMA* 288:2808, 2002.
29. Gordon MS, Ewy GA, Felner JM, et al: Teaching bedside cardiologic examination skills using "Harvey," the cardiology patient simulator, *Med Clin North Am* 64:305, 1980.
30. Sajid AW, Ewy GA, Felner JM, et al: Cardiology patient simulator and computer-assisted instruction technologies in bedside teaching, *Med Educ* 24:512, 1990.
31. Jones JS, Hunt SJ, Carlson SA, et al: Assessing bedside cardiologic examination skills using "Harvey," a cardiology patient simulator, *Acad Emerg Med* 4:980, 1997.
32. Waugh RA, Mayer JW, Ewy GA, et al: Multimedia computer-assisted instruction in cardiology, *Arch Intern Med* 155:197, 1995.
33. Euliano T, Good ML: Simulator training in anesthesia growing rapidly, *J Clin Monit* 13:53, 1997.
34. Good ML: Patient simulation for training basic and advanced clinical skills, *Med Educ* 37(Suppl 1):14, 2003.
35. Murray DJ, Boulet JR, Kras JF, et al: Acute care skills in anesthesia practice: A simulation-based resident performance assessment, *Anesthesiology* 101:1084, 2004.
36. Blum MG, Powers TW, Sundaresan S: Bronchoscopy simulator effectively prepares junior residents to competently perform basic clinical bronchoscopy, *Ann Thorac Surg* 78:287, 2004.
37. Schwid HA, Rooke GA, Ross BK, et al: Use of a computerized advanced cardiac life support simulator improves retention of advanced cardiac life support guidelines better than a textbook review, *Crit Care Med* 27:821, 1999.
38. Saliterman SS: A computerized simulator for critical-care training: New technology for medical education, *Mayo Clin Proc* 65:968, 1990.
39. Grogan EL, Stiles RA, France DJ, et al: The impact of aviation-based teamwork training on the attitudes of health-care professionals, *J Am Coll Surg* 199:843, 2004.
40. Holzman RS, Cooper JB, Gaba DM, et al: Anesthesia crisis resource management: Real-life simulation training in operating room crises, *J Clin Anesth* 7:675, 1995.
41. Henriksen K: Simulation and team training, *Qual Saf Health Care* 13(Suppl 1):i1, 2004.
42. Sedlack RE, Kolars JC, Alexander JA: Computer simulation training enhances patient comfort during endoscopy, *Clin Gastroenterol Hepatol* 2:348, 2004.
43. Schwid HA, Rooke A, Carline J, et al: Evaluation of anesthesia residents using mannequin-based simulation, *Anesthesiology* 97:1434, 2002.
44. American Medical Association: *The Physician's Recognition Award and Credit System: The AMA definition of CME.* Available at: http://www.ama-assn.org/ama1/pub/upload/mm/455/pra2006.pdf. Accessed March 2, 2010.
45. American Board of Anesthesiology: *Maintenance of certification frequently asked questions.* Available at: http://www.theaba.org/FAQ/moc. Accessed March 2, 2010.
46. Schwartz AJ: Learning cardiothoracic anesthesia. In Thys DM, editor: *Textbook of Cardiothoracic Anesthesiology*, New York, 2001, McGraw-Hill, pp 11–23.

SELECTED READINGS

Barrows HS: *Simulated (Standardized) Patients and Other Human Simulations*, Chapel Hill, NC, 1987, Health Sciences Consortium.
Bunker JP, editor: *Education in Anesthesiology*, New York, 1967, Columbia University Press.
Chin C, Schwartz AJ: Teaching Pediatric Cardiac Anesthesiology. In Lake CL, Booker PD, editors: *Pediatric Cardiac Anesthesia*, Philadelphia, 2005, Lippincott Williams & Wilkins, pp 755–765.
Comroe JH: Exploring the heart. In *Discoveries in Heart Disease and High Blood Pressure*, New York, 1983, WW Norton.
Jason H, Westberg J: *Instructional Decision-Making Self-Study Modules for Teachers in the Health Professions (Preview Package)*, National Center for Faculty Development. Miami, FL, 1980, University of Miami School of Medicine.
Lear E, editor: *Virtual reality in patient simulators*, Am Soc Anesthesiol Newsletter, 61(October), 1997.
Lyman RA: Disaster in pedagogy, *N Engl J Med* 257:504, 1957.
McCauley KM, Brest A: *McGoon's Cardiac Surgery: An Interprofessional Approach to Patient Care*, Philadelphia, 1985, FA Davis.
Miller GE: Adventure in pedagogy, *JAMA* 162:1448, 1956.
Miller GE: *Educating Medical Teachers*, Cambridge, MA, 1980, Harvard University Press.
Schwartz AJ: Teaching and learning congenital cardiac anesthesia. In Andropoulos DB, Stayer SA, Russell LA, editors: *Anesthesia for Congenital Heart Disease*, Armonk, NY, 2005, Futura.

41

Transesophageal Echocardiography
Training and Certification

FEROZE MAHMOOD, MD | ADAM B. LERNER, MD

KEY POINTS

1. Transesophageal echocardiography (TEE) can have significant diagnostic and therapeutic impact during both cardiac and noncardiac surgery.
2. The use of perioperative TEE and its potential impact on patient care developed in advance of training and credentialing guidelines.
3. An understanding of key definitions and terms as well as the processes related to certification in perioperative TEE is somewhat complicated but important.
4. The evolution of current guidelines related to training and certification in perioperative TEE occurred in a stepwise fashion over a span of more than two decades.
5. New technologies related to TEE training, such as simulator-based models, continue to evolve and are increasingly being incorporated into training curricula.

The introduction of transesophageal echocardiography (TEE) into the perioperative arena in the mid-1980s heralded a new era in the care of surgical patients and offered a new dimension to the role of anesthesiologists.[1] Soon after its introduction, it became clear that perioperative TEE had the potential for significant impact on the care for both cardiac and noncardiac surgical patients.[2-4] Because of its minimally invasive nature and a high diagnostic potential, TEE has been used by practitioners from multiple specialties, for example, cardiologists, anesthesiologists, and critical care physicians. The therapeutic impact of TEE on preoperative surgical decision making soon was established, and it was recognized that it has the potential to offer improvements in patient care and, perhaps, eventual improvements in outcomes. However, there is the possibility for patient harm from misdiagnosis or from a poor understanding of the limitations of the technology and its application. The introduction of any new technology or technique into clinical practice, which can have such a dramatic impact on patient management, requires proper training and experience. The effectiveness of this expertise should be demonstrable by, among other things, significant training and experience, objective and validated measurement tools such as examinations, and demonstration of continued clinical activity. It was from these basic principles that the development of a certification process for perioperative TEE was born.

The debate surrounding the credentialing and certification for TEE is not unique to this technology. Often, the introduction and acceptance of technology into clinical practice outpace the efforts to legislate the credentialing requirements. Several other clinical techniques (e.g., laparoscopic surgical techniques and percutaneous angioplasty) were widely adopted clinically before credentialing and certification could be established.[5] Perioperative TEE also has been rapidly accepted and deployed as an essential monitor in the cardiac operating rooms (ORs) before training and certification guidelines could be adequately developed. Despite being in clinical practice for more than two decades, a survey conducted among the membership of the Society of Cardiovascular Anesthesiologists (SCA) in 2001 showed that of the nearly 2000 members, less than 30% had any formalized training in TEE, and less than 50% reported having any specific credentialing requirements at their hospitals.[6] Although there have been considerable improvements in perioperative TEE training programs, there is considerable room for improvement, and the majority of the clinical institutions, which include major academic centers, do not have specific credentialing requirements for anesthesiologists to use this monitoring modality.

The importance of collaboration between anesthesiologists and cardiologists was acknowledged in the 1996 American Society of Anesthesiologists/Society of Cardiovascular Anesthesiologists (ASA/SCA) guidelines for training and certification in TEE.[5,7] It was believed that because it was impractical for cardiologists to be present in the OR all the time, it was imperative for anesthesiologists to learn to perform and interpret intraoperative TEE examinations. To encourage more widespread use of TEE, the guidelines also stated that TEE should not be performed for making extremely focused examinations and narrow diagnoses, but broadly as a monitor to assist in cardiac surgical procedures. In addition to specifically describing the evidence of the therapeutic utility of TEE in clinical situations, the indications were analyzed in the context of the patient, the procedure, and the clinical setting[7] (Boxes 41-1 and 41-2). The ASA/SCA guidelines recommended the following fundamental principles for optimal physician training in perioperative TEE[5,7]:

1. Experience and knowledge of the indications, applicability, and use of different echocardiographic techniques and principles for diagnosis of cardiovascular disorders
2. Knowledge of the basic principles of ultrasound physics and instrumentation
3. The need for specific training in the field of echocardiography over and above core residency training
4. Commitment to a continuing medical education program to keep abreast of the latest developments in the field of echocardiography; although not mandated, it is expected that the specified training must be over and above the core anesthesia residency training, *or* a
5. Minimum of 24 months of clinical experience dedicated to the perioperative care of surgical patients

DEFINITIONS

Because of the rapidly changing landscape of the training and certification requirements and because of multiple ambiguities, it often is confusing to follow the terminology used for echocardiography training and certification. This section provides the standard definitions of the most commonly used terms.

Perioperative Echocardiography

According to current guidelines, perioperative echocardiography is defined as TEE, epicardial, or epiaortic echocardiography performed

1173

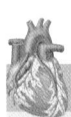

BOX 41-1. INDICATIONS FOR TRANSESOPHAGEAL ECHOCARDIOGRAPHY

Category I indications: Supported by the strongest evidence or expert opinion. Transesophageal echocardiography (TEE) is frequently useful in improving clinical outcomes in these settings and is often indicated, depending on individual circumstances (e.g., patient risk and practice setting).

- Intraoperative evaluation of acute, persistent, and life-threatening hemodynamic disturbances in which ventricular function and its determinants are uncertain and have not responded to treatment
- Intraoperative use in valve repair
- Intraoperative use in congenital heart surgery for most lesions requiring cardiopulmonary bypass
- Intraoperative use in repair of hypertrophic obstructive cardiomyopathy
- Intraoperative use for endocarditis when preoperative testing was inadequate or extension of infection to perivalvular tissue is suspected
- Preoperative use in unstable patients with suspected thoracic aortic aneurysms, dissection, or disruption who need to be evaluated quickly
- Intraoperative assessment of aortic valve function in repair of aortic dissections with possible aortic valve involvement
- Intraoperative evaluation of pericardial window procedures
- Use in intensive care unit for unstable patients with unexplained hemodynamic disturbances, suspected valve disease, or thromboembolic problems (if other tests or monitoring techniques have not confirmed the diagnosis or patients are too unstable to undergo other tests)

Category II indications: Supported by weaker evidence and expert consensus; TEE may be useful in improving clinical outcomes in these settings, depending on individual circumstances, but appropriate indications are less certain.

- Perioperative use in patients with increased risk for myocardial ischemia or infarction
- Perioperative use in patients with risk for hemodynamic disturbances
- Intraoperative assessment of valve replacement

- Intraoperative assessment of repair of cardiac aneurysms
- Intraoperative evaluation of removal of cardiac tumors
- Intraoperative detection of foreign bodies
- Intraoperative detection of air emboli during cardiotomy, heart transplant operations, and upright neurosurgical procedures
- Intraoperative use during intracardiac thrombectomy
- Intraoperative use during pulmonary embolectomy
- Intraoperative use for suspected cardiac trauma
- Preoperative assessment of patients with suspected acute thoracic aortic dissections, aneurysms, or disruption
- Intraoperative use during repair of thoracic aortic dissections without suspected aortic valve involvement
- Intraoperative detection of aortic atheromatous disease or other sources of aortic emboli
- Intraoperative evaluation of pericardectomy, pericardial effusions, or evaluation of pericardial surgery
- Intraoperative evaluation of anastomotic sites during heart and/or lung transplantation
- Monitoring placement and function of assist devices

Category III indications: Little current scientific or expert support; TEE is infrequently useful in improving clinical outcomes in these settings, and appropriate indications are uncertain.

- Intraoperative evaluation of myocardial perfusion, coronary artery anatomy, or graft patency
- Intraoperative use during repair of cardiomyopathies other than hypertrophic obstructive cardiomyopathy
- Intraoperative use for uncomplicated endocarditis during noncardiac surgery
- Intraoperative monitoring for emboli during orthopedic procedures
- Intraoperative assessment of repair or thoracic aortic injuries
- Intraoperative use for uncomplicated pericarditis
- Intraoperative evaluation or pleuropulmonary diseases
- Monitoring placement of intra-aortic balloon pumps, automatic implantable cardiac defibrillators, or pulmonary artery catheters
- Intraoperative monitoring of cardioplegia administration

From Practice guidelines for perioperative transesophageal echocardiography. A report by the American Society of Anesthesiologists and the Society of Cardiovascular Anesthesiologists Task Force on Transesophageal Echocardiography. *Anesthesiology* 84:986–1006, 1996.

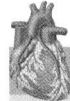

BOX 41-2. COGNITIVE REQUIREMENTS FOR PERIOPERATIVE TRANSESOPHAGEAL ECHOCARDIOGRAPHY

Basic Training
Cognitive Skills
Knowledge of the physical principles of echocardiographic image formation and blood velocity measurement
Knowledge of the operation of ultrasonographs, including all controls that affect the quality of data displayed
Knowledge of the equipment handling, infection control, and electrical safety associated with the techniques of perioperative echocardiography
Knowledge of the indications, contraindications, and potential complications for perioperative echocardiography
Knowledge of the appropriate alternative diagnostic techniques
Knowledge of the normal tomographic anatomy as revealed by perioperative echocardiographic techniques
Knowledge of the commonly encountered blood flow velocity profiles as measured by Doppler echocardiography
Knowledge of the echocardiographic manifestations of native valvular lesions and dysfunction
Knowledge of the echocardiographic manifestations of cardiac masses, thrombi, cardiomyopathies, pericardial effusions, and lesions of the great vessels
Detailed knowledge of the echocardiographic presentations of myocardial ischemia and infarction

Detailed knowledge of the echocardographic presentations of normal and abnormal ventricular function
Detailed knowledge of the echocardiographic presentations of air embolization

Technical Skills
Ability to operate ultasonographs including the primary controls affecting the quality of the displayed data
Ability to insert a TEE probe safely in the anesthetized, tracheally intubated patient
Ability to perform a comprehensive TEE examination and differentiate normal from markedly abnormal cardiac structures and function
Ability to recognize marked changes in segmental ventricular contraction indicative of myocardial ischemia or infarction
Ability to recognize marked changes in global ventricular filling and ejection
Ability to recognize air embolization
Ability to recognize gross valvular lesions and dysfunction
Ability to recognize large intracardiac masses and thrombi
Ability to detect large pericardial effusions
Ability to recognize common echocardiographic artifacts
Ability to communicate echocardiographic results effectively to health care professionals, the medical record, and patients
Ability to recognize complications of perioperative echocardiography

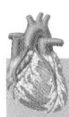

BOX 41-2. COGNITIVE REQUIREMENTS FOR PERIOPERATIVE TRANSESOPHAGEAL ECHOCARDIOGRAPHY—CONT'D

Advanced Training
Cognitive Skills
All the cognitive skills defined under basic training
Detailed knowledge of the principles and methodologies of qualitative and quantitative echocardiography
Detailed knowledge of native and prosthetic valvular function, including valvular lesions and dysfunction
Knowledge of congenital heart disease (if congenital practice is planned, then this knowledge must be detailed)
Detailed knowledge of all other diseases of the heart and great vessels that is relevant in the perioperative period (if pediatric practice is planned, then this knowledge may be more general than detailed)
Detailed knowledge of the techniques, advantages, disadvantages, and potential complications of commonly used cardiac surgical procedures for treatment of acquired and congenital heart disease

Detailed knowledge of other diagnostic methods appropriate for correlation with perioperative echocadiography

Technical Skills
All the technical skills defined under basic training
Ability to acquire or direct the acquisition of all necessary echocardiographic data, including epicardial and epiaortic imaging
Ability to recognize subtle changes in segmental ventricular contraction indicative of myocardial ischemia or infarction
Ability to quantify systolic and diastolic ventricular function and to estimate other relevant hemodynamic parameters
Ability to quantify normal and abnormal native and prosthetic valvular function
Ability to assess the appropriateness of cardiac surgical plans
Ability to identify inadequacies in cardiac surgical interventions and the underlying reasons for the inadequacies
Ability to aid in clinical decision making in the operating room

Adapted from Practice guidelines for perioperative transesophageal echocardiography. A report by the American Society of Anesthesiologists and the Society of Cardiovascular Anesthesiologists Task Force on Transesophageal Echocardiography. *Anesthesiology* 84:986–1006, 1996.

on surgical patients immediately before, during, or after surgery.[7,8] Transthoracic echocardiography, although sometimes performed on surgical patients, is not considered a "perioperative" technique. Thus, the guidelines do not apply to transthoracic echocardiography–related procedures and image acquisition techniques.

Basic Training

At the basic level of training, the trainee should have knowledge of the principles of ultrasound and image acquisition, be able to place a TEE probe, operate the equipment, and conduct an examination. Although independent work is expected, all examinations performed by the basic-level trainee have to be supervised and interpreted under the guidance of an advanced-level echocardiographer together with the availability of a periodic assessment program. It also was recommended that anesthesiologists trained as basic echocardiographers should be able to use the TEE for establishing diagnoses within the customary practice of anesthesiology[7] (Box 41-3).

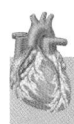

BOX 41-3. BASIC AND ADVANCED LEVEL ECHOCARDIOGRAPHER

	Basic	Advanced
Minimum number of examinations	150	300
Minimum number personally performed	50	150
Program director qualifications	Advanced perioperative echocardiography training	Advanced perioperative echocardiography training plus at least 150 additional perioperative TEE examinations
Program qualifications	Wide variety of perioperative applications of echocardiography	Full spectrum of perioperative applications of echocardiography

From Cahalan MK, Abel M, Goldman M, et al: American Society of Echocardiography and Society of Cardiovascular Anesthesiologists task force guidelines for training in perioperative echocardiography. *Anesth Analg* 94:1384–1388, 2002.

Advanced Training

An advanced-level trainee should have performed at least 300 comprehensive TEE examinations under supervision; in addition, the trainee should have performed 150 examinations independently. The training has to be comprehensive and broad-based with a significant component of independent activities. Such a training process should have a formal and informal evaluation program as well. Furthermore, the echocardiographic examinations performed during basic training can be counted toward completion of advanced training. An anesthesiologist who has advanced TEE training should be able to use TEE to its full diagnostic potential and use it for establishing diagnoses that can possibly impact the planned surgical procedure[7] (see Box 41-3).

Credentialing

Credentialing is the process by which a physician is granted clinical privileges by a local health care organization. Each health care organization by law is free to establish and enforce its own credentialing requirements.

Testamur Status

A testamur status is achieved by demonstration of a passing grade in the examination of special competence in perioperative TEE administered by the National Board of Echocardiography (NBE).[2] For those physicians who cannot be certified to be advanced examiners (explained later), testamur status can be maintained indefinitely (Figure 41-1).

Certification/Diplomate Status

The certification process of the NBE consists of:
1. Successful completion of perioperative TEE examination
2. Current license to practice medicine
3. Current medical board certification
4. Specific training in perioperative care of surgical patients with cardiovascular disorders

The basic and advanced TEE certifications are discussed in greater detail later in the chapter (Figures 41-2 and 41-3). The certification process of the NBE encompasses not only TEE-related training and experience, but has been applied to transthoracic echocardiography and stress echocardiography (Figures 41-4 to 41-7).

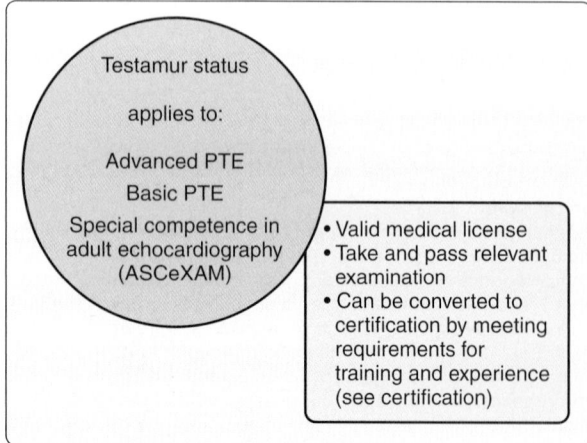

Figure 41-1 **Testamur status.** PTE, perioperative transesophageal echocardiography.

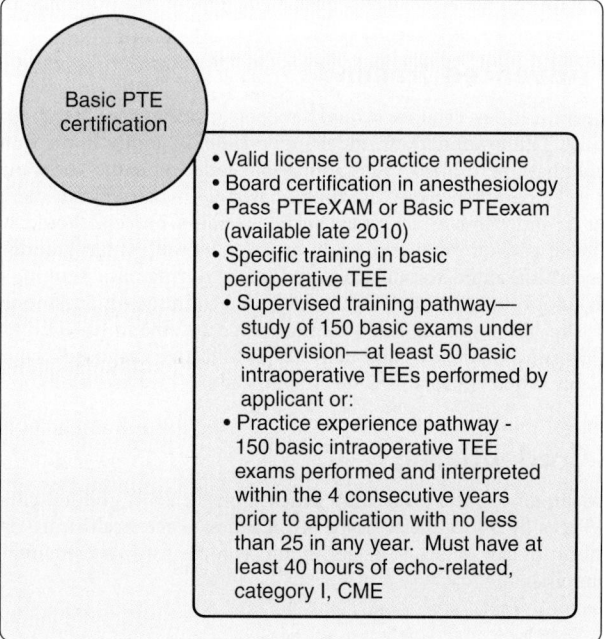

Figure 41-2 **Basic Perioperative Transesophageal Echocardiography (PTE) Certification requirements.** TEE, transesophageal echocardiography.

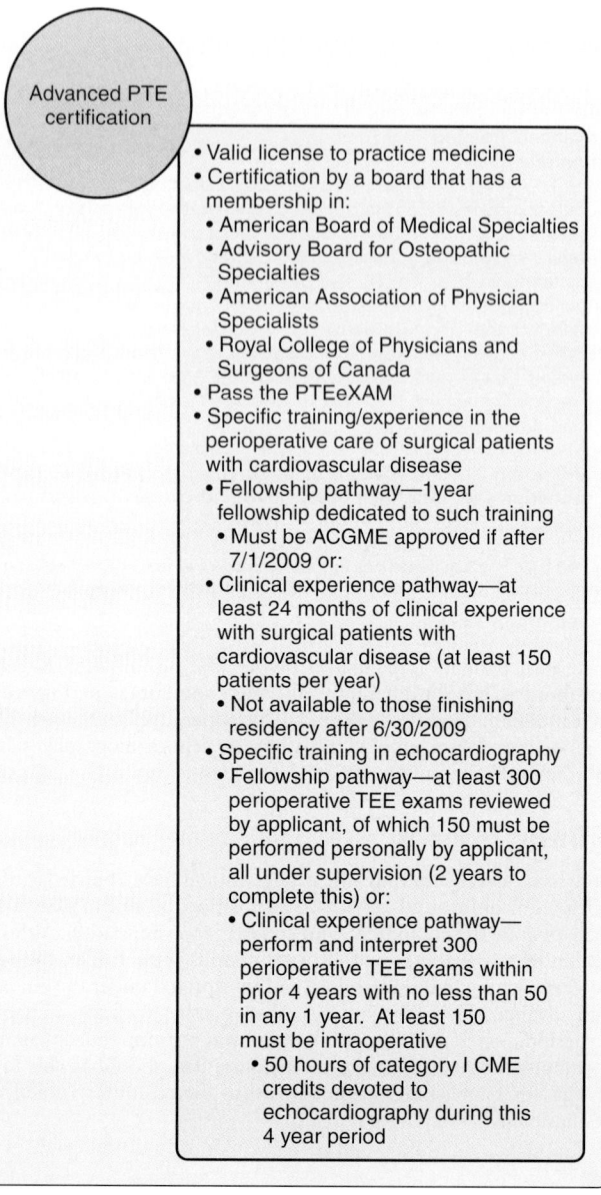

Figure 41-3 **Advanced Perioperative Transesophageal Echocardiography (PTE) Certification requirements.**

PERIOPERATIVE TRANSESOPHAGEAL ECHOCARDIOGRAPHY TRAINING

Since its introduction, there has been considerable controversy about the level of training required to be proficient and competent in performing perioperative TEE. Introduction and ready acceptance of TEE in the cardiac ORs led to a situation in which TEE had to be adopted by anesthesiologists who had already finished their training. They not only had to train themselves by "on-the-job" experience, but had to develop training guidelines for in-training residents and fellows. Because of the lack of a specific testing mechanism, the expertise was established by demonstration of exposure to a specific number of TEE examinations. There was significant debate about the optimum time/number of examinations required to gain adequate training to be a "competent examiner"—that is, the duration of specific training period versus its

comprehensiveness and the total number of examinations versus the variety of pathologies examined.[9,10] As a result of the aforementioned factors, the requirements for adequate training were initially purposely kept flexible to accommodate different levels of experience of practitioners. Also, the requirements were made less binding and restrictive to accommodate different levels of experience and exposure to echocardiography. It was believed that rather than specifying the number of months or examinations performed, it was equally important that anesthesiologists should have broad-based training in perioperative echocardiography with exposure to a wide variety of cases.[8]

Evolution of Training Guidelines

The training guidelines for echocardiography have evolved over time from time-limited experience requirements to achieve an incremental expertise in echocardiography from Level I to III[11–13] to the present situation, when use of TEE is being encouraged for all anesthesiologists (cardiac and noncardiac), and there are suggestions to include TEE

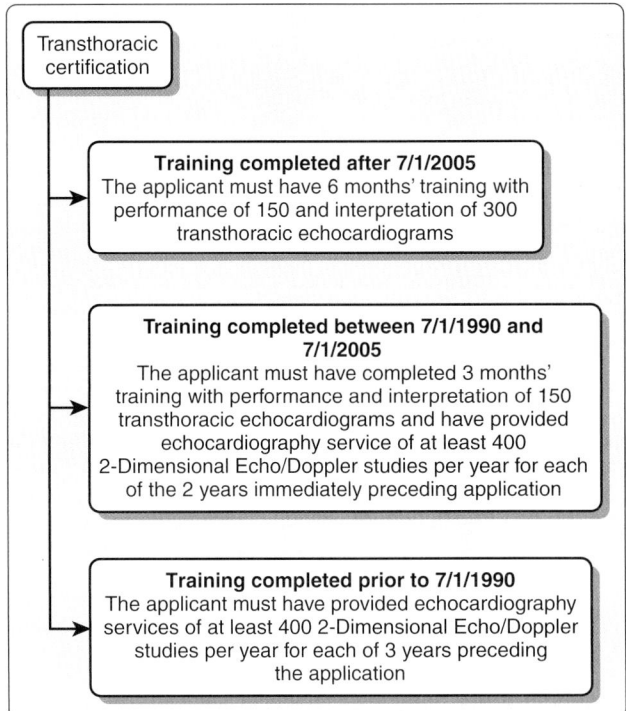

Figure 41-4 Requirements for certification in transthoracic echocardiography.

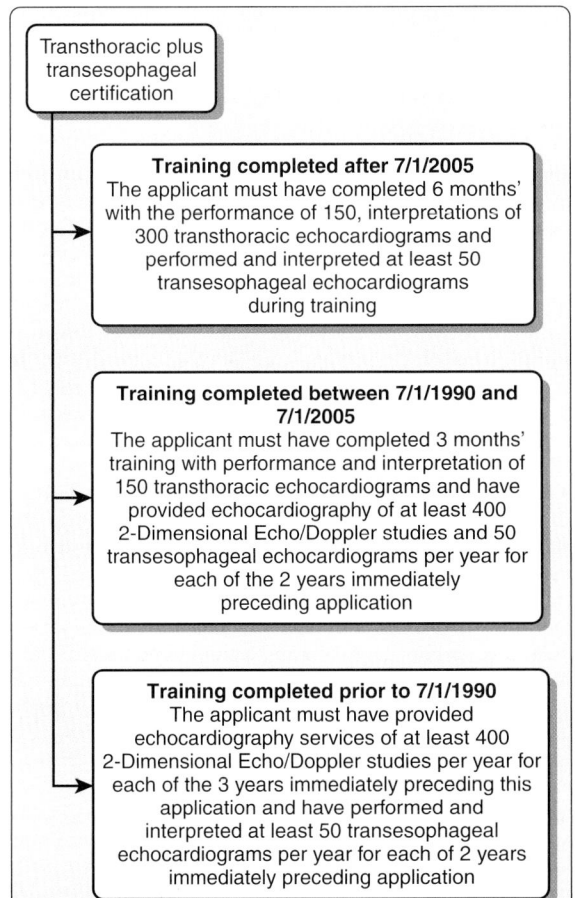

Figure 41-5 Requirements for certification in transthoracic and transesophageal echocardiography.

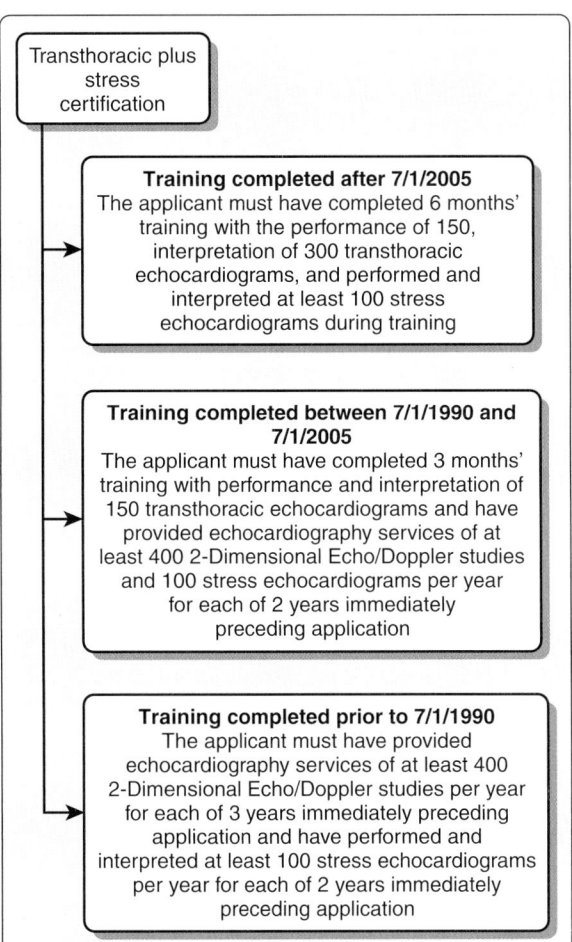

Figure 41-6 Requirements for certification in transthoracic and stress echocardiography.

education as part of the core anesthesia residency training. Over time, the increasing utilization of intraoperative TEE has led to a blurring of specialty lines with anesthesiologists assuming a greater role in performing TEE examinations in the perioperative period, a task originally performed by cardiologists. With the redefined role of anesthesiologists as the "perioperative echocardiographers," the ASA/SCA published their own specific recommendations for perioperative echocardiography for anesthesiologists already using TEE. These guidelines laid down not only the indications and contraindications but also the necessary cognitive and technical skills required to perform a perioperative TEE examination[7] (see Boxes 41-1 and 41-2). Furthermore, rather than defining the expertise of the echocardiographers as Level I, II, or III examiners, as in earlier guidelines, the terms *basic-* and *advanced-level* examiners were used (see Box 41-3). A basic-level echocardiographer is defined as a physician capable of making a decision as to when and how to perform a TEE examination, whereas an advanced-level examiner is someone capable of making independent decisions based on TEE findings, which can potentially change the course of the procedure (see Box 41-3). Because there was a lack of specific training programs for anesthesiologists to acquire TEE skills, the guidelines recommended commercially available educational materials, workshops, and mentorship from experienced echocardiographers to gain expertise.

After considerable thought and deliberation, the initial ASA/SCA practice guidelines were further updated by the ASA/SCA in 2002.[8] Whereas the initial guidelines recommended only establishment of training programs,[7] the updated document described the specifics of the training program environment, program director's qualifications, and mandated the inclusion of TEE training in the

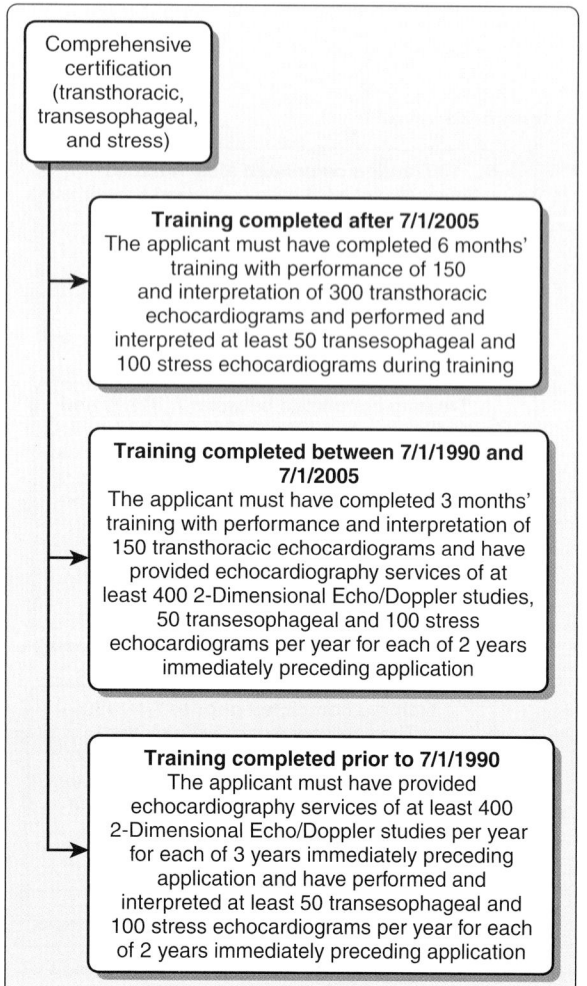

Comprehensive certification (transthoracic, transesophageal, and stress)

Training completed after 7/1/2005
The applicant must have completed 6 months' training with performance of 150 and interpretation of 300 transthoracic echocardiograms and performed and interpreted at least 50 transesophageal and 100 stress echocardiograms during training

Training completed between 7/1/1990 and 7/1/2005
The applicant must have completed 3 months' training with performance and interpretation of 150 transthoracic echocardiograms and have provided echocardiography services of at least 400 2-Dimensional Echo/Doppler studies, 50 transesophageal and 100 stress echocardiograms per year for each of 2 years immediately preceding application

Training completed prior to 7/1/1990
The applicant must have provided echocardiography services of at least 400 2-Dimensional Echo/Doppler studies per year for each of 3 years immediately preceding application and have performed and interpreted at least 50 transesophageal and 100 stress echocardiograms per year for each of 2 years immediately preceding application

Figure 41-7 Requirements for comprehensive certification (transthoracic, transesophageal, and stress echocardiography).

established cardiac anesthesia fellowship programs. It was also recommended that, over time, as in cardiology residency programs, specific TEE training fellowships also should be established for anesthesiologists.[8] Furthermore, in the revised guidelines, epiaortic and epivascular echocardiography examinations also were included as perioperative echocardiography techniques. The updated guidelines have recommended a total of 150 completed TEE examinations, of which 50 are to be performed personally for basic-level trainees, and a total of 300 TEE examinations, of which 150 are to be performed personally for an advanced trainee.[8] Later, the recommendations made by the ASA/SCA updated guidelines (see Box 41-3)[8] also were adopted by the American Heart Association/American College of Cardiology (AHA/ACC) clinical competency statement on echocardiography.[14-16]

In 2006, the Canadian Society of Echocardiography and the Cardiovascular Section of the Canadian Society of Anesthesiologists comprehensively defined the roles of basic and advanced echocardiographers, as well as the training program requirements for basic- and advanced-level echocardiographers.[17,18] These guidelines extended the training requirements and expectations of the diagnostic potential laid out in the ASA/SCA guidelines of 2002[8] for different levels of examiners. A qualified director of a training program in perioperative echocardiography, the training program environment, availability of resources, and the presence of a continuing medical education program also were mentioned as necessary ingredients for an echocardiography training environment.[17,18] The Canadian guidelines have

gone a step further and, in addition to the type of echocardiographic examination, also have identified specific diagnoses expected from basic- and advanced-level examiners. This is significant progress in being more specific as compared with the initial ASA/SCA guidelines,[8] in which only broad expectations were laid down of the depth and comprehensiveness of a perioperative TEE examination from basic- and advanced-level examiners. The Canadian guidelines, however, have increased the expected number of examinations personally performed and interpreted by the trainees (100 for the basic-level and 200 for an advanced-level trainee).[17,18] These TEE studies also may include examinations performed outside the OR in the intensive care unit. Furthermore, these guidelines also have set a time limit of 1 year to complete these TEE training requirements.[17,18]

It is obvious from the earlier discussion that the training expectations and requirements have and will continue to evolve as the technology improves. Equipment costs and lack of training opportunities have been the major impediments to the widespread acceptance and use of this technology in cardiac and noncardiac surgery.[19] The invasive nature of TEE, cumbersome credentialing, and licensing requirements also preclude a "hands-on" experience at continuing medical education workshops and observership-based training programs. Although anesthesia residents are expected to have an introduction to the basic TEE examination during their accredited training, it is a not a mandated part of the anesthesia residency curriculum. Since the accreditation of cardiac anesthesia fellowship programs, TEE training has been formalized with months dedicated to intraoperative echocardiography. The inclusion of TEE as part of an accredited cardiac anesthesia fellowship is the first step toward standardization of training in perioperative echocardiography. Over the next few years, the expectations are likely to change dramatically, and expertise in perioperative echocardiography probably will be considered a core competency in a cardiac anesthesia fellowship.

Training with Transesophageal Echocardiography Simulators

Over the years, many technologic advances have been tried to bridge the gap between the patient and virtual reality. Simulation is becoming a particularly attractive training method for techniques that require manual dexterity. Although simulation is an established technique of learning in the health care industry, no simulator was available for TEE training until recently.[20] The complexity of cardiac structure, valvular function, and synchronization of a real TEE probe with a virtual model of the heart made such an endeavor cost-ineffective or prohibitive. As a result of many technologic breakthroughs and collaborative efforts of physicians, software engineers, and special-effects professionals, a TEE simulator was made available for commercial use in 2008 (Figure 41-8). As a result of this innovation, it is now possible to learn the basic TEE examination outside the OR with a TEE simulator and reduce the initial learning curve.[20] Currently, the simulation technology consists of normal cardiac anatomy and physiology only, and disease states cannot be simulated anatomically or physiologically (Figure 41-9). At the current rate of technology development, it may soon be possible to learn "normal" anatomy, physiology, probe manipulations, and image orientation techniques on a TEE simulator, while concentrating on "abnormal" in the OR. This methodology of learning has the potential to significantly improve TEE training and education for the anesthesia residents of the future. However, the TEE simulator is quite expensive and is available for training in only a few major academic centers in the United States.

Recently, another simulator was introduced by Vimedix that has the capability of performing transthoracic and TEE examinations on a three-dimensional solid model of the heart (Figure 41-10). The simulator also is capable of Doppler interrogation and hemodynamic calculations. In addition, this simulator has the ability to simulate pathologic processes—for example, pericardial tamponade, biventricular systolic dysfunction, and valvular abnormalities (Figure 41-11). The

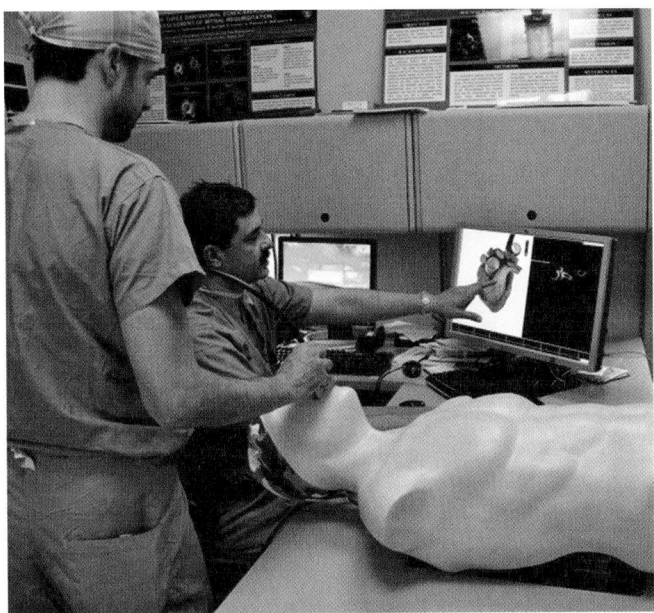

Figure 41-8 Transesophageal echocardiography simulator.

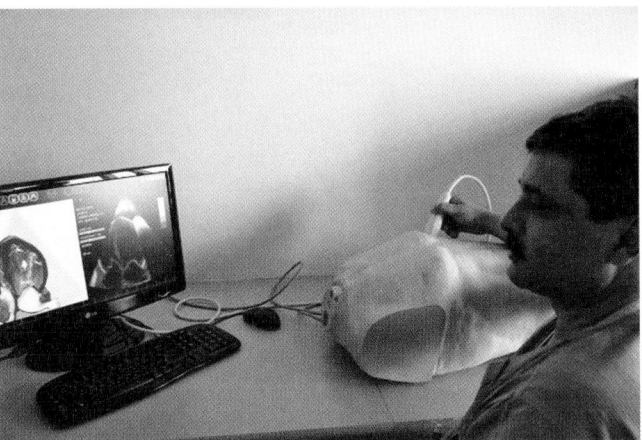

Figure 41-10 Transthoracic echocardiography simulator.

availability of simulated abnormalities can revolutionize the training process and opens the door for novel methods of training and standardized testing.

HISTORY OF THE DEVELOPMENT OF THE CERTIFICATION PROCESS

In 1987, the American Society of Echocardiography (ASE) published its first recommendations on the knowledge, nature, and experience, as well as the type of training site, that were deemed as optimal for training physicians as echocardiographers[11] (see Figure 41-12). In this publication, the ASE identified three levels of training: basic training, advanced training, and director of echocardiographic laboratory training. Basic training (Level I) was an introductory phase that did not aim to allow for independent performance or interpretation of echocardiographic examinations. Advanced training (Level II) sought to develop the knowledge and skills that would

allow for independent practice under the supervision of a laboratory director. Echocardiographic laboratory director training (Level III) sought to prepare the physician to supervise others and to perform specialized echocardiographic procedures, which included perioperative TEE. For each level, requirements for the duration of training and the number of examinations performed and interpreted were set. As discussed earlier, though somewhat altered, this theme of levels in training, knowledge base, and expectations has persisted through the current model of certification. In 1992, the ASE modified these recommendations to relate specifically to TEE, and in 1995, the ACC reaffirmed them.[12,13]

In 1993, in addition to establishing recommendations for training, the ASE appointed a committee to develop and administer an examination in echocardiography that would be known as the ASEeXAM. Furthermore, an entity known as ASEeXAM, Inc. was established as a separate tax-exempt corporation independent from the ASE to avoid a conflict of interest. The primary objective of the examination was to "provide practicing echocardiographers the opportunity to demonstrate special competence in echocardiography."[21] Its other objectives were to set a standard for a knowledge base related to echocardiography, to stimulate continuing education, and to attempt to identify weaknesses and deficiencies in training. The National Board of Medical Examiners was chosen by the ASE to help develop an objective and valid test. The content of the examination consisted of multiple-choice

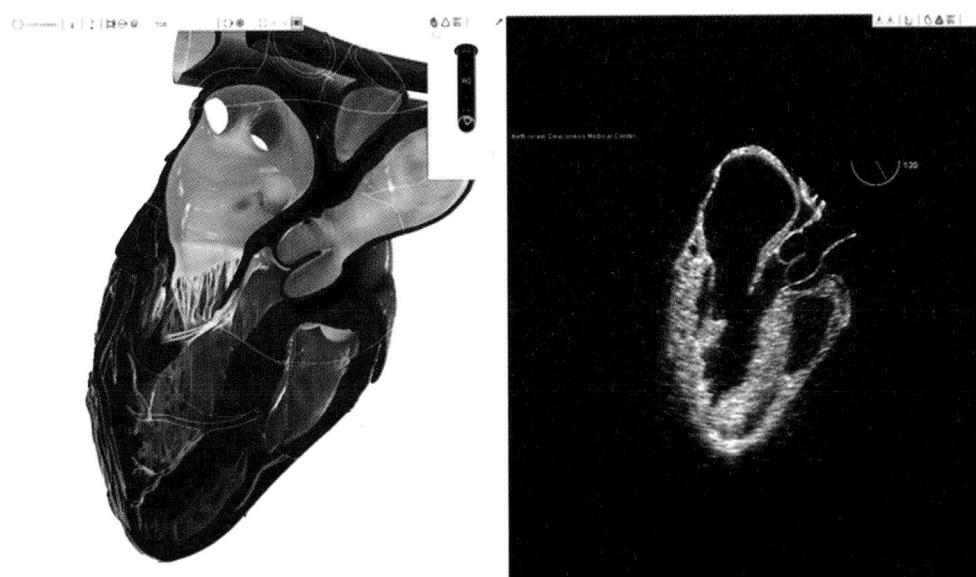

Figure 41-9 A simultaneously displayed anatomic image of the heart with a midesophageal long-axis echocardiographic image obtained with the simulator. The view is rotated to 120°.

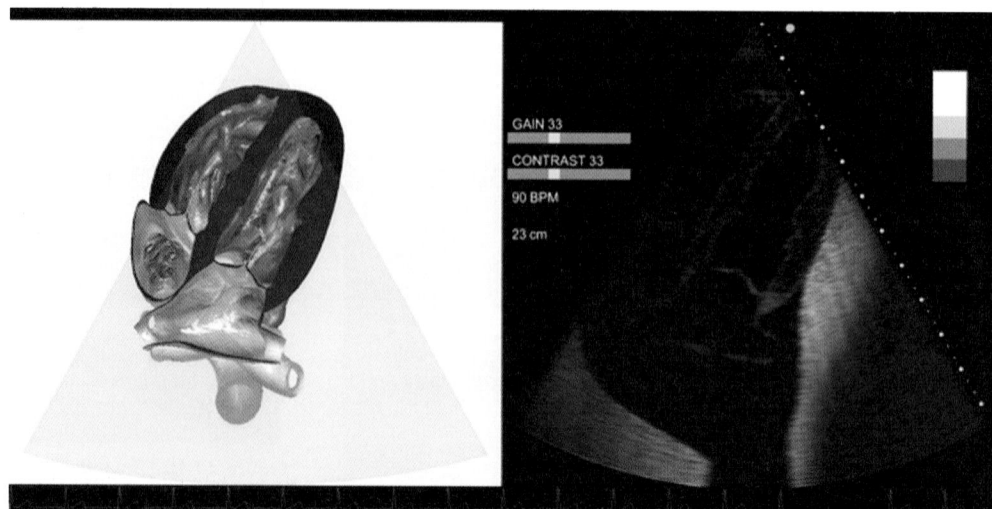

Figure 41-11 Simultaneously obtained echocardiographic and anatomic image obtained from a transthoracic simulator.

questions covering the topics of physical principles, instrumentation, valvular heart disease, chamber size and function, congenital heart disease, and a few other miscellaneous subjects. Perioperative TEE was represented only as a small subtopic. After a field test in 1995, the first operational ASEeXAM was administered in 1996. The test was available to all licensed physicians regardless of field of expertise. Only 21 of the 373 examinees who took this examination (6%) were anesthesiologists. The pass rate was only 59% for all examinees and only 43% among anesthesiologists. Those who passed the examination were given the status of "testamur."[21]

In 1995, following the lead of the ASE, the SCA created its own task force to develop an examination that focused on perioperative TEE (PTE). The SCA was, to some degree, motivated by the concern that the ASEeXAM format functionally excluded anesthesiologists from demonstrating their proficiency in PTE.[5] The SCA also decided to hire the National Board of Medical Examiners to help develop and validate the test. The test was called the PTEeXAM and was administered for the first time in 1998. The examination was open to all licensed physicians, but actual examinees were almost exclusively anesthesiologists. The pass rate on the first examination was 76%.[22] As with the ASEeXAM, examinees who passed were given the status of "testamur." In 1996, the ASA and SCA published guidelines relating to the practice of TEE.[7] These guidelines served mainly to establish recommendations concerning the appropriate indications for and the contraindications against performing TEE. No recommendations were made as to the duration of training or specific amounts of experience needed to reach either of these levels. At that time, the ASA/SCA committee lacked a consensus as to the best training pathway for PTE within the realm of anesthesiology.

During the process of developing examinations and training guidelines, the leadership of the SCA and ASEeXAM, Inc. had discussions regarding their parallel processes. There was justifiable concern on both sides that their two examinations would end up competing with one another, and that this would lead to confusion on the part of echocardiographers, hospital administrators, and third-party payers. Furthermore, if some sort of merger could be arranged that would satisfy the goals of both groups, administrative and other efficiencies could lead to significant cost savings. An agreement was reached and in December 1998, ASEeXAM Inc. was renamed the National Board of Echocardiography (NBE).[2] The Board of Directors of the NBE was structured to include nine directors, three of whom were cardiac anesthesiologists. The board was given the responsibility of overseeing two separate examination committees. One committee was given the charge of maintaining the ASEeXAM, whereas the other oversaw the PTE examination. In 1999, the NBE administered its first pair of examinations. The ASEeXAM was changed to the ASCeXAM.

Certification

After several years of administering these examinations, the NBE next sought to address the issue of offering NBE certification (Figure 41-12). Certification combined successful completion of an NBE examination with the passing of set thresholds related to actual echocardiographic experience or training, or both. These requirements are demonstrated

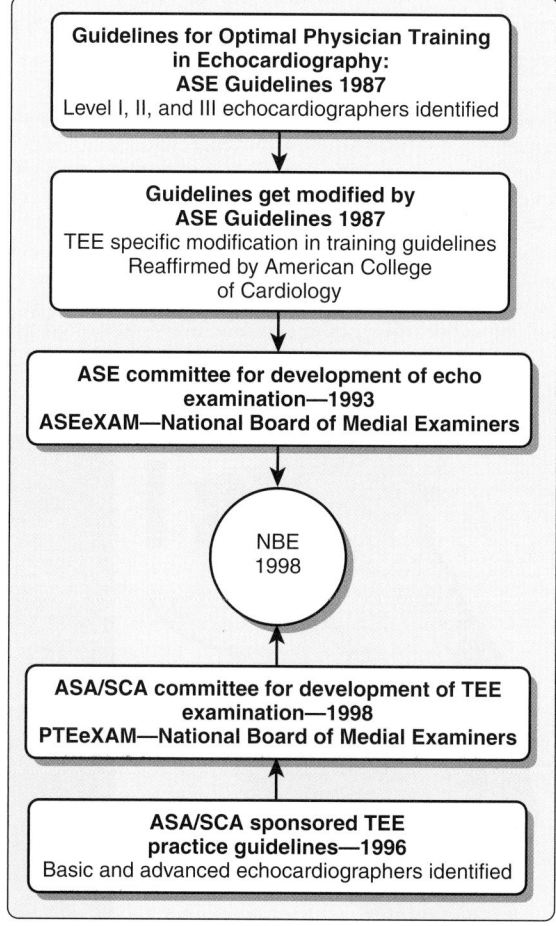

Figure 41-12 Timeline of the development of the echocardiography certification process. ASA/SCA, American Society of Anesthesiologists/Society of Cardiovascular Anesthesiologists; ASE, American Society of Echocardiography; TEE, transesophageal echocardiography.

in Figures 41-2 and 41-3. Certification for the ASCeXAM began in 2001 and was based on the experience criteria developed by the ASE and ACC in the early to mid 1990s (see Figures 41-2 to 41-5). As mentioned earlier, the 1996 ASA/SCA task force did not develop thresholds for experience to distinguish between basic and advanced PTE. In 2002, a task force of SCA and ASE members developed these criteria.[8] This allowed for certification centered around the PTEeXAM in 2004. Physicians who successfully met the requirements for certification were given the status of "diplomate." Both the "diplomate" and "testamur" statuses are time-limited statuses and are valid for 10 years from the date of successful completion of the appropriate examination. The first recertification examination for the ASCeXAM was offered in 2005, and first ecertification for the PTEeXAM was given in 2007.

Basic Certification

In 2010, the NBE offered the first examination on basic PTE and first certification in basic PTE. The development of the basic PTE pathway was done in direct cooperation with the ASA. With the addition of the basic pathway, the former PTEeXAM pathway has now become the advanced PTEeXAM. The development of the basic PTE pathway was developed from the 2002 ASA/SCA guidelines discussed previously.[8] The basic PTE pathway is meant to demonstrate competence for anesthesiologists who use TEE as a monitor during anesthesia. This pathway does not provide a measure of competence for the use of TEE as a diagnostic tool to affect the conduct of surgical procedures because this is an advanced skill.

In 2009, the NBE moved all examinations to computer-based testing centers. It was hoped that this format would reduce costs to both the examinees and the NBE. In addition, this may allow for more standardized viewing of echocardiographic images presented during the examination and can allow more flexibility on dates for administration.

CLINICAL COMPETENCE VERSUS CERTIFICATION

Clinical Experience versus Testing

Even before the institution of an official ASCeXAM[21] and the PTEeXAM[22] by the ASE, it had been demonstrated that experienced echocardiographers performed better on a multiple-choice examination than less experienced practitioners.[23] It was recommended by the society that such tests could be used for periodic quality-assurance programs. Because most training guidelines recommend a specific number of cases to be performed to achieve a certain level, they do not account for individual rates of learning and case-mix variations in a particular program. Therefore, it was recommended that an achievement-based testing system rather than a numerical number of cases should determine the competency to perform perioperative TEE.[23] There is no requirement by the NBE to document actual performance of perioperative TEE as a prerequisite to take the PTEeXAM. Therefore, it is quite possible that individuals may be able to pass the examination without any significant hands-on experience and, thus, may be construed as "experts" without the necessary experience.[24] It also has been suggested that the PTEeXAM should be offered only to physicians who are actually performing perioperative TEE examinations.

Clinical Competence and Testamur Status

The requirements of the NBE for different examinations and certification application are freely available on their website (http://www. echoboards.org/). Although the American Board of Anesthesiology governs the certification process for anesthesiologists, it has never sought to require certification of individual techniques within the scope of the practice.[7] It was recommended in the initial guidelines that if the certification in preoperative TEE was to be pursued, it should be done through a collaborative and a multidisciplinary process. Although the NBE examination has been administered for more than a decade, a passing score on the examination is not a requisite for demonstration of competence

in clinical echocardiography by the ASA/SCA and AHA/ACC guidelines.[8,14-16] Similarly, a considerable number of practitioners use TEE at an advanced level but have not gone through the NBE examination process. A mandatory requirement to demonstrate a passing grade on this examination for competence in echocardiography could also possibly have excluded these experienced and advanced examiners from performing perioperative TEE examinations. Achievement of a passing grade on the PTEeXAM does not imply that the practitioner has achieved the necessary technical skills to perform preoperative TEE examinations independently and, therefore, should not be used to substitute for clinical experience.[18]

Basic Certification

To circumvent the exclusionary effects of a restrictive policy and to promote the use of TEE by general anesthesiologists, the NBE also has offered a basic-level certification in perioperative echocardiography (see Figure 41-2). In this effort, the NBE has recognized that there may be a significant number of practitioners who may not be taking the PTEeXAM because they are not performing enough perioperative TEE examinations to satisfy the NBE requirement to be certified. Basic certification, as offered by the NBE, implies the ability to use the TEE for nondiagnostic monitoring purposes, especially during life-threatening emergencies. The ASA and SCA also have begun a joint initiative to conduct "basic echocardiography" courses throughout the year and at major annual meetings to introduce TEE to general anesthesiologists. These introductory courses and workshops are geared toward basic-level echocardiographers and are designed to enable a basic understanding of the principles of echocardiography. After 2 years of this initiative, the first basic certification examination was held in 2010.

The current requirements for advanced certification have a grandfather clause, that is, the practice experience pathway, to offer certification via the practice experience pathway for physicians who graduated before 2009. This is another opportunity for practitioners who are not formally trained, but perform TEE regularly, to become certified after passing the PTEeXAM. In addition to obtaining a passing score on the PTEeXAM, the practice experience pathway requires demonstration of continued clinical activity and involvement in care of patients with cardiovascular disorders. The Canadian guidelines actually have mandated the demonstration of a passing grade on the PTEeXAM to qualify to be classified even as a basic-level echocardiograher, and passing the examination is considered the first step in becoming an echocardiographer.[18] It is obvious that the training and certification processes in perioperative echocardiography are in evolution. The accredited cardiac anesthesia fellowship programs have incorporated dedicated months of TEE training in their curriculum. Unlike cardiology, no fellowship programs are dedicated to perioperative echocardiography.

Maintenance of Certification

The testamur and the certification diplomas given by the NBE are time-limited, and although not mandated, a recertification examination is strongly encouraged by the NBE. The current guidelines recommend 50 comprehensive examinations personally performed and interpreted by the practitioner to maintain an adequate level of competence in perioperative TEE.[5,14-18] Additional components of ongoing training include, but are not limited to, attendance at conferences and workshops to stay abreast of the latest techniques and advances, case conferences, and case reviews. Provision of such opportunities is considered a responsibility of the training program. The Canadian guidelines, however, recommend that the director level of expertise requires performance of 75 comprehensive TEE examinations annually.[17,18]

ACKNOWLEDGMENT

We acknowledge the support and guidance provided by Greg Hartman, MD, Professor of Anesthesia, Dartmouth-Hitchcock Medical Center, Manchester, NH, in preparation of this manuscript and providing educational materials.

REFERENCES

1. de Bruijn NP, Clements FM, Kisslo JA: Intraoperative transesophageal color flow mapping: Initial experience, *Anesth Analg* 66:386–390, 1987.
2. Eltzschig HK, Rosenberger P, Loffler M, et al: Impact of intraoperative transesophageal echocardiography on surgical decisions in 12,566 patients undergoing cardiac surgery, *Ann Thorac Surg* 85:845–852, 2008.
3. Minhaj M, Patel K, Muzic D, et al: The effect of routine intraoperative transesophageal echocardiography on surgical management, *J Cardiothorac Vasc Anesth* 21:800–804, 2007.
4. Schulmeyer MC, Santelices E, Vega R, et al: Impact of intraoperative transesophageal echocardiography during noncardiac surgery, *J Cardiothorac Vasc Anesth* 20:768–771, 2006.
5. Aronson S, Thys DM: Training and certification in perioperative transesophageal echocardiography: A historical perspective, *Anesth Analg* 93:1422–1427, 2001.
6. Morewood GH, Gallagher ME, Gaughan JP, et al: Current practice patterns for adult perioperative transesophageal echocardiography in the United States, *Anesthesiology* 95:1507–1512, 2001.
7. Practice guidelines for perioperative transesophageal echocardiography. A report by the American Society of Anesthesiologists and the Society of Cardiovascular Anesthesiologists Task Force on Transesophageal Echocardiography, *Anesthesiology* 84:986–1006, 1996.
8. Cahalan MK, Abel M, Goldman M, et al: American Society of Echocardiography and Society of Cardiovascular Anesthesiologists task force guidelines for training in perioperative echocardiography, *Anesth Analg* 94:1384–1388, 2002.
9. Cahalan MK, Foster E: Training in transesophageal echocardiography: In the lab or on the job? *Anesth Analg* 81:217–218, 1995.
10. Savage RM, Licina MG, Koch CG, et al: Educational program for intraoperative transesophageal echocardiography, *Anesth Analg* 81:399–403, 1995.
11. Pearlman AS, Gardin JM, Martin RP, et al: Guidelines for optimal physician training in echocardiography. Recommendations of the American Society of Echocardiography Committee for Physician Training in Echocardiography, *Am J Cardiol* 60:158–163, 1987.
12. Pearlman AS, Gardin JM, Martin RP, et al: Guidelines for physician training in transesophageal echocardiography: Recommendations of the American Society of Echocardiography Committee for Physician Training in Echocardiography, *J Am Soc Echocardiogr* 5:187–194, 1992.
13. Stewart WJ, Aurigemma GP, Bierman FZ, et al: Guidelines for training in adult cardiovascular medicine. Core Cardiology Training Symposium (COCATS). Task Force 4: Training in echocardiography, *J Am Coll Cardiol* 25:16–19, 1995.
14. Quinones MA, Douglas PS, Foster E, et al: ACC/AHA clinical competence statement on echocardiography: A report of the American College of Cardiology/American Heart Association/ American College of Physicians-American Society of Internal Medicine Task Force on Clinical Competence, *J Am Coll Cardiol* 41:687–708, 2003.
15. Quinones MA, Douglas PS, Foster E, et al: ACC/AHA clinical competence statement on echocardiography: A report of the American College of Cardiology/American Heart Association/ American College of Physicians-American Society of Internal Medicine Task Force on clinical competence, *J Am Soc Echocardiogr* 16:379–402, 2003.
16. Quinones MA, Douglas PS, Foster E, et al: American College of Cardiology/American Heart Association clinical competence statement on echocardiography: A report of the American College of Cardiology/American Heart Association/American College of Physicians—American Society of Internal Medicine Task Force on Clinical Competence, *Circulation* 107:1068–1089, 2003.
17. Beique F, Ali M, Hynes M, et al: Canadian guidelines for training in adult perioperative transesophageal echocardiography. Recommendations of the Cardiovascular Section of the Canadian Anesthesiologists' Society and the Canadian Society of Echocardiography, *Can J Cardiol* 22:1015–1027, 2006.
18. Beique F, Ali M, Hynes M, et al: Canadian guidelines for training in adult perioperative transesophageal echocardiography. Recommendations of the Cardiovascular Section of the Canadian Anesthesiologists' Society and the Canadian Society of Echocardiography, *Can J Anaesth* 53:1044–1060, 2006.
19. Mahmood F, Christie A, Matyal R: Transesophageal echocardiography and noncardiac surgery, *Semin Cardiothorac Vasc Anesth* 12:265–289, 2008.
20. Bose R, Matyal R, Panzica P, et al: Transesophageal echocardiography simulator: A new learning tool, *J Cardiothorac Vasc Anesth* 23:544–548, 2009.
21. Weyman AE, Butler A, Subhiyah R, et al: Concept, development, administration, and analysis of a certifying examination in echocardiography for physicians, *J Am Soc Echocardiogr* 14:158–168, 2001.
22. Aronson S, Butler A, Subhiyah R, et al: Development and analysis of a new certifying examination in perioperative transesophageal echocardiography, *Anesth Analg* 95:1476–1482, 2002.
23. Konstadt SN, Reich DL, Rafferty T: Validation of a test of competence in transesophageal echocardiography, *J Cardiothorac Vasc Anesth* 10:311–313, 1996.
24. Oxorn D: Certification in perioperative TEE, *Anesth Analg* 96:1844, 2003.

Note: Page numbers followed by *b* indicate boxes, *f* indicate figures and *t* indicate tables.